Volume Two

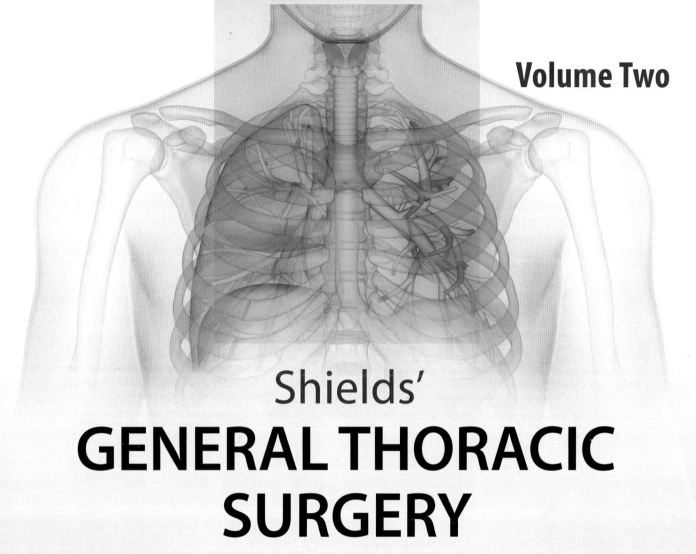

Shields'
GENERAL THORACIC
SURGERY

8th Edition

EDITED BY

Joseph LoCicero III, MD
Professor Emeritus of Surgery
SUNY Downstate
Brooklyn, New York
Physician Consultant
Mobile County Health Department
Mobile, Alabama

Yolonda L. Colson, MD, PhD
Michael A. Bell Distinguished Chair in Healthcare
   Innovation
Professor of Surgery
Harvard Medical School
Brigham and Women's Hospital
Boston, Massachusetts

Richard H. Feins, MD
Professor of Surgery
Division of Cardiothoracic Surgery
University of North Carolina at Chapel Hill
Chapel Hill, North Carolina

Gaetano Rocco, MD, FRCSEd
Professor
Chief, Division of Thoracic Surgery
Instituto Nazionale Tumori, IRCCS, Pascale Foundation
Naples, Italy

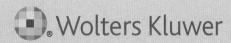
. Wolters Kluwer

Philadelphia • Baltimore • New York • London
Buenos Aires • Hong Kong • Sydney • Tokyo

Acquisitions Editor: Keith Donnellan
Development Editor: Sean McGuire
Development Editor: Brendan Huffman
Editorial Coordinator: Jennifer DiRicco
Editorial Coordinator: Dave Murphy
Marketing Manager: Dan Dressler
Production Project Manager: David Saltzberg
Design Coordinator: Elaine Kasmer
Manufacturing Coordinator: Beth Welsh
Prepress Vendor: Aptara, Inc.

8th edition

Copyright © 2019 Wolters Kluwer.

9 8 7 6 5 4 3 2 1

Printed in The United States of America

Library of Congress Cataloging-in-Publication Data

Names: LoCicero, Joseph, III, 1948- editor. | Feins, Richard H., editor. |
    Colson, Yolonda L., editor. | Rocco, Gaetano, MD, editor.
Title: Shields' general thoracic surgery / [edited by] Joseph LoCicero III,
    Richard H. Feins, Yolonda L. Colson, Gaetano Rocco.
Other titles: General thoracic surgery.
Description: 8th edition. | Philadelphia : Wolters Kluwer, [2019] | Preceded
    by General thoracic surgery / edited by Thomas W. Shields ... [et al.].
    7th ed. c2009. | Includes bibliographical references and index.
Identifiers: LCCN 2017051947 | ISBN 9781451195224
Subjects: | MESH: Thoracic Surgical Procedures | Thoracic Neoplasms–surgery
Classification: LCC RD536 | NLM WF 980 | DDC 617.5/4059–dc23
LC record available at https://lccn.loc.gov/2017051947

LWW.com

Edward J. Bergeron, MD
Munson Medical Center
Traverse City, Michigan

Laureline Berteloot, MD
Radiologist
Department of Pediatric Imaging
Necker-Enfants Malades Hospital
Paris, France

Sanjeev Bhalla, MD
Section Chief
Professor of Radiology
Cardiothoracic Imaging
Mallinckrodt Institute of Radiology
Washington University
St. Louis, Missouri

Shanda H. Blackmon, MD, MPH
Associate Professor
Department of Surgery
Division of Thoracic Surgery
Mayo Clinic
Rochester, Minnesota

Eugene H. Blackstone, MD
Head of Clinical Investigations
The Sydell and Arnold Miller Family Heart &
    Vascular Institute
Staff member
Department of Thoracic and Cardiovascular
    Surgery
Quantitative Health Sciences and Transplant
    Center
Cleveland Clinic
Cleveland, Ohio

Antonio Bobbio, MD, PhD
Praticien Hospitalier
Service de Chirurgie Thoracique
Hôpital Cochin, APHP
Paris, France

Daniel J. Boffa, MD
Associate Professor
Department of Surgery
Yale School of Medicine
New Haven, Connecticut

Timothy Brand, MD
Department of Cardiothoracic Surgery
University of North Carolina at Chapel Hill
Chapel Hill, North Carolina

Alejandro C. Bribriesco, MD
Associate Staff
Department of Thoracic and Cardiovascular
    Surgery
Cleveland Clinic
Cleveland, Ohio

Lisa M. Brown, MD, MAS
Assistant Professor
Division of Cardiothoracic Surgery
UC Davis Health
Sacramento, California

Andrew Brownlee, MD
Fellow
Section of Cardiothoracic Surgery
University of Chicago Medicine
Chicago, Illinois

Alessandro Brunelli, MD
Consultant Thoracic Surgeon
Honorary Clinical Associate Professor
Department of Thoracic Surgery
St. James's University Hospital
Leeds, United Kingdom

Raphael Bueno, MD
Chief
Division of Thoracic Surgery
Brigham and Women's Hospital
Boston, Massachusetts

Timothy F. Burns, MD, PhD
Assistant Professor
Department of Medicine
Division of Hematology Oncology
University of Pittsburgh School of Medicine
Pittsburgh, Pennsylvania

Peter H. Burri, MD
Professor Emeritus of Anatomy
Institute of Anatomy
University of Bern
Bern, Switzerland

Bryan M. Burt, MD
Associate Professor of Surgery
Department of Surgery
Baylor College of Medicine
Houston, Texas

Shamus R. Carr, MD, FACS
Assistant Professor
Department of Surgery
Division of Thoracic Surgery
University of Maryland School of Medicine
Baltimore, Maryland

Philip Carrott, MD
Assistant Professor
Section of Thoracic Surgery
University of Michigan
Ann Arbor, Michigan

Ernest G. Chan, MD
Department of Cardiothoracic Surgery
University of Pittsburgh Medical Center
Pittsburgh, Pennsylvania

Patrick G. Chan, MD
Department of Cardiothoracic Surgery
University of Pittsburgh Medical center
Pittsburgh, Pennsylvania

John Holt Chaney, MD
Attending Physician
Lexington, Kentucky

Andrew C. Chang, MD
John Alexander Distinguished Professor
Head of the Section of Thoracic Surgery
University of Michigan
Ann Arbor, Michigan

Stephanie Chang, MD
Cardiothoracic Surgery Fellow
Department of Surgery
Washington University in St. Louis
St. Louis, Missouri

Delphine L. Chen, MD
Associate Professor of Radiology, Medicine,
    and Biomedical Engineering
Mallinckrodt Institute of Radiology
Washington University School of Medicine
St. Louis, Missouri

Aaron M. Cheng, MD
Associate Professor
Department of Surgery
Division of Cardiothoracic Surgery
Co-Director
UWMC Cardiothoracic ICU
University of Washington
Seattle, Washington

Mala R. Chinoy, PhD, MBA
Professor
Department of Biochemistry and
    Molecular Biology
Penn State College of Medicine
Hershey, Pennsylvania

Priscilla Chiu, MD, PhD
Assistant Professor
Department of Surgery
University of Toronto
Staff Surgeon
Division of General and Thoracic Surgery
The Hospital for Sick Children
Toronto, Ontario, Canada

Cliff K. C. Choong, MBBS, FRCS, FRACS
Associate Professor in Surgery
Consultant Thoracic Surgeon
Monash University School of Rural Health
Latrobe Regional Hospital
Victoria, Australia

Anna Maria Ciccone, MD, PhD
Assistant Professor
Division of Thoracic Surgery
Sapienza University of Rome
Rome, Italy

Graham A. Colditz, MD, DrPH
Niess-Gain Professor of Surgery
Washington University School of Medicine
St. Louis, Missouri

Stéphane Collaud, MD, MSc
Department of Thoracic and Vascular Surgery
    and Heart-Lung Transplantation
Paris-Sud University
Marie Lannelongue Hospital
Le Plessis-Robinson, France

Willy Coosemans, MD, PhD
Clinic Head
Department of Thoracic Surgery
University Hospitals Leuven
Leuven, Belgium

Traves D. Crabtree, MD
Professor of Surgery
Southern Illinois University School of Medicine
Springfield, Illinois

Gerard J. Criner, MD
Professor and Chair
Department of Thoracic Medicine and
    Surgery
Lewis Katz School of Medicine at Temple
    University
Philadelphia, Pennsylvania

Richard S. D'Agostino, MD
Assistant Clinical Professor of Cardiothoracic
    Surgery
Tufts University School of Medicine
Boston Massachusetts
Chair
Division of Thoracic and Cardiovascular
    Surgery
Lahey Hospital and Medical Center
Burlington, Massachusetts

Walid Leonardo Dajer-Fadel, MD
Associate Professor
Department of Cardiothoracic Surgery
General Hospital of Mexico
Mexico City, Mexico

Thomas D'Amico, MD
Gary Hock Endowed Professor of Surgery
Chief, Section of General Thoracic Surgery
Program Director, Thoracic Surgery
Duke University Medical Center
Durham, North Carolina

Gail E. Darling, MD, FRCSC
Professor of Thoracic Surgery
University of Toronto
University Health Network, Toronto
    General Hospital
Toronto, Ontario, Canada

Philippe Dartevelle, MD
Professor of Thoracic and Cardiovascular
    Surgery
University Paris Sud
Marie Lannelongue Hospital
Le Plessis-Robinson, France

Hiroshi Date, MD
Professor and Chairman
Department of Thoracic Surgery
Kyoto University Graduate School of
    Medicine
Kyoto, Japan

Jonathan D'Cunha, MD, PhD
Associate Professor of Surgery
Vice Chairman
Research and Education
Chief
Division of Lung Transplantation/Lung
    Failure
Surgical Director, ECMO
Program Director
Thoracic Surgery Traditional Residency
Program Director
Advanced Lung/Heart Failure Fellowship
Department of Cardiothoracic Surgery
University of Pittsburgh Medical Center
Pittsburgh, Pennsylvania

Herbert Decaluwé, MD, PhD
Department of Thoracic Surgery
University Hospitals Leuven
Leuven, Belgium

Malcolm M. DeCamp, MD
Fowler McCormick Professor of Surgery
Northwestern University Feinberg School
    of Medicine
Chief, Division of Thoracic Surgery
Northwestern Memorial Hospital
Chicago, Illinois

Tracey Dechert, MD, FACS
Assistant Professor of Surgery
Boston University School of Medicine
Division of Trauma and Surgical Critical Care
Boston Medical Center
Boston, Massachusetts

Sebastián Defranchi, MD, MBA
Staff General Thoracic Surgeon
Chair, Patient Safety Department
Chair, Support Services Department
Hospital Universitario Fundación Favaloro
Ciudad de Buenos Aires, Argentina

Pierre Delaere, MD, PhD
Professor
Department of ENT, Head and Neck Surgery
University Hospitals Leuven
Leuven, Belgium

Paul De Leyn, MD, PhD
Professor
Chief, Department of Surgery
University Hospitals Leuven
Leuven, Belgium

Lorenzo Del Sorbo, MD
Assistant Professor
Interdepartmental Division of Critical
    Care Medicine
University of Toronto
University Health Network, Toronto
    General Hospital
Toronto, Ontario, Canada

Steven R. DeMeester, MD
Thoracic and Foregut Surgery
Division of General and Minimally Invasive
    Surgery
The Oregon Clinic
Portland, Oregon

Todd L. Demmy, MD
Professor of Oncology
Department of Thoracic Surgery
Roswell Park Cancer Institute
Professor
Department of Surgery
University of Buffalo, State University of
    New York
Buffalo, New York

Willem Adriaan den Hengst, MD, PhD
Resident
Department of Thoracic and Vascular Surgery
Antwerp University Hospital
Antwerp, Belgium

Chadrick E. Denlinger, MD
Associate Professor
Department of Surgery
Medical University of South Carolina
Charleston, South Carolina

Marc de Perrot, MD, MSc, FRCSC
Associate Professor of Surgery
Division of Thoracic Surgery
University of Toronto
University Health Network, Toronto
    General Hospital
Toronto, Ontario, Canada

Lieven P. Depypere, MD, FEBTS
Associate Clinical Head
Department of Thoracic Surgery
University Hospitals Leuven
Leuven, Belgium

Mathieu Derouet, PhD
Scientific Associate
Department of Thoracic Surgery
University Health Network
Toronto, Ontario, Canada

Daniele Diso, MD, PhD
Associate Professor
Department of Thoracic Surgery,
Sapienza University of Rome
Rome, Italy

Laura Donahoe, MD
Thoracic Surgeon
University of Toronto
University Health Network
Toronto General Hospital
Toronto, Ontario, Canada

Dean M. Donahue, MD
Assistant Professor
Department of Thoracic Surgery
Massachusetts General Hospital
Harvard Medical School
Boston, Massachusetts

Jessica S. Donington, MD, MSCR
Associate Professor
Department of Cardiothoracic Surgery
NYU School of Medicine
New York, New York

Frank D'Ovidio, MD, PhD
Associate Professor
Section General Thoracic Surgery
Department of Surgery
Columbia University
Attending Surgeon
NewYork-Presbyterian Hospital
New York, New York

Nigel E. Drury, PhD, FRCS(CTh)
Clinician Scientist & Consultant in
    Cardiothoracic Surgery
Birmingham Children's Hospital
Birmingham, United Kingdom

Lingling Du, MD
Department of Hematology and Medical
    Oncology
Ochsner Clinic Foundation
New Orleans, Louisiana

Mark R. Dylewski, MD
Chief of Thoracic Surgery
Miami Cancer Institute
Baptist Health of South Florida
Miami, Florida

Janet Edwards, MD, MPH
Assistant Professor
Division of Thoracic Surgery
Cumming School of Medicine at University
    of Calgary
Calgary, Alberta

Melanie A. Edwards, MD
Assistant Professor
Division of Cardiothoracic Surgery
Saint Louis University School of Medicine
Saint Louis, Missouri

Dominic Emerson, MD
Fellow
Cardiac Surgery
Cedars-Sinai Medical Center
Los Angeles, California

Elie Fadel, MD, PhD
Chief
Department of Thoracic and Vascular Surgery
    and Heart-Lung Transplantation
Hopital Marie Lannelongue and Université
    Paris Sud
Le Plessis-Robinson, France

Pierre-Emmanuel Falcoz, MD, PhD, FECTS
Department of Thoracic Surgery
Strasbourg University Hospital
Strasbourg, France

Farhood Farjah, MD, MPH
Associate Professor
Division of Cardiothoracic Surgery
University of Washington
Seattle, Washington

Richard H. Feins, MD
Professor of Surgery
Division of Cardiothoracic Surgery
University of North Carolina at Chapel Hill
Chapel Hill, North Carolina

Stanley C. Fell†
Professor of Cardiothoracic Surgery
Albert Einstein College of Medicine
Bronx, New York

Mark K. Ferguson, MD
Professor
Department of Surgery
University of Chicago Pritzker School of Medicine
Chicago, Illinois

Felix G. Fernandez, MD, MSc
Associate Professor of Surgery
General Thoracic Surgery
Emory University School of Medicine
Atlanta, Georgia

Hiran C. Fernando, MBBS, FRCS
Professor of Surgery
Virginia Commonwealth University
Richmond, Virginia
Inova Fairfax Medical Campus
Falls Church, Virginia

Pasquale Ferraro, MD
Professor
Department of Surgery
Chief
Division of Thoracic Surgery
Alfonso Minicozzi and Family Chair in
    Thoracic Surgery and Lung Transplantation
Centre Hospitalier de l'Université de Montréal
Montreal, Quebec

Raja M. Flores, MD
Chairman and Professor
Department of Thoracic Surgery
Icahn School of Medicine at Mount Sinai
New York, New York

Seth Force, MD
Professor
Department of Surgery
Emory University School of Medicine
Atlanta, Georgia

Richard K. Freeman, MD, MBA
System Chief Medical Officer
St Vincent Health
Indianapolis, Indiana

Joseph S. Friedberg, MD, FACS
Professor
University of Maryland School of Medicine
Thoracic Surgeon-in-Chief
Department of Surgery
Division of Thoracic Surgery
University of Maryland Medical System
Baltimore, Maryland

Henning A. Gaissert, MD
Associate Professor of Surgery
Harvard Medical School
Visiting Surgeon
Massachusetts General Hospital
Boston, Massachusetts

Sidhu P. Gangadharan, MD
Chief
Division of Thoracic Surgery and
    Interventional Pulmonology
Beth Israel Deaconess Medical Center
Associate Professor of Surgery
Harvard Medical School
Boston, Massachusetts

Perry Gerard, MD, FACR
Professor of Radiology and Medicine
Vice Chairman of Radiology
Director of Radiology IT
New York Medical College
Director of Nuclear Medicine and PET-CT
Westchester Medical Center
Valhalla, New York

Rafael Garza-Castillon, MD
Thoracic Surgery Fellow
Department of Thoracic Surgery
Brigham and Women's Hospital
Boston, Massachusetts

Ritu R. Gill, MD, MPH
Assistant Professor
Department of Radiology
Beth Israel Deaconess Medical Center
Harvard Medical School
Boston, Massachusetts

Erin A. Gillaspie, MD
Assistant Professor
Department of Thoracic Surgery
Vanderbilt University Medical Center
Nashville, Tennessee

†Deceased

Jason P. Glotzbach, MD
Assistant Professor
Division of Cardiothoracic Surgery
University of Utah
Salt Lake City, Utah

Diego Gonzalez-Rivas, MD, FECTS
Director Uniportal VATS Training Program
Department of Thoracic Surgery
Shanghai Pulmonary Hospital
Shanghai, China

Andrei-Bogdan Gorgos, MD
Associate Professor
Department of Radiology
University of Montreal
Montreal, Quebec

Dominique Gossot, MD
Head of Thoracic Department—IMM
Curie-Montsouris Thorax Institute
Paris, France

Ramaswamy Govindan, MD
Professor of Medicine
Anheuser-Busch Endowed Chair in
    Medical Oncology
Director, Section of Oncology
Division of Oncology
Washington University School of Medicine
St. Louis, Missouri

Gabriele Simone Grasso, MD
Department of Medicine and Surgery
University of Milano-Bicocca
Milan, Italy

Christina L. Greene, MD
Integrated Cardiac Resident
Department of Cardiothoracic Surgery
Stanford University School of Medicine
Standford, California

Yosef Jose Greenspon, MD, FACS, FAAP
Assistant Professor
Department of Pediatrics
Division of Surgery
Cardinal Glennon Children's Hospital
St. Louis University School of Medicine
St. Louis, Missouri

Sean C. Grondin, MD, MPH, FRCSC, FACS
Professor and Head
Department of Surgery
Cumming School of Medicine at University
    of Calgary
Calgary Zone Clinical Department Head
Alberta Health Services
Foothills Medical Centre
Calgary, Alberta

Federica Grosso, MD
Department of Oncology
SS Antonio e Biagio General Hospital
Alessandria, Italy

Shawn S. Groth, MD, MS
Assistant Professor
Department of Surgery
Baylor College of Medicine
Houston, Texas

Dominique Grunenwald, MD, PhD
Professor Emeritus
Department of Thoracic and Cardiovascular
    Surgery
Pierre and Marie Curie University
Paris, France

Claude Guinet, MD
Radiologist
Department of Radiology
Paris Center University Hospital
Paris, France

Julian Guitron, MD
Associate Professor
Department of Surgery
Division of Thoracic Surgery
University of Cincinnati
Cincinnati, Ohio

Jinny S. Ha, MD
Cardiothoracic Surgery Fellow
Division of Thoracic Surgery
Johns Hopkins Hospital
Baltimore, Maryland

Hironori Haga, MD
Department of Pathology
Kyoto University Hospital
Kyoto, Japan

Semih Halezeroğlu, MD, FETCS
Professor and Chief
Department of Thoracic Surgery
Acibadem University School of Medicine
Istanbul, Turkey

Matthew G. Hartwig, MD, MHS
Associate Professor of Surgery
Division of Thoracic Surgery
Duke University Health System
Durham, North Carolina

Dominik Harzheim, MD
Department of Pneumology and Critical Care
Thoraxklinik, University of Heidelberg
Heidelberg, Germany

Stephen Hazelrigg, MD
Professor and Chairman
Department of Cardiothoracic Surgery
Southern Illinois University School of
    Medicine
Springfield, Illinois

Mark W. Hennon, MD
Assistant Professor
Department of Surgery
University at Buffalo, State University of
    New York
Assistant Professor of Oncology
Department of Thoracic Surgery
Roswell Park Cancer Institute
Buffalo, New York

Claudia I. Henschke, PhD, MD
Department of Radiology
Icahn School of Medicine at Mount Sinai
New York, New York

Felix J. F. Herth, MD, PhD, FCCP, FERS
CMO
Department of Pneumology and Critical
    Care Medicine
Thoraxklinik, University of Heidelberg
Heidelberg, Germany

Nicholas R. Hess, MD
Resident
Department of Cardiothoracic Surgery
University of Pittsburgh Medical Center
Pittsburgh, Pennsylvania

Maxime Heyndrickx, MD
Department of Thoracic Surgery
University Hospital of Caen
Caen, France

Wayne Hofstetter, MD
Professor of Surgery and Deputy Chair
Department of Thoracic and Cardiovascular
    Surgery
University of Texas MD Anderson Cancer Center
Houston, Texas

Young K. Hong, MD
Surgical Oncology and
    Hepatopancreatobiliary Fellow
Department of Surgery
Louisville, Kentucky

Yinin Hu, MD
Resident
Department of Surgery
University of Virginia
Charlottesville, Virginia

James Huang, MD
Associate Attending Surgeon
Thoracic Service, Department of Surgery
Memorial Sloan Kettering Cancer Center
New York, New York

Miriam Huang, MD
Clinical Assistant Professor
Department of Surgery
Jacobs School of Medicine & Biomedical
    Sciences
University of Buffalo
Buffalo, New York

Dedication to Dr. Thomas W. Shields

This 8th edition of General Thoracic Surgery marks the first time Dr. Shields has not been an active member of the editorial directors, yet his influence on the text remains strong. His lifelong interest in lung cancer began in 1951 with a fellowship at the Palmer Memorial Hospital, the cancer building that was part of Deaconess Hospital, now Beth Israel Deaconess Medical Center. His experiences with the thoracic surgeon, dynamic and controversial Richard Overholt inspired him to begin a lifelong study into thoracic lymphatic drainage and lesser pulmonary resections. He traveled the globe gathering data from leading centers making strong bonds with many international colleagues. Using this wealth of knowledge, he compiled the first edition of General Thoracic Surgery published in 1972, updating it every few years.

Dr. Shields was a legend to the surgical students and residents of Northwestern University up to the time of his death in 2010. His devotion to clear communication of thought made him a tough taskmaster. His advocacy of evidence-based practice often made him a lightning rod among his colleagues. We hope that this edition continues the tradition of enhancing our understanding and practice of thoracic surgery through assimilation of knowledge and expertise from around the world.

—JLIII

Dedication to Dr. Carolyn E. Reed, MD

This 8th edition of General Thoracic Surgery is dedicated in part to our friend and colleague, Dr. Carolyn E. Reed who was an editor of the 7th edition and was working on this edition until her untimely death.

Dr. Reed was an outstanding clinician, teacher, and researcher. Her impact on the field of thoracic surgery was extraordinary. While maintaining a busy clinical practice at the Medical University of South Carolina, she made a major impact on our knowledge of diseases of the chest and how to treat them. She was an NIH-funded researcher and investigator on numerous important national clinical trials. She served our specialty as the first woman chair of the American Board of Thoracic Surgery and the first woman president of the Southern Thoracic Surgical Association. Also, she served as vice-chair of the Residency Review Committee for Thoracic Surgery, treasurer of the Society of Thoracic Surgeons, treasurer of Women in Thoracic Surgery, council member of the American Association for Thoracic Surgery, board member of the Joint Council for Thoracic Surgical Education and the Thoracic Surgery Foundation for Research and Education. Posthumously, she was unanimously elected the first woman president of the Society of Thoracic Surgeons.

After her love for providing care to her patients, Dr. Reed's passion was imparting knowledge to her students and residents. It is our hope that this edition of General Thoracic Surgery will make a fitting completion to her obligations, which were such a large part of her life and that those who use it will continue to experience the wonder of being her student.

—RHF

To my family and to all succeeding generations of knowledge-seeking, innovative healers around the world to whom we entrust our future health.

—JLIII

To the men and women of Thoracic Surgery who have dedicated their lives to the treatment of diseases of the chest. It is a specialty that has embraced the research and new technologies required to serve our patients at the highest level and the spirit of professionalism that is the envy of all of medicine. And to the teachers of Thoracic Surgery who devote themselves day in and day out to ensuring that there will always be outstanding chest surgeons.

—RHF

To Gina and Raffaele, sempiternal source of energy and inspiration. Amor gignit amorem.

—GR

To my father for teaching me to dream big, my mother for making hard work and fortitude part of my DNA, my patients for giving me purpose, my collaborator Mark Grinstaff for the gift of creativity and friendship, my husband Gray for providing unlimited love and support and believing in the impossible every day, my two daughters, Karinne and Azuri, and all of my trainees for opening my eyes to the amazing potential of the next generation, and my special team that keeps everything running and makes my work enjoyable.

—YLC

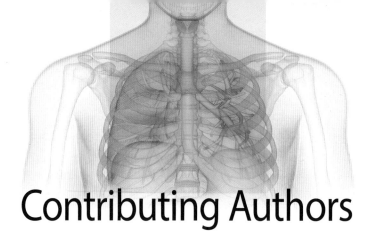

Contributing Authors

Ghulam Abbas, MD, MHCM, FACS
Chief, Division of Thoracic Surgery
West Virginia University School of Medicine
Morgantown, West Virginia

Jay Acharya, MD
Assistant Professor
Department of Radiology
Keck Medicine of USC
Los Angeles, California

Usman Ahmad, MD
Assistant Professor of Surgery
Staff Surgeon, Thoracic Surgery
Cleveland Clinic
Cleveland, Ohio

Marco Alifano, MD, PhD
Full Professor
Department of Thoracic Surgery
Paris Descartes University
Paris Center University Hospital
Paris, France

Mark S. Allen, MD
Professor of Surgery
Division of General Thoracic Surgery
Mayo Clinic
Rochester, Minnesota

Nasser K. Altorki, MB, BCh
Professor of Thoracic Surgery
Department of Cardiothoracic Surgery
Weill Cornell Medical College
New York Presbyterian Hospital
New York, New York

Isabel Alvarado-Cabrero, MD, PhD
Department of Pathology
Mexican Oncology Hospital, IMSS
Mexico City, Mexico

Rafael Andrade, MD, MHA
Associate Professor
Chief, Division of Thoracic and Foregut
    Surgery
University of Minnesota
Minneapolis, Minnesota

Marco Anile, MD, PhD
Associate Professor
Department of Thoracic Surgery
Sapienza University of Rome
Rome, Italy

Beatrice Aramini, MD, PhD
Assistant Professor
Department of Medical and Surgical Sciences
    for Children and Adults
Division of Thoracic Surgery
University of Modena and Reggio Emilia
Modena, Italy

Saeed Arefanian, MD
General Surgery Resident
Department of Surgery
Washington University in St. Louis
St. Louis, Missouri

Amrita K. Arneja, MD
Neuroradiology Fellow
Department of Radiology
Mount Sinai Health System
New York, New York

Oscar Arrieta-Rodriguez, MD, MSc
Department Coordinator
Thoracic Oncology Unit
Instituto Nacional de Cancerología
México City, México

Hisao Asamura, MD
Professor of Surgery
Chief
Division of Thoracic Surgery
Keio University School of Medicine
Tokyo, Japan

Hugh G. Auchincloss, MD, MPH
Division of Thoracic Surgery
Massachusetts General Hospital
Boston, Massachusetts

Diego Avella Patino, MD
Assistant Professor of Surgery
Division of Cardiac and Thoracic Surgery
University of Missouri
Columbia, Missouri

Lea Azour, MD
Assistant Professor
Department of Radiology
NYU Langone Medical Center
New York, New York

Carl L. Backer, MD
Professor of Surgery
Northwestern University Feinberg School
    of Medicine
Division Head
Cardiovascular-Thoracic Surgery
Ann & Robert H. Lurie Children's Hospital
    of Chicago
Chicago, Illinois

Patrick Bagan, MD
Head of Department
Unit of Thoracic and Vascular Surgery
Victor Dupouy Hospital
Argenteuil, France

Erin E. Bailey, MD
General Surgeon
Department of Surgery
Graham Health System
Canton, Illinois

Brian P. Barrick, MD, DDS
Professor
Department of Anesthesiology
University of North Carolina at Chapel Hill
Chapel Hill, North Carolina

Thomas L. Bauer II, MD
Associate Professor of Surgery
Hackensack Meridian School of Medicine at
    Seton Hall University
South Orange, New Jersey
Hackensack Meridian Health Jersey Shore
    University Medical Center
Neptune, New Jersey

Egidio Beretta, MD, PhD
Department of Medicine and Surgery
University of Milano-Bicocca
Milan, Italy

Charles B. Huddleston, MD
Professor
Department of Surgery
St. Louis University School of Medicine
St. Louis, Missouri

Jessica L. Hudson, MD, MPHS
Surgical Resident
Department of Surgery
Washington University
St. Louis, Missouri

Mark D. Iannettoni, MD, MBA
W. Randolph Chitwood, Jr., MD,
    Distinguished Chair in Cardiovascular
    Sciences
Professor and Chief
Division of Thoracic and Foregut Surgery
Program Director
Thoracic Surgery Residency
Chief
Cardiovascular Service Line
East Carolina Heart Institute at Vidant
    Medical Center
Greenville, North Carolina

Carlos Ibarra-Pérez, MD
Master and Doctor in Medical Sciences
University of México
Honorary Consultant in Thoracic Surgery
Instituto Nacional de Cardiología Ignacio
    Chavez
México City, Mexico

Kendra Iskander, MD, MPH
General Surgeon
St. Joseph Hospital
Eureka, California

Dawn E. Jaroszewski, MD, MBA, FACS
Professor of Surgery
Department of Cardiothoracic Surgery
Mayo Clinic
Phoenix, Arizona

Leila Jazayeri, MD
Plastic and Reconstructive Surgeon
Kaiser Permanente San Leandro Medical
    Center
San Leandro, California

Scott B. Johnson, MD
Division Chief, General Thoracic Surgery
Department of Cardiothoracic Surgery
UT Health San Antonio
San Antonio, Texas

David W. Johnstone, MD
Division of Cardiothoracic Surgery
Medical College of Wisconsin
Milwaukee, Wisconsin

David R. Jones, MD
Professor and Chief
Thoracic Surgery Service
Fiona and Stanly Druckenmiller Chair for
    Lung Cancer Research
Memorial Sloan Kettering Cancer Center
New York, New York

Erkan Kaba, MD
Assistant Professor
Department of Thoracic Surgery
Istanbul Bilim University
Istanbul, Turkey

Mohamed K. Kamel, MD
Clinical Fellow
Department of Cardiothoracic Surgery
Weill Cornell Medical College
New York Presbyterian Hospital
New York, New York

Neil Kapadia, MD
Assistant Professor
Department of Radiology
Temple University
Philadelphia, Pennsylvania

Brian J. Karlovits, DO
Director of Clinical Operations
Assistant Professor
Department of Radiation Oncology
UPMC Hillman Cancer Center—Shadyside
Pittsburgh, Pennsylvania

Shaf Keshavjee, MD, FRCSC, FACS
Professor, Division of Thoracic Surgery
University of Toronto
James Wallace McCutcheon Chair in Surgery
Surgeon in Chief
University Health Network
Toronto, Ontario, Canada

Onkar V. Khullar, MD
Assistant Professor
Division of Cardiothoracic Surgery
Emory University School of Medicine
Atlanta, Georgia

Biniam Kidane, MD, MSc, FRCSC
Assistant Professor
Section of Thoracic Surgery
Department of Surgery
University of Manitoba
Winnipeg, Manitoba

Min P. Kim, MD
Associate Professor
Chief, Division of Thoracic Surgery
Department of Surgery
Houston Methodist Hospital
Houston, Texas

Jacob A. Klapper, MD
Assistant Professor of Surgery
Duke University Hospital
Durham, North Carolina

Patrick Kohtz, MD
Resident
Department of Surgery
University of Colorado Anschutz Medical
    Campus
Aurora, Colorado

Rupesh Kotecha, MD
Department of Radiation Oncology
Cleveland Clinic, Taussig Cancer Institute
Cleveland, Ohio
Department of Radiation Oncology
Miami Cancer Institute
Baptist Health South Florida
Miami, Florida

Vasileios Kouritas, MD, PhD, CTh
Cardiothoracic Surgeon
Department of Thoracic Surgery
St. James's University Hospital
Leeds, United Kingdom

Benjamin D. Kozower, MD, MPH
Professor
Department of Surgery
Washington University School of Medicine
St. Louis, Missouri

Seth B. Krantz, MD
Division of Thoracic Surgery
NorthShore University HealthSystem
Evanston, Illinois
Clinical Assistant Professor
Department of Surgery
University of Chicago Pritzker School of
    Medicine
Chicago, Illinois

Mark J. Krasna, MD
Clinical Professor of Surgery
Rutgers New Jersey Medical School
Newark, New Jersey
Hackensack Meridian School of Medicine at
    Seton Hall University
South Orange, New Jersey

Daniel Kreisel, MD, PhD
Professor of Surgery, Pathology and
    Immunology
Surgical Director, Lung Transplant Program
Washington University School of Medicine
St. Louis, Missouri

Alexander Krupnick, MD
Department of Surgery
Division of CT Surgery
University of Virginia
Charlottesville, Virginia

Kiran Lagisetty, MD
Assistant Professor
Section of Thoracic Surgery
Department of Surgery
University of Michigan
Ann Arbor, Michigan

Francesca Lanfranconi, MD, PhD
Research Officer
Institute of Sport, Exercise and Active Living
 (ISEAL)
Victoria University
Melbourne, Australia

Jacob C. Langer, MD
Professor of Surgery
University of Toronto
Pediatric Surgeon
The Hospital for Sick Children
Toronto, Ontario, Canada

Nathaniel B. Langer, MD, MSc
Department of Thoracic and Vascular Surgery
 and Heart-Lung Transplantation
Marie Lannelongue Hospital
Le Plessis-Robinson, France

Michael Lanuti, MD
Associate Professor of Surgery
Harvard Medical School
Director of Thoracic Oncology
Division of Thoracic Surgery
Massachusetts General Hospital
Boston, Massachusetts

Rossano Lattanzio, MD, PhD, Dr.
Researcher
Department of Medical, Oral and
 Biotechnological Sciences
University "G. d'Annunzio"
Chieti, Italy

Christine Lau, MD, MBA
Professor of Surgery
Chief, Division of Thoracic Surgery
University of Virginia
Charlottesville, Virginia

Kelvin Lau, MA(Oxon), DPhil(Oxon), FRCS(CTh)
Chief of Thoracic Surgery
St. Bartholomew's Hospital
London, United Kingdom

Richard S. Lazzaro, MD, FACS
Associate Professor of Cardiothoracic Surgery
Department of Cardiothoracic Surgery
Donald and Barbara Zucker School of
 Medicine at Hofstra/Northwell
Chief
Division of Thoracic Surgery
Lenox Hill Hospital
Director, Robotic Thoracic Surgery
Northwell Health
New York, New York

Dong-Seok Daniel Lee, MD
Assistant Professor
Department of Thoracic Surgery
Mount Sinai Health System
New York, New York

Toni Lerut, MD, PhD
Emeritus Professor of Surgery
Emeritus Chairman, Department of
 Thoracic Surgery
University Hospitals Leuven, Gasthuisberg
 Campus
Leuven, Belgium

Gunda Leschber, MD
Head of Department of Thoracic Surgery
ELK Berlin Chest Hospital
Berlin, Germany

Kunwei Li, MD
Department of Radiology
Icahn School of Medicine at Mount Sinai
New York, New York

Moishe Liberman, MD, PhD
Director, CETOC
Associate Professor of Surgery
Division of Thoracic Surgery
University of Montreal
Montreal, Quebec

Michael J. Liptay, MD
Professor and Chairman
Department of Cardiovascular and
 Thoracic Surgery
Rush University Medical Center
Chicago, Illinois

Virginia R. Litle, MD
Professor of Surgery
Chief of Thoracic Surgery
Boston University
Boston, Massachusetts

Joseph LoCicero III, MD
Professor Emeritus of Surgery
SUNY Downstate Medical Center
Brooklyn, New York
Consultant
Mobile County Health Department
Mobile, Alabama

Jason Michael Long, MD, MPH
Assistant Professor
Department of Surgery
UNC Medical Center
Chapel Hill, North Carolina

Christine Lorut, MD
Unit of Pneumology
Hôpital Cochin, APHP
Paris, France

Donald E. Low, MD, FACS, FRCS(C)
Head of Thoracic Surgery and Thoracic
 Oncology
Department of General, Thoracic and
 Vascular Surgery
Virginia Mason Medical Center
Seattle, Washington

James D. Luketich, MD, FACS
Henry T. Bahnson Professor and Chairman
Department of Cardiothoracic Surgery
Chief, Division of Thoracic and Foregut
 Surgery
University of Pittsburgh School of Medicine
Pittsburgh, Pennsylvania

Audrey Lupo, MD, PhD
Department of Pathology
Hôpitaux Universitaires Paris Centre
Paris, France

Ronson J. Madathil, MD
Acting Assistant Professor
Division of Cardiothoracic Surgery
University of Washington
Seattle, Washington

Mitchell J. Magee, MD, MS
Chief
Division of Thoracic Surgery
Medical City Dallas Hospital
Dallas, Texas

Raja Mahidhara, MD
Thoracic Surgery
St Vincent Health
Indianapolis, Indiana

J. Shawn Mallery, MD
Associate Professor of Medicine
Department of Medicine
Division of Gastroenterology, Hepatology and
 Nutrition
University of Minnesota
Minneapolis, Minnesota

Mirella Marino, MD
Department of Pathology
Regina Elena National Cancer Institute
Rome, Italy

M. Blair Marshall, MD, FACS
Professor of Surgery
Chief, Division of Thoracic Surgery
Department of Surgery
MedStar Georgetown University Hospital
Washington, District of Columbia

Gilbert Massard, MD
Professor
Department of Thoracic Surgery and Lung
 Transplantation
Strasbourg University Hospital
Strasbourg, France

Douglas J. Mathisen, MD
Hermes C. Grillo Professor of Surgery
Harvard Medical School
Chief
General Thoracic Surgery
Massachusetts General Hospital
Boston, Massachusetts

Giulio Maurizi, MD
Division of Thoracic Surgery
Sapienza University of Rome
Sant'Andrea Hospital
Rome, Italy

Donna E. Maziak, MDCM, MSc, FRCSC, FACS
Professor
University of Ottawa
Surgical Oncology Division of Thoracic
    Surgery
Ottawa Hospital—General Campus
Ottawa, Ontario

Daniel P. McCarthy, MD, MBA
Assistant Professor
Department of Surgery
University of Wisconsin
Madison, Wisconsin

Paul Michael McFadden, MD
Professor of Clinical Cardiothoracic Surgery
Surgical Co-Director of Lung Transplantation
Division of Cardiothoracic Surgery
Department of Surgery
University of Southern California
Los Angeles, California

Rachel L. Medbery, MD
Thoracic Surgery Fellow
Department of Surgery
Division of Cardiothoracic Surgery
Emory University School of Medicine
Atlanta, Georgia

Robert A. Meguid, MD, MPH, FACS
Associate Professor
Section of General Thoracic Surgery
Division of Cardiothoracic Surgery
Department of Surgery
University of Colorado Anschutz Medical Campus
Aurora, Colorado

Babak J. Mehrara, MD
Professor and Chief, Plastic and
    Reconstructive Surgery Service
William G. Cahon Chair in Surgery
Memorial Sloan Kettering Cancer Center
New York, New York

Steven J. Mentzer, MD
Professor of Surgery
Brigham and Women's Hospital
Harvard Medical School
Boston, Massachusetts

Robert E. Merritt, MD
Associate Professor of Surgery
Director
The Division of Thoracic Surgery
The Ohio State UnviersityWexner Medical
    Center
Columbus, Ohio

Giuseppe Miserocchi, MD
Professor of Physiology and Biophysics
Department of Medicine and Surgery
University Milano-Bicocca
Milan, Italy

John D. Mitchell, MD
Courtenay C. and Lucy Patten Davis Endowed
    Chair in Thoracic Surgery
Professor and Chief, Section of General
    Thoracic Surgery
Division of Cardiothoracic Surgery
University of Colorado Anschutz Medical
    Campus
Aurora, Colorado

Kamran Mohiuddin, MD
Director Clinical Research
Einstein Medical Center
Philadelphia, Pennsylvania

Elie Mouhayar, MD
Associate Professor of Medicine
Department of Cardiology
University of Texas MD Anderson
    Cancer Center
Houston, Texas

Michael S. Mulligan, MD
Professor of Surgery
Chief
Division of Cardiothoracic Surgery
University of Washington
Seattle, Washington

Michael S. Mulvihill, MD
Resident in Surgery
Department of Surgery
Duke University Medical Center
Durham, North Carolina

Sudish C. Murthy, MD, PhD, FACS, FCCP
Department of Thoracic and Cardiovascular
    Surgery
Cleveland Clinic
Cleveland, Ohio

Philippe Nafteux, MD, PhD
Clinical Head
Department of Thoracic Surgery
University Hospitals Leuven
Leuven, Belgium

Chaitan K. Narsule, MD
Assistant Professor
Department of Surgery
Boston University School of Medicine
Boston, Massachusetts

Basil Nasir, MBBCh
Division of Thoracic Surgery
Centre Hospitalier de l'Université de
    Montréal
Montreal, Quebec

Keith S. Naunheim, MD
The Vallee and Melba Willman Chair
    of Surgery
Chief of Thoracic Surgery
Department of Surgery
Saint Louis University School of Medicine
St. Louis, Missouri

Calvin S. H. Ng, BSc, MD, FRCSEd(CTh), FCCP
Associate Professor
Department of Surgery
The Chinese University of Hong Kong
Hong Kong, SAR, China

Daniel G. Nicastri, MD
Assistant Professor
Department of Thoracic Surgery
Icahn School of Medicine at Mount Sinai
New York, New York

Francis C. Nichols, MD
Professor of Surgery
Consultant General Thoracic Surgery
Mayo Clinic
Rochester, Minnesota

David M. Notrica, MD, FACS, FAAP
Associate Professor
University of Arizona College of Medicine
Tuscan, Arizona
Associate Professor of Surgery
Mayo Clinic School of Medicine
Division of Pediatric Surgery
Phoenix Children's Hospital
Phoenix, Arizona

Daniel Ocazionez, MD
Assistant Professor
Department of Diagnostic and Interventional
    Imaging
University of Texas HSC at Houston
Houston, Texas

Matthias Ochs, MD
Professor and Chair
Institute of Functional and Applied Anatomy
Hannover Medical School
Hannover, Germany

John A. Odell, MBChB, FRCS(Ed), FACS
Emeritus Professor of Surgery
Mayo Clinic
Jacksonville, Florida

Amaia Ojanguren, MD, PhD
Associate Professor of Surgery
University of Lleida
Division of Thoracic Surgery
Arnau de Vilanova University Hospital
Lleida, Spain
Institut Catala de la Salut
Barcelona, Spain

Anne Olland, MD, PhD
Associate Professor
Department of Thoracic Surgery
Strasbourg University Hospital
Strasbourg, France

Mark Onaitis, MD
Associate Professor of Surgery
University of California San Diego
La Jolla, California

Raymond P. Onders, MD
Professor and Chief of General Surgery
Case Western Reserve University School
    of Medicine
University Hospitals Cleveland Medical Center
Cleveland, Ohio

Isabelle Opitz, MD
Associate Professor
Department of Thoracic Surgery
University Hospital Zurich
Zurich, Switzerland

Asishana Osho, MD, MPH
Clinical Fellow
Department of Surgery
Massachusetts General Hospital
Harvard Medical School
Boston, Massachusetts

Berker Özkan, MD
Associate Professor
Department of Thoracic Surgery
Istanbul Medical School
Istanbul University
Istanbul, Turkey

**Siddharth Padmanabhan, MBBS,
LLB, BCom**
Resident
Latrobe Regional Hospital
Victoria, Australia

Hao Pan, MD
Chief Resident
Department of Cardiothoracic Surgery
UT Health San Antonio
San Antonio, Texas

**Kostas Papagiannopoulos, MD, MMED
THORAX (CTH)**
Honorary Senior Lecturer
Leeds University
Department of Thoracic Surgery
St. James's University Hospital
Leeds, United Kingdom

Nadeem Parkar, MD
Chief
Section of Thoracic and Cardiac Imaging
Assistant Professor of Radiology
Assistant Professor of Internal Medicine
Saint Louis University School of Medicine
Saint Louis, Missouri

G. Alexander Patterson, MD
Joseph C. Bancroft Professor of Surgery
Division of Cardiothoracic Surgery
Washington University
St. Louis, Missouri

Edoardo Pescarmona, MD
Department of Pathology
Regina Elena National Cancer Institute
Rome, Italy

Adrienne A. Phillips, MD, MPH
Assistant Professor of Medicine
Department of Medicine
Division of Hematology and Medical
    Oncology
Weill Cornell Medical College
New York, New York

Joseph D. Phillips, MD
Assistant Professor
Department of Surgery
Dartmouth-Hitchcock Medical Center
Lebanon, New Hampshire

Anthony L. Picone, MD, PhD, MBA
Professor of Oncology
Department of Thoracic Surgery
Roswell Park Cancer Institute
Buffalo, New York

Eitan Podgaetz, MD, MPH, FACS
Associate Professor
Texas A&M University
Director of Minimally Invasive
    Thoracic Surgery
Center for Thoracic Surgery
Baylor University Medical Center
Dallas, Texas

Cecilia Pompili, MD
Thoracic Surgeon
Leeds Institute of Cancer and Pathology
University of Leeds
St James's University Hospital
Leeds, United Kingdom

Jeffrey L. Port, MD
Professor of Clinical Cardiothoracic Surgery
Weill Cornell Medical College
Associate Attending
New York Presbyterian Hospital
New York, New York

Ciprian Pricopi, MD
Department of Thoracic Surgery
Georges Pompidou European Hospital
Paris, France

Varun Puri, MD, MSCI
Associate Professor
Department of Surgery
Washington University
St. Louis, Missouri

Joe B. Putnam, Jr., MD, FACS
Medical Director
Baptist MD Anderson Cancer Center
Jacksonville, Florida

Siva Raja, MD, PhD, FACS
Professional Staff, Thoracic Surgery
Surgical Director, Center for Esophageal
    Diseases
Heart and Vascular Institute
Cleveland Clinic Foundation
Cleveland, Ohio

Arvind Rajagopal, MBBS
Assistant Professor
Department of Anesthesiology
Rush University Medical Center
Chicago, Illinois

Ravi Rajaram, MD, MSc
General Surgery Resident
Department of Surgery
Northwestern University Feinberg School
    of Medicine
Chicago, Illinois

**Pala Babu Rajesh, FRCS Ed, FRCS CTh,
FRCS Eng**
Consultant Thoracic Surgeon
Regional Department of Thoracic Surgery
Birmingham Heartlands Hospital
Birmingham, United Kingdom

Prabhakar Rajiah, MBBS, MD, FRCR
Associate Professor of Radiology
Associate Director of Cardiac CT and MRI
Department of Radiology, Cardiothoracic
    Radiology
UT Southwestern Medical Center
Dallas, Texas

Karthik Ravi, MD
Assistant Professor of Medicine
Department of Gastroenterology and Hepatology
Mayo Clinic
Rochester, Minnesota

Rishindra M. Reddy, MD
Associate Professor
Department of Surgery, Section of
  Thoracic Surgery
University of Michigan
Ann Arbor, Michigan

James Regan, MD
Department of Surgery
Southern Illinois University School of
  Medicine
Springfield, Illinois

Jean-François Regnard
Professor of Thoracic Surgery
Head
Department of Thoracic Surgery
Paris Descartes University
Hôpital Cochin, APHP
Paris, France

Janani S. Reisenauer, MD
Department of Pulmonary Medicine
Division of Thoracic Surgery
Mayo Clinic
Rochester, Minnesota

Erino A. Rendina, MD
Chief, Division of Thoracic Surgery
Sapienza University of Rome
Rome, Italy

Carlos S. Restrepo
Professor of Radiology
Director of Cardiothoracic Radiology
UT Health San Antonio
San Antonio, Texas

David Rice, MB, BCh, BAO, FRCSI
Department of Thoracic and Cardiovascular
  Surgery
University of Texas MD Anderson Cancer
  Center
Houston, Texas

Thomas W. Rice, MD
Professor
Department of Surgery
Cleveland Clinic Lerner College of
  Medicine
Section Head, Department of Thoracic
  Surgery
Cleveland Clinic
Cleveland, Ohio

Marc Riquet, MD, PhD
Professor
Department of Thoracic Surgery
Georges Pompidou European Hospital
Paris, France

Valerie W. Rusch, MD
Professor
Department of Surgery
Weill Cornell Medical College
Chief, Thoracic Service
William G. Cahan Chair
Department of Surgery
Memorial Sloan-Kettering Cancer Center
New York, New York

Michele Salati, MD, PhD
Unit of Thoracic Surgery
University Hospital Ancona United Hospitals
Ancona, Italy

Mary Salvatore, MD
Associate Professor
Department of Radiology
Mount Sinai Health System
New York, New York

Pamela Samson, MD
Resident Physician
Department of Surgery
Washington University in St. Louis
St. Louis, Missouri

Nicola Santelmo, MD
Hôpital Civil de Strasbourg
Strasbourg, France

Inderpal (Netu) S. Sarkaria, MD
Vice Chairman, Clinical Affairs
Department of Cardiothoracic Surgery
University of Pittsburgh School of Medicine
University of Pittsburgh Medical Center
Pittsburgh, Pennsylvania

Giorgio V. Scagliotti
Professor of Medical Oncology
Department of Oncology
University of Turin
Torino, Italy

Eric Sceusi, MD
Thoracic Surgeon
Piedmont Heart Institute
Atlanta, Georgia

Lara Schaheen, MD
Chief Resident
Department of Cardiothoracic Surgery
University of Pittsburgh Medical Center
Pittsburgh, Pennsylvania

Philip Maximilian Scherer, MD
Assistant Professor of Radiology
University of Central Florida College of
  Medicine
Florida Hospital
Orlando, Florida
Radiology Specialists of Florida
Maitland, Florida

Colin Schieman, MD, FRCSC
Clinical Associate Professor
Residency Program Director
Section of Thoracic Surgery
Cumming School of Medicine at University
  of Calgary
Calgary, Alberta

David S. Schrump, MD, MBA, FACS
Senior Investigator and Chief
Thoracic and General Surgical Oncology Branch
Center for Cancer Research
National Cancer Institute
Bethesda, Maryland

Matthew J. Schuchert, MD
Associate Professor
Department of Cardiothoracic Surgery
University of Pittsburgh Medical Center
Pittsburgh, Pennsylvania

Christopher W. Seder, MD
Assistant Professor
Department of Cardiovascular and Thoracic
  Surgery
Rush University Medical School
Chicago, Illinois

Agathe Seguin-Givelet, MD, PhD
Department of Thoracic
Curie-Montsouris Thorax Institute
Paris, France

Joanna Sesti, MD
Department of Cardiothoracic Surgery
Robert Wood Johnson Barnabas Health System
Livingston, New Jersey

Farid M. Shamji, MBBS, FRCSC, FACS
Professor of Surgery
Division of Thoracic Surgery
University of Ottawa
Ottawa Hospital—General Campus
Ottawa, Ontario, Canada

Jason P. Shaw, MD
Chief
Department of General Thoracic Surgery
Maimonides Medical Center
Brooklyn, New York

David D. Shersher, MD
Assistant Professor
Department of Surgery
Cooper Medical School of Rowan University
MD Anderson Cancer Center
Camden, New Jersey

Thomas W. Shields, MD, DSc (Hon.)[†]
Professor Emeritus of Surgery
Northwestern University Feinberg School of
  Medicine
Chicago, Illinois

†Deceased

Joseph B. Shrager, MD
Professor of Cardiothoracic Surgery
Stanford University School of Medicine
Chief, Division of Thoracic Surgery
Stanford Cancer Institute
Stanford, California

Antonios C. Sideris
Research Fellow
Division of Thoracic Surgery
Brigham and Women's Hospital
Harvard Medical School
Boston, Massachusetts
Resident
Department of General Surgery
Cleveland Clinic Foundation
Cleveland, Ohio

Alan D. L. Sihoe, MA(Cantab), FRCSEd(CTh), FCSHK, FHKAM, FCCP
Clinical Associate Professor
Department of Surgery
Chief of Thoracic Surgery
The University of Hong Kong
HKU Shenzhen Hospital
Hong Kong, China

Mark A. Socinski, MD
Executive Medical Director
Member, Thoracic Oncology Program
Florida Hospital Cancer Institute
Orlando, Florida

Joshua R. Sonett, MD
Professor and Chief
Thoracic Surgery
Columbia University
New York Presbyterian Hospital
New York, New York

Nathaniel J. Soper, MD, FACS
Loyal and Edith Davis Professor and Chair
Department of Surgery
Northwestern University Feinberg School
   of Medicine
Chief of Surgery
Northwestern Medicine
Chicago, Illinois

James E. Speicher, MD
Assistant Professor
Department of Cardiovascular Sciences
Division of Thoracic and Foregut Surgery
East Carolina University
Greenville, North Carolina

Jonathan D. Spicer, MD, PhD, FRCS
Assistant Professor
Division of Thoracic Surgery
Dr. Ray Chiu Distinguished Scientist in
   Surgical Research
McGill University
Montreal, Canada

Laurence N. Spier
Chief
Division of Thoracic Surgery
NYU-Winthrop University Hospital
Mineola, New York

Sandra Starnes, MD
Professor of Surgery
John B. Flege Chair in Cardiothoracic Surgery
University of Cincinnati College of Medicine
Cincinnati, Ohio

Kevin L. Stephans, MD
Associate Professor
Department of Radiation Oncology
Cleveland Clinic, Taussig Cancer Center
Cleveland, Ohio

Joel Miller Sternbach, MD, MBA
Bechily-Hodes Fellow in Esophagology
Department of Surgery
Northwestern University, Feinberg School of
   Medicine
Chicago, Illinois

Hon Chi Suen, MBBS, FRCSEd, FRCS, RCPS(Glasg), FCSHK, FACS, DABThS, DABS
President
Center for Cardiothoracic Surgery, Inc.
St. Louis, Missouri

David J. Sugarbaker, MD
Professor and Chief
Division of Thoracic Surgery
Baylor College of Medicine
Houston, Texas

Kei Suzuki, MD
Assistant Professor
Department of Surgery
Boston Medical Center
Boston, Massachusetts

Scott J. Swanson, MD
Director
Minimally Invasive Thoracic Surgery
Vice Chair
Cancer Affairs
Brigham and Women's Hospital
Chief Surgical Office
Dana Farber Cancer Institute
Professor of Surgery
Harvard Medical School
Boston, Massachusetts

Gunturu N. Swati, MD
Government Medical College Akola
Visiting student
Icahn School of Medicine at Mount Sinai
   Hospital
New York, New York

Ezra N. Teitelbaum, MD, MEd
Assistant Professor of Surgery and Medical
   Education
Department of Surgery
Northwestern University, Feinberg School of
   Medicine
Chicago, Illinois

Sara Tenconi, MD
Consultant Thoracic Surgeon
Sheffield Teaching Hospitals
United Kingdom

Michael Thomas, MD
Assistant Professor
Department of Surgery
Southern Illinois University School of
   Medicine
Springfield, Illinois

Pascal A. Thomas, MD
Professor and Chief
Department of Thoracic Surgery
North University Hospital–Aix-Marseille
   University
Marseille, France

Prashanthi N. Thota, MD, FACG
Medical Director
Esophageal Center
Director
Center for Swallowing and Motility Disorders
Digestive Disease & Surgery Institute
Cleveland Clinic
Cleveland, Ohio

Alper Toker, MD
Head
Department of Thoracic Surgery
Istanbul University, Istanbul Faculty of
   Medicine
Istanbul, Turkey

Victor F. Trastek, MD
Director of Science of Healthcare Delivery
College of Healthcare Solutions
Arizona State University
Phoenix, Arizona
Consultant in Leadership and Professionalism
Mayo Clinic
Scottsdale, Arizona

H. Adam Ubert, MD
Attending Cardiothoracic Surgeon
Department of Cardiovascular Medicine
Charleston Area Medical Center
Charleston, West Virginia

Eric Vallières, MR, FRCSC
Surgical Director of the Lung Cancer Program
Medical Director
Division of Thoracic Surgery
Swedish Cancer Institute
Seattle, Washington

Victor van Berkel, MD, PhD
Associate Professor
Department of Cardiovascular and Thoracic
  Surgery
University of Louisville School of Medicine
Louisville, Kentucky

Koen van Besien, MD, PhD
Director, Stem Cell Transplant Program
Division of Hematology/Oncology
Weill Cornell Medical College
New York, New York

Dirk Van Raemdonck, MD, PhD
Professor of Surgery
KU Leuven University
Head of Transplant Center
University Hospitals Leuven
Leuven, Belgium

Paul E. Y. Van Schil, MD, PhD
Chair
Department of Thoracic and Vascular
  Surgery
Antwerp University Hospital and Antwerp
  University
Antwerp, Belgium

Hans Van Veer, MD
Assistant Clinic Head
Department of Thoracic Surgery
University Hospitals Leuven
Leuven, Belgium

Ara A. Vaporciyan, MD, FACS
Professor and Chairman
Department of Thoracic and Cardiovascular
  Surgery
University of Texas MD Anderson Cancer
  Center
Houston, Texas

Nirmal K. Veeramachaneni, MD
Department of Thoracic Surgery
University of Kansas Medical Center
Kansas City, Kansas

Federico Venuta, MD
Professor of Thoracic Surgery and Chief
Sapienza University of Rome
Policlinico Umberto I
Rome, Italy

Gregory Videtic, MD, CM, FRCPC, FACR
Professor of Medicine
Cleveland Clinic Lerner College of Medicine
Staff Physician
Department of Radiation Oncology
Cleveland Clinic
Cleveland, Ohio

Carlos Vigliano, MD
Associate Professor
Instituto de Medicina Traslacional, Trasplante
  y Bioingeniería (IMeTTyB)
Favaloro University–CONICET
Chief
Department of Pathology
University Hospital Favaloro Foundation
Buenos Aires, Argentina

Liza Villaruz, MD
Assistant Professor of Medicine
Department of Medicine
University of Pittsburgh School of Medicine
Pittsburgh, Pennsylvania

Robin Vos, MD, PhD
Department of Respiratory Medicine, Lung
  Transplant and Respiratory Intermediate
  Care Unit University Hospitals Leuven,
  Gasthuisberg Campus
Assistant Professor of Medicine
Department of Chronic Diseases, Metabolism
  and Ageing (CHROMETA)
Lab of Respiratory Diseases, KU
Leuven, Belgium

David Waller, FRCS(CTh)
Consultant Thoracic Surgeon
St. Bartholomew's Hospital
London, United Kingdom

Garrett L. Walsh, MD
Professor of Surgery
Department of Thoracic and Cardiovascular
  Surgery
University of Texas MD Anderson Cancer
  Center
Houston, Texas

Saiama N. Waqar, MBBS, MSCI
Assistant Professor of Medicine
Division of Oncology
Washington University School of Medicine
St. Louis, Missouri

William H. Warren, MD[†]
Professor
Department of Cardiovascular Surgery
Rush University Medical Center
Chicago, Illinois

Thomas J. Watson, MD, FACS
Professor of Surgery
Georgetown University School of Medicine
Regional Chief of Surgery
MedStar Washington
Washington, District of Columbia

Jon O. Wee, MD
Section Chief, Esophageal Surgery
Co-Director of Minimally Invasive Thoracic
  Surgery
Director of Robotics in Thoracic Surgery
Division of Thoracic Surgery
Brigham and Women's Hospital
Boston, Massachusetts

Ewald R. Weibel, MD, DSc(hon)
Professor Emeritus
Institute of Anatomy
University of Bern
Bern, Switzerland

Mark Weir, MBChB
Assistant Professor
Department of Thoracic Medicine and Surgery
Lewis Katz School of Medicine at Temple
  University
Philadelphia, Pennsylvania

Michael J. Weyant, MD
Professor of Surgery
Department of Surgery
Division of Cardiothoracic Surgery
University of Colorado
Aurora, Colorado

Abby White, DO
Division of Thoracic Surgery
Brigham and Women's Hospital
Boston, Massachusetts

Ory Wiesel, MD
Clinical Fellow
Division of Thoracic Surgery
Brigham and Women's Hospital
Harvard Medical School
Boston, Massachusetts

Dennis A. Wigle, MD, PhD
Associate Professor
Division of General Thoracic Surgery
Mayo Clinic
Rochester, Minnesota

Elbert E. Williams, MD
Department of Cardiothoracic Surgery
Mount Sinai Health System
New York, New York

Jennifer L. Wilson, MD
Department of Thoracic Surgery
Beth Israel Deaconess Medical Center
Instructor of Surgery
Harvard Medical School
Boston, Massachusetts

Douglas E. Wood, MD, FACS, FRCSEd
The Henry N. Harkins Professor and Chair
Department of Surgery
University of Washington
Seattle, Washington

†Deceased

Neil McIver Woody, MD, MS
Associate Staff
Department of Radiation Oncology
Cleveland Clinic, Taussig Cancer Institute
Cleveland, Ohio

Cameron Wright, MD
Douglas Mathisen Professor of Surgery
Division of Thoracic Surgery
Massachusetts General Hospital
Harvard Medical School
Boston, Massachusetts

Moritz C. Wyler von Ballmoos, MD, PhD, MPH, FACC
Clinical Associate in Surgery
Division of Cardiothoracic Surgery
Duke University Medical Center
Durham, North Carolina

Alexander Yang, MS
MD Candidate, Class of 2020
GW School of Medicine and Health Sciences
Washington, District of Columbia

Chi-Fu Jeffrey Yang, MD
Resident
Department of Surgery
Duke University
Durham, North Carolina

Stephen C. Yang, MD
The Arthur B. and Patricia B. Modell
    Endowed Chair in Thoracic Surgery
Professor of Surgery and Oncology
The Johns Hopkins Medical Institutions
Baltimore, Maryland

David Yankelevitz, MD
Professor
Department of Radiology
Icahn School of Medicine
New York, New York

Anjana Yeldandi, MD
Associate Professor of Pathology
Northwestern Memorial Hospital
Feinberg Pavilion
Chicago, Illinois

Sai Yendamuri, MD, FACS
Professor and Chair
Department of Thoracic Surgery
Roswell Park Cancer Institute
Buffalo, New York

Jonathan C. Yeung, MD, PhD, FRCSC
Assistant Professor
Division of Thoracic Surgery
University of Toronto
Toronto, Ontario

Akihiko Yoshizawa, MD, PhD
Associate Professor
Department of Diagnostic Pathology
Kyoto University Hospital
Kyoto, Japan

Masaya Yotsukura, MD
Assistant
Division of Thoracic Surgery
Keio University School of Medicine
Tokyo, Japan

David S. Younger, MD, MPH, MS
Clinical Associate Professor
Department of Neurology
School of Medicine and College of Global
    Public Health
New York University
New York City, New York

Yachao Zhang, MD
Department of Radiology
Westchester Medical Center
Valhalla, New York

Ze-Rui Zhao, MD
Department of Surgery
Prince of Wales Hospital
Hong Kong, China

Yifan A. Zheng, MD
Resident
Department of Surgery
Division of Thoracic Surgery
Brigham and Women's Hospital
Harvard Medical School
Boston, Massachusetts

Brittany A. Zwischenberger, MD
Cardiothoracic Surgery Fellow
Division of Cardiovascular and Thoracic
    Surgery
Duke University
Durham, North Carolina

Joseph "Jay" B. Zwischenberger, MD
Johnston-Wright Professor and Chairman
Department of Surgery
University of Kentucky
Lexington, Kentucky

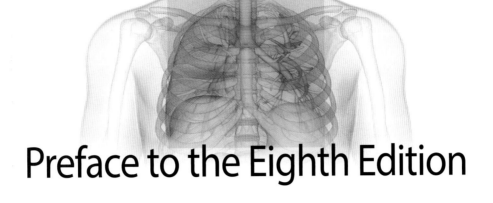

Preface to the Eighth Edition

In the foreword to the first edition of *General Thoracic Surgery* published in 1972, Paul Samson noted that Shields published a text dedicated to the General Thoracic Surgeon to the exclusion of the heart. That occurred at a time when the "romance and appeal which have attended the astounding developments in the surgical treatment of cardiac disease" was skyrocketing.

During the next 40 years of cardiac surgical dominance on the international stage, Shields' book remained focused on the diseases of the lungs, esophagus, chest wall, diaphragm, and mediastinum. The first text, penned by 58 specialists, was encyclopedic in scope and depth. Students and practitioners of this specialty needed no other book. Through its many editions, it carried the same thorough approach and served as the *de facto* bible of the specialty.

Over the decades, other books, atlases and manuals on General Thoracic Surgery have come and gone, but this book has remained the only comprehensive text in continuous publication for the practitioner of thoracic diseases, excluding the heart and great arteries.

In the current digital age, seekers of knowledge no longer rely solely on the static text. They often begin their search for information by scouring the Internet for a variety of media for articles, videos, meeting reports, videos and other tidbits to understand the nuances of a particular disease or procedure. While more dynamic than searching the texts of old, these searches often are hampered by search terms, are disorganized, narrow in scope, and evanescent.

Now, 45 years after the first publication, this edition of *Shields' General Thoracic Surgery* is written by over 150 specialists. It has shed its encyclopedic tradition while maintaining its completeness. It includes dynamic audio and visual content, color coordinated graphics, and analyses of the world's literature and electronic data for the most extensive and concise collection of information for the busy clinician.

For the first time, the edition includes a retrospective into the past with particular attention to the milestones of artificial ventilation and the era of minimal invasion, both of which revolutionized the century-old specialty. It also addresses new topics such as deciphering complex statistical analyses, using efficiently the new World Health Organization's International Classification of Diseases (ICD-10), mining big data sets for specific decision making, and developing and performing effective quality improvement projects for the surgeon's practice and hospital setting.

Long-time users of *Shields* will enjoy the continued comprehensiveness of the chapters. Millennial practitioners will find this transformed edition less ponderous and intimidating than the tomes of the past, yet more thorough and meaningful than imprecise, often fragmented individual electronic searches.

Preface to the First Edition

This volume was prepared to present a comprehensive text on the surgical diseases of the chest wall, pleura, diaphragm, trachea, lung, and mediastinal structures. Initially, an overview of the anatomy and of the physiology of these structures is given. The investigation of the patient's disease and the management of the patient in the perioperative period are considered next. The various operative approaches and the standard surgical procedures are discussed and these are followed by chapters concerned with the disease entities of the aforementioned structures. The major objectives are to present a summation of the current knowledge and the clinical concepts of the surgical management of trauma and diseases of the thorax. The pathophysiologic alterations produced and the corrections of these by appropriate intervention are emphasized throughout. Presentations of the clinical features, pathologic changes, surgical management, operative results, and prognosis of the various disease states are included as an integral part of the whole.

Outstanding surgeons, physicians, and scientists have cooperated in the preparation of the text. As with most multi-authored books, repetition could not be completely eliminated; however, I have tried to keep it at a minimum. In most instances, the repetition serves to emphasize important information relative to the entire subject. Interestingly, conflicting statements are few, and only an occasional footnote has been appended to point out such differences in opinion. This book hopefully will serve as a source of information for the young thoracic surgeon and the person in surgical training. It also should serve as a reference for surgeons, as well as physicians, outside the field of general thoracic surgery who wish to ascertain the current views held by the specialty.

TWS

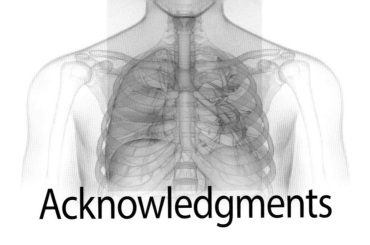

Acknowledgments

Any large textbook such as this one, an army of individuals is required to produce a quality work. The editors appreciate the efforts of the publishers, the artists, and the printers assigned to this project.

Most of all, it is the volunteers who really make the text worthwhile. We thank the authors and co-authors who composed the original content and those who updated the old content. In addition, we thank their administrative assistants who participated in the production of the content.

In particular, the editors wish to acknowledge two volunteers who sacrificed a great deal of personal time and expended their intellectual energy to improve the quality of the book.

From the inception of this edition, Bryan F. Meyers, MD has been a strong advocate and a driving force. He participated in the development of the revised table of contents and in the editor discussions of the revised chapter format. Most importantly, he helped recruit a number of national and international authors.

Special thanks goes to Martha S. LoCicero, MD, who performed substantial copyediting duties in an effort to make the text readable and relevant. She also provided the much needed advice and encouragement over the long development phase of this project.

JLIII

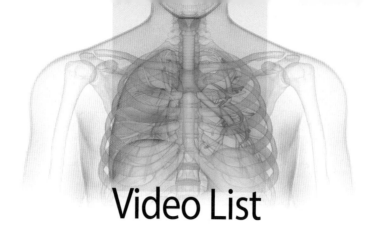

Video List

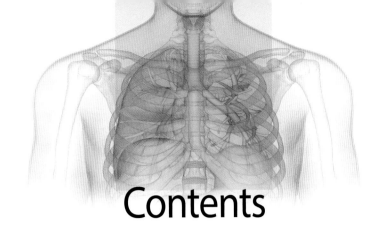

Contents

[†]Deceased

---

†Deceased

CARCINOMA OF THE LUNG

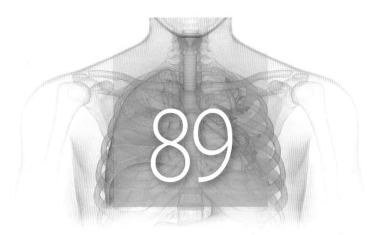

89

Lung Cancer: Epidemiology and Carcinogenesis

Pamela Samson ▪ Graham A. Colditz

LUNG CANCER INCIDENCE AND MORTALITY

Carcinoma of the lung is the leading cause of cancer death in the United States and around the world. The Surveillance, Epidemiology, and End Results (SEER) program estimates that 222,500 people will be diagnosed with lung cancer in 2017, and represent 13.2% of all new cancer cases.[1] The prevalence of lung cancer in the United States is most recently estimated at 408,800 individuals. However, lung cancer continues to cause one quarter (25.9%) of cancer deaths, which is estimated to reach 155,870 in 2015. From 2005 to 2012, the number of lung cancer cases per 100,000 individuals has decreased from 63.0 to 54.5, and the number of lung cancer deaths has decreased from 52.9 to 45.0. Despite these incremental improvements in incidence and deaths, lung malignancy continues to be the largest contributor to cancer mortality—causing more cancer-related deaths than the other most frequent cancers combined (breast, prostate, colorectal, bladder, and melanoma). From 2007 to 2013, only 18.1% of lung cancer patients in the United States survive through 5 years. Currently in the United States, the median age at diagnosis is 70, with almost one-third of cases occurring among individuals aged 65 to 74. Racial disparities in lung cancer diagnosis are also evident, with the highest incidence occurring in African-American males (83.7/100,000 persons). By comparison, the incidence in Caucasian males is 65.9/100,000 persons, Caucasian females 50.8/100,000 persons, and African-American females 49.0/100,000 persons.

Globally, lung cancer has been the most common cancer in the world since 1985. Lung cancer continues to be the most common cancer worldwide in terms of both incidence and mortality.[2] In 2012, lung cancer was the largest single contributor to new cases of cancer diagnosed (1,800,000 new cases, equaling 13% of total new cancer cases) as well as to mortality from cancer (1,600,000 deaths, equaling one-fifth of all cancer deaths). Unlike the improvements in cancer incidence and mortality in the United States, the global incidence and mortality from lung cancer demonstrate increases since 2005. Currently, more than half (58%) of global lung cancer cases occur in developing nations. In a recent retrospective review of global cancer registries, the age-standardized 5-year overall survival from lung cancer ranged from 10% to 20% among both developed and developing countries.[3] The 5-year lung cancer survival exceeded 20% in only three countries: Japan (30%), Israel (24%), and Mauritius (37%). Alternatively, many countries suffer from a 5-year survival rate of less than 10%.

This chapter will focus primarily on a discussion of modifiable risk factors, including tobacco smoking, exposure to occupational carcinogens and ionizing radiation, and diet. The genetic aspects of carcinogenesis will also be discussed.

TOBACCO EXPOSURE

At the turn of the twentieth century, lung cancer was an uncommon disease. In 1912, Adler performed an extensive review of autopsy reports from hospitals in the United States and western European countries and found 374 cases of primary lung cancer. This represented <0.5% of all cancer cases. Adler concluded that "primary malignant neoplasms of the lung are among the rarest forms of disease." Over the next several decades a number of authors in the United States and abroad noted an increase in the incidence of carcinoma of the lung. In a series of 185,434 autopsy cases collected between 1897 and 1930, Hruby and Sweany[4] noted that the incidence of lung cancer had increased disproportionately to the incidence of cancer in general.

In the early decades of the twentieth century, it was postulated that the observed increase in lung cancer might be due to a variety of etiologies, including influenza, tuberculosis, irritating gases, atmospheric pollution from industrial plants and coal fires, and chronic bronchitis. The appreciation that tar could produce lung carcinoma when applied experimentally to the skin of animals raised preliminary concern that inhalation of tar products originating from automobile exhaust or the surface dust of tarred roads could be important factors in the observed rise in lung cancer incidence. As early as 1930, Roffo[5] concluded, from observations made in patients and experimental studies in animals, that tobacco tar liberated from the burning of tobacco was a carcinogenic agent. In 1941, Ochsner and DeBakey[6] stated, in a review of carcinoma of the lung, "It is our definite conviction that the increase in the incidence of pulmonary carcinoma is due largely to the increase in smoking."

In 1950, two landmark epidemiologic studies evaluating the role of tobacco smoking as an etiologic factor in bronchogenic carcinoma were published. Wynder and Graham[7] in the United States reported a case–control study examining 605 cases of lung cancer in men compared with a general male hospital population without cancer. The most striking finding was that 96.5% of lung cancers were found in men who were moderate to heavy smokers for many years, compared with the general population, which had a smoking rate of 73.7%. Several important conclusions were drawn: (a) excessive and prolonged use of tobacco was an important factor in the induction of lung cancer, (b) the occurrence of lung cancer in a nonsmoker was a rare phenomenon, and (c) a lag period of 10 years or more between smoking cessation and the clinical onset of carcinoma could be observed. This report was closely followed by a similar case–control study conducted in the United Kingdom by Doll and Hill.[8] They interviewed 649 male and 60 female lung cancer subjects at 20 London hospitals and compared them with 1,029 patients who had cancer in organs other than the lung and 743 general medical and surgical patients matched for age and sex. In this study, 0.3% of men and 31.7% of women with lung cancer were nonsmokers, compared with 4.2% of men and 53.3% of women without cancer. Like Wynder and Graham, Doll and Hill concluded that an association between carcinoma of the lung and cigarette smoking did indeed exist and that the effect on the development of lung cancer varied with the number of cigarettes smoked.

However, it was not until 1964 that the US Public Health Service published the Surgeon General's landmark report on smoking and health.[9] The principal findings of this report are based largely on prospective cohort studies that demonstrated the following important facts. Cigarette smoking is associated with a 70% increase in the age-specific death rates of men and a lesser increase in the death rates of women. Cigarette smoking is causally related to lung cancer in men. The magnitude of the effect of cigarette smoking far outweighed all other factors leading to lung cancer. The risk of developing lung cancer increases with duration of smoking and the number of cigarettes smoked per day. The report estimates that the average male smoker has an approximately 9- to 10-fold risk of developing lung cancer, whereas heavy smokers have at least a 20-fold risk. Cigarette

smoking is believed to be much more important than occupational exposures in the causation of lung cancer in the general population. Cigarette smoking is the most important cause of chronic bronchitis in the United States. Male cigarette smokers have a higher death rate from coronary artery disease than nonsmoking men.

At the conclusion of the report, the following statement was made: "Cigarette smoking is a health hazard of sufficient importance in the United States to warrant appropriate remedial action." Since the submission of this report, yearly per capita consumption of cigarettes has declined in the United States, although it is estimated that more than one-sixth (17.8%) of Americans still smoke. From a population perspective, there continue to be more male smokers than female (20.5% vs. 15.3%, respectively) and the highest rates of smoking are seen among Native Americans (26.8%) and multiracial individuals (26.8%).[10] In a recent report from the Surgeon General surveying national smoking trends, almost 70% of smokers indicate a desire to stop using tobacco, and over 40% have made at least one quit attempt in the past year.[11]

Cigarette smoke is a complex aerosol composed of both gaseous and particulate compounds. It is broken down into mainstream smoke and sidestream smoke components. Mainstream smoke is produced by inhalation of air through the cigarette and is the primary source of smoke exposure for the smoker. Sidestream smoke is produced from smoldering of the cigarette between puffs and is the major source of environmental tobacco smoke (ETS). The primary substance associated with tobacco addiction is nicotine. Tar is defined as the total particulate matter of cigarette smoke after nicotine and water have been removed. Tar exposure appears to be the major link to lung cancer risk. The Federal Trade Commission determines the nicotine and tar content of cigarettes by measurements made on standardized smoking machines. However, the composition of mainstream smoke can be variable depending on the intensity of inhalation, which differs among individual smokers. Although filter tips decrease the amount of nicotine and tar in mainstream smoke, compression of the tips by lips or fingers has been shown to affect the composition of inhaled smoke.

More than 4,000 individual constituents of cigarette smoke have been identified. Hoffmann and Hoffmann[12] and Burns,[13] in extensive reviews of cigarettes and smoke composition, note that 95% of the weight of mainstream smoke comes from 400 to 500 individual gaseous compounds. The remainder of the weight is made up of >3,500 particulate components. This does not include additives such as flavorings, which are considered trade secrets and are often unknown.

It is clear that mainstream smoke contains a large number of potential carcinogens, including polycyclic aromatic hydrocarbons, aromatic amines, *N*-nitrosamines, and miscellaneous organic and inorganic compounds such as benzene, vinyl chloride, arsenic, and chromium (Table 89.1). Compounds such as the polycyclic aromatic hydrocarbons and *N*-nitrosamines require metabolic activation to reach carcinogenic potential. Detoxification pathways also exist, and the balance between activation and detoxification likely affects individual cancer risk. Radioactive materials such as radon and its decay products, bismuth and polonium, are also present in tobacco smoke.

The agents that appear to be of particular concern in the etiology of carcinoma of the lung are the tobacco-specific *N*-nitrosamines (TSNAs) formed by nitrosation of nicotine during both tobacco processing and smoking. Eight TSNAs have been described, including 4-(methylnitrosamino)-1(3-pyridyl)-1-butanone (NNK), which is known to induce adenocarcinoma of the lung in experimental animal models. Other TSNAs have been linked to cancers of the esophagus, bladder, pancreas, oral cavity, and larynx. Of the TSNAs, NNK appears to be the most important inducer of lung cancer. It has

TABLE 89.1 Tumorigenic Agents in Tobacco and Tobacco Smoke: Evidence for IARC Evaluation of Carcinogenicity

	Processed Tobacco	Mainstream Smoke (Per Cigarette)	
Agent	Per Gram	In Lab Animals	In Humans
PAH			
Benz[a]anthracene		2–70 ng sufficient	NA
Benzo[b]fluoranthene		4–22 ng sufficient	NA
Benzo[j]fluoranthene		6–21 ng sufficient	NA
Benzo[k]fluoranthene		6–12 ng sufficient	NA
Benzo[a]pyrene	0.1–90 mg	20–40 ng sufficient	Probable
Chrysene		40–60 ng sufficient	NA
Dibenz[a,h]anthracene		4 ng sufficient	NA
Dibenz[a,i]pyrene		1.7–3.2 ng sufficient	NA
Dibenzo[a,l]pyrene		Present sufficient	NA
Indeno[1,2,3c,d]pyrene		4–20 ng sufficient	NA
S-Methylchrysene		0.6 ng sufficient	NA
Aza-Arenes			
Quinoline		1 μg NA	NA
Dibenz[a,h]acridine		0.1 ng sufficient	NA
Dibenz[a,j]acridine		3–10 ng sufficient	NA
7H-Dibenzo[c,g]carbazole		0.7 ng sufficient	NA
N-Nitrosamines			
N-Nitrosodimethylamine	ND–215 ng	0.1–180 ng sufficient	NA
N-Nitrosoethylmethylamine		3.13 ng sufficient	NA
N-Nitrosodiethylamine	ND–25 ng	Sufficient	NA
N-Nitrosopyrrolidine	ND–360 ng	1.5–110 ng sufficient	NA
N-Nitrosodiethanolamine	ND–6900 ng	ND–36 ng sufficient	NA
N-Nitrosonornicotine	0.3–89 μg	0.12–3.7 μg sufficient	NA
4-(Methylnitrosamino)-1-(3-pyridyl)-1-butanone	0.2–7 μg	0.08–0.77 μg sufficient	NA
N-Nitrosoanabasine	0.01–1.9 μg	0.14–4.6 μg limited	NA
N-Nitrosomorpholine	ND–690 ng	Sufficient	NA
Aromatic Amines			
2-Toluidine		30–200 ng sufficient	Inadequate
2-Naphthylamine		1–22 ng sufficient	Sufficient
4-Aminobiophenyl		2–5 ng sufficient	Sufficient
Aldehydes			
Formaldehyde	1.6–7.4 μg	70–100 μg sufficient	NA
Acetaldehyde	1.4–7.4 mg	18–1,400 mg sufficient	NA
Crotonaldehyde	0.2–2.4 μg	10–20 μg NA	NA
Miscellaneous Organic Compounds			
Benzene		12–48 μg sufficient	Sufficient
Acrylonitrile		3.2–15 μg sufficient	Limited
1,1-Dimethylhydrazine	60–147 μg	Sufficient NA	
2-Nitropropane		0.73–1.21 μg sufficient	NA
Ethylcarbonate	310–375 ng	20–38 ng sufficient	NA
Vinyl chloride		1–16 ng sufficient	Sufficient
Inorganic Compounds			
Hydrazine	14–51 ng	24–43 ng sufficient	Inadequate
Arsenic	500–900 ng	40–120 ng inadequate	Sufficient
Nickel	2,000–6,000 ng	0–600 ng sufficient	Limited
Chromium	1,000–2,000 ng	4–70 ng sufficient	Sufficient
Cadmium	1,300–1,600 ng	41–62 ng sufficient	Limited
Lead	8–10 μg	Sufficient	Inadequate
Polonium 210	0.2–1.2 pCi	0.03–1.0 pCi NA	NA

IARC, International Agency for Research on Cancer; ND, no data; NA, evaluation has not been done by IARC; PAH, polycyclic aromatic hydrocarbon.
From Burns DM. Tobacco smoking. In: Samet JM, ed. *Epidemiology of Lung Cancer*. New York: Marcel Dekker; 1994:15. Copyright © 1994. Reproduced by permission of Taylor and Francis Group, LLC, a division of Informa plc.

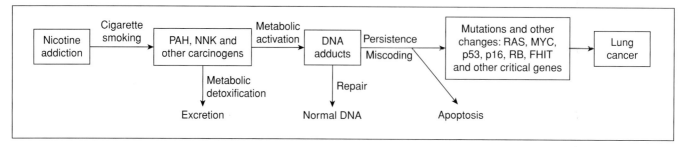

FIGURE 89.1 Schema linking nicotine addiction and lung cancer to tobacco smoke carcinogens and their induction of multiple mutations in critical genes. PAH, polycyclic aromatic hydrocarbons; NNK, 4-(methylnitrosamino)-1-(3-pyridyl)-1-butanone. (From Hecht SS. Tobacco smoke carcinogens and lung cancer. *J Natl Cancer Inst* 1999;91:1194. Reproduced by permission of Oxford University Press.)

carcinogenic effects with both topical and systemic administration. Inhalation of tobacco smoke containing TSNAs results in direct delivery of carcinogens to the lungs. Because these compounds are also absorbed systemically, hematogenous delivery to lung via the pulmonary circulation occurs as well.

Tobacco carcinogens such as NNK can bind to DNA, creating DNA adducts. Repair processes may remove these DNA adducts and restore normal DNA, or cells with damaged DNA may undergo apoptosis. However, failure of the normal DNA repair mechanisms to remove DNA adducts may lead to permanent mutations. As outlined in a schema by Hecht,[14] mutations in critical oncogenes or tumor suppressor genes may contribute to the development of lung cancer (Fig. 89.1).

It is important to note that the dosage of smoke constituents to the smoker can be highly variable, depending not just on the cigarette itself but also on the pattern of smoking. Specifically, the duration and intensity of inhalation, the presence and competence of a filter, and the duration of cooling of the smoke prior to inhalation can all change the composition of smoke. Over the last several decades, the nicotine and tar content of cigarettes has been lowered. However, the primary factor determining the intensity of use of cigarettes is the smoker's nicotine dependence. Thus, although cigarettes now contain less nicotine and tar than previously, smokers tend to smoke more intensively in order to satisfy their nicotine need, with higher puffs per minute and deeper inhalations. In such situations the measurements of tar and nicotine content made by smoking machines may significantly underestimate individual exposure.

Wynder and Hoffmann[15] proposed an intriguing hypothesis as to how low-yield filtered cigarettes might be a contributing factor to the observed increase of adenocarcinoma versus squamous cell carcinoma of the lung over the last several decades. As stated previously, the nicotine-addicted smoker will smoke low-yield cigarettes far more intensively than older nonfiltered higher-yield cigarettes. With deeper inhalation, higher-order bronchi, as opposed to the major bronchi alone, in the peripheral lung will be exposed to carcinogen-containing smoke. These peripheral bronchi lack protective epithelium and are being exposed to carcinogens, including TSNAs linked to the induction of adenocarcinoma. Data from several laboratories, including those of Hoffmann,[12] Belinsky,[16] and Ronai[17] and their colleagues, have documented that NNK is associated with DNA mutations resulting in the activation of K-*ras* oncogenes. Rodenhuis and Slebos[18] reported that K-*ras* oncogene activation has been identified in 24% of human lung adenocarcinomas. Of note, Westra and colleagues[19] have reported that K-*ras* mutations are present in adenocarcinoma of the lung found in ex-smokers, suggesting that such mutations do not revert with the cessation of tobacco smoking. This may in part explain the persistent elevation in lung cancer risk in ex-smokers even years after discontinuing cigarette use.

E-CIGARETTES

Clinical uncertainty also surrounds the emerging use of electronic nicotine delivery systems (or e-cigarettes) and open system vaporizes, sales of which exceeded US $2.5 billion in 2014. More than 40% of current smokers have reported trying e-cigarettes, and some hypothesize that these systems may outsell traditional cigarettes within the next decade. The main components of e-cigarettes include nicotine and flavoring compounds, which are heated and inhaled as a vapor, rather than smoke particulates. However, these devices have been documented to contain carcinogens such as formaldehyde, benzene, toluene, tobacco-specific nitrosamines such as NNK, and polycyclic aromatic compounds (polycyclic aromatic hydrocarbons [PAHs]) albeit in reduced concentrations compared to traditional cigarettes.[20] Of particular concern to public health groups is the popularity of e-cigarettes among adolescents, which has been associated with the use of traditional cigarettes, possibly as a "gateway" product.[21] At this time, these products are sold as tobacco products under the U.S. Food and Drug Administration (FDA) regulation, and the long-term risks of these products are not well characterized at all. It is also unclear if smokers are using these devices as a smoking-cessation "aid" or as a perceived "safer" alternative to traditional cigarettes. In the coming years it will be imperative to study how these products influence smoking-related diseases, including lung cancer.[22]

In 2016, the office of the Surgeon General and the US Health and Human Services published a 250 page document on e-cigarettes concluding, "We know what works to effectively prevent tobacco use among young people. Now we must apply these strategies to e-cigarettes—and continue to apply them to other tobacco products" (E-Cigarette Use Among Youth and Young Adults: A Report of the Surgeon General, 2016, Rockville, MD https://www.surgeongeneral.gov/library/2016ecigarettes/index.html).

There is no doubt that tobacco smoking is the most important modifiable risk factor for lung cancer. It is clear that individual susceptibility is also a factor in carcinogenesis. Although over 80% of lung cancers occur in persons with tobacco exposure, <20% of smokers will ever develop lung cancer. The variability seen in susceptibility is presumably influenced by other environmental factors or by genetic predisposition.

GENETIC FACTORS

A lung cancer risk prediction analysis was developed by Spitz and colleagues[23] that incorporated multiple variables such as smoking history, ETS, occupational exposures to dusts and to asbestos, and family history of cancer. These investigators showed the influence of positive family history of cancer on the risk of lung cancer in

TABLE 89.2 Multivariate Logistic Model for Lung Cancer by Smoking Status

Risk Factor	p Value	OR (95% CI)
Never-Smoker		
ETS (yes versus no)	0.0042	1.80 (1.20–2.89)
Family history (≥2 versus <2)[a]	<0.001	2.00 (1.39–2.90)
Former Smoker		
Emphysema (yes versus no)	<0.001	2.65 (1.95–3.60)
Dust exposure (yes versus no)	<0.001	1.59 (1.29–1.97)
Family history (≥2 versus <2)[a]	<0.001	1.59 (1.28–1.98)
Age stopped smoking		
<42 years	Reference	
42–54 years	0.1110	1.24 (0.95–1.61)
≥54 years	0.0018 (p for trend = 0.017)	1.50 (1.16–1.94)
Current Smoker		
Emphysema (yes)	<0.001	2.13 (1.58–2.88)
Pack-years		
<28	Reference	
28–41.9	0.1932	1.25 (0.89–1.74)
42–57.4	0.0241	1.45 (1.05–2.01)
≥57.5	<0.001 (p for trend <0.001)	1.85 (1.35–2.53)
Dust exposure (yes vs. no)	0.0075	1.36 (1.09–1.70)
Asbestos exposure (yes vs. no)	0.0127	1.51 (1.09–2.08)
Family history[b]		
0	Reference	
≥1	0.0021	1.47 (1.15–1.88)

ETS, environmental tobacco smoke.
[a]Number of first-degree relatives with any cancer.
[b]Number of first-degree relatives with a smoking-related cancer such as lung cancer, renal cancer, cancer of upper digestive tract, esophagus, pancreas, bladder, and cervix.
From Spitz MR, Hong WK, Amos CI, et al. A risk model for prediction of lung cancer. *J Natl Cancer Inst* 2007;99:715–726. Reproduced by permission of Oxford University Press.

never-smokers, former smokers, and current smokers (Table 89.2). Cassidy and colleagues[24] highlighted the significant increased risk of lung cancer specifically for individuals with a family history of early-onset lung cancer (i.e., those <60 years of age) (Table 89.3). Schwartz and colleagues[25] have reviewed the molecular epidemiology of lung cancer, focusing on a number of host susceptibility genetic markers to lung carcinogens. The susceptibility genetic factors included high-penetrance, low-frequency genes and low-penetrance, high-frequency genes, as well as acquired epigenetic polymorphisms. Work by Takemiya[26] and Yamanaka[27] demonstrated the association of lung cancer with rare Mendelian cancer syndromes such as Bloom's and Werner's syndromes, respectively. Studies on familial aggregation have lent support to the idea that there is a hereditary component to the risk of some lung cancers. These familial association approaches have been used to discover high-penetrance, low-frequency genes. A recent meta-analysis involving 32 studies showed a twofold increased risk of lung cancer in individuals with a positive family history of lung cancer. This increased risk associated with family history was still present amongst nonsmokers, as shown by Matakidou and colleagues.[28] Bailey-Wilson and colleagues,[29] using family linkage approaches, reported the first association of familial lung cancer to the region on chromosome 6q23-25 (146 to 164 cM). The addition of smoking history to the effect of this inheritance was associated with a threefold increased risk in lung cancer.

There have also been numerous studies on candidate susceptibility genes that are of low penetrance and high frequency. The approach has been to target genes known to be involved in the absorption, metabolism, and accumulation of tobacco or other carcinogens in lung tissue, with the hypothesis that these genes will affect cancer susceptibility.

TABLE 89.3 Liverpool Lung Project—Multivariate Risk Model Lung Cancer

Risk Factor	p Value	OR (95% CI)
Smoking duration	<0.001	
Never		1.00 reference
1–20 years		2.16 (1.21–3.85)
21–40 years		4.27 (2.62–6.94)
41–60 years		12.27 (7.41–20.30)
>60 years		15.25 (5.71–40.65)
Prior diagnosis of pneumonia	0.002	
No		1.00 reference
Yes		1.83 (1.26–2.64)
Occupational exposure to asbestos	<0.001	
No		1.00 reference
Yes		1.89 (1.35–2.62)
Prior diagnosis of malignant tumor	0.005	
No		1.00 reference
Yes		1.96 (1.22–3.14)
Family history of lung cancer	0.01	
No		1.00 reference
Early onset (<60 years)		2.02 (1.18–3.45)
Late onset (≥60 years)		1.18 (0.79–1.76)

Reprinted by permission from Macmillan Publishers Ltd on behalf of Cancer Research UK: Cassidy A, Myles JP, van Tongeren M, et al. The LLP risk model: an individual risk prediction model for lung cancer. *Br J Cancer* 2008;98:270. Copyright © 2008.

For example, genetic polymorphisms encoding enzymes involved in the activation and conjugation of tobacco smoke compounds such as PAHs, nitrosamines, and aromatic amines have been widely studied. The metabolism of these compounds occurs through either phase I enzymes (oxidation, reduction, and hydrolysis) or phase II (conjugation) enzymes. Some of the frequently studied enzymes in this system include CYP1A1, the glutathione S-transferases (GSTs), microsomal epoxide hydrolase 1 (mEH/EPHX1), myeloperoxidase (MPO), and NAD(P)H quinine oxidoreductase 1 (NQO1). Data on polymorphisms in CYP1A1 and their association with lung cancer risk have been conflicting. A meta-analysis involving 16 studies by Le Marchand and colleagues[30] demonstrated no significant risk associated with the CYP1A1 Ile462Val allele; however, in a pooled analysis, a significant 55% increased risk in whites was observed, especially in women and nonsmokers for squamous cell carcinoma. GST gene products help conjugate electrophilic compounds to the antioxidant glutathione. GSTM1 in its null form occurs in 50% of the population, and studies by Benhamou and colleagues[31] have shown a 17% increased risk of lung cancer in individuals who were GSTM1-null. Amos and colleagues performed a genomewide association scan of tag single nucleotide polymorphisms (SNPs) in histologically confirmed non-small-cell lung cancer (NSCLC) in an effort to identify common low-penetrance alleles that influence lung cancer risk.[32] They identified a susceptibility locus for lung cancer at chromosome 15q25.1, a region containing the nicotinic acetylcholine receptor genes.

Much attention in the past decade has been given to "driver mutations," in a goal to find similar targets to those identified in the causal pathways of colon and breast cancer. The two best characterized at this time in lung cancer include KRAS (Kirsten-Ras) and epidermal growth factor receptor (EGFR) mutations. It is currently estimated that 15% to 25% of NSCLCs possess a KRAS mutation, while 10% to 15% harbor an EGFR mutation. While no current therapies target KRAS mutations directly, randomized controlled trials have evaluated the use of agents (PAS/RAF/MEK-pathway inhibitors) targeting downstream products of KRAS with promising decreases in disease progression. Studies of EGFR have revealed that these mutations are more prevalent in females, persons of East Asian descent, nonsmokers, and those with adenocarcinoma or bronchioalveolar subtype. The presence of EGFR mutations does facilitate additional therapeutic options for the patient—most notably tyrosine kinase inhibitors (TKI). Use of TKI inhibitors compared to conventional chemotherapy in randomized clinical trials has seen a doubling of therapy response rate and progression-free survival.

Results from the many candidate gene polymorphism studies focusing on a single polymorphism in one gene have been mixed. This has led to studies looking at gene–gene interactions, which require even larger study populations. For example, Zhou and colleagues[33] studied the interaction between variants in genes coding for NAT2 (which activates aryl amine cigarette smoke metabolites and deactivates aromatic amines) and mEH (which activates PAHs and deactivates various epoxides). They found significant interactions between NAT2 variants associated with certain acetylation phenotype and mEH variants associated with certain activity level with the risk of lung cancer. For example, a twofold increased risk of lung cancer was observed in 120-pack-year smokers who had the NAT2 slow-acetylation and mEH high-activity genotype. On the other hand, in nonsmokers, a 50% decreased risk of lung cancer was observed among those with the combined NAT2 slow-acetylation and mEH high-activity genotype.

Polymorphisms in genes involved in DNA repair enzymes active in base excision repair (XRCC1, OGG1), nucleotide excision repair (ERCC1, XPD, XPA), double-strand break repair (XRCC3), and different mismatch repair pathways have also been studied in relation to lung cancer risks.[34,35] Chronic inflammation in response to repetitive tobacco exposure has been theorized to be involved in lung tumorigenesis. Genes encoding for the interleukins (IL-1, IL-6, IL-8), the cyclooxygenase enzymes (COX2) involved in inflammation, or the metalloproteases (MMP-1, -2, -3, -12) involved in repair during inflammation have been associated with lung cancer risk. A number of cell cycle–related genes have also been implicated in lung cancer susceptibility. These genes have included tumor suppressor genes $p53$ and $p73$, mouse double minute 2 (MDM2), and the apoptosis genes encoding FAS and FASL.

Wu and colleagues[36] demonstrated that the presence of mutagen sensitivity is associated with an increased risk of lung cancer. Spitz and her group[37] noted that the combined risk for lung cancer was greater in individuals with mutagen sensitivity who smoked than in individuals with either smoking or mutagen sensitivity and greater than that in nonsmokers with mutagen sensitivity alone. DNA adducts, which are pieces of DNA covalently bonded to a cancer-causing chemical such as PAH in cigarette smoke, can be measured as biomarkers to represent the degree of carcinogenesis.[38,39] Several of the lung cancer susceptibility genes mentioned above have been associated with increased DNA adduct levels. Acquired or epigenetic changes to chromosomes can also lead to increased lung cancer susceptibility. These events include changes such as DNA methylation and histone deacetylation and phosphorylation, all of which can affect gene expression and thus carcinogenic potential. Despite numerous genetic association studies, the specific genes responsible for the enhanced risk of lung cancer remain poorly understood. As technology advances, it may be possible to target subgroups identified as genetically at high risk for lung cancer for specific interventions, including intensive efforts at smoking cessation, screening, and prevention programs.

Prevention of smoking initiation would be the most logical intervention because it would prevent the sequence of events leading to cancer outlined in Figure 89.1. However, despite intensive antismoking campaigns and widespread public awareness of the risks associated with smoking, it appears nearly 20% of Americans continue to smoke. Lung cancer risk also appeared to be related to age at smoking cessation. For men who had stopped smoking at age 60, 50, 40, and 30, the cumulative risks of lung cancer by age 70 were 10%, 6%, 3%, and 2%, respectively.[40] Although these statistics appear hopeful, Jemal and colleagues,[41] in an evaluation of data collected by the National Center for Health Statistics in the United States, identified a slowing in the rate of decrease of the birth-cohort trend in lung cancer mortality for whites born after 1950, which they interpreted as a reflection of the impact of increasing teenage smoking. Although there has been some debate as to whether age at initiation of smoking is an independent risk factor for lung cancer, this report would support the report of Wiencke and colleagues[42] that patients in the youngest quartile of age at smoking initiation (7 to 15 years) have the highest DNA adduct levels. Thus, while a frustratingly large percentage of persons in the United States and an increasing number of persons worldwide continue to smoke, efforts to prevent smoking initiation, particularly among children and teenagers, should be supported.

CONTRIBUTION OF OTHER FACTORS

OTHER LUNG DISEASES AND AIRWAY OBSTRUCTIONS

Several nonmalignant lung diseases have been associated with an increased risk of lung cancer. Of these, the strongest association has been shown with chronic obstructive pulmonary disease (COPD). Tobacco smoking is the primary cause of both lung cancer and COPD. A study by Wu and colleagues[38] of women with lung cancer who had never smoked demonstrated a statistically significant association between the presence of airflow obstruction and the development of lung cancer. A recent meta-analysis found that for smokers various pulmonary conditions all demonstrated significant associations with lung cancer, including diagnoses of COPD (relative risk 2.2), chronic bronchitis (1.5), emphysema (2.0), pneumonia (1.4), and tuberculosis (1.8). For never-smokers, the associations remained significant for pneumonia (1.4) and tuberculosis (1.9).[39] A recent pooled analysis from the International Lung Cancer Consortium from 1984 to 2011 found an elevated risk of lung cancer for both smokers and never-smokers that have a diagnosis of emphysema, pneumonia, or tuberculosis.[40]

Several diseases causing pulmonary interstitial fibrosis have also been associated with an increase in lung cancer risk. Hubbard and colleagues[41] evaluated 890 patients with cryptogenic fibrosing alveolitis (CFA, or idiopathic pulmonary fibrosis) and 5,884 control subjects and found that the incidence of lung cancer in study patients was markedly increased even after adjustment for smoking. Patients with CFA had an odds ratio for lung cancer of 8.25 compared with control subjects. An association with lung cancer and other fibrosing diseases such as scleroderma has also been found. In a study of 248 patients with scleroderma reported by Abu-Shakra and colleagues,[42] a 2.1-fold increase in cancer incidence in patients with scleroderma relative to a general population was demonstrated, with the most frequent types being cancer of the lung and breast.

Although the mechanisms by which pulmonary interstitial disease may predispose to malignancy are not clear, various hypotheses have been raised, including malignant transformation related to chronic inflammation, epithelial hyperplasia, and impaired clearance of carcinogens.

GENDER

Since 1950, a >600% increase in lung cancer mortality has been noted in women. Although most of this increase is attributed to the dramatic increase in the prevalence of smoking among women since the 1940s, several disturbing facts have emerged that fuel the controversy as to whether women are more or less susceptible than men to the carcinogenic effects of cigarette smoke. A recent meta-analysis has suggested that male smokers are more susceptible to lung cancer compared to female smokers (RR 1.44).[43] However, caution must be taken with the large meta-analyses such as these—as they often do not account for age of smoking onset (often earlier in men), smoking frequency (often more cigarettes per day in men), and daily use. When considering differences in lung cancer susceptibility to smoking with these considerations, the opposite association (increased susceptibility among women, RR 1.7) has been described.[44]

The observed gender difference in susceptibility may be related to a number of factors, including sex-related differences in nicotine metabolism or in metabolic activation or detoxification of lung carcinogens. Moreover, several reports have commented on gender differences in lung cancer observed at a molecular level. Ryberg[45] and colleagues noted that women with lung cancer have higher DNA adduct levels than men. Patients with higher DNA adduct levels might be anticipated to be more susceptible to carcinogens, which might explain why women appear to develop lung cancer with lower-intensity cigarette exposure. Further, hormonal factors may also play a role in susceptibility. In a case–control study, Taioli and Wynder[46] reported that estrogen replacement therapy was significantly associated with an

increased risk for adenocarcinoma (odds ratio 1.7), while the combination of cigarette smoking and estrogen replacement increased that risk substantially (odds ratio 32.4). Conversely, early menopause (age 40 years or younger) was associated with a decreased risk of adenocarcinoma (odds ratio 0.3).

The second issue is whether cigarette smoking may be associated with a higher risk of the development of nonmalignant lung disease in women than men, including obstructive airway disease. Previous research has suggested that cigarette smoking may be more harmful in its effects on pulmonary function in women than in men.[47] In this study, changes in forced expiratory volume in 1 second (FEV_1) and maximal midexpiratory flow rate (MMFR) and the slope of phase III of the single-breath nitrogen test increased with increasing pack-years more rapidly in women smokers than their male counterparts. These changes were independent of age, height, and weight. Furthermore, Beck and colleagues,[48] in a study of 4,690 whites, found that for a given level of smoking, female subjects demonstrated changes in FEV_1 and maximal expiratory flow at 25% and 50% of vital capacity at a younger age (15 to 24 years) than male subjects (40 to 45 years). Since people with tobacco exposure and spirometric evidence of airway obstruction are at higher risk for developing lung cancer, the suggestion that women may have increased susceptibility to cigarette-induced airway disease may be important in the consideration of their risk for lung cancer as well.

Finally, whereas women may have enhanced susceptibility to the carcinogenic effects of tobacco, it also appears that lung cancer occurs more commonly in nonsmoking women than in nonsmoking men. It has become clear that women never-smokers are more likely than male never-smokers to develop lung cancer. In a case–control study by Zang and Wynder[49] of 1,889 lung cancer subjects and 2,070 control subjects, the proportion of never-smoking lung cancer patients was more than twice as high for women than for men. It is currently estimated that up to one-fifth of all lung cancers in women are among never-smokers. In the past decade, it has become evident that female nonsmokers have a higher prevalence of EGFR mutations, leading historically to an improved treatment response rate with EGFR–TKI therapy.[50] Of note, these EGFR mutations are also more common in patients with adenocarcinoma and patients of East Asian ethnicity. In one comparison of the biological characteristics of lung cancer in female never-smokers and smokers, it was seen that never-smoking women were significantly more likely to have EGFR mutations (50.8% vs. 10.4% in smokers) and a higher percentage of estrogen receptor-α expression (30.1% vs. 10.4% in smokers), also suggesting a scenario where estrogen exposure may influence cancer cell proliferation.[51] Other studies have shown that estrogen receptor-β expression is also higher in women and nonsmokers.[52] While ER-α and ER-β are expressed in lung malignancies of men and women, it is likely the feedback from estrogen exposure that could factor into lung cancer evolution for women disproportionately to men.

RACE AND ETHNICITY

From 1999 to 2011, black males have disproportionately experienced the highest incidence of lung cancer compared to other races.[53] This is then followed by white males, American Indian/Alaska Native, Asian/Pacific Islander, and Hispanic males (Fig. 89.2). For women, the incidence of lung cancer is highest among white females, then black, American Indian/Alaska Native, Asian/Pacific Islander, and Hispanic. The trends for mortality from lung cancer are essentially identical to those for incidence by race (Fig. 89.3). Clinicians and public health officials continue to appropriately investigate cultural differences in tobacco use and exposure as well as outcome differences

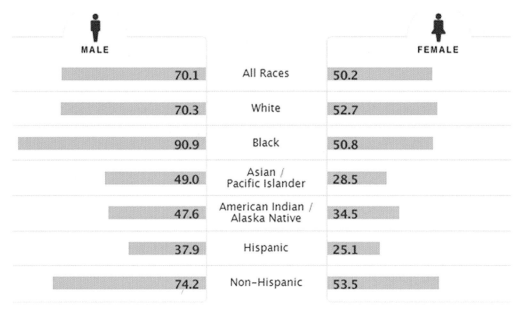

FIGURE 89.2 Number of new lung cancer cases per 100,000 persons by race/ethnicity and gender, 2008–2012, age-adjusted. SEER, V18, Accessed 2017.

according to socioeconomic status, insurance status, and access to care. Previous work has documented health inequalities as persisting in cancer care, including academic centers and Veteran's Affairs hospitals.[54,55] Important work has also been done to examine any biological contributors of cancer causation. Previous work has suggested that even when adjusting for socioeconomic factors and access to care, poorer survival outcomes persist.[56] In one study examining biological characteristics of lung tumors among black and white patients, it was seen that when tumors are examined for any of 26 possible oncogene mutations previously identified in NSCLC as a panel, black patients were less likely to have any mutations found than white patients (68% vs. 59%, respectively).[57] Such findings remind us of the need to continue tumor characterization studies among diverse populations. Previous research from earlier decades had suggested that the popularity of mentholated cigarettes among black smokers

could be a partial explanation for different biological features of lung malignancies in this population; however, recent reviews have called these assumptions into question.[58,59]

For persons of Hispanic ethnicity, large database reviews have revealed that Hispanic white lung cancer patients have improved overall survival when compared to non-Hispanic white patients, and have a slightly higher proportion of bronchioalveolar carcinoma (BAC) compared to other races and ethnicities.[60] As mentioned earlier, persons of East Asian descent have also showed a higher likelihood of expressing EGFR mutations and responding to TKI treatment. In one series, 88% of examined specimens from an East Asian population were found to possess alterations in EGFR, HER2, or ALK.[61] Other studies have confirmed this prevalence in East Asian never-smokers, with 75% demonstrating EGFR mutations, 6% HER2 mutations, and 5% ALK fusions.[62] Therefore the promise of genetic expression

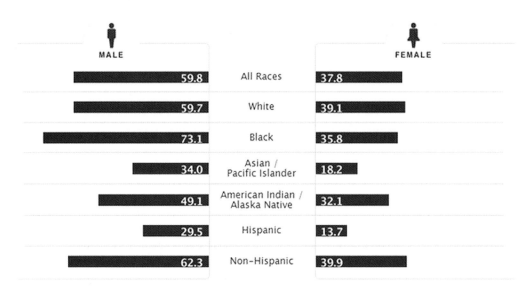

FIGURE 89.3 Number of lung cancer deaths per 100,000 persons by race/ethnicity and gender, 2008–2012, age-adjusted.

assisting in the neoadjuvant or adjuvant treatment of lung cancer is, at this time, closer for some subsets of patients than others.

ENVIRONMENTAL FACTORS

A tremendous amount of epidemiologic work has been directed toward understanding lung carcinogenesis resulting from environmental factors other than tobacco as well as interactions among all these factors. In particular, the combined effects of tobacco smoke with occupational carcinogens have received much attention. An additive or multiplicative risk of lung cancer has been demonstrated when cigarette smoking is present in the setting of exposure to asbestos, radon, arsenic, silica, and nickel, among others. The role of nutrition in cancer development has also increasingly received attention.

ENVIRONMENTAL TOBACCO SMOKE

Because nonsmoking persons exposed to ETS, also known as "second-hand smoke," are observed to have an increased rate of smoke-related problems, including upper respiratory symptoms and eye irritation, and there is an observed increased frequency of respiratory illnesses in children who are so exposed, it logically follows that the acknowledged carcinogenic effect of active tobacco smoking might also be present in those involuntarily exposed. This was initially suggested by reports demonstrating an increased risk of lung cancer in nonsmoking women married to smoking men.[63,64] In 1986, the National Research Council commissioned a review of the effects of ETS and found an overall odds ratio of 1.34 for lung cancer in nonsmokers exposed to household cigarette smoke.[65] Further work has shown that this increased likelihood of lung cancer is present when exposure begins in childhood (between birth and age 25), but later exposure may not have an association to lung cancer.[66] It is currently estimated that globally, second-hand smoke is responsible for approximately 22,000 lung cancer deaths per year.[67]

ETS consists of both mainstream (exhaled) smoke and sidestream smoke from smoldering tobacco (released from the cigarette itself). Both mainstream and sidestream smoke contain vapor-phase compounds (benzene and vinyl chloride) and particulate-phase compounds (aromatic amines and polycyclic aromatic hydrocarbons).[68] Because sidestream smoke is produced at a lower temperature (because it is produced from the smoldering end between puffs), the relative quantities of these particular compounds are different. For example, it has been shown that aromatic amines are actually present in a higher concentration in sidestream smoke.[68] It is estimated that ETS is 85% sidestream smoke, and 15% mainstream smoke.[68]

Metabolites of sidestream and mainstream smoke are found in nonsmokers and can be used as biomarkers for study and monitoring. In collected urine samples, these include cotinine (the primary hepatic metabolite of nicotine) and total NNAL (tNNAL, a known lung carcinogen that is the metabolite of NNK).[69] These metabolites have also been found and documented in blood, saliva, hair, and nails.[69] Furthermore, these urinary and salivary metabolites have been shown to correlate with air nicotine concentrations in smokers' homes.[70] Exposure to particulate matter does not just occur indoors, but has also been documented in open and semi-open settings, as well as residual particles on materials such as walls and furniture (known as "thirdhand smoke").[71,72] Thus, the presence of ETS is pervasive and harmful. The effects of limitations placed on smoking in public places may be of benefit in this regard. However, with approximately 20% of the American adult population still smoking, ETS remains a major public health issue.

ENVIRONMENTAL AIR POLLUTION

Air pollution has become a notable worldwide problem given the current staggering rate of globalization and industrialization. Advances in chemical analytical methods to detect specific pollutants have helped investigators study more accurately the effects of such airborne particulate matter. Early studies by Pershagen and Simonato[73] involving urban–rural comparisons have shown that an "urban factor" is associated with a 10% to 40% increase in lung cancer mortality. A case–control study in Sweden by Nyberg and colleagues (1990) showed a relative risk of lung cancer of 1.44 for individuals exposed to >29.3 $\mu g/m^3$ of NO_2 (as a measure of traffic air pollution) over a period of 21 to 30 years compared with exposures to levels <12.8 $\mu g/m^3$ of NO_2.[74] Two large US cohort studies have suggested that there is an excess risk of lung cancer of about 19% per 10 $\mu g/m^3$ increment in long-term average exposure to fine particulate matter after adjustment for multiple confounding factors.[75,76] Pope and colleagues found, as part of the Cancer Prevention II study, that fine particulate matter and sulfur oxide–related pollution were associated with an 8% increased risk of lung cancer mortality for each 10 $\mu g/m^3$ elevation in long-term average ambient concentration of fine particles <2.5 μm in diameter, or $PM_{2.5}$.[76]

Various potential carcinogenic components are thought to be emitted from different sources of fossil fuel combustion products. Cohen and Pope suggested that there is a gradient of relative risk of lung cancer associated with exposure to combustion products ranging from 7.0 to 22.0 in cigarette smokers, from 2.5 to 10.0 in coke oven workers, from 1.0 to 1.6 in residents of areas with high levels of air pollution, and from 1.0 to 1.5 in nonsmokers exposed to ETS.[77] Diesel exhaust, which is composed of a complex mixture of thousands of gases and fine particles, represents an important component of air pollution. Some of these gaseous components—such as benzene, formaldehyde, and 1,3-butadiene—are suspected or known to cause cancers in humans. Two large independent meta-analyses by Lipsett and Bhatia provided strong support that occupational exposure to diesel exhaust, especially among those involved in the trucking industry, is associated with an approximately 30% to 50% increase in the relative risk of lung cancer.[78,79] These studies provide reasonable grounds for concern that air pollution may increase lung cancer risk, especially in combination with other known risk factors such as active and passive smoking exposures and occupational exposures.

OCCUPATIONAL CARCINOGENS

Several workplace substances have been proven as carcinogens in the lung. The IARC has identified a number of such agents, including arsenic, asbestos, beryllium, cadmium, chloromethyl ethers, chromium, nickel, radon, silica, and vinyl chloride. The occupations associated with exposure to these agents are outlined in Tables 89.7 and 89.8.

ASBESTOS

Asbestos has historically been the most widely recognized occupational cause of lung cancer. Asbestos is a class of naturally occurring fibrous minerals consisting primarily of two groups: serpentine (chrysotile) and amphibole (amosite, crocidolite, tremolite, and others). Used commercially since the late 1800s, their fire-retarding qualities and strength have made them useful in construction and insulating materials. The wide recognition of its carcinogenicity dates to reports in the United Kingdom in the 1950s.[80] Today, it is widely recognized that asbestos exposure can result in a number of pleural and pulmonary manifestations.

Asbestos-related pleural disease may present as effusion, pleurisy, or both. Chronic pleural involvement is manifest as areas of pleural thickening (pleural plaques), usually involving the parietal pleura and often calcified. The relationship between pleural plaques and malignancy has been controversial in previous decades; however, current prospective CT screening programs have found a positive association between pleural plaques and mesothelioma.[81] Currently, the evaluation and follow-up of pleural plaques found on CT remains an active area of discussion.[82]

Inhalation of asbestos fibers can result in parenchymal lung disease, specifically interstitial lung disease ("asbestosis"). All the major types of asbestos can cause interstitial lung disease, although amphibole fibers may be more fibrogenic than chrysotile. The presentation of asbestosis is essentially identical to that of nonspecific interstitial lung disease and idiopathic pulmonary fibrosis. Symptoms typically include dry cough and dyspnea. Physical examination and radiography of the chest are consistent with a bilateral basilar distribution of fibrotic changes. The distinction between asbestosis and nonspecific interstitial lung disease lies in a history of heavy occupational asbestos exposure. In a statement by the American Thoracic Society on the diagnosis of nonmalignant diseases related to asbestosis, the following were considered necessary to the clinical diagnosis of asbestosis: (a) a reliable history of exposure, (b) an appropriate time interval between exposure and detection, and (c) clinical evidence of interstitial lung disease, including chest radiographic abnormality, restrictive pulmonary physiology, abnormal diffusing capacity, and abnormal physical examination consistent with fibrosis.[83]

In a review of the pathogenesis of asbestosis and silicosis, Mossman and Churg note the development of asbestosis occurs above a threshold fiber dose of approximately 25 to 105 fibers per milliliter per year.[84] This threshold dose is usually reached only in workers with heavy occupational exposure, including asbestos insulators, miners, millers, and textile workers. As is the case with other inorganic dusts including silica, the development of interstitial fibrosis usually requires prolonged exposure over months to years. Disease can also follow shorter, more intense exposure, as occurred in shipyard workers employed inside ship compartments during and after World War II. The latency period from exposure to presentation of disease is inversely proportional to exposure level. Therefore, the less the exposure, the longer the latency period. It is important to note that most persons with occupational asbestos exposure never manifest any evidence of interstitial lung disease.

The distinction between asbestos exposure and asbestosis becomes extremely important because of controversy over which represents the actual risk factor for lung cancer. Two reviews discussing the extensive available epidemiologic data illustrate this controversy. Jones and colleagues, in an extensive literature review, highlight several important points.[85] First, it is widely recognized that lung fibrosis of many causes is associated with an increased risk of lung cancer. This is true of idiopathic pulmonary fibrosis as well as interstitial lung disease associated with connective tissue diseases. Second, these authors point to animal experiments in which asbestos-exposed animals that developed lung cancer did so only when they also developed pulmonary fibrosis. Third, pleural plaques, a marker for asbestos exposure, have not proved a reliable marker for increased risk of lung cancer. In contrast, another review of the available medical literature, by Egilman and Reinert,[86] arrives at the opposite conclusion. In their extensive assessment of the available epidemiological data, these authors conclude that "asbestos meets accepted criteria for causation of lung cancer in the absence of clinical or histologic parenchymal asbestosis." Their evaluation of pathologic and epidemiological studies resulted in the conclusion that asbestos can act as a carcinogen independent of the presence of asbestosis.

Whether asbestos exposure alone or asbestosis is the actual risk factor for lung cancer, and whether or not all types of asbestos fibers are carcinogens, tobacco smoking clearly potentiates the observed carcinogenic effect. In a recent review of lung cancer mortality from the Cancer Prevention Study II (CPS II, which includes over 2,000 insulator workers with a history of asbestos exposure), it was found that lung cancer mortality was increased by asbestos exposure in nonsmokers (RR 3.6), by asbestosis in nonsmokers (RR 7.4), and by smoking alone without asbestos exposure (RR 10.3). The combination of lung cancer mortality in smokers exposed to asbestos was additive (RR 14.4), while the combination of smoking and asbestosis was greater than additive (RR = 36.8).[87] Smoking-cessation interventions remain a top priority for those with asbestos exposure or a history of asbestosis, and research from this same series has also suggested a reduction of lung cancer mortality by half within 10 years of quitting.[87] With recognition of the health risks related to asbestos, its use has precipitously declined in the United States since the 1970s (Fig. 89.4). Assuming that occupational exposure continues to decline, in future years the risk of asbestos-related lung cancer will hopefully decrease.

RADON EXPOSURE

Mining is the oldest identified occupation associated with lung cancer. Although the etiologic factors causing the increased lung cancer risk among miners were originally speculated to be dust-related pneumoconioses, the actual carcinogens have been identified as radioactive materials, primarily radon and its decay products. Radon (radon-222) is a naturally occurring decay product of radium-226, itself a decay product of uranium-238 (Table 89.4). Uranium and radium are ubiquitously present in soil and rock, although in highly variable concentration. At usual temperatures, radon is released as a radium decay product as an inert radioactive gas. Radon itself decays with a half-life of 3.82 days into a series of radioisotopes known as radon decay products (or radon daughters) that have half-lives measured in seconds to minutes. These products include polonium-218 and polonium-214, which emit alpha particles. Alpha radiation is highly damaging to tissues. Inhalation of these radon decay products and subsequent alpha particle emission in the lung may cause damage to cells and genetic material. Ultimately, radon decay produces lead-210, which has a half-life of 22 years. The concentration of radon gas in an environment varies depending on two factors: the richness of the source of radium and the degree to which the air around that source is ventilated. Thus, certain sites may be more likely to have a high radon concentration, with the prototypical situation being underground mines with poorly ventilated passageways.

Since Harting and Hesse's[88] 1879 description of lung neoplasms in miners, an increased risk of lung cancer associated with exposure to radon decay products has been demonstrated in a number of different domestic and international population studies of underground miners.[89-95] While not all miners will have an increased risk of lung cancer, both uranium and nonuranium mines may have high radon concentrations, and the risk of lung cancer in such settings is raised. Darby and Samet[96] and Samet and Hornung[97] have emphasized several important points in reviews of these studies.

In general, the relative risk of lung cancer increases with estimated cumulative exposure to radon. The occupational measure

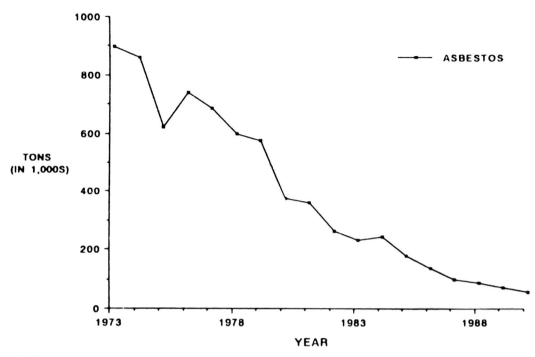

FIGURE 89.4 US asbestos use, 1973–1990. (Modified from Hughes J, Weill H. Asbestos and manmade fibers. In: Samet JM, ed. *Epidemiology of Lung Cancer*. New York: Marcel Dekker; 1994:185. Copyright © 1994. Reproduced by permission of Taylor and Francis Group, LLC, a division of Informa plc.)

of cumulative exposure to radon decay products is the work-level month (WLM). The work level (WL) is any combination of radon decay products in 1 L of air that results in the release of 1.3×105 MV of potential alpha energy. The number of hours worked in a month is defined as 170 hours. The WLM is a product of radon decay product concentration in WL and the duration of working months. In miners with cumulative exposures of 0 to 500 WLM, excess relative risk of lung cancer increases in approximately linear fashion to the amount of exposure. In miners with cumulative exposure of over 1,000 WLMs, the excess relative risk becomes nonlinear and decreases. Darby and Samet[96] suggest that this decrease in excess risk at high cumulative radon exposure may reflect cell sterilization as opposed to genetic mutation.

Excess relative risk reaches a maximum approximately a decade after exposure and then declines with time.

The rate of exposure to radon affects lung cancer risk. Higher excess relative rates per unit exposure are associated with lower average exposure rates. In other words, among miners with equivalent cumulative exposure to radon, those exposed to lower levels for longer periods of time have a higher risk for lung cancer (Table 89.5).

An increased risk of lung cancer is seen in smoking miners compared with nonsmoking miners. The Committee on Biologic Effects of Ionizing Radiation[33] (BEIR IV) concluded in 1988 that radon and smoking increased lung cancer risk in multiplicative fashion. However, a more recent review by Darby and Samet[96] suggests that the two act only additively. In any case, the combination of exposure to the two carcinogens is clearly worse than exposure to either alone.

URANIUM EXPOSURE

Uranium mining has now ceased in the United States. However, radon exposure continues to be an occupational concern in nonuranium mining and underground work in this country as well as in uranium and nonuranium mines around the world. In the United States, occupational exposure to radon is legislatively controlled. Individual exposure records are mandated for all workers in areas where the concentration of radon exceeds 0.3 WLs, with an annual cumulative exposure limit of 4 WLMs. The BEIR IV study[33] estimated that a 40-year exposure at this level would increase a person's lifetime risk of lung cancer twofold. However, this is at best a rough estimate. Continued longitudinal evaluation of occupationally exposed persons is clearly necessary to improve our understanding of the carcinogenic effects of radon.

While miners are exposed to the largest amounts of radiation from radon decay, radon is ubiquitous in the environment, with geographical variation. The National Council on Radiation Protection and Measurements[98] has identified radon and its decay products as the largest component of environmental radiation to persons living in the United States. Furthermore, radon is now recognized as

TABLE 89.4 Principal Decay Products of Radium

Decay Product	Half-Life
Radium 226 ↓	1,620 yrs
Radon 222 ↓	3.82 days
Polonium 218 ↓	3.05 mo
Lead 214 ↓	26.8 mo
Bismuth 214 ↓	19.7 mo
Polonium 214 ↓	0.000164 sec
Lead 210	22 yrs

Adapted from Samet JM. Radon and lung cancer. *J Natl Cancer Inst* 1989;81:745. Reproduced by permission of Oxford University Press.

TABLE 89.5 Relative Risks and Average Exposure Rates in Miners Exposed to Radon

Mining Cohort	Average Radon Exposure Rate (WLM/yr)	Relative Risk of Lung Cancer (% per WLM)	Reference
Malmberget, Sweden (iron)	5	3.6	Radford and Renard[92] (1984)
Ontario, Canada (uranium)	~10	1.3	Muller et al.[116] (1983)
Eldorado Port, Northwest Territories, Canada (uranium)	109	0.27	Howe et al.[93] (1986)

WLM, work-level month.
Modified from Darby SC, Samet JM. Radon. In: Samet JM, ed. *Epidemiology of Lung Cancer*. New York: Marcel Dekker; 1994:223. Copyright © 1994. Reproduced by permission of Taylor and Francis Group, LLC, a division of Informa plc.

the primary source of natural radiation to the bronchial epithelium (Table 89.6). These findings in conjunction with extrapolation of data collected in groups with high occupational radon exposure have escalated concern about the risks of lung cancer related to domestic (also referred to as residential) radon.

The concentration of radon gas in the environment is usually expressed as the number of disintegrations of radon gas in a given volume of air over a given time period. This is usually expressed in Becquerels per cubic meter (Bq/m^3), where $1~Bq/m^3$ equals one disintegration per second per cubic meter of air. Alternatively, radon concentration can be expressed in picocuries per liter (pCi/L); 1 pCi/L is equal to $37~Bq/m^3$. The average concentration of radon gas in the environment is 0.2 pCi/L. In a 1991 survey of homes in the United States, Samet and colleagues[99] reported a mean indoor radon level of approximately 1.25 pCi/L. In this survey, the range of indoor radon levels was quite broad. Most homes had levels only slightly higher than outdoor environmental levels, but a few had levels ranging in excess of 100 pCi/L. The primary factor determining radon gas concentration in homes is the concentration of radium in the surrounding soil and rock. Building materials, well water, and natural gas are less common sources, usually contributing only minimally to indoor radon concentrations. In the United States, the Environmental Protection Agency (EPA) has established "Radon Zones" which account for geographical variation in radon levels based on indoor radon measurements, geology, aerial radioactivity, soil permeability, and foundation type.[100] Zone 1 homes and buildings have a predicted average indoor radon screening level >4 pCi/L, zone 2 has a predicted level between 2 and 4 pCi/L, and zone 3 has a predicted level <2 pCi/L (Fig. 89.5).

A number of studies examining lung cancer risks from domestic exposure have been performed. A meta-analysis of eight such studies was reported by Lubin and Boice.[101] This analysis included 4,263 lung cancer and 6,612 control subjects. The overall estimated relative risk of lung cancer with exposure of $150~Bq/m^3$ was 1.14. This is consistent with extrapolation of risk from studies performed in miners as well as with actual calculated risks in miners with low cumulative radon exposure. It is important to note that this meta-analysis did not demonstrate any greater increase in lung cancer risk than what would be extrapolated from radon exposure in miners. However, Cohen and colleagues have suggested that the effects of low-dose, low-rate radiation have never been adequately evaluated, and contested the assumptions inherent in extrapolation of high radon exposure to domestic situations.[102]

The National Research Council Committee on Health Risks of Exposure to Radon[103] estimates that 1 in 107 bronchial cells will be subject to alpha particle exposures per year. Hei and colleagues[104] have previously shown that the majority of cells survive alpha particle exposure, and a small percent of cells survive multiple exposures to alpha particles. However, while increasing exposure caused increased cell death, the frequency of gene mutations increases in those cells that are repeatedly exposed, but do not die. These findings suggest that environmental and indoor radon exposure is a public health concern in its potential contribution to the development of lung cancer. Thus, further evaluation of the effects of domestic radon on the lung cancer epidemic, and its interaction with smoking, is warranted.

OTHER OCCUPATIONAL CARCINOGENS

A number of other lung carcinogens have been identified relating to a wide array of occupations (see Tables 89.7 and 89.8). Steenland and colleagues[105] from the National Institute for Occupational Safety and

TABLE 89.6 Estimated Annual Average Dose Equivalents From Natural Radiation in the United States

Source of Radiation	Average Annual Dose Equivalent (mSv)				Annual Effective Dose Equivalent Whole Body (mSv)
	Bronchial Epithelium	Other Soft Tissues	Bone Surface	Bone Marrow	
Cosmic	0.27	0.27	0.27	0.27	0.27
Terrestrial gamma	0.28	0.28	0.28	0.28	0.28
Cosmic radionuclides	0.01	0.01	0.01	0.03	0.01
Inhaled radionuclides (mainly radon)	24.00	—	—	—	2.00
Other radionuclides in the body	0.36	0.36	1.10	0.50	0.39
All sources	~25.0	0.9	1.7	1.1	~3.0

Modified from Darby SC, Samet JM. Radon. In: Samet JM, ed. *Epidemiology of Lung Cancer*. New York: Marcel Dekker; 1994:230. Copyright © 1994. Reproduced by permission of Taylor and Francis Group, LLC, a division of Informa plc.

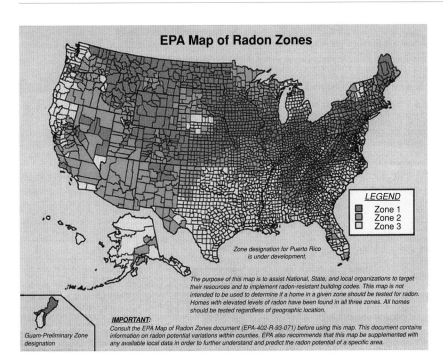

EPA Map of Radon Zones

LEGEND
Zone 1
Zone 2
Zone 3

Zone designation for Puerto Rico is under development.

The purpose of this map is to assist National, State, and local organizations to target their resources and to implement radon-resistant building codes. This map is not intended to be used to determine if a home in a given zone should be tested for radon. Homes with elevated levels of radon have been found in all three zones. All homes should be tested regardless of geographic location.

IMPORTANT: Consult the EPA Map of Radon Zones document (EPA-402-R-93-071) before using this map. This document contains information on radon potential variations within counties. EPA also recommends that this map be supplemented with any available local data in order to further understand and predict the radon potential of a specific area.

Guam-Preliminary Zone designation

FIGURE 89.5 Map of radon zones in the United States. Zone 1 areas (*red*) have a predicted average indoor radon screening level greater than 4 pCi/L. Zone 2 areas (*orange*) have a predicted average indoor radon screening level between 2 and 4 pCi/L, while zone 3 areas (*yellow*) have a screening level less than 2 pCi/L. (United States Environmental Protection Agency, 2015.)

Health (NIOSH) estimated that approximately 9,000 to 10,000 men and 900 to 1,900 women per year in the United States develop lung cancer related to exposure to occupational carcinogens. Although over half of these exposures are related to asbestos, a substantial number remain that are attributable to other exposures. Further, because these figures apply only to known carcinogens, they likely underestimate the actual number of lung cancer cases related to occupational exposures and represent another area in which prevention may play an important role.

DIET

Retinoids, including retinol (vitamin A) and its precursor carotenoids, such as β-carotene, have been the most intensively studied nutritional factors in relation to lung cancer development. One of the most widely cited reports of the effect of diet on the development of cancer was a prospective survey performed by Shekelle and colleagues,[106] of 2,080 men aged 40 to 55. Detailed dietary histories of these men were taken and the cohort was then followed over 19 years. In this study, intake of foods rich in β-carotene was inversely related

TABLE 89.7 Occupational Carcinogens and Associated Occupational Exposures

Known Carcinogen	Occupational Exposure
Arsenic	Copper, lead, or zinc ore smelting Manufacture of insecticides Mining
Asbestos	Asbestos mining Asbestos textile production Brake lining work Cement production Construction work Insulation work Shipyard work
Beryllium	Ceramic manufacture Electronic and aerospace equipment manufacture Mining
Chloromethyl ethers	Chemical manufacturing
Chromium	Chromate production Chromium electroplating Leather tanning Pigment production
Nickel	Nickel mining, refining, electroplating Production of stainless and heat-resistant steel
Polycyclic aromatics	Aluminum production
Hydrocarbon compounds	Coke production Ferrochromium alloy production Nickel-containing ore smelting Roofing
Radon	Mining
Silica	Ceramics and glass industry Foundry industry Granite industry Metal ore smelting Mining and quarrying

TABLE 89.8 Suspected Occupational Carcinogens and Associated Occupational Exposures

Suspected Carcinogen	Occupational Exposures
Acrylonitrile	Textile manufacture Plastics, petrochemical manufacture
Cadmium	Electroplating Pigment production Plastics industry
Formaldehyde	Formaldehyde resin production
Synthetic fibers	Insulation work Insulation production
Vinyl chloride	Plastic production Polyvinyl chloride production

to lung cancer incidence. Subsequent studies, including those by Cade and Margetts[107] and Stryker and colleagues,[108] demonstrated that smokers with the same dietary level of intake have lower serum levels of β-carotene than nonsmokers. These and other studies have suggested that vitamin A and β-carotene may have a protective effect against lung cancer. Byers[109] evaluated 27 such studies published prior to 1994 and concluded that individuals in the lowest quartile of carotene intake had an approximately 50% to 100% increase in lung cancer risk as compared with those in the highest quartile. Thus, by the mid-1990s, the cumulative information suggested that β-carotene and vitamin A might be useful as cancer chemopreventive agents. Three important large-scale epidemiologic studies were performed to investigate this possibility. The Alpha-Tocopherol, Beta Carotene Cancer Prevention (ATBC) Study[110] was a randomized, double-blind, placebo-controlled trial designed to determine whether daily supplementation of α-tocopherol, β-carotene, or both could reduce the incidence of cancers, including cancer of the lung. The study enrolled 29,133 male smokers aged 50 to 60 in Finland. Unexpectedly, a higher than expected mortality, primarily due to lung cancer and heart disease, was observed in the group receiving β-carotene. Omenn and colleagues[111,112] then reported results of the Beta-Carotene and Retinol Efficacy Trial (CARET), also a randomized, double-blind, placebo-controlled study. It was intended to evaluate whether dietary supplementation with β-carotene, vitamin A, or both would decrease the incidence of lung cancer. It enrolled 18,314 men and women felt to be at increased risk for lung cancer (due to either occupational asbestos exposure or smoking history). The CARET study was stopped 21 months early because of "clear evidence of no benefit and substantial evidence of harm." As compared with placebo, the group that received both vitamin A and β-carotene experienced a 17% increase in mortality and a 28% increase in the number of lung cancers.

A third randomized, double-blind, placebo-controlled trial, the Physicians Health Study, reported by Hennekens and colleagues,[113] evaluated the effect of β-carotene in 22,071 male physicians. At the onset of the trial, 11% were current smokers and 39% were former smokers. Over 12 years of follow-up, neither benefit nor harm in terms of malignancy or cardiovascular disease was demonstrated. Of note, the dose of β-carotene in this trial was lower than that in both the ATBC trial and the CARET study.

Ongoing efforts to identify food components that may be protective against cancer continue. On the basis of the findings of the ATBC and CARET trials, the use of supplemental β-carotene and vitamin A should be discouraged. The final word about the role of dietary supplementation in cancer chemoprevention is not out. However, these studies should serve as a reminder that indiscreet and excessive intake of vitamins or other chemicals is potentially harmful.

CONCLUSION

At present, the 5-year survival rate for lung cancer is only 18%. This is in stark contrast to the 5-year survival rates for the other leading causes of cancer death in the United States, including cancers of the colon (65%), skin (melanoma, 92%), breast (89%), and prostate (99%).[114] The role of tobacco as an etiologic factor in lung cancer has been convincingly established. Likewise, ionizing radiation and certain occupational exposures have been recognized as carcinogenic. The challenge in the future will be to modify the impact of these identified external sources of risk while continuing to expand our knowledge of the genetic and molecular basis of carcinogenesis. It is clear that early diagnosis of lung cancer should be considered

imperative, because the 5-year survival rate for treated stage I lung cancer is substantially better than for stages II to IV. With the clinical adoption of low-dose chest computed tomography (LDCT) for high-risk smokers after the results of the National Lung Screening Trial demonstrated a 20% relative reduction in mortality in lung cancer deaths with annual exams, it is hoped that we may see such improvements in the next decade.[115]

At present, with approximately 18% of the American population still smoking cigarettes, continued efforts must be directed at smoking cessation and at preventing people from becoming addicted to smoking. The dismal mortality associated with this disease demands that the medical profession contribute to efforts aimed at limiting its primary cause. If tobacco smoking could be eliminated or at least severely curtailed, we might be able to return lung cancer to its designation by Adler at the turn of the twentieth century as "among the rarest forms of disease."

REFERENCES

1. SEER Fact Sheets. Lung and Bronchus Cancer, 2017. http://seer.cancer.gov/statfacts/html/lungb.html
2. International Agency for Research on Cancer. *World Health Organization. GLOBOCAN 2012: Estimated Cancer Incidence, Mortality and Prevalence Worldwide in 2012.* http://globocan.iarc.fr/Pages/fact_sheets_cancer.aspx
3. Allemani C, Weir HK, Carreira H, et al. Global surveillance of cancer survival 1995–2009: analysis of individual data for 25,676,887 patients from 279 population-based registries in 67 countries (CONCORD-2). *Lancet* 2015;385(9972):977–1010.
4. Hruby A, Sweany H. Primary carcinoma of the lung. *Arch Intern Med* 1933;52:497–540.
5. Roffo A. Leucoplasia tabaquica experimental: *Bol Inst Med Exp Estud Trat Cancer* 1930;7:501.
6. Ochsner A, DeBakey M. Carcinoma of the lung. *Arch Surg* 1941;42:209–258.
7. Wynder EL, Graham EA. Tobacco smoking as a possible etiologic factor in bronchiogenic carcinoma. *JAMA* 1950;143:329–336.
8. Doll R, Hill A. Smoking and carcinoma of the lung. *BMJ* 1950;2:739–748.
9. U.S. Public Health Service. *Smoking and Health: Report of the Advisory Committee to the Surgeon General of the Public Health Service. Publication No. 1103.* Washington, DC: U.S. Department of Health, Education, and Welfare, Public Health Service; 1964.
10. Centers for Disease Control. Smoking and Tobacco Use, 2015. http://www.cdc.gov/tobacco/data_statistics/fact_sheets/fast_facts/
11. U.S. Department of Health and Human Services. The Health Consequences of Smoking—50 Years of Progress: A Report of the Surgeon General, 2014. http://www.surgeongeneral.gov/library/reports/50-years-of-progress/full-report.pdf
12. Hoffmann D, Hoffmann I. The changing cigarette, 1950 to 1995. *J Toxicol Environ Health* 1997;50:307–364.
13. Burns D. Tobacco smoking. In: Samet JA, ed. *Epidemiology of Lung Cancer.* New York: Marcel Dekker; 1994:15.
14. Hecht SS. Tobacco smoke carcinogens and lung cancer. *J Natl Cancer Inst* 1999;91:1194–1210.
15. Wynder E, Hoffman D. Smoking and lung cancer: scientific challenges and opportunities. *Cancer Res* 1994;54:5284–5295.
16. Belinsky SA, Devereux TR, Maronpot RR, et al. Relationship between the formation of promutagenic adducts and the activation of the K-*ras* protooncogene in lung tumors from A/J mice treated with nitrosamines. *Cancer Res* 1989;49:5305–5311.
17. Ronai ZA, Gradia S, Peterson LA, et al. G to A transitions and G to T transversions in codon 12 of the Ki-*ras* oncogene isolated from mouse lung tumors induced by 4-(methylnitrosamino)-1-(3-pyridyl)-1 butanone (NNK) and related DNA methylating and pyridyloxobutylating agents. *Carcinogenesis* 1993;14:2419–2422.
18. Rodenhuis S, Slebos RJ. Clinical significance of K-ras oncogene activation in human lung cancer. *Cancer Res* 1992;52:2665s–2669s.
19. Westra WH, Slebos RJ, Offerhaus GJ, et al. K-ras oncogene activation in lung adenocarcinoma from former smokers. Evidence that K-ras mutations are an early and irreversible event in the development of adenocarcinoma of the lung. *Cancer* 1993;72:432–438.
20. Goniewicz ML, Knysak J, Gawron M, et al. Levels of selected carcinogens and toxicants in vapour from electronic cigarettes. *Tob Control* 2014;23(2):133–139.
21. Barnett TE, Soule EK, Forrest JR, et al. Adolescent electronic cigarette use: associations with conventional cigarette and hookah smoking. *Am J Prev Med* 2015;49(2):199–206.
22. Walton KM, Abrams DB, Bailey WC, et al. NIH electronic cigarette workshop: developing a research agenda. *Nicotine Tob Res* 2015;17(2):259–269.
23. Spitz MR, Hong WK, Amos CI, et al. A risk model for prediction of lung cancer. *J Natl Cancer Inst* 2007;99:715–726.
24. Cassidy A, Myles JP, van Tongeren M, et al. The LLP risk model: an individual risk prediction model for lung cancer. *Br J Cancer* 2008;98:270–276.
25. Schwartz MR, Prysak GM, Bock CH, et al. The molecular epidemiology of lung cancer. *Carcinogenesis* 2007;28:507–518.

26. Takemiya M, Shiraishi S, Teramoto T, et al. Bloom's syndrome with porokeratosis of Mibelli and multiple cancers of the skin, lung and colon. *Clin Genet* 1987;31:35–44.

27. Yamanaka A, Hirai T, Ohtake Y, et al. Lung cancer associated with Werner's syndrome: a case report and review of the literature. *Jpn J Clin Oncol* 1997;27:415–418.

28. Matakidou A, Eisen T, Houlston RS, et al. Systematic review of the relationship between family history and lung cancer risk. *Br J Cancer* 2005;93:825–833.

29. Bailey-Wilson JE, Amos CI, Pinney SM, et al. A major lung cancer susceptibility locus maps to chromosome 6q23-25. *Am J Hum Genet* 2004;75:460–474.

30. Le Marchand L, Guo C, Benhamou S, et al. Pooled analysis of the CYP1A1 exon 7 polymorphism and lung cancer (United States). *Cancer Causes Control* 2003;14:339–346.

31. Benhamou S, Lee WJ, Alexandrie AK, et al. Meta- and pooled analyses of the effects of glutathione S-transferase M1 polymorphisms and smoking on lung cancer risk. *Carcinogenesis* 2002;23;1343–1350.

32. Amos CI, Wu X, Broderick P, et al. Genome-wide association scan of tag SNPs identifies a susceptibility locus for lung cancer at 15q25.1. *Nat Genet* 2008;40;616–622.

33. Zhou W, Liu G, Thurston SW, et al. Genetic polymorphisms in N-acetyltransferase-2 and microsomal epoxide hydrolase, cumulative cigarette smoking, and lung cancer. *Cancer Epidemiol Biomarkers Prev* 2002;11:15–21.

34. Li W, Li K, Zhao L, et al. DNA repair pathway genes and lung cancer susceptibility: a meta-analysis. *Gene* 2014;538(2):361–365.

35. Qian B, Zhang H, Zhang L, et al. Association of genetic polymorphisms in DNA repair pathway genes with non-small cell lung cancer risk. *Lung Cancer* 2011;73(2):138–146.

36. Wu X, Delclos GL, et al. A case-control study of wood dust exposure, mutagen sensitivity, and lung cancer risk. *Cancer Epidemiol Biomarkers Prev* 1995;4:583–588.

37. Spitz MR, Wu X, Lippman S. Markers of susceptibility. In: Roth JA, Cox JD, Hong WK, eds. *Lung Cancer*, 2nd ed. Malden, MA: Blackwell Science; 1998:1.

38. Wu AH, Reynolds P, et al. Previous lung disease and risk of lung cancer among lifetime nonsmoking women in the United States. *Am J Epidemiol* 1995;141:1023–1032.

39. Brenner DR, McLaughlin JR, Hung RJ. Previous lung diseases and lung cancer risk: a systematic review and meta-analysis. *Plos One* 2011;6(3):e17479.

40. Brenner DR, Boffetta P, Duell EJ, et al. Previous lung diseases and lung cancer risk: a pooled analysis from the International Lung Cancer Consortium. *Am J Epidemiology* 2012;176(7):573–585.

41. Hubbard R, Venn A, Lewis S, et al. Lung cancer and cryptogenic fibrosing alveolitis. A population-based cohort study. *Am J Respir Crit Care Med* 2000;161:5–8.

42. Abu-Shakra M, Guillemin F, Lee P. Cancer in systemic sclerosis. *Arthritis Rheum* 1993;36:460–464.

43. Yu Y, Liu H, Zheng S, et al. Gender susceptibility for cigarette smoking-attributable lung cancer: a systematic review and meta-analysis. *Lung Cancer* 2014;85(3):351–360.

44. Zang EA, Wynder EL. Differences in lung cancer risk between men and women: examination of the evidence. *J Natl Cancer Inst* 1996;88(3–4):183–192.

45. Ryberg D, Hewer A, Phillips DH, et al. Different susceptibility to smoking-induced DNA damage among male and female lung cancer patients. *Cancer Res* 1994;54:5801–5803.

46. Taioli E, Wynder EL. Endocrine factors in adenocarcinoma of the lung in women. *J Natl Cancer Inst* 1994;86:869–870.

47. Chen Y, Horne SL, Dosman JA. Increased susceptibility to lung function in female smokers. *Am Rev Respir Dis* 1991;143:1224–1230.

48. Beck GJ, Doyle CA, Schachter EN. Smoking and lung function. *Am Rev Respir Dis* 1981;123:149–155.

49. Zang E, Wynder E. Differences in lung cancer risk between men and women: examination of the evidence. *J Natl Cancer Inst* 1996;88:183–192.

50. Rosell R, Moran T, Queralt C, et al. Screening for epidermal growth factor receptor mutations in lung cancer. *N Engl J Med* 2009;361(10):958–967.

51. Mazieres J, Rouquette I, Lepage B, et al. Specificities of lung adenocarcinoma in women who have never smoked. *J Thorac Oncol* 2013;8:923–929.

52. Wu CT, Chang YL, Shih JY, et al. The significance of estrogen receptor β in 301 surgically treated non-small cell lung cancers. *J Thorac Cardiovasc Surg* 2005;130:979–986.

53. Centers for Disease Control and Prevention. Lung cancer rates by race and ethnicity, http://www.cdc.gov/cancer/lung/statistics/race.htm. Accessed May 2015.

54. Yorio JT, Yan J, Xie Y, et al. Socioeconomic disparities in lung cancer treatment and outcomes persist within a single academic medical center. *Clin Lung Cancer* 2012;13(6):448–457.

55. Samuel CA, Landrum MB, McNeil BJ, et al. Racial disparities in cancer care in the Veterans Affairs health care system and the role of site of care. *Am J Public Health* 2014;104(4):S562–S571.

56. DeSantis C, Naishadham D, Jemal A. Cancer statistics for African Americans, 2013. *CA Cancer J Clin* 2013;63:151–166.

57. Bollig-Fischer A, Chen W, Gadgeel SM, et al. Racial diversity of actionable mutations in non-small cell lung cancer. *J Thorac Oncol* 2015;10(2):250–255.

58. Lee PN. Systematic review of the epidemiological evidence comparing lung cancer risk in smokers of mentholated and unmentholated cigarettes. *BMC Pulm Med* 2011;11(18):1–28.

59. Blot WJ, Cohen SS, Aldrich M, et al. Lung cancer risk among smokers of menthol cigarettes. *J Natl Cancer Inst* 2011;103(10):810–816.

60. Saeed AM, Toonkel R, Glassberg MK, et al. The influence of Hispanic ethnicity on non-small cell lung cancer histology and patient survival: an analysis of the Survival, Epidemiology, and End Results database. *Cancer* 2012;118(18):4495–4501.

61. Sun Y, Ren Y, Fang Z, et al. Lung adenocarcinoma from East Asian never-smokers is a disease largely defined by targetable oncogenic mutant kinases. *J Clin Oncol* 2010;28(30):4616–4620.

62. Li C, Fang R, Sun Y, et al. Spectrum of oncogenic driver mutations in lung adenocarcinomas from East Asian never smokers. *PLoS One* 2011;6(11):e28204.

63. Hirayama T. Non-smoking wives of heavy smokers have a higher risk of lung cancer: a study from Japan. *BMJ* 1981;282:183–185.

64. Trichopoulos D, Kalandidi A, Sparros L, et al. Lung cancer and passive smoking. *Int J Cancer* 1981;27:1–4.

65. National Research Council. *Environmental Tobacco Smoke: Measuring Exposures and Assessing Health Effects*. Washington, DC: U.S. National Research Council, National Academy Press; 1986.

66. Asomaning K, Miller DP, Liu G, et al. Second hand smoke, age of exposure and lung cancer risk. *Lung Cancer* 2008;61:13–20.

67. Oberg M, Jaakkola MS, Woodward A, et al. Worldwide burden of disease from exposure to second-hand smoke: a retrospective analysis of data from 192 countries. *Lancet* 377(9760):8–14.

68. Besaratinia A, Pfeifer GP. Second-hand smoke and human lung cancer. *Lancet Oncol* 2008;9(7):657–666.

69. Avila-Tang E, Al-Delaimy WK, Ashley DL, et al. Assessing secondhand smoke using biological markers. *Tob Control* 2013;22(3):164–171.

70. Martinez-Sanchez JM, Sureda X, Fu M, et al. Secondhand smoke exposure at home: assessment by biomarkers and airborne markers. *Environ Res* 2014;133:111–116.

71. Sureda Z, Fernandez E, Lopez MJ, et al. Secondhand tobacco smoke exposure in open and semi-open settings: a systematic review. *Environ Health Perspect* 2013;121(7):766–773.

72. Ramirez N, Ozel MZ, Lewis AC, et al. Exposure of nitrosamines in thirdhand tobacco smoke increases cancer risk in non-smokers. *Environ Int* 2014;71:139–147.

73. Pershagen G, Simonato L. Epidemiological evidence for the carcinogenicity of air pollutants. In Tomatis L, ed. *Air Pollution and Human Cancer. European School of Oncology Monograph*. Berlin: Springer-Verlag; 1990:63.

74. Nyberg F, Gustavsson P, Järup L, et al. Urban air pollution and lung cancer in Stockholm. *Epidemiology* 2000; 11:487–495.

75. Dockery DW, Pope CA 3rd, Xu X, et al. An association between air pollution and mortality in six U.S. cities. *N Engl J Med* 1993;329:1753–1759.

76. Pope CA 3rd, Burnett RT, Thun MJ, et al. Lung cancer, cardiopulmonary mortality, and long-term exposure to fine particulate air pollution. *JAMA* 2002;287:1132–1141.

77. Cohen AJ, Pope CA III. Lung cancer and air pollution. *Environ Health Perspect* 1995; 1103:219–224.

78. Lipsett MJ, Campleman S. Occupational exposure to diesel exhaust and lung cancer: a meta-anaylsis. *Am J Public Health* 1998;89:1009–1017.

79. Bhatia R, Lopipero P, Smith AH. Diesel exhaust exposure and lung cancer. *Epidemiology* 1998;9:84–91.

80. Doll R. Mortality for lung cancer in asbestos workers. *Br J Ind Med* 1955;12:81–86.

81. Pairon JC, Laurent F, Rinaldo M, et al. Pleural plaques and the risk of pleural mesothelioma. *J Natl Cancer Inst* 2013;105(4):293–301.

82. Roberts HC, Patsios DA, Paul NS, et al. Screening for malignant pleural mesothelioma and lung cancer in individuals with a history of asbestos exposure. *J Thorac Oncol* 2009;4(5):620–628.

83. American Thoracic Society, Medical Section of the American Lung Association. The diagnosis of nonmalignant diseases related to asbestos. *Am Rev Respir Dis* 1986;134:363–368.

84. Mossman BT, Churg A. Mechanisms in the pathogenesis of asbestosis and silicosis. *Am J Respir Crit Care Med* 1998;157:1666–1680.

85. Jones RN, Hughes JM, Weill H. Asbestos exposure, asbestosis, and asbestos-attributable lung cancer. *Thorax* 1996;51(Suppl 2):S19–S23.

86. Egilman D, Reinert A. Lung cancer and asbestos exposure: asbestosis is not necessary. *Am J Ind Med* 1996;30:398–406.

87. Markowitz SB, Levin SM, Miller A, et al. Asbestos, asbestosis, smoking, and lung cancer. New findings from the North American Insulator Cohort. *Am J Respir Crit Care Med* 2013;188(1):90–96.

88. Harting F, Hesse W. Der Lungenkrebs, die Bergkrankheit in den Schneeberger Gruben. *Gesundheitswesen* 1879;31:102–105, 313–337.

89. Samet J. Radon and lung cancer. *J Natl Cancer Inst* 1989;81:745–757.

90. Hornung RW, Meinhardt TJ. Quantitative risk assessment of lung cancer in U.S. uranium miners. *Health Phys* 1987;52:417–430.

91. Archer VE, Gillam JD, Wagoner JK. Respiratory disease mortality among uranium miners. *Ann NY Acad Sci* 1976;271:280–293.

92. Radford EP, Renard KG. Lung cancer in Swedish iron miners exposed to low doses of radon daughters. *N Engl J Med* 1984;310:1485–1494.

93. Howe GR, Nair RC, Newcombe HB, et al. Lung cancer mortality (1950–80) in relation to radon daughter exposure in a cohort of workers at the Eldorado Beaverlodge uranium mine. *J Natl Cancer Inst* 1986;77:357–362.

94. Lubin JH, Qiao YL, Taylor PR, et al. Quantitative evaluation of the radon and lung cancer association in a case control study of Chinese tin miners. *Cancer Res* 1990;50:174–180.

95. Sevc J, Kunz E, Tomásek L, et al. Cancer in man after exposure to radon daughters. *Health Phys* 1988;54:27–46.

96. Darby S, Samet T. Radon. In: Samet JA, ed. *Epidemiology of Lung Cancer*. New York: Marcel Dekker: 1994:219.

97. Samet JM, Hornung RW. Review of radon and lung cancer risk. *Risk Anal* 1990; 10:65–75.

98. National Council on Radiation Protection and Measurements. Evaluation of Occupational and Environmental Exposures to Radon and Radon Daughters in the United States. Report No. 78. Washington, DC: National Academy of Sciences; 1984.

99. Samet JM, Stolwijk J, Rose SL. Summary: international workshop on residential radon epidemiology. *Health Phys* 1991;60:223–227.

100. United States Environmental Protection Agency. EPA Map of Radon Zones, http://www.epa.gov/radon/zonemap.html. Accessed May 2012.

101. Lubin JH, Boice JD Jr. Lung cancer risk from residential radon: meta-analysis of eight epidemiologic studies. *J Natl Cancer Inst* 1997;89:49–57.

102. Cohen BL. How dangerous is low level radiation? *Risk Anal* 1995;15:645–653.

103. National Research Council, Committee on Health Risks of Exposure to Radon (BEIR VI). *Health Effects of Exposure to Radon: Time for Reassessment.* Washington, DC: National Academy of Sciences; 1994.

104. Hei TK, Wu LJ, Liu SX, et al. Mutagenic effects of a single and an exact number of alpha particles in mammalian cells. *Proc Natl Acad Sci USA* 1997;94:3765–3770.

105. Steenland K, Loomis D, Shy C, et al. Review of occupational lung carcinogens. *Am J Ind Med* 1996;29:474–490.

106. Shekelle RB, Lepper M, Liu S, et al. Dietary vitamin A and risk of cancer in the Western Electric study. *Lancet* 1981;2:1185–1190.

107. Cade JE, Margetts BM. Relationship between diet and smoking: is the diet of smokers different? *J Epidemiol Community Health* 1991;45:270 272.

108. Stryker WS, Kaplan LA, Stein EA, et al. The relation of diet, cigarette smoking and alcohol consumption to plasma beta carotene and alpha tocopherol levels. *Am J Epidemiol* 1988;127:283–296.

109. Byers T. Diet as a factor in the etiology and prevention of lung cancer. In: Samet JA, ed. *Epidemiology of Lung Cancer.* New York: Marcel Dekker; 1994:335.

110. Alpha-Tocopherol, Beta Carotene Cancer Prevention Study Group. The effect of vitamin E and beta carotene on the incidence of lung cancer and other cancers in male smokers. *JAMA* 1994;330:1029–1035.

111. Omenn GS, Goodman GE, Thornquist MD, et al. Effects of a combination of beta carotene and vitamin A on lung cancer and cardiovascular disease. *N Engl J Med* 1996;334:1150–1155.

112. Omenn GS, Goodman GE, Thornquist MD, et al. Risk factors for lung cancer and for intervention effects in CARET, the Beta-Carotene and Retinol Efficacy Trial. *J Natl Cancer Inst* 1996;88:1550–1559.

113. Hennekens CH, Buring JE, Manson JE, et al. Lack of effect of long-term supplementation with beta carotene on the incidence of malignant neoplasms and cardiovascular disease. *N Engl J Med* 1996;334:1145–1149.

114. Surveillance, Epidemiology, and End Results Program. http://seer.cancer.gov/statfacts/html. Accessed May 2015.

115. Aberle DR, Adams AM, et al.; The National Lung Screening Trial Research Team. Reduced lung cancer mortality with low-dose computed tomographic screening. *N Engl J Med* 2011;365:395–409.

116. Muller J, Wheeler WC, Gentleman JF, et al. Study of mortality of Ontario miners, 1955–1977. Part 1. Report to Ontario Ministry of Labour, Ontario Workers' Compensation Board, and Atomic Energy Control Board of Canada. 1983, p.84.

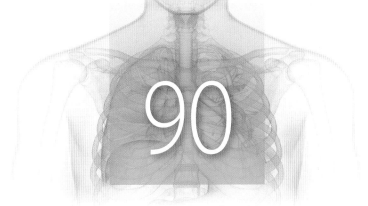

90

Lung Cancer Screening

Douglas E. Wood

INTRODUCTION

Lung cancer is the second most common cause of death in the United States, after heart disease, and the most common cause of cancer death, exceeding that of the next four cancers combined (breast, colon, pancreas, and prostate).[1] In short, lung cancer is an enormous public health concern. Symptoms often do not appear until the disease is advanced, and the symptoms also can be mistaken for other health conditions. Given the individual and population health burden of lung cancer, especially when it is diagnosed at later stages, there is a clear imperative to develop and implement screening strategies for early detection, analogous to those already established for breast, colon, cervical, and prostate cancer.

Although specialists caring for patients with lung cancer have made important incremental improvements in treatment, mortality has remained high due to a disproportionate presentation of lung cancer at an advanced, usually incurable stage. Breast, colon, and prostate cancer all have widely accepted and endorsed screening, and as a result 75% to 95% of these malignancies are diagnosed with local or regional disease that can be treated for potential cure, compared to only 37% of patients diagnosed with lung cancer.[2] In spite of impressive advances in surgery, systemic therapy, and radiation techniques, the biggest opportunity to improve lung cancer survival is to be more effective in identifying early stage disease. Patients operated on for Stage IA tumors now have a survival of approximately 80%.

Patients at risk for lung cancer and their families, have reason to be concerned about a lack of access to lung cancer screening. Lung cancer disproportionately impacts minorities, lower socioeconomic groups, and the elderly, suffers from a stigma of being a self-inflicted disease, and as a result has long suffered from less advocacy and research funding. Institution of a thoughtful, well-implemented national policy supporting lung cancer screening directly responds to the American Cancer Society's 2015 challenge goal "to eliminate disparities in the cancer burden among different segments of the US population."[3]

In the United States, randomized trials, conducted in the late 1970s, examined the value of plain chest radiography with or without sputum cytology for lung cancer screening in men who were active or former smokers.[4] These studies failed to demonstrate a decrease in lung cancer–related mortality in the screened populations. The results of these trials are in contrast to the results of case-controlled studies from Japan and experience with the Early Lung Cancer Action Program (ELCAP) and the International ELCAP (I-ELCAP) demonstrating a benefit associated with screening with low-dose computed tomography (LDCT).[5-7] Owing to these conflicting results, until

recently, the U.S. Preventative Services Task Force (USPSTF) did not recommend either for or against screening and, as a result, insurance coverage for lung cancer screening from both private and government insurers was lacking.

While multiple previous studies of LDCT have demonstrated success in identifying a high proportion of patients with stage I lung cancer, in the absence of a randomized trial they have not alleviated concerns about the biases of uncontrolled studies (i.e., lead-time and overdiagnosis bias), or the unintended harms of screening (false-positive studies and their attendant evaluation).

Lead-time is the length of time between the detection of a disease and its usual clinical presentation and diagnosis. It is the time between early diagnosis with screening and the time in which diagnosis would have been made without screening. Survival statistics can make screening appear to increase survival time, but not actually impact the course of disease if the person dies anyway at a time that previously would have been the usual course without screening. In this situation, screening only identifies disease at an earlier time point, so the length of time between diagnosis and death appears longer, that is, "lead-time bias."

Overdiagnosis bias occurs when screened patients results in an overestimation of survival duration due to inclusion of clinically unimportant disease—subclinical disease that would not become overt before the patient dies of other causes. Both of these could result in *apparent* survival benefit of patients screened for lung cancer in the absence of a randomized trial to evaluate population level effects. Thus, while multiple modern series of low-dose CT demonstrated a high rate of identifying early stage lung cancer and an apparent survival benefit, a high bar for evidence to assure a screening benefit, along with concerns about the unintended consequences of lung cancer screening, both for individual patients and for society, resulted in a continued lack of approval for lung cancer screening amongst major policy groups.

This led to the funding of the National Lung Screening Trial (NLST), the most expensive randomized screening trial of a single cancer ever conducted by the National Cancer Institute. The NLST randomized 53,454 patients at high risk of lung cancer to have an initial LDCT (prevalence scan) followed by two annual LDCT (incidence scans) versus plain chest radiographs at the same time intervals. The study was stopped early due to interim analysis demonstrating a 20% lung cancer mortality benefit for patients in the LDCT arm of the study (Table 90.1).[8] The National Comprehensive Cancer Network (NCCN) and multiple other organizations have subsequently published lung cancer screening guidelines that recommend screening for a high risk population.[9-15] A comprehensive literature survey by the Agency for Healthcare Research and Quality also supported the

TABLE 90.1 National Lung Screening Trial Overview[8]

- Study design: Randomized controlled trial
- Interventions: Three screenings performed over 3 years
  - Control group: Chest x-ray
  - Experimental group: Low-dose CT
- Time frame:
  - Enrollment and screening: 2002–2006
  - Annual follow-up through: 2010
- Primary Outcome: Lung cancer mortality assessed after 5 years of follow-up
- Major eligibility criteria:
  - Age 55–74 years
  - A cigarette smoking history of at least 30 pk-yr
  - Current cigarette smokers and former smokers who quit within 15 years
- Enrollment: 53,454 participants at 33 sites
  - 90% statistical power to detect a 20% reduction in lung cancer mortality
  - Secondary endpoint of all-cause mortality
- Results:
  - ↓ lung cancer mortality: 20%
  - ↓ all-cause mortality: 7%

TABLE 90.2 Current Eligibility for Lung Cancer Screening

- United States Preventive Services Task Force (USPSTF)[17]
  - Requires insurance coverage as a preventive service (no co-pay) for private insurers under the Affordable Care Act
  - Age 55–80 years
  - Current or previous smokers of ≥30 pack-years
  - Previous smokers within 15 years of smoking cessation
- Centers for Medicare and Medicaid Services (CMS or "Medicare")[38]
  - Insurance coverage as a preventive service (no co-pay) for Medicare beneficiaries
  - Age 55–77 years
  - Current or previous smokers of ≥30 pk-yr
  - Previous smokers within 15 years of smoking cessation
  - Requires documentation of shared decision-making
  - Radiology facility and radiologist criteria
  - Submission of lung cancer screening data to national registry

benefit of lung cancer screening[16] and the United States Preventive Services Task Force (USPSTF) recommends LDCT for screening patients age 55 to 80 years with at least 30 pack/year smoking history (unless they have stopped smoking for over 15 years) (Table 90.2).[17]

NCCN GUIDELINES FOR LUNG CANCER SCREENING

Until 2010, NCCN Guidelines regarding lung cancer screening were incorporated within the NCCN Non–Small Cell Lung Cancer Panel and included as a preface to the treatment guidelines for patients with non–small cell lung cancer. In fact, the 2010 guidelines from the Non–Small Cell Lung Cancer Panel stated: "At the present time, the NCCN panel does not recommend the routine use of screening CT as standard clinical practice (category 3). Available data are conflicting and thus, conclusive data from ongoing clinical trials are necessary to define the benefits and risks…" However, increasing interest and publications relating to lung cancer screening led to the establishment of a new panel dedicated to the topic of lung cancer screening. This panel was constituted in late 2009 and early 2010 and consisted of 26 specialists and experts representing thoracic radiology, pulmonary medicine, thoracic surgery, internal medicine, epidemiology, medical oncology, pathology, and a layperson representative.[18]

A combination of workgroup meetings, webinars, and face-to-face meetings led to preliminary drafts of the guidelines. However, the release of the NLST results provided critical and important new information that substantively changed the evidence and the recommendations being considered by the panel. Major revisions of guidelines occurred after the November 2010 NLST results were released, leading to a preliminary draft version of the NCCN Guidelines for lung cancer screening in June 2011 and the final guidelines being published in October 2011, the first major lung cancer screening guidelines to be developed following the publication of the NLST. Annual revisions to the guidelines continue to respond to new data and refine the algorithms used by providers.

The NCCN Guidelines provide a risk assessment to identify and recommend a group of people in whom to recommend lung cancer screening.[10] Relevant history includes smoking status (including

extent, duration, and time from cessation), radon exposure, occupational exposure of agents known to increase lung cancer risk (e.g., asbestos), cancer history (particularly other smoking-related cancers), disease history of chronic obstructive pulmonary disease (COPD) or pulmonary fibrosis, and secondhand smoke exposure. Patients are stratified into high risk, moderate risk, or low risk for the development of lung cancer. Patients stratified as high risk are considered eligible for screening and are recommended to undergo counseling and shared patient–physician decision-making that include a discussion of the benefits and risk of screening before embarking on an annual screening program with low-dose CT. Patients stratified to low or moderate risk are not recommended for routine lung cancer screening.

NCCN high risk patients are stratified into two groups (Table 90.3). The first group is analogous to the inclusion criteria of the NLST. This group is age 55 to 74 years old with at least a 30 pack-year history of smoking, and if not a current smoker, have cessation of smoking period of less than 15 years. The NCCN graded this recommendation as a "Category 1" recommendation due to the high level of evidence

TABLE 90.3 NCCN Risk Categories for Screening

- "NCCN Group 1"—high risk, recommended for shared decision-making for lung cancer screening
  - Age 55–74 years
  - ≥30 pk-yr smoking history
  - ≤15 years smoking cessation
  - Category 1 recommendation
- "NCCN Group 2"—high risk, recommended for shared decision-making for lung cancer screening
  - Age ≥50
  - ≥20 pk-yr smoking history
  - Eligible for definitive therapy
  - Additional risk factors[a]
  - Category 2A recommendation
- NCCN Moderate risk—not recommended for lung cancer screening
  - Age ≥50
  - ≥20 pk-yr smoking history
  - No additional risk factors
- NCCN Low risk—not recommended for lung cancer screening
  - Age <50 or,
  - <20 pk-yr smoking history

[a]Additional risk factors include radon exposure, occupational exposure (e.g., asbestos, silica, beryllium, chromium), cancer history (e.g., survivors of lung cancer, head and neck cancer, other smoking-related cancers), family history of lung cancer in first-degree relatives, disease history (pulmonary fibrosis or chronic obstructive pulmonary disease).

from the NLST and uniform panel consensus. The second group includes patients with risk factors considered to be analogous to the lung cancer risk required for NLST inclusion, as noted above, yet not evaluated within the context of a large randomized trial. The panel considered the wide spectrum of evidence for lung cancer risk factors previously known and published in order to provide guidance to patients and their physicians, as well as to avoid arbitrary exclusion of patients at high risk for developing lung cancer who had not been well-characterized by a randomized trial. This group of patients has frequently been nicknamed the "NCCN Group 2 patients." These are patients ≥50 years of age and ≥20 pack-year smoking history, with at least one additional risk factor for smoking (other than secondhand smoke exposure). For example, a 67-year-old patient with a 25 pack-year smoking history, but also with occupational asbestos exposure would be considered "high risk" within the NCCN Group 2 criteria, but not within NCCN 1 criteria.

The inclusion of these NCCN Group 2 patients into a high-risk group considered eligible for screening has been, perhaps, the most widely discussed and controversial aspect of the NCCN Guidelines. Extensive published data was provided within the manuscript accompanying the guidelines that referenced each of these areas and their contribution to lung cancer risk.[9] The NCCN panel achieved consensus regarding the inclusion of this group as a high-risk category eligible for screening, yet at the lower, 2B level, due to lack of uniformity amongst the panel members themselves. However, in the update of the guidelines in 2015 (version 1.2015) this recommendation was strengthened to a 2A recommendation representing uniform consensus of the NCCN panel. Some guidelines from other groups that have been published subsequently have agreed with and endorsed these NCCN Group 2 patients as being eligible for screening, and have used the NCCN Guidelines as a template for their own recommendations,[14] while others have disagreed and have limited their recommendations for screening to those patients fulfilling only the NLST inclusion criteria.[19] The USPSTF examined a variety of risk models in an effort to optimize recommendations for lung cancer screening.[17] The USPSTF recommendations increased the age range to be considered eligible for screening, similar to the NCCN, but only evaluated the variables of age, smoking exposure, and duration of smoking cessation. Other known risk factors, such as asbestos exposure or underlying pulmonary fibrosis were not evaluated in the USPSTF modeling study.

For patients deemed at high risk for lung cancer and therefore eligible for screening, a clear recommendation is made to invoke the process of "shared decision-making," encouraging an active dialogue between the physician and patient regarding the risks and benefits of lung cancer screening. Shared decision-making is a collaborative process that allows patients and their providers to make health care decisions together, taking into account the best scientific evidence available, as well as the patient's values and preferences. Shared decision-making honors the patient's right to be fully informed of all care options and the potential harms and benefits. This process provides patients with the support they need to make the best individualized care decisions, and is particularly important when it comes to preference-sensitive care, where there is more than one clinically appropriate treatment option, as there is in the case of screening. This also allows the patient's values and preferences to be at the forefront of deciding whether to embark on screening for lung cancer.

OTHER GUIDELINES

After the NLST publication in 2012, and the publication of NCCN lung cancer screening guidelines in 2012, multiple other organizations have provided positive recommendations for lung cancer screening.[9–19] Most of these guidelines used the inclusion criteria of the NLST as the sole group of patients to be considered for screening, based on the view that the NLST provided the only evidence supporting lung cancer screening, and that inclusion of additional patients, including those of similar risk of cancer, was of unknown benefit, and substantial possible harms (Table 90.4).

The only organization who did not endorsed lung cancer screening was the American Academy of Family Physicians (AAFP), who concluded that "the evidence is insufficient to recommend for or against screening for lung cancer with low-dose computed tomography."[20] The AAFP acknowledged the findings of the NLST, but remained concerned about basing recommendations on a single clinical trial, as well as generalizability of screening benefits in the community setting. However, at the foundation of the AAFP position are several important but incorrect assumptions. One of the beliefs by the AAFP panel was that investigators in the NLST benefited from "strict follow-up protocols for lung nodules" that would not be able to replicated in wider clinical practice. However, the opposite is actually the case. In the NLST there was "no standardized, scientifically validated approach to the evaluation of nodules.... no specific evaluation approach was mandated." However, now in an effort to standardize management of screen-detected lung nodules, the NCCN guidelines provide clear algorithms for nodule management based upon size and characteristics, and these are harmonized with the American College

TABLE 90.4 Current Lung Cancer Screening Guidelines

	NLST[8]	USPSTF[17]	CMS[38]	NCCN[9]	ALA[15]	ACCP[13]	AAFP[20]	AATS[14]	CCO[39]	CTFPHC[40]	ESR/ERS[41]
Age	55–74	55–80	55–77	55–74	NS	55–74	No	55–79	55–74	55–74	55–74
Smoking	≥30	≥30	≥30	≥30	NS	≥30	No	≥30	≥30	≥30	≥30
Cessation	≤15	≤15	≤15	≤15	NS	≤15	No	≤15	≤15	≤15	≤15
Other risk factors	No	No	No	Yes	Yes	No	No	Yes	No	No	No
Extended criteria				≥50 ≥20 pk-yr Add risk factor	Risk calculator			≥50 ≥20 pk-yr Add risk factor			

NLST, National Lung Screening Trial; USPSTF, United States Preventive Services Task Force; CMS, Centers for Medicare and Medicaid Services; NCCN, National Comprehensive Cancer Network; ALA, American Lung Association; ACCP, American College of Chest Physicians; AATS, American Association of Thoracic Surgery; CCO, Cancer Care Ontario; CTFPHC, Canadian Task Force on Preventive Health Care; ESR, European Society of Radiology; ERS, European Respiratory Society.

of Radiology (ACR) recently developed Lung-RADS as a standardized reporting and management structure for screen-detected abnormalities. The expectation is that these advances can be applied easily in new and existing lung cancer screening programs with the expectation of a substantial lowering of false-positive findings and invasive evaluations for benign nodules compared to the NLST.

A second concern preventing AAFP endorsement of lung cancer screening was a view that a clinical trial conducted in major medical centers in the United States would not be generalizable to the community at large, resulting in an increase in the unintended harms of excessive testing and poor outcomes from surgery. However, 21% NLST centers were not major academic centers, and an even higher percentage of I-ELCAP centers are community centers, demonstrating that lung cancer screening can be accomplished safely and effectively in diverse practice environments. The Lung Cancer Alliance (LCA), a patient advocacy group dedicated to lung cancer patients, has published a National Framework of Excellence in Lung Cancer Screening[21] that provides clear recommendations on the equipment, facilities, and clinical expertise required to provide lung cancer screening. The ACR has likewise published standards for designation as an ACR Lung Cancer Screening Center.[22] Substantial experience and responsible implementation of standards by professional societies and patient advocacy groups assure a high standard of screening in the community at large.

A third concern expressed by the AAFP representative presenting to the April 30, 2014 Medicare Evidence Development and Clinical Advisory Committee convened to review lung cancer screening, was the view that ongoing screening beyond the 3 years evaluated in the NLST would only increase the number and consequences of false-positive findings, increasing the harms of screening over time. However, again the opposite is true. As presented in the same meeting, and as well known by radiologists and clinicians participating in screening programs, serial screening with LDCT actually decreases the false-positive rate over time. Nodules that are initially deemed "positive" on initial LDCT and are followed with further imaging ultimately become "negative" when they show stability over time, and do not require invasive workup or surgery. Indeed, the accuracy in follow-up scans finding lung cancer is substantially higher due to the presence of previous baseline studies for comparison.

The AAFP is the only specialty group to date not to support lung cancer screening, yet the assumptions and rationale behind this decision appear to be flawed and not correctly recognizing the clinical impact lung cancer screening can have on behalf of the millions of patients at risk of developing lung cancer.

Effective January 1, 2015, USPSTF guidelines now impose a mandate on private insurers under the Affordable Care Act to cover lung cancer screening for this high-risk population. The largest US health care insurer, The Centers for Medicare and Medicaid Services (CMS or "Medicare") were not under the same obligation and initiated an independent National Coverage Analysis to determine policy and coverage for Medicare beneficiaries. The irony was that lung cancer is a disease of the elderly, with 70% of lung cancer diagnoses occurring in the Medicare population. If CMS chose not to cover LDCT for screening, patients in the United States could possibly face the paradox of having coverage for lung cancer screening through age 64, but would no longer be covered as Medicare beneficiaries, just as their risk for lung cancer is peaking. Most believed that this was an untenable policy position, and that CMS would be morally obligated to follow the guidelines published by the USPSTF. A consortium of medical experts led by the ACR, the Society of Thoracic Surgeons (STS), and the LCA worked closely with Medicare administrators to help clarify the benefits and risks of lung cancer screening in the Medicare

population, and to help evaluate and make recommendations regarding widespread national implementation. Medicare followed a short time after USPSTF, providing a positive coverage decision for lung cancer screening in high-risk patients on February 5, 2015. For the first time, patients at risk of lung cancer had access to early detection similar to what has long been available for patients at risk of breast, colon, prostate, and cervical cancers.

CONCERNS ABOUT LUNG CANCER SCREENING

There are legitimate concerns about the unintended harms of lung cancer screening, indeed for any screening or "intervention" for an otherwise healthy patient, and these concerns are important to be addressed in the implementation of screening policy.

Critics of policy supporting lung cancer screening raise legitimate concerns about the unintended harms of screening which must be weighed against the 20% lung cancer mortality benefit conferred to the screened population. In fact, these harms are inherent in screening for any cancer in asymptomatic and otherwise healthy patients. The concerns largely center on false-positive findings that lead to further testing and possibly even invasive procedures, overdiagnosis (treatment of clinically unimportant cancers), morbidity, and mortality of surgery for detected cancers, and the downstream costs of these follow-up tests and procedures. However, the purpose of a large randomized trial such as the NLST is to show the net value of a screening test *after* all the positive and negative effects have been accounted for. In the case of lung cancer screening, the balance was not even close, with a 20% improvement in lung cancer mortality among screened patients. But a closely related concern is the question of generalizability of the results from the NLST to the general community, representing a concern that inferior technique, poor decision-making by physicians, poor outcomes with surgery, and irresponsible implementation may negate the survival benefits conferred by LDCT.

Cancer screening is a little like buying insurance or paying taxes, a large number of people participate and may not directly benefit (or are even harmed to some degree) in order to provide a life-saving benefit for a minority.[23] In screening, this is often characterized as the number needed to screen to save one life from cancer. In the case of lung cancer screening, the NLST demonstrated a need to screen approximately 320 individuals for every life saved. This seems like a lot, and it is; 319 people having testing without mortality benefit. And some of these people may be harmed with additional testing or procedures; yet some may also have benefits less dramatic than life-saving, such as detection of earlier stage cancer that requires less morbid and less expensive treatment. It is important to recognize that these tradeoffs are inherent to any screening program, and in fact are less severe in lung cancer screening than in either breast or colon cancer screening which are widely promoted as important preventive health services. While 320 need to be screened to save one patient from lung cancer, 2,000 need to be screened to avoid a breast cancer death,[24] and 1,200 screened to avoid a colon cancer death.[25]

A legitimate caution in screening programs, including lung cancer screening, is the number of false-positive studies and the consequences of these studies, that is, how many are simply followed with further imaging versus receiving additional testing that may be invasive and risky, or even undergo unnecessary surgery. Mammography results in a 50% incidence of positive findings over 10 years, with 20% of these leading to invasive procedures.[26] Although these unintended negatives of screening are inherent, they can be reasonably mitigated by well-constructed policy and disciplined control within screening programs. First, screening should be limited to a cohort of people at high risk of developing lung cancer, as outlined in the NCCN guidelines,[9] and modeled to create the USPSTF recommendations.[17] Second, an evidence-based algorithmic approach to management of screen detected nodules avoids *ad hoc* follow-up testing and invasive procedures. The NCCN has provided detailed algorithms to guide physicians and patients in the appropriate evaluation of abnormalities detected during screening.[9] Recently, the ACR has published Lung-RADS, a structured reporting and management system modeled after BIRADS which has been used successfully for years in mammography for breast cancer.[27] In the NLST, 96% of abnormal findings were not lung cancer. The vast majority of these (90%) were evaluated by follow-up imaging alone, and only 4% underwent a surgical procedure, the majority of these for patients with lung cancer.[8] Overall, the complication rate of diagnostic follow-up was 1.2%. Eighteen-year experience in the I-ELCAP, only 1.5% of patients had surgical procedures after 31,646 baseline and 37,861 annual repeat CT screenings.[28] Of these, 89% were lung cancer and 91% were stage I disease. It is clear that lung cancer screening can be accomplished with minimal risk from downstream testing, including surgery, with minimally invasive techniques and <5% complication rate in patients without cancer.

A common concern by primary care physicians and other medical specialists is that the primary intervention for a screen-detected early stage lung cancer is surgery, and that surgery for lung cancer is highly morbid and with mortality rates that may negate some of the benefits of early detection. Surgical and anesthetic advances involving preoperative assessment and preparation, minimally invasive surgery, and postoperative care now make lung cancer surgery extremely safe. The STS General Thoracic Surgery Database evaluates outcomes of 850 surgeons at 250 centers in the United States and in patients undergoing pulmonary lobectomy (the most common lung cancer resection) have shown major morbidity in 4.2% of patients, and a mortality rate of 1.7%.[29] Experience with surgery in lung cancer screening programs demonstrate that it is rare in patients with benign lesions, and is accomplished at very low risk of morbidity or mortality.

Another consequence of screening is overdiagnosis, that is, the detection of clinically unimportant cancers that would otherwise not require treatment. Although clinicians long considered this to be trivial, with lung cancers considered universally progressive and fatal, experience with the high sensitivity of modern CT imaging confirms that some patients have very slow growing cancers that may never threaten their life. This is also not unique to lung cancer screening, and is a significant factor for breast, colon, and prostate cancer screening as well. In the study performed on behalf of the USPSTF, models suggest approximately 10% rate of over diagnosis,[16] but Lung-RADS guided management is expected to minimize interventions on even these "benign acting" lung cancers.[26]

In spite of the significant benefits afforded by lung cancer screening, legitimate concerns still exist that impact how policy is implemented and how providers view lung cancer screening as a new preventive service for their patients. Some would caution that the results of the NLST may have overestimated the benefit and underestimated the harm of lung cancer screening due to selection bias of both the patients and the centers involved in the trial. Indeed, in any preventive service there is often a close balance of benefits and harms, with fairly minor perturbations in indications or access shifting these balances. Physicians in particular strive to follow the Hippocratic Oath of "do no harm." However, in preventive services, harm can present in two forms, the unintended negative consequences of evaluation and treatment, but also the denial of preventive services from those who may benefit.

There are two broad strategies for minimizing the harms of lung cancer screening. The first, and the most popular amongst policymakers and preventive service skeptics is to limit access to lung cancer screening by defining very narrow inclusion criteria and limiting the number of centers that can provide lung cancer screening services. This certainly does have the benefit of exposing fewer people to the risks of screening but it has the consequence of using policy to override patient autonomy and shared decision-making, with the potential to disenfranchise and potentially harm patients that are at risk and could benefit from lung cancer screening. A second strategy of minimizing harms is to improve the management of those patients who undergo screening. This includes the creation of evidence-based management algorithms to minimize unnecessary workup of false positives and efficient, standardized workup of possible lung cancer. The second part of the strategy is to assure a high level of expertise in imaging, nodule evaluation, diagnostic strategies, and surgical treatment. This strategy benefits from empowering shared decision-making with patients, and allows us to provide access to patients a similar risk of lung cancer.

SELECTION OF PATIENTS FOR LUNG CANCER SCREENING

One of the most important determinants in lung cancer screening policy and guidelines is the identification of the correct population of patients to be screened. It is also one of the most effective places to limit access in order to minimize harms as a concern of physicians, and to limit healthcare expenditures as an area of concern policymakers. The major policy positions of the USPSTF and CMS have essentially used the inclusion criteria of the NLST, and portray this as a purely "evidence-based decision" due to the lack of additional randomized trials to evaluate other risk factors for lung cancer. However, it is important to realize the strengths and weaknesses of the NLST. What the NLST <u>did</u> do was demonstrate a mortality reduction in patients with a substantial risk factor for lung cancer. However, what the NLST <u>did not</u> do was to define the risk factors for lung cancer. The NLST was a clinical trial, and eligibility criteria were never meant to define the extent of "high risk" or be the basis of public policy. It is important to recognize that the NLST only considered age and smoking history as variables impacting lung cancer risk, and did not consider occupational/environmental exposure, cancer history, family history, or other pulmonary diseases.

The NCCN has frequently been criticized for extending recommendations for lung cancer screening to additional patients beyond those examined in the NLST and approved by USPSTF and Medicare. Some have criticized that the "NCCN Group 2" patients are of lower risk of lung cancer and therefore have substantially less benefit from lung cancer screening. However, this group allows the inclusion of other known risk factors for lung cancer, such as occupational/environmental exposure, cancer history, family history, and disease history.[9] There are decades of research that identify a number of other significant risk factors for lung cancer. Emphysema is an example of a disease process that independently increases lung cancer risk. A large meta-analysis from the International Lung Cancer Consortium demonstrated that emphysema patients have an odds ratio of 2.3 for the risk of lung cancer.[30] Further, there now exist a number of lung cancer risk calculators, and each of these utilize a number of clinical and demographic variables beyond age and smoking history to estimate lung cancer risk.[31,32] Fundamental principles behind the development of the NCCN Group 2 criteria were to qualitatively identify patients at similar risk to those undergoing screening in the NLST, and to allow them to undergo shared decision-making and consideration of screening, recognizing that it would be unlikely for any additional randomized trials to be designed that would individually or cumulatively evaluate these other known risk factors. In fact, this is now been retrospectively validated by the lung cancer screening group at Lahey Clinic. In their large and well-developed screening program, they identified approximately 25% of their screened patients qualifying under NCCN Group 2 criteria, rather than those endorsed by the USPSTF or CMS.[33] McKee and colleagues demonstrated an identical rate of nodule detection and lung cancer diagnosis between the two groups, suggesting a similar lung cancer risk amongst those recommended for screening under NCCN Group 2 guidelines.

Nearly 9 million current and former smokers are eligible for LDCT, with over 12,000 estimated lives saved per year.[34] However, US policy limits eligibility to those essentially fulfilling the inclusion criteria of the NLST clinical trial. While the trial was paramount in showing the mortality benefit of lung cancer screening, it did not purport to define the group of patients at high risk for lung cancer. For purposes of conducting an effective clinical trial, the NLST utilized only age and smoking status as variables to define inclusion, avoiding the complexities of other occupational exposure, cancer history, other diseases, etc. Lung cancer screening guidelines from the NCCN address this limitation by recommending consideration of screening in patients with smoking history and additional risk factors that are estimated to approximate a similar risk of lung cancer as those examined in the NLST.[9] The lung cancer screening program at Lahey Clinic has validated this extended criteria group defined by the NCCN expert panel, showing similar rates of nodule detection and cancer diagnosis in the NCCN group compared to those strictly meeting the NLST criteria.[34] Inclusion of these "NCCN Group 2" criteria patients would expand eligibility to another 2 million Americans, with another possible 3,000 lung cancer deaths averted.

COST-EFFECTIVENESS OF LUNG CANCER SCREENING

No new health care policy should be implemented without thoughtful consideration of the financial impact. Although LDCT screening itself is relatively inexpensive, costs are magnified by downstream testing and procedures in patients with positive findings. Added diagnostic and treatment costs certainly follow the identification of newly diagnosed cancer, or other abnormalities that require evaluation, yet costs of treating early stage lung cancer are much lower than treating later stage disease. The cost-effectiveness analysis of the NLST demonstrated an estimated cost of $52,000 per life-year gained from screening, with potential wide variations based on differing assumptions of screening implemenatation.[35] Independent actuarial analysis by Bruce Pyenson and his colleagues at Milliman, Inc. project lung cancer screening to result in an added cost to commercial insurers of $0.76 per member per month (PMPM), compared to $2.50 PMPM for breast cancer screening and $0.95 PMPM for colon cancer screening.[36] Cost-effectiveness analysis from the same group predicted cost per life-year saved at $19,000 for lung screening, compared to $31,000–51,000 for breast cancer and $19,000–29,000 for colorectal cancer screening.[37] There will be additional information about cost and cost-effectiveness, but current projections are that lung cancer screening is cost-effective, and at lower cost than similar screening programs endorsed for patients in the United States.

CONCLUSION

A primary objective of the American Cancer Society "is to eliminate disparities in the cancer burden among different segments of the US population, defined in terms of socioeconomic status (income, education, insurance status, etc.), race/ethnicity, geographic location, sex, and sexual orientation."[3] American health care policy finally addresses the disparity in access to cancer screening. The NLST has laid the groundwork for current policy, and other investigators and guidelines groups demonstrate that those policies can be extended to further diminish the health care disparities suffered by patients at risk for lung cancer, and the exciting opportunity to save several thousand lives each year.

Professional societies have stepped in to guide both Medicare and physicians on how lung cancer screening can be implemented safely and effectively with a huge benefit in terms of lives saved. The ACR has developed Lung-RADS to ensure uniform reporting of lung nodules with the goal of decreasing the false-positive findings that may lead to unnecessary evaluations. Further, ACR has developed standards for accreditation of centers preforming CT scans to assure high-level and consistent quality in centers performing this study.

NCCN lung cancer screening guidelines provide clear recommendations to physicians and patients about individuals who should be considered for screening, as well as systematic evaluations of any detected abnormalities that can further minimize unnecessary tests and procedures. The guidelines are updated annually as new knowledge becomes available. NCCN guidelines also outline the risks and benefits of screening and now have language supporting shared decision-making between patients and their doctors, so that patients have the best possible information to inform their own choices about lung cancer screening.

The STS has developed and published standards for the surgical management of patients with early stage lung cancer. In addition, the STS maintains the STS National Database, which tracks surgical quality and outcomes in patients undergoing lung cancer operations. The LCA is a vital patient advocacy group that has developed a Centers of Excellence program that helps qualify and identify centers that have the required expertise and facilities for accomplishing lung cancer screening safely and effectively. Finally, the I-ELCAP is an international study that has been performing lung cancer screening for 20 years and has demonstrated that lung cancer screening can be accomplished in a wide diversity of clinical settings, including community centers, and is not dependent upon being performed in large academic medical centers.

REFERENCES

1. American Cancer Society. *Cancer Facts & Figures*. Atlanta, GA: American Cancer Society; 2016.
2. National Cancer Institute. SEER stat fact sheets. https://seer.cancer.gov/statfacts/. Accessed February 19, 2017.
3. American Cancer Society. Cancer Facts and Figures 2014. http://www.cancer.org/research/cancerfactsstatistics/cancerfactsfigures2014/. Accessed September 10, 2014.
4. Garg K, Keith RL, Byers T, et al. Randomized controlled trial with low-dose spiral CT for lung cancer screening: Feasibility study and preliminary results. *Radiology* 2002;225:506–510.
5. Nawa T, Nakagawa T, Kusano S, et al. Lung cancer screening using low-dose spiral CT: results of baseline and 1-year follow-up studies. *Chest* 2002;122:15–20.
6. Sobue T, Moriyama N, et al. Screening for lung cancer with low-dose helical computed tomography: Anti–Lung Cancer Association Project. *J Clin Oncol* 2002;20:911–920.
7. International Early Lung Cancer Action Program Investigators; Henschke CI, Yankelevitz DF, et al. Survival of patients with stage I lung cancer detected on CT screening. *N Engl J Med* 2006;355:1763–1771.
8. National Lung Screening Trial Research Team; Aberle DR, Adams AM, et al. Reduced lung cancer mortality with low-dose computed tomographic screening. *New Engl J Med* 2011;365:395–409.

9. Wood DE, Eapen GA, Ettinger DS, et al. Lung cancer screening. *J Natl Compr Canc Netw* 2012;10:240–265. Update Version 1.2017.

10. National Comprehensive Cancer Network. https://www.nccn.org/professionals/physician_gls/pdf/lung_screening.pdf. Accessed February 19, 2017.

11. Smith RA, Manassaram-Baptiste D, Brooks D, et al. Cancer screening in the United States, 2014: a review of current American Cancer Society guidelines and current issues in cancer screening. *CA Cancer J Clin* 2014;64:30–51.

12. Rocco G, Allen MS, Altorki NK, et al. Clinical statement on the role of the surgeon and surgical issues relating to computed tomography screening programs for lung cancer. *Ann Thorac Surg* 2013;96:445–450.

13. Detterbeck FC, Mazzone PJ, Naidich DP, et al. Screening for lung cancer screening for lung cancer: Diagnosis and management of lung cancer, 3rd ed: American college of chest physicians evidence-based clinical practice guidelines. *Chest* 2013;143(5) (suppl): e78S–e92S.

14. Jaklitsch MT, Jacobson FL, Austin JH, et al. Development of The American Association for Thoracic Surgery guidelines for lung cancer screening using low-dose computed tomography scans for lung cancer survivors and other high-risk groups. *J Thorac Cardiovasc Surg* 2012;144:25–32.

15. American Lung Association. http://www.lung.org/lung-disease/lung-cancer/lung-cancer-screening-guidelines/lung-cancer-screening.pdf. Accessed August 21, 2014.

16. de Koning HJ, Meza R, Plevritis SK, et al. *Benefits and Harms of Computed Tomography Lung Cancer Screening Programs for High-Risk Populations. AHRQ Publication No. 13-05196-EF-2.* Rockville, MD: Agency for Healthcare Research and Quality; 2013.

17. Moyer VA, U.S. Preventive Services Task Force. Screening for lung cancer: US Preventive Services Task Force recommendation statement. *Ann Intern Med* 2014;160:330–338.

18. Wood DE. National Comprehensive Cancer Network (NCCN) Clinical Practice Guidelines for Lung Cancer Screening. *Thorac Surg Clin* 2015;25:185–197.

19. Bach PB, Mirkin JN, Oliver TK, et al. Benefits and harms of CT screening for lung cancer: A systematic review. *JAMA* 2012;307:2418–2429.

20. American Academy of Family Physicians Clinical Preventive Service Recommendation. Lung Cancer. http://www.aafp.org/patient-care/clinical-recommendations/all/lung-cancer.html. Accessed February 19, 2017.

21. Lung Cancer Alliance. National Framework. http://www.lungcanceralliance.org/get-information/am-i-at-risk/national-framework-for-lung-screening-excellence.html. Accessed February 19, 2017.

22. American College of Radiology. ACR Designated Lung Cancer Screening Center. http://www.acr.org/Quality-Safety/Lung-Cancer-Screening-Center. Accessed February 19, 2017.

23. Wood DE. The importance of lung cancer screening with low-dose computed tomography for Medicare beneficiaries. *JAMA Intern Med* 2014;174:2016–2018.

24. Gøtzsche PC, Jørgensen KJ. Screening for breast cancer with mammography. *Cochrane Database Syst Rev* 2013;(6):CD001877.

25. Hewitson P, Glasziou P, Watson E, et al. Cochrane systematic review of colorectal cancer screening using the fecal occult blood test (Hemoccult): an update. *Amer J Gastroenterol* 2008;103:1541–1549.

26. Elmore JG, Barton MB, Moceri VM, et al. Ten-year risk of false positive screening mammograms and clinical breast examinations. *N Engl J Med* 1998;338:1089–1096.

27. American College of Radiology. Lung CT Screening Reporting and Data System (Lung-RADS™). https://www.acr.org/Quality-Safety/Resources/LungRADS. Accessed February 19, 2017.

28. Flores R, Bauer T, Aye R, et al.; I-ELCAP Investigators. Balancing curability and unnecessary surgery in the context of computed tomography screening for lung cancer. *J Thorac Cardiovasc Surg* 2014;147:1619–1626.

29. Data Analysis of The Society of Thoracic Surgeons General Thoracic Database through 12/31/2012, Released May 2013.

30. Brenner DR, Boffetta P, Duell EJ, et al. Previous lung diseases and lung cancer risk: A pooled analysis from the International Lung Cancer Consortium. *Am J Epidemiol.* 2012;176(7):573–585.

31. Lung Cancer Risk Calculators. https://brocku.ca/lung-cancer-risk-calculator. Accessed February 19, 2017.

32. YOUR LUNG CANCER RISK. http://www.shouldiscreen.com/lung-cancer-risk-calculator/. Accessed February 19, 2017.

33. McKee BJ, Hashim JA, French RJ, et al. Experience with a CT screening program for individuals at high risk for developing lung cancer. *J Am Coll Radiol* 2015;12(2): 192–197.

34. Ma J, Ward EM, Smith R, et al. Annual number of lung cancer deaths potentially avertable by screening in the United States. *Cancer* 2013;119:1381–1385.

35. William WC, Gareen IF, Soneji SS, et al.; National Lung Screening Trial Research Team. Cost-effectiveness of CT screening in the National Lung Screening Trial. *N Engl J Med* 2014;371:1793–1802.

36. Pyenson B. Why lung cancer screening makes financial sense: New results from actuarial modeling. *MEDCAC testimony* April 30, 2014. http://www.cms.gov/medicare-coverage-database/details/medcac-meeting-details.aspx?MEDCACId=68. Accessed July 27, 2014.

37. Pyenson BS, Sander MS, Jiang Y, et al. An actuarial analysis shows that offering lung cancer screening as an insurance benefit would save lives at relatively low cost. *Health Affairs* 2012;31:770–779.

38. CMS.gov. Centers for Medicare & Medicaid Services. https://www.cms.gov/medicare-coverage-database/details/nca-decision-memo.aspx?NCAId=274. Accessed February 20, 2017.

39. Roberts H, Walker-Dilks C, Sivjee K, et al. Screening high-risk populations for lung cancer. Toronto, ON, Canada: Cancer Care Ontario; Published April 18, 2013. Program in Evidence-based Care Evidence-based Series No. 15-10.

40. Canadian Task Force on Preventive Health Care; Lewin G, Morissette K, et al. Recommendations on screening for lung cancer. *Canadian Med Assoc J* 2016;188:425–432.

41. Kauczor HU, Bonomo L, Gaga M, et al. ESR/ERS white paper on lung cancer screening. *Eur Respir J* 2015;46:28–39.

91

Investigation and Management of Indeterminate Pulmonary Nodules

Pasquale Ferraro ▪ Andrei-Bogdan Gorgos

INTRODUCTION

With the widespread use of thoracic imaging procedures in a variety of clinical settings such as lung cancer-screening programs, an ever-growing number of indeterminate or solitary pulmonary nodules (SPNs) are being reported. This has led to a significant increase in the number of patients referred to thoracic surgeons to help establish the most appropriate course of action. A seemingly simple clinical problem can in many cases present both a diagnostic and a management challenge due to a wide differential diagnosis and the multitude of diagnostic and therapeutic options available. Ultimately the surgeon must distinguish between benign and malignant processes while offering efficient and cost-effective patient management with minimal discomfort and risk of complications. The objective of any management plan or algorithm is the identification and excision of malignant nodules at the earliest stage possible, in order to optimize the chances for cure and minimize the number of benign nodules unnecessarily removed. Reaching this objective requires a comprehensive and often multidisciplinary approach, which is based on clinical evidence. This chapter reviews the available evidence and provides readers with algorithms that help ensure the most effective management strategy is used with each patient.

CLINICAL HISTORY

The vast majority of SPNs are discovered incidentally in patients who are generally asymptomatic and who undergo testing for some other reason. When first dealing with a reported SPN, obtaining a thorough past and present medical history is an essential component of patient management. The medical history helps identify potential clinical risk factors for lung cancer, while seeking other possible etiologies for an SPN. As seen in Table 91.1, a wide variety of non-neoplastic processes, ranging from infectious to inflammatory, to congenital entities, may present as an SPN. For example, exposure to a potential infectious agent, or signs and symptoms of a systemic condition, can guide the clinician through the investigation and thus improve the diagnostic yield. If an SPN is found on a CT scan of a patient with a recent history of pulmonary infection, repeating the scan 4 to 6 weeks after an appropriate course of antibiotics is certainly warranted, before pursuing with a more invasive needle biopsy and/or surgical excision.

Although uncommon, patients presenting respiratory symptoms such as dyspnea, wheezing, or even mild hemoptysis may in fact

have a small centrally located tumor that can appear as an SPN on imaging. These patients should undergo a complete workup in order to rule out malignancy. Patients with an SPN on CT scan may also present with systemic symptoms such as fatigue, weight loss, and diffuse pain in which case a solitary pulmonary metastasis from an extra thoracic malignancy would be a likely diagnosis. Multiple new pulmonary nodules often represent metastatic disease but may also reflect a reaction to chemotherapeutic agents or secondary infection related to an immune-suppressed state in the setting of malignancy. It is important to note that patients presenting with a lung mass (defined as a focal pulmonary lesion >3 cm) should be managed as an invasive bronchogenic carcinoma until proven otherwise, and proper investigation undertaken.

TABLE 91.1 Differential Diagnosis of Solitary Pulmonary Nodule

Benign Neoplasia	Inflammatory
Hamartoma	Sarcoidosis
Chondroma	Wegner
Fibroma	Rheumatoid arthritis
Lipoma	Amyloidosis
Hemangioma	Microscopic polyangiitis
Leiomyoma	
Neural tumor	**Vascular**
Clear cell tumor	Arteriovenous malformation
Endometriosis	Infarction
	Pulmonary artery aneurysm
Malignant Neoplasia	Pulmonary venous varix
Lung cancer	Hematoma/contusion
Carcinoid tumor	Intrapulmonary lymph node
Metastasis	
Lymphoma	**Congenital**
Teratoma	Lung sequestration
Sarcoma	Bronchial atresia
	Bronchogenic cyst
Infectious	
Fungal	**Miscellaneous**
Parasitic	Rounded atelectasis
Tuberculosis	Infected bulla
Lung abscess	Pulmonary scar
Atypical mycobacteria	Rib fracture
Nocardia	Nipple shadow
Septic emboli	Skin fold
Round pneumonia	Pseudotumor (loculated pleural fluid)

TABLE 91.2 Clinical and Radiologic Features Predicting Malignancy in an SPN

- Older age
- Male gender
- Smoking history (ever vs. never)
- History of prior malignancy
- Hemoptysis
- Nodule diameter
- Presence of spiculation
- Upper lobe location
- Growth rate
- Calcification pattern
- Contrast enhancement on CT scan
- Metabolic activity on PET scan

Whether an SPN is found incidentally or through a lung cancer-screening program, in a patient with or without symptoms, how the individual patient is managed is largely based on the physician's perception. From a practical standpoint, intuitively surgeons try to establish the likelihood or probability that the SPN is cancerous based on knowledge, past experience, and expertise in the field.[1] Combining certain clinical and radiologic features (Table 91.2) facilitates determining the benign or malignant nature of an SPN.[2] The presence, for example, of a significant smoking history, male gender, older age, and a history of prior malignancy are well-established risk factors for lung neoplasia.[3-5] When considering the diameter of an SPN, for example, the risk of malignancy increases with increasing size.

If the probability of malignancy appears high, the patient should undergo a complete workup and an attempt must be made to obtain a tissue sample. Definite tissue diagnosis can be established through different modalities such as bronchoscopy (with or without navigational technique), transthoracic needle biopsy, or surgical excisional biopsy, using a videothoracoscopic technique. A number of factors such as nodule size, location, physician's preference, and the center's expertise influence the choice of procedure as well as the efficacy and diagnostic yield of the technique. Each of these modalities is described in detail in subsequent sections.

INVESTIGATION

IMAGING

The main imaging methods that lead to the discovery of indeterminate lung nodules are the x-ray and CT scan. Multidetector CT (MDCT) is a more sensitive and specific modality for detecting and characterizing such lesions, as compared to conventional x-ray studies. In contrast to the pre-CT scan era, the chest radiograph is nowadays largely used as a general detection method and the vast majority of lesions discovered on such examinations are followed by a complementary CT scan investigation. Radiologic investigations performed for various reasons, such as lung cancer screening in smokers, investigation of certain respiratory conditions (e.g., dyspnea), or cancer (other than lung) workup, regularly detect pulmonary abnormalities of uncertain significance. For example, in a systematic review of 8 lung cancer-screening studies, 8% to 51% of imaging studies demonstrated at least one pulmonary nodule.[6] Once a nodule is found, the principal challenge lies in determining whether it represents cancer or a manifestation of benign disease of no consequence to the patient. Physicians and surgeons must be aware that no single imaging test can confidently predict a newly discovered nodule's benign or

malignant behavior; however, various radiographic features on x-ray and CT scan imaging may provide clues to the nature of the nodule and dictate management.

Indeterminate Nodule CT-Scan Imaging Features—Benign Versus Malignant

By definition, a lung nodule is a rounded opacity, well or poorly defined, with a diameter of up to 3 cm. The size of a nodule is directly related to the likelihood of malignancy in the sense that bigger lesions carry an overall higher cancer risk.

For example, on lung cancer-screening studies, nodules smaller than 5 mm were found to have a malignant rate of 1% or less, whereas nodules larger than 2 cm were cancerous in up to 82% of cases. For nodules between 5 and 10 mm, the observed malignancy risk was between 6% and 28%.[6,7] In patients with a history of known malignancy a higher rate of cancerous nodules is noted (64%); small nodules of less than 5 mm have a chance of malignancy of about 40%.[8]

In terms of consistency, on CT studies, nodules appear as either solid or subsolid (pure ground glass or mixed, i.e., containing ground-glass and solid components) (Fig. 91.1A–C).[9] Many subsolid lesions are due to inflammatory conditions, and they decrease in size or resolve on subsequent imaging studies. Persistent ground-glass lesions, however, carry a high risk of neoplastic or pre-neoplastic behavior, with larger lesions being more likely to represent cancer than their smaller counterparts.[10,11] For example, a study examining the histology of persistent ground-glass nodules that were surgically removed found a 75% incidence of adenocarcinoma and a 6% incidence of atypical adenomatous hyperplasia, with the rest of the cases showing benign organizing pneumonia or nonspecific fibrosis (Fig. 91.1C).[12] Pathologic analysis also demonstrates a higher malignancy rate in subsolid nodules when compared to solid lesions. A 2002 histologic–radiologic correlation study demonstrated a 7% incidence of cancer in solid lesions, compared to 18% and 63% in pure ground-glass and mixed nodules, respectively.[13] Also worthy of note is the fact that a higher solid component of mixed lesions is more strongly correlated with invasive neoplasia.[14]

Calcification patterns are also sought in order to determine the benign or malignant nature of a nodule. Patterns suggestive of a nonmalignant nodule are diffuse, central, laminated, or "popcorn." Calcifications that are punctate, eccentric, or amorphous remain indeterminate, as both malignant and benign lesions may display such features.[15] Fat-containing nodules are virtually always benign and mostly represent pulmonary hamartomas.[16] These lesions may contain calcifications in approximately 20% of cases. A "popcorn" calcification pattern is rare, but when present, it is considered pathognomonic of this entity, and no further workup is needed (Fig. 91.2). Other fat-containing lesions such as lipomas or metastases from liposarcomas and renal cell carcinomas are an extremely rare occurrence.

Generally, benign nodules are well defined, smooth, and round, whereas neoplastic nodules are irregular, lobulated, or spiculated. However, shape alone is not reliable to determine the nature of a nodule, and significant overlap exists.[17] Additional features that increase the likelihood of benignity of small, solid nodules are a polygonal or oval shape, a perifissural location, and a pleural, septal, or vessel attachment.[18-20] It has been postulated that many of the small solid nodules displaying these features represent in fact small intrapulmonary lymph nodes (Fig. 91.3).

Other lung nodule characteristics described on CT scans include cavitation, pseudocavitation (i.e., a "bubbly appearance"), air bronchograms (Fig. 91.4), the "halo" sign (i.e., a ground-glass appearance

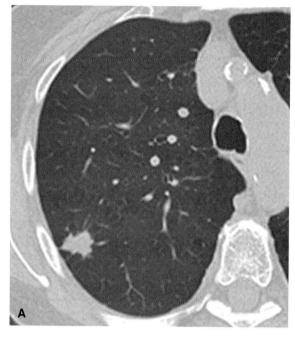
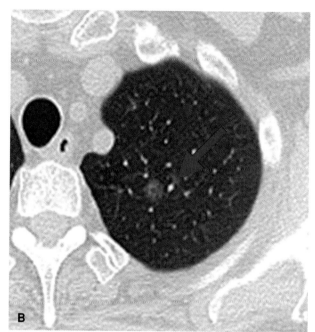
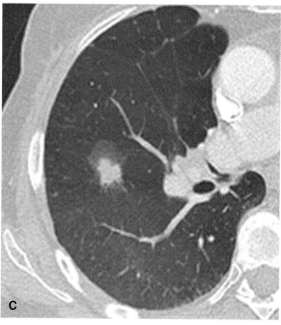

FIGURE 91.1 **A:** Solid peripheral nodule. **B:** Ground-glass opacity. **C:** Mixed nodule.

at the periphery), and the reverse halo sign (i.e., a central ground-glass appearance with a solid periphery). They are common to both benign and malignant processes, and other elements must be used to help determine a nodule's nature. For example, thin-walled cavitary lesions are more frequently associated with a benign entity than their thick-walled counterparts.[21] Lesions that demonstrate air bronchograms and pseudocavitation are more likely malignant,[22] especially in the absence of clinical signs of inflammation. The "halo" sign and "reverse halo" sign have been described with both malignant and benign nodules,[23,24] and interpretation outside of the clinical context can be confusing.

CT scan contrast enhancement has been used as a tool for predicting neoplasia with solid nodules. Generally, malignant nodules will enhance more than 20 HU whereas enhancement of less than 15 HU is a strong predictor of benignity. However, in addition to being relatively time consuming, this technique is subject to certain limitations, since accurate nodule analysis depends on the shape, size, and consistency of the lesion. It is perhaps for these reasons that this method has failed to gain widespread popularity in radiologic practices.[25]

Indeterminate Nodule Growth—Benign Versus Malignant

Serial CT scan examinations allow assessment of nodule growth over time. Based on the mathematical formula for calculating the volume of a sphere, a 25% diameter increase corresponds to an approximate doubling of the total nodule size. In general, volume

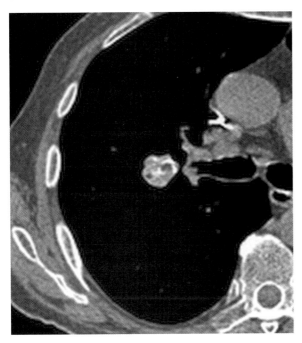

FIGURE 91.2 Benign hamartoma containing fat (intratumoral hypodense areas of density similar to subcutaneous fat) and calcium (hyperdense areas).

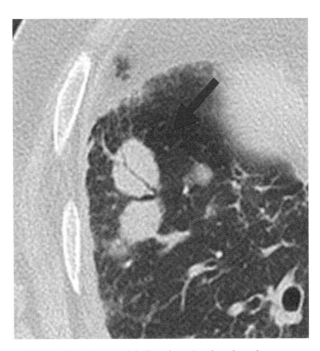

FIGURE 91.4 Neoplastic nodule (lymphoma) with air bronchogram.

doubling in less than 20 days is considered indicative of an inflammatory or infectious process, whereas stability over more than 400 days implies a benign lesion, with granulomas and hamartomas being classic examples. Volume doubling between 20 and 400 days is suspicious for malignancy (Fig. 91.5). In clinical practice, a lung nodule that is stable over a period of 2 years is considered benign[26]; however, caution must be exercised in certain situations. Slow growing tumors, such as low-grade adenocarcinomas, may take a longer

time to double in volume. Therefore, suspicious lesions that demonstrate a subsolid component on CT studies require a more careful evaluation, and when necessary, longer follow-up.[27] Neoplastic lung lesions such as metastases under treatment may display altered patterns of growth, though stability over a period of 2 years is rather unusual. Another pitfall is transient nodule size regression, which has been observed in a small percentage of malignant nodules. This phenomenon occurs presumably due to necrosis and/or fibrosis that can temporarily cause the tumor mass to shrink. In general, decreasing size is associated with a benign nature; however, longer follow-up of truly neoplastic lesions will eventually demonstrate a size progression on subsequent imaging.[28]

Indeterminate Nodule PET—Benign Versus Malignant

Imaging with fluorine-18 (^{18}F)–labeled fluorodeoxyglucose (FDG) positron emission tomography (PET) is the method of choice for evaluating the metabolism of indeterminate pulmonary nodules. Malignant nodules generally metabolize glucose more than their benign counterparts, which translates into a more avid FDG uptake. The standardized uptake value (SUV) is the general quantification method, with a threshold value of 2.5 traditionally accepted to differentiate between neoplasia and a benign process. A visual assessment was proven to be just as accurate.[29] For more accurate imaging, PET technology has been integrated with conventional CT scan image acquisition. Superimposed images allow more precise nodule measurement, characterization, and delineation from neighboring anatomical structures (Fig. 91.6). PET imaging is, however, subject to certain drawbacks. Nodule size for instance is a significant limitation, and accurate characterization of lesions less than 10 mm in size becomes less reliable.[30] Slow growing lesions are another instance where FDG imaging may fail, as a low metabolic activity correlates with little, undetectable glucose uptake. Clinicians must be particularly careful in the case of low-grade tumors, such as adenocarcinomas, carcinoid tumors, low-grade

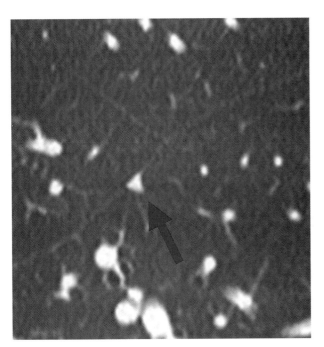

FIGURE 91.3 Benign triangle-shaped, perifissural nodule.

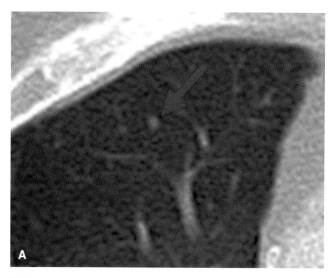
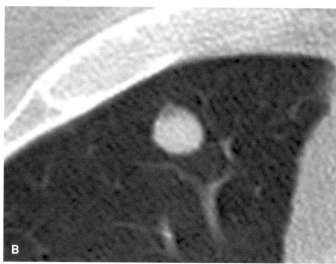

FIGURE 91.5 **A:** Small peripheral 2-mm nodule. **B:** Dramatic size increase on follow-up CT performed 6 months later (melanoma metastasis).

lymphomas, and metastases from renal cancer and certain neoplasias of the mucinous type (e.g., gastrointestinal, breast).[31] The subset of slow growing adenocarcinoma presenting as subsolid nodules often appears hypometabolic and PET imaging for these lesions has a limited utility.[30] Due to their high glucose metabolism, inflammatory lesions are difficult to differentiate from malignant processes, and PET scanning is generally not recommended when acute inflammation is clinically suspected.[31]

INVASIVE INVESTIGATION

Bronchoscopy (ENB, EBUS)

Traditionally, standard bronchoscopy has a limited role in obtaining tissue diagnosis for a peripheral SPN, with a reported yield of 34%

(range 5% to 76%) for lesions less than 20 mm.[32,33] However, the diagnostic yield through endobronchial biopsy, brushings, or washings for central lesions greater than 20 mm or for lesions with a visible bronchogram extending into the nodule may reach 80%, when these features are found.[32,34]

In recent years, the utility of bronchoscopic evaluation of peripheral lesions has been expanded with the development of new techniques such as electromagnetic navigational bronchoscopy (ENB) and radial endobronchial ultrasound (EBUS)–guided biopsies. During navigational bronchoscopy, the pathway to a peripheral lesion is mapped out on the patient's chest CT scan and entered into a computer program. The patient is then placed on an electromagnetic sensing pad and bronchoscopy is performed using a sensing catheter placed through the working channel of a therapeutic bronchoscope. The sensing and steerable catheter is then used to navigate to the lesion and perform

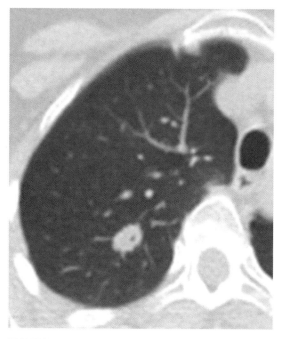
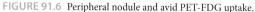
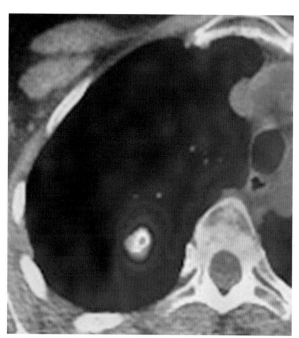

FIGURE 91.6 Peripheral nodule and avid PET-FDG uptake.

a biopsy of the latter. The diagnostic yield for ENB, however, varies greatly ranging from 59% to 85% as reported by a number of authors for SPN measuring on average 22 to 28 mm.[35-38]

By using radial EBUS-guided transbronchial biopsy techniques, diagnostic yields range from 34% to 84%.[39-43] Additionally, the EBUS technique allows visualization of the internal structure of the SPN (homogenous vs. heterogeneous), which may provide insight into the histology of the lesion.[44]

It is important to note that in addition to potentially adding significant cost to the patient workup, both ENB and radial EBUS require substantial resources and extensive training and experience. These techniques are not easily reproducible in less experienced centers and thus cannot be recommended for routine use in patients presenting with an SPN.

Image-Guided Transthoracic Needle Aspiration (TTNA)

A percutaneous image-guided approach provides access to indeterminate lung nodules when histologic diagnosis is deemed necessary. Tissue specimens help establish whether a lesion is benign or malignant and allow cultures to be performed on harvested material when an infectious process is in the differential diagnosis.

The main risks associated with a TTNA procedure are pneumothorax and bleeding (hemoptysis and hemothorax), with infection, gas embolism, and tumor seeding being described as rare occurrences (Fig. 91.7).[45] The main precautions thus relate to the patient's pulmonary reserve and coagulation status. Relatively little has been published on the safety of percutaneous lung biopsies in patients with reduced pulmonary function. Generally, an FEV_1 superior to 1,0 l is considered safe for most pulmonary biopsies; however, particular care must be taken in cases of severe parenchymal disease (e.g., pulmonary fibrosis) that may have less impact on this parameter and yet cause pulmonary reserve impairment (e.g., reduced TLC or DLCO).[46] The risk of pneumothorax varies widely in the medical literature, with most centers reporting an incidence of 20% to 50%,

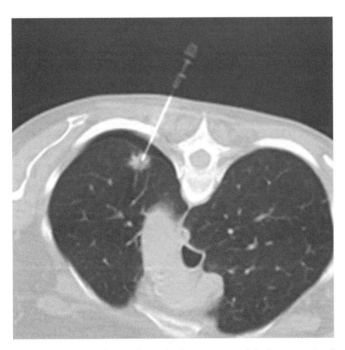

FIGURE 91.7 Lung biopsy (TTNA) of suspicious nodule (note associated iatrogenic pneumothorax).

with a rate of drained pneumothorax of approximately 10%. The great majority of pneumothoraces are treated conservatively or by percutaneous drainage, and severe consequences are very rare.[47] A relatively common complication of lung biopsies is bleeding, with minor hemoptysis or small hemorrhagic pleural effusion accounting for most cases. Massive hemoptysis and hemothorax are reported, and the risk is greatly diminished by selecting patients with appropriate coagulation status.[45]

In general, TTNA procedures are carried out under fluoroscopic x-ray or CT scan guidance, though ultrasound and MRI have both been described in the literature. Fluoroscopic (i.e., real time) imaging is generally useful, since it helps reduce the total intervention time. A coaxial biopsy needle approach is preferred, as it allows multiple passes and specimen collections with a single pleural puncture. The specimen collection is obtained for cytologic or pathologic analysis, depending on center preference and laboratory technical expertise. The size of the needle varies, but generally 17 to 20 G coaxial systems are considered appropriate for most lung lesions.

The yield of percutaneous lung biopsy depends on multiple factors such as nodule and needle size, consistency (e.g., central necrosis), and patient compliance with respiratory motion and lack of movement.

SCREENING

Lung cancer is a pathology that, at least in theory, would be ideally suited for screening: it is the most common, lethal neoplasm. It is detectable in the preclinical phase. Individuals at risk are generally easily identifiable (smokers), and a higher survival is expected for early disease stages. Imaging with chest x-rays and low-dose CT scans as well as noninvasive tests such as sputum analysis have been used to attempt early cancer detection. However, much controversy surrounded this topic over the past decades as researchers struggled to demonstrate the benefits of screening. Pro-advocates argued, based on the assumption that lung cancer survival improvement (as the disease is discovered at an earlier pathologic stage) justifies implementing a screening program. The main counter-rhetoric claimed that the parameter used (i.e., survival) was less than ideal, since it is subject to various biases, and that lung cancer mortality decrease should be rather sought, in order to justify cancer screening.

The first randomized prospective trial that was able to demonstrate a 20% decrease in lung cancer-specific mortality was published in 2011 by the National Lung Cancer Screening Trial (NLCST).[48] Screening of patients with low-dose CT scan of the chest was thus considered appropriate, and numerous scientific bodies around the world have since produced guidelines and recommendations as the movement gains ever more momentum. Some significant questions remain unanswered, however, especially pertaining to optimal screening regimens and cost effectiveness. A particular concern is because of a high number of positive tests (27% for the first two rounds of screening)[49] leading to additional investigative procedures and related (albeit generally minor) complications. An attempt to address this concern was made by the American College of Radiology by developing a standardized reporting system and recommendations (Lung Imaging Reporting and Data System—LungRADS), based on clinical context and lung nodule appearance at imaging, and whose validation is still in progress.[50]

ROLE OF VIDEO-ASSISTED THORACOSCOPIC SURGERY (VATS)

The field of VATS has made significant technical progress over the last 15 years allowing thoracic surgeons to acquire substantial expertise with pulmonary surgery. In contrast to open thoracotomy procedures, the minimally invasive nature of VATS with its numerous advantages in terms of postoperative complications, pain, recovery time, and esthetics has allowed it to become the procedure of choice when dealing with certain thoracic procedures. In the setting of an SPN, VATS not only gives the surgeon a unique opportunity to obtain a histologic diagnosis but also provides definitive treatment for a patient with early stage lung cancer. VATS thus plays an essential role in the management of patients with peripheral SPNs that have a high probability of malignant disease, as the procedure is both efficient and cost effective. VATS also plays an important role in patients with an SPN for which TTNA has failed, in patients with centrally located lesions and a positive PET scan, as well as in patients who request surgery because they are unable to deal with the anxiety caused by an observational approach to an SPN of unknown etiology.

From a technical standpoint, a VATS procedure for an undiagnosed SPN is a straightforward surgery, unless the patient has previously undergone a thoracic operation. The surgery mainly consists of performing an excisional biopsy/wedge resection with negative margins (in order to prevent malignant contamination of the pleural space, should the SPN prove to be cancerous). The results of intra-operative frozen section analysis dictate the remainder of the procedure. Obtaining the proper cultures is obviously important if an infectious process is being considered.

VATS for SPN may be challenging if the nodule is not easily accessible or located at a certain distance from the pleural surface. Suzuki and colleagues, for example, recommended preoperative localization for nodules less than 10 mm in size when situated more than 5 mm from the visceral pleura.[51] Techniques for pre- or intra-operative localization are described below.

PREOPERATIVE LOCALIZATION TECHNIQUES

When nodules are too small or lack sufficient consistency (e.g., ground-glass opacities [GGOs]) to be identified by palpation at thoracotomy, or when the VATS technique is used, the surgeon may opt for preoperative lesion marking. Various methods have been described in the literature, including wire placement,[52,53] lipiodol injection,[54] platinum- and fiber-coated microcoils,[55,56] technetium-99m macroaggregated albumin,[57] and methylene blue.[58] All these techniques involve percutaneous placement of localizing material (e.g., hook wire) or injection of marking substance (e.g., methylene blue) under CT guidance, and reported results are good. Shortcomings of these procedures are generally related to migration or spillage of the material used between the radiologic intervention and surgery and ideally the two are performed in as rapid succession as possible. In addition, complications of the percutaneous nodule marking include adverse effects similar to the ones reported for image-guided lung biopsies: pneumothorax, bleeding, and less frequently, air embolism.

INTRA-OPERATIVE LOCALIZATION TECHNIQUES

A number of authors have reported the use of intra-operative ultrasound imaging at the time of VATS to help locate a small and/or deeply situated SPN. In a series of 18 patients with nodules less than 20 mm, Santambrogio and colleagues successfully identified 100% of SPN intra-operatively.[59] At the authors' institution, a 10-mm VATS ultrasound (5 to 10 MHz) linear probe with a flexible angulating tip is used to detect hyperechoic images in the lung parenchyma intra-operatively. We reported a series of 45 patients with nodules with a mean diameter of 12 mm and situated at a distance from the visceral pleura ranging from 1 to 24 mm. The use of intra-operative VATS ultrasound allowed the surgeon to successfully identify 43 of 46 nodules (93%) without converting to an open thoracotomy[60] (Video 91.1).

ALGORITHMS FOR MANAGEMENT

The task of developing an all-encompassing algorithm dictating the best possible approach for an indeterminate SPN in all patients is not realistic, due to the considerable number of factors involved. Nonetheless, two approaches are generally considered when faced with an indeterminate SPN depending on a lesion's likelihood of malignancy and the patient's ability to deal with the uncertainty of a cancer diagnosis. It should be kept in mind that nodules detected on plain chest x-rays will eventually require CT scan imaging in the great majority of patients. In selected cases where older films are available and demonstrate stability in size and appearance of the nodule over an extended period of time, thus effectively establishing a benign diagnosis, no further action is required. In this section, we present two algorithms that apply to most indeterminate SPNs (Figs. 91.8 and 91.9) and that can guide the surgeon's approach to an indeterminate SPN. The two algorithms dictate clinical management based on the solid versus subsolid nature of the nodule, the size of the nodule, and the probability of cancer.[1,5]

When dealing with solid indeterminate SPNs (Fig. 91.8), the majority of physicians will apply Fleischner Society Guidelines in the management of these patients.[27] These guidelines have gained widespread acceptance over the years and provide rationale for the use of serial CT scan imaging in patient follow-up. Although almost universally applied, it is important to note that these guidelines were developed for SPNs detected incidentally. When the SPN is detected in symptomatic patients or in patients at high risk for cancer, physicians should have a lower threshold for more invasive testing, TTNA, or VATS wedge excision and tissue diagnosis.

In the case of SPNs measuring 8 to 30 mm in diameter, estimating the probability of cancer is an essential objective of patient management (Fig. 91.8). Clinical and radiologic features predicting malignancy in an SPN are summarized in Table 91.2. Hence, in patients at intermediate or high risk for lung cancer, surgical excision by VATS should ultimately be the clinical pathway in most cases. Important considerations include determining the operative risk in older or frail patients, as well as assessing the patient's desire to proceed with an invasive surgical procedure. In patients with a low probability for cancer, serial imaging with or without PET scanning at regular intervals may be deemed appropriate. Obtaining a tissue diagnosis by TTNA or VATS wedge excision is recommended for an SPN in which growth is documented on CT scan, for an SPN with a positive PET scan, as well as for patients who are unable to deal with the uncertainty of waiting and undergoing serial imaging.

The management of patients with a subsolid SPN or GGO is summarized in the algorithm presented in Figure 91.9. The most appropriate course of action must consider a number of factors including

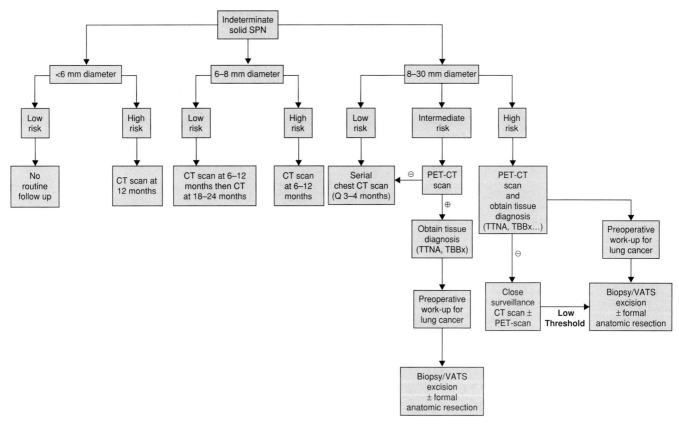

FIGURE 91.8 Management of indeterminate solid solitary pulmonary nodule. (Adapted from Patel VK, Naik SK, Naidich DP, et al. A practical algorithmic approach to the diagnosis and management of solitary pulmonary nodules: part 2: pretest probability and algorithm. *Chest.* 2013;143(3):840–846. Copyright © 2013 The American College of Chest Physicians. With permission.)

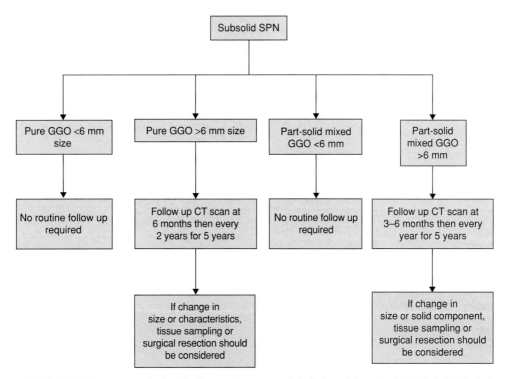

FIGURE 91.9 Management of subsolid solitary pulmonary nodule. (Adapted from Patel VK, Naik SK, Naidich DP, et al. A practical algorithmic approach to the diagnosis and management of solitary pulmonary nodules: part 2: pretest probability and algorithm. *Chest.* 2013;143(3):840–846. Copyright © 2013 The American College of Chest Physicians. With permission.)

the size of the nodule, the characteristics of the nodule, the growth pattern, and the presence of a solid component to the GGO (mixed GGO). Again, in patients with a high probability of cancer, physicians should maintain a low threshold to pursuing the investigation with more invasive testing and TTNA or VATS wedge excision in selected patients.

REFERENCES

1. Gould MK, Donington J, Lynch WR, et al. Evaluation of individuals with pulmonary nodules: when is it lung cancer? Diagnosis and management of lung cancer, 3rd ed: American College of Chest Physicians evidence-based clinical practice guidelines. *Chest* 2013;143(5 Suppl):e93S–e120S. doi:10.1378/chest.12-2351.
2. Patel VK, Naik SK, Naidich DP, et al. A practical algorithmic approach to the diagnosis and management of solitary pulmonary nodules: part 1: radiologic characteristics and imaging modalities. *Chest* 2013;143(3):825–839. doi:10.1378/chest.12-0960.
3. Swensen SJ, Silverstein MD, Ilstrup DM, et al. The probability of malignancy in solitary pulmonary nodules. Application to small radiologically indeterminate nodules. *Arch Intern Med* 1997;157(8):849–855.
4. Gould MK, Ananth L, Barnett PG; Veterans Affairs SNAP Cooperative Study Group. A clinical model to estimate the pretest probability of lung cancer in patients with solitary pulmonary nodules. *Chest* 2007;131(2):383–388.
5. Patel VK, Naik SK, Naidich DP, et al. A practical algorithmic approach to the diagnosis and management of solitary pulmonary nodules: part 2: pretest probability and algorithm. *Chest* 2013;143(3):840–846. doi:10.1378/chest.12-1487.
6. Wahidi MM, Govert JA, Goudar RK, et al. Evidence for the treatment of patients with pulmonary nodules: when is it lung cancer?: ACCP evidence-based clinical practice guidelines (2nd edition). *Chest* 2007;132(3 Suppl):94S–107S.
7. Midthun DE, Swensen SJ, Jett JR, et al. O-127 evaluation of nodules detected by screening for lung cancer with low dose spiral computed tomography. *Lung Cancer* 2003;41(2 Suppl):S40. doi:10.1016/SO169-5002(03)91785-5.
8. Ginsberg MS, Griff SK, Go BD, et al. Pulmonary nodules resected at video-assisted thoracoscopic surgery: etiology in 426 patients. *Radiology* 1999;213(1):277–282.
9. Naidich DP, Bankier AA, MacMahon H, et al. Recommendations for the management of subsolid pulmonary nodules detected at CT: a statement from the Fleischner Society. *Radiology* 2013;266(1):304–317. doi:10.1148/radiol.12120628.
10. Oh JY, Kwon SY, Yoon HI, et al. Clinical significance of a solitary ground-glass opacity (GGO) lesion of the lung detected by chest CT. *Lung Cancer* 2007;55(1):67–73.
11. Lee HY, Lee KS. Ground-glass opacity nodules: histopathology, imaging evaluation, and clinical implications. *J Thorac Imaging* 2011;26(2):106–118.
12. Kim HY, Shim YM, Lee KS, et al. Persistent pulmonary nodular ground-glass opacity at thin-section CT: histopathologic comparisons. *Radiology* 2007;245(1):267–275. Erratum in: *Radiology* 2008;247(1):297.
13. Henschke CI, Yankelevitz DF, Mirtcheva R, et al. CT screening for lung cancer: frequency and significance of part-solid and nonsolid nodules. *AJR Am J Roentgenol* 2002;178(5):1053–1057.
14. Lee HY, Choi YL, Lee KS, et al. Pure ground-glass opacity neoplastic lung nodules: histopathology, imaging, and management. *AJR Am J Roentgenol* 2014;202(3):W224–W233. doi:10.2214/AJR.13.11819.
15. Khan AN, Al-Jahdali HH, Allen CM, et al. The calcified lung nodule: what does it mean? *Ann Thorac Med* 2010;5(2):67–79. doi:10.4103/1817-1737.62469.
16. Bhatia K, Ellis S. Unusual lung tumours: an illustrated review of CT features suggestive of this diagnosis. *Cancer Imaging* 2006;6:72–82.
17. Gurney JW, Lyddon DM, McKay JA. Determining the likelihood of malignancy in solitary pulmonary nodules with Bayesian analysis. Part II. Application. *Radiology* 1993;186(2):415–422.
18. Nair A, Baldwin DR, Field JK, et al. Measurement methods and algorithms for the management of solid nodules. *J Thorac Imaging* 2012;27(4):230–239. doi:10.1097/RTI.0b013e31824f83e1.
19. Xu DM, van der Zaag-Loonen HJ, Oudkerk M, et al. Smooth or attached solid indeterminate nodules detected at baseline CT screening in the NELSON study: cancer risk during 1 year of follow-up. *Radiology* 2009;250(1):264–272. doi:10.1148/radiol.2493070847.
20. Ahn MI, Gleeson TG, Chan IH, et al. Perifissural nodules seen at CT screening for lung cancer. *Radiology* 2010;254(3):949–956. doi:10.1148/radiol.09090031.
21. Woodring JH, Fried AM, Chuang VP. Solitary cavities of the lung: diagnostic implications of cavity wall thickness. *AJR Am J Roentgenol* 1980;135(6):1269–1271.
22. Zwirewich CV, Vedal S, Miller RR, et al. Solitary pulmonary nodule: high-resolution CT and radiologic-pathologic correlation. *Radiology* 1991;179(2):469–476.
23. Lee YR, Choi YW, Lee KJ, et al. CT halo sign: the spectrum of pulmonary diseases. *Br J Radiol* 2005;78(933):862–865.
24. Godoy MC, Viswanathan C, Marchiori E, et al. The reversed halo sign: update and differential diagnosis. *Br J Radiol* 2012;85(1017):1226–1235.
25. Swensen SJ. Functional CT: lung nodule evaluation. *Radiographics* 2000;20(4):1178–1181.
26. Yankelevitz DF, Henschke CI. Does 2-year stability imply that pulmonary nodules are benign? *AJR Am J Roentgenol* 1997;168(2):325–328.
27. MacMahon H, Naidich DP, Goo GM, et al. Guidelines of Management of Incidental Pulmonary Nodules Detected on CT Images: From the Fleischner Society 2017. *Radiology* 2017:284(1).
28. Jennings SG, Winer-Muram HT, Tann M, et al. Distribution of stage I lung cancer growth rates determined with serial volumetric CT measurements. *Radiology* 2006;241(2):554–563.
29. Lowe VJ, Hoffman JM, DeLong DM, et al. Semiquantitative and visual analysis of FDG-PET images in pulmonary abnormalities. *J Nucl Med* 1994;35(11):1771–1776.
30. Nomori H, Watanabe K, Ohtsuka T, et al. Evaluation of F-18 fluorodeoxyglucose (FDG) PET scanning for pulmonary nodules less than 3 cm in diameter, with special reference to the CT images. *Lung Cancer* 2004;45(1):19–27.
31. Chang JM, Lee HJ, Goo JM, et al. False positive and false negative FDG-PET scans in various thoracic diseases. *Korean J Radiol* 2006;7(1):57–69.
32. Rivera MP, Mehta AC; American College of Chest Physicians. Initial diagnosis of lung cancer: ACCP evidence-based clinical practice guidelines (2nd edition). *Chest* 2007;132(3 Suppl):131S–148S.
33. van't Westeinde SC, Horeweg N, Vernhout RM, et al. The role of conventional bronchoscopy in the workup of suspicious CT scan screen-detected pulmonary nodules. *Chest* 2012;142(3):377–384.
34. Lee R, Ost D. Advanced bronchoscopic techniques for diagnosis of peripheral pulmonary lesions. In: John FB, Jr., Praveen M, Atal CM, eds. *Interventional Pulmonary Medicine.* Vol 230. 2nd ed. New York: CRC Press; 2010:186–199.
35. Gildea TR, Mazzone PJ, Karnak D, et al. Electromagnetic navigation diagnostic bronchoscopy: a prospective study. *Am J Respir Crit Care Med* 2006;174(9):982–989.
36. Eberhardt R, Anantham D, Ernst A, et al. Multimodality bronchoscopic diagnosis of peripheral lung lesions: a randomized controlled trial. *Am J Respir Crit Care Med* 2007;176(1):36–41.
37. Pearlstein DP, Quinn CC, Burtis CC, et al. Electromagnetic navigation bronchoscopy performed by thoracic surgeons: one center's early success. *Ann Thorac Surg* 2012;93(3):944–949; discussion 949–50.
38. Bertoletti L, Robert A, Cottier M, et al. Accuracy and feasibility of electromagnetic navigated bronchoscopy under nitrous oxide sedation for pulmonary peripheral opacities: an outpatient study. *Respiration* 2009;78(3):293–300. doi:10.1159/000226128.
39. Chao TY, Chien MT, Lie CH, et al. Endobronchial ultrasonography-guided transbronchial needle aspiration increases the diagnostic yield of peripheral pulmonary lesions: a randomized trial. *Chest* 2009;136(1):229–236. doi:10.1378/chest.08-0577.
40. Eberhardt R, Ernst A, Herth FJ. Ultrasound-guided transbronchial biopsy of solitary pulmonary nodules less than 20 mm. *Eur Respir J* 2009;34(6):1284–1287. doi:10.1183/09031936.00166708.
41. Steinfort DP, Khor YH, Manser RL, et al. Radial probe endobronchial ultrasound for the diagnosis of peripheral lung cancer: systematic review and meta-analysis. *Eur Respir J* 2011;37(4):902–910. doi:10.1183/09031936.00075310.
42. Hsia DW, Jensen KW, Curran-Everett D, et al. Diagnosis of lung nodules with peripheral/radial endobronchial ultrasound-guided transbronchial biopsy. *J Bronchol Interv Pulmonol* 2012;19(1):5–11. doi:10.1097/LBR.0b013e31823fcf11.
43. Narula T, Machuzak MS, Mehta AC. Newer modalities in the work-up of peripheral pulmonary nodules. *Clin Chest Med.* 2013;34(3):395–415. doi:10.1016/j.ccm.2013.06.001.
44. Kurimoto N, Murayama M, Yoshioka S, et al. Analysis of the internal structure of peripheral pulmonary lesions using endobronchial ultrasonography. *Chest* 2002;122(6):1887–1894.
45. Wu CC, Maher MM, Shepard JA. Complications of CT-guided percutaneous needle biopsy of the chest: prevention and management. *AJR Am J Roentgenol* 2011;196(6):W678–W682. doi:10.2214/AJR.10.4659.
46. Kazerooni EA, Hartker FW 3rd, Whyte RI, et al. Transthoracic needle aspiration in patients with severe emphysema. A study of lung transplant candidates. *Chest* 1996;109(3):616–619.
47. Hiraki T, Mimura H, Gobara H, et al. Incidence of and risk factors for pneumothorax and chest tube placement after CT fluoroscopy-guided percutaneous lung biopsy: retrospective analysis of the procedures conducted over a 9-year period. *AJR Am J Roentgenol* 2010;194(3):809–814. doi:10.2214/AJR.09.3224.
48. National Lung Screening Trial Research Team, Aberle DR, Adams AM, et al. Reduced lung-cancer mortality with low-dose computed tomographic screening. *N Engl J Med* 2011;365(5):395–409. doi:10.1056/NEJMoa1102873.
49. Pinsky PF, Gierada DS, Nath PH, et al. National lung screening trial: variability in nodule detection rates in chest CT studies. *Radiology* 2013;268(3):865–873. doi:10.1148/radiol.13121530.
50. Lung CT Screening Reporting and Data System (Lung-RADS). American College of Radiology: acr.org.
51. Suzuki K, Nagai K, Yoshida J, et al. Video-assisted thoracic surgery for small indeterminate pulmonary nodules: indications for preoperative marking. *Chest* 1999;115(2):563–568.
52. Dendo S, Kanazawa S, Ando A, et al. Preoperative localization of small pulmonary lesions with a short hook wire and suture system: experience with 168 procedures. *Radiology* 2002;225(2):511–518.
53. Eichfeld U, Dietrich A, Ott R, et al. Video-assisted thoracoscopic surgery for pulmonary nodules after computed tomography-guided marking with a spiral wire. *Ann Thorac Surg* 2005;79(1):313–316; discussion 316–317.
54. Watanabe K, Nomori H, Ohtsuka T, et al. Usefulness and complications of computed tomography-guided lipiodol marking for fluoroscopy-assisted thoracoscopic resection of small pulmonary nodules: experience with 174 nodules. *J Thorac Cardiovasc Surg* 2006;132(2):320–324.

55. Powell TI, Jangra D, Clifton JC, et al. Peripheral lung nodules: fluoroscopically guided video-assisted thoracoscopic resection after computed tomography-guided localization using platinum microcoils. *Ann Surg* 2004;240(3):481–488; discussion 488–489.

56. Mayo JR, Clifton JC, Powell TI, et al. Lung nodules: CT-guided placement of microcoils to direct video-assisted thoracoscopic surgical resection. *Radiology* 2009;250(2):576–585. doi:10.1148/radiol.2502080442. PubMed PMID: 19188326.

57. Gonfiotti A, Davini F, Vaggelli L, et al. Thoracoscopic localization techniques for patients with solitary pulmonary nodule: hookwire versus radio-guided surgery. *Eur J Cardiothorac Surg* 2007;32(6):843–847.

58. Lenglinger FX, Schwarz CD, Artmann W. Localization of pulmonary nodules before thoracoscopic surgery: value of percutaneous staining with methylene blue. *AJR Am J Roentgenol* 1994;163(2):297–300.

59. Santambrogio R, Montorsi M, Bianchi P, et al. Intraoperative ultrasound during thoracoscopic procedures for solitary pulmonary nodules. *Ann Thorac Surg* 1999; 68(1):218–222.

60. Khereba M, Ferraro P, Duranceau A, et al. Thoracoscopic localization of intraparenchymal pulmonary nodules using direct intracavitary thoracoscopic ultrasonography prevents conversion of VATS procedures to thoracotomy in selected patients. *J Thorac Cardiovasc Surg* 2012;144(5):1160–1165. doi:10.1016/j.jtcvs.2012.08.034. Epub 2012 Sep 12.

92

Pathology of Carcinoma of the Lung

Akihiko Yoshizawa ▪ Hironori Haga ▪ Hiroshi Date

OVERVIEW OF PATHOLOGICAL CLASSIFICATION OF LUNG CARCINOMA

The pathological features of lung carcinoma are extremely heterogeneous at all levels—grossly, microscopically, ultramicroscopically, and molecularly. They depend on the location of the developing tumor, as well as its cell type, grading, and molecular natures. Since 18th century, there have been many attempts to create histologic classifications of lung carcinomas. The first WHO classification for lung carcinoma was published in 1967.[1] This outline remains widely accepted, even today. It includes squamous cell carcinoma (SQCC), adenocarcinoma, small cell lung carcinoma (SCLC), and large cell carcinoma (LCC). Since the 1967 classification, these tumor types have commonly been separated into SCLCs and non–small cell lung carcinomas (NSCLCs or NSCCs), which have different clinical behaviors and treatments. In the current century, many new drugs have been developed for NSCLC. As first demonstrated in 2004,[2,3] lung adenocarcinomas with epidermal growth factor receptor (*EGFR*) gene mutations show significant response to targeted therapy with an EGFR tyrosine-kinase inhibitor (TKI). In addition, patients harboring fusion of the *ALK* gene were reported in 2007,[4,5] and its inhibitor was shown to be dramatically effective for patients with advanced-stage lung adenocarcinoma.[6,7] These discoveries greatly contributed to shifts in treatment for lung adenocarcinoma. On the other hand, treatment with pemetrexed is reported to be more effective for patients with adenocarcinoma or LCC than for patients with SQCC.[8] Moreover, patients with SQCC have a higher risk of developing hemorrhage as a complication if they are treated with bevacizumab, a monoclonal antibody against vascular endothelial growth factor (VEGF).[9] Furthermore, clinical trials are currently being performed to evaluate many other promising drugs that are related to specific molecular targets. Thus, it became necessary to classify NSCLC into categories that would be more appropriate for individual treatments.

In addition, although final determination of the histological subtype of lung carcinoma requires an examination of the resected specimen, this cannot be achieved in practice; because the majority of lung carcinomas are diagnosed at advanced stages, approximately 70% are inoperable. For patients with inoperable lung cancer, appropriate therapeutic options can only be determined from histological diagnoses of small biopsy or cytological specimens. In the context of treatment strategies for patients with lung carcinoma, it also became necessary to devise a new histological classification.

PARADIGM SHIFT IN THE CLASSIFICATION OF LUNG CARCINOMA

The International Association for the Study of Lung Cancer, the American Thoracic Society, and the European Respiratory Society (IASLC/ATS/ERS) have proposed using strategic tissue management to allow histological diagnosis for molecular targeted therapies.[10] As compared with previous classification systems, this approach demonstrates two major shifts. First, a new subclassification of adenocarcinoma was proposed for resected adenocarcinomas. The new subclassification is a significant advance over the earlier WHO classifications, which had some cumbersome features. The details of the new recommendations for resected tumors of lung adenocarcinoma are discussed in the adenocarcinoma section of this chapter. Second, standardized criteria and terminology were proposed for the pathologic diagnosis of lung cancer in small biopsy and cytology specimens. This was the first such attempt in the history of lung cancer classification, and it is therefore presented in detail as follows.

The recommendations describe multiple steps for determining histological diagnosis in small biopsy and cytological specimens under a light microscope (Fig. 92.1).

1. If the SCLC feature is present, SCLC is diagnosed.
2. If clear glandular differentiation or mucin-producing cells are present, adenocarcinoma is diagnosed. Lung adenocarcinomas display specific architectural features (lepidic, acinar, papillary, or micropapillary). If these patterns are identified, it is recommended that they be added to the histological report because they can be associated with radiologic appearance and can be predictors of patient outcomes. Following the same strategy, if clear squamous differentiation is present, SQCC is diagnosed. In this step, ancillary techniques are not always necessary because it is possible to reach a diagnosis based on routine hematoxylin and eosin (H&E) staining in 50% to 70% of cases.
3. If clear glandular differentiation, mucin-producing cells, and squamous differentiation are absent, then most cases are categorized as poorly differentiated carcinoma. In the IASLC/ATS/ERS classification, use of the term "non–small cell lung carcinoma (NSCLC or NSCC)" is recommended at this point. In such cases, additional immunohistochemical (IHC) assessments or mucin staining are recommended. The most accepted markers of lung adenocarcinoma are thyroid transcription factor 1 (TTF-1) and napsin A.[11,12] Regarding markers that can be used to identify differentiation toward SQCC, it has been reported that p40, p63,

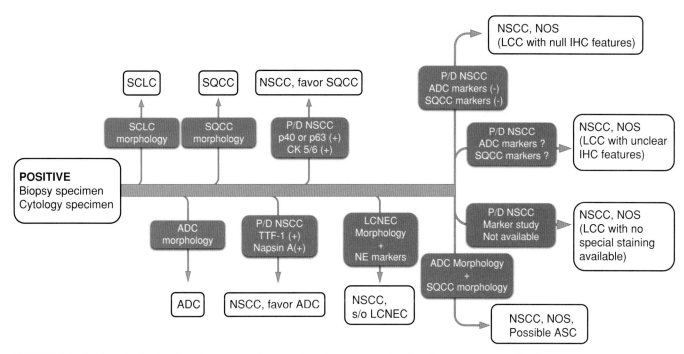

FIGURE 92.1 The algorithm for classifying lung cancer in biopsy and cytology specimens based on the IASLC/ATS/ERS classification. SCLC, small cell lung carcinoma; ADC, adenocarcinoma; SQCC, Squamous cell carcinoma; NE, neuroendocrine; P/D, poorly differentiated; NSCC, non–small cell carcinoma; LCNEC, large cell neuroendocrine carcinoma; ASC, adenosquamous carcinoma; NOS, not otherwise specified; LCC, large cell carcinoma.

and cytokeratin 5/6 are the most specific and sensitive squamous markers.[11,13] Although p63 was originally considered to be good marker for SQCC, recent findings have suggested that it is less specific than p40.[14,15] These antigens continued to be studied actively, and further progress is anticipated; thus, additional markers may be developed in the future to allow more specific and sensitive distinctions between adenocarcinoma and SQCC. At this step of the histological diagnosis process, the categorization "NSCLC, favor adenocarcinoma" is recommended for cases that are positive for an adenocarcinoma maker and/or mucin, but are negative for squamous makers. Conversely, categorization as "NSCLC, favor squamous cell carcinoma" is recommended for cases that are positive for a squamous maker, but are negative for adenocarcinoma makers and/or mucin.

4. The term "non–small cell lung carcinoma, not otherwise specified (NSCLC-NOS)" is only recommended for tumors that lack adenocarcinoma and squamous cell morphology, and express neither adenocarcinoma markers nor squamous markers.

5. Among the tumors in the NSCLC-NOS category, some cases with neuroendocrine (NE) morphology can be identified. IHC staining of NE markers (such as chromogranin A, synaptophysin, and CD56) are additionally recommended for these cases, for example, to detect NE differentiation. When such makers are positive, "NSCLC with NE markers" and/or "large cell neuroendocrine carcinoma (LCNEC)" can be diagnosed, even in small biopsy specimens.

6. In rare settings, cases with both adenocarcinoma and SQCC morphology are present. In such cases, the term "NSCLC with morphological squamous cell and adenocarcinoma patterns" is recommended. These cases can include adenosquamous carcinomas (ASCs). However, the precise diagnosis of ASC should be performed by evaluating entire slides that have been processed from resected tumor, because more than 10% of each component must be present by definition.

The main purpose of this multistep strategy for biopsy or cytology specimens is molecular testing, such as for EGFR, HER2, ALK, ROS1, and RET, because there are targeted drugs that correspond to these gene alterations. Because tumors with *EGFR* mutations are sensitive to specific agents, such as gefitinib and erlotinib, and are mainly identified in cases of adenocarcinoma, the IASLC/ATS/ERS classification notes that *EGFR* mutation tests are recommended for the following tumor classes: adenocarcinoma, NSCLC, favor adenocarcinoma; NSCLC-NOS; and ASC. Additionally, if no mutation of *EGFR* is seen in the tumors, subsequent *ALK* translocation testing is recommended because tumors with this translocation are also sensitive to specific agents, such as crizotinib and alectinib. Although cases with *KRAS* mutations do not have an optional targeted therapy at present, *KRAS* mutation tests are also recommended because mutations in *KRAS* are most frequent in patients from North America and European countries, and can be predictive of these patients' outcomes.

Cytological specimens are superior to biopsy specimens in several ways: they are easier to obtain, they allow rapid onsite evaluation, they impose less of a burden on the patient, and they are more cost-effective. Traditionally, the most important aim of cytology was screening for malignancy. Cytology can provide diagnoses that are equally precise as diagnoses based on small biopsy specimens. Currently, there is an increasing need for cytology because it can also provide simultaneous cell-block sectioning for IHC staining and molecular testing. Further, cytological specimens are the only specimens that can be obtained in some advanced cases. In such cases, the cytological specimen is the only material that is available for diagnosis and molecular testing.

There are several methods of obtaining cytological specimens, such as bronchial washing, bronchial brushing, and transbronchial needle aspiration, and the cytological specimens obtained through each method show similar specific morphology. If such cytological specimens show malignant cells, then classification into four

---

morphologies is recommended, following the same determination algorithm that was described for biopsy specimens: adenocarcinoma, SQCC, SCLC, and undifferentiated carcinoma. For cytological specimens, undifferentiated carcinoma indicates the presence of neither obvious adenocarcinoma, nor SQCC morphology. Specific cytological features of adenocarcinoma, SQCC, and SCLC are discussed in the following sections.

The algorithm for classifying lung cancer is a major component of the IASLC/ATS/ERS document and is also reflected in the subsequent 2015 WHO classification.[10,16] Because therapeutic targets are increasingly being identified outside of adenocarcinoma, a precise diagnosis of lung carcinoma becomes equally important.

ADENOCARCINOMA

DEFINITION AND SUBCLASSIFICATION

Adenocarcinomas account for approximately 30% to 50% of all carcinomas of the lung. In many parts of the world, the incidence of adenocarcinoma is increasing relative to the incidences of SQCC, LCC, and SCLC.[17] By definition, adenocarcinoma is a malignant epithelial tumor with glandular differentiation and/or mucin production. Based on a proposal by the IASLC/ERS/ATS, the expression of pneumocyte markers, such as TTF-1 or napsin A, are included in the definition that was mentioned in the previous section.

The previous WHO classification of lung tumors, which was an upgraded version of the 1999 WHO classification, was published in 2004.[18,19] It includes five usual subtypes of adenocarcinoma (acinar, papillary, bronchioloalveolar, solid with mucin production, and mixed) and several rarer variants (fetal, colloid, mucinous cystadenocarcinoma, signet ring, and clear cell).[19] Although it was used until very recently, many issues in this classification system have been debated.

First, issues with the bronchioloalveolar carcinoma (BAC) subtype have been raised. The term "BAC" has been used since early editions of the WHO classification, and has been defined as adenocarcinoma in which cylindrical tumor cells grow upon the walls of preexisting alveoli.[20] In 1995, Noguchi and colleagues[21] presented a milestone study, in which they reported 100% disease-free survival for small-sized adenocarcinomas with only alveolar replacement growth (which has recently been called a "lepidic growth pattern"). Since their work was published, a growing number of reports have supported Noguchi's concept.[22–24] Based on their reports, the 1999 and 2004 WHO classifications recognized that BAC is a noninvasive adenocarcinoma. However, even after the publications of the 1999 and 2004 WHO classifications, researchers from different parts of the world have continued to report cases of "invasive BAC."[25,26] This has become a source of confusion for pathologists, radiologists, and oncologists.

Second, because lung adenocarcinomas frequently reveal mixed histology (i.e., any combination of lepidic, papillary, acinar, or solid growth patterns), the 1999 WHO classification introduced the entity "adenocarcinoma, mixed subtype," which is defined as a lesion with the combination of more than one histological pattern.[18] However, over 80% of lung adenocarcinomas belonged to this category,[27–29] and this predominance was a key weakness of the 1999 and 2004 WHO classifications of lung adenocarcinoma.

Third, in the 2004 WHO classification, clear cell carcinoma (CCC) and signet ring cell carcinoma are recognized as variants of lung adenocarcinoma. However, data are not available to support any clinical significance to this decision.

TABLE 92.1 Subtyping of Lung Adenocarcinoma

Preinvasive lesions
Atypical adenomatous hyperplasia
Adenocarcinoma in situ (≤3 cm)
  Non-mucinous
  Mucinous
  Mixed mucinous/non-mucinous

Minimally invasive adenocarcinoma (≤3 cm lepidic predominant tumor with ≤0.5 cm invasion)
  Non-mucinous
  Mucinous
  Mixed mucinous/non-mucinous

Invasive adenocarcinoma
Lepidic predominant (lepidic predominant tumor with >0.5 cm invasion)
Acinar predominant
Papillary predominant
Micropapillary predominant
Solid predominant with mucin production

Variants of invasive adenocarcinoma
Invasive mucinous adenocarcinoma (formerly mucinous BAC)
Colloid adenocarcinoma
Fetal (low and high grade) adenocarcinoma
Enteric adenocarcinoma

Finally, several additional growth patterns have been proposed since the publication of the 2004 WHO classification, including micropapillary adenocarcinoma[30–41] and enteric adenocarcinoma.[42,43]

These problems have led the IASLC/ATS/ERS to recommend modifications to the WHO classification (Table 92.1). The details of these modifications are mentioned in the section on microscopic features.

GROSS FEATURES

Most adenocarcinomas of the lung arise in its periphery, whereas up to 13% may be central.[44] The gross features of most peripheral adenocarcinomas reveal pleural puckering, firmness, and a gray-tan colored cut surface (Fig. 92.2A,B). It was observed that many of the tumors arose in conjunction with a lung scar. These so-called "scar carcinomas" had been presumed to arise from or in the scar tissue. However, the studies of Barsky and colleagues[45] and Madri and Carter[46] suggested that the scars were secondary to the desmoplastic properties of the carcinoma, and it is now believed that these tumors do not represent adenocarcinoma arising in a scar. Central necrosis or hemorrhage is not uncommon, but cavitation is rare in lung adenocarcinomas. The periphery of the lesion may be semi-firm with preserved airspaces, corresponding to a probable lepidic or papillary component. Histological acinar or solid patterns cannot usually be discriminated on gross inspection, but most of the cases show a firm tumor without pneumatic airspace. Unlike peripheral adenocarcinomas, central adenocarcinomas often show polypoid endobronchial growth.[47–50] Mucin-rich tumors are characterized by gelatinous and sometimes multiple ill-circumscribed tumors on cut surfaces, which often mimic a gross feature of metastatic colorectal cancer of the lung. Occasionally, peripheral adenocarcinomas spread out over the pleura, thereby mimicking mesothelioma (so-called "pseudomesotheliomatous carcinoma"). Cases with extensive carcinomatous lymphatic permeation and tumor cell embolisms in lymph capillaries are called "lymphangitis carcinomatosa," and are mostly seen in autopsy cases.

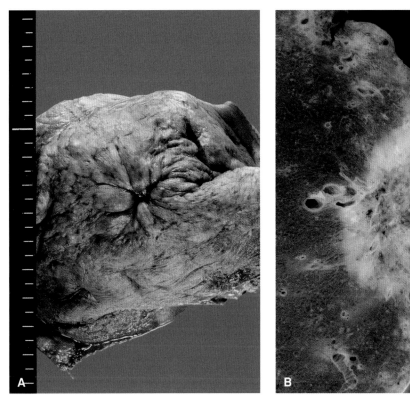

FIGURE 92.2 Invasive adenocarcinoma. Peripheral adenocarcinoma often puckers overlying visceral pleura. **A:** pleural surface; **B:** cut surface.

MICROSCOPIC FEATURES

Lung adenocarcinoma is usually composed of cuboidal to columnar epithelial cells with uniform round nuclei and adequate pink or vacuolated cytoplasm. The cells are arranged in varied following growth patterns: lepidic, acinar or glandular, papillary, micropapillary, and solid. In the IASLC/ATS/ERS proposal,[10] lung adenocarcinomas are divided into four histological categories based on the growth pattern and measurement of the invasive area: preinvasive lesions, which include atypical adenomatous hyperplasia (AAH) and adenocarcinoma in situ (AIS); minimally invasive adenocarcinoma (MIA); invasive adenocarcinoma; and variants. The authors also proposed subclassifying invasive adenocarcinoma according to the most predominant pattern. The new WHO classification of lung adenocarcinoma was published in 2015,[16] based on this proposal.[10] Multiple independent studies have attempted to classify lung adenocarcinomas and validate the classification's clinical significance.[27–29,51–54]

NON-MUCINOUS LEPIDIC GROWTH TUMOR LINEAGE (TRU TYPE ADENOCARCINOMA)

AAH, non-mucinous AIS, non-mucinous MIA, and lepidic-predominant invasive adenocarcinoma (LPA) are considered to reflect a series of steps in the progression of lung adenocarcinoma. The steps go from dysplasia and progression through *in situ* carcinoma, minimally invasive lesions, to invasive carcinomas that have the ability to metastasize (Fig. 92.3). These lesions resemble each other in terms of morphological appearance. They show crowded, uniform, cuboidal to columnar epithelial cells that mimic type II pneumocytes and/or Clara cells with mild to moderate cytological atypia lining on alveolar walls (Fig. 92.4). Yatabe proposed the concept

of a terminal respiratory unit (TRU) to explain this group of lung adenocarcinomas.[55] Tumors in this group are not only similar morphologically, but are also positive for the expression of TTF-1, which is a transcription factor for the peripheral airways that regulates most of the surfactant proteins and Clara cell antigens. Kim and colleagues[56] reported that the cells of this TRU are supplied by common stem cells, supporting the concept of their biological unity. In addition, the clinicopathological features of this tumor group are characterized by significantly higher frequencies in women, never smokers, and those who harbor *EGFR* mutations.[27,57,58] Thus, this tumor group is considered to reflect a unique and important lineage of lung cancer, with potential relevance for treatment.

The differences between non-mucinous AIS, non-mucinous MIA, and LPA are based on the amount of invasive area (Table 92.2). AIS has no invasive area and measures ≤3 cm in diameter, by definition. MIA has small invasive areas (≤5 mm), while LPA is defined as an invasive tumor with a mainly lepidic growth pattern and over 5 mm of invasive area. The rationale for separating these three entities is their prognostic differences. Beginning with the article by Noguchi and colleagues, multiple studies have shown 100% 5-year disease-free survival for patients who had lesions that met the criteria for AIS and were completely resected.[24,52,59–65] Some researchers have also reported lesions that mimic AIS in terms of morphology, but are otherwise inconsistent with the criteria for AIS. In Noguchi et al.'s 1995 report,[21] some small-sized adenocarcinomas with focal vascular or pleural invasion were also associated with 100% disease-free survival. In a study of 100 lung adenocarcinomas measuring ≤3 cm, Suzuki and colleagues[22] reported 100% 5-year survival rates for patients with tumors that had ≤5-mm central fibrosis, 72% 5-year survival rates for patients with tumors that had 6- to 15-mm central fibrosis, and 57% 5-year survival rates for patients

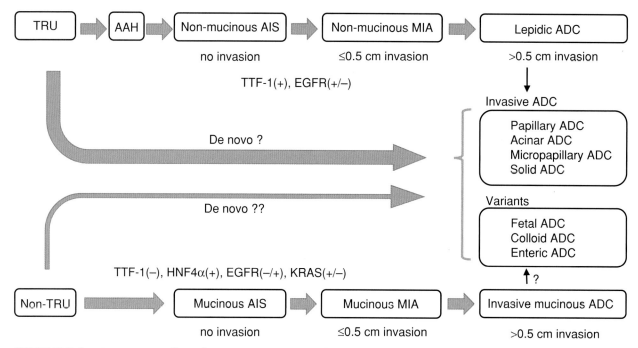

FIGURE 92.3 Stepwise progression of lung adenocarcinoma. AAH, atypical adenomatous hyperplasia; AIS, adenocarcinoma in situ; MIA, minimally invasive adenocarcinoma; ADC, adenocarcinoma; TRU, terminal respiratory unit.

with tumors that had more than 15 mm central fibrosis. Sakurai and colleagues[24] also examined 380 peripheral adenocarcinomas with diameters of ≤2 cm, finding that recurrence developed in only 3.3% of the 91 patients with fibrosis of ≤5 mm and, importantly, that 100% of these patients were alive at 7 years. It is challenging to judge "invasion." The researchers who are cited above recognized vascular invasion, pleural invasion, or active fibrosis as evidence of invasion. However, some pathologists have considered tumor cell proliferation in preserved alveolar structure (such as alveolar floating or filling tumor cells showing a solid/cribriform/papillary pattern) to represent noninvasion. In a large case series of Maeshima and

colleagues,[64] the authors simply measured the area that was not lepidic as the invasive area and reported that adenocarcinomas including a nonlepidic component of 5 mm or less in diameter did not exhibit recurrence. Some other studies based in the United States have also demonstrated high survival rates among patients with tumors showing ≤5 mm of invasion.[52,66] Conversely, some investigators have reported recurrent cases and deaths in patients with lesions that showed minimal invasion.[54,67] In consideration of these various findings, "invasion" is defined as histologic subtypes other than a lepidic pattern and/or myofibroblastic stroma associated with invasive tumor cells, and the new entity MIA was proposed in the IASLC/ATS/ERS classification.[10] In the IASLC/ATS/ERS classification, LPA was additionally introduced as an invasive adenocarcinoma because the recurrence rate of lesions with predominant lepidic growth and over 5 mm of invasion is obviously higher than the recurrence rates of AIS or MIA.[28,29,52]

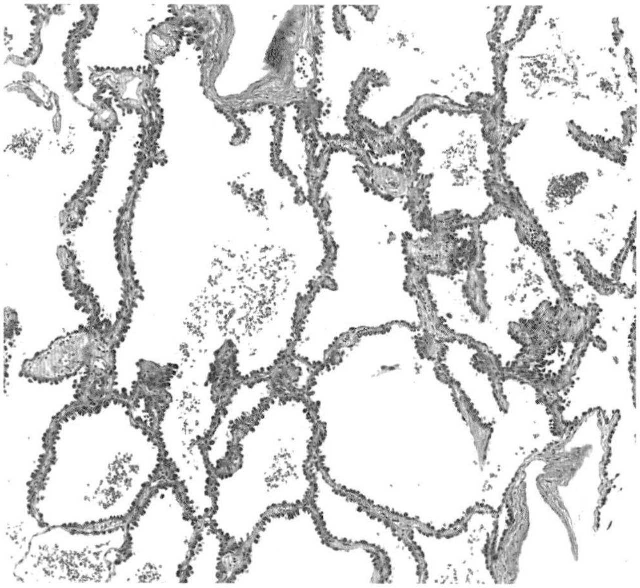

FIGURE 92.4 Adenocarcinoma, lepidic pattern (non-mucinous). Alveolar walls are lined by uniform, cuboidal tumor cells with mild-to-moderate atypia.

TABLE 92.2 Differential Diagnosis of Adenocarcinoma with Lepidic Growth Pattern

	Tumor Size	Invasive Area Size	ly, v, pl	Mucin Producing
AAH	≤0.5 cm	None	Absent	Non-mucinous
AIS	≤3 cm	None	Absent	Non-mucinous/ mucinous/ mixed
MIA	≤3 cm	≤0.5 cm	Absent	Non-mucinous/ mucinous/ mixed
LPA	Any	Over 0.5 cm	Any	Non-mucinous
IMA	Any	Over 0.5 cm	Any	Mucinous

ly, lymphatic invasion; v, vascular invasion; pl, pleural invasion; AAH, atypical adenomatous hyperplasia; AIS, adenocarcinoma in situ; MIA, minimally invasive adenocarcinoma; LPA, lepidic predominant adenocarcinoma; IMA, invasive mucinous adenocarcinoma.

Although the terms "bronchioloalveolar pattern"[68] and "BAC pattern"[27] have been applied to noninvasive areas of a tumor, use of the term "lepidic pattern" is recommended instead in the IASLC/ATS/ERS classification. Use of the term "lepidic pattern" is favored to avoid confusion with "adenocarcinoma in situ," which shows noninvasive growth throughout.

AAH is a proliferation of bronchioloalveolar cells, resembling non-mucinous AIS. AAH has initially been considered as a reactive lesion; however, several studies have noted that the molecular findings of AAH demonstrate a relationship with lung adenocarcinoma. Specifically, the following findings have been reported: *KRAS* mutation,[69,70] *KRAS* polymorphism,[71] *EGFR* mutation,[72,73] p53 expression,[74] loss of heterozygosity,[75] methylation,[76] telomerase overexpression,[77] eukaryotic initiation factor 4E (eIF4E) expression,[78] epigenetic alterations in the WNT pathway,[79] and fragile histidine triad (FHIT) expression.[80] Thus, AAH has been recognized as a precursor to adenocarcinoma in recent years. These lesions have usually been incidentally identified pathologically in lungs resected for adenocarcinoma.[81,82] Rao and Fraire[83] noted that these areas are present in as much as 20% of resected lung cancer specimens as an ill-defined peripheral nodule, and are most often multiple in number. Further, studies have documented these lesions as incidental findings in the adjacent lung parenchyma of 5% to 23% of resected lung adenocarcinomas.[81,82,84–87] Histologically, variable nuclear pleomorphism is present, but is most often mild in nature, without central fibrosis. Kitamura and colleagues[74] have classified these AAHs as low-grade, high-grade, and carcinoma-like; however, this grading system was not recommended in the IASLC/ATS/ERS classification.[10] The most clinical important distinction is the separation of AAH from AIS. AAH is smaller (generally less than 0.5 cm) and shows less cellularity than AIS. Thus, AAH cannot be diagnosed in small biopsy and cytology specimens.

MUCINOUS LEPIDIC GROWTH TUMOR LINEAGE (NON–TRU Type ADENOCARCINOMA)

Clayton initially separated BACs into two cell types: non-mucinous and mucinous.[88] To this day, the concept is continued to be included in the IASLC/ATS/ERS classification. The classification of mucinous lepidic growth-pattern tumors of the lung includes mucinous AIS, mucinous MIA, and invasive mucinous adenocarcinoma (IMA). These tumors are thought to be different from TRU-type adenocarcinomas, based on IHC and genetic profiles.[65,89–91] Their common appearance is characterized by a lepidic growth pattern with cuboidal to tall columnar cells that have basal nuclei and abundant cytoplasmic mucin (Fig. 92.5).

IMA has newly been proposed as a distinct invasive carcinoma, and was formerly named "mucinous BAC." IMA mainly shows a lepidic growth pattern, but can also show the same heterogeneous mixture of lepidic, acinar, papillary, micropapillary, and solid growth as is found in non-mucinous tumors.[92] Alveolar spaces often contain mucin. There is a strong tendency for multicentric, multilobar, and bilateral lung involvement, which may reflect aerogenous spread. When stromal invasion is seen, the malignant cells may show less cytoplasmic mucin and more atypia.[92] In some cases, mixtures of mucinous and non-mucinous components are seen. It is recommended that such cases be described as "mixed invasive mucinous and non-mucinous adenocarcinoma." In 2013, Sugano and colleagues reported that hepatocyte nuclear factor 4 alpha (HNF4α) could serve as a marker of IMA, which is distinct from other adenocarcinomas because of its radiologic, morphologic, and genetic differences.[91] Recently, NRG1 fusions were identified in IMAs and may be considered as a specific gene alteration for IMA.[93,94] IMA is the counterpart to LPA in the category of the TRU lineage.

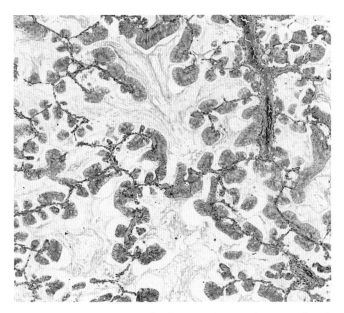

FIGURE 92.5 Adenocarcinoma, lepidic pattern (mucinous). Tumor cells with mucin-rich cytoplasm proliferate on the alveolar walls with extracellular mucin.

Mucinous MIA differs from IMA in terms of all of the following criteria: tumor size (≤3 cm), amount of invasion (≤0.5 cm), solitary nodules, or lack of lymphatic, blood vessel, and pleural invasion. As compared with mucinous MIA and IMA, **mucinous AIS** is defined as a pure lepidic growth-pattern tumor consisting of mucinous columnar cells without any invasive features (Table 92.2, Fig. 92.5). Mucinous AIS and MIA are extremely rare.[52,65] Kadota and colleagues[65] reported no cases of mucinous AIS and only 1 mucinous MIA in their analysis of a large cohort of 864 patients. Thus, these diagnoses need to be made with caution, as most tumors with this histologic appearance will be IMAs.

The term "mucinous AAH" is nonexistent and is considered to be mostly reactive. However, mucinous precancerous lesions have been reported in congenital cystic adenomatoid malformation.[95] Undetermined lesions are often seen in routine practice, even though they may not be mucinous neoplasms.

INVASIVE ADENOCARCINOMA

Over 80% of resected adenocarcinomas are invasive and feature a mixture of two or more histological growth patterns. Thus, even though the term "adenocarcinoma, mixed subtype" appeared in the 1999 and 2004 WHO classifications, it did not provide particularly useful information about tumor morphology. The authors of the IASLC/ATS/ERS classification propose classifying invasive adenocarcinomas according to their predominant patterns: lepidic, acinar, papillary, micropapillary, or solid.[10] To classify the subtypes, Motoi and colleagues[27] first attempted comprehensive histological subtyping in 5% to 10% increments. In 2011, a validation study with a large cohort by Yoshizawa and colleagues[52] demonstrated significant differences in patient outcomes among the histologic subtypes. After the report, studies performed around the world provided better therapeutic and/or prognostic stratification of adenocarcinomas with such mixed growth patterns (Fig. 92.6). These investigations included the work of Russell et al. from Australia, Warth et al. from Germany, Yeh et al. from Taiwan, Yoshizawa et al. from Japan, Gu et al. from China, and Mansuet-Lupo et al. from France.[28,29,53,96–98] In addition, this approach provides novel correlations between histologic subtypes

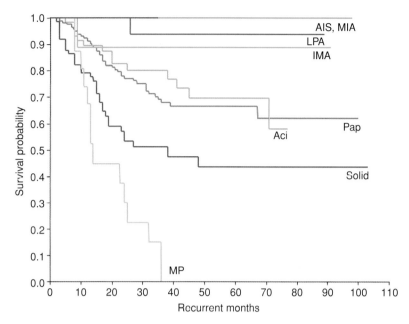

FIGURE 92.6 Disease-free survival for patients with different adenocarcinoma subtypes. The subtypes with favorable prognosis include adenocarcinoma in situ (AIS), minimally invasive adenocarcinoma (MIA), lepidic adenocarcinoma (LPA), followed by acinar adenocarcinoma (Aci), and papillary adenocarcinoma (Pap); solid adenocarcinoma (solid) and micropapillary adenocarcinoma (MP) subtypes are considered to have poorer prognosis. (Modified from Yoshizawa A, Sumiyoshi S, Sonobe M, et al. Validation of the IASLC/ATS/ERS lung adenocarcinoma classification for prognosis and association with EGFR and KRAS gene mutations: Analysis of 440 Japanese patients. *J Thorac Oncol* 2013;8:52–61. Copyright © 2013 International Association for the Study of Lung Cancer. With permission.)

and both molecular and clinical features.[27,28,99–101] Accordingly, the term "adenocarcinoma, mixed subtype" has been discontinued in the most recent WHO classification.

As mentioned in the paragraph on non-mucinous lepidic growth lineage tumors, **lepidic predominant adenocarcinoma** (lepidic adenocarcinoma in the 2015 WHO classification) shows a mainly lepidic growth pattern consisting of type II pneumocytes or Clara cells, and presents at least one invasion focus that measures more than 5 mm in its greatest dimension. Of the five major subtypes of invasive adenocarcinoma, lepidic predominance appears to signify a lesser degree of malignancy than acinar and papillary growth, which are in turn less malignant than micropapillary and solid growth.[29,52]

Acinar predominant adenocarcinoma (acinar adenocarcinoma in the 2015 WHO classification) is characterized mainly by proliferation of glandular structures in the form of acini and tubules (Fig. 92.7). The lining tumor cells are typically cuboidal or columnar,

with or without mucin. Glandular architecture is often observed in the central collapse area of adenocarcinoma, showing a lepidic pattern in the peripheral area. In the IASLC/ATS/ERS classification, considering such structure as invasion is recommended, even when no myofibroblastic stromal reaction is present. Cribriform arrangements are regarded as a pattern of acinar adenocarcinoma.[102,103] However, recent reports have shown that the cribriform pattern appears to be associated with a worse prognosis than the acinar pattern.[104–106]

Papillary predominant adenocarcinoma (papillary adenocarcinoma in the 2015 WHO classification) is characterized by mainly papillary structures supported by fibrovascular cores with complicated secondary and tertiary branches and tuft (Fig. 92.8). The tumor cells are cuboidal or columnar, with either clear or eosinophilic cytoplasm. Mucinous differentiation is rare. Silver and Askin defined papillary adenocarcinoma as a neoplasm with a papillary structure constituting at least 75% of the tumor and concluded

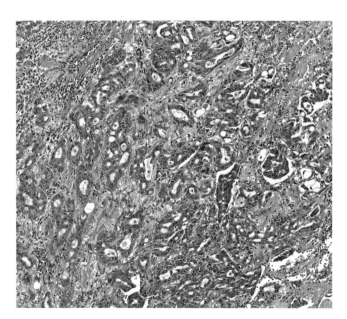

FIGURE 92.7 Invasive adenocarcinoma, acinar pattern. Fused, angulated, or cribriform glands consist of cuboidal tumor cells.

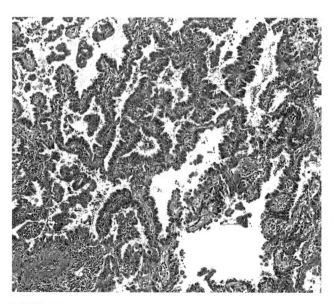

FIGURE 92.8 Invasive adenocarcinoma, papillary pattern. The structures are supported by fibrovascular cores with complicated secondary and tertiary branches and tufts.

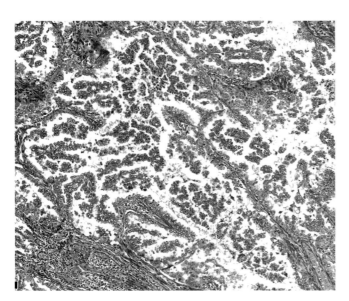

FIGURE 92.9 Invasive adenocarcinoma, micropapillary pattern. Tumor cell clusters show small tufts without fibrovascular cores.

that it is a distinct clinicopathologic entity with considerably worse morbidity and mortality than BAC.[107] On the other hand, some researchers have suggested that papillary predominant adenocarcinoma should be considered as an intermediated grade tumor that shows both a poorer prognosis than AIS–MIA–LPA tumors and a better prognosis than micropapillary- and solid-predominant adenocarcinomas.[28,29,52]

Micropapillary predominant adenocarcinoma (micropapillary adenocarcinoma in the 2015 WHO classification), which was first reported by Amin and colleagues,[30] is a novel entity in 2015 WHO classification. Amin and colleagues studied 35 cases of adenocarcinoma with a micropapillary component and described the pathological details of those cases. In their report, the micropapillary pattern was defined by small papillary tufts lying freely within alveolar spaces or encased within thin walls of connective tissue, representing retracted connective tissue spaces (Fig. 92.9). Following the publication of their work, a number of supporting reports have also been published.[31–41,108] Accordingly, in the IASLC/ATS/ERS classification, micropapillary predominant adenocarcinoma has been proposed as a subtype of invasive adenocarcinoma. Electron microscopy does not show the basement membrane or vascular structures. Although microvilli were observed on the cell surface, their distribution was random. The apical and basal sides of the cells were not clearly delineated and showed intercellular junctions in micropapillary tufts (Fig. 92.10). Since Amin and colleagues[30] reported that the micropapillary component was a possible prognostic factor, many researchers have described adenocarcinoma with micropapillary component as having a significantly poorer prognosis.[31,33–37,39,40] Additionally, some reports have described associations between adenocarcinoma with a micropapillary component and *EGFR* gene mutations.[27,28,38,40,108] In an interesting report, Sumiyoshi and colleagues showed that lung adenocarcinomas with micropapillary components could be controlled with EGFR-TKIs after recurrence because most of the cases harbored *EGFR* mutations, for which EGFR-TKIs were effective.[41]

Solid predominant adenocarcinoma (solid adenocarcinoma in the 2015 WHO classification) is a poorly differentiated adenocarcinoma showing sheets of polygonal cells without intercellular bridges. Tumor cells contain large vesicular nuclei, prominent nucleoli, and

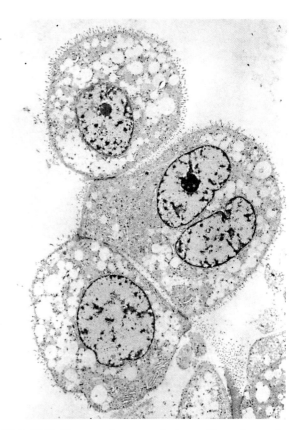

FIGURE 92.10 Electron microscopy of micropapillary adenocarcinoma. Short microvilli appear over entire cell surface; therefore, the apical and basal sides of the cell are not clearly delineated.

moderately abundant cytoplasm in which droplets of mucin can be detected by mucin staining. Solid predominant adenocarcinoma must be distinguished from poorly differentiated SQCC and undifferentiated carcinoma (LCC) because EGFR molecular tests should be performed when the tumor is diagnosed as adenocarcinoma.

VARIANTS

In addition to the five major categories mentioned above, the 2015 WHO classification scheme features four invasive adenocarcinoma variants: IMA, colloid adenocarcinoma, fetal adenocarcinoma, and enteric adenocarcinoma.[16] The new scheme also removes clear cell and signet ring carcinoma as adenocarcinoma subtypes, because neither showed clinical significance.[16] Recent molecular studies have demonstrated that signet ring cell features are associated with particular molecular features, such as *ALK* fusions, *ROS1* fusions, and *RET* fusions.[109–114] Therefore, signet ring cell features still require description.

Historically, "mucinous" tumor of the lung has included a wide variety of tumors: mucinous cyst, mucinous BAC, mucinous carcinoma, mucinous cystadenoma, mucinous multilocular cyst carcinoma, mucinous cystadenocarcinoma, pseudomyxomatous pulmonary adenocarcinoma, mucinous cystic tumor of low malignant potential, mucinous cystic tumor of borderline malignancy, enteric adenocarcinoma, and colloid carcinoma.[19,115–120] In the 2015 WHO classification, colloid adenocarcinoma, IMA (as mentioned above), and enteric adenocarcinoma remain as variants of invasive adenocarcinomas. Although mucinous cystadenocarcinoma is included in the 2004 WHO classification, it belongs to the category of colloid

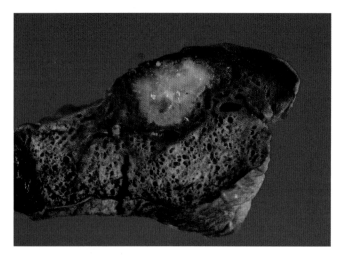

FIGURE 92.11 Colloid adenocarcinoma. The cut surface reveals well-circumscribed, gelatinous tumor.

adenocarcinoma in the 2015 WHO classification. Mucinous cystade-nocarcinoma is particularly rare and probably represents part of the spectrum of colloid adenocarcinoma.

Colloid Adenocarcinoma

Colloid adenocarcinomas are usually solitary peripheral nodules, ranging in size from 1.0 to 5.5 cm in one study.[121] Their cut surfaces demonstrate soft tan-gray mucoid lesions that have well-circumscribed margins, but are not encapsulated (Fig. 92.11). Histologically, colloid adenocarcinoma shows abundant extracellular mucin in pools, which distend the alveolar spaces and destroy their walls The mucin pools contain clusters of mucin-secreting tumor cells, which may consist of goblet cells or other mucin-secreting cells and may form a single layer along fibrous septae. Colloid adenocarcinoma is less frequently found as a pure pattern than as a mixture with other adenocarcinoma histologic subtypes.[42,43,122] Immunohistochemically, colloid adenocarcinomas express CDX2, MUC2, and cytokeratin 20, while staining with cytokeratin 7 and TTF-1 is only focal and weak.[43,89,123] The prognosis of this tumor remains unclear. Colloid adenocarcinoma is often difficult to distinguish from metastatic carcinoma from the gastrointestinal tract, pancreas, breast, or female genital tract. In such cases, clinical correlation is need, but some IHC antigens may also help to distinguish this tumor from metastatic carcinoma.

Fetal Adenocarcinoma

Fetal adenocarcinoma consists of glandular elements with tubules composed of glycogen-rich, nonciliated cells that resemble fetal lung tubules.[19] In 1982, Kradin and colleagues published the first report of fetal adenocarcinoma, describing it as a pulmonary endodermal tumor resembling fetal lung, having a histologic resemblance to the epithelial tubules of the embryonic lung in the first trimester of pregnancy.[124] Although these tumors were originally believed to be a derivation from pulmonary blastoma, they are currently considered to be members of the adenocarcinoma family.[125,126] According to Nakatani's review,[127] these carcinomas constitute a heterogeneous group of adenocarcinomas, ranging from well-differentiated fetal adenocarcinoma to tumors that are more poorly differentiated and more aggressive.[125,128]

Low-grade fetal adenocarcinoma (L-FLAC) and high-grade fetal adenocarcinoma (H-FLAC) are currently recognized in both the 2015 WHO classification and the IASLC/ATS/ERS classification.[10,16] L- and

H-FLAC are distinguished based on the degree of pleomorphism.[127] These tumors present at a wide range of ages, but high-grade tumors tend to affect the elderly, while low-grade tumors more often appear in middle age.[127] Grossly, both types are usually well circumscribed and lobulated. L-FLACs are smaller than H-FLACs (range of sizes: 1 to 10 cm for L-FLACs and 3 to 14 cm for H-FLACs). The cut surfaces of H-FLACs are more heterogeneous because of necrosis; however, they cannot be separated from other invasive adenocarcinomas on the basis of gross findings. Histologically, the neoplastic glands are typically lined by pseudostratified columnar epithelium with uniform oval nuclei and focally glycogen-rich clear cytoplasm (Fig. 92.12). Characteristic morules are commonly observed in L-FLACs, but not in H-FLACs. They consist of solid nests of cells beneath the glandular epithelium with scant benign stroma. The nuclei of morular cells often show clear morphology, which is derived from accumulation of biotin. Biotin is stored in the nuclei of both endometrial cells in pregnancy and endometrioid adenocarcinoma of the female genital tract. Therefore, "pulmonary endometrioid adenocarcinoma" is an alternative term for this tumor.

Unlike metastatic endometrioid adenocarcinoma of the female genital tract, fetal adenocarcinoma of the lung is usually positive for cytokeratin 7 and TTF-1. Immunohistochemically, the epithelial cells in L-FLACs express aberrant nuclear and cytoplasmic staining with beta-catenin. Nakatani et al.[129,130] and Sekine et al.[131] have suggested that upregulation of the WNT signaling pathway is driven by mutations in the beta-catenin gene in L-FLACs, but that this upregulation is not present in H-FLACs, which appear to be distinct from L-FLACs. The cluster cells also express CDX2.[132,133] Along with GATA-6 and TTF-1 reactivity, this CDX2 expression suggests that the structure is simply an immature portion of the developing endodermal branching gland.[133] All L-FLACs and approximately one-third of H-FLACs express NE markers, such as chromogranin A, synaptophysin, and CD56, in glandular and morular cells.[127]

As compared with L-FLACs, H-FLACs feature sheets and disorganized glands with abundant desmoplastic stroma, significant tumor necrosis, and the absence of morules.[127] Most H-FLACs show a mixture of other histological subtypes of lung adenocarcinoma. Recently,

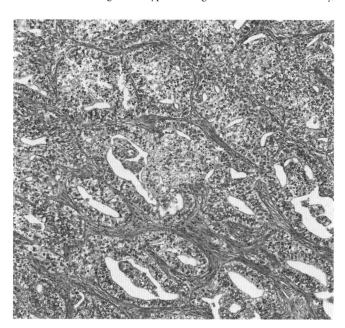

FIGURE 92.12 High-grade fetal adenocarcinoma. Pseudostratified columnar epithelium consists of cells with the uniform oval nuclei and glycogen-rich clear cytoplasm.

Morita and colleagues[133] suggested that H-FLAC is a high-grade lung adenocarcinoma with a fetal lung-like morphology, rather than a specific tumor entity. This suggestion was made because H-FLACs have heterogeneous nonfetal adenocarcinoma morphology and heterogeneous gene mutations, such as in *EGFR* and *KRAS*. The new WHO classification states that H-FLAC typically has at least 50% fetal morphology, and should be considered invasive adenocarcinomas with fetal features when the fetal morphology component accounts for less than 50% of the tumor.[16]

Patients with L-FLAC have a significantly better outcome than patients with H-FLAC.[46,125,127,133] Morita and colleagues[133] reported a 5-year disease-free survival rate of 48.6% and a 5-year overall survival rate of 53.6% in patients with H-FLAC.

Enteric Adenocarcinoma

It is not uncommon to encounter focal enteric differentiation in primary lung adenocarcinoma; however, tumors with more than 50% of this component are extremely rare, and have been calculated to account for approximately 0.1% of cases. In 1991, Tsao and Fraser published the first reported case of a tumor with cytologic characteristics typical of differentiated small intestinal epithelium.[122] On radiological images, its features are similar to those of other invasive lung adenocarcinomas. Li et al.[134] and Maeda et al.[135] have recently noted that these tumors show high FDG-avidity on FDG-PET scans. Grossly, cut surfaces of the tumor feature well-demarcated white-gray masses, with a median size of 3.4 cm (range: 1.5 to 7.0 cm).[42,43,134] Further, yellow punctate necrosis is characteristic, resembling lung metastases from colorectal cancer. Histologically, the tumor is composed of complex glandules, cribriform and solid growth areas with stromal desmoplasia, and necrosis that can share some morphologic features with colorectal adenocarcinoma.[42] The tumors are heterogeneous, with some components that resemble primary lung adenocarcinoma growth. Immunohistochemically, several reports have noted that most enteric adenocarcinomas show positive staining for cytokeratin 7, and that approximately half of all cases show positive staining for TTF-1 and CDX2, which can help to distinguish these tumors from metastatic colorectal adenocarcinoma.[42,43,89,134–136] However, a recent case showed negative staining for cytokeratin 7.[136] Although the IHC profile of enteric adenocarcinoma is not entirely clear, the IASLC/ATS/ERS scheme requires that at least one marker of enteric differentiation is present.[10] It is not known whether there are any distinctive clinical or molecular features of enteric carcinoma, and its prognosis also remains unclear.

CYTOLOGIC FEATURES OF LUNG ADENOCARCINOMA

Cytologic specimens obtained from adenocarcinoma can show several architectural patterns: flat sheets, two to three cell-stratified clusters, pseudopapillary aggregates, lumens in strong stratified clusters, and a honeycomb appearance[137,138] (Fig. 92.13). Small, three-dimensional balls of cells indicate micropapillary structure. Rarely, cases have shown true papillae with central fibrovascular cores. The characteristics of individual tumor cells depend on the tumor cell lineage. TRU-lineage tumor cells typically have lacy cytoplasm and eccentrically located nuclei. Compared with these TRU-lineage tumor cells, tumor cells in mucinous tumors reveal more extracellular mucin and abundant mucin-rich cytoplasm in individual cells. The chromatin pattern of the nuclei varies from finely granular and uniform to hyperchromatic, coarse, and irregularly distributed. The single nucleoli are often well developed.

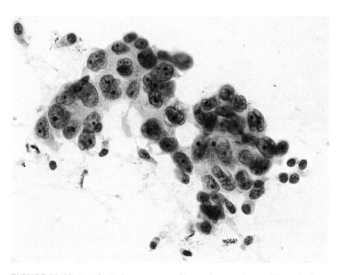

FIGURE 92.13 Cytological appearance of lung adenocarcinoma (Papanicolaou preparation). A flat sheet of tumor cells with the hyperchromatic nuclei and conspicuous nucleoli can be seen.

PROGNOSTIC SIGNIFICANCE OF ADENOCARCINOMA BASED ON NEW IASLC/ATS/ERS CLASSIFICATION

In the new lung adenocarcinoma classification proposed by IASLC/ATS/ERS, lung adenocarcinomas are classified into four histological categories based on the growth pattern and measurement of invasive area: preinvasive lesions, which include AAH and AIS; MIA; 5 invasive adenocarcinomas; and 4 variants as mentioned. Among 514 patients with stage I surgically treated at Memorial Sloan-Kettering Cancer Center, 1 patient with AIS and 13 patients with MIA were identified and they had 100% 5-year disease-free survival.[52] Lepidic predominant ($n = 29$), acinar predominant ($n = 232$), papillary predominant ($n = 143$), micropapillary predominant ($n = 12$), and solid predominant ($n = 67$) revealed 90, 83, 84, 71, 67%, respectively. Similar study was performed using 440 Japanese lung adenocarcinoma patients with all stages surgically treated. Five-year disease-free survival rates were: 100% for AIS ($n = 20$) and MIA ($n = 33$), 93.8% for lepidic predominant adenocarcinoma ($n = 36$), 66.7% for papillary predominant adenocarcinoma ($n = 179$), 69.7% for acinar predominant adenocarcinoma ($n = 61$), 43.3% for solid predominant adenocarcinoma ($n = 78$), and 0% for micropapillary predominant adenocarcinoma ($n = 19$) (Fig. 92.6).

SQUAMOUS CELL CARCINOMA

DEFINITION AND SUBCLASSIFICATION

Histologically, SQCC is defined as malignant epithelial tumor that shows either keratinization and/or intercellular bridges. SQCC was the predominant histological type of lung carcinoma that was observed in smokers during the 1950s, and has been regarded as a tumor of the central bronchi. However, the incidence rates of SQCC in developed countries have reduced along with decreasing rates of tobacco smoking.[139] Consequently, SQCC is no longer the most common type of lung cancer, and peripheral lesions are not uncommon.[140,141] In the 2015 WHO classification, SQCC is divided into three subtypes: keratinizing SQCC, non-keratinizing SQCC, and basaloid SQCC.[16]

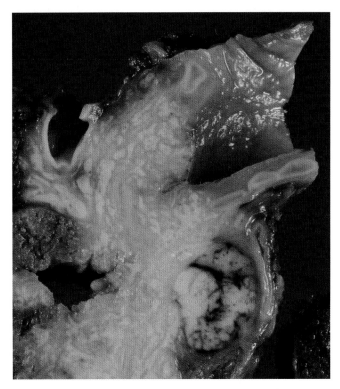

FIGURE 92.14 Gross image of a centrally located squamous cell carcinoma. The tumor presents an endobronchial mass infiltrating to a hilar lymph node.

This subtyping was defined in a similar manner to the subtyping of nasopharyngeal carcinomas in the 2005 WHO classification.[142]

GROSS FEATURES

Cut surfaces of SQCCs are white to gray and often granular or friable. Central cavitation is frequently present in large SQCCs, and mostly includes keratinization, hemorrhage, or necrosis. Central cavitation may occur in 10% to 20% of peripheral lesions.[140] The centrally located lesions usually form polypoid masses and infiltrate through the bronchial wall into the hilar and mediastinal lymph nodes, as well as extrapulmonary organs, such as the mediastinum, large vessels, and the pericardium (Fig. 92.14). The obstructing tumors in the bronchial lumen are often associated with obstructive pneumonitis, distal pulmonary collapse, consolidation, and atelectasis. The peripherally located SQCCs tend to mimic the central lesions. Because small-sized peripheral lesions can cause pleural puckering and invasion into the chest wall, they are sometimes indistinguishable from small-sized adenocarcinoma developing beneath the pleura. Some SQCCs that developed in the apical apex can cause Pancoast syndrome, which is associated with tumor invasion into soft tissue and bone. Preinvasive lesions (squamous dysplasia and carcinoma in-situ) appear as areas characterized by a loss of the normal longitudinal folds of the mucosa of the bronchus. The mucosal area that is involved may be thickened and erythematous.

MICROSCOPIC FEATURES

Keratinizing SQCC presents various amounts of keratinization. It has polygonal or prickle-type cells, stratification, and intercellular bridge formation (Fig. 92.15). Individual tumor cells keratinize, tend to form keratin pearls, or both; the nuclei may be uniform, pleomorphic,

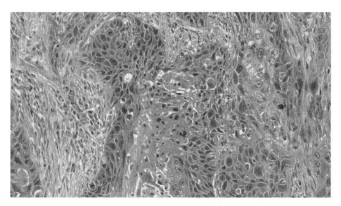

FIGURE 92.15 Keratinizing squamous cell carcinoma. Tumor cells are characterized by keratinization and intracellular bridge formation.

or giant. These findings are very focal in poorly differentiated tumors, while they are easy to identify in well-differentiated tumors. Rarely, squamous cells can take on a spindle shape, which makes the tumor appear histologically sarcomatous.

Non-keratinizing SQCCs are predominantly composed of poorly differentiated cells, with little—but still distinct—evidence of intercellular bridge formation, individual cell keratinization, or both. IHC studies are often required to distinguish these cases from poorly differentiated adenocarcinoma or LCC. Non-keratinizing SQCCs are usually positive for p40, p63, and cytokeratin 5/6, but negative for TTF-1 and napsin A. Tumors without IHC features are not categorized as non-keratinizing SQCC. Regarding histological predictors, Maeshima and colleagues[143] reported that minimal tumor nest is a useful prognostic marker for small-sized SQCC. Takahashi and colleagues[144] noted that the prognosis of patients with fibrous stroma-type tumors was significantly poorer than that of patients with thin stroma-type tumors. Further, they found that the presence of a fibrous stroma was an independent prognostic factor in a multivariate analysis. Both of these reports showed that the degrees of keratinization and tumor differentiation were not associated with prognosis. Recently, Kadota et al.[145] found similar results in a large cohort study that was performed in the United States. The most important aspect of non-keratinizing SQCCs is that they may need to be distinguished from poorly differentiated adenocarcinoma in clinical practice.

Basaloid SQCC is an invasive tumor that is composed of nests with peripheral palisading, and demonstrates focal intercellular bridges or individual cell keratinization (Fig. 92.16). Brambilla and colleagues[146] have described the histological features of this tumor as follows: small, moderately pleomorphic, cuboidal to fusiform cells with hyperchromatic nuclei, granular dense chromatin, inconspicuous nucleoli, scant cytoplasm, and a high mitotic index. In previous WHO classification schemes, this type of carcinoma has been categorized as either poorly differentiated SQCC or LCC, which has confused pathologists and clinicians.[19] Thus, the 2015 WHO classification has defined basaloid carcinoma as a variant of SQCC, requiring >50% basaloid component, even when a keratinizing or nonkeratinizing squamous cell component is present. Immunohistochemically, basaloid SQCC diffusely and strongly expresses squamous makers, such as p40, p63, cytokeratin5/6, and CK14. Kim and colleagues[147] reported that NE markers, such as chromogranin A and synaptophysin, are present in 8.5% of these tumors, but that TTF-1 is never expressed in basaloid SQCC. In small biopsy specimens, it is difficult to distinguish basaloid SQCC from poorly differentiated SQCC, large cell NE carcinoma, small cell lung carcinoma, adenoid cystic carcinoma, and nuclear protein in testis (NUT) midline

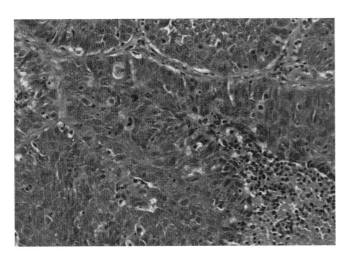

FIGURE 92.16 Basaloid SQCC. A tumor nest is composed of cuboidal and fusiform cancer cells with the scant cytoplasm, which demonstrate peripheral palisading.

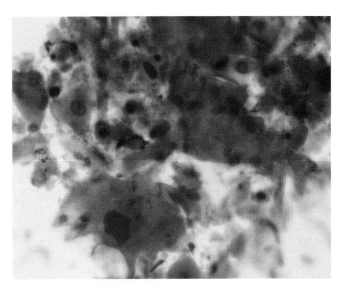

FIGURE 92.17 Cytological appearance of squamous cell carcinoma (Papanicolaou preparation). A brushing smear shows tumor cells of different sizes with the orange cytoplasm indicating keratinization.

carcinoma. Sturm and colleagues[148] reported that high–molecular-weight keratin and p63 staining may help to separate basaloid SQCC from NE tumors, since these antibodies are not seen in NE tumors. Recently, Brambilla and colleagues[149] suggested that IHC analyses of SOX4 and IVL can be used to discriminate basaloid SQCC from nonbasaloid SQCC. Although basaloid SQCC are rare and relevant data are limited, these tumors have been considered to be highly aggressive.[149–151] However, other researchers have concluded that basaloid SQCC does not have a worse prognosis than other non–small cell lung carcinomas.[145,147,152] Thus, the prognostic significance of basaloid SQCC remains controversial.

OBSOLETE VARIANTS

In the newest WHO classification, it was decided that the papillary, small cell, and clear cell variants should no longer be recognized as subtypes of lung SQCC. Sherwin et al.[153] and Dulmet-Brender et al.[154] described exophytic endobronchial squamous carcinoma as an uncommon type of SQCC with a papillomatous, polypoid, or verrucous growth pattern. This subtype was recognized as the papillary variant of SQCC in the previous WHO classification.[19] However, because this type tumor is very rare,[145] and lacks clear prognostic significance, there is sufficient reason to question whether it should be considered a major subtype of SQCC in the WHO classification.

Even though the small cell subtype was included in the 1999 and 2004 WHO classification, it also has a questionable status as a special subtype of SQCC; most tumors of this subtype morphologically mimic basaloid carcinomas, making these subtypes impossible to distinguish. In addition, the term "small cell" could lead clinicians to confuse the diagnosis of these cases with the diagnosis of SQCC.[155]

The 1999 and 2004 WHO classifications also include clear cell SQCC as a variant of SQCC.[18,19] Although up to one-third of pulmonary SQCC feature focal clear cell morphology, tumors that are completely composed of clear cells are extremely rare. Instead, it is important to distinguish the clear cell variant from metastatic tumors from other sites. In addition, the clear cell variant may not have prognostic importance. Based on these considerations, the 2015 WHO classification no longer includes these variants from their earlier classification systems.

Squamous dysplasia and **carcinoma in situ** are precursor lesions of SQCC. Microscopically, carcinoma in situ reveals full-thickness cytologic atypia with an increased nuclear-to-cytoplasmic ratio.

The nuclei are hyperchromatic and mitoses may be present. These changes do not extend beyond the basement membrane.

CYTOLOGIC FEATURES OF SQUAMOUS CELL CARCINOMA

In Papanicolaou staining, keratinized cytoplasm reveals glitter yellow, orange, or red (Fig. 92.17). The cytoplasm of SQCC typically has an opaque or dense, hard appearance, and is less translucent than the cytoplasm of adenocarcinomas. In addition, intercellular bridges are also a representative feature of SQCC. Cells often have round, ovoid, or elongated nuclei, with sharply defined cell borders. The nuclei are usually centrally located and hyperchromatic with inconspicuous nucleoli.

ADENOSQUAMOUS CARCINOMA

ASC is a rare tumor of the lung, accounting for only 0.4% to 4% of non–small cell lung carcinoma (NSCLC).[19] ASCs are defined as tumors composed of an admixture of SQCC and adenocarcinoma (ADC). There has been some debate on the proportion of each component required to make the diagnosis of ASC. Takamori and colleagues reported the requirement at least 5% of the opposite component.[156] Fitzgibbons and Kern made a diagnosis of ASC based on the presence of at least 10% of the other component in each case.[157] The Japan Lung Cancer Society has stated that at least 20% of the tumor should be formed by the less dominant variety.[158] The 2004 WHO classification[19] stipulates that at least 10% of each component should be present in ASC as a matter of practical convenience, and the 2015 WHO classification adheres fundamentally to the 2004 definition of ASC.[16] The exact incidence depends on the chosen cut-off value of each component.

These tumors are more often peripheral than central in location. Although Ishida and colleagues[159] reported an almost equal occurrence in men and women, Shimizu and colleagues,[160] in a much larger series (44 patients vs. 11 patients), reported a marked preponderance in men (35:9). Three-fourths of these tumors were >3 cm in size, with a range of 1.5 to 6.0 cm.

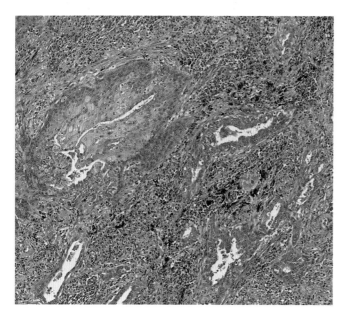

FIGURE 92.18 Adenosquamous carcinoma showing both squamous differentiation (left upper) and glandular differentiation (right lower).

Microscopically, either component may be well, moderately, or poorly differentiated (Fig. 92.18). The squamous cell component was the dominant tumor in the majority of cases in the report by Shimizu and colleagues.[160] Immunohistochemically, pan-keratin stained both the squamous and glandular components, and high–molecular-weight keratin stained primarily the squamous component and not the glandular one. Conversely, low–molecular-weight keratin stained the glandular component slightly more often than the squamous component, but in most cases, it did not stain either component largely. ADC markers, such as TTF-1 and napsin A, are expressed in areas showing glandular differentiation, whereas squamous markers, such as p40, p63, and cytokeratin 5/6, are expressed in the squamous component.[19,161,162] Individual tumor cells usually do not show coexpression of both markers, indicating that the tumor cells of ASC do not bidirectionally differentiate. Molecular studies have tried to address this point of whether ASCs are simple mixes of ADC and SQCC, or if they are highly complex entities at the molecular level. In an experimental study of transcriptome analysis of tumors induced in rats by radon exposure, Bastide and colleagues found that although ASCs consisted of a mix of SQCC and ADC by gene expression, ASCs showed molecular specificities discriminating them from ADC and SQCC.[163] They speculated that ASCs are inherently more complex than admixtures of ADC and SQCC components. The diagnosis of ASC typically does not require IHC analysis with ADC and SQCC markers, because it should be diagnosed only when the discrete differentiated areas are identified within the entire tumor. The IASLC/ATS/ERS multidisciplinary classification of lung carcinoma in small biopsy or cytological specimens recommends making a diagnosis of ASC when both squamous and glandular component are seen. Regarding the tumor grade of ASCs, although there is still insufficient data, cases with undeterminable tumor areas should be graded as poorly differentiated tumors.

ASC is likely to invade blood vessels, and lymph node metastasis occurs in over 50% of patients. The latter was present in 61% of the specimens in Takamori and colleagues' series.[156] The incidence of lymphatic metastasis appears to be greater in patients with a higher percentage of ADC present in the tumor. The cell type of the metastatic disease can vary.

Overall, the prognosis of ASC is poorer than that of either SQCC or ADC. Recently, Maeda and colleagues examined 4,668 patients who underwent resection for primary lung cancer, and found 114 patients (2.4%) with ASC.[164] In their report, the 5-year survival rates were 23.3% for patients with ASC, 58.0% for patients with ADC, and 40.8% for patients with SQCC, and there were statistical differences among the three types. These results support those of many previous studies.[156,157,160,165–168] The reason why ASC tumors behave more aggressively than ADC or SQCC tumors remains unresolved.

The incidence of *EGFR* mutations in ASC is reported to be 13% to 50%.[169–172] However, there are a limited number of studies on the response of ASC lesions to EGFR-TKI therapy.[173–175] The incidence of *KRAS* mutations in ASC is reported to be 4% to 13%.[169,172] *ALK* and *ROS1* rearrangements have also been shown in patients with ASC.[113,176] It should be noted that, at present, molecular tests are needed for patients with ASC as well as for those with ADC.

LARGE CELL CARCINOMA

DEFINITION AND SUBCLASSIFICATION

The concept of LCC has undergone a recent and significant change. According to the 2004 WHO classification, LCC is defined as an undifferentiated NSCLC that lacks the cytological and architectural features of SCLC, ADC, or SQCC.[19] However, even when no histological characteristics of those specific type carcinomas are identified, some cases of LCC demonstrate IHC positivity for napsin A, Clara cell differentiation based on electron microscopy, or *EGFR* mutations by molecular testing. Thus, most traditional LCC is recently considered to be poorly differentiated ADC. In addition, classification of the variants has changed. According to the 2004 WHO classification, there are five variants of LCC: large cell neuroendocrine carcinoma (LCNEC); basaloid carcinoma (BC); lymphoepithelioma-like carcinoma; clear cell carcinoma (CCC); and LCC with rhabdoid phenotype (LCC-RP). Recently, however, BC has been newly classified as a subtype of SQCC, and LCNEC has been newly classified as a subtype of NE carcinoma. Although CCC and LCC-RP have LCC morphology, they are no longer considered subtypes of LCC because undifferentiated carcinoma with entirely clear cell features or with entirely rhabdoid features are extremely rare. Before this paradigm shift, the incidence of the LCC was likely approximately 10%.[177–179] With the new paradigm, the incidence of LCC diminishes to approximately 1%.[17] Over time, and with further molecular classification, the specific designation of LCC might reduce.

GROSS FEATURES

There is no typical gross appearance of LCC. These tumors can occur in either the central or the peripheral zone, although the latter site is somewhat more common. Peripherally located tumors might display cavitation and hemorrhage, but the incidence is less than that seen in peripheral SQCCs (6% vs. 15% to 20%, respectively).

MICROSCOPIC FEATURES

LCCs are composed of stratifying cells without evidence of ADC and SQCC differentiation, such as intercellular bridge formation, keratin production, or glandular formation. Individual cells have enlarged irregular vesicular or hyperchromatic nuclei that might have prominent nucleoli. The cells have abundant cytoplasm and might show a high mitotic rate. In the 2015 WHO classification, LCC is classified into the following three subtypes on the basis of immunohistochemical studies: LCC with null IHC features is undifferentiated carcinoma without expression of markers of ADC or SQCC; LCC with unclear IHC features is undifferentiated carcinoma with a complicated immunoprofile; and LCC with no special staining available is undifferentiated carcinoma with no available IHC studies.

CYTOLOGICAL FEATURES OF LARGE CELL CARCINOMA

Tumor cells of LCC are irregular in size, have abundant cytoplasm and nuclei that show coarse chromatin clumping and prominent nucleoli. In essence, there are no specific cytological features of LCC.

OTHER AND UNCLASSIFIED CARCINOMAS

The 2015 WHO classification includes a new category of "other and unclassified carcinomas," including the following two tumors: lymphoepithelioma-like carcinoma, which was previously considered a type of LCC, and NUT carcinoma.

Lymphoepithelioma-like Carcinoma

Lymphoepithelioma-like carcinoma is an uncommon NSCLC with unique clinical and morphological features. In 1987, Begin and colleagues first reported a primary lung carcinoma that histologically mimicked undifferentiated nasopharyngeal carcinoma and named it lymphoepithelioma-like carcinoma.[180] From 1987 to 2006, more than 150 cases of lymphoepithelioma-like carcinoma have been reported.[181] The characteristics of patients are predominantly young, nonsmoker, and Asian ethnicity. There is a strong association between lymphoepithelioma-like carcinoma and Epstein–Barr virus (EBV) infection,[181–184] and the presence of EBV in the tumor has been demonstrated by PCR for EBV DNA, in-situ hybridization (ISH) studies for EBV DNA and RNA, and immunohistochemistry for EBV-associated proteins. The most characteristic histological feature of this tumor is the infiltration by inflammatory cells, predominantly lymphocytes but also plasma cells, histiocytes, neutrophils, or eosinophils. The demonstration of abundant EBV-encoded small nuclear RNA (EBER) by ISH has become the standard test to show the tumor-specific association of the virus.[181] Most reported cases of this tumor present early and are resectable. Thus, the prognosis of these tumors is thought to be favorable compared to other types of NSCLC.[181,183,184]

NUT-Carcinoma

NUT midline carcinoma is a poorly differentiated SQCC that is genetically defined by rearrangement of the *NUT* gene on chromosome 15q14.[185,186] NUT midline carcinoma typically arises within the midline structures of young individuals; however, it can occur at any age and occasionally outside the midline structures. NUT midline carcinoma of the lung (NC) is extremely rare.[187] The histological features of NCs range from entirely undifferentiated carcinomas to carcinomas with prominent squamous differentiation[188–190] (Fig. 92.19). Immunohistochemically, NCs typically show positivity of pan-cytokeratin and SQCC markers, such as cytokeratin 5/6 and p63. Thus, most cases of NC are initially diagnosed as poorly differentiated SQCC. However, the carcinogenesis of NC is quite different from that of usual SQCC and results from a variety of mutations. Histone acetylation and transcription repression due to *BRD4–NUT* fusion oncogene interference directly causes poorly differentiated carcinomas.[191] Thus, the diagnosis

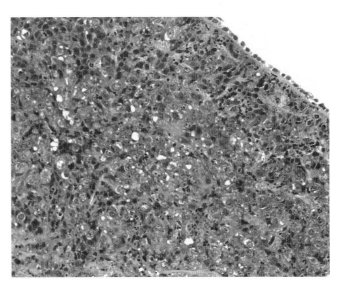

FIGURE 92.19 NUT midline carcinoma. Poorly differentiated tumor cells infiltrate into the bronchial wall.

of NC should be confirmed via IHC staining with the NUT-specific antibody and FISH analysis. NC is an aggressive disease with a median overall survival of 6.7 months.[192] However, the prognosis of NC of the lung remains unclear. Recently, two targeted therapies for NC have emerged.[191,193] IHC or FISH analysis for NC should be considered for pediatric or young adult patients with poorly differentiated SQCC.

CLASSIFICATION OF NEUROENDOCRINE TUMORS OF LUNG

The 2015 WHO classification proposes the following five neuroendocrine tumors of the lung (NETs): (a) diffuse idiopathic pulmonary neuroendocrine cell hyperplasia (DIPNECH), (b) typical carcinoids, (c) atypical carcinoids, (d) LCNECs, and (e) SCLCs.[16] LCNEC was previously classified as a variant of LCC in the 1999 and 2004 WHO classifications.[18,19] However, as many studies show that it is a related lesion of SCLC, LCNEC has been moved to this category from the NSCLC category.

The common histological feature of NETs is NE morphology: nesting architecture, trabecular growth, peripheral palisading patterns, and rosette formation. Moreover, tumors in the category are identified by the presence of one or more of the following substances: (a) neural cell adhesion molecule (CD56), (b) chromogranin A, and (c) synaptophysin. These cells might also be identified by the electron microscopic feature of the presence of neurosecretory granules in the cytoplasm. Travis and colleagues summarized the diagnostic criteria of NE tumors (Table 92.3).[179,194]

DIPNECH is a generalized proliferation of pulmonary NE cells that are confined to the mucosa of airways throughout the lung. It forms diffuse, multifocal, patchy areas that might obstruct the bronchiolar airway, invade locally (Fig. 92.20). The area of growth is slightly enlarged and is referred to as a "tumorlet." Such tumorlets are usually <3 mm in size. Many believe that the DIPNECH lesion is a preinvasive form of typical carcinoid and atypical carcinoid. However, despite this theory, there is no evidence of any connection between DIPNECH and any type of NETs that arises in the lung.

Only the LCNECs and the SCLCs are discussed in this chapter. The typical and atypical carcinoids are presented in Chapter 104.

TABLE 92.3 Criteria for Diagnosis of Neuroendocrine Tumors[18]

Typical Carcinoid

A tumor with carcinoid morphology and <2 mitoses per 2 mm^2 (10 HPF), lacking necrosis and >0.5 cm

Atypical Carcinoid

A tumor with carcinoid morphology with 2–10 mitoses per 2 mm^2 (10 HPF) or necrosis (often punctate)

Large Cell Neuroendocrine Carcinoma (LCNEC)

A tumor with a neuroendocrine morphology (organoid nesting, palisading, rosettes, trabeculae)

High mitotic rate: greater than or equal to 11 per 2 mm^2 (10 HPF), median of 70 per 2 mm^2 (10 HPF)

Necrosis (often large zones)

Cytologic features of a non-small-cell lung carcinoma (NSCLC): large-cell size, low nuclear to cytoplasmic ratio, vesicular or fine chromatin, and/or frequent nucleoli. Some tumors have fine nuclear chromatin and lack nucleoli, but qualify as NSCLC because of large cell size and abundant cytoplasm.

Positive immunohistochemical staining for one or more NE markers (other than neuronspecific enolase) and/or neuroendocrine granules by electron microscopy.

Small Cell Carcinoma (SCLC)

Small size (generally less than the diameter of three small resting lymphocytes)

Scant cytoplasm

Nuclei: finely granular nuclear chromatin, absent or faint nucleoli

High mitotic rate (greater than or equal to 11 per 2 mm^2, median of 80 per 2 mm^2)

Frequent necrosis often in large zones

LARGE CELL NEUROENDOCRINE CARCINOMA

LCNEC was described a fourth subset of NETs of the lung by Travis and colleagues.[195] Most patients with this tumor are heavy-smokers, similar to those with SCLC. Garcia-Yuste and colleagues reported that one-third of these tumors were located centrally and two-thirds peripherally in the lungs.[196] The diagnosis is based on recognition of both NE morphology and the IHC demonstration of at least one specific NE marker.

HISTOLOGIC FEATURES

Grossly, LCNEC is circumscribed with a necrotic, tan-red cut surface,[197] and it usually develops in a peripheral area with a mean size of 3 to 4 cm (range 0.9 to 12 cm).[194,198] Microscopically, the cells of these tumors have NE morphology, including an organoid, trabecular, or palisading pattern (Fig. 92.21). The tumor cells are large, with a low nuclear-to-cytoplasmic ratio and eosinophilic cytoplasm. The nuclei are large with vesicular chromatin and prominent nucleoli, which are distinguishing features from SCLC. Mitotic activity is high with, by definition, more than 10 mitoses per 2 mm^2 (average 60 to 80 mitoses per 2 mm^2). Necrosis is focal or often extensive. When foci of glandular or squamous differentiation might be present, the tumor is considered "combined LCNEC."[194]

IMMUNOHISTOCHEMICAL AND ELECTRON MICROSCOPIC FEATURES

Immunohistochemically, LCNEC tumor cells stain positively for neuron-specific enolase, CEA, and cytokeratins, and stain variably for chromogranin, leu-7, synaptophysin, CD56, and adrenocorticotropic hormone.[195] In 41% to 75% of cases, TTF-1 will be positive.[199,200] The proliferation index by Ki-67 staining is very high, with staining of 50% to 100% of the tumor cells.

Takei and colleagues have suggested the use of three NE markers to identify an LCNEC: neural cell adhesion molecule (CD56), chromogranin A, and synaptophysin.[201] Focal staining by at least one of these three NE markers was deemed to represent a positive NE phenotype. In addition to IHC findings, Travis and colleagues described the electron microscopic features of these tumors, and showed that these tumor cells contain neurosecretory granules and occasionally had glandular differentiation or intercellular junctions.[195] By

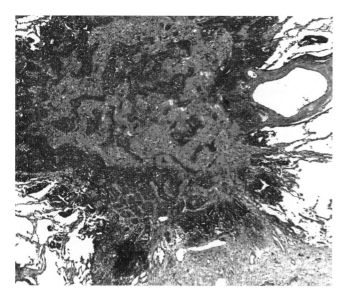

FIGURE 92.20 A tumorlet accompanied by diffuse idiopathic pulmonary neuroendocrine cell hyperplasia (DIPNECH). The tumor shows central fibrous area and ragged, infiltrating edge.

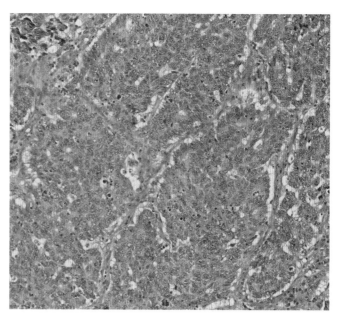

FIGURE 92.21 Large-cell neuroendocrine carcinoma. The tumor has an NE morphology (organoid pattern); tumor cells show a lower nuclear-to-cytoplasmic ratio and prominent nucleoli compared to small cell carcinoma.

definition in the 2004 WHO classification, in addition to identifying NE morphology, it is necessary to stain for NE markers or identify neurosecretory granules by electron microscopy to diagnose LCNEC. The diagnosis of LCNEC is difficult to establish on the basis of small biopsies or cytology, because it is difficult to identify NE morphology and demonstrate NE differentiation by IHC study in such small tissue samples or cytology specimens.[202,203] Careful identification of NE differentiation is necessary to diagnose LCNEC in such specimens.

CLINICAL FEATURES

The clinical course, response to treatment, and prognosis of LCNECs have yet to be determined. However, the majority view suggests that in general, these patients respond poorly to treatment and have a poor prognosis. A review article of NETs of the lung by Travis showed that the clinical outcome for patients with LCNEC tumors was poor, with an overall 5-year survival of 15% to 57%.[203] He concluded that this broad range in the reported outcome might be related to differences in stage distribution, diagnostic criteria, and the extent of surgical staging in the various studies.[196,201,204–212] Several recent studies have shown that LCNEC responds to cisplatin-based chemotherapeutic regimens similar to those used for SCLCs.[213–215] However, as these are retrospective studies of small numbers of patients who received adjuvant therapy following surgery, more validation is needed. Data regarding radiation are insufficient to know whether it is effective in LCNEC.[208]

SMALL CELL LUNG CARCINOMA

Small cell lung carcinomas (SCLCs) grow rapidly and easily metastasize to lymph nodes or other organs; thus, only a few patients with these tumors are considered surgical candidates. Regarding the origin of these lesions, Yesner believes that these tumors arise from the same stem cells that give rise to NSCLC.[216] In contrast, other authors have thought that they arise from basally located NE cells (endodermal Kulchitsky cells) or their precursors. Recently, Yesner's consideration has gained ground because differences are noted between SCLCs and typical and atypical carcinoid (TC/AC), which is thought to arise from Kulchitsky cells. Unlike SCLC or LCNEC, TC/AC often emerges from DIPNECH, TC/AC develops primarily in those who have never smoked, can occur in patients with multiple endocrine neoplasia type (MEN)1, and demonstrates a low frequency of TTF-1 expression. However, the origin of these lesions remains debatable.

The cells of SCLCs have the features of NE cells, including the common expression of amine precursor uptake and decarboxylation cell properties. Although many investigators categorize these tumors as NETs of the lung,[217,218] SCLCs have been considered separately from the other tumors in this category. In the newest WHO classification, however, SCLC is categorized in the NET family because it shares many characteristics with these tumors.

In the 1981 WHO classification (2nd edition), there were three subtypes of SCLC: oat cell carcinoma, intermediate cell type, and combined oat cell carcinoma.[20] However, this categorization was not fully accepted because both the typical oat cell tumors and the intermediate cell tumors have essentially the same clinical behavior.[219–223] Some researchers have suggested that their reported pathologic differences among the subtypes might only be artifacts caused by variations in processing of these tumors for histologic examination.[223] Hirsch and colleagues have classified these tumors as (a) pure SCLC, (b) mixed small cell/large cell carcinoma,

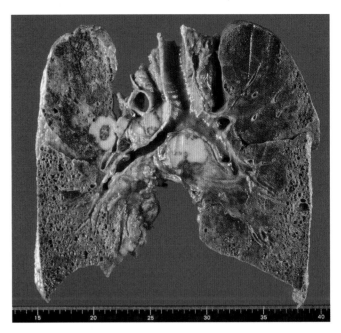

FIGURE 92.22 Small cell carcinoma. The tumor is located in the central area and directly invades the hilar soft part and lymph nodes with metastases into mediastinal lymph nodes (autopsy case).

and (c) combined SCLC with areas of squamous or glandular differentiation. On the basis of the data available at the time, the 2004 WHO classification proposed to subclassify SCLC and combined SCLC, which corresponds to (a) and (b plus c) by Hirsch and colleagues respectively.[19] The frequency of pure SCLC is considered to be approximately 90%, but the truth is unknown because the diagnosis of most SCLC tumors is made only by using small biopsies or cytology specimens.

GROSS FEATURES

The gross observation of SCLC is only possible when the tumor is in a limited stage or when the observation is done at autopsy. It mostly arises in major airways. The tumors are often composed of a mass at the primary site and metastases to the hilar lymph nodes (Fig. 92.22), because they grow very rapidly and metastasize early. The cut surface of SCLCs is typically creamy-white with a soft texture. Central necrosis with cavitation within the tumor or changes in the parenchyma of the lung distal to the tumor occur less frequently than do such changes in SQCCs. The mucosa overlying the tumor in the bronchus is frequently uninvolved, although the normal furrowing of the mucosa might be obliterated.

MICROSCOPIC FEATURES

SCLC is diagnosed histologically primarily based on light microscopy. The tumor cells are round to fusiform and grow in sheets and nests with frequent necrosis that is often extensive (Fig. 92.23). The tumor cells typically have scant cytoplasm and measure less than the diameter of three small resting lymphocytes. The nuclei show molding and are characterized by small, dark, delicate chromatin without prominent nucleoli, characteristics which are more important than cell size in distinguishing SCLC from LCNEC. Tumor nests are supported by a vascular fibrous stroma. The mitotic rate is high, averaging 60 to 80 per 2 mm^2. However, mitoses can be underestimated in

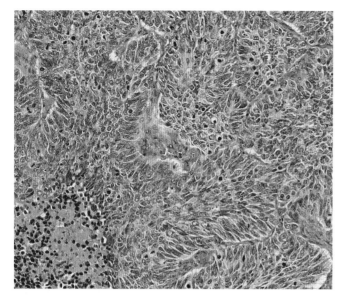

FIGURE 92.23 Small cell lung carcinoma. The tumor is composed of sheets and nests of tumor cells with a high nuclear-to-cytoplasmic ratio demonstrating high mitotic activity.

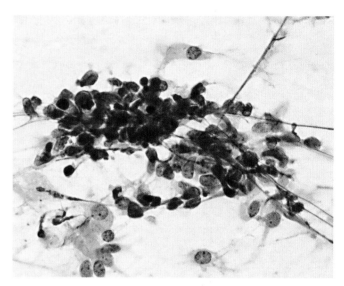

FIGURE 92.24 Cytological appearance of small cell carcinoma (Papanicolaou preparation). Tumor cells have a high nuclear-to-cytoplasmic ratio; the nuclei are characterized by delicate chromatin without the prominent nucleoli. Crush artifact shows a stringy nucleus characteristic for small cell carcinoma.

small biopsy specimens, leading to a mistaken diagnosis of typical or atypical carcinoid if the tumor shows NE morphology. Crushing and distortion of groups of cells, the so-called "crush phenomenon," is characteristic of SCLC, especially in biopsy specimens.

IMMUNOHISTOCHEMICAL AND ELECTRON MICROSCOPIC FEATURES

SCLCs express pan-cytokeratin, such as AE1/AE3, because they are epithelial neoplasms. However, cytokeratin expression in SCLC depends on the subclass. A majority of SCLCs express CK 7, but less frequently than ADC and LCNEC.[224] In contrast, high–molecular-weight CKs, such as CK 1, 5, 10, and 14, which are usually expressed by SQCCs, are not expressed in SCLCs. Approximately 70% to 80% of SCLCs express TTF-1.[199,200] There are several immunohisto-chemically detectable NE antigens: CD56; neuron-specific enolase; protein gene product 9.5; chromogranins; CD57, and synaptophysin. The most widely used in the diagnostic setting of SCLC are chromogranin A, synaptophysin, and CD56. The Ki-67 labeling index of SCLCs is extremely high (80% to 100%). Thus, if the tumor has a low Ki-67 labeling index, it should only carefully be diagnosed as SCLC. Although those IHC antigens are very helpful in the diagnosis of SCLC, Travis emphasized the importance of good quality H&E and cytology specimens to diagnose SCLC.[203]

With the exception of routine H&E and IHC staining, there are some methods to identify NE differentiation. One of the methods is the Glimelius technique, which relies on the binding of silver salts to components of NE substances in the cytoplasm. The other classical method is detection of dense granules in the cytoplasm on electron microscopy.[225,226]

CYTOLOGICAL FEATURES OF SMALL CELL LUNG CARCINOMA

Compared to diagnosis with biopsy specimens, the cytologic diagnosis of SCLC is highly accurate and reliable in most cases due to the crush artifact more commonly seen in biopsy samples than in

cytologic specimens. Tumor cells in the sputum of patients with SCLC appear as single, small groups and have little or no visible cytoplasm, but tumor cells are better preserved in bronchoscopic and FNA samples. Individual SCLC cells are small with round, oval, or spindle-shaped nuclei and scant cytoplasm (Fig. 92.24). Nuclear molding is prominent. Chromatin is uniformly finely divided, and nucleoli are not prominent. Mitotic figures are not as common as might be expected in such proliferative tumors. Necrotic debris is commonly seen in the background.

COMBINED SMALL CELL CARCINOMA

According to the 2004 WHO classification, combined SCLC (combined SCLC) is defined as a tumor composed of an admixture of SCLC and NSCLC, such as ADC, SQCC, LCC, spindle cell carcinoma, or giant cell carcinoma[19] (Fig. 92.25). Adelstein and colleagues noted

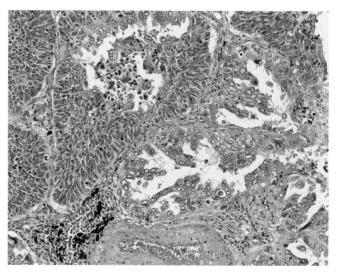

FIGURE 92.25 Combined small cell carcinoma demonstrates both small cell carcinoma area (left upper) and adenocarcinoma area (right lower).

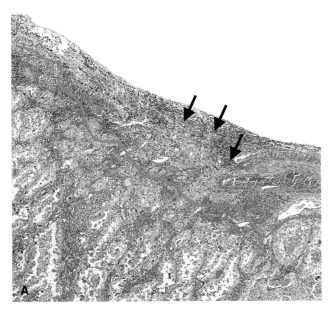
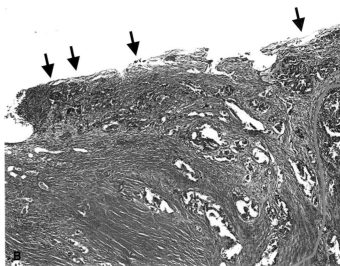

FIGURE 92.26 Visceral pleural invasion. **A:** Tumor cells invade beyond the elastic layer (PL1). **B:** Tumor cells invade the pleural surface (PL2). *Orange lines* and *arrows* indicate the elastic layer and tumor cells, respectively (*Victoria Blue*—H&E staining).

that 10% of their patients with SCLC had a major type of NSCLC present.[227] Nicholson and colleagues reported that combined SCLC might occur in up to 28% of surgically resected cases.[228] Baker at al. and Shepherd et al., as well as others, have observed that the presence of areas of NSCLC in SCLCs tumors increased after chemotherapy.[229,230] In fact, there are times when only NSCLC can be identified in a tumor that was a pure SCLC on the original biopsy specimen. To diagnose combined SCLC, there is no percentage requirement for components of ADC, SQCC, or spindle cell carcinoma, but there should be at least 10% large or giant cells present.[228] When both an SCLC component and an LCNEC component are seen in one tumor, the 2015 WHO classification considers this as combined SCLC rather than combined LCNEC.[16]

PLEURAL INVOLVEMENT BY LUNG CANCER

In the 7th edition of the TNM classification for lung cancer, pleural invasion is classified into the following four categories: PL0, tumor within the subpleural lung parenchyma or superficial invasion into the pleural connective tissue beneath the elastic layer; PL1, tumor invasion beyond the elastic layer; PL2, tumor invasion to the pleural surface; and PL3, tumor invasion into any part of the parietal pleura (Fig. 92.26). Analysis based on a large-scale nationwide Japanese database showed that the overall 5-year survival rates for PL0 (*n* = 3606), PL1 (*n* = 727), PL2 (*n* = 219), and PL3 (*n* = 443) patients were 87%, 77%, 69%, and 54%, respectively. There were significant survival differences between PL0 and PL1, PL1, and PL2, as well as PL2 and PL3.[231]

Pleural lavage cytology (PLC) in the absence of gross pleural seeding with cytologic examination of the cells collected both before and after resection of a lung cancer may identify occult pleural spread. Eagan and colleagues[232] were among the first to note that tumor cells could be present in the pleural cavity in the absence of effusion or gross disease. Since then, numerous studies have shown that PLC status is a prognostic factor for lung cancer.

In general, the frequency of positive PLC is less than 10% among patients with absence of gross pleural seeding. The source of the tumor cells in the pleural space is yet to be determined. Exfoliation of tumor cells, lymphatic invasion within the lung, and vascular invasion have been suggested by the various investigators.[205,233] Once the cells are free within the pleural space, the malignant cell most likely gains access into the general circulation via the parietal pleural lymphatics.

Kameyama et al. extracted the clinicopathological data for 4,171 lung cancer patients who underwent PLC.[234] A total of 217 patients (5.2%) were PLC-positive, which was significantly associated with a higher incidence of adenocarcinoma and advanced disease. Multivariate analysis showed that positive PLC status was an independent factor of poor prognosis. However, PLC findings were not incorporated in the TNM classification.

REFERENCES

1. Kreyberg L, Liebow AA, Uehlinger EA. *Histological Typing of Lung Tumours.* 1st ed. Geneva: World Health Organization; 1967.
2. Paez JG, Janne PA, Lee JC, et al. EGFR mutations in lung cancer: Correlation with clinical response to gefitinib therapy. *Science* 2004;304:1497–1500.
3. Lynch TJ, Bell DW, Sordella R, et al. Activating mutations in the epidermal growth factor receptor underlying responsiveness of non-small-cell lung cancer to gefitinib. *N Engl J Med* 2004;350:2129–2139.
4. Soda M, Choi YL, Enomoto M, et al. Identification of the transforming EML4-ALK fusion gene in non-small-cell lung cancer. *Nature* 2007;448:561–566.
5. Mano H. Non-solid oncogenes in solid tumors: EML4-ALK fusion genes in lung cancer. *Cancer Sci* 2008;99:2349–2355.
6. Kwak EL, Bang YJ, Camidge DR, et al. Anaplastic lymphoma kinase inhibition in non-small-cell lung cancer. *N Engl J Med* 2010;363:1693–1703.
7. Shaw AT, Kim DW, Nakagawa K, et al. Crizotinib versus chemotherapy in advanced ALK-positive lung cancer. *N Engl J Med* 2013;368:2385–2394.
8. Scagliotti GV, Parikh P, von Pawel J, et al. Phase III study comparing cisplatin plus gemcitabine with cisplatin plus pemetrexed in chemotherapy-naive patients with advanced-stage non-small-cell lung cancer. *J Clin Oncol* 2008;26:3543–3551.
9. Sandler A, Gray R, Perry MC, et al. Paclitaxel-carboplatin alone or with bevacizumab for non-small-cell lung cancer. *N Engl J Med* 2006;355:2542–2550.
10. Travis WD, Brambilla E, Noguchi M, et al. International association for the study of lung cancer/american thoracic society/european respiratory society international multidisciplinary classification of lung adenocarcinoma. *J Thorac Oncol* 2011;6: 244–285.
11. Whithaus K, Fukuoka J, Prihoda TJ, et al. Evaluation of napsin A, cytokeratin 5/6, p63, and thyroid transcription factor 1 in adenocarcinoma versus squamous cell carcinoma of the lung. *Arch Pathol Lab Med* 2012;136:155–162.

12. Turner BM, Cagle PT, Sainz IM, et al. Napsin A, a new marker for lung adenocarcinoma, is complementary and more sensitive and specific than thyroid transcription factor 1 in the differential diagnosis of primary pulmonary carcinoma: Evaluation of 1674 cases by tissue microarray. *Arch Pathol Lab Med* 2012;136:163–171.

13. Nicholson AG, Gonzalez D, Shah P, et al. Refining the diagnosis and EGFR status of non-small cell lung carcinoma in biopsy and cytologic material, using a panel of mucin staining, TTF-1, cytokeratin 5/6, and P63, and EGFR mutation analysis. *J Thorac Oncol* 2010;5:436–441.

14. Bishop JA, Teruya-Feldstein J, Westra WH, et al. p40 (DeltaNp63) is superior to p63 for the diagnosis of pulmonary squamous cell carcinoma. *Mod Pathol* 2012; 25:405–415.

15. Nonaka D. A study of DeltaNp63 expression in lung non-small cell carcinomas. *Am J Surg Pathol* 2012;36:895–899.

16. Travis WD, Brambilla E, Burke AP, et al. *WHO Classification of Tumours of the Lung, Pleura, Thymus and Heart.* 4th ed. Geneva: IARC press; 2015.

17. Lewis DR, Check DP, Caporaso NE, et al. US lung cancer trends by histologic type. *Cancer* 2014;120:2883–2892.

18. Travis WD, Colvy TV, Corrin B, et al. *WHO Histological Classification of Tumours, Histological Typing of Lung and Pleural Tumours.* 3rd ed. Berlin: Springer-Verlag; 1999.

19. Travis WD, Brambilla E, Muller-Hermelink HK, et al. *WHO Classification of Tumours, Pathology & Genetics, Tumours of the Lung, Pleura, Thymus and Heart.* Lyon: IARC press; 2004.

20. Kreyberg L. *Histological Typing of Lung Tumours.* 2nd ed. Geneva: World Health Organization; 1981.

21. Noguchi M, Morikawa A, Kawasaki M, et al. Small adenocarcinoma of the lung. Histologic characteristics and prognosis. *Cancer* 1995;75:2844–2852.

22. Suzuki K, Yokose T, Yoshida J, et al. Prognostic significance of the size of central fibrosis in peripheral adenocarcinoma of the lung. *Ann Thorac Surg* 2000;69: 893–897.

23. Yokose T, Suzuki K, Nagai K, et al. Favorable and unfavorable morphological prognostic factors in peripheral adenocarcinoma of the lung 3 cm or less in diameter. *Lung Cancer* 2000;29:179–188.

24. Sakurai H, Maeshima A, Watanabe S, et al. Grade of stromal invasion in small adenocarcinoma of the lung: Histopathological minimal invasion and prognosis. *Am J Surg Pathol* 2004;28:198–206.

25. Ebright MI, Zakowski MF, Martin J, et al. Clinical pattern and pathologic stage but not histologic features predict outcome for bronchioloalveolar carcinoma. *Ann Thorac Surg* 2002;74:1640–1646; discussion 1646–1647.

26. Zell JA, Ou SH, Ziogas A, et al. Epidemiology of bronchioloalveolar carcinoma: Improvement in survival after release of the 1999 WHO classification of lung tumors. *J Clin Oncol* 2005;23:8396–8405.

27. Motoi N, Szoke J, Riely GJ, et al. Lung adenocarcinoma: modification of the 2004 WHO mixed subtype to include the major histologic subtype suggests correlations between papillary and micropapillary adenocarcinoma subtypes, EGFR mutations and gene expression analysis. *Am J Surg Pathol* 2008;32:810–827.

28. Yoshizawa A, Sumiyoshi S, Sonobe M, et al. Validation of the IASLC/ATS/ERS lung adenocarcinoma classification for prognosis and association with EGFR and KRAS gene mutations: Analysis of 440 Japanese patients. *J Thorac Oncol* 2013;8: 52–61.

29. Russell PA, Wainer Z, Wright GM, et al. Does lung adenocarcinoma subtype predict patient survival?: A clinicopathologic study based on the new International Association for the Study of Lung Cancer/American Thoracic Society/European Respiratory Society international multidisciplinary lung adenocarcinoma classification. *J Thorac Oncol* 2011;6:1496–1504.

30. Amin MB, Tamboli P, Merchant SH, et al. Micropapillary component in lung adenocarcinoma: A distinctive histologic feature with possible prognostic significance. *Am J Surg Pathol* 2002;26:358–364.

31. Miyoshi T, Satoh Y, Okumura S, et al. Early-stage lung adenocarcinomas with a micropapillary pattern, a distinct pathologic marker for a significantly poor prognosis. *Am J Surg Pathol* 2003;27:101–109.

32. Roh MS, Lee JI, Choi PJ, et al. Relationship between micropapillary component and micrometastasis in the regional lymph nodes of patients with stage I lung adenocarcinoma. *Histopathology* 2004;45:580–586.

33. Makimoto Y, Nabeshima K, Iwasaki H, et al. Micropapillary pattern: A distinct pathological marker to subclassify tumours with a significantly poor prognosis within small peripheral lung adenocarcinoma (</= 20 mm) with mixed bronchioloalveolar and invasive subtypes (Noguchi's type C tumours). *Histopathology* 2005;46:677–684.

34. Tsutsumida H, Nomoto M, Goto M, et al. A micropapillary pattern is predictive of a poor prognosis in lung adenocarcinoma, and reduced surfactant apoprotein A expression in the micropapillary pattern is an excellent indicator of a poor prognosis. *Mod Pathol* 2007;20:638–647.

35. Kawakami T, Nabeshima K, Makimoto Y, et al. Micropapillary pattern and grade of stromal invasion in pT1 adenocarcinoma of the lung: Usefulness as prognostic factors. *Mod Pathol* 2007;20:514–521.

36. Kamiya K, Hayashi Y, Douguchi J, et al. Histopathological features and prognostic significance of the micropapillary pattern in lung adenocarcinoma. *Mod Pathol* 2008;21:992–1001.

37. Sanchez-Mora N, Presmanes MC, Monroy V, et al. Micropapillary lung adenocarcinoma: A distinctive histologic subtype with prognostic significance. Case series. *Hum Pathol* 2008;39:324–330.

38. Ninomiya H, Hiramatsu M, Inamura K, et al. Correlation between morphology and EGFR mutations in lung adenocarcinomas Significance of the micropapillary pattern and the hobnail cell type. *Lung Cancer* 2009;63:235–240.

39. Nagano T, Ishii G, Nagai K, et al. Structural and biological properties of a papillary component generating a micropapillary component in lung adenocarcinoma. *Lung Cancer* 2010;67:282–289.

40. Zhang J, Liang Z, Gao J, et al. Pulmonary adenocarcinoma with a micropapillary pattern: A clinicopathological, immunophenotypic and molecular analysis. *Histopathology* 2011;59:1204–1214.

41. Sumiyoshi S, Yoshizawa A, Sonobe M, et al. Pulmonary adenocarcinomas with micropapillary component significantly correlate with recurrence, but can be well controlled with EGFR tyrosine kinase inhibitors in the early stages. *Lung Cancer* 2013;81:53–59.

42. Inamura K, Satoh Y, Okumura S, et al. Pulmonary adenocarcinomas with enteric differentiation: Histologic and immunohistochemical characteristics compared with metastatic colorectal cancers and usual pulmonary adenocarcinomas. *Am J Surg Pathol* 2005;29:660–665.

43. Yousem SA. Pulmonary intestinal-type adenocarcinoma does not show enteric differentiation by immunohistochemical study. *Mod Pathol* 2005;18:816–821.

44. Edwards CW. Pulmonary adenocarcinoma: Review of 106 cases and proposed new classification. *J Clin Pathol* 1987;40:125–135.

45. Barsky SH, Huang SJ, Bhuta S. The extracellular matrix of pulmonary scar carcinomas is suggestive of a desmoplastic origin. *Am J Pathol* 1986;124:412–419.

46. Madri JA, Carter D. Scar cancers of the lung: Origin and significance. *Hum Pathol* 1984;15:625–631.

47. Iyoda A, Hiroshima K, Toyozaki T, et al. Clear cell adenocarcinoma with endobronchial polypoid growth. *Pathol Int* 2000;50:979–983.

48. Kodama T, Shimosato Y, Koide T, et al. Endobronchial polypoid adenocarcinoma of the lung. Histological and ultrastructural studies of five cases. *Am J Surg Pathol* 1984;8:845–854.

49. Hishida T, Ishii G, Kodama T, et al. Centrally located adenocarcinoma with endobronchial polypoid growth: clinicopathologic analysis of five cases. *Pathol Int* 2011;61:73–79.

50. Hirata H, Noguchi M, Shimosato Y, et al. Clinicopathologic and immunohistochemical characteristics of bronchial gland cell type adenocarcinoma of the lung. *Am J Clin Pathol* 1990;93:20–25.

51. Girard N, Deshpande C, Lau C, et al. Comprehensive histologic assessment helps to differentiate multiple lung primary nonsmall cell carcinomas from metastases. *Am J Surg Pathol* 2009;33:1752–1764.

52. Yoshizawa A, Motoi N, Riely GJ, et al. Impact of proposed IASLC/ATS/ERS classification of lung adenocarcinoma: prognostic subgroups and implications for further revision of staging based on analysis of 514 stage I cases. *Mod Pathol* 2011;24: 653–664.

53. Warth A, Muley T, Meister M, et al. The novel histologic International Association for the Study of Lung Cancer/American Thoracic Society/European Respiratory Society classification system of lung adenocarcinoma is a stage-independent predictor of survival. *J Clin Oncol* 2012;30:1438–1446.

54. Xu L, Tavora F, Battafarano R, et al. Adenocarcinomas with prominent lepidic spread: Retrospective review applying new classification of the American Thoracic Society. *Am J Surg Pathol* 2012;36:273–282.

55. Yatabe Y, Mitsudomi T, Takahashi T. TTF-1 expression in pulmonary adenocarcinomas. *Am J Surg Pathol* 2002;26:767–773.

56. Kim CF, Jackson EL, Woolfenden AE, et al. Identification of bronchioalveolar stem cells in normal lung and lung cancer. *Cell* 2005;121:823–835.

57. Takeuchi T, Tomida S, Yatabe Y, et al. Expression profile-defined classification of lung adenocarcinoma shows close relationship with underlying major genetic changes and clinicopathologic behaviors. *J Clin Oncol* 2006;24:1679–1688.

58. Shibata T, Hanada S, Kokubu A, et al. Gene expression profiling of epidermal growth factor receptor/KRAS pathway activation in lung adenocarcinoma. *Cancer Sci* 2007;98:985–991.

59. Yamato Y, Tsuchida M, Watanabe T, et al. Early results of a prospective study of limited resection for bronchioloalveolar adenocarcinoma of the lung. *Ann Thorac Surg* 2001;71:971–974.

60. Yamada S, Kohno T. Video-assisted thoracic surgery for pure ground-glass opacities 2 cm or less in diameter. *Ann Thorac Surg* 2004;77:1911–1915.

61. Yoshida J, Nagai K, Yokose T, et al. Limited resection trial for pulmonary ground-glass opacity nodules: Fifty-case experience. *J Thorac Cardiovasc Surg* 2005; 129:991–996.

62. Vazquez M, Carter D, Brambilla E, et al. Solitary and multiple resected adenocarcinomas after CT screening for lung cancer: Histopathologic features and their prognostic implications. *Lung Cancer* 2009;64:148–154.

63. Koike T, Togashi K, Shirato T, et al. Limited resection for noninvasive bronchioloalveolar carcinoma diagnosed by intraoperative pathologic examination. *Ann Thorac Surg* 2009;88:1106–1111.

64. Maeshima AM, Tochigi N, Yoshida A, et al. Histological scoring for small lung adenocarcinomas 2 cm or less in diameter: A reliable prognostic indicator. *J Thorac Oncol* 2010;5:333–339.

65. Kadota K, Villena-Vargas J, Yoshizawa A, et al. Prognostic significance of adenocarcinoma in situ, minimally invasive adenocarcinoma, and nonmucinous lepidic predominant invasive adenocarcinoma of the lung in patients with stage I disease. *Am J Surg Pathol* 2014;38:448–460.

66. Yim J, Zhu LC, Chiriboga L, et al. Histologic features are important prognostic indicators in early stages lung adenocarcinomas. *Mod Pathol* 2007;20:233–241.

67. Borczuk AC, Qian F, Kazeros A, et al. Invasive size is an independent predictor of survival in pulmonary adenocarcinoma. *Am J Surg Pathol* 2009;33:462–469.

68. Lienert T, Serke M, Schonfeld N, et al. Lung cancer in young females. *Eur Respir J* 2000;15:986–990.

69. Westra WH, Baas IO, Hruban RH, et al. K-ras oncogene activation in atypical alveolar hyperplasias of the human lung. *Cancer Res* 1996;56:2224–2228.

70. Sakamoto H, Shimizu J, Horio Y, et al. Disproportionate representation of KRAS gene mutation in atypical adenomatous hyperplasia, but even distribution of EGFR gene mutation from preinvasive to invasive adenocarcinomas. *J Pathol* 2007;212:287–294.

71. Kohno T, Kunitoh H, Shimada Y, et al. Individuals susceptible to lung adenocarcinoma defined by combined HLA-DQA1 and TERT genotypes. *Carcinogenesis* 2010;31:834–841.

72. Yoshida Y, Shibata T, Kokubu A, et al. Mutations of the epidermal growth factor receptor gene in atypical adenomatous hyperplasia and bronchioloalveolar carcinoma of the lung. *Lung Cancer* 2005;50:1–8.

73. Yatabe Y, Kosaka T, Takahashi T, et al. EGFR mutation is specific for terminal respiratory unit type adenocarcinoma. *Am J Surg Pathol* 2005;29:633–639.

74. Kitamura H, Kameda Y, Nakamura N, et al. Atypical adenomatous hyperplasia and bronchoalveolar lung carcinoma. Analysis by morphometry and the expressions of p53 and carcinoembryonic antigen. *Am J Surg Pathol* 1996;20:553–562.

75. Takamochi K, Ogura T, Suzuki K, et al. Loss of heterozygosity on chromosomes 9q and 16p in atypical adenomatous hyperplasia concomitant with adenocarcinoma of the lung. *Am J Pathol* 2001;159:1941–1948.

76. Licchesi JD, Westra WH, Hooker CM, et al. Promoter hypermethylation of hallmark cancer genes in atypical adenomatous hyperplasia of the lung. *Clin Cancer Res* 2008;14:2570–2578.

77. Nakanishi K, Kawai T, Kumaki F, et al. Expression of human telomerase RNA component and telomerase reverse transcriptase mRNA in atypical adenomatous hyperplasia of the lung. *Hum Pathol* 2002;33:697–702.

78. Seki N, Takasu T, Mandai K, et al. Expression of eukaryotic initiation factor 4E in atypical adenomatous hyperplasia and adenocarcinoma of the human peripheral lung. *Clin Cancer Res* 2002;8:3046–3053.

79. Licchesi JD, Westra WH, Hooker CM, et al. Epigenetic alteration of Wnt pathway antagonists in progressive glandular neoplasia of the lung. *Carcinogenesis* 2008;29:895–904.

80. Kerr KM, MacKenzie SJ, Ramasami S, et al. Expression of Fhit, cell adhesion molecules and matrix metalloproteinases in atypical adenomatous hyperplasia and pulmonary adenocarcinoma. *J Pathol* 2004;203:638–644.

81. Carey FA, Wallace WA, Fergusson RJ, et al. Alveolar atypical hyperplasia in association with primary pulmonary adenocarcinoma: A clinicopathological study of 10 cases. *Thorax* 1992;47:1041–1043.

82. Weng SY, Tsuchiya E, Kasuga T, et al. Incidence of atypical bronchioloalveolar cell hyperplasia of the lung: Relation to histological subtypes of lung cancer. *Virchows Arch A Pathol Anat Histopathol* 1992;420:463–471.

83. Rao SK, Fraire AE. Alveolar cell hyperplasia in association with adenocarcinoma of lung. *Mod Pathol* 1995;8:165–169.

84. Nakanishi K. Alveolar epithelial hyperplasia and adenocarcinoma of the lung. *Arch Pathol Lab Med* 1990;114:363–368.

85. Miller RR. Bronchioloalveolar cell adenomas. *Am J Surg Pathol* 1990;14:904–912.

86. Nakayama H, Noguchi M, Tsuchiya R, et al. Clonal growth of atypical adenomatous hyperplasia of the lung: Cytofluorometric analysis of nuclear DNA content. *Mod Pathol* 1990;3:314–320.

87. Nakahara R, Yokose T, Nagai K, et al. Atypical adenomatous hyperplasia of the lung: A clinicopathological study of 118 cases including cases with multiple atypical adenomatous hyperplasia. *Thorax* 2001;56:302–305.

88. Clayton F. Bronchioloalveolar carcinomas. Cell types, patterns of growth, and prognostic correlates. *Cancer* 1986;57:1555–1564.

89. Yatabe Y, Koga T, Mitsudomi T, et al. CK20 expression, CDX2 expression, K-ras mutation, and goblet cell morphology in a subset of lung adenocarcinomas. *J Pathol* 2004;203:645–652.

90. Tsuta K, Ishii G, Nitadori J, et al. Comparison of the immunophenotypes of signet-ring cell carcinoma, solid adenocarcinoma with mucin production, and mucinous bronchioloalveolar carcinoma of the lung characterized by the presence of cytoplasmic mucin. *J Pathol* 2006;209:78–87.

91. Sugano M, Nagasaka T, Sasaki E, et al. HNF4alpha as a marker for invasive mucinous adenocarcinoma of the lung. *Am J Surg Pathol* 2013;37:211–218.

92. Travis WD, Brambilla E, Noguchi M, et al. Diagnosis of lung adenocarcinoma in resected specimens: Implications of the 2011 International Association for the Study of Lung Cancer/American Thoracic Society/European Respiratory Society classification. *Arch Pathol Lab Med* 2013;137:685–705.

93. Fernandez-Cuesta L, Plenker D, Osada H, et al. CD74-NRG1 fusions in lung adenocarcinoma. *Cancer Discov* 2014;4:415–422.

94. Nakaoku T, Tsuta K, Ichikawa H, et al. Druggable oncogene fusions in invasive mucinous lung adenocarcinoma. *Clin Cancer Res* 2014;20:3087–3093.

95. Lantuejoul S, Nicholson AG, Sartori G, et al. Mucinous cells in type 1 pulmonary congenital cystic adenomatoid malformation as mucinous bronchioloalveolar carcinoma precursors. *Am J Surg Pathol* 2007;31:961–969.

96. Yeh YC, Wu YC, Chen CY, et al. Stromal invasion and micropapillary pattern in 212 consecutive surgically resected stage I lung adenocarcinomas: Histopathological categories for prognosis prediction. *J Clin Pathol* 2012;65:910–918.

97. Gu J, Lu C, Guo J, et al. Prognostic significance of the IASLC/ATS/ERS classification in Chinese patients—A single institution retrospective study of 292 lung adenocarcinoma. *J Surg Oncol* 2013;107:474–480.

98. Mansuet-Lupo A, Bobbio A, Blons H, et al. The new histologic classification of lung primary adenocarcinoma subtypes is a reliable prognostic marker and identifies tumors with different mutation status: The experience of a French cohort. *Chest* 2014;146:633–643.

99. Ding L, Getz G, Wheeler DA, et al. Somatic mutations affect key pathways in lung adenocarcinoma. *Nature* 2008;455:1069–1075.

100. Dacic S, Shuai Y, Yousem S, et al. Clinicopathological predictors of EGFR/KRAS mutational status in primary lung adenocarcinomas. *Mod Pathol* 2010;23:159–168.

101. Tsuta K, Kawago M, Inoue E, et al. The utility of the proposed IASLC/ATS/ERS lung adenocarcinoma subtypes for disease prognosis and correlation of driver gene alterations. *Lung Cancer* 2013;81:371–376.

102. Okudela K, Woo T, Mitsui H, et al. Proposal of an improved histological sub-typing system for lung adenocarcinoma—significant prognostic values for stage I disease. *Int J Clin Exp Pathol* 2010;3:348–366.

103. Sica G, Yoshizawa A, Sima CS, et al. A grading system of lung adenocarcinomas based on histologic pattern is predictive of disease recurrence in stage I tumors. *Am J Surg Pathol* 2010;34:1155–1162.

104. Kadota K, Yeh YC, Sima CS, et al. The cribriform pattern identifies a subset of acinar predominant tumors with poor prognosis in patients with stage I lung adenocarcinoma: a conceptual proposal to classify cribriform predominant tumors as a distinct histologic subtype. *Mod Pathol* 2014;27:690–700.

105. Moreira AL, Joubert P, Downey RJ, et al. Cribriform and fused glands are patterns of high-grade pulmonary adenocarcinoma. *Hum Pathol* 2014;45:213–220.

106. Warth A, Muley T, Kossakowski C, et al. Prognostic Impact and Clinicopathological Correlations of the Cribriform Pattern in Pulmonary Adenocarcinoma. *J Thorac Oncol* 2015;10(4):638–644.

107. Silver SA, Askin FB. True papillary carcinoma of the lung: A distinct clinicopathologic entity. *Am J Surg Pathol* 1997;21:43–51.

108. De Oliveira Duarte Achcar R, Nikiforova MN, Yousem SA. Micropapillary lung adenocarcinoma: EGFR, K-ras, and BRAF mutational profile. *Am J Clin Pathol* 2009;131:694–700.

109. Inamura K, Takeuchi K, Togashi Y, et al. EML4-ALK lung cancers are characterized by rare other mutations, a TTF-1 cell lineage, an acinar histology, and young onset. *Mod Pathol* 2009;22:508–515.

110. Rodig SJ, Mino-Kenudson M, Dacic S, et al. Unique clinicopathologic features characterize ALK-rearranged lung adenocarcinoma in the western population. *Clin Cancer Res* 2009;15:5216–5223.

111. Yoshida A, Tsuta K, Nakamura H, et al. Comprehensive histologic analysis of ALK-rearranged lung carcinomas. *Am J Surg Pathol* 2011;35:1226–1234.

112. Takeuchi K, Soda M, Togashi Y, et al. RET, ROS1 and ALK fusions in lung cancer. *Nat Med* 2012;18:378–381.

113. Yoshida A, Kohno T, Tsuta K, et al. ROS1-rearranged lung cancer: A clinicopathologic and molecular study of 15 surgical cases. *Am J Surg Pathol* 2013;37:554–562.

114. Yoshida A, Tsuta K, Wakai S, et al. Immunohistochemical detection of ROS1 is useful for identifying ROS1 rearrangements in lung cancers. *Mod Pathol* 2014;27:711–720.

115. Graeme-Cook F, Mark EJ. Pulmonary mucinous cystic tumors of borderline malignancy. *Hum Pathol* 1991;22:185–190.

116. Davison AM, Lowe JW, Da Costa P. Adenocarcinoma arising in a mucinous cystadenoma of the lung. *Thorax* 1992;47:129–130.

117. Dixon AY, Moran JF, Wesselius LJ, et al. Pulmonary mucinous cystic tumor. Case report with review of the literature. *Am J Surg Pathol* 1993;17:722–728.

118. Kragel PJ, Devaney KO, Meth BM, et al. Mucinous cystadenoma of the lung. A report of two cases with immunohistochemical and ultrastructural analysis. *Arch Pathol Lab Med* 1990;114:1053–1056.

119. Roux FJ, Lantuejoul S, Brambilla E, et al. Mucinous cystadenoma of the lung. *Cancer* 1995;76:1540–1544.

120. Moran CA, Hochholzer L, Fishback N, et al. Mucinous (so-called colloid) carcinomas of lung. *Mod Pathol* 1992;5:634–638.

121. Rossi G, Murer B, Cavazza A, et al. Primary mucinous (so-called colloid) carcinomas of the lung: A clinicopathologic and immunohistochemical study with special reference to CDX-2 homeobox gene and MUC2 expression. *Am J Surg Pathol* 2004;28:442–452.

122. Tsao MS, Fraser RS. Primary pulmonary adenocarcinoma with enteric differentiation. *Cancer* 1991;68:1754–1757.

123. Maeshima A, Miyagi A, Hirai T, et al. Mucin-producing adenocarcinoma of the lung, with special reference to goblet cell type adenocarcinoma: Immunohistochemical observation and Ki-ras gene mutation. *Pathol Int* 1997;47:454–460.

124. Kradin RL, Young RH, Dickersin GR, et al. Pulmonary blastoma with argyrophil cells and lacking sarcomatous features (pulmonary endodermal tumor resembling fetal lung). *Am J Surg Pathol* 1982;6:165–172.

125. Kodama T, Shimosato Y, Watanabe S, et al. Six cases of well-differentiated adenocarcinoma simulating fetal lung tubules in pseudoglandular stage. Comparison with pulmonary blastoma. *Am J Surg Pathol* 1984;8:735–744.

126. Koss MN, Hochholzer L, O'Leary T. Pulmonary blastomas. *Cancer* 1991;67:2368–2381.

127. Nakatani Y, Kitamura H, Inayama Y, et al. Pulmonary adenocarcinomas of the fetal lung type: A clinicopathologic study indicating differences in histology, epidemiology, and natural history of low-grade and high-grade forms. *Am J Surg Pathol* 1998;22:399–411.

128. Mardini G, Pai U, Chavez AM, et al. Endobronchial adenocarcinoma with endometrioid features and prominent neuroendocrine differentiation. A variant of fetal adenocarcinoma. *Cancer* 1994;73:1383–1389.

129. Nakatani Y, Masudo K, Miyagi Y, et al. Aberrant nuclear localization and gene mutation of beta-catenin in low-grade adenocarcinoma of fetal lung type: Up-regulation of the Wnt signaling pathway may be a common denominator for the development of tumors that form morules. *Mod Pathol* 2002;15:617–624.

130. Nakatani Y, Miyagi Y, Takemura T, et al. Aberrant nuclear/cytoplasmic localization and gene mutation of beta-catenin in classic pulmonary blastoma: Beta-catenin immunostaining is useful for distinguishing between classic pulmonary blastoma and a blastomatoid variant of carcinosarcoma. *Am J Surg Pathol* 2004;28:921–927.

131. Sekine S, Shibata T, Matsuno Y, et al. Beta-catenin mutations in pulmonary blastomas: Association with morule formation. *J Pathol* 2003;200:214–221.

132. Wani Y, Notohara K, Nakatani Y, et al. Aberrant nuclear Cdx2 expression in morule-forming tumours in different organs, accompanied by cytoplasmic reactivity. *Histopathology* 2009;55:465–468.
133. Morita S, Yoshida A, Goto A, et al. High-grade lung adenocarcinoma with fetal lung-like morphology: clinicopathologic, immunohistochemical, and molecular analyses of 17 cases. *Am J Surg Pathol* 2013;37:924–932.
134. Li HC, Schmidt L, Greenson JK, et al. Primary pulmonary adenocarcinoma with intestinal differentiation mimicking metastatic colorectal carcinoma: Case report and review of literature. *Am J Clin Pathol* 2009;131:129–133.
135. Maeda R, Isowa N, Onuma H, et al. Pulmonary intestinal-type adenocarcinoma. *Interact Cardiovasc Thorac Surg* 2008;7:349–351.
136. Hatanaka K, Tsuta K, Watanabe K, et al. Primary pulmonary adenocarcinoma with enteric differentiation resembling metastatic colorectal carcinoma: A report of the second case negative for cytokeratin 7. *Pathol Res Pract* 2011;207:188–191.
137. Rodriguez EF, Monaco SE, Dacic S. Cytologic subtyping of lung adenocarcinoma by using the proposed International Association for the Study of Lung Cancer/American Thoracic Society/European Respiratory Society (IASLC/ATS/ERS) adenocarcinoma classification. *Cancer Cytopathol* 2013;121:629–637.
138. Sigel CS, Rudomina DE, Sima CS, et al. Predicting pulmonary adenocarcinoma outcome based on a cytology grading system. *Cancer Cytopathol* 2012;120:35–43.
139. Khuder SA. Effect of cigarette smoking on major histological types of lung cancer: A meta-analysis. *Lung Cancer* 2001;31:139–148.
140. Auerbach O, Garfinkel L. The changing pattern of lung carcinoma. *Cancer* 1991;68:1973–1977.
141. Funai K, Yokose T, Ishii G, et al. Clinicopathologic characteristics of peripheral squamous cell carcinoma of the lung. *Am J Surg Pathol* 2003;27:978–984.
142. Barnes L, Eveson JW, Reichart P, et al. *WHO Classification of Tumours, Pathology & Genetics of Head and Neck Tumours.* Lyon: IARC Press; 2005.
143. Maeshima AM, Maeshima A, Asamura H, et al. Histologic prognostic factors for small-sized squamous cell carcinomas of the peripheral lung. *Lung Cancer* 2006;52:53–58.
144. Takahashi Y, Ishii G, Taira T, et al. Fibrous stroma is associated with poorer prognosis in lung squamous cell carcinoma patients. *J Thorac Oncol* 2011;6:1460–1467.
145. Kadota K, Nitadori J, Woo KM, et al. Comprehensive pathological analyses in lung squamous cell carcinoma: Single cell invasion, nuclear diameter, and tumor budding are independent prognostic factors for worse outcomes. *J Thorac Oncol* 2014;9:1126–1139.
146. Brambilla E, Moro D, Veale D, et al. Basal cell (basaloid) carcinoma of the lung: A new morphologic and phenotypic entity with separate prognostic significance. *Hum Pathol* 1992;23:993–1003.
147. Kim DJ, Kim KD, Shin DH, et al. Basaloid carcinoma of the lung: A really dismal histologic variant? *Ann Thorac Surg* 2003;76:1833–1837.
148. Sturm N, Lantuejoul S, Laverriere MH, et al. Thyroid transcription factor 1 and cytokeratins 1, 5, 10, 14 (34betaE12) expression in basaloid and large-cell neuroendocrine carcinomas of the lung. *Hum Pathol* 2001;32:918–925.
149. Brambilla C, Laffaire J, Lantuejoul S, et al. Lung squamous cell carcinomas with basaloid histology represent a specific molecular entity. *Clin Cancer Res* 2014;20:5777–5786.
150. Moro D, Brichon PY, Brambilla E, et al. Basaloid bronchial carcinoma. A histologic group with a poor prognosis. *Cancer* 1994;73:2734–2739.
151. Moro-Sibilot D, Lantuejoul S, Diab S, et al. Lung carcinomas with a basaloid pattern: A study of 90 cases focusing on their poor prognosis. *Eur Respir J* 2008;31:854–859.
152. Wang LC, Wang L, Kwauk S, et al. Analysis on the clinical features of 22 basaloid squamous cell carcinoma of the lung. *J Cardiothorac Surg* 2011;6:10.
153. Sherwin RP, Laforet EG, Strieder JW. Exophytic endobronchial carcinoma. *J Thorac Cardiovasc Surg* 1962;43:716–730.
154. Dulmet-Brender E, Jaubert F, Huchon G. Exophytic endobronchial epidermoid carcinoma. *Cancer* 1986;57:1358–1364.
155. Travis WD. Pathology of lung cancer. *Clin Chest Med* 2011;32:669–692.
156. Takamori S, Noguchi M, Morinaga S, et al. Clinicopathologic characteristics of adenosquamous carcinoma of the lung. *Cancer* 1991;67:649–654.
157. Fitzgibbons PL, Kern WH. Adenosquamous carcinoma of the lung: A clinical and pathologic study of seven cases. *Hum Pathol* 1985;16:463–466.
158. Society JLC. *General Rules for Clinical and Pathological Recording of Lung Cancer.* 3rd ed. Tokyo: Kanchara; 1987.
159. Ishida T, Kaneko S, Yokoyama H, et al. Adenosquamous carcinoma of the lung. Clinicopathologic and immunohistochemical features. *Am J Clin Pathol* 1992;97:678–685.
160. Shimizu J, Oda M, Hayashi Y, et al. A clinicopathologic study of resected cases of adenosquamous carcinoma of the lung. *Chest* 1996;109:989–994.
161. Jagirdar J. Application of immunohistochemistry to the diagnosis of primary and metastatic carcinoma to the lung. *Arch Pathol Lab Med* 2008;132:384–396.
162. Nobre AR, Albergaria A, Schmitt F. p40: a p63 isoform useful for lung cancer diagnosis—a review of the physiological and pathological role of p63. *Acta Cytol* 2013;57:1–8.
163. Bastide K, Ugolin N, Levalois C, et al. Are adenosquamous lung carcinomas a simple mix of adenocarcinomas and squamous cell carcinomas, or more complex at the molecular level? *Lung Cancer* 2010;68:1–9.
164. Maeda H, Matsumura A, Kawabata T, et al. Adenosquamous carcinoma of the lung: Surgical results as compared with squamous cell and adenocarcinoma cases. *Eur J Cardiothorac Surg* 2012;41:357–361.
165. Naunheim KS, Taylor JR, Skosey C, et al. Adenosquamous lung carcinoma: Clinical characteristics, treatment, and prognosis. *Ann Thorac Surg* 1987;44:462–466.
166. Riquet M, Perrotin C, Lang-Lazdunski L, et al. Do patients with adenosquamous carcinoma of the lung need a more aggressive approach? *J Thorac Cardiovasc Surg* 2001;122:618–619.
167. Nakagawa K, Yasumitu T, Fukuhara K, et al. Poor prognosis after lung resection for patients with adenosquamous carcinoma of the lung. *Ann Thorac Surg* 2003;75:1740–1744.
168. Gawrychowski J, Brulinski K, Malinowski E, et al. Prognosis and survival after radical resection of primary adenosquamous lung carcinoma. *Eur J Cardiothorac Surg* 2005;27:686–692.
169. Toyooka S, Yatabe Y, Tokumo M, et al. Mutations of epidermal growth factor receptor and K-ras genes in adenosquamous carcinoma of the lung. *Int J Cancer* 2006;118:1588–1590.
170. Kang SM, Kang HJ, Shin JH, et al. Identical epidermal growth factor receptor mutations in adenocarcinomatous and squamous cell carcinomatous components of adenosquamous carcinoma of the lung. *Cancer* 2007;109:581–587.
171. Ohtsuka K, Ohnishi H, Fujiwara M, et al. Abnormalities of epidermal growth factor receptor in lung squamous-cell carcinomas, adenosquamous carcinomas, and large-cell carcinomas: Tyrosine kinase domain mutations are not rare in tumors with an adenocarcinoma component. *Cancer* 2007;109:741–750.
172. Jia XL, Chen G. EGFR and KRAS mutations in Chinese patients with adenosquamous carcinoma of the lung. *Lung Cancer* 2011;74:396–400.
173. Mitsudomi T, Kosaka T, Endoh H, et al. Mutations of the epidermal growth factor receptor gene predict prolonged survival after gefitinib treatment in patients with non-small-cell lung cancer with postoperative recurrence. *J Clin Oncol* 2005;23:2513–2520.
174. Shukuya T, Takahashi T, Kaira R, et al. Efficacy of gefitinib for non-adenocarcinoma non-small-cell lung cancer patients harboring epidermal growth factor receptor mutations: A pooled analysis of published reports. *Cancer Sci* 2011;102:1032–1037.
175. Paik PK, Varghese AM, Sima CS, et al. Response to erlotinib in patients with EGFR mutant advanced non-small cell lung cancers with a squamous or squamous-like component. *Mol Cancer Ther* 2012;11:2535–2540.
176. Wang R, Pan Y, Li C, et al. Analysis of major known driver mutations and prognosis in resected adenosquamous lung carcinomas. *J Thorac Oncol* 2014;9:760–768.
177. Shinton NK. The histological classification of lower respiratory tract tumours. *Br J Cancer* 1963;17:213–221.
178. Yesner R, Carter D. Pathology of carcinoma of the lung. Changing patterns. *Clin Chest Med* 1982;3:257–289.
179. Travis WD, Travis LB, Devesa SS. Lung cancer. *Cancer* 1995;75:191–202.
180. Begin LR, Eskandari J, Joncas J, et al. Epstein-Barr virus related lymphoepithelioma-like carcinoma of the lung. *J Surg Oncol* 1987;36:280–283.
181. Ho JC, Wong MP, Lam WK. Lymphoepithelioma-like carcinoma of the lung. *Respirology* 2006;11:539–545.
182. Chan JK, Hui PK, Tsang WY, et al. Primary lymphoepithelioma-like carcinoma of the lung. A clinicopathologic study of 11 cases. *Cancer* 1995;76:413–422.
183. Han AJ, Xiong M, Gu YY, et al. Lymphoepithelioma-like carcinoma of the lung with a better prognosis. A clinicopathologic study of 32 cases. *Am J Clin Pathol* 2001;115:841–850.
184. Chang YL, Wu CT, Shih JY, et al. New aspects in clinicopathologic and oncogene studies of 23 pulmonary lymphoepithelioma-like carcinomas. *Am J Surg Pathol* 2002;26:715–723.
185. Kubonishi I, Takehara N, Iwata J, et al. Novel t(15;19)(q15;p13) chromosome abnormality in a thymic carcinoma. *Cancer Res* 1991;51:3327–3328.
186. French CA, Kutok JL, Faquin WC, et al. Midline carcinoma of children and young adults with NUT rearrangement. *J Clin Oncol* 2004;22:4135–4139.
187. Tanaka M, Kato K, Gomi K, et al. NUT midline carcinoma: Report of 2 cases suggestive of pulmonary origin. *Am J Surg Pathol* 2012;36:381–388.
188. French CA. NUT midline carcinoma. *Cancer Genet Cytogenet* 2010;203:16–20.
189. Evans AG, French CA, Cameron MJ, et al. Pathologic characteristics of NUT midline carcinoma arising in the mediastinum. *Am J Surg Pathol* 2012;36:1222–1227.
190. Suzuki S, Kurabe N, Ohnishi I, et al. NSD3-NUT-expressing midline carcinoma of the lung: First characterization of primary cancer tissue. *Pathol Res Pract* 2015;211(5):404–408.
191. Schwartz BE, Hofer MD, Lemieux ME, et al. Differentiation of NUT midline carcinoma by epigenomic reprogramming. *Cancer Res* 2011;71:2686–2696.
192. Bauer DE, Mitchell CM, Strait KM, et al. Clinicopathologic features and long-term outcomes of NUT midline carcinoma. *Clin Cancer Res* 2012;18:5773–5779.
193. Filippakopoulos P, Qi J, Picaud S, et al. Selective inhibition of BET bromodomains. *Nature* 2010;468:1067–1073.
194. Travis WD, Rush W, Flieder DB, et al. Survival analysis of 200 pulmonary neuroendocrine tumors with clarification of criteria for atypical carcinoid and its separation from typical carcinoid. *Am J Surg Pathol* 1998;22:934–944.
195. Travis WD, Linnoila RI, Tsokos MG, et al. Neuroendocrine tumors of the lung with proposed criteria for large-cell neuroendocrine carcinoma. An ultrastructural, immunohistochemical, and flow cytometric study of 35 cases. *Am J Surg Pathol* 1991;15:529–553.
196. Garcia-Yuste M, Matilla JM, Alvarez-Gago T, et al. Prognostic factors in neuroendocrine lung tumors: A Spanish Multicenter Study. Spanish Multicenter Study of Neuroendocrine Tumors of the Lung of the Spanish Society of Pneumonology and Thoracic Surgery (EMETNE-SEPAR). *Ann Thorac Surg* 2000;70:258–34.
197. Oshiro Y, Kusumoto M, Matsuno Y, et al. CT findings of surgically resected large cell neuroendocrine carcinoma of the lung in 38 patients. *AJR Am J Roentgenol* 2004;182:87–91.
198. Iyoda A, Hiroshima K, Toyozaki T, et al. Clinical characterization of pulmonary large cell neuroendocrine carcinoma and large cell carcinoma with neuroendocrine morphology. *Cancer* 2001;91:1992–2000.
199. Folpe AL, Gown AM, Lamps LW, et al. Thyroid transcription factor-1: Immunohistochemical evaluation in pulmonary neuroendocrine tumors. *Mod Pathol* 1999;12:5–8.

200. Sturm N, Rossi G, Lantuejoul S, et al. Expression of thyroid transcription factor-1 in the spectrum of neuroendocrine cell lung proliferations with special interest in carcinoids. *Hum Pathol* 2002;33:175–182.
201. Takei H, Asamura H, Maeshima A, et al. Large cell neuroendocrine carcinoma of the lung: A clinicopathologic study of eighty-seven cases. *J Thorac Cardiovasc Surg* 2002;124:285–292.
202. Hiroshima K, Abe S, Ebihara Y, et al. Cytological characteristics of pulmonary large cell neuroendocrine carcinoma. *Lung Cancer* 2005;48:331–337.
203. Travis WD. Advances in neuroendocrine lung tumors. *Ann Oncol* 2010;21(Suppl 7): vii65–71.
204. Asamura H, Nakayama H, Kondo H, et al. Lymph node involvement, recurrence, and prognosis in resected small, peripheral, non-small-cell lung carcinomas: Are these carcinomas candidates for video-assisted lobectomy? *J Thorac Cardiovasc Surg* 1996;111:1125–1134.
205. Dresler CM, Fratelli C, Babb J. Prognostic value of positive pleural lavage in patients with lung cancer resection. *Ann Thorac Surg* 1999;67:1435–1439.
206. Iyoda A, Hiroshima K, Baba M, et al. Pulmonary large cell carcinomas with neuroendocrine features are high-grade neuroendocrine tumors. *Ann Thorac Surg* 2002;73:1049–1054.
207. Zacharias J, Nicholson AG, Ladas GP, et al. Large cell neuroendocrine carcinoma and large cell carcinomas with neuroendocrine morphology of the lung: Prognosis after complete resection and systematic nodal dissection. *Ann Thorac Surg* 2003;75:348–352.
208. Paci M, Cavazza A, Annessi V, et al. Large cell neuroendocrine carcinoma of the lung: A 10-year clinicopathologic retrospective study. *Ann Thorac Surg* 2004; 77:1163–1167.
209. Doddoli C, Barlesi F, Chetaille B, et al. Large cell neuroendocrine carcinoma of the lung: An aggressive disease potentially treatable with surgery. *Ann Thorac Surg* 2004;77:1168–1172.
210. Veronesi G, Morandi U, Alloisio M, et al. Large cell neuroendocrine carcinoma of the lung: A retrospective analysis of 144 surgical cases. *Lung Cancer* 2006;53:111–115.
211. Iyoda A, Hiroshima K, Moriya Y, et al. Prognostic impact of large cell neuroendocrine histology in patients with pathologic stage Ia pulmonary non-small cell carcinoma. *J Thorac Cardiovasc Surg* 2006;132:312–315.
212. Iyoda A, Hiroshima K, Nakatani Y, et al. Pulmonary large cell neuroendocrine carcinoma: Its place in the spectrum of pulmonary carcinoma. *Ann Thorac Surg* 2007;84:702–707.
213. Rossi G, Cavazza A, Marchioni A, et al. Role of chemotherapy and the receptor tyrosine kinases KIT, PDGFRalpha, PDGFRbeta, and Met in large-cell neuroendocrine carcinoma of the lung. *J Clin Oncol* 2005;23:8774–8785.
214. Yamazaki S, Sekine I, Matsuno Y, et al. Clinical responses of large cell neuroendocrine carcinoma of the lung to cisplatin-based chemotherapy. *Lung Cancer* 2005;49:217–223.
215. Iyoda A, Hiroshima K, Moriya Y, et al. Prospective study of adjuvant chemotherapy for pulmonary large cell neuroendocrine carcinoma. *Ann Thorac Surg* 2006;82:1802–1807.
216. Yesner R. *Heterogenicity of Small Cell Carcinoma of the Lung.* Austin, TX: University of Texas Press; 1986.
217. Gould VE, Linnoila RI, Memoli VA, et al. Neuroendocrine components of the bronchopulmonary tract: Hyperplasias, dysplasias, and neoplasms. *Lab Invest* 1983;49:519–537.
218. Travis WD. Classification of neuroendocrine tumors of the lung. *Lung Cancer* 1994; 11(Suppl 2):197.
219. Carney DN, Matthews MJ, Ihde DC, et al. Influence of histologic subtype of small cell carcinoma of the lung on clinical presentation, response to therapy, and survival. *J Natl Cancer Inst* 1980;65:1225–1230.
220. Choi H, Byhardt RW, Clowry LJ, et al. The prognostic significance of histologic subtyping in small cell carcinoma of the lung. *Am J Clin Oncol* 1984;7:389–397.
221. Bepler G, Neumann K, Holle R, et al. Clinical relevance of histologic subtyping in small cell lung cancer. *Cancer* 1989;64:74–79.
222. Hirsch FR, Osterlind K, Hansen HH. The prognostic significance of histopathologic subtyping of small cell carcinoma of the lung according to the classification of the World Health Organization. A study of 375 consecutive patients. *Cancer* 1983;52:2144–2150.
223. Hirsch FR, Matthews MJ, Aisner S, et al. Histopathologic classification of small cell lung cancer. Changing concepts and terminology. *Cancer* 1988;62:973–977.
224. Nagashio R, Sato Y, Matsumoto T, et al. Significant high expression of cytokeratins 7, 8, 18, 19 in pulmonary large cell neuroendocrine carcinomas, compared to small cell lung carcinomas. *Pathol Int* 2010;60:71–77.
225. Bensch KG, Corrin B, Pariente R, et al. Oat-cell carcinoma of the lung. Its origin and relationship to bronchial carcinoid. *Cancer* 1968;22:1163–1172.
226. Warren WH, Gould VE, Faber LP, et al. Neuroendocrine neoplasms of the bronchopulmonary tract. A classification of the spectrum of carcinoid to small cell carcinoma and intervening variants. *J Thorac Cardiovasc Surg* 1985;89:819–825.
227. Adelstein DJ, Tomashefski JF Jr, Snow NJ, et al. Mixed small cell and non-small cell lung cancer. *Chest* 1986;89:699–704.
228. Nicholson SA, Beasley MB, Brambilla E, et al. Small cell lung carcinoma (SCLC): A clinicopathologic study of 100 cases with surgical specimens. *Am J Surg Pathol* 2002;26:1184–1197.
229. Baker RR, Ettinger DS, Ruckdeschel JD, et al. The role of surgery in the management of selected patients with small-cell carcinoma of the lung. *J Clin Oncol* 1987;5:697–702.
230. Shepherd FA, Ginsberg RJ, Patterson GA, et al. A prospective study of adjuvant surgical resection after chemotherapy for limited small cell lung cancer. A University of Toronto Lung Oncology Group study. *J Thorac Cardiovasc Surg* 1989;97:177–186.
231. Kawase A, Yoshida J, Miyaoka E, et al. Visceral pleural invasion classification in non-small-cell lung cancer in the 7th edition of the tumor, node, metastasis classification for lung cancer: Validation analysis based on a large-scale nationwide database. *J Thorac Oncol* 2013;8:606–611.
232. Eagan RT, Bernatz PE, Payne WS et al. Pleural lavage after pulmonary resection for bronchogenic carcinoma. *J Thorac Cardiovasc Surg* 1984;88:1000–1003.
233. Aokage K, Yoshida J, Ishii G, et al. The impact of survival of positive intraoperative pleural cytology in patients with non-small-cell lung cancer. *J Thorac Cardiovasc Surg* 2010;139:1246–1252.
234. Kameyama K, Okumura N, Miyaoka E, et al. Prognostic value of intraoperative pleural lavage cytology for non-small cell lung cancer: The influence of positive pleural lavage cytology results on T classification. *J Thorac Cardiovasc Surg* 2014;148:2659–2664.

Ex Vivo Diagnosis of Lung Cancer

Chadrick E. Denlinger ▪ Jacob A. Klapper

INTRODUCTION

Lung cancer remains the leading cause of cancer-related mortality among both men and women in the United States where it accounts for 26.5% of cancer deaths.[1] The most significant contributor to this statistic is the fact that the majority of patients present with advanced stage disease which is associated with a 16% 5-year survival. Several studies have conclusively demonstrated that lung cancer screening with chest radiographs and sputum cytology is not effective for enhancing the early detection of lung cancer.[2–5] However, the National Lung Screening Trial (NLST) demonstrated a 20% reduction in overall mortality among high-risk patients screened with an annual low-dose chest CT scan compared to those screened with annual chest radiographs leading to the adoption of screening programs in many centers.[6] The NLST identified lung nodules in 22% of all screened patients, but only approximately 4% of identified nodules were malignant. The high rate of benign lung nodules and the cost of CT screening of high-risk patients are two concerns associated with the broad application of CT screening programs.

Over the past decade an increasing number of investigations have been conducted that explored additional means, other than radiographic studies, that can be utilized to detect lung cancers and other malignancies. Broadly described as biomarkers, investigators have probed for various genetic, molecular, metabolic, and other means of identifying the presence of cancer in patients who remain asymptomatic. In addition to a wide spectrum of analytes probed, the specimen source also varies widely. Studies have been conducted on samples from peripheral blood, saliva, bronchoalveolar lavage fluid, urine, and biopsies of non-affected central airway. Currently, each of these ex vivo techniques for the identification of lung cancer or risk stratification of known lung nodules lacks sufficient validation for clinical utility, but some will likely enter the clinical realm in the next several years. The following chapter is outlined to demonstrate work that has been conducted to date for each of the respective analyte categories.

MICRORNA

MicroRNAs (miR) are a recently discovered component of the regulatory mechanism impacting the expression of specific target genes. miRs are endogenous short fragments, measuring 18 to 22 nucleotides, of noncoding RNA which are not translated for protein expression. Instead, miRs are antisense strands of RNA that anneal to messenger RNA (mRNA) creating segments of double-stranded RNA which are recognized as viral RNA by the cell and degraded. Some double-stranded RNA are not degraded, but gene translation still blocked because the double-stranded RNA is not able to pass through the ribosome. miRs are initially transcribed as longer segments of primary microRNA that is cleaved by the enzyme slicer/RNAse III in to pre-microRNAs which are further cleaved by the enzyme Dicer into mature miRs (Fig. 93.1). While the specific roles of many miRs are still being investigated in various disease processes, it is known that miRs can act as tumor suppressors or oncogenes and that miR dysregulation participates in cancer development and progression.[7,8] The recognition of altered expression in diseases may prove clinically useful as biomarkers. Numerous different miRs have been implicated as playing oncogenic, tumor suppressor, or mixed roles in the pathogenesis of lung cancers as indicated in Table 93.1.[9] Two important characteristics of miRs regarding their use as biomarkers are that they are readily secreted from cells and they are remarkably stable, unlike full-length RNA that is rapidly degraded by RNAse. For these reasons, miRs have been frequently studied by numerous different investigators looking to establish reliable assays for the early detection of malignancies including lung cancer.

Numerous investigators have evaluated the relative abundances of specific miRs in diseases such as congestive heart failure, aortic aneurysms, cirrhosis, and numerous types of cancer including lung

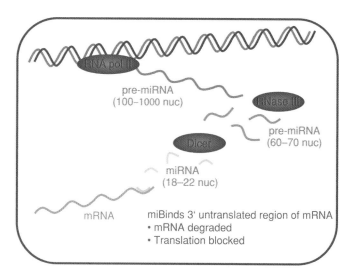

FIGURE 93.1 miRs are initially transcribed from DNA with RNA polymerase as long segments of primary mRNA that are sequentially cleaved by RNAse III and Dicer into pre-miRNA and mature miRNA, respectively. The mature miRNA binds to messenger RNA (mRNA) and inhibits its translation into protein either inducing its degradation or by blocking its binding with ribosomes.

TABLE 93.1 miRs Implicated in the Pathogenesis of Lung Cancer

Oncogenic	Tumor Suppressors			Mixed Oncogenic/ Tumor Suppressor
miR 17 Cluster	Let-7 family			miR 7
miR 17	Let-7a-1	Let-7e	miR-98	miR 31
miR 18a	Let-7a-2	Let-7f-1	miR202	miR 125a
miR 19a	Let-7a-3	Let-7f-2		miR 125b
miR 19b-1	Let-7b	Let-7g		miR 183
miR 20a	Let-7c	Let-7h		miR 182
miR 92a-1	Let-7d	Let-7i		miR 96
miR 21	miR 34/499 family			
miR 221/222	miR 34a	miR 449b		
miR 494	miR 34b/c	miR 449c		
miR 27a	miR 449a			
miR 328	miR 15a			
miR 301	miR 16-1			
miR 93	miR 200 family			
miR 98	miR 200a	miR 429		
miR 197	miR 200b	miR 141		
miR 20	miR 200c			
miR 106	miR 205	miR 15b	miR 16-2	
miR 150	miR 143	miR 145		
	miR 29 Family			
	miR 29a			
	miR 29b			
	miR 29c			
	miR-1	miR-126		
	miR-133	miR-128		
	miR-206	miR-206		

cancer. Recent findings suggest that human plasma contains stable miRs that are available for detection as tumor markers indicating the presence of cancer in patients currently lacking a diagnosis. They may also be useful for indicating cancer recurrence among patients previously treated. In addition, circulating miR concentration profiles may also provide prognostic information through the identification of signature patterns predictive of either a greater or lower risk for cancer recurrence.

Currently, the most frequently studied circulating miR in many cancers including nonsmall-cell lung cancer (NSCLC) is miR-21 which has been shown to relate to cellular proliferation, survival, invasion, and cancer cell migration.[10,11] Numerous studies investigating the prognostic value of miR-21 in tissue-based studies have demonstrated that increased expression of miR-21 correlated with a shorter disease-free and overall survival among patients with cancers of various disease sites, including studies focused exclusively on patients with lung cancer.[12] Furthermore, investigations that assessed miR-21 in serum-based assays also demonstrated its negative prognostic value.[13] Two recent meta-analyses of studies investigating the potential of using circulating miR-21 as a biomarker to determine the presence of cancer identified variable and conflicting results.[14,15] Unfortunately, the conclusions of these analyses were

that the negative and positive predictive values of circulating miR-21 are not sufficient to be of clinical use for the diagnosis or exclusion of cancer.

In a different retrospective study of 11 patients with stage I to II NSCLC undergoing surgical resection, serum levels of 10 different miRs were evaluated (miR-126, miR-150, miR-155, miR-205, miR-21, miR-210, miR-26b, miR-34a, miR-451, and miR-486) and compared to 11 healthy patients.[16] In this analysis only miR-486 and miR-150 were elevated among the patients with NSCLC compared to the healthy control patients who were well matched with regard to age and gender. miR-150 is of particular interest because one of its gene transcript targets is the tumor suppressor p53. Interestingly, miR-21 was not noted to be different between the groups with and without advanced cancer. Furthermore, although the study population was small, trends favoring improved long-term survival were noted among patients with the greatest decline in miR-486 concentrations following surgery. Others have noted that miR-486 expression in advanced stage NSCLC correlates with an increased risk for disease progression, and the authors also correlated expression of miR-486 in tumor tissue with elevated plasma levels of the same miR.[17] These studies suggest that miR-486 may be expressed in lung cancer tissue and detected in peripheral blood.

Others have also related miR expression levels with long-term survival data. miR-210 expression in 60 patients with NSCLC (adenocarcinoma and squamous cell carcinoma) was significantly greater than a comparison group of 30 healthy individuals.[18] Receiver operating characteristic (ROC) curves for miR-210 had an area under the curve of 0.775 for differentiating patients with and without cancer. In addition, patients with more advanced disease stages or lymph node metastases demonstrated a greater elevation of miR-210 expression. Specifically, patients with stage III to IV disease had significantly greater serum levels of miR-210 than patients with stage I to II disease. Furthermore, patients who experienced a strong clinical response to systemic treatment were also observed to have significant decreases in miR-210 expression over the course of their therapy.

miR biomarkers have also been evaluated in bronchoalveolar lavage fluid and sputum for the detection of lung cancers. This carries the intuitive appeal of concentrated markers being present in biologic fluids more directly associated with a presumptive malignant tumor although collection of the bronchoalveolar lavage fluid is more invasive than a blood assay. In a single study comparing sputum and bronchoalveolar lavage fluids, Kim et al. identified a miR panel comprised of miR-21, miR-143 (downregulated), miR-155, miR-210, and miR-372 that classified patients with NSCLC with a sensitivity and specificity of 85.7% and 100%, respectively, using bronchoalveolar lavage fluids.[19] The sensitivity and specificity of the same miR panel in sputum samples were 67.8% and 90%, respectively. Importantly, each patient in this study had stage I or II NSCLC with a mean tumor size of 2.2 cm. A slight majority of these patients had adenocarcinoma histology while the remaining patients had either squamous cell or large cell carcinoma. These results validated a previous study published by the same group of investigators who evaluated the exact same panel of five miRs in the sputum of patients with or without NSCLC.[20]

Although the biomarkers that become elevated rather than depressed in disease states receive the greatest attention because of difficulties conceptualizing how a tumor may have a large enough impact to quench systemic reserves of a given biomarker, some authors have correlated depressed biomarkers with the presence of lung cancer. For example, Li et al. compared systemic levels of miR-148a, miR-148b, and miR-152 of patients with lung cancers of all stages to patients who were either healthy or had other benign lung diseases. Each of these three miRs was depressed among patients with lung cancer compared to the other groups. Furthermore, the greatest depression was observed among patients with larger tumors and patients known to have lymph node metastases.[21] The negative prognostic value of miR-148b among patients with lung cancer was validated in an independent study which demonstrated at the tissue level that downregulation of miR-148b was associated with a greater risk for lymph node metastases and a worse overall survival.[22]

Noting inadequacies of our current staging system for predicting long-term outcomes, investigators have assessed whether or not miR expression may convey additional prognostic information beyond the traditional TNM staging system. Using a broad assessment of serum miR levels in two pilot groups of patients with long and short survival that were well matched with regard to cancer stage and smoking status, more than 100 miRs were identified in each group. miRs with the greatest differential expression between the two groups were then further evaluated in larger training and validation groups using quantitative reverse transcription polymerase chain reaction (qRT-PCR). This revealed four specific miRs (miR-486, miR-30d, miR-1, and miR-499) that were most consistently elevated among patients with a poor long-term survival.[23] Previous studies identified different miRs with prognostic implications when analyzed in resected tissue

specimens. Taken together, these data suggest that miRs measured at the serum level may have prognostic implication.

MIDDLE-SIZED RNA

In addition to miRs, additional small fragments of RNA present in the nucleolus that range in size from 20 to 200 nucleotides which have been called small nucleolar RNAs (snoRNA). Not surprisingly, snoRNAs have also been associated with the development of lung cancer. Comparisons between malignant and adjacent nonmalignant lung tissue have identified differential expression of six different snoRNAs (snoRD33, snoRD66, snoRA73B, snoRD76, snoRD78, and snoRA42) and an even greater list of differentially expressed snoRNAs have been described by others.[24,25] Based on these findings, the same group later measured the levels of each of these snoRNAs in the sputum of a cohort of patients with lung cancer and compared them to a similar group of control patients without cancer.[26] Four of the six snoRNAs had a differential expression between patients with and without cancer and snoRD66 and snoRD78 were the best at discriminating between the two groups with ROC curve area under the curve values of 0.80 and 0.81, respectively. When combined, snoRD66 and snoRD78 had an area under the curve of 0.86 indicating a reasonable ability to discriminating between patients with and without lung cancer.

In a completely independent study, the differential expression of snoRNAs in NSLSC also revealed correlations between specific snoRNAs and long-term survival.[24] Interestingly, the two snoRNAs with the strongest correlation with long-term prognosis were snoRD66 and snoRA78 which were also the best at differentiating between malignant and nonmalignant tissues. While using snoRNAs for the early diagnosis of lung cancer remains in its infancy, collectively these independent studies suggest that they may play some role and they are certainly detectable in readily available biologic fluids such as sputum.

LONG-SEGMENT RNA

Surprisingly, sequencing of the human genome revealed that less than 3% of our DNA is comprised of genes which code for specific known proteins, yet more than 80% of our genome is transcribed into RNA[27] (Fig. 93.2). These transcripts which are not related to translated proteins are appropriately referred to as noncoding RNA.[27] Long noncoding RNAs (lncRNAs) are defined as segments ranging from

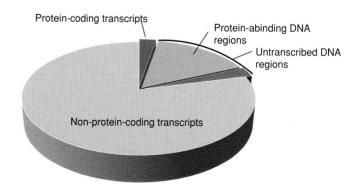

FIGURE 93.2 Approximately 3% of human DNA is transcribed and translated into functional proteins (*red*). Twenty percent of the DNA is not transcribed and the majority of this DNA (*gray*) functions as binding regions for transcription factors. Eighty percent (*pink*) of the DNA is transcribed, but has no recognized protein translation.

200 to 100,000 bases which lack protein coding capability. They are thought to play significant roles in tumor initiation, progression, and metastases by modulating oncogenic and tumor suppressor pathways by mechanisms that remain only partially defined. While miRs have been relatively well studied as they relate to cancers and other diseases, published investigations relating lncRNAs to lung cancer are relatively sparse. This is largely related to technical difficulties with cloning such long segments of RNA, as well as the inherent instability and rapid degradation of long-segment RNAs.

Recently, the recognition of long noncoding RNAs (lncRNAs) was evaluated as potential biomarkers for NSCLC. Some evidence suggests that the lncRNA ANRIL may be involved with the recruitment of the polycomb repressive complex 2 (PRC2) to specific DNA targets for histone methylation, which is a major contributor to epigenetic gene silencing of specific tumor suppressor genes.[28] Others have demonstrated a marked elevation of PVT1, another lncRNA, in NSCLC tissue relative to adjacent nonmalignant lung and bronchial epithelium.[29] Increased expression of PVT1 also correlated positively with increased tumor grade and the presence of lymph node metastases. When PVT1 was selectively targeted in tissue culture with siRNA, cell migration and proliferation were impaired. The importance of lncRNA in cancers is also supported by the fact that more than 8,000 different species of lncRNA have been identified in malignancies.[30] In particular, differential expression of lncRNA in cancers compared to adjacent nonmalignant lung tissue in nonsmoking patients revealed numerous differences.[31] Similarly, Tantai et al. demonstrated that two separate lncRNAs [X-inactive specific transcript (XIST) and HIF1A-AS1] were significantly elevated in lung cancer specimens compared to adjacent nonmalignant lung tissue.[32] Importantly, overexpression in tumors correlated with elevated serum levels in the same patients indicating potential utility as biomarkers. The area under the ROC (AUC) for XIST and HIF1A-AS1 were 0.834 and 0.876, respectively. When the two markers were evaluated in a composite analysis, the two markers were able to discriminate between patients with and without a diagnosis of lung cancer with an AUC of 0.931. Following surgical resection of these early-stage tumors, the authors noted that serum levels of both XIST and HIF1A-AS1 decreased significantly. These studies suggest a potential role for lncRNA in the early detection of lung cancer as well. However, the broad application of these assays may be somewhat limited by the technical challenges inherent in working with long segments of RNA.

PROTEOMICS

Metabolomics is a field of study in cancer detection and prognostication that relates to the end effector protein, lipids, and glycans of cells. In essence, metabolomics studies the culmination and end result of all gene mutations, epigenetic modifications, gene expression driven by extracellular signaling, and the downstream intracellular signal transduction cascades. Metabolomics also relates to the effector proteins which actually determine cellular function. For these reasons, those studying metabolomics suggest that this field of study provides the most meaningful information regarding the biologic behavior of the tumor. The most commonly discussed subset of metabolomics is a field of study known as proteomics which analyzes peptide fragments that can be identified based on the particle's mass and electrical charge. While each peptide fragment may or may not be specifically identified, the analysis of peptide spectra can reliably reveal what proteins had been present in the sample. As with the assessment of RNA, and the identification of certain RNA spectra that may predict the diagnosis of lung cancer, the recognition of the

relative abundance of different peptides has been associated with the presence of malignancies. Another similarity with previously mentioned RNA-based studies, peptide patterns have also been used to provide prognostic information for patients with known cancers.

Numerous examples of proteomics being utilized to help establish the diagnosis of lung cancer in patients and in experimental models are available. For example, serum levels of proteins including S100 calcium binding proteins (S100A2 and S100A6) have been compared between patients with NSCLC and healthy control patients and significant differences between the two groups were identified.[33] Importantly, the majority of the patients enrolled in this study had stage I or II disease indicating that they may be potentially useful among patients with the earliest stages of disease. Although S100A2 has been implicated in the pathogenesis of NSCLC in tissue-based studies, its precise role has not been fully elucidated.[34] As is true with numerous proteomic studies, the precise function of the target protein is not known, but this is not necessary when the assay is being performed solely as a diagnostic marker for lung cancer. Despite the high degree of statistically significant differences between the groups with and without cancer, the areas under the ROC curves for each of the two proteins were 0.646 and 0.668, which limits the clinical applicability of these particular assays.

In an effort to establish a proteomic profile correlating with the earliest detection of lung cancers, Nan et al. evaluated tissue specimens from patients with lung cancers. Using laser capture microdissection to isolate areas of squamous metaplasia or atypical adenomatous hyperplasia, comparisons were made between these regions of premalignancy and nonmalignant adjacent lung parenchyma.[35] Using mass spectrometry, a total of 863 specific proteins were identified, of which 427 were dysregulated in the premalignant tissues. Specific emphasis was placed on focal adhesion kinase and C-terminal Src kinase which were the two most markedly elevated in the premalignant tissues and they may represent molecular modifications in the earliest stages of lung cancer that are potentially identifiable with tissue biopsies.

METABOLOMICS

Over the past decade there has been accumulating evidence that the basic metabolic profile of cancer cells differs from that of normal cells. In particular, malignant cells are more frequently dependent on anaerobic glycolysis rather than aerobic respiration and this is true even in the presence of a normal oxygen tension. This phenomenon is known as the Warburg effect.[36] The reasons for these metabolic alterations in malignant cells, which still retain mitochondria with the capacity for aerobic respiration, are not completely understood. Leading hypotheses, however, include the fact that the preferential catabolism of glucoses to lactate supports biomass accumulation and redox maintenance in proliferating cells.[37] Another metabolic peculiarity that is characteristic of many malignancies is a relative dependence on glutamine which is used as a nitrogen donor for the synthesis of nonessential amino acids (Table 93.2). In addition, glutamine derivatives can be used as substrates for biosynthetic and NAPDH-generating pathways which are essential for maintaining a stable redox balance.[37]

Proton nuclear magnetic resonance (H-NMR) has been utilized to analyze the metabolic profile of peripheral blood samples of patients with NSCLC and compare to blood samples from healthy control individuals. In a comparison of 357 patients with NSCLC and 347 control patients, the metabolic profiles could discriminate between the two groups by performing H-NMR analysis on peripheral blood samples with a sensitivity and specificity of 71% and 89%, respectively.[38] This study included patients with stages I to IV disease and the majority

TABLE 93.2 Serum Amino Acids Correlating With Lung Cancer

Author (Date) ⟶	Rocha (2011)[39]	Puchades-Carrasco (2016)[63]	Maeda (2010)[64]	Miyagi (2011)[65]
Acetate	↓			
Alanine	↓		↑	
Citrate	↓			
Formate	↓			
Glucose	↓	↓		
Glutamine	↓	↑		
Histidine	↓			
Lactate	↑	↑		
Methanol	↓			
Pyruvate	↑			
Tyrosine	↓		↑	
Valine	↓			
Leucine/isoleucine		↑	↑	↑
3-Hydroxybutyrate		↓		
Adipic acid		↓		
Lysine		↑	↑	
N-Acetyl-cystine		↑		
Citrate		↑		
Valine		↑		
Gylcerol		↑		
Creatinine		↑		
Phenylalanine		↓	↑	↑
Prolene			↑	↑
Serine			↑	↑
Gylcine			↑	↓
Methionine			↑	
Ornithine			↑	↑

of patients presented with advanced stages. However, when analyses were performed exclusively on the 76 patients with stage I disease, the sensitivity and specificity were 74% and 78%, respectively. This indicates that the H-NMR analysis of peripheral blood samples has some potential clinical applicability among a patient population for which screening or risk stratification of small pulmonary nodules is most important. In a similar but smaller previous study, H-NMR analysis of peripheral blood samples was performed on patients with stage I to III NSCLC and compared to healthy control patients.[39] Importantly, the majority of patients had stage I disease. Patients with cancer were found to have lower levels of high-density lipoprotein and higher levels of low-density and very low density lipoprotein. In addition, cancer patients had higher levels of lactate and pyruvate, but lower levels of glucose, citrate, formate, and acetate. With different statistical models applied, the most accurate models correctly classified patients with a sensitivity and specificity of 91.5% and 89.2%. These analyses were essentially performed on a training set that included 85 patients with cancer and 78 healthy controls and unfortunately, there was no validation with an independent patient cohort.

Metabolic signatures have also been recognized in exhaled breath samples of patients with lung cancer. In ancient Roman times, the smell of a person's breath was used to help establish certain diagnoses such as diabetes, liver, or renal failure. In recent years, several studies have been completed demonstrating the presence of diagnostic signatures of volatile compounds indicating the presence of lung cancer which are detectable using mass spectrometry. The majority of volatile compounds identified in any individual study have limited congruence with other studies addressing the same question of whether or not a metabolite panel of volatile compounds in exhaled breath can predict the presence of cancer. With this understanding, the volatile compounds that most often are identified across several independent studies include pentane, isoprene, benzene, and decane (Table 93.3).

LIPIDS

Investigations designed to exploit immunotherapeutic strategies for the treatment of lung cancer determined that many malignancies, including lung cancer cells, overexpress the stress-induced heat-shock protein 70 (Hsp70). Not only is the protein expressed to a greater degree in the cytosol of malignant cells, but it is also overexpressed on the cell surface and the protein becomes incorporated in exosomes that are released into the extracellular fluid and blood. Hsp70 is recognized by natural killer cells, which provides the rationale for seeking to exploit this feature for immunotherapy. However, the mere recognition of this protein that is secreted on lipid vesicles also supports investigations evaluating Hsp70 as a biomarker for lung cancer. Gunther et al. compared circulating levels of Hsp70 among 43 (25 squamous cell and 18 adenocarcinoma) patients with lung cancer to 126 healthy control patients. The circulating level of Hsp70, determined by ELISA, was similar between patients with squamous cell cancers and adenocarcinoma. Importantly, the Hsp70 levels of both cancer populations were significantly greater than the healthy control population that was well matched with regard to age and gender.[40]

While the identification of Hsp70 in circulating liposomes may have some potential as a biomarker indicating the presence of lung cancer, there are several aspects that may also limit its application. One such limitation is the fact that the majority of the subjects in clinical studies have advanced stage disease, and it is recognized that the ability to detect Hsp70 in blood correlated with the patients' disease burden.[40,41] This raises the concern that patients with early-stage lung cancer may not have sufficient levels of this tumor marker circulating to differentiate them from healthy patients. Another factor limiting the potential of Hsp70 as biomarker for lung cancer includes the lack of statistical analyses using ROC curves to define a normal Hsp70 value and subsequently to determine the sensitivity and specificity of a serum-based assay. Furthermore, Hsp70 is frequently elevated in inflammatory conditions such as hepatitis and cirrhosis.[42] In addition, Hsp70 may also play a role in inflammatory signaling on the lung such as granulomatous inflammation of *Mycobacterium tuberculosis*.[43] This may limit the use of Hsp70 to determine the nature of small nodules where the two most common diagnoses include cancer and granulomatous disease.

More recently, attention has also been directed toward lipid metabolic profiles that may be unique to malignant cells. In a tissue-based analysis, Marien et al. compared lipid profiles, and in particular phospholipids, of lung cancer specimens to adjacent nonmalignant lung tissues and identified 162 specific lipids with differential expression using mass spectrometry.[44] In this analysis there were 19 individual phospholipids that could discriminate malignant from nonmalignant tissue with an area under the ROC (AUC) of at least 0.90 and 45 phospholipids with an AUC greater than or equal to 0.80. Using linear discriminate analysis to process the data and to evaluate combinations of individual species, a phospholipid profile with an AUC of 0.999

TABLE 93.3 Exhaled Volatile Compounds Correlating With Lung Cancer

Author (Date) ⟶	Phillips (2003)[66]	Machado (2005)[67]	Poli (2005)[68]	Chen (2007)[69]	Fuchs (2010)[70]
Butane	•				
3-Methyl tridecane	•				
7-Methyl tridecane	•				
4-Methyl octane	•				
3-Methyl hexane	•				
Heptane	•				
2-Methyl heptane	•				
Pentane	•	•	•		
5-Methyl decane	•				
Isobutane		•			
Methanol		•			
Ethanol		•			
Acetone		•			
Isoprene		•		•	
Isopropanol		•			
Dimethyl sulfide		•			
Carbon disulfide		•			
Benzene		•	•	•	
Toluene		•			
Ethyl benzene			•		
Xylene			•		
Trimethyl benzene			•		
Toluene			•		
Decane			•	•	
Octane			•		
Penta methyl heptane			•		
Styrene				•	
Undecane				•	
1-Hexene				•	
Hexanol				•	
Propyl benzene				•	
1,2,4-Trimethyl benzene				•	
Heptanal				•	
Methyl cyclopentane				•	
Aldehyde-butanol					•
Formaldehyde					•
Acetaldehyde					•
Pental					•
Hexanal					•

could be developed. These findings have not yet been extrapolated to analyses performed on readily available biologic fluid specimens.

PROTEOGLYCANS

One of the most frequently discussed cell signaling molecules in lung cancer is the epithelial growth factor receptor (EFGR) which is a transmembrane glycoprotein present on most epithelial cells. Importantly, EGFR mutations are responsible for approximately 20% of all lung adenocarcinomas and they represent a treatable molecular target. A soluble form of EGFR (sEGFR) that is comprised of the extracellular domain of EGFR has also been described and is detectable in the serum of patients both with and without cancer. sEGFR is the product of posttranscriptional cleavage or alternative gene splicing. Isoform B arises from proteolytic cleavage of the protein between G625 and M626 and isoform C arises from an alternative mRNA transcript.[45,46] Serum levels of these isoforms appear to be greater among healthy patients and they are decreased among patients with malignancies, including lung cancer.[47] While sEGFR serum levels are significantly lower among patients with lung cancer with a highly significant p value, there is a substantial degree of overlap between individuals with and without cancer giving an area under the ROC curve of only 0.727. Using the ROC curve to establish the optimal cutoff value, the sensitivity and specificity were only 70.4% and 70.3%, respectively. Fortunately, patients' ages, gender, and histologic subtype of NSCLC did not appear to influence the levels of sEGFR.

sEGFR has also been shown to convey both overall prognostic information for patients with lung cancer and predictive response to treatment with erlotinib, an agent that targets the tyrosine kinase domain of EGFR.[48] Interestingly, in this study that included 58 patients being treated with erlotinib, a higher serum level of sEGFR was associated with better progression-free survival and overall survival among patients with stage IIIB or IV NSCLC. Others have found a similar correlation between elevated pretreatment sEGFR concentrations and prolonged progression-free and overall survival rates among larger cohorts of patients treated with either erlotinib or gefitinib for advanced stage NSCLC. The correlation between elevated sEGFR and better long-term survival rates was also true for patients treated with traditional cytotoxic therapy.[49,50]

Correlations between circulating carcinoembryonic antigen (CEA) levels and prognosis are not as consistent. Romero et al. found that an elevated level of CEA was associated with a prolonged overall and progression-free survival among patients with advanced staged NSCLC treated with EGFR inhibitors.[48] Conversely, Kappers et al. in a similar study of patients with advanced NSCLC treated with anti-EGFR agents found that elevated CEA levels were associated with worse clinical outcomes.[49]

Cyfra 21-1 is a fragment of cytokeratin-19 which is detectable in serum that has been evaluated as a potential biomarker for patients with lung cancer. Wieskhopf et al. investigated a cohort of patients with differing histologies to evaluate the performance of Cyfra 21-1 as a biomarker and found that it had a relatively low sensitivity but a high specificity (0.59 and 0.94, respectively) among all patients with NSCLC.[51] Similarly, Cyfra 21-1 could also be used to detect patients with small cell carcinoma with a sensitivity and specificity of 0.19 and 0.94, respectively. Importantly, Cyfra 21-1 expression was the lowest among patients with stage I/II disease compared to stage IIIa or greater which may limit the ability of using this maker to risk stratify patients with small pulmonary nodules. Cyfra 21-1 has also been evaluated for prognostic significance in patients with small cell carcinoma. Using ROC curves to establish a cutoff value of 3.6 ng/mL to differentiate high from low expression, the overall survival rate among patients with high expression of Cyfra 21-1 was significantly worse than in patients with low serum levels.[52]

A recent large study evaluating a panel of serum tumor markers in patients suspected of having lung cancer included a total of 3,144 patients of whom 1,828 (58.1%) were confirmed to have cancer and 1,316 (41.9%) were determined to not have cancer.[53] As expected, the 1,563 (85.5%) of patients with lung cancer had NSCLC subtypes and 265 (14.5%) had small cell carcinoma. The serum of each patient was assessed for CEA, Cyfra-21-1, SCC, CA 153, neuron-specific enolase (NSE), and progastrin releasing peptide (proGRP) and the cutoff values of normal utilized in this study were established previously. The performance of each serum tumor marker among tumors less than 1 cm was reasonable with specificities ranging from 92% to 100%, but the sensitivity of each individual tumor marker was low (0% to 38%). In this panel, CEA and Cyfra 21-1 were the most likely to be positive in patients with either NSCLC or small cell carcinoma. Conversely, NSE and proGRP had the greatest sensitivity for patients with small cell carcinoma, but these markers were poor for patients with NSCLC.

Serum levels of other factors have also been assessed to determine whether or not they convey any diagnostic or prognostic information including VEGF, EGF, IL-6, and TGF but the results appear to be inconclusive at this point.[54]

FIELD EFFECT

Cigarette smoke is the most common environmental factor associated with the development of lung cancer. However, only 10% to 15% of all smokers ever develop lung cancer. An individual's somatic genetic background and subsequent genetic modifications as the result of smoking are likely contributors to malignant transformation of the bronchial epithelium. It is also reasonable to assume that genetic modifications occurring within the bronchial epithelium of central airways are similar to changes occurring throughout the bronchial tree. This concept has been supported by several investigations that have identified genetic changes in the airways of smokers with or without lung cancer that include gene allelic loss, p53 mutations, promoter methylation, enhanced telomerase activity, and altered transcriptional activity.[55–60] Numerous authors have associated genetic modifications within the bronchial epithelium of central airways of cytologic normal cells with the presence or absence of lung cancers located more distally in the airway.

Spira evaluated a panel of 80 gene transcripts using an Affymetrix microarray platform to compare the transcriptome of 60 smoking patients with cancer to 69 smoking patients who did not have cancer.[61] Validation studies utilizing this 80 gene panel found that the biomarker had a 90% sensitivity among patients with stage I lung cancer when used alone and when this probe was combined with cytologic data collected via bronchoscopy, the diagnostic yield increased further by demonstrating a 95% sensitivity and a 95% negative predictive value. This compares favorably to an expected 35% diagnostic yield for traditional bronchoscopic studies for peripheral lesions. Interestingly, genetic changes observed in the central airway epithelial cells were similar to those found in lung cancers even though the predominant cell types analyzed from the bronchial biopsy were ciliated epithelial cells and the primary cell types of origin of lung cancers are glandular cells. These results suggest that genetic modifications induced by smoking that contribute to malignant transformation likely occur throughout the bronchial tree and are not restricted to the specific site where cancers develop.

In addition to assays directed toward the tumor itself, or the detection of a protein or gene product derived from the malignancy, some tumor markers are better characterized to recognizing field effects that may increase the propensity for a malignancy. Therefore, these markers may be utilized to risk stratify patients with lung nodules. Silvestri et al. demonstrated that in a high-risk patient population with suspicious lung nodules, a genetic analysis of epithelial cells from the mainstem bronchus could identify patients with lung cancer.[62] This investigation utilized two different gene classifiers. The first correctly identified 194 of 220 patients with lung cancer (sensitivity 88%) and the second gene classifier correctly identified 237 of 267 patients with lung cancer (sensitivity 89%). The combination of the gene classifiers with diagnostic information obtained from traditional bronchoscopic biopsies, brushes, and bronchial washes increased the sensitivities to 96% and 98% for the two classifiers, respectively, compared to 74% and 76% for bronchoscopy alone. Importantly, when these gene classifiers were applied only to patients with non-diagnostic bronchoscopies, the diagnostic sensitivities were 86% and 92%, respectively. The diagnostic accuracy of the classifier was not influenced by the lesion size or its location (central vs. peripheral) which is particularly important because these factors have a significant influence on the diagnostic yield of bronchoscopy alone.

SUMMARY

Numerous approaches have been utilized in attempt to establish the ex vivo diagnosis of lung cancer. A variety of biological specimen sources have been studied with numerous biological assays. These extensive analyses have yielded a broad array of potential means of diagnosing lung cancer in the earliest stages through minimally invasive means. However, at this time, an assay with sufficient diagnostic accuracy has yet to be developed. We anticipate that future investigations will incorporate results of various assays to establish reliable diagnostic panels that accurately determine the presence or absence of lung cancer in patients.

REFERENCES

1. Siegel RL, Miller KD, Jemal A. Cancer statistics 2016. *CA Cancer J Clin* 2016;66: 7–30.
2. Brett GZ. The value of lung cancer detection by six-month chest radiographs. *Thorax* 1968;23:414–420.
3. Melamed MR, Flehinger RB, Zaman MB, et al. Screening for early lung cancer: results of the Memorial Sloan-Kettering Study in New York. *Chest* 1984;86:44–53.
4. Tockman M. Survival and mortality from lung cancer in a screened population: the Johns Hopkins study. *Chest* 1986;89(suppl):325s–326s.
5. Fontana RS, Sanderson DR, Woolner LB, et al. Screening for lung cancer. A critique of the May Lung Project. *Cancer* 1991;67(4 suppl):1155–1164.
6. The National Lung Screening Trial Research Team. Reduced lung-cancer mortality with low-dose computed tomographic screening. *N Engl J Med* 2011;365:395–409.
7. Lages E, Ipas H, Guttin A, et al. MicroRNAs: molecular features and role in cancer. *Front Biosci (Landmark Ed)* 2012;17:2508–2540.
8. Rothschild SI. Epigenetic therapy in lung cancer—role of microRNAs. *Front Oncol* 2013;19:158.
9. Qi J, Mu D. MicroRNAs and lung cancers: from pathogenesis to clinical implications. *Front Med* 2012;6:134–155.
10. Lu Z, Liu M, Stribinskis V, et al. MicroRNA-21 promotes cell transformation by targeting the programmed cell death 4 gene. *Oncogene* 2008;27:4373–4379.
11. Asangani IA, Rasheed SA, Nikolova DA, et al. MicroRNA-21 (miR-21) post-transcriptionally downregulates tumor suppressor Pdcd4 and stimulates invasion, intravasation and metastasis in colorectal cancer. *Oncogene* 2008;27:2128–2136.
12. Zhu W, Xu B. MicroRNA-21 identified as predictor of cancer outcome: a meta-analysis. *PLoS One* 2014;9:1–7.
13. Wang B, Zhang Q. The expression and clinical significance of circulating microRNA-21 in serum of five solid tumors. *J Cancer Res Clin Oncol* 2012;138: 1659–1666.
14. Wang Y, Gao X, Wei F, et al. Diagnostic and prognostic value of circulating miR-21 for cancer: a systematic review and meta-analysis. *Gene* 2013;533:389–397.
15. Meng X, Xiao C, Zhao Y, et al. Meta-analysis of microarrays: diagnostic value of microRNA-21 as a biomarker for lung cancer. *Int J Biol Markers* 2015;30:e282–e285.
16. Li W, Wang Y, Zhang Q, et al. MicroRNA-486 as a biomarker for early diagnosis and recurrence of non-small cell lung cancer. *PLoS One* 2015;10(8):e0134220.
17. Guo J, Meng R, Li P, et al. A serum microRNA signature as a prognostic factor for patients with advanced NSCLC and its association with tissue microRNA expression profiles. *Mol Med Rep* 2016;13(6):4643–4653. [epub]
18. Li ZH, Zhang H, Yang ZG, et al. Prognostic significance of serum microRNA-210 levels in nonsmall-cell lung cancer. *J Int Med Res* 2013;41:1437–1444.
19. Kim JO, Gazala S, Razzak R, et al. Non-small cell lung cancer detection using microRNA expression profiling of bronchoalveolar lavage fluid and sputum. *Anticancer Res* 2015;35:1873–1880.
20. Roa WH, Kim JO, Razzak R, et al. Sputum microRNA profiling: a novel approach for the early detection of non-small cell lung cancer. *Clin Invest Med* 2012;35:E271.
21. Li L, Chen YY, Li SQ, et al. Expression of miR-148/152 family as potential biomarkers in non-small-cell lung cancer. *Med Sci Monit* 2015;21:1155–1161.
22. Ghasemkhani N, Shadvar S, Masoudi Y, et al. Down-regulated MicroRNA 148b expression as predictive biomarker and its prognostic significance associated with clinicopathological features in non-small-cell lung cancer patients. *Diagn Pathol* 2015;10:164.
23. Hu Z, Chen X, Zhao Y, et al. Serum micro-RNA signatures identified in genome-wide serum micro-RNA expression profiling predict survival of non-small cell lung cancer. *J Clin Oncol* 2010;28:1720–1726.
24. Gao L, Ma J, Mannoor K, et al. Genome-wide small nucleolar RNA expression analysis of lung cancer by next-generation deep sequencing. *Int J Cancer* 2015;136:623–629.
25. Liao J, Yu L, Mei Y, et al. Small nucleolar RNA signatures as biomarkers for non-small cell lung cancer. *Mol Cancer* 2010;9:198.
26. Su J, Liao J, Gao L, et al. Analysis of small nucleolar RNAs in sputum for lung cancer diagnosis. *Oncotarget* 1014;7:5131–5142.
27. Dunham I, Kundaje A, Aldred SF, et al. An integrated encyclopedia of DNA elements in the human genome. *Nature* 2012;489:57–74.
28. Lin L, Gu ZT, Chen WH, et al. Increased expression of the long non-coding RNA ANRIL promotes lung cancer cell metastasis and correlates with poor prognosis. *Diagn Pathol* 2015;10:14.
29. Yang YR, Zang SZ, Zhong CL, et al. Increased expression of the lncRNA PVT1 promotes tumorigenesis in non-small cell lung cancer. *Int J Clin Exp Pathol* 2014;7:6929–6935
30. Martens-Uzunova ES, Bottcher R, Croce CM, et al. Long noncoding RNA in prostate, bladder, and kidney cancer. *Eur Urol* 2014; 65: 1140–1151.
31. Li J, Bi L, Shi Z, et al. RNA sequence analysis of non-small cell lung cancer in female never-smokers reveals candidate cancer-associated long non-coding RNAs. *Pathol Res Pract* 2016;212(6):549–554. [Epub ahead of print]
32. Tantai J, Hu D, Yang Y, et al. Combined identification of long non-coding RNA XIST and HIF1A-AS1 in serum as an effective screening for non-small cell lung cancer. *Int J Clin Exp Pathol* 2015;8:7887–7895.
33. Wang T, Liang Y, Thakur A, et al. Diagnostic significance of S100A2 and S100A6 levels in sera of patients with non-small cell lung cancer. *Tumour Biol* 2016;37(2): 2299–2304. [Epub ahead of print]
34. Hountis P, Matthaios D, Froudarakis M, et al. S100A2 protein and non-small cell lung cancer. The dual role concept. *Tumour Biol* 2014;35:7327–7333.
35. Nan Y, Du J, Ma L, et al. Early candidate biomarkers of non-small cell lung cancer are screened and identified in premalignant lung lesions. *Technol Cancer Res Treat* 2017;16(1):66–74. [Epub ahead of print]
36. Upadhyay M, Samal J, Kandpal M, et al. The Warburg effect: insights from the past decade. *Pharmacol Ther* 2013;137:318–330.
37. Cantor JR, Sabatini DM. Cancer cell metabolism: one hallmark, many faces. *Cancer Discov* 2012;2(10):881–898.
38. Louis E, Adriaensens P, Guedens W, et al. Detection of lung cancer through metabolic changes measured in blood plasma. *J Thorac Oncol* 2016;11:516–523.
39. Rocha CM, Carrola J, Barros AS, et al. Metabolic signatures of lung cancer in biofluids: NMR-based metabonomics of blood plasma. *J Proteome Res* 2011;10:4314–4324.
40. Gunther S, Ostheimer C, Stangl S, et al. Correlation of Hsp70 serum levels with gross tumor volume and composition of lymphocyte subpopulations in patients with squamous cell and adeno non-small cell lung cancer. *Front Immunol* 2015;6:556.
41. Murakami N, Kuhnel A, Schmid TE, et al. Role of membrane Hsp70 in radiation sensitivity of tumor cells. *Radiat Oncol* 2015;10:149.
42. Gehrmann M, Cervello M, Montalto G, et al. Heat shock protein 70 serum levels differ significantly in patients with chronic hepatitis, liver cirrhosis, and hepatocellular carcinoma. *Front Immunol* 2014;5:307.
43. Bulut Y, Michelsen KS, Hayrapetian L, et al. Mycobacterium tuberculosis heat shock proteins use diverse Toll-like receptor pathways to activate pro-inflammatory signals. *J Biol Chem* 2005;280:20961–20967.
44. Marien E, Meister M, Muley T, et al. Non-small cell lung cancer is characterized by dramatic changes in phospholipids. *Int J Cancer* 2015;137:1539–1548.
45. Marianela P, Valle BL, Maihle NJ, et al. Shedding of epidermal growth factor receptor is a regulated process that occurs with overexpression in malignant cells. *Exp Cell Res* 2008:314:2907–2918.
46. Reiter JL, Maihel NJ. Characterization and expression of novel 60 kDa and 110 kDa EGFR isoforms in human placenta. *Ann NY Acad Sci* 2003;995:39–47.
47. Lococo F, Paci M, Rapicetta C, et al. Preliminary evidence on the diagnostic and molecular role of circulating soluble EGFR in non-small cell lung cancer. *Int J Mol Sci* 2015;19:19612–19630.
48. Romero-Ventosa EY, Blanco-Prieto S, González-Piñeiro AL, et al. Pretreatment levels of the serum biomarkers CEA, CYFRA 21-1, SCC and the soluble EGFR and its ligands EGF, TGF-alpha, HB-EGF in the prediction of outcome in erlotinib treated non-small cell lung cancer patients. *Springerplus* 2015;4:171.
49. Kappers I, Vollebergh MA, van Tinteren H, et al. Soluble epidermal growth factor receptor (sEGFR) and carcinoembryonic antigen (CEA) concentration in patients with non-small cell lung cancer: correlation with survival after erlotinib and gefitinib treatment. *Ecancermedicalscience* 2010;4:178.
50. Jantus-Lewintre E, Sirera R, Cabrera A, et al. Analysis of the prognostic value of soluble epidermal growth factor receptor plasma concentration in advanced non-small-cell lung cancer patients. *Clin Lung Cancer* 2011;12:320–327.
51. Wieskopf B, Demangeat C, Purohit A, et al. Cyfra 21-1 as a biologic marker of non-small cell lung cancer. Evaluation of sensitivity, specificity, and prognostic role. *Chest* 1995;108:163–169.
52. Pujol JL, Quantin X, Jacot W, et al. Neuroendocrine and cytokeratin serum markers as prognostic determinants of small cell lung cancer. *Lung Cancer* 2003;39:131–138.
53. Molina R, Marrades RM, Augé JM, et al. Assessment of a combined panel of six serum tumor markers for lung cancer. *Am J Respir Crit Care Med* 2016;193(4): 427–437. [Epub ahead of print]
54. Chakra M, Pujol JL, Lamy PJ, et al. Circulating serum vascular endothelial growth factor is not a prognostic factor of non-small cell lung cancer. *J Thorac Oncol* 2008; 3:1119-1126.
55. Powell CA, Klares S, O'Connor G, et al. Loss of heterozygosity in epithelial cells obtained by bronchial brushing: clinical utility in lung cancer. *Clin Cancer Res* 1999;5:2025–2034.
56. Wistuba II, Lam S, Behrens C, et al. Molecular damage in the bronchial epithelium of current and former smokers. *J Natl Cancer Inst* 1997;89:1366–1373.
57. Franklin WA, Gazdar AF, Haney J, et al. Widely dispersed p53 mutation in respiratory epithelium. A novel mechanism for field carcinogenesis. *J Clin Invest* 1997;100: 2133–2137.
58. Guo M, House MG, Hooker C, et al. Promoter hypermethylation of resected bronchial margins: a field defect of changes? *Clin Cancer Res* 2004;10:5131–5136.
59. Miyazu YM, Miyazawa T, Hiyama K, et al. Telomerase expression in noncancerous bronchial epithelia is a possible marker of early development of lung cancer. *Cancer Res* 2005;65:9623–9627.

60. Spira A, Beane J, Shah V, et al. Effects of cigarette smoke on the human airway epithelial cell transcriptome. *Proc Natl Acad Sci U S A* 2004;101:10143–10148.

61. Spira A, Beane JE, Shah V, et al. Airway epithelial gene expression in the diagnostic evaluation of smokers with suspect lung cancer. *Nat Med* 2007;13:361–366.

62. Silvestri GA, Vachani A, Whitney D, et al. A bronchial genomic classifier for the diagnostic evaluation of lung cancer. *N Engl J Med* 2015;373:243–251.

63. Puchades-Carrasco L, Jantus-Lewintre E, Perez-Rambla C, et al. Serum metabolomics profiling facilitates the non-invasive identification of metabolic biomarkers associated with the onset and progression of non-small cell lung cancer. *Oncotarget* 2016;7:12904–12916.

64. Maeda J, Higashiyama M, Imaizumi A. Possibility of multivariate function composed of plasma amino acid profiles as a novel screening index from non-small cell lung cancer: a case control study. *BMC Cancer* 2010;10:690.

65. Miyagi Y, Higashiyama M, Gochi A, et al. Plasma free amino acid profiling of five types of cancer patients and its application for early detection. *PLoS One* 2011;6:e24143.

66. Phillips M, Cateno RN, Cummin AR, et al. Detection of lung cancer with volatile markers in the breath. *Chest* 2003;123:2115–2123.

67. Machadeo RF, Laskowski D, Deffenderfer O, et al. Detection of lung cancer by sensor array analysis of exhaled breath. *Am J Respir Crit Care Med* 2005;171:1286–1291.

68. Poli D, Carbongnani P, Corradi M, et al. Exhaled volatile organic compounds in patients with non-small cell lung cancer: cross sectional and nested short-term follow up study. *Respir Res* 2005;6:71.

69. Chen X, Xu F, Wang Y, et al. A study of the volatile organic compounds exhaled by lung cancer cells in vitro for breath diagnosis. *Cancer* 2007;110:835–844.

70. Fuchs P, Loeseken C, Schubert JK, et al. Breath gas aldehydes as biomarkers of lung cancer. *Int J Cancer* 2010;126:2663–2670.

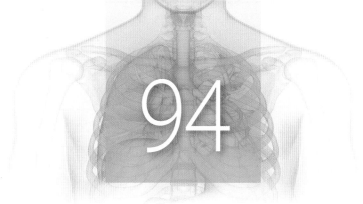

94

Staging of Lung Cancer

Joe B. Putnam, Jr.

INTRODUCTION

The patient with known or suspected lung cancer may present in a number of different ways.[1] Symptoms may or may not be present. The typical evaluation after physical examination includes radiographic studies, clinical characteristics, and radiographic findings. Abnormalities identified should allow the physician to target a specific area or problem for additional investigations. Anatomic and biological considerations such as tumor size, location, and the mechanical effects on other structures, local symptoms (dyspnea, cough, hoarseness, hemoptysis, sputum production), extraneoplastic syndromes, or physical evidence such as clubbing, or signs of metastatic disease (bone pain, neurologic symptoms, facial swelling, etc.) must be considered in determining the diagnosis, and the extent of the disease.[2] Physical examination should focus on the cardiorespiratory system and the cervical and supraclavicular regions to evaluate the presence of supraclavicular (extrathoracic) lymph nodes. Fine-needle aspiration (FNA) of these scalene lymph nodes, or a scalene lymph node biopsy may be required for diagnosis. Diagnosis of lesions in other areas may be obtained by FNA by computed tomography guidance, bronchoscopy with biopsy, or perhaps even open procedures such as minimally invasive thoracic operations. Diagnosis and staging should be obtained by the most direct and least invasive way to ascertain and define the greatest extent or stage of the disease, for example, biopsy of metastatic lesions, evaluation of pleural effusion, or examination of contralateral FDG-PET avid mediastinal lymph nodes.

All components of the evaluation, physical examination, radiographic characteristics, and diagnosis are used to determine the clinical extent of disease. To facilitate staging, characteristics of the tumor (T), the regional and distant lymph nodes (N), or metastatic disease (M) are considered to accurately define the extent of the disease. Biological staging (molecular markers prognostic for survival, as well as predictive for response to therapy) likely will be incorporated into staging systems of the future. Until then, accurate clinical staging followed by a multidisciplinary discussion of the treatment plan is needed. Evaluation and recommendations as appropriate by the surgeon, the medical oncologist, and/or the radiation oncologist before treatment begins ensures optimal treatment recommendations in a timely manner.

To facilitate timely and cost-effective care, various professional societies and organizations have created guidelines for diagnosis, staging, and management for patients with lung cancer.[3–6]

DIAGNOSIS

For each patient with suspected lung cancer, the diagnostic procedure of choice should maximize the likelihood of diagnosis and stage extent of the tumor, minimize unnecessary tests or procedures, and provide the patient with sufficient information to facilitate shared treatment decisions.

SPUTUM CYTOLOGY

Sputum cytology is infrequently used for the diagnosis of lung cancer as other technologies, such as fiberoptic bronchoscopy and transthoracic FNA, have provided more effective yield. Sputum cytology is safe and inexpensive, and when positive, establishes the diagnosis—most commonly with larger central squamous cell cancers.[7] Although the specificity is approximately 99%, the sensitivity is only about 66%[7]—quite low particularly with patients with smaller or peripheral lesions in the absence of symptoms.[1,8] Autofluorescence bronchoscopy may facilitate diagnosis in patients with sputum atypia.[9,10]

BRONCHOSCOPY

Bronchoscopy is commonly used to diagnose, stage, palliate, and sometimes treat lung cancer. The complication rates from flexible bronchoscopy are less than 1% and include but are not limited to bleeding, pneumothorax, cough, hypoxemia, cardiac arrhythmias, and iatrogenic infection. Death is quite rare (<0.05%).[11–14]

Diagnostic techniques such as endobronchial biopsy, brushings, washings, bronchoalveolar lavage, and transbronchial needle aspiration (TBNA) are commonly used in addition to bronchoscopy. In patients with central lesions, fiberoptic bronchoscopy can be the diagnostic procedure of choice with an overall sensitivity of 88%.[1] Fiberoptic bronchoscopy is most effective in tumors which involve the bronchial mucosa or provide extrinsic compression on the bronchus which may be biopsied. Biopsy provides the most effective yield, exceeding that of bronchial washing, or non–ultrasound-guided TBNA. Small peripheral lesions (<2 cm) are more challenging to identify by standard fiberoptic bronchoscopy techniques, although more recent techniques such as navigational bronchoscopy, can locate and biopsy these lesions.[15] For nodules less than 2 cm, the sensitivity of bronchoscopy alone is approximately 34%; for lesions greater than 2 cm, 63%.[1] When all diagnostic tests are used—biopsy, brushings, washings, and TBNA—the sensitivity can approach 80%.[16]

More recently, image-guided biopsy technologies have improved the ability of the interventional pulmonologist biopsy the small peripheral pulmonary nodule. Use of the radial probe endobronchial ultrasound (r-EBUS) with localization of the nodule provided a sensitivity of 73% and a specificity of 100%.[17] In one study, electromagnetic navigational bronchoscopy (ENB) alone achieved 77% sensitivity.[18] These results may not be generalizable. Diagnostic yield of ENB from eight prospective series was 68%.[1] All of the techniques described have a variable clinical performance, and combinations of these techniques may provide better diagnostic yield.[19-21]

TRANSTHORACIC FINE-NEEDLE ASPIRATION

Transthoracic FNA (TTNA) has been increasingly used for diagnosis of peripheral pulmonary nodules using computed tomography for image guidance. Like flexible bronchoscopy, the technique is safe and common postprocedure events include discomfort, mild hemoptysis, hemorrhage (1%), any pneumothorax (15%), and pneumothorax requiring chest tube (6.6%).[22] The risk of pneumothorax depends upon the size of the lesion, location, pleural fusion, size of the biopsy needle, number of insertions and extractions through the lung, and underlying lung diseases such as emphysema or bullous disease.

CT-guided transthoracic FNA has a sensitivity of ≥90%. The false positive rate is only 1% to 2%; however, the false negative rate is high (20% to 30%).[1,23] Confirmation of adequate tissue by a cytopathologist on-site improves the diagnostic effectiveness.[24] Larger amounts of tissue provided by a core biopsy improve diagnostic yield of malignant or benign disease, and facilitate additional tissue availability for molecular studies. A nondiagnostic FNA may simply be a sampling error (false-negative) or may accurately reflect a noncancer diagnosis (true-negative). In patients with a likelihood of cancer, the false negative rate may range between 20% and 30%.[25] If a TTNA is nondiagnostic, additional evaluation, surveillance, or further testing is recommended.

After a nondiagnostic bronchoscopy, a transthoracic FNA may be considered, leaving more invasive approaches such as video-assisted thoracic surgery (VATS) or thoracotomy for subsequent diagnosis, and treatment. The choice of intervention for diagnosis and/or treatment would depend upon the patient's condition, past history, and likelihood of a cancer diagnosis. For patients who are older (greater than 40 years), have a positive smoking history, or history of other cancer; or have radiographic characteristics of larger-sized lesions, spiculation, and upper lobe location, a cancer diagnosis may be more likely. In such patients, an operation may be considered for both diagnosis and treatment. Intraoperative histologic examination can confirm the diagnosis following wedge resection, and before a larger pulmonary resection is performed.

TTNA may be required for diagnosis preoperatively to facilitate discussion of treatment options including alternatives to surgery. Patients at high operative risk (comorbidities, hostile chest, poor physiologic reserve, etc.), likely to have a benign diagnosis, estimated to have a low risk of malignancy, or who prefer to have a diagnosis prior to operative intervention to facilitate preoperative discussion, planning, and management are candidates for this type of diagnostic approach. In patients who are at prohibitive operative risk, a biopsy may be needed to facilitate treatment planning for stereotactic body radiation therapy, chemotherapy, or other local or systemic strategies.

VIDEO-ASSISTED THORACIC SURGERY

In other patients with indeterminate pulmonary nodules, wedge excision can be performed for diagnosis using minimally invasive thoracic surgery techniques such as VATS. Older studies,[26] noted that tumors less than 3 cm in diameter, noncalcified, and located in the outer third of the lung parenchyma were easily identified and resected by VATS. CT scan images are essential to determining the location of the nodule, and in many cases planning the extent of the resection that would be required. If the nodule is located near the visceral pleura, the nodule may be identified visually, or by palpation. Nodules located toward the parenchymal angles of the lobe are more easily identified and resected. Nodules identified on the broad surfaces of the lobes, may require greater resection of lung parenchyma with some deformation of the lung as a consequence of this wedge resection.

Nodules less than 1 cm in size may be more challenging to identify. Although with single lung anesthesia, collapse of the lung, and careful palpation of the area of the nodule identified on CT scan, the surgeon is likely to identify and remove these lesions. Needle localization techniques (transthoracic or endoscopic) can be used, although the coordination of additional modalities will add time to the procedure. These techniques include methylene blue injection in the area, hook wires, radiopaque markers, radiotracer injection localization, and thoracic endosonography to facilitate identification of the area of resection.[27-29]

THORACOTOMY

Open thoracotomy is rarely needed for diagnosis of pulmonary nodules. If a lesion is identified within the central portion of the lobe, a repeat transthoracic FNA or core needle biopsy would be more cost effective than thoracotomy. However, if the diagnosis is needed for a central mass in the operating room, a needle aspiration under direct vision/palpation, or a core needle biopsy could be considered. Care should be taken when a core needle or Tru-Cut needle biopsy is used, as vascular injury involving the pulmonary artery or vein could occur.

STAGING OF LUNG CANCER

The clinical stage of any patient is the clinician's best and final estimate of the extent of the disease prior to the initiation of definitive therapy. As such, the clinical stage is the foundation for all cancer treatment recommendations.

Staging defines the extent of the cancer based upon its anatomic characteristics and the similar survival for patients with those characteristics. Characteristics of the patient's disease can be more clearly understood by using a stage grouping. This can be used to facilitate therapeutic interventions including treatment planning, prognosis, and comparing the results of treatment and clinical investigations. Stage grouping creates a clinical shorthand description of each patient to allow physicians to discuss patients with others, to facilitate exchange of ideas, and to improve treatment outcomes based upon the clinical and pathologic (after resection) stage. Staging should be accurate, cost effective, and reproducible.

The clinician's responsibility is to ensure the highest possible degree of certainty of the clinical stage and use it to recommend the therapy or therapeutic combination of greatest efficacy. Two questions must be answered by the surgeon for each patient: (1) What is the extent of the disease? Where is it? Has it spread? and, (2) Is there an operation which can be performed safely that will effectively treat this disease?

Optimal staging allows the clinician to provide the best recommendations for therapeutic interventions for the patient. In contrast to the clinical stage, obtained from both noninvasive and invasive studies prior to initiation of definitive therapy, the pathological stage is the determination of the extent of the disease based upon histological examination of the resected tissues including the hilar and mediastinal lymph nodes. Staging guidelines for non–small cell carcinoma[30] and small cell carcinoma[31] have been proposed.

The staging system for lung cancer has evolved over the past 40 years. Survival analyses were led by Mountain and colleagues[32,33] and Naruke and colleagues.[34] Definitions of the T characteristic and N characteristic were further refined by Goldstraw and colleagues through the International Association for the Study of Lung Cancer (IASLC) staging project to create a more statistically valid foundation for the 7th edition of the TNM staging system.[35,36]

The American Joint Committee on Cancer (AJCC) and the Union for International Cancer Control (UICC) incorporated these staging system recommendations into an international staging system for lung cancer.[37] New stage grouping were proposed based upon additional data and more refined analyses from the IASLC staging project.

THE CURRENT AJCC 7TH EDITION STAGING SYSTEM

The IASLC embarked upon its lung cancer staging project to include all treatment and diagnostic groups, to collect data for analysis, and to reform future revisions of the staging system.[35] The AJCC 7th edition lung cancer staging reflects the impact of the IASLC lung cancer staging project.[37,38] The IASLC collected over 100,000 NSCLC cases from 23 institutions in 12 countries in Australia, Europe, and the United States treated between 1990 and 2000. Each patient had a minimum of 5 years of follow-up and all treatment modalities were included. Over 81,000 surgical cases were submitted and eligible for analysis. These included 67,725 patients with NSCLC and 13,290 patients with small cell carcinoma. Survival was calculated by the Kaplan–Meier method. Prognostic groups were created using Cox regression analysis and results were both internally and externally validated.[38] Stage groupings were revised to reflect these analyses and internally and externally validated.[36] External validation was assessed against the Surveillance, Epidemiology, and End Results Program Database (SEER). The data collected was retrospective, and an audit of the data was not performed; however, information was provided by credible centers which facilitated data collection, and analysis of a large patient population. Future directions will most certainly include prospective data collection[26,39,40] and proteomic and genomic characteristics.

TUMOR (T)

In the IASLC lung cancer staging project, over 18,000 patients had a T1-T4 tumor with N0 lymph node dissection and an R0 resection.[41] T1 was divided into T1a (≤2 cm) and T1b (>2 to 3 cm). T2 was divided into T2a (>3 to 5 cm) and T2b (>5 to 7 cm). "T2c" would have been >7 cm; however, these patients had a survival that was statistically similar to survival of T3 patients. Therefore lung cancers greater than 7 cm were categorized as T3.

Other T2 descriptors such as visceral pleural invasion and partial atelectasis (less than the entire lung) could not be evaluated statistically because of small number of patients and inconsistent data, but is likely to represent a higher stage characteristic. Nodules in the same lobe were categorized as T3; nodules in a different lobe were categorized as T4; a nodule in a contralateral lobe would be designated as M1a unless there was compelling evidence to suggest synchronous primary tumors.

T3 tumors were characterized as a tumor with invasion into the pleura, pericardium, or diaphragm; an endobronchial tumor less

TABLE 94.1 Recommended Changes for T Characteristic for the 8th Edition TNM Staging System

T1	T1a (≤1 cm); T1b (>1 to ≤2 cm), T1c (>>2 to ≤3cm)
T2	T2a (>3 to ≤4 cm), T2b (>4 to ≤5 cm), or involvement of the main bronchus regardless of distance from the carina, or partial/total atelectasis/pneumonitis.
T3	>5 to ≤7 cm
T4	>7 cm; or diaphragm involvement

From Rami-Porta R, Bolejack V, Crowley J, et al. The IASLC Lung Cancer Staging Project: Proposals for the revisions of the T descriptors in the forthcoming eighth edition of the TNM classification for lung cancer. *J Thorac Oncol* 2015;10:990–1003.

than 2 cm from the carina; or an obstructing tumor causing atelectasis of the entire lung; and as mentioned before, two nodules in the same lobe.

T4 tumors involve the mediastinal structures such as the heart, great vessels, esophagus, and trachea, as well as the vertebral body or the carina. Two nodules, one each in two separate ipsilateral lobes, were characterized as T4.

Pleural metastases or malignant pleural effusion was changed from T4 (in the AJCC 6th edition) to M1 in the AJCC 7th edition. Patients with a malignant pleural effusion, malignant pericardial effusions, or pleural nodules were categorized as M1a, based on poor survival which more closely resembled patients with metastatic disease. Patients with extrathoracic disease were categorized as M1b.

In proposals to revise the 7th edition TNM classification of lung cancer,[42] the IASLC has collected information on 94,708 new patients diagnosed between 1999 and 2010. These data came from 35 sources in 16 countries through an electronic data capture system. 70,967 patients with non–small cell lung cancer, and 6,189 patients with small cell lung cancer were analyzed.[40] The T characteristic will be further refined based upon 1-cm differences for tumors up to 5 cm in size (Table 94.1). Mediastinal pleural invasion will be removed as a T descriptor.[43]

In the forthcoming eighth addition of the TNM classification for non–small cell lung cancer, patients with multiple pulmonary sites of involvement will include more detail. Patients with a second primary lung cancer would be designated with a T, N, and M characteristic for each tumor. Patients with separate tumor nodules would be characterized as T3 in the same lobe, T4 if the same side and different lobe, or M1a if located in a contralateral lobe—with a single N and M designator for all. Multifocal ground-glass tumors are likely to be characterized based on the highest T characteristic based on the size of the largest lesion and either (1) the total number of lesions (e.g., T1b(4)N0M0 for four separate lesions) or (2) simply "m" for multiple lesions (e.g., T1b(m)N0M0).[44,45]

LYMPH NODES (N)

The nodal characteristic and designations did not change in the AJCC 7th edition.[46] Over 67,000 patients had T, N, and M characteristics as well as histologic type and survival. 38,265 patients had clinical nodal and 28,371 patients had pathological nodal staging information. Clinical staging studies included tests such as diagnostic imaging, computed tomography, and mediastinoscopy. Thoracotomy for staging was excluded. Positron emission tomography (PET) was not widely used internationally in this cohort during this time. The lymph node map was proposed combining the Japanese/Naruke and the North American/Mountain lymph node maps.[47] Of special note, the authors proposed radiographic regions for the location of specific mediastinal lymph nodes, particularly for integration with computed tomography, to guide the radiologic staging of patients with NSCLC.

In the forthcoming eighth addition of the TNM classification for lung cancer, the current nodal descriptors and location for both clinical and pathological nodal status (N0 to N3) adequately predict prognosis. Although for lung cancer, nodal status is based on the anatomic location of the involved node, and not on the number of metastatic lymph nodes, future staging models could assess the number of involved nodes and location.[48]

METASTASES (M)

Metastases from NSCLC were divided into M1a and M1b categories.[49] Patients with metastasis to the contralateral lung only were designated as M1a; metastases to regions outside the lung/pleura were designated as M1b. A second nodule in the nonprimary ipsilateral lobe, previously designated as M1, was changed to T4M0. In this situation, the patient received the "benefit of the doubt" approach as this might represent a second primary. There are few features that are definitive for a synchronous primary versus a metastasis. Careful evaluation and then discussion in a multidisciplinary cancer conference will provide the best treatment recommendations.[50]

STAGE GROUPINGS

The TNM definitions (Table 94.2), nodal characteristics (Table 94.3), and stage groupings of the TNM subsets with survival (Table 94.4) are shown. The current international staging system[36] provides the basis for specific patient stage groupings based upon the T, N, and M characteristics as a surrogate for the biologic behavior of the tumor (Fig. 94.1). Proposed changes in the stage grouping for NSCLC for the AJCC eighth edition will be refined based on the proposed changes in definitions as noted above.[42]

Other schematics have been created for the lymph node map[51] and T characteristics.[52]

The mediastinal and regional lymph node classification schema is presented (Fig. 94.2). This map presents a graphic representation of the mediastinal and pulmonary lymph nodes in relation to other thoracic structures for optimal dissection and correct anatomic labeling by the surgeon.

EVALUATION OF T (TUMOR) STAGE

The current changes in the T characteristic reflect the worsening survival as tumor size increases. Computed tomography of the chest and upper abdomen, including the liver and adrenals, typically follows an abnormality identified on plain chest x-rays. Chest roentgenograms (CXRs) and computed tomography of the chest (CT Chest) are the most frequent diagnostic imaging studies performed in patients with chest symptoms. In patients with known or suspected lung cancer, the chest x-ray provides information on the size, shape, density, and location of the primary tumor and its relationship to the mediastinal structures. Although not as sensitive as CT Chest, CXR may identify single or multiple pulmonary nodules, pleural effusions, lung consolidation, bone destruction from metastases, or in more advanced disease, bulky mediastinal lymphadenopathy.

CT Chest provides more detail than the chest x-ray on tumor characteristics, the size, location, and the relationship of the tumor to the mediastinal structures, chest wall, and diaphragm as well as invasion into the vertebrae or other mediastinal structures, and should

TABLE 94.2 T, N, and M Descriptors for Lung Cancer Staging

T (Primary Tumor)

TX	Primary tumor cannot be assessed, or tumor proven by the presence of malignant cells in sputum or bronchial washings but not visualized by imaging or bronchoscopy
T0	No evidence of primary tumor
Tis	Carcinoma in situ
T1	Tumor ≤3 cm in greatest dimension, surrounded by lung or visceral pleura, without bronchoscopic evidence of invasion more proximal than the lobar bronchus (i.e., not in the main bronchus)[a]
	• T1a Tumor ≤2 cm in greatest dimension
	• T1b Tumor >2 cm but ≤3 cm in greatest dimension
T2	Tumor >3 cm but ≤7 cm or tumor with any of the following features (T2 tumors with these features are classified T2a if ≤5 cm):
	• Involves main bronchus, ≥2 cm distal to the carina
	• Invades visceral pleura
	• Associated with atelectasis or obstructive pneumonitis that extends to the hilar region but does not involve the entire lung
	• T2a Tumor >3 cm but ≤5 cm in greatest dimension
	• T2b Tumor >5 cm but ≤7 cm in greatest dimension
T3	Tumor >7 cm or one that directly invades any of the following: chest wall (including superior sulcus tumors), diaphragm, phrenic nerve, mediastinal pleura, parietal pericardium; or
	• tumor in the main bronchus <2 cm distal to the carina[a] but without involvement of the carina; or
	• associated atelectasis or obstructive pneumonitis of the entire lung or
	• separate tumor nodule(s) in the same lobe
T4	Tumor of any size that invades any of the following: mediastinum, heart, great vessels, trachea, recurrent laryngeal nerve, esophagus, vertebral body, carina; or
	• separate tumor nodule(s) in a different ipsilateral lobe

N (Regional Lymph Nodes)

NX	Regional lymph nodes cannot be assessed
N0	Metastasis in ipsilateral peribronchial and/or ipsilateral hilar lymph nodes and intrapulmonary nodes, including involvement by direct extension
N2	Metastasis in ipsilateral mediastinal and/or subcarinal lymph node(s)
N3	Metastasis in contralateral mediastinal, contralateral hilar, ipsilateral or contralateral scalene, or supraclavicular lymph node(s)

M (Distant Metastasis)

MX	Distant metastasis cannot be assessed
M0	No distant metastasis
M1	Distant metastasis
	• M1a Separate tumor nodule(s) in a contralateral lobe;
	• tumor with pleural nodules or malignant pleural (or pericardial) effusion[b]
	• M1b Distant metastasis

[a]The uncommon superficial spreading tumor of any size with its invasive component limited to the bronchial wall, which may extend proximally to the main bronchus, is also classified as T1.
[b]Most pleural (and pericardial) effusions with lung cancer are due to tumor. In a few patients, however, multiple cytopathologic examinations of pleural (pericardial) fluid are negative for tumor, and the fluid is nonbloody and is not an exudate. Where these elements and clinical judgment dictate that the effusion is not related to the tumor, the effusion should be excluded as a staging element and the patient should be classified as T1, T2, T3, or T4.
From Goldstraw P, Crowley J, Chansky K, et al. The IASLC Lung Cancer Staging Project: proposals for the revision of the TNM stage groupings in the forthcoming (seventh) edition of the TNM Classification of malignant tumours. *J Thorac Oncol* 2007;2:706–714. Copyright © 2007 International Association for the Study of Lung Cancer, with permission and Edge SB, Byrd DR, Compton CC, et al. *AJCC Cancer Staging Manual.* 7th ed. New York: Springer; 2009. Reproduced with permission of Springer in the format Book via Copyright Clearance Center.

TABLE 94.3 Lymph Node Map Definitions

N2 nodes—all N2 nodes (single digit designator) lie within the mediastinal pleural envelope.

Highest mediastinal nodes: Nodes lying above a horizontal line at the upper rim of the brachiocephalic (left innominate) vein where it ascends to the left, crossing in front of the trachea at its midline.

1. Upper paratracheal nodes: Nodes lying above a horizontal line drawn tangential to the upper margin of the aortic arch and below the inferior boundary of number 1 nodes.
2. Prevascular and retrotracheal nodes: Pretracheal and retrotracheal nodes may be designated 3A and 3P. Midline nodes are considered to be ipsilateral.
3. Lower paratracheal nodes: The lower paratracheal nodes on the right lie to the right of the midline of the trachea between a horizontal line drawn tangential to the upper margin of the aortic arch and a line extending across the right main bronchus at the upper margin of the upper lobe bronchus and contained within the mediastinal pleural envelope; the lower paratracheal nodes on the left lie to the left of the midline of the trachea between a horizontal line drawn tangential to the upper margin of the aortic arch and a line extending across the left main bronchus at the level of the upper margin of the left upper lobe bronchus, medial to the ligamentum arteriosum and contained within the mediastinal pleural envelope.

Regional (N2) Lymph Node Classification

4. Subaortic (aortopulmonary window): Subaortic nodes are lateral to the ligamentum arteriosum or the aorta or left pulmonary artery and proximal to the first branch of the left pulmonary artery and lie within the mediastinal pleural envelope.
5. Para-aortic nodes (ascending aorta or phrenic): Nodes lying anterior and lateral to the ascending aorta and the aortic arch or the innominate artery, beneath a line tangential to the upper margin of the aortic arch.
6. Subcarinal nodes: Nodes lying caudal to the carina of the trachea, but not associated with the lower lobe bronchi or arteries within the lung.
7. Paraesophageal nodes (below carina): Nodes lying adjacent to the wall of the esophagus and to the right or left of the midline, excluding subcarinal nodes.
8. Pulmonary ligament nodes: Nodes lying within the pulmonary ligament, including those in the posterior wall and lower part of the inferior pulmonary vein.

N1 nodes—all N1 nodes lie distal to the mediastinal pleural reflection and within the visceral pleura.

9. Hilar nodes: The proximal lobar nodes, distal to the mediastinal pleural reflection and the nodes adjacent to the bronchus intermedius on the right; radiographically, the hilar shadow may be created by enlargement of both hilar and interlobar nodes.
10. Interlobar nodes: Nodes lying between the lobar bronchi.
11. Lobar nodes: Nodes adjacent to the distal lobar bronchi.
12. Segmental nodes: Nodes adjacent to segmental bronchi.
13. Subsegmental nodes: Nodes around the subsegmental bronchi.

Reprinted from Mountain CF, Dresler CM. Regional lymph node classification for lung cancer staging. *Chest* 1997;111:1718–1723. Copyright © 1997 The American College of Chest Physicians. With permission.

be performed with contrast, and to include the upper abdomen. CT Chest with contrast provides a better assessment of the relationship of nodule or masses with the vascular structures (pulmonary artery, pulmonary veins, atrium, aorta, great vessels, etc.). Locally advanced tumors may cause significant local problems (pain, dyspnea, neurological impairment, etc.), although CT Chest scans do not consistently define chest wall, mediastinal, or vascular invasion.[53] CT Chest with upper abdomen does delineate size and location of mediastinal lymph nodes, as well as adrenal and liver lesions. CT Chest provides a first step to evaluate the patient for occult metastases. Many

TABLE 94.4 AJCC 7th Edition TNM Stage Groupings[19,35]

Stage	T	N	M	Percent (%) 5-Year Survival	
				Clinical Stage	Path Stage
Occult cancer	TX	N0	M0		not calculated
Stage 0	Tis	N0	M0		not calculated
Stage IA	T1a/b	N0	M0	50	73
Stage IB	T2a	N0	M0	43	58
Stage IIA	T2b	N0	M0	36	46
	T1a/b; T2a	N1	M0		
Stage IIB	T2b	N1	M0	25	36
	T3	N0	M0		
Stage IIIA	Any T1; T2	N2	M0	19	24
	T3	N1/N2	M0		
	T4	N0/N1	M0		
Stage IIIB	T4	N2	M0	7	9
	Any T	N3	M0		
Stage IV	Any T	Any N	M1a/b	2	13

From Goldstraw P, Crowley J, Chansky K, et al. The IASLC Lung Cancer Staging Project:proposals for the revision of the TNM stage groupings in the forthcoming (seventh) edition of the TNM Classification of malignant tumours. *J Thorac Oncol* 2007;2:706–714. Copyright © 2007 International Association for the Study of Lung Cancer, with permission and Edge SB, Byrd DR, Compton CC, et al. AJCC Cancer Staging Manual. 7th ed. New York: Springer; 2009. Reproduced with permission of Springer in the format Book via Copyright Clearance Center.

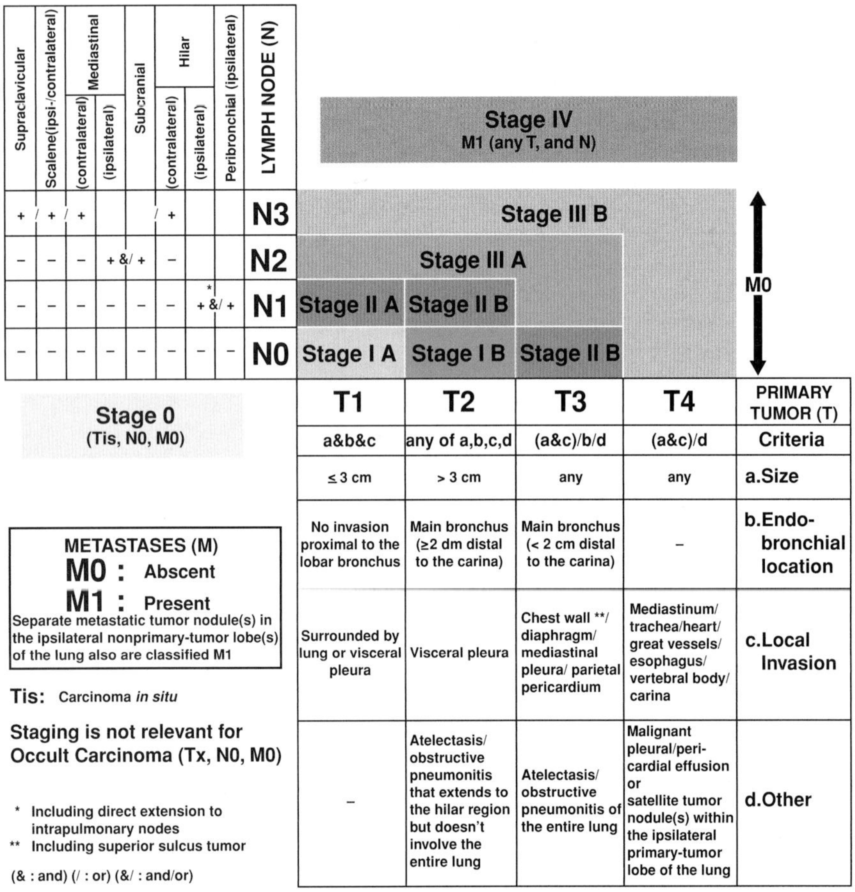

FIGURE 94.1 — TNM staging of lung cancer

Lymph Node (N) classification:

Supraclavicular	Scalene (ipsi-/contralateral)	Mediastinal (contralateral)	Mediastinal (ipsilateral)	Subcranial (ipsilateral)	Hilar (contralateral)	Hilar (ipsilateral)	Peribronchial (ipsilateral)	LYMPH NODE (N)
+	/ + / +				/	+		N3
–	–	–	+ &/ +	–				N2
–	–	–	–	–	–	*+ &/ +		N1
–	–	–	–	–	–	–	–	N0

Stage grid:

- **Stage IV** — M1 (any T, and N)
- N3: **Stage III B**
- N2: **Stage III A**
- N1: **Stage II A** | **Stage II B**
- N0: **Stage I A** | **Stage I B** | **Stage II B**
- M0

Stage 0 (Tis, N0, M0)

Primary Tumor (T) classification:

	T1	T2	T3	T4	PRIMARY TUMOR (T)
	a&b&c	any of a,b,c,d	(a&c)/b/d	(a&c)/d	Criteria
a. Size	≤ 3 cm	> 3 cm	any	any	a. Size
b. Endobronchial location	No invasion proximal to the lobar bronchus	Main bronchus (≥2 dm distal to the carina)	Main bronchus (< 2 cm distal to the carina)	–	b. Endobronchial location
c. Local Invasion	Surrounded by lung or visceral pleura	Visceral pleura	Chest wall **/ diaphragm/ mediastinal pleura/ parietal pericardium	Mediastinum/ trachea/heart/ great vessels/ esophagus/ vertebral body/ carina	c. Local Invasion
d. Other	–	Atelectasis/ obstructive pneumonitis that extends to the hilar region but doesn't involve the entire lung	Atelectasis/ obstructive pneumonitis of the entire lung	Malignant pleural/pericardial effusion or satellite tumor nodule(s) within the ipsilateral primary-tumor lobe of the lung	d. Other

METASTASES (M)
M0 : Absent
M1 : Present
Separate metastatic tumor nodule(s) in the ipsilateral nonprimary-tumor lobe(s) of the lung also are classified M1

Tis: Carcinoma *in situ*

Staging is not relevant for Occult Carcinoma (Tx, N0, M0)

* Including direct extension to intrapulmonary nodes
** Including superior sulcus tumor

(& : and) (/ : or) (&/ : and/or)

FIGURE 94.1 TNM staging of lung cancer. (Reprinted from Lababede O, Meziane MA, Rice TW. TNM staging of lung cancer. *Chest* 1999;115:233–235. Copyright © 1999 The American College of Chest Physicians. With permission.)

abdominal lesions are benign in etiology such as hepatic cysts and adrenal adenoma.

Magnetic resonance imaging (MRI) may complement CT Chest in specific clinical T4 situations where invasion into the chest wall, vertebral body, or vessels are concerned. MRI is not significantly better than CT Chest identification of hilar or mediastinal metastases[53] and is not superior to FDG-PET CT.[54] MRI Chest is especially useful for superior sulcus tumors, or tumors that may involve chest wall, brachial plexus, spinal cord, or vascular structures such as the aorta, subclavian artery, or subclavian vein. In patients where there is a question of invasion, the patient may require exploration as these tumors may abut the structure without invasion.

Positron-emission tomography (PET)[55] is based upon the differential increased metabolism of glucose by cancer cells compared to normal tissues. ^{18}F-flurodeoxyglucose (FDG) is used as a marker. Accumulation of this marker is related to the metabolism of the tissue. Detection of this radioactivity can provide a target lesion for biopsy, or additional investigation. FDG PET may assist in evaluating the local tumor, the mediastinum and its nodal stations, and for the presence of occult metastases.

FDG-PET scans have essentially replaced the nuclear medicine bone scan for evaluation of boney metastases. A PET scan is not a cancer-specific study, as high cellular glucose metabolism is seen in inflammatory processes, fractures, or healing tissues in addition to malignancy.[56,57] Histologic confirmation of suspicious mediastinal lymph node involvement is indicated prior to treatment recommendation. Other thoracic or extrathoracic foci of FDG uptake must be considered for evaluation for histologic evidence of NSCLC. FDG PET coupled with computed tomography may yield increased

sensitivity and specificity in determining the stage of patients with lung cancer before treatment interventions.[36,58] FDG PET is not a sensitive test for brain metastasis. A negative extrathoracic FDG-PET scan carries a low likelihood for metastasis; however, if positive areas are found, additional evaluation (biopsy, etc.) is recommended to confirm the presence of malignant cells. In the absence of confirmed nodal or extrathoracic metastatic disease, resection should be considered.

Patients with multiple suspicious ipsilateral or contralateral pulmonary lesions require additional evaluation to determine cancer nodules in the same lobe (clinical T3), or a separate nodule in an ipsilateral lobe (clinical T4). Concurrent lung cancer and granulomatous disease does exist. Although new nodules in a patient with a primary NSCLC are more likely related to the primary tumor, some patients could have synchronous T1 lesions (e.g., squamous cell and adenocarcinoma) with significant benefit from resection. Contralateral lesions would be evaluated in a similar manner. When in doubt, as to the relationship of the nodules, the benefit should go to the patient and to stage and treat the patient in the way which would provide the best chances of survival.

EVALUATION OF N (NODAL) STAGE

Determination of metastases to mediastinal lymph nodes constitutes a critical point in staging and treatment recommendations.[30] Mediastinal adenopathy (or enlarged lymph nodes) generally are defined as those with a maximal transverse diameter >1 cm in their short axis diameter. Lymph nodes may be enlarged normally from infection (histoplasmosis, previous bronchitis, or pneumonia, etc.) or other

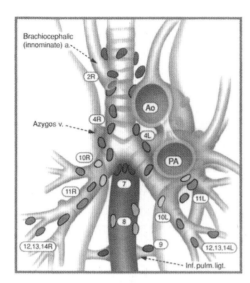

Superior Mediastinal Nodes

- **1** Highest Mediastinal
- **2** Upper Paratracheal
- **3** Pre-vascular and Retrotracheal
- **4** Lower Paratracheal (including Azygos Nodes)

N₂ = single digit, ipsilateral
N₃ = single digit, contralateral or supraclavicular

Aortic Nodes

- **5** Subaortic (A-P window)
- **6** Para-aortic (ascending aorta or phrenic)

Inferior Mediastinal Nodes

- **7** Subcarinal
- **8** Paraesophageal (below carina)
- **9** Pulmonary Ligament

N₁ Nodes

- **10** Hilar
- **11** Interlobar
- **12** Lobar
- **13** Segmental
- **14** Subsegmental

FIGURE 94.2 Lymph node map.

inflammatory processes or disease processes (sarcoid, lymphoma, etc.). Metastasis to lymph nodes may occur in the absence of enlarged mediastinal lymph nodes. Larger lymph nodes are more likely to harbor metastasis than smaller lymph nodes. If mediastinal nodes >1 cm are identified, the patient should be evaluated further by FDG PET or biopsy. Specific imaging techniques[59] such as combined FDG PET + CT can identify nodal lesions as a target for endobronchial ultrasound (EBUS), biopsy, cervical mediastinoscopy (CME), esophageal ultrasound (EUS), VATS, etc. to optimize clinical staging.

Computed tomography has a reported sensitivity for mediastinal lymph node assessment in NSCLC between 57% and 79%, with a positive predictive value of just 56%.[30] No CT size criteria by itself are entirely reliable for the determination of mediastinal lymph node involvement. Although, larger mediastinal lymph nodes can be more easily identified with computed tomography, enlarged lymph nodes (≥1 cm) are more likely to be associated with metastasis (>70%). However, normal size lymph nodes (<1 cm) have a 7% to 15% chance of containing metastases. For patient with known NSCLC, simply having enlarged lymph nodes identified on a CT Chest does not preclude curative resection. CT Chest for evaluation of mediastinal metastases has an overall sensitivity of 57% with specificity of 82%.[60,61] Additional evaluation of the status of enlarged mediastinal lymph nodes by radiologic and invasive mediastinal staging should

be considered prior to any therapeutic decisions. In addition, all decisions regarding operability for local or locally advanced NSCLC must be made by a thoracic surgeon.

In the ACOSOG Z0030 clinical trial[16] PET and CT together were better than either study alone in determining the patient's suitability for resection. The negative predictive value (NPV) of PET for mediastinal node involvement with metastatic NSCLC was 87%, suggesting that invasive mediastinal staging could be considered selectively for patient without enlarged or FDG avid lymph nodes. CT Chest for mediastinal staging in patient with confirmed enlarged mediastinal lymph nodes, demonstrated that 14% of enlarged mediastinal lymph nodes were related to noncancer causes.[30,60] In areas of endemic granulomatous disease, enlarged lymph nodes can be found in even greater percentages of patients. In a patient with early stage disease, normal-sized mediastinal lymph nodes, and no FDG-avid mediastinal lymph nodes, resection with mediastinal lymph node dissection would be recommended. However, if the same patient has a normal-sized, but FDG-avid, mediastinal lymph node, invasive staging would be recommended to complete the patient's clinical staging prior to treatment decisions.

Patients with cStage I tumors without enlarged nodes identified by CT scan are unlikely to have mediastinal nodal metastasis. The false negative rate may approach 8% to 10% and is related to tumor size. Invasive staging is not typically recommended for peripheral T1 lesions without enlarged mediastinal lymph nodes or FDG-PET avid nodes.

Although CT scan can provide a more accurate anatomic characterization of lymph nodes or tumor, the FDG-PET scan supplements that information with metabolic activity. Early results from FDG-PET scans suggested that any FDG avidity was likely to be cancer related; however, because of other disease processes—lymphoma, granulomatous disease, sarcoid—FDG avidity in another itself does not define cancer.[57,62,63] An FDG-PET scan added to a clinically negative mediastinum by CT Chest for T1 tumors is likely to identify occult N2 disease in about 5% of patients based upon the final pathologic staging.[64] Combining CT Chest with FDG PET provides better sensitivity than either test alone (sensitivity 94%, specificity 86%).[65] Despite combinations of CT Chest, FDG-PET scans, or integrated CT/FDG PET, invasive staging is still recommended to confirm mediastinal nodal involvement.[59,66]

In patients with more central tumors, mediastinal lymph nodes with metastasis are more likely. In these patients, or in patients being considered for pneumonectomy, invasive mediastinal staging is appropriate to validate the decision for resection.

In all patients with small cell carcinoma considered for resection, extensive staging by diagnostic imaging including an FDG PET-scan is warranted. In addition, even with a negative FDG-PET scan, mediastinoscopy is warranted given the high incidence of occult mediastinal metastasis.

Invasive staging includes CME or mediastinotomy (Chamberlain procedure), EBUS, or EUS.[67] CME is traditionally indicated in patients with otherwise operable NSCLC with enlarged paratracheal or subcarinal lymph nodes, particularly if the cancer is proximal, pneumonectomy is planned, or if the patient is at increased risk for the planned resection.

A mediastinotomy is used to gain access to the anterior mediastinum and to access the aortopulmonary window area. The operation requires resection of the left second costosternal cartilage to access and evaluate the aortopulmonary window (level 5) or anterior mediastinum (level 6) lymph nodes. The internal mammary artery may be preserved and mobilized away, or may be ligated.

CME has a NPV above 90%, may be performed as an outpatient procedure, and is associated with a low rate of significant complications. When pathological "frozen section" evaluation fails to demonstrate malignant nodal involvement by mediastinoscopy, resection may follow under the same anesthetic. The use of CME regardless of radiographic evidence of nodal involvement (routine mediastinoscopy) is not a cost-effective approach[64] and adds little to the accuracy of staging in patients with an adequate noninvasive preoperative evaluation.[68]

Additional invasive mediastinal techniques however may be helpful.[30,67] EBUS with TBNA may be more sensitive than mediastinoscopy. Combining EBUS and surgical staging may provide greater sensitivity for mediastinal nodal metastases than surgical staging alone and avoid unnecessary thoracotomies.[69,70] VATS techniques can evaluate enlarged level 5 or 6 lymph nodes, and as well, enlarged level 8 or 9 or low level 7 lymph nodes. EUS-guided aspiration can be easily used for transesophageal needles aspiration of subcarinal and AP window lymph nodes.[30]

Specific situations may have identified that CT may have a low predictive value in patients with T3 tumors or central cancers, patients with negative PET in the setting of N1 nodal metastases, or peripheral clinical T1 N0 M0 small cell lung cancer. These patients may have an increased likelihood of N2 metastases and should be considered for invasive mediastinal staging.

EVALUATION OF METASTATIC DISEASE

Extrathoracic or distant metastases (M1b) are common in lung cancer. Beyond a thorough history and physical examination, and standard staging techniques, additional evaluation for metastatic disease is indicated only for selected cases.[30] Where metastatic disease is suspected based on imaging techniques, a tissue diagnosis should be obtained to confirm the presence or absence of metastases.[30,67] Nodules in the contralateral lung are characterized as metastatic disease (M1a) as are malignant pleural effusion and pleural carcinomatosis. The use of adjunctive testing for metastatic disease in the absence of specific clinical findings may be indicated in patients with nonspecific findings suggestive of widespread metastases, such as marked weight loss or severe anemia.

In proposals for the forthcoming AJCC eighth edition of the TNM classification of lung cancer, intrathoracic metastasis (pleural/pericardial effusion, contralateral/bilateral lung nodules or pleural nodules, or combinations, etc.) likely will be grouped as M1a. Patients with single metastasis to a single distant organ would be newly designated as M1b. Multiple distant metastases would be classified as M1c.[71]

A randomized trial by the Canadian Lung Oncology Group compared patients who underwent a clinical evaluation followed by surgery or a full metastatic workup prior to their operation.[72] The endpoints were thoracotomy with recurrence. They recommended that patients with a negative clinical evaluation did not need further testing; that any findings of metastatic disease or other organ specific or nonspecific required further testing; and that N2 disease was a marker for more advanced disease than expected and those patients should undergo extrathoracic staging. The radiologic testing recommended would include brain imaging by CT or MRI and either FDG-PET scan, or abdominal CT and bone scan. Given the more limited use of bone scans, additional testing with brain imaging and whole-body PET would be recommended. An integrated FDG-PET CT scan will include the abdomen as well and can be helpful in localizing FDG avid lesions within the chest, mediastinum, abdomen (liver or adrenals), or bones. Metastatic adrenal involvement may occur in up to 7% of patients at presentation. CT Chest should include the liver and adrenals[73] as minimal additional cost, time, or radiation exposure occurs, and IV contrast is not always required. Indeterminate adrenal lesions on CT may be further evaluated with MRI or with CT-guided percutaneous biopsy.[74]

FDG PET is commonly performed in patients with clinically suspicious lung nodules consistent with lung cancer, or those in whom a diagnosis of lung cancer has been obtained. The PLUS trial randomized patients to conventional evaluation alone or additional evaluation with PET.[75] Patients evaluated with FDG PET had more mediastinal metastasis and distant metastatic disease, FDG PET provided additional information which upstaged the patient which led to other than surgery therapy, and allowed patients to avoid a futile thoracotomy. The process was cost effective as it avoided futile thoracotomy in 20% of patients. The American College of Surgeons Oncology Group Z0050 trial found that FDG PET identified over 6% of patients with unsuspected metastatic disease or second primary malignancy in otherwise resectable patients with NSCLC.[16] False positive distant metastatic disease was also noted in 6.6% of patients and ultimately found to be benign. If PET findings of advanced disease or benign lesions were consistently used, unnecessary thoracotomy could be avoided in up to 20% of patients. PET findings of distant metastatic disease require confirmatory evaluation. A recent randomized trial of whole-body PET in NSCLC staging further supported its role in detecting otherwise undiagnosed metastasis in up to 10% of patients who are otherwise candidates for resection.[53,76]

BRAIN METASTASES

Patients with lung cancer who are neurologically asymptomatic are unlikely to have brain metastases at the time of diagnosis (0% to 10%).[30] In a review of studies of patients with a negative clinical evaluation, the median prevalence of brain metastases was 3% and the median predictive value of a negative clinical evaluation was 97%.[30] In early stage lung cancer, other studies such as CT or MRI of the brain should only be performed if the patient has symptoms such as headache, seizures, or other neurologic dysfunction, etc., or if small cell carcinoma is suspected.[77,78] It is not cost-effective to perform a CT scan of the brain in an otherwise asymptomatic patient who is physiologically fit and stage-appropriate for surgery.[79] MRI brain imaging may be reserved for patients with stage I or II cancer with new neurologic symptom, in all patients with stage III and IV cancer,[30] and for patients with small cell carcinoma, or superior sulcus tumors (Pancoast tumor) as these patients have a higher incidence of occult brain metastases.

Although MRI scan is more sensitive than CT scan of the brain in identifying smaller lesions, it does not appear to be clinically significant in improving survival.[80,81]

Patients with documented mediastinal lymph node metastases (N2) may be at increased risk for brain metastasis[82–84] and should have a CT or MRI of the brain prior to final treatment recommendations.

BONE METASTASIS

Patients with bone metastasis commonly have symptoms of bone pain. Up to 30% of patients in autopsy series may have bone metastasis. In a meta-analysis of 633 patients, bone scans are shown to have the sensitivity of 87% and the specificity of 67%.[65] Although radionuclide bone scan was commonly used in the past to identify bony metastasis, FDG PET has improved diagnostic accuracy compared to bone scan (sensitivity 94.3% vs. 78.1%, $p = 0.001$; specificity 98.8% vs. 97.4%, $p = 0.006$; accuracy 98.3% vs. 95.1%, $p = <0.001$; fewer false positives 1.2% vs. 2.9%; fewer false negatives 5.7% vs. 21.9%).[85] FDG PET is recommended rather than radionuclide bone scan when possible.

ABDOMINAL METASTASIS

CT scan of the chest often includes views of the liver and adrenals. This assessment of the upper abdomen as a component of the chest CT scan is invaluable in identifying these common areas of metastasis. Often metastasis to the adrenal and liver are asymptomatic and identified only by imaging studies.[78] Enlarged adrenals may represent metastasis; however, adrenal adenomas may occur in 2% to 10% of the general population.[86] Assessment of the adrenal may require additional studies including MRI scan. Patients with well-defined low-attenuation lesions suggestive of fat are likely to be benign adenomas. Additional studies such as repeat CT scan with contrast, ultrasound, MRI scan with contrast, or FDG-PET scan may be required.[87] In patients with enlarged and suspicious lesions, percutaneous CT-guided biopsy can establish a diagnosis and stage the patient. Although liver metastasis may occur in patients with lung cancer, other benign liver pathology is common such as hepatic cysts, or hemangiomas. FDG-PET avid liver lesions may represent metastatic disease. A liver biopsy may be required to provide a diagnosis.

TECHNIQUES FOR INTRATHORACIC STAGING

TRANSBRONCHIAL NEEDLE ASPIRATION

TBNA can be performed at the time of bronchoscopy with a catheter-based needle which fits through the working channel of the flexible fiberoptic bronchoscope.[88] Both the primary tumor and mediastinal/hilar lymph nodes can be reached. Time to treatment can be reduced compared to more conventional studies.[89] Multiple factors contribute to sensitivity of this test including needle size, diameter and location of the primary tumor, size and location of the peribronchial and paratracheal lymphadenopathy, and the histology.[90] Larger gauge needles (22-gauge vs. 19) provide more tissue and can increase the diagnostic yield. Lymph nodes in patients with right paratracheal and subcarinal lymphadenopathy are more easily identified and biopsied. On site cytopathology is recommended to confirm a malignant diagnosis and to ensure that sufficient samples are obtained for that diagnosis.[91] TBNA with EBUS guidance for identification and biopsy of lymph nodes provides greater sensitivity to detect and confirm metastases to the paratracheal, subcarinal, and hilar lymph node stations.[92]

TRANSTHORACIC NEEDLE ASPIRATION

Transthoracic needle aspiration is commonly used to obtain a diagnosis of a pulmonary nodule.[93,94] In aggregated analyses of studies examining the use of transthoracic needle biopsy, the prevalence of malignancy is approximately 70% and the median value for nondiagnostic results is about 6%. The median sensitivity for identifying malignancy was $\geq 90\%$ although lower (70% to 82%) for patients with nodules ≤ 15 mm in diameter. A nondiagnostic biopsy will likely to occur in about 20% of patients in a high-prevalence population.[23] A transthoracic needle biopsy is most appropriate when there is a question regarding the clinical probability of cancer, unusual imaging results, patient preferences, or a high likelihood of surgical complications if alternatives to resection would be considered. A nondiagnostic needle biopsy does not mean that there is no cancer; rather, it provides a guide for additional discussion with the patient and family and may serve to reassure some patients, or suggest alternative diagnostic or surveillance strategies for specific patients.[23] TTNA is infrequently used to sample ipsilateral or contralateral mediastinal lymph nodes. Patients with bulky anterior nodal disease, or mediastinal masses, may have a needle biopsy performed for diagnosis. These mediastinal masses are typically fixed between the posterior aspect of the sternum and the great vessels.

CERVICAL MEDIASTINOSCOPY

CME remains the gold standard for assessing metastasis to the mediastinal lymph nodes. This technique as originally promoted by Pearson and colleagues[95] allows exploration and biopsy of lymph nodes within the right and left paratracheal spaces, the anterior tracheal area, the tracheobronchial angles, and anterior superior subcarinal space. Less commonly performed are alternative techniques such as extended CME[96] with extension of the dissection superior and lateral to the aorta extending between the innominate artery and left common carotid artery to approach the para-aortic and AP window lymph nodes (levels 6 and 5 respectively).[97–99]

CME is typically performed with bronchoscopy under general anesthesia as an outpatient procedure, or immediately prior to pulmonary resection. The incision is made just above the sternal notch and carried down to the pretracheal fascia. The mediastinoscope is introduced alongside the trachea to examine the paratracheal spaces, as well as the subcarinal space. Stations 2R and 4R, 2L and 4L, pretracheal nodes in levels 1 and 3, and the anterior subcarinal nodes (level 7) can be accessed via this technique. Other nodes are either too distal (levels 8 and 9) or obstructed by the aorta (levels 5 and 6), and the posterior and inferior subcarinal space is not easily accessed. Typically, five lymph nodes stations are explored (levels 2R, 4R, 2L, 4L, and 7). Identified lymph nodes are biopsied. The paratracheal lymph nodes are easily sampled, particularly on the right side. The false negative rate for paratracheal lymph nodes is about 1% to 2%; and for the subcarinal lymph nodes about 6%. Median sensitivity of CME to detect mediastinal metastasis was approximate 70% with an NPV of approximately 91%.[30]

Complications from CME occur infrequently (~1%). In a series of 2,145 patients, 23 patients experience postoperative events including hemorrhage, 7 (0.33%); vocal cord dysfunction, 12 (0.55%); tracheal injury, 2; and pneumothorax, 2. Only one patient died—following pulmonary artery injury. Five of the seven vascular injuries occurred during biopsy within the 4R region.

Newer technical advances have improved the visualization of the mediastinal lymph nodes. Video mediastinoscopy[100] provides better optical resolution and magnification than the standard mediastinoscope but may be more limiting in the ability to dissect and manipulate the area of dissection. Video-assisted mediastinal lymphadenectomy (VAMLA)[101] has been proposed a modification of CME. The complication rate has been reported at 4% to 6%.[102,103] One advantage is that both the operator, and the assistant can visualize the area being dissected.[104] Transcervical extended mediastinal lymphadenectomy (TEMLA) can potentially acquire more nodal tissue than CME with biopsy; however, this would not be routinely considered for mediastinal staging.[105–107]

ANTERIOR MEDIASTINOTOMY

Originally described by McNeill and Chamberlain,[108] the left anterior (parasternal) mediastinotomy provides access to the aortopulmonary window on the left and to the anterior mediastinum on the right, areas in which CME cannot reach. In either situation, resection of the second costal cartilage is performed sparing the perichondrium. The internal mammary artery is either moved away or ligated. Access to level 5/6 lymph nodes is achieved. Digital exploration can define and target areas of involved nodes. The mediastinoscope can be placed to facilitate biopsy. In patients with left-sided cancers, CME is performed first to exclude contralateral (N3) nodal metastases. Parasternal mediastinotomy has a median sensitivity of 71% for stations 5/6 involvement, and an NPV of 91%.[30,109,110]

VIDEO-ASSISTED THORACOSCOPY

VATS can provide a rapid way to explore the pleural space prior to an open procedure. In early studies, VATS techniques may identify causes of inoperability in up to 8% of cases[111] and can provide access to all nodal stations. On the left, one can achieve access to mediastinal lymph nodes at levels 5, 6, 7, 8, and 9; on the right side, VATS techniques can explore levels 2, 4, 7, 8, and 9. Specific situations may require thoracoscopic techniques rather than mediastinoscopy particularly if enlarged lymph nodes are located distal to the subcarinal space, or along the esophagus, or in areas that are not accessible by other means.

ENDOSCOPIC BRONCHIAL ULTRASOUND

EBUS combines a linear array ultrasound and FNA via the working channel of the bronchoscope to evaluate and stage the mediastinum.[89,112] Guidelines have been proposed for its use.[30,113,114] EBUS FNA is the procedure of choice for endoscopic staging[115] and can be supplemented by EUS.[116] EBUS-FNA can examine all mediastinal, paratracheal, subcarinal, and hilar lymph node areas. EBUS is superior to TBNA and can effectively screen lymph nodes in patients undergoing pulmonary resection with an NPV of 96.3%.[117] The combination of EBUS FNA and EUS FNA provides significant improvements over either study alone.[116] EBUS supplementation of EUS provides better diagnostic ability than EUS supplementation of EBUS.[115] EBUS with FNA can be easily added to standard bronchoscopy procedures. In patients with enlarged or suspicious lymph nodes and a negative EBUS as the first procedure,[118] CME is recommended for completeness of staging prior to pulmonary resection.[69] However, more recent experience with EBUS and EUS has demonstrated that combined EBUS- and EUS-guided biopsies can excess more areas and targets and upstage more patients compared to conventional mediastinoscopy.[119–121] In addition, the use of EUS and EBUS for mediastinal restaging is safe and effective.[122]

ESOPHAGEAL ULTRASOUND

Endoscopic esophageal ultrasonography or EUS complements EBUS for staging the mediastinum.[123] EUS provides a cost-effective way[124] to biopsy periesophageal lymph nodes in levels 9, 8, 5, 6 (which are not accessible by the EBUS), and 7, evaluate for T4 status of certain tumors, and biopsy the left adrenal gland.[125] EUS complements EBUS in that the paratracheal regions (2R, 2L, 4R, 4L) are not identifiable using EUS. In one study, the EBUS bronchoscope was used as a small esophagoscope for examination of the paraesophageal lymph nodes. The proportion of accessible mediastinal lymph node stations by EBUS was 70% and increased to almost 85% by adding the esophageal ultrasonography to the EBUS scope.[126,127] Using endoscopic ultrasound and target lesions identified by CT scan, lymph nodes can be identified and biopsied with high sensitivity (90%) and specificity (97%). With no abnormal mediastinal lymph node identified on computed tomography, the sensitivity was lower (58%). Minor morbidity occurred in 0.8% of patients.[128]

INTRAOPERATIVE STAGING

At the time of operation, an exploration of the chest is required. The tumor should be identified and confirmed. Examination of the pleura diaphragm, and mediastinum for metastases should follow. If possible, palpation of the non–tumor-involved lung should be performed to assess for satellite nodules. Nodules 5 to 6 mm or less may be identified by visual inspection or palpation, which were not identified by the CT scan.

If the tumors involve the chest wall or another component of the thorax, the surgeon must assess resectability. Often tumors may be adherent to the parietal pleura against the chest wall and separable from the chest wall using an extrapleural dissection. If a plane is not clearly defined, chest wall invasion beyond the parietal pleura is likely and a chest wall resection may be required.

Intraoperative palpation of mediastinal lymph nodes may be possible with open thoracotomy. Thoracoscopic techniques preclude palpation of the mediastinum. Regardless of approach, a mediastinal lymph node dissection is recommended for all patients undergoing complete (R0) resection of non–small cell lung cancer. A recent study utilizing the National Cancer Database from the American College of Surgeons Commission on Cancer, demonstrated that with Stage I NSCLC better survival was associated with resecting 10 or more lymph nodes to optimally confirm stage I status. Although this is not a therapeutic intervention, it emphasizes the need for mediastinal lymph node dissection to ensure accuracy by decreasing variability in the mediastinal dissection, and optimizing the accuracy of the pathologic staging.[129]

REFERENCES

1. Rivera MP, Mehta AC, Wahidi MM. Establishing the diagnosis of lung cancer: diagnosis and management of lung cancer, 3rd ed: American College of Chest Physicians evidence-based clinical practice guidelines. *Chest* 2013;143:142S–165S. http://dx.doi.org/10.1378/chest.12-2353.
2. Alberts WM. Introduction to the Third Edition: diagnosis and management of lung cancer, 3rd ed: American College of Chest Physicians evidence-based clinical practice guidelines. *Chest* 2013;143:38S–40S. http://dx.doi.org/10.1378/chest.12-2342.
3. Lim E, Baldwin D, Beckles M, et al. Guidelines on the radical management of patients with lung cancer. *Thorax* 2010;65:1–27. http://dx.doi.org/10.1136/thx.2010.145938.
4. De Leyn P, Dooms C, Kuzdzal J, et al. Revised ESTS guidelines for preoperative mediastinal lymph node staging for non-small-cell lung cancer. *Eur J Cardiothorac Surg* 2014;45:787–798. http://dx.doi.org/10.1093/ejcts/ezu028.
5. Detterbeck FC, Lewis SZ, Diekemper R, et al. Executive summary: diagnosis and management of lung cancer, 3rd ed: American College of Chest Physicians evidence-based clinical practice guidelines. *Chest* 2013;143:7S–37S. http://dx.doi.org/10.1378/chest.12-2377.
6. Ettinger DS, Wood DE, Akerley W, et al. Non-Small Cell Lung Cancer. NCCN Clinical Practice Guidelines in Oncology (NCCN Guidelines). 2016. https://www.nccn.org/professionals/physician_gls/pdf/nscl.pdf9-28-2016.
7. Jay SJ, Wehr K, Nicholson DP, et al. Diagnostic sensitivity and specificity of pulmonary cytology: comparison of techniques used in conjunction with flexible fiber optic bronchoscopy. *Acta Cytol* 1980;24:304–312.
8. Wisnivesky JP, Yung RC, Mathur PN, et al. Diagnosis and treatment of bronchial intraepithelial neoplasia and early lung cancer of the central airways: diagnosis and management of lung cancer, 3rd ed: American College of Chest Physicians evidence-based clinical practice guidelines. *Chest* 2013;143:263S–277S. http://dx.doi.org/10.1378/chest.12-2358.
9. Lam B, Lam SY, Wong MP, et al. Sputum cytology examination followed by autofluorescence bronchoscopy: a practical way of identifying early stage lung cancer in central airway. *Lung Cancer* 2009;64:289–294. http://dx.doi.org/10.1016/j.lungcan.2008.09.016.
10. Sun J, Garfield DH, Lam B, et al. The value of autofluorescence bronchoscopy combined with white light bronchoscopy compared with white light alone in the diagnosis of intraepithelial neoplasia and invasive lung cancer: a meta-analysis. *J Thorac Oncol* 2011;6:1336–1344. http://dx.doi.org/10.1097/JTO.0b013e318220c984.
11. Gilbert C, Akulian J, Ortiz R, et al. Novel bronchoscopic strategies for the diagnosis of peripheral lung lesions: present techniques and future directions. *Respirology* 2014;19:636–644. http://dx.doi.org/10.1111/resp.12301.
12. Dooms C, Seijo L, Gasparini S, et al. Diagnostic bronchoscopy: state of the art. *Eur Respir Rev* 2010;19:229–236. http://dx.doi.org/10.1183/09059180.00005710.
13. El-Bayoumi E, Silvestri GA. Bronchoscopy for the diagnosis and staging of lung cancer. *Semin Respir Crit Care Med* 2008;29:261–270. http://dx.doi.org/10.1055/s-2008-1076746.
14. Ernst A, Silvestri GA, Johnstone D, et al. Interventional pulmonary procedures: guidelines from the American College of Chest Physicians. *Chest* 2003;123:1693–1717. http://dx.doi.org/10.1378/chest.123.5.1693.
15. Arias S, Lee H, Semaan R, et al. Use of Electromagnetic Navigational Transthoracic Needle Aspiration (E-TTNA) for sampling of lung nodules. *J Vis Exp* 2015;e52723. http://dx.doi.org/10.3791/52723.
16. Reed CE, Harpole DH, Posther KE, et al. Results of the American College of Surgeons Oncology Group Z0050 trial: the utility of positron emission tomography in staging potentially operable non-small cell lung cancer. *J Thorac Cardiovasc Surg* 2003;126:1943–1951. http://dx.doi.org/10.1016/j.jtcvs.2003.07.030.
17. Steinfort DP, Vincent J, Heinze S, et al. Comparative effectiveness of radial probe endobronchial ultrasound versus CT-guided needle biopsy for evaluation of peripheral pulmonary lesions: a randomized pragmatic trial. *Respir Med* 2011;105:1704–1711. http://dx.doi.org/10.1016/j.rmed.2011.08.008.
18. Mahajan AK, Patel S, Hogarth DK, et al. Electromagnetic navigational bronchoscopy: an effective and safe approach to diagnose peripheral lung lesions unreachable by conventional bronchoscopy in high-risk patients. *J Bronchology Interv Pulmonol* 2011;18:133–137. http://dx.doi.org/10.1097/LBR.0b013e318216cee6.
19. Mudambi L, Ost DE. Advanced bronchoscopic techniques for the diagnosis of peripheral pulmonary lesions. *Curr Opin Pulm Med* 2016;22:309–318. http://dx.doi.org/10.1097/MCP.0000000000000284.
20. Yarmus LB, Arias S, Feller-Kopman D, et al. Electromagnetic navigation transthoracic needle aspiration for the diagnosis of pulmonary nodules: a safety and feasibility pilot study. *J Thorac Dis* 2016;8:186–194. http://dx.doi.org/10.3978/j.issn.2072-1439.2016.01.47.
21. Eberhardt R, Anantham D, Ernst A, et al. Multimodality bronchoscopic diagnosis of peripheral lung lesions: a randomized controlled trial. *Am J Respir Crit Care Med* 2007;176:36–41. http://dx.doi.org/10.1164/rccm.200612-1866OC.
22. Wiener RS, Schwartz LM, Woloshin S, et al. Population-based risk for complications after transthoracic needle lung biopsy of a pulmonary nodule: an analysis of discharge records. *Ann Intern Med* 2011;155:137–144. http://dx.doi.org/10.7326/0003-4819-155-3-201108020-00003.
23. Gould MK, Donington J, Lynch WR, et al. Evaluation of individuals with pulmonary nodules: when is it lung cancer? Diagnosis and management of lung cancer, 3rd ed: American College of Chest Physicians evidence-based clinical practice guidelines. *Chest* 2013;143:93S–120S. http://dx.doi.org/10.1378/chest.12-2351.
24. Nakajima T, Yasufuku K, Saegusa F, et al. Rapid on-site cytologic evaluation during endobronchial ultrasound-guided transbronchial needle aspiration for nodal staging in patients with lung cancer. *Ann Thorac Surg* 2013;95:1695–1699. http://dx.doi.org/10.1016/j.athoracsur.2012.09.074.
25. Zarbo RJ, Fenoglio-Preiser CM. Interinstitutional database for comparison of performance in lung fine-needle aspiration cytology. A College of American Pathologists Q-Probe Study of 5264 cases with histologic correlation. *Arch Pathol Lab Med* 1992;116:463–470.
26. Giroux DJ, Rami-Porta R, Chansky K, et al. The IASLC Lung Cancer Staging Project: data elements for the prospective project. *J Thorac Oncol* 2009;4:679–683. http://dx.doi.org/10.1097/JTO.0b013e3181a52370.
27. Awais O, Reidy MR, Mehta K, et al. Electromagnetic navigation bronchoscopy-guided dye marking for thoracoscopic resection of pulmonary nodules. *Ann Thorac Surg* 2016;102:223–229. http://dx.doi.org/10.1016/j.athoracsur.2016.02.040.
28. Jackson P, Steinfort DP, Kron T, et al. Practical assessment of bronchoscopically inserted fiducial markers for image guidance in stereotactic lung radiotherapy. *J Thorac Oncol* 2016;11:1363–1368. http://dx.doi.org/10.1016/j.jtho.2016.04.016.
29. Nabavizadeh N, Zhang J, Elliott DA, et al. Electromagnetic navigational bronchoscopy-guided fiducial markers for lung stereotactic body radiation therapy: analysis of safety, feasibility, and interfraction stability. *J Bronchology Interv Pulmonol* 2014;21:123–130. http://dx.doi.org/10.1097/LBR.0000000000000065.
30. Silvestri GA, Gonzalez AV, Jantz MA, et al. Methods for staging non-small cell lung cancer: diagnosis and management of lung cancer, 3rd ed: American College of Chest Physicians evidence-based clinical practice guidelines. *Chest* 2013;143:211S–250S. http://dx.doi.org/10.1378/chest.12-2355.
31. Jett JR, Schild SE, Kesler KA, et al. Treatment of small cell lung cancer: diagnosis and management of lung cancer, 3rd ed: American College of Chest Physicians evidence-based clinical practice guidelines. *Chest* 2013;143:400S–419S. http://dx.doi.org/10.1378/chest.12-2363.
32. Mountain CF. Revisions in the international system for staging lung cancer. *Chest* 1997;111:1710–1717. http://dx.doi.org/10.1378/chest.111.6.1710.
33. Mountain CF, Dresler CM. Regional lymph node classification for lung cancer staging. *Chest* 1997;111:1718–1723. http://dx.doi.org/10.1378/chest.111.6.1718.
34. Naruke T, Suemasu K, Ishikawa S. Lymph node mapping and curability at various levels of metastasis in resected lung cancer. *J Thorac Cardiovasc Surg* 1978;76:832–839.
35. Goldstraw P, Crowley JJ; IASLC International Staging Project. The international association for the study of lung cancer international staging project on lung cancer. *J Thor Oncol* 2006;1:281–286. http://dx.doi.org/10.1016/S1556-0864(15)31581-1.
36. Goldstraw P, Crowley J, Chansky K, et al. The IASLC Lung Cancer Staging Project: proposals for the revision of the TNM stage groupings in the forthcoming (seventh) edition of the TNM Classification of malignant tumours. *J Thorac Oncol* 2007;2:706–714. http://dx.doi.org/10.1097/JTO.0b013e31812f3c1a.
37. Lung. In: Edge SB, Byrd DR, Compton CC, eds. *AJCC Cancer Staging Manual.* 7th ed: Springer; 2009:253–270.
38. Groome PA, Bolejack V, Crowley JJ, et al. The IASLC Lung Cancer Staging Project: validation of the proposals for revision of the T, N, and M descriptors and consequent stage groupings in the forthcoming (seventh) edition of the TNM classification of malignant tumours. *J Thorac Oncol* 2007;2:694–705.
39. Detterbeck FC, Chansky K, Groome P, et al. The IASLC lung cancer staging project: methodology and validation used in the development of proposals for revision of the stage classification of NSCLC in the forthcoming (eighth) edition of the TNM classification of lung cancer. *J Thorac Oncol* 2016;11:1433–1446. http://dx.doi.org/10.1016/j.jtho.2016.06.028.
40. Rami-Porta R, Bolejack V, Giroux DJ, et al. The IASLC lung cancer staging project: the new database to inform the eighth edition of the TNM classification of lung cancer. *J Thorac Oncol* 2014;9:1618–1624. http://dx.doi.org/10.1097/JTO.0000000000000334.
41. Rami-Porta R, Ball D, Crowley J, et al. The IASLC lung cancer staging project: proposals for the revision of the T descriptors in the forthcoming (seventh) edition of the TNM classification for lung cancer. *J Thorac Oncol* 2007;2:593–602. http://dx.doi.org/10.1097/JTO.0b013e31807a2f81.
42. Goldstraw P, Chansky K, Crowley J, et al. The IASLC lung cancer staging project: proposals for revision of the TNM stage groupings in the forthcoming (eighth) edition of the TNM classification for lung cancer. *J Thorac Oncol* 2016;11:39–51. http://dx.doi.org/10.1016/j.jtho.2015.09.009.
43. Rami-Porta R, Bolejack V, Crowley J, et al. The IASLC lung cancer staging project: proposals for the revisions of the T descriptors in the forthcoming eighth edition of the TNM classification for lung cancer. *J Thorac Oncol* 2015;10:990–1003. http://dx.doi.org/10.1097/JTO.0000000000000559.
44. Detterbeck FC, Marom EM, Arenberg DA, et al. The IASLC lung cancer staging project: background data and proposals for the application of TNM staging rules to lung cancer presenting as multiple nodules with ground glass or lepidic features or a pneumonic type of involvement in the forthcoming eighth edition of the TNM Classification. *J Thorac Oncol* 2016;11:666–680. http://dx.doi.org/10.1016/j.jtho.2015.12.113.

45. Detterbeck FC, Nicholson AG, Franklin WA, et al. The IASLC lung cancer staging project: summary of proposals for revisions of the classification of lung cancers with multiple pulmonary sites of involvement in the forthcoming eighth edition of the TNM classification. *J Thorac Oncol* 2016;11:639–650. http://dx.doi.org/10.1016/j.jtho.2016.01.024.
46. Rusch VW, Crowley J, Giroux DJ, et al. The IASLC lung cancer staging project: proposals for the revision of the N descriptors in the forthcoming seventh edition of the TNM classification for lung cancer. *J Thorac Oncol* 2007;2:603–612. http://dx.doi.org/10.1097/JTO.0b013e31807ec803.
47. Rusch VW, Asamura H, Watanabe H, et al. The IASLC lung cancer staging project: a proposal for a new international lymph node map in the forthcoming seventh edition of the TNM classification for lung cancer. *J Thorac Oncol* 2009;4:568–577. http://dx.doi.org/10.1097/JTO.0b013e3181a0d82e.
48. Asamura H, Chansky K, Crowley J, et al. The international association for the study of lung cancer lung cancer staging project: proposals for the revision of the N descriptors in the forthcoming 8th edition of the TNM classification for lung cancer. *J Thorac Oncol* 2015;10:1675–1684. http://dx.doi.org/10.1097/JTO.0000000000000678.
49. Postmus PE, Brambilla E, Chansky K, et al. The IASLC lung cancer staging project: proposals for revision of the M descriptors in the forthcoming (seventh) edition of the TNM classification of lung cancer. *J Thorac Oncol* 2007;2:686–693. http://dx.doi.org/10.1097/JTO.0b013e31811f4703.
50. Detterbeck FC, Franklin WA, Nicholson AG, et al. The IASLC lung cancer staging project: background data and proposed criteria to distinguish separate primary lung cancers from metastatic foci in patients with two lung tumors in the forthcoming eighth edition of the TNM classification for lung cancer. *J Thorac Oncol* 2016;11:651–665. http://dx.doi.org/10.1016/j.jtho.2016.01.025.
51. American Joint Committee on Cancer. AJCC 7th Edition Staging Posters. American Joint Committee on Cancer 2010. Available from: URL: http://www.cancerstaging.org/staging/index.html Notes: ILLUSTRATION. The IASLC *lymph node map* shown ... www.cancerstaging.org/staging/posters/lung12x15.pdf.
52. Rice TW, Murthy SC, Mason DP, et al. A cancer staging primer: lung. *J Thorac Cardiovasc Surg* 2010;139:826–829. http://dx.doi.org/10.1016/j.jtcvs.2009.11.010.
53. Heelan RT, Martini N, Westcott JW, et al. Carcinomatous involvement of the hilum and mediastinum: computed tomographic and magnetic resonance evaluation. *Radiology* 1985;156:111–115. http://dx.doi.org/10.1148/radiology.156.1.4001396.
54. Sommer G, Tremper J, Koenigkam-Santos M, et al. Lung nodule detection in a high-risk population: comparison of magnetic resonance imaging and low-dose computed tomography. *Eur J Radiol* 2014;83:600–605. http://dx.doi.org/10.1016/j.ejrad.2013.11.012.
55. Juweid ME, Cheson BD. Positron-emission tomography and assessment of cancer therapy. *N Engl J Med* 2006;354:496–507. http://dx.doi.org/10.1056/NEJMra050276.
56. Deppen S, Putnam JB, Jr, Andrade G, et al. Accuracy of FDG-PET to diagnose lung cancer in a region of endemic granulomatous disease. *Ann Thorac Surg* 2011;92:428–432. http://dx.doi.org/10.1016/j.athoracsur.2011.02.052.
57. Grogan EL, Deppen SA, Ballman KV, et al. Accuracy of fluorodeoxyglucose-positron emission tomography within the clinical practice of the American College of Surgeons Oncology Group Z4031 trial to diagnose clinical stage I non-small cell lung cancer. *Ann Thorac Surg* 2014;97:1142–1148. http://dx.doi.org/10.1016/j.athoracsur.2013.12.043.
58. Fischer B, Lassen U, Mortensen J, et al. Preoperative staging of lung cancer with combined PET-CT. *N Engl J Med* 2009;361:32–39. http://dx.doi.org/10.1056/NEJMoa0900043.
59. Harders SW, Madsen HH, Hjorthaug K, et al. Mediastinal staging in Non-Small-Cell Lung Carcinoma: computed tomography versus F-18-fluorodeoxyglucose positron-emission tomography and computed tomography. *Cancer Imaging* 2014;14:23. http://dx.doi.org/10.1186/1470-7330-14-23.
60. Toloza EM, Meyers BF, Mackie-McCall L, et al. Prevalence of mediastinal metastases and sensitivity of mediastinoscopy. In: *Potentially Operable Non-Small Cell Lung Cancer Screened By Computerized Tomography and Positron Emission Tomography.* 2006 Annual Meeting. Philadelphia, PA: Abstract; 2006.
61. Fischer BM, Mortensen J, Hansen H, et al. Multimodality approach to mediastinal staging in non-small cell lung cancer. Faults and benefits of PET-CT: a randomised trial. *Thorax* 2011;66:294–300. http://dx.doi.org/10.1136/thx.2010.154476.
62. Deppen SA, Blume JD, Kensinger CD, et al. Accuracy of FDG-PET to diagnose lung cancer in areas with infectious lung disease: a meta-analysis. *JAMA* 2014;312:1227–1236. http://dx.doi.org/10.1001/jama.2014.11488.
63. Deppen SA, Blume JD, Aldrich MC, et al. Predicting lung cancer prior to surgical resection in patients with lung nodules. *J Thorac Oncol* 2014;9:1477–1484. http://dx.doi.org/10.1097/JTO.0000000000000287.
64. Meyers BF, Haddad F, Siegel BA, et al. Cost-effectiveness of routine mediastinoscopy in computed tomography- and positron emission tomography-screened patients with stage I lung cancer. *J Thorac Cardiovasc Surg* 2006;131:822–829. http://dx.doi.org/10.1016/j.jtcvs.2005.10.045.
65. Toloza EM, Harpole L, McCrory DC. Noninvasive staging of non-small cell lung cancer: a review of the current evidence. *Chest* 2003;123:137S–146S. http://dx.doi.org/10.1378/chest.123.1_suppl.137S.
66. Stamatis G. Staging of lung cancer: the role of noninvasive, minimally invasive and invasive techniques. *Eur Respir J* 2015;46:521–531. http://dx.doi.org/10.1183/09031936.00126714.
67. Detterbeck FC, Postmus PE, Tanoue LT. The stage classification of lung cancer: diagnosis and management of lung cancer, 3rd ed: American College of Chest Physicians evidence-based clinical practice guidelines. *Chest* 2013;143:191S–210S. http://dx.doi.org/10.1378/chest.12-2354.
68. Yap KK, Yap KS, Byrne AJ, et al. Positron emission tomography with selected mediastinoscopy compared to routine mediastinoscopy offers cost and clinical outcome benefits for pre-operative staging of non-small cell lung cancer. *Eur J Nucl Med Mol Imaging* 2005;32:1033–1040. http://dx.doi.org/10.1007/s00259-005-1821-0.
69. Annema JT, van Meerbeeck JP, Rintoul RC, et al. Mediastinoscopy vs endosonography for mediastinal nodal staging of lung cancer: a randomized trial. *JAMA* 2010;304:2245–2252. http://dx.doi.org/10.1001/jama.2010.1705.
70. Annema JT, Bohoslavsky R, Burgers S, et al. Implementation of endoscopic ultrasound for lung cancer staging. *Gastrointest Endosc* 2010;71(1):64–70, 70 e1. http://dx.doi.org/10.1016/j.gie.2009.07.027.
71. Eberhardt WE, Mitchell A, Crowley J, et al. The IASLC lung cancer staging project: proposals for the revision of the M descriptors in the forthcoming eighth edition of the TNM classification of lung cancer. *J Thorac Oncol* 2015;10:1515–1522. http://dx.doi.org/10.1097/JTO.0000000000000673.
72. Investigation for mediastinal disease in patients with apparently operable lung cancer. Canadian Lung Oncology Group. *Ann Thorac Surg* 1995;60:1382–1389. http://dx.doi.org/10.1016/S0003-4975(00)02359-6.
73. Chapman GS, Kumar D, Redmond J 3rd., et al. Upper abdominal computerized tomography scanning in staging non-small cell lung carcinoma. *Cancer* 1984;54:1541–1543. http://dx.doi.org/10.1002/1097-0142(19841015)54:8<1541::AID-CNCR2820540812>3.0.CO;2-N.
74. Heinz-Peer G, Honigschnabl S, Schneider B, et al. Characterization of adrenal masses using MR imaging with histopathologic correlation. *AJR Am J Roentgenol* 1999;173:15–22. http://dx.doi.org/10.2214/ajr.173.1.10397092.
75. Verboom P, van TH, Hoekstra OS, et al. Cost-effectiveness of FDG-PET in staging non-small cell lung cancer: the PLUS study. *Eur J Nucl Med Mol Imaging* 2003;30:1444–1449. http://dx.doi.org/10.1007/s00259-003-1199-9.
76. van Tinteren H, Hoekstra OS, Smit EF, et al. Effectiveness of positron emission tomography in the preoperative assessment of patients with suspected non-small-cell lung cancer: the PLUS multicentre randomised trial. *Lancet* 2002;359:1388–1393. http://dx.doi.org/10.1016/S0140-6736(02)08352-6.
77. Balekian AA, Fisher JM, Gould MK. Brain imaging for staging of patients with clinical stage IA non-small cell lung cancer in the national lung screening trial: adherence with recommendations from the choosing wisely campaign. *Chest* 2016;149:943–950. http://dx.doi.org/10.1378/chest.15-1140.
78. Ravenel JG, Mohammed TL, Movsas B, et al. ACR Appropriateness Criteria noninvasive clinical staging of bronchogenic carcinoma. *J Thorac Imaging* 2010;25:W107–W111. http://dx.doi.org/10.1097/RTI.0b013e3181f51e7f.
79. Colice GL, Birkmeyer JD, Black WC, et al. Cost-effectiveness of head CT in patients with lung cancer without clinical evidence of metastases. *Chest* 1995;108:1264–1271. http://dx.doi.org/10.1378/chest.108.5.1264.
80. Davis SD. CT evaluation for pulmonary metastases in patients with extrathoracic malignancy. *Radiology* 1991;180:1–12. http://dx.doi.org/10.1148/radiology.180.1.2052672.
81. Yokoi K, Kamiya N, Matsuguma H, et al. Detection of brain metastasis in potentially operable non-small cell lung cancer: a comparison of CT and MRI. *Chest* 1999;115:714–719. http://dx.doi.org/10.1378/chest.115.3.714.
82. Tarver RD, Richmond BD, Klatte EC. Cerebral metastases from lung carcinoma: neurological and CT correlation. Work in progress. *Radiology* 1984;153:689–692. http://dx.doi.org/10.1148/radiology.153.3.6093189.
83. Ferrigno D, Buccheri G. Cranial computed tomography as a part of the initial staging procedures for patients with non-small-cell lung cancer. *Chest* 1994;106:1025–1029. http://dx.doi.org/10.1378/chest.106.4.1025.
84. Kormas P, Bradshaw JR, Jeyasingham K. Preoperative computed tomography of the brain in non-small cell bronchogenic carcinoma. *Thorax* 1992;47:106–108. http://dx.doi.org/10.1136/thx.47.2.106.
85. Song JW, Oh YM, Shim TS, et al. Efficacy comparison between (18)F-FDG PET/CT and bone scintigraphy in detecting bony metastases of non-small-cell lung cancer. *Lung Cancer* 2009;65:333–338. http://dx.doi.org/10.1016/j.lungcan.2008.12.004.
86. Oliver TW, Bernardino ME, Miller JI, et al. Isolated adrenal masses in nonsmall-cell bronchogenic carcinoma. *Radiology* 1984;153:217–218. http://dx.doi.org/10.1148/radiology.153.1.6473783.
87. Brady MJ, Thomas J, Wong TZ, et al. Adrenal nodules at FDG PET/CT in patients known to have or suspected of having lung cancer: a proposal for an efficient diagnostic algorithm. *Radiology* 2009;250:523–530. http://dx.doi.org/10.1148/radiol.2502080219.
88. Wang KP, Marsh BR, Summer WR, et al. Transbronchial needle aspiration for diagnosis of lung cancer. *Chest* 1981;80:48–50. http://dx.doi.org/10.1378/chest.80.1.48.
89. Navani N, Nankivell M, Lawrence DR, et al. Lung cancer diagnosis and staging with endobronchial ultrasound-guided transbronchial needle aspiration compared with conventional approaches: an open-label, pragmatic, randomised controlled trial. *Lancet Respir Med* 2015;3:282–289. http://dx.doi.org/10.1016/S2213-2600(15)00029-6.
90. Gasparini S, Bonifazi M, Wang KP. Transbronchial needle aspirations vs. percutaneous needle aspirations. *J Thorac Dis* 2015;7:S300–S303. http://dx.doi.org/10.3978/j.issn.2072-1439.2015.11.60.
91. Kinsey CM, Arenberg DA. Endobronchial ultrasound-guided transbronchial needle aspiration for non-small cell lung cancer staging. *Am J Respir Crit Care Med* 2014;189:640–649. http://dx.doi.org/10.1164/rccm.201311-2007CI.
92. Cornwell LD, Bakaeen FG, Lan CK, et al. Endobronchial ultrasonography-guided transbronchial needle aspiration biopsy for preoperative nodal staging of lung cancer in a veteran population. *JAMA Surg* 2013;148:1024–1029. http://dx.doi.org/10.1001/jamasurg.2013.3776.
93. Kothary N, Lock L, Sze DY, et al. Computed tomography-guided percutaneous needle biopsy of pulmonary nodules: impact of nodule size on diagnostic accuracy. *Clin Lung Cancer* 2009;10:360–363. http://dx.doi.org/10.3816/CLC.2009.n.049.

94. Ng YL, Patsios D, Roberts H, et al. CT-guided percutaneous fine-needle aspiration biopsy of pulmonary nodules measuring 10 mm or less. *Clin Radiol* 2008;63:272–277. http://dx.doi.org/10.1016/j.crad.2007.09.003.

95. Pearson FG, Nelems JM, Henderson RD, et al. The role of mediastinoscopy in the selection of treatment for bronchial carcinoma with involvement of superior mediastinal lymph nodes. *J Thorac Cardiovasc Surg* 1972;54:382–390.

96. Ginsberg RJ, Rice TW, Goldberg M, et al. Extended cervical mediastinoscopy. A single staging procedure for bronchogenic carcinoma of the left upper lobe. *J Thorac Cardiovasc Surg* 1987;94:673–678.

97. Freixinet GJ, Garcia PG, de Castro FR, et al. Extended cervical mediastinoscopy in the staging of bronchogenic carcinoma. *Ann Thorac Surg* 2000;70:1641–1643. http://dx.doi.org/10.1016/S0003-4975(00)01825-7.

98. Obiols C, Call S, Rami-Porta R, et al. Extended cervical mediastinoscopy: mature results of a clinical protocol for staging bronchogenic carcinoma of the left lung. *Eur J Cardiothorac Surg* 2012;41:1043–1046. http://dx.doi.org/10.1093/ejcts/ezr181.

99. Witte B, Wolf M, Hillebrand H, et al. Extended cervical mediastinoscopy revisited. *Eur J Cardiothorac Surg* 2014;45:114–119. http://dx.doi.org/10.1093/ejcts/ezt313.

100. Citak N, Buyukkale S, Kok A, et al. Does video-assisted mediastinoscopy offer lower false-negative rates for subcarinal lymph nodes compared with standard cervical mediastinoscopy?. *Thorac Cardiovasc Surg* 2014;62:624–630. http://dx.doi.org/10.1055/s-0033-1358656.

101. Turna A, Demirkaya A, Ozkul S, et al. Video-assisted mediastinoscopic lymphadenectomy is associated with better survival than mediastinoscopy in patients with resected non-small cell lung cancer. *J Thorac Cardiovasc Surg* 2013;146:774–780. http://dx.doi.org/10.1016/j.jtcvs.2013.04.036.

102. Call S, Obiols C, Rami-Porta R, et al. Video-assisted mediastinoscopic lymphadenectomy for staging non-small cell lung cancer. *Ann Thorac Surg* 2016;101:1326–1333. http://dx.doi.org/10.1016/j.athoracsur.2015.10.073.

103. Witte B, Hurtgen M. Video-assisted mediastinoscopic lymphadenectomy (VAMLA). *J Thorac Oncol* 2007;2:367–369. http://dx.doi.org/10.1097/01.JTO.0000263725.89512.d7.

104. Zakkar M, Tan C, Hunt I. Is video mediastinoscopy a safer and more effective procedure than conventional mediastinoscopy? *Interact Cardiovasc Thorac Surg* 2012;14:81–84. http://dx.doi.org/10.1093/icvts/ivr044.

105. Zielinski M. Video-assisted mediastinoscopic lymphadenectomy and transcervical extended mediastinal lymphadenectomy. *Thorac Surg Clin* 2012;22:219–225. http://dx.doi.org/10.1016/j.thorsurg.2011.12.005.

106. Zieliski M. Transcervical extended mediastinal lymphadenectomy: results of staging in two hundred fifty-six patients with non-small cell lung cancer. *J Thorac Oncol* 2007;2:370–372. http://dx.doi.org/10.1097/01.JTO.0000263726.89512.0c.

107. Kuzdzal J, Warmus J, Grochowski Z. Optimal mediastinal staging in non-small cell lung cancer: what is the role of TEMLA and VAMLA? *Lung Cancer* 2014;86:1–4. http://dx.doi.org/10.1016/j.lungcan.2014.07.015.

108. McNeill TM, Chamberlain JM. Diagnostic anterior mediastinotomy. *Ann Thorac Surg* 1966;2:532–539. http://dx.doi.org/10.1016/S0003-4975(10)66614-3.

109. Rami PR. Surgical exploration of the mediastinum by mediastinoscopy, parasternal mediastinotomy and remediastinoscopy: indications, technique and complications. *Ann Ital Chir* 1999;70:867–872.

110. Olak FJ. Parasternal mediastinotomy (Chamberlain procedure). *Chest Surg Clin N Am* 1996;6:31–40.

111. Roviaro G, Varoli F, Rebuffat C, et al. Videothoracoscopic staging and treatment of lung cancer. *Ann Thorac Surg* 1995;59:971–974. http://dx.doi.org/10.1016/0003-4975(95)00029-K.

112. Yasufuku K. Relevance of endoscopic ultrasonography and endobronchial ultrasonography to thoracic surgeons. *Thorac Surg Clin* 2013;23:199–210. http://dx.doi.org/10.1016/j.thorsurg.2013.01.016.

113. Wahidi MM, Herth F, Yasufuku K, et al. Technical aspects of endobronchial ultrasound-guided transbronchial needle aspiration: chest guideline and expert panel report. *Chest* 2016;149:816–835. http://dx.doi.org/10.1378/chest.15-1216.

114. Vilmann P, Clementsen PF, Colella S, et al. Combined endobronchial and esophageal endosonography for the diagnosis and staging of lung cancer: European Society of Gastrointestinal Endoscopy (ESGE) Guideline, in cooperation with the European Respiratory Society (ERS) and the European Society of Thoracic Surgeons (ESTS). *Endoscopy* 2015;47:545–559. http://dx.doi.org/10.1055/s-0034-1392040.

115. Kang HJ, Hwangbo B, Lee GK, et al. EBUS-centred versus EUS-centred mediastinal staging in lung cancer: a randomised controlled trial. *Thorax* 2014;69:261–268. http://dx.doi.org/10.1136/thoraxjnl-2013-203881.

116. Oki M, Saka H, Ando M, et al. Endoscopic ultrasound-guided fine needle aspiration and endobronchial ultrasound-guided transbronchial needle aspiration: are two better than one in mediastinal staging of non-small cell lung cancer? *J Thorac Cardiovasc Surg* 2014;148:1169–1177. http://dx.doi.org/10.1016/j.jtcvs.2014.05.023.

117. Herth FJ, Ernst A, Eberhardt R, et al. Endobronchial ultrasound-guided transbronchial needle aspiration of lymph nodes in the radiologically normal mediastinum. *Eur Respir J* 2006;28:910–914. http://dx.doi.org/10.4065/77.2.155.

118. Um SW, Kim HK, Jung SH, et al. Endobronchial ultrasound versus mediastinoscopy for mediastinal nodal staging of non-small-cell lung cancer. *J Thorac Oncol* 2015;10:331–337. http://dx.doi.org/10.1097/JTO.0000000000000388.

119. Berania I, Kazakov J, Khereba M, et al. Endoscopic mediastinal staging in lung cancer is superior to "Gold Standard" surgical staging. *Ann Thorac Surg* 2016;101:547–550. http://dx.doi.org/10.1016/j.athoracsur.2015.08.070.

120. Liberman M, Sampalis J, Duranceau A, et al. Endosonographic mediastinal lymph node staging of lung cancer. *Chest* 2014;146:389–397. http://dx.doi.org/10.1378/chest.13-2349.

121. Clementsen PF, Skov BG, Vilmann P, et al. Endobronchial ultrasound-guided biopsy performed under optimal conditions in patients with known or suspected lung cancer may render mediastinoscopy unnecessary. *J Bronchology Interv Pulmonol* 2014;21:21–25. http://dx.doi.org/10.1097/LBR.0000000000000028.

122. Szlubowski A, Zielinski M, Soja J, et al. Accurate and safe mediastinal restaging by combined endobronchial and endoscopic ultrasound-guided needle aspiration performed by single ultrasound bronchoscope. *Eur J Cardiothorac Surg* 2014;46:262–266. http://dx.doi.org/10.1093/ejcts/ezt570.

123. Vilmann P, Frost CP, Colella S, et al. Combined endobronchial and esophageal endosonography for the diagnosis and staging of lung cancer: European Society of Gastrointestinal Endoscopy (ESGE) Guideline, in cooperation with the European Respiratory Society (ERS) and the European Society of Thoracic Surgeons (ESTS). *Eur J Cardiothorac Surg* 2015;48:1–15. http://dx.doi.org/10.1093/ejcts/ezv194.

124. Harewood GC, Wiersema MJ, Edell ES, et al. Cost-minimization analysis of alternative diagnostic approaches in a modeled patient with non-small cell lung cancer and subcarinal lymphadenopathy. *Mayo Clin Proc* 2002;77:155–164. http://dx.doi.org/10.4065/77.2.155.

125. Eloubeidi MA, Desmond R, Desai S, et al. Impact of staging transesophageal EUS on treatment and survival in patients with non-small-cell lung cancer. *Gastrointest Endosc* 2008;67:193–198. http://dx.doi.org/10.1016/j.gie.2007.06.052.

126. Hwangbo B, Lee GK, Lee HS, et al. Transbronchial and transesophageal fine-needle aspiration using an ultrasound bronchoscope in mediastinal staging of potentially operable lung cancer. *Chest* 2010;138:795–802. http://dx.doi.org/10.1378/chest.09-2100.

127. Herth FJ, Krasnik M, Kahn N, et al. Combined endoscopic-endobronchial ultrasound-guided fine-needle aspiration of mediastinal lymph nodes through a single bronchoscope in 150 patients with suspected lung cancer. *Chest* 2010;138:790–794. http://dx.doi.org/10.1378/chest.09-2149.

128. Micames CG, McCrory DC, Pavey DA, et al. Endoscopic ultrasound-guided fine-needle aspiration for non-small cell lung cancer staging: a systematic review and metaanalysis. *Chest* 2007;131:539–548. http://dx.doi.org/10.1378/chest.06-1437.

129. Samayoa AX, Pezzi TA, Pezzi CM, et al. Rationale for a minimum number of lymph nodes removed with non-small cell lung cancer resection: correlating the number of nodes removed with survival in 98,970 patients. *Ann Surg Oncol* 2016;23:1005–1011. http://dx.doi.org/10.1245/s10434-016-5509-4.

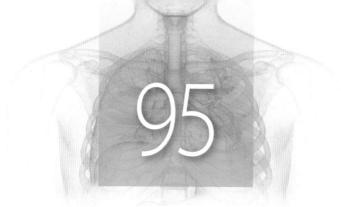

95

Results of Surgical Treatment of Non-Small Cell Lung Cancer

Ernest G. Chan ▪ Patrick G. Chan ▪ Matthew J. Schuchert

INTRODUCTION

Lung cancer is the leading cause of cancer-related mortality worldwide, with an estimated 1.8 million new cases and 1.6 million deaths in 2012, constituting 19% of all cancer deaths.[1] In the United States, lung cancer accounts for a staggering 27% of all cancer-related deaths, with an estimated 158, 080 deaths expected in 2016.[2] This represents approximately as many deaths as the next four causes of cancer-related mortality (colorectal, pancreatic, breast, hepatic) combined. The mean age of presentation is 67 years, but it also afflicts younger patients and is responsible for more life years lost than colorectal, breast, and prostate cancer combined.[3]

The optimal management of patients with non-small cell lung cancer (NSCLC) is dictated by tumor characteristics, clinical stage, as well as, the patient's underlying physiologic status. Patients with clinical stage IA–IIB NSCLC are best managed by anatomic lung resection with mediastinal lymph node sampling or dissection. There is benefit in the use of adjuvant chemotherapy for those patients with nodal involvement (stage IIA or IIB) following complete resection. Patients with advanced NSCLC (stage IIIB or IV) are best managed by chemoradiation (for locoregionally advanced cases, stage IIIB) or chemotherapy only in the case of systemic metastases (stage IV). There is no proven benefit for the routine use of surgery in patients with advanced NSCLC.

Complete (R0) surgical resection of primary NSCLC, along with its lymphatic and vascular supply, constitutes the primary therapeutic approach when technically possible, and affords patients with the best chance for cure. Over the last 75 years, we have witnessed a dramatic evolution of surgical thought in the management of resectable NSCLC. Extent of lung resection has evolved from pneumonectomy to lobectomy, and even segmentectomy in select instances. Standard open techniques have been supplanted by video-assisted thoracic surgery (VATS) as the preferred approach in the setting of early-stage disease. Robotic-assisted and minimally invasive ablative techniques continue to evolve and provide opportunities for surgical innovation. Despite the rapidly changing landscape, the fundamental tenets of complete surgical resection with systematic nodal staging remain the cornerstone of surgical therapy.

In this chapter, the authors explore the results of surgical treatment for NSCLC. The chapter will analyze the expected perioperative outcomes, the modern-day standards of morbidity and mortality as well as the oncological outcomes following surgical resection.

Covered elsewhere are the technical descriptions of lung resections, lung ablative approaches (SBRT, RFA), palliative strategies, as well as results related to small cell lung cancer.

HISTORICAL TRENDS

The first lobectomy for lung cancer is credited to Lothar Heidenhain in 1903, where cancer was detected incidentally during a piecemeal lower lobe resection for bronchiectasis.[4] In 1912, Davies performed the first lobectomy with formal hilar dissection and vascular ligation, though the patient died on the eighth postoperative day secondary to presumed empyema.[5] The first successful single-stage anatomic resection of lung cancer was performed in 1933 by Graham, who performed a pneumonectomy utilizing a mass ligation technique followed by thoracoplasty.[6] Over the next 10 years, pneumonectomy became regarded as the optimal approach for the management of lung cancer, as summarized by Ochsner et al.: "As previously emphasized, it is our firm conviction that any procedure short of total removal of the involved lung is irrational and only by total pneumonectomy can the primary focus as well as the regional lymph nodes be adequately removed."[7] Radical pneumonectomy was regarded as the standard of care and permitted complete excision of the tumor as well as the entire lymphatic supply of the lung,[8] in a manner analogous to the Halstedian approach to breast cancer.[9] Perioperative mortality rates in the largest published series ranged were between 30% and 100%,[10] with reported 3-year survival rates of 24%,[11] but were deemed acceptable in what was otherwise a lethal condition (Table 95.1).

The high attendant morbidity and mortality associated with pneumonectomy, led to the consideration of lesser forms of resection (lobectomy) as a potential alternative.[12] Johnson et al. challenged the need for pneumonectomy in all cases, and theorized that any perceived advantage in survival could be accounted for by differences in patient selection.[13] Bronchoplastic procedures were developed during the late 1940s, culminating in Allison's first successful sleeve lobectomy for a bronchial carcinoma in 1952, as reported by Thomas.[14] Shimkin et al. were the first to provide a direct comparison of outcomes following lobectomy versus pneumonectomy by combining data from the Ochsner and Overholt clinics, and found that extent of disease, more so than extent of resection, dictated differences in survival (Fig. 95.1). They concluded that "more extensive operations increase mortality and do not improve total survival figures."[15] By the late 1950s, lobectomy had surpassed pneumonectomy

TABLE 95.1 Historical Mortality Trends for Resectable NSCLC

Authors	Date	Surgical Approach	Resection Number	Mortality (%)
Graham et al.[6]	1930s	Pneumomectomy	70	31.4
Ochsner et al.[327]	1944	Pneumonectomy	117	25.6
Churchill et al.[16]	1950	Pneumonectomy Lobectomy	114 57	22.8 14.0
Weiss et al.[328]	1974	Pneumonectomy Lobectomy	212 149	17.0 10.1
Ginsberg et al.[329]	1983	Pneumonectomy Lobectomy	569 1,058	6.2 2.9
Romano et al.[330]	1992	Pneumonectomy Lobectomy	1,529 6,569	11.6 4.2
Ginsberg et al.[331]	1995	Lobectomy Sublobar Resection	125 122	1.6 0.8
Wada et al.[332]	1998	Pneumonectomy Lobectomy	586 5,609	3.2 1.2
Harpole et al.[333]	1999	Pneumonectomy Lobectomy	567 2,949	11.5 4.0
Allen et al.[334]	2006	Pneumonectomy Lobectomy Segmentctomy	42 766 70	0 1.3 2.9
Paul et al.[56]	2010	Lobectomy	2,562	1.0
Schuchert et al.[101]	2014	Lobectomy Segmentectomy	312 312	2.5 1.2
Okada et al.[335]	2014	Lobectomy Segmentectomy	479 155	0 0

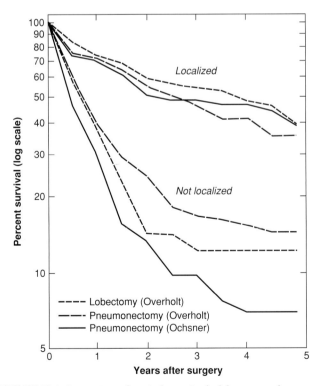

FIGURE 95.1 Comparison of surgical resection by lobectomy and pneumonectomy for localized and nonlocalized NSCLC. (Reprinted from Shimkin MB, Connelly RR, Marcus SC, et al. Pneumonectomy and lobectomy in bronchogenic carcinoma. A comparison of end results of the Overholt and Ochsner clinics. *J Thorac Cardiovasc Surg* 1962;44:503–519. Copyright © 1962 The American Association for Thoracic Surgery. With permission.)

as the preferred method of resection for peripheral lung cancers as a result of the observed reduction in operative morbidity and mortality (15% to 20% vs. 20% to 30%), as well as modest increases in long term survival with lobectomy relative to pneumonectomy (19% vs. 12%) at 5 years (Table 95.1).[16]

Anatomic segmentectomy was first reported by Churchill and Belsey in 1939 for the management of bronchiectasis.[17] The use of segmentectomy for early-stage lung cancer was initially explored by several thoracic surgeons and demonstrated promise as an alternative approach in the management of early-stage lung cancer.[18–21] The Lung Cancer Study group conducted the only randomized study comparing sublobar resection (including segmentectomy and wedge resection) with lobectomy for stage IA NSCLC patients. This study demonstrated that sublobar resection was associated with a threefold increase in local recurrence (17.2% vs. 6.4%) compared with lobectomy.[22] Two years later, another prospective, multicenter nonrandomized study demonstrated a similar trend for increased local recurrence in patients undergoing sublobar resection.[23] These and other studies have firmly established lobectomy as the modern surgical approach of choice in patients with early stage lung cancer.

The increased identification of smaller NSCLC tumors by CT screening protocols in higher-risk surgical patients,[24] however, has led many surgeons to question the appropriateness of lobectomy in all cases.[25,26] A substantial body of literature from Japan, Europe, and the United States has emerged over the last decade that has produced a resurgence of interest in the use of anatomic segmentectomy for patients with small peripheral NSCLC, especially those who might not otherwise tolerate lobectomy.

Over the last 20 years, there has also been a dramatic improvement in surgical instrumentation including the introduction VATS and stapling technology. Roviaro was the first to report a VATS

TABLE 95.2 Perioperative Morbidity and Mortality for Lobectomy

Author	Year	N	Overall Morbidity (%)	Mortality (%)
Watanabe et al.[336]	2004	3,270	NR	1.6
Mckenna et al.[53]	2006	1,100	15.3	0.8
Allen et al.[334]	2006	1,023	38.2	1.4
Paul et al.[56]	2010	2,562	30.4	1%
Kozower et al.[337]	2010	18,800	7.9	2.2
Paul et al.[31]	2013	41,039	49.5	2.1
Paul et al.[338]	2014	6,008	53.1	3
Seder et al.[339]	2016	44,429	NR	1.6

TABLE 95.3 Commonly Encountered Complications During Anatomic Lung Resection

Major Complications	Minor Complications
Respiratory (40%) Atelectasis requiring intervention Pneumonia Respiratory Failure **Pleural (25%)** Empyema Bronchopleural Fistula **Cardiovascular (10%)** Myocardial Infarction Pulmonary Embolism/DVT Heart Failure Stroke **Others (25%)** Post-Op Hemorrhage Chylothorax Miscellaneous	**Respiratory (25%)** Minor Atelectasis Prolonged Air Leak **Cardiovascular (50%)** Arrhythmia **Pleural (25%)** Pneumothorax Effusion

Adapted from Ginsberg RJ. Lung Cancer Surgery: Acceptable Morbidity and Mortality, Expected Results and Quality Control. *Surg Onc* 2002;11:263–266. Copyright © 2002 Elsevier. With permission.

lobectomy in 1992, which has now evolved into the surgical approach of choice, whether performing lobectomy or segmentectomy.[27] The gradual evolution from "big incisions and big resections" to minimally invasive anatomic lobar and sublobar resection techniques, as well as advances in anesthetic and ICU management, has resulted in significant improvement in mortality and perioperative outcomes in the surgical management of lung cancer (Tables 95.1 and 95.4).

PERIOPERATIVE OUTCOMES

Morbidity and Mortality

As noted above, there has been a significant improvement in the morbidity and mortality associated with anatomic lung resection for NSCLC over the last 50 years (Table 95.1). Improvements in ICU care, the introduction of minimally invasive techniques and more sophisticated physiological assessments of potential candidates for surgery have all contributed to better perioperative outcomes. Overall morbidity rates following lobectomy in contemporary series range from 15% to 53%, with an average complication rate of 30% to 40% in most series (Table 95.2). Major complications account for 5% to 10% of all perioperative morbidity.[28] The most common major

complications are respiratory in nature, including pneumonia (4% to 8%)[29] and respiratory failure (3% to 6%).[30] Other major complications include deep vein thrombosis/pulmonary embolism (1% to 2%),[31] chylothorax (1%),[32] and myocardial infarction (1%). The most common minor complications are atrial fibrillation (10% to 15%)[33] and prolonged air leak >5 days (5% to 10%) (Table 95.3).[34] Conversion from VATS to thoracotomy occurs in 4% to 6% of cases. The most common reasons include bleeding, adhesions/hilar fibrosis, and inadequate visualization and exposure.[35] Median length of stay (LOS) following surgery is approximately 6 days for both lobectomy and sublobar resection in most recent series (Table 95.4).

Perioperative mortality (death within 30 days or during the same hospitalization) following lung resection ranges from 1% to 2% for wedge resection, segmentectomy, and lobectomy and from 3% to 7% for pneumonectomy in modern series (Table 95.1). Mortality following lung resection depends upon such factors as patient age and cardiopulmonary status, patient comorbidities, extent of resection, and

TABLE 95.4 Comparison of Wedge Resection Versus Segmentectomy Versus Lobectomy for NSCLC

Author	Year	LOS Wedge	LOS Segment	LOS Lobe	Morbidity Wedge	Morbidity Segment	Morbidity Lobe	Mortality Wedge	Mortality Segment	Mortality Lobe
El-Sherif et al.[96]	2006	6		6	NR		NR	1.4		2.6
Shapiro et al.[340]	2009	NR	4	4	NR	25.8	26.6	NR	0	0.9
De Giacomo et al.[341]	2009	NR	5	10	NR	22.2	29.3	NR	0	1.7
Yamashita et al.[342]	2012	NR	12.2	11.6	NR	19	23	NR	0	0
Zhong et al.[343]	2012	NR	6.1	6.3	NR	12.8	12.3	NR	0	0
Soukiasian et al.[344]	2012	NR	3.8	5.5	NR	37	17	NR	0	0
Schuchert et al.[121]	2012	NR	6	6	NR	35.7	45.7	NR	1.3	2.2
Zhang et al.[345]	2013	NR	7.2	10.4	NR	23.1	28.6	NR	0	0
Zhao et al.[346]	2013	NR	6.2	6.5	NR	8.3	2.2	NR	0	0
McGuire et al.[347]	2013	6.8	NR	7.7	7	NR	12	2.8	NR	1.1
Linden et al.[348]	2014	NR	NR		10.6	21.5		1.2	1.9	
Hwang et al.[349]	2015	NR	6.2	7.1	NR	10.6	17.2	NR	2.10	1.1
Seder et al.[339]	2016	4.0	6.2	7.0	NR	NR	NR	1.2	1.1	1.6

TABLE 95.5 Outcomes Following VATS Versus Open Surgical Anatomic Lung Resection for Treatment of NSCLC

Author	Year	N		LOS (d)		Morbidity (%)		Mortality (%)	
		VATS	Open	VATS	Open	VATS	Open	VATS	Open
Park et al.[350]	2007	122	122	4.9	7.2	17.2	27.9	0	2.5
Whitson et al.[51]	2007	59	88	6.4	7.7	19.3	13.8	NR	NR
Flores et al.[351]	2009	398	343	5	7	24	30	0.2	0.3
Villamizar et al.[55]	2009	382	597	4	5	30	50	2	6
Paul et al.[56]	2010	1,281	1,281	4,0	6	26.2	34.7	0.9	1.0
Gopadalas et al.[352]	2010	759	12,860	9.2	9.3	44.1	43.1	3.4	3.1
Scott et al.[353]	2010	66	686	4.5	7	27.3	47.8	0	1.6
Wang et al.[354]	2010	121	195	6.8	10.2	18.2	23.6	0	0.5
Ilonen et al.[355]	2011	116	212	7.5	10.7	15.5	26.9	2.6	2.8
Paul et al.[31]	2013	10,173	30,866	5	7	46.5	50.4	2.3	1.6
Paul et al.[338]	2014	1,293	4,715	9	6.5	48.7	54.4	1.9	3.3
Boffa et al.[356]	2014	2,745	2,745	4	5	30	36	1.3	1.8
Nwogu et al.[357]	2015	175	175	8	5.4	14.9	25.1	1.7	1.7

prior oncological treatments (e.g., radiation).[36] Site-specific considerations have also been delineated, as with the example of increased mortality risk for right pneumonectomy (especially after neoadjuvant therapy).[37] Major specific causative factors of mortality include pneumonia and respiratory failure, cardiac complications, and pulmonary embolus.[38] Several indices have been validated for estimating the risk of perioperative mortality including general assessments of patient frailty,[39] the Charlson comorbidity index,[40] as well as the National Surgical Quality Improvement Program (NSQIP),[41] and Veteran's Affairs Surgical Quality Improvement Program (VASQIP) risk calculators.[42] Although such indices may be imperfect in estimating true risks observed following lung surgery.[43] Specialty training in thoracic surgery,[44] surgeon volume,[45] and hospital volume[46] have all been linked to reduced mortality following lung resection.

Surgical Approach—VATS Versus Open Techniques

The last 20 years has witnessed a revolution in the fundamental surgical approach to lung cancer, with a shift from standard open techniques to the use of VATS. The published literature suggests that both lobectomy and segmentectomy can be safely performed through either a VATS or open approach. Roviero et al. were the first to report a series of thoracoscopic anatomic lung resections, including patients treated with lobectomy and segmentectomy.[47] The choice between a VATS versus open approach is typically dictated by patient and tumor characteristics, as well as surgeon preference and experience. The efficacy of the VATS approach with wedge resection has been well documented.[25] Formal thoracoscopic segmentectomy has also been performed with excellent results.[48] VATS lobectomy has been associated with decreased postoperatve pain,[49] reduced morbidity and mortality,[50] shorter LOS,[51] and greater discharge independence[52] compared to open techniques (Table 95.5). Long-term results for VATS lobectomy have demonstrated similar morbidity and mortality profiles, as well as equivalent long-term oncologic efficacy when compared with open lobectomy.[53,54]

Onaitis et al. reported a perioperative mortality rate of 1% among 492 patients undergoing VATS lobectomy.[54] McKenna et al. published the largest single-institution series of 1,100 VATS lobectomies. The mortality rate was 0.8%, none of which were attributed to intraoperative complications. In 2009, D'Amico et al. performed a propensity matched analysis of over 1,000 patients undergoing

lobectomy, which demonstrated that the VATS approach was associated with decreased postoperative complication rates (31% vs. 49%), decreased LOS (4 vs. 5 days) and reduced mortality (3% vs. 5%) when compared to an open approach.[55] Similar findings were delineated in a propensity-matched comparison of patients undergoing lobectomy derived from the STS database.[56] No differences have been appreciated in recurrence risk or overall survival whether lobectomy is performed by a VATS or open approach. Given the apparent advantages in perioperative outcomes and the equipoise associated with oncological outcomes, it is highly unlikely that a prospective, randomized trial will ever be performed that definitively compares VATS versus open lobectomy. VATS lobectomy has, thus, gradually superseded standard open techniques in the surgical treatment of uncomplicated stage I NSCLC in most high-volume centers.

Similarly, VATS segmentectomy has been shown to be safe and effective when compared to open segmentectomy techniques.[57] Shiraishi et al. found that VATS segmentectomy was associated decreased length of hospital stay (12 vs. 16 days), with similar morbidity between groups.[58] Atkins et al. similarly noted a shorter hospital stay (VATS = 4.3 vs. Open = 6.8), and found that segmentectomy was associated with improved overall survival compared with open segmentectomy.[59] Schuchert et al. compared 225 segmental resections performed for stage I NSCLC (VATS = 104, Open = 121). There were no reported deaths in those patients undergoing the VATS approach. No differences were observed in operative time, estimated blood loss, mortality, recurrence, or survival between the VATS and Open groups. VATS segmentectomy was associated with a reduced LOS (5 vs. 7 days) and pulmonary complication rate (15.4% vs. 29.8%) compared with the open segmentectomy.[60] Similar to VATS lobectomy, VATS segmentectomy also is emerging as the preferred approach when technically feasible in appropriately selected NSCLC cases that are deemed suitable for segmentectomy.

STAGE IA: LOCALIZED NODE-NEGATIVE NON-SMALL CELL LUNG CANCER

In 2009, the American Joint Committee on Cancer (AJCC) released the updated seventh edition of the TNM Classification System for NSCLC, based on recommendations of the International Association

TABLE 95.6 Oncologic Outcomes Following Segmentectomy Versus Lobectomy for NSCLC

Author	Year	N		Recurrence (%)		Survival (%) *3-Year Survival †5-Year Survival	
		Segment	Lobe	Segment	Lobe	Segment	Lobe
Okada et al.[76]	2006	305	262	14.1	17.2	89.6[†]	89.1[†]
El-Sherif et al.[96]	2006	207	577	29	28.1	40[†]	54[†]
Sienel et al.[358]	2007	48	150	33	17	68[†]	85[†]
Schuchert et al.[60]	2007	182	246	17.6	16.7	80[†]	83[†]
De Giacomo et al.[341]	2009	36	116	25	6.9	66.7[†]	64[†]
Yamashita et al.[342]	2012	90	124	7.7	5.6	75[†]	84[†]
Zhong et al.[343]	2012	39	81	12.8	13.5	79.9[†]	81.0[†]
Kilic et al.[279]	2009	78	106	17	21	46[†]	47[†]
Shapiro et al.[340]	2009	31	113	17.2	20.4	NR	NR
Schuchert et al.[121]	2012	305	594	17.7	20.7	75[†]	76[†]
Zhao et al.[345,346]	2013	36	138	2.8	4.4	NR	NR
Zhang et al.[345]	2013	26	28	NR	NR	65.4*	67.9*
Tsutani et al.[359]	2013	98	383	8.6	12.7	95.7*	93.2*
Landreneau et al.[101]	2014	312	312	20.2	16.7	54[†]	60[†]
Altorki et al.[100]	2014	53	294	19	12	49.1[†]	48[†]
Hwang et al.[349]	2015	94	94	3.2	4.3	96*	94*
Speicher et al.[360]	2016	9,667	29,736	NR	NR	58.2[†]	66.2[†]
Koike et al.[361]	2016	87	87	23	20	84[†]	85[†]
Kodama et al.[362]	2016	80	80	3.7	16.8	97.5[†]	87.7[†]

for the Study of Lung Cancer (IASLC).[21,30,61–64] One of the principal changes in the latest edition is the subclassification of the T descriptor into T1a, T1b, T2a, and T2b tumors based predominantly on tumor size. Tumors that are <3 cm in size and surrounded by lung or visceral pleura without bronchoscopic evidence of invasion more proximal than the lobar bronchus, and without evidence of lymph node metastasis, constitute T1N0M0 lesions (stage IA). By their very nature, such lesions are readily treated by complete (R0) surgical resection and have the best prognosis. Stage IA may be further subdivided based on the T descriptor into T1a (≤2 cm) and T1b (>2 cm but ≤3 cm) tumors.

Anatomic lung resection remains the mainstay of therapy in the setting of early-stage NSCLC.[65] Lobectomy with systematic lymph node sampling or lymphadenectomy constitutes the standard of care, and provides patients with the best chance of cure.[22] As discussed above, for smaller tumors VATS lobectomy represents the preferred approach, when possible, and has been associated with less morbidity, less pain, and improved quality of life metrics compared with thoracotomy. McKenna et al. reported an 84.5% 5-year survival following VATS lobectomy for stage IA NSCLC. Recurrence rates range from 20% to 30% for stage IA tumors (locoregional = 5% to 8%, distant = 15% to 20%). Overall survival for stage IA NSCLC ranges between 70% and 80% at 5 years in most published series (Table 95.6, Fig. 95.2).[61,66–68]

Stage IA NSCLC—Subcentimeter Tumors

With continued technical advances in thoracic imaging and the introduction of CT screening protocols in patient groups at high-risk for lung cancer, smaller and smaller tumors are being identified in clinical practice.[24,69,70] This has led many surgeons to question the necessity of lobectomy in all cases, especially in the case of small, peripheral T1a tumors. This is especially true in the management of subcentimeter

lesions (Fig. 95.3). Emerging data has suggested that sublobar resection techniques (segmentectomy, wedge resection) can achieve outcomes similar to lobectomy in this setting, and may be entirely appropriate in carefully selected smaller, peripheral NSCLC ≤1 cm.[71,72]

Kondo et al. analyzed outcomes in 57 patients with tumors less than 1 cm in diameter including 23 lobectomies, 13 segmentectomies, and 21 wedge resections.[73] There was no difference in cancer-free survival regardless of the resection technique, with an overall 5-year survival of 97%. Miller et al. reviewed the outcomes of 100 patients (71 lobectomies,

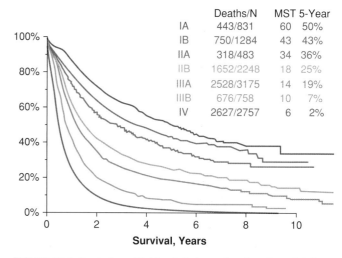

	Deaths/N	MST	5-Year
IA	443/831	60	50%
IB	750/1284	43	43%
IIA	318/483	34	36%
IIB	1652/2248	18	25%
IIIA	2528/3175	14	19%
IIIB	676/758	10	7%
IV	2627/2757	6	2%

FIGURE 95.2 Survival stratified by clinical stage based on Seventh Edition AJCC/UICC Staging System. (Reprinted from Detterbeck FC, Boffa DJ, Tanoue LT. The new lung cancer staging system. *Chest* 2009;136(1):260–271. Copyright © 2009 The American College of Chest Physicians. With permission.)

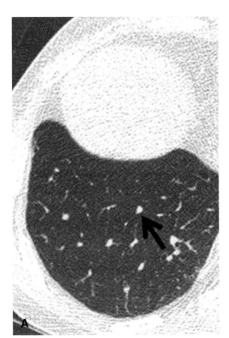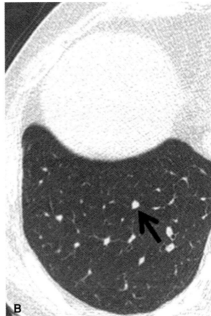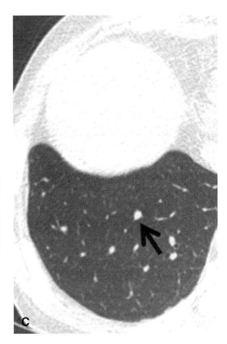

FIGURE 95.3 Subcentimeter Lesion—**A:** Subcentimeter lesion at baseline examination, **B:** 2-year follow up, **C:** 5-year follow-up. (From Shin KE, Lee KS, Yi CA, et al. Subcentimeter lung nodules stable for 2 years at LDCT: long-term follow-up using volumetry. *Respirology (Carlton, Vic)* 2014;19(6):921–928. Copyright © 2014 by John Wiley Sons, Inc. Reprinted by permission of John Wiley & Sons, Inc.)

12 segmentectomies, and 13 wedge resections) with subcentimeter lung cancer and reported an 18% overall recurrence rate. In this study, lobectomy was associated with improved recurrence-free and overall survival compared with limited resection. This result appeared to be driven by significantly reduced disease-free (42%) and overall (27%) survival in the wedge resection group. Of note, no significant differences in recurrence-free or overall survival were seen comparing the lobectomy and segmentectomy groups.[74] Other reports examining sublobar resection in the setting of subcentimeter tumors document no difference in local recurrence or survival.[75,76] Schuchert et al. found that extent of resection (wedge, segment, or lobe) does not appear to have a significant impact on recurrence-free or overall survival rates in subcentimeter lesions.[77] The overall recurrence rate was found to be 9.3%. Locoregional recurrence was 2.8%, much lower than that seen with tumors greater than 1 cm in diameter. Disease-free survival was 88% at 5 years. They noted a low rate of regional nodal involvement encountered in patients with subcentimeter tumors, with three cases of nodal involvement in such patients over a 10-year span. These findings are similar to the reports of Ohta et al.[78] and Sawabata et al.,[79] who also noted a markedly decreased risk of nodal involvement in tumors <1 cm. Risk of nodal involvement in this setting ranges from 0% to 11.1%[80,81] within the reported literature. The increased incidence of well-differentiated adenocarcinoma and bronchoalveolar carcinoma in this cohort compared with tumors >1 cm may also be contributing to the diminished risk of recurrence seen in these patients. Small (<1 cm) ground-glass opacities detected on CT imaging are associated with *in situ* and early cancers that are particularly amenable to sublobar resection when confined to a discrete bronchopulmonary segment.[82] Sublobar resection in this setting allows complete excision of the lesion, while preserving parenchyma in patients who might require future resections,[83] and can achieve exceptional (>90%) 5-year survival.[84,85] Jiang et al. noted shorter survival time among patients undergoing wedge resection when compared to segmentectomy and lobectomy.[86] Sakurai et al. found that solid lesions were associated with a higher recurrence risk in subcentimeter tumors, and advocate lobectomy for these lesions given their worse overall prognosis (88% 5-year survival).[87]

In the absence of a meaningful difference in oncologic outcome between techniques, the reduced operative time, estimated blood loss, LOS, and mortality risk associated with sublobar resection supports the validity of these techniques in the management of small, subcentimeter peripheral tumors. The specific chosen approach should be tailored to individual patient and tumor characteristics, as well as surgeon experience and judgment. New localization techniques such as near-infrared imaging during VATS[88] and methylene blue dye marking via navigational bronchoscopy may enhance the yield of sublobar resection techniques in the setting of subcentimeter lesions.[89] Care should be taken in extrapolating this data to other management strategies, including ablative therapy approaches such as radiofrequency ablation or stereotactic radiosurgery.[90] The data presented here represent a cohort of pathologically confirmed, completely resected subcentimeter tumors. The importance of obtaining an accurate tissue diagnosis, complete (R0) excision with adequate tissue margins, and regional nodal staging must be emphasized.

Stage IA NSCLC—T1aN0 (≤2 cm) Tumors

As highlighted in the discussion regarding subcentimeter tumors above, it has been documented that smaller tumor subsets within the stage IA grouping have a particularly excellent prognosis with surgical therapy. Specifically, tumors ≤2 cm (T1a) have been associated with better outcomes than those between 2 and 3 cm (T1b). Though Ishida et al. found no difference in survival between T1N0 cancers ≤1 cm and tumors 1.1 to 2 cm,[91] Rami-Porta et al. noted that the focal point where survival begins to dichotomize utilizing log-rank analysis was between tumors <2 cm versus those 2 to 3 cm in size (77% vs. 71% at 5 years). They also noted such cut-off points in survival at 3 to 5 cm (58%) and 5 to 7 cm (49%), now currently classified as T2a and T2b tumors. Such clinical observations have led many investigators to evaluate clinical outcomes based on the T1a (<2 cm) and T1b (>2 but ≤3 cm) size categories.[63]

Several recent reports have demonstrated that sublobar resection (anatomic segmentectomy, in particular) may be associated with equivalent recurrence and survival in the setting of small T1a (≤2 cm) tumors. Okada et al. compared the results of extended segmentectomy to lobectomy in patients with T1N0 tumors 2 cm or less in size, documenting equivalent 5-year survival of 87.1% among the segmentectomy patients compared with 87.7% in the lobectomy group.[92] Fernando et al. reported no difference in survival in those patients undergoing lobar or sublobar resection for tumors less than 2 cm.[93] Bando et al. reported on a series of 74 patients with T1N0 NSCLC, and noted locoregional recurrence in only 1.9% of the patients with tumors of 2 cm or less.[94] Carr et al. found that recurrence-free survival was significantly different when comparing T1a and T1b tumors (86% vs. 78%, $p = 0.027$). However, there was no difference noted in recurrence-free survival between patients undergoing segmentectomy or lobectomy in either T classification.[95] Patients that underwent either lobectomy or segmentectomy for stage IA NSCLC experienced an 82% recurrence-free survival.

Stage IA NSCLC—Sublobar Resection Versus Lobectomy

In the only prospective, randomized study performed to date comparing lobectomy with sublobar resection (including wedge resection and segmentectomy) for clinical stage IA NSCLC, the Lung Cancer Study group identified a threefold increase in locoregional recurrence risk among patients undergoing sublobar resection (17.2% vs. 6.4%).[22] As detailed above, sublobar resection (wedge/segment in the case of subcentimeter neoplasms, and anatomic segmentectomy in T1a tumors) has been shown in retrospective studies to achieve similar oncological outcomes when compared with lobectomy for the smaller tumor subsets (T1a) of stage IA NSCLC.

As discussed above, sublobar resection for lung cancer can be performed with a simple wedge resection technique, with appropriate attention being paid to obtaining an adequate surgical margin.[70] With the development of surgical stapling devices, this approach has become the dominant method of sublobar resection employed today.[71] The vast majority of patients treated with sublobar resection in the LCSG study,[22] as well as, in the study by Landreneau et al.[23] underwent simple wedge resection. As discussed above, recurrence

rates with sublobar wedge resections can be up to three times that seen with lobectomy with no apparent difference in 5-year survival.[22,23,96]

Similar to lobectomy, anatomic segmentectomy has been shown to accomplish the fundamental surgical tenets of anatomic R0 resection with systematic nodal staging for NSCLC. It can represent an approach that is both diagnostic and therapeutic in the setting of solitary pulmonary nodules, while at the same time preserving lung parenchyma.[97] This approach is particularly useful in high-risk patients with cardiopulmonary insufficiency, who otherwise might not be able to tolerate a lobectomy.[98] This approach may also be associated with decreased morbidity and mortality risk especially in the elderly and in those with reduced functional status. Segmentectomy may also be a more appropriate choice in the setting of tumors of low malignant potential, where taking more tissue is unlikely to enhance survival.[72] Such studies have rekindled interest in the applicability of sublobar resection for clinical stage I NSCLC, especially stage IA.[99]

Altorki et al. evaluated recurrence and survival among patients undergoing either lobectomy or sublobar resection for clinical stage I NSCLC identified as a solid nodule in the International Early Lung Cancer Action Program. When comparing lobectomy ($n = 347$) to sublobar resection ($n = 53$), the authors found no difference in survival at 10 years (85% vs. 86%, respectively). After adjusting for propensity scores, there was no difference noted between the approaches.[100] In a study evaluating patients with pathological stage I tumors, Schuchert et al. found no difference in recurrence or survival of patients undergoing anatomic segmentectomy versus lobectomy for pathological stage I NSCLC, including patients with stage IA and IB disease.[60] In the largest comparison performed to date, Landreneau et al. reported the results of a propensity-matched comparison of segmentectomy versus lobectomy ($n = 312$ patients/group) for clinical stage IA and IB NSCLC (tumors <5 cm). They found that anatomic segmentectomy can achieve similar perioperative (morbidity and mortality) and oncologic outcomes (recurrence and survival) when compared to lobectomy for clinical stage I disease. Freedom from recurrence at 5 years was 70% for the segmentectomy group (95% CI: [0.63, 0.78]) versus 71% for lobectomy (95% CI: [0.64, 0.78]) (Fig. 95.4). Overall survival at 5 years was 54% in the segmentectomy group (95% CI: [0.47, 0.61])

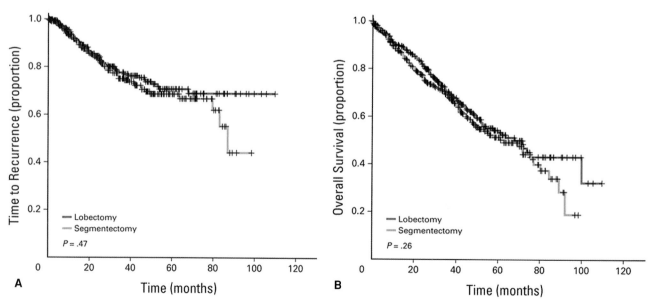

FIGURE 95.4 Kaplan-Meier survival estimates for (**A**) time to recurrence and (**B**) overall survival between propensity score–matched patients undergoing segmentectomy or lobectomy. (From Landreneau RJ, Normolle DP, Christie NA, et al. Recurrence and survival outcomes after anatomic segmentectomy versus lobectomy for clinical stage I non-small-cell lung cancer: a propensity-matched analysis. *J Clin Oncol* 2014;32(23):2449–2455. Reprinted with permission. Copyright © 2014 American Society of Clinical Oncology. All rights reserved.)

versus 60% (95% CI: [0.54, 0.67]) for lobectomy. In multivariate analysis, segmentectomy was not found to be an independent predictor of recurrence (HR: 1.11, 95% CI: 0.87, 1.40) or overall survival (HR = 1.17, 95% CI: 0.89.1.52).[101]

These studies suggest that sublobar resection can potentially achieve similar oncological outcomes compared with lobectomy in carefully selected patients who have undergone careful preoperative staging (Table 95.6). The results of these retrospective studies will need to be validated by currently active prospective, randomized studies in the United States (CALGB 140503) and Japan (JCOG0802/WJOG4607L) comparing sublobar resection versus lobectomy for patients with T1aN0 NSCLC.

Stage IA—Role of Adjuvant Therapy

To date, there is no established additive benefit with the use of induction or adjuvant therapies over resection alone for stage IA disease. Although clinical trials are in progress evaluating novel agents and targeted therapies, including immunotherapy, the use of adjuvant chemotherapy containing cisplatin actually has been shown to have a negative effect on survival for both stages IA and IB, except perhaps in the case of larger tumors (>4 cm—stage IB).[102]

STAGE IB NSCLC

Stage IB NSCLC is defined by lesions >3 cm and ≤5 cm (T2aN0) and/or those with evidence of visceral pleural invasion, as well as those that involve the main bronchus ≥2 cm distal to the carina. Lesions that are associated with atelectasis/obstructive pneumonia extending to hilum but not involving the entire lung, and those that directly cross a fissure and invade an adjacent lobe also fall into this category.[103] Postresection survival rates for pathologic T2aN0 lung cancer have historically ranged from approximately 50% to 65% in most series (Table 95.7).

Stage IB—Tumor Size

Harpole et al. delineated the importance of tumor size in larger node negative NSCLC with the observation that tumors larger than

TABLE 95.7 Survival After Surgical Resection for Stage IB NSCLC

Report	Year	Stage IB (T2N0)	
		N	5-Year Survival (%)
Williams et al.[363]	1981	236	62
Martini et al.[30]	1986	78	65
Roeslin et al.[30]	1987	121	43
Read et al.[21]	1990	327	57
Ichinose et al.[281]	1995	80	67
Mountain[61]	1997	549	57
Inoue et al.[173]	1998	271	65
Jassem et al.[64]	2000	220	53
van Rens et al.[66]	2000	797	46
Naruke et al.[67]	2001	506	60
Fang et al.[274]	2001	702	61
Rena et al.[278]	2002	292	55
Toffalorio et al.[106]	2012	349	71
Bergman et al.[107]	2013	142	54

4 cm had reduced survival when compared to smaller 2- to 4-cm tumors.[104] Carbone et al. noted a statistically significant difference in 5-year survival rates for resected T2N0 cancers between 3 and 5 cm versus those >5 cm: 62% versus 51%, respectively. These authors suggested that NSCLC tumors >5 cm be upgraded to T3.[105] This is in line with the analysis published by Rami-Porta et al. for the IASLC staging reanalysis project.[63] Survival rates for stage IB in the current seventh edition of the Lung Cancer Staging System have improved somewhat, secondary to the re-classification of tumors larger than 5 cm as T2b (stage IIA, >5 and ≤7 cm) and T3 (stage IIB, >7 cm) lesions. In an analysis by Toffalorio et al. of 467 patients with stage IB lesions by sixth edition criteria, stage IB survival as currently classified by seventh edition criteria was 71% at 5 years as compared to 47.7% and 47.4% for reclassified stages IIA and IIB, respectively.[106] In a retrospective study of 222 node-negative patients, Bergman et al. reported an overall 5-year survival rate of 51% in patients with a tumor size >3 cm. When stratified by size utilizing the seventh TNM edition criteria, the 5-year overall survival rates for stages IB, IIA, and IIB were 54%, 51%, and 35%, respectively.[107] These studies highlight the importance of tumor size and the re-classification of the T descriptor emphasized in the seventh edition.

Stage IB—Visceral Pleural Invasion

The presence of visceral pleural invasion is associated with worse outcomes in patients with early-stage (<3 cm) NSCLC,[108] and serves to up-stage patients with node-negative tumors (stage IB).[109,110] Visceral pleural invasion is defined as evidence of penetration of the thick outer elastic lamina by tumor during elastic tissue staining (Fig. 95.5). Visceral pleural invasion is a recognized pathologic variable associated with an increased risk of recurrence and death. Currently, it is the only pathologic variable employed beyond the traditional TNM descriptors.[111]

Harpole et al. found that visceral pleural invasion was a significant predictor of poor outcome, with 5- and 10-year survival rates of 44% and 37%.[104] Similar findings were reported by Ichinose et al.[112] Manac'h et al. noted 5-year survival in 61% of stage I patients without pleural involvement versus 46% of those with pleural invasion.[113] The Lung Cancer Study Group report by Gail et al. noted a 1.66-fold increase in recurrence rates in stage I patients when the visceral pleura was involved by cancer.[114] Extent of pleural involvement has also been shown to contribute to survival. Shimizu et al. reported significantly worse 5-year survival rates in patients with PL1 (invasion beyond the elastic layer or PL2 (invasion to the surface of the visceral pleura) than those with PL0 (tumor does not involve the elastic layer) involvement.[115] Visceral pleural invasion is thus defined by PL1 or PL2 involvement, and is an independent predictor of recurrence and worse survival regardless of tumor size.[109]

Using the prospective multicentre ACOSOG Z0030 trial data set, Fibla et al. identified stage IB tumors with only visceral pleural invasion, tumors between 3 and 5 cm, or both. Five-year survival was significantly worse for the cohort of tumors between 3 and 5 cm with VPI (55.0%) when compared to stage IB status by size (67.2%) or VPI (68.3%) alone.[82] Through a systematic literature search, Jiang et al. found that visceral pleural invasion was a significant adverse prognostic factor in tumors of all sizes.[116]

Stage IB—Impact of Surgical Approach

From the perspective of stage IB status by tumor size (3 to 5 cm), several studies have demonstrated increased recurrence risk with larger tumors (>3 cm) following sublobar resection,[117–119] including anatomic segmentectomy.[96,120,121] Stage IB status by visceral

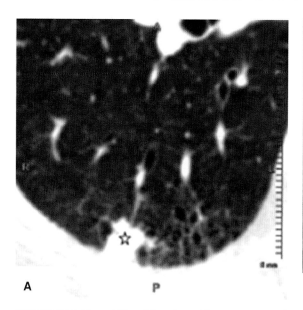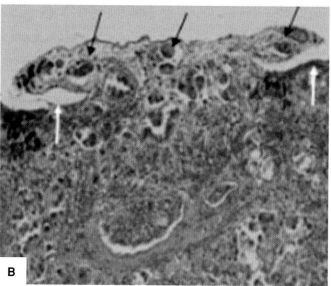

FIGURE 95.5 Visceral Pleural Invasion—Adenocarcinoma with visceral pleural invasion. **A:** 14 mm pulmonary nodule contacting the pleura. **B:** 200× H&E stain. (Reprinted from Ebara K, Takashima S, Jiang B, et al. Pleural invasion by peripheral lung cancer: prediction with three-dimensional CT. *Acad Radiol* 2015;22(3):310–319. Copyright © 2015 Association of University Radiologists. With permission.)

pleural invasion is associated with increased risk of locoregional recurrence and systemic metastases, including intralobar N1 nodal recurrences.[122–124] This finding has raised concerns regarding the extent of resection performed for stage I NSCLC, and has led several authors to advocate lobectomy in all cases with suspected visceral pleural invasion. Schuchert et al. also found that visceral pleural invasion was a significant prognostic variable independently predictive of recurrence (HR: 1.86; 95% CI:1.11 to 3.10, $p = 0.018$), especially following segmentectomy. The reason for the worse prognosis following segmentectomy in the setting of stage IB disease is not entirely clear. It is conceivable that lobectomy permits better surgical margins compared to segmentectomy in relation to these typically larger tumors. It is also possible that increased tumor size is a marker of more aggressive tumor biology, both in terms of local invasiveness (visceral pleural invasion) and a resulting increased propensity for locoregional nodal involvement that is better addressed by lobectomy.[124]

In summary, visceral pleural invasion is an adverse pathologic variable associated with increased recurrence risk following segmentectomy. When larger tumors (3 to 5 cm) or visceral pleural invasion are encountered, lobectomy should be performed.

Stage IB—Role of Adjuvant Chemotherapy

The presence of aggressive pathologic tumor characteristics may provide an indicator for patients with resected stage I disease that might benefit from adjuvant therapy. CALGB 9633 evaluated the outcomes of 344 patients randomized to cisplatin-based chemotherapy following resection of T2N0 tumors versus surgery alone. In an unplanned subgroup analysis, the administration of adjuvant chemotherapy was found to be beneficial for tumors >4 cm in size.[125] In a study evaluating patients from the National Cancer Database, the use of adjuvant chemotherapy in patients with tumors >3 cm was associated with improved median (101.6 vs. 68.2 months) and 5-year survival (67% vs. 55%).[126] These studies suggest that there may be a marginal benefit for adjuvant chemotherapy in the setting of larger tumors >4 cm in size. Plans for adjuvant therapy in this setting are best reviewed in the setting of a multidisciplinary tumor board.

STAGE II NSCLC: N1 ADENOPATHY OR RESECTABLE LOCAL INVASION

The seventh edition of the Lung Cancer Staging System separates stage II NSCLC into two groups: stage IIA, which includes T1N1, T2aN1, and T2bN0 subgroups and stage IIB, which includes T2bN1 and T3N0 designations. Together, the stage II group represents approximately 26% of patients with NSCLC, with IIA accounting for about 10% and IIB 16% of cases. Broadly speaking these groups are comprised of large >5 cm, node negative tumors, or T1-2 lesions with associated N1 disease. Within the stage II groups, T1N1, T2aN1, and T2bN1 represent 8% of the total patient population.[103] Large series, including that of Naruke et al.,[67] and the IASLC database show a 40% to 60% expected 5-year survival after resection. In Naruke's retrospective analysis, 5-year survival after resection for pathologic T1N1, T2N1, and T3N0 were 57.5%, 43.8%, and 46.6%, respectively. After implementing changes to the staging system and incorporating all subgroups, 5-year survival for stages IIA and IIB were found to be 46% and 36%, respectively.[67]

The recognition that larger node-negative tumors over 5 cm were associated with a worse prognosis provided the impetus for shifting these cases from stage IB to stage II (Fig. 95.6). Martini et al. found that tumors <3 cm had a higher survival rates than those >5 cm.[127] Furthermore, Carbone et al. showed that tumors <5 cm had a 5-year survival rate of 51.3% versus 35.1% for tumors >5 cm.[128] Dai et al. analyzed 220 patients with stage II NSCLC. In their cohort, patients with ≤3 cm had a 55.7% 5-year survival rate, while patients with >3 cm had a 45.3% 5-year survival rate.[129] Similar to trends seen in stage I disease, these studies highlight the importance of tumor size on survival in the stage II subgroups.

Lobectomy is the treatment of choice for stage II disease with systematic lymph node sampling or formal lymph node dissection. Sublobar resection is generally not viewed as an appropriate option in these patients. Furthermore, larger IIB lesions tend to be more complicated, frequently requiring full thickness chest wall resections, sleeve resections, or even pneumonectomy.

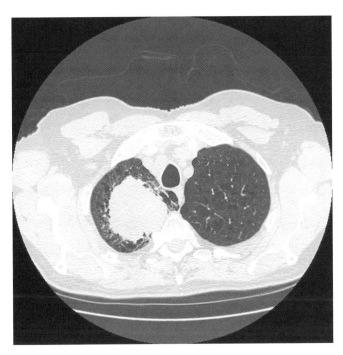

FIGURE 95.6 7 cm mass involving right upper lobe.

Stage IIA—N1 Nodal Involvement

Though stage II is commonly regarded as early stage NSCLC, the fact that it is associated with larger tumors and/or complicated by N1 nodal metastasis translates into lower survival and cure rates compared to stage I, regardless of surgical strategy employed. Survival for pT1N1 patients in the series of van Rens et al. is 52%.[66] The Ludwig Lung Cancer Study Group reported a median survival time of 4.8 years for resected T1N1 patients (as compared with 2.3 years for T2N1).[130] The number of involved lymph nodes may also have an impact on survival in this setting. Wisnivesky et al. showed with the Surveillance, Epidemiology and End Results (SEER) database that a greater number of N1 LNs was associated with significantly worse lung cancer–specific and overall survival.[131] Mean lung cancer–specific survival was 8.8 years, 8.2 years, 6.0 years, and 3.9 years for patients with one, two to three, four to eight, and more than eight positive lymph nodes, respectively. Though this study includes T1 to T3 cases, it highlights that the number of involved lymph nodes may be a potential prognosticator of survival in NSCLC.[131] Similar results are seen in the study by Martini et al., showing that patients with a single malignant node had a 5-year survival rate of 45% as opposed to 31% for those with multiple N1 metastases. Despite these findings, some groups do not show a significant difference in survival comparing single versus multiple N1 lymph node involvement.[132] Wang et al. found that the 5-year survival with ≤1 and >1 lymph nodes involved was 61.0% and 46.9%, respectively, which did not achieve statistical significance in their study.[133] In a similar retrospective study, Nakagawa et al. did not find a survival difference based on the number of involved lymph node stations. In their series, single versus multiple number of involved N1 lymph node stations yielded a 51.9% and 58.5% 5-year survival rate, respectively.[134] Given the disparate findings in these studies, the number of involved N1 lymph nodes has not been found to be a reliable prognostic factor in current staging algorithims.

Intralobar versus extralobar N1 nodal disease also has been suggested to be a prognostic factor in multiple studies. Yano et al. achieved a postresection survival rate of 65% in patients with "lobar" nodal disease (levels 12 and 13), as compared with only 40% when the "hilar" nodes (levels 10 and 11) contained metastatic cancer.[135] Haney et al. retrospectively reviewed their database of stage II resections (n = 230 patients). In their study, extralobar was defined as including lymph nodes from levels 10 and 11 and intralobar included levels 12 to 14. The presence of extralobar (levels 10 and 11) positive lymph nodes was associated with a worse outcome compared to intralobar nodes (level 12 to 14). The median overall survival was 46.9 months for the intralobar cohort and 24.4 months for the extralobar cohort. Interestingly, 24 patients had both intra- and extralobar nodal disease. This cohort fared the same as patients with extralobar disease only.[136] Li et al. showed similar results. Patients with hilar positive lymph nodes had a 35% 5-year survival rate compared to peripheral intralobar positive nodes, which had a 58% 5-year survival rate. In this study, patients with both had poorer outcomes with a 5-year survival of 23%.[137] Likewise, Van Velsen and his group looked into the influences of lymph node involvement on survival rates in T1N1 and T2N1 NSCLC. For T1N1, the overall 5-year survival was 46% in their patient population.[138] They discovered that, like Li et al., lobar N1 metastases had better outcomes than hilar N1 metastases (57% vs. 30%).[139] In addition to this, lymph node involvement by direct extension carried better outcomes than noncontiguous metastases (69% vs. 30%).[138] For their T2N1 group, overall postoperative survival rate at 5 years was 37.8%.[139] Once again, lobar N1 metastases had better outcomes than hilar N1 metastases (65.3% vs. 21%). Patients with hilar metastases also had poorer 5-year survival rates when compared to patients with lymph node involvement by direct extension (21% vs. 44.6%).[139] Riquet et al. also reported improved survival rates for lobar versus hilar N1 (54% vs. 38%) disease. However, there was no difference in survival rates between direct extension versus separate metastasis.[140] To further deduce the differences between nodal involvement, Tanaka et al. divided N1 disease into three groups. They reported postoperative survival for T1-2N1 to be 72% when levels 12 and 13 were affected, 62% for level 11, and 39% for level 10.[141]

With the re-emergence of sublobar resection techniques such as anatomic segmentectomy, the question of what to do with surprise N1 disease during the course of dissection has been raised. Recognizing the increased risk of locoregional recurrence associated with N1 disease,[142] most authors would advocate converting the sublobar resection to lobectomy (assuming the patient's physiological status permits) in cases of surprise N1 nodal involvement detected by frozen section at the time of surgery. In a study by Nomori et al., 15 patients undergoing anatomic segmentectomy were found to have N1or N2 disease intraoperatively. Ten patients (67%) were converted to lobectomy, and five (33%) underwent completion of the segmentectomy only. None of the patients who went on to lobectomy developed a recurrence, whereas 2/5 (40%) of the patients treated by segmentectomy only developed recurrent disease. Interestingly, both of these recurrences were distant, raising the question of aggressive tumor biology as opposed to inadequate local control.[143]

In summary, stage II NSCLC associated with larger tumor sizes (>5 cm) and/or N1 nodal involvement is associated with 5-year survival rates ranging from 25% to 55% in most series, with an average survival of 40% to 45%. Given the larger tumors and nodal involvement inherent in this stage grouping, lobectomy is recommended as the procedure of choice. Central tumors might mandate sleeve resection or even pneumonectomy to achieve an R0 resection.

Stage IIB—T3N0 Disease

T3 tumors are lesions that are >7cm, or any size lesion that invades the chest wall, diaphragm, phrenic nerve, mediastinal pleura, or parietal pericardium. T3 now also includes tumors with ipsilateral intralobar nodules that involve the same lobe as the primary tumor (e.g., satellite nodules). Another subset of T3 tumors are those located within 2 cm of the carina without carinal involvement. Overall 5-year survival rates for T3N0 (stage IIB) involvement range from 22% to 48%, with an average survival between 30% and 35%. In a multi-institutional study, Choi et al. reported a 50% 4-year locoregional relapse-free survival following resection of T3N0 tumors.[144] Naruke[67] and van Rens[66] reported 5-year survival rates of 22% and 33%, respectively. Wisnivesky et al., using the SEER database, reported that 5-year survival rates for T1N1 and T3N0 were not significantly different at 46% and 48%, respectively. In fact, the long-term "cure rate" for T3N0 in their study was better, though not significant compared to T1N1, 33% versus 27%.[145]

Multiple Intralobar Nodules

The seventh edition of the Lung Cancer Staging System has reclassified a second site within the same lobe from T4 to T3, and a second site within the ipsilateral lung from M1 to T4. Determining whether two lesions are separate primaries or if one is metastatic from the other, though not always easy, can often be elucidated by immunohistochemistry and molecular techniques. Deslauriers et al. found that the presence of "satellite nodules" (malignant foci close to the dominant tumor but separate from it) reduced long-term survival by approximately 50% after resection (Fig. 95.7).[146] Nonetheless, the 5-year survival rate of 22% in patients with such nodules represented a much better prognosis than patients previously classified as T4 or M1. Fukuse et al. reported a similarly favorable 5-year survival rate of 26% in 41 cases of resected ipsilateral lesions.[147] Yoshino et al. found a similar late survival in resected unilobar multifocal cases.[148] Pennathur,[149] Rosengart[150] and Okada[151] and their colleagues noted even more favorable results in this cohort of patients, with long-term survival rates of 26, 44%, and 70%, respectively. In the series by Pennathur et al., survival in the node-negative subset was found to be 40%. These positive findings have led the ACCP to issue clinical practice guidelines for satellite

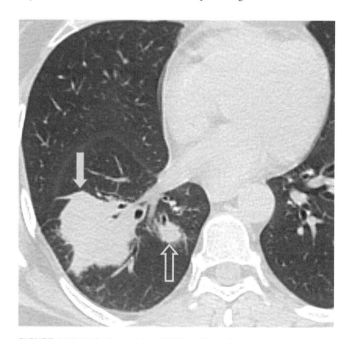

FIGURE 95.7 Right lower lobe NSCLC with ipsilateral intralobar "satellite nodule." (Borrowed from Alonso RC, ed. Non-small cell lung cancer (NSCLC): Review of the seventh edition of the TNM staging system and role of imaging in the staging and follow-up of NSCLC1970. European Congress of Radiology 2011.)

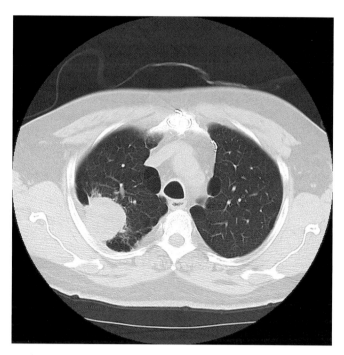

FIGURE 95.8 Right Upper Lobe NSCLC with pleural and potentially chest wall involvement.

nodules acknowledging a good prognosis following surgery. The approach to evaluation and treatment requires no modification than what would be dictated by the primary tumor alone.[152]

Chest Wall Involvement

By far the largest surgical experience with T3N0 tumors involves those invading the parietal pleura or chest wall (Fig. 95.8). It must be stressed that a high proportion of patients in many surgical reports were treated with preoperative or postoperative radiation therapy or both. Despite the chest wall involvement, these patients are surgical candidates for *en bloc* chest wall resection with reconstruction, as appropriate. The major correlatives of long-term survival are node negativity and complete resection. When both criteria are met, long-term survival can be achieved in 29% to 56% of surgical cases, averaging 42%. Efficacy of resection is markedly limited when malignant lymphadenopathy accompanies chest wall invasion (T3N1, stage IIIA). In a series of 334 patients undergoing attempted resection for parietal pleural or chest wall invasion, Downey et al. reported complete R0 resections in 52.4% of their patients. They noted a 5-year survival rate of 32% for a completely resected T3N0 lesion versus 4% in incompletely resected (R1 or R2) patients.[153] Similarly, Burkhart et al. reported a 5-year survival rate of 39% after a complete resection.[154] Lee et al. published their experience with T3 resections secondary to chest wall involvement, and noted a 5-year survival rate of 37.4%. A complete resection drastically affected survival compared to an incomplete resection in their series, 31.7% versus 7.5%. Prognostic factors for survival included extent of resection, tumor size, nodal status, and completeness of resection.[155]

The extent of invasion is divided pathologically into parietal pleural involvement versus extension into muscle and bone. This is often difficult to determine at the time of operation. Kawaguchi et al. examined resected specimens invading only to the parietal pleura versus soft tissue or ribs showing that preoperative CT findings of obvious tumor invasion and complaints of chest pain were independent indicators of deep invasion into soft tissue or ribs. While some tumors may dissect easily off of the chest wall by extrapleural dissection, incomplete resection leads to a markedly reduced survival rate.[156] In patients with T3N0 disease, McCaughan et al. achieved a 5-year survival rate of 62% for parietal pleural T3 as opposed to 35% for muscle and bone invasion, but the difference was not statistically significant.[157] Likewise, Casillas,[158] Elia,[159] and Akay[160] and their colleagues noted no significant difference between patients treated by extrapleural dissection versus full-thickness chest wall resection.

Doddoli et al. strongly suggest that *en bloc* resection be the standard of care for chest wall invasion when technically possible.[161] Albertucci et al. found a significant incidence of incomplete resection and lower survival for extrapleural dissection (33% vs. 50%). Despite this, there are multiple groups that have not noticed a statistically significant difference. Regardless of technique, a complete R0 resection is suggested. Therefore, if there is a lesion attached to parietal pleura by adhesions with superficial invasion, pulmonary resection with an extrapleural dissection can be appropriate in carefully selected cases.

However, if there is any suspicion of formal chest wall involvement, an *en bloc* resection should be performed. Addition of radiotherapy in cases of R1 or R2 residual chest involvement has not been reliably shown to improve disease-free or overall survival.[144]

In summary, NSCLC involving a limited area of the parietal pleura and only superficial invasion may be treated adequately by pulmonary resection combined with extrapleural dissection, but any degree of deeper invasion requires full-thickness *en bloc* chest wall resection. The practical challenge is the definitive identification of the extent of invasion by preoperative and intraoperative assessment. When there is doubt, *en bloc* resection is appropriate.

Superior Sulcus Tumors

Superior sulcus tumors, or Pancoast tumors, are apical lesions that invade the chest wall and thoracic inlet (Fig. 95.9). Due to its location at the apex, frequently these tumors will invade the brachial plexus, subclavian vessels, and the spine. Because of this pattern

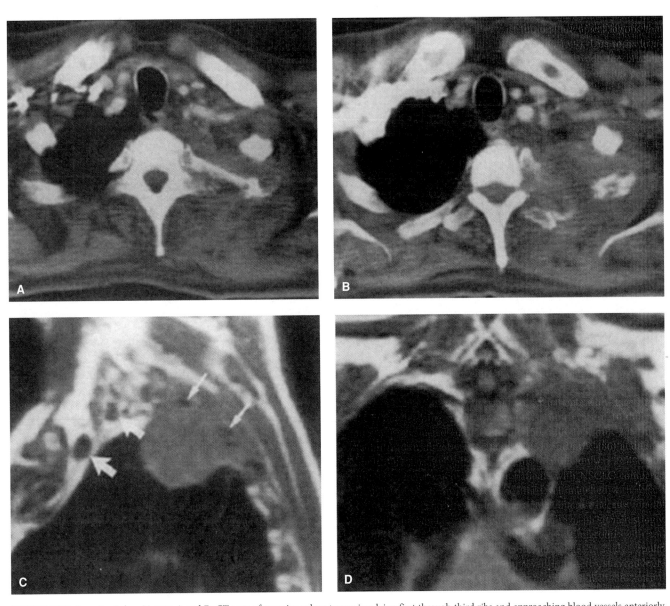

FIGURE 95.9 Superior Sulcus Tumor. **A** and **B:** CT scan of superior sulcus tumor involving first through third ribs and approaching blood vessels anteriorly, **C** and **D:** Perivertebral and mediastinal encroachment. (Reproduced with permission from Heelan RT, Demas BE, Caravelli JF, et al. Superior sulcus tumors: CT and MR imaging. *Radiology* 1989;170(3 Pt 1):637–641.)

of involvement, these are challenging tumors to completely resect because of the need to preserve or reconstruct the neurovascular structures. Patients with these lesions can present with Horner syndrome: miosis, ptosis, and anhidrosis. This indicates the invasion of the stellate ganglion and possibly the nerve root of T1. Preoperative workup with tissue biopsy is important as a small portion of these lesions are small cell carcinomas, which would warrant an alternative therapeutic approach. Careful pre-operative staging is essential in management, including PET-CT imaging and mediastinoscopy. N2 or N3 disease is an absolute contraindication for surgery given the associated poor prognosis.

Shaw and Paulson demonstrated the feasibility of resecting superior sulcus tumors in 1961. They showed that preoperative irradiation followed by surgical resection improved 5-year survival rate to 30%. The extensive early experience of Paulson highlights the limitations of surgery, because only approximately 60% of patients presenting with Pancoast tumors were deemed suitable for treatment pathways including resection.[162] Rusch et al. reported the largest series for resection of superior sulcus tumors ($n = 225$ patients). The majority of patients (55%) received preoperative radiation. Operative mortality was 4%. They noted that for T3N0 superior sulcus lesions, complete resection was achieved in 64% with an associated 5-year survival rate of 46%. However, once disease had progressed to stage III, 5-year survival was only 15%.[163] Attar et al. compared the use of both radiotherapy and chemotherapy in patients with superior sulcus tumors, and evaluated whether preoperative or postoperative treatment mattered. They discovered that preoperative radiation followed by surgery was associated with improved median survival compared to other groups.[164] Subsequently, the Southwest Oncology Group (SWOG) performed a prospective, multi-institutional trial of induction chemoradiotherapy in superior sulcus tumors including T3 and T4 lesions with N0 or N1 disease (Intergroup Trial 0160). Patients received trimodality therapy with two cycles of cisplatin and etoposide with concurrent 45 Gy of radiation. In this study, 92% had a complete resection with 65% showing pathologic complete response or minimal microscopic disease. Two-year survival was 55% for all eligible patients, and 70% for patients who had a complete resection.[165] Wright et al. compared induction chemoradiation versus radiation alone in patients diagnosed with superior sulcus tumors. Complete resection was possible in 80% of the radiation treatment patients versus 93% of the chemoradiation patients. The pathologic response was complete or near complete in 35% of the radiation patients and 87% of the chemoradiation patients. The 4-year survival rates were significantly different (49% for induction radiation and 84% for induction chemoradiation). Local recurrence was also improved in the preoperative induction chemoradiotherapy arm (0% vs. 30% for radiation alone).[166] More recently, Antonoff et al. also showed preoperative chemoradiation frequently resulted in pathologic complete response (32%) supporting the use of neoadjuvant therapy and surgery for superior sulcus tumors.[167] Induction therapy, including combined chemotherapy and radiation therapy, has thus become the standard of care for superior sulcus tumors. This approach offers a better chance at complete resection and improvements in overall survival.

T3 Tumors Invading Structures Other Than Chest Wall

There is limited data regarding stage II lesions that specifically invade other structures such as the mediastinum or those that are in close proximity to the carina. Mediastinal invasion limited to the mediastinal pleura is classified as T3. Pitz et al. found that patients undergoing a complete resection of tumors invading mediastinal pleura

achieved a 25% 5-year survival rate.[168] In a retrospective study, Burt et al. evaluated 225 patients with mediastinal T3 disease. In all patients studied, which also included some patients with mediastinal lymph node invasion (stage III disease), the survival rate was 9%. Among patients with T3N0 disease ($n = 102$), a 5-year survival rate of 19% was achieved. After an incomplete resection (R1 or R2), radiation therapy may improve local control in tumors with mediastinal pleural involvement.[169] Wang et al. studied postoperative radiotherapy for stage II and III incompletely resected NSCLC and survival, including T3 tumors with mediastinal involvement. There was a statistically significant improvement in survival when these patients received postoperative radiation therapy.[170] Recently, Rieber and his colleagues noted similar results.[171]

Diaphragmatic involvement with NSCLC also represents a potentially resectable T3 lesion. There is a paucity of reported surgical experience with this clinical situation. Weksler et al. found only eight cases in a review spanning two decades at Memorial-Sloan Kettering. All four patients with N2 disease died of their lung cancers, with a mean survival of only 92 weeks. Only a single N0 patient was alive at 70 weeks at the time of the report.[172] Inoue et al. reported no 3-year survival in five operated patients with diaphragmatic invasion, despite complete resection and N0–1 status.[173] For unclear reasons, more recent reports suggest an improved outcome. Rocco et al.[174] and Riquet et al.[175] achieved long-term survival in completely resected T3N0 cases with diaphragmatic involvement of 39% and 27%, respectively. Yokoi and colleagues performed combined lung and diaphragmatic resections in 26 cases with T3N0 and 29 cases with T3N1–2 lung cancer. Complete resection of N0 and of N1–2 cases yielded 5-year survival rates of 28% and 18%, respectively.[176] In all of these series, long-term survival is not observed following incomplete resection.

Central tumors within 2 cm from the carina without carinal involvement are also considered stage IIB. Mitchell et al. noted that overall 5-year survival was highest after isolated carinal resection at 51%, compared to 32% for N1 disease and 12% for N2/3 disease.[177] Yamamoto et al. achieved a 28.3% survival rate after carinal resection. Their 5-year survival rate for N0 disease was 50%, and 0% for N1/2 disease.[178] Similar results were shown by Rea et al. who observed a 5-year survival rate of 56% for N0 patients after resection. However, once again, N1 and N2 survival rates were dismal at 17% and 0%, respectively.[179] Lastly, Pitz et al. reported their experience with tumors localized within 2 cm from the carina, and found a 40% 5-year survival rate.[168] Liu et al. noted that 5-year survival becomes dismal if patients have locally advanced lung cancer infiltrating the carina. The 5-year survival rate of patients with primary tracheal and carinal tumors was 55% compared to 16.7% for those with locally advanced lung cancer directly infiltrating the carina.[180]

Patients with these lesions generally require either a sleeve resection with bronchoplastic reconstruction or a pneumonectomy to achieve adequate margins. A sleeve resection should always be considered when possible, given its favorable morbidity profile and preservation of pulmonary function when compared with pneumonectomy. Once again, thorough mediastinal staging is critical to optimize outcomes.

Sleeve Resection Versus Pneumonectomy

Hilar tumors present a challenging clinical scenario for thoracic surgeons given the inherent difficulties in attaining a complete (R0) resection with adequate margins. Generally, these patients will have central tumors that are commonly associated with hilar involvement of the mainstem bronchus or pulmonary artery (Fig. 95.10). Such

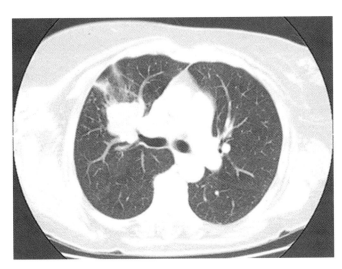

FIGURE 95.10 Hilar lesion requiring right upper lobe sleeve resection.

lesions can be successfully managed by sleeve resection or pneumonectomy. Thomas first described the use of bronchial sleeve resection as a means of conserving lung parenchyma in 1947.[14] Since that time, despite the technical complexities associated with sleeve resection, there has been a gradual increase in the use of this technique given its overall reduced morbidity and mortality profile (Table 95.8), preservation of pulmonary function, and comparable oncological outcomes in relation to pneumonectomy.

Deslauriers et al. analyzed their cohort of 1,230 patients in a single institution who underwent pneumonectomy ($n = 1,046$) or sleeve lobectomy ($n = 184$). The operative mortality was significantly higher in the pneumonectomy group compared to the sleeve lobectomy group, 5.3% versus 1.6%, respectively. In addition to this, 5-year survival was significantly improved for sleeve lobectomy (52%) when compared to pneumonectomy (31%). However, Deslauriers noted that the rates for complete resection were higher for sleeve lobectomy than for pneumonectomy (58 vs. 33%, respectively). When stratifying outcomes by stage I and stage II NSCLC, there was a significant difference favoring sleeve lobectomy compared to pneumonectomy in each group. Finally, site of first recurrence was local in 22% of patients with sleeve lobectomy compared to 35% of patients with pneumonectomy, suggesting that there is no apparent oncological benefit in resecting more lung (e.g., pneumonectomy) as long as an R0 resection can be accomplished.[181] Similar results were reported by Lee et al. In their series, 73 patients underwent sleeve lobectomy and 258 underwent pneumonectomy. Operative mortality was significantly different, 1.4% for sleeve lobectomy versus 10.1% for pneumonectomy. Major complications occurred in approximately 22% of

patients in both groups. The 30-day mortality for sleeve lobectomy was 0% compared to 8.9% for pneumonectomy.[182] Bagan et al. noted similar postoperative complication rates between sleeve resection and pneumonectomy, 28.8% versus 29.9%, respectively. Operative mortality was 12.6% for pneumonectomy versus 2.9% for sleeve lobectomy. Overall 5-year survival was 72.5% for sleeve resection and 53.2% for pneumonectomy.[183] These results were further corroborated by a recent study from Schuchert et al. This was a retrospective review of 253 patients with stage IB-IIB NSCLC, with central disease confined to the inner half of the lung. Patients undergoing sleeve resection with bronchoplasty ($n = 70$) versus lobectomy ($n = 123$) had similar outcomes including overall morbidity (62.9% vs. 45.5%), 30-day mortality (1.4% vs. 0.8%), as well as recurrence-free (24.3% vs. 33.3%) and overall 5-year survival (41% and 45%).[184] In a meta-analysis by Shi et al. of 19 studies comparing sleeve resection versus pneumonectomy, survival at 1, 3, and 5 years favored sleeve lobectomy. Postoperative complications and locoregional recurrences was not significantly different between the two surgical options.[185] Ferguson et al. found that sleeve lobectomy offers a better quality of life and may be more cost effective than pneumonectomy.[186]

In summary, given the overall favorable outcomes associated with sleeve resection when compared to pneumonectomy, sleeve resection should be strongly considered in the surgical management of hilar lesions when technically feasible. Pneumonectomy should be reserved for those cases where an R0 resection can't be accomplished by conventional lobectomy or sleeve lobectomy.

STAGE IIIA NSCLC

Controversy exists regarding the optimal management of patients with stage IIIA NSCLC, which constitutes the "grey zone" between surgical (stage IA–IIB) and nonsurgical (stage IIIB–IV) patient populations. In the seventh edition of the AJCC Staging System for lung cancer, stage IIIA NSCLC is defined as $T_3N_1M_0$, $T_{1-3}N_2M_0$ or $T_4N_{0-1}M_0$. Generally speaking, these are large (>7 cm), central tumors that may be associated with chest wall, mediastinal pleura, or parietal pericardium involvement. There may also be satellite tumor nodules within the same lobe or encroachment upon the mainstem bronchus within 2 cm of the main carina with associated nodal involvement (T3N1 or T3N2 lesions). This stage also encompasses patients with N2 mediastinal lymph node involvement (Fig. 95.11). The addition of the T4 descriptor to stage IIIA in the seventh edition of the AJCC Staging System includes those patients with tumor nodules in different lobes of the ipsilateral lung. As a result of these varying descriptors, there is significant heterogeneity in the underlying tumor characteristics and pattern of disease encountered among patients classified as having stage IIIA NSCLC.

TABLE 95.8 Perioperative Mortality Following Lobectomy, Sleeve Resection, and Pneumonectomy for NSCLC

Author	Year	n	Lobectomy	Sleeve Resection	Pneumonectomy
Ginsberg et al.[329]	1983	2,220	2.9	—	6.2
Romano et al.[330]	1992	12,439	4.2	—	11.6
Suen et al.[364]	1999	7,099	—	5.2	4.9
Deslauriers et al.[181]	2004	1,230	—	1.6	5.3
Allen et al.[334]	2006	1,023	1.3	—	0
Schuchert et al.[121]	2012	253	0.8	1.4	6.7

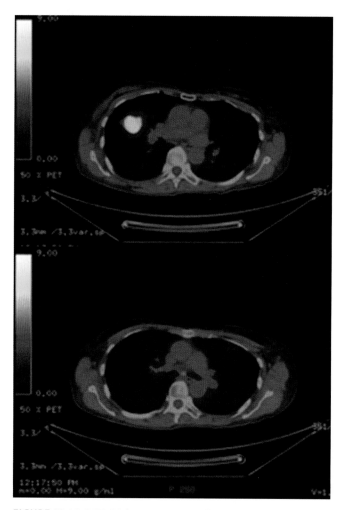

FIGURE 95.11 PET-CT demonstrating a right upper lobe mass with hilar and subcarinal node involvement. (Reprinted from Lin WY, Hsu WH, Lin KH, et al. Role of preoperative PET-CT in assessing mediastinal and hilar lymph node status in early stage lung cancer. *J Chin Med Assocn* 2012;75(5): 203–208. Copyright © 2012 Elsevier. With permission.)

While there are many treatment options for patients with stage IIIA NSCLC, the chances of cure remain quite low (<25%) and a multimodality approach is recommended, frequently employing a combination of chemotherapy, radiation therapy, and surgery in select cases. Treatment options include neoadjuvant therapy followed by surgery, surgery followed by adjuvant chemotherapy, or definitive chemoradiation (platinum-based doublet with 60–70 Gy external beam radiation therapy). No single therapeutic approach is applicable to all patients, and therefore treatment decisions must be made on a case by case basis. Several clinical parameters are useful in helping to stratify patients for the optimal therapeutic approach in this setting, and specifically to determine whether there may be any benefit to surgical resection (Table 95.9).

Histology

Patients with large cell neuroendocrine tumors[187] or pleomorphic carcinomas[188] frequently exhibit aggressive tumor biology, which might be less amenable to complete surgical resection. Metro et al. have demonstrated that locoregionally advanced large cell neuroendocrine carcinomas have a high incidence of systemic metastases (especially brain metastases), and have a worse overall response rate to systemic therapy and overall prognosis than small cell lung cancer.[189]

TABLE 95.9 Factors Influencing Treatment Decisions in Stage IIIA NSCLC

Tumor histology
Single-station or multistation N2 lymph node involvement
Bulky versus nonbulky N2 lymph node involvement
Extracapsular lymph node extension
Resectability of primary tumor ± involved lymph node
Extent of resection required
Physiologic reserve of the patient

When faced with these "bad-acting" histological variants, aggressive attempts at radical surgical resection are unlikely to succeed, and thus consideration should be given to definitive chemoradiation alone in such cases.

Extent of Lymphadenopathy

Bulky mediastinal lymphadenopathy can be defined as lymph nodes measuring greater than 2 to 3 cm in short-axis diameter as measured during CT imaging (Fig. 95.12). Bulky lymphadenopathy has been associated with incomplete surgical resection, and is associated with worse overall outcome compared to nonbulky disease.[190] The number of lymph node stations involved also appears to have an important impact on success of surgical management for stage IIIA NSCLC. Lee and colleagues demonstrated that the 5-year survival of multiple station N2 IIIA (20.4%) was significantly lower than that of single station N2 IIIA (33.8%) disease ($p = 0.016$).[191] Location of lymph nodes also may have some prognostic impact. Single-station N2 involvement in levels 5 and 6 (A-P window/peri-aortic) mediastinal lymph nodes has been associated with improved survival following resection compared to involvement in other lymph node stations. Patterson et al. reported a 42% 5-year survival among patients undergoing surgical resection with isolated subaortic lymph node involvement.[192] Patients with bulky or multi-station lymph node involvement, as well as those that have extracapsular nodal spread are probably best treated by chemoradiation. Patients with nonbulky, single-station nodal involvement without extracapsular spread represent the ideal subgroup with IIIA disease where surgery may be

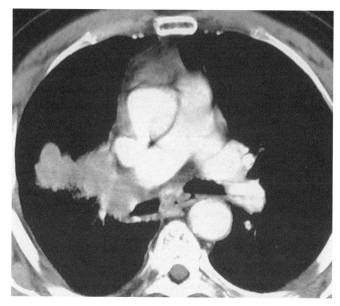

FIGURE 95.12 Hilar lesion with bulky mediastinal lymph node involvement.

considered, in association with either neoadjuvant chemotherapy/chemoradiation or adjuvant chemotherapy.

Neoadjuvant Therapy

The role of neoadjuvant and adjuvant therapy in conjunction with surgery continues to evolve. The use of induction therapy in this setting has been associated with good response rates associated with reduction in tumor volume prior to surgery, and potentially achieving earlier treatment of micrometastatic disease. Furthermore, neoadjuvant chemotherapy regimens tend to be better tolerated with better patient compliance than adjuvant chemotherapy. Induction (neoadjuvant) therapy in the setting of IIIA NSCLC has been explored in several phase III prospective, randomized trials. In these studies, the use of induction chemotherapy was shown to result in a significant increase in median survival compared with surgery alone (21–22 vs. 10 to 14 months) in patients with stage IIIA disease.[193,194] In the largest retrospective study evaluating outcomes in patients with stage IIIA-N2 disease, over 11,000 patients were analyzed from the National Cancer Database. This study found that induction chemoradiation followed by surgery achieved better survival outcomes than surgery followed by adjuvant chemotherapy.[195] Other larger randomized studies have failed to demonstrate a benefit in the setting of stage IB-IIIA disease, with the greatest benefit seen in the stage IB-II subgroups.[196] In a phase III trial investigating the role of neoadjuvant chemotherapy followed by either surgery or radiation therapy (EORTC 08941), no differences were noted in either median or overall survival.[197] In the North American Intergroup trial 0139, Albain et al. also demonstrated no significant survival benefit for patients undergoing induction chemotherapy followed by surgical resection compared with definitive chemoradiation therapy alone (approximate 5-year survival: 27% vs. 20%, respectively; $p = 0.24$) for stage IIIA NSCLC. Interestingly, patients who were resected with lobectomy following induction therapy did have improved survival compared to chemoradiation alone (36% vs. 18%; $p = 0.002$). However, no benefit was seen in patients who were resected with pneumonectomy (22% vs. 24%; $p = $ NS). The high perioperative mortality rate of pneumonectomy following neoadjuvant therapy in this study (26%) appeared to contribute to the worsening survival in this subgroup.[198] The SWOG S9900 trial comparing neoadjuvant chemotherapy plus surgery versus surgery alone for stage IB-IIIA disease similarly showed a high mortality rate (16.7%) among patients undergoing pneumonectomy following induction therapy.[199] Several other studies have reported acceptable mortality rates (5% to 10%) after induction therapy, although these were all retrospective studies.[200–202] These studies have led many investigators to conclude that neoadjuvant therapy followed by surgery should only be considered when complete surgical resection can be accomplished by lobectomy alone.

Surgical Considerations

The fundamental tenets of surgical resection for stage IIIA lung cancer involve a fine balance between complete resection of all tumor and preservation of lung parenchyma in a population with typically poor pulmonary reserve. Lobectomy remains the recommended treatment for resectable disease in patients with adequate physiologic reserve and when R0 resection is achievable.[203] Bronchoplasty and vascular sleeve resections have also been shown to achieve reduced morbidity and mortality when compared to pneumonectomy, with equivalent oncologic outcomes.[204,205] Pneumonectomy is typically reserved for large, bulky, hilar tumors unresectable by lesser means. Mortality rates for pneumonectomy have been reported from 0% to 11.5% in several large recent series (Tables 95.1 and 95.8). Particular

concern has emerged regarding the use of pneumonectomy following neoadjuvant therapy, with documented mortality rates as high as 26%. The negative physiologic effects of pneumonectomy have been well-described and may contribute to the observed higher early mortality rates in this group of patients.[206] Ultimately, the extent of resection should be tailored to individual patient and tumor characteristics to achieve a complete R0 resection with systematic nodal staging. If obtaining complete R0 resection is the primary goal of surgical resection, then it will be necessary to continue to perform pneumonectomy in certain patients in order to provide them with the best chance of cure, despite the observed higher risk and poorer survival results. Thorough preoperative staging, proper patient selection, and improved postoperative care should result in improved outcomes for patients requiring pneumonectomy in the future, and pneumonectomy should continue to be considered an acceptable surgical option for early stage lung cancers with hilar involvement.

T3N1 Disease

The T3N1 subset represents a minority of cases in stage IIIA NSCLC. For individuals with T3N1 tumors, primary surgical resection is recommended followed by adjuvant chemotherapy. An exception to this general strategy would be superior sulcus (Pancoast) tumors, which are treated by chemoradiation first, followed by complete surgical resection. When malignant lymphadenopathy accompanies chest wall invasion, the efficacy of resection is markedly limited. Five-year survival rates in the presence of N1 metastasis range from 8% to 35%, with an average of 19%. With lymphadenopathy and incomplete resection, operation alone is associated with minimal late survival. Downey et al. reported a 5-year survival rate of 27% for completely resected T3N1 compared to 49% for T3N0, and 15% for T3N2 disease. Survival was close to zero for those with incomplete resection.[153] Adjuvant systemic chemotherapy is recommended after complete resection.

T4 Tumors—Synchronous Ipsilateral Nodule in Different Lobe

The presence of separate foci of disease in a different ipsilateral lobe as the primary tumor is currently classified as a T4 lesion. Prognosis is accordingly worse than synchronous intralobar nodules (T3). Okamoto et al. found that ipsilateral nodules in separate lobes were associated with a 5-year survival of only 19.3%, as compared to 54.4% with synchronous intralobar nodules.[207] Okumura and colleagues reported an 11% 5-year survival for synchronous sites in different lobes.[208] Given the marginal outcomes, surgical intervention should only be considered in the context of a multidisciplinary team approach or clinical trial.

T4 Tumors—Mediastinal Invasion

T4 tumors due to mediastinal invasion of vital structures are also now considered as stage IIIA, unless there is documented N2 or N3 nodal involvement (stage IIIB). In properly selected patients, resection is possible. These procedures are technically challenging, and can be associated with increased morbidity and mortality. These lesions include those involving the carina, superior vena cava, heart (mainly the atria), pulmonary artery, aorta, esophagus, and vertebral body.

- Carina: The largest surgical experience with T4 NSCLC involves tumors with carinal involvement. Complete surgical resection typically requires pneumonectomy with bronchoplastic reconstruction (sleeve pneumonectomy), and can be associated with enhanced survival compared with chemoradiation alone. In properly selected patients treated at centers with experience with advanced airway cases, 5-year survival rates of up to 40% have been observed, as reported by Watanabe,[209] Deslauriers,[210] Roviaro,[211] and Mitchell[177] and their colleagues. However, operative mortality remains high. Porhanov et al. reported an operative mortality rate of 16% among 231 carinal resections.[212] Mitchell et al. reported an overall operative mortality of 15% in 60 patients undergoing carinal resection for bronchogenic carcinoma. Overall 5-year survival was 42%.[177] In the largest series reported to date, Yildizeli et al. reported their outcomes in 92 patients undergoing carinal resection with bronchoplastic reconstruction for NSCLC. Overall morbidity was 42.4%. Anastomotic complications with or without bronchopleural fistula occurred in 7.6% of cases. The overall mortality rate was 6.5%. Actuarial 5-year survival was 42.5%.[213] The presence of N2 or N3 disease is associated with a poor prognosis, and is regarded as a contraindication to carinal resection.

- Superior Vena Cava: Lung cancer lesions involving the SVC that are amenable to surgical resection are rare.[214] Involvement can be secondary to a central primary tumor or secondary to malignant mediastinal lymph nodes. Survival following resection of a central tumor is significantly better than resection of lesions secondary to metastatic lymph nodes (36.0% vs. 6.6%).[110] Small series reporting partial tangential resection and primary closure or patching of the superior vena cava (SVC), as well as composite circumferential resection requiring graft reconstruction, have been reported by Dartevelle,[215] Nakahara,[216] and Tsuchiya[217] and their colleagues. Median survival ranges from 8.5 to 40 months.[218] Long-term survival, however, has only been observed and reported in a limited number of cases (one reported by Inoue et al.[219] and 2 of 30 cases in the series of Tsuchiya et al.).[217] Burt et al. reported no long-term survivors among 18 cases of NSCLC invading the SVC and treated by pulmonary resection, brachytherapy, or both.[169] Spaggiari et al. presented their experience with 28 patients who underwent SVC resection and graft replacement for lung cancer. The overall 5-year survival rate was 15%.[220] Misthos et al. found that only one out of nine patients survived 5 years.[221] Patients should undergo thorough preoperative staging, including mediastinoscopy to exclude N2 or greater disease, which portends a poor prognosis. Dartevelle et al. reported long-term results on their preliminary experience in six patients. All six patients had associated malignant lymphadenopathy, and four of the patients received adjuvant radiation. Neither of the two cases with N2 lymph node involvement survived beyond 8 months. Two of the four cases with N1 involvement were reported as alive at 16 and 52 months. In the setting of malignant lymph node involvement, induction therapy may be associated with improved disease-free survival.[222] Bernard et al. reported a 25% 5-year overall survival among eight patients undergoing resection and re-construction.[223] In the largest published series, Yildizeli et al. reported on 39 patients undergoing SVC replacement for NSCLC. Perioperative mortality was 7.7%. Five- and ten-year actuarial survival rates were 29.4% and 22.1%, respectively.[213] In conclusion, long-term favorable outcomes can be obtained with surgery in this subgroup of patients. Thorough preoperative staging and careful patient selection at specialized centers are essential in optimizing outcomes.

- Aorta: Surgical resection of lung neoplasms involving the aorta is rarely performed. The approach commonly involves cardiopulmonary bypass, and outcomes are predominantly limited to technical case reports, as presented by Nakahara,[216] Horita,[224] and Tsuchiya,[217] and their colleagues. Clinical outcomes following aortic resection have been variable. Burt[169] and Bernard[223] and their colleagues each found no long-term survivors in their published series. Klepetko et al. presented five cases of combined left lung and aortic resection; three patients with N2 disease died between 17 and 27 months, and two with pathologic T4N1 disease were alive at 14 and 50 months.[225] Misthos et al. achieved a 30.7% 5-year survival.[221] Kusomoto et al. reported a 44.4% actuarial 5-year survival rate among six patients undergoing concomitant lung and aortic resection.[226] Thoracic aortic endovascular stent graft placement has been introduced as a protective adjunct to lung resection with limited aortic wall involvement, thus avoiding the need for cross-clamping or bypass.[227,228]

- Heart: Cardiac resection (primarily a portion of the atrium) has been rarely reported at the time of lung resection for NSCLC. Hasegawa et al. reviewed the use of cardiopulmonary bypass in 11 patients finding the results to be dismal, with 10/11 (90.9%) ultimately dying of recurrent disease.[229] One patient who had no evidence of recurrence died of aspiration pneumonia 10 months after surgery.[229] Kusomoto et al. also observed a 0% 5-year survival in three patients with concomitant atrial resection.[226] Tsukioka et al. published their experience with partial left atrial resection in patients with primary lung cancer. Complete resection was achieved in 11/12 patients (92%). The overall postoperative 5-year survival rate was 46%. The 5-year survival was better with patients with N0 or N1 disease compared to those with N2 disease (67% vs. 20%, respectively).[230]

- Pulmonary Artery: T4 cancers involving the pulmonary artery trunk are rarely resected. There were no late survivors among seven patients who underwent main pulmonary trunk resection in the series by Tsuchiya et al.[217] In contrast, Rendina,[231] Shrager,[232] and Bernard[223] and their colleagues have clearly demonstrated that tangential or circumferential resection of the right or left proximal pulmonary artery is beneficial in carefully selected cases. Overall late survival rates in these reports were 38%, 48%, and 20%, respectively. The lower figure in Bernard's series is likely due to the inclusion of only patients with intrapericardial pulmonary artery invasion.[223] Ma et al. similarly reported a 37% 5-year survival rate in patients undergoing pulmonary artery reconstruction for stage III NSCLC.[233]

- Esophagus: Combined resection of lung cancer and the esophagus is also very rare. No series with significant results have been reported. The most common method to treat locoregionally advanced lung cancer with esophageal involvement is esophageal stenting as a palliative measure. Esophageal exclusion or retrosternal bypass can be considered as a palliative option in advanced tumors not amenable to stenting.

- Vertebral Body: Although technically feasible in a few instances, as discussed above, the long-term oncological utility of total vertebrectomy is unknown. Grunenwald et al. reported 19 cases of total vertebrectomy or hemivertebrectomy; their 2- and 5-year survival rates were 53% and 14%, respectively.[234] More recently, Mody et al. have reported their experience in 32 cases of T4 tumors with vertebral involvement. Perioperative mortality was 3%. Five-year survival was 40.3%.[235] Adjuvant chemoradiation is commonly employed, and may improve outcomes.[236]

- Multiple Organ Involvement: Composite resections involving the carina, superior vena cava, aorta, heart, esophagus, pulmonary artery, and vertebral body can be performed in an effort to accomplish an R0 resection. Such patients are best evaluated as part of a multidisciplinary approach. The indications for such extended resections must be carefully weighed in the context of expected perioperative complications and mortality rates, the physiological and oncological status of the patient, as well as the expertise of the surgical team.[237] Neoadjuvant chemotherapy (with or without radiation therapy) is frequently employed in these cases, as is adjuvant chemotherapy ± radiation therapy. Current National Comprehensive Cancer Network Guidelines do not recommend surgery for T4 disease associated with N2 or N3 disease (stage IIIB).

Surprise N2 Disease

The identification of unexpected mediastinal lymph node involvement at the time of lung resection (surprise N2 involvement) presents the surgeon with several challenges in the context of intraoperative decision making. Should the planned lung resection be carried out? Should extent of resection to be altered (e.g., segmentectomy vs. lobectomy vs. pneumonectomy)? Should mediastinal lymph nodes be sampled or dissected? There is a general consensus that N2 disease on final pathological evaluation of resected specimens should be followed by adjuvant chemotherapy. Several clinical variables have been shown to portend a positive prognostic impact including the ability to perform a complete (R0) resection, T1,2 primary tumors, single-level nodal involvement and patients with clinical N0 or N1 disease.[238] Planned surgical resections can be carried out in these instances with reasonable oncological outcomes (20% to 45% 5-year survival). Worse outcomes (15% 5-year survival) are seen in patients with multilevel N2 disease, clinical N2 disease by CT, T3/4 tumors, or subcarinal lymph node involvement. Lobectomy is preferred with mediastinal lymph node dissection, when technically possible, and is associated with less mortality than pneumonectomy, and better survival when compared to segmentectomy in the setting of pathological N2 disease. In patients with incidental (occult) N2 disease discovered at the time of surgical resection and in whom complete resection of the primary tumor is technically possible, completion of the planned lung resection with lymphadenectomy is recommended. Adjuvant chemotherapy is also recommended in this setting.

In conclusion, stage IIIA NSCLC represents a heterogeneous group of patients with varying pattern and extent of disease. The optimal treatment strategy for this group as a whole is not well-delineated. Treatments should be individualized based on tumor characteristics, clinical stage, and the patients underlying physiologic status. Neoadjuvant chemoradiation followed by surgery is the standard of care in the management of T3N1 superior sulcus tumors. Patients with large (>7 cm) tumors with N1 nodal involvement, as well as patients with T4 tumors appear to benefit from the addition of adjuvant chemotherapy. Surgical resection following neoadjuvant therapy can be considered in patients with nonbulky, single-station lymph node involvement that can potentially undergo a complete resection. Lobectomy (with or without sleeve resection) is preferred over pneumonectomy following neoadjuvant therapy. When possible, patients with stage IIIA disease should be treated under the auspices of a multidisciplinary committee and/or clinical trial.

STAGE IIIB NSCLC

Stage IIIB NSCLC constitutes approximately 10% to 15% of newly diagnosed NSCLC cases.[131] In the seventh edition of the AJCC/UICC staging system for NSCLC, stage IIIB represents those patients with unresectable T4 tumors (T4N2) and those with contralateral (N3) mediastinal lymph node involvement. T4N0-1 neoplasms, which were historically classified as stage IIIB, are now included in the stage IIIA category. Malignant pleural effusions, also previously classified as stage IIIB, are now re-classified as stage IVA.

Generally speaking, stage IIIB cases are not considered amenable to complete surgical resection, and correspondingly are most commonly treated with definitive concurrent chemoradiation in patients with minimal weight loss and a good performance status.[239] The anticipated 5-year survival of patients falling in this category ranges from 3% to 7%.[103,240] Previous studies have evaluated the role of surgery following induction chemoradiation in a highly selected groups of patients with stage IIIA and IIIB disease.[241,242] In the SWOG 8805 trial, Albain et al. included selected patients with T4 (now stage IIIA) as well as patients with T4N2 and N3 disease (stage IIIB). A total of 34 of the 51 patients classified as IIIB in that study would currently qualify as stage IIIB in the current staging system (T4N2 = 7, N3 = 27). In subset analysis, the T4N0-1 group (now stage IIIA) had improved survival (median survival of 28 vs. 13 months, $p = 0.07$) compared with T4N2 or N3 subgroups. Among the 27 patients with contralateral N3 disease, the 2-year survival was 33% for patients with supraclavicular lymph node involvement versus 0% for those with N3 involvement. In multivariate analysis, the only subgroups associated with a positive prognosis were the T1N2 and T4N0-1 groups (currently stage IIIA). Overall 3-year survival for the stage IIIB cohort was 27%. Barlesi et al. evaluated 60 patients with stage IIIB disease undergoing surgery following neoadjuvant chemoradiation (classified as per the Sixth Edition of the AJCC/UICC Lung Cancer Staging System). The actuarial 5-year survival rate was 16.7% and was not significantly different than the stage IIIA group (17%). Completeness of resection, the presence of vascular invasion and visceral pleural invasion were all independent prognostic variables in multivariate analysis. Current consensus guidelines do not support routine surgical intervention for T4N2 or N3 disease.[242]

Salvage resection can be considered in patients suffering emergent complications (e.g., massive hemoptysis) as a life-saving measure. In addition, surgeons are occasionally consulted regarding patients who have undergone prior definitive chemoradiation for stage IIIB disease, who have demonstrated good response to therapy, and who are left with apparent localized disease on repeat staging. Yang et al. evaluated outcomes of patients undergoing salvage lobectomy after definitive chemoradiation in 31 patients.[243] Of these, five patients were initially classified as stage IIIB disease. Pathological downstaging was noted in 68% of patients in the overall group, with a pathological nodal status of N0 in 90% of patients. The 5-year survival was 36% in this subgroup, compared to 0% in patients with residual nodal disease. This study demonstrates that salvage resection is technically possible in carefully selected patients. Surgical intervention in this setting should only be performed after detailed consideration by a multidisciplinary committee and/or under the auspices of a clinical trial.

STAGE IV NSCLC

It is estimated that 40% of patients with newly diagnosed NSCLC have incurable stage IV disease, which is one of the key factors accounting for the overall poor survival associated with lung cancer.[244] Stage IV lung cancer is divided into patients with malignant pleural effusion (stage IVA) and those with distant metastases (stage IVB). Stage IV disease is generally not successfully treatable by surgical intervention, and systemic chemotherapy constitutes the standard of care in patients with reasonable functional status. Palliative interventions including endobronchial ablation and stenting and management of malignant pleural effusions represent important options in controlling symptoms and optimizing quality of life. These palliative surgical interventions are discussed in detail elsewhere in this text.

Overall 5-year survival in patients with stage IV disease is <5. One clinical scenario where surgical intervention may be associated with improved outcomes is in the setting of solitary metastases involving the brain, adrenal glands, or other extracranial, extra-adrenal sites.[245] The hallmark therapeutic principles involved in considering surgical intervention for patients with solitary foci of metastatic disease from lung cancer include complete resectability of the primary lung tumor, resectability or control by radiation therapy of the metastatic lesion, and no evidence of disease elsewhere.[246] Thorough preoperative staging including PET-CT scan and mediastinoscopy are considered essential in all cases. A long metachronous interval from the time of presentation of the primary lung tumor to the development of solitary metastasis is a positive prognostic feature associated with improved outcomes. In properly selected cases, 5-year survival rates ranging from 10% to 40% have been reported with resection of the primary lesion and metastasectomy.

Intracranial Metastases

Approximately 25% of patients with stage IV NSCLC will have brain metastases (Fig. 95.13). The median survival in the setting of brain metastases in about 2 months when treated with steroids alone, and 3 to 6 months after treatment with whole brain radiation therapy (WBRT).[247] The role of surgical resection in the setting of solitary brain metastases is evolving. There are approximately 35,000 to 40,000 deaths annually associated with symptomatic brain metastases from lung cancer. A solitary lesion is found in nearly half of all patients who present with brain metastases from NSCLC, but most also have extracerebral distant foci or advanced locoregional disease.[248] Although resection or stereotactic radiosurgery (Gamma knife) of the cranial lesion may offer optimal neurologic palliation, pulmonary resection should be undertaken only in cases that would

have been suitable for curative primary resection in the absence of M1 disease, and only after a thorough evaluation to rule out other sites of metastatic disease.

Several series have shown apparent improved survival of about 10% to 20% with removal of a synchronous or metachronous solitary brain metastasis (SBM) and pulmonary resection for otherwise limited NSCLC. The first large experience was reported by Magilligan et al., who found a 5-year survival rate of 21% and a 10-year survival rate of 15% in 41 synchronous and metachronous cases of SBM.[249] In another series of synchronous and metachronous cases, Read et al. reported a 21% 5-year survival rate following complete resection of both the SBM and the primary site in 27 cases, as compared with a median survival rate of only 6.4 months in patients who underwent noncurative resection of either or both sites.[250] Burt et al. reviewed 185 patients who had undergone craniotomy for resection of brain metastases from NSCLC with encouraging survival rates at 1 year (55%), 2 years (27%), 3 years (18%), 5 years (13%), and 10 years (7%). No significant differences in survival were seen when comparing synchronous ($n = 65$) vs. metachronous ($n = 120$) metastatic brain lesions in that study. Complete resection of the primary lung tumor was the most significant factor impacting on survival in patients undergoing cerebral metastasectomy.[251] In a series of 28 patients with synchronous metastasis, Billing et al. noted a 5-year survival rate of 21%,[252] whereas Bonnette et al. reported a lower figure of 11% in 103 cases.[253] Granone et al. reported a 17% 3-year survival rate in 30 cases of synchronous and metachronous brain M1 lesions.[254] Solitary metachronous brain lesions seem to have a better long-term benefit from resection. Although Mussi et al. note only a 6.6% 5-year survival rate for combined resection in synchronous SBM, their reported survival for metachronous lesions was 19%.[255] Favorable

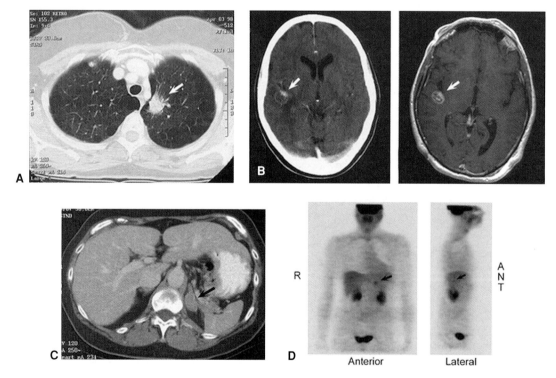

FIGURE 95.13 Multimodality Approach in the Treatment of Solitary Metastases from Non–Small Cell Lung Cancer. **A:** Left upper lobe NSCLC treated by surgical resection. **B:** Solitary brain metastasis diagnosed one year later and treated by GammaKnife. **C:** Subsequent development of a left adrenal mass that increased in size over the course of one year despite chemotherapy. **D:** PET imaging demonstrated an area of intense uptake corresponding to the known adrenal mass, concerning for metastatic disease. The patient underwent a laparoscopic left adrenalectomy with the final pathology identifying metastatic adenocarcinoma from a lung primary. The patient is alive without evidence of disease at 4.5 years status post left upper lobectomy.

TABLE 95.10 Surgical Treatment of Solitary Intracranial Metastases From Non-Small Cell Lung Cancer

Study	Year	n	Regimen	Median Survival (mos)	5-Year Survival (%)
Patchell et al.[256]	1990	25	Surgery/WBXRT	19	25
		23	WBXRT Alone	9	5
Macchiarini et al.[365]	1991	37	Lung Resection and Metastasectomy	27	30
Burt et al.[251]	1992	185	Series of Consecutive Metastasectomy	14	13
Vecht et al.[366]	1993	31	Surgery/WBXRT	11	NR
		32	WBXRT Alone	4	
Mussi et al.[255]	1996	52	Lung Resection and Metastasectomy	19	16
Billing et al.[252]	2001	28	Lung Resection and Metastasectomy	24	21
Bonnette et al.[253]	2001	103	Lung Resection and Metastasectomy	12	11

factors in the setting of synchronous SBM include N0 disease, lower T factor, and adenocarcinoma. Favorable factors in the setting of metachronous SBM include N0 status, lobectomy, and disease-free interval. In the study by Mussi et al., the interval between lung and brain operation was ≥14.5 months. In a randomized trial comparing surgery/whole brain radiotherapy with radiotherapy alone in 25 patients with single brain metastases, the surgery group lived longer (19 vs. 9 months), had fewer locoregional recurrences, and had a better quality of life compared with radiotherapy alone.[256]

Experience has been gained with precision techniques such as stereotactic radiosurgery (Gamma Knife), which is less invasive, can treat areas otherwise inaccessible by surgery, and potentially allows more than one lesion to be treated.[257] Retrospective analyses have failed to delineate a difference in morbidity, mortality, local control, or survival when comparing radiosurgery versus neurosurgery for solitary brain metastases.[258,259] Both modalities are reasonable treatment alternatives as discussed by Fuentes et al. in a Cochrane Systematic Review.[257] There are no currently available prospective studies yet available comparing these modalities. For individuals not eligible for surgery or radiation therapy, the use of tyrosine kinase inhibitors in patients with EGFR muations and ALK rearrangements has been associated with response rates as high as 60% to 80% with complete response rates as high as 40% and median overall survival ranging from 15 to 20 months.[260]

In summary, surgical resection of solitary brain metastases (with or without radiation) or stereotactic radiosurgery can be performed in the presence of a well-controlled or completely resectable primary lung cancer and a negative extensive metastatic workup, with 5-year survival rates ranging from 10% to 20% (Table 95.10).

Adrenal Metastases

Approximately 1/3 of patients dying with NSCLC will have adrenal metastases (Fig. 95.13). Progression of extracranial metastatic disease has been found to be an independent predictor of treatment failure in NSCLC. Several reported case series now demonstrate that aggressive surgical management of isolated adrenal metastases can confer long-term survival. Surgery + chemotherapy appears to increase survival in the setting of synchronous or metachronous adrenal metastases. In a study by Luketich et al. of 14 patients with

solitary synchronous adrenal metastases comparing adrenalectomy/chemotherapy with chemotherapy, median (31 vs. 8.5 months) and 3-year survival (38% vs. 0%) were substantially improved by surgical resection of solitary adrenal metastases in addition to chemotherapy (mitomycin, vinblastine, and cis-platinum).[261] In a retrospective study comparing therapeutic regimens for solitary metachronous adrenal metastases, 18 patients were divided into four groups: Group A (adrenalectomy, 5 patients), Group B (adrenalectomy/chemotherapy, 8 patients), Group C (chemotherapy alone, 2 patients) and Group D (radiation alone, 2 patients). Median survival was greatest in the adrenalectomy/chemotherapy group (19 months) when compared to adrenalectomy alone (14 months), chemotherapy alone (15 months) or radiation alone (8 months). Surgery + adjuvant chemotherapy (paclitaxel/carboplatin) appears to increase survival in metachronous adrenal metastases.[262] Porte et al. identified 11 cases of solitary adrenal metastases in 598 consecutive patients with otherwise operable or resected NSCLC at their institution. Among eight patients with synchronous disease treated by resection, the median survival time was only 10 months, although one patient remained cancer-free at 66 months. Of the three cases of metachronous lesions, two died at 6 and 14 months, and one was alive at 6 months.[263] Porte et al. later reported the outcomes of 43 patients from eight centers. The median survival time was about 16 months for both synchronous and metachronous disease; 2-, 3-, and 4-year survival rates were 29%, 14%, and 11%, respectively.[264] Tanvetyanon et al. reviewed 10 publications contributing 114 patients.[265] They noted that 42% of patients had synchronous metastases and 58% had metachronous metastases. The median disease-free interval for metachronous adrenal metastases was 12 months. Although the median survival was shorter for patients with synchronous metastasis than those with metachronous metastasis (12 months vs. 31 months), the 5-year survival estimates were equivalent, around 25%.[265] Nodal involvement has been associated a worse prognosis.[266]

Surgical resection of solitary adrenal metastases (with adjuvant chemotherapy) can be performed in patients of good performance status where the primary lesion is completely resectable. Adjuvant chemotherapy is recommended following surgery. Patients with nodal involvement should probably not undergo adrenalectomy. In carefully selected patients, 5-year survival rates ranging between 7% and 60% have been reported (Table 95.11).

TABLE 95.11 Surgical Treatment of Adrenal Metastases From Non-Small Cell Lung Cancer

Study	Year	N	Regimen	Median Survival (mos)	5-Year Survival (%)
Luketich et al.[261]	1996	8	Adrenalectomy/Chemo	31	20
		6	Chemo Alone	8.5	0
Beitler et al.[367]	1998	22	Adrenalectomy/Chemo	24	31
Porte et al.[264]	2001	43	Adrenalectomy/Chemo	11	7
Ambrogi et al.[270]	2001	5	Adrenalectomy/Chemo	NR	60
Abdel-Raheem et al.[262]	2002	8	Adrenalectomy/Chemo	19	25
		5	Adrenalectomy Alone	14	0
		2	Chemotherapy Alone	15	0
		2	Radiation alone	8	0
Billing et al.[252]	2001	28	Lung Resection and Adrenalectomy	24	21
Bonnette et al.[253]	2001	103	Lung Resection and Adrenalectomy	12	11
Tanvetyanon et al.[265]	2008	48	Adrenalectomy—Synchronous	12	26
		66	Adrenalectomy—Metachronous	31	25
Raz et al.[266]	2011	20	Adrenalectomy	19	34
		17	Nonsurgical	6	0

Extracranial, Extra-adrenal Metastases

Metastatic disease to organs other than the brain and adrenal glands are rarely amenable to surgical resection. As in the cases of intracranial and adrenal metastases, solitary lesions that are completely resectable (or amenable to stereotactic or external beam radiation) can be treated if the primary site is well-controlled and there are no other signs of disease elsewhere. Splenic,[267] hepatic,[268,269] renal[270] and muscle[271] resections have been reported for solitary metastatic lesions. Luketich et al. reported a 10-year retrospective review of 14 patients who had aggressive treatment of solitary extracranial, extra-adrenal metastases from NSCLC.[272] The sites of metastases included extrathoracic lymph nodes,[6] skeletal muscle,[4] bone,[3] and small bowel.[1] The overall 10-year actuarial survival was 86%. This was a highly selected group with a long metachronous interval of 20 months. In 2001, Downey and Ng reported on a prospective assessment of patients with a solitary synchronous metastasis from lung cancer. Eligible patients were to receive both preoperative and postoperative chemotherapy. Of the 23 patients that were enrolled, only 10 patients ultimately underwent complete resection of both the primary lung tumor and the metastatic site. The median overall survival was 11 months (5-year survival was not reported).[273]

In summary, metastasectomy should be considered in patients with good performance status, a controlled original primary site without signs of additional metastases after an extensive metastatic workup, and a long metachronous interval. If a complete resection of the primary and solitary metastases can be performed in this setting, long-term survival can be achieved (Tables 95.10 and 95.11).

VARIABLES AFFECTING ONCOLOGICAL OUTCOMES

Surgical resection constitutes the primary therapeutic option in the management of early-stage NSCLC. Despite complete (R0) resection, recurrence rates range between 15% and 30%, with 5-year survival ranging from 60 to 70% for stage I disease.[62] The primary T (tumor), N (lymph node), and M (metastasis) descriptors provide the most important prognostic information and stage classification in NSCLC.[61] In addition to the TNM staging system descriptors discussed above, several additional factors including patient age, histologic cell type, central versus peripheral location, surgical margin, angiolymphatic invasion, and tumor-infiltrating lymphocytes (TILs) have been shown to be of prognostic value in predicting recurrence risk in resectable NSCLC.

Age–Lung Resection in the Elderly

Patients diagnosed with lung cancer are often over the age of 65 (median age at the time of diagnosis = 68 years old). According to an analysis of the SEER Program database, patients 70 years or older account for 47% of all lung cancers diagnosed in the United States. Of these, over 80% of cases are stage III or greater.[274] Among patients eligible for lung resection, nearly 62% are 65 years of age or older.[275] These clinical features highlight the importance of age in the clinical decision-making regarding the surgical management of stage IA NSCLC. Tas et al. found that age was a major prognostic factor affecting survival in patients with NSCLC. Patients >60 years of age had significantly lower survival at 1 year (42.5% vs. 67.3%, $p = 0.023$).[276] The interactions associated with age are complex and include a multitude of factors including cardiopulmonary function, underlying medical comorbidities, prior surgery, and performance status. Increasing age is associated with an adverse impact on the above-mentioned variables, which ultimately translates to increased mortality risk with advancing age.

Fernandez et al. showed that surgical treatment for NSCLC was associated with a 2.2% mortality rate in patients ≥65 years old. When further breaking this down by surgery type, mortality rates for wedge resection, segmentectomy, and lobectomy were all similar (3.5% vs. 3.5% vs. 4.3%).[275] Berry et al. reported an operative mortality of 3.8% with a 47% morbidity rate in patients >70 years of age. LOS was increased in patients with at least one complication. Multivariate analysis found age (OR = 1.09, $p = 0.01$), and thoracotomy as surgical approach (OR = 2.21, $p = 0.004$) as independent predictors of morbidity in patients >70 years old.[277] These findings were corroborated by Cattaneo et al. who studied patients >70 years of age who underwent lobectomy for stage I NSCLC. Their results indicate that a VATS approach for lobectomy was associated with a lower rate of complications (28% vs. 45%, $p = 0.04$), LOS (5 days vs. 6 days, $p < 0.001$), and mortality (0% vs. 3%).[50] Therefore, though the elderly population may experience more morbidity following lobectomy in general, proper patient selection and approach may minimize this risk.

Because the elderly patient often presents with multiple comorbidities and can present as a clinically high-risk patient, surgical alternatives to lobectomy should be considered. Several studies have explored the use of sublobar resection for definitive management of stage I NSCLC in the elderly. Ikeda et al. focused on patients aged >80 years old and showed no significant difference in 5-year survival noted in patients with stage I NSCLC undergoing limited surgical resection (58.8%) vs. lobectomy (59.4%).[278] Kilic et al. compared outcomes of patients >75 years of age that underwent either lobectomy (*n* = 106) or anatomic segmentectomy (*n* = 78) for stage I NSCLC. This study demonstrated a reduced morbidity (29.5% vs. 50%) and mortality (1.3 vs. 4.7%) when comparing the anatomical segmentectomy group with the lobectomy group. There was also no difference in locoregional recurrence (6% vs. 4%) or overall survival (49.8% vs. 45.5%) at a median follow-up of 21 and 18 months, respectively.[279] These studies demonstrate that sublobar resection (including segmentectomy) can be effective and potentially beneficial in patients with NSCLC who are high risk due to advanced age.

In 2012, Schuchert et al. compared outcomes following anatomic segmentectomy versus lobectomy for stage I NSCLC. Anatomic segmentectomy was associated with reduced complication (43.6% vs. 58.7%) as well as mortality (0% vs. 7.8%) in patients greater than 80 years old. More importantly, there was no reported difference in recurrence rate during a mean follow-up time of 37 months.[121] Therefore, segmentectomy may be associated with lower mortality and complication rates with the similar recurrence and survival rates among the elderly population, particularly those over the age of 80.

Histology

Squamous cell carcinoma has historically been associated with lower recurrence and death rates per patient per year when compared with nonsquamous or mixed histologies.[114] Read[280] and Ichinose[281] and their colleagues similarly observed an enhanced 5-year survival rate following resection of T1N0 squamous tumors relative to comparable adenocarcinomas. Several other studies, however, have failed to identify a significant difference between squamous and nonsquamous histology.[282,283]

As noted in the discussion on stage IIIA NSCLC, large-cell neuroendocrine carcinoma has been associated with a worse prognosis than other primary NSCLC histologies (adenocarcinoma, squamous cell carcinoma).[284] Iyoda et al. reported a 5-year survival rate of 67% for resected stage I cases as compared to 88% for other stage I histologies.[285] García-Yuste and colleagues noted 5-year survival in only 33% of resected stage I large cell neuroendocrine carcinoma patients.[286] Battafarano et al. noted a significant reduction in freedom from recurrence and overall survival in patients with large cell neuroendocrine carcinomas.[287] In cases of mixed histology containing 10% or more of cells of neuroendocrine differentiation, a lowered survival rate was observed in resected stage I adenocarcinoma patients.[288] Along similar lines, the surgical prognosis for patients with node-negative mixed small cell and non-small cell lesions is also considerably worse than for pure NSCLC. Hage et al. reported 5-year survival rates of 50% and 26% for mixed small cell/non-small cell tumors of pathologic stage IA and IB, respectively, many of which were also treated with preoperative or postoperative chemotherapy.[289]

Ground Glass Opacities and Minimally Invasive Adenocarcinoma

Screening of large populations of at-risk patients has generated a new conundrum. Many lesions discovered at screening are small, peripheral ground-glass lesions that turn out to be adenocarcinoma in situ,

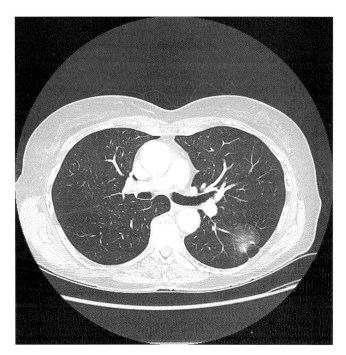

FIGURE 95.14 Ground glass opacity with solid component consistent with adenocarcinoma.

formerly known as bronchioloalveolar carcinoma (BAC), or minimally-invasive adenocarcinomas. A subset of adenocarcinoma of the lung can be classified as ground glass opacities, typically detected as isolated findings on CT imaging (Fig. 95.14). These lesions frequently are comprised of adenocarcinoma in situ/bronchioloalveolar cell carcinoma (BAC) or minimally invasive adenocarcinoma, which generally has a favorable prognosis. Although the 2004 World Health Organization definition of BAC has been narrowed to include only noninvasive lesions composed entirely of BAC, thoracic surgeons have long noted that patients with early-stage pure BAC, mixed BAC and adenocarcinoma, or adenocarcinoma with BAC features fare well with resection.[290] Higashiyama et al. separated 206 resected peripheral adenocarcinomas <2 cm into four groups based on the extent of any BAC component, and found a direct correlation between increased percentage of BAC and survival, with a 100% 5-year survival rate in stage I pure BAC patients.[291] Breathnach et al. reported an 83% survival rate for stage I BAC versus 63% for adenocarcinoma.[292] Sakurai et al. presented a series of T1 (<3 cm) BAC and adenocarcinomas observed over a 10-year period. They noted a 5-year survival rate of 100% among 25 patients with BAC versus a rate of 63.5% among 83 patients with adenocarcinoma.[293]

These radiographic entities were correlated with histology by Noguchi et al. (Noguchi classification). Type A is a localized carcinoma showing replacement growth of alveolar lining epithelial cells with a relatively thin stroma. Type B is a type A lesion that includes a fibrotic foci due to alveolar collapse. Type C GGOs has evidence of fibroblastic proliferation. Types D, E, and F are small advanced adenocarcinomas that are poorly differentiated, tubular and papillary with compressive growth pattern, respectively. In Noguchi's analysis, Types A and B had a 100% 5-year survival rate with no lymph node metastasis, rare vascular and pleural invasion, and a low mitotic rate. Type C and D had 5-year survival rates of 74.8% and 52.4%, respectively.[103]

Surgical approaches include the standard treatment via lobectomy for an isolated GGO. However, many groups have explored the use sublobar resection techniques (wedge resection or segmentectomy) for the management of GGOs, given the lower propensity for metastatic disease with these lesions. Yoshida et al. performed a prospective study of limited resection for pulmonary GGOs 2 cm or smaller. Noguchi type A or B lesions were treated with wedge resection or segmentectomy. In the first 5 years of follow-up, there were no recurrences.[82] In their study, the 5- and 10-year recurrence-free survival was 100% and 92%, respectively. The 5- and 10-year overall survival rates were 100% and 95%.[294] Tsutani et al. published a large series of 239 patients with GGO-dominant tumors. There were no differences in 3-year recurrence-free survival and overall survival when comparing patients who underwent lobectomy, segmentectomy, and wedge resection. In patients with T1a lesions (≤2 cm), there were no lymph node metastasis; however, two of 84 patients with T1b presented with lymph node metastasis. The authors concluded that sublobar resection can be utilized for GGO-dominant tumors with similar results as lobectomy; and that T1a tumors can be safely resected using wedge resection, while T1b tumors are best managed with segmentectomy.[130]

A pure GGO ≤10 mm has an approximately 25% chance of being an adenocarcinoma in-situ and less than a 5% chance of being an adenocarcinoma. If it is >10 mm, the chances become 40% AIS and 20% AC. The likelihood increases to 50% AIS and 25% AC in semisolid GGOs ≤10 mm. If the semisolid GGO is >10 mm, it has a chance of 50% to become an AC.[127]

In summary, solitary cT1aN0M0 ground glass lesions can be managed with sublobar resection. Given the high incidence of multifocality in patients with GGOs, the value of a parenchymal preserving approach is evident. Although lymph node involvement is low in these cases, systematic N1 and N2 node sampling should be performed.

Central Versus Peripheral Location

The location of a tumor within the anatomical confines of a lobe has been shown to be associated with recurrence risk following surgical intervention in patients with stage I NSCLC. Utilizing sixth edition TMN Staging System criteria, Sagawa et al. found that tumor location negated the influence that tumor size had on outcomes. Specifically, in patients with peripheral tumors, 5-year survival was comparable between patients with tumors <2 cm and those with tumors 2 to 3 cm in diameter (83% vs. 80%).[295] Rocha et al. demonstrated lower lobe location as the only significant factor associated with pathological upstaging in early stage NSCLC.[296,297] Central tumor location along with tumor size were identified as independent predictors of occult N2 disease in a study of 224 patients with clinical stage I disease performed by Lee et al.[297] Similarly, Zhang et al. found that central tumor location was the strongest predictor of N2 disease in a review of 530 patients with clinical T1N0 disease by CT.[298] Odell et al. stressed the lack of recognition of the effects of tumor location on outcomes following surgical resection. They noted a clinical to pathological stage shift of 14.4% in their cohort, with the highest proportion of these associated with centrally located clinical stage IB tumors (31.4%). When comparing both stage IA and IB central and peripheral tumors, they noted that though tumor location did not have a significant impact on overall survival ($p = 0.706$), multivariate analysis showed that central location was an independent risk factor for disease recurrence (HR = 1.83, $p = 0.041$).[299] These data indicate a strong correlation between a perihilar, central tumor location and malignant recurrence in clinical stage I NSCLC. This appears to be driven largely by the significant clinical-to-pathological stage shift in these patients. These findings stress the importance of surgery with complete nodal sampling/dissection to achieve a true R0 resection and properly identify those patients with clinical pathological stage shifts in the age of adjuvant systemic therapy.

Surgical Margin

A negative microscopic bronchovascular and parenchymal margin is the primary objective in achieving an R0 resection in the setting of lobectomy and pneumonectomy. What constitutes an adequate margin in the setting of sublobar resection remains unresolved. A negative bronchovascular margin with negative marginal cytology has been suggested to be a reasonable intraoperative approach at margin assessment in this setting.[291] Previous recommendations have implied that 1 cm margins might suffice. More recently, Sawabata et al. have suggested that to minimize local recurrence risk margin distance should be greater than the maximum diameter of the tumor.[79] El-Sherif et al. analyzed the impact of surgical margin in 81 patients undergoing sublobar resection for stage I NSCLC. Tumor margins ≥1 cm were associated with a significantly lower recurrence rate, when compared to margins <1 cm (8 vs. 19%, $p = 0.003$).[300] Schuchert et al. demonstrated that a margin:tumor ratio of less than 1 was associated with a significant increase in recurrence rates compared to ratios ≥1 (25.0% vs. 6.2%; $p = 0.0014$).[60] Detailed preoperative assessment of tumor location and anticipated surgical margin by CT imaging software may enhance surgical decision-making in this setting.[301]

The use of brachytherapy mesh has been evaluated as an adjunct to enhance local control in the setting of sublobar resection, especially in the setting of close surgical margins.[302] Despite promising results in early retrospective series,[303] brachytherapy mesh was not found to enhance local control after longer follow-up.[304] A phase 3 prospective, randomized trial comparing sublobar resection alone versus sublobar resection with brachytherapy mesh (ACOSOG Z4032) demonstrated no improvement in local control with the use of brachytherapy mesh during sublobar resection, even with compromised surgical margins.[305]

Angiolymphatic Invasion

Angiolymphatic invasion is defined as the presence of neoplastic cells within an arterial, venous, or lymphatic lumen during routine histologic evaluation with hematoxylin and eosin stains. Angiolymphatic invasion has been identified as an important prognostic factor in many solid tumors including head and neck,[306] breast,[307] and colon[308] cancers. Angiolymphatic invasion also has been shown to exert an adverse prognostic impact in patients undergoing surgical resection for early-stage lung cancer.[309] Ogawa et al. demonstrated significantly shorter disease-free survival in stage I lung cancers with evidence of blood vessel invasion.[310] Bodendorf and Pechet and their colleagues found that arterial invasion by tumor was associated with a significant reduction in overall 5-year survival, and a significant increase in systemic recurrence.[311,312] Schuchert et al. also found that angiolymphatic invasion was a significant independent risk factor for the development of recurrent disease (28.9% vs. 18.0%, $p = 0.02$) (Fig. 95.15).[313] This adverse pathologic variable may serve to identify patient subsets with "bad-acting" early stage lung cancers that might ultimately benefit from adjuvant therapy protocols, even in the setting of early-stage disease. Clinical trials will be necessary to test this hypothesis.

Tumor Infiltrating Lymphocytes

The presence of a tumor-associated inflammatory infiltrate has been reported as a potentially important prognostic finding in several tumors, including melanoma, renal cell, colorectal, and esophageal cancer. Tumor infiltrating lymphocytes (TILs) also have been shown play an important role in the setting of resected NSCLC. T cell subsets (CD8+ AND CD4+) in particular are felt to represent important constituents of this infiltrate, and have been associated with improved

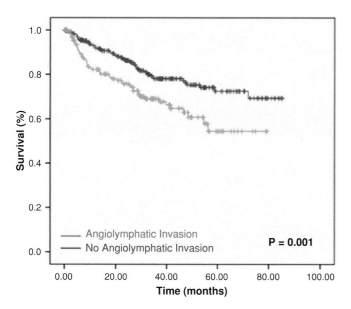

FIGURE 95.15 Recurrence-free survival in patients undergoing resection for clinical stage I NSCLC. Angiolymphatic invasion is associated with increased risk of recurrence and death. (Reprinted from Schuchert MJ, Schumacher L, Kilic A, et al. Impact of Angiolymphatic and Pleural Invasion on Surgical Outcomes for Stage I Non-Small Cell Lung Cancer. *Ann Thorac Surg* 2011;91:1059–1065. Copyright © 2011 The Society of Thoracic Surgeons. With permission.)

survival.[314] In a study of 219 patients undergoing lobectomy for stage I NSCLC, the degree of tumor inflammatory reaction was graded as mild (scattered lymphocytes), moderate, or severe (intimate admixture of inflammatory cells with tumor cells). The presence of moderate-severe TILs was associated with a lower disease recurrence (21 vs. 60%, $p = 0.02$) and improved 5-year disease-free survival (75.6% vs. 35.9%, $p = 0.04$) in tumors >5 cm.[132] In another analysis of 273 patients undergoing resection for clinical stage IA NSCLC (Tumors <2 cm), high levels of TILs were shown to be associated with increased recurrence-free survival (87% vs. 73%, $p = 0.011$), especially in women ($p = 0.016$).[315] It is becoming increasingly recognized that the immune contexture within the region of a tumor exerts a critical influence in immune surveillance and tumor suppression.[316] These observations have fueled the emergence of immunotherapy as a valid treatment option in the treatment of NSCLC. A better understanding of the composition of intratumoral immune subsets as well as mechanisms for enhancing their anti-tumor potential will have a tremendous impact on the 30% to 40% of patients with recurrent lung cancer following surgical resection for stage I disease, and would afford new hope to those suffering from progressive, advanced disease.

FUTURE DIRECTIONS

Robotic Surgery

VATS lobectomy has been associated with several clear benefits over traditional open lobectomy including LOS, postoperative pain, and morbidity. Some investigators have adopted the robotic approach to minimally invasive lung resection surgery (Table 95.12).[317–320] In a study utilizing the STS Database, Louie et al. found that certain quality outcomes including complications, hospital stay (median LOS of 4 days for both groups), 30-day mortality (0.6% vs. 0.8%, $p = 0.4$), and nodal upstaging (8.44% vs. 7.89%, $p = 585$) were all equivalent when comparing robotic and VATS lobectomy. One difference they did note was the longer operative times (186 minutes vs. 173 minutes, $p <0.001$) that have been traditionally associated with robotic approaches in the chest (Table 95.13).[321] Cerfolio et al. investigated the feasibility and surgical techniques required for robotic anatomic segmentectomy. In a cohort of 100 patients undergoing planned pulmonary segmentectomy, only 7% were converted to robotic lobectomy. There were zero conversions to thoracotomy. Median hospital LOS was 3 days. Only 2% of patients experienced major morbidity in the form of pneumonia. There were no 30-day or 90-day mortalities. Of the 79 patients that underwent robotic segmentectomy for lung cancer, with a median follow-up of 30 months, three patients (3.4%) experienced locoregional recurrence in the operated lobe.[322] These results suggest that the use of the robot for anatomic lung resection surgery can be performed safely by an experienced robotic surgeon. The cost:benefit ratio for this approach compared to standard VATS techniques remains to be fully delineated.

Ablative Modalities

Several competing nonsurgical ablative modalities have emerged over the last 10 years for the management of high-risk patients with early-stage NSCLC,[323] including radiofrequency ablation and stereotactic radiosurgery (SRS/SBRT).[324,325] Excellent local control has been reported with SRS/SBRT (85% to 90% for stage I lesions). RFA has been associated with a higher recurrence risk (30% to 40%). Definitions of what constitutes recurrent disease differs substantially between radiation oncology and surgical series, making an informed comparative assessment of the results with SRS/SBRT versus surgery inherently difficult. It should be noted, however, that the early enthusiasm for the remarkable outcomes reported for SRS/SBRT have been curbed somewhat by long-term reports suggesting diminished long-term survival when comparing patients undergoing SBRT versus lobectomy. In a study evaluating outcomes in 13,562 patients with clinical stage I NSCLC who were free of significant comorbidities, Cox proportional hazards analyses suggested that lobectomy was

TABLE 95.12 Perioperative Morbidity and Mortality for Robotic Lung Resection

Author	Year	N	Median Operative Time (minutes)	LOS (d)	Conversion Rate (%)	Overall Morbidity (%)	Mortality (%)
Park et al.[368]	2006	34	218	4.5	12	26	0
Veronesi et al.[320]	2010	54	NR	4.5	13	20	0
Dylewski et al.[318]	2011	200	90	3.0	1.5	26	2
Cerfolio et al.[317]	2011	106	132	2.0	7.7	27	0
Park et al.[319]	2012	325	206	5.0	8	25.2	0.3
Louie et al.[369]	2012	46	213	4.0	2.1	17	0
Louie et al.[321]	2016	1,220	186	4.0	NR	NR	0.6

TABLE 95.13 Surgical Approach: Outcomes Following VATS Versus Robotic Surgical Anatomic Lung Resection for Treatment of NSCLC

Author	Year	N		LOS (d)		Morbidity (%)		Mortality (%)	
		VATS	Robotic	VATS	Robotic	VATS	Robotic	VATS	Robotic
Veronesi et al.[320]	2010	54	54	6	4.5	20.4	18.5	0	0
Cerfolio et al.[317]	2011	318	106	4.0	2.0	27	38	3.1	0
Louie et al.[369]	2012	34	46	4.5	4.0	NR	NR	0	0
Yang et al.[370]	2016	141	172	4.0	4.0	NR	NR	0.7	0

associated with significantly better survival for both T1N0 and T2N0 tumors (p <0.001).[326] The fundamental advantages of surgery over ablative strategies must be carefully considered including complete removal of the tumor (R0 resection), pathologic assessment of surgical margins, the establishment of pathologic regional nodal status and, in this era of increasing enthusiasm for adjuvant systemic therapy, the enhanced ability of surgery to obtain adequate tissue for pharmacogenomic assessment.

REFERENCES

1. Torre LA, Siegel RL, Jemal A. Lung Cancer Statistics. *Adv Exp Med Biol* 2016;893: 1–19.
2. Siegel RL, Miller KD, Jemal A. Cancer statistics, 2016. *CA Cancer J Clin* 2016;66(1): 7–30.
3. Brustugun OT, Moller B, Helland A. Years of life lost as a measure of cancer burden on a national level. *Br J Cancer* 2014;111(5):1014–1020.
4. Sauerbruch F, Nissen R. Zur Erkennung und Behandlung bösartiger Lungengeschwülste. *Arch Klin Chir* 1932;170:118.
5. Davies H. Recent advances in the surgery of the lung and pleura. *Br J Surg* 1913;1(2): 228–258.
6. Graham EA, Singer J. Successful removal of an entire lung for carcinoma of the bronchus. *JAMA* 1933;101(18):1371–1374.
7. Ochsner A, DeBakey M. Surgical considerations of primary carcinoma of the lung. *Surgery* 1940;8(6):992–1023.
8. Ochsner A, DeBakey M. Primary pulmonary malignancy: Treatment by total pneumonectomy; Analysis of 79 collected cases and presentation of 7 personal Cases. *Ochsner J* 1999;1(3):109–125.
9. Halsted WS. I. The Results of Operations for the Cure of Cancer of the Breast Performed at the Johns Hopkins Hospital from June, 1889, to January, 1894. *Ann Surg* 1894;20(5):497–555.
10. Mountain CF, Hermes KE. Surgical treatment of lung cancer. Past and present. *Methods Mol Med* 2003;75:453–487.
11. Bougas JA, Overholt RH. Common factors in lung cancer survivors. *J Thorac Surg* 1956;32(4):508–517; discussion 517–520.
12. Ochsner A. The development of pulmonary surgery, with special emphasis on carcinoma and bronchiectasis. *Am J Surg* 1978;135(6):732–746.
13. Johnson J, Kirby CK, Blakemore WS. Should we insist on radical pneumonectomy as routine procedure in the treatment of carcinoma of the lung? *J Thorac Surg* 1958;36(3):309–315.
14. Thomas CP. The present position relating to cancer of the lung. Lobectomy with sleeve resection. *Thorax* 1960;15:9–11.
15. Shimkin MB, Connelly RR, Marcus SC, et al. Pneumonectomy and lobectomy in bronchogenic carcinoma. A comparison of end results of the Overholt and Ochsner clinics. *J Thorac Cardiovasc Surg* 1962;44:503–519.
16. Churchill E, Sweet R, Soutter L, et al. The surgical management of carcinoma of the lung; A study of the cases treated at the Massachusetts General Hospital from 1930 to 1950. *J Thorac Surg* 1950;20(3):349–365.
17. Churchill ED, Belsey R. Segmental pneumonectomy in bronchiectasis: The lingula segment of the left upper lobe. *Ann Surg* 1939;109(4):481–499.
18. Churchill E, Sweet R, Scannell J, et al. Further studies in the surgical management of carcinoma of the lung; a further study of the cases treated at the Massachusetts General Hospital from 1950 to 1957. *J Thorac Surg* 1958;36(3):301–308.
19. Bonfils-Roberts E, Clagett O. Contemporary indications for pulmonary segmental resections. *J Thorac Cardiovasc Surg* 1972;63(3):433–438.
20. Jensik R, Faber LP, Milloy F, et al. Segmental resection for lung cancer. A fifteen-year experience. *J Thorac Cardiovasc Surg* 1973;66(4):563–572.
21. Read RC, Yoder G, Schaeffer RC. Survival after conservative resection for T1 N0 M0 non-small cell lung cancer. *Ann Thorac Surg* 1990;49(3):391–400.
22. Ginberg R, Rubinstein LV. Randomized trial of lobectomy versus limited resection for T1 no non-small cell lung cancer. *Ann Thorac Surg* 1995;60:615–623.
23. Landreneau RJ, Sugarbaker DJ, Mack MJ, et al. Wedge resection versus lobectomy for stage I (T1 N0 M0) non-small-cell lung cancer. *J Thorac Cardiovasc Surg* 1997;113(4):691–700.
24. Henschke CI, I-ELCAP Investigators. CT screening for lung cancer: Update 2005. *Surg Oncol Clin N Am* 2005;14(4):761–776.
25. Lewis RJ. The role of video-assisted thoracic surgery for carcinoma of the lung: Wedge resection to lobectomy by simultaneous individual stapling. *Ann Thorac Surg* 1993;56(3):762–768.
26. Tang AW, Moss HA, Robertson RJ. The solitary pulmonary nodule. *Eur J Radiol* 2003;45(1):69–77.
27. Roviaro G, Rebuffat C, Varoli F, et al. Videoendoscopic pulmonary lobectomy for cancer. *Surg Laparosc Endosc* 1992;2(3):244–247.
28. Yang J, Xia Y, Yang Y, et al. Risk factors for major adverse events of video-assisted thoracic surgery lobectomy for lung cancer. *Int J Med Sci* 2014;11:863–869.
29. Stéphan F, Boucheseiche S, Hollande J, et al. Pulmonary complications following lung resection: A comprehensive analysis of incidence and possible risk factors. *Chest* 2000;118(5):1263–1270.
30. Heelan RT, Demas BE, Caravelli JF, et al. Superior sulcus tumors: CT and MR imaging. *Radiology* 1989;170(3 Pt 1):637–641.
31. Paul S, Sedrakyan A, Chiu YL, et al. Outcomes after lobectomy using thoracoscopy vs thoracotomy: A comparative effectiveness analysis utilizing the Nationwide Inpatient Sample database. *Eur J Cardiothorac Surg* 2013;43(4):813–817.
32. Kutlu C, Sayar A, Olgac G, et al. Chylothorax: A complication following lung resection in patients with NSCLC. *Thorac Cardiovasc Surg* 2003;51(6):342–345.
33. Onaitis M, D'Amico T, Zhao Y, et al. Risk factors for atrial fibrillation after lung cancer surgery: Analysis of the Society of Thoracic Surgeons general thoracic surgery database. *Ann Thorac Surg* 2010;90(2):368–374.
34. Stolz AJ, Schützner J, Lischke R, et al. Predictors of prolonged air leak following pulmonary lobectomy. *Eur J Cardiothorac Surg* 2005;27(2):334–336.
35. Augustin F, Maier HT, Weissenbacher A, et al. Causes, predictors and consequences of conversion from VATS to open lung lobectomy. *Surg Endosc* 2016;30(6): 2415–2421.
36. Strand TE, Rostad H, Damhuis RA, et al. Risk factors for 30-day mortality after resection of lung cancer and prediction of their magnitude. *Thorax* 2007;62(11): 991–997.
37. Martin J, Ginsberg RJ, Abolhoda A, et al. Morbidity and mortality after neoadjuvant therapy for lung cancer: The risks of right pneumonectomy *Ann Thorac Surg* 2001;72(4):1149–1154.
38. Ginsberg RJ. Lung cancer surgery: Acceptable morbidity and mortality, expected results and quality control. *Surg Oncol* 2002;11(4):263–266.
39. Tsiouris A, Hammoud ZT, Velanovich V, et al. A modified frailty index to assess morbidity and mortality after lobectomy. *J Surg Res* 2013;183(1):40–46.
40. Birim Ö, Kappetein AP, Bogers AJ. Charlson comorbidity index as a predictor of long-term outcome after surgery for nonsmall cell lung cancer. *Eur J Cardiothorac Surg* 2005;28(5):759–762.
41. Jean RA, DeLuzio MR, Kraev AI, et al. Analyzing Risk Factors for Morbidity and Mortality after Lung Resection for Lung Cancer Using the NSQIP Database. *J Am Coll Surg* 2016;222(6):992–1000. e1.
42. Smith T, Li X, Nylander W, et al. Thirty-Day Postoperative Mortality Risk Estimates and 1-Year Survival in Veterans Health Administration Surgery Patients. *JAMA surgery* 2016;151(5):417–422.
43. Samson P, Robinson CG, Bradley J, et al. The National Surgical Quality Improvement Program risk calculator does not adequately stratify risk for patients with clinical stage I non–small cell lung cancer. *J Thorac Cardiovasc Surg* 2016;151(3): 697–705. e1.
44. Tieu B, Schipper P. Specialty matters in the treatment of lung cancer. *Semin Thorac Cardiovasc Surg* 2012;24(2):99–105.
45. Lien YC, Huang MT, Lin HC. Association between surgeon and hospital volume and in-hospital fatalities after lung cancer resections: The experience of an Asian country. *Ann Thorac Surg* 2007;83(5):1837–1843.
46. Lüchtenborg M, Riaz SP, Coupland VH, et al. High procedure volume is strongly associated with improved survival after lung cancer surgery. *J Clin Oncol* 2013; 31(25):3141–3146.
47. Roviaro G, Rebuffat C, Varoli F, et al. Videoendoscopic thoracic surgery. *Int Surg* 1992;78(1):4–9.
48. Nakamura H, Kazuyuki S, Kawasaki N, et al. History of limited resection for non-small cell lung cancer. *Ann Thorac Cardiovasc Surg* 2005;11(6):356–362.
49. Landreneau RJ, Hazelrigg SR, Mack MJ, et al. Postoperative pain-related morbidity: Video-assisted thoracic surgery versus thoracotomy. *Ann Thorac Surg* 1993;56(6): 1285–1289.

50. Cattaneo SM, Park BJ, Wilton AS, et al. Use of video-assisted thoracic surgery for lobectomy in the elderly results in fewer complications. *Ann Thorac Surg* 2008;85(1):231–235; discussion 235–236.
51. Whitson BA, Andrade RS, Boettcher A, et al. Video-assisted thoracoscopic surgery is more favorable than thoracotomy for resection of clinical stage I non-small cell lung cancer. *Ann Thorac Surg* 2007;83(6):1965–1970.
52. Demmy TL, Curtis JJ. Minimally invasive lobectomy directed toward frail and high-risk patients: A case-control study. *Ann Thorac Surg* 1999;68(1):194–200.
53. McKenna RJ Jr, Houck W, Fuller CB. Video-assisted thoracic surgery lobectomy: Experience with 1,100 cases. *Ann Thorac Surg* 2006;81(2):421–425; discussion 425–426.
54. Onaitis MW, Petersen RP, Balderson SS, et al. Thoracoscopic lobectomy is a safe and versatile procedure: Experience with 500 consecutive patients. *Ann Surg* 2006;244(3):420–425.
55. Villamizar NR, Darrabie MD, Burfeind WR, et al. Thoracoscopic lobectomy is associated with lower morbidity compared with thoracotomy. *J Thorac Cardiovasc Surg* 2009;138(2):419–425.
56. Paul S, Altorki NK, Sheng S, et al. Thoracoscopic lobectomy is associated with lower morbidity than open lobectomy: A propensity-matched analysis from the STS database. *J Thorac Cardiovasc Surg* 2010;139(2):366–378.
57. Schuchert MJ, Lamb JR. Thoracoscopic basilar segmentectomy. *Sem Thorac Cardiovasc Surg* 2011;23(1):78–80.
58. Shiraishi T, Shirakusa T, Iwasaki A, et al. Video-assisted thoracoscopic surgery (VATS) segmentectomy for small peripheral lung cancer tumors: Intermediate results. *Surg Endosc* 2004;18(11):1657–1662.
59. Atkins BZ, Harpole DH, Mangum JH, et al. Pulmonary segmentectomy by thoracotomy or thoracoscopy: Reduced hospital length of stay with a minimally-invasive approach. *Ann Thorac Surg* 2007;84(4):1107–1113.
60. Schuchert MJ, Pettiford BL, Keeley S, et al. Anatomic segmentectomy in the treatment of stage I non-small cell lung cancer. *Ann Thorac Surg* 2007;84(3):926–932; discussion 932–933.
61. Mountain CF. Revisions in the International System for Staging Lung Cancer. *Chest* 1997;111(6):1710–1717.
62. Goldstraw P, Crowley J, Chansky K, et al. The IASLC Lung Cancer Staging Project: Proposals for the revision of the TNM stage groupings in the forthcoming (seventh) edition of the TNM Classification of malignant tumours. *J Thorac Oncol* 2007;2(8):706–714.
63. Rami-Porta R, Ball D, Crowley J, et al. The IASLC Lung Cancer Staging Project: Proposals for the revision of the T descriptors in the forthcoming (seventh) edition of the TNM classification for lung cancer. *J Thorac Oncol* 2007;2(7):593–602.
64. Detterbeck FC, Boffa DJ, Tanoue LT. The new lung cancer staging system. *Chest* 2009;136(1):260–271.
65. Ettinger D, Johnson B. Update: NCCN small cell and non-small cell lung cancer Clinical Practice Guidelines. *J Natl Compr Canc Netw* 2005;3 Suppl 1:S17–S21.
66. van Rens MT, de la Riviere AB, Elbers HR, et al. Prognostic assessment of 2,361 patients who underwent pulmonary resection for non-small cell lung cancer, stage I, II, and IIIA. *Chest* 2000;117(2):374–379.
67. Naruke T, Tsuchiya R, Kondo H, et al. Prognosis and survival after resection for bronchogenic carcinoma based on the 1997 TNM-staging classification: The Japanese experience. *Ann Thorac Surg* 2001;71(6):1759–1764.
68. Asamura H, Goya T, Koshiishi Y, et al. A Japanese Lung Cancer Registry study: Prognosis of 13,010 resected lung cancers. *J Thorac Oncol* 2008;3(1):46–52.
69. Wilson DO, Weissfeld JL, Fuhrman CR, et al. The Pittsburgh Lung Screening Study (PLuSS): Outcomes within 3 years of a first computed tomography scan. *Am J Respir Crit Care Med* 2008;178(9):956–961.
70. Wilson DO, Ryan A, Fuhrman C, et al. Doubling times and CT screen–detected lung cancers in the Pittsburgh Lung Screening Study. *Am J Respir Crit Care Med* 2012;185(1):85–89.
71. Pettiford BL, Schuchert MJ, Santos R, et al. Role of sublobar resection (segmentectomy and wedge resection) in the surgical management of non-small cell lung cancer. *Thorac Surg Clin* 2007;17(2):175–190.
72. Schuchert MJ, Pettiford BL, Luketich JD, et al. Parenchymal-sparing resections: Why, when, and how. *Thorac Surg Clin* 2008;18(1):93–105.
73. Kondo D, Yamada K, Kitayama Y, et al. Peripheral lung adenocarcinomas: 10 mm or less in diameter. *Ann Thorac Surg* 2003;76(2):350–355.
74. Miller DL, Rowland CM, Deschamps C, et al. Surgical treatment of non-small cell lung cancer 1 cm or less in diameter. *Ann Thorac Surg* 2002;73(5):1545–1550; discussion 1550–1551.
75. Martin-Ucar AE, Nakas A, Pilling JE, et al. A case-matched study of anatomical segmentectomy versus lobectomy for stage I lung cancer in high-risk patients. *Eur J Cardiothorac Surg* 2005;27(4):675–679.
76. Okada M, Koike T, Higashiyama M, et al. Radical sublobar resection for small-sized non-small cell lung cancer: A multicenter study. *J Thorac Cardiovasc Surg* 2006;132(4):769–775.
77. Schuchert MJ, Kilic A, Pennathur A, et al. Oncologic outcomes after surgical resection of subcentimeter non-small cell lung cancer. *Ann Thorac Surg* 2011;91(6):1681–1687; discussion 1687–1688.
78. Ohta Y, Oda M, Wu J, et al. Can tumor size be a guide for limited surgical intervention in patients with peripheral non-small cell lung cancer? Assessment from the point of view of nodal micrometastasis. *J Thorac Cardiovasc Surg* 2001;122(5):900–906.
79. Sawabata N, Miyaoka E, Asamura H, et al. Japanese lung cancer registry study of 11,663 surgical cases in 2004: Demographic and prognosis changes over decade. *J Thorac Oncol* 2011;6(7):1229–1235.
80. Kishi K, Homma S, Kurosaki A, et al. Small lung tumors with the size of 1cm or less in diameter: Clinical, radiological, and histopathological characteristics. *Lung Cancer* 2004;44(1):43–51.
81. Moriya Y, Iyoda A, Hiroshima K, et al. Clinicopathological analysis of clinical N0 peripheral lung cancers with a diameter of 1 cm or less. *Thorac Cardiovasc Surg* 2004;52(4):196–199.
82. Yoshida J, Nagai K, Yokose T, et al. Limited resection trial for pulmonary ground-glass opacity nodules: Fifty-case experience. *J Thorac Cardiovasc Surg* 2005;129(5):991–996.
83. Roberts PF, Straznicka M, Lara PN, et al. Resection of multifocal non–small cell lung cancer when the bronchioloalveolar subtype is involved. *J Thorac Cardiovasc Surg* 2003;126(5):1597–1601.
84. Kodama K, Higashiyama M, Takami K, et al. Treatment strategy for patients with small peripheral lung lesion (s): Intermediate-term results of prospective study. *Eur J Cardiothorac Surg* 2008;34(5):1068–1074.
85. Koike T, Togashi K, Shirato T, et al. Limited resection for noninvasive bronchioloalveolar carcinoma diagnosed by intraoperative pathologic examination. *Ann Thorac Surg* 2009;88(4):1106–1111.
86. Jiang W, Pang X, Xi J, et al. Clinical outcome of subcentimeter non-small cell lung cancer after surgical resection: Single institution experience of 105 patients. *J Surg Oncol* 2014;110(3):233–238.
87. Sakurai H, Nakagawa K, Watanabe S, et al. Clinicopathologic features of resected subcentimeter lung cancer. *Ann Thorac Surg* 2015;99(5):1731–1738.
88. Keating JJ, Kennedy GT, Singhal S. Identification of a subcentimeter pulmonary adenocarcinoma using intraoperative near-infrared imaging during video-assisted thoracoscopic surgery. *J Thorac Cardiovasc Surg* 2015;149(3):e51–e53.
89. Awais O, Reidy MR, Mehta K, et al. Electromagnetic Navigation Bronchoscopy-Guided Dye Marking for Thoracoscopic Resection of Pulmonary Nodules. *Ann Thorac Surg* 2016;102(1):223–229.
90. Louie AV, Senan S, Dahele M, et al. Stereotactic ablative radiation therapy for subcentimeter lung tumors: Clinical, dosimetric, and image guidance considerations. *Int J Radiat Oncol Biol Phys* 2014;90(4):843–849.
91. Ishida T, Yano T, Maeda K, et al. Strategy for lymphadenectomy in lung cancer three centimeters or less in diameter. *Ann Thorac Surg* 1990;50(5):708–713.
92. Okada M, Sakamoto T, Nishio W, et al. Characteristics and prognosis of patients after resection of nonsmall cell lung carcinoma measuring 2 cm or less in greatest dimension. *Cancer* 2003;98(3):535–541.
93. Fernando HC, Santos RS, Benfield JR, et al. Lobar and sublobar resection with and without brachytherapy for small stage IA non–small cell lung cancer. *J Thorac Cardiovasc Surg* 2005;129(2):261–267.
94. Bando T, Yamagihara K, Ohtake Y, et al. A new method of segmental resection for primary lung cancer: Intermediate results. *Eur J Cardiothorac Surg* 2002;21(5):894–899.
95. Carr SR, Schuchert MJ, Pennathur A, et al. Impact of tumor size on outcomes after anatomic lung resection for stage 1A non–small cell lung cancer based on the current staging system. *J Thorac Cardiovasc Surg* 2012;143(2):390–397.
96. El-Sherif A, Gooding WE, Santos R, et al. Outcomes of sublobar resection versus lobectomy for stage I non-small cell lung cancer: A 13-year analysis. *Ann Thorac Surg* 2006;82(2):408–415; discussion 415–416.
97. Macke RA, Schuchert MJ, Odell DD, et al. Parenchymal preserving anatomic resections result in less pulmonary function loss in patients with Stage I non-small cell lung cancer. *J Cardiothorac Surg* 2015;10(1):49.
98. Donington J, Ferguson M, Mazzone P, et al. American College of Chest Physicians and Society of Thoracic Surgeons consensus statement for evaluation and management for high-risk patients with stage I non-small cell lung cancer. *Chest* 2012;142(6):1620–1635.
99. Schuchert MJ, Abbas G, Pennathur A, et al. Sublobar resection for early-stage lung cancer. *Sem Thorac Cardiovasc Surg* 2010;22(1): 22–31.
100. Altorki NK, Yip R, Hanaoka T, et al. Sublobar resection is equivalent to lobectomy for clinical stage 1A lung cancer in solid nodules. *J Thorac Cardiovasc Surg* 2014;147(2):754–764.
101. Landreneau RJ, Normolle DP, Christie NA, et al. Recurrence and survival outcomes after anatomic segmentectomy versus lobectomy for clinical stage I non-small-cell lung cancer: A propensity-matched analysis. *J Clin Oncol* 2014;32(23):2449–2455.
102. Pignon J-P, Tribodet H, Scagliotti GV, et al. Lung adjuvant cisplatin evaluation: A pooled analysis by the LACE Collaborative Group. *J Clin Oncol* 2008;26(21):3552–3559.
103. Lin WY, Hsu WH, Lin KH, et al. Role of preoperative PET-CT in assessing mediastinal and hilar lymph node status in early stage lung cancer. *J Chin Med Assoc* 2012;75(5):203–208.
104. Harpole DH, Herndon JE, Young WG, et al. Stage I nonsmall cell lung cancer. A multivariate analysis of treatment methods and patterns of recurrence. *Cancer* 1995;76(5):787–796.
105. Carbone E, Asamura H, Takei H, et al. T2 tumors larger than five centimeters in diameter can be upgraded to T3 in non–small cell lung cancer. *J Thorac Cardiovasc Surg* 2001;122(5):907–912.
106. Toffalorio F, Radice D, Spaggiari L, et al. Features and prognostic factors of large node-negative non–small-cell lung cancers shifted to stage II. *J Thorac Oncol* 2012;7(7):1124–1130.
107. Bergman P, Brodin D, Lewensohn R, et al. Validation of the 7th TNM classification for non-small cell lung cancer: A retrospective analysis on prognostic implications for operated node-negative cases. *Acta Oncologica* 2013;52(6):1189–1194.
108. Brewer LA. Patterns of survival in lung cancer. *Chest* 1977;71(5):644–650.
109. Travis WD, Brambilla E, Rami-Porta R, et al. Visceral pleural invasion: Pathologic criteria and use of elastic stains: proposal for the 7th edition of the TNM classification for lung cancer. *J Thorac Oncol* 2008;3(12):1384–1390.

110. Suzuki K, Asamura H, Watanabe S, et al. Combined resection of superior vena cava for lung carcinoma: Prognostic significance of patterns of superior vena cava invasion. *Ann Thorac Surg* 2004;78(4):1184–1189; discussion 1189.

111. Shim HS, Park IK, Lee CY, et al. Prognostic significance of visceral pleural invasion in the forthcoming (seventh) edition of TNM classification for lung cancer. *Lung Cancer* 2009;65(2):161–165.

112. Ichinose Y, Hara N, Ohta M, et al. Is T factor of the TNM staging system a predominant prognostic factor in pathologic stage I non-small-cell lung cancer? A multivariate prognostic factor analysis of 151 patients. *J Thorac Cardiovasc Surg* 1993;106(1):90–94.

113. Manac'h D, Riquet M, Medioni J, et al. Visceral pleura invasion by non-small cell lung cancer: An underrated bad prognostic factor. *Ann Thorac Surg* 2001;71(4):1088–1093.

114. Gail MH, Eagan RT, Feld R, et al. Prognostic factors in patients with resected stage I non-small cell lung cancer. A report from the Lung Cancer Study Group. *Cancer* 1984;54(9):1802–1813.

115. Shimizu K, Yoshida J, Nagai K, et al. Visceral pleural invasion classification in non-small cell lung cancer: A proposal on the basis of outcome assessment. *J Thorac Cardiovasc Surg* 2004;127(6):1574–1578.

116. Jiang L, Liang W, Shen J, et al. The impact of visceral pleural invasion in node-negative non-small cell lung cancer: A systematic review and meta-analysis. *Chest* 2015;148(4):903–911.

117. Jones DR, Daniel TM, Denlinger CE, et al. Stage IB nonsmall cell lung cancers: Are they all the same? *Ann Thorac Surg* 2006;81(6):1958–1962.

118. Kelsey CR, Marks LB, Hollis D, et al. Local recurrence after surgery for early stage lung cancer. *Cancer* 2009;115(22):5218–5227.

119. Birdas TJ, Koehler RP, Colonias A, et al. Sublobar resection with brachytherapy versus lobectomy for stage Ib nonsmall cell lung cancer. *Ann Thorac Surg* 2006;81(2):434–439.

120. Okada M, Nishio W, Sakamoto T, et al. Effect of tumor size on prognosis in patients with non-small cell lung cancer: The role of segmentectomy as a type of lesser resection. *J Thorac Cardiovasc Surg* 2005;129(1):87–93.

121. Schuchert MJ, Awais O, Abbas G, et al. Influence of age and IB status after resection of node-negative non-small cell lung cancer. *Ann Thorac Surg* 2012;93(3):929–935; discussion 935–936.

122. Shimizu K, Yoshida J, Nagai K, et al. Visceral pleural invasion is an invasive and aggressive indicator of non-small cell lung cancer. *J Thorac Cardiovasc Surg* 2005;130(1):160–165.

123. Fujimoto T, Cassivi SD, Yang P, et al. Completely resected N1 non-small cell lung cancer: Factors affecting recurrence and long-term survival. *J Thorac Cardiovasc Surg* 2006;132(3):499–506.

124. Suzuki K, Nagai K, Yoshida J, et al. Predictors of lymph node and intrapulmonary metastasis in clinical stage IA non-small cell lung carcinoma. *Ann Thorac Surg* 2001;72(2):352–356.

125. Strauss GM, Herndon JE, Maddaus MA, et al. Adjuvant paclitaxel plus carboplatin compared with observation in stage IB non-small cell lung cancer: CALGB 9633 with the Cancer and Leukemia Group B, Radiation Therapy Oncology Group, and North Central Cancer Treatment Group Study Groups. *J Clin Oncol* 2008;26(31):5043–5051.

126. Morgensztern D, Du L, Waqar SN, et al. Adjuvant Chemotherapy for Patients with T2N0M0 Non-small-cell Lung Cancer (NSCLC). *J Thorac Oncol* 2016;11(10):1729–1735.

127. Detterbeck FC, Homer RJ. Approach to the ground-glass nodule. *Clin Chest Med* 2011;32(4):799–810.

128. Naidich DP, Bankier AA, MacMahon H, et al. Recommendations for the management of subsolid pulmonary nodules detected at CT: A statement from the Fleischner Society. *Radiology* 2013;266(1):304–317.

129. Kobayashi Y, Mitsudomi T. Management of ground-glass opacities: Should all pulmonary lesions with ground-glass opacity be surgically resected? *Transl Lung Cancer Res* 2013;2(5):354–363.

130. Tsutani Y, Miyata Y, Nakayama H, et al. Appropriate sublobar resection choice for ground glass opacity-dominant clinical stage IA lung adenocarcinoma: Wedge resection or segmentectomy. *Chest* 2014;145(1):66–71.

131. Wisnivesky JP, Yankelevitz D, Henschke CI. Stage of lung cancer in relation to its size: Part 2. Evidence. *Chest* 2005;127(4):1136–1139.

132. Kilic A, Landreneau RJ, Luketich JD, et al. Density of tumor-infiltrating lymphocytes correlates with disease recurrence and survival in patients with large non-small-cell lung cancer tumors. *J Surg Res* 2011;167(2):207–210.

133. Wang L, Liu Y, Xu S. Prognostic factors for surgically managed patients with stage II non-small cell lung cancer. *Int J Clin Exp Med* 2015;8(1):862–868.

134. Nakagawa T, Okumura N, Kokado Y, et al. Retrospective study of patients with pathologic N1-stage II non-small cell lung cancer. *Interact Cardiovasc Thorac Surg* 2007;6(4):474–478.

135. Yano T, Yokoyama H, Inoue T, et al. Surgical results and prognostic factors of pathologic N1 disease in non-small-cell carcinoma of the lung. Significance of N1 level: Lobar or hilar nodes. *J Thorac Cardiovasc Surg* 1994;107(6):1398–1402.

136. Haney JC, Hanna JM, Berry MF, et al. Differential prognostic significance of extralobar and intralobar nodal metastases in patients with surgically resected stage II non-small cell lung cancer. *J Thorac Cardiovasc Surg* 2014;147(4):1164–1168.

137. Li ZM, Ding ZP, Luo QQ, et al. Prognostic significance of the extent of lymph node involvement in stage II-N1 non-small cell lung cancer. *Chest* 2013;144(4):1253–1260.

138. van Velzen E, Snijder RJ, Brutel de la Riviere A, et al. Type of lymph node involvement influences survival rates in T1N1M0 non-small cell lung carcinoma. Lymph node involvement by direct extension compared with lobar and hilar node metastasis. *Chest* 1996;110(6):1469–1473.

139. van Velzen E, Snijder RJ, Brutel de la Riviere A, et al. Lymph node type as a prognostic factor for survival in T2 N1 M0 non-small cell lung carcinoma. *Ann Thorac Surg* 1997;63(5):1436–1440.

140. Riquet M, Manac'h D, Le Pimpec-Barthes F, et al. Prognostic significance of surgical-pathologic N1 disease in non-small cell carcinoma of the lung. *Ann Thorac Surg* 1999;67(6):1572–1576.

141. Tanaka F, Yanagihara K, Otake Y, et al. Prognostic factors in patients with resected pathologic (p-) T1-2N1M0 non-small cell lung cancer (NSCLC). *Eur J Cardiothorac Surg* 2001;19(5):555–561.

142. Fan C, Gao S, Hui Z, et al. Risk factors for locoregional recurrence in patients with resected N1 non-small cell lung cancer: A retrospective study to identify patterns of failure and implications for adjuvant radiotherapy. *Radiat Oncol* 2013;8(1):1.

143. Nomori H, Mori T, Izumi Y, et al. Is completion lobectomy merited for unanticipated nodal metastases after radical segmentectomy for cT1 N0 M0/pN1-2 non-small cell lung cancer? *J Thorac Cardiovasc Surg* 2012;143(4):820–824.

144. Choi Y, Lee IJ, Lee CY, et al. Multi-institutional analysis of T3 subtypes and adjuvant radiotherapy effects in resected T3N0 non-small cell lung cancer patients. *Radiat Oncol J* 2015;33(2):75–82.

145. Wisnivesky JP, Henschke C, McGinn T, et al. Prognosis of Stage II non-small cell lung cancer according to tumor and nodal status at diagnosis. *Lung Cancer* 2005;49(2):181–186.

146. Deslauriers J, Brisson J, Cartier R, et al. Carcinoma of the lung. Evaluation of satellite nodules as a factor influencing prognosis after resection. *J Thorac Cardiovasc Surg* 1989;97(4):504–512.

147. Fukuse T, Hirata T, Tanaka F, et al. Prognosis of ipsilateral intrapulmonary metastases in resected nonsmall cell lung cancer. *Eur J Cardiothorac Surg* 1997;12(2):218–223.

148. Yoshino I, Nakanishi R, Osaki T, et al. Postoperative prognosis in patients with non-small cell lung cancer with synchronous ipsilateral intrapulmonary metastasis. *Ann Thorac Surg* 1997;64(3):809–813.

149. Pennathur A, Lindeman B, Ferson P, et al. Surgical resection is justified in non-small cell lung cancer patients with node negative T4 satellite lesions. *Ann Thorac Surg* 2009;87(3):893–899.

150. Rosengart TK, Martini N, Ghosn P, et al. Multiple primary lung carcinomas: Prognosis and treatment. *Ann Thorac Surg* 1991;52(4):773–779.

151. Okada M, Tsubota N, Yoshimura M, Miyamoto Y. Operative approach for multiple primary lung carcinomas. *J Thorac Cardiovasc Surg* 1998;115(4):836–840.

152. Shen KR, Meyers BF, Larner JM, et al. Special treatment issues in lung cancer: ACCP evidence-based clinical practice guidelines. *Chest* 2007;132(3 suppl):290S–305S.

153. Downey RJ, Martini N, Rusch VW, et al. Extent of chest wall invasion and survival in patients with lung cancer. *Ann Thorac Surg* 1999;68(1):188–193.

154. Burkhart HM, Allen MS, Nichols FC 3rd, et al. Results of en bloc resection for bronchogenic carcinoma with chest wall invasion. *J Thorac Cardiovasc Surg* 2002;123(4):670–675.

155. Lee CY, Byun CS, Lee JG, et al. The prognostic factors of resected non-small cell lung cancer with chest wall invasion. *World J Surg Oncol* 2012;10:9.

156. Kawaguchi K, Mori S, Usami N, et al. Preoperative evaluation of the depth of chest wall invasion and the extent of combined resections in lung cancer patients. *Lung Cancer* 2009;64(1):41–44.

157. McCaughan B, Martini N, Bains M, et al. Chest wall invasion in carcinoma of the lung. Therapeutic and prognostic implications. *J Thorac Cardiovasc Surg* 1985;89(6):836–41.

158. Casillas M, Paris F, Tarrazona V, et al. Surgical treatment of lung carcinoma involving the chest wall. *Eur J Cardiothorac Surg* 1989;3(5):425–429.

159. Elia S, Griffo S, Gentile M, et al. Surgical treatment of lung cancer invading chest wall: A retrospective analysis of 110 patients. *Eur J Cardiothorac Surg* 2001;20(2):356–360.

160. Akay H, Cangir AK, Kutlay H, et al. Surgical treatment of peripheral lung cancer adherent to the parietal pleura. *Eur J Cardiothorac Surg* 2002;22(4):615–620.

161. Doddoli C, D'Journo B, Le Pimpec-Barthes F, et al. Lung cancer invading the chest wall: A plea for en-bloc resection but the need for new treatment strategies. *Ann Thorac Surg* 2005;80(6):2032–2040.

162. Paulson DL. Carcinoma in the superior pulmonary sulcus. *Ann Thorac Surg* 1979;28(1):3–4.

163. Rusch VW, Parekh KR, Leon L, et al. Factors determining outcome after surgical resection of T3 and T4 lung cancers of the superior sulcus. *J Thorac Cardiovasc Surg* 2000;119(6):1147–1153.

164. Attar S, Miller JE, Satterfield J, et al. Pancoast's tumor: Irradiation or surgery? *Ann Thorac Surg* 1979;28(6):578–586.

165. Rusch VW, Giroux DJ, Kraut MJ, et al. Induction chemoradiation and surgical resection for superior sulcus non-small-cell lung carcinomas: long-term results of Southwest Oncology Group Trial 9416 (Intergroup Trial 0160). *J Clin Oncol* 2007;25(3):313–318.

166. Wright CD, Menard MT, Wain JC, et al. Induction chemoradiation compared with induction radiation for lung cancer involving the superior sulcus. *Ann Thorac Surg* 2002;73(5):1541–1544.

167. Antonoff MB, Hofstetter WL, Correa AM, et al. Clinical prediction of pathologic complete response in superior sulcus non-small cell lung cancer. *Ann Thorac Surg* 2016;101(1):211–217.

168. Pitz CC, Brutel de la Riviere A, Elbers HR, et al. Results of resection of T3 non-small cell lung cancer invading the mediastinum or main bronchus. *Ann Thorac Surg* 1996;62(4):1016–1020.

169. Burt ME, Pomerantz AH, Bains MS, et al. Results of surgical treatment of stage III lung cancer invading the mediastinum. *Surg Clin North Am* 1987;67(5):987–1000.

170. Wang EH, Corso CD, Rutter CE, et al. Postoperative radiation therapy is associated with improved overall survival in incompletely resected stage II and III non-small-cell lung cancer. *J Clin Oncol* 2015;33(25):2727–2734.

171. Rieber J, Deeg A, Ullrich E, et al. Outcome and prognostic factors of postoperative radiation therapy (PORT) after incomplete resection of non-small cell lung cancer (NSCLC). *Lung Cancer* 2016;91:41–47.

172. Weksler B, Bains M, Burt M, et al. Resection of lung cancer invading the diaphragm. *J Thorac Cardiovasc Surg* 1997;114(3):500–501.

173. Inoue K, Sato M, Fujimura S, et al. Prognostic assessment of 1310 patients with non–small-cell lung cancer who underwent complete resection from 1980 to 1993. *J Thorac Cardiovasc Surg* 1998;116(3):407–411.

174. Rocco G, Rendina EA, Meroni A, et al. Prognostic factors after surgical treatment of lung cancer invading the diaphragm. *Ann Thorac Surg* 1999;68(6):2065–2068.

175. Riquet M, Porte H, Chapelier A, et al. Resection of lung cancer invading the diaphragm. *J Thorac Cardiovasc Surg* 2000;120(2):417–418.

176. Yokoi K, Tsuchiya R, Mori T, et al. Results of surgical treatment of lung cancer involving the diaphragm. *J Thorac Cardiovasc Surg* 2000;120(4):799–805.

177. Mitchell JD, Mathisen DJ, Wright CD, et al. Clinical experience with carinal resection. *J Thorac Cardiovasc Surg* 1999;117(1):39–52; discussion 52–53.

178. Yamamoto K, Miyamoto Y, Ohsumi A, et al. Surgical results of carinal reconstruction: An alterative technique for tumors involving the tracheal carina. *Ann Thorac Surg* 2007;84(1):216–220.

179. Rea F, Marulli G, Schiavon M, et al. Tracheal sleeve pneumonectomy for non small cell lung cancer (NSCLC): Short and long-term results in a single institution. *Lung Cancer* 2008;61(2):202–208.

180. Liu XY, Liu FY, Wang Z, et al. Management and surgical resection for tumors of the trachea and carina: experience with 32 patients. *World J Surg* 2009;33(12):2593–2598.

181. Deslauriers J, Gregoire J, Jacques LF, et al. Sleeve lobectomy versus pneumonectomy for lung cancer: A comparative analysis of survival and sites or recurrences. *Ann Thorac Surg* 2004;77(4):1152–1156; discussion 1156.

182. Lee ES, Park SI, Kim YH, et al. Comparison of operative mortality and complications between bronchoplastic lobectomy and pneumonectomy in lung cancer patients. *J Korean Med Sci* 2007;22(1):43–47.

183. Bagan P, Berna P, Brian E, et al. Induction chemotherapy before sleeve lobectomy for lung cancer: Immediate and long-term results. *Ann Thorac Surg* 2009;88(6):1732–1735.

184. Schuchert MJ MR, Abbas G, Pitanga A, et al. The Hilar Stage IB-IIB Non-Small Cell Lung Cancer: Differential Morbidity, Mortality and Outcomes Between Lobectomy and Pneumonectomy. *Chest Annual Meeting*, October 23, 2012. Atlanta, Georgia.

185. Shi W, Zhang W, Sun H, et al. Sleeve lobectomy versus pneumonectomy for non-small cell lung cancer: A meta-analysis. *World J Surg Oncol* 2012;10:265.

186. Ferguson MK, Lehman AG. Sleeve lobectomy or pneumonectomy: Optimal management strategy using decision analysis techniques. *Ann Thorac Surg* 2003;76(6):1782–1788.

187. Filosso PL, Rena O, Guerrera F, et al. Clinical management of atypical carcinoid and large-cell neuroendocrine carcinoma: a multicentre study on behalf of the European Association of Thoracic Surgeons (ESTS) Neuroendocrine Tumours of the Lung Working Group. *Eur J Cardiothorac Surg* 2015;48(1):55–64.

188. Mochizuki T, Ishii G, Nagai K, et al. Pleomorphic carcinoma of the lung: Clinico-pathologic characteristics of 70 cases. *Am J Surg Pathol* 2008;32(11):1727–1735.

189. Metro G, Ricciuti B, Chiari R, et al. Survival outcomes and incidence of brain recurrence in high-grade neuroendocrine carcinomas of the lung: Implications for clinical practice. *Lung Cancer* 2016;95:82–87.

190. Gallo AE, Donington JS. The role of surgery in the treatment of stage III non-small-cell lung cancer. *Curr Oncol Rep* 2007;9(4):247–254.

191. Lee JG, Lee CY, Park IK, et al. The prognostic significance of multiple station N2 in patients with surgically resected stage IIIA N2 non-small-cell lung cancer. *J Korean Med Sci* 2008;23(4):604–608.

192. Patterson G, Piazza D, Pearson F, et al. Significance of metastatic disease in subaortic lymph nodes. *Ann Thorac Surg* 1987;43(2):155–159.

193. Roth JA, Atkinson EN, Fossella F, et al. Long-term follow-up of patients enrolled in a randomized trial comparing perioperative chemotherapy and surgery with surgery alone in resectable stage IIIA non-small-cell lung cancer. *Lung Cancer* 1998;21(1):1–6.

194. Rosell R, Gómez-Codina J, Camps C, et al. Preresectional chemotherapy in stage IIIA non-small-cell lung cancer: A 7-year assessment of a randomized controlled trial. *Lung Cancer* 1999;26(1):7–14.

195. Koshy M, Fedewa SA, Malik R, et al. Improved survival associated with neoadjuvant chemoradiation in patients with clinical stage IIIA (N2) non–small-cell lung cancer. *J Thorac Oncol* 2013;8(7):915–922.

196. Depierre A, Milleron B, Moro-Sibilot D, et al. Preoperative chemotherapy followed by surgery compared with primary surgery in resectable stage I (except T1N0), II, and IIIa non-small-cell lung cancer. *J Clin Oncol* 2002;20(1):247–253.

197. van Meerbeeck JP, Kramer GW, Van Schil PE, et al. Randomized controlled trial of resection versus radiotherapy after induction chemotherapy in stage IIIA-N2 non-small-cell lung cancer. *J Natl Cancer Inst* 2007;99(6):442–450.

198. Albain KS, Swann RS, Rusch VW, et al. Radiotherapy plus chemotherapy with or without surgical resection for stage III non-small-cell lung cancer: A phase III randomised controlled trial. *Lancet* 2009;374(9687):379–386.

199. Pisters KM, Vallieres E, Crowley JJ, et al. Surgery with or without preoperative paclitaxel and carboplatin in early-stage non-small-cell lung cancer: Southwest Oncology Group Trial S9900, an intergroup, randomized, phase III trial. *J Clin Oncol* 2010;28(11):1843–1849.

200. Gudbjartsson T, Gyllstedt E, Pikwer A, et al. Early surgical results after pneumonectomy for non-small cell lung cancer are not affected by preoperative radiotherapy and chemotherapy. *Ann Thorac Surg* 2008;86(2):376–382.

201. Sonett JR, Suntharalingam M, Edelman MJ, et al. Pulmonary resection after curative intent radiotherapy (>59 Gy) and concurrent chemotherapy in non-small-cell lung cancer. *Ann Thorac Surg* 2004;78(4):1200–1205; discussion 1206.

202. Weder W, Collaud S, Eberhardt WE, et al. Pneumonectomy is a valuable treatment option after neoadjuvant therapy for stage III non-small-cell lung cancer. *J Thorac Cardiovasc Surg* 2010;139(6):1424–1430.

203. Alberts WM. Diagnosis and management of lung cancer executive summary: ACCP evidence-based clinical practice guidelines (2nd Edition). *Chest* 2007;132(3 Suppl):1s–19s.

204. Deslauriers J, Tronc F, Gregoire J. History and current status of bronchoplastic surgery for lung cancer. *Gen Thorac Cardiovasc Surg* 2009;57(1):3–9.

205. Venuta F, Ciccone AM, Anile M, et al. Reconstruction of the pulmonary artery for lung cancer: Long-term results. *J Thorac Cardiovasc Surg* 2009;138(5):1185–1191.

206. Hsia C, Johnson Jr R. Physiology and morphology of postpneumonectomy compensation. In: Crystal RG, West JB, Weibel ER, et al, eds. *The Lung Scientific Foundations*. 2nd ed. Philadelphia, PA: Lippincott-Raven; 1997:1047–1059.

207. Okamoto T, Iwata T, Mizobuchi T, et al. Surgical treatment for non-small cell lung cancer with ipsilateral pulmonary metastases. *Surg Today* 2013;43(10):1123–1128.

208. Okumura T, Asamura H, Suzuki K, et al. Intrapulmonary metastasis of non–small cell lung cancer: A prognostic assessment. *J Thorac Cardiovasc Surg* 2001;122(1):24–28.

209. Watanabe Y, Shimizu J, Oda M, et al. Results in 104 patients undergoing bronchoplastic procedures for bronchial lesions. *Ann Thorac Surg* 1990;50(4):607–614.

210. Deslauriers J, Mehran RJ, Guimont C, et al. Staging and management of lung cancer: Sleeve resection. *World J Surg* 1993;17(6):712–718.

211. Roviaro GC, Varoli F, Rebuffat C, et al. Tracheal sleeve pneumonectomy for bronchogenic carcinoma. *J Thorac Cardiovasc Surg* 1994;107(1):13–18.

212. Porhanov VA, Poliakov IS, Selvaschuk AP, et al. Indications and results of sleeve carinal resection. *Eur J Cardiothorac Surg* 2002;22(5):685–694.

213. Yildizeli B, Dartevelle PG, Fadel E, et al. Results of primary surgery with T4 non-small cell lung cancer during a 25-year period in a single center: the benefit is worth the risk. *Ann Thorac Surg* 2008;86(4):1065–1075; discussion 1074–1075.

214. Dartevelle P, Macchiarini P, Chapelier A. Technique of superior vena cava resection and reconstruction. *Chest Surg Clin N Am* 1995;5(2):345–358.

215. Dartevelle PG, Chapelier AR, Pastorino U, et al. Long-term follow-up after prosthetic replacement of the superior vena cava combined with resection of mediastinal-pulmonary malignant tumors. *J Thorac Cardiovasc Surg* 1991;102(2):259–265.

216. Nakahara K, Ohno K, Mastumura A, et al. Extended operation for lung cancer invading the aortic arch and superior vena cava. *J Thorac Cardiovasc Surg* 1989;97(3):428–433.

217. Tsuchiya R, Asamura H, Kondo H, et al. Extended resection of the left atrium, great vessels, or both for lung cancer. *Ann Thorac Surg* 1994;57(4):960–965.

218. Lee D-SD, Flores RM. Superior Vena Caval Resection in Lung Cancer. *Thorac Surg Clin* 2014;24(4):441–447.

219. Inoue H, Shohtsu A, Koide S, et al. Resection of the superior vena cava for primary lung cancer: 5 years' survival. *Ann Thorac Surg* 1990;50(4):661–662.

220. Spaggiari L, Thomas P, Magdeleinat P, et al. Superior vena cava resection with prosthetic replacement for non-small cell lung cancer: Long-term results of a multicentric study. *Eur J Cardiothorac Surg* 2002;21(6):1080–1086.

221. Misthos P, Papagiannakis G, Kokotsakis J, et al. Surgical management of lung cancer invading the aorta or the superior vena cava. *Lung Cancer* 2007;56(2):223–227.

222. Shargall Y, de Perrot M, Keshavjee S, et al. 15 years single center experience with surgical resection of the superior vena cava for non-small cell lung cancer. *Lung Cancer* 2004;45(3):357–363.

223. Bernard A, Bouchot O, Hagry O, et al. Risk analysis and long-term survival in patients undergoing resection of T4 lung cancer. *Eur J Cardiothorac Surg* 2001;20(2):344–349.

224. Horita K, Itho T, Ueno T. Radical operation using cardiopulmonary bypass for lung cancer invading the aortic wall. *Thorac Cardiovasc Surg* 1993;41(2):130–132.

225. Klepetko W, Wisser W, Birsan T, et al. T4 lung tumors with infiltration of the thoracic aorta: Is an operation reasonable? *Ann Thorac Surg* 1999;67(2):340–344.

226. Kusumoto H, Shintani Y, Funaki S, et al. Combined resection of great vessels or the heart for non-small lung cancer. *Ann Thorac Cardiovasc Surg* 2015;21(4):332–337.

227. Marulli G, Lepidi S, Frigatti P, et al. Thoracic aorta endograft as an adjunct to resection of a locally invasive tumor: A new indication to endograft. *J Vasc Surg* 2008;47(4):868–870.

228. Mody GN, Janko M, Vasudeva V, et al. Thoracic endovascular aortic stent graft to facilitate aortic resection during pneumonectomy and vertebrectomy for locally invasive lung cancer. *Ann Thorac Surg* 2016;101(4):1587–1589.

229. Hasegawa S, Bando T, Isowa N, et al. The use of cardiopulmonary bypass during extended resection of non-small cell lung cancer. *Interact Cardiovasc Thorac Surg* 2003;2(4):676–679.

230. Tsukioka T, Takahama M, Nakajima R, et al. Surgical outcome of patients with lung cancer involving the left atrium. *Int J Clin Oncol* 2016;21(6):1046–1050.

231. Rendina EA, Venuta F, De Giacomo T, et al. Sleeve resection and prosthetic reconstruction of the pulmonary artery for lung cancer. *Ann Thorac Surg* 1999;68(3):995–1001; discussion 1002.

232. Shrager JB, Lambright ES, McGrath CM, et al. Lobectomy with tangential pulmonary artery resection without regard to pulmonary function. *Ann Thorac Surg* 2000;70(1):234–239.

233. Ma Q, Liu D, Guo Y, et al. Surgical techniques and results of the pulmonary artery reconstruction for patients with central non-small cell lung cancer. *J Cardiothorac Surg* 2013;8:219.

234. Grunenwald DH, Mazel C, Girard P, et al. Radical en bloc resection for lung cancer invading the spine. *J Thorac Cardiovasc Surg* 2002;123(2):271–279.

235. Mody GN, Bravo Iniguez C, Armstrong K, et al. Early Surgical Outcomes of En Bloc Resection Requiring Vertebrectomy for Malignancy Invading the Thoracic Spine. *Ann Thorac Surg* 2016;101(1):231–236; discussion 236–237.

236. Schirren J, Donges T, Melzer M, et al. En bloc resection of non-small-cell lung cancer invading the spine. *Eur J Cardiothorac Surg* 2011;40(3):647–654.

237. Reardon ES, Schrump DS. Extended resections of non-small cell lung cancers invading the aorta, pulmonary artery, left atrium, or esophagus: can they be justified? *Thorac Surg Clin* 2014;24(4):457–464.

238. Detterbeck F. What to do with "Surprise" N2?: intraoperative management of patients with non-small cell lung cancer. *J Thorac Oncol* 2008;3(3):289–302.

239. Jett JR, Schild SE, Keith RL, et al. Treatment of non-small cell lung cancer, stage IIIB: ACCP evidence-based clinical practice guidelines (2nd edition). *Chest* 2007; 132(3 Suppl):266s–276s.

240. Detterbeck FC, Jantz MA, Wallace M, et al. Invasive mediastinal staging of lung cancer: ACCP evidence-based clinical practice guidelines (2nd edition). *Chest* 2007;132(3 Suppl):202s–220s.

241. Albain KS, Rusch VW, Crowley JJ, et al. Concurrent cisplatin/etoposide plus chest radiotherapy followed by surgery for stages IIIA (N2) and IIIB non-small-cell lung cancer: mature results of Southwest Oncology Group phase II study 8805. *J Clin Oncol* 1995;13(8):1880–1892.

242. Barlesi F, Doddoli C, Torre JP, et al. Comparative prognostic features of stage IIIAN2 and IIIB non-small-cell lung cancer patients treated with surgery after induction therapy. *Eur J Cardiothorac Surg* 2005;28(4):629–634.

243. Yang CF, Meyerhoff RR, Stephens SJ, et al. Long-Term Outcomes of Lobectomy for Non-Small Cell Lung Cancer After Definitive Radiation Treatment. *Ann Thorac Surg* 2015;99(6):1914–1920.

244. Socinski MA, Crowell R, Hensing TE, et al.. Treatment of non-small cell lung cancer, stage IV: ACCP evidence-based clinical practice guidelines (2nd edition). *Chest* 2007;132(3 Suppl):277s–289s.

245. Schuchert MJ, Luketich JD. Solitary sites of metastatic disease in non-small cell lung cancer. *Curr Treat Options Oncol* 2003;4(1):65–79.

246. Kozower BD, Larner JM, Detterbeck FC, et al. Special treatment issues in non-small cell lung cancer: Diagnosis and management of lung cancer, 3rd ed: American College of Chest Physicians evidence-based clinical practice guidelines. *Chest* 2013; 143(5 Suppl):e369S–e399S.

247. Soffietti R, Ruda R, Trevisan E. Brain metastases: Current management and new developments. *Curr Opin Oncol* 2008;20(6):676–684.

248. Nayak L, Lee EQ, Wen PY. Epidemiology of brain metastases. *Curr Oncol Rep* 2012;14(1):48–54.

249. Magilligan DJ, Duvernoy C, Malik G, et al. Surgical approach to lung cancer with solitary cerebral metastasis: Twenty-five years' experience. *Ann Thorac Surg* 1986;42(4):360–364.

250. Read RC, Boop WC, Yoder G, et al. Management of nonsmall cell lung carcinoma with solitary brain metastasis. *J Thorac Cardiovasc Surg* 1989;98(5 Pt 2):884–890; discussion 890–891.

251. Burt M, Wronski M, Arbit E, et al. Resection of brain metastases from non-small-cell lung carcinoma. Results of therapy. Memorial Sloan-Kettering Cancer Center Thoracic Surgical Staff. *J Thorac Cardiovasc Surg* 1992;103(3):399–410; discussion 411.

252. Billing PS, Miller DL, Allen MS, et al. Surgical treatment of primary lung cancer with synchronous brain metastases. *J Thorac Cardiovasc Surg* 2001;122(3): 548–553.

253. Bonnette P, Puyo P, Gabriel C, et al. Surgical management of non-small cell lung cancer with synchronous brain metastases. *Chest* 2001;119(5):1469–1475.

254. Granone P, Margaritora S, D'Andrilli A, et al. Non-small cell lung cancer with single brain metastasis: The role of surgical treatment. *Eur J Cardiothorac Surg* 2001;20(2):361–366.

255. Mussi A, Pistolesi M, Lucchi M, et al. Resection of single brain metastasis in non-small-cell lung cancer: prognostic factors. *J Thorac Cardiovasc Surg* 1996;112(1):146–153.

256. Patchell RA, Tibbs PA, Walsh JW, et al. A randomized trial of surgery in the treatment of single metastases to the brain. *N Engl J Med* 1990;322(8):494–500.

257. Kased N, Huang K, Nakamura JL, et al. Gamma knife radiosurgery for brainstem metastases: The UCSF experience. *J Neurooncol* 2008;86(2):195–205.

258. Mariya Y, Sekizawa G, Matsuoka Y, et al. Outcome of stereotactic radiosurgery for patients with non-small cell lung cancer metastatic to the brain. *J Radiat Res* 2010;51(3):333–342.

259. Tian LJ, Zhuang HQ, Yuan ZY. A comparison between cyberknife and neurosurgery in solitary brain metastases from non-small cell lung cancer. *Clin Neurol Neurosurg* 2013;115(10):2009–2014.

260. Dempke WC, Edvardsen K, Lu S, et al. Brain Metastases in NSCLC—are TKIs Changing the Treatment Strategy? *Anticancer Res* 2015;35(11):5797–5806.

261. Luketich JD, Burt ME. Does resection of adrenal metastases from non-small cell lung cancer improve survival? *Ann Thorac Surg* 1996;62(6):1614–1616.

262. Abdel-Raheem MM, Potti A, Becker WK, et al. Late adrenal metastasis in operable non-small-cell lung carcinoma. *Am J Clin Oncol* 2002;25(1):81–83.

263. Porte HL, Roumilhac D, Graziana JP, et al. Adrenalectomy for a solitary adrenal metastasis from lung cancer. *Ann Thorac Surg* 1998;65(2):331–335.

264. Porte H, Siat J, Guibert B, et al. Resection of adrenal metastases from non-small cell lung cancer: A multicenter study. *Ann Thorac Surg* 2001;71(3):981–985.

265. Tanvetyanon T, Robinson LA, Schell MJ, et al. Outcomes of adrenalectomy for isolated synchronous versus metachronous adrenal metastases in non-small-cell lung cancer: A systematic review and pooled analysis. *J Clin Oncol* 2008;26(7): 1142–1147.

266. Raz DJ, Lanuti M, Gaissert HC, et al. Outcomes of patients with isolated adrenal metastasis from non-small cell lung carcinoma. *Ann Thorac Surg* 2011;92(5):1788–1792; discussion 1793.

267. Macheers SK, Mansour KA. Management of isolated splenic metastases from carcinoma of the lung: A case report and review of the literature. *Am Surg* 1992;58(11):683–685.

268. Di Carlo I, Grasso G, Patane D, et al. Liver metastases from lung cancer: Is surgical resection justified? *Ann Thorac Surg* 2003;76(1):291–293.

269. Lindell G, Ohlsson B, Saarela A, et al. Liver resection of noncolorectal secondaries. *J Surg Oncol* 1998;69(2):66–70.

270. Ambrogi V, Tonini G, Mineo TC. Prolonged survival after extracranial metastasectomy from synchronous resectable lung cancer. *Ann Surg Oncol* 2001;8(8): 663–666.

271. Santini M, Vicidomini G, Di Marino MP, et al. Solitary muscle metastasis from lung carcinoma. *J Cardiovasc Surg (Torino)* 2001;42(5):701–702.

272. Luketich JD, Martini N, Ginsberg RJ, et al. Successful treatment of solitary extra-cranial metastases from non–small-cell lung cancer. *Ann Thorac Surg* 1995;60(6): 1609–1611.

273. Downey RJ, Ng KK, Kris MG, et al. A phase II trial of chemotherapy and surgery for non-small cell lung cancer patients with a synchronous solitary metastasis. *Lung Cancer* 2002;38(2):193–197.

274. Ebara K, Takashima S, Jiang B, et al. Pleural invasion by peripheral lung cancer: Prediction with three-dimensional CT. *Acad Radiol* 2015;22(3):310–319.

275. Fernandez FG, Furnary AP, Kosinski AS, et al. Longitudinal Follow-up of Lung Cancer Resection From the Society of Thoracic Surgeons General Thoracic Surgery Database in Patients 65 Years and Older. *Ann Thorac Surg* 2016;101(6): 2067–2076.

276. Tas F, Ciftci R, Kilic L, et al. Age is a prognostic factor affecting survival in lung cancer patients. *Oncology Letters* 2013;6(5):1507–1513.

277. Berry MF, Hanna J, Tong BC, et al. Risk factors for morbidity after lobectomy for lung cancer in elderly patients. *Ann Thorac Surg* 2009;88(4):1093–1099.

278. Alonso RC, ed. Non-small cell lung cancer (NSCLC): Review of the seventh edition of the TNM staging system and role of imaging in the staging and follow-up of NSCLC1970. *European Congress of Radiology*, 2011. doi: http://dx.doi.org/10.1594/ecr2011/C-0313

279. Kilic A, Schuchert MJ, Pettiford BL, et al. Anatomic segmentectomy for stage I non-small cell lung cancer in the elderly. *Ann Thorac Surg* 2009;87(6):1662–1666; discussion 1667–1668.

280. Read RC, Schaefer R, North N, et al. Diameter, cell type, and survival in stage I primary non–small-cell lung cancer. *Arch Surg* 1988;123(4):446–449.

281. Ichinose Y, Yano T, Asoh H, et al. Prognostic factors obtained by a pathologic examination in completely resected non-small cell lung cancer: An analysis in each pathologic stage. *J Thorac Cardiovasc Surg* 1995;110(3):601–605.

282. Agarwal M, Brahmanday G, Chmielewski GW, et al. Age, tumor size, type of surgery, and gender predict survival in early stage (stage I and II) non-small cell lung cancer after surgical resection. *Lung Cancer* 2010;68(3):398–402.

283. Shields TW, Yee J, Conn JH, et al. Relationship of cell type and lymph node metastasis to survival after resection of bronchial carcinoma. *Ann Thorac Surg* 1975;20(5):501–510.

284. Takei H, Asamura H, Maeshima A, et al. Large cell neuroendocrine carcinoma of the lung: A clinicopathologic study of eighty-seven cases. *J Thorac Cardiovasc Surg* 2002;124(2):285–292.

285. Iyoda A, Hiroshima K, Baba M, et al. Pulmonary large cell carcinomas with neuroendocrine features are high-grade neuroendocrine tumors. *Ann Thorac Surg* 2002;73(4):1049–1054.

286. García-Yuste M, Matilla JM, Alvarez-Gago T, et al. Prognostic factors in neuroendocrine lung tumors: A Spanish Multicenter Study. Spanish Multicenter Study of Neuroendocrine Tumors of the Lung of the Spanish Society of Pneumonology and Thoracic Surgery (EMETNE-SEPAR). *Ann Thorac Surg* 2000;70(1):258–263.

287. Battafarano RJ, Fernandez FG, Ritter J, et al. Large cell neuroendocrine carcinoma: An aggressive form of non-small cell lung cancer. *J Thorac Cardiovasc Surg* 2005;130(1):166–172.

288. Hiroshima K, Iyoda A, Shibuya K, et al. Prognostic significance of neuroendocrine differentiation in adenocarcinoma of the lung. *Ann Thorac Surg* 2002;73(6): 1732–1735.

289. Hage R, Elbers J, de la Rivière AB, et al. Surgery for combined type small cell lung carcinoma. *Thorax* 1998;53(6):450–453.

290. Travis WD, Harris C. *Pathology and Genetics of Tumours of the Lung, Pleura, Thymus and Heart.* France: IARC Press; 2004.

291. Higashiyama M, Kodama K, Takami K, et al. Intraoperative lavage cytologic analysis of surgical margins in patients undergoing limited surgery for lung cancer. *J Thorac Cardiovasc Surg* 2003;125(1):101–107.

292. Breathnach O, Kwiatkowski D, Finkelstein D, et al. Bronchioloalveolar carcinoma of the lung: Recurrences and survival in patients with stage I disease. *J Thorac Cardiovasc Surg* 2001;121(1):42–47.

293. Sakurai H, Dobashi Y, Mizutani E, et al. Bronchioloalveolar carcinoma of the lung 3 centimeters or less in diameter: A prognostic assessment. *Ann Thorac Surg* 2004;78(5):1728–1733.

294. Nakao M, Yoshida J, Goto K, et al. Long-term outcomes of 50 cases of limited-resection trial for pulmonary ground-glass opacity nodules. *J Thorac Oncol* 2012;7(10):1563–1566.

295. Sagawa M, Saito Y, Takahashi S, et al. Clinical and prognostic assessment of patients with resected small peripheral lung cancer lesions. *Cancer* 1990;66(12):2653–2657.

296. Rocha AT, McCormack M, Montana G, et al. Association between lower lobe location and upstaging for early-stage non-small cell lung cancer. *Chest* 2004;125(4):1424–1430.

297. Lee PC, Port JL, Korst RJ, et al. Risk factors for occult mediastinal metastases in clinical stage I non-small cell lung cancer. *Ann Thorac Surg* 2007;84(1):177–181.

298. Zhang Y, Sun Y, Xiang J, et al. A prediction model for N2 disease in T1 non–small cell lung cancer. *J Thorac Cardiovasc Surg* 2012;144(6):1360–1364.

299. Odell DD SM, McCormick JN, Wizore JJ, et al. Central Tumor Location for Clinical Stage I Non-Small Cell Lung Cancer (NSCLC): An Underappreciated Negative Prognostic Feature. 39th Annual Meeting – Western Thoracic Surgical Association, June 29, 2013; Coeur d'Alene, ID.

300. El-Sherif A, Fernando HC, Santos R, et al. Margin and local recurrence after sublobar resection of non-small cell lung cancer. *Ann Surg Oncol* 2007;14(8):2400–2405.

301. Chan EG, Landreneau JR, Schuchert MJ, Odell DD, Gu S, Pu J, et al. Preoperative (3-dimensional) computed tomography lung reconstruction before anatomic segmentectomy or lobectomy for stage I non-small cell lung cancer. *J Thorac Cardiovasc Surg.* 2015;150(3):523–528.

302. d'Amato TA, Galloway M, Szydlowski G, Chen A, Landreneau RJ. Intraoperative brachytherapy following thoracoscopic wedge resection of stage I lung cancer. *Chest.* 1998;114(4):1112–1115.

303. Chen A, Galloway M, Landreneau R, et al. Intraoperative 125 I brachytherapy for high-risk stage I non-small cell lung carcinoma. *Int J Radiat Oncol Biol Phys* 1999;44(5):1057–1063.

304. Landreneau JP, Schuchert MJ, Weyant R, et al. Anatomic segmentectomy and brachytherapy mesh implantation for clinical stage I non-small cell lung cancer (NSCLC). *Surgery* 2014;155(2):340–346.

305. Fernando HC, Landreneau RJ, Mandrekar SJ, et al. Impact of brachytherapy on local recurrence rates after sublobar resection: Results from ACOSOG Z4032 (Alliance), a phase III randomized trial for high-risk operable non–small-cell lung cancer. *J Clin Oncol* 2014;32(23):2456–2462.

306. Sparano A, Weinstein G, Chalian A, et al. Multivariate predictors of occult neck metastasis in early oral tongue cancer. *Otolaryngol Head Neck Surg* 2004;131(4):472–476.

307. Livi L, Paiar F, Simontacchi G, et al. Loco regional failure pattern after lumpectomy and breast irradiation in 4,185 patients with T1 and T2 breast cancer. Implications for nodal irradiation. *Acta Oncol* 2006;45(5):564–570.

308. Muller S, Chesner I, Egan M, et al. Significance of venous and lymphatic invasion in malignant polyps of the colon and rectum. *Gut* 1989;30(10):1385–1391.

309. Han H, Silverman JF, Santucci TS, et al. Vascular endothelial growth factor expression in stage I non-small cell lung cancer correlates with neoangiogenesis and a poor prognosis. *Ann Surg Oncol* 2001;8(1):72–79.

310. Ogawa JI, Tsurumi T, Yamada S, et al. Blood vessel invasion and expression of sialyl lewisx and proliferating cell nuclear antigen in stage I non-small cell lung cancer. Relation to postoperative recurrence. *Cancer* 1994;73(4):1177–1183.

311. Bodendorf MO, Haas V, Laberke H-G, et al. Prognostic value and therapeutic consequences of vascular invasion in non-small cell lung carcinoma. *Lung Cancer* 2009;64(1):71–78.

312. Pechet TT, Carr SR, Collins JE, et al. Arterial Invasion Predicts Early Mortality in Stage I Non–Small Cell Lung Cancer. *Ann Thorac Surg* 2004;78(5):1748–1753.

313. Schuchert MJ, Schumacher L, Kilic A, et al. Impact of angiolymphatic and pleural invasion on surgical outcomes for stage I non-small cell lung cancer. *Ann Thorac Surg* 2011;91(4):1059–1065.

314. Hiraoka K, Miyamoto M, Cho Y, et al. Concurrent infiltration by CD8+ T cells and CD4+ T cells is a favourable prognostic factor in non-small-cell lung carcinoma. *Br J Cancer* 2006;94(2):275–280.

315. Horne ZD, Jack R, Gray ZT, et al. Increased levels of tumor-infiltrating lymphocytes are associated with improved recurrence-free survival in stage 1A non-small-cell lung cancer. *J Surg Res* 2011;171(1):1–5.

316. Bremnes RM, Busund L-T, Kilvær TL, et al. The Role of Tumor-Infiltrating Lymphocytes in Development, Progression, and Prognosis of Non-Small Cell Lung Cancer. *J Thorac Oncol* 2016;11(6):789–800.

317. Cerfolio RJ, Bryant AS, Skylizard L, et al. Initial consecutive experience of completely portal robotic pulmonary resection with 4 arms. *J Thorac Cardiovasc Surg* 2011;142(4):740–746.

318. Dylewski MR, Ohaeto AC, Pereira JF. Pulmonary resection using a total endoscopic robotic video-assisted approach. *Semin Thorac Cardiovasc Surg* 2011;23(1):36–42.

319. Park BJ, Melfi F, Mussi A, et al. Robotic lobectomy for non-small cell lung cancer (NSCLC): Long-term oncologic results. *J Thorac Cardiovasc Surg* 2012;143(2):383–389.

320. Veronesi G, Galetta D, Maisonneuve P, et al. Four-arm robotic lobectomy for the treatment of early-stage lung cancer. *J Thorac Cardiovasc Surg* 2010;140(1):19–25.

321. Louie BE, Wilson JL, Kim S, et al. Comparison of Video-Assisted Thoracoscopic Surgery and Robotic Approaches for Clinical Stage I and Stage II Non-Small Cell Lung Cancer Using The Society of Thoracic Surgeons Database. *Ann Thorac Surg* 2016;102;917–924.

322. Cerfolio RJ, Watson C, Minnich DJ, et al. One hundred planned robotic segmentectomies: Early results, technical details, and preferred port placement. *Ann Thorac Surg* 2016;101(3):1089–1096.

323. Fernando HC, Schuchert M, Landreneau R, et al. Approaching the high-risk patient: Sublobar resection, stereotactic body radiation therapy, or radiofrequency ablation. *Ann Thorac Surg* 2010;89(6):S2123–S2127.

324. Pennathur A, Abbas G, Schuchert MJ, et al. eds. *Image-Guided Radiofrequency Ablation for the Treatment of Early-Stage Non-Small Cell Lung Neoplasm in High-Risk Patients. Sem Thorac Cardiovasc Surg* 2010;22(1):53–58.

325. Pennathur A, Luketich JD, Heron DE, et al. Stereotactic radiosurgery/stereotactic body radiotherapy for recurrent lung neoplasm: An analysis of outcomes in 100 patients. *Ann Thorac Surg* 2015;100(6):2019–2024.

326. Rosen JE, Salazar MC, Wang Z, et al. Lobectomy versus stereotactic body radiotherapy in healthy patients with stage I lung cancer. *J Thorac Cardiovasc Surg* 2016;152:44–54.

327. Ochsner A, Dixon JL, DeBakey M. Primary bronchiogenic carcinoma. *Chest* 1945;11(2):97–129.

328. Weiss W. Operative mortality and five-year survival rates in men with bronchogenic carcinoma. *Chest* 1974;66(5):483–487.

329. Ginsberg RJ, Hill LD, Eagan RT, et al. Modern thirty-day operative mortality for surgical resections in lung cancer. *J Thorac Cardiovasc Surg* 1983;86(5):654–658.

330. Romano PS, Mark DH. Patient and hospital characteristics related to in-hospital mortality after lung cancer resection. *Chest* 1992;101(5):1332–1337.

331. Ginsberg RJ, Rubinstein LV. Randomized trial of lobectomy versus limited resection for T1 N0 non-small cell lung cancer. Lung Cancer Study Group. *Ann Thorac Surg* 1995;60(3):615–622.

332. Wada H, Nakamura T, Nakamoto K, et al. Thirty-day operative mortality for thoracotomy in lung cancer. *J Thorac Cardiovasc Surg* 1998;115(1):70–73.

333. Harpole DH Jr, DeCamp MM Jr, Daley J, et al. Prognostic models of thirty-day mortality and morbidity after major pulmonary resection. *J Thorac Cardiovasc Surg* 1999;117(5):969–979.

334. Allen MS, Darling GE, Pechet TT, et al. Morbidity and mortality of major pulmonary resections in patients with early-stage lung cancer: initial results of the randomized, prospective ACOSOG Z0030 trial. *Ann Thorac Surg* 2006;81(3):1013–1019; discussion 1019–1020.

335. Okada M, Mimae T, Tsutani Y, et al. Segmentectomy versus lobectomy for clinical stage IA lung adenocarcinoma. *Ann Cardiothorac Surg* 2014;3(2):153–159.

336. Watanabe S, Asamura H, Suzuki K, et al. Recent results of postoperative mortality for surgical resections in lung cancer. *Ann Thorac Surg.* 2004;78(3):999–1002; discussion 1003.

337. Kozower BD, Sheng S, O'Brien SM, et al. STS database risk models: Predictors of mortality and major morbidity for lung cancer resection. *Ann Thorac Surg* 2010;90(3):875–881.

338. Paul S, Isaacs AJ, Treasure T, et al. Long term survival with thoracoscopic versus open lobectomy: Propensity matched comparative analysis using SEER-Medicare database. *BMJ* 2014;349:g5575.

339. Seder CW, Salati M, Kozower BD, et al. Variation in Pulmonary Resection Practices Between The Society of Thoracic Surgeons and the European Society of Thoracic Surgeons General Thoracic Surgery Databases. *Ann Thorac Surg* 2016;101(6):2077–2084.

340. Shapiro M, Weiser TS, Wisnivesky JP, et al. Thoracoscopic segmentectomy compares favorably with thoracoscopic lobectomy for patients with small stage I lung cancer. *J Thorac Cardiovasc Surg* 2009;137(6):1388–1393.

341. De Giacomo T, Di Stasio M, Diso D, et al. Sub-lobar lung resection of peripheral T1N0M0 NSCLC does not affect local recurrence rate. *Scand J Surg* 2009;98(4):225–228.

342. Yamashita S, Tokuishi K, Anami K, et al. Thoracoscopic segmentectomy for T1 classification of non-small cell lung cancer: a single center experience. *Eur J Cardiothorac Surg* 2012;42(1):83–88.

343. Zhong C, Fang W, Mao T, et al. Comparison of thoracoscopic segmentectomy and thoracoscopic lobectomy for small-sized stage IA lung cancer. *Ann Thorac Surg* 2012;94(2):362–367.

344. Soukiasian HJ, Hong E, McKenna RJ Jr. Video-assisted thoracoscopic trisegmentectomy and left upper lobectomy provide equivalent survivals for stage IA and IB lung cancer. *J Thorac Cardiovasc Surg* 2012;144(3):S23–S26.

345. Zhang L, Ma W, Li Y, et al. Comparative study of the anatomic segmentectomy versus lobectomy for clinical stage IA peripheral lung cancer by video assistant thoracoscopic surgery. *J Cancer Res Ther* 2013;9 Suppl 2:S106–S109.

346. Zhao X, Qian L, Luo Q, et al. Segmentectomy as a safe and equally effective surgical option under complete video-assisted thoracic surgery for patients of stage I non-small cell lung cancer. *J Cardiothorac Surg* 2013;8:116.

347. McGuire AL, Hopman WM, Petsikas D, et al. Outcomes: wedge resection versus lobectomy for non–small cell lung cancer at the Cancer Centre of Southeastern Ontario 1998–2009. *Can J Surg* 2013;56(6):E165–E170.

348. Linden PA, D'Amico TA, Perry Y, et al. Quantifying the safety benefits of wedge resection: A society of thoracic surgery database propensity-matched analysis. *Ann Thorac Surg* 2014;98(5):1705–1711; discussion 1711–1712.

349. Hwang Y, Kang CH, Kim HS, et al. Comparison of thoracoscopic segmentectomy and thoracoscopic lobectomy on the patients with non-small cell lung cancer: A propensity score matching study. *Eur J Cardiothorac Surg* 2015;48(2):273–278.

350. Park BJ, Zhang H, Rusch VW, et al. Video-assisted thoracic surgery does not reduce the incidence of postoperative atrial fibrillation after pulmonary lobectomy. *J Thorac Cardiovasc Surg* 2007;133(3):775–779.

351. Flores RM, Park BJ, Dycoco J, et al. Lobectomy by video-assisted thoracic surgery (VATS) versus thoracotomy for lung cancer. *J Thorac Cardiovasc Surg* 2009;138(1):11–18.

352. Gopaldas RR, Bakaeen FG, Dao TK, et al. Video-assisted thoracoscopic versus open thoracotomy lobectomy in a cohort of 13,619 patients. *Ann Thorac Surg* 2010;89(5):1563–1570.

353. Scott WJ, Allen MS, Darling G, et al. Video-assisted thoracic surgery versus open lobectomy for lung cancer: A secondary analysis of data from the American College

of Surgeons Oncology Group Z0030 randomized clinical trial. *J Thorac Cardiovasc Surg* 2010;139(4):976–981.

354. Wang BY, Liu CC, Shih CS. Short-term results of thoracoscopic lobectomy and segmentectomy for lung cancer in koo foundation sun yat-sen cancer center. *J Thorac Dis* 2010;2(2):64–70.

355. Ilonen IK, Rasanen JV, Knuuttila A, et al. Anatomic thoracoscopic lung resection for non-small cell lung cancer in stage I is associated with less morbidity and shorter hospitalization than thoracotomy. *Acta Oncol* 2011;50(7):1126–1132.

356. Boffa DJ, Dhamija A, Kosinski AS, et al. Fewer complications result from a video-assisted approach to anatomic resection of clinical stage I lung cancer. *J Thorac Cardiovasc Surg* 2014;148(2):637–643.

357. Nwogu CE, D'Cunha J, Pang H, et al. VATS lobectomy has better perioperative outcomes than open lobectomy: CALGB 31001, an ancillary analysis of CALGB 140202 (Alliance). *Ann Thorac Surg* 2015;99(2):399–405.

358. Sienel W, Stremmel C, Kirschbaum A, et al. Frequency of local recurrence following segmentectomy of stage IA non-small cell lung cancer is influenced by segment localisation and width of resection margins–implications for patient selection for segmentectomy. *Eur J Cardiothorac Surg* 2007;31(3):522–527; discussion 527–528.

359. Tsutani Y, Miyata Y, Nakayama H, et al. Oncologic outcomes of segmentectomy compared with lobectomy for clinical stage IA lung adenocarcinoma: Propensity score-matched analysis in a multicenter study. *J Thorac Cardiovasc Surg* 2013;146(2):358–364.

360. Speicher PJ, Gu L, Gulack BC, et al. Sublobar resection for Clinical Stage IA Non-small-cell Lung Cancer in the United States. *Clin Lung Cancer* 2016;17(1):47–55.

361. Koike T, Kitahara A, Sato S, et al. Lobectomy versus segmentectomy in radiologically pure solid small-sized non-small cell lung cancer. *Ann Thorac Surg* 2016;101(4):1354–1360.

362. Kodama K, Higashiyama M, Okami J, et al. Oncologic outcomes of segmentectomy versus lobectomy for clinical T1a N0 M0 non-small cell lung cancer. *Ann Thorac Surg* 2016;101(2):504–511.

363. Williams DE, Pairolero PC, Davis CS, et al. Survival of patients surgically treated for stage I lung cancer. *J Thorac Cardiovasc Surg* 1981;82(1):70–76.

364. Suen HC, Meyers BF, Guthrie T, et al. Favorable results after sleeve lobectomy or Bronchoplasty for bronchial malignancies. *Ann Thorac Surg* 1999;67(6):1557–1562.

365. Macchiarini P, Buonaguidi R, Hardin M, et al. Results and prognostic factors of surgery in the management of non-small cell lung cancer with solitary brain metastasis. *Cancer* 1991;68(2):300–304.

366. Vecht CJ, Haaxma-Reiche H, Noordijk EM, et al. Treatment of single brain metastasis: Radiotherapy alone or combined with neurosurgery? *Ann Neurol* 1993;33(6):583–590.

367. Beitler AL, Urschel JD, Velagapudi SR, et al. Surgical management of adrenal metastases from lung cancer. *J Surg Oncol* 1998;69(1):54–57.

368. Park BJ, Flores RM, Rusch VW. Robotic assistance for video-assisted thoracic surgical lobectomy: Technique and initial results. *J Thorac Cardiovasc Surg* 2006; 131(1):54–59.

369. Louie BE, Farivar AS, Aye RW, et al. Early experience with robotic lung resection results in similar operative outcomes and morbidity when compared with matched video-assisted thoracoscopic surgery cases. *Ann Thorac Surg* 2012;93(5):1598–1604; discussion 1604–1605.

370. Yang HX, Woo KM, Sima CS, et al. Long-term Survival Based on the Surgical Approach to Lobectomy For Clinical Stage I Nonsmall Cell Lung Cancer: Comparison of Robotic, Video-assisted Thoracic Surgery, and Thoracotomy Lobectomy. *Ann Surg* 2016;265(2):431–437.

96

Mediastinal Lymph Node Dissection

Anthony L. Picone ▪ Sai Yendamuri ▪ Todd L. Demmy

INTRODUCTION

Mediastinal lymph node evaluation was recognized as an adjunct in lung cancer treatment dating back to the early descriptions of pneumonectomy and lobectomy surgery.[1,2] Over the decades the variety of approaches to assess mediastinal metastatic disease and their importance in cancer staging has increased greatly. The realization that lymph node positive patients do better with adjuvant therapy alone is impetus enough for the cancer surgeon to perform a careful mediastinal dissection as part of surgical extirpation. This chapter describes the technique of mediastinal lymph node dissection (MLND). Dissection via open thoracotomy is described first, followed by the same dissection performed by VATS. This is then followed by a brief description of transcervical lymph node dissection. These different dissection techniques can be complementary because of their effectiveness at lymph node removal depending on the station. It is important to keep in mind that these dissection techniques do not take away from the importance of interventional diagnostic and staging techniques such as mediastinoscopy, endobronchial ultrasound-guided fine needle aspiration, or transbronchial needle aspiration. Each technique has its own place in the thoracic oncologist's decision-making matrix.[3]

MEDIASTINAL LYMPH NODE MAP

The accurate categorization of lymph node stations is crucial to the staging and treatment of lung cancer. This enables unambiguous communication between investigators in the field. Historically, there have been several lymph node "maps" and revisions to them dating back to the 1960s have been created.[4–7] Unfortunately, this has led to confusion in the literature regarding comparative treatment options and results. The most recent version proposed by the International Association for the Study of Lung Cancer (IASLC) in 2009 has become the accepted standard.[8] Description of lymph node stations in the remainder of this chapter is based on this system that concisely describes precise anatomic boundaries for all lymph nodes especially stations 1 through 10. Figure 96.1 demonstrates the important anatomic boundaries in this revised classification system. In particular, the clarified anatomic location of stations 4, 7, and 10 are utilized in the forthcoming discussion of lymph node dissections. It is important to note that the anatomic dividing line between right-sided and left-sided lymph node stations 2 and 4 (i.e., 2R and

2L; 4R and 4L) is the left lateral wall of the trachea because of the preponderance of drainage to right-sided lymphatics in the superior mediastinum. In addition, the azygous vein, instead of the pleural envelope is used to separate levels 4 and 10 on the right side. In addition, other smaller changes include clarification of the separation between levels 2 and 4 and levels 7 and 10 on the right and levels 5 and 10 on the left.

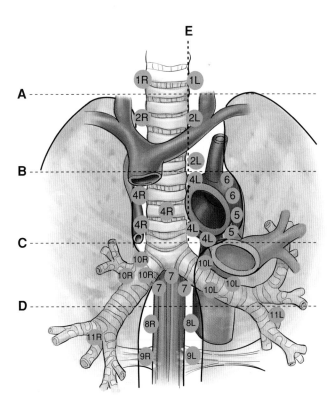

FIGURE 96.1 Important anatomic boundaries for mediastinal lymph node stations; **A:** horizontal line intersects apices of right and left pleural spaces; **B:** horizontal line intersects the caudal margin of brachiocephalic vein with the trachea on the right and the superior border of the aortic arch on the left; **C:** horizontal line intersects the lower border of the azygos vein on the right and the upper rim of the left main pulmonary artery on the left; **D:** horizontal line intersects the lower border of the bronchus intermedius on the right and the border of the lower lobe bronchus on the left. **E:** vertical line at the *left* lateral border of the trachea is the demarcation between the right and left paratracheal regions. (Adapted from Tournoy et al.[9])

MEDIASTINAL LYMPH NODE DISSECTION VERSUS SAMPLING

Assessment of mediastinal lymph nodes improves early stage lung cancer survival rates by excluding cases with unexpected higher stage nodal metastases.[10] Although the optimal total number of lymph nodes resected is uncertain, more stations evaluated and a lower ratio of positive to total lymph nodes sampled predict better outcomes.[11–13] Controversy exists as to whether the systematic removal of one or more lymph nodes from predetermined stations, that is, *mediastinal lymph node sampling* (MLNS), is as effective as the thorough extirpation of all tissue in multiple stations by *MLND*.[14] Several studies have suggested that MLND may provide improved survival over MLNS.[15–17] However, this has not been supported uniformly.[18,19] Moreover, a large randomized trial has demonstrated equivalence of MLNS and MLND in early stage lung cancer.[20] A recent detailed summary of published reports noted that there was no improvement in survival or recurrence rate with MLND in most randomized and nonrandomized studies when patients with all stages were included, but there was evidence of improved median survival in stage 2 and 3a disease.[21] Another interesting report by Hsu and colleagues[22] suggests that stage 1b disease is heterogeneous with long-term outcomes affected by the quality of the MLND. A confounding variable that indirectly supports MLND is the phenomenon of skipping where N2 disease occurs in the absence of N1 metastases. This is attributed to direct mediastinal connection by subpleural lymphatic collectors or the presence of undiagnosed N1 micrometastases.[23,24] Therefore, whether systematic lymph node dissection versus sampling should be performed is still left to the surgeon. It seems clear that both are equivalent in early stage disease. However, in stage 2 and 3 disease, MLND seems to be preferable as there is no downside to it and may confer survival benefit.

Several surgical techniques are currently available to perform either MLNS or MLND as shown in Table 96.1. This chapter will focus on only those techniques that are more commonly employed to perform MLND. The mediastinal regions and stations approachable by these techniques are presented in Figure 96.2. While current studies have demonstrated comparable results for either open thoracotomy versus VATS surgical approach for lymph node dissection,[25–28] both are discussed as a transthoracic method for mediastinal lymph node evaluation. Although several methods for transcervical evaluation of mediastinal lymph nodes exist, the technique of **T**ranscervical **E**xtended **M**ediastinal **L**ymph **A**denectomy (TEMLA) is discussed in some detail as it is comparable to achieving a transthoracic dissection. The extended mediastinoscopy technique is not considered separately as it is rarely performed as such but is mentioned as an element of the TEMLA procedure.[29] Some surgeons believe that current robotic instruments facilitate manipulation and dissection of some lymph node stations but are not presented here.[30] As the robotic technique is dependent on visual cues rather than tactile ones, meticulous dissection of the hilar structures from lymphatic tissue is quite important. This may enhance staging of N1 lymph nodes, but should not affect the yield of N2 lymph nodes much, when compared to VATS techniques.

In considering the extent of MLNS or MLND, the preferential lymphatic drainage pattern based on the location of primary lung neoplasm should be taken into account. These patterns are somewhat reliable for single-station metastases but more advanced disease spreads to multiple stations.[21] Based on several studies,[21,31–33] the likely preferential drainage stations for the various pulmonary lobes are shown in Table 96.2. As a generalization, right lung tumors most frequently metastasize to stations 4R and 7 while left lung tumors most frequently metastasize to stations 5 and 7.[34] It has also been proposed that centrally located tumors from all lobes are more likely to metastasize to station 7 than peripherally located ones.

OPEN MEDIASTINAL LYMPH NODE DISSECTION

Based on the recent IASLC revision of mediastinal lymph node stations, their dissection can be grouped into three main compartments: (1) extrathoracic, (2) right thoracic, and (3) left thoracic.

TABLE 96.1 Categorization of Surgical Mediastinal Lymph Node Evaluative Techniques in the Treatment of Lung Cancer

Approach	Technique Year Described	Consideration
Transcervical	Mediastinoscopy 1959	Original description for a separate staging procedure
	Video Mediastinoscopy 1989	Increased safety and yield of dissection
	Extended Mediastinoscopy 1987	Single-incision technique to assess mediastinal lymph nodes including stations 5 and 6
	Video Assisted Mediastinoscopic Lymph Adenectomy (VAMLA) 2002	Utilized double-bladed mediastinoscope for improved visualization
	Transcervical Extended Mediastinal Lymph Adenectomy (TEMLA) 2005	Maximizes transcervical exposure by use of double-bladed mediastinoscope and sternal retractor
Transthoracic	Open Thoracotomy 1951	Original description of mediastinal lymph node dissection
	Video Assisted Thoracoscopy (VATS) 1994	Minimally invasive approach with results equivalent to open thoracotomy
	Robotic Assisted Thoracoscopy (RATS) 2008	Recent technique with increasing utilization

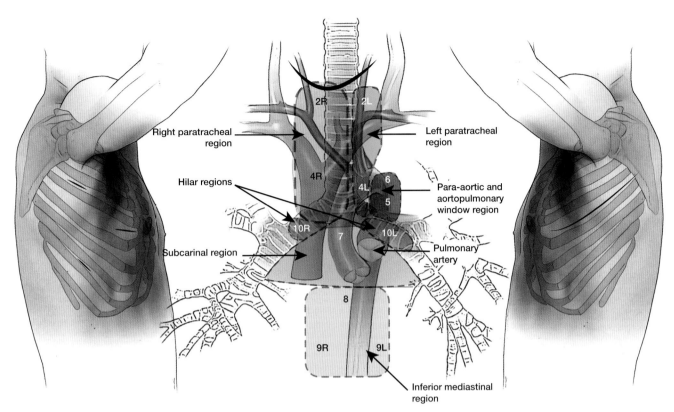

FIGURE 96.2 Techniques for accessing mediastinal compartments; the right paratracheal region can be accessed by either a transthoracic approach (right open thoracotomy or VATS) or a transcervical approach (TEMLA). The hilar N1 lymph nodes (station 10) can similarly be reached by an ipsilateral transthoracic approach or TEMLA. The subcarinal region can be approached from either the right or left transthoracic approach or TEMLA. The left paratracheal region is best approached by TEMLA. The para-aortic and aortopulmonary window region can be approached via a left transthoracic thoracotomy or VATS. An extended dissection during TEMLA can also reach this region. The inferior mediastinal region can be reached by a transthoracic approach (thoracotomy or VATS). TEMLA can access station 8 (paraesophageal) but not stations 9R or 9L.

Only the latter two categories will be considered further as lymph node dissection of N3 (stations 1R, 1L) disease rarely improves outcomes.

RIGHT THORACIC COMPARTMENT

The right compartment contains N2 stations 2R, 4R, 7, 8R, 8L, 9R, and N1 station 10R. While a complete lymph node dissection can

TABLE 96.2 Common Patterns of Mediastinal Lymph Node Metastases

	2R	4R	7	5	6	Other
RUL	*	***				
RML		**	**			
RLL		*	***			basilar segments—also 8 and 9R; superior segment—also 4R
LUL				***	**	inferior lingular segments—6 and 7
LLL			**	*	*	superior segment—7; basilar segments—7, 8, and 9L

*, somewhat likely; **, more likely; ***, most likely.

be achieved for these stations, limited left-sided mediastinal access makes staging for N3 disease difficult, if not impossible. Entry through a standard 5th intercostal space posterolateral thoracotomy incision allows exposure of the right side superior and inferior mediastinum and hilum.

Right Paratracheal Dissection

The borders of this dissection include the trachea posteriorly, the superior vena cava anteriorly, the aortic arch medially, the mediastinal pleura laterally, azygous vein inferiorly, and the thoracic inlet superiorly. Dissection is begun by palpating the right lateral border of the trachea. The superior vena cava lies anterior to the trachea and the esophagus posterior in this region (Fig. 96.3). A vertical incision is then created in the mediastinal pleura along this line from the thoracic inlet superiorly to the azygous vein inferiorly. As dissection is continued into the mediastinal tissue, care must be taken to protect the esophagus posteriorly. The right recurrent laryngeal nerve which lies along the right cervical paratracheal border should not be visible below the level of the thoracic inlet. Vagal fibers arising from the lateral surface of the esophagus, which then innervate the hilar region, are sacrificed.

Superiorly, the 2R lymph node station is exposed. This station is located from the thoracic inlet cephalad to the intersection of the brachiocephalic vein and the trachea caudally (see also Fig. 96.1). These and all other lymph nodes can be harvested either by sharp or blunt dissection. Blood vessels should be controlled preferably by

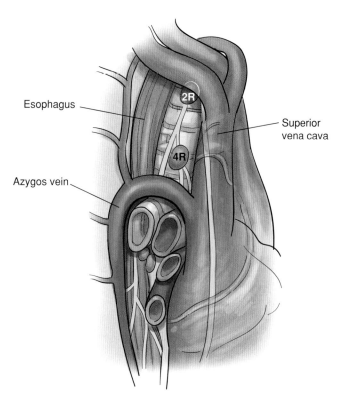

FIGURE 96.3 Right paratracheal region landmarks include the superior vena cava anteriorly, the esophagus posteriorly, the thoracic inlet superiorly, and the azygos vein inferiorly. The right paratracheal lymph node stations can be dissected in continuity. The 2R lymph node station lies cephalad to the intersection point of the caudal margin of the brachiocephalic vein and the trachea while the 4R station lies inferior to this point with the lower boundary being the inferior aspect of the arch of the azygos vein.

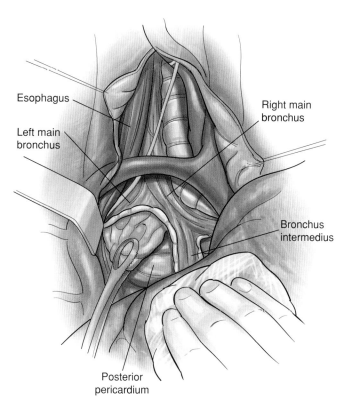

FIGURE 96.4 The subcarinal region contains the subcarinal lymph node packet (station 7) which extends from the carina to the lower border of the bronchus intermedius. The landmarks for this compartment are the right and left main stem bronchi, the posterior aspect of the pericardium anteriorly, and the esophagus posteriorly.

clips or bipolar cautery. Slightly inferiorly and down to the inferior border of the azygous vein, the 4R lymph node station can be similarly harvested. This region known as the right tracheobronchial angle may require mobilization of the vein if it has not been divided already.

Subcarinal and Inferior Mediastinal Dissection

Although not necessary, the division of the azygos vein allows dissection in continuity onto the lateral edge of the right main stem bronchus. Otherwise, dissection can be performed inferior to the vein along the posterior aspect or membranous wall of the right main stem bronchus exposing the subcarinal region (Fig. 96.4). Borders of this dissection include the right and left main stem bronchi, the posterior aspect of the pericardium, which lies anteriorly, and the esophagus which lies posteriorly. Although the right main pulmonary artery lies anterior to the carina, this structure is difficult to reach via a lateral approach (but can be easily injured during a more anterior approach such as mediastinoscopy). This region is highly vascular and requires careful hemostasis, either with clips or with bipolar cautery. This entire packet can be harvested which may contain multiple lymph nodes.

After dissection of the subcarinal region, extension of the pleural incision inferiorly anterior to the esophagus and posterior to the bronchus intermedius will allow entry to the periesophageal or station 8 lymph nodes (Fig. 96.5). These lymph nodes lie on either the left or right side of the esophagus and can be accessed by dissection in the inferior mediastinal periesophageal region. Station 9R lymph

nodes (Fig. 96.6) can be accessed by dividing the inferior pulmonary ligament starting at its diaphragmatic insertion and carefully opening the ligament up to the level of the inferior pulmonary vein. The dissection plane should be in close proximity to the lower lobe lung parenchyma and away from the esophagus. The station 9 lymph nodes are located at the caudal aspect of the inferior pulmonary vein and can be readily harvested.

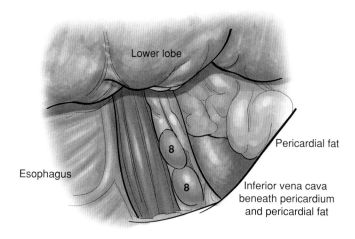

FIGURE 96.5 The inferior mediastinal periesophageal region contains station 8R and 8L lymph nodes. These can be accessed by continuing the dissection along the esophagus inferior to the subcarinal compartment.

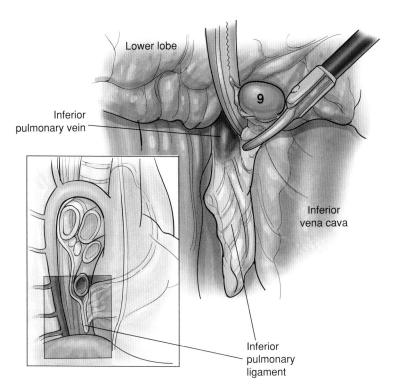

FIGURE 96.6 The station 9 lymph nodes in either the right or left thorax lie at the caudal aspect of the respective inferior pulmonary vein and can be accessed by dividing the inferior pulmonary ligament.

Hilar Node Dissection

Along the lateral and anterior surface of the right main bronchus station, 10R lymph nodes can be found starting at the level of the inferior border of the azygos vein (Fig. 96.7). These N1 hilar lymph nodes continue inferiorly to level of the takeoff of the right upper lobe bronchus (interlobar region). Since this is a very limited region

along the right main stem bronchus, it may be difficult to differentiate between stations 10R and 11R lymph nodes. Access to the latter N1 lymph nodes or interlobar lymph nodes is difficult without first performing pulmonary resection, or at least completing the fissures. The stations 12 (lobar), 13 (segmental), and 14 (subsegmental) lymph nodes are routinely accessed at the pathological examination of pulmonary specimens but they are not part of the surgical dissection. The situation is similar for the corresponding 11L–14L lymph node stations.

LEFT THORACIC COMPARTMENT

The left compartment contains N2 stations 5, 6, 7, 9L and N1 stations 10L. Entry through the 5th intercostal space by posterolateral thoracotomy allows access to the left lateral mediastinum and hilum. Dissection of the left paratracheal region (stations 2L and 4L) is limited by the intervening aortic arch and pulmonary artery. The surgical approach to these stations through a left thoracotomy necessitates mobilization of the aortic arch and its separation from the left main pulmonary artery. This dissection puts the recurrent laryngeal nerve at risk. Stations 5 and 6, however, can be assessed quite easily.

AP Window and Para-Aortic Dissection

Incision of the mediastinal pleura is begun in the vicinity cephalad to the main pulmonary artery and lateral to the aortic arch (Fig. 96.8). The phrenic nerve anterior to and the vagus nerve posterior to the incision must be visualized and protected. The incision is then extended superiorly on to the lateral surface of the aortic arch and upward along the great vessels but does not need to reach the thoracic inlet. In the region of the aortopulmonary window, station 5 lymph nodes (aortopulmonary lymph nodes) can be dissected with care to protect the left recurrent laryngeal nerve as it originates from the vagus nerve and encircles the aortic arch. Slightly cephalad, alongside

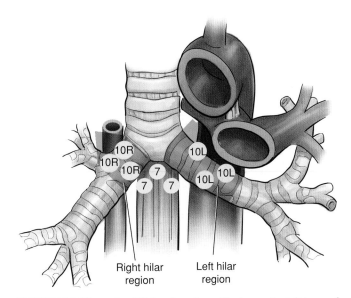

FIGURE 96.7 The station 10R lymph nodes reside along a short distance of the right main stem bronchus from the inferior border of the azygos vein to the interlobar region on its lateral and anterior surface. The station 10L lymph nodes reside along the left main stem bronchus from the upper rim of the main pulmonary artery to the interlobar region on its lateral and anterior surface. Lymph nodes along the proximal portion of the respective hilar arteries and veins are also consider as station 10 (not shown).

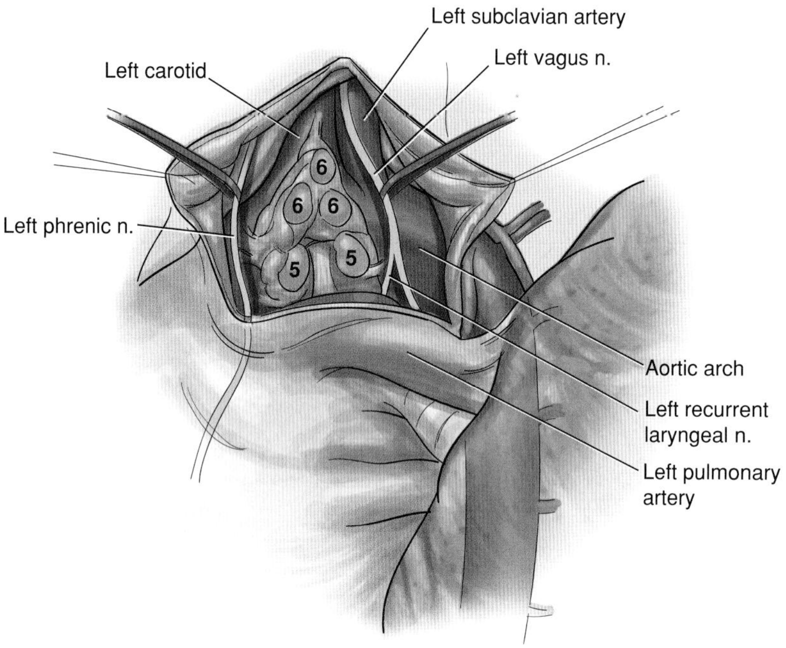

Left subclavian artery

Left carotid

Left vagus n.

6

6 6

5 5

Left phrenic n.

Aortic arch

Left recurrent
laryngeal n.

Left pulmonary
artery

FIGURE 96.8 The aortopulmonary window and para-aortic regions contain stations 5 and 6 lymph nodes, respectively. Landmarks include the main pulmonary artery inferiorly, the aortic arch medially, and the left carotid and subclavian arteries superiorly. The phrenic nerve lies anterior to the line of dissection while the vagus nerve and the recurrent laryngeal branch which encircles the aortic arch lie posterior.

the aortic arch, is the station 6 or para-aortic lymph nodes which can similarly be harvested.

Subcarinal, Inferior Mediastinal, and Hilar Node Dissection

The subcarinal region containing the station 7 lymph nodes is more difficult to access from the left thorax (Fig. 96.9). The left main stem bronchus must be dissected from surrounding structures proximally to the subcarinal region. Traction on the left main stem bronchus greatly

facilitates dissection. When performing a left pneumonectomy, it is helpful to use the dissected left main bronchus for traction before lung amputation. The lymph node packet extends from the carina superiorly to the superior border of the left lower lobe inferiorly. Similar to the right thoracic inferior mediastinal region, the station 9L lymph nodes can be harvested after dividing the inferior pulmonary ligament proximally to the level of the inferior pulmonary vein (Fig. 96.6). Station 8 lymph nodes can be accessed from the left chest but requires mobilization of the esophagus due to impeding anatomic structures including the pericardium, descending aorta, and spine.

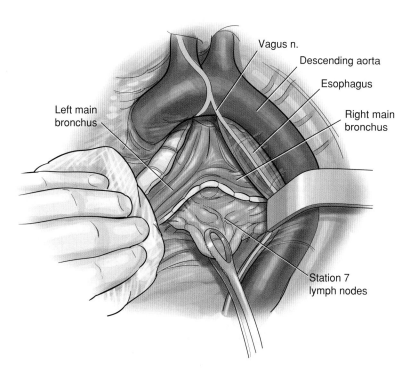

Vagus n.

Descending aorta

Esophagus

Left main
bronchus

Right main
bronchus

Station 7
lymph nodes

FIGURE 96.9 The subcarinal region as seem from the left chest has the same landmarks as previously noted. The station 7 lymph node packet extends from the carina superiorly to the upper border of the left lower lobe inferiorly.

The 10L lymph node station lies along the anterior and lateral surface of the left mainstem bronchus from the upper rim of the main pulmonary artery to the interlobar region inferiorly (Fig. 96.7). The greater length of the left main stem bronchus compared to the right assures dissection of this N1 station without first necessitating lung resection.

VATS MEDIASTINAL LYMPH NODE DISSECTION

Thoracoscopic lymph node dissection has become an accepted surgical method of MLND most often at the time of ipsilateral lung resection. The lymph node stations accessible through either a right- or left-sided VATS procedure are the same as for an open procedure. Similarly, access to lymph node stations 2L and 4L via a right VATS (stage N3 disease) or a left VATS (stage N2 disease) is difficult. A number of permutations (e.g., anterior or posterior) for thoracoscopic access are available and these same ports are generally used for the lymphatic dissection. Other versions of minimally invasive approaches may require special maneuvers to improve exposure (e.g., single-port technique).[35]

RIGHT THORACIC COMPARTMENT

A standard approach for placement of VATS incisions includes two small port incisions, one in the posterior axillary line at the 7th or 8th intercostal space and one in the anterior axillary line at the 5th intercostal space. A third utility incision is placed in the midaxillary line routinely in the 4th intercostal space and extended for a distance of 3 to 4 cm. Either a 5-mm or 10-mm 30-degree or preferably flexible thoracoscope can be placed as shown in Figure 96.10A. Lung retraction if necessary can expose the various regions of the mediastinum. Dissection is performed with the same concern for anatomic structures as in an open procedure. The lack of tactile sensation may make placement of a nasogastric tube helpful in avoiding esophageal injury. The right paratracheal region and its anatomy is well demonstrated in Video 96.1.[36] The diagram shows the location of the stations 3a and 3b lymph nodes for reference but are not included

in the dissection. The en bloc dissection of the right paratracheal 2R and 4R lymph node stations is begun inferior to the azygos vein and carried into the right tracheobronchial angle region. Cephalad to the azygos vein, the mediastinal pleura is incised along its superior rim and along the posterior border of the superior vena cava (Video 96.2).[36] Similar consideration is given to dividing the azygos vein as in the open procedure. Alternatively, because of the vantage point of an inferiorly placed thoracoscope, some surgeons prefer to work beneath a mobile azygos vein and elevate the pleura to dissect the 4R nodes from bottom up. Station 2R superiorly and 4R more inferiorly but cephalad to the lower border of the azygos vein can be either bluntly or sharply dissected. Small blood vessels are controlled best with endoclips or bipolar cautery. As shown, care is taken to protect the vagus nerve. As noted previously, the subcarinal region lies inferior to the azygos vein. A vertical incision in the mediastinal pleura in this location posterior to the right main stem bronchus and bronchus intermedius but just anterior to the esophagus will expose the subcarinal region or station 7 (Video 96.3).[36] The lymph nodes in this region which has the boundaries as noted previously can be completely dissected. Also noted in this video is the relationship of the thoracic duct to the dissection target. The deep boundary which is the left main stem bronchus can be easily recognized as a firm structure which contains the left-sided double-lumen endotracheal tube. Again, continuance of the dissection inferior to this region will expose the station 8 or periesophageal lymph nodes (Video 96.4).[36] The station 9 lymph nodes as noted previously can be accessed after division of the inferior pulmonary ligament (Video 96.5).[36] At times, it is necessary to depress the dome of the diaphragm with an endo instrument to improve exposure of this region while placing cephalad traction on the lower lobe. Station 10R lymph nodes can be dissected as in the open procedure along the anterior and lateral surface of the right main stem bronchus.

LEFT THORACIC COMPARTMENT

A similar set of three access incisions can be used on the left side (Fig. 96.10B). Placement and type of thoracoscope is again the same as for the right-sided VATS procedure. Appropriate lung retraction will expose the aortopulmonary window and para-aortic regions

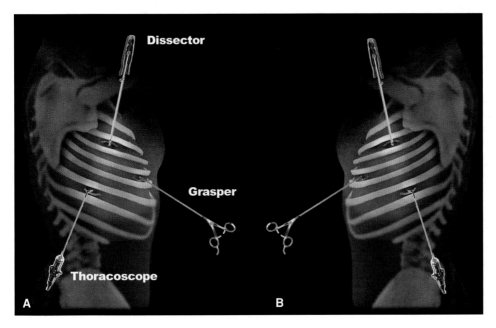

FIGURE 96.10 A three-incision access for a VATS dissection of the mediastinal lymph nodes is shown. The upper mid axillary access incision is routinely extended for 3 cm. The thoracoscope and grasping instruments can be easily switched between incisions. **A:** right chest view; **B:** left chest view.

nicely (lymph node stations 5 and 6, respectively) (Videos 96.6A and B).[36] As in the open procedure, protection of the phrenic and recurrent laryngeal nerves is critical while dissecting these lymph node stations. In particular, when one is using energy. Dissection of the subcarinal region from the left side is shown in Video 96.7.[36] Exposure, as noted previously, requires dissection of the left main stem bronchus and is greatly facilitated by its retraction as demonstrated in the video. This maneuver may cause dislodgment of a left-sided double-lumen endotracheal tube and must be addressed if it occurs. In addition, placing an endoscopic sling around the distal esophagus may also facilitate exposure.

Dissection of stations 9L and 10L can be achieved by similar techniques as those described previously.

TRANSCERVICAL EXTENDED MEDIASTINAL LYMPHADENECTOMY

A newer approach for systematic lymph node dissection is a transcervical approach developed by Zieliński.[37] This approach consists of five steps. First, creation of cervical flaps (Video 96.8): A collar incision is made to a length of 4 to 8 cm along a skin crease. Subplatysmal flaps are made in a plane deep to the external jugular veins after their division. Flaps are raised superiorly as far as possible and inferiorly to the sternal notch. At this time, a retrosternal plane of dissection is established. The strap muscles are then separated in the midline and the thyrothymic ligaments are divided on either side. On the right side, blunt dissection is used to divide the fascia over the innominate artery. During this dissection, level 1 lymph nodes may be harvested. Second, dissection of right paratracheal lymph nodes (Videos 96.9A and B): A retractor is placed to provide sternal lift, with the anesthesiologist taking care to provide adequate neck support. A plane of dissection is developed over the innominate artery to access the right paratracheal lymph node packet. Blunt dissection is used to separate the lymph nodes from the SVC and the trachea. Small vessels can be divided using a bipolar energy device or with clips. Third, subcarinal lymph node dissection (Videos 96.10A and B): A pretracheal plane of dissection is developed akin to that during a mediastinoscopy. The right main pulmonary artery is separated from the trachea. A mediastinoscope with distensible blades is placed in this space. The pulmonary artery is retracted away from the carina using the upper blade of the mediastinoscope. The subcarinal lymph node packet is then dissected with attention paid to obtain hemostasis and avoid injury to the esophagus. Fourth, left paratracheal lymph node dissection (Video 96.11): The left recurrent laryngeal nerve is identified and protected throughout dissection. The left paratracheal lymph node packet is dissected bluntly all the way to the tracheobronchial angle. The use of energy is avoided to prevent recurrent laryngeal nerve injury. Finally, dissection of the aortopulmonary lymph nodes (Video 96.12): A plane of dissection is developed over or under the innominate vein after dissecting it out. This plane is followed above the aortic arch to reach the aortopulmonary lymph node packet. This is then bluntly dissected off and harvested.

TEMLA has a high degree of accuracy for mediastinal staging, especially for pre-resectional staging after neoadjuvant therapy.

CONCLUSION

Lymph node dissection remains an important component of resectional surgery for lung cancer. It is useful for guiding further therapy and may confer a survival advantage. Proper dissection is performed by knowledge of the relevant landmarks as well as structures that must be protected to avoid morbidity. Dissection may be performed via traditional thoracotomy or equally efficiently by several minimally invasive methods. Proficiency in a number of these techniques should help to improve diagnostic accuracy and clinical outcomes for lung cancer patients.

REFERENCES

1. Cahan WG. Radical lobectomy. *J Thorac Cardiovasc Surg* 1960;39:555–572.
2. Cahan WG, Watson WL, Pool JL. Radical pneumonectomy. *J Thorac Surg* 1951; 22(5):449–473.
3. De Leyn P, Dooms C, Kuzdzal J, et al. Revised ESTS guidelines for preoperative mediastinal lymph node staging for non-small-cell lung cancer. *Eur J Cardiothorac Surg* 2014;45(5):787–798.
4. Tisi GM, Friedman PJ, Peters RM. American Thoracic Society. Medical section of the American Lung Association. Clinical staging of primary lung cancer. *Am Rev Respir Dis* 1983;127(5):659–664.
5. Mountain CF, Dresler CM. Regional lymph node classification for lung cancer staging. *Chest* 1997;111(6):1718–1723.
6. Naruke T, Suemasu K, Ishikawa S. Lymph node mapping and curability at various levels of metastasis in resected lung cancer. *J Thorac Cardiovasc Surg* 1978;76(6): 832–839.
7. Zieliński M, Rami-Porta R. Proposals for changes in the Mountain and Dresler mediastinal and pulmonary lymph node map. *J Thorac Oncol* 2007;2(1):3–6.
8. Rusch VW, Asamura H, Watanabe H, et al. The IASLC lung cancer staging project: a proposal for a new international lymph node map in the forthcoming seventh edition of the TNM classification for lung cancer. *J Thorac Oncol* 2009;4(5):568–577.
9. Tournoy KG, Annema JT, Krasnik M, et al., Endoscopic and endobronchial ultrasonography according to the proposed lymph node map definition in the seventh edition of the tumor, node, metastasis classification for lung cancer. *J Thorac Oncol* 2009; 4(12):1576–1584.
10. Ludwig MS, Goodman M, Miller DL, et al. Postoperative survival and the number of lymph nodes sampled during resection of node-negative non-small cell lung cancer. *Chest* 2005;128(3):1545–1550.
11. Legras A, Mordant P, Arame A, et al. Long-term survival of patients with pN2 lung cancer according to the pattern of lymphatic spread. *Ann Thorac Surg* 2014;97(4): 1156–1162.
12. Nwogu CE, Groman A, Fahey D, et al. Number of lymph nodes and metastatic lymph node ratio are associated with survival in lung cancer. *Ann Thorac Surg* 2012;93(5): 1614–1619; discussion 1619–1620.
13. Riquet M, Legras A, Mordant P, et al. Number of mediastinal lymph nodes in non-small cell lung cancer: a Gaussian curve, not a prognostic factor. *Ann Thorac Surg* 2014; 98(1):224–231.
14. Lardinois D, De Leyn P, Van Schil P, et al. ESTS guidelines for intraoperative lymph node staging in non-small cell lung cancer. *Eur J Cardiothorac Surg* 2006;30(5): 787–792.
15. Manser R, Wright G, Hart D, et al. Surgery for early stage non-small cell lung cancer. *Cochrane Database Syst Rev* 2005;(1):CD004699.
16. Wu Y, Huang ZF, Wang SY, et al. A randomized trial of systematic nodal dissection in resectable non-small cell lung cancer. *Lung Cancer* 2002;36(1):1–6.
17. Wright G, Manser RL, Byrnes G, et al. Surgery for non-small cell lung cancer: Systematic review and meta-analysis of randomised controlled trials. *Thorax* 2006;61(7):597–603.
18. Huang X, Wang J, Chen Q, et al. Mediastinal lymph node dissection versus mediastinal lymph node sampling for early stage non-small cell lung cancer: A systematic review and meta-analysis. *PLoS One* 2014;9(10):e109979.
19. Izbicki JR, Passlick B, Pantel K, et al. Effectiveness of radical systematic mediastinal lymphadenectomy in patients with resectable non-small cell lung cancer: results of a prospective randomized trial. *Ann Surg* 1998;227(1):138–144.
20. Darling GE, Allen MS, Decker PA, et al. Randomized trial of mediastinal lymph node sampling versus complete lymphadenectomy during pulmonary resection in the patient with N0 or N1 (less than hilar) non-small cell carcinoma: Results of the American College of Surgery Oncology Group Z0030 Trial. *J Thorac Cardiovasc Surg* 2011;141(3):662–670.
21. D'Andrilli A, Venuta F, Rendina EA. The role of lymphadenectomy in lung cancer surgery. *Thorac Surg Clin* 2012;22(2):227–237.
22. Hsu CP, Hsia JY, Chang GC, et al. Surgical-pathologic factors affect long-term outcomes in stage IB (pT2 N0 M0) non-small cell lung cancer: A heterogeneous disease. *J Thorac Cardiovasc Surg* 2009;138(2):426–433.
23. Prenzel KL, Baldus SE, Mönig SP, et al. Skip metastasis in nonsmall cell lung carcinoma: predictive markers and isolated tumor cells in N1 lymph nodes. *Cancer* 2004;100(9): 1909–1917.
24. Riquet M, Hidden G, Debesse B. Direct lymphatic drainage of lung segments to the mediastinal nodes. An anatomic study on 260 adults. *J Thorac Cardiovasc Surg* 1989;97(4):623–632.
25. Lee HS, Jang HJ. Thoracoscopic mediastinal lymph node dissection for lung cancer. *Semin Thorac Cardiovasc Surg* 2012;24(2):131–141.
26. Palade E, Passlick B, Osei-Agyemang T, et al. Video-assisted vs open mediastinal lymphadenectomy for Stage I non-small-cell lung cancer: results of a prospective randomized trial. *Eur J Cardiothorac Surg* 2013;44(2):244–249; discussion 249.

27. Ramos R, Girard P, Masuet C, et al. Mediastinal lymph node dissection in early-stage non-small cell lung cancer: totally thoracoscopic vs thoracotomy. *Eur J Cardiothorac Surg* 2012;41(6):1342–1348; discussion 1348.

28. Yang H, Li XD, Lai RC, et al. Complete mediastinal lymph node dissection in video-assisted thoracoscopic lobectomy versus lobectomy by thoracotomy. *Thorac Cardiovasc Surg* 2013;61(2):116–123.

29. Silvestri GA, Gonzalez AV, Jantz MA, et al. Methods for staging non-small cell lung cancer: Diagnosis and management of lung cancer, 3rd ed: American College of Chest Physicians evidence-based clinical practice guidelines. *Chest* 2013; 143(5 Suppl):e211S–e250S.

30. Minnich DJ, Bryant AS, Cerfolio RJ. Thoracoscopic and robotic dissection of mediastinal lymph nodes. *Thorac Surg Clin* 2012;22(2):215–218.

31. Cerfolio RJ, Bryant AS. Distribution and likelihood of lymph node metastasis based on the lobar location of nonsmall-cell lung cancer. *Ann Thorac Surg* 2006; 81(6):1969–1973; discussion 1973.

32. Takahashi K, Sasaki T, Nabaa B, et al. Pulmonary lymphatic drainage to the mediastinum based on computed tomographic observations of the primary complex of pulmonary histoplasmosis. *Acta Radiol* 2012;53(2):161–167.

33. Ichinose Y, Kato H, Koike T, et al. Completely resected stage IIIA non-small cell lung cancer: The significance of primary tumor location and N2 station. *J Thorac Cardiovasc Surg* 2001;122(4):803–808.

34. Kotoulas CS, Foroulis CN, et al. Involvement of lymphatic metastatic spread in non-small cell lung cancer accordingly to the primary cancer location. *Lung Cancer* 2004;44(2):183–191.

35. Wang BY, Tu CC, Liu CY, et al. Single-incision thoracoscopic lobectomy and segmentectomy with radical lymph node dissection. *Ann Thorac Surg* 2013;96(3):977–982.

36. Amer K. Systematic mediastinal nodal dissection by VATS. 2012. https://www.youtube.com/watch?v=ORVD7WK6PKs.

37. Zieliński M. The role of transcervical extended mediastinal lymphadenectomy for lung cancer staging. *Expert Rev Med Devices* 2011;8(6):665–667.

Unknown Primary Malignancy Metastatic to Thoracic Lymph Nodes

Marc Riquet ▪ Patrick Bagan

Metastatic lesions from an occult primary site represent 3% to 6% of cancers,[1-4] making carcinoma with an unknown primary the seventh most common malignancy.[2] Lymph nodes are the most common metastatic site and represent 31% to 46% of cases.[3,5-7] Cervical lymph node involvement by squamous cell carcinoma without a primary is the most frequent[3,5,8] and is commonly reported in the "head and neck" literature,[9,10] followed by isolated axillary nodal involvement by adenocarcinoma, almost exclusively affecting the women.[8] In contrast, metastatic cancer in thoracic lymph nodes (peribronchial or/ and hilar [N1] or mediastinal [N2])[11] is rare, or even absent in some series of unknown primaries.[5] It is more commonly reported as "case reports" (Tables 97.1 and 97.2), or more rarely short case series.[12-14] However, metastatic thoracic lymph nodes were mentioned as early as 1970 and represented 1.5% of Holmes and Fouts's unknown primary series.[3] In 2012, whole-body FDG-PET/CT scans performed for the detection of unknown primary demonstrated that 3.7% of patients had thoracic lymph node metastasis.[15]

The metastatic thoracic lymph nodes with unknown primary may be mediastinal or hilar, with the majority being mediastinal. The largest retrospective series on mediastinoscopy did not generally focus on this topic,[16,17] and the metastatic thoracic lymph nodes with unknown primary frequency were probably underestimated. Three series mentioned that 11% to 16% of mediastinal lymph nodes were metastases of an occult primary tumor and only represented small cohorts of 54,[18] 45,[19] and 23[20] patients, respectively. This last cohort consisted of less patients than those collected from the literature in Table 97.2 (n = 30), among whom six were diagnosed by mediastinoscopy and only two were subsequently resected.[21,22] The 16 remaining patients underwent an exploratory thoracotomy for a suspected but never confirmed lung cancer. In a short series of eight patients treated by surgery, a mediastinal lymphadenectomy was performed after mediastinoscopy in only one of them.[14] The suspicion of a lung tumor (n = 3) or hilar adenopathy (n = 4) motivated an exploratory thoracotomy in the other cases.

TABLE 97.1 Intrapulmonary or Hilar Metastatic Lymph Nodes: Reported Cases

Author	Sex/Age	Presentation	Location	Histology	Surgery	Adjuvant Therapy	Follow-up, Months (Status)
Gould[23]	M/57	Hemoptysis, L hilar enlargement	LLL	SCCa	Segmentectomy, LN resection	RT	108 (alive)
Kohdono[24]	M/56	Hoarseness, R hilar enlargement	R hilar	SmCCa	Upper lobe LN resection	None	16 (alive)
Nakamura[25]	M/51	Cough	L hilar (n 11)	SmCCa	LN resection	CT	24 (alive)
Kawasaki[26]	M/69	Routine chest x-ray	R hilar	LCCa	Bilobectomy, LN resection	None	20 (alive)
Kaneko[27]	M/63	Cough and sputum	R hilar	SCCa	R pneumonectomy, LN dissection	None	76 (alive)
Yoshino[28]	M/45	F/U examination	R hilar	AdenoCa	LN dissection	None	35 (alive)
Izumi[29]	M/63	Follow-up for colon cancer	R hilar (n 11 and n 12)	AdenoCa	Upper sleeve lobectomy, LN dissection	None	120 (alive)
Tomita[30]	M/56	Routine medical examination	L hilar	SCCa	LN dissection	None	32 (alive)

Unknown primary malignancy metastatic to thoracic lymph nodes (LN): characteristics of patients with intrapulmonary or hilar LNs (review of the literature). AdenoCa, adenocarcinoma; CT, chemotherapy; F/U, follow-up; L, left; LCCa, large cell carcinoma; LLL, left lower lobe; M, male; n, station number; R, right; RT, radiotherapy; SCCa, squamous cell carcinoma; SmCCa, small cell carcinoma.

TABLE 97.2 Mediastinal Lymph Nodes: Reported Cases

Author	Sex/Age	Presentation	Location	Histology	Surgery	Adjuvant Therapy	Follow-up, Months (Status)
Gould[23]	M/44	Hemoptysis, L hilar enlargement	AP window	UCa	Pneumonectomy LN resection	None	36 (alive, recurrence)
	M/61	F/U, R hilar enlargement	R mediastinum	UCa	LN resection	RT	13 (alive)
Morita[31]	M/56	F/U, mediastinal tumor	R mediastinum	SCCa	Right lower lobectomy, LN resection	None	20 (alive)
Masaki[32]	M/44	Chest pain	R mediastinum	Poorly diff AdenoCa	LN dissection	CT+RT	36 (alive)
Sawada[33]	M/67	Fever, mediastinal LN	R mediastinum	Poorly diff AdenoCa	LN resection	None	23 (alive)
Kohdono[24]	M/67	Hoarseness	L mediastinum	LCCa	LN resection	RT	9 (dead)
	F/58	Hoarseness	L mediastinum	LCCa	Left upper lobectomy LN resection	RT	6 (alive)
Tisdale[34]	M/54	Trousseau's syndrome	R mediastinum	Poorly diff Ca	Mediastinoscopy	CT+RT	NA
	M/50	Trousseau's syndrome	L mediastinum	Poorly diff Ca	Mediastinoscopy	CT+RT	18 (alive) progression/recurrence
Yodonawa[22]	M/65	Mediastinal enlargement	R mediastinum	SCCa	Mediastinoscopy LN resection	RT	12 (alive)
Blanco[35]	M/56	Hemoptysis, subcarinal mass	Mediastinum	SCCa	LN resection	CT + RT	NA (alive)
Sakuraba[36]	M/63	Enlarged R hilus	R mediastinum	SCCa	LN resection	None	34 (lobectomy) 43 (alive)
	M/73	Enlarged L hilus	Mediastinum and L hilar	SCCa	Mediastinoscopy	CT	5 (alive)
	M/57	Mediastinal enlargement	R mediastinum	AdenoCa	LN resection (sternotomy)	RT	5 (alive)
Chen[12]	M/58	Mediastinal enlargement	R mediastinum	AdenoCa	LN resection	CT+RT	33 (alive)
	M/68	Mediastinal enlargement	R mediastinum	SCCa	LN resection	RT	14-pneumonectomy 20 (dead)
	M/59	Mediastinal enlargement	R mediastinum	SCCa	Mediastinoscopy	RT	24 (alive)
	M/65	Mediastinal enlargement	R mediastinum	Clear cell Ca	LN resection (sternotomy)	None	51 (alive)
Ida[37]	F/62	Elevated CEA	NA	AdenoCa	Biopsy (thoracotomy)	Angiotensin II	NA (alive–CEA decreased)
Kamiyoshihara[21]	M/62	Enlarged LN	L hilar	UCa	LN dissection (VATS)	None	8 (alive)
Morita[38]	F/57	Mediastinal mass	R mediastinum	Carcinoma	LN resection (sternotomy)	RT	NA
Adachi[39]	M/78	Elevated CEA level	R mediastinum	Poorly diff AdenoCa	Wedge upper lobe LN resection	RT	6 (alive)
Miwa[13]	M/72	Neck tumor	R mediastinum	Poorly diff SCCa	LN resection	RT	44 (alive)
	M78	No symptom	R mediastinum	Poorly diff AdenoCa	LN resection	RT	82 (alive)
	M/70	No symptom	R mediastinum	Poorly diff SCCa	Biopsy (VATS)	CT+RT	24 (alive)
	M/70	Hoarseness	L mediastinum	UCa	Biopsy (VATS)	CT+RT	33 (alive)

(continued)

TABLE 97.2 Mediastinal Lymph Nodes: Reported Cases (*Continued*)

Author	Sex/Age	Presentation	Location	Histology	Surgery	Adjuvant Therapy	Follow-up, Months (Status)
Shiota[40]	M/68	Cough/chest pain	R mediastinum	AdenoCa	Mediastinoscopy	CT+RT	22 (alive)
Nakano[41]	M/68	No symptoms	B mediastinum	Poorly diff AdenoCa	LN resection (B-VATS)	CT+RT	48 (alive)[a]
Yoshizu[42]	F/71	Mediastinal mass	R mediastinum	Poorly diff AdenoCa	LN resection	NA	24 (alive)
Harada[43]	F/83	Mediastinal mass	R mediastinum	Poorly diff AdenoCa	LN dissection	None	38 (alive, NED)[b]

Unknown primary malignancy metastatic to thoracic lymph nodes (LN): characteristics of patients with mediastinal involved LNs (review of the literature).
[a]the second thoracoscopy was performed after chemotherapy.
[b]mediastinal LN recurrence resected after the first operation.
AdenoCa, adenocarcinoma; AP, aortopulmonary; B, bilateral; CEA, carcinoembryonal antigen; CT, chemotherapy; Diff, differentiated; F, female; F/U, follow-up; L, left; LCCa, large cell carcinoma; LLL, left lower lobe; M, male; n, station number; NA, not available; NED, no evidence of disease; R, right; RT, radiotherapy; SCCa, squamous cell carcinoma; SmCCa, small cell carcinoma; UCa, undifferentiated Ca; VATS, video-assisted thoracoscopic surgery.

The diagnosis traditionally has been obtained by mediastinoscopy. Nowadays a diagnosis can be obtained, in most cases, by endobronchial ultrasound-guided transbronchial needle aspiration (EBUS-TBNA).[44,45] EBUS-TBNA not only may identify metastases in mediastinal lymph nodes, but also in hilar nodes, which may represent up to 26% of lymph node stations biopsied by this technique.[46] Although hilar lymph nodes produce a lower yield (64%) than mediastinal lymph nodes (72%) when examining lymph node specimens,[47] EBUS-guided transbronchial procedures permit avoidance of thoracotomy or thoracoscopy in about two thirds of "N1" patients.[47] This information may be skewed in either direction since most large retrospective series of both mediastinoscopy and EBUS-TBNA do not generally focus on this topic.

Reviews of the literature[8,48,49] state that patients with metastases from an unknown primary malignancy have a median survival of approximately 6 months despite therapy. Some patients with extrathoracic lymph node metastases (axillary, cervical, and inguinal) have had a better outcome with appropriate treatment. However, some patients with isolated metastases to thoracic lymph nodes may have prolonged survival after treatment including surgery, as shown in Tables 97.1 and 97.2. Therefore, awareness of this option is of paramount importance and must be discussed as part of comprehensive care in pre-therapy multidisciplinary tumor board conferences.

Particular characteristics of patients with unknown primary malignancies metastatic to thoracic lymph nodes were described in a short series[14] and 38 other cases available in the literature are given in Tables 97.1 and 97.2. About 21% of patients presented with purely intrapulmonary metastasis (T0N1, Table 97.1) and 79% mediastinal metastasis (N2, Table 97.2).

A specific profile for metastasis may be discerned as follows: mainly male patients (87%), most often right-sided (62.5% and 56.8% for N1 and N2 categories, respectively) and the age interval between 45 and 69 years for N1 patients and 44 and 83 years for N2 patients. Histology was either a squamous cell carcinoma or adenocarcinoma with no undifferentiated tumors for the N1 category. For N2 patients, 53% of cases were based on an aggressive histologic type, poorly or totally undifferentiated. No adjuvant treatment was given in 75% of N1 patients. The majority of N2 patients (76.7%) were treated with surgery, adjuvant treatment being given in 65% of them. The remaining patients underwent chemotherapy, radiotherapy, or both.

No deaths or disease recurrences were observed in N1 patients, in contrast with N2 patients. The latter category had an excess of events (death or recurrence in 23% of cases). The upper mediastinum was always concerned (aortopulmonary 5 and 6 lymph nodes on the left and paratracheal 4R and 2R lymph nodes on the right) except in one case (tracheal bifurcation, station 7). In case of mediastinal metastases, intrapulmonary "N1s" were observed in 20% of cases.

The N1 involvement (alone or associated with N2) was the main cause of lung resections; nine lobectomies and five pneumonectomies were performed. Mediastinal lymph node resection was generally performed by thoracotomy, more rarely by a video-assisted thoracoscopic surgery procedure[21,41,43] and sternotomy.[12,36,38] Resection of intrapulmonary lymph nodes alone was performed in some cases.[14,28,25,30] It may be technically difficult, since this kind of surgery requires a careful dissection to avoid injuring pulmonary vessels as well as lung resection.

Thoracic lymph node metastases are generally observed when the primary malignancy is easily recognized. Mediastinal lymph node metastases of infradiaphragmatic malignancies are possible[50] but rarely appear as isolated secondary sites. Lymph node metastases with a clear-cell carcinoma histology were reported in one patient.[12] A renal cancer origin may be hypothesized in such a case and metastases explained by lymph reflux from the thoracic duct.[51,52] In fact, most metastatic thoracic lymph nodes are due to small-cell or non-small-cell lung cancers, the lymphatic drainage of lungs passing through these lymph nodes (N1 and N2 stations) being commonly involved.[11,53]

Some solitary bulky mediastinal masses can mimic a lymphoma on thoracic computed tomography (CT). These lymphoma-like tumors involving the anterior and middle mediastinum were in fact epithelial cancers, with histology of well- or moderately differentiated adenocarcinoma.[54] As a problem of differential diagnosis, we must exclude some mediastinal masses with a particular histologic profile as mediastinal signet-ring cell carcinomas with a poorly determined cytokeratin distribution.[55]

The hypothesis of thoracic lymph node metastases arising from unknown primary is based on the fact that the patient has no history of a previous cancer (detailed medical history) and that no primary tumor was discovered after a complete physical examination and a thorough workup.[49] Some areas of the guidelines for the diagnosis and management of metastatic malignant disease of unknown primary developed by the National Institute for Health and Clinical Excellence (NICE) in the United Kingdom were summarized and discussed by Taylor et al.[56] The radiological management is essential.[56] Whole-body 18F-fluoro-2-deoxyglucose positron emission tomography/CT is a major diagnostic tool.[15,56,57] Histology is particularly important.[56]

Histologic and immunohistochemical studies of the mediastinal, hilar, or/and peribronchial lymph node metastases are performed to confirm the epithelial nature of the malignant cells, search for the primary site, and eliminate possible endogenous lymph node origin.[23]

Histologic studies are routinely conducted using paraffin-embedded specimens, stained with hematoxylin and eosin (H&E) and periodic acid–Schiff reaction with diastase digestion. For immunohistochemistry, serial paraffin sections are stained with various antibodies: EMA, AE1/AE3, PS100, CD45, p63, CK7, CK20, TTF1, CD117, thyroglobulin, CD5, NCAM, synaptophysin, and PSA. The first four antibodies are used to confirm an epithelial differentiation (EMA+AE1/AE3+) and rule out a melanoma metastasis (PS100+) or a lymphoma (CD45+). If the epithelial differentiation is confirmed, a second set of antibodies is performed. In poorly differentiated lesions, p63 can evidence a squamous cell differentiation, NCAM and synaptophysin neuroendocrine differentiation. Cytokeratin CK7 is found in a wide variety of epithelial structures and adenocarcinomas, including the lung. Its major utility is to exclude colorectal adenocarcinomas (CK7–CK20+). Other gastrointestinal tumors are CK7+CK20+–. Thus, the use of both antigens (CK7/CK20) is valuable in determining the primary site in poorly differentiated adenocarcinomas. TTF1 is a tissue-specific transcription factor expressed in normal lung and thyroid epithelial cells. Therefore it is a very useful immunohistochemical marker in the diagnosis of tumors of lung origin.[58,59] CD5 and CD117 along with p63 positivities hint at a primitive thymic carcinoma. CD117 is also useful to rule out a seminoma. Complementary use of some markers (PSA, thyroglobulin) can rule out other possible primary sites (prostate, thyroid).

Metastatic cancers may remain undiagnosed, with no primary origin, for several reasons. Three main causes are commonly suggested.[24] Firstly, the primary tumor is not large enough to be apparent by current means of clinical, radiologic, or pathologic examination. This suggests that the tumor failed to develop during follow-up. Long-term follow-up is mandatory in such instances because the primary tumor has been shown to become evident long after lymphadenectomy (14 months[12] and 34 months,[36] respectively). Secondly, the primary tumor was removed in the past but unrecognized. This is explained by a previous surgery. However, immunohistochemistry may demonstrate that previously removed tumors were not the primary.[29] Thirdly, the primary tumor may have regressed spontaneously. For example, while it is exceptional to see a lung cancer that "disappears," such instances have been reported by Sperduto et al.,[60] with no lymph nodes involvement, and by Kohdono et al.,[24] thoracic lymph nodes being in the latter case the only metastatic sites.

A fourth hypothesis has been formulated by Gould et al.[23]: that there is no distant primary site and the cancer arises from endogenous cells present within the affected lymph nodes. This has never been demonstrated by recent immunohistochemical studies. However, cancer can arise from mesothelial[61,62] or epithelial inclusions of lymph nodes themselves. The latter event is a common finding in high cervical lymph nodes.[63] Benign glandular inclusions within intrapulmonary lymph nodes have been described by Lin in a fetus[64] and were more recently reported in two adult patients.[14] Such endogenous origin is of paramount importance and requires further research.

Thus, cancer from an unknown primary might be a distinct entity with specific genetic/phenotypic aberrations that define it as "primary metastatic disease." Pentheroudakis et al.[65] reviewed the literature concerning the molecular biology of cancers of unknown primaries (chromosomal abnormalities, oncogenes and oncoproteins, tumor suppressor genes and proteins, angiogenesis). The different results failed to identify an unknown primary-specific molecular signature, leading the authors to suggest that, if it exists, it probably consists of a multigene expression pattern not captured by single-gene studies. More particularly, concerning angiogenesis, it was observed that metastases of squamous cell carcinoma of unknown primary were able to develop a metastatic phenotype and grow at metastatic lymph node sites, and that angiogenesis was redundant for lymph node metastasis.[66] However, emerging studies reviewed by Christiansen and Detmar[67] suggest that tumor-induced lymphangiogenesis promotes metastasis to lymph node and that lymphangiogenic factors act to prepare a premetastatic niche conducive to the establishment of secondary tumors. Ongoing work should focus on lymphangiogenesis in the metastatic lymph nodes of unknown primary[66] and shed new light on that topic.

Patients with metastatic thoracic lymph nodes treated medically have a poor outcome. Surgical treatment either combined with chemotherapy and/or radiation therapy may offer a chance of a cure and an increased survival.[14,18] This was confirmed for both groups of patients (N1 and N2), as shown in Tables 97.1 and 97.2. It compares with increased long-term survival following surgery, as reported for extrathoracic lymph node metastases without primary sites.[5,68–70] The fact that cancer can arise from intranodal epithelial inclusions further supports the validity of surgical removal.

In conclusion, metastatic thoracic lymph nodes with unknown primaries represent a rare entity, but the frequency is probably underestimated. Prolonged survival is obtained by surgery in those cases diagnosed and resected during exploratory thoracotomy. Cases diagnosed by mediastinoscopy or EBUS-guided TBNA are apparently considered to represent metastatic malignancy and hence not amenable to surgery. Attention must be drawn to this entity, as surgery may have a favorable impact on prognosis in those particular cases of unknown primary where lymphadenectomy is possible. To reiterate, it is imperative that resection options be discussed as part of comprehensive care in pre-therapy multidisciplinary tumor board conferences.

REFERENCES

1. Altman E, Cadman E. An analysis of 1,539 patients with cancer of unknown primary site. *Cancer* 1986;57:120–124.
2. Greenlee RT, Murray T, Bolden S, et al. Cancer statistics, 2000. *CA Cancer J Clin* 2000;50:7–33.
3. Holmes FF, Fouts TL. Metastatic cancer of unknown primary site. *Cancer* 1970;26:816–820.
4. Shaw PH, Adams R, Jordan C, et al. A clinical review of the investigation and management of carcinoma of unknown primary in a single center network. *Clin Oncol* 2007;19:87–95.1439.
5. Greager JA, Wood D, Das Gupta TK. Metastatic Cancer from an undetermined primary site. *J Surg Oncol* 1983;23:73–76.
6. Le Chevalier T, Cvitkovic E, Caille P, et al. Early metastatic cancer of unknown primary origin at presentation. A clinical study of 302 consecutive autopsied patients. *Arch Intern Med* 1988;148:2035–2039.
7. Séve P, Billotey C, Broussolle C, et al. The role of 2-deoxy-2-f-18 fluoro-D-glucose positron emission tomography in disseminated carcinoma of unknown primary site. *Cancer* 2007;109:292–299.
8. Pavlidis N, Pentheroudakis G. Cancer of unknown primary site. *Lancet* 2012;379:1428–1435.
9. Aassar OS, Fischbein NJ, Caputo GR, et al. Metastatic head and neck cancer: role and usefulness of FDG PET in locating occult primary tumors. *Radiology* 1999;210:177–181.
10. Greven KM, Keyes JW, Williams DW, et al. Occult primary tumors of the head and neck: lack of benefit from positron emission tomography imaging with 2-(F-18) fluoro-2-deoxy-D-glucose. *Cancer* 1999;86:114–118.
11. Mountain CF, Dresler CM. Regional lymph node classification for lung cancer staging. *Chest* 1997;111:1718–1723.
12. Chen F, Tatsumi A, Nu E, et al. Four cases of cancer of unknown primary site that manifested as mediastinal metastatic lesions (abstract). *Nihon Kokyuki Gakkai Zasshi* 1999;37:1003–1007.
13. Miwa K, Fujioka S, Adachi Y, et al. Mediastinal lymph node carcinoma of an unknown primary site: clinicopathological examination. *Gen Thorac Cardiovasc Syrg* 2009;57:239–243.
14. Riquet M, Badoual C, Le Pimpec Barthes F, et al. Metastatic thoracic lymph node carcinoma with unknown primary site. *Ann Thorac Surg* 2003;75:244–249.
15. Tamam MO, Mulazimoglu M, Guveli TK, et al. Prediction of survival and evaluation of diagnostic accuracy whole body 18F-fluoro-2-deoxyglucose positron emission tomography/computed tomography in the detection carcinoma of unknown primary origin. *Eur Rev Med Pharmacol Sci* 2012;16:2120–2130.

16. Hammoud ZT, Anderson RC, Meyers BF, et al. The current role of mediastinoscopy in the evaluation of thoracic disease. *J Thorac Cardiovasc Surg* 1999;118:894–899.

17. Lemaire A, Nikolic I, Petersen T, et al. Nine-year single center experience with cervical mediastinoscopy: complications and false negative rate. *Ann Thorac Surg* 2006;82:1185–1190.

18. Faure E, Riquet M, Lombe-Weta PM, et al. Malignant mediastinal lymph nodes tumors with unknown primary cancers. *Rev Mal Resp* 2000;17:1095–1099.

19. Couraud L, Houdelette P, Morales F, et al. The role of mediastinoscopy in the diagnosis of pulmonary and mediastinal diseases: review of 400 patients. *Rev Fr Mal Resp* 1979;7:587–590.

20. Thomas de Montpréville V, Dulmet EM, Nashashibi N. Frozen section diagnosis and surgical biopsy of lymph nodes, tumors and pseudotumors of the mediastinum. *Eur J Cardiothorac Surg* 1998;13:190–195.

21. Kamiyoshihara M, Ishikawa S, Kobayashi K, et al. Mediastinal lymph node carcinoma without apparent primary lesion: report of case (abstract). *Kyobu Geka* 2001;54:521–523.

22. Yodonawa S, Mitsui K, Akaogi E, et al. Squamous cell carcinoma of unknown origin affecting mediastinal lymph nodes (abstract). *Nihon Kyobu Shikkan Gakkai Zasshin* 1996;34:1344–1348.

23. Gould VE, Warren WH, Faber P, et al. Malignant cells of epithelial phenotype limited to thoracic lymph nodes. *Eur J Cancer* 1990;26:1121–1126.

24. Kohdono S, Ishidada T, Fukuyama Y, et al. Lymph node cancer of the mediastinal or hilar region with an unknown primary site. *J Surg Oncol* 1995;58:196–200.

25. Nakamura K, Isobe T, Okusaki K, et al. A suspected case of T0N1M0 small cell carcinoma of the lung (abstract). *Nihon Kyobu Shikkan Gakkai Zasshi,* 1994;32:814–818.

26. Kawasaki H, Yoshida J, Yokose T, et al. Primary unknown cancer in pulmonary hilar lymph node with spontaneous transient regression: report of a case. *Jpn J Clin Oncol* 1998;28:405–409.

27. Kaneko K, Yamanda T, Han'uda M, et al. Metastatic squamous cell carcinoma of hilar lymph node with unknown primary site (abstract). *Nihon Kokyuki Gakkai Zasshi* 2000;38:39–44.

28. Yoshino N, Yamaushi S, Hino M, et al. Metastatic thoracic lymph node carcinoma of unknown origin on which we performed two kinds of immunohistochemical examinations. *Ann Thorac Cardiovasc Surg* 2006;12:283–286.

29. Izumi Y, Mukai M, Kikuchi K, et al. Long-term survival after incomplete resection of immunohistochemically diagnosed T0N1 lung cancer: report of a case. *Surg Today* 2006;36:270–273.

30. Tomita M, Matsuzaki Y, Shimizu T, et al. Squamous cell carcinoma of the Hilar Lymph Node with Unknown Primary Tumor: a case report. *Ann Thorac Cardiovasc Surg* 2008;14:242–245.

31. Morita Y, Yamagishi M, Shijubo N, et al. Squamous cell carcinoma of unknown origin in middle mediastinum. *Respiration* 1992;59:344–346.

32. Masaki Y, Yamamoto M, Nishimura H, et al. A case of unknown origin cancer of the mediastinal lymph node. *J Jpn Asso Thoracic Surg* 1992;40:574–577.

33. Sawada M, Ohdama S, Umino T, et al. Metastasis of an adenocarcinoma of unknown origin to mediastinal lymph nodes, and transient regression (abstract). *Nihon Kyobu Shikkan Gakkai Zasshi* 1994;32:867–872.

34. Tisdale JF, Snowden TR, Johnson DR. Case report: Poorly differentiated carcinoma of unknown primary presenting as Trousseau' syndrome. *Am J Med Sci* 1995;309:183–187.

35. Blanco N, Kirgan DM, Little AG. Metastatic squamous cell carcinoma of the mediastinum with unknown primary tumor. *Chest* 1998;114:938–940.

36. Sakuraba M, Mae M, Oonuki T, et al. Mediastinal and hilar lymph node of unknown origin: 3 case reports (abstract). *Nihon Kokyuki Gakkai Zasshi* 1999;37:72–77.

37. Ida K, Kamiya T. Induced hypertensive chemotherapy with angiotensine II found effective for mediastinal lymph node metastases of unknown origin (abstract). *Gan To Kagaku Ryoho* 2000;27:2263–2266.

38. Morita M, Nakai Y, Kakimoto S, et al. Mediastinal lymph node carcinoma with no apparent primary lesion; report of a case (abstract). *Kyobu Geka* 2003;56:1154–1157.

39. Adachi Y, Nakamura H, Nitta S. Mediastinal lymph node adenocarcinoma with unknown primary site: report of a case (abstract). *Kyobu Geka* 2006;59: 5587–5601.

40. Shiota Y, Imai S, Sasaki N, et al. A case of mediastinal lymph node carcinoma of unknown primary site treated with docetaxel and cisplatin with concurrent thoracic radiation therapy. *Acta Med Okayama* 2011;65:407–411.

41. Nakano T, Endo S, Endo T, et al. Multimodal treatment for multistation mediastinal lymph node adenocarcinoma: a case report. *Ann Thorac Cardiovasc Surg* 2012;18: 136–139.

42. Yoshizu A, Kamiya K. Mediastinal lymph node carcinoma of unknown primary site; report of a case (abstract). *Kyobu Geka* 2012;65:507–509.

43. Harada H, Yamashita Y, Kuraoka K, et al. Sequential mediastinal lymphadenectomy of an unknown primary tumor. *Ann Thorac Surg* 2013;95:687–689.

44. Chow A, Oki M, Saka H, et al. Metastatic mediastinal lymph node from an unidentified primary papillary thyroid carcinoma diagnosed by endobronchial ultrasound-guided transbronchial needle aspiration. *Intern Med* 2009;48:1293–1296.

45. Medford ARL. Endobronchial ultrasound-guided transbronchial needle aspiration. *Polskie Arciw Med Wewn* 2010;120:459–466.

46. Rintoul RC, Tournoy KG, El Daly H, et al. EBUS-TBNA for the clarification of PET positive intra-thoracic lymph nodes—an international multi-centre experience. *J Thorac Oncol* 2009;4:44–48.

47. Karunamurthy A, Cai G, Dacic S, et al. Evaluation of endobronchial ultrasound-guided fine-needle aspirations (EBUS-FNA). *Cancer Cytopathol* 2014;122: 23–32.

48. Ghosh L, Dahut R, Kakar S, et al. Management of patients with metastatic cancer of unknown primary. *Curr Probl Surg* 2005;42:12–66.

49. Pavlidis N, Briasoulis E, Hainsworth J, et al. Diagnostic and therapeutic management of cancer of an unknown primary. *Eur J Cancer* 2003;39:1990–2005.

50. Mahon TG, Libshitz HI. Mediastinal metastases of infradiaphragmatic malignancies. *Eur J Radiol* 1992;15:130–134.

51. Assouad J, Riquet M, Berna P, et al. Intrapulmonary lymph nodes metastases and renal cell carcinoma. *Eur J Cardiothorac Surg* 2007;31:132–134.

52. Reinke RT, Higgins CB, Niwayama G, et al. Bilateral pulmonary hilar lymphadenopathy. An unusual manifestation of metastatic renal cell carcinoma. *Radiology* 1976;121:49–53.

53. Rouvière H. Lymphatic vessels of the lungs and intrathoracic lymph nodes. *Ann Anat Pathol* 1929;6:113–158.

54. Sorgho-Lougue LC, Luciani A, Kobeiter H, et al. Adenocarcinomas of unknown primary (ACUP) of the mediastinum mimicking lymphoma: CT findings at diagnosis and follow-up. *Eur J Radiol* 2006;59:42–48.

55. Kusakari C, Soda H, Nakamura Y, et al. Mediastinal signet-ring cell carcinoma of unknown primary: long-term survival by treatment with S-1, a novel derivative of 5-fluorouracil. *Lung Cancer* 2007;56:139–141.

56. Taylor MB, Bromham NR, Arnold SE. Carcinoma of unknown primary: key radiological issues from the recent National Institute for Health and Clinical Excellence guidelines. *Br J Radiol.* 2012;85:661–671.

57. Hundahl Moller AK, Loft A, Kiil Berthelsen A, et al. 18F-FDG PET/CT as a diagnostic tool in patients with extracervical carcinoma of unknown primary site: a literature review. *Oncologist* 2011;16:446–451.

58. Hammar S. Metastatic adenocarcinoma of unknown primary origin. *Hum Pathol* 1998;29:1393–1402.

59. Ordonez NG. Thyroid transcription factor-1 is a marker of lung and thyroid carcinomas. *Adv Anat Pathol* 2000;7:123–127.

60. Sperduto P, Vaezy A, Bridgman A, et al. Spontaneous regression of squamous cell lung carcinoma with adrenal metastasis. *Chest* 1988;94:887–889.

61. Isolato PA, Veinot JP, Jabi M. Hyperplastic mesothelial cells in mediastinal lymph node sinuses with extranodal lymphatic involvement. *Arch Pathol Lab Med* 2000; 124:609–613.

62. Parkash V, Vidwans M, Carter D. Benign mesothelial cells in mediastinal lymph nodes. *Am J Surg Pathol* 1999;23:1264–1269.

63. Lymph nodes. In: Rosai J, ed. *Ackerman's Surgical Pathology,* 8th ed. St. Louis, MO: Mosby; 1996:1661–1773.

64. Lin CS. Benign glandular inclusions. *Am J Surg Pathol* 1980;4:413.

65. Pentheroudakis G, Briasoulis E, Pavlidis N. Cancer of unknown primary site: missing primary or missing biology? *Oncologist* 2007;12:418–425.

66. Agarwal B, Das P, Naresh KN, et al. Angiogenic ability of metastatic squamous carcinoma in the cervical lymph nodes from unknown primary tumours. *J Clin Path* 2011;64:765–770.

67. Christiansen A, Detmar M. Lymphangiogenesis and Cancer. *Genes Cancer* 2011;2: 1146–1158.

68. Didolkar MS, Fanous N, Elias EG, et al. Metastatic carcinomas from occult primary tumors. A study of 254 patients. *Ann Surg* 1977;186:625–630.

69. Guarischi A, Keane TJ, Elhakim T. Metastatic inguinal nodes from an unknown primary neoplasm. *Cancer* 1987;59:572–577.

70. Lefebvre JL, Coche-Dequeant B, Ton Van J, et al. Cervical lymph nodes from an unknown primary tumor in 190 patients. *Am J Surg* 1990;60:443–446.

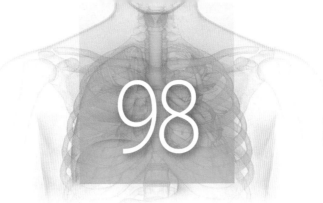

98

Adjuvant Chemotherapy for Non-Small-Cell Lung Cancer

Lingling Du ▪ Ramaswamy Govindan ▪ Saiama N. Waqar

INTRODUCTION

Lung cancer is the leading cause of cancer-related mortality in the United States.[1] Non-small-cell lung cancer (NSCLC) comprises of 87% of all lung cancer cases.[2] Approximately 30% of patients with NSCLC present with early stage disease, while another 30% had locally advanced disease at diagnosis.[3] Surgery provides the chance of cure in nonmetastatic NSCLC. However, even in the setting of complete surgical resection, the 5-year survival rate was only 60% for stage I NSCLC, and plummets to 25% for stage IIIA disease.[4] The distant relapse rate increases as related to a higher stage of disease, with a 5-year distant relapse rate of 15% for stage IA and 60% for stage IIIA NSCLC, respectively.[4] These data suggest that NSCLC might be a systemic disease with micrometastasis even at early stages. A systemic approach such as chemotherapy may improve outcome especially in patients with higher stage of resected NSCLC. Over the past few decades, researchers have examined the role of adjuvant therapy in resected NSCLC. The major clinical trials are reviewed in this chapter.

EARLY STUDIES ON ADJUVANT CHEMOTHERAPY

Early studies evaluated the role of adjuvant CAP (cyclophosphamide, doxorubicin, and cisplatin) in resected NSCLC.[5,6] These trials failed to show a survival benefit. The NSCLC Collaborative Group published their meta-analysis in 1995.[7] This study evaluated the role of chemotherapy in all stages of NSCLC, and included the data of 4,357 patients from 14 randomized trials of surgery with or without chemotherapy. In studies of cisplatin-based regimens, there was a trend toward better survival with chemotherapy compared to surgery alone (HR, 0.87; 95% CI 0.74–1.02; $p = 0.08$). However, this benefit was not statistically significant.

MAJOR CLINICAL TRIALS ON ADJUVANT CHEMOTHERAPY

Several large randomized studies using platinum with newer chemotherapeutic agents have demonstrated survival benefit of adjuvant chemotherapy (Table 98.1). The Adjuvant Lung Project Italy (ALPI) trial is a phase III study examining the efficacy of adjuvant MVP (mitomycin, vindesine, cisplatin) chemotherapy.[8] Patients with completely resected stage I to IIIA NSCLC were enrolled. A total of 1,209 patients were randomized to three cycles of postoperative MVP every 3 weeks versus observation. Sixty-nine percent of patients received all three planned cycles of chemotherapy. Adjuvant radiotherapy was allowed and administered in 82% of patients in the control group, and 65% of patients in the MVP group. Chemotherapy caused grade 3 and 4 neutropenia in 28% of patients. The ALPI trial failed to reveal a survival benefit of adjuvant MVP. The hazard ratio of chemotherapy was 0.96 for overall survival (OS; 95% CI 0.81–1.13; $p = 0.589$) and 0.89 for progress-free survival (PFS; 95% CI 0.76–1.03; $p = 0.128$).

TABLE 98.1 Major Trials of Adjuvant Chemotherapy						
Trial	Stage	No. of Pts	Study Arm	5-yr Survival Rate (%)	HR (95% CI)	p Value
ALPI[8]	I–IIIA	606	MVP		0.96 (0.81–1.13)	0.589
		603	Observation			
IALT[10]	I–IIIA	932	Cis + Etoposide/vinca alkaloids	44	0.86 (0.76–0.98)	<0.03
		935	Observation	40		
NCIC JBR.10[12]	IB–II	242	Cis + Vinorelbine	69	0.69 (0.52–0.91)	0.04
		240	Observation	54		
ANITA[13]	IB–IIIA	407	Cis + Vinorelbine	51	0.80 (0.66–0.96)	0.017
		433	Observation	43		
CALGB 9633[18]	IB	173	Carbo + Paclitaxel	60	0.83 (0.64–1.08)	0.12
		171	Observation	58		

No., number; pts, patients; yr, year; MVP, mitomycin, vindesine, cisplatin; cis, cisplatin; carbo, carboplatin.

The International Adjuvant Lung Cancer Trial (IALT) was the first large randomized study that demonstrated a survival advantage of adjuvant chemotherapy.[10] A total of 1,867 patients with resected stage I to IIIA NSCLC were randomly assigned to cisplatin-based chemotherapy or observation. Etoposide was given as the other agent in 56.5% of patients, vinorelbine in 26.8%, vinblastine in 11%, and vindesine in 5.8%. At a median follow-up of 56 months, adjuvant chemotherapy conferred a significantly prolonged survival, with an absolute benefit of 4% in 5-year survival rate (44.5% with chemotherapy vs. 40.4% with observation; HR, 0.86; 95% CI 0.76–0.98; p <0.03). The disease-free survival (DFS) also favored the chemotherapy arm, with a 5-year DFS rate of 39.4% (vs. 34.3% with observation; HR, 0.83; 95% CI 0.74–0.94; p <0.003). However, with a longer follow-up of 7.5 years, the initial survival advantage was no longer statistically significant in a later updated report (OS: HR, 0.91; 95% CI, 081–1.02; p = 0.10).[11]

The National Cancer Institute of Canada Clinical Trials Group (NCIC-CTG) North American Intergroup JBR.10 trial is one of the landmark studies establishing the role of adjuvant cisplatin and vinorelbine as the standard treatment for resected NSCLC.[12] This study randomly assigned 482 patients with resected stage IB to II NSCLC to four cycles of cisplatin (50 mg/m^2 on days 1 and 8) and vinorelbine (25 mg/m^2 weekly) every 4 weeks or observation. Radiotherapy was not allowed in the study. Adjuvant chemotherapy was commonly associated with neutropenia, fatigue, anorexia, constipation, and neuropathy. Seven percent of patients experienced febrile neutropenia. Grade 3 or greater nonhematologic toxicities were less common (<10%). The 5-year survival rate was significantly higher in the chemotherapy group than the control arm with an absolute increment of 15% (69% vs. 54%; p = 0.03). The hazard ratio was 0.69 for overall survival (95% CI 0.52–0.91; p = 0.04) and 0.60 for relapse-free survival (95% CI 0.45–0.97; p <0.001).

The Adjuvant Navelbine International Trialist Association (ANITA) trial is another pivotal study that revealed superior survival outcome of adjuvant cisplatin and vinorelbine over surgery alone.[13] Patients with resected stage IB–IIIA NSCLC were randomized to four cycles of postoperative cisplatin (100 mg/m^2 on day 1) and vinorelbine (30 mg/m^2 weekly) every 4 weeks versus observation. A total of 840 patients were recruited. Neutropenia was again the most common side effects experienced in 92% of patients. Nine percent of patients had febrile neutropenia. Deaths due to toxicities were recorded in 2% of patients. Despite these adverse events, adjuvant cisplatin and vinorelbine provided a sustained absolute benefit in survival rate, which was 8.6% at 5 years, and 8.4% at 7 years.

To consolidate the findings in previous randomized studies, the Lung Adjuvant Cisplatin Evaluation (LACE) meta-analysis[14] included five large trials of adjuvant cisplatin-based chemotherapy: ALPI,[8] IALT,[10] Big Lung Trial,[15] NCIC JBR.10,[12] and ANITA.[13] Data of 4,584 patients from the five studies were analyzed. Postoperative chemotherapy conferred a substantially better survival, with a hazard ratio of 0.89 for overall survival (95% CI 0.82–0.96; p = 0.005). The absolute benefit in 5-year survival rate was 5.4%. DFS was also improved with chemotherapy, with a hazard ratio of 0.84 (95% CI 0.78–0.91; p <0.001). Patients with stage II and III NSCLC derived significant benefit from adjuvant chemotherapy (stage II: HR, 0.83; 95% CI 0.73–0.95; stage III: HR, 0.83; 95% CI 0.72–0.94). In contrast, chemotherapy did not improve the survival outcome in patients with stage I disease. In fact, stage IA NSCLC even showed a trend toward worse survival with adjuvant chemotherapy (stage IA: HR, 1.40; 95% CI 0.95–2.06; stage IB: HR, 0.93; 95% CI 0.78–1.10). Among different chemotherapy regimens, cisplatin plus vinorelbine were associated with a better outcome compared to the combination of all other regimens (OS: p = 0.04; DFS: p = 0.02; post hoc analysis).

The LACE meta-analysis provided solid evidence of the benefit with adjuvant chemotherapy in patients with resected stage II and III NSCLC.

Cisplatin and vinorelbine also became the standard regimen with the most compelling evidence of its benefit. However, this regimen is associated with various side effects, especially high rates of neutropenia. Studies have explored the efficacy of other drugs that are associated with lesser toxicity. Pemetrexed is an antifolate agent targeting multiple enzymes essential in DNA synthesis and folate metabolism. In the metastatic setting, pemetrexed significantly prolongs the overall survival in patients with nonsquamous NSCLC.[16] The TREAT study is a phase II randomized trial comparing the combination of cisplatin and pemetrexed with cisplatin plus vinorelbine.[17] It randomized patients with resected stage IB–IIIA NSCLC to four cycles of either cisplatin (75 mg/m^2 on day 1) and pemetrexed (500 mg/m^2 on day 1) every 3 weeks or cisplatin (50 mg/m^2 on days 1 and 8) and vinorelbine (25 mg/m^2 weekly) every 4 weeks. The primary endpoint was the clinical feasibility rate, defined as no grade 4 neutropenia or thrombocytopenia, no grade 3 or 4 febrile neutropenia or nonhematologic toxicity, and no premature withdrawal or death. A total of 132 patients were assigned to the treatments, with 57% harboring a nonsquamous histology. The feasibility rates were superior in the cisplatin/pemetrexed group compared to cisplatin/vinorelbine (95.5% vs. 75.4%, p = 0.001). Ninety percent of the planned doses were delivered in the cisplatin/pemetrexed group, whereas in the cisplatin/vinorelbine group, only 66% of the planned cisplatin doses and 64% of the planned vinorelbine doses were administered (p <0.0001). At a mean follow-up of approximately 4 months, there was no difference in overall survival and PFS between the two arms. But the follow-up time is by all means too short to reveal any concrete survival benefits. This study supported the feasibility and the better tolerability of pemetrexed given in the adjuvant setting in resected NSCLC.

ISSUES WITH STAGE IB NSCLC

The role of adjuvant chemotherapy in patients with stage IB NSCLC remains to be elucidated. While the NCIC JBR.10 trial enrolling patients with stage IB and II NSCLC did not show a survival improvement with chemotherapy in patients with stage IB disease (p = 0.79), it also suggested that the effect of treatment does not depend on the stage of disease (p for difference in treatment efficacy according to disease stage = 0.13).[12] In the LACE meta-analysis, patients with stage IB NSCLC did not benefit from the addition of adjuvant chemotherapy (HR, 0.93; 95% CI 0.78–1.10).[14]

The Cancer and Leukemia Group B (CALGB) 9633 study was specifically designed to evaluate the role of adjuvant chemotherapy in patients with resected stage IB NSCLC.[18] A total of 344 patients were randomized to adjuvant carboplatin (area under the curve [AUC] 6/mL/min) and paclitaxel (200 mg/m^2) every 3 weeks for four cycles versus observation. Treatment was generally well tolerated. Only 35% of patients had grade 3 or 4 neutropenia. There were no treatment-related deaths reported. Survival was similar between the two groups (HR, 0.83; 95% CI 0.64–1.08; p = 0.12). However, subgroup analysis suggested a survival advantage of adjuvant chemotherapy in patients with tumors ≥4 cm (HR, 0.69; 95% CI 0.48–0.99; p = 0.043). In an updated report with a median follow-up of 9 years, the survival benefit of chemotherapy remained statistically insignificant.[19] Furthermore, the initial advantage observed in patients with tumors ≥4 cm did not hold up either, with a hazard ratio of 0.77 for OS (90% CI 0.57–1.04; p = 0.079). However, the interpretation of these results needs discretion. The study was underpowered due to poor accrual, and the subgroup analyses were not preplanned. Also, it should be noted that the sample size of patients with tumors ≥4 cm was very small, with 99 patients in the chemotherapy arm and 97 in the control arm, respectively. Therefore, the effect of adjuvant chemotherapy in patients with stage IB disease remains undefined.

CISPLATIN VERSUS CARBOPLATIN

Cisplatin was traditionally deemed to be slightly better than carboplatin in prolonging survival in metastatic NSCLC but with a different toxicity profile.[20] However, whether cisplatin is more superior than carboplatin in the adjuvant setting is unclear. A retrospective study compared the efficacy of carboplatin with cisplatin among patients 65 years or older using data from the Surveillance Epidemiology End Results (SEER) Medicare database.[21] A total of 636 patients who underwent resection for stage II–IIIA NSCLC and received adjuvant platinum-based chemotherapy were included. Cisplatin was administered in 16% of patients, while carboplatin was given in 77%. Seven percent of patients who received both cisplatin and carboplatin were excluded in the comparison. Those who received carboplatin had a lower rate of infection and emesis. Carboplatin and cisplatin provided comparable survival benefit, with a hazard ratio of 0.91 for carboplatin (95% CI 0.70–1.18). To date, there has been no randomized trial that directly compares carboplatin to cisplatin.

UFT-BASED CHEMOTHERAPY

Uracil–tegafur (UFT) is a combination of tegafur and uracil that is orally available. Tegafur is a prodrug, which is metabolized to 5-FU. It is given in combination with uracil, which is an inhibitor of dihydropyrimidine dehydrogenase, an enzyme that degrades 5-FU.[22] In Japan, multiple randomized trials have examined the effect of adjuvant UFT in patients with resected NSCLC.[23–27] The West Japan Study Group (WJSG) for Lung Cancer Surgery group first demonstrated a survival benefit of adjuvant UFT.[24] In this study, a total of 323 patients with completely resected stage I to III NSCLC were randomized to three groups: cisplatin/vindesine/UFT, UFT alone, or observation. The 5-year survival was 60.6% for the cisplatin/vindesine/UFT arm, 64.1% for the UFT arm, and 49.0% for the observation arm, respectively. Adjuvant UFT significantly improved survival outcome, with a hazard ratio of 0.55 for UFT versus observation (95% CI 0.36–0.86; $p = 0.009$), and 0.64 for cisplatin/vindesine/UFT versus observation (95% CI 0.42–0.97; $p = 0.037$).

A meta-analysis examined data from six trials comparing adjuvant UFT to observation alone.[28] The majority of patients had stage I NSCLC. Both the 5- and 7-year survival rate favored the UFT group. Five-year survival rate was 81.5% with adjuvant UFT compared to 77.2% with observation ($p = 0.011$). Seven-year survival rate was 76.5% with UFT versus 69.5% with observation ($p = 0.001$). The overall hazard ratio for postoperative UFT was 0.74 (95% CI 0.61–0.88; $p = 0.001$). A subgroup analysis of node-negative patients revealed that the survival benefit was more prominent in patients with T1b tumors (HR 0.62; 95% CI 0.42–0.90; log-rank $p = 0.011$), but not statistically significant in those with T1a disease (HR 0.84; 95% CI 0.58–1.23).[29] Although adjuvant UFT is recommended in Japan for the T1b subgroup of stage IA and stage IB NSCLC, it should be noted that there have been no studies of UFT conducted outside of Japan. Due to the potential pharmacogenomic differences among different populations, the use of UFT is not recommended outside of Japan.

ROLE OF ADJUVANT RADIATION WITH OR WITHOUT CHEMOTHERAPY

Studies have evaluated the impact of postoperative radiation on reducing the recurrence and improving the outcome of NSCLC. The Postoperative Radiotherapy (PORT) meta-analysis included ten randomized trials with a total of 2,232 patients.[30] Adjuvant radiation was found to have a detrimental effect on survival compared to surgery alone, with a hazard ratio of 1.18 ($p = 0.001$). Postoperative radiation

conferred an 18% increase in the relative risk of death over surgery alone. It did not provide any benefit in reducing either local or distant recurrence (HR 1.13 for local and 1.14 for distant recurrence, respectively; $p = 0.02$ for both). However, subgroup analysis of the ANITA trial suggested that patients with N2 disease derived a survival benefit from adjuvant radiotherapy in both the chemotherapy and the observation groups.[13] The five-year survival rate with and without radiotherapy was 47% and 56% in the chemotherapy arm, and 21% and 17% in the control arm, respectively.

Several randomized trials compared the combination of chemotherapy and radiation either sequentially or concurrently to radiation alone after resection for NSCLC.[31–33] To date, there has been no clear evidence that the combination of chemotherapy and radiotherapy in the adjuvant setting offers survival benefit in resected NSCLC. Therefore, the combination of chemotherapy and radiotherapy is not recommended for routine use in completely resected NSCLC. The ongoing phase III EORTC Lung Adjuvant Radiation Therapy Trial (LUNGART) trial is designed to evaluate the role of adjuvant radiation using current radiotherapy techniques in patients with resected N2 disease (NCT00410683). Patients are randomly assigned to either conformal postoperative radiation or observation after completing adjuvant chemotherapy.

CLINICAL IMPACT OF AGE

Lung cancer is a malignancy of the elderly, with a median age of 70 at diagnosis.[34] An important question in treating elderly patients with completely resected NSCLC is weighing the benefits against the risks of chemotherapy, especially given that some patients may be cured by surgery alone. One issue in interpreting studies of this population is that many studies define patients >65 years of age as elderly, which is not the clinical scenario faced by oncologists in the practice. A retrospective analysis of elderly patients (defined as age >65 years) in the NCIC JBR.10 study revealed that adjuvant chemotherapy still benefits this group of patients (HR for OS, 0.61; 95% CI 0.38–0.98; $p = 0.04$).[35] Elderly patients received fewer doses of chemotherapy ($p = 0.014$ for vinorelbine and 0.006 for cisplatin, respectively), and are less likely to complete treatment ($p = 0.03$). However, treatment-related toxicities, hospitalizations, or death were not significantly different between young and elderly patients. Similarly, the LACE meta-analysis group suggested that elderly patients derive significant benefit from adjuvant chemotherapy. They compared the effect of postoperative chemotherapy among three age groups: young (age <65), midcategory (age 65 to 69), and elderly (age ≥70).[36] There was no statistically significant interaction between age and survival outcome with adjuvant chemotherapy ($p = 0.26$). Elderly patients received lower doses of cisplatin and fewer cycles of chemotherapy. They seemed to experience more grade 4 and greater toxicities, but this was not statistically significant (1.9% for the elderly, 1.4% for the midcategory, 0.7% for the young; $p = 0.24$).

A retrospective study using the Ontario Cancer Registry analyzed data of 6,304 patients with resected NSCLC.[37] Elderly patients were defined as age ≥70 years. The rate of treatment with adjuvant chemotherapy among elderly patients increased from 3.3% between 2001 and 2003 to 16.2% between 2004 and 2006. Cisplatin was administered in 70% of evaluable elderly patients, while 28% received carboplatin. Hospitalization rates were not significantly different between young (28.0% for patients <70 years of age) and elderly patients (27.8% for patients ≥70 years of age; $p = 0.54$). The 4-year survival rate of elderly patients rose from 47.1% for those diagnosed between 2001 and 2003 to 49.9% for those diagnosed between 2004 and 2006 ($p = 0.01$). This was in accordance with the increased use of adjuvant chemotherapy during the same period. The improvement of survival was observed in all subgroups of elderly patients except for those of age ≥80 years. This study concluded that elderly patients (age ≥70 years) benefit from adjuvant chemotherapy, and tolerate the treatment similarly as those <70 years of age. Thus, the decision of chemotherapy should not be based solely upon age. Older patients with good performance status and stage II or III resected NSCLC should be offered adjuvant chemotherapy. However, whether patients of age ≥80 years benefit from postoperative chemotherapy is unclear.

BIOMARKERS PREDICTIVE OF OUTCOME

Multiple studies have attempted to retrospectively identify biomarkers that can predict treatment outcome and guide the decision of adjuvant chemotherapy in resected NSCLC. Molecular markers that have been examined include excision repair cross-complementation group 1 protein (ERCC1), cell cycle regulators p27, tumor suppressor p53 and its encoding gene *TP53*, β-tubulin class III (TUBB3), and MutS homologue 2 (MSH2).[9,38–44] Low expression of ERCC1 was found to be associated with better outcome with adjuvant cisplatin-based chemotherapy. Among patients in the IALT trial who had low ERCC1 expression in their tumors, those treated with chemotherapy had a better survival compared to those in the control group (median OS 56 vs. 42 months; $p = 0.002$).[9]

The Spanish Lung Cancer Group Trial (SCAT) explored the role of Breast Cancer Type 1 (BRCA1) gene expression in predicting benefits from different chemotherapy regimens.[45] Patients with resected node-positive NSCLC were randomly assigned to the control arm or to the experimental arm. Cisplatin and docetaxel are given in the control arm. In the experimental arm, chemotherapy regimens were decided based upon the expression of BRCA1. Patients with low BRCA1 expression received cisplatin and gemcitabine; those with intermediate expression got cisplatin and docetaxel; patients with high BRCA1 expression received docetaxel alone. A total of 500 patients were randomized. At a median follow-up of 30 months, neither OS nor DFS was significantly different between the control and experimental arm. In patients with high BRCA1 expression, there was a trend toward improved survival for patients treated with cisplatin and docetaxel in the control group compared to those who received docetaxel alone in the experimental arm (HR, 0.73; $p =$ not significant). This study does not support tailoring adjuvant chemotherapy regimens according to BRCA1 expression. Other studies have also evaluated the predictive value of several gene signatures in resected NSCLC.[46–48] However, to date, none of the biomarkers or gene signatures has established a definitive role in predicting benefit from adjuvant chemotherapy. Several problems limit the use of these molecular markers in the clinical practice. Most gene expression–based signatures utilized fresh frozen tissue specimens to develop the assay, whereas tumor tissues in the clinical settings are more commonly formalin-fixed paraffin embedded samples. The rate of nucleic acid degradation varies between different preparations of tissues, which make these less reliable. Another issue with biomarker testing is the heterogeneity of tumors. Different areas, even within the same tumor, may have significant discrepancy in expressing the molecular markers, thus making the interpretation of the results difficult.

ROLE OF ADJUVANT-TARGETED THERAPY

So far, one of precision medicine's greatest accomplishments in lung cancer has been the marked improvement in survival and quality of life with the use of molecular-targeted therapy in selected patients whose tumors harbor specific gene abnormalities. Inhibitors targeting the epidermal growth factor receptor (EGFR), anaplastic lymphoma kinase (ALK), and vascular endothelial growth factor (VEGF) have been approved in the treatment of metastatic NSCLC.[49–51]

EGFR-TARGETED THERAPY

EGFR is a transmembrane receptor that is expressed in over 90% of lung cancers. Ligand binding to a single-chain EGFR leads to dimerization, receptor dimerization, and signaling through tyrosine kinase activity, resulting in the activation of multiple pathways involved in cell proliferation, survival, and metastases.[52] Activating mutations involving exons 18 to 21 of the EGFR tyrosine kinase domain are seen in 10% of lung cancers, and predict for response to treatment with tyrosine kinase inhibitors, such as gefitinib, erlotinib, or afatinib.[53,54] These mutations are seen more often in patients who are never-smokers, in women, adenocarcinoma histology, and East Asian ethnicity.[55]

Given the significant benefit of tyrosine kinase inhibitors in the metastatic setting, attempts are being made to incorporate these agents in the curative therapy following surgery. The NCIC BR.19 study is a phase III trial examining the effect of adjuvant gefitinib for 2 years versus placebo in patients with resected stage IB to IIIA NSCLC.[56] The study initially planned to enroll 1,242 patients, but was closed prematurely after 502 patients were accrued. This was prompted by the announcement of potentially detrimental effect with adjuvant gefitinib compared to placebo in stage III NSCLC treated with chemoradiation from the SWOG 0023 study.[57] Since this study was designed prior to the established role of adjuvant chemotherapy as a standard of care, only 87 patients received chemotherapy. In the NCIC BR.19 trial, patients who received adjuvant gefitinib did not derive significant DFS or OS benefit from treatment. There was even a trend toward worse outcome with gefitinib compared to placebo (median OS 5.1 years with gefitinib vs. not yet reached with placebo; HR, 1.24; 95% CI 0.94–1.64; $p = 0.14$). However, this study was underpowered due to premature closure, enrolled patients unselected based on *EGFR* mutation status, and patients in the gefitinib group only receiving treatment for 5 months as opposed to the planned 2 years. Therefore, these results should be interpreted cautiously.

The RADIANT study is a phase III trial exploring the efficacy of adjuvant erlotinib compared to placebo in patients with stage IB–IIIA resected NSCLC with EGFR positive by IHC or FISH.[58] A total of 161 out of the 973 study patients had activating mutations in *EGFR*.[59] For the overall study population, the survival outcome was not significantly different between the erlotinib arm and the placebo arm. In the subgroup of patients with activating *EGFR* mutations, adjuvant erlotinib demonstrated a trend toward better DFS compared to placebo, but the OS was not significantly different (HR, 1.09; 95% CI 0.56–2.16; $p = 0.815$).

The SELECT study is a phase II trial investigating the role of adjuvant erlotinib in *EGFR* mutation-positive NSCLC.[60] Thirty-six patients with resected stage I–IIIA *EGFR* mutated NSCLC received a 2-year course of erlotinib after the completion of standard chemotherapy and/or radiotherapy. Treatment was generally well tolerated, with no grade 4 or 5 adverse events or pneumonitis. At a median follow-up of 2.5 years, the 2-year DFS rate was 94%. This result is encouraging compared to the historical 2-year DFS rate of 72% to 75% in previous phase III studies.[18]

ALK-TARGETED THERAPY

ALK fusion genes result from inversion within chromosome 2p, leading to the N-terminal portion of the echinoderm microtubule-associated protein-like 4 (EML4) gene being fused to the intracellular kinase domain of ALK.[61] Other gene partners for ALK fusion include TGF, KIF5B, and KLC1.[62] ALK fusion proteins activate multiple signaling pathways including the mitogen-activated protein kinase (MAPK) and phosphoinositide 3-kinase (PI3K).[63] ALK gene fusion are more commonly seen in younger patients, men, never-smokers, and adenocarcinoma histology. The prevalence of ALK gene fusions is between 3% and 7% in NSCLC. Crizotinib and ceritinib are inhibitors of ALK that have been approved by the FDA for treatment of ALK-positive metastatic NSCLC.[64,65]

The ongoing Adjuvant Lung Cancer Enrichment Marker Identification and Sequencing Trials (ALCHEMIST) are a constellation of clinical trials designed for patients with early stage nonsquamous NSCLC harboring EGFR mutations or ALK gene fusion (NCT02194738). To be eligible for the study, patients should have completed standard surgical resection and adjuvant chemotherapy with or without radiation. Their tumors are tested for activating EGFR mutations and ALK gene fusion. Those with EGFR mutated tumors are randomized to or placebo for up to 2 years, whereas those with ALK-positive tumors are randomly assigned to crizotinib or placebo for 2 years. The results of the ALCHEMIST studies should help unveil the role of adjuvant-targeted therapy in patients with EGFR-mutated or ALK-positive NSCLC.

VEGF-TARGETED THERAPY

VEGF is an endothelial cell-targeted mitogen that induces angiogenesis.[66] The expression of VEGF is found in a variety of solid tumors, including lung carcinomas.[67] Bevacizumab is a humanized monoclonal antibody that inhibits angiogenesis by targeting VEGF.[68] In advanced NSCLC, the addition of bevacizumab to carboplatin and paclitaxel provided substantial benefit in prolonging survival compared to carboplatin and paclitaxel alone.[51] The ECOG 1505 study (NCT00324805) is a phase III trial designed to evaluate the role of bevacizumab in the adjuvant setting. Patients with resected stage IB to IIIA NSCLC are randomized to chemotherapy alone or with the addition of bevacizumab every 21 days for 1 year. The chemotherapy regimens used included cisplatin in combination with one of the following: vinorelbine, docetaxel, gemcitabine or pemetrexed. This study did not meet its primary endpoint of improved OS with the addition of bevacizumab. In addition, there was no difference in outcomes based on chemotherapy regimen used, though cisplatin and pemetrexed use was associated with least grade 3-5 toxicity compared to the other regimens used.[69] This trial is estimated to complete data collection in 2018.

ROLE OF ADJUVANT IMMUNOTHERAPEUTICS

One of the practice-changing advancements in the treatment of cancers over the past decade is the emergence of immunotherapeutic agents. Immune surveillance has an important role in suppressing tumor growth and development. This is apparent in patients who are on immunosuppression such as transplant recipients, who have increased incidence of lung cancers. Immunotherapy strategies aim to aid recognition of the cancer as "foreign" by the immune system, stimulating the immune response and deinhibiting the mechanism of immune tolerance. Immunotherapeutics that are under investigation in lung cancer include antigen-specific and whole cell cancer vaccines as well as immune checkpoint inhibitors. The immune checkpoints are pathways that lead to self-tolerance through the dampening of immune response. These include cytotoxic T-lymphocyte antigen (CTLA-4) and the programmed death receptor 1 (PD1), both of which have been targeted in lung cancer. CTLA-4 regulates early T cell activity primary in the lymphoid system and competes with CD28 for binding to B7.1 and B7.2. This binding inhibits the T cells through blocking the costimulatory signal from B7/CD28 interaction. PD1 inhibition occurs at the site of the tumor. PD1 is upregulated on activated T cells, and upon recognition of the tumor via T cell receptor, PD1 is engaged by programmed death ligand 1 (PDL1) which is produced in the tumor microenvironment and leads to T cell inactivation. The inhibition of

the PD1 pathway has become an innovative approach to treat refractory squamous NSCLC.[70] Efforts have also been ongoing in evaluating this approach in the adjuvant setting. The NCIC BR31 study is a phase III trial that examines the anti-PD1 inhibitor MEDI4736. Patients with completely resected stage IB (≥4 cm) to IIIA NSCLC are randomly assigned to receive MEDI4736 or placebo for 1 year. Postoperative chemotherapy is allowed, but radiotherapy is not permissible. Tumors are not mandatory to have positive PDL1 expression. The results of the study will help identify the role of adjuvant PDL1 inhibitor in both PDL1-positive and -negative NSCLC tumors.

The ALCHEMIST study was amended to add an additional therapeutic immunotherapy sub-study (ANVIL). Patients whose tumors are EGFR wild-type and ALK fusion negative, and who are candidates for immunotherapy are randomized to receive up to a year of adjuvant nivolumab (an anti-PD1 agent) or observation after completion of their standard of care adjuvant chemotherapy and or radiation (NCT02595944). Recruitment is ongoing.

Recently the results of a window of opportunity study of neoadjuvant nivolumab were reported at the ASCO 2017 Annual Meeting. A total of 22 patients with resectable stage IB-IIIA NSCLC were treated with 2 doses of nivolumab 3 mg/kg over 4 weeks prior to surgery. The primary endpoint of the study was major pathologic response, defined as less than 10% viable tumor cells in the resection specimen and was observed in 43% of cases.[71]

The Lung Cancer Mutation Consortium (LCMC3) is an ongoing study evaluating the role of 2 doses of neoadjuvant atezolizumab, an anti-PD-L1 agent, in patients with resectable stage IB-IIIA NSCLC, also with the primary endpoint of major pathologic response (NCT02927301). This study does allow a year of adjuvant atezolizumab in patients who undergo surgery, and have completed their standard of care adjuvant chemotherapy and or radiation as indicated.

The melanoma antigen family A3 (MAGE-A3) protein is expressed on approximately 33% of resected NSCLC.[72] The recMAGE-A3 + AS15 cancer immunotherapeutic (MAGE-A3 CI) belongs to a class of drugs known as antigen-specific immunotherapeutics (ASCIs) that target MAGE-A3.[73] In a phase II randomized study, adjuvant treatment with MAGE-A3 CI in patients with resected stage IB and II NSCLC that were MAGE-A3 expression positive was associated with better DFS compared to placebo (HR, 0.73 95% CI, 0.45–1.16).[74] Based on these findings, the phase III randomized placebo-controlled MAGRIT trial was designed to test MAGE-A3 CI in the adjuvant setting for patients with resected stage IB–IIIA NSCLC and have positive MAGE-A3 expression.[75] The MAGRIT trial was the largest lung cancer clinical trial to date with a planned enrollment of 2,270 participants. The three coprimary endpoints were DFS in the overall and in the no-adjuvant chemotherapy group and DFS in patients with a predictive gene signature. Treatment with the MAGE-A3 immunotherapeutic did not increase DFS compared to placebo in the overall patient population (median DFS 60.5 vs. 57.9 months; HR 1.024, 95% CI 0.891–1.177; $p = 0.7379$), or in patients that did not receive adjuvant chemotherapy (median DFS 58.0 vs. 56.9 months for MAGE-A3 CI and placebo groups, respectively; HR 0.970, 95% CI 0.797–1.179; p = 0.7572).[76]

A Japanese phase III study examined the effect of postoperative immunotherapy in combination with chemotherapy.[77] A total of 103 patients with resected stage IB to stage IV NSCLC were randomly assigned to chemotherapy with or without immunotherapy, which consisted of autologous activated killer T cells and dendritic cells harvested from patients' regional lymph nodes. The addition of immunotherapy demonstrated a significant advantage in survival, with a 5-year DFS rate of 56.8% (vs. 26.2% with chemotherapy alone; HR, 0.42; 95% CI 0.24–0.74; $p = 0.0027$), and a 5-year OS rate of 81.4% (vs. 48.3% with chemotherapy alone; HR, 0.23; 95% CI 0.09–0.56; $p = 0.0013$). However, these results need to be interpreted with

TABLE 98.2 Ongoing Clinical Trials of Adjuvant Immunotherapeutics

ClinicalTrials .gov Identifier	Study Drug	Ph	Stage	Study Arms	Primary Endpoint	Comment
NCT02595944	Nivolumab	III	IB (4 cm or larger)–IIIA	Nivolumab, observation	OS and/or DFS	Includes both PD-L1 positive and PD-L1 negative tumors
NCT00455572	GSK1572932A	I	IB–IIIA, unresectable stage III	a: concurrent cis/vino and IT b: sequential cis/vino followed by IT c: IT alone for pts not eligible for CT d: IT alone for unresectable stg III after CRT	Immune response, toxicities	MAGE-A3+ tumors
NCT01853878	PRAME IT	II	IA T1b–IIIA	PRAME IT Placebo	DFS	PRAME+ tumors
NCT02273375	MEDI4736	III	IB–IIIA	MEDI4736 Placebo	DFS	PDL1+ tumors
NCT00006470	Tumor vaccine	II	II–IIIA	Monoclonal antibody 11D10/3H1 anti-idiotype vaccine+RT	Immune response, toxicities	
NCT01143545	K562-GM vaccine	I	Resected NSCLC	K562+celecoxib+cyclophosphamide	Toxicities	
NCT01909752	DRibble vaccine	II	III	DRibble+Cyc DRibble+Cyc+imiquimod DRibble+Cyc+GM-CSF	Regimen that has strongest antibody response	After definitive treatment for stage III disease

Ph, phase; cis, cisplatin; vino, vinorelbine; IT, immunotherapy; CT, chemotherapy; stg, stage; CRT, chemoradiation therapy; MAGE-A3, melanoma antigen family A3; PRAME, preferentially expressed antigen of melanoma; DFS, disease-free survival; RT, radiotherapy; PD-L1, programmed death-ligand 1; Cyc, cyclophosphamide; GM-CSF, granulocyte macrophage colony-stimulating factor.

caution, given that one-fifth of the study population had advanced NSCLC, and the chemotherapy regimens used were widely heterogeneous. The role of adjuvant immunotherapeutic awaits to be verified in large, well-designed clinical trials. Ongoing clinical trials of adjuvant immunotherapies are summarized in Table 98.2.

CONCLUSION

After decades of investigation, several large randomized trials have demonstrated a clear survival advantage with adjuvant chemotherapy in resected NSCLC. Postoperative platinum-based chemotherapy provides survival benefit for patients with resected stage II and III disease. Its role in stage IB disease remains controversial. Cisplatin and vinorelbine is the regimen that shows strong evidence of improving survival outcome in large clinical studies. Pemetrexed has also emerged as an alternative to vinorelbine in the adjuvant setting, given its favorable toxicity profile and efficacy in the advanced setting. Carboplatin and cisplatin confer similar survival benefit in retrospective studies, but there has been no prospective trials comparing these two agents in the adjuvant setting. Elderly patients with good performance status do derive a benefit from postoperative chemotherapy. The role of molecular-targeted therapy and immunotherapeutics is being explored. With recent advancements of targeted agents and immunotherapy, adjuvant treatment incorporating innovative approaches may provide more survival benefit in patients with resected NSCLC.

REFERENCES

1. Siegel RL, Miller KD, Jemal A. Cancer statistics, 2015. *CA Cancer J Clin* 2015;65:5–29.
2. Govindan R, Page N, Morgensztern D, et al. Changing epidemiology of small-cell lung cancer in the United States over the last 30 years: analysis of the surveillance, epidemiologic, and end results database. *J Clin Oncol* 2006;24:4539–4544.
3. Morgensztern D, Ng SH, Gao F, et al. Trends in stage distribution for patients with non-small cell lung cancer: a National Cancer Database survey. *J Thorac Oncol* 2010;5:29–33.
4. Pisters KM, Le Chevalier T. Adjuvant chemotherapy in completely resected non-small-cell lung cancer. *J Clin Oncol* 2005;23:3270–3278.
5. Holmes EC, Gail M. Surgical adjuvant therapy for stage II and stage III adenocarcinoma and large-cell undifferentiated carcinoma. *J Clin Oncol* 1986;4:710–715.
6. Niiranen A, Niitamo-Korhonen S, Kouri M, et al. Adjuvant chemotherapy after radical surgery for non-small-cell lung cancer: a randomized study. *J Clin Oncol* 1992;10:1927–1932.
7. Chemotherapy in non-small cell lung cancer: a meta-analysis using updated data on individual patients from 52 randomised clinical trials. Non-small Cell Lung Cancer Collaborative Group. *BMJ* 1995;311:899–909.
8. Scagliotti GV, Fossati R, Torri V, et al. Randomized study of adjuvant chemotherapy for completely resected stage I, II, or IIIA non-small-cell Lung cancer. *J Natl Cancer Inst* 2003;95:1453–1461.
9. Olaussen KA, Dunant A, Fouret P, et al. DNA repair by ERCC1 in non-small-cell lung cancer and cisplatin-based adjuvant chemotherapy. *N Engl J Med* 2006;355:983–991.
10. Arriagada R, Bergman B, Dunant A, et al. Cisplatin-based adjuvant chemotherapy in patients with completely resected non-small-cell lung cancer. *N Engl J Med* 2004;350:351–360.
11. Arriagada R, Dunant A, Pignon JP, et al. Long-term results of the international adjuvant lung cancer trial evaluating adjuvant Cisplatin-based chemotherapy in resected lung cancer. *J Clin Oncol* 2010;28:35–42.
12. Winton T, Livingston R, Johnson D, et al. Vinorelbine plus cisplatin vs. observation in resected non-small-cell lung cancer. *N Engl J Med* 2005;352:2589–2597.
13. Douillard JY, Rosell R, De Lena M, et al. Adjuvant vinorelbine plus cisplatin versus observation in patients with completely resected stage IB-IIIA non-small-cell lung cancer (Adjuvant Navelbine International Trialist Association [ANITA]): a randomised controlled trial. *Lancet Oncol* 2006;7:719–727.
14. Pignon JP, Tribodet H, Scagliotti GV, et al. Lung adjuvant cisplatin evaluation: a pooled analysis by the LACE Collaborative Group. *J Clin Oncol* 2008;26:3552–3559.
15. Waller D, Peake MD, Stephens RJ, et al. Chemotherapy for patients with non-small cell lung cancer: the surgical setting of the Big Lung Trial. *Eur J Cardiothorac Surg* 2004;26:173–182.
16. Scagliotti GV, Parikh P, von Pawel J, et al. Phase III study comparing cisplatin plus gemcitabine with cisplatin plus pemetrexed in chemotherapy-naive patients with advanced-stage non-small-cell lung cancer. *J Clin Oncol* 2008;26:3543–3551.
17. Kreuter M, Vansteenkiste J, Fischer JR, et al. Randomized phase 2 trial on refinement of early-stage NSCLC adjuvant chemotherapy with cisplatin and pemetrexed versus cisplatin and vinorelbine: the TREAT study. *Ann Oncol* 2013;24:986–992.
18. Strauss GM, Herndon JE 2nd, Maddaus MA, et al. Adjuvant paclitaxel plus carboplatin compared with observation in stage IB non-small-cell lung cancer: CALGB 9633 with the Cancer and Leukemia Group B, Radiation Therapy Oncology Group, and North Central Cancer Treatment Group Study Groups. *J Clin Oncol* 2008;26:5043–5051.
19. Strauss GM, Wang XF, Maddaus M, et al. Adjuvant chemotherapy (AC) in stage IB non-small cell lung cancer (NSCLC): Long-term follow-up of Cancer and Leukemia Group B (CALGB) 9633. *J Clin Oncol* 2011;29.
20. Rosell R, Gatzemeier U, Betticher DC, et al. Phase III randomised trial comparing paclitaxel/carboplatin with paclitaxel/cisplatin in patients with advanced non-small-cell lung cancer: a cooperative multinational trial. *Ann Oncol* 2002;13:1539–1549.

21. Gu F, Strauss GM, Wisnivesky JP. Platinum-based adjuvant chemotherapy (ACT) in elderly patients with non-small cell lung cancer (NSCLC) in the SEER-Medicare database: Comparison between carboplatin- and cisplatin-based regimens. *J Clin Oncol* 2011;29.

22. Tanaka F. UFT (tegafur and uracil) as postoperative adjuvant chemotherapy for solid tumors (Carcinoma of the lung, stomach, colon/rectum, and breast): Clinical evidence, mechanism of action, and future direction. *Surg Today* 2007;37:923–943.

23. Kato H, Ichinose Y, Ohta M, et al. A randomized trial of adjuvant chemotherapy with uracil-tegafur for adenocarcinoma of the lung. *N Engl J Med* 2004;350:1713–1721.

24. Wada H, Hitomi S, Teramatsu T. Adjuvant chemotherapy after complete resection in non-small-cell lung cancer. West Japan Study Group for Lung Cancer Surgery. *J Clin Oncol* 1996;14:1048–1054.

25. Imaizumi M; Study Group of Adjuvant Chemotherapy for Lung C. Postoperative adjuvant cisplatin, vindesine, plus uracil-tegafur chemotherapy increased survival of patients with completely resected p-stage I non-small cell lung cancer. *Lung Cancer* 2005;49:85–94.

26. Nakagawa M, Tanaka F, Tsubota N, et al. A randomized phase III trial of adjuvant chemotherapy with UFT for completely resected pathological stage I non-small-cell lung cancer: the West Japan Study Group for Lung Cancer Surgery (WJSG)—the 4th study. *Ann Oncol* 2005;16:75–80.

27. Nakagawa K, Tada H, Akashi A, et al. Randomised study of adjuvant chemotherapy for completely resected p-stage I-IIIA non-small cell lung cancer. *Br J Cancer* 2006;95:817–821.

28. Hamada C, Tanaka F, Ohta M, et al. Meta-analysis of postoperative adjuvant chemotherapy with tegafur-uracil in non-small-cell lung cancer. *J Clin Oncol* 2005;23:4999–5006.

29. Hamada C, Tsuboi M, Ohta M, et al. Effect of postoperative adjuvant chemotherapy with tegafur-uracil on survival in patients with stage IA non-small cell lung cancer: an exploratory analysis from a meta-analysis of six randomized controlled trials. *J Thorac Oncol* 2009;4:1511–1516.

30. Burdett S, Stewart L; Group PM-a. Postoperative radiotherapy in non-small-cell lung cancer: update of an individual patient data meta-analysis. *Lung Cancer* 2005;47:81–83.

31. Lad T, Rubinstein L, Sadeghi A. The benefit of adjuvant treatment for resected locally advanced non-small-cell lung-cancer. *J Clin Oncol* 1988;6:9–17.

32. Keller SM, Adak S, Wagner H, et al. A randomized trial of postoperative adjuvant therapy in patients with completely resected stage II or IIIA non-small-cell lung cancer. Eastern Cooperative Oncology Group. *N Engl J Med* 2000;343:1217–1222.

33. Dautzenberg B, Chastang C, Arriagada R, et al. Adjuvant radiotherapy versus combined sequential chemotherapy followed by radiotherapy in the treatment of resected nonsmall cell lung carcinoma. A randomized trial of 267 patients. GETCB (Groupe d'Etude et de Traitement des Cancers Bronchiques). *Cancer* 1995;76:779–786.

34. Hayat MJ, Howlader N, Reichman ME, et al. Cancer statistics, trends, and multiple primary cancer analyses from the Surveillance, Epidemiology, and End Results (SEER) Program. *Oncologist* 2007;12:20–37.

35. Pepe C, Hasan B, Winton TL, et al. Adjuvant vinorelbine and cisplatin in elderly patients: National Cancer Institute of Canada and Intergroup Study JBR.10. *J Clin Oncol* 2007;25:1553–1561.

36. Fruh M, Rolland E, Pignon JP, et al. Pooled analysis of the effect of age on adjuvant cisplatin-based chemotherapy for completely resected non-small-cell lung cancer. *J Clin Oncol* 2008;26:3573–3581.

37. Cuffe S, Booth CM, Peng Y, et al. Adjuvant chemotherapy for non-small-cell lung cancer in the elderly: a population-based study in Ontario, Canada. *J Clin Oncol* 2012;30:1813–1821.

38. Bepler G, Olaussen KA, Vataire AL, et al. ERCC1 and RRM1 in the international adjuvant lung trial by automated quantitative in situ analysis. *Am J Pathol* 2011;178:69–78.

39. Filipits M, Pirker R, Dunant A, et al. Cell cycle regulators and outcome of adjuvant cisplatin-based chemotherapy in completely resected non-small-cell lung cancer: the International Adjuvant Lung Cancer Trial Biologic Program. *J Clin Oncol* 2007;25:2735–2740.

40. Tsao MS, Aviel-Ronen S, Ding K, et al. Prognostic and predictive importance of p53 and RAS for adjuvant chemotherapy in non small-cell lung cancer. *J Clin Oncol* 2007;25:5240–5247.

41. Ma X, Rousseau V, Sun H, et al. Significance of TP53 mutations as predictive markers of adjuvant cisplatin-based chemotherapy in completely resected non-small-cell lung cancer. *Mol Oncol* 2014;8:555–564.

42. Seve P, Lai R, Ding K, et al. Class III beta-tubulin expression and benefit from adjuvant cisplatin/vinorelbine chemotherapy in operable non-small cell lung cancer: analysis of NCIC JBR.10. *Clin Cancer Res* 2007;13:994–999.

43. Pierceall WE, Olaussen KA, Rousseau V, et al. Cisplatin benefit is predicted by immunohistochemical analysis of DNA repair proteins in squamous cell carcinoma but not adenocarcinoma: theranostic modeling by NSCLC constituent histological subclasses. *Ann Oncol* 2012;23:2245–2252.

44. Kamal NS, Soria JC, Mendiboure J, et al. MutS homologue 2 and the long-term benefit of adjuvant chemotherapy in lung cancer. *Clin Cancer Res* 2010;16:1206–1215.

45. Massuti B, Cobo M, Rodriguez-Paniagua JM, et al. Randomized phase III trial of customized adjuvant chemotherapy (CT) according BRCA-1 expression levels in patients with node positive resected non-small cell lung cancer (NSCLS) SCAT: A Spanish Lung Cancer Group trial (Eudract:2007–000067–15; NCTgov: 00478699). *ASCO Meeting Abstracts* 2015;33:7507.

46. Zhu CQ, Ding K, Strumpf D, et al. Prognostic and predictive gene signature for adjuvant chemotherapy in resected non-small-cell lung cancer. *J Clin Oncol* 2010;28:4417–4424.

47. Tang H, Xiao G, Behrens C, et al. A 12-gene set predicts survival benefits from adjuvant chemotherapy in non small cell lung cancer patients. *Clin Cancer Res* 2013;19:1577–1586.

48. Chen DT, Hsu YL, Fulp WJ, et al. Prognostic and predictive value of a malignancy-risk gene signature in early-stage non-small cell lung cancer. *J Natl Cancer Inst* 2011;103:1859–1870.

49. Shepherd FA, Rodrigues Pereira J, Ciuleanu T, et al. Erlotinib in previously treated non-small-cell lung cancer. *N Engl J Med* 2005;353:123–132.

50. Kwak EL, Bang YJ, Camidge DR, et al. Anaplastic lymphoma kinase inhibition in non-small-cell lung cancer. *N Engl J Med* 2010;363:1693–1703.

51. Sandler A, Gray R, Perry MC, et al. Paclitaxel-carboplatin alone or with bevacizumab for non-small-cell lung cancer. *N Engl J Med* 2006;355:2542–2550.

52. Ciardiello F, Tortora G. EGFR antagonists in cancer treatment. *N Engl J Med* 2008;358:1160–1174.

53. Rosell R, Carcereny E, Gervais R, et al. Erlotinib versus standard chemotherapy as first-line treatment for European patients with advanced EGFR mutation-positive non-small-cell lung cancer (EURTAC): a multicentre, open-label, randomised phase 3 trial. *Lancet Oncol* 2012;13:239–246.

54. Zhou C, Wu YL, Chen G, et al. Erlotinib versus chemotherapy as first-line treatment for patients with advanced EGFR mutation-positive non-small-cell lung cancer (OPTIMAL, CTONG-0802): a multicentre, open-label, randomised, phase 3 study. *Lancet Oncol* 2011;12:735–742.

55. Shigematsu H, Lin L, Takahashi T, et al. Clinical and biological features associated with epidermal growth factor receptor gene mutations in lung cancers. *J Natl Cancer Inst* 2005;97:339–346.

56. Goss GD, O'Callaghan C, Lorimer I, et al. Gefitinib versus placebo in completely resected non-small-cell lung cancer: results of the NCIC CTG BR19 study. *J Clin Oncol* 2013;31:3320–3326.

57. Kelly K, Chansky K, Gaspar LE, et al. Phase III trial of maintenance gefitinib or placebo after concurrent chemoradiotherapy and docetaxel consolidation in inoperable stage III non-small-cell lung cancer: SWOG S0023. *J Clin Oncol* 2008;26:2450–2456.

58. Kelly K, Altorki NK, Eberhardt WE, et al. A randomized, double-blind phase 3 trial of adjuvant erlotinib (E) versus placebo (P) following complete tumor resection with or without adjuvant chemotherapy in patients (pts) with stage IB-IIIA EGFR positive (IHC/FISH) non-small cell lung cancer (NSCLC): RADIANT results. *ASCO Meeting Abstracts* 2014;32:7501.

59. Shepherd FA, Altorki NK, Eberhardt WE, et al. Adjuvant erlotinib (E) versus placebo (P) in non-small cell lung cancer (NSCLC) patients (pts) with tumors carrying EGFR-sensitizing mutations from the RADIANT trial. *ASCO Meeting Abstracts* 2014;32:7513.

60. Neal JW, Pennell NA, Govindan R, et al. The Select Study: A Multicenter Phase II Trial Of Adjuvant Erlotinib In Resected Epidermal Growth Factor Receptor (EGFR) Mutation-positive Non-small Cell Lung Cancer (NSCLC). *J Thor Oncol* 2012;7:S209.

61. Soda M, Choi YL, Enomoto M, et al. Identification of the transforming EML4-ALK fusion gene in non-small-cell lung cancer. *Nature* 2007;448:561–566.

62. Shaw AT, Engelman JA. ALK in lung cancer: past, present, and future. *J Clin Oncol* 2013;31:1105–1111.

63. Shaw AT, Solomon B. Targeting anaplastic lymphoma kinase in lung cancer. *Clin Cancer Res* 2011;17:2081–2086.

64. Shaw AT, Yeap BY, Solomon BJ, et al. Effect of crizotinib on overall survival in patients with advanced non-small-cell lung cancer harbouring ALK gene rearrangement: a retrospective analysis. *Lancet Oncol* 2011;12:1004–1012.

65. Shaw AT, Mehra R, Kim D-W, et al. Clinical activity of the ALK inhibitor LDK378 in advanced, ALK-positive NSCLC. *ASCO Meeting Abstracts* 2013;31:8010.

66. Ferrara N. Vascular endothelial growth factor: basic science and clinical progress. *Endocr Rev* 2004;25:581–611.

67. Volm M, Koomagi R, Mattern J, et al. Angiogenic growth factors and their receptors in non-small cell lung carcinomas and their relationships to drug response in vitro. *Anticancer Res* 1997;17:99–103.

68. Mukherji SK. Bevacizumab (Avastin). *AJNR Am J Neuroradiol* 2010;31:235–236.

69. Wakelee HA, Dahlberg SE, Keller SM, et al. E1505: Adjuvant chemotherapy +/− bevacizumab for early stage NSCLC-outcomes based on chemotherapy subsets. *J Clin Oncol* 2016;34(suppl 15):8507–8507.

70. Rizvi NA, Mazieres J, Planchard D, et al. Activity and safety of nivolumab, an anti-PD-1 immune checkpoint inhibitor, for patients with advanced, refractory squamous non-small-cell lung cancer (CheckMate 063): a phase 2, single-arm trial. *Lancet Oncol* 2015;16:257–265.

71. Chaft JE, Forde PM, Smith KN, et al. Neoadjuvant nivolumab in early stage, resectable non-small cell lung cancers. *J Clin Oncol* 2017;35(suppl 15):8508.

72. Vansteenkiste J, Zielinski M, Linder A, et al. Adjuvant MAGE-A3 Immunotherapy in Resected Non-Small-Cell Lung Cancer: Phase II Randomized Study Results. *J Clin Oncol* 2013;31:2396–2402.

73. Jang SJ, Soria JC, Wang L, et al. Activation of melanoma antigen tumor antigens occurs early in lung carcinogenesis. *Cancer Res* 2001;61:7959–7963.

74. Vansteenkiste J, Zielinski M, Linder A, et al. Final results of a multi-center, double-blind, randomized, placebo-controlled phase II study to assess the efficacy of MAGE-A3 immunotherapeutic as adjuvant therapy in stage IB/II non-small cell lung cancer (NSCLC). *J Clin Oncol* 2007;25(18S):7554.

75. database NIoHCT. GSK1572932A Antigen-Specific Cancer Immunotherapeutic as Adjuvant Therapy in Patients With Non-Small Cell Lung Cancer. *Clin Trials.gov identifier* NCT00480025

76. Vansteenkiste JF, Cho BC, Vanakesa T, et al. MAGRIT, a double-blind, randomized, placebo-controlled Phase III study to assess the efficacy of the recMAGE-A3 +AS15 cancer immunotherapeutic as adjuvant therapy in patients with resected MAGE-A3 positive non-small cell lung cancer (NSCLC). *Ann Oncol* 2014;25(suppl_4):iv409–iv416. 10.1093/annonc/mdu347.

77. Kimura H, Matsui Y, Ishikawa A, et al. Randomized controlled phase III trial of adjuvant chemo-immunotherapy with activated killer T cells and dendritic cells in patients with resected primary lung cancer. *Cancer Immunol Immunother* 2015;64:51–59.

99

Radiation for Lung Cancer

Kevin L. Stephans ▪ Rupesh Kotecha ▪ Neil McIver Woody ▪ Gregory Videtic

INTRODUCTION

Radiation plays a prominent role in the definitive and palliative management of lung cancer. Stereotactic body radiotherapy (SBRT) serves as an alternative to surgery for poor-risk and medically inoperable stage I non–small cell lung cancer (NSCLC), while standard external beam radiation may be used as either as neoadjuvant, adjuvant, or definitive therapy in stage III disease. Limited stage (LS) small cell lung cancer (SCLC) is managed with combined chemotherapy and radiation. This chapter will detail the role of external beam radiation in the management of lung cancer.

STAGE I NON–SMALL CELL LUNG CANCER

For patients who are medically inoperable, options include observation, standard radiation, or SBRT. Unless the patient is medically unstable, observation is not favored as historically the rate of death from lung cancer exceeds 50% even in patients whose comorbidities preclude conventional treatment despite their competing health risks.[1,2] Conventional radiation to doses of 60 to 70 Gray (Gy) in 30 to 35 fractions was an option prior to the advent of SBRT; however, local control (LC) for conventional treatments appears to be inferior,[2,3] likely due to delivery of inadequate biologically effective dose (BED) to attain a high rate of tumor control.[4] Furthermore standard fractionated regimens are long and inconvenient, as well as, more expensive in this poor-risk population. Also, multiple randomized studies comparing conventional radiation to SBRT have been abandoned given the overall superior data for SBRT. The effect of SBRT is demonstrated in a Dutch cancer registry study where with the implementation of SBRT, the fraction of stage I NSCLC patients going untreated has declined, while survival in the radiated group has improved simultaneously.[5]

Stereotactic Body Radiation Therapy

SBRT is a radiation technique that allows for the precise delivery of large fractions of radiation by multiple beams guided by a set of coordinates relating to the direct position of the tumor rather than external marks or anatomical structures. The large dose and small treatment margin requires careful delineation of target and nontarget structures, as well as precise management of target motion and treatment set-up. While SBRT is primarily used for medically inoperable stage I NSCLC, other indications include lung oligometastasis[6] and thoracic re-irradiation.[7,8] SBRT is under investigation for poor-risk stage I SCLC,[9,10] operable stage I NSCLC,[11,12] as well as, potentially a boost to conventionally fractionated radiation in locally advanced NSCLC.[13,14]

Delivery of SBRT begins with a treatment planning session in which a patient is immobilized within a custom-created device such as a vacuum bag which conforms to their anatomy typically while supine with arms extended above the head (Fig. 99.1A). Tumor motion is assessed by either 4D CT imaging or fluoroscopy. If there is any significant tumor motion this may be managed by abdominal compression to reduce diaphragmatic excursion, respiratory gating using either controlled breath-hold or surrogates for tumor position (internal or external), or alternatively tumor tracking and

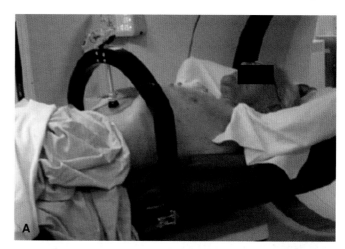

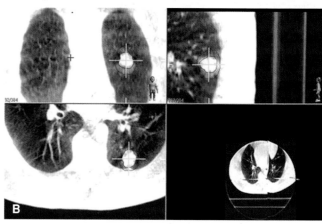

FIGURE 99.1 **A:** Treatment set-up and respiratory immobilization by abdominal compression for SBRT. **B:** Cone-beam CT image acquired at time of treatment confirming alignment of primary target (*red outline*) and surrounding planning target volume (PTV, *purple outline*).

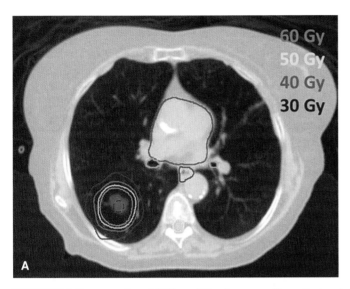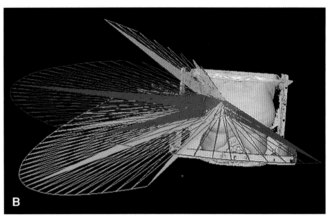

FIGURE 99.2   Representative axial CT scan (**A**) and corresponding patient rendering with beam arrangement (**B**) for a medically inoperable patient with a peripherally located Stage IA (T1bN0M0) lung cancer of the right upper lobe who underwent stereotactic body radiation therapy (SBRT) to a dose of 60 Gy in 3 fractions delivered using 6 MV photons via three noncoplanar arcs. Of note, respiratory excursion for this patient was limited with use of an abdominal hoop compression device. The gross tumor volume (GTV) is represented by the *shaded blue volume*, and the planning target volume (PTV) is represented by the *shaded red volume*. Organs at risk including the heart (*pink*), esophagus (*purple*), spinal cord (*yellow*), and bronchial tree (*green*) are outlined. The representative isodose lines and their corresponding doses are provided in the color legend.

respiratory modeling. Tumor position is directly verified during treatment by cone-beam CT (CBCT) or other similar technology to ensure proper targeting at the time of radiation delivery (Fig. 99.1B). Gross tumor volume (GTV) is defined as all visible tumor on images acquired during simulation with assistance from fused diagnostic images as needed. This is expanded to an internal target volume (ITV) which accounts for any respiratory motion noted on imaging, and finally a planning target volume (PTV) to account for set-up error, deformation and any additional uncertainty during treatment (typically 5 mm).[15,16]

Radiation beam arrangement, using either static beams, intensity modulated beams, or multiple arcs in one or multiple planes, is used to cover the PTV with appropriate radiation dose utilizing a calculation algorithm which accounts for differences in tissue density with the goal of maximizing dose conformality and rapid fall-off (Fig. 99.2). Constraints for radiation dose–volume relationships to nearby sensitive tissues such as the lungs, heart, spinal cord, esophagus, trachea, proximal bronchial tree, vasculature, brachial plexus and ribs/chest wall have been established (Table 99.1),[17] though continue to be refined with increasing experience.

TABLE 99.1 Suggested Normal Tissue Constraints for Stereotactic Body Radiation Therapy

Critical Structure	Max Critical Volume Above Threshold	Three-Fraction Treatment		Five-Fraction Treatment		Toxicity Endpoint
		Threshold Dose (Gy)	Max Point Dose (Gy)[a]	Threshold Dose (Gy)	Max Point Dose (Gy)[a]	
Spinal cord	<10% of subvolume	18.0 (6.0 Gy/fx)	21.9 (7.3 Gy/fx)	23.0 (4.6 Gy/fx)	30 (6 Gy/fx)	Myelitis
Esophagus[b]	<5 cc	17.7 (5.9 Gy/fx)	25.2 (8.4 Gy/fx)	19.5 (3.9 Gy/fx)	35 (7 Gy/fx)	Stenosis or fistula
Brachial plexus	<3 cc	20.4 (6.8 Gy/fx)	24.0 (8.0 Gy/fx)	27.0 (5.4 Gy/fx)	30.5 (6.1 Gy/fx)	Neuropathy
Heart/pericardium	<15 cc	24.0 (8.0 Gy/fx)	30.0 (10.0 Gy/fx)	32.0 (6.4 Gy/fx)	38 (7.6 Gy/fx)	Pericarditis
Great vessels	<10 cc	39.0 (13.0 Gy/fx)	45.0 (15.0 Gy/fx)	47.0 (9.4 Gy/fx)	53 (10.6 Gy/fx)	Aneurysm
Trachea and large bronchus[b]	<4 cc	15.0 (5.0 Gy/fx)	30.0 (10.0 Gy/fx)	16.5 (3.3 Gy/fx)	40 (8 Gy/fx)	Stenosis or fistula
Bronchus-smaller airways	<0.5 cc	18.9 (6.3 Gy/fx)	23.1 (7.7 Gy/fx)	21.0 (4.2 Gy/fx)	33 (6.6 Gy/fx)	Stenosis with atelectasis
Rib	<1 cc	28.8 (9.6 Gy/fx)	36.9 (12.3 Gy/fx)	35.0 (7.0 Gy/fx)	43 (8.6 Gy/fx)	Pain or fracture
Skin	<10 cc	30.0 (10.0 Gy/fx)	33.0 (11.0 Gy/fx)	36.5 (7.3 Gy/fx)	39.5 (7.9 Gy/fx)	Ulceration
Lung (right and left)	1500 cc	11.6 (2.9 Gy/fx)	—	12.5 (2.5 Gy/fx)	—	Basic lung function
	1000 cc	12.4 (3.1 Gy/fx)	—	13.5 (2.7 Gy/fx)	—	Pneumonitis

Gy, Gray; fx, fraction.
[a]Max point dose corresponds to 0.035 cc of tissue or less.
[b]Avoid circumferential radiation.

Radiation dose prescriptions typically range from 30 to 60 Gy in 1 to 8 fractions and are dependent upon tumor location, size, and proximity to sensitive structures. Since BED is very sensitize to radiation fraction size, a linear quadratic formula has been utilized to estimate SBRT BED and overall performs well for comparing dose regimens[18] though alternative models have also been proposed as further data emerges.[19] A phase I dose escalation study established 54 Gy in 3 fractions as the maximum tolerated SBRT dose for peripheral stage I NSCLC.[20] Subsequently, a phase II study led to the identification that while this regimen is well tolerated for peripheral tumors <5 cm in size, this aggressive dose regimen leads to significant risk of toxicity when treating tumors within 2 cm of the trachea and proximal bronchial tree, defined as "central."[21] While this caused some concern in treating such central tumors with SBRT, it is noted that a Japanese series utilizing a lower dose per fraction (10 to 12 Gy) did not report significant toxicity with SBRT for central tumor location.[22–24] Subsequent publications from the Netherlands validated 60 Gy in 8 fractions even for very large central tumors.[25] Several US retrospective series similarly demonstrated the safety of SBRT for central lung lesions with fraction sizes of up to 10 Gy/fraction.[26,27] Recently RTOG 0813, a dose-escalation for SBRT of central lung tumors escalating dose from 50 up to 60 Gy in 5 fractions was completed reaching the highest dose level without interruption with results expected soon.[15]

A dose-response relationship has been consistently identified whereby it appears that improved LC is gained from regimens with BEDs exceeding 100 Gy_{10}, a level which can be attained safely for both peripheral and central tumors.[24,28] More recent publications have examined whether even higher doses with BEDs exceeding 140 to 150 Gy_{10} may further improve control, though results have been somewhat conflicting,[2,29,30] and randomized data will likely be needed to reach a firm conclusion on the ideal SBRT dose-fractionation schedule.

SBRT Outcomes

LC of the index lesion after lung SBRT is typically defined as the absence of tumor progression within 1 cm of the primary tumor site, and has historically ranged from 90% to 98%.[12,22–24,31–34] This is in step with prospective surgical series showing a loco-regional failure rate of 5% to 7% for lobectomy and 8% to 17% for sublobar resection.[35,36] A pooled meta-analysis of 40 SBRT studies totaling 4,850 patients and 23 surgical studies (lobar or sublobar resection, 7,071 patients in total) likewise suggests LC by this definition is similar.[33] It is important to note that identifying local failure after SBRT is more challenging than after lobectomy given that significant postradiation fibrosis arising in many patients might lead to overestimation of local failure. And, the inability to rule out the presence of a small number of viable tumor cells within fibrosis and the comparatively shorter follow-up of SBRT series might result in underestimation of local failure (Fig. 99.3).[37] Furthermore, LC in surgical series is more often reported as loco-regional control. When accounting for lobar failure,

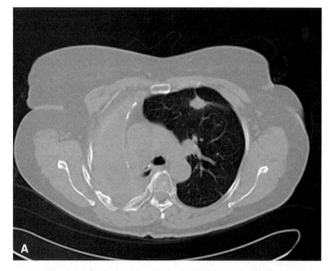

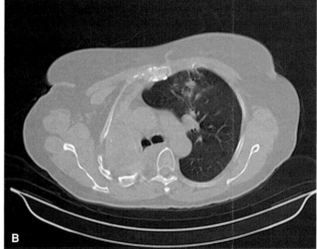

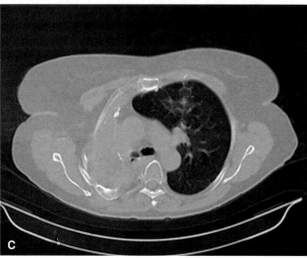

FIGURE 99.3 Medically inoperable patient with a history of a right pneumonectomy for two metachronous lung cancers who subsequently developed a Stage I (T1N0M0) lung cancer of the left upper lobe and was treated with stereotactic body radiation therapy (SBRT). Axial CT of the chest at the time of SBRT (**A**) demonstrated a spiculated nodule in the left-upper lobe which had decreased in size and was surrounded by a patchy linear infiltrate 6 months after SBRT (**B**). Follow-up axial CT scan of the chest performed 1 year after SBRT showed significant reduction in size of the nodule, almost indistinguishable from the background of patchy, ill-defined interstitial infiltrate surrounding the treated region (**C**).

LC in SBRT series drops slightly. RTOG 0236, a landmark prospective trial of SBRT utilizing 60 Gy in 3 fractions (estimated 54 Gy in 3 fractions with heterogeneity corrections) for peripheral stage I NSCLC, demonstrated 3-year LC of 97.6%, lobar control of 90.6%, locoregional control of 87.2%, and a 22.1% rate of distant recurrence.[34] Of note, the reported incidence of nodal failure after SBRT is surprisingly lower than the expected rate of nodal upstaging after surgical nodal dissection for clinical stage I lung cancer,[38] though may still be slightly higher than that seen in surgical series.[39] Increasing quality of pretreatment imaging as well as availability of nonsurgical nodal staging techniques, only modestly used in most SBRT series, may also impact the incidence of nodal failure going forward.

In comparison to surgical series, SBRT for stage I NSCLC is typically associated with lower reported overall survival (OS). This is likely in large part due to patient selection given the predominance of medically inoperable patients and high rates of death due to comorbid conditions in SBRT series.[33,39,40] It is supported by the observation that after performing multivariate adjustment or propensity score–based analysis SBRT, OS is typically similar to surgical cohorts.[33,39,40] Notably small series of SBRT in medically operable patients have yielded excellent OS.[11,12] The previously noted pooled analysis also demonstrated a relationship between OS and the percent of operable patients within individual SBRT series, which when curve-fit to surgical series also suggested the potential for similar OS in equally operable patients.[33] Ultimately however, modeling data cannot replace clinical data, and with no long-term series of sufficient volume for SBRT in operable patients in the United States population, surgery should remain the standard of care for operable patients in this country.

Patient Selection

Patients with NSCLC frequently present with medical comorbidities related to risk factors for their disease such as smoking and environmental exposure. Clinically they fall on a spectrum from medically inoperable to those at low risk for surgical complications and mortality. It also applies to those at risk for quality-of-life changes with surgery and patients in good health with minimal surgical risk. Shared multidisciplinary decision making is the key to selection so that choice of therapy matches the patient's disease, medical risk profile, and patient goals. Established models to estimate risk of surgical morbidity and mortality are critical in assigning patients to operative versus nonoperative approaches.[41] Operable patients with low-surgical risk should undergo lobectomy. As surgical risk for both morbidity and mortality rises based on patient comorbidities, consideration of SBRT becomes more appropriate. The identification of the ideal threshold for a change to SBRT is highly controversial, though

modeling studies have suggested this may be around a surgical mortality risk level of 3.5% to 4%, above which SBRT may be more cost-effective.[42,43] To absolutely establish this level, better data comparing surgical to SBRT outcomes is needed, though this does approximate our institutional selection. Beyond purely control and risk-based patient selection, another challenging group from a decision-making perspective are elderly but medically operable patients who in the last decades of life may value simplicity of therapy, quality-of-life, and avoidance of risk equally heavily as outcomes. Prospective quality of life studies suggest SBRT to be associated with excellent preservation of physical function, avoidance of dyspnea, social well-being, and emotional function,[44] whereas surgical series suggest persistence of pain, dyspnea, fatigue, and some reduced physical function from baseline lasting 8 to 24 months after surgery.[45] While surgery remains the standard for such medically operable patients, it is important to weigh how differences in outcome and risk fit into a patient's priorities while still remaining objective overall. Physically fit but elderly patients who may value the simplicity of a nonoperative approach or prioritize quality-of-life and risk management above small differences in oncologic outcome represent a challenge in decision making. The dynamics of the above interactions with the spectrum of operability in lung cancer make patient selection extremely challenging.

Toxicity

SBRT is overall well tolerated, even in the medically inoperable population. Patients may experience fatigue for 4 to 6 weeks following treatment (Fig. 99.4).[44] Pulmonary function is well conserved[46] with generally <3% risk of radiation pneumonitis.[12,22–24,31–34] Even patients with extremely compromised pulmonary function exhibiting OS outcomes at or above the mean,[47,48] suggest there is no clear lower limit to pulmonary function for SBRT provided patients are medically stable. Although, criteria for whom no treatment is the best approach are still needed. Neuropathic pain and rib fractures may occur with 10% to 25% of treatments to targets abutting the chest wall, though symptoms are generally modest and potentially less common than in surgical series. More significant chest wall pain, skin ulcers, brachial plexopathy, and bronchial or esophageal fistulas have been reported, though are extremely uncommon and risk is modifiable during the planning process when properly identified.[49]

STAGE II NSCLC

Stage II NSCLC is uncommon, and almost universally treated surgically with adjuvant chemotherapy. The high radiation dose levels

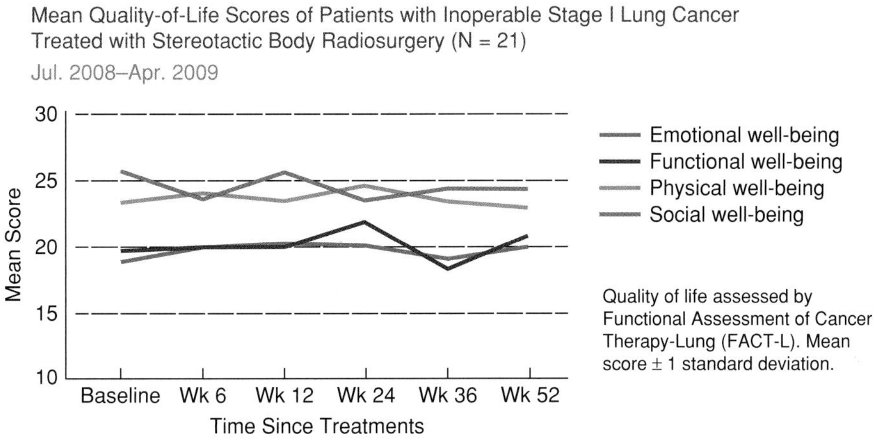

Mean Quality-of-Life Scores of Patients with Inoperable Stage I Lung Cancer Treated with Stereotactic Body Radiosurgery (N = 21)

Jul. 2008–Apr. 2009

FIGURE 99.4 Prospective quality-of-life study demonstrating maintenance of physical, functional, mental and emotional well-being after treatment with SBRT for stage I NSCLC. (From Videtic GM, Reddy CA, Sorenson L. A prospective study of quality of life including fatigue and pulmonary function after stereotactic body radiotherapy for medically inoperable early-stage lung cancer. *Support Care Cancer* 2013;21:211–218. Copyright © Springer-Verlag 2012. With permission of Springer.)[44]

given with SBRT which are needed to attain adequate rates of LC have not been documented to be safe for treatment of nodal stations in the hilum or mediastinum with significant cross-sectional radiation to sensitive structures. This necessitates the use of fractionated radiation in this setting delivering lower BED. Patients unable to tolerate surgical resection can be treated with concurrent or sequential chemoradiation, or radiation alone if unable to tolerate the addition of chemotherapy. Similar dose and targeting strategies, as those discussed below for stage III disease, apply in this setting.

T3N0 disease represents a distinct subset of stage II NSCLC. The use of radiation in surgically managed T3N0 NSCLC is controversial and data is limited. As R0 resection is associated with improved survival,[50] neoadjuvant radiation might be considered if downstaging is needed for complete resection; however, with advances in reconstruction after surgery this scenario is rare. No randomized trials of postoperative radiation in T3N0 have been reported. One small retrospective review suggests possible benefit while two larger series do not. Thus, the main indication for postoperative radiation in this setting should be limited to positive surgical margins.[51] Medically inoperable patients with chest wall invasion (T3N0) whose tumors measured <5 cm were within the eligibility of RTOG 0236.[34] However, none were enrolled, and the decision for SBRT versus conventional radiation to 60 to 70 Gy in 30 to 35 fractions with or without chemotherapy based on comorbidities remains controversial.

STAGE III NSCLC

Potentially Operable Stage IIIA NSCLC

The most significant branch in the decision-tree for stage III NSCLC is whether to proceed with trimodality therapy versus nonoperative therapy. For resectable stage IIIA patients, the evaluation of operability should always include a multidisciplinary evaluation including a thoracic surgeon, pulmonologist, medical oncologist, and radiation oncologist. Evaluation of resectability is made by the thoracic surgeon, and operability by the multidisciplinary team lead by pulmonology, thoracic surgery, and possibly cardiology based on evaluation of the expected operative risk based on established models.[41] The LC rate of nonoperative therapy is typically inferior to that attained by the addition of surgical resection.[52,53] This is due to the limitations of normal tissue toxicity on radiation dose when including significant portions of the mediastinum. Comparisons of phase II series of operative and nonoperative patients are not reliable given significant differences in the patient populations included in these series. Allocation of therapy for resectable stage IIIA NSCLC remains controversial as two randomized trials in this patient population have not demonstrated a clear advantage to either approach. The Intergroup 0139 study randomized 396 patients with technically resectable clinically staged IIIA (N2) NSCLC to either: (1) definitive RT to 61 Gy concurrent with two cycles of PE (cisplatin 50 mg/m^2 d1,8,29,36, etoposide 50 mg/m^2 d1–5,29–33) or (2) the same chemotherapy concurrent with radiation to 45 Gy followed by resection.[53] Progression-free survival (PFS) was improved by the addition of surgical resection. However, there was no benefit to OS in the entire series of patients. However, it is important to note that in a subset analysis of patients undergoing lobectomy, there was a doubling of survival (18% vs. 36% at 5 years) in patients undergoing trimodality therapy compared to those undergoing definitive chemoradiation alone. A second randomized study, EORTC 08941, showed no difference in PFS or OS for trimodality therapy compared to chemoradiation (in this case sequential chemotherapy followed by radiation).[54] In both of these trials the rate of operative mortality was relatively high, and beyond that reported in series from experienced

centers. As such the authors support the strategy of offering trimodality therapy to patients with low expected surgical morbidity and mortality, while deferring to definitive nonoperative therapy in the remainder of patients. While LC is improved by resection the predominant pattern of failure remains distant, and one must carefully balance the risks of resection against the improvements of escalating local therapy in this patient population.

Neoadjuvant Chemoradiation or Neoadjuvant Chemotherapy Alone?

For stage IIIA patients being offered operative therapy there is also some controversy over proceeding with neoadjuvant chemoradiation, the standard of the Intergroup trial, versus neoadjuvant chemotherapy alone, reserving radiation for adjuvant therapy as pathologically indicated. Results of two somewhat underpowered randomized trials suggest that neoadjuvant chemoradiation improves rates of complete resection and mediastinal downstaging, as well as, a possibly clinical response without clearly improving PFS or OS.[55,56] The addition of neoadjuvant radiation does add slightly more hematologic toxicity and esophagitis, though no clear differences in surgical complications or mortality.[55,56] Confounding these results is the fact that patients in the neoadjuvant chemo arm of the larger GLCCG study received adjuvant radiation, such that this is really a trial of neoadjuvant chemotherapy with either neoadjuvant or adjuvant radiation. RTOG 0412 was a phase III trial comparing neoadjuvant cisplatin and docetaxel with or without thoracic radiotherapy to 50.4 Gy, with both arms receiving adjuvant docetaxel following surgical resection. Unfortunately, this trial was abandoned due to lack of patient accrual. SAKK-16/00 and NCCCTS-06-164 are ongoing randomized trials investigating this question

Induction Chemoradiation Regimens

Induction chemoradiation is classically delivered as 45 Gy in 25 fractions with concurrent cisplatinum and etoposide as per SWOG 8805 (Fig. 99.5A–C).[57] This backbone has also been used for the treatment of Pancoast tumors with 5-year OS >50% in a phase II cooperative group study for node negative patients.[58,59] Alternative induction regimens including twice daily fractionation have also been used with success. Given that rates of mediastinal downstaging have consistently correlated with OS after neoadjuvant chemoradiation, high-dose induction regimens have been explored to treat the mediastinum to upward of 60 Gy in 30 fractions. While early results do confirm excellent mediastinal downstaging, OS has been modest and some potential for increased toxicity compared to standard regimens has been reported. This approach is being investigated in the currently active trial RTOG 0839 investigating 60 Gy in 30 fractions plus a randomization with or without concurrent panitumumab.[60]

Postoperative Radiation

While four randomized trials have confirmed a survival advantage for the addition of adjuvant chemotherapy for resected stage II–III NSCLC,[61–65] adjuvant radiation has a more limited range of indications. Historically, the PORT meta-analysis suggested a survival detriment for postoperative radiation in stages I and II NSCLC. The included studies were based on predominately utilizing large-field 2D planned external beam radiation. These were often on low energy or Cobalt-60-based treatment platforms.[66] Cardiac and pulmonary complications from this wide-field radiation are hypothesized to have offset the LC benefit. A more modern Italian study recently did suggest possible survival advantage to small field (bronchial stump only) radiation in stage I NSCLC,[67] though this has not been duplicated

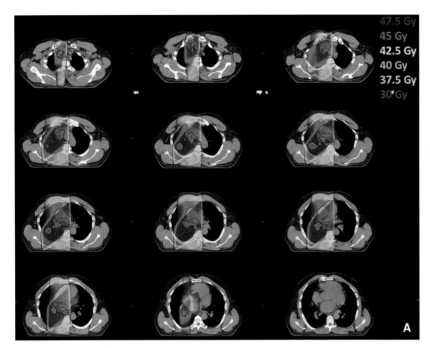
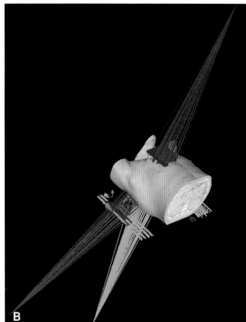

47.5 Gy
45 Gy
42.5 Gy
40 Gy
37.5 Gy
30 Gy

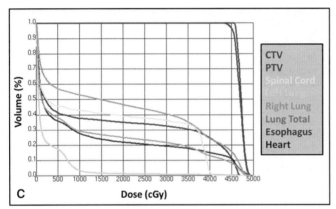

CTV
PTV
Spinal Cord
Left Lung
Right Lung
Lung Total
Esophagus
Heart

FIGURE 99.5 A: Representative axial CT scans of the gross tumor volume (GTV, *green outline*) and clinical target volume (CTV, *blue outline*) in a patient with a Stage IIIA (T1bN2M0) adenocarcinoma of the right upper lobe undergoing induction chemoradiation therapy to a dose of 45 Gy in 25 fractions of 1.8 Gy/fraction using 10 MV photons via 3 fields followed by right upper lobectomy and mediastinal lymph node dissection. Organs at risk are also outlined including the heart (*red*) and esophagus (*purple*). Dose distribution shown in color wash format with the corresponding doses as identified in the color legend. **B:** Patient rendering with beam arrangement for the treatment plan displayed in Figure 99.5. As can be visualized in this rendering, three radiotherapy fields were used to encompass the treatment volume including an anterior (*red*), posterior (*green*), and posterior oblique field (*blue*). **C:** Dose–volume histogram. The clinical target volume (CTV) includes the gross disease and areas of microscopic extension of disease and the planning target volume (PTV) includes a margin to account for set-up reproducibility error. Organs-at-risk for lung cancer patients include the spinal cord, total lung, esophagus, and heart. In addition to a qualitative analysis of the dose distribution, close examination of the minimum, maximum, and specific volume constraints are examined to ensure that a radiation therapy treatment plan maximizes the dose of radiation therapy to the tumor volume and minimizes the dose of radiation therapy to normal organs in the field.

and postoperative radiation is not indicated after complete resection of stage I or II NSCLC.

In stage III N2+ resected NSCLC the Lung Cancer Study Group (included in PORT meta-analysis) did demonstrate improved LC for postoperative radiation.[66,68] Furthermore, a subset analysis of a randomized adjuvant chemotherapy study,[69] and reviews of the Surveillance, Epidemiology, and End Results Program (SEER) and National Cancer Database[70,71] also suggest the potential for a survival advantage when modern techniques are utilized in the setting of resected stage III NSCLC.

Postoperative radiation is typically delivered sequentially after completion of chemotherapy. In the setting of positive margins concurrent

delivery is an alternative.[72] The target volume for postoperative radiation is the bronchial stump and hilum, as well as, known clinically and pathologically involved mediastinal nodal stations. Intervening nodal stations may be covered as well. The recommended dose is 50 Gy in 25 fractions for patients with negative margins. The dose should be increased to 54 to 60 Gy in 27 to 30 fractions in the setting of a close or positive margin.

Nonoperative Stage IIIA and IIIB NSCLC

The standard of care for nonoperative stage IIIA NSCLC is concurrent chemotherapy and radiation to a dose of 60 Gy in 30 fractions.[73]

Several randomized trials, including RTOG 94-10,[74] as well as a meta-analysis,[75] have suggested improved outcomes with OS increasing by approximately 6% when concurrent chemotherapy can be integrated. For patients unable to tolerate concurrent therapy, sequential chemotherapy followed by radiation is an alternative. Those unable to receive chemotherapy may be treated with radiation alone. When delivering sequential therapy or radiation alone there may be a benefit to dose escalation or altered radiation fractionation. RTOG 8311 demonstrated an improved outcome with 69.6 Gy in 1.2 Gy fractions given twice daily compared to daily radiation. Separate studies suggested a benefit to three times daily radiation over standard therapy.[76–78] Such hyperfractionated regimens may be logistically challenging for poor risk patients, and hypofractionated regimens such as 45 Gy in 15 fractions,[79] or split course therapy delivering two courses of 30 Gy in 10 fractions can be considered.[80] A meta-analysis has suggested a 2.5% OS benefit at 5 years for the use of altered fractionation when concurrent chemotherapy is not able to be administered.[81]

In contrast, neither altered fractionation,[74] nor dose escalation beyond 60 Gy in 30 fractions, appears to offer an advantage in the setting of concurrent chemoradiation. While retrospective series,[82] pooled analyses of consecutive RTOG phase II and III trials,[83] and a Chinese randomized trial[84] suggested possible benefit to dose escalation, the modern landmark study RTOG 0617 clearly demonstrated no advantage. Potentially there is some detriment to dose escalation beyond 60 Gy in 30 fractions.[85] RTOG 0617 enrolled 544 patients randomizing between 60 Gy in 30 fractions and 74 Gy in 37 fractions. OS was notably decreased in the high-dose arm. An association between higher cardiac dose and lower survival was likewise noted, but has not been validated. A second randomization of the addition of cetuximab to standard concurrent carboplatinum- and paclitaxel-based chemotherapy also increased toxicity without an improvement in OS. Rather than uniform dose escalation, newer studies such as RTOG 1106, are now testing whether advanced imaging and adaptive radiation replanning using an isotoxicity model may provide a vehicle for increasing the intensity of therapy to maximize LC.[86] As well, RTOG 1308 will re-examine dose escalation using protons, which have a unique and potentially advantageous dose distribution compared to photons.[87]

The target volume for definitive radiation has evolved substantially over time. Early trials used 2D x-ray-based approaches to radiation targeting treating standard comprehensive fields delineated by bony anatomy. Even after moving to CT-based 3D treatment planning, most historical radiation regimens included coverage of both the known tumor volume as well as "elective nodal radiation." This means the coverage of lymph nodes are beyond those clearly identified on imaging and pathology. More modern studies have focused treatment on only known involved sites. And, it has been noted that isolated failure in nonradiated elective nodal regions is quite rare (<5%),[88–90] and as such can likely be omitted to reduce field size, normal tissue exposure, and hopefully toxicity. A Chinese randomized study of standard dose elective nodal radiation compared to dose-escalated involved site radiation likewise demonstrated a benefit to smaller treatment fields.[84] Given uncommon failure in elective nodal regions, combined with higher rates of in-field failure focusing treatment on identified sites of disease only, is the approach endorsed by modern guidelines.[52,84,88]

PALLIATION OF METASTATIC NSCLC

The primary indications for radiation in metastatic NSCLC are for the palliation of symptomatic metastasis, or treatment of central nervous system disease where penetration of chemotherapy is poor. Patients with solitary brain metastasis who have only stage I thoracic disease may benefit from consolidative chest radiation or SBRT.[91] Otherwise, asymptomatic patients with stage IV disease should be referred for systemic therapy or palliative care alone outside of a clinical trial setting. The use of SBRT to treat isolated progression in sites of developing resistance in patients with mutations that have pharmacologic targets is a promising area of research.[92] Early reports of SBRT to sites of progression on first-line therapy of oligo-metastatic NSCLC have also been provocative.[93,94] However, they need further investigation and clarification before becoming part of the standard of care.

For patients presenting with symptomatic chest disease several randomized trials have investigated the role of 30 Gy in 10 fractions compared to more hypofractionated approaches such as 17 Gy in 2 fractions 1 week apart.[95,96] This demonstrates that thoracic symptoms can be treated safely and effectively by simple treatment schedules with no symptom relief benefit to higher radiation doses. Selected patients with good performance status may see modest survival benefits from higher-dose palliative regimens (30 Gy/10 fraction equivalent or higher). But this is at the expense of moderately higher esophageal toxicity rates.[96] Although these randomized clinical trials of palliative RT for lung cancer have been conducted in patients with NSCLC, the treatment approaches and results from such studies are readily applicable to the patient with symptoms related to SCLC.

Bone metastasis can likewise be treated by a range of dose fractionation schedules with equal symptomatic relief. A Cochrane review of 11 prospective randomized studies of single versus multiple fraction palliative radiation regimens including 3,435 patients with bone metastases across multiple primary tumor sites showed no difference in response rate, though it did suggest lower need for retreatment (7% vs. 22%) and the risk of pathologic fracture (1.6% vs. 3%) for multiple fraction regimens.[97] These small differences should be taken into account. However, for patients with poor overall prognosis, the efficiency of single fraction regimens may be desirable.

Brain metastasis from NSCLC and SCLC are typically treated with surgery followed by radiation. Otherwise radiation alone gives poor penetration of chemotherapy beyond the blood–brain barrier. Outcomes for patients can be estimated using the Graded Prognostic Assessment (GPA) specific to NSCLC.[98] For patients with high GPA reflected by a limited number of lesions, good performance status, and absence of progressive extracranial disease, the choice of stereotactic radiosurgery (SRS) versus whole brain radiation (WBRT) with or without an SRS boost is controversial. Recently, the trend has shifted to primary SRS. This may lead to improvements in LC, reduced rates of neurotoxicity, and improvements in quality of life.[99] This is supported by the most recent National Comprehensive Cancer Network (NCCN) guidelines, even for patients with multiple lesions. However, it leaves patients at risk for distant intracranial failure. For those who have received WBRT, an SRS boost may be considered for patients with specific disease features, such as presence of a single lesion, large metastasis, or for those with an excellent performance status.[100,101] Given the fatigue, memory changes, alopecia, and other side effects of WBRT, efforts have been made to find strategies to reduce toxicity. In separate studies the drug memantine,[102] and more strikingly hippocampal-avoiding WBRT delivered utilizing hippocampal-sparing intensity-modulated radiation, may reduce neurocognitive toxicity. RTOG 0933 is a nonrandomized phase II trial investigating the feasibility of hippocampal-sparing WBRT for brain metastasis. It demonstrated no evidence for increased failure rates with a mean relative decline of memory by delayed recall of only 7% at 4 months compared to historical controls of 30% for similar dose regimens delivered by opposed lateral beams.[103]

SMALL CELL LUNG CANCER

Limited Stage SCLC

Given the propensity for even LS-SCLC to be a regional and systemic disease it is not surprising that a study from the prechemotherapy era of the 1960s demonstrates improved outcomes with regional radiation compared to surgical resection.[104] Even with the introduction of chemotherapy in the 1980s, a number of randomized trials have shown that the addition of thoracic radiation to chemotherapy reduces intrathoracic failures by approximately one-half (75% to 90% with chemotherapy alone, compared to 30% to 60% when thoracic radiation is added to chemotherapy).[105] Meta-analyses have similarly confirmed that the addition of thoracic radiation confers an OS benefit of 5% for patients treated with combined modality therapy compared to chemotherapy alone.[106,107] Meta-analysis investigating the timing of radiation have suggested that starting treatment with cycle 1 or 2 of platinum-based chemotherapy appears to confer the greatest advantage.[107–109]

The optimal radiation dose-fractionation regimen is not yet known. The US standard of care is most often 45 Gy given in 30 fractions of 1.5 Gy delivered twice daily over 3 weeks concurrent with the first of two of four cycles of Etoposide and Cisplatinum chemotherapy. This is based on a randomized study demonstrating superior survival with this regimen compared to 45 Gy in 25 fractions delivered once daily over 5 weeks.[110] It is not clear whether this advantage was due to twice daily versus daily treatment, faster completion of treatment in a disease where resistant clones may repopulate rapidly, or to a higher BED in the twice daily arm (or a combination of these factors). Of note, the rate of grade 3 and higher esophagitis in the twice daily arm was increased (11% vs. 27%) in particular for patients over the age of 70. Remarkably, similar phase 2 outcomes have been reported for regimens of 40 Gy in 15 fractions given with the second cycle of chemotherapy,[108] a hybrid of daily and twice daily radiation delivering 61.2 Gy in 5 weeks, 7 weeks of daily radiation to 66 to 70 Gy in 33 to 35 fractions.[112] Randomized trials comparing many of the above regimens are underway both in the United States and the United Kingdom.[113,114]

Prophylactic Cranial Irradiation

SCLC has high affinity for the brain. While only 10% of patients present with brain metastasis at initial diagnosis, approximately half will develop brain metastasis over the course of their disease. Given this risk, prophylactic cranial irradiation (PCI) was investigated as a means to address microscopic tumor burden at presentation. PCI has been shown to reduce the risk of brain metastasis (58.6% vs. 33.3%) and improve OS (15.3% vs. 20.7% at 3 years) in patients with LS-SCLC.[115] As the meta-analysis suggested, a dose-response relationship for reduction in the rate of brain metastasis occurred. A subsequent randomized trial was completed to assess radiation dose escalation. A PCI dose of 25 Gy in 10 fractions (compared to 36 Gy in daily or twice daily fractions) was determined to remain the standard of care with the lowest rates of toxicity and equivalent OS to other regimens.[116] A similar magnitude benefit was seen in the 15% of patients with extensive stage (ES) SCLC compared to those with LS-SCLC and the role of PCI in ES-SCLC was explored. In 2007, the EORTC reported the results of a phase III trial randomizing ES-SCLC patients with any response after standard first-line systemic therapy to PCI or observation.[117] At 1 year, the PCI patients were found to have a lower rate of symptomatic brain metastases (15% vs. 40%) and improved 1-year (27% vs. 13%) and median (6.7 months vs. 5.4 months) OS. Criticism of this study includes the fact that there was no baseline brain imaging prior to PCI such that a percentage of patients may have had active

gross brain disease (albeit subclinial) at the time of PCI. Nonetheless, the findings of this study suggest that PCI should be considered in ES-SCLC as well. Though given that this remains mostly an incurable disease with a very modest OS benefit to PCI, the toxicity of therapy must be kept in mind during patient selection for ES-SCLC. While the toxicity of PCI is modest, patients do note several months of fatigue, as well as lasting short-term memory and balance changes. Future plans are to explore technology such as hippocampal-sparing WBRT as discussed above for PCI for LS-SCLC.

Extensive Stage SCLC

Historically the standard of care for ES-SCLC has been six cycles of Etoposide and Cisplatinum chemotherapy without a clear role for radiation aside from palliation of symptomatic recurrent disease. While several smaller studies did not demonstrate benefit, a 1999 randomized trial by Jeremic and colleagues suggested improved 5-year OS (9.1% vs. 3.7%) with the addition of accelerated hyperfractionated thoracic RT (54 Gy/36 BID fractions over 18 days) with concurrent daily carboplatin/etoposide. This is compared to chemotherapy alone for patients with a complete response of distant sites and at least a partial response of local disease after three cycles of induction chemotherapy.[118,119] This result prompted further investigation into the role of consolidative chest radiation for ES-SCLC. Recently reported, the EORTC randomized 498 patients with ES-SCLC and at least a partial response to four to six cycles of chemotherapy to consolidative chest radiation (without treatment of metastasis) to a dose of 30 Gy in 10 fractions together with PCI compared to PCI alone.[119] While the primary endpoint of 1-year OS was not statistically significantly improved (33% for thoracic RT compared to 28% for the control group), 2-year OS was improved (13% vs. 3%) while progression was also reduced. RTOG 0937 was a second cooperative group study investigating the role of consolidative radiation to the primary and metastatic sites for patients with partial response to four or fewer sites of disease along with PCI. This study was closed in early 2015 prior to completing accrual when interim analysis revealed that the study had crossed the futility boundary for the primary endpoint of improving OS. Furthermore, there was a disproportion of high-grade toxicity in the experimental arm.[120] RTOG 0937 did treat the primary site to a higher dose than the EORTC study and also mandated coverage of the metastatic sites in addition to the primary. Pending the final results of RTOG 0937 aggressive multiple-field radiation after response to chemotherapy in ES-SCLC is not recommended. However, more conservative consolidation of the primary site to a dose of 30 Gy in 10 fractions may be considered in select patients.

FUTURE DIRECTIONS

With the advent of biologically targeted therapy, investigation is needed into how best to integrate and sequence these agents in combination with radiation. Furthermore, research into radiation resistance and normal tissue sensitivity may bring significant improvement in patient selection for radiation versus other therapies through personalized medicine. Finally, as systemic therapy improves, there will be an increasing population of patients with oligo-progressive disease. In the future, there may be patients who may benefit from stereotactic ablation of single sites of progression performed in combination with continuation of otherwise successful systemic therapy.

REFERENCES

1. McGarry RC, Song G, des Rosiers P, et al. Observation-only management of early stage, medically inoperable lung cancer: Poor outcome. *Chest* 2002;121:1155–1158.

2. Koshy M, Malik R, Mahmood U, et al. Stereotactic body radiotherapy and treatment at a high volume facility is associated with improved survival in patients with inoperable stage I non-small cell lung cancer. *Radiother Oncol* 2015;114:148–154.

3. Grutters JP, Kessels AG, Pijls-Johannesma M, et al. Comparison of the effectiveness of radiotherapy with photons, protons and carbon-ions for non-small cell lung cancer: A meta-analysis. *Radiother Oncol* 2010;95:32–40.

4. Martel MK, Ten Haken RK, Hazuka MB, et al. Estimation of tumor control probability model parameters from 3-D dose distributions of non-small cell lung cancer patients. *Lung Cancer* 1999;24:31–37.

5. Palma D, Visser O, Lagerwaard FJ, et al. Impact of introducing stereotactic lung radiotherapy for elderly patients with stage I non-small-cell lung cancer: A population-based time-trend analysis. *J Clin Oncol* 2010;28:5153–5159.

6. Tree AC, Khoo VS, Eeles RA, et al. Stereotactic body radiotherapy for oligometastases. *Lancet Oncol* 2013;14:e28–e37.

7. Liu H, Zhang X, Vinogradskiy YY, et al. Predicting radiation pneumonitis after stereotactic ablative radiation therapy in patients previously treated with conventional thoracic radiation therapy. *Int J Radiat Oncol Biol Phys* 2012;84:1017–1023.

8. Hearn JW, Videtic GM, Djemil T, et al. Salvage stereotactic body radiation therapy (SBRT) for local failure after primary lung SBRT. *Int J Radiat Oncol Biol Phys* 2014; 90(2):402–406.

9. Videtic GM, Stephans KL, Woody NM, et al. Stereotactic body radiation therapy-based treatment model for stage I medically inoperable small cell lung cancer. *Pract Radiat Oncol* 2013;3:301–306.

10. Shioyama Y, Nakamura K, Sasaki T, et al. Clinical results of stereotactic body radiotherapy for stage I small-cell lung cancer: A single institutional experience. *J Radiat Res* 2013;54:108–112.

11. Onishi H, Shirato H, Nagata Y, et al. Stereotactic body radiotherapy (SBRT) for operable stage I non-small-cell lung cancer: Can SBRT be comparable to surgery? *Int J Radiat Oncol Biol Phys* 2011;81:1352–1358.

12. Lagerwaard FJ, Verstegen NE, Haasbeek CJ, et al. Outcomes of stereotactic ablative radiotherapy in patients with potentially operable stage I non-small cell lung cancer. *Int J Radiat Oncol Biol Phys* 2012;83:348–353.

13. Feddock J, Arnold SM, Shelton BJ, et al. Stereotactic body radiation therapy can be used safely to boost residual disease in locally advanced non-small cell lung cancer: A prospective study. *Int J Radiat Oncol Biol Phys* 2013;85:1325–1331.

14. Karam SD, Horne ZD, Hong RL, et al. Dose escalation with stereotactic body radiation therapy boost for locally advanced non small cell lung cancer. *Radiat Oncol* 2013;8:179.

15. RTOG 0813. Seamless phase I/II study of stereotactic lung radiotherapy (SBRT) for early-stage, centrally located, non-small cell lung cancer (NSCLC) in medically inoperable patients, http://www.rtog.org/ClinicalTrials/ProtocolTable/StudyDetails.aspx?study=0813. Accessed May 14, 2015.

16. RTOG 0915. A randomized phase II study comparing 2 Stereotactic Body Radiation Therapy (SBRT) schedules for medically inoperable patients with stage I peripheral non-small cell lung cancer, http://www.rtog.org/ClinicalTrials/ProtocolTable/StudyDetails.aspx?study=0915. Accessed May 14, 2015.

17. Benedict SH, Yenice KM, Followill D, et al. Stereotactic body radiation therapy: The report of AAPM task group 101. *Med Phys* 2010;37:4078–4101.

18. Park C, Papiez L, Zhang S, et al. Universal survival curve and single fraction equivalent dose: Useful tools in understanding potency of ablative radiotherapy. *Int J Radiat Oncol Biol Phys* 2008;70:847–852.

19. Kavanagh BD, Newman F. Toward a unified survival curve: In regard to Park et al. (*Int J Radiat Oncol Biol Phys* 2008;70:847–852) and Krueger et al. (*Int J Radiat Oncol Biol Phys* 2007;69:1262–1271). *Int J Radiat Oncol Biol Phys* 2008;71:958–959.

20. Timmerman R, Papiez L, McGarry R, et al. Extracranial stereotactic radioablation: Results of a phase I study in medically inoperable stage I non-small cell lung cancer. *Chest* 2003;124:1946–1955.

21. Timmerman R, McGarry R, Yiannoutsos C, et al. Excessive toxicity when treating central tumors in a phase II study of stereotactic body radiation therapy for medically inoperable early-stage lung cancer. *J Clin Oncol* 2006;24:4833–4839.

22. Uematsu M, Shioda A, Suda A, et al. Computed tomography-guided frameless stereotactic radiotherapy for stage I non-small cell lung cancer: A 5-year experience. *Int J Radiat Oncol Biol Phys* 2001;51:666–670.

23. Nagata Y, Takayama K, Matsuo Y, et al. Clinical outcomes of a phase I/II study of 48 gy of stereotactic body radiotherapy in 4 fractions for primary lung cancer using a stereotactic body frame. *Int J Radiat Oncol Biol Phys* 2005;63:1427–1431.

24. Onishi H, Shirato H, Nagata Y, et al. Hypofractionated stereotactic radiotherapy (HypoFXSRT) for stage I non-small-cell lung cancer: Updated results of 257 patients in a Japanese multi-institutional study. *J Thorac Oncol* 2007;2:S94–S100.

25. Haasbeek CJ, Lagerwaard FJ, Slotman BJ, et al. Outcomes of stereotactic ablative radiotherapy for centrally located early-stage lung cancer. *J Thorac Oncol* 2011;6: 2036–2043.

26. Senthi S, Haasbeek CJ, Slotman BJ, et al. Outcomes of stereotactic ablative radiotherapy for central lung tumours: A systematic review. *Radiother Oncol* 2013;106:276–282.

27. Chang JY, Li QQ, Xu QY, et al. Stereotactic ablative radiation therapy for centrally located early stage or isolated parenchymal recurrences of non-small cell lung cancer: How to fly in a "no fly zone". *Int J Radiat Oncol Biol Phys* 2014;88:1120–1128.

28. Kestin L, Grills I, Guckenberger M, et al. Dose-response relationship with clinical outcome for lung stereotactic body radiotherapy (SBRT) delivered via online image guidance. *Radiother Oncol* 2014;110:499–504.

29. Zhang J, Yang F, Li B, et al. Which is the optimal biologically effective dose of stereotactic body radiotherapy for stage I non-small-cell lung cancer? A meta-analysis. *Int J Radiat Oncol Biol Phys* 2011;81:e305–e316.

30. Mehta N, King CR, Agazaryan N, et al. Stereotactic body radiation therapy and 3-dimensional conformal radiotherapy for stage I non-small cell lung cancer: A pooled analysis of biological equivalent dose and local control. *Pract Radiat Oncol* 2012;2:288–295.

31. Lagerwaard FJ, Haasbeek CJ, Smit EF, et al. Outcomes of risk-adapted fractionated stereotactic radiotherapy for stage I non-small-cell lung cancer. *Int J Radiat Oncol Biol Phys* 2008;70:685–692.

32. Fakiris AJ, McGarry RC, Yiannoutsos CT, et al. Stereotactic body radiation therapy for early-stage non-small-cell lung carcinoma: Four-year results of a prospective phase II study. *Int J Radiat Oncol Biol Phys* 2009;75:677–682.

33. Zheng X, Schipper M, Kidwell K, et al. Survival outcome after stereotactic body radiation therapy and surgery for stage I non-small cell lung cancer: A meta-analysis. *Int J Radiat Oncol Biol Phys* 2014;90:603–611.

34. Timmerman R, Paulus R, Galvin J, et al. Stereotactic body radiation therapy for inoperable early stage lung cancer. *JAMA* 2010;303:1070–1076.

35. Ginsberg RJ, Rubinstein LV. Randomized trial of lobectomy versus limited resection for T1 N0 non-small cell lung cancer. Lung cancer study group. *Ann Thorac Surg* 1995;60:615–622; discussion 622–623.

36. Fernando HC, Landreneau RJ, Mandrekar SJ, et al. Impact of brachytherapy on local recurrence rates after sublobar resection: Results from ACOSOG Z4032 (alliance), a phase III randomized trial for high-risk operable non-small-cell lung cancer. *J Clin Oncol* 2014;32:2456–2462.

37. Huang K, Palma DA, IASLC Advanced Radiation Technology Committee. Follow-up of patients after stereotactic radiation for lung cancer: A primer for the nonradiation oncologist. *J Thorac Oncol* 2015;10:412–419.

38. Marwaha G, Reddy C, Stephans K, et al. Lung SBRT: Regional nodal failure is not predicted by tumor size. *J Thorac Oncol* 2014;9:1693–1697.

39. van den Berg LL, Klinkenberg TJ, Groen HJ, et al. Patterns of recurrence and survival after surgery or stereotactic radiotherapy for early stage NSCLC. *J Thorac Oncol* 2015;10:826–831.

40. Crabtree TD, Denlinger CE, Meyers BF, et al. Stereotactic body radiation therapy versus surgical resection for stage I non-small cell lung cancer. *J Thorac Cardiovasc Surg* 2010;140:377–386.

41. Smetana GW, Lawrence VA, Cornell JE, et al. Preoperative pulmonary risk stratification for noncardiothoracic surgery: Systematic review for the American college of physicians. *Ann Intern Med* 2006;144:581–595.

42. Puri V, Crabtree TD, Kymes S, et al. A comparison of surgical intervention and stereotactic body radiation therapy for stage I lung cancer in high-risk patients: A decision analysis. *J Thorac Cardiovasc Surg* 2012;143:428–436.

43. Louie AV, Rodrigues G, Hannouf M, et al. Stereotactic body radiotherapy versus surgery for medically operable stage I non-small-cell lung cancer: A Markov model-based decision analysis. *Int J Radiat Oncol Biol Phys* 2011;81:964–973.

44. Videtic GM, Reddy CA, Sorenson L. A prospective study of quality of life including fatigue and pulmonary function after stereotactic body radiotherapy for medically inoperable early-stage lung cancer. *Support Care Cancer* 2013;21:211–218.

45. Kenny PM, King MT, Viney RC, et al. Quality of life and survival in the 2 years after surgery for non small-cell lung cancer. *J Clin Oncol* 2008;26:233–241.

46. Stanic S, Paulus R, Timmerman RD, et al. No clinically significant changes in pulmonary function following stereotactic body radiation therapy for early- stage peripheral non-small cell lung cancer: An analysis of RTOG 0236. *Int J Radiat Oncol Biol Phys* 2014;88:1092–1099.

47. Henderson M, McGarry R, Yiannoutsos C, et al. Baseline pulmonary function as a predictor for survival and decline in pulmonary function over time in patients undergoing stereotactic body radiotherapy for the treatment of stage I non-small-cell lung cancer. *Int J Radiat Oncol Biol Phys* 2008;72:404–409.

48. Stephans KL, Djemil T, Reddy CA, et al. Comprehensive analysis of pulmonary function test (PFT) changes after stereotactic body radiotherapy (SBRT) for stage I lung cancer in medically inoperable patients. *J Thorac Oncol* 2009;4: 838–844.

49. Shultz DB, Diehn M, Loo BW, Jr. To SABR or not to SABR? Indications and contraindications for stereotactic ablative radiotherapy in the treatment of early-stage, oligometastatic, or oligoprogressive non-small cell lung cancer. *Semin Radiat Oncol* 2015;25:78–86.

50. Rusch VW, Parekh KR, Leon L, et al. Factors determining outcome after surgical resection of T3 and T4 lung cancers of the superior sulcus. *J Thorac Cardiovasc Surg* 2000;119:1147–1153.

51. Scott WJ, Howington J, Movsas B, et al. Treatment of stage II non-small cell lung cancer. *Chest* 2003;123:188S–201S.

52. Machtay M, Paulus R, Moughan J, et al. Defining local-regional control and its importance in locally advanced non-small cell lung carcinoma. *J Thorac Oncol* 2012;7:716–722.

53. Albain KS, Swann RS, Rusch VW, et al. Radiotherapy plus chemotherapy with or without surgical resection for stage III non-small-cell lung cancer: A phase III randomised controlled trial. *Lancet* 2009;374:379–386.

54. van Meerbeeck JP, Kramer GW, Van Schil PE, et al. Randomized controlled trial of resection versus radiotherapy after induction chemotherapy in stage IIIA-N2 non-small-cell lung cancer. *J Natl Cancer Inst* 2007;99:442–450.

55. Sauvaget J, Rebischung JL, Vannetzel JM. Phase III study of neo-adjuvant MVP versus MVP plus chemo-radiotherapy in stage III NSCLC. *J Clin Oncol (Meeting Abstracts)* 2000.

56. Thomas M, Rube C, Hoffknecht P, et al. Effect of preoperative chemoradiation in addition to preoperative chemotherapy: A randomised trial in stage III non-small-cell lung cancer. *Lancet Oncol* 2008;9:636–648.

57. Albain KS, Rusch VW, Crowley JJ, et al. Concurrent cisplatin/etoposide plus chest radiotherapy followed by surgery for stages IIIA (N2) and IIIB non-small-cell lung cancer: Mature results of southwest oncology group phase II study 8805. *J Clin Oncol* 1995;13:1880–1892.

58. Rusch VW, Giroux DJ, Kraut MJ, et al. Induction chemoradiation and surgical resection for non-small cell lung carcinomas of the superior sulcus: Initial results of southwest oncology group trial 9416 (intergroup trial 0160). *J Thorac Cardiovasc Surg* 2001;121:472–483.

59. Kernstine KH, Moon J, Kraut MJ, et al. Trimodality therapy for superior sulcus non-small cell lung cancer: Southwest oncology group-intergroup trial S0220. *Ann Thorac Surg* 2014;98:402–410.

60. RTOG 0839. Randomized phase II study of pre-operative chemoradiotherapy +/- panitumumab (IND #110152) followed by consolidation chemotherapy in potentially operable locally advanced (stage IIIA, N2+) non-small cell lung cancer, http://www.rtog.org/ClinicalTrials/ProtocolTable/StudyDetails.aspx?study=0839. Accessed May 14, 2015.

61. Winton T, Livingston R, Johnson D, et al. Vinorelbine plus cisplatin vs. observation in resected non-small-cell lung cancer. *N Engl J Med* 2005;352:2589–2597.

62. Douillard JY, Rosell R, De Lena M, et al. Adjuvant vinorelbine plus cisplatin versus observation in patients with completely resected stage IB-IIIA non-small-cell lung cancer (adjuvant navelbine international trialist association [ANITA]): A randomised controlled trial. *Lancet Oncol* 2006;7:719–727.

63. Pignon JP, Tribodet H, Scagliotti GV, et al. Lung adjuvant cisplatin evaluation: A pooled analysis by the LACE collaborative group. *J Clin Oncol* 2008;26:3552–3559.

64. Strauss GM, Herndon JE, 2nd, Maddaus MA, et al. Adjuvant paclitaxel plus carboplatin compared with observation in stage IB non-small-cell lung cancer: CALGB 9633 with the cancer and leukemia group B, radiation therapy oncology group, and north central cancer treatment group study groups. *J Clin Oncol* 2008;26:5043–5051.

65. Arriagada R, Dunant A, Pignon JP, et al. Long-term results of the international adjuvant lung cancer trial evaluating adjuvant cisplatin-based chemotherapy in resected lung cancer. *J Clin Oncol* 2010;28:35–42.

66. PORT Meta-Analysis Trialists Group. Postoperative radiotherapy for non-small cell lung cancer. *Cochrane Database Syst Rev* 2003;(1):CD002142.

67. Trodella L, Granone P, Valente S, et al. Adjuvant radiotherapy in non-small cell lung cancer with pathological stage I: Definitive results of a phase III randomized trial. *Radiother Oncol* 2002;62:11–19.

68. Weisenberger TH. Effects of postoperative mediastinal radiation on completely resected stage II and stage III epidermoid cancer of the lung. The lung cancer study group. *N Engl J Med* 1986;315:1377–1381.

69. Douillard J, Rosell R, De Lena M, et al. Impact of postoperative radiation therapy on survival in patients with complete resection and stage I, II, or IIIA non-small-cell lung cancer treated with adjuvant chemotherapy: The adjuvant navelbine international trialist association (ANITA) randomized trial. *Int J Radiat Oncol Biol Phys* 2008;72:695–701.

70. Lally BE, Zelterman D, Colasanto JM, et al. Postoperative radiotherapy for stage II or III non-small-cell lung cancer using the surveillance, epidemiology, and end results database. *J Clin Oncol* 2006;24:2998–3006.

71. Robinson C, Patel AP, Bradley JD, et al. Postoperative radiotherapy for pathologic N2 Non–Small-cell lung cancer treated with adjuvant chemotherapy: A review of the national cancer data base. *J Clin Oncol* 2015;33:870–876.

72. Keller SM, Adak S, Wagner H, et al. A randomized trial of postoperative adjuvant therapy in patients with completely resected stage II or IIIA non-small-cell lung cancer. Eastern cooperative oncology group. *N Engl J Med* 2000;343:1217–1222.

73. Rodrigues G, Choy H, Bradley J, et al. Definitive radiation therapy in locally advanced non-small cell lung cancer: Executive summary of an american society for radiation oncology (ASTRO) evidence-based clinical practice guideline. *Pract Radiat Oncol* 2015;5:141–148.

74. Curran WJ, Jr, Paulus R, Langer CJ, et al. Sequential vs. concurrent chemoradiation for stage III non-small cell lung cancer: Randomized phase III trial RTOG 9410. *J Natl Cancer Inst* 2011;103:1452–1460.

75. Auperin A, Le Pechoux C, Rolland E, et al. Meta-analysis of concomitant versus sequential radiochemotherapy in locally advanced non-small-cell lung cancer. *J Clin Oncol* 2010;28:2181–2190.

76. Saunders MI, Rojas A, Lyn BE, et al. Experience with dose escalation using CHARTWEL (continuous hyperfractionated accelerated radiotherapy weekend less) in non-small-cell lung cancer. *Br J Cancer* 1998;78:1323–1328.

77. Belani CP, Choy H, Bonomi P, et al. Combined chemoradiotherapy regimens of paclitaxel and carboplatin for locally advanced non-small-cell lung cancer: A randomized phase II locally advanced multi-modality protocol. *J Clin Oncol* 2005;23:5883–5891.

78. Cox JD, Azarnia N, Byhardt RW, et al. A randomized phase I/II trial of hyperfractionated radiation therapy with total doses of 60.0 Gy to 79.2 Gy: Possible survival benefit with greater than or equal to 69.6 Gy in favorable patients with radiation therapy oncology group stage III non-small-cell lung carcinoma: Report of radiation therapy oncology group 83-11. *J Clin Oncol* 1990;8:1543–1555.

79. Amini A, Lin SH, Wei C, et al. Accelerated hypofractionated radiation therapy compared to conventionally fractionated radiation therapy for the treatment of inoperable non-small cell lung cancer. *Radiat Oncol* 2012;7:33.

80. Slotman BJ, Njo KH, de Jonge A, et al. Hypofractionated radiation therapy in unresectable stage III non-small cell lung cancer. *Cancer* 1993;72:1885–1893.

81. Mauguen A, Le Pechoux C, Saunders MI, et al. Hyperfractionated or accelerated radiotherapy in lung cancer: An individual patient data meta-analysis. *J Clin Oncol* 2012;30:2788–2797.

82. Sibley GS, Mundt AJ, Shapiro C, et al. The treatment of stage III nonsmall cell lung cancer using high dose conformal radiotherapy. *Int J Radiat Oncol Biol Phys* 1995;33:1001–1007.

83. Machtay M, Bae K, Movsas B, et al. Higher biologically effective dose of radiotherapy is associated with improved outcomes for locally advanced non-small cell lung

carcinoma treated with chemoradiation: An analysis of the radiation therapy oncology group. *Int J Radiat Oncol Biol Phys* 2012;82:425–434.

84. Yuan S, Sun X, Li M, et al. A randomized study of involved-field irradiation versus elective nodal irradiation in combination with concurrent chemotherapy for inoperable stage III nonsmall cell lung cancer. *Am J Clin Oncol* 2007;30:239–244.

85. Bradley JD, Paulus R, Komaki R, et al. Standard-dose versus high-dose conformal radiotherapy with concurrent and consolidation carboplatin plus paclitaxel with or without cetuximab for patients with stage IIIA or IIIB non-small-cell lung cancer (RTOG 0617): A randomised, two-by-two factorial phase 3 study. *Lancet Oncol* 2015;16:187–199.

86. RTOG 1106/ACRIN 6697. Randomized phase II trial of individualized adaptive radiotherapy using during-treatment FDG-PET/CT and modern technology in locally advanced non-small cell lung cancer (NSCLC), http://www.rtog.org/ClinicalTrials/ProtocolTable/StudyDetails.aspx?study=1106. Accessed May 14, 2015.

87. RTOG 1308. Phase III randomized trial comparing overall survival after photon versus proton chemoradiotherapy for inoperable stage II-IIIB NSCLC, http://www.rtog.org/ClinicalTrials/ProtocolTable/StudyDetails.aspx?study=1308. Accessed May 14, 2015.

88. Rosenzweig KE, Sura S, Jackson A, et al. Involved-field radiation therapy for inoperable non small-cell lung cancer. *J Clin Oncol* 2007;25:5557–5561.

89. Belderbos JS, Kepka L, Spring Kong FM, et al. Report from the international atomic energy agency (IAEA) consultants' meeting on elective nodal irradiation in lung cancer: Non-small-cell lung cancer (NSCLC). *Int J Radiat Oncol Biol Phys* 2008;72:335–342.

90. Chang JY, Kestin LL, Barriger RB, et al. ACR appropriateness criteria(R) nonsurgical treatment for locally advanced non-small-cell lung cancer: Good performance status/definitive intent. *Oncology (Williston Park)* 2014;28:706–710, 712, 714 passim.

91. Bonnette P, Puyo P, Gabriel C, et al. Surgical management of non-small cell lung cancer with synchronous brain metastases. *Chest* 2001;119:1469–1475.

92. Gan GN, Weickhardt AJ, Scheier B, et al. Stereotactic radiation therapy can safely and durably control sites of extra-central nervous system oligoprogressive disease in anaplastic lymphoma kinase-positive lung cancer patients receiving crizotinib. *Int J Radiat Oncol Biol Phys* 2014;88:892–898.

93. Iyengar P, Kavanagh BD, Wardak Z, et al. Phase II trial of stereotactic body radiation therapy combined with erlotinib for patients with limited but progressive metastatic non-small-cell lung cancer. *J Clin Oncol* 2014;32:3824–3830.

94. Ashworth AB, Senan S, Palma DA, et al. An individual patient data metaanalysis of outcomes and prognostic factors after treatment of oligometastatic non-small-cell lung cancer. *Clin Lung Cancer* 2014;15:346–355.

95. Rosenzweig KE, Chang JY, Chetty IJ, et al. ACR appropriateness criteria nonsurgical treatment for non-small cell lung cancer: Poor performance status or palliative intent. *J Am Coll Radiol* 2013;10:654–664.

96. Rodrigues G, Videtic GMM, Sur R, et al. Palliative thoracic radiotherapy in lung cancer: An American society for radiation oncology evidence-based clinical practice guideline. *Pract Radiat Oncol* 2011;1:60–71.

97. Johnstone C, Lutz ST. External beam radiotherapy and bone metastases. *Ann Palliat Med* 2014;3:114–122.

98. Sperduto PW, Kased N, Roberge D, et al. Summary report on the graded prognostic assessment: An accurate and facile diagnosis-specific tool to estimate survival for patients with brain metastases. *J Clin Oncol* 2012;30:419–425.

99. Sahgal A, Aoyama H, Kocher M, et al. Phase 3 trials of stereotactic radiosurgery with or without whole-brain radiation therapy for 1 to 4 brain metastases: Individual patient data meta-analysis. *Int J Radiat Oncol Biol Phys* 2015;91:710–717.

100. Andrews DW, Scott CB, Sperduto PW, et al. Whole brain radiation therapy with or without stereotactic radiosurgery boost for patients with one to three brain metastases: Phase III results of the RTOG 9508 randomised trial. *Lancet* 2004;363:1665–1672.

101. Sperduto PW, Shanley R, Luo X, et al. Secondary analysis of RTOG 9508, a phase 3 randomized trial of whole-brain radiation therapy versus WBRT plus stereotactic radiosurgery in patients with 1–3 brain metastases; Poststratified by the graded prognostic assessment (GPA). *Int J Radiat Oncol Biol Phys* 2014;90:526–531.

102. Brown PD, Pugh S, Laack NN, et al. Memantine for the prevention of cognitive dysfunction in patients receiving whole-brain radiotherapy: A randomized, double-blind, placebo-controlled trial. *Neuro Oncol* 2013;15:1429–1437.

103. Gondi V, Pugh SL, Tome WA, et al. Preservation of memory with conformal avoidance of the hippocampal neural stem-cell compartment during whole-brain radiotherapy for brain metastases (RTOG 0933): A phase II multi-institutional trial. *J Clin Oncol* 2014;32:3810–3816.

104. Thorax. In: Edge SB, Byrd DR, Compton CC, Fritz AG, Greene FL, Trotti A., eds. AJCC Cancer Staging Handbook. 7th ed. New York, NY: Springer; 2010:299–323.

105. Kepka L, Sprawka A, Casas F, et al. Radiochemotherapy in small-cell lung cancer. *Expert Rev Anticancer Ther* 2009;9:1379–1387.

106. Warde P, Payne D. Does thoracic irradiation improve survival and local control in limited-stage small-cell carcinoma of the lung? A meta-analysis. *J Clin Oncol* 1992;10:890–895.

107. Pignon JP, Arriagada R, Ihde DC, et al. A meta-analysis of thoracic radiotherapy for small-cell lung cancer. *N Engl J Med* 1992;327:1618–1624.

108. Murray N, Coy P, Pater JL, et al. Importance of timing for thoracic irradiation in the combined modality treatment of limited-stage small-cell lung cancer. The national cancer institute of Canada clinical trials group. *J Clin Oncol* 1993;11:336–344.

109. Andrews DW. Should surgery followed by whole-brain radiation therapy be the standard treatment for single brain metastasis? *Nat Clin Pract Oncol* 2008;5:572–573.

110. Nieder C, Astner ST, Grosu A, et al. The role of postoperative radiotherapy after resection of a single brain metastasis. Combined analysis of 643 patients. *Strahlenther Onkol* 2007;183:576–580.

111. Komaki R, Paulus R, Ettinger DS, et al. Phase II study of accelerated high-dose radiotherapy with concurrent chemotherapy for patients with limited small-cell lung cancer: Radiation therapy oncology group protocol 0239. *Int J Radiat Oncol Biol Phys* 2012;83:e531–e536.

112. Bogart JA, Herndon JE, 2nd, Lyss AP, et al. 70 Gy thoracic radiotherapy is feasible concurrent with chemotherapy for limited-stage small-cell lung cancer: Analysis of cancer and leukemia group B study 39808. *Int J Radiat Oncol Biol Phys* 2004;59:460–468.

113. Faivre-Finn C, Falk S, Ashcroft L, et al. Protocol for the CONVERT trial-Concurrent ONce-daily VErsus twice-daily RadioTherapy: An international 2-arm randomised controlled trial of concurrent chemoradiotherapy comparing twice-daily and once-daily radiotherapy schedules in patients with limited stage small cell lung cancer (LS-SCLC) and good performance status. *BMJ Open* 2016;6:e009849.

114. CALGB 30610/RTOG 0538: Phase III comparison of thoracic radiotherapy regimens in patients with limited small cell lung cancer also receiving cisplatin and etoposide, http://www.rtog.org/ClinicalTrials/ProtocolTable.aspx. Accessed May 14, 2015.

115. Auperin A, Arriagada R, Pignon JP, et al. Prophylactic cranial irradiation for patients with small-cell lung cancer in complete remission. Prophylactic cranial irradiation overview collaborative group. *N Engl J Med* 1999;341:476–484.

116. Le Pechoux C, Dunant A, Senan S, et al. Standard-dose versus higher-dose prophylactic cranial irradiation (PCI) in patients with limited-stage small-cell lung cancer in complete remission after chemotherapy and thoracic radiotherapy (PCI 99-01, EORTC 22003-08004, RTOG 0212, and IFCT 99-01): A randomised clinical trial. *Lancet Oncol* 2009;10:467–474.

117. Slotman B, Faivre-Finn C, Kramer G, et al. Prophylactic cranial irradiation in extensive small-cell lung cancer. *N Engl J Med* 2007;357:664–672.

118. Spira A, Ettinger DS. Extensive-stage small-cell lung cancer. *Semin Surg Oncol* 2003;21:164–175.

119. Jeremic B, Shibamoto Y, Nikolic N, et al. Role of radiation therapy in the combined-modality treatment of patients with extensive disease small-cell lung cancer: A randomized study. *J Clin Oncol* 1999;17(7):2092–2099.

120. RTOG 0937. Randomized phase II study comparing prophylactic cranial irradiation alone to prophylactic cranial irradiation and consolidative extra-cranial irradiation for extensive disease small cell lung cancer (ED-SCLC), http://www.rtog.org/ClinicalTrials/ProtocolTable/StudyDetails.aspx?study=0937&mode=broadcasts&ptid=387. Accessed May 14, 2015.

Multimodality Therapy for Non-Small Cell Lung Cancer

Onkar V. Khullar ▪ Seth Force

With recent advancements in therapies for non-small cell cancer (NSCLC), contemporary management has become increasingly multidisciplinary, often involving thoracic surgeons, pulmonologists, medical oncologists, radiation oncologists, and interventional radiologists. Multimodality therapies have allowed us to extend care to patients who previously had little to no treatment options. Due to the complexity of managing patients with lung cancer in this modern era, both the National Comprehensive Cancer Network and the American College of Chest Physicians now recommend utilizing a multidisciplinary tumor board to provide optimal, multimodality treatment options for patients.[1,2] However, despite the increasing utilization of interdisciplinary care, there remains considerable confusion regarding the various roles of multimodality therapy in the management of NSCLC. To this point, two independent surveys commissioned in 2012 to query medical oncologists and thoracic surgeons noted considerable variability in the management of stage IIIA NSCLC. In fact, not only were there differences across specialty lines, but there was also notable lack of consensus even within individual specialties.[3,4]

In order to provide optimal care for the lung cancer patient, the role of surgery and the judgment of thoracic surgeons remains critical as surgical resection remains the mainstay therapy for stages I–IIIA. Therefore, it is necessary for the thoracic surgeon to be involved in or aware of the care of all patients with potentially resectable disease and surgeons must be intimately familiar with all possible therapies in each treatment modality. With that goal in mind, this chapter will review the current options and standards for multimodality therapy in the care of the patient with NSCLC.

approaches such as wedge and segmental resections is beyond the scope of this chapter. Regardless of whether a sublobar or lobar resection is employed, the surgeon's first priority should always be to obtain a complete resection with negative microscopic (R0) margins. While not as clearly delineated as in more advanced stages, there is certainly a role for multimodality therapy in stage I NSCLC (Table 100.1).

The role for preoperative biopsy, while admittedly not required in most situations, should be discussed as a multidisciplinary team including surgeons, radiologists, and pulmonologists. Peripheral lesions in patients being considered for surgical resection rarely require preoperative biopsy to confirm a diagnosis of cancer. A relatively high false negative biopsy rate and the low morbidity associated with thoracoscopic wedge resection has resulted in a diminished role for percutaneous biopsy. Further, there is some suggestion of increased pleural recurrence and metastases following resection that has been performed after a percutaneous biopsy.[6] While results of these retrospective series are conflicting about the potential harm, percutaneous biopsy is typically an unnecessary, invasive procedure in this setting of a clinically suspicious and peripheral stage I lesion.

On the other hand, a preoperative biopsy may be warranted for central lesions that would otherwise require a less desirable "diagnostic lobectomy" for surgical resection, particularly in marginal surgical candidates or in patients for whom the clinical evidence for a cancer seems weaker. Review by a multidisciplinary team in this situation can be beneficial in deciding the optimal approach for diagnosis: percutaneous transthoracic needle biopsy, transbronchial biopsy, or surgical resection. Electromagnetic navigation bronchoscopy (ENB) is a promising interdisciplinary technology

STAGE I NON-SMALL CELL LUNG CANCER

ADJUNCTS TO SURGICAL THERAPY

Despite improvements in adjuvant chemotherapy and other targeted therapies, the mainstay therapy for early stage lung cancer remains surgical resection.[1] The gold standard surgical therapy in medically appropriate patients remains anatomic lobectomy. This recommendation is based on a randomized trial completed by the Lung Cancer Study Group (LCSG) in 1995.[5] However, for the subgroup of patients with clinical stage I ground glass lesions smaller than 2 cm and adenocarcinoma in situ, it appears that sublobar surgical approaches may be appropriate. Further discussion of the utility of sublobar surgical

---

TABLE 100.1 Multimodality Therapy for Stage I NSCLC

- Surgical resection ± brachytherapy[a]
- Intraoperative fluoroscopic localization with preoperative transthoracic or transbronchial fiducial marking
- Potentially adjuvant platinum-based chemotherapy for tumors >4 cm
- Alternatives to resection for high-risk candidates
  - Stereotactic body radiotherapy
  - Radiofrequency ablation

[a]Results of ACOSOG Z4032 show no improvement in locoregional recurrence with use of I125 brachytherapy except potentially in the setting of positive surgical margins.
Data from Fernando HC, Landreneau RJ, Mandrekar SJ, et al. Impact of brachytherapy on local recurrence rates after sublobar resection: Results from ACOSOG Z4032 (Alliance), a phase III randomized trial for high-risk operable non-small-cell lung cancer. *J Clin Oncol* 2014;32(23):2456–2462.

by which lesions deep within lung parenchyma can be biopsied. A recent meta-analysis of 17 studies, including over 1,100 patients, found a sensitivity and specificity of 82% and 100% with this technique.[15] In addition to biopsy, ENB can simultaneously be used for fiducial marker placement which may guide either fluoroscopic intraoperative localization of tumors or stereotactic body radiotherapy (SBRT).

While surgical resection is the generally accepted primary therapy, there are several additional treatment options available to patients that should be considered, particularly in patients with inadequate lung function to tolerate pulmonary resection. The primary concern in choosing the optimal treatment for early stage NSCLC is the prevention of locoregional recurrence. Despite what is felt to be a curative treatment, an unacceptably high number of patients will develop recurrent disease. Results from LCSG showed local recurrence rates of 7% after lobectomy and 18% after sublobar resection for stage I lung cancer.[7] Several retrospective case series have shown similar results, and recurrence rates are even higher for stage Ib and II disease.[1] Thus, one important goal of multimodality therapies, in general, at this early stage, is the prevention of locoregional recurrence. To this end, several therapies have been studied as potential adjuncts to surgical resection: intraoperative fluoroscopic tumor localization, brachytherapy, local radiation, and adjuvant chemotherapy.

Frequently, subcentimeter ground-glass lesions can be difficult to localize/palpate thoracoscopically. The authors have recently reported a multidisciplinary technique for intraoperative localization using intraoperative fluoroscopy.[7] In this technique, gold fiducials were percutaneously inserted in a peritumoral location with CT guidance prior to surgery. Intraoperative fluoroscopy was then utilized to identify and localize the lesion. Using this method, the pulmonary nodule was successfully resected in 98% of cases (57 of 58 patients), 20% of whom were identified as having primary lung cancer. Procedure-related complications occurred in three patients, and included fiducial embolization, fiducial migration, and intraparenchymal hematoma. Alternatively, the fiducial may be placed using ENB instead of CT-guided needle placement. This relatively simple multidisciplinary technique can be used to identify small, semisolid, and difficult-to-identify lesions.

The use of brachytherapy mesh applied at the time of sublobar resection has previously been proposed in a attempt to prevent recurrence with mixed results. Brachytherapy is a method by which radioactive iodine-125 (I125) seeds are incorporated into the lung staple line after surgical resection, with either suture or a manufactured Vicryl mesh impregnated with I125 seeds. Intraoperative brachytherapy would have the theoretical advantages of 100% patient compliance with minimal radiation injury to surrounding tissues. One retrospective review of 291 patients with T1N0 NSCLC found local recurrence after sublobar resection with brachytherapy approached that of lobectomy (3.3%), thus prompting further prospective study.[8] ACOSOG Z4032 was a phase III trial in which high-risk surgical patients were randomized to undergo sublobar resection with or without brachytherapy.[9] Unfortunately, no difference in local recurrence (HR = 1.01, p = 0.91) was found between the two cohorts. Similarly, no difference was identified between the groups in overall survival (OS). However, a trend was noted in favor of the brachytherapy arm in a very small subset of patients with positive staple line cytology (HR = 0.22, p = 0.24), leading the authors to propose that the lack of difference, despite the intriguing retrospective data that inspired the study, may have been due to much closer attention to parenchymal margin status in trial patients. Given these results, if a negative margin can be obtained surgically, it is difficult to recommend use of brachytherapy.

ALTERNATIVES TO SURGICAL THERAPY

In general, radiotherapy is not recommended in patients with completely resected pathologic stage I NSCLC. However, in the unusual circumstance of a patient being a nonsurgical candidate, alternative local therapies can be utilized for local tumor control. Most commonly these include conventional radiotherapy, SBRT, and radiofrequency ablation (RFA). OS rates with conventional radiotherapy have historically been quite poor (5% to 30%) when compared with surgical resection, and should no longer be considered for primary therapy in early stage lung cancer patients. SBRT, on the other hand, focuses intense doses of radiation (up to 60 Gy) conformed tightly to the site of disease in a relatively few fractions, minimizing spread to surrounding tissues. Modern technology allows for image-guided, focused delivery of high dose radiotherapy while compensating for respiratory tumor motion. As a result, SBRT is generally well tolerated with minimal side effects, with local control rates in nonoperative patients reported as high as 90%. The Radiation Therapy Oncology Group (RTOG) 0236 trial enrolled 59 patients with peripherally located NSCLC <5 cm treated with SBRT at a dose of 54 Gy. Results of this study showed excellent rates of local control with only one failure, an OS rate of 56%, and a 3-year disease-free survival rate of 48%.[10] Given these results, SBRT is considered the standard primary therapy for early stage NSCLC in nonoperative patients. However, distant recurrence occurred in 22% patients, likely a result of understaging from lack of lymph node evaluation. To date there is no prospective study comparing SBRT with surgical resection. Therefore, surgical resection remains the standard therapy in the majority of patients who are appropriate operative candidates. If SBRT is felt to be appropriate, surgeons can still play a contributing role in planning the radiation field for patients who are selected to have SBRT for treatment of their cancer. In this way, surgeons can maintain a role in the decision-making process for treating higher-risk patients.

Other nonsurgical therapies for local tumor control includes RFA, where a high-frequency electric current is directly applied in order to coagulate and necrose the tumor. An RFA probe is percutaneously applied to the tumor using CT guidance typically under general anesthesia. As a result, it is difficult to utilize for larger, central tumors. Unfortunately, after administration of RFA it is often difficult to assess treatment response as a residual mass is still present on imaging, often with an increased inflammatory response for the first 3 months after RFA administration. Serial CT imaging can be used to evaluate for tumor growth as can PET-CT scans. Recently published results of the ACOSOG Z4033 trial, a prospective multicenter observational study, has shown 2-year survival similar to that of SBRT (70%).[11] However, local recurrence was noted in 19 of 51 patients, with the 2-year recurrence-free survival only 60%. In addition, survival was notably worse in patients with tumors larger than 2 cm. This prospective study confirms the findings of several other retrospective, single-institution, case series.[12] Given these findings, the preference of many centers is to utilize SBRT for inoperable patients.

ADJUVANT THERAPY

The use of adjuvant therapies, including chemotherapy and radiation, for NSCLC has been extensively studied. Adjuvant radiation therapy for stages I and II is generally not recommended as there has been no identified benefit.[13] However, in select subgroups of patients, cisplatin-based chemotherapy regimens may provide a modest survival benefit. Several well-known prospective trials, along with the lung adjuvant cisplatin evaluation (LACE) meta-analysis, have evaluated the use of platinum-based adjuvant chemotherapy regimens.[14] While these studies do suffer from variability in treatment protocols and surgical approaches (nearly one-third of patients in LACE underwent pneumonectomy), some generalizable conclusions can be drawn. For example, the majority of studies agree that there is no role for adjuvant chemotherapy for T1 (<3 cm) N0 NSCLC. In fact, results of LACE, a meta-analysis including the five largest prospective trails of cisplatin-based chemotherapy, suggest a possible deleterious effect with the use of adjuvant therapy in that early cohort (HR = 1.4, 95% CI 0.95–2.06).

Unfortunately, there is no clear consensus recommendation regarding the use of adjuvant therapy for larger tumors (>3 cm) with negative lymph nodes (stage IB). Two large randomized studies have been specifically designed to answer this question: CALBG 9633[15] and JBR 10[16]. While initial analysis of these studies favored the use of adjuvant chemotherapy for patients with stage IB, late follow-up in both studies demonstrated no benefit ultimately with no difference in survival identified. However, an unplanned subgroup analysis did identify a potential survival benefit in patients with tumors larger than 4 cm. As a result, it is a common practice for patients with T1b tumors >4 cm to meet with an oncologist to discuss benefits of adjuvant therapy. In addition, with the reclassification of tumors >5 cm to stage II, further study is needed to determine if these patients would benefit from adjuvant chemotherapy. Further details regarding the use of adjuvant therapy will be discussed later in this chapter.

Finally, several ongoing studies are evaluating the use of targeted therapies with immunotherapies and/or tyrosine kinase inhibitors (TKIs) in the adjuvant setting for patients with stage I–III disease. Until the results of these studies (RADIANT, SELECT, TASTE, ADJUVANT, and ALCHEMIST) are available, the use of these therapies in the multimodality setting for stages I–IIIA should be restricted to patients enrolled in these clinical trials. It is an increasingly common practice to send all tumor samples for genetic mutational testing for assistance in future treatment planning in the event of progression of disease.

STAGE II NON-SMALL CELL LUNG CANCER

As there is still a significant possibility of curative resection along with improved survival when compared with alternative therapies, surgical resection remains the mainstay in treatment of patients with Stage II NSCLC. All patients with this stage of disease should be evaluated by a thoracic surgeon along with a multidisciplinary team. Anatomic lobar resection with lymphadenectomy remains the primary treatment in the majority of patients.[1] However, multimodality therapy plays an important role in both staging and adjuvant therapy (Table 100.2).

CLINICAL AND PATHOLOGIC STAGING

Given the presence of larger tumors or hilar nodal disease, a significant proportion of patients with clinical stage II disease will be

TABLE 100.2 Multimodality Therapy for Stage 2 NSCLC

- Mediastinoscopy, thoracoscopy, and endobronchial ultrasound for mediastinal staging
- Surgical resection
- Adjuvant platinum-based chemotherapy
- Neoadjuvant platinum-based chemotherapy in selected cases
- Mutation targeted therapy in clinical trials

upstaged to stage IIIA after surgical resection due to occult mediastinal metastases. Therefore, it is important to accurately stage the mediastinum in these patients, an area in which there is an important role for multidisciplinary management. Mediastinal lymph nodes can be assessed with one or more of the following tests/procedures: PET-CT, endobronchial ultrasound (EBUS), mediastinoscopy, or thoracoscopy. The sensitivity and specificity of PET-CT scanning for mediastinal disease has been reported in one review to be 84% and 89%, respectively.[17] Therefore, we do not routinely perform further preoperative invasive mediastinal lymph node sampling unless there is clinical concern for occult metastases, or if a pneumonectomy may be required. Yet, despite a negative PET-CT, occult hilar disease is identified on final pathology as often as 10% to 20% of the time, stressing the importance of, at a minimum, mediastinal lymph node sampling at the time of resection. If mediastinal nodal metastases are suspected, nodal tissue can be sampled either transbronchially with EBUS or surgically with cervical mediastinoscopy or thoracoscopy. Several studies have confirmed the accuracy and reliability of EBUS compared with surgical sampling, and either modality may be used with confidence.[18] Further detailed discussion of EBUS is covered elsewhere in this book.

ADJUVANT THERAPY

Beyond staging, there is an important role for multimodality therapies at this disease stage, specifically in regards to adjuvant chemotherapy. In stage II patients with negative regional nodal disease (tumors larger than 5 cm) the role of SBRT is unclear. Local tumor control rates in tumors of this size are unknown as the majority of studies examining SBRT include only patients with clinical stage I disease. RFA or cryotherapy are generally not considered, as local control becomes quite poor in tumors larger than 3 cm. Further, regional lymph node metastases are significantly more likely in tumors of this size, making surgical lymphadenectomy paramount for appropriate staging and selection of patients for adjuvant therapy. There is little utility for radiotherapy alone in patients with locoregional lymph node metastases (N1 or 2) as the importance of local tumor control is significantly less in this setting, and may, in fact, be detrimental. One meta-analysis showing significantly worse hazard for death in patients with stages I and II disease after radiotherapy.[13] However, in the truly inoperable patient, radiotherapy can be considered in patients exhibiting symptoms of local tumor growth, such as hemoptysis or chest wall and arm pain.

Despite minimal role for radiation therapy in stage II disease, there is a role for chemotherapy. While the optimal chemotherapy regimen for NSCLC remains to be determined, there does appear to be a small but significant benefit in OS after adjuvant therapy for patients with stage II and III disease. The LACE meta-analysis identified a 5.4% OS benefit favoring chemotherapy.[14] Most studies have used platinum-based doublets, typically with cisplatin with a vinca alkaloid.

Unfortunately, adjuvant chemotherapy therapy is significantly limited by patient compliance, particularly after pneumonectomy. 24% of patients in the LACE meta-analysis were able to complete only two or fewer cycles of chemotherapy out of the prescribed three to four cycles, most commonly due to patient refusal or toxicity.[14] A few studies have examined the use of neoadjuvant chemotherapy in an attempt to improve compliance with and completion of chemotherapy regimens.[19,20] The NATCH trial, a prospective randomized study comparing preoperative chemotherapy + surgery, postoperative chemotherapy + surgery, and surgery alone in stage I and II patients, found a significantly higher likelihood of starting the prescribed chemotherapy regimen when given preoperatively (97% vs. 66%).[19] However, no difference in OS was identified between the two groups. On the other hand, a recent meta-analysis of 15 studies including stages I–IIIa found an absolute survival improvement in 5-year survival of 5% with the use of preoperative chemotherapy over surgery alone, regardless of stage, or a 13% reduction in the relative risk of death.[20] Overall, while induction therapy may provide little benefit over adjuvant therapy, it is clear that compliance with induction therapy is better when compared to adjuvant therapy. In general, while adjuvant chemotherapy is considered standard, induction therapy could be considered for large, locally advanced stage II tumors where resectability is in question, after which patients should be restaged to assess for any tumor response which may aid in surgical resection.

STAGE IIIA NON-SMALL CELL LUNG CANCER

Multimodality therapy is arguably most important in the management of stage IIIA NSCLC (Table 100.3). Therefore, most centers recommend that patients with stage IIIA disease be routinely discussed at a multidisciplinary tumor board (discussed further below), as staging and management will require the collaboration of surgery, pulmonology, pathology, medical oncology, and radiation oncology.

CLINICAL AND PATHOLOGIC STAGING

With the routine use of PET scanning, many patients with stage III disease are diagnosed via clinical staging. Pathologic evaluation of mediastinal lymph nodes is necessary to confirm staging, and can be performed using any of the aforementioned modalities. If PET imaging is concerning for mediastinal nodal metastases, our institutional preference is to confirm a pathologic diagnosis with EBUS, rather than with cervical mediastinoscopy, as this makes future mediastinal restaging significantly easier. The accuracy of such combined staging techniques (PET and biopsy) is over 90%. Once neoadjuvant therapy, as discussed below, is completed, confirmation of mediastinal clearance can then be accomplished with cervical mediastinoscopy. This algorithm avoids the need for a "redo" mediastinoscopy which can be technically challenging due to scarring and inflammation from the initial surgery. Alternatively, if mediastinoscopy is used initially for staging, thoracoscopy can be used for restaging to avoid entering the same mediastinal tissue planes. Thoracoscopy has the advantage of allowing sampling of level 5 and 6 lymph nodes on the left. The disadvantage of this route is the inability to sample contralateral mediastinal lymph nodes. Finally, even if PET-CT is negative, patients with T3 and T4 tumors should still undergo pathologic mediastinal staging given a positive predictive value of only 60% for PET alone.

TREATMENT STRATEGY

Treatment of patients with stage IIIA disease hinges on the specific status of mediastinal lymph nodes, as this stage represents a

heterogeneous population of disease. Surgery alone has poor results and has little role as isolated therapy given the presence of extrapulmonary disease. Further, in patients with multistation, bulky, infiltrative N2 disease there is likely little role for surgical resection in any setting. Optimal therapy for stage IIIA NSCLC with bulky N2 disease is concurrent cisplatin-based chemotherapy and radiotherapy, a class IA ACCP recommendation based on multiple phase 3 randomized controlled trials.[21] However, all patients should be evaluated by a thoracic surgeon to confirm the presence of bulky mediastinal disease. The typical radiation dose is 60 to 70 Gy and should be given concurrently with chemotherapy, if tolerated. While concurrent therapy has been associated with higher rates of local adverse events, such as esophagitis and pneumonitis when compared with sequential therapy, it has resulted in a slight improvement in OS.[22] Overall, rates of systemic metastases remains high and 5-year survival low (5% to 15%) in such patients. On the other side of the spectrum of stage IIIA disease are patients with occult N2 metastases incidentally noted on pathologic examination after surgical resection, a relatively uncommon occurrence given the accuracy of mediastinal staging as previously discussed. Such patients should be evaluated for adjuvant chemotherapy or chemoradiotherapy and can look forward to relatively favorable survival (25% to 35%) among the IIIa cohort. Results from the LACE meta-analysis showed a significant benefit for adjuvant cisplatin-based chemotherapy in patients with pathologic stage III after surgical resection (HR = 0.83).[14]

Patients with single station mediastinal lymph node invasion (N2), or local T3 invasion (chest wall or pleura) with N1 nodal disease should be considered for multimodality therapy with concurrent neoadjuvant chemoradiation therapy followed by surgery in order to optimize cure rates. Following neoadjuvant therapy, restaging using standard imaging should be performed to assess for treatment response, along with pathologic restaging of the mediastinum. If there has not been progression of disease, surgical resection should be considered. T4 lesions with local invasion into select surrounding structures, including the SVC, recurrent laryngeal nerve, and vertebral body, can be considered for surgical resection and induction therapy. In general, however, the majority of T4 lesions invading the great vessels, trachea, esophagus, and carina, are typically unresectable aside from select scenarios.

Lastly, in patients with single station, non-bulky N2 disease, trimodality therapy with neoadjuvant chemotherapy and radiation, followed by surgical resection should be considered. This recommendation is based on the Intergroup trial INT0139, a phase III trial of patients with ipsilateral N2 NSCLC, randomized patients to induction chemotherapy (cisplatin and etoposide) and radiotherapy (45 Gy), followed by either resection or additional radiation, followed by additional chemotherapy.[23] In regard to OS, no difference was identified between induction plus surgery and induction plus more radiation in the overall cohort (5-year survival 27% vs. 20%, respectively), though progression-free survival was better in the induction plus resection cohort (HR = 0.77). In addition, OS was significantly improved for patients who underwent lobectomy, but not pneumonectomy. Of the 155 patients who underwent resection, 54 were pneumonectomies. Furthermore, of the 16 perioperative mortalities, 14 were after pneumonectomy. As a result, the investigators concluded that trimodality therapy with induction chemoradiation therapy should be considered in patients with ipsilateral N2 disease who could be resected with lobectomy only. These results were confirmed in a recent retrospective analysis of over 11,000 patients with clinical stage IIIA undergoing surgical resection.[24] Treatment with neoadjuvant chemotherapy (HR = 0.66) and with lobectomy (HR = 0.72) were both associated with significantly improved OS. A single institution retrospective series of 136 patients who underwent

TABLE 100.3 Multimodality Therapy for Stage 3A NSCLC

- Endobronchial ultrasound vs. mediastinoscopy
- Neoadjuvant chemotherapy
- Neoadjuvant radiation therapy
- Surgical resection
- Adjuvant chemotherapy
- Mutation targeted therapy in clinical trials

resection after induction therapy did not identify a difference in survival between lobectomy (n = 105) and pneumonectomy (n = 31).[25] Overall, caution should be used if pneumonectomy, especially a right pneumonectomy, is needed after induction therapy in order to accomplish complete resection.

It must be stressed that all patients being considered for trimodality therapy should be evaluated by a thoracic surgeon prior to initiation of induction therapy in order to determine if surgical resection would be possible, or if patients should be treated with definite chemoradiation. In addition, if trimodality therapy is being considered, it is important to regulate the dose of radiation utilized to less than 60 Gy. In one retrospective analysis, radiation doses of 60 Gy or higher was associated with significantly higher rates of postoperative complications with no difference in OS.[26] Further, in a randomized trial of 232 patients with stage IIIA disease, comparing induction therapy with chemoradiation versus chemotherapy alone, both followed by surgery, Pless et al.[27] found no difference in median and 3-year survival. This led the authors to conclude that the inclusion of radiation with induction therapy may not be necessary, as the driver of long-term survival was systemic, and not local, disease. Ultimately, patients with stage IIIA NSCLC should be evaluated by a multidisciplinary team led by the thoracic surgeon for multimodality treatment, as this will play a central role in both staging and treatment of such patients.

STAGE IIIB AND IV NON-SMALL CELL LUNG CANCER

There is little role for resection for patients with advanced stage lung cancer. Local disease control, with either surgical resection or radiation, has little impact on OS in the setting of distant spread of disease (Table 100.4). A few studies have examined the utility of surgical resection in carefully selected patients.[21,28] The SWOG 8805 trial, a phase II study examining trimodality therapy with chemoradiation followed by surgical resection and then consolidation chemotherapy if incompletely resected, in stage IIIA (n = 75) and IIIB (n = 51) patients interestingly found equivalent survival (27% vs. 24%) between the two stages after this treatment regimen.[28] Notably, T4 N0-1 patients benefited the most of all subgroups. At the time of the study, these tumors were classified as stage IIIB. However, under the most recent AJCC 7th edition staging, these tumors are now classified as stage IIIA. At this time, there is no role for surgical resection in patients with N3 disease, and such patients should be evaluated for definitive chemotherapy. In addition, there is no proven role for palliative surgical resection in the presence of distant spread. Patients with acute, life-threatening hemoptysis or recurrent, postobstructive pulmonary infections can be considered for radiation therapy if quality of life can be preserved postoperatively. However, expectations must be carefully discussed with the patient, given the high likelihood of a poor outcome regardless of treatment plan. The

TABLE 100.4 Multimodality Therapy for Stage IIIB and Stage 4 NSCLC

- Palliative chemotherapy
- Surgical resection for select oligometastatic disease including isolated brain metastasis, adrenal lesion, or satellite pulmonary nodule in contralateral lung
- Tube thoracostomy or talc pleurodesis for malignant effusion
- Targeted therapies
- Palliative and hospice care

overall median survival of patients with metastatic disease is less than 10 months.

An exception to this guideline, though, appears to be fit patients with oligometastatic disease, including synchronous or metachronous isolated brain metastasis, adrenal metastasis, or a satellite pulmonary nodules in the absence of mediastinal lymph node metastases or other evidence of distant spread. Again, such patients should be carefully and thoroughly discussed at a multidisciplinary "Tumor Board." If treated with multimodality therapy, including resection of both the primary cancer and the isolated metastases, followed by adjuvant chemotherapy, these patients may enjoy considerable prolongation of life. For example, multimodality therapy including a thoracic surgeon, a neurosurgeon, medical, and radiation oncologists can result in a significant survival benefit in patients with isolated brain metastases. Resection of the primary NSCLC and brain metastasis, followed by adjuvant chemotherapy, median survival in retrospective case series has been reported as high as 24 months with a 5-year survival of 20%.[29] Prognostic factors associated with improved survival included adenocarcinoma histology, N0 mediastinal lymph node status, and longer interval between presentation of the primary cancer and brain metastases. This again stresses the importance of mediastinal lymph node evaluation with a multimodality approach including PET-CT imaging, EBUS, and/or cervical mediastinoscopy. If patients are unable to undergo surgical resection of a brain metastases, alternative approaches include whole brain radiation and cerebral stereotactic radiosurgery.

Special consideration should also be given to patients with bilateral pulmonary lesions. Under the most recent AJCC staging guidelines, the presence of satellite pulmonary nodules within a different lobe on the ipsilateral lung is considered a T4 lesion, whereas lesions in the contralateral lung is considered M1a. Further, it is often difficult to determine if such lesions represent metastatic spread or a second primary malignancy. In retrospective series, surgical resection of both sites resulted in median survival as high as 25 months with a 5-year survival of an incredible 38%.[30] It is the authors' practice to resect such lesions with staged surgeries, ideally with anatomic resections if adequate pulmonary function is present. Such patients should be considered for multimodality therapy with adjuvant chemotherapy. Additional, careful evaluation of mediastinal lymph nodes must be considered, as the presence of lymphatic metastases is again a significant negative prognostic factor. Such patients with contralateral synchronous lesions and mediastinal adenopathy probably should not be considered for surgical resection and should be referred for definitive chemoradiotherapy. Combinations of resection and SBRT have potential in the class of patients with contralateral but node negative lesions. A resection and lymphadenectomy on the larger lesions, followed by SBRT to the smaller lesion, might prove to be a good balance between aggressive and conservative for some patients.

Lastly, patients with otherwise node negative lung cancer, but isolated adrenal lesions, should also be considered for dual resection and chemotherapy. It is often difficult to determine if these adrenal lesions truly represent a metastasis versus a benign lesion such as an adenoma. Careful discussion of such cases with a radiologist and potentially an interventional radiologist or laparoscopic adrenal surgeon is needed as MRI imaging can be helpful in determining if the lesion is neither benign nor malignant, though often a tissue diagnosis will be needed. This can be obtained with either image-guided percutaneous biopsy or with laparoscopy. Left gland lesions may also be accessible for FNA using endoscopic ultrasound. If metastatic cancer is confirmed, such patients should still be evaluated by a thoracic surgeon for possible multimodality therapy. In a pooled analysis of 114 patients, resection of both sites resulted in a 5-year survival of 25%, suggesting there is a role for surgical resection and adjuvant chemotherapy in such patients.[31]

Unfortunately, only a small percentage of patients with stage IV NSCLC will present with oligometastasis. Typically, the primary goal for any therapy in the setting of metastatic lung cancer should be focused on prolonging life and/or improving quality of life, depending on the wishes of the patient.[32] Multimodality treatment with a thoracic surgeon, medical oncologist, radiation oncologist, and palliative care physicians can be extremely beneficial. Palliative surgical procedures such talc pleurodesis and the insertion of an indwelling, flexible thoracostomy tube can be considered for patients with malignant, symptomatic pleural effusions. Palliative chemotherapy using cisplatin-based doublets has been shown to significantly improve OS.[33,34] The use of targeted biologic therapies such as TKIs (erlotinib or gefitinib) and antiangiogenic agents (bevacizumab), has been shown to improve progression-free survival. Therefore, current guidelines recommend that all patients with stage IV NSCLC with adenocarcinoma histology undergo molecular testing for mutation analysis. If a mutation is present, targeted therapies should be considered for first-line therapy.[32,35]

MULTIDISCIPLINARY TUMOR BOARD

Clearly, multimodality treatment of patients with NSCLC can be complex, cumbersome, and time consuming. As mentioned earlier, the use of a multidisciplinary tumor board in formulating a comprehensive treatment plan for patients is recommended by the National Comprehensive Cancer Network and American College of Chest Physicians, and can considerably simplify this process.[1,2] While there is no definitive data confirming that the use of such meetings does improve survival, a recently published study surveying over 1,600 oncologists and surgeons found that frequent physician participation in tumor boards was at least associated with higher rates or patient participation in clinic trials and higher rates of curative-intent surgery in patients with stage I and II NSCLC.[36] Similarly, a retrospective analysis of a tertiary care center found that after initiating a multidisciplinary conference, adherence to NCCN treatment guidelines improved by 16% and rates of multidisciplinary evaluation improved by 34%.[37] Finally, a recent observational study found that treatment recommendations changed in 40% of patients with lung cancer after discussion at a multidisciplinary conference.[38] With complexity of contemporary lung cancer management, it comes as no surprise that case discussion among several providers of varying backgrounds can have such a positive effect on treatment plans. We, therefore, strongly recommend the use of multidisciplinary tumor boards or, if this is not possible, a discussion among a multidisciplinary team of providers, when determining optimal treatment plans for patients.

SUMMARY

In summary, with new, more effective therapies available for all stages of lung cancer, the management of lung cancer is becoming increasingly complex. Such treatments involve a number of medical disciplines, including thoracic surgery, pulmonology, medical oncology, radiation oncology, radiology, interventional radiology, palliative care, and occasionally neurosurgery. Multimodality therapies have resulted in both improved survival and quality of life for patients with lung cancer. Yet, with so many different specialties involved, the role of the thoracic surgeon as a "Captain of the Ship" has become even more important and central to the care of patients with NSCLC.

REFERENCES

1. Howington JA, Blum MG, Chang AC, et al. Treatment of stage I and II non-small cell lung cancer: Diagnosis and management of lung cancer, 3rd ed: American College of Chest Physicians evidence based clinical practice guidelines. *Chest* 2013;143(5 Suppl): e278S–e313S.
2. Ettinger DS, Wood DE, Akerley W, et al. Non-small cell lung cancer, version 1.2015. *J Natl Compr Canc Netw* 2014;12(12):1738–1761.
3. Veeramachaneni NK, Feins RH, Stephenson BJ, et al. Management of stage IIIA non-small cell lung cancer by thoracic surgeons in North America. *Ann Thorac Surg* 2012;94(3):922–926; discussion: 926–928.
4. Tanner NT, Gomez M, Rainwater C, et al. Physician preferences for management of patients with stage IIIA NSCLC: Impact of bulk of nodal disease on therapy selection. *J Thorac Oncol* 2012;7(2):365–369.
5. Ginsberg RJ, Rubinstein LV. Randomized trial of lobectomy versus limited resection for T1 N0 non-small cell lung cancer. Lung Cancer Study Group. *Ann Thorac Surg* 1995;60(3):615–622; discussion: 622–623.
6. Asakura K, Izumi Y, Yamauchi Y, et al. Incidence of pleural recurrence after computed tomography-guided needle biopsy in stage I lung cancer. *PLoS One* 2012;7(8): e42043.
7. Sancheti MS, Lee R, Ahmed SU, et al. Percutaneous fiducial localization for thoracoscopic wedge resection of small pulmonary nodules. *Ann Thorac Surg* 2014;97(6): 1914–1918; discussion: 1919.
8. Fernando HC, Santos RS, Benfield JR, et al. Lobar and sublobar resection with and without brachytherapy for small stage IA non-small cell lung cancer. *J Thorac Cardiovasc Surg* 2005;129(2):261–267.
9. Fernando HC, Landreneau RJ, Mandrekar SJ, et al. Impact of brachytherapy on local recurrence rates after sublobar resection: Results from ACOSOG Z4032 (Alliance), a phase III randomized trial for high-risk operable non-small-cell lung cancer. *J Clin Oncol* 2014;32(23):2456–2462.
10. Timmerman R, Paulus R, Galvin J, et al. Stereotactic body radiation therapy for inoperable early stage lung cancer. *JAMA* 2010;303(11):1070–1076.
11. Dupuy DE, Fernando HC, Hillman S, et al. Radiofrequency ablation of stage IA non-small cell lung cancer in medically inoperable patients: Results from the American College of Surgeons Oncology Group Z4033 (Alliance) trial. *Cancer* 2015;121(19): 3491–3498.
12. Bilal H, Mahmood S, Rajashanker B, et al. Is radiofrequency ablation more effective than stereotactic ablative radiotherapy in patients with early stage medically inoperable non-small cell lung cancer? *Interact Cardiovasc Thorac Surg* 2012;15(2):258–265.
13. Group PM-aT. Postoperative radiotherapy for non-small cell lung cancer. *Cochrane Database Syst Rev* 2000;(2):CD002142.
14. Pignon JP, Tribodet H, Scagliotti GV, et al. Lung adjuvant cisplatin evaluation: A pooled analysis by the LACE Collaborative Group. *J Clin Oncol* 2008;26(21): 3552–3559.
15. Strauss GM, Herndon JE, 2nd, Maddaus MA, et al. Adjuvant paclitaxel plus carboplatin compared with observation in stage IB non-small-cell lung cancer: CALGB 9633 with the Cancer and Leukemia Group B, Radiation Therapy Oncology Group, and North Central Cancer Treatment Group Study Groups. *J Clin Oncol* 2008;26(31):5043–5051.
16. Butts CA, Ding K, Seymour L, et al. Randomized phase III trial of vinorelbine plus cisplatin compared with observation in completely resected stage IB and II non-small-cell lung cancer: updated survival analysis of JBR-10. *J Clin Oncol* 2010;28(1): 29–34.
17. Toloza EM, Harpole L, McCrory DC. Noninvasive staging of non-small cell lung cancer: a review of the current evidence. *Chest* 2003;123(1 Suppl):137S–146S.
18. Toloza EM, Harpole L, Detterbeck F, et al. Invasive staging of non-small cell lung cancer: A review of the current evidence. *Chest* 2003;123(1 Suppl):157S–166S.
19. Felip E, Rosell R, Maestre JA, et al. Preoperative chemotherapy plus surgery versus surgery plus adjuvant chemotherapy versus surgery alone in early-stage non-small-cell lung cancer. *J Clin Oncol* 2010;28(19):3138–3145.
20. Non-small cell Meta-analysis Collaborative Group. Preoperative chemotherapy for non-small-cell lung cancer: a systematic review and meta-analysis of individual participant data. *Lancet* 2014;383(9928):1561–1571.
21. Ramnath N, Dilling TJ, Harris LJ, et al. Treatment of stage III non-small cell lung cancer: Diagnosis and management of lung cancer, 3rd ed: American College of Chest Physicians evidence-based clinical practice guidelines. *Chest* 2013;143(5 Suppl): e314S–e340S.
22. Belani CP, Choy H, Bonomi P, et al. Combined chemoradiotherapy regimens of paclitaxel and carboplatin for locally advanced non-small-cell lung cancer: A randomized phase II locally advanced multi-modality protocol. *J Clin Oncol* 2005;23(25):5883–5891.
23. Albain KS, Swann RS, Rusch VW, et al. Radiotherapy plus chemotherapy with or without surgical resection for stage III non-small-cell lung cancer: A phase III randomised controlled trial. *Lancet* 2009;374(9687):379–386.
24. Samson P, Patel A, Crabtree TD, et al. Multidisciplinary treatment for stage IIIA non-small cell lung cancer: Does institution type matter? *Ann Thorac Surg* 2015;100: 1773–1779.
25. Paul S, Mirza F, Port JL, et al. Survival of patients with clinical stage IIIA non-small cell lung cancer after induction therapy: age, mediastinal downstaging, and extent of pulmonary resection as independent predictors. *J Thorac Cardiovasc Surg* 2011;141(1):48–58.
26. Bharadwaj SC, Vallieres E, Wilshire CL, et al. Higher versus standard preoperative radiation in the trimodality treatment of stage IIIa lung cancer. *Ann Thorac Surg* 2015;100(1):207–214.
27. Pless M, Stupp R, Ris HB, et al. Induction chemoradiation in stage IIIA/N2 non-small-cell lung cancer: A phase 3 randomised trial. *Lancet* 2015;386(9998):1049–1056.

28. Albain KS, Rusch VW, Crowley JJ, et al. Concurrent cisplatin/etoposide plus chest radiotherapy followed by surgery for stages IIIA (N2) and IIIB non-small-cell lung cancer: mature results of Southwest Oncology Group phase II study 8805. *J Clin Oncol* 1995;13(8):1880–1892.

29. Billing PS, Miller DL, Allen MS, et al. Surgical treatment of primary lung cancer with synchronous brain metastases. *J Thorac Cardiovasc Surg* 2001;122(3):548–553.

30. De Leyn P, Moons J, Vansteenkiste J, et al. Survival after resection of synchronous bilateral lung cancer. *Eur J Cardiothorac Surg* 2008;34(6):1215–1222.

31. Tanvetyanon T, Robinson LA, Schell MJ, et al. Outcomes of adrenalectomy for isolated synchronous versus metachronous adrenal metastases in non-small-cell lung cancer: a systematic review and pooled analysis. *J Clin Oncol* 2008;26(7):1142–1147.

32. Socinski MA, Evans T, Gettinger S, et al. Treatment of stage IV non-small cell lung cancer: Diagnosis and management of lung cancer, 3rd ed: American College of Chest Physicians evidence-based clinical practice guidelines. *Chest* 2013;143(5 Suppl): e341S–e368S.

33. Chemotherapy in non-small cell lung cancer: a meta-analysis using updated data on individual patients from 52 randomised clinical trials. Non-small Cell Lung Cancer Collaborative Group. *BMJ* 1995;311(7010):899–909.

34. Schiller JH, Harrington D, Belani CP, et al. Comparison of four chemotherapy regimens for advanced non-small-cell lung cancer. *N Engl J Med* 2002;346(2):92–98.

35. Mok TS, Wu YL, Thongprasert S, et al. Gefitinib or carboplatin-paclitaxel in pulmonary adenocarcinoma. *N Engl J Med* 2009;361(10):947–957.

36. Kehl KL, Landrum MB, Kahn KL, et al. Tumor board participation among physicians caring for patients with lung or colorectal cancer. *J Oncol Pract* 2015;11(3):e267–e278.

37. Freeman RK, Van Woerkom JM, Vyverberg A, et al. The effect of a multidisciplinary thoracic malignancy conference on the treatment of patients with lung cancer. *Eur J Cardiothorac Surg* 2010;38(1):1–5.

38. Schmidt HM, Roberts JM, Bodnar AM, et al. Thoracic multidisciplinary tumor board routinely impacts therapeutic plans in patients with lung and esophageal cancer: A prospective cohort study. *Ann Thorac Surg* 2015;99(5):1719–1724.

101

Novel Therapeutic Strategies for Non-Small Cell Lung Cancer

Saeed Arefanian ▪ Stephanie Chang ▪ Alexander Krupnick

OVERVIEW

Conventional therapy consisting of a combination of chemotherapy, radiation, and/or surgery is the mainstay for treatment of non-small cell lung cancer (NSCLC). However, recent advances in understanding the biology of lung cancer has led to increased potential targets for lung cancer treatment. This chapter will focus on the genetic and immunologic factors in lung cancer development, as well as the emerging therapeutic adjuvants that can be used in clinical practice.

GENETIC TARGETS

LUNG CANCER RESULTS FROM GENOMIC INSTABILITY AND ALTERATION OF SOMATIC GENES

The origin of cancer as a product of alterations in normal pathways controlling cell growth and differentiation was not appreciated until the 1970s. Two concomitant discoveries by Nowell and Hungerford at the University of Pennsylvania and Bishop and Varmus at the University of California San Francisco defined cancer as a result of genetic modifications passed down through somatic DNA.[1] They further discovered that mutated DNA leads to malignant transformation due to alteration or overproduction of an otherwise naturally occurring protein. Bishop and Varmus showed that DNA coding for a viral oncogene was similar to DNA present in every normal cell.[2] Thus, the realization that life-threatening malignancies represents nothing more than a modification of normal cellular processes is a relatively recent phenomenon.

A conceptual framework for understanding how cancer-specific alterations result in a malignant phenotype was subsequently established by Hanahan and Weinberg.[3,4] They described several defining hallmarks of cancer, and postulated that these were acquired through a multistep mutational process leading to the development and progression of cancer. Such hallmarks include sustained signaling resulting in cellular proliferation, evasion of normally occurring growth suppression, resistance to cell death, as well as replicative immortality (Fig. 101.1). All these hallmarks identify unique characteristics of cancer that differentiate it from normal tissues. Most importantly, all these hallmarks result from the alteration and ongoing instability of the genome.

ONCOGENE ADDICTION CAN BE TARGETED FOR RATIONAL THERAPY OF SELECT MALIGNANCIES

The oncogene addiction theory proposed in early 2000s provided experimental support for the notion that certain tumors, despite their wide array of genetic mutations, depend on one dominant oncogene for survival. It has been shown experimental inactivation of a single gene can hinder the growth and induce apoptosis of cancer cell lines *in vitro*.[5-7] This discovery initiated extreme excitement in the cancer community, suggesting that a personalized "magic bullet" may pave the way to a cure. This notion was further propagated by the clinical success of imatinib, (Gleevec, Novartis), a small tyrosine kinase inhibitor (TKI) targeting constitutive activation of Abelson (ABL) tyrosine kinase that results from the balanced translocation between the long arms of chromosome 9 (9q34) and of chromosome 22 (22q11). Interestingly, the fusion protein known as BCR-ABL, or the Philadelphia chromosome, was the discovery at the University of Pennsylvania by Nowell and Hungerford who helped pave the way for the notion that cancer is a genetically driven disease.[1] In phase I trial, the majority of the patients with chronic Philadelphia chromosome positive chronic myeloid leukemia (CML) demonstrated disease regression after a single treatment.[8] Such responses were evident even in patients with the aggressive form of the disease, known as blast crisis.[9] Furthermore, significant numbers of patients with CML were cured through blockade of this single oncogenic pathway. The clinical success of CML treatment through inhibition of a single dominant oncogene created large enthusiasm for identifying and characterizing driver oncogenes in many cancers.

RATIONAL IDENTIFICATION OF DRIVER ONCOGENES CAN NOW REPLACE PRIOR EFFORTS OF EMPIRIC OR HISTOLOGICALLY DRIVEN THERAPY

Initial Efforts in Targeting Tyrosine Kinase

The epithelial growth factor receptor (EGFR) family consists of four transmembrane receptor tyrosine kinases (ErbB-1, HER-2/ErbB-2, ErbB-3, ErbB-4) that form signaling homo- or heterodimers after binding their respective ligand. This system normally functions in the maintenance and growth of epithelial tissues. Expression and overexpression of these receptors is detected in multiple epithelial cancers, especially NSCLC of the squamous histology.[10] Based on

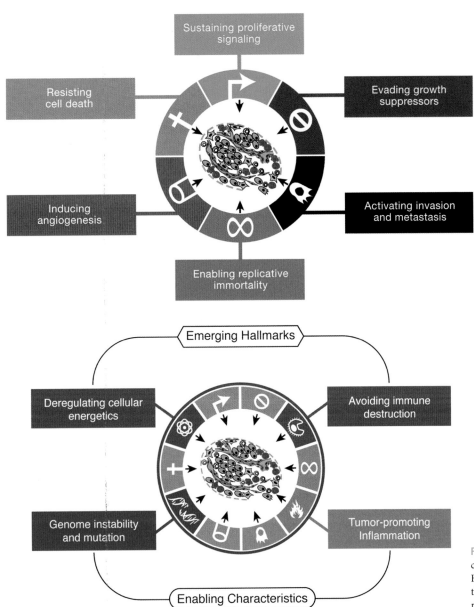

FIGURE 101.1 Hallmark characteristics of cancer. (Reprinted from Figs. 101.1 and 101.3 of Hanahan D, Weinberg RA. Hallmarks of cancer: the next generation. *Cell* 2011;144:646–674. Copyright © 2011 Elsevier. With permission.)

such histologic identification, it was assumed that excessive signaling through this pathway was an instrumental driver mutation in lung cancer, especially squamous cell lung cancer. In the 1990s, small molecules were developed to block signaling through this pathway by interfering with the intracellular tyrosine kinase domains of the EGFR family members. Two of these compounds, namely gefitinib and erlotinib (Iressa and Tarceva, manufactured by AstraZeneca and OSI Pharmaceuticals, respectively) were tested in phase I and II clinical trials.[11,12] Both compounds were designed to competitively interfere with ATP binding in the catalytic cleft of the intracellular portion of the molecule. Ten to twenty percent of patients who had previously received chemotherapy demonstrated a response to these TKIs, but, to the surprise of the investigators, responses did not occur in patients with squamous histology.[11–13] In fact, responses were most prominent in females from Asian countries who were never smokers with adenocarcinoma with bronchioalveolar features. Further investigation demonstrated that mutations clustering within the tyrosine kinase domain targeted by these first generation TKIs, rather than EGFR expression levels, were the critical determinant of

response.[14,15] Such specific mutations were simply more common in never smoking women of Asian origin.

Identification of Other Biologic Targets

Partially based on the realization that serendipitous matching of patient mutations to the appropriate targeted therapy was not a rational approach to for the design of clinical trials, the National Institute of Health started The Cancer Genome Atlas (TCGA) project in 2005 in order to catalogue mutations associated with and responsible for specific human malignancies. This incredible wealth of data has shed light on the mutational profile of lung and other cancers. Recent TCGA data specifically examined the mutational landscape of squamous and adenocarcinoma of the lung compared to 10 other common cancers, focusing on somatic variants of expressed genes.[16] This analysis revealed several unique aspects of lung cancer. While most malignancies average one mutation per megabase, lung cancer had the highest mutational rate, with as many as 8.15 mutations/megabase (Fig. 101.2). Unlike the case for breast or

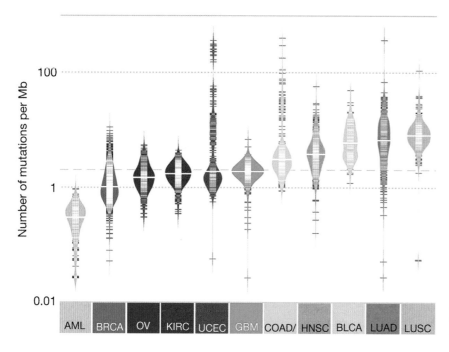

ovarian cancer, a large number of mutations were nonsynonymous, that is, resulting in an amino acid change altering protein structure or function. This was most commonly due to the characteristic C to A transversion mutation associated with cigarette smoke.[17] Other mutations, such as those in the Kelch-like ECH-associated protein 1 (Keap1), an intracellular stress-sensor, were most prevalent in lung cancer compared to others. Mutations in the tumor protein 53 tumor suppressor gene (TP53) were evident across the full spectrum of malignancies.

Expansion of TCGA allowed for further analysis of lung adenocarcinoma, such as specific and combined exome sequencing, protein analysis, and the analysis of DNA coding for expressed proteins, with sequencing of messenger RNA, microRNA, methylation patterns of DNA. Eighteen somatic mutations, particularly ones affecting protein structure and function, were specifically prevalent in lung adenocarcinoma. These include the TP53 mutation common to most cancers, as well as mutations in Kirsten rat sarcoma viral oncogene homolog (Kras) and epidermal growth factor receptor (EGFR), which were already known to be driver mutations contributing to growth of

adenocarcinoma (Fig. 101.3).[18] However, such detailed analysis identified several novel candidate driver genes previously unappreciated as playing a role in lung cancer (Fig. 101.4). While not completely evident at the genomic level, the combination of RNA and protein analysis further demonstrated the critical role of the receptor tyrosine kinase/Rat sarcoma small GTPase/RAF proto-oncogene serine/threonine-protein kinase pathway (RTK/RAS/RAF pathway for short), with its activation in as many as 76% of all lung adenocarcinomas (Fig. 101.5). Similar analysis of lung squamous cell carcinoma revealed a different pattern of mutations with alteration of the PI3-kinase pathway, NOTCH1 signaling as well as HLA-A pathway of antigen presentation (Fig. 101.6).[19] Both squamous and adenocarcinoma had mutations in the TP53 tumor suppression pathway.

Targeting ALK/ROS1 Tyrosine Kinases

In addition to EGFR, several key driver mutations have gained importance in the understanding and treatment of lung cancer. A fusion protein of chromosome 2, rearranging the anaplastic lymphoma

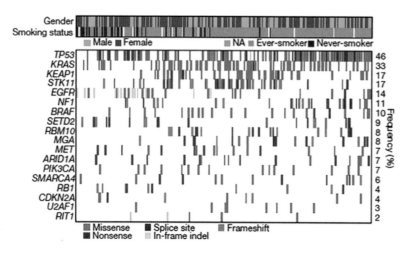

FIGURE 101.3 Frequency and nature of common mutations in lung adenocarcinoma. (Reprinted by permission from Macmillan Publishers Ltd: Cancer Genome Atlas Research Network. Comprehensive molecular profiling of lung adenocarcinoma. *Nature* 2014;511:543–550. Copyright © 2014.)

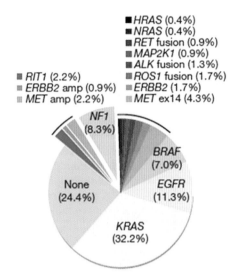

FIGURE 101.4 Distribution of common driver mutations in lung adenocarcinoma. (Reprinted by permission from Macmillan Publishers Ltd: Cancer Genome Atlas Research Network. Comprehensive molecular profiling of lung adenocarcinoma. *Nature* 2014;511:543–550. Copyright © 2014.)

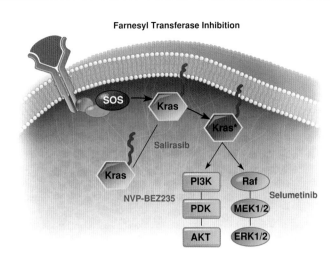

FIGURE 101.5 Kras signaling cascade and possible inhibitors.

tyrosine kinase (ALK) with the echinoderm microtubule-associated protein-like 4 (EML4), results in a driver mutation responsible for 2% to 4% of all NSCLC.[20–22] Such recombination occurs at several "hot spots," specifically intron 13 of EML4 to intron 19 of ALK, after an inversion mutation in chromosome 2, and fusion of exons 1 to 13 of EML4 to exons 20 to 29 of ALK.[20,23–26] Epidemiologically, the ALK-EML4 translocation is similar to EGFR mutations and is mostly present in never smoking young female patients.[23,27–32] In fact, the two mutations in EGFR and AML4-ALK are nearly mutually exclusive in this patient population.[23,25,29,32–37] C-ros oncogene 1 (ROS1) is another receptor with tyrosine kinase activity and high homology with ALK. Constitutive activation of ROS1 occurs due to rearrangement and fusion of the kinase domain with multiple partners, most commonly CD74.[38] This rearrangement has been reported

in 1.2% to 2.6% of lung adenocarcinoma specifically young, Asian nonsmokers.[39–41]

Crizotinib, or Xalkori, is a TKI approved by the FDA for ALK and ROS1 fusion-positive lung cancer. Similar to other TKIs, it competitively inhibits the ATP-binding pocket of select tyrosine kinases to prevent constitutive signaling. Early and late phase clinical trials have demonstrated a significant survival advantage with the addition of crizotinib to standard therapy. An open label phase III trial published in 2013 (Profile 1007) demonstrates doubling in progression-free survival of patients treated with Crizotinib compared to chemotherapy in patients with locally advanced or metastatic lung cancer who had already received prior treatment.[42] Further data in chemotherapy naïve patients demonstrates that Crizotinib is also effective as first-line therapy (Profile 1014).[43] While Crizotinib was developed as a kinase inhibitor for the ALK mutation, it has shown good results for tumors with ROS1 rearrangement as well.[40] Advances in such TKI approaches have yielded other second-line compounds that offer activity once Crizotinib resistance develops.[44]

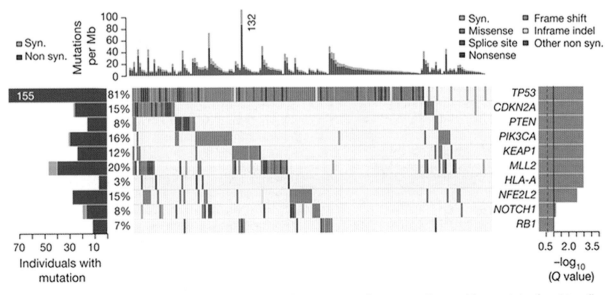

FIGURE 101.6 Frequency and nature of common mutations in lung squamous cell carcinoma. (Reprinted by permission from Macmillan Publishers Ltd: Cancer Genome Atlas Research Network. Comprehensive genomic characterization of squamous cell lung cancers. *Nature* 2012;489:519–525. Copyright © 2012.)

Targeting Kras

As a member of the RAS proto-oncogene family, Kras encodes a G protein that is important in cell proliferation and survival. The protein exists in two forms, either as inactive GDP-bound or activated GTP-bound.[45] Since GTPase activity is required for changing the activated form to the GDP-bound inactivated form in a quiescent cell, mutations that decrease the GTPase activity of the protein translates into increases in signaling and, consequently, increases in the cell proliferation and growth.[46] Activation of Kras is the most common mutation in lung adenocarcinoma, but is rare in small cell or squamous cell carcinoma. It is also more prevalent in males and smokers.[22] Interestingly, single nucleotide substitutions resulting in one amino acid change have different epidemiologic origins. The G to T transversion in codon 12, for example, is a common mutation in smokers, while the G to A transition is common in nonsmokers. Alterations of KRAS are mutually exclusive with other defined driver mutations, including EGFR, ALK, and ROS1.[47]

Despite the near ubiquitous role of Kras mutations in lung adenocarcinoma (Fig. 101.3), clinical trials targeting this pathway have been disappointing. The enzyme farnesyl transferase plays a critical role in posttranslational modification of a number of G proteins, including Kras. Direct targeting of mutant Kras in lung cancer with farnesyl transferase inhibitors was attempted as part of a phase II clinical trial.[48] Despite consistent inhibition of farnesylation, no clinical efficacy was documented. Disruption of Kras function in other models, such as pancreatic cancer, has also been attempted. Salirasib, for example, is an S-trans, transfarnesylthiosalicylic acid derivative that can act as a rather specific and nontoxic Ras antagonist. It functions by dislodging Ras from its membrane anchorage domains, accelerating its degradation.[49] Safety and activity was documented in both preclinical and clinical models.[50]

Unlike the case for tyrosine kinases, efforts in directly targeting Kras activity are hampered by its extremely high, picomolar, affinity for GTP/GDP and the absence of any known allosteric regulatory sites.[51] In 2013, investigators from the University of California, San Francisco, reported the first successful set of small molecules that irreversibly bind to a common oncogenic mutant form of Kras, with the substitution of amino acid at position 12 from glycine (G) to a cysteine (C) (KrasG12C). Interestingly, the compounds depend on the mutant cysteine for binding and have been successful in preventing mutant Kras binding to downstream effectors in *in vitro* culture models.[52] Translation of such therapy to clinically relevant protocols, however, is still far away.

Targeting Pathways Downstream of Kras

Based on the difficulties of inhibiting constitutive Kras activity directly, clinical trials targeting activation of this pathway in malignant cells have focused on downstream inhibitors (Fig. 101.5). RAF-MAPK and PI3K-AKT represent the two major signaling pathways downstream of Kras. The genetically engineered mouse model of Kras-driven lung cancer was instrumental in testing the combination of the MAPK inhibitor Selumetinib and pan-PI3K-AKT inhibitor NVP-BEZ235.[53] As of 2015, several phases IB and II clinical trials are open targeting both of these pathways (NCT01363232, NCT01390818, NCT00996892). An alternative strategy combining docetaxel-based cytotoxic chemotherapy with selumetinib has demonstrated efficacy in increasing progression-free survival in Kras-mutant lung cancer patients who had failed first-line therapy.[54]

Targeting p53

Tumor protein 53, or p53, is a DNA-binding transcription factor that is almost ubiquitously expressed in multiple organisms to regulate many aspects of cell function and survival.[55,56] Under normal conditions, p53 remains quiescent and is rapidly degraded. At times of cellular stress, including malignant transformation, p53 is stabilized with increasing intracellular levels mediating transcription of pro-apoptotic factors, mediators of cell cycle arrest, as well as cellular senescence. For these reasons, p53 has been named the "guardian of the genome."[57] Not surprisingly, it is mutated in most human cancers including roughly 50% of lung cancer (Fig. 101.3). All mutations that arise in p53 result in loss of its wild-type activity, and also exerts a "dominant negative" effect, which interferes with function of any remaining wild-type p53.[58] Despite this seemingly obvious target for tumor therapy efforts to curtail the dominant negative effect of mutant p53 or restore its wild-type function has proven difficult. During a broad screen of low–molecular-weight compounds, the small–molecular-weight compound PRIMA-1 (2,2-bis(hydroxymethyl)-1-azabicyclo(2,2,2) octan-3-one) (APR-017, Aprea AB, Sweden) was discovered to be able to restore tumor suppressive properties of mutant p53.[59] Phase I safety trials demonstrated that these compounds were well tolerated with minimal adverse side effects. Cell cycle arrest, upregulation of p53 target genes, and tumor cell apoptosis confirmed that p53 function was at least partially restored by the administration of PRIMA derivatives.[60] Phase II clinical trials to advance this therapy are currently in progress.[61]

Direct p53 replacement as therapy for lung cancer underwent significant advancement in the 1990s and early 2000s by Jack Roth and the MD Anderson group. Based on preclinical animal models, direct injection of p53-expressing retrovirus into NSCLC was performed as a phase I safety trial.[62] No major toxicity was evident, and tumor regression occurred in three out of the nine patients in the trial. Based on the dangers associated with retroviral vectors, further clinical testing was performed using adenoviral-mediated delivery. Several larger phase I and II trials in both lung, head, and neck, as well as liver cancer confirmed safety of this approach, but demonstrated only minimal efficacy of this therapy.[63–65] Nevertheless adenoviral p53 replacement is approved for use in China (Gendicine, Shenzhen SiBiono GeneTech.). Clearly, further trials that combine p53 replacement with complementary overlapping strategies are necessary to fully take advantage of this approach.

IMMUNOTHERAPY

OVERVIEW OF THE IMMUNE SYSTEM

The mammalian immune system has evolved to provide host defense against a constant onslaught of pathogens present in the external environment. Evolutionary adaptation has created a complex network of cellular and anatomic barriers that, in mammals, can be broadly divided into two arms consisting of the innate and adaptive immune system (Fig. 101.7). The innate immune system consists of rapid-acting nonspecific components that recognize stress ligands present on infected, transformed, and dying cells. Leukocytes of the innate immune system include macrophages, neutrophils, dendritic cells, mast cells, eosinophils, basophils, and natural killer (NK) cells. NK cells specifically have a prominent evolutionary role in tumor clearance, as it can lyse transformed cells without prior sensitization. Phylogenetically this arm of the immune system can be found in most multicellular organisms.

The adaptive immune system has evolved in higher organisms starting with jawed fishes.[66] Unlike the innate immune system, the adaptive immune response exhibits slower kinetics, but has the potential for the formation of long-term memory and recall responses. The

**Innate immunity
(rapid response)**

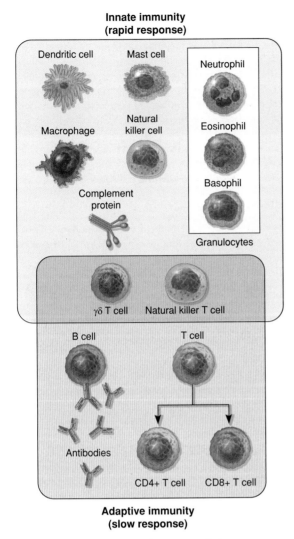

**Adaptive immunity
(slow response)**

FIGURE 101.7 Cellular components of the innate and adaptive immune system.

adaptive immune system consists of the humoral and the cellular components comprised of B and T lymphocytes respectively. The production of antibodies, which mediate recognition and targeting of foreign antigens for destruction, are directed by B lymphocytes and characterize the humoral immune response. The cell-mediated response includes helper (CD4+) and cytotoxic (CD8+) T lymphocytes that can act through direct cytotoxicity, as well as potentiation of the immune response through cytokine production. Unlike pattern recognition of stress ligands and danger signals, the adaptive immune response relies of the presentation of foreign antigen by professional antigen presenting cells in the context of major histocompatibility complex I and II (MHC I and II). Consequently, during development, T lymphocytes must undergo positive selection, ensuring that the T cell receptor is capable of recognizing self-MHC, as well as negative selection, ensuring that those clones recognizing self-antigen are deleted. This process of negative selection, while important for normal immune function in eliminating autoreactive cells, also hinders immune-based therapy, since malignancies essentially represent altered self.

IMMUNOTHERAPY FOR LUNG CANCER

The clinical use of immunotherapy for treatment of malignancy can be traced to the late 1800s, when a New York surgeon, Coley, treated

patients with a mixture of inactivated bacterial products known as "Coley's toxin."[67] This treatment most likely caused nonspecific immune activation, but it led to prominent regression of certain tumors in select patients. Since that time, improved understanding of the tumor immune response and of tumor antigens has resulted in more refined immunotherapy. Most immunotherapy for solid organ malignancies focuses on manipulation of the adaptive arm of the immune system. Such protocols can be generally broken up two separate strategies of (1) passive immunotherapy, specifically the administration of an immunologic agents made outside the body to directly attack tumors and; (2) active immunotherapy aimed to stimulate an antitumor immune response by the existing immune system. While great advances in passive immunotherapy have been made in the form of expansion and activation of tumor infiltrating lymphocytes, chimeric antigen receptor T cells (CARTs),[68] or lytic antibodies,[69] all current efforts at immunotherapy for lung cancer have been in the form of active immunization.

Both squamous and adenocarcinoma of the lung have the highest mutational rates of all solid tumors (Fig. 101.2). These mutations not only result in the activation of driver oncogenes and silencing of tumor suppressors, but also lead to the expression of antigenic proteins not normally present in adult tissues. Such tumor-associated antigens (TAA) consist of novel proteins that arise as a consequence of amino acid substitution, embryonic proteins not present in the adult, or cancer-testes antigens normally hidden from the immune system.[70] Recently, this notion has been extended to multiple other housekeeping proteins that demonstrate unique and patient-specific patterns of mutation.[71,72] Genetic screening of lung cancer has identified several targets for immunotherapy.

MAGE-A3

Melanoma-Associated Antigen A3, or MAGE-A3 is a tumor-associated antigen that is normally only expressed in human testicular cells,[73] but is also present in malignancies including 35% to 50% of NSCLC.[74] Administration of a MAGE-A3 peptide vaccine with an adjuvant as a form of active immunotherapy has been shown to have early efficacy in malignant melanoma,[75] stimulating interest in its use as a potential target for NSCLC. MAGE-A3 contains epitopes that can be presented by both MHC Class I and Class II, allowing for CD4+ and CD8+ T cell activation.[76] A vaccine targeting MAGE-A3 was evaluated in an international randomized phase II trial of lung cancer patients with stage IB or stage II tumors after surgical resection.[77] The MAGE-A3 antigen was expressed on all patients enrolled in the trial. This study showed a trend toward increased disease-free interval, disease-free survival, and overall survival, but these were not statistically significant. A phase III trial named MAGE-A3 as Adjuvant Non-Small Cell Lung Cancer Immunotherapy (MAGRIT) examined the effect of the vaccine on stage IB to IIIA patient with NSCLC whose tumors expressed MAGE-A3. Despite its initial promise in the phase II, the treatment with the vaccine did not result in any differences in disease-free survival, which was the primary endpoint of the trial.[78]

Mucin 1

Mucin 1 (MUC1) is a transmembrane protein expressed on epithelial cells and overexpressed in 74% to 86% of NSCLCs.[79] The MUC1 protein plays a role in inhibiting T cell proliferation, as well as being an antiadhesion molecule involved in tumor cell migration and carcinogenesis.[80,81] There are currently two vaccines targeting MUC1: L-BLP25 and TG4010. L-BLP25 is a liposomal vaccine that may facilitate antigen-specific T cell proliferation in addition to increased interferon-gamma secretion.[82] A phase IIB trial examined patients with stage IIIB or IV NSCLC who had disease stabilization after first-line treatment. The vaccine arm demonstrated increased mean survival time of 17.4 months in patients receiving L-BLP25 compared to 13 months in the control arm. Specifically, in patients with stage IIIB disease, the difference in median survival time was increased to 30.6 months after vaccination compared to 13.3 months in the control arm.[83,84] There have been two subsequent phase III trials looking at L-BLP25: Stimulating Targeted Antigenic Response To NSCLC (START) and Stimuvax Trial in Asian NSCLC Patients: Stimulating Immune Response (INSPIRE). START evaluated stage III patients who had some response or disease stabilization after chemoradiation therapy. This study demonstrated no significant difference in the overall survival (25.6 months in the L-BLP25 arm compared to 22.3 months in the control).[85] Criticisms of the START trial, including the lack of biomarker assessment for MUC-1 expression, have led some to question its conclusions. The INSPIRE trial has the same patient population as the START trial, but is still underway at the time of this writing (https://clinicaltrials.gov).

TG4010 is a recombinant viral vector that expresses both MUC1 and the immunostimulatory cytokine interleukin-2 (IL-2),[87] whose effect has been studied in a phase IIB trial, which examined untreated stage IIIB and IV patients. The first arm contained patients given TG4010 therapy in combination with chemotherapy, while those in the second arm were administered TG4010 until disease progression, followed by combination with chemotherapy. Patients in the first arm demonstrated an increase in partial response, but demonstrated no difference in the overall median survival or 1 year survival as a whole.[86] In a similar phase IIB trial, untreated patient with stage IIIB and IV NSCLC were randomized to chemotherapy or chemotherapy with TG4010. The addition of TG4010 significantly increased the response rate to chemotherapy, and was also associated with increased 6-month progression-free survival (55% in chemotherapy + TG4010 vs. 35% in chemotherapy alone).[87]

PRAME

Preferentially Expressed Antigen of Melanoma, or PRAME is an antigen initially found to be expressed in melanoma, but is also present in NSCLC and other malignancies. It is normally expressed in ovaries, endometrium, kidneys, and the adrenal medulla.[88] Its role in tumor immunology has yet to be fully elucidated, though likely has to do with evasion of the retinoic acid receptor pathway.[89] A phase II trial, PRAME as Adjuvant Immunotherapy In Resected non-Small Cell Lung Cancer (PEARL), assessed the efficacy of the liposomal vaccine to this TAA. The patient population included resected Stage I-IIIA NSCLC, with PRAME expression and disease-free survival as the primary end point. It is currently closed and still acquiring follow-up data.[61]

IMMUNE EVASION OF MUCOSAL BARRIER ORGANS CREATES DIFFICULTIES IN IMMUNOTHERAPY FOR LUNG CANCER

Mucosal barrier organs, such as the lung, stomach, and intestine, are constantly exposed to the external environment and thus have developed unique immunologic strategies to downregulate immune responses to what is perceived as normal environmental antigen.[90–92] Animal data from our laboratory has demonstrated that cancer within the lung can lead to T cell inactivation. Identical delivery of the same tumor to another location in the body does not lead to similar levels of T cell dysfunction.[93] Basic understanding of immunologic mechanism contributing to mucosal and tumor-specific immune evasion,

however, has revolutionized recent approaches to lung cancer immunotherapy. Within the last several decades, the role of defined receptors in the downregulation of immune responses has resulted in a new approach to immunologic control of cancer. Surface presentation of cytotoxic lymphocyte antigen-4 (or CTLA-4) and programmed death ligand-1 (PD-L1) by antigen presenting cells has been defined as a powerful evolutionary mechanism to downregulate and control the immune response.[94,95] Multiple other negative co-stimulatory receptors have been discovered in the last several years as well (Fig. 101.8).[96] Such immunologic "checkpoints" have evolved to prevent unwarranted activation of the immune system. Both humans and mice with mutations in these pathways suffer from autoimmune disease.[97]

Check-Point Blockade

Check-point blockade immunotherapy has revolutionized our ability to reverse tumor-mediated immunosuppression and represents the most impressive advance in immunotherapy in the last decade. Ipilimumab (Yervoy, Bristol-Myers Squibb) is a monoclonal antibody that can successfully block the negative inhibitory effects of CTLA-4.[98] In both chemotherapy naïve patients, as well as those who have failed chemotherapy, ipilimumab has been demonstrated to extend overall survival and improve performance in patients with melanoma. This drug has recently obtained FDA-approval for treatment of melanoma.[99,100] While fewer studies have evaluated the role of ipilimumab in NSCLC, a phase II clinical trial demonstrated a modest survival advantage setting the stage for future randomized trials.[101] In this trial, patients with no prior systemic therapy who have Stage IIIB, Stage IV, or recurrent disease, were randomly assigned to either chemotherapy with paclitaxel and carboplatin alone or chemotherapy with ipilimumab. Those in the chemotherapy and ipilimumab arm were treated either concurrently or with chemotherapy prior to ipilimumab administration. Progression free survival was increased in the group that receiving phased ipilimumab, but not the concurrent group, indicating a potential target for immunotherapy in NSCLC. Currently, a randomized phase III trial is in progress, which compares chemotherapy alone to chemotherapy with phased ipilimumab in patients with NSCLC.[102]

Programmed Cell Death Receptor-1

Programmed cell death receptor-1 (PD-1) is also an important regulator of T cell activation and interacts with its ligand PD-L1. Expression of this ligand on NSCLC is associated with poor prognosis.[103] Nivolumab (Opdivo, Bristol-Myers Squibb), a human monoclonal antibody targeting PD-1, has been evaluated in multiple solid organ malignancies, including NSCLC and melanoma. A phase I trial evaluated patients with advanced NSCLC, as well as other tumors, with a response rate of 14% among all doses of nivolumab and rates as high as 32% at some doses.[104] Responses correlated with tumor cell expression of PD-L1. NSCLC patients that responded had a specifically long duration of mean response of 74 months. Currently, there are multiple active clinical trials studying nivolumab, including two phase III trials evaluating it as a second-line therapy in NSCLC, and one phase III trial comparing nivolumab to chemotherapy as first-line therapy in patients with PD-L1 positive tumors.[102,105] Preliminary results of one phase III trial evaluating nivolumab in combination with platinum-based chemotherapy in stage IIIB and IV NSCLC demonstrated an overall objective response rate of 45% and a 1-year survival rate of 59% to 87%.[105] Another monoclonal antibody for PD-1 blockade, pembrolizumab (Keytruda, Merck), has been deemed safe in patients with PD-L1–expressing NSCLC with an approximate 23% rate of response.[102] Further trials with pembrolizumab are pending.

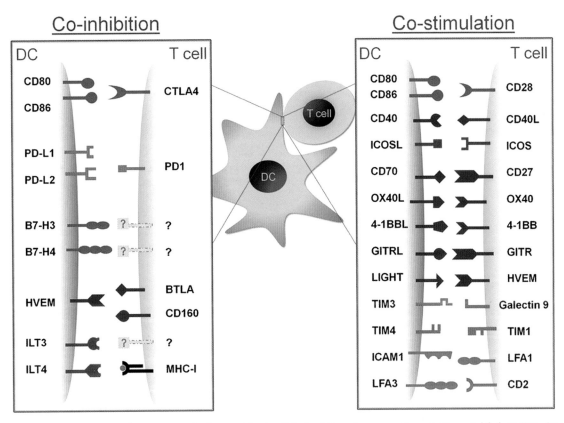

FIGURE 101.8 Positive and negative co-stimulatory molecules. DC, dendritic antigen presenting cell. (From Bakdash G, Sittig SP, van Dijk T, et al. The nature of activatory and tolerogenic dendritic cell-derived signal II. *Front Immunol*, http://dx.doi.org/10.3389/fimmu.2013.00053. Accessed February 28, 2013.)

There have also been trials evaluating antibodies targeting the ligand, PD-L1. A phase I trial was conducted with MPDL3280A (Genentech), a monoclonal antibody to PD-L1, in patients with NSCLC, melanoma, and other solid malignancies. For NSCLC, the response rate was 23%, with 24-week progression-free survival of 44% in squamous and 46% in nonsquamous lung cancer.[106] Further examination of PD-L1 blockade are currently underway.

ROLE OF THE INNATE IMMUNE SYSTEM IN LUNG CANCER IMMUNOTHERAPY

While most immunotherapy focuses on the manipulation of the adaptive arm of the immune system, the innate arm also is also a potentially powerful target for controlling malignancies. NK cells have evolved to recognize patterns of stress receptors expressed on malignant and virally transformed cells. Low cytotoxic activity of NK cells can be linked to an overall cancer susceptibility[107,108] and inherent function of this cell population can be prognostically linked to the treatment-related outcome of lymphoma.[109-111] Interestingly data from our institution has demonstrated that, similar to lymphoma, NK cells rather than T or B lymphocytes, play a critical role in controlling the progression and therapy of lung cancer in murine models.[93,112] Such findings beg the question of whether the reversal of NK dysfunction may be a viable therapeutic strategy for lung cancer.

IL-2 is a cytokine with pleiotropic effects, and is essential for the activation of multiple cells, specifically NK cells.[113] Its potential therapeutic role in NSCLC is only recently being investigated. One study has demonstrated that patients with Stage III/IV NSCLC who respond to paclitaxel-ifosfamide-cisplatin chemotherapy have significantly increased IL-2 levels in their serum compared to poor responders.[114] Higher IL-2 levels were also associated with increased median survival (26 months in higher IL-2 vs. 7.5 months in lower IL-2). Such data begs the question whether, similar to the FDA-approved use of high dose IL-2 for malignant melanoma and renal cell carcinoma, exogenous administration of this cytokine could be used for immunotherapy of lung cancer. Research in murine models has demonstrated that poor lung cancer–specific cytotoxicity of NK cells can be reversed by exogenous IL-2.[93] In small early clinical trials IL-2 therapy does show promise in the treatment of NSCLC. A nonrandomized phase II trial evaluated the effect of gefitinib, a TKI, with and without concomitant subcutaneous IL-2 in patients with recurrent of metastatic NSCLC. The addition of IL-2 increased overall survival (6.9 months in gefitinib alone vs. 20.1 months in gefitinib + IL-2).[115] Several phase 1 trials evaluating the effective of IL-2 combined with other therapy are currently underway.[61]

SUMMARY

Historically, the diagnosis of lung cancer led to a cancer-related survival of 6 months to 1 year in the majority of patients. Recent advances in genetic profiling of lung cancer have led to rational use of targeted therapy and prolongation of survival in patients with select driver mutations. Unlike the case for malignant melanoma, historic attempts at immune-based therapy have failed. Recent understanding of lung cancer–related immunosuppression has revolutionized check-point blockade immunotherapy, with lung cancer patients now representing a major portion of those enrolled in such clinical trials. Additionally, targeting NK cells through IL-2 administration is another potential target for NSCLC treatment. Further work in basic understanding of

Kras inhibition and restoration of p53 function offers the possibility for long-term control or even cure of this disease.

REFERENCES

1. Nowell PC, Hungerford DA. Chromosome studies on normal and leukemic human leukocytes. *J Nat Cancer Inst* 1960;25:85–109.
2. Stehelin D, Varmus HE, Bishop JM, et al. DNA related to the transforming gene(s) of avian sarcoma viruses is present in normal avian DNA. *Nature* 1976;260:170–173.
3. Hanahan D, Weinberg RA. The hallmarks of cancer. *Cell* 2000;100:57–70.
4. Hanahan D, Weinberg RA. Hallmarks of cancer: the next generation. *Cell* 2011;144:646–674.
5. Weinstein IB. Disorders in cell circuitry during multistage carcinogenesis: the role of homeostasis. *Carcinogenesis* 2000;21:857–864.
6. Jain M, Arvanitis C, Chu K, et al. Sustained loss of a neoplastic phenotype by brief inactivation of MYC. *Science* 2002;297:102–104.
7. Weinstein IB. Addiction to oncogenes—the Achilles heal of cancer. *Science* 2002;297:63–64.
8. Druker BJ, Talpaz M, Resta DJ, et al. Efficacy and safety of a specific inhibitor of the BCR-ABL tyrosine kinase in chronic myeloid leukemia. *N Engl J Med* 2001;344:1031–1037.
9. Druker BJ, Sawyers CL, Kantarjian H, et al. Activity of a specific inhibitor of the BCR-ABL tyrosine kinase in the blast crisis of chronic myeloid leukemia and acute lymphoblastic leukemia with the Philadelphia chromosome. *N Engl J Med* 2001;344:1038–1042.
10. Rusch V, Baselga J, Cordon-Cardo C, et al. Differential expression of the epidermal growth factor receptor and its ligands in primary non-small cell lung cancers and adjacent benign lung. *Cancer Res* 1993;53:2379–2385.
11. Kris MG, Natale RB, Herbst RS, et al. Efficacy of gefitinib, an inhibitor of the epidermal growth factor receptor tyrosine kinase, in symptomatic patients with non-small cell lung cancer: a randomized trial. *JAMA* 2003;290:2149–2158.
12. Perez-Soler R, et al. Determinants of tumor response and survival with erlotinib in patients with non–small-cell lung cancer. *J Clin Oncol* 2004;22:3238–3247.
13. Fukuoka M, et al. Multi-institutional randomized phase II trial of gefitinib for previously treated patients with advanced non-small-cell lung cancer (The IDEAL 1 Trial) [corrected]. *J Clin Oncol* 2003;21:2237–2246.
14. Paez JG, Chachoua A, Hammond LA, et al. EGFR mutations in lung cancer: correlation with clinical response to gefitinib therapy. *Science* 2004;304:1497–1500.
15. Lynch TJ, Bell DW, Sordella R, et al. Activating mutations in the epidermal growth factor receptor underlying responsiveness of non-small-cell lung cancer to gefitinib. *N Engl J Med* 2004;350:2129–2139.
16. Kandoth C, et al. Mutational landscape and significance across 12 major cancer types. *Nature* 2013;502:333–339.
17. Ding L, et al. Somatic mutations affect key pathways in lung adenocarcinoma. *Nature* 2008;455:1069–1075.
18. Cancer Genome Atlas Research Network. Comprehensive molecular profiling of lung adenocarcinoma. *Nature* 2014;511:543–550.
19. Cancer Genome Atlas Research Network. Comprehensive genomic characterization of squamous cell lung cancers. *Nature* 2012;489:519–525.
20. Choi YH, Ekholm D, Krall J, et al. Identification of a novel isoform of the cyclic-nucleotide phosphodiesterase PDE3A expressed in vascular smooth-muscle myocytes. *Biochem J* 2001;353:41–50.
21. Solomon B, Varella-Garcia M, Camidge DR. ALK gene rearrangements: a new therapeutic target in a molecularly defined subset of non-small cell lung cancer. *J Thorac Oncol* 2009;4:1450–1454.
22. Cooper WA, Lam DC, O'Toole SA, et al. Molecular biology of lung cancer. *J Thorac Dis* 2013;5(Suppl 5):S479–S490.
23. Koivunen JP, Kim J, Lee J, et al. Mutations in the LKB1 tumour suppressor are frequently detected in tumours from Caucasian but not Asian lung cancer patients. *Br J Cancer* 2008;99:245–252.
24. Soda M, Choi YL, Enomoto M, et al. Identification of the transforming EML4-ALK fusion gene in non-small-cell lung cancer. *Nature* 2007;448:561–566.
25. Choi YL, Soda M, Yamashita Y, et al. EML4-ALK mutations in lung cancer that confer resistance to ALK inhibitors. *N Engl J Mede* 2010;363:1734–1739.
26. Shaw AT, Solomon B. Targeting anaplastic lymphoma kinase in lung cancer. *Clin Cancer Res* 1;17:2081–2086.
27. Lindeman NI, Cagle PT, Beasley MB, et al. Molecular testing guideline for selection of lung cancer patients for EGFR and ALK tyrosine kinase inhibitors: guideline from the College of American Pathologists, International Association for the Study of Lung Cancer, and Association for Molecular Pathology. *J Thorac Oncol* 2013;8:823–859.
28. Shaw AT, Yeap BY, Mino-Kenudson M, et al. Clinical features and outcome of patients with non-small-cell lung cancer who harbor EML4-ALK. *J Clin Oncol* 2009;27:4247–4253.
29. Selinger CI, Rogers TM, Russell PA, et al. Testing for ALK rearrangement in lung adenocarcinoma: a multicenter comparison of immunohistochemistry and fluorescent in situ hybridization. *Mod Pathol* 2013;26:1545–1553.
30. Rodig SJ, Mino-Kenudson M, Dacic S, Yeap BY, et al. Unique clinicopathologic features characterize ALK-rearranged lung adenocarcinoma in the western population. *Clin Cancer Res* 2009;15:5216–5223.
31. Sakairi Y, Nakajima T, Yasufuku K, et al. EML4-ALK fusion gene assessment using metastatic lymph node samples obtained by endobronchial ultrasound-guided transbronchial needle aspiration. *Clin Can Res* 2010;16:4938–4945.

32. Wong DW, Leung EL, So KK, et al. The EML4-ALK fusion gene is involved in various histologic types of lung cancers from nonsmokers with wild-type EGFR and KRAS. *Cancer* 2009;115:1723–1733.
33. Yip PY, Yu B, Cooper WA, et al. Patterns of DNA mutations and ALK rearrangement in resected node negative lung adenocarcinoma. *J Thorac Oncol* 2013;8:408–414.
34. Inamura K, Takeuchi K, Togashi Y, et al. EML4-ALK lung cancers are characterized by rare other mutations, a TTF-1 cell lineage, an acinar histology, and young onset. *Mod Pathol* 2009;22:508–515.
35. Sasaki T, Koivunen J, Ogino A, et al. A novel ALK secondary mutation and EGFR signaling cause resistance to ALK kinase inhibitors. *Cancer Res* 2011;71:6051–6060.
36. Sholl LM, Weremowicz S, Gray SW, et al. Combined use of ALK immunohistochemistry and FISH for optimal detection of ALK-rearranged lung adenocarcinomas. *J Thorac Oncol* 2013;8:322–328.
37. Tiseo M, Gelsomino F, Boggiani D, et al. EGFR and EML4-ALK gene mutations in NSCLC: a case report of erlotinib-resistant patient with both concomitant mutations. *Lung Cancer* 2011;71:241–243.
38. Davies KD, Le AT, Theodoro MF, et al. Identifying and targeting ROS1 gene fusions in non-small cell lung cancer. *Clin Cancer Res* 2012;18:4570–4579.
39. Chin LP, Soo RA, Soong R, et al. Targeting ROS1 with anaplastic lymphoma kinase inhibitors: a promising therapeutic strategy for a newly defined molecular subset of non-small-cell lung cancer. *J Thorac Oncol* 2012;7:1625–1630.
40. Bergethon K, et al. ROS1 rearrangements define a unique molecular class of lung cancers. *J Clin Oncol* 2012;30:863–870.
41. Takeuchi K, Soda M, Togashi Y, et al. RET, ROS1 and ALK fusions in lung cancer. *Nat Med* 2012;18:378–381.
42. Shaw AT, Kim DW, Nakagawa K, et al. Crizotinib versus chemotherapy in advanced ALK-positive lung cancer. *N Engl J Med* 2013;368:2385–2394.
43. Solomon BJ, Mok T, Kim DW, et al. First-line crizotinib versus chemotherapy in ALK-positive lung cancer. *N Engl J Med* 2014;371:2167–2177.
44. Zou HY, Li Q, Engstrom LD, et al. PF-06463922 is a potent and selective next-generation ROS1/ALK inhibitor capable of blocking crizotinib-resistant ROS1 mutations. *Proc Nat Acad Sci Am* 2015;112:3493–3498.
45. Downward J. Targeting RAS signalling pathways in cancer therapy. *Nat Rev Cancer* 2003;3:11–22.
46. Karnoub AE, Weinberg RA. Ras oncogenes: split personalities. *Nat Rev Mol Cell Biol* 2008;9:517–531.
47. Sequist LV, Heist RS, Shaw AT, et al. Implementing multiplexed genotyping of non-small-cell lung cancers into routine clinical practice. *Ann Oncol* 2011;22:2616–2624.
48. Adjei AA, Mauer A, Bruzek L, et al. Phase II study of the farnesyl transferase inhibitor R115777 in patients with advanced non-small-cell lung cancer. *J Clin Oncol* 2003;21:1760–1766.
49. Weisz B, Giehl K, Gana-Weisz M, et al. A new functional Ras antagonist inhibits human pancreatic tumor growth in nude mice. *Oncogene* 1999;18:2579–2588.
50. Laheru D, Shah P, Rajeshkumar NV, et al. Integrated preclinical and clinical development of S-trans, trans-Farnesylthiosalicylic Acid (FTS, Salirasib) in pancreatic cancer. *Invest New Drugs* 2012;30:2391–2399.
51. John J, Sohmen R, Feuerstein J, et al. Kinetics of interaction of nucleotides with nucleotide-free H-ras p21. *Biochemistry* 1990;29:6058–6065.
52. Ostrem JM, Peters U, Sos ML, et al. K-Ras(G12C) inhibitors allosterically control GTP affinity and effector interactions. *Nature* 2013;503:548–551.
53. Engelman JA, Chen L, Tan X, et al. Effective use of PI3K and MEK inhibitors to treat mutant Kras G12D and PIK3CA H1047R murine lung cancers. *Nat Med* 2008;14:1351–1356.
54. Janne PA, Shaw AT, Pereira JR, et al. Selumetinib plus docetaxel for KRAS-mutant advanced non-small-cell lung cancer: a randomised, multicentre, placebo-controlled, phase 2 study. *Lancet Oncol* 2013;14:38–47.
55. Chang C, Simmons DT, Martin MA, et al Identification and partial characterization of new antigens from simian virus 40-transformed mouse cells. *J Virol* 1979;31:463–471.
56. Levine AJ, Momand J, Finlay CA. The p53 tumour suppressor gene. *Nature* 1991;351:453–456.
57. Lane DP. Cancer. p53, guardian of the genome. *Nature* 1992;358:15–16.
58. Hollstein M, Sidransky D, Vogelstein B, et al. p53 mutations in human cancers. *Science* 1991;253:49–53.
59. Bykov VJ, Issaeva N, Shilov A, et al. Restoration of the tumor suppressor function to mutant p53 by a low-molecular-weight compound. *Nat Med* 2002;8:282–288.
60. Lehmann S, Bykov VJ, Ali D, et al. Targeting p53 in vivo: a first-in-human study with p53-targeting compound APR-246 in refractory hematologic malignancies and prostate cancer. *J Clin Oncol* 2012;30:3633–3639.
61. https://www.clinicaltrials.gov
62. Roth JA, Nguyen D, Lawrence DD, et al. Retrovirus-mediated wild-type p53 gene transfer to tumors of patients with lung cancer. *Nat Med* 1996;2:985–991.
63. Yang ZX, Wang D, Wang G, et al. Clinical study of recombinant adenovirus-p53 combined with fractionated stereotactic radiotherapy for hepatocellular carcinoma. *J Cancer Res Clin Oncol* 2010;136:625–630.
64. Tazawa H, Kagawa S, Fujiwara T. Advances in adenovirus-mediated p53 cancer gene therapy. *Expert Opin Biol Ther* 2013;13:1569–1583.
65. Yoo GH, Moon J, LeBlanc M, et al. A phase 2 trial of surgery with perioperative INGN 201 (Ad5CMV-p53) gene therapy followed by chemoradiotherapy for advanced, resectable squamous cell carcinoma of the oral cavity, oropharynx, hypopharynx, and larynx: report of the Southwest Oncology Group. *Arch Otolaryngol Head Neck Surg* 2009;135:869–874.
66. Li J, Barreda DR, Zhang YA, et al. B lymphocytes from early vertebrates have potent phagocytic and microbicidal abilities. *Nat Immunol* 2006;7:1116–1124.

67. Coley WB. The treatment of malignant tumors by repeated inoculations of erysipelas: with report of ten original cases. *Am J Med Sci* 1893;105:487–511.

68. Hinrichs CS, Rosenberg SA. Exploiting the curative potential of adoptive T-cell therapy for cancer. *Immunol Rev* 2014;257:56–71.

69. Zappasodi R, de Braud, Di Nicola, et al. Lymphoma Immunotherapy M: Current Status. *Front Immunol* 2015;6:448.

70. Gjerstorff MF, Andersen MH, Ditzel HJ. Oncogenic cancer/testis antigens: prime candidates for immunotherapy. *Oncotarget* 2015;6:15772–15787.

71. Gubin MM, Zhang X, Schuster H, et al. Checkpoint blockade cancer immunotherapy targets tumour-specific mutant antigens. *Nature* 2014;515:577–581.

72. Carreno BM, Zhang X, Schuster H, et al. Cancer immunotherapy. A dendritic cell vaccine increases the breadth and diversity of melanoma neoantigen-specific T cells. *Science* 2015;348:803–808.

73. Muscatelli F, Walker AP, De Plaen E, et al. Isolation and characterization of a MAGE gene family in the Xp21.3 region. *Proc Nat Acad Sc Am* 1995;92:4987–4991.

74. Sienel W, Varwerk C, Linder A, et al. Melanoma associated antigen (MAGE)-A3 expression in Stages I and II non-small cell lung cancer: results of a multi-center study. *Eur J Cardiothorac Surg* 2004;25:131–134.

75. Kruit W, Suciu S, Dreno B, et al. Active immunization toward the MAGE-A3 antigen in patients with metastatic melanoma: Four-year follow-up results from a randomized phase II study (EORTC16032-18031). *J Clin Oncol* 2011;29(suppl 15);8535–8535.

76. Schultz ES, Lethé B, Cambiaso CL, et al. A MAGE-A3 peptide presented by HLA-DP4 is recognized on tumor cells by CD4+ cytolytic T lymphocytes. *Cancer Res* 2000;60:6272–6275.

77. Vansteenkiste J, Zielinski M, Linder A, et al. Adjuvant MAGE-A3 immunotherapy in resected non-small-cell lung cancer: phase II randomized study results. *J Clin Oncol* 2013;31:2396–2403.

78. Vansteenkiste J, Cho B, Vanakesa T, et al. MAGRIT, a double-blind, randomized, placebo-controlled Phase III study to assess the efficacy of the recMAGE-A3 + AS15 cancer immunotherapeutic as adjuvant therapy in patients with resected MAGE-A3-positive non-small cell lung cancer (NSCLC). *Ann Oncol* 2014;25: iv409–iv416.

79. Ho SB, Niehans GA, Lyftogt C, et al. Heterogeneity of mucin gene expression in normal and neoplastic tissues. *Cancer Res* 1993;53:641–651.

80. Agrawal B, Longenecker BM. MUC1 mucin-mediated regulation of human T cells. *Int Immunol* 2005;17:391–399.

81. Shen Q, Rahn JJ, Zhang J, et al. MUC1 initiates Src-CrkL-Rac1/Cdc42-mediated actin cytoskeletal protrusive motility after ligating intercellular adhesion molecule-1. *Mol Cancer Res* 2008;6:555–567.

82. Szyszka-Barth K, Ramlau K, Gozdzik-Spychalska J, et al. Actual status of therapeutic vaccination in non-small cell lung cancer. *Contemp Oncol (Pozn)* 2014;18:77–84.

83. Butts C, Maksymiuk A, Goss G, et al. Updated survival analysis in patients with stage IIIB or IV non-small-cell lung cancer receiving BLP25 liposome vaccine (L-BLP25): phase IIB randomized, multicenter, open-label trial. *J Cancer Res Clin Oncol* 2011;137:1337–1342.

84. Butts C, Murray N, Maksymiuk A, et al. Randomized phase IIB trial of BLP25 liposome vaccine in stage IIIB and IV non-small-cell lung cancer. *J Clin Oncol* 2005;23:6674–6681.

85. Butts C, Socinski MA, Mitchell PL, et al. Tecemotide (L-BLP25) versus placebo after chemoradiotherapy for stage III non-small cell lung cancer (START): a randomised, double-blind, phase 3 trial. *Lancet Oncol* 2014;15:59–68.

86. Ramlau R, Quoix E, Rolski J, et al. A phase II study of Tg4010 (Mva-Muc1-Il2) in association with chemotherapy in patients with stage III/IV Non-small cell lung cancer. *J Thorac Oncol* 2008;3:735–744.

87. Quoix E, Ramlau R, Westeel V, et al. Therapeutic vaccination with TG4010 and first-line chemotherapy in advanced non-small-cell lung cancer: a controlled phase 2B trial. *Lancet Oncol* 2011;12:1125–1133.

88. Ikeda H, Lethé B, Lehmann F, et al. Characterization of an antigen that is recognized on a melanoma showing partial HLA loss by CTL expressing an NK inhibitory receptor. *Immunity* 1997;6:199–208.

89. Epping MT, Wang L, Edel MJ, et al. The human tumor antigen PRAME is a dominant repressor of retinoic acid receptor signaling. *Cell* 2005;122:835–847.

90. Limmer A, Ohl J, Wingender G, et al. Cross-presentation of oral antigens by liver sinusoidal endothelial cells leads to CD8 T cell tolerance. *Eur J Immunol* 2005;35: 2970–2981.

91. Holt PG, Oliver J, Bilyk N, et al. Downregulation of the antigen presenting cell function(s) of pulmonary dendritic cells in vivo by resident alveolar macrophages. *J Exp Med* 1993;177:397–407.

92. McMenamin C, Holt PG. The natural immune response to inhaled soluble protein antigens involves major histocompatibility complex (MHC) class I-restricted CD8+ T cell-mediated but MHC class II-restricted CD4+ T cell-dependent immune deviation resulting in selective suppression of immunoglobulin E production. *J Exp Med* 1993;178: 889–899.

93. Chang S, Lin X, Higashikubo R, et al. Unique pulmonary antigen presentation may call for an alternative approach toward lung cancer immunotherapy. *Oncoimmunology* 2013;2:e23563.

94. McAdam AJ, Schweitzer AN, Sharpe AH. The role of B7 co-stimulation in activation and differentiation of CD4+ and CD8+ T cells. *Immunol Rev* 1998;165:231–247.

95. Ishida Y, Agata Y, Shibahara K, et al. Induced expression of PD-1, a novel member of the immunoglobulin gene superfamily, upon programmed cell death. *EMBO J* 1992;11:3887–3895.

96. McGrath MM, Najafian N. The role of coinhibitory signaling pathways in transplantation and tolerance. *Front Immunol* 2012;3:47.

97. Francisco LM, Sage PT, Sharpe AH. The PD-1 pathway in tolerance and autoimmunity. *Immunol Rev* 2010;236:219–242.

98. Leach DR, Krummel MF, Allison JP. Enhancement of antitumor immunity by CTLA-4 blockade. *Science* 1996;271:1734–1736.

99. Robert C, Thomas L, Bondarenko I, et al. Ipilimumab plus dacarbazine for previously untreated metastatic melanoma. *N Engl J Med* 2011;364:2517–2526.

100. Hodi FS, O'day SJ, McDermott DF, et al. Improved survival with ipilimumab in patients with metastatic melanoma. *N Engl J Med* 2010;363:711–723.

101. Lynch TJ, Bondarenko I, Luft A, et al. Ipilimumab in combination with paclitaxel and carboplatin as first-line treatment in stage IIIB/IV non-small-cell lung cancer: results from a randomized, double-blind, multicenter phase II study. *J Clin Oncol* 2012;30: 2046–2054.

102. Johnson DB, Rioth MJ, Horn L. Immune checkpoint inhibitors in NSCLC. *Curr Treat Options Oncol* 2014;15:658–669.

103. Mu CY, Huang JA, Chen Y, et al. High expression of PD-L1 in lung cancer may contribute to poor prognosis and tumor cells immune escape through suppressing tumor infiltrating dendritic cells maturation. *Med Oncol* 2011;28:682–688.

104. Topalian SL, Hodi FS, Brahmer JR, et al. Safety, activity, and immune correlates of anti-PD-1 antibody in cancer. *N Engl J Med* 2012;366:2443–2454.

105. Antonia SJ, Brahmer JR, Gettinger S, et al., Nivolumab (anti-PD-1; BMS-936558, ONO-4538) in combination with platinum-based doublet chemotherapy (PT-DC) in advanced non-small-cell lung cancer (NSCLC). *J Clin Oncol* 2014;32(suppl 5): abstr 8113.

106. Soria J, Cruz C, Bahleda R, et al. Clinical activity, safety and biomarkers of PD-L1 blockade in non-small cell lung cancer (NSCLC): Additional analyses from a clinical study of the engineered antibody MPDL3280A (anti-PDL1). Presented at ECC 2013. Abstract 3408.

107. Tursz T, Dokhelar MC, Lipinski M, et al. Low natural killer cell activity in patients with malignant lymphoma. *Cancer* 1982;50:2333–2335.

108. Imai K, Matsuyama S, Miyake S, et al. Natural cytotoxic activity of peripheral-blood lymphocytes and cancer incidence: an 11-year follow-up study of a general population. *Lancet* 2000;356:1795–1799.

109. Baumann MA, Milson TJ, Patrick CW, et al. Correlation of circulating natural killer cell count with prognosis in large cell lymphoma. *Cancer* 1986;57: 2309–2312.

110. Mehta BA, Satam MN, Advani SH, et al. In vitro modulation of natural killer cell activity in non-Hodgkin's lymphoma patients after therapy. *Cancer Immunol Immunother* 1989;28:148–152.

111. Fischer L, Penack O, Gentilini C, et al. The anti-lymphoma effect of antibody-mediated immunotherapy is based on an increased degranulation of peripheral blood natural killer (NK) cells. *Exp Hematol* 2006;34:753–759.

112. Kreisel D, Gelman AE, Higashikubo R, et al. Strain-specific variation in murine natural killer gene complex contributes to differences in immunosurveillance for urethane-induced lung cancer. *Cancer Res* 2012;72:4311–4317.

113. Meropol NJ, Porter M, Blumenson LE, et al. Daily subcutaneous injection of low-dose interleukin 2 expands natural killer cells in vivo without significant toxicity. *Clin Cancer Research* 1996;2:669–677.

114. Koufos N, Michailidou D, Xynos ID, et al. Modulation of peripheral immune responses by paclitaxel-ifosfamide-cisplatin chemotherapy in advanced non-small-cell lung cancer. *J Cancer Res Clin Oncol* 2013;139:1995–2003.

115. Bersanelli M, Buti S, Camisa R, et al. Gefitinib plus interleukin-2 in advanced non-small cell lung cancer patients previously treated with chemotherapy. *Cancers (Basel)* 2014;6:2035–2048.

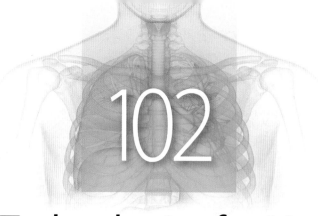

102

Emerging Technologies for Management of Lung Cancer in Patients With Marginal Physiologic Function

Kendra Iskander ▪ Hiran C. Fernando

Lung cancer continues to be a significant public health issue in the United States and worldwide. Annually, over 200,000 new cases of lung cancer are diagnosed in the United States and an estimated 159,000 Americans are expected to die from lung cancer in 2014, accounting for approximately 27% of all cancer deaths.[1] If lung cancer is identified at an early stage, then lobectomy with curative intent is possible. Unfortunately, a large number of patients will not be candidates for lobectomy or any type of resection because of comorbid diseases and marginal physiologic function. Over the last 20 years, significant treatment advances have been made in managing such high-risk lung cancer patients, so that therapy with curative intent with minimal risk is now possible.

Generally, patients can be considered to fall into three risk categories: (1) average-risk operable, who will usually be offered lobectomy; (2) high-risk operable, where lobectomy is considered not to be an option, but a sublobar resection is considered still feasible; and (3) medically inoperable, where any type of resection is felt to not be feasible, and so alternative local therapy is used.

Currently, there are no well-established guidelines for defining which patients are high risk and who is medically inoperable. Historically, pulmonary function tests (PFTs) have been most useful in guiding physicians between operative and nonoperative management strategies. However, previous studies have shown that even in patients with significant emphysema and marginal PFTs, resection may still be feasible.[2]

Differential ventilation/perfusion scans or quantitative CT scans can also be useful in helping to determine operability as described in the American College of Chest Physicians practice guidelines on the evaluation of patients for lung resection.[3] In addition to PFTs, other critical elements to consider include cardiac function, age, and oxygen saturation. At a 2003 meeting of the American College of Surgeons Oncology Group, two studies were developed for high risk or medically inoperable patients with lung cancer.[4] To allow inclusion of multiple factors in addition to pulmonary function, the investigators developed major and minor criteria.[4] Patients had to meet a minimum of one major or two minor criteria to be classified as high risk. To be defined as medically inoperable, patients had to meet the same criteria but also required evaluation by an approved thoracic surgeon, who deemed the patient to not be a candidate for any resection. The criteria for these studies are as follows:

Major Criteria: $FEV_1 \leq 50\%$ or DLCO $\leq 50\%$

Minor Criteria: Age >75 years, FEV or DLCO 50% to 60%, Pulmonary hypertension, Ejection fraction <40%, paO_2 <55 mm Hg, pCO_2 >45 mm Hg.

It should be emphasized that these criteria were designed to enable inclusion into these surgical trials. There are patients who meet these criteria, but who, based on performance status and tumor characteristics, may still be optimally treated with even lobar resection. Similarly, there are patients who exceed the physiologic criteria defined for inclusion in these studies, but who will not be candidates for any form of resection. This underscores the need for evaluation of such patients in a multidisciplinary setting that includes an experienced thoracic surgeon in the evaluation process.

In the following chapter, we review options for patients deemed to be high-risk operable, as well as those deemed medically inoperable.

HIGH-RISK OPERABLE PATIENTS

Lobectomy has been the treatment of choice for stage 1 NSCLC due to the decreased rate of local recurrence. This standard is largely the result of a randomized study by Ginsberg et al.[5] which showed a threefold rate of recurrence among patients with T_1N_0 NSCLC treated with sublobar resection as compared to lobectomy. As a result, sublobar resection by segmentectomy or wedge resection for stage 1 NSCLC is currently considered a compromise option reserved for patients deemed to be high risk.[6] Table 102.1 shows outcomes in patients with stage I NSCLC treated with sublobar resection. However, based on the results of several studies from Japan and the detection of ever smaller tumors from screening programs, sublobar resection is currently being investigated as an option for average-risk patients with small peripheral tumors.

Ultimately, the rationale for performing a sublobar resection is to decrease the amount of lung removed relative to the amount of healthy lung remaining. Harada et al.[14] demonstrated that in patients undergoing segmentectomy versus lobectomy postoperative lung function correlated with the extent of lung resection. In another study comparing lobectomy to segmentectomy for stage I NSCLC, significant declines were seen in forced vital capacity, forced expiratory volume in 1 second and diffusing capacity after lobectomy, but

TABLE 102.1 Result of Sublobar Resection for Stage 1 NSCLC

Author (yr)	Modality	Number Studied	Median Survival Time (yrs)	2-yr Survival %	3-yr Survival %	5-yr Survival %
Deng (2014)[7]	Sublobar	212	4.2	89.5	76.1	67.3
Crabtree (2014)[8]	Sublobar	458	2.8	74.1	67.6	58.6
Altorki (2014)[9]	Sublobar	53	5.1	88.6	79.2	52.8
Park (2012)[10]	Sublobar	248	n/a	98	93	90
Keenan (2004)[11]	Sublobar	54	n/a	86	74	62
Koike (2003)[12]	Sublobar	74	n/a	n/a	91	89
LCSG (1995)[5]	Sublobar	122	n/a	80	78	44
Read (1990)[13]	Sublobar	113	n/a	n/a	n/a	84

after segmentectomy significant decline was only seen in diffusing capacity.[11]

The principal concern with sublobar resection is with its oncologic effectiveness. One issue is the adequacy of lymph node evaluation. If lymph node sampling or dissection is not performed there is a high likelihood of under staging. This will be more of an issue after wedge resection rather than segmentectomy, since it is likely that parenchymal lymph nodes will be removed during the bronchial and vessel dissection required for segmentectomy. A recent analysis from a prospective study of sublobar resection confirmed this concept in that patients undergoing wedge resection had a lower yield of lymph nodes and lymph node stations sampled compared to segmentectomy.[15] As a result there was also a higher incidence of nodal upstaging (9% vs. 1%) in patients who underwent segmentectomy. The same study also demonstrated that parenchymal margin was also smaller after a wedge resection. Margin size has been demonstrated to impact outcomes as reported in a study by El-Sherif et al.[16] In the study a greater parenchymal margin decreased the rate of recurrence. Local recurrence was 14.6% with a margin <1 cm versus 7.5% with a margin >1 cm.[16]

Another way of assessing margins is by looking at staple line cytology. This was evaluated in a study by Sawabata et al.[17] where the staple line of the resected specimen was run across a slide to look for malignant cells. Interestingly, there were patients who had positive staple line cytology, yet negative histology. There was a 47% positive staple line cytology rate, while standard histologic techniques identified positive margins in only 20%.[17] In these patients with positive cytology there was a 57% rate of relapse versus 0% in patients with negative cytology margins.

One method of improving surgical margins that has been investigated is the use of adjuvant intraoperative brachytherapy. There are two common methods of successfully performing the brachytherapy.[18,19] In the first technique, polyglactin sutures containing iodine-125 (^{125}I) seeds (Oncura, Princeton, NJ) are placed 5 mm away from and parallel to the staple line on each side of the resection margin. The suture strands are then fixed to the lung surface with several 3.0 silk or polyglactin sutures placed 1 to 2 cm apart. A second technique involves creating a polyglycolic mesh implant containing suture strands of the isotope ^{125}I. The ^{125}I suture can be woven into a piece of vicryl mesh at 1-cm intervals at the time of surgery, or the implant can also be ordered directly from the manufacturers. The mesh is then sutured over the staple line. The dosimetry goal of the brachytherapy is to deliver 100 Gy at 5 to 7 mm intervals along the central axis of the resection margin.

The radioactive mesh method was first reported in 1998 and demonstrated that at 7 months postoperatively no patients had pneumonitis on surveillance CT scan.[19] These two methods offered 100%

compliance in delivering localized radiation over a complex three-dimensional area to the desired location and was safe for patients. In comparison, external beam radiotherapy can be challenging to deliver after surgery with concerns related to compliance with the outpatient radiation schedule in these compromised patients as well as the additional risks of radiation injury to healthy areas of lung.[18]

A significant concern with brachytherapy is the possibility of radiation exposure to the health care team. Smith et al.[20] addressed these concerns by looking at intraoperative radiation exposures during implantation of brachytherapy mesh. Diodes were placed on the patient, surgeon's hands, and the radiation oncologist during the creation and implantation of the mesh. The overall radiation dose to each person was 2 mrem, one-third the dose of a single chest radiograph. Therefore, brachytherapy can be performed with minimal risk.

An additional concern is that brachytherapy can affect pulmonary function and dyspnea in the high-risk patient group undergoing a sublobar resection.[21] Fernando et al. reported no significant difference in percentage change in DLCO or dyspnea score from baseline to 3 months for patients treated with sublobar resection with or without brachytherapy. Multivariable regression analysis (adjusted for baseline values) showed no significant impact of treatment arm, tumor location (upper vs. other lobe), or surgical approach (video-assisted thoracoscopic surgery vs. thoracotomy) on 3-month FEV_1, DLCO, and dyspnea score. The authors concluded that adjuvant intraoperative brachytherapy in conjunction with sublobar resection did not significantly worsen pulmonary function or dyspnea at 3 months in a high-risk population with NSCLC nor was it associated with increased perioperative pulmonary adverse events.

Initial retrospective studies using adjuvant brachytherapy were encouraging with reduced local recurrence rates reported. Santos et al. reported an 18.6% rate of local recurrence with sublobar resection alone. With the addition of brachytherapy, the local recurrence rate was decreased to 2%.[22] Another retrospective study by Fernando et al.[23] of 124 patients undergoing sublobar resection of which half were treated with mesh brachytherapy showed a local recurrence rate of 17.2% for those without adjuvant treatment and 3.3% for those with brachytherapy. Strongly supporting the use of brachytherapy was a study by Birdas et al.[24] examining stage 1B NSCLC patients treated with either lobectomy versus sublobar resection with mesh brachytherapy. Of these 167 patients the local recurrence rates were comparable between the two groups, 3.2% versus 4.8%, respectively.

The initial success from these reports led to the development of a prospective randomized trial comparing sublobar resection alone to sublobar resection with brachytherapy.[25] The study population included high-risk operable patients with NSCLC ≤3 cm. The primary end point was time to local recurrence. Surprisingly, there was no significant difference in time to local recurrence or survival which was a secondary endpoint. Local recurrences occurred in 12.1% of patients at 3 years of follow-up, lower than many other reports of sublobar resection. This suggested that surgeons participating in this prospective trial may have paid closer attention to parenchymal margins. Supporting this idea was that when the authors compared outcomes between arms in patients with compromised margins, only 14 patients (6.6%) had positive staple line cytology. This group had the strongest trend toward favoring the use of brachytherapy in that local recurrence occurred in 10% of the patients treated with brachytherapy compared to 25% in patients treated with sublobar resection alone.

In summary, despite encouraging early data the routine use of brachytherapy is not supported. The benefit of brachytherapy is most likely in those patients who have compromised margins following sublobar resection and this patient group is challenging to predict preoperatively.

MEDICALLY INOPERABLE PATIENTS

STEREOTACTIC BODY RADIATION THERAPY

Previously, the standard of care for these patients was external beam radiation therapy. However, in compromised patients, this can be challenging to deliver effectively. Results of external beam radiation for stage I NSCLC have generally been poor, but studies have also demonstrated that in medically inoperable patients external beam radiation is associated with better lung cancer specific survival compared to no treatment.[26]

Over the last 10 to 15 years stereotactic body radiation therapy (SBRT) has emerged as an excellent therapeutic option for the medically inoperable patient with NSCLC. Outcomes in patients with stage I NSCLC treated with SBRT are outlined in Table 102.1. An issue with treating lung tumors, particularly if small, is that these move with respiration. Ensuring delivery of radiation to the tumor and minimizing injury to healthy lung can therefore be challenging. To overcome the physiologic respiratory motion of the lung, multiple techniques have been employed. The simplest method to achieve this is with breath holding to limit the motion of the lung.[27] A second method called respiratory gaiting integrates the patient's breathing with modulating the radiation beam. To achieve this technique, a CT scan while the patient is breathing is obtained to locate the exact location of the tumor at multiple time points during the respiratory cycle. The timing of the radiation exposure is then modulated to focus at the point in the respiratory cycle in which maximal tumor exposure is possible.

Dynamic tracking is a third method utilizing the CyberKnife Stereotactic Radiosurgery System (Accuray, Sunnyvale, CA). This system has a linear accelerator to deliver the radiation on a mobile robotic arm. Image-guided cameras focus on gold tumor markers that are placed prior to therapy adjacent to the neoplasm. Lung and chest wall expansion and recoil are evaluated as well. Using this method, a precise location of the tumor in space can be captured and radiation can be delivered at any point in the respiratory cycle with the robotic arm.

With improved target accuracy and using multiple planes of radiation, much higher radiation doses can be delivered compared to external beam radiation therapy.[28] Traditional external beam radiation treatment plans involving fractions delivered over several weeks may deliver around 60 Gy. SBRT is typically delivered over 1 to 5 fractions. Although dosing is not quite comparable a single dose of 20 Gy delivered by SBRT is equivalent to 60 Gy dosing by conventional external beam radiation.[28] Many treatment plans allow for a biologic effective dose of over 100 Gy and the higher radiation doses provided by SBRT can result in improved local control and survival. For instance, Onishi et al.[29] showed that patients who received a dose of <100 Gy (biologic equivalent dose) had a 69% survival while those that had a dose >100 Gy (biologic equivalent dose) had an 88% survival at 5 years.

A recent large study examined SBRT in 100 consecutive medically inoperable patients with lung cancer.[30] All patients in this study were evaluated by a thoracic surgeon and were not candidates for surgical resection due to poor pulmonary function, previous therapy including failed resection, or the patient refused an operation. Forty-six patients had a primary lung neoplasm (NSCLC), 35 patients had recurrent cancer, and 19 had pulmonary metastases. Patients underwent three fractions of 20 Gy. Placement of the tumor markers resulted in 26% of patients requiring a chest tube. The median overall survival was 24 months with a 50% probability of 2-year survival. For patients with primary lung cancer 44% of those survived at 2 years while 84% with metastatic disease lived. The authors concluded that stereotactic surgery for lung neoplasm is safe and provides an alternative for medically inoperable patients. Table 102.2 demonstrates results in patients with stage I NSCLC treated with SBRT.

Another issue with SBRT is the risk of significant complications when large doses of radiation are used close to the central airways. In a phase II study involving 70 patients, excessive toxicity (including some grade 5 complications) was seen with high radiation doses for central tumors.[35] Studies are in progress to evaluate optimal dosimetry with SBRT for such tumors.

Probably the most important trial in North America for SBRT in the multicenter prospective study is RTOG0236.[33] This multicenter study involved 55 evaluable patients with biopsy-proven NSCLC. At 34.4 months median follow-up, the primary tumor control was 97.6%. The 3-year overall survival was 55.8% with a median survival of 48 months. These and other excellent results in medically inoperable patients have led some investigators to recommend SBRT for

TABLE 102.2 Result of Stereotactic Body Radiation Therapy for Stage 1 NSCLC

Author (yr)	Modality	Number Studied	Median Survival Time (yrs)	2-yr Survival %	3-yr Survival %	5-yr Survival %
Davis (2015)[31]	SBRT	59	2.3	60	n/a	n/a
Shibamoto (2012)[32]	SBRT	180	3	n/a	69	52.2
Timmerman (2010)[33]	SBRT	55	4	72	55.8	n/a
Stephans (2009)[34]	SBRT	86	n/a	52	48	n/a
Timmerman (2006)[35]	SBRT	70	2.7	54.7	36	30
Onishi (2004)[29]	SBRT	245	2	88.9	56	47

the high-risk operable patient, perhaps replacing the standard of sublobar resection.[36]

However, there are concerns with making these conclusions. Definitions of local recurrence and control are not similar between surgical and SBRT studies. In addition, the patients even in multicenter studies are not similar.[4,37]

Underscoring this potential problem is a report by Crabtree et al.[8] that compared survival between patients undergoing SBRT and surgical resection. Patients were matched based on age, tumor size, comorbidity score, FEV_1, and tumor location. Overall 3-year survival was 52% for the SBRT group and 68% for the resection group.

In summary, SBRT is an evolving and rapidly developing field in lung cancer. It provides an aggressive therapy to a focal area with reduced complications and is an important treatment modality in the medically inoperable patient.

PERCUTANEOUS THERMAL ABLATION

Radiofrequency ablation (RFA) is a minimally invasive treatment alternative for lung cancer. It has been successfully used in primary and metastatic tumors in high-risk surgical candidates.[38] The benefit of this treatment modality is the capacity to heat tissue to a lethal temperature in a specific anatomic location, thereby reducing damage to surrounding tissue. RFA first became popular in treating hepatic tumors.[39] Typically, the procedure is performed by interventional radiologists or by thoracic surgeons in the CT scan suite, although in some instances these are performed in the OR. General anesthesia may or may not be used and is dependent on the operator. A target ablation size 1.0 cm greater than the maximum diameter of the tumor is used in essence creating a thermal margin. RFA utilizes an alternating current that passes from a generator to the patient and so electrosurgical grounding pads are required to be placed on the patient. As the alternating currents move from the electrode placed in the tumor, frictional heating of the tissue around the electrode in the tumor occurs. Once local temperature reaches over 60°C, there is instantaneous cell death. Most systems will achieve even higher temperatures than this level.

There are multiple systems currently available on the market and they function by a similar technique as described. Boston Scientific (Natick, Massachusetts), RITA (RITA Medical Systems, Fremont, California), and Valleylab (Boulder, Colorado) each make their own RF device. The Boston Scientific and RITA probes consist of single needle with an expandable tip that expands within the targeted tumor. The Valleylab probe consists of a single needle or three parallel needles that are placed into the target tumor. The Valleylab probes are internally cooled, which helps to prevent tissue charring around the probe, allowing more effective heating and larger area of tissue destruction. A

pilot study showed that having an expandable probe provides a larger overall treated volume with more spherical ablated area.[40]

Generally RFA is a low-risk procedure, with the most common complication being pneumothorax. A multicenter study of 493 patients reported pneumothorax in 30% of patients and pleural effusion in 10% of patients.[41] It should be emphasized however that despite the incidence of pneumothorax, the risks of grade 3 or higher complications as categorized by the Common Terminology for Adverse Events is low, and in fact similar to that reported after SBRT. A multicenter prospective trial that involved 52 patients was recently reported.[4] Grade 3 to 5 adverse events occurred in 11.5% of patients. There were two grade 3 pneumothoraces, and the only grade 4 and 5 complications that occurred were felt to be related to the patients' co-morbid disease rather than attributable to the RFA procedure.

Generally, the literature involving RFA has not been as strong as that supporting SBRT. The studies have usually involved single centers, smaller cohorts of patients that include both lung cancer and patients with pulmonary metastases, and often shorter follow-up. Table 102.3 demonstrates results in patients with stage I NSCLC treated with RFA. A study by Simon et al.[38] involved 153 patients of whom 75 had stage I NSCLC that was treated with RFA. The median survival was 29 months with a 1-, 2-, 3-, 4-, and 5-year survival rates of 78%, 57%, 36%, 27%, and 27%, respectively. A key finding of their study was the difference in local control of tumors less than 3 cm in size. Patients with smaller tumors <3 cm treated with RFA had a 1-year survival rate of 83% and 5-year survival rate of 47%. In the RAPTURE (RFA of pulmonary tumors response evaluation trial) study, RFA was used for lung lesions <3.5 cm in diameter in 107 patients.[42] The 2-year survival was 48%, and median survival was 21 months in this trial. Investigators from the Massachusetts General Hospital also reported on 31 patients with NSCLC treated with RFA.[43] The median survival in this study was 30 months, and 2- and 4-year survivals were 78% and 47%, respectively. In the multicenter study of RFA discussed above, 2-year survival was 71.2 and was even higher in patients with tumors less than 2 cm at 84%.[4]

Other thermal methods of ablation are now being reported for peripheral lung cancers. These include microwave ablation (MWA) or cryoablation (CRYO). MWA systems operate at much higher frequencies compared to RFA. The frequency typically used of RFA is 470 kHz, in comparison to MWA medical systems that operate at either 945 MHz or 2.45 GHz. There are several theoretical advantages with the use of MWA; these include higher intratumoral temperatures, larger ablation volumes, reduced treatment times, and deeper penetration of the MWA field compared with RFA.[49] Our group previously reported an animal study using MWA.[50] MWA was effective in creating areas of 100% nonviability, which potentially could lead to better local control in clinical practice.

TABLE 102.3 Result of Radiofrequency Ablation Therapy for Stage 1 NSCLC

Author (yr)	Modality	Number Studied	Median Survival Time (yrs)	2-yr Survival %	3-yr Survival %	5-yr Survival %
Lanuti (2012)[44]	RF	45	3.8	n/a	67	31
Ambrogi (2011)[45]	RF	59	2.8	n/a	40	25
Lanuti (2009)[43]	RF	34	2.5	78	n/a	n/a
Hiraki (2007)[46]	RF	20	3.7	67–93	n/a	n/a
Simon (2007)[38]	RF	75	2.9	57	36	27
Pennathur (2007)[47]	RF	18	n/a	68	n/a	n/a
Fernando (2005)[48]	RF	9	n/a	88.9	n/a	n/a

TABLE 102.4 Result of Cryotherapy and Microwave Ablation for Stage 1 NSCLC

Author (yr)	Modality	Number Studied	Median Survival Time (yrs)	2-yr Survival %	3-yr Survival %	5-yr Survival %
Moore (2015)[51]	Cryo	45	n/a	n/a	78	67
Yang (2014)[52]	Micro	47	2.8	63	43	16
Yamauchi (2012)[53]	Cryo	22	5.6	88	88	n/a
Wolf (2008)[54]	Micro	50	1.9	55	45	n/a

Currently there are two commercially available CRYO systems in the United States. These are the Cryohit (Galil Medical, Yokneam, Israel) and Cryocare (Endocare, Irvine, CA, USA) systems. Both systems are argon gas–based systems. An advantage of cryotherapy is that an ice-ball will occur as the ablation is being delivered. The ice-ball development can be followed real-time with CT imaging, which is helpful in monitoring the progress of a treatment. A disadvantage with the CRYO and some of the MWA systems is that multiple applicators are required for successful ablation of tumors. It can be challenging to place multiple probes simultaneously into pulmonary tumors in an appropriate orientation because of displacement by the ribs around the tumor.

Currently the literature supporting the use of MWA and CRYO for NSCLC is even more limited than that for RFA. Table 102.4 demonstrates results in patients with stage I NSCLC treated with either CRYO or MWA. Although encouraging groundwork exists, prospective studies with comparison to either RFA/SBRT are needed to better establish the role of these alternative ablation modalities.

BRONCHOSCOPIC ABLATION

Over the last decade, electromagnetic navigation bronchoscopy (ENB) has been introduced into clinical practice.[55] ENB allows a surgeon to pass a bronchoscope or catheter into the periphery of the lung using the guidance of virtual bronchoscopy created by these systems. Primarily this technology is used to obtain a tissue diagnosis, place fiducials to guide SBRT, or to inject dye into small peripheral lesions to guide VATS resections.[55] It may soon be possible to combine bronchoscopic navigation with placement of a flexible ablation probe directly into a tumor. Potentially this could allow diagnosis and treatment in the same setting.

This approach was reported in a study from Japan.[56] In this study ten patients had ablation immediately prior to planned resection. Three probe sizes (5 mm, 8 mm, and 10 mm active tip) were used. The larger probe sizes were also water cooled. They demonstrated that the technique could be performed safely and that larger volumes of ablation were achieved with increasing probe size. The same group subsequently reported on two patients who received bronchoscopic ablation as their only form of therapy for NSCLC.[57] The patients were free of recurrence for 4 and 3.5 years. Although very preliminary, these reports may represent the next evolution in minimally invasive therapy for lung cancer.

CONCLUSIONS

Patients with early stage lung cancer, who have marginal physiologic function, should not be denied therapy. A number of therapeutic options now exist, and careful evaluation in a multidisciplinary setting that includes an experienced thoracic surgeon in this process is vital. For the high-risk but operable patient sublobar resection should still be considered the standard of care. For the medically inoperable patient

SBRT or ablation can be offered; however, the relative advantages and disadvantages of these therapies still need to be determined.

REFERENCES

1. Cancer Facts and Figures; American Cancer Society 2014;15.
2. DeRose JJ, Jr., Argenziano M, El-Amir N, et al. Lung reduction operation and resection of pulmonary nodules in patients with severe emphysema. *Ann Thorac Surg* 1998;65:314–318.
3. Colice GL, Shafazand S, Griffin JP, et al.; American College of Chest Physicians. Physiologic evaluation of the patient with lung cancer being considered for resectional surgery: ACCP evidenced-based clinical practice guidelines (2nd edition). *Chest* 2007;132:161S–177S.
4. Crabtree T, Puri V, Timmerman R, et al. Treatment of stage I lung cancer in high-risk and inoperable patients: Comparison of prospective clinical trials using stereotactic body radiotherapy (RTOG 0236), sublobar resection (ACOSOG Z4032), and radiofrequency ablation (ACOSOG Z4033). *J Thorac Cardiovasc Surg* 2013;145:692–699.
5. Ginsberg RJ, Rubinstein LV. Randomized trial of lobectomy versus limited resection for T1 N0 non-small cell lung cancer. Lung Cancer Study Group. *Ann Thorac Surg* 1995; 60:615–622; discussion 622–623.
6. Landreneau RJ, Sugarbaker DJ, Mack MJ, et al. Wedge resection versus lobectomy for stage I (T1 N0 M0) non-small-cell lung cancer. *J Thorac Cardiovasc Surg* 1997;113: 691–698; discussion 698–700.
7. Deng B, Cassivi SD, de Andrade M, et al. Clinical outcomes and changes in lung function after segmentectomy versus lobectomy for lung cancer cases. *J Thorac Cardiovasc Surg* 2014;148:1186–1192, e1183.
8. Crabtree TD, Puri V, Robinson C, et al. Analysis of first recurrence and survival in patients with stage I non-small cell lung cancer treated with surgical resection or stereotactic radiation therapy. *J Thorac Cardiovasc Surg* 2014;147:1183–1191; discussion 1191–1182.
9. Altorki NK, Yip R, Hanaoka T, et al. Sublobar resection is equivalent to lobectomy for clinical stage 1A lung cancer in solid nodules. *J Thorac Cardiovasc Surg* 2014;147: 754–762; discussion 762–764.
10. Park BJ, Melfi F, Mussi A, et al. Robotic lobectomy for non-small cell lung cancer (NSCLC): Long-term oncologic results. *J Thorac Cardiovasc Surg* 2012;143:383–389.
11. Keenan RJ, Landreneau RJ, Maley RH, Jr., et al. Segmental resection spares pulmonary function in patients with stage I lung cancer. *Ann Thorac Surg* 2004;78:228–233; discussion 228–233.
12. Koike T, Yamato Y, Yoshiya K, et al. Intentional limited pulmonary resection for peripheral T1 N0 M0 small-sized lung cancer. *J Thorac Cardiovasc Surg* 2003;125: 924–928.
13. Read RC, Yoder G, Schaeffer RC. Survival after conservative resection for T1 N0 M0 non-small cell lung cancer. *Ann Thorac Surg* 1990;49:391–398; discussion 399–400.
14. Harada H, Okada M, Sakamoto T, et al. Functional advantage after radical segmentectomy versus lobectomy for lung cancer. *Ann Thorac Surg* 2005;80:2041–2045.
15. Kent M, Landreneau R, Mandrekar S, et al. Segmentectomy versus wedge resection for non-small cell lung cancer in high-risk operable patients. *Ann Thorac Surg* 2013;96: 1747–1754; discussion 1754–1755.
16. El-Sherif A, Fernando HC, Santos R, et al. Margin and local recurrence after sublobar resection of non-small cell lung cancer. *Ann Surg Oncol* 2007;14:2400–2405.
17. Sawabata N, Matsumura A, Ohota M, et al.; Thoracic Surgery Study Group of Osaka University. Cytologically malignant margins of wedge resected stage I non-small cell lung cancer. *Ann Thorac Surg* 2002;74:1953–1957.
18. Shennib H, Bogart J, Herndon JE, et al.; Cancer, Leukemia Group B, Eastern Cooperative Oncology Group. Video-assisted wedge resection and local radiotherapy for peripheral lung cancer in high-risk patients: The Cancer and Leukemia Group B (CALGB) 9335, a phase II, multi-institutional cooperative group study. *J Thorac Cardiovasc Surg* 2005;129:813–818.
19. d'Amato TA, Galloway M, Szydlowski G, et al. Intraoperative brachytherapy following thoracoscopic wedge resection of stage I lung cancer. *Chest* 1998;114:1112–1115.
20. Smith RP, Schuchert M, Komanduri K, et al. Dosimetric evaluation of radiation exposure during I-125 vicryl mesh implants: Implications for ACOSOG z4032. *Ann Surg Oncol* 2007;14:3610–3613.
21. Fernando HC, Landreneau RJ, Mandrekar SJ, et al. The impact of adjuvant brachytherapy with sublobar resection on pulmonary function and dyspnea in high-risk patients with operable disease: Preliminary results from the American College of Surgeons Oncology Group Z4032 trial. *J Thorac Cardiovasc Surg* 2011;142:554–562.
22. Santos R, Colonias A, Parda D, et al. Comparison between sublobar resection and 125Iodine brachytherapy after sublobar resection in high-risk patients with Stage I non-small-cell lung cancer. *Surgery* 2003;134:691–697; discussion 697.

23. Fernando HC, Santos RS, Benfield JR, et al. Lobar and sublobar resection with and without brachytherapy for small stage IA non-small cell lung cancer. *J Thorac Cardiovasc Surg* 2005;129:261–267.

24. Birdas TJ, Koehler RP, Colonias A, et al. Sublobar resection with brachytherapy versus lobectomy for stage Ib nonsmall cell lung cancer. *Ann Thorac Surg* 2006;81: 434–438; discussion 438–439.

25. Fernando HC, Landreneau RJ, Mandrekar SJ, et al. Impact of brachytherapy on local recurrence rates after sublobar resection: Results from ACOSOG Z4032 (Alliance), a phase III randomized trial for high-risk operable non-small-cell lung cancer. *J Clin Oncol* 2014;32:2456–2462.

26. Wisnivesky JP, Bonomi M, Henschke C, et al. Radiation therapy for the treatment of unresected stage I-II non-small cell lung cancer. *Chest* 2005;128:1461–1467.

27. Liu HH, Balter P, Tutt T, et al. Assessing respiration-induced tumor motion and internal target volume using four-dimensional computed tomography for radiotherapy of lung cancer. *Int J Radiat Oncol Biol Phys* 2007;68:531–540.

28. Kreuter M, Vansteenkiste J, Griesinger F, et al. Trial on refinement of early stage non-small cell lung cancer. Adjuvant chemotherapy with pemetrexed and cisplatin versus vinorelbine and cisplatin: the TREAT protocol. *BMC Cancer* 2007;7:77.

29. Onishi H, Araki T, Shirato H, et al. Stereotactic hypofractionated high-dose irradiation for stage I nonsmall cell lung carcinoma: Clinical outcomes in 245 subjects in a Japanese multiinstitutional study. *Cancer* 2004;101:1623–1631.

30. Pennathur A, Luketich JD, Heron DE, et al. Stereotactic radiosurgery for the treatment of lung neoplasm: Experience in 100 consecutive patients. *Ann Thorac Surg* 2009;88:1594–1600; discussion 1600.

31. Davis JN, Medbery C 3rd, Sharma S, et al. Stereotactic body radiotherapy for early-stage non-small cell lung cancer: clinical outcomes from a National Patient Registry. *J Radiat Oncol* 2015;4:55–63.

32. Shibamoto Y, Hashizume C, Baba F, et al. Stereotactic body radiotherapy using a radiobiology-based regimen for stage I nonsmall cell lung cancer: A multicenter study. *Cancer* 2012;118:2078–2084.

33. Timmerman R, Paulus R, Galvin J, et al. Stereotactic body radiation therapy for inoperable early stage lung cancer. *JAMA* 2010;303:1070–1076.

34. Stephans KL, Djemil T, Reddy CA, et al. A comparison of two stereotactic body radiation fractionation schedules for medically inoperable stage I non-small cell lung cancer: the Cleveland Clinic experience. *J Thorac Oncol* 2009;4:976–982.

35. Timmerman R, McGarry R, Yiannoutsos C, et al. Excessive toxicity when treating central tumors in a phase II study of stereotactic body radiation therapy for medically inoperable early-stage lung cancer. *J Clin Oncol* 2006;24:4833–4839.

36. Louie AV, Senan S. Treatment for high-risk patients with early-stage non-small-cell lung cancer. *J Clin Oncol* 2015;33:377.

37. Fernando HC. Reply to A.V. Louie et al. *J Clin Oncol* 2015;33:378.

38. Simon CJ, Dupuy DE, DiPetrillo TA, et al. Mayo-Smith WW: Pulmonary radiofrequency ablation: Long-term safety and efficacy in 153 patients. *Radiology* 2007, 243:268–275.

39. Curley SA, Izzo F, Delrio P, et al. Radiofrequency ablation of unresectable primary and metastatic hepatic malignancies: Results in 123 patients. *Ann Surg* 1999;230: 1–8.

40. Denys AL, De Baere T, Kuoch V, et al. Radio-frequency tissue ablation of the liver: In vivo and ex vivo experiments with four different systems. *Eur Radiol* 2003;13:2346–2352.

41. Steinke K, Sewell PE, Dupuy D, et al. Pulmonary radiofrequency ablation—an international study survey. *Anticancer Res* 2004;24:339–343.

42. Lencioni R. Radiofrequency ablation of pulmonary tumors response evaluation (RAPTURE) trail. Proceedings of the Society of Interventional Radiology 2005.

43. Lanuti M, Sharma A, Digumarthy SR, et al. Radiofrequency ablation for treatment of medically inoperable stage I non-small cell lung cancer. *J Thorac Cardiovasc Surg* 2009;137:160–166.

44. Lanuti M, Sharma A, Willers H, et al. Radiofrequency ablation for stage I non-small cell lung cancer: management of locoregional recurrence. *Ann Thorac Surg* 2012;93: 921–927; discussion 927–988.

45. Ambrogi MC, Fanucchi O, Cioni R, et al. Long-term results of radiofrequency ablation treatment of stage I non-small cell lung cancer: a prospective intention-to-treat study. *J Thorac Oncol* 2011;6:2044–2051.

46. Hiraki T, Gobara H, Iishi T, et al. Percutaneous radiofrequency ablation for clinical stage I non-small cell lung cancer: Results in 20 nonsurgical candidates. *J Thorac Cardiovasc Surg* 2007;134:1306–1312.

47. Pennathur A, Luketich JD, Abbas G, et al. Radiofrequency ablation for the treatment of stage I non-small cell lung cancer in high-risk patients. *J Thorac Cardiovasc Surg* 2007;134:857–864.

48. Fernando HC, De Hoyos A, Landreneau RJ, et al. Radiofrequency ablation for the treatment of non-small cell lung cancer in marginal surgical candidates. *J Thorac Cardiovasc Surg* 2005;129:639–644.

49. Vogl TJ, Naguib NN, Lehnert T, et al. Radiofrequency, microwave and laser ablation of pulmonary neoplasms: Clinical studies and technical considerations—review article. *Eur J Radiol* 2011;77:346–357.

50. Santos RS, Gan J, Ohara CJ, et al. Microwave ablation of lung tissue: Impact of single-lung ventilation on ablation size. *Ann Thorac Surg* 2010;90:1116–1119.

51. Moore W, Talati R, Bhattacharji P, et al. Five-year survival after cryoablation of stage I non-small cell lung cancer in medically inoperable patients. *J Vasc Interv Radiol* 2015;26:312–319.

52. Yang X, Ye X, Zheng A, et al. Percutaneous microwave ablation of stage I medically inoperable non-small cell lung cancer: clinical evaluation of 47 cases. *J Surg Oncol* 2014;110:758–763.

53. Yamauchi Y, Izumi Y, Hashimoto K, et al. Percutaneous cryoablation for the treatment of medically inoperable stage I non-small cell lung cancer *PLOS One* 2012;7:e332223.

54. Wolf FJ, Grand DJ, Machan JT, et al. Microwave ablation of lung malignancies: Effectiveness, CT findings, and safety in 50 patients. *Radiology* 2008;247:871–879.

55. Eberhardt R, Anantham D, Herth F, et al. Electromagnetic navigation diagnostic bronchoscopy in peripheral lung lesions. *Chest* 2007;131:1800–1805.

56. Tanabe T, Koizumi T, Tsushima K, et al. Comparative study of three different catheters for CT imaging-bronchoscopy-guided radiofrequency ablation as a potential and novel interventional therapy for lung cancer. *Chest* 2010;137:890–897.

57. Koizumi T, Kobayashi T, Tanabe T, et al. Clinical experience of bronchoscopy-guided radiofrequency ablation for peripheral-type lung cancer. *Case Rep Oncol Med* 2013; 2013:515160.

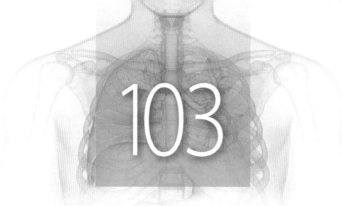

Small-Cell Lung Cancer

Liza Villaruz ▪ Brian J. Karlovits ▪ Timothy F. Burns ▪ Mark A. Socinski

INTRODUCTION

Lung cancer is the leading cause of cancer mortality in the United States and worldwide.[1] An estimated 224,210 new cases of lung cancer were diagnosed in 2014 in the United States alone, and 159,260 lung cancer deaths are estimated to occur.[1] Small-cell lung cancer (SCLC) represents approximately 15% of the cases of lung cancer.[2] The incidence of SCLC is decreasing within the United States, probably owing to a decrease in the prevalence of smoking.[2] Among women, the incidence of SCLC is increasing, which reflects an increase in the prevalence of smoking among women approximately a generation ago.[2] While tobacco use is the most common etiologic agent associated with SCLC, other such agents including exposure to asbestos, radon, uranium mining, and bis-chloromethyl ether have also been associated with SCLC.[3] Cases of SCLC in lifelong non-smokers have been reported, but the pathology should be carefully reviewed to confirm the diagnosis. SCLC is characterized by rapid growth, the high prevalence of early metastases to the mediastinal lymph nodes and distant sites, and high response rate (RR) to standard chemotherapy. Without treatment, the prognosis is very poor, and the median survival of patients who do not receive treatment is estimated to be 2 to 4 months.[4]

BIOLOGY AND GENETICS

Originally described in 1926 as "oat cell carcinoma" because of the histologic appearance of the cells under the microscope, the biology of SCLC is distinct from adenocarcinoma or squamous cell carcinoma of the lung in that its cell of origin has neuroendocrine features.[5-7] SCLC belongs to a larger group of neuroendocrine tumors of the lung, which range from low-grade typical carcinoids to intermediate-grade atypical carcinoids to high-grade neuroendocrine tumors, including large-cell neuroendocrine carcinoma and SCLC.[8,9] SCLC is associated with an extremely high mutation rate (an average of 7.4 mutations per mega base pair), largely owing to an association with smoking. Given the success in identifying and targeting oncogenic driver mutations in non-small cell lung cancer (NSCLC), there is a strong interest in identifying similar targetable drivers in SCLC. These efforts have been limited in part by the traditional difficulty in obtaining large biopsy samples, and therefore it has not been possible for the cancer genome atlas (TCGA) to undertake a sequencing effort in SCLC.[10] In stark contrast to NSCLC in which over a thousand tumors have undergone whole exome sequencing, whole exome sequencing data exists for less than a 100 SCLC tumors.[11,12] Despite these limitations, many of the major genomic changes in

SCLC have been defined. Mutations in the tumor suppressors, TP53 (70% to 90%) and RB1 (100%) are present in almost all SCLC cases. Recurrent mutations have also been identified in CREBBP, EP300, and MLL genes that encode histone modifiers.[12] In addition, recent studies have identified MYC family member alterations in almost 20% of SCLC, amplification of the stem cell transcription factor SOX2 in almost 27% of SCLC, and amplification of FGFR1 in 6% of SCLC.[11,12]

STAGING

The proper staging of patients with SCLC determines the prognosis and treatment paradigm to be used. The most commonly used staging system is the two-stage system developed in the 1950s by Veterans Administration Lung Study Group (VALSG) for patients with inoperable lung cancer.[13] Limited-stage (LS) disease is defined as disease confined to one hemithorax, including tumors with local extension and ipsilateral supraclavicular nodes, if they are able to be encompassed in the same radiation portal as the primary tumor. All other disease, including malignant pleural or pericardial effusions, the presence of contralateral hilar or supraclavicular lymph nodes, or extrathoracic disease is classified as extensive-stage (ES) disease. Despite the simplicity of this staging system, areas of controversy and ambiguity exist.[14] In 1989, the International Association for the Study of Lung Cancer (IASLC) issued a consensus report that expanded the definition of LS disease to include contralateral mediastinal and supraclavicular nodes and ipsilateral pleural effusion, regardless of whether cytology is positive or negative. In clinical practice, most physicians blend the VALSG and IASLC criteria by considering contralateral mediastinal and ipsilateral supraclavicular lymph node involvement as LS disease on a patient to patient basis, based on the ability to include these regions in a safe radiation port.

The Radiation Therapy Oncology Group (RTOG) and the Eastern Cooperative Oncology Group (ECOG) have defined LS disease as disease confined to one hemithorax and exclude patients with malignant effusion or contralateral hilar or supraclavicular lymphadenopathy.[15] The National Comprehensive Cancer Network (NCCN) defines LS as disease confined to the ipsilateral hemithorax that can be safely treated with definitive radiation doses and excludes T3–4 tumors due to multiple lung nodules that are too extensive or have tumor or nodal volume that is too large to be encompassed within a tolerable radiation field.[16] The European Organization for Research and Treatment of Cancer (EORTC) defines LS disease as disease that involves <50% of the maximum transverse diameter of the thorax on a chest x-ray before starting chemotherapy.[17]

TABLE 103.1 Standard Staging Test

1. CT of the chest, abdomen, and pelvis or CT of the chest through the liver and adrenal glands
2. Bone scan
3. MRI or CT scan with contrast of the brain
4. If pleural effusions are present, thoracentesis should be performed with cytologic evaluation
5. Bone marrow biopsy in patients with nucleated RBCs on peripheral smear or unexplained thrombocytopenia or neutropenia

CT, computed tomography; RBC, red blood cell; MRI, magnetic resonance imaging.

Recently, it was been suggested that the newly revised TNM staging classification for lung cancer according to the American Joint Committee on Cancer (AJCC) 7th edition replace the VALSG staging system.[18] This recommendation is based on a prognostic analysis of 8,088 SCLC patients in the IASLC database, in whom the overall clinical stages I to IV according to the AJCC 7th edition groupings were predictive of overall survival (OS).[19] In this staging system, patients with pleural effusions are considered to have stage IV M1a disease. Interestingly, patients with ES disease exclusively on the basis of a pleural effusion had an intermediate survival between patients with LS disease and patients with ES disease with other metastatic sites, regardless of the pleural fluid cytology.[19]

The most frequent staging procedures are listed in Table 103.1. There can be significant variability on the staging procedures performed, because once a patient is determined to have ES disease, the utility of detecting additional sites of metastases may be limited and may not change the treatment paradigm. However, if the patient potentially has LS disease, a meticulous workup for distant metastases should be performed. This includes a bone scan to evaluate for osseous metastases, computed tomography (CT) of the abdomen to evaluate for liver and/or adrenal metastases, and a magnetic resonance imaging (MRI) or CT scan with contrast of the brain to detect brain metastases. If a patient potentially has LS disease and a pleural effusion, he or she should undergo a thoracentesis with cytologic evaluation to determine whether there is a malignant pleural effusion. While most pleural effusions in patients with SCLC are due to tumor, patients in whom multiple cytologic evaluations are negative for tumor, in whom the pleural fluid is nonbloody and transudative, the effusion should be excluded as a staging element.[16] Previously, bone marrow biopsy has been included as part of the staging workup; however, that is no longer routinely required. Bone marrow biopsy should be reserved for patients who have LS disease and have a hematologic abnormality that is suspicious for bone marrow involvement or an unexplained neutropenia or thrombocytopenia.[16] An elevated lactate dehydrogenase (LDH) has prognostic value, but it is not routinely included in the staging workup.[20]

Positron emission tomography (PET) scans with 18-fluoro-2-deoxy-D-glucose (FDG) have revealed superior sensitivity for detecting distant metastases in patients with NSCLC, and greater specificity for adrenal and bone lesions.[21-23] A number of trials have investigated PET-scan staging in SCLC, but most of these trials have been performed at a single institution with a limited number of patients (≤120).[24-31] Based on the preliminary evidence from these trials, PET-scan staging has been found to have greater sensitivity in the detection of intra- and extrathoracic nodal involvement and distant metastases. A number of patients on these trials had their treatment plans changed owing to the detection of occult distant metastatic disease or changes in the radiation field to include intrathoracic lymph nodes with suspected malignant involvement. In two prospective trials from the Netherlands the utility of staging imaging and the implications on radiation treatment planning were evaluated.[32,33] In the first, the radiation field definition was based on CT alone; excluding elective nodal coverage led to an unacceptably high rate of isolated nodal failure (11%).[32] Conversely, integrating PET staging to guide radiation field design to the involved disease alone was associated with isolated nodal failure of 3%, illustrating the value of PET in limiting radiation fields to involved disease alone and reducing potential lung toxicity.[33] The current evidence-based medicine guidelines from the American College of Chest Physicians (ACCP) and NCCN recommend the use of PET scanning in patients with clinical suspicion for LS-SCLC.[4]

SURGICAL TREATMENT

The current standard treatment for LS-SCLC is the combination of chemotherapy and radiation therapy. However, specific subsets of patients with LS-SCLC may benefit from surgical resection. In addition to these subsets, the SCLC histology can be an incidental finding at the time of surgery. An assessment of the role of surgical resection is complicated by the fact surgery is performed in only a small minority of patients, and these patients frequently receive additional chemo- and/or radiotherapy. There is also concern that the patients who are considered surgical candidates may have a biologically more indolent disease or would be considered good prognosis candidates for chemoradiotherapy. Many of the case series or retrospective reviews of surgical therapy have included heterogeneous patient populations and were also performed before currently available staging procedures. Thus, a significant percentage of the patients who underwent surgery would have had metastatic disease detected with the current staging tests. Most of the interest in surgical resection in SCLC involves a subset of patients with LS-SCLC who present without evidence of mediastinal nodal involvement (stages I and II) or who are suspected of having a mixed histology of SCLC and NSCLC and have residual disease after chemoradiotherapy.

Several retrospective reviews have demonstrated long-term survival of patients with SCLC treated with surgery alone (Table 103.2).[34-37] A randomized trial performed by the British Medical Research Council randomized operable patients (n = 144) to radiotherapy or surgical resection.[38] The median survival was significantly longer on the radiotherapy arm in comparison to the surgical arm, 10 months versus 7 months, respectively (P = 0.04). This trial required bronchoscopic biopsy to confirm the diagnosis. Therefore, there was a high prevalence of centrally located tumors and, given the staging methods available at the time, undoubtedly many patients had distant disease at the time of surgical resection. On the surgical arm, only 48% of patients underwent surgical resection, raising doubts about the feasibility of surgical resection in LS-SCLC. The results of this trial discouraged surgical resection as the primary therapy for LS-SCLC.

The high prevalence of occult micrometastatic disease even in patients with early-stage disease and the high rate of distant failure led to interest in combining surgical resection and chemotherapy. Several retrospective reviews have investigated the survival of patients after a combination of surgical resection and chemotherapy and/or radiotherapy (Table 103.2).[39-43] A retrospective review of patients who were treated with chemotherapy before and after surgical resection at the University of Toronto (n = 119) revealed a median survival of 111 weeks and a 5-year OS rate of 39%.[44] The 5-year OS rates for patients with pathologic stage I (n = 35), stage II (n = 36), and stage III (n = 48) disease were 51%, 28%, and 19%, respectively. A separate retrospective analysis investigating the long-term survival (defined as ≥3 years) of 37 patients who underwent resection in comparison with 127 who did not undergo surgical resection revealed a

TABLE 103.2 Role of Surgery in Limited Stage Small-Cell Lung Cancer

First Author	No. of Patients	Treatment	Median Survival Time (mo)	5-Year Survival Rate (%)
Davis[34]	118	Surgery	18	20
Sorensen[37]	71	Surgery		12
Shore[36]	40	Surgery		27
Shah[35]	28	Surgery	34	43
Shields[43]	132	S→Chemo/RT	11	23
Karrer[39]	112	S→Chemo/PCI	37	p 51[a]
Lucchi[40]	92	S→Chemo	24	32
Shepherd[42]	63	S→Chemo/RT	19	31
Osterlind[41]	52	S→Chemo		p 25[b]
Lad[48]	70	Chemo→S/RT/PCI	15	10
Shepherd[49]	38	Chemo→S/RT/PCI	21	36
Eberhardt[46]	32	Chemo→RT→S	36	46
Holoye[47]	22	Chemo→S	25	33
Williams[50]	21	Chemo→S/PCI		
Shepherd[54]	28	Salvage[c]	24	28

[a]Reported as 3-year survival.
[b]Reported as 3.5-year survival.
[c]Salvage therapy consisted of surgical resection for patients with persisted or locally recurrent disease after chemo ± RT.
S, surgery; RT, radiation therapy; PCI, prophylactic cranial irradiation.

long-term survival rate of 35% in patients who underwent resection and 6% in those who did not.[45] All but one of the resected patients received chemotherapy, and all patients who did not undergo resection received chemoradiotherapy. The 5-year OS rate of patients with stage I disease (n = 13) was 64.2% and for stage II (n = 10), 42.5%. This survival data in patients with stage I and II disease have raised the possibility that surgery may have a role in the treatment of early-stage patients with SCLC.

Several other studies have investigated the role of preoperative or neoadjuvant chemotherapy.[46–50] The use of preoperative chemotherapy may result in earlier treatment of distant micrometastatic disease and facilitate surgical resection by shrinking intrathoracic disease. A phase II trial at the University of Toronto (n = 72) prospectively evaluated the role of preoperative chemotherapy in patients with LS-SCLC.[49] The overall RR was 80%, and 57 patients (79%) were candidates for surgical resection, but only 38 patients underwent surgical resection. The median survival time for surgically resected patients was 91 weeks, and the projected 5-year survival rate was 36%. Patients with pathologic stage I had a significantly longer survival time than patients with stage II or III disease. A second phase II trial (n = 40), which investigated preoperative chemotherapy, revealed an overall RR of 87%, and 11 patients underwent thoracotomy and 8 underwent resection.[51] Additional trials revealed a benefit to the combination of surgical resection after induction chemotherapy.[49,52–54]

In order to investigate the benefit of surgical resection after induction chemotherapy, the Lung Cancer Study Group (LCSG) performed a prospective randomized trial in which patients receiving five cycles of chemotherapy were randomized to radiotherapy to the chest and brain or surgical resection.[48] Patients were required to have at least a partial response, have pure small-cell histologic features, and be appropriate candidates for surgical resection. Of the 328 patients enrolled, 217 patients achieved a response (66%) and 146 patients were randomized (44% of all patients). Of the patients randomized to surgical resection, 83% (n = 58) underwent surgical resection

and 77% underwent complete resection (n = 54). The nodal status did not influence unresectability rates but the pretreatment T status influenced the unresectability rates. The unresectability rates for pretreatment T3, T2, and T1 were 40%, 16%, and 6%, respectively. There was no difference in survival between the treatment arms (P = 0.78) with a median survival for all patients of 12 months and 16 months for patients who were randomized. The results of this trial do not support the use of surgical resection after induction chemotherapy.

More recently, the role of surgery has been analyzed in several population-based studies. In 14,179 patients with LS-SCLC identified in the US Surveillance, Epidemiology, and End Results (SEER) registry between 1998 and 2002, 863 patients underwent surgery, in whom median survival was 28 months and 5-year OS rate 34.6% compared with a median survival of 13 months and a 5-year OS rate 9.9% in patients who did not undergo surgery (P < 0.001).[55] Patients undergoing surgery more commonly had T1 or T2 disease (P < 0.001). The median survival for patients with localized disease was 42 months versus 15 months in favor of surgery with a 5-year OS rate of 44.8% versus 13.7% (P < 0.001). For patients with regional disease, the median survival was 22 months versus 12 months in favor of surgery with a 5-year OS rate of 26.3% versus 9.3% (P < 0.001). Patients with N2 disease had a statistically significant survival benefit from the addition of post-op radiotherapy (PORT). Survival was 16 months for surgery alone versus 22 months with PORT. In a separate analysis of 1,560 patients with stage I SCLC in the SEER database treated from 1988 to 2004, 247 patients underwent lobectomy, 121 had local tumor excision/ablation, 10 had a pneumonectomy, and surgery was unknown in 21. In patients undergoing lobectomy without radiation therapy, the 3- and 5-year OS was 58.1% and 50.3%, respectively. In patients undergoing lobectomy with radiation therapy, 3- and 5-year OS was 64.9% and 57.1%, respectively.[56] Most recently, survival was estimated in 28,621 cases of potentially resectable SCLC in the National Cancer Data Base (NCDB), of whom 2,476 patients (9%) underwent surgery of the primary site with curative intent.[29] The 5-year OS was 51%, 25%, and 18% for clinical stages I, II, and IIIA, respectively. The addition of surgery to chemotherapy was associated with decreased likelihood of death (hazard ratio: 0.57, 95% confidence interval [CI]: 0.47–0.68), indicating a potential role for surgical resection as part of initial treatment with chemotherapy in selected patients with LS-SCLC.

While these large population-based studies support the role of surgery in select patients with stage I SCLC after diligent systemic and mediastinal staging, it is important to note the retrospective design of these studies and the inability to account for possible confounding by selection of patients with inherently better prognosis. The ACCP guidelines state that in patients with clinical stage I SCLC, who are being considered for curative intent surgical resection, invasive mediastinal staging, and extrathoracic imaging (head CT/MRI and PET or CT with bone scan) should be performed. SCLC has a greater propensity for mediastinal nodal metastases, and it is notable that the false-negative rate of mediastinoscopy in SCLC has been reported to be as high as 16%.[57] In patients who have stage I SCLC after thorough staging, surgical resection is suggested over nonsurgical management (Grade 2C) and in patients who have undergone curative intent surgery, adjuvant platinum-based chemotherapy should be given.[18] Patients who undergo surgical resection and receive systemic chemotherapy should then be considered for thoracic radiation therapy (TRT) to reduce the rate of local relapse and consideration of prophylactic cranial irradiation (PCI).[15] The other clinical scenario, when surgical resection is considered, is when a patient has a mixed histology with SCLC and NSCLC and achieves a significant response but has residual disease. The purpose of the surgical resection is to treat the residual NSCLC optimally.

The NCCN guidelines state that patients with T1 or T2 tumors should undergo mediastinoscopy or endoscopic evaluation of the mediastinum and, if negative, should undergo surgical resection, preferably a lobectomy with mediastinal nodal dissection or sampling.[16] Postoperatively, all patients should receive chemotherapy, and patients with involvement of the mediastinum should receive concurrent chemotherapy and mediastinal radiation therapy.[16]

Limited-Stage SCLC

A recent analysis revealed that the percentage of patients who were classified as having LS disease is approximately 40%.[2] The vast majority of patients with LS disease will be treated with a combination of chemotherapy and radiation.[58] The 5-year survival rate from the United States NCDB from 1985 to 2000 with this treatment approach is approximately 15%.[59] In 2000, some 50% of the cases of LS-SCLC were in women, and 45% were in patients aged ≥70 years.[59]

The treatment paradigm of chemotherapy and radiation has been developed through multiple clinical trials over the last several decades. Treatment of LS-SCLC with chemotherapy alone results in poor local control rates, with intrathoracic failure occurring in 75% to 90% of patients.[60] The addition of TRT significantly reduced the rate of intrathoracic failures to 30% to 60% but did not consistently result in an improvement in OS in individual clinical trials.[60] In 1992, two separate meta-analyses were published establishing the role of TRT in the treatment of LS-SCLC.[61,62] Pignon et al.[61] evaluated 13 randomized trials of LS-SCLC, which included 2,410 patients, and the relative risk (RR) of death in the chemoradiotherapy group compared with the chemotherapy-alone group was 0.86 (95% CI, 0.78–0.94; $P = 0.001$). This corresponded to a 14% reduction in mortality and an absolute improvement in OS at 3 years of 5.4% ± 1.4%. No clear benefit was noted in the indirect comparison of early versus late TRT or sequential versus nonsequential strategies. Warde and

Payne[62] evaluated 11 randomized trials, and their analysis revealed an OS benefit for the addition of TRT to chemotherapy (odds ratio [OR] for 2-year survival = 1.53; 95% CI 1.30–1.76; $P < 0.001$); the absolute difference in the 2-year survival rate was 5.4%. Data related to intrathoracic tumor control was available in 9 of the 11 trials, and when the addition of TRT was analyzed, it was found to have improved intrathoracic tumor control by 25.3% (OR for treatment effect on local control = 3.02; 95% CI 2.80–3.24; $P < 0.0001$). The risk for treatment-related deaths was 1.2% (95% CI, 0.6%–3.0%). The consistent findings of these two meta-analyses established the role of TRT in the treatment of LS-SCLC and demonstrated that improvements in local control could result in improvements in OS. Cisplatin and etoposide (EP) and cyclophosphamide, doxorubicin, and vincristine (CAV) have demonstrated equal efficacy in ES disease. However, cisplatin and etoposide can be administrated concurrently with TRT, which has made it the preferred treatment paradigm in LS-SCLC.

Once the therapeutic benefit of TRT had been established, investigations into dose, fractionation schedule, and the timing of TRT were initiated. Because SCLC is a radiosensitive tumor, historically, relatively modest doses of TRT have been employed (45 to 50 Gy) in daily 1.8- to 2-Gy fractions. However, despite the high RR, the durability of the responses was poor. Intensifying the radiotherapy dose by accelerating the delivery of TRT was one of the initial treatment strategies investigated (Table 103.3). Turrisi et al.[63] investigated treatment with 45 Gy in 5 weeks (1.8 Gy for 25 fractions) versus 45 Gy in 3 weeks (1.5 Gy twice daily for 30 fractions) beginning with the first of four cycles of EP. The 5-year survival rate was 26% with the accelerated schedule versus 16% with the conventional one ($P = 0.04$). The major toxicity observed with accelerated in comparison to conventional TRT was an increased rate of grade 3/4 esophagitis, 32% and 16%, respectively. There was a significant improvement in overall local tumor control, defined as local, as well as, local plus distant recurrence, in the accelerated treatment arm. Despite the superior survival observed on the twice-daily treatment arm, this treatment has not been widely adopted. A review of practice patterns by Movsas et al. revealed that 10% of patients with LS-SCLC received twice-daily therapy and 80% of patients received once-daily TRT.[64] The higher rate of severe esophagitis and the inconvenience of twice-daily TRT may deter the widespread implementation of this treatment. In a pooled analysis of patients assigned to receive daily radiotherapy to 70 Gy on three consecutive CALGB LS-SCLC trials (39808, 30002, and 30206), the rate of grade 3 or greater esophagitis was 23%. The median OS for the pooled population was 19.9 months, and 5-year OS rate was 20%, indicative of similar survival between 70 Gy (2 Gy daily) compared with 45 Gy (1.5 Gy twice daily[65]). CALGB 30610 is a randomized phase III clinical trial that is currently investigating optimal radiotherapy dose and schedule in LS-SCLC. The study was originally designed as a 3-arm trial comparing chemotherapy given concurrently with 45 Gy/1.5 Gy twice daily versus 70 Gy/2 Gy daily versus 61.2 Gy/1.8 Gy daily. In a prespecified interim analysis, the 70 Gy arm was selected over the 61.2 Gy arm based upon a comparison of treatment-related toxicity. Hence, the ongoing trial is comparing concurrent chemotherapy with either the 45 Gy twice-daily or 70 Gy once-daily radiation doses and schedule.

In a North Central Cancer Treatment Group (NCCTG) trial, TRT was delayed until the fourth cycle and was delivered as 48 Gy in 32 fractions with a 2.5-week treatment break after the initial 24 Gy (vs. 50.4 Gy in 28 fractions on the control arm). This study did not demonstrate an advantage of split-course twice-daily radiotherapy (Table 103.3).[66] The total time to complete TRT was similar between the two arms, but the treatment break may have affected the efficacy of the accelerated treatment arm by allowing for repopulation. A

TABLE 103.3 Select Phase III Trials of Once-Daily Versus Twice-Daily Radiotherapy

First Author	No.	TRT Dose	Chemotherapy	Local Failure (%)	Median Survival Time (mo)	5-Year Overall Survival Rate (%)
Turrisi[63]						
Once daily	206	45 Gy[a]	Cisplatin/etoposide × 4	52	19	16
Twice daily	211	45 Gy[a]	Cisplatin/etoposide × 4	36	23	26
Schild[66]						
Once daily	131	50.4 Gy[b]	Cisplatin/etoposide × 6	40	20.6[c]	21
Twice daily	130	24 Gy in 16 fractions		36	20.6	22
		2.5-wk break				
		24 Gy in 16 fractions				
		Total dose = 48 Gy				
Schild[68]	76	30 Gy in 20 fractions[d]	Cisplatin/etoposide × 6	34	20	24
		2-wk break				
		30 Gy in 20 fractions				
		Total dose 60 Gy				

[a]Chemotherapy and thoracic radiation therapy (TRT) started on cycle 1.
[b]Patients received three cycles of cisplatin/etoposide and were then randomized to once-daily versus twice-daily TRT. Patients received TRT concurrent with cycles 4 and 5.
[c]Median survival time from time of randomization. Overall survival time for all patients (N = 311) 20.9 months.
[d]TRT was given with cycles 4 and 5 of chemotherapy.

retrospective review by Canadian investigators corroborated this by showing that significant treatment breaks may counteract the potential benefit of more intensified TRT.[67] Another consideration was that the TRT was initiated on cycle 1 in the trial by Turrisi et al. and cycle 4 (week 12) in this NCCTG trial. A more recent NCCTG single arm phase II clinical trial investigated TRT given concurrently with cycles 4 and 5 of chemotherapy as 30 Gy/1.5 Gy twice daily, followed by a 2-week break, followed by completion of 30 Gy/1.5 Gy twice daily.[68] This TRT regimen was associated with a reasonable 5-year survival rate of 24% with a 5-year cumulative incidence of in-field treatment failure of 34% (Table 103.3).

Debate persists about the optimal timing of TRT, and at least five meta-analyses have been published related to this subject.[69–73] The meta-analysis by Fried et al.[70] revealed a survival advantage for early (defined as within 9 weeks of starting chemotherapy) versus late TRT, and this advantage was more pronounced when cisplatin-based therapy and more intensified TRT were used. A separate systemic review by Pijls-Johannesma et al.[72] defined TRT as starting within 30 days after the start of chemotherapy and did not find a significant difference in OS at 2 or 5 years between early and late radiotherapy. However, when trials that used platinum-based chemotherapy were analyzed, significantly higher 2- and 5-year survival rates were observed with early TRT. A separate analysis by Spiro et al.[73] suggested that the benefit of TRT was present only if the delivery of concurrent chemotherapy was not compromised. A separate and interesting analysis investigated the impact of time from start to completion of TRT on OS.[74] This analysis revealed that completing therapy in <30 days was associated with an improved 5-year survival rate (RR = 0.62; 95% CI 0.49–0.80; P = 0.0003).[74] The collective data from these meta-analyses favors the initiation of early TRT, often defined as TRT delivered within the first three cycles of chemotherapy, and support the use of platinum-based therapy. It also appears important that treatment breaks for TRT be kept to a minimum and that the delivery of chemotherapy should not be compromised.

Just as there have been significant investigations into modifying the TRT in LS disease, there has been investigation into integrating

novel therapeutic agents into the treatment of LS-SCLC (Table 103.4). In general, these trials have involved the addition or substitution of a newer agent into the standard EP treatment platform. The most commonly investigated agents have been paclitaxel, irinotecan, topotecan, and ifosfamide, and the TRT doses have ranged from 42 to 63 Gy delivered in once- or twice-daily fractions in phase II trials.[64,72,74–82] With the exception of the integration of irinotecan into LS-SCLC by Japanese investigators, none of these phase II trials, unfortunately, have revealed promising enough survival data to warrant further exploration in a phase III trial.[64,77] The Japanese Clinical Oncology Group Trial 0202 compared three cycles of EP with three cycles of irinotecan/cisplatin (IP) after an initial cycle of EP with 45 Gy of twice-daily TRT and demonstrated similar OS between the two groups. Toxicities were as expected with more grade 3 or 4 diarrhea occurring in the cisplatin/irinotecan group.[83]

In addition to these trials, there have been several trials that have investigated the integration of "targeted" agents into the treatment of LS-SCLC. In SCLC, the expression of matrix metalloproteinases has been associated with poor survival,[79] and thus SCLC was a logical disease to investigate the role of matrix metalloproteinase inhibitors (MMPIs) such as marimastat and BAY12-9566. A phase III trial evaluating 532 patients with SCLC, of whom 279 had LS-SCLC, compared maintenance marimastat to placebo.[82] Patients who demonstrated a response to chemotherapy were randomized to marimastat or placebo for 2 years. The progression-free survival (PFS) and OS times were similar between the two treatment arms. An interim analysis of treatment with BAY12-9566 in SCLC (n = 327) revealed a significantly shorter time to disease progression in the BAY12-9566 treatment arm compared with placebo.[81] These trials indicate that MMPIs are unlikely to have a significant role of the treatment of SCLC. A phase II study of tirapazamine, which has selective cytotoxicity for hypoxic cells, in combination with cisplatin and etoposide with TRT (SWOG 0222), demonstrated a promising PFS and OS with acceptable toxicity in patients with LS-SCLC, but was halted early due to excess toxicity of tirapazamine in a head and neck cancer trial.[84] Bec2 is an anti-idiotypic antibody that mimics GD3, a ganglioside

TABLE 103.4 New Chemotherapy Approaches in LS-SCLC

First Author	No. of Patients	Chemotherapy	TRT	2-Year Survival Rate (%)	Median Survival Time (mo)
Kubota[77]	31	Cisplatin/etoposide × one cycle then cisplatin/irinotecan	45 Gy BID cycle 1	41	20.2
Mitsuoka[64]	51	Cisplatin/etoposide × one cycle then cisplatin/irinotecan	45 Gy BID cycle 1	51	NR
Bremnes[75]	39	Paclitaxel/cisplatin/etoposide	42 Gy BID cycle 3	37	21
Levitan[78]	31	Paclitaxel/cisplatin/etoposide	45 Gy BID cycle 1	47	22.3
Sandler[117]	63	Paclitaxel/cisplatin/etoposide	63 Gy BID cycle 3	NR	NR
Ettinger[128]	53	Paclitaxel/cisplatin/etoposide	45 Gy BID cycle 1	54.7	24.7
Glisson[129]	67	Ifosfamide/etoposide/cisplatin	45 Gy BID cycle 1	50	23.7
Bogart[130]	63	Paclitaxel/topotecan/carboplatin	70 Gy BID cycle 3	48	22.4
Baas[88]	38	Paclitaxel/etoposide/cisplatin	45 Gy BID cycle 2	47	19.5
Hanna[76]	53	Ifosfamide/cisplatin/etoposide	45 Gy BID cycle 1	36	15.1
Woo[131]	44	Ifosfamide/cisplatin/etoposide	40 Gy BID cycle 1	NR	22.5
Kubota[83]	258	Cisplatin/etoposide x one cycle, followed by:	45 Gy BID cycle 1		
		Cisplatin/etoposide	NR	3.2	
		Cisplatin/irinotecan	NR	2.8	

LS-SCLC, limited-stage small-cell lung cancer; TRT, thoracic radiotherapy; NR, not reported.

that has been shown to be overexpressed in approximately 60% of the SCLC tissues examined. A randomized phase III clinical trial compared Bec2/bacilli Calmette–Guérin (BCG) vaccination versus observation in LS-SCLC patients with response after chemoradiotherapy. There was no improvement in survival, PFS, or quality of life in the vaccination arm (OS 16.4 and 14.3 months in the observation and vaccination arms, respectively; $P = 0.28$), though a trend toward prolonged survival was noted among vaccinated patients who developed a humoral response, suggesting more study may be warranted of vaccines in LS-SCLC that produce a more robust immunologic response.[85] A randomized phase II trial investigated whether treatment with vandetanib, an inhibitor of vascular endothelial and epidermal growth factor receptors, could prolong PFS in responding patients with SCLC. Of the 107 patients enrolled, 46 had LS-SCLC and 61 had ES-SCLC. In preplanned subset analysis, LS patients had a trend toward longer survival with vandetanib therapy in comparison with placebo, but this did not reach statistical significance.[86]

There has also been interest in integrating bevacizumab, a monoclonal antibody against vascular endothelial growth factor (VEGF), into the treatment of LS-SCLC. A phase II study investigated treatment with carboplatin, irinotecan, and bevacizumab with TRT followed by bevacizumab for up to 6 months in patients with stable or responding disease.[87] Among the first 29 patients, there were two with a confirmed and a third with a suspected tracheoesophageal fistula. Two of the three cases were fatal, and all occurred during the maintenance phase of bevacizumab in the context of persistent esophagitis. The study was closed to further accrual.[87] This trial illustrates the intricacies of integrating a novel agent that may have a unique set of toxicities into a multimodality treatment paradigm.

Another frequent issue of debate in the treatment of LS-SCLC is about substitution of carboplatin for cisplatin in LS-SCLC. Several phase II trials have reported on using carboplatin-based treatments.[88–90] A recent study looking into 1,603 patients with LS-SCLC in the SEER-Medicare lung cancer database demonstrated comparable OS and lung cancer–specific survival between patients treated

with concurrent chemoradiotherapy with either cisplatin or carboplatin.[91] However, there are limited phase III trial data about the efficacy of carboplatin, and because treatment for LS-SCLC is potentially curative, the current standard of care is cisplatin-based therapy in LS-SCLC unless the patient is intolerant or has a contraindication to cisplatin-based therapy.

Extensive-Stage Disease

The majority of patients who have SCLC will present with ES disease where the primary treatment is chemotherapy.[2] Despite a very high initial response to a variety of chemotherapeutic agents, patients inevitably develop resistance to chemotherapy, and the OS in patients with ES-SCLC remains poor. The median survival observed on clinical trials remains 7 to 10 months, and less than 5% of patients live beyond 2 years.[92] The combination of EP was developed 25 years ago and remains the standard therapy in Europe and the United States.[93,94] The substitution of carboplatin for cisplatin has been evaluated in phase III trials, and treatment with carboplatin has similar efficacy and superior tolerability.[95–98] Carboplatin is frequently used in patients with poor performance status or in elderly patients to reduce the incidence of nausea, vomiting, ototoxicity, and nephrotoxicity. Several trials have investigated a variety of strategies including: increasing dose intensity or total dose of chemotherapy; consolidation, alternating, and maintenance of chemotherapy; or integrating high-dose chemotherapy with peripheral stem cell rescue into the treatment paradigm of ES-SCLC. No novel treatment paradigm has consistently demonstrated a significant improvement in OS.[95,99–106]

There has been increasing interest in the investigation of novel agents into the treatment of ES-SCLC. A phase III trial performed by the Japanese Clinical Oncology Group compared IP every 28 days versus EP every 21 days in patients with ES-SCLC (n = 230). An interim analysis revealed that patients who were treated with IP in comparison with patients treated with EP experienced a longer median survival (12.8 months vs. 9.8 months, respectively; $P = 0.002$) (Table 103.5). The 1- and 2-year survival rates with IP and EP were

TABLE 103.5 Select Phase III Trials in ES-SCLC

First Author	No. of Patients	Treatment Comparison	Median Survival Time	1-Year Overall Survival Rate (%)
Noda[80]	230	Cisplatin 80 mg/m^2 day 1 + etoposide 100 mg/m^2 days 1, 2, and 3 every 21 days	9.4 mo	37.7
		vs.		
		Cisplatin 60 mg/m^2 day 1 + irinotecan 60 mg/m^2 days 1, 8, and 15 every 28 days	12.8 mo	58.4
Hanna[76]	331	Cisplatin 60 mg/m^2 day 1 + etoposide 120 mg/m^2 days 1, 2, and 3 every 21 days	10.2 mo	35
		vs.		
		Cisplatin 30 mg/m^2 days 1 and 8 + irinotecan 65 mg/m^2 days 1 and 8 every 21 days	9.3 mo	35
Eckardt[100]	784	Cisplatin 80 mg/m^2 day 1 + etoposide 100 mg/m^2 days 1, 2, and 3 every 21 days	40.3 wks	31
		vs.		
		Cisplatin 80 mg/m^2 day 5 + topotecan 1.7 mg/m^2 days 1 to 5	39.3 wks	31
Hermes[101]	209	Carboplatin AUC = 4 + irinotecan (175 mg/m^2)	8.5 mo	34
		vs.		
		Carboplatin AUC = 4 + etoposide 120 mg/m^2 PO days 1 to 5	7.1 mo	24
Lara[107]		Cisplatin 60 mg/m^2 day 1 + irinotecan 60 mg/m^2 days 1, 8, and 15 every 28 days	9.9 mo	41
		vs.		
		Cisplatin 80 mg/m^2 day 1 + etoposide 100 mg/m^2 days 1 to 3 every 21 days	9.1 mo	34
Satouchi[108]		Cisplatin 60 mg/m^2 day 1 + irinotecan 60 mg/m^2 days 1, 8, and 15 every 28 days	17.7 mo	68.3
		vs.		
		Cisplatin 60 mg/m^2 day 1 + amrubicin 40 mg/m^2 days 1, 2, and 3 and every 21 days.	15 mo	63.9

ES-SCLC, extensive-stage small-cell lung cancer; AUC, area under the curve using the Chatelut equation.

58.4% versus 27.7%, respectively, and 19.5% versus 5.2%, respectively. The IP combination was associated with a higher-grade 3/4 diarrhea than EP (16% vs. 0%, respectively). The day 15 irinotecan was not administered 50% of the time due to toxicity.

A North American trial (Table 103.5) compared EP with IP is ES-SCLC (n = 331), but the IP schedule used in the North American trial was cisplatin (30 mg/m^2) on days 1, 8 and irinotecan (65 mg/m^2) on days 1, 8 every 21 days.[76] The schedule of IP differed in order to increase dose intensity, in response to the poor compliance with the day 15 irinotecan administration. The IP and EP groups had a similar median time to progression (4.1 vs. 4.6 months, respectively) and OS (median survival time, 9.3 months, vs. 10.2 months, respectively; P = 0.74). The IP arm in comparison with the EP arm was associated with significantly more vomiting and diarrhea but significantly less neutropenia, febrile neutropenic anemia, and thrombocytopenia. Potential explanations for the discordant results between the two trials include the different schedule of irinotecan therapy, pharmacogenomic differences between the North American and Japanese patient populations (specifically differences in polymorphisms of UDP-glucuronosyltransferase [UGT1A1], an enzyme that metabolizes irinotecan), and molecular differences in lung cancer between the two populations. The Southwest Oncology Group (SWOG) trial S0124 compared EP and IP using the schedule used in the trial by Noda et al. and also failed to confirm the previously reported survival benefit observed with IP in Japanese patients. EP and IP had comparable efficacy, with less hematologic and greater gastrointestinal toxicity with IP. Underlying polymorphisms in ABCB1 (which is involved in membrane transport) and UGT1A1 were associated with IP-related diarrhea and neutropenia, respectively, emphasizing the potential importance of pharmacogenomics in interpreting irinotecan trials in SCLC.[107] A Norwegian Lung Cancer Group and Swedish Lung Cancer Study Group compared carboplatin (area under the curve [AUC] = 4) using the Chatelut formula[11] with irinotecan (175 mg/m^2) every 21 days (n = 105) or etoposide (120 mg/m^2 orally on days 1 to 5) (n = 104) in ES-SCLC.[101] The median survival times observed for carboplatin/irinotecan versus carboplatin/etoposide were 8.5 and 7.1 months, respectively (P = 0.02), and the hazard ratio for OS was 1.41 (95% CI, 1.06–1.87), favoring the carboplatin/irinotecan treatment arm.

Another recent phase III trial compared EP every 21 days versus cisplatin (60 mg/m^2 on day 5) and oral topotecan (1.7 mg/m^2/day on days 1 to 5) every 21 days (n = 784).[99] The median survival time observed with cisplatin/topotecan was similar to that with EP (39.3 weeks vs. 40.3 weeks), and the 1-year survival rate in both groups was 31% (95% CI, 27%–36%). The difference met the predefined criterion of ≤10% absolute difference for noninferiority of cisplatin/topotecan relative to EP. Treatment with cisplatin/topotecan was associated with a lower rate of grade 3/4 neutropenia but with a higher rate of grade 3/4 anemia and thrombocytopenia.

Carboplatin/pemetrexed had shown promising survival results and a low rate of hematologic toxicity in a phase II trial, and a phase III trial comparing carboplatin/pemetrexed versus carboplatin/etoposide with the primary endpoint of noninferiority for survival was initiated.[79] An interim analysis in December 2007, after 700 patients had been enrolled, revealed that carboplatin/pemetrexed would not meet the primary endpoint of noninferiority in OS in comparison with carboplatin/etoposide. The Data Monitoring Committee recommended stopping the trial on grounds of futility. A randomized phase III trial (JCOG 0509) compared amrubicin plus cisplatin (AP) with IP in chemotherapy naïve patients with ES-SCLC. This study was halted at a second interim analysis due to futility. In an updated survival analysis, AP was associated with inferior median OS and PFS and higher rates of grade 4 neutropenia and grade 3 and 4 febrile neutropenia compared with IP.[108]

While the majority of patients achieve good disease control initially, patients with SCLC usually experience relapse within 6 months of first-line chemotherapy and often do not respond to subsequent chemotherapy. As such, the development of maintenance strategies to delay cancer progression and prolong survival after initial chemotherapy for ES-SCLC has been an area of interest. A phase III clinical trial evaluated the role of four cycles of maintenance topotecan versus observation in patients with stable or responding disease after induction with EP. In 223 patients randomized to maintenance topotecan versus observation, topotecan was associated with improvement in PFS compared with observation (3.6 months vs. 2.3 months, respectively; $P < 0.001$), but no improvement in OS (8.9 months vs. 9.3 months, respectively; $P = 0.43$).[109] The high frequency of chemotherapy-refractory SCLC after initial chemotherapy may partially explain the lack of survival benefit from a topotecan maintenance strategy. More recently, the randomized phase II Cancer and Leukemia Group B (CALGB) 30504 trial evaluated maintenance sunitinib, a multitargeted small molecule tyrosine kinase inhibitor with selectivity for the vascular endothelial growth factor receptor (VEGFR), in patients with ES-SCLC with stable or responsive disease after initial chemotherapy with platinum/etoposide. This trial met its primary endpoint demonstrating a PFS benefit with maintenance sunitinib (2.1 months with placebo compared with 3.7 months with sunitinib; HR 1.62; $P = 0.02$), but did not demonstrate prolongation in OS. Three complete responses were noted in patients receiving sunitinib. Ten of thirteen patients evaluable after crossover from placebo to sunitinib benefited from stable disease, suggestive of a sunitinib crossover effect in refractory SCLC that might have affected the OS analysis.[110]

In patients with ES-SCLC who respond to chemotherapy and receive PCI, intrathoracic disease control is a significant issue with roughly 90% patients experiencing disease progression within the thorax within 1 year of diagnosis.[111] The role of TRT in these select patients with ES-SCLC was evaluated in two phase III clinical trials. The first by Jeremic et al.,[112] randomized 109 patients who had intrathoracic response and complete distant response to further EP alone or accelerated hyperfractionated radiotherapy (54 Gy in 36 twice-daily fractions over 18 days) with carboplatin and etoposide. Patients receiving TRT had an improved median survival (17 vs. 11 months) and 5-year OS (9.9 vs. 3.7%) over those that did not. More recently, Slotman et al.[113] randomized 498 patients with responsive disease undergoing PCI to receive either TRT (30 Gy in 10 fractions) or no TRT. No severe adverse side effects were noted. While this study did not meet the primary endpoint of improved 1-year OS

with TRT compared with control (33% vs. 28%, respectively; HR 0.84; $p = 0.066$), 2-year OS was significantly prolonged (13% vs. 3%, respectively; $p = 0.004$) with TRT, and progression was less likely in the TRT group than in the control group (HR 0.73; $p = 0.001$). These studies would suggest that TRT may influence long-term survival in a subset of patients with ES-SCLC with responsive disease to first-line therapy.

SECOND-LINE THERAPY

Given the fact that all patients will inevitably experience progression, there has been interest in second-line chemotherapy. In the second-line treatment of ES-SCLC, patients are frequently divided into chemotherapy-refractory versus chemotherapy-sensitive groups, based on whether they experience progression of their disease within 60 or 90 days of completing first-line chemotherapy. The only agent approved by the U.S. Food and Drug Administration (FDA) is topotecan. This approval was based on a phase III trial (n = 211) that compared topotecan 1.5 mg/m^2 daily for 5 days every 21 days versus cyclophosphamide (1,000 mg/m^2), adriamycin (45 mg/m^2), and vincristine (CAV) 2 mg on day 1 every 21 days.[63] The two therapies demonstrated similar RRs, time to tumor progression, and OS. However, the proportion of patients who experienced symptom improvement was greater in the topotecan group than in the CAV group in four of the eight symptoms evaluated. Topotecan was associated with a lower rate of grade 4 neutropenia but a higher rate of grade 4 thrombocytopenia and grade 3/4 anemia. A subsequent phase III trial (n = 309) demonstrated similar efficacy and tolerability of oral and intravenous topotecan in relapsed chemotherapy-sensitive (defined as >90 days after the end of chemotherapy) SCLC.[100]

A subsequent phase III trial compared treatment with oral topotecan versus best supportive care (BSC) in patients with relapsed SCLC (n = 141).[102] The median survival times observed in the oral topotecan versus the BSC arms were 25.9 weeks versus 13.9 weeks, respectively (HR = 0.64, 95% CI 0.45–0.90; $P = 0.01$). Importantly, the survival advantage was observed in both patients with resistant disease (defined as progression ≤60 days) and patients with sensitive disease (defined as progression >60 days). For the patients with resistant disease (defined as progression ≤60 days), the median survival on topotecan was 23.2 weeks (95% CI, 10.7–30.9) compared with 13.2 weeks (95% CI, 7.0–21.0) on BSC. Patients treated with topotecan had a slower deterioration in quality of life and greater symptom control. This trial supported the use of oral topotecan in both chemotherapy-sensitive and chemotherapy-refractory disease.

The efficacy of amrubicin versus topotecan as second-line treatment of SCLC was the subject of a randomized phase III clinical trial. In 637 randomized patients with both sensitive and refractory SCLC, median OS did not differ with amrubicin versus topotecan (7.5 months vs. 7.8 months, respectively; HR 0.880; $P = 0.170$), though in refractory patients, median OS was 6.2 and 5.7 months, respectively (HR 0.77; $P = 0.047$). While amrubicin was associated with improvements in PFS (4.1 months vs. 3.5 months, respectively: HR 0.802; $P = 0.018$), and ORR (31.1% vs. 16.9%, respectively; OR 2.223; $p = 0.001$) compared with topotecan, the gains in survival in the refractory population were modest, and amrubicin has failed to gain approval in the treatment of ES-SCLC in the United States. Rates of anemia, leukopenia, and thrombocytopenia were lower with amrubicin than with topotecan, whereas febrile neutropenia occurred more frequently with amrubicin. Amrubicin-treated patients experienced significantly more grade 3 and 4 infections. However, significantly fewer patients in this arm required transfusions.[114]

Recently, there has been significant interest in the role of immune checkpoint therapy in ES-SCLC. Pembrolizumab and nivolumab, anti–PD-1 monoclonal antibodies designed to block the interaction between PD-1 and its ligands PD-L1 and PD-L2, have shown significant antitumor activity in multiple advanced malignancies. In a phase I clinical trial of pembrolizumab in patients with previously treated ES-SCLC with PD-L1–positive tumors by immunohistochemistry, responses were noted in 7 of 20 patients (ORR 35%). Responses tended to occur early in the course of treatment (median time to response 8.6 weeks) and were durable with the majority of responders on treatment for 16 or more weeks with ongoing benefit.[115] A phase I/II clinical trial evaluated nivolumab and the combination of nivolumab and ipilimumab, an anti-CTLA monoclonal antibody, in previously treated patients with ES-SCLC and any PDL1 status (n = 70), a third of whom had platinum-refractory disease. Both nivolumab and nivolumab/ipilimumab were well tolerated, though precipitation of a paraneoplastic syndrome (three patients; limbic encephalitis) and autoimmune disease (1 patient; myasthenia gravis) were noted. Nivolumab and nivolumab/ipilimumab were associated with RRs of 18% and 32.6%, and median OS of 4.4 months and 8.2 months, respectively. Responses were noted in both platinum-sensitive and platinum-refractory disease, occurred rapidly, and appear to be durable.[116] Although these early phase data is encouraging, more clinical data is needed to validate immune checkpoint inhibition as a therapeutic strategy in ES-SCLC.

TARGETED THERAPIES IN ES-SCLC

There has also been significant interest in integrating targeted therapies into the treatment of ES-SCLC. Early efforts focused on incorporating antiangiogenic agents into standard chemotherapy regimens. A series of phase III trials were undertaken with thalidomide either in patients who responded to their first two cycles of chemotherapy,[103] or in combination with the initial chemotherapy followed by thalidomide maintenance.[104] These trials failed to demonstrate a definitive survival benefit, and it is unlikely that thalidomide will have a significant role in the treatment of SCLC.

The humanized monoclonal antibody, bevacizumab, which targets VEGF-A has also been examined in ES-SCLC. The ECOG trial investigated bevacizumab in combination with EP (n = 61), and the combination led to a median survival of 11.1 months.[117] The Cancer and Leukemia Group B (CALGB) trial investigated bevacizumab in combination with IP (n = 68), and the combination led to a median survival of 11.7 months.[118] The Sarah Cannon Research Institute investigated bevacizumab in combination with carboplatin and irinotecan (n = 51), and the median survival time observed was 10.9 months.[119] The SALUTE clinical trial was a randomized phase II clinical trial (n = 102) assessing the efficacy of bevacizumab in combination with platinum/etoposide as initial therapy in ES-SCLC. Bevacizumab was associated with improved PFS compared with placebo (5.5 months compared with 4.4 months, respectively; HR 0.53; 95% CI, 0.32 to 0.86), but no significant OS advantage (9.4 vs. 10.9 months for bevacizumab and placebo groups, respectively).[120] A randomized phase II/III clinical trial (IFCT 0802) evaluated the efficacy of bevacizumab in combination with initial chemotherapy with the primary endpoint of RR. In this clinical trial, 74 patients with responsive disease after two cycles of platinum-based chemotherapy were randomized to an additional four cycles of chemotherapy with or without bevacizumab. The percentage of still-responding patients after four cycles, did not differ between the chemotherapy alone arm (89.2%) versus the chemotherapy plus bevacizumab arm (91.9%;

$P = 1.00$). Neither PFS nor OS differed significantly between treatment arms (PFS, 5.5 vs. 5.3 months; OS, 13.0 and 11.1 months, in the chemotherapy alone and chemotherapy plus bevacizumab groups, respectively). As the addition of bevacizumab did not increase the proportion of patients responding after four cycles of therapy, this study did not proceed to the phase III portion of the study.[121] The addition of bevacizumab to chemotherapy in ES-SCLC is no longer an area of active investigation. However, as discussed above, there remains significant interest in the maintenance setting for utilizing the multi-targeted tyrosine kinase inhibitor, sunitinib, which works at least in part through inhibiting the VEGF receptor.

As previously discussed, *MYC* family member alterations are found in almost 20% of SCLC.[11,12] Interestingly, preclinical studies have suggested that *MYC* amplified tumors may be more sensitive to aurora kinase inhibitors,[122] and a phase 2 trial in SCLC testing monotherapy treatment with the aurora kinase inhibitor, alisertib, demonstrated promising activity (RR 21%).[123] The combination of alisertib in combination with paclitaxel is currently being explored in SCLC (NCT02038647). In addition, the stem cell transcription factor *SOX2* is amplified in almost 27% of SCLC, and there is strong interest in targeting stem cell pathways in SCLC including several trials targeting the NOTCH signaling pathway (NCT01859741). Finally, amplification of *FGFR1* was found in 6% of SCLC and may be targetable with currently available FGFR inhibitors.[11]

In addition, proteomic studies in SCLC have suggested a critical role for the DNA repair proteins, CHK1 and PARP1.[124] Interestingly, single agent activity has been observed with PARP inhibitor monotherapy in SCLC patients,[125] and currently there are several ongoing trials testing PARP inhibitors either alone or combination with first-line (cisplatin/etoposide) or second-line (temodar) cytotoxic therapy.[10] In summary, current efforts in targeted therapy for SCLC are focused on targeting mutational subsets of SCLC (*MYC* amplified, *FGRF1* amplification), stem cell pathways, or critical DNA repair pathways required for survival of the SCLC.

PROPHYLACTIC CRANIAL IRRADIATION

Brain metastases are a frequent problem in patients with SCLC. Approximately 10% to 15% of patients will have brain metastases at the time of diagnosis, and the cumulative incidence of brain metastases at 3 years for patients with LS-SCLC in complete remission is as high as 50% to 60%.[56] Owing to the frequent development of brain metastases, PCI was evaluated in at least seven randomized controlled trials.[4] Although a clear survival benefit could not be demonstrated in the individual trials, a meta-analysis of the seven trials by Auperin et al. revealed a significant survival benefit to PCI for patients with a radiographic complete response with 3-year survival rates increased from 15.3% to 20.7% ($P < 0.01$).[4] PCI was shown to reduce the incidence of brain metastases by 50%. This meta-analysis suggested that PCI is best delivered after completion of the chemotherapy. As the majority of patients included in the meta-analysis had LS-SCLC (85.8%), it established PCI as the standard of care for patients with LS-SCLC. There is some ambiguity, though, regarding the need for a complete response as these trials used chest radiographs to assess response, and as such many physicians have interpreted a CT-based favorable response as adequate for PCI.

Given a persistent risk of brain metastases following PCI and the wide-ranging radiation doses included in the Auperin meta-analysis, an Intergroup study[111] attempted to address these issues by randomizing 720 patients with LS-SCLC to a higher dose using a hyperfractionation schedule (36 Gy delivered at 1.5 Gy twice daily) versus a standard dose (25 Gy delivered at 2.5 Gy once daily). There was no significant reduction in the incidence of brain metastases between the two arms, and in fact the higher-dose arm resulted in inferior 2-year survival (37 vs. 42%) with greater neurotoxicity defined by the Hopkins Verbal Learning Test. Based on this, PCI at 25 Gy in 10 fractions remains the standard of care in LS-SCLC.

A phase III trial also investigated the role of PCI in patients with ES-SCLC who have responded to four to six cycles of chemotherapy.[111] The primary endpoint was time to symptomatic brain metastases, and patients were randomly assigned to PCI (n = 143) or observation (n = 143). Patients receiving PCI in comparison with the patients on the observation arm had a lower rate of symptomatic brain metastases (HR = 0.27, 95% CI 0.16–0.44; $P < 0.001$), and increased median OS to 6.7 versus 5.4 months, respectively ($P = 0.003$). The 1-year survival rate from the time of randomization in the PCI group was 27.1% (95% CI, 19.4–35.5) versus 13.3% (95% CI, 8.1–19.9), and the HR for death in PCI group was 0.68 (95% CI, 0.52–0.88). No significant differences were found in role, cognitive, or emotional functioning or quality of life between the two groups. This trial demonstrated that PCI in ES-SCLC provides significant clinical benefit with an acceptable rate of toxicity. A meta-analysis of 16 randomized clinical trials involving 1,983 patients of whom 1,021 were submitted to PCI and 962 were not, overall mortality was 4.4% lower in patients treated with PCI compared with those who were not (OR = 0.73; $p = 0.01$). This decrease in mortality was noted among the patients with a complete response after induction chemotherapy (OR = 0.68; 95% CI: 0.50-0.93; $p = 0.02$) and in both LS-SCLC (OR 0.73; $p = 0.03$) and ES-SCLC (OR 0.48; $p = 0.02$) patients, suggesting a benefit with PCI across disease stages and especially in patients with a complete response after induction chemotherapy.[126]

More recently, a randomized phase III clinical study conducted in Japan evaluated PCI (25 Gy/10 fractions) versus observation in patients with ES-SCLC and responsive disease after initial platinum-doublet chemotherapy. The study was terminated at a preplanned interim analysis after accrual of 162 patients because of futility. The median OS was 10.1 and 15.1 months for PCI and observation, respectively (HR = 1.38; $P = 0.091$). While PCI significantly reduced the risk of brain metastases compared with observation (32.4% vs. 58.0% at 12 months; $P < 0.001$), PFS was comparable between the two arms (2.2 vs. 2.4 months, respectively; HR = 1.12, 95% CI = 0.82–1.54).[116] In contrast to the prior trial of PCI in patients with ES-SCLC, the Japanese trial required an MRI prior to enrollment to ensure absence of brain metastases, suggesting the prior benefit of PCI seen in ES-SCLC might actually have been due to treatment of nonradiographically detected brain metastases.

FUTURE DIRECTIONS

While treatment of LS-SCLC with a combination of chemotherapy and radiation has curative potential, the overwhelming majority of patients eventually succumb to recurrent disease. Similar, patients with ES-SCLC have a high initial RR to chemotherapy. However, the median survival remains modest owing to the rapid development of chemotherapy resistance and subsequent progression of disease. Given the recalcitrance of SCLC, the National Cancer Institute recently developed a scientific framework for the improvement of treatment for patients with SCLC.[127] The framework highlighted the importance of tissue collection efforts to perform further comprehensive genomic profiling of clinically annotated SCLC specimens to improve our understanding of the frequency, distribution, and range of molecular abnormalities in SCLC at diagnosis and relapse; also, to establish cell line and mouse models that facilitate study of the clinical behavior of SCLC. This will hopefully lead to the development of novel therapeutic approaches targeting molecular vulnerabilities of SCLC and further the study of mechanisms underlying both the high initial RRs of SCLC and the rapid emergence of resistance to drug and radiation treatment.

REFERENCES

1. Siegel RL, Miller KD, Jemal A. Cancer statistics, 2015. *CA Cancer J Clin* 2015;65: 5–29.
2. Govindan R, Page N, Morgensztern D, et al. Changing epidemiology of small-cell lung cancer in the United States over the last 30 years: analysis of the surveillance, epidemiologic, and end results database. *J Clin Oncol* 2006;24:4539–4544.
3. Steenland K. Epidemiology of occupation and coronary heart disease: research agenda. *Am J Ind Med* 1996;30:495–499.
4. Samson DJ, Seidenfeld J, Simon GR, et al. Evidence for management of small cell lung cancer: ACCP evidence-based clinical practice guidelines (2nd edition). *Chest* 2007;132:314S–323S.
5. Barnard W. The nature of the "oat-celled sarcoma" of the mediastinum. *J Pathol Bacteriol* 1926;29:241–244.
6. Franklin WA, Noguchi M, Gonzalez A. Molecular and cellular pathology of lung cancer: Small cell lung carcinoma. In: Pass H, Carbone DP, Johnson DH, et al., eds. *Principles & Practice of Lung Cancer: The Official Reference Text of the IASLC.* 4th ed. Philadelphia, PA: Lippincott Williams & Wilkins; 2010:299–302.
7. Stovold R, Meredith SL, Bryant JL, et al. Neuroendocrine and epithelial phenotypes in small-cell lung cancer: implications for metastasis and survival in patients. *Br J Cancer* 2013;108:1704–1711.
8. World Health Organization Classification of Tumours. *Pathology and Genetics of Tumours of the Lung, Pleura, Thymus and Heart.* Lyon, France: IARC Press; 2004.
9. Brambilla E, Travis WD, Colby TV, et al. The new World Health Organization classification of lung tumours. *Eur Respir J* 2001;18:1059–1068.
10. Byers LA, Rudin CM. Small cell lung cancer: where do we go from here? *Cancer* 2015;121:664–672.
11. Rudin CM, Durinck S, Stawiski EW, et al. Comprehensive genomic analysis identifies SOX2 as a frequently amplified gene in small-cell lung cancer. *Nat Genet* 2012; 44:1111–1116.
12. Peifer M, Fernandez-Cuesta L, Sos ML, et al. Integrative genome analyses identify key somatic driver mutations of small-cell lung cancer. *Nat Genet* 2012;44: 1104–1110.
13. Zelen M. Keynote address on biostatistics and data retrieval. *Cancer Chemother Rep* 1973;34:31–42.
14. Micke P, Faldum A, Metz T, et al. Staging small cell lung cancer: Veterans Administration Lung Study Group versus International Association for the Study of Lung Cancer—what limits limited disease? *Lung Cancer* 2002;37:271–276.
15. Morris DE, MA S, Detterbeck F. Limited stage small cell lung cancer. In: Detterbeck F, Rivera M, MA S, et al, eds. *Diagnosis and Treatment of Lung Cancer: An Evidence-Based Guide for the Practicing Clinician.* Philadelphia, PA: Saunders; 2001.
16. Ettinger DS, Wood DE, Akerley W, et al. Non-small cell lung cancer, version 1.2015. *J Natl Compr Canc Netw* 2014;12:1738–1761.
17. Gregor A, Cull A, Stephens RJ, et al. Prophylactic cranial irradiation is indicated following complete response to induction therapy in small cell lung cancer: results of a multicentre randomised trial. United Kingdom Coordinating Committee for Cancer Research (UKCCCR) and the European Organization for Research and Treatment of Cancer (EORTC). *Eur J Cancer* 1997;33:1752–1758.
18. Jett JR, Schild SE, Kesler KA, et al. Treatment of small cell lung cancer: Diagnosis and management of lung cancer, 3rd ed: American College of Chest Physicians evidence-based clinical practice guidelines. *Chest* 2013;143:e400S–e419S.
19. Shepherd FA, Crowley J, Van Houtte P, et al. The International Association for the Study of Lung Cancer lung cancer staging project: proposals regarding the clinical staging of small cell lung cancer in the forthcoming (seventh) edition of the tumor, node, metastasis classification for lung cancer. *J Thorac Oncol* 2007;2:1067–1077.
20. Albain KS, Crowley JJ, LeBlanc M, et al. Determinants of improved outcome in small-cell lung cancer: an analysis of the 2,580-patient Southwest Oncology Group data base. *J Clin Oncol* 1990;8:1563–1574.
21. Detterbeck FC, Falen S, Rivera MP, et al. Seeking a home for a PET, part 2: Defining the appropriate place for positron emission tomography imaging in the staging of patients with suspected lung cancer. *Chest* 2004;125:2300–2308.
22. MacManus MP, Hicks RJ, Matthews JP, et al. High rate of detection of unsuspected distant metastases by pet in apparent stage III non-small-cell lung cancer: implications for radical radiation therapy. *Int J Radiat Oncol Biol Phys* 2001;50:287–293.
23. Weder W, Schmid RA, Bruchhaus H, et al. Detection of extrathoracic metastases by positron emission tomography in lung cancer. *Ann Thorac Surg* 1998;66:886–892; discussion 892–883.
24. Blum R, MacManus MP, Rischin D, et al. Impact of positron emission tomography on the management of patients with small-cell lung cancer: preliminary experience. *Am J Clin Oncol* 2004;27:164–171.
25. Bradley JD, Dehdashti F, Mintun MA, et al. Positron emission tomography in limited-stage small-cell lung cancer: a prospective study. *J Clin Oncol* 2004;22:3248–3254.
26. Brink I, Schumacher T, Mix M, et al. Impact of [18F]FDG-PET on the primary staging of small-cell lung cancer. *Eur J Nucl Med Mol Imaging* 2004;31:1614–1620.

27. Kamel EM, Zwahlen D, Wyss MT, et al. Whole-body (18)F-FDG PET improves the management of patients with small cell lung cancer. *J Nucl Med* 2003;44:1911–1917.
28. Schumacher T, Brink I, Mix M, et al. FDG-PET imaging for the staging and follow-up of small cell lung cancer. *Eur J Nucl Med* 2001;28:483–488.
29. Combs SE, Hancock JG, Boffa DJ, et al. Bolstering the case for lobectomy in stages I, II, and IIIA small-cell lung cancer using the National Cancer Data Base. *J Thorac Oncol* 2015;10:316–323.
30. Azad A, Chionh F, Scott AM, et al. High impact of 18F-FDG-PET on management and prognostic stratification of newly diagnosed small cell lung cancer. *Mol Imaging Biol* 2010;12:443–451.
31. van Loon J, Offermann C, Bosmans G, et al. 18FDG-PET based radiation planning of mediastinal lymph nodes in limited disease small cell lung cancer changes radiotherapy fields: a planning study. *Radiother Oncol* 2008;87:49–54.
32. van Loon J, De Ruysscher D, Wanders R, et al. Selective nodal irradiation on basis of (18)FDG-PET scans in limited-disease small-cell lung cancer: a prospective study. *Int J Radiat Oncol Biol Phys* 2010;77:329–336.
33. Flanagan FL, Dehdashti F, Siegel BA, et al. Staging of esophageal cancer with 18F-fluorodeoxyglucose positron emission tomography. *AJR Am J Roentgenol* 1997; 168:417–424.
34. Davis S, Wright PW, Schulman SF, et al. Long-term survival in small-cell carcinoma of the lung: a population experience. *J Clin Oncol* 1985;3:80–91.
35. Shah SS, Thompson J, Goldstraw P. Results of operation without adjuvant therapy in the treatment of small cell lung cancer. *Ann Thorac Surg* 1992;54:498–501.
36. Shore DF, Paneth M. Survival after resection of small cell carcinoma of the bronchus. *Thorax* 1980;35:819–822.
37. Sorensen HR, Lund C, Alstrup P. Survival in small cell lung carcinoma after surgery. *Thorax* 1986;41:479–482.
38. Fox W, Scadding JG. Treatment of oat-celled carcinoma of the bronchus. *Lancet* 1973;2:616–617.
39. Karrer K, Shields TW, Denck H, et al. The importance of surgical and multimodality treatment for small cell bronchial carcinoma. *J Thorac Cardiovasc Surg* 1989;97:168–176.
40. Lucchi M, Mussi A, Chella A, et al. Surgery in the management of small cell lung cancer. *Eur J Cardiothorac Surg* 1997;12:689–693.
41. Osterlind K, Hansen M, Hansen HH, et al. Influence of surgical resection prior to chemotherapy on the long-term results in small cell lung cancer. A study of 150 operable patients. *Eur J Cancer Clin Oncol* 1986;22:589–593.
42. Shepherd FA, Evans WK, Feld R, et al. Adjuvant chemotherapy following surgical resection for small-cell carcinoma of the lung. *J Clin Oncol* 1998;6:832–838.
43. Shields TW, Higgins GA, Jr., Humphrey EW, et al. Prolonged intermittent adjuvant chemotherapy with CCNU and hydroxyurea after resection of carcinoma of the lung. *Cancer* 1982;50:1713–1721.
44. Shepherd FA, Ginsberg RJ, Feld R, et al. Surgical treatment for limited small-cell lung cancer. The University of Toronto Lung Oncology Group experience. *J Thorac Cardiovasc Surg* 1991;101: 385–393.
45. Hara N, Ichinose Y, Kuda T, et al. Long-term survivors in resected and nonresected small cell lung cancer. *Oncology* 1991;48:441–447.
46. Eberhardt W, Stamatis G, Stuschke M, et al. Prognostically orientated multimodality treatment including surgery for selected patients of small-cell lung cancer patients stages IB to IIIB: long-term results of a phase II trial. *Br J Cancer* 1991;81:1206–1212.
47. Holoye PY, McMurtrey MJ, Mountain CF, et al. The role of adjuvant surgery in the combined modality therapy of small-cell bronchogenic carcinoma after a chemotherapy-induced partial remission. *J Clin Oncol* 1990;8:416–422.
48. Lad T, Piantadosi S, Thomas P, et al. A prospective randomized trial to determine the benefit of surgical resection of residual disease following response of small cell lung cancer to combination chemotherapy. *Chest* 1994;106:320S–323S.
49. Shepherd FA, Ginsberg RJ, Patterson GA, et al. A prospective study of adjuvant surgical resection after chemotherapy for limited small cell lung cancer. A University of Toronto Lung Oncology Group study. *J Thorac Cardiovasc Surg* 1989;97:177–186.
50. Williams CJ, McMillan I, Lea R, et al. Surgery after initial chemotherapy for localized small-cell carcinoma of the lung. *J Clin Oncol* 1987;5:1579–1588.
51. Prager RL, Foster JM, Hainsworth JD, et al. The feasibility of adjuvant surgery in limited-stage small cell carcinoma: a prospective evaluation. *Ann Thorac Surg* 1984;38:622–626.
52. Baker RR, Ettinger DS, Ruckdeschel JD, et al. The role of surgery in the management of selected patients with small-cell carcinoma of the lung. *J Clin Oncol* 1987;5: 697–702.
53. Meyer JA, Comis RL, Ginsberg SJ, et al. Phase II trial of extended indications for resection is small cell carcinoma of the lung. *J Thorac Cardiovasc Surg* 1982;83: 12–19.
54. Shepherd FA, Ginsberg R, Patterson GA, et al. Is there ever a role for salvage operations in limited small-cell lung cancer? *J Thorac Cardiovasc Surg* 1991;101:196–200.
55. Schreiber D, Rineer J, Weedon J, et al. Survival outcomes with the use of surgery in limited-stage small cell lung cancer: should its role be re-evaluated? *Cancer* 2010;116: 1350–1357.
56. Yu JB, Decker RH, Detterbeck FC, et al. Surveillance epidemiology and end results evaluation of the role of surgery for stage I small cell lung cancer. *J Thorac Oncol* 2010;5:215–219.
57. Inoue M, Nakagawa K, Fujiwara K, et al. Results of preoperative mediastinoscopy for small cell lung cancer. *Ann Thorac Surg* 2010;70:1620–1623.
58. Socinski MA, Bogart JA. Limited-stage small-cell lung cancer: the current status of combined-modality therapy. *J Clin Oncol* 2007;25:4137–4145.
59. Gaspar LE, Gay EG, Crawford J, et al. Limited-stage small-cell lung cancer (stages I-III): observations from the National Cancer Data Base. *Clin Lung Cancer* 2005;6: 355–360.
60. Faivre-Finn C, Lorigan P, West C, et al. Thoracic radiation therapy for limited-stage small-cell lung cancer: unanswered questions. *Clin Lung Cancer* 2005;7:23–29.
61. Pignon JP, Arriagada R, Ihde DC, et al. A meta-analysis of thoracic radiotherapy for small-cell lung cancer. *N Engl J Med* 1992;327:1618–1624.
62. Warde P, Payne D. Does thoracic irradiation improve survival and local control in limited-stage small-cell carcinoma of the lung? A meta-analysis. *J Clin Oncol* 1992; 10:890–895.
63. Turrisi AT, 3rd, Kim K, Blum R, et al. Twice-daily compared with once-daily thoracic radiotherapy in limited small-cell lung cancer treated concurrently with cisplatin and etoposide. *N Engl J Med* 1999;340:265–271.
64. Mitsuoka S, Kudoh S, Takada Y, et al. Phase II study of cisplatin, etoposide and concurrent thoracic radiotherapy (TRT) followed by irinotecan and cisplatin in patients with limited stage small-cell lung cancer (SCLC); updated results of WJTOG9902. *J Clin Oncol* 2004;22(14 suppl):7044.
65. Salama JK, Hodgson L, Pang H, et al. A pooled analysis of limited-stage small-cell lung cancer patients treated with induction chemotherapy followed by concurrent platinum-based chemotherapy and 70 Gy daily radiotherapy: CALGB 30904. *J Thorac Oncol* 2013;8:1043–1049.
66. Schild SE, Bonner JA, Shanahan TG, et al. Long-term results of a phase III trial comparing once-daily radiotherapy with twice-daily radiotherapy in limited-stage small-cell lung cancer. *Int J Radiat Oncol Biol Phys* 2004;59:943–951.
67. Videtic GM, Fung K, Tomiak AT, et al. Using treatment interruptions to palliate the toxicity from concurrent chemoradiation for limited small cell lung cancer decreases survival and disease control. *Lung Cancer* 2001;33:249–258.
68. Schild SE, Bonner JA, Hillman S, et al. Results of a phase II study of high-dose thoracic radiation therapy with concurrent cisplatin and etoposide in limited-stage small-cell lung cancer (NCCTG 95-20-53). *J Clin Oncol* 2007;25:3124–3129.
69. De Ruysscher D, Pijls-Johannesma M, Vansteenkiste J, et al. Systematic review and meta-analysis of randomised, controlled trials of the timing of chest radiotherapy in patients with limited-stage, small-cell lung cancer. *Ann Oncol* 2006;17:543–552.
70. Fried DB, Morris DE, Poole C, et al. Systematic review evaluating the timing of thoracic radiation therapy in combined modality therapy for limited-stage small-cell lung cancer. *J Clin Oncol* 2004;22:4837–4845.
71. Huncharek M, McGarry R. A meta-analysis of the timing of chest irradiation in the combined modality treatment of limited-stage small cell lung cancer. *Oncologist* 2004;9:665–672.
72. Pijls-Johannesma M, De Ruysscher D, Vansteenkiste J, et al. Timing of chest radiotherapy in patients with limited stage small cell lung cancer: a systematic review and meta-analysis of randomised controlled trials. *Cancer Treat Rev* 2007;33:461–473.
73. Spiro SG, James LE, Rudd RM, et al. Early compared with late radiotherapy in combined modality treatment for limited disease small-cell lung cancer: a London Lung Cancer Group multicenter randomized clinical trial and meta-analysis. *J Clin Oncol* 2006;24:3823–3830.
74. De Ruysscher D, Pijls-Johannesma M, Bentzen SM, et al. Time between the first day of chemotherapy and the last day of chest radiation is the most important predictor of survival in limited-disease small-cell lung cancer. *J Clin Oncol* 2006;24:1057–1063.
75. Bremnes RM, Sundstrom S, Vilsvik J, et al. Norwegian Lung Cancer Study G. Multicenter phase II trial of paclitaxel, cisplatin, and etoposide with concurrent radiation for limited-stage small-cell lung cancer. *J Clin Oncol* 2001;19:3532–3538.
76. Hanna N, Bunn PA, Jr., Langer C, et al. Randomized phase III trial comparing irinotecan/cisplatin with etoposide/cisplatin in patients with previously untreated extensive-stage disease small-cell lung cancer. *J Clin Oncol* 2006;24:2038–2043.
77. Kubota K, Nishiwaki Y, Sugiura T, et al. Pilot study of concurrent etoposide and cisplatin plus accelerated hyperfractionated thoracic radiotherapy followed by irinotecan and cisplatin for limited-stage small cell lung cancer: Japan Clinical Oncology Group 9903. *Clin Cancer Res* 2005;11:5534–5538.
78. Levitan N, Dowlati A, Shina D, et al. Multi-institutional phase I/II trial of paclitaxel, cisplatin, and etoposide with concurrent radiation for limited-stage small-cell lung carcinoma. *J Clin Oncol* 2001;18:1102–1109.
79. Michael M, Babic B, Khokha R, et al. Expression and prognostic significance of metalloproteinases and their tissue inhibitors in patients with small-cell lung cancer. *J Clin Oncol* 1999;17:1802–1808.
80. Noda K, Nishiwaki Y, Kawahara M, et al. Irinotecan plus cisplatin compared with etoposide plus cisplatin for extensive small-cell lung cancer. *N Engl J Med* 2002; 346:85–91.
81. Rigas J, Denham CA, Rinaldi D, et al. Randomized placebo-controlled trials of the matrix metalloproteinase inhibitor (MMPI), BAY12-9566 as adjuvant therapy for patients with small cell and non-small cell lung cancer. *Proc Am Soc Clin Oncol* 2003;22:525.
82. Shepherd FA, Giaccone G, Seymour L, et al. Prospective, randomized, double-blind, placebo-controlled trial of marimastat after response to first-line chemotherapy in patients with small-cell lung cancer: a trial of the National Cancer Institute of Canada-Clinical Trials Group and the European Organization for Research and Treatment of Cancer. *J Clin Oncol* 2002;20:4434–4439.
83. Kubota K, Hida T, Ishikura S, et al. Etoposide and cisplatin versus irinotecan and cisplatin in patients with limited-stage small-cell lung cancer treated with etoposide and cisplatin plus concurrent accelerated hyperfractionated thoracic radiotherapy (JCOG0202): a randomised phase 3 study. *Lancet Oncol* 2014;15:106–113.
84. Le QT, Moon J, Redman M, et al. Phase II study of tirapazamine, cisplatin, and etoposide and concurrent thoracic radiotherapy for limited-stage small-cell lung cancer: SWOG 0222. *J Clin Oncol* 2009;27:3014–3019.
85. Giaccone G, Debruyne C, Felip E, et al. Phase III study of adjuvant vaccination with Bec2/bacille Calmette-Guerin in responding patients with limited-disease small-cell lung cancer (European Organisation for Research and Treatment of Cancer 08971-08971B; Silva Study). *J Clin Oncol* 2005;23:6854–6864.

86. Arnold AM, Seymour L, Smylie M, et al. Phase II study of vandetanib or placebo in small-cell lung cancer patients after complete or partial response to induction chemotherapy with or without radiation therapy: National Cancer Institute of Canada Clinical Trials Group Study BR.20. *J Clin Oncol* 2007;25:4278–4284.

87. https://www.gene.com/download/pdf/avastin_te_letter.pdf

88. Baas P, Belderbos JS, Senan S, et al. Concurrent chemotherapy (carboplatin, paclitaxel, etoposide) and involved-field radiotherapy in limited stage small cell lung cancer: a Dutch multicenter phase II study. *Br J Cancer* 2006;94:625–630.

89. Spigel D, Hainsworth J, Burris HA, 3rd, et al. Long-term follow-up of limited stage small cell lung cancer patients treated with carboplatin-based chemotherapy and radiotherapy by the Minnie Pearl Cancer Research Network (MPCRN). *J Clin Oncol* 2004;22(14 suppl):7222.

90. Sunpaweravong P, Magree L, Rabinovitch R, et al. A phase I/II study of docetaxel, etoposide, and carboplatin before concurrent chemoradiotherapy with cisplatin and etoposide in limited-stage small cell lung cancer. *Invest New Drugs* 2006;24:213–221.

91. Kim E, Biswas T, Koroukian SM, et al. Comparison of cisplatin-versus carboplatin-based concurrent chemoradiation for limited-stage small cell lung cancer using SEER-Medicare data. *J Clin Oncol* 2014;32:5s (suppl; abstr 7596).

92. El Maalouf G, Rodier JM, Faivre S, et al. Could we expect to improve survival in small cell lung cancer? *Lung Cancer* 2007;57(Suppl 2):S30–S34.

93. Evans WK, Feld R, Osoba D, et al. VP-16 alone and in combination with cisplatin in previously treated patients with small cell lung cancer. *Cancer* 1984;53:1461–1466.

94. Roth BJ, Johnson DH, Einhorn LH, et al. Randomized study of cyclophosphamide, doxorubicin, and vincristine versus etoposide and cisplatin versus alternation of these two regimens in extensive small-cell lung cancer: a phase III trial of the Southeastern Cancer Study Group. *J Clin Oncol* 1992;10:282–291.

95. Ardizzoni A, Tjan-Heijnen VC, Postmus PE, et al. Standard versus intensified chemotherapy with granulocyte colony-stimulating factor support in small-cell lung cancer: a prospective European Organization for Research and Treatment of Cancer-Lung Cancer Group Phase III Trial-08923. *J Clin Oncol* 2002;20:3947–3955.

96. Giaccone G, Dalesio O, McVie GJ, et al. Maintenance chemotherapy in small-cell lung cancer: long-term results of a randomized trial. European Organization for Research and Treatment of Cancer Lung Cancer Cooperative Group. *J Clin Oncol* 1993;11:1230–1240.

97. Gregor A, Drings P, Burghouts J, et al. Randomized trial of alternating versus sequential radiotherapy/chemotherapy in limited-disease patients with small-cell lung cancer: a European Organization for Research and Treatment of Cancer Lung Cancer Cooperative Group Study. *J Clin Oncol* 1997;15:2840–2849.

98. Skarlos DV, Samantas E, Kosmidis P, et al. Randomized comparison of etoposide-cisplatin vs. etoposide-carboplatin and irradiation in small-cell lung cancer. A Hellenic Co-operative Oncology Group study. *Ann Oncol* 1994;5:601–607.

99. Eckardt JR, von Pawel J, Papai Z, et al. Open-label, multicenter, randomized, phase III study comparing oral topotecan/cisplatin versus etoposide/cisplatin as treatment for chemotherapy-naive patients with extensive-disease small-cell lung cancer. *J Clin Oncol* 2006;24:2044–2051.

100. Eckardt JR, von Pawel J, Pujol JL, et al. Phase III study of oral compared with intravenous topotecan as second-line therapy in small-cell lung cancer. *J Clin Oncol* 2007;25:2086–2092.

101. Hermes A, Bergman B, Bremnes RM, et al. A randomized phase III trial of irinotecan plus carboplatin versus etoposide plus carboplatin in patients with small cell lung cancer, extensive disease (SCLC-ED): IRIS Study. *J Clin Oncol* 2007;25(18S):abstract 7523.

102. O'Brien ME, Ciuleanu TE, Tsekov H, et al. Phase III trial comparing supportive care alone with supportive care with oral topotecan in patients with relapsed small-cell lung cancer. *J Clin Oncol* 2006;24:5441–5447.

103. Pujol JL, Breton JL, Gervais R, et al. A prospective randomized phase III, double-blind, placebo-controlled study of thalidomide in extended-disease (ED) SCLC patients after response to chemotherapy (CT): an intergroup study FNCLCC Cleo04-IFCT 00-01. *J Clin Oncol* 2006;24(18S):abstract 7057.

104. Siow-Ming L, Woll PJ, James LE, et al. A phase III randomised, double blind, placebo controlled trial of etoposide/carboplatin with or without thalidomide in advanced SCLC. *J Clin Oncol* 2007;2(S Suppl 4): abstract PRS-04.

105. Socinski MA, Weissman C, Hart LL, et al. Randomized phase II trial of pemetrexed combined with either cisplatin or carboplatin in untreated extensive-stage small-cell lung cancer. *J Clin Oncol* 2006;24:4840–4847.

106. von Pawel J, Schiller JH, Shepherd FA, et al. Topotecan versus cyclophosphamide, doxorubicin, and vincristine for the treatment of recurrent small-cell lung cancer. *J Clin Oncol* 1999;17:658–667.

107. Lara PN, Jr., Natale R, Crowley J, et al. Phase III trial of irinotecan/cisplatin compared with etoposide/cisplatin in extensive-stage small-cell lung cancer: clinical and pharmacogenomic results from SWOG S0124. *J Clin Oncol* 2009;27:2530–2535.

108. Satouchi M, Kotani Y, Shibata T, et al. Phase III study comparing amrubicin plus cisplatin with irinotecan plus cisplatin in the treatment of extensive-disease small-cell lung cancer: JCOG 0509. *J Clin Oncol* 2014;32:1262–1268.

109. Schiller JH, Adak S, Cella D, et al. Topotecan versus observation after cisplatin plus etoposide in extensive-stage small-cell lung cancer: E7593–a phase III trial of the Eastern Cooperative Oncology Group. *J Clin Oncol* 2001;19:2114–2122.

110. Ready NE, Pang HH, Gu L, et al. Chemotherapy with or without maintenance sunitinib for untreated extensive-stage small-cell lung cancer: A randomized, double-blind, placebo-controlled phase II study-CALGB 30504 (Alliance). *J Clin Oncol* 2015;33:1660–1665.

111. Slotman B, Faivre-Finn C, Kramer G, et al. Prophylactic cranial irradiation in extensive small-cell lung cancer. *N Engl J Med* 2007;357:664–672.

112. Jeremic B, Shibamoto Y, Nikolic N, et al. Role of radiation therapy in the combined-modality treatment of patients with extensive disease small-cell lung cancer: A randomized study. *J Clin Oncol* 1999;17:2092–2099.

113. Slotman BJ, van Tinteren H, Praag JO, et al. Use of thoracic radiotherapy for extensive stage small-cell lung cancer: a phase 3 randomised controlled trial. *Lancet* 2015;385: 36–42.

114. von Pawel J, Jotte R, Spigel DR, et al. Randomized phase III trial of amrubicin versus topotecan as second-line treatment for patients with small-cell lung cancer. *J Clin Oncol* 2014;32:4012–4019.

115. Ott PA, Elez Fernandez ME, Hiret S, et al. Pembrolizumab (MK-3475) in patients (pts) with extensive small-cell lung cancer (SCLC): Preliminary safety and efficacy results from KEYNOTE-028. *J Clin Oncol* 2015;33(suppl): abstr 7502.

116. Antonia S, Bendell JC, Taylor MH, et al. Phase I/II study of nivolumab with or without ipilimumab for treatment of recurrent small cell lung cancer (SCLC): CA209-032. *J Clin Oncol* 2015;33(suppl; abstr 7503).

117. Sandler A, Szwaric S, Dowlati A, et al. A phase II study of cisplatin (P) plus etoposide (E) plus bevacizumab (B) for previously untreated extensive stage small cell lung cancer (SCLC) (E3501): A trial of the Eastern Oncology Group. *J Clin Oncol* 2011;25(18S):abstract 7564.

118. Ready NE, Dudek AZ, Pang HH, et al. Cisplatin, irinotecan, and bevacizumab for untreated extensive-stage small-cell lung cancer: CALGB 30306, a phase II study. *J Clin Oncol* 2011;29:4436–4441.

119. Spigel DR, Greco FA, Zubkus JD, et al. Phase II trial of irinotecan, carboplatin, and bevacizumab in the treatment of patients with extensive-stage small-cell lung cancer. *J Thorac Oncol* 2009;4:1555–1560.

120. Spigel DR, Townley PM, Waterhouse DM, et al. Randomized phase II study of bevacizumab in combination with chemotherapy in previously untreated extensive-stage small-cell lung cancer: results from the SALUTE trial. *J Clin Oncol* 2011;29:2215–2222.

121. Pujol JL, Lavole A, Quoix E, et al. Randomized phase II-III study of bevacizumab in combination with chemotherapy in previously untreated extensive small-cell lung cancer: results from the IFCT-0802 trial†. *Ann Oncol* 2015;26:908–914.

122. Targeted therapies: Alisertib tested in patients with solid tumours. *Nat Rev Clin Oncol* 2015;12:312.

123. Melichar B, Adenis A, Lockhart AC, et al. Safety and activity of alisertib, an investigational aurora kinase A inhibitor, in patients with breast cancer, small-cell lung cancer, non-small-cell lung cancer, head and neck squamous-cell carcinoma, and gastro-oesophageal adenocarcinoma: a five-arm phase 2 study. *Lancet Oncol* 2015;16:395–405.

124. Byers LA, Wang J, Nilsson MB, et al. Proteomic profiling identifies dysregulated pathways in small cell lung cancer and novel therapeutic targets including PARP1. *Cancer Discov* 2012;2:798–811.

125. Wainberg ZA, Rafii S, Ramanathan RK, et al. Safety and antitumor activity of the PARP inhibitor BMN673 in a phase 1 trial recruiting metastatic small-cell lung cancer (SCLC) and germline BRCA-mutation carrier cancer patients. *J Clin Oncol* 2014;32(5S):(suppl; abstr 7522).

126. Viani GA, Boin AC, Ikeda VY, et al. Thirty years of prophylactic cranial irradiation in patients with small cell lung cancer: a meta-analysis of randomized clinical trials. *J Bras Pneumol* 2012;38:372–381.

127. https://deainfo.nci.nih.gov/advisory/ctac/workgroup/SCLC/SCLC%20Congressional%20Response.pdf

128. Ettinger DS, Berkey BA, Abrams RA, et al. Radiation Therapy Oncology Group 9609. Study of paclitaxel, etoposide, and cisplatin chemotherapy combined with twice-daily thoracic radiotherapy for patients with limited-stage small-cell lung cancer: A Radiation Therapy Oncology Group 9609 phase II study. *J Clin Oncol* 2005;23(22):4991–4998.

129. Glisson B, Scott C, Komaki R, et al. Cisplatin, ifosfamide, oral etoposide, and concurrent accelerated hyperfractionated thoracic radiation for patients with limited small-cell lung carcinoma: results of radiation therapy oncology group trial 93-12. *J Clin Oncol* 2000;18(16):2990–2995.

130. Bogart JA, Herndon II JE, Lyss AP, et al. 70 Gy thoracic radiotherapy is feasible concurrent with chemotherapy for limited-stage small-cell lung cancer: Analysis of Cancer and Leukemia Group B study 39808. *Int J Radiat Oncol Biol Phys* 2004;59(2):460–468.

131. Woo IS, Park YS, Kwon SH, et al. A phase II study of VP-16-fosfamide-cisplatin combination chemotherapy plus early concurrent thoracic irradiation for previously untreated limited small cell lung cancer. *Jpn J Clin Oncol* 2000;30(12):542–546.

OTHER TUMORS OF THE LUNG

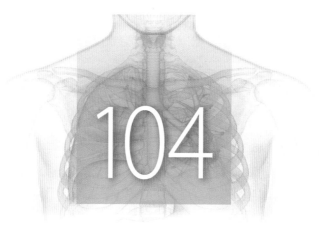

104

Carcinoid Tumors

Joanna Sesti ▪ Jessica S. Donington

HISTORY

The recognition of the neuroendocrine basis of bronchopulmonary neuroendocrine tumors (BPNETs) is credited to Friedrich Feyrter, who was the first to describe a diffuse syncytium of neuroendocrine cells distributed through the body, including the lungs. For many years the distinction between small cell carcinomas and carcinoids, which were thought to be benign, remained controversial. Throughout the 1960s to 1970s, advances in histopathology allowed scientists to clarify the notion of well-differentiated carcinoid tumors representing one end of the spectrum with typical small cell carcinomas at the other.[1] In 1972, Arrigoni et al.[2] published an article describing a new subgroup termed *atypical* carcinoids, which overall had more malignant features than well-differentiated carcinoids. It was thought that *atypical* carcinoids represented the link between the two ends of the spectrum; this notion became widely accepted in the 1980s.[1]

CLASSIFICATION

In 1977, Gould[3] proposed a new classification system for BPNETs, which advocated doing away with the term bronchial adenoma, since it did not adequately represent the malignant nature of all carcinoid tumors. This classification system would undergo multiple revisions until in 1998. Travis and colleagues[4,5] sought to simplify the field by grouping all BPNETs into four categories: *typical carcinoids, atypical carcinoids, large cell neuroendocrine tumors, and small cell neuroendocrine tumors*. Nevertheless, the definitive classification scheme was not formalized until 2004 when the World Health Organization (WHO)

defined a system that allowed pathologists around the world to define BPNETs uniformly (Table 104.1).[6] This system redefined the cutoff of atypical carcinoids from 2 to 5 mitoses/2 mm^2 to 2 to 10 mitoses/ 2 mm^2 (10 HPFs), and included necrosis or architectural disruption. This change yielded a classification system with better prognostic significance by reassigning approximately 30% of carcinoid tumors, and

TABLE 104.1 World Health Organization Classification Systems of Pulmonary Neuroendocrine Tumors[7,8]

Tumor Type	Criteria
Typical carcinoid	NE features <2 mitoses/2 mm^2 hotspot no evidence of necrosis
Atypical carcinoid	NE features 2–10 mitoses/2 mm^2 hotspot evidence of necrosis or architectural disruption
Large cell	NE features >10 mitoses/2 mm^2 hotspot Large zones of necrosis Cells arranged in organoid nests with peripheral palisading Large tumor cells with distinct nuclei, and strong chromogranin staining
Small cell	NE features >10 mitoses/2 mm^2 Small tumor cells with scant cytoplasm Dense, hyperchromatic, granular chromatin Nucleoli are absent or inconspicuous

NE, neuroendocrine.

as a result improved survival for both typical carcinoids and atypical carcinoids (10-year survival of 87% vs. 73% for typical carcinoids and 35% vs. 9% for atypical carcinoids).[7]

In the recently published 2015 edition of the WHO Classification of Lung tumors[9] further refinements to the neuroendocrine tumor classifications were made. There was increased attention to the role of immunohistochemistry (IHC) in diagnosis, especially related to small biopsy specimens.[10] Ki-67 (the product of *MK167* gene mapping to 10q26.2 gene involved in cell proliferation) which is expressed as a labeling index (percent of positive tumor cells) is used primarily to help separate high-grade neuroendocrine tumors (large cell neuroendocrine and small cell neuroendocrine) from bronchopulmonary carcinoids, but is not recommended as a means for differentiating typical carcinoids and atypical carcinoids. The Ki-67 expression index for small cell neuroendocrine tumors are usually >50%, while that for large cell neuroendocrine are approximately 40% (range 25% to 52%), <20% in atypical carcinoids, and <2% in typical carcinoids. The 2015 WHO classification also placed increased specification on the process for counting mitosis, due to the recognition that it is the most important criteria for separating typical carcinoids and atypical carcinoids, and for separating these from small cell and large cell neuroendocrine tumors.[11] It is now specified that mitosis should be counted in "hotspots," the areas of highest activity and in 2 mm^2 area rather than 10 HPFs. In tumors that are near the cutoffs of 2 or 20 mitosis per 2 mm^2, at least three 2 mm^2 areas should be counted and the mean used for determining mitotic rate.[10] They also specified that mitotic rate and necrosis status should be included in pathology reports.

CLINICAL PRESENTATION

Demographics

Small cell neuroendocrine tumors are the most common BPNET, representing approximately 14% of lung cancers.[12] Large cell neuroendocrine tumors account for approximately 3% of lung cancers, and carcinoid tumors 1% to 2%. Atypical carcinoids are the rarest accounting for 0.1% to 0.2% of all lung cancers.[13] In general, patients with carcinoid tumors tend to be younger with a median age of 48 years.[14,15] There is a bimodal distribution with peaks at approximately 35 and 55 years of age, the significance of which is that younger patients are unlikely to present with atypical carcinoids (<10% in patients <30 years of age) (Fig. 104.1).[16–18]

Carcinoids are evenly spread between men and women, with an average incidence of 50% in women (46% to 58%) across various studies.[15,19–26] No association exists between smoking and typical carcinoid tumors. Although some evidence suggest a link between smoking and the incidence of atypical carcinoids,[25,27,28] other

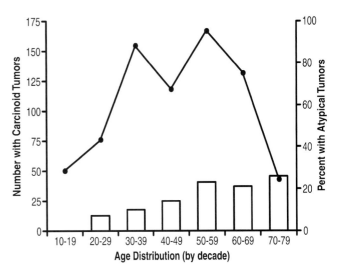

FIGURE 104.1 Age distribution of patients with bronchial carcinoid tumors (*line graph*) and percentage of carcinoid tumors that are atypical by decades of age (*bar graph*). Data is based on reports using the old (1972) classification system.[3] (From Kiser AC, Detterbeck FC. Carcinoid and mucoepidermoid tumors. In Detterbeck FC, Rivera MP, Socinski MA, et al., eds. *Diagnosis and Treatment of Lung Cancer: An Evidence-Based Guide for the Practicing Clinician.* Philadelphia, PA: Saunders; 2001:379–393. Copyright © 2001 Elsevier. With permission.)

studies show a similar proportion of smokers to that of the general population.[18,22,29–32]

Symptoms

Approximately half of patients with BPNETs are asymptomatic. In those patients with symptoms, cough, recurrent pneumonia, and hemoptysis represent the overwhelming complaints (Table 104.2). Central carcinoids often present with symptoms related to obstruction like obstructive pneumonia, wheezing, and hemoptysis. Peripheral carcinoids lack the inherent obstructive characteristics of central carcinoids and as a result are usually discovered incidentally in asymptomatic patients.[33] Due to the large proportion of young and never smoking patients and patients with no symptoms or nonspecific symptoms, diagnosis of carcinoids can be delayed. While older series report low rates of diagnosis within 1 year,[34] one could speculate that with the recent approval of low dose CT for lung cancer screening, these numbers would improve.

Paraneoplastic Syndromes

Carcinoid syndrome is characterized by episodic flushing and diarrhea. Carcinoid syndrome occurs in approximately 2% to 7% of thoracic neuroendocrine tumors, but only 1% to 3% of bronchopulmonary

TABLE 104.2 Symptoms Associated With Bronchopulmonary Carcinoid Tumors

Study	Asymptomatic (%)	Recurrent Pneumonia (%)	Cough (%)	Hemoptysis (%)	Pain (%)	Dyspnea (%)	Wheezing (%)
Filosso et al.[35]	48	17	21	21	11	1	1
Ducrocq et al.[36]	27	29	10	24	1	1	1
Fink et al.[27]	30	41	35	23	—	—	—
Rea et al.[23]	16	29	17	14	3	2	—

carcinoids. This is a much lower rate than mid-gut carcinoids, a result of the fact that bronchopulmonary carcinoids have decreased serotonin production.[37] An elevated level of urinary 5-hydroxyindoleacetic acid (5-HIAA) is commonly found in patients with symptoms.[21,38] Secondary to the high levels of monoamine oxidase in pulmonary tissue, carcinoid syndrome is almost exclusively seen in the setting of liver metastasis.[27,39] Interestingly, although true carcinoid syndrome is rare, milder forms, seen more frequently with isolated symptoms of flushing and diarrhea are more frequent with one study of 126 patients showing rates of 12% and 10%, respectively.[40] Right-sided valvular disease has been noted rarely with pulmonary carcinoid tumors.[39] Carcinoid crisis, a life-threatening complication of carcinoid syndrome, manifested by flushing, confusion, coma, and either hypotension or hypertension can be precipitated by diagnostic or therapeutic interventions, including initiation of chemotherapy.[38]

Cushing syndrome is also reported with pulmonary neuroendocrine tumors. The evaluation of Cushing syndrome requires three major steps: (1) confirmation of high cortisol levels, (2) differentiation between adrenal or ectopic sources, and (3) identifying the potential ectopic source (pituitary vs. others).[37] Some of the more common ectopic sources of Cushing syndrome include the pituitary gland small cell neuroendocrine bronchopulmonary carcinoid tumors, thymus, gastrointestinal tract pheochromocytomas, and, medullary thyroid carcinoma.[37] Most common symptoms of Cushing syndrome include: increase in body weight (70%), hypertension (78%), menstrual irregularities or amenorrhea (78%), hirsutism (75%), osteopenia/osteoporosis (75%), and hypokalemia (71%).[41] Pulmonary neuroendocrine tumors are a common source of Cushing syndrome, but is only reported in a small percent of patients with pulmonary neuroendocrine tumors. In a series of 90 patients at the National Institute of Health, bronchopulmonary carcinoids were the underlying etiology of Cushing syndrome in approximately 38%.[41] On the other hand, in a series of patients with bronchopulmonary carcinoids, Cushing syndrome was present in 1% to 6% of patients.[15,21,36,38,42] CT and MRI are able to localize the pulmonary source in the majority of patients, and so are required in patients diagnosed with Cushing syndrome.[41,42]

Other syndromes associated with bronchopulmonary carcinoid tumors which have been reported include acromegaly (excessive growth hormone),[15,38] and hyperparathyroidism (parathyroid hormone).[43]

Tumor Location

The anatomic distribution of typical or atypical carcinoids is slightly different with approximately 85% of typical carcinoids occupying a central location (typically defined as visible by bronchoscopy) versus only 15% of atypical carcinoids (Table 104.3).[15,23,32] As far as the bronchial distribution of both central typical carcinoids and atypical carcinoids, approximately 75% are found within lobar or segmental bronchi. Main bronchus and tracheal carcinoids are less common (right main stem: 6%, left main stem: 8%, tracheal 0.7%).[14]

TABLE 104.3 Peripheral Versus Central Distribution of Typical and Atypical Carcinoid Tumors

Study	Central			Peripheral		
	N	TC %	AC %	N	TC %	AC %
Garcia-Yuste et al.[15]	439	88	12	222	82	18
Rea et al.[23]	195	75	25	57	49	51
Daddi et al.[32]	44	93	7	43	88	12

N, number; TC, typical carcinoid; AC, atypical carcinoid.

DIAGNOSTIC TESTS AND STAGING

Chest X-Ray

Chest x-rays are not particularly sensitive or specific for bronchopulmonary carcinoid tumors. Evidence of atelectasis, a central mass, or a peripheral mass is appreciated in 40%, 25%, and 30% of patients, respectively.[44] There is no way to distinguish between atypical carcinoids and typical carcinoids on chest x-ray. All in all, chest x-ray does not form an essential part in the diagnostic workup of carcinoid tumors.

Computed Tomography

Radiographically, peripheral carcinoids are typically homogenous, round, and sharply demarcated masses, which is in stark contrast to primary lung malignancies that present as spiculated or ground glass lesions, but not unique enough to differentiate from other benign lesions. Central lesions are often associated with atelectasis and postobstructive pneumonitis. Carcinoids tend to have indolent growth patterns, which makes examination of old films important. Although, CT cannot reliably distinguish between typical carcinoids and atypical carcinoids, the importance of CT evaluation resides in the ability to appreciate extrabronchial involvement of central carcinoids, and define the relationship of the tumor to nearby vessels with the use of intravenous contrast.

Although little data exists looking at the ability of CT alone to predict lymph node involvement in a bronchopulmonary carcinoid, one study by Chughtai et al.[45] of 40 patients documented a sensitivity of 67%, specificity of 97%, false negative rate of 6%, and a false positive rate of 20%. Data from NSCLC studies suggest a false negative rate between 20% and 25% in central tumors and those with N1 enlargement (>1 cm); on the other hand, peripheral cN0 tumors have much lower false negative rates (<10%). As a result, current guidelines recommend mediastinal lymph node evaluation in patients with large, central tumors, and in patients with enlarged hilar or mediastinal lymph nodes.

^{18}F Fluorodeoxyglucose Positron Emission Tomography

^{18}F Fluorodeoxyglucose (FDG) is a glucose analogue that is useful in detecting malignancy because it is taken up by cells with high glucose metabolism. As a result, tumors with high proliferative indices can be identified, while those that are slow growing are more difficult to discern. The indolent nature of carcinoids, especially typical carcinoids, has made the use of ^{18}F FDG positron emission tomography (PET) somewhat controversial. While original studies suggested low detection rates for both typical or atypical carcinoids, subsequent studies have challenged this notion.[46] Table 104.4 lists recent studies which have shown high levels of detection, specifically with a SUVmax cutoff level of 1.5 and 2.5. Due to the more aggressive nature of atypical carcinoids, one could assume a higher level of sensitivity of PET CT versus typical carcinoids.[47–53] Finally, SUVmax values have been linked to survival in both typical carcinoids and atypical carcinoids; nevertheless, the exact relationship needs further investigation.[47,51]

^{68}Ga DOTA-Peptides Positron Emission Tomography

Somatostatin is a peptide hormone that functions in cell proliferation through its interaction with G-protein-coupled somatostatin receptors (SSTRs). Pulmonary neuroendocrine tumors have been shown to have a high density of SSTRs, which correlates with the degree of tumor differentiation (typical carcinoids have the highest level of expression).[54] Tracers like ^{68}Ga DOTA-peptides, have allowed imaging

TABLE 104.4 ^{18}F FDG PET Scan in the Evaluation of Bronchopulmonary Carcinoid Tumors

Author	Year	N Typical	N Atypical	Average Peak SUV	Detection Rate (%) SUV ≥ 2.5	Detection Rate (%) SUV ≥ 1.5
Wartski et al.[53]	2004	1	1	7.7	100	100
Kruger et al.[51]	2006	12	1	3.1	60	93
Daniels et al.[48]	2007	11	5	N/R	75	N/R
Chong et al.[47]	2007	2	5	4.0	85	100
Kayani et al.[50]	2009	11	2	3.0	80	100
Jindal et al.[49]	2011	13	7	4.8	70	75
Stefani et al.[52]	2013	24	7	6.6	52	96
Overall		74	22	4.8	74	94

N, number; SUV, standard uptake value.

of the SSTRs using PET scanners. Although different ^{68}Ga DOTA-peptides have variable affinities for different SSTRs, a clinical application has not been identified yet.[54] One of the major advantages of ^{68}Ga DOTA-peptides over ^{18}F FDG is that it is not dependent on the metabolic activity of the cells. As the previous section highlighted, bronchopulmonary carcinoids are indolent tumors and tend to have lower metabolic activity, which hinders the diagnostic potential of ^{18}F FDG PET/CT. Finally, ^{68}Ga DOTA-peptides PET/CT has superior resolution and localization abilities compared to 111 (^{111}In) pentetreotide receptor scintigraphy (otherwise known as a somatostatin scan).[50] Table 104.5 summarizes some of the literature evaluating its use in bronchopulmonary carcinoids.[49,50,55,56] In select studies, ^{68}Ga DOTA-peptides PET/CT has demonstrated a higher level of sensitivity than either somatostatin scans or of ^{18}F FDG PET/CT.[57,58] Further analysis is needed to define the role of this promising study in the diagnosis and staging of bronchopulmonary carcinoids.

The combined use of ^{68}Ga DOTA-peptides PET/CT and ^{18}F FDG PET/CT has been explored. Kumar and colleagues[55] found that typical carcinoids had slight ^{18}F FDG and high ^{68}Ga DOTA uptake, while atypical carcinoids had moderate ^{18}F FDG and high ^{68}Ga DOTA uptake. Jindal et al.[49] showed higher ^{68}Ga DOTA uptake in typical carcinoids and higher ^{18}F FDG uptake in atypical carcinoids. Overall, the most common pattern of dual uptake for dual-tracer PET/CT is a high ^{68}Ga DOTA and low ^{18}F FDG for typical carcinoids, and low or moderate ^{68}Ga DOTA and high ^{18}F FDG uptake for atypical carcinoids.[54]

Octreotide Scan

Although commonly used in the evaluation of abdominal carcinoids, only two-thirds of bronchopulmonary carcinoids are SSTR-positive.[59]

TABLE 104.5 ^{68}Ga DOTA-peptides PET Scan in the Evaluation of Bronchopulmonary Carcinoid Tumors

Author	Year	N Typical	N Atypical	Detection Rate (%)
Kumar et al.[55]	2009	3		100
Kayani et al.[50]	2009	11	2	100
Jindal et al.[49]	2011	13	7	95
Venkitaraman et al.[56]	2014	21	5	96
Total/Average		48	14	97

Further complicating its routine use in bronchopulmonary carcinoids, octreotide scans have been found to be positive in the vast majority of NSCLC and SCLC as well as in patients with pneumonia, sarcoidosis, granuloma, and lymphoma.[59,60] Few studies have documented sensitivity for primary bronchopulmonary carcinoid tumors of 81% to 100% and a false positive rate of 19%.[59,61,62] As far as its ability to detect lymph node involvement, octreotide scans have a sensitivity of 88% to 100% and a false negative rate of 22%.[59,62]

Endobronchial Biopsy

Bronchoscopy is the primary diagnostic test for patients with suspected bronchopulmonary carcinoids. The typical description of a carcinoid tumor is a smooth, rounded, and reddish-brown lesion often covered by bronchial mucosa (Fig. 104.2). Although, endobronchial biopsy of bronchopulmonary carcinoid tumors has been discouraged in the past due to concerns for uncontrollable hemorrhage, several studies have shown it to be a safe procedure with a risk profile similar to other bronchoscopic procedures. Table 104.6 summarizes the incidence of minor and major bleeding during endobronchial biopsy of suspected carcinoid tumors in several studies.[16,17,20,23,27,28,35,36,63–66] The data suggests that bronchoscopic biopsy of carcinoid tumors does not carry an increased risk of significant bleeding as once was thought.

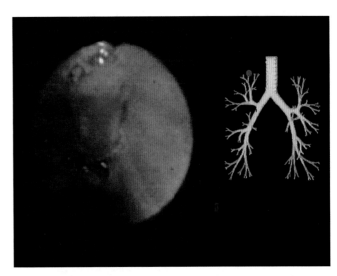

FIGURE 104.2 Bronchoscopic image of typical carcinoid protruding from right upper lobe bronchus.

TABLE 104.6 Results of Endobronchial Biopsy in Patients With Bronchopulmonary Carcinoid Tumors

Study	N	# Biopsies	Bleeding Events	Major Bleeding Events[a]
Rea et al.[23]	252	195	0	0
Cardillo et al.[63]	163	89	0	0
Fink et al.[27]	142	72	0	0
Ducrocq et al.[36]	139	102	2	0
Filosso et al.[35]	126	75	0	0
McCaughn et al.[28]	12	25	3	0
Bertelsen et al.[16]	82	60	2	0
Hurt and Bates[17]	79	61	2	0
Marty-Ané et al.[64]	79	37	0	0
Francioni et al.[65]	69	48	4	0
Todd et al.[66]	69	23	6	0
Stamatis et al.[20]	227	190	—	4
Total	1,439	977	19 (1.9%)	4 (0.3%)

[a]Major bleeding events defined as patients who required operative treatment or blood products.
N, number of patients.

The diagnostic ability of endobronchial biopsy is between 70% and 80% in patients whom adequate biopsies were obtained.[16,17,20,23,27,28,35,36,63–66] In addition, the ability to determine the correct subtype per the WHO guidelines (atypical vs. typical carcinoids) requires a fairly large piece of well-preserved tumor (2 mm²). For this reason, it is not surprising that identification of the correct subtype with endobronchial biopsy occurs only 40% to 50% of the time.[35,64,67] In general, endobronchial biopsy of pulmonary bronchial tumors is safe and yields a reasonable number of diagnoses despite its limitations in establishing the correct subtype.

Transthoracic Biopsy

Transthoracic needle biopsy (TTNB) is usually reserved for peripheral tumors. Unfortunately, the same issue which limits the diagnostic potential of endobronchial biopsy (the large amount of tissue necessary to generate a clear diagnosis) also affects TTNB. The ability to identify a carcinoid tumor by TTNB is approximately 40% (23% to 80%).[25,27,45,63,68] Even more concerning, the ability to distinguish the carcinoid subtype is 10% to 20% lower.[25,68] In conclusion, although in some cases TTNB may be diagnostic, a negative result is not particularly helpful.

EVALUATION OF PATIENTS

General

Endobronchial tumors in lobar or segmental bronchi in young patients (<40 years of age) have a very high likelihood of being carcinoid tumors. Other possibilities include squamous cell carcinoma, which are uncommon in young patients; adenoid cystic carcinomas, which are commonly found in the trachea; and finally, mucoepidermoid tumors, which have similar presentations but management is quite similar. For this reason, diagnosis of central carcinoids can be made without a biopsy.

Peripheral carcinoids tend to be round and sharply demarcated. Their slow growth and no- or low-level FDG avidity helps to distinguish them from other lung tumors. The vast majority of intrathoracic

carcinoids are primary bronchopulmonary tumors. A solitary pulmonary metastasis from an extrathoracic source is very rare, especially in the absence of liver involvement, and so there is no need to search for an extrathoracic primary site.

Determining the histologic subtype is important since the evaluation and treatment is different between atypical carcinoids and typical carcinoids. Parameters such as age, central versus peripheral location, and nodal status can be used to predict the histologic subtype. Typical carcinoids represent >90% of carcinoid tumors in younger patients, while in patients >50 years old the number is approximately 80% to 85%. Central tumors are more likely to represent a typical carcinoid (~85%), as opposed to peripheral tumors (~70%). Over 90% of patients with typical carcinoids do not have nodal involvement.

Central, cN0

In patients who present with a suspected bronchopulmonary carcinoid tumor that is central and without nodal involvement one can assume it is a primary bronchopulmonary typical carcinoid unless the lesions present with rapid growth patterns, in an older patient (>50), or with multiple lesions. These patients also have a very low risk of distant disease, and therefore further imaging workup is not necessary in patients with a negative clinical examination and central N0 carcinoid tumor found on CT. In addition, preoperative invasive mediastinal staging is not required due to low frequency of involvement. Finally, in light of the fact that 85% of central carcinoids and 85% of N0 carcinoids are typical carcinoids, tissue diagnosis is unlikely to change diagnosis and management. In the case of a central, N0 carcinoid, one can proceed directly to surgical treatment.

Central; cN1 or N2

Patients who present with central, node-positive bronchopulmonary carcinoids have a 50% chance of having an atypical carcinoids. Patients with N1 disease have a 36% chance of atypical histology versus N2 at 63% (Fig. 104.3). Differentiation between typical carcinoids and atypical carcinoids is challenging on small biopsy and therefore large biopsy by

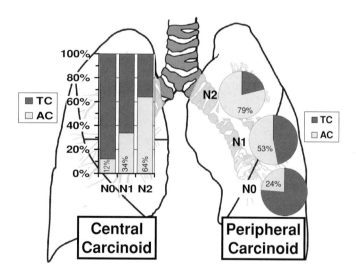

FIGURE 104.3 Calculated proportion of typical and atypical carcinoid tumors among bronchial carcinoid tumors by location and pathologic nodal status. The calculations are based on the following data and assumptions: (1) Typical carcinoids account for 83% of all central carcinoids, 69% of all peripheral carcinoids (Table 104.2). (2) For a typical or atypical carcinoid, the nodal distribution is as reported in Table 104.4. The assumption is made that the rate of nodal involvement is the same for a typical or atypical carcinoid whether the tumor is central or peripheral.

mediastinoscopy is required. While mediastinal nodal involvement with typical histology may not alter treatment decisions, atypical histology and N2 involvement is associated with poor prognosis and a multidisciplinary approach to treatment is needed. Atypical carcinoids are more prone to present with distant metastasis, and so evaluation for clinically asymptomatic distant metastasis is recommended. While the general consensus for bronchopulmonary carcinoids with N2 favors resection with adjuvant chemotherapy, neoadjuvant approaches have been discussed and no direct comparisons of approaches exists.

Peripheral; cN0

Approximately 24% of peripheral, cN0 carcinoid tumors are atypical. Due to the low incidence of atypical carcinoids in this population and nodal involvement, routine preoperative mediastinal staging is not recommended. The rate of distant metastasis in these patients is also quite low (<5%), which also argues against routine screening in clinically asymptomatic patients prior to resection.

Peripheral; cN1 or cN2

Patients who present with a peripheral carcinoid and cN1 or cN2 disease have a 53% and 79% chance of having an atypical carcinoids, respectively. As argued previously, for central, node-positive disease, patients with peripheral node-positive disease should be considered for pretreatment invasive mediastinal staging if there is a consideration for neoadjuvant therapy. Rates of distant metastasis are also elevated in this group and so evaluation with brain MRI, PET, or bone scan, and octreotide scanning should be considered in cN1 disease and strongly recommended for cN2 disease.

TREATMENT, PROGNOSIS, AND OUTCOMES

General Aspects

Surgical resection is the treatment of choice for bronchopulmonary carcinoid tumors, with the aim of complete tumor removal while preserving as much lung parenchyma as possible. Survival rates following resection for typical carcinoids are excellent, 5- and 10-year are >90%; survival for atypical carcinoids is not as good, with 5- and 10-year survivals of 75% and 56%, respectively (Table 104.7).[7,15,25,32,35,63] While deaths are due to recurrence in approximately one in four patients with typical carcinoids, this number is doubled in atypical carcinoids.

The surgical approach to resection can range from a simple wedge of a peripheral lesion to pneumonectomy. Parenchymal-sparing bronchoplastic procedures have become the preferred approach for central tumors. These are valuable treatment options when applicable.[69] One study showed an increase in bronchial sleeve resections of 40% to 65%. Along similar lines, segmental resections for peripheral tumors have increased from 26% to 60% since 1980.[70] Between 5% and 20% of typical carcinoids and 30% to 70% of atypical carcinoids metastasize to lymph nodes; therefore, complete mediastinal lymph node sampling or dissection is recommended at the time of resection.[29] Recurrence after resection of bronchopulmonary carcinoid tumors is uncommon, especially for typical carcinoids. Studies looking at patterns of recurrence have shown the vast majority of recurrences to be distant (10% to 13% local versus 74% to 78% distant).[36,64,70–72] This highlights the fact that, albeit indolent, carcinoid tumors have metastatic potential.

TABLE 104.7 Survival Rate, Pattern of Recurrence and Cause of Death for Typical and Atypical Bronchopulmonary Carcinoid Tumors

Author	N	Survival (%)		Recurrence (%)		Cause of Death (%)	
		5 yrs	10 yrs	Local	Distant	Other	Recurrence
Typical							
Garcia-Yuste et al.[15]	569	97	92	0.88	1.58	65	35
Rea et al.[23]	174	97	93	0	3.4	N/R	N/R
Cardillo et al.[63]	121	99	—	1.6[a]		83	17
Mezzetti et al.[25]	88	92	90	11[a]		—	7
Daddi et al.[32]	79	96	92	N/R	N/R	N/R	N/R
Filosso et al.[35]	75	97	93	5.5[a]		(89)[b]	(11)[b]
Travis et al.[7]	51	87	87	N/R	N/R	N/R	N/R
Overall	**1,157**	**95**	**91**	**5.5**		**74**	**26**
Atypical							
Garcia-Yuste et al.[15]	92	78	67	3.26	16.3	25	75
Rea et al.[23]	78	78	64	0	17.9	—	—
Cardillo et al.[63]	42	70	—	−26[a]		33	67
Mezzetti et al.[25]	10	71	60	−50[a]		—	30
Daddi et al.[32]	8	87	60	N/R	N/R	N/R	N/R
Filosso et al.[35]	38	77	53	19.5[a]		(89)[b]	(11)[b]
Travis et al.[7]	62	56	35	N/R	N/R	N/R	N/R
Overall	**330**	**75**	**56**	**24**		**29**	**57**

[a]Local and distant recurrence pooled.
[b]Typical and atypical carcinoid pooled.
N, number; N/R, not reported.

Peripheral Tumors

Peripheral carcinoids have a higher probability of being atypical histology. Due to the low yield of transthoracic biopsy and the inability of frozen sections to accurately distinguish between typical carcinoids and atypical carcinoids, one could argue to proceed directly with lobar resection. The extent of resection for peripheral typical carcinoids remains a point for discussion, as they have low malignant potential and some argue that limited resection should suffice, but, in a 2012 survey by the European Society for Thoracic Surgery (ESTS), 88% of surgeons felt anatomic resection by segmentectomy or lobectomy was preferred in patients with adequate pulmonary reserve compared to only 11% who considered wedge an adequate surgical option.[73] Although, more radical pulmonary resection were once considered necessary, a propensity-matched analysis which included atypical carcinoids found that extent of resection does not impact overall survival.[74] Ninety-five percent of those surveyed by the ESTS responded that a pneumonectomy should be avoided whenever possible.[73] Intraoperative mediastinal staging should conform to standards for other NSCLCs. For typical carcinoids, complete resection and mediastinal dissection is sufficient, even if nodal disease is present, but patients with atypical carcinoids and N1 or N2 involvement should be considered for adjuvant chemotherapy.

Central

Central node negative tumors have a strong propensity to be typical histology and therefore parenchymal-sparing procedures are strongly favored, especially since these are frequently younger patients who have excellent long-term survival.[75] Parenchymal-sparing resections (bronchial sleeve resections and sleeve lobectomy) have shown equivalent survival when compared to lobectomy and pneumonectomy; survival at 5, 10, and 15 years were 91%, 89%, and 78% for standard resections, which was comparable to conservative resections, 95%, 95%, and 88%, respectively.[30,36,76,77] Most recommend a clear surgical margin by frozen section,[20,64] but little evidence exists to define what constitutes an adequate margin of resection. Some suggest a margin of 0.5 mm, but follow-up data is lacking.[67] In general, a negative frozen section is considered sufficient for typical carcinoids, but evidence suggests a margin of ≥1 cm should be achieved for atypical carcinoids.[78]

Patients with central carcinoid tumors and mediastinal nodal involvement are more challenging. For typical carcinoids, similar to peripheral tumors, negative resection and mediastinal lymph node dissection appear to be adequate therapy. Adjuvant radiation or chemotherapy is generally not recommended because survival rates are >90%.[15] But the ideal therapy for central atypical carcinoids with nodal involvement is less clear. Some advocate more extensive resections (lobectomy and pneumonectomy) to decrease risk of local recurrence. These patients should undergo workup for metastatic disease prior to initiation of treatment. The role of radiotherapy is not well defined, but studies have shown the response rate to chemotherapy is similar for atypical carcinoids and NSCLC.[79] Although, no consensus exists regarding administration of neoadjuvant or adjuvant chemotherapeutic agents in these cases, the high risk of distant recurrence in atypical, N+ disease argues that one or the other would be beneficial.

SPECIAL SITUATIONS

Endobronchial Resection for Typical Carcinoids

Although endobronchial resection was previously reserved for patients with insufficient reserve to tolerate a standard resection, several studies have validated this as a reasonable option for patients with endobronchial typical carcinoids. Selection of patients for endobronchial resection is important, as many carcinoids thought to be endobronchial can involve areas outside the airway. Nevertheless, with good adequate patient selection, initial bronchoscopic treatment was able to fully eradicate tumors in approximately 45% of patients in some series.[80,81] Recurrence rates are approximately 5% after intervals of 7 to 10 years, and fortunately, most of these patients were candidates for resection.[81] Overall and disease-free 10-year survival after endobronchial resection was 84% and 94%, respectively.[82] Cryotherapy can also be used safely as an effective endobronchial adjunct to decrease recurrence.[83] Endoscopic resection of endobronchial carcinoids seems to be a viable option in carefully selected patients, but robust functional imaging is recommended to rule out extraluminal or nodal spread. For those with pneumonitis or sever infection distal to a proximal obstructing tumor, endobronchial resection to open the airway and allow the infection to clear can be performed in preparation for a more definitive parenchymal-sparing procedure.[14]

Tumorlets

Tumorlets are carcinoid tumors that measure <5 mm in greatest diameter and are found in 7% to 10% of patients with bronchopulmonary carcinoids. They are more common in older women, and can have either typical or atypical histology.[45,84] Although a trend toward worse survival is seen (60% at 5 years), tumorlets should not be considered metastatic disease in patients with carcinoid tumors, especially older women.[45] Treatment of a patient with a primary carcinoid and additional tumorlets is resection.

METASTATIC AND NONRESECTABLE CARCINOID TUMORS

A wide variety of therapeutic strategies have been developed for treatment of metastatic carcinoid tumors from varied primary sources, including the lung. These include: resection; radiofrequency ablation; liver transplant; bioactive agents (somatostatin analogues and interferon), standard chemotherapy; targeted agents (everolimus, sunitinib, and bevacizumab),[85] and targeted radiotherapy using a variety of isotopes.[86] Chemotherapy regimens are commonly similar to those used for SCLC with response rates of 20% to 30%.[79,87,88] The recent analysis of the RADIANT-2 study showed that median progression-free survival for patients on everolimus plus octreotide was 13.6 months compared with 5.6 months with octreotide alone (HR 0.72; 95% CI, 0.31–1.68).[89] Although this study was small, it is one of the largest trials examining systemic therapy in BP carcinoids.

Peptide receptor radionuclide therapy is a promising new technique that relies on the presence of SSTRs on the surface of neuroendocrine tumors, to which an isotopically labeled radio-peptide can be directed. The radio-peptide allows direct delivery into the intracellular compartment of the tumor.[90] Results of two phase I/II studies were reported in 2004 and included a small subset (11 patients) with BP carcinoids. After completion of treatment with[91] Y-octreotide, one had partial remission and eight showed stabilization of disease.[91] In a more recent series of 1,109 patients treated with[91] Y-octreotide, 84 had bronchopulmonary carcinoids, with an objective response in the bronchopulmonary carcinoid group 28.6%.[92]

The value of standard radiation therapy (RT) is unclear due to the fact that it is almost always used in combination with other therapies. Nevertheless, an improvement was seen in 14% to 25% of patients receiving chemotherapy and thoracic RT[79,88] and in 11% (1/9) receiving RT to metastatic sites.[88]

The multiplicity of treatment regimens for metastatic bronchopulmonary carcinoids attests to the fact that not one has been found to be significantly superior to the others. It is reasonable to consider chemotherapy or RT in patients with locally advanced or metastatic bronchopulmonary carcinoid tumors. A regimen decided upon by a multidisciplinary group will likely be the most useful. Further randomized trials are needed, but difficult to perform to the rarity of the problem.

FOLLOW-UP

The indolent nature of bronchopulmonary carcinoids requires long-term follow-up. Recurrences for typical and atypical carcinoids have been described with 10 years and 5 years, respectively.[15,30,35,36,64,93] It is unclear if early detection results in a better outcome when it comes to recurrences. In some cases it has resulted in cure,[48] but more commonly only palliative therapy is possible. Survival with palliative therapies is about 2 to 3 years.[35,79]

It is thus generally recommended that patients undergo surveillance for recurrent disease for at least 20 years. While the surveillance interval can be spread out for typical carcinoids, closer monitoring is recommended for atypical carcinoids, more similar to that for resected NSCLC. A thorough history and physical looking for evidence of distant recurrence and a chest x-ray should be obtained. Liver, mediastinum, and abdominal lymph nodes, lung, cutaneous, and bone metastasis are reported and require evaluation. Any suspicious areas found on preliminary workup should be followed up with either CT or PET. Since most recurrences are distant, bronchoscopy is generally not necessary.

SUMMARY

Bronchopulmonary carcinoid tumors are a well-described group of neoplasms. They are indolent by nature but by no means benign. A presumptive diagnosis of a bronchopulmonary carcinoid tumor can be made in many patients based on clinical and radiographic characteristics without the need for a biopsy. Nevertheless, if necessary, endobronchial biopsy via bronchoscopy is safe with a low risk of bleeding.

The histologic classification of carcinoid tumors has been continuously refined by the WHO. Treatment algorithms can be altered by the histology of a carcinoid. Typical tumors have better survival and lower incidence of recurrence. Central or peripheral tumors that are clinically N0 are most likely typical carcinoids, and require no further imaging or invasive testing. In patients with clinically positive N1 or N2 tumors, mediastinoscopy and metastatic workup are considered as these have a higher likelihood of being atypical carcinoids.

Surgical resection is the mainstay of treatment, with excellent survival in both typical carcinoids and atypical carcinoids. As long as an R0 resection can be completed there is no evidence to suggest a sublobar resection or other parenchymal-sparing options are inferior to a lobectomy or pneumonectomy for treatment of either typical carcinoids or atypical carcinoids. For those with pN2 and an atypical carcinoids, adjuvant or neoadjuvant treatment should be discussed in a multidisciplinary manner. Treatment of locally advanced or metastatic disease requires further investigation, but promising regimens exist. Given the indolent nature of bronchopulmonary carcinoids, surveillance is necessary for a protracted period of time (20 years).

REFERENCES

01. Modlin IM, Bodei L, Kidd M. A historical appreciation of bronchopulmonary neuroendocrine neoplasia: Resolution of a carcinoid conundrum. *Thorac Surg Clin* 2014;24:235–255.
02. Arrigoni MG, Woolner LB, Bernatz PE. Atypical carcinoid tumors of the lung. *J Thorac Cardiovasc Surg* 1972;64:413–421.
03. Gould VE. Neuroendocrinomas and neuroendocrine carcinomas: APUD cell system neoplasms and their aberrant secretory activities. *Pathol Annu* 1977;12 Pt 2:33–62.
04. Travis WD, Gal AA, Colby TV, et al. Reproducibility of neuroendocrine lung tumor classification. *Hum Pathol* 1998;29:272–279.
05. Travis WD, Linnoila RI, Tsokos MG, et al. Neuroendocrine tumors of the lung with proposed criteria for large-cell neuroendocrine carcinoma. An ultrastructural, immunohistochemical, and flow cytometric study of 35 cases. *Am J Surg Pathol* 1991;15:529–553.
06. Travis WD, Brambilla E, Konrad Muller-Hermlink H, et al. *World Health Organization Classification of Tumours. Pathology and Genetics of Tumours of the Lung, Pleura, Thymus, and Heart.* Lyon (France): IARC Press; 2004.
07. Travis WD, Rush W, Flieder DB, et al. Survival analysis of 200 pulmonary neuroendocrine tumors with clarification of criteria for atypical carcinoid and its separation from typical carcinoid. *Am J Surg Pathol* 1998;22:934–944.
08. Travis WD. Pathology and diagnosis of neuroendocrine tumors: Lung neuroendocrine. *Thorac Surg Clin* 2014;24:257–266.
09. Travis WD, Brambilla E, Burke AP, et al. *WHO Classification of Tumours of the Lung, Pleura, Thymus and Heart.* 4th ed. Lyon: International Agency for Research on Cancer; 2015.
10. Travis WD, Brambilla E, Nicholson AG, et al. The 2015 World Health Organization classification of lung tumors: Impact of genetic, clinical and radiologic advances since the 2004 classification. *J Thorac Oncol* 2015;10:1243–1260.
11. Travis WD, Brambilla E, Burke AP, et al. Introduction to the 2015 World Health Organization Classification of Tumors of the Lung, Pleura, Thymus, and Heart. *J Thorac Oncol* 2015;10:1240–1242.
12. Surveillance Epidemiology, and End Results (SEER) Program. *Lung cancer histolgoically confirmed SEER 18 registries resarach data plus Hurricane Katrina impacted Louisiana cases 1973-2010, November 2012; total US County Attributes. April 2013 edition. 2014.* Available at: www.seer.cancer.gov. National Cancer Institute, DCCPS, Surveillance Research Program, Surveillanc Systems Branch.
13. Chen LC, Travis WD, Krug LM. Pulmonary neuroendocrine tumors: What (little) do we know? *J Natl Compr Canc Netw* 2006;4:623–630.
14. Detterbeck FC. Management of carcinoid tumors. *Ann Thorac Surg* 2010;89:998–1005.
15. Garcia-Yuste M, Matilla JM, Cueto A, et al. Typical and atypical carcinoid tumours: analysis of the experience of the Spanish Multi-centric Study of Neuroendocrine Tumours of the Lung. *Eur J Cardiothorac Surg* 2007;31:192–197.
16. Bertelsen S, Aasted A, Lund C, et al. Bronchial carcinoid tumours. A clinicopathologic study of 82 cases. *Scand J Thorac Cardiovasc Surg* 1985;19:105–111.
17. Hurt R, Bates M. Carcinoid tumours of the bronchus: A 33 year experience. *Thorax* 1984;39:617–623.
18. Paladugu RR, Benfield JR, Pak HY, et al. Bronchopulmonary Kulchitzky cell carcinomas. A new classification scheme for typical and atypical carcinoids. *Cancer* 1985;55:1303–1311.
19. Vadasz P, Palffy G, Egervary M, et al. Diagnosis and treatment of bronchial carcinoid tumors: Clinical and pathological review of 120 operated patients. *Eur J Cardiothorac Surg* 1993;7:8–11.
20. Stamatis G, Freitag L, Greschuchna D. Limited and radical resection for tracheal and bronchopulmonary carcinoid tumour. Report on 227 cases. *Eur J Cardiothorac Surg* 1990;4:527–532; discussion 533.
21. Soga J, Yakuwa Y. Bronchopulmonary carcinoids: An analysis of 1,875 reported cases with special reference to a comparison between typical carcinoids and atypical varieties. *Ann Thorac Cardiovasc Surg* 1999;5:211–219.
22. Schrevens L, Vansteenkiste J, Deneffe G, et al. Clinical-radiological presentation and outcome of surgically treated pulmonary carcinoid tumours: A long-term single institution experience. *Lung Cancer* 2004;43:39–45.
23. Rea F, Rizzardi G, Zuin A, et al. Outcome and surgical strategy in bronchial carcinoid tumors: Single institution experience with 252 patients. *Eur J Cardiothorac Surg* 2007;31:186–191.
24. Rea F, Binda R, Spreafico G, et al. Bronchial carcinoids: A review of 60 patients. *Ann Thorac Surg* 1989;47:412–414.
25. Mezzetti M, Raveglia F, Panigalli T, et al. Assessment of outcomes in typical and atypical carcinoids according to latest WHO classification. *Ann Thorac Surg* 2003;76:1838–1842.
26. Kurul IC, Topcu S, Tastepe I, et al. Surgery in bronchial carcinoids: experience with 83 patients. *Eur J Cardiothorac Surg* 2002;21:883–887.
27. Fink G, Krelbaum T, Yellin A, et al. Pulmonary carcinoid: Presentation, diagnosis, and outcome in 142 cases in Israel and review of 640 cases from the literature. *Chest* 2001;119:1647–1651.
28. McCaughan BC, Martini N, Bains MS. Bronchial carcinoids. Review of 124 cases. *J Thorac Cardiovasc Surg* 1985;89:8–17.
29. Gustafsson BI, Kidd M, Chan A, et al. Bronchopulmonary neuroendocrine tumors. *Cancer* 2008;113:5–21.
30. Ferguson MK, Landreneau RJ, Hazelrigg SR, et al. Long-term outcome after resection for bronchial carcinoid tumors. *Eur J Cardiothoracic Surg* 2000;18:156–161.
31. El Jamal M, Nicholson AG, Goldstraw P. The feasibility of conservative resection for carcinoid tumours: Is pneumonectomy ever necessary for uncomplicated cases? *Eur J Cardiothorac Surg* 2000;18:301–306.

32. Daddi N, Ferolla P, Urbani M, et al. Surgical treatment of neuroendocrine tumors of the lung. *Eur J Cardiothorac Surg* 2004;26:813–817.

33. Detterbeck FC. Clinical presentation and evaluation of neuroendocrine tumors of the lung. *Thorac Surg Clin* 2014;24:267–276.

34. Martensson H, Bottcher G, Hambraeus G, et al. Bronchial carcinoid: An analysis of 91 cases. *World J Surg* 1987;11:356–364.

35. Filosso PL, Rena O, Donati G, et al. Bronchial carcinoid tumors: surgical management and long-term outcome. *J Thorac Cardiovasc Surg* 2002;123:303–309.

36. Ducrocq X, Thomas P, Massard G, et al. Operative risk and prognostic factors of typical bronchial carcinoid tumors. *Ann Thorac Surg* 1998;65:1410–1414.

37. Ferone D, Albertelli M. Ectopic Cushing and other paraneoplastic syndromes in thoracic neuroendocrine tumors. *Thorac Surg Clin* 2014;24:277–283.

38. Davila DG, Dunn WF, Tazelaar HD, et al. Bronchial carcinoid tumors. *Mayo Clin Proc* 1993;68:795–803.

39. Ricci C, Patrassi N, Massa R, et al. Carcinoid syndrome in bronchial adenoma. *Am J Surg* 1973;126:671–677.

40. Harpole DH, Jr., Feldman JM, Buchanan S, et al. Bronchial carcinoid tumors: A retrospective analysis of 126 patients. *Ann Thorac Surg* 1992;54:50–54; discussion 54–55.

41. Ilias I, Torpy DJ, Pacak K, et al. Cushing's syndrome due to ectopic corticotropin secretion: Twenty years' experience at the National Institutes of Health. *J Clin Endocrinol Metab* 2005;90:4955–4962.

42. Limper AH, Carpenter PC, Scheithauer B, et al. The Cushing syndrome induced by bronchial carcinoid tumors. *Ann Intern Med* 1992;117:209–214.

43. Docherty HM, Heath DA. Multiple forms of parathyroid hormone-like proteins in a human tumour. *J Mol Endocrinol* 1989;2:11–20.

44. Kaiser AC DF. Carcinoid and mucoepidermoid tumors. In: Detterbeck FC, Rivera MP, Socinski MA, et al., eds. *Diagnosis and Treatment of Lung Cancer: An Evidence-Based Guide for the Practicing Clinician*. Philadelphia, PA: Saunders; 2001:379–393.

45. Chughtai TS, Morin JE, Sheiner NM, et al. Bronchial carcinoid–twenty years' experience defines a selective surgical approach. *Surgery* 1997;122:801–808.

46. Erasmus JJ, McAdams HP, Patz EF Jr., et al. Evaluation of primary pulmonary carcinoid tumors using FDG PET. *AJR Am J Roentgenol* 1998;170:1369–1373.

47. Chong S, Lee KS, Kim BT, et al. Integrated PET/CT of pulmonary neuroendocrine tumors: diagnostic and prognostic implications. *AJR Am J Roentgenol* 2007;188: 1223–1231.

48. Daniels CE, Lowe VJ, Aubry MC, et al. The utility of fluorodeoxyglucose positron emission tomography in the evaluation of carcinoid tumors presenting as pulmonary nodules. *Chest* 2007;131:255–260.

49. Jindal T, Kumar A, Venkitaraman B, et al. Evaluation of the role of [18F]FDG-PET/CT and [68Ga]DOTATOC-PET/CT in differentiating typical and atypical pulmonary carcinoids. *Cancer Imaging* 2011;11:70–75.

50. Kayani I, Conry BG, Groves AM, et al. A comparison of 68Ga-DOTATATE and 18F-FDG PET/CT in pulmonary neuroendocrine tumors. *J Nucl Med* 2009;50:1927–1932.

51. Kruger S, Buck AK, Blumstein NM, et al. Use of integrated FDG PET/CT imaging in pulmonary carcinoid tumours. *J Intern Med* 2006;260:545–550.

52. Stefani A, Franceschetto A, Nesci J, et al. Integrated FDG-PET/CT imaging is useful in the approach to carcinoid tumors of the lung. *J Cardiothorac Surg* 2013;8:223.

53. Wartski M, Alberini JL, Leroy-Ladurie F, et al. Typical and atypical bronchopulmonary carcinoid tumors on FDG PET/CT imaging. *Clin Nucl Med* 2004;29:752–753.

54. Lococo F, Treglia G, Cesario A, et al. Functional imaging evaluation in the detection, diagnosis, and histologic differentiation of pulmonary neuroendocrine tumors. *Thorac Surg Clin* 2014;24:285–292.

55. Kumar A, Jindal T, Dutta R, et al. Functional imaging in differentiating bronchial masses: An initial experience with a combination of (18)F-FDG PET-CT scan and (68)Ga DOTA-TOC PET-CT scan. *Ann Nucl Med* 2009;23:745–751.

56. Venkitaraman B, Karunanithi S, Kumar A, et al. Role of 68Ga-DOTATOC PET/CT in initial evaluation of patients with suspected bronchopulmonary carcinoid. *Eur J Nucl Med Mol Imaging* 2014;41:856–864.

57. Gabriel M, Oberauer A, Dobrozemsky G, et al. 68Ga-DOTA-Tyr3-octreotide PET for assessing response to somatostatin-receptor-mediated radionuclide therapy. *J Nucl Med* 2009;50:1427–1434.

58. Hofmann M, Maecke H, Borner R, et al. Biokinetics and imaging with the somatostatin receptor PET radioligand (68)Ga-DOTATOC: preliminary data. *Eur J Nucl Med* 2001;28:1751–1757.

59. Granberg D, Sundin A, Janson ET, et al. Octreoscan in patients with bronchial carcinoid tumours. *Clin Endocrinol (Oxf)* 2003;59:793–799.

60. Lau SK, Johnson DS, Coel MN. Imaging of non-small-cell lung cancer with indium-111 pentetreotide. *Clin Nucl Med* 2000;25:24–28.

61. Musi M, Carbone RG, Bertocchi C, et al. Bronchial carcinoid tumours: A study on clinicopathological features and role of octreotide scintigraphy. *Lung Cancer* 1998;22:97–102.

62. Yellin A, Zwas ST, Rozenman J, et al. Experience with somatostatin receptor scintigraphy in the management of pulmonary carcinoid tumors. *Isr Med Assoc J* 2005;7:712–716.

63. Cardillo G, Sera F, Di Martino M, et al. Bronchial carcinoid tumors: nodal status and long-term survival after resection. *Ann Thorac Surg* 2004;77:1781–1785.

64. Marty-Ane CH, Costes V, Pujol JL, et al. Carcinoid tumors of the lung: Do atypical features require aggressive management? *Ann Thorac Surg* 1995;59:78–83.

65. Francioni F, Rendina EA, Venuta F, et al. Low grade neuroendocrine tumors of the lung (bronchial carcinoids)–25 years experience. *Eur J Cardiothorac Surg* 1990;4: 472–476.

66. Todd TR, Cooper JD, Weissberg D, et al. Bronchial carcinoid tumors: Twenty years' experience. *J Thorac Cardiovasc Surg* 1980;79:532–536.

67. Warren WH, Faber LP, Gould VE. Neuroendocrine neoplasms of the lung. A clinico-pathologic update. *J Thorac Cardiovascr Surg* 1989;98:321–332.

68. Nicholson SA, Ryan MR. A review of cytologic findings in neuroendocrine carcinomas including carcinoid tumors with histologic correlation. *Cancer* 2000;90: 148–161.

69. Anile M, Diso D, Rendina EA, et al. Bronchoplastic procedures for carcinoid tumors. *Thorac Surg Clin* 2014;24:299–303.

70. Schreurs AJ, Westermann CJ, van den Bosch JM, et al. A twenty-five-year follow-up of ninety-three resected typical carcinoid tumors of the lung. *J Thorac Cardiovasc Surg* 1992;104:1470–1475.

71. Garcia-Yuste M, Matilla JM, Alvarez-Gago T, et al. Prognostic factors in neuroendocrine lung tumors: a Spanish Multicenter Study. Spanish Multicenter Study of Neuroendocrine Tumors of the Lung of the Spanish Society of Pneumonology and Thoracic Surgery (EMETNE-SEPAR). *Ann Thorac Surg* 2000;70:258–263.

72. Warren WH, Gould VE. Neuroendocrine neoplasms of the lung. A 10 year perspective of their classification. *Zentralbl Pathol* 1993;139:107–113.

73. Caplin ME, Baudin E, Ferolla P, et al. Pulmonary neuroendocrine (carcinoid) tumors: European Neuroendocrine Tumor Society expert consensus and recommendations for best practice for typical and atypical pulmonary carcinoids. *Ann Oncol* 2015;26:1604–1620.

74. Yendamuri S, Gold D, Jayaprakash V, et al. Is sublobar resection sufficient for carcinoid tumors? *Ann Thorac Surg* 2011;92:1774–1778; discussion 1778–1779.

75. Oberg K, Hellman P, Ferolla P, et al.; ESMO Guidelines Working Group. Neuroendocrine bronchial and thymic tumors: ESMO Clinical Practice Guidelines for diagnosis, treatment and follow-up. *Ann Oncol* 2012;23 Suppl 7:vii120–23.

76. Maurizi G, Ibrahim M, Andreetti C, et al. Long-term results after resection of bronchial carcinoid tumour: evaluation of survival and prognostic factors. *Interact Cardiovasc Thorac Surg* 2014;19:239–244.

77. Fox M, Van Berkel V, Bousamra M 2nd, et al. Surgical management of pulmonary carcinoid tumors: Sublobar resection versus lobectomy. *Am J Surg* 2013;205: 200–208.

78. Schmid S, Aicher M, Csanadi A, et al. Significance of the resection margin in bronchopulmonary carcinoids. *J Surg Res* 2016;201:53–58.

79. Wirth LJ, Carter MR, Janne PA, et al. Outcome of patients with pulmonary carcinoid tumors receiving chemotherapy or chemoradiotherapy. *Lung Cancer* 2004;44:213–220.

80. Brokx HA, Paul MA, Postmus PE, et al. Long-term follow-up after first-line bronchoscopic therapy in patients with bronchial carcinoids. *Thorax* 2015;70(5):468–472.

81. Brokx HA, Risse EK, Paul MA, et al. Initial bronchoscopic treatment for patients with intraluminal bronchial carcinoids. *J Thorac Cardiovasc Surg* 2007;133:973–978.

82. Luckraz H, Amer K, Thomas L, et al. Long-term outcome of bronchoscopically resected endobronchial typical carcinoid tumors. *J Thorac Cardiovasc Surg* 2006;132: 113–115.

83. Bertoletti L, Elleuch R, Kaczmarek D, et al. Bronchoscopic cryotherapy treatment of isolated endoluminal typical carcinoid tumor. *Chest* 2006;130:1405–1411.

84. Aubry MC, Thomas CF Jr., Jett JR, et al. Significance of multiple carcinoid tumors and tumorlets in surgical lung specimens: Analysis of 28 patients. *Chest* 2007;131: 1635–1643.

85. Stevenson R, Libutti SK, Saif MW. Novel agents in gastroenteropancreatic neuroendocrine tumors. *JOP* 2013;14:152–154.

86. Kwekkeboom DJ, Mueller-Brand J, Paganelli G, et al. Overview of results of peptide receptor radionuclide therapy with 3 radiolabeled somatostatin analogs. *J Nucl Med* 2005;46 Suppl 1:62S–66S.

87. Forde PM, Hooker CM, Boikos SA, et al. Systemic therapy, clinical outcomes, and overall survival in locally advanced or metastatic pulmonary carcinoid: A brief report. *J Thorac Oncol* 2014;9:414–418.

88. Granberg D, Eriksson B, Wilander E, et al. Experience in treatment of metastatic pulmonary carcinoid tumors. *Ann Oncol* 2001;12:1383–1391.

89. Fazio N, Granberg D, Grossman A, et al. Everolimus plus octreotide long-acting repeatable in patients with advanced lung neuroendocrine tumors: Analysis of the phase 3, randomized, placebo-controlled RADIANT-2 study. *Chest* 2013;143: 955–962.

90. Bodei L, Cremonesi M, Kidd M, et al. Peptide receptor radionuclide therapy for advanced neuroendocrine tumors. *Thorac Surg Clin* 2014;24:333–349.

91. Bodei L, Cremonesi M, Zoboli S, et al. Receptor-mediated radionuclide therapy with 90Y-DOTATOC in association with amino acid infusion: a phase I study. *Eur J Nucl Med Mol Imaging* 2003;30:207–216.

92. Imhof A, Brunner P, Marincek N, et al. Response, survival, and long-term toxicity after therapy with the radiolabeled somatostatin analogue [90Y-DOTA]-TOC in metastasized neuroendocrine cancers. *J Clin Oncol* 2011;29:2416–2423.

93. Thomas CF Jr., Tazelaar HD, Jett JR. Typical and atypical pulmonary carcinoids: Outcome in patients presenting with regional lymph node involvement. *Chest* 2001;119:1143–1150.

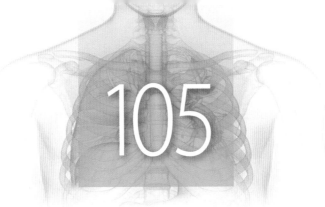

105

Adenoid Cystic Carcinoma and Other Primary Salivary Gland–Type Tumors of the Lung

Richard S. D'Agostino

The submucosal serous and mucous glands of the tracheobronchial tree are similar to those of the major and minor salivary glands and can give rise to morphologically and biologically analogous tumors. Adenoid cystic carcinoma, mucoepidermoid carcinoma, epithelial–myoepithelial carcinoma, pleomorphic adenoma, acinic cell carcinoma, and oncocytoma have in prior years been included with carcinoid tumors under the misleading and antiquated rubric *bronchial adenomas*. Unlike true adenomas, adenoid cystic carcinoma, mucoepidermoid carcinoma, epithelial–myoepithelial carcinoma, and acinic cell carcinoma are malignant lesions. Although their growth rate is often indolent, local invasion and lymph node metastases ultimately may occur, and in some cases biologic behavior is aggressive. Pleomorphic adenoma and oncocytoma can behave in a benign or malignant fashion. The 2015 World Health Organization Classification of Lung Tumors[82] codifies mucoepidermoid carcinoma, adenoid cystic carcinoma, epithelial–myoepithelial carcinoma, and pleomorphic adenoma under the histologic grouping of "salivary gland-type tumors."

These noncarcinoid, salivary gland–type tumors of the lung are uncommon and constitute less than 2% of all primary lung neoplasms.

ADENOID CYSTIC CARCINOMA

Adenoid cystic carcinoma, formerly called cylindroma, most often arises in the salivary glands. Less frequent primary sites include the lung, breast, skin, uterine cervix, esophagus, and prostate.

PATHOLOGY

The majority of pulmonary adenoid cystic carcinomas develop centrally in the trachea and major bronchi. These otherwise uncommon tumors account for 25% to 50% of all primary tracheal malignancies. Dalton and Gatling[1] and Inoue and colleagues,[2] among others, reported instances of primary adenoid cystic carcinoma arising peripherally and suggested that this may be the case in approximately 10% of patients. Peripheral lesions, however, are more likely to represent metastases from an extrathoracic primary site. Synchronous hematogenous metastases at the time of initial presentation are rarely encountered. However, Maziak and colleagues[3] and Prommegger

and Salzer[4] noted late metachronous hematogenous metastases in 44% and 55% of their patients, respectively. On macroscopic inspection, adenoid cystic carcinoma appears white, pink, or light tan and is either polypoid or annular. The overlying mucosa is usually intact, although ulceration may occur. Direct transluminal extension is the rule. Malignant submucosal and perineural infiltration is common and often extends a considerable distance proximally and distally from the main tumor mass (Fig. 105.1).

Adenoid cystic carcinomas are histologically similar regardless of their primary site. The following three patterns are recognized: cribriform, tubular, and solid. The cribriform or cylindromatous subtype is the classic finding (Fig. 105.2). Nests and columns of small rounded or polyhedral cells arranged in a sieve-like pattern surround gland-like spaces filled with periodic acid–Schiff–positive material. The tubular pattern is defined by cords of polygonal cells containing central ducts that are separated from surrounding stroma. The solid or basaloid pattern is morphologically the least differentiated

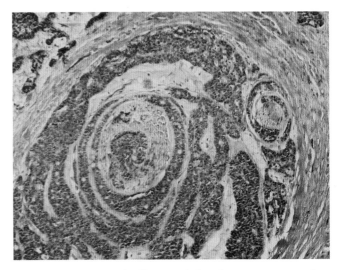

FIGURE 105.1 Perineural infiltration of adenoid cystic carcinoma is characteristic of this tumor and is the route of extension toward the mediastinum. (Courtesy of Bruce Tronic.)

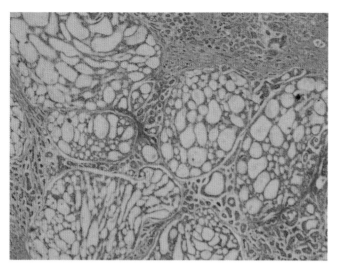

FIGURE 105.2 Adenoid cystic carcinoma with the typical cribriform or cylindromatous pattern.

and consists of sheets of small cuboidal cells with prominent mitoses and occasional small clusters of larger polygonal cells. An individual tumor can display more than one pattern (Fig. 105.3). Nomori and colleagues[5] found that tumors with solid elements are associated with an aggressive clinical course and with the appearance of distant metastases more often than with other patterns. However, Albers and colleagues[6] found histologic grade to be an inconclusive prognostic factor. Moran[7] noted that the immunohistochemical profile of adenoid cystic carcinoma is dominated by the myoepithelial cell proliferation. These tumor cells showed positive staining with both wide-spectrum and low-molecular-weight keratin as well as with vimentin and actin antibodies. Reactivity to S-100 protein has been variable. Staining for glial fibrillary acidic protein was uniformly negative. This latter finding can be used to distinguish adenoid cystic

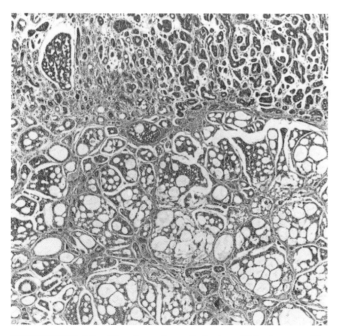

FIGURE 105.3 Adenoid cystic carcinoma in the bronchial submucosa. The tumor is growing in a basaloid pattern beneath the intact ciliated epithelium. In the deeper zone, it displays the classic cribriform pattern.

carcinoma from pleomorphic adenoma, a tumor that also has a prominent myoepithelial cell component. Although the histopathologic features of adenoid cystic carcinoma are usually distinctive enough to allow for definitive diagnosis by routine light microscopy, this tumor can be confused with adenocarcinoma, especially when faced with a small biopsy specimen. In such situations, the demonstration of a myoepithelial cell immunophenotype supports the diagnosis of adenoid cystic carcinoma. Lin and colleagues[8] found eight of nine patients with tracheobronchial adenoid cystic carcinoma negative for the biomarkers p53, HER-2/neu, and COX-2. The one patient positive for HER-2/neu developed distant metastases 4 years postoperatively. Albers and colleagues[6] noted all 13 tumors in their series to stain positively for c-kit protein (CD117, a type III tyrosine kinase receptor) but could find no correlation between histologic grade and Ki-67 (a marker for cell proliferation) activity.

CLINICAL FEATURES

Adenoid cystic carcinoma typically occurs in patients 40 to 50 years of age, but it has been reported in persons ranging in age from 18 to 82 years. Men and women are affected nearly equally, with a slight male predominance. There is no known association with tobacco use or environmental toxins. Because they are located centrally and are often not apparent on chest radiographs, most tumors are detected only after they produce symptoms. Patients generally describe one or more of the following problems: dyspnea, cough, hemoptysis, wheezing, hoarseness, stridor, or recurrent pneumonias. In some cases, significant tracheal or main bronchial obstruction occurs early and can be life threatening. However, in many instances the intraluminal component is relatively small despite extensive submucosal and extraluminal spread. This pattern, coupled with typically slow growth, can produce an insidious presentation. An interval of several months to years may elapse between the onset of symptoms and the establishment of a diagnosis. Gaissert and colleagues[9] noted mean symptom duration of 24 months prior to diagnosis. Some patients are treated for prolonged periods for an erroneous diagnosis of asthma or chronic obstructive lung disease. The physical examination may demonstrate diminished or absent breath sounds because of complete obstruction of a lobe or an entire lung, a unilateral wheeze from partial blockage of a main bronchus, or stridor produced by tracheal involvement, but also may be negative. Peripheral adenopathy and clubbing are not features of adenoid cystic carcinoma.

RADIOGRAPHIC FEATURES

Owing to the central location of most tumors, the chest radiograph may appear normal, but can show atelectasis of a lobe or an entire lung. A hilar or mediastinal mass may be present. Subtle changes in airway contour occasionally are noted, particularly with lesions of the intrathoracic trachea. On the other hand, tumor masses in the cervical trachea are often easily appreciated on plain neck radiographs (Fig. 105.4). Computed tomography (CT) accurately defines both intraluminal and transverse extraluminal tumor and is helpful in detecting metastases to the lung or pleura. However, single detector CT scan consistently underestimates the longitudinal extent of airway involvement because of partial volume averaging and the tendency for submucosal tumor extension. Magnetic resonance imaging, with its ability to image multiple anatomic planes and to provide variably weighted images has been reported to be superior to single detector CT for delineating the extent of both submucosal infiltration and mediastinal involvement.[10,11] In the current era, multidetector CT

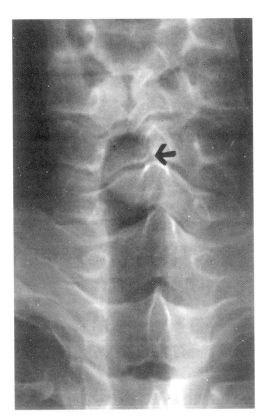

FIGURE 105.4 Anteroposterior neck radiograph shows an endotracheal mass (*arrow*). Biopsy confirmed adenoid cystic carcinoma.

scan with multiplanar image reconstruction is the imaging study of choice. It allows for rapid image acquisition and excels in defining both the longitudinal and lateral extent of tumor.[12] Nevertheless, multidetector CT is a poor predictor of perineural and mediastinal fat invasion. Campistron and colleagues,[13] in 2008, reported a singular case of bronchial adenoid cystic carcinoma with a synchronous histologically proven metastasis to the liver, detected by positron emission tomography ([18]FDG PET-CT) and proposed that [18]FDG PET-CT be considered in the initial staging of these tumors. Salivary gland tumors are similar to other indolent lung tumors, such as carcinoid tumors and well-differentiated adenocarcinomas, in that they show variable uptake of [18]FDG. However, ElNayal and colleagues[14] have shown that a greater degree of FDG uptake is associated with the presence of nodal disease.

DIAGNOSIS

Because adenoid cystic carcinomas usually are covered by normal bronchial epithelium, cytologic examination of the sputum is generally unrewarding unless the overlying respiratory epithelium has been eroded. Except for the unusual circumstance of a peripherally situated lesion, these tumors are identified at bronchoscopy, and the diagnosis is established by transmucosal biopsy. The typical bronchoscopic appearance is that of a broad-based polypoidal mass partially or completely obstructing the airway (Fig. 105.5). Alternatively, the tumor may appear as a diffuse, submucosal infiltration causing luminal distortion and obstruction. Although Attar and colleagues,[15] among others, reported substantial bleeding after biopsy of bronchial tumors in some patients, hemorrhage appears to be more of a problem with carcinoid and mucoepidermoid tumors than with adenoid cystic carcinomas. Care must be taken with large

intraluminal tumors as instrumentation may lead to acute airway compromise from swelling, bleeding, or secretions. The rigid bronchoscope provides a greater degree of control in such instances and also can be used to core out obstructing tumors. These situations are best managed under a general anesthetic and in close coordination with the anesthesiologist. The extent of tracheal involvement should be thoroughly assessed both visually and with transmucosal biopsies to determine the length of trachea available for reconstruction.

TREATMENT

The treatment of choice is resection when feasible. Airway stents and radiation therapy should not be employed as initial therapeutic maneuvers in otherwise resectable patients. Gaissert and colleagues[9] were able to perform resection in 75% of their patients. Contraindications to resection were most often due to the length of airway involvement and to the extent of regional disease. It cannot be overemphasized that submucosal and perineural infiltration commonly extends beyond macroscopic tumor boundaries. Intraoperative frozen section examination of resection margins should be performed routinely as a method of ensuring adequate tumor clearance. Conlan and colleagues,[16] Grillo and Mathisen,[17] and Gaissert and colleagues[9] found that tumor spread to hilar and mediastinal lymph nodes does not preclude long-term survival. In the case of tracheal resections, Grillo and Mathisen[17] stressed that lymph nodes adjacent to the tumor should be resected and distant nodes sampled, but that extensive dissection should be avoided because it may jeopardize anastomotic healing. They also pointed out that, in some cases, one must accept a microscopically positive margin rather than extend the resection and produce tension on the suture line. Resection should not be performed when it would result in grossly positive peritracheal margins or when the length of tracheal involvement prevents safe reconstruction. Tumors involving a lobar bronchus can often be managed with lobectomy, using bronchoplastic techniques where applicable. However, submucosal spread in the main-stem bronchus may mandate a pneumonectomy. Adenoid cystic carcinomas arising in a bronchial location have been shown to have a greater propensity for lymph node metastases[18] suggesting that

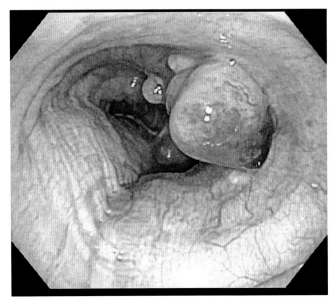

FIGURE 105.5 Bronchoscopic view of a polypoid adenoid cystic carcinoma of the distal trachea and carina. (Courtesy of Daniel Raymond, Cleveland Clinic Foundation.)

extensive lymphadenectomy be employed at the time of resection. Extensive tracheal or carinal involvement presents more complex situations. Gaissert and colleagues[9] noted carinal involvement in 41 of 101 patients with an associated perioperative mortality of 16% for carinal resection during the 40-year span of their study. Although perioperative mortality has decreased in recent years, the risks of resection must be considered carefully because treatment methods other than resection can provide effective palliation for long periods. Grillo and Mathisen,[17] Pearson and colleagues,[19] and Perelman and colleagues[20] described their extensive experience with these situations. The techniques of bronchial sleeve lobectomy and tracheal and carinal resections are discussed in other chapters. Wurtz and colleagues[21] reported a single series of five adenoid cystic and one mucoepidermoid carcinoma treated with aortic allograft replacement of the trachea and carina. Although complete microscopic resection was achieved in 83% of these extensive tumors, significant complications were seen in five patients. As microscopic resection margins can be effectively treated with more traditional therapies, further advances are necessary before tracheal replacement can be considered in the management of these tumors.

Most adenoid cystic carcinomas are radiosensitive and radiation therapy is the primary treatment for extensive inoperable cancers and for patients in whom resection carries an unacceptable risk. Fields and colleagues[22] noted that in patients treated with external beam radiation therapy alone, the rate of complete response was significantly related to a tumor dose of 60 Gy or more; currently tumor doses between 55 and 65 Gy are commonly employed. Endoluminal high dose-rate brachytherapy is another method that appears to have a palliative role. Harms and colleagues[23] and Carvalho and colleagues,[24] among others, have reported successful primary tumor control with high dose-rate brachytherapy as a supplement to external beam radiotherapy, although late tracheitis and stenosis necessitated tracheal stent in some of their patients. Given the surgically close or microscopically positive margins for many resected patients, external beam radiation therapy is now utilized routinely as an adjunct to resection. Gaissert and colleagues,[9] among others, have employed doses between 45 and 65 Gy beginning 6 to 8 weeks following resection. Limited experience with preoperative neoadjuvant radiation therapy has been reported in the past.[19,25] For some patients with unresectable or recurrent disease, tumor debulking by neodymium:yttrium–aluminum–garnet (Nd:YAG) laser ablation, with or without concomitant airway stenting, may provide satisfactory palliation.[26,27] Treatment may be affected with the fiberoptic and/or rigid bronchoscope although the latter is favored by most clinicians because it allows easier tumor debulking by morcellation, rapid control of hemorrhage, and protection of the contralateral airway if so needed. Laser photocoagulation and radiation therapy are often used in combination for the palliation of symptoms related to adenoid cystic carcinoma and can be associated with prolonged survival.[6,28] Laser ablation should be considered before radiation therapy in patients with critical proximal airway obstruction because irradiation in this setting may produce enough edema to cause asphyxia. Because of the rarity of these tumors, reliable data regarding the efficacy of systemic chemotherapy for pulmonary adenoid cystic carcinoma is scant. A systematic review of published data regarding chemotherapy for primary or metastatic adenoid cystic carcinoma involving any body site suggests that combination therapy with cisplatin and an anthracycline may offer some value in palliation.[29]

PROGNOSIS

Because adenoid cystic carcinoma tends to grow slowly, prolonged survival with persistent disease is not unusual. Local recurrence can occur many years after complete resection. As noted, purely palliative therapy may offer long-term, symptom-free survival. Carter and Eggleston[30] compiled the results of several studies including patients who were treated both definitively and palliatively and noted that the 5-, 10-, and 20-year survival rates were 85%, 55%, and 20%, respectively. Studies of patients who have undergone resection for central adenoid cystic carcinomas, often with adjuvant radiation therapy, document favorable results. Perelman and Koroleva[25] reported a 66% survival rate at 5 years and a 56% survival rate at 15 years. Maziak and colleagues[3] reported survival rates of 79% at 5 years and 51% at 10 years for 32 patients treated with primary resection. Twenty-six of these patients received adjuvant radiation therapy. Six unresectable patients treated with radiation therapy alone had an average survival of 6 years. These investigators found a statistically nonsignificant trend for an increased 10-year survival rate in those patients who underwent complete resection (69% vs. 39% for incomplete resection). Webb and colleagues[31] noted a 10-year survival of 30% in a series of 19 patients that included patients with both incident and recurrent disease. Kanematsu and colleagues[32] noted local recurrence-free survival rates of 91% at 5 years and 76% at 10 years in 11 patients who underwent resection. Included in that group were six patients with residual microscopic tumor, five of whom received postoperative radiation therapy. Zhao and colleagues[18] treated 82 patients with resection and noted overall survival rates 91% and 56% at 5 and 10 years, respectively. Importantly, they found a greater propensity for lymph node metastases and poorer disease-free survival in patients whose tumor arose in a bronchial, rather than tracheal, location. Grillo and Mathisen[17] reported that, during their 27-year study period, only 7 of 60 patients who underwent surgery (12%) died of their tumors. Gaissert and colleagues,[9] in an update of that experience, demonstrated 5- and 10-year survival rates of 52% and 29% for completely resected patients but only 33% and 10% for unresectable patients. Logistic multivariate analysis identified both complete resection and negative margins but not lymph node status to be associated with superior 10-year survival.

MUCOEPIDERMOID CARCINOMA

Mucoepidermoid carcinoma, first reported by Smetana and colleagues,[33] is an uncommon lesion that accounts for less than 0.2% of all lung neoplasms but is the most common salivary-gland–type cancer seen in the lung. It is the second-most common primary malignant epithelial pulmonary tumor seen in children. It is morphologically similar to the mucoepidermoid tumor of the salivary glands.

PATHOLOGY

Like their salivary gland counterparts, bronchial mucoepidermoid carcinomas are classified as high- or low-grade lesions on the basis of their histologic appearance. Most mucoepidermoid carcinomas arise beyond the carina, usually mainstem bronchi but occasionally in lobar or segmental airways. Unlike adenoid cystic carcinoma, tracheal involvement is uncommon. Most tumors appear grossly as intrabronchial polypoid masses without a significant extraluminal component. Penetration of the bronchial wall and a more infiltrative growth pattern are usually associated with the high-grade malignant tumors.

Histologically, mucoepidermoid carcinomas show varying mixtures of clear non–mucus secreting columnar cells and mucus-rich goblet cells (Fig. 105.6) admixed with basaloid, transitional, and epidermoid cells. An ultrastructural and immunohistochemical study of 16 bronchial mucoepidermoid tumors[34] supports a ductal unit origin

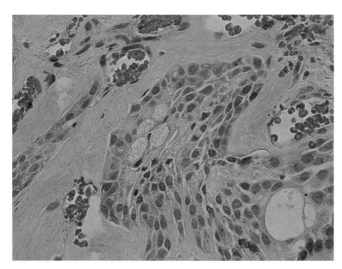

FIGURE 105.6 Low-grade mucoepidermoid carcinoma. Squamous nests with focal glandular lumen and cytoplasmic mucin droplets. (Courtesy of Bruce Tronic.)

without a myoepithelial component. Although low-grade malignant tumors can have mixed cystic and solid histologic characteristics, the cystic component usually predominates. Although mild cytologic atypia can be seen, mitoses are rare. Microscopic invasion of the bronchial submucosa is common, but extension into pulmonary parenchyma is unusual. High-grade tumors more commonly show areas of solid growth, but mixed solid and cystic or predominantly glandular growth can be seen (Fig. 105.7). Cellular atypia, mitotic activity, areas of necrosis, and abrupt transition from one cell type to another are characteristic. The high-grade variant of mucoepidermoid carcinoma occasionally can be difficult to distinguish from adenosquamous carcinoma of the lung. Klacsmann and colleagues[35] proposed several criteria by which this differentiation can be made. The diagnostic confusion is compounded by infrequent reports, such as that of Barsky and colleagues,[36] of mucoepidermoid tumors with

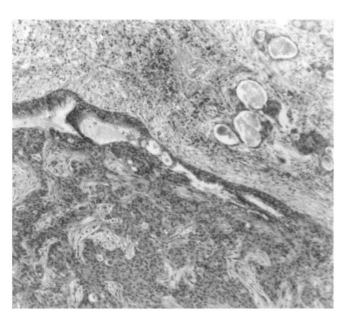

FIGURE 105.7 High-grade mucoepidermoid carcinoma showing solid nests of squamous cells with foci of glandular elements and mucin production (**upper right**).

low-grade histologic features that clinically behave in an aggressive fashion. Shilo and colleagues[37] noted six cases of low-grade pulmonary mucoepidermoid carcinoma associated with an intense lymphoplasmacytic infiltrate. They pointed out that this histologic variant could be confused with low-grade lymphoma. All six tumors were immunoreactive with CK7 and negative for TTF-1 and CK20.

CLINICAL FEATURES

Although some investigators have noted an equal dispersion among sexes, Turnbull and colleagues[38] and Vadasz and Egervary[39] have noted that men are affected two to three times as frequently as women. The average age of patients in published series varies widely from 35 to 53 years, with patients as young as 3 years and as old as 78 years having been reported. Yousem and Hochholzer[40] found that more than 50% of low-grade lesions occurred in patients younger than 30 years of age, whereas the majority of high-grade tumors were found in people over 30 years of age. As with adenoid cystic carcinoma, there is no apparent relationship to tobacco use or exposure to environmental toxins. Most patients present with cough, dyspnea, wheezing, hemoptysis, or obstructive pneumonia. The average duration of symptoms is between 8 and 18 months, but some individuals report symptoms for many years. An occasional patient is asymptomatic. The occurrence of pain, weight loss, or other constitutional symptoms suggests a more aggressive or disseminated tumor. The results of physical examination may be normal, or signs of partial or total airway obstruction may be noted.

RADIOGRAPHIC FEATURES

The radiographic appearance of mucoepidermoid carcinoma is similar to that described for adenoid cystic tumors. The chest radiograph results may be normal or may show signs of whole lung, lobar, or segmental obstruction with or without an associated proximal mass. A distinct well-circumscribed or lobulated intraluminal mass, however, is generally identified by CT scan (Fig. 105.8), which may also demonstrate significant destruction of chronically obstructed parenchymal areas (Fig. 105.9). CT scan is also valuable for assessing local invasion and nodal metastases in cases of high-grade tumors. Mucoepidermoid carcinoma rarely presents as an isolated peripheral pulmonary nodule or mass. High-resolution CT scanning has demonstrated marked heterogeneous enhancement which appears to correlate histologically with more densely vascularized mucin

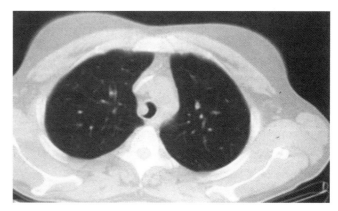

FIGURE 105.8 CT scan shows a well-circumscribed mass arising from the lateral tracheal wall with no apparent extraluminal component. Biopsy documented a low-grade mucoepidermoid carcinoma.

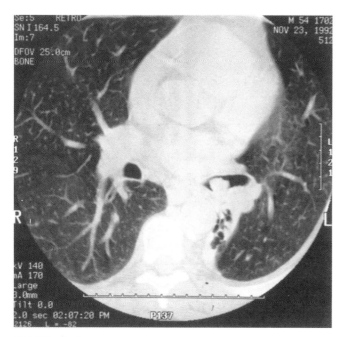

producing areas of the tumor.[41] Variable detection of pulmonary mucoepidermoid carcinoma by ^{18}F-FDG PET has been noted.[42,43]

DIAGNOSIS

As with adenoid cystic tumors, the diagnosis of mucoepidermoid carcinoma is made most often by bronchoscopic biopsy. The lesions are typically covered by normal respiratory mucosa and bronchial brushings and washings are usually nondiagnostic. The tumors appear as soft, well-demarcated polypoid masses and generally have a small base. Conlan and colleagues[16] reported hemorrhage following biopsy in 2 of 12 patients in their series, but neither required special measures for control.

TREATMENT

Most patients present with low-grade tumors that are either localized or minimally invasive. These lesions are best treated by complete resection, often using bronchoplastic techniques to conserve as much normal lung as possible. Hilar and mediastinal node sampling is also performed. Metastasis to hilar or mediastinal lymph nodes is unusual in low-grade tumors. Patients with the high-grade variant should also be managed with resection, but can show hilar and mediastinal node involvement in up to 50% of cases. Occasionally, patients with low-grade tumors are found to have microscopically positive margins after resection. The management and ultimate fate of such patients is unclear. Recurrent disease is associated with high-grade tumors and for some patients reoperation and reresection has been used successfully.[40,44,45]

The role of radiation therapy, either as the primary therapy or postoperative adjuvant treatment, is uncertain. It is commonly employed as postoperative adjuvant treatment in the setting of higher-grade histology and/or nodal metastases. However, Turnbull and colleagues[38] as well as Heitmiller and colleagues[44] noted that radiation therapy may be ineffective in altering the course of high-grade

tumors. As with adenoid cystic carcinoma, there is limited data regarding the efficacy of chemotherapy. Recent investigation[46] has shown that an EGFR mutation is present in 40% of pulmonary mucoepidermoid carcinomas and suggests that these tumors may be a target for tyrosine kinase inhibitors. Endobronchial laser and brachytherapy should be considered for palliation of obstructive symptoms in some patients, but clinical experience with these methods in mucoepidermoid carcinoma is minimal.

PROGNOSIS

Patients with low-grade tumors who undergo complete resection can be expected to be cured of their disease. In contrast, Turnbull,[38] Heitmiller,[44] and Leonardi[47] and their colleagues, all reported 100% mortality rates at 11 to 28 months in cases of high-grade mucoepidermoid carcinoma. Similarly, Vadasz and Egervary[39] noted a 31% 5-year survival rate in 29 patients with high-grade tumors, and all five of their patients with mediastinal lymph node involvement died within 5 years. Gaissert and colleagues[48] noted an 83% 10-year survival rate for 12 resected patients, but both of their two unresected patients died within 5 years. The prognosis is intermediate for patients with low-grade tumors who have undergone operation but have microscopically involved bronchial resection margins. The role of adjuvant treatment in this group is unknown. Serial radiographic and bronchoscopic surveillance is indicated to detect local recurrence.

EPITHELIAL–MYOEPITHELIAL CARCINOMA

Primary pulmonary epithelial–myoepithelial carcinoma is an exceedingly rare low-grade malignant tumor that has been recognized as a distinct entity only in the past two decades.[49] In prior times it had been variably referred to as "adenomyoepithelioma," "epithelial–myoepithelial tumor," and "malignant mixed tumor comprising epithelial and myoepithelial cells." Fewer than 40 cases have been described in the literature. The average patient age is middle age but it has been reported in a patient as young as 7 years.[50] The typical patient complains of a protracted cough, dyspnea, or episodes of pneumonia. As with other lung tumors of salivary gland origin, patients may be mistakenly treated for asthma-like conditions prior to the establishment of the correct diagnosis. There does not appear to be any sex predilection and there is no apparent relationship to tobacco exposure or environmental toxins.

Plain chest radiographs often are normal, especially in the setting of nonobstructing or partially obstructing lesions. Computed tomographic scans typically show an endobronchial mass located in a lobar or main stem bronchus. Tracheal and peripheral pulmonary locations have been reported.[51,52] When faced with a peripheral pulmonary epithelial–myoepithelial carcinoma, the possibility of metastatic disease from the salivary gland must be considered, as distant metastases can be seen in up to 25% of primary salivary tumors and can occur a decade or more after initial diagnosis. Bronchoscopic examination demonstrates a polypoid endobronchial mass usually 15 to 50 mm in size, white/tan to gray in color, and with a gelatinous to solid texture. The lesions are typically well-circumscribed, unencapsulated, and the overlying bronchial epithelial surface is intact. Nguyen and colleagues[53] and Fulford and colleagues,[54] among others, have elucidated the histology and immunohistochemistry of these neoplasms. Microscopically, these tumors demonstrate a biphasic cell population with an inner layer of duct forming epithelial cells and an outer layer of myoepithelial cells. The epithelial cells stain positively for cytokeratin and epithelial membrane antigen and are actin and S-100 negative. The myoepithelial cells stain strongly for S-100 protein, smooth muscle actin, and vimentin. It has been suggested that the myoepithelial component may drive the biologic behavior of these tumors.[55] Song and colleagues,[56] reporting on their series of five patients, noted a single instance of metastatic disease in the only patient to demonstrate a predominantly myoepithelial differentiation.

These tumors are treated by complete resection, which for the majority of patients can be effected by lobectomy. Centrally situated tumors may require pneumonectomy. Metastasis to a peribronchial lymph node with associated lymphovascular and perineural invasion has been reported in a single case,[53] although the long-term fate of that patient is unknown. Salivary gland epithelial–myoepithelial carcinoma can exhibit late local recurrence and on rare occasions distant metastatic disease. The long-term fate of primary pulmonary epithelial–myoepithelial carcinoma is undefined due to rarity of the tumor and short follow-up periods in reported cases.

PLEOMORPHIC ADENOMA

Pleomorphic adenoma, also known as mixed tumor of salivary gland type, is rarely encountered in the lung and tracheobronchial tree. Payne and colleagues[57] were the first to report two cases of pleomorphic adenoma arising in bronchial glands. Since then, only a small number of cases have been encountered.[58–61] Patients typically range in age from 35 to 74 years, although a case has been reported in a patient as young as 8 years. There is no apparent gender predilection. Symptoms of bronchial obstruction such as cough, dyspnea, and wheezing are most common, but some patients have had fever, weight loss, and pleural effusion. Other patients are asymptomatic, and the lesion is discovered incidentally. Chest radiographs can show a pulmonary mass, postobstructive atelectasis or pneumonitis, or an associated pleural effusion. Reported tumors have ranged in size from 2 to 16 cm. Macroscopically, these tumors are soft to rubbery in texture and have a gray–white myxoid appearance. Most parenchymal tumors are well circumscribed. Endobronchial tumors present as a polypoid mass with some degree of bronchial obstruction.

Histologically, these are biphasic neoplasms showing admixtures in varying proportions of epithelial and stromal elements (Fig. 105.10). Moran and colleagues[58] have identified three distinct

histologic patterns: (a) the "classical" mixed tumor with prominent glandular component and chondromyxoid stroma; (b) the solid variant with few glandular structures and predominant solid sheets of myoepithelial cells set against a myxoid background; and (c) obvious cytologic features of malignancy with trabeculae of myoepithelial cells set in a prominent myxoid background. Immunohistochemically, the epithelial and myoepithelial components react with S-100, AE1/AE3, and cytokeratin antibodies and the myoepithelial cells with antibodies against vimentin and muscle-specific actin.[58,61] Reactivity to both high-molecular-weight keratin and TTF-1 has also been reported.[62]

Because these tumors can be benign or malignant, careful histopathologic evaluation is mandatory. The therapeutic goal is complete surgical resection. Most of the reported patients were treated with lobectomy, bilobectomy, or pneumonectomy. Patients with small circumscribed and completely resected lesions with benign histologic features have done well. However, patients with large, infiltrative lesions and histologic features of malignancy tend to develop recurrent and/or metastatic disease. Carcinoma developing in association with a primary or recurrent benign pleomorphic adenoma has been described.[63]

ACINIC CELL CARCINOMA

Fechner and colleagues[64] were the first to report a primary pulmonary neoplasm that was histologically and ultrastructurally identical to acinic cell carcinomas arising in the salivary glands. Since then, less than 20 other instances of this entity have been reported. These tumors usually occur in adults, but reported ages of patients range from 4 to 75 years. There is no apparent sex predilection. These lesions can present as an endobronchial or endotracheal mass or as a peripheral nodule and range in size between 1 and 4.5 cm. Presenting symptoms correspond to the size and location of the tumor. Endobronchial lesions produce symptoms of bronchial obstruction such as cough or wheezing. Peripheral lesions may be totally asymptomatic and discovered as incidental radiographic findings. Macroscopically, these tumors are usually well circumscribed, although not encapsulated, and tan-white or yellow in color.

Histologically, four different growth patterns are recognized: solid, acinar, microcystic, and papillary-cystic (Fig. 105.11). In addition,

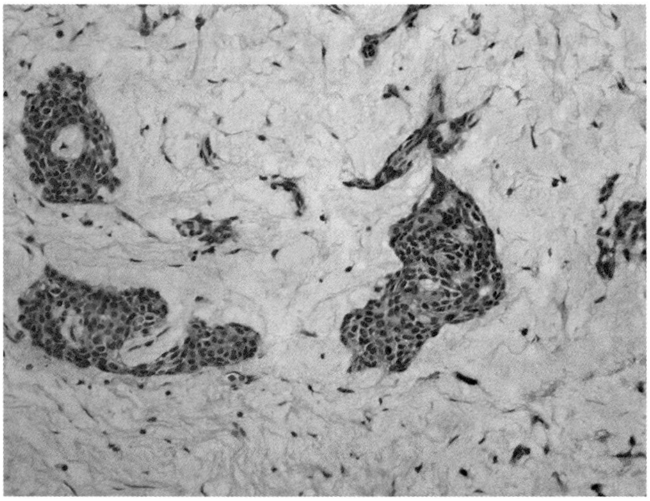

FIGURE 105.10 Pleomorphic adenoma. Nests of benign myoepithelial cells embedded in a myxoid stroma. (Courtesy of Bruce Tronic.)

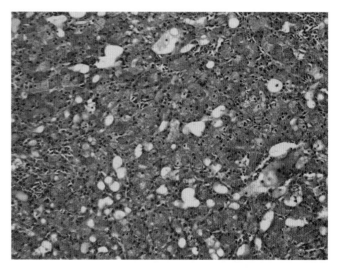

FIGURE 105.11 Acinic cell carcinoma showing a solid growth pattern. (Courtesy of Bruce Tronic.)

oncocytic, clear, and vacuolated cell populations are observed. In a detailed pathologic analysis of five pulmonary acinic cell carcinomas, Moran and colleagues[65] found these lesions to stain positively with low-molecular-weight and broad-spectrum keratin antibodies as well as epithelial membrane antigen antibodies. Stains for vimentin, S-100 protein, chromogranin, and lysozyme were uniformly negative. Electron microscopy shows abundant zymogen-type cytoplasmic granules characteristic of acinar-type secretory cells. These ultrastructural and immunohistochemical characteristics can be of use in differentiating pulmonary acinic cell carcinomas from other morphologically similar primary and metastatic lung tumors. Rare instances of combined carcinoid and acinic cell carcinoma have been reported[66,67] suggesting that neuroendocrine and acinic components may have a common stem cell origin.

Most reported cases have been managed by primary surgical resection, including segmentectomy, lobectomy, bilobectomy, and tracheal resection. The results of treatment appear to be excellent because there have been no reported deaths from this lesion. Ansari and colleagues[68] reported endoscopic laser tumor ablation to improve airway patency before tracheal resection. Horowitz and Kronenberg[69] reported a case of tracheal acinic cell carcinoma removed through the bronchoscope with electrocauterization of the tumor base. This patient has been followed for 8 years without evidence of recurrence. Ukoha and colleagues[70] reported a case of primary pulmonary acinic cell carcinoma metastatic to interlobar lymph nodes. The patient was treated with lobectomy, mediastinal lymphadenectomy, and adjuvant radiation therapy and was without recurrence 20 months postoperatively. Chuah and colleagues[71] reported a second such patient with metastasis to one hilar node, treated initially with lobectomy, who developed a metastasis to the paravertebral sulcus 20 months following resection.

ONCOCYTOMA

Oncocytoma is the most infrequently occurring of all salivary gland–type pulmonary neoplasms, and only a handful of cases have been documented. This tumor is composed of oncocytes, a descriptive term for epithelial cells with abundant granular eosinophilic cytoplasm and relatively small nuclei. A variety of organelles can impart an eosinophilic granular appearance to the cytoplasm by light microscopy, and a true oncocytoma is defined by the sole ultrastructural criterion of marked mitochondrial hyperplasia. The cause of the mitochondrial hyperplasia is unknown. Oncocytes are normally found in mature organs forming part of the lining epithelium of glandular ducts and acini. They have been found in the salivary glands, thyroid, buccal mucosa, breast, trachea, kidney, and gastrointestinal tract as well as in other locations. According to Hamperl,[72] oncocytes represent a special metaplastic transformation of epithelial cells, and their numbers increase in frequency with the advancing age of the individual. Tashiro and colleagues[73] demonstrated immunoreactivity to cytokeratin and vimentin but not to alpha-actin. Oncocytomas are different from oncocytic carcinoids, which demonstrate biphasic populations of oncocytic and carcinoid cells or the presence of neurosecretory granules by electron microscopy.

Fechner and Bentinck[74] reported the first case of a true pulmonary oncocytoma confirmed by electron microscopy. Subsequent isolated instances of pulmonary oncocytoma have been reported by others.[75–80] These patients ranged in age from 16 to 68 years and most were men. The presenting symptoms have been cough, pneumonitis, or chest discomfort. One patient's tumor was discovered as an incidental radiographic finding. Chest radiographs can show a well-circumscribed parenchymal mass or an area of infiltrate distal to an obstructed bronchus. These tumors are yellowish tan or reddish brown in color. Patients were treated with local excision or with lobectomy, and there have been no reported instances of recurrence. Nielsen[81] reported the only case of bronchial oncocytoma with an infiltrative growth pattern and a microscopic metastasis to a parabronchial lymph node. The patient underwent lobectomy and remained without recurrence 2 years later.

REFERENCES

1. Dalton L, Gatling RR. Peripheral adenoid cystic carcinoma of the lung. *South Med J* 1990;83:577–579. http://dx.doi.org/10.1097/00007611-199005000-00026
2. Inoue H, Iwashita A, Kanegae H, et al. Peripheral pulmonary adenoid cystic carcinoma with substantial submucosal extension to the proximal bronchus. *Thorax* 1991;46:147–148. http://dx.doi.org/10.1136/thx.46.2.147
3. Maziak DE, Todd TR, Keshavjee SH, et al. Adenoid cystic carcinoma of the airway: thirty-two-year experience. *J Thorac Cardiovasc Surg* 1996;112:1522–1531. http://dx.doi.org/10.1016/S0022-5223(96)70011-9
4. Prommegger R, Salzer GM. Long-term results of surgery for adenoid cystic carcinoma of the trachea and bronchi. *Eur J Surg Oncol* 1998;24:440–444. http://dx.doi.org/10.1016/S0748-7983(98)92465-9
5. Nomori H, Kaseda S, Kobayashi K, et al. Adenoid cystic carcinoma of the trachea and main-stem bronchus. A clinical, histopathologic, and immunohistochemical study. *J Thorac Cardiovasc Surg* 1988;96:271–277.
6. Albers E, Lawrie T, Harrell JH. Tracheobronchial adenoid cystic carcinoma: a clinicopathologic study of 14 cases. *Chest* 2004;125:1160–1165. http://dx.doi.org/10.1378/chest.125.3.1160
7. Moran CA. Primary salivary gland-type tumors of the lung. *Semin Diagn Pathol* 1995;12:106–122.
8. Lin CM, Li AF, Wu LH, et al. Adenoid cystic carcinoma of the trachea and bronchus—a clinicopathologic study with DNA flow cytometric analysis and oncogene expression. *Eur J Cardiothorac Surg* 2002;22:621–625. http://dx.doi.org/10.1016/S1010-7940(02)00406-2
9. Gaissert HA, Grillo HC, Shadmehr MB, et al. Long-term survival after resection of primary adenoid cystic and squamous cell carcinoma of the trachea and carina. *Ann Thorac Surg* 2004;78:1889–1897. http://dx.doi.org/10.1016/j.athoracsur.2004.05.064
10. Shanley DJ, Daum-Kowalski R, Embry RL. Adenoid cystic carcinoma of the airway: MR findings. *AJR* 1991;156:1321–1322. http://dx.doi.org/10.2214/ajr.156.6.1851382
11. Akata S, Ohkubo Y, Park J, et al. Multiplanar reconstruction MR image of primary adenoid cystic carcinoma of the central airway (MPR of central airway adenoid cystic carcinoma). *Clin Imaging* 2001;25:332–336. http://dx.doi.org/10.1016/S0899-7071(01)00317-5
12. Kwak SH, Lee KS, Jeong YJ, et al. Adenoid cystic carcinoma of the airways: helical CT and histopathologic correlation. *AJR* 2004;183:277–281 http://dx.doi.org/10.2214/ajr.183.2.1830277
13. Campistron M, Rouquette I, Courbon F, et al. Adenoid cystic carcinoma of the lung: interest of 18FDG PET/CT in the management of an atypical presentation. *Lung Cancer*, 2008; 59:133–136. http://dx.doi.org/10.1016/j.lungcan.2007.06.002
14. ElNayal A, Moran CA, Fox PS, et al. Primary salivary gland-type lung cancer: Imaging and clinical predictors of outcome. *AJR* 2013;201:W57–W63. http://dx.doi.org/10.2214/AJR.12.9579
15. Attar S, Miller JE, Hankins J, et al. Bronchial adenoma: a review of 51 patients. *Ann Thorac Surg* 1985;40:126–435. http://dx.doi.org/10.1016/S0003-4975(10)60004-5
16. Conlan AA, Payne WS, Woolner LB, et al. Adenoid cystic carcinoma (cylindroma) and mucoepidermoid carcinoma of the bronchus. Factors affecting survival. *J Thorac Cardiovasc Surg* 1978;76:369–377.
17. Grillo HC, Mathisen DJ. Primary tracheal tumors: treatment and results. *Ann Thorac Surg* 1990;49:69–77. http://dx.doi.org/10.1016/0003-4975(90)90358-D
18. Zhao Y, Zhao H, Fan L, et al. Adenoid cystic carcinoma in the bronchus behaves more aggressively than its tracheal counterpart. *Ann Thorac Surg* 2013;96:1998–2005. http://dx.doi.org/10.1016/j.athoracsur.2013.08.009
19. Pearson FG, Thompson DW, Weissberg D, et al. Adenoid cystic carcinoma of the trachea. *Ann Thorac Surg* 1974;18:16–29. http://dx.doi.org/10.1016/S0003-4975(10)65713-X
20. Perelman MI, Koroleva N, Birjukov J, et al. Primary tracheal tumors. *Semin Thorac Cardiovasc Surg* 1996;8:400–402.
21. Wurtz A, Porte H, Conti M, et al. Surgical techniques and results of tracheal and carinal replacement with aortic allografts for salivary-gland type carcinoma. *J Thorac Cardiovasc Surg* 2010;140:387-393. http://dx.doi.org/10.1016/j.jtcvs.2010.01.043
22. Fields JN, Rigaud G, Emani BN. Primary tumors of the trachea. Results of radiation therapy. *Cancer* 1989;63:2429–2433. http://dx.doi.org/10.1002/1097-0142(19890615)63:12%3C2429::AID-CNCR2820631210%3E3.0.CO;2-0
23. Harms W, Latz D, Becker H, et al. Treatment of primary tracheal carcinoma: the role of external and endoluminal radiotherapy. *Strahlenther Onkol* 2000;176:22–27. http://dx.doi.org/10.1007/PL00002300
24. Carvalho HA, Figueredo V, Pedreira WL, et al. High dose-rate brachytherapy as a treatment option in primary tracheal tumors. *Clinics* 2005;60:299–304. http://dx.doi.org/10.1590/S1807-59322005000400007
25. Perelman MI, Koroleva NS. Primary tumors of the trachea. In Grillo H, Eschapasse H, eds. *International Trends in General Thoracic Surgery*. Vol. 2. Philadelphia, PA: Saunders, 1987:91–106.

26. Diaz-Jimenez JP, Canela-Cardona M, Maestre-Alcacer J. Nd:YAG laser photoresection of low-grade malignant tumors of the tracheobronchial tree. *Chest* 1990;97:920–922. http://dx.doi.org/10.1378/chest.97.4.920

27. Lee JH, Jung EJ, Jeon K, et al. Treatment outcomes of patients with adenoid cystic carcinoma of the airway. *Lung Cancer* 2011;72:244–249. http://dx.doi.org/10.1016/j.lungcan.2010.08.011

28. Personne C, Colchen A, Leroy M, et al. Indications and technique for endoscopic laser resections in bronchology: a critical analysis based upon 2,284 resections. *J Thorac Cardiovasc Surg* 1986;91:710–715.

29. Laurie SA, Ho AL, Fury MG, et al. Systemic therapy in the management of metastatic or locally recurrent adenoid cystic carcinoma of the salivary glands: a systematic review. *Lancet Oncol* 2011;12:815–825. http://dx.doi.org/10.1016/S1470-2045(10)70245-X

30. Carter D, Eggleston J. *Atlas of Tumor Pathology, Fasicle 17: Tumors of the Lower Respiratory Tract.* Washington, DC: Armed Forces Institute of Pathology, 1980.

31. Webb BD, Walsh GL, Roberts DB, et al. Primary tracheal malignant neoplasms: The University of Texas MD Anderson Cancer Center experience. *J Am Coll Surg* 2006;202:237–246. http://dx.doi.org/10.1016/j.jamcollsurg.2005.09.016

32. Kanematsu T, Yohena T, Uehara T, et al. Treatment outcome of resected and nonresected primary adenoid cystic carcinoma of the lung. *Ann Thorac Cardiovasc Surg* 2002;8:74–77. http://www.atcs.jp/pdf/2002 8 2/74.pdf

33. Smetana HF, Iverson L, Swann LL. Bronchogenic carcinoma, an analysis of 100 autopsy cases. *Mil Surg* 1952;111:335–351.

34. Sanchez-Mora N, Parra-Blanco V, Cebollero-Presmanes M, et al. Mucoepidermoid tumors of the bronchus. Ultrastructural and immunohistochemical study. Histogenic correlations. *Histol Histopathol* 2007;22:9–13. http://www.hh.um.es/pdf/Vol_22/22_1/Maricchiolo-22-79-83-2007.pdf

35. Klacsmann PG, Olson JL, Eggleston JC. Mucoepidermoid carcinoma of the bronchus. *Cancer* 1979;43:1720–1733. http://dx.doi.org/10.1002/1097-0142(197905)43:5%3C1720::AID-CNCR2820430523%3E3.0.CO;2-Q

36. Barsky SH, Martin SE, Matthews M, et al. "Low-grade" mucoepidermoid carcinoma of the bronchus with "high-grade" biological behavior. *Cancer* 1983;51:1505–1509. http://dx.doi.org/10.1002/1097-0142(19830415)51:8%3C1505::AID-CNCR2820510825%3E3.0.CO;2-9

37. Shilo K, Foss RD, Franks TJ, et al. Pulmonary mucoepidermoid carcinoma with prominent tumor-associated lymphoid proliferation. *Am J Surg Pathol* 2005;29:407–411. http://dx.doi.org/10.1097/01.pas.0000151616.14598.e7

38. Turnbull AD, Huvos AG, Goodner JT, et al. Mucoepidermoid tumors of bronchial glands. *Cancer* 1971;28:539–544. http://dx.doi.org/10.1002/1097-0142(197109)28:3%3C539::AID-CNCR2820280302%3E3.0.CO;2-G

39. Vadasz P, Egervary M. Mucoepidermoid bronchial tumors: a review of 34 operated cases. *Eur J Cardiothorac Surg* 2000;17:566–569. http://dx.doi.org/10.1016/S1010-7940(00)00386-9

40. Yousem SA, Hochholzer L. Mucoepidermoid tumors of the lung. *Cancer* 1987;60:1346–1352. http://dx.doi.org/10.1002/1097-0142(19870915)60:6%3C1346::AID-CNCR2820600631%3E3.0.CO;2-0

41. Ishizumi T, Tateishi U, Watanabe S, et al. Mucoepidermoid carcinoma of the lung: high-resolution CT and histopathologic findings in five cases. *Lung Cancer* 2008;60:125–131. http://dx.doi.org/10.1016/j.lungcan.2007.08.022

42. Kinoshita H, Shimotake T, Furukawa T, et al. Mucoepidermoid carcinoma of the lung detected by positron emission tomography in a 5 year old girl. *J Pediatr Surg* 2005;40:E1–E3. http://dx.doi.org/10.1002/1097-0142(19870915)60:6%3C1346::AID-CNCR2820600631%3E3.0.CO;2-0

43. Shin SS, Lee KS, Kim BT, et al. Focal parenchymal lung lesions showing a potential of false-positive and false-negative interpretations on integrated PET/CT. *AJR* 2006;186:639–648. http://dx.doi.org/10.2214/AJR.04.1896

44. Heitmiller RF, Mathisen DJ, Ferry JA, et al. Mucoepidermoid lung tumors. *Ann Thorac Surg* 1989;47:394–399. http://dx.doi.org/10.1016/0003-4975(89)90380-9

45. Kang DY, Yoon YS, Kim HK, et al. Primary salivary gland-type lung cancer:sugical outcomes. *Lung Cancer* 2011;72:250–254. http://dx.doi.org/10.1016/j.lungcan.2010.08.021

46. Han SW, Kim HP, Jeon YK, et al. Mucoepidermoid carcinoma of lung:potential target of EGFR-directed treatment. *Lung Cancer* 2008;61:30–34.http://dx.doi.org/10.1016/j.lungcan.2007.11.014

47. Leonardi HK, Jung-Legg Y, Legg MA, et al. Tracheobronchial mucoepidermoid carcinoma. Clinicopathological features and results of treatment. *Ann Thorac Cardiovasc Surg* 1978;76:431–438.

48. Gaissert HA, Grillo HC, Shadmehr MB, et al. Uncommon primary tracheal tumors. *Ann Thorac Surg* 2006;82:268–273. http://dx.doi.org/10.1016/j.athoracsur.2006.01.065

49. Wilson RG, Moran CA. Epithelial-myoepithelial carcinoma of the lung: immunohistochemical and ultrastructural observations and review of the literature. *Hum Pathol* 1997;28:631–634. http://dx.doi.org/10.1016/S0046-8177(97)90088-5

50. Rosenfeld A, Schwartz D, Garzon S, et al. Epithelial-myoepithelial carcinoma of the lung. A case report and review of the literature. *J Pediatr Hematol Oncol* 2009;31:206–208. http://dx.doi.org/10.1097/MPH.0b013e3181978e62

51. Munoz G, Felipo F, Marquina I, et al. Epithelial-myoepithelial tumor of the lung: a case report referring to its molecular histogenesis. *Diagn Pathol* 2011;6:71–75. http://dx.doi.org/10.1186/1746-1596-6-71

52. Cho SH, Park SD, Ko TY, et al. Primary epithelial myoepithelial lung carcinoma. *Korean J Thorac Cardiovasc Surg* 2014;47:59–62. http://dx.doi.org/10.5090/kjtcs.2014.47.1.59

53. Nguyen CV, Suster S, Moran CA. Pulmonary epithelial-myoepithelial carcinoma: a clinicopathologic and immunohistochemical study of 5 cases. *Human Pathology* 2009;40:366–373. http://dx.doi.org/10.1016/j.humpath.2008.08.009

54. Fulford LG, Kamata Y, Okudera K, et al. Epithelial-myopeithelial carcinomas of the bronchus. *Am J Surg Pathol* 2001;25:1508–1514. http://dx.doi.org/10.1097/00000478-200112000-00006

55. Pelosi G, Fragetta F. Epithelial-myoepithelial carcinomas of the bronchus (letter). *Am J Surg Pathol* 2002;26:950–951 http://dx.doi.org/10.1097/00000478-200207000-00016

56. Song DH, Choi IH, Ha SY, et al. Epithelial-myoepithelial carcinoma of the tracheo-bronchial tree: the prognostic role of myoepithelial cells. *Lung Cancer* 2014;83:416-419. http://dx.doi.org/10.1016/j.lungcan.2014.01.005

57. Payne WS, Schier J, Woolner LB. Mixed tumors of the bronchus (salivary gland type). *J Thorac Cardiovasc Surg* 1965;49:663–668.

58. Moran CA, Suster S, Askin FB, et al. Benign and malignant salivary gland-type mixed tumors of the lung. Clinicopathologic and immunohistochemical study of eight cases. *Cancer* 1994;73:2481–2490. http://dx.doi.org/10.1002/1097-0142(19940515)73:10%3C2481::AID-CNCR2820731006%3E3.0.CO;2-A

59. Fitchett J, Luckraz H, Gibbs A, et al. A rare case of primary pleomorphic adenoma in main bronchus. *Ann Thorac Surg* 2008:86;1025–1026. http://dx.doi.org/10.1016/j.athoracsur.2008.02.073

60. Kamiyoshihara M, Ibe T, Takeyoshi I. Pleomorphic adenoma of the main bronchus in an adult treated using a wedge bronchiectomy. *Gen Thoracic Cardiovascular Surge* 2009;57:43-45. http://dx.doi.org/10.1007/s11748-008-0319-7

61. Gakidis I, Mihos PT, Chatziantoniou C, et al. A large neglected pleomorphic asdemoa of the lung:report of a rare case. *Asian Cardiovasc Thorac Ann* 2014;22:620–622. http://dx.doi.org/10.1177/0218492313479959

62. Mejean-Lebreton F, Barnoud R, de la Roche E, et al. Benign salivary gland–type tumors of the bronchus: expression of high molecular weight cytokeratins. *Ann Pathol* 2006;26:30–34. http://dx.doi.org/10.1016/S0242-6498(06)70658-7

63. Weissferdt A, Moran CA. Pulmonary salivary-gland tumors with features of malignant mixed tumor (carcinoma ex pleomorphic adenoma). *Am J Clin Pathol* 2011;136:793–798. http://dx.doi.org/10.1309/AJCP50FBZWSACKIP

64. Fechner RE, Bentinck BA, Askew JB. Acinic cell tumor of the lung: a histologic and ultrastructural study. *Cancer*1972;29:501–508. http://dx.doi.org/10.1002/1097-0142(197202)29:2%3C501::AID-CNCR2820290241%3E3.0.CO;2-B

65. Moran CA, Suster S, Koss MN. Acinic cell carcinoma of the lung ("Fechner tumor"). A clinicopathologic, immunohistochemical and ultrastructural study of five cases. *Am J Surg Pathol* 1992;16:1039–1050. http://dx.doi.org/10.1097/00000478-199211000-00002

66. Rodriguez J, Diment J, Lombardi L, et al. Combined typical carcinoid and acinic cell tumor of the lung: a heretofore unreported occurrence. *Hum Pathol* 2003;34:1061–1065. http://dx.doi.org/10.1053/S0046-8177(03)00347-2

67. Sano A, Takeuchi E, Hebisawa A, et al. Combined typical carcinoid and acinic cell tumor of the lung. *Interact Cardiovasc Thorac Surg* 2011;12:311–312. http://dx.doi.org/10.1510/icvts.2010.258186

68. Ansari MA, Marchevsky A, Strick L, et al. Upper airway obstruction secondary to acinic cell carcinoma of the trachea: use of Nd:YAG laser. *Chest* 1996;110:1120–1122. http://dx.doi.org/10.1378/chest.110.4.1120

69. Horowitz Z, Kronenberg J. Acinic cell carcinoma of the trachea. *Auris Nasus Larynx* 1994;21:193–195. http://dx.doi.org/10.1016/S0385-8146(12)80144-1

70. Ukoha OO, Quartararo P, Carter D, et al. Acinic cell carcinoma of the lung with metastasis to lymph nodes. *Chest* 1971;115:591–544. http://dx.doi.org/10.1378/chest.115.2.591

71. Chuah KL, Yap WM, Tan HW. Recurrence of pulmonary acinic cell carcinoma. *Arch Pathol Lab Med* 2006;130:932–933. http://www.archivesofpathology.org/doi/pdf/10.1043/1543-2165%282006%29130%5B932%3AROPACC%5D2.0.CO%3B2

72. Hamperl H. Benign and malignant oncocytoma. *Cancer* 1962;15:1019–1027. http://dx.doi.org/10.1002/1097-0142(196209/10)15:5%3C1019::AID-CN-CR2820150519%3E3.0.CO;2-5

73. Tashiro Y, Iwata Y, Nabae T, et al. Pulmonary oncocytoma: report of a case in conjunction with an immunohistochemical and ultrastructural study. *Pathol Int* 1995;45:448–451. http://dx.doi.org/10.1111/j.1440-1827.1995.tb03483.x

74. Fechner RE, Bentinck BA. Ultrastructure of bronchial oncocytoma. *Cancer* 1973;31:1451–1457. http://dx.doi.org/10.1002/1097-0142(197306)31:6%3C1451::AID-CNCR2820310621%3E3.0.CO;2-L

75. Santos-Briz A, Terron J, Sastre R, et al. Oncocytoma of the lung. *Cancer* 1977;40:1330–1336. http://dx.doi.org/10.1002/1097-0142(197709)40:3%3C1330::AID-CNCR2820400350%3E3.0.CO;2-K

76. Fernandez MA, Nyssen J. Oncocytoma of the lung. *Can J Surg* 1982;25:332–333.

77. Cwierzyk TA, Glasberg SS, Virshup MA, et al. Pulmonary oncocytoma. Report of a case with cytologic, histologic and electron microscopic study. *Acta Cytol* 1985;29:620–623.

78. Tesluk H, Dajee A. Pulmonary oncocytoma. *J Surg Oncol* 1985;29:173–175. http://dx.doi.org/10.1002/jso.2930290308

79. deAquino RT, Magliari ME, Saad R, et al. Bronchial oncocytoma. *Sao Paulo Med J* 2000;118:195–197. http://dx.doi.org/10.1590/S1516-31802000000600009

80. Burrah R, Kini U, Correa M, et al. Pulmonary oncocytoma: a rare case. *Asian Cardiovasc Thorac Ann* 2006;14:e113–e114.

81. Nielsen AL. Malignant bronchial oncocytoma: case report and review of the literature. *Hum Pathol* 1985;16:852–854. http://dx.doi.org/10.1016/S0046-8177(85)80260-4

82. Travis WD, Brambilla E, Burke AP, Marx A, Nicholson AG. *WHO Classification of Tumours of the Lung, Pleura, Thymus and Heart.* Lyon: International Agency for Research on Cancer, 2015.

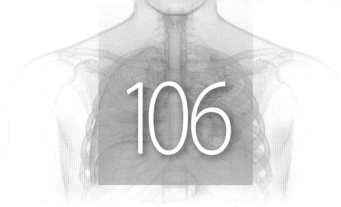

Benign Tumors of the Lung

Virginia R. Litle ■ Ghulam Abbas

Benign tumors of the lung are infrequently encountered. Martini and Beattie[1] reported that <1% of the lung tumors resected at Memorial Sloan-Kettering Hospital were benign. Chan and colleagues[2] pointed out that the benign lung tumors probably accounted for less than 5% of all primary lung tumors. In the older literature, during the 1960s and less so in the 1970s, most of the adenomas were carcinoid tumors or cylindromas, which is another name for adenoid cystic carcinoma. The change in terminology makes it difficult to evaluate the older literature. In this chapter, there is no discussion of either of these lung tumors, since they are not benign. Benign tumors may be derived from all cell types present in the lung and may be either parenchymal or endobronchial in location.

No standardized classification of benign lung tumors exists. The authors took the liberty of creating classifications (Table 106.1 for solitary tumors and Table 106.2 for multiple tumors) mostly derived from the World Health Organization (WHO) classification of tumors and including the lung group authored by Travis and colleagues and the soft tissue group authored by Fletcher and colleagues.[3,4] Since the pulmonary hamartoma is the most common of the benign tumors, we elected to discuss this entity first and to discuss the remaining entities in the order in which they appear in the two classification tables of solitary and multiple benign pulmonary tumors (Tables 106.1 and 106.2).

Some of the tumors in this section were considered benign, but in some cases, they may recur or metastasize. These tumors include pleomorphic adenoma, myoepithelioma and adenomyoepithelioma, solitary fibrous tumor, inflammatory myofibroblastic tumor, and benign metastasizing leiomyoma.

TABLE 106.1 Benign Solitary Tumors of the Lung

Epithelial Tumors
Papilloma
  Squamous cell papilloma (exophytic or inverted types)
  Glandular papilloma
  Mixed squamous cell and glandular papilloma
Adenoma
  Alveolar adenoma
  Papillary adenoma (type II pneumocyte or Clara cell adenoma)
  Adenoma of salivary gland type
    Pleomorphic adenoma
    Mucous gland adenoma
    Oncocytoma
    Myoepithelioma and adenomyoepithelioma
  Mucinous cystadenoma

Soft Tissue Tumors
Adipocytic
  Angiomyolipoma
  Lipoma
Fibroblastic/myofibroblastic
  Fibromyxoma
  Inflammatory fibrous polyp
  Inflammatory myofibroblastic tumor (inflammatory pseudotumor)
  Solitary fibrous tumor (localized fibrous mesothelioma)
Smooth muscle
  Leiomyoma

Pericytic
  Glomus tumor
Vascular
  Hemangioma
  Lymphatic lesions (solitary intrapulmonary lymphangioma)
Cartilaginous
  Chondroma
Osseous
  Osteoma
Peripheral nerve sheath and related lesions
  Granular cell tumor
  Meningioma
  Neurofibroma
  Schwannoma
  Psammomatous melanotic schwannoma
Paraganglionic
  Paraganglioma
  Gangliocytic paraganglioma

Miscellaneous Tumors
Clear cell tumor (sugar tumor)
Hamartoma
Myelolipoma
Nodular amyloidoma
Sclerosing hemangioma
Teratoma
Thymoma

From Fletcher CDM, Unni KK, Mertens F, eds. *World Health Organization Classification of Tumours. Pathology and Genetics of Tumours of Soft Tissue and Bone.* Lyon: IARC Press; 2002:10; Travis WD, Brambilla E, Müller-Hermelink HK, Harris CC. *World Health Organization Classification of Tumours. Pathology and Genetics of Tumours of the Lung, Pleura, Thymus and Heart.* Lyon: IARC Press; 2004:10.

TABLE 106.2 Benign Multiple Tumors of the Lung

Multiple tumors
    Benign metastasizing leiomyomas
    Cystic fibrohistiocytic tumor (metastatic dermatofibroma)
    Pulmonary capillary hemangiomatosis
    Pulmonary hyalinizing granuloma
    Pulmonary lymphangioleiomyomatosis

From Fletcher CDM, Unni KK, Mertens F, eds. *World Health Organization Classification of Tumours. Pathology and Genetics of Tumours of Soft Tissue and Bone.* Lyon: IARC Press; 2002:10; Travis WD, Brambilla E, Müller-Hermelink HK, Harris CC. *World Health Organization Classification of Tumours. Pathology and Genetics of Tumours of the Lung, Pleura, Thymus and Heart.* Lyon: IARC Press; 2004:10.

HISTORICAL PERSPECTIVE

Steele[5] published a review of the resection of 887 pulmonary nodules. The nodules could be subdivided as follows: granulomas (53.4%), malignant tumors (35.6%), hamartomas (7.3%), miscellaneous tumors (2.5%), and pleural or chest wall tumors (1%). Shortly thereafter, Aletras and colleagues[6] discussed 16 "benign" lung tumors that consisted of the following: 8 adenomas (subdivided into 90% carcinoid tumor and 10% pleomorphic adenoma), 5 hamartomas, 1 schwannoma, 1 arteriovenous fistula, and 1 fibroma (probably a solitary fibrous tumor). Arrigoni and colleagues[7] reported 130 cases of benign lung tumors from the Mayo Clinic. The tumors they reported could be classified as follows: hamartoma (76.9%), benign fibrous mesothelioma (probably solitary fibrous tumor) (12.3%), xanthoma and inflammatory pseudotumors (5.4%), and other (5.4%). In these early series, the pulmonary hamartoma is clearly the most common benign tumor.

Since the early papers mentioned above, other series of benign lung tumors have appeared. Between 1974 and 1988, Mitsudomi and colleagues[8] resected 36 benign tumors or tumor-like lesions out of 721 thoracotomies. The tumors were hamartoma (58%), inflammatory pseudotumor (25%), and sclerosing hemangioma (16%). Otani and colleagues[9] reported, in their 20-year experience with benign lung tumors, that the most common ones were hamartoma (54%), sclerosing hemangioma (18%), bronchogenic cyst (13.6%), leiomyoma (9%), and adenoma (4.5%). In conclusion, the hamartoma is the most common benign tumor of the lung. Allen[10] in his review of rare solitary benign lung tumors, agreed that the hamartoma was the most common.[11] In one series, the patients who underwent resection for focal pulmonary lesions that were thought to be malignant but then were benign were distributed as follows: granulomas in 65%, hamartoma 12%, pneumonia or pneumonitis in 10%, fibrosis in 4%, and other in 9%.[11] The category of other lesions includes abscess, aspergilloma, amyloid, bronchogenic cyst, carcinoid tumorlet, clear cell tumor, inflammatory pseudotumor, meningioma, mesothelial hyperplasia, necrosis, and rheumatoid nodule. Again, pulmonary hamartoma remains the most common benign solitary tumor.

HAMARTOMA

Pulmonary hamartomas are benign neoplasms composed predominantly of chondroid or chondromyxoid tissue intermixed with variable portions of other mesenchymal components, including fat, myxoid fibrous connective tissue, smooth muscle, and bone (Fig. 106.1). Clefts of normal respiratory epithelial cells represent entrapment by the expanding mesenchymal growth. The 2015 WHO Classification

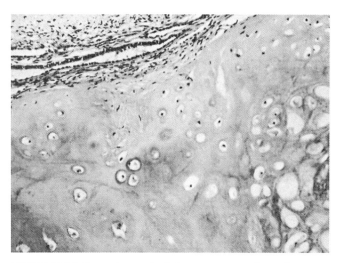

FIGURE 106.1 Photomicrograph of a hamartoma. Note the predominance of cartilage cells.

of Tumors of the Lung, Pleura, Thymus and Heart classifies the hamartomas of lung as pulmonary hamartomas.[12] In contrary to the hamartomas of the other part of the body which are not considered neoplasms, pulmonary hamartomas have an International Classification of Diseases for Oncology code as multiple genetic studies have established that they are true neoplasms.

CLINICAL FEATURES

Pulmonary hamartomas are the most common benign pulmonary tumor of the lung and account for 4% to 7% of all solitary pulmonary nodules. They are found more commonly in men with a preponderance of 2:1 to 3:1 and the peak incidence is in the fifth to seventh decades of life, though no age group is exempt.[13] They are usually asymptomatic and discovered incidentally but may present with hemoptysis, cough, chest tightness, and repeated respiratory infections. They typically present as solitary, small (<4 cm), well-circumscribed, peripheral nodules but infrequently are found centrally or endobronchially. Le Roux[14] recorded an incidence of 8% of endobronchial hamartomas in 27 patients. Gjevre and colleagues,[13] however, noted an incidence of only 1.4% in 215 cases of hamartoma seen at the Mayo Clinic. The true incidence undoubtedly lies somewhere between these two percentages. The location distribution is equal among all lobes.[15] Slow growth is not unusual but doubling time is well below that of malignant lesions. Hansen and colleagues[16] reported that the size of the hamartoma could increase by an average of 3.2 ± 2.6 mm per year. They conducted a study on 89 patients with pulmonary hamartomas. Forty patients had a needle biopsy with a sensitivity of 85%. Seventy-five patients (84%) underwent surgical resection and 15 patients underwent surveillance scans. During a 4-year follow-up of these 15 patients, there was an average increase of 3.2 ± 2.6 mm per year in the size of the hamartoma.

RADIOLOGY

The characteristic radiographical appearance of a hamartoma is a solitary, peripheral, well-circumscribed, smooth or slightly lobulated lung nodule. Calcification is present in 10% to 30% of lesions and fat density is present up to 50% of nodules, both being presented in 19% of pulmonary hamartomas.[17] The presence of fat in the nodule

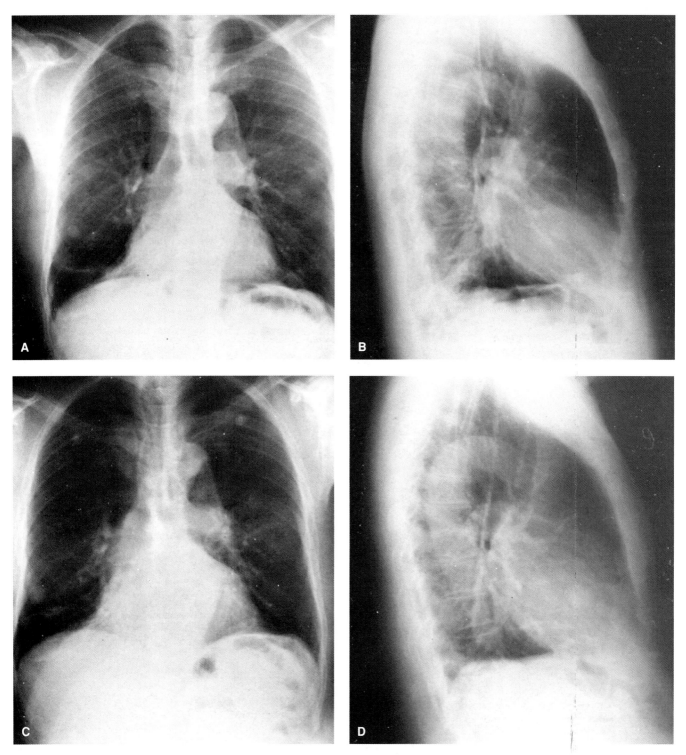

FIGURE 106.2 **A:** Posteroanterior radiograph of calcified lesion overlying aortic knob on the left. **B:** Lateral radiograph shows the lesion to be in the anterior segment of the left lung. **C:** CT scan showing calcification within the mass. **D:** Enhanced CT scan revealing popcorn-like calcifications in the mass, typical of a hamartoma.

is considered diagnostic and biopsy or resection can be avoided. In summary, a less than 4 cm peripheral well-circumscribed nodule with popcorn-like calcification and fat on CT is diagnostic for pulmonary hamartoma unless proven otherwise (Fig. 106.2).[18]

Magnetic resonance imaging (MRI) is an additional diagnostic tool that can be useful when a discrete pulmonary nodule demonstrates neither fat nor calcification on CT scan. The MRI image identifies

(particularly the T2-weighted images) the common cleft-like structure of a pulmonary hamartoma and can provide confidence in the diagnosis.[19]

Endobronchial hamartomas are usually undetectable radiographically except when distal parenchymal lung changes (e.g., atelectasis, obstructive pneumonia, or abscess formation) suggest an obstructing, endobronchial lesion.[13]

PATHOLOGY

On gross examination, hamartomas have a gray lobulated or bosselated surface. On cut section, they have a gray appearance. There may be some gritty yellow areas that represent calcifications. On microscopic examination, hamartomas are composed of lobulated masses of mature cartilage with other mesenchymal elements that include adipose tissue, smooth muscle, bone, and fibrovascular as well as fibromyxoid tissue.[20] Frequently there are cleft-like spaces between the lobules of cartilage that are lined by respiratory epithelium. Pulmonary hamartomas have a high frequency of the translocation t(3;12)(q27-28;q14-15), resulting in gene fusion of the high mobility group protein gene *HMGA2* and the *LPP* gene. The *HMGA2–LPP* fusion gene usually consists of exons 1–3 of *HMGA2* and exons 9–11 of *LPP* and seems to be expressed in all tumors with this translocation.[21–24]

DIAGNOSIS

The above-mentioned specific radiological features, if present, are considered to be diagnostic for a pulmonary hamartoma and observation is recommended. Tissue diagnosis may be necessary if malignancy is suspected.

The CT-guided fine needle aspiration (FNA) is the best modality to obtain tissue for diagnosis of the peripheral pulmonary nodules. It can be diagnostic up to 85% of cases.[25] Typically a needle biopsy will reveal fibromyxomatous tissue, which stains metachromatically with Giemsa or Wright's stain, and fragments of low columnar epithelium.

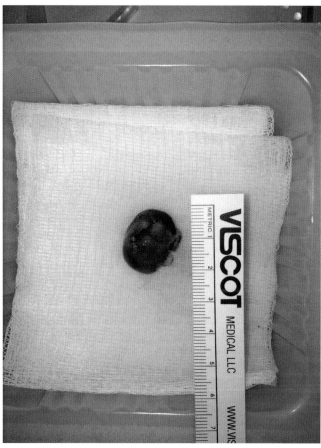

FIGURE 106.4 Two-centimeter endotracheal hamartoma after bronchoscopic excision.

When fragments of cartilage are present cytologically, the aspiration is diagnostic of a hamartoma. Recently navigational bronchoscopy-guided transbronchial biopsy has been shown to be an alternate to percutaneous biopsy, though less accurate then percutaneous CT-guided FNA.[26] Beside FNA, core needle biopsy, forceps biopsy, and brushing can be performed using navigational bronchoscopy. The navigational bronchoscopy has a much higher yield if CT shows an accessible small airway leading to the nodule.

Endobronchial ultrasound (EBUS) is another useful modality for evaluation of the lesions in proximity of the tracheobronchial tree.[27] EBUS findings of calcification may aid in the diagnosis. Furthermore, EBUS-guided transbronchial FNA can be performed to obtain tissue for diagnosis.[28]

Bronchoscopic appearance and biopsy of endobronchial lesions is usually diagnostic. Flexible or rigid bronchoscopy is indicated for patients with pulmonary symptoms to evaluate for endobronchial lesions, which usually reveal a smooth, fleshy, pedunculated, polypoid mass, tan or pink in appearance (Fig. 106.3).[29] Bronchoscopic extraction of an endobronchial or endotracheal lesion can be diagnostic and therapeutic (Fig. 106.4).

TREATMENT

If the diagnosis is confirmed by needle biopsy or CT and MRI findings are diagnostic then no further intervention is needed unless there are unusual circumstances. Slow growth is expected, so follow-up with serial annual low-dose CT scan is recommended.

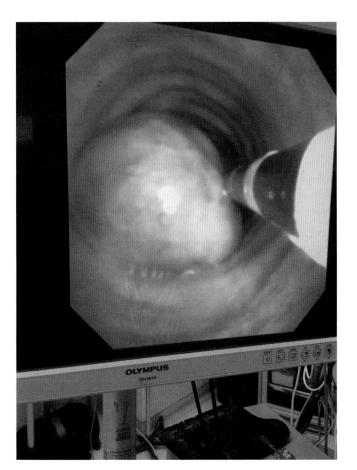

FIGURE 106.3 Bronchoscopic view of an endotracheal hamartoma five centimeters distal to cords.

Resection with thoracoscopy is also diagnostic and therapeutic. This can be approached with video-assisted thoracoscopic surgery (VATS) or robotically. Most lesions are small and peripherally located, and are easily amenable for a wedge resection with negative margin. Multiple studies have shown that wedge resection is associated with a very low recurrence rate.[13,15,16,25,30,31] Deeper lesions, which still can be handled with wedge resection but not easily palpable during VATS, can be marked transbronchially up to the visceral pleura using methylene blue dye through navigational bronchoscopy.[32] Alternately, CT-guided coil or hook wire can be inserted preoperatively to facilitate intraoperative identification and resection.[33] VATS or robotic-assisted segmentectomy or subsegmentectomy should be performed for deeper lesions. Rarely lobectomy will be necessary for more central lesions. Alternatively, muscle-sparing thoracotomy and palpation-assisted resection may be necessary.

Bronchoscopic resection through flexible or rigid bronchoscopy, using variety of energy sources, is an accepted and preferred approach for endobronchial hamartomas. In a retrospective study of 135 patients with hamartomas, Kim et al.[34] reported successful bronchoscopic resection of 15 endobronchial hamartomas via bronchoscopic interventions and concluded that it is a safe and preferred approach. Mondello and colleagues[35] used electrocautery snare via flexible bronchoscope to resect an endobronchial hamartoma. They suggested that flexible bronchoscope may be advantageous as compared to rigid bronchoscope due to its maneuvering ability and magnified image. Lee and colleagues[36] reported use of cryoablation via bronchoscope to resect bronchial hamartoma. There have been reports of use of electrocautery or argon plasma coagulator for bronchoscopic resection of hamartoma.[37] Several authors have reported using neodymium:yttrium-aluminum-garnet (Nd:YAG) laser to resect endobronchial lesions including hamartomas. Most of these lesions can be therapeutically resected endobronchially with very low incidence of recurrence. Repeat laser ablation and resection can be performed for recurrent lesions.[38]

Parenchymal preserving bronchial (bronchial sleeve) resection and bronchoplasty may be necessary for the lesions not completely removeable endobronchially.[39,40] When the definitive diagnosis confirms the benign nature of endobronchial tumors, bronchoplasty should be the operation of choice whenever possible. The type of bronchoplastic procedure, sleeve resection, bronchoplasty with resection or transverse bronchoplasty should be chosen on an individual basis after careful assessment of the location and extension of the lesion.

MALIGNANCY ASSOCIATED WITH HAMARTOMA

Although in past there have been several reports of malignancy occurring in hamartomas, no real evidence exists to support the development of malignancy in a hamartoma. However, of interest in this regard is the possible association of hamartoma with synchronous or metachronous bronchogenic carcinoma of malignant change.

Karasik and colleagues[31] reported that a bronchial carcinoma (synchronous or metachronous) was identified 6.3 times more often in patients with a hamartoma than would be expected in the normal population. They suggested that an etiologic relationship was present. Van den Bosch and colleagues,[41] however, who identified six synchronous and five metachronous bronchial carcinomas in a series of 154 patients with hamartomas (an incidence of 7%), believed the association was essentially coincidental. Ribet and colleagues[42] in their series, recorded that three patients had an associated bronchial carcinoma, a 6.6-fold increase in the number of cases normally expected. These authors came to the same conclusion that there was an etiologic relationship present, as had Karasik and colleagues.

In a recent study, the authors compare resection of hamartomas with surveillance.[43] They analyzed 61 patients with asymptomatic needle biopsy-proven peripheral pulmonary hamartoma. Forty-one patients had a 5-year follow-up without developing new symptoms or malignant transformation. The study concluded that it is reasonable to follow pulmonary hamartomas. In summary, there is no convincing evidence of malignant transformation or association of hamartomas with lung cancer. Hence, it is safe to observe asymptomatic hamartomas.

OTHER SOLITARY BENIGN TUMORS

Since the hamartoma is the most common of all the solitary benign tumors, it is discussed first. Thereafter, the tumors are discussed in the order in which they are listed in Tables 106.1 and 106.2. Table 106.3 shows those tumors that are mainly endobronchial. Benign tumors of epithelial and soft tissue origin as well as the miscellaneous tumor are rare. Many of these tumors may be either endobronchial or peripheral in location but generally have a greater predilection for one of the two locations. The symptomatology depends on whether a bronchus is irritated or a bronchial lumen is occluded partially or completely by an endobronchial lesion. The peripherally located tumors usually are asymptomatic.

EPITHELIAL TUMORS

PAPILLOMA

The subject of pulmonary papillomas is confusing, because multiple squamous papillomas may occur in the upper respiratory tract and larynx and may involve the lungs. Occasionally, there is some overlap between the squamous papillomas of recurrent respiratory papillomatosis (RRP) and solitary squamous papillomas. Older discussions and classifications described a disease that begins in the larynx and pharynx with latter involvement of the tracheobronchial tree and lungs.

TABLE 106.3 Solitary Tumors of the Lung That May Be in an Endobronchial Location

Epithelial Tumors
Papilloma
　Squamous cell papilloma
　Glandular papilloma
　Mixed squamous cell and glandular papilloma
Adenoma
　Pleomorphic adenoma
　Mucous gland adenoma

Soft Tissue Tumors
Adipocytic
　Lipoma
Fibroblastic/myofibroblastic
　Inflammatory myofibroblastic tumor
　Fibrous polyp
Cartilaginous
　Chondroma
Peripheral nerve sheath tumors and related lesions
　Granular cell tumor
　Neurofibroma
Paraganglionic
　Gangliocytic paraganglioma

According to Derkay and Wiatrak,[44] upper respiratory papillomatosis is due to infection with the human papillomaviruses (HPV) types 6 and 11. The squamous papillomas may recur and they may involve the tracheobronchial tree and the lungs. When the squamous papillomas recur, the disease becomes known as RRP. RRP can be divided into two forms: a juvenile onset form and an adult onset form. The juvenile form usually has its onset in the teen years, but it can start as early as the first year of life. The adult form tends to present in the third and fourth decades. Pulmonary squamous papillomas should be viewed as a separate entity from RRP.

Squamous Papilloma

A papilloma is a benign epithelial neoplasm composed of multiple fronds of papillary squamous epithelium. It usually has a thin fibrovascular core. The majority of papillomas are exophytic, but a few inverted ones have been described. An inverted papilloma grows downward toward the underlying stroma and is thus called inverted rather than exophytic.

Flieder and colleagues[45] comprehensively reviewed the subject of solitary pulmonary papillomas—including the squamous, glandular, and mixed papillomas—with 14 cases of their own and 27 cases from the literature. They described 27 patients with squamous cell papillomas, with five being their own patients. The patients ranged in age from 28 to 74 years with a median age of 54 years. There were 23 men and 4 women; 6 had a history of smoking. Five of their patients were symptomatic, with hemoptysis, recurrent pneumonia, and wheezing; three of their five patients had radiographic abnormalities, including one with a hilar mass and two with postobstructive pneumonia and bronchiectasis. In the 27 cases, the papillomas were equally distributed between the left and the right lungs. The tumors ranged in size from 0.7 to 9.0 cm. On microscopic examination, the lesions were composed of papillary arborizing connective tissue stalks lined by keratinizing or nonkeratinizing squamous epithelium. Of the five patients, one had a tumor that was positive for HPV types 6 and 11 but negative for 16, 18, 31, 33, and 51. Two other patients were tested and were negative for all of the previously listed types of human papillomavirus. All five patients were alive and well with the follow-up periods ranging from 3 months to 16 years.

HPV is probably the cause of most of these lesions. Popper and colleagues[46] demonstrated that HPV types 11 and 6 were associated with benign papillomas, whereas types 16 or 18, sometimes in combination with type 31, 33, or 35, were found in papillomas of patients who developed squamous cell carcinoma. Katial and colleagues[47] reported an endobronchial squamous papilloma that was positive for types 6 and 11 but negative for 16, 18, 31, 33, and 35. Kawaguchi and colleagues[48] reported a solitary squamous papilloma of the right upper lobe that contained HPV type 11. Lam and colleagues[49] reported HPV 6b in an atypical squamous papilloma of the trachea.

Iwata and colleagues[50] reported an inverted Schneiderian papilloma in the right lower lobe of the lung. This tumor is noteworthy because few inverted papillomas are reported in the lung, and it was associated with elevated serum levels of carcinoembryonic antigen and squamous cell carcinoma–associated antigen. Once the lesion was removed, the levels returned to almost normal. HPV types 6, 11, 16, and 18 were not detected in the tumor.

Miura and colleagues[51] pointed out that treatment should be conservative, but patients may require further surgery if they develop a malignancy. They suggested that if the lesion is limited to a small area, it could be treated with photodynamic therapy, Nd:YAG laser, or with the less expensive argon plasma coagulator.[52] Cryotherapy has been described to successfully ablate tracheal papilloma.[53] Nevertheless,

these patients should be followed. These aforementioned lesions are usually removed endoscopically, or occasionally, a bronchotomy or sleeve resection may be necessary. When irreversible parenchymal damage distal to the lesion is present, surgical resection of the destroyed lung tissue also is required.

Glandular Papilloma

A glandular papilloma is a benign papillary tumor lined by ciliated or nonciliated columnar epithelial cells. A synonymous term is *columnar cell papilloma*. According to Flieder and colleagues,[54] these are extremely rare endobronchial tumors that occur at a median age of 68 years with no predilection for sex. Patients may present with obstructive symptoms, such as wheezing or hemoptysis. On microscopic examination, the tumor can have thick arborizing stromal stalks covered by glandular epithelium. These tumors are benign, but they may recur following incomplete resection.

Mixed Squamous Cell and Glandular Papilloma

A mixed squamous cell and glandular papilloma is a benign endobronchial papillary tumor showing a mixture of squamous and glandular epithelium. A synonymous term is *transitional cell papilloma*, and this is what Colby and colleagues[55] called it in their description. These are extremely rare tumors with only 18 cases reported in the world literature.[56] The tumors have an equal sex distribution and the median age is 64 years. Patients may have obstructive symptoms. The histology shows fibrovascular cores that lined by both squamous and glandular epithelium. Complete resection appears to be curative.[54,56]

ADENOMA

Alveolar Adenoma

An alveolar adenoma is a benign, well-circumscribed peripheral lung tumor. It may be mistaken for a lymphangioma. Yousem and Hochholzer[57] reported six patients with alveolar adenomas. They were mostly women and ranged in age from 45 to 74 years. Most of the lesions were found on routine chest radiography. Radiographically, Fujimoto and colleagues[58] describe alveolar adenomas as peripheral, well-circumscribed solitary nodules. MRI shows the nodules to have a cystic space with fluid and thin rim enhancement. Cavazza and Hartman and their colleagues[59,60] also described alveolar adenomas as showing a cystic component. Halldorsson and colleagues[61] report a positron emission tomography (PET) scan and the lesion showed no uptake. On excision, the tumors averaged 2 cm in diameter and were easily shelled out from the adjacent pulmonary parenchyma. On histologic examination, the tumors are composed of spaces lined by a low cuboidal epithelium with underlying connective tissue stroma that may be myxoid. Cavazza and colleagues[59] describe adipose tissue in the lesion as well as the mesenchymal cells immunostaining for S-100. Halldorsson and colleagues[61] report that the epithelial cells immunostain for cytokeratin CK7 and CK20 as well as thyroid transcription factor 1 (TTF-1). Five of the six patients were alive and well at the end of a 12-month follow-up period, with one patient lost to follow-up. Saito and colleagues[62] described a case of an alveolar adenoma.

Bohm and colleagues[63] as well as Oliveira and colleagues[64] have each described an additional case of alveolar adenoma. Both groups believe that it is a distinct lung neoplasm. Burke and colleagues[65] reviewed 17 cases and performed a variety of immunohistochemical stains on the tumors. They concluded that alveolar adenomas were benign neoplasms consisting of an admixture of alveolar epithelium, mostly type 2 pneumocytes, and septal mesenchymal tissue, fibroblasts, or fibroblast-like cells. Oliveira and colleagues[64] speculate that the lesion is derived from a primitive mesenchymal cell with the capacity to differentiate toward a type 2 pneumocyte lineage. In contrast, Bohm and colleagues[63] believe the neoplasm is derived from a benign proliferation of both the type 2 pneumocytes and the septal mesenchyme. Cavazza and colleagues[59] performed microsatellite analysis on the epithelial and mesenchymal components of an alveolar adenoma and found alterations of the epithelial cells but not the mesenchymal ones. These findings suggest that the tumor is derived from the epithelial cells.

Papillary Adenoma (Type II Pneumocyte Adenoma or Clara Cell Adenoma)

A papillary adenoma is a rare benign papillary neoplasm that is thought to arise from a multipotential stem cell that differentiates toward type II pneumocytes, Clara cells, or ciliated respiratory epithelial cells. Synonyms for this lesion include *Clara cell adenoma, bronchiolar papilloma, bronchiolar adenoma, type II pneumocyte adenoma,* and *papillary adenoma of type II pneumocytes.* Spencer and colleagues described two cases. Fantone and Noguchi and their colleagues[66-68] described papillary adenomas of the lung that had ultrastructural differentiation toward type 2 pneumocytes (lamellar bodies) and Clara cells (membrane-bound, electron-dense granules). Hegg, Sanchez-Jimenez, Fukuda, Mori, and Dessy and their colleagues[69-73] have all added additional cases to the literature.

The patients range in age from 2 months to 60 years, and the tumor may occur in either gender. The lesions are usually detected in asymptomatic patients on routine chest imaging. On gross examination, the tumors are usually described as well-demarcated white nodules in the lung periphery. Microscopic examination shows a papillary architecture with prominent fibrovascular cores. The epithelial cells, lining the cores, are predominantly cuboidal with basal nuclei and eosinophilic cytoplasm. Sheppard and colleagues[74] point out that the surface cells immunostain with TTF-1. Ultrastructurally, Clara cells and type II pneumocytes are identified. The differential diagnosis includes alveolar adenoma, papillary bronchioloalveolar carcinoma, papillary variant of sclerosing hemangioma, papillary variant of carcinoid tumor, and metastatic carcinoma. Resection appears to be curative, with all of the patients surviving for at least 2 to 10 years. Mori and colleagues,[72] using morphometry with 12-dimensional cluster analysis, found a resemblance of some of the cells to type II pneumocyte adenocarcinoma, but their patient was alive with no evidence of recurrence at 3 years. Dessy and colleagues[73] described two cases of this lesion with infiltrative features. They also found two other cases in the literature with infiltrative features. They proposed changing the name to peripheral papillary tumor of undetermined malignant potential.

Adenoma of Salivary Gland Type: Pleomorphic Adenoma

A pleomorphic adenoma is a benign tumor showing both epithelial and connective tissue differentiation. These tumors contain glands and myoepithelial cells that are usually set in a cartilaginous stroma and are also known as benign mixed tumors. A carcinoma arising in a pleomorphic adenoma is known as carcinoma ex pleomorphic adenoma. Jin and Park, Ang, and Tanigaki and colleagues[75-77] have reported individual cases of pulmonary pleomorphic adenomas.

Sakamoto and colleagues[78] reported one case of pleomorphic adenoma in the lung and reviewed six other reported cases. The patients ranged in age from 47 to 74 years with equal sex distribution. The

clinical symptoms can include included pneumonia and cough. Moran and colleagues[79] described eight patients with pleomorphic adenomas in which two were malignant. They concluded that size at presentation, extent of local infiltration, and mitotic activity were the most reliable prognostic features. Moran[80] summarized the findings in 16 patients with pleomorphic adenomas. His mostly female patients ranged in age from 35 to 74 years. Hara and colleagues[81] described the radiologic findings. On chest CT, the tumor was a well-circumscribed partly lobulated nodule without calcifications. The mass was enhanced heterogeneously. On MRI, the mass showed low- to intermediate-signal intensity of T1-weighted images and heterogeneous intermediate intensity on T2-weighted images. The tumors could be either endobronchial or parenchymal in location, but no predilection occurred for a particular lung or segment. On microscopic examination, the pulmonary tumors do not have as prominent a cartilaginous stroma as do the salivary gland tumors. Treatment is surgical excision. These patients require long-term follow-up. Some lesions seem to have the ability to recur and metastasize, and they are difficult to identify histologically.

Tracheal pleomorphic adenomas have been reported. Most of these are single case reports, including those of Kim, Baghai-Wadji, and Aribas and their colleagues.[82-84] The three patients ranged in age from 8 to 42 years. All three patients were symptomatic and thought to have asthma as they presented with dyspnea. Two of the tumors were in the trachea and one involved the carina and right bronchus. In two of the cases, the tumors ranged from 1.5 to 2 cm in greatest dimension. The histology revealed glands in a chondromyxoid stroma. Surgery is the treatment of choice. As with the pulmonary pleomorphic adenomas, these patients should also receive long-term follow-up, because some lesions seem to have the ability to recur and metastasize.

Adenoma of Salivary Gland Type: Mucous Gland Adenoma

A mucous gland adenoma is an extremely rare benign exophytic tumor of the bronchus that is derived from the mucous glands of the bronchus. The tumor must be composed of cystic glands, be superficial to the cartilaginous plate, be in the bronchus, and have some normal bronchial seromucous glands. The tumor is also known as mucous gland cystadenoma, bronchial cystadenoma, bronchial adenoma arising in mucous glands, mucous cell adenoma, polyadenoma, adenomatous polyp, and adenoma of mucous gland type.

Mucous gland adenoma has been described by Weinberger and colleagues[85] as well as by Gilman, Weiss and Ingram, Kroe and Pitcoc, Emory and colleagues, and Edwards and Matthews.[85-90] England and Hochholzer[91] reported 10 additional cases. Their patients ranged in age from 25 to 67 years. Historically, this lesion tends to occur twice as often in men as in women, but these authors found a slight predominance in women. The symptoms are cough, fever, recurrent pneumonia, and hemoptysis. The chest radiograph may also show obstructive pneumonitis, postobstructive atelectasis, and, on rare occasion, a solitary peripheral lesion. Kwon and colleagues[92] reported the CT findings in two patients, which consisted of a well-defined mass with an air meniscus sign or abutting the bronchus, suggesting an intraluminal location. The lesion occurs equally between the right and left sides and more often is found in the major bronchi of the middle and lower lobes. On gross examination, the tumors varied in size from 0.8 to 6.8 cm. The tumors projected into the lumen of the bronchus. They were usually encapsulated by a thin membrane and easily separated from the bronchus. The cut surface is cystic with mucus within the cystic space.

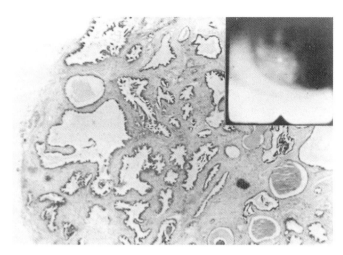

FIGURE 106.5 Low-power photomicrograph of a mucous gland adenoma. **Inset** shows the endoscopic appearance.

Endoscopically, they appear as firm pink masses with intact overlying epithelium (Fig. 106.5). Histologically, they are composed of numerous small mucus-filled cysts lined by well-differentiated mucous epithelium (Fig. 106.6). The major differential diagnosis is low-grade mucoepidermoid carcinoma. Even though these lesions rarely have a stalk, they can be completely removed endoscopically by curettage, cryotherapy, or laser ablation, as reported by Ishida and colleagues.[93] Thoracotomy and surgical resection are indicated only when distal lung has been destroyed or endoscopic removal is contraindicated or incomplete. Complete removal of these tumors endoscopically or surgically results in a permanent cure.

Adenoma of Salivary Gland Type: Oncocytoma

An oncocytoma is an extremely rare benign exophytic tumor of the bronchus that is composed of oncocytic cells. The tumor is also known as oxyphilic adenoma or oncocytic adenoma. Fechner and Bentinck[94] have described the pulmonary oncocytoma. There have been multiple single case reports of pulmonary or tracheal oncocytomas.[95–101]

The patients in the above reported cases ranged in age from 16 to 75 years with a slight male predominance. Most of the patients

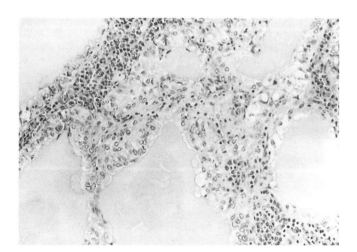

FIGURE 106.6 High-power photomicrograph of a mucous gland adenoma consisting of cysts of various diameters lined by columnar mucous cells. A chronic inflammatory reaction separates the tubules.

were asymptomatic, but some complained of cough, hemoptysis, chest pain, and dyspnea. The chest radiographs may show obstructive pneumonitis with an infiltrate or a solitary peripheral lesion although the case reported by Laforga and Aranda[97] had multiple nodules. The solitary lesions were randomly distributed in the lungs. On gross examination, the tumors were well circumscribed and varied in size from 1.5 to 3.5 cm in greatest dimension. The cut surface was yellow tan to reddish brown to pink. On microscopic examination, the tumors have ovoid cells with small uniform nuclei and abundant finely granular eosinophilic cytoplasm. On electron microscopy, the cytoplasm shows mitochondrial hyperplasia. The treatment is surgical resection.

Adenoma of Salivary Gland Type: Myoepithelioma and Adenomyoepithelioma

The existence of this entity is confusing because of the terminology. Yousem and Nicholson[102] consider the terms adenomyoepithelioma, myoepithelioma, epithelial–myoepithelial tumor, epimyoepithelial carcinoma, epithelial–myoepithelial tumor of unproven malignant potential and malignant mixed tumor comprising epithelial and myoepithelial cells to be synonyms with epithelial–myoepithelial carcinoma, which is viewed as a low-grade carcinoma. Chang and colleagues[103] have described a pneumocytic adenomyoepithelioma, which is discussed at the end of this section.

Myoepithelial cells are flat cells that lie between the epithelial cells of a gland and the basement membrane. They are usually found in the salivary glands and are thought to have contractile properties. The older concept of myoepitheliomas was of a benign tumor. Kilpatrick and Limon[104] also view these lesions as low-grade malignancies and grouped them with the parachordoma and mixed tumors of soft tissue. The tumors are discussed in this section because they have traditionally been viewed as benign.

Strickler and colleagues described a pulmonary myoepithelioma, and Tsuji and Pelosi and their colleagues described adenomyoepitheliomas or, as Pelosi and colleagues preferred to call them, pulmonary epithelial–myoepithelial tumor of unproven malignant potential (PEMTUMP).[105–107] They prefer this term because at present these tumors appear benign.

The myoepithelioma described by Strickler and colleagues[105] was an incidental finding on a chest radiograph in a man in his 60s. On gross examination, the lesion was 3.3 cm in greatest dimension, had tan-yellow-white surfaces and well-demarcated margins. On microscopic examination, it was composed of spindle cells that immunostained for S-100 and actin but not keratin. On electron microscopy, the tumor contained filaments consistent with myofilaments. Cagirici and colleagues[108] described a myoepithelioma in a 54-year-old woman. She presented with exertional dyspnea, cough, and intermittent pleuritic chest pain. A chest radiograph showed a peripheral 2-cm mass in the left lower lobe. Grossly, the tumor was white-gray with well-demarcated margins. Microscopically it consisted of uniform spindle-shaped cells that immunostained for S-100 and smooth muscle actin but not desmin, synaptophysin, or CD34. The patient underwent a wedge resection and was disease-free at 2-year follow-up.

Pelosi and colleagues reported a PEMTUMP and reviewed the six cases in the world's literature, including the one described by Tsuji and colleagues.[106,107] In the review, the patients ranged from 47 to 66 years of age. Tumors ranged in size from 1.3 to 16 cm. The cut surfaces were tan-yellow-white and the tumors were randomly distributed throughout both lungs. Radiographically, the lesions were solid nodules. On microscopic examination, the tumors showed a biphasic pattern composed of glands (epithelial cells) and spindle cells (myoepithelial cells). The epithelial cells stained strongly for keratin and weakly for S-100. In contrast, the myoepithelial cells stained strongly for S-100 and actin but weakly for keratin. Overall, the patients did well, but some were lost to follow-up. The longest follow-up was 36 months. None of these patients are known to have died from their disease. Surgery appears curative, but follow-up is advised.

Chang and colleagues[103] described five cases of pneumocytic adenomyoepithelioma. They view it as a tumor that shows epithelial myoepithelial and pneumocytic differentiation. Their five patients were all women and ranged in age from 52 to 63 years. The history was available for three patients. Two were asymptomatic with the lesion being incidentally discovered on a chest radiograph. The other patient complained of chest pain and dyspnea. The tumors did not show a preferred location and they measured between 0.8 and 2.6 cm in greatest dimension. Microscopically, all five tumors showed a double-layered glandular formation and all were close to a small caliber airway. The epithelial cells showed immunostaining for keratin, epithelial membrane antigen (EMA), and TTF-1. In contrast, the myoepithelial cells showed immunostaining for smooth muscle actin, S-100 and p63, but were negative for keratin. The treatment is surgical. The follow-up period is up to 6.5 years with no recurrence; however, one patient had multiple bilateral nodules and has been followed for only 5 months.

MUCINOUS CYSTADENOMA

According to Colby and colleagues,[55] a mucinous cystadenoma is a "unilocular cystic lesion whose fibrous wall is lined by well-differentiated, presumably benign columnar mucinous epithelium." This lesion was first described by Sambrook Gowar and later by Dail, Kragel, Dixon, and Roux and their colleagues; Graeme-Cook and Mark and Dail have further described this entity.[109–114] These lesions occur in both men and women, who are usually smokers in their 50s and 60s. Most of these tumors are discovered as asymptomatic peripheral masses on routine chest radiography.

On gross examination, the mass is a unilocular cyst filled with clear gelatinous material. On microscopic examination, a fibrous cyst wall is lined by mucinous epithelium. Occasionally, the wall is thinned, and the mucin extravasates into the adjacent pulmonary parenchyma. The cysts should be examined completely because they may have areas of borderline malignancy or adenocarcinoma. The treatment for these lesions is complete resection, and the prognosis of the benign tumors is excellent.

Mann and colleagues[115] reported the local recurrence of a mucinous cystic tumor of borderline malignancy 4 years after its initial resection. They suggested that a mucinous cystic tumor with any histologic identification of evidence of even early malignant features should undergo a lobectomy as the procedure of choice rather than a more limited excision.

SOFT TISSUE TUMORS

ADIPOCYTIC ANGIOMYOLIPOMA

Angiomyolipoma is benign tumor of adipose tissue that contains blood vessels, adipose tissue, and smooth muscle. Marcheix and colleagues[116] reported one in the lung of a 63-year-old asymptomatic woman who presented with a chest radiograph that showed a nodule in the right lower lobe. A CT scan showed a nonenhancing nodule

with a fat-like density and no calcifications. The lesion was hypermetabolic on PET scan. Microscopically it was unencapsulated and composed of mature fat with thick-walled blood vessels and smooth muscle cells. These tumors stain with desmin and HMB-45 antibodies. The patient had no history of tuberous sclerosis or lymphangioleiomyomatosis (LAM). The angiomyolipoma is now included in the perivascular epithelioid cell tumor family (PEComas). This includes mesenchymal derived tumors positive for both smooth muscle and melanocytic markers.[117] These tumors can be associated with tuberous sclerosis and can be benign but also malignant.

LIPOMA

Lipomas are benign tumors of mature adipose tissue, which may occur in either an endobronchial or a parenchymal location. Lipomas arise most often from the wall of the tracheobronchial tree (80%) and have potential to cause life-threatening obstruction.[118] Bango and Yokozaki and their colleagues[119,120] have urged CT examination to determine the extent of pulmonary involvement. They also suggest bronchoscopic laser vaporization of the tumor as the treatment of choice, although a local resection by bronchotomy or sleeve resection may be required.

Muraoka and colleagues[121] reported 64 cases of endobronchial lipomas from the Japanese literature. Fifty patients were men and 14 were women and they had a mean age of 60 years. The majority of the patients were symptomatic (75%), with the symptoms consisting of sputum, cough, hemoptysis, fever, and dyspnea. The tumors ranged in size from 0.3 to 6.5 cm in greatest dimension. On microscopic examination, the tumors were composed of mature adipose tissue. Surgical procedures—including pneumonectomy (4), lobectomy (24), bilobectomy (8), and bronchotomy (4)—were required in 57.9%. Bronchoscopic removal by Nd:YAG laser (17), electrosurgical resection (5), or a combination of both (5) was carried out in the other 42% of patients. Bronchoscopic removal is preferred whenever possible.

Civi and colleagues[122] reported a case of a peripheral lipoma and reviewed the world literature where they found eight additional cases. There was a male predominance, with seven men and two women; the ages ranged from 44 to 71 years. One patient was asymptomatic and the remaining eight had symptoms that consisted of sputum, cough, fever, hemoptysis, chest pain, dyspnea, wheezing, and right arm paresthesia. On gross examination, the tumors ranged from 1.3 cm to 7.8 cm in greatest dimension. On microscopic examination, the tumor should consist of mature fat; however, their tumors contained occasional giant cells with multiple pleomorphic nuclei. These could represent floret-like giant cells, as are seen in pleomorphic lipomas. Treatment is surgical resection.

FIBROBLASTIC/MYOFIBROBLASTIC PULMONARY MICROCYSTIC FIBROMYXOMA

A pulmonary microcystic fibromyxoma is thought to be a benign tumor of the lung composed of myxoid connective tissue with microcyst formation. The only well-known myxoid tumor of the lung is the myxoid variant of a pulmonary hamartoma. Shilo and colleagues[123] described three cases of this tumor. Their patients consisted of two women and one man ages 45 to 65 years. All were symptomatic and the lesion was found incidentally, with no evidence of an extrapulmonary primary on evaluation. Chest radiographs showed a nodule. On gross examinations, the nodules varied in size from 1 to 2.3 cm in greatest dimension and were described as brownish to white-tan. On microscopic examination, the tumors were composed of bland stellate cells with the formation of microcysts. No mitosis or necrosis was present. Immunohistochemically, the cells were positive for vimentin but negative for keratin, TTF-1, and various other markers. All of the patients are well, with follow-up ranging from 18 to 72 months. The treatment was surgical removal.

INFLAMMATORY FIBROUS POLYP

A polyp is a mass of tissue protruding from an epithelial surface that is composed mostly of underlying connective tissue and covered by ciliated columnar epithelium with possible areas of squamous metaplasia. The stalk is usually composed of loose connective tissue with capillaries and an infiltrate of plasma cells, lymphocytes, and eosinophils. These can mimic a malignancy and can be confused with the bronchial fibroepithelial polyp, which is glistening white and firm and uncommon like most of these endobronchial lesions.[124] On rare occasions, there can be multiple polyps. A synonym is *inflammatory endobronchial polyp*. Patients may present with symptoms of obstruction, such as wheezing or recurrent infections. Dinçer and colleagues[125] point out that some of the etiologic factors include foreign-body aspiration, prolonged mechanical ventilation, asthma, chronic sinusitis, chronic smoke inhalation, and mycobacterial infections. Inflammatory polyps tend to be more common in adults, but they can also involve children. Arguelles and Blanco[126] described an asthmatic 10-year-old boy who had multiple bronchial polyps. Roberts and colleagues[127] described multiple endobronchial polyps in a girl with a history of cystic fibrosis who at the age of 12 years underwent a resection. McShane and colleagues[128] described three infants and a 12-year-old boy with endobronchial polyps. All of the infants had histories of intubation and McShane and colleagues postulated that the polyps may have resulted from irritation of the endotracheal tube or the suctioning of the patients. There was no history of intubation in the 12 years old.

In adults, endobronchial polyps may be secondary to a variety of causes. Some of the less common causes include a case secondary to tuberculosis as described by Nishi and colleagues.[129] The mycobacteria were identified in the polyp by special stain. Another case is reported by Asano and colleagues,[130] who describe polyps in a woman with disseminated *Mycobacterium intracellulare*. In this instance, the organisms were not identified in the polyp by special stains. Naber and colleagues[131] described endobronchial polyps in lung transplant patients that were secondary to cytomegalovirus. The virus could be identified in the polyp following immunohistochemical staining.

INFLAMMATORY MYOFIBROBLASTIC TUMOR (INFLAMMATORY PSEUDOTUMOR)

Coffin and Fletcher, in the WHO classification, define inflammatory myofibroblastic tumor as an intermediate (rarely metastasizing) soft tissue tumor with a variety of histologic appearances.[132] *Inflammatory myofibroblastic tumor* is probably the most accepted term for this tumor, but the term *inflammatory pseudotumor* is still widely used. Other synonyms include *plasma cell granuloma, fibrous histiocytoma, fibroxanthoma, histiocytoma, xanthoma, xanthofibroma, xanthogranuloma, mast cell granuloma, pseudosarcomatous myofibroblastic tumor,* and, incorrectly, *sclerosing hemangioma.* Pulmonary fibrous histiocytoma is considered to be inflammatory myofibroblastic tumor. Moran and Suster[133] reviewed this tumor and called it an inflammatory pseudotumor. It is discussed here because generally it is viewed as a benign tumor. Originally, it was thought to be a reactive fibrohistiocytic process that took place after an inflammatory or

infectious event. Gomez-Roman and colleagues[134] described human herpesvirus-8 as being expressed in inflammatory pseudotumors, suggesting an etiologic possibility. The tumor is now being considered a neoplasm for several reasons. Melloni and colleagues[135] point out that the tumor can be locally aggressive, relapse, and give rise to distal metastases. In addition, the tumor contains cytogenetic abnormalities, with rearrangement of the anaplastic lymphoma kinase (ALK) gene on chromosome 2p23, resulting in the overexpression of ALK-1 protein. ROS1 gene fusion may also be seen; thus, there may be a role for cytogenetic studies for further classification.[136]

This varied histologic picture creates confusion in both the diagnosis of the tumor and in its classification. Matsubara and colleagues[137] postulated that these tumors originate as an organizing intra-alveolar pneumonia and described three histologic patterns. These patterns were (a) organizing pneumonia type, (b) fibrous histiocytoma pattern, and (c) lymphoplasmacytic type. Subsequently, Colby and colleagues[55] divided the inflammatory pseudotumors into two major groups, according to their histology: (a) fibrohistiocytic and (b) plasma cell granuloma. Most recently, Coffin and Fletcher[132] divided the histologic patterns into three types: (a) compact spindle cell pattern, (b) hypocellular fibrous pattern, and (c) a scar-like pattern. Given the varied histologic pattern, it is generally very difficult to make the diagnosis preoperatively either by bronchial biopsy, lung needle biopsy or FNA.

Melloni, Coffin, Sakurai, and Kobashi and their colleagues[135,138–140] have all published a series of cases about inflammatory myofibroblastic tumors. All of the series discuss the radiology, but Kim and colleagues[141] focus on the CT features of these tumors. Of these reports, the one of Coffin and colleagues[138] is probably the most interesting, because they report 59 patients with inflammatory myofibroblastic tumors whose tumors had either histologic atypia or clinical aggressiveness. The 59 cases could be divided as follows: classic morphology (5 cases), atypical histologic features (21 cases), local recurrence (27 cases), and/or metastasis (6 cases). These tumors originated in the following sites: abdomen and pelvis 64%, lung 22%, head and neck 8%, and extremities 5%. The patients ranged in age from 3 weeks to 74 years, with a mean age of 13.2 years and median age of 11 years.

Agrons and colleagues[142] described the chest radiographs of patients with inflammatory myofibroblastic tumors as showing a solitary, peripheral, sharply circumscribed mass, usually in one of the lower lobes. Kim and colleagues[141] described the CT findings. They found the tumors could be divided into four locations: tracheal, bronchial, central, and parenchymal. All the tumors were well defined and round to ovoid. Some of the tumors showed mild enhancement with contrast. Most of the nodules showed homogeneous enhancement with a few showing heterogeneous enhancement. Intratumoral calcifications were seen in one patient.

Coffin and colleagues[138] described the gross pathologic appearance of these tumors as a circumscribed solitary or multinodular mass with a white to tan cut surface. Hemorrhage and necrosis were present in a few cases. The tumors ranged in size from 1.2 to 22 cm in greatest dimension with a mean of 7.8 cm. On microscopic examination, 16 had typical histologic features (5 ordinary, 8 recurrent, and 3 metastatic) and 43 had atypical histologic features (21 atypical, 19 recurrent, and 3 metastatic). The typical histology consisted of spindle cells with inflammatory cells such as plasma cells, macrophages, lymphocytes, and eosinophils. Some of the atypical features included hypercellularity, necrosis, abundant large ganglion-like cells, cellular and nuclear pleomorphism, anaplastic giant cells, and atypical mitosis. Yousem and colleagues[143] describe the pulmonary tumors as being immunohistochemically positive for vimentin and smooth muscle actin and rarely positive for desmin. About 40% of the cases stain for ALK-1. The tumors do not stain for myogenin, myoglobin, CD117 (cKit), or S-100.

SOLITARY FIBROUS TUMOR (FIBROMA AND LOCALIZED FIBROUS MESOTHELIOMA)

A solitary fibrous tumor is a mesenchymal tumor probably originating from fibroblasts. Guillon and colleagues,[144] in the WHO classification, consider it an intermediate tumor that rarely metastasizes rather than one that is benign or malignant. This is usually a pleural tumor and cases in the lung are single case reports. Colby and colleagues[55] prefer the term intrapulmonary localized fibrous tumor; other synonyms include localized mesothelioma, fibrous mesothelioma, solitary fibrous mesothelioma, pleural fibroma, subserosal fibroma, and submesothelial fibroma. This tumor is more extensively discussed in the chapter on mediastinal mesenchymal tumors (Chapter 172).

Fridlington, Sagawa, Baliga, and Patsios and their colleagues[145–148] have all reported intrapulmonary solitary fibrous tumors. The patients in these reports range in age from 42 to 72 years. One patient presented with symptomatic hypoglycemia as well as bilateral digital clubbing and coarsened facial features. In all of the patients, the chest radiographs showed nodules with no preference for any lobe. On CT scan, there was a well-defined nodule with soft tissue attenuation with intense contrast enhancement.

On gross examination, the tumors ranged in size from 1.2 to 20 cm in greatest dimension and were well circumscribed. The cut surfaces were usually pink-white with a whorled surface. On microscopic examination, the tumor was composed of cellular and hypocellular areas with spindle cells. These tumors have a histologic appearance identical to that of a localized fibrous tumor of the pleura (see Chapter 65). In these tumors, the immunohistochemical stains for CD34 and vimentin are usually positive, whereas CD99 and bcl-2 are variable positive. The treatment of choice is surgical resection. In the patient of Fridlington and colleagues,[145] the hypoglycemia went away and the skin changes resolved after excision. Otherwise, the cases did not have long-term follow-up. Most such patients will be cured by surgical excision. Since this tumor can metastasize on rare occasions, the patients need to be followed.[149]

SMOOTH MUSCLE LEIOMYOMA

Leiomyomas are benign tumors of smooth muscle. They account for about 2% of the benign tumors of the lung. They may occur in the trachea, bronchus, or pulmonary parenchyma (Table 106.4). The distribution is approximately equal between a tracheobronchial and a parenchymal location.[7,150–152] The tumor is most often discovered in young and middle-aged adults and is more common in women. In women who have had a uterine leiomyoma removed in the past, it is difficult if not impossible to differentiate a true pulmonary leiomyoma from a benign metastasizing leiomyoma from the original uterine tumor; thus, meticulous follow-up is necessary.

TABLE 106.4 Leiomyoma of the Lower Respiratory Tract

Site	No. of Cases	Percentage
Trachea	12	17.6
Bronchus	22	32.3
Parenchyma	34	50.0

Reproduced from White SH, Ibrahim NB, Forrester-Wood CP, et al. Leiomyomas of the lower respiratory tract. *Thorax* 1985;40:306–311, with permission from BMJ Publishing Group Ltd.

The parenchymal lesions are solitary masses of varying size. Gotti and colleagues[153] described one that was a multiloculated mass associated with a large pedunculated cyst that occupied the upper third of the left pleural space. These authors also noted other reports of "leiomyomas" associated with cyst formation, but most if not all of these were in patients with leiomyomatosis (see later in this chapter under "Multiple Benign Tumors"). Ko and colleagues[154] reported the first calcified endobronchial leiomyoma in the left main bronchus near the carina in a 65-year-old man who presented with cough, sputum production, and fever. The tumor was composed of spindle-shaped cells consistent with smooth muscle and the immunohistochemical staining was positive for desmin and smooth muscle actin. The patient had the tumor removed by laser surgery and recovered. Bilgin and colleagues[155] also reported an endobronchial leiomyoma in a 43-year-old woman who had a normal uterus. She presented with cough and increased sputum production for 2 years and underwent an inferior right bilobectomy for palliative therapy.

Surgical resection is the treatment of choice. In selected patients with endobronchial lesions without distal destroyed lung tissue, laser resection of the tumor may be possible. Archambeaud-Mouveroux and colleagues[156] reported successful management of a benign bronchial leiomyoma by endoscopic use of a Nd:YAG laser. Endobronchial resection without the use of laser is also satisfactory[157] and in some cases a sleeve resection may be indicated for the endobronchial lesion.[158] Peripheral leiomyoma may be resected with VATS.[159]

PERICYTIC GLOMUS TUMOR

According to Marchevsky, glomus tumors (glomangiomas) are derived from the cells of a special arteriovenous shunt, the Suquet-Hoyer canal.[160] They are generally located in the nail beds as well as the pads of the fingers and toes. They are involved in temperature control. On rare occasions, these tumors may be found in the lung as a solitary nodule. Yilmaz and colleagues[161] as well as Zhang and England[162] have each reported individual cases of pulmonary glomus tumors. Koss and Gaertner and their colleagues[163,164] reported a total of seven cases of glomus tumors of the lung. The patients ranged in age from 20 to 67 years. There were six men and one woman. For the most part, they were asymptomatic. Most of the lesions were in the right lung, but one was in the left mainstem bronchus and one was in the parenchyma of the left lung. On chest radiography, pulmonary glomus tumors appear as solitary nodules. Ueno and colleagues[165] described the CT and MRI findings of a case. On unenhanced CT, they saw a well-delineated mass with no calcification or fat attenuation. After contrast injection, the periphery of the mass was enhanced but the center was poorly enhanced. On MRI, the majority of the mass showed an isointense signal relative to skeletal muscle on T1-weighted images and a relatively high intensity signal on T2-weighted images. However, the center of the mass showed high intensity on both T1- and T2-weighted images.

These tumors should be distinguished from hemangiopericytomas, carcinoids, paragangliomas, and smooth muscle tumors. All of the cases were treated surgically. Two patients were lost to follow-up, but the other five patients were followed for 6 months to 5 years, and all were free of disease.

VASCULAR CAVERNOUS HEMANGIOMA

A cavernous hemangioma is a benign vascular tumor that is extremely uncommon in the lung. Most of the literature is based on single case reports. In some instances, the cavernous hemangiomas may be multiple. Galliani and colleagues[166] described a cavernous hemangioma in a 10-week-old male infant. They emphasized that if such a lesion is a true arteriovenous malformation, the possibility of hereditary hemorrhagic telangiectasia (Rendu-Osler-Weber disease) should be considered. Silverman and colleagues[167] studied patients with pulmonary venous malformations by MRI imaging. They concluded that by using their criteria, MRI imaging was an excellent noninvasive modality for evaluating these lesions.

Maeda, Sirmali, and their colleagues[168–172] have both reported solitary cavernous hemangiomas, whereas others have reported multiple cavernous hemangiomas. Radiographically, multiple lesions can look similar to metastatic cancer. The patients of Maeda, Sirmali, and their colleagues[168,169] were both 54-year-old men with one asymptomatic and the other complaining of hemoptysis. In the asymptomatic one, the CT scan showed an ill-defined mass, 4 by 3 cm, with tiny calcifications in the left lung hilum; in the other there was a well-defined mass 4 by 3 cm in the left upper lobe. Both showed dilated blood vessels on histology and both underwent surgical excision. The cases of Kobayashi and colleagues[170] and Fine and Whitney[171] were in a 15-year-old girl and an 84-year-old man. Both had multiple vascular lesions.

LYMPHATIC LESIONS

Lymphatic lesions of the lung and thorax are rare and, according to Faul and colleagues,[173] who have recently reviewed the subject, can be divided into four basic categories (Table 106.5): (a) lymphangioma, (b) lymphangiectasis, (c) lymphangiomatosis, and (d) lymphatic dysplasia, as well as some additional categories that are not listed in the table. The occurrence of a solitary intrapulmonary lymphangioma is rare. The lesion is usually a small peripheral nodule, and can be diffuse.[174] However, high-resolution CT (HRCT) usually shows the lesion to be cystic with a smooth border. The tumor, as a rule, is asymptomatic but occasionally may be associated with dyspnea, as in the case in a child reported by Kim and colleagues[175] and an infant as reported by Lee and colleagues.[176] It may cause hemoptysis, as reported by Holden and colleagues.[177] A pneumothorax may also be seen with these cystic lesions. Pathologically, the mass is composed of benign-appearing contiguous interconnecting lymphatic spaces, as described by Langston and Askin.[178] A small number of cases have been reported in the past several years (1994 to 2003) by Takemura, Takahara, Wilson, and Nagayasu and their colleagues.[179–182] Treatment consists of limited but complete surgical removal by one of the many appropriate surgical techniques. The outlook for success is excellent.

TABLE 106.5 Pulmonary Disorders of the Lymphatic System

Lymphangioma
  Capillary
  Cavernous
  Cystic
Lymphangiectasis
  Primary (congenital)
  Secondary
Lymphangiomatosis
  Single organ involvement (e.g., diffuse pulmonary lymphangiomatosis)
  Multiple organ involvement
  Lymphatic dysplasia syndromes
  Other lymphatic disorders

Modified from Faul JL, Berry GJ, Colby TV, et al. Thoracic lymphangiomas, lymphangiectasis, lymphangiomatosis, and lymphatic dysplasia syndrome. *Am J Respir Crit Care Med* 2000;161(3 Pt 1):1037–1046.

In the article of Faul and colleagues,[173] the authors clearly define the other three entities. Pulmonary lymphangiectasis is found in a primary and secondary form. The primary form is usually found in neonates, and it causes a severe respiratory failure that is usually fatal.[183] The secondary form results from a pathologic process that impairs lymph drainage and increases lymph production. Histologically, the visceral pleura has a network of dilated capillaries. Lymphangiomatosis is the presence of multiple lymphangiomas. Histologically, the lesions resemble solitary lymphangiomas. This disease frequently presents in late childhood and is equally distributed between males and females. Patients with pulmonary involvement have a poor prognosis. The last group of diseases is the lymphatic dysplasia syndrome. This entity includes primary lymphedema syndromes, congenital chylothorax, idiopathic effusions, and the yellow nail syndrome. Lymphatic dysplasia consists of a primary lymphedema with prominent fibrous septation in the subcutaneous fat. The condition is more frequent in women than men. Clinically, patients develop recurrent chest infections, pleural effusions, and bronchiectasis. Their prognosis is related to the severity of the bronchiectasis.

CARTILAGINOUS PULMONARY CHONDROMA

A chondroma is a benign tumor composed of mature hyaline cartilage. In the lung, there are two types of cartilaginous tumors. One is the pulmonary hamartoma, which is usually composed of cartilage, fat, connective tissue, and smooth muscle, as described at the beginning of this chapter. The other is the pulmonary chondroma that is associated with Carney's triad. Whether a third type of pulmonary cartilaginous tumor exists is debatable, according to Wick and Mills.[184]

Carney's triad is not to be confused with Carney syndrome or Carney complex. Carney and colleagues[185] described Carney complex that might also be called the LAMB syndrome (lentigines, atrial myxoma, mucocutaneous myxomas, and blue nevi) or the NAME syndrome (nevi, atrial myxoma, myxoid neurofibroma, and ephelides). The major features described by Carney and colleagues[185] were (a) single or multiple cardiac myxomas, (b) myxoid tumors at various cutaneous and mucosal sites, (c) myxoid mammary fibromatosis, (d) multiple lentigines/freckles, and (e) rare endocrine tumors. Since that original description, Carney[186] recognized that psammomatous melanotic schwannoma was also a component of Carney syndrome. Simansky and colleagues[187] reported one patient with this tumor in the lung and we have chosen to discuss it later under the peripheral nerve sheath and related lesions section.

Carney and colleagues[188–191] described Carney's triad. The triad originally consisted of pulmonary chondromas, functional extra-adrenal paraganglioma, and a gastrointestinal stromal tumor. The triad usually occurred in women under 30 years of age and the tumors could be multiple. Some patients had only two of the tumors, and it became acceptable to make the diagnosis if only two of the tumors were present and not the full triad. In 1999, Carney described other tumors that also occurred with the triad; these included nonfunctioning adrenal cortical adenomas, esophageal leiomyomas, and esophageal and small bowel gastrointestinal tumors. Scopsi and colleagues[192] did not think that the triad was inherited in a familial fashion.

In 2002, Carney and Stratakis[193] described a familial syndrome of paragangliomas and gastrointestinal stromal tumors that were distinct from Carney's triad. This new syndrome lacked the pulmonary chondromas as well as the female predominance. In contrast, it showed an autosomal dominant mode of transmission and a predominance of the paragangliomas.

Rodriguez and colleagues[194] reviewed the pathology of chondromas seen in Carney's triad and compared them to the pathology of pulmonary hamartomas. They described pulmonary chondromas from 41 patients with Carney's triad and compared them with 123 patients with pulmonary hamartomas. The patients with Carney's triad had a mean age of 24.8 years with a female predominance. The tumors were often multiple and could be either central or peripheral.[195] In contrast, the mean age of the patients with pulmonary hamartomas was 58.9 years. Patients were mostly men. The tumors were usually solitary and could be in a central or peripheral location. On gross examination, the pulmonary chondromas were well circumscribed or bosselated with a gray or white cut surface. On microscopic examination, the pulmonary chondromas of Carney's triad were composed almost exclusively of cartilage with myxoid change and were usually calcified or ossified. They were delineated from the adjacent pulmonary tissue by a fibrous pseudocapsule. On the other hand, the pulmonary hamartomas contained several different tissue components including adipose tissue, smooth muscle, and fibromyxoid stroma as well as entrapped epithelium.

OSSEOUS OSTEOMA

An osteoma is a benign tumor of bone that is usually found in the skull. Markert and colleagues[196] report a case of a 39-year-old man with a history of multiple myeloma who was treated with a bone marrow transplant. About 2 years and several months following the transplant, the patient's myeloma relapsed. In preparation for a second marrow transplant, a chest radiograph revealed a well-circumscribed tumor in the right upper lobe of the lung. The lobe was subsequently resected. On histologic examination, the tumor was found to be composed of mature lamellar bone trabeculae with fat and fibrous tissue as well as entrapped bronchioles between the trabeculae. It was well encapsulated by fibrous tissue. The authors speculate that the tumor's presence may have something to do with the previous bone marrow transplant and that the tumor represented an extraskeletal osteoma.

PERIPHERAL NERVE SHEATH TUMORS AND RELATED LESIONS

Granular Cell Tumors (Myoblastomas)

Granular cell tumors are rare, benign tumors composed of large cells with a granular eosinophilic cytoplasm. Synonyms include *granular cell myoblastoma, granular cell schwannoma,* and *granular cell nerve sheath tumor.* Some of these tumors may be endobronchial and cause obstructive symptoms with distal atelectasis.[197,198] Lui and colleagues[199] reviewed the features of the endobronchial granular cell tumors. Deavers and colleagues[200] reviewed a series of 20 cases. Their patients ranged in age from 20 to 57 years and were evenly divided between men and women. In approximately half of the patients, the tumors were incidental findings. The other patients had symptoms secondary to obstruction, which included postobstructive pneumonia and atelectasis. Hemoptysis can occur. The chest radiographs showed lobar infiltration, coin lesions, and lobar atelectasis. Some patients had findings caused by other diseases. Solitary lesions were present in 75% of the patients. Multiple pulmonary lesions were present in 10% (two patients). Three other patients (15%) had a solitary pulmonary lesion in addition to the presence of multiple skin tumors.

On gross examination, the tumors ranged in size from 0.3 to 5.0 cm. They are usually located in an endobronchial position but may occur in the parenchyma. The cut surfaces of the tumor may be tan-white, pink, or yellow. They are usually circumscribed but not encapsulated. On microscopic examination, the tumors are composed of large cells with an abundant pink granular cytoplasm. The tumor cells immunostain for S-100. Cutlan and Eltorky[201] described three granular cell tumors that were associated with malignancies (mucoepidermoid carcinoma, squamous cell carcinoma, and adenocarcinoma).

The treatment is conservative resection except in those few patients with an associated malignant lesion. Complete resection is curative, although these tumors may recur. Asymptomatic patients may be followed. Epstein and Mohsenifar[202] used Nd:YAG laser to treat an obstructing granular cell tumor and suggested this might be an effective tool for treating these cases in certain instances. Argon beam coagulator has also been used via bronchoscopy.[52] Surgical resection of the tumor and any associated damaged lung tissue may be required.

Meningioma, Pulmonary

A meningioma is derived from meningothelial (arachnoid) cells. Meningiomas in the pulmonary parenchyma can be primary or metastatic. Most pulmonary meningiomas are reported as single case reports.[203–206] Spinelli and colleagues[207] have suggested that this tumor may arise from meningothelial-like nodules found in the lungs.

Patients with pulmonary meningiomas are more often women ages 24 to 74. Patients generally present with an asymptomatic nodule on chest radiography. Meirelles and colleagues[206] reported a pulmonary meningioma to be positive on PET scan, mimicking a carcinoma. Grossly, the tumor is usually a well-circumscribed, round, gray-to-white nodule ranging in size from 1.7 to 6.0 cm. Multiple lesions occur rarely, as reported by Ueno and de Perrot and their colleagues.[165,208] Microscopically, the tumors are composed of meningothelial cells with psammoma bodies. Electron microscopically, the tumors contain interdigitating cell membranes and desmosomes. The tumor cells immunohistochemically stain consistently with vimentin and variably with EMA but not with keratin, S-100, or neuron-specific enolase. Cerebral meningiomas immunostain for progesterone receptor, but pulmonary lesions do not appear to have been stained for this marker. Moran and colleagues[209] concluded that vimentin and EMA are the most reliable immunologic markers of these tumors. The treatment is surgical excision and the prognosis is excellent. Unfortunately, a primary pulmonary meningioma may be malignant. Two cases have been reported, one by Erlandson and one by Prayson and Farver.[210,211] The fate of the former patient is unknown, but the second patient had a rapid downhill course and had both local and distant disease within 5 months. Thus, of the 29 cases reviewed by Cesario and colleagues,[204] the incidence of possible malignancy is very low at 6.8%.

Cases of metastatic meningioma from the cranium to the lung have been reported.[212–215] A patient in whom a pulmonary meningioma is diagnosed should be examined to exclude an intracranial lesion.

Neurofibroma

Neurofibromas are benign tumors of the nerve sheath composed of Schwann, perineural-like, and fibroblastic cells. Neurofibromas are rare tracheal tumors and occur mainly in an endobronchial location. In a recent review of the literature, Hsu and colleagues[216] identified 23 other cases of tracheobronchial neurofibromas. The patients ranged from 8 to 64 years with a 2:1 male-to-female ratio. The symptoms were obstructive and treatment surgical. Willmann and colleagues[217] reported a case associated with neurofibromatosis type 1. Batori and colleagues[218] reported an intrapulmonary case. Surgical resection or endobronchial ablation is indicated as dictated by the extent and location of the tumor. Suzuki and colleagues[219] reported the treatment of two tracheobronchial neurofibromas with Nd:YAG laser ablation.

Schwannoma

A schwannoma is a benign neurogenic tumor composed entirely of Schwann cells. Synonyms include *neurilemoma* and *neurinoma*. Neurogenic tumors may be difficult to classify because of degenerative changes.[220] In this case, a special stain for S-100 may be helpful because the neurogenic tumor stains positively. Righini and colleagues[221] reported a primary polypoid tracheal schwannoma in a 51-year-old woman who presented with cough and dyspnea. She underwent a partial resection of the trachea with an anastomosis. Three years later, she was alive and well.

Psammomatous Melanotic Schwannoma

Simansky and colleagues[187] reported the occurrence of a psammomatous melanotic schwannoma in the lung. This tumor may be part of Carney syndrome and is mentioned previously in the section on cartilaginous lesions (pulmonary chondromas). These authors incorrectly listed 25 cases of this tumor in a review of the literature. On further review, all of the cases were nonmelanotic (see reading references, "Schwannomas").

The psammomatous melanotic schwannoma is most commonly found in the costovertebral area of the thorax arising from a neurogenic structure. It may be associated with myxomas, skin pigmentation, and endocrine overactivity, as it was in the aforementioned case reported by Simansky and colleagues.[187] On immunohistochemical studies, the psammomatous melanotic schwannoma is positive for S-100 protein, vimentin, and HMB-45 and negative for the presence of chromogranin, synaptophysin, and keratin. Treatment is surgical removal.

Paraganglionic Pulmonary Paraganglioma

Paragangliomas are tumors arising from neuroectodermally derived paraganglionic tissue. These tumors are usually benign, but malignant cases have been reported. These tumors are usually named by their location; synonyms include *chemodectoma, glomus jugulare tumor, carotid body tumor,* and *aortic body tumor.* Aubertine and Flieder[222] reported a case and critically reviewed past case reports that may have been carcinoids. They point out that the terminology is confusing and these lesions should not be confused with minute chemodectomas of the lung, now known as minute meningothelial nodules. On microscopic examination, the tumor cells are ovoid with abundant cytoplasm and surrounded by vascular channels. The cells immunostain positive for chromogranin A and synaptophysin but not for keratin. The sustentacular cells immunostained for S-100. A year after surgery, this patient was alive and well.

Rarely, a pulmonary paraganglioma, although its histologic features are those of a benign lesion, may metastasize to the regional lymph nodes and thus would be considered malignant.[223-225] Resection by VATS can be curative with consideration of adjuvant radiation therapy.[226]

Pulmonary Gangliocytic Paraganglioma

Gangliocytic paraganglioma is a rare tumor that is usually found in the duodenum. It is composed of three types of cells: (a) ganglion-like cells, (b) neuroendocrine cells, and (c) Schwann cells. It is thought to represent either a hyperplastic or neoplastic proliferation. Nearly all duodenal cases have a benign course despite the presence

of lymph node metastasis. Hironaka and colleagues[227] reported the first case of one of these tumors occurring in the lung, while Kee and colleagues[228] reported a second one in a 54-year-old woman. Both were in an endobronchial location and caused obstructive symptoms. The patient of Kee and colleagues[228] was a 75-year-old man who complained of right anterior chest pain. The chest radiograph revealed atelectasis of the right middle and lower lobes of the lung. A CT scan showed a 1.5-cm endobronchial mass almost occluding the bronchus at the lower portion of the truncus intermedius. The patient underwent a bilobectomy of the right middle and lower lobes. There was no lymph node involvement. Grossly, the yellow polypoid tumor measured 1.6 cm in greatest dimension. Microscopically, the tumor consisted of three cell types. The first was a round endocrine cell with an oval nuclei, stippled chromatin, and eosinophilic cytoplasm. These cells had a Zellballen arrangement. The second was a large ganglion-like cell. The third was a spindle-shaped cell (Schwann cells). Immunohistochemically, the endocrine cells stained with cytokeratin (CAM 5.2), synaptophysin, and chromogranin. The ganglion-like cells stained with neurofilaments. The spindle-shaped cells stained with S-100 and neurofilaments. This staining pattern is consistent with the respective cells. The endocrine cells also stained for alpha-human chorionic gonadotropin (α-HCG), calcitonin, and somatostatin. The ganglion-like cells stained with somatostatin. The treatment is surgical resection.

MISCELLANEOUS TUMORS

CLEAR CELL TUMOR (SUGAR TUMOR) OF THE LUNG

Nicholson[229] defines clear cell tumors or sugar tumors of the lung as benign tumors that probably arise from the perivascular epithelioid cells. The tumor was first reported by Liebow and Castleman,[230] who later described a series of 12 cases. Most of the patients are between 40 and 60 years old with an equal distribution between men and women. The patients are usually asymptomatic with lesion being discovered on a routine chest radiograph. Santana, Kavunkal and colleagues reported cases that presented with hemoptysis, and Gora-Gebka and colleagues reported a case that presented with systemic symptoms.[231-233] The chest radiographs and CT scan usually show a well-demarcated nodule. On gross examination, the tumor is well demarcated with a gray to red surface. On microscopic examination, the tumor is composed of cells with a clear cytoplasm. The cells contain glycogen which stains purple with a PAS stain and the color disappears after treatment with diastase. The typical immunohistochemical staining is focal positive staining with S-100 and HMB-45 and negative staining for cytokeratin (CK) 7. Adachi and colleagues[234] reported a case that stained for CD1a, raising the possibility that these tumors arise from Langerhans cells. Excision is curative.

Leong and Meredith[235] stressed the necessity of differentiating these benign lesions from the numerous malignant "clear cell" tumors that can be encountered in the lung, such as metastatic renal cell carcinoma or a primary clear cell carcinoma. The aforementioned authors suggest that the immunohistochemical features are most important in distinguishing these various tumors (Table 106.6).

PULMONARY MYELOLIPOMA

Myelolipoma is a benign tumor composed of an admixture of mature adipose tissue and hematopoietic cells (myeloid, erythroid, megakaryocytic, and, at times, lymphoid tissues) that commonly occurs

TABLE 106.6 Immunophenotype of Common Clear Cell Tumors of the Lung

	CK	VIM	Chgn	HMB45	S-100
Sugar tumor	–	+	–	+	+
Clear cell carcinoma	+	±	–	–	–
Clear cell carcinoid	+	–	+	–	–
Renal cell carcinoma	+	+	–	–	±

CK, broad-spectrum cytokeratin; VIM, vimentin; Chgn, chromogranin; HMB45, melanosome-associated protein; S100, S100 protein.
Reprinted from Leong AS-Y, Meredith DJ. Clear cell tumors of the lung. In Corrin B, eds. *Pathology of Lung Tumors*. New York: Churchill Livingstone; 1997:159. Copyright © 1997 Elsevier. With permission.

in the adrenal gland. It is a rare primary pulmonary parenchymal neoplasm. Sato and colleagues[236] reported a case and reviewed the literature. Their summary showed that the patients were between 45 and 81 years of age with a mean age of 60 years, and there was a predominance of men. The patients were all asymptomatic. The chest radiograph showed a nodule. The tumors were randomly distributed in the lungs with all but one being >2.5 cm in greatest dimension. On gross examination, the tumors showed a yellow-brown cut surface. On microscopic examination, the tumors showed mature fat and hematopoietic cells with the trilineage of normal bone marrow. The diagnosis may be established with FNA. The treatment may be expectant, although conservative surgical excision may be elected if major growth or symptoms occur.

NODULAR AMYLOID

Nodular amyloid is an extracellular deposition of protein fibrils. Abbas points out that although amyloid has a uniform appearance, it is not composed of a single protein but rather of at least 15 distinct ones.[237] The three most common ones are (a) AL (amyloid light chain), which is derived from plasma cells and contains immunoglobulin light chains; (b) AA (amyloid-associated), which is a unique nonimmunoglobulin protein synthesized by the liver; and (c) Aβ (Abeta) amyloid, found in the cerebral lesions of Alzheimer's disease. A less common one is ATTR (amyloid transthyretin), found in senile systemic amyloidosis.

Gillmore and Hawkins classified respiratory amyloidosis as comprising four types: laryngeal, tracheobronchial, nodular parenchymal, and diffuse alveolar septal parenchymal (Table 106.7).[238] Nodular amyloid is the focus of this discussion, and it is believed to originate from either a local production of amyloid protein plasma cells or a focal deposition in a patient with systemic amyloidosis. Recent case reports include those of Kawashima, Niepolski, Pitz, Calatayud, and Suzuki and their colleagues.[219,239–242] Higuchi and colleagues[243] collected 34 cases of primary nodular pulmonary amyloidosis from the Japanese literature and added a case of their own. Sixteen of the patients had single lesions and 19 had multiple lesions. The patients ranged in age from young to old, but most tend to be in the sixth and seventh decades of life and both sexes are affected equally. Patients are usually asymptomatic, and the amyloid tumors are discovered on incidental chest radiography. Surgical resection is considered curative. Multiple myeloma does not appear to be frequently associated with these lesions, but the patients should be evaluated for the possibility of this disease.

On histology, the tumors are composed of dense eosinophilic material that may show a peripheral lymphoplasmacytic infiltrate and multinucleated giant cells. A Congo red stain will turn the material red. Under polarizing light, the Congo red stain will show an apple green birefringence. An attempt should be made to identify whether the protein is AA or AL. Lim and Dacic and their colleagues[244,245] addressed the issue between nodular amyloid and lymphoma. Lim and colleagues[244] concluded that marginal-zone lymphomas of the mucosa-associated lymphoid tissue (MALT) type could be found in association with nodular amyloid. Dacic and colleagues[245] described histologic and immunohistologic observations that could be employed to separate nodular amyloid from malignant lymphoma. The lymphomas were identified by lymphatic tracking of lymphocytes, pleural infiltration, and sheet-like masses of plasma cells.

Immunohistochemically, the lymphomas showed a B-cell population with light-chain restriction. A treatment consists of observation once the diagnosis has been established or surgical excision. Ross and Magro[246] recommend surgical excision for AL nodular amyloid with assessment for extrapulmonary disease.

SCLEROSING HEMANGIOMA

A sclerosing hemangioma is a benign lung tumor of undetermined histogenesis. The tumor was originally thought to be of vascular

TABLE 106.7 Respiratory Tract Amyloid Syndromes

Amyloid Type	Distribution of Amyloid (Radiology ± Bronchoscopy)	Clinical Significance
AL	**Laryngeal**	Nodular or diffuse infiltrative form.
		Usually localized, sometimes extending into tracheobronchial tree, associated with focal clonal immunocyte[a] dyscrasia.
	Tracheobronchial	Nodular or diffuse infiltrative form. Amyloid deposits usually confined to respiratory tract in association with focal clonal immunocyte dyscrasia.
	Parenchymal Nodular	Solitary or multiple nodules, usually confined to respiratory tract in association with focal clonal immunocyte dyscrasia.
	Diffuse alveolar septal	
	Intrathoracic lymphadenopathy	Usually a manifestation of systemic AL amyloidosis.
ATTR, AA, others	**Parenchymal diffuse alveolar septal**	Usually an incidental histologic finding. Clinically evident disease and radiologic abnormalities extremely rare.

[a]Immunocyte is any cell in the lymphoid series that can react with an antigen to produce an antibody or participate in cell-mediated reactions.
AL, amyloid light chain; ATTR, amyloid transthyretin; AA, amyloid associated.
Reproduced from Gillmore JD, Hawkins PN. Amyloidosis and the respiratory tract. *Thorax* 1999;54:444–451, with permission from BMJ Publishing Group Ltd.

origin, hence the name. Synonyms include *pneumocytoma* and *papillary pneumocytoma*. Yoo and colleagues[247] postulated that the two cell types seen in the tumor probably derive from a single primitive respiratory epithelial cell type and then differentiate into more and less differentiated type II pneumocytes.

The tumor was originally described by Liebow and Hubbell.[248] Katzenstein and colleagues[249] described 51 cases that Liebow and Hubbell reviewed after their initial description in 1956. These authors noted that the patients ranged in age from 15 to 69 years, with an average age of 42 years. Eighty-four percent of the patients were women. The tumor is more common in Asian populations, such as Japanese. Most (78%) of the patients were asymptomatic. Those who were symptomatic complained of hemoptysis, vague chest pain, or both. On radiographic study, the sclerosing hemangioma appears as a solitary nodule that is found more often in one of the lower lobes (Fig. 106.7). Sugio and Iyoda and colleagues respectively described an additional 10 and 26 cases of this tumor with similar clinical findings to those of Katzenstein and colleagues.[249–251] More than 95% of these tumors are peripheral and solitary. In their review of 100 of these tumors, Devouassoux-Shisheboran and colleagues found that four were located in the pleura and one each endobronchially and in the mediastinum.[252]

On gross examination, sclerosing hemangiomas appear well circumscribed and the cut surfaces can have a mottled yellow-white appearance. Histologically, these tumors are composed of four architectural patterns, with tumors showing varying combinations of the patterns. The four patterns are (a) papillary, (b) sclerotic, (c) solid, and (d) hemorrhagic. The tumors are composed of two cell types that are (a) surface cells that are cuboidal in shape and (b) round (polygonal) cells in the stroma. Calcifications may be present but are rare. A few are associated with a tumorlet, but no carcinoids have been described. Of all of the sclerosing hemangiomas reported (probably in the range of up to 200 cases), 10 patients (2%) have been reported to have had metastatic spread of the sclerosing hemangioma to one or several bronchial or hilar lymph nodes. Katakura and colleagues[253] summarized these cases. Even those patients with metastatic disease appear to have a favorable prognosis. Nodal dissection is indicated when both of these findings are present.

TERATOMA

Teratomas are benign tumors that originate from more than one germ cell line. They usually arise along the midline and it is extremely rare to see one in the lung. The age of presentation ranges from 10 to 68 years. Symptoms are nonspecific and include chest pain, fever, cough, hemoptysis, weight loss, pneumonia, and bronchiectasis. Trichoptysis is strong evidence of a teratoma. Chest radiograph usually shows a lobulated mass, but there may be cavitation or areas of consolidation. CT scan may show discrete areas of soft tissue with a high fat content and punctuate calcifications. Cut section through the tumor may show a cystic space filled with yellow sebaceous material. Histologic examination shows skin, fat and neural tissue. The treatment is surgical. The prognosis is excellent.

THYMOMA, PRIMARY PULMONARY

A thymoma is an intrapulmonary neoplasm identical to mediastinal thymomas and is thought to arise from ectopic thymic rests in the lung. Myers and colleagues[254] reviewed the subject and found 25 cases of intrapulmonary thymoma. The patients ranged in age from 14 to 77 years with a median age of 50 years. The tumors were

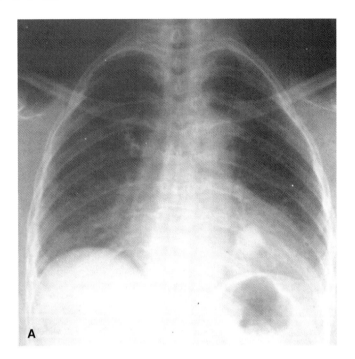

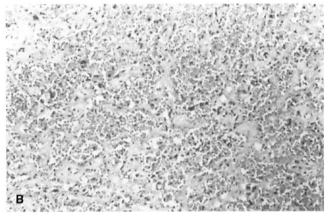

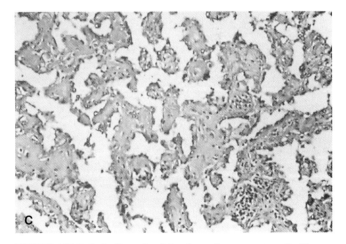

FIGURE 106.7 **A:** Radiograph of the chest of an asymptomatic 63-year-old woman with a mass in the left lower lung field that had been present for >5 years. Recent growth was noted. Removal and histologic examination of the mass revealed a sclerosing hemangioma. **B:** Low-power photomicrograph of the sclerosing hemangioma. Dense solid areas contain typical polygonal cells. **C:** High-power photomicrograph shows papillary areas with the fibrovascular cores lined by cuboidal cells.

almost equally distributed between men and women. Most of the patients were asymptomatic and the lesions were discovered incidentally on chest radiograph. Of the 25 patients, 9 were symptomatic with hemoptysis, recurrent pneumonia, and chest pain. Four patients had paraneoplastic syndromes, such as myasthenia gravis or Good's syndrome (hypogammaglobulinemia associated with thymoma). The lesions were fairly randomly distributed between the lungs and the lobes. Most were solitary and peripheral, although a few were multifocal and some were localized to the hilum. The tumors ranged in size from 1.5 to 12.8 cm.

On gross examination, intrapulmonary thymomas may be solid or cystic and have a variable color. On microscopic examination, the tumors may have broad bands of collagen with a mixture of bland epithelial cells and lymphocytes. Martini and Beattie[1] used different immunohistochemical studies to determine the nature of the epithelial cells in six of their eight cases.[255] These cells had positive results for keratin and the EMA but negative results for vimentin, desmin, actin, and S-100 protein. The patients do well following surgical resection. Myers and colleagues[254] felt that patients should be managed surgically and that radiotherapy may be of some value in incompletely resected cases. Patients with paraneoplastic syndromes tended to fare worse than the others. The patients should be followed long term because of the risk of late local recurrence.

MULTIPLE BENIGN TUMORS

Benign Metastasizing Leiomyoma

Benign metastasizing leiomyoma is the name given to solitary or multiple nodules of benign-appearing smooth muscle in the lung. These nodules are thought to come from uterine leiomyomas. The lesions could represent (a) a uterine leiomyoma colonizing the lung, (b) metastatic low-grade leiomyosarcoma, and (c) primary pulmonary leiomyomatosis. Patton and colleagues[256] measured the telomere lengths of pulmonary lesions and the uterine leiomyomas. They concluded that the lung nodules are clonally derived from benign-appearing uterine leiomyomas. Nucci and colleagues[257] performed cytogenetic analysis on metastasizing leiomyomas and found consistent chromosomal aberrations. They concluded that these tumors were a genetically distinct entity that probably arose from uterine leiomyomas.

Pitts and colleagues[258] reviewed benign metastasizing leiomyomas. They usually occur in women who have undergone uterine surgery for leiomyomas and may occur years after surgery. Most of the patients are asymptomatic and the lesions are usually discovered on a chest radiograph performed for some other reason. Abramson and colleagues[259] thought that the disease was characterized radiographically by numerous well-defined, randomly distributed pulmonary nodules. On CT, the lesions are randomly distributed through the lungs and range in size from 0.1 to 4.2 cm in greatest dimension. On gross examination, the tumor should be firm and white with a fairly well-defined border. Histology reveals that the tumor is composed of bland spindle cells with oval nuclei and eosinophilic cytoplasm. The cells are usually in a pattern of interlacing fascicles and there may be entrapped respiratory epithelium. The tumors will immunostain for estrogen and progesterone receptors as well as desmin and caldesmon.

Since the tumors contain estrogen and progesterone receptors, they may be treated with a combination of surgery, hormonal manipulation, and chemotherapy. Jacobson and colleagues[260] treated a patient with goserelin, a luteinizing hormone–releasing hormone analog, and showed improvement in the patient's blood gas analyses and chest radiograph. Regression of these tumors can occur after oophorectomy. Säynäjäkangas and colleagues[261] treated a patient

with tamoxifen and showed through CT scans that the nodules did not enlarge and new ones did not appear.

Cystic Fibrohistiocytic Tumor (Metastatic Dermatofibroma)

A cystic fibrohistiocytic tumor is a rare spindle cell proliferation in the lung. Osborn, Gu, and their colleagues[262,263] have both reviewed the topics. The lesion is now believed to represent metastases from a skin dermatofibroma (cellular fibrous histiocytomas). Joseph and colleagues[264] first described two cases of cystic fibrohistiocytic tumors of the lungs. Gu and colleagues[263] summarized 13 cases from the literature. The patients ranged in age from 19 to 65 years with an average age of 36 years and a male predominance. They had a variety of complaints, including hemoptysis, pneumonia, pneumothorax, dyspnea, and fatigue. Some were asymptomatic. Most had a history of the removal of a skin dermatofibroma. The time interval from the removal of the skin lesion until the appearance of the lung disease ranged from 23 to 1.5 years. The chest radiograph showed multiple bilateral nodular opacities with some of them containing cystic change. Microscopic examination of the tumors showed variably dilated airspaces lined by cuboidal epithelium and underlying spindle cells with a storiform pattern. The disease appears to be indolent, as most patients were alive with disease at time interval of 1 to 20 years after diagnosis.

Pulmonary Capillary Hemangiomatosis

Yi[265] reviewed pulmonary capillary hemangiomatosis and defined the disease as a proliferation of capillaries in the alveolar septa, the bronchial and venous walls, pleura, and even regional lymph nodes. Tron and colleagues[266] agree with this definition. The nature of this process is poorly understood and it could be reactive, hamartomatous, or neoplastic. The disease occurs equally in men and women ranging from 6 to 71 years old. Clinical symptoms include progressive shortness of breath, pleuritic chest pain, and frequent hemoptysis. Later, these patients may develop signs of cor pulmonale and elevated pulmonary artery pressure. According to El-Gabaly and colleagues,[267] the chest radiographs show a diffuse bilateral reticulonodular pattern. CT scan shows enlarged pulmonary arteries and multiple small bilateral poorly defined nodular opacities. Histology shows a proliferation of capillary-like endothelium-lined blood vessels in the alveolar walls and interlobular septa as well as the peribronchial and perivascular connective tissue. The treatment is bilateral lung transplant or heart–lung transplant. Faber and colleagues[268] treated a patient with bilateral lung transplantation. Assaad and colleagues[269] found an overexpression of platelet-derived growth factor (PDGF)–β gene and PDGF receptor-β gene.

Pulmonary Hyalinizing Granuloma

Pulmonary hyalinizing granuloma is a benign tumor that is composed of dense hyalinized connective tissue. The etiology is unknown, but the tumor has been associated with infectious, neoplastic, autoimmune diseases as well as sclerosing mediastinitis and retroperitoneal fibrosis. Many of the descriptions are single case reports.[270–272]

The two largest series are those of Engleman and colleagues, who first described the entity, and Yousem and Hochholzer.[273,274] The tumors are usually multiple,[275] although Na and colleagues[276] described one that was solitary. The tumor occurs between 19 and 77 years of age with a mean age of 44 years. The lesions are equally distributed between men and women. Patients may be asymptomatic or complain of cough, shortness of breath, chest pain, or weight loss. The chest radiographs usually demonstrate multiple bilateral, ill-defined pulmonary nodules or masses. The lesions are nodular and vary from a few millimeters to 15 cm in greatest dimension. On gross examination, the nodules have a white surface and are well circumscribed. On microscopic examination, the tumors are composed of dense bands of collagen and there may be a lymphoplasmacytic infiltrate around the periphery of the nodule. Treatment is surgical.

PULMONARY LYMPHANGIOLEIOMYOMATOSIS

Pulmonary LAM was first reported by Lutenbacher in a woman with tuberous sclerosis (Fig. 106.8).[277] Cohen and colleagues[278] describe LAM as occurring in two forms: (a) sporadic (S-LAM) or (b) associated with tuberous sclerosis (TCS-LAM).

LAM and tuberous sclerosis are linked by mutations in two tumor suppressor genes, TSC1 and TCS2. Tuberous sclerosis is an autosomal dominant neurocutaneous disorder where the patients have mental retardation, seizures, subungual fibromas, angiofibromas, and shagreen patches on their skin.

Incidence

Johnson[279] estimated that sporadic lymphangioleiomyomatosis (S-LAM) had a prevalence of about 1 in 1 million people in the general population. In contrast, approximately 40% of adult females with tuberous sclerosis (TSC-LAM) had signs of LAM.

Pathogenesis

The exact pathogenesis of LAM is not known, but in the last few years, several clues have emerged as to what might be causing the disease. According to Goncharova and Krymskaya,[280] there is a loss of function of the tumor suppressor genes tuberous sclerosis complex 1 and 2 (TSC1 and TSC2) through either a somatic or genetic mutation. These genes are involved in a signal transduction pathway. The disease is thought to develop by a two-hit mechanism. The first hit is a mutation of either TSC1 or TSC2 and the second is a loss of heterozygosity (LOH) with a loss of function of the TSC1 or TSC2 proteins. Both genes are negative regulators of the mammalian target of rapamycin (mTOR)/p70 S6 kinase (S6K1) signaling pathway. The loss of the proteins produced by TSC1 (hamartin) or TSC2 (tuberin)

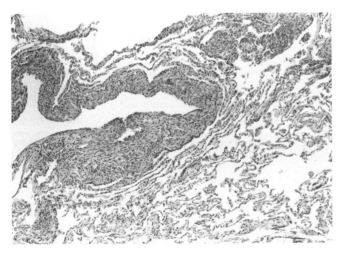

FIGURE 106.8 Photomicrograph of a section of lung in a patient with lymphangioleiomyomatosis. Note the accumulation of muscle cells that appear immature and are clustered randomly in the alveolar walls and around the small bronchi and blood vessels.

appear to lead to an activation of the signaling pathway with subsequent LAM cell proliferation.

Clinical Features

Taylor and colleagues[281] described the typical patient with LAM as a woman of childbearing age. Cohen and colleagues[278] pointed out that older women (>40 years) are being diagnosed with LAM and this diagnosis should be considered in an older woman with dyspnea. Ryu and colleagues[282] reported on the characteristics of 230 women enrolled in the LAM registry of the National Heart, Lung and Blood Institute (NHLBI). Of the 230 patients enrolled in the registry 196 (85.2%) were sporadic (S-LAM) and 34 (14.8%) were tuberous sclerosis–associated (TSC-LAM). For both groups, the average age of enrollment was 44.5 years. About 40% were postmenopausal and 87% were white. The primary events or conditions that led to diagnosis were (a) a spontaneous pneumothorax (35.8%), (b) other pulmonary symptoms (dyspnea or wheezing) (28.4%), (c) abnormal chest radiograph (19.7%), (d) pleural effusion (2.6%), and (e) renal angiomyolipoma (3.9%). Laboratory tests—including complete blood count, serum chemistries with liver enzymes, and urinalysis—revealed no abnormalities. Young and colleagues raised the possibility that elevated levels of serum vascular endothelial growth factor-D (VEGF-D) may be useful in diagnosing S-LAM.[283] Glassberg[284] described the pulmonary function tests of these patients as showing a combination of restrictive and obstructive changes including an elevated total lung capacity, increased residual volume, and reduced forced expiratory volume at 1 second. In addition, the carbon monoxide diffusing capacity is reduced and the arterial blood gas reveals hypoxemia without hypercapnia.

Radiology

Bearz and colleagues[285] point out that the radiologic findings are important for the diagnosis of LAM. The early chest radiographs show diffuse slight hyperinflation with linear opacities in the lung bases. Later, there is a reticulonodular pattern that progresses to a honeycomb pattern. On CT scan, the lungs show numerous thin-walled cysts, with the HRCT scans being very helpful in establishing the diagnosis. The CT findings have been described by Swensen and Müller and their colleagues. The HRCT findings consist of numerous, variable-sized cysts surrounded by normal-appearing lung parenchyma.[286,287] The cysts usually vary between 0.2 and 2 cm in size but may be as large as 6 cm. Müller and colleagues noted that usually the smaller the size of the cysts, the milder the disease.[287] The cysts are distributed equally throughout the lung, but occasionally the lower lobes appear to be more involved.

Pathology

On gross examination, the end-stage lung of LAM will show multiple cysts with a honeycomb pattern. On microscopic examination, Taveira-DaSilva and colleagues[288] describe the lung as showing multiple cysts and the proliferation of two types of LAM cells that form nodules in the lung. One cell type has a spindle shape and the other has a round shape or is epithelioid. Immunohistochemically, both types of cells stain with smooth muscle antigens, such as desmin and smooth muscle actin. The round cells will also stain with HMB45. Immunostains also reveal the presence of estrogen and progesterone receptors. The dilated alveoli or cysts usually contain hemosiderin-laden macrophages. In addition to the cystic destruction of the lung, the growth of these LAM cells leads to the obstruction of airways and lymphatics with the formation of cystic lymphatic spaces. The destructive lung changes eventually lead to a loss of pulmonary function.

Treatment

In LAM, the lung disease and other complications—such as pneumothorax, chylothorax, and renal angiomyolipomas—need to be treated. The clinical observations that the disease presents in premenopausal women and that it may be exacerbated by oral contraceptives, pregnancy, and the onset of menses as well as the presence of tissue estrogen and progesterone receptors suggest that hormones play a role in the progression of this disease. Juvet and colleagues[289] point out that these observations have led to a variety of hormone-based treatments, with the current most common treatment being the administration of progesterone. They also point out that there is as yet no definite evidence that this therapeutic approach is effective, with some reports showing benefit and others not. Tamoxifen has been used but appears to worsen the disease in some patients. Lung transplantation is the ultimate treatment. Chen and colleagues[290] describe the recurrence of the LAM cells in the transplanted lung.

As described in the section on pathogenesis, rapamycin (sirolimus) may inhibit the signal transduction pathway and stop or slow the LAM cells from proliferating. Bissler and colleagues describe the use of rapamycin for the treatment of the pulmonary disease and the angiomyolipomas.[291] The treatment showed a decrease in the size of the angiomyolipomas and some improvement in pulmonary function. The FEV_1 and the FVC both improved; however, total lung capacity and carbon monoxide diffusing capacity did not. The decline in lung function may be stabilized with mTOR inhibitors like rapamycin; however, referral for lung transplantation should be considered for those with worsening function. Unfortunately, LAM has been reported to occur in the transplanted lungs after a long postoperative interval.[292]

Moses and colleagues[293] described the use of doxycycline in the treatment of the lung. They attribute lung parenchymal destruction to the presence of matrix metalloproteinases (MMPs), which cause proteolysis of tissue. Doxycycline is an MMP inhibitor, and the presence of MMPs can be measured in the urine. They describe a 66-year-old woman with LAM whose pulmonary function improved after taking the drug and her urinary MMPs decreased.

Of the complications, the first time a patient has a pneumothorax, it should be treated with pleurodesis, because recurrent pneumothoraces are likely.[294] The chylothorax should be treated by obliteration of the pleural space or ligation of the thoracic duct. Johnson[279] suggests that the renal angiomyolipomas should be followed depending on their size.[279] These tumors may result in a spontaneous peritoneal hemorrhage which is a serious complication for the patient.

Finally, these patients are generally advised not to become pregnant, as pregnancy may exacerbate the lung disease, leading to a pneumothorax or a chylous pleural effusion. The patients are also advised against air travel owing to the risk of a pneumothorax, dyspnea, and chest pain. Pollock-BarZiv and colleagues[295] emphasize that the decision to travel must be individualized.

REFERENCES

1. Martini N, Beattie EJ. Less common tumors of the lung. In: Shields TW, ed. *General Thoracic Surgery*. 2nd ed. Philadelphia, PA: Lea & Febiger; 1983:780.
2. Chan AL, Shelton DK, Yoneda KY. Unusual primary lung neoplasms. *Curr Opin Pulm Med* 2001;7(4):234–241.
3. Travis WD, Brambilla E, Muller-Hermelink HK, et al. *World Health Organization Classification of Tumours. Pathology and Genetics of Tumours of the Lung, Pleura, Thymus and Heart*. Lyon: IARC Press; 2004.
4. Fletcher CD, Unni KK, Mertens F. *World Health Organization Classification of Tumours. Pathology and Genetics of Tumours of Soft Tissue and Bone*. Lyon: IAC Press; 2002.
5. Steele JD. The solitary pulmonary nodule. report of a cooperative study of resected asymptomatic solitary pulmonary nodules in males. *J Thorac Cardiovasc Surg* 1963;46:21–39.
6. Aletras A, Bjoerk VO, Fors B, et al. "Benign" bronchopulmonary neoplasms. *Dis Chest* 1963;44:498–504.
7. Arrigoni MG, Woolner LB, Bernatz PE, et al. Benign tumors of the lung. A ten-year surgical experience. *J Thorac Cardiovasc Surg* 1970;60(4):589–599.
8. Mitsudomi T, Kaneko S, Tateishi M, et al. Benign tumors and tumor like lesions of the lung. *Int Surg* 1990;75(3):155–158.
9. Otani Y, Yoshida I, Kawashima O, et al. Benign tumors of the lung: a 20-year surgical experience. *Surg Today* 1997;27(4):310–312.
10. Allen JS. Rare solitary benign tumors of the lung. *Semin Thorac Cardiovasc Surg* 2003;15:315–322.
11. Smith MA, Battafarano RJ, Meyers BF, et al. Prevalence of benign disease in patients undergoing resection for suspected lung cancer. *Ann Thorac Surg* 2006;81(5):1824–1828; discussion 1828–1829.
12. Travis WD, Brambilla E, Nicholson AG, et al. The 2015 World Health Organization classification of lung tumors: impact of genetic, clinical and radiologic advances since the 2004 classification. *J Thorac Oncol* 2015;10(9):1243–1260.
13. Gjevre JA, Myers JL, Prakash UB. Pulmonary hamartomas. *Mayo Clin Proc* 1996;71(1):14–20.
14. Le Roux BT. Pulmonary 'hamartomata'. *Thorax* 1964;19:236–243.
15. Lien YC, Hsu HS, Li WY, et al. Pulmonary hamartoma. *J Chin Med Assoc* 2004;67(1):21–26.
16. Hansen CP, Holtveg H, Francis D, et al. Pulmonary hamartoma. *J Thorac Cardiovasc Surg* 1992;104(3):674–678.
17. Thomas JW, Staerkel GA, Whitman GJ. Pulmonary hamartoma. *AJR Am J Roentgenol* 1999;172(6):1643.
18. Siegelman SS, Khouri NF, Leo FP, et al. Solitary pulmonary nodules: CT assessment. *Radiology* 1986;160(2): 307–312.
19. Park KY, Kim SJ, Noh TW, et al. Diagnostic efficacy and characteristic feature of MRI in pulmonary hamartoma: comparison with CT, specimen MRI, and pathology. *J Comput Assist Tomogr* 2008;32(6): 919–925.
20. Tomashefski JF Jr. Benign endobronchial mesenchymal tumors: their relationship to parenchymal pulmonary hamartomas. *Am J Surg Pathol* 1982;6(6):531–540.
21. Fletcher JA, Pinkus GS, Weidner N, et al. Lineage-restricted clonality in biphasic solid tumors. *Am J Pathol* 1991;138(5):1199–1207.
22. Dal Cin P, Kools P, De Jonge I, et al. Rearrangement of 12q14-15 in pulmonary chondroid hamartoma. *Genes Chromosomes Cancer* 1993;8(2):131–133.
23. Xiao S, Lux ML, Reeves R, et al. HMGI(Y) activation by chromosome 6p21 rearrangements in multilineage mesenchymal cells from pulmonary hamartoma. *Am J Pathol* 1997;150(3):901–910.
24. Kazmierczak B, Meyer-Bolte K, Tran KH, et al. A high frequency of tumors with rearrangements of genes of the HMGI(Y) family in a series of 191 pulmonary chondroid hamartomas. *Genes Chromosomes Cancer* 1999;26(2):125–133.
25. Hamper UM, Khouri NF, Stitik FP, et al. Pulmonary hamartoma: diagnosis by transthoracic needle-aspiration biopsy. *Radiology* 1985;155(1):15–18.
26. Makris D, Scherpereel A, Leroy S, et al. Electromagnetic navigation diagnostic bronchoscopy for small peripheral lung lesions. *Eur Respir J* 2007;29(6):1187–1192.
27. Yasufuku K, Nakajima T, Chiyo M, et al. Endobronchial ultrasonography: current status and future directions. *J Thorac Oncol* 2007;2(10):970–979.
28. Hata Y, Isobe K, Sasamoto S, et al. Pulmonary hamartoma diagnosed by convex probe endobronchial ultrasound-guided transbronchial needle aspiration (EBUS-TBNA). *Intern Med* 2010;49(12):1171–1173.
29. Rai SP, Patil AP, Saxena P, et al. Laser resection of endobronchial hamartoma via fiberoptic bronchoscopy. *Lung India* 2010;27(3):170–172.
30. Guo W, Zhao YP, Jiang YG, et al. Surgical treatment and outcome of pulmonary hamartoma: a retrospective study of 20-year experience. *J Exp Clin Cancer Res* 2008;27:8.
31. Karasik A, Modan M, Jacob CO, et al. Increased risk of lung cancer in patients with chondromatous hamartoma. *J Thorac Cardiovasc Surg* 1980;80(2):217–220.
32. Tay JH, Wallbridge PD, Larobina M, et al. Electromagnetic navigation bronchoscopy-directed pleural tattoo to aid surgical resection of peripheral pulmonary lesions. *J Bronchology Interv Pulmonol* 2016; 23(3):245–250.
33. Hanauer M, Perentes JY, Krueger T, et al. Pre-operative localization of solitary pulmonary nodules with computed tomography-guided hook wire: report of 181 patients. *J Cardiothorac Surg* 2016;11:5.
34. Kim SA, Um SW, Song JU, et al. Bronchoscopic features and bronchoscopic intervention for endobronchial hamartoma. *Respirology* 2010;15(1):150–154.
35. Mondello B, Lentini S, Buda C, et al. Giant endobronchial hamartoma resected by fiberoptic bronchoscopy electrosurgical snaring. *J Cardiothorac Surg* 2011;6:97.
36. Lee SH, Kim KT, Yi EJ, et al. Endoscopic cryosurgical resection of pulmonary hamartoma with flexible bronchoscopy. *Korean J Thorac Cardiovasc Surg* 2011; 44(4):307–310.
37. Jura JB, Dillard TA. Complete resection of endobronchial hamartoma by electrocautery and argon plasma ablation via fiberoptic bronchoscopy. *Chest* 2003;124(Suppl 4):289S–290S.
38. Scarlata S, Graziano P, Lucantoni G, et al. Endoscopic treatment of primary benign central airway tumors: Results from a large consecutive case series and decision making flow chart to address bronchoscopic excision. *Eur J Surg Oncol* 2015;41(10):1437–1442.
39. Jalal A, Jeyasingham K. Bronchoplasty for malignant and benign conditions: a retrospective study of 44 cases. *Eur J Cardiothorac Surg* 2000;17(4):370–376.
40. Tomos P, Karaiskos T, Lahanas E, et al. Transverse bronchoplasty of the membranous wall after resection of an endobronchial hamartoma. *Ann Thorac Surg* 2007; 83(2):703–704.
41. van den Bosch JM, Wagenaar SS, Corrin B, et al. Mesenchymoma of the lung (so called hamartoma): a review of 154 parenchymal and endobronchial cases. *Thorax* 1987;42(10):790–793.

42. Ribet M, Jaillard-Thery S, Nuttens MC. Pulmonary hamartoma and malignancy. *J Thorac Cardiovasc Surg* 1994;107(2):611–614.

43. Sinner WN. Fine-needle biopsy of hamartomas of the lung. *AJR Am J Roentgenol* 1982;138(1):65–69.

44. Derkay CS, Wiatrak B. Recurrent respiratory papillomatosis: a review. *Laryngoscope* 2008;118(7):1236–1247.

45. Flieder DB, Koss MN, Nicholson A, et al. Solitary pulmonary papillomas in adults: a clinicopathologic and in situ hybridization study of 14 cases combined with 27 cases in the literature. *Am J Surg Pathol* 1998;22(11):1328–1342.

46. Popper HH, el-Shabrawi Y, Wöckel W, et al. Prognostic importance of human papilloma virus typing in squamous cell papilloma of the bronchus: comparison of in situ hybridization and the polymerase chain reaction. *Hum Pathol* 1994; 25(11):1191–1197.

47. Katial RK, Ranlett R, Whitlock WL. Human papilloma virus associated with solitary squamous papilloma complicated by bronchiectasis and bronchial stenosis. *Chest* 1994;106(6):1887–1889.

48. Kawaguchi T, Matumura A, Iuchi K, et al. Solitary squamous papilloma of the bronchus associated with human papilloma virus type 11. *Intern Med* 1999;38(10): 817–819.

49. Lam CW, Talbot AR, Yeh KT, et al. Human papillomavirus and squamous cell carcinoma in a solitary tracheal papilloma. *Ann Thorac Surg* 2004;77(6):2201–2202.

50. Iwata T, Inoue K, Nishiyama N, et al. Pulmonary inverted Schneiderian papilloma causing high serum levels of carcinoembryonic antigen and squamous cell carcinoma-associated antigen: report of a case. *Surg Today* 2007;37(9):790–793.

51. Miura H, Tsuchida T, Kawate N, et al. Asymptomatic solitary papilloma of the bronchus: review of occurrence in Japan. *Eur Respir J* 1993;6(7): 1070–1073.

52. Miller SM, Bellinger CR, Chatterjee A. Argon plasma coagulation and electrosurgery for benign endobronchial tumors. *J Bronchology Interv Pulmonol* 2013; 20(1):38–40.

53. Yildirim F, Turk M, Demircan S, et al. Tracheal papilloma treated with cryotherapy and interferon-alpha: A case report and review of the literature. *Case Rep Pulmonol* 2015:356796.

54. Flieder D. Glandular papillomas. In: Travis WD, Muller-Hermelink HK, eds. *World Health Organization Classification of Tumours. Pathology and Genetics of Tumours of the Lung, Pleura, Thymus and Heart*. Lyon: IARC Press; 2004:80.

55. Colby TV, Koss Michael N, Travis WD. *Atlas of Tumor Pathology: Tumors of the Lower Respiratory Tract*. Washington DC: Armed Forces Institute of Pathology; 1995:61.

56. Kozu Y, Maniwa T, Ohde Y, et al. A solitary mixed squamous cell and glandular papilloma of the lung. *Ann Thorac Cardiovasc Surg* 2014;20 (Suppl): 625–628.

57. Yousem SA, Hochholzer L. Alveolar adenoma. *Hum Pathol* 1986;17(10):1066–1071.

58. Fujimoto K, Müller NL, Sadohara J, et al. Alveolar adenoma of the lung: computed tomography and magnetic resonance imaging findings. *J Thorac Imaging* 2002;17(2):163–166.

59. Cavazza A, Paci M, De Marco L, et al. Alveolar adenoma of the lung: a clinicopathologic, immunohistochemical, and molecular study of an unusual case. *Int J Surg Pathol* 2004;12(2):155–159.

60. Hartman MS, Epstein DM, Geyer SJ, et al. Alveolar adenoma. *Ann Thorac Surg* 2004;78(5):1842–1843.

61. Halldorsson A, Dissanaike S, Kaye KS. Alveolar adenoma of the lung: a clinicopathological description of a case of this very unusual tumour. *J Clin Pathol* 2005;58(11):1211–1214.

62. Saito EH, de Aaraujo LR, Carneiro LH, et al. Alveolar adenoma. *J Bras Pneumol* 2006;32(3):267–269.

63. Bohm J, Fellbaum C, Bautz W, et al. Pulmonary nodule caused by an alveolar adenoma of the lung. *Virchows Arch* 1997;430(2):181–184.

64. Oliveira P, Moura Nunes JF, Clode AL, et al. Alveolar adenoma of the lung: further characterization of this uncommon tumour. *Virchows Arch* 1996;429(2–3):101–108.

65. Burke LM, Rush WI, Khoor A, et al. Alveolar adenoma: a histochemical, immunohistochemical, and ultrastructural analysis of 17 cases. *Hum Pathol* 1999;30(2): 158–167.

66. Spencer H, Dail DH, Arneaud J. Non-invasive bronchial epithelial papillary tumors. *Cancer* 1980;45(6):1486–1497.

67. Fantone JC, Geisinger KR, Appelman HD. Papillary adenoma of the lung with lamellar and electron dense granules. An ultrastructural study. *Cancer* 1982; 50(12):2839–2844.

68. Noguchi M, Kodama T, Shimosato Y, et al. Papillary adenoma of type 2 pneumocytes. *Am J Surg Pathol* 1986;10(2):134–139.

69. Hegg CA, Flint A, Singh G. Papillary adenoma of the lung. *Am J Clin Pathol* 1992; 97(3):393–397.

70. Sanchez-Jimenez J, Ballester-Martínez A, Lodo-Besse J, et al. Papillary adenoma of type 2 pneumocytes. *Pediatr Pulmonol* 1994;17(6):396–400.

71. Fukuda T, Ohnishi Y, Kanai I, et al. Papillary adenoma of the lung. Histological and ultrastructural findings in two cases. *Acta Pathol Jpn* 1992;42(1):56–61.

72. Mori M, Chiba R, Tezuka F, et al. Papillary adenoma of type II pneumocytes might have malignant potential. *Virchows Arch* 1996;428(3):195–200.

73. Dessy E, Braidotti P, Del Curto B, et al. Peripheral papillary tumor of type-II pneumocytes: a rare neoplasm of undetermined malignant potential. *Virchows Arch* 2000;436(3):289–295.

74. Sheppard MN, Burke L, Kennedy M. TTF-1 is useful in the diagnosis of pulmonary papillary adenoma. *Histopathology* 2003;43(4):404–405.

75. Jin HY, Park TS. Pulmonary pleomorphic adenoma: report of a rare case. *Korean J Intern Med* 2007;22(2):122–124.

76. Ang KL, Dhannapuneni VR, Morgan WE, et al. Primary pulmonary pleomorphic adenoma. An immunohistochemical study and review of the literature. *Arch Pathol Lab Med* 2003;127(5):621–622.

77. Tanigaki T, Shoyama Y, Iwasaki M, et al. Pleomorphic adenoma in the lung. *Monaldi Arch Chest Dis* 2002;57(1):30–32.

78. Sakamoto H, Uda H, Tanaka T, et al. Pleomorphic adenoma in the periphery of the lung. Report of a case and review of the literature. *Arch Pathol Lab Med* 1991;115(4):393–396.

79. Moran CA, Suster S, Askin FB, et al. Benign and malignant salivary gland-type mixed tumors of the lung. Clinicopathologic and immunohistochemical study of eight cases. *Cancer* 1994;73(10):2481–2490.

80. Moran CA. Primary salivary gland-type tumors of the lung. *Semin Diagn Pathol* 1995;12(2):106–122.

81. Hara M, Sato Y, Kitase M, et al. CT and MR findings of a pleomorphic adenoma in the peripheral lung. *Radiat Med* 2001;19(2):111–114.

82. Kim KH, Sung MW, Kim JW, et al. Pleomorphic adenoma of the trachea. *Otolaryngol Head Neck Surg* 2000;123(1 Pt 1):147–148.

83. Baghai-Wadji M, Sianati M, Nikpour H, et al. Pleomorphic adenoma of the trachea in an 8-year-old boy: a case report. *J Pediatr Surg*, 2006;41(8):e23-e26.

84. Aribas OK, Kanat F, Avunduk MC. Pleomorphic adenoma of the trachea mimicking bronchial asthma: report of a case. *Surg Today* 2007;37(6):493–495.

85. Weinberger MA, Katz S, Davis EW. Peripheral bronchial adenoma of mucous gland type; clinical and pathologic aspects. *J Thorac Surg* 1955;29(6):626–635.

86. Gilman RA, Klassen KP, Scarpelli DG. Mucous gland adenoma of bronchus; report of a case with histochemical study of secretion. *Am J Clin Pathol* 1956;26(2):151–154.

87. Weiss L, Ingram M. Adenomatoid bronchial tumors. A consideration of the carcinoid tumors and the salivary tumors of the bronchial tree. *Cancer* 1961;14:161–718.

88. Kroe DJ, Pitcock JA. Benign mucous gland adenoma of the bronchus. *Arch Pathol* 1967;84(5):539–542.

89. Emory WB, Mitchell WT Jr, Hatch HB Jr. Mucous gland adenoma of the bronchus. *Am Rev Respir Dis* 1973;108(6):1407–1410.

90. Edwards CW, Matthews HR. Mucous gland adenoma of the bronchus. *Thorax* 1981;36(2):147–148.

91. England DM, Hochholzer L. Truly benign "bronchial adenoma." Report of 10 cases of mucous gland adenoma with immunohistochemical and ultrastructural findings. *Am J Surg Pathol* 1995;19(8):887–899.

92. Kwon JW, Goo JM, Seo JB, et al. Mucous gland adenoma of the bronchus: CT findings in two patients. *J Comput Assist Tomogr* 1999;23(5):758–760.

93. Ishida T, Kamachi M, Hanada T, et al. Mucous gland adenoma of the trachea resected with an endoscopic neodymium:yttrium aluminum garnet laser. *Intern Med* 1996;35(11):890–893.

94. Fechner RE, Bentinck BR. Ultrastructure of bronchial oncocytoma. *Cancer* 1973; 31(6):1451–1457.

95. Fernandez MA, Nyssen J. Oncocytoma of the lung. *Can J Surg* 1982;25(3):332–333.

96. Tesluk H, Dajee A. Pulmonary oncocytoma. *J Surg Oncol* 1985;29(3):173–175.

97. Laforga JB, Aranda FI. Multicentric oncocytoma of the lung diagnosed by fine-needle aspiration. *Diagn Cytopathol* 1999;21(1):51–54.

98. Santos-Briz A, Terrón J, Sastre R, et al. Oncocytoma of the lung. *Cancer* 1977; 40(3):1330–1336.

99. de Jesus MG, Poon TP, Chung KY. Pulmonary oncocytoma. *N Y State J Med* 1989; 89(8):477–480.

100. Van Genechten M, Schelfout K, Germonpré PR, et al. Benign oncocytoma of the trachea. *Ann Thorac Surg* 2005;80(1):e3–e4.

101. Burrah R, Kini U, Correa M, et al. Pulmonary oncocytoma: a rare case. *Asian Cardiovasc Thorac Ann* 2006;14(6):e113–e114.

102. Yousem SA, Nicholson AG. Epithelial-myoepithelial carcinoma. In: Travis WD, Muller-Hermelink HK, Brambilla E, et al. eds. *World Health Organization Classification of Tumours. Pathology and Genetics of Tumours of the Lung, Pleura, Thymus and Heart, B.E*. Lyon: IARC Press; 2004:67.

103. Chang T, Husain AN, Colby T, et al. Pneumocytic adenomyoepithelioma: a distinctive lung tumor with epithelial, myoepithelial, and pneumocytic differentiation. *Am J Surg Pathol* 2007;31(4):562–568.

104. Kilpatrick SE, Limon J. Mixed tumor/myoepithelioma/parachordoma. In: Fletcher CDM, Mertens F, eds. *World Health Organization Classification of Tumours. Pathology and Genetics of Tumours of Soft Tissue and Bone, U.K*. Lyon: IARC Press; 2002: 198–199.

105. Strickler JG, Hegstrom J, Thomas MJ, et al. Myoepithelioma of the lung. *Arch Pathol Lab Med* 1987;111(11):1082–1085.

106. Tsuji N, Tateishi R, Ishiguro S, et al. Adenomyoepithelioma of the lung. *Am J Surg Pathol* 1995;19(8):956–962.

107. Pelosi G, Fraggetta F, Maffini F, et al. Pulmonary epithelial-myoepithelial tumor of unproven malignant potential: report of a case and review of the literature. *Mod Pathol* 2001;14(5):521–526.

108. Cagirici U, Sayiner A, Inci I, et al. Myoepithelioma of the lung. *Eur J Cardiothorac Surg* 2000;17(2):187–189.

109. Sambrook Gowar FJ. An unusual mucous cyst of the lung. *Thorax* 1978;33(6): 796–799.

110. Dail DH. Uncommon tumors. In: Tumors HS, Dail DH, Colby TV, eds. *Pulmonary Pathology*: New York: Springer-Verlag; 1994:1279.

111. Kragel PJ, Devaney KO, Meth BM, et al. Mucinous cystadenoma of the lung. A report of two cases with immunohistochemical and ultrastructural analysis. *Arch Pathol Lab Med* 1990;114(10):1053–1056.

112. Dixon AY, Moran JF, Wesselius LJ, et al. Pulmonary mucinous cystic tumor. Case report with review of the literature. *Am J Surg Pathol* 1993;17(7):722–728.

113. Roux FJ, Lantuéjoul S, Brambilla E, et al. Mucinous cystadenoma of the lung. *Cancer* 1995;76(9):1540–1544.

114. Graeme-Cook F, Mark EJ. Pulmonary mucinous cystic tumors of borderline malignancy. *Hum Pathol* 1991;22(2):185–190.

115. Mann GN, Wilczynski SP, Sager K, et al. Recurrence of pulmonary mucinous cystic tumor of borderline malignancy. *Ann Thorac Surg* 2001;71(2):696–697.

116. Marcheix B, Brouchet L, Lamarche Y, et al. Pulmonary angiomyolipoma. *Ann Thorac Surg* 2006;82(4):1504–1506.

117. Thway K, Fisher C. PEComa: morphology and genetics of a complex tumor family. *Ann Diagn Pathol* 2015;19(5):359–368.

118. Wu BR, Chen CH, Liao WC, et al. Life-threatening tracheal benign tumor: lipoma. *Intern Med* 2016;55(12):1677–1678.

119. Bango, A, Colubi L, Molinos L, et al. Endobronchial lipomas. *Respiration* 1993;60(5):297–301.

120. Yokozaki M, Kodama T, Yokose T, et al. Endobronchial lipoma: a report of three cases. *Jpn J Clin Oncol* 1996;26(1):53–57.

121. Muraoka M, Oka T, Akamine S, et al. Endobronchial lipoma: review of 64 cases reported in Japan. *Chest* 2003;123(1):293–296.

122. Civi K, Ciftçi E, Gürlek Olgun E, et al. Peripheral intrapulmonary lipoma: a case report and review of the literature. *Tuberk Toraks* 2006;54(4):374–377.

123. Shilo K, Miettinen M, Travis WD, et al. Pulmonary microcystic fibromyxoma: Report of 3 cases. *Am J Surg Pathol* 2006;30(11):1432–1435.

124. Casalini E, Cavazza A, Andreani A, et al. Bronchial fibroepithelial polyp: a clinico-radiologic, bronchoscopic, histopathological and in-situ hybridisation study of 15 cases of a poorly recognised lesion. *Clin Respir J* 2015;11(1):43–48.

125. Dinçer I, Demir A, Akin H, et al. A giant endobronchial inflammatory polyp. *Ann Thorac Surg* 2005;80(6):2353–2356.

126. Arguelles M, Blanco I. Inflammatory bronchial polyps associated with asthma. *Arch Intern Med* 1983;143(3):570–571.

127. Roberts C, Devenny AM, Brooker R, et al. Inflammatory endobronchial polyposis with bronchiectasis in cystic fibrosis. *Eur Respir J* 2001;18(3):612–615.

128. McShane D, Nicholson AG, Goldstraw P, et al. Inflammatory endobronchial polyps in childhood: clinical spectrum and possible link to mechanical ventilation. *Pediatr Pulmonol* 2002;34(1):79–84.

129. Nishi J, Yoshinaga M, Noguchi H, et al. Bronchial polyp in a child with endobronchial tuberculosis under fiberoptic bronchoscopic observation. *Pediatr Int* 2000;42(5):573–576.

130. Asano T, Itoh G, Itoh M. Disseminated Mycobacterium intracellulare infection in an HIV-negative, nonimmunosuppressed patient with multiple endobronchial polyps. *Respiration* 2002;69(2):175–177.

131. Naber JM, Palmer SM, Howell DN. Cytomegalovirus infection presenting as bronchial polyps in lung transplant recipients. *J Heart Lung Transplant* 2005;24(12):2109–2113.

132. Coffin CM, Fletcher J. Inflammatory myofibroblastic tumour, In: Fletcher CDM, Mertens F, eds. *World Health Organization Classification of Tumours. Pathology and Genetics of Tumours of Soft Tissue and Bone,* U.K. Lyon: IARC Press; 2002:91.

133. Moran CA, Suster S. Unusual non-neoplastic lesions of the lung. *Semin Diagn Pathol* 2007;24(3):199–208.

134. Gomez-Roman JJ, Sánchez-Velasco P, Ocejo-Vinyals G, et al. Human herpesvirus-8 genes are expressed in pulmonary inflammatory myofibroblastic tumor (inflammatory pseudotumor). *Am J Surg Pathol* 2001;25(5):624–629.

135. Melloni G, Carretta A, Ciriaco P, et al. Inflammatory pseudotumor of the lung in adults. *Ann Thorac Surg* 2005;79(2):426–432.

136. Antonescu CR, Suurmeijer AJ, Zhang L, et al. Molecular characterization of inflammatory myofibroblastic tumors with frequent ALK and ROS1 gene fusions and rare novel RET rearrangement. *Am J Surg Pathol* 2015;39(7):957–967.

137. Matsubara O, Tan-Liu NS, Kenney RM, et al. Inflammatory pseudotumors of the lung: progression from organizing pneumonia to fibrous histiocytoma or to plasma cell granuloma in 32 cases. *Hum Pathol* 1988;19(7):807–814.

138. Coffin CM, Hornick JL, Fletcher CD. Inflammatory myofibroblastic tumor: comparison of clinicopathologic, histologic, and immunohistochemical features including ALK expression in atypical and aggressive cases. *Am J Surg Pathol* 2007;31(4):509–520.

139. Sakurai H, Hasegawa T, Watanabe Si, et al. Inflammatory myofibroblastic tumor of the lung. *Eur J Cardiothorac Surg* 2004;25(2):155–159.

140. Kobashi Y, Fukuda M, Nakata M, et al. Inflammatory pseudotumor of the lung: clinicopathological analysis in seven adult patients. *Int J Clin Oncol* 2006;11(6):461–466.

141. Kim TS, Han J, Kim GY, et al. Pulmonary inflammatory pseudotumor (inflammatory myofibroblastic tumor): CT features with pathologic correlation. *J Comput Assist Tomogr* 2005;29(5):633–639.

142. Agrons GA, Rosado-de-Christenson ML, Kirejczyk WM, et al. Pulmonary inflammatory pseudotumor: radiologic features. *Radiology* 1998;206(2):511–518.

143. Yousem SA, Tazelaar HD, Manabe T, et al. Inflammatory myofibroblastic tumor. In: Travis WD, Muller-Hermelink HK, et al. eds. *World Health Organization Classification of Tumours. Pathology and Genetics of Tumours of the Lung, Pleura, Thymus and Heart, B.E.* Lyon: IARC Press; 2004:105–106.

144. Guillon L, Fletcher JA. Extrapleural SFT and hemangiopericytoma. In: Fletcher CDM, Mertens F, eds. *World Health Organization Classification of Tumours. Pathoogy and Genetics of Tumours of Soft Tissue and Bone,* U.K. Lyon; IARC Press; 2002:86–90.

145. Fridlington J, Weaver J, Kelly B, et al. Secondary hypertrophic osteoarthropathy associated with solitary fibrous tumor of the lung. *J Am Acad Dermatol* 2007;57(5 Suppl):S106–S110.

146. Sagawa M, Ueda Y, Matsubara F, et al. Intrapulmonary solitary fibrous tumor diagnosed by immunohistochemical and genetic approaches: report of a case. *Surg Today* 2007;37(5):423–425.

147. Baliga M, Flowers R, Heard K, et al. Solitary fibrous tumor of the lung: a case report with a study of the aspiration biopsy, histopathology, immunohistochemistry, and autopsy findings. *Diagn Cytopathol* 2007;35(4):239–244.

148. Patsios D, Hwang DM, Chung TB. Intraparenchymal solitary fibrous tumor of the lung: an uncommon cause of a pulmonary nodule. *J Thorac Imaging* 2006;21(1):50–53.

149. Zhanlong M, Haibin S, Xiangshan F, et al. Variable Solitary Fibrous Tumor Locations: CT and MR Imaging Features. *Medicine (Baltimore)* 2016;95(13):e3031.

150. Hurt R. Benign tumours of the bronchus and trachea, 1951–1981. *Ann R Coll Surg Engl* 1984;66(1):22–26.

151. Yellin A, Rosenman Y, Lieberman Y. Review of smooth muscle tumours of the lower respiratory tract. *Br J Dis Chest* 1984;78(4):337–351.

152. White SH, Ibrahim NB, Forrester-Wood CP, et al. Leiomyomas of the lower respiratory tract. *Thorax* 1985;40(4):306–311.

153. Gotti G, Haid MM, Paladini P, et al. Pedunculated pulmonary leiomyoma with large cyst formation. *Ann Thorac Surg* 1993;56(5):1178–1180.

154. Ko SM, Han SB, Lee SK, et al. Calcified endobronchial leiomyoma. *Br J Radiol* 2007;80(953):e91–e93.

155. Bilgin S, Yilmaz A, Okur E, et al. Primary endobronchial leiomyoma: a case report. *Tuberk Toraks* 2004;52(3):272–274.

156. Archambeaud-Mouveroux F, Bourcereau J, Fressinaud C, et al. Bronchial leiomyoma: report of a case successfully treated by endoscopic neodymium-yttrium aluminum garnet laser. *J Thorac Cardiovasc Surg* 1988;95(3):536–538.

157. Kim KH, Suh JS, Han WS. Leiomyoma of the bronchus treated by endoscopic resection. *Ann Thorac Surg* 1993;56(5):1164–1166.

158. Koledin M, Koledin B, Ilincić D, et al. A case of endobronchial leiomyoma treated by sleeve resection of the right upper lobe bronchus. *Vojnosanit Pregl* 2016;73(2):208–210.

159. Fu Y, Li H, Tian B, et al. Pulmonary benign metastasizing leiomyoma: a case report and review of the literature. *World J Surg Oncol* 2012;10:268.

160. Marchevsky AM. Lung tumors derived from ectopic tissues. *Semin Diagn Pathol* 1995;12(2):172–184.

161. Yilmaz A, Bayramgurler B, Aksoy F, et al. Pulmonary glomus tumour: a case initially diagnosed as carcinoid tumour. *Respirology* 2002;7(4):369–371.

162. Zhang Y, England DM, Primary pulmonary glomus tumor with contiguous spread to a peribronchial lymph node. *Ann Diagn Pathol* 2003;7(4):245–248.

163. Koss MN, Hochholzer L, Moran CA. Primary pulmonary glomus tumor: a clinicopathologic and immunohistochemical study of two cases. *Mod Pathol* 1998;11(3):253–258.

164. Gaertner EM, Steinberg DM, Huber M, et al. Pulmonary and mediastinal glomus tumors—report of five cases including a pulmonary glomangiosarcoma: a clinicopathologic study with literature review. *Am J Surg Pathol* 2000;24(8):1105–1114.

165. Ueno M, Fujiyama J, Yamazaki I, et al. Cytology of primary pulmonary meningioma. report of the first multiple case. *Acta Cytol* 1998;42(6):1424–1430.

166. Galliani CA, Beatty JF, Grosfeld JL. Cavernous hemangioma of the lung in an infant. *Pediatr Pathol* 1992;12(1):105–111.

167. Silverman JM, Julien PJ, Herfkens RJ, et al. Magnetic resonance imaging evaluation of pulmonary vascular malformations. *Chest* 1994;106(5):1333–1338.

168. Maeda, R., Isowa N, Sumitomo S, et al. Pulmonary cavernous hemangioma. *Gen Thorac Cardiovasc Surg* 2007;55(4):177–179.

169. Sirmali M, Isowa N, Sumitomo S, et al. A pulmonary cavernous hemangioma causing massive hemoptysis. *Ann Thorac Surg* 2003;76(4):1275–1276.

170. Kobayashi A, Ohno S, Bando M, et al. Cavernous hemangiomas of lungs and liver in an asymptomatic girl. *Respiration* 2003;70(6):647–650.

171. Fine SW, Whitney KD. Multiple cavernous hemangiomas of the lung: a case report and review of the literature. *Arch Pathol Lab Med* 2004;.128(12):1439–1441.

172. Miyamoto U, Tominaga M, Tomimitsu S, et al. A case of multiple pulmonary cavernous hemangioma. *Respirol Case Rep* 2015;3(1):29–32.

173. Faul JL, Berry GJ, Colby TV, et al. Thoracic lymphangiomas, lymphangiectasis, lymphangiomatosis, and lymphatic dysplasia syndrome. *Am J Respir Crit Care Med* 2000;161(3 Pt 1):1037–1046.

174. Lim HJ, Han J, Kim HK, et al. A rare case of diffuse pulmonary lymphangiomatosis in a middle-aged woman. *Korean J Radiol* 2014;15(2):295–299.

175. Kim WS, Lee KS, Kim I, et al. Cystic intrapulmonary lymphangioma: HRCT findings. *Pediatr Radiol* 1995;25(3):206–207.

176. Lee CH, Kim YD, Kim KI, et al. Intrapulmonary cystic lymphangioma in a 2-month-old infant. *J Korean Med Sci* 2004;19(3):458–461.

177. Holden WE, Morris JF, Antonovic R, et al. Adult intrapulmonary and mediastinal lymphangioma causing haemoptysis. *Thorax* 1987;42(8):635–636.

178. Langston C, Askin FB. Pulmonary distress in the neonate, infant and child. In: Thurlbeck WM, ed. *Pathology of the Lung.* 2nd ed. New York: Thieme Medical Publishers; 1995.

179. Takemura T, Watanabe M, Takagi K, et al. Thoracoscopic resection of a solitary pulmonary lymphangioma: report of a case. *Surg Today* 1995;25(7):651–653.

180. Takahara T, Morisaki Y, Torigoe T, et al. Intrapulmonary cystic lymphangioma: report of a case. *Surg Today* 1998;28(12):1310–1312.

181. Wilson C, Askin FB, Heitmiller RF. Solitary pulmonary lymphangioma. *Ann Thorac Surg* 2001;71(4):1337–1338.

182. Nagayasu T, Hayashi T, Ashizawa K, et al. A case of solitary pulmonary lymphangioma. *J Clin Pathol* 2003;56(5):396–398.

183. Ferreira CR, Sibre V, Schultz R, et al. Congenital generalized lymphangiectasia: a rare developmental disorder for non-immune fetal hydrops. *Autops Case Rep* 2015;5(4):27–33.

184. Wick MR, Tazelaar HD, Mills SE. Benign and borderline tumors of the lungs and pleura. In: Leslie KO, ed. *Practical Pulmonary Pathology a Diagnostic Approach,* W.M. Philadelphia, PA: Churchill Livingstone; 2005:689.

185. Carney JA, Gordon H, Carpenter PC, et al. The complex of myxomas, spotty pigmentation, and endocrine overactivity. *Medicine (Baltimore)* 1985;64(4):270–283.

186. Carney JA. Psammomatous melanotic schwannoma. A distinctive, heritable tumor with special associations, including cardiac myxoma and the Cushing syndrome. *Am J Surg Pathol* 1990;14(3):206–222.

187. Simansky DA, Aviel-Ronen S, Reder I, et al. Psammomatous melanotic schwannoma: presentation of a rare primary lung tumor. *Ann Thorac Surg* 2000;70(2):671–672.

188. Carney JA, Sheps SG, Go VL, et al. The triad of gastric leiomyosarcoma, functioning extra-adrenal paraganglioma and pulmonary chondroma. *N Engl J Med* 1977;296(26):1517–1518.

189. Carney JA. The triad of gastric epithelioid leiomyosarcoma, functioning extra-adrenal paraganglioma, and pulmonary chondroma. *Cancer* 1979;43(1):374–382.

190. Carney JA. The triad of gastric epithelioid leiomyosarcoma, pulmonary chondroma, and functioning extra-adrenal paraganglioma: a five-year review. *Medicine (Baltimore)* 1983;62(3):159–169.

191. Carney JA. Gastric stromal sarcoma, pulmonary chondroma, and extra-adrenal paraganglioma (Carney Triad): natural history, adrenocortical component, and possible familial occurrence. *Mayo Clin Proc* 1999;74(6):543–552.

192. Scopsi L, Collini P, Muscolino G. A new observation of the Carney's triad with long follow-up period and additional tumors. *Cancer Detect Prev* 1999;23(5):435–443.

193. Carney JA, Stratakis CA. Familial paraganglioma and gastric stromal sarcoma: a new syndrome distinct from the Carney triad. *Am J Med Genet* 2002;108(2):132–139.

194. Rodriguez FJ, Aubry MC, Tazelaar HD, et al. Pulmonary chondroma: a tumor associated with Carney triad and different from pulmonary hamartoma. *Am J Surg Pathol* 2007;31(12):1844–1853.

195. Ishii H, Akiba T, Marushima H, et al. A case of bilateral multiple pulmonary chondroma: necessity of follow-up for Carney's triad. *Gen Thorac Cardiovasc Surg* 2012;60(8):534–536.

196. Markert E, Gruber-Moesenbacher U, Porubsky C, et al. Lung osteoma—a new benign lung lesion. *Virchows Arch* 2006;449(1):117–120.

197. Vaos G, Zavras N, Priftis K, et al. Bronchial granular cell tumor in a child: impact of diagnostic delay on the type of surgical resection. *J Pediatr Surg* 2006;41(7):1326–1328.

198. Miyake M, Tateishi U, Maeda T, et al. Bronchial granular cell tumor: a case presenting secondary obstructive changes on CT. *Radiat Med* 2006;24(2):154–157.

199. Lui RC, McKenzie FN, Kim YD, et al. Primary endobronchial granular cell myoblastoma. *Ann Thorac Surg* 1989;48(1):113–115.

200. Deavers M, Guinee D, Koss MN, et al. Granular cell tumors of the lung. Clinicopathologic study of 20 cases. *Am J Surg Pathol* 1995;19(6):627–635.

201. Cutlan RT, Eltorky M. Pulmonary granular cell tumor coexisting with bronchogenic carcinoma. *Ann Diagn Pathol* 2001;5(2):74–79.

202. Epstein LJ, Mohsenifar Z. Use of Nd:YAG laser in endobronchial granular cell myoblastoma. *Chest* 1993;104(3):958–960.

203. Robinson G. Pulmonary meningioma. Report of a case with electron microscopic and immunohistochemical findings. *Am J Clin Pathol* 1992;97(6):814–817.

204. Cesario A, Galetta D, Margaritora S, et al. Unsuspected primary pulmonary meningioma. *Eur J Cardiothorac Surg* 2002;21(3):553–555.

205. Picquet J, Valo I, Jousset Y, et al. Primary pulmonary meningioma first suspected of being a lung metastasis. *Ann Thorac Surg* 2005;79(4):1407–1409.

206. Meirelles GS, Ravizzini G, Moreira AL, et al. Primary pulmonary meningioma manifesting as a solitary pulmonary nodule with a false-positive PET scan. *J Thorac Imaging* 2006;21(3):225–227.

207. Spinelli M, Claren R, Colombi R, et al. Primary pulmonary meningioma may arise from meningothelial-like nodules. *Adv Clin Path* 2000;4(1):35–39.

208. de Perrot M, Kurt AM, Robert J, et al. Primary pulmonary meningioma presenting as lung metastasis. *Scand Cardiovasc J* 1999;33(2):121–123.

209. Moran CA, Hochholzer L, Rush W, et al. Primary intrapulmonary meningiomas. a clinicopathologic and immunohistochemical study of ten cases. *Cancer* 1996;78(11):2328–2333.

210. Erlandson RA. *Diagnostic Transmission Electron Microscopy of Human Tumors.* New York: Masson; 1981.

211. Prayson RA, Farver CF. Primary pulmonary malignant meningioma. *Am J Surg Pathol* 1999;23(6):722–726.

212. Wende S, Bohl J, Schubert R, et al. Lung metastasis of a meningioma. *Neuroradiology* 1983;24(5):287–291.

213. Miller DC, Ojemann RG, Proppe KH, et al. Benign metastasizing meningioma. Case report. *J Neurosurg* 1985;62(5):763–766.

214. Kodama K, Doi O, Higashiyama M, et al. Primary and metastatic pulmonary meningioma. *Cancer* 1991;67(5):1412–1417.

215. Leemans, J, Van Calenbergh F, Sciot R, et al. Pulmonary metastasis of a meningioma presenting as a solitary pulmonary nodule: 2 case reports. *Acta Clin Belg* 2016;71(2):107–110.

216. Hsu HS, Wang CY, Li WY, et al. Endotracheobronchial neurofibromas. *Ann Thorac Surg* 2002;74(5):1704–1706.

217. Willmann JK, Weishaupt D, Kestenholz PB, et al. Endotracheal neurofibroma in neurofibromatosis type 1: an unusual manifestation. *Eur Radiol* 2002;12(1):190–192.

218. Batori M, Lazzaro M, Lonardo MT, et al. A rare case of pulmonary neurofibroma: clinical and diagnostic evaluation and surgical treatment. *Eur Rev Med Pharmacol Sci* 1999;3(4):155–157.

219. Suzuki H, Sekine Y, Motohashi S, et al. Endobronchial neurogenic tumors treated by transbronchial electrical snaring and Nd-YAG laser abrasion: report of three cases. *Surg Today* 2005;35(3):243–246.

220. McCluggage WG, Bharucha H. Primary pulmonary tumours of nerve sheath origin. *Histopathology* 1995;26(3):247–254.

221. Righini CA, Lequeux T, Laverierre MH, et al. Primary tracheal schwannoma: one case report and a literature review. *Eur Arch Otorhinolaryngol* 2005;262(2):157–160.

222. Aubertine CL, Flieder DB. Primary paraganglioma of the lung. *Ann Diagn Pathol* 2004;8(4):237–241.

223. Hangartner JR, Loosemore TM, Burke M, et al. Malignant primary pulmonary paraganglioma. *Thorax* 1989;44(2):154–156.

224. Skodt V, Jacobsen GK, Helsted M. Primary paraganglioma of the lung. Report of two cases and review of the literature. *APMIS* 1995;103(7-8):597–603.

225. Lemonick DM, Pai B, Hines GL. Malignant primary pulmonary paraganglioma with hilar metastasis. *J Thorac Cardiovasc Surg* 1990;99(3):563–564.

226. Huang X, Liang QL, Jiang L, et al. Primary pulmonary paraganglioma: a case report and review of literature. *Medicine (Baltimore)* 2015;94(31):e1271.

227. Hironaka M, Fukayama M, Takayashiki N, et al. Pulmonary gangliocytic paraganglioma: case report and comparative immunohistochemical study of related neuroendocrine neoplasms. *Am J Surg Pathol* 2001;25(5):688–693.

228. Kee AR, Forrest CH, Brennan BA, et al. Gangliocytic paraganglioma of the bronchus: a case report with follow-up and ultrastructural assessment. *Am J Surg Pathol* 2003;27(10):1380–1385.

229. Nicholson AG. Clear cell tumor. In: Travis WD, Muller-Hermelink HK, Curtis CH, et al. eds. *World Health Organization Classification of Tumours. Pathology and Genetics of Tumours of the Lung, Pleura, Thymus and Heart, B.E.* Lyon: IARC Press; 2004.

230. Liebow AA, Castleman B. Benign clear cell ("sugar") tumors of the lung. *Yale J Biol Med* 1971;43(4-5):213–222.

231. Santana AN, Nunes FS, Ho N, et al. A rare cause of hemoptysis: benign sugar (clear) cell tumor of the lung. *Eur J Cardiothorac Surg* 2004;25(4):652–654.

232. Kavunkal AM, Pandiyan MS, Philip MA, et al. Large clear cell tumor of the lung mimicking malignant behavior. *Ann Thorac Surg* 2007;83(1):310–312.

233. Gora-Gebka M, Liberek A, Bako W, et al. The "sugar" clear cell tumor of the lung-clinical presentation and diagnostic difficulties of an unusual lung tumor in youth. *J Pediatr Surg* 2006;41(6):e27–e29.

234. Adachi Y, Kitamura Y, Nakamura H, et al. Benign clear (sugar) cell tumor of the lung with CD1a expression. *Pathol Int*, 2006;56(8):453–456.

235. Leong AS-Y, Meredith DJ. Clear cell tumors of the lung. In: Corrin B, ed. *Pathology of Lung Tumors.* New York: Churchill Livingstone: 1997:159.

236. Sato N, Sagara Y, Shiraishi Y, et al. Two cases of parenchymal pulmonary leiomyoma. *J Jpn Assoc Chest Surg* 1997;11.

237. Abbas AK. Diseases of immunity. In: Kumar V, Fausto N, eds. *Robbins and Cotran Pathologic Basis of Disease.* 7th ed. Philadelphia, PA: Elsevier Saunders: 2005:259.

238. Gillmore JD, Hawkins N. Amyloidosis and the respiratory tract. *Thorax* 1999;54(5):444–451.

239. Kawashima T, Nishimura H, Akiyama H, et al. Primary pulmonary mucosa-associated lymphoid tissue lymphoma combined with idiopathic thrombocytopenic purpura and amyloidosis in the lung. *J Nippon Med Sch*, 2005;72(6):370–374.

240. Niepolski L, Grzegorzewska AE, Szymas J. Nodular pulmonary amyloidosis and Sjogren's syndrome in a patient treated with intermittent hemodialysis. *Hemodial Int* 2007;11(4):406–410.

241. Pitz MW, Gibson IW, Johnston JB. Isolated pulmonary amyloidosis: case report and review of the literature. *Am J Hematol* 2006;81(3):212–213.

242. Calatayud J, Candelas G, Gómez A, et al. Nodular pulmonary amyloidosis in a patient with rheumatoid arthritis. *Clin Rheumatol* 2007;26(10):1797–1798.

243. Higuchi M, Gunji T, Suzuki H, et al. A case of primary nodular pulmonary amyloidosis. *J Jpn Assoc Chest Surg* 1997;11(1):34–39.

244. Lim JK, Lacy MQ, Kurtin PJ, et al. Pulmonary marginal zone lymphoma of MALT type as a cause of localised pulmonary amyloidosis. *J Clin Pathol* 2001;54(8):642–646.

245. Dacic S, Colby TV, Yousem SA. Nodular amyloidoma and primary pulmonary lymphoma with amyloid production: a differential diagnostic problem. *Mod Pathol* 2000;13(9):934–940.

246. Ross P Jr, Magro CM. Clonal light chain restricted primary intrapulmonary nodular amyloidosis. *Ann Thorac Surg* 2005;80(1):344–347.

247. Yoo SH, Jung KC, Kim JH, et al. Expression patterns of markers for type II pneumocytes in pulmonary sclerosing hemangiomas and fetal lung tissues. *Arch Pathol Lab Med* 2005;129(7):915–919.

248. Liebow AA, Hubbell DS. Sclerosing hemangioma (histiocytoma, xanthoma) of the lung. *Cancer* 1956;9(1):53–75.

249. Katzenstein AL, Gmelich JT, Carrington CB. Sclerosing hemangioma of the lung: a clinicopathologic study of 51 cases. *Am J Surg Pathol* 1980;4(4):343–356.

250. Sugio K, Yokoyama H, Kaneko S, et al. Sclerosing hemangioma of the lung: radiographic and pathological study. *Ann Thorac Surg* 1992;53(2):295–300.

251. Iyoda A, Hiroshima K, Shiba M, et al. Clinicopathological analysis of pulmonary sclerosing hemangioma. *Ann Thorac Surg* 2004;78(6):1928–1931.

252. Devouassoux-Shisheboran M, Hayashi T, Linnoila RI, et al. A clinicopathologic study of 100 cases of pulmonary sclerosing hemangioma with immunohistochemical studies: TTF-1 is expressed in both round and surface cells, suggesting an origin from primitive respiratory epithelium. *Am J Surg Pathol* 2000;24(7):906–916.

253. Katakura H, Sato M, Tanaka F, et al. Pulmonary sclerosing hemangioma with metastasis to the mediastinal lymph node. *Ann Thorac Surg* 2005;80(6):2351–2353.

254. Myers O, Kritikos N, Bongiovanni M, et al. Primary intrapulmonary thymoma: a systematic review. *Eur J Surg Oncol* 2007;33(10):1137–1141.

255. Moran CA, Suster S, Fishback NF, et al. Primary intrapulmonary thymoma. A clinicopathologic and immunohistochemical study of eight cases. *Am J Surg Pathol* 1995;19(3):304–312.

256. Patton KT, Cheng L, Papavero V, et al. Benign metastasizing leiomyoma: clonality, telomere length and clinicopathologic analysis. *Mod Pathol* 2006;19(1):130–140.

257. Nucci MR, Drapkin R, Dal Cin P, et al. Distinctive cytogenetic profile in benign metastasizing leiomyoma: pathogenetic implications. *Am J Surg Pathol* 2007;31(5):737–743.

258. Pitts S, Oberstein EM, Glassberg MK. Benign metastasizing leiomyoma and lymph-angioleiomyomatosis: sex-specific diseases? *Clin Chest Med* 2004;25(2):343–360.
259. Abramson S, Gilkeson RC, Goldstein JD, et al. Benign metastasizing leiomyoma: clinical, imaging, and pathologic correlation. *AJR Am J Roentgenol* 2001;176(6):1409–1413.
260. Jacobson TZ, Rainey EJ, Turton CW. Pulmonary benign metastasising leiomyoma: response to treatment with goserelin. *Thorax* 1995;50(11):1225–1226.
261. Saynajakangas O, Maiche AG, Liakka KA. Multiple progressive pulmonary leio-myomatous metastases treated with tamoxifen—a case report with a review of the literature. *Acta Oncol* 2004;43(1):113–114.
262. Osborn M, Mandys V, Beddow E, et al. Cystic fibrohistiocytic tumours presenting in the lung: primary or metastatic disease? *Histopathology* 2003;43(6):556–562.
263. Gu M, Sohn K, Kim D, et al. Metastasizing dermatofibroma in lung. *Ann Diagn Pathol* 2007;11(1):64–67.
264. Joseph MG, Colby TV, Swensen SJ, et al. Multiple cystic fibrohistiocytic tumors of the lung: report of two cases. *Mayo Clin Proc* 1990;65(2):192–197.
265. Yi ES. Tumors of the pulmonary vasculature. *Cardiol Clin* 2004;22(3):431–440, vi–vii.
266. Tron V, Magee F, Wright JL, et al. Pulmonary capillary hemangiomatosis. *Hum Pathol* 1986;17(11):1144–1150.
267. El-Gabaly M, Farver CF, Budev MA, et al. Pulmonary capillary hemangiomatosis imaging findings and literature update. *J Comput Assist Tomogr* 2007;31(4):608–610.
268. Faber CN, Yousem SA, Dauber JH, et al. Pulmonary capillary hemangiomatosis. A report of three cases and a review of the literature. *Am Rev Respir Dis* 1989;140(3):808–813.
269. Assaad AM, Kawut SM, Arcasoy SM, et al. Platelet-derived growth factor is increased in pulmonary capillary hemangiomatosis. *Chest* 2007;131(3):850 855.
270. Pinckard JK, Rosenbluth DB, Patel K, et al. Pulmonary hyalinizing granuloma associated with Aspergillus infection. *Int J Surg Pathol* 2003;11(1):39–42.
271. Esme H, Ermis SS, Fidan F, et al. A case of pulmonary hyalinizing granuloma associated with posterior uveitis. *Tohoku J Exp Med* 2004;204(1):93–97.
272. Winger DI, Spiegler P, Trow TK, et al. Radiology-Pathology Conference: pulmo-nary hyalinizing granuloma associated with lupus-like anticoagulant and Morvan's Syndrome. *Clin Imaging* 2007;31(4):264–268.
273. Engleman P, Liebow AA, Gmelich J, et al. Pulmonary hyalinizing granuloma. *Am Rev Respir Dis* 1977;115(6):997–1008.
274. Yousem SA, Hochholzer L. Pulmonary hyalinizing granuloma. *Am J Clin Pathol* 1987;87(1):1–6.
275. Duzgun N, Kurtipek E, Esme H, et al. Pulmonary Hyalinizing Granuloma Mimicking Metastatic Lung Cancer. *Case Rep Pulmonol* 2015;2015:610417.
276. Na KJ, Song SY, Kim JH, et al. Subpleural pulmonary hyalinizing granuloma presenting as a solitary pulmonary nodule. *J Thorac Oncol* 2007;2(8):777–779.
277. Lutembacher R. Dysembryomes metatypique des reins. Carcinose submiliare aigue poumon avec emphyseme generalise et double pneumothorax. *Ann Med Intern (Paris)* 1918;5:435.
278. Cohen MM, Pollock-BarZiv S, Johnson SR. Emerging clinical picture of lymph-gioleiomyomatosis. *Thorax* 2005;60(10):875–879.
279. Johnson SR. Lymphangioleiomyomatosis. *Eur Respir J* 2006;27(5):1056–1065.
280. Goncharova EA, Krymskaya VP. Pulmonary lymphangioleiomyomatosis (LAM): progress and current challenges. *J Cell Biochem* 2008;103(2):369–382.
281. Taylor JR, Ryu J, Colby TV, et al. Lymphangioleiomyomatosis. clinical course in 32 patients. *N Engl J Med* 1990;323(18):1254–1260.
282. Ryu JH, Moss J, Beck GJ, et al. The NHLBI lymphangioleiomyomatosis registry: characteristics of 230 patients at enrollment. *Am J Respir Crit Care Med* 2006;173(1):105–111.
283. Young LR, Inoue Y, McCormack FX. Diagnostic potential of serum VEGF-D for lymphangioleiomyomatosis. *N Engl J Med* 2008;358(2):199–200.
284. Glassberg MK. Lymphangioleiomyomatosis. *Clin Chest Med* 2004;25(3):573–582, vii.
285. Bearz A, Rupolo M, Canzonieri V, et al. Lymphangioleiomyomatosis: a case report and review of the literature. *Tumori* 2004;90(5):528–531.
286. Swensen SJ, Hartman TE, Mayo JR, et al. Diffuse pulmonary lymphangiomatosis: CT findings. *J Comput Assist Tomogr* 1995;19(3):348–352.
287. Muller NL, Chiles C, Kullnig P. Pulmonary lymphangiomatosis: correlation of CT with radiographic and functional findings. *Radiology* 1990;175(2):335–339.
288. Taveira-DaSilva AM, Steagall WK, Moss J. Lymphangioleiomyomatosis. *Cancer Control* 2006;13(4):276–285.
289. Juvet SC, Hwang D, Downey GP. Rare lung diseases I—Lymphangioleiomyomatosis. *Can Respir J* 2006;13(7):375–380.
290. Chen F, Bando T, Fukuse T, et al. Recurrent lymphangioleiomyomatosis after living-donor lobar lung transplantation. *Transplant Proc* 2006;38(9):3151–3153.
291. Bissler JJ, McCormack FX, Young LR, et al. Sirolimus for angiomyolipoma in tuberous sclerosis complex or lymphangioleiomyomatosis. *N Engl J Med* 2008;358(2):140–151.
292. Zaki KS, Aryan Z, Mehta AC, et al. Recurrence of lymphangioleiomyomatosis: Nine years after a bilateral lung transplantation. *World J Transplant* 2016;6(1):249–254.
293. Moses MA, Harper J, Folkman J. Doxycycline treatment for lymphangioleio-myomatosis with urinary monitoring for MMPs. *N Engl J Med* 2006;354(24):2621–2622.
294. Khoja AM, Duggal D, Keni A, et al. Palliative management of lymphangioleiomyo-matosis: Using video-assisted thoracoscopic surgery. *J Bronchology Interv Pulmonol* 2014;21(1):54–57.
295. Pollock-BarZiv S, Cohen MM, Downey GP, et al. Air travel in women with lymph-angioleiomyomatosis. *Thorax* 2007;62(2):176–80.

SUGGESTED READINGS

General

Churg A. Tumors of the lung. In: Thurlbeck W, ed. *Pathology of the Lung*. New York: Thieme; 1988:311–423.
Dunnill MS. Rare pulmonary tumors. In: Dunnill MS, ed. *Pulmonary Pathology*. 2nd ed. New York: Churchill Livingstone; 1987:413.
Hasleton PS. Benign tumors and their malignant counterparts. In Hasleton PS, ed. *Spencer's Pathology of the Lung*. 5th ed. New York: McGraw-Hill, 1996:875–986.
Mackay B, Lukeman JM, Ordonez NG. *Tumors of the Lungs*. Philadelphia, PA: Saunders; 1991.
Madewell JE, Feigin DS. Benign tumors of the lung. *Semin Roentgenol* 1977;12:175–186.
Marchesky AM, ed. *Surgical Pathology of Lung Neoplasms*. New York: Marcel Dekker; 1990.
Spencer H. Rare pulmonary tumors. In: Spencer H, ed. *Pathology of the Lung*, 4th ed. New York: Pergamon Press; 1985:933.

Connective Tissue Tumors, Benign

Orlowski TM, Stasiak K, Kolodziej J. Leiomyoma of the lung. *J Thorac Cardiovasc Surg* 1978;76:257–261.
Schraufnagel DE, Morin JE, Wang NS. Endobronchial lipoma. *Chest* 1979;75:97–99.

Epithelial Tumors

Spencer H, Dail DH, Arneaud J. Noninvasive bronchial epithelial papillary tumors. *Cancer* 1986;45:1486–1497.

Granular Cell Myoblastoma—Granular Cell Tumor

O'Connell DJ, MacMahon H, DeMeester TR. Multicentric tracheobronchial and oesophageal granular cell myoblastoma. *Thorax* 1978;33:596–602.
Valenstein SL, Thurer RJ. Granular cell myoblastoma of the bronchus: case report and literature review. *J Thorac Cardiovasc Surg* 1978;76:465–468.

Hamartoma

Becker RM, ViLorio J, Chiu C. Multiple pulmonary myomatous hamartomas in women. *J Thorac Cardiovasc Surg* 1976;71:631–632.
Bennett LL, Lesar MS, Tellis CJ. Multiple calcified chondrohamartomas of the lung: CT appearance. *J Comput Assist Tomogr* 1985;9:180–182.
Hansen CP, Holtveg H, Francis D, et al. Pulmonary hamartoma. *J Thorac Cardiovasc Surg* 1992;104:674–678.
Koutras P, Urschel HC Jr, Paulson DL. Hamartoma of the lung. *J Thorac Cardiovasc Surg* 1971;61:768–776.
Minasian H. Uncommon pulmonary hamartomas. *Thorax* 1977;32:360–364.
Petheram IS, Heard BE. Unique massive pulmonary hamartoma: case report with review of hamartoma treated at Brompton Hospital in 27 years. *Chest* 1979;75:95–97.
Ramzy I. Pulmonary hamartomas: cytologic appearances of fine-needle aspiration biopsy. *Acta Cytol* 1976;20:15–19.
Shah JP, Chaudhry KU, Huvos AG, et al. Hamartomas of the lung. *Surg Gynecol Obstet* 1973;136:406–408.
Spencer H. Hamartomas, blastoma and teratoma of the lung. In Spencer H, ed. *Pathology of the Lung*. 4th ed. New York: Pergamon Press; 1985:1061.
Tomashefski JF Jr. Benign endobronchial mesenchymal tumors: their relationship to parenchymal pulmonary hamartomas. *Am J Surg Pathol* 1982;6:531–540.

Inflammatory Myofibroblastic Tumor (Previously Known as Fibrous Histiocytoma, Benign)

Agrons GA, Rosado-de-Christenson ML, Kirejczyk WM, et al. Pulmonary inflammatory pseudotumor: radiologic features. *Radiology* 1988;206:511–518.
Aisner SC, Albin RJ, Templeton PA, et al. Endobronchial fibrous histiocytoma. *Ann Thorac Surg* 1995;60:710–712.
Berardi RS, Lee SS, Chen HP, et al. Inflammatory pseudotumors of the lung. *Surg Gynecol Obstet* 1983;156:89–96.
Bueno R, Wain JC, Wright CD, et al. Bronchoplasty in the management of low-grade airway neoplasms and benign bronchial stenoses. *Ann Thorac Surg* 1996;62:824–828; discussion 828-9.
Cohen MC, Kaschula ROC. Primary pulmonary tumors in childhood: a review of 31 years experience and the literature. *Pediatr Pulmonol* 1992;14:222–232.
Conforti S, Bonacina E, Ravini M, et al. A case of fibrous histiocytoma of the trachea in an infant treated by endobronchial Nd:YAG laser. *Lung Cancer* 2007;57:112–114.
Doski JJ, Priebe CJ Jr, Driessnack M, et al. Corticosteroids in the management of unre-sected plasma cell granuloma (inflammatory pseudotumor) of the lung. *J Pediatr Surg* 1991;26:1064–1066.
Duncan JD, Greenberg SD, Mattox KL, et al. Benign fibrous histiocytoma: a rare endo-bronchial neoplasm. *Int Surg* 1986;71:110–111.
Imperato JP, Folkman J, Sagerman RH, et al. Treatment of plasma cell granuloma of the lung with radiation therapy. A report of two cases and a review of the literature. *Cancer* 1986;57:2127–2129.

Ishida T, Oka T, Nishino T, et al. Inflammatory pseudotumor of the lung in adults: radiographic and clinicopathological analysis. *Ann Thorac Surg* 1989;48:90–95.

Tagge E, Yunis E, Chopyk J, et al. Obstructing endobronchial fibrous histiocytoma: potential for lung salvage. *J Pediatr Surg* 1991;26:1067–1069.

Viguera JL, Pujol JL, Reboiras SD, et al. Fibrous histiocytoma of the lung. *Thorax* 1976;31:475–479.

Lymphangioleiomyomatosis

Graham ML, Spelsberg TC, Dines DE, et al. Pulmonary lymphangiomyomatosis: with particular reference to steroid-receptor assay studies and pathologic correlation. *Mayo Clin Proc* 1984;59:3–11.

Luna CM, Gené R, Jolly EC, et al. Pulmonary LAM associated with tuberous sclerosis: treatment with tamoxifen and tetracycline pleurodesis. *Chest* 1985;88:473–475.

Pseudotumors

Bahadori H, Liebow AA. Plasma cell granulomas of the lung. *Cancer* 1973;31:191–208.

Graham ML, Spelsberg TC, Dines DE, et al. Pulmonary lymphangiomyomatosis: with particular reference to steroid-receptor assay studies and pathologic correlation. *Mayo Clin Proc* 1984;59:3.

Spencer H. The pulmonary plasma cell/histiocytoma complex. *Histopathology* 1984;8:903–916.

Spoto G Jr, Rossi NP, Allsbrook WC. Tracheobronchial plasma cell granuloma. *J Thorac Cardiovasc Surg* 1977;73:804–806.

Warter A, Satge D, Roeslin N. Angioinvasive plasma cell granuloma of the lung. *Cancer* 1987;59:435–443.

Schwannomas, Benign

Bosch X, Ramírez J, Font J, et al. Primary intrapulmonary benign schwannoma. A case with ultrastructural and immunohistochemical confirmation. *Eur Respir J* 1990;3:234–237.

Higashimoto Y, Ohata M, Kobayashi H, et al. A case of primary intrapulmonary benign schwannoma. *Nihon Kyobu Shikkan Gakkai Zasshi* 1991;29:360–364.

Michel JL, de Montpreville V, Bobichon I, et al. Endo- and exo-bronchial schwannoma treated by resection-anastomosis of the left bronchial stump. *Rev Mal Respir* 1995;12:628–630.

Nesbitt JC, Vega DM, Burke T, et al. Cellular schwannoma of the bronchus. *Ultrastruct Pathol* 1996;20:349–354.

Roviaro G, Montorsi M, Varoli F, et al. Primary pulmonary tumours of neurogenic origin. *Thorax* 1983;38:942–945.

Uchiyama Y, Minami H, Yamashita M, et al. A case of intrapulmonary schwannoma and a review of the Japanese literature. *Nippon Kyobu Geka Gakkai Zasshi* 1989;37:1238–1241.

Umeki S, Kato H, Tsukiyama K, et al. A case of intrapulmonary schwannoma that should be distinguished from lung cancer. *Nippon Kyobu Shikkan Gakkai Zasshi* 1990;28:1635–1639.

Vascular Tumors

Forsee JH, Mahon HW, James LA. Cavernous hemangioma of the lung. *Ann Surg* 1950;131:418–423.

Paul KP, Börner C, Müller KM, et al. Capillary hemangioma of the right main bronchus treated by sleeve resection in infancy. *Am Rev Respir Dis* 1991;143:876–879.

Wodehouse GE. Hemangioma of the lung: a review of four cases. *J Thorac Cardiovasc Surg* 1948;17:408–415.

Uncommon Primary Malignant Tumors of the Lung

Sebastián Defranchi ■ Carlos Vigliano

The World Health Organization (WHO) published in 2015 an updated classification of Tumors of the Lung, Pleura, Thymus, and Heart.[1] In this last edition, most of the uncommon primary malignant tumors of the lungs are classified into one of the following categories: (1) epithelial tumors, (2) mesenchymal tumors, (3) lymphohistiocytic tumors, and (4) tumors of ectopic origin (Table 107.1). The use of immunohistochemistry in resected specimens to fully classify lung cancer and genetic profiling, are two of the most significant changes introduced in the new classification.

Out of 80 rare pulmonary neoplasms seen at the Mayo Clinic in a 11-year review (1980 to 1990), Miller and Allen reported that 41% were non-Hodgkin's lymphomas, 20% were carcinosarcomas,

TABLE 107.1 Uncommon Primary Malignant Tumors of the Lung

Epithelial Tumors
Sarcomatoid Carcinomas
Pleomorphic carcinoma
Spindle cell carcinoma
Giant cell carcinoma
Carcinosarcoma
Pulmonary blastoma
Others and Unclassified Carcinomas
Lymphoepithelioma-like carcinoma
NUT carcinoma

Mesenchymal Tumors
Malignant PEComa
Epithelioid hemangioendothelioma
Pleuropulmonary blastoma
Synovial sarcoma
Pulmonary artery intimal sarcoma
Pulmonary myxoid sarcoma with EWSR1-CREB1 translocation
Myoepithelial carcinoma
Other mesenchymal tumors

Lymphohistiocytic Tumors
Extranodal marginal zone lymphoma of mucosa-associated lymphoid tissue (MALT lymphoma)
Diffuse large B-cell lymphoma
Intravascular large B-cell lymphoma

Tumors of Ectopic Origin
Intrapulmonary thymoma
Melanoma

15% were mucoepidermoid carcinomas (these tumors are discussed in Chapter 20), and 18% were sarcomas; the remaining were either malignant melanomas or blastomas. In this series, the main features were a median age of 60 years, a predominant surgical option (79%), and a 5-year survival of 39%.[2]

EPITHELIAL TUMORS

SARCOMATOID CARCINOMAS

Sarcomatoid carcinoma is a generic term used to classify a group of non-small cell lung carcinomas that show components of sarcoma. Five types of sarcomatoid carcinomas are included in the 2015 WHO classification: (1) pleomorphic carcinoma, (2) spindle cell carcinoma, (3) giant cell carcinoma, (4) carcinosarcoma, and (5) pulmonary blastoma.

Usually, the pathologic diagnosis of these tumors is very difficult and even not recommended on small biopsies or needle cytology. In particular, the diagnosis of pleomorphic carcinoma, spindle cell carcinoma, and giant cell carcinoma should be done based on the histological evaluation of the entire surgical specimen.

Nakajima et al.[3] described the immunohistochemistry pattern in 37 patients with resected sarcomatoid carcinomas. In this series, most sarcomatoid carcinomas were pleomorphic, spindle, and giant cell carcinomas. All cases were positive for one or two cytokeratins (CAM5.2 or AE1/AE3) and 65% were positive for the epithelial membrane antigen (EMA). Vimentin was positive in the sarcomatoid elements of the tumor in 89% of the specimens. Pathologic stage higher than I and the presence of affected lymph nodes were found to be adverse prognostic factor.

Molecular testing is recommended on sarcomatoid carcinomas. The already known genetic abnormalities are used to select which test should be performed. For example, a pleomorphic carcinoma showing an adenocarcinoma differentiation should be tested for epidermal growth factor receptor (EGFR) mutations and ALK-MET rearrangement. Conversely, k-ras mutations have been found in up to 38% of patients with sarcomatoid carcinoma.[4]

In a series of 75 patients, 58 had a pleomorphic carcinoma, 7 presented only a mixture of spindle and giant cells, 10 had a pure spindle cell cancer, and 3 cases, only giant cells. Of the remaining four patients, three had a carcinosarcoma whereas one had a pulmonary blastoma.[5]

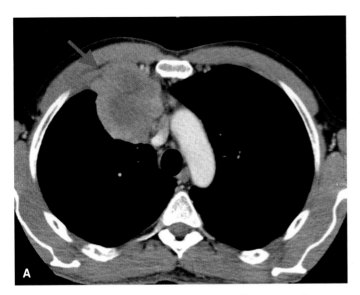 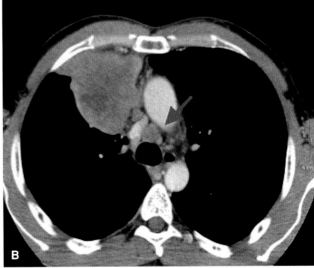

FIGURE 107.1 Pleomorphic carcinoma. **A:** Chest wall invasion can be seen across the intercostal space. **B:** 4R adenopathy.

Sarcomatoid carcinomas are more prevalent in male smokers and the mean age of diagnosis is similar to the one of non-small cell lung cancer (NSCLC) of 62 years.[6] These tumors usually present with cough, dyspnea, or hemoptysis; chest wall invasion is not unusual. They are aggressive tumors with a very poor prognosis, which depends on the extension of the disease (Fig. 107.1).

In a report from the MD Anderson Cancer Center on 63 patients with sarcomatoid carcinomas, a 5-year survival rate of 24.5% was noted.[6] The authors performed a propensity match analysis between 63 patients with NSCLC and the 63 with sarcomatoid carcinomas. The latter included pleomorphic, spindle cell, and giant cell carcinoma subtypes. They found that survival was significantly better in patients with similar stage NSCLC counterparts. The median survival rate for patients with sarcomatoid carcinomas was 14.4 months, compared to 80.3 months of patients with NSCLC. On multivariate analysis, patients with sarcomatoid carcinomas presented with higher stage pathological T status. There were not survivors at 5 years in patients with stage III tumors.

Pleomorphic Carcinoma

According to the new WHO classification, pleomorphic carcinoma is a poorly differentiated adenocarcinoma, squamous cell carcinoma, or undifferentiated non-small cell cancer (NSCC) that contains at least 10% spindle and/or giant cells or a carcinoma consisting only of spindle and giant cells.[1] Worth of note in the new WHO classification is the use of the term NSCC for carcinomas that show no clear signs of squamous or adenocarcinoma differentiation morphologically or by immunohistochemistry.[1]

Ro,[7] Fishback,[8] Chang,[9] Rossi,[5] Raveglia,[10] and Chen[11] and their colleagues have described 12, 78, 16, 58, 20, and 26 cases of pleomorphic carcinomas, respectively (Table 107.2). Not all series were homogenous since most included spindle cell carcinomas, giant cell carcinomas, or a combination of both. In earlier reports, sarcomatoid components were referred as malignant fibrous histiocytoma (MFH)-like patterns (Figs. 107.2 and 107.3).

As a rule, the non-small-cell carcinomatous elements are sparse in relationship to the tumor volume. In this setting, the prevalence of each carcinoma component may vary, being adenocarcinoma, the most commonly found (Table 107.2).

The stroma of the tumor can be fibrous or myxoid. Areas of necrosis are common. The tumors express focal staining for cytokeratins and a diffused stain for vimentin (Fig. 107.2). Rossi et al.[5] utilized the thyroid transcription factor-1 (TTF-1) and CK7 to verify the pulmonary origin of these tumors. They found that 55% of 20 specimens were positive for TTF-1 while 70% were positive for CK staining; surfactant protein A staining was negative in all specimens.[5]

Chang et al.[12] studied the status and implications of EGFR mutations in pleomorphic carcinomas of the lung. EGFR mutations were found in up to 24% of patients with pleomorphic carcinomas. In the

TABLE 107.2 Histologic Composition of Pleomorphic Carcinomas in Different Series

First Author	Year	Number of PCs	Type of Carcinoma				
			SQ	Adeno	Large-Cell	Other	S/G
Ro et al.[7]	1992	12	3	4	3	2	0
Fishback et al.[8]	1994	78	6	18	35	2	17
Nakajima et al.[3]	1999	37	8	19	5	5	34
Chang et al.[9]	2001	16	4	9	0	3	0
Rossi et al.[5]	2003	58	12	14	18	7	7
Raveglia et al.[10]	2004	20	2	2	2	0	14
Yuki et al.[15]	2007	45	8	25	12	0	11

SQ, squamous cell carcinoma; Adeno; adenocarcinoma; S/G, spindle/giant cell carcinoma.

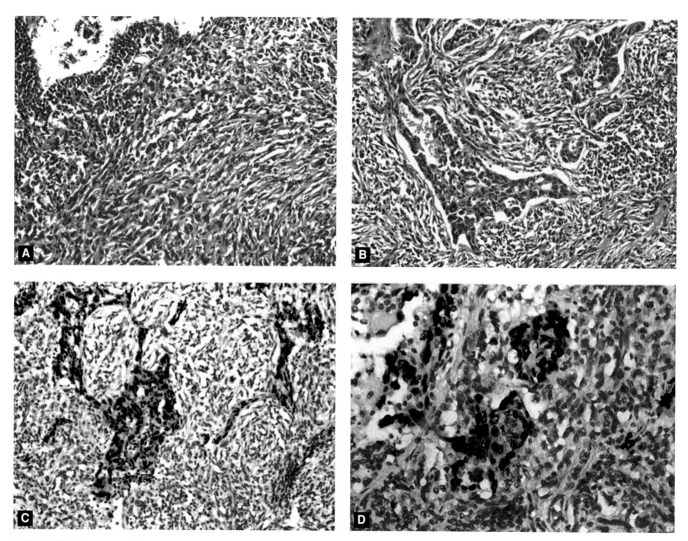

FIGURE 107.2 Sarcomatoid carcinoma. **A:** Sarcomatoid carcinoma infiltrating bronchial wall. **B:** Biphasic pleomorphic carcinoma showing an overtly carcinomatous component admixed with a spindle cell sarcomatoid component (H&E ×200). **C:** Positive cytokeratin 7 immunostaining in carcinomatous component. **D:** Positive nuclear immunostaining for TTF-1 in neoplastic cells (×400).

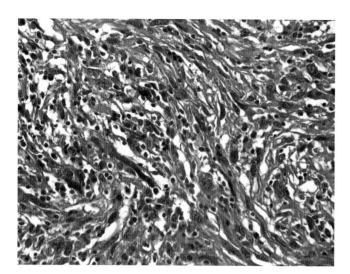

FIGURE 107.3 Sarcomatoid carcinoma composed of spindle cell type showing a fascicular pattern of atypical spindle cells (H&E ×400).

study of Kaira et al.,[13] mutations were found in exons 19 and 21 in patients with pleomorphic carcinoma and adenocarcinoma components. However, only a short-term duration response to gefitinib (a tyrosine kinase inhibitor) was documented. In this series, a high Ki-67 index was found (a median value of 67%), showing active cellular proliferation.

Pleomorphic carcinomas occur in men more commonly than in women; patients are usually in the sixth or seventh decades of life and have been chronic heavy smokers. These tumors are usually not incidental findings since most of the patients present with symptoms (chest pain, cough, or hemoptysis).[8] Pleomorphic carcinomas are often found in the upper lobes, more in the right lung than in the left lung. The tumor may be endobronchial in location, but most of these lesions arise in the pulmonary parenchyma as a solid mass. Chang et al.[9] reported that the tumors could also be cavitary. CT scan findings include lung nodules or more frequently masses of up to 10 cm in diameter with low-density areas suggesting necrosis.[14] In PET-CT scans they appeared as hyper metabolic masses with peak standardized uptake value (SUV) of up to 26.[13]

Lymph node disease, chest wall involvement and mediastinal invasion are common features of these tumors. As a result, a significant proportion of patients present with clinical stage III[3,6,8] requiring extended resections to achieve R0.[14]

Yuki et al.[15] observed that pN1 disease was present in 11.1% and pN2 involvement was present in 26.7% of their 45 patients. In patients without nodal involvement, vascular invasion was present in 16 of 28 patients (57.1%). Distant metastasis was common in the postoperative period.

Surgical resection, when possible, is the treatment of choice; in a retrospective series of 60 patients, survival was significantly longer when an R0 resection was performed (compared to an R1 resection).[14] The 3- and 5-year survival rates in this series were 47.7% and 25.6%, respectively. Survival rates were significantly better in patients in whom R0 resection was achieved and no lymph node metastases were found. In the study of Kaira et al., the median survival for patients that underwent lung resection was 8.5 months; the median survival was not reached for the patients that did not have surgical resection.[13] Standard anatomic procedures and extended chest wall, bronchial, and mediastinal resections have been reported. Anatomic resections with mediastinal lymph node dissection should be preferred over lesser resections as the procedures of choice. However, it should be noted that only a small number of patients would present with small lesions treatable by minor lung resections.

Some have suggested that postoperative chemotherapy be added. There are, however, no data to support its use. In Chang et al.[12] series, the average survival was 5 months. Most of the patients in their series died from early distant metastasis (bone, brain, adrenal glands and even unusual sites such as esophagus, jejunum, rectum, or kidney). Raveglia et al.[10] noted that over two-thirds of their patients were dead within a year and only two of the remaining six were alive and well at 32 and 21 months, respectively. In the series of patients, eight (12%) patients survived longer than 5 years. By univariate analysis, size greater than 5 cm, stage higher than I, and the presence of metastases or lymph node involvement were risk factors for decreased survival.

Palliative chemotherapy was investigated and retrospectively reported in 13 patients by Bae et al.[16] Patients received chemotherapy regimens known to be active for the treatment of advanced NSCLC. No patient showed treatment response and progression after a second-line regimen was the rule. The median survival upon the initiation of chemotherapy was 5 months,[16] a similar finding to Chang's report.[13]

Spindle Cell Carcinoma

In this variant of sarcomatoid carcinoma, spindle shaped cells are predominantly seen, identical to the spindle cell component of the pleomorphic carcinoma. However, no specific pattern of carcinoma can be recognized.[1] The epithelial derivation of the spindle cell may be established by immunohistochemistry demonstration of the presence of positivity to cytokeratins or by the electronic microscopic identification of epithelial differentiation.

Some series of patients with pleomorphic sarcoma include a small number of patients with pure spindle cell carcinomas.[3,5,8,10] Histologically, Rossi et al.[5] found that some of the cells were "cigar-shaped" and arranged in long fascicles in some tumors; in others, the tumor cells were more elongated, had atypical nuclei, and grew in long fascicles presenting with a suggestive herringbone pattern.[5] The two aforementioned patterns suggested leiomyosarcoma and fibrosarcoma, respectively. A third pattern was composed of uniform spindle cells intermingled with lymphocytes, plasma cells, and eosinophils. This pattern suggested an inflammatory pseudotumor or a follicular dendritic cell sarcoma. Both Raveglia et al.[10] and Rossi et al.[5]

demonstrated that an admixture of giant cells could be present in a number of these tumors but that pure tumors of spindle (sarcomatoid) cells or giant cells do occur. Fishback et al.[8] and Rossi et al.[5] reported 7 and 10 pure spindle cell carcinomas in their series, respectively. Immunohistochemically, the spindle cells are usually positive for cytokeratins in approximately 75% of the cases reported by Ro[7] and 100% by Raveglia[10] and their colleagues, respectively. The spindle cells are also positive for vimentin. In addition, Rossi et al.[5] found that over half of these tumors were positive for TTF-1, a marker associated with the pulmonary origin of these cells. Finally, 70% of the tumors were positive for CK 7, which is strongly expressed in various epithelia, including the lung.

Spindle cell carcinomas most often occur in middle-aged adults (i.e., 45 to 65 years of age). The tumors are more often found in men, former or current smokers and in a peripheral location in the lungs. Some tumors can involve the bronchus, with endobronchial extension in 40% of their cases. The upper rather than the lower lobes are more likely to be the site of the tumor.[10]

Cough and hemoptysis were common symptoms in the reported patients. In Rossi's series,[5] eight of the ten patients had stage I disease. The remaining four were divided between stages IIb and IIIa.

Complete surgical resection and mediastinal lymph node dissection represent the treatment of choice. The value of pre- or postoperative irradiation and/or chemotherapy is unknown. These tumors are aggressive and most patients have recurrent disease within months of definitive treatment (Fig. 107.4). However, long-term survival does occur. This was recorded in 14% of the patients in Ro et al.[7] series. The only significant feature that suggests possible long-term survival is the presence of stage I disease at the time of treatment.

Giant Cell Carcinoma

Giant cell carcinoma is made almost exclusively of giant cells, with no differentiated carcinomatous elements.[1] Pure giant cell carcinomas are made up of large, bizarre, pleomorphic and multinucleated tumor giant cells. The lesion microscopically is often discohesive and infiltrated by inflammatory cells, especially by neutrophils. This inflammatory cell infiltration suggests a strong local immune response against the tumor. However, they behave very aggressively.

Programmed death-1 (PD-1) is a membrane receptor found on T-cells and macrophages. PD-1 modulates their activity once these cells are activated. Tumors with the over expression of PD-1 receptor ligand called programmed death ligand-1 (PD-L1) are believed to escape the immune-mediated responses by prematurely activating T cell and macrophage's PD-1, thereby inducing cell death. Velcheti

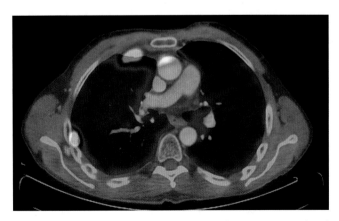

FIGURE 107.4 Pleomorphic carcinoma. PET-CT showing recurrent pleural and chest wall disease after surgical resection.

et al.[17] found that 9 out of 13 sarcomatoid carcinomas studied were positive for PD-L1 (69.2%); 10 cases of giant cell carcinoma were included in this series, with 6 (60%) testing positive for PD-L1. PD-L1 levels were significantly higher than in NSCLC.

Three pure giant-cell carcinomas were reported in an early report by Fishback et al.[8] Another three cases were recorded in the report by Rossi et al.[5] These tumors are very aggressive and rapidly fatal.

Carcinosarcoma

A carcinosarcoma is defined as a malignant neoplasm composed of both malignant epithelial (usually squamous or adenocarcinoma) and differentiated sarcoma elements. The sarcoma component should show differentiation into specific heterologous mesenchymal tissues, such as bone, cartilage, or striated muscle, but not fibroblasts. The purpose of this definition was to separate carcinosarcoma from spindle cell carcinoma. Carcinosarcomas are believed to originate from a sarcomatoid transformation of a carcinoma[18]; they are considered clonal tumors.[1]

The more common presenting symptoms are cough and hemoptysis. Chest pain, fever, and malaise may also occur. Meade et al.[19] described a patient with associated pulmonary osteoarthropathy. Patients with a peripheral tumor may be asymptomatic. Surgical resection, when possible, is the indicated treatment.[2]

Nappi et al.[20] reviewed 21 cases of carcinosarcomas and spindle cell carcinomas. They noted that both of these tumors tended to behave in an aggressive fashion, with 20 of their patients dying within 2 years and only 1 patient alive with no evidence of disease at 21 months. Metastases to the regional lymph nodes and to distant organs, especially to the brain, are common. In most series, however, most of the patients die within the first year of resection.[21–24] Approximately 16% to 23% of patients may survive 5 years or longer. However, in the series reported by Miller and Allen,[2] a 5-year survival rate of only 6% was recorded. Koss et al. studied 66 cases of carcinosarcomas.[25] The patients had a mean age of 65 years with a ratio of men to women of 7.25:1.[25] The tumors usually presented in the upper lobes and many measured >7 cm in its greatest dimension; the majority (62%) were endobronchial or central, with 38% being peripheral in location.[25] The 5-year survival rate was 21.3%; only tumor size >6 cm appeared to be adversely related to survival.[25] Similar findings were reported in other series, with a median survival of 1 year.[26]

Pulmonary Blastoma

Pulmonary blastoma is a biphasic tumor composed of an epithelial component resembling well-differentiated fetal adenocarcinoma and a primitive mesenchymal stroma. Albeit not required to make the diagnosis, these foci may show osteosarcoma, chondrosarcoma, or rhabdomyosarcoma differentiation.[1] The first pulmonary blastoma was reported by Barnard[27] who named this tumor "embryoma." Spencer[28] reviewed Barnard's case, added three cases of his own, and renamed the tumor "pulmonary blastoma."

The epithelial component found in pulmonary blastoma is low-grade fetal adenocarcinoma forming tubules lined by pseudostratified columnar cells with small and uniform nucleus. Focally, the glandular cells may show polymorphism. The mesenchymal component appears as oval cells with high nuclear-cytoplasmic ratio. They have the tendency to differentiate in fibroblasts-like cells embedded in the surrounding myxoid matrix.[1] Immunohistochemistry shows diffuse positivity in the epithelial component for CK7, cytokeratin AE1/AE3, carcinoembryonic antigen and TTF-1. Focally, these cells are positive for chromogranin A, synaptophysin, Clara cell antigen, vimentin, and polypeptide hormones. The mesenchymal component is diffusely positive for vimentin and muscle-specific actin. Cytokeratin AE1/AE3 is only focally positive in the mesenchymal component.[1,29]

Larsen and Sorensen described malignant glands and either an adult sarcomatous or embryonic mesenchyme.[30] Bodner and Koss[31] studied nine pulmonary blastomas for mutations in the p53 gene. They found a mutation in five of nine (42%) pulmonary blastomas. In the pulmonary blastomas, both the epithelial and mesenchymal components showed the mutation, suggesting a common origin from a single clone of cells.

Macher-Goeppinger et al. studied the expression of EGFR, HER2, c-KIT, and β-catenin in five patients with pulmonary blastoma.[32] Mutations in EGFR, c-KIT, k-ras, and the β-catenin gene (CTNNB1) were also studied.[32] EGFR expression was observed in all PBs, but only one patient presented a mutation in this gene.[32] In addition, c-KIT and HER-2 were not overexpressed and k-ras and c-KIT were not mutated. However, all patients presented mutation in the β-catenin gene (CTNNB1).[32] Aberrant β-catenin nuclear/cytoplasmic localization by immunostaining has been reported.[33] Activating mutations of CTNNB1 were associated with the activation of the Wnt pathway; the Wnt pathway regulates key aspects of cell determination, differentiation, and organogenesis during development.[34] In other case report, a high expression of PD-L1 was noted, suggesting the presence of a target for novel treatments.[35]

Larsen and Sorensen[30] reviewed the subject of pulmonary blastomas and reported on a total of 156 cases, estimating their incidence to be only 0.5% of all pulmonary neoplasms. The ratio of men to women was approximately 2:1 and the median age was 40 years.[30] The most common clinical complaints were cough, hemoptysis, and dyspnea. In a large percentage of cases, the chest radiographs revealed a unilateral pulmonary mass randomly located in the lung. The tumors were peripheral or hilar, and some involved both regions.[30] Results of clinical laboratory tests were nonspecific. Sputum cytology was negative in the six patients from which it was obtained. Bronchoscopy and fine-needle aspiration (FNA) were variably helpful in the diagnosis of the tumor.[30]

The biphasic blastomas ranged in size from 2 to 27 cm, with a mean of 10.2 cm. In patients with biphasic pulmonary blastoma, tumors <5 cm in greatest dimension carried a more favorable prognosis than that noted with larger tumors. In a case report, PET-CT demonstrated increased fluorodeoxyglucose uptake within the mass with an SUV max of 22.1.[29] In 2002, Zaida et al.[36] identified three biphasic pulmonary blastomas in just over 11 years at a regional center in Wales. All three patients had advanced disease. Two received only chemotherapy or radiotherapy; both were dead within less than a year. The third patient underwent neoadjuvant chemotherapy followed by surgical resection and postoperative chemotherapy for a stage IIIb blastoma located in the left lower lobe. At 32 months, there was no evidence of disease. Thus these authors have recommended intensive chemotherapy and surgical resection as treatment of choice.[36]

OTHER AND UNCLASSIFIED CARCINOMAS

Lymphoepithelioma-like Carcinoma

The first patient with a lymphoepithelioma-like carcinoma of the lung was described by Begin et al.[37] It is a tumor that is characterized by the presence of a poorly differentiated carcinoma mixed with a marked lymphocyte infiltration; Epstein–Barr virus (EBV) is thought to have a role in the pathogenesis of this disease.[1] Most of the published case reports of lymphoepithelioma-like carcinomas of the lung have occurred in patients of Asian descent, especially those from southeastern China. Han et al.[38] reviewed 3,663 consecutive cases of lung carcinoma in southern China and found 32 cases that met the criteria for lymphoepithelioma-like carcinoma. They tested these 32 cases as well as 19 nonlymphoepithelioma-like carcinoma by *in situ* hybridization and immunohistochemistry for EBV-encoded small nonpolyadenylated RNA (EBER) which is found in the nucleus of the epithelial component of the tumor. Of the 32 cases, 30 (94%) were positive for EBER as opposed to none of the 19 control patients.[38] They concluded that EBV infection might have an essential role in the development of pulmonary lymphoepithelioma-like carcinoma.[38]

Chang et al.[39] found similar results in 23 patients and also thought that EBV probably played a role in the genesis of these malignancies. These authors also observed that the tumors expressed bcl-2, which probably gave the infected cells a growth advantage.[39] Latent membrane protein-1 (LMP1) expression as well as *p*53 and C-*erb*-B-2 expression was extremely low in these tumors.[39]

Microscopic findings include a syncytial pattern of growth, large vesicular nucleus, prominent nucleoli, and a marked infiltration of lymphocytes. The tumor cells show positivity for cytokeratin AE1/AE2, CK5/7, p40, and p63, suggesting a squamous origin.[1] Lymphoid cells are CD3+ T cells and CD20 B cells.

Most of the lung lesions are solitary masses; occasionally, lymph node metastases may be present, as in the patient reported by Frank et al.[40] Wöckel et al.,[41] who reviewed 30 cases published in the literature, noted that lymph node metastasis was present in 25% of the patients. They also pointed out that hematologic metastasis was uncommon, and if it did occur, it was confined most often to the skeletal system.

The usual therapy for these unusual tumors has been surgical resection. Curcio,[42] Frank,[40] Chang[39] and their colleagues added intensive chemotherapy after the initial resection. The rationale of adding adjuvant chemotherapy is based on the study of Al-Sarraf et al.,[43] who reported the superiority of chemotherapy versus radiation therapy with locally advanced nasopharyngeal carcinoma which, in a fashion similar to lymphoepithelioma-like carcinoma of the lung, also shows a lymphocyte infiltrate. Chang et al.[39] recommended the use of gemcitabine and cisplatin. In early-stage pulmonary disease, the short-term survival rate with surgery alone has been satisfactory, but the long-term prognosis is yet unknown. Likewise, the value of chemotherapy as an adjunct in patients with resected pulmonary lymphoepithelioma-like carcinoma remains unknown. Han et al.[44] subsequently compared the long-term survival of their 32 cases of pulmonary lymphoepithelioma-like carcinoma with 84 cases of pulmonary nonlymphoepithelioma-like carcinoma. They found that pulmonary lymphoepithelioma-like carcinomas had a better prognosis in stages II, III, and IV than did a typical NSCLC.[44]

NUT Carcinoma

Nuclear protein of the testis (NUT) midline carcinomas (NMC) are epithelial neoplasms characterized by a chromosomal rearrangement in the NUT gene. The NUTM1 gene is located in chromosome 15q14 and translocated on different genes. The most frequent translocation occurs with the gene BRD4 located on chromosome 19q13.1.[45]

The description and characterization of NMC is relatively new. One of the first reports of a patient with an NMC was done in 1999 on a 12-year-old girl that was originally treated for sore throat. Upon progression of the symptoms, an ulcerating mass in the epiglottis was found. Given the unusual presentation and pathologic features seen on the biopsy, cytogenetic analysis of the tumor was done and a translocation between the chromosome 15 and 19 was found.[46]

NMCs are very rare; they can occur in different parts of the body but the head, neck, and mediastinum are the most common sites.[47] Pathologically, NMCs present as undifferentiated carcinomas or might show prominent squamous differentiation.[1] The diagnosis is done with the use of an immunohistochemical antibody that binds to NUT protein when overexpressed. Sholl et al. reported on the largest series of NMCs consisting of nine patients.[48] The mean age of presentation was 41 years and most patients were symptomatic. Smoking history was not significant. The tumors were centrally located with a preference for the lower and right lobes. All tumors presented as masses of 5 cm in diameter or more with concomitant hilar and mediastinal lymphadenopathies. Bone metastases were common at presentation. In addition, metabolic uptake was significant on PET-CT.[48]

A monomorphic proliferation of intermediate-sized epithelioid cells with high nuclear to cytoplasmatic ratio, and small amounts of pale cytoplasm were the prominent pathological features. Moreover, immunohistochemistry showed diffuse positivity for p63.[1,48]

As these tumors present as locally advanced disease or as M1b disease, they are not resected. Prognosis is very poor despite the use of chemotherapy or radiotherapy, with all patients dying within 5 months.[48]

MESENCHYMAL TUMORS

MALIGNANT PECOMA

PEComatous tumors are included as an individual category under the mesenchymal tumors classification in the last edition of the WHO classification of lung tumors.[1] A PEComa is a mesenchymal tumor that originates from perivascular epithelioid cells (PEC). The PEComa category includes three tumors: (1) lymphangioleiomyomatosis (LAM) which is now considered a clonal destructive disease with invasive and metastatic potential; (2) PEComa, benign, which includes the clear cell "sugar" tumor; and (3) a malignant variant of PEComa. Malignant PEComas are extremely rare, with only few cases reported in the literature.[49–52]

They present as a round lung nodule or mass, usually located in the periphery of the lung and show significant enhancement upon the administration of contrast, due, at least in part, to the rich vascularization. In one report, a moderate SUV uptake was noted in a patient that developed PEComa metastatic lesions in both lungs.[53]

PECs show a clear to granular cytoplasm and a centrally round to oval nucleus. Atypia is mild, if present; immunohistochemically, PEC expresses myogenic and melanocytic markers, such as HMB45, HMSA-1, MelanA/Mart1, microphthalmia transcription factor (Mitf) and actin.[54] Its immunoreactivity for vimentin is usually inconspicuous.[54] If feasible, surgical resection is the treatment of choice.

EPITHELIOID HEMANGIOENDOTHELIOMA

Epithelioid hemangioendothelioma is a low-grade sclerosing angiosarcoma that occurs in the lung as well as the liver, bone, soft tissue, and other sites. It usually has a clinical behavior reminding both hemangioma and angiosarcoma. This vascular lesion was first described by Dail and Liebow[55] in 1975. Later, Dail et al. reviewed 19 additional cases.[56] They initially called this tumor an intravascular bronchioloalveolar tumor (IVBAT). Weiss and Enzinger[57] described 41 cases of an identical tumor occurring in soft tissue and proposed the term "epithelioid hemangioendothelioma" (PHE), which has become widely accepted. Weiss et al.[58] published a combined review of lesions in soft tissue, lung, liver, and bone. Since then, individual case reports have appeared in the literature. Wenisch and Lulay[59] reported that, in the lung, these tumors occur in patients who are 4 to 70 years of age, with one-third of the patients less than 30 years of age. The tumor occurs four times more frequently in women than in men. Most of the patients are asymptomatic or complain of a non-productive cough. PHE can present as a single lung nodule or more frequently as multiple nodules on imaging.[60] Ross et al.[61] note that the chest radiographs and CT scans reveal many small (<1 cm in diameter) nodular densities in both lung fields. PET-CT metabolic activity is variable. According to Moran and Suster,[62] these tumors have a tendency to fill the alveoli in a polypoid fashion and are characterized by proliferation of round-to-oval epithelial endothelioid cells which contain abundant cytoplasm with oval nuclei embedded in a hyaline matrix. In addition, the cells are immunohistochemically positive for endothelial markers: CD34, CD31, and Factor VIII. Nuclear Fli-1, a protein that is expressed in endothelial cells, has also been recently considered useful for the diagnosis of PEH.[63] Weibel-Palade bodies may be seen infrequently on electron microscopic examination.

The average survival after diagnosis is 4.6 years. Lymph node metastases are uncommon with only a 9% incidence reported by Cronin and Arenberg.[64] Conversely, distant metastases are more frequently found, with an incidence of 39% in 31 cases reported by Bagan et al.[60] In this series, the liver was involved in six patients, the bone in three, the brain in two, and the bowel in one.[60] Kitaichi et al.[65] reviewed 21 patients with epithelioid hemangioendothelioma and found three subsets of patients who had a poor prognosis. These patients had either pleural effusions, tumors with a spindle cell component, or pleuritis with the presence of extra pleural tumor cells. Bagan et al.[60] reviewed the findings of 75 patients in the English and French literature and added five cases of their own. The data were essentially the same as just presented. They did, however, separate the patients into two groups: (a) asymptomatic with only a pulmonary nodule or nodules and (b) symptomatic patients due to vascular endothelial cell proliferation resulting in alveolar hemorrhage, hemoptysis, hemorrhagic pleural effusion, or the presence of anemia. Patients in the first group had a satisfactory prognosis with a median survival of 180 months whereas patients in the second group had a much poorer survival. Of all of the poor prognostic features, the presence of hemoptysis and pleural effusion were the most ominous with respiratory failure being a usual cause of death.[60]

Treatment should be determined according to the extent of the disease in the lungs and the presence or absence of distant metastases, especially if the liver is involved. Multicentric disease should also be considered as hemangioendothelioma can occur in the lungs and liver at the same time. When a single or few nodules are present, surgical resection should be contemplated. Lerut et al.[66] have reported satisfactory outcomes following liver transplantation in selected patients. Bagan et al.[60] suggested the possibility of lung transplantation in highly selected patients with extensive bilateral pulmonary disease. The same author[60] briefly discussed the use of various drugs in the management of these tumors. Interferon α2a, azathioprine, steroids, carboplatin, and etoposide have been used with variable and unpredictable results. As noted, death from pulmonary insufficiency is the usual course of this disease, although distant metastatic disease may likewise be a relatively common cause.

Lau et al. reported in 2011 the findings from a self-reported database from the International Hemangioendothelioma, Epithelioid Hemangioendothelioma, and Related Vascular Disorders (HEARD)

Support Group.[67] Overall, 206 patients with a median age at diagnosis of 38 years, were analyzed. The liver was the most common affected organ (99 patients), followed by the lungs (89 patients); the overall 5-year survival rate was 73%. Males and patients older than 55 years carried a worse prognosis. As in other studies, the presence of hemoptysis and pleural effusion significantly affected survival.[67]

PLEUROPULMONARY BLASTOMA

Priest et al.[68] reported 50 cases of pleuropulmonary blastomas, including 11 previously reported by Manivel et al.[69] They classified the lesions as types I, II, and III based on whether the lesions were cystic (type I), cystic and solid (type II), or solid (type III). Their patients ranged in age from newborn to 12 years. They found that each type tended to occur at a different age. Type I (7 patients) presented at an average age of 10 months. Type II (24 patients) presented at an average age of 34 months. Type III (19 patients) presented at an average age of 44 months.[68] Overall, there were 24 boys and 26 girls. Their symptoms included respiratory distress, fever, chest or abdominal pain, and malaise. The chest radiographs showed densities, sometimes with cystic formation. On gross examination, the tumors ranged in size from 2 to 28 cm and weighed ≤1,100 g.[68] The appearance ranged from cystic to solid, with grey, soft surfaces. On microscopic examination, type I tumors had multiloculated cysts separated by thin septa and lined by respiratory mucosa. Beneath the epithelium, there were round to spindle-shaped immature cells. Some of these cells had the appearance of rhabdomyoblasts. In some cases, spindle cells are lacking and considered as regressed type I tumors or type Ir. Type II and III tumors had mixed sarcomatous and blastomatous elements. Rhabdomyoblasts and chondroblasts could be identified in the sarcomatous areas.[68] The immunohistochemical studies show that the neoplastic cells are reactive to vimentin. Desmin is expressed in rhabdomyoblasts and helps in their identification in type I tumors. Areas of chondroid differentiation might show positivity for S100. Cytokeratin and TTF-1 are found in the respiratory mucosa that lines the tumor.[1]

Indolfi et al.[70] described 11 additional patients with pleuropulmonary blastoma. In this series, there were seven boys and four girls; most of the patients were children younger than 5 years with a median age of 32 months. The most common presenting symptom was respiratory distress. The treatment for these lesions is surgical excision followed by chemotherapy and rarely by radiation therapy. The thorax was a common site of recurrence. The central nervous system and bone were also common metastatic sites.[70] MRI is recommended to rule out central nervous system disease.

Pleuropulmonary blastomas are known to have an identified genetic basis in up to 40% of cases, called pleuropulmonary blastoma family tumor and dysplasia syndrome or DICER1. Patients with the DICER1 syndrome have an increased risk of developing testis, ovarian, lung, and thyroid tumors.[1]

At the last follow-up in Priest et al.[68] study of 50 patients, 26 were disease-free, 23 had died of their disease, and 1 was alive with disease. Although statistically there did not seem to be a survival advantage of one type, the data seemed to suggest that patients with type I tumor may have a survival advantage over those with type II or III. While overall 2-year survival was 72%, the 2-year survival rates for type I, II, and III were 80%, 73%, and 48%, respectively.[68] An aggressive treatment plan including surgery, if feasible, followed by chemotherapy with ifosfamide, vincristine, actinomycin D, and doxorubicin is recommended in most cases. However, this tumor remains an aggressive neoplasm of early childhood, despite advances in adjuvant therapy.[71]

SYNOVIAL SARCOMA

Hartel et al. reported in 2007 a case series with 60 patients diagnosed with primary pulmonary and mediastinal synovial sarcomas.[72] Synovial sarcomas have been classified as monophasic and biphasic; the monophasic subtype is characterized only by elongated spindle cells arranged in dense cellular fascicles whereas the biphasic includes also an epithelial component. Tornkvist et al.[73] discussed the unique chromosomal translocation observed in synovial sarcoma. The translocation is t (X; 18) (p 11.2;q 11.2) resulting from the fusion of the SYT gene on chromosome 18 with the SSX gene on chromosome X. The fusion is known as the SYT-SSX fusion.

In Hartel's report,[72] subtyping of SYT/SSX1 and SSX2 was performed. In their report, the mean age at diagnosis was 42 years (29 males and 27 females); treatment included anatomic and wedge resections. Almost half of the patients in their series were dead at 5 years. CT scan showed pleural-based tumors and homogenous or heterogeneous enhancement; pleural effusions were common. At MRI, a triple sign is described: bright, dark, and grey, representing tumor, hemorrhage, and necrosis, respectively. Mean tumor size was 7.5 cm; 88% were monophasic and 12% biphasic. Dense cellularity, interlacing fascicles, hyalinized stroma were the most common microscopic features.[72] A chromosomal translocation t (x; 18) was found in 92% of the cases including fusion type SYT/SSX1 in 58% of the patients and SYT/SSX2 in 42%. SYT/SSX1 translocations occurred in younger patients and carried a worse prognosis than SYT/SSX2.[72] Conversely, younger age (less than 25 years old), tumor size of less than 5 cm and absence of poorly differentiated lesions are considered positive prognosticators.[74]

Zeren,[75] Essary[76] and their colleagues reported on 25 and 12 primary pulmonary sarcomas with features of monophasic synovial sarcoma, respectively. In both studies, these tumors were seen slightly more often in women than in men and had a median size of 4.2 cm.[75,76] The patients in Zeren's study had an age between 30 and 50 years, while the age range in Essary's study was 20 to 72 years.[75,76] Clinical symptoms included chest pain, cough, dyspnea, and hemoptysis. The tumors were either peripheral or central in location and appeared to be well circumscribed but not encapsulated; they all had histological and ultrastructural features of monophasic synovial sarcoma.[75]

Okamoto et al. described the immunohistochemical and molecular findings in 11 patients with pulmonary synovial sarcomas.[77] All cases presented at least one epithelial marker, either AE1/AE3, CAM5.2, or EMA, appearing scattered in small groups of cells or on individual cells. In addition, S-100 was focally or diffusely positive in 83% of cases, while blc-2 was in 72%. α-SMA and desmin were negative in all cases. β-catenin was diffusely positive in two of eleven cases and other seven cases showed focal and moderate expression; an aberrant expression in the cytoplasm and/or nuclei was also observed. In all Okamoto's cases, the fusion gene could be amplified: SYT/SSX1 was identified in nine cases and SYT/SSX2 in two cases.

In all patients surgical removal is suggested as the treatment of choice. The prognosis of the patients with this rare tumor is undetermined but is suspected to be poor.

PULMONARY ARTERY INTIMAL SARCOMA

A pulmonary trunk sarcoma is a primary lesion arising within the pulmonary artery or, as Mandelstramm[78] described, from the pulmonary valve of the heart. In reviews by Wackers et al.,[79] Bleisch and Kraus,[80] Baker and Goodwin,[81] and Goldblum and Rice[82] as well as by Emmert-Buck[83] and Nonomura[84] and their colleagues, undifferentiated sarcoma, leiomyosarcoma, and fibrosarcoma make

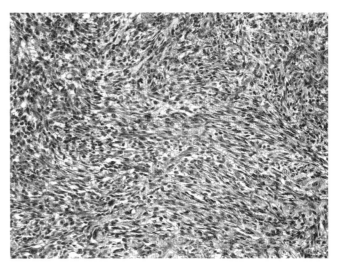

FIGURE 107.5 Pulmonary artery intimal leiomiosarcoma (H&E ×100).

up for the majority of the cell types of these intravascular tumors but also include pleomorphic rhabdomyosarcoma and epithelioid angiosarcoma. Burke and Virmani,[85] based on the results of immunohistochemistry, concluded that most pulmonary artery sarcomas were derived from intimal cells with myofibroblastic differentiation. Both Ko et al.[86] and Leone et al.[87] described leiomyosarcomas in the pulmonary vein (Fig. 107.5).

Large vessel sarcomas may spread distally within the vascular tree or extend outside the vessel to invade the surrounding lung parenchyma. The tumor may appear at any age. In the reported series, the age range was 20 to 80 years, with an average of 50 years.[79,80,84,85] There is a slight predominance of these large vessel sarcomas in women. Common symptoms include chest pain and dyspnea, and one-third of the patients may also have cough, hemoptysis, and palpitations. As these symptoms mimic those of pulmonary embolism, it is not unusual for these patients to be treated for pulmonary embolism before definite diagnosis. The absence of a procoagulant state, an elevated erythrocyte sedimentation rate, anemia, and weight loss, point at the diagnosis of PA sarcoma which is usually established several months since the onset of symptoms. Pulmonary hypertension with proximal dilatation of the vessels is a constant feature; right-sided heart failure ensues as a late manifestation of the disease.[93] Several authors[88–89] reported the radiographic features of PA sarcoma which usually include a lobulated perihilar mass and multiple defects within the pulmonary artery observed at angiography. CT and MRI may help to determine the extent of the disease. In fact, CT scan usually shows hyperdense lesions with nonhomogeneous attenuation from hemorrhage into the tumor. The presence of an irregular mass inside the pulmonary artery, arising from the pulmonary valve and extending distally in the pulmonary vasculature, is characteristic[90] (Fig. 107.6). Mader et al.[91] believe that MRI is the imaging modality of choice for these lesions because it is noninvasive and gives an excellent definition of the heart, pericardium, mediastinum, and lungs. MRI can also delineate both the extent and location of the lesion. Cox et al. agreed with this assessment and believed the imaging findings are quite specific.[92] Parish et al.,[93] in addition to discussing the MRI and CT features of nine cases, suggested that transesophageal echocardiography might also be useful in evaluating pulmonary trunk sarcomas. Simpson and Mendelson agreed that the new imaging modalities, including helical CT and MRI, are useful in making the diagnosis.[94] In the three reported patients, PA sarcoma typically enhanced with gadolinium administration, which is very

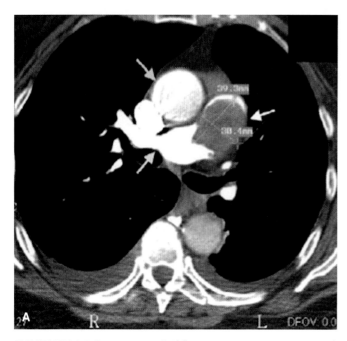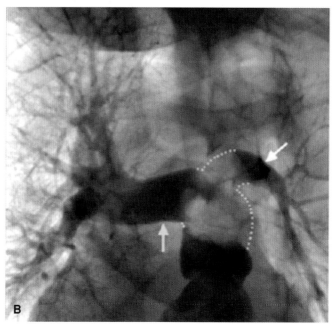

FIGURE 107.6 Pulmonary artery (PA) leiomiosarcoma. **A:** CT angiogram showing a filling defect in the PA trunk (*white arrow*); *yellow arrow* marks the right PA, *light blue arrow* marks the ascending aorta. **B:** PA angiogram showing the filling defect.

useful to differentiate a tumor from PE, and demonstrated increased glucose uptake at PET-CT.

Treatment is surgical resection. Several authors[95,96] reported cases in which these tumors were successfully resected. Kruger et al.[97] reported prolonging survival with resection followed by adjuvant therapy.

Blackmon et al.[98] reviewed 77 patients from the literature and added eight patients from their own series. Their patients had resection through median sternotomy and cardiopulmonary bypass. Homograft pulmonary artery replacement, valve replacement, and pneumonectomy were required in five, three, and five patients, respectively. Median survival was 71 months and 5-year survival was 72% for their eight patients. When their series was combined with the 77 patients from the literature, median survival and 5-year survival were 36.5 months and 49.2%, respectively. Survival was much worse for those patients in which a complete tumor resection could not be achieved.[98] For this reason, Blackmon et al. recommended to consider radical surgery if the patient has a good cardiopulmonary reserve, there is no disease outside the chest, the amount of disease is preoperatively considered technically resectable at imaging and the patient would tolerate a pneumonectomy if necessary. They also recommend chemotherapy (Adriamycin and ifosfamide for two cycles) for those patients that are stable enough to wait for resection after chemotherapy, as multimodality treatment improved survival.[98]

Mussot et al. report a median survival of 17 months after pulmonary endarterectomy in a surgical series of 31 resected patients[90] with a 30-day mortality rate of 13%. Another paper by Wong et al.[99] did not show that pulmonary endarterectomy increased survival in 14 patients that underwent surgery compared to patients that did not have surgery. Three patients died in the postoperative period. Symptoms improved in all patients that survived surgery. The median overall survival in this series of 20 patients was 17 months. They did find a trend toward improved survival in those patients that underwent surgery plus chemotherapy and radiotherapy postoperatively.[99]

Genoni et al. described four patients who underwent resection for pulmonary trunk sarcomas.[100] One had a thromboendarterectomy of

the pulmonary trunk with adjuvant radiation therapy and remained disease-free after 3 years. One tumor was resected, but the patient developed metastases. After chemotherapy, the metastases disappeared and the patient remained alive and well 1 year later. The other two patients died within 2 months of surgery. One died as the result of a tumor mass in the inferior vena cava and the other died of cerebral metastases. Mayer et al. reported the results of resection in seven patients with pulmonary artery sarcomas.[101] None of the patients died in the perioperative period. Four patients were dead after 19 months due to metastatic disease or recurrent tumor; two patients were alive after 21 and 35 months despite the presence of metastatic pulmonary disease. One patient was alive at 62 months with no evidence of recurrent disease.[101]

PULMONARY MYXOID SARCOMA WITH EWSR1-CREB1 TRANSLOCATION

Pulmonary myxoid sarcoma with EWSR1-CREB1 translocation is an infrequent lung tumor that was recently described.[102] The recurrent fusion gene, EWSR1-CREB1 is a distinctive pathologic feature.[102] Thway et al. reported a case series of 10 patients who, at presentation, were mostly symptomatic with a mean age of 45 years.[102] All tumors affected the pulmonary parenchyma with an endobronchial component described in most patients. Tumors usually measure up to 4 cm and have a lobulated architecture. Microscopically, cords of polygonal, spindle, or stellate cells within myxoid stroma, similar to extraskeletal myxoid chondrosarcoma can be seen. Cellular atypia is mild to moderate; mitosis is demonstrated in the range of less than 5 up to 32 mitosis per 2 mm^2.[1] Necrosis tends to be focal in up to 50% of cases.[1]

Tumors were immunoreactive only for vimentin; EMA was only positive focally. In Thway series, the EWSR1-CREB1 fusion gene was found in seven of nine cases tested by reverse transcription-polymerase chain reaction and direct sequencing. Patients, in whom complete resection is achieved, remained disease-free.

MYOEPITHELIAL CARCINOMA

Myoepithelial tumors occur as an endobronchial mass that causes respiratory symptoms. It is a very rare tumor, with less than 15 cases reported. The tumor cells are epithelioid or spindle with uniform nucleus and clear or eosinophilic cytoplasm.[1] Treatment is based on surgical resection according to the extension of the disease.

OTHER MESENCHYMAL TUMORS

Other mesenchymal tumors can occur in the lung, are classified as soft tissue tumors and resemble the counterparts that occur in any other part of the body.[1] In fact, primitive mesenchymal cells are present in every organ of the human body. In the lung, tumors of mesenchymal origin may arise from the stromal elements of the bronchial or vascular wall or from the interstices of lung parenchyma. These tumors usually expand toward the lung parenchyma; occasionally they extend into the lumen of a bronchus. Only rarely do they invade and break through the bronchial epithelium. As a result, these tumors do not exfoliate cells, and diagnosis by cytological examination tracheobronchial washings is uncommon. Grossly, the tumor usually appears as a well-circumscribed and encapsulated mass in the lung parenchyma. They generally spread by local invasion. Peripheral lesions may invade the adjacent pleura and chest wall; only rarely they cavitate. They can metastasize by way of the circulation and rarely by lymphatic invasion. As Watson and Anlyan[103] have noted, metastases to distant organs are usually late manifestations of the disease process. Microscopically, these tumors present a wide range of cellular differentiation.

Primary pulmonary sarcomas occur at almost any age, with equal frequency in males and females. Fadhli et al.[104] report an age range of 4 to 83 years. The tumors occur with equal frequency in either lung. Many patients are asymptomatic, and lesions are detected only on a routine radiograph of the chest. Symptomatic patients most commonly experience chest pain, cough, dyspnea, and hemoptysis. Fever, fatigue, anorexia, and weight loss usually are late manifestations of the disease. On radiographs of the chest, the tumor usually appears as a sharply demarcated mass density within the lung substance at the hilum or in the lung periphery. The lesions are usually solitary. Martini et al.[105] reported that these tumors vary in diameter from 1 to 15 cm or more, with an average diameter of 6 to 7 cm. Peripheral tumors invading the chest wall may be associated with varying degrees of pleural effusion. Tumors obstructing a bronchus (~15%) may result in distal parenchymal changes.[105]

Keel et al.[106] have reported a study of 26 primary pulmonary sarcomas. The tumors were distributed as follows: seven MFHs (27%), six synovial sarcomas (23%), three malignant peripheral nerve sheath tumors (12%), three leiomyosarcomas (12%), two angiosarcomas (8%), two intimal sarcomas (8%), two fibrosarcomas (8%), and one epithelioid hemangioendothelioma (4%). The patients ranged in age from 18 to 75 years, with a mean age of 48 years. The tumors ranged in size from 0.9 cm to filling the entire hemithorax. The tumors were distributed almost equally between the two lungs, with one being bilateral, two in the pulmonary artery, and one in a location that was not stated. In a follow-up study of 23 of these patients by Bacha et al.,[107] it was recorded that three patients were unresectable. Conversely, 13 patients were treated by surgical resections that included lobectomies, bilobectomies, sleeve resections, a carinal resection, and a chest wall resection whereas 4 underwent radical pneumonectomies, and 3 an extended resection with the use of cardiopulmonary bypass.[107] Postoperatively, 11 patients received chemotherapy and 8 had radiation therapy.[107] At a follow-up ranging from 2 to 183 months with a mean of 48 months, the outcomes on 22 patients

were reported.[107] Overall, 14 patients were free of disease, 2 were alive with disease, 6 died of disease, and 1 died of surgical complications. The size and grade did not correlate with the survival but the completeness of the resection did. Thus, these authors concluded that patients with pulmonary sarcomas may have an acceptable survival rate if the resection is complete.

In another study of primary lung sarcomas, Magne et al.[108] reported on nine patients—five women and four men, ranging in age from 35 to 73 years with a median of 63 years. Common symptoms were chest pain (four patients) and dyspnea (four patients). All underwent surgery, with three having incomplete resections. The tumors ranged in size from 2 to 15 cm; they consisted of four MSHs, three leiomyosarcomas, one fibrosarcoma, and one myxoid liposarcoma. Five patients received adjuvant chemotherapy (containing anthracyclin and ifosfamide) and three received adjuvant radiation therapy. The median overall survival was 36 months. In the three patients with incomplete resections, the median survival was 47 months. Two patients underwent a second procedure for the management of recurrence, and each had a satisfactory long-term survival (58 and 83 months, respectively).[108] This good long-term survival for patients with resected recurrence emphasizes the importance of close follow-up for these patients. The important prognostic factors are low grade, small tumor size, and initial complete resection.

Pulmonary Fibrosarcoma

Combining together patients from the series of Guccion and Rosen[109] and Nascimento et al.[110] yields a total of 22 cases of primary pulmonary fibrosarcomas. The patients ranged in age from 23 to 69 years, with an average age of 47 years. There were 16 (72%) men and 6 (27%) women. This bias might exist because one of the studies is from the Armed Forces Institute of Pathology. These fibrosarcomas may occur in either an endobronchial or a parenchymal location. The endobronchial tumors were almost always symptomatic. The symptoms ranged from none to chest pain, cough, hemoptysis, and shortness of breath.[109,110] McLigeyo et al.[111] reported a pulmonary fibrosarcoma in a 50-year-old woman who presented with hypoglycemia and hypertrophic pulmonary osteoarthropathy. In the reported series, most patients were treated mainly by surgical excision.[109,110] A few patients received radiation therapy and chemotherapy in an adjuvant setting. In Guccion and Rosen's[109] series, several patients were lost to follow-up, but the majority of the followed-up patients died of their disease. Those patients with endobronchial lesions seemed to survive longer. In the nine cases of Nascimento et al.,[110] seven died from their disease within 3 months to 18 years after treatment and two were alive at 7 and 18 years following treatment. The patient who survived 18 years had an endobronchial lesion. The one who survived 7 years had a parenchymal tumor.

Pulmonary fibrosarcoma is rare in children. Kuhnen et al.[112] described a pulmonary spindle cell tumor in a newborn that they believed to be a fibrosarcoma. Prognosis is thought to be excellent after resection of such a lesion. Picard et al.[113] resected a bronchial fibrosarcoma by a sleeve resection of the left upper lobe in an 8-year-old boy; the patient was alive and well 2 years after resection. Goldthorn et al.[114] described a cavitating fibrosarcoma in a 11-year-old girl who underwent a resection followed by chemotherapy. She had a 36-month disease-free survival. Picard et al.,[113] in their review of bronchopulmonary fibrosarcomas, noted that at least 28 cases have been recorded in children; 6 were newborns and the others ranged in age from 1 month to 19 years. Each gender was approximately equally affected, as were the two lungs. According to Hancock et al.,[115] these tumors account for 9.6% of the cases of pediatric lung

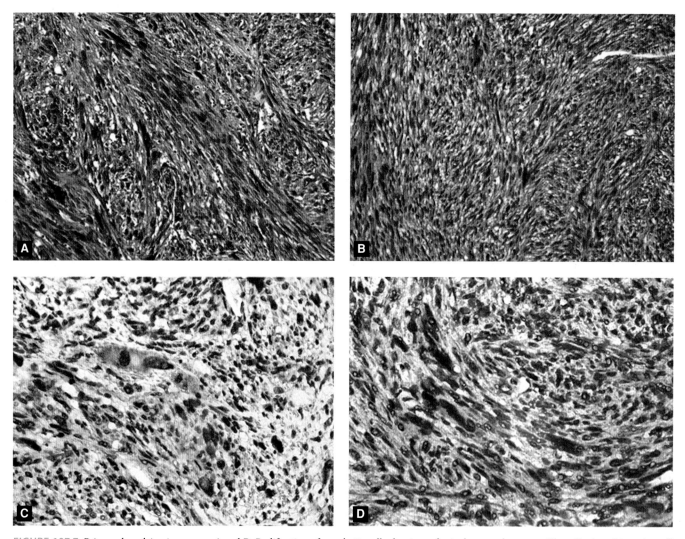

FIGURE 107.7   Primary lung leiomiosarcoma. **A** and **B:** Proliferation of neoplastic cells showing a fascicular growth pattern. The cells show "cigar shaped" nuclei with eosinophilic cytoplasm. **C:** Cytoplasmatic smooth muscle actin positivity. **D:** Intense cytoplasmatic smooth muscle actin positivity.

tumors. In children, the tumor is low-grade and the prognosis is relatively satisfactory with an early survival rate of approximately 78%. Complete surgical resection is the procedure of choice. The roles of radiation therapy and chemotherapy are unknown.

Pulmonary Leiomyosarcoma

Guccion and Rosen[109] as well as Nascimento et al.[110] and Moran et al.[116] have reported a total of 41 cases of pulmonary leiomyosarcomas. These patients ranged in age from a newborn to 91 years, with an average of 51 years. There were 29 men and 12 women, for a gender ratio of 2.4:1. The symptoms ranged from none to cough, chest pain, dyspnea, and hemoptysis. The chest radiographs usually showed a solitary homogeneous density with sharply lobulated borders. Cavitation was observed in some of the leiomyosarcomas, as noted by Lillo-Gil et al.[117] The tumors were randomly distributed in all the lobes of both lungs. On gross examination, the leiomyosarcoma may be in an endobronchial, parenchymal, or subpleural location and is usually well-circumscribed, firm, and grey-white. Areas of necrosis or hemorrhage may exist. Microscopically, the tumor comprises spindle cells with broad fascicles that intersect at right angles. Distant metastases may occur to the lung and not infrequently the adrenal glands are involved (Figs. 107.7 and 107.8).

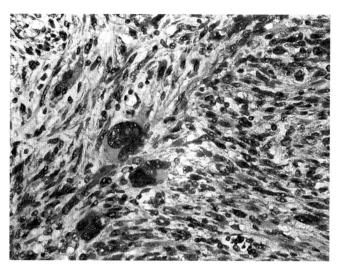

FIGURE 107.8   Primary lung leiomiosarcoma showing smooth muscle actin positivity (high power field, ×400).

Moran et al.[116] divided the pulmonary leiomyosarcomas into low-grade, intermediate-grade, and high-grade malignancy. The low-grade neoplasms have a well-developed fascicular pattern. The cells have "cigar-shaped" nuclei without much atypia, eosinophilic cytoplasm, and 1 to 3 mitoses per 10 high power fields (HPFs). The intermediate-grade tumors have a fairly well-preserved fascicular pattern but are more cellular. The cells have more atypical hyperchromatic nuclei. Mitoses are increased to 3 to 8 per 10 HPFs. Areas of hemorrhage and necrosis are not apparent. High-grade tumors show a more solid cellular proliferation with less of a fascicular pattern. The cells are markedly pleomorphic with large hyperchromatic nuclei and prominent nucleoli. Mitoses are increased to 8 to 12 per 10 HPFs, and areas of hemorrhage and necrosis are present. Immunostaining shows that most of the tumors (75%) stain for smooth muscle actin.[116]

Treatment is surgical removal of the tumor. Shimizu et al.[118] resected a primary pulmonary leiomyosarcoma and a hepatic metastasis in a single-stage procedure. Whether such aggressive intervention is appropriate is questionable. A small number (three) of extensive leiomyosarcomas of the lung that involved the heart or great vessels have been excised completely with support of cardiopulmonary bypass.[119] All three patients tolerated well the procedures, had an uneventful postoperative course and at a follow-up of 15, 61, and 216 months were found to be alive and well.[119] Likewise, patients with other sarcomas of the lung appear to do well with this radical approach when careful selection criteria are applied and the resection of the tumor is complete. However, when a pneumonectomy is required, the mortality may be as high as 22%.[119] The results obtained in this series are in contrast to the dismal results when cardiopulmonary bypass is used to support the resection of extensive non-small-cell lung cancer associated with lymph node metastases. Three such patients were recorded in the same report and the survival was only 4, 6, and 26 months. Byrne[120] and Park[121] and their colleagues, among others, have reported variable results with this approach. Proper selection of patients is a most important key for success.

As a rule the prognosis is poor, with the majority of the patients dying of the disease, although a few patients have survived for more than 10 years.[119] Muscolino et al.[122] reported successful resections and long-term survivals (7 years) in two patients with low-grade bronchial leiomyosarcoma. This report supports the conclusion of Moran et al.[116] that the grade of the tumor was one of the more important factors in determining the patient's prognosis.

Pulmonary Rhabdomyosarcoma

Rhabdomyosarcomas are malignant tumors of skeletal muscle and may occur in various age groups and in either sex. The majority of the cases occur in infants and children from the ages of 1.5 years to 14 years, but Przygodzki et al.[123] have described three cases in men ranging in age from 57 to 78 years. Comin et al.[124] reported a primary pulmonary rhabdomyosarcoma in a 62-year-old patient. The symptoms depend on whether the lesion is endobronchial or parenchymal. According to d'Agostino et al.,[125] many of the rhabdomyosarcomas that arise in children are associated with cystic adenomatous malformations. The chest radiographs usually show a mass that may contain cysts. The computed tomographic (CT) scan shows a soft tissue mass that may be cystic. Pathologically, the tumors have reddish grey surfaces with hemorrhagic and necrotic areas. On microscopic examination, the cells may be arranged in fascicles or may be randomly organized. The nuclei are hyperchromatic with a nucleolus and eosinophilic cytoplasm. Cross striations within the cytoplasm can be demonstrated with a phosphotungstic acid hematoxylin stain. The cells will usually immunostain for desmin, actin (HHF-35), sarcomeric actin, troponin-T, and vimentin.

Treatment is surgical resection, and according to Schiavetti et al.,[126] it is usually combined with chemotherapy and radiation therapy in an adjuvant setting. McDermott et al.[127] pointed out that these patients were predisposed to develop cerebral metastases. The patient of Comin et al.[124] underwent a left pneumonectomy followed by radiation. He was alive and free of disease at 9 months. In the younger age group, approximately one-third of the patients died or were living with disease, and approximately two-thirds were alive with no evidence of disease at varying periods of follow-up. Noda et al.[128] noted that serum neuron-specific enolase was helpful in detecting metastasis and disease recurrence in a patient with alveolar rhabdomyosarcoma of the lung.

Malignant Fibrous Histiocytoma

A MFH is usually found in the extremities or retroperitoneum in adults. It occurs infrequently in the lung and is less common than pulmonary fibrosarcomas and leiomyosarcomas. Yousem and Hochholzer[129] reviewed 22 cases that they identified from the files of the Armed Forces Institute of Pathology. McDonnell et al.[130] reported one case of pulmonary MFH and reviewed 15 other cases they found in the literature. Halyard et al.[131] reported 4 cases and reviewed 49 cases that have appeared in the English-language literature. The patients in these three reports ranged in age from 18 to 80 years, with an average age of 55 years. There was a slight preponderance of men and the most common clinical symptoms were cough, chest pain, weight loss, and hemoptysis.[131] Hypoglycemia and hypertrophic pulmonary osteoarthropathy also were observed in a few patients.[131] Hermann et al.[132] reported on a 57-year-old man with spontaneous hypoglycemia associated with this tumor, with a markedly high level of insulin growth factor 2 (IGF-2), suppressed levels of insulin, as well as C-peptide associated with low levels of growth hormone and IGF-1. Following resection of the tumor, insulin and C-peptide both returned to normal and the IGF-1/IGF-2 ratio increased to the normal reference range. In most instances, the chest radiograph showed a mass lesion, usually a large solid noncavitary mass. Calcification in the mass is rarely seen. The tumors appear to be distributed randomly between both lungs. Microscopically, most of the tumors were storiform (pleomorphic), and a few were of the myxoid or inflammatory type. Tian et al.[133] reported seven cases seen in 11 years in their thoracic unit in Shanyang, China. The findings were similar in all respects to those in the aforementioned reports.

The primary therapeutic approach to these tumors is complete surgical excision followed by radiation therapy or chemotherapy if either is clinically indicated. Saga et al.[134] suggest the neoadjuvant as well as the postoperative use of chemotherapy (i.e., cisplatin with vindesine) in patients with large bulky lesions. Poor prognostic indicators are an advanced stage at the time of diagnosis, extension of the tumor into the chest wall or mediastinum, metastasis beyond the thorax, or incomplete excision. Halyard et al.[131] reported that eight patients in their report had survived more than 5 years after surgical excision with or without adjuvant therapy, for a survival rate of 15%. Lane et al.[135] reported a similar survival rate; 14% (one patient) at 48 months in seven patients after surgical resection of the tumor.

Pulmonary Chondrosarcoma

Morgan and Salama[136] reported a case of pulmonary chondrosarcoma, an extremely rare tumor, and reviewed the literature. The eight patients identified with primary pulmonary chondrosarcoma ranged in age from 23 to 73 years, with an average age of 46 years. The lesions were distributed equally between the sexes. Colby et al.[137] noted that fewer than 20 chondrosarcomas of the lung have been reported. The clinical symptoms in the order of frequency were cough, chest pain, and dyspnea. The tumor seemed to be more common in the left lung. Radiologically, these tumors have shown areas of calcification or ossification. These tumors were solid masses, but Parker et al.[138] described a patient in whom the CT scan and magnetic resonance imaging (MRI) mimicked a bronchogenic cyst.

The outlook is poor in most patients. Local recurrence and distant metastases commonly occur, as noted by Morgenroth et al.[139] and Hayashi et al.[140] Huang et al.[141] reported the successful surgical resection of mesenchymal chondrosarcoma of the lung and noted the immunohistochemical features of diffuse positivity against vimentin for all components and reaction to S-100 limited to the cartilaginous areas. The tumor was negative to cytokeratins, EMA, leukocyte common antigen, and a panel of neuroendocrine markers. The only other case of mesenchymal chondrosarcoma of the lung in the literature that we could find was that reported by Kurotaki et al.[142]

Pulmonary Osteosarcoma

Primary pulmonary osteosarcoma is rare. Loose et al.[143] reported two cases and found nine other cases in the literature. According to their experience, for a lesion to be considered an extraosseous osteosarcoma, it should adhere to the following criteria: (a) the tumor must be composed of a uniform pattern of sarcomatous tissue that excludes the possibility of a malignant mixed mesenchymal tumor, (b) osteoid or bone must be formed by the sarcoma, and (c) a primary osseous tumor must be excluded.[143] The patients ranged in age from 35 to 83 years, with a mean of 61 years. The tumors were seen equally in men and women. The most common clinical symptom was chest pain. The sarcomas were distributed approximately equally in the right and left lungs. When possible, the tumor should be resected although the prognosis is poor. Seven patients in the collected series died of their disease, two patients died of other diseases, and three patients were alive within 2 to 14 months of follow-up.[143] Several additional case reports of osteosarcomas have appeared in the literature in the early 1990s. Petersen[144] reported on a 70-year-old man with a large lung mass. A technetium 99m–methylene diphosphonate bone scan revealed an abnormal area in the region of the left lower lung, but not in the skeleton. On the lobectomy specimen, the lesion was diagnosed as an osteosarcoma. Connolly et al.[145] described a 93-year-old man whose chest radiograph showed a densely calcified lung lesion. On needle biopsy, it proved to be an osteosarcoma. The patient died at home, and the family refused an autopsy. Bhalla et al.[146] described a 58-year-old man with a cavitary lesion that was thought to be an abscess. The CT scan showed an irregular cavity with a partially calcified thick wall. A repeat scan 3 weeks later showed increasing calcifications and a marked increase in size. The patient was treated with drainage and antibiotics but without improvement. At autopsy, the mass was a pulmonary osteosarcoma. Chapman et al.[147] reported a case of pulmonary osteosarcoma in a 33-year-old woman. She survived for 42 months after pneumonectomy, adjuvant chemotherapy, and irradiation but developed widespread metastatic disease. Her tumor showed an overexpression of bcl-2, which is an antiapoptotic protein, and cyclin D1, which drives cells from the G1 phase of the cell cycle to the S phase. Both markers have been associated with resistance to chemotherapy. In addition, the tumor showed a higher level of genomic aberrations than do skeletal osteosarcomas.

Pulmonary Liposarcoma

A primary liposarcoma is one of the sarcomas that very rarely occur in the lung. Krygier et al.[148] described a patient with a pleomorphic liposarcoma whose disease ran a rapidly fatal course despite aggressive treatment. These investigators also noted 11 other cases of primary liposarcomas of the lung that had been reported in the literature. The most common type of liposarcoma was the myxomatous variety, as reported by Hochberg and Crastnopol[149] and others. The most successful treatment is complete surgical resection when possible.

Neurogenic Sarcoma

A neurogenic sarcoma is a malignant proliferation of Schwann cells. Other synonyms for this lesion include *malignant schwannoma* and *neurofibrosarcoma*. Roviaro et al.[150] described an example of a primary pulmonary malignant schwannoma in a 27-year-old man. The patient was symptomatic, with weight loss and chest pain. A large well-defined mass in the right lower lung field was identified on radiographic studies of the chest. Histologically, the tumor consisted of immature fusiform cells in sheets and cords. Mitotic figures were common. Some of the cells tended to form fascicles with a reticular pattern resembling that of a neurofibroma. The final diagnosis was that of a malignant schwannoma. Recurrence of the tumor occurred shortly after resection, and the patient died of the malignant process 4 months after the surgical resection. A second patient was reported by Rowlands et al.[151] A primary malignant melanotic schwannoma of the right upper lobe bronchus was identified in a 27-year-old man. A sleeve lobectomy was performed, and on histologic examination the morphology of the tumor was characteristic of a melanotic schwannoma. Areas of both Antoni A and B pattern were present, and varying numbers of melanosomes at different levels of maturation were readily demonstrated. Mitotic figures were scanty. The patient developed a cerebral metastasis and was terminal 14 months after the initial diagnosis.

McCluggage and Bharucha[152] subsequently reported two additional cases and reviewed the literature. Their patients were 34 and 45 years of age; one was a man and the other a woman. Both presented with dyspnea and chest pain. On gross examination, one tumor was 8 cm and the other 10 cm in diameter. One was a white, circumscribed mass that had a whirled appearance on cut section. The other was also white but contained necrotic areas. On microscopic examination, the smaller tumor had a benign appearance with a fibrous capsule and spindle cells with irregular wavy nuclei. The larger tumor was highly cellular with necrosis. It had pleomorphic cells and multinucleated giant cells with easily identified mitotic figures. Immunostaining revealed that both tumors were focally positive for S-100 protein and diffusely positive for vimentin. They were negative for desmin, carcinoembryonic antigen, and CAM 5.2, a keratin. The tumor was resected in both patients, but each patient subsequently developed metastatic disease.

Primary Pulmonary Ganglioneuroblastoma

Primary ganglioneuroblastoma of the lung is rare. Only few cases have been reported in the English-language literature. Cooney[153] reported the first case, which occurred in a 47-year-old man. The patient presented with cough and was found to have a 5-cm mass in the right lower lobe on radiographs of the chest. The tumor was removed by a lower bilobectomy. On examination of the specimen, the tumor abutted the segmental bronchi, but no intrabronchial tumor was noted. Microscopically the tumor had a fibrous capsule that enclosed a rim of mature ganglioneuromatous tissue containing mature and immature ganglion cells that surrounded a central core composed of primitive neuroblastoma. Vascular invasion of the tumor was evident. Cooney suggested that the tumor arose within a sympathetic component of the posterior pulmonary plexus. Reportedly, the patient was living and well 2½ years after the surgical resection.[153]

Two other cases of primary pulmonary ganglioneuroblastoma were recorded by Hochholzer et al.[154] Both patients were adult women, and in each the tumor extended from an adjacent bronchus. The first patient was 38 years old and had the signs and symptoms of an advanced multiple endocrine neoplasia (MEN) type 1 syndrome. Blood chemistries supported the diagnosis. There were also radiographic findings of a 3-cm infrahilar mass and two small peripheral nodules in the right lung. The patient died within several days of admission, and the autopsy revealed the perihilar mass to be a typical ganglioneuroblastoma with direct invasion of two adjacent hilar lymph nodes but no intrabronchial extension. One of the peripheral masses was a carcinoid tumorlet and the other was a metastatic islet cell tumor of the pancreas. An islet cell tumor of the tail of the pancreas, a tumor of a parathyroid gland, and a cystic tumor of the pituitary gland were also present. The thyroid gland was normal. The second patient was 20 years old and essentially asymptomatic, but radiographs of the chest revealed a mass in the left upper lobe. A left upper lobectomy was performed and the mass, 5 by 5 cm in size, histologically was a typical ganglioneuroblastoma abutting and invading the bronchial lumen. No lymph node involvement was seen. Immunohistochemical studies revealed focal staining for neurofilament protein and S-100 protein and diffuse staining for neuron-specific enolase. The staining for chromogranin, keratin, and glial fibrillary acidic protein was negative. The patient was alive without metastatic or locally recurrent disease, 1 year after the surgical resection.

Although the eventual prognosis has yet to be determined, the primary pulmonary neuroblastomas to date appear to have a low malignant potential. Surgical resection is the treatment of choice.

Primary Malignant "Triton" Tumor of the Lung

A malignant neurogenic tumor with rhabdomyoblastic differentiation is known as a triton tumor (ectomesenchymoma). Triton tumors are more commonly found in the soft tissues whereas their occurrence in the lung is rare. In the thorax these tumors are more commonly located in the mediastinum. Moran et al.[155] have described two such tumors that originated in the lung. One patient was a 3-year-old child and the other a 53-year-old man. Both patients had a large intrapulmonary mass, and each presented with marked dyspnea. Both lesions were removed by pneumonectomy. The tumors were characterized by atypical spindle cell proliferation in an abundant myxoid stroma. Areas of focal rhabdomyoblastic differentiation were present and were characterized by large cells with occasional cytoplasmic cross striations. Immunohistochemically, focal reaction to S-100 protein was present in the atypical spindle cells and a strong reaction to desmin and myoglobin was present in the rhabdomyoblastic areas. The course of the tumor was rapidly fatal in the child, and there is no follow-up information on the man.

Malignant Mesenchymoma

Malignant mesenchymoma is a sarcoma composed of two or more cellular elements, excluding fibrous tissue. Domizio et al.[156] reported a case arising from a cyst in a 4-year-old boy. The boy had a history of pulmonary cyst in the right lower lobe diagnosed when he was 6 months old by chest radiograph; he had a clinical history of anorexia, recurrent dry cough, and night sweats. He was anemic with an elevated erythrocyte sedimentation rate. At the time of admission, the chest radiograph showed an opaque right hemithorax with an air-fluid level in the right midlung field and the mediastinum shifted to the left. He underwent a right lower lobectomy. On gross examination, the lobe was replaced by a necrotic tumor. The viable outer rim was composed of yellowish-grey gelatinous nodules with an area of

central necrosis. Microscopically, the tumor was composed of large anaplastic cells with numerous multinucleate giant cells. There were areas of rhabdomyosarcoma and chondrosarcoma. A cystic lesion was also present with multiple cystic spaces lined by epithelial cells. The patient was treated with chemotherapy and radiation therapy and was free of disease at short-term follow-up.

LYMPHOHISTIOCYTIC TUMORS

In the 2015 WHO classification of lung tumors, a category has been created to include the so-called lymphohistiocytic tumors. Three malignant lung tumors are included in this category: Extranodal marginal zone lymphoma of mucosa-associated lymphoid tissue (MALT lymphoma), diffuse large B-cell lymphoma and intravascular large B-cell lymphoma.

EXTRANODAL MARGINAL ZONE LYMPHOMAS OF MUCOSA-ASSOCIATED LYMPHOID TISSUE (MALT LYMPHOMA)

According to Koss,[157] most of the non-Hodgkin's lymphomas that originate in the lung are low grade and derived from B cells. They are thought to be derived from MALT, which is composed of lymphoid tissue within the bronchial mucosa. MALT of the bronchus is supposed to be acquired as a consequence of the presence of chronic inflammation of the airway, such as the induced by smoking, autoimmune disease, or infection. This system is thought to have a role in dealing with inhaled antigens. In various series, the low-grade lymphomas constitute the majority (50% to 70%) of the primary lung lymphomas. Lung MALT lymphomas are low-grade, slow growing tumors that usually have an indolent course. In different series, long-term survival is very good, with 10-years survival rates of up to 50%.[158,159]

These lesions are proliferations of small lymphocytes and plasmocytoid lymphocytes surrounding reactive follicles. Infiltration of bronchial or bronchiolar epithelium with lymphocytes is characteristic of MALT lymphoma, which is called lymphoepithelial lesion. Reactive follicular hyperplasia is usually demonstrated. The neoplastic cells are monoclonal B cell lymphocytes that stain for CD20 or CD79a and are negative for CD10, CD23, and Bcl-6. They are also positive for Bcl-2. Ki-67 is usually less than 20%. Once the diagnosis is established by tissue biopsy, nodal disease should be ruled out elsewhere by a body CT, or preferably by PET-CT. Bone marrow biopsy is recommended to rule out bone marrow involvement.[160] The absence of extrapulmonary involvement at the time of diagnosis or during the next 3 months after initial diagnosis, in presence of a clonal lymphocytic lung proliferation as described above, complete the diagnosis of primary lung lymphoma.

Cytogenetically, the most common finding is a translocation, t (11;18) (q21; q21), which is present in about one-third of cases, followed by t (14;18) (p32; q21). These tumors may have a heavy-chain gene rearrangement. Both translocations affect the MALT1 gene. The cellular pathway that is affected with these translocations is the NF-κB pathway.

The staging system usually reported for primary lymphoma of the lung is the Ann Arbor pulmonary lymphoma staging system, which is shown in Table 107.3.[158]

Ferraro et al. from the Mayo Clinic reported in 2000 a series of 48 patients with primary Non-Hodgkin Lymphoma of the lung that underwent some kind of thoracic surgical procedure.[158] MALT lymphomas were found in 73% of this group of patients. Patients were aged between 15 and 85 years old (mean age 61.8 years) and

TABLE 107.3 Ann Arbor Pulmonary Lymphoma Staging System

Stage IE: Lung only, could be bilateral
Stage II 1E: Lung and hilar lymph nodes
Stage II 2E: Lung and mediastinal lymph nodes
Stage II 2EW: Lung and chest wall or diaphragm
Stage III: Lung and lymph nodes below the diaphragm
Stage IV: Diffuse lymphoma

56% were female. Symptoms were present in 62% of patients, being cough, fatigue, and weight loss the most common. Pulmonary infiltrates or a pulmonary mass were the most common radiographic findings. Bronchoscopy had a low yield for the diagnosis of pulmonary lymphoma (18%), a finding also supported by other papers.[161] An R0 resection was possible in 40% of patients. The rest of the patients had biopsies or were found to have extensive and unresectable thoracic disease. Most patients were staged as IE and 54% got postoperative chemotherapy.

Kurtin et al. found 29% of their patients to have autoimmune diseases. Additionally, they tested 28 of their 50 patients for a monoclonal gammopathy and found it in 12 patients (43%).[162]

King et al. described the imaging studies of 24 patients with pulmonary MALT lymphoma.[163] They found multiple lesions in 19 out of 24 patients (79%), solitary lesions in 4 out of 24 patients (17%), and a diffuse pulmonary infiltrate in 1 patient (4%). Associated high-resolution CT (HRCT) scans revealed air bronchograms, airway dilatation, a positive angiogram sign, and a halo of ground glass shadowing at the margins of the lesion. Other observations included peribronchovascular thickening, hilar and mediastinal lymph node enlargement, and pleural effusions or thickening (Fig. 107.9). Up to 50% of patients are asymptomatic and the lung MALT lymphoma is incidentally discovered on imaging.

The prognosis of primary MALT lymphomas is good. Koss et al.[164] reported a 5-year survival rate of 70%. Miller and Allen recorded a similar 86% survival rate at 5 years in their series of 22 patients with small-cell lymphomas of the lung.[2] Kennedy et al.[165] reported a median survival rate of 9.75 years in their group of 12 patients. In the series of Fiche et al., the patients with small-cell lymphomas had

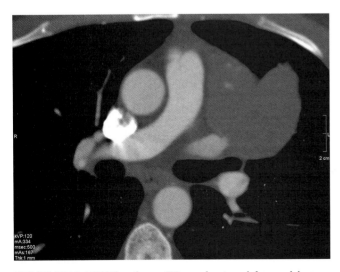

FIGURE 107.9 MALT lymphoma. CT scan showing a left upper lobe mass which required a left upper lobectomy to be resected. Pathology showed a MALT B-cell lymphoma.

a 93.6% survival rate at 5 years and a 60% survival rate at 10 years.[166] Ferraro et al. reported actuarial survival rates at 1, 5, and 10 years of 91%, 68%, and 53%, respectively, regardless of therapy.[158] A review of the Surveillance Epidemiology and End-Results (SEER) database of 326 patients, reported a median overall survival of 112 months and 7.5 years disease-specific survival rate of 85%.[167]

Treatment options include initial observation, surgery, chemotherapy, radiation therapy, or a combination of such modalities. Graham et al. at the Massachusetts General Hospital recorded a series of primary pulmonary lymphomas (PPLs).[168] Most of the 18 patients (78%) had MALT lymphomas, two of which progressed to large-cell lymphoma, a high-grade malignancy. Complete surgical resection, if achievable, is considered to be definitive and no further therapy is indicated.[168] Otherwise, if the resection is incomplete, chemotherapy should be added to the treatment regimen. Drugs such as rituximab, chlorambucil, and cyclophosphamide, vincristine, and prednisolone (CVP) may be used. With recurrent disease, more aggressive regimens such as cyclophosphamide, doxorubicin, vincristine, and prednisone (CHOP), or Adriamycin, bleomycin, vinblastine, and decarbonize (ABVD) may be employed. Radiation therapy alone may be used after an incomplete resection or in the management of a recurrence.[168]

Zinzani et al. treated 17 patients with biopsy-proven lung MALT lymphomas with fludarabine- and mitoxantrone-containing regimens and a complete response was found in 82.3% of patients. The authors advocate for the use of this regimen as first-line therapy in the treatment of lung MALT lymphomas.[169] Similarly, Kim et al. reported a high rate of objective response in eight patients treated with single-agent chlorambucil or CVP combination regimen.[161]

Although there are no definite guidelines about the role of surgery in lung MALT lymphomas, surgery is advocated in many cases as in the Mayo Clinic or Massachusetts General Hospital's series. As in many cases an invasive diagnostic approach is necessary due to the low diagnostic yield of nonsurgical tissue samples, surgery has a very important role in the diagnosis and treatment of this disease. Ferraro et al. recommend that any resectable lung lesion should be approached as such and a complete lung resection and mediastinal lymph node staging performed. In unresectable lesions, surgery (minimally invasive if possible) is reserved to obtain a tissue biopsy. However, the authors do not recommend performing extensive resections as pneumonectomy to treat lung MALT lymphomas as the extent of resection did not improve survival in their patients.[158]

Recurrence can occur in up to 50% of cases, being the lymph nodes the most common site of recurrence. Although surgery could be considered to treat recurrences, chemotherapy is preferred in this setting.

DIFFUSE LARGE B-CELL LYMPHOMA

Diffuse large B-cell lymphoma (DLBCL) is a less common type of primary lung lymphoma. It is a lymphoma that consists of a diffuse proliferation of B cells with a nuclear size equal or exceeding the size of a macrophage's nucleus, or more than twice the size of a normal appearing lymphocyte. The neoplastic B cells express CD20 and CD79a.[1]

In the series of PPLs reported by Toh and Ang,[170] 2 out of 11 patients (18%) had a large-cell lymphoma. Tamura et al.,[171] in a similar study, found 3 of 24 (12.5%) were large-cell lymphomas. Kim et al. reported 24 patients with PPLs, 9 of which were diagnosed with DLBCL.[161]

Patients with large-cell lymphoma are usually in their fifth and sixth decades of life. Men and women are affected almost equally and patients are usually symptomatic. Symptoms include cough, chest pain, dyspnea, fever, and weight loss. Tumors tend to occur in the upper lobes but also may be found in the other lobes, and even the entire lung may be involved. The chest radiographs show an infiltrate or nodules similar to those seen in patients with MALT lymphoma. On histologic examination, the tumors are composed of cells with large nuclei and prominent nucleoli. Hilar lymph nodes are frequently involved. Chest wall and pleural involvement have been noted. Cavitation may occur with the mixed (large and small) cell types. After establishing the diagnosis, the treatment of choice is chemotherapy in combination with radiation therapy. Despite chemotherapy is the treatment of choice, sometimes resective surgery is performed to establish a definite diagnosis.[158,161]

In the report of Kurtin et al., eight of the nine patients received various regimens of chemotherapy.[162] These large-cell tumors are more aggressive than MALT lymphomas, and the prognosis is correspondingly poorer. However, the survival data for DLBCL of the lung is less clear because fewer cases have been reported.

Although complete responses are frequent, relapses are also common.[161] L'Hoste et al. reported late recurrence in 53% of their patients. Recurrences can occur within months or many years after the initial treatment.[172] Cordier et al. reported no survivors out of nine patients by the end of 4 years.[173] In general, these patients do not survive as long as patients with MALT lymphomas as shown Kim et al.[161] Kurtin et al. estimated an overall survival rate at 1, 3, and 5 years of 77.8% for patients with large-cell lymphomas; at 10 years, the survival rate was 51.9%.[162]

Despite an initial response to appropriate therapy, patients with aids and primary large-cell lymphoma have a poorer prognostic outlook, the presence of prior or concurrent opportunistic infection is particularly harmful in these patients. Ray et al.[174] described 12 cases of AIDS-related PPL occurring between 1986 and 1996. Their patients ranged in age from 32 to 56 years, with an average age of 38 years. The ratio of men to women was 11:1. The symptoms were cough, dyspnea, and chest pain, with most of the patients having B symptoms, such as fever, weight loss, or night sweats. The mean time from human immunodeficiency virus (HIV) seropositive to the discovery of the lymphoma was 5 years. The patients were treated with various regimens of chemotherapy. The median survival was 4 months, with all 12 patients dying by 17 months. This report implicates EBV in the pathogenesis of these lymphomas.[174]

INTRAVASCULAR LARGE B CELL LYMPHOMA

Intravascular large B cell lymphoma (ILBCL) is an aggressive subtype of extranodal DLBCL. The hallmark of this type of tumor is the lymphoma cells inside the blood vessels, especially in the capillaries.[1] The neoplastic lymphocytes found inside the vessels are large cells with vesicular nuclei and prominent nucleoli. Mitosis are often times seen. Neoplastic cells are positive for B cell markers as CD29 and CD79a. It can present as a diffuse lung disease with hypoxemia or pulmonary hypertension. Ground glass opacities are other forms of radiological presentation. Treatment is with chemotherapy. Rituximab has been reported as a useful drug, but the prognosis is poor.[1]

The true incidence of pulmonary lymphomas other than B-cell type is unknown. Immunophenotyping using immunohistochemistry is valuable in defining the lineage of origin. To differentiate between a reactive process and a T cell malignant disease, monoclonality of the T cells needs to be demonstrated by TCR gene rearrangement. Compared with pulmonary B cell lymphoma, the outcome of

patients affected by non–B cell lymphoma of the lung is much worse (Fig. 107.10).

TUMORS OF ECTOMPIC ORIGIN

INTRAPULMONARY THYMOMA

Intrapulmonary thymomas are epithelial neoplasms that occur in the lung and are similar to their counterparts in the thymus.[1] They are thought to originate from ectopic thymic tissue in the lung. They can present with respiratory symptoms or be found as incidental lung nodules or masses. Paraneoplastic syndromes as myasthenia gravis can be found in patients suffering from intrapulmonary thymomas. Surgical resection is the treatment of choice when it is localized in the lung.[1]

PRIMARY LUNG MELANOMA

At the Mayo Clinic, Miller and Allen[2] reviewed 80 patients with rare pulmonary neoplasms over a 10-year span. Only three patients had pulmonary melanoma, which represents 0.03% of their 10,134 patients with lung cancer. Jennings et al.[175] described a primary malignant melanoma of the lower respiratory tract and summarized another 19 cases in the literature. They used the following criteria to exclude other possible primary sites: (a) no previously removed skin lesion, particularly pigmented; (b) no ocular tumors removed and no enucleation; (c) solitary tumor; (d) morphologic tumor characteristics compatible with a primary tumor; (e) no demonstrable melanoma in other organs at the time of removal; and (f) autopsy without primary melanoma demonstrated elsewhere, especially the skin or the eyes. The differentiation of a primary melanoma from a melanin-containing carcinoid tumor is necessary in all cases. The immunohistochemical and ultrastructural differences between these two tumors (Table 107.4) may be helpful in this regard (Fig. 107.11). In the 20 reported cases reviewed by Jennings et al.[175] the patients ranged in age from 29 to 80 years, with almost equal distribution between men and women. In four patients, the melanoma arose in either the trachea or the tracheal carina, whereas in the remaining 16 patients, the melanoma arose in bronchial sites involving any one of the lobes of the lungs. The clinical symptoms, physical findings, and radiographic features were not described for many of these patients, although melanomas arising in the bronchus behave clinically like a primary lung carcinoma with resulting bronchial obstruction. Marchevsky[176] pointed out that bronchial melanomas are morphologically similar to those of the skin and mucosa. Lung melanomas, also immunostain for S100 protein, Melan A, and HMB-45 but not for neuroendocrine markers, which helps separate them from carcinoids. Wilson and Moran[177] also described the immunohistochemistry for seven primary pulmonary melanomas. They found these tumors to be positive for S-100, HMB-45, and vimentin, but negative for cytokeratin, CAM 5.2 (a keratin), and chromogranin. If a melanoma is encountered and no history or evidence of a simultaneous or previous primary lesion can be elicited, resection should be performed if possible. Treatment instituted in the cases reported in the literature ranged from no therapy to resection of the entire lung. Eight patients died of their disease, six were free of disease for as long as 11 years, and two other patients were free of disease at 12 and 19 months. Ost et al. described an additional case of pulmonary melanoma and concluded that aggressive surgical

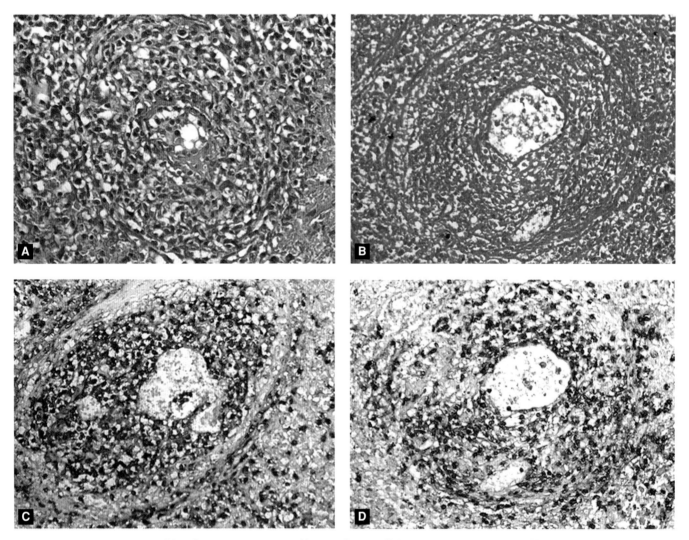

FIGURE 107.10 Angiocentric T-cell lymphoma. **A:** Angiocentric infiltration of tumor cells (H&E). **B:** Giemsa. **C** and **D:** Diffuse positivity to CD3 cells.

TABLE 107.4 Differentiation of a Primary Melanoma of the Lung and a Melanin-Containing Carcinoid

Primary Melanoma		Melanin-Containing Carcinoid
Ultrastructural Features		
Cytoplasmic organelles		Abundant mitochondria
Smooth endoplastic reticulum		Desmosomes
Pigment-Laden Bodies		
No neurosecretory granules		Neurosecretory granules present
Immunohistochemical Features		
+++	S-100 protein	±
−	Neuron-specific enolase	+++
−	Calcitonin	+++
−	Keratin	+
−	Epithelial membrane antigen	+
−	Chromogranin A	++
+++	HMB-45	NR

±, present or absent; +++, strongly positive; ++, moderately positive; +, present; NR, not recorded.

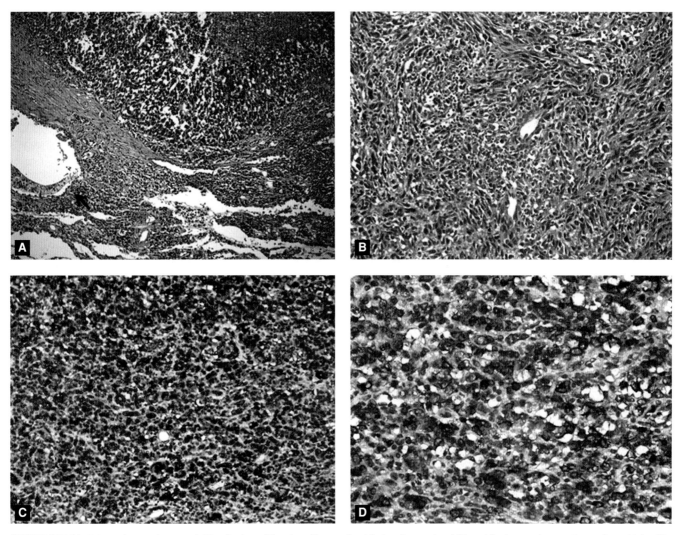

FIGURE 107.11   Primary lung melanoma. **A:** Neoplastic proliferation of large cells with abundant eosinophilic and finely granular cytoplasm; a bronchial wall is marked by the *arrow* (H&E, ×100). **B:** Marked cellular atypia and large nucleoli are seen (H&E, ×200). **C:** Diffuse staining for Melan A (×200). **D:** diffuse staining for Melan A (×400).

resection, regardless of lymph node involvement, offered the best long-term survival.[178]

REFERENCES

1. Travis WD, Brambilla E, Burke AP, et al. *WHO Clasiffication of Tumors of the Lung, Pleura, Thymus and Heart.* Lyon: International Agency for Research on Cancer; 2015.
2. Miller DL, Allen MS. Rare pulmonary neoplasms. *Mayo Clin Proc* 1993;68:492.
3. Nakajima M, Kasai T, Hashimoto H, et al. Sarcomatoid Carcinoma of the Lung: a clinicopathological study of 37 cases. *Cancer* 1999;86:608–616.
4. Italiano A, Cortot AB, Ilie M, et al. EGFR and KRAS status of primary sarcomatoid carcinomas of the lung: implications for anti-EGFR treatment of a rare lung malignancy. *Int J Cancer* 2009;125(10):2479–2482.
5. Rossi G, Cavazza A, Sturm N, et al. Pulmonary carcinomas with pleomorphic, sarcomatoid or sarcomatous elements: a clinicopathologic and immunohistochemical study of 75 cases. *Am J Surg Pathol* 2003;27:311–324.
6. Martin LW, Correa AM, Ordonez NG, et al. Sarcomatoid carcinoma of the lung: a predictor of poor prognosis. *Ann Thorac Surg* 2007;84:973–980.
7. Ro JY, Oxen JL, Lee JS, et al. Sarcomatoid carcinoma of the lung. Immunohistochemical and ultrastructural studies of 14 cases. *Cancer* 1992;69:376–386.
8. Fishback NF, Travis WD, Moran CA, et al. Pleomorphic (spindle/giant cell) carcinoma of the lung. Clinicopathologic correlation of 78 cases. *Cancer* 1994;73:45.
9. Chang Y-L, Lee YC, Shih JY, et al. Pulmonary pleomorphic (spindle) cell carcinoma: peculiar clinicopathologic manifestations different from ordinary non-small carcinoma. *Lung Cancer* 2001;34:91–97.
10. Raveglia F, Mezzetti M, Panigalli T, et al. Personal experience in surgical management of pulmonary pleomorphic carcinoma. *Ann Thorac Surg* 2004;78:1742–1747.
11. Chen F, Sonobe M, Sato T, et al. Clinicopathological characteristics of surgically resected pulmonary pleomorphic carcinoma. *Eur J Cardiothorac Surg* 2012;41: 1037–1042.
12. Chang YL, Wu CT, Shih JY, et al. EGFR and p53 status of pulmonary pleomorphic carcinoma: implications for EGFR tyrosine kinase inhibitors therapy of an aggressive lung malignancy. *Ann Surg Oncol* 2011;18:2952–2960.
13. Kaira K, Horie Y, Ayabe E, et al. Pulmonary Pleomorphic Carcinoma: A Clinicopathological Study Including EGFR Mutation Analysis. *J Thorac Oncol* 2010;5: 460–465.
14. Ji C, Zhong C, Fang W, et al. Surgical treatment for pulmonary pleomorphic carcinoma: A retrospective study of 60 patients. *Thorac Cancer* 2014;5:250–254.
15. Yuki T, Sakuma T, Ohbayashi C, et al. Pleomorphic carcinoma of the lung: a surgical outcome. *J Thorac Cardiovasc Surg* 2007;84:399–404.
16. Bae H, Min H, Lee, Se, et al. Palliative chemotherapy for pulmonary pleomorphic carcinoma. *Lung Cancer* 2007;58:112–115.
17. Velcheti V, Rimm D, Schalper K. Sarcomatoid Lung Carcinomas Show High Levels of Programmed Death Ligand-1 (PD-L1). *J Thorac Oncol* 2013;8:803–805.
18. Kimino K, Nakasone T, Kishikawa M. A case of so-called pulmonary carcinosarcoma. *J Jpn Assoc Chest Surg* 1996;10:833–837.
19. Meade P, Moad J, Fellows D, et al. Carcinosarcoma of the lung with hypertrophic pulmonary osteoarthropathy. *Ann Thorac Surg* 1991;51:488–490.
20. Nappi O, Glasner SD, Swanson PE, et al. Biphasic and monophasic sarcomatoid carcinomas of the lung. A reappraisal of "carcinosarcomas" and "spindle-cell carcinomas." *Am J Clin Pathol* 1994;102:331–340.
21. Ishida T, Tateishi M, Kaneko S, et al. Carcinosarcoma and spindle cell carcinoma of the lung. Clinicopathologic and immunohistochemical studies. *J Thorac Cardiovasc Surg* 1990;100:844–852.
22. Grahmann PR, Swoboda L, Bonnet R, et al. Carcinosarcomas of the lung. Three case reports and literature review. *Thorac Cardiovasc Surg* 1993;41:312–317.

23. Berho M, Moran CA, Suster S. Malignant mixed epithelial/mesenchymal neoplasms of the lung. *Semin Diagn Pathol* 1995;12:123–139.

24. Wick MR, Ritter JH, Humphrey PA. Sarcomatoid carcinomas of the lung: a clinicopathologic review. *Am J Clin Pathol* 1997;108:40–53.

25. Koss MN, Hochholzer L, Frommelt RA. Carcinosarcoma of the lung: a clinicopathologic study of 66 patients. *Am J Surg Pathol* 1999;23:1514.

26. Davis M, Eagan R, Weiland L, et al. Carcinosarcoma of the lung: Mayo Clinic experience and response to chemotherapy. *Mayo Clin Proc* 1984;59:598–603.

27. Barnard WG. Embryoma of lung. *Thorax* 1952;7:299–301.

28. Spencer H. Pulmonary blastoma. *J Pathol* 1961;82:161–166.

29. Smyth R, Fabre A, Dodd J, et al. Pulmonary blastoma: a case report and review of the literature. *BMC Res Notes* 2014;7:294.

30. Larsen H, Sorensen JB. Pulmonary blastoma: a review with special emphasis on prognosis and treatment. *Cancer Treat Rev* 1996;22:145–160.

31. Bodner SM, Koss MN. Mutations in the p53 gene in pulmonary blastomas: immunohistochemical and molecular studies. *Hum Pathol* 1996;27:1117–1123.

32. Macher-Goeppinger S, Penzel R, Roth W, et al. Expression and mutation analysis of EGFR, c-KIT, and β-catenin in pulmonary blastoma. *J Clin Pathol* 2011;64: 349–353.

33. Nakatani Y, Miyagi Y, Takemura T, et al. Aberrant nuclear/cytoplasmic localization and gene mutation of beta-catenin in classic pulmonary blastoma: beta-catenin immunostaining is useful for distinguishing between classic pulmonary blastoma and a blastomatoid variant of carcinosarcoma. *Am J Surg Pathol* 2004;28:921–992.

34. Koyima Y, Habas R. Wnt signal transduction pathways. *Organogenesis* 2008;4: 68–75.

35. Bosch-Barrera J, Holguin F, Baldó X, et al. Neoadjuvant Chemoradiotherapy Treatment for a Classic Biphasic Pulmonary Blastoma with High PD-L1 Expression. *Anticancer Res* 2015;35:4871–4875.

36. Zaida A, Zamvar V, Macbeth F, et al. Pulmonary blastoma: medium-tern results from a regional center. *Ann Thorac Surg* 2002;73:1572–1575.

37. Begin LR, Eskandari J, Joncas J, et al. Epstein-Barr virus related lymphoepithelioma-like carcinoma of the lung. *J Surg Oncol* 1987;36:280–283.

38. Han AJ, Xiong M, Zong YS. Association of Epstein-Barr virus with lymphoepithelioma-like carcinoma of the lung in southern China. *Am J Clin Pathol* 2000;114:220–226.

39. Chang Y-L, Wu CT, Shih JY, et al. New aspects in clinicopathologic and oncogene studies of 23 pulmonary lymphoepithelioma-like carcinomas. *Am J Surg Pathol* 2002;26:715–723.

40. Frank MW, Shields TW, Joob AW, et al. Lymphoepithelioma-like carcinoma of the lung. *Ann Thorac Surg* 1997;64:1162–1164.

41. Wöckel W, Höfler G, Popper HH, et al. Lymphoepithelioma-like lung carcinomas. *Pathologe* 1997;18:147–152.

42. Curcio LD, Cohen JS, Paz IB, et al. Primary lymphoepithelioma-like carcinoma of the lung in a child. Report of an Epstein-Barr virus–related neoplasm. *Chest* 1997;111:250–251.

43. Al-Sarraf M, LeBlanc M, Giri PG, et al. Superiority of chemoradiation vs. radiotherapy in patients with locally advanced nasopharyngeal cancer. *Proc Am Soc Clin Oncol* 1996;15:313.

44. Han AJ, Xiong M, Gu YY, et al. Lymphoepithelioma-like carcinoma of the lung with a better prognosis. A clinicopathologic study of 32 cases. *Am J Clin Pathol* 2001;115:841–850.

45. French CA. Demystified molecular pathology of NUT midline carcinomas. *J Clin Pathol* 2010;63:492–496.

46. French C. NUT Midline Carcinoma. *Cancer Genet Cytogenet* 2010;203:16–20.

47. Stelow E. A Review of NUT Midline Carcinoma. *Head and Neck Pathol* 2011;5:31–35.

48. Sholl L, Nishimo M, Pakharel S, et al. Primary Pulmonary NUT Midline Carcinoma: Clinical, Radiographic, and Pathologic Characterizations. *J Thorac Oncol* 2015;10:951–959.

49. Ye T, Chen H, Hu H, et al. Malignant clear cell sugar tumor of the lung: patient case report. *J Clin Oncol* 2010;28:e626–e628.

50. Sale GE, Kulander BG. "Benign" clear-cell tumor (sugar tumor) of the lung with hepatic metastases ten years after resection of pulmonary primary tumor. *Arch Pathol Lab Med* 1988;112:1177–1178.

51. Parfitt JR, Keith JL, Megyesi JF, et al. Metastatic PEComa to the brain. *Acta Neuropathol* 2006;112:349–351.

52. Yan B, Yau EX, Petersson F. Clear cell "sugar" tumour of the lung with malignant histological features and melanin pigmentation—the first reported case. *Histopathology* 2011;58:498–500.

53. Lim H, Lee H, Han J, et al. Uncommon of the uncommon: Malignant Perivascular Epithelioid Cell Tumor of the Lung. *Korean J Radiol* 2013;14:692–696.

54. Martignoni G, Pea M, Reghellin D. PEComas: the past, the present and the future. *Virchows Arch* 2008;452:119–132.

55. Dail D, Liebow AA. Intravascular bronchioalveolar tumor (abstract). *Am J Pathol* 1975;78:6a–7a.

56. Dail DH, Liebow AA, Gmelich JT, et al. Intravascular, bronchiolar, and alveolar tumor of the lung (IVBAT). An analysis of twenty cases of a peculiar sclerosing endothelial tumor. *Cancer* 1983;51:452–464.

57. Weiss SW, Enzinger FM. Epithelioid hemangioendothelioma: a vascular tumor often mistaken for a carcinoma. *Cancer* 1982;50:970–981.

58. Weiss SW, Ishak KG, Dail DH, et al. Epithelioid hemangioendothelioma and related lesions. *Semin Diagn Pathol* 1986;3:259–287.

59. Wenisch HJC, Lulay M. Lymphogenous spread of an intravascular bronchioloalveolar tumour. Case report and review of the literature. *Virchows Arch [A]* 1980;387: 117–123.

60. Bagan P, Hassan M, Barthes FL, et al. Prognostic factors and surgical indications of epithelioid hemangioendo-thelioma: a review of the literature. *Ann Thorac Surg* 2006;82:2010–2013.

61. Ross GJ, Violi L, Friedman AC, et al. Intravascular bronchioloalveolar tumor: CT and pathologic correlation. *J Comput Assist Tomogr* 1989;13:240–243.

62. Moran CA, Suster S. Tumors of lungs and pleura. In: Fletcher CDM, ed. *Diagnostic Histopathology of Tumors*. 2nd ed. New York: Churchill Livingston; 2000:171.

63. Mehtaa S, Dasb A, Barnardc N. Metastatic Pulmonary Epithelioid Hemangioendothelioma: A case report and review of the literature. *Respir Med Case Rep* 2012;7:17–20.

64. Cronin P, Arenberg D. Pulmonary epithelioid hemangioendothelioma: an unusual case and review of the literature. *Chest* 2004;125:789–793.

65. Kitaichi M, Nagai S, Nishimura K, et al. Pulmonary epithelioid haemangioendothelioma in 21 patients, including three with partial spontaneous regression. *Eur Respir J* 1998;12:89–96.

66. Lerut J P, Orlando G, Sempoux C, et al. Hepatic haemangioendothelioma in adults: excellent outcome following liver transplantation. *Transpl Int* 2004;17: 202–207.

67. Lau K, Massad M, Pollak C, et al. Clinical Patterns and Outcome in Epithelioid Hemangioendothelioma With or Without Pulmonary Involvement: Insights From and Internet Resgistry in the Study of a Rare cancer. *Chest* 2011;140:1312–1318.

68. Priest JR, et al. Pleuropulmonary blastoma: a clinicopathologic study of 50 cases. *Cancer* 1997;80:147.

69. Manivel JC, Priest JR, Watterson J, et al. Pleuropulmonary blastoma. The so-called pulmonary blastoma of childhood. *Cancer* 1988;62:1516–1526.

70. Indolfi P, Casale F, Carli M, et al. Pleuropulmonary blastoma: management and prognosis of 11 cases. *Cancer* 2000;89:1396–1401.

71. Khan A, El Borai A, Alnoaiji M. Pleuropulmonary Blastoma: A case report and Review of the Literature. *Case Rep Pathol* 2014; article ID 509086, 6 pages.

72. Hartel P, Fanburg-Smith J, Frazier A, et al. Primary pulmonary and mediastinal synovial sarcoma: a clinicopathologic study of 60 cases and comparison with five prior studies. *Mod Pathol* 2007;20:760–796.

73. Tornkvist M, Brodin B, Bartolazzi A, et al. A novel type of SYT/SSX fusion: methodological and biological implications. *Mod Pathol* 2002;15:679–685.

74. Bergh P, Meis-Kindblom J, Gherlinzoni F, et al. Synovial Sarcoma: Identification of Low and High Risk Groups. *Cancer* 1999;85:2596–607.

75. Zeren H, Moran CA, Suster S, et al. Primary pulmonary sarcomas with features of monophasic synovial sarcoma: a clinicopathological, immunohistochemical, and ultrastructural study of 25 cases. *Hum Pathol* 1995;26:474–480.

76. Essary LR, Vargas SO, Fletcher CDM. Primary pleuropulmonary synovial sarcoma: reappraisal of a recently described anatomic subset. *Cancer* 2002;94:459.

77. Okamoto S, Hisaoka M, Daa T, et al. Primary Pulmonary Synovial Sarcoma: A Clinicopathologic, Immunohistochemical, and Molecular Study of 11 Cases. *Hum Pathol* 2004;35:850–856.

78. Mandelstramm M. Über primary Neubildung des Herzens. *Virchows Arch [A]* 1923;245:43.

79. Wackers FJ, Van Der Schoot JB, Hamper JF. Sarcoma of the pulmonary trunk associated with hemorrhagic tendency. A case report and review of the literature. *Cancer* 1969;23:339–351.

80. Bleisch VR, Kraus FT. Polypoid sarcoma of the pulmonary trunk: analysis of the literature and report of a case with leptomeric organelles and ultrastructural features of rhabdomyosarcoma. *Cancer* 1980;46:314–324.

81. Baker PB, Goodwin RA. Pulmonary artery sarcomas: a review and report of a case. *Arch Pathol Lab Med* 1985;109:35–39.

82. Goldblum JR, Rice TW. Epithelioid angiosarcoma of the pulmonary artery. *Hum Pathol* 1995;26:1275–1277.

83. Emmert-Buck MR, Stay EJ, Tsokos M, et al. Pleomorphic rhabdomyosarcoma arising in association with the right pulmonary artery. *Arch Pathol Lab Med* 1994;118:1220–1222.

84. Nonomura A, Kurumaya H, Kono N, et al. Primary pulmonary artery sarcoma: report of two autopsy cases studied by immunohistochemistry and electron microscopy, and review of 110 cases reported in the literature. *Acta Pathol Jpn* 1988;38:883–896.

85. Burke AP, Virmani R. Sarcomas of the great vessels. A clinicopathologic study. *Cancer* 1993;71:1761–1773.

86. Ko TM, Mayer DA, Tsapogas MJ, et al. Leiomyosarcoma of the pulmonary vein. *J Cardiovasc Surg (Torino)* 1996;37:421–423.

87. Leone O, Piana S, Cenacchi G, et al. Leiomyosarcoma of the pulmonary vein: case report with immunohistochemical and ultrastructural findings. *Gen Diagn Pathol* 1996;142:235–240.

88. Moffat RE, Chang CHJ, Slaven JE. Roentgen considerations in primary pulmonary artery sarcoma. *Radiology* 1972;104:283–288.

89. Britton PD. Primary pulmonary artery sarcoma—a report of two cases, with special emphasis on the diagnostic problems. *Clin Radiol* 1990;41:92–94.

90. Mussot S, Ghigna M, Mercier O, et al. Restrospective institutional study of 31 patients treated for pulmonary artery sarcoma. *Eu J Cardiothorac Surg* 2013;43: 787–793.

91. Mader MT, Poulton TB, White RD. Malignant tumors of the heart and great vessels: MR imaging appearance. *Radiographics* 1997;17:145–153.

92. Cox JE, Chiles C, Aquino SL, et al. Pulmonary artery sarcomas: a review of clinical and radiologic features. *J Comput Assist Tomogr* 1997;21:750–755.

93. Parish JM, Rosenow EC, Swensen SJ, et al. Pulmonary artery sarcoma. Clinical features. *Chest* 1996;110:1480–1488.

94. Simpson WL Jr, Mendelson DS. Pulmonary artery and aortic sarcomas: cross-sectional imaging. *J Thorac Imaging* 2000;15:290–294.

95. Head HD, Flam MS, John MJ, et al. Long-term palliation of pulmonary artery sarcoma by radical excision and adjuvant therapy. *Ann Thorac Surg* 1992;53:332–334.
96. Redmond ML, Shepard JW, Gaffey TA, et al. Primary pulmonary artery sarcoma. A method of resection. *Chest* 1990;98:752–753.
97. Kruger I, Borowski A, Horst M, et al. Symptoms, diagnosis, and therapy of primary sarcomas of the pulmonary artery. *Thorac Cardiovasc Surg* 1990;38:91–95.
98. Blackmon S, Rice D, Correa A, et al. Management of primary pulmonary artery sarcomas. *Ann Thorac Surg* 2009;87:977–984.
99. Wong H, Gounaris I, McCormack A, et al. Presentation and management of pulmonary artery sarcoma. *Clin Sarcoma Res* 2015;5:3.
100. Genoni M, Biraima AM, Bode B, et al. Combined resection and adjuvant therapy improves prognosis of sarcomas of the pulmonary trunk. *J Cardiovasc Surg (Torino)* 2001;42:829–833.
101. Mayer E, Kriegsmann J, Gaumann A, et al. Surgical treatment of pulmonary artery sarcoma. *J Thorac Cardiovasc Surg* 2001;121:77–82.
102. Thway K, Nicholson A, Lawson K, et al. Primary pulmonary myxoid sarcoma with EWSR1-CREB1 fusion: a new tumor entity. *Am J Surg Pathol* 2011;35:1722–1732.
103. Watson WL, Anlyan AJ. Primary leiomyosarcoma: a clinical evaluation of six cases. *Cancer* 1954;7:250–258.
104. Fadhli HA, Harrison AW, Shaddock SH. Primary pulmonary leiomyosarcoma. *Dis Chest* 1965;48:431–433.
105. Martini N, Hajdu SI, Beattie EJ Jr. Primary sarcoma of lung. *J Thorac Cardiovasc Surg* 1971;61:33–38.
106. Keel SB, Bacha E, Mark EJ, et al. Primary pulmonary sarcoma: a clinicopathologic study of 26 cases. *Mod Pathol* 1999;12:1124–1131.
107. Bacha EA, Wright CD, Grillo HC, et al. Surgical treatment of primary pulmonary sarcomas. *Eur J Cardiothorac Surg* 1999;15:456–460.
108. Magne N, Porsin B, Pivot X, et al. Primary lung sarcomas: long survivors obtained with iterative complete surgery. *Lung Cancer* 2001;31:241–245.
109. Guccion JG, Rosen SH. Bronchopulmonary leiomyosarcoma and fibrosarcoma: a study of 32 cases and review of the literature. *Cancer* 1972;30:836–847.
110. Nascimento AG, Unni KK, Bernatz PE. Sarcomas of the lung. *Mayo Clin Proc* 1982;57:355–359.
111. McLigeyo SO, Mbui J, Kungu A, et al. Fibrosarcoma of the lung with extrapulmonary manifestations: case report. *East Afr Med J* 1995;72:465–467.
112. Kuhnen C, Harms D, Niessen KH, et al. Congenital pulmonary fibrosarcoma. Differential diagnosis of infantile pulmonary spindle cell tumors [in German]. *Pathologe* 2001;22:151–156.
113. Picard E, Udassin R, Ramu N, et al. Pulmonary fibrosarcoma in childhood: fiber-optic bronchoscopic diagnosis and review of the literature. *Pediatr Pulmonol* 1999;27:347–350.
114. Goldthorn JF, Duncan MH, Kosloske AM, et al. Cavitating primary pulmonary fibrosarcoma in a child. *J Thorac Cardiovasc Surg* 1986;91:932–934.
115. Hancock BJ, Di Lorenzo M, Youssef S, et al. Childhood primary pulmonary neoplasms. *J Pediatr Surg* 1993;28:1133–1136.
116. Moran CA, Suster S, Abbondanzo SL, et al. Primary leiomyosarcomas of the lung: a clinicopathologic and immunohistochemical study of 18 cases. *Mod Pathol* 1997b;10:121–128.
117. Lillo-Gil R, Albrechtsson U, Jakobsson B. Pulmonary leiomyosarcoma appearing as a cyst. Report of one case and review of the literature. *Thorac Cardiovasc Surg* 1985;33:250–252.
118. Shimizu J, Sasaki M, Nakamura Y, et al. Simultaneous lung and liver resection for primary pulmonary leiomyosarcoma. *Respiration* 1997;64:179–181.
119. Weibe K. Extended pulmonary resection of advanced thoracic malignancies with support of cardiopulmonary bypass. *Eur J Cardiothorac Surg* 2006;29:571–577.
120. Byrne JG, Leacche M, Agnihotri AK, et al. The use of cardiopulmonary bypass during resection of locally advanced thoracic malignancies. *Chest* 2004;125:1581–1586.
121. Park J B, Bacchetta M, Bains MS, et al. Surgical management of thoracic malignancies invading the heart and great vessels. *Ann Thorac Surg* 2004;78:1024–1030.
122. Muscolino G, Bedini AV, Buffa PF. Leiomyosarcoma of the bronchus: report of two cases of resection with long-term follow-up. *J Thorac Cardiovasc Surg* 2000;119(4 part 1):853–854.
123. Przygodzki RM, Moran CA, Suster S, et al. Primary pulmonary rhabdomyosarcomas: a clinicopathologic and immunohistochemical study of three cases. *Mod Pathol* 1995;8:658–661.
124. Comin CE, Santucci M, Novelli L, et al. Primary pulmonary rhabdomyosarcoma: report of a case in an adult and review of the literature. *Ultrastruct Pathol* 2001;25:269–273.
125. d'Agostino S, Bonoldi E, Dante S, et al. Embryonal rhabdomyosarcoma of the lung arising in cystic adenomatoid malformation: case report and review of the literature. *J Pediatr Surg* 1997;32:1381–1383.
126. Schiavetti A, Dominici C, Matrunola M, et al. Primary pulmonary rhabdomyosarcoma in childhood: clinico-biologic features in two cases with review of the literature. *Med Pediatr Oncol* 1996;26:201–207.
127. McDermott VG, Mackenzie S, Hendry GM. Case report: primary intrathoracic rhabdomyosarcoma: a rare childhood malignancy. *Br J Radiol* 1993;66:937–941.
128. Noda T, Todani T, Watanabe Y, et al. Alveolar rhabdomyosarcoma of the lung in a child. *J Pediatr Surg* 1995;30:1607–1608.
129. Yousem SA, Hochholzer L. Malignant fibrous histiocytoma of the lung. *Cancer* 1987;60:2532–2541.
130. McDonnell T, Kyriakos M, Mazoujian G, et al. Malignant fibrous histiocytoma of the lung. *Cancer* 1988;61:137–145.
131. Halyard MY, Camoriano JK, Culligan JA, et al. Malignant fibrous histiocytoma of the lung. Report of four cases and review of the literature. *Cancer* 1996;78:2492–2497.
132. Hermann BL, Saller B, Kiess W, et al. Primary malignant fibrous histiocytoma of the lung: IGF-II producing tumor induces fasting hypoglycemia. *Exp Clin Endocrinol Diabetes* 2000;108:515–518.
133. Tian D, Yin H, Zhao H, et al. Results of surgical treatment of primary pulmonary malignant fibrous histiocytoma. *J Jpn Assoc Chest Surg* 1997;11:631.
134. Saga K, Sato T, Abiko M, et al. A case of primary malignant fibrous histiocytoma of the lung (in Japanese). *Kyobu Geka* 2001;54:191–194.
135. Lane KL, Shannon RJ, Weiss SW. Hyalinizing spindle cell tumor with giant rosettes: a distinctive tumor closely resembling low-grade fibromyxoid sarcoma. *Am J Surg Pathol* 1997;21:1481–1488.
136. Morgan AD, Salama FD. Primary chondrosarcoma of the lung. Case report and review of the literature. *J Thorac Cardiovasc Surg* 1972;64:460–466.
137. Colby TV, Koss MN, Travis WD. Miscellaneous mesenchymal tumors. In *Atlas of Tumor Pathology, Tumors of the Lower Respiratory Tract*. Fascicle 13. Third Series. Washington, DC: Armed Forces Institute of Pathology; 1995:384.
138. Parker LA, Molina PL, Bignault AG, et al. Primary pulmonary chondrosarcoma mimicking bronchogenic cyst on CT and MRI. *Clin Imaging* 1996;20:181–183.
139. Morgenroth A, Pfeuffer HP, Viereck HJ, et al. Primary chondrosarcoma of the left inferior lobar bronchus. *Respiration* 1989;56:241–244.
140. Hayashi T, Tsuda N, Iseki M, et al. Primary chondrosarcoma of the lung. A clinico-pathologic study. *Cancer* 1993;72:69–74.
141. Huang H-Y, Hsieh MJ, Chen WJ, et al. Primary mesenchymal chondrosarcoma of the lung. *Ann Thorac Surg* 2002;73:1960–1962.
142. Kurotaki H, Tateoka H, Takeuchi M, et al. Primary mesenchymal chondrosarcoma of the lung. A case report with immunohistochemical and ultrastructural studies. *Acta Pathol Jpn* 1992;42:364–371.
143. Loose JH, El-Naggar AK, Ro JY, et al. Primary osteosarcoma of the lung. Report of two cases and review of the literature. *J Thorac Cardiovasc Surg* 1990;100:867–873.
144. Petersen M. Radionuclide detection of primary pulmonary osteogenic sarcoma: a case report and review of the literature. *J Nucl Med* 1990;31:1110–1114.
145. Connolly JP, McGuyer CA, Sageman WS, et al. Intrathoracic osteosarcoma diagnosed by CT scan and pleural biopsy. *Chest* 1991;100:265–267.
146. Bhalla M, Thompson BG, Harley RA, et al. Primary extraosseous pulmonary osteogenic sarcoma: CT findings. *J Comput Assist Tomogr* 1992;16:974–976.
147. Chapman AD, Pritchard SC, Yap WW, et al. Primary pulmonary osteosarcoma: case report and molecular analysis. *Cancer* 2001;91:779–784.
148. Krygier G, Amado A, Salisbury S, et al. Primary lung liposarcoma. *Lung Cancer* 1997;17:271–275.
149. Hochberg L, Crastnopol P. Primary sarcoma of the bronchus and lung. *Arch Surg* 1956;73:74–98.
150. Roviaro G, Montorsi MA, Varoli FE, et al. Primary pulmonary tumours of neurogenic origin. *Thorax* 1983;38:942–945.
151. Rowlands D, Edwards C, Collins F. Malignant melanotic schwannoma of the bronchus. *J Clin Pathol* 1987;40:1449–1455.
152. McCluggage WG, Bharucha H. Primary pulmonary tumors of nerve sheath origin. *Histopathology* 1995;26:247–254.
153. Cooney TP. Primary pulmonary ganglioneuroblastoma in an adult: maturation, involution and the immune response. *Histopathology* 1981;5:451–463.
154. Hochholzer L, Moran CA, Koss MN. Primary pulmonary ganglioneuroblastoma: a clinicopathologic and immunohistochemical study of two cases. *Ann Diagn Pathol* 1998;2:154–158.
155. Moran CA, Suster S, Koss MN. Primary malignant "triton" tumour of the lung. *Histopathology* 1997;30:140–144.
156. Domizio P, Liesner RJ, Mireaux CD, et al. Malignant mesenchymoma associated with a congenital lung cyst in a child: case report and review of the literature. *Pediatr Pathol* 1990;10:785–797.
157. Koss MN. Pulmonary lymphoid disorders. *Semin Diagn Pathol* 1995;12:158–171.
158. Ferraro P, Trastek VF, Adlakha H, et al. Primary non-Hodgkin's lymphoma of the lung. *Ann Thorac Surg* 2000;69:993–997.
159. Parissis H. Forty years literature review of primary lung lymphoma. *J Cardiothorac Surg* 2011;6:23.
160. Cadranel J, Wislez M, Antoine M. Primary pulmonary lymphoma. *Eur Respir J* 2002;20:750–762.
161. Kim J, Lee S, Park J, et al. Primary Pulmonary Non-Hodgkin's Lymphoma. *Jpn J Clin Oncol* 2004;34:510–514.
162. Kurtin PJ, Myers JL, Adlakha H, et al. Pathologic and clinical features of primary pulmonary extranodal marginal zone B-cell lymphoma of MALT type. *Am J Surg Pathol* 2001;25:997–1008.
163. King LJ, Padley SP, Wotherspoon AC, et al. Pulmonary MALT lymphoma: imaging findings in 24 cases. *Eur Radiol* 2000;10:1932–1938.
164. Koss MN, Hochholzer L, Nichols PW, et al. Primary non-Hodgkin's lymphoma and pseudolymphoma of the lung: a study of 161 patients. *Hum Pathol* 1983;14:1024–1038.
165. Kennedy JL, Nathwani BN, Burke JS, et al. Pulmonary lymphomas and other pulmonary lymphoid lesions. A clinicopathologic and immunologic study of 64 patients. *Cancer* 1985;56:539–552.
166. Fiche M, Capron F, Berger F, et al. Primary pulmonary non-Hodgkin's lymphomas. *Histopathology* 1995;26:529.
167. Stefanovic A, Morgensztern D, Fong T, et al. Pulmonary marginal zone lymphoma: A single centre experience and review of the SEER database. *Leuk Lymphoma* 2008;49:1311–1320.
168. Graham BB, Mathisen DJ, Mark EJ, et al. Primary pulmonary lymphoma. *Ann Thorac Surg* 2008;80:1248–1253.

169. Zinzani P, Pellegrini C, Gandolfi L, et al. Extranodal marginal zone B-cell lymphoma of the lung: experience with fludarabine and mitoxantrone-containing regimens. *Hematol Oncol* 2013;31:183–188.

170. Toh HC, Ang PT. Primary pulmonary lymphoma—clinical review from a single institution in Singapore. *Leuk Lymph* 1997;27:153–163.

171. Tamura A, Komatsu H, Yanai N, et al. Primary pulmonary lymphoma: relationship between clinical features and pathologic findings in 24 cases. The Japan National Chest Hospital Study Group for Lung Cancer. *Jpn J Clin Oncol* 1995;25:140–152.

172. L'Hoste RJ, Filippa DA, Lieberman PH, et al. Primary pulmonary lymphomas. A clinicopathologic analysis of 36 cases. *Cancer* 1984;54:1397–1406.

173. Cordier JF, Chailleux E, Lauque D, et al. Primary pulmonary lymphomas. A clinical study of 70 cases in nonimmunocompromised patients. *Chest* 1993;103:201–208.

174. Ray P, Antoine M, Mary-Krause M, et al. AIDS-related primary pulmonary lymphoma. *Am J Respir Crit Care Med* 1998;158:1221–1229.

175. Jennings TA, Axiotis CA, Kress Y, et al. Primary malignant melanoma of the lower respiratory tract. Report of a case and literature review. *Am J Clin Pathol* 1990;94:649–655.

176. Marchevsky AM. Lung tumors derived from ectopic tissues. *Semin Diagn Pathol* 1995;12:172–184.

177. Wilson RW, Moran CA. Primary melanoma of the lung: a clinicopathologic and immunohistochemical study of eight cases. *Am J Surg Pathol* 1997;21:1196–1202.

178. Ost D, Joseph C, Sogoloff H, et al. Primary pulmonary melanoma: case report and literature review. *Mayo Clin Proc* 1999;74:62–66.

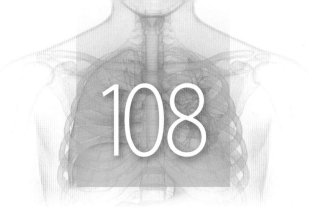

108

Pulmonary Metastases

Paul E. Y. Van Schil ▪ Willem Adriaan den Hengst ▪ Mark S. Allen ▪ Joe B. Putnam, Jr.

Secondary tumors to the lung represent lung metastases from a primary tumor inside or outside the chest. They are a manifestation of systemic disease, and secondary lymph node involvement may also occur heralding a poor prognosis. The role of surgery for lung metastases remains controversial as there are no large randomized trials showing a survival advantage for patients undergoing surgical resection.[1] On the other hand, in surgical series the best long-term survival is obtained compared with other treatment modalities or conservative management, but the question remains whether this is solely due to selection bias or whether there is a real survival benefit. What is clear from surgical series is that complete resection yields the best overall and disease-free survival but this can only be obtained in a minority of patients presenting with lung metastases. In case of resectable lung metastases, 5-year survival rates of 30% to 40% may generally be obtained.[2] However, a substantial number of patients will develop recurrent disease inside the chest demonstrating that micrometastases that go undetected at the initial procedure will determine long-term outcome.

As currently high-grade evidence is lacking, every patient with pulmonary metastases should be discussed within an experienced, multidisciplinary team, and best available treatment should be determined on an individual basis. Surgery, radiotherapy, or combined modality treatment is indicated in selected cases. As lung metastases may occur in a younger patient population compared to primary lung cancer, a lot of effort is currently made to improve long-term results and new treatment modalities are developed.

In this chapter, history of surgery for lung metastases is briefly described followed by pathology, symptoms, diagnosis, and specific treatment modalities with main emphasis on surgical techniques and results. Subsequently, specific histologic types of primary tumors in adults and children are addressed as well as recurrent pulmonary metastases. Prognostic factors are analyzed and lastly, promising novel treatment strategies are discussed.

HISTORICAL PERSPECTIVE

Probably, the first case of documented lung metastases dates from 1786 described in the *Case Books* of John Hunter.[3] The primary cancer was a malignant tumor of the femur and the patient died of widespread pulmonary deposits only 7 weeks after the leg was amputated. A sublobar resection for a metastasis of a sarcoma of the leg was reported in 1927 by Tudor Edwards.[4] The patient had undergone amputation of the leg 6 years earlier at the Royal Brompton Hospital in London. A famous case is described by Barney and Churchill who reported one of the first long-term survivors of pulmonary

metastasectomy after resection of a metastasis from a patient with metastatic renal cell cancer.[5] After nephrectomy for local control of the primary tumor, the patient underwent resection of the metastasis. The operation took place in 1933 and the patient survived for 23 years eventually dying of an unrelated cause. Alexander and Haight reviewed the first large series (25 patients) of those who had resection of metastases from carcinoma and sarcoma.[6] They concluded that patients who could withstand the resection and in whom no other metastases were evident could undergo resection. Mannix described in 1953, for the first time, resection of multiple pulmonary metastases from a patient with osteochondroma of the tibia.[7] Only one nodule was identified on the preoperative chest radiograph. In 1965 N. Thomford had already published a series of 205 patients who underwent pulmonary metastasectomy.[8] A surprisingly 5-year survival rate of 30.3% was reported, which is similar to results today.

Few attempts were made at multiple or repetitive resections for pulmonary metastases until Martini and colleagues in 1971 described the value of resecting multiple metastases and the associated survival advantage of multiple resections (multiple sequential operations) for treatment of osteogenic sarcoma.[9] Selection criteria have been proposed by many; however, Putnam and Roth noted that unresectability may be the sole exclusion criterion.[10] Resections of solitary and multiple pulmonary metastases from numerous primary neoplasms have been performed with long-term survival in 20% to 40% of patients, as shown by Pastorino and colleagues.[2]

Autopsy studies have demonstrated that about one-third of patients with cancer die with pulmonary metastases and that a small percentage die with metastases confined solely to the lungs. Metastases from osteogenic and soft tissue sarcomas commonly occur only in the lungs, as shown by Potter and colleagues.[11] Less commonly, patients with other solid organ neoplasms from melanoma, breast, or colon have isolated pulmonary metastases, but these metastases may represent favorable tumor biology and a treatable subset of such patients. In the absence of extrathoracic metastases, patients with isolated and resectable pulmonary metastases should undergo complete resection in an attempt to prolong survival although no high-grade evidence is available. Even in the presence of extrathoracic metastases as, for example, synchronous liver and lung metastases from a colorectal cancer, selected individual patients with complete resection may have a survival advantage. Limitations on the number of metastases resected with benefit have not as yet been determined; however, the greater the number of radiographically identified metastases before resection, or the larger the number palpated in the operating room, the greater likelihood that micrometastases exist and that the lesions are unresectable (Fig. 108.1). Early and potentially aggressive recurrence is likely. Multidisciplinary evaluation

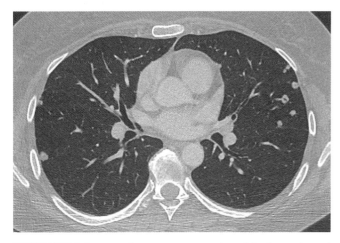

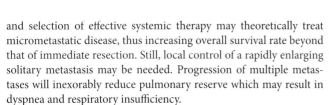

FIGURE 108.1 Patient with numerous metastatic nodules from colorectal cancer. Due to diffuse pulmonary involvement this patient was considered to be inoperable.

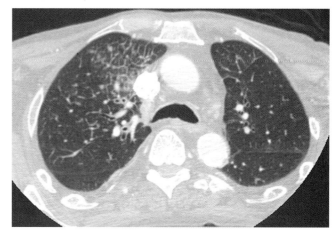

FIGURE 108.2 Patient with carcinomatous lymphangitis, most pronounced on the right side.

and selection of effective systemic therapy may theoretically treat micrometastatic disease, thus increasing overall survival rate beyond that of immediate resection. Still, local control of a rapidly enlarging solitary metastasis may be needed. Progression of multiple metastases will inexorably reduce pulmonary reserve which may result in dyspnea and respiratory insufficiency.

PATHOLOGY

Malignant tumors may metastasize by hematogenous, lymphatic, and aerogenous routes or by direct invasion. Underlying tumor biology and host resistance determine mechanisms of spread, location of metastases, and extent of growth. Hematogenous metastases are most frequently found in the capillary beds of the lung, liver, brain, and bone. Clumps of tumor cells that metastasize to the lung parenchyma may be trapped or preferentially adhere to the underlying capillary endothelium. A complicated tumor–host interaction occurs and most of these tumor emboli die; however, some may permeate the endothelium and grow. Tumor cells may travel by lymphatics and occupy a discrete position within the lung parenchyma, or they may diffusely involve the entire lung (e.g., lymphangitic spread of breast carcinoma or other metastatic adenocarcinomas) (Fig. 108.2). Depending on the primary histology (usually related to adenocarcinoma or squamous cell carcinoma primary tumors), metastases can develop in draining pulmonary lobar, hilar, or mediastinal nodes heralding a poor prognosis. Direct invasion of metastases into other structures may occur as the metastasis grows. Resection of the pulmonary metastasis and the contiguous structure is recommended. Putnam and colleagues noted that extended resection may achieve local control and survival benefit if complete resection of metastases can be achieved with negative margins.[12] Finally, aerogenous spread of tumor from one site within the lung to another may occur and recent data show that this mechanism is probably underrecognized. In primary lung adenocarcinoma this has been described as "spread through alveolar spaces" or STAS.[13] Imaging features are found to be helpful to differentiate aerogenous spread from hematogenous and lymphatic metastases.[14] It should also be recognized that many tumors are largely heterogeneous and that, within a specific tumor, clonal evolution may occur resulting in subclones with newly acquired genetic alterations and mutations giving rise to "many tumors in one" with different metastatic potentials.[15] Chen

and colleagues evaluated EGFR mutation heterogeneity and found the highest discordance rate in patients with multiple pulmonary nodules which might explain the mixed tumor response to tyrosine kinase inhibitors.[16] To make it even more complex, Sardari Nia et al. demonstrated that different growth patterns may be present between the primary tumor and distant metastases.[17] In a study of 24 patients with lung metastases from a clear cell renal cancer a non-angiogenic, alveolar growth pattern adopting the local vasculature was detected in 33% of cases which might explain resistance to antiangiogenic therapy.

SYMPTOMS

Symptoms rarely occur from pulmonary metastases. Therefore diagnosis of metastases is routinely made on follow-up imaging after primary tumor resection. Palliation for pain is rarely needed because the parietal pleura is infrequently involved by parenchymal metastases. A distinction must be made between pleural-based and parenchymal-based metastases before resection. Few (<5%) patients with metastases present with symptoms of dyspnea, pain, cough, or hemoptysis. Bocklage and colleagues noted that patients with metastases from angiosarcoma would present with these symptoms, having lasted from a few weeks to months.[18] Rarely, patients with peripheral sarcomatous metastases may develop pneumothorax from disruption of the peripheral pulmonary parenchyma. Srinivas and Varadhachary have suggested that patients with a primary malignancy and a pneumothorax should be evaluated for lung metastases.[19]

DIAGNOSIS

Pulmonary metastases may appear on imaging examinations as solitary or multiple nodules and as well-circumscribed or diffuse opacities; they may be miliary or massive in appearance, as described by Snyder and Pugatch.[20] Still, the radiographic findings of patients with pulmonary nodules may be nonspecific and represent a wide spectrum of benign or malignant processes. The surgeon must consider other, more locally related diagnoses such as histoplasmosis, tuberculosis, or other malignant diseases such as lung cancer in these patients. There are no pathognomonic radiographic criteria for metastatic disease. However, multiple, small, well-circumscribed peripheral nodules in the patient with a known primary malignancy are very likely to be metastatic disease. The Fleischner Society published specific guidelines for management of small solid nodules and, more recently, also evaluation of subsolid lesions.[21,22] A practical algorithmic approach to diagnosis and management of solitary pulmonary nodules was described by Patel and colleagues.[23,24]

In the Lung Metastasectomy Project established by the European Society of Thoracic Surgeons (ESTS), imaging requirements for patients with lung metastases were proposed.[25] Due to its high sensitivity, computed tomography (CT) is considered the standard imaging modality for evaluation of pulmonary nodules. A helical CT scan with 3- to 5-mm reconstruction thickness is recommended and it should be performed within 4 weeks of pulmonary metastasectomy. If positron emission tomography (PET) is available, it is mainly recommended to detect extrathoracic metastatic sites especially if there is a high uptake of the fluorodeoxyglucose (FDG) isotope in the primary tumor. In approximately 10% to 15% of patients extrathoracic involvement may be detected which will change management strategy. In a survey of current practice amongst ESTS members published by Internullo and colleagues in 2008, helical CT is most frequently used (74%) while PET scanning is used as an additional examination in less than 50%.[26]

High-resolution CT of the chest may achieve resolution of pulmonary abnormalities 2 to 3 mm in diameter. Metastases may appear at this size, but also sequelae of infections such as granulomas or other pulmonary parenchymal changes may produce these small indeterminate lesions. In some countries granulomatous disease from histoplasmosis is prevalent and clinical correlation with the radiographic size and number of the lesions, location, and physical and radiographic characteristics must be considered.

The accuracy of chest CT in detecting pulmonary metastases was evaluated by Parsons et al. in two studies.[27,28] In the most recent one, 53 patients underwent 60 pulmonary metastasectomies. Adequate clinical history and focused documentation on helical CT were available. Preoperative helical CT was entirely correct in 19% of cases meaning that there were no missed metastases or false-positive lesions. In total, metastases were missed by CT in 46% of cases. A similar study was performed by Althagafi and colleagues who reported 215 pulmonary metastasectomies performed by thoracotomy with careful lung palpation.[29] The number of nodules found on preoperative CT was compared to the final number of lesions on the pathology report. Ipsilateral, non-imaged malignant lung metastases were found in 36% of cases and the number was highest for mesenchymal tumors. These studies demonstrate that manual lung palpation by an open approach is still required when a complete resection of all detectable lung metastases is the final aim. This is also advocated by the Lung Metastasectomy Working Group.[25]

Magnetic resonance imaging (MRI) may be as sensitive as CT for identifying pulmonary metastases, but it adds little additional information, as observed by Feuerstein and Wyttenbach and their colleagues.[30,31] MRI is not routinely recommended for evaluation of patients with pulmonary metastases limited to the pulmonary parenchyma but it may provide complementary information to CT in planning resection for metastases involving the posterior mediastinum, neural foramina, or great vessels, as recommended by Wyttenbach and colleagues.[31]

Franzius and colleagues compared FDG PET with helical chest CT to detect pulmonary metastases arising from malignant bone tumors.[32] FDG PET had a sensitivity of 50%, a specificity of 98%, and an accuracy of 87%, compared with spiral chest CT of 75%, 100%, and 94%, respectively. The authors concluded that helical chest CT is superior to FDG PET in detecting pulmonary metastases from primary bone tumors.

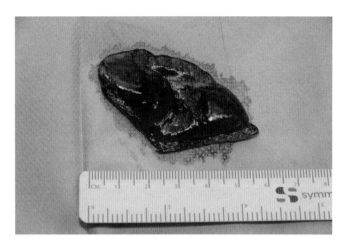

FIGURE 108.3 Wedge excision in a patient with presumed lung metastasis from colorectal cancer. Pathology showed intrapulmonary lymph node.

In a review by Fortes and colleagues of 84 patients who underwent 106 resections, at least one nodule was PET-positive in 68%.[33] The true-positive rate was 66.6% and the false-negative rate was 33.3% for all nodules. Veronesi and colleagues noted that glucose uptake by FDG PET and angiogenesis were independent biologic features in patients with pulmonary metastasis from the various neoplasms and that this may suggest future antiangiogenic therapies.[34]

Benign granulomatous diseases may mimic metastases; however, in patients with a prior diagnosis of malignancy, new and multiple nodules are most likely metastases. Fine-needle aspiration or thoracoscopic wedge excision may be helpful for diagnosis or staging of pulmonary nodules in high-risk patients (Fig. 108.3). Clinical stage I or II primary nonsmall-cell lung cancer (NSCLC) may be indistinguishable from a solitary metastasis, particularly if the original tumor was squamous cell carcinoma or adenocarcinoma. For these two histologies specifically or in patients in whom an NSCLC cannot be excluded, lobectomy and a systematic mediastinal lymph node dissection, provided the patient has sufficient pulmonary reserve, would be a procedure of choice. In patients with lymphangitic spread of cancer and dyspnea, biopsy may be required to differentiate neoplasm from infection.

Although helical chest CT is considered the standard examination, the surgeon must select the radiographic imaging or scanning techniques that will provide the necessary and complete clinical information required for treatment-planning decisions. Woodard and colleagues have suggested several factors that may influence the surgeon's choice of radiographic studies.[35] These factors include (a) identifying the size, location, and characteristics of pulmonary nodules or metastases; (b) characterizing the solitary squamous cell carcinoma (or adenocarcinoma) metastasis from a primary NSCLC; (c) evaluating for extrathoracic metastatic disease (other sites of hematogenous spread, metastasis to regional lymph nodes, or other tumors); and (d) evaluating the potential for local invasion.

METASTASIS OR PRIMARY BRONCHIAL CARCINOMA

Pulmonary metastases from sarcomas or other distinctive nonpulmonary neoplasms are easy to diagnose. Solitary carcinomatous metastasis from breast or colon cancers and squamous cell carcinoma metastasis from head and neck primary tumors are more difficult to distinguish from primary lung carcinoma. Patients with ≥2 pulmonary nodules can be considered to have metastases. Treatment may be similar. In tumors without a propensity for bilaterality (e.g., nonsarcomatous histology), a unilateral approach may be optimal.

Historically, a comparison of the primary neoplasm and the lung nodule using light microscopy has been the only method for determining origin of the lung nodule or neoplasm. Electron microscopy, as studied by Herrera and colleagues, or specific molecular or genetic characteristics may identify the origin of these neoplasms more precisely.[36] Monoclonal antibodies may assist in discriminating between primary bronchial adenocarcinoma and colon carcinoma metastatic to the lung, as described by Ghoneim and colleagues.[37] Comprehensive histologic assessment may be helpful to differentiate multiple lung primaries from metastatic disease as described by Girard and colleagues.[38]

To determine the nature of the new pulmonary nodules, Lefor and colleagues developed algorithms for patients with squamous cell carcinoma of the head and neck region who developed such nodules after treatment.[39] Characteristics of metastases and of primary lung carcinoma were examined in an attempt to better direct subsequent therapy. Yet since the genotype of malignant tumors is unstable, a definitive molecular technique to differentiate metastases from a primary tumor is not available. Clinical judgment is useful in these circumstances.

TREATMENT OF PULMONARY METASTASES

Most patients with pulmonary metastases have multiple sites of metastases or unresectable pleural or pulmonary metastases. In these patients, treatment is directed systemically for control of the disease and to palliate symptoms. Although radiation therapy or chemotherapy is frequently used, inconsistent response rarely leads to control or cure. Chemotherapy as initial therapy for these "systemic metastases" and resection as "salvage" may provide better results than resection alone. Where the primary tumor is controlled and metastases are confined to the lungs, resection of all visualized or palpable metastases may be considered. Complete resection of isolated pulmonary metastases is generally associated with improved survival regardless of primary histology, although no high-level evidence from controlled trials is currently available. A randomized trial in patients with pulmonary metastases from colorectal carcinoma is currently open for inclusion randomizing patients between surgery and conservative management when they are in a grey transition zone defined by the presence of several metastases or a short disease-free interval (DFI).[40]

CHEMOTHERAPY

Chemotherapy has not been used routinely for treatment of resectable pulmonary metastases. However, with the exception of the patient with only one metastasis or with a few metastases and a long DFI, occult micrometastases may commonly exist. For example, in sarcomas, control of the primary tumor may be achieved in various ways; however, later occurrence of pulmonary metastases from existing micrometastases at the time of control of the primary results in decreased survival compared with patients who do not have occult metastases. Even with multiple resections, complete eradication of all micrometastases may be unachievable. Use of chemotherapy or other targeted therapies to assist in the control of micrometastases may be valuable for systemic control, which may enhance the local control achieved by resection. The traditional measure of post-resection survival and post-resection

disease-free survival may be inadequate when resection is considered as salvage after chemotherapy for pulmonary metastases. A more fitting measure of survival should include "survival from diagnosis including radiologic diagnosis of metastases." The duration of chemotherapy, the extent of response, the histology of the primary malignancy, and the fitness of the patient all affect the timing of resection and potentially long-term outcomes.

Over the last decades, the survival rate in patients with osteosarcoma has improved from 20% to approximately 60% to 70%. Limb-sparing procedures have replaced amputation. Neoadjuvant chemotherapy with a variety of agents has been instituted. The incidence of pulmonary metastases in patients with primary osteogenic sarcoma treated with surgical resection and adjuvant chemotherapy has dramatically declined compared with treatment of the primary osteogenic sarcoma with surgery alone, as shown by Skinner, Goorin, and Pastorino and their colleagues.[41–43] Hirota and colleagues have observed that newer agents are increasingly being incorporated into chemotherapeutic strategies.[44] Nonetheless, Ferguson and colleagues confirmed that relapse still remains a significant problem in these patients.[45] In their report, carboplatin as induction therapy was followed by resection and postoperative multidrug chemotherapy in 37 patients. No patient had a complete response. Patients with metastases confined to the lungs were more likely to survive than were patients with distant bone metastases. Salvage treatment with resection alone for pulmonary metastasis generates an actuarial survival rate of only about 30%. Salvage chemotherapy with resection may be effective in prolonging survival in patients who develop pulmonary metastases from osteogenic sarcoma, as described by Marina and Pastorino and their colleagues.[46,47] However, more effective systemic therapies are necessary.

The results of preoperative chemotherapy (high-dose methotrexate, cisplatin, doxorubicin, and ifosfamide) followed by surgery and additional postoperative chemotherapy have been examined. Goorin and colleagues found that the combination of etoposide and high-dose ifosfamide as an induction regimen for patients with pulmonary metastasis from osteosarcoma can be effective despite significant myelosuppression, infection, and renal toxicity.[48] Bacci and colleagues noted that in 16 patients chemotherapy was given, followed by simultaneous resection of the primary and metastatic tumors.[49] Complete resection was accomplished in 15 patients. However, five patients died within a few months as a result of undetectable metastatic disease. Survival was strongly correlated with the chemotherapy effects (necrosis) in the primary tumor and in the metastases. Improved survival with combined modality therapy (chemotherapy followed by salvage surgery) was achieved compared with historic results.

Salah and Toubasi recently reported a series of 25 patients with metastatic osteosarcoma who achieved complete remission following resection of lung metastases.[50] Most patients received peri-operative chemotherapy. Five-year overall survival rate was 30%. Negative prognostic factors in univariate analysis included chondroblastic subtype, post-chemotherapy necrosis <90%, metastasis detected during neoadjuvant or adjuvant chemotherapy, and visceral pleural invasion. In multivariate analysis only chondroblastic subtype was significant.[50]

Chemotherapy alone may be insufficient. Jaffe and colleagues examined the role of chemotherapy in 31 patients with osteogenic sarcoma.[51] Only three patients were cured with chemotherapy alone, while four patients underwent resection. No viable tumor was found in the resected mass. New therapies are needed for better treatment of osteogenic sarcoma. Until then, combinations of chemotherapy and local control (resection) will be needed. Glasser and colleagues noted that histologic response to chemotherapy (percentage of necrosis) was the only independent predictor of enhanced survival in a study of 279 patients with stage II osteogenic sarcoma.[52]

Based on the effects of chemotherapy in the treatment of primary sarcoma, the effective use of such chemotherapy as planned induction therapy before resection of metastatic disease remains more elusive. Lanza and colleagues examined the response of soft tissue sarcoma metastases that were treated with chemotherapy before surgery.[53] Patients were graded as having complete, partial, or no response or progression from the chemotherapy. Survival could not be predicted based on response to chemotherapy alone.

An optimal therapeutic strategy may be to combine systemic and local control, particularly in those patients with recurrent disease (pulmonary metastasis). Chemotherapeutic agents with activity in primary soft tissue sarcoma are limited. According to Benjamin and Patel and their colleagues, doxorubicin and ifosfamide are the two most active chemotherapeutic agents for soft tissue sarcoma and have a positive dose–response profile.[54,55] Resection of pulmonary metastases after optimizing response to chemotherapy may enhance overall local and systemic control, resulting in improvements in overall and disease-free survival. This therapeutic model appears to provide a synergistic benefit over and above that which can be achieved with either surgery alone or with chemotherapy alone. Doxorubicin and ifosfamide have been used in a dose-intensive manner with resulting improved response rates, decreased time to progression, and improved survival, particularly in patients treated for higher-risk primary extremity soft tissue sarcoma. This regime for pulmonary metastases from soft tissue sarcoma provides similar survival benefits to regimes for other malignancies. Patients with a biologic response to chemotherapy before resection may have some benefit in receiving the same combination of chemotherapy after resection. Newer, non-doxorubicin-based regimes include gemcitabine and docetaxel; ifosfamide and etoposide; and lastly, cyclophosphamide and topotecan.[56] In a series of 66 patients with high-grade extremity and truncal soft tissue sarcomas treated with peri-operative chemotherapy, negative margins were obtained in 89% of cases.[57] Distant 5-year recurrence-free survival was 64%. A recent review concluded that in patients with localized soft tissue sarcoma who have a likelihood of recurrent disease, systemic therapy should be strongly considered.[56] In this way, response evaluation to induction chemotherapy becomes possible tailoring subsequent therapy.

Other characteristics may suggest effectiveness or lack of effectiveness for various chemotherapeutic agents. Dhaini and colleagues evaluated human P450 isoenzymes, specifically CYP3A4/5, which aid in the metabolism and detoxification of carcinogens and chemotherapy.[58] The authors found that patients with distant metastases were more likely to have elevated expression of CYP3A4/5 within the primary tumor biopsy specimen than patients without metastatic disease ($p = 0.0004$). The authors concluded that high levels of this human cytochrome P450 isoenzyme may be a marker to predict metastases or limited survival in patients with primary osteogenic sarcoma. Cyclooxygenase II (COX-II) enzyme levels did not correlate with primary or metastatic disease and survival, as noted by Dickens and colleagues.[59]

A recommended practice is to consider patients with soft tissue sarcoma with one or two isolated lung lesions based on high-resolution CT of the chest and a long DFI for immediate surgery. For patients with more than two lesions, chemotherapy (adriamycin, ifosfamide) could be used to assess a biologic response. When maximal response has been achieved, resection can be performed followed by additional chemotherapy. For initially unresectable metastases, chemotherapy may provide a response sufficient to allow surgical resection, after which additional chemotherapy may be considered.

If chemotherapy is unsuccessful, surgery may be considered for palliation of symptoms. In marginal patients in whom chemotherapy provided only a minimal response or no change, surgery may be considered for local control of the metastases. Occasionally, metastases may grow to enormous size, compressing the heart and mediastinum (a "tumor thorax" or "tumor tamponade") with the same consequences of tension pneumothorax or hemothorax. Chemotherapy is not commonly effective in this situation, given the need for urgent mechanical intervention. A heroic attempt at resection may be required but is infrequently performed.

RADIATION THERAPY

Although initially radiation therapy was used to palliate symptoms of advanced metastases (e.g., extensive pleural involvement, bone metastases), over the last decade new sophisticated techniques have been introduced which allow precise application of high doses of oligofractionated radiotherapy. Techniques similar to stereotactic brain radiotherapy are currently applied to primary lung cancer and lung metastases.[60] As high doses are precisely delivered to the tumor, this is also called "ablative" radiotherapy. However, in specific regions as the bases of the lower lobes, control of tumor motion during respiration is critical. Several methods have been developed to achieve this as breath holding, abdominal compression devices, respiratory gating, and tumor-tracking systems.

In a recent review, Shultz and colleagues addressed the current role of stereotactic radiotherapy for pulmonary oligometastases and oligometastatic lung cancer.[60] For oligometastatic disease 1-year local control rates of 70% to 95% are reported with 1- or 2-year progression-free survival rates ranging from 25% to 70%. However, no global recommendations can be made as most series include a heterogeneous spectrum of primary tumors. Different radiation schedules were used resulting in quite variable outcomes. Precise response evaluation is difficult to evaluate but for surgical series, number of metastases and DFI seem to be important.

Several concerns remain when applying these newer techniques to the lung parenchyma: precise histology is not always obtained limiting the validity of the results, thorough lymph node evaluation is not performed, and response criteria have not been precisely defined.[61] As radiotherapy induces an inflammatory reaction in the irradiated field, criteria are difficult to determine, especially when PET scanning is used to judge response. So currently, metastasectomy is still considered the standard therapeutic option on the condition that a complete resection can be obtained. Stereotactic radiotherapy and other local treatment modalities as radiofrequency ablation are mainly reserved for patients who are functionally or technically unresectable, those with recurrent disease after a previous resection, and those with incomplete resection or positive margins.[60] In some patients with recurrent or progressive local disease after stereotactic radiotherapy, the so-called "salvage" surgery may be considered.[62]

SURGERY

In selected patients with resectable pulmonary metastases and absence of extrathoracic metastases, complete resection is generally associated with improved long-term survival regardless of histology. In even more highly selected patients with extrathoracic metastases controlled or resected, excision of isolated pulmonary metastases may be considered to remove all known disease. An example of such a patient is one with colorectal carcinoma who has previously had hepatic metastases resected and is now discovered to have pulmonary metastases. In these patients, the thoracic surgeon may take advantage of the tumor biology, which limits metastases to the liver and lung. These patients have enhanced long-term survival compared with those with unresectable metastases. However, this may be partly due to patient selection as no randomized controlled trials are available, clearly demonstrating a survival advantage of surgery.[1]

SELECTION OF PATIENTS FOR RESECTION

Patients with isolated pulmonary metastases may be selected for resection. Clinical criteria have been proposed to identify and select patients who can benefit optimally from resection of their pulmonary metastases by McCormack, Mountain, and Pastorino and their colleagues as well as by Putnam and Roth[2,10,63,64] (Table 108.1). Unfortunately, most patients with metastases do not benefit from surgery because of one or more of the following reasons: (a) a biologically aggressive tumor characterized by extensive disease, (b) a short DFI between control of their primary tumor and identification of pulmonary metastases, and (c) rapid metastatic growth.

In patients being considered for resection, physical examination, radiographic examination, and physiologic assessment are performed to estimate the extent of resection and determine whether the planned procedure may be safely performed. Extensive cardiac and pulmonary assessments are emphasized, especially in patients with bilateral disease or recurrent metastases after a previous operation. In patients with preoperative chemotherapy or in those in whom pulmonary compromise is expected, a spectrum of pulmonary function tests are performed. These tests include spirometry with and without bronchodilators, diffusion capacity for carbon monoxide (DL_{CO}), and oxygen consumption testing ($\dot{V}o_2$). Echocardiography and an exercise stress test may also be needed.

In the operating room, the latest chest CT scan is displayed prominently. After bronchoscopy, a double-lumen endotracheal tube is placed and used for anesthetic gas delivery. The operated lung is deflated followed by careful manual palpation. All suspicious nodules are identified and subsequently removed. Every nodule is resected with a margin of normal tissue. Nodules should not be "shelled out" because viable tumor cells remain on the periphery of the resected area. The margin should be adequate. Even when the margin is negative, microscopic cells may remain. Higashiyama and colleagues prospectively evaluated 51 patients with pulmonary metastases with an intraoperative lavage cytology technique for the surgical margin.[65] They found that 11% of patients had a positive cytology at the margin despite having a rim of normal tissue. Additional tissue was then resected. Localized micrometastases may be present in some patients despite a macroscopically negative margin. This may contribute to subsequent local recurrence. In general, the decision as to the adequacy of margin is the surgeon's alone. After resection, the lung parenchyma may become distorted around the nodule, thereby giving the illusion of a positive or close margin to the pathologist. If a mechanical stapling device is used, the pathologist commonly discards the staple line prior to evaluating the "stapled" parenchymal margin. It is important for the pathologist to note the width of the excised mechanical stapling line and to include it in the pathology report. Lymph node metastases herald a poorer prognosis.

Earlier in 2001 Loehe et al. demonstrated in a prospective study that there was a trend toward improved survival in patients undergoing lung resection for metastases when mediastinal nodes were not involved.[66] In 2004, Ercan and colleagues reported on their experience with 70 patients who had had a complete mediastinal lymphadenectomy during pulmonary metastasectomy.[67] These investigators found that 28.6% of their patients had involvement in the lymph

TABLE 108.1 Excision of Pulmonary Metastases

Criteria for resection of pulmonary metastases:
  Pulmonary nodules consistent with metastases
  Control of primary tumor
  All nodules potentially resectable with planned surgery
  Adequate postoperative pulmonary reserve anticipated
  No extrathoracic metastases
Other indications for partial or complete resection of pulmonary metastases:
  Need to establish a diagnosis
  Remove residual nodules after chemotherapy
  Obtain tissue for tumor markers or immunohistochemical studies
  Decrease tumor burden

nodes and that such involvement was a significant prognostic factor for poor outcome (3-year survival without nodal involvement, 69%, vs. 38% with nodal involvement). Szöke et al. reported a series of 24 patients who underwent resection of lung metastases from colorectal cancer and in 33.3% of cases positive mediastinal lymph nodes were detected.[68] The proportion of positive lymph nodes was higher for central lung metastases (62.5%) compared to peripheral ones (18.8%). The Lung Metastasectomy Working Group recommends to perform a systematic lymph node dissection and indicated that videomediastinoscopy may play a role in more accurate staging of patients with lung metastases.[69]

Is there a limit to the number of metastases that can be resected with associated survival benefit? In the large retrospective database reported by Pastorino and colleagues, a significant survival difference was found between patients with only one metastasis and those with more than one metastasis.[2] Other authors who have been tempted to address this specific question include Putnam, Girard, and Robert and their colleagues.[70–72] In general, only unresectability as defined by the thoracic surgeon should be considered as an absolute contraindication to resection. As the numbers of metastases increase, the potential for occult micrometastatic disease also increases, reflecting biologically more aggressive behavior. Although the surgeon may be able to extirpate all identifiable disease mechanically by visual inspection and palpation, the surgeon typically cannot identify or extirpate microscopic disease. The biology of patients with excessive numbers of metastases (but yet still "resectable") is not changed by resection. Balancing the advantages of mechanical resection with the need for control of micrometastatic disease may be best accomplished in a multidisciplinary center with a multidisciplinary conference of all potential treating physicians.

Pneumonectomy is rarely indicated for lung metastases although long-term survival may be obtained in highly selected patients with reported 5-year survival rates ranging from 20% to 45%.[73,74] Even resections of lung metastases after pneumonectomy have been described reaching the limits of our surgical treatment.[75] Pneumonectomy may also be considered for mechanical palliation of mediastinal compression from "tumor thorax," as shown by Putnam and Grunenwald and their colleagues.[12,76]

SURGICAL TECHNIQUES AND INCISIONS

Surgical access for resection includes single muscle-sparing anterolateral or posterolateral thoracotomy, staged bilateral thoracotomies, median sternotomy, bilateral anterior thoracotomy with transverse sternotomy (the clamshell incision) and minimally invasive techniques consisting of video-assisted thoracoscopic (VATS) or robotic procedures.

TABLE 108.2 Advantages and Disadvantages of Various Surgical Resections

Procedure	Advantages	Disadvantages	Lymph Node Dissection
Median sternotomy	Bilateral thoracic explorations with one incision	Resection of lesions posterior and medial (near the hila) may be difficult	Nodal sampling (bilateral)
	Less patient discomfort	Difficult exposure to the left lower lobe in patients with obesity, congestive heart failure, or chronic obstructive pulmonary disease (increased thoracic anteroposterior diameter)	Feasible but visceral and paravertebral regions difficult to reach
Transverse sternotomy or clamshell	Bilateral thoracic explorations with one incision	Larger incision	Systematic nodal dissection (bilateral)
	Good exposure to all aspects of both right and left thoraces	Patient discomfort	All lymph node regions accessible
	Access to both right and left hila and to left lower lobe		
Posterolateral thoracotomy	Standard approach (shorter incision with anterolateral approach)	Patient discomfort	Systematic nodal dissection (unilateral)
	Excellent exposure of the hemithorax	Only one hemithorax may be explored per operation	All ipsilateral lymph node regions can be reached
		A second operation is needed for bilateral metastases	
Video-assisted thoracic surgery	Potentially less immunosuppressive	Unable to fully evaluate metastases in the lung parenchyma	Nodal sampling (unilateral)
	Excellent visualization	Late chest wall port recurrences	Some regions more difficult to access as posterior hilum and subcarinal region
	Excellent exposure for visceral pleural metastases	Does not identify occult nodules which are not visible	
	May identify unresectable metastases, extrapleural disease, pleural studding, etc.		

Patients with bilateral metastases may be safely explored with either a median sternotomy or staged bilateral thoracotomies, as noted by Johnston and Roth and colleagues.[77,78] The incisions chosen do not influence patient survival if all metastases are resected. Various advantages and disadvantages are unique to each approach, also regarding systematic lymph node dissection (Table 108.2).

In the previously mentioned survey of current practice amongst ESTS members published by Internullo et al., the choice of surgical approach was addressed.[26] In case of clinically unilateral disease, anterolateral thoracotomy, thoracoscopy (VATS), and sternotomy are preferred by 36.3%, 28.8%, and 1.4% of responders, respectively. If clinically bilateral disease is present, bilateral staged thoracotomy is most frequently used (66.2%) followed by sternotomy (16.9%) and bilateral sequential thoracotomy in one stage (19.3%).

Patients with sarcomas and unilateral nodules often have multiple and bilateral metastases discovered during the operation. Bilateral metastases may occur in 38% to 60% of patients with preoperative unilateral sarcomatous metastasis. Post-resection survival rates after median sternotomy or bilateral staged thoracotomies and complete resection are similar.

Despite the previous discussion, for selected cases with unilateral disease, bilateral exploration may not be necessary. High-resolution CT or integrated PET-CT scanning may assist in this determination. Younes and colleagues[79] evaluated the role of ipsilateral thoracotomy in patients with unilateral pulmonary metastasis for contralateral disease-free survival and overall survival. They noted that there was no significant difference in survival in patients who had recurrence in the contralateral lung compared with those who had bilateral metastases on admission. They suggested that delaying the contralateral thoracotomy did not affect survival. Also the Lung Metastasectomy Working Group did not favor routine bilateral exploration in case of unilateral disease on chest CT scan.[80]

LASER-ASSISTED RESECTION

Laser-assisted pulmonary resection, described by Kodama, Branscheid, Miyamoto, Landreneau, Mineo, and Rolle and their colleagues, using the neodymium:yttrium-aluminum garnet (Nd:YAG) laser, may provide an effective means of resecting pulmonary metastases.[81–86] Use of the laser may enhance preservation of lung parenchyma with less distortion. Bovie electrocautery may also spare lung parenchyma by removing the metastases with minimal distortion of remaining lung (cautery excision). Air leaks, if they occur, can be sealed by oversewing the parenchymal defect or by the use of fibrin glue. Disadvantages of laser resection may include longer operating time and a potential for prolonged postoperative air leaks. Newer laser technologies have been developed. Rolle and colleagues described a specific 1,318-nm Nd:YAG laser for better and more precise incisions into the parenchyma with concurrent coagulation and sealing of the lung tissue.[86] A 5-mm rim of tissue destruction is achieved.

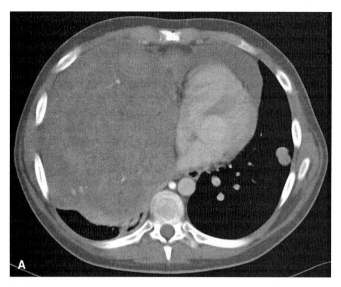
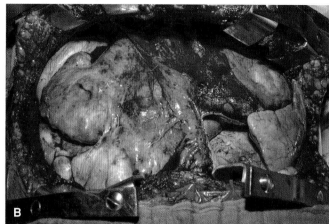

FIGURE 108.4 Twenty-one-year-old patient with extragonadal germ cell tumor with lung metastasis on left side (**A**). Patient was not responsive to chemotherapy anymore and salvage surgery was performed by clam shell incision to remove the mediastinal tumor and lung metastases (**B**).

In a prospective randomized trial conducted by Mineo and colleagues, use of the Nd:YAG laser for resection of lung metastases was examined in 45 patients.[85] The authors identified that the use of the laser reduced hospital stay, air leak, and tissue loss; however, a survival advantage was not proved.

Osei-Agyemang and colleagues reported a retrospective series of 301 patients operated for lung metastases with use of Nd:YAG laser in 20.6% of cases.[87] Although the number of resected lesions was higher in the laser group, no differences were observed in long-term survival.

The use of the laser for resection of pulmonary metastases is oncologically equal to other techniques and may provide advantages by preserving lung tissue and minimizing associated surgical trauma. On the other hand, complete and in-depth pathologic examination is not possible and evaluation of margins cannot be performed if the metastasis has been obliterated, or the margin destroyed as a planned component of the laser resection.

MEDIAN STERNOTOMY AND CLAMSHELL INCISION

For the median sternotomy incision, the patient is positioned supine with the entire anterior thorax exposed from the neck to the umbilicus and laterally to each anterior axillary line. The sternum is divided longitudinally. The pulmonary ligament is divided on each side to mobilize the lung completely. The lungs are sequentially deflated and palpated. Metastases are identified and resected, and then the deflated lung is reinflated. The deflated right lung may be brought completely into the field, attached by only the hilar structures. Exposure of the left lower lobe may be more difficult than exposure of the other lobes because of the overlying heart. With appropriate gentle traction on the pericardium, the left lower lobe can be exposed quite readily and brought into the operative field. Various techniques to better visualize the lung may be used, such as surgical packs behind the hilum of the deflated lung to elevate the parenchyma, or an internal mammary artery retractor to expose basilar tumors or posterior hilar left lower lobe masses. In certain circumstances visualization can be supplemented by the use of video thoracoscopy. Relative contraindications to median sternotomy include obesity, chronic obstructive pulmonary disease, elevated hemidiaphragm (particularly on the left), and

cardiomegaly. Patients with metastases involving the left hilum or the posterior or medial portions of the left lower lobe may benefit from bilateral staged thoracotomies rather than median sternotomy. A median sternotomy in these situations may compromise completeness of resection and injure lung parenchyma or create a need for greater pulmonary resection than would be otherwise required.

The transverse sternotomy or "clamshell incision," as described by Bains and colleagues, is a modification of the median sternotomy incision.[88] Originally, this approach developed from the early days of carinal surgery and was later rediscovered for access to enhance bilateral sequential single-lung transplantation. A curvilinear incision is made under the breasts or pectoral muscles. The pectoral muscles are elevated to gain access to the fourth intercostal space bilaterally, whereupon the chest is entered and the incision carried to the sternum bilaterally. The most lateral aspect of the incision may curve superiorly toward the axilla. The sternum is divided transversely at the level of the fourth intercostal space with a Gigli or oscillating saw. After placement of a chest retractor for both the right and left thorax, the chest is opened, giving excellent exposure to the right and left thorax, hilum, and mediastinum (Fig. 108.4A,B). Advantages of this approach include better exposure of the left hilum posteriorly and the left lower lobe. Extensive lymph node dissection is feasible. Disadvantages include a large, painful incision and some difficulty with sternal reconstruction and stabilization, although insertion of Kirschner wires inside the sternal medulla facilitates sternal repositioning and healing.

THORACOTOMY

A thoracotomy is the classical approach to pulmonary resection for carcinoma of the lung. Compared to sternotomy, a posterolateral thoracotomy with division of the latissimus dorsi muscle or an anterolateral muscle-sparing thoracotomy with preservation of this muscle may provide better exposure for metastases located more medially or more posteriorly near the hilum on the left side. An ipsilateral systematic lymph node dissection is also easier to accomplish. In addition, for patients with bulky metastases, a posterolateral thoracotomy provides good access for faster resection and optimal sparing of lung parenchyma. The surgeon is typically limited to operating in one hemithorax. Although feasible, bilateral sequential thoracotomies are rarely performed in the same patient at the same operation.

The vertical axillary thoracotomy may also be considered. Margaritora and colleagues have described their experience with staged axillary thoracotomy.[89] Hospitalization was short (3.2 days). Operative trauma was minimal, as was postoperative pain. The interval between the two staged procedures was about 24 days.

Bilateral anterior thoracotomy as described by d'Amato and colleagues may also be used.[90] Bilateral minithoracotomy with video assistance was used as an alternative to the other surgical approaches to the chest.

VIDEO-ASSISTED AND ROBOTIC THORACIC SURGERY

VATS resection using high-resolution video imaging may be helpful for the diagnosis, staging, and resection of metastases. Its usefulness is limited, however, because metastases can be identified generally only on the surface of the lung or the outer 10% to 20%, depending on size. Metastases within the lung parenchyma may be undetectable with this technique. In one early report, Landreneau and colleagues have described minimal morbidity and no mortality in 61 patients who underwent 85 thoracoscopic pulmonary resections.[91] Lesions were small (<3 cm) and located in the outer one-third of the lung parenchyma. Metastases in 18 patients were resected through thoracoscopy in this series. VATS was the only procedure performed in these patients. Thoracoscopy may readily be used for diagnosis of metastatic disease, as stated by McCormack and colleagues, but its use in the definitive treatment of metastatic disease is more controversial. In an elegant study, McCormack and colleagues prospectively evaluated VATS resection for the treatment of pulmonary metastases.[92] Patients were screened with CT, and VATS was performed on all patients. Under the same anesthetic, thoracotomy or median sternotomy was performed. The authors found more nodules at thoracotomy than had been noted at the VATS procedure. Limitations of the study were the inclusion of patients with multiple metastases or prior sarcoma histology, and screening with older CT scans. A similar study was performed in the Netherlands by Mutsaerts and colleagues.[93] Twenty-eight patients evaluated by chest CT underwent VATS resection of lung metastases followed by confirmatory thoracotomy. Accuracy of VATS was highest in case of a solitary lesion <3 cm and located in the lung periphery on CT scan. In case more than one lung lesion was present on CT scan, in four out of five cases additional lesions were detected by manual palpation during thoracotomy. This was confirmed by a recent, observer-blinded study performed by Eckardt and Licht.[94] In 89 patients 140 suspicious nodules were present on chest CT. By VATS 87% of lesions could be localized. During thoracotomy 67 additional nodules were found of which 22 (33%) were metastases.

Landreneau and colleagues recorded their experience in 80 patients with colorectal metastasis who underwent thoracoscopic resection of pulmonary metastasis.[95] A single lesion was removed in 60 patients, and two or more lesions were removed in 20 patients. The overall 5-year survival rate was 30.8%. The authors required that all lesions identified on CT be identified at thoracoscopy; or the minimally invasive approach would be abandoned. If location of the lesion compromised a complete resection, conversion to thoracotomy was performed. Accurate, high-resolution CT is critical for the selection of patients for minimally invasive techniques, as reported by Nakajima and colleagues.[96] Lin and colleagues also noted that the results appeared comparable to historical results by open thoracotomy.[97] The need for high-resolution helical CT scanning was crucial

for patient selection. In addition, conversion to an open procedure was recommended when preoperative lesions were not identified or when surgical margins would be compromised.

To balance the need for palpation of the lung parenchyma in addition to minimizing trauma with thoracoscopy, Mineo and colleagues retrospectively evaluated transxiphoid palpation of both lungs during VATS for lung metastasis.[98] Bilateral palpation was performed in 65 of 74 patients. Twenty-three radiographically undetected malignant lesions were identified. The authors recommended that this technique be considered as a blended approach to minimize thoracic trauma while providing for palpation of the lung parenchyma.

At present, VATS can be advocated for diagnosis or staging of the extent of metastases or for resection of metastases in highly selected patients with a solitary nodule on helical chest CT and nonsarcomatous histology. Patients with sarcomatous histology frequently (40–60%) have occult metastases, which may be better palpated and resected with open thoracotomy. Today, with high-resolution CT, metastases may be identified while quite small (3–4 mm, etc.). In the absence of other metastases, patients with one or two lesions compatible with metastasis could be treated with VATS resection; however, palpation would not be possible to identify occult metastases. Patients and physicians would need to balance the risks and benefits of this approach in consideration of the patient's projected overall course. In patients with solitary metastasis from solid tumor adenocarcinoma or squamous cell carcinoma, careful consideration must be given to excluding primary lung carcinoma, which would require lobectomy and systematic mediastinal lymph node dissection for optimal care. Complications of VATS may include not resecting all metastases, positive margins, or pleural seeding with extraction of the metastasis.[99–101]

Recently, robotic surgery has been introduced providing excellent three-dimensional visualization of the operative field in conjunction with highly flexible robotic arms allowing accurate surgery by a minimally invasive approach. However, no comparative studies are currently available and its real contribution for resection of lung metastases remains to be determined.

Follow-up on all patients is necessary at regular intervals because the likelihood of recurrence remains for a long period of time.

RESULTS OF RESECTION OF PULMONARY METASTASES

As large, prospective controlled trials are not available at the present time, the results of pulmonary metastasectomy require critical analysis of factors that may potentially influence survival. Analysis of results should be based on review or study of single primary histology (breast, colon, melanoma) or similar histology (e.g., soft tissue sarcomas) and sufficient numbers of patients. Prognostic indicators have been reviewed to assess their influence singularly and in combination on post-resection survival in patients with pulmonary metastases and to assist clinically in describing appropriate patients for resection of pulmonary metastases. Age, gender, histology, grade, location of the primary tumor, stage of primary tumor, DFI between resection of the primary tumor and the appearance of the metastasis, number of nodules on preoperative radiologic studies, unilateral or bilateral metastases, tumor doubling time (TDT), and synchronous or metachronous metastases may be evaluated preoperatively. Postoperatively, extent and completeness of resection, technique of resection, nodal spread, number of metastases and location, re-resection, post-thoracotomy disease-free survival, and overall survival may also be considered in selecting patients for resection of pulmonary metastasis.

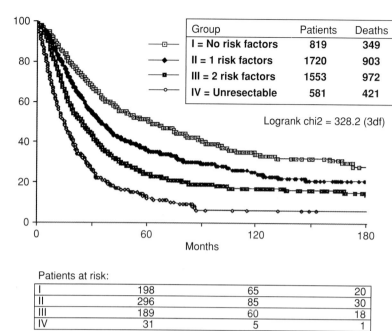

Group	Patients	Deaths
I = No risk factors	819	349
II = 1 risk factors	1720	903
III = 2 risk factors	1553	972
IV = Unresectable	581	421

Logrank chi2 = 328.2 (3df)

Patients at risk:

I	198	65	20
II	296	85	30
III	189	60	18
IV	31	5	1

FIGURE 108.5 Survival of the four prognostic groups determined in the retrospective analysis of 5,206 cases published by Pastorino and colleagues[2]: group I, resectable, no risk factors (disease-free interval [DFI] ≥36 months and single metastasis); group II, resectable, one risk factor (DFI <36 months or multiple metastases); group III, resectable, two risk factors (DFI <36 months and multiple metastases); and group IV, unresectable. (Reprinted from Pastorino U, Buyse M, Friedel G, et al. Long-term results of lung metastasectomy: prognostic analyses based on 5206 cases. *J Thorac Cardiovasc Surg* 1997;113(1):37–49. Copyright © 1997 The American Association for Thoracic Surgery. With permission.)

Pastorino and colleagues reviewed the long-term results of resection of pulmonary metastases based on an International Registry of Lung Metastases.[2] This International Registry was established in 1991 based on 5,206 patients with pulmonary metastases and treatment collected from Europe, the United States, and Canada. It is still the largest database that is currently available. Various clinical characteristics were compared in a retrospective yet consistent and controlled manner. Eighty-eight percent of these patients had complete resection. A solitary metastasis was resected in 2,383 patients; multiple lesions were resected in 2,726. Epithelial histology predominated (2,260 patients), followed by sarcoma (2,173), germ cell (363), and melanoma (328). With a median follow-up of 46 months, actuarial survival was 36% at 5 years, 26% at 10 years, and 22% at 15 years. For incomplete resection, actuarial survival was 15% at 5 years. The multivariate analysis showed several favorable prognostic indicators: resectable metastases, germ cell tumors, DFI of ≥36 months, and a solitary metastasis. In this international and multi-institutional study, the overall operative mortality rate was 1%; the mortality rate was 2.4% after incomplete resections and 0.8% after complete resections.

The most frequently performed operation was unilateral thoracotomy (58% of patients). Bilateral exploration was performed through either bilateral synchronous or staged thoracotomy (11%) or median sternotomy (27%). Thoracoscopy was performed in only 2% of patients. Wedge resections (67%), segmentectomy (9%), lobectomy or bilobectomy (21%), and pneumonectomy (4%) were performed. Only 26% of patients had ≥4 metastases. Only 9% had ≥10 metastases, and 3% had ≥20. Multiple metastases were most commonly resected in sarcomas (64%), germ cell tumors (57%), epithelial tumors (43%), and melanoma (39%). Metastases to the mediastinal lymph nodes were uncommon but only a minority of patients had a formal lymph node dissection. Overall, 3% had redo surgery, 15% had two operations, 4% had three operations, and 1% had four or more operations. The maximum number of resections performed on a single patient was seven.

The authors proposed a system by which patients can be grouped into prognostic categories. These would include three parameters: (a) resectability, (b) DFI, and (c) number of metastases. In patients with resectable lesions, a DFI <36 months and multiple metastases

were found to be independent risk factors. In resectable patients, therefore, three clinically distinct groups could be identified: group I, no risk factors, DFI of ≥36 months, single metastasis; group II, one risk factor, DFI <36 months, or multiple metastases; and group III two risk factors, DFI <36 months, and multiple metastases. Group IV consisted of all the unresectable patients. The authors noted that median survival was 61 months for group I, 34 months for group II, 24 months for group III, and 14 months for group IV (Fig. 108.5). The discriminate power of the model was appropriate for epithelial tumors, soft tissue sarcomas, and melanomas.

The value of this International Registry of Lung Metastases lies in its large collection of patient characteristics. These clinically identifiable characteristics may be reexamined and analyzed for various hypotheses. The limitations of such a registry lie in not accounting for variables in the biologic behavior of these metastases. This variable behavior may be explained by molecular characteristics on which the clinical features are based. This clinical database has been used to evaluate the value of resection of pulmonary metastases from various histologies as well as other clinical and molecular characteristics that may be valuable in selecting patients for optimal care of their metastases.

Another large, more recent, single-center experience which was also a retrospective study was reported by Casiraghi and colleagues.[102] In total, 708 pulmonary metastasectomies were performed in 575 patients. Mean DFI was 46.6 months. An open resection was performed in 97% of patients. Overall 5-year survival rate for patients who underwent complete resection was 46%. Multivariate analysis showed complete resection, germ cell tumors, and DFI ≥36 months to be significant positive factors in relation to survival. Not significant were the number of metastases, number of metastasectomies, and presence of lymph node metastases. However, it should be indicated that lymph node evaluation was only performed in 50% of patients.

EXTENDED RESECTION OF PULMONARY METASTASES

Of all patients undergoing resection of pulmonary metastases, <3% require an extended resection. Pneumonectomy or other extended

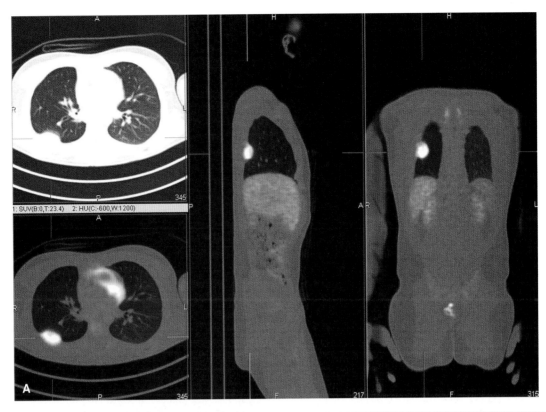

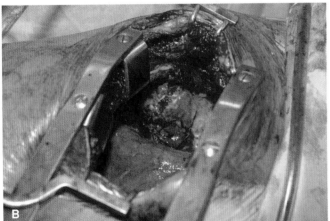

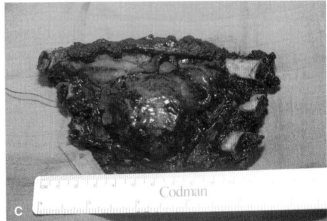

FIGURE 108.6 Twenty-one-year-old patient with undifferentiated cerebral tumor presenting with large chest wall metastasis on PET-CT scan (**A**) necessitating chest wall resection (**B,C**).

resection of pulmonary metastases may be performed safely in highly selected patients with associated long-term disease-free survival (Fig. 108.6A–C). Pneumonectomy or en bloc resection of pulmonary metastases with chest wall or other thoracic structures, such as diaphragm, pericardium, or superior vena cava, has been performed in a small number of patients with good results, as noted by Putnam and colleagues.[12] Nineteen patients had a pneumonectomy, and 19 patients had other extended resection. The 5-year actuarial survival rate was 25%. The mortality rate was 5%, and these deaths occurred in patients having pneumonectomy, often after multiple prior wedge resections for metastases.

In a French study by Spaggiari and colleagues, 42 patients were treated for pulmonary metastases over 10 years: 29 patients underwent pneumonectomy for sarcoma, 12 for carcinoma, and 1 for a lipoma.[103] Most tumors were centrally located. Two postoperative

deaths occurred. Four patients had major complications. Five patients (12%) had recurrences in the contralateral lung. The median survival time was only 6.3 months, and the 5-year survival rate was 16%. Given that the standard surgical mortality rate for operations for pulmonary metastases is <1%, mortality for pneumonectomy should be considered in planning operations for patients with large, centrally located metastases. Although mortality for pneumonectomy for pulmonary metastases corresponds to mortality for other histologies, the 5-year survival rate of only 16% should prompt strict preoperative selection criteria. The authors suggest that young patients, those with a long DFI, and those with normal carcinoembryonic antigen (CEA) levels (for patients with metastases from colorectal carcinoma) be considered for pneumonectomy for pulmonary metastases.

Koong and colleagues also examined the value of pneumonectomy for metastases by retrospective review of the International Registry of Lung Metastases.[74] Of the 5,206 patients enrolled, 133 (2.6%) had undergone pneumonectomy for pulmonary metastases between 1962 and 1994. Of these patients, 84% underwent complete resection, and the 30-day mortality rate was 3.6%. The 5-year survival rate was 20% with complete resection. For incomplete resection, the peri-operative mortality rate was 19%, and most did not survive beyond 5 years. The authors identified favorable prognostic factors of (a) single metastasis, (b) negative mediastinal lymph nodes, and (c) complete resection (R0). The authors concluded that pneumonectomy may be performed safely with adequate long-term survival.

These studies reveal that pneumonectomy is rarely indicated for pulmonary metastases. All the above series represent a highly selected group of patients and although the results are encouraging, pneumonectomy should be used only in rare circumstances as the surgical treatment of metastatic disease. Most if not all prognostic variables should be favorable before recommending pneumonectomy.

Larger or rapidly growing metastases may compress the mediastinum, or a uniquely positioned metastasis may impinge on or invade cardiac structures or great vessels. The use of cardiopulmonary bypass or other cardiovascular surgical techniques may allow resection of these metastases with palliation of symptoms and the potential for cure. Vaporciyan and colleagues reviewed a single-institution experience of resection with cardiopulmonary bypass of metastatic noncardiac primary malignancies.[104] Patients with inferior vena cava tumors were excluded. Nine patients with sarcomas required cardiopulmonary bypass because their tumors directly involved the heart and the great vessels. The mortality rate was 11%. Of the 11 patients who underwent resection with curative intent, 10 had a complete resection. The use of cardiopulmonary bypass may be considered in highly selected patients, particularly when complete resection is anticipated.

Intra-atrial extension of sarcoma through the pulmonary veins is rare but may also be safely treated with pulmonary resection (pneumonectomy and resection of the tumor from the left atrium). Careful palpation of the involved vein can be performed intraoperatively, but excessive manipulation can result in tumor embolization. Extracorporeal cardiopulmonary support is required for a complete, safe resection, as noted by Heslin and Shuman and their colleagues.[105,106]

OSTEOGENIC SARCOMA

Goorin and colleagues and Huth and Eilber reported that pulmonary metastases from osteogenic sarcoma may occur in up to 80% of patients who relapse after treatment for their primary neoplasm, whether or not they receive adjuvant chemotherapy.[42,107] Chest CT is commonly used to identify patients with potential metastases. The positive predictive value for chest CT may be limited. Often, the surgeon finds twice the number of nodules than otherwise would be expected simply on the basis of preoperative CT of the chest, as described by Picci and colleagues.[108] Resection as initial therapy for solitary metastasis, resection as salvage after chemotherapy for these pulmonary metastases, and multiple repeat thoracotomies may all be considered in selecting an optimal therapeutic strategy (Fig. 108.7).

Meyer and colleagues reported that because metastases from osteogenic sarcoma are often isolated to the lungs, resection may render a significant number of patients disease-free and enhance long-term survival.[109] The 5-year survival rate may range up to 40%, as shown by Snyder and Belli and their colleagues.[110,111] Patients may have benefit regardless of the time of identification of lung metastases. In one Japanese study, Tsuchiya and colleagues noted that a longer DFI was associated with improved 5-year survival.[112] Still, 2-year survival

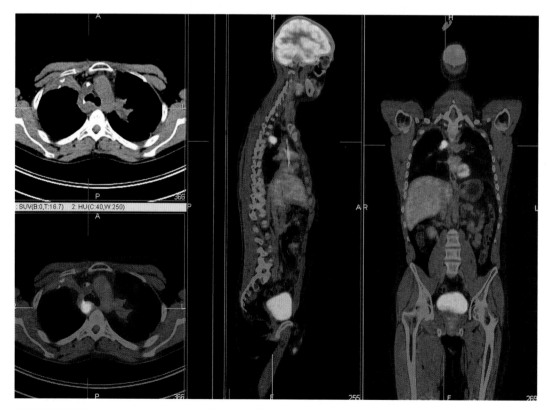

FIGURE 108.7 Patient with osteosarcoma of tibia who underwent several interventions for lung metastases. During follow-up a new metastasis was detected on posterior side of right main bronchus which was removed by sternotomy followed by postoperative radiotherapy.

from the time of identification of pulmonary metastases ranged from 24% to 33% for patients with lung metastases identified at initial presentation, during preoperative chemotherapy, or during postoperative chemotherapy. Patients with lung metastases that occurred or were identified after completion of chemotherapy had a 2-year overall survival of 40% and a 5-year survival rate of 31%. However, in a small study, Yonemoto and colleagues evaluated 117 patients with osteogenic sarcoma of the extremity; 9 patients had pulmonary metastases at presentation.[113] Patients who were treated with chemotherapy and aggressive resection had a 5-year survival rate of 64%.

A more critical point of view was formulated by Treasure et al. who performed a systematic review of the reported outcomes of the Thames Cancer Registry data regarding bone and soft tissue sarcoma.[114] An analysis was made of a total of 1,357 pulmonary metastasectomies performed between 1980 and 2006; 43% of patients also had a subsequent metastasectomy. Five-year survival rates after a first metastasectomy were 34% for sarcoma and 25% for soft tissue sarcoma. A better prognosis was noted with fewer metastases and a longer DFI. These survival rates were higher than those observed among unselected registry data. However, the authors conclude that there is insufficient evidence to attribute this to the metastasectomy itself.[114]

Carter, Jaffe, and Putnam and their colleagues have evaluated survival and prognostic factors in patients with pulmonary metastases from osteogenic sarcoma.[115–117] In a series from the National Institutes of Health, Putnam and colleagues evaluated 80 patients with osteogenic sarcoma of the extremity.[117] Of these, 43 patients developed pulmonary metastases and 39 underwent one or more thoracic explorations for resection of their metastases. The 5-year survival rate was 40%. Various prognostic factors were analyzed. Three or fewer nodules, longer DFI, resectable metastases, and the fewer metastases identified and resected were associated with longer post-thoracotomy survival. Resection was not possible if >16 nodules were identified on preoperative tomograms. A multivariate analysis did not find any combination of factors to be more predictive than the number of nodules identified on preoperative tomograms. Heij and colleagues reported 40 children with osteogenic sarcoma and demonstrated that incomplete excision, lack of primary tumor control, and progression and development of metastases during treatment were all negative prognostic factors.[118] Surprisingly, in resectable patients, the number of metastases, DFI, unilateral versus bilateral metastases, preoperative and postoperative adjuvant treatment, and the number of thoracotomies performed were not significant prognostic factors.

Mizuno and colleagues reported a retrospective series of 58 pulmonary metastasectomies in 52 patients with a complete resection rate of 92%.[119] VATS was performed in 59%. Median follow-up was 33 months with a 5-year survival rate of 50.9%; recurrent disease after a first metastasectomy was observed in 36 patients (62%) and 20 underwent repeated resection with a 5-year survival rate of 49.7%. In multivariate analysis complete resection and number of metastatic nodules were significant prognostic factors.[119]

Chemotherapy may prevent or cure micrometastatic disease not amenable to surgery, as stated by Belli and colleagues.[111] Most patients with osteogenic sarcoma of the extremities are treated with neoadjuvant chemotherapy and limb salvage, as proposed by Bacci, Goorin, and Ferrari and their colleagues.[48,120,121] On the other hand, patients treated with adjuvant chemotherapy after local control (typically with a limb salvage procedure) will show a different pattern of systemic relapse. Likewise, such a therapeutic approach was not shown to decrease event-free survival by Goorin and colleagues.[122] All patients received 44 weeks of combination chemotherapy. They also reported that presurgical chemotherapy (for 10 weeks) did not improve event-free survival compared with immediate surgery. Voute

and colleagues have suggested that combination chemotherapy—such as cisplatin and doxorubicin, or cisplatin, ifosfamide, and doxorubicin—would be active in patients with osteogenic sarcoma.[123] Miniero and colleagues have suggested that high-dose chemotherapy and autologous peripheral blood stem cell transplantation could be considered as a promising regimen for patients with metastatic osteogenic sarcoma, particularly those who were not cured by conventional chemotherapy.[124]

Chemotherapy may assist in treating newly diagnosed metastatic osteogenic sarcoma, as recommended by Ferguson and colleagues.[45] However, response may be difficult to assess, given the calcified matrix of these metastases.

A recent study evaluated factors that are predictive for survival following complete surgical remission of pulmonary metastasis in a multimodality setting.[50] Common practice constitutes multiagent chemotherapy, consisting of cisplatin and doxorubicin or ifosfamide-containing regimens, prior to pulmonary metastasectomy, and delivery of adjuvant chemotherapy postoperatively. In a series of 62 patients with metastatic osteosarcoma, 25 achieved complete remission after resection of the pulmonary metastases. Five-year overall and disease-free survival rates were 30% and 21%, respectively. In univariate analysis, chondroblastic subtype, post-chemotherapy necrosis <90% in the primary tumor, metastases detected during chemotherapy, and visceral pleural invasion were negative prognostic factors. In multivariate analysis only chondroblastic subtype remained significant.

SOFT TISSUE SARCOMAS

Soft tissue sarcomas comprise a family of nonossifying malignant neoplasms arising from mesenchymal connective tissues that can metastasize to the lungs, as described by Hoos and colleagues.[125] Potter and colleagues demonstrated that, as with osteogenic sarcomas, local recurrence is common (20%) and metastases are predominantly to lungs as shown in Figure 108.8A–C.[11]

Billingsley and colleagues performed a multifactorial analysis of 994 patients with primary extremity soft tissue sarcoma treated at the Memorial Sloan-Kettering Cancer Center; 230 patients had recurrences.[126] In the cases where disease recurred, 73% (169 of 273) of recurrences appeared initially within the lungs. Median survival after recurrence of metastases was 11.6 months. Multivariate analysis identified resection of metastatic disease, DFI, the presence of local recurrence, and age >50 years as significant prognostic indicators. Primary tumor characteristics did not have an association with survival after resection of pulmonary metastases. In general, a longer DFI of >6 months and three or fewer metastases were associated with a higher overall 5-year survival.

In a retrospective study of the European Organization for Research and Treatment of Cancer (EORTC)—Soft Tissue and Bone Sarcoma Group, van Geel and colleagues noted a 5-year overall survival rate of 38% after complete resection of pulmonary metastases.[127] Negative margins, younger age (<40 years), and lower-grade tumors (grade 1 or 2) were associated with improved survival compared with that of patients without these characteristics.

In patients with histologically documented pulmonary metastases from soft tissue sarcomas treated at the National Cancer Institute, Jablons and colleagues showed that significant preoperative predictors of enhanced survival included TDT >20 days, <4 nodules on preoperative tomograms, and DFI >12 months.[128] Predictive ability for better survival was improved when all three prognostic factors were combined. These patients represent those who will have the best response (i.e., prolonged post-resection survival) to pulmonary

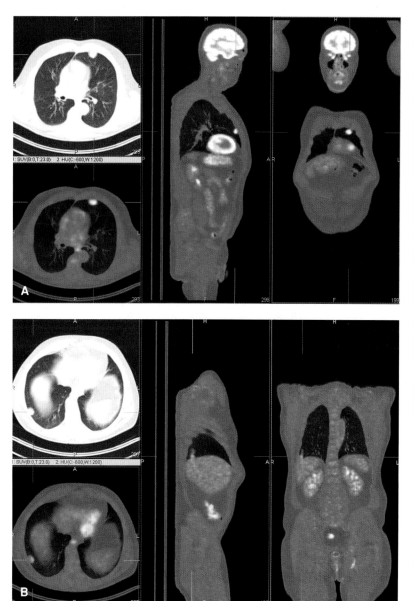

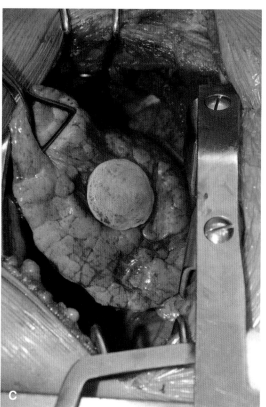

FIGURE 108.8 Patient with myxofibrosarcoma of left leg who presented with bilateral lung metastases in close contact with chest wall (**A,B**) which were treated by staged thoracotomies in association with isolated lung perfusion (**C**). No invasion of chest wall was present.

metastasectomy. Casson and colleagues evaluated determinants of 5-year survival in 58 patients who had complete resection and were followed until death or for a minimum of 5 years.[129] Favorable prognostic factors included TDT >40 days, unilateral disease, three or fewer nodules identified on preoperative tomograms, two or fewer metastases resected, and tumor histology (median survival, 33 months for malignant fibrous histiocytoma vs. 17 months for all others). Using multivariate analysis, the number of nodules (at least four) was the most significant adverse prognostic indicator. The addition of tumor histology (malignant fibrous histiocytoma) improved the predictive ability of this model. The absolute 5-year survival rate was 25% (15 of 58 patients).

Resection of recurrent pulmonary metastases from soft tissue sarcoma is associated with improved post-resection survival compared with that of patients with unresectable metastases. Pogrebniak and colleagues evaluated 43 patients who had two or more resections.[130] In 31 completely resectable patients (72%), median survival was 25 months, whereas incompletely resectable or unresectable patients had a median survival of only 10 months. A longer DFI (≥18 months) was also associated with prolonged disease-free

survival. Increased age and female gender were associated with an increased risk for death from disease in resected patients with recurrent pulmonary metastases in contrast to initially isolated pulmonary metastases. Casson and colleagues noted that among 39 patients with recurrent pulmonary metastases from adult soft tissue sarcomas, resectable patients and those with only one metastasis had the best post-resection survival.[129]

Results of systemic chemotherapy as single-modality therapy for metastatic soft tissue sarcoma remain poor. Median survival ranges from 13 to 16 months, as reported by Weh and Elias and their colleagues.[131,132] The role of adjuvant chemotherapy remains unproven but it can be considered in patients with localized soft tissue sarcoma who have a high likelihood of recurrent disease.[56] Woll and colleagues reported 351 patients who were randomized between adjuvant chemotherapy consisting of doxorubicin and ifosfamide, and no additional chemotherapy after resection of high-grade sarcomas.[133] No survival benefit of adjuvant chemotherapy could be demonstrated. However, the patient population was quite heterogeneous and the authors indicate that future studies should focus on patients with large, grade III extremity sarcomas. In patients with chemosensitive tumors, neoadjuvant chemotherapy might be considered to evaluate response to chemotherapy and improve recurrence-free survival.[56] Look Hong and colleagues published a series of 66 patients with soft tissue sarcoma who were treated with neoadjuvant chemotherapy consisting of mesna, adriamycin, ifosfamide, and dacarbazine (MAID) followed by surgical resection and postoperative chemotherapy with or without radiotherapy.[57] Negative surgical margins were obtained in 89% of patients. Five-year overall and disease-specific survival rates were 86% and 89%, respectively.

Soft tissue sarcomas are rare tumors and multidisciplinary management in high-volume centers is recommended to determine optimal staging and treatment.

COLORECTAL NEOPLASMS

Colorectal metastases commonly spread to local or regional nodes or to the liver through the portal venous system. Colorectal metastases may also occur initially as pulmonary metastases.

Criteria for resection of lung metastases from colorectal cancer are not different from other primary tumors. These include that the primary tumor has been treated adequately, complete resection of all metastases is feasible, cardiopulmonary evaluation shows no contraindication for the planned resection, and extrapulmonary metastases, if present, can be completely eradicated. In case of synchronous metastases resection can be performed simultaneously or as staged procedures. The precise survival advantage of resection of lung metastases from colorectal cancer has not been established yet, but its role is further evaluated in a randomized trial that is currently open for inclusion.[40] Hopefully, this trial will provide a better insight into indications and outcome of lung metastasectomy.

The distinction between a single metastasis from colorectal carcinoma and a primary NSCLC is typically made by histology and specific markers. An example of a patient with a history of colorectal cancer and multiple pulmonary nodules with different histologic characteristics is presented in Video 108.1, also demonstrating isolated lung perfusion. Molecular markers specific for metastases or lung carcinoma may aid in distinguishing a metastatic tumor from a primary lung carcinoma.[38] Complete resection, where possible, should be considered. Screening of serum CEA may be helpful in all patients with prior diagnosis of colorectal carcinoma. Although TTF-1 and SP-A are good markers of NSCLC, better markers for colorectal metastases to the lung are needed. Barbareschi and colleagues evaluated nuclear CDX-2 transcription factor.[134] This factor is expressed in normal epithelium and in most colorectal adenocarcinomas. They found this to be a sensitive and specific marker for colorectal metastases to the lung. CD transcription factor was identified in 88 of 90 specimens of primary and metastatic colorectal carcinoma, and it was not identified in primary NSCLC.

Patients with pulmonary metastases from colorectal carcinoma may be resected safely with low morbidity and mortality and long-term survival. In a large series from the Mayo Clinic, McAfee and colleagues presented 139 patients who underwent resection of pulmonary metastases from colorectal carcinoma with an operative mortality rate of 1.4%.[135] The overall 5-year survival rate was 30.5%, and the median follow-up was 7 years. Patients with a solitary pulmonary metastasis and those with a preoperative CEA level <4.0 ng/mL had better post-thoracotomy survival than other patients. Of interest was that longer DFI and diameter of metastases <3 cm were not associated with improved survival. Higashiyama and colleagues described a strong association between prethoracotomy serum CEA and survival.[136] Patients with a high prethoracotomy serum CEA were more likely to have extrathoracic metastases. The authors recommend evaluation for extrathoracic metastases in patients with a high prethoracotomy serum CEA.

In a systematic review of prognostic factors for survival after resection of lung metastases in patients with colorectal cancer, Gonzalez and colleagues evaluated 25 studies published between 2000 and 2011 which included at least 40 patients.[137] In total 2,925 patients were analyzed. Significant factors that were predictive of poor survival include a short DFI, multiple lung metastases, positive hilar or mediastinal lymph nodes, and elevated prethoracotomy CEA level. In contrast, a history of previously resected liver metastases was not found to be significant.

Salah and colleagues performed a pooled analysis of 1,112 metastasectomies performed in 927 patients who were extracted from eight studies performed between 1983 and 2008.[138] Following a first lung resection 5-year survival rate was 54.3%. Multivariate analysis identified three poor prognostic factors: DFI <36 months, multiple lung metastases, and elevated CEA level. Peri-operative chemotherapy and previous resection of liver metastasis were not significant in this analysis.

Other predictors of survival have been studied; the role of the adhesion molecule CD44 variant 9 and its relationship to pulmonary metastases from colorectal cancer was examined in 42 patients by Goi and colleagues.[139] The overall survival rate was 35%. Patients with elevated CD44 variant 9 had a higher rate of pulmonary metastases (88%) than patients in whom CD44 variant 9 was normal (the rate of metastases was only 42%).

Pulmonary metastases may develop after resection of hepatic metastases. In these patients, complete resection of pulmonary metastases may be associated with improved survival. Labow and colleagues noted a 3-year survival rate of 60% in the resected group versus 31% in the nonresected group.[140] Patients in this study met the standard criteria for resection of pulmonary metastases, and there was no concurrent extrapulmonary disease. In a French study by Regnard and colleagues, the authors examined 43 patients who had undergone complete resection of hepatic metastasis and then subsequently developed pulmonary metastases.[141] The median survival time was 19 months, and the 5-year survival rate was estimated to be 11%. Patients with a CEA >5 ng/mL had a significantly lower probability of survival than did those with lower levels (<5 ng/mL [$p = 0.0018$]). Follow-up for these patients should include imaging examinations and serum CEA, as proposed by Ike and colleagues.[142] Poorer survival is found in patients who cannot be completely resected or who are denied operation because their disease is deemed to be unresectable. Of the total population of patients with colorectal metastases, those with completely resectable lung or hepatic metastases represent a small percentage and are the ones with the most favorable "biology" of the tumor. The surgeon can take advantage of this biologically favorable subset of patients. With sequential and complete resection of both lung and hepatic metastases, survival may be enhanced.

In a recent, pooled analysis of patients who underwent resection of lung metastases after previously resected liver metastases, Salah and colleagues analyzed 146 patients from five studies performed between 1983 and 2009.[143] Five-year overall and recurrence-free survival rates from date of pulmonary metastasectomy were 54.4% and 29.3%, respectively. In multivariate analysis only the presence of positive thoracic lymph nodes proved to be significant with a hazard ratio of 4.9.

To evaluate prognostic factors in patients undergoing repeat resection of pulmonary oligometastatic disease from colorectal cancer, Salah and colleagues identified 148 patients operated between 1983 and 2008.[144] Operative mortality was 0.7% following the second metastasectomy and 2.7% after subsequent metastasectomies. Five-year overall survival rate was 57.9% from the second metastasectomy on. Independent factors heralding a poor prognosis were >2 metastatic nodules and a maximum diameter of the largest nodule ≥3 cm.

Chemotherapy has become an important treatment modality for metastatic colorectal cancer. For advanced disease, combination chemotherapy consisting of 5-fluorouracil (5-FU), leucovorin and oxaliplatin (FOLFOX), or 5-FU, leucovorin, and irinotecan (FOLFIRI) is most widely used with median overall survival rates ranging between 14.7 and 20.0 months.[145–147] By addition of cetuximab in selected patients, median overall survival time increases to 23.5 months.[147]

In case of liver metastases that are considered for surgical resection, peri-operative combination chemotherapy with the FOLFOX regimen is recommended.[145] However, the optimal treatment schedule has not been determined yet.

In patients undergoing pulmonary metastasectomy the role of neoadjuvant or adjuvant chemotherapy is less clear as no convincing evidence is currently available supporting its use in daily practice. For this reason every patient with lung metastases from colorectal cancer should be discussed within a multidisciplinary tumor board including a thoracic surgeon to determine the optimal treatment strategy.

BREAST CARCINOMA

Metastatic breast cancer has been defined as a systemic disease with metastases occurring in multiple sites.[148] Treatment is typically systemic, by chemotherapy, hormonal or other therapy, or palliative. In a minority of patients, resection of isolated pulmonary metastases may be considered although the level of evidence is low.[149] As with other primary tumors, favorable prognostic factors are fewer metastases and a longer DFI.[148] Patanaphan and colleagues have reported 145 patients with metastatic breast carcinoma (145 of 558, or 26%); the major sites of metastases were bone (51%), lung (17%), brain (16%), and liver (6%).[150] Overall median survival was 12 months for patients with lung metastases, who were mostly treated with either palliative chemotherapy, irradiation, or both. Lanza and colleagues studied 44 women with a prior history of breast cancer who underwent pulmonary resection for new pulmonary lesions.[151] Seven patients were excluded who had benign nodules (three patients) or unresectable metastases (four patients). In 37 resectable patients, the actuarial 5-year survival rate was 50%. DFI >12 months was associated with a longer median survival time (82 months) and 5-year survival rate (57%) compared with patients with a DFI of <12 months (15 months median, 0% 5-year survival; $p = 0.004$). Estrogen receptor–positive status tended to be associated with a longer post-thoracotomy survival ($p = 0.098$). Other favorable prognostic factors included positive receptor status of the primary tumor (improved 3-year survival rate of 61%) compared with negative receptor status (38% 3-year survival rate). Bathe and coauthors described the distant sites of failure following ablation of liver and lung metastases.[152] They recommend that adjuvant therapy with significant activity against visceral metastasis might enhance survival. Resection of solitary metastasis, according to Friedel and colleagues, provided a 35% 5-year survival rate, as compared with 0% after resection of ≥5 metastases.[153] Simpson and colleagues noted that favorable selection of patients increased survival up to 62% at 5 years.[154]

Staren and colleagues evaluated 33 patients treated with surgical resection of pulmonary metastases from breast carcinoma and compared the results to those of 30 patients treated primarily with systemic chemotherapy and hormonal therapy.[155] Patients having complete resection of metastases had a longer median survival than did patients with medical therapy, particularly when single nodules were compared (58 months vs. 34 months median survival). The 5-year

survival rate in patients treated with some surgical resection was 36%, compared with 11% in patients treated only medically. A review by Bodzin and colleagues[26] confirms these findings. Friedel and colleagues reviewed the results of resection in 467 patients with isolated metastases from breast cancer.[156] The 5-year survival rate was 38%. The authors note that DFIs of ≥36 months were associated with a 5-year survival rate of 45%. Patients with solitary metastases did better than those with multiple metastases, although the data were not statistically significant.

TESTICULAR NEOPLASMS

Nonseminomatous testicular tumors can be diagnosed by the occurrence of new pulmonary nodules identified on chest radiograph or by chest CT scan.[157,158] Metastatic testicular seminoma most commonly is identified as mediastinal nodal enlargement which is best evaluated by high-resolution chest CT.[159]

These tumors are particular sensitive to chemotherapy which represents the primary treatment modality. Surgery is indicated to remove residual or newly occurring metastases, also for diagnostic purposes. In such lesions not only persisting cancer can be present but also tumor necrosis or transformation to mature teratoma which may equally grow to a significant volume. Specific tumor markers are important to evaluate response to chemotherapy. The latter has been maximized when there is no further reduction in size of the nodules. Most patients require retroperitoneal lymph node dissections (69%), although thoracotomies may be required in 18%. Kulkarni and Carsky and their colleagues evaluated 80 patients with germ cell tumors and lung metastases treated with chemotherapy and subsequent surgery.[160,161] In this series, 35% (28 patients) achieved complete response after chemotherapy; 45% (36 patients) with partial response underwent surgery for resection of residual metastases. The residual disease was in the abdomen (17 patients), the lungs (15 patients), or both (4 patients); 27 of 36 patients (75%) achieved complete response after both chemotherapy and surgery. Carter and colleagues noted that extensive pulmonary metastases (unresectable metastases) were a predictor of ultimate treatment failure.[162] In contrast, Gels and colleagues reported a 10-year survival rate of 82.2% after chemotherapy and resection of residual retroperitoneal and pulmonary tumors.[163] Morbidity after surgical resection was minimal.

Liu and colleagues evaluated the role of pulmonary metastasectomy for testicular germ cell tumors over a 28-year period.[164] The typical patient was young (median age 27 years). Preoperative tumor markers were normal in most patients, and patients with multiple metastases predominated. About half the patients had synchronous presentation of their metastases. Complete resection was generally possible. Most of these patients had already undergone chemotherapy. Viable metastasis was present in 44% of the patients; in the remainder, there was no viable tumor (mature teratoma and fibrosis or necrosis were equally represented). Twenty-five percent had metastasis to other sites after resection of their pulmonary metastasis. The overall 5-year survival rate was 68%; for the patients diagnosed after 1985, the survival rate was 82%. The authors noted that extrathoracic metastases (nonpulmonary visceral sites) as well as the presence of viable tumor in the resected specimens were adverse prognostic indicators. Patients with metastases outside the pulmonary parenchyma, elevated tumor markers, and a viable tumor had a worse prognosis. Parenchymal resection not only removed all identifiable disease but also provided a measure of the effectiveness of the chemotherapy treatment.

Schnorrer and colleagues described 28 patients with pulmonary metastases from germ cell or testicular neoplasms who were treated with bleomycin, etoposide, and cisplatin.[165] An overall complete response was achieved in 21 patients (75%); in 11 of these, a complete response was achieved after chemotherapy alone. Resection of residual mass was necessary in 12 patients with normalized serum markers. Resection of the residual mass was recommended for histology and may modify subsequent treatment. The overall cure rate was 89.3%.

In one multi-institutional study of 215 patients, Steyerberg and colleagues evaluated the potential to predict necrosis, mature teratoma, or cancer in the residual pulmonary masses.[166] Necrosis (54%) and mature teratoma (33%) predominated, whereas cancer occurred in 13%. The authors recommended that retroperitoneal lymph node dissection be performed before thoracotomy because the pathology found during the latter dissection was a strong predictor of pathology at thoracotomy.

GYNECOLOGIC NEOPLASMS

Various authors—including Niwa, Anderson, Chauveinc, Shiromizu, and Bouros and their colleagues—have discussed the role of pulmonary resection as well as other therapy for the treatment of metastatic uterine and cervical malignancies.[167–171] Fuller and colleagues from the Massachusetts General Hospital reviewed a 40-year experience of treating patients with pulmonary metastases from gynecologic cancer.[172] The 5-year survival rate was 36%. Lesions <4 cm in diameter and a DFI >36 months were associated with prolonged survival. Shiromizu and colleagues confirmed that a smaller size (2.8 cm average) of the metastasis, a smaller number of metastases (one to three), and no lymph node metastasis were important favorable prognostic factors.[171]

In a series of 133 patients with uterine malignancies reported by Anraku and colleagues, 5-year survival rates in women with squamous cell carcinoma, cervical adenocarcinoma, and endometrial carcinoma were 47%, 40%, and 76%, respectively.[173] Leitao and colleagues reviewed 41 patients with recurrent uterine leiomyosarcoma; 18 patients had distant metastases, 6 had both local and distant metastases, and 17 had local recurrence.[174] Thoracic resection was performed in 13 patients. The authors noted that DFI and complete resection were predictors of improved survival. Kumar and colleagues reviewed 97 patients with metastatic gestational trophoblastic disease; chemotherapy was the treatment of choice.[175] Selective thoracotomy in patients with solitary lung metastases reduced the treatment time and need for further aggressive chemotherapy. The overall 2-year survival rate after diagnosis was 65%. A DFI of <1 year was associated with poorer survival. Barter and colleagues studied 2,116 patients with primary cervical malignancy between 1969 and 1984 and found 88 patients (88 of 2,116, or 4.16%) with pulmonary lesions consistent with metastases.[176] Prognosis was poor with chemotherapy only (median survival 8 months), and only 2 of 88 were long-term survivors. Imachi and colleagues identified 50 of 817 patients (6.1%) treated for carcinoma of the uterine cervix who developed pulmonary metastases; 81% of these patients had local recurrence or other metastases, and chemotherapy was given.[177] The authors suggest that surgery may be considered for patients with pulmonary metastases without extrathoracic metastases.

Resection of pulmonary metastases from squamous cell carcinoma of the uterine cervix has also been described by Fuller and Seki and their coinvestigators.[172,178] The role of chemotherapy for treatment of endometrial cancer is evolving, although there is no standard chemotherapy regimen for patients with metastatic disease. Niwa and colleagues have reported on patients who underwent chemotherapy with paclitaxel and carboplatin.[167] The multiple lung metastases

either disappeared or remained as scars after six courses. The patients have remained disease-free for 28 and 7 months, respectively.

RENAL CELL CARCINOMA

Various series have examined the value of resection of pulmonary metastases from renal cell carcinoma. Several recent collected series have demonstrated the safety and efficacy of resection of metastatic renal cell carcinoma. Pfannschmidt and colleagues noted that complete resection of the pulmonary metastases, absence of primary tumor recurrence, and absence of other extrathoracic metastatic disease were associated with a 5-year survival rate of 36.9%.[179] In patients with complete resection, the 5-year survival rate was 41.5%, compared with 22.1% for patients with an incomplete resection. Multivariate analysis demonstrated that the number of pulmonary metastases, the involvement of lymph nodes with regional metastases, and the length of the DFI were overall predictors of survival. Similar findings were confirmed by Piltz and Friedel and their colleagues as well as by Fischer and Schmid.[180–182]

Schott and colleagues reported 39 patients (4.1%) with pulmonary metastases after nephrectomy for renal carcinoma in 938 patients.[183] Patients with pulmonary metastases <2 cm in diameter and limited to one site had prolonged survival and DFI compared with other patients. Pogrebniak and colleagues from the National Cancer Institute reported 23 patients who underwent resection of pulmonary metastases from renal cell carcinoma, of which 18 had previous interleukin-2–based immunotherapy.[184] The patients who underwent resection (15 of 23, or 65%) had a longer survival (mean 49 months; median not reached) than did the patients who did not receive resective surgery (median 16 months; $p = 0.02$). Post-resection survival did not depend on the number of nodules seen on CT, resected nodules, or the DFI. Complete resection was the most important factor associated with 5-year survival, as described by Fourquier and van der Poel and their colleagues.[185,186] Murthy and colleagues confirmed that larger number and size of metastatic nodules, increasing number of lymph node metastases, shorter DFI, and diminished preoperative forced vital capacity were negative prognostic factors.[187]

MELANOMA

The overall biologic behavior of melanoma cannot be predicted. Most commonly, pulmonary metastases occur in addition to other regional (lymphatic) or visceral sites, and overall long-term survival is poor. In the rare patient who presents with isolated pulmonary metastases, resection may be associated with long-term survival as shown in Figure 108.9A,B.[188,189] Five-year survival rates range from 4.5% to 25%. In a large series of 1,521 patients with stage IV melanoma, the 5-year survival rate was only 4% (median survival 8.3 months), as reported by Barth and colleagues.[190] PET scans may be effective for screening for extrathoracic metastases in patients with potentially isolated pulmonary metastases. Patients who underwent resection of radiologically isolated pulmonary metastases had a 5-year survival rate of 22.1%; and those who underwent a PET scan preoperatively had significantly better 5-year survival, as noted by Dalrymple-Hay and colleagues.[191] As observed in the retrospective database of Pastorino, patients with recurrent disease after resection of lung metastases from melanoma will mostly have extrathoracic recurrences not amenable to surgical resection.[2] Allen and Coit found that patients with early recurrence (within 1 year), multiple metastases, and incompletely resected metastases will have poor survival.[192]

Gorenstein and colleagues evaluated 56 patients with histologically proven pulmonary metastases from melanoma. The overall

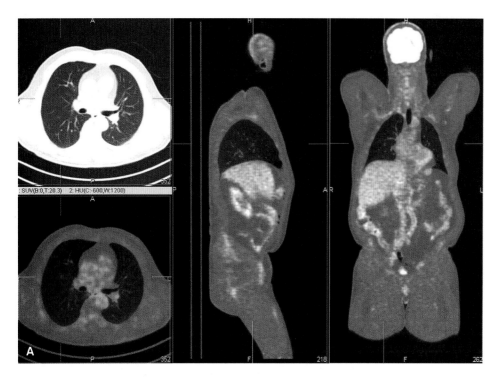

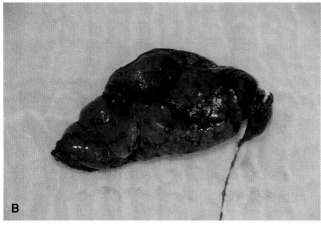

FIGURE 108.9 Patient with history of melanoma of right scapula. During follow-up multiple chest nodules were detected on PET-CT scanning (**A**). Besides one lung metastasis multiple hyaline nodules were found which were not metastatic (**B**).

post-resection survival rate was 25% at 5 years.[193] Patients with earlier primary stage melanoma and those with metastases to the lungs as the first site of metastasis had longer post-resection survival than did other patients. Location of the primary tumor, histology, thickness, Clark level, nodal metastases, metastasis doubling time, and type of resection of the primary tumor were not associated with improved post-resection survival.

Lewis and Harpole evaluated pulmonary metastases in 945 patients in a population of 7,564 melanoma patients.[194,195] Bilateral as well as multiple metastases were present in most of these patients. Multivariate predictors of survival included complete resection, DFI, chemotherapy, two or fewer metastases, negative lymph nodes, and histologic type. The 5-year survival for all 7,564 patients was 4%, in contrast to a 20% 5-year survival rate in patients with resection of the pulmonary metastases.

SQUAMOUS CELL CARCINOMA

Squamous cell carcinomas of the aerodigestive tract may occur in one or multiple areas. In patients with a primary squamous cell carcinoma outside the lung, pulmonary metastases or a separate primary lung cancer may occur. Secondary lung neoplasms may be resected with survival benefit, as emphasized by Nibu and colleagues.[196] They found an overall 5-year survival rate of 32% in patients undergoing complete resection of squamous cell carcinoma metastases resulting from a primary tumor of the head and neck. A solitary pulmonary nodule correlated with improvement in survival. Finley and colleagues described factors associated with improved survival in patients with squamous cell carcinoma metastases from head and neck cancers.[197] These included complete resection, control of primary, early stage of head and neck primary, one nodule on chest radiograph, and longer DFI (>2 years) from primary resection. Complete resection of all malignant disease was associated with a 5-year survival rate of 29%. The number of nodules was not significantly associated with survival. However, in eight patients with >1 nodule, median survival was 2 years, and there were no 5-year survivors. Therefore the benefits of resection of multiple pulmonary metastases from head and neck primary squamous cell carcinoma are not completely clear and no prospective randomized evidence is currently available.

When imaging examinations reveal a solitary pulmonary lesion after treatment of primary squamous cell carcinoma elsewhere in the body, the origin of the pulmonary lesion remains questionable. The lesion may represent a solitary metastasis, a primary bronchial carcinoma, or a benign process. In patients with a prior diagnosis of NSCLC, the lesion would be considered a metastasis if with similar histology and within 2 years of original resection or a new primary if >2 years from original resection. The recommended treatment for such a solitary lesion is bronchoscopy, thoracic exploration, and an excisional biopsy. If a squamous cell carcinoma is identified, a lobectomy and systematic mediastinal lymph node dissection should be performed, particularly if there is any question that the lesion could be a second primary neoplasm. In patients with compromised pulmonary function, a sublobar resection may be indicated.[198]

Lefor and colleagues attempted to correlate primary carcinomas of the head and neck with subsequent development of pulmonary metastases or second primary lung carcinomas.[39] They used an algorithm that considered the DFI, histology, radiographic findings, and characteristics of the lung lesion as well as the identification of mediastinal lymphadenopathy. The authors recommend that indeterminate lesions be treated as primary lung carcinomas (e.g., lobectomy and mediastinal lymph node dissection) because this provides the best local control of the disease as well as the potential for cure. Leong and colleagues proposed a way of distinguishing metastases of squamous cell carcinoma of the head and neck from primary squamous cell carcinoma of the lung.[199] In 16 patients, deletion of loci on chromosomal arms 3p and 9p was compared with the primary head and neck squamous cell carcinoma and the solitary squamous cell carcinoma in the lung. Similar (concordant) patterns of loss suggest metastases; however, three patients' tumors had different (discordant) patterns of loss, pointing to separate primary neoplasms. The authors suggest that microsatellite analysis can be applied to the patient with multiple tumors for additional refinement of the site of origin. Such knowledge may influence subsequent therapy.

CHILDHOOD TUMORS

Primary tumors of childhood—such as hepatoma, neuroblastoma, hepatoblastoma, osteogenic sarcoma, Ewing's sarcoma, and rhabdomyosarcoma—commonly spread to the lungs; however, with the exception of osteogenic sarcoma, other sites of metastatic disease are frequent. Chemotherapy remains the major treatment modality for metastases in multiple sites in children. Pulmonary resection for metastases may be required for initial or salvage therapy, to document metastases in the lungs, to assess the tumor's response to chemotherapy or the viability of the remaining tumor, and to enhance post-resection survival in children with resectable metastases.

Hepatoblastoma

Hepatoblastoma may metastasize to the lungs in about 44% of patients, as described by Uchiyama, Karnak, and Perilongo and their colleagues.[200–202] Improved survival in patients with hepatoblastoma requires a multidisciplinary treatment program including resection of the hepatoblastoma in the liver, combination chemotherapy (cisplatin based), and resection of isolated pulmonary metastases. The latter has been found to be a safe procedure with a positive impact on patient's prognosis although surgical aspects or guidelines for resection of lung metastases have not been clearly established.[203]

Combination chemotherapy is recommended by Katzenstein and Nishimura and their coinvestigators.[204,205] Perilongo and colleagues described a prospective single-arm study of preoperative cisplatin and doxorubicin for patients presenting with metastases from hepatoblastoma followed by surgical resection and two more courses of adjuvant chemotherapy.[202] In this study, conducted by the International Society of Pediatric Oncology, 31 of 154 patients presented with metastases. Five-year overall survival rate was 57%. The authors recommended the aforementioned therapeutic strategy for systemic and local control in these children. The International Society of Pediatric Oncology also reported 40 children with hepatocellular carcinoma; this study was published by Czauderna and colleagues.[206] Metastatic disease was identified in 31% of these patients and was associated with a worse survival compared with children with hepatoblastoma.

Wilms' Tumor

Patients with Wilms' tumor may present with pulmonary metastases at the time of diagnosis or as a relapse after initial treatment, as recorded by Macklis and colleagues.[207] Early diagnosis using chest CT scan may identify metastases in up to 36% of patients, as shown by Wilimas and colleagues.[208] Pulmonary metastases may be resected safely from children with Wilms' tumor (Fig. 108.10A,B), as emphasized by de Kraker, di Lorenzo, and Fuchs and colleagues.[203,209,210] Green and colleagues described 211 patients entered in one of the

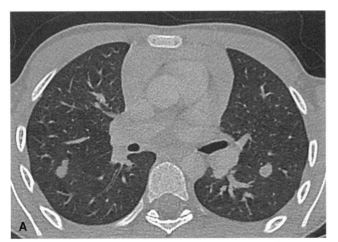
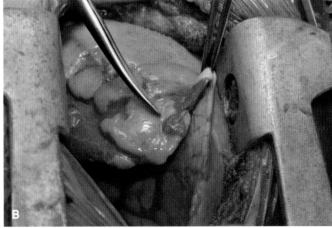

FIGURE 108.10 Ten-year-old patient with history of nephrectomy for Wilms' tumor. Bilateral lung metastases were present on chest CT scan (**A**) which were removed by staged thoracotomies preceded by systemic chemotherapy (**B**).

three National Wilms' Tumor Studies whose initial relapse was in the lungs and who showed no survival advantage to resection of pulmonary metastases over treatment with chemotherapy and whole-lung irradiation.[211] Combination therapy, including surgery, radiation, and chemotherapy, may be applied. Godzinski and colleagues noted that 4-year disease-free survival with pulmonary metastasis reached 83% with such therapy.[212]

Ewing's Sarcoma

Ewing's sarcoma metastasizes preferentially to the lungs in children and may be resected as described by Bacci and Fuchs.[203,213] Lanza and colleagues examined patients with resectable pulmonary metastases from Ewing's sarcoma.[214] These patients had prolonged survival (actuarial 5-year survival 15%; median 28 months) compared with patients who were explored but found to have unresectable metastases (no survivors beyond 22 months; median survival 12 months; $p = 0.0047$). Patients with ≤4 metastases had better survival than patients with >4 nodules. Lung irradiation may aid in prolonging survival, according to Spunt and Dunst and their colleagues.[215,216] Spunt and colleagues noted a 5-year survival rate of 37.3%.[215] The European Intergroup Cooperative Ewing's Sarcoma Studies reported 114 patients with Ewing's sarcoma who underwent peri-operative chemotherapy and local treatment for the primary tumor.[217] Whole-lung radiation therapy (15 to 18 Gy) was given to 75 patients; 63% of first relapses involved the lung. Adverse risk factors included poor chemotherapy response of the primary tumor, bilateral metastases, and no lung irradiation, as reported by Paulussen and colleagues.[217,218]

Osteogenic Sarcoma

Osteogenic sarcoma metastasizes preferentially to the lungs and may be resected with associated survival benefit (see prior discussion on osteogenic sarcoma in this chapter). Resection of pulmonary metastases from osteogenic sarcoma is associated with prolonged post-resection survival, as noted by La Quaglia as well as by Bacci and Hirano and their colleagues.[49,219,220] Adjuvant therapy, such as chemotherapy, as proposed by Goorin and colleagues, or lung irradiation, as proposed by Burgers and Whelan and their colleagues, may also be valuable, particularly for micrometastases.[48,221,222] Snyder and colleagues have suggested that post-resection survival may be as high as 39% at 5 years.[110] La Quaglia found that 80% of patients without distant metastases at presentation had long-term survival with treatment including chemotherapy, as compared with only 20% before 1970.[219]

In a review of 39 patients with a single pulmonary metastasis treated at three major centers, recurrent osteosarcoma occurred at a median of 2.5 years after the initial diagnosis.[223] Median age at diagnosis was 14.6 years. All patients underwent metastasectomy and 31% also received chemotherapy; 10-year post-relapse event-free and overall survival were 33% and 53%, respectively. Chemotherapy had no added benefit in this particular group of patients.

Kaste and colleagues reviewed 32 patients with synchronous primary and pulmonary metastases.[224] Only one patient had a solitary bone metastasis without lung metastases. Chest CT was used to identify synchronous pulmonary metastases. The authors note that the number of nodules and the lobes of the lung involved were predictors of survival.

RECURRENT PULMONARY METASTASES

If pulmonary metastases recur in the lungs after initial complete resection, repeat resection (one or more times) can be performed

(Fig. 108.7). Patients may be selected by the same criteria as presented in Table 108.1. In the retrospective international database of Pastorino, patients with recurrent disease after previous metastasectomy were analyzed separately.[2] In case of colorectal carcinoma or sarcoma, most patients presented with single or multiple recurrent metastases inside the chest in contrast to patients with melanoma who presented with extrathoracic recurrences in the majority of cases. In general, 5-year survival rate after a second pulmonary metastasectomy was still 44%, but these are highly selected patients presenting with tumors with a favorable biologic behavior. Kandioler and colleagues reported 35 patients who had undergone reoperation for pulmonary metastasis.[225] The 5- and 10-year survival rates were 48% and 28%, respectively. A DFI >1 year was a favorable prognostic factor. There was no survival advantage associated with histology, whether epithelial carcinoma, osteosarcoma, or soft tissue sarcoma.

Several studies have reviewed results of multiple resections for recurrent pulmonary metastases. Rizzoni and colleagues have described 29 patients with recurrent pulmonary metastases from soft tissue sarcomas with two or more resections of pulmonary metastases.[226] Patients with favorable tumor biology (resectable metastases, longer TDT, ≤3 nodules, and DFI of >6 months) had longer survival. There was no operative mortality, and complications occurred in only 7.5%. Median survival was 14.5 months, and the overall 5-year survival rate was 22%. Resectable patients had a median survival of 24 months. Casson and colleagues confirmed these findings in 39 patients with adult soft tissue sarcomas.[129] Thirty-four patients were resectable (median survival time 28 months; 5-year survival rate about 32%). Unresectable patients had a median survival of 7 months. Median survival after resection of a solitary recurrent metastasis was 65 months, as compared with patients with ≥2 nodules (14 months median; $p = 0.01$). Weiser and colleagues reviewed patients who relapsed after complete resection of isolated pulmonary metastases.[227] The post-thoracotomy disease-specific survival following re-resection was 42.8 months (estimated 5-year survival rate 36%). The authors noted three independent prognostic factors associated with favorable outcomes: (a) one or two nodules, (b) size ≤2 cm, and (c) lower-grade primary tumor histology. Patients without good prognostic factors had a median disease-specific survival of 10 months. The authors suggest that re-exploration and resection of recurrent pulmonary metastases from sarcoma could be beneficial with improvements in survival. Patients with poor prognostic factors will have worse survival and should be considered for alternative or investigational therapies. In the report by Casiraghi and colleagues, the number of metastasectomies did not statistically influence long-term survival.[102]

Repeat resection of pulmonary metastasis may salvage a subset of pediatric patients with sarcomatous histologies. These pediatric sarcomas include osteogenic sarcoma, nonrhabdomyosarcomatous soft tissue sarcoma, and Ewing's sarcoma. At the National Cancer Institute, Temeck and colleagues described 70 patients who underwent at least one reoperation between 1965 and 1995.[228] Osteosarcoma predominated, with 36 patients. Single-wedge resection was the most common operation performed (84%). The authors note that complete resection was the most important and favorable prognostic factor. Patients with complete resection had improved survival compared with those who were incompletely resected. Median survival was 2.3 years. In resectable patients, median survival was 5.6 years, compared with 0.7 year in unresectable patients ($p <0.0001$). From this review, the authors conclude that an aggressive surgical approach in patients with small numbers of lesions, longer DFI, and the ability to obtain a complete resection is warranted and associated with prolonged survival.

PROGNOSTIC INDICATORS

Predictors for improved survival have been studied retrospectively for various tumor types to identify selected patients who will benefit from pulmonary metastasectomy. These prognostic indicators are clinical, biologic, and molecular criteria that describe the biologic interaction between the metastases and the patient and their association with prolonged survival. These prognostic indicators may be used to identify patients who are most likely to benefit from resection of pulmonary metastases.

Analysis of prognostic indicators in groups of patients with pulmonary metastases from heterogeneous tumors describes prolonged survival in patients with resectable metastases. Complete resection, longer DFI, longer TDT, fewer numbers of metastases, or solitary metastasis are prognostic indicators generally associated with prolonged post-resection survival. Prognostic indicators should be studied in patients with the same primary tumor to define their association with post-resection survival. A wide variability exists in the characteristics of pulmonary metastases from different primary neoplasms and the subsequent survival of patients with these metastases. The study of prognostic indicators from the same primary neoplasm yields the most precise information on association with post-resection survival. Age and gender do not usually influence post-thoracotomy survival and generally should not be considered prognostic factors.

COMPLETE RESECTION

Complete resection consistently correlates with improved post-thoracotomy survival for patients with pulmonary metastases. If pulmonary metastases cannot be completely removed, the post-thoracotomy survival rate is less than that for patients who underwent complete resection. This is clearly shown in the International Registry published by Pastorino and colleagues indicating complete resection as a major prognostic factor.[2] However, in contrast to lung cancer, no precise criteria exist to define complete R0, microscopically incomplete R1, macroscopically incomplete R2, or uncertain resections while performing lung metastasectomy.

LOCATION AND STAGE OF PRIMARY TUMOR

Post-resection survival is not usually influenced by the specific anatomic location of the primary tumor. Post-resection survival in patients with more advanced primary neoplasms does not usually differ from that in patients with earlier-stage disease. Although initial or primary stage may suggest the biologic aggressiveness of the tumor, it has little impact on subsequent survival in patients with isolated pulmonary metastases.

DISEASE-FREE INTERVAL

The initial DFI extends from resection of the primary tumor until pulmonary metastases or other metastases are detected. A short DFI may indicate a more virulent tumor with a poor prognosis. Metastases may be multiple and grow rapidly. A longer DFI may represent a less biologically aggressive tumor and correlates with a longer post-resection survival. The DFI may also be defined as the time between resection of the pulmonary metastases and recurrence of metastases in the lungs or elsewhere. DFIs of >12 months are usually associated with improved survival. A DFI >36 months was an independent predictor of survival in the International Registry of Lung Metastases, as shown by Pastorino and colleagues.[2]

NUMBER OF NODULES ON PREOPERATIVE RADIOGRAPHIC STUDIES

High-resolution CT is currently the preferred examination in patients with suspected pulmonary metastases due to its high sensitivity. However, as discussed previously in the section "Diagnosis," specificity is lower as nodules may or may not represent metastases. Theoretically, earlier detection and treatment of metastases could improve survival. Laterality (unilateral or bilateral) of pulmonary metastases does not directly influence post-resection survival; the number of nodules is a more precise prognostic indicator.

NUMBER OF METASTASES RESECTED

The number of metastases resected may be associated with DFS and overall survival. Complete resection is needed. In general, the number of metastases resected exceeds the total number of nodules identified on preoperative radiographic studies. Careful palpation of lung parenchyma will identify more nodules than would be otherwise suspected based on preoperative studies, especially in patients with osteogenic or soft tissue sarcomas. These nodules may be benign or malignant and must be resected in order to have histologic confirmation of the status. Not all nodules on preoperative chest radiographic studies are malignant, as discussed previously in the section "Diagnosis."

TUMOR DOUBLING TIME

TDT is based on original observations by Collins and colleagues and was applied for lung metastases by Joseph and colleagues.[229–231] TDT has been analyzed for multiple tumor types and is calculated by measuring the same metastasis on similar studies (e.g., serial chest radiographs), which are separated by a minimum of 10 to 14 days. The most rapidly growing nodule is selected. The TDT can be easily calculated by plotting changing diameters of pulmonary metastases on semilogarithmic paper; however, graphical error may be present. A mathematical formula may be used to precisely calculate TDT:

$$TDT = time \times 0.231/\ln (\text{second diameter/first diameter})$$

where time is the difference in days between the first diameter measurement and the second diameter measurement and ln is the natural logarithm.

Errors may occur in the calculation of TDT because not all metastases grow at the same rate. Different growth rates between tumor nodules may reflect heterogeneity of metastases from the primary. The TDT may indirectly reveal the underlying biologic nature of the metastases and therefore influence the patient's post-resection survival.

Pulmonary metastases initially grow exponentially, and with increased size, the growth rate diminishes. Laird described growth kinetics which considered a gradual diminution in TDT with time and increased size of the metastasis.[232] The specific growth rate may be difficult to determine because classical radiographs demonstrate a 3D structure in two dimensions. Tumor volume calculations may better describe the TDT in selected patients, as described by Belshi and Eggli et al.[233,234] In addition, the growth rate measured over a few weeks represents only a brief period in the lifetime of the metastasis. Although this growth rate is presumed to be linear, it may not always follow this pattern, and TDT reflects only growth during the interval measured. Volumetric assessment has also been described by Vogel and colleagues to evaluate response after chemotherapy allowing more precise measurements.[235]

ENDOBRONCHIAL OR NODAL METASTASES

Involvement of mediastinal lymph nodes from pulmonary metastases is probably underreported as not in all series a consistent lymph node dissection has been performed. As discussed previously in the section "Selection of Patients for Resection," hilar or mediastinal lymph node involvement heralds a poorer prognosis. Udelsman and colleagues note that patients with endobronchial metastases from adult soft tissue sarcomas have a short post-resection survival.[236] Seven of 11 patients with endobronchial metastases lived ≤6 months.

MULTIVARIATE ANALYSIS OF PROGNOSTIC FACTORS

Use of multivariate analysis may allow more accurate prediction of post-resection survival and better patient selection. Separate prognostic variables may be combined to enhance the predictive value for survival. Jablons and colleagues found the DFI, gender, resectability, and truncal location in patients with pulmonary metastases from soft tissue sarcomas to be the best predictors of post-thoracotomy survival.[128] Putnam and colleagues noted that DFI >12 months, TDT >20 days, and ≤4 nodules on preoperative full-lung tomograms as multivariate prognostic indicators were the best predictors of post-thoracotomy survival in patients with pulmonary metastases from soft tissue sarcomas.[70] Roth and colleagues compared prognostic indicators in patients with osteogenic sarcoma and soft tissue sarcoma.[237] When combined, the TDT, number of metastases on preoperative full-lung tomograms, and DFI improved predictive ability over any single indicator or pair of indicators. Multivariate analysis in the International Registry published by Pastorino and colleagues showed incomplete resection, DFI <36 months, >1 lung metastasis, and specific histologic types as melanoma to be significant negative factors in relation to survival.[2]

NOVEL TREATMENT STRATEGIES

Thoracic surgeons take full advantage of the unique and fortuitous tumor biology represented by the patient with isolated and resectable pulmonary metastases. Despite better-refined and more aggressive resection techniques, enhanced selection of patients, and evolving multidisciplinary care, only a minority of patients with isolated pulmonary metastases undergo resection. Better therapy must include treatment for macroscopic disease as well as occult or microscopic disease.

Various strategies have been proposed to treat metastases more effectively isolated to the lung. Systemic (intravenous) chemotherapy has been discussed in the context of specific histology. New and experimental techniques include identification of molecular markers that would serve to identify metastases and their organ of origin as well as their potential responsiveness to systemic chemotherapy. Identification of these characteristics may lead to specific gene replacement strategy or chemotherapy aimed at certain genetic products. Directed regional drug delivery can be accomplished through various routes, including inhalation, chemoembolization, or isolated single- or double-lung perfusion or infusion. Recently,

the general concept of synthetic lethality directed at multiple pathways seems a promising therapeutic approach which may also be applied to lung metastases.[238]

MOLECULAR CHARACTERISTICS FOR TARGETED THERAPY

Molecular events associated with pulmonary metastases have been identified in patients with osteogenic sarcoma as recently reported by Zhou and colleagues.[239] Amplification of the MDM2 gene (the human homolog of a murine p53-binding protein) may regulate p53 protein function by inactivating the protein and deregulating or enhancing tumor growth as described in a recent review by Iwamuka and Agarwal.[240] Ladanyi and colleagues noted no detectable MDM2 gene amplification in the primary osteogenic sarcoma, compared with its presence in 14% of metastases.[241] Amplification of MDM2 may be associated with metastases and tumor progression in osteogenic sarcoma. However, Sugano and colleagues found a decrease of MDM2 gene amplification in metastatic colorectal cancer showing that the precise function of MDM2 is still not fully understood.[242]

Changes in Ki-67 activity are associated with worse survival and tumor progression, as shown by Hernandez-Rodriguez and colleagues.[243] They evaluated 38 patients with immunohistochemical analysis. Fifteen of 17 patients who expressed Ki-67 developed pulmonary metastases and had a higher mortality rate. The author recommended using Ki-67 as a prognostic molecular marker for pulmonary metastases in patients with osteogenic sarcoma. This is further supported by a study of Matsumoto and colleagues, who reported that the combined use of vascular endothelial growth factor A (VEGF-A) and Ki-67 can predict outcome in osteosarcoma metastases.[244] At the end of their study, all patients with negative VEGF-A and Ki-67 expression were alive whereas all patients who had positive VEGF-A and Ki-67 died within 5 years.

Reduced expression of KAI1/CD82 is associated with poor prognosis and metastasis. Arihiro and Inai reviewed the role of KAI1 and its relationship to metastases and prognosis.[212] At least 67% of benign bone tumors and 36% of osteogenic sarcomas express this metastasis-suppressor gene. Only one of four patients with osteogenic sarcoma metastatic to the lung was positive for KAI1/CD82. A marked reduction of KAI1/CD82 was reported for metastatic melanoma by Tang and colleagues, suggesting it to be a prognostic marker in melanoma patients.[245] The reduction of KAI1/CD82 is also found in many other tumor types like prostate, breast, and ovarian cancer.

Pollock and colleagues noted that in soft tissue sarcomas, mutations of the p53 gene, a tumor-suppressor gene, may provide for uncontrolled cell growth.[246] Restoration of normal p53 ("wild-type") levels to soft tissue sarcomas may provide more controlled cell growth or even programmed cell death (apoptosis). In one in vitro study, transduction of wild-type p53 into soft tissue sarcomas bearing mutated p53 genes altered the malignant potential of the tumor. After transduction, transfected cells expressed wild-type p53, decreased cell proliferation, and decreased colony formation in soft agar, and demonstrated decreased tumor formation in severe combined immunodeficient mice in vivo.[246] The ability to restore wild-type p53 function in soft tissue sarcoma in vitro and in these mice may ultimately be considered as future therapy for patients with soft tissue sarcomas.

Targets for gene transfer may include chemotherapy-resistant tumors or tumors with a greater propensity for metastatic spread. Scotlandi and colleagues noted that overexpression of the MDR1 gene product P-glycoprotein, which is a multidrug transport protein, is an important predictor of poor prognosis in osteosarcoma patients treated with chemotherapy.[247] A rodent model of osteogenic sarcoma with a high propensity for pulmonary metastasis has been developed by Asai and colleagues.[248] In this metastatic tumor model, matrix metalloproteinase-2 (MMP-2) activity increased, as did VEGF messenger RNA (mRNA). As mentioned previously, the combined increase of VEGF-A and Ki-67 had a negative effect on survival in patients with osteosarcoma.[244]

Patients with tumors that exhibit overexpression of P-glycoprotein develop resistance to chemotherapeutic agents. In these patients, the MDR phenotype is not de novo more aggressive (i.e., more metastatic); however, the poor outcome of patients with the MDR phenotype associated with P-glycoprotein overexpression is related to the cells' lack of response to cytotoxic drugs. A doxorubicin sensitivity assay recommended by Kumta and colleagues may be a better determinant of improved chemotherapy responsiveness and subsequent clinical outcome than P-glycoprotein.[249] One potential mechanism of resistance to doxorubicin may lie in the ability to regulate MDR1 RNA levels after administration of doxorubicin, as shown by Abolhoda and coinvestigators.[250]

Attenuation of insulin-like growth factor (IGF) activation may also improve survival, as proposed by Beech and colleagues.[251] Activation of the IGF-1 receptor decreases the systemic response to doxorubicin. In vitro studies have demonstrated that activation of the IGF-1 receptor enhances tumor resistance to doxorubicin. Inhibition of IGF-1 receptor activation may be an effective adjunct to conventional chemotherapy as reported by Olmos and colleagues.[252]

Increased expression of erbB-2 or gene amplification has been associated with poor survival in patients with osteogenic sarcoma, as shown by Onda and colleagues.[253] In this study, 42% of patients with osteogenic sarcoma had metastases that expressed erbB-2 and correlated with early development of pulmonary metastasis and poor survival. ErbB-2, therefore, may enhance tumor growth and promote metastases. These authors recommended that erbB-2 be considered a prognostic factor for patients with osteosarcoma. Murine models for "suicide gene therapy" treatment of osteogenic sarcoma cells have been developed by Seto and colleagues.[254] However, differences between the primary tumor and the metastases from osteosarcoma may exist. Akatsuka and colleagues examined the relationship between erbB-2 and survival in patients with osteogenic sarcoma.[255] Eighty-one patients with osteogenic sarcoma in the extremities were treated with resection and chemotherapy; 61% of the patients had high levels of expression of erbB-2. Patients with higher levels of expression had improved DFS and overall survival. Patients with decreased levels had a worse prognosis.

Other gene products have been proposed for transfer into pulmonary metastases. Benjamin and colleagues have proposed treatment of pulmonary metastases using bolus intravenous injections of Ad-OC-E1 in patients who had exhausted all chemotherapy regimens of greater effectiveness.[256] The adenoviral vector Ad-OC-E1a (OCaP1) contains a murine osteocalcin (OC) promoter to regulate the production of the adenoviral E1a protein.

LOCOREGIONAL CHEMOTHERAPY TREATMENTS

Novel drug delivery systems may enhance chemotherapy treatment effects by increasing drug concentration in lung tissues and minimizing systemic effects and toxicity of such treatment, as noted by Putnam and Van Schil and colleagues.[257,258] In many patients, surgery has been used as sole therapy or as salvage treatment after maximal chemotherapy response has been achieved. Systemic toxicity may limit the amount of chemotherapy given to an individual patient. Regional drug delivery to the lungs minimizes systemic drug delivery,

thus preventing systemic toxicity; however, this technique substantially increases the drug delivered to the lung over a short period. Several techniques have been reported to achieve highly efficient locoregional chemotherapeutic treatment, of which isolated lung perfusion, selective pulmonary artery perfusion, and chemoembolization are the most thoroughly investigated. The technique of clinical isolated lung perfusion as performed at the Antwerp University Hospital, Belgium, is shown in Videos 108.1 and 108.2.

Preclinical studies by Weksler and coinvestigators in rodents with experimental pulmonary metastases from a methylcholanthrene-induced syngeneic sarcoma have shown that chemotherapy may be delivered regionally to pulmonary tissue in significantly higher concentrations than by systemic delivery.[259,260] Minimal to no systemic toxicity was noted. In this model, isolated single-lung perfusion with doxorubicin was safe and effective. A simple microsurgical technique was performed in rats. After left thoracotomy, the pulmonary artery and veins were isolated and clamped. The lung was flushed before infusing doxorubicin. The infusion occurred over 10 minutes. Then, the drug was flushed out before the cannulas were removed and circulation was restored. A perfusion concentration of 255 mg/L caused less general toxicity than a systemic dose equivalent to 75 mg/m². The extraction ratio was 58%, and pulmonary tissue concentration of doxorubicin was 25-fold higher than with the systemic dose. The technique was also effective. Nine of 10 animals treated at 320 mg/L had complete eradication of metastases from an implanted methylcholanthrene-induced sarcoma. Other chemotherapeutic agents have been used, including melphalan and gemcitabine by Van Putte and colleagues and paclitaxel by Schrump and colleagues.[261-263] So far, only melphalan has shown to be effective against pulmonary metastases from both sarcoma and adenocarcinoma in animal models, as shown by Den Hengst and Hendriks and colleagues.[264-266]

Initial clinical studies of lung perfusion by Pass and Johnston and their colleagues have shown higher drug concentrations in pulmonary tissue, although clinical tumor response has been mixed.[267,268] Johnston and colleagues have described a continuous perfusion of the lungs with doxorubicin (single lung) as a safe experimental procedure and subsequently applied their technique clinically.[268] Drug concentrations in normal lung and tumor generally increased with higher drug dosages. Two of eight patients had major complications: one patient developed pneumonia and sternal dehiscence and another developed respiratory failure 4 days after lung perfusion. No objective responses occurred (none of four patients with sarcomas). Continuous perfusion with a pump circuit offers some theoretical advantages but may be mechanically complex.

Pass and colleagues examined isolated single-lung perfusion with tumor necrosis factor-alpha, interferon-alpha, and moderate hyperthermia for patients with unresectable pulmonary metastases.[267] No hospital deaths occurred, and a short-term (<6-month) decrease in nodule size was noted in 3 of 15 patients. Schroder and colleagues reported on four patients with sarcoma metastases treated with hyperthermic (41°C) isolated lung perfusion with cisplatin 70 mg/m².[269] No systemic toxicity was noted. One patient developed noncardiogenic edema of the lung, and the systemic cisplatin levels were continuously low. In a phase I study, Burt and colleagues examined the role of isolated lung perfusion with a dose escalation of doxorubicin.[270] The authors noted that drug concentrations in the treated lung correlated with the drug delivered. There was no cardiac or systemic toxicity. There were minimal or undetectable blood levels of the drug. One patient had no ventilation or perfusion in the lung after receiving 80 mg/m² of doxorubicin. No partial or complete responses were noted, although one patient developed stable disease for a period of time. The authors determined a maximum tolerated dose of 40 mg/m^2 in this isolated lung perfusion model. Similar findings were noted by Putnam and colleagues.[258]

Ratto and colleagues introduced the concept of combining resection of lung metastases with isolated lung perfusion as additional or adjuvant treatment.[271] In a series of six patients, platinum was administered in the perfusion circuit, which was found to be feasible and safe. Hendriks and colleagues reported a phase I trial in which melphalan was used in combination with pulmonary metastasectomy.[272] The maximum tolerated dose was set after this trial at 45 mg of melphalan at a perfusion temperature of 42°C. This phase I trial was followed by an extension trial, reported by Grootenboers and colleagues who concluded that the maximum tolerated dose was 45 mg of melphalan at a perfusion temperature of 37°C.[273] The long-term follow-up of these two trials (in total 23 patients) was reported by Den Hengst and colleagues, showing that isolated lung perfusion with melphalan has no long-term negative effect on pulmonary function and no long-term pulmonary toxicity.[274] As such, this technique is used as adjuvant treatment for resectable pulmonary metastases in order to reduce the local recurrence rate in the operated lung. So far, only one phase II trial has been published of isolated lung perfusion with melphalan for the treatment of resectable lung metastases. In this multicenter trial, reported by Den Hengst and colleagues, lung perfusion with melphalan was combined with pulmonary metastasectomy for the treatment of lung metastases from osteosarcoma, soft tissue sarcoma, and colorectal carcinoma.[275] A dose of 45 mg of melphalan was given at a perfusion temperature of 37°C; perfusion time was 30 minutes, followed by a 5 minute wash-out. In total 50 patients were included, of which 30 had colorectal carcinoma as primary tumor. Twelve patients had staged bilateral perfusions. There was no peri-operative mortality and acceptable short-term morbidity. After a median follow-up of 24 months, 18 patients died (2 of unrelated cause) and 30 patients had recurrent disease. The 3-year overall survival and disease-free survival were 57 ± 9% and 36 ± 8%, respectively. Survival data for colorectal cancer and sarcoma patients are provided in Table 108.3. This trial showed an intrapulmonary recurrence rate in the operated lung of 23% which is lower than the 48% to 66% reported by Pastorino and colleagues.[2] This finding suggests that isolated lung perfusion may be a valuable tool in the future in combined modality treatment of lung metastases.

Although the benefits of isolated lung perfusion are promising, it remains an invasive technique, which has to be combined with thoracotomy and one-lung ventilation. Therefore, less invasive techniques are currently explored. Selective pulmonary artery perfusion is an endovascular technique to apply high-dose chemotherapy by a minimally invasive technique. In this way, this procedure can be used repeatedly and also be applied in patients who cannot tolerate one-lung ventilation or have initially inoperable lung metastases. To enhance local uptake of the chemotherapeutic agent, a balloon is inflated in the pulmonary artery, causing blood flow occlusion. So far, only animal studies have been published using this technique. Furrer, Krueger, and colleagues used this technique with doxorubicin in a pig model, showing similar lung concentration levels as in isolated lung perfusion.[276,277] Van Putte and colleagues used gemcitabine in both a rodent and pig model, showing high lung levels of gemcitabine.[278,279] Den Hengst and colleagues reported the use of selective pulmonary artery perfusion with melphalan in a rodent model with pulmonary sarcoma metastases.[264] In this study the authors compared selective perfusion with isolated lung perfusion and systemic injection of melphalan. They found that selective pulmonary artery perfusion and isolated lung perfusion are equally effective and are both superior to intravenous melphalan in achieving high lung levels of melphalan, as well as in eliminating pulmonary metastases and improving survival.

As an alternative technique, chemoembolization with degradable starch microspheres loaded with carboplatin has been studied in an animal model by Schneider and colleagues.[280,281] The use of degradable microspheres allows for higher concentrations in the lung parenchyma during the degradation phase of the treatment. Vogl and colleagues used chemoembolization with palliative intention in 52 patients with unresectable lung metastases.[282] The tumor-feeding pulmonary arteries were selectively injected with lipiodol, mitomycin C, and microspheres under guidance of a pulmonary artery balloon catheter. Patients received repetitive treatment ranging from 2 to 10 sessions. Treatment was well tolerated without any major side effects or complications. Partial response was noted in 16 cases, stable disease in 11, and progressive in 25 cases. No follow-up studies were yet reported regarding this technique.

Brooks and coinvestigators have described effective in vivo delivery of gene products using a herpes virus factor.[283] They confirm that such treatment in a rat model of sarcomatous pulmonary metastasis can reduce tumor burden.

INHALATIONAL THERAPY

Inhalational therapy or inhalational administration of chemotherapy, gene products, or other biologic compounds (e.g., interleukin-2 [IL-2]) has been actively investigated by various authors, mainly for metastatic renal cell carcinoma and melanoma as described by Huland and colleagues.[284] Intratracheal instillation of macrophage-activating lipopeptide-2 served as an immunotherapeutic agent

TABLE 108.3 Survival Data According to Pathologic Diagnosis

	3-Year OS	4-Year OS	MST[a]	3-Year DFS	4-Year DFS	Median TTP[a]	3-Year PPFS	4-Year PPFS	Median TTLPP[a]
All patients	57 ± 9%	49 ± 11%	44 (95% CI 30–58)	36 ± 8%	36 ± 8%	16 (95% CI 7–25)	79 ± 6%	63 ± 15%	NR
CRC	62 ± 13%	62 ± 13%	NR	41 ± 11%	41 ± 11%	21 (95% CI 2–40)	72 ± 8%	72 ± 8%	NR
Sarcoma	48 ± 12%	32 ± 15%	30 (95% CI 8–51)	27 ± 10%	27 ± 10%	8 (95% CI 6–10)	90 ± 7%	45 ± 32%	44 (95% CI 11–77)

[a]Months.
CRC, colorectal cancer; NR, not reached; OS, overall survival; DFS, disease-free survival; MST, median survival time; TTP, time to progression; PPFS, pulmonary progression-free survival; TTLPP, time to local pulmonary progression.
Reprinted from den Hengst WA, Hendriks JM, Balduyck B, et al. Phase II multicenter clinical trial of pulmonary metastasectomy and isolated lung perfusion with melphalan in patients with resectable lung metastases. *J Thorac Oncol* 2014;9(10):1547–1553. Copyright © 2014 International Association for the Study of Lung Cancer. With permission.

against mammary adenocarcinoma, as noted by Shingu and colleagues in a murine model and by Hershey and colleagues in a canine model.[285,286] Aerosolized liposome-encapsulated paclitaxel was effective in reducing renal cell carcinoma metastases in a murine model developed by Koshkina and colleagues.[287] A mouse model of intranasal IL-2 gene delivery for effective treatment of pulmonary metastases from osteogenic sarcoma has been created by Jia and colleagues.[288] They used polyethylenimine (PEI), a polycationic DNA carrier, for gene product delivery. Mice treated had fewer and smaller pulmonary metastases than animals not treated. The authors noted high concentrations in the tumor area and observed minimal systemic toxicity. Enk and colleagues found that inhalational therapy with IL-2 in patients with pulmonary metastases from melanoma was safe and could be given with concurrent chemotherapy.[289] IL-2 aerosolized liposomes were also well tolerated, as reported by Skubitz and Anderson.[290] Posch and colleagues used low-dose IL-2 inhalation for the prevention of recurrence of pulmonary melanoma metastases after resection.[291] After a median follow-up of 25.7 months, no intrapulmonary recurrences occurred in the five patients they treated this way. Guma and colleagues found an improved survival in mice with osteosarcoma pulmonary metastases treated with aerosol IL-2 in combination with natural killer cells.[292] The use of inhaled gemcitabine caused an upregulation of Fas expression, which induced apoptosis in pulmonary osteosarcoma metastases in a mice model, as reported by Gordon and Kleinerman.[293]

BIOLOGIC MODIFIERS

Liposome-encapsulated muramyl tripeptide (L-MTP-E) activates macrophages to become tumoricidal. This strategy may be valuable in patients with chemoresistant tumors. After treatment, plasma levels of cytokines are increased. Monocyte-mediated cytotoxicity is also increased. L-MTP-E therapy may be therapeutically effective, as shown by Kleinerman and colleagues.[294,295] In a report from Meyers and colleagues, the use of L-MTP-E as additional treatment may reduce the risk of recurrence and death in patients with metastatic osteosarcoma.[296]

Investigations of DOTAP:cholesterol liposomes, protamine sulfate, and plasmid DNA construct (LPD) by Whitmore and colleagues have shown increased antitumor activity by the lipopolyplex alone as well as the LPD.[297] The mechanism of action suggests a systemic proinflammatory cytokine response.

RADIOFREQUENCY ABLATION

Radiofrequency ablation (RFA) provides controlled thermal destruction of tumors or other tissue and has been examined in several recent reviews. RFA has been applied to malignant liver tumors as described by Curley, the kidney by Finelli, Matin, and their colleagues, and the lung by Dupuy, Zhu, and colleagues.[298–301] The safe and effective use of interstitial thermal therapy (RFA) for the treatment of lung neoplasms was examined in preclinical models that reproducibly created thermal injuries in normal lung parenchyma. These lesions were affected by conductive heat loss through air, blood flow, and bronchi. Use of RFA techniques is still experimental for local control of pulmonary metastases. Limitations of RFA for lung metastases include potential injury to vascular or bronchial structures, generation of heat that must be dissipated, and failure to control or ablate all viable tumor, as described by Steinke and colleagues.[302] Usually, no precise histology is obtained and response evaluation is difficult to determine. An alternative technique to RFA

is microwave ablation utilizing electromagnetic waves resulting in coagulation necrosis.[303]

As pulmonary metastases have variable consistency, they may be difficult to penetrate with the large needle necessary to carry the ablation tines. Yan and colleagues described 55 "nonsurgical" patients who underwent RFA for colorectal pulmonary metastases.[304] Eligibility criteria included <7 nodules (30 were solitary), no nodule could be adjacent to bronchi or pulmonary vessel, and the primary cancer had to be under control. The median interval from the primary cancer to lung RFA was 25 months, and only four patients had poor performance status. Mean age was 62 years and the median number of pulmonary metastases ablated per patient was 2. A repeat RFA was performed in 24% of the patients. Complications occurred in 42% of patients, of which 16 were pneumothoraces and 9 of these required a chest tube. After a follow-up of 24 months, 21 of the 55 patients demonstrated local progression. Overall survival at 2 years was only 34%, and no patient who had a hilar lesion or a lesion ≥3 cm survived past 24 months.

Vogl and colleagues applied microwave ablation in 130 lesions observed in 80 patients.[303] Successful ablation was obtained in 73% of cases. For lesions <3 cm, success rate was 82% but for lesions >3 cm, only 25%. For peripheral lesions, ablation proved to be successful in 80% of cases in contrast to 50% for centrally located nodules. Two-year survival rate was 75%.

Percutaneous RFA was administered in 27 patients presenting with a total of 49 pulmonary metastases from colorectal carcinoma by Hiraki and colleagues.[305] A CT-guided approach was applied in 41 RFA sessions. Pneumothorax occurred in 20 of the latter patients (49%) but only 3 (7.3%) needed a chest tube. Primary effectiveness rate after 3 years was 56% and 3-year overall survival 48%. An interesting study was performed by Schneider and colleagues applying bipolar or multipolar RFA in 32 patients followed by resection by open thoracotomy.[306] Wedge resection or lobectomy was done together with a mediastinal lymph node dissection. Complete necrosis was present in 38%, scattered vital tumor in 50%, and incomplete ablation defined as >20% remaining vital tumor tissue in 13%. RFA was found to be technically feasible and safe but its curative concept is questioned due to the high rate of remaining viable tumor cells.

Palussière and colleagues attempted single-session RFA for bilateral lung lesions in 67 patients.[307] Single session was not possible in 40 patients (60%), mainly due to occurrence of pneumothorax. So, single session could be applied in 27 patients (40%) for treatment of 66 lung metastases. Overall incidence of pneumothorax was 67%. Median time to progression was 9.5 months and median overall survival time 26 months.

When applying RFA or stereotactic radiotherapy, no histologic confirmation of malignancy is usually present, there is no lymph node sampling, and for this reason, no precise tumor staging. This results in an unclear selection of patients for adjuvant therapy. With a percutaneous technique, palpation of lung parenchyma to ensure no additional lesions are present is not possible. Although survival and palliation may be improved, their use in operable patients remains controversial as discussed by Van Schil.[62] No randomized studies exist directly comparing these techniques to classical surgical resection. Because there is no clear definition of complete resection with these techniques, their use should presently be limited to functionally inoperable patients till randomized evidence becomes available. It should also be noted that salvage surgery performed after non-resectional therapies represents a major challenge for thoracic surgeons in many cases.[62] Further prospective studies are required to determine the precise results and long-term outcome of salvage surgery after non-resectional therapies.

REFERENCES

1. Treasure T, Internullo E, Utley M. Resection of pulmonary metastases: a growth industry. *Cancer Imaging* 2008;8:121–124.
2. Pastorino U, Buyse M, Friedel G, et al. Long-term results of lung metastasectomy: prognostic analyses based on 5206 cases. *J Thorac Cardiovasc Surg* 1997;113(1):37–49.
3. Hunter J, Allen E, Turk JL, et al. *The Case Books of John Hunter FRS.* Royal Society of Medicine Services; 1993.
4. Pastorino U, Treasure T. A historical note on pulmonary metastasectomy. *J Thorac Oncol* 2010;5(6 Suppl 2):S132–S133.
5. Barney JD CE. Adenocarcinoma of the kidney with metastasis to the lung cured by nephrectomy and lobectomy. *J Urol* 1939;42:269–1276.
6. Alexander J, Haight C. Pulmonary resection for solitary metastatic sarcomas and carcinomas. *Surge Gynecol Obstet* 1947;85(2):129–146.
7. Mannix EP, Jr. Resection of multiple pulmonary metastases fourteen years after amputation for osteochondrogenic sarcoma of tibia; apparent freedom from recurrence two years later. *J Thorac Surg* 1953;26(5):544–549.
8. Thomford NR, Woolner LB, Clagett OT. The surgical treatment of metastatic tumors in the lungs. *J Thorac Cardiovasc Surg* 1965;49:357–363.
9. Martini N, Huvos AG, Mike V, et al. Multiple pulmonary resections in the treatment of osteogenic sarcoma. *Ann Thorac Surg* 1971;12(3):271–280.
10. Putnam JB, Jr, Roth JA. Prognostic indicators in patients with pulmonary metastases. *Semin Surg Oncol* 1990;6(5):291–296.
11. Potter DA, Glenn J, Kinsella T, et al. Patterns of recurrence in patients with high-grade soft-tissue sarcomas. *J Clin Oncol* 1985;3(3):353–366.
12. Putnam JB, Jr, Suell DM, Natarajan G, et al. Extended resection of pulmonary metastases: Is the risk justified? *Ann Thorac Surg* 1993;55(6):1440–1446.
13. Onozato ML, Kovach AE, Yeap BY, et al. Tumor islands in resected early-stage lung adenocarcinomas are associated with unique clinicopathologic and molecular characteristics and worse prognosis. *Am J Surg Pathol* 2013;37(2):287–294.
14. Gaikwad A, Souza CA, Inacio JR, et al. Aerogenous metastases: a potential game changer in the diagnosis and management of primary lung adenocarcinoma. *Am J Roentgenol* 2014;203(6):W570–W582.
15. Govindan R. Cancer. Attack of the clones. *Science* 2014;346(6206):169–170.
16. Chen ZY, Zhong WZ, Zhang XC, et al. EGFR mutation heterogeneity and the mixed response to EGFR tyrosine kinase inhibitors of lung adenocarcinomas. *Oncologist* 2012;17(7):978–985.
17. Sardari Nia P, Hendriks J, Friedel G, et al. Distinct angiogenic and non-angiogenic growth patterns of lung metastases from renal cell carcinoma. *Histopathology* 2007;51(3):354–361.
18. Bocklage T, Leslie K, Yousem S, et al. Extracutaneous angiosarcomas metastatic to the lungs: clinical and pathologic features of twenty-one cases. *Mod Pathol* 2001;14(12):1216–1225.
19. Srinivas S, Varadhachary G. Spontaneous pneumothorax in malignancy: a case report and review of the literature. *Ann Oncol* 2000;11(7):887–879.
20. Snyder BJ, Pugatch RD. Imaging characteristics of metastatic disease to the chest. *Chest Surgery Clin N Am* 1998;8(1):29–48.
21. MacMahon H, Austin JH, Gamsu G, et al. Guidelines for management of small pulmonary nodules detected on CT scans: a statement from the Fleischner Society. *Radiology* 2005;237(2):395–400.
22. Naidich DP, Bankier AA, MacMahon H, et al. Recommendations for the management of subsolid pulmonary nodules detected at CT: a statement from the Fleischner Society. *Radiology* 2013;266(1):304–317.
23. Patel VK, Naik SK, Naidich DP, et al. A practical algorithmic approach to the diagnosis and management of solitary pulmonary nodules: part 1: radiologic characteristics and imaging modalities. *Chest* 2013;143(3):825–839.
24. Patel VK, Naik SK, Naidich DP, et al. A practical algorithmic approach to the diagnosis and management of solitary pulmonary nodules: part 2: pretest probability and algorithm. *Chest* 2013;143(3):840–846.
25. Detterbeck FC, Grodzki T, Gleeson F, et al. Imaging requirements in the practice of pulmonary metastasectomy. *J Thorac Oncol* 2010;5(6 Suppl 2):S134–S139.
26. Internullo E, Cassivi SD, Van Raemdonck D, et al. Pulmonary metastasectomy: a survey of current practice amongst members of the European Society of Thoracic Surgeons. *J Thorac Oncol* 2008;3(11):1257–1266.
27. Parsons AM, Detterbeck FC, Parker LA. Accuracy of helical CT in the detection of pulmonary metastases: Is intraoperative palpation still necessary? *Ann Thorac Surg* 2004;78(6):1910–1916; discussion 1916–1918.
28. Parsons AM, Ennis EK, Yankaskas BC, et al. Helical computed tomography inaccuracy in the detection of pulmonary metastases: can it be improved? *Ann Thorac Surg* 2007;84(6):1830–1836.
29. Althagafi KT, Alashgar OA, Almaghrabi HS, et al. Missed pulmonary metastasis. *Asian Cardiovasc Thorac Ann* 2014;22(2):183–186.
30. Feuerstein IM, Jicha DL, Pass HI, et al. Pulmonary metastases: MR imaging with surgical correlation–a prospective study. *Radiology* 1992;182(1):123–129.
31. Wyttenbach R, Vock P, Tschappeler H. Cross-sectional imaging with CT and/or MRI of pediatric chest tumors. *Eur Radiol* 1998;8(6):1040–1046.
32. Franzius C, Daldrup-Link HE, Sciuk J, et al. FDG-PET for detection of pulmonary metastases from malignant primary bone tumors: comparison with spiral CT. *Ann Oncol* 2001;12(4):479–486.
33. Fortes DL, Allen MS, Lowe VJ, et al. The sensitivity of 18F-fluorodeoxyglucose positron emission tomography in the evaluation of metastatic pulmonary nodules. *Eur J Cardiothorac Surg* 2008;34(6):1223–1227.
34. Veronesi G, Landoni C, Pelosi G, et al. Fluoro-deoxy-glucose uptake and angiogenesis are independent biological features in lung metastases. *Br J Cancer* 2002;86(9):1391–1395.
35. Woodard PK, Dehdashti F, Putman CE. Radiologic diagnosis of extrathoracic metastases to the lung. *Oncology (Williston Park)* 1998;12(3):431–438; discussion 441–442, 444.
36. Herrera GA, Alexander CB, Jones JM. Ultrastructural characterization of pulmonary neoplasms. II. The role of electron microscopy in characterization of uncommon epithelial pulmonary neoplasms, metastatic neoplasms to and from lung, and other tumors, including mesenchymal neoplasms. *Surv Synth Pathol Res* 1985;4(2):163–184.
37. Ghoneim AH, Brisson ML, Fuks A, et al. Monoclonal anti-CEA antibodies in the discrimination between primary pulmonary adenocarcinoma and colon carcinoma metastatic to the lung. *Mod Pathol* 1990;3(5):613–618.
38. Girard N, Deshpande C, Lau C, et al. Comprehensive histologic assessment helps to differentiate multiple lung primary nonsmall cell carcinomas from metastases. *Am J Surg Pathol* 2009;33(12):1752–1764.
39. Lefor AT, Bredenberg CE, Kellman RM, et al. Multiple malignancies of the lung and head and neck. Second primary tumor or metastasis? *Arch Surg* 1986;121(3):265–270.
40. Treasure T, Fallowfield L, Lees B. Pulmonary metastasectomy in colorectal cancer: the PulMiCC trial. *J Thorac Oncol* 2010;5(6 Suppl 2):S203–S206.
41. Skinner KA, Eilber FR, Holmes EC, et al. Surgical treatment and chemotherapy for pulmonary metastases from osteosarcoma. *Arch Surg* 1992;127(9):1065–1070; discussion 1070–1071.
42. Goorin AM, Shuster JJ, Baker A, et al. Changing pattern of pulmonary metastases with adjuvant chemotherapy in patients with osteosarcoma: results from the multi-institutional osteosarcoma study. *J Clin Oncol* 1991;9(4):600–605.
43. Pastorino U, Gasparini M, Tavecchio L, et al. The contribution of salvage surgery to the management of childhood osteosarcoma. *J Clin Oncol* 1991;9(8):1357–1362.
44. Hirota T, Konno K, Fujimoto T, et al. [Combined multimodal therapy for osteosarcoma–neoadjuvant chemotherapy]. *Gan To Kagaku Ryoho Cancer Chemother* 1999;26(8):1068–1075.
45. Ferguson WS, Harris MB, Goorin AM, et al. Presurgical window of carboplatin and surgery and multidrug chemotherapy for the treatment of newly diagnosed metastatic or unresectable osteosarcoma: Pediatric Oncology Group Trial. *J Pediatr Hematol Oncol* 2001;23(6):340–348.
46. Marina NM, Pratt CB, Rao BN, et al. Improved prognosis of children with osteosarcoma metastatic to the lung(s) at the time of diagnosis. *Cancer* 1992;70(11):2722–2727.
47. Pastorino U, Gasparini M, Valente M, et al. Primary childhood osteosarcoma: the role of salvage surgery. *Ann Oncol* 1992;3(Suppl 2):S43–S46.
48. Goorin AM, Harris MB, Bernstein M, et al. Phase II/III trial of etoposide and high-dose ifosfamide in newly diagnosed metastatic osteosarcoma: a Pediatric Oncology Group trial. *J Clin Oncol* 2002;20(2):426–433.
49. Bacci G, Mercuri M, Briccoli A, et al. Osteogenic sarcoma of the extremity with detectable lung metastases at presentation. Results of treatment of 23 patients with chemotherapy followed by simultaneous resection of primary and metastatic lesions. *Cancer* 1997;79(2):245–254.
50. Salah S, Toubasi S. Factors predicting survival following complete surgical remission of pulmonary metastasis in osteosarcoma. *Mol Clin Oncol* 2015;3(1):157–162.
51. Jaffe N, Carrasco H, Raymond K, et al. Can cure in patients with osteosarcoma be achieved exclusively with chemotherapy and abrogation of surgery? *Cancer* 2002;95(10):2202–2210.
52. Glasser DB, Lane JM, Huvos AG, et al. Survival, prognosis, and therapeutic response in osteogenic sarcoma. The Memorial Hospital experience. *Cancer* 1992;69(3):698–708.
53. Lanza LA, Putnam JB, Jr., Benjamin RS, et al. Response to chemotherapy does not predict survival after resection of sarcomatous pulmonary metastases. *Ann Thorac Surge* 1991;51(2):219–224.
54. Benjamin RS, Wiernik PH, Bachur NR. Adriamycin: a new effective agent in the therapy of disseminated sarcomas. *Med Pediatr Oncol* 1975;1(1):63–76.
55. Patel SR, Vadhan-Raj S, Burgess MA, et al. Results of two consecutive trials of dose-intensive chemotherapy with doxorubicin and ifosfamide in patients with sarcomas. *Am J Clin Oncol* 1998;21(3):317–321.
56. Ravi V, Patel S, Benjamin RS. Chemotherapy for soft-tissue sarcomas. *Oncology (Williston Park)* 2015;29(1):43–50.
57. Look Hong NJ, Hornicek FJ, Harmon DC, et al. Neoadjuvant chemoradiotherapy for patients with high-risk extremity and truncal sarcomas: a 10-year single institution retrospective study. *Eur J Cancer* 2013;49(4):875–883.
58. Dhaini HR, Thomas DG, Giordano TJ, et al. Cytochrome P450 CYP3A4/5 expression as a biomarker of outcome in osteosarcoma. *J Clin Oncol* 2003;21(13):2481–2485.
59. Dickens DS, Kozielski R, Leavey PJ, et al. Cyclooxygenase-2 expression does not correlate with outcome in osteosarcoma or rhabdomyosarcoma. *J Pediatr Hematol Oncol* 2003;25(4):282–285.
60. Shultz DB, Filippi AR, Thariat J, et al. Stereotactic ablative radiotherapy for pulmonary oligometastases and oligometastatic lung cancer. *J Thorac Oncol* 2014;9(10):1426–1433.
61. Van Schil PE. Results of surgery for lung cancer compared with radiotherapy: do we speak the same language. *J Thorac Oncol.* 2013;8(2):129–130.
62. Van Schil PE. Salvage surgery after stereotactic radiotherapy: a new challenge for thoracic surgeons. *J Thorac Oncol* 2010;5(12):1881–1882.
63. McCormack PM, Bains MS, Beattie EJ, Jr., et al. Pulmonary resection in metastatic carcinoma. *Chest* 1978;73(2):163–166.
64. Mountain CF, McMurtrey MJ, Hermes KE. Surgery for pulmonary metastasis: a 20-year experience. *Ann Thorac Surg* 1984;38(4):323–330.
65. Higashiyama M, Kodama K, Takami K, et al. Intraoperative lavage cytologic analysis of surgical margins as a predictor of local recurrence in pulmonary metastasectomy. *Arch Surg* 2002;137(4):469–474.

66. Loehe F, Kobinger S, Hatz RA, et al. Value of systematic mediastinal lymph node dissection during pulmonary metastasectomy. *Ann Thorac Surg* 2001;72(1):225–229.
67. Ercan S, Nichols FC, 3rd, Trastek VF, et al. Prognostic significance of lymph node metastasis found during pulmonary metastasectomy for extrapulmonary carcinoma. *Ann Thorac Surg* 2004;77(5):1786–1791.
68. Szoke T, Kortner A, Neu R, et al. Is the mediastinal lymphadenectomy during pulmonary metastasectomy of colorectal cancer necessary? *Interact Cardiovasc Thorac Surg* 2010;10(5):694–698.
69. Garcia-Yuste M, Cassivi S, Paleru C. Thoracic lymphatic involvement in patients having pulmonary metastasectomy: incidence and the effect on prognosis. *J Thorac Oncol* 2010;5(6 Suppl 2):S166–S169.
70. Putnam JB, Jr., Roth JA, Wesley MN, et al. Analysis of prognostic factors in patients undergoing resection of pulmonary metastases from soft tissue sarcomas. *J Thorac Cardiovasc Surg* 1984;87(2):260–268.
71. Girard P, Baldeyrou P, Le Chevalier T, et al. Surgical resection of pulmonary metastases. Up to what number? *Am J Resp Critic Care Med* 1994;149(2 Pt 1):469–476.
72. Robert JH, Ambrogi V, Mermillod B, et al. Factors influencing long-term survival after lung metastasectomy. *Ann Thorac Surg* 1997;63(3):777–784.
73. Hendriks JM, van Putte B, Romijn S, et al. Pneumonectomy for lung metastases: report of ten cases. *Thorac Cardiovasc Surg* 2003;51(1):38–41.
74. Koong HN, Pastorino U, Ginsberg RJ. Is there a role for pneumonectomy in pulmonary metastases? International Registry of Lung Metastases. *Ann Thorac Surg* 1999;68(6):2039–2043.
75. Grunenwald D, Spaggiari L, Girard P, et al. Lung resection for recurrence after pneumonectomy for metastases. *Bull Cancer* 1997;84(3):277–281.
76. Grunenwald D, Spaggiari L, Girard P, et al. Completion pneumonectomy for lung metastases: Is it justified? *Eur J Cardiothorac Surg* 1997;12(5):694–697.
77. Johnston MR. Median sternotomy for resection of pulmonary metastases. *J Thorac Cardiovasc Surg* 1983;85(4):516–522.
78. Roth JA, Pass HI, Wesley MN, et al. Comparison of median sternotomy and thoracotomy for resection of pulmonary metastases in patients with adult soft-tissue sarcomas. *Ann Thorac Surg* 1986;42(2):134–138.
79. Younes RN, Gross JL, Deheinzelin D. Surgical resection of unilateral lung metastases: Is bilateral thoracotomy necessary? *World J Surg* 2002;26(9):1112–1116.
80. Molnar TF, Gebitekin C, Turna A. What are the considerations in the surgical approach in pulmonary metastasectomy? *J Thorac Oncol* 2010;5(6 Suppl 2):S140–S144.
81. Kodama K, Doi O, Higashiyama M, et al. Surgical management of lung metastases. Usefulness of resection with the neodymium:yttrium-aluminum-garnet laser with median sternotomy. *J Thorac Cardiovasc Surg* 1991;101(5):901–908.
82. Branscheid D, Krysa S, Wollkopf G, et al. Does ND-YAG laser extend the indications for resection of pulmonary metastases? *Eur J Cardiothorac Surg* 1992;6(11):590–596; discussion 597.
83. Miyamoto H, Masaoka T, Hayakawa K, et al. [Application of the Nd-YAG laser for surgical resection of pulmonary metastases]. *Kyobu Geka* 1992;45(1):56–59.
84. Landreneau RJ, Hazelrigg SR, Johnson JA, et al. Neodymium:yttrium-aluminum garnet laser-assisted pulmonary resections. *Ann Thorac Surg* 1991;51(6):973–977; discussion 977–978.
85. Mineo TC, Ambrogi V, Pompeo E, et al. The value of the Nd:YAG laser for the surgery of lung metastases in a randomized trial. *Chest* 1998;113(5):1402–1407.
86. Rolle A, Koch R, Alpard SK, et al. Lobe-sparing resection of multiple pulmonary metastases with a new 1318-nm Nd:YAG laser—first 100 patients. *Ann Thorac Surg* 2002;74(3):865–869.
87. Osei-Agyemang T, Palade E, Haderthauer J, et al. Pulmonale Metastasektomie: Analyse technischer und onkologischer Ergebnisse bei 301 Patienten mit Fokus auf die Laserresektion [Pulmonary metastasectomy: an analysis of technical and oncological outcomes in 301 patients with a focus on laser resection]. *Zentralbl Chir* 2013;138(Suppl 1):S45–S51.
88. Bains MS, Ginsberg RJ, Jones WG, 2nd, et al. The clamshell incision: an improved approach to bilateral pulmonary and mediastinal tumor. *Ann Thorac Surg* 1994;58(1):30–32; discussion 33.
89. Margaritora S, Cesario A, Galetta D, et al. Staged axillary thoracotomy for bilateral lung metastases: an effective and minimally invasive approach. *Eur J Cardiothorac Surg* 1999;16(Suppl 1):S37–S39.
90. d'Amato T, Santucci TS, Macherey RS, et al. Bilateral anterior minithoracotomy with video assistance for lung volume reduction surgery and pulmonary metastasectomy. *Surg Endosc* 2002;16(2):364–346.
91. Landreneau RJ, Hazelrigg SR, Ferson PF, et al. Thoracoscopic resection of 85 pulmonary lesions. *Ann Thorac Surg* 1992;54(3):415–419; discussion 419–420.
92. McCormack PM, Bains MS, Begg CB, et al. Role of video-assisted thoracic surgery in the treatment of pulmonary metastases: results of a prospective trial. *Ann Thorac Surg* 1996;62(1):213–216; discussion 216–217.
93. Mutsaerts EL, Zoetmulder FA, Meijer S, et al. Outcome of thoracoscopic pulmonary metastasectomy evaluated by confirmatory thoracotomy. *Ann Thorac Surg* 2001;72(1):230–203.
94. Eckardt J, Licht PB. Thoracoscopic or open surgery for pulmonary metastasectomy: an observer blinded study. *Ann Thorac Surg* 2014;98(2):466–469; discussion 469–470.
95. Landreneau RJ, De Giacomo T, Mack MJ, et al. Therapeutic video-assisted thoracoscopic surgical resection of colorectal pulmonary metastases. *Eur J Cardiothorac Surg* 2000;18(6):671–676; discussion 676–677.
96. Nakajima J, Takamoto S, Tanaka M, et al. Thoracoscopic surgery and conventional open thoracotomy in metastatic lung cancer. *Surg Endoscopy* 2001;15(8):849–853.
97. Lin JC, Wiechmann RJ, Szwerc MF, et al. Diagnostic and therapeutic video-assisted thoracic surgery resection of pulmonary metastases. *Surgery* 1999;126(4):636–641; discussion 641–642.
98. Mineo TC, Ambrogi V, Mineo D, et al. Transxiphoid hand-assisted videothoracoscopic surgery. *Ann Thorac Surg* 2007;83(6):1978–1984.
99. Walsh GL, Nesbitt JC. Tumor implants after thoracoscopic resection of a metastatic sarcoma. *Ann Thorac Surg* 1995;59(1):215–216.
100. Ang KL, Tan C, Hsin M, Goldstraw P. Intrapleural tumor dissemination after video-assisted thoracoscopic surgery metastasectomy. *Ann Thorac Surg* 2003;75(5):1643–1645.
101. Downey RJ, McCormack P, LoCicero J, 3rd. Dissemination of malignant tumors after video-assisted thoracic surgery: a report of twenty-one cases. The Video-Assisted Thoracic Surgery Study Group. *J Thorac Cardiovasc Surg* 1996;111(5):954–960.
102. Casiraghi M, De Pas T, Maisonneuve P, et al. A 10-year single-center experience on 708 lung metastasectomies: the evidence of the "International Registry of Lung Metastases." *J Thorac Oncol* 2011;6(8):1373–1378.
103. Spaggiari L, Grunenwald DH, Girard P, et al. Pneumonectomy for lung metastases: indications, risks, and outcome. *Ann Thorac Surg* 1998;66(6):1930–1933.
104. Vaporciyan AA, Rice D, Correa AM, et al. Resection of advanced thoracic malignancies requiring cardiopulmonary bypass. *Eur J Cardiothorac Surg* 2002;22(1):47–52.
105. Heslin MJ, Casper ES, Boland P, et al. Preoperative identification and operative management of intraatrial extension of lung tumors. *Ann Thorac Surg* 1998;65(2):544–546.
106. Shuman RL. Primary pulmonary sarcoma with left atrial extension via left superior pulmonary vein. En bloc resection and radical pneumonectomy on cardiopulmonary bypass. *J Thorac Cardiovasc Surg* 1984;88(2):189–192.
107. Huth JF, Eilber FR. Patterns of recurrence after resection of osteosarcoma of the extremity. Strategies for treatment of metastases. *Arch Surg* 1989;124(1):122–126.
108. Picci P, Vanel D, Briccoli A, et al. Computed tomography of pulmonary metastases from osteosarcoma: the less poor technique. A study of 51 patients with histological correlation. *Ann Oncol* 2001;12(11):1601–1604.
109. Meyer WH, Schell MJ, Kumar AP, et al. Thoracotomy for pulmonary metastatic osteosarcoma. An analysis of prognostic indicators of survival. *Cancer* 1987;59(2):374–379.
110. Snyder CL, Saltzman DA, Ferrell KL, et al. A new approach to the resection of pulmonary osteosarcoma metastases. Results of aggressive metastasectomy. *Clin Orthop Relat Res* 1991;(270):247–253.
111. Belli L, Scholl S, Livartowski A, et al. Resection of pulmonary metastases in osteosarcoma. A retrospective analysis of 44 patients. *Cancer* 1989;63(12):2546–2550.
112. Tsuchiya H, Kanazawa Y, Abdel-Wanis ME, et al. Effect of timing of pulmonary metastases identification on prognosis of patients with osteosarcoma: the Japanese Musculoskeletal Oncology Group study. *J Clin Oncol* 2002;20(16):3470–3477.
113. Yonemoto T, Tatezaki S, Ishii T, et al. Prognosis of osteosarcoma with pulmonary metastases at initial presentation is not dismal. *Clin Orthop Relat Res* 1998;(349):194–199.
114. Treasure T, Fiorentino F, Scarci M, et al. Pulmonary metastasectomy for sarcoma: a systematic review of reported outcomes in the context of Thames Cancer Registry data. *BMJ Open* 2012;2(5).
115. Carter SR, Grimer RJ, Sneath RS, et al. Results of thoracotomy in osteogenic sarcoma with pulmonary metastases. *Thorax* 1991;46(10):727–731.
116. Jaffe N, Smith E, Abelson HT, Frei E, 3rd. Osteogenic sarcoma: alterations in the pattern of pulmonary metastases with adjuvant chemotherapy. *J Clin Oncol* 1983;1(4):251–254.
117. Putnam JB, Jr., Roth JA, Wesley MN, et al. Survival following aggressive resection of pulmonary metastases from osteogenic sarcoma: analysis of prognostic factors. *Ann Thorac Surg* 1983;36(5):516–523.
118. Heij HA, Vos A, de Kraker J, et al. Prognostic factors in surgery for pulmonary metastases in children. *Surgery* 1994;115(6):687–693.
119. Mizuno T, Taniguchi T, Ishikawa Y, et al. Pulmonary metastasectomy for osteogenic and soft tissue sarcoma: Who really benefits from surgical treatment? *Eur J Cardiothorac Surg* 2013;43(4):795–799.
120. Bacci G, Ferrari S, Longhi A, et al. Pattern of relapse in patients with osteosarcoma of the extremities treated with neoadjuvant chemotherapy. *Eur J Cancer* 2001;37(1):32–38.
121. Ferrari S, Briccoli A, Mercuri M, et al. Postrelapse survival in osteosarcoma of the extremities: prognostic factors for long-term survival. *J Clin Oncol* 2003;21(4):710–715.
122. Goorin AM, Schwartzentruber DJ, Devidas M, et al. Presurgical chemotherapy compared with immediate surgery and adjuvant chemotherapy for nonmetastatic osteosarcoma: Pediatric Oncology Group Study POG-8651. *J Clin Oncol* 2003;21(8):1574–1580.
123. Voute PA, Souhami RL, Nooij M, et al. A phase II study of cisplatin, ifosfamide and doxorubicin in operable primary, axial skeletal and metastatic osteosarcoma. European Osteosarcoma Intergroup (EOI). *Ann Oncol* 1999;10(10):1211–1218.
124. Miniero R, Brach del Prever A, Vassallo E, et al. Feasibility of high-dose chemotherapy and autologous peripheral blood stem cell transplantation in children with high grade osteosarcoma. *Bone Marrow Transplant* 1998;22(Suppl 5):S37–S40.
125. Hoos A, Lewis JJ, Brennan MF. Weichgewebssarkome–prognostische faktoren und multimodale therapie [Soft tissue sarcoma: prognostic factors and multimodal treatment]. *Chirurg* 2000;71(7):787–794.
126. Billingsley KG, Lewis JJ, Leung DH, et al. Multifactorial analysis of the survival of patients with distant metastasis arising from primary extremity sarcoma. *Cancer* 1999;85(2):389–395.
127. van Geel AN, Pastorino U, Jauch KW, et al. Surgical treatment of lung metastases: The European Organization for Research and Treatment of Cancer-Soft Tissue and Bone Sarcoma Group study of 255 patients. *Cancer* 1996;77(4):675–682.

128. Jablons D, Steinberg SM, Roth J, et al. Metastasectomy for soft tissue sarcoma. Further evidence for efficacy and prognostic indicators. *J Thorac Cardiovasc Surg* 1989;97(5):695–705.

129. Casson AG, Putnam JB, Natarajan G, et al. Efficacy of pulmonary metastasectomy for recurrent soft tissue sarcoma. *J Surg Oncol* 1991;47(1):1–4.

130. Pogrebniak HW, Roth JA, Steinberg SM, et al. Reoperative pulmonary resection in patients with metastatic soft tissue sarcoma. *Ann Thorac Surg* 1991;52(2):197–203.

131. Weh HJ, Zugel M, Wingberg D, et al. Chemotherapy of metastatic soft tissue sarcoma with a combination of adriamycin and DTIC or adriamycin and ifosfamide. *Onkologie* 1990;13(6):448–452.

132. Elias A, Ryan L, Sulkes A, et al. Response to mesna, doxorubicin, ifosfamide, and dacarbazine in 108 patients with metastatic or unresectable sarcoma and no prior chemotherapy. *J Clin Oncol* 1989;7(9):1208–1216.

133. Woll PJ, Reichardt P, Le Cesne A, et al. Adjuvant chemotherapy with doxorubicin, ifosfamide, and lenograstim for resected soft-tissue sarcoma (EORTC 62931): a multicentre randomised controlled trial. *Lancet Oncol* 2012;13(10):1045–1054.

134. Barbareschi M, Murer B, Colby TV, et al. CDX-2 homeobox gene expression is a reliable marker of colorectal adenocarcinoma metastases to the lungs. *Am J Surg Pathol* 2003;27(2):141–149.

135. McAfee MK, Allen MS, Trastek VF, et al. Colorectal lung metastases: results of surgical excision. *Ann Thorac Surg* 1992;53(5):780–785; discussion 785–786.

136. Higashiyama M, Kodama K, Higaki N, et al. Surgery for pulmonary metastases from colorectal cancer: the importance of prethoracotomy serum carcinoembryonic antigen as an indicator of prognosis. *Jpn J Thorac Cardiovasc Surg* 2003; 51(7):289–296.

137. Gonzalez M, Poncet A, Combescure C, et al. Risk factors for survival after lung metastasectomy in colorectal cancer patients: a systematic review and meta-analysis. *Ann Surg Oncol* 2013;20(2):572–579.

138. Salah S, Watanabe K, Welter S, et al. Colorectal cancer pulmonary oligometastases: pooled analysis and construction of a clinical lung metastasectomy prognostic model. *Ann Oncol* 2012;23(10):2649–2655.

139. Goi T, Koneri K, Katayama K, et al. Evaluation of clinicopathological factors and the correlation between the adhesion molecule CD44 variant 9 expression and pulmonary metastases from colorectal cancers. *Int Surg* 2002;87(2):130–136.

140. Labow DM, Buell JE, Yoshida A, et al. Isolated pulmonary recurrence after resection of colorectal hepatic metastases—Is resection indicated? *Cancer J* 2002;8(4):342–327.

141. Regnard JF, Grunenwald D, Spaggiari L, et al. Surgical treatment of hepatic and pulmonary metastases from colorectal cancers. *Ann Thorac Surg* 1998;66(1): 214–218; discussion 218–219.

142. Ike H, Shimada H, Ohki S, et al. Results of aggressive resection of lung metastases from colorectal carcinoma detected by intensive follow-up. *Dis Colon Rectum* 2002;45(4):468–473; discussion 473–475.

143. Salah S, Ardissone F, Gonzalez M, et al. Pulmonary metastasectomy in colorectal cancer patients with previously resected liver metastasis: pooled analysis. *Ann Surg Oncol* 2015;22(6):1844–1850.

144. Salah S, Watanabe K, Park JS, et al. Repeated resection of colorectal cancer pulmonary oligometastases: pooled analysis and prognostic assessment. *Ann Surg Oncol* 2013;20(6):1955–1961.

145. Kim HK, Cho JH, Lee HY, et al. Pulmonary metastasectomy for colorectal cancer: How many nodules, how many times? *World J Gastroenterol* 2014;20(20):6133–6145.

146. de Gramont A, Figer A, Seymour M, et al. Leucovorin and fluorouracil with or without oxaliplatin as first-line treatment in advanced colorectal cancer. *J Clin Oncol* 2000;18(16):2938–2947.

147. Van Cutsem E, Kohne CH, Lang I, et al. Cetuximab plus irinotecan, fluorouracil, and leucovorin as first-line treatment for metastatic colorectal cancer: updated analysis of overall survival according to tumor KRAS and BRAF mutation status. *J Clin Oncol* 2011;29(15):2011–2019.

148. Garcia-Yuste M, Cassivi S, Paleru C. Pulmonary metastasectomy in breast cancer. *J Thorac Oncol.* 2010;5(6 Suppl 2):S170–S171.

149. Ruiterkamp J, Ernst MF. The role of surgery in metastatic breast cancer. *Eur J Cancer* 2011;47(Suppl 3):S6–S22.

150. Patanaphan V, Salazar OM, Risco R. Breast cancer: metastatic patterns and their prognosis. *South Med J* 1988;81(9):1109–1112.

151. Lanza LA, Natarajan G, Roth JA, et al. Long-term survival after resection of pulmonary metastases from carcinoma of the breast. *Ann Thorac Surg* 1992;54(2): 244–247; discussion 248.

152. Bathe OF, Kaklamanos IG, Moffat FL, et al. Metastasectomy as a cytoreductive strategy for treatment of isolated pulmonary and hepatic metastases from breast cancer. *Surg Oncol* 1999;8(1):35–42.

153. Friedel G, Linder A, Toomes H. The significance of prognostic factors for the resection of pulmonary metastases of breast cancer. *Thorac Cardiovasc Surg* 1994; 42(2):71–75.

154. Simpson R, Kennedy C, Carmalt H, et al. Pulmonary resection for metastatic breast cancer. *Aust N Z J Surg* 1997;67(10):717–719.

155. Staren ED, Salerno C, Rongione A, et al. Pulmonary resection for metastatic breast cancer. *Arch Surg* 1992;127(11):1282–1284.

156. Friedel G, Pastorino U, Ginsberg RJ, et al. Results of lung metastasectomy from breast cancer: prognostic criteria on the basis of 467 cases of the International Registry of Lung Metastases. *Eur J Cardiothorac Surg* 2002;22(3):335–344.

157. Lien HH, Lindskold L, Fossa SD, et al. Computed tomography and conventional radiography in intrathoracic metastases from non-seminomatous testicular tumor. *Acta Radiol* 1988;29(5):547–549.

158. Tesoro-Tess JD, Pizzocaro G, Zanoni F, et al. Reliability of diagnostic imaging after orchiectomy alone in follow-up of clinical stage I testicular carcinoma: excessive cost with potential risk. *Lymphology* 1987;20(3):161–165.

159. Williams MP, Husband JE, Heron CW. Intrathoracic manifestations of metastatic testicular seminoma: a comparison of chest radiographic and CT findings. *Am J Roentgenol* 1987;149(3):473–475.

160. Kulkarni RP, Reynolds KW, Newlands ES, et al. Cytoreductive surgery in disseminated non-seminomatous germ cell tumours of testis. *Br J Surg* 1991;78(2):226–269.

161. Carsky S, Ondrus D, Schnorrer M, et al. Germ cell testicular tumours with lung metastases: chemotherapy and surgical treatment. *Int Urol Nephrol* 1992;24(3): 305–311.

162. Carter GE, Lieskovsky G, Skinner DG, et al. Reassessment of the role of adjunctive surgical therapy in the treatment of advanced germ cell tumors. *J Urol* 1987;138(6): 1397–1401.

163. Gels ME, Hoekstra HJ, Sleijfer DT, et al. Thoracotomy for postchemotherapy resection of pulmonary residual tumor mass in patients with nonseminomatous testicular germ cell tumors: aggressive surgical resection is justified. *Chest* 1997;112(4):967–973.

164. Liu D, Abolhoda A, Burt ME, et al. Pulmonary metastasectomy for testicular germ cell tumors: a 28-year experience. *Ann Thorac Surg* 1998;66(5):1709–1714.

165. Schnorrer M, Ondrus D, Carsky S, et al. Management of germ cell testicular cancer with pulmonary metastases. *Neoplasma* 1996;43(1):47–50.

166. Steyerberg EW, Keizer HJ, Messemer JE, et al. Residual pulmonary masses after chemotherapy for metastatic nonseminomatous germ cell tumor. Prediction of histology. ReHiT Study Group. *Cancer* 1997;79(2):345–355.

167. Niwa K, Kometani K, Sekiya T, et al. Complete remission of uterine endometrial cancer with multiple lung metastases treated by paclitaxel and carboplatin. *Int J Clin Oncol.* 2002;7(3):197–200.

168. Anderson TM, McMahon JJ, Nwogu CE, et al. Pulmonary resection in metastatic uterine and cervical malignancies. *Gynecol Oncol* 2001;83(3):472–476.

169. Chauveinc L, Deniaud E, Plancher C, et al. Uterine sarcomas: the Curie Institut experience. Prognosis factors and adjuvant treatments. *Gynecol Oncol* 1999;72(2):232–237.

170. Bouros D, Papadakis K, Siafakas N, et al. Natural history of patients with pulmonary metastases from uterine cancer. *Cancer* 1996;78(3):441–4477.

171. Shiromizu K, Kasamatsu T, Takahashi M, et al. A clinicopathological study of postoperative pulmonary metastasis of uterine cervical carcinomas. *J Obstet Gynaecol Res* 1999;25(4):245–249.

172. Fuller AF, Jr., Scannell JG, Wilkins EW, Jr. Pulmonary resection for metastases from gynecologic cancers: Massachusetts General Hospital experience, 1943–1982. *Gynecol Oncol* 1985;22(2):174–180.

173. Anraku M, Yokoi K, Nakagawa K, et al. Pulmonary metastases from uterine malignancies: results of surgical resection in 133 patients. *J Thorac Cardiovasc Surg* 2004; 127(4):1107–1112.

174. Leitao MM, Brennan MF, Hensley M, et al. Surgical resection of pulmonary and extrapulmonary recurrences of uterine leiomyosarcoma. *Gynecol Oncol* 2002;87(3): 287–294.

175. Kumar J, Ilancheran A, Ratnam SS. Pulmonary metastases in gestational trophoblastic disease: a review of 97 cases. *Br J Obstet Gynaecol* 1988;95(1):70–74.

176. Barter JF, Soong SJ, Hatch KD, et al. Diagnosis and treatment of pulmonary metastases from cervical carcinoma. *Gynecol Oncol* 1990;38(3):347–351.

177. Imachi M, Tsukamoto N, Matsuyama T, et al. Pulmonary metastasis from carcinoma of the uterine cervix. *Gynecol Oncol* 1989;33(2):189–192.

178. Seki M, Nakagawa K, Tsuchiya S, et al. Surgical treatment of pulmonary metastases from uterine cervical cancer. Operation method by lung tumor size. *J Thorac Cardiovasc Surg* 1992;104(4):876–881.

179. Pfannschmidt J, Hoffmann H, Muley T, et al. Prognostic factors for survival after pulmonary resection of metastatic renal cell carcinoma. *Ann Thorac Surg* 2002;74(5):1653–1657.

180. Piltz S, Meimarakis G, Wichmann MW, et al. Long-term results after pulmonary resection of renal cell carcinoma metastases. *Ann Thorac Surg* 2002;73(4):1082–1027.

181. Friedel G, Hurtgen M, Penzenstadler M, et al. Resection of pulmonary metastases from renal cell carcinoma. *Anticancer Res* 1999;19(2C):1593–1596.

182. Fischer CG, Schmid H. Operative therapy in disease progression and local recurrence of renal cell carcinoma. *Urol Int* 1999;63(1):10–15.

183. Schott G, Weissmuller J, Vecera E. Methods and prognosis of the extirpation of pulmonary metastases following tumor nephrectomy. *Urol Int* 1988;43(5): 272–274.

184. Pogrebniak HW, Haas G, Linehan WM, et al. Renal cell carcinoma: resection of solitary and multiple metastases. *Ann Thorac Surg* 1992;54(1):33–38.

185. Fourquier P, Regnard JF, Rea S, et al. Lung metastases of renal cell carcinoma: results of surgical resection. *Eur J Cardiothorac Surg* 1997;11(1):17–21.

186. van der Poel HG, Roukema JA, Horenblas S, et al. Metastasectomy in renal cell carcinoma: a multicenter retrospective analysis. *Eur Urol* 1999;35(3):197–203.

187. Murthy SC, Kim K, Rice TW, et al. Can we predict long-term survival after pulmonary metastasectomy for renal cell carcinoma? *Ann Thorac Surg* 2005; 79(3):996–1003.

188. Ollila DW, Morton DL. Surgical resection as the treatment of choice for melanoma metastatic to the lung. *Chest Surg Clin N Am* 1998;8(1):183–196.

189. Caudle AS, Ross MI. Metastasectomy for stage IV melanoma: For whom and how much? *Surg Oncol Clin N Am* 2011;20(1):133–144.

190. Barth A, Wanek LA, Morton DL. Prognostic factors in 1,521 melanoma patients with distant metastases. *J Am Coll Surg.* 1995;181(3):193–201.

191. Dalrymple-Hay MJ, Rome PD, Kennedy C, et al. Pulmonary metastatic melanoma—the survival benefit associated with positron emission tomography scanning. *Eur J Cardiothorac Surg* 2002;21(4):611–614; discussion 614–615.

192. Allen PJ, Coit DG. The role of surgery for patients with metastatic melanoma. *Curr Opin Oncol* 2002;14(2):221–226.

193. Gorenstein LA, Putnam JB, Natarajan G, et al. Improved survival after resection of pulmonary metastases from malignant melanoma. *Ann Thorac Surg* 1991;52(2):204–210.

194. Harpole DH, Jr., Johnson CM, Wolfe WG, et al. Analysis of 945 cases of pulmonary metastatic melanoma. *J Thorac Cardiovasc Surg* 1992;103(4):743–748; discussion 748–750.

195. Lewis CW, Jr., Harpole D. Pulmonary metastasectomy for metastatic malignant melanoma. *Semin Thorac Cardiovasc Surg* 2002;14(1):45–48.

196. Nibu K, Nakagawa K, Kamata S, et al. Surgical treatment for pulmonary metastases of squamous cell carcinoma of the head and neck. *Am J Otolaryngol* 1997;18(6):391–395.

197. Finley RK, 3rd, Verazin GT, Driscoll DL, et al. Results of surgical resection of pulmonary metastases of squamous cell carcinoma of the head and neck. *Am J Surg* 1992;164(6):594–598.

198. Sihoe AD, Van Schil P. Non-small cell lung cancer: when to offer sublobar resection. *Lung Cancer* 2014;86(2):115–120.

199. Leong PP, Rezai B, Koch WM, et al. Distinguishing second primary tumors from lung metastases in patients with head and neck squamous cell carcinoma. *J Natl Cancer Inst* 1998;90(13):972–927.

200. Uchiyama M, Iwafuchi M, Naito M, et al. A study of therapy for pediatric hepatoblastoma: prevention and treatment of pulmonary metastasis. *Eur J Pediatr Surg* 1999;9(3):142–145.

201. Karnak I, Emin Senocak M, Kutluk T, et al. Pulmonary metastases in children: an analysis of surgical spectrum. *Eur J Pediatr Surg* 2002;12(3):151–158.

202. Perilongo G, Brown J, Shafford E, et al. Hepatoblastoma presenting with lung metastases: treatment results of the first cooperative, prospective study of the International Society of Paediatric Oncology on childhood liver tumors. *Cancer* 2000;89(8):1845–1853.

203. Fuchs J, Seitz G, Handgretinger R, et al. Surgical treatment of lung metastases in patients with embryonal pediatric solid tumors: an update. *Semin Pediatr Surg* 2012;21(1):79–87.

204. Katzenstein HM, London WB, Douglass EC, et al. Treatment of unresectable and metastatic hepatoblastoma: a pediatric oncology group phase II study. *J Clin Oncol* 2002;20(16):3438–3444.

205. Nishimura S, Sato T, Fujita N, et al. High-dose chemotherapy in children with metastatic hepatoblastoma. *Pediatr Int* 2002;44(3):300–305.

206. Czauderna P, Mackinlay G, Perilongo G, et al. Hepatocellular carcinoma in children: results of the first prospective study of the International Society of Pediatric Oncology group. *J Clin Oncol* 2002;20(12):2798–2804.

207. Macklis RM, Oltikar A, Sallan SE. Wilms' tumor patients with pulmonary metastases. *Int J Radiat Oncol Biol Phys* 1991;21(5):1187–1193.

208. Wilimas JA, Douglass EC, Magill HL, et al. Significance of pulmonary computed tomography at diagnosis in Wilms' tumor. *J Clin Oncol* 1988;6(7):1144–1146.

209. de Kraker J, Lemerle J, Voute PA, et al. Wilm's tumor with pulmonary metastases at diagnosis: the significance of primary chemotherapy. International Society of Pediatric Oncology Nephroblastoma Trial and Study Committee. *J Clin Oncol* 1990;8(7):1187–1190.

210. Di Lorenzo M, Collin PP. Pulmonary metastases in children: results of surgical treatment. *J Pediatr Surg* 1988;23(8):762–765.

211. Green DM, Breslow NE, Ii Y, et al. The role of surgical excision in the management of relapsed Wilms' tumor patients with pulmonary metastases: a report from the National Wilms' Tumor Study. *J Pediatr Surg* 1991;26(6):728–733.

212. Godzinski J, Tournade MF, De Kraker J, et al. The role of preoperative chemotherapy in the treatment of nephroblastoma: the SIOP experience. Societe Internationale d'Oncologie Pediatrique. *Semin Urol Oncol* 1999;17(1):28–32.

213. Bacci G, Briccoli A, Picci P, et al. Metachronous pulmonary metastases resection in patients with Ewing's sarcoma initially treated with adjuvant or neoadjuvant chemotherapy. *Eur J Cancer* 1995;31A(6):999–1001.

214. Lanza LA, Miser JS, Pass HI, et al. The role of resection in the treatment of pulmonary metastases from Ewing's sarcoma. *J Thorac Cardiovasc Surg* 1987;94(2):181–187.

215. Spunt SL, McCarville MB, Kun LE, et al. Selective use of whole-lung irradiation for patients with Ewing sarcoma family tumors and pulmonary metastases at the time of diagnosis. *J Pediatr Hematol Oncol* 2001;23(2):93–98.

216. Dunst J, Paulussen M, Jurgens H. Lung irradiation for Ewing's sarcoma with pulmonary metastases at diagnosis: results of the CESS-studies. *Strahlenther Onkol* 1993;169(10):621–623.

217. Paulussen M, Ahrens S, Craft AW, et al. Ewing's tumors with primary lung metastases: survival analysis of 114 (European Intergroup) Cooperative Ewing's Sarcoma Studies patients. *J Clin Oncol* 1998;16(9):3044–3052.

218. Paulussen M, Ahrens S, Burdach S, et al. Primary metastatic (stage IV) Ewing tumor: survival analysis of 171 patients from the EICESS studies. European Intergroup Cooperative Ewing Sarcoma Studies. *Ann Oncol* 1998;9(3):275–281.

219. La Quaglia MP. Osteosarcoma. Specific tumor management and results. *Chest Surg Clin N Am* 1998;8(1):77–95.

220. Hirano J, Okumura S, Omoto K, et al. [Prognosis for the cases after resection of pulmonary metastasis of osteosarcoma]. *Kyobu Geka Jpn J Thorac Surg* 2003;56(1):4–8.

221. Burgers JM, van Glabbeke M, Busson A, et al. Osteosarcoma of the limbs. Report of the EORTC-SIOP 03 trial 20781 investigating the value of adjuvant treatment with chemotherapy and/or prophylactic lung irradiation. *Cancer* 1988;61(5):1024–1031.

222. Whelan JS, Burcombe RJ, Janinis J, et al. A systematic review of the role of pulmonary irradiation in the management of primary bone tumours. *Ann Oncol* 2002;13(1):23–30.

223. Daw NC, Chou AJ, Jaffe N, et al. Recurrent osteosarcoma with a single pulmonary metastasis: a multi-institutional review. *Br J Cancer* 2015;112(2):278–282.

224. Kaste SC, Pratt CB, Cain AM, et al. Metastases detected at the time of diagnosis of primary pediatric extremity osteosarcoma at diagnosis: imaging features. *Cancer* 1999;86(8):1602–1608.

225. Kandioler D, Kromer E, Tuchler H, et al. Long-term results after repeated surgical removal of pulmonary metastases. *Ann Thorac Surg* 1998;65(4):909–912.

226. Rizzoni WE, Pass HI, Wesley MN, et al. Resection of recurrent pulmonary metastases in patients with soft-tissue sarcomas. *Arch Surg* 1986;121(11):1248–1252.

227. Weiser MR, Downey RJ, Leung DH, Brennan MF. Repeat resection of pulmonary metastases in patients with soft-tissue sarcoma. *J Am Coll Surg* 2000;191(2):184–190; discussion 190–191.

228. Temeck BK, Wexler LH, Steinberg SM, et al. Reoperative pulmonary metastasectomy for sarcomatous pediatric histologies. *Ann Thorac Surg* 1998;66(3):908–912; discussion 913.

229. Collins VP, Loeffler RK, Tivey H. Observations on growth rates of human tumors. *Am J Roentgenol, Radium Ther Nucl Med* 1956;76(5):988–1000.

230. Joseph WL, Morton DL, Adkins PC. Variation in tumor doubling time in patients with pulmonary metastatic disease. *J Surg Oncol* 1971;3(2):143–149.

231. Joseph WL, Morton DL, Adkins PC. Prognostic significance of tumor doubling time in evaluating operability in pulmonary metastatic disease. *J Thorac Cardiovasc Surg* 1971;61(1):23–32.

232. Laird AK, Barton AD. Cell proliferation in precancerous liver: linear growth curve. *Nature* 1960;188:417–418.

233. Belshi R, Pontvert D, Rosenwald JC, et al. Automatic three-dimensional expansion of structures applied to determination of the clinical target volume in conformal radiotherapy. *Int J Radiat Oncol Biol Phys* 1997;37(3):689–696.

234. Eggli KD, Close P, Dillon PW, et al. Three-dimensional quantitation of pediatric tumor bulk. *Pediatr Radiol* 1995;25(1):1–6.

235. Vogel MN, Schmucker S, Maksimovic O, et al. Reduction in growth threshold for pulmonary metastases: an opportunity for volumetry and its impact on treatment decisions. *Br J Radiol* 2012;85(1015):959–964.

236. Udelsman R, Roth JA, Lees D, et al. Endobronchial metastases from soft tissue sarcoma. *J Surg Oncol* 1986;32(3):145–149.

237. Roth JA, Putnam JB, Jr., Wesley MN, et al. Differing determinants of prognosis following resection of pulmonary metastases from osteogenic and soft tissue sarcoma patients. *Cancer* 1985;55(6):1361–1366.

238. McLornan DP, List A, Mufti GJ. Applying synthetic lethality for the selective targeting of cancer. *N Engl J Med* 2014;371(18):1725–1735.

239. Zhou W, Hao M, Du X, et al. Advances in targeted therapy for osteosarcoma. *Discov Med* 2014;17(96):301–307.

240. Iwakuma T, Agarwal N. MDM2 binding protein, a novel metastasis suppressor. *Cancer Metast Rev* 2012;31(3–4):633–640.

241. Ladanyi M, Cha C, Lewis R, et al. MDM2 gene amplification in metastatic osteosarcoma. *Cancer Res* 1993;53(1):16–18.

242. Sugano N, Suda T, Godai TI, et al. MDM2 gene amplification in colorectal cancer is associated with disease progression at the primary site, but inversely correlated with distant metastasis. *Genes Chromosomes Cancer* 2010;49(7):620–629.

243. Hernandez-Rodriguez NA, Correa E, Sotelo R, et al. Ki-67: a proliferative marker that may predict pulmonary metastases and mortality of primary osteosarcoma. *Cancer Detect Prev* 2001;25(2):210–215.

244. Matsumoto I, Oda M, Yachi T, et al. Outcome prediction of pulmonary metastasectomy can be evaluated using metastatic lesion in osteosarcoma patients. *World J Surg* 2013;37(8):1973–1980.

245. Tang Y, Cheng Y, Martinka M, et al. Prognostic significance of KAI1/CD82 in human melanoma and its role in cell migration and invasion through the regulation of ING4. *Carcinogenesis* 2014;35(1):86–95.

246. Pollock R, Lang A, Ge T, et al. Wild-type p53 and a p53 temperature-sensitive mutant suppress human soft tissue sarcoma by enhancing cell cycle control. *Clin Cancer Res* 1998;4(8):1985–1994.

247. Scotlandi K, Serra M, Nicoletti G, et al. Multidrug resistance and malignancy in human osteosarcoma. *Cancer Res* 1996;56(10):2434–2439.

248. Asai T, Ueda T, Itoh K, Yoshioka K, et al. Establishment and characterization of a murine osteosarcoma cell line (LM8) with high metastatic potential to the lung. *Int J Cancer* 1998;76(3):418–422.

249. Kumta SM, Zhu QS, Lee KM, et al. Clinical significance of P-glycoprotein immunohistochemistry and doxorubicin binding assay in patients with osteosarcoma. *Int Orthop* 2001;25(5):279–282.

250. Abolhoda A, Wilson AE, Ross H, et al. Rapid activation of MDR1 gene expression in human metastatic sarcoma after in vivo exposure to doxorubicin. *Clin Cancer Res* 1999;5(11):3352–3356.

251. Beech DJ, Perer E, Helms J, et al. Insulin-like growth factor-I receptor activation blocks doxorubicin cytotoxicity in sarcoma cells. *Oncol Rep* 2003;10(1):181–184.

252. Olmos D, Tan DS, Jones RL, et al. Biological rationale and current clinical experience with anti-insulin-like growth factor 1 receptor monoclonal antibodies in treating sarcoma: twenty years from the bench to the bedside. *Cancer J* 2010;16(3):183–194.

253. Onda M, Matsuda S, Higaki S, et al. ErbB-2 expression is correlated with poor prognosis for patients with osteosarcoma. *Cancer* 1996;77(1):71–78.

254. Seto M, Yamazaki T, Sonoda J, et al. Suppression of tumor growth and pulmonary metastasis in murine osteosarcoma using gene therapy. *Oncol Rep* 2002;9(2):337–340.

255. Akatsuka T, Wada T, Kokai Y, et al. ErbB2 expression is correlated with increased survival of patients with osteosarcoma. *Cancer* 2002;94(5):1397–1404.

256. Benjamin R, Helman L, Meyers P, et al. A phase I/II dose escalation and activity study of intravenous injections of OCaP1 for subjects with refractory osteosarcoma metastatic to lung. *Human Gene Ther* 2001;12(12):1591–1593.

257. Van Schil PE. Surgical treatment for pulmonary metastases. *Acta Clin Belg* 2002;57(6):333–339.

258. Putnam JB, Jr. New and evolving treatment methods for pulmonary metastases. *Semin Thorac Cardiovasc Surg* 2002;14(1):49–56.

259. Weksler B, Schneider A, Ng B, et al. Isolated single lung perfusion in the rat: an experimental model. *J Appl Physiol (1985)* 1993;74(6):2736–2739.

260. Weksler B, Lenert J, Ng B, et al. Isolated single lung perfusion with doxorubicin is effective in eradicating soft tissue sarcoma lung metastases in a rat model. *J Thorac Cardiovasc Surg* 1994;107(1):50–54.

261. Van Putte BP, Hendriks JM, Romijn S, et al. Single-pass isolated lung perfusion versus recirculating isolated lung perfusion with melphalan in a rat model. *Ann Thorac Surg* 2002;74(3):893–898; discussion 898.

262. Van Putte BP, Hendriks JM, Romijn S, et al. Isolated lung perfusion with gemcitabine in a rat: pharmacokinetics and survival. *J Surg Res* 2003;109(2):118–122.

263. Schrump DS, Zhai S, Nguyen DM, et al. Pharmacokinetics of paclitaxel administered by hyperthermic retrograde isolated lung perfusion techniques. *J Thorac Cardiovasc Surg* 2002;123(4):686–694.

264. Den Hengst WA, Hendriks JM, Van Hoof T, et al. Selective pulmonary artery perfusion with melphalan is equal to isolated lung perfusion but superior to intravenous melphalan for the treatment of sarcoma lung metastases in a rodent model. *Eur J Cardiothorac Surg* 2012;42(2):341–347; discussion 347.

265. Hendriks JM, Van Schil PE, De Boeck G, et al. Isolated lung perfusion with melphalan and tumor necrosis factor for metastatic pulmonary adenocarcinoma. *Ann Thorac Surg* 1998;66(5):1719–1725.

266. Hendriks JM, Van Schil PE, Van Oosterom AA, et al. Isolated lung perfusion with melphalan prolongs survival in a rat model of metastatic pulmonary adenocarcinoma. *Eur Surg Res* 1999;31(3):267–271.

267. Pass HI, Mew DJ, Kranda KC, et al. Isolated lung perfusion with tumor necrosis factor for pulmonary metastases. *Ann Thorac Surg* 1996;61(6):1609–1617.

268. Johnston MR, Minchen RF, Dawson CA. Lung perfusion with chemotherapy in patients with unresectable metastatic sarcoma to the lung or diffuse bronchioloalveolar carcinoma. *J Thorac Cardiovasc Surg* 1995;110(2):368–373.

269. Schroder C, Fisher S, Pieck AC, et al. Technique and results of hyperthermic (41 degrees C) isolated lung perfusion with high-doses of cisplatin for the treatment of surgically relapsing or unresectable lung sarcoma metastasis. *Eur J Cardiothorac Surg* 2002;22(1):41–46.

270. Burt ME, Liu D, Abolhoda A, et al. Isolated lung perfusion for patients with unresectable metastases from sarcoma: a phase I trial. *Ann Thorac Surg* 2000;69(5):1542–1549.

271. Ratto GB, Toma S, Civalleri D, et al. Isolated lung perfusion with platinum in the treatment of pulmonary metastases from soft tissue sarcomas. *J Thorac Cardiovasc Surg* 1996;112(3):614–622.

272. Hendriks JM, Grootenboers MJ, Schramel FM, et al. Isolated lung perfusion with melphalan for resectable lung metastases: a phase I clinical trial. *Ann Thorac Surg* 2004;78(6):1919–1926; discussion 1926–1927.

273. Grootenboers MJ, Hendriks JM, van Boven WJ, et al. Pharmacokinetics of isolated lung perfusion with melphalan for resectable pulmonary metastases, a phase I and extension trial. *J Surg Oncol* 2007;96(7):583–589.

274. Den Hengst WA, Van Putte BP, Hendriks JM, et al. Long-term survival of a phase I clinical trial of isolated lung perfusion with melphalan for resectable lung metastases. *Eur J Cardiothorac Surg* 2010;38(5):621–627.

275. den Hengst WA, Hendriks JM, Balduyck B, et al. Phase II multicenter clinical trial of pulmonary metastasectomy and isolated lung perfusion with melphalan in patients with resectable lung metastases. *J Thorac Oncol* 2014;9(10):1547–1553.

276. Furrer M, Lardinois D, Thormann W, et al. Cytostatic lung perfusion by use of an endovascular blood flow occlusion technique. *Ann Thorac Surg* 1998;65(6):1523–1528.

277. Krueger T, Kuemmerle A, Kosinski M, et al. Cytostatic lung perfusion results in heterogeneous spatial regional blood flow and drug distribution: evaluation of different cytostatic lung perfusion techniques in a porcine model. *J Thorac Cardiovasc Surg* 2006;132(2):304–311.

278. Van Putte BP, Hendriks JM, Romijn S, et al. Pharmacokinetics after pulmonary artery perfusion with gemcitabine. *Ann Thorac Surg* 2003;76(4):1036–1040; discussion 1040.

279. van Putte BP, Grootenboers M, van Boven WJ, et al. Selective pulmonary artery perfusion for the treatment of primary lung cancer: improved drug exposure of the lung. *Lung Cancer* 2009;65(2):208–213.

280. Schneider P, Foitzik T, Pohlen U, et al. Temporary unilateral microembolization of the lung—a new approach to regional chemotherapy for pulmonary metastases. *J Surg Res* 2002;107(2):159–166.

281. Schneider P, Kampfer S, Loddenkemper C, et al. Chemoembolization of the lung improves tumor control in a rat model. *Clin Cancer Res* 2002;8(7):2463–2468.

282. Vogl TJ, Lehnert T, Zangos S, et al. Transpulmonary chemoembolization (TPCE) as a treatment for unresectable lung metastases. *Eur Radiol* 2008;18(11):2449–2455.

283. Brooks AD, Ng B, Liu D, et al. Specific organ gene transfer in vivo by regional organ perfusion with herpes viral amplicon vectors: implications for local gene therapy. *Surgery* 2001;129(3):324–334.

284. Huland E, Heinzer H, Huland H, et al. Overview of interleukin-2 inhalation therapy. *Cancer J Sci Am* 2000;6(Suppl 1):S104–S112.

285. Shingu K, Kruschinski C, Luhrmann A, et al. Intratracheal macrophage-activating lipopeptide-2 reduces metastasis in the rat lung. *Am J Respir Cell Mol Biol* 2003;28(3):316–321.

286. Hershey AE, Kurzman ID, Forrest LJ, et al. Inhalation chemotherapy for macroscopic primary or metastatic lung tumors: proof of principle using dogs with spontaneously occurring tumors as a model. *Clin Cancer Res* 1999;5(9):2653–2659.

287. Koshkina NV, Waldrep JC, Roberts LE, et al. Paclitaxel liposome aerosol treatment induces inhibition of pulmonary metastases in murine renal carcinoma model. *Clin Cancer Res* 2001;7(10):3258–3262.

288. Jia SF, Worth LL, Densmore CL, et al. Eradication of osteosarcoma lung metastases following intranasal interleukin-12 gene therapy using a nonviral polyethylenimine vector. *Cancer Gene Ther* 2002;9(3):260–266.

289. Enk AH, Nashan D, Rubben A, et al. High dose inhalation interleukin-2 therapy for lung metastases in patients with malignant melanoma. *Cancer* 2000;88(9):2042–2046.

290. Skubitz KM, Anderson PM. Inhalational interleukin-2 liposomes for pulmonary metastases: a phase I clinical trial. *Anticancer Drugs* 2000;11(7):555–563.

291. Posch C, Weihsengruber F, Bartsch K, et al. Low-dose inhalation of interleukin-2 bio-chemotherapy for the treatment of pulmonary metastases in melanoma patients. *Br J Cancer* 2014;110(6):1427–1432.

292. Guma SR, Lee DA, Ling Y, et al. Aerosol interleukin-2 induces natural killer cell proliferation in the lung and combination therapy improves the survival of mice with osteosarcoma lung metastasis. *Pediatr Blood Cancer* 2014;61(8):1362–1368.

293. Gordon N, Kleinerman ES. Aerosol therapy for the treatment of osteosarcoma lung metastases: targeting the Fas/FasL pathway and rationale for the use of gemcitabine. *J Aerosol Med Pulm Drug Deliv* 2010;23(4):189–196.

294. Kleinerman ES. Biologic therapy for osteosarcoma using liposome-encapsulated muramyl tripeptide. *Hematol Oncol Clin N Am* 1995;9(4):927–938.

295. Kleinerman ES, Gano JB, Johnston DA, et al. Efficacy of liposomal muramyl tripeptide (CGP 19835A) in the treatment of relapsed osteosarcoma. *Am J Clin Oncol* 1995;18(2):93–99.

296. Meyers PA, Chou AJ. Muramyl tripeptide-phosphatidyl ethanolamine encapsulated in liposomes (L-MTP-PE) in the treatment of osteosarcoma. *Adv Exp Med Biol* 2014;804:307–321.

297. Whitmore M, Li S, Huang L. LPD lipopolyplex initiates a potent cytokine response and inhibits tumor growth. *Gene Ther* 1999;6(11):1867–1875.

298. Curley SA. Radiofrequency ablation of malignant liver tumors. *Ann Surg Oncol* 2003;10(4):338–347.

299. Finelli A, Rewcastle JC, Jewett MA. Cryotherapy and radiofrequency ablation: pathophysiologic basis and laboratory studies. *Curr Opin Urol* 2003;13(3):187–191.

300. Matin SF. Laparoscopic approaches to urologic malignancies. *Curr Treat Options Oncol* 2003;4(5):373–383.

301. Dupuy DE, Mayo-Smith WW, Abbott GF, et al. Clinical applications of radiofrequency tumor ablation in the thorax. *Radiographics* 2002;22 Spec No:S259–S269.

302. Steinke K, Glenn D, King J, et al. Percutaneous pulmonary radiofrequency ablation: difficulty achieving complete ablations in big lung lesions. *Br J Radiol* 2003;76(910):742–725.

303. Vogl TJ, Naguib NN, Gruber-Rouh T, et al. Microwave ablation therapy: clinical utility in treatment of pulmonary metastases. *Radiology* 2011;261(2):643–651.

304. Yan TD, King J, Sjarif A, et al. Treatment failure after percutaneous radiofrequency ablation for nonsurgical candidates with pulmonary metastases from colorectal carcinoma. *Ann Surg Oncol* 2007;14(5):1718–1726.

305. Hiraki T, Gobara H, Iishi T, et al. Percutaneous radiofrequency ablation for pulmonary metastases from colorectal cancer: midterm results in 27 patients. *J Vasc Intervent Radiol* 2007;18(10):1264–1269.

306. Schneider T, Reuss D, Warth A, et al. The efficacy of bipolar and multipolar radiofrequency ablation of lung neoplasms—results of an ablate and resect study. *Eur J Cardiothorac Surg* 2011;39(6):968–973.

307. Palussiere J, Gomez F, Cannella M, et al. Single-session radiofrequency ablation of bilateral lung metastases. *Cardiovasc Intervent Radiol* 2012;35(4):852–829.

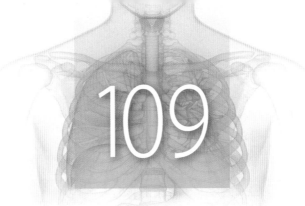

109

Pulmonary Malignancies in the Immunocompromised Host

David S. Schrump

INTRODUCTION

The concept of cancer immune surveillance was initially proposed by Ehrlich in 1909[1] and subsequently refined by Burnett, who postulated that "genetic changes must be common in somatic cells and a proportion of these changes will represent a step toward malignancy. It is an evolutionary necessity that there should be some mechanism for eliminating or inactivating such potentially dangerous mutant cells and that this mechanism is of immunologic character."[2] More recently the concept of immuno-editing has been proposed to explain the selection process by which pluripotent cancer cells which are not initially eliminated by immune surveillance establish a dynamic equilibrium with the host immune system and ultimately escape from dormancy as immuno-resistant clones leading to clinical manifestations of malignancy.[3,4]

The concepts of cancer immune surveillance and immuno-editing are supported by convincing laboratory as well as clinical observations. For instance, mice with severe combined immunodeficiency exhibit significantly higher frequencies of spontaneous tumors and increased susceptibilities to carcinogen-induced malignancies.[5,6] Chemically induced sarcomas established in wild-type and RAG-2-deficient mice which lack T and B cells grow at the same rate when injected into RAG-2-deficient mice. The majority of sarcomas from RAG-2-deficient mice are rejected when inoculated into wild-type mice, yet virtually all sarcomas from wild-type mice grow progressively when transferred to other wild-type mice due to prior immunoselection.[7] Patients with primary immunodeficiencies or immunosuppression resulting from infection or organ transplantation are at significantly increased risk of developing a variety of cancers induced by viral agents or environmental exposures.[4] These observations, as well as recent clinical trials demonstrating impressive and durable responses to immune checkpoint inhibitors in patients with malignancies (including lung cancers) not traditionally viewed as immunogenic,[8,9] provide compelling evidence for cancer immune surveillance and immuno-editing in humans. This chapter will focus on pulmonary malignancies arising in people who are immunocompromised as a result of infection with human immunodeficiency virus (HIV), as well as patients who are pharmacologically immunosuppressed following hematopoietic cell or solid organ transplantation.

HIV/AIDS

Discovered three decades ago, human immunodeficiency virus (HIV) is the etiologic agent of acquired immunodeficiency syndrome (AIDS). Since the beginning of the HIV epidemic, approximately 71 million people have been infected by nine major genetic variants with differing susceptibilities to antiretroviral drugs, and nearly 34 million people have died of the disease[10] (http://www.who.int/gho/hiv/en/). Globally, an estimated 37 million people were living with HIV in 2014. Presently, 0.8% of adults aged 15 to 49 years worldwide are living with HIV, although the burden of the epidemic varies considerably between countries and regions. Sub-Saharan Africa remains most severely affected, with nearly 1 in every 20 adults living with HIV; this region accounts for approximately 70% of people living with HIV worldwide (http://www.unaids.org/sites/default/files/media_asset/20150714_FS_MDG6_Report_en.pdf).

The introduction of highly active antiretroviral therapy (HAART) has significantly altered the clinical course of HIV/AIDS.[11] In essence, these agents have converted HIV/AIDS from a uniformly fatal illness to a chronic disease. Presently, life expectancies of people living with HIV/AIDS (PLWHA) who are receiving HAART are comparable to HIV(–) individuals.[12] Nevertheless, despite HAART, HIV continues to disrupt innate as well as adaptive host immunity as evidenced by aberrant expression of inflammatory mediators, dysregulation of proliferation and apoptosis of lymphoid cells, and persistent low-level retroviral replication in the intestines and lungs.[10]

As a result of HAART, AIDS-defining cancers (ADC) including Kaposi sarcoma (KS) and non-Hodgkin lymphoma (NHL), which may occasionally be seen in the lungs, have steadily decreased, whereas non-AIDS-defining cancers (NADC), such as anal and hepatocellular carcinomas and lung cancers, have increased.[13] Presently NADC account for more than 50% of all malignancies in HIV-infected patients.[14] Although related in part to aging, the increased risk of NADC in PLWHA has also been attributed to HIV-mediated immunodeficiency with simultaneous immune activation/inflammation resembling age-related immune senescence, non-HIV cancer risk factors such as smoking and oncogenic viral infections, and a combination of ill-defined environmental and genetic factors.[10,15,16]

AIDS-DEFINING CANCERS

Kaposi Sarcoma

Among the first ADC to be described, KSs are not true sarcomas but instead are multicentric angioproliferative spindle cell neoplasms induced by latent human herpesvirus 8 (HHV8; Kaposi sarcoma herpes virus [KSHV]) co-infection and chronic inflammation.[17,18] Four types of KS have been defined: classic, endemic, transplant-associated, and AIDS-related. In PLWHA, systemic immune activation and HHV8 infection in lymphatic endothelial cells promote expression of numerous growth factors as well as pro-inflammatory and pro-angiogenic cytokines that drive neoplastic transformation.[18–20] Whereas the incidence of KS has decreased by two-thirds (15.2 to 4.9 per 1,000 patient-years) following introduction of HAART,[21] this disease still remains the second most common tumor associated with HIV infections worldwide and is the most common AIDS-related cancer in sub-Saharan Africa where sero-prevalence of HHV8 is high and access to HAART is limited.[18,20] In developed countries, KSs are primarily seen in persons who have previously undiagnosed HIV or have only recently commenced HAART.[22]

KS typically involves skin, nasopharynx, lymph nodes, and visceral organs, particularly the GI tract and lungs. Approximately 50% of all KS patients will have GI involvement which is often asymptomatic at the time of diagnosis. The vast majority (85% to 95%) of KS with pulmonary involvement occurs in association with cutaneous disease; however, up to 15% of patients with pulmonary KS have no skin involvement.[19,23] Although occasionally asymptomatic, patients with pulmonary KS frequently present with bronchospasm, dyspnea, and a barking cough with or without fever.[20,23] Radiographically, pulmonary KS is characterized by the presence of diffuse bilateral nodules, bronchovascular thickening, pseudo-alveolar masses with air bronchograms, flame-like infiltrates, and pleural effusions.[11,24,25] Such infiltrates can also be seen in patients with opportunistic infections. Gallium–thallium radionuclide scans may be useful for distinguishing pulmonary KS from infection since KS lesions do not take up gallium, but do take up thallium.[26] These parenchymal findings are often but not always associated with the presence of reddish-purple endobronchial lesions frequently at airway bifurcations.[27] In such cases, bronchoscopy can establish the diagnosis; nearly 50% of patients will have evidence of alveolar hemorrhage in BAL fluids. Pleural fluid analysis is generally nondiagnostic, since most effusions associated with pulmonary KS are due to secondary infections.[11] Patients in whom endobronchial lesions are not detected require biopsy of parenchymal disease. Diagnosis is established by histologic evidence of a spindle cell neoplasm which is positive for panendothelial surface markers as well as intracellular HHV8 latency-associated nuclear antigen (LANA).[18]

Pulmonary KS may run a rapidly progressive course especially in patients who are severely immunocompromised.[20] Initial treatment of pulmonary KS involves administration of HAART to decrease inflammation, inhibit HIV replication, and improve immune response to HHV8 if not already initiated.[20,28] Patients with symptomatic and rapidly progressive KS need chemotherapy.[29] Antiviral drugs (such as ganciclovir) are not effective since they treat the lytic—not the latent phase of HHV8 infection. Pegylated liposomal doxorubicin or liposomal daunorubicin are first-line agents; paclitaxel, which has been associated with increased systemic toxicities, is frequently used for recurrence following anthracycline therapy.[18] A recent review of six randomized trials and three observational studies demonstrated no significant differences in outcomes following treatment with liposomal doxorubicin, liposomal daunorubicin, or paclitaxel.[30] In regions where HAART, liposomal drug preparations, and paclitaxel are unavailable, therapy may be based on doxorubicin, bleomycin, and vincristine (ABV).[31] A variety of immune modulatory drugs including interferon alfa, interleukin-12, thalidomide, and lenalidomide, as well as inhibitors of VEGF signaling may also be considered for recurrent disease.[18–20]

In the pre-HAART era, median survival of patients with KS was 2 to 6 months with survival being associated with extent of disease and CD4 counts, as well as the presence of systemic illness and B symptoms.[20] Survival of patients with KS has increased in the HAART era; presently, survival appears to be most dependent on extent of tumor involvement and systemic illness rather than magnitude of immunosuppression.[19] Nevertheless, prognosis remains poor for patients with pulmonary KS[11]—particularly those manifesting immune reconstitution inflammatory syndrome (IRIS)—a condition characterized by paradoxical clinical deterioration in the context of immune recovery during antiretroviral therapy.[32,33] In the HAART era, overall survival of HIV-infected patients with pulmonary KS is 49% compared to 82% for PLWHA who have KS without pulmonary involvement.[34]

Non-Hodgkin Lymphoma

One of the leading ADC in the pre-HAART era, the incidence of NHL has decreased significantly in the HAART era (from 6.2% to 3.2%).[35] NHL is a heterogeneous group of T- and B-cell neoplasms; the majority of NHL in PLWHA are B-cell neoplasms, with diffuse large B-cell lymphomas (DLBCL) or Burkitt lymphomas being the most common.[20] Two major types of DLBCL are seen in PLWHA.[36] Centroblastic DLBCL are usually seen in patients with mild immunosuppression. Histologically, these neoplasms have a germinal center phenotype; approximately 30% of these neoplasms are associated with Epstein–Barr virus (EBV) infection.[20] Tumor cells do not express LMP1 but typically exhibit rearrangements of BCL6.[37] Immunoblastic DLBCL are generally seen in patients with advanced immunosuppression. These lymphomas exhibit a non-germinal center B-cell activation phenotype; 90% of these neoplasms are associated with EBV infection, and lymphoma cells express LMP1 and EBNA2.[20,37] Following introduction of HAART, there has been a marked decrease in the prevalence of immunoblastic NHL in PLWHA.[11]

Most often seen in the lungs as a manifestation of disease originating elsewhere,[11,38] NHL may occasionally present as primary pulmonary lymphoma (PPL; defined as lungs being the sole site of lymphomatous parenchymal disease with or without hilar disease at diagnosis and for three subsequent months).[39] In contrast to PPLs in HIV-negative patients which tend to be low-grade B-cell neoplasms,[40] PPLs in PLWHA are typically high-grade B-cell lymphomas with latent EBV infection.[11,41] Similar to the pathogenesis of KS, diminished immune surveillance as a result of chronic immunosuppression and increased systemic inflammation induced by HIV infection promote development of NHL in PLWHA.[20]

HIV-infected individuals with pulmonary NHL typically present with pleuritic or pneumonic disease and are usually symptomatic with cough, dyspnea, tachypnea, and a variety of B symptoms.[11] CT scans demonstrate diffuse, bilateral pulmonary nodules predominantly at the bases often without hilar/mediastinal lymphadenopathy, as well as pleural effusions.[42] Serum and pleural fluid lactated dehydrogenase (LDH) levels are typically elevated. Diagnosis can be established by transbronchial or percutaneous biopsies or cytologic evaluation of pleural fluid.[38] Standard treatment for pulmonary DLBCL in PLWHA includes cyclophosphamide, doxorubicin, vincristine, prednisone (CHOP) with or without rituximab (CHOP-R), or CHOP-R with etoposide (EPOCH-R). In the HAART era, outcomes for PLWHA and DLBCL are similar to HIV-negative DLBCL patients with response rates of 50% to 70% and overall survival rates ranging from 56% to 67%.[20] Autologous hematopoietic stem cell transplantation may be considered for treatment of relapsing DLBCL in patients with HIV infections that are under control.[43]

Primary effusion lymphomas (PEL) are rare B-cell NHL that can present as pleural (60% to 90%), pericardial (up to 30%), or peritoneal (30% to 60%) effusions without an obvious associated mass.[44,45] Typically, B cells in these neoplasms are co-infected with HHV8 and EBV[36] and exhibit gene expression signatures between those of multiple myeloma and EBV-associated immunoblastic lymphomas.[46,47] Due to the low incidence of PEL (1% to 4% of all lymphomas in PLWHA),[18] no standard of care has been established. HAART should be started immediately if not already initiated. In contrast to other NHL in PLWHA, PEL do not respond well to standard chemotherapeutic agents. Presently, prognosis of HIV-infected patients with PEL is poor; median survival is approximately 2 to 9 months, and 2-year overall survival is approximately 36% for patients receiving treatment with CHOP or related regimens.[45] Recent studies suggest that targeted agents including the proteasome inhibitor, bortizumab, and rapamycin (an inhibitor or m-TOR signaling), as well antiviral agents such as cidofovir and ganciclovir, may improve survival of patients with PEL.[18,20,48]

NON-AIDS-DEFINING CANCERS

Multicentric Castleman Disease

Although not a NADC per se,[49] Castleman disease is a lymphoproliferative disorder frequently observed in PLHA.[23] Two forms of Castleman disease have been described based on histologic criteria.[36] The plasma cell variant is usually multicentric and is characterized by plasma cell proliferation with preservation of nodal architecture. The hyaline vascular variant is unicentric and characterized by abnormal germinal centers and hyalinized vessels.[23,36] Multicentric Castleman disease (MCD; plasma cell variant) is typically seen in PLWHA.[20] Immunoblasts in the mantle zone of lymph nodes from these patients harbor HHV8, and it is believed that MCD is a manifestation of the lytic phase of HHV8 infection in these cells.[36] The majority of HIV-infected patients with MCD also have KS,[20] and MCD significantly increases risk of NHL in these individuals.[50] Patients typically present with fatigue, fever, splenomegaly, and lymphadenopathy. One-third of cases have pulmonary involvement.[20] Radiographically, MCD is associated with interstitial pneumonitis with or without pleural effusion and hilar/mediastinal lymphadenopathy; common CT findings include diffuse reticulo-nodular interstitial infiltrates, interlobar septal and peribronchovascular thickening, and pleural effusions.[51] Severity of symptoms and overall prognosis appear to coincide with high systemic levels of pro-inflammatory cytokines such as interleukin-6 (IL-6), and elevated levels of HHV8 in peripheral blood.[52–54] There does not appear to be an association between MCD and HIV viral load or CD4 counts.[55] Bronchoscopy is rarely necessary; diagnosis is established by histologic examination of a lymph node biopsy.[56]

In contrast to the incidence of KS which has decreased, the incidence of MCD has increased in the HAART era.[57] These findings suggest that immunosuppression predisposes to KS but not MCD. Presently there is no standard of care for HHV8-associated MCD.[18] Treatment should be directed toward correcting immunodeficiency with HAART, inhibiting the lymphoid proliferation and controlling HHV8 infection.[23,56] HAART should be commenced if not already

initiated. Typical regimens include CHOP or ABV, as well as immune modulatory agents, and antibodies against IL-6 or CD20 (altizumab and rituximab, respectively).[20,58] Recent studies suggest that rituximab alone can mediate clinical and radiographic improvements in the majority of HIV-infected patients with MCD and decrease risk of NHL in these individuals.[59] Exacerbation of KS may occur with rituximab alone[56]; hence R-CHOP may be a better option for patients with good performance status (PS) who have concomitant KS and MCD. Survival of patients with HIV-infected patients with MCD has improved dramatically in the HAART era, with recent data indicating 5-year survival of 77% since 2005.[60]

Lung Cancer

Patterns of cancer risk in PLWHA appear to be similar to individuals undergoing solid organ transplants (SOTs).[61] These observations suggest that immune suppression predisposes to NADC, including lung cancers which presently rank among the most frequent and most lethal NADC in PLWHA. Despite these observations, current studies have not consistently demonstrated associations between severity of immunodeficiency and lung cancer risk in PLWHA. The lack of prospectively collected data and comparable comparison groups limits adjustments for confounding variables that influence lung cancer risk among various studies. Shiels et al.[62] performed a meta-analysis of 18 studies including 625,716 HIV-infected individuals and observed a lung cancer standardized incidence ratio (SIR) of 2.6 (95% CI 2.1 to 3.1). Hou et al.[63] conducted an extensive analysis of 65 population-based studies examining incidence and risk of lung cancer in HIV-infected patients. Whereas no Chinese articles met criteria for review, the analysis included studies from five continents including Europe, North America, Australia, Asia, and Africa. SIRs or adjusted incidence rate ratios (IRRs) were 0.7 to 6.9 in the United States, 1.5 to 3.4 in Europe, and 5.0 in Africa. Whereas risks of lung cancer were higher in females and younger patients, more lung cancers occurred in males and older patients. A Veterans Administration Cohort study (VACS) including 37,294 HIV-infected patients and 75,750 uninfected individuals demonstrated that HIV infection was associated with a 1.7-fold (95% CI 1.5 to 1.9) increased risk of lung cancer after controlling for age, sex, race/ethnicity, smoking, prior bacterial pneumonia, and COPD.[64]

In a prospective Danish population-based cohort study, 5053 HIV-positive patients were evaluated relative to 50,530 HIV-negative patients. The adjusted IRR in PLWHA was 2.38 (95% CI 1.61 to 3.53).[65] Parents of these patients also had an increased risk of lung cancer (IRRs = 1.31 and 1.35 for fathers and mothers, respectively), suggesting that genetic variables contribute to lung cancer development in PLWHA. Another prospective study involving 2,495 IV drug users (IVDU) demonstrated that HIV infection was associated with a 2.3-fold increase in lung cancer risk after adjusting for age, gender, and average number of cigarettes smoked per day.[66]

Increased risk of lung cancer in HIV-infected patients may be related to smoking which is—two to three times more prevalent in this population; 40% to 70% of HIV-infected patients are smokers or former smokers.[15,67] Chronic inflammation[15] also appears to be a significant contributing factor; in transgenic murine models, HIV infection does not induce lung cancers in the absence of inflammation.[68] Other factors contributing to increased lung cancer risk in PLWHA include recurrent pneumonias,[69] as well as HIV-driven emphysema/COPD.[15,67,70]

If immune dysregulation with loss of immune surveillance predisposes to lung cancer in HIV-infected individuals, then lung cancer risk should correlate with magnitude and duration of immune suppression; furthermore, pharmacologic interventions which decrease systemic HIV load and restore immune function should reduce lung cancer risk in PLWHA.[16,32,71] Numerous studies have examined these issues with conflicting results (reviewed in Almodovar,[10] Dubrow et al.,[16] and Sigel et al.[70]). For example, Frish et al.[72] observed that lung cancer risk was highest at the time of an AIDS diagnosis (relative risk = 10) with the lowest risk observed in distant pre-AIDS period (>25 months), suggesting that immunodeficiency contributes to lung cancer development in PLWHA. Consistent with these findings, Silverberg et al.[73] observed that relative risk of lung cancer in HIV-infected individuals was significantly increased if CD4 counts were less than 200/μL. In contrast, a more recent Swiss HIV cohort study revealed no association between lung cancer risk and either CD4 count, viral load, or history of AIDS-related pulmonary diagnosis after adjusting for smoking.[74]

Patel and colleagues[75] analyzed data from two large prospective studies that included 54,780 HIV-positive patients in 13 regions in the United States. They compared lung cancer incidence between 1992 and 2003 and identified 140 lung cancers (overall SIR = 3.3). The SIR in pre-HAART era was 3.5, compared to 3.8 and 3.6 in early and late HAART eras, respectively. In another study involving 5,238 HIV-infected patients in Baltimore relative to a control population (Detroit) in the SEER database, Engels and colleagues[76] observed that the incidence of lung cancer rose across three periods corresponding to pre-HAART (1989 to 1994), early HAART (1995 to 1999), and late HAART (2000 to 2003) eras; SIRs were 1.7, 5.2, and 5.3, respectively ($P = 0.02$).

Other studies have found opposite results. An analysis of 375,933 patients in six American states between 1980 and 2002 demonstrated that lung cancer incidence decreased in the HAART era compared to the pre-HAART era (SIR 3.3 from 1996 to 2002 vs. 2.6 from 1990 to 1995).[77] Hleyhel et al.[78] evaluated risk of NADC in 85,504 HIV-infected individuals in France during three eras: 1997 to 2000, 2001 to 2004, and 2005 to 2009. Lung cancer risk fell during the combined antiretroviral therapy (cART) era. Among those with CD4(+) cell recovery, lung cancer risk was close to the general population. Using the SEER Registry, Robbins et al.[79] observed a 52% excess of lung cancer in HIV-infected individuals relative to controls. In another recent study involving 86,620 HIV-infected subjects and 196,987 controls entered between 1996 and 2009, Silverberg et al.[80] estimated only a 1.2-fold higher cumulative incidence of lung cancer by age 75 in HIV-infected versus noninfected patients (3.4%; 95% CI 3.1 to 3.7 vs. 2.8%; 95% CI 2.5 to 3.0). Their model predicted no calendar trends in cumulative incidence of lung cancer; however, a declining hazard rate (HR) trend of lung cancer was observed in HIV-infected patients, which was similar to that predicted for noninfected controls. The authors concluded that these findings were consistent with general population trends related to decreasing prevalence of cigarette smoking. As such, discrepancies regarding results of these and other studies examining HIV and lung cancer risk may be related to differences in eras and patient populations, as well as declining rates of competing causes of death, aging populations that would otherwise be more prone to develop lung cancer, and possibly persistent subtle deficiencies in immune surveillance despite normalization of CD4 counts by HAART.[15,32] Whereas some antiretroviral agents are potential mutagens, to date there have been no consistent associations between specific drugs and lung cancer risk in PLWHA.

The average age of HIV-infected patients diagnosed with lung cancer is 38 to 57 years compared to 70 years of age in non–HIV-infected patients. Although these findings suggest more rapid evolution of malignancies in PLWHA, the discrepancy appears due primarily to differences in age of the HIV population relative to uninfected controls rather than premature aging in PLWHA.[15]

A recent prospective Veterans Aging Cohort study of HIV-infected individuals and demographically matched HIV(–) veterans revealed no significant differences in age at diagnosis of a number of major diseases including lung cancer in HIV-infected versus uninfected individuals.[81] The majority lung cancers in PLWHA are adenocarcinomas; up to 85% of these cases are diagnosed in advanced age. As such, the higher prevalence of lung cancers in PLWHA cannot be attributed to increased surveillance since the stage distribution in HIV-positive patients is similar to that of HIV-negative individuals.

A number of studies have sought to examine outcomes of HIV-infected patients with lung cancer. Bearz and colleagues[82] evaluated 68 HIV-infected patients with lung cancer; 34 patients were diagnosed in the pre-HAART era and 34 were diagnosed in the HAART era. PS was significantly worse in patients diagnosed in the pre-HAART era; 47% of patients in the pre-HAART era received chemotherapy with or without radiation compared to 79.4% in post-HAART era ($P = 0.004$). The median overall survival in the pre-HAART era was 3.8 months versus 7 months in the HAART era ($P = 0.01$). In a retrospective cohort study comparing 22 HIV-infected lung cancer patients with 2,430 lung cancer patients with HIV unspecified status resected at Johns Hopkins University Hospital from 1985 to 2009, Hooker and colleagues[83] noted that 30-day mortality rates did not differ between HIV-infected and HIV unspecified patients. However, survival rates were significantly lower in HIV patients undergoing surgery relative to controls. In addition, patients with CD4 counts less than 200/μL had worse survivals. More recent studies have confirmed that survival of HIV-infected patients with lung cancers has increase somewhat in the HAART era primarily due to improved PS and ability to receive stage-appropriate care. A more recent retrospective review of the Dat'AIDS cohort including 52 patients (90% stage III/IV) demonstrated a median overall survival of 12 months.[84] CD4 count equal or greater than 200/μl, PS < 2, and HAART were significantly associated with increased survival in multivariate analysis. Presently there appears to be no consistent association between lung cancer prognosis and class of antiretroviral agents (protease inhibitor, nucleoside reverse transcriptase (RT) inhibitor, non-nucleoside RT inhibitor). However, protease inhibitors have been significantly associated with grade 4 hematologic toxicities in patients receiving chemotherapy.[84]

Rengan et al.[85] used the SEER Registry to identify 322 HIV-infected patients and 71,976 noninfected patients with NSCLC diagnosed between January 2000 and December 2005. The authors observed no significant differences regarding stage-related survivals in HIV-infected versus control patients. Median survival of HIV-infected patients with stage I or II cancers who underwent surgery was 50 months (95% CI 42.0 to unestimable) versus 58 months (95% CI 57.0 to 60.0) for controls ($P = 0.88$). Using the same SEER Registry linked to Medicare claims, Siegel et al.[86] identified 267 HIV-infected lung cancer patients and 1,428 noninfected lung cancer patients. There were no differences regarding stages at presentation or percent of patients receiving stage-appropriate treatment. However, lung cancer–specific survivals were significantly worse in HIV-infected patients compared to similarly staged control patients. The authors postulated that differences in their findings compared to those of Rengan and colleagues[85] were due to the use of different algorithms for identifying HIV infection in the two studies, and contamination of the HIV cohort in the Rengan study by individuals who were suspected of having HIV infection but were ultimately found not to have this disease.

Increased lung cancer mortality in HIV-infected patients despite appropriate treatment for their malignancies has also been noted in several additional studies. Marcus et al.[87] reported a HR of 1.3 for lung cancers–specific mortality in HIV patients relative to matched controls. In a study using linked cancer and HIV registries in six states, Coghill et al.[88] observed that after adjusting for cancer treatment, HIV infection remained associated with increased cancer-specific mortality for several NADC including lung cancer (HR for lung cancer mortality 1.28; 95% CI: 1.14 to 1.44). Despite these clinical findings, there presently is no molecular evidence that HIV infection predisposes to more aggressive lung cancers.

Using the National Cancer Data Base, Suneja et al.[89] evaluated outcomes of 3,045 HIV-infected cancer patients relative to 1,087,648 HIV(–) cancer patients in the United States diagnosed between 2003 and 2011. Eighty-eight percent of HIV(+) patients had a previous diagnosis of AIDS with median CD4 counts of 144 cells/µL at the time of cancer diagnosis. The adjusted odds ratio (OR) for lung cancer was 2.18 (95% CI: 1.80 to 2.64). IV drug abusers, older patients, blacks, and those with CD4 counts less than the median were more likely not to receive standard care. HIV-infected patients were more likely to have disseminated disease at the time of cancer diagnosis, which could have affected PS or comorbidities that may have rendered them poor candidates for treatment; furthermore, socioeconomic status and insurance issues may have limited access of HIV-infected patients to healthcare. Even when the analysis was restricted to patients with local stage cancers for whom standard care was potentially curative, HIV infection was associated with lack of standard treatment for lung cancer (OR = 2.43; 95% CI: 1.46 to 4.03).

More recently these authors extended their analysis to include 10,265 HIV-infected cancer patients and 2,219,232 HIV-negative cancer patients.[90] HIV-infected patients were more likely to not receive treatment for a variety of malignancies including lung cancer (adjusted OR for lung cancer: 2.46; 95% CI: 2.19 to 2.76, P <0.001). These differences were not attributable to higher comorbidities scores in HIV-infected patients. Notably approximately 65% of HIV-infected patients had Medicaid, Medicare, or no insurance, whereas nearly 75% of HIV-uninfected patients had private insurance. Predictors of lack of cancer treatment included black race as well as Medicare and Medicaid or no insurance. However, insurance issues alone cannot fully account for the disparities, since privately insured HIV-infected lung cancer patients were significantly more likely not to receive cancer therapy relative to HIV-negative lung cancer patients with private insurance (23% vs. 10%, adjusted OR 2.47; 95% confidence interval 1.89 to 3.22, P <0.001). These disparities in cancer treatment appear to be due to a variety of complex factors including exclusion of HIV-infected patients from investigational studies hence limited direct evidence of drug efficacy in these individuals; lack of standard guidelines for therapy; potential for significant drug interactions between HAART regimens and chemotherapeutic agents[91,92]; overall complexity of simultaneously treating HIV/AIDS and lung cancer[70,84,91]; reluctance of physicians to offer potentially toxic therapy to HIV-infected patients; as well as access to healthcare.[90]

The increased risk of lung cancer and lung cancer mortality in HIV-infected individuals, which does not appear to be entirely accounted for by cigarette smoking, suggests that these patients should be enrolled in lung cancer screening programs.[93] Of concern, however, is the fact that underlying lung disease, which in some studies has been associated with increased lung cancer risk in PLWHA, may result in more false-positive scans and unnecessary interventions in these patients. Sigel et al.[94] evaluated incident nodules identified by CT scans from 160 HIV-infected patients and 139 uninfected individuals between 2009 and 2012 in a multi-institutional Examinations of HIV Associated Lung Emphysema (EXHALE) study. Using National Lung Screening Trial (NLST) criteria, HIV status did not alter the proportion of CT scans interpreted as positive (29% in HIV-infected vs. 24% in uninfected patients; $p = 0.3$). However, HIV-infected patients with CD4+ counts less than 200 cells/µL

were significantly more likely to have positive scans. Despite these findings, evaluations triggered by abnormal scans were not significantly different in HIV-infected versus uninfected patients.

Makinson et al.[95] conducted a French multicenter study involving 442 HIV-positive smokers age 40 years or older with 20 or more pack-year history of smoking, and CD4 T lymphocyte nadir less than 300/dL screened between February 2011 and June 2012. All patients underwent a single round of CT scans. Median age of these patients was 49 years; 84% were male, and median tobacco exposure was 30 pack-years. Median nadir of CD4 T-cell count was 168/dL indicative of a prior state of significant immunosuppression. Ninety patients (21%) had a positive scan, 15 of whom (17%) underwent invasive diagnostic procedures. NSCLC was diagnosed in nine patients during initial screening (2%); six of these patients (66%) had early-stage carcinomas. An additional patient developed stage IV small cell lung cancer (SCLC) after CT screening. Eight of the lung cancers were detected in patients less than 55 years of age.

Findings from this French study compare favorably to results of the randomized American NLST,[96] which enrolled patients with heavier tobacco exposure (all patients had exposures equal to or greater than 30 pack-years). Positive scans were observed in 27.3% of initial scans, and surgery was performed in 4.2% of patients. Prevalence of lung cancer was 1.1%; 158 of the 292 lung cancers (58%) detected by CT scans were stage I tumors.

Hulbert et al.[97] conducted a prospective trial involving CT screening of 224 HIV-infected persons from 2006 to 2013. Eligibility criteria included age greater or equal to 25 years, cigarette exposure equal to or greater than 20 pack-years, and HIV infection. Patients underwent baseline CT scans, and up to three additional annual scans. The authors used a modification of International-Early Lung Cancer Action Project (I-ELCAP) and NSLT criteria for defining suspicious nodules. Only one incident lung cancer was observed in 678 person-years. Of note, only 30% to 50% of those eligible completed their subsequent annual scans either because they were lost to follow-up or were noncompliant. This experience suggests that low-dose CT screening for lung cancer may be challenging to implement effectively for inner city HIV populations with limited social support. Nevertheless, given the associations between HIV infection, cigarette smoking, and lung cancer risk as well as mortality, CT screening for lung cancers in PLWHA should be the focus of larger prospective clinical trials.

HEMATOPOIETIC CELL AND SOLID ORGAN TRANSPLANTS

Post-Transplant Lymphoproliferative Disorders

Post-transplant lymphoproliferative disorders (PTLD) constitute a heterogeneous group of diseases which presently rank among the most deadly complications of allo-hematopoietic cell and solid organ transplantation.[98,99] The majority (~80%) of PTLD are due to primary EBV infection or reactivation and impaired antiviral immunity as a result of iatrogenic immunosuppression. EBV-seronegative patients have markedly higher (10 to 76 fold) risk of developing PTLD[98,100,101]; as such, the incidence of PTLD is increased in children due to higher rates of primary EBV infection.[102] PTLD are seen in 0.5% to 2.5% of patients undergoing allo-hematopoietic cell transplantation (allo-HCT), most commonly 2 to 6 months post-transplant.[103,104] In contrast, PTLD are observed in approximately 20% of small bowel transplant recipients, 10% of lung transplant patients, 6% of heart transplant patients, and approximately 3% of liver and renal transplant recipients with median onset of 30 to 40 months post-transplant.[99,102,105–107] EBV-negative PTLD typically present 50 to 60 months post-transplant and appear to be more aggressive malignancies.[98,108,109] Currently, PTLD are the most common causes of cancer-related mortality in adult SOT recipients.[98] The vast majority of PTLD are of recipient origin.[110]

Significant risk factors for PTLD in allo-HCT recipients include T-cell depletion of the donor product, age greater than 50, EBV serology, HLA mismatch, and severity of graft-versus-host disease.[98,99,111] In contrast, risk factors for PTLD in SOT recipients include EBV status, age at transplantation, type of organ transplant, and intensity as well as duration of immunosuppression; other risk factors include cytomegalovirus (CMV), HHV8, and hepatitis C infection (98,99). The incidence of PTLD is significantly higher in the first year post-transplant, particularly for heart and lung recipients.[112]

Currently PTLD are classified into four major histologic categories based on WHO criteria.[113] Early lesions are typically seen in the first post-transplant year and are characterized either by polyclonal plasmacytic hyperplasia or infectious mononucleosis-like lymphoid proliferations with preservation of nodal architecture. Polymorphic PTLD are polyclonal lymphoid proliferations associated with effacement of nodal architecture or extranodal mass. Monomorphic PTLD (the most common type of PTLD) are comprised of monoclonal proliferations constituting T or B cell lymphomas, the most frequent of which are DLBCL. Classic Hodgkin lymphoma, the least common type of PTLD, usually presents late following transplantation and is histologically identical to classical Hodgkin lymphoma.[98]

The timing of PTLD following transplant may be associated with patterns of disease presentation and prognosis. For example, PTLD occurring less than year post lung transplant tend to present in the chest with involvement of the allograft or mediastinal lymph nodes and less systemic dissemination; these malignancies more often are polymorphic and more responsive to reduction of immunosuppression (RIS). In contrast, late occurring PTLD in lung recipients tend to present with GI tract involvement and more systemic disease; these neoplasms are more commonly monomorphic and less responsive to RIS.[114,115] Additional studies have confirmed that early PTLD are typically associated with primary EBV infection in EBV-seronegative hosts and are CD20 positive with a higher incidence of graft involvement.[116]

Signs and symptoms of PTLD relate to organs involved and may include fever, night sweats, dyspnea/cough, tender lymphadenopathy, abdominal discomfort, and, infrequently, neurologic deficits.[98,99] Chest x-rays and CT scans frequently demonstrate parenchymal infiltrates and nodules, with mediastinal or retroperitoneal lymphadenopathy.[98,99,114] More than 70% of PTLD in lung transplant recipients present as intrathoracic disease, 50% of which are solitary pulmonary nodules.[112,114,117–119] FDG-PET scans are useful for identifying systemic sites of disease.[120] Diagnosis is established by excisional or core needle biopsies with histologic, immunologic, and cytogenetic phenotyping, as well as fluorescence in-situ hybridization (FISH) analysis of EBV RNA sequences; additional diagnostic studies include EBV, HIV, and hepatitis serologies.[98]

Treatment of PTLD includes RIS (which alone may be effective in early PTLD[121,122]). Antiviral drugs such as intravenous ganciclovir or oral valganciclovir typically are ineffective in EBV-seropositive recipients, although some experts use them to reduce de novo infection of more B lymphocytes.[123] Additional therapies include rituximab with or without concurrent chemotherapy (i.e., CHOP or EPOCH), as well as adoptive immunotherapy using T cells genetically engineered to recognize EBV antigens.[80,98,121,124]

Given the potential mortality associated with PTLD, many centers monitor EBV loads in transplant recipients with aggressive initiation of therapy based on viral DNA copy numbers and EBV status.[121] Such assays have utilized serum, plasma, or PBMC as sources of DNA, and hence may differ in monitoring lytic versus latent phases of EBV infection.[99,111,123] Whereas no standardized monitoring and intervention criteria have been established, most transplant centers monitor EBV loads and preemptively intervene in EBV-seronegative SOT patients with increasing EBV loads or other EBV-seropositive SOT recipients with rising EBV loads in association with fever, lymphadenopathy, hepatosplenomegaly, increased LDH, or extranodal disease. Preemptive treatments may also be initiated for allo-HCT recipients >50 years of age or those who received T-cell depleting regimens or HLA-mismatched grafts.

Aggressive monitoring of EBV loads with adjustments of immunosuppression and initiation of chemotherapy most likely has contributed to the decrease in incidence of PTLD in the modern era. Additional efforts have focused on identification of risk factors associated with response to therapy and survival of patients with PTLD.[125,126] A recent study demonstrated that an International Prognostic Index based on five variables (age greater than 60 years, stage of tumor, PS, extranodal disease, and serum LDH) as well as type of transplant and response to rituximab monotherapy accurately stratified patients with rapidly growing lymphomas into high- versus low-risk cohorts; notably, recipients of thoracic organ transplants who did not respond to rituximab monotherapy were at very high risk of disease progression and death following subsequent CHOP-based therapy.[127]

PTLD can be particularly challenging in patients with heart and/or lung transplants. Kumarasinghe et al.[128] conducted a retrospective review of all patients undergoing heart and lung transplantation at a single institution between January 1984 and December 2001 and diagnosed with PTLD between January 1984 and December 2013. Seventy of 1,490 patients with heart or heart–lung transplants (4.7%) developed PTLD, including 41 of 763 (5.3%) heart, 22 of 709 (3.1%) lung, 6 of 79 (7.6%) heart–lung, and of 14 (7.1%) heart–kidney recipients. Median age at transplant was 42 years, and median age at diagnosis of PTLD was 50 years. Notably, the incidence of PTLD decreased from 7.2% during 1984 to 1990 to 1.99% during 2006 to 2010, a phenomenon which the authors attributed to decreased use of cytolytic agents such as antithymocyte globulin (ATG), improved surveillance, and prophylactic antiviral treatment following transplantation.

Early PTLD was observed in 31% of patients; approximately 75% of all PTLD were monomorphic DLBCL. All patients were initially treated by RIS, and one-third of patients received antiviral therapy; 36% achieved a CR. Patients receiving rituximab had a 50% CR rate, whereas 22% had no response. Patients receiving non-rituximab–based chemotherapy had a 40% CR rate, with an additional 40% having no response to therapy. The overall CR rate was 46%. Five-year OS for patients with PTLD was 29%. Survival of patients treated with rituximab was 51% compared to 26% for patients in the non-rituximab group; this difference was not statistically significant due to low numbers of patients. Five- and 10-year survival rates for patients with PTLD were significantly worse than patients without PTLD (60% vs. 68% and 34% vs. 51%, respectively; $p = 0.0029$). Multivariate analysis revealed that bone marrow involvement, hypoalbuminemia, and no response within 1 to 3 months of treatment were associated with poor survival.

The high mortality rate for patients with PTLD observed in the aforementioned study is consistent with results from other single-institution studies. Muchtar et al.[129] identified 9 cases of PTLD in 338 patients (2.7%; 95% confidence interval, 0.94% to 4.38%) who underwent lung or heart–lung transplantation between 1997 and 2012. An additional patient transplanted at another hospital was referred to the authors' institution for treatment of PTLD. Median time from transplantation to PTLD was 41 months. Three patients had early

PTLD. All patients were treated initially by RIS, and an additional regimen, which typically was chemotherapy with or without rituximab. One patient underwent wedge resection of the lung graft. Eight (80%) patients had a complete response whereas 2 (20%) patients had progressive disease. With a median follow-up of 17 months, eight patients (including seven complete responders) died as a result of chronic rejection (n = 5), disease progression (n = 1), treatment-related toxicity (n = 1), or second primary malignancy (n = 1). Overall survival of 2 years after diagnosis of PTLD was 34% (95% CI: 9% to 62%). Wudihikarn et al.[118] reported a median survival of 10 months and 75% mortality rate in 32 patients who developed PTLD following lung or heart–lung transplantation between 1985 and 2008. Kremer et al.[117] reported a median survival of 18.6 months for 35 patients who developed PTLD following lung transplantation between 1991 and 2011. Consistent with findings of Kumarasinghe and colleagues, the incidence of PTLD fell dramatically during the study period. These findings, together with advances in prevention, detection, and treatment of PTLD,[99,121,123] suggest that mortality rates associated with these neoplasms may decrease as well in the future.

In a recent analysis using the United Network for Organ Sharing (UNOS) database, Hayes et al.[130] observed 120 cases of PTLD among 14,487 patients (0.83%) who received heart transplants between 2006 and 2013. Patients who developed PTLD had significantly worse survivals compared to those who did not have PTLD (HR 4.95; 95% CI: 3.7 to 6.5). Propensity score matching confirmed worse survival in patients with PTLD compared to those who did not develop PTLD (HR = 2.667; 95% CI: 1.04 to 6.82; $p = 0.040$). Collectively these data suggest that despite the decreasing frequency of PTLD following thoracic organ transplants, PTLD still pose significant mortality risks and should be prevented if possible and aggressively treated when diagnosed.

Kaposi Sarcoma

Rarely seen in patients who have undergone hematopoietic transplants,[131] KS are more typically observed in recipients of SOT,[132] presumably due to the increased immunosuppression required to prevent rejection in these individuals. Although the overall incidence of KS in recipients of SOTs is low, the absolute risk is up to 200 fold higher in these individuals compared to the normal population.[17,133] Overall risk of KS in transplant recipients tends to reflect the prevalence of HHV8 infection worldwide.[133] In general, the risk of KS following SOT increases with increasing age at transplantation, HLA mismatch—particularly HLA-A and HLA-B alleles, aggressiveness of immunosuppression, and male gender.[134–136] Eighty percent of KS occur in patients who were seropositive prior to transplantation.[137] Opportunistic infections such as pneumocystis carinii may increase risk of KS post-transplant.[137] KS has been associated with essentially all immune suppression drugs including ATG, corticosteroids, purine synthesis inhibitors, and especially calcineurin inhibitors, which appear to decrease time to KS.[137,138] Whereas up to 90% of post-transplant KS have cutaneous manifestations, KS may also affect lymph nodes (20%), GI tract (50%), and lungs (20%).[133] Pulmonary involvement tends to occur in advanced disease and typically presents with progressive dyspnea, hypoxia, and hypocapnia with diffuse bilateral interstitial infiltrates with or without pleural effusions.[139] Flame-like parenchymal infiltrates observed in HIV-associated pulmonary KS have not been described in transplant patients. As with AIS-related KS, diagnosis of transplantation-associated KS is established by tissue biopsy. Presently, serologic assays for anti-KS antibodies or polymerase chain reaction (PCR) quantitation of HHV8 viral DNA loads appear to correlate with disease burden, yet are not sufficiently developed for routine monitoring of KS or for predicting occurrence of KS in transplant recipients.[133,140]

Mbulaiteye et al.[134] identified 65 KS cases among 234,127 SOT recipients in the United States from 1993 to 2003. Most cases occurred within 2 years after transplantation; increased risk was associated with age of recipient, male gender, Hispanic recipient, non-US citizen, and HLA-A and HLA-B mismatch. No association was observed between KS risk and specific immunosuppressive regimens. In an additional study, Piselli et al.[141] evaluated risk of KS in a large Italian cohort receiving SOT from 1970 to 2006, corresponding to 33,621 patient-years; primary risk factors of KS included male gender, older age at transplantation, and recipient of lung allograft.

Treatment of KS includes decreasing immunosuppression as much as possible while avoiding allograft rejection.[133] Approximately 20% of KS patients exhibit remission after tapering immunosuppression.[134] In general, cutaneous and visceral sites of disease tend to respond in parallel. Patients receiving calcineurin inhibitors should be switched to sirolimus, an inhibitor of mammalian target of rapamycin (mTOR) signaling with immunosuppressive as well as antineoplastic activities.[142,143] Patients not responding to these interventions—particularly those with progressive pulmonary or pleural involvement—should be considered for chemotherapy using liposomal doxorubicin, liposomal daunorubicin, or paclitaxel; similar to HIV-related KS, antiviral agents are not effective in post-transplant KS.[133] Recent studies demonstrating impaired HHV8-specific cellular immune responses in immunosuppressed patients with KS[144] support the development of vaccines to boost immunity to HHV8 in these individuals.

Whereas post-transplant KS with visceral involvement was associated with a 56% mortality rate in a large series extending from 1993 to 2003,[134] advances in diagnosis and treatment of these patients most likely has improved in the more modern era; however, such data are not presently available. Nevertheless, KS with pulmonary involvement can be particularly challenging in thoracic organ transplant recipients. Sleiman et al.[145] reported a case of KS involving the recipient's trachea and bronchus but not the lung allograft that completely regressed after decreasing immunosuppression. Sahseberg-Studer et al.[146] reported a case of KS involving the skin and graft in an HHV8-seropositive patient receiving a lung from a seronegative donor presenting 8 months post-transplant that was fatal. More recently, Sathy et al.[147] observed KS involving the grafts in two HHV8-seropositive recipients of double lung transplants from seronegative donors; one patient had KS involving both lungs, whereas the other had cutaneous as well as visceral KS with pulmonary and pleural involvement. Both cases were rapidly progressive and fatal despite RIS and initiation of chemotherapy. Patel et al.[148] reported their experience with concomitant KS and MCD in a heart transplant recipient who succumbed despite aggressive manipulation of immunosuppression, and initiation of antiviral agents as well as rituximab.

Lung Cancer

Secondary solid malignancies account for 5% to 10% of all late deaths in patients with hematopoietic cell transplants, with the risk steadily increasing after the fifth post-transplant year.[149] Risk factors for secondary malignancies in these patients include age at transplantation, genetic predisposition (i.e., Fanconi anemia), total body irradiation, chronic graft-versus-host disease, and immunosuppressive regimens.[150,151] Whereas a variety of neoplasms including oral, salivary, esophageal, liver, and reproductive cancers are more frequent in recipients of allo-HCT relative to control populations, lung cancers are quite uncommon in these individuals.[152,153] Erhardt et al.[150] observed only 4 lung cancers among 146 solid malignancies in 23,471 recipients of allogeneic bone marrow transplants; median survival of these patients was only 3 months.

Pharmacologic immunosuppression after SOTs creates an HIV-like state, which is associated with increased risk of a variety of malignancies. Using data from the Transplant Cancer Match Study linking US transplantation registry with 14 regional and state cancer registries, Hall et al.[154] estimated the cumulative risk of cancer after transplantation for two periods (1987 to 1999 and 2000 to 2008) relative to cancers in non-transplant patients in the SEER registry. The 5-year cumulative incidence was higher for the second period (4.4% vs. 4.2%; $p = 0.006$) due to decreased risk of competing events such as graft failure, re-transplantation, or death. Five-year cumulative risks of colon, lung, and kidney cancer were higher among transplant patients. In a large cohort study, Engels et al.[132] evaluated the spectrum of cancer risk in US SOT patients using data linked from the US Scientific Registry of Transplant Recipients from 1987 to 2008 and 13 regional or state cancer registries. A total of 175,732 SOTs (58% kidney; 22% liver; 10% heart; 4% lung) were performed during this period. Overall cancer risk was elevated with a SIR of 2.10 (95% CI: 2.06 to 2.14). Lung cancer risk was elevated (SIR 1.97; 95% CI: 1.86 to 2.08) for all transplants and was highest in lung transplants (SIR 6.13). Increased lung cancer risk was also noted for other SOTs including kidney, liver, and heart (SIRs 1.46, 1.95, 2.67, respectively). Recent analysis has indicated that SRTR cancer data are substantially incomplete; as such this database may underestimate true cancer incidence in transplant patients.[155]

Using the US Organ Procurement Transplant Network/United Network of Organ Sharing database containing 193,905 patients receiving organs between 1999 and 2008, Sampaio et al.[156] observed lung cancer incidences of 1.12%, 2.18%, 3.24%, and 5.94% in recipients of kidney, liver, and heart, and lung transplants, respectively; the incidence of lung cancer exceeded the incidence of PTLD (5.72%) in lung transplant recipients. Shiels et al.[157] evaluated data on 15 cancer types diagnosed between 1996 and 2010 using studies that linked US cancer registries with transplant and HIV registries; 8,411 of 4.5 million cancer cases were diagnosed in PLWHA, whereas 7,322 of 6.4 million cancer cases occurred in transplant patients. Relative to non-immunosuppressed patients, PLWHA tended to be diagnosed with late-stage lung cancers (OR 1.13), whereas transplant patients tended to be diagnosed with earlier stage tumors (OR 0.54), possibly due to enhanced surveillance.

Increased lung cancer risk in lung recipients appears primarily due to smoking-related diseases such as COPD and emphysema that led to the transplants. The majority of lung cancers arise in the remaining native lung; however, some cancers particularly those diagnosed within 6 months post-transplant may be due to occult cancer arising in the explanted lung.[158] Occasionally, cancers may arise in the transplanted organ. Chen et al.[159] used Y chromosome FISH techniques to evaluate origin of cancer in six NSCLC arising in gender-mismatched kidney or heart transplant patients; all of the cancers were derived from recipient cells. Dickson et al.[160] observed lung cancer in 9 of 131 (6.9%) patients receiving single lung transplants and 0 of 131 (0%) propensity matched double lung transplant patients diagnosed at a mean of 52 months post-transplant. All tumors arose in native lungs. Six of the nine tumors were squamous cell carcinomas, and overall 5-year survival was 25%. Multivariate analysis demonstrated that single versus double lung transplant was a significant risk factor for post-transplant lung cancer (RR 5.31; 95% CI: 4.01 to 7.02, $P <0.0001$); smoking history and age at transplant were not significant risk factors. In an additional study, Minai et al.[161] identified 13 lung cancers arising in 12 patients who were among 520 individuals (2.3%) receiving lung transplants between 1990 and 2006 at the

Cleveland Clinic. Time from transplant to lung cancer diagnosis was 119 (21 to 416) weeks. Eleven patients had COPD and all had more than 30 pack-year history of cigarette smoke exposure. Eleven of the 13 cancers arose in native lungs. Two metachronous cancers arose in a lung transplanted from a donor with >50 pack-year cigarette exposure. Eight of the 12 patients had stage IV disease, and one was medically inoperable. Three patients (including the one with metachronous primaries in the transplanted lung) underwent lobectomy with one postoperative death. Resection of the second primary in the transplanted lung was not possible, and this patient ultimately died of disease. Overall survival at 2 years for the 12 patients was 17%.

Yserbyt et al.[162] examined incidence and outcomes of lung cancers diagnosed in 494 patients receiving lung and heart–lung transplants between January 2000 and June 2011. Nine of 101 (8.9%) single lung transplant recipients and 4 of 393 (1.0%) double lung transplant patients developed lung cancers at a mean of 41 ± 27 months post-transplant. All had a history of cigarette smoking. Nine patients had locally advanced or metastatic disease at diagnosis. Patients with early-stage tumors had a median survival of 21 months compared to 6 months for patients with locally advanced or metastatic disease.

Whereas single-institution studies have suggested SOT patients who develop lung cancer have very poor survivals, stage-specific outcomes of these patients in the modern era have not been clearly established. Using the SEER Registry linked to Medicare claims, Sigel et al.[163] identified 597 lung cancer patients 65 years of age or older who previously had received kidney, liver, heart, or lung transplants and compared outcomes of these patients with 114,410 lung cancer patients with no transplant history. Transplant patients had earlier stage at diagnosis ($p = 0.002$) and were more likely to have squamous cell carcinomas ($p = 0.02$). Whereas a history of non-lung SOT was associated with poor overall survival relative to control ($p <0.05$), survival of lung transplant recipients with lung cancer was no different than matched patients without prior lung transplant after accounting for competing causes of death. These recent findings suggest that pharmacologic immunosuppression per se does not significantly impact clinical progression of NSCLC and that if possible lung transplant patients should receive stage-specific standard of care treatment for their malignancies.

Similar trends have been identified in heart transplant patients. Dorent and colleagues[164] observed a 2.2% incidence of lung cancer at 16 years post-transplant in patients undergoing heart transplants from 1982 to 1998. Fourteen lung cancer cases were identified among 756 heart transplant patients. Smoking was the only variable that correlated with lung cancer risk. Thirteen patients had NSCLC whereas one had SCLC. Eight of the 13 NSCLC patients underwent surgery, with 7 alive at 52 ± 31 months post-diagnosis. There was no apparent effect of immunosuppression on survival of lung cancer patients.

Rinaldi and colleagues[165] identified 12 lung cancer cases among 475 patients undergoing heart transplants between 1985 and 1998 at a single institution in Italy. Multivariate analysis revealed no impact of immunosuppression regimens on lung cancer risk; however, younger age at transplantation was associated with increased risk of this neoplasm. Lung cancer patients had an 83% mortality rate. In another retrospective single-institution analysis, Bagan et al.[166] reported their surgical experience with 25 heart transplant recipients diagnosed with lung cancer at a median of 88 months post-transplant. All patients had significant smoking histories. Surgeries included 23 lobectomies and 2 wedge resections; morbidity was 28% (primarily infection-related) and 3 patients died in the postoperative period. Median survival of 18 stage I patients was 58.6 months compared to 13.5 months for patients with stage II or higher disease. These data suggest that surgery for early-stage lung cancer is feasible in heart transplants patients.

In an additional retrospective study, Mohammadi and colleagues[167] identified 19 cases of lung cancer in 829 recipients of heart transplants and compared outcomes of these patients with a case-matched heart transplant control group. Median time from transplant to lung cancer diagnosis was 68.8 ± 42.4 months. A history of smoking was the only risk factor identified for lung cancer. Fourteen patients were asymptomatic and had cancer detected either by routine CXR (10 patients) or CT scans (4 patients); the remaining five patients were symptomatic at presentation. All lung cancer patients were males. Not surprisingly there was a trend for cancers to be larger and to have nodal involvement in patients with lung cancers initially detected by CXR or those presenting with symptoms. The majority of patients in the CXR and the symptomatic groups died of disease, while all of the patients with cancers detected by CT scans were alive with a follow-up ranging from 10 to 85 months. These authors advocated routine use of chest CT scans for surveillance of heart transplant recipients.

Bruschi et al.[168] identified 22 lung cancers among 660 patients (3.3%) undergoing heart transplant between 1985 and 2006 diagnosed at a mean of 73.7 ± 30 months post-transplant; 91% of the lung cancer patients were male. Eleven (50%) had stage III/IV disease. Ten patients underwent surgery (nine lobectomies and one wedge resection) with median survival time of 70.4 months and 5-year overall survival of 56% compared to a 33% 1-year survival for inoperable patients. The authors concluded that survival of heart transplant patients undergoing surgery for early-stage NSCLC was acceptable and advocated the use of CT screening for early detection of lung cancers in heart transplant recipients.

Crespo et al.[169] identified 102 lung cancers in 4,357 patients (2%) undergoing heart transplants in Spain between 1984 and 2008; these cancers were diagnosed at a mean of 6.4 years post-transplant. Lung cancer incidence rose with increasing age at heart transplant and was higher in males and patients with pre-transplant smoking history. Potentially curative surgery was performed in 21 of 28 operable cases, with 2-year survival rates of 70% for these patients versus 16% for patients with inoperable disease.

In a more recent study, Maio and colleagues[170] evaluated the incidence and outcomes of cancers occurring in 633 recipients of organ transplants in the Israel Penn International Transplant Tumor Registry (1980 to 2007) relative to 1,282,984 patients in the SEER Registry (1988 to 2004); 179 of these malignancies (25%) were NSCLC including 30 (17%) stage I, 15 (80%) stage II, 29 (16%) stage III, and 105 (59%) stage IV tumors; 48 of these patients (28%) had previously received heart or lung transplants, whereas the remaining patients were liver or kidney recipients. With the exception of stage II patients in the transplant cohort who had survival worse than the respective controls (possibly due to low numbers), stage-specific survivals of transplant patients with lung cancer were no different than survivals of the respective control groups. Notably, 74% of patients in the transplant cohort presented with locally advanced or metastatic disease. These findings, together with recent I-ELCAP and NLST data, support the use of low-dose CT scans for surveillance in SOT recipients—particularly those with other risk factors for lung cancer.

CONCLUSIONS

HAART has converted HIV infection from a uniformly fatal disease to a chronic illness. As a result, the frequencies of ADC such as KS and NHL have decreased whereas NADC including pulmonary carcinomas have increased. Presently it is unclear if controlled HIV infection and decreased systemic inflammation will impact lung cancer risk independent of cigarette smoking, the major risk factor contributing to increased prevalence of lung cancer in PLWHA. Further studies are necessary to define lung cancer risk and mortality in HIV-infected individuals in the modern era. Current efforts should focus on curtailing cigarette abuse in order to reduce lung cancer incidence and mortality in PLWHA who are aging, and as such may be prone to such malignancies. Studies are in progress to define molecular signatures of lung cancer in HIV-infected patients; such analyses may identify novel mechanisms contributing to HIV-associated lung cancers, as well as potential therapeutic targets in these neoplasms. Additional efforts should focus on reducing disparities regarding access to treatment for HIV-infected patients with lung cancer.

Advances in immunosuppression as well as early detection and treatment of PTLD and KS have resulted in decreased frequencies of these potentially lethal complications in transplant patients. Recipients of SOT, particularly thoracic organs are at increased risk of lung cancer, presumably due to antecedent cigarette abuse and immunosuppression. Double lung transplants could be considered as a measure to decrease lung cancer risk; however, given limited organ supply, this may not be feasible. As such, SOT recipients as well as PLWHA should either be enrolled in prospective trials or routinely monitored for lung cancer using low-dose CT scans and I-ELCAP or NLST algorithms.

The fact that patterns of cancer risk in PLWHA and transplant recipients are similar strongly suggests that lung cancers in these patients are to some extent the result of deficient immune surveillance. The relative effects of HIV infection and organ transplantation on immune surveillance and immuno-editing of malignancies are the focus of ongoing laboratory and clinical investigation.

REFERENCES

1. Ehrlich P. Über den jetzigen stand der chemotherapie. *Ber Dtsch Chem Ges* 1909;42(1):17–47.
2. Burnet FM. The concept of immunological surveillance. *Prog Exp Tumor Res* 1970;13:1–27.
3. Muenst S, Laubli H, Soysal SD, et al. The immune system and cancer evasion strategies: therapeutic concepts. *J Intern Med* 2016;279(6):541–562.
4. Corthay A. Does the immune system naturally protect against cancer? *Front Immunol* 2014;5:197.
5. Mapara MY, Sykes M. Tolerance and cancer: mechanisms of tumor evasion and strategies for breaking tolerance. *J Clin Oncol* 2004;22(6):1136–1151.
6. Swann JB, Smyth MJ. Immune surveillance of tumors. *J Clin Invest* 2007;117(5):1137–1146.
7. Shankaran V, Ikeda H, Bruce AT, et al. IFNgamma and lymphocytes prevent primary tumour development and shape tumour immunogenicity. *Nature* 2001;410(6832):1107–1111.
8. Santarpia M, Giovannetti E, Rolfo C, et al. Recent developments in the use of immunotherapy in non-small cell lung cancer. *Expert Rev Respir Med* 2016;10(7):781–798.
9. McGranahan N, Furness AJ, Rosenthal R, et al. Clonal neoantigens elicit T cell immunoreactivity and sensitivity to immune checkpoint blockade. *Science* 2016;351(6280):1463–1469.
10. Almodovar S. The complexity of HIV persistence and pathogenesis in the lung under antiretroviral therapy: challenges beyond AIDS. *Viral Immunol* 2014;27(5):186–199.
11. Lambert AA, Merlo CA, Kirk GD. Human immunodeficiency virus-associated lung malignancies. *Clin Chest Med* 2013;34(2):255–272.
12. van Sighem AI, Gras LA, Reiss P, et al.; ATHENA national observational cohort study. Life expectancy of recently diagnosed asymptomatic HIV-infected patients approaches that of uninfected individuals. *AIDS* 2010;24(10):1527–1535.
13. Rubinstein PG, Aboulafia DM, Zloza A. Malignancies in HIV/AIDS: from epidemiology to therapeutic challenges. *AIDS* 2014;28(4):453–465.
14. Engels EA, Biggar RJ, Hall HI, et al. Cancer risk in people infected with human immunodeficiency virus in the United States. *Int J Cancer* 2008;123(1):187–194.
15. Brickman C, Palefsky JM. Cancer in the HIV-infected host: epidemiology and pathogenesis in the antiretroviral era. *Curr HIV/AIDS Rep* 2015;12(4):388–396.
16. Dubrow R, Silverberg MJ, Park LS, et al. HIV infection, aging, and immune function: implications for cancer risk and prevention. *Curr Opin Oncol* 2012;24(5):506–516.
17. Grulich AE, Vajdic CM. The epidemiology of cancers in human immunodeficiency virus infection and after organ transplantation. *Semin Oncol* 2015;42(2):247–257.
18. Bhutani M, Polizzotto MN, Uldrick TS, et al. Kaposi sarcoma-associated herpesvirus-associated malignancies: epidemiology, pathogenesis, and advances in treatment. *Semin Oncol* 2015;42(2):223–246.

19. La Ferla L, Pinzone MR, Nunnari G, et al. Kaposi's sarcoma in HIV-positive patients: the state of art in the HAART-era. *Eur Rev Med Pharmacol Sci* 2013; 17(17):2354–2365.

20. Pinzone MR, Berretta M, Cacopardo B, et al. Epstein-Barr virus- and Kaposi sarcoma-associated herpesvirus-related malignancies in the setting of human immunodeficiency virus infection. *Semin Oncol* 2015;42(2):258–271.

21. Fishback NF, Travis WD, Moran CA, et al. Pleomorphic (spindle/giant cell) carcinoma of the lung. A clinicopathologic correlation of 78 cases. *Cancer* 1994;73(12): 2936–2945.

22. Yanik EL, Napravnik S, Cole SR, et al. Incidence and timing of cancer in HIV-infected individuals following initiation of combination antiretroviral therapy. *Clin Infect Dis* 2013;57(5):756–764.

23. Borie R, Cadranel J, Guihot A, et al. Pulmonary manifestations of human herpesvirus-8 during HIV infection. *Eur Respir J* 2013;42(4):1105–1118.

24. Khalil AM, Carette MF, Cadranel JL, et al. Intrathoracic Kaposi's sarcoma. CT findings. *Chest* 1995;108(6):1622–1626.

25. Chou SH, Prabhu SJ, Crothers K, et al. Thoracic diseases associated with HIV infection in the era of antiretroviral therapy: clinical and imaging findings. *Radiographics* 2014;34(4):895–911.

26. Lee VW, Fuller JD, O'Brien MJ, et al. Pulmonary Kaposi sarcoma in patients with AIDS: scintigraphic diagnosis with sequential thallium and gallium scanning. *Radiology* 1991;180(2):409–412.

27. Gruden JF, Huang L, Webb WR, et al. AIDS-related Kaposi sarcoma of the lung: radiographic findings and staging system with bronchoscopic correlation. *Radiology* 1995;195(2):545–552.

28. Barski A, Cuddapah S, Cui K, et al. High-resolution profiling of histone methylations in the human genome. *Cell* 2007;129(4):823–837.

29. Krown SE. Highly active antiretroviral therapy in AIDS associated Kaposi's sarcoma: implications for the design of therapeutic trials in patients with advanced, symptomatic Kaposi's sarcoma. *J Clin Oncol* 2004;22(3):399–402.

30. Gbabe OF, Okwundu CI, Dedicoat M, et al. Treatment of severe or progressive Kaposi's sarcoma in HIV-infected adults. *Cochrane Database Syst Rev* 2014;8: CD003256.

31. Mosam A, Shaik F, Uldrick TS, et al. A randomized controlled trial of highly active antiretroviral therapy versus highly active antiretroviral therapy and chemotherapy in therapy-naive patients with HIV-associated Kaposi sarcoma in South Africa. *J Acquir Immune Defic Syndr* 2012;60(2):150–157.

32. Cribbs SK, Fontenot AP. The impact of antiretroviral therapy on lung immunology. *Semin Respir Crit Care Med* 2016;37(2):157–165.

33. Bower M, Nelson M, Young AM, et al. Immune reconstitution inflammatory syndrome associated with Kaposi's sarcoma. *J Clin Oncol* 2005;23(22):5224–5228.

34. Palmieri C, Dhillon T, Thirlwell C, et al. Pulmonary Kaposi sarcoma in the era of highly active antiretroviral therapy. *HIV Med* 2006;7(5):291–293.

35. International Collaboration on HIV and Cancer. Highly active antiretroviral therapy and incidence of cancer in human immunodeficiency virus-infected adults. *J Natl Cancer Inst* 2000;92(22):1823–1830.

36. Cesarman E. Gammaherpesviruses and lymphoproliferative disorders. *Annu Rev Pathol* 2014;9:349–372.

37. Carbone A, Vaccher E, Gloghini A, et al. Diagnosis and management of lymphomas and other cancers in HIV-infected patients. *Nat Rev Clin Oncol* 2014;11(4): 223–238.

38. Eisner MD, Kaplan LD, Herndier B, et al. The pulmonary manifestations of AIDS-related non-Hodgkin's lymphoma. *Chest* 1996;110(3):729–736.

39. Koss MN. Malignant and benign lymphoid lesions of the lung. *Ann Diagn Pathol* 2004;8(3):167–187.

40. Pina-Oviedo S, Weissferdt A, Kalhor N, et al. Primary pulmonary lymphomas. *Adv Anat Pathol* 2015;22(6):355–375.

41. Ray P, Antoine M, Mary-Krause M, et al. AIDS-related primary pulmonary lymphoma. *Am J Respir Crit Care Med* 1998;158(4):1221–1229.

42. Allen CM, Al-Jahdali HH, Irion KL, et al. Imaging lung manifestations of HIV/AIDS. *Ann Thorac Med* 2010;5(4):201–216.

43. Diez-Martin JL, Balsalobre P, Re A, et al. Comparable survival between HIV+ and HIV−non-Hodgkin and Hodgkin lymphoma patients undergoing autologous peripheral blood stem cell transplantation. *Blood* 2009;113(23):6011–6014.

44. Nador RG, Cesarman E, Chadburn A, et al. Primary effusion lymphoma: a distinct clinicopathologic entity associated with the Kaposi's sarcoma-associated herpes virus. *Blood* 1996;88(2):645–656.

45. Boulanger E, Gerard L, Gabarre J, et al. Prognostic factors and outcome of human herpesvirus 8-associated primary effusion lymphoma in patients with AIDS. *J Clin Oncol* 2005;23(19):4372–4380.

46. Klein U, Gloghini A, Gaidano G, et al. Gene expression profile analysis of AIDS-related primary effusion lymphoma (PEL) suggests a plasmablastic derivation and identifies PEL-specific transcripts. *Blood* 2003;101(10):4115–4121.

47. Jenner RG, Maillard K, Cattini N, et al. Kaposi's sarcoma-associated herpesvirus-infected primary effusion lymphoma has a plasma cell gene expression profile. *Proc Natl Acad Sci U S A* 2003;100(18):10399–10404.

48. Carbone A, Gloghini A. KSHV/HHV8-associated lymphomas. *Br J Haematol* 2008; 140(1):13–24.

49. Krishnan S, Schouten JT, Jacobson DL, et al. Incidence of non-AIDS-defining cancer in antiretroviral treatment-naive subjects after antiretroviral treatment initiation: an ACTG longitudinal linked randomized trials analysis. *Oncology* 2011;80(1–2): 42–49.

50. Oksenhendler E, Boulanger E, Galicier L, et al. High incidence of Kaposi sarcoma-associated herpesvirus-related non-Hodgkin lymphoma in patients with HIV infection and multicentric Castleman disease. *Blood* 2002;99(7):2331–2316.

51. Guihot A, Couderc LJ, Rivaud E, et al. Thoracic radiographic and CT findings of multicentric Castleman disease in HIV-infected patients. *J Thorac Imaging* 2007;22(2):207–211.

52. Staskus KA, Sun R, Miller G, et al. Cellular tropism and viral interleukin-6 expression distinguish human herpesvirus 8 involvement in Kaposi's sarcoma, primary effusion lymphoma, and multicentric Castleman's disease. *J Virol* 1999; 73(5):4181–4187.

53. Cannon JS, Nicholas J, Orenstein JM, et al. Heterogeneity of viral IL-6 expression in HHV-8-associated diseases. *J Infect Dis* 1999;180(3):824–828.

54. Menke DM, Chadburn A, Cesarman E, et al. Analysis of the human herpesvirus 8 (HHV-8) genome and HHV-8 vIL-6 expression in archival cases of Castleman disease at low risk for HIV infection. *Am J Clin Pathol* 2002;117(2):268–275.

55. Mylona EE, Baraboutis IG, Lekakis LJ, et al. Multicentric Castleman's disease in HIV infection: a systematic review of the literature. *AIDS Rev* 2008;10(1): 25–35.

56. Oksenhendler E. HIV-associated multicentric Castleman disease. *Curr Opin HIV AIDS* 2009;4(1):16–21.

57. Powles T, Stebbing J, Bazeos A, et al. The role of immune suppression and HHV-8 in the increasing incidence of HIV-associated multicentric Castleman's disease. *Ann Oncol* 2009;20(4):775–779.

58. Gerard L, Berezne A, Galicier L, et al. Prospective study of rituximab in chemotherapy-dependent human immunodeficiency virus associated multicentric Castleman's disease: ANRS 117 CastlemaB Trial. *J Clin Oncol* 2007;25(22):3350–3356.

59. Gerard L, Michot JM, Burcheri S, et al. Rituximab decreases the risk of lymphoma in patients with HIV-associated multicentric Castleman disease. *Blood* 2012;119(10): 2228–2233.

60. Hoffmann C, Schmid H, Muller M, et al. Improved outcome with rituximab in patients with HIV-associated multicentric Castleman disease. *Blood* 2011; 118(13):3499–3503.

61. Grulich AE, van Leeuwen MT, Falster MO, et al. Incidence of cancers in people with HIV/AIDS compared with immunosuppressed transplant recipients: a meta-analysis. *Lancet* 2007;370(9581):59–67.

62. Shiels MS, Cole SR, Kirk GD, et al. A meta-analysis of the incidence of non-AIDS cancers in HIV-infected individuals. *J Acquir Immune Defic Syndr* 2009;52(5): 611–622.

63. Hou W, Fu J, Ge Y, et al. Incidence and risk of lung cancer in HIV-infected patients. *J Cancer Res Clin Oncol* 2013;139(11):1781–1794.

64. Sigel K, Wisnivesky J, Gordon K, et al. HIV as an independent risk factor for incident lung cancer. *AIDS* 2012;26(8):1017–1025.

65. Engsig FN, Kronborg G, Larsen CS, et al. Lung cancer in HIV patients and their parents: a Danish cohort study. *BMC Cancer* 2011;11:272.

66. Shiels MS, Cole SR, Mehta SH, et al. Lung cancer incidence and mortality among HIV-infected and HIV-uninfected injection drug users. *J Acquir Immune Defic Syndr* 2010;55(4):510–515.

67. Triplette M, Crothers K, Attia EF. Non-infectious pulmonary diseases and HIV. *Curr HIV/AIDS Rep* 2016;13(3):140–148.

68. Kawabata S, Heredia A, Gills J, et al. Impact of HIV on lung tumorigenesis in an animal model. *AIDS* 2015;29(5):633–635.

69. Shebl FM, Engels EA, Goedert JJ, et al. Pulmonary infections and risk of lung cancer among persons with AIDS. *J Acquir Immune Defic Syndr* 2010;55(3):375–379.

70. Sigel K, Pitts R, Crothers K. Lung malignancies in HIV infection. *Semin Respir Crit Care Med* 2016;37(2):267–276.

71. Gingo MR, Morris A. Pathogenesis of HIV and the lung. *Curr HIV/AIDS Rep* 2013; 10(1):42–50.

72. Frisch M, Biggar RJ, Engels EA, et al. Association of cancer with AIDS-related immunosuppression in adults. *JAMA* 2001;285(13):1736–1745.

73. Silverberg MJ, Chao C, Leyden WA, et al. HIV infection, immunodeficiency, viral replication, and the risk of cancer. *Cancer Epidemiol Biomarkers Prev* 2011;20(12): 2551–2559.

74. Clifford GM, Lise M, Franceschi S, et al. Lung cancer in the Swiss HIV Cohort Study: role of smoking, immunodeficiency and pulmonary infection. *Br J Cancer* 2012;106(3):447–452.

75. Patel P, Hanson DL, Sullivan PS, et al. Incidence of types of cancer among HIV-infected persons compared with the general population in the United States, 1992–2003. *Ann Intern Med* 2008;148(10):728–736.

76. Engels EA, Brock MV, Chen J, et al. Elevated incidence of lung cancer among HIV-infected individuals. *J Clin Oncol* 2006;24(9):1383–1388.

77. Engels EA, Pfeiffer RM, Goedert JJ, et al. Trends in cancer risk among people with AIDS in the United States 1980–2002. *AIDS* 2006;20(12):1645–1654.

78. Hleyhel M. Risk of non-AIDS-defining cancers among HIV-1-infected individuals in France between 1997 and 2009: results from a French cohort. *AIDS* 2014; 28(14):2109–2118.

79. Robbins HA, Pfeiffer RM, Shiels MS, et al. Excess cancers among HIV-infected people in the United States. *J Natl Cancer Inst* 2015;107(4):pii: dju503.

80. Silverberg MJ, Lau B, Achenbach CJ, et al. Cumulative incidence of cancer among persons with HIV in North America: a cohort study. *Ann Intern Med* 2015;163(7): 507–518.

81. Althoff KN, McGinnis KA, Wyatt CM, et al. Comparison of risk and age at diagnosis of myocardial infarction, end-stage renal disease, and non-AIDS-defining cancer in HIV-infected versus uninfected adults. *Clin Infect Dis* 2015;60(4):627–638.

82. Bearz A, Vaccher E, Martellotta F, et al. Lung cancer in HIV positive patients: the GICAT experience. *Eur Rev Med Pharmacol Sci* 2014;18(4):500–508.

83. Hooker CM, Meguid RA, Hulbert A, et al. Human immunodeficiency virus infection as a prognostic factor in surgical patients with non-small cell lung cancer. *Ann Thorac Surg* 2012;93(2):405–412.

84. Makinson A, Tenon JC, Eymard-Duvernay S, et al. Human immunodeficiency virus infection and non-small cell lung cancer: survival and toxicity of antineoplastic chemotherapy in a cohort study. *J Thorac Oncol* 2011;6(6):1022–1029.

85. Rengan R, Mitra N, Liao K, et al. Effect of HIV on survival in patients with non-small-cell lung cancer in the era of highly active antiretroviral therapy: a population-based study. *Lancet Oncol* 2012;13(12):1203–1209.

86. Sigel K, Crothers K, Dubrow R, et al. Prognosis in HIV-infected patients with non-small cell lung cancer. *Br J Cancer* 2013;109(7):1974–1980.

87. Marcus JL, Chao C, Leyden WA, et al. Survival among HIV-infected and HIV-uninfected individuals with common non-AIDS-defining cancers. *Cancer Epidemiol Biomarkers Prev* 2015;24(8):1167–1173.

88. Coghill AE, Shiels MS, Suneja G, et al. Elevated cancer-specific mortality among HIV-infected patients in the United States. *J Clin Oncol* 2015;33(21):2376–2383.

89. Suneja G, Shiels MS, Angulo R, et al. Cancer treatment disparities in HIV-infected individuals in the United States. *J Clin Oncol* 2014;32(22):2344–2350.

90. Suneja G, Lin CC, Simard EP, et al. Disparities in cancer treatment among patients infected with the human immunodeficiency virus. *Cancer* 2016;122(15):2399–2407.

91. Makinson A, Pujol JL, Le Moing V, et al. Interactions between cytotoxic chemotherapy and antiretroviral treatment in human immunodeficiency virus-infected patients with lung cancer. *J Thorac Oncol* 2010;5(4):562–571.

92. Pillai VC, Venkataramanan R, Parise RA, et al. Ritonavir and efavirenz significantly alter the metabolism of erlotinib—an observation in primary cultures of human hepatocytes that is relevant to HIV patients with cancer. *Drug Metab Dispos* 2013;41(10):1843–1851.

93. Sharma D, Newman TG, Aronow WS. Lung cancer screening: history, current perspectives, and future directions. *Arch Med Sci* 2015;11(5):1033–1043.

94. Sigel K, Wisnivesky J, Shahrir S, et al. Findings in asymptomatic HIV-infected patients undergoing chest computed tomography testing: implications for lung cancer screening. *AIDS* 2014;28(7):1007–1014.

95. Makinson A, Eymard-Duvernay S, Raffi F, et al. Feasibility and efficacy of early lung cancer diagnosis with chest computed tomography in HIV-infected smokers. *AIDS* 2016;30(4):573–582.

96. Church TR, Black WC, Aberle DR, et al. Results of initial low-dose computed tomographic screening for lung cancer. *N Engl J Med* 2013;368(21):1980–1991.

97. Hulbert A, Hooker CM, Keruly JC, et al. Prospective CT screening for lung cancer in a high-risk population: HIV-positive smokers. *J Thorac Oncol* 2014;9(6):752–759.

98. Singavi AK, Harrington AM, Fenske TS. Post-transplant lymphoproliferative disorders. *Cancer Treat Res* 2015;165:305–327.

99. Dharnidharka VR, Webster AC, Martinez OM, et al. Post-transplant lymphoproliferative disorders. *Nat Rev Dis Primers* 2016;2:15088.

100. Walker RC, Marshall WF, Strickler JG, et al. Pretransplantation assessment of the risk of lymphoproliferative disorder. *Clin Infect Dis* 1995;20(5):1346–1353.

101. Dharnidharka VR, Lamb KE, Gregg JA, et al. Associations between EBV serostatus and organ transplant type in PTLD risk: an analysis of the SRTR National Registry Data in the United States. *Am J Transplant* 2012;12(4):976–983.

102. Taylor AL, Marcus R, Bradley JA. Post-transplant lymphoproliferative disorders (PTLD) after solid organ transplantation. *Crit Rev Oncol Hematol* 2005;56(1):155–167.

103. Landgren O, Gilbert ES, Rizzo JD, et al. Risk factors for lymphoproliferative disorders after allogeneic hematopoietic cell transplantation. *Blood* 2009;113(20):4992–5001.

104. Juvonen E, Aalto SM, Tarkkanen J, et al. High incidence of PTLD after non-T-cell-depleted allogeneic haematopoietic stem cell transplantation as a consequence of intensive immunosuppressive treatment. *Bone Marrow Transplant* 2003;32(1):97–102.

105. Cockfield SM. Identifying the patient at risk for post-transplant lymphoproliferative disorder. *Transpl Infect Dis* 2001;3(2):70–78.

106. Burns DM, Crawford DH. Epstein-Barr virus-specific cytotoxic T-lymphocytes for adoptive immunotherapy of post-transplant lymphoproliferative disease. *Blood Rev* 2004;18(3):193–209.

107. Parker A, Bowles K, Bradley JA, et al. Diagnosis of post-transplant lymphoproliferative disorder in solid organ transplant recipients—BCSH and BTS Guidelines. *Br J Haematol* 2010;149(5):675–692.

108. Leblond V, Davi F, Charlotte F, et al. Posttransplant lymphoproliferative disorders not associated with Epstein-Barr virus: a distinct entity? *J Clin Oncol* 1998;16(6):2052–2059.

109. Nelson BP, Nalesnik MA, Bahler DW, et al. Epstein-Barr virus-negative post-transplant lymphoproliferative disorders: a distinct entity? *Am J Surg Pathol* 2000;24(3):375–385.

110. Kinch A, Cavelier L, Bengtsson M, et al. Donor or recipient origin of posttransplant lymphoproliferative disorders following solid organ transplantation. *Am J Transplant* 2014;14(12):2838–2845.

111. Rasche L, Kapp M, Einsele H, et al. EBV-induced post transplant lymphoproliferative disorders: a persisting challenge in allogeneic hematopoetic SCT. *Bone Marrow Transplant* 2014;49(2):163–167.

112. Bakker NA, van Imhoff GW, Verschuuren EA, et al. Presentation and early detection of post-transplant lymphoproliferative disorder after solid organ transplantation. *Transplant Int* 2007;20(3):207–218.

113. Allen U, Preiksaitis J. Epstein-Barr virus and posttransplant lymphoproliferative disorder in solid organ transplant recipients. *Am J Transplant* 2009;9(Suppl 4):S87–S96.

114. Neuringer IP. Posttransplant lymphoproliferative disease after lung transplantation. *Clin Dev Immunol* 2013;2013:430209.

115. Armitage JM, Kormos RL, Stuart RS, et al. Posttransplant lymphoproliferative disease in thoracic organ transplant patients: ten years of cyclosporine-based immunosuppression. *J Heart Lung Transplant* 1991;10(6):877–886; discussion 886–887.

116. Ghobrial IM, Habermann TM, Macon WR, et al. Differences between early and late posttransplant lymphoproliferative disorders in solid organ transplant patients: are they two different diseases? *Transplantation* 2005;79(2):244–247.

117. Kremer BE, Reshef R, Misleh JG, et al. Post-transplant lymphoproliferative disorder after lung transplantation: a review of 35 cases. *J Heart Lung Transplant* 2012;31(3):296–304.

118. Wudhikarn K, Holman CJ, Linan M, et al. Post-transplant lymphoproliferative disorders in lung transplant recipients: 20-yr experience at the University of Minnesota. *Clin Transplant* 2011;25(5):705–713.

119. Bakker NA, van Imhoff GW, Verschuuren EA, et al. Early onset post-transplant lymphoproliferative disease is associated with allograft localization. *Clin Transplant* 2005;19(3):327–334.

120. Bakker NA, Pruim J, de Graaf W, et al. PTLD visualization by FDG-PET: improved detection of extranodal localizations. *Am J Transplant* 2006;6(8):1984–1985.

121. Petrara MR, Giunco S, Serraino D, et al. Post-transplant lymphoproliferative disorders: from epidemiology to pathogenesis-driven treatment. *Cancer Lett* 2015;369(1):37–44.

122. Marques HH, Shikanai-Yasuda MA, dAzevedo LS, et al. Management of post-transplant Epstein-Barr virus-related lymphoproliferative disease in solid organ and hematopoietic stem cell recipients. *Rev Soc Bras Med Trop* 2014;47(5):543–546.

123. San-Juan R, Comoli P, Caillard S, et al. Epstein-Barr virus-related post-transplant lymphoproliferative disorder in solid organ transplant recipients. *Clin Microbiol Infect* 2014;20(Suppl 7):109–118.

124. Park EK, Takahashi K, Hoshuyama T, et al. Global magnitude of reported and unreported mesothelioma. *Environ Health Perspect* 2011;119(4):514–518.

125. Fox CP, Burns D, Parker AN, et al. EBV-associated post-transplant lymphoproliferative disorder following in vivo T-cell-depleted allogeneic transplantation: clinical features, viral load correlates and prognostic factors in the rituximab era. *Bone Marrow Transplant* 2014;49(2):280–286.

126. Ghobrial IM, Habermann TM, Maurer MJ, et al. Prognostic analysis for survival in adult solid organ transplant recipients with post-transplantation lymphoproliferative disorders. *J Clin Oncol* 2005;23(30):7574–7582.

127. Trappe RU, Choquet S, Dierickx D, et al. International prognostic index, type of transplant and response to rituximab are key parameters to tailor treatment in adults with CD20-positive B cell PTLD: clues from the PTLD-1 trial. *Am J Transplant* 2015;15(4):1091–1100.

128. Kumarasinghe G, Lavee O, Parker A, et al. Post-transplant lymphoproliferative disease in heart and lung transplantation: defining risk and prognostic factors. *J Heart Lung Transplant* 2015;34(11):1406–1414.

129. Muchtar E, Kramer MR, Vidal L, et al. Posttransplantation lymphoproliferative disorder in lung transplant recipients: a 15-year single institution experience. *Transplantation* 2013;96(7):657–663.

130. Hayes D, Jr., Tumin D, Foraker RE, et al. Posttransplant lymphoproliferative disease and survival in adult heart transplant recipients. *J Cardiol* 2016;2017;69(1):144–148.

131. Sala I, Faraci M, Magnano GM, et al. HHV-8-related visceral Kaposi's sarcoma following allogeneic HSCT: report of a pediatric case and literature review. *Pediatr Transplant* 2011;15(1):E8–E11.

132. Engels EA, Pfeiffer RM, Fraumeni JF, Jr., et al. Spectrum of cancer risk among US solid organ transplant recipients. *JAMA* 2011;306(17):1891–901.

133. Lebbe C, Legendre C, Frances C. Kaposi sarcoma in transplantation. *Transplant Rev (Orlando)* 2008;22(4):252–261.

134. Mbulaiteye SM, Engels EA. Kaposi's sarcoma risk among transplant recipients in the United States (1993–2003). *Int J Cancer* 2006;119(11):2685–2691.

135. Tessari G, Naldi L, Boschiero L, et al. Incidence and clinical predictors of Kaposi's sarcoma among 1721 Italian solid organ transplant recipients: a multicenter study. *Eur J Dermatol* 2006;16(5):553–537.

136. Shepherd FA, Maher E, Cardella C, et al. Treatment of Kaposi's sarcoma after solid organ transplantation. *J Clin Oncol* 1997;15(6):2371–2377.

137. Frances C, Mouquet C, Marcelin AG, et al. Outcome of kidney transplant recipients with previous human herpesvirus-8 infection. *Transplantation* 2000;69(9):1776–1779.

138. Guba M, Graeb C, Jauch KW, et al. Pro- and anti-cancer effects of immunosuppressive agents used in organ transplantation. *Transplantation* 2004;77(12):1777–1782.

139. Restrepo CS, Martinez S, Lemos JA, et al. Imaging manifestations of Kaposi sarcoma. *Radiographics* 2006;26(4):1169–1185.

140. Pellet C, Chevret S, Frances C, et al. Prognostic value of quantitative Kaposi sarcoma–associated herpesvirus load in posttransplantation Kaposi sarcoma. *J Infect Dis* 2002;186(1):110–113.

141. Piselli P, Busnach G, Citterio F, et al. Risk of Kaposi sarcoma after solid-organ transplantation: multicenter study in 4,767 recipients in Italy, 1970–2006. *Transplant Proc* 2009;41(4):1227–1230.

142. Hernandez-Sierra A, Rovira J, Petit A, et al. Role of HHV-8 and mTOR pathway in post-transplant Kaposi sarcoma staging. *Transplant Int* 2016;29(9):1008–1016.

143. Campistol JM, Schena FP. Kaposi's sarcoma in renal transplant recipients–the impact of proliferation signal inhibitors. *Nephrol Dial Transplant* 2007;22(Suppl 1):i17–i22.

144. Lambert M, Gannage M, Karras A, et al. Differences in the frequency and function of HHV8-specific CD8 T cells between asymptomatic HHV8 infection and Kaposi sarcoma. *Blood* 2006;108(12):3871–3880.

145. Sleiman C, Mal H, Roue C, et al. Bronchial Kaposi's sarcoma after single lung transplantation. *Eur Respir J* 1997;10(5):1181–1183.

146. Sachsenberg-Studer EM, Dobrynski N, Sheldon J, et al. Human herpes-virus 8 seropositive patient with skin and graft Kaposi's sarcoma after lung transplantation. *J Am Acad Dermatol* 1999;40(2 Pt 2):308–311.

147. Sathy SJ, Martinu T, Youens K, et al. Symptomatic pulmonary allograft Kaposi's sarcoma in two lung transplant recipients. *Am J Transplant* 2008;8(9):1951–1956.

148. Patel A, Bishburg E, Zucker M, et al. Concomitant Kaposi sarcoma and multicentric Castleman's disease in a heart transplant recipient. *Heart Lung* 2014;43(6):506–509.

149. Socie G, Rizzo JD. Second solid tumors: screening and management guidelines in long-term survivors after allogeneic stem cell transplantation. *Semin Hematol* 2012;49(1):4–9.

150. Ehrhardt MJ, Brazauskas R, He W, et al. Survival of patients who develop solid tumors following hematopoietic stem cell transplantation. *Bone Marrow Transplant* 2016;51(1):83–88.

151. Adhikari J, Sharma P, Bhatt VR. Risk of secondary solid malignancies after allogeneic hematopoietic stem cell transplantation and preventive strategies. *Future Oncol* 2015;11(23):3175–3185.

152. Rizzo JD, Curtis RE, Socie G, et al. Solid cancers after allogeneic hematopoietic cell transplantation. *Blood* 2009;113(5):1175–1183.

153. Yokota A, Ozawa S, Masanori T, et al. Secondary solid tumors after allogeneic hematopoietic SCT in Japan. *Bone Marrow Transplant* 2012;47(1):95–100.

154. Hall EC, Pfeiffer RM, Segev DL, et al. Cumulative incidence of cancer after solid organ transplantation. *Cancer* 2013;119(12):2300–2308.

155. Yanik EL, Nogueira LM, Koch L, et al. Comparison of cancer diagnoses between the US solid organ transplant registry and linked central cancer registries. *Am J Transplant* 2016;16(10):2986–2993.

156. Sampaio MS, Cho YW, Qazi Y, et al. Posttransplant malignancies in solid organ adult recipients: an analysis of the U.S. National Transplant Database. *Transplantation* 2012;94(10):990–998.

157. Shiels MS, Copeland G, Goodman MT, et al. Cancer stage at diagnosis in patients infected with the human immunodeficiency virus and transplant recipients. *Cancer* 2015;121(12):2063–2071.

158. Olland AB, Falcoz PE, Santelmo N, et al. Primary lung cancer in lung transplant recipients. *Ann Thorac Surg* 2014;98(1):362–371.

159. Chen W, Brodsky SV, Zhao W, et al. Y-chromosome status identification suggests a recipient origin of posttransplant non-small cell lung carcinomas: chromogenic in situ hybridization analysis. *Hum Pathol* 2014;45(5):1065–1070.

160. Dickson RP, Davis RD, Rea JB, et al. High frequency of bronchogenic carcinoma after single-lung transplantation. *J Heart Lung Transplant* 2006;25(11):1297–1301.

161. Minai OA, Shah S, Mazzone P, et al. Bronchogenic carcinoma after lung transplantation: characteristics and outcomes. *J Thorac Oncol* 2008;3(12):1404–1409.

162. Yserbyt J, Verleden GM, Dupont LJ, et al. Bronchial carcinoma after lung transplantation: a single-center experience. *J Heart Lung Transplant* 2012;31(6):585–590.

163. Sigel K, Veluswamy R, Krauskopf K, et al. Lung cancer prognosis in elderly solid organ transplant recipients. *Transplantation* 2015;99(10):2181–2189.

164. Dorent R, Mohammadi S, Tezenas S, et al. Lung cancer in heart transplant patients: a 16-year survey. *Transplant Proc* 2000;32(8):2752–2754.

165. Rinaldi M, Pellegrini C, D'Armini AM, et al. Neoplastic disease after heart transplantation: single center experience. *Eur J Cardiothorac Surg* 2001;19(5):696–701.

166. Bagan P, Assouad J, Berna P, et al. Immediate and long-term survival after surgery for lung cancer in heart transplant recipients. *Ann Thorac Surg* 2005;79(2):438–442.

167. Mohammadi S, Bonnet N, Leprince P, et al. Long-term survival of heart transplant recipients with lung cancer: the role of chest computed tomography screening. *Thorac Cardiovasc Surg* 2007;55(7):438–441.

168. Bruschi G, Conforti S, Torre M, et al. Long-term results of lung cancer after heart transplantation: single center 20-year experience. *Lung Cancer* 2009;63(1):146–150.

169. Crespo-Leiro MG, Villa-Arranz A, Manito-Lorite N, et al. Lung cancer after heart transplantation: results from a large multicenter registry. *Am J Transplant* 2011;11(5):1035–1040.

170. Miao Y, Everly JJ, Gross TG, et al. De novo cancers arising in organ transplant recipients are associated with adverse outcomes compared with the general population. *Transplantation* 2009;87(9):1347–1359.

THORACIC TRAUMA

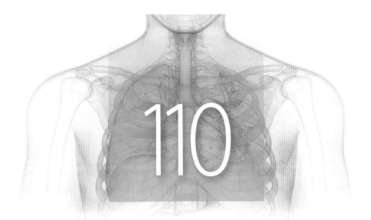

Blunt and Penetrating Injuries of the Chest Wall, Pleura, Diaphragm, and Lungs

Hao Pan ▪ Scott B. Johnson

INTRODUCTION

Thoracic trauma often results in devastating injury with a high morbidity and mortality. Trauma is known to be the leading cause of death in the first four decades of life.[1] Of the 805 facilities participating in the American College of Surgeons (ACS) National Trauma Data Bank (NTDB), trauma-related mortality accounted for 34,622 deaths in the United States in 2012. Chest trauma is second only to head trauma as the most common causes of traumatic deaths. However, it should also be noted that the vast majority of thoracic injuries can usually be treated with relatively simple maneuvers.[2] Blunt trauma from motor vehicle crashes accounts for 70% to 80% of thoracic injuries. In a study by Kulsretha, of the 1,359 consecutive patients admitted at a level I trauma center, 48.7% presented with rib fractures; 2.1% with flail chest; 5.4% with sternal fracture(s)/dislocation(s); and 20.4% with pneumothorax and/or hemothorax. Of their overall 9.4% mortality, noncardiac thoracic injuries accounted for 36.7% of the total deaths.[3]

Involvement of a thoracic surgeon is often warranted to address specific injuries or management concerns. It is imperative that any thoracic trauma be evaluated in the setting of the patient's overall condition, since one's attention can easily be diverted toward more obvious injuries at the exclusion of subtle, yet perhaps more fatal ones (e.g., patients who have suffered severe head injury). Commonly this scenario involves a critically ill patient that may require multiple consultants and imaging modalities providing competing priorities. It must be remembered that trauma of the thoracic cavity is not exempt from any of the basic treatment tenets as described by the Advanced Trauma Life Support (ATLS) algorithms beginning with a primary and secondary survey.[4] As with all patients who have sustained major trauma, a diligent, thorough, and thoughtful approach in their diagnosis and treatment is necessary if a successful outcome is to be achieved.

INDICATIONS FOR IMMEDIATE INTERVENTION

During the primary survey, as outlined by the ATLS algorithm, immediate assessment and stabilization of the airway, breathing, and circulation should be completed in an efficient and expeditious manner.[4] Upon arrival to the emergency department (ED), the primary objective is to identify and address any life-threatening injuries. Oftentimes, many of these primary maneuvers will be lifesaving and based purely on clinical exam or presentation without radiographic interpretation. The following secondary survey identifies additional injuries in a systematic manner. However, when approaching thoracic injuries, special attention should be given to the neck veins, the appearance/motion of the chest wall, palpation, chest percussion, and breath sounds. Due to the critical nature of trauma patients, success in the management of thoracic injuries rests upon a high index of suspicion, prompt recognition, and aggressive management by the treating physician.

Only a small percentage of trauma patients require an emergency department thoracotomy (EDT) which is defined as a thoracotomy

TABLE 110.1 Indications for Emergency Department Thoracotomy
1. Acute pericardial tamponade with impending loss of vital signs
2. Exsanguinating intrathoracic hemorrhage
3. Witnessed arrest unresponsive to resuscitation

TABLE 110.2 Indications for Urgent Thoracotomy
1. Chest drainage >1,500 mL initial or >250 mL/hr for 4+ hrs
2. Large unevacuated hemothorax
3. Cardiac tamponade
4. Chest wall defect with ventilatory compromise
5. Massive air leak with incomplete lung expansion
6. Great vessel injury with hemodynamic instability

performed in the ED for patients arriving in extremis or an attempt to temporize exsanguinating injuries until they can be dealt with in the operating room. Current indications to perform EDT include severe penetrating or blunt injury with recent witnessed loss of signs of life (SOL) and persistent and/or severe hemorrhagic shock.[5] In many instances the cause of hemodynamic instability is not known. Therefore a high level of suspicion, guided by chest tube drainage, and ultrasound findings in the ED might be the only premise for a bedside thoracotomy.[6]

When EDT is required, the surgeon should keep in mind the indications (Tables 110.1 and 110.2), mechanism of injury (MOI), and the radiographic findings to guide the incision and exploration. Rhee and colleagues reported on 25 years of published data on the mortality after EDT for both blunt and penetrating injury.[7] They examined 4,620 patients from 24 studies who underwent EDT with an associated overall survival rate of 7.4%. The investigators found that the major factors influencing outcomes were the MOI, location of major injury (LOMI), and whether there were SOL. Survival was 8.8% for penetrating injuries and only 1.4% for blunt injuries. The survival rate for isolated thoracic injuries was 10.7%, whereas it was only 0.7% in patients with multiple injuries. The survival rate was the highest at 19.4% for those with isolated penetrating cardiac injuries. Whether or not SOL were present was important: survival rate was 11.5% when present and only 2.6% when not present. The absence of SOL in the field yielded a survival rate of only 1.2%. In summary, despite a relatively low survival rate, EDT should still be done in appropriately selected patients, especially those with witnessed loss of SOL, particularly those with isolated, penetrating wounds to the chest.

BLEEDING

Hemothorax is second only to rib fractures as the most common finding in patients presenting with thoracic trauma and is present in approximately 25% of these patients. In life-threatening situations with hemodynamic instability chest tube placement can be a rapid, therapeutic, and often diagnostic procedure. Not only can chest tube placement diagnose bleeding, but it can also be helpful in diagnosing and treating air leaks. Bleeding can arise from the chest wall, lung parenchyma, major thoracic vessels, heart, and/or diaphragm. Frequently chest tube insertion is done without any imaging if clinical signs or instability are present. Most commonly, a 24- or 28-Fr thoracostomy tube is used. The generally accepted criteria for thoracic exploration are initial drainage of 1,500 mL at the time of chest tube placement, which is considered a massive hemothorax, or continued drainage of 250 mL/hr over the next 4 hours.[4] A small or moderate-size hemothorax that stops bleeding immediately after placement of a tube thoracostomy can usually be managed conservatively. If the patient becomes hemodynamically unstable at any time and an intrathoracic source is suspected, emergent thoracotomy should be considered, regardless of chest tube drainage. A chest radiograph (CXR) should be obtained after tube thoracostomy to ensure proper position and evacuation of the pleural space.

CARDIOVASCULAR COLLAPSE

Indications for the use of EDT that appear in the literature range from vague to quite specific. This has led to a joint position statement from the national association of EMS physicians and the ACS committee on trauma regarding the guidelines for withholding or termination of resuscitation in prehospital traumatic cardiopulmonary arrest.[8] Adherence to these algorithms (Fig. 110.1) has been well proven as they reliably predict mortality and patients who are potentially salvageable based on prehospital physiologic status.[9,10] When EDT is employed however, the purpose is to evacuate any pericardial tamponade, control hemorrhage, allow for open cardiac massage, cross-clamp the descending thoracic aorta to redistribute blood flow, and limit sub-diaphragmatic hemorrhage.[11] Cross-clamping the descending aorta however can be difficult and cause more harm if not done properly. Although helpful in redirecting needed blood flow to more critical areas of the body, it is not absolutely necessary to perform and should be abandoned if it becomes too difficult or time-consuming. Tamponade should be released, massive pulmonary bleeding controlled with staplers, clamps, or manual compression, and cardiac injuries treated. If under pressure, air in the mediastinum can also cause tamponade which may be fatal if not addressed appropriately.[12]

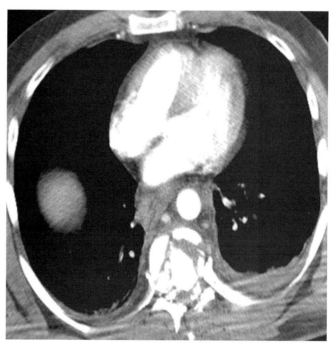

FIGURE 110.1 Axial CT chest of patient in MVC with a shattered thoracic spine vertebral body.

MASSIVE AIR LEAK

This potentially lethal injury is relatively rare, found in 2.5% to 8% of blunt thoracic trauma patients.[13–15] However, subcutaneous emphysema, large persistent air leak after tube thoracostomy, and continued pneumothorax should alert the clinician to the presence of major tracheobronchial injury (TBI). TBI has become more easily diagnosed with the advent of multidetector computed tomography (MDCT). However, failure to diagnose it expeditiously may lead to death or long-term disability.[13] A massive air leak through a lacerated lung can result in inadequate ventilation and hypoxemia. Typically, the more proximal the injury, the more severe the decompensation becomes. Subcutaneous emphysema results when air dissects along the bronchi and pulmonary vessels into the mediastinum and into the subcutaneous space of the neck and face. Usually the severity of the emphysema parallels the severity of the injury.

A high level of suspicion and urgent thoracotomy should be considered when facing rapid progression of subcutaneous air or mediastinal emphysema, signs of mediastinitis, or there is difficulty with mechanical ventilation due to the injury itself.[16] When facing a decompensating patient in the ED, a classic left-sided EDT may be suboptimal for a suspected right TBI. Therefore, it is important to remember to direct any early surgical intervention toward the suspected site of injury. Airway management may require selectively bypassing the injury by means of endobronchial intubation into the distal uninjured bronchus with a single-lumen or double-lumen endotracheal tube. Tube exchange and lung separation to maintain oxygenation can be challenging for seriously injured patients. Lee and colleagues described using a bronchial blocker to stabilize respiratory dynamics in the setting of massive air leak before induction and tube exchange.[17] Such isolation maneuvers can also facilitate single-lung ventilation if thoracotomy and surgical repair are undertaken.[6,18] Hypoventilation in patients with massive air leaks can significantly complicate ventilator management. In patients who fail standard mechanical ventilation, continuous oscillation therapy and airway pressure release ventilation (APRV) may be effective in reducing barotrauma and improving both oxygenation and ventilation.[19] APRV allows the patient to "overbreathe" throughout the respiratory cycle and thus reduces the likelihood of barotrauma from the patient "fighting the ventilator." In addition, consistent high airway pressures increase alveolar recruitment, consequently preventing shunt in patients with severe hypoxia due to parenchymal injury. Major TBI should be repaired once the basic trauma surveys have been completed and the patient has been stabilized.

DIAGNOSTIC STUDIES

Imaging modalities have become an integral part of the trauma evaluation. Chest radiography is the most common initial study, usually obtained while the trauma team completes the physical evaluation. Bedside ultrasonography (US) is now routinely used in emergent settings in the ED.[20] It aids in the diagnosis of pericardial effusion, pneumothorax, and intra-abdominal fluid. In most instances it replaces the diagnostic peritoneal lavage (DPL). However, computed tomography (CT) allows more detailed assessment of injuries so long as the patient remains hemodynamically stable.

Diagnostic imaging plays a key role in the identification of injuries and their management in patients who have sustained chest trauma. The modern era of radiologic imaging has drastically changed the approach and clinical endpoints during the work-up in previously vague scenarios. The information gleaned from these studies not only serves to tailor individual therapy, but also can frequently determine overall prognosis and outcome. A CXR is generally the initial study of choice as it is an easily accessible and quick modality. It can provide basic data to help identify major intrathoracic abnormalities that can lead to instability as further studies are pursued. MDCT is now being used with increasing frequency in major trauma centers and becoming part of the diagnostic trauma algorithm.[21–23] CT can be an extraordinarily valuable resource as it can be completed quickly and provide valuable data in the assessment of aortic, pulmonary, airway, skeletal, and diaphragmatic injuries. Magnetic resonance imaging (MRI) has a limited role in the initial evaluation of patients with suspected chest trauma. Similar to CT, patients undergoing MRI must be stable, but it requires significantly more time to complete and the emergent nature of trauma patients and contraindication of certain metal implants often preclude this population. However, in selected patients who are hemodynamically stable, MRI may be particularly useful for the evaluation of both spinal and diaphragmatic injuries.[24,25] Other imaging modalities employed to provide additional data in the setting of thoracic trauma include echocardiography, angiography, bronchoscopy, and video-assisted thoracoscopic surgery (VATS), which can be both diagnostic and therapeutic.

PLAIN CHEST RADIOGRAPH

The portable CXR is the most appropriate initial radiographic study as it is an easily accessible and quick modality to obtain while the trauma team completes the physical evaluation. The ATLS guidelines of the ACS also include CXRs as a routine adjunct to the primary trauma survey. Most life-threatening or major injuries can be detected and treated based on the clinical exam and CXR alone. Ideally, CXR should be obtained upright if possible as the supine position combined with expiratory artifacts and the magnification effect of a short beam distance may make the mediastinum appear more widened than it actually is. CXR has a 98% negative predictive value and is therefore quite useful when normal. It is important to consider the CXR as a screening exam since it is rarely diagnostic of any one specific injury. Although plain upright CXR remains one of the basic imaging studies routinely performed, it has several limitations (such as diagnosis of diaphragmatic injury, which is often missed). In addition, preexisting diaphragmatic eventration or an elevated, paralyzed hemidiaphragm may erroneously suggest acute diaphragmatic injury when there is none present. Although a CXR can be a very useful screen imaging test to obtain, there is a growing body of literature which suggests that in the presence of a completely normal physical exam a CXR may be unnecessary.[26,27]

CHEST COMPUTED TOMOGRAPHY

CT is a highly sensitive imaging modality to detect thoracic injuries after blunt chest trauma and is clearly superior to CXR in visualizing lung contusions, pneumothorax, and hemothorax. Modern MDCT can yield well-defined detail of the chest wall and the major intrathoracic organs using both sagittal and coronal reconstructions and can be helpful in planning surgical strategy. CT imaging can alter the initial management in a significant number of patients with suspected chest trauma. It has also been shown to detect unexpected injuries and abnormalities leading to altered management and improved survival in trauma patients.[28–30] Historically, CT has been very useful in screening for major intrathoracic aortic injury. Studies have demonstrated that, in cases where there is a normal mediastinum with no hematoma showing an intact aorta surrounded by a normal fat pad, CT has essentially a 100% negative predictive value for aortic injury.[31–33]

CT can be extraordinarily useful for detecting hemopericardium, hemothorax from any cause, injury to the brachiocephalic vessels, pneumothorax, rib fractures, pulmonary contusion, as well as, sternal fractures.[34] It can also be useful in detecting pneumomediastinum caused by pulmonary injury, TBI, esophageal rupture, or iatrogenic injury from barotrauma or traumatic intubation. In studies comparing CT with CXR, CT demonstrated serious injuries in 65% of patients with no injury seen on CXR. These injuries included pulmonary contusion, pneumothorax, hemothorax, diaphragmatic rupture, foreign body, and sternal fracture.[23,35] Even in patients without suspected chest trauma, CT of the abdomen, which commonly includes the lower portion of the thorax, can often demonstrate an intrathoracic injury, that when seen should spur further investigation of the chest.[36] It is also important to systematically examine entire image series so that unsuspecting injuries are not missed. This can help identify other injuries that should be prioritized and addressed (Figs. 110.1 and 110.2).

With the advent of high-resolution CT, diagnosis of injuries has drastically improved. CT has been shown to be useful in delineating the extent of pulmonary contusions and identifying those at high risk for acute pulmonary failure.[37–40] Several scoring systems based upon the combination of the area involved by CT imaging and Glasgow Coma Scale (GCS) have been developed to determine the probability for the need for mechanical ventilation and for the development of acute respiratory distress syndrome (ARDS), pneumonia, prolonged intensive care unit length of stay (LOS), and/or death.[39,40]

Three-dimensional CT has also been shown to be useful in diagnosing and determining the severity of sternal fractures.[41] Axial, coronal, and sagittal CT reconstructions can now reliably image traditionally difficult-to-image diagnoses, such as penetrating diaphragmatic injuries, with sensitivity and specificity of 82% to 87% and 72% to 99%, respectively.[42,43] Advancement of technology has now spawned new investigational algorithms that include fast, multi-slice CT scanners that could potentially incorporate bedside tomography

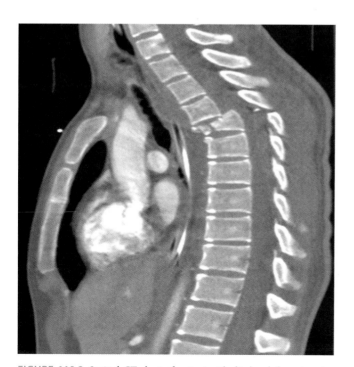

FIGURE 110.2 Sagittal CT chest of patient with displaced thoracic spine vertebral body fracture.

into the secondary survey.[44] In the setting of thoracic trauma, CT was found to change the treatment modality in 83% of patients.[45]

ULTRASOUND

Bedside US is now routine. It aids in the diagnosis of pericardial effusion, pneumothorax, and intra-abdominal fluid. In most instances it replaces the DPL. As its resolution has improved with time, bedside thoracic US is now a more sensitive screening test than CXR for the detection of pneumothorax in adult patients with blunt chest trauma.[46] Specifically, the "stratosphere sign" is seen when air separates the visceral and parietal pleura and lung sliding is absent, indicating pneumothorax.[47,48] In addition to aiding diagnoses, US can provide confirmation of line and tube placement.

Transthoracic echocardiogram (TTE) has become an effective noninvasive screening modality for diagnosing pericardial effusion in the trauma setting. The potential for a relative novice to produce adequate quality images and quantify ejection fraction has been proven and may allow for consistent urgent cardiothoracic assessment.[49] Although subxiphoid pericardial window is considered the gold standard for confirmation of the diagnosis of pericardial tamponade, conventional two-dimensional TTE has been shown to reveal as little as 50 mL of blood within the pericardium and simultaneously provide hemodynamic and structural details.[50,51] Lopez et al. showed that TTE can detect and distinguish hemopericardium from other effusions of lower echogenicity.[52] Because TTE is a rapid examination that can be performed in the ED, it can reduce the time to diagnosis and therefore facilitate earlier therapeutic intervention resulting in improved survival.[53,54] Used appropriately, US can reduce unnecessary diagnostic and therapeutic interventions.[55] Additionally, TTE has been shown to identify cardiac sources of hemodynamic instability unrelated to tamponade.[56] TTE also provides rapid, repeatable, and multisystem assessment to guide diagnosis and management of thoracic injuries. The anatomic and hemodynamic information it yields can match or exceed the speed and utility of existing tests such as CXR or central venous pressure determination.[57] Thus TTE is a very useful adjunctive screening mechanism and ongoing assessment tool that can be used to evaluate both penetrating and blunt thoracic injuries.

BRONCHOSCOPY

Flexible bronchoscopy is a highly effective diagnostic and therapeutic tool. It can be performed quickly with minimal sedation. Indications to perform bronchoscopy include suspected bronchial obstruction, foreign body, TBI, massive hemoptysis, continuous air leak/subcutaneous emphysema, toxic inhalation/burn injury, and iatrogenic injuries to the membranous trachea. The procedure can be done using either the standard hollow metal (rigid) or the flexible fiberoptic bronchoscope. Rigid bronchoscopy is usually performed under general anesthesia and is often used for clearing major airways of bulky obstructing lesions such as tumors, foreign bodies, or blood clots. Flexible bronchoscopy, on the other hand, can be done readily at the bedside, even in non-intubated patients. Bronchoscopy can help secure airways and guide placement of endotracheal tubes. When examining for suspected injuries and one is found, the entire tracheobronchial tree should still be examined so that additional injuries are not missed.

Bronchoscopy remains the gold standard in diagnosing a multitude of thoracic trauma injuries including TBI. It can also provide valuable information with regard to surgical planning, although findings may be subtle or nonspecific.[58] Bronchoscopy for massive hemoptysis may reveal hemorrhage associated with pulmonary contusion and prompt the placement of a double-lumen endotracheal tube or balloon catheter for tamponade. Hemorrhage isolated to one lobe or segment may also be contained with a bronchial blocker.[59] Bronchoscopy for lung, lobar, or segmental collapse may also reveal aspirated material, thick secretions, or mucous plugging.[60]

When there is clinical suspicion for TBI or upper airway injury it is also useful to pull back the endotracheal tube over the bronchoscope to visualize the upper trachea and subglottic apparatus. It is critical while doing this to safely maintain an airway and have all personnel and instruments readily available if reintubation is required. Serial bronchoscopies in the setting of acute trauma to the thorax, specifically blunt trauma, have also been well described. The decision to perform bronchoscopy should rely on clinical judgment but be readily considered in the trauma setting when an indication exists. Since it can be done with little risk, the clinician should have a low threshold to perform it: generally speaking, if one thinks of doing it, it probably should be done.

VIDEO-ASSISTED THORACOSCOPIC SURGERY

Since the advent of sophisticated video technology and optics, VATS has evolved as an important tool in thoracic surgery. While thoracoscopic procedures have been used for many years, newer technical advances as well as increasing surgeon familiarity with minimally invasive surgery have made VATS increasingly popular and useful. Thoracic surgeons have attempted to minimize the extent of thoracic exploration for chest injuries since 1946.[61–63] However, it was not until 1993 that the use of modern VATS was reported by Ochsner and his group.[64] A recent meta-analysis found that when compared to open thoracotomy, VATS is a better treatment for hemodynamically stable patients with chest trauma with improved perioperative outcomes and less complications.[65] VATS has been recommended for a variety of therapeutic purposes following chest trauma, such as hemostasis of bleeders, evacuation of clotted hemothorax, repair of lung laceration, wedge lung resection, repair of diaphragmatic laceration, control of air leak, removal of foreign body, and decortication of empyema. Contraindications to VATS include obliterated pleural spaces, inability to tolerate single-lung ventilation, hemodynamic instability, circulatory shock, and life-threatening thoracic injury. The majority of reports advocate the early use of VATS (within 5 days) after trauma since there may be more operative difficulties if VATS is delayed.[66]

Similar to the randomized studies comparing VATS to open thoracotomy for elective thoracic surgery, some of its advantages include faster patient recovery, shorter LOS, and decreased pain. Infection, atelectasis, and pneumonia are reported complications of both VATS and open thoracotomy, and perioperative mortality rate has not been found to be significantly different between the two. Early VATS may decrease LOS and cost when compared with tube thoracostomy in patients with blunt chest trauma and retained hemothorax.[67]

SPECIFIC INJURIES

TRAUMATIC ASPHYXIA

Traumatic asphyxia or "Perthes syndrome" occurs as a result of sudden or severe compression injury of the thorax or upper abdomen, most often associated with severe blunt trauma secondary to crush injury. Entrapment of children under automatic garage doors is a prime example.[68] The true incidence of traumatic asphyxia is unknown; however, there are scattered case reports involving either the elderly or the very young.[69,70] The diagnosis is usually made by MOI and physical examination. Generally, the clinical manifestations are a by-product of excessive venous pressures. Characteristic signs include bulbar conjunctival hemorrhage, facial/cervical cyanosis, and temporary loss of vision due to retinal edema.[71,72] The facial and upper chest petechiae become most prominent a few hours after the initial injury. Neurologic sequelae are common and are thought to be secondary to anoxic injury, as well as possible cerebral edema and hemorrhage. The exact pathophysiology is thought to be due to a crushing injury applied to the mediastinum, which causes a high-pressure retrograde flow of blood from the right atrium into the valveless innominate and jugular venous system. In addition, a sudden reflexive inspiration is thought to occur against a closed glottis, which may transiently elevate intrathoracic pressures. This results in sudden and rapid venous hypertension of the valveless cervicofacial system.

Among survivors, traumatic asphyxia is generally self-limited and supportive treatment is recommended. Specific therapy for traumatic asphyxia is based on physiologic techniques to decrease intracranial pressure, including elevation of the head of the bed and oxygen therapy. The need to treat other critical associated injuries may take priority. Commonly these can include head injuries, pulmonary contusions, blunt abdominal trauma, rib fractures, brachial and radial nerve injuries, hemothorax, and pneumothorax.[73] The majority of fatalities are usually from associated injuries and their complications, but can also be directly related to prolonged compression causing massive, irreversible neurologic insult from the resultant apnea and hypoxia. The long-term prognosis of patients with traumatic asphyxia is generally good after discharge if able to survive the initial insult. Lee et al. demonstrated that despite severity of injury, no long-term disability was detected at an average follow-up of 4.4 years and all had returned to work or school.[74] No long-term survivors demonstrated residual cyanosis, petechiae, swelling, or neurologic sequelae.

MEDIASTINAL AND SUBCUTANEOUS EMPHYSEMA

Traumatic injuries to the upper airway, tracheobronchial tree, esophagus, or lung parenchyma can all lead to mediastinal and subcutaneous emphysema. Physical exam, CXR, or CT commonly demonstrates these injuries. Typically, the severity of the emphysema is directly related to the severity of the trauma. Air dissects along the bronchi and pulmonary vessels into the mediastinum and may migrate into the subcutaneous space of the neck and face, sometimes reaching from the torso down to the inguinal ligament and external genitalia. Judicious use of bronchoscopy and esophagoscopy is recommended should there be any sign of worsening by clinical or radiographic criteria. Decompression incisions in the skin are rarely if ever indicated.

PNEUMOTHORAX

Pneumothorax is generally the result of either a blunt or penetrating injury to the pleura. A pneumothorax develops when a defect forms within either the visceral or the mediastinal pleura, allowing air to enter the pleural space. Traumatic causes are often secondary to stab wounds, projectile injuries, or rib fractures. With penetrating chest trauma, air can enter the pleural space either through the chest wall externally or through the visceral pleura from the tracheobronchial tree internally. In blunt trauma, a pneumothorax may develop if the visceral pleura is lacerated by a rib fracture or alveolar rupture. Once the alveolus is ruptured, air enters the interstitial space and/or dissects the visceral pleura toward the mediastinum. Iatrogenic procedures account for a significant proportion of pneumothoraces. The most common causes in descending order are thoracentesis, followed by subclavian venipuncture and positive pressure ventilation.[75] In addition, iatrogenic pneumothorax can cause substantial morbidity and even result in mortality.[76] Posttraumatic pneumothorax may be missed during initial assessment of critically injured patients. Consequently, a CXR should always be obtained as early as possible during the secondary survey. In traumatic pneumothorax, chest tube drainage is recommended, even for small collections of air, particularly with the change in respiratory physiology caused by positive pressure ventilation.[77]

All types of pneumothorax may progress to tension physiology; the incidence is approximately 1% to 3% of spontaneous pneumothoraces. Tension pneumothorax can be a rapidly progressive condition; therefore, early identification is essential and immediate decompression should be performed when suspected on clinical grounds. Tension pneumothorax is a clinical diagnosis, which may appear as severe respiratory distress, distended neck veins, deviated trachea away from the side of tension, absent breath sounds, or tympany to percussion on the affected side (Fig. 110.3). As the ipsilateral lung collapses, the increased pressure causes the mediastinum to shift toward the contralateral side, compresses the contralateral lung, and impairs the venous return to the right atrium. Once the diagnosis is made, treatment should not be delayed for confirmatory radiograph. Immediate relief of a tension pneumothorax is of the essence to avoid cardiovascular collapse and possible death.

Immediate release of a tension pneumothorax can be accomplished by placing a needle into the pleural space to allow pressure in the pleura to equilibrate with the atmosphere. A 14- or 16-gauge long needle is introduced in the midclavicular line at the second intercostal space (ICS) (identified by palpating the angle of Louis). This temporizing

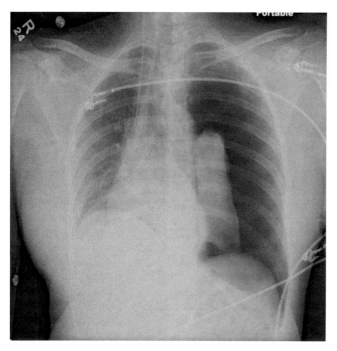

FIGURE 110.3 Tension pneumothorax. Note a completely collapsed left lung and rightward mediastinal shift away from side of the pneumothorax.

measure relieves the compression of the underlying lung as well as the distortion of vital mediastinal structures, such as the superior and inferior vena cavae, allowing better venous blood return to the heart. While this measure simply turns a tension pneumothorax into an open, non-tension pneumothorax, it allows for immediate blood return to the heart, ultimately preventing cardiovascular collapse.

Open pneumothorax caused by traumatic communication between the pleural space and the atmosphere may cause "sucking chest wounds," if the wound diameter approaches two-thirds of that of the trachea. This is most often found in patients either impaled by an object or injured by gunshot wound. This is a life-threatening emergency, as air will preferentially enter the pleural space during respiration, resulting in loss of negative intrathoracic pressure. The resultant open pneumothorax leads to collapse of the ipsilateral lung as well as ineffective ventilation of the contralateral lung due to mediastinal shifting, resulting in profound hypoventilation. Such wounds are often associated with other devastating intrathoracic injuries. A temporary "three-way dressing" should be applied to the wound at the scene of the injury in an attempt to improve ventilation. This involves placing a plastic sheet taped shut on three sides, leaving the fourth side unsealed in hopes of creating a one-way valve dressing. This will theoretically allow air to egress, potentially reinflating the lung while keeping air from entering the pleural cavity. Upon arrival to the trauma bay, a chest tube is placed away from the site of injury to re-expand the lung and the wound is covered with an impermeable dressing. Most wounds will require operative debridement and removal of foreign bodies (if present). Closure of the wounds may be accomplished by mobilizing surrounding tissues. However, large defects may require rotational or free musculocutaneous flaps with pectoralis, latissimus dorsi, or rectus abdominis muscle flaps used. The use of synthetic materials such as Marlex, Gore-Tex, or methylmethacrylate may be necessary but runs the risk for infection secondary to the inevitable contamination associated with the injury when used in traumatic situations.

A high index of suspicion for a tension pneumothorax should be maintained in ventilated patients with chest wall trauma receiving general anesthesia with sudden deterioration, particularly if they require increasing peak inspiratory pressures.[77,78] Some surgeons routinely insert thoracostomy tubes in multiply injured patients with rib fractures, even without clear evidence of a pneumothorax to prevent development of a tension pneumothorax. While this type of aggressive strategy is not necessary, careful monitoring and aggressive management is essential in case the patient's cardiopulmonary status deteriorates.

HEMOTHORAX

Hemothorax is second only to rib fractures as the second most common complication seen in patients with chest trauma with an incidence of approximately 25%. Hemothorax is often associated with penetrating chest injury or chest wall blunt trauma with bony injury. On examination, patients generally have decreased breath sounds and dullness to percussion over the affected side with associated dyspnea and tachypnea. Depending on the amount of blood loss, there may also be concomitant hemodynamic shock. The major cause of significant hemothorax is lung laceration or bleeding from an injured intercostal vessel or internal thoracic artery. CXR may not reveal a fluid collection of less than 300 mL. US can be rapidly performed by the surgeon carrying out the initial evaluation of the injured patient and has been found to be comparable to CXR for accuracy in the detection of hemothorax which may expedite diagnosis and treatment.[79–81] A slight reverse Trendelenburg position of the patient is helpful in identifying smaller hemothoraces that otherwise are easily missed. More commonly, a hemothorax is confirmed and quantified on CT when CXR or US is abnormal or nonspecific.[82] Small hemothoraces generally seal themselves within a few days. Accumulation of more than 1,500 mL of blood within a pleural space is considered massive and more commonly seen on the left side, secondary to aortic rupture (blunt trauma) or pulmonary hilar or major vessel injury (penetrating trauma). Massive hemothorax can lead to hemodynamic instability including hypotension and circulatory collapse. Neck veins may be flat or distended depending upon the balance between blood loss and intrathoracic pressure. A mediastinal shift with tracheal deviation is typically away from the side of blood accumulation.

Adequate management mandates complete evacuation of the blood collection. Intrathoracic bleeding recognized in the ED should be treated with a closed-tube thoracostomy. Most commonly, a 24- or 28-Fr thoracostomy tube is placed anterior to the mid-axillary line at the fifth or sixth ICS. There is no clear evidence that chest tube size impacts efficacy of drainage, rate of complications including retained hemothorax, need for additional tube drainage, or invasive procedures.[83] Furthermore, tube size does not appear to affect the discomfort perceived by patients at the site of insertion. A CXR should routinely be obtained after placing a tube thoracostomy to check the position of the tube and ensure that the pleural space has been adequately drained.

When to perform a thoracic exploration based on amounts of chest tube drainage is a matter of debate. However, the generally accepted criteria by ATLS are initial drainage of 1,500 mL at the time of chest tube placement or continued drainage of 250 mL/hr for the next 4 hours. If the patient is hemodynamically unstable at any time, and intrathoracic bleeding is suspected as the cause, emergent thoracotomy should be done regardless of chest tube output. A moderate-size hemothorax (500 to 1,500 mL) that stops bleeding immediately after a tube thoracostomy can often be managed conservatively with a closed drainage system. Parenchymal injuries generally abate on their own because of low pulmonary vasculature pressures and high concentrations of tissue thromboplastin within the lung.[84] If emergent thoracotomy is indicated, adequate exposure of the entire hemithorax is required.

Retained hemothorax is associated with high rates of empyema and pneumonia. Therefore, open evacuation should be considered to reduce the risk of empyema and prevent the formation of a fibrous peel (resulting in lung entrapment). In most cases this can be done electively if the bleeding has stopped. VATS should only be considered in the stable patient and can be useful in evacuating retained hemothorax and exploring for ongoing bleeding when other measures fail. However, the surgeon should not hesitate to convert to open thoracotomy for exposure or drainage if VATS is suboptimal. Coselli and colleagues presented their experience with hemothoraces in 14,300 patients with blunt or penetrating thoracic trauma, in which 1.1% developed residual organized hemothorax or empyema: 25.2% of this group underwent early evacuation with no mortality and an average LOS of only 10 days.[85] However, when progression to empyema occurred, the mortality rate increased to 9.5% with an average LOS of 37.9 days.

VATS should be considered as primary treatment in stable patients with retained hemothorax since it can be performed with relatively high success rates, and a conversion to open thoracotomy can always be done if needed. More than one procedure may be necessary. A large prospective, multicenter AAST study found that 26.5% of patients undergoing VATS for retained hemothoraces required two procedures, 5.4% required three procedures, and thoracotomy was ultimately required in 20.4% of the patients.[86] Possible sources of intrathoracic bleeding include intercostal vessels, internal

thoracic arteries, pulmonary parenchyma, major pulmonary vessels, the heart, and/or the great vessels. Among patients with posttraumatic retained hemothorax, the incidence of developing an empyema was 26.8%. Independent predictors of empyema development include rib fractures, Injury Severity Score (ISS) of 25 or higher, and the need for additional interventions for evacuation.[87,88]

RIB FRACTURES

Rib fractures are common and are often associated with other injuries. Rib fractures themselves usually cause minor problems; however, they often are a marker of more serious injury. Pulmonary contusion often accompanies the rib fractures and may be more clinically relevant. A study by Flagel et al. reviewing the NTDB showed that 13% of those patients with a diagnosis of one or more fractured ribs developed significant chest wall related complications and the need for mechanical ventilation. The overall mortality rate for patients with rib fractures was 10% and the mortality rate increased significantly (P <0.02) for each additional rib fracture independent of patient age. The mortality rate increased from 5.8% for a single rib fracture to 10% for five fractured ribs. In addition, the mortality rate increased dramatically for six, seven, and eight or more fractured ribs to 11.4%, 15%, and 34.4%, respectively. The same pattern was seen for developing pneumonia, ARDS, pneumothorax, aspiration pneumonia, and empyema.[89]

The utility of epidural analgesic catheters in patients who have sustained rib fractures remains controversial. In a prospective, randomized controlled trial, Bulger and colleagues randomized patients with three or more rib fractures to either receive epidural anesthesia or intravenous opioids for pain control. They found that the groups were comparable in mean age, ISS, Chest Abbreviated Injury Scale, and mean number of rib fractures. The epidural group had a greatly reduced rate of pneumonia and duration of mechanical ventilation.[90] However, Carrier et al. performed a systematic review and a meta-analysis of randomized controlled trials of epidural analgesia in adult patients with traumatic rib fractures and found no significant benefit of epidural analgesia on mortality, intensive care unit (ICU) stay, or overall LOS when compared to other analgesic modalities. They did notice a trend in decreased duration of mechanical ventilation with the use of thoracic epidural analgesia and local anesthetics, however.[91] A recent multi-site prospective study containing 5,043 patients found that trauma centers are more likely to place epidural catheters in patients with rib fractures and that epidural catheter placement was associated with a significantly decreased mortality in patients with blunt thoracic injury with three or more rib fractures.[92] Several studies support the more liberal use of continuous epidural analgesia in severe chest wall injuries to improve outcomes.[93–95]

Treatment of rib fractures is largely supportive care, based on the tenets of judicious fluid use, pulmonary toilet, and aggressive pain control. Uncontrolled pain may result in chest wall splinting and chronic hypoventilation. Adequate pain control is mandatory to allow early mobilization, deep inspiratory efforts, and coughing in order to avoid secondary complications. Pulmonary physiotherapy, nasotracheal suctioning, and prompt bronchoscopy should be instituted in patients unable to clear secretions. Management of pain due to rib fractures can be difficult since there is a delicate balance between adequate pain control and oversedation, particularly when using oral or intravenous narcotics. When this poses a problem the clinician can employ several other modalities including epidural analgesia, intercostal nerve blocks, intrapleural catheter analgesia, and even transcutaneous electrical nerve stimulation. Intercostal nerve blocks require repeated administration with the risk for pneumothorax on each injection; however, this may be obviated with the placement of indwelling pain catheters with slow release reservoirs. Truitt et al. found that continuous intercostal nerve block placed in the extrathoracic paraspinous space significantly improved pulmonary function, pain control, and shortened LOS in patients with rib fractures.[96] After acute pain is managed, pain control can be transitioned to transdermal analgesia supplemented by oral analgesics and anti-inflammatory agents.

The age of the patient should be taken into particular account in the setting of rib fractures, as well as their location. It has been shown that rib fractures occurring in the very young should alert the clinician to possible non-accidental trauma (NAT). Barsness et al. found that in children younger than 3 years of age, the positive predictive value of a rib fracture as an indicator of NAT was 95%.[97] It is also important to note that rib fractures in children are relatively rare following cardiopulmonary resuscitation (CPR). In a study by Maguire et al., out of 923 children who underwent CPR, only 3 children sustained rib fractures, all of which had anterior fractures (two midclavicular and one costochondral).[98] In their systematic review of the literature, CPR performed by both medical and nonmedical personnel was never the cause of a posterior rib fracture in a child.

With regard to the elderly, there is a consensus that rib fractures are associated with an increased mortality and that a higher number of rib fractures correlate with worse outcome. One study further classified that the term "elderly" should be used liberally since patients over the age of 45 with more than four rib fractures were more severely injured and at significantly increased risk of adverse outcomes as compared to a younger cohort.[99] A near linear relationship between age and complications has been shown with elderly patients who sustain approximately twice the morbidity and mortality after blunt chest trauma with rib fractures compared to younger patients with similar injuries.[100] Battle et al. systematically reviewed 29 articles up to 2010 and found that the risk factors for mortality in patients sustaining blunt chest wall trauma were patient age of 65 years or older, three or more rib fractures, and the presence of preexisting disease, especially cardiopulmonary disease.[101] The development of pneumonia postinjury was also a significant risk factor for mortality. Consequently, it is well accepted that older patients have worse outcomes following blunt chest trauma with rib fractures than younger ones.[102]

The location and morphology of the rib fracture is also important. It has been shown that left-sided rib fractures are associated with splenic injuries and right-sided fractures are associated with liver injuries. Although isolated rib fractures have an associated incidence of vascular injury of only 3%, historical data identified that first rib fractures in association with multiple rib fractures have a 24% incidence of associated vascular injury.[103] More recent data from the Mayo Clinic randomly selected 185 out of 1,894 patients who had undergone a chest CT angiogram with first and/or second rib fractures and compared them to those without.[104] Although this was a purely retrospective, randomly selected cohort study with different levels of injury they determined that no subset of rib fracture seen on spine CT was associated with an elevated risk of major vessel injury. Therefore, the previous axiom that first and second rib fractures should prompt further evaluation to rule out aortic injury may not hold true. Nevertheless, the constellation of rib fractures and widened mediastinum, upper-extremity pulse deficit, subclavian groove fracture, brachial plexus injury, and expanding hematoma may be best studied with a contrasted CT instead of the classic subclavian artery and aortic arch arteriography. Morphology of rib fractures, specifically sharp, jagged cortices, has been associated with penetration of the underlying thoracic organs due to the transient phenomenon

of severe deformation of the chest cavity. Clinical suspicion for secondary penetrating cardiac and thoracic aortic injury should be high in traumas involving high-energy injuries such as pedestrian versus motor vehicle causing deformity of the chest cavity.[105–107] There have been documented cases of sudden death associated with rib fragments lacerating the aorta, and, consequently, some propose an early operation for patients who have multiple, jagged rib fractures in the left chest.[108,109]

FLAIL CHEST

Instability of the chest wall results from multiple adjacent rib fractures and/or disruption of costochondral junctions, thereby allowing that portion of the chest wall to move independently during respiration. The strict definition of flail chest is the fracture of at least four consecutive ribs in two or more places; however, the functional definition is an incompetent segment of chest wall large enough to impair respiratory dynamics. The chest wall segment floats unattached to any bony structure resulting in paradoxical chest wall motion. Consequently, the negative pressure generated by inspiration within the thorax is dissipated by movement of the flail segment inward. This causes simultaneous equilibration of the intrathoracic pressure which leads to a reduction in vital capacity (VC) and ineffective ventilation. This, along with the any associated pulmonary contusion, may lead to the development of ARDS. Major mortality and morbidity of flail chest can be attributed to the resultant hypoventilation/hypoxia that occurs.

The force needed to create a flail segment depends on the compliance of the ribs. Subsequently, elderly patients may sustain significant chest injuries from low-energy impact, whereas in one study only 0.95% of children developed flail chest even after severe thoracic trauma.[110] The literature has reported an incidence as high as 9.3% of all rib fractures and 6% of all blunt traumas presenting as flail injuries.[111] Pulmonary contusion, which is common in the setting of flail chest, can cause a significant decrease in oxygen diffusion to a variable portion of the ipsilateral lung.

Basic tenets for the management of flail chest center around early and aggressive intervention. Adequate analgesia is of paramount importance in patient recovery and may contribute to the return of normal respiratory mechanics. Early mechanical ventilatory support providing positive pressure remains the gold standard against which all other forms of treatment are measured. In 1956, Avery et al. coined this type of treatment as "internal pneumatic stabilization."[112] Positive pressure ventilation forces the flail segment to rise and fall synchronously with the remainder of the chest wall. However, prolonged mechanical ventilation is associated with the development of pneumonia and poorer outcomes. Patients not mechanically ventilated may greatly benefit from humidified air, aggressive pulmonary physiotherapy with incentive spirometry, deep breathing and coughing several times each hour, deep suctioning in patients unable to clear secretions, and judicious use of bronchoscopy to remove any retained secretions promptly. This cohort of unintubated patients should be closely observed, while they undergo constant pain management and aggressive pulmonary therapy. A recent review of 3,467 patients with flail chest from the NTDB demonstrated more than 99% of patients were treated nonoperatively and only 8% received epidural catheters.[113] Given the high rates of morbidity and mortality in patients with a flail chest, the authors recommended alternate methods of treatment, including more consistent use of epidural catheters for pain and/or surgical fixation.

Treatment of the unstable chest wall remains controversial. However, a mounting body of literature has developed in the last few decades regarding operative fixation of flail segments (Fig. 110.4).

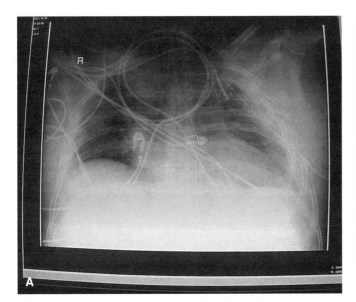

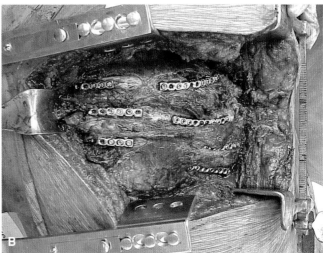

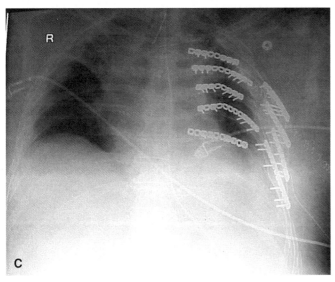

FIGURE 110.4 **A:** CXR demonstrating a left-sided flail chest. **B:** Intraoperative picture demonstrating operative fixation. **C:** CXR demonstrating successful fixation of the flail chest.

Surgical stabilization has been associated with a faster ventilator wean, shorter ICU stay, lower hospital cost, and faster recovery of pulmonary function in a select group of patients with flail chest.[114] Basic indications for fixation are persistent pain, severe chest wall instability, progressive decline in pulmonary function, or inability to separate from the ventilator despite optimal mechanical and pharmacologic management. Open fixation is also indicated for flail chest when thoracotomy is performed for other concomitant injuries. Leinicke et al. performed a meta-analysis including 538 patients and found that with operative fixation, patients with flail chest had a significantly reduced duration of mechanical ventilation, lower LOS, mortality, incidence of pneumonia, and tracheostomy.[115] A prospective, randomized study in 2013 compared operative fixation with current best practice mechanical ventilator management and found significantly shorter ICU stay and ventilation requirements in the operative arm with no differences in spirometry at 3 months or quality of life at 6 months.[116] Another study found that in the 77.8% of patients who underwent open fixation, ventilatory support lasted for a mean of 3.1 days compared with 7.2 days in the nonoperative group. The mortality rate in the surgical group was 11.1%, compared with 27% for the nonsurgical group.[111]

One prospective study by Lardinois et al. covered a decade of experience with patients that underwent operative fixation of severe anterolateral flail chests and evaluated their pulmonary function tests at 6 months.[117] They found a significantly better recorded versus predicted VC and forced expiratory volume in 1 second (FEV1). The median ratio of the recorded and predicted total lung capacity (TLC) was shown to be significantly higher than 0.85, indicating prevention of pulmonary restriction. Another prospective, randomized study also found improved percent forced vital capacity (FVC) was higher in the operatively fixated group at 1 month and later.[118] This study also found reduced medical cost, which has become a growing concern. This was further substantiated by Bhatnagar and colleagues, who sought to determine if open reduction and internal fixation of ribs for flail chest was a cost-effective means for managing these patients.[119] They found that not only did patients significantly improve clinically, but that surgical fixation remained the most cost-effective strategy with cost savings averaging $8,400 per patient. When surveyed, the majority of surgeons report that rib and sternal fracture repair is indicated in selected patients. However, a much smaller proportion indicated that they had experience performing this procedure.[120] Although the published literature on surgical fixation has been rapidly growing, this technique remains unfamiliar to most surgeons. It is suspected that surgical fixation of flail chest will become the standard of care in the future as barriers to this underutilized surgical procedure are overcome.[120,121]

Historically reported mortality from flail chest was 30% to 40% in the mid-1970s; in the modern era this rate has improved to 16%.[113] However, flail chest continues to cause significant morbidity including pneumonia, prolonged respiratory failure, increased LOS, ARDS, and sepsis. Head injury presenting with flail chest has a particularly poor prognosis. Patients presenting with concurrent head injury and flail chest require more ventilatory support, require longer ICU stay, and have worse outcomes in almost every category when compared to those without a head injury.[113] Patients with rib fractures also experience considerable long-term disability and lose an average of 70 days of work or usual activity during their recovery.[122] Long-term morbidity develops in up to 60% of patients with the most common being persistent chest wall pain or deformity, and 20% to 60% of patients never return to full-time employment.[123,124]

LUNG CONTUSION

Pulmonary contusion is a common injury following blunt chest wall trauma, resulting in profound ventilation/perfusion mismatch and significant left-to-right shunting. Mortality ranges between 10% and 25%. Hemorrhage and interstitial edema result from injury to the lung parenchyma. This is thought to be caused by a combination of alveolar stretching, parenchymal tearing, and concussive forces. Clinical symptoms, including respiratory distress with hypoxemia and hypercarbia, may take 12 to 24 hours after injury to fully develop, and tends to peak at about 72 hours.[125] Lung injury in the absence of identifiable rib fractures typically presents with diffuse injury, whereas rib fractures and flail chest are associated with localized injury. Hypoxemia, although nonspecific, is the most common clinical finding associated with pulmonary contusion. Typical CXR findings in the appropriate clinical setting remain the mainstay of diagnosis. Typical findings usually demonstrate a focal or diffuse consolidative process that does not follow anatomical segments or lobes. Pulmonary contusion may not become radiographically apparent up to 48 hours post-injury, with an average delay of 6 hours. However, CT scan has been demonstrated to identify the presence of pulmonary contusion almost immediately post-injury.[126-129] In addition, 3D CT reconstruction can help estimate the total volume of injured lung present.[38,130]

Pulmonary contusion commonly results in prolonged mechanical ventilation.[39,102,131] It has been shown that when pulmonary contusion involves 28% or more of the total lung volume, most if not all patients will require mechanical ventilation; however, the need for mechanical ventilatory support is unlikely when 18% or less of the lung volume is involved.[102,132] Underlying principles of treatment include managing any associated rib fractures, providing adequate pain control and aggressive pulmonary physiotherapy, and limiting fluid administration. Hypervolemia may worsen fluid extravasation into the alveolar spaces and worsen parenchymal consolidation in the setting of compromised capillary permeability. However, under-resuscitation should also be avoided, as this may lead to thickened secretions, worsened cardiac output, and shunting. Fluid administration in these patients is often a difficult balancing act, requiring sound clinical judgment. Treatment is generally supportive. Steroids and prophylactic antibiotics are generally not indicated in the treatment of uncomplicated pulmonary parenchymal injuries. Close respiratory monitoring and frequent clinical examination are important since respiratory failure occurs usually within the first few hours post-injury. Once diagnosed and coexistent injuries are treated, the patient should be transferred to a monitored bed.

Pulmonary toilet should be achieved through several mechanisms, including nasotracheal suctioning, chest physiotherapy, and postural drainage. This minimizes atelectasis and helps clear bronchial secretions. If the patient is unable to clear secretions adequately, selective bronchoscopy can be helpful. Supportive therapy for pulmonary contusion is essentially the same as for patients with flail chest and rib fractures, especially when considering these injuries often coincide. Mechanical ventilation can minimize edema and increase functional residual capacity, in turn decreasing shunting and improving hypoxemia. Positioning patients with the injured lung in the nondependent position may also improve oxygenation, especially in patients refractory to other measures.[133] Positive end expiratory pressure (PEEP) is used to overcome the closing pressure of the alveoli. However, it should be carefully titrated to ensure adequate oxygenation as excessive PEEP may actually worsen the shunt as the increased pressure is transmitted to the capillary level of gas exchange. Stretch secondary to overdistention from increased volume administration should particularly be avoided since this can extend the area of injury.

Atelectasis can lead to infectious pneumonia, which often contributes to worsening hypoxia after the initial couple of days post-injury. Furosemide can be helpful in managing fluid balance in patients with pulmonary contusion and may have additional benefit beyond its diuretic effect.[134] ARDS can complicate pulmonary contusion in 5% to 20% of cases and long-term pulmonary dysfunction is a common chronic disability.[125,135,136] Dyspnea may affect as many as 90% of patients during the first 6 months after pulmonary contusion. In addition, functional reserve capacity has been found to be diminished as late as 4 years after injury with the majority of patients demonstrating subtle changes on CT.[136]

PULMONARY HEMATOMA

Pulmonary hematoma may be difficult to differentiate from pulmonary contusion because of the surrounding intraparenchymal hemorrhage. However, a hematoma typically develops into a discrete mass with distinct margins within 24 to 48 hours after the injury. CT scans can be helpful in distinguishing between contusion and hematoma. In most cases, the hematoma itself does not interfere with gas exchange and is reabsorbed in time. Only rarely may such a hematoma become secondarily infected and present as an abscess requiring drainage, or require operative intervention for other reasons.

STERNAL FRACTURE

Sternal fractures have been shown to decrease the stability of the thorax in cadavers.[137] A large, level I trauma center found that over a 10-year period the incidence of sternal fracture was 0.33%.[138] The most common MOI was motor vehicle collision (68%) followed by auto versus pedestrian (18%). Interestingly sternal fractures were found to be present in 14% to 26% of medical autopsy cases that had received chest compressions prior to death.[139,140] Associated injuries are common in patients with sternal fractures: rib fractures occurred in 49.6% to 57.8%; lung contusions in 33.7%; cardiac contusions in 3.6% to 8%; thoracic aortic injuries in 4%; and cardiac lacerations in 2.4%.[138,141] The fracture is typically transverse and is usually located in the upper and mid portions of the body of the sternum. Clinical exam findings that help establish the diagnosis are point tenderness, swelling, and deformity. The gold standard for skeletal imaging in chest trauma is CT, which can often identify sternal fractures otherwise overlooked by lateral CXR.[142,143] MRI plays a minor role but can be useful for further investigation of sternal fractures once the patient has been stabilized. Specifically, it can be particularly useful for identifying secondary osteomyelitis or acute mediastinitis and in evaluating sternoclavicular joint involvement or involvement of other mediastinal structures.[144,145] Older patients (age >55), seat belt wearers, and front-seat vehicle occupants involved in frontal collisions are at greatest risk[138,141,146] for sustaining associated injuries. A recent study comparing over 42,000 trauma admissions over two decades demonstrated an incidence of sternal fracture in 0.64% of all patients.[147] In this series 91% of patients were seat-belted and the cars involved in the more recent years of the study were significantly older and not equipped with airbags. Eighteen percent of patients sustained multiple organ injury, with 11.2% dying at the scene and 2.3% dying in the hospital.

The more serious complications, as well as, deaths that occur in patients with sternal fractures are usually related to associated injuries, such as flail chest, head injury, or pulmonary or cardiac contusion.[148] There have been some early observational studies describing fracture morphology, displacement, and location that can provide important information regarding concomitant injuries.[149,150] Some degree of injury to the myocardium is common; however, its clinical significance and the need for subsequent testing in hemodynamically stable patients are questionable. Many investigators have attempted to evaluate the role of these tests as well as the routine common practice to admit these patients for observation. There is clear evidence that TTE and creatinine kinase assays in the assessment of isolated sternal fractures, particularly with a normal admission electrocardiogram (EKG) and CXR, may not be indicated.[151,152]

Underlying cardiac and aortic injuries are rare but highly lethal and should be screened for on the initial chest CT scan. Much attention has been directed toward isolated sternal fractures without additional injuries and a normal EKG, which has been described as a rather benign prognosis.[153,154] Consistent with these findings, isolated sternal fractures can be managed with rest and analgesia, since the diagnosis of a sternal fracture is not an independent predictor of morbidity or mortality. Management algorithms for isolated sternal fractures continue to be an area of interest.[155] After appropriate exclusion of critical injuries, the majority of patients can be observed or safely discharged home as long as the following criteria are met: (1) the injury is not a high-velocity impact; (2) the fracture is not severely displaced; (3) there are no clinically significant associated injuries; and (4) complex analgesics are not required.[138] Recent studies demonstrate the widespread, continued practice of routine admission for patients with isolated sternal fractures for observation, even though evidence appears to suggest that this is unnecessary.[156,157]

Treatment of sternal fractures is most often conservative and consists of good pain control and appropriate pulmonary hygiene similar to that for rib fractures.[151,158] This usually results in complete bony union. Indications for operative sternal fixation are lacking but should be judged individually. Generally accepted criteria for operative fixation include (1) severely displaced fractures; (2) severe pain; (3) sternal instability compromising pulmonary or cardiac function; and/or (4) nonunion of the sternum due to a pseudarthrosis sterni.[157,159] Operative techniques include internal fixation using plating systems or wires, usually through a midline incision. Sternal fixation is often performed in a delayed fashion. Given the potential loss of thoracic spinal stability after sternal fracture, restoration of the thoracic cage with sternal fixation theoretically supports an aggressive approach. However, there continues to be a lack of consensus among surgeons on when and if to operate on these injuries, in addition to

a lack of randomized trials demonstrating optimal treatment. Only a small percentage of patients (2% in one series) actually underwent sternal fixation.[160]

MAJOR PULMONARY PARENCHYMAL INJURY

Major parenchymal lacerations following blunt injuries are rare. They are typically associated with rupture of the visceral pleura and may lead to significant mortality and morbidity. Bleeding from the injured alveolar and pulmonary circulation can lead to both shock (due to intrathoracic hemorrhage) and suffocation if the patient's blood floods the airway.[161] Prognosis is significantly worsened by the presence of hemorrhagic shock, defined as systolic blood pressure below 80 mm Hg at hospital arrival and/or 1000 mL or more of blood loss though the chest tube within 2 hours of arrival.[162]

Most pulmonary parenchymal injuries are initially treated with chest tube drainage. Bronchoscopy should be performed when massive hemoptysis or a continuous air leak is present. Hemorrhage isolated to one lobe or segment may be contained with a bronchial blocker.[59,161,163] Resuscitation in the ED requires a team-based approach. Occasionally, an anterolateral EDT is necessary to provide hilar control of the injury with cardiac massage if needed. Simultaneously, volume resuscitation and maximal ventilatory support can be provided. Profound ventilation/perfusion mismatch and significant left-to-right shunting may be present. Initial management and need for operative therapy are guided by hemodynamic status, lung expansion, size of air leak, chest tube output, and any available radiologic imaging that may help determine the urgency of the intervention needed.[164,165]

The goals of surgery are to stop bleeding, repair and prevent air leaks, and debride any devitalized lung tissue. The preferred incision is a lateral or posterolateral thoracotomy, although a transverse sternotomy or even clamshell incision may be necessary to provide adequate exposure.[163] The initial step is to obtain control of the ipsilateral hilum by hand or finger pressure. Other methods may encompass cross-clamping[166,167] or the use of a Rumel tourniquet.[168] Intrapericardial dissection of the hilar vessels may be necessary. Endoscopic surgical staplers are the most effective means of rapid and consistent control of both air leaks and hemorrhage while also preserving lung function.[163,164,166] Techniques for controlling bleeding pulmonary parenchyma is the tractotomy or nonanatomic stapled resection.[166,169,170] In the case of a penetrating wound to the lung with massive bleeding a tractotomy can be performed to expose the culprit vessel(s) (Fig. 110.5). Localized bleeding or bronchial leaks in the tract can then be identified and controlled with suture. Mortality rates after tractotomies have been reported between 0% and 17%.[166,169,171–173] When local measures fail or are not possible, a nonanatomic wedge resection or lobectomy may be required to provide control of bleeding. Proximal lesions may require extensive resection, including pneumonectomy; however, mortality is proportional to the amount of lung tissue resected.[169] A 15-year retrospective review conducted at a level I trauma center found mortality rates for pneumorrhaphy to be 23.9%; for tractotomy, 9.1%; for wedge resection, 20%; lobectomy, 35%; and pneumonectomy, 69.7%.[174] Morbidities include ARDS, pneumonia, empyema, ischemia of the stapled tissue, recurrent bleeding, and bronchopleural fistula.[169,175]

PROXIMAL PULMONARY AND HILAR INJURIES

The high mortality associated with a lobectomy or pneumonectomy after traumatic lung injury is the reason lesser resections should

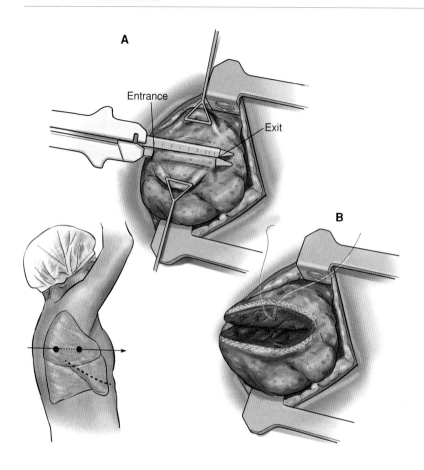

A

Entrance

Exit

B

FIGURE 110.5 **A:** Bleeders are exposed by inserting the stapler into the tract dividing the overlying parenchyma with a surgical stapler. **B:** Active bleeders or air leaks are closed with suture.

always be attempted first, although location of injury can often preclude nonanatomic surgical treatment. Following traumatic pneumonectomy, the combination of elevated peripheral vascular resistance (as seen in hemorrhagic shock), coupled with the sudden direction of the cardiac output in its entirety to the contralateral side is usually poorly tolerated.[176,177] Unfortunately, pneumonectomy may be the only alternative. When this is the case, it should be completed as expeditiously as possible. Blood loss, shock, and end organ malperfusion have all been well documented as independent predictors of mortality.[162,178,179]

Patients presenting with proximal parenchymal and/or hilar injuries have a high mortality and often present in a severely decompensated physiologic state.[176,177,180] Lobectomy can sometimes control the injury; however, if vascular control is not rapidly obtained, a stapled pneumonectomy may be considered as a last resort. This carries an extremely high mortality of more than 60% however and therefore should not be done lightly.[174,178] This high mortality is thought to be due to numerous causes such as acute right heart failure, shock-induced release of thromboxane, and other leukocyte effects on the pulmonary circulation.[181,182] It should be noted that nitric oxide inhalation has been found to be beneficial as a vasodilator in the treatment of ARDS and pulmonary edema after major lung resections.[183,184]

AIR EMBOLISM

In severe chest trauma, specifically penetrating hilar injuries, air embolism may result. Air embolism can be divided into either venous or arterial. The most common cause of venous air embolism is through a peripheral systemic vein. Relatively large amounts of venous air are usually tolerated in this manner where lethal volumes

typically have to approach 5 to 8 mL/kg. Penetrating hilar injuries on the other hand may result in arterial air embolism. Air embolism was first reported in a case series of eight gunshot and stab wounds in 1974 by Thomas and Stevens.[185] The cause of arterial (or systemic) air embolism is most often found at the hilum, where the major vessels are in close proximity to the airways and injury between the two may result in bronchovenous communication. In contrast to venous air embolism, even small amounts of systemic air entering the left side of the heart can be fatal, resulting in hemodynamic instability secondary to ventricular fibrillation and seizure activity.

Air embolism is difficult to recognize. It often presents as catastrophic circulatory collapse, cerebral events, or sudden death in the conscious patient. The clinician must be wary of subtle presentations. The diagnosis should be clinically suspected in patients presenting with pulseless electrical activity. Several diagnostic tools (TTE, Doppler, CT) can detect intracardiac and cerebral air, but are not necessary to confirm the diagnosis.[186] Management of endotracheal pressure is critical in this scenario as gas will easily pass from the pulmonary venous system into the systemic circulation. The patient should receive 100% oxygen, to allow faster absorption of gas emboli secondary to the increased solubility of oxygen.[187] Nitrous oxide increases bubble size and should be avoided. Hypovolemia should also be avoided to reduce the pressure gradient favoring air entry into the pulmonary venous system. Despite aggressive management and prompt recognition, one series of 61 patients with systemic air embolism had a mortality rate of 80% in those that sustained blunt trauma and 48% in those that sustained penetrating trauma.[188] The definitive treatment of systemic air embolism with unilateral lung injury is immediate thoracotomy and hilar control of the injured lung to arrest the continuous passage of air into the coronary, cerebral, and/or other systemic arteries.[188,189]

TRACHEOBRONCHIAL INJURY

TBI can be a challenge to diagnose, manage, and definitively treat. The true incidence is difficult to establish, as a large proportion (30% to 80%) of these patients will die before reaching the hospital.[190] Based on autopsy reports, an estimated 2.5% to 3.2% of patients who die as a result of trauma may have associated TBI.[13,191] More than 80% of TBI occurs within 2.5 cm of the carina.[58,191,192] The majority of patients with TBI present with some degree of respiratory difficulty, and these patients often require emergent measures to secure and control the airway. Early recognition and expeditious surgical intervention can be lifesaving in these otherwise potentially lethal injuries. Orotracheal intubation with or without bronchoscopic guidance is the most common method used. Simply achieving adequate ventilation may require some level of ingenuity and patients with cervical injuries or open neck wounds can be intubated through the open wound in order to secure the airway if necessary.[58]

Common presenting symptoms include dyspnea, voice changes, dysphagia, hoarseness, and pain.[19,193] Initial physical findings in patients with TBI can be subtle. However, physical exam findings may range from minor neck bruising, abrasions, or tachypnea to substantial hematomas, subcutaneous emphysema, inability to phonate, air bubbles from a neck wound, and/or deformity of the thyroid cartilage.[194] Massive air leak and the inability to re-expand the lung after tube thoracostomy are highly indicative of a TBI.[195] Although pneumothorax and pneumomediastinum are nonspecific, disruption of the normal contour of the trachea and overdistention of the endotracheal balloon are virtually pathognomonic.[196] The use of bronchoscopy is mandatory in identifying tracheobronchial injuries and continues to be the gold standard in its diagnosis.[19,193,194] Multi-slice detector CT imaging with multiplanar reconstruction (MPR) and 3D reconstruction can significantly increase diagnostic accuracy to 94% to 100%, which may also help in guiding optimal surgical approach.[196,197] As technology evolves, it has been suggested that bronchoscopy perhaps becomes a confirmatory test only after screening MPR has been performed.[197] Bronchoscopy along with chest CT with MPR and 3D reconstruction of the airway represents the procedure of choice for definitive diagnosis.[194]

In blunt force trauma, the mechanisms that lead to TBI are thought to originate from one of three distinct etiologies: (1) a rapid increase in the airway pressure against a closed glottis by sudden thoracic compression leads to tracheal perforation or rupture of the main bronchi. This mechanism may explain TBI after blunt abdominal injury with sudden displacement of the diaphragm; (2) extensive anteroposterior chest compression forcing the lungs apart laterally and causing distention and rupture of central airway structures near the carina as a result of crush injury; or (3) rapid deceleration with shearing force applied to the fixed portions of the trachea at the junctions of the cricoid or the carina resulting in rupture of the mobile portions of the trachea.[198] Because of these anatomical considerations, more than 80% of all TBI from blunt trauma originates within 2.5 cm of the carina.[192] In only 30% of cases is a definitive diagnosis made within 24 hours of injury. Commonly, the diagnosis is made late, only after pulmonary collapse occurs and sepsis begins.

Although surgical treatment of most TBI is still considered standard of care, conservative treatment can be considered in carefully selected patients. Isolated membranous injuries appear to be more suited for this approach.[199] Generally, the prerequisites for conservative management include small lacerations (<2 cm), a location of the injury that allows the tube's cuff to be inflated distal to the site of the injury, and adequate ventilation using relatively low tidal volumes.[194] Although conservative treatment can be considered,

surgical treatment of TBI should be performed for symptomatic cartilaginous injuries and rapid progression of subcutaneous or mediastinal emphysema, when there are signs of mediastinitis or there is difficulty with mechanical ventilation related to the injury itself.[16] Currently the reported rate of conservative treatment in patients with TBI ranges from 33.3% to 94.4%.[200] Airway management may necessitate bypassing the injury by means of endobronchial intubation into the uninjured bronchus with a single-lumen or double-lumen endotracheal tube. These maneuvers may not only facilitate single-lung ventilation for improved oxygenation but also provide lung isolation for exposure and surgical repair.[18] Furthermore, airway pressures should be minimized in patients with TBI to avoid suture line disruption and/or extension of a known injury.[19]

Since the initial report by Shaw and colleagues, primary repair of TBI has been encouraged and should be done as soon as possible.[13,194,201–203] Double-lumen endotracheal intubation is the method of choice for securing the airway (when possible), although occasionally bronchial blockers may be the only option. Careful and thoughtful discussion with the anesthesiologist regarding airway management ahead of time is mandatory. In addition, the surgical approach should be considered along with whether the insult was blunt or penetrating trauma. The injury can further be characterized as cervical trachea versus intrathoracic trachea versus major bronchi. Most repairs of cervical tracheal injuries can be approached through a collar incision. In patients with injuries high in the mediastinal trachea or with suspected great vessel injury, a median sternotomy may be preferred. When the injury is associated with a unilateral pneumothorax or when a bronchial injury is diagnosed preoperatively, an ipsilateral posterolateral thoracotomy is the incision of choice. For injuries to the mediastinal trachea, an approach via a right posterolateral thoracotomy usually provides good exposure.[19] A high right posterolateral thoracotomy (usually through the third or fourth ICS) can provide excellent exposure of the proximal and mid trachea. An incision through the fifth ICS usually provides excellent exposure of the distal trachea and carina. Because of the heart, aorta, and other anatomical considerations, the proximal left mainstem may actually be best approached through a right thoracotomy.

Most patients can undergo primary repair of their TBI using a tailored surgical technique specific to the injury.[58] After the traumatic margins are debrided, primary repair can be accomplished using simple interrupted, running, or telescoping techniques. The repair should be done with absorbable sutures with the knots tied on the outside to avoid the development of subsequent granulomas that may erode into the lumen.[204,205] Suture lines can be buttressed using pleura, pericardium, mediastinal fat, intercostal muscle, or rotational muscle flaps if necessary.[58,195,206] This may be especially helpful when there is an adjacent injury to the esophagus and separation of suture lines is desired. When a major bronchus is disrupted, lobectomy may be preferred over primary repair, with closure of the bronchial stump debrided back to healthy tissue. With injuries to the mainstem bronchi, primary repair is preferred over pneumonectomy due to the higher mortality associated with performing an emergency pneumonectomy.[176,177,207] Injury to the trachea should be repaired primarily. Tracheostomy through the wound is an alternative if an anterior tracheal injury is present and is less than half of the airway's circumference and/or involves only up to two cartilaginous rings.[208]

Occasionally, injured segments of the trachea are unrepairable. In these cases, resection of the injured segment with primary anastomosis may be necessary. Principles of tracheal resection and reconstruction include the following: (1) the trachea should be mobilized anteriorly and posteriorly given its lateral blood supply; (2) no more than one-half of the trachea (i.e., approximately 8 to 10 tracheal rings) should be resected; and (3) release maneuvers can be performed to minimize tension on the anastomosis including division of the inferior pulmonary ligaments, pericardial release of the pulmonary hilum, cervical flexion, and suprahyoid laryngeal release.[209–211] Of these, cervical flexion is the simplest and perhaps the most effective.[19,58] A suture placed from the chin to the chest ("Grillo stitch" or "guardian suture") in these patients may help to minimize cervical extension in the early postoperative period, but should not be placed too tight. Associated injuries to neighboring structures such as the carotid arteries, jugular veins, cervical spine, and esophagus are not uncommon in these patients and should be meticulously searched for and treated appropriately if found.

Depending on the severity of associated injuries and on airway compromise directly due to TBI, surgical treatment can be either immediate or delayed. Although perhaps inferior to early repair, delayed repair of TBI can be successful, even if performed months out from the original injury and can be treated in a similar fashion.[192] Late complications of untreated TBI are not uncommon and include bronchial stenosis, recurrent pneumonia, and bronchiectasis.[18]

Mortality from traumatic TBI has decreased from 36% before 1950 and 30% in 1966 to 9% in 2001.[18,19,192] Advancement in surgical techniques and improvement in the understanding and treatment of the physiologic abnormalities observed with the more commonly seen associated injuries have undoubtedly contributed to this progress. When early surgical airway repair is performed, 90% of patients with TBI have a good long-term result.[212] In a series by Reece and Shatney, the authors conclude that primary early repair provides the best long-term outcome, with 67% of patients who underwent primary tracheal repair having a significantly superior outcome when compared to those that had a stent or a tracheostomy.[213] Finally, it is estimated that major coexisting injuries can be found in 40% to 100% of all trauma victims with TBI, which can significantly impact the prognosis of these patients.[212,214] Consequently, major morbidity and mortality after TBI is primarily affected by the presence of concomitant injuries. Long-term complications include airway stenosis and phonation problems from injuries to the larynx and recurrent laryngeal nerves.[13,215]

INTUBATION INJURIES OF THE TRACHEA

The incidence of iatrogenic TBI is approximately one event in every 20,000 to 75,000 elective orotracheal intubations, increasing up to 15% when emergently performed. The incidence of TBI is 0.2% to 0.7% for percutaneous tracheostomy.[16,216] Timing of discovery of the injury is an important variable as intraoperative diagnosis varies between 17% and 25% and delayed recognition (up to 10 days after intubation) occurs in 82.4% of patients.[217,218] Post-intubation tracheal injuries are characterized by an insidious onset and a high mortality. Diagnosis requires a high index of suspicion. Subcutaneous emphysema is the most common clinical manifestation, followed by pneumomediastinum, pneumothorax, dyspnea/respiratory distress, and hemoptysis. Diagnostic confirmation is usually made by bronchoscopy. This provides data on the exact location and extent of the injury. It also helps to plan the therapeutic approach and can be used to reposition airway access if necessary.

Injuries are generally longitudinal and are most frequently located in the membranous portion of the trachea, which lacks cartilaginous support. Several risk factors for sustaining an iatrogenic injury to the airway have been described in the literature and can be divided into mechanical versus anatomical variables. Mechanical variables include multiple forced attempts at intubation, inexperience of the health professional, the use of endotracheal tube

introducers or stylets that protrude beyond the tip of the tube, overinflation of the cuff, incorrect position of the tip of the tube, repositioning the tube without deflation of the cuff, and inappropriate size of the endotracheal tube.[218–221] Anatomical factors include congenital tracheal abnormalities, weakness of the membranous trachea, chronic bronchitis and other inflammatory lesions of the tracheobronchial tree, diseases that alter the position of the trachea (mediastinal collections, lymph nodes, or tumors), chronic use of steroids, and advanced age.[13,218,222]

Consensus has not yet been reached on the management of iatrogenic TBI. Early surgical repair has traditionally been the mainstay of treatment; however, conservative treatment has been shown to be effective regardless of etiology, size, or site of the injury. Minambres and colleagues reported a series of 71 patients with post-intubation tracheal injuries that underwent conservative treatment and had a mortality of 14.5%.[218] Some have advocated conservative treatment consisting of antibiotic administration and supportive care when the laceration is <1 to 3 cm in length.[217,218] This decision is largely determined by the local extent of the injury, ventilatory impairment, and ability to isolate the injury. However, surgical treatment is recommended if there is rapid progression of subcutaneous and/or mediastinal emphysema, mediastinitis, or difficulty with ventilation. Depending on the site of the injury, a collar incision, thoracotomy, or partial sternotomy approach may be appropriate. A transtracheal endoluminal approach has been described as a method to repair the membranous trachea (Fig. 110.6).[223–226] This is done by incising the anterior wall of the trachea longitudinally. Both edges of the trachea are retracted laterally and the membranous laceration is repaired, then the anterior wall is closed separately. In cases where there is additional injury to the esophagus, this approach can provide exposure to repair this too and allow the placement of muscle tissue between the esophagus and trachea prior to closure of the trachea.

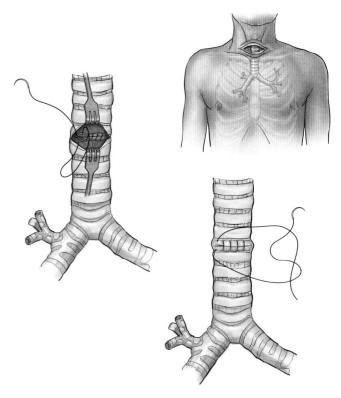

FIGURE 110.6 Anterior transtracheal endoluminal repair of membranous tracheal injury.

SCAPULAR AND CLAVICULAR FRACTURES

Fractures of the scapula are relatively rare injuries that commonly result from severe blunt trauma, specifically motor vehicle accidents. The amount of energy required to cause these injuries explains the 80% to 90% incidence of associated injuries, with a mortality generally ranging approximately 10%.[227–229] In the presence of fractures of the scapula, underlying rib fractures are more common along with an increased ISS and an increased Abbreviated Injury Scale score.[229] Concurrent brachial plexus injuries are common, and therefore a detailed neurovascular examination should be performed. Consensus opinion regarding treatment and operative indications to repair scapular fractures are lacking. Nonoperative management consists of shoulder immobilization with subsequent early range-of-motion exercises. Previously, Jones and colleagues found that despite nonoperative management, all fractures healed, and they found no differences in return to work, pain, or complications.[230] However, others have documented poor functional outcomes following nonoperative management of displaced scapular fractures. Historically, surgeons have been dissuaded to operate on these uncommon fractures because of their complex anatomy, necessary surgical approaches, and fracture patterns. However, open reduction and internal fixation may be indicated when the function of the glenohumeral joint is impaired, fractures extend to the glenoid neck and body, or the scapular neck or body fracture is displaced over 20 mm.[230,231]

In contrast to scapular fractures, clavicular fractures are relatively common and often isolated injuries and are not typically associated with a higher ISS. Treatment by immobilization combined with adequate analgesia is usually effective for most fractures. Operative repair is rarely necessary and is usually reserved for severely displaced fractures.[232] However, in the adolescent population early plate fixation of displaced midshaft clavicle fractures may result in shorter time to union with lower complication rates.[233] Double disruptions of the superior suspensory shoulder complex (commonly referred to as "floating shoulder" injuries) involve midshaft clavicle and scapular neck/body fractures along with a loss of bony attachment of the glenoid. The treatment for this injury has been debated for many years. However, recent studies have demonstrated dramatically improved clinical and functional outcomes of patients who underwent operative fixation of the clavicle fracture only.[234] Damage to the underlying subclavian vessels or the brachial plexus is fortunately rare.

SCAPULOTHORACIC DISSOCIATION

Scapulothoracic dissociation is an infrequent yet devastating injury, which is often the result of high-energy trauma to the shoulder girdle. At least 50% of reported cases are a result of motorcycle accidents.[235] When thrown from a motorcycle, the rider may reflexively hold onto the handle bar, leading to a distraction/sheer force strong enough to dislocate the acromioclavicular joint and tearing the shoulder girdle musculature.[236] Identification of this injury requires a high index of clinical suspicion, based upon the MOI, physical findings, and radiographic findings. Obtaining details regarding the accident scene can be helpful. The degree of injury to the musculoskeletal, neurologic, and vascular structures of the arm and shoulder should be carefully assessed. Clinically, patients usually present with massive soft tissue swelling, shoulder instability, tenderness, pulselessness, weakness, and numbness of the upper extremity. The musculoskeletal portion of the injury usually involves an acromioclavicular separation, displaced clavicular fracture, and/or sternoclavicular disruption.[237] Vascular lesions have been reported in 88% of patients and severe

neurologic injuries occur in 94% of patients.[237] When this injury is suspected, emergent subclavian, axillary, and brachial arteriography may be helpful to evaluate vascular structures, especially if the patient has a pulseless extremity.[235,238,239]

Diagnosis of scapulothoracic dissociation can be made with an anterior/posterior CXR: lateral displacement of the scapula is pathognomonic.[235] Damschen and later Zelle described a classification system based on clinical presentation: Type I is a musculoskeletal injury alone; type IIA is a musculoskeletal injury with vascular injury; type IIB is a musculoskeletal injury with neurologic injury; type III is a musculoskeletal injury with neurologic and vascular injury; and type IV has complete neurologic, vascular, and musculoskeletal avulsion, which is predictive of a poor outcome.[240,241] Such a "flail extremity" has been reported in 52% of patients and generally leads to early amputation in 21% and results in an overall mortality of 10%.[237] In general, patients with this injury often have poor overall outcomes, mostly from associated injuries. Treatment includes arterial and venous ligation to stop exsanguination if present, orthopedic stabilization, and consideration for above elbow amputation electively, specifically if brachial plexus avulsion is present, to allow for a more useful extremity. Early amputation is associated with quicker return to employment and better pain relief, while delay in amputation is associated with myoglobinuria, hyperkalemia, vascular thrombosis, and increased risk for pressure ulcers in the flail extremity.[235] Overall prognosis for limb recovery is poor.

DIAPHRAGMATIC RUPTURE

Patients with diaphragmatic injuries can be classified into two major categories: acute and chronic. The latter encompasses those injuries missed initially and recognized only after being released from the original hospitalization. The cause of diaphragmatic rupture is variable dependent on geography: penetrating trauma is the most common MOI in Montreal and South Africa, whereas in the developed world blunt trauma is the overwhelming cause.[242–244] Virtually all patients with diaphragmatic rupture sustain multiple additional injuries that can often obscure specific signs or symptoms causing a delay in diagnosis. The overall incidence of diaphragmatic rupture varies between 0.36% and 3% and is not initially recognized in up to 69% of severe trauma patients who survive long enough to be admitted to the hospital.[245–247] If a diaphragmatic injury is initially missed, one or more of the abdominal viscera may eventually herniate into the thoracic cavity. This may lead to complications including organ ischemia resulting in significant morbidity and potential mortality. The constant positive pressure of the abdomen combined with the constant negative pressure of the chest naturally provokes visceral herniation and enlargement of the defect over time.

BLUNT DIAPHRAGMATIC INJURIES

Hanna and Okada state that the typical mechanisms that result in diaphragmatic rupture are motor vehicle accidents, falls from great height, motor vehicle crash (MVC) versus pedestrian, and crushing injuries.[244,247] Blunt diaphragmatic injury is variable in the literature; however, the majority of injuries appear to be to the left diaphragm (65% to 86%) with the remainder to the right diaphragm (14% to 35%) and bilateral (1.5%) (with approximately 5% unclassified).[248–250] Blunt trauma to the abdomen increases the transdiaphragmatic pressure gradient between the abdominal compartment and the thorax. This may cause shearing and avulsion of the diaphragm, commonly resulting in a large tear along the central tendon (typically larger than

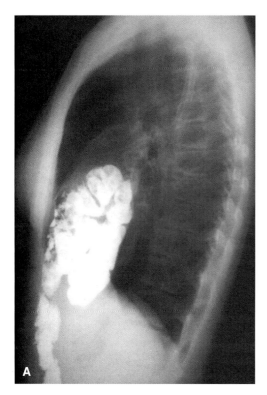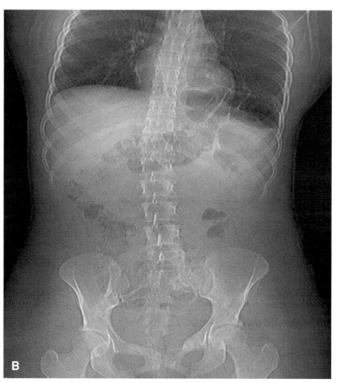

FIGURE 110.7 Delayed presentation of a left diaphragm rupture 8 months after a motor vehicle crash. **A:** Barium enema demonstrating colon herniated into the chest. **B:** Plain film demonstrating colon herniated into the left chest.

a defect caused by penetrating trauma).[251] The large defect created along with the sudden increase in intra-abdominal pressure commonly leads to hollow visceral herniation into the pleural space. The right hemidiaphragm is in direct apposition to the liver, therefore cushioning it from blunt force trauma.[252] Right-sided diaphragmatic rupture has been predominantly associated with high-velocity blunt trauma.[243] Right-sided injuries are usually posterolateral to the central tendon, but the pericardial or central portion of the diaphragm may also tear. Herniation through an acute rupture after blunt injury is about 66% more common than after penetrating injury. The most commonly herniated organs on the left side are the stomach, spleen, small bowel, and infrequently colon (Fig. 110.7). On the right side the presence of the liver minimizes hollow visceral herniation through the diaphragmatic defect. However, when herniation occurs on the right, the liver is usually involved, while the second most common organ to be affected is the colon (Fig. 110.8).[253] Rupture of the right hemidiaphragm is frequently associated with vascular injuries, particularly of the vena cava and hepatic veins.

Diaphragmatic rupture without visceral injury or herniation may be difficult to detect due to a paucity of clinical signs and symptoms. Only a minority of patients present with respiratory distress, cardiac abnormalities, deviated trachea, and/or bowel sounds in the chest. Over 95% of patients have associated injuries, many presenting with hypovolemic shock, sepsis, or traumatic brain injury. Patients with blunt force injury to the diaphragm generally have a median ISS of >40.[243,244,246,250,254] The widely adopted and easily accessible FAST exam in the initial assessment of the trauma patient has prompted several reports that recommend its use to assess diaphragmatic injury.[255–257] An immobile diaphragm or abnormal diaphragmatic motion may indicate rupture. In patients requiring emergency exploration for any other life-threatening injuries, the diagnosis of diaphragmatic rupture is usually made during its thorough inspection

as part of any exploratory laparotomy. Despite improved accessibility to US the reported rate of these injuries initially overlooked remains between 20% and 40%.[255]

Routine CXR can alert the clinician to the diagnosis of diaphragmatic injury with sensitivities ranging from 30% to 62% in the absence

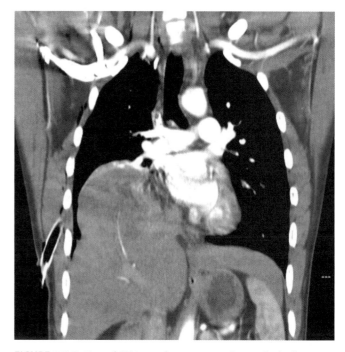

FIGURE 110.8 Coronal CT image demonstrating a large right diaphragmatic rupture with herniation of the liver into the right chest.

of a hernia, and up to 94% in the presence of a hernia.[256,258–260] Common findings include abdominal contents in the thorax, with or without signs of focal constriction (collar sign), nasogastric tube seen in the thorax, >4 cm elevated hemidiaphragm (left > right), and distortion of the diaphragmatic margin.[261] The hernia sac is visualized as a soft tissue opacity, containing visceral gas in the thorax, which is pathognomonic of diaphragmatic rupture. One or more air–fluid levels and radiolucency may be seen in the lower hemithorax as well as shifting of the mediastinum away from the side of the hernia. Occasionally a rounded shadow protruding above the right hemidiaphragm appears on the lateral film, which is highly diagnostic for a right-sided rupture. Non-diagnostic findings such as pneumothorax and hemithorax are also frequently present. The usefulness of CXR is controversial. Beal and colleagues describe CXR as often non-diagnostic in identifying traumatic diaphragmatic injuries. They attributed their low incidence of missed injury to an aggressive approach in the severely injured patient population, where exploratory laparotomy was a routine part of the complete evaluation.[246] Consequently, CXR can be used as part of the initial work-up of a trauma patient. However, it should not be considered as the definitive imaging modality if a diaphragmatic injury is suspected.

In patients who do not require emergent exploration, the diagnosis may be confirmed with barium contrast images of either the upper or lower gastrointestinal tract. CT of the abdomen and thorax is a very useful and reliable tool in the evaluation of diaphragmatic injury.[256,262,263] Killeen and colleagues found that for left-sided injuries the sensitivity was 78% and specificity 100%; for right-sided injuries the sensitivity was 50% and the specificity 100%.[263] Various features seen on CT scan are described as diaphragmatic discontinuity, thickened diaphragm, and the "collar sign," which is constriction of the stomach or colon as it passes through the tear.[264] When the diagnosis remains elusive, despite the common initial investigatory methods, MRI may be helpful, often revealing detailed characteristics of the rupture not otherwise appreciated. Although MRI is not useful in most acute traumatic situations due to its relatively long duration and sensitivity for motion artifact, it can be helpful in selected patients, especially those who present with delayed traumatic diaphragmatic rupture.[256] MRI is more costly in terms of time and resources, yet the diaphragm in its entirety is more clearly revealed on T1-weighted sagittal magnetic resonance images.[265,266] MRI is probably most useful to help distinguish chronic diaphragmatic rupture and herniation from eventration and simple paralytic elevation.

Diaphragmatic rupture should be repaired expeditiously given the risk of respiratory and circulatory compromise. In addition, due to the nature of opposing positive intra-abdominal pressure now communicating with negative intrathoracic pressure, bowel obstruction, incarceration, and strangulation become a significant possibility. In addition, small, relatively easily repairable defects can enlarge over time, causing adhesions within the chest requiring a more invasive approach for later repair. The surgical options to treat diaphragmatic injury include laparoscopy, thoracoscopy, laparotomy, and thoracotomy. Although the hemidiaphragm may be best exposed via an ipsilateral thoracotomy, the type of approach should be unique to each patient. Acute diaphragmatic injuries are best approached through the abdomen, as more than 89% of patients with this injury have an associated intra-abdominal injury or massive bleeding, which commonly originates from a lacerated abdominal organ.[246,248] In addition, adhesions within the chest are usually not an issue in the acute situation, making reduction of intra-abdominal viscera relatively easy through the belly. In contrast, patients with diaphragmatic rupture presenting in the latent phase may develop adhesions between the herniated abdominal and intrathoracic organs, requiring a

thoracotomy approach to reduce. When an abdominal exploration is otherwise not indicated, the decision to perform a thoracotomy versus celiotomy to reduce a chronic traumatic diaphragmatic herniation is a clinical one. A change in approach may become necessary intraoperatively, and it is always wise to prepare both the operating room and the patient for such a possibility ahead of time. Exploratory laparoscopy and thoracoscopy have been successful in diagnosing diaphragmatic tears with a quoted sensitivity and specificity of 100% and have also been shown to be effective in repair of left-sided acute diaphragmatic injuries.[267–269] Once all associated visceral injuries are repaired, the diaphragmatic tear is closed usually with interrupted figure-of-eight large-caliber non-absorbable sutures.[247,250] Prosthetic material is rarely needed with acute blunt trauma injuries.

Diaphragmatic injuries rarely cause death by themselves; however, the mortality rate following blunt injury to the diaphragm ranges from 14% to 40.5%, usually secondary to associated injuries.[243,246,248,250,252,270] In a more recent report on 105 patients, Hanna and colleagues found a mortality of 18%, both for blunt and penetrating ruptures.[244] In this cohort of patients, repeated evaluation for days after injury is necessary to discern injury in patients not requiring laparotomy. Increased mortality was noted in those patients with a higher ISS, head trauma, and rib. A case series by Shah et al. found that mortality was 17% in those in whom the acute diagnosis was made, and the majority of the morbidity in the group that underwent operation was due to pulmonary complications.[248] They further elaborated that the definitive diagnosis depends on a high index of suspicion, careful scrutiny of the radiologic imaging in patients with thoracoabdominal or polytrauma, and meticulous inspection of the diaphragm when operatively exploring for concurrent injuries.

PENETRATING DIAPHRAGMATIC INJURIES

Penetrating diaphragmatic injuries are most often caused by stab or gunshot wounds to the lower chest. Hanna, Okada, and Demetriades described in their respective series of penetrating injuries that stab wounds were the overwhelming cause of injury in 74.2% to 94%, while the rest were from gunshot wounds.[244,247,271] In the differentiation between blunt versus penetrating diaphragmatic injuries there are several distinct differences. The defect in the diaphragm as a result of penetrating trauma is generally significantly smaller when compared to blunt trauma. Hanna and colleagues showed that the mean size of a diaphragmatic defect caused by blunt trauma was 10.6 cm as compared to 3.1 cm caused by penetrating trauma.[244] Another study found that up to 84% of penetrating injuries result in a defect <2 cm, whereas blunt trauma consistently resulted in defects >2 cm with the majority being over 10 cm.[272] Furthermore, herniation of abdominal viscera may be more delayed in cases of penetrating trauma. In the acute setting, abdominal solid organ injury is more common with penetrating injuries.

There are no specific physical signs that necessarily lead to a diagnosis of diaphragmatic injury when there is no associated herniation. The key to an early diagnosis is a high level of suspicion, specifically with injuries located below the nipple line, but in the upper abdomen, flank, or back. The trajectory of missile and projectile injuries should always be thoroughly assessed, as the presence of abdominal complaints in a patient who has sustained a chest wound is strongly suggestive of a diaphragmatic injury, and vice versa. Operative exploration remains the gold standard for diagnosing penetrating diaphragmatic injuries.[43,268] Careful visual and manual evaluation of the surface of the diaphragm is important for their detection.[247] The most common scenario of a missed diaphragmatic injury is a stab wound with no organ herniation that does not warrant surgical exploration, as compared to gunshot wounds of the trunk, which usually mandate emergency exploration.

In the authors' institution it was found that CXR was abnormal in only 57% of the cases in 93 patients with penetrating injuries.[273] In another large study of only penetrating injuries, Demetriades and colleagues found that the diagnostic accuracy of CXR in patients with hollow viscus herniation into the chest was 74%, but in those with uncomplicated diaphragmatic injuries without herniation this figure was only 6%. Contrast studies of the gastrointestinal tract were 100% diagnostic in patients with hollow viscus herniation. More recent reports detailing the use of CT imaging for the identification of penetrating diaphragmatic injuries quote a sensitivity rate of 94% and specificity nearing 100%.[43] After the results were validated with operative evaluation, MDCT was found to have more than a 90% positive predictive value in diagnosing diaphragmatic injury in patients that sustained penetrating torso trauma. Some authors advocate that all penetrating injuries with trajectories suspicious for causing diaphragmatic injury, symptomatic or not, should be explored to provide a complete and meticulous inspection of the diaphragm.[273] Diagnostic laparoscopy has been shown to have a specificity, sensitivity, and negative predictive value of 100%, 87.5%, and 96.8%, respectively.[274–276] Diagnostic thoracoscopy has been shown to have similar results of 90%, 100%, and 100%, respectively.[277–279]

Similar to blunt diaphragm injury, the abdominal approach has been historically favored in the penetrating trauma setting because it permits accurate detection and simple repositioning of herniated abdominal organs, enabling the examination of both diaphragmatic leaflets and repair of associated visceral injuries. However both laparotomy and thoracotomy may be necessary when repair of both supra- and infra-diaphragmatic injuries are required. Okada and colleagues utilized repeated assessments of FAST exams and rate of bleeding from chest drains in patients with severe injuries of the chest and abdomen to determine the order of surgical approach. The order and necessity of surgical approach should be based on suspected injuries and their severities, but should include a thorough examination of the diaphragm regardless. When identified, diaphragmatic injuries can be safely and effectively repaired via thoracoscopy.[279–281] Penetrating injuries to the diaphragm are most amenable to primary repair due to their usual diminutive size.[268]

Diaphragmatic injuries alone are rarely the cause of death. In Hanna and colleagues' series of traumatic diaphragmatic injuries over 13 years they found an overall mortality of 18.1%.[244] However, the major causes of death were traumatic brain injury in 31.6% and hemorrhagic shock in 68.4%. There was no significant difference between the mortality rates of blunt and penetrating injuries. In the patients who died, 100% had associated injuries that required operative intervention, whereas only 74.4% of the survivors had associated injuries requiring operative intervention. Similarly, Symbas et al. found that associated organ injuries resulted in high morbidity and mortality in their series of 185 patients with penetrating injuries that resulted in a mortality of 2.2%.[252] The variables found to be associated with increased risk of death were higher ISS, the presence of hollow viscus injury, and older age.[244]

DELAYED DIAGNOSIS OF DIAPHRAGMATIC HERNIA

Diaphragmatic injuries are relatively easy to miss, especially if the clinician does not follow the trajectory closely or does not adequately inspect the diaphragm when exploring operatively. A chronic diaphragmatic hernia may present at any time from 3 months to 40 years after the initial injury.[243,282] Delayed rupture of a devitalized diaphragmatic muscle theoretically can occur several days after

initial injury. Extubation could precipitate this when the intrathoracic pressure becomes negative.[283] Likely explanations for delayed presentation include that the diaphragmatic defect becomes symptomatic only after herniation occurs or that the defect is discovered incidentally when radiographic evaluations are performed for unrelated reasons. Hanna and colleagues observed the following times for diagnosing diaphragmatic injury: within 6 hours of admission, 90.5%; after 6 hours but within same hospitalization, 6.7%; and late diagnosis (4 months to 3 years), 2.7%.[244] Historically, missed diaphragmatic injuries are more commonly associated with blunt trauma as opposed to penetrating trauma, probably since patients with penetrating trauma are more likely to be operatively explored early. Late hernias resulting from blunt trauma tend to contain multiple abdominal viscera. In order of frequency, Symbas reported that the stomach, followed by the colon, small bowel, omentum, and then the spleen herniate through left-sided defects, whereas the colon and liver commonly herniate through right-sided tears.[252]

Frequent complaints that lead to diagnosis of chronic diaphragmatic hernia are progressive chest pain, abdominal pain, dyspnea, cough, and partial or complete bowel obstruction.[284] Larger hernias are more likely to produce respiratory compromise by reducing the functional VC on the affected side. Smaller hernias that contain a loop of large bowel or stomach may cause partial or complete obstruction. Strangulation of the viscus may develop, just as with any other hernia, and carry an ominous prognosis. Historically, studies to establish the diagnosis were barium by mouth or a barium enema. However, helical CT with axial, sagittal, and coronal reconstruction has been demonstrated to have a sensitivity of 73% and specificity of 90% in this delayed cohort.[285] A high index of suspicion is imperative to accurately diagnose a delayed traumatic diaphragmatic hernia. The patient's medical history, specifically past trauma and timing, plays a pivotal role no matter the severity. Often the patient will have difficulty recalling a history of trauma even though eventually one is obtained.

Once compelling imaging has been established, diagnostic thoracoscopy can be performed as an elective procedure based on the presentation and symptoms of the patient. The operative tenets generally include hernia reduction, repair of the diaphragmatic defect, and pleural drainage. Repair of delayed defects tend to be technically more challenging since the degree of adhesions present in the thoracic cavity tend to be greater and the herniated organs may be more difficult to reduce. A counter incision in the abdomen may be necessary for a complete repair of the diaphragm, or to affect complete reduction of the involved organs, or to ensure proper placement of the organs intra-abdominally when abdominal adhesions or loss of domain may be of issue. The repair of the diaphragmatic defect can usually be accomplished primarily with non-absorbable sutures. Occasionally, biologic and/or permanent mesh placement is necessary for repair of more complex injuries, especially for those chronic defects that have significantly enlarged over time.[268] Combined thoracoscopic and laparoscopic repair has been reported as feasible and effective.[286–288] However, Matthews and colleagues advocate that injuries near the esophageal hiatus are probably best repaired through an open approach.[289] This is largely due to the inability to laparoscopically safely suture-close a transverse diaphragmatic laceration longer than 10 cm anterior to the esophageal hiatus and adjacent to the pericardium. The morbidity and mortality of elective late diaphragmatic hernia repair is generally the same as that of any major operation, yet these risks may vary greatly depending on the anatomy of the hernia, the condition and the extent of the involved viscera, and the urgency of repair. The mortality from elective repair is low but the mortality from ischemic bowel secondary to strangulation may be as high as 80%.[290] Hegarty and colleagues corroborated this increased risk with a series of 25 patients that acutely presented with chronic hernias. Mortality exponentially increased from 20% to 80% among those who developed gangrene and perforation.[291] For this reason elective repair is advocated for most hernias once diagnosed even in the absence of symptoms.

EXTRACORPOREAL MEMBRANE OXYGENATION IN CHEST TRAUMA

Extracorporeal membrane oxygenation (ECMO) has only relatively recently been recognized as an important adjunct in treating patients who develop trauma-associated ARDS. Its benefits include the ability to rewarm, correct acid–base abnormalities, and provide oxygenation and circulatory support when necessary. Initially, ECMO was thought to be relatively contraindicated in cases of polytrauma due to uncontrollable hemorrhage from inaccessible organs. However, there is a growing body of literature to support the use of ECMO in selected trauma patients. Due to vast resource utilization and its ability to sustain life support almost indefinitely, institutions must carefully evaluate their indications and judiciously apply ECMO with a specific endpoint in mind. Attempted salvage of irreversibly severely brain-injured trauma victims should be avoided.

When applied appropriately, ECMO has been shown to be of benefit in both the adult and pediatric aged population.[292-294] The availability to place a patient on veno-venous (VV) ECMO via a single double-lumen cannula (Avalon®, Fa. Maquet, Rastatt, Germany) allows the removal of deoxygenated blood via one lumen with ends in the superior and inferior cava, followed by oxygenation of the blood which is then returned via a second lumen with the port positioned directly across from the tricuspid valve.[295] This essentially delivers preoxygenated blood to the lungs and allows for less aggressive ventilation techniques and lower ventilator pressures, which can promote healing. Such a cannula can be placed at the bedside utilizing transesophageal echocardiography and/or fluoroscopy to guide placement, usually via the right internal jugular vein. Doppler evaluation can help confirm return flow adjacent to the tricuspid valve, thereby minimizing the mixing of oxygenated and deoxygenated blood. The limitation of such a delivery technique is that it lacks support in providing cardiac contractility when primary pump failure is present. However, it does not require the placement of an arterial cannula and therefore has advantages in limiting the need for anticoagulation and potential additional bleeding sources in cases where primary pump failure is not an issue. In addition, the development of smaller, specialized ECMO systems can minimize or even obviate the need for anticoagulation and therefore lessen the potential for hemorrhagic complications.[296] When using heparin-coated cannulas, administering VV ECMO via the single-lumen technique, and utilizing lower systemic anticoagulation regimes, bleeding complications can usually be minimized and when bleeding complications do occur they can usually be treated conservatively. In a German study reviewing their ECMO database registry, Ried and colleagues reported on 26 trauma patients with a mean ISS score of 59 that received treatment with VV ECMO for a mean of 6 days and had an in-hospital mortality of 19%, which was only approximately one-third of the mortality expected from their ISS alone.[297] Obviously this is a very highly selected patient population and should rightly remain so given the vast resource allocation that ECMO demands. ECMO therapy has reportedly been used as rescue therapy even in the presence of coagulopathy and/or brain injury with potential worsening of intracranial bleeding. In a small series by Biderman et al., they reported maintaining high blood flow rates (4 to 5 L/min) to prevent clotting in patients who could not receive heparin. Although the number of

patients in their series was small, their survival rate was 60%.[298] This suggests that ECMO may be considered as potential rescue therapy even in patients with severe disseminated intravascular coagulation or active bleeding, so long as thoughtful hematologic algorithms are constructed and followed.[296,298] Although clear, evidence-based inclusion and exclusion criteria do not yet exist, the use of ECMO in highly selected individuals who develop trauma-associated ARDS appears to be of benefit.

REFERENCES

1. LoCicero J, Mattox KL. Epidemiology of chest trauma. *Surg Clin North Am* 1989; 69(1):15–19.
2. Shorr RM, Crittenden M, Indeck M, et al. Blunt thoracic trauma. Analysis of 515 patients. *Ann Surg* 1987;206(2):200–205.
3. Kulshrestha P, Munshi I, Wait R. Profile of chest trauma in a level I trauma center. *J Trauma* 2004;57(3):576–581.
4. American College of Surgeons. *Advanced Trauma Life Support for Doctors, Student Course Manual*. Chicago, IL: American College of Surgeons; 2004.
5. Schwab CW, Adcock OT, Max MH. Emergency department thoracotomy (EDT). A 26-month experience using an "agonal" protocol. *Am Surg* 1986;52(1):20–29.
6. Phelan HA, Patterson SG, Hassan MO, et al. Thoracic damage-control operation: principles, techniques, and definitive repair. *J Am Coll Surg* 2006;203(6):933–941.
7. Rhee PM, Acosta J, Bridgeman A, et al. Survival after emergency department thoracotomy: review of published data from the past 25 years. *J Am Coll Surg* 2000;190(3):288–298.
8. Hopson LR, Hirsh E, Delgado J, et al. Guidelines for withholding or termination of resuscitation in prehospital traumatic cardiopulmonary arrest: joint position statement of the National Association of EMS Physicians and the American College of Surgeons Committee on Trauma. *J Am Coll Surg* 2003;196(1):106–112.
9. Mollberg NM, Glenn C, John J, et al. Appropriate use of emergency department thoracotomy: implications for the thoracic surgeon. *Ann Thorac Surg* 2011;92(2): 455–461.
10. Martin SK, Shatney CH, Sherck JP, et al. Blunt trauma patients with prehospital pulseless electrical activity (PEA): poor ending assured. *J Trauma* 2002;53(5): 876–880; discussion 880–881.
11. Sersar SI, Alanwar MA. Emergency thoracotomies: two center study. *J Emerg Trauma Shock* 2013;6(1):11–15.
12. Moore AV, Putnam CE, Ravin CE. The radiology of thoracic trauma. *Bull N Y Acad Med* 1981;57(4):272–292.
13. Roxburgh JC. Rupture of the tracheobronchial tree. *Thorax* 1987;42(9):681–688.
14. Angood PB, Attia EL, Brown RA, et al. Extrinsic civilian trauma to the larynx and cervical trachea—important predictors of long-term morbidity. *J Trauma* 1986; 26(10):869–873.
15. De La Rocha AG, Kayler D. Traumatic rupture of the tracheobronchial tree. *Can J Surg* 1985;28(1):68–71.
16. Gómez-Caro Andrés A, Moradiellos Díez FJ, Ausín Herrero P, et al. Successful conservative management in iatrogenic tracheobronchial injury. *Ann Thorac Surg* 2005;79(6):1872–1878.
17. Lee DK, Lim SH, Lim BG, et al. Management of traumatic pneumothorax with massive air leakage: role of a bronchial blocker: a case report. *Korean J Anesthesiol* 2014;67(5):354–357.
18. Chu CP, Chen PP. Tracheobronchial injury secondary to blunt chest trauma: diagnosis and management. *Anaesth Intensive Care* 2002;30(2):145–152.
19. Johnson SB. Tracheobronchial injury. *Semin Thorac Cardiovasc Surg* 2008;20(1): 52–57.
20. Branney SW, Moore EE, Cantrill SV, et al. Ultrasound based key clinical pathway reduces the use of hospital resources for the evaluation of blunt abdominal trauma. *J Trauma* 1997;42(6):1086–1090.
21. Gordic S, Alkadhi H, Hodel S, et al. Whole-body CT-based imaging algorithm for multiple trauma patients: radiation dose and time to diagnosis. *Br J Radiol* 2015;88(1047):20140616.
22. Schueller G, Scaglione M, Linsenmaier U, et al. The key role of the radiologist in the management of polytrauma patients: indications for MDCT imaging in emergency radiology. *Radiol Med* 2015;120(7):641–654.
23. Chardoli M, Hasan-Ghaliaee T, Akbari H, et al. Accuracy of chest radiography versus chest computed tomography in hemodynamically stable patients with blunt chest trauma. *Chin J Traumatol* 2013;16(6):351–354.
24. Rajasekaran S, Kanna RM, Shetty AP. Management of thoracolumbar spine trauma: an overview. *Indian J Orthop* 2015;49(1):72–82.
25. Khatri K, Farooque K, Gupta A, et al. Spinal cord injury without radiological abnormality in adult thoracic spinal trauma. *Arch Trauma Res* 2014;3(3):e19036.
26. Wisbach GG, Sise MJ, Sack DI, et al. What is the role of chest X-ray in the initial assessment of stable trauma patients? *J Trauma* 2007;62(1):74–78; discussion 78–79.
27. Ziegler K, Feeney JM, Desai C, et al. Retrospective review of the use and costs of routine chest x rays in a trauma setting. *J Trauma Manag Outcomes* 2013;7:2.
28. Deunk J, Dekker HM, Brink M. The value of indicated computed tomography scan of the chest and abdomen in addition to the conventional radiologic work-up for blunt trauma patients. *J Trauma* 2007;63(4):757–763.
29. Van Vugt R, Deunk J, Brink M, et al. Influence of routine computed tomography on predicted survival from blunt thoracoabdominal trauma. *Eur J Trauma Emerg Surg* 2011;37(2):185–190.

30. Huber-Wagner S, Biberthaler P, Häberle S, et al. Whole-body CT in haemodynamically unstable severely injured patients—a retrospective, multicentre study. *PloS One* 2013;8(7):e68880.

31. Gavant ML. Helical CT grading of traumatic aortic injuries. Impact on clinical guidelines for medical and surgical management. *Radiol Clin North Am* 1999;37(3):553–574, vi.

32. Patel NH, Stephens KE, Mirvis SE, et al. Imaging of acute thoracic aortic injury due to blunt trauma: a review. *Radiology* 1998;209(2):335–348.

33. Mirvis SE, Shanmuganathan K, Buell J, et al. Use of spiral computed tomography for the assessment of blunt trauma patients with potential aortic injury. *J Trauma* 1998;45(5):922–930.

34. Van Hise ML, Primack SL, Israel RS, et al. CT in blunt chest trauma: indications and limitations. *Radiographics* 1998;18(5):1071–1084.

35. Chen MY, Miller PR, McLaughlin CA, et al. The trend of using computed tomography in the detection of acute thoracic aortic and branch vessel injury after blunt thoracic trauma: single-center experience over 13 years. *J Trauma* 2004;56(4):783–785.

36. Wong H, Gotway MB, Sasson AD, et al. Periaortic hematoma at diaphragmatic crura at helical CT: sign of blunt aortic injury in patients with mediastinal hematoma. *Radiology* 2004;231(1):185–189.

37. Cho SH, Kim EY, Choi SJ, et al. Multidetector CT and radiographic findings of lung injuries secondary to cardiopulmonary resuscitation. *Injury* 2013;44(9):1204–1207.

38. Wang S, Ruan Z, Zhang J, et al. The value of pulmonary contusion volume measurement with three-dimensional computed tomography in predicting acute respiratory distress syndrome development. *Ann Thorac Surg* 2011;92(6):1977–1983.

39. De Moya MA, Manolakaki D, Chang Y, et al. Blunt pulmonary contusion: admission computed tomography scan predicts mechanical ventilation. *J Trauma* 2011;71(6):1543–1547.

40. Strumwasser A, Chu E, Yeung L, et al. A novel CT volume index score correlates with outcomes in polytrauma patients with pulmonary contusion. *J Surg Res* 2011;170(2):280–285.

41. Kehdy F, Richardson JD. The utility of 3-D CT scan in the diagnosis and evaluation of sternal fractures. *J Trauma* 2006;60(3):635–636.

42. Bodanapally UK, Shanmuganathan K, Mirvis SE, et al. MDCT diagnosis of penetrating diaphragm injury. *Eur Radiol* 2009;19(8):1875–1881.

43. Stein DM, York GB, Boswell S, et al. Accuracy of computed tomography (CT) scan in the detection of penetrating diaphragm injury. *J Trauma* 2007;63(3):538–543.

44. Hilbert P, zur Nieden K, Hofmann GO, et al. New aspects in the emergency room management of critically injured patients: a multi-slice CT-oriented care algorithm. *Injury* 2007;38(5):552–558.

45. Błasińska-Przerwa K, Pacho R, Bestry I. The application of MDCT in the diagnosis of chest trauma. *Pneumonol Alergol Pol* 2013;81(6):518–526.

46. Wilkerson RG, Stone MB. Sensitivity of bedside ultrasound and supine anteroposterior chest radiographs for the identification of pneumothorax after blunt trauma. *Acad Emerg Med* 2010;17(1):11–17.

47. Lichtenstein D, van Hooland S, Elbers P, et al. Ten good reasons to practice ultrasound in critical care. *Anaesthesiol Intensive Ther* 2014;46(5):323–335.

48. Kline JP, Dionisio D, Sullivan K, et al. Detection of pneumothorax with ultrasound. *AANA J* 2013;81(4):265–271.

49. Culp BC, Mock JD, Chiles CD, et al. The pocket echocardiograph: validation and feasibility. *Echocardiography* 2010;27(7):759–764.

50. Esmaeilzadeh M, Alimi H, Maleki M, et al. Aortic valve injury following blunt chest trauma. *Res Cardiovasc Med* 2014;3(3):e17319.

51. Ortiz Y, Waldman AJ, Bott JN, et al. Blunt chest trauma resulting in both atrial and ventricular septal defects. *Echocardiography* 2015;32(3):592–594.

52. Lopez-Sendon J, Garcia-Fernandez MA, Coma-Canella I, et al. Identification of blood in the pericardial cavity in dogs by two-dimensional echocardiography. *Am J Cardiol* 1984;53(8):1194–1197.

53. Plummer D, Brunette D, Asinger R, et al. Emergency department echocardiography improves outcome in penetrating cardiac injury. *Ann Emerg Med* 1992;21(6):709–712.

54. Meyer DM, Jessen ME, Grayburn PA. Use of echocardiography to detect occult cardiac injury after penetrating thoracic trauma: a prospective study. *J Trauma* 1995;39(5):902–907; discussion 907–909.

55. Ferrada P, Wolfe L, Anand RJ, et al. Use of limited transthoracic echocardiography in patients with traumatic cardiac arrest decreases the rate of nontherapeutic thoracotomy and hospital costs. *J Ultrasound Med* 2014;33(10):1829–1832.

56. Petkov MP, Napolitano CA, Tobler HG, et al. A rupture of both atrioventricular valves after blunt chest trauma: the usefulness of transesophageal echocardiography for a life-saving diagnosis. *Anesth Analg* 2005;100(5):1256–1258, table of contents.

57. Peterson D, Arntfield RT. Critical care ultrasonography. *Emerg Med Clin North Am* 2014;32(4):907–926.

58. Rossbach MM, Johnson SB, Gomez MA, et al. Management of major tracheobronchial injuries: a 28-year experience. *Ann Thorac Surg* 1998;65(1):182–186.

59. Inoue H, Shohtsu A, Ogawa J, et al. Endotracheal tube with movable blocker to prevent aspiration of intratracheal bleeding. *Ann Thorac Surg* 1984;37(6):497–499.

60. Hara KS, Prakash UB. Fiberoptic bronchoscopy in the evaluation of acute chest and upper airway trauma. *Chest* 1989;96(3):627–630.

61. Jackson AM, Ferreira AA. Thoracoscopy as an aid to the diagnosis of diaphragmatic injury in penetrating wounds of the left lower chest: a preliminary report. *Injury* 1976;7(3):213–217.

62. Jones JW, Kitahama A, Webb WR, et al. Emergency thoracoscopy: a logical approach to chest trauma management. *J Trauma* 1981;21(4):280–284.

63. Martins Castello Branco J. Thoracoscopy as a method of exploration in penetrating injuries of the thorax. *Dis Chest* 1946;12:330–335.

64. Ochsner MG, Rozycki GS, Lucente F, et al. Prospective evaluation of thoracoscopy for diagnosing diaphragmatic injury in thoracoabdominal trauma: a preliminary report. *J Trauma* 1993;34(5):704–709; discussion 709–710.

65. Wu N, Wu L, Qiu C, et al. A comparison of video-assisted thoracoscopic surgery with open thoracotomy for the management of chest trauma: a systematic review and meta-analysis. *World J Surg* 2015;39(4):940–952.

66. Billeter AT, Druen D, Franklin GA, et al. Video-assisted thoracoscopy as an important tool for trauma surgeons: a systematic review. *Langenbecks Arch Surg* 2013;398(4):515–523.

67. Smith JW, Franklin GA, Harbrecht BG, et al. Early VATS for blunt chest trauma: a management technique underutilized by acute care surgeons. *J Trauma* 2011;71(1):102–105; discussion 105–107.

68. Kriel RL, Gormley ME, Krach LE, et al. Automatic garage door openers: hazard for children. *Pediatrics* 1996;98(4 Pt 1):770–773.

69. Pramanik P. Elder homicide by unique combination of different mechanisms of asphyxia. *Int J Appl Basic Med Res* 2015;5(1):61–64.

70. Montes-Tapia F, Barreto-Arroyo I, Cura-Esquivel I, et al. Traumatic asphyxia. *Pediatr Emerg Care* 2014;30(2):114–116.

71. El koraichi A, Benafitou R, Tadili J, et al. [Traumatic asphyxia or Perthe's syndrome. About two paediatric cases]. *Ann Fr Anesth Rèanim* 2012;31(3):259–261.

72. Senoglu M, Senoglu N, Oksuz H, et al. Perthes syndrome associated with intramedullary spinal cord hemorrhage in a 4-year-old child: a case report. *Cases J* 2008;1(1):17.

73. Lee MC, Wong SS, Chu JJ, et al. Traumatic asphyxia. *Ann Thorac Surg* 1991;51(1):86–88.

74. Landercasper J, Cogbill TH. Long-term followup after traumatic asphyxia. *J Trauma* 1985;25(9):838–841.

75. Sassoon CS, Light RW, O'Hara VS, et al. Iatrogenic pneumothorax. etiology and morbidity. Results of a Department of Veterans Affairs Cooperative Study. *Respir Int Rev Thorac Dis* 1992;59(4):215–220.

76. Despars JA, Sassoon CS, Light RW. Significance of iatrogenic pneumothoraces. *Chest* 1994;105(4):1147–1150.

77. Sharma A, Jindal P. Principles of diagnosis and management of traumatic pneumothorax. *J Emerg Trauma Shock* 2008;1:34–41.

78. Roberts DJ, Leigh-Smith S, Faris PD, et al. Clinical presentation of patients with tension pneumothorax: a systematic review. *Ann Surg* 2015;261(6):1068–1078.

79. Sisley AC, Rozycki GS, Ballard RB, et al. Rapid detection of traumatic effusion using surgeon-performed ultrasonography. *J Trauma* 1998;44(2):291–296; discussion 296–297.

80. Rozycki GS, Pennington SD, Feliciano DV. Surgeon-performed ultrasound in the critical care setting: its use as an extension of the physical examination to detect pleural effusion. *J Trauma* 2001;50(4):636–642.

81. Ma OJ, Mateer JR. Trauma ultrasound examination versus chest radiography in the detection of hemothorax. *Ann Emerg Med* 1997;29(3):312–315; discussion 315–316.

82. Brink M, Kool DR, Dekker HM, et al. Predictors of abnormal chest CT after blunt trauma: a critical appraisal of the literature. *Clin Radiol* 2009;64(3):272–283.

83. Inaba K, Lustenberger T, Recinos G, et al. Does size matter? A prospective analysis of 28-32 versus 36-40 French chest tube size in trauma. *J Trauma Acute Care Surg* 2012;72(2):422–427.

84. Sherwood SF, Hartsock RL. *Trauma Nursing from Resuscitation Through Rehabilitation.* 3rd ed. Philadelphia, PA: Saunders; 2002:543–590.

85. Coselli JS, Mattox KL, Beall AC. Reevaluation of early evacuation of clotted hemothorax. *Am J Surg* 1984;148(6):786–790.

86. DuBose J, Inaba K, Demetriades D, et al. Management of post-traumatic retained hemothorax: a prospective, observational, multicenter AAST study. *J Trauma Acute Care Surg* 2012;72(1):11–22; discussion 22–24; quiz 316.

87. DuBose J, Inaba K, Okoye O, et al. Development of posttraumatic empyema in patients with retained hemothorax: results of a prospective, observational AAST study. *J Trauma Acute Care Surg* 2012;73(2):752–757.

88. Karmy-Jones R, Holevar M, Sullivan RJ, et al. Residual hemothorax after chest tube placement correlates with increased risk of empyema following traumatic injury. *Can Respir J* 2008;15(5):255–258.

89. Flagel BT, Luchette FA, Reed RL, et al. Half-a-dozen ribs: the breakpoint for mortality. *Surgery* 2005;138(4):717–723; discussion 723–725.

90. Bulger EM, Edwards T, Klotz P, et al. Epidural analgesia improves outcome after multiple rib fractures. *Surgery* 2004;136(2):426–430.

91. Carrier FM, Turgeon AF, Nicole PC, et al. Effect of epidural analgesia in patients with traumatic rib fractures: a systematic review and meta-analysis of randomized controlled trials. *Can J Anaesth* 2009;56(3):230–242.

92. Gage A, Rivara F, Wang J, et al. The effect of epidural placement in patients after blunt thoracic trauma. *J Trauma Acute Care Surg* 2014;76(1):39–45; discussion 45–46.

93. Wisner DH. A stepwise logistic regression analysis of factors affecting morbidity and mortality after thoracic trauma: effect of epidural analgesia. *J Trauma* 1990;30(7):799–804; discussion 804–805.

94. Mackersie RC, Karagianes TG, Hoyt DB, et al. Prospective evaluation of epidural and intravenous administration of fentanyl for pain control and restoration of ventilatory function following multiple rib fractures. *J Trauma* 1991;31(4):443–449; discussion 449–451.

95. Luchette FA, Radafshar SM, Kaiser R, et al. Prospective evaluation of epidural versus intrapleural catheters for analgesia in chest wall trauma. *J Trauma* 1994;36(6):865–869; discussion 869–870.

96. Truitt MS, Murry J, Amos J, et al. Continuous intercostal nerve blockade for rib fractures: ready for primetime? *J Trauma* 2011;71(6):1548–1552; discussion 1552.

97. Barsness KA, Cha ES, Bensard DD, et al. The positive predictive value of rib fractures as an indicator of nonaccidental trauma in children. *J Trauma* 2003; 54(6):1107–1110.

98. Maguire S, Mann M, John N, et al. Does cardiopulmonary resuscitation cause rib fractures in children? A systematic review. *Child Abuse Negl* 2006;30(7):739–751.

99. Holcomb JB, McMullin NR, Kozar RA, et al. Morbidity from rib fractures increases after age 45. *J Am Coll Surg* 2003;196(4):549–555.

100. Bulger EM, Arneson MA, Mock CN, et al. Rib fractures in the elderly. *J Trauma* 2000;48(6):1040–1046; discussion 1046–1047.

101. Battle CE, Hutchings H, Evans PA. Risk factors that predict mortality in patients with blunt chest wall trauma: a systematic review and meta-analysis. *Injury* 2012;43(1):8–17.

102. Huber S, Biberthaler P, Delhey P, et al. Predictors of poor outcomes after significant chest trauma in multiply injured patients: a retrospective analysis from the German Trauma Registry (Trauma Register DGU®). *Scand J Trauma Resusc Emerg Med* 2014;22(1):52.

103. Gupta A, Jamshidi M, Rubin JR. Traumatic first rib fracture: Is angiography necessary? A review of 730 cases. *Cardiovasc Surg Lond Engl* 1997;5(1):48–53.

104. Khosla A, Ocel J, Rad AE, et al. Correlating first- and second-rib fractures noted on spine computed tomography with major vessel injury. *Emerg Radiol* 2010;17(6):461–464.

105. Kanchan T, Menezes RG, Sirohi P. Penetrating cardiac injuries in blunt chest wall trauma. *J Forensic Leg Med* 2012;19(6):350–351.

106. Park HS, Ryu SM, Cho SJ, et al. A treatment case of delayed aortic injury: the patient with posterior rib fracture. *Korean J Thorac Cardiovasc Surg* 2014;47(4):406–408.

107. Bruno VD, Batchelor TJP. Late aortic injury: a rare complication of a posterior rib fracture. *Ann Thorac Surg* 2009;87(1):301–303.

108. Sata S, Yoshida J, Nishida T, et al. Sharp rib fragment threatening to lacerate the aorta in a patient with flail chest. *Gen Thorac Cardiovasc Surg* 2007;55(6):252–254.

109. El Husseiny M, Karam L, Haddad F, et al. Perforation of the aorta by a rib edge: an unusual complication after chest wall resection. *Ann Vasc Surg* 2012;26(4):574.e15–e17.

110. Nakayama DK, Ramenofsky ML, Rowe MI. Chest injuries in childhood. *Ann Surg* 1989;210(6):770–775.

111. Balci AE, Eren S, Cakir O, et al. Open fixation in flail chest: review of 64 patients. *Asian Cardiovasc Thorac Ann* 2004;12(1):11–15.

112. Avery EE, Benson DW, Morch ET. Critically crushed chests; a new method of treatment with continuous mechanical hyperventilation to produce alkalotic apnea and internal pneumatic stabilization. *J Thorac Surg* 1956;32(3):291–311.

113. Dehghan N, de Mestral C, McKee MD, et al. Flail chest injuries: a review of outcomes and treatment practices from the National Trauma Data Bank. *J Trauma Acute Care Surg* 2014;76(2):462–468.

114. Pettiford BL, Luketich JD, Landreneau RJ. The management of flail chest. *Thorac Surg Clin* 2007;17(1):25–33.

115. Leinicke JA, Elmore L, Freeman BD, et al. Operative management of rib fractures in the setting of flail chest: a systematic review and meta-analysis. *Ann Surg* 2013;258(6):914–921.

116. Marasco SF, Davies AR, Cooper J, et al. Prospective randomized controlled trial of operative rib fixation in traumatic flail chest. *J Am Coll Surg* 2013;216(5):924–932.

117. Lardinois D, Krueger T, Dusmet M, et al. Pulmonary function testing after operative stabilisation of the chest wall for flail chest. *Eur J Cardiothorac Surg* 2001;20(3):496–501.

118. Tanaka H, Yukioka T, Yamaguti Y, et al. Surgical stabilization of internal pneumatic stabilization? A prospective randomized study of management of severe flail chest patients. *J Trauma* 2002;52(4):727–732; discussion 732.

119. Bhatnagar A, Mayberry J, Nirula R. Rib fracture fixation for flail chest: what is the benefit? *J Am Coll Surg* 2012;215(2):201–205.

120. Mayberry JC, Ham LB, Schipper PH, et al. Surveyed opinion of American trauma, orthopedic, and thoracic surgeons on rib and sternal fracture repair. *J Trauma* 2009;66(3):875–879.

121. Richardson JD, Franklin GA, Heffley S, et al. Operative fixation of chest wall fractures: an underused procedure? *Am Surg* 2007;73(6):591–597.

122. Kerr-Valentic MA, Arthur M, Mullins RJ, et al. Rib fracture pain and disability: can we do better? *J Trauma* 2003;54(6):1058–1063; discussion 1063–1064.

123. Beal SL, Oreskovich MR. Long-term disability associated with flail chest injury. *Am J Surg* 1985;150(3):324–326.

124. Landercasper J, Cogbill TH, Lindesmith LA. Long-term disability after flail chest injury. *J Trauma* 1984;24(5):410–414.

125. Cohn SM, Dubose JJ. Pulmonary contusion: an update on recent advances in clinical management. *World J Surg* 2010;34(8):1959–1970.

126. Toombs BD, Sandler CM, Lester RG. Computed tomography of chest trauma. *Radiology* 1981;140(3):733–738.

127. Shin B, McAslan TC, Hankins JR, et al. Management of lung contusion. *Am Surg* 1979;45(3):168–175.

128. Schild HH, Strunk H, Weber W, et al. Pulmonary contusion: CT vs plain radiograms. *J Comput Assist Tomogr* 1989;13(3):417–420.

129. Hankins JR, Attar S, Turney SZ, et al. Differential diagnosis of pulmonary parenchymal changes in thoracic trauma. *Am Surg* 1973;39(6):309–318.

130. Miller PR, Croce MA, Bee TK, et al. ARDS after pulmonary contusion: accurate measurement of contusion volume identifies high-risk patients. *J Trauma* 2001; 51(2):223–228; discussion 229–230.

131. Tyburski JG, Collinge JD, Wilson RF, et al. Pulmonary contusions: quantifying the lesions on chest X-ray films and the factors affecting prognosis. *J Trauma* 1999;46(5):833–838.

132. Wagner RB, Jamieson PM. Pulmonary contusion. Evaluation and classification by computed tomography. *Surg Clin North Am* 1989;69(1):31–40.

133. Voggenreiter G, Neudeck F, Aufmkolk M, et al. Intermittent prone positioning in the treatment of severe and moderate posttraumatic lung injury. *Crit Care Med* 1999;27(11):2375–2382.

134. Trinkle JK, Furman RW, Hinshaw MA, et al. Pulmonary contusion. Pathogenesis and effect of various resuscitative measures. *Ann Thorac Surg* 1973;16(6):568–573.

135. Senanayake EL, Poon H, Graham TR, et al. UK specialist cardiothoracic management of thoracic injuries in military casualties sustained in the wars in Iraq and Afghanistan. *Eur J Cardiothorac Surg* 2014;45(6):e202–e207.

136. Kishikawa M, Yoshioka T, Shimazu T, et al. Pulmonary contusion causes long-term respiratory dysfunction with decreased functional residual capacity. *J Trauma* 1991;31(9):1203–1208; discussion 1208–1210.

137. Watkins R, Watkins R, Williams L, et al. Stability provided by the sternum and rib cage in the thoracic spine. *Spine* 2005;30(11):1283–1286.

138. Recinos G, Inaba K, Dubose J, et al. Epidemiology of sternal fractures. *Am Surg* 2009;75(5):401–404.

139. Lederer W, Mair D, Rabl W, et al. Frequency of rib and sternum fractures associated with out-of-hospital cardiopulmonary resuscitation is underestimated by conventional chest X-ray. *Resuscitation* 2004;60(2):157–162.

140. Black CJ, Busuttil A, Robertson C. Chest wall injuries following cardiopulmonary resuscitation. *Resuscitation* 2004;63(3):339–343.

141. Oyetunji TA, Jackson HT, Obirieze AC, et al. Associated injuries in traumatic sternal fractures: a review of the National Trauma Data Bank. *Am Surg* 2013; 79(7):702–705.

142. Traub M, Stevenson M, McEvoy S, et al. The use of chest computed tomography versus chest X-ray in patients with major blunt trauma. *Injury* 2007;38(1):43–47.

143. Collins J. Chest wall trauma. *J Thorac Imaging* 2000;15(2):112–119.

144. Restrepo CS, Martinez S, Lemos DF, et al. Imaging appearances of the sternum and sternoclavicular joints. *Radiographics* 2009;29(3):839–859.

145. Aslam M, Rajesh A, Entwisle J, et al. Pictorial review: MRI of the sternum and sternoclavicular joints. *Br J Radiol* 2002;75(895):627–634.

146. Hills MW, Delprado AM, Deane SA. Sternal fractures: associated injuries and management. *J Trauma* 1993;35(1):55–60.

147. Knobloch K, Wagner S, Haasper C, et al. Sternal fractures occur most often in old cars to seat-belted drivers without any airbag often with concomitant spinal injuries: clinical findings and technical collision variables among 42,055 crash victims. *Ann Thorac Surg* 2006;82(2):444–450.

148. Buckman R, Trooskin SZ, Flancbaum L, et al. The significance of stable patients with sternal fractures. *Surg Gynecol Obstet* 1987;164(3):261–265.

149. Scheyerer MJ, Zimmermann SM, Bouaicha S, et al. Location of sternal fractures as a possible marker for associated injuries. *Emerg Med Int* 2013;2013:7. Article ID 407589.

150. Von Garrel T, Ince A, Junge A, et al. The sternal fracture: radiographic analysis of 200 fractures with special reference to concomitant injuries. *J Trauma* 2004; 57(4):837–844.

151. Sadaba JR, Oswal D, Munsch CM. Management of isolated sternal fractures: determining the risk of blunt cardiac injury. *Ann R Coll Surg Engl* 2000;82(3):162–166.

152. Yilmaz EN, van Heek NT, van der Spoel JI, et al. Myocardial contusion as result of isolated sternal fractures: a fact or a myth? *Eur J Emerg Med* 1999;6(4):293–295.

153. Celik S, Celik M, Aydemir B, et al. Long-term results of diaphragmatic plication in adults with unilateral diaphragm paralysis. *J Cardiothorac Surg* 2010;5:111.

154. Wright SW. Myth of the dangerous sternal fracture. *Ann Emerg Med* 1993;22(10):1589–1592.

155. Karangelis D, Bouliaris K, Koufakis T, et al. Management of isolated sternal fractures using a practical algorithm. *J Emerg Trauma Shock* 2014;7(3):170–173.

156. Hossain M, Ramavath A, Kulangara J, et al. Current management of isolated sternal fractures in the UK: time for evidence based practice? A cross-sectional survey and review of literature. *Injury* 2010;41(5):495–498.

157. Khoriati AA, Rajakulasingam R, Shah R. Sternal fractures and their management. *J Emerg Trauma Shock* 2013;6(2):113–116.

158. Brookes JG, Dunn RJ, Rogers IR. Sternal fractures: a retrospective analysis of 272 cases. *J Trauma* 1993;35(1):46–54.

159. Hendrickson SC, Koger KE, Morea CJ, et al. Sternal plating for the treatment of sternal nonunion. *Ann Thorac Surg* 1996;62(2):512–518.

160. Athanassiadi K, Gerazounis M, Moustardas M, et al. Sternal fractures: retrospective analysis of 100 cases. *World J Surg* 2002;26(10):1243–1246.

161. Nishiumi N, Nakagawa T, Masuda R, et al. Endobronchial bleeding associated with blunt chest trauma treated by bronchial occlusion with a univent. *Ann Thorac Surg* 2008;85(1):245–250.

162. Nishiumi N, Maitani F, Tsurumi T, et al. Blunt chest trauma with deep pulmonary laceration. *Ann Thorac Surg* 2001;71(1):314–318.

163. Nishiumi N, Inokuchi S, Oiwa K, et al. Diagnosis and treatment of deep pulmonary laceration with intrathoracic hemorrhage from blunt trauma. *Ann Thorac Surg* 2010;89(1):232–238.

164. Stewart KC, Urschel JD, Nakai SS, et al. Pulmonary resection for lung trauma. *Ann Thorac Surg* 1997;63(6):1587–1588.

165. Karmy-Jones R, Jurkovich GJ, Shatz DV, et al. Management of traumatic lung injury: a Western Trauma Association Multicenter review. *J Trauma* 2001;51(6):1049–1053.

166. Wall MJ, Villavicencio RT, Miller CC, et al. Pulmonary tractotomy as an abbreviated thoracotomy technique. *J Trauma* 1998;45(6):1015–1023.

167. Van Natta TL, Smith BR, Bricker SD, et al. Hilar control in penetrating chest trauma: a simplified approach to an underutilized maneuver. *J Trauma* 2009; 66(6):1564–1569.

168. Powell RJ, Redan JA, Swan KG. The hilar snare, and improved technique for securing rapid vascular control of the pulmonary hilum. *J Trauma* 1990;30(2):208–210.

169. Cothren C, Moore EE, Biffl WL, et al. Lung-sparing techniques are associated with improved outcome compared with anatomic resection for severe lung injuries. *J Trauma* 2002;53(3):483–487.

170. Petrone P, Asensio JA. Surgical management of penetrating pulmonary injuries. *Scand J Trauma Resusc Emerg Med* 2009;17:8.

171. Gasparri M, Karmy-Jones R, Kralovich KA, et al. Pulmonary tractotomy versus lung resection: viable options in penetrating lung injury. *J Trauma* 2001;51(6):1092–1095; discussion 1096–1097.

172. Velmahos GC, Baker C, Demetriades D, et al. Lung-sparing surgery after penetrating trauma using tractotomy, partial lobectomy, and pneumonorrhaphy. *Arch Surg* 1999;134(2):186–189.

173. Wall MJ, Hirshberg A, Mattox KL. Pulmonary tractotomy with selective vascular ligation for penetrating injuries to the lung. *Am J Surg* 1994;168(6):665–669.

174. Huh J, Wall MJ Jr, Estrera AL, et al. Surgical management of traumatic pulmonary injury. *Am J Surg* 2003;186(6):620–624.

175. Onat S, Ulku R, Avci A, et al. Urgent thoracotomy for penetrating chest trauma: analysis of 158 patients of a single center. *Injury* 2011;42(9):900–904.

176. Bowling R, Mavroudis C, Richardson JD, et al. Emergency pneumonectomy for penetrating and blunt trauma. *Am Surg* 1985;51(3):136–139.

177. Baumgartner F, Omari B, Lee J, et al. Survival after trauma pneumonectomy: the pathophysiologic balance of shock resuscitation with right heart failure. *Am Surg* 1996;62(11):967–972.

178. Martin MJ, McDonald JM, Mullenix PS, et al. Operative management and outcomes of traumatic lung resection. *J Am Coll Surg* 2006;203(3):336–344.

179. Matsumoto K, Noguchi T, Ishikawa R, et al. The surgical treatment of lung lacerations and major bronchial disruptions caused by blunt thoracic trauma. *Surg Today* 1998;28(2):162–166.

180. Wiencek RG, Wilson RF. Central lung injuries: a need for early vascular control. *J Trauma* 1988;28(10):1418–1424.

181. Richardson JD, Miller FB, Carrillo EH, et al. Complex thoracic injuries. *Surg Clin North Am* 1996;76(4):725–748.

182. Pardy BJ, Dudley HA. Post-traumatic pulmonary insufficiency. *Surg Gynecol Obstet* 1977;144(2):259–269.

183. Mathisen DJ, Kuo EY, Hahn C, et al. Inhaled nitric oxide for adult respiratory distress syndrome after pulmonary resection. *Ann Thorac Surg* 1998;66(6):1894–1902.

184. Rabkin DG, Sladen RN, DeMango A, et al. Nitric oxide for the treatment of postpneumonectomy pulmonary edema. *Ann Thorac Surg* 2001;72(1):272–274.

185. Thomas AN, Stephens BG. Air embolism: a cause of morbidity and death after penetrating chest trauma. *J Trauma* 1974;14(8):633–638.

186. Ho AM, Ling E. Systemic air embolism after lung trauma. *Anesthesiology* 1999; 90(2):564–575.

187. Ho AM. Is emergency thoracotomy always the most appropriate immediate intervention for systemic air embolism after lung trauma? *Chest* 1999;116(1):234–237.

188. Yee ES, Verrier ED, Thomas AN. Management of air embolism in blunt and penetrating thoracic trauma. *J Thorac Cardiovasc Surg* 1983;85(5):661–668.

189. Trunkey DD. Initial treatment of patients with extensive trauma. *N Engl J Med* 1991; 324(18):1259–1263.

190. Burke JF. Early diagnosis of traumatic rupture of the bronchus. *JAMA* 1962; 181:682–686.

191. Lynn RB, Iyengar K. Traumatic rupture of the bronchus. *Chest* 1972;61(1):81–83.

192. Kiser AC, O'Brien SM, Detterbeck FC. Blunt tracheobronchial injuries: treatment and outcomes. *Ann Thorac Surg* 2001;71(6):2059–2065.

193. Corneille MG, Stewart RM, Cohn SM. Upper airway injury and its management. *Semin Thorac Cardiovasc Surg* 2008;20(1):8–12.

194. Prokakis C, Koletsis EN, Dedeilias P, et al. Airway trauma: a review on epidemiology, mechanisms of injury, diagnosis and treatment. *J Cardiothorac Surg* 2014;9:117.

195. Gabor S, Renner H, Pinter H, et al. Indications for surgery in tracheobronchial ruptures. *Eur J Cardiothorac Surg* 2001;20(2):399–404.

196. Scaglione M, Romano S, Pinto A, et al. Acute tracheobronchial injuries: impact of imaging on diagnosis and management implications. *Eur J Radiol* 2006;59(3):336–343.

197. Faure A, Floccard B, Pilleul F, et al. Multiplanar reconstruction: a new method for the diagnosis of tracheobronchial rupture? *Intensive Care Med* 2007;33(12):2173–2178.

198. Welter S. Repair of tracheobronchial injuries. *Thorac Surg Clin* 2014;24(1):41–50.

199. Gómez-Caro A, Ausín P, Moradiellos FJ, et al. Role of conservative medical management of tracheobronchial injuries. *J Trauma* 2006;61(6):1426–1434; discussion 1434–1435.

200. Koletsis E, Prokakis C, Baltayiannis N, et al. Surgical decision making in tracheobronchial injuries on the basis of clinical evidences and the injury's anatomical setting: a retrospective analysis. *Injury* 2012;43(9):1437–1441.

201. Shaw RR, Paulson DL, Kee KL. Traumatic tracheal rupture. *J Thorac Cardiovasc Surg* 1961;(42):281–297.

202. Grover FL, Ellestad C, Arom KV, et al. Diagnosis and management of major tracheobronchial injuries. *Ann Thorac Surg* 1979;28(4):384–391.

203. Baumgartner F, Sheppard B, de Virgilio C, et al. Tracheal and main bronchial disruptions after blunt chest trauma: presentation and management. *Ann Thorac Surg* 1990;50(4):569–574.

204. Barmada H, Gibbons JR. Tracheobronchial injury in blunt and penetrating chest trauma. *Chest* 1994;106(1):74–78.

205. Taskinen SO, Salo JA, Halttunen PE, et al. Tracheobronchial rupture due to blunt chest trauma: a follow-up study. *Ann Thorac Surg* 1989;48(6):846–849.

206. Lyons JD, Feliciano DV, Wyrzykowski AD, et al. Modern management of penetrating tracheal injuries. *Am Surg* 2013;79(2):188–193.

207. Klapper J, Hirji S, Hartwig MG, et al. Outcomes after pneumonectomy for benign disease: the impact of urgent resection. *J Am Coll Surg* 2014;219(3):518–524.

208. Pate JW. Tracheobronchial and esophageal injuries. *Surg Clin North Am.* 1989; 69(1):111–123.

209. Grillo HC, Mathisen DJ, Wain JC. Laryngotracheal resection and reconstruction for subglottic stenosis. *Ann Thorac Surg* 1992;53(1):54–63.

210. Grillo HC. *Surgery of the Trachea and Bronchi.* Raleigh, NC: PMPH-USA; 2004. 912 p.

211. Grillo HC. Surgical anatomy of the trachea and techniques of resection. In: Shields TW, ed. *General Thoracic Surgery.* 5th ed. Philadelphia, PA: Lippincott Williams & Wilkins; 2000:873–883.

212. Karmy-Jones R, Wood DE. Traumatic injury to the trachea and bronchus. *Thorac Surg Clin* 2007;17(1):35–46.

213. Reece GP, Shatney CH. Blunt injuries of the cervical trachea: review of 51 patients. *South Med J* 1988;81(12):1542–1548.

214. Euathrongchit J, Thoongsuwan N, Stern EJ. Nonvascular mediastinal trauma. *Radiol Clin North Am* 2006;44(2):251–258, viii.

215. Balci AE, Eren N, Eren S, et al. Surgical treatment of post-traumatic tracheobronchial injuries: 14-year experience. *Eur J Cardiothorac Surg* 2002;22(6):984–989.

216. Schneider T, Volz K, Dienemann H, et al. Incidence and treatment modalities of tracheobronchial injuries in Germany. *Interact Cardiovasc Thorac Surg* 2009;8(5):571–576.

217. Carbognani P, Bobbio A, Cattelani L, et al. Management of postintubation membranous tracheal rupture. *Ann Thorac Surg* 2004;77(2):406–409.

218. Miñambres E, Burón J, Ballesteros MA, et al. Tracheal rupture after endotracheal intubation: a literature systematic review. *Eur J Cardiothorac Surg* 2009;35(6):1056–1062.

219. Chen EH, Logman ZM, Glass PS, et al. A case of tracheal injury after emergent endotracheal intubation: a review of the literature and causalities. *Anesth Analg* 2001;93(5):1270–1271, table of contents.

220. Evagelopoulos N, Tossios P, Wanke W, et al. Tracheobronchial rupture after emergency intubation. *Thorac Cardiovasc Surg* 1999;47(6):395–397.

221. Marty-Ané CH, Picard E, Jonquet O, et al. Membranous tracheal rupture after endotracheal intubation. *Ann Thorac Surg* 1995;60(5):1367–1371.

222. Wagner A, Roeggla M, Hirschl MM, et al. Tracheal rupture after emergency intubation during cardiopulmonary resuscitation. *Resuscitation* 1995;30(3):263–266.

223. Angelillo-Mackinlay T. Transcervical repair of distal membranous tracheal laceration. *Ann Thorac Surg* 1995;59(2):531–532.

224. Gupta V, Thingnam SK, Kuthe S, Verma GR. A novel surgical technique of repair of posterior wall laceration of thoracic trachea during transhiatal esophagectomy. *Interact Cardiovasc Thorac Surg* 2009;9(2):347–349.

225. Lancelin C, Chapelier AR, Fadel E, et al. Transcervical-transtracheal endoluminal repair of membranous tracheal disruptions. *Ann Thorac Surg* 2000;70(3):984–986.

226. Schneider T, Storz K, Dienemann H, et al. Management of iatrogenic tracheobronchial injuries: a retrospective analysis of 29 cases. *Ann Thorac Surg* 2007;83(6):1960–1964.

227. Armstrong CP, Van der Spuy J. The fractured scapula: importance and management based on a series of 62 patients. *Injury* 1984;15(5):324–329.

228. Veysi VT, Mittal R, Agarwal S, et al. Multiple trauma and scapula fractures: so what? *J Trauma* 2003;55(6):1145–1147.

229. Tadros AM, Lunsjo K, Czechowski J, et al. Multiple-region scapular fractures had more severe chest injury than single-region fractures: a prospective study of 107 blunt trauma patients. *J Trauma* 2007;63(4):889–893.

230. Jones CB, Sietsema DL. Analysis of operative versus nonoperative treatment of displaced scapular fractures. *Clin Orthop* 2011;469(12):3379–3389.

231. Cole PA, Freeman G, Dubin JR. Scapula fractures. *Curr Rev Musculoskelet Med* 2013;6(1):79–87.

232. Altamimi SA, McKee MD; Canadian Orthopaedic Trauma Society. Nonoperative treatment compared with plate fixation of displaced midshaft clavicular fractures. Surgical technique. *J Bone Joint Surg Am* 2008;90(Suppl 2 Pt 1):1–8.

233. Vander Have KL, Perdue AM, Caird MS, et al. Operative versus nonoperative treatment of midshaft clavicle fractures in adolescents. *J Pediatr Orthop* 2010;30(4):307–312.

234. Gilde AK, Hoffmann MF, Sietsema DL, et al. Functional outcomes of operative fixation of clavicle fractures in patients with floating shoulder girdle injuries. *J Orthop Traumatol* 2015;16(3):221–227.

235. Brucker PU, Gruen GS, Kaufmann RA. Scapulothoracic dissociation: evaluation and management. *Injury* 2005;36(10):1147–1155.

236. McCague A, Schulte A, Davis JV. Scapulothoracic dissociation: an emerging high-energy trauma in medical literature. *J Emerg Trauma Shock* 2012;5(4):363–366.

237. Althausen PL, Lee MA, Finkemeier CG. Scapulothoracic dissociation: diagnosis and treatment. *Clin Orthop* 2003;(416):237–244.

238. Nagi ON, Dhillon MS. Traumatic scapulothoracic dissociation. A case report. *Arch Orthop Trauma Surg* 1992;111(6):348–349.

239. Rubenstein JD, Ebraheim NA, Kellam JF. Traumatic scapulothoracic dissociation. *Radiology* 1985;157(2):297–298.

240. Damschen DD, Cogbill TH, Siegel MJ. Scapulothoracic dissociation caused by blunt trauma. *J Trauma* 1997;42(3):537–540.

241. Zelle BA, Pape HC, Gerich TG, et al. Functional outcome following scapulothoracic dissociation. *J Bone Joint Surg Am* 2004;86-A(1):2–8.

242. Matsevych OY. Blunt diaphragmatic rupture: four year's experience. *Hernia* 2008;12(1):73–78.

243. Clarke DL, Greatorex B, Oosthuizen GV, et al. The spectrum of diaphragmatic injury in a busy metropolitan surgical service. *Injury* 2009;40(9):932–937.

244. Hanna WC, Ferri LE, Fata P, et al. The current status of traumatic diaphragmatic injury: lessons learned from 105 patients over 13 years. *Ann Thorac Surg* 2008;85(3):1044–1048.

245. Simpson J, Lobo DN, Shah AB, et al. Traumatic diaphragmatic rupture: associated injuries and outcome. *Ann R Coll Surg Engl* 2000;82(2):97–100.

246. Beal SL, McKennan M. Blunt diaphragm rupture. A morbid injury. *Arch Surg* 1988;123(7):828–832.

247. Okada M, Adachi H, Kamesaki M, et al. Traumatic diaphragmatic injury: experience from a tertiary emergency medical center. *Gen Thorac Cardiovasc Surg* 2012;60(10):649–654.

248. Shah R, Sabanathan S, Mearns AJ, et al. Traumatic rupture of diaphragm. *Ann Thorac Surg* 1995;60(5):1444–1449.

249. Lee WC, Chen RJ, Fang JF, et al. Rupture of the diaphragm after blunt trauma. *Eur J Surg Acta Chir* 1994;160(9):479–483.

250. Tan KK, Yan ZY, Vijayan A, et al. Management of diaphragmatic rupture from blunt trauma. *Singapore Med J* 2009;50(12):1150–1153.

251. Walchalk LR, Stanfield SC. Delayed presentation of traumatic diaphragmatic rupture. *J Emerg Med* 2010;39(1):21–24.

252. Symbas PN, Vlasis SE, Hatcher C. Blunt and penetrating diaphragmatic injuries with or without herniation of organs into the chest. *Ann Thorac Surg* 1986;42(2):158–162.

253. Brown GL, Richardson JD. Traumatic diaphragmatic hernia: a continuing challenge. *Ann Thorac Surg* 1985;39(2):170–173.

254. Peer SM, Devaraddeppa PM, Buggi S. Traumatic diaphragmatic hernia—our experience. *Int J Surg Lond Engl* 2009;7(6):547–549.

255. Thillois JM, Tremblay B, Cerceau E, et al. Traumatic rupture of the right diaphragm. *Hernia* 1998;2(3):119–121.

256. Eren S, Kantarcı M, Okur A. Imaging of diaphragm rupture after trauma. *Clin Radiol* 2006;61(6):467–477.

257. Ammann AM, Brewer WH, Maull KI, et al. Traumatic rupture of the diaphragm: real-time sonographic diagnosis. *Am J Roentgenol* 1983;140(5):915–916.

258. Payne JH Jr, Yellin AE. Traumatic diaphragmatic hernia. *Arch Surg* 1982;117(1):18–24.

259. Waldschmidt ML, Laws HL. Injuries of the diaphragm. *J Trauma* 1980;20(7):587–592.

260. Gelman R, Mirvis SE, Gens D. Diaphragmatic rupture due to blunt trauma: sensitivity of plain chest radiographs. *Am J Roentgenol* 1991;156(1):51–57.

261. Sliker CW. Imaging of diaphragm injuries. *Radiol Clin North Am* 2006;44(2):199–211.

262. Heiberg E, Wolverson MK, Hurd RN, et al. CT recognition of traumatic rupture of the diaphragm. *Am J Roentgenol* 1980;135(2):369–372.

263. Killeen KL, Mirvis SE, Shanmuganathan K. Helical CT of diaphragmatic rupture caused by blunt trauma. *Am J Roentgenol* 1999;173(6):1611–1616.

264. Grant LA, Griffin N. *Grainger & Allison's Diagnostic Radiology Essentials*. Elsevier Health Sciences; 2013. 974.

265. Wataya H, Tsuruta N, Takayama K, et al. Delayed traumatic hernia diagnosed with magnetic resonance imaging. *Jpn J Thorac Dis* 1997;35(1):124–128.

266. Pace ME, Krebs TL. MR imaging of the thoracoabdominal junction. *Magn Reson Imaging Clin N Am* 2000;8(1):143–162.

267. Martin I, O'Rourke N, Gotley D, et al. Laparoscopy in the management of diaphragmatic rupture due to blunt trauma. *Aust N Z J Surg* 1998 Aug;68(8):584–586.

268. Ties JS, Peschman JR, Moreno A, et al. Evolution in the management of traumatic diaphragmatic injuries: a multicenter review. *J Trauma Acute Care Surg* 2014;76(4):1024–1028.

269. Mintz Y, Easter DW, Izhar U, et al. Minimally invasive procedures for diagnosis of traumatic right diaphragmatic tears: a method for correct diagnosis in selected patients. *Am Surg* 2007;73(4):388–392.

270. Ozpolat B, Kaya O, Yazkan R, et al. Diaphragmatic injuries: a surgical challenge. Report of forty-one cases. *Thorac Cardiovasc Surg* 2009;57(6):358–362.

271. Demetriades D, Kakoyiannis S, Parekh D, et al. Penetrating injuries of the diaphragm. *Br J Surg* 1988;75(8):824–826.

272. Wise L, Connors J, Hwang YH, et al. Traumatic injuries to the diaphragm. *J Trauma* 1973;13(11):946–950.

273. Miller L, Bennett EV, Root HD, et al. Management of penetrating and blunt diaphragmatic injury. *J Trauma* 1984;24(5):403–409.

274. Ivatury RR, Simon RJ, Weksler B, et al. Laparoscopy in the evaluation of the intrathoracic abdomen after penetrating injury. *J Trauma* 1992;33(1):101–108; discussion 109.

275. Powell BS, Magnotti LJ, Schroeppel TJ, et al. Diagnostic laparoscopy for the evaluation of occult diaphragmatic injury following penetrating thoracoabdominal trauma. *Injury* 2008;39(5):530–534.

276. Friese RS, Coln CE, Gentilello LM. Laparoscopy is sufficient to exclude occult diaphragm injury after penetrating abdominal trauma. *J Trauma* 2005;58(4):789–792.

277. Bagheri R, Tavassoli A, Sadrizadeh A, et al. The role of thoracoscopy for the diagnosis of hidden diaphragmatic injuries in penetrating thoracoabdominal trauma. *Interact Cardiovasc Thorac Surg* 2009;9(2):195–197; discussion 197–198.

278. Freeman RK, Al-Dossari G, Hutcheson KA, et al. Indications for using video-assisted thoracoscopic surgery to diagnose diaphragmatic injuries after penetrating chest trauma. *Ann Thorac Surg* 2001;72(2):342–347.

279. Martinez M, Briz JE, Carillo EH. Video thoracoscopy expedites the diagnosis and treatment of penetrating diaphragmatic injuries. *Surg Endosc* 2001;15(1):28–32; discussion 33.

280. Mouroux J, Venissac N, Leo F, et al. Surgical treatment of diaphragmatic eventration using video-assisted thoracic surgery: a prospective study. *Ann Thorac Surg* 2005;79(1):308–312.

281. Potaris K, Mihos P, Gakidis I. Role of video-assisted thoracic surgery in the evaluation and management of thoracic injuries. *Interact Cardiovasc Thorac Surg* 2005;4(4):292–294.

282. Dexter JC, Gold PM. Acute onset of dyspnea associated with colonoscopy. *J Am Med Assoc* 1980;244(11):1239–1240.

283. Goh BK, Wong AS, Tay KH, et al. Delayed presentation of a patient with a ruptured diaphragm complicated by gastric incarceration and perforation after apparently minor blunt trauma. *CJEM* 2004;6(4):277–280.

284. Shreck GL, Toalson TW. Delayed presentation of traumatic rupture of the diaphragm. *J Okla State Med Assoc* 2003;96(4):181–183.

285. Sirbu H, Busch T, Spillner J, et al. Late bilateral diaphragmatic rupture: challenging diagnostic and surgical repair. *Hernia* 2005;9(1):90–92.

286. Grushka J, Ginzburg E. Through the 10-mm looking glass: advances in minimally invasive surgery in trauma. *Scand J Surg* 2014;103(2):143–148.

287. Koehler RH, Smith RS. Thoracoscopic repair of missed diaphragmatic injury in penetrating trauma: case report. *J Trauma* 1994;36(3):424–427.

288. Baldassarre E, Valenti G, Gambino M, et al. The role of laparoscopy in the diagnosis and the treatment of missed diaphragmatic hernia after penetrating trauma. *J Laparoendosc Adv Surg Tech A* 2007;17(3):302–306.

289. Matthews BD, Bui H, Harold KL, et al. Laparoscopic repair of traumatic diaphragmatic injuries. *Surg Endosc* 2003;17(2):254–258.

290. Christie DB, Chapman J, Wynne JL, et al. Delayed right-sided diaphragmatic rupture and chronic herniation of unusual abdominal contents. *J Am Coll Surg* 2007;204(1):176.

291. Hegarty MM, Bryer JV, Angorn IB, et al. Delayed presentation of traumatic diaphragmatic hernia. *Ann Surg* 1978;188(2):229–233.

292. Cordell-Smith JA, Roberts N, Peek GJ, et al. Traumatic lung injury treated by extracorporeal membrane oxygenation (ECMO). *Injury* 2006;37(1):29–32.

293. Fortenberry JD, Meier AH, Pettignano R, et al. Extracorporeal life support for posttraumatic acute respiratory distress syndrome at a children's medical center. *J Pediatr Surg* 2003;38(8):1221–1226.

294. Wu SC, Chen WT, Lin HH, et al. Use of extracorporeal membrane oxygenation in severe traumatic lung injury with respiratory failure. *Am J Emerg Med* 2015;33(5):658–662.

295. Gothner M, Buchwald D, Strauch JT, et al. The use of double lumen cannula for veno-venous ECMO in trauma patients with ARDS. *Scand J Trauma Resusc Emerg Med* 2015;23:30.

296. Arlt M, Philipp A, Voelkel S, et al. Extracorporeal membrane oxygenation in severe trauma patients with bleeding shock. *Resuscitation* 2010;81(7):804–809.

297. Ried M, Bein T, Philipp A, et al. Extracorporeal lung support in trauma patients with severe chest injury and acute lung failure: a 10-year institutional experience. *Crit Care Lond Engl* 2013;17(3):R110.

298. Biderman P, Einav S, Fainblut M, et al. Extracorporeal life support in patients with multiple injuries and severe respiratory failure: a single-center experience? *J Trauma Acute Care Surg* 2013;75(5):907–912.

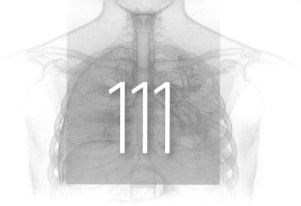

Barotrauma and Inhalation Injuries

Brittany A. Zwischenberger ■ Joseph B. Zwischenberger

Barotrauma, in general, indicates damage to the alveoli due to increased alveolar pressure or overinflation. Barotrauma can present in nonmechanically ventilated patients, such as deep-sea divers, or in mechanically ventilated patients, which contributes to ventilator-induced lung injury (VILI).

Inhalation injury can occur due to aspiration, smoke, caustic inhalants, near drowning, inflammation, infection, airway obstruction, hyperexpansion, or external compressive forces, to name common causes.

Both barotrauma and inhalation injury lead to parenchymal damage, inflammation, and transudation or leakage of fluid that causes decreased gas exchange and pulmonary compliance.

BAROTRAUMA

INTRODUCTION

Barotrauma is damage caused by a difference in pressure between a gas space and the surrounding fluid and body tissue. Barotrauma can present in individuals who experience a sudden change in alveolar pressure as experienced when diving or sudden pressure changes in flight as with airplane aerobatic maneuvers. Barotrauma was historically also used to describe the deleterious effects of positive pressure mechanical ventilation on normal lungs. The more appropriate term, ventilator-induced lung injury (VILI), represents the changes to the alveoli, specifically endothelial and epithelial permeability and inflammation due to positive pressure ventilation on alveoli.[1] VILI is the end result of barotrauma (pressure), volutrauma (hyperexpansion), biotrauma (inflammation), and atelectrauma (atelectasis). Positive pressure ventilation can lead to a decrease in lung compliance and dysfunction of gas exchange, which may accelerate the development or progression of adult respiratory distress syndrome (ARDS). This chapter will focus on the pathogenesis, clinical manifestations, and management of VILI.

NONMECHANICALLY VENTILATED BAROTRAUMA

Briefly, barotrauma in normally (nonmechanically) ventilated individuals, such as divers, is due to Boyle Law, which states that volume and pressure are inversely related in a fixed mass of an ideal gas at constant temperature. For example, as divers encounter increased pressure at greater depths, gas volume is reduced and alveoli are compressed, which can result in capillary damage.[2] Likewise, high alveolar pressure can force gas into the pulmonary capillaries and

generate gaseous emboli. Conversely, as a diver ascends, atmospheric pressure decreases, and the gas volume in the alveoli increases. If patients do not exhale adequately or air-trapping occurs, alveoli will overexpand and rupture or again cause capillary damage. Treatment of barotrauma in nonmechanically ventilated patients is emergent recompression in a hyperbaric oxygen chamber to rebalance the gas and tissue forces.

VILI: EARLY YEARS

Artificial respiration is described as early as 177 A.D., and the potentially deleterious effects of positive pressure ventilation was noted in the 1700s.[3] The description of VILI began in 1939 when Macklin demonstrated that a sudden increase in alveolar pressure may result in a gradient sufficient to disrupt the alveolar wall. The rupture occurs at the junction of the alveolar wall and vascular sheath, and air dissects along the loose connective tissues of the bronchovascular sheath into the pleural or peritoneal spaces or mediastinum and subcutaneous tissue.[4,5] The clinical presentations of pneumothorax, pneumomediastinum, subcutaneous emphysema, and pneumoperitoneum are the end results of the ruptured alveoli and resulting air leakage. Fowler[6] first reported uneven distribution of ventilation in both normal subjects and patients with underlying lung disease. Mead et al.[7] proposed a theoretical model describing the interdependence of alveoli; the pressure exerted on adjacent expanded and collapsed alveoli can lead to excessively high transpulmonary pressures. Later, Greenfield et al.[8] demonstrated surfactant dysfunction due to positive pressure ventilation in a canine model. Finally, Gattinoni et al.[9] introduced the concept of "baby lungs" to describe the decreased functioning alveoli participating in gas exchange in lungs with decreased compliance and atelectasis. The subsequent explosion of studies on what we call VILI today is an elegant story of bench to bedside.

SEMINAL BENCH STUDIES ON VILI

"Respirator lung" was initially believed to be a product of barotrauma. But as the story evolved through bench research, additional injuries caused by positive pressure ventilation became apparent. Volutrauma, atelectrauma, and eventually biotrauma surfaced as our understanding of VILI improved,[10] as depicted in Figure 111.1.

Webb and Tierney[11] demonstrated that positive pressure ventilation produced more injury than just air leaks. Rats with normal lungs were ventilated with peak inspiratory pressure (PIP) of 14, 30, or 45 cm H_2O without pulmonary end-expiratory pressure (PEEP) and then PIP of 30 or 45 cm H_2O with PEEP of 10 cm H_2O. Ventilation

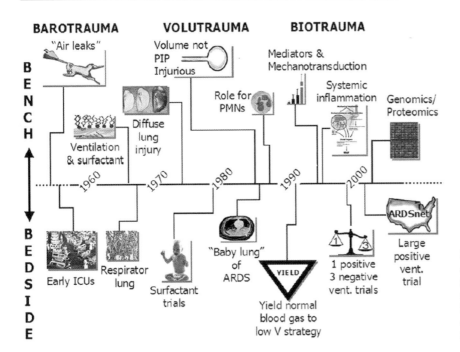

FIGURE 111.1 Time line of important basic science and clinical observations influencing our understanding and of ventilator-induced lung injury and the resulting changes in ventilator support over the years. (From Tremblay LN and Slutsky AS. Ventilator-induced lung injury: From the bench to the bedside. *Intensive Care Med* 2006;32:24–33.)

with high pressures (30 or 45 cm H_2O) produced perivascular edema, and ventilation at higher airway pressures (>45 cm H_2O) without PEEP led to severe lung injury (gross pulmonary edema, severe hypoxia) and death within 35 minutes. PIP of 14 cm H_2O was associated with minimal injury. Finally, PEEP offered protection from alveolar edema in high inspiratory pressure ventilation. Webb and Tierney discussed concerns for "overdistension" of inflated alveoli and reported their shift in management of ventilated patients to avoid high inspiratory pressure and focus on low frequency ventilation with PEEP.

Dreyfuss et al.[12] delineated the role of volutrauma in VILI by modifying ventilator parameters in rats wearing a thoracoabdominal binder to limit chest wall excursion. Rats receiving high tidal volume ventilation, regardless of airway pressure, developed severe lung injury with pulmonary edema, increased alveolar-capillary permeability, and structural changes. Conversely, ventilation with lower tidal volumes, regardless of airway pressure, does not develop ultrastructural changes or signs of alveolar edema or hemorrhage. This study represented a shift in focus from barotrauma (injury due to airway pressure) to volutrauma (injury due to lung volume).

Atelectrauma was highlighted by Muscedere et al.[13] in their study on the role of PEEP in injured rat lungs. The authors ventilated rat lungs with low tidal volumes (5 to 6 mL/kg) with PEEP both above and below the inflection point from the inspiratory pressure–volume curve. Compliance fell dramatically in lungs ventilated with PEEP below the inflection point. The authors concluded that ventilation with PEEP below the inflection point could lead to distal airway collapse and reduced lung compliance. Therefore, the repetitive opening and collapse of alveoli due to insufficient end-expiratory lung volume, or atelectrauma, contributed to VILI.

Biotrauma emerged as another component of VILI. Kawano et al.[14] found that ventilated neutrophil-depleted rabbits developed minimal lung injury. However, lung dysfunction developed upon reinfusion of neutrophils suggested that VILI is mediated, at least in part, by immune cells. Additional inflammatory mediators (tumor necrosis factor [TNF] alpha, interleukin [IL]-6, and IL-10) were identified by Tremblay et al.[15] in bronchoalveolar lavage samples from rats when performed at various ventilation settings.

Stretch-activated signal transduction pathways, that is, integrin receptors, can alter gene expression or alveolar cell structure. Parker et al.[16,17] used gadolinium to inhibit endothelial stretch-activated channels in rats and demonstrated that inhibition of tyrosine kinase attenuates lung injury, while inhibition of phosphotyrosine kinase increases susceptibility of the lungs to VILI. Therefore, ventilator-induced elevated transalveolar pressures caused molecular and cell-mediated microvascular permeability resulting in VILI.[18]

Animal studies also identified predisposing factors to VILI. Age, surfactant dysfunction, aspiration, and underlying lung disease were found to increase susceptibility to VILI.[19–21]

The negative effects of positive pressure ventilation are not limited to the lung. Sheep receiving high tidal volume (50 to 70 mL/kg, PIP 50 cm H_2O) settings had increased mortality due to multisystem organ failure compared to low–tidal volume (10 mL/kg, PIP 15 to 20 cm H_2O) settings.[22] Investigators have demonstrated inflammatory mediators (TNF alpha, IL-6), *Escherichia coli,* and lipopolysaccharides (LPS) in the peripheral circulation suggest that VILI promotes a systemic pro-inflammatory state with translocation of bacteria.[23–25]

SEMINAL BEDSIDE STUDIES ON VILI

In the 1980s, widespread clinical use of computerized axial tomography (CAT) dramatically changed our understanding of ARDS. To our surprise, what appeared by chest x-ray to be opaque lung fields, on CAT were nonhomogeneous lungs, with dense atelectatic lung located in the dependent portions while ventilated hyperinflated lung was seen in the nondependent portions. Gattinoni et al.[9,26] investigated lung compliance, lung volumes, and lung appearance on CAT in patients with acute lung injury ventilated at different levels of PEEP (5, 10, 15 cm H_2O). The authors demonstrated normally aerated, poorly aerated, and nonaerated lung tissue and concluded that ventilation preferentially flows to the normal appearing aerated lung, thus illustrating the concept of "baby lung" (Fig. 111.2).

Use of decreased ventilator pressures and volume to limit lung damage often resulted in CO_2 retention. The term "permissive hypercapnia" was first introduced by Darioli and Perret[27] in 1984 to encourage clinicians to tolerate higher pCO_2 with mild respiratory acidosis

PEEP: 5 cm H₂O   **PEEP: 10 cm H₂O**   **PEEP: 15 cm H₂O**

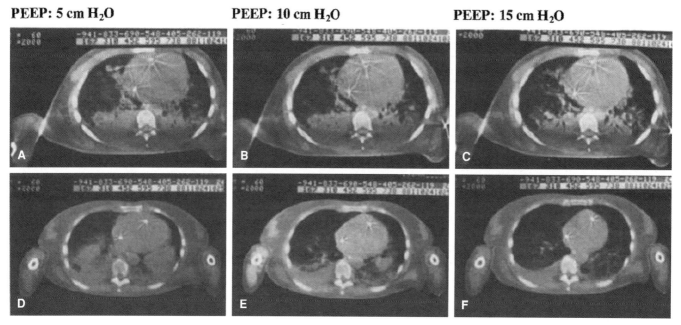

FIGURE 111.2 CT scans illustrating normally aerated, poorly aerated, and nonaerated lung tissue and illustrating the concept of "baby lung." (From Gattinoni L, Mascheroni D, Torresin A, et al. Morphological response to positive end expiratory pressure in acute respiratory failure. Computerized tomography study. *Intensive Care Med* 1986;12:137–142. Copyright © Springer-Verlag 1986. With permission of Springer.)

in order to avoid ventilator induced barotrauma. Patients with status asthmaticus had favorable results when the ventilator was titrated to correct hypoxemia but allowing persistent hypercapnia. Later, Hickling et al.[28] retrospectively demonstrated a reduction in mortality by 60% after implementing a "protective" ventilation strategy with tidal volume 4 to 7 mL/kg and PIP <40 or <30 cm H_2O if possible.

Subsequent landmark prospective randomized trials by Amato et al. also demonstrated a significant survival advantage ($p < 0.001$) and greater rates of weaning from mechanical ventilation ($p < 0.005$) with a low volume/high PEEP strategy (tidal volume <6 mL/kg, PIP <40 cm H_2O, PEEP 15 to 20 cm H_2O, permissive hypercapnia and goal plateau pressure <30 cm H_2O).[29,30] Three additional prospective randomized trials published negative results prompting the landmark, multicenter, prospective randomized trial ARDSNet, which confirmed that low tidal volume (6 mL/kg predicted body weight) and plateau pressure ≤30 cm H_2O offered a 22% relative survival advantage over "traditional" 12 mL/kg and plateau pressure <50 cm H_2O.[31]

Finally, the biotrauma demonstrated in animal models was suggested in human studies with increased inflammatory markers identified in bronchoalveolar lavage and plasma in patients receiving "traditional" ventilation settings (tidal volume 11 mL/kg, PEEP 6 cm H_2O) compared to patients receiving lung protective settings (tidal volume 7 mL/kg, PEEP 15 cm H_2O).[32]

PATHOPHYSIOLOGY

Positive pressure ventilation can lead to a decrease in lung compliance and dysfunctional gas exchange. The following section discusses five different effects of positive pressure ventilation which contribute to VILI: barotrauma, volutrauma, atelectrauma, biotrauma, and systemic (extrapulmonary) manifestations.

Barotrauma, Volutrauma

Barotrauma, lung injury due to high airway pressure, and volutrauma, lung injury due to high tidal volume, are intimately related and

collectively reflect mechanical damage to the lung due to transpulmonary pressure. This injury is due to "high lung volume ventilation." When air flow is zero (end inspiration), the force inflating the lungs is transpulmonary pressure. An alveolus will expand when pressure overcomes the surface tension (P surface), the lung parenchyma (P parenchyma), and the chest wall (P pleura). In other words,

P (transpulmonary) = P (surface + parenchyma) − P (pleura).

A diver, for example, at 10 m below the surface experiences one additional atmosphere of pressure (1034 cm H_2O) against his thorax and must generate enough airway pressure to overcome external force and expand the thorax.[33] Likewise, the oxygen tank must provide one extra atmosphere of pressure to provide air flow and appropriate transpulmonary pressure for oxygenation. While the airway pressure is abnormally high, the tidal volume is physiologic. If the diver emerges to sea level at the elevated airway pressure, however, then the pleural pressure will drop and alveoli will experience pathologic pressures.

Similarly, a trumpet player playing a note can generate airway pressures as high as 150 cm H_2O, yet the respiratory muscles produce a large positive pleural pressure (140 cm H_2O) to counterbalance.[34] The resulting transpulmonary pressure is +10 cm H_2O (Fig. 111.3).

Considering the studies by Dreyfuss et al.,[12] the rats with restricted chest walls (strapped thorax) did not experience lung damage so they tolerated higher airway pressure. Rats with freely expanding chest walls (unstrapped) and relatively low pleural pressures experienced lung damage at high airway pressures due to high transpulmonary pressures. Therefore, airway pressure and pleural pressure can be abnormally high with a normal transpulmonary pressure. Transpulmonary pressure is the summation of the forces acting on the alveoli, or the stress. High transpulmonary pressure can lead to VILI.

Injury due to barotrauma and volutrauma is unpredictable. Underlying lung disease, for example, changes the compliance of the lung. The concept of "baby lung," derived from the appearance of ARDS on CT scans, highlights how respiratory compliance correlates only with the amount of normally aerated tissue versus nonaerated, and ARDS lungs are functionally smaller.[9,35] Likewise, the effect of

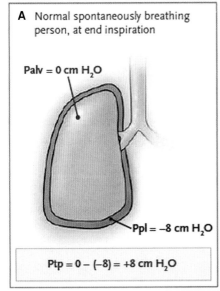

A Normal spontaneously breathing person, at end inspiration

Palv = 0 cm H$_2$O

Ppl = –8 cm H$_2$O

Ptp = 0 – (–8) = +8 cm H$_2$O

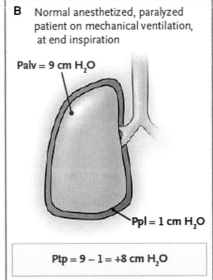

B Normal anesthetized, paralyzed patient on mechanical ventilation, at end inspiration

Palv = 9 cm H$_2$O

Ppl = 1 cm H$_2$O

Ptp = 9 – 1 = +8 cm H$_2$O

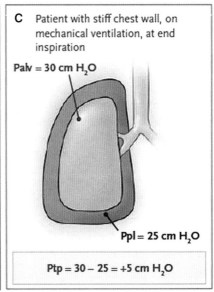

C Patient with stiff chest wall, on mechanical ventilation, at end inspiration

Palv = 30 cm H$_2$O

Ppl = 25 cm H$_2$O

Ptp = 30 – 25 = +5 cm H$_2$O

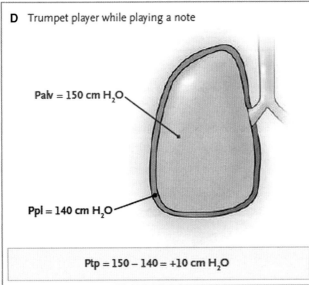

D Trumpet player while playing a note

Palv = 150 cm H$_2$O

Ppl = 140 cm H$_2$O

Ptp = 150 – 140 = +10 cm H$_2$O

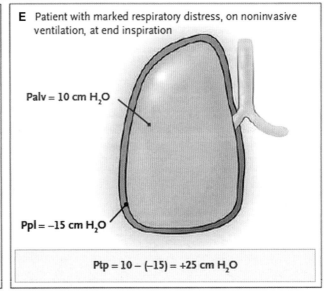

E Patient with marked respiratory distress, on noninvasive ventilation, at end inspiration

Palv = 10 cm H$_2$O

Ppl = –15 cm H$_2$O

Ptp = 10 – (–15) = +25 cm H$_2$O

FIGURE 111.3 **Panel A** shows end inspiration in a patient with normal lung function who is breathing spontaneously; the alveolar pressure (Palv) is 0, and the pleural pressure (Ppl) is negative (−8 cm of water), creating a transpulmonary pressure (Ptp) of +8 cm of water. **Panel B** shows the same lung while the patient undergoes general anesthesia and positive-pressure ventilation with the use of the same tidal volume as in Panel A. The lung would be similarly stretched with a Palv of 9 cm of water and a Ppl of 1 cm of water for a Ptp of +8 cm of water. **Panel C** shows end inspiration in a patient with severe obesity, massive ascites, or pleural effusions, who may have a very stiff chest wall. In such patients, much of the pressure that is applied by the ventilator will be used to distend the chest wall rather than the lung. As such, the plateau pressure may be high, but so will the Ppl, and hence there may not be an increase in Ptp with accompanying lung distention. **Panel D** shows a musician playing a trumpet, which can result in airway pressures of as much as 150 cm of water. However, because of the positive Ppl developed by the respiratory muscles, the pressure across the lung will not exceed normal values. **Panel E** shows a patient with marked dyspnea who is undergoing a type of mechanical ventilation that requires the active contraction of the respiratory muscles to initiate the assisted breath (e.g., noninvasive ventilation or pressure-support ventilation). In such cases, there may be large negative swings in Ppl, leading to a very high Ptp, even though the airway pressure is only 10 cm of water. (From Slutsky AS, Ranieri VM. Ventilator-induced lung injury. *New Eng J Med* 2013;369:2126–2136. Copyright © 2013 Massachusetts Medical Society. Reprinted with permission from Massachusetts Medical Society.)

PEEP is unpredictable. While PEEP can recruit poorly and nonaerated lung, it may injure the aerated regions of the lung by overdistention. Gattinoni's "baby lung" concept supported a clinical shift toward low–tidal volume ventilation.

Biotrauma

Microscopically, positive pressure ventilation imposes mechanical forces on lung tissue that damage cells and promotes a local and systemic inflammatory state.[36,37] Two mechanisms are proposed for

this ventilator-induced inflammatory response. Firstly, positive pressure ventilation can cause direct trauma to the cell causing disruption of cell walls.[38] Secondly, positive pressure ventilation causes cyclic stretching, which can induce pulmonary cells to produce inflammatory cytokines.[39]

Atelectrauma

Atelectrauma refers to the additional lung injury caused by the cyclic opening and closing of alveoli and surfactant dysfunction,

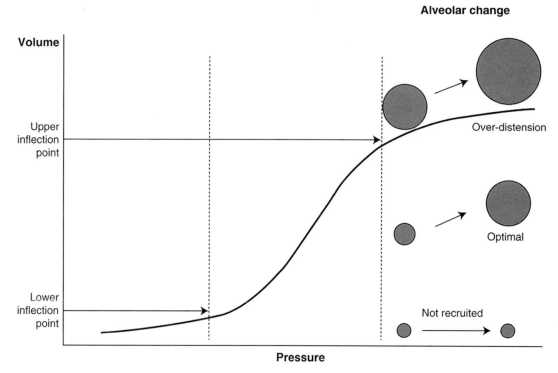

FIGURE 111.4 Pressure–volume curve seen with ventilator management. (From Soni N, Williams P. Positive pressure ventilation: what is the real cost? *Br J Anaesth* 2008;101:446–457. Reproduced by permission of Oxford University Press.)

which leads to epithelial sloughing, hyaline membrane formation, and pulmonary edema. This form of lung injury serves as the platform for proponents of "open up the lung and keep the lung open," or "open lung strategy," highlighting the problem with ventilation at insufficient volumes, or "low–lung volume ventilation."[40] In "low–lung volume ventilation," tidal ventilation starts below and ends above the lower inflection point on the pressure–volume curve (Fig. 111.4).

Laplace's Law, related to pulmonary physiology, states that the pressure to stabilize an alveolus is directly related to the surface tension at the air-liquid interface and inversely related to the radius of the alveolus. Differential inflation of alveoli throughout the lung reflects Laplace's Law: smaller pressures are required to increase the volume of larger alveoli and larger pressures are required to open collapsed alveoli (Fig. 111.5).

Likewise, greater effort (pressure) is required to blow up a deflated balloon, but less effort is required to inflate the balloon once it is open. The opening pressure necessary to overcome the alveolar surface tension is mitigated by surfactant. Likewise, patients with surfactant dysfunction, including SP-B deficiency, require increased force.[33] Similarly, greater pressure is required to keep the alveolar units open, making collapse easier. The challenge to clinicians is to recruit sufficient alveoli for adequate gas exchange while avoiding overinflation of the higher compliant alveoli already open.

CLINICAL MANIFESTATION

VILI leads to poor outcomes.[30,31,43,44] As described above, on a microscopic level, VILI can lead to parenchymal injury with pulmonary

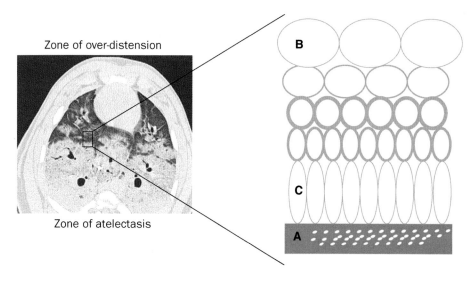

Zone of over-distension

Zone of atelectasis

FIGURE 111.5 Atelectrauma. The interface between collapsed and consolidated lung (**A**) and overdistended lung units (**B**) is heterogeneous and unstable. Depending on ambient conditions this region is prone to cyclic recruitment and derecruitment and localized asymmetrical stretch of lung units (**C**) immediately opposed to regions of collapsed lung. (Reprinted from Pinhu L, Whitehead T, Evans T, et al. Ventilator-associated lung injury. *Lancet* 2003;361:332–340. Copyright © 2003 Elsevier. With permission.)

edema, hyaline membrane formation, remodeling, and induction of a local inflammatory response.[33] VILI can also induce a systemic inflammatory response. Grossly, air leaks due to ruptured alveoli from barotrauma/volutrauma manifest as pneumothorax, pneumomediastinum, subcutaneous emphysema, and pneumoperitoneum. Rarely, air leaks can progress to tension pneumothorax, cardiac tamponade, or air emboli.

VILI does not present in a uniform way, nor is the management as simple as "protective" ventilator strategy. The injury induced by mechanical ventilation is a product of the intensity and duration of positive pressure, and the manifestations are a product of the patient's underlying physiology and disease requiring mechanical ventilation. The clinical management of VILI is an evolving field without a "one size fits all" answer. Below are the current options for the prevention and management of VILI.

CLINICAL MANAGEMENT

Treatment is supportive, with institution of lung-protective ventilator strategies. Pneumothorax is managed with a chest tube. Pneumomediastinum, subcutaneous emphysema, and pneumoperitoneum can usually be monitored for signs of worsening. Importantly, the best treatment for VILI is prevention.

"Protective" Ventilation Strategies

Low–Tidal Volume Ventilation

Low–tidal volume ventilation (6 to 9 mL/kg), compared to traditional volumes (12 to 13 mL/kg), significantly decreases mortality by 22% to 32% in patients with ARDS.[31,45] The ARDSNet study implemented "low–tidal volume ventilation" as a standard of care in critical care and utilizes tidal volume of 6 mL/kg with primary goal of plateau pressure <30 cm H_2O and permissive hypercapnia (pCO_2 "compatible with life" or pH > 7.20).[31]

Important limitations to the ARDSNet study in its application to ventilator standards were inclusion and exclusion criteria. The population included patients with acute lung injury (P/F < 350) and ARDS (P/F < 200). Patients were excluded if they had severe chronic respiratory disease, morbid obesity, burns, a contraindication to hypercapnia or hypoxia (i.e., increased intracranial pressure), or predicted 6-month mortality more than 50%.

A limitation to goal plateau pressures <30 cm H_2O, is in patients with reduced chest wall compliance, most commonly due to obesity.[46] Importantly, plateau pressures may not adequately predict the transpulmonary pressures, chest wall or actual lung distention. Esophageal manometry, which measures pleural pressures and indirectly transpulmonary pressures, may provide insight into more appropriate tidal volumes and plateau pressures for patients with reduced chest wall compliance.

High PEEP

The presence of atelectasis and de-recruited lungs is well documented.[9,47] PEEP given above the inflection point on the pressure–volume curve may improve compliance and minimize repetitive opening and closing of alveoli with subsequent VILI.[13]

The optimal PEEP to deliver is controversial, but recent studies have suggested that higher PEEP increases survival in sicker patients.[48–51] A meta-analysis of three trials (1,136 patients) reported improved survival among patients with ARDS who received higher PEEP; conversely, patients without ARDS who received lower PEEP did not benefit and results suggest patients actually experience harm from higher PEEP.[51]

Recruitment maneuvers aim to inflate de-recruited areas of the lung by applying continuous positive airways pressure for an extended period of time, such as pressure of 35 cm H_2O for 30 seconds. The maneuvers are controversial.[52] A prospective, randomized study of the ARDS Clinical Trials Networks reported variable therapeutic benefits from recruitment maneuvers with side effects including hypotension.[53] Initial improvements in arterial oxygenation (within 2 minutes), became nonsignificant after 15 minutes. Limitations of the study included the use of high PEEP, which may have reduced the potential of recruitment-induced improvements.

High-Frequency Oscillatory Ventilation

High-frequency oscillatory ventilation (HFOV) is an alternative mode of ventilation that delivers rapid breaths per minute (300 to 900) of small tidal volumes, (~70 mL) therefore maintaining a relatively constant airway pressure. Theoretically, maximizing alveolar recruitment and oxygenation and minimizing tidal volumes serves as a lung protective ventilator mode reducing the risk of VILI. While HLOV may reduce treatment failure (refractory hypoxemia, hypercapnia, hypotension, or barotrauma), its impact on survival is unclear.[54,55]

Currently, HFOV is not used as a first-line treatment of ARDS. Two large randomized trials (OSCILLATE and OSCAR) found increased mortality or no difference in mortality, respectively, compared to low–tidal volume ventilation.[56,57] The OSCILLATE trial also highlighted the increased need for sedatives and vasoactive agents in patients treated with HFOV.

HFOV may be appropriate on a case-by-case basis, yet it is generally reserved as a rescue mode.

Adjunctive Strategies

Prone Positioning

Patients refractory to lung protective ventilation strategies may benefit from adjunctive strategies. Prone positioning (face-down) may minimize VILI. Three mechanisms are proposed: first, allowing more homogenous distribution of transpulmonary pressure; second, by "resting" anterior lung units at risk of overdistension; and third, improving ventilation–perfusion mismatch.[38] A recent prospective, randomized controlled trial (PROSEVA) demonstrated that early application of prone positioning in severe ARDS (P/F < 150 mm Hg) improves survival (28-day mortality 16%) compared to supine positioning (mortality 33%).[58] Still, prone positioning remains controversial, and appropriate implementation for VILI is not conclusive.

Extracorporeal Life Support

Extracorporeal life support (ECLS), which includes ECMO and extracorporeal CO_2 removal (ECCO2R), was historically reserved as a salvage therapy in ARDS. Currently, ECLS is finding broadened applications. The landmark CESAR trial demonstrated improved survival at 6 months in patients with severe, but potentially reversible, respiratory failure who received ECMO compared to conventional management.[59] ECMO maintains gas exchange while allowing the lungs rest from high pressure ventilation, thereby minimizing VILI.

Patients with VILI on ECMO can receive positive pressure mechanical ventilation at ultraprotective ventilator pressures. The most common ventilator settings are PEEP 10 cm H_2O, respiratory rate 10 cm H_2O, and mean airway pressure around 16 cm H_2O. Options include a "total rest strategy" with very low–tidal volume and PEEP (2 to 3 mL/kg and 4 to 5cm H_2O, respectively) or "open lung strategy" with higher PEEP (15 to 20 cm H_2O). A recent retrospective multicenter observational study concluded that higher PEEP levels (>12 cm H_2O)

Selection of ECLS Support Level/Configuration

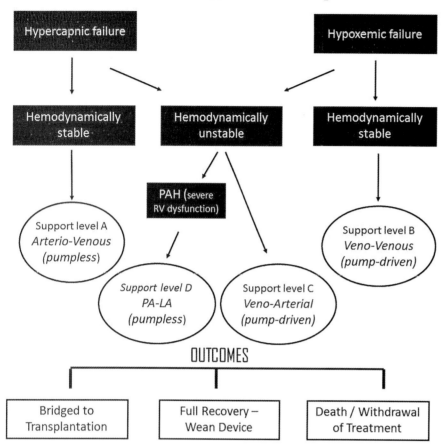

FIGURE 111.6 Algorithm for selection of ECLS support level and configuration. (From Keshavjee S, Cypel M. Extracorporeal life support pre and post lung transplantation. In: Annich GM, Lynch WR, MacLaren G, Wilson JM, Bartlett RH, eds. ECMO. Extracorporeal Cardiopulmonary Support in Critical Care, 4th ed. Ann Arbor, MI: ELSO; 2012:413. With permission.)

during the first 3 days of ECMO were associated with lower mortality compared to lower PEEP (10 to 12 cm H_2O) on multivariate analysis ($p = 0.0006$).[60] Interestingly, Goligher et al. identified a sub-group of ventilated patients, "PEEP responders," on a post hoc analysis of two randomized controlled trials.[49,50,61] PEEP responders demonstrated improved oxygenation and improved mortality with increased PEEP indicating that "one-size-fits-all" ventilation strategies may be inappropriate. Future research will need to investigate whether recruited or nonrecruited (resting) lungs heal faster.

Most recently, Hoopes and others have reported improved outcomes in small series of patients with ARDS utilizing ambulatory ECMO techniques. Both venovenous (especially using double lumen catheter access) and venoarterial ECMO can be configured to allow ambulation.[62–64] Ambulatory ECMO has several real and theoretical advantages. Extubating the patient while on ECMO allows oral hygiene, normal cough, and deep breathing to aid management of secretions while speech allows free communication with staff and family. Finally, ambulation promotes conditioning of respiratory, diaphragm, and large muscle groups. One can assume improved circulation, less pressure sores, less deep venous thrombosis and pulmonary emboli, as well as decreased frailty. One can predict less inflammatory mediators and less pneumonia, less bowel stasis, fever, and urinary tract infections. All very enticing, but the risk/benefit of ambulatory ECMO still needs more validation.

Of equal importance is the application of ambulatory ECMO as a bride to lung transplant or bridge to decision. Hoopes and others have considered ambulatory ECMO as standard of care in patients who deteriorate while awaiting a suitable donor lung.[65,66] This approach

stabilizes the patient and allows conditioning of the recipient. The risk/benefit and costs are all concerns but early results are very promising.[67] Likewise, many are using ECMO as a stabilizing technique to allow diagnostic studies, treatment response, or family discussions to determine treatment strategies—hence, a bridge to decision. Patients with cardiopulmonary failure who are upright, ambulatory, and socially interactive have many reasons for improved outcomes. Further experience is necessary to make firm recommendations.

Current recommendations for device configurations from the Extracorporeal Life Support Organization (ELSO) are outlined in the algorithm in Figure 111.6.

Pharmacologic

Neuromuscular blockade may reduce VILI by mitigating patients that "fight the vent."[38,69] Anti-inflammatory agents may interfere with the inflammatory cascade of VILI.[70] Finally, intravenous injection of mesenchymal stem cells into rats with acute lung injury was found to improve systemic oxygenation and lung compliance and to decrease lung inflammation and histological lung injury.[71]

FUTURE

Current research is investigating better ways to individualize ventilator settings. Again, the ARDSNet protocol describes a generalized approach to ventilation with a set tidal volume (based on ideal body weight), plateau pressure, and PEEP, which fails to account for a patient's lung and chest wall compliance. Measurement of esophageal pressures, and indirectly pleural pressures and transpulmonary pressures, allows clinicians to adjust ventilator settings to reflect the patient's chest wall mechanics.[46,72]

The use of ECMO is growing rapidly, and criteria for ECMO are broadening. Hoopes proposes three criteria for ECMO: (1) any patient with acute lung injury on the ventilator, (2) medical futility is a contraindication, and (3) "failure to rescue" as metrics that are the only quality assessment and performance improvement (QAPI) measures of consequence.[73] These criteria may be perceived as liberal, but early results suggest the bridge to decision approach of early ECMO may yield dramatic improvement in survival, length of stay, and overall cost. Lung injuries do not benefit from paralysis, sedation, mechanical intubation, and nonphysiologic positive pressure ventilation; so, as previously presented, ECMO offers an avenue for extubation and ambulation. Patients must be recoverable; medical futility is an important contraindication for ECMO. Early identification of futility is often elusive when addressing individual patients.

Patient management is also evolving. ECMO on a mechanically ventilated patient can increase morbidity so we push to extubate patients early (within 24 hours) while on ECMO. Anticoagulation is limited or avoided when tolerated or bleeding occurs. Finally, it is important to establish an exit strategy prior to initiating ECMO.

Evidence continues to grow that novel modes of mechanical ventilation, such as neurally adjusted ventilatory assist, are feasible and improve patient physiology and patient ventilator interaction; data on clinical outcomes are limited but supportive. Since there is no optimization of conventional treatments, ECMO should not be reserved only for a patient that has "failed" all conventional treatments.[74]

PREDICTING OUTCOMES

Deciding whether to initiate ECMO for patients with severe ARDS remains a challenging decision and requires balancing the probability of achieving a good outcome in a severely ill patient against the costs (time, labor, expertise, and equipment) associated with employing a scarce and resource-intensive intervention. A prognostic instrument, the RESP (Respiratory ECMO Survival Prediction) score, might assist in clinical decision-making. The RESP score was developed from data in the ELSO registry and was externally validated to predict the probability of survival after initiation of ECMO for severe ARDS.[75] The actual clinical usefulness of the score remains uncertain; the score predicts the probability of survival in patients in whom ECMO is initiated but does not predict whether ECMO initiation will significantly alter the probability of survival.[76]

INHALATION INJURY

Inhalation injury can occur due to smoke, near drowning, aspiration pneumonia, pneumonitis, inflammation plus airway obstruction, etc.

INTRODUCTION

Inhalation injury is a nonspecific term describing injury to the respiratory system due to inhalation of thermal or chemical irritants. Inhalation injuries are associated with significant morbidity and mortality.[76–79] Patients with cutaneous burn plus inhalation injury demonstrated a mortality of 27% to 35% compared to mortality of 4% to 14% in patients with cutaneous burns alone. In other words, burn patients with inhalation injury have at least double the mortality. Shirani et al. elegantly demonstrated the increased incidence of inhalation injury with increasing burn size and the increase in

mortality with inhalation injury as well as inhalation injury complicated by pneumonia.[80] Incidence varies by region and institution, with reports describing inhalation injury in 7% to 20% of burn patients.[76,77,80] Age, percentage of total body surface area (TBSA), and PaO_2/FiO_2 ratio were independent predictors of mortality in patients with inhalation injury.[71,81] Uniformity in diagnostic criteria, scaling of severity, and use of common terminology to describe outcomes is lacking, therefore hindering the development of systematic approaches to treatment and research. Finally, advances in critical care have led to improved survival in burn patients; though similar to VILI, treatment of inhalation injury is primarily supportive.[80]

CLASSIFICATION

Inhalation injuries are broadly classified as direct thermal injury, inhaled chemical irritants, and systemic toxicity due to inhaled gases.[82] *Direct thermal injuries* are restricted to upper airway structures, with the exception of blast injury and steam inhalation. Direct thermal injuries are a result of high temperatures to which the upper airway is exposed. *Inhaled chemicals* cause a local irritation throughout the respiratory tract as a result of the chemical composition of the inhaled substance. *Systemic toxicity* results from inhaled toxins with systemic effects, such as carbon monoxide or cyanide.

CLINICAL PRESENTATION

Upper airway injury due to direct thermal injury presents as massive swelling of the tongue, epiglottis, and aryepiglottic folds with obstruction.[83] Airway edema will evolve with ongoing resuscitation requiring diligent re-examination of the patient's respiratory status. If airway compromise is anticipated, the patient should be considered for intubation for airway protection.

Lower airway injury, due to inhaled chemical irritants damaging epithelial and capillary endothelial cells of the airway, manifests as tracheobronchitis. Mucociliary transport is damaged so bacterial clearance is reduced. Loss of surfactant results in atelectasis. As a local inflammatory response ensues, the lungs develop a diffuse inflammatory exudate and bronchial edema. Patients develop airway obstruction due to inflammation, edema, and spasm. Necrosis of respiratory epithelium places patients at risk of bacterial pneumonia.

The manifestation of the inhalation injury is ultimately a result of the physiochemical properties of the causative agent, amount of smoke inhaled, and pre-existing pulmonary disease.

PATHOPHYSIOLOGY

Direct heat injury is caused by the inhalation of air heated to a temperature of 150°C or higher. The upper airways perform the majority of airway heat exchange thereby protecting the lower airways (subglottic structures) from extremes of heat.

Fires liberate numerous biologically harmful chemicals that can be inhaled and cause injury to the airways. The lungs are initially damaged by incomplete products of combustion, most importantly by aldehydes, oxides of sulfur, and nitrogen. Flames can also liberate numerous biologically harmful chemicals. Common household items and home building materials contribute to the inhalation injury. Ammonia, a product of insulation, clothing, and many fabrics, may combine with water to form ammonium hydroxide, an alkali that produces liquefaction necrosis. Additional by-products include hydrogen chloride (released from plastics), aldehydes (released by wood), nitrogen dioxide (released by

TABLE 111.1 Bronchoscopic Criteria Used to Grade Inhalation Injury

Grade 0 (no injury): absence of carbonaceous deposits, erythema, edema, bronchorrhea, or obstruction

Grade 1 (mild injury): minor or patchy areas of erythema, carbonaceous deposits in proximal or distal bronchi (any or combination)

Grade 2 (moderate injury): moderate degree of erythema, carbonaceous deposits, bronchorrhea, with or without compromise of the bronchi (any or combination)

Grade 3 (severe injury): severe inflammation with friability, copious carbonaceous deposits, bronchorrhea, bronchial obstruction (any or combination)

Grade 4 (massive injury): evidence of mucosal sloughing, necrosis, endoluminal obliteration (any or combination)

From Endorf FW, Gamelli RL. Inhalation injury, pulmonary perturbations, and fluid resuscitation. *J Burn Care Res* 2007;28:80–83. doi: 10.1097/BCR.0B013E31802C889F

cellulose), and carbonyl-chloride (released by polyvinyl chloride) and can contribute to pulmonary edema and pain.

DIAGNOSIS

Diagnostic criteria for inhalation injury are not uniform and are often institution specific. Broadly, diagnosis of inhalation injury requires exposure to caustic inhalants with clinical sequel. Exposure is characterized by mechanism (e.g., flame, electricity, steam), quality (house fire), and quantity (duration of exposure). On physical exam, patients may have facial burns or singed nasal hair, carbonaceous sputum, or evidence of respiratory compromise (O_2 requirements, stridor). Diagnostic studies include bronchoscopy and ^{133}Xe scans. Bronchoscopic findings can be graded using the Abbreviated Injury Score (AIS) criteria proposed by Endorf and Gamelli[84] (Table 111.1).

Overall survival is worse in patients with higher grades of injury as evaluated by bronchoscopic criteria.[84] Depending on institution, diagnosis of inhalation injury may be based on need for intubation and mechanical ventilation, bronchoscopic findings, or nuclear medicine scans (^{133}Xe lung scan). Importantly, respiratory compromise may not manifest for 24 hours so a high index of suspicion must be maintained. Patient responses to exposures vary and are a result of underlying physiology. Likewise, a scoring system for severity of inhalation injury by CT imaging (RADS score) has been developed where normal (0), increased interstitial markings (1), ground glass opacification (2), and consolidation (3) can be combined with clinical findings to better direct level of therapy.[85]

Carbon Monoxide Diagnosis

If carbon monoxide (CO) injury is suspected, a blood sample will be taken to determine the amount of serum CO. Once CO levels increase to 70 parts per million (ppm) and above, symptoms become more noticeable and may include nausea, dizziness, and unconsciousness. Immediate oxygen therapy is required. If the patient can breathe independently, an oxygen mask will be applied; if not, mechanical ventilation will be initiated. If injury from CO exposure is severe, the patient may be placed in a hyperbaric oxygen chamber. The chamber has twice the pressure of normal air and can quickly increase oxygen levels in the blood.[86]

Cyanide Toxicity Diagnosis

Cyanide is a product of combustion found in a variety of common products. Almost any structural fire will have cyanide released.

Injury from cyanide exposure is treatable but requires quick diagnosis. A diagnosis of cyanide toxicity should be considered in patients with rapid collapse or seizures accompanied by metabolic acidosis and decreased oxygen consumption.[87] A variety of tests, including determination of carboxyhemoglobin (HbCO) level by co-oximetry, red blood cell cyanide concentration determined by infrared spectroscopy, and electrocardiogram, will be necessary to determine if cyanide poisoning has occurred. Cyanide toxicity is characterized by a normal arterial oxygen tension and an abnormally high venous oxygen tension, resulting in a decreased arteriovenous oxygen difference (<10%). A high–anion-gap metabolic acidosis is a hallmark of significant cyanide toxicity.[88] Cyanide toxicity occurs at the cellular level and oxygenation alone is not enough.

TREATMENT

The development of a clinical grading system (0 to 4) and the use of modalities such as CAT scan grading (0 to 3) may allow for a more nuanced evaluation of inhalation injury and enhanced ability to prognosticate progressive therapy. Supportive respiratory care remains the primary treatment modality in managing inhalation injury. Progressively aggressive treatment modalities are widely utilized but currently lack evidence-based recommendations. These treatment modalities include bronchodilators, mucolytic agents, inhaled anticoagulants, nonconventional ventilator modes, prone positioning, extracorporeal membrane oxygenation (ECMO), and ambulatory methods.[89,90] Each of these therapies has shown dramatic outcomes in select patient populations. Each, however, is dependent upon patient selection, comorbidities, multiorgan dysfunction, patient compliance, and primary diagnosis. Recent research focusing on molecular mechanisms involved in inhalation injury has increased the number of potential therapies. Inhaled and systemic modification of inflammatory mediators and alveolar tissue response has shown promise in experimental models.

The future will unlikely discover a magic bullet that allows a "one size fits all" approach. Current recommendations focus on supportive care. Only low–tidal-volume ventilator strategies have shown evidence-based efficacy in broad patient populations. Virtually all advanced therapies are limited to select patient populations. Specific diagnostic modalities, patient selection, and cost/risk/benefit relationships must be stratified to direct application of advanced modalities. For example, ECMO (especially ambulatory) is now recommended as a bridge to lung transplant in select patients. ECMO, however, requires expertise, training, specialists and equipment, all of which would impact the cost of healthcare unless thoughtfully applied. All of the therapies mentioned share a common need for proper patient selection. The future will be dictated by quality, safety, and efficacy models based on disease understanding and diagnostics that a given population can afford.

REFERENCES

1. Kuipers MT, van der Poll T, Schultz MJ, et al. Bench-to-bedside review: damage-associated molecular patterns in the onset of ventilator-induced lung injury. *Crit Care* 2011;15:235.
2. Bove AA. Diving medicine. *Am J Resp Crit Care Med* 2014;189:1479–1486.
3. Baker AB. Artificial respiration, the history of an idea. *Med HistoryI* 1971;15:336–351.
4. Macklin CC. Transport of air along sheaths of pulmonic blood vessels from alveoli to mediastinum—clinical implications. *Arch Int Med* 1939;64:913–926.
5. Macklin MT, Macklin CC. Malignant interstitial emphysema of the lungs and mediastinum as an important occult complication in many respiratory diseases and other conditions an interpretation of the clinical literature in the light of laboratory experiment. *Medicine* 1944;23:281–358.
6. Fowler WS. Lung function studies; uneven pulmonary ventilation in normal subjects and in patients with pulmonary disease. *J Appl Physiol* 1949;2:283–299.

111 Barotrauma and Inhalation Injuries   **1457**

7. Mead J, Takishim T, Leith D. Stress distribution in lungs—a model of pulmonary elasticity. *J Appl Physiol* 1970;28:596–608.
8. Greenfield LJ, Ebert PA, Benson DW. Effect of positive pressure ventilation on surface tension properties of lung extracts. *Anesthesiology* 1964;25:312–316.
9. Gattinoni L, Mascheroni D, Torresin A, et al. Morphological response to positive end expiratory pressure in acute respiratory failure. Computerized tomography study. *Intensive Care Med* 1986;12:137–142.
10. Tremblay LN, Slutsky AS. Ventilator-induced lung injury: From the bench to the bedside. *Intensive Care Med* 2006;32:24–33.
11. Webb HH, Tierney DF. Experimental pulmonary edema due to intermittent positive pressure ventilation with high inflation pressures. Protection by positive end-expiratory pressure. *Am Rev Respir Dis* 1974;110:556–565.
12. Dreyfuss D, Soler P, Basset G, et al. High inflation pressure pulmonary edema. Respective effects of high airway pressure, high tidal volume, and positive end-expiratory pressure. *Am Rev Respir Dis* 1988;137:1159–1164.
13. Muscedere JG, Mullen JB, Gan K, et al. Tidal ventilation at low airway pressures can augment lung injury. *Am J Respir Crit Care Med* 1994;149:1327–1334.
14. Kawano T, Mori S, Cybulsky M, et al. Effect of granulocyte depletion in a ventilated surfactant-depleted lung. *J Appl Physiol (1985)* 1987;62:27–33.
15. Tremblay L, Valenza F, Ribeiro SP, et al. Injurious ventilatory strategies increase cytokines and c-fos m-rna expression in an isolated rat lung model. *J Clin Invest* 1997;99:944–952.
16. Parker JC, Ivey CL, Tucker JA. Gadolinium prevents high airway pressure-induced permeability increases in isolated rat lungs. *J Appl Physiol (1985)* 1998;84:1113–1118.
17. Parker JC, Ivey CL, Tucker A. Phosphotyrosine phosphatase and tyrosine kinase inhibition modulate airway pressure-induced lung injury. *J Appl Physiol (1985)* 1998;85(5):1753–1761.
18. Tremblay LN, Slutsky AS. Ventilator-induced injury: From barotrauma to biotrauma. *Proc Assoc Am Phys* 1998;110:482–488.
19. Coker PJ, Hernandez LA, Peevy KJ, Adkins K, Parker JC. Increased sensitivity to mechanical ventilation after surfactant inactivation in young rabbit lungs. *Crit Care Med* 1992;20:635–640.
20. Adkins WK, Hernandez LA, Coker PJ, et al. Age effects susceptibility to pulmonary barotrauma in rabbits. *Crit Care Med* 1991;19:390–393.
21. Dreyfuss D, Soler P, Saumon G. Mechanical ventilation-induced pulmonary edema. Interaction with previous lung alterations. *Am J Respir Crit Care Med* 1995;151:1568–1575.
22. Kolobow T, Moretti MP, Fumagalli R et al. Severe impairment in lung function induced by high peak airway pressure during mechanical ventilation. An experimental study. *Am Rev Respir Dis* 1987;135:312–315.
23. von Bethmann AN, Brasch F, Nusing R, et al. Hyperventilation induces release of cytokines from perfused mouse lung. *Am J Respir Crit Care Med* 1998;157:263–272.
24. Nahum A, Hoyt J, Schmitz L, et al. Effect of mechanical ventilation strategy on dissemination of intratracheally instilled Escherichia coli in dogs. *Crit Care Med* 1997;25:1733–1743.
25. Murphy DB, Cregg N, Tremblay L, et al. Adverse ventilatory strategy causes pulmonary-to-systemic translocation of endotoxin. *Am J Respir Crit Care Med* 2000;162:27–33.
26. Gattinoni L, Pesenti A, Avalli L, et al. Pressure-volume curve of total respiratory system in acute respiratory failure. Computed tomographic scan study. *Am Rev Respir Dis* 1987;136:730–736.
27. Darioli R, Perret C. Mechanical controlled hypoventilation in status asthmaticus. *Am Rev Respir Dis* 1984;129:385–387.
28. Hickling KG, Henderson SJ, Jackson R. Low mortality associated with low volume pressure limited ventilation with permissive hypercapnia in severe adult respiratory distress syndrome. *Intensive Care Med* 1990;16:372–377.
29. Amato MB, Barbas CS, Medeiros DM, et al. Beneficial effects of the "open lung approach" with low distending pressures in acute respiratory distress syndrome. A prospective randomized study on mechanical ventilation. *Am J Respir Crit Care Med* 1995;152:1835–1846.
30. Amato MB, Barbas CS, Medeiros DM, et al. Effect of a protective-ventilation strategy on mortality in the acute respiratory distress syndrome. *New Eng J Med* 1998;338:347–354.
31. Ney L, Kuebler LM. Ventilation with lower tidal volumes as compared with traditional tidal volumes for acute lung injury and the acute respiratory distress syndrome. The acute respiratory distress syndrome network. *New Eng J Med* 2000;342:1301–1308.
32. Ranieri VM, Suter PM, Tortorella C, et al. Effect of mechanical ventilation on inflammatory mediators in patients with acute respiratory distress syndrome: a randomized controlled trial. *JAMA* 1999;282:54–61.
33. Gattinoni L, Protti A, Caironi P, et al. Ventilator-induced lung injury: the anatomical and physiological framework. *Crit Care Med* 2010;38:S539–S548.
34. Slutsky AS, Ranieri VM. Ventilator-induced lung injury. *New Eng J Med* 2013;369:2126–2136.
35. Gattinoni L, Pesenti A. The concept of "baby lung". *Intensive Care Med* 2005;31:776–784.
36. Pugin J. Molecular mechanisms of lung cell activation induced by cyclic stretch. *Crit Care Med* 2003;31:S200–S206.
37. Uhlig S. Ventilation-induced lung injury and mechanotransduction: Stretching it too far? *Am J Physiol Lung Cell Mol Physiol* 2002;282:L892–L896.
38. Terragni P, Ranieri VM, Brazzi L. Novel approaches to minimize ventilator-induced lung injury. *Curr Opin Crit Care* 2015;21:20–25.
39. Vlahakis NE, Schroeder MA, Limper AH, et al. Stretch induces cytokine release by alveolar epithelial cells in vitro. *Am J Physiol* 1999;277:L167–L173.
40. Lachmann B. Open up the lung and keep the lung open. *Intensive Care Med* 1992;18:319–321.

41. Soni N, Williams P. Positive pressure ventilation: what is the real cost? *Br J Anaesth* 2008;101:446–457.
42. Pinhu L, Whitehead T, Evans T, et al. Ventilator-associated lung injury. *Lancet* 2003;361:332–340.
43. Stewart TE, Meade MO, Cook DJ, et al. Evaluation of a ventilation strategy to prevent barotrauma in patients at high risk for acute respiratory distress syndrome. Pressure- and Volume-Limited Ventilation Strategy Group. *New Eng J Med* 1998;338:355–361.
44. Ricard JD, Dreyfuss D, Saumon G. Ventilator-induced lung injury. *Eur Respir J Suppl* 2003;42:2s–9s.
45. Jardin F, Fellahi JL, Beauchet A, et al. Improved prognosis of acute respiratory distress syndrome 15 years on. *Intensive Care Med* 1999;25:936–941.
46. Talmor D, Sarge T, O'Donnell CR, et al. Esophageal and transpulmonary pressures in acute respiratory failure. *Crit Care Med* 2006;34:1389–1394.
47. Crotti S, Mascheroni D, Caironi P, et al. Recruitment and derecruitment during acute respiratory failure: A clinical study. *Am J Respir Critical Care Med* 2001;164:131–140.
48. Brower RG, Lanken PN, MacIntyre N, et al. Higher versus lower positive end-expiratory pressures in patients with the acute respiratory distress syndrome. *New Eng J Med* 2004;351:327–336.
49. Meade MO, Cook DJ, Guyatt GH, et al. Ventilation strategy using low tidal volumes, recruitment maneuvers, and high positive end-expiratory pressure for acute lung injury and acute respiratory distress syndrome: A randomized controlled trial. *JAMA* 2008;299:637–645.
50. Mercat A, Richard JC, Vielle B, et al. Positive end-expiratory pressure setting in adults with acute lung injury and acute respiratory distress syndrome: A randomized controlled trial. *JAMA* 2008;299:646–655.
51. Briel M, Meade M, Mercat A, et al. Higher vs lower positive end-expiratory pressure in patients with acute lung injury and acute respiratory distress syndrome: Systematic review and meta-analysis. *JAMA* 2010;303:865–873.
52. Gattinoni L, Carlesso E, Brazzi L, et al. Positive end-expiratory pressure. *Curr Opin Crit Care* 2010;16:39–44.
53. Brower RG, Morris A, MacIntyre N, et al.; ARDS Clinical Trials Network, National Heart, Lung, and Blood Institute, National Institutes of Health. Effects of recruitment maneuvers in patients with acute lung injury and acute respiratory distress syndrome ventilated with high positive end-expiratory pressure. *Crit Care Med* 2003;31:2592–2597.
54. Sud S, Sud M, Friedrich JO, et al. High frequency oscillation in patients with acute lung injury and acute respiratory distress syndrome (ARDS): Systematic review and meta-analysis. *BMJ* 2010;340:c2327.
55. Gu XL, Wu GN, Yao YW, et al. Is high-frequency oscillatory ventilation more effective and safer than conventional protective ventilation in adult acute respiratory distress syndrome patients? A meta-analysis of randomized controlled trials. *Crit Care* 2014;18:R111.
56. Young D, Lamb SE, Shah S, et al. OSCAR Study Group. High-frequency oscillation for acute respiratory distress syndrome. *New Eng J Med* 2013;368:806–813.
57. Ferguson ND, Cook DJ, Guyatt GH, et al.; OSCILLATE Trial Investigators; Canadian Critical Care Trials Group. High-frequency oscillation in early acute respiratory distress syndrome. *New Eng J Med* 2013;368:795–805.
58. Guerin C, Reignier J, Richard JC, et al.; PROSEVA Study Group. Prone positioning in severe acute respiratory distress syndrome. *New Eng J Med* 2013;368:2159–2168.
59. Peek GJ, Mugford M, Tiruvoipati R, et al.; CESAR trial collaboration. Efficacy and economic assessment of conventional ventilatory support versus extracorporeal membrane oxygenation for severe adult respiratory failure (Cesar): A multicentre randomised controlled trial. *Lancet* 2009;374:1351–1363.
60. Schmidt M, Stewart C, Bailey M, et al. Mechanical ventilation management during extracorporeal membrane oxygenation for acute respiratory distress syndrome: A retrospective international multicenter study. *Crit Care Med* 2015;43:654–664.
61. Goligher EC, Kavanagh BP, Rubenfeld GD, et al. Oxygenation response to positive end-expiratory pressure predicts mortality in acute respiratory distress syndrome. A secondary analysis of the lovs and express trials. *Am J Respir Crit Care Med* 2014;190:70–76.
62. Hayes D Jr, Kukreja J, Tobias JD, et al. Ambulatory venovenous extracorporeal respiratory support as a bridge for cystic fibrosis patients to emergent lung transplantation. *Semin Thorac Cardiovasc Surg* 2012;24:232–234.
63. Abrams DC, Brodie D, Rosenzweig EB, et al. Upper-body extracorporeal membrane oxygenation as a strategy in decompensated pulmonary arterial hypertension. *Pulm Circ* 2013;3:432–435.
64. Wang D, Zhou X, Liu X, et al. Wang-Zwische double lumen cannula-toward a percutaneous and ambulatory paracorporeal artificial lung. *ASAIO J* 2008;54:606–611.
65. Hoopes CW, Kukreja J, Golden J, et al. Extracorporeal membrane oxygenation as a bridge to pulmonary transplantation. *J Thorac Cardiovasc Surg* 2013;145:862–867.
66. Lehr CJ, Zaas DW, Cheifetz IM, et al. Ambulatory extracorporeal membrane oxygenation as a bridge to lung transplantation: walking while waiting. *Chest* 2015;147:1213–1218.
67. Bain JC, Turner DA, Rehder KJ, et al. Economic outcomes of extracorporeal membrane oxygenation with and without ambulation as a bridge to lung transplantation. *Respir Care* 2016;61:1–7.
68. Keshavjee S, Cypel M. Extracorporeal life support pre and post lung transplantation. In: Annich GM, Lynch WR, MacLaren G, et al., eds. ECMO. Extracorporeal Cardiopulmonary Support in Critical Care, 4th ed. Ann Arbor, MI: ELSO; 2012:413.
69. Papazian L, Forel JM, Gacouin A, et al.; ACURASYS Study Investigators. Neuromuscular blockers in early acute respiratory distress syndrome. *New Eng J Med* 2010;363:1107–1116.
70. Uhlig S, Uhlig U. Pharmacological interventions in ventilator-induced lung injury. *Trends Pharmacol Sci* 2004;25:592–600.

71. Curley GF, Hayes M, Ansari B, et al. Mesenchymal stem cells enhance recovery and repair following ventilator-induced lung injury in the rat. *Thorax* 2012;67: 496–501.

72. Soroksky A, Esquinas A. Goal-directed mechanical ventilation: Are we aiming at the right goals? A proposal for an alternative approach aiming at optimal lung compliance, guided by esophageal pressure in acute respiratory failure. *Crit Care Res Prac* 2012;2012:597932

73. Hoopes CW. ECMO for respiratory failure: patient selection, surgical approach, and patient management. Presented at American Association of Thoracic Surgeons (AATS) 2015 Annual Meeting. Available at: http://webcast.aats.org/2015/Presentations_2/608/04252015/1000-Optimal%20Therapi1/1015_Hoopes_C/1015_Hoopes_AATS.pdf

74. Diaz-Guzman E, Zwischenberger JB, Thannickal VJ, et al. Extracorporeal membrane oxygenation for acute respiratory failure in adults: The need for pulmonary INTERMACS. *Am J Respir Crit Care Med* 2014;190:1321–1322.

75. Schmidt M, Bailey M, Sheldrake J, et al. Predicting survival after extracorporeal membrane oxygenation for severe acute respiratory failure. The Respiratory Extracorporeal Membrane Oxygenation Surviv.al Prediction (RESP) score. *Am J Respir Crit Care Med* 2014;189:1374–1382.

76. Goligher EC, Doufle G, Fan E. Update in mechanical ventilation, sedation, and outcomes 2014. *Am J Respir Crit Care Med* 2015;191:1367–1373.

77. Tredget EE, Shankowsky HA, Taerum TV, et al. The role of inhalation injury in burn trauma. A Canadian experience. *Ann Surg* 1990;212:720–727.

78. Smith DL, Cairns BA, Ramadan F, et al. Effect of inhalation injury, burn size, and age on mortality: A study of 1447 consecutive burn patients. *J Trauma* 1994;37: 655–659.

79. Colohan SM. Predicting prognosis in thermal burns with associated inhalational injury: A systematic review of prognostic factors in adult burn victims. *J Burn Care Res* 2010;31:529–539.

80. Shirani KZ, Pruitt BA, Jr., Mason AD, Jr. The influence of inhalation injury and pneumonia on burn mortality. *Ann Surg* 1987;205:82–87.

81. Wearn C, Hardwicke J, Kitsios A, et al. Outcomes of burns in the elderly: Revised estimates from the Birmingham burn centre. *Burns* 2015;41:1161–1168.

82. Woodson LC. Diagnosis and grading of inhalation injury. *J Burn Care Res* 2009;30: 143–145.

83. Dries DJ, Endorf FW. Inhalation injury: epidemiology, pathology, treatment strategies. *Scand J Trauma Resusc Emerg Med* 2013;21:31.

84. Endorf FW, Gamelli RL. Inhalation injury, pulmonary perturbations, and fluid resuscitation. *J Burn Care Res* 2007;28:80–83.

85. Oh JS, Chung KK, Allen A, et al. Admission chest CT complements fiberoptic bronchoscopy in prediction of adverse outcomes in thermally injured patients. *J Burn Care Res* 2012;33:532–538.

86. Kealey GP. Carbon monoxide toxicity. *J Burn Care Res* 2009;30:146–147.

87. Baskin SI, Brewer TG. Cyanide poisoning. In: Sidell FR, Takafuji ET, Franzi DR, eds. *Med Aspects of Chemical and Biological Warfare*. Washington, DC: Department of the Army, Office of the Surgeon General; 1997:271–286.

88. Baud FJ, Borron SW, Mégarbane B, et al. Value of lactic acidosis in the assessment of the severity of acute cyanide poisoning. *Crit Care Med* 2002;30:2044–2050.

89. Walker PF, Buehner MF, Wood LA, et al. Diagnosis and management of inhalation injury: an updated review. *Crit Care* 2015;19:351.

90. Sen S, Greenhalgh D, Palmieri T. Review of burn research for the year 2010. *J Burn Car Res* 2012;33:577–586.

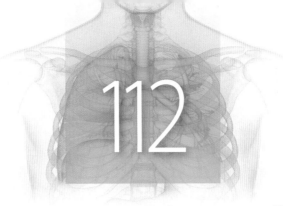

112

Acute Respiratory Distress Syndrome

Ronson J. Madathil ▪ Aaron M. Cheng ▪ Michael S. Mulligan

Our understanding of the relationship between injury, inflammation, and pulmonary dysfunction has been evolving rapidly over the last two centuries. First published in 1819, René Laennec's *A Treatise on the Diseases of the Chest and on Mediate Auscultation* discusses an "idiopathic anasarca of the lungs" as well as "the great affinity… between inflammation and the dropsical diathesis" in the setting of critical illness.[1] By 1892, in his classic text, *The Principles and Practice of Medicine: Designed for the Use of Practitioners and Students of Medicine,* Osler[2] noted that "pneumonia follows traumatism with great frequency, more particularly injury of the chest," which was described by Litten as "contusions-pneumonia." This association between trauma and pulmonary dysfunction would be seen in practice manyfold with the advent of world war. In 1913 with World War I, Pasteur[3] described the entity of "acute massive collapse" of the lung and stressed its relation to trauma. In 1945 with World War II, Majors Burford and Burbank[4] of the Army Medical Corps built on Pasteur's work and called attention to "traumatic wet lung" and the accompanying increase in the "normal amount of interstitial and intra-alveolar fluid" that left the bronchopulmonary tree "not only [with] more fluid to rid itself of, but…less capable of doing so." By the time of the Vietnam War, terms like "shock lung," "wet lung," "stiff lung," "Da Nang lung," "pump lung," and "postperfusion lung" were being used to describe postresuscitation pulmonary dysfunction after circulatory shock in both military and civilian arenas.[5] Finally in 1967, Ashbaugh and colleagues[6] defined "respiratory distress syndrome" as the final common pathway of "alveolar instability" leading to "loss of compliance, refractory cyanosis, and microscopic atelectasis." In 1971, Petty and Ashbaugh[7] coined the term "Adult Respiratory Distress Syndrome" and outlined the basics of its clinical features and principles of management, some of which continue to prove useful today. In 1994, the American-European Consensus Conference (AECC) established definitions and criteria that allowed for the inclusion of children into studies of this syndrome, and thus the modern term of "Acute Respiratory Distress Syndrome" (ARDS) was born.[8]

DEFINITION OF ARDS

In 2012, the Berlin definition of ARDS replaced the 1994 AECC definition of ARDS. Given that much the available evidence regarding ARDS is based on the AECC definition, both definitions are provided herein. The AECC definition included criteria for ARDS and the creation of the term "Acute Lung Injury" (ALI) to describe cases in which the criteria for ARDS were met but in which the hypoxemia was less severe (i.e., P_aO_2/F_iO_2 ≤300 mm Hg vs. P_aO_2/F_iO_2 ≤200 mm Hg). In addition to hypoxia, the other criteria were acute onset, the presence of bilateral infiltrates on chest radiography, and the absence of a cardiogenic cause of the pulmonary edema as defined by a pulmonary artery occlusion pressure (PAOP) less than 18 mm Hg or a lack of clinical evidence for elevated left atrial pressures (Table 112.1).[8]

The definition provided by the 1994 AECC was widely adopted by the clinical and research community. However, despite improvements in the ability to care for patients with ARDS, after 18 years of research and clinical experience it became evident that the AECC definition was lacking. Issues such as the failure to define the period of time that qualifies as "acute onset," the variability in determining the presence of hydrostatic edema, the reality that P_aO_2/F_iO_2 determination is sensitive to the patient's ventilator settings at time of measurement, and the inconsistencies in chest radiograph interpretation were major drivers to restructure the definition of ARDS (Table 112.2).[9]

The major changes introduced by the 2012 Berlin definition of ARDS are that the pulmonary capillary occlusion pressure criterion

TABLE 112.1 Acute Lung Injury and Acute Respiratory Distress Syndrome

	Timing of Onset	Oxygenation	Chest Radiography	Evaluation of Cardiogenic Causation
Acute lung injury	Acute	P_aO_2/F_iO_2 ≤300 mm Hg regardless of positive end-expiratory pressure	Bilateral infiltrates	PAOP[a] ≤18 mm Hg or absence of clinical evidence of elevated left atrial pressure
Acute respiratory distress syndrome	Acute	P_aO_2/F_iO_2 ≤200 mm Hg regardless of positive end-expiratory pressure	Bilateral infiltrates	PAOP[a] ≤18 mm Hg or absence of clinical evidence of elevated left atrial pressure

[a]PAOP, pulmonary artery occlusion pressure.
Adapted from Bernard GR, Artigas A, Brigham KL, et al. The American-European Consensus Conference on ARDS. Definitions, mechanisms, relevant outcomes, and clinical trial coordination. *Am J Respir Crit Care Med* 1994;149:818–824.

TABLE 112.2 The AECC Definition—Limitations and Berlin's Methods of Addressing These

	AECC Definition	AECC Limitations	Method to Address Limitations
Timing of onset	Acute onset	"Acute" is undefined	"Acute" time frame defined
ALI Category	All patients with P_aO_2/F_iO_2 ≤300 mm Hg	Misinterpreted as P_aO_2/F_iO_2 = 201 to 300, leading to confusing ALI/ARDS term	3 Mutually exclusive subgroups of ARDS by severity; ALI term removed
Oxygenation	P_aO_2/F_iO_2 ≤300 mm Hg (regardless of PEEP)	Inconsistency of P_aO_2/F_iO_2 ratio due to the effect of PEEP and/or F_iO_2	Minimal PEEP level added across subgroups F_iO_2 effect less relevant in severe ARDS group
Chest radiography	Bilateral infiltrates observed on frontal chest radiograph	Poor interobserver reliability of chest radiograph interpretation	Chest radiograph criteria clarified Example radiographs created
PAOP[a]	PAOP[a] ≤18 mm Hg when measured or no clinical evidence of left atrial hypertension	High PAOP[a] and ARDS may coexist Poor interobserver reliability of PAOP and clinical assessments of left atrial hypertension	PAOP[a] requirement removed Hydrostatic edema not the primary cause of respiratory failure Clinical vignettes created to help exclude hydrostatic edema
Risk Factor	None	Not formally included in definition	Included When none identified, need to objectively rule out hydrostatic edema

[a]PAOP, pulmonary artery occlusion pressure.

Adapted with permission from The ARDS Definition Task Force. Acute respiratory distress syndrome: The Berlin definition. *JAMA* 2012;307(23):2526–2533. Copyright © 2012 American Medical Association. All rights reserved.

is removed, and that the term ALI is dropped in favor of a "mild-moderate-severe" grading system for ARDS based on level of hypoxia with some standardization of ventilator settings. Thus, mild ARDS is defined as a P_aO_2/F_iO_2 from 200 to 300 mm Hg at a PEEP/CPAP ≥5 cm H_2O, moderate ARDS as a P_aO_2/F_iO_2 from 100 to 200 mm Hg at a PEEP ≥5 cm H_2O, and severe ARDS as a P_aO_2/F_iO_2 <100 mm Hg at a PEEP ≥5 cm H_2O. Additionally, the term "acute onset" is defined as one week, chest imaging is allowed to include CT scanning, and the rule out of a cardiogenic cause of pulmonary dysfunction (e.g., by echocardiography) is required only if there is no ARDS risk factor present (Tables 112.3 and 112.4). Other variables were considered, such as dead space and lung compliance measurements; however, there were no significant differences in the ability of these additional variables to enhance the predictive validity of the weight-adjusted criteria when evaluated based on the available data, so a simpler definition of ARDS based solely on oxygenation was chosen.[9]

brain injury has been revised upward from 21% to 25% based on the 2012 Berlin definition.[10] More modifications based upon the Berlin definition are likely forthcoming.

In 2005, the incidence of ARDS in the United States, based on a multicenter prospective population-based cohort study, estimated that each year in the United States there are 190,600 cases of ALI, which are associated with 74,500 deaths and 3.6 million hospital days with an age-adjusted incidence of 86.2 per 100,000 person-years and an in-hospital mortality rate of 38.5%. The incidence of ALI increased with age from 16 per 100,000 person-years for those aged 15 to 19 years to 306 per 100,000 person-years for those aged 75 to 84 years. Mortality increased with age from 24% for patients aged 15 to 19 years to 60% for patients aged 85 years or older.[11]

The incidence of ARDS outside of the United States appears to be lower. The incidence in Europe is reported to be 7.1% overall and 15.8% in patients admitted with all-cause respiratory failure and

EPIDEMIOLOGY OF ARDS

It is important to note that much of the currently available data regarding the incidence of ARDS is based on the 1994 AECC definition of ARDS and ALI. The incidence of ARDS following traumatic

TABLE 112.3 Risk Factors for ARDS

Direct Pulmonary Insults	Indirect Pulmonary Insults
Pneumonia	Non-pulmonary sepsis
Aspiration of gastric contents	Major trauma
Inhalational injury	Pancreatitis
Pulmonary contusion	Severe burns
Pulmonary vasculitis	Non-cardiogenic shock
Drowning	Drug overdose
	Multiple transfusions or transfusion-associated acute lung injury (TRALI)

Adapted with permission from The ARDS Definition Task Force. Acute respiratory distress syndrome: The Berlin definition. *JAMA* 2012;307(23):2526–2533. Copyright © 2012 American Medical Association. All rights reserved.

TABLE 112.4 The Berlin Definition of ARDS

Timing	Within 1 week of a known clinical insult or new or worsening respiratory symptoms
Chest Imaging[a]	Bilateral opacities—not fully explained by effusions, lobar/lung collapse, or nodules
Origin of edema	Respiratory failure not fully explained by cardiac failure or fluid overload. Need objective assessment (e.g., echocardiography) to exclude hydrostatic edema if no risk factor present
Oxygenation[b]	
Mild	P_aO_2/F_iO_2 from 200–300 mm Hg with PEEP/CPAP ≥5 cmH_2O
Moderate	P_aO_2/F_iO_2 from 100–200 mm Hg with PEEP ≥5 cmH_2O
Severe	P_aO_2/F_iO_2 <100 mm Hg with PEEP ≥5cm H_2O

[a]Refers to chest radiograph or CT scan.
[b]If altitude is higher than 1000 m, the correction factor should be calculated as follows: P_aO_2/F_iO_2 × (barometric pressure/760).

Adapted with permission from The ARDS Definition Task Force. Acute respiratory distress syndrome: The Berlin definition. *JAMA* 2012;307(23):2526–2533. Copyright © 2012 American Medical Association. All rights reserved.

16.1% in those requiring mechanical ventilation.[12] ICU and hospital mortalities are 22.6% and 32.7% for ALI, and 49.4% and 57.9% for ARDS, respectively.[13] In Australia, the incidence is 34 cases per 100,000 person-years with a mortality rate of 28% for ALI.[12]

PATHOPHYSIOLOGY OF ARDS

In healthy tissue, a careful balance of forces governs the exchange of fluid and protein between the plasma in the capillary, the surrounding interstitium, and the draining lymphatics to keep a given organ optimally functioning. In 1896, Starling[14] proposed that the volumetric flow of fluid across the capillary wall is governed by a net imbalance of hydrostatic and oncotic forces ($\Delta P_{hydrostatic}$ and $\Delta P_{oncotic}$, respectively). Although Starling never described the mathematical relationship between these forces in his original work (this was done later by Iverson and Johansen in 1929), the equation used today bears his name.[15] The steady-state relationship between fluid flow across an idealized semi-permeable capillary membrane and these forces is shown in the following, simplified Starling equation:

$$J_v = K_f \times (\Delta P_{hydrostatic} - \Delta P_{oncotic}) \quad (1)$$

where J_v is the net fluid flux between compartments (by convention, a positive number represents net flow out of the capillary lumen and a negative number represents net flow into the capillary lumen) and K_f is the filtration coefficient, which is a product of the permeability of the endothelial membrane (L_p) and the surface area available for movement of fluid (A). Refining Equation 1 with this product and expanding $\Delta P_{hydrostatic}$ and $\Delta P_{oncotic}$ to demonstrate those forces whose effect is to direct fluid out of the capillary lumen (the capillary

hydrostatic pressure and the interstitial oncotic pressure) and those whose effect is to direct fluid into the capillary lumen (the capillary oncotic pressure and the interstitial hydrostatic pressure) reveals the following, expanded Starling equation:

$$J_v = L_p A \times [(P_c - P_i) - \sigma(\pi_c - \pi_i)], \quad \text{where } 0 \le \sigma \le 1 \quad (2)$$

where P_c and P_i are the respective capillary and interstitial hydrostatic pressures, π_c and π_i are the respective capillary and interstitial oncotic pressures, and σ is the reflection coefficient of the capillary membrane to proteins (which ranges from 0 if completely protein permeable to 1 if completely protein impermeable).[15]

The original model is meant to describe a capillary-tissue–lymphatic system as shown in Figure 112.1. It assumes an idealized capillary whose wall is a homogenous single layer with a reflection coefficient close to 1, thus leaving the proteins mostly in the capillary lumen and the interstitium filled with what is mathematically treated as a nearly protein-free ultrafiltrate. This model also posits that at the proximal (arterial) end of the capillary, the net filtration gradient is directed outward and that as the hydrostatic pressure falls along the length of the capillary, the gradient becomes directed inward at the distal (venous) end of the capillary as the fluid is returned to the capillary lumen driven primarily by the oncotic pressure gradient. The overaccumulation of fluid in the interstitium, and thus tissue edema, is prevented by this net filtration reversal and lymphatic removal.[15,16] Since its introduction, further measurements and studies have since shown that many of the assumptions of the traditional model are incorrect, and that this single layer model is far too simple for the more complex structure and interplay of the capillary, interstitial space, and lymphatics—particularly in the context of organ tissue-type and tissue state (e.g., inflamed).[17–23]

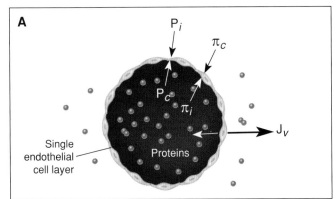

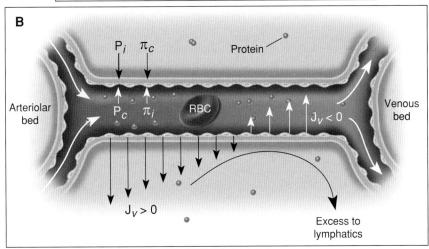

FIGURE 112.1 Classic Starling Capillary-Tissue–Lymphatic System Model. J_v, net filtration, positive value out of capillary, negative value into capillary; P_c, hydrostatic pressure of the capillary; P_i, hydrostatic pressure of the interstitium; π_c, oncotic pressure of the capillary; π_i, oncotic pressure of the interstitium. **A:** Cross-section of classic model capillary with Starling forces and their direction. **B:** Depiction of classic Starling Capillary-Tissue–Lymphatic System Model with Starling forces and demonstration of net filtration change over length of capillary.

Regarding the structure of the capillary itself, the capillary wall is not a homogenous single layer, but rather an outer layer of endothelial cells whose luminal surface is lined with an inner layer of the capillary wall called the glycocalyx. This is a 60 to 750 nm thick hydrated gel layer formed from glycosaminoglycans (GAGs) and other glycoproteins (e.g., sialic acids) that serves as a filtration barrier (Fig. 112.2). The glycocalyx forms protrusions into the lumen ("hairy tufts")

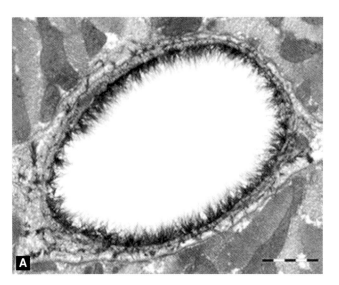

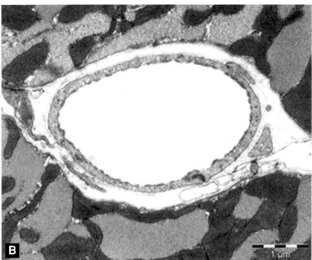

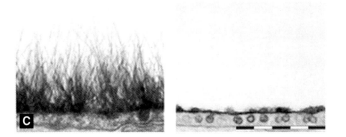

FIGURE 112.2 **A:** Electron micrograph of normal rat capillary cross-section. **B:** After hyaluronidase treatment to remove the glycocalyx layer. **C:** Detail of normal capillary wall with intact glycocalyx (left) and without (right). It is notable that a far greater proportion of the capillary wall thickness is actually glycocalyx and not the endothelial cell layer. (From van den Berg BM, Vink H, Spaan JA. The endothelial glycocalyx protects against myocardial edema. *Circ Res* 2003;92(6):592–594. doi: 10.1161/01.RES.0000065917.53950.75.)

which allow it to serve as a size-selective and charge-selective molecular sieve to plasma proteins, and yet remain permeable to water and small solutes such as oxygen and other nutrient metabolites.[17] The endothlial cells are also separated by intercellular clefts. These clefts can be closed partially or nearly completely by junctional strands which further modulate the selectivity of the whole barrier.[17,18] This selectivity differs depending on the type of tissue in which the capillary is present. Thus, the capillary reflection coefficient is not fixed close to 1 as is assumed in the classical model, but rather to a tissue-specific (e.g., kidney, lung, brain, etc.) and context-sensitive value (e.g., inflammation, variations in autoregulated smooth muscle controlled filtration, etc.) thereby rendering the interstitium not entirely protein-free.[19]

Instead, it has been shown that almost 50% of the body's albumin content is extravascular and that the directly measured oncotic pressure of the interstitium is approximately 30% to 60% of that of plasma.[20,21] The interstitium is not simply a nearly protein-free ultrafiltrate of plasma, but rather a dynamic system that consists of three phases: a free-flowing fluid phase, a gel phase composed of polyanionic GAGs, and a collagen matrix.[19,21] Interstitial albumin is confined to the fluid phase and its concentration is governed by water and albumin flux across the capillary. The GAGs of the gel phase have sodium ions bound to them which results in a net osmotic effect that promotes capillary filtration. The collagen matrix provides an opposing hydrostatic pressure. The net effect of these forces combined with those occurring in the capillary has been demonstrated to be that in the majority of the body's capillary beds, net filtration occurs throughout the entire length of the capillary.[18] This is contrary to the assumed reversal of filtration thought to occur in the traditional model. To prevent edema then, the accumulation from the continual net filtration of fluid and protein from the capillary to the interstitial space is returned to the intravascular space primarily by lymphatic drainage (Fig. 112.3).[18,21]

The original model and Starling's equation fall short of accurately describing this multicompartment, multilayer system. Newer and more sophisticated mathematical models have been proposed to account for these additional findings. One such model proposed by Facchini and colleagues attempts to account for the glycocalyx as a second layer in addition to the capillary cell wall to describe the total solvent (fluid) fluxes (J_v) and solute (protein) fluxes (J_s), thus revealing the following equations:

$$J_v = \int_0^{2\pi} q_v(r)(r+\xi)d\theta = -2\Pi(r+\xi)_p\left(\frac{dp}{dr} - \sigma\frac{d\Pi}{dr}\right) \quad (3)$$

$$J_s = \int_0^{2\pi} q_s(r)(r+\xi)d\theta = -2\pi(r+\xi)\Pi\left[_p(\sigma-1)\frac{dp}{dr} + (_p\sigma - _d)\frac{d\Pi}{dr}\right]$$

$$(4)$$

where the basic overall form still mirrors that of the original Starling equation (Equation 2),[17] but it is evident that a full modeling of this system will be complex, and even then, it will have to be tailored to specific tissue types and tissue states.

Particularly in the lungs, this complex system is a bit unique. As part of the right-sided, low pressure half of the cardiac system, the alveolar capillaries have a relatively low hydrostatic pressure compared to other capillary beds in the body that are perfused by the left-sided, higher pressure half of the cardiac system. Despite this, the pulmonary bed is relatively robust in its ability to withstand edema formation, requiring at least a 15 mm Hg increase in the filtration gradient before edema can be appreciated.[15] Augmentation of lymphatic flow and the increased interstitial hydrostatic pressure

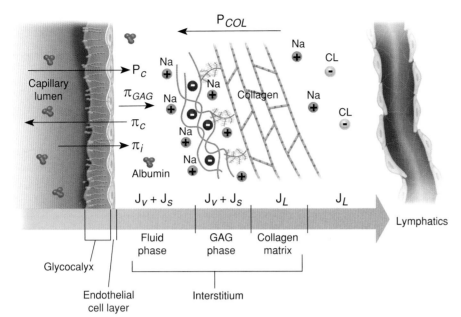

FIGURE 112.3 Updated Capillary Glycocalyx–Triphasic Interstitium-Lymphatic Model. J_v, net capillary fluid flow; J_s, net capillary solute flow; J_L, net lymphatic flow; P_c, hydrostatic pressure of the capillary; P_{COL}, hydrostatic pressure of the interstitial collagen matrix; π_c, oncotic pressure of the capillary; π_i, oncotic pressure of the interstitial free fluid phase; π_{GAG}, oncotic pressure of the interstitial GAGs in the gel phase. An integrated and updated representation of the capillary-tissue–lymphatic model. In the steady state, net lymphatic flow (J_L) must equal net capillary flow ($J_v + J_s$) to prevent tissue edema. Note also how the interstitium consists of three unique phases with their own associated forces: a free-flowing fluid phase, a gel phase composed of polyanionic GAGs, and a collagen matrix.

(which will decrease the overall outward filtration gradient) protect the lungs from edema at lower pressures.[24] In cases of acute increases in pulmonary capillary pressures, edema formation can begin at pressures of 18 mm Hg due to overwhelming the clearance ability of the lymphatic system. In cases of chronic increases (e.g., chronic heart failure), edema may not be seen until pulmonary capillary pressures of >25 mm Hg as the lymphatic system has had time to adapt.[25] Additionally, the alveolar capillaries are more protein-permeable than other capillary beds resulting in a smaller oncotic pressure gradient.[15,26] This has a protective effect in pro-edema states like chronic hypoalbuminemia where the increased protein permeability allows for equilibration of the luminal and interstitial albumin concentrations, thus mitigating pulmonary edema even when the hypoalbuminemia is low enough to cause peripheral edema.[27] In the setting of acute crystalloid administration where there is little time for interstitial albumin to equilibrate, not surprisingly, pulmonary edema occurs far more easily.

In ARDS, these systems are thrown out of balance. In particular, the functions of the glycocalyx in the capillaries of the pulmonary tissue are disrupted and result in the pathophysiologic manifestations of ARDS: augmented neutrophil adhesion, increased protein and fluid permeability, and dysfunctional NO signaling and vasorelaxation (Fig. 112.4).[28,29] The glycocalyx serves as a natural barrier between circulating neutrophils and the pulmonary endothelium and interstitium. Studies of patients with inflammatory diseases like septic shock demonstrate high plasma concentrations of circulating GAG fragments suggestive of glycocalyx degradation. This degradation has been shown to be associated with activation of endothelial heparinase, which acts on heparin sulfate (the major GAG component of the glycocalyx), leading to glycocalyx degradation and subsequent exposure of pulmonary endothelial surface adhesion molecules (e.g., ICAM-1, VCAM-1) that assist in the adherence and extravasation of circulating activated neutrophils.[28]

Unlike in the systemic capillary beds, in the pulmonary capillary bed, the glycocalyx GAGs do not appear to serve as a passive barrier to fluid and protein.[28] Rather, it is the degradation of the non-GAG components (sialic acids) that results in the increased protein and fluid permeability of the pulmonary endothelium. Whether this is

due to their structural effects or alterations in signaling is unclear, though it appears that use of particular neuraminidases to degrade sialic acids was actually associated with increases in barrier function suggesting more of a signaling role.[28,29] Thus, the idea that the glycocalyx serves as a passive barrier to protein and fluid is not the complete picture.

The signaling functions of the glycocalyx may also play a part in the alterations of NO signaling and vasorelaxation seen in ARDS. The heparin sulfate and hyaluronic acid GAGs of the glycocalyx are key components in the translation of vascular luminal shear stress into NO-regulated vasodilation, a process known as mechanotransduction.[28,29] In vitro studies have demonstrated a NO-dependent increase in vascular permeability in the setting of increased vascular flow/shear stress. This effect was lost after treatment with heparinase-III suggesting that the heparin sulfates of the glycocalyx serve as a vascular pressure transducer to the endothelial cells. Nonetheless, the characteristic interstitial edema, protein leakage, and ultimately decreased lung compliance seen in ARDS may be at least partially attributable to the degradation of the glycocalyx that occurs during inflammatory states.[28,29]

Since Starling's model, the physiology of the pulmonary vascular bed has proved to be remarkably more complex and nuanced than originally conceived. The importance of the draining lymphatics, the triphasic interstitium, and the glycocalyx and its interactions with the endothelium may have important implications in the design of future treatments of ARDS. Modulation, in addition to preservation and restoration of the glycocalyx, may be necessary to attenuate the pathologic manifestations of ARDS. For example, basic science proof-of-concept models have already been developed utilizing biomimetic polymers to bind to the glycocalyx of lung endothelium and augment barrier function in an effort to reduce permeability to protein and fluid flux into the interstitium.[30,31] This has implications in the setting of conditions that put patients at risk for ARDS like sepsis, trauma, pulmonary resection, and perhaps even in the setting of lung transplantation. The lymphatics of the donor lungs are not in continuity with those of the recipient, thus leaving the only major exit for the fluid and protein accumulated in the interstitium due to ischemia–reperfusion injury efflux back into the pulmonary vasculature. Until

A The glycocalyx under normal conditions.

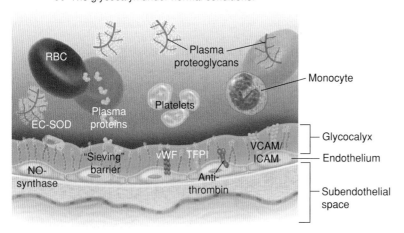

B The glycocalyx under stressed conditions (e.g., sepsis, ARDS, ischemia-reperfusion injury, etc.).

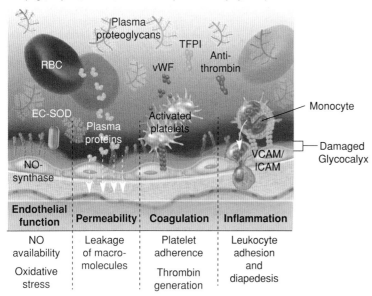

Endothelial function	Permeability	Coagulation	Inflammation
NO availability	Leakage of macro-molecules	Platelet adherence	Leukocyte adhesion and diapedesis
Oxidative stress		Thrombin generation	

FIGURE 112.4 The Effects of Damage to the Glycocalyx. **A:** The glycocalyx under normal conditions. **B:** The glycocalyx under stressed conditions (e.g., sepsis, ARDS, ischemia-reperfusion injury, etc.).

such interventions are clinically available, an overall conservative-fluid strategy with judicious use of vasopressors to address minor dips in systemic blood pressure rather than a traditional aggressive volume-resuscitation strategy is likely the best approach.

MANAGEMENT OF ARDS

The main principle in ARDS management is to provide the patient adequate pulmonary support, in a manner that minimizes iatrogenic injury, and also to arrest and prevent further insult to other organ systems while correcting the underlying causes and drivers of the ARDS. The foundation of this principle is the observation that only a minority of ARDS patients die from respiratory failure alone whereas a majority die from their primary illness or from secondary complications such as sepsis and multisystem organ failure.[32–34] At the time Ashbaugh and colleagues[6] coined the term "respiratory distress syndrome," mortality rates for ARDS were around 50%. Though the specific mortality rates are difficult to quote as they vary between observational versus randomized trials. Since that time mortality

rates for ARDS generally have been declining.[35] A specific cause for this decline is unclear. The reasons are likely multifactorial and the result of a variety of improvements in understanding and subsequent management strategies.

VENTILATOR STRATEGIES

The details of conventional ventilator management are covered in Chapter 41. In ARDS, conventional management strategies often prove to be inadequate as the syndrome progresses. While there is some supporting data regarding the use of negative pressure ventilation in the management of ARDS,[36] the vast majority of data and experience is with positive pressure ventilation. Since positive pressure ventilation is nonphysiologic by definition,[37–39] and the pathophysiology of ARDS renders the lungs particularly susceptible to injury from the ventilator itself,[40] the focus of ventilator management strategies for ARDS is on minimizing the harmful effects of the ventilator on the lungs while still providing adequate oxygenation. Major harmful pulmonary effects associated with the ventilator are shown in Table 112.5.

TABLE 112.5 Deleterious Effects of Various Ventilator Strategies

Oxygen Toxicity—hyperoxia leading to absorptive atelectasis and reactive oxygen species (ROS) that cause injury ranging from tracheobronchitis to diffuse alveolar damage (DAD) that is histologically indistinguishable from ARDS.[41–43]

Barotrauma—gross pulmonary air leaks (pneumothorax, pneumomediastinum, pneumoperitoneum, and/or subcutaneous emphysema) due to rupture from the excessive differential between the alveolar pressure and that of the bronchovascular sheath.[44,45]

Volutrauma—alveolar overdistension leading to alveolar strain. This excessive end-inspiratory alveolar stretch from large ventilator-delivered lung volumes can result in edema and DAD.[46,47]

Atelectrauma/Cyclical Atelectasis—repeated collapse and re-expansion of alveoli between ventilatory breaths can result in significant cytokine release causing inflammation and edema.[48–50]

Biotrauma—release of inflammatory mediators from the lung causing inflammation, edema, and DAD. This occurs as a primary consequence of positive-pressure ventilation itself as well as secondary consequence, or "final common pathway," of harmful ventilator effects described above.[51,52] In the setting of the abnormal and increased capillary permeability that occurs in ARDS, these mediators may cross over into the systemic circulation which could contribute to the multisystem organ failure seen in ARDS patients.[53–56]

The consequence of this collection of deleterious effects from the ventilator is known as ventilator-associated lung injury (VALI),[57–59] and while it is often clinically indistinguishable from ARDS (unless barotrauma is present), it more than likely worsens outcomes when present in ARDS patients.[60,61]

What does improve outcomes of ARDS patients is the early application and adherence to a strategy of low tidal volume ventilation (LTVV) which is also known as lung protective ventilation (LPV). The rationale of this approach is to use smaller tidal volumes to reduce alveolar overdistension thereby reducing VALI. In 2000, the results of the ARDSnet (ARMA) trial were published which compared the outcomes of 861 mechanically ventilated ARDS patients randomly assigned to two different initial tidal volumes: a conventional tidal volume goal of 12 mL/kg predicted body weight (PBW) versus an LTVV goals of 6 mL/kg PBW. The tidal volumes were then adjusted to maintain plateau pressures below a certain level ($\leq$50 cm H_2O in the conventional group and $\leq$30 cm H_2O in the LTVV group). The study was stopped early due to the demonstration of a lower mortality in the LTVV group compared to the conventional group (31.0% vs. 39.8%, p <0.007). Additionally, the LTVV group had more ventilator-free days (12 vs. 10 days, p <0.007) and were more likely to be breathing off of the ventilator by day 28 (65.7% vs. 55.0%, p <0.001) when compared with the conventional group.[62] This observed mortality benefit of LTVV over conventional ventilation has since been strongly supported by additional studies.[63,64]

Two analyses of the same cohort of over 480 patients have demonstrated that strict adherence to the strategy is required to fully realize the benefits of LTVV. In the first analysis, an increase of initial tidal volume by 1 mL/kg PBW conferred a 23% increase in mortality (adjusted HR 1.23; 95% CI 1.06–1.44; P = 0.008), and each additional 1 mL/kg PBW after the initial tidal volume was associated with a 15% increase in mortality (adjusted HR 1.15; 95% CI 1.02–1.29; P = 0.019).[65] In the second analysis, when compared with no adherence to the LTVV strategy, the estimated absolute risk reduction

(ARR) in 2-year mortality for a prototypical patient with 50% adherence to LTVV was 4.0% (0.8% to 7.2%, P = 0.012) and with 100% adherence was 7.8% (1.6% to 14.0%, P = 0.011).[66] An intervention shown to promote early application and adherence is implementation in the ICU of a written protocol for LTVV which is associated with enhanced compliance in ARDS patients.[67]

Application of LTVV can be achieved either by volume- or pressure-controlled modes of positive pressure mechanical ventilation. Generally speaking, assuming that the patient's lung mechanics and effort are stable from breath to breath, a volume-control mode should produce a stable airway pressure and a pressure-control mode should deliver stable tidal volumes. In practice, it is probably easiest to achieve goal LTVV using a volume-control mode of ventilation with careful airway pressure monitoring and the desired tidal volume set by the clinician; however, a pressure-control mode may be used by titrating the pressure to achieve a 6 mL/kg PBW tidal volume. Ultimately, the ideal mode is best determined by patient response and clinician comfort with the applied mode of ventilation to achieve proper adherence to the LTVV strategy.

To further minimize VALI, the LTVV strategy can be combined with the use of applied positive end-expiratory pressure (PEEP) into a strategy known as open lung ventilation (OLV). While the LTVV serves to minimize alveolar overdistension, the applied PEEP is meant to reduce the number of alveoli subject to cyclical atelectasis thus maintaining a more consistently "open lung." Volutrauma and atelectrauma are the two biggest contributors to VALI,[68] and the OLV strategy is intended to attenuate their effects. Studies of the OLV strategy have demonstrated a mortality benefit. In one Brazilian multicenter trial, 53 ARDS patients were randomized to either conventional ventilation or OLV. Conventional ventilation was defined as tidal volumes of 12 mL/kg PBW, the lowest PEEP for acceptable oxygenation, and maintenance of a P_aCO_2 of 35 to 38 mm Hg. OLV was defined as tidal volumes of 6 mL/kg PBW, PEEP titrated to end-expiratory pressures above the lower inflection point on the static pressure–volume curve, driving pressures <20 cm H_2O above PEEP, preferential use of pressure-limited ventilatory modes, and P_aCO_2 was allowed to rise if necessary to maintain the strategy (i.e., permissive hypercapnia [PHC]). The OLV group had a lower 28-day mortality (38% vs. 71%, P <0.001), higher rates of weaning from mechanical ventilation (66% vs. 29%, P <0.005), and lower rates of barotrauma despite the higher PEEP and mean airway pressures (7% vs. 42%, P <0.02).[69] In another multicenter randomized-controlled study from Spain, 103 ARDS patients were randomized to either conventional ventilation (tidal volumes 9 to 11 mL/kg PBW, PEEP >5 cm H_2O) or OLV (tidal volumes 5 to 8 mL/kg PBW, PEEP set 2 cm above the lower inflection point of the pressure volume curve of the respiratory system on day 1). The trial was stopped early due to meeting predetermined efficacy criteria. All outcomes were better in the OLV group versus the conventional ventilation group: ICU mortality (32% vs. 53.3%, p <0.040), hospital mortality (34% vs. 55.5%, p <0.041), ventilator-free days at day 28 (10.90 vs. 6.02, p <0.008), and mean difference in the number of additional organ failures (0.3 vs. 1.2, p <0.001).[70] While the OLV appears to be a superior strategy to conventional ventilation, what is unclear from these studies is whether there is added mortality benefit gained from the higher PEEP component or if the demonstrated mortality benefit is derived entirely from the LTVV component.

To address this issue, three large multicenter randomized controlled trials have tested higher versus lower PEEP combined with a baseline LTVV strategy in both groups: the Assessment of Low tidal Volume and elevated End-expiratory volume to Obviate Lung Injury trial (ALVEOLI trial),[71] the Expiratory Pressure trial (ExPress trial),[72] and the Lung Open Ventilation Study trial (LOVS trial).[73] While the ExPress trial did show an improvement using a high PEEP (OLV) compared with a low PEEP (LTVV) strategy in ventilator-free days (7 vs. 3 days, $P = 0.04$) and organ failure-free days (6 vs. 2 days, $P = 0.04$),[74] individually none of these studies demonstrated an improvement in mortality with OLV versus LTVV. However, when the data from these studies were combined as a meta-analysis using an individual patient analysis, there was a modest mortality benefit for patients with Berlin-defined moderate or severe ARDS (i.e., patients with P_aO_2 <200 mm Hg) using an OLV versus LTVV strategy (34.1% vs. 39.1%, $P = 0.049$), as well as ventilator-free days at day 28 (12 vs. 7 days, p <0.004).[75] Thus, while there may not necessarily be as clear a mortality benefit of OLV over LTVV as compared with LTVV over conventional ventilation, there appears to be clinical utility, and little harm, realized from employing an OLV strategy, particularly in moderate and severe ARDS patients.

The idea of using applied PEEP in ARDS has been around since Ashbaugh's original description of ARDS.[6] Physiologically, it increases the end-expiratory lung volume (EELV), but this can happen in one of two ways. Ideally, applied PEEP increases EELV by reopening collapsed lung (recruitment) and preventing re-collapse (de-recruitment and atelectrauma). However, in a patient that has a paucity of recruitable lung, the observed increase in EELV is due to increased inflation of already opened alveoli which may lead to overdistension and volutrauma.[68] The challenge is then to determine which patients will respond beneficially to applied PEEP and those that will not. There is a large variability, anywhere from 0% to >50% in one study, in the amount of recruitable lung in the ARDS patient population.[76] The various OLV studies used different approaches to determine PEEP, but none made valid individual patient assessments of recruitability and optimal PEEP determination.[74,77,78] This may be the reason for the small net effect observed in improving mortality.[79] Given the heterogeneity of ARDS patients and their amount of recruitable lung, determining a valid method by which to individualize PEEP to patients would seem to be a reasonable goal.

A variety of clinical techniques have been devised and examined to determine the optimal PEEP in an individual ARDS patient:[80] multiple pressure–volume curves analysis,[60,81–85] measurement of lung volume by nitrogen washout/wash-in,[86,87] transpulmonary pressure estimation by transesophageal pressure measurement,[74,77–79,88,89] use of lung ultrasound,[80] and use of simple oxygenation response to titrate PEEP.[78,79,82,90,91] Though more suited to research study, CT scan–derived PEEP selection has also been examined,[90] and even though it provides the most direct way to assess recruitability (by visual analysis), lung recruitability and CT scan–derived PEEP were unrelated. In other words, to overcome the compressive forces and to lift up the thoracic cage, a similar PEEP level is required in higher and lower recruiters to keep the whole lung open (16.8 ± 4 cm H_2O vs. 16.6 ± 5.6 cm H_2O, $P = 1$).[92]

Given that there is some evidence to indicate that high PEEP is beneficial in some ARDS patients, a better means to individualize therapy using a bedside method to assess lung recruitability would seem necessary. Although reasonably founded in the basics of pulmonary physiology and each with some measure of supporting data, when compared, none of the aforementioned methods has stood out as the ideal clinically preferred means to select the "right" PEEP for a given ARDS patient. While it is clear that more study is required before a given method can be fully endorsed. That is a patient-specific, individually determined level that avoids atelectrauma, provides maximal compliance, maximal oxygenation, and the lowest dead space all without volutrauma and without affecting hemodynamics. There is also the feeling that a more appreciable reality that "the

best PEEP" may not actually exist.[93] Based on current understanding of pulmonary physiology and ARDS pathophysiology as well as the available data regarding the various ventilation and PEEP titration strategies, a sensible approach to determining initial ventilator settings in an ARDS patient that reasonably compromises between oxygenation, hemodynamics, and cyclical atelectasis (dependent on lung recruitability, which is correlated to ARDS severity) would be to employ a LTVV strategy using low PEEP (5–10 cm H_2O) in mild ARDS, moderate PEEP (10–15 cm H_2O) in moderate ARDS, and high PEEP (15–20 cm H_2O) in severe ARDS.[94,95]

PERMISSIVE HYPERCAPNIA

The focus of ventilator management strategies for ARDS is on minimizing the harmful effects of the ventilator on the lungs while still providing adequate oxygenation. With the clearly demonstrated benefits of LTVV, it becomes important to understand how to deal with the physiologic consequences of its application. One of the commonly encountered consequences of the lower tidal volumes in the LTVV strategy is a reduction in minute ventilation leading to an increase in P_aCO_2 (hypercarbia) with an accompanying decrease in pH (acidemia). Though physiologically linked, P_aCO_2 and pH can be independently managed to some degree. The strategy that accepts this state of iatrogenic hypercarbia with acidemia management in exchange for protective alveolar hypoventilation with lower alveolar pressure to minimize alveolar overdistension is known as permissive hypercapnia (PHC).[96,97]

To attenuate the degree of hypercapnia and acidemia, the highest respiratory rate as limited by auto-PEEP should be chosen.[98] To minimize dead space ventilation, both the ventilator tubing should be made as short as is reasonably possible and a heated humidifier should be used instead of a heat and moisture exchanger.[99,100] If despite these interventions, the P_aCO_2 continues to rise, the rate at which the P_aCO_2 is allowed to rise should be gradual. Ideally it should occur at a rate <10 mm Hg/hr and even slower if the P_aCO_2 >80 mm Hg, which will allow for the robust extracellular and intracellular adaptive mechanisms to adjust appropriately.[101] These systems can confer the ability to tolerate extraordinarily high P_aCO_2 levels—even as high as 373 mm Hg—without adverse outcome.[102]

There is no consensus as to whether the resultant acidemia should be corrected, and if so, how and to what degree. It is interesting to note that in the ARMA trial showing the benefit of maintaining a plateau pressure <30 cm H_2O with LTVV, the patient pH was corrected to a value of 7.38 by day 1 with sodium bicarbonate infusions and ventilator rate increases,[82] whereas in three trials that showed no benefit to LTVV, the patients had pH values of 7.29,[103] 7.28,[104] and 7.34[105] by day 1.[106] This by no means provides hard evidence to warrant strict correction of pH to normal. Reasons not to correct the pH to normal include the potential for benefit from hypercapnic acidemia and potential for harm from buffering it.[107,108] Buffering with sodium bicarbonate can worsen hypercapnia and increase intracellular acidity,[109] and a large change in serum bicarbonate generally results in only a modest increase in pH for a given P_aCO_2 thus making the required amount of bicarbonate to be administered in the setting of hypercarbia prohibitive.[94,110–112] Use of an agent other than sodium bicarbonate such as Carbicarb, or tris-hydroxymethyl aminomethane (THAM or tromethamine) should mitigate some of these issues as they provide buffering capacity without CO_2 production.[113,114] A reasonable goal then, would be to maintain a pH of at least 7.15 to 7.20 using either Carbicarb or THAM preferentially and only sodium bicarbonate if necessary.[109]

There is a fair amount of data to suggest that moderate hypercapnia (often independent of acidemia) is protective in lung disease by directly reducing stretch-induced inflammation and VALI, limiting lung ischemia–reperfusion injury, providing protection in early pneumonia and early sepsis, attenuating pulmonary vascular remodeling in pulmonary hypertension, and inhibiting increased alveolar capillary permeability in a variety of pulmonary disease states.[99] Despite these potential benefits, hypercapnia is no panacea either. There are also data showing that it may slow lung epithelial and cellular repair following stretch injury, increase bacterial dissemination, impair neutrophils in prolonged sepsis, exacerbate pulmonary hypertension, right ventricular dysfunction, and decrease alveolar fluid clearance.[115] However in the context of ARDS, there have been no clinical trials to examine the direct effects of PHC on ARDS patients. A secondary analysis of the ARMA trial demonstrated that hypercapnic acidosis was associated with reduced 28-day mortality in the conventional ventilation group, but not in the LTVV group, after controlling for comorbidities and severity of lung injury.[116] While this may suggest that there is an independent benefit to PHC in protecting the lung whose observable effect was perhaps overshadowed by the protective effect on LTVV in the intervention group, since this was a *post hoc* analysis of a study designed primarily to examine the effects of LTVV and not PHC on ARDS. The determination of a relationship between PHC and overall lung protection in the clinical setting cannot be made.

NEUROMUSCULAR BLOCKADE

ARDS patients are often plagued with issues of ventilator dyssynchrony and chest wall elastance resulting in increased work of breathing and carbon dioxide production as well as decreased oxygenation. While neuromuscular blockade has been shown to improve oxygenation in ARDS,[109] it also is associated with complications such as increased neuromuscular weakness in critically ill patients.[117] Despite these conflicting initial observations, meta-analysis of three major studies demonstrates that short-term (<48 hours) infusion of cisatracurium besylate consistently reduced the risk of death at 28 days, death at ICU discharge, death at hospital discharge. It also reduced the risk of barotrauma without affecting the duration of mechanical ventilation or the risk of ICU-acquired weakness for critically ill adults with moderate to severe ARDS being treated with LTVV.[118]

FLUID MANAGEMENT

Due to the impaired lymphatic drainage and increased vascular permeability that is present in ARDS, an ARDS patient is more likely to develop pulmonary edema for any given hydrostatic pressure, including when euvolemic. With this premise in mind, a conservative fluid strategy has been suggested as an intervention to reduce the amount of pulmonary edema in ARDS patients.

The Fluid and Catheter Treatment Trial (FACTT) by the ARDS-net group examined this idea. Using central venous pressure (CVP) or PAOP to determine volume status, 1,000 ARDS patients were randomized into two groups governed by explicit protocols: a fluid-conservative group (goal CVP <4 mm Hg or PAOP <8 mm Hg) and a fluid-liberal group (goal CVP 10 to 14 mm Hg or PAOP 14 to 18 mm Hg), both treated for 7 days. During the study, the cumulative fluid balance over 7 days was −136 ± 491 mL in the fluid-conservative group and 6,992 ± 502 mL in the fluid-liberal group (P <0.001). Although there was no significant difference in 60-day mortality, the fluid-conservative group compared with the fluid-liberal group demonstrated improved lung function and lower lung injury scores

over the first 7 days. During the first 28 days, they demonstrated a higher number of ventilator-free days (14.6 ± 0.5 vs. 12.1 ± 0.5, P <0.001) and days not in the ICU (13.4 ± 0.4 vs. 11.2 ± 0.4, P <0.001) without an increase in the incidence or prevalence of shock during the study or the use of dialysis during the first 60 days (10% vs. 14%, P = 0.06).[119] The fluid-conservative FACTT protocol is complex. Since FACTT, a simplification of the fluid-conservative protocol known as FACTT Lite was created and examined retrospectively, and though it had a greater cumulative fluid balance than FACTT's fluid conservative protocol, it had equivalent clinical and safety outcomes.[120]

While a CVP <4 mm Hg or PAOP <8 mm Hg is a reasonable goal to target from an ARDS standpoint, from a clinical point of view, preservation of end-organ perfusion trumps ARDS management. During FACTT, mean CVP and PAOP remained well above the target goals in the fluid-conservative management group, highlighting how difficult these goals are to achieve even in the setting of a trial.[121] Another adjunct to potentially improve fluid balance would be the use of albumin instead of crystalloid, particularly in combination with furosemide. Based on limited data, the use of albumin appears to improve oxygenation and fluid balance in early ARDS (<72 hours) with no change in mortality.[115,122]

PRONE POSITIONING

For decades, mechanical ventilation in the prone position has been used as alternative to the supine position to improve oxygenation in patients with pulmonary disease and ARDS in particular. The exact mechanism of this effect is uncertain and likely multifactorial. The most important mechanisms are likely improved gas exchange, decreased lung compression from intrathoracic and abdominal contents, and improved perfusion resulting in better V/Q matching and decreased shunt fraction.[123-128] In 2013, a multicenter prospective randomized controlled trial enrolled 466 patients with severe ARDS to either undergo prone-positioning sessions of at least 16 hours within the first 12 to 24 hours or to be left in the supine position. The 28-day mortality rate was lower in the prone group compared with the supine group (16.0% vs. 32.8%, P <0.001), with a hazard ratio of 0.39 (95% CI 0.25 to 0.63). Unadjusted 90-day mortality was also lower in the prone group (23.6% vs. 41.0%, P <0.001), with a hazard ratio of 0.44 (95% CI 0.29 to 0.67). The incidence of complications did not differ significantly between the groups, except for the higher incidence of cardiac arrests in the supine group.[129]

A separate meta-analysis in 2015, which included the aforementioned 2013 study, found that prone positioning compared to supine positioning tended to reduce the mortality rates in ARDS patients (41% vs. 47%, RR 0.90, 95% CI 0.82 to 0.98, P = 0.02). This effect was not found to be statistically significant due to the moderate–high heterogeneity of the studies included in the meta-analysis (I^2 61%, P = 0.01). Subgroup analysis demonstrated that the mortality rates for LPV (RR 0.73, 95% CI, 0.62 to 0.86, P = 0.0002) and duration of prone positioning >12 hours (RR 0.75, 95% CI 0.65 to 0.87, P <0.0001) were reduced in the prone position and that the heterogeneity was low (I^2 46%, P = 0.12). It also found that while prone positioning was not associated with an increase in cardiac events or ventilator-associated pneumonia, it was associated with an increased incidence of pressure sores (RR 1.23, 95% CI, 1.07 to 1.41) and endotracheal tube dislocation (RR 1.33, 95% CI 1.02 to 1.74). The authors concluded that prone positioning for ARDS patients should be prioritized over other invasive procedures because related life-threatening complications are rare.[130] Another meta-analysis in 2015 independently confirmed this nonsignificant trend toward reduced mortality (OR

0.76, 95% CI 0.54 to 1.06; $P = 0.11$, I^2 63%), and the authors reached the same conclusions.[131] In centers with the experience and available resources to handle the complications of prone positioning, this may be a reasonable recommendation; however, additional randomized controlled studies are required to confirm the benefits of prone position in ARDS before it can be said that it should be widely adopted by all centers.

INHALED PULMONARY VASODILATORS

The loss of alveolar units coupled with the pulmonary vascular dysregulation in ARDS leads to an increase in ventilation–perfusion mismatching. The appeal of inhaled pulmonary vasodilators (e.g., nitric oxide, prostacyclin) is that they selectively dilate vessels in the remaining well-ventilated areas of lung by virtue of their inhaled delivery thereby improving ventilation–perfusion matching, which results in improved oxygenation. Also, adding to their appeal are their extremely short half-lives, which limits their effects to the pulmonary bed and usually avoids systemic effects like hypotension.

The use of inhaled nitric oxide in ARDS has been debated for some time. It has been studied in a number of randomized clinical trials and examined in several meta-analyses.[132] None of these studies demonstrated a mortality benefit to the use of nitric oxide in ARDS with only a transient improvement in oxygenation, and at least one meta-analysis, suggested an increase in renal impairment with the use of nitric oxide.[133,134] In the most recent meta-analysis from 2014, the authors concluded that nitric oxide does not reduce mortality in adults or children with ARDS, whether it be mild–moderate ARDS (RR 1.12, 95% CI 0.89 to 1.42; $p = 0.33$; $n = 740$, 7 trials, I^2 0%) or severe ARDS (RR 1.01, 95% CI 0.78 to 1.32; $p = 0.93$; $n = 329$, 6 trials, I^2 0%).[135]

The data for prostacyclin use in ARDS mirrors that of inhaled nitric oxide in that it has not been shown to improve mortality or other patient outcomes but does improve oxygenation and reduces pulmonary arterial pressure.[121] Based on these data, the routine use of inhaled pulmonary vasodilators in ARDS cannot be recommended, but they may be reasonably used as a temporizing rescue therapy in cases of refractory severe hypoxia.

EXTRACORPEAL INTERVENTION

Since the 1960s, extracorporeal techniques have been suggested as a potential supportive treatment in respiratory failure.[136,137] Early studies demonstrated poor results with high morbidity and mortality rates. This was probably due to a number of reasons, not the least of which were hemorrhagic complications related to early ECMO circuits and the use of mechanical ventilation strategies that were not truly lung protective (pre-LTVV era).[138–140] Nevertheless, based on this evidence, the use of ECMO in ARDS was thought to be not justifiable outside of the clinical research setting.

Then in 2009, the results of the Conventional ventilation, or ECMO, for Severe Adult Respiratory Failure (CESAR) trial were published. This was a United Kingdom multicenter randomized control trial involving 180 patients who were assigned 1:1 to LTVV with ECMO or LTVV alone. Of the 90 patients in the LTVV-ECMO group, 68 (75%) received ECMO. The study demonstrated that survival to 6 months without disability was better in the LTVV-ECMO group compared with the LTVV group (63% vs. 47%, RR 0.69, 95% CI 0.05 to 0.97, $p = 0.03$). Referral to consideration for treatment by ECMO treatment also led to a gain of 0.03 quality-adjusted life-years (QALYs) at 6-month follow-up, and a lifetime model predicted

the cost per QALY of ECMO to be £19,252 ($19,000). The authors concluded that it was both advisable and economical to recommend for the transfer of adult patients with severe but potentially reversible respiratory failure with a Murray score >3.0 or pH <7.20 while optimally managed, to a center with an ECMO-based management protocol to significantly improve survival without severe disability.[141]

That same year, the H1N1 influenza A pandemic resulted in a sudden increase in the occurrence of rapid-onset, severe ARDS. The profound refractory hypoxemia spurred a resurgence in the use of ECMO as a rescue therapy, but this time combined with protective ventilation. Registry data from national and international sources suggested that the early use of ECMO produced favorable results in those patients with severe hypoxemia.[142–144] These results, combined with the favorable results of the CESAR trial, have led to the recommendation by various individuals and panels that ECMO be included, at least as a rescue therapy, in the treatment algorithm for ARDS.[9,68,145,146] Nonetheless, in 2015, a systematic review was performed that examined the relevant trials on the application of ECMO. Unfortunately, study data could not be pooled for meta-analysis due to heterogeneity given the remarkable advances in ventilator and ECMO techniques, especially after the year 2000. This review demonstrated that data on use of ECMO in patients with acute respiratory failure, while encouraging, remains inconclusive with no appreciable decrease in mortality.[147]

In 1978, a new extracorporeal technique known as extracorporeal carbon dioxide removal ($ECCO_2R$) was devised to address the hypercapnia that accompanied low-frequency positive pressure ventilation (LFPPV) that was thought to reduce barotrauma at the time by reducing respiratory rates to 1 to 2 breaths/min while maintaining tidal volumes of 10 to 15 mL/kg.[133] While LFPPV gave way to LTVV, $ECCO_2R$ still remains a potentially promising means of addressing the hypercapnia that accompanies LTVV. This would allow for more aggressive, ultraprotective tidal volumes (<4 to 6 mL/kg PBW) to reduce plateau pressure even lower than 30 cm H_2O which retrospective analysis of the ARDSNet database suggests may be beneficial.[148] As with ECMO, newer generation devices have been developed with lower priming volumes and more efficient gas exchange. The major difference with ECMO is that lower flow rates are necessary with $ECCO_2R$ (300 to 1,000 mL/min vs. 3,000 to 5,000 mL/min) which is adequate for CO_2 removal.[80] This allows for smaller cannulas and devices, and the potential to make $ECCO_2R$ for CO_2 removal as widely available as continuous renal replacement therapy (CRRT) is currently for fluid and solute removal. Studies of $ECCO_2R$ in ARDS are limited, but promising. A prospective cohort study in 2009 demonstrated that in ARDS patients with persistent plateau pressures of 28 to 30 cm H_2O despite treatment with an LTVV strategy of 6 mL/kg PBW for 72 hours who had then achieved a lower plateau pressure with refractory hypercapnic acidosis after tidal volume reduction to 4 mL/kg PBW, the use of $ECCO_2R$ for 72 hours was associated with a reduction of P_aCO_2 (from 73.6 ± 11.1 to 47.2 ± 8.6 mm Hg, P <0.001), sufficient to normalize arterial pH (from 7.20 ± 0.02 to 7.38 ± 0.04, P <0.001). This allowed for continued use of ultraprotective tidal volumes of 3.7 to 4.6 mL/kg PBW which maintained the reduced plateau pressures and may have allowed for the reduction in pulmonary cytokine concentrations also observed in this group.[149]

Since this study, a randomized control trial of 79 patients who were assigned to either ultraprotective LTTV (3 mL/kg PBW) with $ECCO_2R$ or standard LTTV (6 mL/kg PBW) showed significantly improved 60-day ventilator-free days in a subgroup of patients (those with severe ARDS) compared to control (40.9 ± 12.8 days vs. 28.2 ± 16.4 days, $p = 0.033$). There was a significant reduction in analgesic and sedative use, significantly reduced IL-6 levels, and an increased ratio of spontaneous breathing compared to control. Notably, due to enrollment limitations, the study did not reach the pre-specified sample size which may have to contribute to negative finding of the primary outcome of a reduction of the period of mechanical ventilation within 28 or 60 days or the intensive care and hospital stay. Thus, this necessitates the subgroup analysis.[150]

In extreme cases of severe ARDS where end-organ perfusion is compromised due to profound refractory hypoxia and/or hypercapnia with acidosis, ECCO$_2$R and ECMO offer an intellectually appealing means of rescue for the otherwise salvageable patient. It is in the less severe cases that more data is necessary to determine whether application of ECCO$_2$R or ECMO would provide benefit over traditional ARDS therapies. Study design could be challenging as some part of this theoretical benefit may be indirect due to the unique ability of these extracorporeal techniques to be combined with other advances in care. These are advances such as early mobilization and reduced sedative/paralytic use, known to reduce ICU morbidity and perhaps mortality. Should the data be positive, proper application and maintenance of these combined therapies will require highly trained staff and coordination across multiple disciplines, which will likely initially limit these techniques to specialized centers of excellence.

OUTCOMES OF ARDS

Among survivors of ARDS, morbidity is common and usually evident on discharge. This may be due to the underlying cause of the ARDS or due to prolonged ICU/hospital stay. Though the lungs are the primary site of the disease, the systemic nature of ARDS leaves no major organ system spared from potential negative effect.

Neurocognitive morbidity and psychiatric illness appear to be common among ARDS survivors. Nearly all aspects of neurocognitive function appear to be affected, such as short- and long-term memory, attention, concentration, visuospatial abilities, and language. The reported incidence of neurocognitive dysfunction ranges from 40% to 100% in ARDS survivors early after discharge, and this high incidence persists out to 12 months (34% to 78%).[151-153] In regards to psychiatric illness, a spectrum of disorders has been observed, most notably anxiety, depression, and PTSD. The incidence of at least one of these psychiatric illnesses has been reported as 62% to 66% with the incidence of two or more of these psychiatric illnesses in 42% of ARDS survivors.[50,154]

The effects of ARDS on the physical conditioning of its survivors are profound. In one study, the incidence of impaired physical function was 66% at 2 years.[52] In particular, the persistence of this morbidity is remarkable with one prospective cohort of 109 survivors demonstrating impaired 6-minute walk tests results of 66% of predicted at 1 year and 76% of predicted at 5 years.[155]

Despite being the primary organ affected by ARDS, the lungs manage to make some reasonable measure of recovery in most ARDS survivors. In one study, on discharge, approximately 80% of the patients demonstrated reduced diffusing capacity, 20% had airflow obstruction, and 20% had chest restriction.[156] At 6 months, lung volumes and spirometry should measure within 80% of predicted values, and at 5 years, diffusion capacity should also normalize.[53,54,157] Fortunately, very few patients end up requiring supplemental oxygen.[54]

Overall, survivors of ARDS often continue to deal with the ramifications of their illness well beyond its in-hospital resolution. In one study, mortality at 1 year was greater than in-hospital mortality (41% vs. 24%, respectively, $P <0.0001$). This was mainly predicted by comorbidities, advanced age, and discharge to a facility.[158] On the other hand, another study demonstrated that of those ARDS patients who were working at the time of their acute illness, 77% returned to work and 94% of these patients returned to their original work, usually with a gradual transition back to work involving a modified work schedule or job retraining.[53] Predictably, it is those patients with good reserve prior to their acute illness that are best able to recover from ARDS.

REFERENCES

1. Laennec RTH, Forbes SJ. *A Treatise on the Diseases of the Chest and on Mediate Auscultation.* 3rd ed. London, England: Thomas & George Underwood; 1829:179–180.
2. Osler W. *The Principles and Practice of Medicine: Designed for the Use of Practitioners and Students of Medicine.* New York: D. Appleton and Company; 1892:512.
3. Pasteur W. Massive collapse of the lung. (Syn. active lobar collapse). *Br J Surg* 1913;1:587–601.
4. Burford TH, Burbank B. Traumatic wet lung; observations on certain physiologic fundamentals of thoracic trauma. *J Thorac Surg* 1945;14:415–424.
5. Fishman AP. Shock Lung: A Distinctive Nonentity. *Circulation* 1973;47:921–923.
6. Ashbaugh DG, Bigelow DB, Petty TL, et al. Acute Respiratory Distress in Adults. *Lancet* 1967;290:319–323.
7. Petty TL, Ashbaugh DG. The adult respiratory distress syndrome: Clinical features, factors influencing prognosis and principles of management. *Chest* 1971;60(3):233–239.
8. Bernard GR, Artigas A, Brigham KL, et al. The American-European Consensus Conference on ARDS. Definitions, mechanisms, relevant outcomes, and clinical trial coordination. *Am J Respir Crit Care Med* 1994;149:818–824.
9. The ARDS Definition Task Force*. Acute respiratory distress syndrome: The Berlin Definition. *JAMA* 2012;307(23):2526–2533.
10. Aisiku IP, Yamal JM, Doshi P, et al. The incidence of ARDS and associated mortality in severe TBI using the Berlin definition. *J Trauma Acute Care Surg* 2016;80(2):308–312.
11. Rubenfeld GD, Caldwell E, Peabody E, et al. Incidence and outcomes of acute lung injury. *N Engl J Med* 2005;353:1685–1693.
12. MacCallum NS, Evans TW. Epidemiology of acute lung injury. *Curr Opin Crit Care* 2005;11(1):43–49.
13. Brun-Buisson C, Minelli C, Bertolini G, et al. Epidemiology and outcome of acute lung injury in European intensive care units. *Intens Care Med* 2004;30:51–61.
14. Starling EH. On the absorption of fluids from the connective tissue spaces. *J Physiol* 1896;19(4):312–326.
15. Taylor AE. Capillary fluid filtration: Starling forces and lymph flow. *Circ Res* 1981; 49: 557–575.
16. Wiederhielm CA. Dynamics of capillary fluid exchange: A nonlinear computer simulation. *Microvasc Res* 1979;18(1):48–82.
17. Facchini L, Bellin A, Toro EF. A mathematical model for filtration and macromolecule transport across capillary walls. *Microvasc Res* 2014;94:52–63.
18. Levick JR, Michel CC. Microvascular fluid exchange and the revised Starling principle. *Cardiovasc Res* 2010;87(2):198–210.
19. Reed RK, Rubin K. Transcapillary exchange: role and importance of the interstitial fluid pressure and the extracellular matrix. *Cardiovasc Res* 2010;87(2):211–217.
20. Woodcock TE, Woodcock TM. Revised Starling equation and the glycocalyx model of transvascular fluid exchange: an improved paradigm for prescribing intravenous fluid therapy. *Br J Anaesth* 2012;108(3):384–394.
21. Bhave G, Neilson EG. Body fluid dynamics: back to the future. *J Am Soc Nephrol* 2011;22(12):2166–2181.
22. Renkin, EM. B. W. Zweifach Award lecture. Regulation of the microcirculation. *Microvasc Res* 1985;30(3):251–263.
23. Effros RM, Parker JC. Pulmonary vascular heterogeneity and the Starling hypothesis. *Microvasc Res* 2009;78(1):71–77.
24. Taylor AE. The lymphatic edema safety factor: the role of edema dependent lymphatic factors (EDLF). *Lymphology* 1990;23(3):111–123.
25. Szidon JP. Pathophysiology of the congested lung. *Cardiol Clin* 1989;7(1):39–48.
26. Crandall ED, Staub NC, Goldberg HS, et al. Recent developments in pulmonary edema. *Ann Intern Med* 1983;99(6):808–822.
27. Zarins CK, Rice CL, Peters RM, et al. Lymph and pulmonary response to isobaric reduction in plasma oncotic pressure in baboons. *Circ Res* 1978;43(6):925–930.
28. Yang Y, Schmidt EP. The endothelial glycocalyx: an important regulator of the pulmonary vascular barrier. *Tissue Barriers* 2013;1(1):pii: 23494.
29. Collins SR, Blank RS, Deatherage LS, et al. Special article: the endothelial glycocalyx: emerging concepts in pulmonary edema and acute lung injury. *Anesth Analg* 2013;117(3):664–674.
30. Giantsos KM, Kopeckova P, Dull RO. The use of an endothelium-targeted cationic copolymer to enhance the barrier function of lung capillary endothelial monolayers. *Biomaterials* 2009;30(29):5885–5891.
31. Giantsos-Adams K, Lopez-Quintero V, Kopeckova P, et al. Study of the therapeutic benefit of cationic copolymer administration to vascular endothelium under mechanical stress. *Biomaterials* 2011;32(1):288–294.
32. Stapleton RD, Wang BM, Hudson LD, et al. Causes and timing of death in patients with ARDS. *Chest* 2005;128(2):525–532.
33. Montgomery AB, Stager MA, Carrico CJ, et al. Causes of mortality in patients with the adult respiratory distress syndrome. *Am Rev Respir Dis* 1985;132(3):485–489.

34. Suchyta MR1, Clemmer TP, Elliott CG, et al. The adult respiratory distress syndrome. A report of survival and modifying factors. *Chest* 1992;101(4):1074–1079.

35. Phua J, Badia JR, Adhikari NK, et al. Has mortality from acute respiratory distress syndrome decreased over time?: A systematic review. *Am J Respir Crit Care Med* 2009;179(3):220–227.

36. Raymondos K, Molitoris U, Capewell M, et al. Negative- versus positive-pressure ventilation in intubated patients with acute respiratory distress syndrome. *Crit Care* 2012;16(2):R37.

37. Soni N, Williams P. Positive pressure ventilation: what is the real cost? *Br J Anaesth* 2008;101(4):446–57.

38. Robb J. Physiological changes occurring with positive pressure ventilation: Part one. *Intensive Crit Care Nurs* 1997;13(5):293–307.

39. Robb J. Physiological changes occurring with positive pressure ventilation: Part Two. *Intensive Crit Care Nurs* 1997;13(6):357–364.

40. Gammon RB, Shin MS, Buchalter SE. Pulmonary barotrauma in mechanical ventilation. Patterns and risk factors. *Chest* 1992;102(2):568–572.

41. Thomson L, Paton J. Oxygen toxicity. *Paediatr Respir Rev* 2014;15(2):120–123.

42. Lumb AB, Walton LJ. Perioperative oxygen toxicity. *Anesthesiol Clin* 2012;30(4):591–605.

43. Davis WB, Rennard SI, Bitterman PB, et al. Pulmonary oxygen toxicity. Early reversible changes in human alveolar structures induced by hyperoxia. *N Engl J Med* 1983;309(15):878–883.

44. Rouby JJ, Lherm T, Martin de Lassale E, et al. Histologic aspects of pulmonary barotrauma in critically ill patients with acute respiratory failure. *Intensive Care Med* 1993;19(7):383–389.

45. Maunder RJ, Pierson DJ, Hudson LD. Subcutaneous and mediastinal emphysema. Pathophysiology, diagnosis, and management. *Arch Intern Med* 1984; 144(7):1447–1453.

46. Webb HH, Tierney DF. Experimental pulmonary edema due to intermittent positive pressure ventilation with high inflation pressures. Protection by positive end-expiratory pressure. *Am Rev Respir Dis* 1974;110(5):556–565.

47. Dreyfuss D, Saumon G. Role of tidal volume, FRC, and end-inspiratory volume in the development of pulmonary edema following mechanical ventilation. *Am Rev Respir Dis* 1993;148:1194–1203.

48. Chu EK, Whitehead T, Slutsky AS. Effects of cyclic opening and closing at low- and high-volume ventilation on bronchoalveolar lavage cytokines. *Crit Care Med* 2004;32(1):168–174.

49. Muscedere, JG, Mullen JB, Gan K, et al. Tidal ventilation at low airway pressures can augment lung injury. *Am J Respir Crit Care Med* 1994;149:1327–1334.

50. Dueck R. Alveolar recruitment versus hyperinflation: A balancing act. *Curr Opin Anaesthesiol* 2006;19(6):650–654.

51. Tremblay LN, Slutsky AS. Ventilator-induced lung injury: from the bench to the bedside. *Intensive Care Med* 2006;32(1):24–33.

52. Tremblay LN, Slutsky AS. Ventilator-induced injury: from barotrauma to biotrauma. *Proc Assoc Am Physicians* 1998;110(6):482–428.

53. von Bethmann AN, Brasch F, Nüsing R, et al. Hyperventilation induces release of cytokines from perfused mouse lung. *Am J Respir Crit Care Med* 1998;157:263–272.

54. Slutsky AS, Tremblay LN. Multiple system organ failure. *Am J Respir Crit Care Med* 1998;157:1721–1725.

55. Ranieri VM, Suter PM, Tortorella C, et al. Effect of mechanical ventilation on inflammatory mediators in patients with acute respiratory distress syndrome: a randomized controlled trial. *JAMA* 1999;282(1):54–61.

56. Stüber F, Wrigge H, Schroeder S, et al. Kinetic and reversibility of mechanical ventilation-associated pulmonary and systemic inflammatory response in patients with acute lung injury. *Intensive Care Med* 2002;28(7):834–841.

57. Slutsky AS, Ranieri VM. Ventilator-induced lung injury. *N Engl J Med* 2013; 369(22):2126–2136.

58. Parker JC, Hernandez LA, Peevy KJ. Mechanisms of ventilator-induced lung injury. *Crit Care Med* 1993;21(1):131–143.

59. International Consensus Conferences in Intensive Care Medicine: Ventilator-associated Lung Injury in ARDS. This official conference report was cosponsored by the American Thoracic Society, The European Society of Intensive Care Medicine, and The Societé de Réanimation de Langue Française, and was approved by the ATS Board of Directors, July 1999. *Am J Respir Crit Care Med* 1999;160(6):2118–2124.

60. Jonson B, Richard JC, Straus C, et al. Pressure-volume curves and compliance in acute lung injury: evidence of recruitment above the lower inflection point. *Am J Respir Crit Care Med* 1999;159(4 Pt 1):1172–1178.

61. Villar J. Ventilator or physician-induced lung injury? *Minerva Anestesiol* 2005;71(6):255–258.

62. The Acute Respiratory Distress Syndrome Network. Ventilation with lower tidal volumes as compared with traditional tidal volumes for acute lung injury and the acute respiratory distress syndrome. *N Engl J Med* 2000;342(18):1301–1308.

63. Putensen C, Theuerkauf N, Zinserling J, et al. Meta-analysis: ventilation strategies and outcomes of the acute respiratory distress syndrome and acute lung injury. *Ann Intern Med* 2009;151(8):566–576.

64. Petrucci N, De Feo C. Lung protective ventilation strategy for the acute respiratory distress syndrome. *Cochrane Database Syst Rev* 2013;2:CD003844.

65. Needham DM, Yang T, Dinglas VD, et al. Timing of low tidal volume ventilation and intensive care unit mortality in acute respiratory distress syndrome. A prospective cohort study. *Am J Respir Crit Care Med* 2015;191(2):177–185.

66. Needham DM, Colantuoni E, Mendez-Tellez PA, et al. Lung protective mechanical ventilation and two year survival in patients with acute lung injury: prospective cohort study. *BMJ* 2012;344:e2124.

67. Umoh NJ, Fan E, Mendez-Tellez PA, et al. Patient and intensive care unit organizational factors associated with low tidal volume ventilation in acute lung injury. *Crit Care Med* 2008;36(5):1463–1468.

68. Rittayamai N, Brochard L. Recent advances in mechanical ventilation in patients with acute respiratory distress syndrome. *Eur Respir Rev* 2015;24(135):132–140.

69. Amato MB, Barbas CS, Medeiros DM, et al. Effect of a protective-ventilation strategy on mortality in the acute respiratory distress syndrome. *N Engl J Med* 1998;338(6):347–354.

70. Villar J, Kacmarek RM, Pérez-Méndez L, et al. A high positive end-expiratory pressure, low tidal volume ventilatory strategy improves outcome in persistent acute respiratory distress syndrome: a randomized, controlled trial. *Crit Care Med* 2006;34(5):1311–1318.

71. Brower RG, Lanken PN, MacIntyre N, et al.; National Heart, Lung, and Blood Institute ARDS Clinical Trials Network. Higher versus lower positive end-expiratory pressures in patients with the acute respiratory distress syndrome. *N Engl J Med* 2004;351(4):327–336.

72. Mercat A, Richard JC, Vielle B, et al.; Expiratory Pressure (Express) Study Group. Positive end-expiratory pressure setting in adults with acute lung injury and acute respiratory distress syndrome: a randomized controlled trial. *JAMA* 2008;299(6):646–655.

73. Meade MO, Cook DJ, Guyatt GH, et al.; Lung Open Ventilation Study Investigators. Ventilation strategy using low tidal volumes, recruitment maneuvers, and high positive end-expiratory pressure for acute lung injury and acute respiratory distress syndrome: a randomized controlled trial. *JAMA* 2008;299(6):637–645.

74. Brochard L. Measurement of esophageal pressure at bedside: pros and cons. *Curr Opin Crit Care* 2014;20(1):39–46.

75. Briel M, Meade M, Mercat A, et al. Higher vs lower positive end-expiratory pressure in patients with acute lung injury and acute respiratory distress syndrome: systematic review and meta-analysis. *JAMA* 2010;303(9):865–873.

76. Gattinoni L, Caironi P, Cressoni M, et al. Lung recruitment in patients with the acute respiratory distress syndrome. *N Engl J Med* 2006;354(17):1775–1786.

77. Keller SP, Fessler HE. Monitoring of oesophageal pressure. *Curr Opin Crit Care* 2014;20(3):340–346.

78. Chiumello D, Guérin C. Understanding the setting of PEEP from esophageal pressure in patients with ARDS. *Intensive Care Med*. 2015;41(8):1465–1467.

79. Gulati G, Novero A, Loring SH, et al. Pleural pressure and optimal positive end-expiratory pressure based on esophageal pressure versus chest wall elastance: incompatible results. *Crit Care Med* 2013;41(8):1951–1917.

80. Bouhemad B, Brisson H, Le-Guen M, et al. Bedside ultrasound assessment of positive end-expiratory pressure-induced lung recruitment. *Am J Respir Crit Care Med* 2011;183(3):341–347.

81. Richard JC, Brochard L, Vandelet P, et al. Respective effects of end-expiratory and end-inspiratory pressures on alveolar recruitment in acute lung injury. *Crit Care Med* 2003;31(1):89–92.

82. Maggiore SM, Jonson B, Richard JC, et al. Alveolar derecruitment at decremental positive end-expiratory pressure levels in acute lung injury: comparison with the lower inflection point, oxygenation, and compliance. *Am J Respir Crit Care Med* 2001;164(5):795–801.

83. Ranieri VM, Giuliani R, Fiore T, et al. Volume-pressure curve of the respiratory system predicts effects of PEEP in ARDS: "occlusion" versus "constant flow" technique. *Am J Respir Crit Care Med* 1994;149(1):19–27.

84. Eissa NT, Ranieri VM, Corbeil C, et al. Analysis of behavior of the respiratory system in ARDS patients: effects of flow, volume, and time. *J Appl Physiol (1985)* 1991;70(6):2719–2729.

85. Hata JS, Togashi K, Kumar AB, et al. The effect of the pressure-volume curve for positive end-expiratory pressure titration on clinical outcomes in acute respiratory distress syndrome: a systematic review. *J Intensive Care Med* 2014;29(6):348–356.

86. Dellamonica J, Lerolle N, Sargentini C, et al. PEEP-induced changes in lung volume in acute respiratory distress syndrome. Two methods to estimate alveolar recruitment. *Intensive Care Med* 2011;37(10):1595–1604.

87. Dellamonica J, Lerolle N, Sargentini C, et al. Accuracy and precision of end-expiratory lung-volume measurements by automated nitrogen washout/washin technique in patients with acute respiratory distress syndrome. *Crit Care* 2011;15(6):R294.

88. Buytendijk, HJ. *Intraesophageal Pressure and Lung Elasticity* [Dissertation Thesis]. Groningen: University of Groningen; 1949.

89. Talmor D, Sarge T, Malhotra A, et al. Mechanical ventilation guided by esophageal pressure in acute lung injury. *N Engl J Med* 2008;359(20):2095–2104.

90. Santa Cruz R, Rojas JI, Nervi R, et al. High versus low positive end-expiratory pressure (PEEP) levels for mechanically ventilated adult patients with acute lung injury and acute respiratory distress syndrome. *Cochrane Database Syst Rev* 2013;6:CD009098.

91. Goligher EC, Kavanagh BP, Rubenfeld GD, et al. Oxygenation response to positive end-expiratory pressure predicts mortality in acute respiratory distress syndrome. A secondary analysis of the LOVS and ExPress trials. *Am J Respir Crit Care Med* 2014;190(1):70–76.

92. Cressoni M, Chiumello D, Carlesso E, et al. Compressive forces and computed tomography-derived positive end-expiratory pressure in acute respiratory distress syndrome. *Anesthesiology* 2014;121(3):572–581.

93. Gattinoni L, Carlesso E, Cressoni M. Selecting the "right" positive end-expiratory pressure level. *Curr Opin Crit Care* 2015;21(1):50–57.

94. Hasselbalch, Karl Albert. *Die Berechnung der Wasserstoffzahl des Blutes aus der freien und gebundenen Kohlensäure desselben, und die Sauerstoffbindung des Blutes als Funktion der Wasserstoffzahl*. Julius Springer; 1916.

95. Gattinoni L, Carlesso E, Brazzi L, et al. Friday night ventilation: a safety starting tool kit for mechanically ventilated patients. *Minerva Anestesiol* 2014;80(9):1046–1057.

96. Hickling KG, Henderson SJ, Jackson R. Low mortality associated with low volume pressure limited ventilation with permissive hypercapnia in severe adult respiratory distress syndrome. *Intensive Care Med* 1990;16(6):372–327.

97. Tuxen DV. Permissive hypercapnic ventilation. *Am J Respir Crit Care Med* 1994;150(3):870–874.
98. Richecoeur J, Lu Q, Vieira SR, et al. Expiratory washout versus optimization of mechanical ventilation during permissive hypercapnia in patients with severe acute respiratory distress syndrome. *Am J Respir Crit Care Med* 1999;160(1):77–85.
99. Contreras M, Masterson C, Laffey JG. Permissive hypercapnia: what to remember. *Curr Opin Anaesthesiol* 2015;28(1):26–37.
100. Prin S, Chergui K, Augarde R, et al. Ability and safety of a heated humidifier to control hypercapnic acidosis in severe ARDS. *Intensive Care Med* 2002;28(12):1756–1760.
101. Feihl F, Perret C. Permissive hypercapnia. How permissive should we be? *Am J Respir Crit Care Med* 1994;150(6 Pt 1):1722–1737.
102. Garg SK. Permissive hypercapnia: Is there any upper limit? *Indian J Crit Care Med* 2014;18(9):612–614.
103. Stewart TE, Meade MO, Cook DJ, et al. Evaluation of a ventilation strategy to prevent barotrauma in patients at high risk for acute respiratory distress syndrome. Pressure- and Volume-Limited Ventilation Strategy Group. *N Engl J Med* 1998;338(6):355–361.
104. Brochard L, Roudot-Thoraval F, Roupie E, et al. Tidal volume reduction for prevention of ventilator-induced lung injury in acute respiratory distress syndrome. The Multicenter Trail Group on Tidal Volume reduction in ARDS. *Am J Respir Crit Care Med* 1998;158(6):1831–1838.
105. Brower RG, Shanholtz CB, Fessler HE, et al. Prospective, randomized, controlled clinical trial comparing traditional versus reduced tidal volume ventilation in acute respiratory distress syndrome patients. *Crit Care Med* 1999;27(8):1492–1498.
106. Tobin MJ. Culmination of an era in research on the acute respiratory distress syndrome. *N Engl J Med* 2000;342(18):1360–1361.
107. Laffey JG, Kavanagh BP. Carbon dioxide and the critically ill—too little of a good thing? *Lancet* 1999;354(9186):1283–1286.
108. Laffey JG, Engelberts D, Kavanagh BP. Buffering hypercapnic acidosis worsens acute lung injury. *Am J Respir Crit Care Med* 2000;161(1):141–146.
109. Gainnier M, Roch A, Forel JM, et al. Effect of neuromuscular blocking agents on gas exchange in patients presenting with acute respiratory distress syndrome. *Crit Care Med* 2004;32(1):113–119.
110. Albert MS, Dell RB, Winters RW. Quantitative displacement of acid-base equilibrium in metabolic acidosis. *Ann Intern Med* 1967;66(2):312–322.
111. Engel K, Dell RB, Rahill WJ, et al. Quantitative displacement of acid-base equilibrium in chronic respiratory acidosis. *J Appl Physiol* 1968;24(3):288–295.
112. Kellum JA. Determinants of blood pH in health and disease. *Crit Care* 2000;4(1):6–14.
113. Shapiro JI, Elkins N, Logan J, et al. Effects of sodium bicarbonate, disodium carbonate, and a sodium bicarbonate/carbonate mixture on the PCO2 of blood in a closed system. *J Lab Clin Med* 1995;126(1):65–69.
114. Nahas GG, Sutin KM, Fermon C, et al. Guidelines for the treatment of acidaemia with THAM. *Drugs* 1998;55(2):191–224.
115. Uhlig C, Silva PL, Deckert S, et al. Albumin versus crystalloid solutions in patients with the acute respiratory distress syndrome: a systematic review and meta-analysis. *Crit Care* 2014;18(1):R10.
116. Kregenow DA, Rubenfeld GD, Hudson LD, et al. Hypercapnic acidosis and mortality in acute lung injury. *Crit Care Med* 2006;34(1):1–7.
117. Watling SM, Dasta JF. Prolonged paralysis in intensive care unit patients after the use of neuromuscular blocking agents: a review of the literature. *Crit Care Med* 1994;22(5):884–893.
118. Alhazzani W, Alshahrani M, Jaeschke R, et al. Neuromuscular blocking agents in acute respiratory distress syndrome: a systematic review and meta-analysis of randomized controlled trials. *Crit Care* 2013;17(2):R43.
119. National Heart, Lung, and Blood Institute Acute Respiratory Distress Syndrome (ARDS) Clinical Trials Network; Wiedemann HP, Wheeler AP, Bernard GR, et al. Comparison of two fluid-management strategies in acute lung injury. *N Engl J Med* 2006;354(24):2564–2575.
120. Grissom CK, Hirshberg EL, Dickerson JB, et al.; National Heart Lung and Blood Institute Acute Respiratory Distress Syndrome Clinical Trials Network. Fluid management with a simplified conservative protocol for the acute respiratory distress syndrome. *Crit Care Med* 2015;43(2):288–295.
121. Fuller BM, Mohr NM, Skrupky L, et al. The use of inhaled prostaglandins in patients with ARDS: A systematic review and meta-analysis. *Chest* 2015;147(6):1510–1522.
122. Oczkowski SJ, Mazzetti I. Colloids to improve diuresis in critically ill patients: a systematic review. *J Intensive Care* 2014;2:37.
123. Pelosi P, Brazzi L, Gattinoni L. Prone position in acute respiratory distress syndrome. *Eur Respir J* 2002;20(4):1017–1028.
124. Albert RK, Hubmayr RD. The prone position eliminates compression of the lungs by the heart. *Am J Respir Crit Care Med* 2000;161(5):1660–1665.
125. Malbouisson LM, Busch CJ, Puybasset L, et al. Role of the heart in the loss of aeration characterizing lower lobes in acute respiratory distress syndrome. CT Scan ARDS Study Group. *Am J Respir Crit Care Med* 2000;161(6):2005–2012.
126. Jozwiak M, Teboul JL, Anguel N, et al. Beneficial hemodynamic effects of prone positioning in patients with acute respiratory distress syndrome. *Am J Respir Crit Care Med* 2013;188(12):1428–1433.
127. Nyrén S, Mure M, Jacobsson H, et al. Pulmonary perfusion is more uniform in the prone than in the supine position: scintigraphy in healthy humans. *J Appl Physiol (1985)* 1999;86(4):1135–1141.
128. Henderson AC, Sá RC, Theilmann RJ, et al. The gravitational distribution of ventilation-perfusion ratio is more uniform in prone than supine posture in the normal human lung. *J Appl Physiol (1985)* 2013;115(3):313–324.
129. Guérin C, Reignier J, Richard JC, et al.; PROSEVA Study Group. Prone positioning in severe acute respiratory distress syndrome. *N Engl J Med* 2013;368(23):2159–2168.
130. Park SY, Kim HJ, Yoo KH, et al. The efficacy and safety of prone positioning in adults patients with acute respiratory distress syndrome: a meta-analysis of randomized controlled trials. *J Thorac Dis* 2015;7(3):356–367.
131. Mora-Arteaga JA, Bernal-Ramírez OJ, Rodríguez SJ. The effects of prone position ventilation in patients with acute respiratory distress syndrome. A systematic review and metaanalysis. *Med Intensiva* 2015;39(6):352–365.
132. Niven DJ, Stelfox HT. Inhaled nitric oxide in patients with acute respiratory distress syndrome: an end to the debate? *Crit Care Med* 2014;42(2):472–473.
133. Gattinoni L, Kolobow T, Tomlinson T, et al. Low-frequency positive pressure ventilation with extracorporeal carbon dioxide removal (LFPPV-ECCO2R): an experimental study. *Anesth Analg* 1978;57(4):470–477.
134. Afshari A, Brok J, Møller AM, et al. Inhaled nitric oxide for acute respiratory distress syndrome (ARDS) and acute lung injury in children and adults. *Cochrane Database Syst Rev* 2010;(7):CD002787.
135. Adhikari NK, Dellinger RP, Lundin S, et al. Inhaled nitric oxide does not reduce mortality in patients with acute respiratory distress syndrome regardless of severity: systematic review and meta-analysis. *Crit Care Med* 2014;42(2):404–412.
136. Ty TC, Sarkozy E, Dobell AR, et al. Experimental respiratory insufficiency. Attempted correction with membrane oxygenator. *Arch Surg* 1965;91(6):881–883.
137. Awad JA, Brassard A, Roy J, et al. Arteriovenous perfusion with the disc oxygenator. Treatment of acute respiratory failure. *Arch Surg* 1969;99(1):69–74.
138. Anderson H 3rd, Steimle C, Shapiro M, et al. Extracorporeal life support for adult cardiorespiratory failure. *Surgery* 1993;114(2):161–172; discussion 172–173.
139. Morris AH, Wallace CJ, Menlove RL, et al. Randomized clinical trial of pressure-controlled inverse ratio ventilation and extracorporeal CO2 removal for adult respiratory distress syndrome. *Am J Respir Crit Care Med* 1994;149(2 Pt 1):295–305.
140. Zapol WM, Snider MT, Hill JD, et al. Extracorporeal membrane oxygenation in severe acute respiratory failure. A randomized prospective study. *JAMA* 1979;242(20):2193–2196.
141. Peek GJ, Mugford M, Tiruvoipati R, et al.; CESAR trial collaboration. Efficacy and economic assessment of conventional ventilatory support versus extracorporeal membrane oxygenation for severe adult respiratory failure (CESAR): a multicentre randomised controlled trial. *Lancet* 2009;374(9698):1351–1363.
142. Australia and New Zealand Extracorporeal Membrane Oxygenation (ANZ ECMO) Influenza Investigators, Davies A, Jones D, Bailey M, et al. Extracorporeal membrane oxygenation for 2009 influenza A(H1N1) acute respiratory distress syndrome. *JAMA* 2009;302(17):1888–1895.
143. Noah MA, Peek GJ, Finney SJ, et al. Referral to an extracorporeal membrane oxygenation center and mortality among patients with severe 2009 influenza A(H1N1). *JAMA* 2011;306(15):1659–1668.
144. Pham T, Combes A, Rozé H, et al.; REVA Research Network. Extracorporeal membrane oxygenation for pandemic influenza A(H1N1)-induced acute respiratory distress syndrome: a cohort study and propensity-matched analysis. *Am J Respir Crit Care Med* 2013;187(3):276–285.
145. Brodie D, Bacchetta M. Extracorporeal membrane oxygenation for ARDS in adults. *N Engl J Med* 2011;365(20):1905–1914.
146. Richard C, Argaud L, Blet A, et al. Extracorporeal life support for patients with acute respiratory distress syndrome: report of a Consensus Conference. *Ann Intensive Care* 2014;4:15.
147. Tramm R, Ilic D, Davies AR, et al. Extracorporeal membrane oxygenation for critically ill adults. *Cochrane Database Syst Rev* 2015;1:CD010381.
148. Hager DN, Krishnan JA, Hayden DL, et al.; ARDS Clinical Trials Network. Tidal volume reduction in patients with acute lung injury when plateau pressures are not high. *Am J Respir Crit Care Med* 2005;172(10):1241–1245.
149. Terragni PP, Del Sorbo L, Mascia L, et al. Tidal volume lower than 6 ml/kg enhances lung protection: role of extracorporeal carbon dioxide removal. *Anesthesiology* 2009;111(4):826–835.
150. Bein T, Weber-Carstens S, Goldmann A, et al. Lower tidal volume strategy (≈3 ml/kg) combined with extracorporeal CO2 removal versus 'conventional' protective ventilation (6 ml/kg) in severe ARDS: the prospective randomized Xtravent-study. *Intensive Care Med* 2013;39(5):847–856.
151. Hopkins RO, Weaver LK, Pope D, et al. Neuropsychological sequelae and impaired health status in survivors of severe acute respiratory distress syndrome. *Am J Respir Crit Care Med* 1999;160(1):50–56.
152. Mikkelsen ME, Christie JD, Lanken PN, et al. The adult respiratory distress syndrome cognitive outcomes study: long-term neuropsychological function in survivors of acute lung injury. *Am J Respir Crit Care Med* 2012;185(12):1307–1315.
153. Pandharipande PP, Girard TD, Jackson JC, et al.; BRAIN-ICU Study Investigators. Long-term cognitive impairment after critical illness. *N Engl J Med* 2013; 369(14):1306–1316.
154. Bienvenu OJ, Colantuoni E, Mendez-Tellez PA, et al. Depressive symptoms and impaired physical function after acute lung injury: a 2-year longitudinal study. *Am J Respir Crit Care Med* 2012;185(5):517–524.
155. Herridge MS, Tansey CM, Matté A, et al.; Canadian Critical Care Trials Group. Functional disability 5 years after acute respiratory distress syndrome. *N Engl J Med* 2011;364(14):1293–1304.
156. Orme J Jr, Romney JS, Hopkins RO, et al. Pulmonary function and health-related quality of life in survivors of acute respiratory distress syndrome. *Am J Respir Crit Care Med* 2003;167(5):690–694.
157. Herridge MS, Cheung AM, Tansey CM, et al.; Canadian Critical Care Trials Group. One-year outcomes in survivors of the acute respiratory distress syndrome. *N Engl J Med* 2003;348(8):683–693.
158. Wang CY, Calfee CS, Paul DW, et al. One-year mortality and predictors of death among hospital survivors of acute respiratory distress syndrome. *Intensive Care Med* 2014 Mar;40(3):388–396.

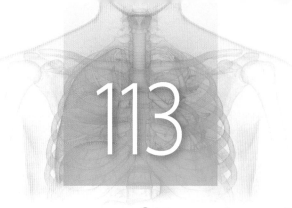

113

Management of Foreign Bodies of the Aerodigestive Tract

Sandra Starnes ▪ Julian Guitron

FOREIGN BODIES OF THE AIRWAY

Foreign body aspiration is a serious and potentially fatal event. The first extraction of an airway foreign body was performed in 1897 by Gustav Killian, an otolaryngologist from Germany widely recognized as the father of bronchoscopy. He removed a pork bone from the right mainstem bronchus actually using a rigid esophagoscope.[1] Chevalier Jackson, another otolaryngologist, developed the first lighted rigid bronchoscope along with several bronchoscopic forceps in the early 1900s. He established the basic principles of treating airway foreign bodies, many of which remain valid today.[2] The flexible bronchoscope was introduced decades later in the 1960s by Shigeto Ikeda.[3,4]

Foreign body aspiration can occur at any age; however, it is most prevalent in children. While the majority of the literature focuses on the pediatric population, most of the principles of management can be applied to the adult population. The key to successful management includes a prompt diagnosis and a thoughtful, stepwise treatment plan that anticipates common challenges and involves the most experienced personnel available.

EPIDEMIOLOGY AND ETIOLOGY

Up to 75% of the cases of foreign body aspirations occur in children younger than 3 years of age.[5,6] The high incidence in this age group reflects the tendency of children to explore the world using their mouth while they talk, run, or play. In addition, these children have not developed a full posterior dentition and have immature neuromuscular mechanisms for swallowing and airway protection. Males account for around 60% of cases in children.[5] The spectrum of foreign bodies aspirated varies by country, due to factors such diet and traditions of the population. Organic materials account for 68% to 86% of aspirated objects, with nuts and seeds being the most common.[5,7]

There are very few published series of foreign body aspiration in adults, with most reports comprising small numbers of patients. Mean age ranges from 48 to 65 with males comprising 60% to 69% of the cases.[8-10] Risk factors that play a role in many, but not all, cases of foreign body aspiration in adults include neurologic dysfunction, alcoholism, and dental manipulation. Organic materials represent 59% to 84% of objects aspirated, with bones being the most common.[8-10]

CLINICAL SIGNS AND SYMPTOMS

The most common presentation of airway foreign bodies includes an initial choking episode followed by cough and dyspnea. Three stages of symptoms result from aspiration. Immediately after a foreign body is aspirated, one observes violent paroxysms of coughing, choking, and gagging. Acute airway obstruction may result either from the foreign body obstructing airflow, or from laryngospasm. If the patient survives the initial phase and the foreign body is still present, a second phase of variable length ensues. During the second phase, the foreign body becomes lodged, reflexes fatigue, and the immediate reflexive symptoms subside. This stage is the most problematic. Many patients have their retained foreign bodies diagnosed late or even overlooked. It is during this second stage that clinicians are falsely reassured by the absence of signs and symptoms and are inclined to minimize the possibility of the presence of a foreign body. In the third phase, a chronically retained foreign body may lead to obstruction, erosion, or infection. Signs may include fever, cough, and hemoptysis. Complications include atelectasis, pneumonia, or lung abscess.

History of a witnessed choking episode can be elicited in 60% to 76% of children[11-13]; however, parents may downplay the significance of such an event or not recall the incident until after the foreign body has been extracted. Older children are often reluctant to admit to such an episode out of fear of being punished. Nonetheless, around 6% to 9% of children present with critical respiratory distress.[12,13]

The current medical practice of treating an asthmatic or "croupy" child with antibiotics or corticosteroids may obscure signs and symptoms that normally would be expected with a retained foreign object. Clearing of symptoms with these agents cannot always be assumed to be diagnostic of a specific disease process. The fact that a wheeze disappears or a pneumonic process temporarily clears may merely mean that the patient's reaction to a foreign body has been controlled temporarily. The recurrence of symptoms after completing the therapy should heighten a physician's suspicion of an aspirated foreign body.

A history suggestive of foreign body aspiration (choking episode) is less common in adults (38% to 55%) likely due to larger airways, and critical respiratory distress is rare.[8,10] Adult patients often present later with complications such as atelectasis, recurrent pneumonia, chronic cough, or hemoptysis. Foreign body aspiration may not be suspected until found on bronchoscopy.

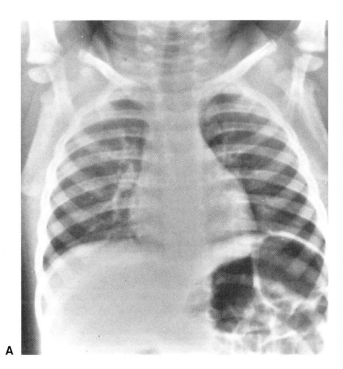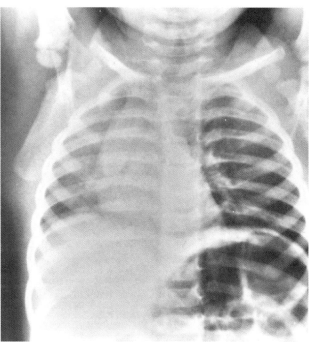

A   B

FIGURE 113.1 **A:** Anteroposterior radiograph of the chest during inspiration. **B:** Anteroposterior radiograph of the chest during expiration. Note the trapping of air in the left lung field, caused by a peanut in the left mainstem bronchus.

In children, foreign bodies are found in the right bronchial tree in 52% to 58% of cases, left bronchial tree in 33% to 40% of cases, and trachea in 5% to 7% of cases.[5,11,14] In adults, they are found in the right bronchial tree in 67% to 76% of cases, in the left bronchial tree in 16% to 32% of cases, and very rarely in the trachea.[8,10]

DIAGNOSIS

Chest radiography (CXR) is the standard initial test when foreign body aspiration is suspected in stable patients. Only 8% to 16% of foreign bodies are radiopaque.[5] Indirect findings suggestive of a foreign body include air trapping, atelectasis, or infiltrate. CXR may be normal in 13% to 29% of cases in both children and adults,[5,10,14] with abnormalities identified more commonly with a delay in diagnosis. Inspiratory and expiratory images may be helpful to detect air trapping. Jackson[15] described the pathophysiology behind the radiographic diagnosis of radiolucent bronchial foreign bodies. Initially, the object creates a bypass valve, which allows ingress and egress of air. At this stage, radiography results are normal. As edema of the surrounding bronchial wall develops, a one-way valve is created. On inspiration, the bronchus dilates and permits ingress of air. However, on expiration, the bronchus constricts and seals around the foreign body blocking the egress of air. Thus, air trapping (obstructive emphysema) results. Radiographically, when a check valve is created, the inspiratory film is normal, whereas the expiratory film shows hyperinflation of the affected lung and shift of the mediastinum to the opposite side (Fig. 113.1). If inspiratory and expiratory films are not possible because a child is tachypnic or uncooperative, lateral decubitus chest films or fluoroscopy may also identify air trapping. Eventually, when enough edema develops to block both ingress and egress of air, a stop valve is created. Obstructive atelectasis is seen radiographically. This late complication usually takes days or weeks to develop.

Many reports have evaluated the sensitivity and specificity of various clinical and diagnostic findings in documented cases of foreign body aspiration in order to avoid unnecessary bronchoscopy in those without foreign bodies. Heyer[11] evaluated the predictive value of clinical, radiologic, and laboratory findings in 160 children with suspected foreign body aspiration, of which 122 had actual foreign bodies. CXR was abnormal in 74% of the entire group, 86% of those with proven foreign bodies, and 37% of those without foreign bodies. Predictors of foreign body aspiration in multivariant analysis were focal hyperinflation on CXR, witnessed choking crisis, and white blood cell count >10,000/μL. All patients who had all three risk factors were found to have a foreign body on bronchoscopy, whereas, only 16% of those without any of the findings had a foreign body.

Chest computed tomography (CT) with or without virtual bronchoscopy is commonly used in the adult population and has also been described in children. In a series of 1,024 children with foreign body aspiration, 141 (14%) had a normal CXR. These patients underwent chest CT and 89% of the scans were abnormal.[12] The few series evaluating CT in children with suspected foreign body aspiration have shown that a negative CT virtually rules out a foreign body; however, false positives may occur in up to 30% of cases.[16,17] In the majority of cases, CT is unnecessary in children and careful judgment is needed to avoid unnecessary radiation exposure.

TREATMENT

Aspirated foreign bodies rarely present as acute emergencies in both the pediatric and adult population. Supraglottic, glottic, and tracheal foreign bodies are more likely to cause acute emergent situations with severe respiratory distress. These patients may progress to a complete obstruction and must be managed as true airway emergencies. Bronchial foreign bodies usually do not result in an emergency situation unless there is hypoxia due to complete obstruction of one of the main bronchi. These patients must also be taken to the operating room emergently for extraction. In stable patients, the ideal treatment is the prompt endoscopic removal once the appropriate planning and

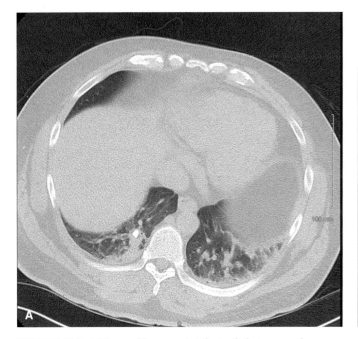

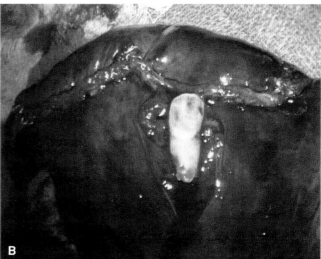

FIGURE 113.2 A 39-year-old man aspirated a tooth during an oral surgery procedure. Two attempts at removal by an otolaryngologist and a pulmonologist failed, resulting in the tooth being pushed further down into the peripheral airway. The tooth was ultimately removed surgically with a thoracoscopic wedge resection under fluoroscopic guidance. **A:** A chest CT demonstrating the tooth in the distal airway with postobstructive consolidation. **B:** Operative photo showing a wedge resection specimen from the lung with the tooth extracted.

resources are in place and contingency preparations have been made for possible complications. Poorly planned interventions without experienced individuals and proper equipment will likely lead to failure and an increased risk of complications (Fig. 113.2). In the absence of a life-threatening situation, the intervention requires thorough and thoughtful planning. In a study of 151 children at Great Ormond Street Hospital for Children who underwent bronchoscopy at the next available time during regular working hours with the normal dedicated team, there was no difference in complications between those treated on the same day versus the next day.[18]

Dried Beans or Peas

Dried beans or peas present a particular situation unique to most other foreign bodies. When a bronchus is obstructed by a dried bean for more than 24 hours, absorbed moisture can cause swelling that can even result in rupture of the capsule (Fig. 113.3). As the bean swells, the airway becomes increasingly obstructed and the space between bean and bronchial wall tightens, obliterating the space for the forceps to reach past, making the extraction extremely difficult. This may be a situation where the use of a cryoprobe could be very helpful as will be discussed further on in this chapter. Most children raised on farms are taught from a young age not to play near large containers of dried beans or peas so as to prevent drowning and asphyxiation.

Preoperative Preparation

When foreign body aspiration is not an acute emergency, the surgeon gathers as much information as possible from the patient or family and ensures that all necessary equipment and personnel are available before the patient enters the operating room. It is extremely helpful to know what the foreign body is. Most adults will be able to describe the object. In children, the parents may know or suspect what the foreign body might be. If it does not result in undo delay, they are asked to

return home to obtain a duplicate. If this is not possible, they are asked to draw the object as accurately as possible. Knowledge of whether it is an organic or inorganic object, the size, shape, and whether it has any edges is helpful. When a duplicate object can be obtained, it is tested to determine which bronchoscope and forceps are best suited for extraction. Communication with the nursing team and anesthesiologist is essential. In any airway procedure, the surgeon must take the

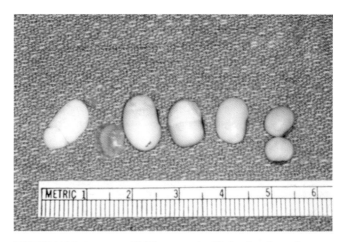

FIGURE 113.3 An 8-year-old fell into a trailer filled with soybeans; he essentially drowned, aspirating multiple soybeans, four of which are seen on the left. The two soybeans on the right were brought in by his father for comparison. They contained approximately 13% moisture when harvested from the field and are about half the size of the moisture-swollen beans that were extracted from the child's tracheobronchial tree. Despite preoperative cyanosis, the patient recovered without sequelae. (From Holinger LD. Foreign bodies of the airway and esophagus. In: Holinger LD, Lusk RP, Green CG, eds. *Pediatric Laryngology and Bronchoesophagology*. Philadelphia, PA: Lippincott—Raven; 1997:236. With permission.)

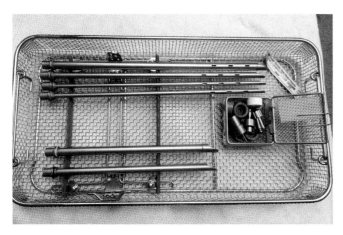

FIGURE 113.4 Example of a rigid bronchoscopy set. Different diameter scopes are color coded for ease of assemblage. Notice the tracheoscopes are shorter without side orifices while the bronchoscopes do have them for ventilation when the distal opening is at the mainstem bronchus with only partial opening for air flow.

time to discuss the interventional steps to be followed with the anesthesiologist and develop a mutually agreed upon plan for anesthetic and airway management. A plan for orderly removal of the object is discussed with each member of the team, and his or her role in that plan is delineated clearly.

Instrumentation

A full bronchoscopy set must be available and functioning properly (Fig. 113.4). Failure to remove a foreign body or loss of a patient can never be excused by the lack of proper equipment. If a full range of rigid scopes and foreign body forceps is not available, the procedure should not be attempted. Rigid bronchoscopes are available in a range of sizes (7 to 14 mm diameter in adults and 2.5 to 6 mm diameter in pediatrics) and lengths. In general, the shortest, widest bronchoscope that can reach the foreign body atraumatically is chosen. Ideally, two laryngoscopes and two bronchoscopes are lighted and readied; should a light fail or a forceps become jammed in the scope, a backup is immediately available. A lighted rod-lens telescope is used for a magnified view. An optical forceps can often be helpful. A variety of instruments, including grasping forceps and suction catheters, should be available for extraction of the object.

In the author's experience, the flexible cryoprobe has become a useful additional tool in the armamentarium for extractions. Cryoextraction refers to the removal of a foreign body by means of a flexible cryoprobe which freezes the object and surrounding secretions to be pulled out en bloc. Organic foreign bodies and some inorganic ones can be removed with this technique, which will be described further on in this chapter.

Anesthesia

In children, preoperative sedation is generally avoided. Instead, the parents, anesthesiologist, and nursing staff help keep the child calm before induction to avoid dislodgment of the foreign body because of crying.

General anesthesia is used for of foreign body extractions with particular considerations. Spontaneous respiration during the intervention is preferred over apneic techniques. If the patient is completely paralyzed, he or she becomes entirely dependent on a well-sealed airway for ventilation and oxygenation. In the setting of a rigid bronchoscopy, the seal is only partial, allowing the patient to gently move

air which creates a safety net, particularly should the airway become momentarily lost. Topicalization of the upper airway is of paramount importance, commonly initiated in the preoperative area by nebulization of lidocaine and instructing the patient to inhale both through the nose and mouth. The larynx and trachea are sprayed with topical 4% lidocaine before the bronchoscope is introduced. Our preference is to administer a low-dose short-acting paralytic agent to intubate the trachea with the rigid bronchoscope. Once in the airway, all efforts are placed into obtaining an appropriate seal to ventilate the patient while spontaneous respiration returns. Lidocaine can also be administered through the bronchoscope to prevent coughing. Positive-pressure ventilation, particularly "bagging," is avoided because this tends to drive the foreign body further distally. An inhalational agent is intermittently delivered through the closed system of the rigid bronchoscope in addition to short-acting intravenous anesthetics. During the actual attempts at extraction, 100% oxygen is given through the bronchoscope. If spontaneous respiration is not possible due to bronchial hyperactivity, a short-acting, nondepolarizing muscle relaxant may be used with ventilation maintained at lower tidal volumes during extraction attempts.

Technique

Rigid bronchoscopy is the preferred technique for foreign body removal, especially in children. A flexible scope can be used in the initial airway inspection to locate the position of the foreign body. It is also useful in patients who cannot extend their neck or with peripherally located objects. Flexible bronchoscopy is used for extraction more commonly in adults, with reports ranging from 56% to 100% of cases using a flexible scope.[8,10,19]

Once the bronchoscope has been advanced into the trachea, ventilation is established with very close communication with the anesthesia team to determine periods where efforts are placed on ventilation alternating with attention focused on the extraction efforts. Jet ventilation can also be used if available as it allows ventilation through the open bronchoscopic system almost simultaneously with the extraction efforts. The tracheobronchial tree is inspected completely, because multiple foreign bodies are present in up to 9% of cases.[20] All secretions are suctioned out to ensure optimal respiratory function when the involved side is inspected. The location of the foreign body is approached slowly and carefully to avoid overriding or displacement. Care is taken to avoid driving the foreign body further down. Suction is used to remove secretions from around the foreign body, but it is not typically used in the attempt at extraction.

The endoscopist must resist the impulse to seize the foreign body as soon as it is discovered. Before any attempt at extraction, a careful study is made to determine the size, shape, position, probable location of unseen parts, and relation to surrounding structures. As determined by the appearance of the presenting part combined with the knowledge obtained from the radiographic studies, the endoscopist may suspect that sharp points are buried deep within the mucosa or outside the wall in the mediastinum. When the most favorable position for grasping has been ascertained, the closed forceps is inserted through the scope. All manipulation is gentle and delicate. The forceps is advanced until it lightly touches the foreign body; the endoscope is then withdrawn a short distance to permit the forceps blades to be opened if necessary. The forceps blades are advanced until the tips pass the equator of the object; then they are closed. The tip of the scope is advanced against the foreign body, which is held against the tube opening. The grasp of the forceps is maintained firmly with the right hand while all traction for withdrawal is made by the left hand. The thumb of the left hand firmly clamps the forceps to lock the relationship between the forceps and the scope during extraction so that the three units are extracted as one. The bronchoscope keeps the vocal cords apart until the foreign body has exited the glottis. Just before exiting the glottis, the foreign body is rotated to the sagittal plane, which is the largest diameter of the laryngeal lumen.

After removal of a foreign body from the tracheobronchial tree, the laryngoscope is reinserted and a second pass is made with the bronchoscope. Retained secretions are aspirated, and the entire bronchial tree is rechecked to be certain that no fragments or other objects remain and there is no obvious airway injury. Granulation tissue is resected as necessary, and bleeding can be controlled with a topical vasoconstrictive agent.

In the rare circumstance that a spherical foreign body cannot be removed, a Fogarty catheter may be lubricated and passed through the bronchoscope distal to the object. The balloon is then inflated and withdrawn in order to dislodge the object proximally and allow its extraction. It may be necessary to create a temporary tracheostomy for extraction in case the object cannot pass through the glottis. This would be most likely in the pediatric population. If an object cannot be removed, a thoracotomy may be necessary. Lobectomy may be required in patients with long-standing foreign bodies and chronic obstruction resulting in a destroyed lung.

Special techniques have been developed for the extraction of pointed objects. The first priority during the extraction procedure is to localize the point. The point is released and sheathed within the scope. It often is necessary to accomplish this by first moving the object distally to disengage the point, then advancing the scope over the object rather than pulling the object into the tube. Long, pointed objects typically lodge with the point facing upward. This occurs even if the object enters point first. The point becomes engaged by the mucosa and the object tumbles, then proceeds with the point trailing (Fig. 113.5).

Special techniques for long pointed objects include aligning the bronchus to approach the object by its long axis. Biplane fluoros-

copy may be of assistance in this situation. Magnets have also been used. Tacks, nails, and large-headed foreign bodies in the tracheobronchial tree are released, sheathed, and removed with an inward rotation method that is used for pins and needles with imbedded points. A side-grasping forceps captures the object at the point. A corkscrew motion is used to push the pin distally while rotating it clockwise, freeing the point and aligning the shaft with the long axis of the forceps. The scope is then advanced over the point to sheath it for extraction. When a point cannot be sheathed, the foreign body may be withdrawn with the point trailing. A rotation forceps allows a point to rotate and trail.

Fluoroscopic assistance may be used for radiopaque foreign bodies in the upper lobe, pins in the lung periphery, and sharp or irregular foreign bodies, such as dental bridgework. For accurate localization, simultaneous biplane fluoroscopy is required; it may be available only in a special procedures room within the radiology department. The technique is deceptively simple but extremely hazardous because the fluoroscope does not visualize the tissues that lie between the forceps blades and the foreign body.

As a foreign body is brought out through the larynx, the lateral pressure of the vocal folds may strip it from the forceps' grasp (stripping off). Because complete airway obstruction may ensue, a prompt, efficient response is required. The airway is re-established immediately by removing the object or by pushing it down into the bronchus in which it had been lodged, allowing ventilation of the good lung. A foreign body lost in the trachea is usually carried into the uninvolved bronchus. This occurs because the previously obstructed lung or lobe moves little air and is edematous or narrowed by granulation tissue. This may create an emergency because the patient's only functional lung is completely obstructed. The object must be removed immediately or relocated into the other bronchus. If the foreign body cannot be visualized readily, it may be found next to the scope; below the vocal folds; or in the mouth, hypopharynx, or nasopharynx.

Once the foreign body is relocated, it is regrasped and extracted. "Stripping off" may result from factors related to the forceps or the foreign body itself. Forceps factors include faulty application of the forceps, use of the wrong forceps for the problem, mechanically imperfect forceps, and poorly adjusted or poorly constructed forceps. Three foreign body factors can lead to stripping off: poor orientation of the foreign body (solution: rotate 90 degrees at the vocal folds); insecure grasp of the foreign body (solution: sheath the foreign body with the end of the bronchoscope and lock the forceps against the bronchoscope with the left thumb); and a foreign body too large for the laryngeal lumen (solution: fragment the foreign body or remove it through a tracheotomy).

Foreign body retrieval by cryoprobe is feasible mostly with organic objects. Early experience with cryoextraction involved mucous plugs and blood clots that are otherwise difficult to grasp. The tip of the probe freezes by activating the trigger pedal and 5 to 10 seconds of time are allowed for cryoadhesion to take place at which point the probe is pulled back en bloc with the object. Organic objects such as chicken bones present adequate cryoadhesion for retrieval while only few inorganic foreign bodies do (Fig. 113.6).[21] Particular attention must be paid to the mucosal walls of the involved airway. The freezing block should not involve normal tissue as it could be stripped off when the probe and foreign body are pulled back for extraction (Video 113.1). In our experience, using the flexible bronchoscope through the rigid one permits sufficient precision to center the foreign body at the tip of the probe, and once the frozen bloc is achieved, the flexible scope is retrieved into the rigid one as described above and both scopes along with the object are pulled

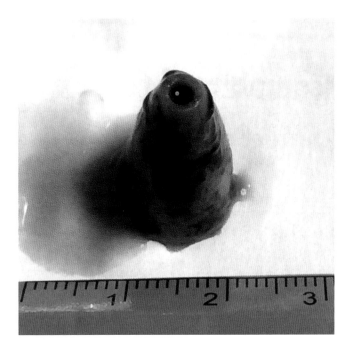

FIGURE 113.5 Pen cap that had been logged in the right lower lobe bronchus for 10 years with only a few episodes of pneumonia. Notice the opening at the tip were the ink cartridge normally would protrude, likely allowed some degree of flow of air and secretions.

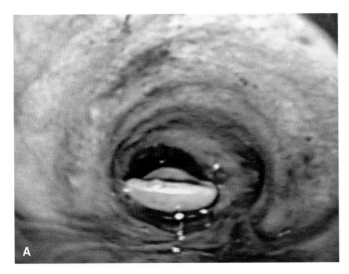

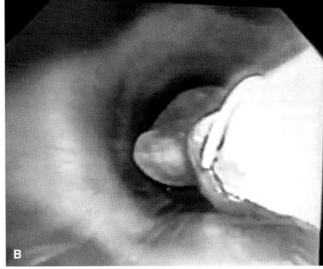

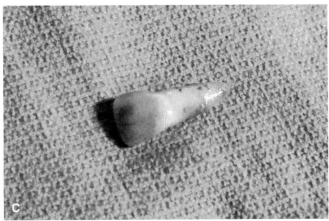

FIGURE 113.6 **A:** Incisor tooth aspirated just hours prior to the extraction and lodged in the bronchus intermedius. **B:** After several failed attempts with various forceps and catheters, the flexible cryoprobe was used successfully. The picture shows the moment the frozen tooth and probe enter the rigid scope. Frozen tooth, flexible and rigid bronchoscopes were retrieved en bloc. **C:** Incisor tooth shown on the back table after cryoextraction.

out of the patient. The probe with the object, still within the flexible scope, is then submerged in saline for thawing and assessment of the removed item at the back table by an assistant while the endoscopist focuses on securing the airway.

POSTOPERATIVE TREATMENT

After endoscopic foreign body extraction, the patient is usually admitted to the hospital for overnight observation. Antibiotics are prescribed only if there was a preoperative diagnosis of pneumonia. On the day after the procedure, if the patient is afebrile and the lungs are clear to auscultation, the patient is discharged home. However, if the patient remains febrile or has persistent pulmonary signs or symptoms, CXR is performed and appropriate therapeutic measures are taken.

RESULTS AND COMPLICATIONS

Successful extraction of foreign bodies with bronchoscopy is between 93.7% and 99.7%.[13,14,22] Tracheostomy has been reported in <0.01%, either due to the foreign body being too large for extraction or laryngeal edema.[13] Mortality has been reported to be 0.21% to 0.8%.[5,13,14] In a large series of 1,428 children with foreign body aspiration in China between 1985 and 2007, the foreign body was successfully removed by rigid bronchoscopy in 99.7%. Tracheostomy was required in four patients and one patient required thoracotomy.

Mortality in this series was 0.21% due to hypoxia. Two of these cases involved dried beans.[14]

Intraoperative complications include failure to remove the object requiring either tracheostomy or thoracotomy for removal, airway injury, bleeding, and hypoxia. Postoperative complications include laryngeal edema, bronchospasm, bleeding, atelectasis, pneumonia, and pneumothorax. In a review of 504 foreign body removals in children and adults, 42 complications occurred. Patients who initially underwent a bronchoscopy elsewhere and those requiring longer procedure times had a higher incidence of complications.[23]

Traumatic laryngitis and laryngeal edema are treated with elevation of the head of the bed, humidity, racemic epinephrine, and high-dose corticosteroids. When laryngeal edema is anticipated, corticosteroid therapy should be initiated in the operating room. Laryngeal edema is proportional to the time the bronchoscope is in the larynx, the trauma of the procedure, and the size of the bronchoscope in relation to the size of the larynx. To prevent laryngeal edema, smaller bronchoscopes that pass easily through the larynx are preferred, although there may be an air leak with positive-pressure ventilation.

Repetition of any endoscopic procedure after an unsuccessful attempt at removal is avoided until laryngeal symptoms resolve; 3 to 7 days is usually adequate. It is wise to use this waiting period in patients who have had previous attempts at endoscopic extraction elsewhere. The presence of severe respiratory obstruction is an obvious exception to these guidelines.

If the initial attempt at endoscopic extraction is unsuccessful because of granulation tissue with bleeding and purulent bronchitis, the patient should be treated for approximately 3 days with intravenous and nebulized dexamethasone and intravenous antibiotics. Such treatment has resulted in dramatic resolution of the granulation tissue before endoscopic extraction has been reattempted.

FOREIGN BODIES IN THE ESOPHAGUS

EPIDEMIOLOGY AND ETIOLOGY

Foreign body ingestions are reasonably common and potentially serious events. Most foreign bodies retained in the GI tract are found in the esophagus. While mortality is very rare, foreign bodies in the esophagus can cause the highest morbidity because of the potential for perforation and associated mediastinitis. Since retentions lasting greater than 24 hours are associated with the highest rates of complications, all esophageal foreign bodies should be managed on an urgent basis. Esophageal foreign bodies can be divided into inorganic or "true foreign bodies" and organic foreign bodies such as food bolus impaction.

Esophageal foreign bodies can occur at any age with a mean ranging from 34 to 50 in most series. There tends to be a bimodal distribution with a mean age of around 4 years in the pediatric population and 50 to 60 in the adult population. There is a slight male predominance ranging from 56% to 63%.[24–32] Foreign body impaction in adults is most commonly a food bolus, typically meat, followed by bones. Children tend to have inorganic or "true foreign bodies," with coins being the most common.[24,27,30–32] Risk factors for true foreign body impaction include mental retardation, alcohol intoxication, or underlying psychiatric problems. Further, edentulous adults are at risk of foreign body ingestions, particularly of their dental prostheses. Underlying esophageal pathology such as strictures or Schatzki rings, motility disorders, malignancy, or previous esophageal surgery, is a common finding with food bolus impactions. However, the rate of underlying pathology varies widely among series, ranging from 6% to 50%.[24,25,27,28,30,32,33] Eosinophilic esophagitis is being increasingly recognized as an underlying pathology associated with esophageal foreign body, particularly food bolus impaction. Guidelines for the diagnosis of eosinophilic esophagitis defined by the American Gastroenterological Association include: symptoms of esophageal dysfunction, ≥15 eosinophils in one high-power field, and lack of response to high-dose proton pump inhibitors or a normal pH study.[34] The true incidence of eosinophilic esophagitis in patients who present with esophageal foreign bodies is unclear given that most patients do not have esophageal biopsies at the time of presentation. In a study of 548 patients, eosinophilic esophagitis was found in 9% of cases and 12% of patients with food bolus impactions; however, only 27% of patients undergoing endoscopy had an esophageal biopsy. Eosinophilic esophagitis was associated with male gender, younger age, and Caucasian race and was the strongest predictor of recurrent esophageal foreign body impaction.[27]

The location of retained esophageal foreign bodies varies depending on the object ingested, the age of the patient, and the presence of underlying pathology. The upper esophagus, especially at the level of the cricopharyngeus muscle, is the most common location (60% to 80%) for esophageal foreign body impaction, particularly in children.[25,28,33]

CLINICAL SIGNS AND SYMPTOMS

Typical symptoms of esophageal foreign body impaction include dysphagia and odynophagia. Odynophagia may be due to persistent inflammation triggered by the foreign body, but it can also indicate significant mucosal injury by an object that has already passed. Other symptoms may include chest pain, excessive salivation, regurgitation, and vomiting. An inability to tolerate salivary secretions indicates complete esophageal obstruction and requires urgent treatment. Respiratory symptoms such as cough, dyspnea, or stridor can be seen with aspiration of food or saliva secondary to the esophageal obstruction, concomitant aspiration of a foreign body, or extrinsic compression of the trachea by the esophageal object. In addition to the nature and timing of the foreign body ingestion, the history should include details of any previous esophageal abnormalities such as dysphagia, other episodes of foreign body impaction, esophageal or oropharyngeal surgery, caustic injury, radiation, or prior dilation. This information allows the physician to anticipate the likely underlying pathology and level of obstruction.

On physical examination, older children and adults may be able to identify the material swallowed and point to a particular area of discomfort, although few patients are able to localize the level of impaction reliably. Patients are more precise when the impaction occurs proximal to the cricopharyngeus. On the other hand, localization of the "foreign body sensation" to the mid- or lower sternum usually indicates esophageal rather than pharyngeal retention. Focalization to the suprasternal notch can be seen with either pharyngeal or esophageal retention. Particular attention should be paid to crepitus, tenderness, or erythema in the neck, each of which suggests an oropharyngeal or cervical esophageal perforation. Perforations at the level of the esophagogastric junction may occur distal to the diaphragmatic hiatus with peritoneal rather than pleural contamination. Therefore, a thorough abdominal examination should include signs of peritonitis or bowel obstruction, both of which would preclude endoscopic management.

DIAGNOSIS

Radiographic evaluation typically starts with plain films of the neck and chest which can locate most artificial objects and steak bones as well as to evaluate for the presence of mediastinal or peritoneal free air. However, chicken or fish bones, plastic, wood, and most glass are radiolucent. Both anteroposterior and lateral views should be obtained and can differentiate an esophageal from a tracheal foreign body. Barium or water-soluble contrast studies should generally be avoided. Oral contrast agents place patients at increased risk for aspiration during endoscopy and also make endoscopic extraction of retained foreign bodies more difficult. In addition, the hypertonicity of Gastrografin in particular carries a significant risk for pulmonary edema if this agent is aspirated. Moreover, a normal radiographic examination does not generally preclude the need for endoscopy in a symptomatic patient. One setting where oral contrast studies can be useful is in confirming the presence of an esophageal perforation suspected by examination or radiology findings. CT scans may be useful in identifying some foreign bodies not visualized on plain films and to diagnose complications such as perforation (Fig. 113.7). In light of a suspicious clinical history and/or persistent symptoms, endoscopic evaluation should be performed even with negative imaging.

TREATMENT

While many foreign bodies may pass spontaneously, objects impacted in the esophagus should be dealt with in a timely fashion. Urgent endoscopy is recommended for certain situations including high-grade esophageal obstruction, disc batteries located in the esophagus,

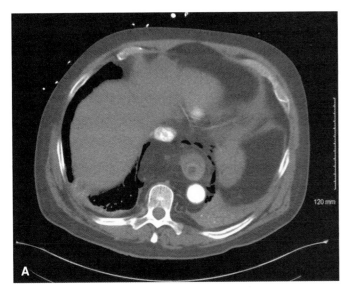 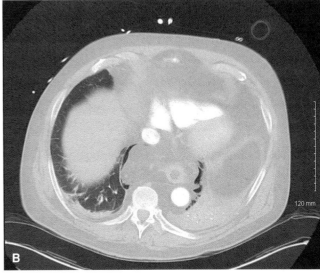

FIGURE 113.7 A 67-year-old man presented with a food impaction. He underwent an endoscopy at an outside hospital and was found to have a food bolus completely obstructing the esophagus. This was attempted to be removed; however, there was concern for a perforation at the time. A CT was obtained which showed a large amount of mediastinal air around the esophagus. There was evidence of food impaction in the distal esophagus. On endoscopy, he was found to have an impacted food bolus at the gastroesophageal junction. He underwent extraction of the food bolus and placement of an esophageal stent. **A:** Mediastinal windows demonstrating the impacted food bolus in the distal esophagus. **B:** Lung windows demonstrated pneumomediastinum.

and sharp objects.[35] In other situations, patients without significant symptoms can be managed on a more elective basis. However, foreign bodies should not be allowed to remain in the esophagus for more than 24 hours due to the increase in complications.[35] Assessment of the patient's airway status is critical and patients with high-grade proximal obstructions may require endotracheal intubation.

Rigid esophagoscopy or direct laryngoscopy should be used initially for impacted objects proximal to the level of the hypopharynx and cricopharyngeus muscle. Flexible endoscopy is used for objects in the mid and lower esophagus and can be done with sedation or general anesthesia. A variety of instruments should be available for extraction, including rat-tooth and alligator forceps, a polypectomy snare, baskets, short and long overtubes, and a foreign body protector hood (Fig. 113.8). If possible, a practice session with a similar object outside of the patient before endoscopy may be helpful. Snares and forceps are most useful for sharp objects, whereas retrieval nets and baskets seem to be most effective for small, blunt objects. The use of an overtube provides several advantages including airway protection, ease of repeated insertion of the endoscope during extraction of multiple foreign bodies or piecemeal extraction of a food bolus, and protection of the esophageal mucosa during the removal of sharp objects (Fig. 113.9). Esophageal intubation with an overtube carries the risk of hypopharyngeal injury. Passage of the overtube may not be feasible in the setting of a very proximal foreign body obstruction. In addition, bypassing the upper esophageal sphincter with an overtube interferes with air distention, making visualization of the esophageal lumen more difficult. Short overtubes can be used for airway protection and to shield the upper esophagus and pharynx, while longer overtubes confer additional protection for the distal esophagus and lower esophageal sphincter. While longer overtubes are more cumbersome to use, they are particularly helpful for the removal of sharp objects located in the stomach. Protector hoods are typically less cumbersome than overtubes and more comfortable for patients; these devices are particularly useful for the removal of objects from the stomach that may injure the lower esophageal sphincter during extraction.

Inorganic "True" Foreign Bodies

Coins are the most commonly ingested artificial objects, particularly in the pediatric population. Laryngoscopic or endoscopic extraction is generally the preferred approach. A period of expectant management for the asymptomatic patient with a coin lodged in the esophagus who has no known underlying pathology can be considered, as many, do pass spontaneously.[35] A study of 168 asymptomatic patients under 21 years of age observed varying rates of spontaneous passage depending on the location of impaction: 14% if in the proximal third,

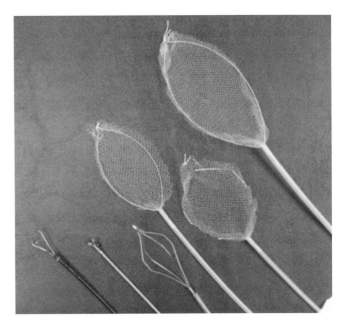

FIGURE 113.8 Devices used for endoscopic management of esophageal foreign body and food impaction. From **left** to **right:** Tripod retrieval device, rat-tooth forceps, polyp retrieval basket, Roth net (standard oval, octagonal, large).

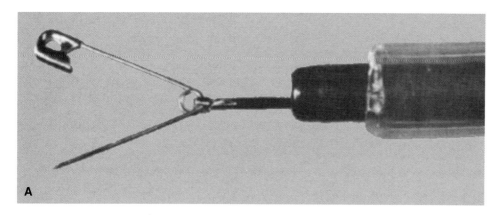

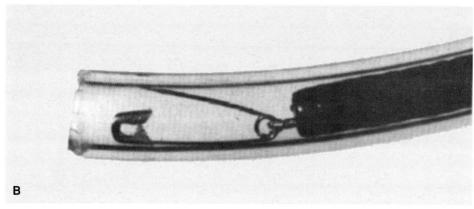

FIGURE 113.9 Technique for extraction of an open safety pin (**A**) demonstrating the importance of having the sharp point trail behind as the pin is pulled into an overtube (**B**).

43% if in the middle third, and 67% if in the distal third.[36] Given the higher rate of complications after 24 hours, expectant management should be limited to no longer than 18 hours. Once a coin has reached the stomach, it will typically pass spontaneously and can be observed with serial x-rays.

Sharp objects present unique challenges and may be inorganic or organic such as bones. Removal can be accomplished by forceps or snares. To reduce the risk of mucosal lacerations with extraction, the sharp end of the object should be pointed distally when grasped and extracted with the sharp end trailing behind. Otherwise, an overtube or protector hood can be used as described above. While many sharp objects pass through the GI tract uneventfully, a sharp object identified in the esophagus should be removed emergently given the high risk of complications. If feasible, endoscopic removal of any sharp object should be attempted if it is localized in the stomach or proximal duodenum.[35]

Disk or button batteries usually pass spontaneously, although case reports have described liquefaction necrosis and perforation related to the extrusion of concentrated potassium hydroxide from alkaline batteries. Esophageal injury can also result from pressure necrosis or low-voltage electrical burns. Urgent endoscopic removal of all batteries located in the esophagus is recommended due to the risk of complications.[35] The use of a basket or net is recommended. Rat-tooth or grasping forceps should be avoided owing to the risk of battery puncture, with resultant leakage of caustic contents. If a battery has already passed into the stomach, endoscopic retrieval can be reserved for those that remain in the stomach on repeat radiography at 48 hours or those with diameter greater than 20 mm.

Cocaine wrapped in plastic or latex condoms ("body packing") is usually, but not always, seen on plain radiographs or CT scans. Since rupture and leakage of contents can be lethal, endoscopic extraction is not recommended.[35] Conservative management is generally advised, with surgical intervention for signs of obstruction, packet rupture, or lack of progression on serial imaging.

Organic Foreign Bodies

The impaction of a food bolus or bone is the most common cause of esophageal foreign body in the adult population as discussed above. These patients typically present minutes to hours after swallowing a bolus of food and feeling a foreign body sensation in the chest. Patients may have varying degrees of esophageal obstruction and present with worsening neck or chest pain in conjunction with excess salivation. Urgent treatment is indicated in those with severe symptoms or patients who are unable to swallow their own secretions. While mild symptoms often resolve spontaneously, endoscopic intervention is indicated within 24 hours to reduce the risk of complications.

Endoscopic intervention is usually successful in removing a food bolus. A variety of techniques can be used. Forceps, snares, or nets can be used successfully for extraction. The bolus can also be pushed into the stomach. It is preferred that the distal lumen of the esophagus is visualized beyond the bolus to rule out an obstructing lesion such as a tumor or tight stricture to lessen the risk of perforation. In some cases, disruption of the retained food into small pieces can facilitate removal or passage into the stomach. When the food bolus cannot be completely retrieved with a net and several intubations appear necessary, an overtube can be employed as described above.

In patients with an underlying stricture, dilation is safe at the time of the initial food disimpaction in the absence of significant mucosal injury on endoscopy. Given the emergence of eosinophilic esophagitis as an important cause of food impaction, this diagnosis should be considered in patients with a food bolus impaction without apparent underlying pathology, especially in those with repeat food bolus

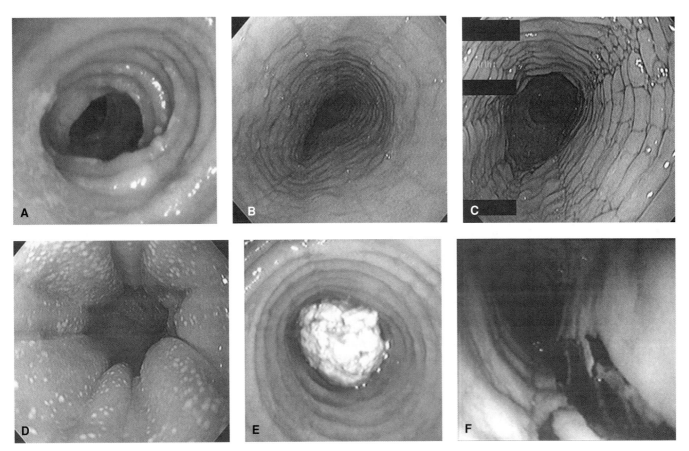

FIGURE 113.10   Endoscopic features of eosinophilic esophagitis. **A:** Concentric mucosal rings with luminal narrowing. **B:** Longitudinally oriented linear furrows. **C:** Mucosal edema and longitudinal furrows. **D:** Punctate white exudates represent eosinophilic microabscess formation and can mimic candidal esophagitis. **E:** Food impaction in a patient with eosinophilic esophagitis. **F:** Linear tear following esophageal dilation in a patient with eosinophilic esophagitis.

impactions. Typical endoscopic features include "corrugated" or "ringed" appearance to the mucosa, longitudinal furrowing, whitish exudates, smaller caliber esophagus, and edema (Fig. 113.10). Multiple, concentric mucosal rings and longitudinal furrowing are the most common endoscopic features in adults. Mucosal fragility, or the "crepe paper" esophagus, as well as mucosal exudates that can mimic candidal esophagitis are less common but more specific endoscopic signs. Eosinophilic esophagitis may occur in the absence of apparent endoscopic abnormalities, emphasizing the importance of mucosal biopsies when there is clinical suspicion. Owing to the patchy distribution of esophageal eosinophilia, a minimum of five biopsies should be obtained from the proximal and distal esophagus.[34] Since esophageal dilation in patients with eosinophilic esophagitis may have a higher rate of esophageal perforation, medical therapy should be tried first.[34] Treatment in adults most commonly involves the use of topical steroids, while elimination of dietary antigens has proven effective in the pediatric population.

Several noninvasive approaches to esophageal food impactions have been studied with varying success. Proteolytic enzymes such as papain ("meat tenderizers") are not recommended due to the potential of severe complications, including perforation and death.[35] Glucagon, by relaxing smooth muscle, including the lower esophageal sphincter, may allow spontaneous passage of a food bolus. It is usually administered as a 1-mg intravenous bolus. Since glucagon appears to be a safe, noninvasive option, a trial of this agent prior to proceeding with endoscopic management is reasonable; although, reported success rates are low.[24]

Results and Complications

Endoscopic intervention is successful in 93% to 99% of cases.[30,32,37,38] If endoscopic retrieval fails, there are several options. Often the first endoscopic attempt is done under sedation by gastroenterology. In these cases, extraction under general anesthesia by the thoracic surgeon either using flexible or rigid endoscopy is often successful. Surgical removal is required in approximately 1% of cases.[28] Mortality is low, with most large series reporting no mortality.[28,30]

Complications include mucosal laceration and bleeding which can typically be managed conservatively. Perforation has been reported in 1% to 4% of cases and appears more common with rigid esophagoscopy.[37,38] If recognized early, placement of a covered esophageal stent is successful in most cases. Particular attention must be paid to adequate pleural drainage if involved. After stent placement, one should routinely obtain an esophagogram to ensure that the leak is sealed. Patients are discharged on a soft diet and the stent is typically removed 6 to 8 weeks later. In patients with significant mediastinal contamination, or any signs of sepsis surgical repair and wide drainage is necessary.

REFERENCES

1. Killian G. Direct endoscopy of the upper air-passages and oesophagus: its diagnosis and therapeutic value in the search for and removal of foreign bodies. *J Laryngol Rhinol Otol* 1902;17:461.
2. Jackson C, Jackson CL. *Diseases of the Air and Food Passages of Foreign Body Origin*. Philadelphia, PA: Saunders; 1936.
3. Ikeda S. *Atlas of Flexible Bronchofiberscopy*. Baltimore, MD: University Park Press; 1974.

4. Ikeda S. The flexible bronchofiberscope. *Keio J Med* 1968;17:1–16.

5. Fidkowski CW, Zheng H, Firth PG. The anesthetic considerations of tracheobronchial foreign bodies in children: a literature review of 12,979 cases. *Anesth Analg* 2010;111:1016–1025.

6. Foltran F, Ballali S, Rodriguez H, et al. Inhaled foreign bodies in children: a global perspective on their epidemiological, clinical, and preventive aspects. *Pediatr Pulmonol* 2013;48:344–351.

7. Kaushal P, Brown DJ, Lander L, et al. Aspirated foreign bodies in pediatric patients, 1968–2010: a comparison between the United States and other countries. *Int J Pediatr Otorhinolaryngol* 2011;75:1322–1326.

8. Debelijak A, Sorli J, Music E, et al. Bronchoscopic removal of foreign bodies in adults: experience with 62 patients from 1974–1998. *Eur Respir J* 1999;14:792–795.

9. Baharloo F, Veychkemans F, Francis C, et al. Tracheobronchial foreign bodies: presentation and management in children and adults. *Chest* 1999;115:1357–1362.

10. Mise K, Savicevic AJ, Pavlov N, et al. Removal of tracheobronchial foreign bodies in adults using flexible bronchoscopy: experience 1995–2006. *Surg Endosc* 2009;23:1360–1364.

11. Heyer CM, Bollmeier ME, Rossler L, et al. Evaluation of clinical, radiologic, and laboratory prebronchoscopy findings in children with suspected foreign body aspiration. *J Pediatr Surgery* 2006;41:1882–1888.

12. Gang W, Zhengxia P, Hongbo L, et al. Diagnosis and treatment of tracheobronchial foreign bodies in 1024 children. *J Pediatr Surg* 2012;47:2004–2010.

13. Sahin A, Meteroglu F, Eren S, et al. Inhalation of foreign bodies in children: experience of 22 years. *J Trauma Acute Care Surg* 2013;74:658–663.

14. Hui H, Na L, Zhijun CJ, et al. Therapeutic experience from 1428 patients with pediatric tracheobronchial foreign body. *J Pediatr Surg* 2008;43:718–721.

15. Jackson C, Jackson Cl. *Bronchoesophagology*. Philadelphia, PA: Saunders; 1950.

16. Hitter A, Hullo E, Durand C, et al. Diagnostic value of various investigations in children with suspected foreign body aspiration. *Europ Annals of Otorhinolaryngol, Head and Neck Dis* 2011;128:248–252.

17. Adaleti I, Kurugogla S, Ulus S, et al. Utilization of low-dose multidetector ct and virtual bronchoscopy in children with suspected foreign body aspiration. *Pediatr Radiol* 2007;37:33–40.

18. Mani N, Soma M, Massey S, et al. Removal of inhaled foreign bodies—middle of the night or the next morning? *Int J Pediatr Otorhinolaryngol* 2009;73:1085–1089.

19. Ramos MB, Fernandez-Villar A, Rivo JE, et al. Extraction of airway foreign bodies in adult: experience from 1987–2008. *Interactive Cardiovasc Thorac Surg* 2009;9:402–405.

20. Hughes CA, Barody FM, March BR. Pediatric tracheobronchial foreign bodies: historical review from the Johns Hopkins Hospital. *Ann Otol Rhinol Laryngol* 1996;105:555–561.

21. Fruchter O, Kramer MR. Retrieval of various foreign bodies by flexible bryoprobe: in vitro feasibility study. *Clin Resp J* 2015;9(2):176–179.

22. Zerella JT, Dimler M, Mcgill LC, et al. Foreign body aspiration in children: value of radiography and complications of bronchoscopy. *J Pediatr Surg* 1998;33:1651–1654.

23. Zaytoun GM, Rouadi PW, Baki H. Endoscopic management of foreign bodies in the tracheobronchial tree: predictive factors for complications. *Otolaryngol Head Neck Surg* 2000;123:311–316.

24. Crockett SD, Sperry SLW, Miller CB, et al. Emergency care of esophageal foreign body impactions: timing, treatment modalities and resource utilization. *Dis Esophagus* 2013;26:105–112.

25. Chen T, Wu HF, Shi Q, et al. Endoscopic management of impacted esophageal foreign bodies. *Dis Esophagus* 2013;26:799–806.

26. Williams P, Jameson S, Bishop P, et al. Esophageal foreign bodies and eosinophilic esophagitis—the need for esophageal mucosal biopsy: a 12-year survey across pediatric subspecialties. *Surg Endosc* 2013;27:2216–2220.

27. Sperry SL, Crockett SD, Miller CB, et al. Esophageal foreign body impactions: epidemiology, time trends, and the impact of the increasing prevalence of eosinophilic esophagitis. *Gastrointest Endosc* 2011;74:985–991.

28. Wu WT, Chui CT, Kuo CJ, et al. Endoscopic management of suspected esophageal foreign body in adults. *Dis Esophagus* 2011;24:131–137.

29. Nadir A, Sahin E, Nadir I, et al. Esophageal foreign bodies: 177 cases. *Dis Esophagus* 2011;24:6–9.

30. Li ZS, Sun ZX, Zou DW, et al. Endoscopic management of foreign bodies in the upper gi tract: experience with 1088 cases in china. *Gastrointest Endosc* 2006;64:485–492.

31. Balci AE, Eren S, Eren MN. Esophageal foreign bodies under cricopharyngeal level in children: an analysis of 1116 cases. *Interactive Cardiovasc Thorac Surg* 2004;3:14–18.

32. Mosca S, Manes G, Martino R, et al. Endoscopic management of foreign bodies in the upper gastrointestinal tract: report on a series of 414 adult patients. *Endoscopy* 2001;33:692–696.

33. Athanassiadi K, Gerazounis M, Metaxas E, et al. Management of esophageal foreign bodies: a retrospective review of 400 cases. *Eur J Cardiothorac Surg* 2002;21:653–656.

34. Furuta GT, Liacouras CA, Collins MH, et al. Eosinophilic esophagitis in children and adults: a systemic review and consensus recommendations for diagnosis and treatment. *Gastroenterology* 2007;133:1342–1363.

35. Ikenberry SO, Jue TL, Anderson MA, et al. Management of ingested foreign bodies and food impactions. *Gastrointest Endosc* 2011;73:1085–1091.

36. Waltzman ML, Baskin M, Wypij D, et al. A randomized clinical trial of the management of esophageal coins in children. *Pediatrics* 2005;116:614–619.

37. Yan X, Zhou L, Lin S, et al. Therapeutic effect of esophageal foreign body extraction management: flexible versus rigid endoscopy in 216 adults of Beijing. *Med Sci Monit* 2014;20:2054–2060.

38. Gmeiner D, Von Rahden BH, Meco C, et al. Flexible versus rigid endoscopy for treatment of foreign body impaction in the esophagus. *Surg Endosc* 2007;21:2026–2029.

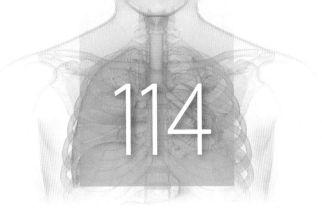

114

Blunt and Penetrating Injuries of the Esophagus

Tracey Dechert ▪ Virginia R. Litle

As within many areas of medicine, the first writing of esophageal injury dates back to ancient times. A case report titled "A Gaping Wound of the Throat Penetrating the Gullet" was one of many case reports in the Edwin Smith Papyrus, which was written in ancient Egypt between 4,000 and 5,000 years ago.[1] In more recent history, the first report of a tracheoesophageal fistula after blunt trauma was reported in 1936, and several years later, the first case of successful management of an esophageal perforation with drainage was described in 1947.[2,3]

Traumatic esophageal injuries are an uncommon entity present in only 0.14% to 1% of patients following noniatrogenic injury.[4,5] Damage to the esophagus is usually caused by penetrating trauma but it remains a rare injury even in busy urban trauma centers that have a large volume of penetrating trauma, with most busy centers seeing an average of 2 to 9 patients/year.[6–10] Although the overall prevalence of the injury remains low, penetrating esophageal injuries carry high morbidity and mortality, with a particular concern focused on the thoracic esophagus. In a recent analysis of the National Trauma Data Bank, 227 patients were studied from 107 centers.[11] Overall mortality in patients with traumatic esophageal injury was found to be 44%, with 92% of these deaths taking place in less than 24 hours, most commonly due to the result of severe associated injuries. Significant predictors of esophageal-related complications were age and abbreviated injury score of the abdomen/pelvis >3. The only significant predictor of mortality was injury severity score, with esophageal-related complications not significantly impacting mortality. Young black men sustaining gunshot wounds to the chest represent the highest risk demographic with morbidity rates in that subset reaching 46% and a mortality rate of 20%.[5]

Sheely and colleagues published a 22-year experience with over 700 patients who sustained penetrating neck trauma.[12] Thirty-nine patients (5.6%) had a cervical esophageal injury. Of note, these 39 patients had 55 associated injuries with the trachea being the additional structure most often injured. Papers in other smaller studies examining transcervical gunshot wounds also reveal a low incidence of esophageal trauma. In a study of 34 patients with transcervical gunshot wounds, two patients (6%) were found to have an esophageal injury.[13] In a similar study with 97 patients published a few years later, 6% of the patients had an aerodigestive injury.[14] In a larger study examining patients who sustained a gunshot wound to the chest, the authors reported a 0.7% incidence of intrathoracic esophageal injuries in 1,961 patients.[15]

Penetrating esophageal trauma occurs most commonly in the cervical esophagus.[16,17] In a study describing penetrating injuries to the esophagus, 45/77 (58%) patients sustained an injury to the cervical esophagus. Gunshot wound was the most common mechanism, occurring in 75% of patients.[16] In over 559 patients with esophageal perforation treated at the University of Pennsylvania, only 9% were attributable to trauma. Of those patients with traumatic esophageal perforation, penetrating injuries to the cervical esophagus represented the most common location and mechanism.[18] Similar results were noted in a multicenter study from American Association for the Surgery of Trauma.[17] In 2001, that group performed a retrospective study over a 10.5-year period which included 34 institutions. Four hundred and five patients with known penetrating esophageal injuries were studied, with bullet or shotgun wounds reported as the predominant mechanism (78.8%), and stab wounds representing the next most common mechanism (18.5%). The cervical esophagus was again the most commonly injured part with 56.5% of study patients sustaining this injury. The thoracic esophagus was injured in 30% of patients and the abdominal esophagus had the lowest rate of injury (17%) with 3.5% of patients having combined injuries.

Esophageal injury following blunt chest trauma is extremely rare, 0.1 to 0.001%.[19] Causes of blunt trauma can include motor vehicle accidents and even the Heimlich maneuver. Among all patients with an esophageal perforation, traumatic esophageal rupture is the specific cause in 4% to 14% of patients.[20,21] However, these esophageal perforations and ruptures are usually due to iatrogenic injury caused by diagnostic or therapeutic procedures or penetrating injury, not blunt trauma.[22] Similar to the pattern of injury in penetrating trauma patients, blunt cervical esophageal injury is more common than thoracic esophageal trauma.[19] There are various factors that contribute to the rarity of blunt thoracic esophageal injury. The esophagus has a protected location deep in the posterior mediastinum with easy mobility due to a lack of tethering. The esophagus is also protected by the rigid hard shell of the human chest. The force required to cause blunt thoracic esophageal injury may be so high that most such patients could succumb to associated injuries prior to receiving care.

Blunt traumatic injury is often associated with trauma to the upper abdomen and in this case, as in Boerhaave Syndrome, perforation occurs in the weakest area of the esophagus.[23] The force to the epigastrium forces gastric contents rapidly into the esophagus causing a linear tear with leakage of contents into the pleural space or mediastinum.

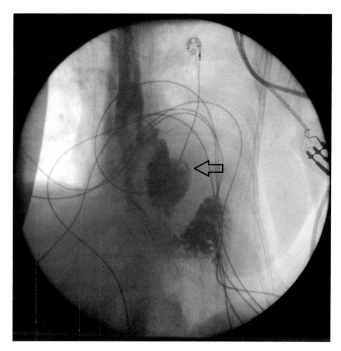

FIGURE 114.1 Extravasation of gastrografin contrast from a distal esophageal perforation (*arrow*) after contrast injection via a nasogastric tube.

The distal esophageal rupture with spillage of gastric contents into the chest usually occurs on the left side (Fig. 114.1) and is complicated by contamination of the mediastinum (Fig. 114.2A) and left pleural space (Fig. 114.2B) as seen on chest computed tomography. However, perforation can also occur when the esophagus is trapped between the sternum and thoracic vertebrae in association with fracture or compression of thoracic vertebra.[24,25] Another potential mechanism that can lead to esophageal injury in blunt trauma results from the disruption of the esophageal blood supply leading to ischemia and subsequent perforation. This mechanism is possible in patients who sustain deceleration–traction forces.[25]

In a retrospective study examining 3,606 trauma admissions over a 1-year period, Beal found five patients with blunt esophageal injury, estimating an incidence of this injury in major blunt trauma to be 0.001%.[19] An accompanying meta-analysis found 96 total reported cases since 1900. The most common mechanism of trauma was motor vehicle collision. The cervical and upper thoracic esophagus was the site of perforation in 82% of the cases.

Given the low incidence of esophageal injury after trauma and the vague and nonspecific signs and symptoms of early esophageal injury, there must be a high index of suspicion raised for esophageal injury in all trauma patients—especially those who sustain penetrating or severe blunt trauma to the neck, chest, or abdomen. More importantly, a delay in diagnosis leads to increased morbidity and mortality.[17,26–28]

The clinical presentation of patients with esophageal injury depends on many factors—the mechanism of injury, the location and size of the injury, the degree of contamination, the length of time between the injury and detection, and the presence of severe associated injuries.[29] The lack of a specific symptom complex increases the difficulty of diagnosis and there are several clinical scenarios for which the suspicion of an esophageal injury must be explored. An esophageal injury should be suspected in a blunt trauma patient with left hemothorax or pneumothorax in the absence of rib fractures. In patients with transmediastinal gunshot wounds, an esophageal injury should be suspected if the wound trajectory or a bullet or fragment is found close to the esophagus. An injured patient exhibiting signs of shock that are disproportionate to their apparent injuries may have an undiagnosed esophageal injury.

Patients with esophageal injury may present with a constellation of symptoms, but pain is the most common. The character of the pain may be different depending on the location of the injury. With injury to the cervical esophagus, pain is typically less severe but the patient may have neck ache and/or stiffness. In thoracic esophageal injury, severe chest pain on the side of the injury is common. Injury to the abdominal esophagus may result in sharp epigastric pain that is unrelenting if the injury is anterior or a dull epigastric pain that radiates to the back in a posterior perforation. In a study that examined esophageal injuries from all causes during a 50-year period, pain was

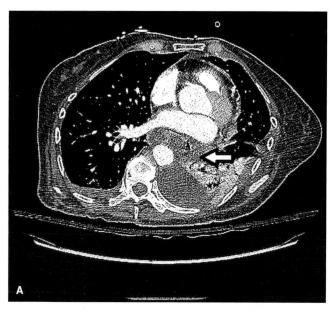
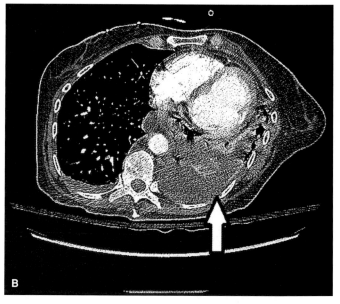

FIGURE 114.2 Chest computed tomography showing (**A**) mediastinal air and fluid collection (*arrow*) and (**B**) left pleural effusion after distal esophageal blunt trauma.

the most common symptom, described in 71% of patients.[30] Other common signs and symptoms included fever (51%), dyspnea (24%), and crepitus (22%).

The mechanism of injury, along with specific clinical signs and symptoms, can assist with the diagnosis of an esophageal injury. In a study examining mandatory versus selective exploration for penetrating neck trauma, Meyer and colleagues noted that cervical esophageal injuries could be diagnosed on clinical grounds alone in 68% of their 120 patients.[29] Another study found that patients who sustained gunshot wounds or stab wounds presented with signs or symptoms suggestive of an esophageal injury in 100% or 50% of cases, respectively.[31]

However, many trauma patients who have mechanisms concerning to esophageal injury are moderately or severely injured and thus are intubated in the trauma bay where a thorough history with detailed complaints is not possible and the physical examination is compromised due to intubation and sedation. Further confounding the diagnosis is the fact that many of the clinical signs, such as dysphagia, hematemesis, stridor, or epigastric tenderness are unreliable due to the high prevalence of other major injuries to the respiratory tract, the vasculature, and the central nervous system.[18] Esophageal injuries may not be suspected as these common symptoms could be attributable to other more obvious injuries. Given the proximity of the esophagus to major vessels and other mediastinal structures, the concern for other associated potentially life-threatening injuries are a more immediate focus and the esophageal injury may be overlooked or the diagnosis delayed.

Diagnostic imaging is standard during the primary survey-resuscitation phase in all patients with significant blunt trauma and in many patients with penetrating trauma to the torso. Findings on the initial chest x-rays, in addition to history and examination findings, may raise suspicion for an esophageal injury. The most common chest radiograph findings of esophageal perforation are left pleural effusion (66% of cases) and cervical or mediastinal emphysema (60%) (Fig. 114.3).[32] Other findings on conventional radiographs include

pneumothorax or pneumoperitoneum, depending on the location of perforation and duration of injury. A nasogastric tube may be suspected to be outside the esophagus on standard chest radiography. It is important to note that although chest radiograph is suggestive in 90% of patients with esophageal perforation, it may also be normal immediately after the injury.[33] Han and colleagues reported that radiographic evidence of mediastinal emphysema requires at least 1 hour after the initial injury to become discernable, while pleural effusion and mediastinal widening can be evolving over several hours after the injury.[33]

EVALUATION AND MANAGEMENT

Management of traumatic injury follows similar principles as those used for treating iatrogenic injury or Boerhaave syndrome. The challenge with traumatic injury is that the patients are often less stable because of associated major injuries to great vessels, heart, lungs, and airway. The principles of management of the suspected esophageal injury are summarized in Table 114.1.

Blunt cervical injuries are rare but just as with penetrating cervical injuries from a stab wound or gunshot wound, treatment includes direct visualization of the esophagus with an endoscope. After confirming an injury, a left neck exploration would be indicated for possible repair of the injury and drainage of the site. After debridement of contaminated tissue, primary repair can be carried out with an inner layer of interrupted or running absorbable 4-0 sutures and outer interrupted 3-0 silk sutures. There is no evidence to support stenting traumatic cervical esophageal injuries, although an analogous situation might be a cervical anastomotic leak after an esophagectomy, where stenting has a suggested role.[34] The risks of stenting proximally include impingement on the glottis, migration of the stent, and tissue in-growth with subsequent injuries caused at the time of stent removal. The absence of reports on stenting cervical esophageal trauma likely reflects the rare incidence of blunt cervical esophageal trauma and current acceptance of exploration, repair, and drainage as primary management strategies. Neck exploration is typically indicated in penetrating cervical esophageal trauma for controlling sepsis, debridement, and primary repair. Quite commonly, a drain is placed.

For both blunt and penetrating thoracic esophageal injuries, the management principles in Table 114.1 are commonly followed. An upper endoscopy is required to pinpoint the location of the injury, and concerns about injury exacerbation occurring with the flexible

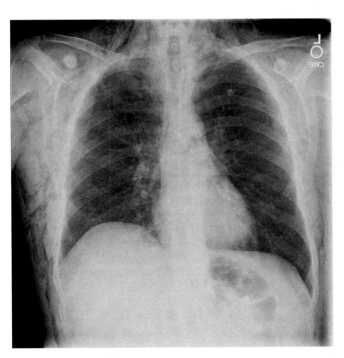

FIGURE 114.3 A chest radiograph demonstrating pneumomediastinum and extensive subcutaneous emphysema after blunt chest trauma.

TABLE 114.1 Principles of Management of Traumatic Esophageal Perforation

Fluid resuscitation

Broad-spectrum antibiotics to cover gram-negative rods, gram-positive cocci, anaerobes, and yeast

Identify site of injury
  Gastrografin swallow
  Thin barium swallow
  Chest and abdominal computed tomography
  Upper flexible endoscopy

Drain
  Closed suction
  Thoracostomy

Nutrition
  Enteral
  Parenteral

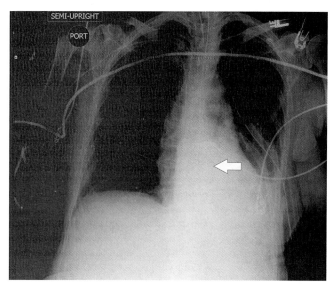

FIGURE 114.4 Self-expanding metal stent (*arrow*) covering distal esophageal blunt trauma perforation.

fiberoptic endoscope have not proven true. For the hemodynamically stable patient with a contained perforation which drains spontaneously back into the esophagus, arguments can be made for watchful waiting versus the use of a temporary completely covered self-expanding metal stent (Fig. 114.4). For patients with evidence of sepsis into the left chest, an approach including thoracotomy, debridement, repair of the injury, tissue buttressing, and drainage is indicated. For intra-abdominal perforation, a laparotomy with repair, drainage, gastrostomy for decompression, and jejunostomy tube for nutrition are appropriate. Indications for esophageal diversion with cervical esophagostomy and gastrostomy tube would include profoundly devitalized tissue unsuitable for primary repair and/or sepsis control. In a setting of concomitant injuries and hemodynamic instability, primary esophagectomy is not advised and likewise diversion may be carried out if the goal of repair, drainage, and control of sepsis is not possible.

REFERENCES

1. Breasted JH, ed. *The Edwin Smith Surgical Papyrus*. Chicago, IL: University of Chicago Press; 1930;46:312.
2. Vinson PP. External trauma as a cause of lesions of the oesophagus. *Am J Digest Dis Nutr* 1936;3:457–459.
3. Frink NW. Spontaneous rupture of the esophagus: report of a case with recovery. *J Thorac Surg* 1947;16:291–297.
4. Riley RD, Miller PR, Meredith JW. Injury to the esophagus, trachea and bronchus. In Moore EE, Feliciano DV, Mattox KL, eds. *Trauma*. New York: McGraw-Hill; 2004:539.
5. Makhani M, Midani D, Goldberg A, et al. Pathogenesis and outcomes of traumatic injuries of the esophagus. *Dis Esophagus* 2014;27:630–636.
6. Rohman M, Ivatury RR. Esophagus. In: Ivatury RR, Cayten CG, eds. *Textbook of Penetrating Trauma*. Baltimore, MD: Williams & Wilkins; 1996:555.
7. Oparah SS, Mandal AK. Operative management of penetrating wounds of the chest in civilian practice: review of indications in 125 consecutive patients. *J Thorac Cardiovasc Surg* 1979;77:162–168.
8. Symbas PN, Hatcher CR, Vlasis SE. Esophageal gunshot injuries. *Ann Surg* 1980;191:703–707.
9. Cheadle W, Richardson JD. Options in management of trauma to the esophagus. *Surg Gynecol Obstet* 1982;155:380–384.
10. Hatzitheofilou C, Strahlendorf C, Kakoyiannis S. Penetrating external injuries of the oesophagus and pharynx. *Br J Surg* 1993;80:1147–1149.
11. Patel MS, Malinoski DJ, Zhou L, et al. Penetrating oesophageal injury: a contemporary analysis of the National Trauma Data Bank. *Injury* 2013;44:48–55.
12. Sheely CH, Mattox KL, Beall AC, et al. Penetrating wounds of the cervical esophagus. *Am J Surg* 1975;130:707–711.
13. Hirshberg A, Wall MJ, Johnston RH, et al. Transcervical gunshot injuries. *Am J Surg* 1994;167:309–312.
14. Demetriades D, Theodorou D, Cornwell E, et al. Transcervical gunshot injuries: mandatory operation is not necessary. *J Trauma* 1996;40:758–760.
15. Cornwell EE, Kennedy F, Ayad IA, et al. Transmediastinal gunshot wounds: a reconsideration of the role of aortography. *Arch Surg* 1996;131:949–952.
16. Defore WW Jr, Mattox KL, Hansen HA, et al. Surgical management of penetrating injuries of the esophagus. *Am J Surg* 1977;134(6):734–738.
17. Asensio JA, Chahwan S, Forno W, et al. Penetrating esophageal injuries: multicenter study of the American Association for the Surgery of Trauma. *J Trauma* 2001;50:289–296.
18. Brinster CJ, Singhal S, Lee L, et al. Evolving options in the management of esophageal perforation. *Ann Thorac Surg* 2004;77(4):1475–1483.
19. Beal SL, Pottmeyer EW, Spisso JM. Esophageal perforation following external blunt trauma. *J Trauma* 1988;28(10):1425–1432.
20. Eroglu C, Can KI, Karaoganogu N, et al. Esophageal perforation: the importance of early diagnosis and primary repair. *Dis Esophagus* 2004;17(1):91–94.
21. Gupta NM, Kamen L. Personal management of 57 consecutive patients with esophageal perforation. *Am J Surg* 2004;187(1):58–63.
22. Kuhlman JE, Pozniak MA, Collins J, et al. Radiographic and CT findings of blunt chest trauma: aortic injuries and looking beyond them. *Radiographica* 1998;18(5):1085–1106.
23. Blencowe NS, Strong S, Hollowood AD. Spontaneous oesophageal rupture. *BMJ* 2013;346:f3095.
24. Monzon JR, Ryan B. Thoracic esophageal perforation secondary to blunt trauma. *J Trauma* 2000;49:1129–1131.
25. Stothert JC Jr, Buttorff J, Kaminski DL. Thoracic esophageal and tracheal injury following blunt trauma. *J Trauma* 1980;20(11):992–995.
26. Shaker H, Elsayed H, Whittle I, et al. The influence of the "golden 24-h rule" on the prognosis of oesophageal perforation in the modern era. *Eur J Cardiothorac Surg* 2010;38(2):216–222.
27. Brewer LA, 3rd, Carter R, Mulder GA, et al. Options in the management of perforations of the esophagus. *Am J Surg* 1986;152(1):62–69.
28. Bladergroen MR, Lowe JE, Postlethwait RW. Diagnosis and recommended management of esophageal perforation and rupture. *Ann Thorac Surg* 1986;42(3):235–239.
29. Meyer JP, Barrett JS, Schuler JJ, et al. Mandatory vs selective exploration for penetrating neck trauma. *Arch Surg* 1987;122:592–597.
30. Nesbitt JC, Sawyers JL. Surgical management of esophageal perforation. *Am Surg* 1987;53:183–191.
31. Weigelt JA, Thal ER, Snyder WH III, et al. Diagnosis of penetrating cervical esophageal injuries. *Am J Surg* 1987;154:619–622.
32. Shanmuganathan K, Matsumoto J. Imaging of penetrating chest trauma. *Radiol Clin North Am* 2006;44(2):335–338, viii.
33. Han SY, McElvein RB, Aldrete JS, et al. Perforation of the esophagus: correlation of site and cause with plain film findings. *AJR Am J Roentgenol* 1985;145:537–540.
34. Speer E, Dunst CM, Shada A, Reavis KM, Swanstrom LL. Covered stents in cervical anastomoses following esophagectomy. *Surg Endosc* 2016;30:3297–3303.

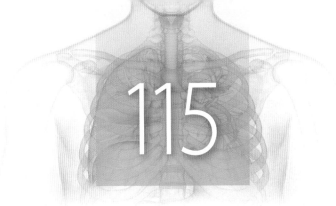

115

Esophageal Perforation

Raja Mahidhara ▪ Richard K. Freeman

INTRODUCTION

Esophageal perforation is a relatively uncommon clinical emergency with significant morbidity and mortality. Recognition and initiation of treatment is often delayed as symptoms may mimic other disorders such as myocardial infarction, aortic dissection, pneumonia, pneumothorax, pulmonary embolism, dyspeptic syndromes, or an acute abdomen. Patients susceptible to esophageal perforation commonly have intrinsic esophageal pathology which may complicate repair and comorbidities which increase perioperative risk. The lack of a serosal investment can make repair of a perforation technically challenging. This is especially true in the setting of inflammation and infection where leak rates following repair near 20% are reported at experienced centers.[1,2] Despite advances in antimicrobial therapy, surgical critical care, and imaging techniques, care of patients with esophageal perforation remains a challenge even for the most experienced thoracic surgeons (Table 115.1).

Optimal treatment of an esophageal perforation depends on the location, timing of presentation, and underlying esophageal pathology. Primary repair of an esophageal perforation has been the standard treatment in the absence of severe distal obstructive pathology such as undilatable peptic stricture, end-stage achalasia, or malignancy. Over the last decade, however, combined endoscopic and minimally invasive strategies, that fulfill the basic principles of management and circumvent the additional burden of more extensive surgery in this critically ill patient population, has been recognized as an alternative treatment in selected patients.[3,4]

ETIOLOGY

The esophagus is prone to perforation at anatomical and pathologic sites of narrowing. The three natural anatomic points of narrowing are at the level of the cricopharyngeus muscle, at the aortic knob near the left mainstream bronchus, and at the esophagogastric junction.

TABLE 115.1 Basic Principles in the Management of Esophageal Perforation

1. Prompt evaluation with an index high of suspicion
2. Hemodynamic resuscitation
3. Antimicrobial therapy
4. Control of the perforation site
5. Relief of distal obstruction
6. Drainage of infected spaces
7. Enteral nutrition.

Other potential areas of weakness related to intrinsic esophageal pathology include stricture, ulcer, or malignancy and may occur anywhere along the course of the esophagus. In a review of case series comprising over 1,100 patients, perforation occurred in the cervical esophagus in 23.3% of cases, in the thoracic esophagus in 66.1% and in the abdomen in 10.2%.[5]

Iatrogenic injury from endoscopy or echocardiography accounts for 54% to 59% of esophageal perforations. The overall rate of perforation after esophagoscopy is 0.03%. This risk increases 100 fold to 16% after interventional procedures including sclerotherapy, variceal banding, cryotherapy, radiofrequency ablation, or dilation, especially after therapeutic endomucosal resection. Spontaneous perforations account for 15% to 20% of cases and occur equally frequently in the thorax and abdomen. Foreign body ingestion (10% to 12%), trauma (9% to 12%), intraoperative injury (1%), and malignancy (1%) are less frequent causes.[6]

DIAGNOSIS

The diagnosis of esophageal perforation begins with a high index of suspicion, as there are no pathognomonic signs or symptoms. The cause and location of esophageal perforation dictate the features of the clinical presentation. A history of instrumentation, caustic or foreign body ingestion, emesis, or trauma in the appropriate clinical setting should raise the level of suspicion.

The most common presenting symptoms are pain (70%), fever (44%), dyspnea (26%), and subcutaneous emphysema (25%).[7] Perforation in the cervical esophagus may present with inability to swallow salivary secretions, dysphagia, odynophagia, and/or neck stiffness. Perforation in the chest may present with pleuritic, midepigastric, or substernal pain while perforation in the abdomen can present with the spectrum of symptoms associated with an acute abdomen.

A chest roentgenogram may show a widened mediastinum, pneumomediastinum, subcutaneous emphysema, pleural effusion, or pneumothorax. However, none of these abnormalities are recognized in up to a third of cases.[8] Computer-assisted tomography is often obtained in the evaluation of chest and/or pain. Findings associated with esophageal perforation include, but are not limited to, hydropneumomediastinum mediastinal, dilated esophagus, extravasation of oral contrast, esophageal fistula, pleural effusion, ascites, and hydropneumothorax (Fig. 115.1). Thoracentesis, most often performed before the diagnosis of esophageal perforation is considered, may yield turbid pleural fluid with high levels of amylase, low pH (<6.0), or undigested food particles. A pleural effusion showing multimicrobial infection is highly suspicious for being caused by an esophageal perforation.

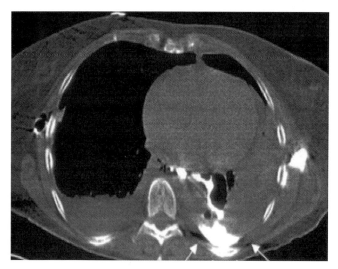

FIGURE 115.1 CT scan of an esophageal perforation with mediastinitis and pleural effusion.

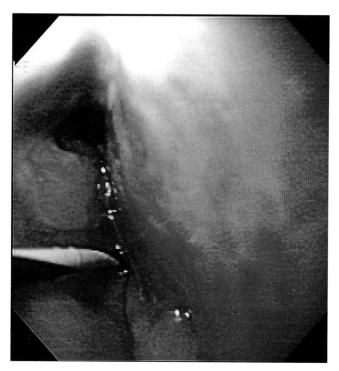

FIGURE 115.2 Endoscopic picture of an esophageal perforation.

Directed evaluation of the esophagus begins with a contrast study. Water-soluble contrast agents like Gastrografin or nonionic agents such as Omnipaque are advocated for the initial screening of suspected patients with perforation because of their rapid absorption if extravasation occurs into mediastinal, pleural, or peritoneal spaces. However, such agents have a positive predictive value of only 50% of cervical and 75% to 80% of thoracic perforations.[9] Therefore, an esophagram using water soluble or nonionic agents that does not reveal a leak should be immediately followed by a study with barium which has an accuracy of greater than 90% for esophageal perforation. Water-soluble agents should be avoided in patients at risk for aspiration because of the risk of pneumonitis. A thin solution of barium may be used instead. Barium which has extravasated into the mediastinum does not appear to complicate immediate operative debridement.[10]

For patients who are hemodynamically unstable or unable to swallow, flexible esophagoscopy under anesthesia in an operative setting has a sensitivity of 100% and specificity of 83% (Fig. 115.2).[11] Endoscopy also allows the surgeon to evaluate the extent of injury and to consider endoluminal treatment options. A percutaneous endoscopic gastrostomy can also be placed if indicated.

NONOPERATIVE THERAPY

It should be noted that observation alone should be differentiated from nonoperative therapy. Observation alone is reserved only for moribund patients unlikely to survive any operative intervention because of substantial delays in the recognition of perforation or because of underlying comorbidities. Criteria for nonoperative therapy was first described by Cameron et al.[12] for the treatment of contained leaks identified by esophagram in seven patients. These criteria have been modified with further accumulation of clinical experience (Table 115.2).[13,14]

Patients are managed with the strict cessation of any oral intake, parenteral nutrition, and intravenous antibiotics for 5 to 7 days after which contrast esophagram is repeated. Operative intervention should be immediately available with any signs of clinical deterioration. Successful nonoperative therapy has been reported in 80% to 90% of these highly selected cases that meet the strict inclusion criteria noted above.[13,14]

OPERATIVE REPAIR

Primary Repair

Certain common principles apply to any surgical repair of an esophageal perforation regardless of the anatomic location. These include debridement of all devitalized tissue, generous incision of the muscular layers of the esophagus to expose the proximal and distal extent of the mucosal injury and two-layer repair of the perforation. Interrupted, absorbable 4-0 suture is used for the mucosal repair while interrupted nonabsorbable suture is used to approximate the muscularis. An alternative stapled technique has also been reported.[15] Every effort is made to avoid narrowing of the esophagus especially with long longitudinal repairs. This may require a myotomy on the opposite wall of the esophagus to allow a tension-free closure of the muscularis and/or repair over a bougie.

Distal obstruction must be addressed at the time of surgery to reduce the chance of a postrepair leak.[16] Strictures can be dilated with Maloney dilators guided by the surgeon's hand in the operative field. Savary dilators can be used over a guide wire with fluoroscopy.

For patients with known or suspected achalasia, a Heller myotomy should be considered at the time of perforation repair. The myotomy should be performed on the opposite wall (180 degrees) of the

TABLE 115.2 Factors Associated With Success of Nonoperative Management

1. Recent perforation
2. Contained perforation (does not disseminate widely into pleural or peritoneal spaces)
3. Prompt drainage back into the esophageal lumen on esophagram
4. No evidence of malignancy, obstruction, or stricture distal to the perforation
5. No evidence of sepsis
6. Minimal symptoms

esophagus from the site of perforation. The decision as to whether to perform a complete or partial fundoplication after Heller myotomy should be carefully considered. Often there is little reliable information about the patient's baseline esophageal motility and swallowing function in this setting. Fundoplication may therefore cause a functional obstruction in patients with an undiagnosed disorder of esophageal motility putting the primary repair at risk.

When there has been a delay in diagnosis greater than 24 hours or substantial extraluminal contamination from the leakage of fluid and debris has occurred, the integrity of the repair can be enhanced with the use of a vascularized, pedicled flap onto the suture line. The most commonly used rotational flap in the chest is an intercostal muscle. Other options include the serratus anterior, latissimus dorsi, pericardial fat pad, or diaphragm for thoracic leaks. The strap muscles of the neck can be used for cervical perforation repairs. Omentum, a limb of small intestine (serosal patch) or a portion of the gastric fundus (Thal patch), may be used in the abdomen.

Drains are placed in the neck, pleura, mediastinum, and abdomen as indicated by the site of injury. A plan for enteral nutrition should also be made at the time of the initial surgery. Nasoenteric feeding tubes can be placed under direct endoscopic vision past the injury and through the pylorus. Percutaneous endoscopic or radiologic gastrostomy with extension of a tube past the pylorus is also readily available at most centers. Care must be taken to avoid the greater curvature of the stomach and proximity to the right gastroepiploic artery in case the stomach is subsequently needed as a conduit. If this is not felt to be safe or possible, then operative gastrostomy and/or jejunostomy should be performed.

Cervical Esophageal Perforation

Perforations of the cervical esophagus are almost always treated with a transcervical primary repair. In the supine position with a shoulder roll, the neck is extended and the face is turned to the right. A left oblique incision is made along the anterior border of the sternocleidomastoid muscle from the cricoid to the sternal notch. The carotid sheath is retracted laterally while the larynx and trachea are retracted medially. Care should be taken if self-retaining retractors are used to avoid excessive tension which may cause injury to the recurrent laryngeal nerve. The middle thyroid vein and omohyoid muscle should be divided. Blunt dissection of the prevertebral space is done to mobilize the esophagus and bring it into the operative field. Early after injury and if severe inflammation has not developed, blunt dissection of the tracheoesophageal groove may further enhance mobilization of the esophagus into the field. After the injury is visualized a myotomy is performed to expose the extent of injury and the mucosa is repaired as described above. Strap muscles are mobilized as needed for coverage. Closed suction drains are placed in the mediastinum though some advocate use of passive drainage with a Penrose to avoid negative pressure on the suture line. The platysma is loosely approximated with interrupted absorbable suture and the skin is closed.

In cases when the site or extent of perforation is not well visualized, drainage alone is done with acceptable outcomes. This may be with closed suction drains or open drainage if there is a high degree of contamination or necrosis of soft tissue in the field. In such cases, careful image monitoring should be performed to recognize any progression of infection in to the mediastinum.

Intrathoracic Esophageal Perforation

The level of the perforation of the thoracic esophagus dictates the surgical approach. Injuries in the midesophagus are best approached by a right thoracotomy. An injury proximal to the carina is best exposed by a 4th interspace incision while injury distal to the carina

is approached by a 5th or 6th interspace incision. An esophageal injury near the esophagogastric junction is most commonly exposed using a left posterolateral thoracotomy through the 6th interspace.

Prior to entering the thoracic cavity, a posteriorly based intercostal muscle flap can be harvested as a potential buttress for primary repair. The lung is decorticated. The inferior pulmonary ligament is divided and the posterior mediastinal pleura is widely incised. Exposure of the esophagus for injuries proximal to the carina is facilitated by division of the azygos vein. The mediastinum is debrided and the perforation is localized and repaired as note above. A nasogastric tube may be guided into the stomach with the aid of the surgeon. The chest is copiously irrigated and chest tubes are placed.

Intra-abdominal Esophageal Perforation

An upper midline laparotomy is the preferred approach to repair of the intra-abdominal esophagus. The incision may be extended or a bilateral subcostal incision may also be employed if body habitus is large or if other pathology must be addressed. The left triangular ligament of the liver is divided and the left lobe of the liver is retracted medially to expose the hiatus of the diaphragm. The gastrohepatic and the gastrocolic ligament are incised and the lesser sac is opened. Short gastric vessels of the stomach are divided to mobilize the fundus of the stomach. The peritoneal investment of the crus of the diaphragm is incised taking care to avoid injury to the muscle. The phrenoesophageal ligament is incised and the esophagogastric junction is encircled to deliver the cardia of the stomach and the lower esophagus into the field. Blunt dissection of the lower esophagus in the mediastinum facilitates debridement of that space and allows for better exposure of the injury. The perforation is identified, exposed, and repaired as noted above. Distal obstruction should be simultaneously addressed. A fundoplication and repair of a patulous hiatus of the diaphragm may be considered for patients with reflux or with stigmata of severe reflux like an ulcer or a stricture. Care must be taken, however, to avoid creating an iatrogenic obstruction.

Esophagectomy and Diversion Procedures

Primary repair of esophageal perforation is contraindicated in the setting of a distal obstruction, or end-stage esophageal disease that cannot reasonably be relieved at the time of repair. Examples include malignancy, achalasia with sigmoid esophagus, and undilatable peptic stricture from reflux disease. Traditional operative options include esophagectomy or diversion and drainage.

Esophagectomy can be performed from a transthoracic or transhiatal approach. Advantages of the transhiatal approach are avoidance of the additional morbidity of thoracotomy, reconstruction in the neck avoids placing an anastomosis in an inflamed surgical field, an anastomotic leak can be managed well nonoperatively, and postoperative swallowing function is excellent. Advantages of the transthoracic approach are that there is less tension on an intrathoracic anastomosis and that other thoracic pathology including decortication and drainage of the mediastinum can be more effectively accomplished. While the potential for significant morbidity exists with this approach, Orringer notes that conservative procedures for a perforation with pre-existing esophageal disease inflict more morbidity than resection which eliminates the source of sepsis and the underlying disease.[17]

Diversion and drainage is indicated when the patient is unstable, repair is not possible due to the size of the defect and friability of surrounding tissues or if pre-existing esophageal disease is present that cannot be effectively simultaneously treated. The principles of diversion included control and drainage of extraluminal contamination, proximal diversion of the esophagus with cervical esophagostomy, and gastric diversion with gastrostomy and jejunostomy for feeding. The intrathoracic esophagus is resected when possible, but may be left in situ if the patient is hemodynamically unstable.

While many techniques for esophageal diversion have been described, typically a thoracotomy is performed to resect the esophagus and to debride and drain the mediastinum. The esophagus is transected proximal to perforation, taking care to leave as much length as possible, and distally at the esophagogastric junction. A gastrostomy and jejunostomy are also performed.

For proximal diversion, the cervical esophagus is exposed and isolated as noted in the section on primary repair. The esophagus is bluntly and circumferentially dissected and encircled with a Penrose drain at the thoracic inlet taking care to avoid injury to the recurrent laryngeal nerve in the tracheoesophageal groove. The esophagus is mobilized as far distally as possible. The authors use a mediastinoscope to directly visualize blunt mobilization of the esophagus under the left mainstem bronchus to the level of the subcarinal space. The loop of esophagus is delivered into the field and either a side or end esophagostomy is created.

For end esophagostomy, the esophagus is transected as far distally as possible. If using a cervical approach, a subcutaneous tunnel is fashioned over the clavicle and pectoralis onto a flat portion of the chest to facilitate stoma appliance placement and preserve esophageal length. If a transthoracic approach is used, the distal esophagus can be matured through an intercostal incision to the infraclavicular anterior chest wall.

Reconstruction of the alimentary tract for oral feedings is typically done 6 months later. The gastric remnant, colon, or jejunum may be used commonly by a substernal approach. These procedures can result in significant morbidity and mortality and often result in less than acceptable functional results for the patient.[18]

Endoluminal Therapy for Esophageal Perforation

An ideal treatment for an esophageal leak would be one that minimized the negative impact of the treatment on the patient while fulfilling the traditional goals of therapy previously outlined. However, a principle component of such a treatment model has been missing: a simple, reliable method for sealing even relatively large perforations without the need for thoracotomy and/or celiotomy. Taking advantage of advances in biomaterials, a generation of esophageal stents has been developed over the last decade that share the characteristics of ease of insertion, a minimal requirement for esophageal dilation, and the ability to form an occlusive seal within the lumen of the esophagus.

The evolution of treating patients with an esophageal perforation or fistula with an esophageal stent began in patients who either were exceedingly high risk for an operative repair or had undergone a previous operative repair that failed. We found that this technique resulted in 95% of these leaks being sealed without further surgery.[19] Encouraged by these results, we and others went on to evaluate esophageal stent placement for acute iatrogenic and spontaneous perforations as well as patients experiencing an esophageal perforation in association with an esophageal or gastric malignancy and found similar results.

The authors' current technique is to place all esophageal stents for an esophageal perforation or fistula in the operating room using general anesthesia and fluoroscopy following flexible esophagoscopy (Fig. 115.2). The approach has been to oversize the stent both in length and diameter. This has had a beneficial effect on stent migration and on the ability to seal a leak relatively quickly.

Adequate drainage of infected areas is also simultaneously achieved either by video-assisted thoracoscopy, laparoscopy, or image-guided percutaneous drainage. Between 20% and 60% of patients require

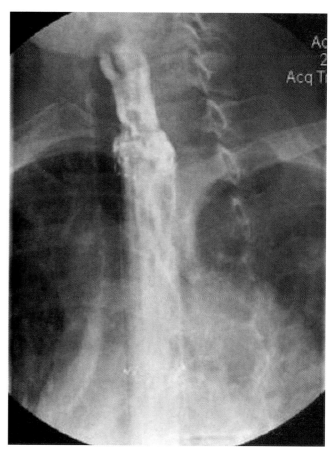

FIGURE 115.3 Chest roentgenogram of an esophageal stent occluding a perforation.

such a procedure at the time of stent placement. A mechanism for enteral nutrition should also be contemplated while the patient is anesthetized in the operating room.

Leak occlusion is confirmed by a contrast esophagram a minimum of 24 hours after stent placement or when the patient is able to participate in the examination (Fig. 115.3). In the absence of a continued leak, an oral diet is initiated.

It is the intention to remove all patients' esophageal stents following a sufficient amount of time to allow the leak to seal. This is individualized for each patient taking into consideration the resolution of any indications of systemic infection. Stent removal is also carried out in the operating room under general anesthesia. Flexible esophagoscopy is performed before and after stent removal and an esophagram is performed before oral intake is resumed.

Experience has led the authors to remove stents much earlier than we did in initial series. This is due to a better understanding of how these leaks seal and then heal; adherence to adjacent structures creating a watertight seal followed by eventual tissue in-growth and repair. Several reports of significant complications related to indwelling esophageal stents including tracheoesophageal fistulae, aortoesophageal fistulae, and bowel obstruction resulting from stent migration have also prompted the authors to routinely consider stent removal after 10 to 14 days.[20]

As with any surgical procedure, success is often as dependent upon the care afterward as the procedure itself. This is no different for esophageal stent placement for acute perforation or fistula. The thoracic surgeon should direct the care of these patients just as if they had undergone an operative repair. This is not only important in making sure patients who fail stent therapy receive timely operative intervention,

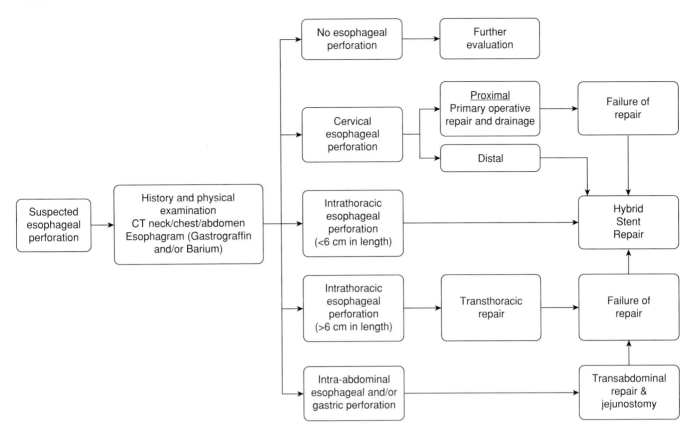

FIGURE 115.4 Treatment algorithm for esophageal perforation.

but is essential in determining that all associated areas of intrathoracic or intra-abdominal infection are recognized and promptly treated.

Similarly, despite esophageal stent placement being tolerated better by patients than a traditional operative repair, the systemic inflammatory response and/or sepsis often produced in these patients require that they be cared for with the same vigilance. This includes appropriate fluid resuscitation, antimicrobial therapy, and cardio-pulmonary support administered in a critical care environment. An integral part of this process is planning a route for enteral nutrition at the time of stent placement. Our preference has been to place a percutaneous endoscopic gastrostomy just prior to esophageal stent placement if the patient does not have another form of enteral access and has not undergone esophagectomy. This can be placed to gravity drainage for the first 24 hours, eliminating the need for a nasogastric tube with feedings initiated thereafter.

CHOICE OF TREATMENT

Esophageal stent placement for acute perforation or fistula has sig-nificantly changed our practice as well as other thoracic surgeons around the world. We now consider nearly all such patients for stent placement as initial therapy (Fig. 115.4). Notable exceptions are patients with a perforation of the cervical esophagus, a perforation that traverses the gastroesophageal junction, an esophageal injury greater than 6 cm in length and esophageal injuries recognized during another operative procedure or in a patient that will require an immediate thoracotomy for an associated injury. Esophageal stent placement also appears to be an optimal therapy for patients who have undergone an operative repair of an esophageal perforation which has failed.[21] Esophageal stents can also be placed to reinforce an operative repair in the setting of severe inflammation as described

by Keeling et al.[22] A perforation in an area of malignancy should not be considered a contraindication to stent placement as long as the stent relieves any obstruction distal to the perforation.

A recent propensity-matched comparison of patient with an acute esophageal perforation treated with either surgical repair or stent placement was published. This investigation found that esophageal stent placement for the treatment of an acute esophageal perforation appears to be as effective as surgical repair. Stent placement, however, resulted in a shorter length of stay, lower rates of morbidity, and lower costs when compared to traditional surgical repair (Table 115.3).

TABLE 115.3 A Comparison of Outcomes for the Two Treatment Cohorts

	OR	SR	p
N	30	30	
ICU stay (mean days)	4 ± 3	2 ± 1	0.001
Total length of stay (mean days)	11 ± 7	6 ± 3	0.0007
Oral intake (mean days)	8 ± 7	3 ± 2	0.0004
Leak following initial repair	6 (20%)	5 (17%)	1
Reoperative repair	4 (13%)	1 (3%)	0.35
Stent migration		4 (13%)	
Morbidity	13 (43%)	4 (17%)	0.02
Mortality	2 (7%)	1 (3%)	1
Readmission	5 (17%)	2 (7%)	0.4
Dysphagia	8 (27%)	2 (7%)	0.08

ICU, intensive care unit; LTAC, long-term acute care center; OR, operative repair; SR, stent repair.

OUTCOMES

Most data regarding esophageal perforation are derived from single institution case series with small numbers of patients. While it is difficult to make conclusions based on outcomes from individual reports, several case reviews performed over current and historical eras provide insight into the natural history of this disease and its optimal treatment.

MORBIDITY

Early morbidity after surgical intervention is primarily related to leak at the site of repair. Overall, failure of primary repairs occurs in approximately 20% of cases.[1,2] Time interval from presentation to repair and whether the repair was reinforced with muscle appear to be important factors in the success of the repair. In a series of 28 patients treated with reinforced primary repair by Wright et al.,[23] the overall postrepair leak rate was 28%. In subset analysis, patients who presented within 24 hours of the onset of symptoms experienced a postrepair leak rate of 13.3%, all of which were contained and required no further operative treatment. By contrast, the postrepair leak rate was 67% in patients who presented after 24 hours.

The anastomotic leak after esophagectomy performed for esophageal perforation is low. In a series of 25 patients treated with transhiatal esophagectomy after perforation because of severe intrinsic esophageal pathology, there was a leak rate of only 4%.[17] Altorjay and colleagues[24] also reported a series of 27 patients treated with transthoracic esophagectomy with an anastomotic leak rate of only 7%.

A delay in treatment also appears to increase the overall risk of complications following esophageal perforation. In a recent series by Linden and colleagues,[25] a significant complication occurred in 20% of patients treated within 24 hours in contrast to a complication rate of 61% for patients treated after a delay of greater than 24 hours after presentation. Other complications including pneumonia, empyema, respiratory failure, abscess, and sepsis also appear more frequently in patients who experience a delay in their diagnosis and treatment.

Data on swallowing function after repair of esophageal perforation is limited. In a series of 42 patients by Iannettoni et al.,[26] over half required dilation for dysphagia following operative repair of an esophageal perforation. Sawyer et al.[27] similarly reported that two-thirds of patients required dilation after repair. Stent placement may result in a lower rate of postrepair stenosis and dysphagia when compared to traditional operative repair.

MORTALITY

The overall reported mortality after esophageal perforation ranges between 12% and 22%.[5,6,23,28] The location and cause of injury, underlying esophageal pathology, delay in presentation, and method of treatment are all factors that influence the rate of morbidity and mortality. Perforation in the cervical esophagus is associated with the lowest rate of mortality reported at 6%. Perforation in the thoracic esophagus has a reported mortality of 11% to 27% while injury occurring of the intra-abdominal esophagus results in a mortality rate of 13% to 21%.

Mortality also varies by the etiology of perforation. Spontaneous perforation is associated with the highest mortality at a rate of 14% to 36%. This is statistically higher than mortality after iatrogenic injury (14% to 19%) or trauma (7% to 14%). This elevated rate of mortality in patients experiencing a spontaneous esophageal perforation appears to be related to patient comorbidities, a frequent delay in diagnosis and treatment, and a higher rate of sepsis at presentation.[3] The differences in mortality seen between injury sites is likely related

to the summation of differences in etiology, detection, ease of repair, and extent of contamination.

The time interval between the development of symptoms, diagnosis, and treatment has traditionally been recognized as an important factor in not only the rate of mortality of patients with an esophageal perforation but also the success of primary repair. A delay in treatment of greater than 24 hours after onset of symptoms may be the most significant determinant in mortality after perforation. Mortality ranges from 7% to 14% if treatment is initiated prior to 24 hours after the onset of symptoms regardless of location or cause but increases to 20% to 35% if the time interval is greater than 24 hours.[5,6,23,28]

When comparing different surgical and nonsurgical interventions from case series, interpretation of mortality rates is limited. In a pooled analysis of over 700 patients, nearly half underwent primary repair with a mortality of 12%. Mortality from esophagectomy was 17% while rates from diversion and drainage alone were substantially higher at 24% and 36%, respectively. Nonoperative therapy was unsuccessful in 18% of cases.[5]

Esophageal stent placement for primary therapy esophageal perforation has been utilized and reported with increasing frequency over the last 10 years. The addition of minimally invasive techniques to drain the abdomen, pleural cavities, and mediastinum fulfills the criteria of source control, drainage and enteral nutrition. An analysis of 7 series comprising 159 patients demonstrated an overall mortality rate of 14%.[29] In a meta-analysis of 75 studies reported since 2000, primary repair was associated with a pooled mortality of 9.5%, esophagectomy 13.8%, other intervention (diversion or t-tube repair) with 20.0% and esophageal stenting with 7.3%.[30]

SUMMARY

Esophageal perforation is a relatively uncommon thoracic emergency with a relatively high morbidity and mortality. Principles of therapy include prompt evaluation, hemodynamic resuscitation, antimicrobial therapy, control of the perforation site, drainage of infection, and enteral nutrition. Though differences in outcome seem to depend in part on the etiology and location of perforation, prompt recognition and treatment are crucial in limiting morbidity and mortality as seen in the dramatic differences in results between patients repaired within 24 hours of perforation and those repaired later than 24 hours after perforation.

Several treatment strategies are available to the thoracic surgeon in managing esophageal perforations. Nonoperative therapy may be successful in highly selected patients that meet stringent inclusion criteria. At the other extreme, esophagectomy is most commonly reserved for the patient with a perforation in the setting of underlying esophageal pathology that cannot be resolved. Esophageal diversion is reserved for patients who have either failed operative or endoscopic treatment of their perforation and are not reasonable candidates for esophagectomy.

Primary repair when possible has long been the gold standard in the management of esophageal perforation. Basic principles for a successful repair include complete exposure of the injury, two-layer interrupted closure, relief of distal obstruction, and pedicled tissue reinforcement. Accumulating evidence over the past 10 years has shown that endoluminal therapy with removable covered esophageal stents may be a reasonable alternative to primary repair in selected cases.

REFERENCES

1. Ferguson MK, Reeder LB, Olak J. Outcome after failed initial therapy for rupture of the esophagus or intrathoracic stomach. *J Gastrointest Surg* 1997;1(1):34–39.
2. Whyte RI, Iannettoni MD. Orringer MB Intrathoracic esophageal perforation. The merit of primary repair. *J Thorac Cardiovasc Surg* 1995;109(1):140–144; discussion 144–146.

3. Freeman RK, Van Woerkom JM, Vyverberg A, et al. Esophageal stent placement for the treatment of spontaneous esophageal perforations. *Ann Thorac Surg* 2009;88(1):194–198.

4. David EA, Kim MP, Blackmon SH. Utility of removable esophageal covered self-expanding metal stents for leak and fistula management. *Am J Surg* 2011;202(6):796–801; discussion 936–937.

5. Hasimoto CN, Cataneo DC, Eldib R, et al. Efficacy of surgical versus conservative treatment in esophageal perforation: a systematic review of case series studies. *Acta Cir Bras* 2013;28(4):266–271.

6. Brinster CJ, Singhal S, Lee L, et al. Evolving options in the management of esophageal perforation. *Ann Thorac Surg* 2004;77(4):1475–1483.

7. Freeman RK, Ascioti AJ, Mahidhara R. Treatment strategies for unresectable esophageal carcinoma. *Surg Clinics North Am* 2012;92:1337–1351.

8. Han SY, McElvein RB, Aldrete JS, et al. Perforation of the esophagus: correlation of site and cause with plain film findings. *AJR AM J Roentgenol* 1985:145(3):537–540.

9. Foley MH, Ghahremani GG, Rogers LF. Reappraisal of contrast media used to detect upper gastrointestinal perforations: comparison of ionic water-soluble media with barium sulfate. *Radiology* 1982;144(2):231–237.

10. Gollub MJ, Bains MS. Barium sulfate: a new (old) contrast agent for diagnosis of postoperative esophageal leaks. *Radiology* 1997;202(2):360–362.

11. Horwitz B, Krevsky B, Buckman RF Jr, et al. Endoscopic evaluation of penetrating esophageal injuries. *Am J Gastroenterol* 1993;88(8):1249–1253.

12. Cameron JL, Kieffer RF, Hendrix TR, et al. Selective nonoperative management of contained intrathoracic esophageal disruptions. *Ann Thorac Surg* 1979;27(5):404–408.

13. Altorjay A, kiss J, Voros A, et al. Nonoperative management of esophageal perforations. Is it justified? *Ann Surg* 1997;225(4):415–421.

14. Bradley L, Miller JI, Mansour KA. Esophageal perforation: emphasis on management. *Ann Thorac Surg* 1996;61(5):1447–1451; discussion 1451–1452.

15. Whyte RI, Iannettoni MD, Orringer MB. Intrathoracic esophageal perforation. The merit of primary repair. *J Thorac Cardiovasc Surg* 1995;109(1):140–146.

16. Moghissi K, Pender D. Instrumental perforation of the oesophagus and their management. *Thorax* 1988;(43):642–646.

17. Orringer MB, Stirling MC. Esophagectomy for esophageal disruption. *Ann Thorac Surg* 199049(1):35–42; discussion 42–43.

18. Di Pierro FV, Rice TW, DeCamp MM, et al. Esophagectomy and staged reconstruction. *Eur J Cardiothorac Surg* 2000;17:702–709.

19. Freeman RK, Ascioti, Wozniak TC. Postoperative esophageal leak management with the Polyflex esophageal stent. *J Thorac Cardiovasc Surg* 2007;133(2):333–338.

20. Freeman RK, Ascioti, AJ, Dake M, et al. An assessment of the optimal time for removal of esophageal stents used in the treatment of an esophageal anastomotic leak or perforation. *Ann Thorac Surg* 2015;100(2):422–428.

21. Freeman RK, Ascioti, AJ, Dake M, et al. An analysis of esophageal stent placement for persistent leak after the operative repair of intrathoracic esophageal perforation. *Ann Thorac Surg* 2014;97:1755–1720.

22. Keeling WB, Miller DL, Lam GT, et al. Low mortality after treatment for esophageal perforation: A single-center experience. *Ann Thorac Surg* 2010;90:1669–1673.

23. Wright CD, Mathisen DJ, Wain JC, et al. Reinforced primary repair of thoracic esophageal perforation. *Ann Thorac Surg* 1995;60(2):245–258.

24. Altorjay A, Kiss J, Voros A, et al. The role of esophagectomy in the management of esophageal perforations. *Ann Thorac Surg* 1998;65(5):1433–1436.

25. Linden PA, Bueno R, Mentzer SJ, et al. Modified T-tube repair of delayed esophageal perforation results in a low mortality rate similar to that seen with acute perforations. *Ann Thorac Surg* 2007;38(3):1129–1133.

26. Iannettoni MD, Vlessis AA, Whyte RI, et al. Functional outcome after surgical treatment of esophageal perforation. *Ann Thorac Surg* 1997;64(6):1606–1609.

27. Sawyer R, Phillips C, Vakil N. Short- and long-term outcome of esophageal perforation. *Gastrointest Endosc* 1995;41(2):130–134.

28. Jones WG, Ginsberg RJ. Esophageal perforation: a continuing challenge. *Ann Thorac Surg* 1992;53(3):534–543.

29. Biancari F, D'Andrea V, Paone R, et al. Current treatment and outcome of esophageal perforations in adults: systematic review and meta-analysis of 75 studies. *World J Surg* 2013;37(5):1051–1059.

30. Desari BV, Neely D, Kennedy A, et al. The role of esophageal stents in the management of esophageal anastomotic leaks and benign esophageal perforations. *Ann Surg* 2014;259(5):852–860.

UNDERSTANDING STATISTICAL ANALYSIS AND MEDICAL DECISION MAKING

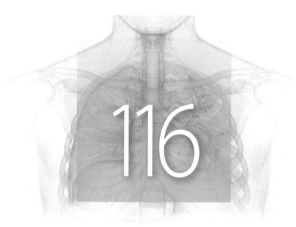

Statistics and Medical Decision Making for the Surgeon

Mark K. Ferguson

INTRODUCTION

Surgical decision making is an art form that relies as much on training and experience as it does on medical evidence. Decisions as we understand them today require balancing risks of complications and potential benefits of operations, and should include a patient's expectations and desires in the recommendation. Prior to the middle and late twentieth century, individual practitioners rarely accumulated sufficient procedural volume and outcomes data to generate algorithms with which to guide decisions. The experiential/anecdotal nature of these processes dominated practice from the earliest recorded interventions until well into the twentieth century.

Only in the recent history of thoracic surgery do we have high-quality evidence that guides our practice in a few highly selected areas. For example, although it was recognized since the time of Hippocrates that treatment of empyema could be life-saving, formal study of empyema management wasn't instituted until the formation of the Empyema Commission during World War I.[1–3] Although Morriston Davies demonstrated the feasibility of performing a lobectomy using

anatomic dissection in 1912[4] and Graham succeeded in a similar venture for pneumonectomy some 21 years later,[5] techniques of lung resection were quite varied for another half century. The randomized trial of lobectomy versus parenchymal sparing resection for lung cancer treatment, initiated by the Lung Cancer Study Group 70 years after Davies' milestone, was among the first to critically assess surgical techniques for lung cancer therapy.[6] Despite the fact that the feasibility of esophageal cancer resection was demonstrated in 1913,[7] it wasn't until nearly a century later that randomized trials of surgical approaches to this disease were performed.[8–10]

Evidence informing surgical judgment in thoracic surgery accumulates slowly. Recognition of comorbidities and the importance of organ system function, especially cardiopulmonary function, in assessing potential surgical candidates began in the 1950s. The early work of Gaensler in identifying the fraction of expired lung volume per time was essential in determining which patients were candidates for surgery for tuberculosis.[11,12] Similar work on diffusing capacity that same decade predated the general recognition of this value as a risk factor for lung surgery by more than 30 years.[13,14] Exercise capacity, which simultaneously assessed cardiac and pulmonary function, was recognized only shortly thereafter as a more comprehensive tool

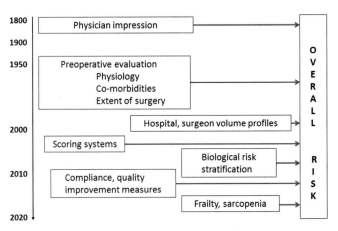

FIGURE 116.1 Increasing sophistication of surgical risk estimation over time.

for assessing operative risk, and has only recently been accepted in algorithms for evaluation of lung resection candidates.[15,16]

The process of defining risk increased in sophistication over many decades, and expanded beyond pure physiologic data (Fig. 116.1). In the early twenty-first century the availability of information on institution size, procedural volume, surgeon volume, and institution infrastructure was identified as important in outcomes for higher risk procedures.[17,18] Similarly, individual surgeons' training, practice pattern, and volume data helped expand the number of factors that were recognized as being related to surgical outcomes.[19-23] Identification of genetic and molecular influences on inflammation, healing, and immune function advanced our understanding further and provided targets for mitigation of risk.[24-28] Most recently, frailty and sarcopenia have been identified as important contributors to adverse postoperative outcomes.[29-31]

Using such data, the development of risk scoring systems has flourished since the 1990s, when large datasets became available for analysis. Risk scores are now incorporated into national databases for use in risk estimation, informed discussions with patients and their families, and benchmarking institutional and surgeon performance. The Society of Thoracic Surgeons (STS) has developed a risk score for major lung resection,[32] as have the European Society of Thoracic Surgeons (Euroscore)[33] and the French Thoracic Society with its Epithor score.[34] Other risk scores that are in use, even though they are not formally sanctioned by national medical societies, include the revised cardiac risk index for thoracic surgery (ThRCRI),[35] a risk score for pulmonary complications after esophagectomy,[36] and a score predicting the likelihood of intensive care unit readmission after major lung resection,[37] to name a few.

Predictive scores that are most accurate arise from single-institution or single-surgeon datasets, and usually are not very generalizable. The most widely applicable predictive scores are generated from large datasets. However, such scores lack the ability to accommodate highly specific patient characteristics, and thus are most useful for evaluating groups of patients rather than individual patients. Applying a validated risk score to an individual patient may provide a general idea as to that patient's relative risk, but may not be ideal for determining specific risk. Surgical judgment remains the predominant method of assessing overall risk and the probability of specific adverse events. Judgment ideally is based on factual knowledge and accumulated experience.

There is growing and diverse information on outcomes and risk that a surgeon can draw on for decision making. How these elements are used individually and collectively, and what some of the pitfalls in their use are, are discussed in this chapter.

EVIDENCE-BASED MEDICINE

For most of the history of clinical surgery, surgeon experience was the key to risk assessment. The limited data that were reported were typically single-institution or single-surgeon based and were subject to numerous biases. Many developing surgeons learned through observation in teaching clinics and surgical amphitheaters, such as those of Billroth and Kocher in the late nineteenth century, as well as Murphy in the early twentieth century (Fig. 116.2).[38] As standards for data collection, analysis, and reporting improved, surgeons began to weigh published results as being at least as important as individual experience and expert dictum in their assessments. The explosion of surgical journals and published reports in the late twentieth and early twenty-first centuries created challenges to clinical surgeons. Keeping abreast of the current literature became difficult, even as subspecialization and super specialization was increasingly common. Fortunately, meta-analytic techniques, first popularized in the 1970s in education research, were available for assessing outcomes of clinical medical research.[39] These techniques help synthesize information to assist clinicians in interpreting large numbers of publications that often have disparate results. The methodology forms the basis of the Cochrane Collaboration, which is a valuable resource enabling physicians to utilize evidence-based conclusions in their clinical practice.[40]

The volume of evidence is only one factor making synthesis of published data manageable. Another important factor is the quality of evidence. A number of methods for assigning quality have been used since the 1980s, with the most popular method being the GRADE system.[41] This system categorizes evidence quality into four levels (Table 116.1). The highest quality evidence usually comes from large randomized controlled trials, meta-analyses, and carefully performed reviews, and indicates the likelihood that reported risks and outcomes approach the actual risks and outcomes.

In the 1980s, a series of reports assessed the use of evidence in medicine and identified substantial variations in clinical practice and lack of alignment of clinical practice with published evidence, such as was reported for the use of coronary angiography.[42] These findings helped trigger interest in the use of published evidence to inform

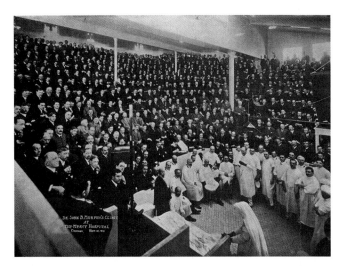

FIGURE 116.2 An example of an early 20th century surgical amphitheater, in which learners, sometimes numbering in the tens or hundreds, observed operations performed live. (Courtesy of the National Library of Medicine (http://resource.nlm.nih.gov/101433151).)

TABLE 116.1 Levels of Evidence According to GRADE[41]

Evidence Level	Description	Interpretation
High quality	The authors are very confident that the estimate that is presented lies very close to the true value	There is very low probability of further research completely changing the presented conclusions
Moderate quality	The authors are confident that the presented estimate lies close to the true value, but it is also possible that it may be substantially different	Further research may completely change the conclusions
Low quality	The authors are not confident in the effect estimate and the true value may be substantially different	Further research is likely to change the presented conclusions completely
Very low quality	The authors do not have any confidence in the estimate and it is likely that the true value is substantially different from it	New research will most probably change the presented conclusions completely

medical practice more rigorously. A structure for evidence-based recommendations was initially developed by Eddy and others in the late 1980s and early 1990s.[43,44] The two elements of evidence-based medicine are explicit evaluation of evidence and application of the evaluation to education and individual patient decision making through specific recommendations rated according to their strength.[41] Recommendations are categorized as strong or weak using the following criteria: the balance between positive and negative outcomes; the quality of evidence; values and preferences; and costs.

GUIDELINES AND STANDARDS OF CARE

Using evidence-based techniques, a number of organizations have developed information intended to guide physicians in the management of common problems. These usually take the form of guidelines, which are nonbinding suggestions for clinical practice based on medical evidence and developed through a formal consensus process. Examples of guidelines for the specialty of thoracic developed by professional organizations include those issued by the National Comprehensive Cancer Network (NCCN),[45] the American Association for Thoracic Surgery (AATS),[46] and the STS.[47] Other guidelines are developed by informal groups created to develop a guideline for a single defined topic, such as those for managing Barrett's esophagus with high-grade dysplasia[48] or Barrett's esophagus with low-grade dysplasia,[49] or the effort to better define adverse outcomes after esophagectomy.[50]

In contrast, standards consist of expected practices that are generally accepted. From a medical-legal standpoint, standard of care is defined as practice that should be followed by a reasonably prudent practitioner given a specific set of clinical circumstances. Standards may arise from a number of sources, including local government, individual hospitals, and professional societies. Standards in clinical surgery are typically very basic, such as the mandate for obtaining informed consent prior to performing an operation or the prohibition of itinerant surgery. Compliance with guidelines is discretionary, whereas compliance with standards is mandatory.

Compliance with guidelines is not always ensured. Surgeons are relatively unfamiliar with guidelines for cancer care and don't use guidelines to help in decision making very often compared to their medical oncologist counterparts.[51] In fact, guidelines can be very useful to the practicing surgeon, especially in instances when the surgeon is evaluating a complex or unfamiliar situation. Following them rigorously, however, should be avoided. There should always be a place for surgeon judgment in making recommendations to individual patients, which should largely be based on the patient's risk, values, and preferences.

RISK ASSESSMENT

When a surgeon assesses risk using an algorithm specific to the contemplated operation, and then applies that assessment to an individual patient, that surgeon combines the art and science of surgery. The successful surgeon uses science, judgment, and patient preferences in order to balance expected outcomes against anticipated risk. Risk assessment is composed of knowledge of specific risk factors and how they influence outcomes, an understanding of predictive scores and whether and how they apply to the individual patient, and surgeon experience. Typical elements involved in risk assessment include physiologic evaluation, assessment of comorbidities, technical challenges, cancer stage, possible complications, effects on quality of life, overall life expectancy, and patient enthusiasm for the possible intervention. The influence of surgeon- and patient-related factors on subsequent decision making should be understood. Patients' preferences with regard to outcomes are often discordant with those of surgeons.[52] In fact, results that are considered by clinicians to be metrics of good surgical outcomes are often not highly regarded by patients facing major surgery, whose primary concern is long-term quality of life (Table 116.2).

Risk assessment should be a deliberate, conscious act rather than one that is accomplished by rote or on the basis of intuition. Sometimes assessments for common problems are so repetitive and second

TABLE 116.2 Mal-alignment of Surgeon and Patient Perspectives on Outcomes of Interest[52]

Surgeon Perspective	Patient Perspective
R0 resection	Extent of surgery unimportant
Low morbidity	Complications, including pneumonia, need for therapeutic bronchoscopy, and need for ventilator support for up to 1 mo, are acceptable as long as recovery is likely
No mortality	Pain control is important
Short hospital duration of stay	Length of stay of little importance
No readmission	Substantially reduced activity levels unacceptable
No chronic postoperative pain	Fear of long-term supplemental oxygen need
Improvement in targeted clinical condition	Quality of life is primary focus

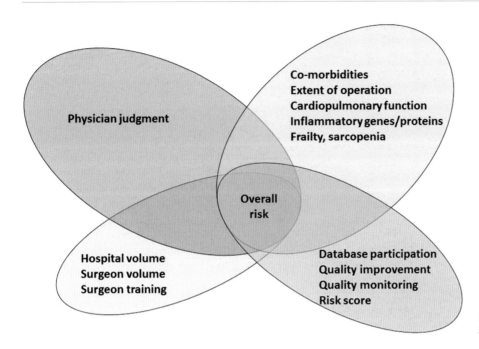

Co-morbidities
Extent of operation
Cardiopulmonary function
Inflammatory genes/proteins
Frailty, sarcopenia

Physician judgment

Overall risk

Hospital volume
Surgeon volume
Surgeon training

Database participation
Quality improvement
Quality monitoring
Risk score

FIGURE 116.3 Overlapping components of risk assessment.

nature that they are performed unconsciously. It is important to avoid this pitfall, as crucial elements regarding an individual patient's risk profile may be missed. Explicitly stating results of crucial elements of the risk assessment and discussing these with the patient and the surgical team may help in achieving mindful risk assessment. The use of checklists and creation of elements in the electronic medical record may assist in reinforcing conscious evaluations. The most important element in risk assessment is physician judgment that results from a deliberate evaluation of relevant factors (Fig. 116.3).

CLINICAL DECISION MAKING

THE SURGEON'S PERSPECTIVE

The mandate of the surgeon is to balance expected risk and anticipated outcomes of therapy to optimize the patient's overall condition and outlook. This is usually done in consultation with the patient and the patient's family, with the intent of understanding the patient's values and preferences. However, challenges in communication between the surgeon and patient often obscure the patient's understanding and desires. Such challenges may be related to, among other factors, social, cultural, racial, educational, and relational differences.

Surgeons traditionally have taken a paternalistic approach to decision making. Historically, many patients have accepted this approach, being uncomfortable with challenging the surgeon's authority, knowledge, experience, and confidence. Attitudes toward physicians evolved during the late twentieth and early twenty-first centuries, and empiric trust has eroded, being replaced with a variety of attitudes reflected by a range of behaviors from intelligent questioning to suspicion and distrust. In this challenging environment, surgeons fare best when they summarize facts, describe accepted guidelines for therapy, demonstrate findings on imaging and other staging and preoperative testing to patients and their families, and explain the reasoning for their recommendations.

Surgeon decision making may be influenced by external factors, including metrics that are now available as part of public reporting of outcomes. The introduction of mandatory reporting in New York

State in 1989 was followed by reporting efforts regionally, nationally, and internationally. It triggered behavioral changes in cardiac surgeons, having negatively influenced morale in the specialty that may have induced cardiothoracic surgeons to seek employment in other countries after training in a country that mandated public reporting.[53] More importantly, surgeons, particularly those experiencing higher-than-average operative mortality rates, appeared to decrease their frequency of performing surgery on high-risk patients, possibly restricting access of sicker patients to potentially curative therapy.[54,55]

A number of factors may unconsciously, and perhaps inappropriately, influence surgeon judgment. For procedures that are performed infrequently, surgeons tend to rely on published outcomes information and overweigh the possibility of complications. In contrast, surgeons tend to rely on their experience in judging risk if they have performed an operation many times, resulting in reliance on a relatively small sample size and underweighing the risk of complications. Adverse patient events that immediately precede a surgical decision for a different patient are also important, as these events tend to make a surgeon's decision making more conservative.[56] Interestingly, when experiencing a track history of very good outcomes, a person's natural tendency is to become less conservative in decision making, which leads to worsening of overall outcomes. This may be part of the explanation for the frequently observed zero mortality paradox in surgery.[57]

A surgeon's attitude toward risk may also importantly influence decision making. The stereotypical surgeon is confident, is comfortable making decisions with limited data, and does not frequently second-guess these decisions. These characteristics may not be optimal for the delivery of high-quality surgical care. One factor associated with increased rates of reoperations and readmissions included a "macho" attitude, which accounted for nearly 20% of the variation in these rates.[58] Other attitudes in surgeons that were of concern included impulsive behavior, elevated self-confidence, and an anti-authority outlook. When evaluated with regard to personality types, risk tolerance is related to the qualities thinking, extrovert, and perception.[59] Risk aversion was associated with feeling, introvert, and judgment qualities. Knowledge of these innate or learned characteristics may help surgeons understand their decision-making behavior.

THE PATIENT'S PERSPECTIVE

Arguably the most important voice in the decision-making process is that of the patient. There is growing interest in patients taking more responsibility for their health care decisions, especially with regard to interventions such as major surgery that carry substantial risk. Surgical paternalism, which historically has been the primary mechanism of such decisions, is giving way to patients' desires to better understand and participate in the decision-making process.[60] Patients and their families are increasingly knowledgeable about their diagnoses, procedures, and surgeons, and their questions are more numerous and are often better informed. The Internet, social networking, and public reporting systems have made information, whether accurate or not, more plentiful and accessible.

A number of factors influence the ability of a patient to participate effectively in the decision-making process, including differences in culture, ethnicity, gender, religious beliefs, degree of education and intelligence, numerosity, and cognitive abilities.[61–65] A surgeon's understanding of the challenges that these factors bring to the decision-making process can enhance the patient experience. This requires use of language appropriate to the patient's level of education, avoidance of assumptions regarding religious beliefs or culturally based myths related to complications or outcomes of surgery, and use of clear examples that illustrate anticipated outcomes or the risk of complications rather than simply stating percentages, which are often misunderstood. Taking appropriate time to educate patients so they have a shared basic understanding of the underlying assumptions and goals regarding their health problem and potential treatment plan enables the patients and their families to become more effectively involved in their health care decisions. The use of videos, informational pamphlets, or counseling from the physician's team and the patient's community can help save time and reduce misunderstanding during the patient–physician encounter. The different factors to consider, and their potential outcomes, can sometimes be illustrated graphically in ways that resonate with patients.[66] Decision aids have been shown to be very effective in helping physicians and patients understand the patient's values and desires and in improving patients' satisfaction with their treatment decision. Unfortunately, no such tools are currently available for common thoracic diseases or procedures other than lung transplantation.[67]

Patients sometimes make non-intuitive and potentially harmful decisions when offered therapeutic options for serious diagnoses. An experiment conducted among healthy people asked individuals to choose between treatment or observation for a non-aggressive cancer.[68] In one scenario, in which the 5-year mortality rate for the cancer when untreated was 5% and the risk of dying as a result of surgery was 10%, 65% of participants elected to have surgery. Part of the explanation may be in lack of numerosity among the subjects. However, another likely explanation is that individuals have an urge to pursue active therapy in the face of a potentially lethal diagnosis, regardless of whether that therapy is beneficial. This tendency should be kept in mind when discussing therapeutic options with patients.

SHARED DECISION MAKING

Shared decision making is the process by which the physician and the patient, often along with the patient's family and possibly community members, have relatively balanced roles in selecting from among treatment options. Engaging the patient and the patient's support system in decision making when fateful decisions must be made is paramount in patient-centered care. Many times there is only one logical treatment choice, such as the administration of antibiotics

TABLE 116.3 Surgery- Versus Patient-Centered Indicators of Quality and Safety[70]

Surgery Centered	Patient Centered
Freedom from complications	Respect for the patient's values, preferences, and expressed needs
Physical comfort, including pain management	Coordinated and integrated care
Short duration of hospital stay	Clear, high-quality information and education for the patient and family
Discharge to home	Physical comfort, including pain management
Freedom from readmission	Emotional support and alleviation of fear and anxiety
Rapid surgical recovery and return to normal activities	Involvement of family members and friends, as appropriate
Maintained or improved quality of life	Continuity, including through care-site transitions
Cure of disease or prolongation of life	Access to care

for sepsis. However, under most circumstances there is more than one reasonable therapeutic option. The process of shared decision making requires that both parties share information.[69] The surgeon informs the patient of the treatment options, their likely benefits, and their potential risks. The patient informs the surgeon of his or her values and preferences. Involving the patient in decision making adds value to the process and helps align patient interests with metrics of successful surgical intervention (Table 116.3).[70] Physicians generally support shared decision making, but implementation of this process is not easy. Patients are sometimes reluctant to participate, surgeons must learn to yield their authority and to communicate better, and systems need to be developed that provide additional resources and the time that is required for successful shared decision making.

USING PUBLISHED EVIDENCE IN SURGICAL DECISION MAKING

Key to determining risk and communicating with patients is an understanding of how to interpret published results. This requires a basic knowledge of statistical methods and their reporting. Surgeons should understand statistics because such knowledge is key to determining whether the design, analysis, and reporting of results are correct. One review of publications on the quality of medical literature concluded that there were " . . . few journal articles that are scientifically sound in terms of reporting usable data and providing even moderately strong support for their inferences."[71] Another review identified errors in the use of even the most simple statistics in over 25% of journal articles.[72]

Typical questions a clinician should consider when reading a clinical paper include: Was the question posed correctly? Were there sufficient patients to address the question? Are the results really positive/negative? Is there any evidence of experimental bias? Are there alternative interpretations of the findings that the authors failed to consider? Understanding key elements of a scientific report is vital to interpreting reported outcomes. The publication should specify or describe key elements in design, research methods, analysis, and reporting (Table 116.4).[73]

TABLE 116.4 Elements That Should Be Included in Published Clinical Research Papers[73]

Study Design
Rationale for study
Specific question or hypothesis
Retrospective, prospective
Observational, interventional
Type of clinical trial
Phase 1
Phase 2
Phase 3

Research Methods
Time period of study
Inclusion/exclusion criteria
Source of subjects
Rationale for sample sizes (power calculation)
Statement regarding study registration with https://clinicaltrials.gov/ if appropriate

Data Analysis
Specific tests performed
Methodology for all except the most common tests, including underlying assumptions
Software used for analyses
Statement of how missing data were managed
State what parameters are reported (median and range or quartiles, etc., mean and standard deviation, etc.)

Results Reporting
CONSORT diagram, if appropriate
Summary of population characteristics and, if appropriate, subpopulation characteristics
Outcomes of analyses related to hypothesis or central question
Specific p-values reported for each comparison (use of NS for not significant is not appropriate)
Associations such as linear regression or simple correlation should be presented with scatter plots
Survival curves should have censoring indicators for smaller studies and should include numbers of patients at risk at appropriate intervals.
Categorical data should be presented as counts and percentages
Ordinal variables should not be reported as mean and standard deviation, but as counts and percentages
Regression models should be reported in full so that all covariates that were considered in the model are evident

STATISTICAL ANALYSES COMMON TO SURGICAL STUDIES

The following section offers a very basic description of statistical techniques commonly used in clinical medicine that surgeons should have some familiarity with. The information is framed from the perspective of the practicing clinician, and is provided as much as possible in nontechnical language. Technical terms are provided for reference and clarity (Table 116.5).

REPORTING GROUP CHARACTERISTICS

Group characteristics are typically included as the first dataset in a clinical report. If more than one group is included in the study, characteristics of each group and the study population as a whole should be presented. For categorical data, numbers of patients or events

and their relevant percentages should be listed; listing percentages without stating the number from which they were derived is not appropriate. For continuous data, reporting the mean and standard deviation is appropriate unless the data are skewed (not distributed in a bell-curve pattern), in which case reporting the median and the 25th and 75th percentiles provides a better picture of the data. Ordinal variables should be depicted as counts and percentages, not as mean and standard deviation.

EXPERIMENTAL DESIGN CONSIDERATIONS

It is important to understand the methodology of clinical study design for a number of reasons; in this section the focus will be on identifying sample sizes needed to reach reliable conclusions. Shortcomings in this element of design often prevent identification of meaningful results, or can lead to incorrect conclusions, even when all other aspects of the study are designed well. The key elements to understand are power, sample size, and effect size.[74] For many clinical studies it is important to determine the likelihood (α) of a false-positive result, or type I error, which occurs when statistical significance is declared when it does not exist. It is equally important to determine the likelihood (β) of a false-negative result, or type II error, which occurs when no significance is identified even though it exists. Finally, the size of the effect, or the extent of the differences in outcomes between groups, must be estimated or derived from prior studies. These values help estimate the required sample size, which is key to determining whether a study can enroll sufficient patients to be meaningful, is essential for budgeting purposes, and is important in knowing whether an existing database is sufficiently large to draw conclusions.

The statistical significance criterion, α, is an indication of how unlikely it is that significance will be identified when, in fact, no significant difference between groups exists. Most commonly α is set at 0.05 (a 5% chance of a false-positive result), but values of 0.01 or less are sometimes used. In most studies we desire a small risk of type II error (β; or a false-negative result). The complement of this $(1-\beta)$ is referred to as the power of the test, which arbitrarily is typically set at 80%. The effect size can vary greatly depending on the clinical question posed. For example, the IALT trial of postoperative adjuvant chemotherapy after complete resection of nonsmall cell lung cancer was designed based on an effect size, or difference in outcomes between groups, of 5% (improvement from 50% to 55% survival at 5 years).[34] The sample size is determined based on α, β, and the effect size; larger sample sizes provide greater statistical power. In the adjuvant chemotherapy study, α was set at 0.05 and β was set at 0.90, which resulted in a sample size for the study of 3,300 patients.

DETERMINING WHETHER VARIABLES ARE RELATED

It is often of interest to assess the relationship of one clinical variable to another, or of an outcome to a clinical variable. For example, identifying a relationship between increasing age and increasing operative mortality may be informative for patient selection. Other reasons to identify such relationships include the confounding nature of correlated variables when performing multivariable analyses, which makes regression coefficients unstable and difficult to interpret. Simple identification of a relationship between two variables or a variable and an outcome is not meaningful, and searching widely for relationships is frowned upon. Data analyses, in general, should be hypothesis-driven and not performed in a post hoc manner. It is also important to understand that if a variable is related to an outcome of interest, this does not imply causation. Thus, stating

TABLE 116.5 Common Statistical Terms and Their Definitions

Term	Definition
Categorical data	Data that can be assigned to one of a limited and fixed number of values or categories
Ordinal data	Data assigned to categories that are ordered and for which the distance between categories is not known
Continuous data	Data that can take any numerical value
Normal distribution	Data that, when graphed according to their increasing values and the frequencies of those values, are symmetric around a central value (bell curve) with the mean, median, and mode all equal
Power	The probability of accepting the alternative hypothesis over the null hypothesis when the alternative hypothesis is true. It is affected by the sample size, the magnitude of the effect of interest, and the choice of statistical significance threshold
Effect size	A quantitative measure of the strength of a statistical outcome that helps understand its substantive rather than its statistical significance
Null hypothesis	A default statement, or initial assumption, that there is no difference between two groups
Type I error	Incorrect rejection of a true null hypothesis (a "false-positive" conclusion)
Type II error	Incorrect acceptance of a false null hypothesis (a "false-negative" conclusion)
Statistical significance	The numerical threshold (significance level, α) below which it is assumed that the null hypothesis is false, commonly set at 5%
Correlation coefficient	A measure (r) of the strength and direction of the linear relationship between two variables; ranges from -1 to 1
Coefficient of determination	Denoted as r^2; it represents the proportion of change in a dependent variable that is due to an independent variable; ranges from 0 to 1
Linear regression	A method of modeling a linear relationship between a dependent variable (Y) and an independent variable (X)
Multivariable regression	A method for identifying and quantifying the unique contributions of multiple factors to a single outcome of interest
Chi-squared test (χ^2 test)	An evaluation of the distribution of categorical variables in an A × B table that assesses the degree to which the expected distribution is not observed
Fisher's exact test	An evaluation of the distribution of categorical variables in a 2 × 2 table that assesses the degree to which the expected distribution is not observed
Propensity score	The probability of receiving an intervention that is conditional on covariates that determine receipt of the intervention
t-test	A method of determining whether two groups of values have different mean values
Analysis of variance (ANOVA)	A method of comparing the means of more than two groups of values
Standard deviation	A measure of the spread of a group of normally distributed values
Odds ratio	A relative measure of effect that allows comparison of an intervention group to a placebo/comparator group. The numerator is the odds of an event in the intervention group, the denominator is the odds of that event in the placebo/comparator group, yielding an odds ratio
Relative risk	The ratio of the probability of an event in an intervention or affected group to the probability of that event in a placebo group
Confidence interval	An estimated range of values calculated from a dataset that is likely to include an unknown value from a similar dataset. The confidence level for the interval determines the likelihood that the confidence interval will contain the unknown value; common choices for confidence levels are 0.90, 0.95, and 0.99
Kaplan–Meier method	A statistical approach for generating survival curves from lifetime data, typically used to assess the fraction of patients alive for a certain amount of time after an intervention
Log rank test	A method of comparing survival curves for two groups of individuals
Cox proportional hazards modeling	A method of assessing the effects of several variables on a time-related event such as survival
Hazard ratio	The ratio of the hazard rates of mortality or other time-related event for an intervention group (numerator) and a placebo/comparator group (denominator)
Quality-adjusted life-year (QALY)	A measure combining the quality and quantity of life. The degree of disease burden is estimated as a percentage of perfect health and multiplied by time lived. One QALY is 1 yr lived in perfect health
Incremental cost-effectiveness ratio (ICER)	The difference in costs between two interventions divided by the difference in their effectiveness. A measure of cost-effectiveness of an intervention
Decision analysis	A field of study and a group of statistical methods for formally outlining and quantifying outcomes of important decisions and factors that affect them
Receiver operating characteristic (ROC) analysis	A method of illustrating the performance of a binary classification. Threshold values for creating the binary classification are varied, and the resultant true-positive and false-positive rates in observed data are plotted
Bootstrapping	A method of iterative random sampling from a dataset, with replacement, to enable assignment of measures of accuracy to the parameters of the dataset
Meta-analysis	A technique for increasing the reliability of research by combining results of all similar trials or experiments

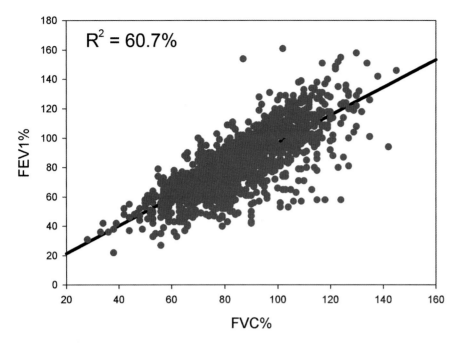

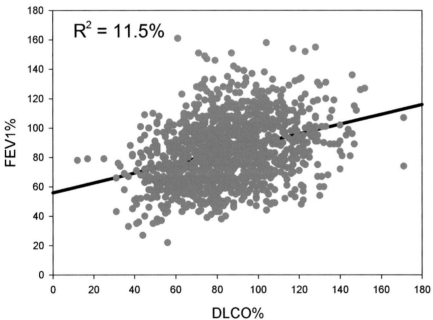

FIGURE 116.4 An example of linear regression plots comparing the relationships between pulmonary function variables. There is a high coefficient of determination (R^2) between forced expiratory volume in the first second (FEV1%) and forced vital capacity (FVC%; *top panel*); in contrast, the coefficient of determination between FEV1% and diffusing capacity (DLCO%; *bottom panel*) is small.

that "a change in X resulted in a change in Y" implies causation. It is preferable to state that "a change in X was associated with a change in Y." Causation may be inferred from a clinical perspective, but is not implicit from a statistical perspective.

Methods for determining relatedness of continuous variables include calculation of a correlation coefficient and regression analysis. Pearson's correlation coefficient (r) is a measure of the linear relationship between two continuous variables, and is expressed as a value between –1 and 1. The closer to 1, the greater the linear relationship between the two variables. The closer to –1, the greater the inverse relationship between the two variables. This test does not require knowing or hypothesizing how the two variables are related—whether one is independent and the other is dependent, for example. If variables are related but not in a linear manner, the correlation coefficient may be close to zero, and would not be a reliable

indicator of the true relationship. Inspection of a scatter plot may assist in assessing this.[75]

Simple regression analysis evaluates the relationship between a response (dependent) variable and a predictor (independent) variable. This method assesses the direction, size, and statistical significance of the relationship between the two variables. As with correlation, linear regression is informative only for variables that have a linear relationship (Fig. 116.4). The method permits calculation of an expected value for the dependent variable based on a known value for the independent variable. The coefficient of determination (R^2) is a measure of how much the independent variable accounts for variation in the dependent variable. In datasets in which two variables have a high degree of correlation (e.g., r = 0.90), the amount of variability in the response variable accounted for by the predictor variable is also high (in this example, 81%). Nonlinear regression examining the relationship between two

Mortality from lung cancer among men aged 40 to 70

	Current smokers	Never smokers	Total
Dead incidence	5,630 (3,827 expected)	147 (1,950 expected)	5,777
Alive incidence	11,121 (12,924 expected)	8,389 (6,585 expected)	19,510
Total	16,751	8,536	25,287

Chi-Squared = 3261.988, DF = 1, p value < 0.0001

FIGURE 116.5 Chi-squared analysis of the distribution of smoking history and lung cancer mortality demonstrating a strong statistical relationship between the two. (Data from Hjellvik V, Selmer R, Gjessing HK, et al. Body mass index, smoking, and risk of death between 40 and 70 years of age in a Norwegian cohort of 32,727 women and 33,475 men. *Eur J Epidemiol* 2013;28:35–43.)

variables can be calculated using a variety of other mathematical relationships. Multiple regression can also be performed using two or more independent variables.

Assessing potential relationships between categorical variables requires statistical methods such as the chi-squared test (χ^2 test) and Fisher's exact test. The chi-squared test assumes that the characteristics of two or more variables are independently normally distributed; the test can be used to assess this assumption. For example, if one were to assess two variables in a population such as smoking status and lung cancer mortality, those with a smoking history would have a much higher incidence of lung cancer mortality than nonsmokers, thus demonstrating the relationship (lack of independence) of the two variables (Fig. 116.5).[76] In contrast, examining the prevalence of obesity related to smoking status likely would not reveal important differences in distribution (Fig. 116.6).[76] Fisher's exact test addresses similar issues but is limited to a 2×2 matrix and is more appropriate for datasets in which there are small numbers in some of the cells in the matrix.

CREATING COMPARABLE GROUPS FROM LARGE DATASETS

Among the most common challenges in clinical reporting are those that are created when examining outcomes between groups that have different characteristics. Randomized trials simplify the assessment

Incidence of obesity related to smoking status among men

	Current smokers	Never smokers	Total
Not obese	15,804 (15,781 expected)	947 (969 expected)	16,751
Obese	8,020 (8,042 expected)	516 (494 expected)	8,536
Total	23,824	1,463	25,287

Chi-Squared = 1.591, DF = 1, p value = 0.207

FIGURE 116.6 Chi-squared analysis of the distribution of obesity and lung cancer mortality, demonstrating the absence of a strong statistical relationship between the two. (Data from Hjellvik V, Selmer R, Gjessing HK, et al. Body mass index, smoking, and risk of death between 40 and 70 years of age in a Norwegian cohort of 32,727 women and 33,475 men. *Eur J Epidemiol* 2013;28:35–43.)

of treatment effects by creating groups that are likely to be comparable in most important respects. In contrast, retrospective and observational studies frequently involve comparisons between groups that may be quite different. This may be a result of varying time periods of intervention, biases in patient selection or treatment assignment, variations in clinical management or treating surgeons, or different baseline characteristics between groups of interest. Controlling for these differences is essential in performing fair comparisons between groups.

Methods that have been used to meet these challenges include matching patients for sex and age or a few other important clinical variables using "nearest neighbor" techniques. While potentially useful, these methods are often biased against the treatment group and don't incorporate a sufficient number of clinical variables to permit creation of truly similar groups. A better alternative is the use of propensity score matching, which weights clinical variables based on their degree of association with the outcome variable.[77,78] Covariates are selected that have the potential to predict outcomes or to influence treatment selection. Two critical elements must be assumed in the process: The covariates selected for estimating propensity scores contain all of the information relevant to the outcomes, and the possibility of a patient receiving either treatment option is realistic. A propensity score is estimated for each patient and represents the probability of being assigned to the specific treatment being investigated. The patients in each group ("control" and "treatment") are then matched to each other based on these scores, typically using nearest neighbor or other statistical techniques. The resulting groups are often much smaller in number than the original groups, as some patients in one group will not have a match in the other group. The clinical characteristics of each matched group must be compared to verify that the patient pools are similar before an analysis of the treatment effect size and statistical significance is performed (Table 116.6).[79]

COMPARING ACUTE OUTCOMES BETWEEN GROUPS

Acute outcomes for patients (a categorical variable) can be assessed for their relationship to other categorical variables (such as the incidence of postoperative complications and mortality), ordinal variables (such as changes in dysphagia score after esophageal surgery), and continuous variables (such as changes in physiologic variables in response to interventions). For each type of variable a variety of statistical tests are available for assessing the effects of an intervention. Categorical variables are usually compared using the χ^2 test or Fisher's exact test as described earlier.

Continuous variables are classified as to whether they are normally distributed. The characteristic of a normal distribution is that the means of many random samples taken from the population for that variable will distribute into a bell-shaped curve. This may be true even if the population being sampled appears to be skewed. Having a normal distribution indicates that the mean and standard deviation can be determined and may be used to calculate confidence intervals (CIs). Parametric tests for normally distributed continuous variables include t-tests and analysis of variance (ANOVA). When a population is not normally distributed, nonparametric tests are appropriate. These include the Spearman correlation test, the Mann–Whitney test for comparing two independent means, and the Kruskal–Wallis test for comparing >2 independent means.

Assessment of a continuous dependent variable (such as postoperative forced vital capacity) according to a categorical independent variable having two states (such as VATS vs. open surgery) is done with a t-test. A t-test examines whether the population means of two groups are different. If the means of the dependent variable are

TABLE 116.6 An Example of Propensity Score Matching to Achieve Comparable Groups Using Characteristics of Patients Undergoing Either Open or Minimally Invasive (VATS) Lobectomy[79]

Variable	Unmatched			Matched		
	Open (N = 26,050)	VATS (N = 2,721)	P-value	Open (N = 2,721)	VATS (N = 2,721)	P-value
Male	69.3%	58.2%	<0.0001	57.6%	58.2%	NS
Site			<0.0001			NS
RUL	35.6%	32.1%		35.8%	32.1%	
RML	6.1%	9.2%		7.0%	9.2%	
RLL	16.3%	17.4%		16.6%	17.4%	
LUL	24.6%	21.9%		23.9%	21.9%	
LLL	16.5%	17.4%		15.4%	17.4%	
Elective surgery	98.9%	99.7%	<0.0001	99.2%	99.7%	NS
ECOG PS			<0.0001			NS
0	45.5%	57.7%		59.2%	57.7%	
1	39.0%	32.4%		31.6%	32.4%	
≥2	8.3%	5.7%		5.5%	5.7%	
Heart failure	0.7%	1.1%	0.035	0.9%	1.1%	NS
Diabetes	2.2%	3.9%	<0.0001	3.3%	3.9%	NS
Induction chemotherapy	11.1%	4.4%	<0.0001	5.1%	4.4%	NS

VATS, video-assisted thoracic surgery; NS, not statistically significant; RUL, right upper lobe; RML, right middle lobe; RLL, right lower lobe; LUL, left upper lobe; LLL, left lower lobe; ECOG PS, Eastern Cooperative Oncology Group performance status.

unrelated (in this case, a patient has either VATS or open surgery, making each group independent of the other), a two-sample t-test is appropriate. If the values of the dependent variables are related, such as if pre- and postoperative function is being compared within the same patient group, a paired t-test is performed. The paired t-test is often more powerful than a two-sample t-test because the variation between groups is eliminated. For example, if the first 12 digits of the Fibonacci series are listed in two columns (1, 1, 2, 3, 5, 8, 13, . . .), the first beginning with 1 and the other beginning with 0, the unpaired and paired t-tests yield the same means (31.3, 19.3) and standard deviations (44.5, 27.5) for each column. However, the p-values for the two tests differ importantly (0.437, 0.032).

Examining values of a continuous dependent variable (postoperative vital capacity) according to a categorical independent variable having more than two states (such as racial group or BMI category) can be performed with multiple t-tests. However, the process of multiple comparisons (an independent variable having three categories would require three comparisons: A vs. B, B vs. C, A vs. C) increases the probability of identifying a statistically significant outcome purely by chance. This type of multiple comparisons requires an adjustment of the p-value for which statistical significance is claimed based on the number of comparisons. In this example, the stated threshold for significance (0.05) is divided by the number of comparisons among groups (3) to yield a new significance threshold (0.0167) for this situation (Bonferroni correction; the correction factor is: $(x(x - 1))/2$ where x is the number of comparisons). Failure to adjust the threshold can potentially lead to a type I error (see earlier).

Prior to performing multiple comparisons, it's useful to explore the dataset using a more omnibus test such as ANOVA. ANOVA is a method of comparing means among groups in conjunction with the variations among and between groups. If ANOVA does not produce significant differences among the groups, then multiple t-tests will not yield significant differences between groups. If ANOVA does produce a

significant value, then the pairwise comparisons can be used to determine between which groups the differences exist. Alternatively, use of an automated single-step procedure that incorporates multiple comparisons, such as the Tukey–Kramer method, may be considered.

For situations in which a large number of comparisons are performed, the Bonferroni correction and similar techniques will likely be too conservative. In such situations many investigators now use computerized resampling methods that entail hundreds or thousands of recursive testing help eliminate the possibility of type I errors. Examples include bootstrapping and Monte Carlo simulations (see later).

Outcomes for two continuous variables can be evaluated after transforming one or both variables from continuous to categorical variables. This process creates increased statistical power, especially for smaller datasets, but is associated with loss of fidelity. For example, evaluating BMI as a continuous independent variable in its relationship to postoperative pulmonary complications after lung resection reveals a complex curve indicating increased risk at the extremes of BMI (Fig. 116.7).[80] In contrast, using categories of BMI that dichotomize patients as ≤25 (normal and underweight) or >25 (overweight and obese) fails to reveal the increased risk associated with being in underweight or obese III categories. The transformations, when performed, ideally are based on published clinical thresholds of interest, on predetermined mathematical descriptors such as median, or on values determined by receiver operating characteristic (ROC) analysis (see later).

Continuous variables are otherwise evaluated with regression techniques, which are described in a previous section. Such techniques may include linear or nonlinear equations to achieve a best-fit line for two continuous variables. Prediction errors for individual comparisons commonly result, as most biologic processes don't rigorously conform to expectations. These errors, known as residuals, represent the distance of the observed values from the predicted values. The goal of the process is to minimize the sum of the residuals. Graphing the residuals is often helpful in identifying where the concentration of

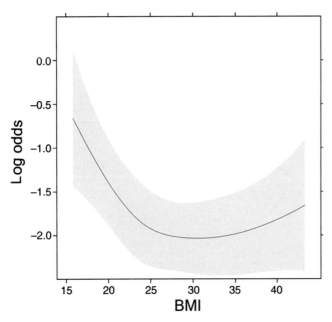

FIGURE 116.7 The complex relationship between BMI and postoperative pulmonary complications after lung resection is clearly evident when using BMI as a continuous variable; it is likely that dichotomizing BMI into [normal or underweight] versus [overweight or obese] would not permit identification of the relationships. (From Ferguson MK, Im HK, Watson S, et al. Association of body mass index and outcomes after major lung resection. *Eur J Cardiothorac Surg* 2014;45:e94–e99. Reproduced by permission of European Association for Cardiothoracic Surgery.)

prediction error is greatest, which helps the investigator understand the behavior of the interaction between the variables.

IDENTIFYING FACTORS ASSOCIATED WITH SHORT-TERM OUTCOMES

When considering clinical decisions, it is often useful to assess the association of specific clinical factors with acute postoperative outcomes such as surgical complications, duration of hospital stay, or the need for reintervention. A method of expressing the relationship of a clinical parameter to outcomes is the odds ratio (OR). The OR is a measure of effect size and is typically used to express outcomes of logistic regression analyses. An example of this is the OR of postoperative pulmonary complications in patients with renal failure (exposed group) compared to those with normal renal function (nonexposed group) after lobectomy for lung cancer; the OR for pulmonary complications in patients with renal insufficiency is 1.53.[81] Note that OR does not connote a causative role for the clinical factor related to the outcome, only that a statistical association exists. It is most commonly used in case-controlled studies. The statistical significance of OR requires an understanding of the spread of values, typically expressed as the 95% CI, which is defined as: $CI = \log(\text{risk ratio}) \pm SE \times z_\alpha$, where SE is the standard error and z_α is the standard score for the chosen level of significance.

Another method of assessing the incidence of clinical parameters in different populations is the relative risk (RR; risk ratio) in one population (exposed group; intervention group) compared to another population (nonexposed group; comparator). This method can be applied to a binary outcome, and is most amenable to events that are expected to have a low frequency. An RR equal to 1 indicates that there is no difference in risk between the groups. An RR <1 means that the event is less likely to occur in the exposed group than the nonexposed group, and an RR >1 indicates that the event

is more likely to occur in the exposed group than the nonexposed group. RR is most appropriately used in randomized controlled trials and when calculating outcomes from a large population sample, as in epidemiologic work.

There is often confusion between OR and RR in clinical literature. The two are mathematically related. RR is a more intuitive measure, indicating that, at an RR of 1.5, the population of interest has a predicted event rate that is 50% higher than the comparator. The OR is more difficult to understand by nonstatisticians, and an OR cannot be interpreted as representing a 50% increased risk of an event. OR often has the feature of offering a more attractive (larger) effect size than the RR, and thus is sometimes selected to express outcomes because of this. However, it is more accurate to use RR in most situations other than for case-referent studies, particularly when expressing outcomes of logistic regression analyses.[82,83]

COMPARING SURVIVAL OR INCIDENCE OUTCOMES BETWEEN GROUPS

Survival analysis is used to evaluate time to an event, such as death, time to reoperation, or time to disease recurrence. Survival is typically not directly observed: events are not recorded in real time, and individuals often have not experienced an event by the time the analysis is performed. These characteristics require that some data are "censored." Data for a subject are right censored when the subject has not experienced the event by the time the data are analyzed, when an event has occurred at an unspecified time but after a known date, or when a subject is lost to follow-up. Data are left censored when an event has occurred prior to a known date but the actual date is unknown. Typically survival is assessed using the Kaplan–Meier method.

The Kaplan–Meier method is a nonparametric technique that permits a step-wise graphical representation of survival. The graph is marked by events (death, recurrence, censoring) resulting in a vertical decrease in the curve, between which the horizontal segments of the curve represent periods during which survival is assumed to be constant (Fig. 116.8).

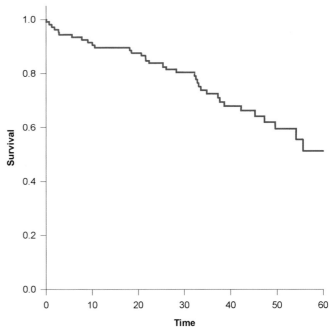

FIGURE 116.8 An example of a Kaplan–Meier survival curve depicting outcomes after resection for pathologic stage I nonsmall cell lung cancer.

To assess potential differences in survival between groups, different Kaplan–Meier survival curves may be compared using the log rank test. This test compares the distribution of survival times between two or more groups. X^2 distribution is used to assess the statistical significance of the differences. Note that the treatment group assignment and time are the only variables affecting outcomes in this analysis. Identification of other factors that may be involved in time-related outcomes requires Cox proportional hazards modeling (see later).

IDENTIFYING FACTORS ASSOCIATED WITH SURVIVAL

As part of clinical decision making, it is often helpful to know what clinical factors influence long-term outcomes. In the case of malignancy, cancer stage and resectability are usually associated with survival. Other factors that help determine survival may not be intuitive. One method for exploring whether a clinical variable affects survival is Cox proportional hazards modeling. In this technique, the effect of a specified amount of change in a covariate is related to an increase/decrease in the rate of the outcome. For example, use of adjuvant postoperative chemotherapy increased the 5-year survival rate after complete resection of nonsmall cell lung cancer by 4.1%; this was associated with a hazard ratio for mortality in the chemotherapy group of 0.86 (95% CI 0.76 to 0.98; p <0.03) compared to the control group.[84] An example comparing survival among multiple categories is illustrated in Figure 116.9.[85] The clinical factor does not have to be categorical or binary—outcomes may be related to a continuous variable, which typically result in a logarithmic rate of change in the hazard function.

Outcomes of Cox analyses are often expressed as hazard ratios (HR). The hazard ratio is the ratio of the hazard rates of two explanatory variables related to an outcome or event of interest. In a fictitious example, if the long-term mortality rate after open lobectomy is twice as high as the long-term mortality rate after VATS lobectomy, the HR for open lobectomy is 2.

The utility of Cox proportional hazard modeling is dependent on the proportional hazards assumption, which states that the hazard for one individual must be proportional to the hazard of another individual. This assumption should be tested routinely when using Cox modeling; an easy method is to visually examine the survival curves in question, verifying that the distance between the curves is constant over time. The assumption is clearly violated if the survival curves cross. It is usually necessary to adjust the model for other known covariates related to the outcome in order to determine whether the covariate of interest is independently related to the outcome.

COST-EFFECTIVE ANALYSIS

In analyzing outcomes of competing interventions, it is useful not only to know the differences in clinical effectiveness, but to also know the relative costs of each (to the individual, institution, health care system, society, etc.). Specific outcomes of interest are identified, and the relative cost of each intervention is tabulated. Cost-effectiveness is expressed as a ratio, with the denominator representing the health outcome (e.g., gains in life-years) and the numerator indicating the cost associated with the health gain. A common method of expressing outcomes is using cost per quality-adjusted life-year (QALY), in which the life-years gained are adjusted by the quality of life experienced during that time using a scale of 0 (death) to 1 (perfect health). Whether an intervention is cost-effective is sometimes determined by its ICER, or incremental cost-effectiveness ratio. A typical threshold for an acceptable ICER, from a societal perspective, is $50,000 per QALY gained. For reference, ICERs for examples of accepted medical care are: $31,000 for breast cancer screening[86]; $11,000 for colon cancer screening with fecal occult blood testing[87]; $81,000 for lung cancer screening with computed tomography[88]; $100,000 for heart transplantation[89]; and $175,000 for lung transplantation.[90]

While the concept of this type of analysis is straightforward, the data collection and analyses offer important challenges. These include accurate identification of costs (medical, patient time away from work, family time away from work, etc.), the time frame of analysis, and accurate estimates of quality of life during various time frames included in the analyses. Costs must also be adjusted for the time frame in which they are incurred, usually using factors such as the consumer price index or a similar price index specific for health care costs. The National Lung Screening Trial (NLST) provides an instructive example of how outcomes may change when underlying assumptions are only slightly changed: using different incremental costs and incremental QALYs yielded ICERs ranging from $32,000 to $615,000 per QALY gained.[88]

MODELING OUTCOMES

For some physicians the concepts of ORs or ICER are abstract and may be difficult to apply to a specific clinical scenario. Decision-analytic techniques are often used to provide more concrete methods of illustrating the benefits and costs of potential outcomes. Modeling of outcomes incorporates options for management and estimates the likelihood of outcomes using probabilities that are usually derived from published literature. The process is often represented graphically using diagrams and decision trees. A typical decision tree includes two or more treatment choices for a defined patient population with a defined clinical problem. Outcomes for each choice are identified and are assigned probabilities. Costs may be assigned to the different interventions, and values such as life-years gained and quality of life can be assigned to the outcomes.

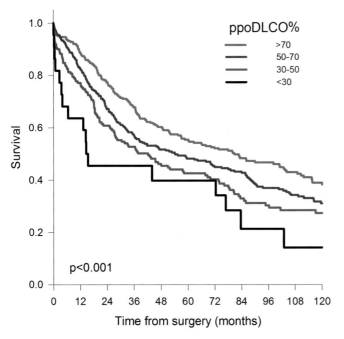

FIGURE 116.9 Kaplan–Meier survival curves comparing outcomes according to postoperative predicted diffusing capacity (ppoDLCO%), compared using Cox proportional hazard modeling. (From Ferguson MK, Watson S, Johnson E, et al. Predicted postoperative lung function is associated with all-cause long-term mortality after major lung resection for cancer. *Eur J Cardiothorac Surg* 2014;45:660–664. Reproduced by permission of European Association for Cardiothoracic Surgery.)

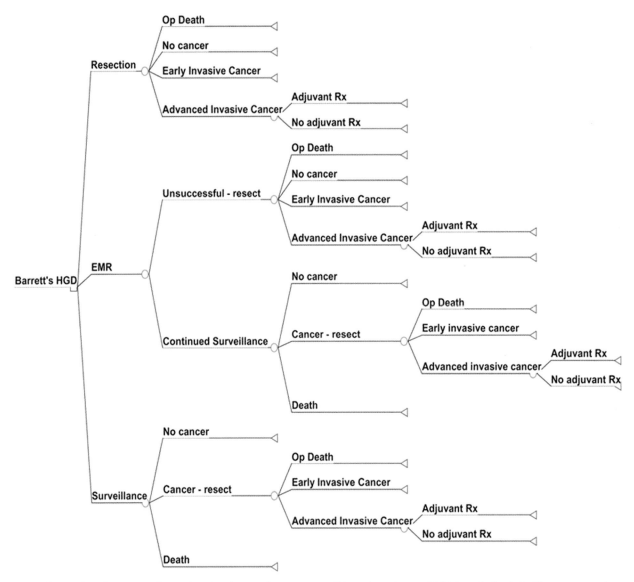

FIGURE 116.10 A decision tree designed to identify optimal management of Barrett's esophagus with high-grade dysplasia. Management options include endoscopic surveillance, esophageal resection, or endoscopic mucosal resection. Branching at nodes (*green circles*) represents possible outcomes.

Using the probabilities, costs, and values, the model is run, resulting in each treatment having an outcome metric that can be compared to the other treatment(s). This can assist the clinician in selecting the treatment with the optimal outcome. An example of a simple decision-analytic tree (Fig. 116.10) illustrates choices for management of a patient with Barrett's esophagus who was found to have high-grade dysplasia.

Decision trees can be simple, but to capture a clinical scenario more accurately it may be necessary to create very intricate decision trees. It is often useful to employ techniques that capture complex real-world outcomes rather than simply defined outcomes. For example, a patient who undergoes complex therapies followed by a long recovery period experience a series of health states from well (prior to the development of the clinical problem) to death (at the extreme, resulting from complications of treatment, the clinical problem itself, unrelated problems, etc.) and every type of health state in between. Transitions from one health state to another are often nonlinear (Fig. 116.11). The process of capturing information about health states and how individuals transition between them as a feature of decision analysis is termed Markov modeling.

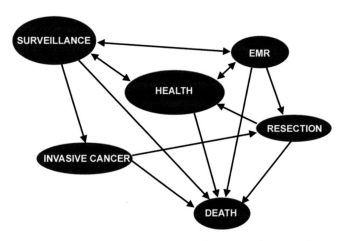

FIGURE 116.11 Transitions from one clinical state to another are nonlinear, reflecting typical variations in patient experiences, and are used in Markov modeling. The clinical states represent possible outcomes in management of Barrett's esophagus with high-grade dysplasia identified in Figure 116.10.

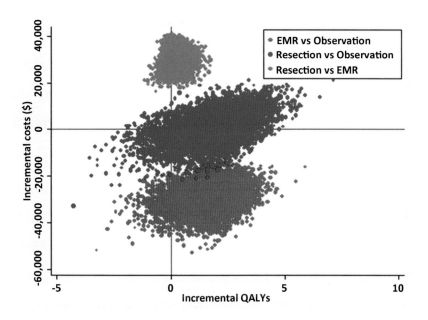

FIGURE 116.12 An example of probabilistic modeling for management of Barrett's esophagus with high-grade dysplasia as illustrated in Figure 116.10. Rather than yielding point estimates of outcomes, the range of possible outcomes for each management option is illustrated by a cloud.

More complex modeling can be accomplished by creating ranges of values for events and disease states rather than providing point estimates. As the model is run, it is possible to randomly select values for each variable from within the stated range. Multiple iterations of this process, typically in the thousands, provide a range of possible outcomes that may more accurately reflect the variability in biologic and human behavior (Fig. 116.12). One version of this type of probabilistic modeling is the Monte Carlo simulation method, which is typically used in conjunction with Markov modeling in clinical outcomes research.

TEST EFFECTIVENESS

It is often useful for the clinician to be able to assess the effectiveness of a predictive algorithm or a clinical test in making decisions about their patients. Examples include how well a lab value correlates with a diagnosis of interest, and how accurately a risk score predicts the incidence of an adverse outcome. A common method of assessing the performance of a binary classifier, such as a laboratory test with a cutoff value separating normal from abnormal, is ROC analysis. This creates a graphical representation of the performance of the test by plotting the true-positive rate (sensitivity) against the false-positive rate (1 – specificity) as discriminating (cutoff) values for the test are varied. The resultant plot is in the shape of a curve that is separated from an imaginary line representing outcomes of random choice; if the curve extends up and to the left, the outcomes for the predictive variable are better than a random guess (Fig. 116.13). The maximum distance of the curve from the point of perfect discrimination, which maximizes the value of sensitivity + specificity, can be used to choose an optimum cutoff value for the classifier. The area under the curve (AUC; C-statistic) can also be calculated and is interpreted by some as an approximation of the accuracy of the test (Fig. 116.14).[91] An AUC of 0.8 or better is typically the threshold used to determine that a test is effective. Differences in AUC, compared using 95% CIs, may be used to discriminate between the utility of one classifier versus another in predicting an outcome.

Predictive algorithms are often developed to help clinicians assess the likelihood of an event for an individual patient by inserting that patient's characteristics into the algorithm and calculating a risk score. Risk scores are typically generated from large datasets that may or may not represent the population from which an individual patient is derived. Validation of a predictive algorithm using a variety of different populations is useful in assessing its generalizability.[35,91–94] One method for validating an algorithm using a new dataset is the Hosmer–Lemeshow test (Fig. 116.15). The predicted rate of an outcome for each category of patients in the new dataset is compared to the observed rate of the outcome for each category; lack of statistical significance between the outcomes suggests that the algorithm is valid for discriminating the frequency of outcomes among groups of patients and is accurate in predicting the rate of outcomes for each group.[91]

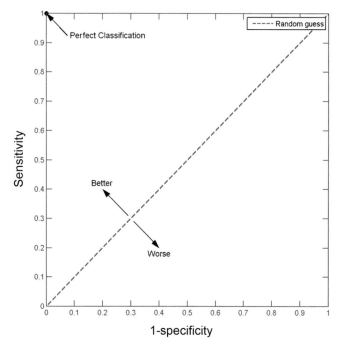

FIGURE 116.13 An illustration of important landmarks in a receiver operator characteristic display.

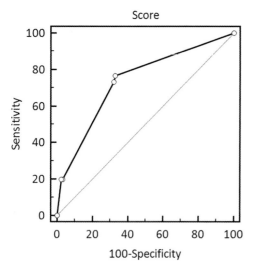

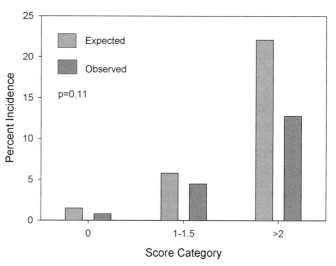

FIGURE 116.14 A receiver operating characteristic (ROC) curve for the utility of a predictive score for prolonged air leak after thoracoscopic lung resection. (From Ferguson MK, Celauro AD, Vigneswaran WT. Validation of a modified scoring system for cardiovascular risk associated with major lung resection. *Eur J Cardiothorac Surg* 2012;41:598–602. Reproduced by permission of European Association for Cardiothoracic Surgery.)

FIGURE 116.15 An example of a Hosmer–Lemeshow test comparing expected to observed event rates in the validation of a predictive score for broncho-pleural fistula after lung resection. (From Ferguson MK, Celauro AD, Vigneswaran WT. Validation of a modified scoring system for cardiovascular risk associated with major lung resection. *Eur J Cardiothorac Surg* 2012;41:598–602. Reproduced by permission of European Association for Cardiothoracic Surgery.)

MAKING INFERENCES FROM REPEATED SAMPLING OF DATA

At times it is useful to perform multiple evaluations of single datasets through repeated sampling methods such as bootstrapping in order to make inferences from those data. Examples include computation of CIs, selection of variables for use in multivariable analyses, and validation of model construction.[95] To perform bootstrapping, sampling from a dataset is performed to create multiple new datasets, each of which represents a new sample. Sampling is usually performed with replacement (individuals who are selected from the original sample are eligible to be selected again in creating the new sample; the sample size can be as large as the original sample); under special circumstances sampling without replacement (individuals can only be selected once from the original sample) is used, but of necessity results in a smaller sample size. Resampling may be performed hundreds or thousands of times depending on the analysis being performed (Fig. 116.16).[95] Statistical analyses are then performed

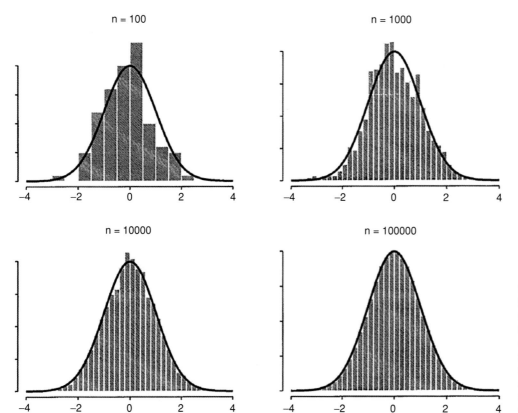

FIGURE 116.16 An example of how increasing the number of resampling events (bootstrapping) can progressively approximate the underlying distribution of a sample. (Reprinted from Grunkemeier GL, Wu Y. Bootstrap resampling methods: something for nothing? *Ann Thorac Surg* 2004;77:1142–1144. Copyright © 2004 The Society of Thoracic Surgeons. With permission.)

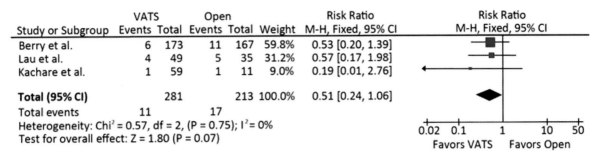

FIGURE 116.17 This forest plot identifies the effect size (*squares*) and confidence interval (*horizontal lines*) of individual studies as well as the summary effect (*diamond*). Heterogeneity (I^2) is also reported. (From Zhang R, Ferguson MK. Video-assisted versus open lobectomy in patients with compromised lung function: a literature review and meta-analysis. *PLoS One* 2015;10:e0124512.)

on each sample, generating a series of outcomes that approaches the "true" distribution of the outcomes present in the initial sample.

SYNTHESIZING RESULTS FROM MULTIPLE STUDIES

It is often the case that published studies are inconclusive; sometimes the range of error is too great to achieve statistical significance, or perhaps definite conclusions are stated but the sample size is too small or does not represent a general population. In such instances, meta-analysis to assess results of multiple conceptually similar studies can be very useful. Meta-analyses create pooled estimates of outcomes, which increase the statistical power of any conclusions, and can also identify outliers among results of different studies. Knowledge of the characteristics of a good-quality meta-analysis is helpful in judging the utility of the results.

The process of a meta-analysis should be appropriately structured to help ensure that the results are accurate. The first step is a clear statement of the problem or question. A structured literature search is then conducted, which ideally utilizes the skills of a trained professional. Individual studies are selected based on pre-established criteria that may include study size, structure, and quality. Statistical techniques for meta-regression are selected based on the type and quality of the data abstracted from the selected studies. The results are typically reported in a forest plot, which is a graphical representation of the strength of the effects of individual studies (represented by the size of squares representing individual studies) accompanied by a line indicating the associated CI of the effect (Fig. 116.17).[96] These are plotted against a line of no effect. The summary effect is represented by a diamond, the lateral extent of which indicates the CI. The heterogeneity (I^2) of the studies is also reported, indicating the extent to which the effects among the studies differ.

REFERENCES

1. Dunham EK. An application to empyema of the principles underlying the use of antiseptics. *Ann Surg* 1918;68:148–151.
2. Graham EA, Bell RD. Open pneumothorax: its relation to the treatment of empyema. *Am J Med Sci* 1918;156:839–871.
3. Aboud FC, Verghese AC. Evarts Ambrose Graham, empyema, and the dawn of clinical understanding of negative intrapleural pressure. *Clin Infect Dis* 2002;15;34: 198–203.
4. Davies MH. Recent advances in the surgery of the lung and pleura. *Br J Surg* 1913; 1:228–258.
5. Graham EA, Singer JJ. Successful removal of an entire lung for carcinoma of the bronchus. *JAMA* 1933;101:1371–1374.
6. Ginsberg RJ, Rubinstein LV. Randomized trial of lobectomy versus limited resection for T1 N0 non-small cell lung cancer. Lung Cancer Study Group. *Ann Thorac Surg* 1995;60:615–623.
7. Torek F. The first successful case of resection of the thoracic portion of the oesophagus for carcinoma. *Surg Gynecol Obstet* 1913;16:614.
8. Hulscher JB, van Sandick JW, de Boer AG, et al. Extended transthoracic resection compared with limited transhiatal resection for adenocarcinoma of the esophagus. *N Engl J Med* 2002;347:1662–1669.
9. Biere SS, van Berge Henegouwen MI, Maas KW, et al. Minimally invasive versus open oesophagectomy for patients with oesophageal cancer: a multicentre, open-label, randomised controlled trial. *Lancet* 2012;379(9829):1887–1892.
10. Li B, Xiang J, Zhang Y, et al. Comparison of Ivor-Lewis vs Sweet esophagectomy for esophageal squamous cell carcinoma: a randomized clinical trial. *JAMA Surg* 2015;150:292–298.
11. Gaensler EA. Analysis of the ventilatory defect by timed capacity measurements. *Am Rev Tuberc* 1951;64:256–278.
12. Gaensler EA, Cugell DW, Lindgren I, et al. The role of pulmonary insufficiency in mortality and invalidism following surgery for pulmonary tuberculosis. *J Thorac Surg* 1955;29:163–187.
13. McIlroy MB, Bates DV. Respiratory function after pneumonectomy. *J Thorac Surg* 1956;11:303–311.
14. Curtis JK, Rasmussen HK, Wright F, et al. Studies of pulmonary function before and after pulmonary surgery. III. Breathholding carbon monoxide diffusion of each lung before and after pneumonectomy. *J Thorac Cardiovasc Surg* 1963;45:166–174.
15. Brunelli A, Charloux A, Bolliger CT, et al.; European Respiratory Society and European Society of Thoracic Surgeons Joint Task Force on Fitness for Radical Therapy. ERS/ESTS clinical guidelines on fitness for radical therapy in lung cancer patients (surgery and chemo-radiotherapy). *Eur Respir J* 2009;34:17–41.
16. Brunelli A, Kim AW, Berger KI, et al. Physiologic evaluation of the patient with lung cancer being considered for resectional surgery: diagnosis and management of lung cancer, 3rd ed: American College of Chest Physicians evidence-based clinical practice guidelines. *Chest* 2013;143(Suppl 5):e166S–e190S.
17. Bach PB, Cramer LD, Schrag D, et al. The influence of hospital volume on survival after resection for lung cancer. *N Engl J Med* 2001;345:181–188.
18. Birkmeyer JD, Siewers AE, Finlayson EV, et al. Hospital volume and surgical mortality in the United States. *N Engl J Med* 2002;346:1128–1137.
19. Birkmeyer JD, Stukel TA, Siewers AE, et al. Surgeon volume and operative mortality in the United States. *N Engl J Med* 2003;349:2117–2127.
20. Dimick JB, Goodney PP, Orringer MB, et al. Specialty training and mortality after esophageal cancer resection. *Ann Thorac Surg* 2005;80:282–286.
21. Farjah F, Flum DR, Varghese TK Jr, et al. Surgeon specialty and long-term survival after pulmonary resection for lung cancer. *Ann Thorac Surg* 2009;87:995–1006.
22. Phillips JD, Merkow RP, Sherman KL, et al. Factors affecting selection of operative approach and subsequent short-term outcomes after anatomic resection for lung cancer. *J Am Coll Surg* 2012;215:206–215.
23. Freeman RK, Dilts JR, Ascioti AJ, et al. A comparison of quality and cost indicators by surgical specialty for lobectomy of the lung. *J Thorac Cardiovasc Surg* 2013;145: 68–74.
24. Bogar L, Molnar Z, Tarsoly P, et al. Serum procalcitonin level and leukocyte antisedimentation rate as early predictors of respiratory dysfunction after oesophageal tumour resection. *Crit Care* 2006;10:R110.
25. Amar D, Zhang H, Park B, et al. Inflammation and outcome after general thoracic surgery. *Eur J Cardiothorac Surg* 2007;32:431–434.
26. Kim JY, Hildebrandt MA, Pu X, et al. Variations in the vascular endothelial growth factor pathway predict pulmonary complications. *Ann Thorac Surg* 2012;94: 1079–1085.
27. Bagan P, Berna P, De Dominicis F, et al. Nutritional status and postoperative outcome after pneumonectomy for lung cancer. *Ann Thorac Surg* 2013;95:392–396.
28. Cagini L, Andolfi M, Leli C, et al. B-type natriuretic peptide following thoracic surgery: a predictor of postoperative cardiopulmonary complications. *Eur J Cardiothorac Surg* 2014;46:e74–e80.
29. Tsiouris A, Hammoud ZT, Velanovich V, et al. A modified frailty index to assess morbidity and mortality after lobectomy. *J Surg Res* 2013;183:40–46.
30. Sheetz KH, Zhao L, Holcombe SA, et al. Decreased core muscle size is associated with worse patient survival following esophagectomy for cancer. *Dis Esophagus* 2013;26:716–722.
31. Hodari A, Hammoud ZT, Borgi JF, et al. Assessment of morbidity and mortality after esophagectomy using a modified frailty index. *Ann Thorac Surg* 2013;96:1240–1245.

32. Kozower BD, Sheng S, O'Brien SM, et al. STS database risk models: predictors of mortality and major morbidity for lung cancer resection. *Ann Thorac Surg* 2010;90:875–883.

33. Brunelli A, Varela G, Van Schil P, et al.; ESTS Audit and Clinical Excellence Committee. Multicentric analysis of performance after major lung resections by using the European Society Objective Score (ESOS). *Eur J Cardiothorac Surg* 2008;33:284–288.

34. Bernard A, Rivera C, Pages PB, et al. Risk model of in-hospital mortality after pulmonary resection for cancer: a national database of the French Society of Thoracic and Cardiovascular Surgery (Epithor). *J Thorac Cardiovasc Surg* 2011;141:449–458.

35. Ferguson MK, Saha-Chaudhuri P, Mitchell JD, et al. Prediction of major cardiovascular events after lung resection using a modified scoring system. *Ann Thorac Surg* 2014;97:1135–1140.

36. Reinersman JM, Allen MS, Deschamps C, et al. External validation of the Ferguson pulmonary risk score for predicting major pulmonary complications after oesophagectomy. *Eur J Cardiothorac Surg* 2016;49(1):333–338.

37. Brunelli A, Ferguson MK, Rocco G, et al. A scoring system predicting the risk for intensive care unit admission for complications after major lung resection: a multicenter analysis. *Ann Thorac Surg* 2008;86:213–218.

38. Wangensteen OH, Wangensteen SD. *The Rise of Surgery: From Empiric Craft to Scientific Discipline*. Minneapolis, MN: University of Minnesota Press; 1978; 453–473.

39. O'Rourke K. An historical perspective on meta-analysis: dealing quantitatively with varying study results. *J R Soc Med* 2007;100:579–582.

40. http://www.cochrane.org/. Accessed September 5, 2015.

41. http://www.gradeworkinggroup.org/index.htm. Accessed September 5, 2015.

42. Chassin MR, Kosecoff J, Solomon DH, et al. How coronary angiography is used: clinical determinants of appropriateness. *JAMA* 1987;258:2543–2547.

43. Eddy DM. Practice policies: guidelines for methods. *JAMA* 1990;263:1839–1841.

44. Eddy DM. Guidelines for policy statements. *JAMA* 1990;263:2239–2243.

45. http://www.nccn.org/. Accessed September 5, 2015.

46. http://aats.org/guidelines/. Accessed September 8, 2015.

47. http://www.sts.org/quality-research-patient-safety/research/practice-guidelines. Accessed September 5, 2015.

48. Bennett C, Vakil N, Bergman J, et al. Consensus statements for management of Barrett's dysplasia and early-stage esophageal adenocarcinoma, based on a Delphi process. *Gastroenterology* 2012;143:336–346.

49. Bennett C, Moayyedi P, Corley DA, et al. BOB CAT: a large-scale review and Delphi consensus for management of barrett's esophagus with no dysplasia, indefinite for, or low-grade dysplasia. *Am J Gastroenterol* 2015;110:662–682.

50. Low DE, Alderson D, Cecconello I, et al. International consensus on standardization of data collection for complications associated with esophagectomy: Esophagectomy Complications Consensus Group (ECCG). *Ann Surg* 2015;262:286–294.

51. Jagsi R, Huang G, Griffith K, et al. Attitudes toward and use of cancer management guidelines in a national sample of medical oncologists and surgeons. *J Natl Compr Canc Netw* 2014;12:204–212.

52. Cykert S, Kissling G, Hansen CJ. Patient preferences regarding possible outcomes of lung resection: what outcomes should preoperative evaluations target? *Chest* 2000;117:1551–1559.

53. Westaby S, Baig K, De Silva R, et al. Recruitment to UK cardiothoracic surgery in the era of public outcome reporting. *Eur J Cardiothorac Surg* 2015;47:679–683.

54. Romano PS, Marcin JP, Dai JJ, et al. Impact of public reporting of coronary artery bypass graft surgery performance data on market share, mortality, and patient selection. *Med Care* 2011;49:1118–1125.

55. Shahian DM, Edwards FH, Jacobs JP, et al. Public reporting of cardiac surgery performance: Part 1—history, rationale, consequences. *Ann Thorac Surg* 2011; 92(Suppl 3):S2–S11.

56. Hertwig R, Barron G, Weber EU, et al. Decisions from experience and the effect of rare events in risky choice. *Psychol Sci* 2004;15:534–539.

57. Dimick JB, Welch HG. The zero mortality paradox in surgery. *J Am Coll Surg* 2008; 206:13–16.

58. Kadzielski J, McCormick F, Herndon JH, et al. Surgeons' attitudes are associated with reoperation and readmission rates. *Clin Orthop Relat Res* 2015;473:1544–1551.

59. Contessa J, Suarez L, Kyriakides T, et al. The influence of surgeon personality factors on risk tolerance: a pilot study. *J Surg Educ* 2013;70:806–812.

60. Wilson CT, Woloshin S, Schwartz LM. Choosing where to have major surgery: who makes the decision? *Arch Surg* 2007;142:242–246.

61. Mead EL, Doorenbos AZ, Javid SH, et al. Shared decision-making for cancer care among racial and ethnic minorities: a systematic review. *Am J Public Health* 2013; 103:e15–e29.

62. Cykert S, Dilworth-Anderson P, Monroe MH, et al. Factors associated with decisions to undergo surgery among patients with newly diagnosed early-stage lung cancer. *JAMA* 2010;303:2368–2376.

63. Lathan CS, Neville BA, Earle CC. The effect of race on invasive staging and surgery in non-small-cell lung cancer. *J Clin Oncol* 2006;24:413–418.

64. Cykert S, Phifer N. Surgical decisions for early stage, non-small cell lung cancer: which racially sensitive perceptions of cancer are likely to explain racial variation in surgery? *Med Decis Making* 2003;23:167–176.

65. Dalton AF, Bunton AJ, Cykert S, et al. Patient characteristics associated with favorable perceptions of patient-provider communication in early-stage lung cancer treatment. *J Health Commun* 2014;19:532–544.

66. https://hbr.org/2015/10/measuring-and-communicating-health-care-value-with-charts. Accessed June 21, 2017.

67. Austin CA, Mohottige D, Sudore RL, et al. Tools to promote shared decision making in serious illness: a systematic review. *JAMA Intern Med* 2015;175:1213–1221.

68. Fagerlin A, Zikmund-Fisher BJ, Ubel PA. Cure me even if it kills me: preferences for invasive cancer treatment. *Med Decis Making* 2005;25:614–619.

69. Charles C, Gafni A, Whelan T. Shared decision-making in the medical encounter: what does it mean? (or it takes at least two to tango). *Soc Sci Med* 1997;44:681–692.

70. Gerteis M, Edgman-Levitan S, Daley J, et al. *Through the Patient's Eyes*. San Francisco, CA: Jossey-Bass; 1993.

71. Williamson JW, Goldschmidt PG, Colton T. The quality of medical literature: an analysis of validation assessments. In: Bailar JC, Mosteller F, eds. *Medical Uses of Statistics*. 1st ed. Waltham, MA: NEJM Books; 1986:370–391.

72. Glantz SA. It is all in the numbers. *J Am Coll Cardiol* 1993;21:835–837.

73. Hickey GL, Dunning J, Seifert B, et al.; EJCTS and ICVTS Editorial Committees. Statistical and data reporting guidelines for the European Journal of Cardio-Thoracic Surgery and the Interactive CardioVascular and Thoracic Surgery. *Eur J Cardiothorac Surg* 2015;48:180–193.

74. Grunkemeier GL, Jin R. Power and sample size: how many patients do I need? *Ann Thorac Surg* 2007;83:1934–1939.

75. Anscombe FJ. Graphs in statistical analysis. *Am Stat* 1973;27:17–21.

76. Hjellvik V, Selmer R, Gjessing HK, et al. Body mass index, smoking, and risk of death between 40 and 70 years of age in a Norwegian cohort of 32,727 women and 33,475 men. *Eur J Epidemiol* 2013;28:35–43.

77. McMurry TL, Hu Y, Blackstone EH, et al. Propensity scores: methods, considerations, and applications in the Journal of Thoracic and Cardiovascular Surgery. *J Thorac Cardiovasc Surg* 2015;150:14–19.

78. Deb S, Austin PC, Tu JV, et al. A review of propensity-score methods and their use in cardiovascular research. *Can J Cardiol* 2016;32(2):259–265.

79. Falcoz PE, Puyraveau M, Thomas PA, et al.; ESTS Database Committee and ESTS Minimally Invasive Interest Group. Video-assisted thoracoscopic surgery versus open lobectomy for primary non-small-cell lung cancer: a propensity-matched analysis of outcome from the European Society of Thoracic Surgeon database. *Eur J Cardiothorac Surg* 2016;49(2):602–609.

80. Ferguson MK, Im HK, Watson S, et al. Association of body mass index and outcomes after major lung resection. *Eur J Cardiothorac Surg* 2014;45:e94–e99.

81. Ferguson MK, Gaissert HA, Grab JD, et al. Pulmonary complications after lung resection in the absence of chronic obstructive pulmonary disease: the predictive role of diffusing capacity. *J Thorac Cardiovasc Surg* 2009;138:1297–1302.

82. Nurminen M. To use or not to use the odds ratio in epidemiologic analyses? *Eur J Epidemiol* 1995;11:365–371.

83. Holcomb WL, Chaiworapongsa T, Luke DA, et al. An odd measure of risk: use and misuse of the odds ratio. *Obstet Gynecol* 2001;98:685–688.

84. Arriagada R, Bergman B, Dunant A, et al.; International Adjuvant Lung Cancer Trial Collaborative Group. Cisplatin-based adjuvant chemotherapy in patients with completely resected non-small-cell lung cancer. *N Engl J Med* 2004;350:351–360.

85. Ferguson MK, Watson S, Johnson E, et al. Predicted postoperative lung function is associated with all-cause long-term mortality after major lung resection for cancer. *Eur J Cardiothorac Surg* 2014;45:660–664.

86. Pharoah PD, Sewell B, Fitzsimmons D, et al. Cost effectiveness of the NHS breast screening programme: life table model. *BMJ* 2013;346:f2618.

87. van Ballegooijen M, Habbema JDF, Boer R, et al. *A Comparison of the Cost-Effectiveness of Fecal Occult Blood Tests with Different Test Characteristics in the Context of Annual Screening in the Medicare Population*. Rockville, MD: Agency for Healthcare Research and Quality (US); 2003. Available at https://www.ncbi.nlm.nih.gov/books/NBK285640/

88. Black WC, Soneji SS, Sicks JD, et al.; National Lung Screening Trial Research Team. Cost-effectiveness of CT screening in the National Lung Screening Trial. *N Engl J Med* 2014;371:1793–1802.

89. Long EF, Swain GW, Mangi AA. Comparative survival and cost-effectiveness of advanced therapies for end-stage heart failure. *Circ Heart Fail* 2014;7:470–478.

90. Vasiliadis HM, Collet JP, Penrod JR, et al. A cost-effectiveness and cost-utility study of lung transplantation. *J Heart Lung Transplant* 2005;24:1275–1283.

91. Ferguson MK, Celauro AD, Vigneswaran WT. Validation of a modified scoring system for cardiovascular risk associated with major lung resection. *Eur J Cardiothorac Surg* 2012;41:598–602.

92. Brunelli A, Varela G, Salati M, et al. Recalibration of the revised cardiac risk index in lung resection candidates. *Ann Thorac Surg* 2010;90:199–203.

93. Brunelli A, Cassivi SD, Fibla J, et al. External validation of the recalibrated thoracic revised cardiac risk index for predicting the risk of major cardiac complications after lung resection. *Ann Thorac Surg* 2011;92:445–448.

94. Pforr A, Pagès PB, Baste JM, et al.; Epithor Project (French Society of Thoracic and Cardiovascular Surgery). A predictive score for bronchopleural fistula established using the French database Epithor. *Ann Thorac Surg* 2016;101(1):287–293.

95. Grunkemeier GL, Wu Y. Bootstrap resampling methods: something for nothing? *Ann Thorac Surg* 2004;77:1142–1144.

96. Zhang R, Ferguson MK. Video-assisted versus open lobectomy in patients with compromised lung function: a literature review and meta-analysis. *PLoS One* 2015; 10:e0124512.

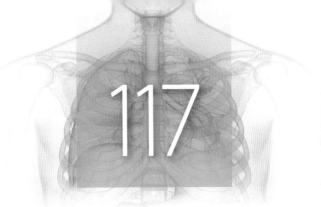

Clinical Practice Guidelines in General Thoracic Surgery

Robert E. Merritt

INTRODUCTION

In recent years, the Society of Thoracic Surgeons (STS) has constructed numerous practice guidelines based on evidence-based medicine derived from a complete review of current published studies on various topics. The clinical practice guidelines are intended to provide thoracic surgeons with guidance on the management of various clinical issues in Thoracic Surgery.[1] Clinical practice guidelines can be defined as consensus statements that include evidence-based recommendations that are provided to improve patient outcomes. In most cases, a panel of experts performs a systematic review of the literature and determines the benefits of management options based on the quality and strength of the supporting clinical data derived from clinical research studies. The strength of the practice guideline recommendation is directly linked to the strength of supporting clinical data. The strongest clinical guideline recommendations are usually directly coupled with well-designed randomized clinical trials. In addition to the STS, the American Association of Thoracic Surgery (AATS), the American College of Chest Physicians (ACCP), and the National Comprehensive Cancer Network (NCCN) have published clinical practice guidelines that are relevant to the management of thoracic diseases, such as lung cancer. This chapter will review the current clinical practice guidelines in General Thoracic Surgery.

METHODS FOR WRITING CLINICAL PRACTICE GUIDELINES

The scope of a clinical practice guideline and the specific questions that need to be addressed must be clearly defined by the panel of clinical experts who are assembled for review of the current published research studies. The literature search strategy should include searches of PubMed/MEDLINE, EMBASE, AMED, and Cochrane databases. The relevant articles need to be reviewed with rigor and validated prior to inclusion. The AGREE II instrument was developed to assess and validate the overall quality of clinical practice guidelines.[2] The AGREE II instrument evaluates clinical guidelines for biases, external validation, and feasibility for clinical practice.

Clinical guidelines should offer an assessment of the validity of each clinical recommendation. The strength of the recommendation is directly linked to the quality of the evidence in the published literature that supports the clinical guideline. The Grading of Recommendations, Assessment, Development, and Evaluation (GRADE) system provides a framework which can be utilized to determine the strength and quality of evidence that supports an individual clinical guideline.[3] Level IA represents a strong recommendation and high quality of evidence which is derived from randomized controlled clinical trials which are well designed. Level 1B represents a strong recommendation; however, the quality of evidence is from randomized controlled clinical trials with flawed methodology and spurious results. Level 1C represents a strong recommendation which is supported by a low level of evidence from observational studies or seriously flawed randomized controlled clinical trials. Level 2A represents a weak recommendation with high-quality evidence from a well-designed randomized controlled clinical trial. Level 2B represents a weak recommendation supported by moderate quality of evidence such as a poorly designed randomized, controlled clinical trial with inconsistent results. Finally, level 2C represents a weak recommendation with low-quality evidence derived from observational studies.

CURRENT CLINICAL PRACTICE GUIDELINES IN THORACIC SURGERY

Diagnosis and Staging of Esophageal Cancer

Esophageal Cancer remains among one of the most lethal forms of cancer in the world with an estimated 16,640 cases diagnosed a year and 14,500 deaths a year.[4] Despite advances in treatment, esophageal cancer remains one of the most lethal cancers with an overall 5-year survival rate of 15%. A taskforce is assembled through the Workforce on Evidence Based Surgery and General Thoracic Surgery Workforce of the STS to perform a systematic review on the diagnosis and staging of esophageal cancer.[5] The executive summary for diagnosis and staging of esophageal cancer is as follows.

1. Flexible endoscopy with biopsy is the primary method for the diagnosis of esophageal carcinoma. (Class I recommendation: level of evidence B.)
2. For early stage esophageal carcinoma, computed tomography of the chest and abdomen is an optional test for staging. (Class I recommendation: level of evidence B.)
3. For locoregional esophageal cancer, computed tomography of the chest and abdomen is the recommended test for clinical staging. (Class I recommendation: level of evidence B.)
4. For locoregional esophageal cancer, positron emission tomography (PET) is a recommended test for staging. (Class I recommendation: level of evidence B.)

5. For early stage esophageal cancer, positron emission tomography (PET) is an optional test for clinical staging. (Class II B recommendation: level of evidence B.)

6. In the absence of metastatic disease, endoscopic ultrasonography is recommended to improve the accuracy of clinical staging. (Class IIA recommendation: level of evidence B.)

7. Endoscopic mucosal resection (EMR) should be considered as a diagnostic/staging tool for small, discrete nodules or areas of dysplasia when the disease appears limited to the mucosa or submucosa as assessed by endoscopic ultrasonography. (Class II A recommendation: level of evidence B.)

8. For locally advanced (T3/T4) adenocarcinoma of the esophagogastric junction infiltrating the anatomic cardia, or Siewert type III esophagogastric tumors, laparoscopy is recommended to improve the accuracy of staging. (Class IIB recommendation: level of evidence C.)

Management of Barrett Esophagus With High-Grade Dysplasia

The management of Barrett esophagus with high-grade dysplasia remains controversial. The previous standard of care had been esophagectomy; however, endoscopic ablative therapies have become more commonplace in the management of Barrett esophagus with high-grade dysplasia. Endoscopic treatment options that obviate the need for esophagectomy include endoscopic surveillance, mucosal ablation, and endoscopic mucosal resection. The STS Guideline for the management of Barrett esophagus was divided into four main components: (1) endoscopic surveillance; (2) mucosal ablation; (3) endoscopic mucosal resection; and (4) esophagectomy.[6]

Endoscopic surveillance is clearly justified because the progression of metaplasia to adenocarcinoma is a widely accepted paradigm for esophageal carcinogenesis.[7] Surveillance is performed to detect early progression of Barrett esophagus to esophageal carcinoma. There are no randomized clinical trials comparing endoscopic biopsy methods for Barrett esophagus; however, a biopsy performed every 1 cm to 2 cm in four quadrants within the Barrett segment has become the standard.[8] The frequency of endoscopic surveillance for Barrett esophagus with high-grade dysplasia has been described as 3 to 6 months.[7,9]

Mucosal Ablative Therapies and Endoscopic Mucosal Ablation

Photodynamic therapy and radiofrequency ablation are the most common endoscopic ablative therapies that have been used for Barrett esophagus with high-grade dysplasia. The following recommendations from the STS are listed below:

1. The level of evidence for photodynamic therapy for ablation of residual intestinal metaplasia after endoscopic mucosal resection of a small intramucosal carcinoma in high-risk patients is class III (B).

2. Photodynamic therapy should be considered for the eradication of high-grade dysplasia in patients at high risk for undergoing esophagectomy. (Class III recommendation: level of evidence B.)

3. Radiofrequency ablation may be considered to treat patients with Barrett's intestinal metaplasia. (Class III recommendation: level of evidence B.)

4. Radiofrequency ablation may be effective for ablation of high-grade dysplasia; however, further clinical trials are necessary. (Class III recommendation: level of evidence B.)

5. It is reasonable to use endoscopic mucosal resection to excise discrete esophageal mucosal nodules that are small, flat, or

polyploidy in nature, and not invading deeper than the submucosa. Due to the multifocality of Barrett esophagus, a concomitant mucosal ablative procedure is frequently required to assure complete eradication of disease. (Class III recommendation: level of evidence B.)

The optimal management of Barrett esophagus with high-grade dysplasia remains controversial. Endoscopic surveillance requires strict adherence to established biopsy protocols and expert histologic interpretation. Mucosal ablative therapies are appropriate for high-risk patients and include photodynamic therapy and radiofrequency ablation. Endoscopic mucosal resection can be useful for evaluating nodules within a Barrett segment. Esophagectomy is still considered the standard approach for the definitive management of high-grade dysplasia and intramucosal adenocarcinoma at experienced centers. The use of ablative therapy and endoscopic mucosal resection for high-grade dysplasia will require additional clinical investigation.

Practice Guideline for Multimodality Management of Esophageal Carcinoma

The STS Workforce of Evidence Based Surgery comprised clinical guidelines for the management of esophageal cancer based on clinical stage.[10] In recent years, multimodality therapy has become the standard treatment for locally advanced esophageal carcinoma. The summary of the practice guideline recommendations are listed below.

1. After neoadjuvant therapy, patients without metastatic disease, in whom surgical resection can be safely performed, should receive esophageal resection. (Class I recommendation: level of evidence A.)

2. Patients with potentially curable, locally advanced esophageal cancer should be cared for in a multidisciplinary setting. (Class I recommendation: level of evidence B.)

3. Restaging studies after neoadjuvant therapy are recommended before resection to rule out interval development of distant metastatic disease. (Class I recommendation: level of evidence B.)

4. Endoscopic ultrasound restaging for residual local disease is inaccurate and can be omitted. (Class IIA recommendation: level of evidence B.)

5. A positron emission tomography scan is recommended for restaging after neoadjuvant therapy to detect interval development of distant metastatic disease. (Class IIA recommendation: level of evidence B.)

6. Neoadjuvant platinum-based doublet chemotherapy alone is beneficial before resection for patients with locally advanced esophageal adenocarcinoma. (Class IIA recommendation: level of evidence A.)

7. Neoadjuvant chemoradiation therapy should be used for locally advanced squamous cell cancer and either neoadjuvant chemotherapy or chemoradiation therapy of locally advanced adenocarcinoma; multimodality therapy has advantages over surgical resection alone. (Class IIA recommendation: level of evidence A.)

8. Patients with adenocarcinoma who have not received neoadjuvant therapy should be considered for adjuvant chemoradiotherapy if the pathologic specimen reveals regional lymph node disease. (Class IIA recommendation: level of evidence B.)

9. Radiotherapy as a monotherapy before resection is not recommended. (Class III recommendation: level of evidence A.)

Prophylaxis and Management of Atrial Fibrillation With General Thoracic Surgery Patients

Atrial fibrillation occurs between 12% and 44% of patients who undergo either a pulmonary resection or esophagectomy.[11] Despite a large body of literature on the management of atrial fibrillation in general thoracic surgery patients, there were no practice guidelines available. The STS Workforce of Evidence Based Surgery developed practice recommendations from an expansive review of the literature.[11] The American Association for Thoracic Surgery also released clinical guidelines for the prevention and management of perioperative atrial fibrillation and flutter.[12] The STS clinical guideline recommendations are listed below:

1. Patients taking beta-blockers before general thoracic surgery should have beta-blockade continued in the postoperative period. (Class I recommendation: level of evidence B.)
2. Patients with hemodynamically stable and symptomatically acceptable postoperative atrial fibrillation should receive a trial of rate control lasting approximately 24 hours. (Class I recommendation: level of evidence B.)
3. Patients with hemodynamically stable and symptomatically acceptable postoperative atrial fibrillation should receive a trial of rate control lasting approximately 24 hours. (Class I recommendation: level of evidence B.)
4. A selective beta-1 blocking agent is recommended as the initial drug for rate control in the absence of moderate–severe chronic obstructive pulmonary disease or active bronchospasm. (Class I recommendation: level of evidence B.)
5. Diltiazem should be the first agent used in the presence of moderate–severe chronic pulmonary disease or active bronchospasm. (Class I recommendation: level of evidence B.)
6. Patients with hemodynamically stable but symptomatically intolerable atrial fibrillation should be chemically cardioverted, with electrical cardioversion if chemical cardioversion fails. (Class I recommendation: level of evidence C.)
7. Amiodarone prophylaxis is reasonable to reduce the incidence of atrial fibrillation after general thoracic surgery (excluding pneumonectomy), according to strict dosing regimens. For patients undergoing pulmonary lobectomy, the recommended dose is 1,050 mg by continuous infusion over the first 24 hours after surgery, followed by 400 mg orally daily for 6 days. (Class III recommendation: level of evidence B.)
8. Diltiazem prophylaxis is reasonable in most patients undergoing major pulmonary resection who are not taking a beta-blocker preoperatively. The dose should be adjusted to avoid hypotension. (Class III recommendation: level of evidence B.)
9. Magnesium supplementation is reasonable to augment the prophylactic effects of other medications. (Class III recommendation: level of evidence B.)
10. For patients with fewer than two risk factors for stroke and patients considered not suitable for warfarin who have postoperative atrial fibrillation that recurs or persists for more than 48 hours, aspirin, 325 mg daily, is reasonable if aspirin is not contraindicated. (Class III recommendation: level of evidence A.)
11. For patients with two or more risk factors for stroke (age >75 years, hypertension, impaired ventricular function, prior stroke or transient ischemic attack) who have postoperative atrial fibrillation that recurs or persists for more than 48 hours, anticoagulation therapy is reasonable if not otherwise contraindicated. (Class III recommendation: level of evidence A.)

Lung Cancer Screening Guidelines

Lung cancer is the leading cause of cancer-related mortality in the United States with over 159,000 deaths annually.[13] Most lung cancer cases present in the later stages which result in poor overall survival rates despite therapeutic intervention. Early detection may offer a survival advantage when the lung cancers are discovered in the earliest stage which can be treated with a potentially curative surgical resection. The results from the National Lung Screening Trial supported the use of low-dose computed tomography to screen individuals at high risk for lung cancer.[14] The NCCN released clinical practice guidelines for lung cancer screening in 2011.[15] Lung cancer screening with low-dose computed tomography was recommended for patients aged 55 to 80 years old with a 30 pack-year or more history of smoking. This level of evidence is 1B due to the results of multiple randomized clinical trials assessing low-dose computed tomography lung cancer screening in high-risk groups. The NCCN guidelines also recommended low-dose computed tomography lung cancer screening for patients aged 50 years or older and a 20 pack-year or more history of smoking tobacco, and one additional risk factor, such as a family history of lung cancer and radon exposure. This is a level 2A recommendation because evidence was derived from nonrandomized clinical studies and observational data. Routine lung cancer screening is not recommended in low-risk populations which include patients aged less than 50 years and a less than a 20 year pack-year smoking history which is a level 2A recommendation.

Clinical Practice Guidelines for Stage I and Stage II Non–Small Cell Lung Cancer

The surgical management of stage I and stage II non–small cell lung cancer (NSCLC) is always undergoing constant evolution. The areas of debate center on intraoperative lymph node staging (lymph node sampling versus dissection), the role of sublobar resection for smaller tumors, and the use of minimally invasive techniques for anatomical resection, such as robotics and video-assisted techniques. The use of postoperative chemotherapy and radiation has also been included in practice guidelines for the management of early stage lung cancer. The ACCP have devised clinical practice guidelines for the management of stage I and stage II NSCLC.[16] The summary of the guidelines are listed below:

1. For patients with clinical stage I and II NSCLC and no medical contraindication to operative intervention, surgical resection is recommended. (Grade of recommendation, 1A.)
2. In patients with stage I and II NSCLC, who are medically fit for surgical resection, lobectomy or greater resection are recommended rather than sublobar resections (wedge resection or segmentectomy). (Grade of recommendation, 1A.)
3. For patients with completely resected stage IA NSCLC, the use of adjuvant chemotherapy is not indicated. (Grade of recommendation, 1A.)
4. For patients with completely resected stage II NSCLC and good performance status, the use of platinum-based adjuvant chemotherapy is recommended. (Grade of recommendation, 1A.)
5. For patients with clinical stage I and II NSCLC, it is recommended that they be evaluated by a thoracic surgical oncologist with expertise in lung cancer, even if they are being considered for nonsurgical options. (Grade of recommendation, 1B.)
6. In patients with stage I NSCLC who may tolerate operative intervention but not a lobectomy due to diminished pulmonary function, sublobar resection is recommended. (Grade of recommendation, 1B.)
7. The use of video-assisted thoracic surgery (VATS) by surgeons experienced in these techniques is an acceptable alternative to open thoracotomy. (Grade of recommendation, 1B.)
8. An intraoperative systematic mediastinal lymph node sampling or dissection should be performed for accurate pathologic staging. (Grade of recommendation, 1B.)

9. In patients with centrally located or locally advanced lung cancers, sleeve lobectomy is preferred over pneumonectomy for complete resection. (Grade of recommendation, 1B.)
10. For patients with N1 lymph node metastases, sleeve lobectomy is preferred over pneumonectomy to achieve a complete resection. (Grade of recommendation, 1B.)
11. For patients with completely resected stage IB NSCLC, the use of adjuvant chemotherapy is not recommended. (Grade of recommendation, 1B.)
12. For patients with stage I and II NSCLC who are not surgical candidates or refuse surgery, curative intent fractionated radiotherapy is recommended. (Grade of recommendation, 1B.)
13. For patients with completely resected stage IA and IB NSCLC, postoperative radiotherapy is associated with decreased survival and is not recommended. (Grade of recommendation, 1B.)

CONCLUSION

The STS, the AATS, the ACCP, and the NCCN have derived a series of clinical practice guidelines for the management of esophageal cancer, Barrett esophagus, atrial fibrillation, early stage lung cancer, the staging and diagnosis of esophageal cancer, and lung cancer screening with low-dose computed tomography. These guidelines are intended to provide evidenced-based clinical recommendations; however, they are not intended to be clinical mandates. Thoracic surgeons must astutely assess the quality of the literature that supports the clinical guideline before accepting the guideline as the current standard of care. The guidelines should serve as a reference point to assist thoracic surgeons in clinical decision making in the surgical management of a variety of complex disease processes. The clinical practice guidelines provide a comprehensive review of the current literature and the perspective of a consortium of experts in thoracic surgery, oncology, radiology, gastroenterology, and pulmonary medicine.

REFERENCES

1. Edwards FH, Ferguson TB. The Society of Thoracic Surgeons practice guidelines. *Ann Thorac Surg* 2004;77:1140–1141.
2. Haroon M, Ranmal R, McElroy H, et al. Developing clinical guidelines: how much rigour is required? *Arch Dis Child Educ Pract Ed* 2015;100(2):89–96.
3. Atkins D, Best D, Briss PA, et al. Grading quality of evidence and strength of recommendations. *BMJ* 2004;327:1490.
4. Cancer facts and figures 2014. American Cancer Society. http://www.cancer.org/research/cancerfacts/cancer-facts-and figures 2014. Accessed June 24, 2015.
5. Varghese Jr. TK, Hofstetter WL, Risk NP, et al. The Society of Thoracic Surgeons guidelines on the diagnosis and staging of patients with esophageal cancer. *Ann Thorac Surg* 2013;97:346–356.
6. Fernando HC, Murthy SC, Hofstetter W, et al. The Society of Thoracic Surgeons practice guideline series: guidelines for the management of Barrett's esophagus with high-grade dysplasia. *Ann Thorac Surg* 2009;87:1993–2002.
7. Hameeteman W, Tygat GN, Houthoff HJ, et al. Barrett's esophagus: development of dysplasia and adenocarcinoma. *Gastroenterology* 1989;96:1249–1256.
8. Reid BJ, Blount PL, Feng Z, et al. Optimizing endoscopic biopsy detection of early cancers in Barrett's high-grade dysplasia. *Am J Gastroenterol* 2000;95:3089–3096.
9. Schnell TG, Sontag SJ, Chejfec G, et al. Long-term nonsurgical management of Barrett's high-grade dysplasia. *Gastroenterology* 2001;120:1607–1619.
10. Little AG, Lerut AE, Harpole DH, et al. The Society of Thoracic Surgeons practice guidelines on the role of multimodality treatment for cancer of the esophagus and gastroesophageal junction. *Ann Thorac Surg* 2014;98:1880–1885.
11. Fernando HC, Jaklitsch MT, Walsh GL, et al. The Society of Thoracic Surgeons practice guideline on the prophylaxis and management of atrial fibrillation associated with general thoracic surgery: executive summary. *Ann Thorac Surg* 2011;92:1144–1152.
12. Frendl G, Sodickson AC, Chung MK, et al. 2014 AATS guidelines for the prevention and management of perioperative atrial fibrillation and flutter for thoracic surgical procedures. *J Thorac Cardiovasc Surg* 2014;148:e153–e193.
13. Siegel R, Ma J, Zou A, et al. Cancer Statistics, 2014. *Cancer J Clin* 2014;64:9–29.
14. National Lung Screening Trial Research Team, Aberle DR, Adams AM, et al. Reduced lung-cancer mortality with low-dose computed tomographic screening. *N Engl J Med* 2011;365:395–409.
15. Wood DE, Kazerooni E, Baum SL, et al. Lung cancer screening, version 1.2015. *J Natl Compr Canc Netw* 2015;13:23–34.
16. Scott WJ, Howington J, Feigenberg S, et al. Treatment of non-small cell lung cancer stage I and stage II: ACCP evidence-based clinical practice guidelines (2nd ed.). *Chest* 2007;132:234S–242S.

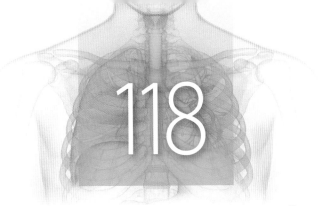

Rationale for and Use of Large National Databases

Yinin Hu ▪ Varun Puri ▪ Benjamin D. Kozower

INTRODUCTION

From late in the twentieth century until now, the medical community has witnessed the transition from single-institutional reports comprised of hundreds of patients to Cochrane meta-analyses summarizing thousands of patients, and ultimately to national administrative and clinical database queries including tens of thousands of patients. Cardiothoracic surgery has been a leader in the use of robust databases largely because coronary artery bypass grafting (CABG) was one of the most common and expensive surgical procedures performed. Surgeons, hospitals, insurance companies, government, and other stakeholders were all using different data sources to measure CABG outcomes and compare providers. The Society of Thoracic Surgeons (STS) National Database is a robust, risk-adjusted database established in 1989 as an initiative for quality improvement and patient safety among cardiothoracic surgeons. As a result, the STS database has come to be acknowledged by other specialties, government and consumer groups, and third-party payers as the gold-standard clinical data analysis registry.

The importance of collating and analyzing large groups of patients, now accepted as self-evident, was not broadly recognized until the 1970s. Lindberg described that the development of storage mechanisms for patient medical history and integrating those systems within a hospital ranked among the most complex of medical innovations.[1] However, even this level of complexity is no longer adequate to satisfy the appetite of today's evidence-based practitioner. Elementary statistics dictates that the ability to discern associations between two or more clinical features is greatly affected by sample size. Thus, for uncommon features and small effect sizes, single-hospital records of patient history may not provide adequate power for meaningful study. In addition, reliance upon single-institution data inevitably leads to questions of generalizability.

Frawley and colleagues define *databases* as a logically integrated collection of data organized to facilitate the storage, modification, and retrieval of information.[2] The authors describe two processes integral to the extraction of knowledge from databases: identifying an interesting pattern and describing the pattern concisely and meaningfully. Computer-based databases first arose in the 1950s, when physicians brought patient records to a central computer for processing. Communication between computers through telephone lines in the 1960s allowed concurrent data processing from multiple sites. By the 1980s, the emergence of microcomputers saw massive expansion of storage capacity. As computer access became widely available in the 1990s, electronic medical records (EMRs) crept into clinical practice. Finally, in the 2000s, advancements in informatics and coding facilitated the automated collection of data from EMR to bring medical databases to their current state.[3]

CLASSIFICATION

Medical databases are considered *primary* if data are collected initially for the direct purposes of the user; and are considered *secondary* if data are derived from other primary databases for objectives not originally tied to the data collection.[4] For example, a hospital's EMR may be considered a primary database, as the repository of data is used by clinicians and other providers during patient care. A database like the STS, which employs professional data abstractors who comb through EMRs in order to accumulate clinical data for quality-control and research purposes, is an example of a secondary database.

Databases may be further divided into clinical, claims, biosurveillance, medical knowledge, and other subcategories, based on their primary objectives. Broadly, clinical databases are used primarily to lend insight into patient care. Administrative databases have the primary objective of arranging payments for claims of provided clinical services. Many of these use discharge abstracts and are considered administrative databases. Biosurveillance databases aim to track epidemiological patterns of clinical features, for example, to maintain records of adverse drug events or potential infectious epidemics. Finally, medical knowledge databases collate data from a variety of sources including textbooks and other publications in order to communicate information and expand medical exploration.[3] This chapter will focus on the use of clinical and administrative databases to improve quality of care and lend evidence to medical decision making.

Michalski and colleagues describe two primary purposes of clinical databases: (1) to identify features and patterns through descriptive analyses and (2) to derive classification rules through predictive analyses.[5] These databases are characterized by large volumes of clinically relevant patient-level data and are typically designed to facilitate retrieval and analyses for clinical objectives. Such databases can be specialized to focus on disease-specific, therapy-specific, or population-specific data, and their scope can vary from single provider to international. They can even be designed exclusively for research purposes, in which case data are commonly extracted from

TABLE 118.1 Features of Administrative and Clinical Database Categories

| | Single Institution | | Multi-Institution | |
	Research Database	Hospital Database	Administrative Database	National Clinical Database
Features				
Purpose	Research	Quality/research/reimbursement	Reimbursement	Quality/research
Origin	Individual investigators	Hospital	Public	Clinical societies
Support	Private/public	Private	Public	Public/clinical societies
Quality of Data				
Comprehensiveness	++	+++	––	++
Completeness	+++	+	++	++
Data accuracy	+++	+++	–	++
Potential bias	–	+++	––	+
Patients				
Sample size	–––	––	+++	++
Rare disease	+++	–––	++	+
Heterogeneity	––	+	+++	+
Generalizability	–––	–	+++	+
Pragmatism				
Accessibility	++	+++	+++	–
Independence	++	+++	++	–
Cost	–––	++	+	+

(+), strength; (–), weakness.

other primary medical databases to address one or more specific, clinically relevant questions. Because clinical databases support such broad purposes, the degree of detail and breadth of information contained within each database varies greatly. Typically, they are designed with clinical decision making in mind, and therefore contain accurate information on patient history, comorbidities, laboratory values, functional testing, and outcomes.

Administrative databases are records of transactions that are purported to have occurred between patients and providers, and their data are derived from bills (claims) submitted to public or private insurance organizations. Although not designed for clinical purposes, these databases do have several strengths, namely, they are anonymous (and therefore do not require patient authorization for use), inexpensive, widely available, associated with cost structures, and typically contain very large population samples. However, administrative databases are limited by their primary objective: payment. Reimbursements are usually classified based on the International Classification of Diseases (ICD-CM) coding system. Diagnoses, procedures, and events that are not reimbursed are therefore often inadequately captured. For example, because pediatric immunizations may be bundled into standard outpatient visits, they may be underreported in administrative databases. Chronic diseases and comorbidities are often underreported because each provider interaction is usually classified by one reimbursement diagnosis. Not infrequently, the billing diagnosis for a provider interaction may not be the primary reason for the visit, but rather the code which could provide the highest reimbursement supported by the medical record.[6] Acknowledging that individual databases within each category may vary greatly; a simplified overview of the characteristics, strengths, and weakness of clinical and administrative databases is presented in Table 118.1.

RATIONALE

QUALITY IMPROVEMENT

The use of multi-institutional outcomes to stimulate improvement in patient quality of care is a movement born in the second half of the nineteenth century. In a letter to the International Statistical Congress in 1860, Florence Nightingale advocated for the collection of hospital statistics for comparative outcomes assessment. This was later expanded upon by a proposal for the expansion of outcomes data for surgical operations in 1863.[7] The next great leap in medical transparency took place in the United States with the 1986 publication of hospital mortality rates by the Health Care Financing Administration, a predecessor of the Centers for Medicare and Medicaid Services.[8] This early report heralded the advent of several subsequent initiatives, including those implemented by the STS, the Veterans Administration, and state-specific groups. From the outset, these databases saw important applications in outcomes reporting, risk adjustment, and resource utilization.

Beginning in the late 1980s, public demand for transparency led to the use of databases for outcomes reporting. In 1991, *Newsweek* sued the New York State Department of Health to obtain outcomes for coronary artery bypass (CABG) linked to individual surgeons. The movement was reinforced by the Supreme Court of New York, which dictated that the public was entitled to this clinical information.[9] The quality implications of public reporting of cardiac surgical outcomes in New York have been studied extensively. Public reporting of CABG report cards was associated with a 41% decline in risk-adjusted CABG mortality rate in New York.[10] Through an innovative trial that studied public report cards for myocardial infarction and heart failure, Tu and colleagues demonstrated that public reporting was associated with a reduction in 30-day myocardial infarction mortality, but did not significantly impact adherence to process measures.[11] Whether these associations were truly due to incentives driven by public reporting or simply an effect of institutional feedback is unclear. Northern New England had similar trends in declining mortality over the same period as New York.[12] Unlike New York, New England had instituted a system of confidential feedback reports for providers and collaborative policies that promoted best-practice dissemination. Work by Guru and colleagues mirrored these findings, noting that postoperative mortality following CABG decreased 29% in Ontario following institution of confidential reporting, but that no further reduction was associated with a subsequent transition to public reporting.[13]

To date, there is no national system that reports cardiothoracic surgical outcomes for all hospitals and individual surgeons in the United States. In contrast, the Heart Surgery in Great Britain website (http://heartsurgery.healthcarecommission.org.uk) covers all public cardiac units and nearly 200 individual surgeons. However, 37 states and the District of Columbia mandate reporting for inpatient hospital data at the state level.[14] These reports may include actual mortality rates or categorical outcomes such as "higher than expected"

or "lower than expected." While some states including California and New Jersey construct reports through clinical data from the STS database, others may use administrative data alone. The impact of these state-level public reports appears substantial. In New York, patients who chose top-performing providers had approximately half the chance of dying as those who chose a provider from the bottom quartile, and surgeons with high mortality rates were more likely to retire or leave practice than lower-mortality counterparts.[15]

One of the primary critiques of early public outcomes reporting was the inadequacy of patient-level risk adjustment. Early attempts to assess illness severity of patients for CABG did not adequately represent patient comorbidities or physiologic measures such as ejection fraction, emergent procedures, or the need for intra-aortic balloon pump.[16] Great strides have taken place since that time, particularly within the STS database, which now risk-adjusts for patients undergoing CABG through a 24-variable algorithm that uses Bayes theorem.[17] Due to a lack of present-on-admission information, risk adjustment using administrative databases provides an added challenge. Two common comorbidity metrics designed specifically to interpret administrative data are the Charlson and Elixhauser indices (Table 118.2).[18,19] Elixhauser, the more recent of the two, is notable in that it was designed for databases lacking present-on-admission flags

TABLE 118.2 Comparison of the Charlson and Elixhauser Comorbidity Indices

System	Charlson (Weight)	Elixhauser
Cardiovascular	Myocardial infarct (1) Congestive heart failure (1) Peripheral vascular disease (1)	Congestive heart failure Peripheral vascular disorder Arrhythmia Valvular disease Hypertension Coagulopathy Blood loss anemia Deficiency anemia
Pulmonary	Chronic pulmonary disease (1)	Chronic pulmonary disease Pulmonary circulation disorder
GI/HPB	Ulcer (1) Mild liver disease (1) Moderate/severe liver disease (3)	Peptic ulcer disease excluding bleeding Liver disease
Metabolic	Diabetes (1) Diabetes with end organ damage (2)	Diabetes, uncomplicated Diabetes, complicated Hypothyroidism Obesity Weight loss
GU	Moderate/severe renal disease (2)	Renal failure Fluid/electrolyte disorders
Neurologic	Cerebrovascular disease (1) Hemiplegia (2) Dementia (1)	Paralysis Other neurologic
Oncologic	Any tumor (2) Lymphoma (2) Metastatic solid tumor (6) Leukemia (2)	Solid tumor without metastases Lymphoma Metastatic cancer
Other	Connective tissue disease (1) AIDS (6)	AIDS Rheumatoid arthritis/collagen vascular disease Alcohol abuse Drug abuse Psychosis Depression

entirely. As both sets of comorbidities miss a number of clinically relevant chronic conditions, numerous modifications have been proposed.[20,21] In a systematic review of comparative studies on administrative data, Sharabiani and colleagues summarized the predictive performance of several common risk-adaptation indexes, noting in particular that index performance differed substantially based on whether the predictive outcome was short- or long-term mortality.[22]

Administrative and clinical databases can both lend to studies on resource utilization. Clinical databases are often the source for outcomes following interventions of interest, while national administrative databases frequently provide both reliable records of provider interactions and generalizable cost structures for decision analyses. For example, early postoperative readmissions are often viewed as indicators of suboptimal quality of care and have come under increasing scrutiny as a potential target for health-care resource reduction.[23] Using the administrative Medicare Provider Analysis and Review (MEDPAR) files, Shih assessed the reliability of postoperative readmission following CABG as a quality measure across 1,210 hospitals.[24] Concluding that relatively few hospitals had case volumes adequate to make readmission rate a meaningful and reliable quality metric, the authors argued against the use of readmission as an indicator of quality in cardiac surgery. The Medicare administrative database has also been used to demonstrate an absence of variability—following risk adjustment—in readmission rates following pulmonary resection for cancer.[25] In aggregate, studies such as these have potential implications in the United States for national policy-level decisions affecting how health-care dollars are and will be distributed.

RESEARCH

The utility of large national databases in facilitating clinically relevant research cannot be overstated. These resources offer the opportunity for large-scale, population-based research with existing, archived data, and avoid limitations of other epidemiological studies such as nonresponse and drop-out. Because they are often abstracted from multi-institutional clinical records and anonymized by a third party, database research is often exempt from institutional review. Perhaps the greatest strength of national databases is their sheer sample size, which supports wide-ranging research methodologies ranging from descriptive epidemiology to prognostic modeling, propensity matching, and cohort investigations.[26]

There are few circumstances in which the power of a large sample size is felt more readily than in the study of rare diseases. In the United States, a rare disease is defined as a disorder with a prevalence of less than 200,000 people.[27] The public promotion of studies investigating therapeutics targeting rare diseases is captured by the Orphan Drug Act of 1983. Among the many diseases that have benefited from the law's incentivizing policies are important pulmonary therapies such as epoprostenol for pulmonary hypertension, tobramycin for pseudomonal infections in the setting of cystic fibrosis, and aprotinin for prophylaxis against perioperative blood loss. Integral to today's rare diseases research effort is the data management coordinating center (DMCC), which develops data management systems for the collection, storage, and analysis of data for rare diseases across numerous institutions.[28] International rare disease patient registries are some of the most progressive large database efforts; these registries are anticipated to help formulate research hypotheses, recruit subjects for clinical trials, and survey the effect of recently approved interventions.[29]

An equally important advantage of large national databases—particularly administrative databases—is the consistency with which they may capture long-term patient outcomes. While single-institutional registries and cohort studies require costly prospective follow-up

with substantial drop-out and nonresponse rates, databases such as the MEDPAR file that store provider claims will often track clinical interactions throughout a patient's lifetime. For example, postoperative outcomes are often tracked by departmental registries to 30 days following discharge. Thereafter, particularly for high-volume cardiothoracic surgery centers, patients often follow up with or are readmitted to hospitals different from the operating hospital. In a recent study using the Surveillance, Epidemiology, and End Results-Medicare (SEER-Medicare) database, we found that more than one in four postoperative readmissions following lung resection were to facilities that did not perform the original operation.[25] These readmissions would have likely been missed by clinical databases focusing only on readmissions to operating providers. Fernandez and colleagues recently used the same database to show the association between early readmission and long-term survival following esophagectomy, taking advantage of longitudinal outcomes not available through departmental records or even the STS database.[30]

LIMITATIONS AND PITFALLS

ETHICAL PITFALLS

Use of large national databases for quality monitoring or research purposes is not without significant limitations and potential pitfalls. While limitations are frequently stated in peer-reviewed research publications, the societal impact of quality monitoring using national databases may be equally—if not more—problematic. When the New York State Department of Health developed the Cardiac Surgery Reporting System—the first physician-specific mortality report of its kind—substantial concerns arose regarding the internal consistency of risk factor coding instruments.[31] Because the mortality reports were risk-adjusted, providers could "game the system" by up-coding patient comorbidities and surgical complexity to manipulate publically perceived outcomes. Even more concerning is the incentivization of unwarranted denial of care to high-risk patients and other risk-aversion tactics. Omoigui and colleagues noted an increase in high-risk transfers to the Cleveland Clinic from New York after the latter region introduced public report cards.[32] Survey studies in the same period demonstrated reduced willingness to operate on high-risk patients and difficulties in referring this population to surgeons.[33,34] However, not all studies show the same reactionary patterns. For example, Hannan and colleagues found a higher proportion of high-risk patients in states with public reporting than in those that did not.[35] Whether this finding was due to a true absence of risk aversion or the presence of up-coding strategies in regions with public reporting is unclear.

QUALITY OF DATA

There are several caveats to the use of large databases in research. National databases are often expensive to acquire, and the volume and organization of data are such that a dedicated, trained statistician is usually necessary to interpret and analyze the information. Independent of resource requirements, the quality of data within national databases is also variable. Because administrative databases exist to support billing and claims, nonessential data for billing may be excluded and very disparate clinical entities are often grouped together under a single code. Despite mandated reporting of some quality measures independent of billing processes, more and more data will likely be excluded from administrative databases as the Center for Medicare and Medicaid Services (CMS) progressively extends its do-not-pay list.[6] As a result, reductions in the prevalence of chronic diseases, readmissions, and other under-claimed features recorded in administrative databases in the near future may not reflect true epidemiologic patterns. For clinical databases, it is imperative to know if they are audited and what their accuracy rates are when interpreting the results of a study.

Financial and quality incentives for up-coding also impact research reliability. Up-coding for the purpose of increasing hospital reimbursement is known as "code creep." In 1999, Psaty and colleagues studied 485 patients with a discharge diagnosis of heart failure and found that more than one-third of patients did not have clinical records to support the diagnosis.[36] They concluded that up-coding for heart failure alone was costing Medicare $993 million annually. Up-coding may also occur to manipulate perceived quality. Siregar and colleagues prospectively studied cardiac surgery patients across the Netherlands using the EuroSCORE risk-adjustment metric to assess the potential effect of up-coding on provider quality measures. They concluded that misclassification of high-risk patients by as little as a 1.1-fold increase in EuroSCORE can greatly influence perceived provider performance.[37]

To characterize information reliability, numerous studies have scrutinized the concordance across databases and between databases and medical records. Broadly, these studies have found that accuracy of administrative data varies based on the objectivity of the service or diagnosis in question. In a study of the validity of the Complications Screening Program—a system that screens for in-hospital complications by abstracting data from discharge records, McCarthy and colleagues found that 9% to 37% of screened complications did not have substantiating clinical records, including postoperative pneumonia (20%), postoperative deep vein thrombosis (33%), and wound infection (37%). Quan and colleagues reviewed 1,200 medical charts across three Canadian hospitals in detail to measure the validity of the existing administrative database based on ICD-9 procedure codes and found that agreement was high for major procedures (cholecystectomy, appendectomy, colectomy, etc.), while less than half of minor procedures (radiography, computerized tomography, coronary angiography, endotracheal intubation, etc.) had greater than 50% agreement between the administrative database and detailed review.[38] In a direct comparison between Medicare and SEER files regarding treatment of cancer, Cooper and colleagues found high concordance for major surgical resections (≥85%) but lower agreement for biopsies and local excisions (≤50%). There were even greater inconsistencies in the capturing of radiation therapy and chemotherapy.[39] Taken in aggregate, these studies suggest that administrative databases may be reliable for major interventions and events such as major surgery, readmission, and death, but not for comorbidities, complications, and minor treatments.

METHODOLOGICAL PITFALLS

There are potential pitfalls regarding the ways by which large patient samples may be used in research. Daly and colleagues summarized the fundamentals of basic biostatistics by demonstrating that significance level (p-value), the smallest clinically meaningful difference, and the statistical power are all interrelated.[40] Just as a small clinical study may not be able to demonstrate statistical significance despite a measurable difference in treatment outcome, a study of extremely large samples can generate statistically significant results for clinically meaningless differences in observed effects. A classic example lies in the thyroid cancer literature. In a study of more than 50,000 patients using the National Cancer Database (NCDB), Bilimoria and colleagues concluded that papillary thyroid cancers ≥1 cm in size

should undergo total thyroidectomy (rather than lobectomy) due to improved survival (p = 0.04). While the hazard ratio of lobectomy was 1.31, the absolute risk difference at 5 years was less than 1%, and less than 3% at 10 years.[41] When reviewing studies with sample sizes in the tens of thousands, any result with a borderline level of significance (p ≈ 0.05) should prompt a thoughtful interpretation of the clinical significance of absolute risk differences.

Another common and flawed methodology is to conduct data-driven—rather than hypothesis-driven—statistical analyses. Also known as "data-mining" or "fishing," such tactics take advantage of the reverence with which many readers regard statistical significance (p <0.05). Statistical inference logic is based on the rejection of a null hypothesis if the observed data are unlikely under the null hypothesis. However, by increasing the number of hypotheses tested, a researcher increases the likelihood of witnessing a rare event, and therefore increases the likelihood of making a type 1 error. From a practical perspective, if a researcher investigates 20 variables related to an outcome, 1 of them is likely to be significant purely by chance (5% or p = 0.05). A classic approach to adjust for this error is to use a lower p-value through calculations such as a Bonferroni correction (to test for n hypotheses on a set of data, test each hypothesis at a significance level of $1/n$ times what it would be for a single hypothesis).[42] A more fitting approach is to perform hypothesis-driven research, by which multiplicity is avoided by only testing hypotheses that are clinically meaningful.

SUMMARY OF MAJOR NATIONAL DATABASES

In this section, features of several commonly used national databases are summarized, and examples of cardiothoracic research conducted using each database are provided. A summary of the features, of each database is provided in Table 118.3.

MEDPAR

Features

The MEDPAR file contains data from claims for services provided to Medicare beneficiaries admitted to certified inpatient hospitals and skilled nursing facilities.[43] Managed care organization data are excluded. Each record in MEDPAR represents an inpatient stay. Data include beneficiary demographics, diagnosis codes, surgeries, and dates of care. Death records are tracked for up to 3 years following the most recent inpatient discharge. Records also include the facility that provides each service. MEDPAR has been used for medical research since the 1980s; its current file includes data from the years 1999 through 2013. Acquisition of identifiable data requires review by the Research Data Assistance Center and CMS.

Examples of Research

Welke and colleagues conducted a comparative study between the STS's National Cardiac Database (NCD) and MEDPAR.[44] The group identified Medicare beneficiaries undergoing cardiac surgery between 1993 and 2001 within MEDPAR Part A files using ICD-9 codes and a comparison patient sample within NCD over the same period. For hospitals that matched across both databases, MEDPAR captured a smaller proportion of patients aged 65 and older (likely due to growth of Medicare-managed care). MEDPAR coded fewer comorbidities than NCD. Annual in-hospital mortality rates for

TABLE 118.3 Major Databases Relevant to Thoracic Surgery

	Type	Coverage	Diseases	Patient Data	Pathology Data	Treatments	Outcomes[a]	Research Topics
MEDPAR	Admin	Medicare inpatients	All	Demographics	Diagnosis codes	Hospitalizations Length of stay Surgeries Facilities Total charge	3 yrs	Cost-effectiveness Long-term outcomes
SEER	Admin	Regional (28% national)	Cancer	Demographics	Diagnosis codes Staging Pathologic subtypes Multiple primaries	Surgery Chemo/radiation	Survival Progression Cause of death	Epidemiology Predictive models
NIS	Admin	All inpatients	All	Demographics Comorbidities	Diagnosis codes	Hospital features Length of stay Total charge	Discharge status	Cost-effectiveness Short-term outcomes Provision of care
NCDB	Admin	Accredited facilities (70% national)	Cancer	Demographics	Diagnosis codes Staging Histology	Detailed cancer treatment profile	Long term	Long-term outcomes
NSQIP	Clinical	>500 facilities 8-day sampling cycle	All	Demographics Comorbidities	Diagnosis codes	Detailed surgical treatment profile	30-day mortality/ morbidity	Quality of care Perioperative outcomes
STS-GTSD	Clinical	>230 facilities	Thoracic	Demographics Physiologic testing Comorbidities	Diagnosis codes Staging Histology	Detailed surgical treatment profile	30-day mortality/ morbidity	Quality of care Perioperative outcomes

[a]Most databases with long-term outcomes also retain short-term outcome measures.

CABG were similar between the two databases, with less than 1% difference for the majority of hospitals. However, postoperative mortality (in-hospital plus 30-day mortality) was higher in the MEDPAR database, highlighting its ability to capture deaths that occur prior to discharge, but more than 30 days following an operation.

MEDPAR has been used to study both quality and cost in general thoracic surgery. Using data from 1998 to 1999, Goodney and colleagues characterized three classes of surgeon providers for pulmonary resection: general surgeons, cardiothoracic surgeons, and noncardiac thoracic surgeons. General surgeons were found to have a 7.6% adjusted operative mortality rate, compared to 5.6% and 5.8% for cardiothoracic and noncardiac thoracic surgeons, respectively. A significant difference persisted when analyses were restricted to high-volume hospitals (>45 resections annually).[45] In a cost-analysis study, Cipriano and colleagues identified more than 60,000 lung cancer patients through SEER-Medicare to estimate costs for various phases of treatment. While outpatient costs were derived from a variety of sources including the National Claims History, the Outpatient Standard Analytical File, and durable medical equipment files, inpatient costs were drawn exclusively from MEDPAR.[46]

SURVEILLANCE, EPIDEMIOLOGY, AND END RESULTS

Features

The SEER program is sponsored by the National Cancer Institute and comprises population-based tumor registries collecting information on all incident cancer cases across a limited number of regions in the United States. Data are organized by incident case, and include patient demographics, date of diagnosis, cancer characteristics, treatments provided, vital status follow-up, and cause of death. Notably absent from SEER are modes of screening and diagnosis, patient comorbidities, and long-term disease status. Furthermore, treatments provided greater than 4 months following an initial cancer diagnosis are not recorded.[47] Data collection began in 1973 and has progressively expanded in coverage; however, even the most recent registry (SEER 18) includes only 28% of the US population.[48] Earlier registries (SEER 9) cover a smaller fraction of patients, but with more years of available data. Beginning with SEER 9, the Multiple Primary-Standardized Incidence Ratios (MP-SIR) method was made available to perform multiple primary analyses, providing the ability to link two cancers epidemiologically and draw etiologic inferences. In 1991, SEER became substantially more relevant to outcomes research through linkage with MEDPAR data. Patients are matched by social security number, name, gender, and date of birth.[49]

Examples of Research

In its original unlinked form, SEER is optimized for epidemiologic studies of disease incidence and prognosis. Hamid and colleagues used SEER to study the survival outcomes of Asian pacific islanders with nonsmall-cell lung cancer (NSCLC). Assessing over 150,000 incident cases between 2004 and 2010, the group concluded that, compared to non-Hispanic whites, Asian pacific islanders were diagnosed earlier, were more likely to undergo surgical treatment, and had superior survival for stage I, II, and IV disease.[50] To characterize the independent impact of tumor size on survival for NSCLC, Zhang and colleagues modeled overall survival using SEER-derived risk factors including demographics, histology, and primary tumor extension. In 15 of 16 subgroups categorized by tumor extension and node status, tumor size was found to be significantly predictive of overall survival under multivariable analysis.[51]

After linking with MEDPAR claims data, SEER offers unique opportunities to capture outcomes following operations for cancer. In two studies on lung resection outcomes for NSCLC, our group found that 90-day mortality was double that at 30 days, and that readmission within 30 days is associated with a sixfold increase in the rate of subsequent mortality.[25,52] Fernandez and colleagues used SEER-Medicare data to show that readmission following esophagectomy for esophageal cancer has an impact not just on early outcomes, but on long-term survival as well.[30]

NATIONAL INPATIENT SAMPLE (NIS)

Features

The NIS (at times, also called the Nationwide Inpatient Sample) was developed as a part of the Healthcare Cost and Utilization Project, sponsored by the Agency for Healthcare Research and Quality. The largest publicly available all-payer inpatient medical database in the United States, the NIS was redesigned in 2012 to be organized by discharge, rather than by hospital.[53] Data within NIS are composed of a 20% sample of discharges from participating hospitals, stratified by hospital characteristics such as teaching/nonteaching, region, and rural/urban. Unlike SEER, NIS represents more than 95% of the US population. Unlike MEDPAR, state and hospital identifiers are not provided, thus limiting its applications for quality-of-care research. NIS data include patient demographics, diagnoses, procedures, hospital characteristics, total charges, discharge status, length of stay, and comorbidities.

Examples of Research

Highlighting the comprehensive nature of the NIS database in general thoracic surgery is a study by our group in 2012. Comparing esophagectomies across three databases—NIS, STS's General Thoracic Database (GTDB), and National Surgical Quality Initiative Program (NSQIP)—the study showed that GTDB and NSQIP only represented small minorities of the total estimated resections nationwide.[54] Because NIS has a large catchment, cost assessments using this database are also some of the most generalizable. Gopaldas and colleagues used the 2004 and 2006 NIS database to compare outcomes and hospitalization costs of video-assisted thoracoscopic (VATS) versus open lobectomies. The authors noted that, although the VATS group had a higher intraoperative complication rate, clinical outcomes and hospitalization costs were similar across the two groups.[55]

The NIS is also conducting research on trends in provision of care. Taking advantage of NIS's inclusion of low-volume centers and availability of hospital characteristics, Al-Refaie and colleagues studied the population of patients who received cancer surgery at low-volume hospitals. The group discovered that patients who were minorities, had nonprivate insurance, and had more comorbidities were more likely to receive complex cancer operations (including esophagectomies and lung resections) at low-volume hospitals.[56] In a study of national discharges between 2001 and 2012, Ford noted that the hospitalization rate for lung cancer decreased, while the average charge per hospitalization increased. Meanwhile, age-adjusted hospitalizations for chronic obstructive pulmonary disease did not change.

These findings indicated that, despite expansive antismoking efforts, the health-care burden of smoking-related illness had not subsided.[57]

NATIONAL CANCER DATA BASE

Features

The NCDB was created in 1989 and is jointly sponsored by the American College of Surgeons and the American Cancer Society. Unlike SEER, which has a geographically based coverage, NCDB only collects hospital registry data from 1,500 Commission on Cancer-accredited facilities. The included data represent approximately 70% of incident cancer cases nationwide.[58] Importantly, these data include all incident cancer patients and not just patients receiving a surgical procedure as seen with NSQIP or STS. Data are submitted by the accredited facilities using standardized criteria and include patient demographics, cancer stage, histology, treatment, and outcomes. Due to its original purpose to evaluate patient management and compare cancer care outcomes, NCDB is ideally suited to study cancer treatment practice profiles, create survival reports, and conduct quality-of-care research. At present, the NCDB is accessible only to members of the American College of Surgeons. For access, researchers must apply for a Participant User File (PUF), which contains de-identified patient-level data that do not identify hospitals or providers. The NCDB also has in place extensive processes to ensure de-identification, thus, geographic data are very broad (New England, Middle Atlantic, etc.), no specific date items are provided, and each accredited facility is given a unique facility identifier.

Examples of Research

Although NCDB includes more incident cases than SEER, it does not necessarily represent the most generalizable population. For example, in a comparison of breast, colorectal, lung, and prostate cancer cases between the two databases in 1992, NCDB contained nearly six times the number of lung cancer cases as SEER. The NCDB was also more complete in its reporting of lung cancer laterality and staging. However, SEER data were more complete regarding the Hispanic heritage of patients across all cancer types and also included a greater proportion of Asian-American and American Indian patients.[59]

The most common use of NCDB data is to compare long-term outcomes across different cancer treatments for specific disease subgroups.[60,61] Mikell and colleagues queried NSCLC patients with N2 disease treated with chemotherapy to assess factors associated with survival. Under multivariable Cox proportional hazards analysis, postoperative radiotherapy was associated with improved overall survival. Here, the unique advantages of NCDB data—consistent staging, long-term outcomes, and comprehensive treatment records—were employed effectively.[62] The NCDB also contains more comprehensive surgical data than SEER. Hancock and colleagues used the database's records of surgical margin status to study the impact of adjuvant therapy among NSCLC patients, concluding that administration of both adjuvant chemotherapy and radiation is associated with improved outcomes among margin-positive patients regardless of stage.[63]

NATIONAL SURGICAL QUALITY IMPROVEMENT PROGRAM (NSQIP)

Features

Born out of the Veterans Affairs (VA) medical system's National VA Surgical Risk Study, NSQIP did not begin to capture data from non-VA hospitals until 1999. After an initial pilot study of 18 hospitals, the program was extended to additional hospitals in 2004 and is now open to all private sector hospitals that meet minimum participation requirements. Among these requirements is the employment of one or more dedicated Surgical Clinical Reviewers trained to collect clinical data including patient risk factors and 30-day mortality and morbidity. Data quality is verified through regular audits.[64] Unlike other databases, NSQIP samples consecutive operative cases within each facility based on an 8-day cycle. Sampling protocol is also varied based on procedure type and facility case volume. Serving its original objective of improving surgical quality, NSQIP allows each participating facility to compare its risk-adjusted mortality and complication rates to the aggregate of other NSQIP hospitals. Like the NCDB, NSQIP data for research are made available through extensively de-identified PUFs.

Examples of Research

The ability of NSQIP to track and potentially improve surgical outcomes was studied by Lucas and Pawlik in 2014, who assessed a variety of surgical procedures including esophagectomy. Postoperative mortality rates across the procedures ranged from 1.1% (proctectomy) to 4.3% (hepatectomy); postoperative morbidity varied substantially as well. From 2006 to 2011, risk-adjusted rate of complications following esophagectomy decreased (OR 0.87), yet there was a trend in increasing perioperative mortality. Importantly, however, the dataset only captured 83 post-esophagectomy deaths over the span of 6 years, demonstrating the potential shortcoming in sample size of NSQIP relative to other databases.[65] Corroborating these equivocal findings is work by Etzioni and colleagues, who studied risk-adjusted complication and mortality rates across 113 academic hospitals over the span of 2009 to 2013. Roughly half of hospitalizations were to NSQIP participant facilities. No significant differences in risk-adjusted mortality or complication rate were noted when comparing NSQIP to non-NSQIP hospitals.[66] The authors concluded that there is not yet evidence that the NSQIP reporting system has resulted in widespread quality improvement.

Due to its high level of detail in capturing patient comorbidities, operative characteristics, and short-term postoperative morbidity and mortality, NSQIP is well suited for risk factor modeling despite its comparatively smaller sample size relative to NCDB and NIS. Mungo and colleagues stratified patients receiving pulmonary resection based on body mass index to determine the relationship between obesity and postoperative outcomes. While obese patients had longer operative times than normal weight patients, risk-adjusted 30-day mortality, serious morbidity, and average length of stay were not significantly different between the two groups.[67] Differences in surgical approach are also captured by NSQIP. Comparing transhiatal to Ivor-Lewis esophagectomy, Papenfuss and colleagues demonstrated longer operative times, increased need for postoperative blood transfusion, and more frequent reoperation with the transthoracic approach. However, rates of serious complication and 30-day mortality were not different between the two groups.[68]

SOCIETY OF THORACIC SURGEONS

Features

Commonly regarded as the flagship national clinical repository for cardiothoracic surgery, the STS database is comprised of three specialty-specific databases: the adult cardiac surgery database (ACSD),

the general thoracic surgery database (GTDB), and the congenital heart surgery database (CHSD). The oldest and largest, ACSD, arose from the concern of the STS regarding the methodology of the Health Care Financing Administration's 1986 comprehensive report of identifiable hospital mortality rates.[69] The ACSD, first available to STS members in 1989,[70] now covers more than 95% of cardiac surgery programs in the United States. The hallmarks of ACSD are detailed clinical data (including comorbidities, concurrent therapies, and physiologic parameters), risk-adjusted quality indicators for common cardiac operations, and in-hospital/30-day outcomes. Voluntary public reporting for ACSD participants began in 2010. The GTDB was not formally implemented until 2002. As of 2013, the GTDB includes more than 800 cardiothoracic and general surgeons. Given the relatively smaller volumes of general thoracic procedures compared to cardiac operations, reporting periods are based on a 3-year window and results are provided to GTDB members semiannually. Like the ACSD, the GTDB includes risk-adjustment models using demographics, comorbidities, and physiologic parameters and focuses on short-term endpoints of length of stay, mortality, and morbidity.[71,72] The smallest of the three databases, the CHSD is nevertheless the largest database tracking pediatric congenital heart disease outcomes, with 109 participant hospitals and over 300 surgeons.[73] Acknowledging the smaller and more geographically scattered nature of the congenital cardiac provider community, the CHSD was instrumental in collaboration between medical and surgical specialists, adopting common nomenclature, and developing standardized quality assessment tools. An important feature of STS is that individual institutions are responsible for the data collection and reporting process. The substantial cost associated with self-reporting is one of the principal barriers to complete penetrance among across all surgical providers, especially smaller-volume institutions.

The Duke Clinical Research Institute (DCRI) has been the data warehouse for the STS database since 1999. Researchers interested in working with raw STS data files must collaborate with DCRI for registry expertise, statistical analysis, and project management. The STS databases have traditionally been operative databases with in-hospital/30-day follow-up. Recently, these databases have been linked with Medicare files to provide long-term outcomes that will be integral to comparative effectiveness research, predictive modeling efforts, and patient decision making.[74] Details for using STS data are available on line at http://www.sts.org/quality-research-patient-safety/research/publications-and-research/access-data-sts-national-database.

Examples of Research

The accuracy of the STS-GTDB compares favorably to most other surgical databases. An independent firm was contracted in 2011 to audit 5% of randomly selected participant sites on accuracy of lobectomy records reported in the GTDB. Across 10 sites and 559 cases, agreement rate and overall data accuracy each approached 95%.[75] The adult and congenital databases also have data accuracy rates of 95%. While quality of data in GTDB appears reliable, generalizability is commonly criticized. Welke and colleagues reported that hospitals participating in the NCD (precursor to STS-ACSD) were more likely to be larger, not-for-profit academic institutions, recorded higher case volumes, and had lower mortality rates overall.[44] We reported post-esophagectomy in-hospital mortality rates of 3.2% in GTDB, compared to 2.6% in NSQIP and 6.1% in NIS. GTDB also had a lower median length of stay than both alternative databases.[54] Perioperative mortality, defined as death before discharge or within 30 days of an operation, is reportedly 2.2% within GTDB,[71] compared to 4.1% within SEER-Medicare.[52]

Despite its concerns regarding generalizability, the GTDB provides unique opportunities to study clinically detailed questions using highly accurate data. For example, Taylor and colleagues identified patients with marginal pulmonary function through the GTDB and assessed rates of complication and survival following lobectomy for cancer. Adjusting for other factors, marginal pulmonary function was not found to be an independent predictor of major complication or early mortality.[76] The group concluded that, for carefully selected patients with marginal pulmonary function, lobectomy remains a viable surgical option to treat NSCLC. To study the accuracy of clinical staging, Crabtree and colleagues identified patients with stage T2 N0 esophageal cancer and determined the rates of up-staging and down-staging with surgery. The group found that 26% of patients were down-staged, while nearly half were up-staged at the operation. Because T2 N0 is a threshold for induction therapy, the group concluded that the accuracy of preoperative clinical staging should be further refined.[77]

CONCLUSIONS

Large national databases offer unique opportunities for quality monitoring, reporting, and research. While strengths differ across specific systems, common advantages over single-institution databases are patient sample size, accumulation of rare diseases, and generalizability. When conducting research, investigators must be mindful of the relative strengths and weaknesses of the database(s) to be used. Administrative databases contain useful cost data, long-term follow-up, and a relatively complete account of a small selection of variables. Specialty-specific clinical databases provide more detail for each patient or procedure, but may not capture long-term outcomes and have variable generalizability. Nevertheless, as a relatively recent and progressively growing tool in the armamentarium of the surgeon-investigator, large national databases have been essential contributors to our understanding of surgical outcomes, provision of care, and quality.

REFERENCES

1. Lindberg DA. *The Growth of Medical Information Systems in the United States.* Lexington, MA: Lexington Books, 1979.
2. Frawley WJ, Piatetsky-Shapiro G, Matheus CJ. *Knowledge discovery in databases: an overview.* AI Mag 1992;13:57–70.
3. Collen MF. *Computer Medical Databases: The First Six Decades (1950–2010).* London: Springer-Verlag London, 2012.
4. Gliklich RE, and Dreyer NA. *Registries for Evaluating Patient Outcomes: A User's Guide.* Rockville, MD: Agency for Healthcare Research and Quality, 2010.
5. Michalski RS, Baskin AB, Spackman KA. A logic-based approach to conceptual database analysis. *Med Inform (Lond)* 1982;8:187–195.
6. Ferver K, Burton B, Jesilow P. The use of claims data in healthcare research. *Open Public Health J* 2009;2:11–24.
7. McDonald L. Florence Nightingale and the early origins of evidence-based nursing. *Evid Based Nurs* 2001;4:68–69.
8. Fink A, Yano EM, Brook RH. The condition of the literature on differences in hospital mortality. *Med Care* 1989;27:315–336.
9. Griffith BP, Hattler BG, Hardesty RL, et al. The need for accurate risk-adjusted measures of outcome in surgery. Lessons learned through coronary artery bypass. *Ann Surg* 1995;222:593–598; discussion 598–599.
10. Hannan EL, Kilburn H Jr, Racz M, et al. Improving the outcomes of coronary artery bypass surgery in New York State. *JAMA* 1994;271:761–766.
11. Tu JV, Donovan LR, Lee DS, et al. Effectiveness of public report cards for improving the quality of cardiac care: the EFFECT study: a randomized trial. *JAMA* 2009;302:2330–2337.
12. Ghali WA, Ash AS, Hall RE, et al. Statewide quality improvement initiatives and mortality after cardiac surgery. *JAMA* 1997;277:379–382.
13. Guru V, Fremes SE, Naylor CD, et al.; Cardiac Care Network of Ontario. Public versus private institutional performance reporting: what is mandatory for quality improvement? *Am Heart J* 2006;152:573–578.
14. Steinbrook R. Public report cards—cardiac surgery and beyond. *N Engl J Med* 2006;355:1847–1849.
15. Jha AK, Epstein AM. The predictive accuracy of the New York State coronary artery bypass surgery report-card system. *Health Aff (Millwood)* 2006;25:844–855.
16. Kouchoukos NT, Anderson RP, Fosburg RG, et al. Report of the Ad Hoc Committee on physician-specific mortality rates for cardiac surgery. *Ann Thorac Surg* 1993;56:1200–1202.
17. Edwards FH, Clark RE, Schwartz M. Coronary artery bypass grafting: the Society of Thoracic Surgeons National Database experience. *Ann Thorac Surg* 1994;57:12–19.
18. Charlson ME, Pompei P, Ales KL, et al. A new method of classifying prognostic comorbidity in longitudinal studies: development and validation. *J Chronic Dis* 1987;40:373–383.
19. Elixhauser A, Steiner C, Harris DR, et al. Comorbidity measures for use with administrative data. *Med Care* 1998;36:8–27.
20. Deyo RA, Cherkin DC, Ciol MA. Adapting a clinical comorbidity index for use with ICD-9-CM administrative databases. *J Clin Epidemiol* 1992;45:613–619.
21. van Walraven C, Austin PC, Jennings A, et al. A modification of the Elixhauser comorbidity measures into a point system for hospital death using administrative data. *Med Care* 2009;47:626–633.
22. Sharabiani MT, Aylin P, Bottle A. Systematic review of comorbidity indices for administrative data. *Med Care* 2012;50:1109–1118.
23. Centers for Medicare & Medicaid Services Readmissions Reduction Program. 2013.
24. Shih T, Dimick JB. Reliability of readmission rates as a hospital quality measure in cardiac surgery. *Ann Thorac Surg* 2014;97:1214–1218.
25. Hu Y, McMurry TL, Isbell JM, et al. Readmission after lung cancer resection is associated with a 6-fold increase in 90-day postoperative mortality. *J Thorac Cardiovasc Surg* 2014;148(5):2261–2267.e1.
26. Baron JA, Weiderpass E. An introduction to epidemiological research with medical databases. *Ann Epidemiol* 2000;10:200–204.
27. Groft SC. Rare diseases research: expanding collaborative translational research opportunities. *Chest* 2013;144:16–23.
28. Griggs RC, Batshaw M, Dunkle M, et al. Clinical research for rare disease: opportunities, challenges, and solutions. *Mol Genet Metab* 2009;96:20–26.
29. Rubinstein YR, Groft SC, Bartek R, et al. Creating a global rare disease patient registry linked to a rare diseases biorepository database: Rare Disease-HUB (RD-HUB). *Contemp Clin Trials* 2010;31:394–404.
30. Fernandez FG, Khullar O, Force SD, et al. Hospital readmission is associated with poor survival after esophagectomy for esophageal cancer. *Ann Thorac Surg* 2015;99:292–297.
31. Green J, Wintfeld N. Report cards on cardiac surgeons. Assessing New York State's approach. *N Engl J Med* 1995;332:1229–1232.
32. Omoigui NA, Miller DP, Brown KJ, et al. Outmigration for coronary bypass surgery in an era of public dissemination of clinical outcomes. *Circulation* 1996;93:27–33.
33. Burack JH, Impellizzeri P, Homel P, et al. Public reporting of surgical mortality: a survey of New York State cardiothoracic surgeons. *Ann Thorac Surg* 1999;68:1195–1200; discussion 1201–1202.
34. Schneider EC, Epstein AM. Influence of cardiac-surgery performance reports on referral practices and access to care. A survey of cardiovascular specialists. *N Engl J Med* 1996;335:251–256.
35. Hannan EL, Sarrazin MS, Doran DR, et al. Provider profiling and quality improvement efforts in coronary artery bypass graft surgery: the effect on short-term mortality among Medicare beneficiaries. *Med Care* 2003;41:1164–1172.
36. Psaty BM, Boineau R, Kuller LH, et al. The potential costs of upcoding for heart failure in the United States. *Am J Cardiol* 1999;84:108–109, A9.
37. Siregar S, Groenwold RH, Versteegh MI, et al. Gaming in risk-adjusted mortality rates: effect of misclassification of risk factors in the benchmarking of cardiac surgery risk-adjusted mortality rates. *J Thorac Cardiovasc Surg* 2013;145:781–789.
38. Quan H, Parsons GA, Ghali WA. Validity of procedure codes in International Classification of Diseases, 9th revision, clinical modification administrative data. *Med Care* 2004;42:801–809.
39. Cooper GS, Yuan Z, Stange KC, et al. Agreement of Medicare claims and tumor registry data for assessment of cancer-related treatment. *Med Care* 2000;38:411–421.
40. Daly LE Confidence intervals and sample sizes: don't throw out all your old sample size tables. *BMJ* 1991;302:333–336.
41. Bilimoria KY, Bentrem DJ, Ko CY, et al. Extent of surgery affects survival for papillary thyroid cancer. *Ann Surg* 2007;246:375–381; discussion 381–384.
42. Drummond M, O'Brien B. Clinical importance, statistical significance and the assessment of economic and quality-of-life outcomes. *Health Econ* 1993;2:205–212.
43. CMS Medicare Provider Analysis and Review (MEDPAR) File. 2015
44. Welke KF, Peterson ED, Vaughan-Sarrazin MS, et al. Comparison of cardiac surgery volumes and mortality rates between the Society of Thoracic Surgeons and Medicare databases from 1993 through 2001. *Ann Thorac Surg* 2007;84:1538–1546.
45. Goodney PP, Lucas FL, Stukel TA, et al. Surgeon specialty and operative mortality with lung resection. *Ann Surg* 2005;241:179–184.
46. Cipriano LE, Romanus D, Earle CC, et al. Lung cancer treatment costs, including patient responsibility, by disease stage and treatment modality, 1992 to 2003. *Value Health* 2011;14:41–52.
47. Warren JL, Klabunde CN, Schrag D, et al. Overview of the SEER-Medicare data: content, research applications, and generalizability to the United States elderly population. *Med Care* 2002;40:IV-3–18.
48. National Cancer Institute SEER*Stat Databases: November 2013 Submission. 2015, 2014.
49. Potosky AL, Riley GF, Lubitz JD, et al. Potential for cancer related health services research using a linked Medicare-tumor registry database. *Med Care* 1993;31:732–748.
50. Hamid MS, Shameem R, Gafoor K, et al. Non-small-cell lung cancer clinicopathologic features and survival outcomes in Asian Pacific Islanders residing in the United States: a SEER analysis. *J Cancer Epidemiol* 2015;2015:269304.

51. Zhang J, Gold KA, Lin HY, et al. Relationship between tumor size and survival in non-small cell lung cancer (NSCLC): an analysis of the Surveillance, Epidemiology, and End Results (SEER) registry. *J Thorac Oncol* 2015;10(4):682–690.

52. Hu Y, McMurry TL, Wells KM, et al. Postoperative mortality is an inadequate quality indicator for lung cancer resection. *Ann Thorac Surg* 2014;97:973–979.

53. Healthcare Cost and Utilization Project. *Overview of the National (Nationwide) Inpatient Sample (NIS)*. Rockville, MD: Agency for Healthcare Research and Quality; 2016:2014.

54. Lapar DJ, Stukenborg GJ, Lau CL, et al. Differences in reported esophageal cancer resection outcomes between national clinical and administrative databases. *J Thorac Cardiovasc Surg* 2012;144:1152–1157.

55. Gopaldas RR, Bakaeen FG, Dao TK, et al. Video-assisted thoracoscopic versus open thoracotomy lobectomy in a cohort of 13,619 patients. *Ann Thorac Surg* 2010;89: 1563–1570.

56. Al-Refaie WB, Muluneh B, Zhong W, et al. Who receives their complex cancer surgery at low-volume hospitals? *J Am Coll Surg* 2012;214:81–87.

57. Ford ES. Hospital discharges, readmissions, and emergency department visits for chronic obstructive pulmonary disease or bronchiectasis among US adults: findings from the Nationwide Inpatient Sample 2001–2012 and Nationwide Emergency Department Sample 2006–2011. *Chest* 2014;147(4):989–998.

58. American College of Surgeons Commission on Cancer National Cancer Data Base PUF. 2015, 2008.

59. Mettlin CJ, Menck HR, Winchester DP, et al. A comparison of breast, colorectal, lung, and prostate cancers reported to the National Cancer Data Base and the Surveillance, Epidemiology, and End Results Program. *Cancer* 1997;79:2052–2061.

60. Robinson CG, Patel AP, Bradley JD, et al. Postoperative radiotherapy for pathologic n2 non-small-cell lung cancer treated with adjuvant chemotherapy: a review of the national cancer data base. *J Clin Oncol* 2015;33.870–876.

61. Patel AP, Crabtree TD, Bell JM, et al. National patterns of care and outcomes after combined modality therapy for stage IIIA non-small-cell lung cancer. *J Thorac Oncol* 2014;9:612–621.

62. Mikell JL, Gillespie TW, Hall WA, et al. Postoperative radiotherapy is associated with better survival in non-small cell lung cancer with involved N2 lymph nodes: results of an analysis of the National Cancer Data Base. *J Thorac Oncol* 2015;10: 462–471.

63. Hancock JG, Rosen JE, Antonicelli A, et al. Impact of adjuvant treatment for microscopic residual disease after non-small cell lung cancer surgery. *Ann Thorac Surg* 2015;99:406–413.

64. American College of Surgeons NSQIP History. 2015, 2015.

65. Lucas DJ, Pawlik TM. Quality improvement in gastrointestinal surgical oncology with American College of Surgeons National Surgical Quality Improvement Program. *Surgery* 2014;155:593–601.

66. Etzioni DA, Wasif N, Dueck AC, et al. Association of hospital participation in a surgical outcomes monitoring program with inpatient complications and mortality. *JAMA* 2015;313:505–511.

67. Mungo B, Zogg CK, Hooker CM, et al. Does obesity affect the outcomes of pulmonary resections for lung cancer? A National Surgical Quality Improvement Program analysis. *Surgery* 2015;157(4):792–800.

68. Papenfuss WA, Kukar M, Attwood K, et al. Transhiatal versus transthoracic esophagectomy for esophageal cancer: a 2005–2011 NSQIP comparison of modern multicenter results. *J Surg Oncol* 2014;110:298–301.

69. Shahian DM, Jacobs JP, Edwards FH, et al. The Society of Thoracic Surgeons National Database. *Heart* 2013;99:1494–1501.

70. Clark RE. It is time for a national cardiothoracic surgical data base. *Ann Thorac Surg* 1989;48:755–756.

71. Kozower BD, Sheng S, O'Brien SM, et al. STS database risk models: predictors of mortality and major morbidity for lung cancer resection. *Ann Thorac Surg* 2010;90:875–881; discussion 881–883.

72. Wright CD, Kucharczuk JC, O'Brien JC, et al.; Society of Thoracic Surgeons General Thoracic Surgery Database. Predictors of major morbidity and mortality after esophagectomy for esophageal cancer: a Society of Thoracic Surgeons General Thoracic Surgery Database risk adjustment model. *J Thorac Cardiovasc Surg* 2009; 137:587–595; discussion 596.

73. Jacobs JP, Jacobs ML, Mavroudis C, et al. Nomenclature and databases for the surgical treatment of congenital cardiac disease—an updated primer and an analysis of opportunities for improvement. *Cardiol Young* 2008;18(Suppl 2):38–62.

74. Jacobs JP, Edwards FH, Shahian DM, et al. Successful linking of the Society of Thoracic Surgeons adult cardiac surgery database to Centers for Medicare and Medicaid Services Medicare data. *Ann Thorac Surg* 2010;90:1150–1156; discussion 1156–1157.

75. Magee MJ, Wright CD, McDonald D, et al. External validation of the Society of Thoracic Surgeons General Thoracic Surgery Database. *Ann Thorac Surg* 2013;96: 1734–1739; discussion 1738–1739.

76. Taylor MD, LaPar DJ, Isbell JM, et al. Marginal pulmonary function should not preclude lobectomy in selected patients with non-small cell lung cancer. *J Thorac Cardiovasc Surg* 2014;147:738–744; discussion 744–746.

77. Crabtree TD, Kosinski AS, Puri V, et al. Evaluation of the reliability of clinical staging of T2 N0 esophageal cancer: a review of the Society of Thoracic Surgeons database. *Ann Thorac Surg* 2013;96:382–390.

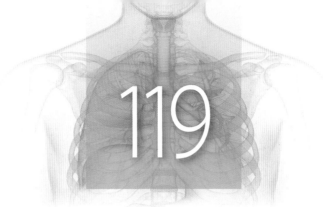

119

ICD-10: Implications for Future Clinical Research and Reporting

Melanie A. Edwards ▪ Keith S. Naunheim

HISTORY OF DISEASE CLASSIFICATION SYTEMS

The first efforts to classify and systematize human disease came with a publication by Francois Bossier De Lacroix who listed ten major disease classes which, in total, contained approximately 2,400 individual maladies.[1] Subsequent efforts by William Cullen in Edinburgh (the *Synopsis Nosologiae Methodica*) and John Graunt in London (the London Bills of Mortality) were qualitative classification works used primarily on a regional basis (Fig. 119.1). However in 1837 the General Register Office of England and Wales appointed William Farr

to oversee and then report on the official classification of diseases.[2] During his career he strove to standardize not just the qualitative but also the quantitative aspects of disease, stressing epidemiology, and statistical analysis. Farr also wanted to work collaboratively to institute an international standard for such information and was eventually successful in 1855 at the Paris Congress of International Statistical Congress. At that meeting the Congress adopted a list of 139 headings in hopes that it would become the worldwide standard to describe the totality of diseases in mankind. This was the first such effort toward international standardization.

Currently, most civilized countries use the International Classification of Disease (ICD) system. This had its origins in 1891 in Vienna when Jacques Bertillon, the Chief of Statistical Services of the City of Paris, was charged with updating the disease classification schema on behalf of the International Statistical Institute (successor to the International Statistical Congress). The new schema was presented at their annual meeting in Chicago in 1893 and over the ensuing years was adopted sporadically by multiple cities, regions, and countries. However, in 1900, France convened the first conference on the International List of Causes of Death with delegates from 26 countries for the purpose of international standardization. A detailed classification schema including 179 groups was agreed upon and adopted, thus essentially becoming the ICD-1 system. It was planned that revisions would occur every 10 years and in fact they did occur in 1909 (ICD-2), 1920 (ICD-3), 1929 (ICD-4), and in 1938 (ICD-5), at which time 200 disease classifications were identified. In 1946, the ICD classification system update was entrusted to the Interim Commission of the World Health Organization (WHO). The WHO not only modernized the classification schema but also sought to define a structure for the tabulation and publication of morbidity and mortality statistics so as to enable international comparisons of mortality. This revision, recognized now as ICD-6, was followed by revisions in 1955 (ICD-7) and 1965 (ICD-8). The ICD-9 revision began in Geneva in 1975 and was an effort to provide additional detail by expanding the prior three-digit system to 4 and 5 digits for those countries wishing to utilize additional details in their tabulations. This allowed for classification, not only of the underlying disease, but also for the manifestation of that disease in a specific organ or site. This classification system was finalized in 1977 and adopted in the United States in 1979.[1]

Because of the ongoing rapid advances in medical knowledge and technology, there soon emerged criticisms that ICD-9 was quickly becoming obsolete and in 1989 the ICD-10 revision was instituted

FIGURE 119.1 Title page of John Graunt's Bills of Mortality which cataloged the cases of death annually in London.

and began to be adopted by countries throughout the world. The United States, however, continued using the ICD-9 system throughout the end of the 20th and well into the 21st century.

RATIONALE FOR ICD UPDATE

While the conversion from the ICD-9 to ICD-10 diagnostic classification system had been proposed in the United States for at least two decades, there was resistance to change on the part of most health care players including providers, hospitals, and third-party payers. However, in 2013, the federal government, through the offices of the Centers for Medicare & Medicaid Services (CMS) mandated the conversion with a completion date in 2104. After much turmoil and public comment this conversion was delayed for a year but eventually took place on October 1, 2015. The rationale offered by CMS for this mandate was identical to the arguments made for all prior conversions, for example, that extant ICD system no longer accurately depicted the practice of medicine due to advances in knowledge and technology. ICD-9 was purported to provide only limited and generalized data which often proved inaccurate with regard to the clinical diagnoses and hospital procedures. The public health community felt that updating to ICD-10 would provide the granularity and specificity necessary to ensure accuracy in coding both diagnoses and procedures.

METHODOLOGIC CHANGES DURING CONVERSION

This greater granularity and specificity reported with ICD-10 is the result of a wholesale redesign of the classification system. Like ICD-9, ICD-10 consisted of two separate classification systems, the diagnosis codes (ICD-10-CM) and the hospital procedure codes (ICD-10-PCS). Currently 27 nations utilize the ICD-10-CM diagnostic classification system; this includes all of North America, China, Japan, Australia/ New Zealand, all of Western Europe, and the Nordic countries as well as approximately half of countries in South American. The ICD-10-PCS procedure coding system is used only in the United States for reimbursement purposes. Table 119.1 outlines the major differences between the old and new classification systems both with regard to diagnosis and procedure codes.

The new, more complex classification methodology allows for markedly increased granularity. The system includes the ability to code for disease site (arm, leg, trunk), laterality (left vs. right), and the evolutionary phase of the injury (initial encounter, subsequent encounter, sequela). In addition, ICD-10 provides for classification of a panoply of causation with regard to the nature of the injury (collision, burn, laceration, bites, etc.), the agent of injury (such as orcas, spiders, in-laws, military water craft among others) and the locale in which the injury occurred (swimming pool, basement, opera theater, driveway to name just a few). This surge in granularity results in a vastly increased number of codes. The permutations made possible by this increased coding capability results in an increase in the absolute number of diagnostic codes from about 14,000 options to over 68,000 options while the procedure codes rise from 3,800 to 72,000 potential hospital procedure codes. This marked increase in both number and complexity makes it very difficult for one to map equivalent diagnosis codes between the two ICD systems. There are at least 225 examples of a single ICD-9 code mapping to 50 or more ICD-10 codes and 119 instances where one ICD-9 code will map to over 100 ICD-10 codes.[3]

PURPORTED ADVANTAGES

Proponents of ICD-10 insist the increased number of digits in this new coding schema provides the granularity and complexity that is necessary to depict the world of medicine and surgery in the 21st century. The specificity of ICD-10 will allow for coding even the most unusual morbid occurrences (Fig. 119.2). It also makes possible the future addition of diagnosis and procedure codes as new conditions are recognized and new procedures devised. Such expansion was not possible in the ICD-9 system which was limited to only five digits.

The intended benefit of such new granularity and specificity is the ability to improve the efforts of the health care delivery system on many fronts including quality metric improvement, public health surveillance, organizational modeling of quality and productivity as well as international comparison of disease incidence and results as most other countries already use ICD-10. The new methodology is also purported to provide benefit in the reimbursement arena due to increased accuracy of coding for coverage determinations which is supposed to result in fewer claim denials, obviate the need for claim adjudication and reduce the opportunity for health care fraud.

TABLE 119.1 Comparison of ICD-9 and ICD-10 Methodology	
ICD-9-CM (Diagnosis)	**ICD-10-CM (Diagnosis)**
3 to 5 digits	3 to 7 digits
Decimal after the third digit	Decimal after the third digit
First digit is alpha or numeric	First digit always alpha
Digit 2 through 5 numeric	Digit 2 is numeric
	Digit 3 through 7 alpha or numeric
ICD-9-PCS (Procedure)	**ICD-10-PCS (Procedure)**
3 to 4 digits	7 digits
All digits numeric	Decimal after the third digit
First digit is alpha or numeric	Each digit alpha or numeric
Decimal after second digit	No decimal

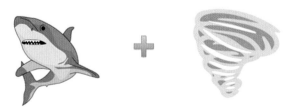

ICD10 CODES FOR INJURY DURING SHARKNADO

W56.42
Struck by shark

X37.1XXA
Tornado, initial encounter

FIGURE 119.2 Appropriate diagnostic codes for injury sustained when struck by a shark falling from the sky during a sharknado.

But in addition to all these intended advantages, it has been proposed that the increased complexity will greatly improve and foster better research based on the ICD system. Proponents suggest that ICD-10 will improve society's ability to measure outcomes, efficacy, and costs of new medical procedures and technology. For example, ICD-10 coding for behavioral risks such as smoking, poor dietary habits, and lack of exercise could potentially prove to be important prognostic factors with regard to clinical outcomes. The suggestion is that detailed coding of more specific comorbidities such as "E11.51 Type 2 diabetes mellitus with circulatory complications with diabetic peripheral angiopathy without gangrene," once factored into risk algorithms, may also lead to better risk adjustment and clinical decision making.

POTENTIAL DISADVANTAGES

The remarkable increase in the volume and complexity of both diagnostic and procedure codes in the ICD-10 system has caused consternation amongst practitioners. There are now approximately 340 codes for diabetes and its related conditions and effects. These are the permutations which occurred following subcategorization of diabetes type (type 1, type 2, drug induced, disease, pregnancy induce, and other), adequacy of control (hypoglycemia, hyperglycemia, ketoacidosis), the affected organ systems (ophthalmologic, neurologic, renal, cutaneous, vascular, gastrointestinal), and the multiple complications that arise in each (i.e., for the eye—proliferative retinopathy, nonproliferative retinopathy [mild, moderate, or severe], macular edema, cataracts, and combinations of the above). General medical practitioners have decried the volume and complexity of such coding as they are often caring for patients with four or five such chronic conditions, each of which is supposed to be coded with similar specificity. Such activities require increased time and effort at the computer terminal, and the cumulative effect in patient, after patient leads to more work of documentation with less time for patient care. In fact, a recent study found that for every 1 hour of time devoted to clinical care, a physician spends additional 2 hours completing the electronic health record (EHR) and paper work.[4]

In the realm of CT surgery, there are 60 separate codes for chronic stable myocardial ischemia dealing with permutations of pathophysiology (aneurysm, coronary artery aneurysm, coronary dissection, atherosclerosis), vessel type (native or autologous graft), graft type (artery or vein) symptoms (with/without angina), vasoactivity (with/without spasm), and specific patient (transplanted vs. native heart) among others. Unfortunately, current EHR systems have been designed to mandate physician coding of diagnoses at multiple time points throughout a hospital stay including the time of admission, the performance of a procedure, and at the time of discharge. These are "hard stop" entries meaning that these activities (admission, operative reporting, discharge) **cannot** proceed until an ICD-10 code is inserted by the clinician recording in the chart. Thus, the doctor is forced to make an entry in order to continue delivering care. In the present era, physicians are harried and hurried continuously throughout the day, and many, if not most, resent the idea that they have to function not only as the caregiver but also as a data entry clerk. Rather than spend the time and effort delving through screen after screen of ICD-10 codes to identify the single most appropriate code among the scores, if not hundreds, of options, most doctors, whether hospitalists or surgeons, will default to a general diagnosis ("diabetes mellitus" or "chronic myocardial ischemia") and that code will be entered in the vast majority of charts. This brings into question the accuracy and the utility of the information being entered.

Apologists for the ICD-10 system will counter that the professional coders working in the hospital or the practice can and will make the appropriate corrections at the time of discharge but that assumes that coders have the knowledge and experience to make the distinction between different versions of the same disease. Most will not have the ability to discern the nuances of different sorts of diabetic retinopathies and the acumen to pick up the presence or absence of, as well as the reported severity of, macular edema on the retinal exam. The issue becomes even more complex in teaching hospitals where residents and medical students insert daily notes, many of which contain suggested diagnoses and conditions that, due to the inexperience of the trainees, may or may not be valid. Yet such "diagnoses" could and, in many instances, will likely be noted and coded by the nonmedical coding personnel responsible for entering the ICD-10 information. The ICD-10 system is no different than any other data categorization platform; the more complex and granular the system becomes, the greater the chance for mistaken entries and inaccuracies.

In truth, ICD-10 is not an entity that can be judged in isolation, but rather must be evaluated as a piece of a complex data entry/analysis model that includes the ICD-10 schema itself, the EHR platform in all its iterations and all the personnel responsible for data entry. Valid conclusions and decisions can only be gleaned from analysis of ICD-10 data if the clinical information is identified, appropriately interpreted, and then assigned the correct codes; failure in any one of these tasks dooms any subsequent analysis to failure. The failing may occur due to the complexity of the classification scheme (ICD-10), limitations of the data entry platform (EHR) or due to the faults and frailties of the humans responsible for inputting correct data. To quote the old computer programmer aphorism—"Garbage in . . . garbage out." This would appear to be a major weakness of the ICD-10 system, a flaw it shares with many if not most other administrative databases. For this reason, many clinicians suggest that clinical databases or registries should form the foundation for clinical research in the future.

ADMINISTRATIVE VERSUS CLINICAL DATABASES

High-quality clinical databases and registries prove to be far better for clinical research than administrative ones and their primary advantages include:

1. Standard definitions—in a clinical database, specific definitions exist for comorbidities and endpoints such as congestive heart failure or renal insufficiency or pneumonia. This allows for accuracy in coding by data managers who usually have a medical background. Such hard definitions are rare in most administrative databases with the result that comorbidity and/or complications will be coded with highly variable levels of accuracy and/or consistency.
2. Structured data—much of the coding of comorbidities and complications in ICD 10 will be performed from extracting those specifics from free text entries into the medical record. This requires some interpretation and judgment so that free text can be "translated" into data endpoints and elements which have not been prospectively designed into the structure of the database.
3. Clinically trained data managers—most personnel managing data in clinical registries have a medical background and can understand nuances in medical technology/terminology. In addition, they are trained in rules for assigning diagnoses and outcomes

according to specified definitions. Institutional coders, while well trained in coding terminology, generally have no medical background and assign diagnoses and outcomes in response to key words within the chart which may or may not correlate with the actual patient's condition.

4. Validated data—high-quality clinical registries are regularly audited for accuracy, something that rarely, if ever, occurs in institutional administrative databases and almost never with EHRs.

Can such differences significantly affect the results of research? Shahian et al.[5] compared the results of the validated clinical registry to a contemporaneous state administrative database in patients undergoing coronary artery bypass grafting (CABG). The authors demonstrated a 27% difference in the volume of CABG procedures as well as a 40% over estimation of hospital mortality by the administrative database. This and many similar articles suggest that conclusions derived solely from analysis using administrative databases should be taken with a grain of salt. One should then ask, how accurate has ICD-10 proven to be in those countries currently employing it.

ACCURACY OF ICD-10: EARLY RESULTS

In America, ICD-10 has only been in use for a year and so objective or definitive results are not available from this country. However, the early subjective opinions regarding those results do not appear to be encouraging. The American Health Information Management Association (AHIMA) reported on a survey performed on four hundred randomly selected coding professionals, 156 of whom responded. The survey sought opinions regarding whether ICD-10 had resulted in the expected improvements in coding accuracy. Unfortunately, 88% of respondents felt it had not improved (61% unchanged, 27% worsened) while only 11% felt accuracy had increased. Many proponents of ICD-10 suggested that with the new system and computerized coding tools, coder productivity would also improve. The AHIMA survey also inquired regarding coder productivity and 68% of coder's opined that productivity had suffered while 26% reported no change and only 6% suggested productivity had improved.[6]

In order to obtain any objective data regarding the precision and accuracy of ICD-10 performance, it is necessary to turn to the international community where that system has been in use for a decade or more. Perhaps the best results reported came from the Czech Republic where investigators utilized ICD-10 codes (I60 subarachnoid hemorrhage, I61 intracerebral hemorrhage, I63 cerebral infarction, I64 stroke not specified as hemorrhage or infarction, G45 transient ischemic attack) in an attempt to identify patient's with stroke and transient ischemic attacks cases in their national hospital registry. ICD-10 codes were compared with hospital discharge summaries that were examined independently by two clinical reviewers. For the five individual ICD-10 codes, diagnosis was confirmed as correct between 1% to 92% of the time (average 82%) with the worst accuracy in I64 (stroke not specified as hemorrhage or infarction) with a 1% accuracy and G45 (transient ischemic attack) which was correctly coded 49% of the time. The most accurate coding was for I60 (subarachnoid hemorrhage) and I61 (intracerebral hemorrhage) both of which were coded adequately 91% of the time.[7]

Somewhat less encouraging results were reported from Canada where ICD-10 coding for sepsis was assessed in 1,001 intensive care unit patients, 604 of whom had documented sepsis. Although the specificity of ICD-10 classification system was high at 99%, the sensitivity was only 46%, suggesting that the utilization of only ICD-10 information would miss over half the cases of sepsis. The authors

proposed an ICD-10 coded algorithm which proved to increase sensitivity up to 72% of cases but this occurred a cost of a decreased specificity which fell to 85%.[8]

Similar ICD-10 analyses have been reported from France regarding acute coronary syndrome,[9] Denmark regarding colon cancer,[10] and Thailand dealing with comorbidity identification.[11] In each country, ICD-10 codes proved to be distinctly inaccurate in a disturbingly high percentage of cases. In many instances, authors reported that algorithms and models could be designed utilizing multiple ICD-10 codes and that such algorithms often improved the sensitivity of results, but always at the cost of decreased specificity. However, neither the raw code matching nor the algorithmic models reported in these articles could approach the 96% accuracy rate reported by the external audit agency for the Society of Thoracic Surgeons National Clinical Database (David Shahian, personal communication).

All the above literature suggests that, despite the increased granularity and specificity of the ICD system, it will not prove to be of sufficient accuracy to perform high-quality clinical research, no matter what coding models or algorithms are employed. Clinical registries and databases which utilize standard definitions, clinical data managers, and structured data (with accuracy verified via audit) are likely to be the best tools for ongoing clinical inquiry for the foreseeable future. The results from analyzing such rigorously collected clinical data can and should be used for the purpose of clinical decision-making, a claim that cannot be made for the ICD-10 data.

ICD-10 RESEARCH OPPORTUNITIES

There are many types of research, both qualitative and quantitative, which can be potentially performed using the ICD classification system including epidemiologic, sociologic, economic, demographic, and clinical. Cardiothoracic (CT) surgeons can be, and are involved in all these different types of research efforts, but clinical research takes precedence for most. It is important for all researchers to understand that in America, the ICD-9 classification system, although originally conceived and utilized for clinical purposes, had evolved during the latter half of the 20th century into an administrative database utilized primarily for reimbursement and clerical purposes by third party-payers and hospitals. Very little, if any, clinical research in the field of CT surgery was based on the ICD classification system.

The new ICD-10 system will also be used for reimbursement and administrative tasks but its "improvements" in granularity and specificity are intended to increase its clinical utility as well. That being said, researchers must keep in mind that it continues to be an administrative database, not a true clinical database or registry. As noted above, its intrinsic weaknesses include the fact that it is integrated into an EHR designed for administrative rather than clinical inquiry and that data are entered either by nonmedically trained personnel and/or by medical personnel often with limited time to provide detailed and specific coding information in all cases. This is very different from what occurs in a clinical database and such differences likely will have profound effects on the utility and validity of results from research projects based on ICD-10 methodology.

Health care has not been exempt from the explosion of "big data" in recent years and it may seem intuitive that having more information, such as can be provided by ICD-10, would lead to more informed decision-making, improved quality, and overall better patient care. However, all the criticisms pertinent to "big data" outside the health care realm are also pertinent to it inside the medical arena. First and foremost, "big data" is good for detecting correlation but generally poor at identifying cause and effect. Another drawback is the staggering volume of data available for analysis which can easily result in the identification of correlations that are simply due to random chance and have no clinical utility.

Another limitation is that any inherent biases which exist within the data will inexorably lead to false or inaccurate conclusion upon analysis. Since the ICD classification system has evolved into a de facto reimbursement tool, literally hundreds of billions of dollars change hands on the basis of the data entered therein. Thus, it is a reasonable concern that there may be some level of "upcoding" to optimize reimbursement. Such systematic data alteration would lead to inaccurate coding and obviously less than completely accurate conclusions once analysis is undertaken.

Keeping in mind the inherent weaknesses of an administrative database, ICD-10 might have some value for clinical research in those areas where robust clinical databases do not exist. Researchers will need to critically assess the extent to which ICD-10 data is appropriate to answer the clinical questions posed when designing research studies. It may be best suited as an initial investigative resource to examine the prevalence of less common disease processes or discover changes within disease-related demographic profiles. In this vein, it is possible that epidemiologic data could be leveraged to prepare for and respond to public health emergencies. Also, because ICD-10 system has the capacity to expand and accommodate new diagnosis and procedure codes, as new technology is introduced it might be possible to link the clinical data pertinent to that technology to cost and resource utilization data. This could theoretically make it possible to not only track the utilization but also to assess the efficacy of new procedures or technology.

FUTURE IMPROVEMENTS

The promise of ICD-10 to improve health care delivery can only be met by leveraging the advantages of the system while critically assessing its limitations and redesigning our health information systems to address those limitations. The two most important issues to address are the difficulty of data acquisition due to the lack of system interoperability and the serious concern regarding data validity and accuracy.

The ability of administrators and researchers to connect to a centralized EHR within health care delivery organizations could streamline access to data for quality improvement and clinical research. Having nationwide, pooled data would expand the impact and relevance of such investigations, but that ideal is nowhere near reality at present. Reconfiguring systems to improve accessibility to ICD-10 derived data within a system or region is often impractical due to cost and privacy concerns, as well as other administrative challenges. There are well over a hundred EHR systems available and, by intentional proprietary design, virtually none of them are compatible with one another. Even hospitals utilizing the same brand of EHR software are often unable to exchange information due to their utilization of different versions. Thus, the total body of useful medical data is fragmented across hundreds of thousands of sites across the country. Until the greater medical community addresses this issue of EHR interoperability, the full potential of ICD-10 to

inform clinical and policy decisions, both regionally and nationally, will never be realized.

Similarly, as outlined in a previous section, there are system-wide deficiencies with regard to the accuracy and validity of ICD-10 data being entered into the EHR. In the current iteration, data quality is a major limitation. The optimal value of ICD-10 cannot be achieved unless investments are made in health information systems with regard to input processes that ensure the accuracy of ICD-10 data. An international group has proposed a set of methodological research priorities for the use of ICD-10 in clinical research. Among the 13 proposals is a prospective study that would compare standard medical record inputs (from which much of the ICD-10 coding is derived) to real-time assessments by an independent clinician, thus quantifying the accuracy, or lack thereof, of the medical record as a data source.[12] The authors also suggest the development of internal consistency safeguards (e.g., prostatectomy coding for a woman would be prohibited) as well as data definition standardization, both nationally and internationally. Other measures such as creating enhanced education and training standards for coders (to reduce variability in coding) and performing regular audits, as is done in clinical databases, are interventions that could significantly improve the validity of ICD-10 data for clinical research.[12]

If these issues are adequately addressed, one would hope to produce a more accurate, user-friendly and accessible system which will be a valuable tool in addressing epidemiologic, social, demographic, and economic issues in health care. However, even such an improved system will likely prove to be insufficient in areas where nuanced clinical analysis is required to make ongoing care decisions. In such instances, clinical data registries will still be the optimal resource to allow for high-quality patient care decisions.

REFERENCES

1. Knibbs GH. The international classification of disease and causes of death and its revision. *Med J Aust* 1929;1:2–12.
2. First annual report. London: Registrar General of England and Wales. *Journal of the Statistical Society of London*, 1839;2(4):269–274.
3. Manchikanti L, Falco FJ, Hirsch JA. Ready or not! Here comes ICD 10. *J Neurointervent Surg* 2013;5:86–91.
4. Sinsky C, Colligan L, Li L, et al. Allocation of physician time in ambulatory practice: a time and motion study in 4 specialties. *Ann Intern Med* 2016;165:753–760.
5. Shahian DM, Silverstein T, Lovett AF, et al. Comparison of clinical and administrative data sources for hospital coronary artery bypass graft surgery report cards. *Circulation* 2007;115:1518–1527.
6. Perceived Effects of ICD10 Coding on Productivity and Accuracy Among Coding Professionals. http://www.ahimafoundation.org/downloads/pdfs/CodingProductivity_Final-6-10-16.pdf
7. Sedova P, Brown RD, Zvolsky M, et al. Validation of stroke diagnosis in the National Registry of Hospitalized Patients in the Czech Republic. *J of Stroke Cerebrovasc Dis* 2015;24:2032–2038.
8. Jolley RJ, Quan H, Jette N, et al. Validation and optimization of an ICD-10 coded case definition for sepsis using administrative health data. *BMJ Open* 2015;5(12):e009487.
9. Bezin J, Girodet PO, Rambelomanana S, et al. Choice of ICD-10 codes for the identification of acute coronary syndrome in the French hospitalization database. *Fundam Clin Pharmacol* 2015;29:586–591.
10. Helqvist L, Erichsen R, Gammelager H, et al. Quality of the Danish ICD-10 colorectal cancer diagnosis codes in the Danish national registry of patients. *Eur J Cancer Care* 2012;21:722–727.
11. Rattanaumpawan R, Wongkamhla T, Thamilikitkul V. Accuracy of ICD-10 coding system for identifying comorbidities and infectious conditions using data from a Thai university hospital administrative database. *J Med Assoc Thai* 2016;99:368–373.
12. De Coster C, Quan H, Finlayson A, et al. Identifying priorities in methodological research using ICD-9-CM and ICD-10 administrative data: report from an international consortium. *BMC Health Serv Res* 2006;6:77.

120

Instruments and Resources for Quality Improvement in Thoracic Surgery

Farhood Farjah ▪ Douglas E. Wood

INTRODUCTION

Surgeons have a long history of leading quality improvement (QI) efforts, and the health care system has a long history of resisting it. The fabled story of Ernest Amory Codman, MD[1] provides an excellent case study of the duality of American Medicine. Around a 100 years ago, Codman—a surgeon at the Massachusetts General Hospital—systematically tracked his patients' demographics, diagnoses, treatments, and 1-year outcomes. He was one of the first, if not the first, to institute a morbidity and mortality conference. Codman boldly proposed a plan to his peers and administrators to evaluate surgeon competence, and subsequently lost his privileges. He then established his own hospital and helped found the American College of Surgeons (ACS) and its Hospital Standardization Program—the latter organization ultimately becoming the Joint Commission. Codman's leadership and courage inspired substantial progress in QI, and yet a century later health care stakeholders with competing interests do not universally accept QI as an imperative.

Of course, one of the greatest barriers to implementing QI is the lack of a universal definition. In 1990, the Institute of Medicine (IOM) proposed the following definition for health care quality: "The degree to which health services for individuals and populations increase the likelihood of desired health outcomes and are consistent with current professional knowledge."[2] Nearly a decade later, the IOM provided a more granular description of quality through six aims—safety, effectiveness, patient-centeredness, timeliness, efficiency, and equity. Despite these well-intended efforts to define it, the task of measuring and improving quality remains challenging and sometimes elusive.

The prime motivation for thoracic surgeons to pursue QI are outcomes that are worse than expected, as well as inexplicable variability in care in the community-at-large. For instance, a national study revealed that only a minority of operated lung cancer patients underwent invasive mediastinal staging, and a majority of those who underwent mediastinoscopy had no lymph node tissue submitted for pathologic analysis.[3] Variability in short- and long-term outcomes after pulmonary resection for lung cancer has been observed across hospitals and surgeons.[4–12] Disparities in care have also been documented among surgically managed lung cancer patients.[13–16] These observations have motivated QI initiatives in thoracic surgery that aim to reduce unjustified variability in care and improve patient-centered outcomes.

The purpose of this chapter is to summarize bedrock principles of quality measurement, assessment, and improvement as well as highlight several examples of thoracic surgery specific initiatives.

QUALITY MEASUREMENT

Avedis Donabedian, M.D. put forth a model for measuring the quality of health care delivery consisting of structure, process, and outcomes.[17] It is the most widely used framework for studying care delivery, measuring quality, and implementing QI interventions. This section will provide definitions and examples of processes, structures, and outcomes as well as highlight some of the advantages and disadvantages of each from the perspective of measurement and implementation.

Process

Processes-of-care refer to a health care-related activity provided for or on behalf of a patient. In other words, processes describe the use of diagnostics, therapeutics, and/or supportive measures. Specific examples in thoracic surgery include the use of positron-emission tomography (PET) for lung cancer staging[18–22] or lung-volume reduction surgery (LVRS) for severe emphysema.[23] Processes-of-care are relatively easy to measure, are not influenced by case-mix, may serve as a surrogate for measuring long-term outcomes, and are potentially actionable from a surgeon's perspective. The disadvantages of processes-of-care are that they seldom have a well-established causal link to outcomes that is supported by evidence from randomized trials; appropriateness of use is difficult to assess because the denominator (patients with an indication and without a contraindication) is difficult to measure; and patient compliance is necessary but not mandatory because of the ethical principal of autonomy.

Structure

Structures-of-care refers to the context in which a patient receives care. In other words, structure refers to the environment defined by facilities, equipment, health care personnel, reimbursement, health care policy, and cultural and sociopolitical characteristics of a population. Specific examples in thoracic surgery include hospital and surgeon volume[4–6] and surgeon specialty.[7–10] The key advantage and disadvantage of structures is that they are easy to measure but difficult to modify, respectively.

Outcome

Outcomes refer to the effect of care delivery on patients, populations, the health care system, and society. Patient-centered outcomes are those that matter the most to patients. Examples include survival after lung or esophageal cancer resection, health-related quality-of-life (HRQOL), cancer recurrence, pain, functional status, decisional-regret, and satisfaction. Patient-centered outcomes that can only be reported by the patient (e.g., HRQOL) and are called patient-reported outcomes and are measured using standardized and validated instruments (i.e., questionnaires or interviews). An example of the distinction between patient-centered and patient-reported outcomes is that cancer recurrence is important to patients but recurrence can be measured through medical record review and is therefore not a patient-reported outcome. Because health care delivery also affects individuals and groups other than the patient, it is important to clearly understand the perspective (i.e., patient, surgeon, health care system, societal) of any outcome-based analysis. It is also important to understand that outcomes may account for varying concepts. For instance, the effectiveness of pulmonary resection for lung cancer is often measured in terms of overall survival, whereas safety is often measured in terms of morbidity and mortality. Other concepts captured through outcomes measurement include resource utilization (e.g., length-of-stay [LOS], readmission), costs, HRQOL, patient satisfaction, and value (e.g., health benefits divided by costs). The advantage of measuring outcomes is that they are the most easily interpreted measure of quality because they represent the "bottom-line." In some cases, for example, in-patient death, outcomes are very easy to measure. Conversely, they can be difficult to measure. For instance, survival measurement requires time and money for complete follow-up, and HRQOL requires a validated instrument, patient cooperation, and resources to collect data. Another disadvantage of outcomes assessment is that they require statistical adjustments for variation in case-mix and to discriminate between signal and noise. The added burden of collecting additional clinical variables for the purposes of risk-adjustment and hiring statisticians is expensive. Furthermore, surgeons, hospitals, and other stakeholders must "buy-in" to the adequacy of the risk-adjustment strategy before they will use the information to change care delivery.

QUALITY ASSESSMENT

Quality measurement naturally leads to the desire to assess whether a hospital and/or surgeon is a high-quality provider. When structures-of-care are used to measure quality, a provider is judged by whether or not he possesses desired structural attributes (e.g., high-volume, staffed by board-certified thoracic surgeons) of a high-quality center. In contrast, when process utilization and/or outcomes are used to measure quality, individual performance can be compared to other hospitals and/or an established benchmark. Variation in performance (i.e., process utilization and/or outcomes) may arise from three factors—chance, case-mix, and differential care delivery.[24] The role of statistics in the QI setting is to mitigate the influence of chance and account for variation in case-mix.

Chance

Outcomes associated with esophagectomy provide a good case example of how chance complicates quality assessment. The average operative mortality rate for esophagectomy among participants in the Society of Thoracic Surgeons General Thoracic Surgery Database (STS-GTSD) was 2.7%.[25] Imagine a hospital that performed

50 esophagectomies in 1 year with zero deaths. Although it would appear that this hypothetical hospital has outstanding outcomes, the influence of chance precludes making such a conclusion. Based on the "rules of three" ($100 \times 3/n$)[26]—which estimates the upper bound of a 95% confidence interval—the operative mortality rate of this hospital could be as high as 6% ($100 \times 3/50$). In other words, a 0% mortality rate could simply represent a lucky year for this center rather than its true performance. Without more cases, one cannot rule out the possibility that this hospital is a good (zero death) or bad (mortality two times greater than the average) outlier.

The signal-to-noise ratio is influenced heavily by procedural volume and the event rate of interest (e.g., operative mortality). An analysis of seven operations, including cardiovascular, orthopedic, and high-risk oncologic procedures, revealed that only coronary artery bypass-grafting (CABG) is performed frequently enough to distinguish signal (i.e., quality) from noise (i.e., chance) despite a low event rate and with only 3 years of data collection.[27] Despite higher associated event rates for pulmonary resection and esophagectomy, average procedural volumes are too low at any one center to discriminate provider performance. Statistical techniques using Bayesian methodology (also known as reliability adjustment) have been adopted to combat the problem of chance.[28,29] The simplest conceptualization of this technique is that it "shrinks" estimates toward the known average event rate. In the esophagectomy example earlier, the 0% mortality would have been "adjusted" for the volume of cases at that hospital in 1 year such that the "reliability-adjusted" mortality rate would be somewhere between 0% and 2.7%. These methods are used by several organizations evaluating quality including the STS-GTSD,[10] the American College of Surgeons' National Surgical Quality Improvement Program (ACS-NSQIP),[30] and Medicare.

Case-mix

Case-mix refers has to do with the notion that some hospitals and surgeons care for sicker patients, and as a consequence their outcomes will be unfairly judged. There is no question that sicker patients have worse outcomes and possibly in ways that are not modifiable. However, the degree to which case-mix actually varies from center to center in an impactful way is far less clear. There has been no systematic effort to describe variation in case-mix across hospitals performing thoracic surgery, or its potential impact on judging performance. A provocative study of publicly available cardiac surgery report cards from New York and Pennsylvania demonstrated that risk-adjustment had no bearing on hospital rankings relative to using unadjusted outcomes.[31] While these findings do not resonate with experienced cardiothoracic surgeons, they are important to consider. The consequence of pursuing risk-adjustment is the burden and expense of increased data collection. Using ACS-NSQIP data, investigators have shown that it is possible to minimize the number of variables collected for risk-adjustment without compromising the validity of performance rankings.[32] For the time being, in order to ensure provider "buy-in" and participation in systematic QI, risk-adjustment using clinical registry data remains the gold standard. Currently, the STS-GTSD and ACS-NSQIP both use statistical techniques to adjust for potential variation in case-mix across centers.[11,30,33]

QUALITY IMPROVEMENT

Quality measurement and assessment requires an intervention to change care delivery and outcomes. When judging quality using structures-of-care metrics, the commonly recommended intervention is regionalization—centralization of care to limited specific centers or providers based on a priori determined criteria (e.g., high-volume esophagectomy hospital). Alternatively, when measuring individual performance (i.e., process utilization and risk-adjusted outcomes), the commonly recommended intervention is to "raise the tide" with an eye toward "floating all boats"—a broad set of interventions intended to mitigate suboptimal care delivery and outcomes without limiting care to specific centers or providers. This section outlines the pros and cons of varying QI interventions.

Regionalizing Thoracic Surgical Care

Harold Luft, PhD suggested regionalizing surgical care because of an association between volume and short-term outcomes. This suggestion was reinvigorated at the turn of the 21st century by John D. Birkmeyer, MD when he demonstrated associations between hospital and surgeon volume and short-term outcomes among patients undergoing high-risk-operations including pulmonary resection and esophagectomy.[4,5] Around the same time, other investigators had shown that higher hospital volume was also associated with higher long-term survival among lung cancer patients.[6] These observations dovetailed with the efforts of the LeapFrog Group—a coalition of employers advocating for higher quality health care. The significance of LeapFrog was that even in the absence of enforceable health policy, this powerful employer-based coalition could steer patients to higher volume centers for these operations. Although no federal health policy emerged as a result of these studies, the LeapFrog Group pursued its vision and hospitals started reporting and marketing their compliance with LeapFrog metrics.

Shortly after publication of these high-profile volume–outcome studies, a body of evidence emerged demonstrating an association between specialization in thoracic surgery and better short- and long-term outcomes among lung cancer patients.[8-10] One recent study suggests that care provided by thoracic surgeons was associated with lower rates of mortality and "failure-to-rescue" for esophagectomy compared to general surgeons.[34] All investigations demonstrated these associations independent of volume and/or other hospital characteristics (e.g., teaching status, bed size). Regionalization based on surgeon-specialty is as an alternative to regionalization based on hospital characteristics.

Regionalization offers a relatively quick solution for suboptimal care and outcomes, but it is controversial and has potential limitations. Subsequent studies have demonstrated that the volume–outcome relationship is sensitive to statistical and modeling techniques.[35-37] Others have criticized volume–outcome studies because they were conducted using administrative databases that have a limited number of clinical variables for risk-adjustment. Although not the focus of the study, an STS-GTSD investigation evaluating a surrogate measure for morbidity and mortality using robust clinical registry data for risk-adjustment did not identify a relationship between volume and outcome.[33] Other lines of evidence suggest that regionalization may paradoxically worsen population-level outcomes. Interviews with Medicare beneficiaries who had undergone high-risk operations, including lung resection, revealed that half would not change hospitals even if there was an alternative center nearby with a 1% lower mortality rate.[38] These findings raised the possibility that regionalization could result in patients—particularly those in rural areas or living far from high-quality centers or providers—being "forced" into choosing between traveling to receive care or not receiving any treatment at all. Other investigators found that low-volume centers more commonly care for marginalized patients, and suggested that a policy of regionalization that does not explicitly mention a plan for caring for these patients may in fact increase disparities in care.[39]

Another issue with volume-based referral is uncertainty about hospitals and surgeons having the capacity to accommodate an influx of patients. Finally, there are substantial political barriers at the clinician and hospital level to regionalization. Thoracic surgical procedures are a source of significant revenue. Many surgeons and hospitals are unlikely to willingly give up this source of revenue, at least not under the predominantly fee-for-service care delivery model in the United States (US). Some have suggested that health care reform could change this perspective.[40]

Over a decade's worth of time has allowed for an assessment of the impact of volume-based regionalization, driven by political and market forces, on outcomes. Two national studies show that over time more patients were cared for by higher volume centers and that operative mortality rates are improving over time for several operations including lung and esophageal resection.[41,42] For pulmonary resection, improvements in outcomes over time could not be attributed to the shifts in care to higher volume centers because operative mortality rates were decreasing across all hospitals. For esophagectomy, one study suggested that shift in care to higher volume centers were partially responsible for better outcome over times,[41] but the other study found no such relationship.[42] The potential impact of specialty-based regionalization has not been evaluated recently. An older investigation reported that between 1992 and 2002 the proportion of patients cared for by general surgeons decreased by just under 5%.[9] The impact of spontaneous specialty-based regionalization is unknown but unlikely to be significant, again because hospitals and surgeons are unwilling to give up revenue under a fee-for-service model. Overall, the available evidence in favor of regionalizing thoracic oncologic care is at best controversial, although regionalization has not been implemented in an organized manner.

Successful regionalization requires enforceable health policy backed by multistakeholder support and surveillance systems to monitor for any potential unintended consequences of centralized care. Organ transplantation is one example of regionalized care in the US. Because of the great disparity between need and availability of organs, legislation was created to ensure the safe and equitable allocation, distribution, and transplantation of organs. Registry participation is mandatory and allows for tracking of both transplanted and nontransplanted patients. Transplant centers are required to participate in QI activities and are subjected to random site visits by various auditors. Outcomes by center and organ are reported and available to the public. Another example of regionalization in the US is LVRS for severe emphysema. In an unusual move, the Center for Medicare and Medicaid Services (CMS) partnered with the National Health, Lung, and Blood Institute to conduct a multicenter randomized trial of LVRS versus medical therapy for severe emphysema.[23] A subgroup of patients benefited from LVRS and as a result CMS-created policy that limited reimbursement for LVRS to centers and surgeons who participated in the trial or were a lung transplant center. These two examples from end-stage lung disease demonstrate the complexity of regionalizing care in the US.

Raising the Tide

Raising-the-tide is a multifaceted approach to improving outcomes and represents the bulk of actual QI efforts in thoracic surgery. It is motivated by the belief that optimal care delivery and outcomes *can be* achieved in all settings; however, raising the tide does not necessarily assume that optimal care and outcomes *will be* achieved in all settings. This belief and assumption hint at the need of a feedback loop where standards are determined, adherence is measured, benchmarked performance data is returned to the hospital and/or surgeon, and action is taken to improve performance. Most QI interventions do not address all aspects of the feedback loop. Furthermore, several components of the feedback loop require significant assumptions—for instance, standards and benchmarks can be defined and agreed upon in a multistakeholder fashion and that a clear line of action exists to remedy suboptimal performance. For these reasons, raising-the-tide is considered by many to be a "weak intervention." Nonetheless, raising-the-tide is more likely to be acceptable to the broadest range of stakeholders, and therefore most likely to be implemented into real-world practice.

One broad example of raising-the-tide is through codification of best practices and defining quality metrics. Groups of physicians have come to together to publish practice guidelines. Examples include the National Comprehensive Cancer Network (NCCN), American College of Chest Physicians (ACCP), STS, and the American Association for Thoracic Surgery (AATS). The National Quality Forum (NQF) is a nonprofit, membership-based organization that is led by many different stakeholders including hospital and health system administrators, business leaders, physicians, payers, and health policy experts. These organizations review the available evidence and seek consensus-based recommendations. Codification of best practices and defined quality metrics facilitates measurement of processes, structures, and outcomes, but the impact of doing so on quality is largely unknown. A national cohort study of temporal trends in the management of lung cancer patients reported a steady decline in resection rates among early-stage patients that could not be explained by increasing age and/or comorbidities.[43] This result was puzzling because it coincided with increased dissemination of practice guidelines by the NCCN and ACCP over the period of study, and increased dissemination of guidelines was expected to increase resection rates. Unfortunately, limitations of the data source precluded an understanding of why resection rates declined. A qualitative study of clinicians and administrators from Ontario reported on the barriers to achieving guideline-concordant lung cancer care, including lack of organizational support by clinical administrative leadership, uncertainty about the generalizability of trial results in the community-at-large, and the physician–patient dynamic.[44] These examples highlight some of the challenges of codification of best practices and defining quality metrics as a stand-alone approach to raising-the-tide.

Another example of an approach to raising-the-tide is benchmarked performance feedback using national databases. The STS-GTSD is the predominant mechanism for feedback to hospitals performing general thoracic surgery. ACS-NSQIP also provides feedback to hospitals to performing pulmonary and esophageal surgery, although the set of complications measured are not specific to thoracic surgical patients. Participation is voluntary for both the STS-GTSD and ACS-NSQIP. The impact of the STS-GTSD has not yet been evaluated, but an analysis of the STS Adult Cardiac Database demonstrated steadily improving observed-to-expected mortality rates over a 10-year period after the implementation of the STS database.[45] In contrast, the impact of ACS-NSQIP on general and vascular surgery patients was recently reported in two high-profile studies.[46,47] Key findings from both studies were that outcomes improved over time for all hospitals regardless of participation in a national database and that participation in ACS-NSQIP was not associated with improved outcomes or lower costs of care. These latter studies highlight why performance feedback alone may be insufficient for impactful QI.

Following the footsteps of cardiac surgery, locoregional initiatives to improve thoracic surgical quality are rapidly emerging as yet another means of raising-the-tide. The idea of a regional QI collaborative in cardiac surgery was first implemented in New England and subsequently in Washington, Michigan, Virginia, Alabama, and Minnesota.[48–54] A pre-/postimplementation study in New England

revealed declining mortality rates,[48] and a pre-/postinvestigation of Alabama's mortality rates compared to another state and national estimates demonstrated a larger improvement over time.[51] Locoregional QI initiatives have the advantage of engaging relevant stakeholders to overcome challenges and seize opportunities that make sense locally. A strong sense of community, collaboration, and cooperation is necessary despite competition within a common marketplace. For example, in Michigan, feedback on internal mammary artery (IMA) utilization rates, sites visits, and the sharing of information between surgeons was associated with an increase in IMA use over time and to levels greater than the national rate as reported by the STS.[52] Because of the success of regional cardiac surgery QI initiatives, similar locoregional programs have been developed in thoracic surgery. Two states—Washington and Michigan—now have regional QI collaboratives in general thoracic surgery.[12,55] Several health systems—Providence Health and Services[56] and the Catholic Health Initiative (personal communication Bahirathan Krishnadasan)—are also developing locoregional QI programs that measure evidence-based, consensus-driven metrics with feedback on performance and system-level support to drive changes in care delivery. Another program—called ProvenCare Lung Cancer (discussed in greater depth later in the chapter)—was developed on a national level for implementation at the individual hospital level.

Transparency through public reporting is another example of an attempt to raise-the-tide. Leaders in cardiac surgery have invoked an ethical responsibility to promote patient autonomy as the primary reason to pursue public reporting of quality measures.[57] Whether or not public reporting actually improves quality remains an area of ongoing interest. After the release of publicly available outcomes data for CABG in New York State, risk-adjusted mortality rates declined.[58] However, in nearby Massachusetts, there was a similar decline in risk-adjusted mortalities despite the absence of statewide outcomes reporting system.[59] Furthermore, apparent improvement in outcomes in New York may have been due in part to migration of high-risk patients out of the state. A survey of New York surgeons indicated that nearly a third refused to operate on certain patients because of public reporting,[60] and a study of referral patterns and case-mix showed an increase in high-risk patients from New York State to Cleveland Clinic.[61] Finally, it is important to consider whether or not patients would use this information to make health care decisions. A survey of Medicare beneficiaries who underwent high-risk surgery reported that the reputation of the surgeon and hospital was the most important factor influencing their decision about where to receive care, and that comparative hospital data was the least important factor.[38] Similarly, a 2008 Kaiser Family Foundation Study reported that a majority of patients would choose a hospital familiar with them rather than a higher-rated facility.[62] Overall, there remains uncertainty about the impact of public reporting on quality and outcomes. A composite metric for voluntary public reporting of outcomes in thoracic surgery was recently developed but has not yet been implemented.[63]

PRACTICAL CONSIDERATIONS

Unintended Consequences

QI should be viewed as a health care intervention—no different than a diagnostic test, drug, and/or operation—with benefits, risks, alternatives, and costs. The principle of "first do no harm" is just as relevant in QI as it is thoracic surgical care. Fortunately, there is no evidence that current QI initiatives in thoracic surgery have caused harm, but there are concerns that underscore the importance of thoughtful QI.

Improving One Outcome May Worsen Another

Attempts to improve one outcome may paradoxically worsen another. For example, for many years, there has been an interest in decreasing LOS as a means of increasing the value of surgical care. Over time the average LOS is decreasing while readmission rates are increasing.[64,65] Two investigative groups using two independent data sources showed a similar phenomenon—a U-shaped relationship between LOS and readmission rates.[65,66] In other words, above a threshold LOS—4 days in one study and 5 days in the other—as the LOS increases so does the readmission rate, presumably correlating because longer admissions are a consequence of sicker patients who are therefore readmitted more frequently. However, below this threshold, as LOS decreases, the readmission rate increases. These observations provide empirical evidence of what most experienced thoracic surgeons know already—if you push a patient out of the hospital too early, they will bounce back. These findings suggest that an attempt to decrease the average LOS beyond an "optimized" point may inadvertently increase readmissions. As of 2015, the CMS began limiting reimbursement for unplanned readmissions after treatment for acute myocardial infarction (AMI), congestive heart failure, pneumonia, and acute exacerbation of chronic obstructive pulmonary disease or for patients readmitted for elective total hip or knee arthroplasty. This policy could curb attempts to decrease LOS. Surgeons and hospitals actively attempting to drive down their mean LOS would benefit from a surveillance system that also tracks their readmission rates. Whether or not LOS and readmissions are in fact good quality measures is a matter of debate, but their U-shaped relationship provides a simple example of how improving one outcome may worsen another. This limitation of QI can be remedied by measuring all relevant and interacting outcomes, although doing so comes with the added expense of data collection and analysis.

Improving Quality Measures But Not Quality

One way to improve apparent performance but not quality is to game the system. Upcoding or "coding creep" refers to providers inappropriately documenting risk factors.[57] Doing so systematically will likely result in a surgeon's or hospital's patients appearing to be sicker (i.e., higher risk) than they really are. The consequence of having apparently sicker patients is that the expected mortality rate increases. If actual mortality rates remain unchanged, then it would appear that the observed-to-expected mortality rate has improved. Understandably, if surgeons and hospitals are aware of performance monitoring and have traditionally been lousy documenters of comorbid conditions, they would naturally be motivated to improve their documentation. Though appropriate, it can be excessive, and/or lead to the phenomenon of improving observed-to-expected mortality rates over time without meaningful changes or improvements in care delivery and outcomes. Another way to game the system is to simply not operate on high-risk patients and transfer them to another hospital, state, or region, as was the case in New York State after adoption of public report cards.[60,61] The types of gaming described here can be remedied in two ways. Regular and random audits of data accuracy and validity can deter inappropriate and/or excessive upcoding. National surveillance systems of patients, care, and outcomes can monitor for risk-avoidance on the part of surgeons, hospitals, and health systems.

Another way to improve quality metrics but not quality is through the use of surrogate endpoints. Surrogate measures offer advantages to direct measurement in terms of feasibility, expense, and timeliness. However, in the scientific world, they can also lead to erroneous inference. A classic example is measuring the frequency of premature ventricular contractions (PVCs) as a surrogate for sudden death and cardiac-related mortality in the setting of AMI. Many studies had showed that the antiarrhythmic drug flecainide suppressed PVCs effectively. Unfortunately, the Cardiac Arrhythmia Suppression Trial demonstrated that flecainide also significantly increased the risk of early death through unknown mechanisms.[67] This and other examples have motivated the Federal Drug Administration to have a higher level of scrutiny for surrogate measures of efficacy in drug trials.[68] Similarly, in QI, surrogate endpoints can lead to erroneous inference. For example, a quality metric—prolonged LOS greater than 14 days—was developed in the early phases of the STS General Thoracic Database as a surrogate measure for major morbidity and mortality after lung resection.[33] The motivation for this measure was to have an event that occurs frequently enough to allow for stable comparisons of performance that exclude the possibility of chance (see earlier discussion). Although well-intended, there was a suspicion that perhaps many important postoperative adverse events were in fact missed by the metric prolonged LOS. A subsequent single institution study revealed that prolonged LOS missed 80% of postoperative inpatient complications of which an overwhelming majority required additional inpatient therapies.[69] This finding coupled with another national study showing declining prolonged LOS rates over time[65] in the absence of performance measurement raised the possibility that apparent improvement in prolonged LOS might not reflect better quality care. In other words, unknown forces were driving down the proportion of patients with prolonged LOS, but a majority of these patients may still be experiencing complications significant enough to warrant additional inpatient care. The potential disadvantages of surrogate measures can be remedied by simply avoiding their use or extending a higher level of scrutiny during development and validation.

Sustainability

QI, like many other activities in life, is threatened by its sustainability. Two specific threats include burden and relevance.

Participation in QI is both time and resource intensive. For example, at a minimum, surgeons and hospitals must set aside time to scour QI reports, develop projects to improve care and outcomes, and then implement them into practice. Much time and energy is needed to coordinate recurring local meetings, and to attend regional or national meetings. This time burden is amplified when there are numerous different sources of information about quality, and numerous "people to answer to." In some cases, clinicians themselves abstract and input raw clinical data into registries, but in most cases chart abstractors and data entry personnel are required to complete this task. Financial burden arises from the salary and benefits for such personnel as well as costs from the data vendor and national database. For example, it is estimated that participation in ACS-NSQIP costs upward of $100,000 a year.[24] Individual hospitals shoulder these expenses. Time and expense are significant barriers to the sustainability of QI efforts.

Many have argued that because complications result in increased health care costs, QI will pay for itself; however, health economists and thought leaders have challenged this notion on the basis that traditional economics do not apply to health care.[40] Specifically, there is information asymmetry between "buyers" and "suppliers" of health services. Furthermore, third-party payers and employers distort relationships traditionally defined as buyers and sellers resulting in buyers, sellers, suppliers, and recipients of health care. Finally, the costs of poor quality care are typically shifted. For instance, a particularly bad year of complications and high expenses may translate into higher insurance premiums for next year's beneficiaries. With health care reform, it seems like accountable care organizations will shoulder the burden of poor quality care and therefore be motivated to pursue QI. The Veteran's Affairs Administration and Health Maintenance Organizations are examples of where the payer is the provider of health care and are incentivized to improve quality. Of course, it is debatable whether these care delivery systems in fact provide better care. Although health economics is well beyond the scope of this chapter, it is important to recognize that it is far from clear that hospitals (and surgeons) alone should invest in QI.

There are several approaches that may mitigate the burden of QI on providers and health systems. Specialists could attempt to consolidate QI efforts eliminating redundancy in data collection and analysis. National databases could sponsor studies that seek to minimize the number of variables needed for risk-adjustment without affecting model performance (i.e., development and validation of parsimonious risk-models). Measurement and analysis could be anchored around standards put forth by practice guidelines and outcomes and quality metrics determined by multistakeholder, nonprofit organizations. To further minimize the burden of data collection and analysis, initiatives might choose to take on quality gaps in sequence rather than in parallel—in other words measuring a limited set of process and outcome measures on a revolving basis. Regional collaboratives may expedite the resolution of quality gaps, and seek metrics that are pertinent to the local community. Finally, the case for QI should be made taking into consideration the many relevant perspectives that naturally arise from having many different stakeholders—patients, physicians, other providers, hospitals, insurers, and employers. Historically, QI has been driven by surgeons and is not surprisingly surgeon-centric. An attempt to broaden quality metrics to appeal to many stakeholders will increase the odds of engagement and financial support of QI projects.

QUALITY IMPROVEMENT INITIATIVES IN THORACIC SURGERY

Society of Thoracic Surgeons

The Society of Thoracic Surgeons (STS) is a professional organization committed to enhancing the ability of cardiothoracic surgeons to provide the highest quality patient care through education, research, and advocacy. Four specific ways the STS promotes quality are (1) defining structure, process, and outcome measures, (2) maintaining a national database for feedback performance, (3) developing and disseminating practice guidelines, and (4) supporting other national QI efforts.

The quality metrics identified by the STS have been endorsed or are under review for endorsement by the National Quality Forum. Participation in a systematic national database for general thoracic surgery is one structure-of-care metric. Process-of-care measures include recording of clinical stage and performance status for pulmonary resection and esophagectomy. Outcome measures for lung resection include risk-adjusted LOS >14 days[33] and risk-adjusted morbidity and mortality.[11] For esophagectomy, the outcome measure is risk-adjusted morbidity and mortality.[25] Although public reporting of general thoracic surgery outcomes has not been adopted by the STS, a composite measure of morbidity and mortality was recently developed for this purpose.[63]

The STS General Thoracic Surgery Database (STS-GTSD) is a national clinical registry with participation open to any surgeon (i.e., general thoracic, cardiac, general, and/or vascular surgeon) who performs general thoracic surgery as part of their practice. Between 2002 and 2008, the STS-GTSD had information on only 8% of all patients undergoing lung resection nationally,[70] but this period of time represents early implementation of the database. Over 9 years,

the number of participating sites increased from just under 20 to over 200 centers.[70] More recent estimates suggest that 25% to 50% of all pulmonary resections are now captured by the STS-GTSD. Every 6 months, a report is generated and sent to each participating site. The report includes aggregate information about patient characteristics, procedures, operative volume, outcomes, and of course the quality metrics described earlier. Recently, an independent audit of random sites was performed and revealed 95% accuracy without evidence of purposeful omission or gaming.[71] Prior to this audit, an important criticism of the STS-GTSD was that the validity of this voluntary database had not been established. This audit refutes these concerns. Because of the voluntary nature of STS-GTSD participation, it is not surprising that the outcomes of participants appear to be better than that of the nation as a whole.[70] Greater national participation is expected to yield greater opportunities for QI.

The STS also publishes practice guidelines for general thoracic surgery. Available topics include diagnosis and staging of patients with esophageal cancer,[72] multimodality treatment for cancer of the esophagus and gastroesophageal junction,[3] and management of Barrett esophagus with high-grade dysplasia.[73] The Workforce on Evidence-Based Surgery is tasked with identifying subject matter, exhaustive review of the literature, and consensus-based generation of recommendations.

Finally, the STS has supported other national QI initiatives. Choosing Wisely is an initiative of the American Board of Internal Medicine (ABIM) Foundation that fundamentally seeks to promote conversations between providers and patients about evidence-based practice, avoidance of duplicative tests, freedom from harm, and necessity. A physician charter on professionalism, published in 2002 and subsequently endorsed by 130 medical specialties, was "put into practice" through funding from the ABIM Foundation. Each specialty was tasked with creating a list of "things patients and providers should question" using the following criteria: limited to items that fall within the purview of the specialty; supported by evidence; thoroughly documented and publicly available upon request; frequently ordered/costly; easy for a lay person to understand; and measurable/actionable. STS Workforce Chairs from Adult Cardiac and Vascular Surgery, General Thoracic Surgery, and Evidence-Based Surgery were called upon to help create the specialty specific draft recommendations for Choosing Wisely. A survey of STS members from the US was conducted to obtain member feedback on these draft items. Concurrently, a systematic review of the literature was performed. A total of eight evidentiary statements were presented to the STS Executive Committee resulting in the approval of five specialty-specific recommendations.[74] Two of these recommendations were specific to general thoracic surgery and they are: patients who have no cardiac history and good functional status do not require preoperative stress testing before noncardiac thoracic surgery; and patients with suspected or biopsy-proven stage I nonsmall cell lung cancer do not require brain imaging before definitive care in the absence of neurologic symptoms.

ProvenCare Lung Cancer

ProvenCare Lung Cancer is a nationally developed QI initiative that is intended to be deployed at local institutions in a tailored fashion.[75] The idea originated from the Geisinger Health System—an integrated health care delivery system—in 2005 and was developed to mitigate variability in care for patients undergoing CABG. Based on the principles of reliability science (standardization, error proofing, and failure mode redesign), clinical work flows were re-engineered, effective feedback mechanisms were built, and multistakeholder institutional commitment was sought from administrators and providers alike. The success of this intervention led to similar projects for percutaneous coronary intervention, total hip replacement, and cataract surgery. Although successful in this integrated health system, the generalizability of this intervention had not been evaluated.

In 2009, the Geisinger Health System and the American College of Surgeons Commission on Cancer partnered to host an inaugural meeting with representatives from a variety of hospital settings (e.g., academic and community hospitals, electronic and paper medical records, individual and group practices) performing pulmonary resection for lung cancer. The goal was to develop, implement, and evaluate ProvenCare Lung Cancer at these sites to demonstrate the feasibility and value of using this model of QI outside the Geisinger Health System and for different disease population. The standard components of ProvenCare Lung Cancer are a patient engagement contract and a 38-point all-or-nothing process-of-care checklist spanning care elements from the initial to the postoperative clinic visit. These processes-of-care were selected based on consensus among experts and published evidence. Each system was then responsible for identifying physician champion, local institutional stakeholder engagement, implementation of a feedback system, and a mechanism to remedy noncompliance. Ultimately, 12 centers participated in ProvenCare Lung Cancer. All 12 also participated in the STS-GTSD which will eventually allow for a pre-/postimplementation comparison of risk-adjusted outcomes. Between 2010 and 2012, overall compliance with the checklist across all centers increased from approximately 40% to 90% (unpublished data). These preliminary findings suggest that a nationally developed QI project can be successfully implemented with local modifications to ensure reliable delivery of thoracic oncologic surgical care. Future plans are to expand this model from a surgical-based to a disease-based QI intervention ensuring reliable delivery of care across the entire cancer continuum from lung cancer screening to posttreatment surveillance.

FUTURE DIRECTIONS

It is no doubt hard to predict the future of thoracic surgical QI, but there are two broad directions worth considering as there are already inklings of change in our field.

One new direction is disease-based QI. Perhaps the easiest way to describe this approach to QI is to consider the denominator. Instead of the denominator including only operated lung cancer patients, the denominator would include all patients with confirmed or suspected nonsmall cell lung cancer. This approach to QI is impactful in two ways. By moving "proximally" on the cancer care continuum, more individuals reap the potential benefits of QI. A simple conceptualization of the cancer care continuum is prevention, screening, diagnosis/staging, treatment, and survivorship/end-of-life care. More "proximal" aspects of the care continuum have a larger denominator. For example, up to 94 million former or current smokers are eligible for smoking cessation and lung cancer screening, whereas only 240,000 new patients per year are diagnosed with lung cancer.[76] Roughly 60,000 (~25%) undergo resection. Ensuring high-quality, evidence-based prevention and screening will likely reach more people than ensuring high-quality treatment. Another perhaps more important way that disease-based QI makes an impact is by revealing the most egregious departures from optimal care. Patients with suspected or confirmed nonsmall cell lung cancer should undergo rigorous pretreatment staging. Most would agree that an overstaged patient falsely presumed to have advanced disease and a deprived curative-intent resection is a terrible departure from ideal care. Evaluating only surgical patients

precludes an understanding of how many patients are inappropriately deprived optimal treatments. Moving "proximally" to evaluate a larger denominator consisting of patients with suspected or confirmed potentially resectable lung cancer allows QI initiatives to fully realize their potential in positively influencing individuals and the general population. ProvenCare Lung Cancer is currently developing a set of quality metrics and interventions that will tackle the entire continuum of lung cancer care from diagnosis to treatment and end-of-life care. It is evident that leaders within thoracic surgery are already steering QI toward a disease-based rather than treatment-based model of QI.

The other new direction for QI is the adoption of evidence-based QI interventions. As stated throughout this chapter, most QI initiatives do not have a high-level of evidence to support them. Most rely on expert opinion and observational data with limitations relating to inadequate comparators and/or adjustment for confounding variables. Unfortunately, there is a growing body of evidence that suggests that QI efforts do not impact outcomes and some cases may have unintended consequences.[77] In an era of threatened sustainability, stakeholders—particularly those who make financial investments and surgeons and other providers who invest their valuable time—may increasingly demand a higher level of evidence before adopting QI initiatives. Fortunately, robust methods exist to respond to this demand. Specifically, clustered randomized trials are uniquely suited to test hypotheses about the superiority of QI initiatives over usual care. In a clustered randomized trial, a hospital or health system is randomized to the intervention rather than the patient. This approach avoids the challenges, confusion, and concerns of applying QI to some but not all patients within one health system. When it is strongly believed that a QI will benefit patients—and therefore there may be ethical reasons why a region might not want to withhold the intervention—there is still an opportunity to evaluate the impact of the QI initiative. A clustered step-wedge trial design allows all hospitals or health systems to eventually adopt the QI intervention, but each hospital or system is randomized in terms of the timing of adoption.[78] This study design allows for robust inference about the effect of a QI intervention on patient outcomes without denying the intervention to patients and providers. Thoracic surgeons have an opportunity generate the highest level of evidence to support their QI initiatives in the same manner in which they have generated high levels of evidence to support their clinical interventions.

REFERENCES

1. Neuhauser D. Ernest Amory Codman MD. *Qual Saf Health Care* 2002;11:104–105.
2. Lohr KN. *Medicare: A Strategy for Quality Assurance, Volume I.* Washington, DC: The National Academies Press; 1990.
3. Little AG, Rusch VW, Bonner JA, et al. Patterns of surgical care of lung cancer patients. *Ann Thorac Surg* 2005;80:2051–2056; discussion 2056.
4. Birkmeyer JD, Siewers AE, Finlayson EV, et al. Hospital volume and surgical mortality in the United States. *N Engl J Med* 2002;346:1128–1137.
5. Birkmeyer JD, Stukel TA, Siewers AE, et al. Surgeon volume and operative mortality in the United States. *N Engl J Med* 2003;349:2117–2127.
6. Bach PB, Cramer LD, Schrag D, et al. The influence of hospital volume on survival after resection for lung cancer. *N Engl J Med* 2001;345:181–188.
7. Silvestri GA, Handy J, Lackland D, et al. Specialists achieve better outcomes than generalists for lung cancer surgery. *Chest* 1998;114:675–680.
8. Goodney PP, Lucas FL, Stukel TA, et al. Surgeon specialty and operative mortality with lung resection. *Ann Surg* 2005;241:179–184.
9. Farjah F, Flum DR, Varghese TK, Jr, et al. Surgeon specialty and long-term survival after pulmonary resection for lung cancer. *Ann Thorac Surg* 2009;87:995–1004; discussion 1005–1006.
10. Schipper PH, Diggs BS, Ungerleider RM, et al. The influence of surgeon specialty on outcomes in general thoracic surgery: A national sample 1996 to 2005. *Ann Thorac Surg* 2009;88:1566–1572; discussion 1572–1573.
11. Kozower BD, Sheng S, O'Brien SM, et al. STS database risk models: Predictors of mortality and major morbidity for lung cancer resection. *Ann Thorac Surg* 2010;90:875–881; discussion 881–883.

12. Farjah F, Varghese TK, Costas K, et al. Lung resection outcomes and costs in Washington State: A case for regional quality improvement. *Ann Thorac Surg* 2014; 98:175–181; discussion 182.

13. Bach PB, Cramer LD, Warren JL, et al. Racial differences in the treatment of early-stage lung cancer. *N Engl J Med* 1999;341:1198–1205.

14. Farjah F, Wood DE, Yanez III ND, et al. Racial disparities among patients with lung cancer who were recommended operative therapy. *Arch Surg* 2009;144:14–18.

15. Lathan CS, Neville BA, Earle CC. The effect of race on invasive staging and surgery in non-small-cell lung cancer. *J Clin Oncol* 2006;24:413–418.

16. Cykert S, Dilworth-Anderson P, Monroe MH, et al. Factors associated with decisions to undergo surgery among patients with newly diagnosed early-stage lung cancer. *JAMA* 2010;303:2368–2376.

17. Donabedian A. Evaluating the quality of medical care. *Milbank Mem Fund Q* 1966;44: 166–206.

18. Maziak DE, Darling GE, Inculet RI, et al. Positron emission tomography in staging early lung cancer: A randomized trial. *Ann Intern Med* 2009;151:221–228.

19. Fischer B, Lassen U, Mortensen J, et al. Preoperative staging of lung cancer with combined PET-CT. *N Engl J Med* 2009;361:32–39.

20. van Tinteren H, Hoekstra OS, Smit EF, et al. Effectiveness of positron emission tomography in the preoperative assessment of patients with suspected non-small-cell lung cancer: The PLUS multicentre randomised trial. *Lancet* 2002;359:1388–1392.

21. Herder GJ, Kramer H, Hoekstra OS, et al. Traditional versus up-front [18F] fluorode-oxyglucose-positron emission tomography staging of non-small-cell lung cancer: A Dutch cooperative randomized study. *J Clin Oncol* 2006;24:1800–1806.

22. Viney RC, Boyer MJ, King MT, et al. Randomized controlled trial of the role of positron emission tomography in the management of stage I and II non-small-cell lung cancer. *J Clin Oncol* 2004;22:2357–2362.

23. Fishman A, Martinez F, Naunheim K, et al. A randomized trial comparing lung-volume-reduction surgery with medical therapy for severe emphysema. *N Engl J Med* 2003;348:2059–2073.

24. Birkmeyer JD, Dimick JB. Understanding and reducing variation in surgical mortality. *Annu Rev Med* 2009;60:405–415.

25. Wright CD, Kucharczuk JC, O'Brien SM, et al.; Society of Thoracic Surgeons General Thoracic Surgery Database. Predictors of major morbidity and mortality after esophagectomy for esophageal cancer: A Society of Thoracic Surgeons General Thoracic Surgery Database risk adjustment model. *J Thorac Cardiovasc Surg* 2009; 137:587–595; discussion 596.

26. Hanley JA, Lippman-Hand A. If nothing goes wrong, is everything all right? Interpreting zero numerators. *JAMA* 1983;249:1743–1745.

27. Dimick JB, Welch HG, Birkmeyer JD. Surgical mortality as an indicator of hospital quality: The problem with small sample size. *JAMA* 2004;292:847–851.

28. Dimick JB, Staiger DO, Birkmeyer JD. Ranking hospitals on surgical mortality: The importance of reliability adjustment. *Health Serv Res* 2010;45:1614–1629.

29. MacKenzie TA, Grunkemeier GL, Grunwald GK, et al. A primer on using shrinkage to compare in-hospital mortality between centers. *Ann Thorac Surg* 2015;99:757–761.

30. Cohen ME, Ko CY, Bilimoria KY, et al. Optimizing ACS NSQIP modeling for evaluation of surgical quality and risk: Patient risk adjustment, procedure mix adjustment, shrinkage adjustment, and surgical focus. *J Am Coll Surg* 2013;217:336–346.e1.

31. Dimick JB, Birkmeyer JD. Ranking hospitals on surgical quality: Does risk-adjustment always matter? *J Am Coll Surg* 2008;207:347–351.

32. Dimick JB, Osborne NH, Hall BL, et al. Risk adjustment for comparing hospital quality with surgery: How many variables are needed? *J Am Coll Surg* 2010;210:503–508.

33. Wright CD, Gaissert HA, Grab JD, et al. Predictors of prolonged length of stay after lobectomy for lung cancer: A Society of Thoracic Surgeons General Thoracic Surgery Database risk-adjustment model. *Ann Thorac Surg* 2008;85:1857–1865; discussion 1865.

34. Gopaldas RR, Bhamidipati CM, Dao TK, et al. Impact of surgeon demographics and technique on outcomes after esophageal resections: A nationwide study. *Ann Thorac Surg* 2013;95:1064–1069.

35. Kozower BD, Stukenborg GJ. Hospital esophageal cancer resection volume does not predict patient mortality risk. *Ann Thorac Surg* 2012;93:1690–1696; discussion 1696–1698.

36. Kozower BD, Stukenborg GJ. The relationship between hospital lung cancer resection volume and patient mortality risk. *Ann Surg* 2011;254:1032–1037.

37. French B, Farjah F, Flum DR, et al. A general framework for estimating volume-outcome associations from longitudinal data. *Stat Med* 2012;31:366–382.

38. Schwartz LM, Woloshin S, Birkmeyer JD. How do elderly patients decide where to go for major surgery? Telephone interview survey. *BMJ* 2005;331:821.

39. Liu JH, Zingmond DS, McGory ML, et al. Disparities in the utilization of high-volume hospitals for complex surgery. *JAMA* 2006;296:1973–1980.

40. Flum DR, Pellegrini CA. The business of quality in surgery. *Ann Surg* 2012;255:6–7.

41. Finks JF, Osborne NH, Birkmeyer JD. Trends in hospital volume and operative mortality for high-risk surgery. *N Engl J Med* 2011;364:2128–2137.

42. Learn PA, Bach PB. A decade of mortality reductions in major oncologic surgery: the impact of centralization and quality improvement. *Med Care* 2010;48:1041–1049.

43. Farjah F, Wood DE, Yanez D 3rd, et al. Temporal trends in the management of potentially resectable lung cancer. *Ann Thorac Surg* 2008;85:1850–1855; discussion 1856.

44. Brouwers MC, Makarski J, Garcia K, et al. A mixed methods approach to understand variation in lung cancer practice and the role of guidelines. *Implement Sci* 2014;9:36.

45. Grover FL, Shroyer AL, Hammermeister K, et al. A decade's experience with quality improvement in cardiac surgery using the Veterans Affairs and Society of Thoracic Surgeons national databases. *Ann Surg* 2001;234:464–472; discussion 472–474.

46. Osborne NH, Nicholas LH, Ryan AM, et al. Association of hospital participation in a quality reporting program with surgical outcomes and expenditures for Medicare beneficiaries. *JAMA* 2015;313:496–504.

47. Etzioni DA, Wasif N, Dueck AC, et al. Association of hospital participation in a surgical outcomes monitoring program with inpatient complications and mortality. *JAMA* 2015;313:505–511.

48. O'Connor GT, Plume SK, Olmstead EM, et al. A regional intervention to improve the hospital mortality associated with coronary artery bypass graft surgery. The Northern New England Cardiovascular Disease Study Group. *JAMA* 1996;275:841–846.

49. Arom KV, Petersen RJ, Orszulak TA, et al. Establishing and using a local/regional cardiac surgery database. *Ann Thorac Surg* 1997;64:1245–1249.

50. Goss JR, Whitten RW, Phillips RC, et al. Washington State's model of physician leadership in cardiac outcomes reporting. *Ann Thorac Surg* 2000;70:695–701.

51. Holman WL, Allman RM, Sansom M, et al. Alabama coronary artery bypass grafting project. *JAMA* 2001;285:3003–3010.

52. Johnson SH, Theurer PF, Bell GF, et al. A statewide quality collaborative for process improvement: Internal mammary artery utilization. *Ann Thorac Surg* 2010;90:1158–1164; discussion 1164.

53. Speir AM, Rich JB, Crosby I, et al. Regional collaboration as a model for fostering accountability and transforming health care. *Semin Thorac Cardiovasc Surg* 2009;21: 12–19.

54. Prager RL, Armenti FR, Bassett JS, et al. Cardiac surgeons and the quality movement: The Michigan experience. *Semin Thorac Cardiovasc Surg* 2009;21:20–27.

55. The Michigan Society of Thoracic and Cardiovascular Surgeons. Quality Collaborative. http://www.mstcvsqualitycollaborative.org/. Accessed March 10, 2015.

56. Providence Health and Services. Thoracic Surgery Initiative. http://oregon.providence. org/our-services/p/providence-cancer-center-annual-report-2012/spotlight-thoracic/. Accessed March 10, 2015.

57. Shahian DM, Edwards FH, Jacobs JP, et al. Public reporting of cardiac surgery performance: Part 1—history, rationale, consequences. *Ann Thorac Surg* 2011;92:S2–S11.

58. Hannan EL, Kilburn H, Jr., Racz M, et al. Improving the outcomes of coronary artery bypass surgery in New York State. *JAMA* 1994;271:761–766.

59. Ghali WA, Ash AS, Hall RE, et al. Statewide quality improvement initiatives and mortality after cardiac surgery. *JAMA* 1997;277:379–382.

60. Burack JH, Impellizzeri P, Homel P, et al. Public reporting of surgical mortality: A survey of New York State cardiothoracic surgeons. *Ann Thorac Surg* 1999;68:1195–1200; discussion 1201–1202.

61. Omoigui NA, Miller DP, Brown KJ, et al. Outmigration for coronary bypass surgery in an era of public dissemination of clinical outcomes. *Circulation* 1996;93:27–33.

62. 2008 Update on Consumers' Views of Patient Safety and Quality Information: Summary & Chartpack. Anonymous. http://kff.org/other/poll-finding/2008-update-on-consumers-views-of-patient. Accessed March 14, 2015.

63. Kozower BD, O'Brien SM, Kosinski AS, et al. The society of thoracic surgeons composite score for rating program performance for lobectomy for lung cancer. *Ann Thorac Surg* 2016;101:1379–1386; discussion 1386–1387.

64. Memtsoudis SG, Besculides MC, Zellos L, et al. Trends in lung surgery: United States 1988 to 2002. *Chest* 2006;130:1462–1470.

65. Farjah F, Wood DE, Varghese TK, et al. Health care utilization among surgically treated Medicare beneficiaries with lung cancer. *Ann Thorac Surg* 2009;88:1749–1756.

66. Freeman RK, Dilts JR, Ascioti AJ, et al. A comparison of length of stay, readmission rate, and facility reimbursement after lobectomy of the lung. *Ann Thorac Surg* 2013;96: 1740–1745; discussion 1745–1746.

67. Echt DS, Liebson PR, Mitchell LB, et al. Mortality and morbidity in patients receiving encainide, flecainide, or placebo. The Cardiac Arrhythmia Suppression Trial. *N Engl J Med* 1991;324:781–788.

68. Fleming TR. Surrogate endpoints and FDA's accelerated approval process. *Health Aff (Millwood)* 2005;24:67–78.

69. Farjah F, Lou F, Rusch VW, et al. The quality metric prolonged length of stay misses clinically important adverse events. *Ann Thorac Surg* 2012;94:881–888.

70. LaPar DJ, Bhamidipati CM, Lau CL, et al. The society of thoracic surgeons general thoracic surgery database: Establishing generalizability to national lung cancer resection outcomes. *Ann Thorac Surg* 2012;94:216–221; discussion 221.

71. Magee MJ, Wright CD, McDonald D, et al. External validation of the society of thoracic surgeons general thoracic surgery database. *Ann Thorac Surg* 2013;96:1734–1739; discussion 1738–1739.

72. Varghese TK, Jr, Hofstetter WL, Rizk NP, et al. The society of thoracic surgeons guidelines on the diagnosis and staging of patients with esophageal cancer. *Ann Thorac Surg* 2013;96:346–356.

73. Fernando HC, Murthy SC, Hofstetter W, et al. The Society of Thoracic Surgeons practice guideline series: guidelines for the management of Barrett's esophagus with high-grade dysplasia. *Ann Thorac Surg* 2009;87:1993–2002.

74. Wood DE, Mitchell JD, Schmitz DS, et al. Choosing wisely: Cardiothoracic surgeons partnering with patients to make good health care decisions. *Ann Thorac Surg* 2013;95: 1130–1135.

75. Katlic MR, Facktor MA, Berry SA, et al. ProvenCare lung cancer: A multi-institutional improvement collaborative. *CA Cancer J Clin* 2011;61:382–396.

76. Siegel R, Naishadham D, Jemal A. Cancer statistics, 2012. CA. *Cancer J Clin* 2012;62: 10–29.

77. Fullerton DA, Sundt TM. Process versus outcome: The sugar window. *Ann Thorac Surg* 2014;98:1902–1904.

78. Brown CA, Lilford RJ. The stepped wedge trial design: A systematic review. *BMC Med Res Methodol* 2006;6:54.

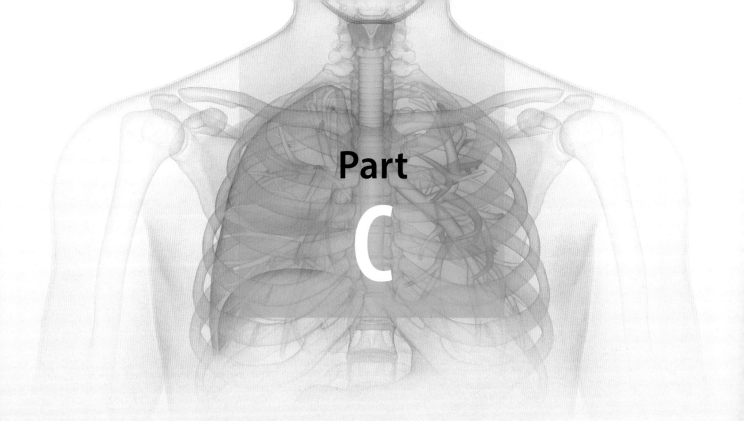

Part

C

THE ESOPHAGUS

STRUCTURE OF THE ESOPHAGUS

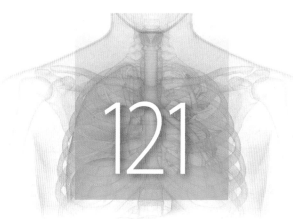

121

Embryology of the Aerodigestive Tract

Steven J. Mentzer

In adults, the trachea (anterior) is intimately juxtaposed to the esophagus (posterior). The posterior membranous trachea and the longitudinal muscle of the esophagus are only separable by a potential space. The intimate proximity reflects a common embryologic relationship, but the separation reflects distinct function and morphology.

The trachea, the primary conduit for ventilating air, develops cartilaginous rings anteriorly and longitudinal smooth muscle posteriorly. Air passing through the nose and nasal turbinates is warmed and humidified. The conditioned air passes through a tracheal lumen that is lined with ciliated pseudostratified columnar epithelium and a mucin layer apparently designed to trap particulates and facilitate mucociliary clearance.

In contrast, the food passing from the oropharynx to the esophagus is conditioned by mastication and salivary enzymes. Deglutition ensures that the food bolus is passed from the hypopharynx to the esophagus—bypassing the interposed tracheal opening. The circular and longitudinal smooth muscle of the esophagus facilitates peristalsis and the propulsion of the food bolus into the stomach. The epithelial lining is characterized by stratified squamous keratinized epithelium apparently designed as a protective layer for the proximal gastrointestinal tract.

Despite these functional distinctions, the esophagus and trachea share a common embryologic origin. In human embryogenesis, 3 to 4 weeks of gestation is a phase involving significant growth and regionalization. At the beginning of this developmental phase, the esophagus is a proximal region of the foregut—a simple epithelial tube of endoderm surrounded by mesenchyme. By 4 weeks of gestation, a ventral tracheal bud appears in the foregut. The tracheal bud grows into the ventral mesenchyme. As the tracheal bud elongates, the esophageal region of the foregut and the ventral tracheal bud separate through a dynamic process of septation and elongation.

ESOPHAGEAL EMBRYOLOGY

Between 4 and 5 weeks of gestation, the esophageal foregut matures and elongates. The proximal and distal portions of the esophagus lengthen creating a discrete tube connecting the pharynx to the dilated gastric primordium. The surrounding mesoderm contributes to the circular muscle by the 6th week of gestation; longitudinal muscle begins forming by 9 weeks. The splanchnic mesenchyme surrounding the lower esophagus appears to be responsible for the distinct smooth muscle anatomy and function of the lower esophagus, the lower esophageal sphincter, and cardia. By 7 weeks of gestation, the esophagus attains its birth length of 8 to 10 cm.[1]

The blood supply and innervation of the esophagus also reflects early development. The blood supply of the esophagus is primarily derived from the 4th branchial arch which produces both the subclavian artery and the aorta. Branches of the subclavian artery, including the inferior thyroid artery, supply the cervical esophagus. Branches of the aorta supply the thoracic esophagus. Neural crest cells migrate in waves to form the enteric plexus. Parasympathetic innervation of the esophagus is supplied by the vagus nerve. Sympathetic innervation is supplied by the thoracic sympathetic plexus and the celiac plexus.

Although the mesoderm contributes the components of the esophageal wall, the endoderm is responsible for the esophageal epithelium and submucosal glands. In the initial phases of development, the esophageal lining is stratified columnar epithelium. During development the lining becomes cuboidal and ciliated.

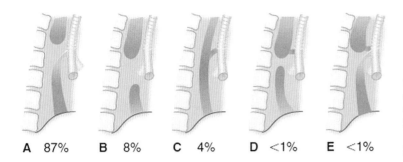

A 87% B 8% C 4% D <1% E <1%

FIGURE 121.1 Schematic diagram of the five most commonly encountered forms of esophageal atresia and tracheoesophageal fistula. (Reprinted from Herbst JJ. Gastrointestinal tract. In: Behrman RE, Kleigman RM, Nelson WE, et al., eds. *Nelson Textbook of Pediatrics*. 14th ed. Philadelphia, PA: WB Saunders; 1992:942. Copyright © 1992 Elsevier. With permission.)

Only after birth does the esophagus acquire a stratified squamous epithelium.

ESOPHAGEAL ATRESIA AND TRACHEOESOPHAGEAL FISTULA

After the development of the medial ventral diverticulum, the primitive foregut is divided into the esophagus and trachea. The process of tracheoesophageal septation and elongation are associated with primarily two congenital malformations: esophageal atresia and tracheoesophageal fistula (TEF). Although esophageal atresia and TEFs may exist as separate anomalies, the vast majority of patients have combined malformations (Fig. 121.1).

Esophageal atresia without a tracheal fistula is observed in 5% to 10% of patients with congenital tracheoesophageal disorders. Esophageal atresia typically involves a proximal blind esophageal pouch and a distal esophageal remnant near the diaphragm. Possibly a result of misdirected elongation, the result is a relatively long segment of missing esophagus. When primary repair fails or the defect does not permit the restoration of esophageal continuity, reconstruction of esophageal atresia requires an interposition graft—typically, the interposition of stomach, colon, or small intestine.[2]

In all cases of TEF, the tracheal conduit to the main stem bronchi is intact. Despite a patent airway lumen, structural abnormalities in the trachea at the site of the fistula, such as tracheomalacia and a loss of normal ciliated epithelium, can occur. These congenital problems are often associated with ongoing morbidity later in life.

In contrast to esophageal atresia, all cases of TEF involve fistulous communication between the esophagus and trachea; however, the communication can arise between different segments of the esophagus. The most common TEF, approximately 85% of congenital TEF, involves a blind proximal pouch and the distal esophageal segment communicating with the trachea (Gross type C). In this configuration, positive pressure ventilation results in ineffective pulmonary expansion and overdistension of the upper gastrointestinal tract.

Other configurations of TEF are less common. Esophageal atresia with a proximal TEF occurs approximately 5%, TEF without esophageal atresia 4%, and esophageal atresia with fistulas to both pouches (H-type fistula) occurs in approximately 1% of TEF. The various configurations of TEF are believed to reflect failure of embryologic septation during the early phases (weeks 3 to 4) of tracheal and esophageal development.

VACTERL

Approximately 25% to 35% of patients with congenital tracheoesophageal disorders have other anomalies. The most common anomalies are cardiac (35%), genitourinary (25%), gastrointestinal (25%), and skeletal (15%). The common occurrence of any combination of these anomalies has led to identification of a *vertebral, anal, cardiac, tracheoesophageal, renal, and limb* (VACTERL) association. The extent to which these associations are nonrandom is debated, but more recent studies suggest that the VACTERL associations may be due to defective midline blastogenesis.

ESOPHAGEAL STENOSIS AND WEBS

Controversy surrounds the potential congenital basis of other esophageal disorders. Esophageal stenosis and webs, most commonly occurring in the middle and distal esophagus, may not be diagnosed until adulthood. Because stenosis and webs can be acquired, it is unclear how many of these disorders are congenital. Regardless of their developmental origins, stenoses and webs are rare and not associated with other congenital anomalies.

LUNG EMBRYOLOGY

During the early development of the lung, between 3 and 4 weeks of gestation, the tracheoesophageal septum deepens and there is progressive separation of the trachea and the esophagus. Although the mechanism of separation is not well understood, a failure of separation results in a variety of developmental anomalies including laryngeal clefts, tracheoesophageal fistulae, esophageal atresia, and tracheal atresia.

The lung anlage arises from the ventral outpouching of the foregut. At 26 to 28 days, the ventral tracheal bud divides to form two epithelial lined lung buds. As these lung buds extend into the surrounding mesenchyme, the buds form the main bronchi and eventually the left and right lung. The five lobar bronchi are identifiable by 32 days and all segmental bronchi have formed by 36 days of gestation.[3]

Histologically, the embryonic (25 to 35 days) and pseudoglandular (35 days to 16 weeks) stages of lung development are characterized by the elaboration of primitive-appearing conducting airways. The presence of primitive airways in the surrounding mesenchyme gives the histologic impression of glands—hence, the name "pseudoglandular" stage. Club and goblet cells are present in the proximal airways.

The creation of the branching airway system reflects a robust developmental program. The endodermal lung buds progressively grow into the surrounding mesoderm in a dichotomous branching pattern; that is, a branching system that divides a single bronchus into two relatively equal "daughter" branches. Occasionally, a parent bronchus will divide into three daughter branches in a pattern known as trichotomy. The human upper bronchial tree, in comparison to other species, is one of the most symmetrical trees with respect to airway diameter and angle of branching.[4] This branching system is often described as bipodial/tripodial. In contrast, rodents have an asymmetric branching pattern that is referred to as a monopodial system. The reasons for species differences in airway geometry are unknown, but these differences have practical implications for animal models of inhalational therapeutics and airborne toxicology.

The branching pattern in the lung is a remarkable developmental process. The airways form a hierarchical continuum that extends from the trachea to the alveoli. The first 15 generations of branching airways are composed of conducting tubes; the subsequent eight generations combine conducting airways with alveolar gas exchange units.[5] Despite some irregularity in the branching pattern, the progressive reduction in diameter and length of each generation of the airway is remarkably similar at each level. This so-called "self-similarity" reflects fractal relationships within the lung and the appearance of an optimally designed space-filling tree.[6]

The efficiency in the design of the branching tree is associated with few developmental anomalies. One of the more common anomalies is a right upper lobe orifice that originates, not in the right mainstem bronchus, but rather in the distal trachea. Because ungulates have a cranial lobe with an orifice in the distal trachea, this anomaly is colloquially referred to as a "pig bronchus." The incidence of a tracheal bronchus is estimated to be between 0.1% and 2%.[3]

The development of the branching pattern in the lung—a process referred to as branching morphogenesis—is a striking developmental program because of its complexity and reproducibility. Branching morphogenesis is particularly intriguing as it can occur in explanted tissues in vitro. It has been known for years that the interaction between the epithelial lung bud and the surrounding mesenchyme regulates branching morphogenesis. More recently, molecular studies have shown that the reciprocal epithelial–mesenchymal interactions are associated with an array of signaling molecules. Each of these molecules appears to be influenced by negative regulators, response thresholds, and positional dependency.[7]

Molecular families including fibroblast growth factor (Fgf), bone morphogenic protein (Bmp), and Sonic hedgehog (Shh) appear to be important signaling pathways in branching morphogenesis. It appears that at least the first 15 to 16 branch generations in the human lung are genetically "hardwired" with tight molecular control.[8] The last eight generations, including the lung containing the alveoli and gas exchange surface area, appear to be more adaptive to the anatomy and function of the peripheral lung. It is not surprising that these peripheral airways appear to be the regions of the lung responsible for remodeling during adult lung growth.[9]

The canalicular stage of lung development, between 16 and 24 weeks, marks a dramatic change in lung morphology. The surrounding mesenchyme associated with the pseudoglandular stage is significantly reduced, creating the appearance of primitive septa between airways. The thinning of the mesenchyme is associated with blood vessel formation. The presence of blood vessels within the thinning septa creates the appearance of "canals" forming in the thinning mesenchyme.

Further thinning of the septa and dilatation of the primitive airspaces creates "saccular" airspaces that characterize human lung development between 24 weeks and 36 weeks. The distal lung tissues surrounding the saccular airspaces are referred to as the primary septa of the lung (Fig. 121.2A).[10] The canalicular and saccular stages of lung development are associated with the appearance of type I and type II cells in the developing distal airspaces.

Maturation and thinning of the primary septa coincide with liquid distention of the airways. By midgestation, liquid is produced by the pulmonary epithelium. Because of glottic closure, fluid retained in the lung maintains lung expansion by creating a positive pressure gradient between the lumen of the airway and the amniotic cavity.[11]

How much mechanical fluid distention contributes to regulating the morphologic changes in the canalicular and saccular stages of lung development is unknown, but decreased fluid (oligohydramnios) results in pulmonary hypoplasia. Conversely, tracheal occlusion—for example, by tracheal ligation—increases lung distention. Experimental studies by Adzick and colleagues[12] suggest that tracheal ligation increases lung distention, lung dry weight, branching morphogenesis, and lung vessel growth.

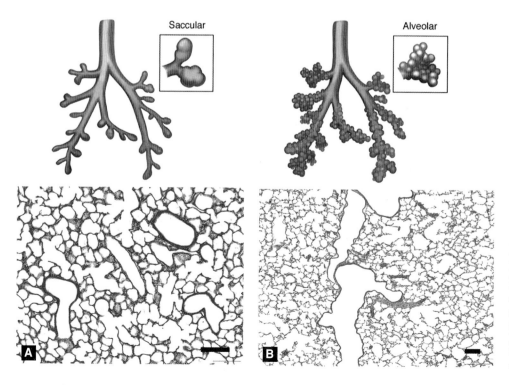

FIGURE 121.2 The saccular and alveolar stages of mammalian lung development. **A:** The saccular stage is characterized by large airspaces and thickened septa; these are called the primary septa. **B:** By the alveolar phase of lung development, so-called secondary septa create partitions in the distal airspaces that become the walls of alveoli. Histology shows rat lung development. (Reproduced with permission from Valenzuela CD, Wagner WL, Bennett RD, et al. Extracellular assembly of the elastin cable line element in the developing lung. *Anat Rec*; 2017; 300(9):1670–1679. Copyright © 2017 by John Wiley Sons, Inc. Reprinted by permission of John Wiley & Sons, Inc.) Bar = 100 um.

Fetal breathing movements are another mechanical and potentially adaptive influence on lung growth. In addition to liquid distention, fetal breath movements have been observed in long-gestation mammals such as humans and sheep. In humans, fetal breath movements are prominent in the third trimester. The absence of fetal breath movements has been noted as a primary mechanism of lung growth failure in human fetuses.[13] In experimental animals, high cervical cord transection or bilateral phrenic nerve transection results in hypoplastic lungs. Although the precise developmental function of fetal breath movements is unclear, the influence of fetal breath movements appears to be additive to the effects of fluid distension.

Another clinical condition associated with mechanical impairment of the lung is congenital diaphragmatic hernia (CDH). CDH most commonly occurs through a patent left-sided pleuroperitoneal canal (foramen of Bochdalek). Population studies indicate a birth prevalence of 3.3 per 10,000 total births.[14] CDH is a significant cause of perinatal morbidity and mortality. CDH has a 1-year mortality of 45%; the mortality is largely a result of pulmonary hypoplasia and pulmonary hypertension.[15]

An arrest of the normal adaptive stages of lung development leads to the clinical condition known as bronchopulmonary dysplasia (BPD). The two major pathologic features of PBD are alveolar hypoplasia and altered microvascular maturation.[16] The absence of well-developed alveolar walls, containing gas exchange capillaries, leads to the clinical presentation of hypoxia and respiratory insufficiency. The histology of BPD is reminiscent of the saccular stage of lung development before the preterm alveolar stage.

The alveolar stage (36 to 38 weeks) involves the creation of alveolar walls or septations in the primitive primary septa (Fig. 121.2B). The alveolar stage of lung development can be conceptualized as the conversion of wide primitive corridor to a narrower corridor surrounded by many small "rooms." The walls of these rooms are partitions that are "lifted" from the primary septa. The partitions form the walls of alveoli and are referred to as secondary septa. Secondary septa appear to be lifted from the primary septa by an elaborate elastin and collagen cable system.[17] The elastin/collagen cable is a helical structure in the distal airways that appears to be important not only in lung development, but also in lung remodeling and regeneration.

Progressive lung growth results in proximal–distal patterning in the airways. In proximal airways, club and goblet cells populate the lining of the lung. Distal airways are populated by type I and type II lung cells. Although the lineage relationship between the cell types is still unknown, a variety of context-specific factors appear to influence cell phenotype and cell differentiation. The potential role of progenitor cells and stem cells in contributing to lung development and population of the airways is an area of active investigation.

An intriguing region of the lung apparently involved in cell reconstitution is the junction of the columnar epithelium of the proximal airways with the squamoid epithelium of the distal airspaces. This region of the lung, called the bronchioalveolar duct junction (BADJ), appears to be actively involved in repopulating the airways after injury. In animal models, a common injury model is parenterally administered naphthalene. The function of both self-renewal and reconstitution of the airspaces have been ascribed to "bronchioalveolar stem cells" (BASC). In humans, a lung injury with a direct effect on distal airways and BADJ is "coal miners' lung" or pneumoconiosis.[18] More recently, the BADJ has been implicated in the development of minimally-invasive adenocarcinomas increasingly recognized in nonsmokers.[19]

Perinatally, the commonest presentation of congenital lung lesions is an abnormal antenatal ultrasound scan. The most frequent diagnoses are congenital cystic adenomatoid malformation (CAM), broncho-

pulmonary sequestration. Less common lesions include congenital lobar emphysema and bronchogenic cysts.[20]

CYSTIC ADENOMATOID MALFORMATION

Congenital CAMs are histologically characterized by multicystic areas of dilated distal airspaces and absent secondary alveolar septa. The multicystic areas are in communication with normal proximal airways; typically, these areas have a normal blood supply. Patients with a large malformation volume ratio have a significantly greater risk of hydrops fetalis. Most patients, however, are asymptomatic and have an excellent outcome. In asymptomatic patients, surgery between 3 and 6 months of age has been recommended to lower the risk of infection and allow for compensatory lung growth.

PULMONARY SEQUESTRATIONS

By definition, pulmonary sequestrations are regions that are isolated from surrounding parenchyma. Pulmonary sequestrations are generally divided into two types: intralobar (15%) and extralobar (85%) sequestrations. Intralobar sequestrations are found in otherwise normal lung tissue and are typically associated with chronic infection. Classically, intralobar sequestrations are found in the medial and posterior basilar segments of the lower lobe and are supplied by an enlarged artery arising in the inferior pulmonary ligament and venous drainage is via the pulmonary veins. In contrast, extralobar sequestrations are enveloped in a pleural covering and are completely isolated from surrounding lung tissue. In most cases, the extralobar sequestrations are found within the lower chest. The sequestration is often supplied by an enlarged aberrant artery arising from the aorta below the diaphragm and venous drainage is typically via systemic veins to the right atrium, vena cava, or azygous. In the postnatal period, children presenting with an extralobar sequestration may have associated developmental anomalies such as CDH.

CONGENITAL LOBAR EMPHYSEMA

Congenital lobar emphysema is typically identified as lobar hyperinflation leading to mediastinal shift associated with hemodynamic and respiratory compromise. The etiology of the hyperinflation is attributable to intrinsic and extrinsic causes. Intrinsic causes are related to gas trapping as a result of abnormal bronchial airways, mucosal growth or regions of hypercompliant parenchyma. Extrinsic causes of gas trapping include compression from vascular or lung malformations. Congenital lobar emphysema must be considered in a neonate with respiratory distress and signs of tension pneumothorax.

BRONCHOGENIC CYST

Bronchogenic cysts are typically unilocular cysts of various sizes filled with mucous or fluid. The cysts, more generally classified as foregut cysts, are lined by pseudostratified ciliated columnar respiratory epithelium and frequently contain cartilage. Bronchogenic cysts are usually found in the mediastinum, although they may be found anywhere in the thoracic cavity. Bronchogenic cysts are usually asymptomatic, but large cysts can be associated with mass-effect on intrathoracic structures. Bronchogenic cysts are usually treated with simple excision.

REFERENCES

1. Skandalakis JE, Ellis H. Embryologic and anatomic basis of esophageal surgery. *Surg Clin-North Am* 2000;80:85–155.
2. Loukogeorgakis SP, Pierro A. Replacement surgery for esophageal atresia. *Eur J Pediatr Surg* 2013;23:182–190.
3. Desir A, Ghaye B. Congenital abnormalities of intrathoracic airways. *Radiol Clin N Am* 2009;47:203–225.
4. Schlesinger RB, McFadden LA. Comparative morphometry of the upper bronchial tree in 6 mammalian-species. *Anat Rec* 1981;199:99–108.
5. Weibel ER. Functional morphology of lung parenchyma. In: *Handbook of Physiology, The Respiratory System, Mechanics of Breathing.* Wiley-Blackwell; 1986: 89–111.
6. Mandelbrot BB. *The Fractal Geometry of Nature.* New York: Freeman; 1977.
7. Chuang PT, McMahon AP. Branching morphogenesis of the lung: new molecular insights into an old problem. *Trends Cell Biol* 2003;13:86–91.
8. Morrisey EE. Balancing the developmental niches within the lung. *Proc Natl Acad Sci* 2013;110:18029–18030.
9. Butler J, Loring SH, Patz S, et al. Evidence for adult lung growth in humans. *N Engl J Med* 2012;367:244–247.
10. Valenzuela CD, Wagner WL, Bennett RD, et al. Extracellular assembly of the elastin cable line element in the developing lung. *Anat Rec* 2017; In press.
11. Harding R, Hooper SB. Regulation of lung expansion and lung growth before birth. *J Appl Physiol* 1996;81:209–224.
12. Adzick NS, Harrison MR, Glick PL, et al. Experimental pulmonary hypoplasia and oligohydramnios—relative contributions of lung fluid and fetal breathing movements. *J Pediatr Surg* 1984;19:658–665.
13. Hooper SB, Wallace MJ. Role of the physicochemical environment in lung development. *Clin Exp Pharmacol Physiol* 2006;33:273–279.
14. Torfs CP, Curry CJ, Bateson TF, et al. A population-based study of congenital diaphragmatic hernia. *Teratology* 1992;46:555–565.
15. Balayla J, Abenhaim HA. Incidence, predictors and outcomes of congenital diaphragmatic hernia: a population-based study of 32 million births in the United States. *J Matern Fetal Neonatal Med* 2014;27:1438–1444.
16. Coalson JJ. Pathology of bronchopulmonary dysplasia. *Semin Perinatol* 2006;30:179–184.
17. Wagner W, Bennett RD, Ackermann M, et al. Elastin cables define the axial connective tissue system in the murine lung. *Anat Rec* 2015;298:1960–1968.
18. Duguid JB, Lambert MW. Pathogenesis of coal miners pneumoconiosis. *J Pathol Bacteriol* 1964;88:389–403.
19. Rowbotham SP, Kim CF. Diverse cells at the origin of lung adenocarcinoma. *Proc Natl Acad Sci U S A* 2014;111:4745–4746.
20. Stanton M, Njere I, Ade-Ajayi N, et al. Systematic review and meta-analysis of the postnatal management of congenital cystic lung lesions. *J Pediatr Surg* 2009;44: 1027–1033.

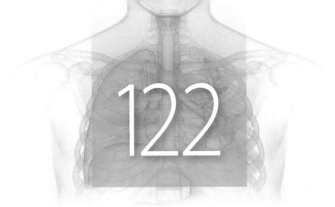

122

Anatomy of the Esophagus

Thomas J. Watson

The esophagus is a muscular tube extending from the pharynx to the stomach and bordered by two sphincters. It holds one primary responsibility: the aboral transport of ingested food, liquid, and saliva. Prevention of reflux of gastric contents is inherent to this task. Unlike other portions of the gastrointestinal tract, the esophagus has no known endocrine, exocrine, immunologic, digestive, absorptive, or secretory roles.

The esophagus starts as a continuation of the pharynx, is normally 20 to 30 cm in length in adults, and terminates at the cardia of the stomach. With the head in its normal anatomic position and the neck in neutral flexion, the transition from pharynx to esophagus begins at the inferior edge of the cricoid cartilage opposite the lower border of the sixth cervical vertebra (Fig. 122.1). The esophagus descends along the front of the vertebral column, through the superior and posterior mediastinum, then passes through the diaphragm and enters the abdomen, ending at the gastroesophageal junction opposite the 11th thoracic vertebra. The esophagus normally is anchored firmly

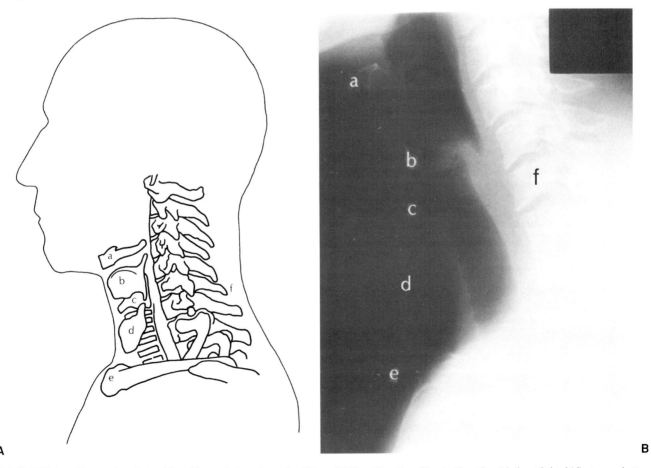

A   **B**

FIGURE 122.1 **A:** Topographic relationships of the cervical esophagus: hyoid bone (*a*), thyroid cartilage (*b*), cricoid cartilage (*c*), thyroid gland (*d*), sternonclavicular joint (*e*), C6 (*f*). **B:** Lateral radiographic appearance.

to the cricoid cartilage at its upper end and to the diaphragm at its lower end. Flexion and extension of the neck or deglutition move these points of fixation in a cranial direction for the distance of one vertebral body. The general orientation of the esophagus is vertical with several curves in its course. At its commencement it is situated in the midline with deviation to the left side as far as the root of the neck. It gradually passes to the midline again at the level of the 5th thoracic vertebra, and finally inclines to the left as it passes forward to the esophageal hiatus in the diaphragm. The esophagus also demonstrates anteroposterior flexures corresponding to the curvatures of the cervical and thoracic portions of the vertebral column.

RADIOGRAPHIC, ENDOSCOPIC, AND MANOMETRIC ANATOMY OF THE ESOPHAGUS

Radiographically, the appearance of the esophagus corresponds to its normal anatomy. On the anteroposterior radiograph, the esophagus lies in the midline with a deviation to the left in the lower portion of the neck and upper portion of the thorax. It returns to the midline in the midportion of the thorax near the bifurcation of the trachea (Fig. 122.2A). In the lower portion of the thorax, the esophagus again deviates to the left upon entry into the abdominal cavity through the diaphragm.

On the lateral radiograph, the esophagus follows the posterior curve of the vertebral column, except the lower thoracic portion, where it curves anteriorly to pass through the diaphragmatic hiatus (Fig. 122.2B). This posterior curve and its terminal left anterior deviation are of particular importance in the performance of rigid diagnostic and therapeutic esophagoscopy. During this procedure, the position of the patient should allow full extension of the cervical and thoracic spine so that the rigid scope can be manipulated safely through the terminal arc. As a result of these anatomic configurations,

the distal esophagus is the second most common site of iatrogenic esophageal perforation during rigid endoscopy, the first being the narrow entrance of the esophagus at the level of the cricopharyngeus.

There are three areas of normal anatomic narrowing in the esophagus that are commonly seen during esophagoscopy or contrast esophagogram. The most superior narrowing is caused by the cricopharyngeus muscle at the anatomical border of the pharynx and proximal esophagus. This is the narrowest point of the esophagus with an average luminal diameter of 1.5 cm and is the most common site of iatrogenic perforation. The crossing of the left main stem bronchus and the aortic arch results in anterior and left lateral esophageal wall indentation causing the second narrowing of the esophagus, with an average luminal diameter of 1.6 cm. The most distal narrowing of the esophagus is at the diaphragmatic hiatus and is caused by the physiologic lower esophageal sphincter. There is great variation of the luminal diameter at this point, depending upon the normal distention of the esophagus by the passage of a food bolus, with measurements ranging from 1.6 to 2.5 cm.

The shape of the native, resting esophagus is determined by its contiguous structures as well as by the body cavities it traverses. As assessed by barium esophagography, the cervical esophagus is flattened due to compression by surrounding structures; the thoracic portion is more rounded due to the negative pressure environment of the thorax; and the abdominal portion is again flattened, due to positive intra-abdominal pressure. Just above the level of the diaphragm, the esophagus develops a distinct dilatation, perhaps due to outflow resistance imposed by the lower esophageal sphincter as well as a relative lack of buttressing by adjacent organs.

Measurements obtained during endoscopic examination (Fig. 122.3) reveal the average distance from the incisor teeth to the top of the stomach to be 38 to 40 cm in men and 2 cm shorter in women. These distances are proportionately shorter in children, being 18 cm at birth, 22 cm at the age of 3 years, and 27 cm at an age of 10. In men, the length of the esophagus from the cricopharyngeus muscle to the gastroesophageal junction ranges from 23 to 30 cm with an average of

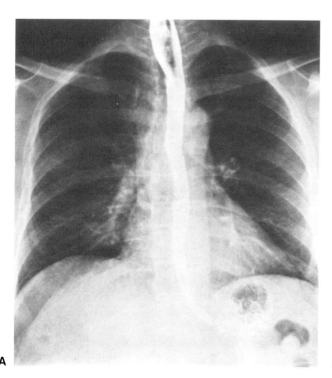
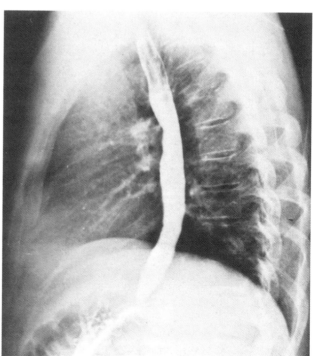

A   B

FIGURE 122.2 Barium esophagogram. **A:** Anteroposterior view. **B:** Lateral view.

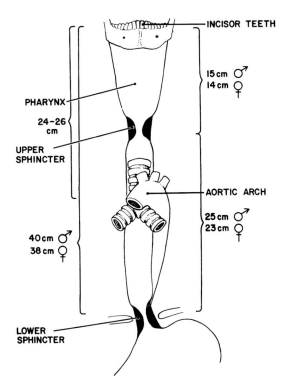

FIGURE 122.3 Important clinical endoscopic measurements of the esophagus in adults.

ANATOMIC RELATIONS OF THE ESOPHAGUS

RELATIONSHIP OF THE ESOPHAGUS TO THE HYPOPHARYNX

The esophagus serves as a conduit between the pharynx and the stomach. The pharyngeal musculature consists of three overlapping, broad, flat, fan-shaped constrictors (Fig. 122.5). The superior constrictor arises mainly from the medial pterygoid plate, the middle constrictor arises from the hyoid bone, and the inferior constrictor arises from the thyroid and cricoid cartilages. These muscles originate bilaterally, joining with their counterparts in the posterior midline to create a median posterior raphe.

The upper orifice to the esophagus is collared by the cricopharyngeus muscle. This muscle originates from both edges of the cricoid cartilage and forms a continuous transverse muscle band without an interruption by a median posterior raphe. The fibers of this muscle blend inseparably with those of the inferior pharyngeal constrictor above and the inner circular muscles of the cervical esophagus below. The cricopharyngeus can be conceptualized as an inferior extension of the inferior constrictor muscle. The inferior constrictor, thus, has two parts: an upper, or retrothyroid, portion with diagonal fibers and a lower, or retrocricoid, portion with transverse fibers. These two parts of the same muscle possess quite distinct functions, the upper portion acting in a propulsive fashion to move a swallowed bolus from the pharynx into the esophagus and the lower portion serving as an upper esophageal sphincter.

25 cm. In women, the range is from 20 to 26 cm with an average of 23 cm. The distance from the incisor teeth to the cricopharyngeus muscle is 15 cm in men and 14 cm in women. The bifurcation of the trachea and the indentation of the aortic arch range between 24 and 26 cm from the incisor teeth. When planning potential esophageal surgery, it is helpful to locate intraluminal tumors, strictures, or other pathology in reference to the incisors, to help guide a decision regarding a right or left thoracotomy approach and avoid interference with the aortic arch.

Esophageal length may be determined by manometric assessment. The distance between the bottom of the upper esophageal sphincter and the top of the lower esophageal sphincter represents esophageal body length and varies according to the height of the individual (Fig. 122.4).

RELATIONSHIP OF THE CERVICAL ESOPHAGUS TO STRUCTURES AND FASCIAL PLANES OF THE NECK

The cervical portion of the esophagus is approximately 5 cm long and is situated with the trachea and the main substance of the thyroid gland in front, and the vertebral column and longus colli muscles behind. The esophagus is separated from these structures by loose areolar tissue. On either side, the esophagus is in relation with the common carotid artery sheaths and parts of the thyroid lobes.

The esophagus descends between the trachea and the vertebral column from the level of the 6th cervical vertebra posteriorly, and the suprasternal notch anteriorly, to the level of the interspace between the 1st and 2nd thoracic vertebrae. The recurrent laryngeal nerves lie in the right and left tracheoesophageal grooves. Due to the slight left cervical esophageal deviation, the left recurrent nerve lies closer

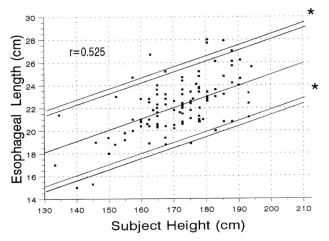

FIGURE 122.4 Nomogram of subject's height versus esophageal length.

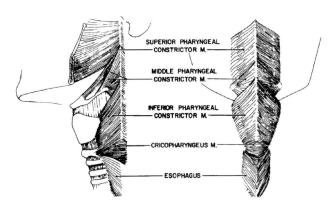

FIGURE 122.5 External muscles of the pharynx.

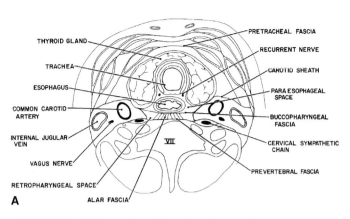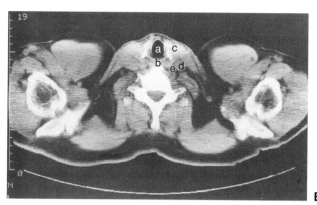

FIGURE 122.6 **A:** Cross-section of the neck at the level of the thyroid isthmus. **B:** Computed tomographic appearance viewed from above: trachea (*a*), esophagus (*b*), left thyroid lobe (*c*), internal jugular vein (*d*), common carotid artery (*e*).

to the esophagus than the right nerve, which takes the more lateral course around the right subclavian artery.

The cervical fascial planes formed by the pretracheal fascia anteriorly, the prevertebral fascia posteriorly, and the fascia of the carotid sheaths laterally, cause two potential spaces in the neck: a paraesophageal space containing the thyroid gland, larynx, trachea, and pharynx, and a retroesophageal space (Fig. 122.6). The latter, a continuous space from the base of the skull to the superior mediastinum, is of particular clinical importance due to the potential for spread of infection originating in the neck into the mediastinum.

RELATIONSHIP OF THE THORACIC ESOPHAGUS TO MEDIASTINAL STRUCTURES

The thoracic portion of the esophagus is approximately 20 cm long and, proximally, is situated in the superior mediastinum between the trachea and the vertebral column, slightly to the left of midline. From the thoracic inlet to the tracheal bifurcation, the thoracic esophagus remains in intimate relation with the posterior wall of the trachea and the prevertebral fascia. Just above the tracheal bifurcation, the esophagus passes behind and to the right of the aortic arch, and descends in the posterior mediastinum along the right side of the descending aorta. This anatomic positioning of the aortic arch can cause a notch indentation in the left lateral esophageal wall noticeable on contrast

esophagogram or upper endoscopy. Immediately below this point, the esophagus crosses both the bifurcation of the trachea and the left main stem bronchus, due to the deviation of the terminal portion of the trachea to the right by the aorta (Fig. 122.7). From that point distally, the esophagus passes along the posterior extent of the subcarinal lymph nodes, and then descends behind the pericardium adjacent to the left atrium to reach the diaphragmatic hiatus (Fig. 122.8).

The right lateral surface of the thoracic esophagus is covered completely by the parietal pleura, except at the level of the 4th thoracic vertebra, where the azygos vein turns anteriorly over the esophagus to join the superior vena cava. The left lateral surface of the upper portion of the esophagus is covered anterolaterally by the left subclavian artery and posterolaterally by the parietal pleura. The distal esophagus lies to the right of the descending thoracic aorta, which then disappears behind the esophagus at the level of the 8th thoracic vertebra. The left lateral esophageal wall from this point distally is covered only with the parietal pleura of the mediastinum. Due to the absence of structural support, the left lateral distal esophagus is a common site of esophageal perforation in Boerhaave syndrome. From the bifurcation of the trachea downward, both the vagal nerves and the esophageal nerve plexus lie on the muscular wall of the esophagus.

The thoracic esophagus is adjacent to the trachea, the left main bronchus, the pericardium, and the diaphragm in front, and the vertebral column, the longus colli muscles, the right aortic intercostal

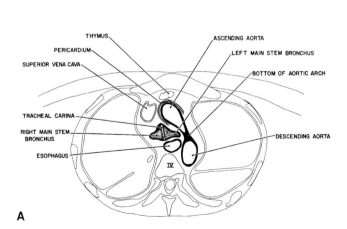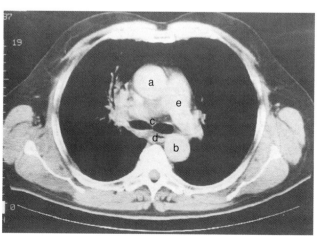

FIGURE 122.7 **A:** Cross-section of the thorax at the level of the tracheal bifurcation. **B:** CT appearance viewed from above: ascending aorta (*a*), descending aorta (*b*), tracheal carina (*c*), esophagus (*d*), pulmonary artery (*e*).

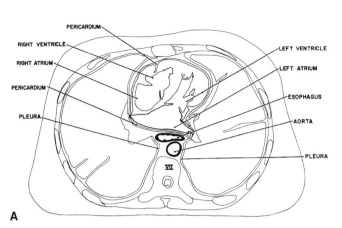

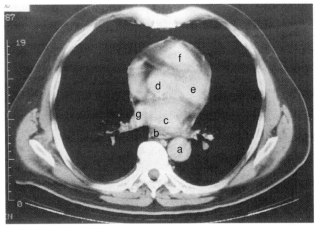

FIGURE 122.8 **A:** Cross-section of the thorax at mid-left atrial level. **B:** CT appearance viewed from above: aorta (*a*), esophagus (*b*), left atrium (*c*), right atrium (*d*), left ventricle (*e*), right ventricle (*f*), pulmonary vein (*g*).

arteries, the thoracic duct, the hemiazygos veins, and the distal thoracic aorta behind. The inferior vena cava, while not in apposition to the esophagus, lies anterior and to its right. The thoracic duct passes through the hiatus on the anterior surface of the vertebral column behind the aorta and under the right crus. In the thorax, the duct is situated dorsal to the esophagus between the azygos vein on the right and the descending thoracic aorta on the left. From the level of the 4th and 5th thoracic vertebrae upward, the thoracic duct gradually crosses to the left and is located between the esophagus and the left parietal pleura, dorsal to the aortic arch and the intrathoracic part of the subclavian artery. In the neck, it turns more laterally from the esophagus to join the venous system at the junction of the left subclavian and left internal jugular veins.

RELATIONSHIP OF THE TERMINAL ESOPHAGUS TO THE DIAPHRAGMATIC HIATUS AND STOMACH

The muscular fibers forming the crura of the diaphragm arise by tendinous bands from the anterolateral surface of the first three or four lumbar vertebrae and their intervening fibrocartilages (Fig. 122.9). The right crus is longer and thicker than the left and the inferior

extension of its fibers gives rise to the ligament of Treitz. The upper abdominal aorta lies at the base of the diaphragmatic hiatus just anterior to the vertebral bodies. The celiac and superior mesenteric arteries, as they arise from the upper abdominal aorta, separate the muscle bundles of the right and left crura. In many situations, a well-demarcated median arcuate ligament unites the two crura anterior to the aorta just above the celiac artery. The ligament is usually, though not always, a well-defined ligamentous structure.

The anatomy of the esophageal hiatus is quite variable. The most common variant presents as the formation of both the right and left margins of the hiatus by the right crus. As it ascends, the right crus divides into superficial and deep muscle layers, forming the muscular rim of the right and left edges of the esophageal hiatus, respectively. The left crus ascends vertically to the left margin of the hiatus. This configuration, however, is found in only about half of individuals, and many alternate anatomical arrangements exist.

As the esophagus passes through the diaphragmatic hiatus, it is surrounded by the phrenoesophageal membrane, a fibroelastic ligament that arises from the subdiaphragmatic fascia as a continuation of the transversalis fascia (Fig. 122.10). The phrenoesophageal membrane divides at the lower margin of the esophageal hiatus into a stout elongated ascending leaf surrounding the terminal segment of the esophagus in a tent-like manner and into a shorter, thin, descending leaf, which merges as the visceral peritoneal gastric covering. The upper leaf of the membrane is attached in a circumferential manner

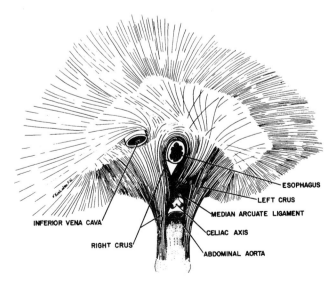

FIGURE 122.9 The diaphragm and esophageal hiatus seen from below.

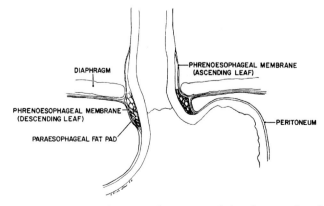

FIGURE 122.10 Attachments and structure of the phrenoesophageal membrane.

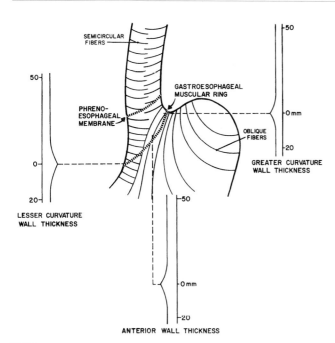

FIGURE 122.11 The inner muscular fiber arrangement and muscular thickness at the cardia. (Adapted from Liebermann-Meffert D, Allgöwer M, Schmid P, et al. Muscular equivalent of the lower esophageal sphincter. *Gastroenterology* 1979;76:31. Copyright © 1976 AGA Institute. With permission.)

around the esophagus 1 to 2 cm above the level of the hiatus. The ring of fatty tissue between the upper leaf of the membrane and the cardia is interspersed with fibers from the lower leaf of the membrane. These fibers blend in with elastic-containing adventitia of the distal 2 cm of esophagus and cardia of the stomach making up the abdominal esophageal portion, which is subjected to the positive pressure environment of the abdomen.

The abdominal portion of the esophagus is about 1.25 cm long and abuts the posterior surface of the left lobe of the liver. This segment is somewhat conical with its base applied to the upper orifice of the stomach, known as the antrum cardiacum. Only its front and left aspects are covered by peritoneum. At the gastroesophageal junction, the outer longitudinal muscle fibers of the esophagus are continuous with the corresponding longitudinal muscle fibers of the stomach. The inner circular fibers interlace with, and eventually are replaced by, the inner oblique gastric fibers arising in the direction of the gastric fundus (Fig. 122.11). Just distal to the upper phrenoesophageal membrane insertion, the gastric muscular wall becomes thicker due to increased density of the esophageal circular musculature on the lesser curvature side and the gastric oblique musculature on the greater curvature side. The line of maximal muscular thickness has an oblique orientation such that it is situated more cephalad on the greater curvature side than on the lesser curvature side. The muscle mass is also asymmetric, with more thickness on the greater curvature side. The physiology of this asymmetric oblique muscle thickening is thought to contribute to the antireflux mechanism. The manometrically defined lower esophageal high-pressure zone is situated in this region, and the length of the high-pressure zone is similar to the length of the thickening. Other anatomical factors contributing to competency of the cardia as an antireflux barrier include the rosette-like configuration of the gastric mucosa at the gastroesophageal junction, the sharp angle between the lower esophagus and the gastric fundus, as well as the phrenoesophageal membrane and its attachments to the esophageal hiatus.

MUSCULATURE OF THE ESOPHAGUS

The upper 2 to 6 cm of the esophagus contains only striated muscle fibers. Progressing more distally, smooth muscle fibers gradually become more abundant, such that at a distance of 4 to 8 cm from the superior end, or at the junction of the upper and lower two-thirds of the esophagus, smooth muscle normally constitutes 50% of the esophageal muscle mass. From this point downward, smooth muscle gradually replaces the striated muscle completely. Because most of the clinically significant esophageal motility disorders involve only the smooth muscle, their effects on esophageal function are maximal in the lower two-thirds of the esophagus. In addition, when a surgical esophageal myotomy is indicated, the incision usually needs only to extend this distance.

The musculature of the esophagus can be divided into an outer longitudinal and an inner circular layer. The longitudinal muscle fibers originate from a cricoesophageal tendon arising from the dorsal upper edge of the anteriorly located cricoid cartilage. The two bundles of muscles diverge and meet in the midline on the posterior wall of the esophagus about 3 cm below the cricoid (Fig. 122.5). From this point on, a layer of longitudinal muscle fibers covers the entire circumference of the esophagus. This configuration of the longitudinal muscle fibers around the most proximal part of the esophagus leaves a V-shaped area in the posterior wall covered only with circular muscle fibers. In the upper one-third of the esophagus, the longitudinal muscle layer is thicker on the lateral surface than on the ventral or dorsal surfaces. In the lower two-thirds, the longitudinal layer becomes more uniform, and its overall thickness decreases distally. The course of the longitudinal muscle fibers is that of an elongated spiral, turning to the left around one quarter of the esophageal circumference (90 degrees) as they descend.

The circular muscle layer of the esophagus is thicker than the outer longitudinal layer. These circular fibers run horizontally only in the isolated and retracted esophagus. In situ, their course is elliptical, spiraling with an orientation that varies according to the level of the esophagus. In the cervical portion, the highest point of the ellipse is dorsal. In the upper thoracic portion, the highest point is right lateral, while behind the heart the highest point is ventral. In the abdomen, the fibers are nearly horizontal. The arrangement of both the longitudinal and circular muscle fibers makes the peristalsis of the esophagus assume a worm-like drive as opposed to segmental and sequential squeezing. As a consequence, severe motor abnormalities of the esophagus assume a spiraling corkscrew-like pattern on the barium swallow radiograph.

ARTERIAL BLOOD SUPPLY OF THE ESOPHAGUS

The cervical portion of the esophagus receives its main blood supply from the inferior thyroid artery with smaller accessory branches from the common carotid, subclavian, and superficial cervical arteries. The thoracic portion receives its blood supply from the bronchial arteries, with 75% of individuals having one right-sided and one or two left-sided branches. Typically, two esophageal branches arise directly from the distal thoracic aorta. The upper branch is usually the shorter of the two, originating at the level of the 6th or 7th thoracic vertebra. The lower branch is longer and originates at the level of the 8th or 9th thoracic vertebra. The abdominal portion of the esophagus receives its blood supply mainly from esophageal branches of the left gastric and inferior phrenic arteries (Fig. 122.12). On entering the wall of

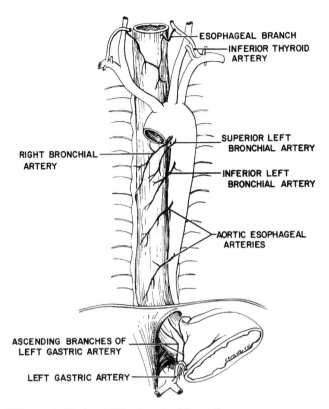

FIGURE 122.12 Arterial blood supply of the esophagus.

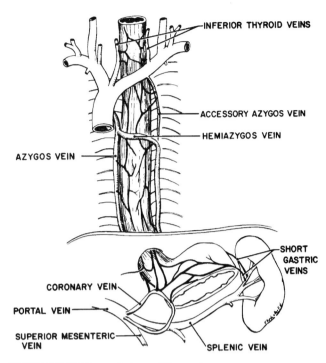

FIGURE 122.13 Venous drainage of the esophagus.

the esophagus, the arteries assume a T-shaped division to form longitudinal anastomoses, giving rise to an intramural vascular network in the muscular and submucosal layers. As a consequence of this abundant collateral network, the esophagus can be mobilized from the stomach to the level of the aortic arch without fear of devascularization and ischemic necrosis. However, caution should be exercised in extensively mobilizing the esophagus in patients who have had a previous thyroidectomy and ligation of the inferior thyroid arteries proximal to the origin of the esophageal branches.

VENOUS DRAINAGE OF THE ESOPHAGUS

Blood from the capillaries of the esophagus flows into a submucosal venous plexus and then into a periesophageal venous plexus from which the esophageal veins originate. In the cervical region, the esophageal veins empty into the inferior thyroid vein; in the thoracic region, into the bronchial, azygos, or hemiazygos veins; and in the abdominal region, into the coronary vein (Fig. 122.13). The submucosal venous networks of the esophagus and stomach are in continuity with each other and, in patients with portal venous obstruction, this communication functions as an important collateral pathway for portal blood to enter the superior vena cava via the azygos system.

NERVE SUPPLY OF THE ESOPHAGUS

The constrictor muscles of the pharynx receive branches from the pharyngeal plexus, which is on the posterolateral surface of the middle constrictor muscle. This plexus is formed by pharyngeal branches of the vagus nerves, with a small contribution from the 9th and 11th cranial nerves (Fig. 122.14). The complete parasympathetic innervation of the esophagus is provided by the vagus nerves.

The cricopharyngeal sphincter and the cervical portion of the esophagus receive their vagal innervation from branches of both recurrent laryngeal nerves. The right recurrent nerve arises at the lower margin of the subclavian artery, the left at the lower margin of the aortic arch. They both swing dorsally around these vessels and ascend in the groove between the esophagus and trachea, giving branches to each. Damage to these nerves not only interferes with the function of the vocal cords, but also interferes with the function of the

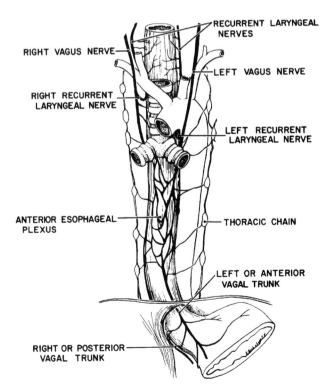

FIGURE 122.14 Innervation of the esophagus.

cricopharyngeal sphincter and the motility of the cervical esophagus, causing a predisposition to pulmonary aspiration on swallowing.

The upper thoracic esophagus receives its vagal innervation from branches of the left recurrent laryngeal nerve and by direct branches from both vagus nerves as they descend through the superior mediastinum. The lower thoracic esophagus is innervated by the esophageal plexus located directly on both the anterior and posterior esophageal walls. This plexus is formed by fibers from both vagus nerves after they pass behind the hilum of the lung and turn medially to reach the esophagus. The esophageal plexus also receives fibers from the thoracic sympathetic chain. The left vagus nerve splits before the esophageal plexus to form two branches: the first branch runs through the ventral esophageal plexus and constitutes the main element of the anterior or left abdominal vagal trunk; the second branch runs around the left esophageal wall, to join the dorsal esophageal plexus, and contributes to the formation of the posterior or right abdominal vagal trunk. As a result of the intertwining of fibers from both the left and right vagus nerves in the esophageal plexus, both the left or anterior and right or posterior abdominal vagal trunks contain fibers of the original left and right vagus nerves. The average distance above the diaphragm at which the left or anterior vagal trunk becomes a single nerve is 5.13 cm, and the right or posterior vagal trunk is 3.7 cm.

The preganglionic sympathetic fibers supplying the esophagus take origin from the 4th to the 6th spinal cord segments and terminate in the cervical and thoracic sympathetic ganglia. The pharyngeal plexus receives sympathetic fibers that arrive directly from the superior cervical ganglion via vagus nerves. The postganglionic fibers reach the esophagus via nerve branches that veer off from the cervical and thoracic sympathetic chain: some reach the esophageal wall directly, while others join the vagus trunks. Thus, the vagus nerves caudal to their entrance into the neck always contain a number of postganglionic sympathetic fibers. The distal esophageal segments also receive direct sympathetic fibers from the celiac ganglion. These fibers reach the esophagus via the periarterial plexus around the left gastric and phrenic arteries.

Afferent visceral sensory pain fibers from the esophagus end without synapse in the first four segments of the thoracic spinal cord by using a combination of sympathetic and vagal pathways. These pathways are also occupied by afferent visceral sensory fibers from the heart, which explains the frequent overlap in symptomatology between the esophagus and the heart.

LYMPHATIC DRAINAGE OF THE ESOPHAGUS

The detailed lymphatic anatomy of the esophagus and its lymphatic drainage is discussed in Chapter 123.

SUGGESTED READINGS

Abel W. The arrangement of the longitudinal and circular musculature at the upper end of the oesophagus. *J Anat Physiol* 1913;47:381.

Arey LB, Tremaine MJ. The muscle content of the lower esophagus of man. *Anat Rec* 1933;56:315.

Bowden RE, El-Ramli HA. The anatomy of the oesophageal hiatus. *Br J Surg* 1967;54:983.

Butler H. The veins of the oesophagus. *Thorax* 1951;6:276.

Demel R. The blood supply of the esophagus: a study of surgery of the esophagus (Die Gefassversorgung der Speiserohre. Ein Beitrag zur Oesophaguschirurgie). *Arch Klin Chir* 1924;128:453.

Eliska O. Phreno-oesophageal membrane and its role in the development of hiatal hernia. *Acta Anat (Basel)* 1973;86:137.

Keith A. A demonstration on diverticula of the alimentary tract of congenital or of obscure origin. *BMJ* 1910;1:376.

Liebermann-Meffert D, Allgöwer M, Schmid P, et al. Muscular equivalent of the lower esophageal sphincter. *Gastroenterology* 1979;76:31.

Lindner HH, Kemprud E. A clinicoanatomical study of the arcuate ligament of the diaphragm. *Arch Surg* 1971;103:600.

Shapiro AL, Robillard GL. Gastroesophageal vagal and sympathetic innervation: in relation to an anatomic approach to combined gastric vagal sympathectomy. *J Int Coll Surg* 1950a;13:318.

Shapiro AL, Robillard GL. The esophageal arteries: their configurational anatomy and variations in relation to surgery. *Ann Surg* 1950b;131:171.

Swigart LL, Siekert RG. The esophageal arteries: an anatomic study of 150 specimens. *Surg Gynecol Obstet* 1950;90:234.

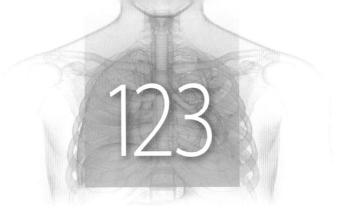

123

Lymphatic Drainage of the Esophagus

Thomas L. Bauer II ■ Mark J. Krasna

INTRODUCTION

Understanding the rich lymphatic drainage of the esophagus is very relevant to thoracic surgeons both in terms of staging and in planning esophagectomy in the management esophageal cancer. This chapter will review lymphatic anatomy related to the esophagus, esophageal cancer staging, and treatment in relation to lymphatic spread. Curative surgical and radiation therapies are based on this understanding.

ANATOMY

The lymphatic drainage of the esophagus is longitudinal and intramural through a rich lymphatic network as first described by Sakata in 1903.[1] The longitudinal submucosal network tends to drain superiorly from the upper third and inferiorly from the distal third.[2] Collecting trunks originating from the submucosal network intermittently pierce the muscularis propria to drain into regional lymph nodes (Fig. 123.1).[3] They are able to penetrate the esophageal wall through transverse, ascending, or descending pathways of variable length. However, this physiology is difficult to confirm, and very well may be altered by lymphatic obstruction from inflammation or tumor infiltration. Thus the true direction of flow in any given disease state is difficult to confirm.

LYMPH NODE ANATOMY AND MAPPING

Standardization of lymph node location facilitates clinical trials, research, and communication when managing esophageal cancer. The most commonly used maps are the Japanese system,[4] which originated from a gastric cancer nodal mapping system, and the system first described by Casson and colleagues[5] (Fig. 123.2) based on the lymph node map for lung cancer. The latter has been adopted by the American Joint Committee on Cancer for esophageal cancer staging; thus the discussion will focus on the current 7th edition AJCC system. This regional node map utilizes the mediastinal stations originally described by Naruke and co-workers[6] for lung cancer for levels 1 to 9. There are station modifications for esophageal cancer staging which include 3P (posterior) for paraesophageal lymph nodes above the tracheal bifurcation, and station 8 is divided into middle and lower paraesophageal lymph nodes. Stations 15 through 20 are demonstrated in Figure 123.2.

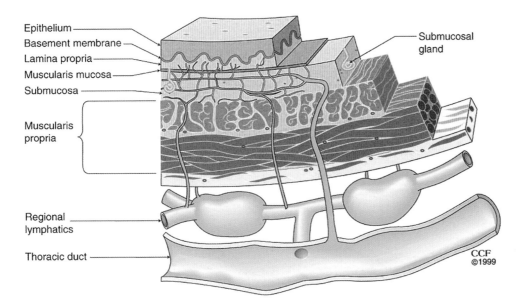

Epithelium
Basement membrane
Lamina propria
Muscularis mucosa
Submucosa
Muscularis propria
Regional lymphatics
Thoracic duct
Submucosal gland

CCF
©1999

FIGURE 123.1 The lymphatic anatomy of the esophagus. Lymphatics enter the mucosa to lie just below the basement membrane of the epithelium and drain the lamina propria and muscularis mucosa. The submucosa is richly supplied with an interconnecting network of lymphatic channels that run the length of the esophagus. Lymphatics intermittently pierce the muscularis propria to drain into regional lymph nodes or directly into the thoracic duct. (Reprinted with permission from the Cleveland Clinic Foundation.)

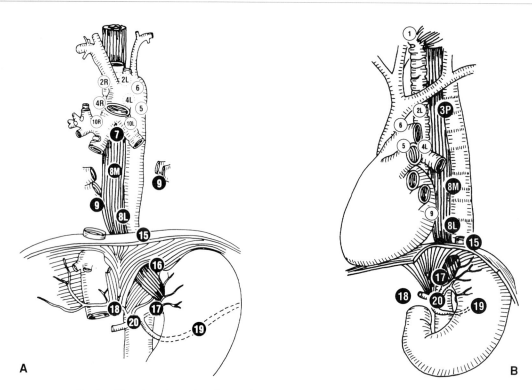

Regional lymph node stations for staging esophageal cancer, from front (A) and side (B).

1	Supraclavicular nodes	Above suprasternal notch and clavicles
2R	Right upper paratracheal nodes	Between intersection of caudal margin of innominate artery with trachea and the apex of the lung
2L	Left upper paratracheal nodes	Between top of aortic arch and apex of the lung
3P	Posterior mediastinal nodes	Upper paraesophageal nodes, above tracheal bifurcation
4R	Right lower paratracheal nodes	Between intersection of caudal margin of innominate artery with trachea and cephalic border of azygous vein
4L	Left lower paratracheal nodes	Between top of aortic arch and carina
5	Aortopulmonary nodes	Subaortic and para-aortic nodes lateral to the ligamentum arteriosum
6	Anterior mediastinal nodes	Anterior to ascending aorta or innominate artery
7	Subcarinal nodes	Caudal to the carina of the trachea
8M	Middle paraesophageal lymph nodes	From the tracheal bifurcation to the caudal margin of the inferior pulmonary vein
8L	Lower paraesophageal lymph nodes	From the caudal margin of the inferior pulmonary vein to the esophagogastric junction
9	Pulmonary ligament nodes	Within the inferior pulmonary ligament
10R	Right tracheobronchial nodes	From cephalic border of azygous vein to origin of RUL bronchus
10L	Left tracheobronchial nodes	Between carina and LUL bronchus
15	Diaphragmatic nodes	Lying on the dome of the diaphragm, and adjacent to or behind its crura
16	Paracardial nodes	Immediately adjacent to the gastroesophageal junction
17	Left gastric nodes	Along the course of the left gastric artery
18	Common hepatic nodes	Along the course of the common hepatic artery
19	Splenic nodes	Along the course of the splenic artery
20	Celiac nodes	At the base of the celiac artery

FIGURE 123.2 American Joint Commission on Cancer esophageal staging, nodal designation. (Reprinted from Casson AG, Rusch VW, Ginsberg RJ, et al. Lymph node mapping of esophageal cancer. *Ann Thorac Surg* 1994;58(5):1569–1570. Copyright © 1994 The Society of Thoracic Surgeons. With permission.)

The recurrent laryngeal nerve (RLN) node is a station described at the cervical base continuous to the upper mediastinum. Its role is not clearly understood but some authors have demonstrated that this indicates which patients should have a three-field node dissection performed for middle and upper third thoracic squamous tumors.[7,8] Others have demonstrated that the number of nodes involved is of greater significance than the presence or absence of cancer in the RLN.[9] Although three-field lymphadenectomy is not widely accepted in the West; recent data suggests that perhaps greater attention should be paid to cervical node disease, irrespective of the location of the primary tumor.[11]

Nagaraja and colleagues[12] performed a meta-analysis of articles evaluating the use of sentinel lymph nodes in the management of esophageal cancer. The overall detection rate was 93% with a negative predictive value of 77%. The high rate of skip metastasis of 50% to 60% in lymph nodes, supports sentinel node mapping and potentially extended lymphadenectomies.[13]

CLINICAL IMPLICATIONS—PATTERNS OF METASTATIC SPREAD IN ESOPHAGEAL CANCER

The overall incidence of metastases to lymph nodes in carcinoma of the esophagus ranges between 45% and 70% in different series.[10,11,14,15] Depth of penetration is the greatest predictor of nodal involvement but location and histology impact nodal spread as well. Standardized nodal stations allows for proper surgical resection by applying known anatomic boundaries to the resection.

T STATUS

The more extensive the tumor invasion, the greater the probability of nodal involvement. Esophageal wall invasion, or T status, was identified by Rice and colleagues[14] as a significant predictor of lymph node involvement. Merkow et al.[17] demonstrated that 5% of T1A esophageal cancers have nodal metastasis in the national cancer database. Likelihood of lymph node involvement for T1, T2, T3, and

TABLE 123.1 Prevalence of Nodal Metastases by T Status

T Status	% With N1 Involvement	Odds Ratio for N1 Involvement Compared With T1
T1	10.8%	1
T1a	2.6%	1
T1b	22.2%	1
T2	43.2%	6
T3	77.2%	23
T4	66.7%	35

Reprinted from Rice TW, Zuccaro G Jr, Adelstein DJ, et al. Esophageal carcinoma: depth of tumor invasion is predictive of regional lymph node status. *Ann Thorac Surg* 1998;65:787–792. Copyright © 1998 The Society of Thoracic Surgeons. With permission.

T4 increases from 1× to 6×, 23×, and 35×, respectively (Table 123.1). Similar findings are found by other authors.[16]

TUMOR LOCATION

Most Western surgeons complete the same lymphadenectomy regardless of whether the cancer is in the middle or distal esophagus. There continue to be proponents of transhiatal (limited intrathoracic nodal resection) versus Ivor Lewis (thoracic nodal dissection) versus McKeown resection (thoracic +/− cervical lymphadenectomy). These decisions tend to be based more in personal biases than tumor location. As the number of minimally invasive esophagectomies increases, it is likely that the number of transhiatal approaches will decrease and be replaced with minimally invasive approaches that include thoracic lymphadenectomy. This again, will be based most likely on surgeon preference rather than tumor location.

Figure 123.3 shows the pattern of spread by histologic type and location looking at T1 esophageal cancers. Tumors in all locations of both histologic types have been demonstrated to spread to cervical, thoracic, and abdominal locations. Lerut and colleagues performed three-field esophagectomies on 174 patients (96 adenocarcinoma, 78 squamous). A total of 12% of patients had an increase in their TNM

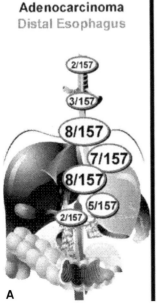

Adenocarcinoma
Distal Esophagus

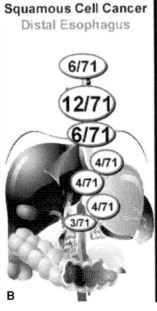

Squamous Cell Cancer
Distal Esophagus

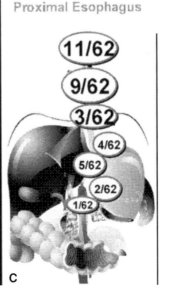

Squamous Cell Cancer
Proximal Esophagus

A   B   C

FIGURE 123.3 Topographic distribution of lymph node metastases shown as the number of patients with positive nodes at the specified regions in relation to the total number of patients in the group. All patients are pT1a or pT1b. **A:** Patients with early adenocarcinoma (all but two located below the level of the tracheal bifurcation). **B:** Early esophageal squamous cell cancer located below the level of the tracheal bifurcation. **C:** Early esophageal squamous cell cancer located at or above the level of the tracheal bifurcation. In patients with lymph node metastases at more than one location, all locations are shown. (From Stein HJ. Early esophageal cancer: Pattern of lymphatic spread and prognostic factors for long-term survival after surgical resection. *Ann Surg* 2005;242:566–573.)

classification by performing the cervical lymphadenectomy. In spite of this, the role of the cervical field lymphadenectomy in distal third adenocarcinomas was still felt to be investigational.[11]

HISTOLOGY

Squamous cell carcinomas and adenocarcinomas differ in terms of etiology, epidemiologically, metastatic potential, treatment response, and progression.[17] In T1 tumors, squamous cell tumors have nodal metastases in 10% of intramucosal and 50% of submucosal cancers. However, for adenocarcinomas, intramucosal tumors rarely have nodal metastases and intramucosal rates are 13% to 44%.[14,19,20]

Stein et al.[21] reported the prevalence of nodal metastases after esophagectomy for early stage tumors. For squamous tumors, 2/26 (7.7%) Tla lesions had nodal metastases, and 39 of 107 (36.4%) lb neoplasms had positive nodes. For adenocarcinoma, 0/70 had nodal involvement with Tla status, and 18 of 87 (21%) with lb.

NEW HORIZONS

PREOPERATIVE STAGING

The most recent NCCN guidelines recommend CT scan with IV and oral contrast of the chest and abdomen. If there is no evidence of metastatic disease then PET-CT, and endoscopic ultrasound are recommended to adequately stage patients preoperative. PET-CT is also recommended by the NCCN as well as the most recent guideline from STS for restaging after induction therapy.[21] The correct staging of patients with EUS-guided FNA of visualized nodal disease facilitates the use of preoperative chemoradiation which improves survival.

EXTENT OF LYMPH NODE RESECTION

Although the number of identified lymph nodes is decreased after induction therapy, adequate lymphadenectomy is important.[22] Altorki and colleagues[23] demonstrated improved survival with the removal of increased numbers of lymph nodes in patients that did not receive induction therapy. Using Cox regression modeling, Peyre et al.[24] demonstrated that the optimum number of nodes resected was 23.

The NCCN Guidelines Version 2.2015 recommends that at least 15 regional lymph nodes be resected to adequately stage patients who have not had preoperative chemoradiation based on Risk et al.'s[18] analysis of the Worldwide Esophageal Cancer Consortium (WECC). Their study demonstrated no link between extent of lymphadenectomy in Tis esophageal cancer patients. Patients with six or less positive nodes benefited from more extended nodal resections. They further identified optimum number of nodes resected based on T level for both adenocarcinoma and squamous cell carcinoma in N0M0 patients. Using standardized variable importance (VIMP), Risk and colleagues calculated the optimum number of nodes to be resected in a large cancer consortium based on tumor type and depth.

Optimum Nodal Resection based on T level[18]

	Adenocarcinomas	Squamous Cell Carcinoma
Tis	No link	No link
T1	10	12
T2	15	22
T3/4	31	42

MICROSTAGING OF LYMPH NODES

Standard lymph node evaluation is done by hematoxylin and eosin staining. Several immunohistochemical staining regimens have demonstrated increased detection rates.

Tanabe et al.[25] evaluated lymph node–associated superficial squamous cell carcinoma with AE1/AE3. In 78 patients, 34 had no detectable disease in the lymph nodes, 12 and 34 had disease detected by IHC and H and E, respectively. Heeren et al.[26] studied GEJ esophageal cancers in 148 patients. Sixty patients were identified as N0 by H and E staining but an additional 30% would have been upstaged by AE1/AE3 IHC staining.

STAGING SYSTEM REVISIONS

The AJCC staging for lymph nodes currently lists N0 as no regional nodal metastasis; N1 as metastasis in 1 to 2 regional lymph nodes; N2 as metastasis in 3 to 6 regional lymph nodes; and N3 as metastasis in 7 or more regional lymph nodes.[27]

Finally, knowledge of nodal involvement before treatment begins would allow possible fine tuning of radiation fields. Likewise, it can help preoperative surgeons to discuss whether a more radical resection or extensive lymphadenectomy should be undertaken.

CONCLUSION

Understanding the relationships of lymph nodes to esophageal carcinoma allows for accurate staging and management of these complex patients. Correctly assessing the presence of nodal disease with CT/PET and EUS with FNA provides therapy tailored to the patient's specific stage and tumor location. While various surgical approaches are utilized the minimally invasive approach is becoming increasingly more accepted as the standard approach at high volume esophageal centers. Finally, the extent of lymphadenectomy impacts patient survival. Esophageal surgeons should be well studied in this area and strive for complete lymph node resections as described in this chapter.

REFERENCES

1. Sakata K. Ueber die Lymphgef'asse des: Oesophagus und fiber seine regionaren Lymphdrfisen mit Berficksichtigung der Verbreitung' des Carcinoms. *Mitt Grenzgeb Medizin* 1903;11:629–656.
2. Liebermann-Meffert D. Anatomy, embryology, and histology. In: Pearson FG, Cooper JD, Deslaurier J, et al., eds. *Esophageal Surgery*. 2nd ed. New York: Churchill Livingstone; 2002:8–31.
3. Orringer MB. Transhiatal esophagectomy without thoracotomy. In Shields TW, LoCicero J, Ponn RB, et al., eds. *General Thoracic Surgery*. 6th ed. Philadelphia, PA: LWW; 2004.
4. Japanese Society for Esophageal Diseases. Guide lines for the clinical and pathologic studies on carcinoma of the esophagus. *Jpn J Surg* 1976;6:69–78.
5. Casson AG, Rusch VW, Ginsberg RJ, et al. Lymph node mapping of esophageal cancer. *Ann Thorac Surg* 1994;58:1569–1570.
6. Naruke T, Suemasu K, Ishikawa S. Lymph node mapping and curability at various levels of metastasis in resected lung cancer. *J Thorac Cardiovasc Surg* 1978;76:832–839.
7. Tabira Y. Recurrent nerve nodal involvement is associated with cervical nodal metastasis in thoracic esophageal carcinoma. *J Am Coll Surg* 2000;191:232–237.
8. Ueda Y, Shiozaki A, Itoi H, et al. Intraoperative pathological investigation of recurrent nerve nodal metastasis can guide the decision whether to perform cervical lymph node dissection in thoracic esophageal cancer. *Oncol Rep* 2006;16: 1061–1066.
9. Wu J, Chen QX, Zhou XM, et al. Does recurrent laryngeal nerve lymph node metastasis really affect the prognosis in node-positive patients with squamous cell carcinoma of the middle thoracic esophagus? *BMC Surg* 2014;14:43.
10. Hosch SB, Stoecklein NH, Pichlmeier U, et al. Esophageal cancer: The mode of lymphatic tumor cell spread and its prognostic significance. *J Clin Oncol* 2001;19:1970–1975.
11. Lerut T. Three-field lymphadenectomy for carcinoma of the esophagus and gastroesophageal junction in 174 Ro resections: Impact on staging, disease-free survival, and outcome: A plea for adaptation of TNM classification in upper-half esophageal carcinoma. *Ann Surg* 2004;240:962–972.

12. Nagaraja V, Eslick GD, Cox MR. Sentinel lymph nodes in oesophageal cancer- a systemic review and meta-analysis. *J Gastrointest Oncol* 2014;5(2):127–141.

13. Ando N, Ozawa S, Kitagawa Y, et al. Improvement in the results of surgical treatment of advanced squamous esophageal carcinoma during 15 consecutive years. *Ann Surg* 2000;232(2):225–232.

14. Rice TW, Zuccaro G, Jr., Adelstein DJ, et al. Esophageal carcinoma: Depth of tumor invasion is predictive of regional lymph node status. *Ann Thorac Surg* 1998;65:787–792.

15. Schurr PG, Yekebas EF, Kaifi JT, et al. Lymphatic spread and microinvolvement in adenocarcinoma of the esophago-gastric junction. *J Surg Oncol* 2006;94:307–315.

16. Nigro JJ, DeMeester SR, Hagen JA, et al. Node status in transmural esophageal adenocarcinoma and outcome after en bloc esophagectomy. *J Thorac Cardiovasc Surg* 1999;117:960–968.

17. Merkow RP, Bilimoria KY, Keswani RN, et al. Treatment trends, risk of lymph node metastasis, and outcomes for localized esophageal cancer. *J Natl Cancer Inst* 2014; 106(7):pii: dju133.

18. Risk NP, Ishwaran H, Rice T, et al. Optimum lymphadenectomy for esophageal cancer. *Ann Surg* 2000;251:46–50.

19. Rohatgi PR, Swisher SG, Correa AM, et al. Comparison of clinical stage, therapy response, and patient outcome between squamous cell carcinoma and adenocarcinoma of the esophagus. *Int J Gastrointest Cancer* 2005;36:69–76.

20. Buskens CJ, Westerterp M, Lagarde SM, et al. Prediction of appropriateness of local endoscopic treatment for high-grade dysplasia and early adenocarcinoma by EUS and histopathologic features. *Gastrointest Endosc* 2004;60:703–710.

21. Stein HJ, Feith M, Bruecher BL, et al. Early esophageal cancer: Pattern of lymphatic spread and prognostic factors for long term survival after surgical resection. *Ann Surg* 2005;242:566–573.

22. Little AG, Lerut AE, Harpole DH, et al. The society of thoracic surgeons practice guidelines on the role of multimodality treatment for cancer of the esophagus and gastroesophageal Junction. *Ann Thorac Surg* 2014;98:1880–1885.

23. Altorki NK, Zhou XK, Stiles B, et al. Total number of resected lymph nodes predicts survival in esophageal cancer. *Ann Surg* 2008;248(2):221–226.

24. Peyre CG, Hagen JA, DeMeester SR, et al. The number of lymph nodes removed predicts survival in esophageal cancer: An international study on the impact of extent of surgical resection. *Ann Surg* 2008 248(4):549–556.

25. Tanabe T, Nishimaki T, Watanabe H, et al. Immunohistochemically detected micrometastasis in lymph nodes from superficial esophageal squamous cell carcinoma. *J Surg Oncol* 2003;82(3):153–159.

26. Heeren PA1, Kelder W, Blondeel I, et al. Prognostic value of nodal micrometastases in patients with cancer of the gastro-oesophageal junction. *Eur J Surg Oncol* 2005;31(3):270–276.

27. American Joint Committee on Cancer. *AJCC Cancer Staging Manual 7th Edition 2010.*

PHYSIOLOGY OF THE ESOPHAGUS

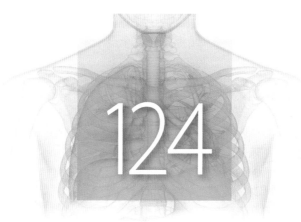

124

Anatomy, Physiology, and Physiologic Studies of the Esophagus

Siva Raja ▪ Prashanthi N. Thota ▪ Sudish C. Murthy

The esophagus is a surprisingly complex organ for such a simple hollow viscus that serves solely to shuttle food and saliva from pharynx to stomach in a unidirectional manner. Its rather unfortified anatomic structure belies its central role at the beginning of the digestive tract. Although endoscopic ultrasound can identify five distinct layers, this somewhat overstates the relatively primitive construction of the esophagus. Despite some rather cumbersome nomenclature (Fig. 124.1), there are fundamentally three important anatomic boundaries: (1) the mucosa, consisting of stratified squamous cells with deeper glands; (2) the submucosa, an intervening areolar tissue plane through which course the lymphatic and vascular supply to and from the mucosa; and (3) the muscularis (propria), a dense

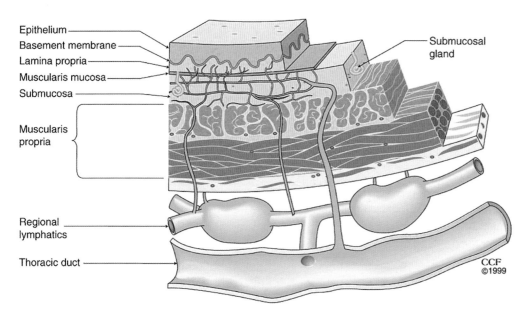

Epithelium
Basement membrane
Lamina propria
Muscularis mucosa
Submucosa

Muscularis propria

Regional lymphatics

Thoracic duct

Submucosal gland

CCF ©1999

FIGURE 124.1 Architecture of the body of the esophagus with lymphatic drainage also demonstrated. (Copyright © Cleveland Clinic Foundation.)

muscular shell split into a much thicker inner circular layer and a more attenuated outer longitudinal layer. The muscular component varies as the organ courses distally, with striated muscle principally present in the cervical region and gradually transitioning to smooth muscle as the organ courses through the thorax. There is no serosal covering of the organ, underscoring the relative ease with which spontaneous perforation can occur.

This is, however, where the simplicity ends and the complexity begins. The organ must propel food in an aboral direction only, while often distending significantly to permit passage of a food bolus.[1] There are both entry (upper esophageal sphincter [UES]) and exit (lower esophageal sphincter [LES]) that are tightly regulated with time-related relaxation and contraction orchestrated by the initiation of a swallow. Finally, the organ must defend itself from gastroesophageal reflux. Herein lies the beauty of its construction and orchestration of its function.

From both anatomic and physiologic standpoints, the esophagus can be separated into two segments: cervical and thoracic. The functional difference between the two seems indistinguishable, and there appears to be seamless integration of peristalsis across the length of the organ despite the difference in composition of the muscular component as the organ descends. There are, however, subtle differences in disease presentations based on the anatomic segment of the esophagus affected and its specific lymphatic drainage pattern.

When considering esophageal physiology and derangements thereof, a more practical understanding is best appreciated by considering the esophagus as comprising three anatomic components: the UES, esophageal body, and LES. The vast majority of benign diseases of the esophagus revolve around dysfunction at one or more of these foci. These three regions align anatomically with the cervical, thoracic, and abdominal portions of the esophagus, and consequently, interactions with the unique surrounding environment around each modify (and can magnify) disease presentation.

THE UPPER ESOPHAGEAL SPHINCTER

The UES is not defined by any unique anatomic distinguishing feature, although several do exist. It is principally identified as a high-pressure zone separating the pharynx from the esophagus. As such, it is the gate keeper for entrance of a food bolus into the esophagus and the last bastion of defense against regurgitation or reflux of swallowed food coming from below.

It is, in part, composed of the cricopharyngeus muscle, which likely serves as the dominant contributor to the high pressures measured in the region.[2,3] However, that the high-pressure zone of the UES measures some three times the width of the cricopharyngeus muscle suggests important contributions from other structures.[4,5] Investigations have led to the suspicion that a component of tonic contraction exists and meaningfully contributes to resting UES tone as denervated UES still retains an increased closing pressure.[6] The concept that an important passive elastic component of the UES exists has been forwarded by some and is supported by animal studies.[6,7]

It might be best to consider that the UES is an amalgam of striated muscle, cartilage, and aponeurotic tissue.[8] This curious construction presumably accounts for the asymmetric geometric dimensions and inherent difficulties in accurate anatomic categorization. Because of its presumed singular striated muscle component, its innervation originates in the nucleus ambiguus of the brainstem.[9]

When contracted, the UES clearly maintains a pressure barrier segregating the pharynx from the esophagus. Interestingly, UES tone is impacted by body posture as well as the volume, composition, and

velocity of esophageal contents, including those that are refluxing.[8] Faster rates of esophageal pressure change resulting from an admixture of both air and liquid in refluxate favor relaxation of the UES, and this appears to correlate with the role of facilitator that it plays in both eructation and emesis.[8,10]

As expected, relaxation of the UES occurs at the onset of swallowing. This is closely followed by a subsequent re-contraction of the UES to perhaps twice its resting pressure, which then subsides and allows for regression of UES tone back toward baseline shortly thereafter. This wave of contraction then progresses down the esophagus as the primary peristaltic wave.[2]

THE BODY OF THE ESOPHAGUS

The body of the esophagus is identified as that region between the UES and LES. Luminal construction is similar across the entire length of the esophagus, with the exception of the gradual change of muscle type from striated to smooth. This is consistent with the transition of a swallow from voluntary to involuntary action once initiated. From a practical standpoint, moving the food bolus distally is the only function of the body, as there is no clear regulatory function.

Once a swallow is initiated, a relatively orderly, though not constant, peristaltic wave is created. Surprisingly, the speed of the wave varies, being relatively slow after deglutination and further slowing in the mid-body, only to accelerate toward the LES, where it then slows again.[2] Not all initiated peristaltic waves are actually completed, as dry swallows result in one-third of aborted peristaltic waves in normal controls.[2] Nonetheless, a properly initiated swallow should result in a normal peristaltic wave traveling the entire length of the esophageal body in about 10 seconds.

The phenomenon of secondary peristalsis refers to peristaltic waves that are not initiated by deglutination. The stimulus for their genesis is presumed to be esophageal distention or irritation. The amplitude of waves measured manometrically is indistinguishable from primary peristalsis. This might represent a housekeeping-type function perhaps clearing refluxate and saliva from the lumen.[2]

Neurologic control of peristalsis is complex. The striated muscle component falls under central jurisdiction of the swallowing center in the brainstem, and this is thought to be the sole source of neurologic input.[11] There is a sequential, hierarchical activation of lower motor neurons in the nucleus ambiguus to effect peristalsis in the striated muscle of the esophagus.

Regulation of peristalsis in the smooth muscle of the body is far more complicated. Two distinct mechanisms are likely at play. First, there appears to be a local (peripheral) neurologic mechanism. This intramural system seems to be responsible for local control in a manner similar to that observed in the small intestine, with peristalsis initiated as a response to lumen distention. However, the precise causality is a bit more convoluted. There is a curious inhibition of contraction and not excitation that is noted with direct electrical stimulation. This is followed by a subsequent rebound contraction that occurs promptly after cessation of the stimuli and is supported clinically by esophageal deflation, after distention, eliciting this rebound contraction phenomenon.[11,12] This suggests that local *inhibitory* nerves are responsible for some part of esophageal smooth muscle peristalsis.[11]

Unfortunately, this is not where the story ends. There is also a central neurologic component of smooth muscle contraction. This became evident when it was recognized that cervical vagotomy abolished smooth muscle peristalsis.[11] However, the mode of central activation is not quite the same as with striated muscle control. There is non-orchestrated, non-sequential, simultaneous activation of myenteric plexus neurons (instead of an organized, hierarchical input) that, though critical, still presumably leaves peristalsis under primary control of the local nerve net.[11]

Finally, the complex interplay of excitatory and inhibitory signals controlling peristalsis and esophageal motor function is facilitated through nitric oxide (NO). This molecule seems to be the most important inhibitory neurotransmitter. It has been speculated that both excitatory and inhibitory pathways supply myenteric plexuses and that during peristalsis, inhibitory myenteric neurons are activated first and soon after followed by the peristaltic wave.[11] Interestingly, inhibitors of NO synthase seem to increase the speed of the peristaltic wave.[11,13] An appreciation of this inhibitory pathway is critical when considering diseases such as achalasia.

THE LOWER ESOPHAGEAL SPHINCTER

The LES was initially considered a nebulous region at the distal end of the esophagus. There were few easily appreciated recognizable features distinguishing the region, and the lack of landmarks led to difficulty in its characterization. Early definitions suggested that the LES was simply a high-pressure zone that relaxed during swallowing and sat just above the gastroesophageal junction.[14,15] Thankfully, we now have a much better sense of the LES, as anatomic, morphologic, and functional analyses have clarified our understanding of the region (Fig. 124.2).

The LES is primarily considered on a functional basis, with anatomic concerns relegated to a somewhat lesser importance unless needed to explain aberrant function. To date, it has proven difficult to determine what precise mechanism controls and modulates the baseline resting tone of the LES. Neurologic control mediated through the vagus nerve has fallen out of favor during the past decade. In its place has risen the concept of a myogenic basis for LES basal tone regulation, dependent on numerous hormones and neurotransmitters in the local milieu.[11]

Regardless of the resting tone, once deglutination is initiated, there is an element of central control that allows for appropriate time-related relaxation of the LES to permit completion of the peristaltic wave to the stomach. There are neural pathways from the caudal and rostral parts of the dorsal motor nucleus (DMN) of the vagus nerve that, upon swallowing, activate inhibitory neurons first. This causes a simultaneous inhibition of the entire esophagus. There appears to be a gradient of duration of inhibition across the length of the organ, as

the inhibitory signal is far more protracted in the more distal parts of the esophagus than proximal. As the inhibition subsides, beginning in the cephalad portion of the organ, there is a sequential activation of excitatory neurons in the rostral DMN that provokes contractility and propulsion of the food bolus.[11]

Relaxation of the LES starts within seconds of initiation of the swallow and lasts a surprisingly long time (about 5 minutes). Local post-ganglionic neurons release nitric oxide as the dominant inhibitor. In addition, isolated relaxation of the LES can occur. This is considered a vaso-vagal reflux that involves only the inhibitory neural pathway and not the excitatory. This reflex is important for eructation and emesis and can be initiated by gastric distention.

Finally, in addition to the smooth muscle component of the LES, there is likely some contribution to both resting tone and relaxation by the diaphragmatic hiatus. There is disagreement about how important this anatomic structure actually is as part of the antireflux barrier. The role of the diaphragm *pinchcock* has been studied, and some have suggested that the striated muscle fibers at the hiatus that envelop the LES form an *external* LES.[11,16] The control mechanism remains somewhat elusive, however. Finally, the angle of His (the angle at which the esophagus enters the stomach) has been long understood as being a potent mechanical component of the antireflux mechanism of the LES, but the exact mechanism of this benefit remains poorly understood.

PHYSIOLOGY AND PATHOLOGY

This focused review of esophageal physiology becomes relevant only when disease processes affecting the esophagus are being considered. To that end, benign acquired esophageal pathology largely falls into two broad categories: disruption of its antireflux capacity (gastroesophageal reflux disease [GERD]) or disturbances of motor function (esophageal dysmotility). Hence, further understanding of the testing modalities that facilitate an in-depth understanding of physiologic and pathologic states of the above-mentioned categories is essential in any discussion of esophageal function or dysfunction. Specifically, we will now discuss pH testing and manometry as they pertain to the antireflux capacity and motor function of the esophagus. Familiarity with the unique physiologic assessments of each of these elements will galvanize a more focused understanding of the surgical physiology of the esophagus (Table 124.1).

GASTROESOPHAGEAL REFLUX DISEASE

A primary function of the LES is to prevent retrograde escape of gastric contents, which include the acidic milieu of the stomach. The loss of the high-pressure zone that is the hallmark of the LES for anatomic or functional reasons can result in abnormal exposure of the esophagus to acid. Abnormal acid exposure can be seen as a result of a loss of LES tone, loss of peristalsis of the esophagus, or increased intra-gastric pressure from gastroparesis. This is known as GERD and is a common disorder in the United States. Classic symptoms of GERD include heartburn and regurgitation. The atypical or extra-esophageal symptoms of GERD include chest pain, hoarseness, recurrent sore throat, dental caries, bronchospasm, wheezing, chronic cough, or recurrent chest infections. Unfortunately, disorders such as achalasia, cholelithiasis, gastritis, gastric or duodenal ulcer, and coronary artery disease all can produce symptoms that mimic GERD. Consequently, the diagnosis of GERD on the basis of symptoms alone is neither sensitive nor specific.

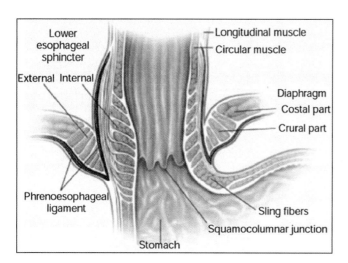

FIGURE 124.2 Anatomy of the lower esophageal sphincter.

TABLE 124.1 Surgical Physiology of the Esophagus

	Upper Esophageal Sphincter (UES)	Esophageal Body	Lower Esophageal Sphincter (LES)
Location	Cervical esophagus	Thoracic esophagus	Esophageal hiatus
Muscle type	Skeletal	Skeletal with gradual transition to smooth muscle	Smooth muscle (skeletal muscle comprises the external sphincter)
Neurologic control	Central and elastic recoil	Peripheral and central	Peripheral and central
Resting tone	Yes	No	Yes
Classic motor diseases	Hypertensive: Zenker's diverticulum	Hypertensive: Jackhammer esophagus type III achalasia	Hypertensive: types 1–III achalasia epiphrenic diverticulum Hypotensive: GERD

Classic approaches to the diagnosis of GERD were to identify reflux with barium radiography or to reproduce the symptoms with an acid-perfusion or Bernstein test.[17] Endoscopy is commonly performed in patients with reflux symptoms, and although the presence of erosive esophagitis is quite specific, it also lacks sensitivity for less severe reflux.[18] However, many patients with GERD, especially those with respiratory manifestations, do not have esophagitis. With the introduction of potent acid-suppressing medications, another common practice has been to treat patients with reflux symptoms with a proton pump inhibitor; if the symptoms improve, a presumptive diagnosis of GERD is made. All of the above-mentioned modalities lack the sensitivity to reliably detect abnormal esophageal acid exposure and GERD. As such, reliance on these tests alone has led many a patient and surgeon down the road of ineffective medical and surgical therapy.

The most reliable way to diagnose GERD is to document increased esophageal exposure to gastric acid with ambulatory 24-hour pH monitoring. This technique allows clinicians to quantitate esophageal acid exposure and diagnose reflux disease when acid exposure exceeds the upper limits of normal. Consequently, 24-hour pH monitoring has emerged as the test with the greatest sensitivity and specificity for the diagnosis of gastroesophageal reflux and is currently considered the "gold standard."[19] It can be performed with the standard trans-nasal catheter or with newer wireless systems that are catheter free after deployment of the monitoring device.

24-HOUR ESOPHAGEAL pH MONITORING

Antireflux therapy can be successful only to the extent that the patient's symptoms are due to reflux disease. A multivariate analysis of factors predicting outcome after laparoscopic Nissen fundoplication showed that an abnormal 24-hour pH score predicted the best result.[20] Other significant predictors of a good outcome in this analysis were the presence of typical reflux symptoms and substantial symptomatic improvement with preoperative acid-suppression medication. When patients had all three factors in their favor, a good to excellent outcome was achieved in 97.4%. The purpose of monitoring esophageal pH is to detect the presence of increased esophageal exposure to refluxed acidic gastric contents.

It is important to emphasize that 24-hour esophageal pH monitoring is merely a means of measuring esophageal exposure to gastric juice. To define abnormal exposure, normal exposure was first determined in a group of asymptomatic volunteers. Normally, gastric pH is in the range of 1 to 2, and the intraluminal pH of the esophagus

is between 4 and 7. A dip in the continuously measured esophageal pH <4 has become the most commonly used threshold for determining a reflux episode. In 1974, Johnson and DeMeester[21] reported the results of 24-hour pH monitoring in the following manner: (1) cumulative reflux time, expressed as the percentage of *total monitored time*; (2) percentage of time monitored *upright*; (3) percentage of time monitored *supine*; (4) frequency of reflux episodes, expressed as the *number of reflux episodes* per 24 hours; (5) duration of reflux episodes, expressed as the *number of episodes longer than 5 minutes*; and (6) the *length in minutes of the longest episode*. This report identified these six components of a 24-hour pH record that could be specifically analyzed. A value greater than 14.72 for a composite score of these six components is considered to be abnormal.

PERFORMANCE OF THE STUDY

It is important to standardize the test so that it is performed the same way in all patients. Patients should be encouraged to be as active as they normally are during the study. All medications that affect the pH of the stomach or the motility of the foregut should be stopped before the study. Although there is some lack of consensus between institutions, we recommend cessation of proton pump inhibitors for 7 days, H2 blockers and pro-motility agents for 48 hours, and antacids for 6 hours prior to testing.

CATHETER AND CATHETER-LESS SYSTEMS

Traditionally, the 24-hour pH study has been performed with a catheter passed down the nose, which is left in place for the duration of the study. The location was calculated by manometric guidance to be 5 cm above the LES. However, despite the small catheter size, many patients have difficulty tolerating it for the entire 24-hour period. Consequently, catheter-less systems (Bravo® probe, OMOM® probe) have essentially replaced the old trans-nasal catheter in the developed world. The device can be placed endoscopically 5 cm above the LES. This system uses a capsule containing the pH probe, a transmitter, and a battery, all in a small device that is attached to the esophageal mucosa with a special pin (Fig. 124.3). The device transmits pH data to a storage device worn on the belt. Generally, the capsule falls off after several days and is passed out via the gastrointestinal tract. In addition, it allows 48 to 96 hours of pH data to be collected and analyzed. In addition to the obvious advantage of patient tolerance and compliance with routine activity, the additional time (24 hours vs. 48 to 96 hours) increases the sensitivity of the test.

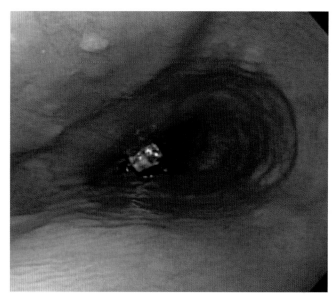

FIGURE 124.3 Bravo probe in the esophagus.

Also, one can perform monitoring of pre- and post-therapy to see the effect of therapy. The disadvantages are cost, possible chest pain, and premature dislodgment of the sensor.[22]

pH TESTING

Patients are asked to keep a diary during the pH study and to document meal periods as well as any symptoms they experience. Only water is allowed between meals, and any episodes of water drinking must be written in the diary. Acidic foods such as carbonated beverages are generally forbidden to eliminate false-positive results. Although it is important to evaluate the patient in the most physiologic conditions possible, it is probably prudent to avoid conditions that are known to exacerbate reflux and therefore may influence the results of the study. Such conditions include vigorous exercise, alcohol drinking, or cigarette smoking. A normal pH study is shown in Figure 124.4.

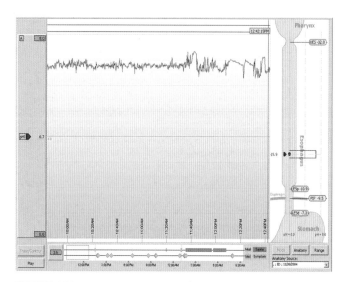

FIGURE 124.4 Representative output from a patient with normal acid exposure.

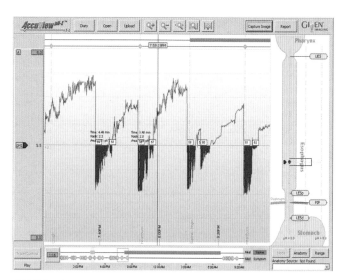

FIGURE 124.5 Representative output from a patient with abnormal acid exposure.

RESULTS OF pH TESTING IN GERD

In early disease, the sphincter is competent except during periods of stress, which occur with eating and gastric distention. A pH tracing in these patients typically demonstrates frequent episodes of reflux limited primarily to the upright, postprandial period (Fig. 124.5). Bi-positional reflux—that is, reflux in both the upright and supine positions—is associated with more advanced disease and usually indicates that function of the LES is severely impaired. Pure supine reflux is rare. Intermittent, prolonged reflux episodes on the 24-hour pH tracing suggest delayed esophageal clearance, particularly if they occur in the upright position.

GERD AND SPECIAL CIRCUMSTANCES

In several specific circumstances, 24-hour esophageal pH monitoring can be useful to assist in determining whether reflux is a potential cause of a patient's symptoms. These circumstances include monitoring in patients with unexplained chest pain, recurrent pulmonary infections, and adult-onset asthma.

REFLUX AND UNEXPLAINED CHEST PAIN

As many as 10% of patients with GERD have chest pain as their only symptom. Furthermore, exercise can induce reflux, and patients may present with exercise-induced chest pain that further confuses the etiology. Given the concern that heart disease is responsible for the chest pain, these patients often undergo an extensive cardiac evaluation before consideration is given to an esophageal etiology for the symptoms. When a cardiac etiology was ruled out, nearly 50% of patients with unexplained chest pain were found to have increased esophageal acid exposure on pH testing.[23] In addition to reflux, esophageal motor disorders can produce chest pain, perhaps as a consequence of "esophageal claudication." Other studies have used ambulatory motility monitoring to demonstrate that noncardiac chest pain episodes in some patients were immediately preceded by a markedly increased frequency of esophageal contractions, which were mostly simultaneous, double-peaked or multi-peaked, of high (>180 mm Hg) amplitude, or of prolonged duration (>7 seconds).[24]

REFLUX AND RESPIRATORY SYMPTOMS

Reflux has long been recognized as a potential cause of respiratory symptoms. In 1892, Sir William Osler noted that his asthma patients would often worsen if they ate a large meal in the evening instead of at noon. A 24-hour pH monitoring study demonstrated in patients with asthma that 80% had abnormal reflux independent of bronchodilator usage.[25] In any asthmatic patient, the quandary is whether reflux is the cause or merely an incidental finding to the asthma. It is unknown what percentage of the 13 to 15 million asthmatic individuals in the United States have asthma precipitated or exacerbated by episodes of reflux and which patients should have detailed reflux testing. However, several clinical settings have been identified that are highly suggestive of a reflux etiology for airway symptoms, and patients with asthma who fit into one or more of these settings should be evaluated for reflux disease. These clinical settings include recurrent pneumonia, especially in the mid-lung fields; severe broncho-pulmonary disease in a nonsmoker without obvious allergic triggers; onset of bronchial asthma in late childhood or adult life; asthma symptoms that are worse after eating a large meal or drinking alcohol; nocturnal asthma; and difficult-to-control asthma. Symptoms that may be associated with reflux-induced laryngeal irritation include chronic throat clearing, recurrent hoarseness, or frequent sore throats.

The potential association between reflux and respiratory symptoms is rarely missed in patients who present with one or more of the classic reflux symptoms (heartburn, regurgitation, or dysphagia) in addition to their respiratory complaints. However, many patients present with exclusively respiratory complaints, such as intermittent wheezing, chronic cough or throat clearing, episodes of nocturnal choking, apneic spells, hoarseness, laryngitis, or recurrent pneumonia. In these patients the potential association with GERD is frequently overlooked and a high index of suspicion is necessary to make the diagnosis. In this population, objective testing with 24- or 48-hour pH monitoring can help support the association of their respiratory symptoms with their GERD.

Merely documenting abnormal esophageal acid exposure on 24-hour pH monitoring in patients with respiratory symptoms is inadequate to conclude that reflux is the cause of the respiratory symptoms. In some patients there are other causes of the respiratory symptoms, such as sinusitis, postnasal drip, or allergic conditions, and while reflux may exacerbate the respiratory symptoms, it may not be the sole cause. Further, respiratory conditions themselves may induce or exacerbate reflux. The relationship between the respiratory event and a reflux episode can help differentiate patients with reflux and respiratory symptoms in whom correction of reflux is likely to alleviate some or much of the respiratory complaint. Determining this relationship is best done by ambulatory esophageal pH monitoring. A study of 128 patients with GERD and airway-related symptoms after laparoscopic antireflux surgery showed a resolution or improvement of respiratory symptoms in about 60% of the patients. In the same cohort, typical symptoms such as heartburn and regurgitation improved in >90% of the patients. This highlights the less than perfect association of respiratory symptoms of GERD with surgical intervention for GERD.[26]

Last, an area of recent interest is in patients with end-stage pulmonary disease, such as COPD, interstitial pulmonary fibrosis, and the post-lung transplant population.[27] Our work identified pre-transplant GERD as predictor of worse early allograft function after lung transplantation.[28] Further, in a review of the Duke University experience, patients who had an antireflux operation before or early after lung transplantation had improved graft function and increased survival compared with all other patients.[29] These findings confirm the important relationship between gastroesophageal reflux and chronic lung disease and suggest that patients with end-stage lung disease awaiting lung transplant should be evaluated with pH testing.

BILE REFLUX

Duodenogastric reflux has been recognized as an independent clinical entity. Attempts to detect or diagnose duodenogastric reflux relied on the endoscopic presence of gastritis, gastric or esophageal sampling for bile salts, and nuclear medicine radionuclide scans. Studies using impedance technology have conclusively documented that effective acid suppression with proton pump inhibitors merely changes the character of the refluxed material from acid to weak acid or alkaline, but the overall number of reflux events remains unchanged.[30] Duodenogastric reflux is frequently sporadic; as a consequence, these tests lack sensitivity. Currently the best method to detect both acid reflux and non- or weak acid reflux events is combined pH and impedance testing. The importance of weak acid reflux in causing persistent symptoms in patients on proton pump inhibitor therapy is increasingly being recognized, as is the fact that only antireflux surgery reliably eliminates both acid and non- or weak acid reflux events.[31,32]

HISTORY OF ESOPHAGEAL MANOMETRY

Esophageal manometry is the gold standard test for evaluation of esophageal peristaltic function of the esophageal body and that of the adjoining sphincters. The concept was developed in the 1950s and confined to research laboratories until development of the water-perfused manometry system, which consisted of water-perfused catheters, a pneumo-hydraulic pump, and pressure transducers, in the mid-1970s.[14,33,34] The early manometry systems were fraught with the disadvantages of widely spaced pressure sensors and inaccurate evaluation of LES relaxation due to cephalad movement of the LES relative to the sensor. To circumvent this latter problem, a 6-cm-long Dent sleeve sensor was introduced in 1976.[35] These conventional catheters had pressure sensors every 3 to 5 cm and necessitated pull-through maneuvers and repeated repositioning for data acquisition. In the 1990s, by increasing the number of pressure sensors to every 1 cm along the length of the catheter, high-resolution esophageal manometry (HREM) came into existence, facilitating simultaneous pressure measurements of both the sphincters and along the entire length of the esophagus.[36] This led to the development of esophageal pressure topography (EPT), a simplified visual display of enormous manometric data using sophisticated computer algorithms. EPT plots incorporate time on the x-axis and esophageal position on the y-axis, with warmer colors representing high pressures and cooler colors representing low pressures.[37]

Currently, there are two main types of manometry catheters available: (1) water-perfused catheters connected to an external transducer, water pump, and a data recorder and (2) solid-state catheters with internal micro-transducers. The latter are sensitive to rapid pressure changes and hence are more useful for evaluation of UES than water-perfused catheters. Due to the ease of data acquisition and superior diagnostic accuracy, HREM has gradually replaced conventional manometry for assessing esophageal function. A further advancement is a three-dimensional HREM which provides a digitally created three-dimensional image of the esophagus, which may be especially useful when assessing the UES, which has asymmetrical muscular anatomy.[38]

TECHNIQUE OF PERFORMING HREM

Patients are advised to fast for at least 6 hours and avoid medications that alter esophageal motility, such as caffeine, calcium channel blockers, nitrates, prokinetics, loperamide, α-adrenergic antagonists, opiate agonists or antagonists, anticholinergics, and tricyclic antidepressants. After obtaining consent, the manometry catheter is inserted transnasally and positioned to record from the hypopharynx to the stomach, with at least three sensors in the stomach. The standard protocol includes a 30-second baseline recording without swallowing followed by 10 5-mL water swallows separated by 20- to 30-second intervals in the supine position. Instead of a line tracing, the HREM data are displayed as an EPT or a Clouse plot, which is a three-dimensional spatiotemporal plot depicting esophageal pressure amplitude from pharynx to stomach.

COMPONENTS OF HREM-EPT PLOT

Anatomic sphincters: The UES and LES are visualized within EPT plot as high-pressure zones in the proximal and distal end of the esophagus, respectively.

Esophageal body: Peristalsis consists of sequential contractions demarcated by three pressure troughs (proximal, middle, and distal). The first contractile segment is the striated portion of the proximal esophagus, while the fourth contractile segment is the LES. The second and third contractile segments comprise most of the esophageal body. Figure 124.6 depicts the EPT plot of a normal swallow.

Transition zone: A proximal trough that corresponds to transition from extrinsically controlled striated muscle to intrinsically dominated smooth muscle.

Respiratory inversion point: The location at which the inspiratory esophagogastric junction (EGJ) pressure becomes less than the expiratory EGJ pressure. This is the point of transition from intrathoracic to intraabdominal environment.

Isobaric contour: A line on a pressure topography plot where the pressure is equal to a specific value, for example, 20 mm Hg. The 20 mm Hg isobaric contour includes areas where pressure exceeds 20 mm Hg and excludes areas of lesser pressure.

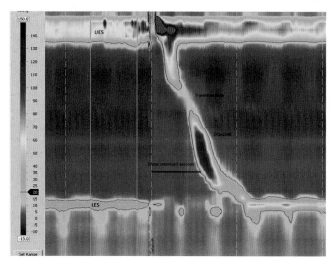

FIGURE 124.6 Normal EPT plot.

Intrabolus pressure: This corresponds to abnormal pressurization to >30 mm Hg. It is "panesophageal" if it extends from the UES to EGJ (as in achalasia type II), "compartmentalized" if it extends from the contractile front to the EGJ, and "EGJ pressurization" if it is restricted between the LES and CD in conjunction with hiatal hernia.

CHICAGO CLASSIFICATION

The advent of HREM with EPT led to the development of new metrics and parameters for assessment of esophageal motility disorders and forms the foundation of the Chicago Classification, which continues to be updated (the latest version 3).[39–41] In addition to the parameters presented above, the other metrics used in the Chicago Classification are as follows:

1. **Integrated relaxation pressure (IRP):** The average minimum EGJ pressure for 4 seconds of relaxation (contiguous or noncontiguous) within 10 seconds of upper sphincter relaxation. The upper limit of normal is less than 15 mm.

2. **Distal contractile integral (DCI):** A measure of the peristaltic vigor of the distal esophageal contraction. The DCI is a product of the mean distal contractile amplitude × length of the distal esophagus × contractile duration.

3. **Contractile deceleration point (CDP):** The inflection point where the peristaltic wave slows down in the distal esophagus. It is located within 3 cm of the LES. This landmark defines a transition from esophageal peristaltic clearance to emptying of the phrenic ampulla on fluoroscopy.

4. **Distal latency (DL):** The interval between UES relaxation and the CDP. Normal is more than 4.5 seconds.

5. **Peristaltic breaks:** Breaks of more than 5 cm or a 20-mm isobaric contour are considered abnormal, whereas breaks of less than 3 cm can be encountered in normal subjects.

6. **Contractile force velocity (CFV):** The peristaltic velocity of esophageal body between proximal trough and CDP on a 30-mm isobaric contour. Normal velocity is up to 8 cm/s. The clinical significance of rapid contractions with normal latency is not known.

7. **EGJ morphology:** Both LES and crural diaphragm (CD) contribute to EGJ pressure. Depending on the relative locations of LES and CD, which are best evaluated during inspiration, the EGJ can be classified into the following morphologic types (Fig. 124.7A–D):

   Type I: Complete overlap between LES and CD with no separation.

   Type II: Minimal but discernible LES–CD separation, but the nadir pressure between the peaks is still positive. This represents an intermediate condition between normal and a hiatal hernia.

   Type III: More than a 2-cm separation between LES and CD.

   III A: The pressure inversion point is proximal to the CD.

   III B: The pressure inversion point is proximal to the LES.

8. **EGJ function:** A novel metric, esophagogastric junction contractile integral (EGJ-CI), has been proposed as a means to evaluate EGJ antireflux barrier function. Similar to DCI of esophageal body, the upper and lower margins of the EGJ were enclosed in a DCI tool box. The duration of the box is three consecutive respiratory cycle and the threshold isobaric contour is set at 2 mm Hg above the gastric pressure. The value computed with the DCI tool in mm Hg s cm is then divided by the duration of the three respiratory cycles (in seconds), yielding EGJ-CI units of mm Hg cm. A value below 13 is considered a defective EGJ-CI. Patients with a defective EGJ-CI more frequently have positive impedance-pH monitoring

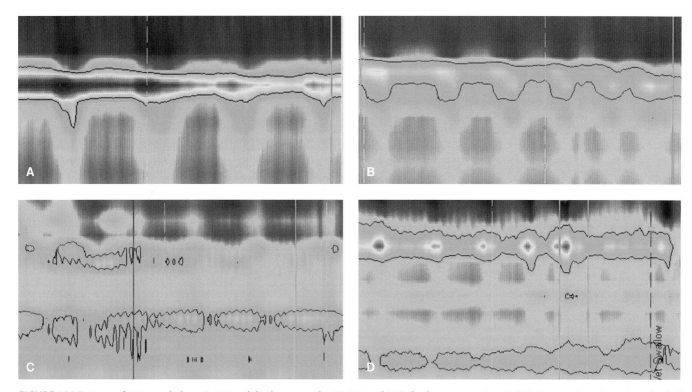

FIGURE 124.7 Types of EGJ morphology. **A:** LES and diaphragm overlap. **B:** Minimal LES–diaphragm separation. **C:** IIIA: Pressure inversion point at level of diaphragm. **D:** IIIB: Pressure inversion point at level of LES.

or esophageal mucosal lesions at endoscopy (p <0.05 and p <0.05, respectively) than patients with a normal EGJ-CI. An EGJ-CI cut-off value of 5 mm Hg cm identified GERD at impedance-pH (sensitivity 89%, specificity 63%).[42]

9. **UES evaluation:** Due to the rapidity of contraction, complex anatomy, and radial asymmetry of the UES, its evaluation is challenging and best done with a HREM solid-state catheter.[43] The parameters evaluated are basal UES pressure, UES relaxation time, nadir pressure during UES relaxation, UES coordination with pharyngeal contraction, amplitude of pharyngeal contraction, and intrabolus pressure. However, the values are not standardized. It is useful in the evaluation of patients presenting with oropharyngeal dysphagia.

STEPWISE APPROACH TO DIAGNOSIS OF ESOPHAGEAL MOTILITY DISORDERS USING CHICAGO CLASSIFICATION

Diagnosis of esophageal motility begins with assessment of the EGJ. The first step is to ensure that the catheter has passed below the diaphragm, as evidenced by the pressure inversion point. Sometime, the catheter tip does not pass below the diaphragm and remains coiled inside large hiatal hernia sacs. In these instances, LES can still be evaluated. LES relaxation is assessed by LES-IRP. A median pressure over 15 mm Hg is considered abnormal relaxation.

When there is 100% aperistalsis, a lower cut-off value of 10 mm Hg is used to diagnose achalasia type I. If there is panesophageal pressurization to more than 30 mm Hg in two or more swallows, achalasia type II is considered irrespective of LES-IRP.[41] Type III achalasia is characterized by lack of normal peristalsis and premature contractions ≥20% of the swallows. EGJ outflow obstruction is diagnosed when there is elevated median LES-IRP with sufficient

evidence of peristalsis and criteria for types I to III achalasia are not met (Fig. 124.8A–D).

Each individual swallow is assessed and classified as normal, failed, weak, hypercontractile, or premature based on the criteria listed in Table 124.2 and Figure 124.9A–E.

TABLE 124.2 Characterization of Esophageal Contractility

Contraction Vigor	
Failed	DCI <100 mm Hg s cm
Weak	DCI >100 mm Hg s cm, but <450 mm Hg s cm
Ineffective	Failed or weak
Normal	DCI >450 mm Hg s cm but <8,000 mm Hg s cm
Hypercontractile	DCI ≥8,000 mm Hg s cm
Contraction Pattern	
Premature	DL <4.5 s
Fragmented	Large break (>5 cm length) in the 20-mm Hg isobaric contour with DCI >450 mm Hg s cm
Intact	Not achieving the above diagnostic criteria
Intrabolus Pressure Pattern (30-mm Hg Isobaric Contour Referenced to Atmospheric)	
Panesophageal pressurization	Uniform pressurization of >30 mm Hg extending from the UES to the EGJ
Compartmentalized esophageal pressurization	Pressurization of >30 mm Hg extending from the contractile front to the EGJ
EGJ pressurization	Pressurization restricted to zone between the LES and CD in conjunction with LES–CD separation
Normal	No bolus pressurization >30 mm Hg

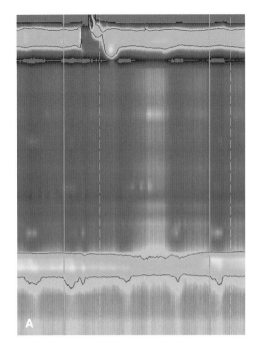
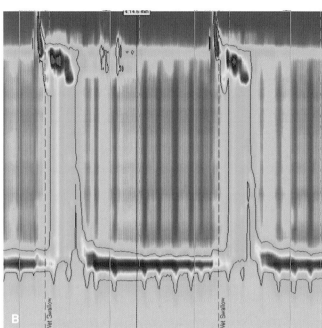
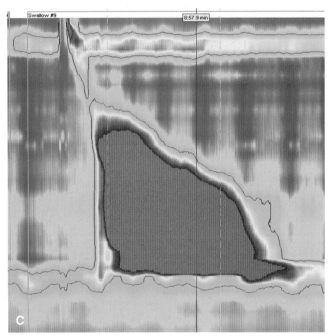
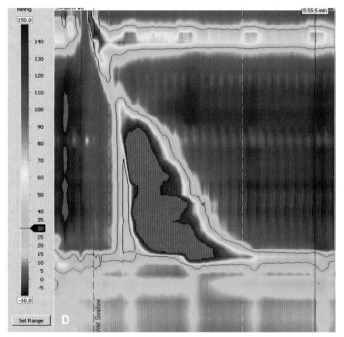

FIGURE 124.8 Types of achalasia. Type I (**A**), type II (**B**), type III (**C**), EG junction obstruction (**D**).

Any pressurization patterns are noted in the report for additional interpretation.

These findings are all utilized to fit classification criteria for a manometric diagnosis per the Chicago Classification, as presented in Table 124.3.

VARIATIONS IN PROTOCOL

Upright Posture

The study is typically performed in the supine position to negate the effect of gravity on bolus transit.[44] The upright position is more physiologic and better tolerated by patients with regurgitation and at high risk of aspiration. The changes noted in upright position are lower

CFV, higher DCI, and shorter transition zone. Normal values have been established.[45]

Solid Boluses

Solid boluses may trigger esophageal dysmotility more than small liquid swallows and may increase the diagnostic yield of esophageal motor disorders in patients reporting dysphagia. Slower CFV, longer DL, and stronger DCI were seen for the solid compared to liquid swallows.[46] In one study, 7/18 (39%) patients had a change in diagnosis based on HRM studies during or after the test meal that altered clinical management, with the majority responding well to specific treatment directed at the cause of symptoms. HRM measurements during a test meal are more sensitive to clinically

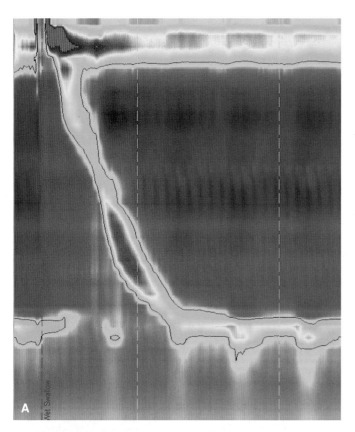

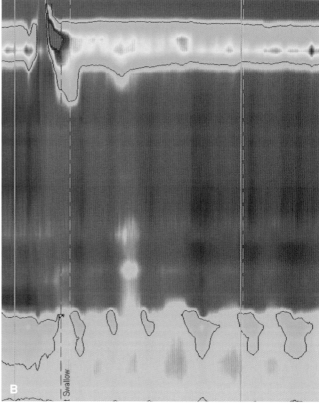

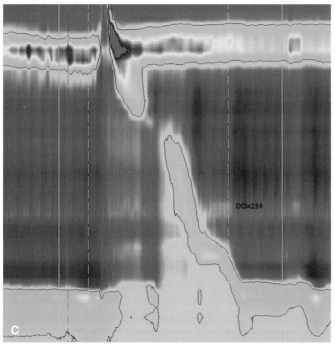

FIGURE 124.9 Types of swallows. Normal swallow (**A**), failed swallow (**B**), weak swallow (**C**), premature contraction (**D**), hypercontractile swallow (**E**). (*continued*)

relevant dysfunction, identify the cause of symptoms, and guide effective management as determined by clinical outcomes at 2-year follow-up.[47]

Peristaltic Reserve Assessed by Multiple Rapid Swallows

Multiple rapid swallows (MRS) can be used as a supplemental test to evaluate peristaltic reserve in ineffective esophageal motility. MRS

consists of administering five 2-mL water swallows separated by 2- to 3-second intervals during which peristaltic activity is inhibited. This is followed by an augmented contraction. In a cohort study of GERD patients prior to fundoplication, the DCI of augmented contraction following MRS was compared to the mean DCI of the prior 10 test swallows. The DCI ratio (DCI after MRS/mean DCI of the 10 swallows) was greater than 1 in 64% of patients without post-fundoplication dysphagia, 44% of patients with early dysphagia, and

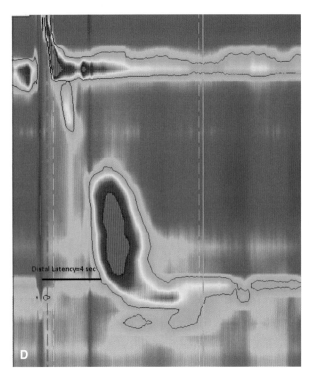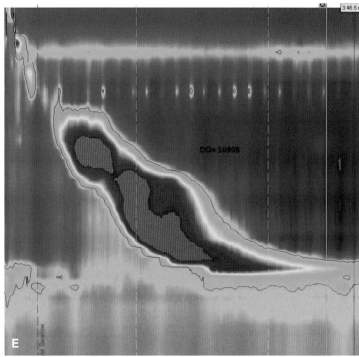

FIGURE 124.9 (*Continued*)

TABLE 124.3 Chicago Classification Version 3

Achalasia and EGJ Outflow Obstruction	Criteria
Type I achalasia (classic achalasia)	Elevated median IRP (>15 mm Hg) 100% failed peristalsis (DCI <100 mm Hg) Premature contractions with DCI values less than 450 mm Hg s cm satisfy criteria for failed peristalsis
Type II achalasia (with esophageal compression)	Elevated median IRP (>15 mm Hg), 100% failed peristalsis (DCI <100 mm Hg), panesophageal pressurization with ≥20% of swallows
Type III achalasia (spastic achalasia)	Elevated median IRP (>15 mm Hg), no normal peristalsis, premature (spastic) contractions with DCI >450 mm Hg s cm with ≥20% of swallows May be mixed with panesophageal pressurization
EGJ outflow obstruction	Elevated median IRP (>15 mm Hg), sufficient evidence of peristalsis such that criteria for types I–III achalasia are not met
Major Disorders of Peristalsis (Not Encountered in Normal Subjects)	
Absent contractility	• Normal median IRP, 100% failed peristalsis • Achalasia should be considered when IRP are borderline and when there is evidence of esophageal pressurization • Premature contractions with DCI values less than 450 mm Hg s cm meet criteria for failed peristalsis
Distal esophageal spasm	Normal median IRP, ≥20% premature contractions with DCI >450 mm Hg s cm. Some normal peristalsis may be present
Hypercontractile esophagus (jackhammer)	At least two swallows with DCI >8,000 mm Hg s cm. Hypercontractility may involve, or even be localized to, the LES
Minor Disorders of Peristalsis	
Ineffective esophageal motility (IEM)	≥50% ineffective swallows Ineffective swallows can be failed or weak (DCI <450 mm Hg s cm) Multiple repetitive swallow assessment may be helpful in determining peristaltic reserve
Fragmented peristalsis	≥50% fragmented contractions with DCI >450 mm Hg s cm
Normal Esophageal Motility	Not fulfilling any of the above classifications

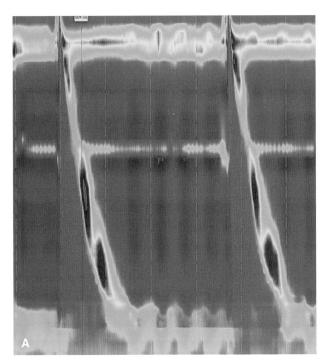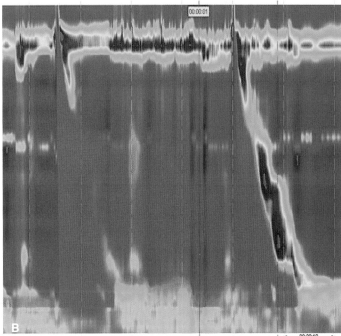

FIGURE 124.10 Impedance pictures. Normal bolus transit (**A**). Incomplete bolus transit (**B**).

11% of patients with late dysphagia after fundoplication (p <0.02). A DCI ratio >0.85 had a 67% sensitivity and 64% specificity in predicting late postoperative dysphagia.[48]

24-Hour Ambulatory Esophageal Manometry

The 24-hour ambulatory manometry was first reported in 1985 for evaluation of esophageal motility disorders in patients with noncardiac chest pain.[49] Compared with standard manometry, ambulatory esophageal manometry led to a change in the diagnosis in a substantial portion of patients with symptoms suggestive of a primary esophageal motor disorder.[50] In patients with non-obstructive dysphagia, normal peristaltic contractions were lacking during the meal periods. In patients with noncardiac chest pain, ambulatory motility monitoring showed the abnormal motor activity characterized by an increased frequency of simultaneous, double- and triple-peaked, high-amplitude, and long-duration contractions immediately preceding the pain episodes. In patients with GERD, ambulatory motility monitoring showed that the contractility of the esophageal body deteriorates with increasing severity of esophageal mucosal injury, compromising the clearance function of the esophageal body. In a recent study of 59 patients with noncardiac chest pain who underwent 24-hour impedance and ambulatory HREM, 37.3% had their symptoms explained by abnormalities on pH-impedance monitoring and 6.8% by ambulatory manometry.[51] HREM, using the Chicago Classification v3.0 criteria alone, did not identify any of the four patients with esophageal spasm on ambulatory manometry. However, taking into account other abnormalities, such as simultaneous (rapid) or repetitive contractions, HREM had a sensitivity of 75% and a specificity of 98.2% for the diagnosis of esophageal spasm. Therefore, in patients with noncardiac chest pain, ambulatory 24-hour manometry has a low additional diagnostic yield.

Impedance Testing

In contrast to standard manometry, esophageal manometry with impedance testing can assess both contraction and bolus clearance and direction, either antegrade or retrograde. Impedance measures changes in resistance of alternating electrical current passing through pairs of metal rings on a catheter. The HREM impedance catheters have 12 to 18 pairs of impedance-measuring rings and 32 to 36 pressure sensors. The impedance-detected swallows are considered complete if bolus entry occurs at the most proximal sensor and passes completely through the most distal one (Fig. 124.10A). Impedance is considered abnormal if more than 30% of liquid swallows show incomplete bolus transit (Fig. 124.10B) or more than 40% of viscous swallows show incomplete bolus transit. Impedance monitoring is abnormal in all patients with severe motor abnormalities such as achalasia and scleroderma, but abnormal in approximately half of patients with ineffective esophageal motility or diffuse esophageal spasm.[52] In a study of 576 consecutive patients who underwent manometry and impedance, 158 had normal manometry but abnormal impedance and were more likely to present with dysphagia.[53] Abnormal bolus transit for viscous, liquid, and both types of swallow was found in 60%, 19%, and 21%, respectively. Therefore, in patients with non-obstructive dysphagia and normal manometry, impedance testing will identify a subset of patients with impaired bolus transit. Esophageal manometry with impedance has been used to evaluate patients with chronic belching, suspected rumination syndrome, and suspected aerophagia.[54,55]

Impedance Planimetry/Endoflip Technology

Impedance planimetry is a technique that measures cross-sectional area of the esophagus in response to its distention and is used to evaluate esophageal distensibility and sensitivity. This technique has been used to study esophageal stiffness in eosinophilic esophagitis and to assess visceral hyperalgesia in patients with functional chest pain.[56,57] The functional luminal imaging probe (EndoFLIP; Crospon Ltd., Galway, Ireland) is used to provide real-time and dynamic information on EGJ distention that is visualized as cylinders of different diameters, based on cross-sectional area and pressure measurements (Fig. 124.11). Using this technique, Kwiatek et al. have shown that

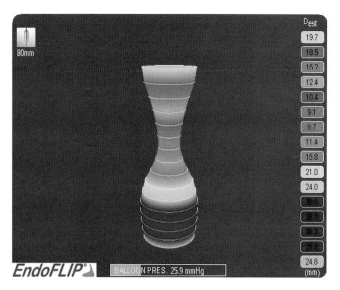

FIGURE 124.11 Endoflip® pictures.

the EGJ was two to three times more distensible in GERD patients than controls and normalized after fundoplication.[58] It can be also be used intra-operatively to assess adequacy of myotomy in achalasia patients[59] and as a smart bougie to assess tightness of wrap during fundoplication surgery.[60] It is used to guide further management in achalasia patients with suboptimal response to initial treatment.[61] Endoflip can also provide information regarding UES compliance without the need for fluoroscopy.[62] Thus far, impedance planimetry has demonstrated itself a useful research tool but its clinical utility is uncertain at this point.

SUMMARY

The anatomy and physiology of the esophagus are complex, and a better understanding is achieved when examined in the context of pathologic dysfunction. Esophageal dysmotility and GERD are some of the most common conditions and can often coexist in the same patient. This brief treatise is intended to provide the foundation to better understand an in-depth exploration of GERD and esophageal motility disorders such as achalasia in the coming sections.

REFERENCES

1. Cundall D, Tuttman C, Close M. A model of the anterior esophagus in snakes, with functional and developmental implications. *Anat Rec (Hoboken)* 2014;297(3):586–598.
2. Duranceau AC, Ferraro P. Physiology and physiologic studies of the esophagus. In: Shields TW, LoCicero J, Reed CE, et al. eds. *General Thoracic Surgery*. Philadelphia, PA: Lippincott Williams & Wilkins; 2009:1691–1706.
3. Jones CA, Hammer MJ, Hoffman MR, et al. Quantifying contributions of the cricopharyngeus to upper esophageal sphincter pressure changes by means of intramuscular electromyography and high-resolution manometry. *Ann Otol Rhinol Laryngol* 2014;123(3):174–182.
4. Welch RW, Luckmann K, Ricks PM, et al. Manometry of the normal upper esophageal sphincter and its alterations in laryngectomy. *J Clin Invest* 1979;63(5):1036–1041.
5. Winans CS. The pharyngoesophageal closure mechanism: a manometric study. *Gastroenterology* 1972;63(5):768–777.
6. Airdar O. Dados sebre a aque tetonica muscular da porcao inicial do es ofago humano. *Arquiv Cirurg Clin Exp* 1943(7):548.
7. Asoh R, Goyal RK. Manometry and electromyography of the upper esophageal sphincter in the opossum. *Gastroenterology* 1978;74(3):514–520.
8. Ahuja NK, Chan WW. Assessing upper esophageal sphincter function in clinical practice: a primer. *Curr Gastroenterol Rep* 2016;18(2):7.
9. Cunningham ET Jr, Sawchenko PE. Central neural control of esophageal motility: a review. *Dysphagia* 1990;5(1):35–51.
10. Babaei A, Dua K, Naini SR, et al. Response of the upper esophageal sphincter to esophageal distension is affected by posture, velocity, volume, and composition of the infusate. *Gastroenterology* 2012;142(4):734–743.e7.

11. Goyal RK, Chaudhury A. Physiology of normal esophageal motility. *J Clin Gastroenterol* 2008;42(5):610–619.
12. Christensen J, Lund GF. Esophageal responses to distension and electrical stimulation. *J Clin Invest* 1969;48(2):408–419.
13. Yamato S, Hirano I, Goyal RK. Effect of galanin and galanin antagonists on peristalsis in esophageal smooth muscle in the opossum. *Am J Physiol Gastrointest Liver Physiol* 2000;279(4):G719–G725.
14. Butin JW, Olsen AM, Moersch HJ, et al. A study of esophageal pressures in normal persons and patients with cardiospasm. *Gastroenterology* 1953;23(2):278–293.
15. Ingelfinger FJ, Kramer P, Sanchez GC. The gastroesophageal vestibule, its normal function and its role in cardiospasm and gastroesophageal reflux. *Am J Med Sci* 1954;228(4):417–425.
16. Mittal RK, Rochester DF, McCallum RW, Electrical and mechanical activity in the human lower esophageal sphincter during diaphragmatic contraction. *J Clin Invest* 1988;81(4):1182–1189.
17. Bernstein LM, Baker LA. A clinical test for esophagitis. *Gastroenterology* 1958;34(5):760–781.
18. Muthusamy VR, Lightdale JR, Acosta RD, et al. The role of endoscopy in the management of GERD. *Gastrointest Endosc* 2015;81(6):1305–1310.
19. Patti MG. An evidence-based approach to the treatment of gastroesophageal reflux disease. *JAMA Surg* 2016;151(1):73–78.
20. Campos GM, Peters JH, DeMeester TR, et al. Multivariate analysis of factors predicting outcome after laparoscopic Nissen fundoplication. *J Gastrointest Surg* 1999;3(3):292–300.
21. Johnson LF, Demeester TR. Twenty-four-hour pH monitoring of the distal esophagus. A quantitative measure of gastroesophageal reflux. *Am J Gastroenterol* 1974;62(4):325–332.
22. Lee JS. Is wireless capsule pH monitoring better than catheter systems? *J Neurogastroenterol Motil* 2012;18(2):117–119.
23. DeMeester TR, O'Sullivan GC, Bermudez G, et al. Esophageal function in patients with angina-type chest pain and normal coronary angiograms. *Ann Surg* 1982;196(4):488–498.
24. Stein HJ, DeMeester TR, Eypasch EP, et al. Ambulatory 24-hour esophageal manometry in the evaluation of esophageal motor disorders and noncardiac chest pain. *Surgery* 1991;110(4):753–761; discussion 761–763.
25. Sontag SJ, O'Connell S, Khandelwal S, et al. Most asthmatics have gastroesophageal reflux with or without bronchodilator therapy. *Gastroenterology* 1990;99(3):613–620.
26. Kaufman JA, Houghland JE, Quiroga E, et al. Long-term outcomes of laparoscopic antireflux surgery for gastroesophageal reflux disease (GERD)-related airway disorder. *Surg Endosc* 2006;20(12):1824–1830.
27. Patti MG, Vela MF, Odell DD, et al. The intersection of GERD, aspiration, and lung transplantation. *J Laparoendosc Adv Surg Tech A* 2016;26(7):501–505.
28. Murthy SC, Nowicki ER, Mason DP, et al. Pretransplant gastroesophageal reflux compromises early outcomes after lung transplantation. *J Thorac Cardiovasc Surg* 2011;142(1):47–52.e3.
29. Cantu E 3rd, Appel JZ 3rd, Hartwig MG, et al. J. Maxwell Chamberlain Memorial Paper. Early fundoplication prevents chronic allograft dysfunction in patients with gastroesophageal reflux disease. *Ann Thorac Surg* 2004;78(4):1142–1151; discussion 1142–1151.
30. Vela MF, Camacho-Lobato L, Srinivasan R, et al. Simultaneous intraesophageal impedance and pH measurement of acid and nonacid gastroesophageal reflux: effect of omeprazole. *Gastroenterology* 2001;120(7):1599–1606.
31. Castell DO, Mainie I, Tutuian R, Non-acid gastroesophageal reflux: documenting its relationship to symptoms using multichannel intraluminal impedance (MII). *Trans Am Clin Climatol Assoc* 2005;116:321–333; discussion 333–334.
32. Mainie I, Tutuian R, Agrawal A, et al. Combined multichannel intraluminal impedance-pH monitoring to select patients with persistent gastro-oesophageal reflux for laparoscopic Nissen fundoplication. *Br J Surg* 2006;93(12):1483–1487.
33. Stef JJ, Dodds WJ, Hogan WJ, et al. Intraluminal esophageal manometry: an analysis of variables affecting recording fidelity of peristaltic pressures. *Gastroenterology* 1974;67(2):221–230.
34. Arndorfer RC, Stef JJ, Dodds WJ, et al. Improved infusion system for intraluminal esophageal manometry. *Gastroenterology* 1977;73(1):23–27.
35. Dent J. A new technique for continuous sphincter pressure measurement. *Gastroenterology* 1976;71(2):263–267.
36. Clouse R, Parks T, Haroian L, et al. Development and clinical validation of a solid-state high-resolution pressure measurement system for simplified and consistent esophageal manometry. *Am J Gastroenterol* 2003;98:S32–S33.
37. Clouse RE, Staiano A. Topography of the esophageal peristaltic pressure wave. *Am J Physiol* 1991;261(4 Pt 1):G677–G684.
38. Meyer JP, Jones CA, Walczak CC, et al. Three-dimensional manometry of the upper esophageal sphincter in swallowing and nonswallowing tasks. *Laryngoscope* 2016;126(11):2539–2545.
39. Pandolfino JE, Ghosh SK, Rice J, et al. Classifying esophageal motility by pressure topography characteristics: a study of 400 patients and 75 controls. *Am J Gastroenterol* 2008;103(1):27–37.
40. Bredenoord AJ, Fox M, Kahrilas PJ, et al. Chicago Classification Criteria of esophageal motility disorders defined in high resolution esophageal pressure topography. *Neurogastroenterol Motil* 2012;24(suppl 1):57–65.
41. Kahrilas PJ, Bredenoord AJ, Fox M, et al. The Chicago Classification of esophageal motility disorders, v3.0. *Neurogastroenterol Motil* 2015;27(2):160–174.
42. Tolone S, De Bortoli N, Marabotto E, et al. Esophagogastric junction contractility for clinical assessment in patients with GERD: a real added value? *Neurogastroenterol Motil* 2015;27(10):1423–1431.

43. Bhatia SJ, Shah C. How to perform and interpret upper esophageal sphincter manometry. *J Neurogastroenterol Motil* 2013;19(1):99–103.
44. Roman S, Damon H, Pellissier PE, et al. Does body position modify the results of oesophageal high resolution manometry? *Neurogastroenterol Motil* 2010;22(3):271–275.
45. Sweis R, Anggiansah A, Wong T, et al. Normative values and inter-observer agreement for liquid and solid bolus swallows in upright and supine positions as assessed by esophageal high-resolution manometry. *Neurogastroenterol Motil* 2011;23(6):509. e198.
46. Zhang X, Xiang X, Tu L, et al. Esophageal motility in the supine and upright positions for liquid and solid swallows through high-resolution manometry. *J Neurogastroenterol Motil* 2013;19(4):467–472.
47. Sweis R, Anggiansah A, Wong T, et al. Assessment of esophageal dysfunction and symptoms during and after a standardized test meal: development and clinical validation of a new methodology utilizing high-resolution manometry. *Neurogastroenterol Motil* 2014;26(2):215–228.
48. Shaker A, Stoikes N, Drapekin J, et al. Multiple rapid swallow responses during esophageal high-resolution manometry reflect esophageal body peristaltic reserve. *Am J Gastroenterol* 2013;108(11):1706–1712.
49. Maas LC, Gordon RK, Penner D, et al. 24-hour ambulatory manometry in diagnosis of esophageal motor disorders causing chest pain. *South Med J* 1985;78(7):810–813.
50. Stein HJ, DeMeester TR. Indications, technique, and clinical use of ambulatory 24-hour esophageal motility monitoring in a surgical practice. *Ann Surg* 1993;217(2):128–137.
51. Barret M, Herregods TV, Oors JM, et al. Diagnostic yield of 24-hour esophageal manometry in non-cardiac chest pain. *Neurogastroenterol Motil* 2016;28(8):1186–1193.
52. Tutuian R, Castell DO. Combined multichannel intraluminal impedance and manometry clarifies esophageal function abnormalities: study in 350 patients. *Am J Gastroenterol* 2004;99(6):1011–1019.
53. Koya DL, Agrawal A, Freeman JE, et al. Impedance detected abnormal bolus transit in patients with normal esophageal manometry. Sensitive indicator of esophageal functional abnormality? *Dis Esophagus* 2008;21(6):563–569.
54. Bredenoord AJ, Weusten BL, Sifrim D, et al. Aerophagia, gastric, and supragastric belching: a study using intraluminal electrical impedance monitoring. *Gut* 2004;53(11):1561–1565.
55. Tutuian R, Castell DO. Rumination documented by using combined multichannel intraluminal impedance and manometry. *Clin Gastroenterol Hepatol* 2004;2(4):340–343.
56. Kwiatek MA, Hirano I, Kahrilas PJ, et al. Mechanical properties of the esophagus in eosinophilic esophagitis. *Gastroenterology* 2011;140(1):82–90.
57. Nasr I, Attaluri A, Hashmi S, et al. Investigation of esophageal sensation and biomechanical properties in functional chest pain. *Neurogastroenterol Motil* 2010;22(5):520–526. e116.
58. Kwiatek MA, Pandolfino JE, Hirano I, et al. Esophagogastric junction distensibility assessed with an endoscopic functional luminal imaging probe (EndoFLIP). *Gastrointest Endosc* 2010;72(2):272–278.
59. Mccoy E, Snape W, Lin MS, et al. EndoFLIP* in comparison to high-resolution manometry and Eckardt score in the assessment of achalasia prior to intervention. *Am J Gastroenterol* 2015;110:S701–S702.
60. Ilczyszyn A, Botha AJ. Feasibility of esophagogastric junction distensibility measurement during Nissen fundoplication. *Dis Esophagus* 2014;27(7):637–644.
61. Ngamruengphong S, von Rahden BH, Filser J, et al. Intraoperative measurement of esophagogastric junction cross-sectional area by impedance planimetry correlates with clinical outcomes of peroral endoscopic myotomy for achalasia: a multicenter study. *Surg Endosc* 2016;30(7):2886–2894.
62. Regan J, Walshe M, Rommel N, et al. New measures of upper esophageal sphincter distensibility and opening patterns during swallowing in healthy subjects using EndoFLIP(R). *Neurogastroenterol Motil* 2013;25(1):e25–e34.

DIAGNOSTIC STUDIES OF THE ESOPHAGUS

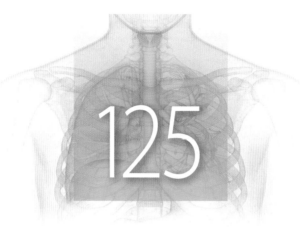

125

Radiologic Evaluation of the Esophagus

Beatrice Aramini ▪ Frank D'Ovidio

In the new millennium, imaging remains an important aspect in evaluating patients with esophageal diseases. Although the barium esophagogram has fallen into disuse in many institutions, supplanted by endoscopy and manometry, it remains an essential tool in evaluating patients with esophageal symptoms, especially dysphagia.[1] The videofluoroscopic examination is the principal technique for demonstrating a wide range of functional and structural lesions of the pharynx and esophagus. This method is a simple, cost-effective technique for demonstrating esophageal lesions that typically manifest with dysphagia or odynophagia and combines with digital radiography while the patient is drinking a suspension of barium sulfate.

Because of the ubiquitous use of endoscopy, the barium esophagogram has been relegated to the museum in many institutions. As a result, many recent radiology trainees have not been adequately instructed in the proper performance and interpretation of this examination in patients with esophageal disease. Furthermore, in the past 25 years some gastrointestinal (GI) radiologists have stressed the mucosal aspect of the examination in an attempt to compete with endoscopy. This has led to an emphasis on aspects of the examination that are of less importance to the gastroenterologist and esophageal surgeon and a de-emphasis on those aspects of the examination that are helpful.[1]

In addition to the conventional barium esophagography, several other imaging techniques are currently available for evaluation of the esophagus. The selection of an appropriate examination requires a tailored approach based on clinical information about the character and duration of symptoms; their relationships to coexistent systemic diseases; or any previous surgical, diagnostic, or therapeutic procedures

involving the esophagus. This chapter provides an overview of the radiologic modalities used for the demonstration and differential diagnosis of various functional or organic disorders affecting the esophagus.

RADIOGRAPHIC METHODS OF EXAMINATION

PLAIN CHEST RADIOGRAPHY

Normally, the esophagus is not seen roentgenologically unless outlined by residual air or retained food from a pathologic process. This is partly because the esophagus collapses during its resting phase, whereas the upper and lower esophageal sphincters (LESs) maintain their tonic contraction to prevent aspiration of air and retrograde flow of gastric contents into the esophagus.

The esophagus is best examined in the prone right anterior oblique (RAO) or left posterior oblique (LPO) positions. Additional views in the upright and supine postures in the oblique, anteroposterior (AP), and posteroanterior (PA) positions are very valuable. Films in full inspiration are most commonly used. Moreover, films exposed during the Müller (after a forced expiration, an attempt at inspiration is made with closed mouth and nose or closed glottis, whereby the negative pressure in the chest and lungs is made very subatmospheric) and Valsalva maneuvers may have their applicability; in particular, Müller for varices and Valsalva for herniae. Special postures, such as Trendelenburg or in the bending-over position may be required to demonstrate hiatal hernia or regurgitation. Nevertheless, the standard PA and lateral chest radiographs may provide significant clues to the diagnosis of an underlying pathology when the esophageal lumen contains an abnormal collection of air, fluid, or food particles or harbors an ingested radiopaque object.

On chest radiography, diffuse mediastinal widening in the absence of a normal gas collection in the gastric fundus might be a manifestation of a dilated esophagus, usually containing a foamy mixture of air, food, or secretions. These features are highly suggestive of achalasia but may also be seen with a peptic stricture or infiltrating tumor of the gastroesophageal junction (GEJ). Carcinoma of the esophagus may also be visible on chest films as a soft tissue mass thickening the esophagopleural stripe, indenting the trachea, or causing mediastinal adenopathy and pulmonary metastasis. Furthermore, plain radiographs of the chest and neck play an important role in the diagnosis of ingested foreign bodies and suspected esophageal perforation.[2,3]

SINGLE-CONTRAST ESOPHAGRAM WITH BARIUM

The barium examination of the esophagus requires a tailored and flexible approach by the radiologist.[4–6] The pharynx and esophagus are made visible on x-ray film by a liquid suspension called barium sulfate (barium) that is considered as the standard contrast material for opacification of the esophageal lumen (Figs. 125.1 to 125.4). Barium is

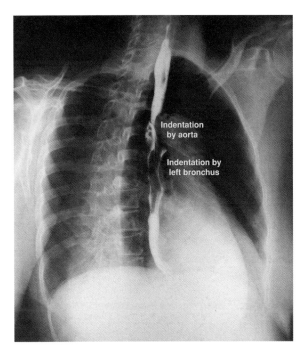

FIGURE 125.1 X-ray barium view of normal esophagus.

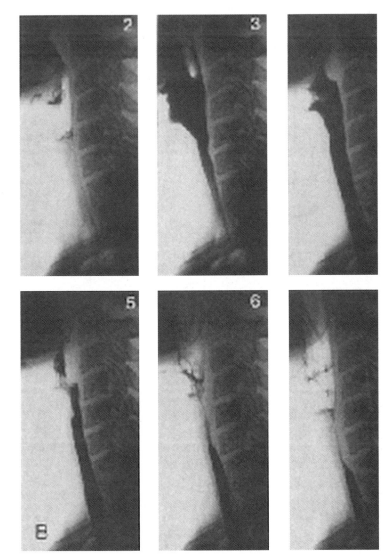

FIGURE 125.2 X-ray hypopharynx and cervical esophagus during swallowing.

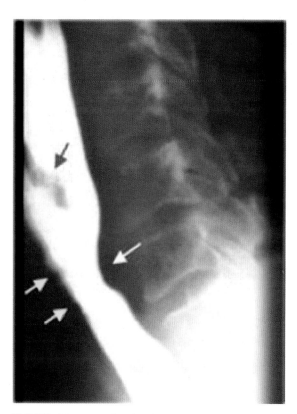 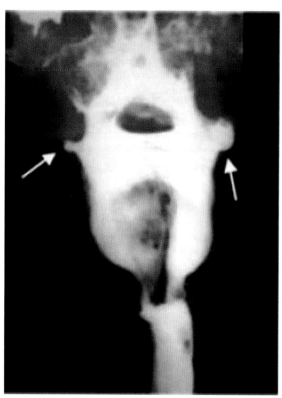

FIGURE 125.3 Particular of the hypopharynx. **Left:** Lateral view: Epiglottis (*red arrow*). Post cricoid impression (*yellow arrows*). Crico-pharyngeus impression (*white arrow*). **Right:** AP-view: Small lateral pharyngeal pouches (*arrows*).

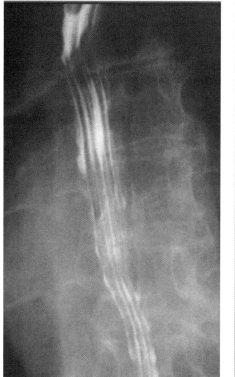 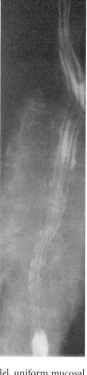

FIGURE 125.4 Esophageal mucosa: normal thin, parallel, uniform mucosal folds.

a dry, white, chalky, inert metallic powder that is mixed with water to make a thick, milkshake-like drink. Barium is an x-ray absorber and appears white on x-ray film. It is composed by a colloidal suspension of micropulverized barium sulfate in water. Commercial products of various densities and viscosities are available. They usually contain flavoring agents as well as chemical additives such as aluminum hydroxide, sorbitol, and methylcellulose to create a clearer picture. When swallowed, a barium drink coats the inside walls of the pharynx and esophagus so that the swallowing motion, inside wall lining, and size and shape of these organs is visible on x-ray (Fig. 125.1).

A barium swallow may be performed separately or as part of an upper gastrointestinal (UGI) series, which evaluates the esophagus, stomach, and duodenum (first part of the small intestine).

There are three phases in the examination: (1) examination of the esophagus while fully dilated; (2) examination of the mucosa of the esophagus; and (3) examination of the normal dynamics, especially during extremes of respiratory action.[7–10]

Radiologic examination of the esophagus is performed under fluoroscopic observation. In conventional single-contrast esophagography, the patient is first examined in the upright and then in the recumbent position while taking sequential swallows of a relatively dilute mixture of barium sulfate in water (40% to 80% weight per volume).

Images of the well-distended esophagus are obtained, including views of the gastroesophageal segment during suspended respiration, which accentuates any existing hiatal hernia or Schatzki ring. In infants, a nursing bottle is used for oral administration of nonionic, isotonic iodinated contrast material, but controlled instillation through a soft feeding tube is recommended if esophageal atresia or tracheoesophageal fistula (TEF) is suspected.

The uniform tubular shape of the opacified esophageal lumen and the repetitive nature of its peristaltic activity permit an accurate fluoroscopic analysis of both motility and structural changes. In addition, a permanent digital record of the observed normal or pathologic findings is routinely obtained. Continuous dynamic recording is the preferred technique for the evaluation of pharyngeal and esophageal motility. The fluoroscopic study of esophageal peristalsis and motility disorders is conducted with the patient in the prone-oblique position. The horizontal placement eliminates the interference of gravity with the passage of contrast material and permits better visibility of the esophagus by projecting it away from the thoracic spine. The patient is instructed to swallow one mouthful of barium at a time. The initiated primary peristaltic wave appears as a lumen-obliterating contraction that propagates distally at 2 to 4 cm per second. In normal adults, the bolus transit through the 20- to 24-cm long esophagus, and is completed in 6 to 8 seconds. Patients with esophageal dysmotility, however, usually show considerable retention and delayed clearing of barium. The associated fluoroscopic findings are decreased incidence and amplitude of peristaltic waves after deglutition, failure of the initiated contraction to progress distally, and repetitive nonpropulsive waves, commonly referred to as tertiary contractions.

The use of barium with x-rays contributes to the visibility and the study of various characteristics of the pharynx and esophagus, in particular *the phrenic ampulla*, which is the lower end of the esophagus; *the vestibule,* which is the distal end of the esophagus; and the *esophagogastric junction (EGJ).*

Phrenic Ampulla

The phrenic ampulla represents a physiologic dilatation of the lower end of the thoracic esophagus seen when the esophagus is fully opacified. It is best observed in full-sustained inspiration in RAO position, following ingestion of several mouthfuls of thick barium paste (Fig. 125.5).[7]

The phrenic ampulla is a pear-shaped structure with narrowed portion (apex) uppermost and the upper limit quite variable

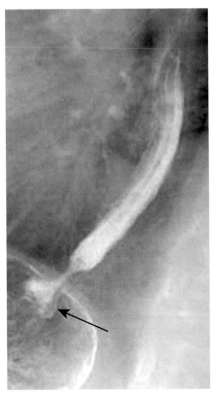

(Fig. 125.5). The base may resemble the base of a triangle. This probably occurs in a slightly redundant esophagus and represents the base of the phrenic ampulla resting flatly against the diaphragm at the site of the esophageal hiatus. The level of the base of the phrenic ampulla in the prone RAO position may vary from 0 to 2 cm above the dome of the diaphragm, and closely corresponds to the site of the esophageal hiatus on deep inspiration.

The size of the phrenic ampulla varies with the thickness and amount of ingested barium and with the tone of the esophagus. It is usually larger and more globular in older patients and after a standard meal. Peristaltic waves may change the size of the phrenic ampulla due to compression of the bolus against a contracted vestibule or by retrograde flow. As the vestibule opens, the phrenic ampulla empties rapidly, usually leaving no residue in thoracic esophagus (Fig. 125.6).

Thick barium may require a number of secondary peristaltic contractions as the phrenic ampulla becomes progressively smaller. The phrenic ampulla is always located above the level of the esophageal hiatus, and is actually a dilated esophageal segment due to accumulated barium held up above the level of the contracted vestibule.[7]

Vestibule

The normally contracted distal end of the esophagus is the vestibule. It occasionally becomes the abdominal segment of the esophagus, although its location is normally within esophageal hiatus. Its position varies with respiration, being chiefly abdominal in full inspiration. It lies within upper and lower attachments of the phrenoesophageal membrane. In an esophagus essentially empty except for a thin coating of barium, there is hardly any change in the mucosal pattern of the vestibular segment, although at times there is some coarsening of its folds and some slight narrowing in its entire length as compared with the thoracic esophagus (especially on full inspiration).[2,6]

In a full esophagus and while the patient is drinking liquid barium, the vestibule is open and cannot be distinguished from the reminder of the esophagus. However, the level of the esophageal hiatus can occasionally be seen as a fixed area of narrowing due to the mechanical limitation of its size. If patient stops drinking and is requested to breathe deeply, the vestibule contracts and the phrenic ampulla forms above the area of the contracted vestibule.[3]

As the phrenic ampulla empties, the vestibule fills and occasionally at this point two physiologic dilatations may be detected for a brief interval, corresponding to the emptying phrenic ampulla and the filling vestibular segment. Some stasis of barium also may occur in the vestibule for a short time, resulting in a small dilated pouch seen either in inspiration or expiration. The stasis occurs directly above the level of the EGJ, and thus can be differentiated from retained barium in the phrenic ampulla or in a small hiatal hernia.[6]

The Esophagogastric Junction

The EGJ is at the level of Lerche's constrictor cardia and near the lower attachment of the phrenoesophageal membrane.[11] It can be easily identified in the prone RAO position if the stomach is not excessively filled with the barium and air. In the RAO position the fundus of the stomach is usually filled with air, which acts as a double contrast medium for maximum visualization of the vestibular segment. The dilatation and contraction of the lower vestibular segment at the EGJ may be seen occasionally as a ring of varying size.[11,12] Herniation of the gastric mucosa into the lower esophagus and invagination of the esophagus have been described as prograde prolapse.[13]

Ott[14] and Aksglaede and colleagues[7] have reported that in contrast to the dilated atonic esophageal body in achalasia, both the entity of nutcracker esophagus and diffuse esophageal spasm are

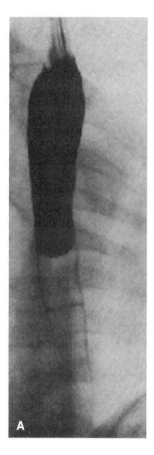
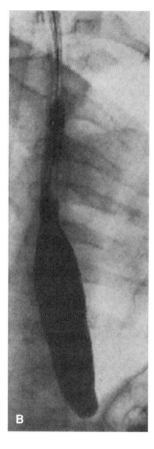
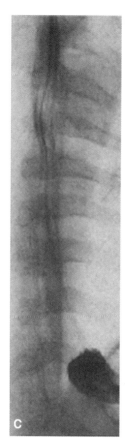

FIGURE 125.6 Normal esophagogram in right anterior oblique position, taken at three different intervals after swallowing. Immediately after deglutition the filled esophagus appears as a continuous radiopaque column (**A**); shows the peristaltic wave trailing the barium column and obliterating the esophageal lumen (**B**). In (**C**) only a small amount of barium coating the mucosal folds is left.

characterized by recurrent high-amplitude contractions that cause dysphagia and cramping retrosternal pain. In this context it should also be noted, as pointed out by Ott[15] and Richter[16] and their colleagues, that functional and organic abnormalities of the esophagus are common sources of noncardiac chest pain, and barium esophagography can provide the correct diagnosis.

ESOPHAGRAM WITH WATER-SOLUBLE IODINATED CONTRAST MEDIA

Iodinated water-soluble preparations—such as Gastrografin (Bracco Diagnostics, Princeton, NJ) or Hypaque (Amersham Health, Princeton, NJ)—have been used in instances of suspected esophageal perforation and anastomotic leakage. These aqueous contrast media are readily absorbed after extravasation into the mediastinal soft tissues and pleural or peritoneal spaces, but they rarely define the anatomy of the defect clearly. As documented by Foley[17] and Buecker[12] and their colleagues, the mucosal tears and transmural perforations of the esophagus are better diagnosed with barium than with iodinated contrast media. These researchers have pointed out that 25% to 50% of esophageal perforations are unrecognizable or inadequately shown during initial evaluation with water-soluble agents because their low density and rapid diffusion into the surrounding tissues impairs an optimal mucosal coating and visualization of extraluminal leakage. Furthermore, the aspiration of such iodinated hypertonic solutions into the lungs can lead to pulmonary edema and chemical pneumonitis, particularly among patients with esophageal dysmotility or obstruction. Brick and colleagues[6] as well as Ghahremani[18] has pointed out that nonionic low-osmolality contrast media—such as Omnipaque (Amersham Health, Princeton, NJ) or Isovue (Bracco Diagnostics, Princeton, NJ)—may be used safely. Much more recently,

the use of CT oral contrast esophagography followed by an esophagographic chest CT has made the argument for their utilization moot.

DOUBLE-CONTRAST ESOPHAGOGRAPHY

Double-contrast esophagography permits an accurate demonstration of mucosal abnormalities that are usually the hallmark of inflammatory or neoplastic processes. The patient first ingests an effervescent agent and then rapidly gulps the high-density barium in the upright, LPO position in order to obtain double-contrast views of the esophagus. For this purpose, carbon dioxide released by ingested effervescent agents, such as citrocarbonate granules, is used together with swallowed air. This serves as a radiolucent intraluminal gas collection to expand the lumen and provide a detailed view of the esophageal inner surface. Any areas of narrowing or rigidity are also better recognized when the otherwise pliable esophageal wall is maximally stretched.

Double-contrast radiography of the normal esophagus typically shows a smooth, featureless mucosa and the well-demarcated walls of this tubular structure (Fig. 125.7). The longitudinal folds of the esophagus become visible when the esophagus is collapsed or when there is mild esophagitis of the distended esophagus. Transverse striations of the esophagus, the so-called feline esophagus, are seen in patients with reflux disease; this is caused by contraction of the longitudinally oriented muscularis mucosae. Some patients develop dilated submucosal glands, and when these fill with barium, they appear as multiple small outpouchings on esophagrams, simulating ulcerations.

The patient is then placed in a recumbent, right-side down position for double-contrast views of the gastric cardia and fundus. The cardia can often be recognized by the presence of three or four stellate folds that radiate to a central point at the GEJ, also known as the cardiac rosette.[19]

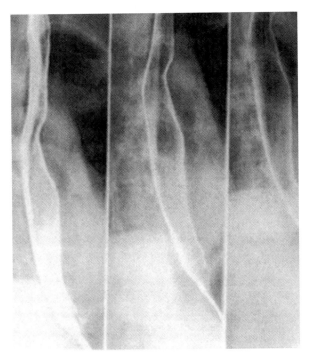

FIGURE 125.7 Normal double-contrast esophagram.

After the double-contrast phase of the examination is completed, the patient is placed in the prone, RAO position and asked to take discrete swallows of a low-density barium suspension in order to evaluate esophageal motility. Esophageal dysmotility is considered to be present when abnormal peristalsis is detected on two or more of five separate swallows.[20] The patient then rapidly gulps the low-density barium suspension to optimally distend the esophagus in order to rule out rings or strictures that could be missed on the double-contrast phase of the examination. Finally, the patient is turned from a supine to a right lateral position to assess for spontaneous gastroesophageal reflux or for reflux induced by a Valsalva maneuver.

The purpose of barium studies in patients with reflux symptoms is not simply to document the presence of hiatal hernia or gastroesophageal reflux, but rather to detect morphologic sequelae of reflux, including reflux esophagitis, peptic strictures, Barrett esophagus, and esophageal adenocarcinoma.

SOLID-BOLUS TEST

Subtle areas of narrowing and symptomatic lower esophageal rings can be evaluated by the use of commercially available barium tablets 12.5 mm in diameter or marshmallows of predetermined size. Ott et al.[21] and Ghahremani et al.[22] have reported that this permits more accurate measurement of the narrowed lumen and its functional significance.

VIDEOFLUOROGRAPHIC SWALLOW STUDY

In the past 20 years, radiography and manometry have been combined to study bolus displacement in the esophagus related to LES and peristaltic dysfunction in patients with gastroesophageal reflux disease (GERD).[23–27] Other imaging techniques such as scintigraphy have been used to visualize and quantify bolus transport in esophageal disorders.[28,29] The distribution and movement of both liquid and air components of a swallowed bolus have been studied in healthy subjects using computerized tomography.[30] Moreover, the passage of

gas from the stomach to the esophagus can now be detected by intraluminal impedance to take into account gas and liquid reflux during transient LES relaxation.[31,32]

The videofluoroscopic swallow study is the most commonly utilized instrumental assessment tool to determine the nature and extent of an oropharyngeal swallowing disorder. The studies are captured using fluoroscopy in video or digitized format that allows detailed analysis of the oropharyngeal swallowing process. The videofluoroscopic swallow study does not diagnose the etiology of the swallowing disorder; instead, it determines the details of oropharyngeal swallow dysfunction and helps guide decisions regarding behavioral swallow therapy based on those findings.

A video imaging chair is primarily used. However, sometimes the study is performed with the patient in the standing position for a faster study, when it is safe and acceptable to the patient. The upright positioning may be precluded because of medical conditions such as low blood pressure, acute stroke, spinal cord injury bracing, or other skeletal limitations. Under such circumstances, the patient can also be placed in the side-lying position or in the patient's representative eating position.

Whenever possible, the patient is seated as upright as possible. All studies are started with the patient in the lateral view where aspiration is most efficiently detected, and then finished with an anterior–posterior view to assess swallow symmetry and vocal cord function. Observation of vocal cord movement on pronouncement of the vowel /ah/ by the patient is often used as the end point of the study.

With fluoroscopy, anatomic structures and landmarks are identified with mechanism at rest without contrast.

A standard protocol is utilized for administration of radiopaque material (usually barium) mixed with liquid and food of varying consistencies in smaller to larger amounts and thinner to thicker viscosities as tolerated. The typical protocol utilizes thin liquid, thick liquid (nectar), puree, and solid (graham cracker cookie) coated with puree as our standard administration, but this is altered pending any unique circumstance or request from patient or staff. Examination of the esophagus is at the discretion of the radiologist.

RADIOGRAPHIC FINDINGS IN ESOPHAGEAL MOTILITY DISORDERS

Achalasia

Achalasia cardia is one of the common causes of motor dysphagia, involving the lower two-thirds (smooth muscle segment) of the esophagus. Though the disease was first described more than 300 years ago, exact pathogenesis of this condition still remains enigmatic. It seems to be caused by degeneration of intramural myenteric plexus neurons. This results in impaired LES relaxation and loss of peristaltic sequencing of the esophageal contractions, producing symptoms of dysphagia, chest pain, and regurgitation.[33,34]

By definition, an assessment of esophageal motor function is essential in the diagnosis of achalasia. Barium esophagram and esophagogastroduodenoscopy (EGD) (Fig. 125.8) are complementary tests to manometry in the diagnosis and management of achalasia.

However, neither EGD nor barium esophagram alone is sensitive enough to make the diagnosis of achalasia with certainty. EGD may be supportive of a diagnosis of achalasia in only one-third of patients, whereas esophagram may be nondiagnostic in up to one-third of patients.[35] Thus, "normal" findings on EGD or esophagram in patients suspected of having achalasia should prompt esophageal motility testing. However, in patients with classic endoscopic and/or esophagram findings, esophageal motility would be considered supportive to confirm the diagnosis.

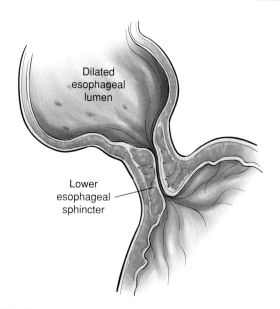

FIGURE 125.8 Gross appearance of esophagus in classical achalasia.

The classic features are esophageal dilatation, aperistalsis, impaired esophageal emptying in the upright position, and symmetric tapering at the GEJ (bird's beak appearance). Aperistalsis results in failure to clear barium bolus from the esophagus in the supine position, and subsequent barium boluses.[36] In the upright position, retained food and saliva cause a heterogeneous air–fluid level at the top of the barium column. This upright position also can be used to assess barium emptying.[37] Healthy subjects should empty a barium bolus challenge of 150 to 250 mL within 1 to 2 minutes. Most patients with achalasia have residual barium in the esophagus at the end of 5 minutes. In early disease, the esophagus may be minimally dilated and, with the distal tapering at the GEJ, may be confused for a peptic stricture (Fig. 125.9A). However, a careful fluoroscopic evaluation of esophageal peristalsis always finds evidence of simultaneous contractions and failure of the primary esophageal wave to clear the esophagus of barium.[36,38] As the disease progresses, the esophagus become more dilated generally in the range of 3 to 8 cm, sometimes with a sigmoid-like left angle deviation of the distal esophagus (Fig. 125.9B). In chronic endstage cases, the esophagus, called "idiopathic megaesophagus," becomes massively dilated (>9 cm), and may resemble a sigmoid colon with stool (the inhomogeneous barium from the residual food) (Fig. 125.9C). In classic achalasia, the distal esophagus has a smooth tapering resembling a bird's beak (Fig. 125.9B). Conventional diagnostic criteria for achalasia are impaired EGJ relaxation, absence of

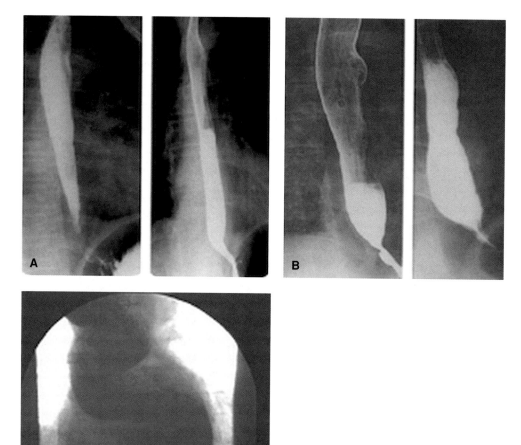

FIGURE 125.9 Radiographic view of achalasia subtypes. GI **A:** Initial esophagram of patient with early achalasia and no esophageal dilation. **B:** Patient after 2 years of nonoperative treatment. Note significant esophageal dilation and air–fluid level compared to pretreatment. **C:** End-stage achalasia with sigmoid or megaesophagus. (From Motility online (May 2006) | doi:10.1038/gimo53).

normally propagated peristaltic contractions, and absence of a structural explanation (e.g., tumor, stricture) for these abnormalities.[35,39]

However, the radiographic achalasia classification have been compared to the manometric test which is essential in making the diagnosis with the vast majority of patients exhibiting the classic findings of incomplete LES relaxation and aperistalsis of the esophageal body. Nowhere has the evolution of high-resolution manometry had more impact than in the diagnosis of achalasia. In 2008, Pandolfino et al.[40] recognized three distinct manometric patterns of esophageal body contractility in achalasia: (1) no significant pressurization; (2) rapidly propagated compartmentalized pressurization, either localized to the distal esophagus or present across the entire length of the esophagus; and (3) rapidly propagated pressurization attributable to spastic contractions. Although all three subtypes had impaired EGJ relaxation and aperistalsis, they each represent a distinct pathophysiologic scenario and possibly an explanation for some of the observed variability in treatment response.

The manometric finding of aperistalsis and incomplete LES relaxation without evidence of a mechanical obstruction solidifies the diagnosis of achalasia in the appropriate setting.[39]

Diffuse Esophageal Spasm

Diffuse spasm is a neuromuscular motor disorder of the esophagus characterized by substernal distress or dysphagia or both (Fig. 125.10).[41,42]

It is thought to be characterized on barium studies by intermittently absent or weakened primary esophageal peristalsis with simultaneous, lumen-obliterating, nonperistaltic contractions that compartmentalize the esophagus, producing a classic corkscrew appearance.[43–46]

The swallow-induced contractions may be normotensive, hypotensive, or hypertensive. LES relaxation is usually normal, although minor degrees of LES relaxation dysfunction may be present. With an appropriate technique, aimed at discovering motility disorders (examination of the patient in a recumbent position using a sufficient amount of contrast material, and cinematographic or video recording of several swallows), abnormalities will usually be found in patients with diffuse spasm. In some patients, an otherwise normal examination may yield markedly abnormal results if it is carried out during an attack of pain.[47]

Hypertensive Peristalsis, Isolated LES Hypertension, and Hypercontracting LES

The classic description of diffuse esophageal spasm on barium studies includes the presence of repetitive, simultaneous, lumen-obliterating nonperistaltic contractions that compartmentalize the esophagus, producing a distinctive corkscrew appearance.[43–45]

The radiographic reports provided a relatively detailed assessment of esophageal motility in patients. Primary peristalsis is intermittently absent or weakened. Weakened peristalsis is defined radiographically as delayed propagation or variable disruption of the peristaltic stripping wave as it traversed the esophagus, often associated with incomplete clearance of barium from the esophagus when the peristaltic wave reached the GEJ. In contrast, absent peristalsis is defined radiographically as a complete absence of a peristaltic stripping wave in the esophagus. In general, peristalsis is considered abnormal if an abnormal peristaltic wave or esophageal aperistalsis is observed on fluoroscopy on two or more of five separate swallows of low-density barium in the prone RAO position, as described previously by Ott et al.[20] The strength of any nonperistaltic contractions has been

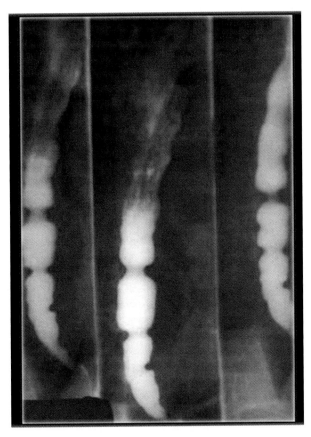

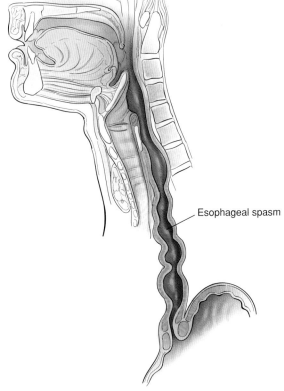

Esophageal spasm

FIGURE 125.10 Diffuse esophageal spasm.

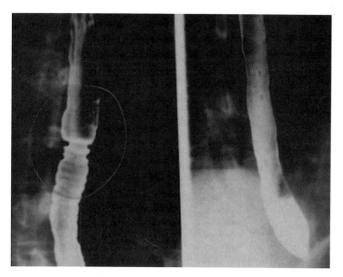

FIGURE 125.11 Hypercontracting LES.

classified either as mild, moderate, or severe (i.e., lumen-obliterating or nearly lumen-obliterating).

However, hypertensive peristalsis (also termed "nutcracker esophagus"), isolated LES hypertension, and hypercontracting LES diagnosis (Fig. 125.11) are characterized by the combination of radiologic and manometric findings. Other techniques (endoscopy, intraluminal pH measurements, etc.) are used to detect other conditions such as organic obstruction or reflux. It should be emphasized that both hypertensive peristalsis and isolated LES hypertension are manometric abnormalities and not clinical entities with predictable functional sequelae. Indeed, these manometric abnormalities may be transient phenomena related to stress (including the stress associated with esophageal intubation). Isolated hypertensive LES and hypercontracting LES may have similar pathophysiology as the hypertensive peristalsis.[46]

Scleroderma of the Esophagus

Scleroderma esophagus is part of a connective tissue disorder, which leads to atrophy of esophageal smooth muscle with consequent loss of LES tone and esophageal peristalsis (Fig. 125.12). It is one of the most important secondary motor disorders to affect the esophagus.[47]

Barium studies may demonstrate a normal stripping wave that clears the upper esophagus, but stops at the level of the aortic arch. This can be attributed to the striated muscle that composes the upper third of the esophagus. In the lower two-thirds, muscular contractions are weak and uncoordinated and eventually progress to aperistalsis. When in the recumbent position, barium remains static in the dilated, atonic esophagus. In contrast to achalasia, when the patient is seated upright the barium readily flows through the widely patent and dysfunctional LES. Related findings may include the presence of a hiatal hernia, reflux esophagitis, and peptic strictures.

Esophageal Varices

Esophageal varices may be classified as "uphill" or "downhill" (Fig. 125.13). Uphill are caused by portal hypertension with increased pressure with portal venous system transmitted upward via dilated esophageal collaterals to the superior vena cava. In contrast, downhill varices are caused by superior vena cava obstruction with downward flow via dilated esophageal collaterals to the portal venous system and inferior vena cava.[48]

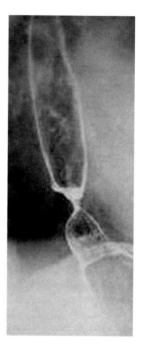

FIGURE 125.12 Esophageal scleroderma with also a 3 cm long hiatal hernia. (Courtesy of Dr F.I. Habib.)

Using a thin-barium technique, radiographic appearances of esophageal varices were described first by Wolf[49] in his 1928 paper, "Die Erkennug von osophagus varizen im rontgenbilde," or "Radiographic detection of esophageal varices." In 1931, Schatzki established the basis for the modern-day fluoroscopic detection of esophageal varices by refining positional and physiologic maneuvers to optimize visualization.

Barium swallow examination is not a sensitive test, and it must be performed carefully with close attention to the amount of barium used and the degree of esophageal distention. These images may help in detecting only 50% of esophageal varices. In 1993, Ginai AZ et al.[50] defined three parameters used for evaluation of varices at barium swallow:

1. *the Length.* The length of the varices was measured on the radiographs in centimeters. The highest level to which the varices in the esophagus could be visualized was taken as the proximal limit and the level just above the EGJ as the distal limit;
2. *the Width.* The maximum width of the mucosal folds representing varices was measured in millimeters on the radiographs;
3. *the Tortuosity.* Some degree of subjectivity is impossible to exclude when examining this parameter. The tortuosity of the folds was defined as: no tortuosity (−), slight (+), moderate (+ +) and severe (+ + +).

However, today more sophisticated imaging with computed tomography (CT) scanning, magnetic resonance imaging (MRI), magnetic resonance angiography (MRA), and endoscopic ultrasonography (EUS) plays an important role in the evaluation of portal hypertension and esophageal varices.[51–55]

Pouches and Diverticula

An esophageal diverticulum is a pouch that protrudes outward in a weak portion of the esophageal lining. This pocket-like structure can appear anywhere in the esophageal lining between the throat and stomach.[56]

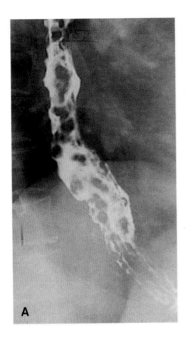 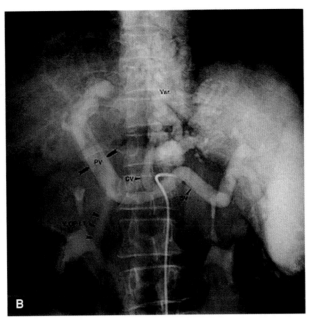

FIGURE 125.13 Image (**A**) depicts multiple varices on esophagram. Image (**B**) is an angiographic demonstration of cavernous transformation of the portal vein (PV) with reversal of blood flow through the coronary veins (CV) and splenic vein (SV) producing esophageal varices (Var).

Esophageal diverticula (pleural of diverticulum) are classified by their location within the esophagus[57]:

- Zenker diverticula (pharyngoesophageal) is the most common type of diverticula of the esophagus. Zenker diverticula are usually located in the back of the throat, just above the esophagus (Fig. 125.14A,B);
- Midthoracic diverticula, in the mid-chest (Fig. 125.15);
- Epiphrenic diverticula, above the diaphragm (Fig. 125.16).

Diagnostic modalities for pharyngeal and esophageal diverticula include barium swallow, upper endoscopy, esophageal manometry, and CT scan, or any combination of the above. CT scan can be especially helpful in the evaluation of traction diverticulum by providing definitions of the adjacent anatomic structures in the mediastinum. The differential diagnosis for oropharyngeal dysphagia includes iatrogenic causes such as tracheostomy, neck surgery, laryngectomy, and malignancy.

The barium swallow is a very helpful examination in the diagnosis of each of the diverticular conditions. A Zenker diverticulum is a pharyngeal outpouching readily seen in the cervical region (Fig. 125.14A,B). A midthoracic or traction diverticulum is typically a small, wide-mouth pouch located near the tracheal bifurcation (Fig. 125.15). An epiphrenic diverticulum, on the other hand, appears as a large globular pouch, often associated with abnormal esophageal contractions, as demonstrated in Figure 125.16.

Hiatal Hernia

Hiatal hernia is defined as the protrusion of all parts of the stomach (rarely other viscera) into the thoracic cage through the esophageal hiatus (Fig. 125.17).[30]

According to Johnson,[31] a hiatal hernia is shown best by combining respiratory movements with firm manual compression of the upper abdomen while maximal force is exerted at the end of expiration. Hafter[58] recommends the prone RAO position in full expiration, with abdominal compression by a ballow or pillow. Wolf[59] also recommends the prone RAO position. The Trendelenburg position with films exposed in full inspiration/expiration, or Valsalva may also be used. Abdominal compression may be added. The prone Trendelenburg position may also be attempted

with the patient in the RAO position, and the table tilted cephalad 45 degrees.

There are two main types of hiatal hernia: the sliding (type I) and the paraesophageal (type II).[60]

Poppel et al.[61] described three subtypes of sliding hiatus hernia: (1) concentric short esophagus, in which the EGJ is at the apex of the herniated pocket and the herniation is symmetrical; (2) eccentric short esophagus, in which there is upward displacement of the EGJ with the herniated stomach off to one side; (3) redundant esophagus, in which the esophagus is long and lying to one side of the herniated stomach.[60] Today, we recognize two additional types such as the combined sliding and paraesophageal, also called type III, and the fixed also called type IV.[62]

As the upward migration of the vestibular segment progresses to the stage of gastric herniation, the notches corresponding to the upper attachment fade and become more and more part of the phrenic ampulla. The lower point of attachment of the phrenoesophageal membrane now becomes more prominent. The size of the vestibular segment diminishes. However, in the dilated stage, three pockets may now be identified representing phrenic ampulla, vestibule, and actual hernia.

The following additional roentgenologic findings may be present (Figs. 125.18 and 125.19): (1) flattening of the base of the hernial pocket, above the esophageal hiatus, if the esophageal hiatus is not too wide; (2) stasis of barium in the herniated segment above the esophageal hiatus; (3) absent peristaltic waves in the herniated pocket; (4) irregularly shaped pouch as compared to the smooth, pear-shaped phrenic ampulla; (5) identifiable gastric mucosal folds within the pouch; (6) localization of the EGJ above the diaphragm; (7) upward pull of the gastric mucosal folds through the esophageal hiatus; (8) retrograde filling of a herniated pouch; and (9) a small fundus of stomach.[60]

Recently, the radiologic classification of hiatal hernia has been considered by the position of the GEJ respect to the gastric folds (Fig. 125.20).[63] In *normal EGJ*, the EGJ is located below the diaphragm, at the apex of the angle of His; in *sliding hiatal hernia*, the EGJ rises above the esophageal hiatus, together with a portion of the fundus of the stomach, while the patient is in a prone position and straining, although it recedes within the abdomen in the upright position. In *hiatal insufficiency*, in the upright position, the

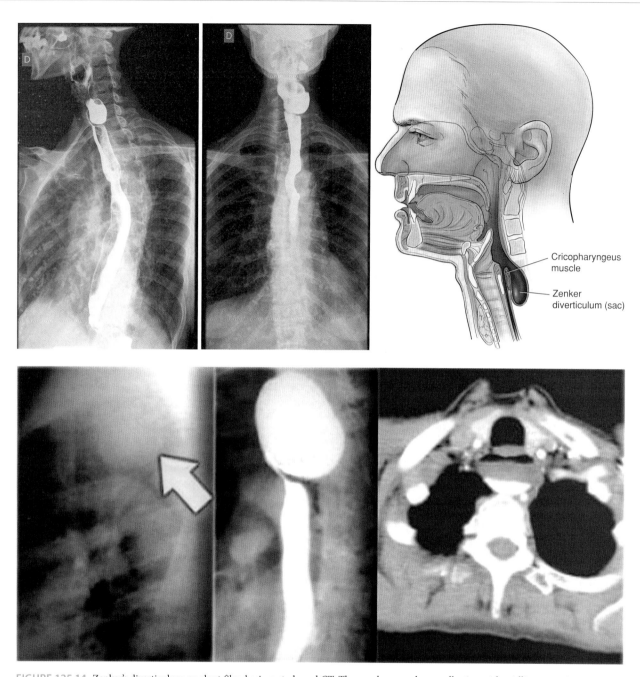

Cricopharyngeus muscle

Zenker diverticulum (sac)

FIGURE 125.14 Zenker's diverticulum on chest film, barium study and CT. The esophagram shows collection with midline posterior origin just above cricopharyngeus protruding lateral, usually to left, and caudal with enlargement (*arrow*).

esophagus is straightened, the angle of His is widened, and the EGJ is at the level of the diaphragmatic hiatus (hiatal notch); the intra-abdominal esophageal segment has disappeared; in **concentric hiatal hernia**, in the upright position, the esophagus is straightened, the EGJ is located above the diaphragm, and the gastrocardial folds display a "tent-shaped" appearance.

In patients with **short esophagus**, in the upright position, the esophagus is straight and rigid, the EGJ is fixed far above the diaphragm, and it may be stenotic; the intrathoracic stomach has a "funnel- or bell-shaped" appearance.

In **massive incarcerated gastric hiatal hernia**, in the orthostatic position, a great portion of the stomach is fixed in the chest with a bottleneck appearance of the transhiatal portion; the esophagus may be straightened or curled.

Reflux Esophagitis

Reflux esophagitis is by far the most common inflammatory disease involving the esophagus. This condition is characterized on single-contrast esophagograms by thickened folds, marginal ulcerations, and decreased dispensability, even if such findings are detected only in patients with advance disease. Double-contrast esophagrams have a sensitivity approaching 90% for the diagnosis of reflux esophagitis and is considered the radiologic technique of choice for patients with suspected GERD.

Early reflux esophagitis may be manifested by a finely nodular or granular appearance of the mucosa with poorly defined radiolucency that fades peripherally as a result of mucosal edema and inflammation (Fig. 125.21).[64,65]

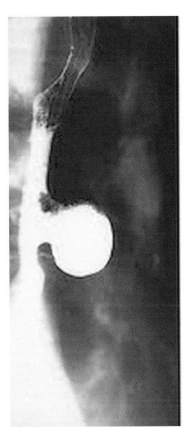
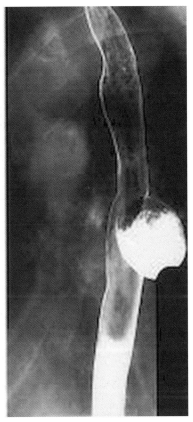
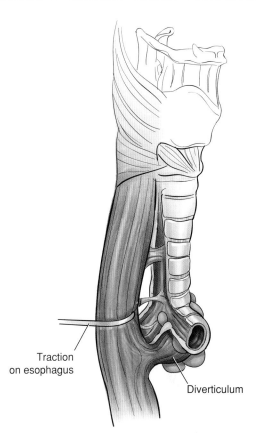

Traction
on esophagus

Diverticulum

FIGURE 125.15 Midthoracic diverticulum.

With more advanced disease, barium studies may reveal shallow ulcers and erosions in the distal esophagus. The ulcers may have a punctate, linear, or stellate configuration, and are frequently associated with surrounding halos of edematous mucosa, radiating folds, or sacculation of the adjacent esophageal wall (Fig. 125.22).[65]

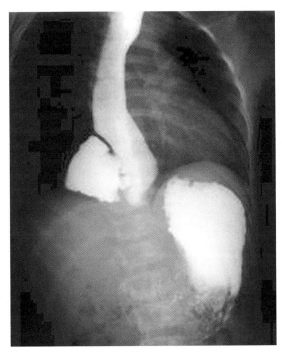

FIGURE 125.16 Epiphrenic diverticulum.

Barrett Esophagus

Barrett esophagus is characterized by progressive columnar metaplasia of the distal esophagus caused by chronic gastroesophageal reflux and reflux esophagitis (Fig. 125.23). In the presence of a hiatal hernia or gastroesophageal reflux, a mid-esophageal stricture or ulcers are thought to be highly suggestive of Barrett esophagus. However, the classic radiologic signs of Barrett esophagus are seen in only 5% to 10% of all patients with Barrett esophagus.[66,67] Other common findings in Barrett esophagus, such as reflux esophagitis and peptic strictures, are often present in patients with uncomplicated reflux disease who do not have Barrett esophagus. As result, many investigators have traditionally believed that esophagography has limited value in diagnosing Barrett esophagus, although other investigators have shown that double-contrast esophagography can be a useful imaging test for Barrett esophagus in patients with reflux symptoms.[68] However, a larger group of patients at moderate risk for Barrett esophagus because of esophagitis or peptic strictures in the distal esophagus should be undergo endoscopy, based on severity of symptoms, age, and overall health of the patient.

INFECTIOUS ESOPHAGITIS

Candida Esophagitis

Candida albicans is the most common cause of infectious esophagitis. It usually occurs as an opportunistic infection in immunocompromised patients, particularly those with acquired immunodeficiency syndrome (AIDS). Single-contrast barium studies have limited value in detecting Candida esophagitis because of the superficial nature of the disease; in contrast, double-contrast barium studies have a

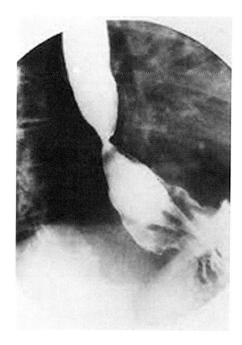

FIGURE 125.17 Hiatal hernia.

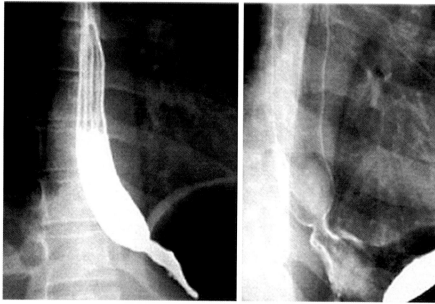

FIGURE 125.18 Sliding hiatus hernia.

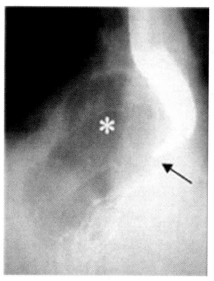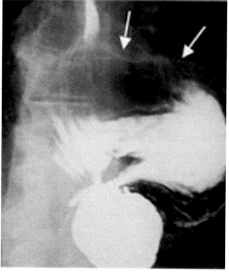

FIGURE 125.19 Paraesophageal hiatus hernia. On the far left gas filled gastric fundus (*asterisk*) protrudes through hiatus but the GE junction (*arrow*) is below diaphragm. Next to it a paraesophageal hernia with most of 'upside down' stomach in chest with greater curvature (*arrows*) flipped up.

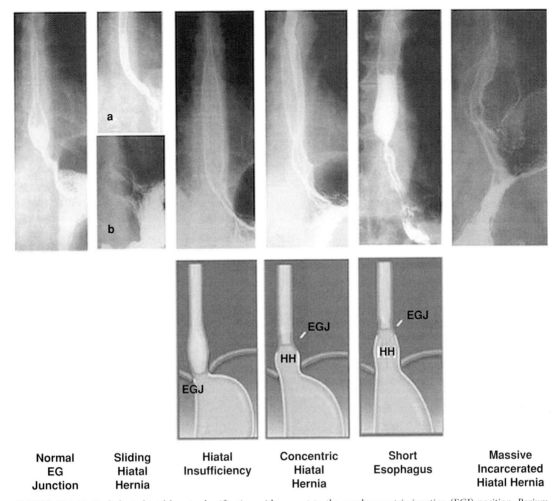

| Normal EG Junction | Sliding Hiatal Hernia | Hiatal Insufficiency | Concentric Hiatal Hernia | Short Esophagus | Massive Incarcerated Hiatal Hernia |

FIGURE 125.20 Radiologic hiatal hernia classification with respect to the esophagogastric junction (EGJ) position. Barium swallow. *Black outline* is the esophageal wall; *white outline* is the gastric wall. HH, Hiatal hernia; EGJ, Esophagogastric junction of the esophagus. (From Mattioli S, D'Ovidio F, Pilotti V, et al. Hiatus hernia and intrathoracic migration of esophagogastric junction in gastroesophageal reflux disease. *Dig Dis Sci* 2003;48:1823–1831. Copyright © 2003 Plenum Publishing Corporation. With permission of Springer.)[64]

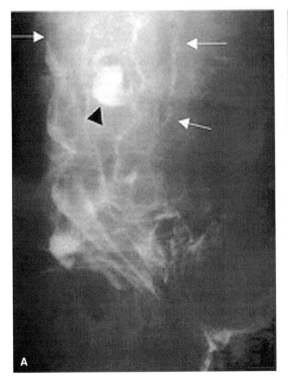

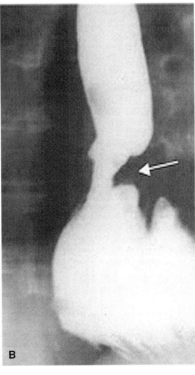

FIGURE 125.21 A: Air-contrast esophagram shows thick esophageal mucosal folds (*arrows*) and an ulcer (*arrowhead*) due to GERD. **B:** Single contrast esophagram shows stricture (*arrow*) and sliding hiatus hernia.

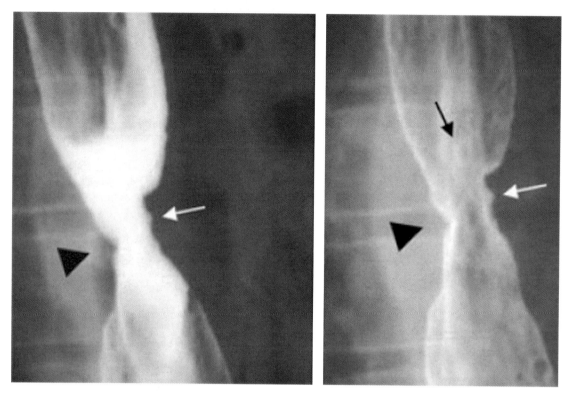

FIGURE 125.22 On the left irregular stricture (*arrowhead*) and erosions (*arrows*) due to GERD.

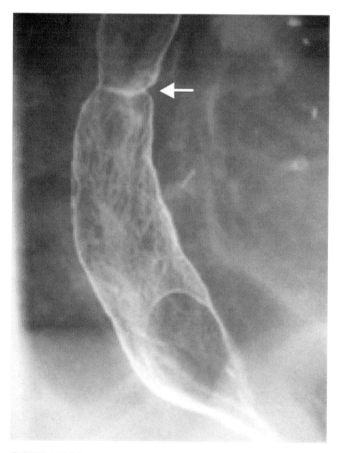

FIGURE 125.23 A patient with a Barrett esophagus. The reticular mucosa is characteristic of Barrett columnar metaplasia, especially with the associated web-like (*arrow*) stricture.

sensitivity of about 90% in diagnosing Candida esophagitis in relation to endoscopy,[69,70] primarily because of the ability to demonstrate mucosal plaques with this technique (Fig. 125.24).

Herpes Esophagitis

The herpes simplex virus is another cause of infectious esophagitis. Most patients with this condition are immunocompromised, but herpes esophagitis may occasionally develop as an acute, self-limited disease in otherwise healthy patients.[71]

On double-contrast studies, small esophageal vesicles that subsequently rupture to form discrete, punch-out ulcers on the mucosa may be associated with this infection.[72,73] The ulcers can have a punctate, stellate, or volcano-like appearance and are often surrounded by radiolucent mounds of edema (Fig. 125.25).

Cytomegalovirus Esophagitis

Cytomegalovirus esophagitis is another cause of infectious esophagitis that occurs primarily in patients with AIDS (Fig. 125.26). Main features of CMV esophagitis on double-contrast studies are one or more giant, flat ulcers that are several centimeters or more length.[73]

The ulcers may have an ovoid or diamond-shaped configuration and are often surrounded by a thin radiolucent rim of edematous mucosa.

Drug-Induced Esophagitis

Tetracycline and its derivative, doxycycline, are two of the agents more commonly responsible for a drug-induced esophagitis in the United States, but other offending medications include potassium chloride, quinidine, aspirin, or other nonsteroidal anti-inflammatory drugs and alendronate (Fig. 125.27).[74] Patients affected typically

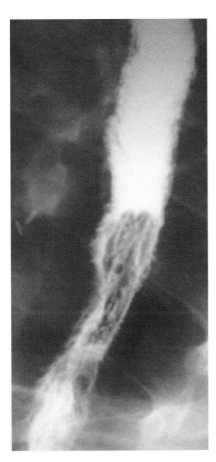

FIGURE 125.24   The barium study shows numerous fine erosions and small plaques due to *Candida albicans* in immunocompromised patient.

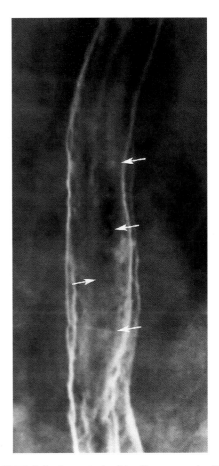

FIGURE 125.25 Infectious esophagitis. Herpes esophagitis. Double-contrast esophagram shows small, discrete ulcers (*arrows*) in the midesophagus on a normal background mucosa. Note the radiolucent mounds of edema surrounding the ulcers. In the appropriate clinical setting, this appearance is highly suggestive of herpes esophagitis, since ulceration in candidiasis almost always occurs on a background of diffuse plaque formation.

ingest the medications with little or no water and immediately before going to bed. Prolonged contact of the esophageal mucosa causes focal contact esophagitis. The radiographic findings depend on the nature of the offending medication. Tetracycline and doxycycline are associated with the development of small, superficial ulcers in the upper and midesophagus indistinguishable from those in herpes esophagitis.[75,76]

Idiopathic Eosinophilic Esophagitis

Idiopathic eosinophilic esophagitis has been recognized as an increasingly common inflammatory condition of the esophagus, occurring predominantly in young men with long-standing dysphagia and recurrent food impactions, often associated with an atopic history and a peripheral eosinophilia (Fig. 125.28).[77] The diagnosis can be confirmed on endoscopic biopsy specimens showing more than 20 eosinophils per high-power field.[77,78]

The diagnosis on barium studies may be suggested by the presence of segmental esophageal strictures, sometimes associated with distinctive ring-like indentations, producing a so-called "ringed-esophagus."[79]

Radiation Esophagitis

A radiation dose of 5,000 cGy or more to the mediastinum may cause severe injury to the esophagus. This condition may be manifested by ulceration or by a granular appearance of the mucosa and decreased distensibility resulting from edema and inflammation of the irradiated segment.[80]

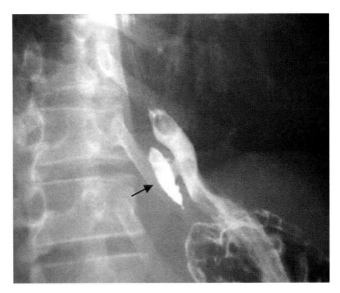

FIGURE 125.26 An AIDS patient with an infectious esophagitis due to Cytomegalovirus. Such giant ulcers (*arrow*) can also be due to HIV alone.

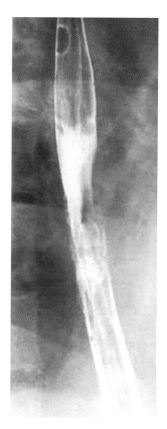

FIGURE 125.27 Doxycycline-induced esophagitis.

Caustic Esophagitis

Accidental or intentional ingestion of lye or other caustic agents can lead to a severe form of esophageal injury characterized by marked esophagitis and stricture formation (Fig. 125.29). A water soluble contrast should be used because of the risk of esophageal perforation. Such studies may reveal marked edema, spasm, and ulceration of the affected esophagus, and in some cases, esophageal disruption (Fig. 125.29).[81]

Fistulae

The most common result of the esophageal-airway fistula comes from a direct invasion of the tracheobronchial tree by advanced esophageal carcinoma (Fig. 125.30). Such fistulae have been reported in 5% to 10% of all patients with esophageal cancer, often occurring after treatment with radiation therapy.[82]

Other causes of esophageal-airway fistulae include esophageal instrumentation, trauma, foreign bodies, and surgery.

Affected patients typically present with violent episodes of coughing and choking during deglutition. When an esophageal-airway fistula is suspected on clinical grounds, barium should be used instead of water-soluble contrast agents, because the hyperosmolar agents may cause severe pulmonary edema if a fistula is present.[82]

Esophageal Perforation

If untreated, perforation of the thoracic esophagus is associated with mortality rate of nearly 100% because of fulminant mediastinitis.[82]

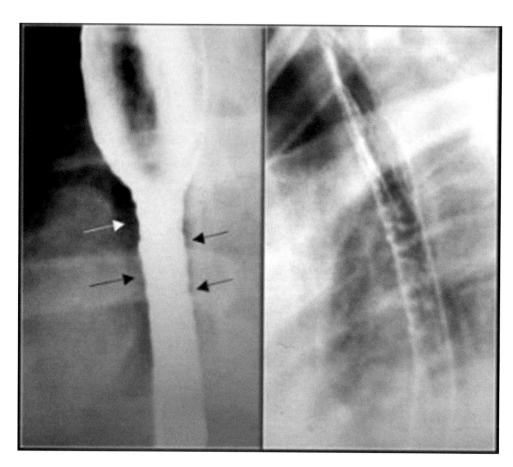

FIGURE 125.28 A patient with eosinophilic esophagitis. There is diffuse distal narrowing and corrugated margins (*arrows*) due to ring-like indentations, that are characteristic of eosinophilic esophagitis.

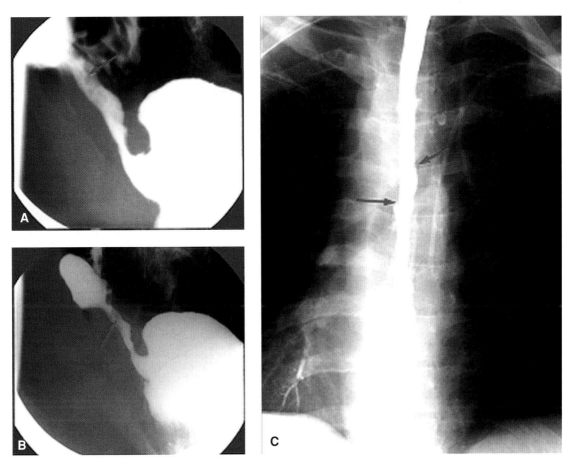

FIGURE 125.29 (**A**) and (**B**) both depict ulcerations of the distal esophageal mucosa secondary to lye ingestion (*arrow*). (**C**) depicts irregular narrowing of the esophagus with ulcerations (*arrows*).

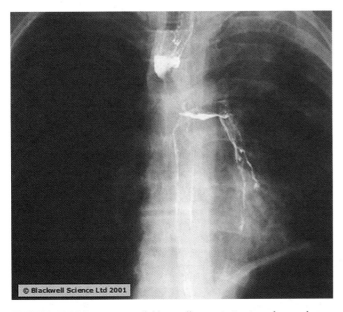

FIGURE 125.30 A water-soluble swallow examination shows obstruction of the esophagus by a stricture at the level of the aortic arch, with some of the contrast entering the left bronchial tree via a fistula. The mechanism needs to be distinguished from aspiration of contrast into the airway. The patient also has a left phrenic nerve palsy. (Republished with permission of John Wiley & Sons, Inc. from Vallance R. *An Atlas of Diagnostic Radiology in Gastroenterology*. Oxford: Blackwell Science; 1998, permission conveyed through Copyright Clearance Center, Inc.)

The most common cause of esophageal perforation is endoscopy, accounting up to 75% of cases,[82] although other causes include foreign bodies, food impactions, penetrating and blunt trauma, esophageal dilation, and spontaneous esophageal perforation resulting from a sudden, rapid increase in intraluminal esophageal pressure (Boerhaave syndrome). The presence of mediastinal gas on CT should be highly suggestive of esophageal perforation; however, CT is unreliable to determine the site of perforation.

Esophagography is often performed on patients with suspected esophageal perforation. Some patients may have free leaks into the mediastinum (Fig. 125.31).

TUMORS

BENIGN TUMORS

Benign tumors and cysts of the esophagus are rare, particularly when compared with other esophageal lesions such as carcinoma and reflux esophagitis.[83]

Leiomyomas

Leiomyomas are rare benign esophageal neoplasms with an indolent clinical course. Symptoms mimic that of esophageal cancer. Esophagoscopy and EUS are the main diagnostic methods. Symptomatic and large leiomyomas should be treated surgically while small,

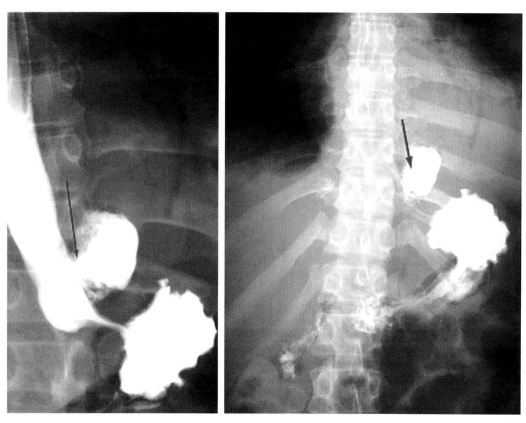

FIGURE 125.31 These images on esophagram depict contrast extravasation from the distal esophagus in a patient with spontaneous perforation of the esophagus. *Arrows* show the point of extravasation.

asymptomatic lesions may be managed by regular follow-up and repeated endoscopies.[83–86]

Leiomyomas are rare in the cervical region; over 80% are in the thoracic portion of the esophagus below the level of the aortic arch. Approximately 40% are in the middle third and 48% in the lower third.[83,84]

The characteristics of leiomyomas of the esophagus as demonstrated by barium x-ray studies were described in detail by Schatzki and Hawes,[87] and subsequently by other radiologists.

The intramural leiomyoma produces in profile a smooth, semilunar defect with intact mucosa and sharp borders. The abrupt sharp angle where the tumor meets the normal esophageal wall both proximally and distally is characteristic although not pathognomonic. Usually about half of the tumor mass appears to project into the lumen. Mucosal folds over the tumor will be obliterated as seen in the direct plane, but may be seen on the opposite wall, a finding called the smear effect. The barium column may split or fork at the level of the tumor.

Delay in passage of the barium or proximal dilatation are seldom seen with the usual lesion (Fig. 125.32). The larger tumors, especially in the lower esophagus and at the cardia, may cause apparent flattening of the esophageal lumen which will appear narrowed in one plane and widened in the opposite. Gross irregularity, deformity, and angulation may be seen in the esophagogastric leiomyoma (Fig. 125.33).[86]

Polyps

A polyp is a mass of tissue protruding abnormally from the mucous membrane (protective lining of epithelial cells for secretion and absorption) of the esophagus (Fig. 125.34). Esophageal polyps are a rare condition and affects about 0.5% of the population. Esophagus is the muscular tube connecting the mouth with the stomach (Fig. 125.34). Most polyps are benign but some can get malignant.

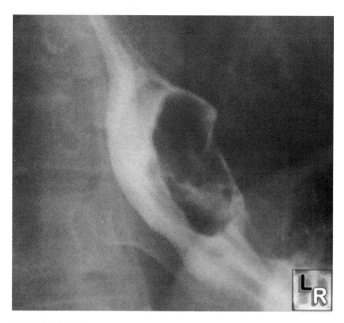

FIGURE 125.32 Leiomyoma of the esophagus.

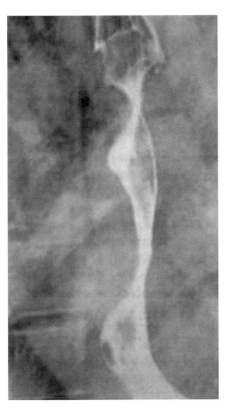

FIGURE 125.33 Barium contrast x-ray of the chest reveals a long segment of circumferential soft tissue mass encircling the esophagus.

MALIGNANT TUMORS

Esophageal carcinoma constitutes about 1% of all cancers in the United States and 7% of all GI tumors.[88] Early dissemination of tumor occurs because the esophagus lacks a serosa, so there is no anatomic barrier to prevent these cancers from spreading rapidly into the mediastinum. Patients with esophageal carcinoma usually present with dysphagia, but this is a late finding that develops after the tumor has invaded the esophageal wall, periesophageal lymphatics, or other mediastinal structures.

Double-contrast esophagography has a sensitivity of greater than 95% in the detection of esophageal cancer,[89] a number comparable to the endoscopic sensitivity of 95% to 100% when brushings and biopsy specimens are obtained.[90] Early esophageal cancers are usually small protruded lesions less than 3.5 cm in size.

These tumors may manifest on double contrast studies as plaque-like lesions (often containing flat central ulcers) (Fig. 125.35), sessile polyps with a smooth or slightly lobulated contour, or focal irregularities of the esophageal wall.[91]

Adenocarcinoma

Early adenocarcinomas may also manifest as a localized area of wall flattening or irregularity within a pre-existing peptic stricture.[91] Superficial spreading carcinoma is another form of early esophageal cancer characterized by poorly defined nodules or plaques that merge with one another, producing a confluent area of disease (Fig. 125.36).[91,92]

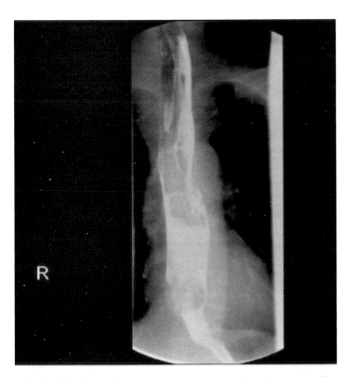

FIGURE 125.34 Radiologic view of esophageal polyps. Barium swallow showed an enlarged esophagus, with a large endoluminal filling defect and irregular luminal filling by the barium contrast.

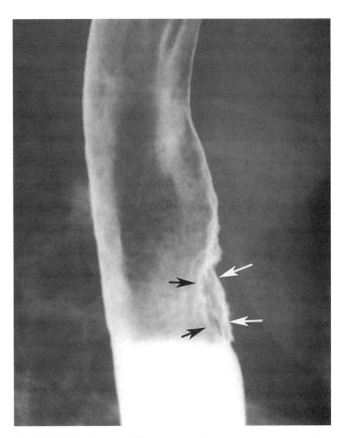

FIGURE 125.35 Upright LPO spot image from double-contrast esophagography shows early esophageal cancer in profile as a plaque-like lesion (*black arrows*) with flat central ulcer (*white arrows*) on left lateral wall of the midesophagus.

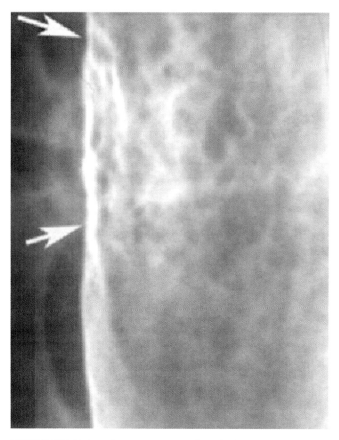

FIGURE 125.36 Upright LPO spot image from double-contrast esophagography shows superficial spreading carcinoma as focal area of mucosal nodularity (*arrows*) in midesophagus, without a discrete mass. Note how nodules merge with one another, producing a confluent area of disease.

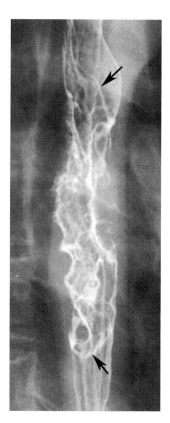

FIGURE 125.37 Upright LPO spot image from double-contrast esophagography shows advanced infiltrating carcinoma as irregular area of narrowing, with mucosal nodularity, ulceration, and shelf-like margins (*arrows*) in midesophagus.

Advanced esophageal carcinomas usually appear on barium studies as infiltrating, polypoid, ulcerative, or, less commonly, varicoid lesions.[90] Infiltrating carcinomas manifest as irregular luminal narrowing with mucosal nodularity or ulceration and abrupt shelf-like borders (Fig. 125.37). Polypoid carcinomas appear as lobulated intraluminal masses or polypoid ulcerated masses (Fig. 125.38). Primary ulcerative carcinomas are seen as giant meniscoid ulcers surrounded by a radiolucent rind of tumor.[93] Finally, varicoid carcinomas are those in which submucosal spread of tumor produces thickened, tortuous, longitudinal defects (Fig. 125.39) that mimic the appearance of varices.[94] Varicoid tumors have a fixed configuration, however, whereas varices change in size and shape at fluoroscopy. Also, varices rarely cause dysphagia because they are soft and compressible. Thus, it is usually possible to differentiate these conditions on the basis of the clinical and radiographic findings.

Squamous Cell Carcinoma

Squamous cell carcinoma and adenocarcinoma of the esophagus cannot be reliably differentiated on barium studies. Nevertheless, squamous cell carcinoma tends to involve the upper or middle part of the esophagus (Fig. 125.40), whereas adenocarcinoma is located mainly in the distal esophagus. Unlike squamous cell carcinoma, adenocarcinoma also has a marked tendency to invade the gastric cardia or fundus and composes as many as 50% of all malignant tumors that involve the GEJ.[95,96]

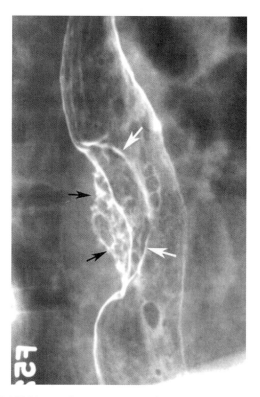

FIGURE 125.38 Upright LPO spot image from double-contrast esophagography shows advanced esophageal carcinoma as polypoid mass (*white arrows*) with a large area of ulceration (*black arrows*) on the right posterolateral wall of the distal esophagus (small rounded defects abutting mass are air bubbles).

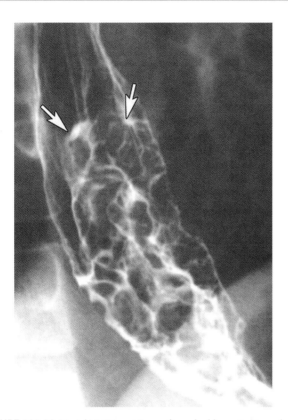

FIGURE 125.39 Upright LPO spot image from double-contrast esophagography shows varicoid carcinoma as lobulated submucosal lesion in the distal esophagus that could be mistaken for varices. However, this lesion had a fixed appearance at fluoroscopy and an abrupt proximal demarcation (*arrows*) from normal esophagus.

EVALUATION OF THE ESOPHAGUS BY OTHER IMAGING TECHNIQUES

COMPUTED TOMOGRAPHY

Although CT has a well-defined role in the evaluation of esophageal malignancies, its utility in nonmalignant conditions is still evolving. Fluoroscopic esophagography and endoscopy are the most commonly used investigations for benign esophageal lesions and provide excellent mucosal visualization.

CT is the technique of choice for investigating thoracic complications due to esophageal diseases.[97] It is a useful first-line imaging tool in patients with esophageal diseases presenting with nonspecific chest pain. Furthermore, benign esophageal diseases may be found incidentally on a thoracic CT. Disadvantages of CT include the inability to demonstrate mucosal details, inadequate esophageal distension, and nonspecificity of certain findings such as wall thickening.[97]

On CT normal esophageal view, the paraesophageal fat is visualized as an interface between the esophagus and adjacent vascular, cardiac, and connective tissue structures. The cervical esophagus lies near the midline, posterior to and occasionally indenting the trachea. It usually does not contain air. As the esophagus enters the thorax, it lies posterior and slightly to the left of the trachea, and the esophagotracheal fat pad is often thin. More inferiorly, the esophagus is situated close to the posterior surface of the left mainstem bronchus, descending thoracic aorta, and thoracic spine. Tumors, adenopathy, and aneurysms can all displace and invade the esophagus.

Small amounts of intraesophageal air are seen in approximately 65% of normal individuals. Megibow[98] recorded that the presence of an air–fluid level, fluid-filled lumen, or lumen caliber >10 mm usually indicates obstruction or severe esophageal dysmotility. Although

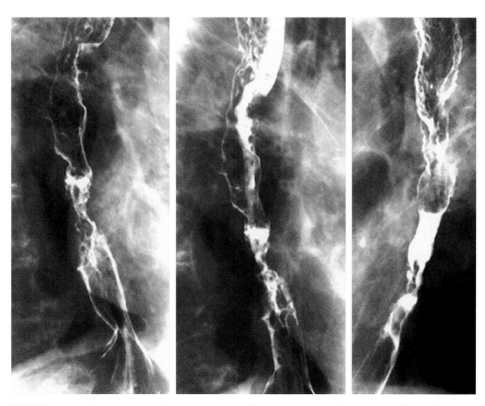

FIGURE 125.40 The esophagram shows a squamous cell carcinoma with Schatzi ring and filling defects proximal to the ring.

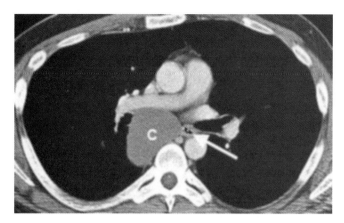

FIGURE 125.41 Esophageal duplication cyst (C). The *arrow* shows the esophagus.

there are no normal standards for the cross-sectional diameter of the collapsed esophagus, the wall thickness of a distended esophagus should not exceed 3 mm.

Esophageal Benign Diseases

Duplication Cysts

The esophagus is the second most common site of GI duplication.[99] Most patients are asymptomatic and the usual presentation is an incidental mediastinal mass detected on a plain radiograph. CT usually shows a homogeneous, well-defined, thin-walled, noncommunicating cyst abutting the esophagus (Figs. 125.41 and 125.42). Complications, such as bleeding and infections, can result in hyperdense contents and mural thickening. Differentials include bronchogenic cyst, lymphangioma, and neurenteric cyst.

Foreign Bodies

Foreign bodies are a commonly encountered problem in emergency departments, especially in children, the elderly, and patients with learning difficulties. Food boluses and coins are the most common foreign bodies in the adult and pediatric population, respectively.[100,101] Other common foreign bodies include fish and chicken bones, and dentures. Initial imaging includes plain radiographs of the neck, chest, and abdomen for identification of a radio-opaque foreign body as well as its potential complications. However, CT allows for more definitive localization. CT appearances depend on the type of foreign body ingested (Fig. 125.43). The sites of impaction include the cervical esophagus, GEJ, and at the site of a previous stricture. It is especially useful for radiolucent foreign bodies that may not be detected on radiographs and for evaluation of potential endoscopy blind spots in the hypopharynx and cervical esophagus. CT is also useful to assess potential complications such as perforation and mediastinitis.

Esophageal Injury and Perforation

CT is considered to be the preferred imaging modality in esophageal emergencies.[99,100] Esophageal wall thickening and defect and

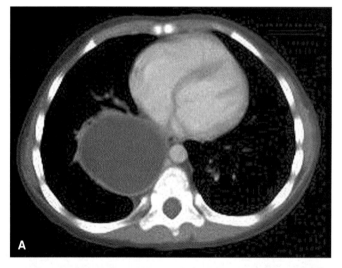

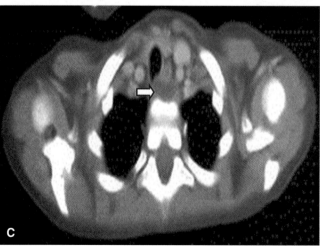

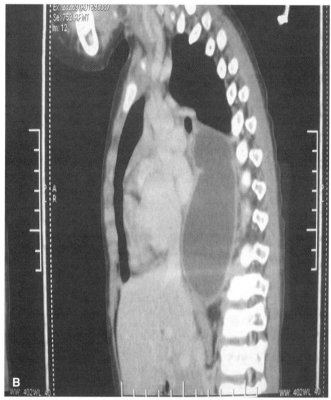

FIGURE 125.42 Computed tomography scan of esophageal duplication cysts. (**A**) Transverse and (**B**) sagittal views of the large-sized cyst; and (**C**) transverse view of the small-sized cyst (*white arrow*). (From Zhefeng Zhang, Feng Jin, Hao Wu, et al. Double esophageal duplication cysts, with ectopic gastric mucosa: a case report. *J Cardiothorac Surg* 2013;8:221.)

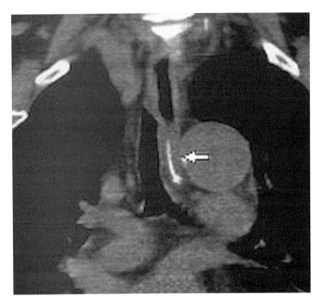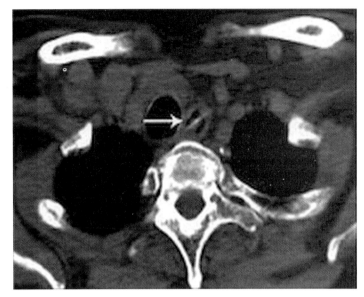

FIGURE 125.43 CT image of the thorax showing a fish bone (*arrow*). (From Venkatesh SH, Venkatanarasimha Karaddi NK. CT findings of accidental fish bone ingestion and its complications. *Diagn Interv Radiol.* 2016;22(2):156–160.)

periesophageal fluid and air on CT are signs that suggest esophageal perforation.[100–103] Because the esophagus is wrapped in the mediastinum, esophageal fluid content leakage might be trapped near the perforator.[104]

The technique of choice for visualization of esophageal injury is esophagography.[96]

Although esophagography is better for detecting the site of the leak, CT can detect a small amount of mediastinal gas, which in the appropriate clinical context, is indicative of an esophageal perforation. It is especially useful in patients in whom esophagograms are either negative or difficult to perform. It can also be used to investigate patients with penetrating injury to assess other mediastinal structures and lungs, and to rule out nonesophageal causes in patients with atypical symptoms.

CT findings vary with the severity of the injury. Partial thickness tears are usually occult on CT.

Occasionally, there may be subtle findings, such as esophageal wall thickening, extraluminal air, or hemorrhage, at the site of mucosal injury. Intramural hematomas and dissections are rarer forms of injury that usually resolve within a few days or weeks.

Concentric or eccentric esophageal wall thickening with increased density of mural contents is seen in a hematoma.[105] An intramural dissection is seen as a mucosal flap with submucosal air or contrast medium. Findings in a full-thickness perforation include contrast medium leak, an esophageal wall defect, periesophageal fluid collections (Fig. 125.44), and mediastinal air (Fig. 125.45).[106,107] Involvement of the mediastinum can be seen as fat stranding and inflammatory soft tissue, fluid collections, and abscesses (Fig. 125.46). Pleuropulmonary involvement is characterized either by pleural effusion, empyema, pneumothorax, lung consolidation, abscess, or, pleuropulmonary fistulas.

Fistulas

Fistulas can be congenital or acquired.[108] The advent of CT has revolutionized diagnostic imaging and many authors have advocated the use of CT scan in preoperative evaluation of EA/TEF (esophageal atresia/TEF) patients, as it is a quick noninvasive procedure that precisely delineates the anatomy of the TEF and accurately assesses the inter-pouch gap.[109–116] It also delineates the

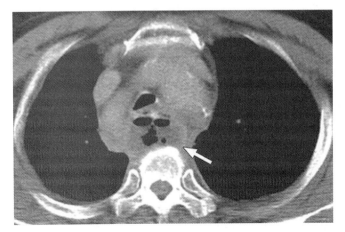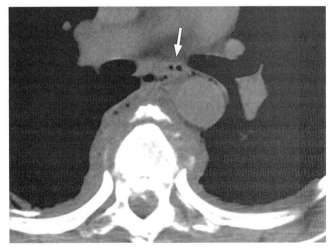

FIGURE 125.44 CT image shows periesophageal fluid collection with air in thoracic segment (*arrow*). (From Wu CH, Chen CM, Chen CC, et al. Esophagography after pneumomediastinum without CT findings of esophageal perforation: is it necessary? *Am J Roentgenol* 2013;201:977–984.)

FIGURE 125.45 CT image shows periesophageal infiltration with air (*arrow*).

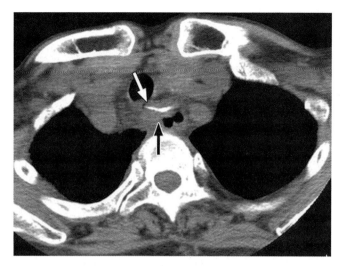

FIGURE 125.46 CT image shows esophageal injury caused by fish bone (*white arrow*) with periesophageal infiltration as well as periesophageal air collection (*black arrow*).

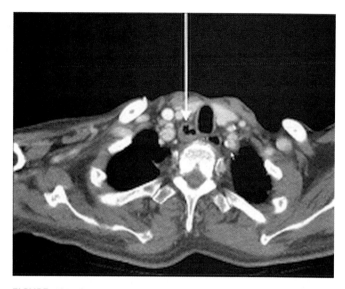

FIGURE 125.48 Transverse chest CT scan revealed the lower neck area midesophagus. *Arrow* shows the communication of the esophagus with trachea.

spatial relationships of the two esophageal pouches and the TEF with the aid of 3D images.[109–116] These anatomical factors in many instances may influence the mortality and long-term morbidity in these patients and also guide the preoperative and postoperative strategies.

The CT findings depend on the type of fistulous communication. The fistula itself may be seen as an air or contrast medium-containing track. Indirect signs are usually more common, for example, contrast medium, air, and water within the pleural cavity in an esophagopleural fistula. CT is also useful for evaluating thoracic complications of fistulas (Figs. 125.47 and 125.48).

Esophageal Diverticulum

As described in the previous paragraph, diverticula may be classified based on their location (pharyngoesophageal junction, mid and

distal esophagus), mechanism (pulsion and traction), or the layers forming the wall of the out-pouching (true, false, and intramural) (Fig. 125.49). True diverticula contain all layers of the esophageal wall, whereas false diverticula contain the mucosa and submucosa (Figs. 125.50 and 125.51).

Achalasia

Achalasia is increasingly being detected incidentally during CT scans (Fig. 125.52). Patients with uncomplicated achalasia demonstrate a dilated thin-walled esophagus filled with fluid/food debris. Overall CT has little role in directly assessing patients with achalasia, but is useful in assessing common complications. Careful assessment of the wall of the esophagus should be undertaken to identify any focal regions of thickening which may indicate malignancy. The lungs should be inspected for evidence of aspiration.

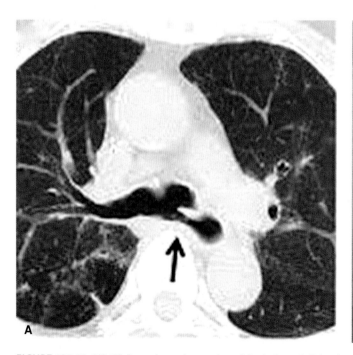

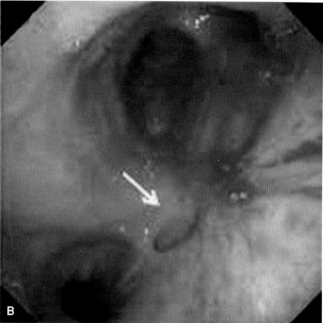

FIGURE 125.47 (**A**) CT shows the tracheoesophageal fistula (*arrow*); (**B**) endoscopic view of the tracheaoesophageal fistula (*arrow*).

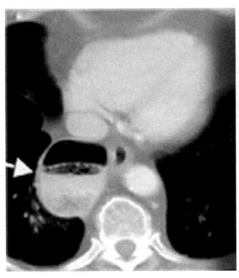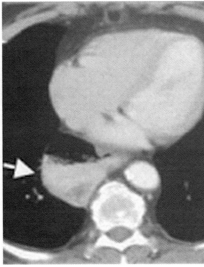

FIGURE 125.49 CT view of a large epiphrenic diverticulum. The CT demonstrates a large diverticulum (*arrow*) extends to the right just above diaphragm. (From Rajesh U, Naware SS. Large Epiphrenic Diverticulum of Esophagus. *Med J Armed Forces India* 2008;64(3):291–292.)

Hiatal Hernia

CT scan may be useful in an urgent situation for patients with suspected complications from a volvulized paraesophageal hernia.[117] The hernia site and any herniated organs within the chest cavity are clearly visualized in most cases. Multislice CT with sagittal, coronal, and 3D reformatted images has increased the sensitivity of CT for the detection of hiatal hernia.[118] If intestinal obstruction and strangulation occur, dilated intestinal segments will be visualized with air–fluid levels within the chest cavity and abdomen. Cephalad migration of the GEJ or gastric fundus through the hiatus can be clearly visualized on oral contrast-enhanced CT images.

Benign Tumors

Benign tumors account for one-fifth of all esophageal neoplasms and include squamous papillomas, gastrointestinal stromal tumor (GISTs); fibrovascular polyps; and other mesenchymal tumors, such as fibromas, neurofibromas, and haemangiomas.[119] GISTs are the most common benign submucosal esophageal neoplasms.[120,121] These are usually asymptomatic but may present with dysphagia. On CT, GISTs are usually seen as an incidental finding or detected in the setting of workup for a mediastinal mass. CT may show a well-defined, homogeneous, soft-tissue mass abutting the esophagus (Fig. 125.53). Differentiating GISTs from other benign and malignant esophageal neoplasms based on CT findings alone may be difficult.[122]

Leiomyomas

Although leiomyoma of the esophagus is relatively rare, it is the most common benign tumor involving this structure. In a series of 7,459 autopsies, Moersch and Harrington[123] detected only 44 benign tumors of the esophagus.

Thirty-two (73%) of these, however, were leiomyomas. In a series of 103 benign esophageal tumors obtained from surgical and autopsied patients, Totten et al.[83] found 46 (45%) of 103 tumors to be leiomyomas. According to the reported CT findings, esophageal leiomyomas are smoothly marginated, round or ovoid masses of muscle attenuation,

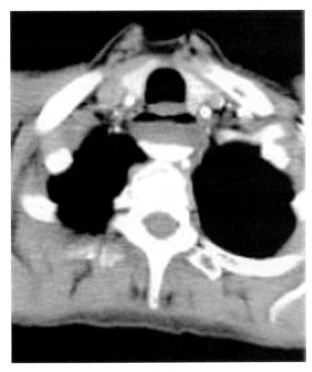

FIGURE 125.50 Zenker diverticulum on CT.

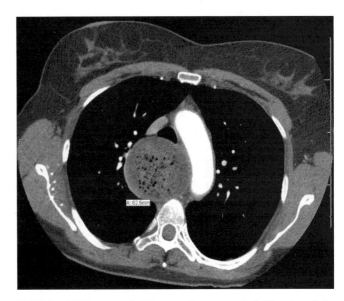

FIGURE 125.51 An axial CT image showing marked dilatation of the esophagus in a person with achalasia.

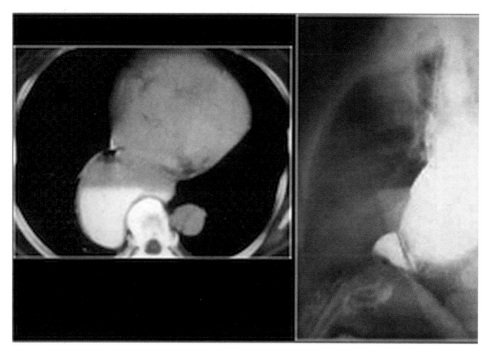

FIGURE 125.52 On the left another patient with achalasia.

lying intramurally or eccentrically within the esophageal wall (Fig. 125.54). Surrounding mediastinal fat is not usually disrupted.[122,124] In Carillas et al.,[125] enhanced scans showed that tumor attenuation was homogeneously low or iso and, characteristically, the same even when contrast medium was administered. These findings of homogeneity and slight enhancement contrast with those of uterine leiomyomas, which show recognizable enhancement and heterogeneity owing to calcification, hyaline and cystic degeneration, infection or necrosis.[125] This difference in the degree of enhancement is presumed to be due to the relatively small vascular supply of the esophageal tumors.

Malignant Tumors

CT is recommended for initial imaging following confirmation of malignancy at pathologic analysis, primarily to rule out

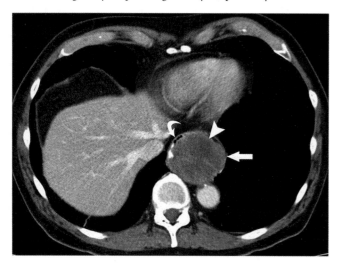

FIGURE 125.53 View of CT esophageal GIST. Axial image from a contrast-enhanced CT scan demonstrates a hypoattenuating well-circumscribed mildly enhancing intraluminal mass in the lower esophagus (*arrow*). Note subtle low attenuation area of necrosis within the mass (*arrowhead*). Compressed lumen of the esophagus containing small amount of oral contrast is seen (*curved arrow*).

unresectable or distant metastatic disease.[126] The normal esophageal wall is usually less than 3 mm thick at CT when the esophagus is distended[127]; any wall thickness greater than 5 mm is considered abnormal.[128] Asymmetric thickening of the esophageal wall is a primary but nonspecific CT finding of esophageal cancer (Figs. 125.55 and 125.56). CT is limited in determining the exact depth of tumor infiltration of the esophageal wall. In most comparative studies, the accuracy of CT for assessment of T stage is lower than that of endoscopic ultrasound (EUS).[129,130] CT is unable to adequately help differentiate between T1, T2, and T3 disease (Figs. 125.57 and 125.58), a distinction that is important when considering the use of neoadjuvant chemotherapy and radiation therapy.[131] Exclusion of T4 disease, as indicated by the preservation of fat planes between the esophageal cancer and adjacent structures, is the most important role of CT in the determination of T status (Fig. 125.59).[132]

The CT criteria for local invasion include (*a*) loss of fat planes between the tumor and adjacent structures in the mediastinum, and (*b*) displacement or indentation of other mediastinal structures. Aortic invasion is suggested if 90 degrees or more of the aorta is in contact with the tumor[133] or if there is obliteration of the triangular fat space between the esophagus, aorta, and spine adjacent to the primary tumor (Fig. 125.60).[134] A tracheobronchial fistula or tumor extension into the airway lumen is a definite sign of tracheobronchial invasion. Displacement of the trachea or bronchus, or indentation of the posterior wall of the trachea or bronchus by the tumor, have also proved accurate in predicting tracheobronchial invasion (Fig. 125.60).[133,135] Pericardial invasion is suspected if pericardial thickening, pericardial effusion, or indentation of the heart with loss of the pericardial fat plane is seen.

With the advent of multidetector CT, along with significant advances in three-dimensional imaging techniques, CT has become more valuable in the evaluation of T staging of esophageal cancer.

The microscopic spread of esophageal cancer is frequently far more extensive than the macroscopic boundaries of the tumor. CT estimates of tumor length made with multiplanar reformatted images are more accurate than those made with axial scans alone (Fig. 125.57). Multiplanar reformatted images are also useful in

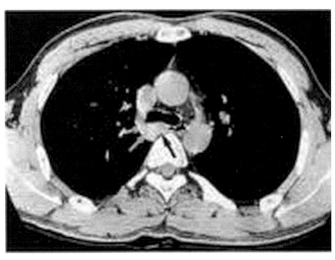
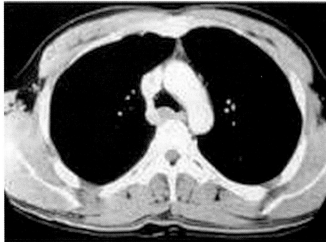

FIGURE 125.54 Esophageal leiomyoma in a 47-year-old man with no subjective symptoms.

evaluating esophageal cancer at the EGJ, which is difficult to evaluate with axial scans alone (Fig. 125.60).

PET and CT/PET

Current preoperative staging techniques, such as CT, are of limited accuracy, and invasive procedures often are used for better assessment of the stage of the disease.[136] Beginning in the mid-1990s, positron emission tomography (PET) has been evaluated as a method for the staging of esophageal and gastric cancer. In the past few years, combined PET/CT scanners have been rapidly replacing conventional

PET for the evaluation of oncologic patients. Although there are still only limited data regarding the use of PET/CT in esophageal and gastric cancers, the combination of these two modalities is expected to improve the accuracy of image interpretation, and thus lead to better management of cancer patients.[137,138]

However, CT is limited for detection of early-stage (T1 and T2) tumors and for differentiating malignant from benign causes of esophageal wall thickening. The accuracy of CT is further limited by the diminished amount of mediastinal fat in many patients with esophageal cancer, who often have sustained significant weight loss

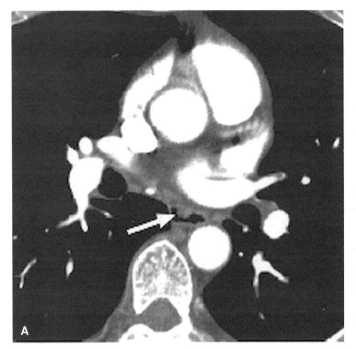
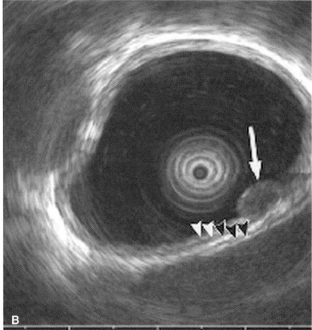

FIGURE 125.55 T1 N0 M0 (stage I) SCC of the midesophagus in a 52-year-old man. **A:** Contrast material–enhanced CT scan obtained at the level of the left superior pulmonary vein shows a small, nodular protruding lesion (*arrow*). **B:** Endoscopic US image clearly depicts a polypoid lesion (*arrow*) with extension into the second (hypoechoic) deep mucosal layer. Note the normal alternating hyper- and hypoechoic architecture of the esophageal wall (*arrowheads*). The first layer is hyperechoic and represents the interface between balloon and superficial mucosa, the second layer (hypoechoic) represents the lamina propria and muscularis mucosae, the third layer (hyperechoic) represents the submucosa, the fourth layer (hypoechoic) represents the muscularis propria, and the fifth layer (hyperechoic) represents the interface between the serosa and surrounding tissues.

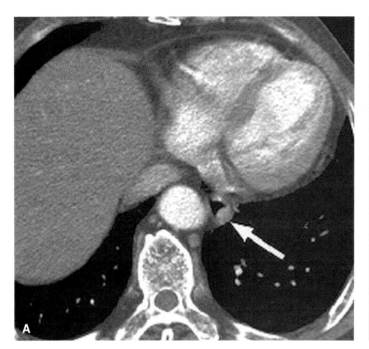
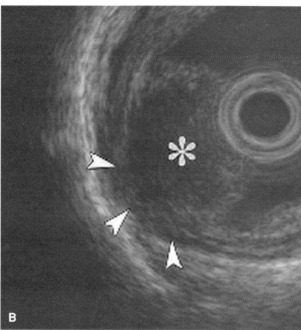

FIGURE 125.56 T2 N0 M0 (stage IIA) SCC of the lower esophagus in a 61-year-old man. **A:** Contrast-enhanced CT scan obtained at the level of the left ventricle shows an eccentric, nodular esophageal lesion (*arrow*). **B:** Endoscopic US image shows a mural nodule (*) with penetration into the fourth (hypoechoic) layer of the esophageal wall (muscularis propria) (*arrowheads*).

by the time of presentation. In addition, accurate assessment of the local extent of the tumor may be hindered by partial-volume averaging consequent to the close proximity of the tumor to the pulsating aorta or heart.[139] FDG-PET can detect esophageal cancer before it becomes evident on CT, but PET is limited in its ability to determine the extent of tumor spread through the esophageal wall or tumor invasion of the adjacent structures. This limitation results chiefly from the poorer resolution of PET by comparison with anatomic imaging methods and its limited delineation of normal anatomic structures. A heterogeneous pattern of FDG uptake at the primary site, especially when it has irregular margins, is suggestive of local extension of the tumor into the surrounding soft tissues. Several investigators have shown that FDG-PET has a higher sensitivity than CT for detection of primary esophageal cancer (83% to 100% vs. 67%

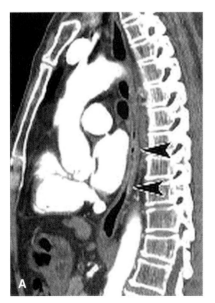
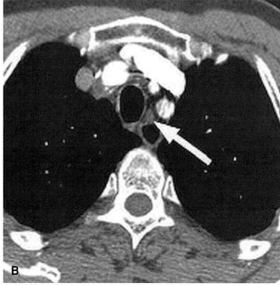
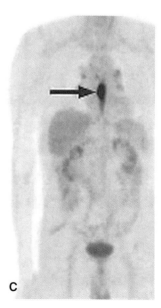

FIGURE 125.57 T3 N1 M0 (stage III) SCC of the midesophagus in a 64-year-old man. No clear-cut esophageal abnormality was seen at axial CT. **A:** Sagittal reformatted CT image clearly shows the extent of esophageal wall thickening with enhancement (*arrowheads*) at the level of the left atrium. **B:** Axial CT scan obtained at the level of the left innominate vein shows a left upper paratracheal lymph node 5 mm in diameter (*arrow*), a finding that was subsequently confirmed to be a metastatic lymph node. **C:** Coronal PET scan shows intense FDG uptake in the primary tumor (*arrow*). The lymph node in the left paratracheal region (cf **B**) is not seen (false-negative finding).

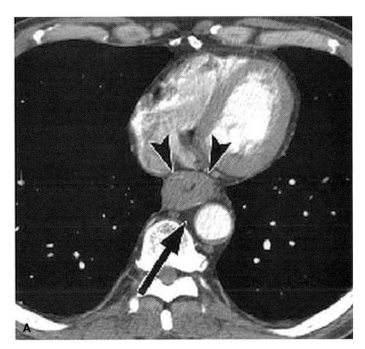

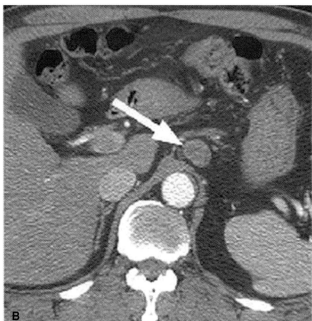

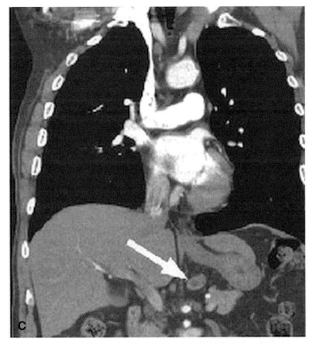

FIGURE 125.58 T3 N1 M0 (stage III) SCC of the middle and lower esophagus in a 66-year-old man. **A:** Axial CT scan obtained at the level of the left ventricle shows diffuse esophageal wall thickening. Note the preservation of the fat plane (*arrowheads*) between the mass and the heart, and the triangular fat space (*arrow*) between the esophagus, aorta, and spine adjacent to the primary tumor, findings that are consistent with T3 disease. **B:** Axial CT scan shows an enlarged lymph node (*arrow*). **C:** Coronal CT scan shows a lymph node (*arrow*) that is localized to the left gastric region (a finding indicative of N1 disease) rather than the celiac region (M1a disease). Note that the lymph node is cephalad to the origin of the celiac artery and can be identified adjacent to the branches of the celiac axis rather than adjacent to the celiac artery itself.

to 92%) (Fig. 125.61).[140–148] The one exception was a study utilizing a partial-ring PET scanner without attenuation correction of images, where PET was found to have a lower sensitivity than CT (84% vs. 97%).[149] In most studies, false-negative results of PET occurred in patients with small T1 lesions. Physiologic uptake of FDG in the normal esophagus may also be a limitation in detection of small or well-differentiated tumors.

PET/CT provides incremental staging information, changes management in one-third of patients and has powerful prognostic stratification in the primary staging of esophageal cancer. It should be incorporated in routine clinical practice for staging of patients with esophageal cancer. The relatively high survival of patients with locally advanced disease on PET/CT indicates that these patients

may have benefitted from more aggressive and more appropriately planned multimodality treatment.

Although PET scans are approved for staging and restaging of esophageal cancer, they may not be the best option for evaluating patients after chemoradiation. That was the conclusion of a study presented at the Gastrointestinal Cancers Symposium.[150] PET is widely used to assess patient response to both chemotherapy and chemoradiation in patients with esophageal cancer. And several studies have shown that the imaging technique can be used to detect new sites of metastatic disease. Yet few studies have looked at the impact radiation has on such posttreatment scans, or whether PET imaging unnecessarily highlights a significant number of noncancerous aberrations, the assessment of which can delay treatment or cause unnecessary morbidity.[150]

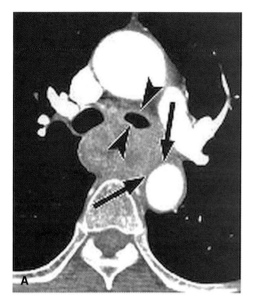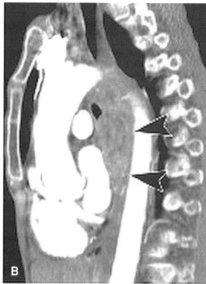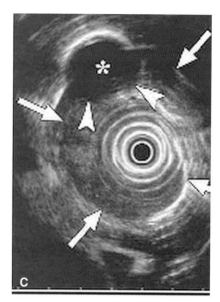

FIGURE 125.59 T4 N1 M0 (stage III) SCC of the midesophagus in a 61-year-old man. **A:** Contrast-enhanced CT scan obtained at the level of the mainstem bronchi shows marked esophageal wall thickening with tumor extension into the periesophageal fat. Note the diffuse wall thickening and narrowing of the left main bronchus (*arrowheads*). There is loss of the normal fat plane (*arrows*) between the esophagus and the thoracic aorta, a finding that is suggestive of aortic invasion. **B:** Sagittal reformatted CT image shows a broad interface (*arrowheads*) between the esophageal mass and the thoracic aorta. **C:** Endoscopic US image shows loss of the interface (*arrowheads*) between the esophageal mass (*arrows*) and the thoracic aorta (*), a finding that is also suggestive of aortic invasion.

ESOPHAGEAL ENDOSONOGRAPHY

EUS is an endoscopic technique that provides highly accurate imaging of mucosal, submucosal, and periluminal structures.[151] It is often used for the preoperative staging of GI malignancies such as esophageal, gastric, pancreatic, and rectal cancers for which it has an accuracy of 90%, 88%, and 90%, respectively, when performed with experienced hands.[152–156] EUS has an important role in predicting treatment response after neoadjuvant therapy.

EUS and EUS-FNA represent the most accurate method for locoregional staging of esophageal carcinoma, and should be performed for local staging in those patients who are good surgical candidates and other imaging techniques (CT, PET) have demonstrated no distant metastases. The presence of EUS as an adjunct for staging is mandatory in busy thoracic surgery practices.

Currently available echoendoscopes operate at different ultrasound frequencies (5, 7.5, 12, and 20 MHz), allowing one to visualize the esophageal wall as a five-layer structure (first hyperechoic layer: superficial mucosa, second hypoechoic layer: deep mucosa, third hyperechoic layer: submucosa, fourth hypoechoic layer: muscularis propria, and fifth hyperechoic layer: adventitia).[157] Based on these special characteristics, EUS allows to assess the degree of tumor infiltration into the wall layers and subsequently to determine the tumor stage (T stage).[157]

However, the muscularis mucosa cannot be visualized with dedicated echoendoscopes (Fig. 125.62).[158,159] High-frequency miniprobes (20 MHz) provide a more detailed visualization, allowing one to delineate nine layers in the esophageal wall (first and second layer: superficial mucosa [hyper and hypoechoic, respectively]; third layer: lamina propria [hyperechoic]; fourth layer: muscularis mucosa [hypoechoic]; fifth layer: submucosa [hyperechoic]; sixth, seventh, and eighth layer: [hypo-, hyper-, and hypoechoic, respectively] inner circular muscle and outer longitudinal muscle of the muscularis propria with intermuscular connective tissue; ninth layer: adventitia [hyperechoic]).[158,159] Visualization of the muscularis mucosa is

important when evaluating superficial lesions and nonsurgical alternatives are being considered. However, if the muscularis mucosa is involved by tumor, lymph node metastases may be present in up to 10% of patients and EMR should not be performed with a curative intent (Fig. 125.63).[160,161]

One of the major criticisms of EUS and EUS-FNA is that the technique depends on the operator who performs the examination. Several studies have investigated the degree of inter- and intraobserver agreement for EUS staging of esophageal carcinoma.[162–164]

In summary, tumor stage, degree of experience, as well as technical factors (balloon overinflation, oblique scanning, and inadequate use of higher scanning frequencies) have been postulated as the main causes for errors among inexperienced endosonographers.[160,163,165]

MAGNETIC RESONANCE IMAGING

Esophageal MRI is compromised by respiratory and cardiac motion. The esophagus is most often imaged in the body coil because the respiratory artefacts produced by a surface coil positioned on the rib cage can be difficult to eliminate. Respiratory artefacts can be minimized by respiratory compensation and single-breath-hold pulse sequences. In addition, cardiac gating and gradient moment nulling help reduce artefacts from great vessel and cardiac pulsation. Spatially selective presaturation pulses on spin-echo sequences also minimize artefacts from flowing blood, as Semelka and colleagues[166] noted in Semelka's textbook *Abdominal and Pelvic MRI*.

The esophagus appears as a low-signal-intensity structure contrasted by high-signal-intensity fat on T1-weighted images. On T2-weighted images, the muscular wall of the esophagus has low signal intensity, whereas intraluminal contents have high signal intensity. According to Semelka and colleagues,[166] the muscular wall of the esophagus enhances moderately after the injection of intravenous gadolinium diethylenetriamine penta-acetic acid (Gd-DTPA).

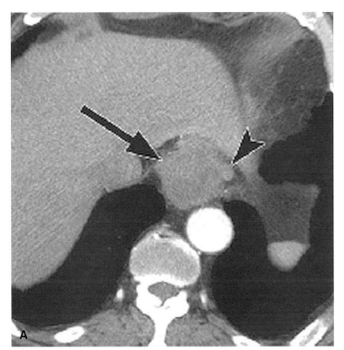

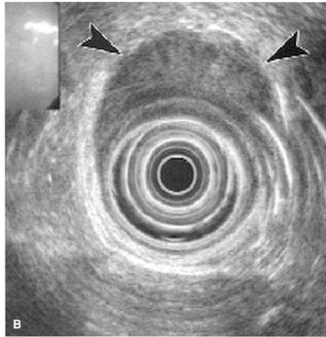

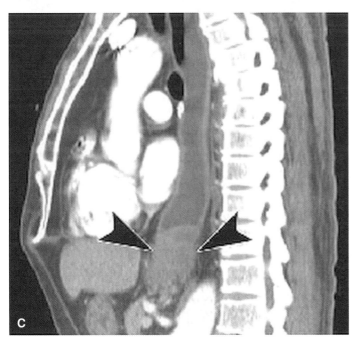

FIGURE 125.60 T3 N0 M0 (stage IIA) SCC of the lower thoracic esophagus with involvement of the gastroesophageal junction in a 61-year-old man. **A:** Axial CT scan obtained just above the hiatus shows a mass that involves the lower esophagus, along with periesophageal fat infiltration (*arrow*). A periesophageal lymph node (*arrowhead*) is also noted, a finding that was subsequently confirmed to be benign. **B:** Endoscopic US image shows that the mass has infiltrated all the layers of the esophageal wall and into the adventitia (*arrowheads*). **C:** Sagittal CT scan clearly shows tumor involvement of the lower esophagus, gastroesophageal junction, and part of the heart (*arrowheads*).

Although not a primary means of imaging the esophagus, MRI can serve as an alternative technique to CT and represents an important supplemental imaging method.

In conclusion, barium esophagography has optimal sensitivity for the detection of lesions when a double-contrast technique is used. Such technique requires that the patient be able to stand upright, which may not be possible with patients who are debilitated. For bulkier obstructive lesions, an air-contrast technique may not be possible, and a detailed mucosal examination may not be achieved distal to the obstruction.

A notable limitation of CT in diagnosis involves the characterization of lymph nodes. With CT scans, size criteria are used to determine possible metastatic involvement; however, lymph nodes may be enlarged because of infectious or inflammatory etiologies. Conversely, subcentimeter lymph nodes may harbor metastatic tumor.

Ultrasonographic examinations are highly operator dependent. Limitations of EUS with the standard Olympus diagnostic echoendoscope (13 mm in diameter) include an inability to pass the malignant stricture with the transducer. This limitation results in an incomplete examination, which occurred in 40% of patients reported by Massari et al.[165] However, the use of a dedicated 8-mm-diameter esophagoprobe for EUS allows complete examination in most patients.

With PET, the resolution and cost remain the primary limitations. Subcentimeter foci of tumor metabolism may not be detected.

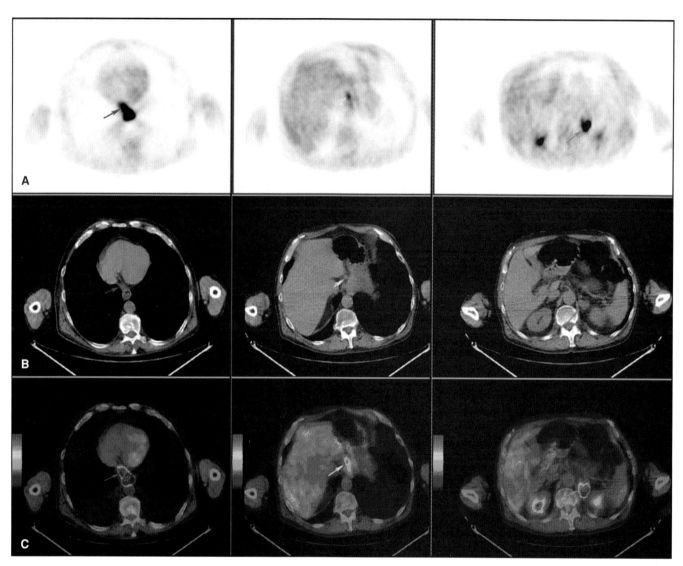

FIGURE 125.61 PET (**A**), coregistered CT (**B**), and fused PET/CT (**C**) images in a patient undergoing primary staging for a lower esophageal cancer. PET/CT demonstrated intense ^{18}F-FDG activity in the primary tumor and metastatic nodal disease in a periesophageal (*red arrows*) and a left gastric node (*yellow arrows*), which were not considered pathologically enlarged on prior staging dedicated CT. A left adrenal lesion was of indeterminate etiology on CT but was intensely ^{18}F-FDG–avid compatible with a distant metastasis (*orange arrows*). Planned curative surgery was avoided and the patient received palliative treatment. The left adrenal metastasis was confirmed by progressive enlargement on serial imaging.

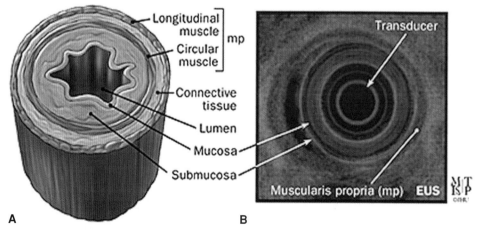

FIGURE 125.62 A: Normal anatomy of the esophageal wall; **B:** Endoscopic ultrasonography (EUS) image.

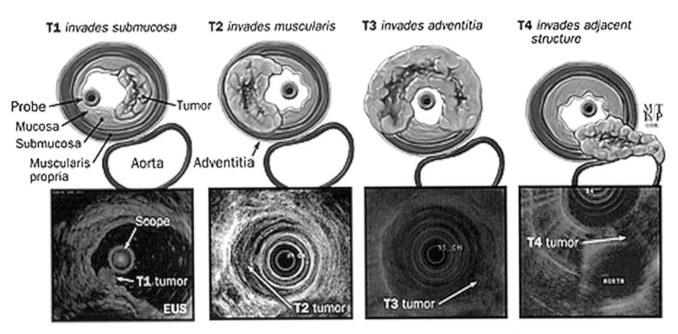

FIGURE 125.63 Esophageal carcinoma staging progression from T1 to T4 with corresponding endoscopic ultrasonography images.

REFERENCES

1. Patterson A, Pearson FG, Cooper JD, et al. *Pearson's Thoracic and Esophageal Surgery.* 3rd ed. Philadelphia, PA: Churchill Livingstone/Elsevier; 2008.
2. Antoch G, Freudenberg LS, Stattaus J, et al. Whole-body positron emission tomography–CT: optimized CT using oral and IV contrast materials. *AJR Am J Roentgenol* 2002;179:1555–1560.
3. Balzarini L, Potepan P, Musumeci RN. Diagnosis and staging of esophageal carcinoma by magnetic resonance imaging. In Meyers MA, ed. *Neoplasms of the Digestive Tract: Imaging, Staging, and Management.* Philadelphia, PA: Lippincott-Raven; 1998:49–59.
4. Levine MS, Rubesin SE, Ott DJ. Update on esophageal radiology. *AJR Am J Roentgenol* 1990;155:933–941.
5. Laufer I. Barium studies of the upper gastrointestinal tract. In Gore RM, Levine MS, eds. *Textbook of Gastrointestinal Radiology.* 2nd ed. Philadelphia, PA: Saunders; 2000:272–284.
6. Brick SH, Caroline DF, Lev-Toaff AS, et al. Esophageal disruption: evaluation with iohexol esophagography. *Radiology* 1988;169:141–143.
7. Aksglaede K, Funch-Jensen P, Vestergaard H, et al. Diagnosis of esophageal motor disorders: a prospective study comparing barium swallow, food barium mixture, and continuous swallows with manometry. *Gastrointest Radiol* 1992;17:1–4.
8. Ghahremani GG. Ingested foreign bodies: radiological diagnosis and management. In Thompson WM, ed. *Common Problems in Gastrointestinal Radiology.* Chicago: Year Book Medical; 1989;152:63–72.
9. Ghahremani GG. Esophageal trauma. *Semin Roentgenol* 1994;29:387–400.
10. Baker ME, Einstein DM, Herts BR, et al. Gastroesophageal reflux disease: integrating the barium esophagram before and after antireflux surgery. *Radiology* 2007;243(2):329–339.
11. Brucher BL, Weber W, Bauer M, et al. Neoadjuvant therapy of esophageal squamous cell carcinoma: response evaluation by positron emission tomography. *Ann Oncol* 2001;233:300–309.
12. Buecker A, Wein BB, Neuerburg JM, et al. Esophageal perforation: comparison of use of aqueous and barium-containing contrast media. *Radiology* 1997;202:683–686.
13. Choi JY, Lee KH, Shim YM, et al. Improved detection of individual nodal involvement in squamous cell carcinoma of the esophagus by FDG-PET. *J Nucl Med* 2000;41:808–815.
14. Ott DJ. Esophageal motility disorders. *Semin Roentgenol* 1994;29:321–331.
15. Ott DJ, Abernethy WB, Chen MY, et al. Radiologic evaluation of esophageal motility in 170 patients with chest pain. *AJR Am J Roentgenol* 1990;155:983–985.
16. Richter JE, Bradley LA, Castell DO. Esophageal chest pain: current controversies in pathogenesis, diagnosis, and therapy. *Ann Intern Med* 1989;110:66–78.
17. Foley MJ, Ghahremani GG, Rogers LF. Reappraisal of contrast media used to detect upper gastrointestinal perforations: comparison of ionic water-soluble media with barium sulfate. *Radiology* 1982;144:231–237.
18. Ghahremani GG. Radiologic evaluation of suspected gastrointestinal perforations. *Radiol Clin North Am* 1993;31:1219–1234.
19. Herlinger H, Grossman R, Laufer I, et al. The gastric cardia in double-contrast study: its dynamic image. *AJR Am J Roentgenol* 1980;135:21–29.
20. Ott DJ, Chen YM, Hewson EG, et al. Esophageal motility assessment with synchronous video tape fluoroscopy and manometry. *Radiology* 1989;173:419–422.
21. Ott DJ, Kelley TF, Chen MY, et al. Evaluation of the esophagus with a marshmallow bolus: clarifying the cause of dysphagia. *Gastrointest Radiol* 1991;16:1–4.
22. Ghahremani GG, Weingardt JP, Curtin KR, et al. Detection of occult esophageal narrowing with barium tablet during chest radiography. *Clin Imaging* 1996;20:184–190.
23. Wilkins T, Gillies RA, Thomas AM, et al. The prevalence of dysphagia in primary care patients: a hamesnet research network study. *J Am Board Fam Med* 2007;20:144–150.
24. Karkos PD, Papouliakos S, Karkos CD, et al. Current evaluation of the dysphagic patient. *Hippokratia* 2009;13:141–146.
25. Allen JE, White C, Leonard R, et al. Comparison of esophageal screen findings on videofluoroscopy with full esophagram results. *Head Neck* 2012;34:264–269.
26. Chen CL, Orr WC. Comparison of esophageal motility in patients with solid dysphagia and mixed dysphagia. *Dysphagia* 2005;20:261–265.
27. Cho TK, Choi MG, Oh SN, et al. Comparisons of bolus transit patterns identified by esophageal impedance to barium esophagram in patients with dysphagia. *Dis Esophagus* 2012;25:17–25.
28. Costa MMB, Nova JLL, Carlos MT, et al. Videofluoroscopy - a new method. *Radiol Bras* 1992;25:11–8.
29. Costa MMB. Estudo qualitativo da deglutição pelo método videofluoroscópico. In: Furkim AM, Santini CRQS. *Disfagias Orofaríngeas.* São Paulo: Pró-Fono; 2008:173–188.
30. Costa MMB. Videofluoroscopy: the gold standard exam for studying swallowing and its dysfunction. *Arq Gastroenterol* 2010;47:327–328.
31. Johnson HD. Active and passive opening of the cardia and its relation to the pathogenesis of hiatus hernia. *Gut.* 1966;7(4):392–401.
32. Gullung JL, Hill EG, Castell DO, et al. Oropharyngeal and esophageal swallowing impairments: their association and the predictive value of the modified barium swallow impairment profile and combined multichannel intraluminal impedance-esophageal manometry. *Ann Otol Rhinol Laryngol* 2012;121:738–745.
33. Jones DB, Mayberry JF, Rhodes J, et al. Preliminary report of an association between measles virus and achalasia. *J Clin Pathol* 1983;36:655–657.
34. Holloway RH, Wyman JB, Dent J. Failure of transient lower oesophageal sphincter relaxation in response to gastric distension in patients with achalasia: evidence for neural mediation of transient lower oesophageal sphincter relaxations. *Gut* 1989;30:762–767.
35. Pandolfino JE, Kahrilas PJ. AGA technical review on the clinical use of esophageal manometry. *Gastroenterology* 2005;128:209–224.
36. Schima W, Ryan JM, Harisinghani M, et al. Radiographic detection of achalasia: diagnostic role of video fluoroscopy. *Clin Radiol* 1998;53:372–375.
37. DeOliveira JMA, Birgisson S, Doinoff C, et al. Timed-barium swallow: a simple technique for evaluating esophageal emptying in patients with achalasia. *AJR Am J Roentgenol* 1997;169:473–479.
38. Stewart ET. Radiographic evaluation of the esophagus and its motor disorders. *Med Clin North Am* 1981;65:1173–1190.
39. Spechler SJ, Castell DO. Classification of oesophageal motility abnormalities. *Gut* 2001;49:145–151.
40. Pandolfino JE, Kwiatek MA, Nealis T, et al. Achalasia: a new clinically relevant classification by high-resolution manometry. *Gastroenterology* 2008;135(5):1526–1533.
41. Kramer P. Diffuse esophageal spasm. In: Bayless TM. *Modern Treatment. Management of Esophageal Disease.* New York: Harper & Row; 1970:1151–1162.

42. Creamer B. Motor disturbances of the esophagus. In: Handbook of physiology, sect. 6, Alimentary canal, vol. IV, Motility, ed. C. F. CODE. Washington, DC: Amer. Physiol. Soc; 1968:2331–2343.

43. Chen YM, Ott DJ, Hewson EG, et al. Diffuse esophageal spasm: radiographic and manometric correlation. *Radiology* 1989;170:807–810.

44. Laufer I. Motor disorders of the esophagus. In: Levine MS, ed. *Radiology of the Esophagus*. Philadelphia, PA: Saunders; 1990:229–246.

45. Miller LS, Parkman HP, Schiano TD, et al. Treatment of symptomatic nonachalasia esophageal motor disorders with botulinum toxin injection at the lower esophageal sphincter. *Dig Dis Sci* 1996;41(10):2025–2031.

46. Bloomston M, Serafini F, Rosemurgy AS. Videoscopic Heller myotomy as first-line therapy for severe achalasia. *Am Surg* 2001;67(11):1105–1109.

47. Ebert EC. Esophageal disease in scleroderma. *J Clin Gastroenterol* 2006;40(9): 769–775.

48. Levine MS. Varices. In: Gore RM, Levine MS, eds. *Textbook of Gastrointestinal Radiology*. 2nd ed. Philadelphia, PA: WB Saunders; 2000:452–463.

49. Wolf G. Die Erkennug von osophagus varizen im rontgenbilde. *Fortsch Roentgenstr Nuklearmed Ergenzungsband* 1928;37:890–893.

50. Ginai AZ, Van Buuren HR, Hop WC, et al. Oesophageal varices: how reliable is a barium swallow?. *Br J Radiol* 1993;66:322–326.

51. In: Gazelle GS, Saini S, Mueller PR, eds. *Hepatobiliary and Pancreatic Radiology: Imaging and Intervention*. New York: Thieme Medical Pub; 1998:294–317.

52. Gore RM, Levine MS, eds. *Textbook of Gastrointestinal Radiology*. 2nd ed. Philadelphia, PA: WB Saunders Co; 2000:454–463.

53. Lee JKT, Sagel SS, Stanley RJ, et al, eds. *Computed Body Tomography with MRI Correlation* Philadelphia, PA: Lippincott Williams & Wilkins; 1998:645–646.

54. Lefkovitz Z, Cappell MS, Kaplan M, et al. Radiology in the diagnosis and therapy of gastrointestinal bleeding. *Gastroenterol Clin North Am* 2000;29(2):489–512.

55. Pieters PC, Miller WJ, DeMeo JH. Evaluation of the portal venous system: complementary roles of invasive and noninvasive imaging strategies. *Radiographics* 1997;17(4):879–895.

56. Hammon JW Jr., Rice RP, Postlethwait RW, et al. Esophageal intramural diverticulosis: a clinical and pathological survey. *Ann Thorac Surg* 1974;17(3):260–267.

57. Watemberg S, Landau O, Avrahami R. Zenker's diverticulum: reappraisal. *Am J Gastroenterol* 1996;91(8):1494–1498.

58. Hafter E. Hiatal hernia. *Digestive diseases and sciences. Am J Dig Dis* 1958;3(12):901–915.

59. Wolf B. Roentgenologic examination of the esophagus. *Am J Gastroenterol* 1957;2:443.

60. Zaino C, Poppel MW, Jacobson HG, et al. *The Lower Esophageal Vestibular Complex*. Springfield, IL: Charles C. Thomas Publisher, 1963.

61. Poppel M, Zaino C, Lentino W. Roentgenologic study of the lower esophagus and esophagogastric junction. *Radiology* 1955;64:690–700.

62. Skandalakis LJ, Skandalakis JE. *Surgery of the Oesophagus*. Edinburgh: Churchill Livingstone; 1988.

63. Mattioli S, Lugaresi ML, Costantini M. The short esophagus: intraoperative assessment of esophageal length. *J Thorac Cardiovasc Surg* 2008;136:834–841.

64. Mattioli S, D'Ovidio F, Pilotti V, et al. Hiatus hernia and intrathoracic migration of esophagogastric junction in gastroesophageal reflux disease. *Dig Dis Sci* 2003;48(9):1823–1831.

65. Levine MS. Gastroesophageal reflux disease. In: Gore RM, Levins MS, eds. *Textbook of Gastrointestinal Radiology*. 2nd ed. Philadelphia, PA: WB Sauders; 2000:329–349.

66. Levine MS, Kressel HY, Caroline DF, et al. Barrett esophagus: reticular pattern of the mucosa. *Radiology* 1983;147:663–667.

67. Chen YM, Gelfand DW, Ott DJ, et al. Barrett esophagus as an extension of severe esophagitis: analysis of radiologic signs in 29 cases. *AJR Am J Roentgenol* 1985;145:275–281.

68. Gilchrist AM, Levine MS, Carr RF, et al. Barrett's esophagus: diagnosis by double-contrast esophagography. *AJR Am J Roentgenol* 1988;150:97–102.

69. Levine MS, Macones AJ, Laufer I. Candida esophagitis: accuracy of radiographic diagnosis. *Radiology* 1985;154:581–587.

70. Vahey TN, Maglinte DDT, Chernish SM. State-of-the-art barium examination in opportunistic esophagitis. *Dig Dis Sci* 1986;31:1192–1195.

71. Shortsleeve MJ, Levine MS. Herpes esophagitis in otherwise healthy patients: clinical and radiographic findings. *Radiology* 1992;182:859–861.

72. Levine MS, Loevner LA, Saul SH, et al. Herpes esophagitis: sensitivity of double contrast esophagography. *AJR Am J Roentgenol* 1988;151:57–62.

73. Balthazar EM, Megibow AJ, Hulnick D, et al. Cytomegalovirus esophagitis in AIDS: radiographic features in 16 patients. *AJR Am J Roentgenol* 1987;149:919–923.

74. Kikendall JW, Friedman AC, Oyewole MA, et al. Pill-induced esophageal injury: case reports and review of the medical literature. *Dig Dis Sci* 1983;28:174–182.

75. Creteur V, Laufer I, Kressel HY, et al. Drug-induced esophagitis detected by double contrast radiography. *Radiology* 1983;147:365–368.

76. Bova JG, Dutton NE, Goldstein HM, et al. Medication-induced esophagitis: diagnosis by double-contrast esophagography. *AJR Am J Roentgenol* 1987;148:731–732.

77. Fox VL, Nurko S, Furuta GT. Eosinophilic esophagitis: it's not just kid 's stuff. *Gastrointest Endosc* 2002;56:260–270.

78. Munitiz V, Martinez de Haro LF, Ortiz A, et al. Primary eosinophilic esophagitis. *Dis Esophagus* 2003;16:165–168.

79. Zimmerman SL, Levine MS, Rubesin SE, et al. Idiopathic eosinophilic esophagitis in adults: the ringed esophagus. *Radiology* 2005;236:159–165.

80. Collazzo LA, Levine MS, Rubesin SE, et al. Acute radiation esophagitis: radiographic findings. *AJR Am J Roentgenol* 1997;169:1067–1070.

81. Levine MS. Other esophagitides. In: Gore RM, Levine MS, eds. *Textbook of Gastrointestinal Radiology*. 2nd ed. Philadelphia, PA: WB Saunders; 2000:364–386.

82. Levine MS. Miscellaneous abnormalities of the esophagus. In: Gore RM, Levine MS, eds. *Textbook of Gastrointestinal Radiology*. 2nd ed. Philadelphia, PA: WB Saunders; 2000:465–483.

83. Totten RS, Stout AP, Humphreys GH II, et al. Benign tumors and cysts of the esophagus. *J Thorac Surg* 1953;25:606–622.

84. Lewis B, Maxfield RG. Leiomyoma of the esophagus. Case report and review of the literature. *Int Abstr Surg* 1954;99:105–128.

85. Storey CF, Adams WC Jr. Leiomyoma of the esophagus. A report of 4 cases and review of the surgical literature. *Am J Surg* 1956;91:3–23.

86. Boyd DP, Hill LD. Benign tumors of the esophagus. *Ann Surg* 1954;139(3): 312–324.

87. Schatzki R, Hawes LE. Tumors of the esophagus below the mucosa and their roentgenological differential diagnosis. *Rev Gastroenterol* 1950;17:991–1014.

88. Livstone EM, Skinner DB. Tumors of the esophagus. In: Berk JE, ed. *Bockus Gastroenterology*. 4th ed. Philadelphia, PA: Saunders; 1985:818–840.

89. Levine MS, Chu P, Furth EE, et al. Carcinoma of the esophagus and esophagogastric junction: sensitivity of radiographic diagnosis. *AJR Am J Roentgenol* 1997;168:1423–1426.

90. Levine MS, Halvorsen RA. Carcinoma of the esophagus. In: Gore RM, Levine MS, eds. *Textbook of Gastrointestinal Radiology*. 2nd ed. Philadelphia, PA: Saunders; 2000:403–433.

91. Levine MS, Dillon EC, Saul SH, et al. Early esophageal cancer. *AJR Am J Roentgenol* 1986;146:507–512.

92. Itai Y, Kogure T, Okuyama Y, et al. Superficial esophageal carcinoma: radiological findings in double-contrast studies. *Radiology* 1978;126:597–601.

93. Gloyna RE, Zornoza J, Goldstein HM. Primary ulcerative carcinoma of the esophagus. *AJR Am J Roentgenol* 1977;129:599–600.

94. Yates CW, LeVine MA, Jensen KM. Varicoid carcinoma of the esophagus. *Radiology* 1977;122:605–608.

95. Levine MS, Caroline D, Thompson JJ, et al. Adenocarcinoma of the esophagus: relationship to Barrett mucosa. *Radiology* 1984;150:305–309.

96. Keen SJ, Dodd GD, Smith JL. Adenocarcinoma arising in Barrett esophagus: pathologic and radiologic features. *Mt Sinai J Med* 1984;51:442–450.

97. Jagmohan P, Goh PS. Benign oesophageal diseases: a review of the CT findings. *Clin Radiol* 2013;68:859–867.

98. Megibow AJ. CT of the gastrointestinal tract: techniques and principles of interpretation. In Gore RM, Levine MS, eds. *Textbook of Gastrointestinal Radiology*. 2nd ed. Philadelphia, PA: Saunders; 2000:77–85.

99. Macpherson RI. Gastrointestinal tract duplications: clinical, pathologic, aetiologic and radiologic considerations. *RadioGraphics* 1993;13:1063–1080.

100. Mosca S, Manes G, Martino R, et al. Endoscopic management of foreign bodies in the upper gastrointestinal tract: report on a series of 414 adult patients. *Endoscopy* 2001;33:692–696.

101. Li ZS, Sun ZX, Zou DW, et al. Endoscopic management of foreign bodies in the upper-GI tract: experience with 1088 cases in China. *Gastrointest Endosc* 2006;64: 485–492.

102. Halber MD, Daffner RH, Thompson WH. CT of the oesophagus: i. Normal appearance. *AJR Am J Roentgenol* 1979;133:1047–1050.

103. Macchi V, Porzianto A, Bardini R, et al. Rupture of ascending aorta secondary to oesophageal perforation by fish bone. *J Forensic Sci* 2008;52:1181–1184.

104. Wu CH, Chen CM, Chen CC, et al. Esophagography after pneumomediastinum without CT findings of esophageal perforation: is it necessary?. *AJR Am J Roentgenol* 2013;201:977–984.

105. Restrepo CS, Lemos DF, Ocazionez D, et al. Intramural haematoma of the oesophagus: a pictorial essay. *Emerg Radiol* 2008;15:13–22.

106. De Lutio di Castelguidone E, Merola S, Pinto A, et al. Oesophageal injuries: spectrum of multidetector row CT findings. *Eur J Radiol* 2006;59:344–348.

107. De Lutio di Castelguidone E, Pinto A, Merola S, et al. Role of spiral and multislice computed tomography in the evaluation of traumatic and spontaneous oesophageal perforation. *Radiol Med* 2005;109:252–259.

108. Garge S, Rao KLN, Bawa M. The role of preoperative CT scan in patients with tracheoesophageal fistula: A review. *J Pediatr Surg* 2013;48:1966–1971.

109. Mahalik SK, Sodhi KS, Narasimhan KL, et al. Role of preoperative 3D CT reconstruction for evaluation of patients with esophageal atresia and tracheoesophageal fistula. *Pediatr Surg Int* 2012;28(10):961–966.

110. Su P, Huang Y, Wang W, et al. The value of preoperative CT scan in newborns with type C esophageal atresia. *Pediatr Surg Int* 2012;28(7):677–80.

111. Ratan SK, Varshney A, Mullick S, et al. Evaluation of neonates with esophageal atresia using chest CT scan. *Pediatr Surg Int* 2004;20(10):757–761.

112. Fitoz S, Atasoy C, Yagmurlu A, et al. Three dimensional CT of congenital esophageal atresia and distal tracheoesophageal fistula in neonates: preliminary results. *AJR Am J Roentgenol* 2000;175(5):1403–1407.

113. Lam WW, Tam PK, Chan FL, et al. Esophageal atresia and tracheal stenosis: use of three-dimensional CT and virtual bronchoscopy on neonates, infants, and children. *AJR Am J Roentgenol* 2000;174(4):1009–1012.

114. Tam PK, Chan FL, Saing H. Diagnosis and evaluation of esophageal atresia by direct sagittal CT. *Pediatr Radiol* 1987;17(1):68–70.

115. Johnson JF, Sueoka BL, Mulligan ME, et al. Tracheoesophageal fistula: diagnosis with CT. *Pediatr Radiol* 1985;15(2):134–135.

116. Luo CC, Lin JN, Wang CR. Evaluation of oesophageal atresia without fistula by three-dimensional computed tomography. *Eur J Pediatr* 2002;161(11):578–580.

117. Kohn GP, Price RR, DeMeester SR, et al. Guidelines for the management of hiatal hernia. *Surg Endosc* 2013;27:4409–4428.

118. Eren S, Ciris F. Diaphragmatic hernia: diagnostic approaches with review of the literature. *Eur J Radiol* 2005;54:448–459.

119. Ming SC. Tumours of oesophagus and stomach. *Atlas of Tumour Pathology, Fascicle 7*. Washington, DC: Armed Forces Institute of Pathology; 1973:16–23.

120. Plachta A. Benign tumours of the oesophagus: review of the literature and report of 99 cases. *Am J Gastroenterol* 1962;38:639–652.

121. Goldstein HM, Zornoza J, Hopens T. Intrinsic diseases of the adult oesophagus: benign and malignant tumours. *Semin Roentgenol* 1981;16:183–197.

122. Megibow AJ, Balthazar EJ, Hulnick DH, et al. CT evaluation of gastrointestinal leiomyomas and leiomyosarcomas. *AJR Am J Roentgenol* 1985;144:727–731.

123. Moersch HJ, Harrington SW. Benign tumor of the esophagus. *Ann Otol* 1944;53:800–817.

124. Gallinger S, Steinhardt MI, Goldger M. Giant leiomyoma of the esophagus. *Am J Gastroenterol* 1983;78:708–711.

125. Carillas J, Joseph RC, Guerra JJ. CT appearance of uterine leiomyomas. *RadioGraphics* 1990;10:999–1007.

126. Kim TJ, Kim HY, Lee KW, et al. Multimodality assessment of esophageal cancer: preoperative staging and monitoring of response to therapy. *RadioGraphics* 2009;29(2):403–421.

127. Noh HM, Fishman EK, Forastiere AA, et al. CT of the esophagus: spectrum of disease with emphasis on esophageal carcinoma. *RadioGraphics* 1995;15: 1113–1134.

128. Desai RK, Tagliabue JR, Wegryn SA, et al. CT evaluation of wall thickening in the alimentary tract. *RadioGraphics* 1991;11:771–783.

129. Wakelin SJ, Deans C, Crofts TJ, et al. A comparison of computerised tomography, laparoscopic ultrasound and endoscopic ultrasound in the preoperative staging of oesophago-gastric carcinoma. *Eur J Radiol* 2002;41:161–167.

130. Wallace MB, Nietert PJ, Earle C, et al. An analysis of multiple staging management strategies for carcinoma of the esophagus: computed tomography, endoscopic ultrasound, positron emission tomography, and thoracoscopy/laparoscopy. *Ann Thorac Surg* 2002;74:1026–1032.

131. Berger AC, Scott WJ. Noninvasive staging of esophageal carcinoma. *J Surg Res* 2004;117:127–133.

132. Rice TW. Clinical staging of esophageal carcinoma. CT, EUS, and PET. *Chest Surg Clin N Am* 2000;10:471–485.

133. Picus D, Balfe DM, Koehler RE, et al. Computed tomography in the staging of esophageal carcinoma. *Radiology* 1983;146:433–438.

134. Takahashi S, Takeuchi N, Shiozaki H, et al. Carcinoma of the esophagus: CT vs MR imaging in determining resectability. *AJR Am J Roentgenol* 1991;156:297–302.

135. Halvorsen RA Jr., Magruder-Habib K, Foster WL Jr., et al. Esophageal cancer staging by CT: long-term follow-up study. *Radiology* 1986;161:147–151.

136. Dehdashti F, Siegel BA. PET and PET/CT imaging in esophageal and gastric cancers. *Positron Emission Tomography* 2006:165–180.

137. Bar-Shalom R, Yefremov N, Guralnik L, et al. Clinical performance of PET/CT in evaluation of cancer: additional value for diagnostic imaging and patient management. *J Nucl Med* 2003;44:1200–1209.

138. Antoch G, Saoudi N, Kuehl H, et al. Accuracy of whole-body dual modality fluorine-18-2-fluoro-2-deoxy-D-glucose positron emission tomography and computed tomography (FDG-PET/CT) for tumor staging in solid tumors: comparison with CT and PET. *J Clin Oncol* 2004;22:4357–4368.

139. Duignan JP, McEntee GP, O'Connell DJ, et al. The role of CT in the management of carcinoma of the oesophagus and cardia. *Ann R Coll Surg Engl* 1987;69:286–288.

140. Flanagan FL, Dehdashti F, Siegel BA, et al. Staging of esophageal cancer with FDG-PET. *AJR Am J Roentgenol* 1997;168:417–424.

141. Block MI, Sundaresan SR, Patterson GA, et al. Improvement in staging of esophageal cancer with the addition of positron emission tomography. *Ann Thorac Surg* 1997;64:770–777.

142. Kole AC, Plukker JT, Nieweg OE, et al. Positron emission tomography for staging oesophageal and gastroesophageal malignancy. *Br J Cancer* 1998;74:521–527.

143. Luketich JD, Schauer P, Meltzer CC, et al. The role of positron emission tomography in staging esophageal cancer. *Ann Thorac Surg* 1997;64:765–769.

144. Rankin SC, Taylor H, Cook GJR, et al. Computed tomography and positron emission tomography in the pre-operative staging of oesophageal carcinoma. *Clin Radiol* 1998;53:659–665.

145. Yeung HWD, Macapinlac HA, Mazumdar M, et al. FDG-PET in esophageal cancer: incremental value over computed tomography. *Clin Positron Imaging* 1999;2(5):255–260.

146. Flamen P, Lerut A, Van Cutsem E, et al. Utility of positron emission tomography for the staging of patients with potentially operable esophageal carcinoma. *J Clin Oncol* 2000;18:3202–3210.

147. McAteer D, Wallis F, Couper G, et al. Evaluation of 18F-FDG positron emission tomography in gastric and oesophageal carcinoma. *Br J Radiol* 1999;72:525–529.

148. Räsänen JV, Sihvo EIT, Knuuti J, et al. Prospective analysis of accuracy of positron emission tomography, computed tomography, and endoscopic ultrasonography in staging of adenocarcinoma of the esophagus and the esophagogastric junction. *Ann Surg Oncol* 2003;10:954–960.

149. Meltzer CC, Luketich JD, Friedman D, et al. Whole-body FDG positron emission tomographic imaging for staging esophageal cancer comparison with computed tomography. *Clin Nucl Med* 2000;25:882–887.

150. Morosini D. Post-chemo PET scans may not be optimal in esophageal cancer. *Oncology Times* 2008;30(7):45.

151. Sun F, Chen T, Han J, et al. Staging accuracy of endoscopic ultrasound for esophageal cancer after neoadjuvant chemotherapy: a meta-analysis and systematic review. *Dis Esophagus* 2015;28:757–771. doi: 10.1111/dote.12274.

152. Vazquez-Sequeiros E. Optimal staging of esophageal cancer. *Ann Gastroenterol* 2010;23(4):230–236.

153. Pera M, Cameron AJ, Trastek VF, et al. Increasing incidence of adenocarcinoma of the esophagus and esophagogastric junction. *Gastroenterology* 1993;104:510–513.

154. Blot WJ, Devesa SS, Kneller RW, et al. Rising incidence of adenocarcinoma of the esophagus and gastric cardia. *JAMA* 1991;265:1287–1289.

155. Forastiere AA, Heitmiller RF, Kleinberg L. Multimodality therapy for esophageal cancer. *Chest* 1997;112:195S–200S.

156. Pommier RF, Vetto JT, Ferris BL, et al. Relationships between operative approaches and outcomes in esophageal cancer. *Am J Surg* 1998;175:422–425.

157. Kimmey MB, Martin EW, Haggitt RC, et al. Histological correlates of gastrointestinal endoscopic ultrasound images. *Gastroenterology* 1989;96:433–441.

158. Hasegawa N, Niwa Y, Arisawa T, et al. Preoperative staging of superficial esophageal carcinoma: comparison of an ultrasound probe and standard endoscopic ultrasonography. *Gastrointest Endosc* 1996;44:388–393.

159. Murata Y, Suzuki S, Ohta M, et al. Small ultrasonic probes for determination of depth 2 of superficial esophageal cancer. *Gastrointest Endosc* 1996;44:23–28.

160. Tajima Y, Nakanishi Y, Ochiai A, et al. Histopathologic findings predicting lymph node metastasis and prognosis of patients with superficial esophageal carcinoma: analysis of 240 surgically resected tumors. *Cancer* 2000;88:1285–1293.

161. Tio TL. Diagnosis and staging of esophageal carcinoma by endoscopic ultrasonography. *Endoscopy* 1998;30:A33–A40.

162. Catalano MF, Sivak MV Jr., Bedford RA, et al. Observer variation and reproducibility of endoscopic ultrasonography. *Gastrointest Endosc* 1995;41:115–120.

163. Palazzo L, Burtin P. Interobserver variation in tumor staging. *Gastrointest Endosc Clin North Am* 1995;5:559–567.

164. Fockens PF, Van den Brande J, van Dullemen HM, et al. Endosonographic T-staging of esophageal carcinoma: a learning curve. *Gastrointest Endosc* 1996;44:58–62.

165. Massari M, Cioffi U, De Simone M, et al. Endoscopic ultrasonography for preoperative staging of esophageal carcinoma. *Surg Laparosc Endosc* 1997;7:162–165.

166. Semelka RC, Brown MA, Altun E. Gastrointestinal tract. In Semelka RC, ed. *Abdominal–Pelvic MRI*. New York: Wiley-Liss; 2002:319–372.

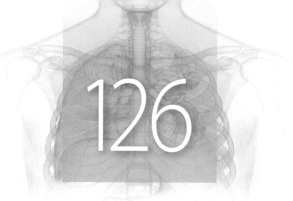

126

Endoscopy of the Esophagus

Donna E. Maziak ▪ Farid M. Shamji

INTRODUCTION

Diseases of the esophagus present fewer difficult clinical problems than elsewhere in the alimentary tract. This is due to its relative simplicity—a hollow muscular tube, about 23 to 25 cm long, stretching from the pharynx to the stomach and having specialized sphincters at each end with different functions; a true anatomic sphincter at the proximal end and a physiological sphincter at the distal end. It is readily accessible to investigation by barium contrast x-rays, computerized scan with oral contrast, esophagogastroscopy, and esophageal function studies with high-resolution manometry and 24-hour pH or 24-hour impedance pH studies.

The esophagus has relatively simple function in health; it conveys the bolus of food to the stomach by active peristalsis within 6 to 8 seconds rather than by gravity alone. Bolus transit can be impaired when there is an abnormality of neuromuscular mechanism as in achalasia, ineffective esophageal motility (IEM) disorder, or diabetic autonomic neuropathy; due to intrinsic disease in the wall of the esophagus as in connective tissue disorders, eosinophilic esophagitis (EoE), chronic reflux esophagitis and peptic stricture formation, fixed hiatus hernia, benign and malignant neoplasm, and caustic ingestion; or due to extrinsic pressure from a mass in the thoracic inlet or in the middle and posterior mediastinum.

Sensations from the esophagus readily reach consciousness. Heartburn is an intense and unpleasant substernal burning sensation, which lasts for a few seconds to minutes, and is due to the corrosive effect of regurgitating gastric juice. Severe substernal pain, identical to that of coronary artery disease, can arise from distension of the lower esophagus by reflux of gastric contents, secondary esophageal spasm, or by primary hypercontractile esophageal motility disturbance. Difficulty in swallowing, as a sensation, is a precise symptom that must never be ignored. It is ominous in early or later life and often infers cancer. Fixed hiatus hernia, EoE, and achalasia of the cardia can be benign causes of dysphagia.

CLINICAL PRESENTATION OF ESOPHAGEAL DISEASES

The three symptoms indicating presence of esophageal disease—frequent episodes of severe heart burn due to pathological reflux disorder, atypical substernal chest pain that cannot be distinguished from customary angina by patients, and difficulty in swallowing—require special attention to clinical history before proceeding to focused investigations. The entire length of the esophagus is not accessible for physical examination because the esophagus, except for 2 cm in the neck posterior to the trachea and 3 cm in the abdomen within the tunnel of the diaphragmatic crura, is deep in the posterior mediastinum behind the heart; even the proximal and distal portion cannot be examined by hand. It is required that correct diagnosis be established from clinical history and specific investigations before appropriate treatment can be recommended. The investigations to be performed must support the clinical diagnosis. Accurate diagnosis is usually possible if the taking of a careful clinical history is combined with a thorough radiographic examination with a solid bolus of barium. This is followed by direct inspection of the interior of the esophagus by endoscopy which is often necessary. Functional assessment of esophagus requires high-resolution manometry and 24-hour esophageal acid pH study, 24-hour impedance pH study or reflux testing with wireless Bravo system for 24 to 96 hours.

A BRIEF HISTORY OF ENDOSCOPY AND ITS APPLICATION

Endoscopy (EGD) is used widely for the diagnosis and treatment in esophageal, gastric, and small bowel disorders. In 2009, approximately 7 million EGD procedures were performed in the USA at a cost of $12.3 billion.[1] In the first decade of the new millennium, there was a 50% increase in the utilization of the EGD. With this, is an ever-expanding increase in the indications and utilization of EGD, with an even greater and more invasive application?

RIGID ESOPHAGOSCOPY

The instrument and the technique as we now know was the work of Johann von Mikulicz (most outstanding surgeon of his time after his mentor Billroth) and J. Leiter (instrument maker) in 1881.[2] This was preceded by the work of A. Kussmaul in 1865 who studied a sword—swallower in order to design modification of his original instrument to access the stomach.[3] Mikulicz was quick to recognize in 1881 that much patience, considerable skill, and minimal pressure without undue force were critical to avoid damage in the cricopharyngeal sphincter. The clinical observations made by Mikulicz during endoscopy speaks well of his skill and clinical acumen. He observed physiological nature of the esophagus and pathological entities such as foreign bodies, cancer, and esophageal obstruction from extrinsic pressure due to the lung, mediastinal nodal metastases, and even descending thoracic aortic aneurysm.

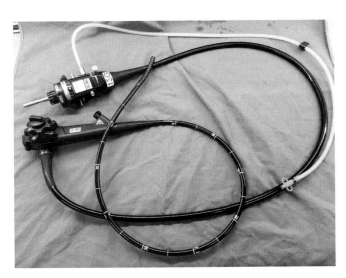

FIGURE 126.1 Flexible esophagogastroscopy.

FLEXIBLE ESOPHAGOGASTROSCOPY

The word endoscopy is derived from Greek and it means within (endo) and skopien (to view). The development of fiber optic endoscope and the use of the first prototype instrument to look at the inside of his own stomach by Basil Hirschowitz in 1957 are credited to Hopkins and Kapany of the Imperial College in London (they dealt with advances in fiber optics) and Basil Hirschowitz, Marvin Pollard, C. Wilbur Peters, and Larry Curtis (University of Michigan, Ann Arbor), designing and perfecting glass fibers.[4] It was in October 1960 when the first production model was developed and considered acceptable for clinical use as fiberscope. It was not until 1968 and later that it became, with controllable tip model and proper channel size for suction and instillation of air or water to facilitate insufflating the stomach and keeping the lens clear and obtain biopsy specimens, adequate length, flexibility, and acceptable scope diameter that widespread use became a reality. Diagnostic accuracy of the esophageal mucosal diseases has been enhanced by the advances in the technology (Fig. 126.1).

PERCUTANEOUS ENDOSCOPIC GASTROSTOMY

Gastrocutaneous fistulae arising spontaneously or after penetrating injury were subject of interest for studying digestion by Jacob Helm in 1803 and gastric secretion by William Beaumont in 1822.[5] Therapeutic human gastrostomy for providing nutrition or for gastric outlet obstruction came into existence in 1849, first successfully performed by Charles Sedillot.[6] It became a popular and useful operation, and in the beginning it carried substantial morbidity and mortality. Percutaneous "incisionless" gastrostomy was developed in the pediatric patients by Jeffrey Ponsky and Michael Gauderer in 1980.[7] Since then it has become safe and effective operation in hospitalized patients, patients requiring head and neck operations for cancer, and for patients with severe neurological disorders with inability to swallow without aspiration.

ENDOSCOPIC ULTRASOUND

Endoscopic ultrasound (EUS) utilizes the principle of ultrasonic transducers and detectors based on the fundamental observations of flying bats at night without striking obstacles (guidance system was auditory rather than visual from observation made in 1794 by L. Spallanzani) and discovery of piezoelectric effect (Pierre and Jacques Curie in 1880 experimenting with oscillating current across quartz crystal and generating sound waves).[8] Experimental observation of gall stones by George Ludwig led to the successful identification of the layers of the bowel wall by John J. Wild.[9] Doppler ultrasound, to quantify flow as well as tissue characteristics was followed by development of internal probes by R Uchida and Hiroki Watanabe.[10,11] Current types of EUS equipment support pulse and color Doppler functions as well as fine needle aspiration of the submucosal tumors and mediastinal lymph nodes. Staging of esophageal cancer has been enhanced for the two descriptors: T status (depth of mural invasion) and N status (lymphatic spread), very important now in the planning of the standard of care for esophageal cancer by induction treatment before resection.

VIDEO CAPSULE ENDOSCOPY

Video capsule endoscopy (VCE) was first introduced in clinical practice in 2001 for diseases of the small bowel. In 2004, an esophageal capsule was introduced and is being used in clinical applications.[12] VCE involves a capsule containing a video camera, a sensing system with sensor pads, data recorder and battery pack, and a work station with a computer. The main indications are for screening of Barrett esophagus and of esophageal varices. However, the sensitivity of esophageal VCE has been quite variable, ranging from 60% to 100% in Barrett esophagus and from 50% to 89% for erosive esophagitis.

ABSOLUTE REQUIREMENTS BEFORE CONDUCTING ENDOSCOPIC EXAMINATION OF THE ESOPHAGUS

Attention to details in the taking of careful clinical history combined with a thorough radiographic examination and exercising good judgment, considerable endoscopic skills and recognizing the virtue of patience during endoscopy, and blessed with knowledge of esophageal diseases are the absolute requirements for any surgeon, otolaryngologist, or gastroenterologist in order to perform safe and effective endoscopic examination of the esophagus, stomach, and first and second part of duodenum proximal to the Ampulla of Vater. The examination may be for establishing diagnosis, for endoscopic mucosal resection (EMR) for metaplastic and dysplastic Barrett epithelium, for assessing the results of medical and surgical treatment, for planning Botox injection or pneumatic dilatation in achalasia, for therapeutic removal of foreign bodies, dilating benign strictures, or insertion of esophageal stents, or for Per oral endoscopic myotomy (POEM) for achalasia.

It is unwise to proceed to endoscopy without first conducting a thorough direct inspection of mouth and oropharynx; inflammatory or neoplastic lesions, or neurological cause should be ruled out. Equally important is the clinical examination of the neck (searching for goiter or enlarged lymph nodes), chest, and abdomen (epigastric mass). The esophagus is not accessible to physical examination due to its location and course. It begins just behind the cricoid cartilage in the neck at the level of the sixth cervical vertebra as a continuation of the hypopharynx. It descends through the neck (in the thoracic inlet posterior to the trachea), thorax (in the mediastinum behind the trachea first and then the heart) and diaphragm (in the esophageal hiatus). This the reason why thorough radiographic studies are essential before endoscopic examination; beginning with chest x-ray looking for mass in the lung or the mediastinum, esophageal dilatation, and for evidence of aspiration pneumonia; CT chest and upper abdomen with oral contrast enhancement for detailed assessment of the esophagus and its regional anatomy and relationship in the mediastinum; and from the barium swallow, the anatomical assessment of the embryological foregut derivatives—esophagus, stomach, and proximal duodenum to guide safe endoscopic examination and minimize the risk of aspiration pneumonia and inadvertent esophageal perforation.

MANDATORY PROCEDURAL PROTOCOL IN ENDOSCOPY OF THE ESOPHAGUS

It is recognized that the risk to the patient undergoing endoscopic examination must be minimal and acceptable to the institution ultimately responsible for the care of the patient. The physician has a responsibility to comply with professional standards of practice and participate in quality improvement assurance program.

It requires that the responsible physician has received proper training in endoscopic examination of the esophagus, in both diagnostic and therapeutic. For this to be so, it is necessary to understand how the endoscope works and the general principles of endoscopy. The physician must have knowledge of preprocedural clinical evaluation of the patient's history and physical findings in order to minimize the risk of adverse outcomes. This is important in the use of sedation for the procedure and equally important in understanding the pharmacology of drugs used for conscious sedation. The physician performing the endoscopy is responsible in ensuring that patient preparation is correct to improve safety and success of the procedure. Adverse events inherent with endoscopic procedures to be avoided are hypoxemia, hemodynamic instability, pulmonary aspiration, and inadvertent esophageal perforation. Safety prevails and the risk to the patient should be minimized.

The physician responsible for the endoscopy must be well educated in the use of biopsy forceps, different types of dilators in current use for the esophageal stricture, techniques of safe pneumatic dilatation and Botox injection, different types of stents available, and techniques for insertion and retrieval. More advanced endoscopic skills include percutaneous endoscopic gastrostomy (PEG), POEM, EMR, EUS as well as a vast array of emerging technologies.

ENDOSCOPY IN THE ASSESSMENT OF ESOPHAGEAL DISEASES

The clinical problems for which diagnostic endoscopic examination of esophagus is required are discussed below:

PATHOLOGIC GASTROESOPHAGEAL REFLUX DISEASE

Chronic damage to the squamous esophageal mucosa by frequent spontaneous, postural, and postprandial back flow of gastric contents—acid, pepsin, bile, and conjugated bile salts—into the esophagus may result in ulcerative esophagitis, formation of esophageal peptic stricture, and formation of specialized intestinal metaplasia representing Barrett esophagus. It is the formation of Barrett epithelium which is now of major health concern because it carries the rising risk of malignant change to adenocarcinoma. The complications developing in Barrett epithelium include true peptic ulcer which can penetrate,

perforate and bleed, and malignant transformation from low-grade to high-grade dysplasia, carcinoma in-situ, and finally invasive adenocarcinoma. The cell of origin of intestinal metaplasia is unknown. The mechanism whereby gastric refluxate triggers metaplasia and why this occurs in some but not all individuals with GERD is unknown. The transcription factor CDX2 induced by conjugated bile salts penetrating into the deeper layers of mucosa when squamous epithelium is rendered permeable by refluxing acid is believed to play a role in promoting intestinal metaplasia.

Barrett epithelium is an acquired condition caused by chronic gastroesophageal reflux disease. It has well-recognized association with adenocarcinoma of the esophagus, the incidence of which continues to increase in North America, Europe, and Australia. Studies show that the incidence of this cancer has increased sixfold between 1975 and 2001 accompanied by an increase in mortality from 2 to 15 deaths per million. The 5-year survival rate for this cancer is low when it is clinically detected at the stage when it is advanced disease. Therefore, it is required that the presence of this premalignant metaplastic, specialized intestinal epithelium be documented in all high-risk individuals and search is made for early neoplastic change in dysplasia and early mucosal adenocarcinoma: those at risk are white obese male patients over the age of 50 years who have long standing reflux disorder beginning at an earlier age, increased duration of reflux symptoms, and increased severity of nocturnal reflux symptoms.

The necessity of esophageal mucosal biopsy to confirm visual pathology identified by barium study or endoscopy is important in management. It is the confirmation of presence or absence of Barrett epithelium and neoplastic transformation within it that is necessary for management and this is only possible by careful endoscopic examination in screening or surveillance protocols such as schematic representation in Prague classification; this uses C descriptor (indicating circumferential extent of metaplasia) and M descriptor (indicating the maximum extent of metaplasia), and random and targeted mucosal biopsies according to the Seattle protocol (four-quadrant biopsies at 2-cm intervals every 2 years if only metaplasia is present and four-quadrant biopsies at 1-cm intervals once a year when low-grade dysplastic changes are noted in the Barrett epithelium).[13,14] In order to make meaningful gain in achieving high cure rate, the malignant change must be detected early before cancer invades deep into the submucosa and gains foothold in the lymphatics and venous plexus. This is where attention to details during endoscopy becomes vital. It begins with a physician who is well trained in conventional and advanced endoscopic techniques and diligently follows the defined endoscopic protocols of documentation of mucosal abnormalities and obtains and appropriately labels the mucosal biopsies. After this, it will depend on the expertise of the pathologist for histological interpretation and guidance. The importance of pathology in the management of metaplastic and dysplastic Barrett epithelium cannot be underestimated. Finally, it will be up to the knowledgeable foregut surgeon and gastroenterologist to coordinate complete care of the patients (Fig. 126.2).

Several advanced endoscopic diagnostic technologies for Barrett esophagus for imaging and endotherapy are now available and knowledge of application of these is necessary. Conventional white-light video endoscopy of the esophagus for detection of early premalignant lesions in Barrett esophagus, dysplasia, and carcinoma in situ, has limitation and miss rates are high. This is unacceptable in modern times if cure for esophageal cancer is to become a reality.

Two different types of electronically enhanced endoscopic imaging technologies have evolved for both detection and accurate characterization and confirmation of early precursor preneoplastic lesions.

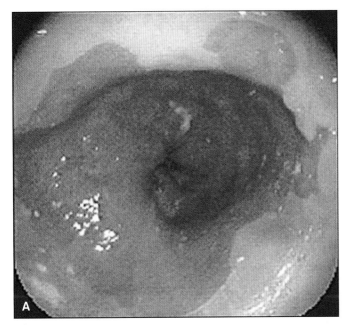

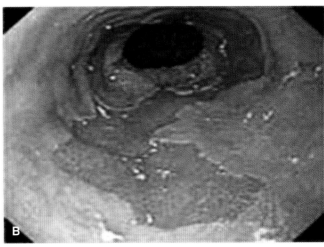

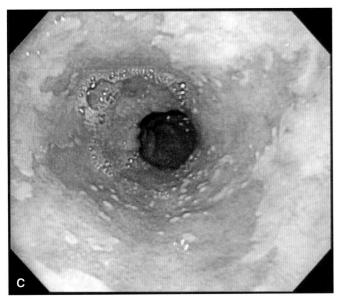

FIGURE 126.2 Applying Prague Classification, all images represent C2M5, 2 cm circumferential extent of metaplasia and 5 cm maximal extent of metaplasia from the true gastroesophageal junction.

The advantage is promising real-time "optical biopsy." One type is broad field enhancement techniques with narrow band imaging (NBI), autofluorescence imaging (AFI), and endoscopic trimodal imaging (ETMI). The second type is high-resolution imaging with confocal laser endomicroscopy (CLE), optical coherence tomography (OCT), contact light microscopy (CLM), and volumetric laser endomicroscopy (Nvision VLE). These techniques require specific endoscopic training for competency.

Broad Field Enhancement

Narrow Band Imaging

This technology was developed by Gono and colleagues[15] in 1999 by collaboration of Olympus Corporation and Japanese National Cancer Center. Using optical filters instead of dyes to narrow the bandwidths (415 and 540 nm) of white light to blue-green light (415 and 540 nm) for superficial penetration and the ability to visualize mucosal capillaries and subepithelial vascular patterns, it is possible to detect early changes of angiogenesis associated with the development of dysplasia

and intramucosal cancer in Barrett epithelium. NBI has high sensitivity and specificity (94% to 100% and 75% to 99%) for detection of neoplasia. Fewer biopsies per patient are required by using this technology; mean 8.5 biopsy samples per case with standard resolution endoscopy versus mean 4.7 biopsy specimens per case with NBI-directed biopsy.

Autofluorescence Imaging

The intent of AFI endoscopy is to increase the diagnostic yield in surveillance endoscopy to detect dysplastic changes in Barrett epithelium. The technique utilizes the differences in fluorescence emission to distinguish different tissue types. It depends on interactions of incident short wavelength blue light (390 to 470 nm) with endogenous tissue "fluorophores" (stroma) producing emission of fluorescent light of a longer wavelength that is captured by the endoscope and processor. The optical signals produced depend on the structure and composition of the tissues being excited. Neoplasia, changes the composition of the stromal tissue, resulting in loss of fluorescence (magenta) whereas normal tissues emit green fluorescence. AFI has a 91% sensitivity and 43% specificity.[16]

Endoscopic Trimodal Imaging

ETMI combines high-definition white light endoscopy (HD-WLE) with virtual chemoendoscopy with NBI and AFI for detection of high-grade dysplasia and early cancer in Barrett epithelium. Curvers and colleagues[17] reported on use of ETMI in 2010 and found that targeted detection rate was better (65% vs. 45%) but overall neoplasia detection rate was similar (84% vs. 72%). Unfortunately, it had the disadvantage of more false positives (71% vs. 53%). The total ETMI time was 20 minutes compared to HD-WLE 12 minutes.

High Resolution Imaging

Confocal Laser Endomicroscopy

This is endoscope based by Pentax (pCLE) and probe based by Mauna Kea Tech (pCLE), permitting real-time subcellular imaging with enhanced specificity of esophageal mucosa and in vivo histopathology during endoscopy.[18] It allows detailed submucosal analysis. This has the advantage of replacing conventional biopsies. It focuses on increased spatial resolution with illumination and detection systems on the same plane and avoiding contamination by light scattering from other planes. Images are obtained by excitation of fluorescent molecule using intravenous contrast agent (Fluorescein 1.0 to 5.0 mL of 10% solution). CLE has been combined with NBI for detection of subtle mucosal abnormalities and localized lesions and in vivo histology in Barrett esophagus. Both sensitivity and specificity are very high, and detection of presence of neoplastic lesions is more accurate; the sensitivity and specificity for the prediction of nondysplastic Barrett epithelium is 98% and 94% and for neoplastic changes it is 93% and 98%.

Optical Coherence Tomography

OCT is based on similar principles of interferometry and ultrasound using near-infrared light to produce high-resolution images of esophageal mucosa in vivo.[19] Contrast medium is not used and there is no tissue contact. It permits up to 2-mm depth tissue penetration and provides 2- to 4-μm spatial resolution and cross-sectional imaging. It is unable to sample large areas rapidly. Clinical application is limited because of intensity of back scattered light at various depths. It has 68% sensitivity and 82% specificity. Positive predicted value is 53% and negative predicted value is 89%.

Nvision—Volumetric Laser Endomicroscopy

VLE-Fourier domain interferometry is 100 times faster than traditional OCT (time domain interferometry).[20] VLE provides high-resolution, cross-sectional, and real-time imaging of tissue: resolution of 7 microns, imaging depth of 3 mm into tissue, and volumetric imaging of >10,000 mm³ in less than 90 seconds. Optical probe enables volumetric (circumferential and longitudinal) scan over 6 cm length.

Endocystoscopy

This requires first administering mucolytic agent N-acetyl cysteine and then spraying 0.5% methylene blue (MB) with a spray catheter, and 2 minutes later the mucosa is washed off.[21] MB binds to absorptive epithelium present in Barrett intestinal metaplasia. In Barrett epithelium, the two areas of interest are to identify intestinal epithelium (positive staining) and to detect dysplasia by negative staining. The aim is to obtain targeted mucosal biopsies. There is limited data in Barrett esophagus to support wide use because the dysplasia detection rate is similar with MB versus four-quadrant biopsy. MB may be useful in identifying apparent or possible short-segment Barrett esophagus.

SCREENING AND SURVEILLANCE OF BARRETT EPITHELIUM

Metaplastic Barrett epithelium is acquired as the consequence of chronic gastroesophageal reflux disorder. The refluxate responsible is in the gastric juice consisting of acid, pepsin, bile acids, and conjugated bile salts. It is the unpredictable progression to dysplasia in Barrett epithelium that is worrisome for subsequent development of adenocarcinoma of the esophagus. Careful assessment with endoscopy is not only essential but mandatory, and mucosal biopsies must be obtained for histological confirmation of the abnormal epithelium starting at the cardia of the stomach at the esophagogastric junction (EGJ) and extending proximally for the entire length of the columnar mucosa. The hallmark of Barrett epithelium is the presence of goblet cells in the biopsied mucosa reported by the pathologist. The correct endoscopic technique is four-quadrant mapping mucosal biopsies taken according to the Seattle protocol at 1-cm intervals for dysplastic Barrett epithelium and at 2-cm intervals for metaplastic Barrett epithelium with a 2-mm cup biopsy forceps; each biopsy site at each level is to be marked separately.[14] For future reference, schematic representation in Prague classification using C descriptor (indicating circumferential extent of metaplasia) and M descriptor (indicating the maximum extent of metaplasia) must be recorded.[13] The guidelines for frequency of surveillance of Barrett epithelium have been defined according to the presence of metaplasia, low-grade dysplasia, high-grade dysplasia, and carcinoma in situ. Added to the surveillance endoscopy is the accepted method of EMR of the dysplastic Barrett epithelium for detecting intramucosal and invasive submucosal adenocarcinoma, both important in T staging of esophageal adenocarcinoma and frontline treatment of mucosal adenocarcinoma without lymphatic spread. The technique of EMR is described as focal EMR, multiband mucosectomy (MBM), widespread EMR (w-EMR), and complete Barrett's eradication (CBE-EMR). The advantages of EMR are physical removal of dysplastic epithelium or intramucosal adenocarcinoma and accurate focal pathologic T staging. The disadvantages are risk of bleeding, perforation, stricture formation all likely related to lack of expertise and not paying attention to details. The good prognostic factors in EMR pathology are lesion size <2 cm, well-differentiated carcinoma, lesion limited to mucosa (m type), and no vascular and lymphatic invasion.

The guidelines for frequency of surveillance of Barrett epithelium have been defined according to the presence of metaplasia, low-grade dysplasia, high-grade dysplasia, and carcinoma in situ. The use of chromoendoscopy, enhanced endoscopic imaging for targeted biopsies, and VCE all show promise in surveillance.

Morphological classification from endoscopic appearance of superficial cancer suggesting that invasion is limited to the mucosa or submucosal (T0) was accepted in a joint meeting in 2002 in Paris and is referred to as The Paris Classification (Figs. 126.3 and 126.4).[22]

Morphologic Appearance	Type
Protruding	
Pedunculated	0–Ip
Sessile	0–Is
Non-protruding and non-excavated	
Slightly elevated	0–IIa
Completely flat	0–IIb
Depressed	0–IIc
Excavated	0–III

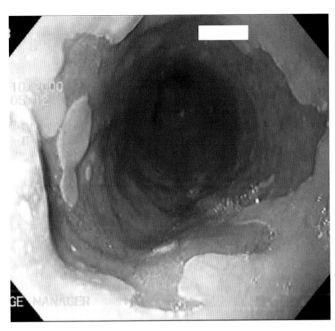

FIGURE 126.3 Barrett esophagus.

ENDOSCOPIC ABLATION MODALITIES FOR DYSPLASTIC BARRETT EPITHELIUM

Endoscopic therapy for BE includes techniques that ablate the mucosa (photodynamic therapy [PDT], multipolar coagulation, argon plasma coagulator [APC], radiofrequency energy, cryotherapy with either liquid nitrogen or carbon dioxide) and others that resect the mucosa, either endoscopic mucosal (EMR) or submucosal resection (ESD). EMR is often applied in situations of a short segment of dysplastic BE, superficial esophageal carcinoma in situ, and for esophageal squamous carcinoma. Ablative techniques are usually reserved for dysplastic mucosa only.

Argon Plasma Coagulator (APC) was originally developed as a hemostatic device and it has been used for ablating mucosa in Barrett esophagus. Several investigators have reported good results. Esophageal perforation is to be avoided by preventing the probe becoming embedded into the mucosa when the current is being applied to the target lesion. The risk of perforation and stricture formation is increased when high output power in the range of 80 to 90 W is used.

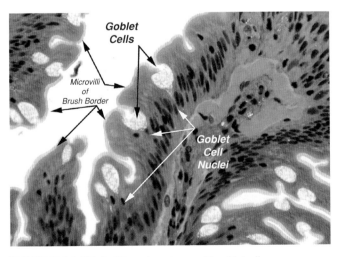

FIGURE 126.4 H & E of Barrett esophagus with goblet cells.

While improved outcomes have been described in the treatment of Barrett esophagus with high-grade dysplasia, the treatment was ineffective in intramucosal cancer.

Photodynamic Therapy (PDT) for treatment of early esophageal cancers began in 1961. It requires the use of photosensitizing drug Photofrin II (2 mg/kg body weight) which is activated by light of specific wavelength (red light of 630-nm wavelength) 48 hours after administration allowing enough time for the drug to concentrate into the tumor tissue. The disadvantages of PDT are cutaneous photosensitivity, severe chest pain, complications of pleural effusion, atrial fibrillation, and esophageal stricture, and inability to stage the mucosal disease.

Endoscopic Mucosal Resection (EMR) is now widely used for metaplastic Barrett epithelium that has progressed to dysplasia and early intramucosal cancer. The technique demands excellent endoscopic skills and understanding of cancer surgery. Application of EMR increased after the Japanese pioneers recognized that the procedure was safe in good hands and that vascular invasion and lymphatic spread were extremely rare when the cancer was superficial intraepithelial or confined to the upper two-thirds of the mucosa; the 5-year survival approached 100% when the disease was entirely in the outer mucosa.[23] It was only when the cancers penetrated into the bottom one-third of the mucosa did vascular invasion or lymphatic metastasis become apparent in 25% of the patients; with deeper invasion into submucosa, the 5-year survival decreased to 55% to 59%. It is not only the learning and mastering different EMR techniques that is important but also the details of the techniques have to be followed rigorously guided by protocol by the endoscopists each time. In most cases, EMR is now used for staging as a prelude to further treatment or as definitive treatment. The characteristics of superficial esophageal cancers which are amenable to EMR cap techniques with favorable outcomes are size <2.0 cm; depth of penetration that is superficial to muscularis mucosa; grade of cancer that is well-differentiated; and in appearance it is polypoid, elevated, or flat. It is required that maximum gastric acid suppression is enforced after the procedure and that surveillance is maintained. The average diameter of resected mucosa for pathologic examination is about 1 cm and the mucosal defect left behind is about 2 to 3 cm in diameter. Esophageal stricture formation after EMR is not a major concern.

Endoscopic Submucosal Dissection (ESD) has the advantage over EMR in that it permits en bloc complete resection of the neoplastic tissue without the fear of leaving behind cancer at the margins of resection and improves cure rate in early cancer.[24] It is a technically demanding procedure beginning with first marking the area to be resected with 3-mm margin using cautery followed by forming a submucosal bleb with a specific solution (different types are available) before careful controlled dissection proceeds in the submucosal plane. The dissection technique can be very demanding taking up to 2 hours and several "knives" are available; both needle knife and IT knife have the advantage of easier use without increased risk of penetrating the full thickness of the esophageal wall. Submucosal dissection is maintained in the plane superficial to the muscularis propria layer.

It has become recognized and accepted that endoscopic treatment for early esophageal cancer in properly staged patients is a viable alternative to esophagectomy. Careful depth staging is by assessing the depth of penetration of cancer in the esophageal wall. This is essential and it is best done by EMR or ESD. After complete mucosal resection, the specimen is best analyzed by two independent pathologists for depth of invasion. Cancer that has invaded beyond muscularis mucosa is at increased risk of lymphatic metastases and requires further treatment; and esophagectomy would be the best option.

DYSPHAGIA

Difficulty in swallowing is a precise symptom that must never be ignored. It is ominous in middle and later life if it is brief in duration and progressive in severity resulting in progressive weight loss, and often spells cancer. Incarcerated hiatus hernia, achalasia, scleroderma, and EoE are benign causes of dysphagia. Watching the patient eat or drink may provide an important diagnostic clue. Rabbit-like movements of the jaw caused by fear of letting food leave the mouth are typical of high esophageal obstruction. Intermittent dysphagia and regurgitation of undigested food just swallowed and saliva, and trick movements such as attempts to breathe out forcibly through a closed glottis to force obstructed food bolus through the unrelaxed lower esophageal sphincter (LES), and some associated weight loss suggests presence of achalasia. Early satiety, postprandial discomfort, postural regurgitation, and heart burn indicate presence of fixed hiatus hernia and associated gastroesophageal reflux disease. Accurate diagnosis is usually possible if the taking of a careful history is combined with a thorough radiographic examination followed by direct inspection of the interior of the esophagus by esophagoscopy and targeted and random mucosal biopsy. Esophageal function test is necessary for confirming diagnosis of disturbance of esophageal motility as in achalasia or scleroderma, hypertensive LES characterized as EGJ obstruction, IEM disorder, and collagen vascular disorder such as scleroderma. Endoscopy is a mandatory examination in patients who have abnormal esophageal motility study suggesting presence of achalasia but accompanied by pathological weight loss; in such cases, pseudoachalasia secondary to an obstructing small gastroesophageal cancer must be ruled out with absolute certainty; esophageal manometry cannot distinguish between classical achalasia and pseudoachalasia.

Endoscopy is indicated to determine the underlying etiology, exclude malignant and premalignant conditions, assess the need for therapy, and perform dilation. Dilation allows for immediate and sustainable relief of symptoms. Peptic strictures account for up to 80% of all benign strictures, but has been decreasing because of the use of proton pump inhibitors. There are various techniques of dilation, including the weighted push type mercury or tungsten-filled bougies with both radial and axial forces (e.g., Maloney, Hurst), polyvinyl wire-guided dilators (e.g., Savary-Gilliard, American), and balloon dilators (which exert a radial force only). Steroid injection into benign strictures, before or after the dilations, may improve outcomes and decrease the need for repeat dilations.

Esophageal resection for cancer is recognized to offer the best chance for cure if detected early and often with combination of induction chemoradiotherapy. However, locoregional tumor recurrence at the anastomosis occurs often in these patients causing progressive dysphagia and inanition. Insertion of permanent expandable metallic esophageal stent by endoscopy has become the accepted method of achieving palliation. Similarly, temporary esophageal stent insertion is now frequently used for nutritional support during induction therapy for cancer and for managing anastomotic leaks after esophagectomy for 4 to 6 weeks duration.

Esophageal stent insertion is not without complications. Major complications are perforation, aspiration pneumonia, bleeding, severe pain, and erosion into the aorta or proximal airways. Minor complications are mild retrosternal chest pain and gastroesophageal reflux disorder.

RECURRENT DYSPHAGIA AFTER PREVIOUS SURGERY

Endoscopy is a must investigation in patients who are complaining of esophageal symptoms after having undergone operation on the esophagus or stomach. Knowledge of altered anatomy of the foregut after the operation is essential in symptomatic patients and endoscopy should be preceded by barium contrast study to determine the need of additional studies. The demand for endoscopic assessment has increased in recent times because of ever increasing complications of bariatric surgery, laparoscopic fundoplication failures after repair of hiatus hernia and for gastroesophageal reflux disorder, complication of leak from the site of resection of epiphrenic diverticulum, anastomotic complications after esophagectomy and gastrectomy, and misdiagnosis leading to inappropriate operation for benign esophageal disorders. Clinical wisdom, recognition of the need for appropriate supplementary investigations, and thorough understanding of the altered anatomy inherent with each specific operation are essential in proper management of the new problem.

ENDOSCOPIC PALLIATION WITH ESOPHAGEAL STENT INSERTION

Endoscopic placement of esophageal stent has now become a frequent routine procedure in four clinical situations:

1. In patients with inoperable malignant stricture for compassion, comfort, relief of dysphagia, and to maintain nutrition for the duration of life.
2. As a temporary measure in patients with malignant stricture to maintain nutrition while receiving induction oncologic treatment before planned resection.
3. As a temporary intervention for 4 to 6 weeks in patients who have developed two complications at the anastomosis, which are leak and stricture.
4. Temporarily in patients with benign, refractory strictures requiring repeated dilations. Plastic or fully covered metal stents are used in these circumstances.

The advances made in the manufacture of reliable esophageal stents, ease and safety of insertion without general anesthesia, and low risk of complications of erosion, perforation, blockage, and migration have made endoscopic palliation less formidable. This is so important in patients whose life span is shortened to several months by advanced inoperable esophageal cancer that is causing near-total esophageal obstruction or has fistulized into the proximal airways, and the need for comfort and maintenance of oral nutrition are very important.

Esophageal malignant stricture dilatation produces palliation in swallowing for a period that is brief and last for 1 to 2 weeks only and has to be repeated often and has an increased risk of perforation. More durable palliation for improved quality of swallowing is obtained with covered self-expanding metal stents (Ultraflex, Boston Scientific) requiring sedation, minimal dilatation, and fluoroscopy for accurate placement.[25] It has an easy-to-use delivery system and can be used as distal release for distal obstruction or proximal release for proximal obstruction. For the obstructing cancer in the lower third esophagus and gastroesophageal junction, the preferred stent is with built-in antireflux valve for the prevention of gastroesophageal reflux.

Invasion by proximal esophageal cancer and fistulization into the proximal airways shortens life to matter of weeks from aspiration pneumonia and malignant cachexia. Esophageal by-pass operations are not necessary anymore with the advent of current covered easy-to-insert esophageal stents.

INCARCERATED LARGE FIXED HIATUS HERNIA

It is not an infrequent occurrence that an elderly patient presents with acute chest or epigastric pain, with or without vomiting or

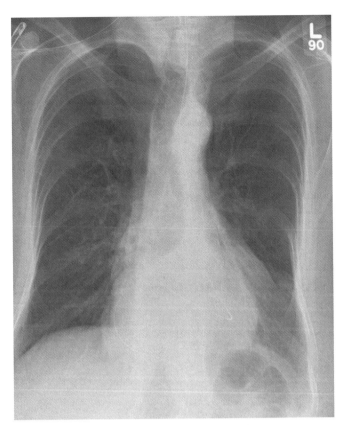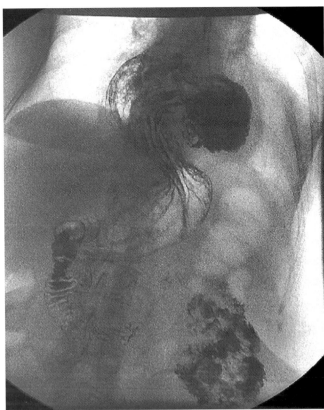

FIGURE 126.5 Plain radiograph (**A**) and with oral contrast (**B**) demonstrating a large fixed hernia with vovulus.

retching, or with coffee-ground emesis or fresh blood hematemesis in the emergency room and is found to have a fixed hiatus hernia. The patient after ruling out acute coronary syndrome or pulmonary embolism is often discharged home only to return repeatedly with similar complaints before the correct diagnosis of symptomatic hiatus hernia is made. Similarly, a patient may be seen by the family physician complaining of difficulty with swallowing for which medical therapy with proton pump inhibitor and prokinetic drug is prescribed without investigations. Sometimes, a patient known to have a large fixed hiatus hernia receives supplemental iron therapy for extended duration for undiagnosed iron deficiency anemia without considering that such recognized fixed hiatus hernia may be responsible for slow occult chronic blood loss from congested gastric mucosa in the herniated stomach. In all these clinical scenarios, careful endoscopy assessment is essential and to be performed urgently or electively as required by urgency of the situation. In patient suspected to have possible strangulation of hiatus hernia, viability of the herniated stomach must be assessed quickly by endoscopy for confirming the diagnosis and planning appropriate surgical treatment. Endoscopic reduction is reserved for gastric volvulus in patients that are not surgical candidates for repair (Fig. 126.5).

PLACEMENT OF PERCUTANEOUS GASTROSTOMY TUBE

This has become one of the most frequently performed operations in patients who require nutritional support and are unable to swallow solid foods and liquids without the risk of pulmonary aspiration, frequently witnessed in patient with neurological diseases. It can be performed with an endoscope and under local sedation as a day procedure. Quite often it is electively inserted for nutritional support in

patients undergoing head and neck cancer operations. PEG tubes may also be extended into the small intestine by passing a jejunal extension tube through the PEG tube and into the jejunum via the pylorus. A gastrostomy can also be used to treat volvulus of the stomach, where the tube is used for gastropexy, with adhering the stomach to the abdominal wall, preventing twisting of the stomach. A PEG tube can be used in providing gastric or postsurgical drainage as well.

ATYPICAL CHEST PAIN

Atypical chest pain is a common complaint and often presents as a major diagnostic problem because it can be due to heart disease or esophageal disease. Both diseases are common and they may present simultaneously and certain components of their presentation are similar. The pain is recognized as being atypical from of its unusual distribution or unusual precipitating and relieving factors. It is the physician who will call it atypical when the description of the complaint differs from his concept of the frequent typical characterization according to origin from the specific site. Inaccuracy in diagnosis has the potential of resulting in serious consequences from inappropriate therapy.

Heartburn is a typical symptom of gastroesophageal reflux disorder. It is an intense and unpleasant typical substernal burning sensation which lasts for a few seconds to minutes. It may occur when lying horizontally or upright, and often after meals. It is usually relieved immediately by antacids. It is a common symptom of hiatus hernia; it is due to corrosive effect of regurgitating gastric juice (hydrochloric acid, pepsin, bile acids, and conjugated bile salts) against which the squamous esophageal mucosa has no protection. Endoscopy may be normal or it may reveal mucosal findings of reflux-related damage to esophageal mucosa: chronic esophagitis, peptic stricture formation, columnar-lined esophagus, and Barrett epithelium. Symptoms do not correlate with the degree of esophageal damage that can occur. There are two commonly used classifications systems for documenting disease severity, the Los Angeles and the Savary-Miller classification.[26,27] The Los Angeles system has the advantage of having shown good intra- and interobserver agreement and the severity of esophagitis correlates with the extent of esophageal acid exposure on 24-hour pH monitoring.

Atypical chest pain, not related to ischemic heart disease, on the other hand is difficult to evaluate and it may arise in the esophagus. One reason is reflux disorder resulting in peptic esophagitis; other reasons are secondary esophageal spasm or distension of esophagus induced by the refluxing bolus. Primary hypercontractile esophageal motility disorder, previously described as nutcracker esophagus or distal esophageal spasm, has known to cause episodic central chest pain. After assessment by endoscopy, it will depend on esophageal manometry and 24-hour pH study to determine the nature of underlying disorder.

EOSINOPHILIC ESOPHAGITIS

EoE is increasing in prevalence and detection and it was rarely recognized before 1990. An allergic immune reaction involving both IgE- and T-cell–mediated hypersensitivity to inhaled aeroallergens and ingested food allergens is incriminated in its pathogenesis.[28] This causes a dense eosinophilic infiltrate into the epithelial lining of the esophagus. Secondary causes of esophageal eosinophilia must be excluded.

Specific criteria need to be present to make this diagnosis. EoE is a clinicopathological disorder diagnosed taking into consideration both clinical and pathological information without either of these parameters interpreted in isolation, and defined by specific criteria which are clinical features of esophageal dysfunction, dysphagia and food impactions; and endoscopic findings of esophageal wall thickening, luminal narrowing, furrowing, and stricture, formation of rings (trachealization). Esophageal mucosal biopsy characteristically shows intraepithelial eosinophils (greater than 15 per hpf in areas of

peak density), eosinophilic microabscesses (defined as a collection of four or more EOs within the epithelium), a particular affiliation of intraepithelial eosinophils to aggregate in the surface layers of the epithelium (surface layering), surface sloughing of squamous cells and intraepithelial eosinophils, and intraepithelial eosinophils degranulation.

This is a specific diagnosis established only from recognizable endoscopy features and mucosal biopsies obtained according to the defined guidelines. Between two and four mucosal biopsies should be obtained from both the proximal and distal esophagus to maximize the likelihood of detecting eosinophilia. There appears to be an increased risk for mucosal tearing during endoscopy, which may translate into perforation. Biopsies of the gastric antrum and duodenum should be taken if there is a suspicion of eosinophilic gastroenteritis (Fig. 126.6).

THERAPEUTIC ENDOSCOPY

Foreign bodies must always be considered as a cause of dysphagia. There is usually a history of choking during a meal, though this may not be obtained from small children, or in psychotic patients. It is not infrequent to see patients coming to the emergency room complaining of food bolus obstruction in the presence or absence of clinical history to suggest pre-existing esophageal disorder. Urgent endoscopy for removal of the foreign body is in order. Flexible esophagoscopy under sedation should be attempted first before resorting to rigid esophagoscopy under general anesthesia in the operating room. Different types of retrieval forceps should be available. Caution is advised when use of balloon dilators or push-through dilators becomes necessary since this entails risk of esophageal perforation and fluoroscopy should be used to reduce the risk.

CAUSTIC INGESTION

Emergency endoscopy is indicated to examine the oral cavity, pharynx, larynx, and the esophagus down to the most proximal site of

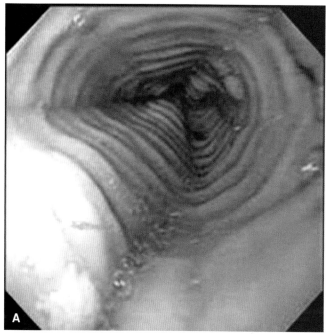

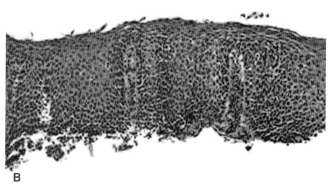

FIGURE 126.6 Eosinophilic esophagitis. **A:** Esophagus with trachealization. **B:** H & E showing mucosal biopsy with intraepithelial eosinophils.

mucosal injury in order to confirm the diagnosis and the extent of the corrosive damage. Thereafter, the need for repeat endoscopy is dictated by patient's recovery during hospitalization. The examination will need to be repeated after 7 to 10 days and at this time, to examine the entire esophagus, stomach, and proximal duodenum. Therapeutic endoscopy for dilatation of esophageal strictures may be required at regular intervals thereafter.

There is a recognized increased risk of squamous cell carcinoma developing late after lye ingestion with incidence ranging between 2.3% and 6.2%. The cancer is located more commonly in the midesophagus. Since it is a late complication of lye ingestion, endoscopic surveillance is recommended for several decades after ingestion.

ESOPHAGEAL PERFORATION

Free or contained esophageal perforations, spontaneous or iatrogenic in origin, should be assessed with endoscopy immediately before undertaking emergency operation. The information important in management and should be obtained from the endoscopic examination must include confirmation of perforation, the level of perforation and its size, and presence or absence of intrinsic esophageal disease. This information is necessary in making therapeutic decision to repair the perforation or to resect esophagus immediately and delayed reconstruction; or, to consider insertion of temporary esophageal stent insertion for 4 to 6 weeks. In this situation, it is best to perform the endoscopy with minimal air insufflation to avoid gastric distension and tension pneumomediastinum, and tension pneumothorax.

PER ORAL ENDOSCOPIC ESOPHAGEAL MYOTOMY

Nonsurgical management of achalasia for relief of distal esophageal functional obstruction due to nonrelaxing LES has been with pneumatic dilatation or Botox injection. Unfortunately, there is a risk of esophageal perforation of <5% with pneumatic dilatation and improvement in swallowing occurs in about 80%. Botox injection into the LES at four sites results in improved swallowing in 75% to 80% and improvement is not durable requiring repeat Botox injection after 6 months.

POEM was introduced in the management of achalasia 4 years ago in Japan and has become popular worldwide as experience is increasing.[29] It was recognized in porcine model that selective subtotal needle-knife incision of only the circular muscle layer of the muscularis propria from within the submucosal working space could be safely performed. The technique is now increasingly used to lower the LES pressure in minimally invasive surgery. The technique involves the creation of a 2-cm long mucosal incision in the esophagus, 14 cm proximal to the LES. A submucosal tunnel is created from the incision to the LES with dissection of the circular muscle fibers over the distal 7 cm of the esophagus and the proximal 2 cm of the gastric cardia. The mucosal incision is then clipped closed. Preliminary results are good with a low complication rate but it is too early to comment on long-term results. The wide application of endoscopy is the reason for emphasizing the importance of proper training in endoscopy and its safe use in different situations.

ENDOLUMINAL TREATMENT FOR REFLUX DISEASE

Laparoscopic fundoplication remains the gold standard in surgical interventions for reflux disease in both adults and children. However, patients and physicians continue to search for less invasive

approaches by means of endoscopy. Currently, there are two devices reported to create an incisionless fundoplication. The first is EsophyX, where once the endoscope is positioned, the instrument is deployed in the stomach and used to create a full-thickness plication secured by fasteners made of polypropylene, placed 3 to 5 cm about the GE junction that aids in the serosa-to-serosa fusion.[30] Numerous published series have reported mixed results, with very brief follow-up.

The second device, Stretta, makes use of radiofrequency (RF) treatment for reflux disease.[31,32] It uses specialized catheters and RF to remodel the musculature of the LES and gastric cardia, leading to a reduction in tissue compliance and transient LES relaxations. This translates into restoration of the natural barrier function of the LES and reduces spontaneous regurgitation caused by transient inappropriate relaxation of the sphincter. Multiple prospective clinical trials and randomized trials have shown excellent safety and efficacy of this procedure. Long-term outcome to 48 months has shown a decrease or elimination of proton pump inhibitors with improvement in quality of life and symptom scores.

ESOPHAGEAL DIVERTICULA

Pulsion "pressure" diverticula are usually pharyngeal and not esophageal. They are acquired and not congenital, and seen more common in old age. They develop on the posterior wall between the upper and lower divisions of the inferior pharyngeal constrictor muscle where the lumen is narrow, with the cricoid cartilage in front. Assessment with endoscopy, and only after barium study, should be performed with utmost care to avoid iatrogenic perforation. A rare complication to be ruled out by endoscopy is cancer developing in the diverticulum when a fixed filling defect is seen on barium study. Epiphrenic "pressure" diverticulum is seen in the distal 10 cm of the esophagus, resulting from esophageal motility disorder such as achalasia or from peptic esophageal stricture. Endoscopy becomes an integral part of assessment.

ESOPHAGITIS

Acute esophagitis is the natural consequence of swallowing injurious substances such as foreign bodies, caustic acid (coagulative mural necrosis) and alkali (liquefactive mural necrosis), digital batteries, and corrosives like iron (e.g., when children mistake ferrous sulfate tablets for sweets). Inflammatory changes with necrosis of the mucous membrane occur in severe cases and stricture formation results if the patient survives.

Chronic esophagitis is frequently due to reflux disorder and hiatus hernia, for the esophagus is lined by squamous epithelium and is not equipped to withstand the corrosive effect of regurgitating gastric juice. Chronic esophagitis also follows reflux of bile and conjugated bile salts.

Antibiotics and immunosuppression may cause dysphagia, especially in those weakened by prolonged illness, treatment of cancer with chemotherapy, chronic corticosteroid therapy, and AIDS. This is due to moniliasis (thrush), which is usually visible in the mouth and pharynx.

RECURRENT ASPIRATION PNEUMONIA

Esophagus should be considered as a cause of recurrent pneumonia from unsuspected recurrent tracheobronchial aspiration. Oral contrast study with water-soluble medium Omnipaque should be followed by endoscopy. The esophageal conditions to look for are pharyngoesophageal diverticulum, disorder of the cricopharyngeus muscle such as mitochondrial myopathy, inherited oculopharyngeal muscular dystrophy, achalasia, esophageal stricture, and gastric outlet obstruction due to peptic ulcer disease or recalcitrant pylorospasm after esophagectomy for cancer.

HEMATEMESIS AND MELENA

The pathological causes to search for urgent endoscopy include esophageal varices complicating liver cirrhosis and portal hypertension, erosive esophagitis, Barrett's ulcer in the columnar-lined esophagus, intrathoracic stomach and peptic ulcer. Having ruled these out on endoscopy, it is necessary to consider other possibilities such as aortoduodenal fistula complicating aortic surgery or aneurysm. Noninvasive therapy is administered for bleeding varices and peptic ulcer at endoscopy.

DYSPEPSIA

Dyspepsia is defined as pain or other symptoms (excluding dysphagia) in the upper abdomen or lower part of the chest associated with eating. Accounts of dyspepsia often give a long list of causes which are traditional; thus unhygienic eating habits or irregular mode of life are often blamed, though without justification. Gastritis and peptic ulcer are most likely, but sometimes organic cause cannot be found and symptoms are psychosomatic. Causes of dyspepsia are many and the only conditions that can be diagnosed by endoscopy are diseases of the upper gastrointestinal tract: esophagitis, fixed hiatus hernia, and associated reflux disorder or volvulus, neoplasm, peptic ulcer, and gastritis.

ESOPHAGEAL CANCER

Malignancies of the esophagus are diagnosed by endoscopy with mucosal biopsies in 96% of cases. Strictures and obstructing cancers may prevent visualization of the entire length, and brush cytology may be used in these instances. Ultrathin endoscopes may also help in these situations. Detecting early stage carcinoma may be improved with adjunct techniques such as chromoendoscopy, narrowband imaging, confocal microscopy, spectroscopy, and magnification endoscopy.

Further staging information may be established by involving EUS and fine needle aspiration in conjunction with cross-sectional imaging. EUS has been shown to be superior in both the local tumor and nodal staging over CT scans. EUS for restaging after neoadjuvant chemoradiation is often being used to determine the effectiveness of the treatment before surgery.

Endoscopic curative therapy can be used in mucosal cancers, both by resection and ablation techniques. EMR and ESD permit targeted removal, and permit large tissue specimens for diagnosis and accurate staging. Ablation techniques for intramucosal carcinoma include PDT, cryotherapy, argon plasma coagulation, heater probe treatment, brachytherapy, and radiofrequency ablation. Insertion of expandable stents provides good palliation for obstructing tumors and covering of tracheoesophageal fistulas.

CONCLUSION

From 1881, when Von Mikulicz combined the three essential components of the endoscope, the electric light source, an optical system, and a tubular endoscopic body to 1957 when Hirschowitz introduced the fiberoptic endoscope, many advances have been made since then to revolutionize endoscopy from diagnostic to therapeutic.

It cannot be forgotten that medicine is both an art and science. To practice it well, it requires the physician to be learned both in wisdom and understanding and recognition of maladies. The precise and intelligent recognition and appreciation of minor differences is the real essential factor in all successful medical diagnosis.

The management of esophageal disorders requires physicians to have a thorough understanding of pathophysiology and pathogenesis of these disorders. Mastery in endoscopic examination is essential but second to the first requirement that is the power of observation, detection of visual pathologic changes, and correlation of pathologic biopsies to the functional loss.

The practicing thoracic surgeon must acquire the necessary expertise in safe conduct of endoscopy, both diagnostic and therapeutic, and familiarize with the advances made in order to maintain the standard of care and lead the way in its evaluation and implementation.

REFERENCES

1. Peery AF, Dellono ES, Lund J, et al. Burden of gastrointestinal disease in the United States: 2012 update. *Gastroenterology* 2012;143:1179–1187; e1–e3.
2. Kielan W, Lazarkiewicz B, Grzebieniak Z, et al. Jan Mikulicz-Radecki: one of the creators of world surgery. *Keio J Med* 2005;54(1):1–7.
3. Johnson SK, Naidu RK, Ostopowicz RC, et al. Adolf Kussmaul: distinguished clinician and medical pioneer. *Clin Med Res* 2009;7(3):107–112.
4. Hirshowitz BI. Endoscopic examination of the stomach and duodenal cap with the fibroscope. *Lancet* 1961;277:1074–1078.
5. Beaumont W. *Experiments and observations on the gastric juice and physiology of digestion*. Edinburgh: Maclachlan and Stewart; 1838.
6. Billmann F. A pioneer in medicine and surgery: Charles Sedillot. *Int J surg* 2012;10(9):542–546.
7. Ponsky JL. The development of the PEG: How it was. *J Interv Gastroenterol* 2011;1(2):88–89.
8. Curie J, Curie P. Development via compression of electric polarization in hemihedral crystals with inclined faces. *Bul Soc Min de France* 1880;3:90–93.
9. Wild JJ, Neal D. Use of high-frequency ultrasonic waves for detecting changes of texture in living tissues. *Lancet* 1951;1:655–657.
10. Uchida R, Hagiware Y, Irie T. Electro-scanning ultrasound diagnostic equipment. *Jap Med El* 1971;58(141):833–837.
11. Watenabe H, Ingaie D, tanahashi Y, et al. Development and application of a new equipment for transrectal ultrasonography. *J Clin Ultrasound* 1974;2:91–98.
12. Sharma P, Wani S, Rastugi A, et al. The diagnostic accuracy of esophageal capsule endoscopy in patients with gastrointestinal reflux disease and Barrett's esophagus: a blinded, prospective study. *Am J Gastroenterol* 2008;103:525–532.
13. Sharma P, Dent J, Armstrong D, et al. The development and validation of an endoscopic grading system for Barrett's esophagus; the Prague C & M criteria. *Gastroenterology* 2006;131:1392–1399.
14. Berstein De, Barkin JS, Reiner DK, et al. Standard biopsy forceps versus large-capacity forceps with and without needles. *Gastrointest Endosc* 1995;41:573–576.
15. Gono K, Obi T, Yamaguchi M, et al. Appearance of enhanced tissue features in narrow-band endoscopic imaging. *J Biomed Opt* 2004;9(3):568–577.
16. Kara MA, Peters FP, Fockens P, et al. Endoscopic video-autofluorescence imaging followed by narrow band imaging for detecting early neoplasia in Barrett's esophagus. *Gastrointest Endosc* 2006;64(2):170–185.
17. Curvers WL, van Vilsteren FG, Baak LC, et al. Endoscopic trimodal imaging versus standard video endoscopy for detection of early Barrett's neoplasm: a multicenter, randomized crossover study in general practice. *Gastrointest Endosc* 2011;75(2):195–203.
18. Kiesslich R, Goetz M, Vietu M, et al. Confocal laser endomicroscopy. *Gastrointest Endosc Clin N Am* 2005;15(4):715–731.
19. Lightdale CJ. Optical coherence tomography in Barrett's esophagus. *Gastrointest Endosc Clin N Am* 2013;23(3):549–563.
20. Bertani H, Frazzoni M, Dabizzi E, et al. Improved detection of incident dysplasia by probe-based confocal laser endomicroscopy in a Barrett's esophagus surveillance program. *Dig Dis Sci* 2013;58:188–193.
21. Inoue H, Sasajima K, Sugaya S, et al. Endoscopic in vivo evaluation of tissue atypia in the esophagus using a newly designed integrated endocytoscope: a pilot trial. *Endoscopy* 2006;38(09):891–895.
22. The Paris endoscopic classification of superficial neoplastic lesions: esophagus, stomach and colon. *Gastrointest Endosc* 2003;58(6):S3–S43.
23. Gotoda T, Yanagigawa A, Sasuko M, et al. Incidence of lymph node metastasis form early gastric cancer: estimation with a large number of cases at 2 large centers. *Gastric Cancer* 2000;3(4):219–225.

24. Ishihara R, Yamamoto S, Hanaoka N, et al. Endoscopic submucosal dissection for superficial Barrett's esophageal cancer in the Japanese state and perspective. *Ann Trans Med* 2014;2(3):177–184.

25. Hindy P, Hong J, Lam-Tsai Y, et al. A comprehensive review of esophageal stents. *Gastroenterol Hepatol* 2012;8(8):526–534.

26. Lundell LR, Dent J, Bennett JR, et al. Endoscopic assessment of esophagitis: clinical and functional correlates and further validation of the Los Angeles classification. *Gut* 1999;45:172–180.

27. Monnier P, Savary M. Contribution of endoscopy to gastro-oesophageal reflux disease. *Scand J Gastroenterol* 1984;106:26–32.

28. Furuta GT, Liacouras CA, Collins MH, et al. Eosinophilic esophagitis in children and adults: a systemic review and consensus recommendations for diagnosis and treatment. *Gastroenterol* 2007;133(4):1342–1363.

29. Inoue H, Minami H, Kobayash Y, et al. Per-oral endoscopic myotomy (POEM) for esophageal achalasia. *Endoscopy* 2010;10:265–271.

30. Cadiere GB, Rajan A, Rqibate M, et al. Endoluminal fundoplication (ELF)—evolution of EsophyX, a new surgical device for transoral surgery. *Minim Invasive Ther Allied Technol* 2006;15:348–355.

31. Arts J, Sifrim D, Rutgeerts P, et al. Influence of radiofrequency energy to the lower oesophageal junction (the Stretta procedure) on symptoms, acid exposure, and esophageal sensitivity to acid perfusion in gastroesphageal reflux disease. *Dig Dis Sci* 2007;52(9):2170–2177.

32. Triadafilopoulos G. Changes in GERD symptom scores correlate with improvement in esophageal acid exposure after the Stretta procedure. *Surg Endoscop* 2004;18(7):1038–1044.

127

Esophageal Ultrasound

J. Shawn Mallery ▪ Rafael Garza-Castillon ▪ Eitan Podgaetz ▪ Rafael Andrade

INTRODUCTION

Endoscopic ultrasound (EUS) was first described as an imaging tool for the gastrointestinal tract in 1980.[1,2] The indications for EUS quickly expanded to imaging and EUS-guided fine-needle aspiration (EUS-FNA) of upper gastrointestinal and mediastinal pathology,[3–13] and in 1996 EUS-FNA was introduced for the diagnosis and staging of lung cancer.[14] Over time, EUS has also very gradually developed into a therapeutic tool with applications such as EUS-guided drainage, access, and local therapy. In addition to advancements in 2D EUS imaging that provide extraordinary detail of the wall of the gastrointestinal tract and surrounding structures, forward-viewing EUS, contrast-enhanced EUS, and 3D EUS have emerged as a potential diagnostic tools, but have not yet gained widespread clinical application.[2,15–17]

This chapter focuses on the clinical application of EUS for patients with esophageal and other thoracic diseases.

BASIC PRINCIPLES AND EQUIPMENT

Basic ultrasound (US) concepts merit mention to guide the reader through this chapter.

ULTRASOUND, ECHOGENICITY, AND DOPPLER EFFECT

Medical US is the use of high-frequency (>20 kHz) sound waves to image anatomic structures.[3] Echogenicity is the tissue's ability to bounce sound waves. Tissues with high echogenicity (e.g., bone) tend to bounce off sound waves, the US image will appear in shades of gray. Low echogenicity tissue has high water content and little ability to reflect sound waves, the US image is typically dark or even black. The differential echogenicity of tissues is the principle for an US image. As a result of water's very low echogenicity when compared to air, a fluid-filled balloon surrounding the US transducer can reduce the echogenicity between the US probe and the GI wall and enhance image quality (Fig. 127.1A,B).

As a general rule, high-frequency US (e.g., 12 to 30 MHz) has little tissue penetration, but provides excellent detail of the tissue in the immediacy of the US transducer. High-frequency EUS is excellent to image the GI tract mucosa and wall layers. Lower frequency EUS (e.g., 5 to 12 MHz) has deep tissue penetration and is best suited to image structures further away from the wall of the GI tract and to guide needle biopsies.

The Doppler effect is a difference in sound wave frequency caused by motion[4] and in medical US imaging this effect can be used to

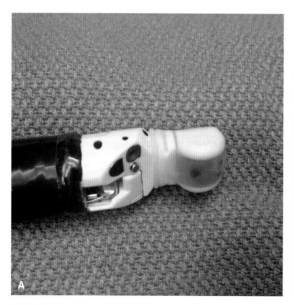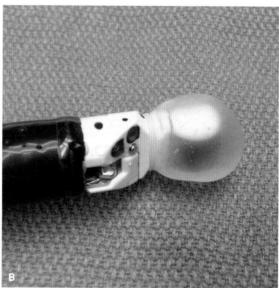

FIGURE 127.1 Tip of EUS scope with deflated balloon (**A**), and with water-inflated balloon to optimize image quality (**B**).

provide a graphic image of blood flow. The main purpose of Doppler color flow imaging in EUS is to help the operator differentiate between vascular and nonvascular structures.

BASIC ENDOSCOPIC ULTRASOUND EQUIPMENT

A detailed discussion of EUS equipment is beyond the focus of this chapter and the interested reader is referred elsewhere.[5]

The basic equipment components for EUS are an endoscope with videoendoscopic, suction, and insufflation capabilities; an US transducer; and an US imaging console. The US transducer may be an integral part of the tip of a specialized endoscope or may be placed as a probe through the biopsy channel of a standard videoendoscope.

Three main types of EUS imaging devices exist. The first two types are standard EUS endoscopes with integrated US transducer configurations for either radial-array or linear-array US imaging. Radial US transducers provide a 360-degree view in the axial plane, that is, cross-sectional images perpendicular to the long axis of the endoscope and GI tract as in an axial CT scan (Fig. 127.2). Linear US transducers provide a sector- or wedge-shaped image in the longitudinal plane (along the long axis) of the endoscope (Fig. 127.3). The third type of probes are "through-the-scope" radial high-frequency miniprobes, that are placed through the biopsy channel of a videoendoscope (Fig. 127.4). Standard radial imaging is purely diagnostic with no tissue sampling capabilities, while linear US is the imaging modality used for US-guided tissue sampling (Fig. 127.5A,B).

A needle advanced through the biopsy port of a linear EUS device will remain within the imaging plane and be visualized for its entire length as a bright (hyperechoic) linear structure which may be carefully guided toward the tissue or organ of interest (Fig. 127.5B). Linear array echoendoscopes are available in both diagnostic and therapeutic forms, with the therapeutic devices offering larger biopsy channels which allow the placement of larger therapeutic devices such as stents; this larger channel diameter is more relevant to nonmediastinal applications such as the drainage of pancreatic fluid collections. The therapeutic echoendoscopes by necessity have larger outer diameters. All of the EUS endoscopes provide video-endoscopic visualization, however the camera is directed obliquely rather than the typical forward view of a standard endoscope. As such, passage of the device is somewhat more challenging, the operator must place the echoendoscope with

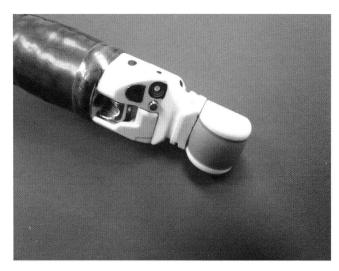

FIGURE 127.3 Tip of EUS scope with linear US transducer (*orange*) to provide a sector view.

great care through the upper esophageal sphincter, strictures, and stenotic tumors.

Historically, the majority of endosonographers performed initial examinations using the radial device and then used a linear device only when a structure requiring tissue sampling was identified. More recently, however, many endosonographers are primarily using linear devices for the entirety of the exam in order to save time and avoid the need for duplicate examinations.

EUS miniprobes are designed to be passed through the working channel of a standard endoscope or bronchoscope. These devices may be useful in the evaluation of small focal luminal abnormalities which may be difficult to locate with standard echoendoscopes, since the probe can be directly positioned adjacent to the lesion of interest under end-viewing endoscopic guidance. In addition, these probes utilize higher-frequency imaging between 12 and 30 MHz (with individual probes using only a single frequency). Miniprobes are particularly useful for the evaluation of small nodules within the esophageal wall such as early cancers or small subepithelial tumors. The higher frequencies allow more precise definition of esophageal wall layers. Although miniprobes may also be advanced through tightly stenotic esophageal cancers, their higher frequency (and thus limited depth of penetration) typically provides inadequate depth of imaging to determine accurate T-classification for these typically thick, higher stage lesions.

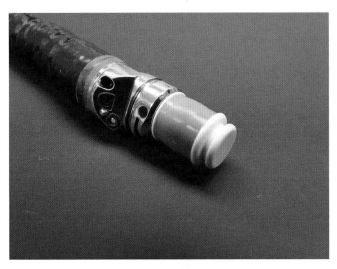

FIGURE 127.2 Tip of EUS scope with radial US transducer (*orange*) to provide a 360-degree view.

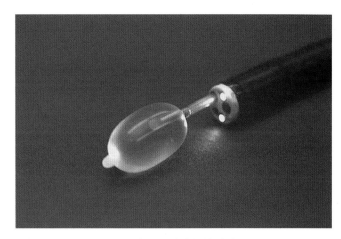

FIGURE 127.4 A "through-the-scope" radial high-frequency miniprobe.

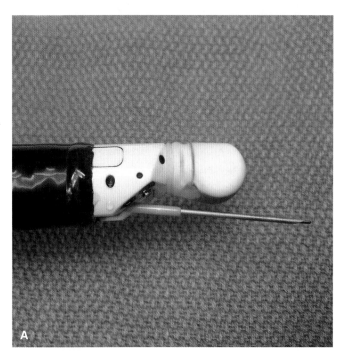

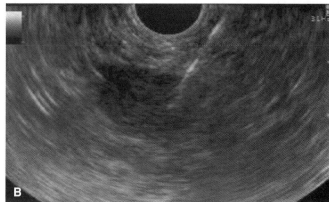

FIGURE 127.5 Linear EUS scope with biopsy needle (**A**), EUS image of biopsy needle within a left adrenal nodule (**B**).

TECHNIQUE

EUS examination may be performed under moderate IV sedation, monitored anesthesia care, or general anesthesia depending on the preference of the physician and/or patient, comorbidities and the sensitivity of the patient to IV sedatives. Typically, the patient is in the left lateral decubitus position and the endoscopist stands at the left side of the bed. However, when a procedure is performed under general anesthesia and particularly with bronchoscopy in the same setting, it is preferable for the patient to be supine and to work from the head of the bed. Diagnostic endoscopy is commonly performed prior to passage of the EUS device in order to localize any potential sites of stenosis (which are difficult to assess with the oblique-viewing echoendoscopes). The degree of any identified stenosis is also assessed. Passage of a standard echoendoscope requires a lumen of at least 15 mm in diameter and difficulty passing a standard endoscope indicates that passage of the echoendoscope will not be immediately possible. Under these circumstances a limited EUS examination of the proximal portion of the tumor may often be sufficient in either identifying at T3 disease or lymph node (LN) metastasis. Alternatively, more complete imaging may also be possible in this setting with the smaller caliber endobronchial US device, which can allow imaging of the entire length of a stenotic tumor, as well as the mediastinum distal to the mass, common upper abdominal LN locations (including celiac, left gastric, and gastrohepatic ligament), much of the left lobe of the liver and the left adrenal gland. The authors do not advocate dilation of a malignant stenosis with the only goal of obtaining a complete EUS examination. The use of minimal dilation with extreme caution should only be justified if it is necessary for therapeutic reasons and if the operator is extremely experienced. Perforation at the site of an esophageal cancer is a devastating complication.

Following diagnostic endoscopy, the echoendoscope is passed under direct (but oblique) endoscopic visualization. The endoscope is then advanced into the stomach and/or duodenum and sonographic examination begun. It is the authors' typical practice to perform complete abdominal examination whenever possible even in the setting of previously identified mediastinal disease. This may be valuable in many situations, because in the setting of mediastinal malignancy, further evaluation could identify hepatic, adrenal, or abdominal LN metastases. These locations are all readily amenable to EUS-guided needle aspiration.

As mentioned previously, air has high echogenicity and US imaging cannot be performed through air. The intervening air between the GI wall and transducer must be eliminated to obtain adequate imaging. This is accomplished by suctioning of the surrounding air, flexing the endoscope to place the transducer in direct contact with the wall, and/or inflating a water balloon around the transducer (Fig. 127.1A,B). However, these techniques may result in compression of the esophageal wall layers which may interfere with T-classification of early esophageal neoplasms or determination of the wall layer of origin for intramural subepithelial tumors. In this situation, an appropriate acoustic interface may be obtained by instilling water into the esophageal lumen allowing visualization of the esophageal wall without touching the wall with the transducer. Esophageal water instillation, particularly in a nonintubated patient, should only be performed in reverse Trendelenburg position and with oral suction immediately available to reduce the risk of aspiration.

RADIAL EUS

For radial EUS, the mediastinal examination may be performed by simply slowly withdrawing the echoendoscope from the GE junction to the esophageal inlet. The US image orientation is typically adjusted to provide a standard orientation, which is roughly analogous to axial CT images, with either the aorta placed at a 5 o'clock position or the spine at 6 o'clock.

LINEAR EUS

For linear EUS, complete examination is begun at the GE junction by performing a complete 360-degree rotation of the echoendoscope.

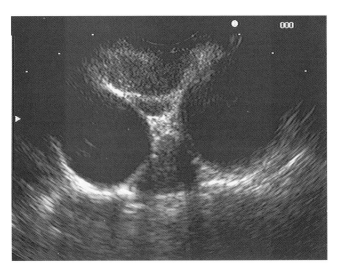

FIGURE 127.6 Left paratracheal LN (station 4L; closer to EUS transducer, top) and aortopulmonary LN (station 5; bottom). Aorta: hypoechoic circle on right of image. Pulmonary artery: hypoechoic circle on left of image.

The echoendoscope is then withdrawn approximately 2 to 3 cm and the scope again rotated 360 degrees. Imaging is continued in this manner until the endoscope balloon reaches the thoracic inlet. In this manner, it is possible to visualize the aortic arch and descending thoracic aorta, the main and left pulmonary arteries, the azygos vein and azygos arch, and LN stations adjacent to the esophagus. This includes many nodes in stations 2R and 2L (some are not seen due to intervening air in the trachea), station 4L, station 7, station 8, and station 9. The triangular space between the esophageal wall, aortic arch, and pulmonary artery is often inaccurately referred to in GI literature as the aortopulmonary (AP) window (station 5), but is actually the left lower paratracheal space (station 4L). The AP window is seen by EUS deep to the point of closest approximation of the aortic arch and pulmonary artery. Nodes in this location are sometimes accessible for EUS-guided sampling if there is sufficient space between the two arterial structures or with transpulmonary artery puncture (Fig. 127.6). LNs in station 6 (preaortic) can be sampled by transaortic puncture by very experienced operators; however, authors advise against transaortic puncture since the aorta is a high-pressure vessel. Imaging of the anterior mediastinum, including pretracheal nodes, is not possible via EUS due to artifact from the intervening trachea. These nodes are readily imaged by EBUS. The evaluable regions of the mediastinum by EUS and EBUS overlap and the two technologies are complementary. Combining both EUS and EBUS allows evaluation of virtually the entire middle and posterior mediastinum.

EUS-GUIDED TISSUE SAMPLING

A variety of specially designed needles ranging from 25 gauge to 19 gauge as well as special core biopsy needles are available by multiple manufacturers. The distal tips of these needles have a roughened surface to improve sonographic visualization and appear as a bright white linear structure in the sonographic view. These needles are attached to handle assemblies which are advanced down the biopsy channel of the echoendoscope (Fig. 127.5A). For needle aspiration, the structure of interest is positioned sonographically near the center of the (linear array) US image (Fig. 127.5B), and the needle tip is then advanced through the esophageal wall into the structure of

interest under continuous sonographic visualization. Doppler imaging may be used prior to puncture to exclude significant intervening vasculature. Once a sample has been obtained, the needle contents are then expressed either onto a microscope slide for immediate bedside interpretation or into the appropriate specimen solution (typically formalin, unless viable cells are needed for lymphoma evaluation or cultures are requested). Additional passes are then performed, ideally with guidance from onsite cytologic (rapid onsite evaluation [ROSE]) interpretation for adequacy. Techniques for sampling, preferred needle gauge, and preferred needle design vary significantly from operator to operator. Typically three to five passes are performed. If preliminary cytology suggests inadequate cellularity, needle gauge may be changed, core biopsy attempted, or another site sampled. Antibiotic prophylaxis is generally not recommended for EUS-FNA with the exception of sampling cystic structures (typically pancreatic cysts).

RAPID ONSITE EVALUATION

ROSE of cytologic specimens by experienced cytopathologists is key for immediate decision making and streamlines patient care; ROSE of mediastinal LN by experienced cytopathologists is congruent with final cytopathologic interpretation in 95% of cases.[18–21] The cytologic evaluation is just as important as the operator's skill; without skilled cytopathologists it is not possible to achieve the necessary diagnostic accuracy to properly guide therapy.

EUS MINIPROBES

Miniprobes are small radial EUS probes that can be placed through the working channel of a standard upper GI videoendoscope (Fig. 127.4). To examine small mucosal abnormalities, the miniprobe must be advanced past the tip of the videoendoscope and placed adjacent to the lesion (Fig. 127.7). To optimize the image, air must be suctioned out of the lumen and intraluminal water instillation may be required with the abovementioned precautions.

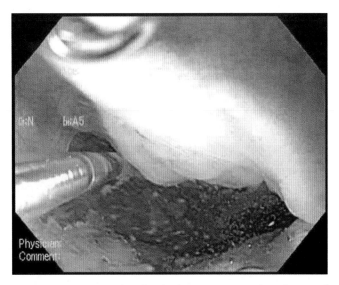

FIGURE 127.7 Miniprobe placed adjacent to an esophageal mucosal nodule. The esophagus has been partially filled with water to optimize imaging (the head of the bed must be elevated to minimize the risk of aspiration, see text).

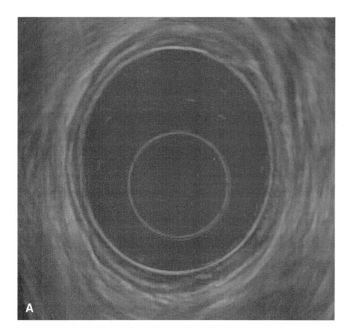

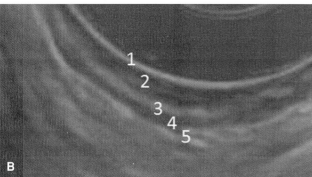

FIGURE 127.8 **A:** Normal esophageal mucosa (radial EUS, 7.5 MHz). **B:** Magnified view of the normal five layers of the esophageal mucosa (see text).

EUS EVALUATION OF ESOPHAGEAL DISEASE

NORMAL ANATOMY OF THE ESOPHAGEAL WALL

The anatomic layers of the esophageal wall are best evaluated with radial EUS and in particular with high-frequency radial EUS. Standard 7.5 MHz radial EUS imaging of the esophageal wall reveals five layers (Fig. 127.8A,B):

1. Interface between intraluminal fluid and the superficial mucosa (hyperechoic, white)
2. Deep mucosa including lamina propria and muscularis mucosae (hypoechoic, dark)
3. Submucosa (hyperechoic, white)
4. Muscularis propria (hypoechoic, dark)
5. Adventitia or interface with surrounding mediastinal structures (hyperechoic, white)

High-frequency (≥20 MHz) radial miniprobe imaging provides greater detail and reveals nine layers (Fig. 127.9).

1. Interface between intraluminal fluid and the superficial mucosa (hyperechoic, white)
2. Deep mucosa (hypoechoic, dark)
3. Interface between mucosa and muscularis mucosae (hyperechoic, white)
4. Muscularis mucosae (hypoechoic, dark)
5. Submucosa (hyperechoic, white)
6. Inner circular muscle (hypoechoic, dark)
7. Connective tissue between two esophageal muscle layers (hyperechoic, white)
8. Outer longitudinal muscle (hypoechoic, dark)
9. Adventitia or interface with surrounding mediastinal structures (hyperechoic, white)

High-frequency miniprobe imaging of the esophageal wall is useful to evaluate and classify early mucosal tumors.

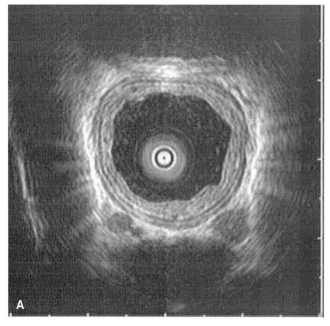

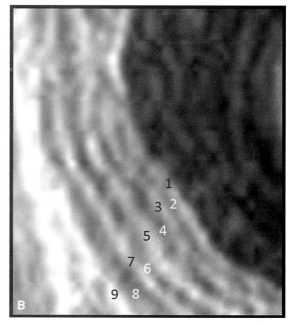

FIGURE 127.9 **A:** Normal esophageal mucosa (high-frequency radial EUS, >20 MHz). **B:** Magnified view of the normal nine layers of the esophageal mucosa on high-frequency radial EUS (see text).

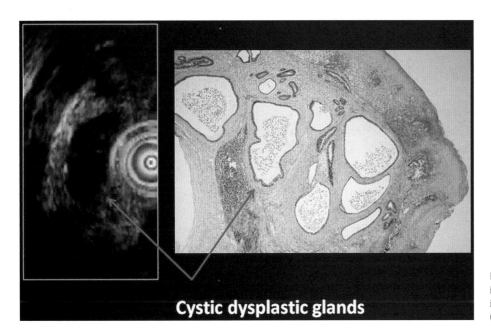

Cystic dysplastic glands

FIGURE 127.10 High-frequency radial EUS image of intramucosal cysts (**right**) representing dilated glands with high-grade dysplasia (**left:** matching micrograph).

BARRETT ESOPHAGUS WITH HIGH-GRADE DYSPLASIA/CARCINOMA IN SITU AND INTRAMUCOSAL CARCINOMA

The clinical utility of high-frequency EUS for the evaluation of high-grade dysplasia/carcinoma in situ (HGD/Tis) and intramucosal carcinoma (IMC/pT1a) in Barrett esophagus (BE) has been challenged, and endoscopic mucosal resection (EMR) is currently the favored diagnostic technique in these patients.[6,7] The key finding that must be assessed by high-frequency EUS is the absence or presence of submucosal invasion (i.e., pT1a vs. pT1b), since submucosal invasion is a key determinant of the risk of LN metastases. The role of high-frequency EUS in the distinction between the different depths of mucosal and submucosal invasion is beyond the scope of this chapter, and at this stage still of limited clinical relevance.

EUS IN Tis, T1M ESOPHAGEAL CANCER

The ultrasonographic appearance of uT0 (Tis) consists of hypoechoic abnormalities exclusively within the mucosa (no invasion of lamina propria, high-frequency EUS layers 1 to 3) (Fig. 127.10).

ESOPHAGEAL CANCER

Esophageal cancer should be thoroughly staged with EUS if the information obtained via EUS is essential to proper staging. Consequently, it is important to determine the key staging information that will guide therapy. Since EUS is a tool used primarily for local staging of esophageal cancer (i.e., T and N status), it is of value mostly in stage I to III disease. In patients post chemotherapy or chemoradiation therapy, EUS is of limited use and accuracy (Table 127.1).

T Stage

EUS plays an important role as a guide to therapy. In general terms, and in the absence of nodal disease, patients with T1 (confined to mucosa or submucosa) and most T2 tumors (invading into muscularis propria) can proceed directly to endoscopic therapy (T1a) or surgery (T1a–T2) while patients with T3 tumors should receive planned multimodal therapy.[8]

T1

T1 tumors are confined to mucosa or submucosa and the main role of EUS is to differentiate between mucosal and submucosal invasion, since therapy may differ. However, EMR plays a more reliable role in the precise level of invasion in early T1 lesions (see above) (Fig. 127.11).

T2 and T3

T2 tumors invade into the muscularis propria (Fig. 127.12) and T3 tumors invade into the adventitia (Fig. 127.13). In clinical practice, and in the absence of nodal disease, EUS plays a very important role in the differentiation between T2 and T3 tumors. Although the best treatment T3 tumors is still a matter of discussion, patients with T2

TABLE 127.1 Diagnostic Accuracy of EUS Staging in Esophageal Cancer

T (Tumor)	
Pretreatment	
Overall	72–84%[15–17,21–24]
Superficial tumors, HFUS[a]	73–80%[10,11,25]
Nodular BE, nodular BE (HFUS)	64–79%[13,26]
T1mm vs. T1sm (HFUS)	≈20%[22,25,27,28]
T1 vs. T2 (standard EUS)[b29,30]	50–60%[27]
T3/4 (standard EUS)	74%[15]
Posttreatment	
Overall	29–50%[31–35]
N (Lymph Node)	
Pretreatment	
EUS only	66–89%[15,21,23–25,30,36–39]
EUS + FNA	87–100%[13,15,16,21,24,39–42]
Posttreatment	
Overall	58–62%[31–35]

[a]HFUS, high-frequency US, 15–30 MHz.
[b]In patients staged as T2N0M0 can be as low as 19–39%.
Standard EUS, 5–12 MHz.

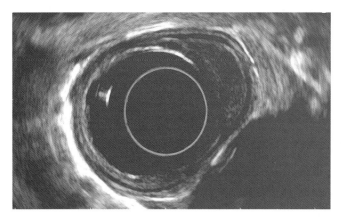

FIGURE 127.11 T1 tumor (at 2 o'clock) with preserved hyperechoic submucosal layer.

tumors tend to proceed directly to surgery, while patients with T3 tumors are generally treated with multimodal therapy protocols.

T4

The invasion of adjacent mediastinal structures by EUS indicates a T4 tumor. Importantly, EUS can differentiate between potentially resectable T4 tumors (T4a [invasion into pericardium, pleura, diaphragm]) (Fig. 127.14) and nonresectable T4 tumors (T4b [invasion into heart, great vessels, airway, etc.]) (Fig. 127.15).

N Stage

Periesophageal LNs can be evaluated by EUS for shape, size, echogenicity, borders, and number. The accuracy of EUS imaging alone for N staging is limited (Table 127.1); however, EUS provides helpful information that must be considered in conjunction with other clinical staging modalities (CT, PET). Once periesophageal LN (mediastinal LN stations, celiac LN) are visualized (Fig. 127.16A,B), the operator must describe the following characteristics to help guide N staging:

1. Shape: oval (benign) versus round (malignant)
2. Size: 10 mm (short axis) is the normal upper limit of mediastinal and celiac LN
3. Echogenicity: heterogeneous with hyperechoic center (suggests benign) versus homogenous and hypoechoic (likely malignant)
4. Borders: less well-defined (benign) versus sharp (malignant)
5. Number of LN: staging of nodal disease from N1 to N3

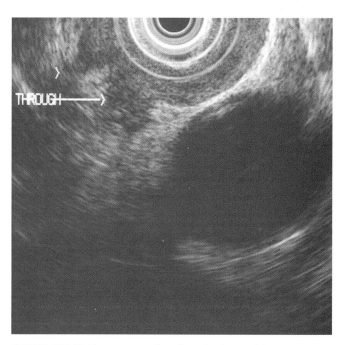

FIGURE 127.13 T3 tumor invading through adventitial layer into periesophageal fat (arrow).

FNA improves the diagnostic accuracy of LN staging (Table 127.1); however, FNA is not indicated in peritumoral LN. Peritumoral LN are likely to be interpreted as malignant on cytopathology, since traversing the tumor with the needle increases the likelihood of a false positive result.

In summary, EUS N stage determination has to be factored in with clinical and radiologic findings. Although EUS is a useful N staging tool, the limited accuracy of imaging alone, and the impossibility of accurate sampling of peritumoral LN emphasize the importance of the clinician as the interpreter of all available staging information (clinical, radiologic, and EUS).

M Stage

The role of EUS in metastatic disease is quite limited, since EUS can image only the immediate vicinity of the esophagus. However, EUS

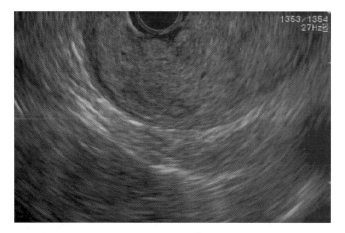

FIGURE 127.12 T2 tumor with invasion of muscularis propria but preserved outer hyperechoic adventitial layer.

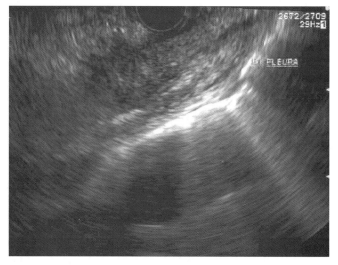

FIGURE 127.14 T4a tumor invading into pleura.

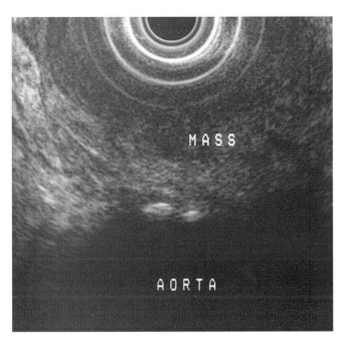

FIGURE 127.15 T4b tumor invading the aortic wall (no visible tissue plane between the mass and the aortic wall).

can be helpful in the definitive documentation of metastatic disease in the liver (Fig. 127.17), adrenal gland (Fig. 127.5B), and pleural lining (Fig. 127.18).

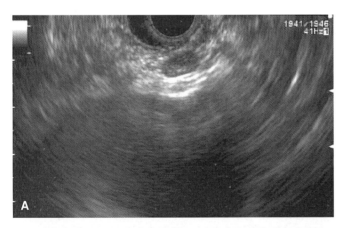

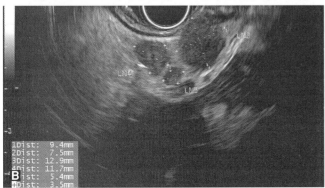

FIGURE 127.16 **A:** Single periesophageal LN with indeterminate EUS features (<10 mm short axis, oval, fuzzy borders, but mostly hypoechoic; see text). **B:** Multiple periesophageal LN with EUS features of malignancy (>10 mm short axis, hypoechoic, round, sharp borders; see text).

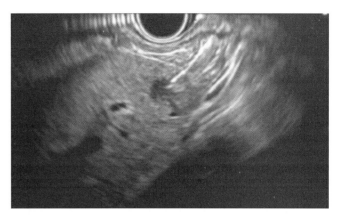

FIGURE 127.17 EUS-FNA of a 5 mm liver metastasis (left lobe of the liver).

EUS EVALUATION OF SUBEPITHELIAL TUMORS OF THE ESOPHAGUS

A variety of tumors may arise from within the wall of the esophagus deep to the mucosal layer. Collectively these are referred to as subepithelial tumors. The term submucosal tumor is also often used; however, this implies an origin in the submucosal layer of the esophageal wall, which is not always the case. These lesions are identified endoscopically as protruding masses covered by grossly normal overlying mucosa (Fig. 127.19). At times there may be central ulceration; however, the majority of mucosa is normal. These lesions may be either premalignant or malignant and further evaluation is generally recommended. EUS is uniquely suited for this purpose.

Depending upon the size of the endoscopic lesion, EUS imaging may be performed using either standard echoendoscopes or through-the-scope miniprobes. As was previously discussed, very small lesions may be difficult to localize with echoendoscopes and better seen with miniprobes. The goals of the EUS examination are three-fold: to determine the echogenicity of the lesion (hypoechoic, anechoic, or hyperechoic), to identify a layer of origin if possible, and to obtain material for a cytologic or histologic diagnosis when necessary. Anechoic lesions are completely black sonographically which typically implies a fluid-filled structure/cyst. These lesions may produce distal acoustic enhancement which confirms the fluid-filled nature. Hypoechoic lesions are dark gray but not completely black. Hyperechoic lesions are bright white and lighter that the surrounding tissue. Determination of echogenicity and layer of origin will narrow the differential diagnosis and is occasionally diagnostic.

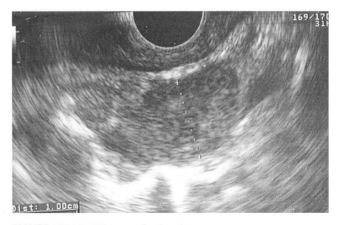

FIGURE 127.18 EUS image of a pleural metastasis.

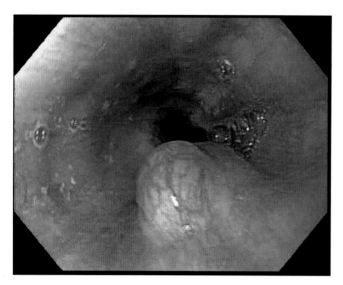

FIGURE 127.19 Endoscopic view of a subepithelial esophageal lesion with normal overlying mucosa.

POTENTIAL LESIONS BY LAYER OF ORIGIN

Layer 2: Deep Mucosa

Lesions arising in layer 2 are nearly always hypoechoic. The finding of a hypoechoic lesion arising in layer 2 in the esophagus would most commonly indicate either leiomyoma or gastrointestinal stromal tumor (GIST). In the esophagus, leiomyoma is far more common, while gastric lesions are statistically most likely to be GISTs. In addition, most GISTs arise from layer 4 rather than layer 2, although this is at times difficult to determine. Differential would also include granular cell tumors, other mesenchymal tumors such as gastrointestinal autonomic nerve tumors (GANTs) or Schwannoma, or carcinoid tumors (which are uncommon in the esophagus).

Anechoic lesions are typically assumed to be cystic, in which case these may indicate either mucoid retention cysts or duplication cysts (Fig. 127.20). Duplication cysts may have a variety of sonographic appearances and may be located either within or adjacent to the esophageal wall. At times, particularly when large, they may contain visible wall layers including a distinct hyperechoic muscular wall which may be contiguous with layer 4 of the esophageal wall. Although classically thought to be hypoechoic, leiomyomas may often appear entirely anechoic and be misinterpreted as cysts (Fig. 127.21).

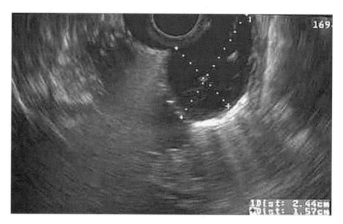

FIGURE 127.21 Anechoic leiomyoma that can be misinterpreted as a cyst without EUS-FNA.

This can be clarified by performing directed needle aspiration (which will fail to collapse the lesion in the instance of leiomyoma).

Hyperechoic lesions in layer 2 are very uncommon. These may indicate lipoma, although lipoma is much more common in layer 3. Rare lymphomas may result in hyperechoic thickening of layer 2. Fibromas and granulomas may occasionally also present with this appearance.

Tissue sampling of lesions in layer 2 may be accomplished several ways. Repeated forceps biopsy in the same location ("tunnel biopsy") will often allow sampling deep to the overlying mucosa and obtain diagnostic material. Smaller lesions may simply be endoscopically resected via suction mucosal resection. Larger lesions may be sampled via FNA or biopsy as discussed previously.

Layer 3: Submucosa

Hypoechoic lesions in the esophageal submucosa are relatively uncommon and may represent granular cell tumors or rare carcinoids and neurogenic tumors (Fig. 127.22).

Hyperechoic lesions in esophageal submucosa are nearly always lipomas. Rarely lymphoma may have this appearance.

Anechoic lesions in the submucosa are cystic lesions. As stated before, these may represent congenital duplication cysts or mucoid retention cysts.

Hyperechoic and anechoic lesions in layer 3 generally do not require tissue sampling, as a reasonably reliable diagnosis can be made based on the sonographic appearance. Hypoechoic lesions may

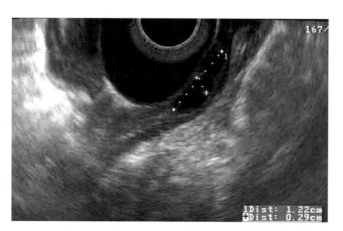

FIGURE 127.20 Deep mucosal cyst.

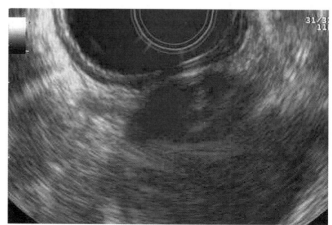

FIGURE 127.22 Tumor arising from submucosa.

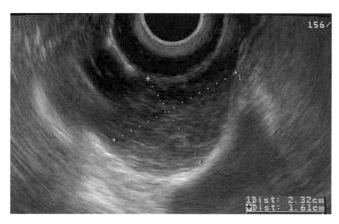

FIGURE 127.23 Gastrointestinal stromal tumor (GIST) arising from the deep mucosa (layer 2).

be definitively diagnosed by tissue sampling as per layer 2 lesions, utilizing either tunnel forceps biopsy, mucosal resection or needle aspiration/biopsy depending on the size of the lesion.

Layer 4: Muscularis Propria

Virtually all subepithelial tumors arising in layer 4 are mesenchymal neoplasms, and the vast majority of these are GISTs (Fig. 127.23). As stated previously, most leiomyomas will arise from layer 2 rather than layer 4; however, this layer of origin may be at times difficult to determine. Other mesenchymal neoplasms such as GANTs remain in the differential diagnosis.

Rarely, hypoechoic tumors in layer 4 may indicate esophageal metastases from nonesophageal primary lesions, such as breast cancer. This diagnosis is suggested by a prior clinical history of malignancy, rapid development of dysphagia, and an irregular/serrated deep margin of the mass.

Nearly all layer 4 lesions are hypoechoic. Very rarely hyperechoic lesions may occur in the setting of lymphoma, metastases, or neurogenic tumors.

The finding of a lesion in layer 4 generally warrants tissue diagnosis to exclude clinically important lesions such as GIST or metastasis. This tissue diagnosis requires needle aspiration/biopsy. EMR using standard methods would result in esophageal perforation and leak, and tunnel forceps biopsy in this setting is of generally low yield. Although newer endoscopic techniques for resection of these lesions via submucosal tunneling (endoscopic submucosal dissection [ESD]) are being developed, they are still not considered standard and are beyond the scope of this review.

INDICATIONS

Endoscopic esophageal US is primarily a diagnostic tool; however, over the past decade, EUS has also gradually emerged as a potential therapeutic tool.

DIAGNOSTIC EUS

The first common sense steps are to determine if a patient is clinically fit to undergo EUS and whether EUS will alter the management of the patient. After proper clinical assessment of a patient, the disease type and the anatomic location of a pathologic process dictate the indications for diagnostic EUS.

ESOPHAGEAL PATHOLOGY

As described in specific sections, EUS is a valuable tool for the diagnosis and staging of a variety of benign and malignant esophageal disease processes. Although the indications for each specific disease process may vary, as a general rule, the esophageal lumen should be patent. The diagnostic accuracy of EUS after neoadjuvant or definitive chemotherapy or chemoradiation therapy is generally poor (*see Results*, Table 127.1), and in the authors' opinions, routine diagnostic EUS after treatment just adds potential morbidity and cost to the patient's evaluation and treatment. In addition, the presence of a malignant stricture demands great caution from the EUS operator, since undue dilation may lead to esophageal perforation. It is preferable to forego EUS or obtain basic relevant EUS information on a tumor, than to cause a tumor perforation. The authors cannot stress enough the devastating consequences of a perforated esophageal cancer.

EXTRAESOPHAGEAL PATHOLOGY

Endoscopic esophageal US is useful to evaluate abnormalities in many of the organs and structures immediately adjacent to the esophagus. The clinician must be adept at identifying these structures and their relation to the esophagus to decide whether EUS evaluation is appropriate.

Proximal Esophagus

Although the cervical and thoracic inlet vasculature, thyroid gland, trachea, and spine are accessible for EUS imaging, EUS plays almost no clinical role in the assessment or management of cervical disease processes.

Proximal Intrathoracic Esophagus

The proximal intrathoracic esophagus (above the carina) allows imaging and EUS-guided access to many periesophageal structures:

- The aorta, proximal aortic arch, and origin of arch vessels
- Pulmonary artery
- The spine
- The azygos vein
- The thoracic duct
- Trachea
- Paratracheal LN
- Aortopulmonary and para-aortic LN
- Posterior mediastinum
- Upper lobes of the lungs

Disease processes that affect central mediastinal LNs and the posterior mediastinum can be accurately evaluated with EUS-FNA. In addition, centrally located lung lesions (>1 cm, within 0 to 5 cm from the esophageal wall) are also accessible for EUS-FNA in selected cases.[43] EUS imaging is also valuable to determine whether a pathologic process invades major vessels.

Distal Intrathoracic Esophagus

The distal intrathoracic esophagus (below the carina) provides EUS access to:

- The subcarinal LN
- The posterior mediastinum
- The left atrium and left ventricle
- The pulmonary artery

- The pulmonary veins
- The descending aorta
- The spine
- The left lobe of the liver
- The inferior vena cava and hepatic veins
- Lower lobes of the lungs
- Lower pleural spaces

The use of EUS in the distal intrathoracic esophagus follows the same principles as in the proximal intrathoracic esophagus.

Intra-abdominal Esophagus and Proximal Stomach

The intra-abdominal esophagus and proximal stomach allow evaluation of:

- The left lobe of the liver
- The aorta
- The celiac trunk
- The left adrenal gland
- The hepatic artery
- The splenic artery
- Gastrohepatic ligament
- LN within or adjacent to these structures

In the intra-abdominal esophagus and proximal stomach, EUS plays a role primarily to stage esophageal or lung malignancies.

Evaluation of the gastric wall, pancreas, biliary system, and spleen are beyond the scope of this chapter.

Therapeutic EUS

Over the past decade, a very gradual development of EUS-guided therapeutic interventions has emerged and holds promise for a select group of patients (see Section on Therapeutic EUS).

RESULTS

Endosonographic equipment is continuously improving and endoscopists are gaining more experience, leading to increased diagnostic capabilities for a variety of diseases overtime. The performance of EUS will depend on numerous factors including type and frequency of the probe used, operator experience, the anatomic location of the lesion being studied, the presence of stenosis, and whether or not it is complemented by FNA among other factors. It is an operator dependent procedure and requires a learning curve. The transducer located at the tip of the EUS emits US waves at various frequencies. The standard echoendoscope probe has a frequency between 5 and 12 MHz and displays the esophageal wall as a five-layer structure.[10,11] As an alternative, high-frequency ultrasound (HFUS) probes can be introduced through the working channel of standard endoscopes, working at frequencies between 15 and 30 MHz and displaying the esophagus as a nine-layer structure.[10,12,13] Procedures done with HFUS improve the image resolution of the esophageal wall layers in tradeoff with scanning depth, especially for LN assessment.[11,22]

ESOPHAGEAL CANCER

EUS provides reliable assessment of the T and N stage of esophageal carcinoma. It may also identify lesions missed by other imaging modalities. The diagnostic performance of EUS with respect to esophageal cancer will depend on assessment of T, N, or M stage,

presence of BE, location of the tumor (upper, middle, or lower esophagus), and whether patients received neoadjuvant therapy (NAT) or not. Correct staging is of paramount importance since it guides further therapy including endoscopic, neoadjuvant, surgical, or palliative therapies.[22] The overall diagnostic accuracy of EUS for T-staging varies depending on the series, but has usually been found in the range of 72% to 84%.[15–17,21–24] Time elapsed between EUS and surgery has also been studied, with longer waiting times for surgery impacting deleteriously the accuracy of initial EUS staging compared to pathologic staging as the gold standard.[36]

TUMOR ASSESSMENT IN BARRETT ESOPHAGUS AND HIGH-GRADE DYSPLASIA

EUS performance has been studied for tumor assessment in the setting of BE with HGD. Changes that are commonly observed in the setting of BE are due to chronic inflammation and metaplastic changes. Musculofibrous anomaly is characterized by thickening of the muscularis mucosa (MM), smooth muscle hypertrophy that extends into the lamina propria, and fibrosis. Duplication of the MM has also been observed in a number of patients.[44,45] Carcinoma has been reported in around 30% of esophagectomy specimens in patients with HGD.[26] Due to the radical differences in treatment modalities and prognosis between intramucosal and invasive carcinomas, correct classification of T and N stages is critical in patients with and without BE. EUS cannot reliably differentiate between benign and malignant wall thickening in the setting of BE and HGD. Moreover, the sensitivity and accuracy of EUS for submucosal tumor invasion is low, especially in the presence of nodular BE, even with the use of HFUS.[6,13,22,26,37,46] In this setting, HFUS has been found to have a diagnostic accuracy around 64% to 79%.[13,26] EMR after EUS has increased accuracy for staging patients with IMCs, especially in the presence of nodular BE.[6,12,22,27,45,47] MM duplication and musculofibrous anomaly may lead to diagnostic misinterpretation with respect to intramucosal or invasive adenocarcinoma in EMR specimens, and may also lead to EUS overstaging.[44,45,48] The most important application of EUS in BE appears to involve the characterization of deeper invading carcinomas and LN status assessment, which may preclude the use of endoscopic ablative therapies.[26,48]

T STAGE FOR INTRAMUCOSAL AND EARLY INVASIVE ESOPHAGEAL CANCER

EUS can be challenging when performed in the setting of superficial esophageal lesions. Lesion localization with the side-viewing echoendoscope may be troublesome. The water-filled balloon can become overdistended and compress the lesion and this in turn can affect appropriate tumor staging.[22] Studies have shown that EUS alone cannot reliably differentiate between T1mm and T1sm stage, with reported accuracy to distinguish between these two around 20%, and understaging being the matter of greatest concern.[22,25,27,28] This limitation is thought to arise from the difficulty in assessing submucosal involvement secondary to peritumoral edema (which may result in overstaging) or not being able to identify involvement beyond the MM (resulting in understaging).[11,27] HFUS for superficial cancers has a reported overall accuracy around 73% to 80%, especially for tumors located in the tubular part of the esophagus, but the accuracy in tumors at the gastroesophageal junction is much lower.[10,11,25,49,50] EMR has been suggested as an adjunct for EUS in early esophageal cancer due to low accuracy of the latter when performed alone.[27,37,38]

The limitations in accuracy of HFUS in BE and early intraepithelial lesions, have led experts to question the need for EUS, since EMR is more reliable.[6,7] As a general rule, EUS does not seem to have a role in nonnodular Barrett since EUS changes the staging in only 4% of patients according to a recent meta-analysis.[51] In patients with nodular Barrett, EMR appears to have greater utility as a diagnostic tool than EUS.[6,7] In addition, EMR may have a therapeutic role for intramucosal tumors without evidence of LN involvement (although a small fraction will have LN involvement on pathology) in patients in which surgery is prohibitive. Continued careful surveillance of any residual Barrett mucosa is required.[27,37,38] The diagnostic accuracy of the standard echoendoscope to distinguish between T1 and T2 tumors is estimated to be around 50% to 60%.[27] cT2N0M0 tumors are a controversial subgroup; although the majority of these staged with standard EUS receive appropriate therapy, there is an important subset of patients who are clinically understaged.[16,29,40,52–54] Forty to fifty-five percent of patients classified as cT2N0M0 will have malignant LN involvement on the pathologic specimen.[53] EUS accuracy in patients with T2N0M0 tumors has been found to be as low as 13% to 39%.[29,30]

T STAGE OF LOCALLY ADVANCED ESOPHAGEAL CANCER

EUS accuracy for T stage in advanced disease has been estimated to be close to 74%.[15] It has been reported to decrease in the setting of strictures requiring dilation, which can be present in up to 30% to 45% of cases.[15,55] If the echoendoscope does not pass a stricture, it is suggested that the procedure be aborted and that these patients be treated as having locally advanced disease with NAT.[11,23] There is no increased diagnostic yield when trying to pass these stenotic segments and the risk of perforation increases.[23] Some authors have observed miniprobe HFUS to be more reliable for staging impassable tumors.[15] A study addressed the potential for metastatic spread when dilation is attempted and did not find any correlation.[56]

N STAGE OF ESOPHAGEAL CANCER

The likelihood of LN metastases correlates with the extent of tumor penetration into the esophageal wall layers. There is a very low probability for intramucosal tumors to have LN involvement (2% to 6%). Tumors that invade into the submucosa or beyond have a higher probability of LN involvement (20% to 50%).[6,25,48] LN echo features used to determine malignant involvement are hypoechoic structure, sharply demarcated border, rounded contour, and size greater than 10 mm.[15,41,57] These features have been shown to have an additive effect. When all features are present, the accuracy is close to 100% for predicting malignant involvement; however, all four criteria are uncommonly found.[41,42,57] The accuracy for EUS for N stage mostly range from 66% to 89%.[15,21,23–25,30,36–39] Miniprobe HFUS have been found to be less reliable for LN assessment.[37] Nevertheless, there have been studies reporting accuracy of 100% using miniprobe HFUS for nodal involvement.[15] Malignant LN involvement may escape detection in some patients, so certain refinements in diagnostic capabilities have been suggested. The addition of FNA to EUS has been shown to be superior to LN echo features alone, increasing accuracies up to 87% to 100%, although this will depend on the location and accessibility of the suspicious LNs and timely specimen review by the cytopathologist.[13,15,16,21,24,39–42] The sensitivity also improves with the addition of FNA from 84.7% to 96.7%.[39] The accuracy of EUS-FNA

for detecting metastasis to celiac lymph nodes (CLNs) is good and ranges from 85.7% to 98%.[21,42]

M STAGE OF ESOPHAGEAL CANCER

The performance of EUS for detecting metastatic disease is relatively poor. This may be explained by the difficulty in assessing the air-filled lungs and the lateral segments of the right hepatic lobe. EUS is usually performed after documenting the absence of detectable metastatic disease with the use of positron-emission tomography (PET), computed tomography (CT) scans, or a combination of these. EUS can detect (and confirm with FNA) focal hepatic metastases that are initially missed by CT scan, which is a rare occurrence but has a major impact on management and prognosis.[38]

STAGING BEFORE AND AFTER NEOADJUVANT THERAPY

EUS staging before NAT does not reliably predict which patients will ultimately have a complete pathologic response.[58] There have been various studies to determine the role of EUS for restaging after NAT, and to assess whether it is capable of determining responders from nonresponders. The results have been poor, with accuracies for assessing pathologic T and N stages as low as 29% to 50% and 58% to 62%, respectively.[31–35] Inflammation and fibrosis are thought to play an important role in the poor performance of preoperative EUS to detect downstaging in patients who received NAT.[31,33–35,38] EUS overstaging after NAT has been observed with rates as high as 49%, especially for patients who achieve complete pathologic response, although understaging has also been reported.[33,35] In conclusion, EUS should not be routinely used for restaging esophageal cancer after NAT.[31–35,38] A decrease of 50% or greater of the maximal cross-sectional area of the tumor appears to be more reliable for determining response to treatment after NAT, and also correlates better with survival in this setting.[33,34,38]

TUMOR LOCATION

The diagnostic performance of EUS decreases as tumor location changes from the upper esophagus toward the GEJ. Tumors located in the tubular esophagus are better staged than those near the GEJ.[11,13,25] This difference is believed to result from the difficulty in creating an adequate acoustic interface when tumors are near to the GEJ.[10,12] This finding might explain the greater statistically nonsignificant accuracy for squamous cell carcinomas than adenocarcinomas.[22]

EUS IN THE EARLY DETECTION OF POSTOPERATIVE RECURRENCE

The detection of early postoperative anastomotic recurrence may be difficult, since the symptoms may be very similar to those of a benign stricture or postoperative dysmotility. Moreover, the site of recurrence with respect to the layers of the esophagus may me deeper to the mucosa or extramural, making endoscopic biopsies problematic or unreliable. EUS is a useful tool in the setting of anastomotic recurrence, having a sensitivity over 90%, higher than either endoscopy or CT. False positives do occur, with fibrotic changes playing an important role in misinterpretation. EUS-FNA helps improve the specificity in this setting. EUS surveillance may detect a significant percentage of recurrences in an asymptomatic stage.[38]

CORRELATION BETWEEN EUS STAGING AND SURVIVAL IN ESOPHAGEAL CANCER

The association between EUS staging information and survival has been analyzed and reported in various studies.[38,59] These have shown an important correlation between EUS-guided findings of advanced T or N status (with more than three peritumoral LNs), the presence of CLN involvement, and their association with poor survival.[38,59] Receipt of EUS by itself is a predictor of improved 1-, 3-, and 5-year survival compared to patients that do not receive EUS.[60] This finding is very likely related to the more precise staging of patients, which leads to appropriate stage-specific therapies.[60] Common barriers for receiving EUS are cost and accessibility.

Benign Tumors

Less than 1% of clinically identified esophageal tumors are benign, but because they are asymptomatic, they may be more common than previously reported.[61] These benign tumors include squamous papillomas, fibrovascular polyps, duplication and bronchial cysts, granular cell tumors, lipomas, leiomyomas, and hemangiomas among others, with some of these lesions having malignant variants. Leiomyomas are the most common benign esophageal tumors and represent around 70% of cases.[61,62] Esophagoscopy has improved for the identification of extramucosal benign tumors of the esophagus but is not a good tool for classification. Intramural and paraesophageal tumors are very difficult to distinguish by this technique. In this clinical situation, EUS has proved to be an essential diagnostic tool, with its ability to classify tumors by layer of origin, size, borders, and echogenicity among others features.[61] EUS-FNA may not provide sufficient cellular architectural information for the differentiation of leiomyomas and leiomyosarcomas. Benign esophageal tumors are typically asymptomatic, and when they are found to have typical EUS characteristics, observation with EUS is indicated. Resection is indicated when they become symptomatic.[61]

Gastrointestinal Stromal Tumors

GISTs affecting the esophagus are extremely rare and account for approximately 1% of cases.[21,63] A correct diagnosis is challenging, since conventional imaging techniques and biopsies during esophagoscopy may not have good accuracy.[64] EUS helps determine the location, echoendoscopic features, and size of subepithelial tumors. GISTs are characterized by their hypoechoic appearance, normal endoscopic and endosonographic mucosa, and are found to arise from the fourth hypoechoic endosonographic layer.[21,64] Invasive GISTs are characterized endosonographically by irregular extraluminal borders, cystic areas, echogenic foci, and size greater than 3 cm.[64] Studies concerning the performance of EUS for GISTs are performed mostly for lesions involving the stomach, since this is the most common location. EUS has an accuracy around 64% and 80%, respectively, for the differentiation of malignant and benign subepithelial lesions.[64] Characterizing small, early-stage subepithelial lesions may be difficult due to the absence of well-established echoendoscopic features. FNA, when added, may increase accuracy in the study of these subepithelial lesions, but has limitations associated to the firm nature of these tumors, low cytologic yield, and force required to penetrate the tumors.[62,64] The accuracy of EUS and EUS-FNA for diagnosing potentially aggressive GISTs is 78% and 91%, respectively.[21]

Lung Nodules and Masses

EUS-FNA is reliable and safe for the evaluation of pulmonary nodules and masses in proximity to the esophagus.[21,43] Biopsy of intraparenchymal centrally located pulmonary lesions that are not adjacent to the esophagus or central airways may be more challenging.[43] Endobronchial ultrasound-guided transbronchial needle aspiration (EBUS-TBNA) and EUS-FNA are techniques that can aid in the diagnosis and sampling of these lesions.[43] The diagnostic accuracy of EUS-FNA and EBUS-TBNA for assessment of centrally located lesions in proximity to the esophagus or central airways is in the range of 86% to 94%. For those patients with central lesions not in immediate proximity to the airway or esophagus (Fig. 127.24A,B), the diagnostic accuracy of EBUS-TBNA and EUS-FNA is 93.8%, with a low complication rate.[43]

Lung Cancer Staging

EUS-FNA is a helpful diagnostic and staging tool for patients with lung cancer, and together with mediastinoscopy and endobronchial ultrasonography with transbronchial needle aspiration (EBUS-TBNA), is part of an armamentarium of complementary diagnostic tools.[20]

Mediastinal LN staging with EUS imaging alone is unreliable,[42,65] staging EUS must be performed with FNA. EUS provides access to mediastinal lymph node (MLN) stations 2R, 2L, 4L, 7, 8, and 9), the left adrenal gland, and the liver for staging. Experienced operators may also sample MLN station 5 (Fig. 127.6) via a transpulmonary artery or transaortic puncture (discouraged by the authors since the aorta is a high-pressure vessel), and sometimes even the right adrenal gland (Fig. 127.25A,B).[18,19] In addition, EUS may provide information on lung tumor resectability by determination of aortic or esophageal invasion (Fig. 127.26A,B).

Technique

In patients with lung nodules, lung tumors, mediastinal lymphadenopathy, or mediastinal masses, EUS can be performed as described in the technique section of this chapter. Alternatively, EUS can be performed at the time of EBUS with the EBUS scope. The authors first perform EBUS and then EUS with the EBUS scope to access additional MLNs if needed. However, the EBUS scope is not an appropriate tool to transpulmonary artery puncture, adrenal gland FNA, or liver evaluation. In general terms, the authors use the EBUS scope only for EUS evaluation of MLNs; if the need to sample a lung lesion, the adrenal gland, or the liver is anticipated, the authors use the EUS scope.

Results

A systematic review and meta-analysis of 1,201 patients from 18 reports of EUS-FNA for NSCLC staging found a pooled sensitivity of 83% (95% CI: 78% to 87%) and a pooled specificity of 97% (95% CI, 96% to 98%). In eight studies, the diagnostic performance of EUS-FNA was evaluated exclusively in patients with abnormal MLNs on imaging, with papers that evaluated EUS-FNA in patients without abnormal MLNs on imaging, with a sensitivity of 90% (95% CI, 84% to 94%) and a specificity of 97% (95% CI, 95% to 98%). However, four articles evaluated the diagnostic performance of EUS-FNA in patients without abnormal MLNs on imaging and the pooled sensitivity was only 58% (95% CI, 39% to 75%) (Table 127.2).[65–69]

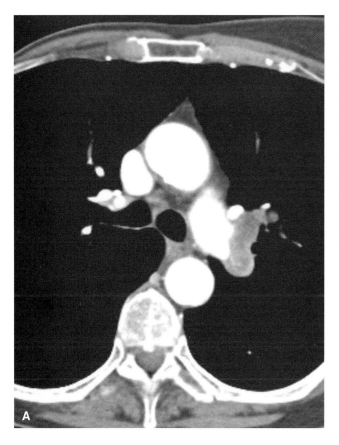

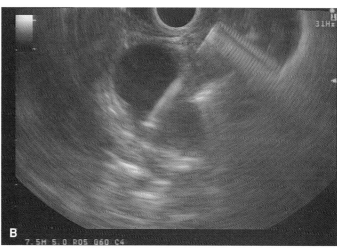

FIGURE 127.24 Left upper lobe mass. **A:** CT scan. **B:** EUS-FNA with transpulmonary artery approach.

In our experience, EUS is helpful when access or visualization of MLN stations is difficult via EBUS, since the esophagus has a more pliable wall than the tracheobronchial tree, and air within the tracheobronchial tree can result in poor transmission of US waves. Also, EBUS-TBNA of MLNs from patients with centrally located squamous cell cancers with widespread airway dysplasia or carcinoma in situ may result in false positive findings; EUS-FNA reduces that risk, but false positives may still occur.[70]

EUS-FNA AND EBUS-FNA

The combination of EUS-FNA and EBUS-TBNA provides near complete mediastinal staging without a skin incision. Several small studies have been published on the use of the combination of EBUS-FNA and EUS-FNA for NSCLC staging; excellent sensitivity (93%), NPV (97%), and accuracy (99%) have been reported.[71,72]

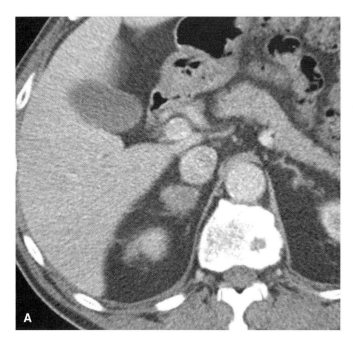

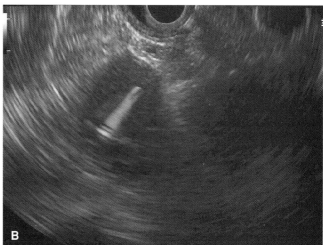

FIGURE 127.25 Right adrenal gland metastasis. **A:** CT scan, the duodenum does not appear in the immediacy of the lesion; however, endoscopic manipulation allowed for a safe FNA window. **B:** EUS-FNA of right adrenal metastasis (Right kidney in left upper hand corner, inferior vena cava to the right of the lesion).

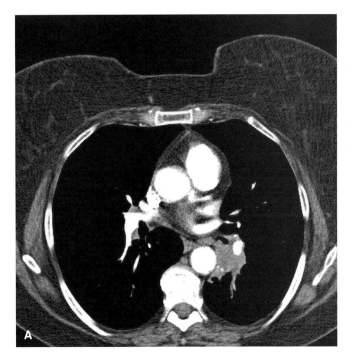

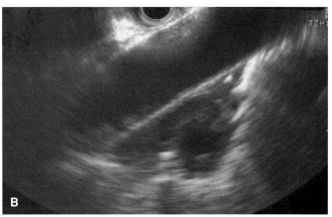

FIGURE 127.26 Left lower lobe lung cancer. **A:** CT scan cannot determine the presence or absence of aortic wall invasion. **B:** EUS demonstrates a clear layer between the tumor and the aortic wall. On real-time imaging the tumor could be seen sliding along the wall of the aorta.

EUS-FNA AND MEDIASTINOSCOPY

The addition of EUS to mediastinoscopy improves diagnostic accuracy by detecting N2/N3 disease or mediastinal invasion that may be missed in up to 16% of patients who undergo mediastinoscopy alone.[70] The combination of EUS and mediastinoscopy is superior to either diagnostic procedure alone, with combined sensitivity of 86%, specificity of 97%, negative predictive value of 93%, and diagnostic accuracy of 93%.[70]

EUS FOR RESTAGING OF THE MEDIASTINUM

Repeat mediastinoscopy is the gold standard in patients with NSCLC who require restaging after NAT. Repeat mediastinoscopy in experienced centers is associated with lower diagnostic performance than initial mediastinoscopy (NPV of 79% to 85%).[73–77]

TABLE 127.2 Diagnostic Performance of EUS in Lung Lesions and Lung Cancer Staging

Lung Lesion	
EUS (± EBUS)	86–94%[21,43]
Mediastinal Lymph Node	
EUS, sensitivity (pooled)	76–98%[18,19,66,70]
EUS, specificity (pooled)	96–98%%[18,19,66,70]
EUS + EBUS, sensitivity	93%[71,72]
EUS + EBUS, NPV	97%[71,72]
EUS + Med[a], sensitivity	86%[70]
EUS + Med[a], specificity	97%[70]

[a]Mediastinoscopy.

The diagnostic efficacy of EUS-FNA alone for mediastinal restaging has been assessed in small series (<30 patients), with reported NPV of 67% to 91.7%.[78,79]

The combination of EUS-FNA and EBUS-TBNA in restaging the mediastinum in a series of 106 patients after NAT for NSCLC had a sensitivity of 67%, specificity of 96%, PPV of 95%, NPV of 73%, and accuracy of 81%. The diagnostic performance of the combination of EUS-FNA and EBUS-TBNA was better than of either individual procedure.[80] In patients with NSCLC who require restaging after NAT the clinician must tailor the diagnostic approach according to the individual patient's needs and circumstances.

MEDIASTINAL CYSTS AND PRIMARY MEDIASTINAL TUMORS

Mediastinal cysts mostly consist of congenital or acquired thymic cysts and foregut duplication cysts. EUS-FNA is an adequate tool to ascertain the cystic nature of these lesions and obtain tissue for pathologic analysis. Acute mediastinitis is a potential complication when performing EUS-FNA for the diagnosis of these cystic lesions.[21] Malignant lymphoma is the most common primary neoplasm that affects the mediastinum, and can often be sampled by EUS-FNA. However, the ability to perform all necessary tests on a needle sample is not uniformly reliable. Other primary neoplasms of the mediastinum that may be characterized with the use of EUS include neurogenic tumors (Fig. 127.27A,B), extra-adrenal paragangliomas, mesenchymal tumors, and metastatic germ-cell neoplasms.[21]

COMPLICATIONS

The overall complication rate for esophageal EUS is extremely low. However, there is a small risk for serious complications including perforations with the echoendoscope, with an estimated incidence of cervical esophageal perforation around 0.03% to 0.06%, and Killian's triangle is the site at greatest risk for injury.[81] The complication rate for EUS-FNA is low ranging from 0.5% to 2.3%.[21,39,65,82] Complications

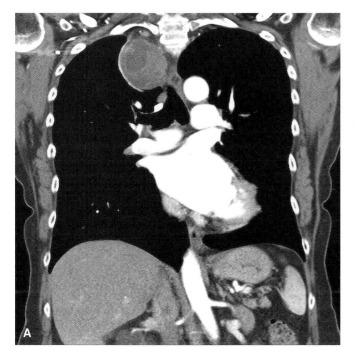

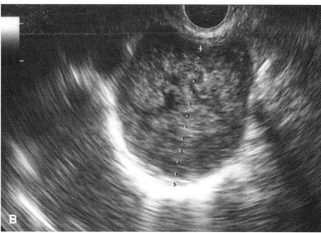

FIGURE 127.27 Right apical Schwannoma. **A:** CT scan. **B:** EUS.

consist primarily of infection and bleeding, and more rarely perforation, peritonitis, mediastinitis, acute portal vein thrombosis, and aspiration pneumonia.[21,39,82,83] Tumor seeding during EUS-FNA is difficult to assess as a result of surgical resection removing the needle pathway and the effects of chemotherapy on tissues.[21] Dilation of stenotic tumors for the passage of the echoendoscope increases the risk of perforation, and is reported to be as high as 24%.[23]

EUS-FNA VERSUS PET IN ESOPHAGEAL CANCER STAGING

Traditionally multiple modalities, such as EUS, PET, and CT, are required for esophageal staging workup. Multiple modalities, such as EUS, PET, and CT, are required for esophageal staging workup. Accurate staging of esophageal cancer generally requires a combination of EUS-FNA and PET/CT.

A meta-analysis showed that EUS-FNA has a higher sensitivity for initial staging of locoregional disease,[84] while FDG (fluorine-18 fluorodeoxyglucose)-PET-CT scans have better diagnostic performance for staging of distant nodal or organ metastases. The combination of EUS-FNA and PET-CT has better staging accuracy[85] than either of these modalities alone.

After chemoradiotherapy, PET-CT has better staging accuracy and is a better predictor of survival than EUS, since the staging accuracy of EUS in this setting is poor. (Table 127.1).[86,87]

In summary, EUS is more sensitive than PET-CT for initial staging of locoregional disease, while PET-CT is more accurate for initial staging of metastatic disease. In patients after chemotherapy or chemoradiation therapy, PET-CT is the main restaging and monitoring modality, and EUS only plays a very limited role.

THERAPEUTIC EUS

While EUS was developed as a diagnostic modality, it has gradually gained a role as a therapeutic tool. Interventional EUS has been primarily evaluated for benign and malignant pancreatic pathology and other upper abdominal diseases. Therapeutic options include drainage of fluid collections or abscesses,[88–96] gastropexy in Roux-en-Y patients,[97] to guide natural orifice transluminal endoscopic surgery (NOTES)[98–100] or peroral endoscopic myotomy (POEM),[101] radiofrequency ablation,[102–104] brachytherapy and fiducial marker placement,[105,106] injection of therapeutic agents (e.g., ethanol),[107,108] botulinum toxin A,[109,110] immunotherapy,[111–115] oncolytic viruses,[116–119] and high-intensity focused ultrasound (HIFU).[120–125] Only few of these reports actually address therapeutic EUS for esophageal[101,109,110] or intrathoracic interventions.[98,106]

EUS AND THE ROLE OF THE THORACIC SURGEON

Thoracic surgeons play a key role in the evaluation and management of patients with thoracic diseases. Institutional circumstances tend to dictate if thoracic surgeons have the opportunity to train in and practice EUS. In some practices, thoracic surgeons are the primary EUS operators for patients with thoracic diseases, while in most scenarios thoracic surgeons perform little or no EUS. Regardless of the level of technical ability in EUS, it is very important for thoracic surgeons to understand the exact indications, results, and limitations of EUS as to properly integrate EUS in the care of patients. The primary question to ask is not who should perform EUS in patients with thoracic diseases; the answer is obviously the operator who is most skilled. The main issue is to understand how to best ensure that our patients get the highest quality of care. In the authors' opinions, the best care places the patient in the center and the providers form a team to optimize that patient's care. The key questions to ask are:

1. Does EUS provide the information needed to care for a patient?
2. Is EUS the least invasive approach to evaluate a particular patient?
3. Is a negative result from EUS-FNA acceptable given the limitations of the NPV of FNA?
4. Does EUS fit in the most efficient quality-oriented care of a patient?

Thoracic surgeons should play a key role to answer the above questions. Whether a thoracic surgeon is the indicated EUS operator in a particular setting is secondary. Nonetheless, the authors believe that the value of thoracic surgeons learning and practicing EUS lies more in thinking outside of traditional thoracic surgery practice boundaries. The evolution of thoracic surgical practice depends on how much one wishes to step outside of established comfort zones.

CONCLUSION/SUMMARY

Endoscopic esophageal US is a versatile and established diagnostic tool for the evaluation of patients with thoracic diseases. The role of therapeutic EUS in patients with thoracic diseases is in its early phases and may be promising for a select group of patients.

REFERENCES

1. DiMagno EP, Buxton JL, Regan PT, et al. Ultrasonic endoscope. *Lancet* 1980;1(8169):629–631.
2. Mekky MA. Endoscopic ultrasound in gastroenterology: From diagnosis to therapeutic implications. *World J Gastroenterol* 2014;20(24):7801–7807.
3. Encyclopaedia Britannica. Ultrasound diagnosis. http://www.britannica.com/topic/ultrasound.
4. Encyclopaedia Britannica. The Doppler effect. http://www.britannica.com/science/Doppler-effect.
5. Gress F, Savides TJ, eds. *Endoscopic Ultrasonography*. Wiley-Blackwell. 2016:1–214.
6. Bulsiewicz WJ, Dellon ES, Rogers AJ, et al. The impact of endoscopic ultrasound findings on clinical decision making in Barrett's esophagus with high-grade dysplasia or early esophageal adenocarcinoma. *Dis Esophagus* 2014;27(5):409–417. doi:10.1111/j.1442-2050.2012.01408.x.
7. Pouw RE, Heldoorn N, Herrero LA, et al. Do we still need EUS in the workup of patients with early esophageal neoplasia? A retrospective analysis of 131 cases. *Gastrointest Endosc* 2011;73(4):662–668. doi:10.1016/j.gie.2010.10.046.
8. NCCN Guidelines. Esophageal and esophagogastric junction cancers. *NCCN Clin Pract Guidelines Oncol* 2016:1–129.
9. Prasad P, Wittmann J, Pereira SP. Endoscopic ultrasound of the upper gastrointestinal tract and mediastinum: Diagnosis and therapy. *Cardiovasc Intervent Radiol* 2006;29(6):947–957. doi:10.1007/s00270-005-0184-z.
10. May A, Günter E, Roth F, et al. Accuracy of staging in early oesophageal cancer using high resolution endoscopy and high resolution endosonography: a comparative, prospective, and blinded trial. *Gut* 2004;53(5):634–640. doi:10.1136/gut.2003.029421.
11. Meister T, Domagk D, Heinzow H, et al. Miniprobe endoscopic ultrasound accurately stages esophageal cancer and guides therapeutic decisions in the era of neoadjuvant therapy: results of a multicenter cohort analysis. *Surg Endosc* 2013;27(8):2813–2819. doi:10.1007/s00464-013-2817-7.
12. Chemaly M, Scalone O, Durivage G, et al. Miniprobe EUS in the Pretherapeutic Assessment of Early Esophageal Neoplasia. *Endoscopy* 2008;40(1):2–6. doi:10.1055/s-2007-966958.
13. Seerden T, Larghi A. Staging of early adenocarcinoma in Barrett's esophagus. *Gastrointest Endosc Clin N Am* 2011;21(1):53–66. doi:10.1016/j.giec.2010.09.006.
14. Pedersen BH, Vilmann P, Folke K, et al. Endoscopic ultrasonography and real-time guided fine-needle aspiration biopsy of solid lesions of the mediastinum suspected of malignancy. *Chest* 1996;110(2):539–544. doi:10.1378/chest.110.2.539.
15. Shimpi RA, George J, Jowell P, Gress FG. Staging of Esophageal Cancer by EUS: Staging Accuracy Revisited. *Gastrointest Endosc* 2007;66(3):475–482. doi:10.1016/j.gie.2007.03.1051.
16. Crabtree TD, Yacoub WN, Puri V, et al. Endoscopic ultrasound for early stage esophageal adenocarcinoma: implications for staging and survival. *Ann Thorac Surg* 2011;91(5):1509–1516. doi:10.1016/j.athoracsur.2011.01.063.
17. Pfau PR, Perlman SB, Stanko P, et al. The role and clinical value of EUS in a multimodality esophageal carcinoma staging program with CT and positron emission tomography. *Gastrointest Endosc* 2007;65(3):377–384. doi:10.1016/j.gie.2006.12.015.
18. Groth SS, Andrade RS. Endobronchial and endoscopic ultrasound-guided fine-needle aspiration: a must for thoracic surgeons. *Ann Thorac Surg* 2010;89(6):S2079–S2083. doi:10.1016/j.athoracsur.2010.03.018.
19. Cameron SE, Andrade RS, Pambuccian SE. Endobronchial ultrasound-guided transbronchial needle aspiration cytology: a state of the art review. *Cytopathol* 2010;21(1):6–26. doi:10.1111/j.1365-2303.2009.00722.x.
20. Andrade RS, Groth SS, Rueth NM, et al. Evaluation of mediastinal lymph nodes with endobronchial ultrasound: the thoracic surgeon's perspective. *J Thorac Cardiovasc Surg* 2010;139(3):578–583. doi:10.1016/j.jtcvs.2009.11.017.
21. Bardales RH, Stelow EB, Mallery S, et al. Review of endoscopic ultrasound-guided fine-needle aspiration cytology. *Diagn Cytopathol* 2006;34(2):140–175. doi:10.1002/dc.20300.
22. Attila T, Faigel DO. Role of endoscopic ultrasound in superficial esophageal cancer. *Dis Esophagus* 2009;22(2):104–112.
23. Worrell SG, Oh DS, Greene CL, et al. Endoscopic ultrasound staging of stenotic esophageal cancers may be unnecessary to determine the need for neoadjuvant therapy. *J Gastrointest Surg* 2014;18(2):318–320. doi:10.1007/s11605-013-2398-8.
24. Pech O, Günter E, Dusemund F, et al. Accuracy of endoscopic ultrasound in preoperative staging of esophageal cancer: results from a referral center for early esophageal cancer. *Endoscopy* 2010;42(06):456–461. doi:10.1055/s-0029-1244022.
25. Rampado S, Bocus P, Battaglia G, et al. Endoscopic ultrasound: accuracy in staging superficial carcinomas of the esophagus. *Ann Thorac Surg* 2008;85(1):251–256. doi:10.1016/j.athoracsur.2007.08.021.
26. Savoy A, Wallace M. EUS in the management of the patient with dysplasia in Barrett's esophagus. *J Clin Gastroenterol* 2005;39(4):263–267.
27. Maish MS, DeMeester SR. Endoscopic mucosal resection as a staging technique to determine the depth of invasion of esophageal adenocarcinoma. *Ann Thorac Surg* 2004;78(5):1777–1782. doi:10.1016/j.athoracsur.2004.04.064.
28. Bergeron E, Lin J, Chang A, et al. Endoscopic ultrasound is inadequate to determine which t1/t2 esophageal tumors are candidates for endoluminal therapies. *J Thorac Cardiovasc Surg* 2013;147(2):765–771. doi:10.1016/j.jtcvs.2013.10.003.
29. Sancheti M, Fernandez F. Management of T2 esophageal cancer. *Surg Clin N Am* 2012;92(5):1169–1178. doi:10.1016/j.suc.2012.07.003.
30. Tekola BD, Sauer BG, Wang AY, et al. Accuracy of endoscopic ultrasound in the diagnosis of t2n0 esophageal cancer. *J Gastrointest Cancer* 2014;45(3):342–346.
31. Heinzow HS, Seifert H, Tsepetonidis S, et al. Endoscopic ultrasound in staging esophageal cancer after neoadjuvant chemotherapy—results of a multicenter cohort analysis. *J Gastrointest Surg* 2013;17(6):1050–1057. doi:10.1007/s11605-013-2189-2.
32. Schneider PM, Metzger R, Schaefer H, et al. Response evaluation by endoscopy, rebiopsy, and endoscopic ultrasound does not accurately predict histopathologic regression after neoadjuvant chemoradiation for esophageal cancer. *Ann Surg* 2008;248(6):902–908.
33. Misra S, Choi M, Livingstone AS, et al. The role of endoscopic ultrasound in assessing tumor response and staging after neoadjuvant chemotherapy for esophageal cancer. *Surg Endosc* 2012;26(2):518–522. doi:10.1007/s00464-011-1911-y.
34. Kalha I, Kaw M, Fukami N, et al. The accuracy of endoscopic ultrasound for restaging esophageal carcinoma after chemoradiation therapy. *Cancer* 2004;101(5):940–947. doi:10.1002/cncr.20429.
35. Griffin JM, Reed CE, Denlinger CE. Utility of restaging endoscopic ultrasound after neoadjuvant therapy for esophageal cancer. *Ann Thorac Surg* 2012;93(6):1855–1860. doi:10.1016/j.athoracsur.2011.12.095.
36. Fisher JM, Pohl H, Gordon SR, et al The impact of time elapsed between endoscopic ultrasound and esophagectomy on concordance of ultrasonographic and pathologic staging of esophageal malignancy. *Dig Dis Sci* 2011;56(10):2987–2991. doi:10.1007/s10620-011-1719-6.
37. Bergeron EJ, Lin J, Chang AC, et al. Endoscopic ultrasound is inadequate to determine which t1/t2 esophageal tumors are candidates for endoluminal therapies. *J Thorac Cardiovasc Surg* 2014;147(2):765–771; discussion: 771–773. doi:10.1016/j.jtcvs.2013.10.003.
38. Mallery S, Van Dam J. EUS in the evaluation of esophageal carcinoma. *Gastrointest Endosc* 2000;52(6):S6–S11. doi:10.1067/mge.2000.110722.
39. Puli SR, Reddy J, Bechtold M, et al. Staging accuracy of esophageal cancer by endoscopic ultrasound: a meta-analysis and systematic review. *World J Gastroenterol* 2008;14(10):1479–1412. doi:10.3748/wjg.14.1479.
40. Eloubeidi MA, Cerfolio RJ, Bryant AS, et al. Efficacy of endoscopic ultrasound in patients with esophageal cancer predicted to have n0 disease. *Eur J Cardio-Thorac Surg* 2011;40:636–641. doi:10.1016/j.ejcts.2010.12.054.
41. Parmar KS, Zwischenberger JB, Reeves AL, et al. Clinical impact of endoscopic ultrasound-guided fine needle aspiration of celiac axis lymph nodes (M1a disease) in esophageal cancer. *Ann Thorac Surg* 2002;73(3):916–920. doi:10.1016/S0003-4975(01)03560-3.
42. Chen VK, Eloubeidi MA. Endoscopic ultrasound-guided fine needle aspiration is superior to lymph node echofeatures: a prospective evaluation of mediastinal and peri-intestinal lymphadenopathy. *Am J Gastroenterol* 2004;99(4):628–633. doi:10.1111/j.1572-0241.2004.04064.x.
43. Dincer E, Gliksberg E, Andrade R. Endoscopic ultrasound and/or endobronchial ultrasound-guided needle biopsy of central intraparenchymal lung lesions not adjacent to airways or esophagus. *Endoscopic Ultrasound* 2015;4(1):40–44. doi:10.4103/2303-9027.151332.
44. Lewis J, Wang K, Abraham S. Muscularis mucosae duplication and the musculofibrous anomaly in endoscopic mucosal resections for Barrett esophagus. *Am J Surg Pathol* 2008;32(4):566–571. doi:10.1097/PAS.0b013e31815bf8c7.
45. Mandal RV, Forcione DG, Brugge WR, et al. Effect of tumor characteristics and duplication of the muscularis mucosae on the endoscopic staging of superficial barrett esophagus-related neoplasia. *Am J Surg Pathol* 2009;33(4):620–625. doi:10.1097/PAS.0b013e31818d632f.
46. Waxman I, Raju GS, Critchlow J, et al. High-Frequency probe ultrasonography has limited accuracy for detecting invasive adenocarcinoma in patients with Barrett's esophagus and high-grade dysplasia or intramucosal carcinoma: a case series. *Am J Gastroenterol* 2006;101(8):1773–1779. doi:10.1111/j.1572-0241.2006.00617.x.
47. Larghi A, Lightdale CJ, Memeo L, et al. EUS followed by EMR for staging of high-hrade dysplasia and early cancer in Barrett's esophagus. *Gastrointest Endosc* 2005;62(1):16–23. doi:10.1016/S0016-5107(05)00319-6.
48. Ortiz J, Konda V, Chennat J, et al. Is endoscopic ultrasound (EUS) necessary in the pre-therapeutic assessment of Barrett's esophagus with early neoplasia? *J Gastrointest Oncol* 2012;3(4):314–321. doi:10.3978/j.issn.2078-6891.2012.038.
49. Dhupar R, Rice RD, Correa AM, et al. Endoscopic ultrasound estimates for tumor depth at the gastroesophageal junction are inaccurate: implications for the

liberal use of endoscopic resection. *Ann Thoracic Surg* 2015;100(5):1812–1816. doi:10.1016/j.athoracsur.2015.05.038.

50. Pech O, Günter E, Ell C. Endosonography of high-grade intra-epithelial neoplasia/early cancer. *Best Pract Res Clin Gastroenterol* 2009;23(5):639–647. doi:10.1016/j.bpg.2009.05.010.

51. Qumseya BJ, Brown J, Abraham M, et al. Diagnostic performance of EUS in predicting advanced cancer among patients with Barrett's esophagus and high-grade dysplasia/early adenocarcinoma: systematic review and meta-analysis. *Gastrointest Endosc* 2015;81(4):865–874.e2. doi:10.1016/j.gie.2014.08.025.

52. Kountourakis P, Correa AM, Hofstetter WL, et al. Combined modality therapy of cT2N0M0 esophageal cancer. *Cancer.* 2011;117(5):925–930. doi:10.1002/cncr.25651.

53. Hardacker TJ, Ceppa D, Okereke I, et al. Treatment of clinical T2N0M0 esophageal cancer. *Ann Surg Oncol* 2014;21(12):3739–3743. doi:10.1245/s10434-014-3929-6.

54. Crabtree TD, Kosinski AS, Puri V, et al. Evaluation of the reliability of clinical staging of T2 N0 esophageal cancer: A review of the Society of Thoracic Surgeons Database. *Ann Thorac Surg* 2013;96(2):382–390. doi:10.1016/j.athoracsur.2013.03.093.

55. Kelly S, Harris KM, Berry E, et al. A systematic review of the staging performance of endoscopic ultrasound in gastro-oesophageal carcinoma. *Gut* 2001;49(4):534–539.

56. Hancock SM, Gopal DV, Frick TJ, et al. Dilation of malignant strictures in endoscopic ultrasound staging of esophageal cancer and metastatic spread of disease. *Diagnost Therap Endosc* 2011;2011(10):1–6. doi:10.1155/2011/356538.

57. Catalano MF, Sivak MV Jr., Rice T, et al. Endosonographic features predictive of lymph node metastasis. *Gastrointest Endosc* 1994;40(4):442–446. doi:10.1016/S0016-5107(94)70206-3.

58. Mallery S, DeCamp M, Bueno R, et al. Pretreatment staging by endoscopic ultrasonography does not predict complete response to neoadjuvant chemoradiation in patients with esophageal carcinoma. *Cancer* 1999;86(5):764–769. doi:0.1002/(SICI)1097-0142(19990901)86:53.0.CO;2-W.

59. Eloubeidi MA, Wallace MB, Hoffman BJ, et al. Predictors of survival for esophageal cancer patients with and without celiac axis lymphadenopathy: impact of staging endosonography. *Ann Thorac Surg* 2001;72(1):212–219. doi:10.1016/S0003-4975(01)02616-9.

60. Wani S, Das A, Rastogi A, et al. Endoscopic ultrasonography in esophageal cancer leads to improved survival rates: results from a population-based study. *Cancer* 2015;121(2):194–201. doi:10.1002/cncr.29043.

61. Rice TW. Benign esophageal tumors: Esophagoscopy and endoscopic esophageal ultrasound. *Semin Thorac Cardiovasc Surg* 2003;15(1):20–26. doi:10.1016/S1043-0679(03)00035-2.

62. Stelow EB, Stanley MW, Mallery S, et al. Endoscopic ultrasound-guided fine-needle aspiration findings of gastrointestinal leiomyomas and gastrointestinal stromal tumors. *Am J Clin Pathol* 2003;119(5):703–708. doi:10.1309/UWUVQ0010D9W0HPN.

63. Kukar M, Kapil A, Papenfuss W, et al. Gastrointestinal stromal tumors (gists) at uncommon locations: a large population based analysis. *J Surg Oncol* 2015;111(6):696–701. doi:10.1002/jso.23873.

64. Karaca C, Turner BG, Cizginer S, et al. Accuracy of EUS in the evaluation of small gastric subepithelial lesions. *Gastrointest Endosc* 2010;71(4):722–727. doi:10.1016/j.gie.2009.10.019.

65. Jacobson BC, Hirota WK, Goldstein JL, et al. The role of EUS for evaluation of mediastinal adenopathy. *Gastrointest Endosc* 2003;58(6):819–821. doi:10.1016/S0016-5107(03)01996-5.

66. Micames CG, McCrory DC, Pavey DA, et al. Endoscopic ultrasound-guided fine-needle aspiration for non-small cell lung cancer staging. *Chest* 2007;131(2):539–548. doi:10.1378/chest.06-1437.

67. Cerfolio RJ, Bryant AS, Eloubeidi MA. Routine mediastinoscopy and esophageal ultrasound fine-needle aspiration in patients with non-small cell lung cancer who are clinically N2 negative. *Chest* 2006;130(6):1791–1795. doi:10.1378/chest.130.6.1791.

68. Block MI. Transition from mediastinoscopy to endoscopic ultrasound for lung cancer staging. *Ann Thorac Surg* 2010;89(3):885–890. doi:10.1016/j.athoracsur.2009.11.034.

69. Block MI, Tarrazzi FA. Invasive mediastinal staging—endobronchial ultrasound, endoscopic ultrasound, and mediastinoscopy. *Semin Thorac Cardiovasc Surg* 2013;25(3):218–227. doi:10.1053/j.semtcvs.2013.10.001.

70. Annema JT. Endoscopic ultrasound added to mediastinoscopy for preoperative staging of patients with lung cancer. *JAMA* 2005;294(8):931–936. doi:10.1001/jama.294.8.931.

71. Wallace MB. Minimally invasive endoscopic staging of suspected lung cancer. *JAMA* 2008;299(5):540–546.

72. Vilmann P, Krasnik M, Larsen SS, et al. Transesophageal endoscopic ultrasound-guided fine-needle aspiration (EUS-FNA) and endobronchial ultrasound-guided transbronchial needle aspiration (EBUS-TBNA) biopsy: a combined approach in the evaluation of mediastinal lesions. *Endoscopy* 2005;37(9):833–839. doi:10.1055/s-2005-870276.

73. Call S, Rami-Porta R, Obiols C, et al. Repeat mediastinoscopy in all its indications: experience with 96 patients and 101 procedures. *Eur J Cardiothorac Surg* 2011;39(6):1022–1027. doi:10.1016/j.ejcts.2010.10.019.

74. Marra A, Hillejan L, Fechner S, et al. Remediastinoscopy in restaging of lung cancer after induction therapy. *J Thorac Cardiovasc Surg* 2008;135(4):843–849. doi:10.1016/j.jtcvs.2007.07.073.

75. Van Schil P, van der Schoot J, Poniewierski J, et al. Remediastinoscopy after neoadjuvant therapy for non-small cell lung cancer. *Lung Cancer* 2002;37(3):281–285. doi:10.1016/S0169-5002(02)00101-0.

76. Mateu-Navarro M, Rami-Porta R, Bastús-Piulats R, et al. Remediastinoscopy after induction chemotherapy in non-small cell lung cancer. *Ann Thorac Surg* 2000;70(2):391–395. doi:10.1016/S0003-4975(00)01437-5.

77. De Leyn P. Prospective comparative study of integrated positron emission tomography-computed tomography scan compared with remediastinoscopy in the assessment of residual mediastinal lymph node disease after induction chemotherapy for mediastinoscopy-proven stage iiia-n2 non-small-cell lung cancer: a leuven lung cancer group study. *J Clin Oncol* 2006;24(21):3333–3339. doi:10.1200/JCO.2006.05.6341.

78. Annema J. Mediastinal restaging: EUS-FNA offers a new perspective. *Lung Cancer* 2003;42(3):311–318. doi:10.1016/S0169-5002(03)00364-7.

79. Stigt JA, Oostdijk AH, Timmer PR, et al. Comparison of EUS-guided fine needle aspiration and integrated PET-CT in restaging after treatment for locally advanced non-small cell lung cancer. *Lung Cancer* 2009;66(2):198–204. doi:10.1016/j.lungcan.2009.01.013.

80. Szlubowski A, Zieli ski M, Soja J, et al. Accurate and safe mediastinal restaging by combined endobronchial and endoscopic ultrasound-guided needle aspiration performed by single ultrasound bronchoscope. *Eur J Cardiothorac Surg* 2014;46(2):262–266. doi:10.1093/ejcts/ezt570.

81. Eloubeidi MA, Tamhane A, Lopes TL, et al. Cervical esophageal perforations at the time of endoscopic ultrasound: a prospective evaluation of frequency, outcomes, and patient management. *Am J Gastroenterol* 2009;104(1):53–56. doi:10.1038/ajg.2008.21.

82. Puli SR, Reddy JB, Bechtold ML, et al. Accuracy of endoscopic ultrasound in the diagnosis of distal and celiac axis lymph node metastasis in esophageal cancer: a meta-analysis and systematic review. *Dig Dis Sci* 2008;53(9):2405–2414. doi:10.1007/s10620-007-0152-3.

83. Cârţână T, Sâftoiu A, Popescu C, et al. Delayed peritonitis after endoscopic ultrasound-guided fine-needle aspiration of a metastatic celiac lymph node. *Endoscopy* 2011;43(S 02):E122–E123. doi:10.1055/s-0030-1256158.

84. Van Vliet EP, Heijenbrok-Kal MH, Hunink MG, et al. Staging investigations for oesophageal cancer: a meta-analysis. *Br J Cancer* 2008;98(3):547–557. doi:10.1038/sj.bjc.6604200.

85. Lowe VJ, Booya F, Fletcher JG, et al. Comparison of positron emission tomography, computed tomography, and endoscopic ultrasound in the initial staging of patients with esophageal cancer. *Mol Imaging Biol* 2005;7(6):422–430. doi:10.1007/s11307-005-0017-0.

86. Cerfolio RJ, Bryant AS, Ohja B, et al. The accuracy of endoscopic ultrasonography with fine-needle aspiration, integrated positron emission tomography with computed tomography, and computed tomography in restaging patients with esophageal cancer after neoadjuvant chemoradiotherapy. *J Thorac Cardiovasc Sur* 2005;129(6):1232–1241. doi:10.1016/j.jtcvs.2004.12.042.

87. Swisher SG, Maish M, Erasmus JJ, et al. Utility of PET, CT, and EUS to identify pathologic responders in esophageal cancer. *Ann Thorac Surg* 2004;78(4):1152–1160. doi:10.1016/j.athoracsur.2004.04.046.

88. Seewald S, Imazu H, Omar S, et al. EUS-guided drainage of hepatic abscess. *Gastrointest Endosc* 2005;61(3):495–498. doi:10.1016/S0016-5107(04)02848-2.

89. Seewald S, Brand B, Omar S, et al. EUS-guided drainage of subphrenic abscess. *Gastrointest Endosc* 2004;59(4):578–580. doi:10.1016/S0016-5107(03)02878-5.

90. Shami VM, Talreja JP, Mahajan A, et al. EUS-guided drainage of bilomas: a new alternative? *Gastrointest Endosc* 2008;67(1):136–140. doi:10.1016/j.gie.2007.07.040.

91. Kahaleh M, Wang P, Shami VM, et al. Drainage of gallbladder fossa fluid collections with endoprosthesis placement under endoscopic ultrasound guidance: a preliminary report of two cases. *Endoscopy* 2005;37(4):393–396. doi:10.1055/s-2005-860998.

92. Ponnudurai R, George A, Sachithanandan S, et al. Endoscopic ultrasound-guided drainage of a biloma: a novel approach. *Endoscopy* 2006;38(2):199–199. doi:10.1055/s-2006-925143.

93. Lee SS, Park DH, Hwang CY, et al. EUS-guided transmural cholecystostomy as rescue management for acute cholecystitis in elderly or high-risk patients: a prospective feasibility study. *Gastrointest Endosc* 2007;66(5):1008–1012. doi:10.1016/j.gie.2007.03.1080.

94. Choi J-H, Lee SS. Endoscopic ultrasonography-guided gallbladder drainage for acute cholecystitis: from evidence to practice. *Dig Endosc* 2014;27(1):1–7. doi:10.1111/den.12386.

95. Kwan V, Eisendrath P, Antaki F, et al. EUS-guided cholecystenterostomy: a new technique (with videos). *Gastrointest Endosc* 2007;66(3):582–586. doi:10.1016/j.gie.2007.02.065.

96. Baron TH, Topazian MD. Endoscopic transduodenal drainage of the gallbladder: implications for endoluminal treatment of gallbladder disease. *Gastrointest Endosc* 2007;65(4):735–737. doi:10.1016/j.gie.2006.07.041.

97. Attam R, Leslie D, Arain M, et al. EUS-guided sutured gastropexy for transgastric ERCP (ESTER) in patients with Roux-en-Y gastric bypass: a novel, single-session, minimally invasive approach. *Endoscopy* 2015;47(07):646–649. doi:10.1055/s-0034-1391124.

98. Fritscher-Ravens A. EUS-guided NOTES Interventions. *Gastrointest Endosc Clin N Am* 2008;18(2):297–314. doi:10.1016/j.giec.2008.01.009.

99. Elmunzer BJ, Schomisch SJ, Trunzo JA, et al. EUS in localizing safe alternate access sites for natural orifice transluminal endoscopic surgery: initial experience in a porcine model. *Gastrointest Endosc* 2009;69(1):108–114. doi:10.1016/j.gie.2008.04.030.

100. Jeong SU. Forward-viewing endoscopic ultrasound-guided NOTES interventions: A study on peritoneoscopic potential. *World J Gastroenterol* 2013;19(41):7160. doi:10.3748/wjg.v19.i41.7160.

101. Minami H, Inoue H, Isomoto H, et al. Clinical application of endoscopic ultrasonography for esophageal achalasia. *Dig Endosc* 2015;27(S1):11–16. doi:10.1111/den.12432.

102. Goldberg SN, Mallery S, Gazelle GS, et al. EUS-guided radiofrequency ablation in the pancreas: results in a porcine model. *Gastrointest Endosc* 1999;50(3):392–401. doi:10.1053/ge.1999.v50.98847.

103. Carrara S, Arcidiacono P, Albarello L, et al. Endoscopic ultrasound-guided application of a new internally gas-cooled radiofrequency ablation probe in the liver and spleen of an animal model: a preliminary study. *Endoscopy* 2008;40(09):759–763. doi:10.1055/s-2008-1077520.

104. Carrara S, Arcidiacono P, Albarello L, et al. Endoscopic ultrasound-guided application of a new hybrid cryotherm probe in porcine pancreas: a preliminary study. *Endoscopy* 2008;40(4):321–326. doi:10.1055/s-2007-995595.

105. Varadarajulu S, Trevino J, Shen S, et al. The use of endoscopic ultrasound-guided gold markers in image-guided radiation therapy of pancreatic cancers: a case series. *Endoscopy* 2010;42(05):423–425. doi:10.1055/s-0029-1243989.

106. Pishvaian AC, Collins B, Gagnon G, et al. EUS-guided fiducial placement for cyberknife radiotherapy of mediastinal and abdominal malignancies. *Gastrointest Endosc* 2006;64(3):412–417. doi:10.1016/j.gie.2006.01.048.

107. Levy MJ, Chari ST, Wiersema MJ. Endoscopic ultrasound-guided celiac neurolysis. *Gastrointest Endosc Clin N Am* 2012;22(2):231–247. doi:10.1016/j.giec.2012.04.003.

108. Harada N, Wiersema MJ, Wiersema LM. Endosonography-guided celiac plexus neurolysis. *Gastrointest Endosc Clin N Am* 1997:237–245. doi:10.1016/S0016-5107(96)70047-0.

109. Maiorana A, Fiorentino E, Genova EG, et al. Echo-guided injection of botulinum toxin in patients with achalasia: initial experience. *Endoscopy* 1999;31(2):S3–S4.

110. Ciulla A, Cremona F, Genova G, et al. Echo-guided injection of botulinum toxin versus blind endoscopic injection in patients with achalasia: final report. *Minerva Gastroenterol Dietol* 2013;59(2):237–240.

111. Chang KJ, Nguyen PT, Thompson JA, et al. Phase I clinical trial of allogeneic mixed lymphocyte culture (cytoimplant) delivered by endoscopic ultrasound-guided fine-needle injection in patients with advanced pancreatic carcinoma. *Cancer* 2000;88(6):1325–1335. doi:10.1002/(SICI)1097–0142(20000315)88:6.3.0.CO;2-T.

112. Hirooka Y, Itoh A, Kawashima H, et al. A combination therapy of gemcitabine with immunotherapy for patients with inoperable locally advanced pancreatic cancer. *Pancreas* 2009;38(3):69–74. doi: 10.1097/MPA.0b013e318197a9e3.

113. Akiyama Y, Maruyama K, Nara N, et al. Antitumor effects induced by dendritic cell-based immunotherapy against established pancreatic cancer in hamsters. *Cancer Letters* 2002;184(1):37–47. doi:10.1016/S0304-3835(02)00189-1.

114. Yu JS. Vaccination with tumor lysate-pulsed dendritic cells elicits antigen-specific, cytotoxic t-cells in patients with malignant glioma. *Cancer Res* 2004;64(14):4973–4979. doi:10.1158/0008–5472.CAN-03–3505.

115. Irisawa A, Takagi T, Kanazawa M, et al. Endoscopic ultrasound-guided fine-needle injection of immature dendritic cells into advanced pancreatic cancer refractory to gemcitabine. *Pancreas* 2007;35(2):189–190. doi:10.1097/01.mpa.0000250141.25639.e9.

116. Senzer N, Mani S, Rosemurgy A, et al. TNFerade biologic, an adenovector with a radiation-inducible promoter, carrying the human tumor necrosis factor alpha gene: a phase i study in patients with solid tumors. *J Clin Oncol* 2004;22(4):592–601. doi:10.1200/JCO.2004.01.227.

117. Mulvihill S, Warren R, Venook A, et al. Safety and feasibility of injection with an e1b-55 kda gene-deleted, replication-selective adenovirus (onyx-015) into primary carcinomas of the pancreas: a phase i trial. *Gene Ther* 2001;8(4):308–315. doi:10.1038/sj.gt.3301398.

118. Hecht J, Bedford R, Abbruzzese J, et al. A phase I/II trial of intratumoral endoscopic ultrasound injection of onyx-015 with intravenous gemcitabine in unresectable pancreatic carcinoma. *Clin Can Res* 2003;9:555–561.

119. Hecht JR, Farrell JJ, Senzer N, et al. EUS or percutaneously guided intratumoral tnferade biologic with 5-fluorouracil and radiotherapy for first-line treatment of locally advanced pancreatic cancer: a phase i/ii study. *Gastrointest Endosc* 2012;75(2):332–338. doi:10.1016/j.gie.2011.10.007.

120. Lubbe AS, Bergemann C. Ultrasound therapy for malignant tumors: a conceptual assessment. *J Clin Ultrasound*. 1994;22(2):113–117. doi:10.1002/jcu.1870220208.

121. Sanghvi NT, Syrus J, Foster RS, et al. Noninvasive surgery of prostate tissue by high-intensity focused ultrasound: an updated report. RR Anderson, KE Bartels, LS Bass, et al., eds. *Eur J Ultrasound* 1999;9:19–29. doi:10.1117/12.386253.

122. Uchida T, Sanghvi NT, Gardner TA, et al. Transrectal high-intensity focused ultrasound for treatment of patients with stage t1b-2n0m0 localized prostate cancer: a preliminary report. *Urology* 2002;59(3):394–398. doi:10.1016/S0090–4295(01)01624-7.

123. Sanghvi NV, Hawes RH. High-intensity focused ultrasound. *Gastrointest Endosc Clin N Am* 1994;4(2):383–395.

124. Prat F, Chapelon JY, Arefiev A, et al. High-Intensity focused ultrasound transducers suitable for endoscopy: feasibility study in rabbits. *Gastrointest Endosc* 1997;46(4):348–351. doi:10.1016/S0016-5107(97)70124-X.

125. Melodelima D, Prat F, Fritsch J, et al. Treatment of esophageal tumors using high intensity intraluminal ultrasound: first clinical results. *J Translat Med* 2008;6(1):28–10. doi:10.1186/1479-5876-6-28.

OPERATIVE PROCEDURES IN THE MANAGEMENT OF ESOPHAGEAL DISEASE

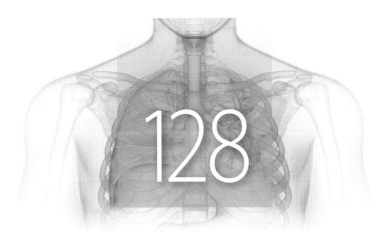

128

Operative Strategies for Esophageal Dysmotility Disorders

Chaitan K. Narsule ■ Hiran C. Fernando

INTRODUCTION

Esophageal motility disorders affect the motor function of any or all portions of the esophageal body. These disorders normally present with noncardiac chest pain and/or dysphagia. Over time, esophageal dysmotility can cause the development of pulsion diverticula such as those seen at the junction of the pharynx and esophagus (Zenker's diverticulum) and at the distal esophagus (epiphrenic diverticulum). As a result, patients may also present with symptoms such as the regurgitation of undigested food, halitosis, and even aspiration.

In this chapter, we describe traditional and contemporary approaches to the operative management of esophageal dysmotility disorders. Specific focus will be directed to the management of achalasia and esophageal diverticula (particularly Zenker's diverticula). Operations for all of these diseases follow an extensive workup that routinely involves endoscopy, manometry, a barium esophagram, and sometimes a 24-hour pH probe study. While medical management will not specifically be addressed, it suffices that intervention for primary esophageal dysmotility disorders follows a trial-and-error period of medical and nonsurgical therapies, including treatments

for spasm (nitrates, calcium channel blockers, botulinum toxin), gastroesophageal (GE) reflux (proton pump inhibitors or histamine-2 receptor blockers), or pneumatic dilation.

ACHALASIA

Achalasia is the most common esophageal dysmotility disorder. It is characterized by aperistalsis of the esophageal body and incomplete relaxation of the lower esophageal sphincter (LES), which is due to the loss of inhibitory activity—and intact excitatory activity—of the sphincter. The onset of symptoms is usually subtle, and patients typically present after having symptoms that have persisted sometimes for years prior to presentation. Most patients present with dysphagia and regurgitation of food contents. Weight loss, chest pain, heartburn, and cough are also associated with achalasia. While chest x-rays may demonstrate an air–fluid level in the posterior mediastinum or absence of a gastric bubble, the diagnosis is best established by a barium esophagram that demonstrates a bird's beak appearance of the GE junction, manometry demonstrating the findings described above, and endoscopy to rule out pseudoachalasia. Endoscopic ultrasonography can be a useful adjunct, particularly if pseudoachalasia related to an underlying cancer is in question. Following this workup, several operative interventions are available for the management of achalasia.

LAPAROSCOPIC HELLER MYOTOMY

A laparoscopic Heller myotomy is the conventional treatment of choice for achalasia. In our experience, two 12-mm laparoscopic ports are first placed through the left and right rectus abdominus sheath at a point that is approximately one-third of the distance between the xiphoid process and the umbilicus. (Alternatively, after obtaining initial laparoscopic access through the right rectus sheath with a 12-mm Hasson trocar, the second port placed through the left rectus sheath can be a 5-mm trocar.) Additionally, two 5-mm trocars are placed bilaterally at the mid-clavicular line and just below the costal margins. Also, a fifth trocar that is 5 mm in size is placed below the right costal margin, near the mid-axillary line. This trocar accommodates a flexible laparoscopic articulated triangular liver retractor which is used to retract the left lateral segment of the liver anteriorly to expose the gastrohepatic ligament and the intra-abdominal esophagus and is fixed in place using an external retractor clamping system (Fig. 128.1).

The gastrohepatic ligament is incised and completely divided to the esophageal hiatus of the diaphragm using a laparoscopic coagulation shears. Next, the phrenoesophageal ligament is incised. If a posterior (Toupet) fundoplication is planned, the esophagus must be completely mobilized away from the left and right crura of the diaphragm. Additionally, mobilization of the fundus with division of the short gastric vessels is necessary to ensure that there is no tension on the fundoplication. Our preference, however, is to perform a partial anterior (Dor) fundoplication. This procedure does not require circumferential dissection around the esophagus, and usually does not require division of the short gastric vessels. Additionally, if a small mucosal perforation occurs during the myotomy, the mucosa can be repaired and an overlying anterior fundoplication will help to buttress this repair. Regardless of the fundoplication approach selected, the key step in dissection is mobilization of the fat pad overlying the GE junction. This step allows for the clear identification of the GE junction to facilitate an adequate myotomy that extends along the distal esophagus and onto the stomach.

Prior to performing the myotomy, a dilute epinephrine solution is injected into the esophageal muscle at the GE junction. This facilitates the creation of the myotomy by (1) minimizing the small amount of bleeding that can occur at the myotomy site and (2) helping to define

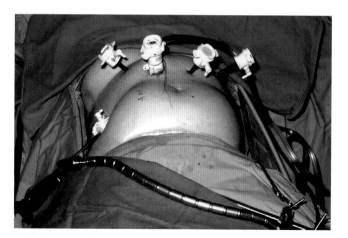

FIGURE 128.1 Port placement and set up for a laparoscopic Heller myotomy.

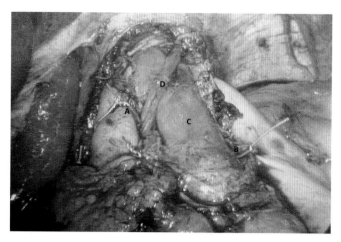

FIGURE 128.2 Toupet fundoplication after myotomy; *A,* fundus sutured to right side of myotomized esophagus; *B,* fundus sutured to left side of myotomized esophagus; *C,* mucosa after performing myotomy; and *D,* anterior vagus nerve.

the plane between the muscle and the underlying mucosa because of localized distension of the muscle. Either hook electrocautery or the laparoscopic coagulation shears can be used to start the myotomy. However, once the dissection plane is started, the myotomy is often easy to extend by simply retracting bilaterally on the muscle edges. The most complicated part of the dissection is inferiorly, where it is necessary to extend the myotomy onto the proximal stomach. Here, the muscular fibers tend to be thinner and the muscular-mucosa plane is more difficult to define. However, it is important to divide the muscular sling fibers in this area.

Once the myotomy is completed, a partial fundoplication is performed. For a Dor fundoplication, the fundus is brought anteriorly over the myotomized esophagus. The first suture is placed between the fundus, the muscle at the superior edge of the myotomized esophagus, and top of the right crura. Typically, 2-0 nonabsorbable sutures are used. Additional sutures are placed between the fundus and the muscular edges of the esophagus to the (patient's) right side of the myotomy. Sutures are also placed to anchor the superior margin of the fundus to the anterior margin of the diaphragmatic hiatus. This completes the Dor fundoplication.

For a Toupet fundoplication, a retroesophageal window is created with careful dissection behind the posterior vagus nerve, which is protected and preserved. Following division of the short gastric vessels, the posterior aspect of the fundus—nearest to the short gastric vessels—is delivered posterior to the intra-abdominal esophagus through the retroesophageal window. The back of the fundus is sutured to the crura using interrupted nonabsorbable 2-0 sutures. If required, the crura can be reapproximated first; however, this is often not necessary since there is usually no significant hiatal hernia or diaphragmatic defect. Finally, the myotomized edges of the esophagus are sutured to both the left and right aspects of fundus (Fig. 128.2). In creating the posterior fundoplication, it is helpful to have a bougie or a gastroscope in place to minimize narrowing of the GE junction.

Our practice is to obtain a barium esophagram on the first postoperative day to delineate the anatomy and rule out an esophageal leak. With a negative study, patients are transitioned to clear liquids, undergo nutritional education, and are then discharged home.

The utility of fundoplication with Heller myotomy was studied in a prospective, randomized, double-blinded clinical trial reported in 2004 by Richards and colleagues.[1] Forty-three patients were enrolled, with 21 patients undergoing myotomy alone and 22 patients undergoing myotomy with Dor fundoplication. The addition of the Dor fundoplication significantly reduced the incidence of postoperative GE reflux (9.1% vs. 47.6% without Dor fundoplication, p = 0.005) and was not associated with any significant differences in postoperative dysphagia or LES pressure. It is our preference to include a partial fundoplication with each Heller myotomy procedure.

ROBOT-ASSISTED HELLER MYOTOMY

Robot-assisted Heller myotomy using the da Vinci Si robot (Intuitive Surgical, Inc., Sunnyvale, CA) has emerged as an alternative to conventional laparoscopic esophagomyotomy for the treatment of achalasia. Our port placement approach is demonstrated in Figure 128.3. We have found that it is preferable to place the ports in a slightly more inferior position away from the hiatus, which allows for greater mobility for the robotic instruments within the abdomen. However, the ports are still easily adaptable to a standard laparoscopic approach and instrumentation, should conversion from a robot-assisted approach to a laparoscopic approach be necessary. Conversion to laparotomy has never been required in our practice.

In the robot-assisted Heller myotomy procedure, following the induction of anesthesia and endotracheal intubation, the operating table is turned 45 degrees toward the patient's right side in order to accommodate the array of robotic arms that are positioned directly over the head and left shoulder of the patient. The anesthesiologist remains at the head of the table, but also to the patient's right side. Our port insertion scheme is as follows: a 12-mm port is placed through the left rectus sheath at a level between the xiphoid process and the umbilicus (or slightly lower, depending on the patient's body habitus) which will accommodate the robot camera. Two robotic 8-mm ports are placed below the left and right costal margins at the mid-clavicular lines, as indicated in Figure 128.3. Additional ports include a 5-mm port for the liver retractor (placed below the right costal margin along the anterior axillary line) and a standard 12-mm assistant port used for suctioning, retraction, clip placement, and injection of epinephrine solution, prior to performing the myotomy.

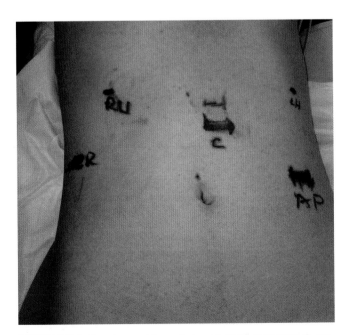

FIGURE 128.3 Port placement for a robot-assisted Heller myotomy. C, camera port; LH, robotic left-hand port; RH, robotic right-hand port; LIVER, port for triangular liver retractor; AP, assistant port.

This is placed inferior to both the camera port and the robotic left arm (on the left side of the patient's abdomen).

Next, the robot arm array is docked onto the ports. The camera arm is placed through the 12-mm port in the left rectus sheath. Then, robot arms no. 1 and no. 2 are attached to the left and right subcostal mid-clavicular ports and will serve as the surgeon's main working ports. The approach for Heller myotomy is then identical to that for the laparoscopic approach. We have found that the magnified stereoscopic, three-dimensional view from the da Vinci robot's laparoscope is very helpful to clearly differentiate between the outer longitudinal and circular muscular layers of the esophagus and the underlying esophageal mucosa and facilitates a safe and complete myotomy. Since the robotic ultrasonic shears have only limited degrees of freedom of movement, robotic hook electrocautery is used to perform the myotomy in combination with traction as described above in the laparoscopic approach.

Several institutional series exist comparing the outcomes of a robot-assisted Heller myotomy to the laparoscopic approach. Horgan and colleagues reported on a retrospective review of three institutions at which patients underwent robotic-assisted (n = 59) or laparoscopic (n = 62) Heller myotomy for achalasia.[2] This series demonstrated a learning curve with the robot-assisted approach as the operative time was significantly shorter for the laparoscopic group (122 ± 44 vs. 141 ± 49 minutes, p <0.05) for the first half of the cases reviewed, but reportedly was not different in the comparison of the last 30 cases. Though there was no mortality associated with this experience, there was a higher rate of esophageal perforations in the laparoscopic group when compared to the robot-assisted group (16% vs. 0%).

Melvin and colleagues reported their cumulative 4-year experience with robotic-assisted Heller myotomy and partial fundoplication in 2005 with favorable results.[3] One hundred four patients were included, and a learning curve was demonstrated with the mean operating time decreasing from 162.63 minutes during the first 2 years of the study to 113.50 minutes during the last 2 years of the study (p = 0.0001). Additionally, no esophageal perforations occurred, one patient required conversion to an open approach, and no patients required reoperation. Similarly, Huffman and colleagues reported their experience of 61 consecutive patients undergoing either laparoscopic or robot-assisted Heller myotomy over a 6-year period.[4] While there was no operative mortality in either group, there was a higher rate of esophageal perforations in the laparoscopic group compared to the robot-assisted group (8% vs. 0%) and increased operative time associated with the robotic cases (355 ± 23 vs. 287 ± 9 minutes for the laparoscopic cases).

Despite these studies favoring the robot-assisted approach, Shaligram and colleagues reported a multi-center retrospective review of open, laparoscopic, and robotic Heller myotomy for achalasia.[5] In comparing patients who underwent laparoscopic and robot-assisted Heller myotomy, there was no difference between the groups in terms of mortality, morbidity, intensive care unit admissions, length of stay, or 30-day readmissions. Cost was, however, significantly higher for the robot-assisted myotomy group compared to the laparoscopic myotomy group ($9,415 ± 5,515 vs. $7,441 ± 7,897, p = 0.0028).

PER-ORAL ESOPHAGEAL MYOTOMY

Per-oral esophageal myotomy (POEM) is an endoscopic approach to achalasia that was first reported in 2008 and is rapidly becoming an accepted alternative for the operative treatment of achalasia. Patients who undergo this procedure do so in an operating room setting and under general anesthesia.

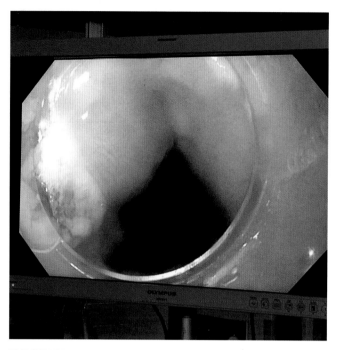

FIGURE 128.4 Mucosotomy at the beginning of a POEM procedure.

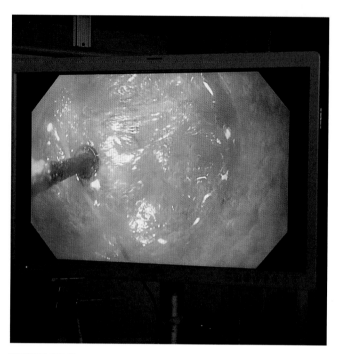

FIGURE 128.5 Creating the submucosal tunnel during a POEM procedure.

A standard endoscope, with a dissecting cap in place, is used. However, instead of air insufflation, carbon dioxide insufflation through the gastroscope is required. Additional flexible instruments are also needed to create the mucosotomy, submucosal tunnel, and subsequent myotomy that will be described below. Examples of instruments commonly used include the triangle-tip knife (Olympus Waltham, Ma, USA, KD-640-L), the hybrid knife (ERBE), an injecting needle (e.g., Olympus NM-400L-0423), and hemostatic graspers (Olympus FD-411UR). Following endoscopy of the foregut, at a point approximately 10 cm proximal to the GE junction, a submucosal injection is delivered containing a mixture of saline and indigo carmine or methylene blue which helps expand the submucosal layer in preparation for a mucosotomy. A 2-cm mucosotomy is then made using electrocautery, and the deeper circular muscle fibers are identified (Fig. 128.4). Next, a submucosal tunnel is developed (Fig. 128.5) with blunt dissection, insufflation with carbon dioxide gas, hydro-dissection into the submucosa, and electrocautery to a point approximately 2 cm beyond the GE junction onto the gastric cardia. The gastroscope is then retracted proximally to a point approximately 2 to 4 cm below the initial mucosotomy site. The circular muscle fibers are then divided using electrocautery in a proximal to distal manner; the longitudinal muscle fibers are left intact (Fig. 128.6). Once completed, esophagogastroscopy is performed to confirm that the endoscope can pass smoothly through the GE junction and that the proximal gastric mucosa has a blanched appearance on retroflexion (corresponding to the distal limit of the dissection). These findings demonstrate that an adequate myotomy has been performed. Finally, the mucosotomy is closed using endoscopic clips or the Apollo OverStitch (Apollo Endosurgery Inc., Austin, TX). As this technique is gaining traction in the United States, other groups have begun applying this technique to the management of giant mid-esophageal diverticula with early success in a limited number of patients.[6]

Studies comparing POEM with laparoscopic Heller myotomy exist in the literature; however, none are randomized. Bhayani and colleagues reported on their experience of 101 patients who underwent either laparoscopic Heller myotomy with a partial fundoplication (n = 64) or POEM (n = 37).[7] Median operative time (149 vs. 120 minutes, p <0.001) and hospitalization (2.2 vs. 1.1 days, p <0.0001) were higher for the patients undergoing laparoscopic myotomy and postoperative morbidity was similar. Although postoperative resting pressures were higher in the POEM group (16 vs. 7.1 mm Hg, p = 0.006) compared to the laparoscopic myotomy patients, post-myotomy relaxation pressures and distal esophageal contraction amplitudes were not significantly different between the groups. Additionally, Kumagai and colleagues published their series

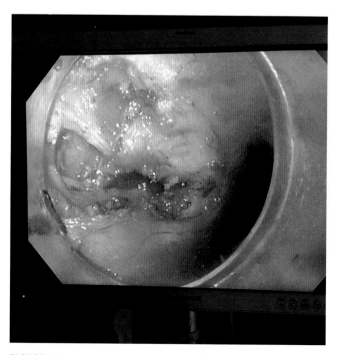

FIGURE 128.6 Starting the myotomy for a POEM procedure.

comparing 42 patients who underwent POEM with 41 patients who underwent laparoscopic Heller myotomy.[8] There was no significant difference in esophageal emptying, as assessed by a timed barium esophagram, in their series. Also, longer operation times and younger patients were independent predictors of treatment failure after POEM.

A specific advantage of the POEM technique is that it is possible to create a long myotomy of the thoracic esophagus. This has led to an expanded use of POEM outside of treating achalasia, to include treating diseases such as diffuse esophageal spasm and nutcracker esophagus.[9]

THORACIC MYOTOMY (OPEN VS. THORACOSCOPIC)

Currently, esophagomyotomy for achalasia or diffuse esophageal spasm is infrequently performed through a thoracic approach. Nevertheless, in situations where a patient has undergone a laparoscopic or open abdominal approach or when a patient has diffuse esophageal spasm that is refractory to medical therapy, an open or video-assisted approach through the left chest can be effective in resolving a patient's symptoms and allow for a long-segment esophagomyotomy without disruption of the phrenoesophageal ligament.

Double-lumen endotracheal intubation and positioning in the right lateral decubitus position with the left lung deflated is required. A left thoracotomy is performed through the seventh intercostal space. With division of the inferior pulmonary ligament and cephalad retraction of the deflated left lung, the mediastinal pleura over the esophagus is incised. Identification of the esophagus is expedited with the placement of a nasogastric tube.

For achalasia, a longitudinal incision is made through both of the outer muscular (longitudinal and circular) layers of the esophagus with exposure of the external mucosal surface. This incision is extended cephalad for a total of 5 to 7 cm, or at least 2 cm above the transition point of dilation of the proximal esophagus. The myotomy is also extended caudally to the GE junction. Next, the muscular fibers are gently, but bluntly, mobilized to expose the mucosa to approximately 50% of its circumference to prevent a recurrence.

Occasionally, the mucosa can inadvertently be entered. If this happens, the mucosa is primarily repaired. This repair is then tested with the insufflation of air through the nasogastric tube, under warm saline instilled within the pleural cavity. For complex injuries to the mucosa, the myotomy can be closed over the injury and a new myotomy can be performed elsewhere. For diffuse esophageal spasm, the esophagomyotomy can be extended as far cephalad as possible (up to the esophageal segment next to the aortic arch).

A thoracoscopic approach can also be undertaken instead of a thoracotomy. A 10-mm port is placed in seventh intercostal space at the level of the anterior axillary line, followed by another 10-mm port in the mid-axillary line, as far down caudally as can be seen with thoracoscopic guidance near the costophrenic recess. Additionally, a posterior 5-mm port is placed approximately four fingerbreaths below the inferior angle of the scapula, and a final 10-mm port is placed at approximately the fourth intercostal space and mid-axillary line. With cephalad retraction on the deflated left lung, the inferior pulmonary ligament is incised. A thoracoscopic fan retractor can also be used to carefully place downward traction on the left hemidiaphragm to expose the mediastinal pleura overlying the esophagus. This pleura is incised, dissection is carried out around the esophagus, and the esophagus is encircled with a Penrose drain. Lateral traction on the Penrose drain allows for its mobilization during esophagomyotomy. Hook electrocautery is then utilized to achieve the desired amount of myotomy.

ZENKER'S DIVERTICULUM

Although esophageal diverticula near the larynx was first described in 1769,[10] this pathology has been associated with Zenker following his report on a series of almost 30 patients with this condition.[11] Zenker's diverticulum is a pseudodiverticulum that occurs when the esophageal mucosa expands through the esophageal muscular wall in Killian's triangle (bordered proximally by the oblique fibers of the inferior pharyngeal constrictor muscle and distally by the transverse fibers of the cricopharyngeus muscle), the transition zone between the hypopharynx and the esophagus. It is considered to be a pulsion diverticulum caused by dysfunction of the cricopharyngeus muscle leading to its decreased compliance. This decreased compliance, in turn, leads to higher intraluminal pressure whenever a food bolus passes through this segment of the alimentary tract. It is believed that this mechanism causes the formation of the pulsion diverticulum in the triangle, proximal to the cricopharyngeus muscle.

The dysphagia associated with these pathologic changes is the main symptom of Zenker's diverticulum. Others include the regurgitation of food pieces, choking, halitosis, globus sensation, the presence of abnormal noises during deglutition, aspiration, and other ear, nose, and throat symptoms. This condition occurs more commonly in elderly patients than in younger patients. Also, several investigators have reported that more than half of all patients with Zenker's diverticulum have additional associated upper gastrointestinal pathology (i.e., GE reflux, hiatal hernia, etc.) that should be identified upon presentation.

For symptomatic patients, treatment of Zenker's diverticulum is indicated. Fortunately, open and endoscopic options for managing this pathology are available.

OPEN REPAIR OF ZENKER'S DIVERTICULUM

Open Zenker's diverticulectomy is typically undertaken through the left neck. Following induction of anesthesia and endotracheal intubation, the head is positioned facing the right side and care is taken to carefully pad all pressure points. Following prepping and draping of the left neck, an incision is made anterior to the left sternocleidomastoid muscle. This wound is deepened through the platysma and the sternocleidomastoid muscle is retracted laterally to expose the omohyoid muscle, which crosses the field from medial to lateral. As the diverticulum is located deep to this muscle, this muscle is divided. Next, the carotid sheath and hypoglossal nerve are identified and retracted laterally. The thyroid gland is exposed medially in its position just deep to the strap muscles, and it is retracted medially. The middle thyroid vein is identified, ligated, and divided. Additionally, if the inferior thyroid artery appears within the wound and crosses the esophagus to provide perfusion inferiorly to the left thyroid lobe, it may need to be ligated and divided to provide appropriate esophageal exposure (though often this is not necessary).

The diverticulum usually emerges in the posterior aspect of Killian's triangle, between the pharyngeal constrictor and the cricopharyngeus muscles. It is typical that the dependent portion of the diverticulum descends between the posterior wall of the esophagus and the prevertebral fascia. The diverticulum should be mobilized. The neck of the diverticulum, which is usually present at the level of the cricoid cartilage, must be carefully exposed. If the neck anatomy is complicated by previous operative scarring or radiation, the placement of an esophageal bougie can help clarify anatomy (though this is not routinely necessary), but care must be taken to avoid perforation of the diverticulum with the bougie. With retraction of the diverticulum cephalad, the transverse fibers of the cricopharyngeus muscle will be seen just below in the inferior-most aspect of the neck of the diverticulum.

Next, a cricopharyngeal myotomy is performed. A right-angle clamp is placed between the cricopharyngeus muscle and the mucosa. The clamp is elevated in the posterior midline, and the transverse muscle fibers are divided for a length of approximately 5 to 6 cm. Thereafter, the cricopharyngeus muscle is elevated from the underlying esophageal mucosa with careful blunt dissection. The mucosa is then seen as bulging out from the myotomy.

For very small diverticula, following myotomy, often only a small amount of bulging mucosa is seen which may potentially obviate the need for a diverticulectomy. For larger diverticula, it is common to perform a diverticulectomy using a linear stapler across the neck of the diverticulum, which is quick and simple though occasionally associated with a self-limited salivary fistula. Alternatively, some surgeons prefer performing a diverticulopexy. In this procedure, the most dependent portion of the diverticula is turned upside down and suspended from the prevertebral fascia of the cervical spine. The diverticulopexy forces the diverticula to drain by gravity into the esophagus. It is the author's preference to proceed with diverticulectomy if an open procedure is selected due to its ease and very low rate of associated complications.

ENDOSCOPIC TRANS-ORAL STAPLING

Endoscopic trans-oral stapling is the minimally invasive alternative approach to treating a patient with a Zenker's diverticulum. Its advantages include a completely natural-orifice approach obviating the need for an open operative approach, potentially a shorter operative time, and decreased hospital length of stay. Patients without limitations in neck extension, micrognathia, or prominent front teeth are ideal candidates. It should be emphasized that patients with small diverticula are not candidates for this approach since it is necessary to completely divide the cricopharyngeus muscle endoscopically, and this will not be possible with small diverticula.

Patients undergo trans-oral stapling while under general anesthesia. Ideally, a small endotracheal tube is used. The patient's neck is hyperextended and supported accordingly. Next, flexible endoscopy is performed to evaluate the size of the diverticulum and for any other associated esophageal or gastric pathology. With the endoscope in the stomach, a guidewire is advanced through the scope and into the stomach, and it is left in place as the endoscope is withdrawn. Following this, a Weerda rigid endoscope (Karl Storz, Tuttlingen, Germany) is placed trans-orally to expose the true esophageal lumen and the lumen of the Zenker's diverticulum. Through this exposure, the diverticulum can be probed, irrigated, and suctioned in order to clear it of any debris. A 5-mm rigid video endoscope can be used to enhance visualization through the Weerda endoscope.

In order to deliver the hypertrophic cricopharyngeus muscle (sometimes called a "cricopharyngeus bar") into the stapler, a traction suture is placed into the septum between the true esophageal lumen and the diverticulum (Fig. 128.7). We use a full-length 2-0 polyester Endo-Stitch (Covidien, Minneapolis, MN). Next, an Endo-GIA stapler of 30 mm size (US Surgical, Norwalk, CT) is used for stapling. For this procedure, the anvil is purposely modified by shortening of the tip to ensure that the stapler will staple and cut all the way to the most dependent portion of the diverticulum. The stapler is inserted through the rigid endoscope, with the anvil oriented into the diverticulum (Fig. 128.8). With traction on the traction suture to elongate the cricopharyngeal bar, the stapler is positioned. It is used

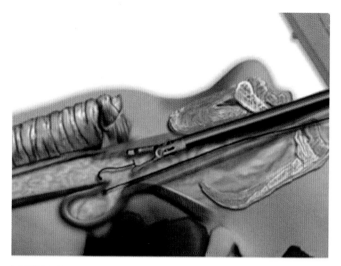

FIGURE 128.7 Placement of a trans-oral Endo-Stitch through the cricopharyngeal bar.

to staple the bar all the way to the bottom of the diverticulum. In our experience, one staple firing is usually sufficient; however, for larger diverticula additional staplings can be performed as needed. Thereafter, the rigid endoscope is removed and a completion flexible endoscopy is performed to confirm hemostasis, an intact staple line, and complete division of the cricopharyngeal bar. Following extubation, the patient is typically admitted for observation, and a barium esophagram is obtained on the first postoperative day. Thereafter, patients are started on a clear liquid diet and advanced and are usually discharged to home in 1 to 2 days.

Modern series of the trans-oral stapling technique for the management of Zenker's diverticulum have demonstrated favorable outcomes. In 2007, Morse and colleagues reported a 10-year retrospective review in which 47 patients with Zenker's diverticulum underwent either an open (N = 19) or endoscopic (N = 28) procedure.[12] Twenty-four of the 28 patients successfully underwent trans-oral stapling, with the remaining 4 undergoing conversion to the open approach. Notably, operative time was significantly less for the trans-oral stapling group (1.57 vs. 2.35 hours for the open group). Also, both the trans-oral stapling group and the open group had equivalent improvements in their dysphagia scores.

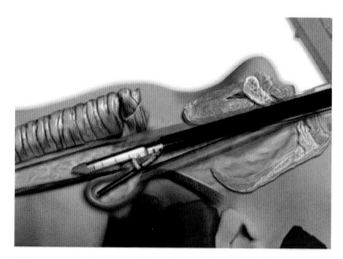

FIGURE 128.8 Placement of the stapler into the Zenker's diverticulum for trans-oral stapling.

Approaches that obviate the need for a rigid endoscope have been described. Pescarus and colleagues have reported a 67-month retrospective experience in which a flexible high-resolution gastroscope with an endoscopic cap was used to achieve division mucosotomy followed by a 5 to 10 mm myotomy beyond the diverticulum tip, all with needle knife or hook cautery; mucosal reapproximation was completed using endoclips.[13] In this series, 26 patients underwent flexible endoscopic myotomy and there were significant short-term (at 1 month) and long-term improvements in dysphagia, regurgitation, cough, and aspiration.

In addition, rates of symptom recurrence have been reported in several series. Chiari and colleagues reported on their series of transoral stapling of Zenker's diverticulum in which 39 of 46 patients were successfully treated.[14] Notably, there was resolution of dysphagia to solids in 71.1% of patients and to liquids in 84.7% of patients. Moreover, there was resolution of regurgitation in 76.3% of patients. With a median follow-up of 11 months, resolution of dysphagia persisted in 92% of patients, and resolution of regurgitation persisted in 89% of patients. Only 12% required re-intervention for recurrent symptoms. In addition, Chang et al. evaluated the outcomes of their series involving 159 cases of endoscopic stapling for Zenker's diverticulum.[15] In this cohort of patients, 98% had improved or complete resolution of symptoms with a mean hospital stay of less than 1 day, immediate resumption of a diet, and a rate of significant complications at 2% (without mortality). At a mean follow-up of 32.2 months, there was a recurrence of symptoms in 11.8% of patients.

DISTAL ESOPHAGEAL DIVERTICULUM

Esophageal diverticula are generally rare entities that are characterized primarily by anatomic location. Epiphrenic diverticula are typically pulsion diverticula occurring in the distal esophagus and often related to an underlying motility disorder. Mid-esophageal diverticula are usually traction diverticula occurring secondary to inflammatory diseases. Traditionally, operations for these diverticula have been performed by an open approach. However, operative morbidity can be significant and so operative intervention is usually reserved for those patients with significant symptoms.[16]

As experience with minimally invasive surgery for other esophageal disorders has increased, centers have reported the use of minimally invasive approaches for treating esophageal diverticula.[17,18] For epiphrenic diverticula, our initial approach had been similar to that for laparoscopic esophageal myotomy as described above. From the abdominal approach, the distal esophagus and diverticulum were exposed. Since the diverticulum is a mucosal outpouching without a muscular covering, its location was used as the proximal limit of a myotomy which was then extended distally onto the stomach. However, because of esophageal leaks noted with our initial experience, this approach was modified. In our current practice, the neck of the diverticulum is exposed and the diverticulum is resected with a laparoscopic stapler. The esophageal muscle is then closed over this staple line, and the myotomy is performed on the side opposite to the diverticulum. A partial fundoplication is also performed.

In some cases, the diverticulum cannot be safely exposed and resected from a laparoscopic approach, and so a combined laparoscopic and right thoracoscopic approach may be necessary. Increasingly, for larger diverticula and mid-esophageal diverticula, we use a right thoracoscopic approach only (Fig. 128.9). A 10-mm port is placed in the seventh or eighth intercostal space anteriorly for the initial thoracoscopic evaluation. Another 10-mm port is placed

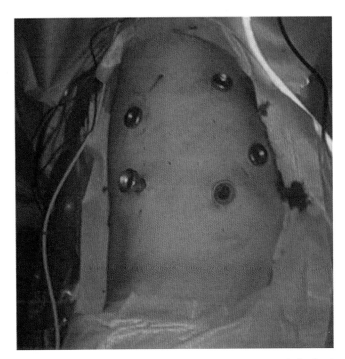

FIGURE 128.9 Port placement for right thoracoscopic approach for distal esophageal diverticulectomy.

in the eighth intercostal space posteriorly. A 5-mm port is placed posteriorly, below the inferior angle of the scapula. Another 5-mm port is placed two or three interspaces above the camera port, and a final 10-mm port is placed higher to allow for the use of a fan-shaped lung retractor. The surgeon will stand posterior to the patient, and two assistants stand anterior to the patient.

The esophagus will be mobilized above and below the diverticulum, and the origin of the diverticulum will be exposed. An endoscopic 45-mm reticulating stapler is placed across the neck of the diverticulum and used for diverticulectomy (Fig. 128.10). Placement of a bougie is helpful to stabilize the esophagus during the dissection and also to minimize narrowing of the esophageal lumen during stapling of the diverticulum. After resection of the diverticulum, the esophageal muscle is reapproximated over the staple line and a myotomy is created away from the staple line. If necessary, the patient can be brought back for a staged laparoscopy to extend the myotomy distally and/or to add a partial fundoplication; however, this is not necessary in most cases.

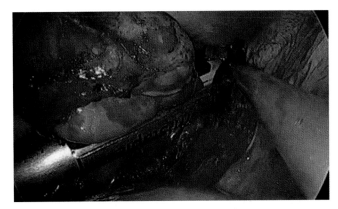

FIGURE 128.10 Stapled diverticulectomy of a distal esophageal diverticulum through a right thoracoscopic approach.

CONCLUSIONS

The management of esophageal motility disorders has undergone significant evolution over the past 15 years. Traditional open approaches with thoracotomy or laparotomy have been replaced in many centers with minimally invasive approaches. These also continue to evolve, for instance, from a thoracoscopic approach to a laparoscopic or robotic approach for achalasia and, more recently, to a completely endoscopic approach. Despite the procedure used, the surgeon should carefully evaluate each patient, confirm the diagnosis, and be certain that the patient is truly symptomatic in order to justify operative repair.

REFERENCES

1. Richards WO, Torquati A, Holzman MD, et al. Heller myotomy versus Heller myotomy with Dor fundoplication for achalasia: a prospective randomized double-blind clinical trial. *Ann Surg* 2004;240(3):405–412
2. Horgan S, Galvani C, Gorodner MV, et al. Robotic-assisted Heller myotomy versus laparoscopic Heller myotomy for the treatment of esophageal achalasia: multicenter study. *J Gastrointest Surg* 2005;9(8):1020–1029.
3. Melvin WS, Dundon JM, Talamini M, et al. Computer-enhanced robotic telesurgery minimizes esophageal perforation during Heller myotomy. *Surgery* 2005, 138(4):553–558.
4. Huffmanm LC, Pandalai PK, Boulton BJ, et al. Robotic Heller myotomy: a safe operation with higher postoperative quality-of-life indices. *Surgery* 2007;142(4):613–618.
5. Shaligram A, Unnirevi J, Simorov A, et al. How does the robot affect outcomes? A retrospective review of open, laparoscopic, and robotic Heller myotomy for achalasia. *Surg Endosc* 2012;26(4):1047–1050.
6. Mou Y, Zeng H, Wang Q, et al. Giant mid-esophageal diverticula successfully treated by per-oral endoscopic myotomy. *Surg Endosc* 2016;30(1):335–338.
7. Bhayani NH, Kurian AA, Dunst CM, et al. A Comparative study on comprehensive, objective outcomes of laparoscopic Heller myotomy with per-oral endoscopic myotomy (POEM) for achalasia. *Ann Surg* 2014;259:1098–1103.
8. Kumagai K, Tsai JA, Thorell A, et al. Per-oral endoscopic myotomy for achalasia. Are results comparable to laparoscopic Heller myotomy? *Scand J Gastroenterol* 2015;50(5):505–512.
9. Sharata AM, Dunst CM, Pescarus R, et al. Peroral endoscopic myotomy (POEM) for esophageal primary motility disorders: analysis of 100 consecutive patients. *J Gastrointest Surg* 2015;19(1):161–170.
10. Ludlow A. A case of obstructed deglutition from a preternatural bag formed in the pharynx. In: Johnson W, Caldwell T, eds. *Medical Observations and Inquiries by a Society of Physicians in London.* London: London Medical Society; 1769;85–101.
11. Zenker FA, von Ziemssen H. Krankheiten des Oesophagus. In: von Ziemssen H, ed. *Handbuch des speciellen Pathologie und Therapie.* Leipzig: FC Vogel; 1877;1–87.
12. Morse CR, Fernando HC, Ferson PF, et al. Preliminary experience by a thoracic service with endoscopic transoral stapling of cervical (Zenker's) diverticulum. *J Gastrointest Surg* 2007;11:1091–1094.
13. Pescarus R, Shlomovitz E, Sharata AM, et al. Trans-oral cricomyotomy using a flexible endoscope: technique and clinical outcomes. *Surg Endosc* 2016;30(5):1784–1789. ePub, accepted July 13, 2015.
14. Chiari C, Yeganehfar W, Scharitzer M, et al. Significant symptomatic relief after transoral endoscopic staple-assisted treatment of Zenker's diverticulum. *Surg Endosc* 2003;17:596–600.
15. Chang CY, Payyapilli RJ, Scher RL. Endoscopic staple diverticulostomy for Zenker's diverticulum: review of literature and experience in 159 consecutive cases. *Laryngoscope* 2003;113:957–965.
16. Benacci JC, Deschamps C, Trastek VF, et al. Epiphrenic diverticulum: results of surgical treatment. *Ann Thorac Surg* 1993;55:1109–1114.
17. Fernando HC, Luketich JD, Samphire J, et al. Minimally invasive operation for esophageal diverticula. *Ann Thorac Surg* 2005;80:2076–2081.
18. Zaninotto G, Parise P, Salvador R, et al. Laparoscopic repair of epiphrenic diverticulum. *Semin Thorac Cardiovasc Surg* 2012;24:218–222.

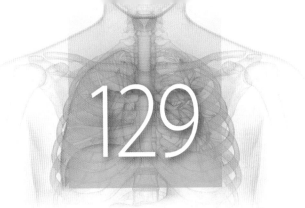

Surgical Techniques for the Treatment of Reflux Disease

Antonios C. Sideris ▪ Yifan A. Zheng ▪ Abby White ▪ Raphael Bueno

INTRODUCTION

As many as 1-in-3 North Americans experience gastroesophageal reflux disease (GERD).[1] This increasing disease burden, in the era of minimally invasive surgery and improved medical therapy with proton pump inhibitors (PPIs), makes it especially important to identify patients who will benefit the most from surgical therapy. How GERD is defined is also important. The American Gastroenterological Association defines GERD as reflux that causes "troublesome symptoms and/or complications."[2] Care must be taken to avoid diagnosis of reflux based solely on imaging findings in the absence of symptoms. GERD represents a spectrum of disease, which ranges from mild symptoms controlled with over-the-counter medications and lifestyle modifications to stricture and malignancy. GERD may also be accompanied by anatomic abnormalities such as a hiatal hernia.

PHYSIOLOGY AND PATHOLOGY

The pathophysiologic basis of reflux disease lies in an impaired balance between protective and damaging mechanisms of the esophagus and gastroesophageal junction (GEJ), ultimately leading to abnormally prolonged contact of caustic gastric contents with the esophageal mucosa.

PROTECTIVE MECHANISMS

Protective mechanisms can be subdivided into three main categories: anatomical barriers, esophageal luminal clearance, and intrinsic mucosal resistance to injury.

The anatomical barrier remains the most critical defense against GERD, and is comprised of the lower esophageal sphincter (LES) and the extrinsic components of the diaphragmatic apparatus. The LES is not a true anatomical sphincter; rather it corresponds to a functional area of elevated luminal pressure, identified by intraluminal manometry that extends along the most distal 2 to 4 cm of the esophagus. A pronounced circular muscle may be identified at this area along with increased vessel and connective tissue density compared to the rest of the organ. The LES shows a resting pressure of 15 to 30 mm Hg, unevenly distributed and distinctly different from the intraluminal pressure of the rest of the esophagus and the stomach. Under normal circumstances, the sphincter remains tonically contracted—an intrinsic property of the muscle itself which is further enhanced by extrinsic innervation. Constriction is mediated by acetylcholine whereas nitric oxide is thought to be the mediator of relaxation that occurs after swallowing. Resting pressure varies between individuals and may be further influenced by multiple factors, including the inspiratory cycle, positional changes, various foods, endogenous hormones, and pharmacologic agents (Table 129.1).

The second component of the anatomical barrier is the diaphragmatic apparatus, which consists of the diaphragmatic crural fibers, the extrinsic pressure from the anatomical compartment surrounding the LES and the angle of His. More specifically, the diaphragm encircles the esophagus in a pincer-like configuration. During inspiration or independent increases in intraabdominal pressure, crural fibers contract along the body of the diaphragm, causing an increase in LES pressure. Additionally, the esophageal opening is oriented obliquely within the diaphragm, creating an acute angle (termed *angle of His*) at the point where the esophagus connects into the gastric cardia. As the intra-abdominal and intra-gastric pressures increase, the stomach wall is pressed against the LES along the angle of His, augmenting the sphincter's efficiency. Moreover, the presence of the phrenoesophageal ligament acts to support the LES and ensure its proper position while affording some movement. Finally, the mucosal folds of the gastric cardia serve as functional flap valves that enhance the sphincter's action during contraction.

The second line of defense against reflux involves clearance of caustic agents (acid, pepsin, bile) from the esophageal lumen. Normally, swallowing initiates a primary peristaltic wave which propels the food bolus along the esophagus. Secondary peristalsis in the absence of pharyngeal contraction is stimulated by the presence of acidic contents in the distal esophagus. Finally, positional changes may affect luminal clearance, and the upright position is thought to accelerate clearance by gravity. Clearance is further enhanced by the buffering action of salivary and other esophageal secretions (normal salivation is about 1 L/day).

The last barrier is the inherent resistance to tissue injury. Mucosal defenses can be subcategorized into pre-epithelial and epithelial. Pre-epithelial defenses involve mainly superficial mucous and bicarbonate production forming a protective layer, which is poorly developed in the esophagus. The most important factor at the microscopic level, however, is the epithelial resistance itself, which consists of tight cellular junctions that impede intercellular hydrogen ion

TABLE 129.1 Substances that Influence Lower Esophageal Sphincter Pressure

	Increase LESP	Decrease LESP
Hormones	Gastrin, motilin, substance P	Secretin, cholecystokinin, glucagon, gastric inhibitory polypeptide, vasoactive intestinal polypeptide, progesterone
Neural Agents	Alpha-adrenergic agonists, beta-adrenergic antagonists, cholinergic agonists	Alpha-adrenergic antagonists, beta-adrenergic agonists, cholinergic antagonists, serotonin
Medications	Metoclopramide, domperidone, prostaglandin F2α, cisapride	Nitrates, calcium channel blockers, theophylline, morphine, meperidine, diazepam, barbiturates
Foods	Protein	Fat, chocolate, ethanol, peppermint

Reprinted from Kahrilas PJ. Gastroesophoageal reflux disease and its complications. In: Feldman M, ed. Sleisenger & Fordtran's Gastrointestinal and Liver Disease. 6th ed. Philadelphia, PA: WB Saunders Company; 1998:498–516. Copyright © 1998 Elsevier. With permission.

diffusion and hence protect against injury. Finally, evidence suggests that esophageal epithelial cells may extrude hydrogen ions by upregulation of the expression of Na/H and Cl/HCO3 exchangers. Age, nutritional status, cigarette smoking, and alcohol consumption may adversely affect the mucosal ability to resist injury.

MECHANISMS OF INJURY

The primary mechanisms of injury causing GERD can be grouped into three main categories: transient LES relaxations (tLESRs), hypoactive LES, and anatomic dysfunction of the gastroesophageal apparatus. tLESRs are vagally stimulated, nonswallow induced relaxations that are not followed by lower esophageal peristaltic waves. They allow venting of swallowed gas and are largely regarded as part of the physiologic mechanism of belching in both normal subjects and GERD patients. In fact, the discerning characteristic between the two populations may only be a higher percentage of tLESR associated with gastric reflux in patients compared to their normal counterparts.[3] tLESRs are considered the main culprit in mild cases. However, they contribute to only about one-third of episodes associated with severe disease, where a more prominent association with a hypotensive LES exists. In such advanced cases, reflux may be caused by a strain-induced opening secondary to increased intra-abdominal pressure or may be an unprovoked reflux, accentuated by the concomitant esophageal hypomotility.[4]

The presence of a hiatal hernia as an independent cause of reflux is still debated as only a subset of patients with hiatal hernia suffer from GERD. Nevertheless, once present, it alters the normal configuration of the LES and the diaphragmatic apparatus, increasing susceptibility to reflux if other factors coexist. Additionally, the intrathoracic portion of the stomach may form an abnormal "pouch" interposed between the LES and the diaphragm, facilitating reflux into the esophagus once the LES relaxes. Of note, a large proportion of patients with hiatal hernias suffer from concomitant distal esophageal motility impairment which further aggravates the problem.

Secondary causes of reflux include a long list of conditions such as Zollinger–Ellison syndrome, scleroderma, and other connective tissue diseases, prior gastric surgery, and delayed gastric emptying such as in idiopathic or diabetic gastroparesis or in gastric outlet obstruction.[4]

SURGICAL INDICATIONS AND CONTRAINDICATIONS

The spectrum of indications for operative intervention in patients with GERD has been shifting in recent years. Until recently, the most

common reason for surgical management has been disease progression refractory to medical treatment, owing mainly to the lack of effective medications. With the introduction and widespread use of PPIs that provide excellent relief for the majority of patients with reflux, disease progression is noted only in a fraction of the population—5-year progression was found to be 5.9% in nonerosive reflux disease, 12.1% in Los Angeles (LA) grade A/B patients and 19.7% in LA grade C/D patients with no evidence of Barrett esophagus at baseline (Table 129.2).[5]

In fact, given the rarity of disease progression with appropriate medical care, one should maintain a very high index of suspicion for the presence of an alternative diagnosis.[6,7] Complications of GERD not responding to medical therapy (esophagitis, stricture, recurrent aspiration, or pneumonia) remain appropriate surgical indications.

The presence of Barrett esophagus with or without low-grade dysplasia in the setting of symptomatic reflux is generally acceptable as a clear indication for antireflux surgery.[8] However, there is no consensus on whether antireflux surgery can prevent progression of dysplasia in asymptomatic Barrett's. Although there have been many reports of regression of Barrett esophagus after surgical treatment of reflux disease,[9] the benefit of surgical over medical management to date remains inconclusive.[10] Furthermore, there is a paucity of data on the outcomes of combining newer therapeutic modalities for Barrett's (radiofrequency ablation, endomuscular resection) with an antireflux procedure.[11,12] If surgical management is chosen, endoscopic surveillance should be continued postoperatively according to the patient's preoperative pathological changes.[13]

At present, the majority of patients seeking surgical consultation consists of those who fail to comply with medical management, do not wish to be maintained on medications long-term, or exhibit intolerance or interference of PPIs with other prescribed regimens. Indeed, the rising cost of the medications and the need for frequent

TABLE 129.2 The Los Angeles Classification of Esophagitis

Grade A	One (or more) mucosal break no longer than 5 mm, that does not extend between the tops of two mucosal folds
Grade B	One (or more) mucosal break more than 5 mm long that does not extend between the tops of two mucosal folds
Grade C	One (or more) mucosal break that is continuous between the tops of two or more mucosal folds but which involves less than 75% of the circumference
Grade D	One (or more) mucosal break which involves at least 75% of the esophageal circumference

Reproduced from Lundell LR, Dent J, Bennett JR, et al. Endoscopic assessment of oesophagitis: clinical and functional correlates and further validation of the Los Angeles classification. *Gut* 1999;45(2):172–180, with permission from BMJ Publishing Group Ltd..

TABLE 129.3 Prevalence of Symptoms Occurring More Than Once Per Week Among 1,000 Patients with GERD

Symptom	Prevalence (%)
Heartburn	80
Regurgitation	54
Abdominal pain	29
Cough	27
Dysphagia for solids	23
Hoarseness	21
Belching	15
Bloating	15
Aspiration	14
Wheezing	7
Globus	4

Reprinted from Yates RB, Oelschlager BK. Surgical treatment of gastroesophageal reflux disease. *Surg Clin North Am* 2015;95(3):527–553. Copyright © 2015 Elsevier. With permission.

follow-ups with dose adjustments pose a challenge, especially to young and otherwise fit patients who desire a definitive solution to their problem. Additionally, there has been significant concern regarding potential interaction between PPI intake and clopidogrel metabolism, potentially leading to increased adverse cardiovascular and gastrointestinal bleeding complications. However, no definitive evidence has been found to date, and the issue remains controversial.[14,15] Other clinically relevant PPI interactions include diazepam, phenytoin, carbamazepine, HIV protease inhibitors (increase plasma levels), and warfarin (decrease INR). Finally, decreased magnesium absorption secondary to prolonged PPI use may lead to interference and exacerbation of hypomagnesemia in patients taking medications such as digoxin and diuretics. These patients should be closely monitored for their magnesium levels.

There are very few absolute contraindications for the fundoplication operation. Most contraindications are severe comorbidities that make the patient a poor surgical candidate. Relative contraindications for the laparoscopic approach include the presence of multiple previous upper abdominal operations, while a severely foreshortened esophagus and the presence of a giant paraesophageal hernia may require modification of the procedure. Patients with BMI ≥35 may be better served by a bariatric procedure such as a Roux-en-Y operation which achieves the dual goal of symptomatic relief and weight reduction with improvement of comorbidities; such benefits become less evident in patients with BMI 30 to 35.[13,16] In the morbidly obese population with GERD symptomatology, another bariatric operation such as sleeve gastrectomy or gastric banding is strongly discouraged.

PREOPERATIVE EVALUATION

A thorough preoperative evaluation to confirm the diagnosis and to assess the extent of the problem is paramount for successful management of patients with GERD. The evaluation begins with a thorough history and physical examination. Typical symptoms include heartburn, dysphagia, or regurgitation, whereas cough, nonallergic/nocturnal asthma, hoarseness, and sore throat are considered atypical (Table 129.3). Studies have shown that surgical intervention is more successful in alleviating typical symptoms (Table 129.4).[6,7,17–19] The pattern (timing, patient position, etc.) and duration of symptomatology along with previous therapy and response to medical treatment must be evaluated. Preexisting comorbidities and prior surgeries should be reviewed, especially in delineating the esophageal anatomy for surgical planning.

TABLE 129.4 Predictors of Airway Symptom Response to Laparoscopic Antireflux Surgery

Preoperative Symptom/Finding[c]	Improvement n (%)[a]	No Improvement n (%)[b]	p Value	Symptom	Improvement in Symptom Frequency n (%)	Patients Reporting Symptom as "Better" n (%)
Heartburn	83 (90)	34 (94)	0.44	Cough (n = 108)	76 (70)	80 (74)
Regurgitation	41 (45)	17 (47)	0.79	Hoarseness (n = 82)	57 (70)	54 (66)
Abdominal pain	34 (37)	16 (44)	0.44	Wheezing (n = 37)	25 (69)	25 (69)
Bloating	43 (47)	19 (53)	0.54	Sore Throat (n = 41)	28 (68)	29 (70)
Primary symptom respiratory	32 (35)	13 (36)	0.80	Dyspnea (n = 31)	15 (48)	20 (65)
UGI reflux	55 (60)	15 (16)	0.36			
Hiatal hernia (EGD or UGI)	65 (71)	24 (67)	0.66			
Esophagitis	34 (37)	17 (47)	0.29			
EGD Barrett esophagus	10 (11)	3 (8)	0.90			
Normal peristalsis	75 (82)	29 (81)	0.34			
Distal esophageal amplitude low	5 (5)	4 (11)	0.30			
Distal acid exposure abnormal	81 (88)	29 (81)	0.21			
Pharyngeal reflux present	5 (5)	1 (3)	0.02			

UGI, upper gastrointestinal; EGD, esophagogastroduodenoscopy.
Improvement was defined as improvement of the primary preoperative airway symptom by one number on the numeric frequency scale.
[a]92 improved.
[b]36 did not improve.
[c]Variable was present before LARS.
From Kaufman JA, Houghland JE, Quiroga E, et al. Long-term outcomes of laparoscopic antireflux surgery for gastroesophageal reflux disease (GERD)-related airway disorder. *Surg Endosc* 2006;20(12):1824–1830. Copyright © 2006 Springer Science+Business Media, Inc. With permission of Springer.

1. upper endoscopy
2. esophageal motility evaluation by conventional/high-resolution manometry
3. 24-hour pH monitoring
4. anatomic imaging modality of the upper gastrointestinal tract

TABLE 129.6 Composite Reflux (DeMeester) Score[22]

Components
Percent of total time pH <4
Percent of upright time pH <4
Percent of supine time pH <4
Total number of episodes pH <4
Number of episodes pH <4 lasting >5 minutes
Number of minutes of longest episode pH <4

Score
<14.7 indicates absence of reflux (95% confidence interval)

Adapted from Johnson LF, Demeester TR. Twenty-four-hour pH monitoring of the distal esophagus. A quantitative measure of gastroesophageal reflux. *Am J Gastroenterol* 1974;62(4):325–332.

Regardless of how thorough the history and physical examination may be, they should not be considered sufficient evidence to support the diagnosis of GERD.[20] Further evaluation should be completed with (1) upper endoscopy, (2) esophageal motility evaluation by conventional or high-resolution manometry, (3) 24-hour pH monitoring and (4) an anatomic imaging modality of the upper gastrointestinal tract (Table 129.5).

ANATOMIC EXAMINATIONS

Upper Gastrointestinal Series

A barium esophagogram or, preferably, a video esophagogram should be obtained in every patient considered for antireflux surgery. It is essential to delineate the anatomy of the esophagus and to identify anatomical abnormalities, such as a hiatal hernia, esophageal diverticula, or anatomic strictures. Multiple views in patients with hiatal hernias in the supine and upright positions may also reveal the presence of a foreshortened esophagus if the hernia fails to reduce upon sitting.

A carefully obtained video esophagogram may suggest the presence of occult motility disorders of the esophagus, such as achalasia, localized or diffuse spasm, or impaired peristalsis. It can also assist in confirming the diagnosis by showing moderate or severe reflux or spontaneous retrograde flow of gastric contrast to the level of the clavicles.

Esophagogastroduodenoscopy

An upper endoscopy should also be performed in any patient in whom operative intervention is considered. It can provide visual evidence of mucosal inflammation, intestinal metaplasia in Barrett esophagus, hiatal hernia and the presence of strictures or other pathology such as cancer. Biopsies should also be obtained in all patients, as early abnormalities may not be readily apparent by inspection only. The presence of Barrett esophagus with dysplasia should be ruled out, as this could alter the operative plan to an ablative procedure or resection. The location of the GEJ relative to the diaphragm and the degree of esophagitis/stricture are noted because of the potential for a foreshortened esophagus that may warrant Collis gastroplasty. One additional use of the preoperative EGD is for correct placement of the pH probe or the manometry catheter.

PHYSIOLOGIC EXAMINATIONS

Esophageal Manometry

Esophageal manometry, conventional or high-resolution, is the gold standard for assessing LES function and esophageal peristalsis. A large percentage of patients with GERD may have manometric evidence of LES impairment (approximately 60%) or esophageal dysmotility, which varies with the severity of the underlying esophagitis (25% in mild vs. 48% in severe esophagitis).[21] The primary goals of the procedure are (1) to rule out contraindications to standard fundoplications such as achalasia, diffuse esophageal spasm, nutcracker esophagus, hypertensive LES, or scleroderma, (2) to determine the strength and coordination of esophageal peristaltic waves and (3) to assess LES length, location, and pressure at rest and during swallowing. The results of this test are essential to proper surgical planning because patients who undergo complete fundoplication have a median increase of 12 mm Hg in the outflow resistance of the LES that requires sufficient esophageal contractions to overcome. A potential pitfall of high-resolution manometry is that it may inaccurately estimate the overall and intraabdominal length of the LES as well as the LES position, thereby increasing the likelihood of an inaccurate pH result.[23] The presence of low amplitude or disordered esophageal contractions should signal the need for a partial fundoplication or even a nonoperative approach to avoid debilitating postoperative dysphagia.

Esophageal pH Monitoring

Twenty-four-hour esophageal pH monitoring is considered the "gold standard" for the diagnosis of gastroesophageal reflux and is crucial for correlating patients' symptoms to reflux events, especially in those with nonerosive GERD. Correct positioning of the probe is critical for the accuracy of the test—it should be placed 5 cm above the manometrically confirmed upper edge of the LES. Measurements are used to calculate the composite reflux score (DeMeester score, Table 129.6), with a result ≥14.7 signifying pathologic reflux (accuracy 96%).[24] Extending the monitoring period for 48 hours has been shown to increase accuracy and sensitivity by up to 22%.[25] Recently, the Esophageal Diagnostic Advisory Panel recommended that all patients, especially those with nonerosive esophagitis, who are being evaluated for possible surgical intervention, undergo pH testing after being off acid suppression for 7 days to allow for proper interpretation of the results. Any H2-blockers should also be stopped for 3 days prior to testing. The only group that may be exempt consists of those with Los Angeles grade C or D esophagitis, after excluding pill esophagitis and achalasia.[20] Patients who cannot tolerate cessation of acid suppression may be evaluated by esophageal impedance testing, which can detect any type of reflux episode, regardless of pH. A helpful algorithm interpreting the results is depicted in Figure 129.1.

Gastric Emptying

Occasionally, surgical candidates will complain of significant postprandial bloating, abdominal distention, and nausea and should be evaluated for gastroparesis. Alternatively, significant amounts of retained food may be noted during the preoperative EGD, thereby prompting an evaluation for disorders of gastric emptying. Undiagnosed gastroparesis may lead to postoperative gas-bloat symptoms and/or wrap failure. The Esophageal Diagnostic Advisory Panel recommends that a gastric emptying study (nuclear scintigraphy with

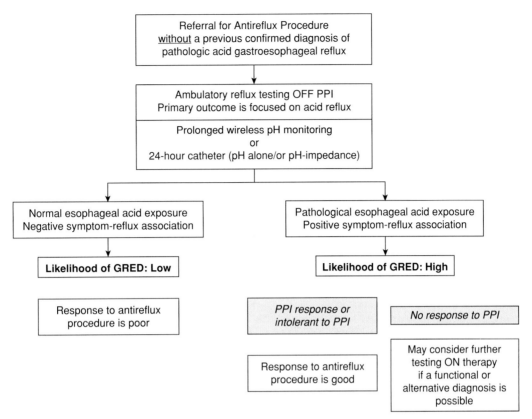

FIGURE 129.1 Approach to the patient being evaluated for antireflux surgery. (From Jobe BA, Richter JE, Hoppo T, et al. Preoperative diagnostic workup before antireflux surgery: an evidence and experience-based consensus of the esophageal diagnostic advisory panel. *J Am Coll Surg* 2013;217(4):586–597. Reprinted with permission from the Journal of the American College of Surgeons.)

radioactive Tc-99m or In-111) be performed selectively in this population, extending the monitoring period to 4 hours. In normal subjects, 50% of the gastric emptying is completed by 15 to 90 minutes for liquids and 45 to 100 minutes for solids.[20]

SURGICAL TREATMENT OPTIONS

The main factors that a surgeon must weigh fall under three categories: (1) operative approach (open vs. minimally invasive, transabdominal vs. transthoracic); (2) extent of fundoplication (complete vs. partial); and (3) need for additional procedures, such as esophageal lengthening procedures.

Since the introduction of minimally invasive fundoplication in the early 1990s by Dallemagne's group, the technique has evolved to become the standard of care. The minimally invasive approach is preferred in almost all patients with very few exceptions, because it has been shown to yield similar outcomes with a better safety profile, shorter hospital stays, and faster return to work.[26–42] The main indications for the open approach include inability to complete the minimally invasive operation safely, a need for open abdominal operation for concurrent intraabdominal pathology, and the occasional very complex case of reoperation following previously failed fundoplication(s), although these may be done laparoscopically in specialized centers.[43] Nevertheless, the prudent surgeon always maintains a low threshold for conversion to an open procedure, especially early on in the learning curve.

Most fundoplications are currently performed transabdominally. The thoracic approach is used in the event of an extremely hostile abdomen or if a thoracotomy is required for another reason and an antireflux operation is indicated as well. Recently, some groups have attempted to perform robotically assisted fundoplication with good short-term outcomes. However, long-term data are still warranted before a recommendation can be made regarding this technique.[44–46]

Currently, the vast majority of patients treated in the United States undergo a complete (360 degrees) fundoplication. In contrast, European centers most commonly create a partial wrap, usually via a Toupet fundoplication. Several randomized trials have failed to definitively demonstrate that one approach yields superior outcomes over the other.[47–61] The current thinking is that patients who do not exhibit concurrent esophageal dysmotility would benefit more from a complete fundoplication, because it decreases the frequency of reflux episodes more effectively. However, due to a higher resistance to flow, it is associated with a higher incidence of postoperative dysphagia; hence a partial wrap may be better suited for patients with suspected or confirmed esophageal dysmotility.

Regardless of the operative approach that is chosen, the main goals of restoring the functional and mechanical competence of the GEJ barrier are the same and should be understood and observed by all esophageal surgeons.[62] One must permanently restore at least 2 cm of intraabdominal esophagus. It has been clearly demonstrated that distal esophageal resistance to resting intraabdominal pressure is directly proportional to its abdominal length. Sufficient mobilization should be encouraged; if this proves to be inadequate, a neoesophagus can be constructed by an esophageal lengthening procedure.

By itself, restoration of the intra-abdominal esophagus is insufficient to relieve GERD. Therefore, the GEJ should be further reinforced to resist increases of intragastric and intra-abdominal pressure

TABLE 129.7 Steps in Fundoplication

1. Identification of the right and left vagus
2. Preservation of the hepatic branch of the vagus
3. Mobilization of the gastric fundus facilitated by division of the short gastric vessels
4. Crural closure
5. Bougie for esophageal diameter calibration
6. Short wrap (≤2 cm)

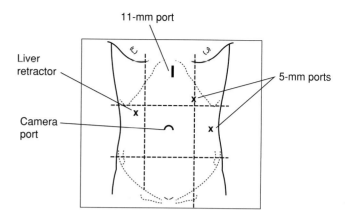

FIGURE 129.2 Placement of laparoscopic ports for fundoplication.

particularly after the obligatory dissection of all crural connections. This reinforcement is achieved by creating a fundoplication around the lower abdominal esophagus, in order to augment the resting LES pressures. Only the fundus of the stomach and not the body should be included in the fundoplication, because only the former relaxes upon swallowing. Should the body of the stomach be inadvertently included in the wrap, a lack of relaxation may prevent the food bolus from being propelled into the stomach, with resulting dysphagia. Finally, the diaphragmatic crura need to be adequately approximated to avoid creation of an iatrogenic paraesophageal hernia.

In all approaches, certain intraoperative steps are followed to standardize and improve the outcomes.[63,64] These include the identification and preservation of the left and right vagus, the mobilization of the fundus of the stomach, closure of the diaphragmatic crura, and the creation of a short, floppy wrap over a bougie (Table 129.7).

MINIMALLY INVASIVE FUNDOPLICATION

COMPLETE FUNDOPLICATION (NISSEN)

Minimally invasive Nissen fundoplication is currently considered the standard of care and is the most commonly performed antireflux operation. However, the procedure may be exceptionally challenging in certain patients, such as those with extreme obesity where related organomegaly may obscure the field, or those with multiple previous upper abdominal surgeries with associated adhesion formation that alters the planes and the consistency of the tissues. Adhesions and obesity can also impair the achievement of adequate pneumoperitoneum. Patients with severe COPD may also not tolerate CO_2 pneumoperitoneum at all. Finally, in our practice, the presence or suspicion of ischemic stomach (an extremely rare circumstance) constitutes a relative contraindication to laparoscopic fundoplication (Table 129.8).

Patient Positioning and Trocar Placement

The operation is performed under general anesthesia. Appropriate perioperative antibiotics are administered and a Foley catheter is placed for bladder decompression. An EGD is routinely performed to reassess the anatomy and an orogastric tube is inserted for gastric

TABLE 129.8 The Major Steps of Nissan Fundoplication

1. Placement of ports for intraabdominal access
2. Circumferential hiatal dissection and reduction of any paraesophageal hernia
3. Division of the short gastric arteries
4. Dissection of the esophagus into the mediastinum to free up length
5. Evaluation of esophageal length and lengthening if indicated
6. Closure of the hiatus
7. Creation of a short, shoe-shined floppy wrap

decompression during the operation. The patient's arms are tucked at the sides. The operation can be completed in the supine or the lithotomy position; we favor the latter. Meticulous attention is paid to properly securing the patient in order to avoid slippage, nerve compression, and injuries intraoperatively. The surgeon stands between the patient's legs with the first assistant to the patient's right.

A 11-mm supraumbilical incision is made and intraperitoneal access is obtained via the Hassan technique for the camera port. Alternatively, an optical trocar entry may be attempted, especially in the case of prior abdominal operations. Once access is confirmed, pneumoperitoneum is established via a CO_2 insufflator to a maximal pressure of 15 to 19 mm Hg. A 30-degree or deflectable tip laparoscope is inserted and inspection of the peritoneal cavity is performed, with special attention to identification of trocar or access related injuries. Subsequently, all ports are placed under direct vision (Fig. 129.2). A 5-mm trocar is placed in the left subcostal margin at the midclavicular line. An assistant port using a 5-mm trocar is placed in the left anterior axillary line at the same level as the camera port. A 11-mm subxiphoid port is then placed and finally a 5-mm right subcostal port is placed along the midclavicular line for the liver retractor. During and immediately after port insertion, all interfering adhesions should be meticulously mobilized. The patient is then positioned in steep reverse-Trendelenburg for the remainder of the operation.

Initial Dissection

A self-retaining liver retractor is inserted and the left lateral lobe of the liver is retracted away from the operative field. The assistant grasps the esophageal fat pad and gently retracts it anteriorly, caudally and medially, toward the patient's right whereas a second grasper gently lifts the gastrosplenic ligament laterally, exposing the short gastric arteries. Dissection starts 10 to 15 cm distal to the angle of His, at a point cephalad to the gastroepiploic vessels. After the lesser sac is opened, the surgeon sequentially divides the short gastric vessels and all other attachments until the fundus has been completely mobilized. We prefer to divide the two peritoneal leaves separately. Complete mobilization of the gastric fundus is especially important to ensure formation of a tension-free wrap.

Attention is then turned to the dissection of the gastrohepatic ligament. The assistant grasps the esophageal fat pad and gently retracts it anteriorly, caudally and laterally, toward the patient's left. With this maneuver, the gastrohepatic ligament is exposed and divided along the lesser curvature at the clear portion (*pars flaccida*), proceeding cephalad until the left crus is identified. Every attempt should be made to leave the peritoneal covering of the crura in place, in our experience this has been shown to greatly increase the strength of the tissue during the hiatal closure step of the repair. The surgeon should be cautious to avoid inadvertent division of the replaced left hepatic artery (present in 5% of patients and provides most of the blood perfusion to the left hepatic lobe) which may cross the dissection path transversely. However, if needed it can usually be divided with impunity. Other structures that may be found in this area include vagal branches, which should be avoided, and an accessory left hepatic artery which may be divided without consequence. Once the right crus is reached, the anterior layer of the phrenoesophageal membrane is divided and the crural pillar exposed. Very gently, with the help of blunt dissection, an instrument is introduced between the right crus and the esophagus, and the distal esophagus is gently swept to the left. The esophagus is recognized by its longitudinal muscle fibers, its course and the presence of the posterior vagus nerve which is usually found in the 9 to 6 o'clock position. The dissection then proceeds bluntly around the esophageal hiatus along the median arcuate ligament toward the left. Care is exercised to avoid injury to the anterior vagus nerve and its branches. The left crus is similarly dissected and the phrenoesophageal ligament divided. The vagus nerves are protected. Subsequently, using traction and counter traction with a closed instrument, the esophagus is elevated and a large retroesophageal window is developed.

After both crural pillars are dissected and the phrenoesophageal membrane has been divided up to the crural decussations, if a hiatal hernia is present, it is reduced into the abdomen and the sac is amputated. If the pleura is inadvertently injured, the anesthesia team should be promptly notified. This type of pneumothorax rarely requires placement of a chest tube and can be managed intraoperatively by increasing airway pressure and simultaneously lowering the pressure of the pneumoperitoneum. The esophagus should be dissected free of attachments 3 to 5 cm into the mediastinum to secure sufficient length.

The surgeon proceeds with assessment of the abdominal esophageal length without tension. The true GEJ is identified by the characteristic confluence of the longitudinal esophageal muscle fibers to the muscle fibers of the stomach. At rest, there must be at least 2 to 3 cm of intraabdominal esophagus. If the patient has a foreshortened esophagus, a Collis gastroplasty is performed to avoid the risk of a failed Nissen due to inadequate esophageal length.

Hiatal Closure

It is our practice to proceed with hiatal closure even if there is no hiatal hernia identified initially, because the hiatus is always widened during the dissection.

The esophagus is gently retracted using a Kittner retractor and the hiatal opening is visualized. The crura are sewn together with 0-ethibond sutures, and calibrated with a 52 Maloney dilator. We start caudally and gradually advance cephalad, placing sutures in 0.5 to 0.75 cm intervals. Usually, three simple interrupted sutures are sufficient. We favor a looser closure to avoid obstruction, by leaving approximately 1 to 1.5 cm of space posteriorly and allowing the esophagus to rest in its normal position. The bougie is retracted to 25 cm from the incisors until required again to calibrate the wrap.

Fundoplication

The esophagus is again retracted anteriorly to expose the retroesophageal window. A reticulating grasper is advanced through the window from the patient's right to the left. The most cephalad point along the greater curvature, indicated by the line of short gastric vessels, is grasped and gently retracted behind the esophagus and to the right. Subsequently, the most apical part of the anterior surface of the great curvature is grasped and brought anterior to the esophagus and to

the right. Using Babcock clamps, the two edges are grasped together and the bougie dilator is again gently advanced into the stomach. A "shoeshine" maneuver is performed to assess for correct orientation with proper tension and no excess redundancy of the wrap. If the fundus is well mobilized, the wrap will remain in that position without spontaneously retracting. The short gastric vessels are expected to line up along the lateral edge of the wrap, indicating correct orientation without twisting of the fundus.

We then proceed with securing the fundoplication with the Maloney dilator used for calibration. Our preference is to use the Endo Stitch device for this portion of the operation. We create two to three 0 sutures, passed from the left to the right side, taking 1 cm of gastric wall. We allow for a wrap length of 2 to 2.5 cm. Initial sutures are placed from the stomach to the esophagus and to the stomach again. The last stitch is from gastric wall to gastric wall. Care should be exercised to ensure that all bites remain seromuscular and that no mucosa is included, to avoid mucosal ischemia and delayed perforation.

Once satisfied with the wrap, the bougie is gently removed, and the anesthesia team introduces a nasogastric tube (NGT) under visual guidance. We inspect the abdominal cavity for hemostasis. The ports are sequentially removed under direct vision and the 11-mm incisions are closed in layers, approximating the fascial layer with the aid of the Carter-Thomason instrument. Finally, the skin is closed and the patient is extubated in the operating room.

PARTIAL FUNDOPLICATION (TOUPET)

In patients with high suspicion (very foreshortened esophagus, long-standing hiatal hernia, advanced esophagitis) or documentation of esophageal dysmotility, we prefer to perform a partial Toupet fundoplication, by creating a 270-degree posterior wrap.

From a technical standpoint, all steps of the procedure are identical to the minimally invasive Nissen fundoplication (see previous section) except for the formation of the wrap. Once the hiatus is properly exposed and dissected, and the fundus is completely mobilized, the esophagus is retracted anteriorly with the assistance of a Penrose drain or a Kittner to expose the retroesophageal window. A reticulating instrument is passed through the window in a right-to-left direction and the most cephalad point along the posterior greater curvature is grasped and brought to the right of the esophagus, where it should lay without spontaneously retracting once the grasp is released. We leave approximately 90-degrees of anterior esophageal wall unwrapped and secure the lip of the posterior wrap to the anterolateral esophagus with three or four interrupted 0 sutures, taking care to only include the seromuscular layers without inclusion of the mucosa in the knot. The right crus is included in securing the wrap.

OPEN FUNDOPLICATION

Except in very rare circumstances, we always attempt to start the operation laparoscopically and convert to open if unable to safely proceed. One added benefit of the laparoscopic-first approach in our experience has been that abdominal insufflation greatly facilitates mediastinal dissection, especially if a paraesophageal hernia is present.

The core principles and steps of the open fundoplication are very similar to that of its minimally invasive counterpart. The positioning differs in that the right arm may be extended or tucked, while the left is tucked at the side to optimize ergonomics and access to critical structures. A shallow reverse Trendelenburg position is maintained throughout the operation. The peritoneal cavity is accessed via an upper midline incision, which may be extended as needed to the lower abdomen. Once the abdomen is entered, meticulous adhesiolysis is performed to allow for complete abdominal exploration and recognition of the proper landmarks and planes. The falciform ligament is ligated using two 0-silk sutures and divided, and the left triangular ligament is incised. A fixed upper body retractor is placed to expose the esophageal hiatus and to elevate the left costal margin, while a self-retaining malleable retractor is utilized for lateral displacement of the left liver lobe. Esophageal dissection and mobilization of the GEJ is then completed as in the minimally invasive operation. Once the entire circumference of the distal esophagus has been mobilized, taking particular care to identify and protect the vagal trunks, the surgeon places a finger behind the esophagus to guide the Penrose drain around the esophagus at the hiatus. As in laparoscopic fundoplication, the abdominal length of the esophagus is assessed: if at least 2 to 3 cm of intraabdominal esophagus cannot be achieved at rest without undue tension, an esophageal lengthening procedure is performed.

After the "shoeshine" maneuver, a 360-degree wrap is secured. The bougie is exchanged for a 18Fr NGT. The surgeon should be able to pass his/her fifth finger between the wrap and the esophagus, indicating that the wrap is not too tight. In partial (Toupet) fundoplication, the edge of the wrap is secured along the anterior-right aspect of the distal esophageal wall. A 2- to 2.5-cm 270-degree posterior wrap is created, so that only a 90-degree anterior esophageal area is left uncovered. The posterior wrap is then secured with interrupted 2-0 sutures to the right crural pillar and the lateral aspect of the anterior leaf of the wrap is secured to the left crural pillar.

TRANSTHORACIC COMPLETE FUNDOPLICATION (NISSEN)

A transthoracic Nissen may be performed in patients necessitating a thoracotomy for concomitant disease or in patients with a severely foreshortened esophagus. Esophageal mobilization is arguably superior via the thoracic approach. However, a thoracotomy is painful and appropriate measures for pain control and pulmonary toilet should be instituted even in the preoperative period.

Intubation with a double-lumen endotracheal tube is performed to isolate and deflate the left lung. The patient is placed in the right lateral decubitus position and a left posterolateral thoracotomy is performed along the seventh intercostal space. The mediastinal pleura overlying the esophagus is divided and the esophageal bed exposed. Next, we divide the inferior pulmonary ligament to ensure optimal exposure. The esophagus is completely mobilized from the level of the carina to the hiatus, taking care to avoid entry into the right pleural space. Both vagi are identified and preserved coursing longitudinally along the organ. Aortic branches are carefully divided. Once the esophagus is completely mobilized, a Penrose drain is placed around the esophagus to assist with operative exposure.

The length of the esophagus is assessed and an esophageal lengthening procedure is completed if needed (see description of Collis gastroplasty below). Additionally, if a hiatal hernia is identified, it is reduced and the sac is carefully dissected from both crura and excised. Division of the phrenoesophageal membrane at the level of the hiatus is performed and the hiatus is enlarged bluntly. Next, the GEJ and the gastric fundus are mobilized by division of the pars flaccida of the gastrohepatic ligament to the right and sequential division of the short gastric arteries along the gastrosplenic ligament to the left. Retroesophageal dissection is also performed. The right and left crura are approximated posteriorly with two to four permanent sutures, which remain untied until the fundoplication is completed. The fundus is brought into the left chest. A 56–60-Fr bougie is gently

introduced into the stomach along the lesser curvature. We create a 360-degree floppy Nissen fundoplication around the distal esophagus. The wrap is secured with two to three interrupted permanent 2-0 sutures. Each suture is submucosal and is passed from wrap to esophagus to wrap again. The bougie is removed and the fundoplication returned to the abdomen. The previously placed crural sutures are secured, closing the hiatus. To minimize the change of postoperative dysphagia, the surgeon confirms the looseness of the hiatal closure by gauging with an index finger. A 28-Fr thoracostomy tube is placed and the thoracotomy incision closed in layers.

BELSEY-MARK IV FUNDOPLICATION

Belsey's transthoracic approach has undergone many modifications to become today's Belsey-Mark IV fundoplication, often performed in conjunction with the Collis gastroplasty (Fig. 129.3).[65] The gastroplasty allows for the return of the GEJ to its subdiaphragmatic location without undue tension. The Belsey fundoplication and Collis gastroplasty as described by Pearson and Henderson[66] is now relegated to a specific subset of patients with GERD undergoing surgical treatment. Because of its transthoracic approach, the Belsey operation is good for (1) the obese patient where the laparoscopic intra-abdominal approach is limited by insufflation pressure, or (2) the re-operative patient that has had extensive abdominal surgery. The Belsey fundoplication is a partial wrap that is suited for patients with abnormal esophageal motility because it is less likely to contribute to postoperative dysphagia.

Patient Positioning and Operative Access

Anesthetic induction and the preincision preparations are similar to those in the patient undergoing a transthoracic Nissen fundoplication. The patient is placed in the right lateral decubitus position with appropriate padding at the pressure points on the body. The operative bed is then flexed to open the left intercostal spaces.

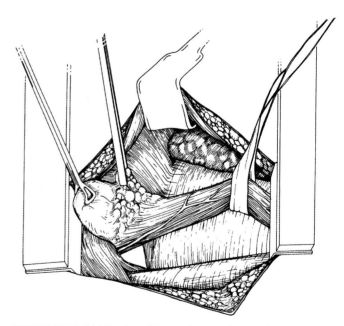

FIGURE 129.3 Mobilization of the esophagus and stomach through a left posterolateral thoracotomy. The esophagus, gastroesophageal fat pad, stomach, diaphragmatic hiatus, aorta, pericardium, and lung are depicted. The fundus of the stomach is drawn through the hiatus into the chest with a Babcock clamp. The forceps is on the fat pad at the gastroesophageal junction, which is then dissected. (From Luketich J. *Master Techniques in Surgery: Esophageal Surgery.* Philadelphia, PA: Lippincott Williams & Wilkins; 2014. With permission.)

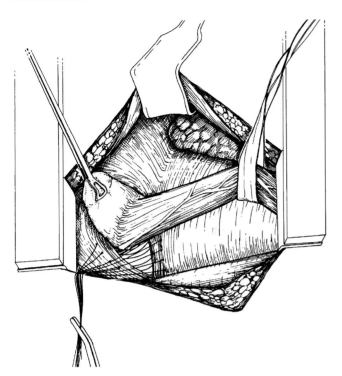

FIGURE 129.4 A transthoracic exposure showing the fat pad removed and anterior retraction of the esophagus with placement of the crural sutures for closure of the posterior hiatus. (From Luketich J. *Master Techniques in Surgery: Esophageal Surgery.* Philadelphia, PA: Lippincott Williams & Wilkins; 2014. With permission.)

Dissection and Mobilization of the Esophagus and Stomach

A muscle sparing thoracotomy is created at the sixth or seventh intercostal space (Figs. 129.3 and 129.4). A rib cutter may be used to shingle a part of a rib posteriorly for better exposure. Next, the inferior pulmonary ligament is divided with electrocautery and the lung is retracted superiorly, to provide exposure of the esophagus.

A Penrose drain is looped around the esophagus and used to apply gentle traction while a circumferential dissection is performed at the level of the inferior pulmonary vein. The bilateral vagus nerves are identified as well as any hernia sac. If a hernia sac is present, it is dissected from the hiatus circumferentially and then divided to provide entry into the abdomen. The crura are then dissected free. The gastrohepatic omentum is divided and two or three of the highest short gastric vessels may be ligated and divided to fully mobilize the gastric fundus and allow the stomach to be freely delivered into the chest. Three to five sutures are placed in the crura for eventual closure of the enlarged hiatus, but left untied. The fat pad is dissected off the GEJ beginning posterolaterally and just to the left of the posterior vagus nerve. The dissection continues anteriorly with careful mobilization of the anterior vagus nerve and ligation of any small vessels.

Creation of the Wrap

A partial 270-degree wrap is created with three rows of horizontal mattress sutures (Figs. 129.5 to 129.7). The middle horizontal mattress suture of each row must straddle the oversewn gastroplasty staple line. The first row and second row of sutures create the fold and subsequent apposition of the fundus to the esophagus. One row of sutures is placed in the esophagus, the other on the adjacent fundus. The third row of sutures is created by passing the needles of the untied sutures through the hiatus and then back up through the diaphragm,

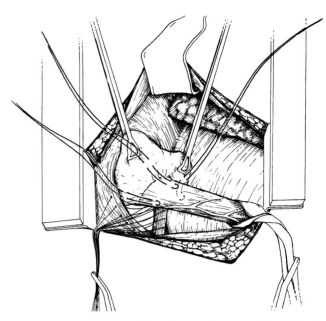

FIGURE 129.5 Construction of a Belsey 240-degree partial fundoplication showing placement of the first row of sutures 1.5 to 2 cm above the gastroesophageal junction. Particular attention must be given to placement of the right lateral suture as detailed in the text. (From Luketich J. *Master Techniques in Surgery: Esophageal Surgery.* Philadelphia, PA: Lippincott Williams & Wilkins; 2014. With permission.)

being careful to maintain the 270-degree spacing of the wrap. These sutures are left untied. The GEJ with its 270-degree fundoplication is then placed in a subdiaphragmatic location and the sutures are tied to maintain this position. The previously placed crural sutures are now tied. The enlarged hiatus is closed but allows enough space for

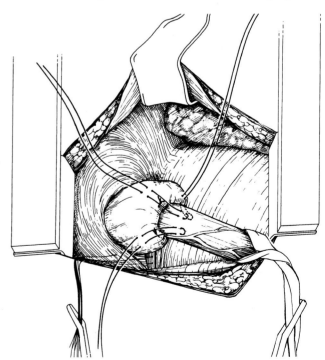

FIGURE 129.6 Continued construction of the Belsey 240-degree partial fundoplication showing placement of the second row of sutures 2 cm above the row of previously tied sutures. (From Luketich J. *Master Techniques in Surgery: Esophageal Surgery.* Philadelphia, PA: Lippincott Williams & Wilkins; 2014. With permission.)

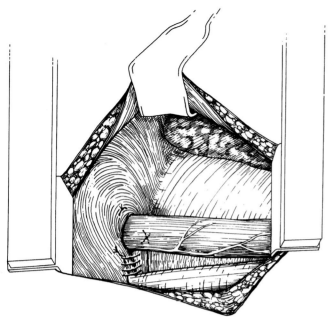

FIGURE 129.7 A completed Belsey 240-degree partial fundoplication showing the right and left crura approximated after tying the previously placed crural sutures. The positions of the tied holding sutures are also shown. (From Luketich J. *Master Techniques in Surgery: Esophageal Surgery*. Lippincott Williams & Wilkins; 2014. With permission.)

a finger to be passed next to the esophagus. A NGT is placed with surgical field guidance, the chest is irrigated, and a chest tube is placed. The lung is re-expanded and the thoracotomy is closed in the standard fashion. The patient is then extubated.

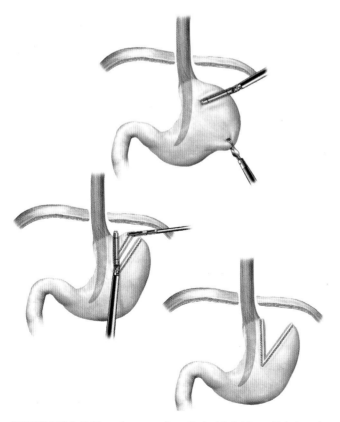

FIGURE 129.8 Collis wedge gastroplasty. (Luketich J. *Master Techniques in Surgery: Esophageal Surgery*. Lippincott Williams & Wilkins; 2014.)

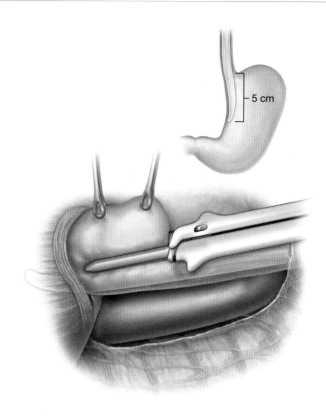

FIGURE 129.9 A Collis type gastroplasty to functionally lengthen the esophagus in preparation for a Collis–Nissen procedure is depicted. It is important to firmly press the stapler and dilator against the lesser curve of the stomach so the diameter of the created gastric tube (the neoesophagus) is not larger than the diameter of the esophagus. (From Luketich J. *Master Techniques in Surgery: Esophageal Surgery*. Lippincott Williams & Wilkins; 2014. With permission.)

COLLIS GASTROPLASTY

A Collis gastroplasty is often performed in the presence of a foreshortened esophagus (Figs. 129.8 and 129.9). The rationale for such an operation is that inadequate abdominal esophageal length has been shown to place undue tension on the wrap, which may lead to higher incidence of wrap failure by slippage, disruption, or herniation.[67] The pathogenesis of short esophagus is multifactorial, stemming from chronic inflammation with eventual fibrosis and contracture of the esophagus as well as from external displacement and eventual deformation from a large hiatal hernia.[68] We perform this procedure if any suspicion of inadequate esophageal length or undue tension remains after the completion of hiatal dissection. There is a higher risk of staple line leak associated with this procedure. As with all antireflux operations, except in very rare circumstances, most of the esophageal lengthening procedures performed by our group are completed in a minimally invasive fashion. Given the requirement for more extensive dissection, the operation should be attempted by more experienced operators. A thorough understanding of thoracic esophageal anatomy is of utmost importance for proper transhiatal mediastinal mobilization, always keeping in mind the anatomic relationship of the esophagus with vital nearby structures, such as the left and right vagus nerves, the aorta and its esophageal branches, the posterior membranous wall of the left main stem bronchus, the azygos vein, the pleura and the pericardium.

Complete mobilization usually adds 3 to 4 cm of distal esophageal length in the majority of patients. The orogastric tube is removed and a size 52-Fr bougie is carefully advanced to the stomach and positioned along the lesser curvature for a distance of about

10 cm. The gastric fundus is grasped extended laterally with two noncrushing instruments, one positioned along the edge of the greater curvature as close to the angle of His as possible and another one a few centimeters more distally. A reticulating Endo-GIA stapler (blue load) is fired three times, removing a wedge-shaped fundic portion close to the cardia. The remaining portion of the fundus is used to perform the appropriate fundoplication (Nissen or Toupet) as described previously.

A Collis gastroplasty is very commonly performed in patients undergoing a Belsey fundoplication, given that severe esophageal foreshortening is one of the main indications for this antireflux operation. A Bougie is carefully passed into the stomach by the anesthesiologist. The fundus is retracted and a stapler is passed between the cardia and the fundus, parallel to the bougie, and fired to create an additional 4 to 5 cm of esophageal length. Any longer of a gastroplasty length is not recommended as this segment of neoesophagus will not have normal esophageal motility. The gastroplasty staple line may be oversewn but not necessarily given the high quality of current stapling devices.

REOPERATION FOR FAILED FUNDOPLICATION

Failed fundoplication with recurrence of reflux symptomatology represents a challenge for both the patient and the surgeon. Reoperation in the upper abdomen can be a daunting task for the inexperienced surgeon, especially considering the added difficulty of hiatal dissection and the higher risk of bleeding and perforation; referral to tertiary centers should be considered when appropriate. If recurrence consists primarily of heartburn well controlled by PPIs, a redo fundoplication can be postponed. If an anatomically correctable source is identified in a patient presenting with dysphagia or regurgitation, an antireflux reoperation can be part of the therapeutic algorithm.[69] Reoperative fundoplications can be successfully completed with minimally invasive techniques reliably in expert hands with good results.[43,70]

Meticulous, systematic adhesiolysis is of utmost importance. The left liver lobe is commonly found firmly adhered to the anterior leaf of the previous wrap and must be separated for proper hiatal exposure. It is acceptable to cut through a liver capsule rather than injure the stomach. The surgeon should frequently reassess the anatomy to be sure that dissection is performed along the correct anatomical plane. When dissecting near the prior fundoplication and esophagus, sharp dissection is preferred to avoid thermal injury to the esophagus. Once the anatomy is clearly established and mobilized, the previous fundoplication must be fully reversed to restore the normal anatomy and facilitate a complete assessment of the root cause of the initial failure. The hiatal opening is repaired in the usual fashion with biological mesh if necessary. Finally, we proceed with securing a new fundoplication.

INTRAOPERATIVE COMPLICATIONS

Intraoperative complications specific for antireflux operations include bleeding due to splenic injury, gastric or esophageal perforation, and pneumothorax. Significant intraoperative bleeding is unusual with proper technique and usually originates from branches of the left gastric or the short gastric arteries. Splenic injury has been reported in up to 8% to 10% of open antireflux procedures but is lower with the minimally invasive approach. Significant bleeding from the left upper quadrant must always prompt evaluation for potential splenic injury, especially in cases where the gastrosplenic ligament is very

short and the spleen is very closely opposed to the gastric fundus. If such injury is suspected, attempts to control the bleeding by direct pressure should be initiated. Hemostatic agents may be used; a splenectomy is rarely required. However, if the bleeding persists and more than 2 units of red cells are transfused or the patient shows signs of hemodynamic instability, one should not hesitate to proceed with splenectomy. This can be completed laparoscopically or may necessitate conversion to an open procedure.

Another operative complication is esophageal or gastric perforation, which has an incidence of 0% to 4% that is influenced by the type of procedure and the experience of the operator. Perforation is higher in redo operations and in patients undergoing transthoracic repair. Meticulous dissection with careful identification of the planes and structures and gentle handling of the tissues is of utmost importance in avoiding such injuries, especially in the case of reoperations. Careful inspection of the esophagus and the stomach upon completion of the fundoplication and prior to closure of the incision(s) may help prevent undiagnosed injuries that lead to delayed identification of leaks. We generally leave a drain in patients undergoing redo procedures to monitor for leaks.

Pneumothorax is an intraoperative complication due to violation of the pleura during hiatal dissection and esophageal mobilization. It occurs in less than 2% of operations. In the abdominal approach, given that the injury is usually localized to the pleura without lung violation, chest tube placement is rarely needed.

When intraoperative complications are encountered, converting from a minimally invasive fundoplication to an open procedure may be warranted. Conversion rates up to 25% have been reported, but this rate is usually less than 5% in the hands of surgeons experienced with thoracoscopy and laparoscopy.

POSTOPERATIVE CARE

After surgery, the patient is maintained on intravenous fluids with strict avoidance of volume overload as this may lead to pulmonary and bowel edema. The head of the bed is kept at an elevation of 20 to 30 degrees and the NGT is placed to low wall suction. The patient is given an intravenous PPI and patient-controlled anesthesia (PCA). A postoperative chest x-ray is ordered to assess for pneumothorax and accurate positioning of the NGT. However, a NGT is not routinely required in uncomplicated cases.

On postoperative day 1, the NGT is removed and the patient is begun on sips of clear liquids. A swallow study may be obtained on postoperative day 1 or 2 to rule out leaks. The patient is subsequently advanced to a clear liquid diet and then to a full liquid diet as tolerated. PCA may be discontinued and the patient placed on oral analgesics. Early ambulation is encouraged.

The patient is discharged on postoperative day 2 or 3 and he/she is maintained on the full liquid diet until their 2-week follow-up appointment. The diet is then advanced as tolerated and the patient is counselled to avoid certain foods such as bread which may lead to impaction at the level of the fundoplication. Consultation with a nutritionist may help the patient learn and adhere to the postsurgery diet.

POSTOPERATIVE COMPLICATIONS

The main postoperative complications include dysphagia, gas-bloat syndrome, increased flatulence, and wrap failure. Mild postoperative dysphagia is reported by up to 80% of patients in the early postoperative period. Transient and mild dysphagia is often due to the localized inflammation and edema at the surgical site and, therefore, is self-limited. As long as patients achieve adequate hydration, they are managed expectantly. Intermittent dysphagia is noted by 10% of patients for up to 2 years postoperatively, whereas only 2% of patients report severe, debilitating symptoms.[71,72] With persistent or worsening dysphagia, other causes such as a slipped or tight wrap or crural closure, impacted food, or undiagnosed esophageal motility disorder must be considered. Postoperative dysphagia may be treated with dilations or a conversion from a Nissen to a partial fundoplication if operative management is warranted. An observation period of at least 12 months is advisable before proceeding with another operation.

Gas-bloat syndrome refers to the inability to belch or vomit, leading to air trapping and postprandial gastric distention with associated discomfort. Creation of a short, floppy fundoplication minimizes the risk of this complication, along with adherence to an appropriate postoperative diet, with avoidance of carbonated beverages and avoidance of aerophagia. In the majority of cases, this is also a self-limiting complication, but in long-standing debilitating cases conversion to a partial wrap may be required. Prior to undertaking reoperative surgery for bloating, however, one must investigate the presence of confounding factors. Undiagnosed gastroparesis may have been present preoperatively or may have occurred as a consequence of intraoperative vagal injury. A gastric emptying study should be obtained. In such cases, a pyloroplasty, either alone or as a component of the reoperative surgery, may be warranted.

The aforementioned complications are pertinent to both open and minimally invasive operations, but the incisional hernia is more likely to occur after the open approach. Open surgery is complicated by the development of incisional hernias in up to 26% of patients[40,46] compared to a 1% to 4% probability of a port incision hernia.[40,46,73]

OUTCOMES

The learning curve for each procedure varies and it is estimated that at least 15 to 30 thoracoscopic/laparoscopic antireflux operations should be performed under supervision by an experienced surgeon prior to attempting to perform one independently. Mortality has been reported to be as low as 0% to 1% in large series and serious morbidity ranges between 2% and 10%.[40,46]

Open Nissen fundoplication has achieved 90% success in controlling reflux symptoms at 10 years.[74] Open Belsey-Mark IV fundoplication has also achieved a high success rate of 85% to 95% symptom control at 5 years[75] and other fundoplication operations have demonstrated similar rates of reflux relief. In more recent years, minimally invasive approaches to these procedures have produced results comparable to their open counterparts.[38,76,77] There is no definitive evidence that the minimally invasive approach is technically superior to the open approach, but because of potential advantages such as shortened length of hospital stay and decreased postoperative pain, minimally invasive antireflux procedures are the preferred approach.

After fundoplication, patients have reported significantly improved or normalized quality of life, including elimination of symptoms.[78] The success of the fundoplication depends on adequate calibration around the bougie of the tightness of the wrap (if it is a complete 360-degree wrap), with a tendency toward a looser wrap to avoid dysphagia while maintaining reflux control. However, recurrence can occur early or late in the postoperative course.

The main reasons for recurrence are improper preoperative work-up, wrong operative indications, and improper execution of the operative steps.[69] Of the 10% to 20% of fundoplication patients

in whom reflux will recur, a minority will require a second antireflux procedure. Failure of the fundoplication is often related to reherniation through the esophageal hiatus or a "slipped" fundoplication. One of the most common reasons for wrap reherniation is the presence of an unrecognized shortened esophagus, which is present in 20% to 40% of reoperations.[67,79] Suspicion must be high in patients with new onset of substernal or epigastric pain. "Slipped" fundoplication is often due to unrecognized misplacement of the wrap over the gastric cardia instead of around the true GEJ[67] and is commonly due to surgeon inexperience or lack of adherence to proper surgical technique. Both conditions require reoperation, after careful preoperative evaluation.

The success rate with secondary procedures is decreased at 70% to 85% and even lower in the percentage that require tertiary operations.[70,80] A majority of GERD recurrences can be managed with antireflux medications and those that warrant a second operation may be approached via a minimally invasive method regardless of the approach used in the primary operation.

REFERENCES

1. El-Serag HB, Sweet S, Winchester CC, et al. Update on the epidemiology of gastro-oesophageal reflux disease: a systematic review. *Gut* 2014;63(6):871–880.
2. Kahrilas PJ, Shaheen NJ, Vaezi MF. American Gastroenterological Association Medical Position Statement on the management of gastroesophageal reflux disease. *Gastroenterology* 2008;135(4):1383–1391.
3. Mittal RK, McCallum RW. Characteristics and frequency of transient relaxations of the lower esophageal sphincter in patients with reflux esophagitis. *Gastroenterology* 1988;95(3):593–599.
4. Kahrilas PJ. GERD pathogenesis, pathophysiology, and clinical manifestations. *Cleve Clin J Med* 2003;70(suppl 5):S4–S19.
5. Malfertheiner P, Nocon M, Vieth M, et al. Evolution of gastro-oesophageal reflux disease over 5 years under routine medical care–the ProGERD study. *Aliment Pharmacol Ther* 2012;35(1):154–164.
6. Campos GM, Peters JH, DeMeester TR, et al. Multivariate analysis of factors predicting outcome after laparoscopic Nissen fundoplication. *J Gastrointest Surg* 1999;3(3):292–300.
7. Davis CS, Baldea A, Johns JR, et al. The evolution and long-term results of laparoscopic antireflux surgery for the treatment of gastroesophageal reflux disease. *JSLS* 2010;14(3):332–341.
8. Yau P, Watson DI, Devitt PG, et al. Laparoscopic antireflux surgery in the treatment of gastroesophageal reflux in patients with Barrett esophagus. *Arch Surg* 2000;135(7):801–805.
9. Chang EY, Morris CD, Seltman AK, et al. The effect of antireflux surgery on esophageal carcinogenesis in patients with barrett esophagus: a systematic review. *Ann Surg* 2007;246(1):11–21.
10. Wassenaar EB, Oelschlager BK. Effect of medical and surgical treatment of Barrett's metaplasia. *World J Gastroenterol* 2010;16(30):3773–3779.
11. Bennett C, Moayyedi P, Corley DA, et al. BOB CAT: A large-scale review and delphi consensus for management of Barrett's esophagus with no dysplasia, indefinite for, or low-grade dysplasia. *Am J Gastroenterol* 2015;110(5):662–682; quiz 683.
12. DeMeester SR. Barrett's oesophagus: treatment with surgery. *Best Pract Res Clin Gastroenterol* 2015;29(1):211–217.
13. Stefanidis D, Hope WW, Kohn GP, et al. Guidelines for surgical treatment of gastroesophageal reflux disease. *Surg Endosc* 2010;24(11):2647–2669. http://www.sages.org/publications/guidelines/guidelines-for-surgical-treatment-of-gastroesophageal-reflux-disease-gerd/
14. Dunn SP, Steinhubl SR, Bauer D, et al. Impact of proton pump inhibitor therapy on the efficacy of clopidogrel in the CAPRIE and CREDO trials. *J Am Heart Assoc* 2013;2(1):e004564.
15. Cardoso RN, Benjo AM, DiNicolantonio JJ, et al. Incidence of cardiovascular events and gastrointestinal bleeding in patients receiving clopidogrel with and without proton pump inhibitors: an updated meta-analysis. *Open Heart* 2015;2(1):e000248.
16. Patterson EJ, Davis DG, Khajanchee Y, et al. Comparison of objective outcomes following laparoscopic Nissen fundoplication versus laparoscopic gastric bypass in the morbidly obese with heartburn. *Surg Endosc* 2003;17(10):1561–1565.
17. Bresadola V, Dado G, Favero A, et al. Surgical therapy for patients with extraesophageal symptoms of gastroesophageal reflux disease. *Minerva Chir* 2006;61(1):9–15.
18. Kaufman JA, Houghland JE, Quiroga E, et al. Long-term outcomes of laparoscopic antireflux surgery for gastroesophageal reflux disease (GERD)-related airway disorder. *Surg Endosc* 2006;20(12):1824–1830.
19. Worrell SG, DeMeester SR, Greene CL, et al. Pharyngeal pH monitoring better predicts a successful outcome for extraesophageal reflux symptoms after antireflux surgery. *Surg Endosc* 2013;27(11):4113–4118.
20. Jobe BA, Richter JE, Hoppo T, et al. Preoperative diagnostic workup before antireflux surgery: an evidence and experience-based consensus of the Esophageal Diagnostic Advisory Panel. *J Am Coll Surg* 2013;217(4):586–597.

21. Kahrilas PJ, Dodds WJ, Hogan WJ, et al. Esophageal peristaltic dysfunction in peptic esophagitis. *Gastroenterology* 1986;91(4):897–904.
22. Johnson LF, Demeester TR. Twenty-four-hour pH monitoring of the distal esophagus. A quantitative measure of gastroesophageal reflux. *Am J Gastroenterol* 1974;62(4):325–332.
23. Ayazi S, Hagen JA, Zehetner J, et al. The value of high-resolution manometry in the assessment of the resting characteristics of the lower esophageal sphincter. *J Gastrointest Surg* 2009;13(12):2113–2120.
24. Fuchs KH, DeMeester TR, Albertucci M. Specificity and sensitivity of objective diagnosis of gastroesophageal reflux disease. *Surgery* 1987;102(4):575–580.
25. Tseng D, Rizvi AZ, Fennerty MB, et al. Forty-eight-hour pH monitoring increases sensitivity in detecting abnormal esophageal acid exposure. *J Gastrointest Surg* 2005;9(8):1043–1051.
26. Laine S, Rantala A, Gullichsen R, et al. Laparoscopic vs conventional Nissen fundoplication. A prospective randomized study. *Surg Endosc* 1997;11(5):441–444.
27. Bais JE, Bartelsman JF, Bonjer HJ, et al. Laparoscopic or conventional Nissen fundoplication for gastro-oesophageal reflux disease: randomised clinical trial. The Netherlands Antireflux Surgery Study Group. *Lancet* 2000;355(9199):170–174.
28. Heikkinen TJ, Haukipuro K, Bringman S, et al. Comparison of laparoscopic and open Nissen fundoplication 2 years after operation. A prospective randomized trial. *Surg Endosc* 2000;14(11):1019–1023.
29. Nilsson G, Larsson S, Johnsson F. Randomized clinical trial of laparoscopic versus open fundoplication: blind evaluation of recovery and discharge period. *Br J Surg* 2000;87(7):873–878.
30. Luostarinen M, Virtanen J, Koskinen M, et al. Dysphagia and oesophageal clearance after laparoscopic versus open Nissen fundoplication. A randomized, prospective trial. *Scand J Gastroenterol* 2001;36(6):565–571.
31. Wenner J, Nilsson G, Öberg S, et al. Short-term outcome after laparoscopic and open 360 degrees fundoplication. A prospective randomized trial. *Surg Endosc* 2001;15(10):1124–1128.
32. Chrysos E, Tsiaoussis J, Athanasakis E, et al. Laparoscopic vs open approach for Nissen fundoplication. A comparative study. *Surg Endosc* 2002;16(12):1679–1684.
33. Ackroyd R, Watson DI, Majeed AW, et al. Randomized clinical trial of laparoscopic versus open fundoplication for gastro-oesophageal reflux disease. *Br J Surg* 2004;91(8):975–982.
34. Catarci M, Gentileschi P, Papi C, et al. Evidence-based appraisal of antireflux fundoplication. *Ann Surg* 2004;239(3):325–337.
35. Nilsson G, Wenner J, Larsson S, et al. Randomized clinical trial of laparoscopic versus open fundoplication for gastro-oesophageal reflux. *Br J Surg* 2004;91(5):552–559.
36. Franzen T, Anderberg B, Wirén M, et al. Long-term outcome is worse after laparoscopic than after conventional Nissen fundoplication. *Scand J Gastroenterol* 2005;40(11):1261–1268.
37. McHoney M, Eaton S, Wade A, et al. Inflammatory response in children after laparoscopic vs open Nissen fundoplication: randomized controlled trial. *J Pediatr Surg* 2005;40(6):908–913.
38. Draaisma WA, Rijnhart-de Jong HG, Broeders IA, et al. Five-year subjective and objective results of laparoscopic and conventional Nissen fundoplication: a randomized trial. *Ann Surg* 2006;244(1):34–41.
39. Hakanson BS, Thor KA, Thorell A, et al. Open vs laparoscopic partial posterior fundoplication. A prospective randomized trial. *Surg Endosc* 2007;21(2):289–298.
40. Salminen PT, Hiekkanen HI, Rantala AP, et al. Comparison of long-term outcome of laparoscopic and conventional nissen fundoplication: a prospective randomized study with an 11-year follow-up. *Ann Surg* 2007;246(2):201–206.
41. Broeders JA, Rijnhart-de Jong HG, Draaisma WA, et al. Ten-year outcome of laparoscopic and conventional Nissen fundoplication: randomized clinical trial. *Ann Surg* 2009;250(5):698–706.
42. Peters MJ, Mukhtar A, Yunus RM, et al. Meta-analysis of randomized clinical trials comparing open and laparoscopic anti-reflux surgery. *Am J Gastroenterol* 2009;104(6):1548–1561.
43. Wakeam E, Wee J, Lebenthal A, et al. Does BMI predict recurrence or complications after reoperative reflux surgery? Review of a single center's experience and a comparison of outcomes. *J Gastrointest Surg* 2014;18(11):1965–1973.
44. Cadiere GB, Himpens J, Vertruyen M, et al. Evaluation of telesurgical (robotic) NISSEN fundoplication. *Surg Endosc* 2001;15(9):918–923.
45. Morino M, Pellegrino L, Giaccone C, et al. Randomized clinical trial of robot-assisted versus laparoscopic Nissen fundoplication. *Br J Surg* 2006;93(5):553–558.
46. Qu H, Liu Y, He QS. Short- and long-term results of laparoscopic versus open anti-reflux surgery: a systematic review and meta-analysis of randomized controlled trials. *J Gastrointest Surg* 2014;18(6):1077–1086.
47. Thor KB, Silander T. A long-term randomized prospective trial of the Nissen procedure versus a modified Toupet technique. *Ann Surg* 1989;210(6):719–724.
48. Lundell L, Abrahamsson H, Ruth M, et al. Lower esophageal sphincter characteristics and esophageal acid exposure following partial or 360 degrees fundoplication: results of a prospective, randomized, clinical study. *World J Surg* 1991;15(1):115–120.
49. Lundell L, Abrahamsson H, Ruth M, et al. Long-term results of a prospective randomized comparison of total fundic wrap (Nissen-Rossetti) or semifundoplication (Toupet) for gastro-oesophageal reflux. *Br J Surg* 1996;83(6):830–835.
50. Jobe BA, Wallace J, Hansen PD, et al. Evaluation of laparoscopic Toupet fundoplication as a primary repair for all patients with medically resistant gastroesophageal reflux. *Surg Endosc* 1997;11(11):1080–1083.
51. Laws HL, Clements RH, Swillie CM. A randomized, prospective comparison of the Nissen fundoplication versus the Toupet fundoplication for gastroesophageal reflux disease. *Ann Surg* 1997;225(6):647–653.
52. Hagedorn C, Lonroth H, Rydberg L, et al. Long-term efficacy of total (Nissen-Rossetti) and posterior partial (Toupet) fundoplication: results of a randomized clinical trial. *J Gastrointest Surg* 2002;6(4):540–545.
53. Zornig C, Strate U, Fibbe C, et al. Nissen vs Toupet laparoscopic fundoplication. *Surg Endosc* 2002;16(5):758–766.
54. Chrysos E, Tsiaoussis J, Zoras OJ, et al. Laparoscopic surgery for gastroesophageal reflux disease patients with impaired esophageal peristalsis: total or partial fundoplication? *J Am Coll Surg* 2003;197(1):8–15.
55. Patti MG, Robinson T, Galvani C, et al. Total fundoplication is superior to partial fundoplication even when esophageal peristalsis is weak. *J Am Coll Surg* 2004;198(6):863–869.
56. Nakadi IE, Melot C, Closset J, et al. Evaluation of da Vinci Nissen fundoplication clinical results and cost minimization. *World J Surg* 2006;30(6):1050–1054.
57. Guerin E, Betroune K, Closset J, et al. Nissen versus Toupet fundoplication: results of a randomized and multicenter trial. *Surg Endosc* 2007;21(11):1985–1990.
58. Booth MI, Stratford J, Jones L, et al. Randomized clinical trial of laparoscopic total (Nissen) versus posterior partial (Toupet) fundoplication for gastro-oesophageal reflux disease based on preoperative oesophageal manometry. *Br J Surg* 2008;95(1):57–63.
59. Mickevicius A, Endzinas Z, Kiudelis M, et al. Influence of wrap length on the effectiveness of Nissen and Toupet fundoplication: a prospective randomized study. *Surg Endosc* 2008;22(10):2269–2276.
60. Strate U, Emmermann A, Fibbe C, et al. Laparoscopic fundoplication: Nissen versus Toupet two-year outcome of a prospective randomized study of 200 patients regarding preoperative esophageal motility. *Surg Endosc* 2008;22(1):21–30.
61. Shaw JM, Bornman PC, Callanan MD, et al. Long-term outcome of laparoscopic Nissen and laparoscopic Toupet fundoplication for gastroesophageal reflux disease: a prospective, randomized trial. *Surg Endosc* 2010;24(4):924–932.
62. DeMeester TR, Peters JH, Bremner CG, et al. Biology of gastroesophageal reflux disease: pathophysiology relating to medical and surgical treatment. *Annu Rev Med* 1999;50:469–506.
63. Dunnington GL, DeMeester TR. Outcome effect of adherence to operative principles of Nissen fundoplication by multiple surgeons. The Department of Veterans Affairs Gastroesophageal Reflux Disease Study Group. *Am J Surg* 1993;166(6):654–657.
64. Patti MG, Arcerito M, Feo CV, et al. An analysis of operations for gastroesophageal reflux disease: identifying the important technical elements. *Arch Surg* 1998;133(6):600–606; discussion 606–607.
65. Stylopoulos N, Rattner DW. The history of hiatal hernia surgery: from Bowditch to laparoscopy. *Ann Surg* 2005;241(1):185–193.
66. Pearson FG, Henderson RD. Long-term follow-up of peptic strictures managed by dilatation, modified Collis gastroplasty, and Belsey hiatus hernia repair. *Surgery* 1976;80(3):396–404.
67. Awais O, Luketich JD, Schuchert MJ, et al. Reoperative antireflux surgery for failed fundoplication: an analysis of outcomes in 275 patients. *Ann Thorac Surg* 2011;92(3):1083–1089.
68. Terry M, Smith CD, Branum GD, et al. Outcomes of laparoscopic fundoplication for gastroesophageal reflux disease and paraesophageal hernia. *Surg Endosc* 2001;15(7):691–699.
69. Patti MG, Allaix ME, Fisichella PM. Analysis of the Causes of Failed Antireflux Surgery and the Principles of Treatment: A Review. *JAMA Surg* 2015;150(6):585–590.
70. Makdisi G, Nichols FC, 3rd, Cassivi SD, et al. Laparoscopic repair for failed antireflux procedures. *Ann Thorac Surg* 2014;98(4):1261–1266.
71. Hunter JG, Swanstrom L, Waring JP. Dysphagia after laparoscopic antireflux surgery. The impact of operative technique. *Ann Surg* 1996;224(1):51–57.
72. Peters JH, DeMeester TR, Crookes P, et al. The treatment of gastroesophageal reflux disease with laparoscopic Nissen fundoplication: prospective evaluation of 100 patients with "typical" symptoms. *Ann Surg* 1998;228(1):40–50.
73. O'Boyle CJ, Watson DI, Jamieson GG, et al. Division of short gastric vessels at laparoscopic nissen fundoplication: a prospective double-blind randomized trial with 5-year follow-up. *Ann Surg* 2002;235(2):165–170.
74. DeMeester TR, Bonavina L, Albertucci M, et al. Nissen fundoplication for gastroesophageal reflux disease. Evaluation of primary repair in 100 consecutive patients. *Ann Surg* 1986;204(1):9–20.
75. Skinner DB, Belsey RH. Surgical management of esophageal reflux and hiatus hernia. Long-term results with 1,030 patients. *J Thorac Cardiovasc Surg* 1967;53(1):33–54.
76. McKernan JB, Champion JK. Minimally invasive antireflux surgery. *Am J Surg* 1998;175(4):271–276.
77. Salminen P, Hurme S, Ovaska J. Fifteen-year outcome of laparoscopic and open Nissen fundoplication: a randomized clinical trial. *Ann Thorac Surg* 2012;93(1):228–233.
78. Barrat C, Capelluto E, Catheline JM, et al. Quality of life 2 years after laparoscopic total fundoplication: a prospective study. *Surg Laparosc Endosc Percutan Tech* 2001;11(6):347–350.
79. Horvath KD, Swanstrom LL, Jobe BA. The short esophagus: pathophysiology, incidence, presentation, and treatment in the era of laparoscopic antireflux surgery. *Ann Surg* 2000;232(5):630–640.
80. Khajanchee YS, O'Rourke R, Cassera MA, et al. Laparoscopic reintervention for failed antireflux surgery: subjective and objective outcomes in 176 consecutive patients. *Arch Surg* 2007;142(8):785–901.

130

Techniques of Esophagectomy

Toni Lerut

Milestones in Surgery for Esophageal Carcinoma

1913—F. Torek: first successful transthoracic resection of the esophagus[1]

1913—W. Denk: cadaver and experimental animal studies on the transhiatal resection of the esophagus[2]

1933—T. Ohsawa: first report on transthoracic esophageal resection and esophagogastrostomy[3]

1933—G. Turner: first transhiatal resection[4]

1938—W. Adams and D. Phemister: first single-stage transthoracic resection and reconstruction in the United States[5]

1946—I. Lewis: esophageal resection and esophagogastrostomy via a right thoracotomy and laparotomy[6]

1976—K. McKeown: description of three-hole esophagectomy[7]

1978—M. Orringer: popularizes transhiatal esophagectomy in the Western hemisphere[8]

1992—A. Cushieri: first report on thoracoscopic esophagectomy[9]

2003—J. Luketich: popularizes total thoracoscopic and laparoscopic esophagectomy[10]

In 1913 Franz Torek[1] published a report on the first successful transthoracic resection of the esophagus. Reconstruction was not attempted and the patient received enteral nutrition via a rubber tube connecting the proximal esophagostomy with a gastrostomy; she lived for 13 years after her resection.

Other attempts were made in the following years, but most failed due to lack of appropriate technology to adequately ventilate the lungs during surgery. Only after the introduction of safe orotracheal intubation in the late 1920s, by Rowbotham[11] and Magill,[12] could surgeons safely undertake such complex operations as transthoracic esophagectomy. Over the following decades, pioneers such as Ohsawa,[3] Grey Turner,[4] Adam and Phemister,[5] Sweet,[13] Ivor Lewis,[6] McKeown,[7] and Belsey[14] further developed and refined the surgical techniques that we continue to use today. However, postoperative mortality remained high well past 1970. Better insight regarding medical operability and improved perioperative management hallmarked the 1980s and 1990s, and operative mortality was successfully decreased to less than 5%,[15] with current figures around 1% to 2% in many centers of excellence.

Better selection of oncologic operability through the introduction of CT scan, PET scan, and echo-endoscopy has resulted in a marked decrease of futile exploratory thoracotomies. Improved surgical techniques in conjunction with the advent of induction therapy helped increase R0 resection rates in locally advanced (T3) carcinoma, reaching >90% in many published series.

As a result of these advances, long-term survival has significantly improved over the last several decades, reaching an overall 5-year survival today of approximately 35% to 45%.[16]

Although high-grade dysplasia and T1a carcinoma are frequently treated with nonsurgical approaches, that is, EMR (endoscopic mucosal resection),[17] and particularly for squamous cell carcinoma, definitive chemoradiotherapy,[18] surgery remains the cornerstone of curative therapy for cancer of the esophagus and gastroesophageal junction (GEJ).

PRINCIPLES OF SURGERY

Surgery for esophageal carcinoma and carcinoma of the GEJ is considered to be one of the most complex interventions performed on the digestive tract. Indeed, the complexity of surgical resection is heightened by the intimate anatomic relationship of the esophagus with the trachea, the mainstem bronchi, and, more distally, the pericardium, aorta, and diaphragm. A malignancy arising from the esophagus may easily invade any of these adjacent critical structures, thus rendering the cancer unresectable. Additionally, lymphatic dissemination occurs early and negatively impacts overall survival. Lymph node metastases are found in less than 5% of intramucosal tumors, but are present in 30% to 40% of submucosal tumors, and over 80% of transmural tumors.[19] Furthermore, the number of involved nodes increases with tumor volume.[20] The esophageal wall is characterized by an extensive submucosal lymphatic plexus, which allows early dissemination and gives rise to "skip" metastases (i.e., lymph nodes adjacent to the primary tumor are not affected, but more distant lymph nodes contain metastases).[21]

Macroscopic, as well as microscopic, complete resection (R0) is the ultimate goal of esophagectomy for cancer. As a result, optimal preoperative staging and individual case presentation and discussion at the multidisciplinary tumor board are of paramount importance. In cases of suspicious lymph nodes (cN+) and/or transmural tumor extension (cT3-4), a multimodality treatment plan including induction chemo ± radiotherapy is commonly used in most centers today.

Although the pattern of lymphatic dissemination is often difficult to reliably predict, carcinomas of the proximal and middle thirds of the esophagus tend to metastasize to the cervical region, and more distal tumors and those of the GEJ tend to metastasize to the lymph nodes around the celiac trunk. Positive nodal disease is not necessarily a contraindication for surgery if the metastatic lymph nodes are deemed resectable and within the region of the primary tumor. These may include lymph nodes near the celiac trunk for tumors in the distal third of the esophagus or cervical lymph nodes for tumors in the middle or proximal portions of the esophagus.

Resection is ill-advised when a macroscopically incomplete resection is expected, typically due to invasion of adjacent structures and/or non-resectable metastases. Absolute contraindications for esophagectomy include local tumor invasion of non-resectable neighboring structures (T4), carcinomatosis peritonei, hematogenous metastases involving solid organs, or non-resectable metastatic lymph nodes.

Given the challenges of achieving complete tumor resection (R0) and the early and sometimes unpredictable pattern of lymphatic dissemination, the optimal operative approach and the extent of surgery remain a matter of debate.

EXTENT OF OPERATION

Radical En Bloc Resection

The concept of extensive en bloc resection was reported in 1963,[22] but its associated mortality of more than 20% discouraged general acceptance. Skinner[23] and Akiyama[24] reintroduced the concept of en bloc resection combined with extensive lymphadenectomy. Ultimately, they were able to reduce operative mortality to 5%, with 5-year survival rates of 18% and 42%, respectively. The radical en bloc resection, as opposed to the standard resections, aims at performing a wide as possible peritumoral with an en bloc lymph node resection of the middle and distal thirds of the posterior mediastinum.[23]

Two-Field Lymph Node Dissection

The early lymphatic dissemination of tumor to the upper mediastinum and abdomen via the submucosal plexus was the reason Japanese researchers developed a meticulous two-field lymphadenectomy. This incorporates a wide local excision of the primary tumor as well as a lymphadenectomy of the entire posterior mediastinum, including the subcarinal nodes and nodes along the left recurrent nerve and brachiocephalic trunk. In the abdomen it includes the lymph nodes along the celiac trunk, common hepatic and splenic arteries, as well as the lesser gastric curvature and lesser omentum.[24]

Three-Field Lymph Node Dissection

About 20% of patients with a distal esophageal tumor present with metastasis in the cervical region.[25] This finding led to development of the three-field lymph node dissection. In addition to the aforementioned removal of the thoracic and abdominal nodes, the cervical lymph nodes are also dissected out in this operation. Typically this includes the paraesophageal nodes, the nodes lateral to the carotid vessels, and the supraclavicular nodes.

OPERATIVE APPROACHES

Transthoracic

Esophageal tumors situated in the proximal and middle thirds of the intrathoracic esophagus are typically approached via the right thoracic cavity. In contrast, for distal tumors and tumors of the GEJ, a left-sided approach provides optimal exposure. Double-lumen endotracheal intubation with intra-operative deflation of the lung at the operative side facilitates dissection in the posterior mediastinum. The most common transthoracic approaches are the Ivor Lewis (two hole)[6] and McKeown (three hole)[7] which are right-sided approaches that involve a right thoracotomy in combination with a laparotomy, as well as a left-sided approach via left thoracophrenolaparotomy in conjunction with a cervical incision, as described by Sweet[13] and Belsey.[14]

Transhiatal

The first transhiatal esophageal resection was performed by Grey Turner in 1933.[4] It was reintroduced by Akiyama[26] in Japan in the 1970s and was mainly used in the surgical treatment of hypopharyngeal carcinoma. Orringer[8] introduced this approach in the Western hemisphere for surgical management of cancers of the thoracic esophagus and GEJ in an effort to reduce postoperative mortality, which was still generally above 10% at the time.

Minimally Invasive Esophagectomy

In an effort to limit the physiologic stress of esophagectomy while preserving the principle of en bloc resection, a minimally invasive approach to esophageal resection has evolved in the last 20 to 30 years. The credit for the first thoracoscopic resection goes to Cushieri in 1992[9] with Luketich[10] later popularizing the total thoracoscopic laparoscopic esophagectomy. The most frequent indications for MIE are Barrett's high-grade dysplasia or small tumors (T1a or T1b without suspicious nodes),[27] although technical advances are expanding MIE into treatment of more advanced cancers as well.[28] In recent years there has also been increasing interest in performing esophagectomy via a robotic approach.[29]

AREAS OF CONTROVERSY

Over the years, controversy has persisted over the degree of resection and extent of lymphadenectomy. Those who believe that lymph node involvement equates to systemic disease often advocate for a simple resection and reconstruction typically through a transhiatal approach.[8] Others believe that the natural course of the disease may be influenced in a positive way by radical esophagectomy and extensive (two- or three-field) lymphadenectomy, typically performed through a transthoracic approach.[23] Hulscher et al.[30] published a randomized trial comparing outcomes following a limited transhiatal resection versus transthoracic resection with extended en bloc lymph node dissection for adenocarcinoma of the esophagus and GEJ. Although there was no statistically significant difference overall, there was a clear long-term trend favoring the more extensive resection, particularly for adenocarcinoma of the distal esophagus.[31]

An equally debatable topic in this field pertains to what constitutes the minimum number of lymph nodes to remove to achieve an adequate lymphadenectomy. There are also no prospective randomized trials to answer this question. It has been suggested that 23 nodes is the optimal number of nodes to be removed,[32] whereas the World Wide Esophageal Cancer Collaboration (WECC) has suggested 10 nodes for T1 cancers, 20 nodes for T2, and 30 nodes for T3 tumors.[33] With respect to considering the third field (cervical lymphadectomy), the Japanese data[34] suggest that it may offer a survival advantage, particularly for patients with supra-carinal tumors. The Japanese data are supported by a recent meta-analysis by Ye.[35] Altorki[36] reported a 5-year survival of 40% in squamous cell carcinoma, and Lerut[25] reported a 5-year survival of 28%, after three-field lymphadenectomy in patients with middle third squamous cell carcinoma and positive cervical lymph nodes.

Perhaps even more important is the influence of hospital volume. An increasing number of publications suggest a potential benefit associated with centralization of esophagectomies to high-volume centers.[37]

In this chapter several acknowledged expert surgeons describe in detail the various surgical approaches to esophagectomy, reflecting on their personal insights and practices in the surgical treatment of cancer of the esophagus and GEJ.

REFERENCES

1. Torek F. The first successful case of resection of the thoracic portion of the esophagus for carcinoma. *Surg Gynecol Obstet* 1913;16:614–617.
2. Denk W. Zur Radikaloperation des Oesophaguskarzinoms (vorläufige Mittelung). *Zentralbl Chir* 1913;40:1065–1068.
3. Ohsawa T. Esophageal surgery (in Japanese). *Nippon Geka Gakkai Zasshi* 1933;34:1318–1590.
4. Turner GG. Excision of the thoracic oesophagus for carcinoma with reconstruction of an extrathoracic gullet. *Lancet* 1933;ii:315–316.
5. Adams W, Phemister DB. Carcinoma of the lower thoracic esophagus. Report of a successful resection and esophago-gastrostomy. *J Thorac Surg* 1938;7:621–627.
6. Lewis I. The surgical treatment of carcinoma of the oesophagus with special reference to a new operation for growths of the middle third. *Br J Surg* 1946;34(133):18–31.
7. Mc Keown KC. Total three-stage esophagectomy for cancer of the esophagus. *Br J Surg* 1976;63(4):259–262.
8. Orringer MB. Esophagectomy without thoracotomy. *J Thorac Cardiovasc Surg* 1978;76(5):643–654.
9. Cushieri A. Endoscopic oesophagectomy through a right thoracoscopic approach. *J R Coll Edinb* 1992;37(1):7–11.
10. Luketich JD, Alvelo-Rivera M, Buenaventura PO, et al. Minimally invasive esophagectomy: outcomes in 222 patients. *Ann Surg* 2003;238(4):486–494.
11. Rowbotham S. Laryngeal intubation in anaesthetics. *Br Med J* 1923;1(3261):1090–1091.
12. Magill W. Endotracheal anesthesia. *Proc R Soc Med* 1928;22(2):83–88.
13. Sweet RH. Carcinoma of the esophagus and cardiac end of the stomach: immediate and late results of treatment by resection of primary esophagogastric anastomosis *JAMA* 1947;135:485–490.
14. Belsey RH. Surgical exposure of the esophagus. In: Skinner DBJ, Belsey RH, eds. *Management of Esophageal Disorders*. Philadelphia, London, Toronto, Montreal, Sydney, Tokyo: WB Saunders Company; 1988:192–201, 757.
15. Jamieson GG, Mathew G, Ludemann R, et al. Postoperative mortality following oesophagectomy and problems in reporting its rate. *Br J Surg* 2004;91(8):943–947.
16. Lerut T, Moons J, Coosemans W, et al. Multidisciplinary treatment of advanced cancer of the esophagus and gastroesophageal junction: a European center's approach. *Surg Oncol Clin N Am* 2008;17:485–502, vii–viii.
17. Pouw RE, Wirths K, Eisendrath P, et al. Efficacy of radiofrequency ablation combined with endoscopic resection for Barrett's esophagus with early neoplasia. *Clin Gastroenterol Hepatol* 2010;8(1):23–29.
18. Stahl M, Stuschke M, Lehmann N, et al. Chemoradiation with and without surgery in patients with locally advanced squamous cell carcinoma of the esophagus. *J Clin Oncol* 2005;23(10):2310–2317.
19. Clark GW, Peters JH, Ireland AP, et al. Nodal metastasis and sites of recurrence after en bloc esophagectomy for adenocarcinoma. *Ann Thorac Surg* 1994;58:646–654.
20. Akiyama H, Tsurumaru M, Kawamura T, et al. Principles of surgical treatment for carcinoma of the esophagus: analysis of lymph node involvement. *Ann Surg* 1981;194:438–446.
21. Nishimaki T, Suzuki T, Kanda T, et al. Extended radical esophagectomy for superficially invasive carcinoma of the esophagus. *Surgery* 1999;125(2):142–147.
22. Logan A. The surgical treatment of carcinoma of the esophagus and cardia. *J Thorac Cardiovasc Surg* 1963;46:150–161.
23. Skinner DB. En bloc resection for neoplasms of the esophagus and cardia. *J Thorac Cardiovasc Surg* 1983;65:59–71.
24. Akiyama H, Tsurumaru M, Udagawa H, et al. Radical lymph node dissection for cancer of the thoracic esophagus. *Ann Surg* 1994;220:364–373.
25. Lerut T, Nafteux P, Moons J, et al. Three-field lymphadenectomy for carcinoma of the esophagus and gastroesophageal junction in 174 R0 resections: impact on staging, disease-free survival, and outcome: a plea for adaptation of TNM classification in upper-half esophageal carcinoma. *Ann Surg* 2004;240(6):962–972.
26. Akiyama H, Hiyama M, Miyazono H. Total esophageal reconstruction after extraction of the esophagus. *Ann Surg* 1975;182(5):547–552.
27. Nafteux P, Moons J, Coosemans W, et al. Minimally invasive oesophagectomy: a valuable alternative to open oesophagectomy for the treatment of early oesophageal and gastro-oesophageal junction carcinoma. *Eur J Cardiothorac Surg* 2011;40(6):1455–1463.
28. Luketich JD, Pennathur A, Awais O, et al. Outcomes after minimally invasive esophagectomy: review of over 1000 patients. *Ann Surg* 2012;256(1):95–103.
29. Weksler B, Sharma P, Moudgill N, et al. Robot-assisted minimally invasive esophagectomy is equivalent to thoracoscopic minimally invasive esophagectomy. *Dis Esophagus* 2012;25(5):403–409.
30. Hulscher JB, van Sandlick JW, de Boer AG, et al. Extended transthoracic resection compared with limited transhiatal resection for adenocarcinoma of the esophagus. *N Engl J Med* 2002;347(21):1662–1669.
31. Omloo JM, Lagarde SM, Hulscher JB, et al. Extended transthoracic resection compared with limited transhiatal resection for adenocarcinoma of the mid/distal esophagus: five-year survival of a randomized clinical trial. *Ann Surg* 2007;246(6):992–1000; discussion 1000–1001.
32. Peyre CG, Hagen JA, DeMeester SR, et al. The number of lymph nodes removed predicts survival in esophageal cancer: an international study on the impact of extent of surgical resection. *Ann Surg* 2008;248(4):549–556.
33. Rizk NP, Ishwaran H, Rice TW, et al. Optimum lymphadenectomy for esophageal cancer. *Ann Surg* 2010;251(1):46–50.
34. Kato H, Watanabe H, Tachimori Y, et al. Evaluation of neck lymph node dissection for thoracic esophageal carcinoma. *Ann Thorac Surg* 1991;51:931–935.
35. Ye T, Sun Y, Zhang Y, et al. Three field or two field resection for thoracic esophageal cancer: a meta-analysis. *Ann Thorac Surg* 2013;96(6):1933–1941.
36. Altorki N, Kent M, Ferrara C, et al. Three-field lymph node dissection for squamous cell and adenocarcinoma of the esophagus. *Ann Surg* 2002;236(2):177–1783.
37. Birkmeyer JD, Siewers AE, Finlayson EV, et al. Hospital volume and surgical mortality in the United States. *N Engl J Med* 2002;346:1128–1137.

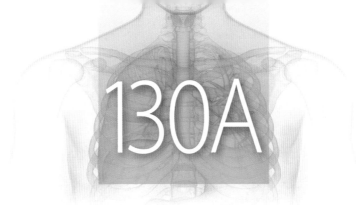

130A

Transthoracic Resection of the Esophagus

Philippe Nafteux ■ Willy Coosemans ■ Lieven P. Depypere ■ Hans Van Veer ■ Toni Lerut

INTRODUCTION

The evolution of esophageal cancer surgery has been remarkable. Indeed, from an era where surgery was mainly performed for symptom relief with cure being seen almost as an accident, to today's focus on surgery for curative intent to offer a genuine chance at long-term survival in nearly half of the treated patients, has been a long, difficult, but rewarding journey. In 1913, Franz Torek, an American surgeon with German roots who studied and worked in New York, was the first to successfully perform a transthoracic esophagectomy. His patient survived for almost 13 years after the operation.[1] Although the tumor was successfully resected, the patient lived with an externally reconstructed gastrointestinal conduit. Further evolution was dominated by others: Adams and Phemister[2] performed a one-stage esophagectomy with an intrathoracic esophagogastrostomy through a left thoracotomy and phrenotomy in Chicago in 1938, and Ivor Lewis defined in 1946 that the side chosen for the operation should be the one that yields the better exposure. He resected distal and gastroesophageal junction (GEJ) tumors via the left thoracoabdominal approach, while middle third tumors were approached from the right side in combination with a laparotomy.[3] In all cases, the anastomosis was made in the chest: Logan and later Skinner and DeMeester's en bloc resection, Akiyama et al.[4,5] demonstrated the importance of meticulous and extensive two- (and three-) field lymphadenectomy, McKeown[6] described a total three-stage esophagectomy in 1976. In an attempt to particularly reduce pulmonary complications seen after open transthoracic esophagectomy, the McKeown and, by extension, the Ivor Lewis approach are considered the basis of less invasive approaches using thoracoscopy and laparoscopy, and the creation of an intrathoracic or cervical anastomosis which is claimed to have a more favorable functional and oncologic outcome.[7–10]

INDICATION, ADVANTAGES, AND DISADVANTAGES

Although minimally invasive esophagectomy is typically performed via a right thoracoscopy, the location of the tumor has significant influence on the best approach of choice in open surgery. A right-sided approach is the preferred approach for (supra)carinal tumors and infracarinal tumors with suspicious paratracheal lymph nodes.

Although a minimally invasive resection also approaches the thoracic esophagus from the right side and values the same oncologic principles, the open right-sided approach is generally preferred over a minimal invasive approach in the case of a bulky tumor with possible adherence to the membranous part of the trachea, as can be expected in cases of salvage surgery after definitive chemoradiotherapy. In such cases, a minimally invasive esophagectomy might pose more risk of injury to the trachea when compared to the tactile feedback offered during an open procedure.

In contrast, a left thoracoabdominal approach is more appropriate for esophageal tumors below the level of the carina or tumors of the GEJ. This approach facilitates reconstruction in case a total gastrectomy needs to be performed. It also allows extensive lymph node dissection in the upper abdomen and permits further dissection along the left side of the abdominal aorta down to the left common iliac artery. Through this approach a cervical esophagogastric anastomosis is perfectly feasible, albeit that the supra-aortic part of the esophagus has to be mobilized bluntly. However, this approach does not allow for a true high paratracheal lymphadenectomy from within the chest and therefore, this needs to be completed via a cervical approach when deemed necessary. So, if one is intending to perform a paratracheal lymph node dissection, a right-sided approach is to be preferred.

The location of the anastomosis is not only dependent on the location of the tumor but also on the surgeon's preference. Leakage from the cervical anastomosis is reported to occur more frequently, due to the fact that the anastomosis is created further away from the feeding blood vessels of the gastric tube and thus is in the watershed region, as compared to an intrathoracic anastomosis. However, based on current available literature, complication rates between intrathoracic and cervical anastomosis seem to be comparable in retrospective series in terms of frequency and related morbidity and mortality.[11,12]

On the other hand, a cervical leak can usually be better controlled and will perhaps cause less sepsis in comparison to a leaking anastomosis in the upper-mid mediastinum which then drains into the lower chest. Thus, a cervical anastomosis often allows a more conservative approach to a leak as compared to an intrathoracic leak.

PREPARATION FOR SURGERY

Patients are prepared for surgery with an epidural catheter placed at the 7th thoracic intervertebral space under local anesthetic. An

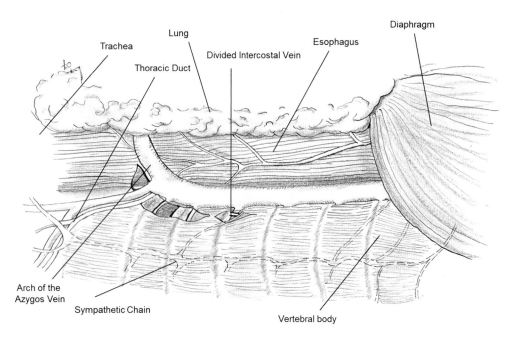

FIGURE 130A.1 View of esophagus by right thoracotomy.

arterial line is preferentially placed in the radial artery of the right arm. After induction with propofol, and starting sevoflurane for general anesthesia, the patient is intubated with a right- or left-sided double lumen endotracheal tube or a single lumen endotracheal tube with a right- or left-sided bronchial blocker according to the side of access. The double lumen tube is more commonly used because of the ease of access once the tube is in place and the faster collapse of the lung in comparison to the use of a bronchial blocker.

Next, a central line is preferably placed in the right subclavian vein. By doing so, the surgical field is not compromised in the case of a left cervicotomy or even a bilateral cervicotomy when a three-field lymphadenectomy is indicated. The subclavian position decreases the risks of colonization from the surgical site and so possibly central line infections as compared to a jugular central line.[13] Lastly, a catheter is inserted to monitor urine output during and after the intervention.

The patient is positioned in the left or right lateral decubitus on a bean bag to stabilize the positioning. Attention is paid to prevent decubitus lesions and nerve damage by padding the lower leg, knee, and foot. The lower leg is flexed, the upper is positioned straight. Under the left axilla, a cotton roll, axillary role, or plexus pillow is placed and the right arm is positioned in an arm support. The right hemichest is then draped after disinfection with an iodine alcoholic solution. To reduce the occurrence of surgical site infections, the skin in the surgical field is also draped with an incisional foil.

TECHNIQUES

RIGHT-SIDED APPROACH

We classically advocate a three-hole approach (McKeown) with the patient positioned in left lateral decubitus for the thoracic part of the operation and in a supine position for the laparotomy and cervicotomy. Some centers prefer a two-hole approach (Ivor-Lewis), placing the anastomosis high in the apex of the chest and thus omitting a cervicotomy.

The thoracotomy is performed by entering the 5th intercostal space and a view on the whole thoracic esophagus is obtained by retracting the right lung (Fig. 130A.1). The right inferior pulmonary ligament is transected (Fig. 130A.2), facilitating retraction of the lung. The azygos vein (Fig. 130A.3) is ligated and divided. The esophagus is mobilized with all its surrounding soft tissue (Fig. 130A.4). This is performed as a so-called en bloc resection all periesophageal tissues, thoracic duct, subcarinal (Fig. 130A.5) and paraesophageal lymph nodes as one single entity together with the esophagus. All branches of the azygos vein and arterial branches for the esophagus coming off the aorta have to be divided and ligated or clipped. Great

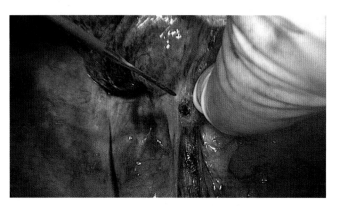

FIGURE 130A.2 Division of the inferior pulmonary ligament.

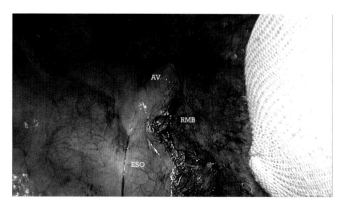

FIGURE 130A.3 Incision of the pleura along the pulmonary hilum with identification of structures. AV, azygos vein; RMB, right main bronchus; ESO, esophagus.

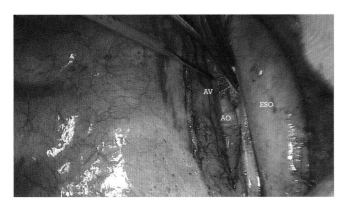

FIGURE 130A.4 Mobilization of the esophagus along the azygos vein. AV, azygos vein; AO, aorta; E, esophagus.

care is taken not to damage the membranous part of the airways (Fig. 130A.6). The dissection of the esophagus is performed down into the hiatus esophagei and cranially up into the basis of the neck. The thoracic duct is isolated in the top of the chest and above the diaphragm. It is subsequently clipped and transected (Fig. 130A.7). After completion of these steps, the paratracheal nodes are removed separately, starting by dissecting the right paratracheal region and removing all fatty and lymphatic tissues. The dissection is continued alongside the right recurrent nerve (Fig. 130A.8) up to the neck where the lymph nodes at the level of the brachiocephalic trunk extending into the base of the neck are removed. If those nodes are proven malignant on frozen section, a three-field lymphadenectomy (i.e., adding the cervical field) will be performed. It is also important that the lymph nodes in the aortopulmonary window and alongside the left recurrent nerve are dissected away from these structures, taking care not to damage them. After closure of the chest and turning the patient supine, a laparotomy is performed using a midline or a bisubcostal incision according to the surgeon's preference. Mobilizing the left hepatic lobe facilitates access to the hiatus in order to finalize the dissection of the esophagus (Fig. 130A.9). In general, a gastric tube is usually used to restore continuity, and it must be prepared accordingly. The greater curve is mobilized, preserving the right gastroepiploic vessels by dividing its branches for the greater omentum as well as the short gastric vessels. The lesser omentum is opened and after dividing the hepatic branches of the vagal nerves,

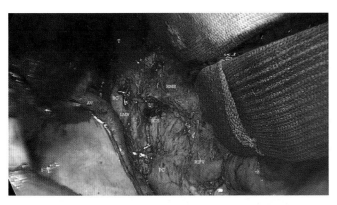

FIGURE 130A.5 View of the tracheal bifurcation with the mobilized esophagus retracted. AV, divided azygos vein; PC, pericardium; T, trachea; RMB, right main bronchus; LMB, left main bronchus; SCS, subcarinal space; RIPV, right inferior pulmonary vein; BC, bronchial cuff of double lumen tube in the left main bronchus; VC, vertebral column.

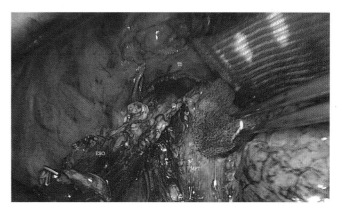

FIGURE 130A.6 Mobilization of the proximal esophagus away from the membranous part of the trachea. MPT, membranous part of trachea; ESO, mobilized esophagus; TI, thoracic inlet.

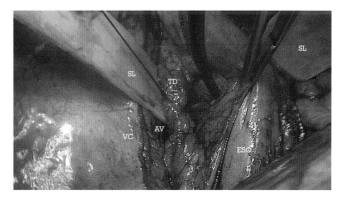

FIGURE 130A.7 Mobilization of the thoracic duct, with clips on the distal duct. AV, azygos vein; TD, thoracic duct; ESO, esophagus; VC, vertebral column; SL, sling.

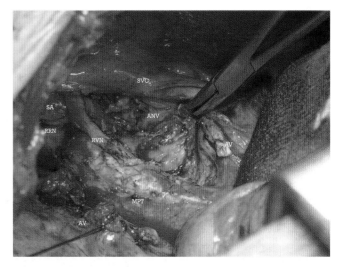

FIGURE 130A.8 View of the emptied right paratracheal compartment after the nodes are removed. MPT, membranous part of the trachea; RVN, right vagus nerve; AV, azygos vein (ligated); SVC, superior vena cava; RRN, right recurrent nerve; ANV, anonymous vein; SA, subclavian artery.

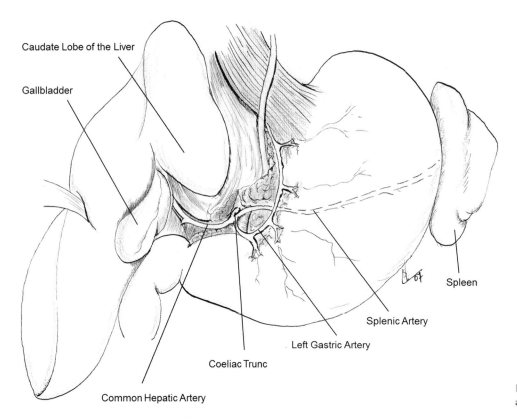

Caudate Lobe of the Liver

Gallbladder

Spleen

Splenic Artery

Left Gastric Artery

Coeliac Trunc

Common Hepatic Artery

FIGURE 130A.9 View of the upper abdominal compartment.

the dissection is continued toward the hiatus esophagei. The phreno-oesophageal ligament is incised exposing the abdominal and distal esophagus. If required for oncologic reasons a muscular rim of the esophageal hiatus is resected as well. The right gastric artery is divided at a level close to the pylorus. The left gastric artery and vein are dissected and ligated with resection of all lymphatic and fatty tissues surrounding them. A 4 cm diameter gastric tube is fashioned using linear staplers (Fig. 130A.10A,B). The lymph node dissection continues by removing all nodes starting from the celiac axis, and along the splenic artery into the splenic hilum. To the right all the lymph nodes and soft tissue along the common hepatic artery are cleared, the limit being the inferior vena cava and portal vein. This equals a so-called DII lymphadenectomy (Fig. 130A.11).

The gastric tube is then fixed to the lesser curvature with two stay sutures in order to be able to pull the gastric tube into the mediastinum from the neck.

For the Ivor-Lewis procedure, the operation is started in the abdomen followed by thoracic dissection and finally anastomosis at the top of the chest. The principles of the resection are comparable with the Mc Keown procedure described above.

LEFT-SIDED APPROACH

A thoracoabdominal approach (thoracophrenotomy) provides excellent exposure to both the upper abdomen and mediastinum. It is used for tumors of the distal esophagus and GEJ.

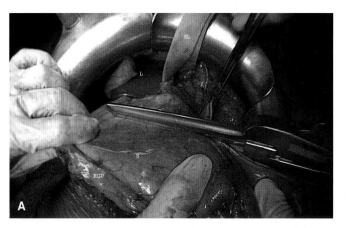

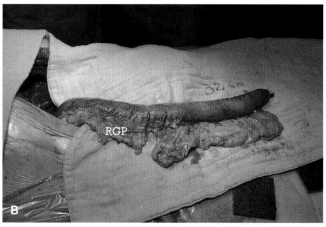

FIGURE 130A.10 **A, B:** Creation of the gastric tube using a linear stapling device. S, stomach; RGP, right gastroepiploic pedicle; L, liver; SL, sling around abdominal esophagus.

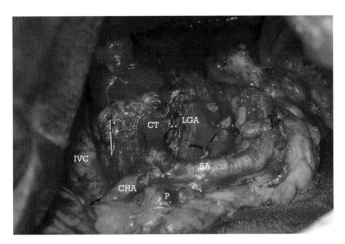

FIGURE 130A.11 View of the stump of the left gastric artery and neighboring vessels after lymphadenectomy. LGA, left gastric artery stump; CT, celiac trunk; CHA, common hepatic artery; SA, splenic artery; IVC, inferior vena cava; P, pancreas.

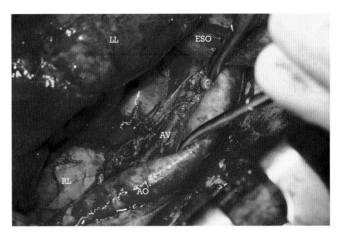

FIGURE 130A.13 Thoracic esophageal dissection. Ao, descending aorta; AV, azygos vein; LL, left lung; RL, right lung; ESO, esophagus. Part of the right pleura has been resected en bloc with the esophagus.

The operation is performed with the patient placed in right lateral position with the left hip rolled slightly toward the back to facilitate abdominal exposure. A posterolateral thoracotomy through the 6th intercostal space is extended across the costal margin slightly into the abdomen and is combined with a peripheral phrenotomy (leaving a diaphragmatic rim of 2 cm on the chest wall which will permit closure of the diaphragm) and thus preserving the phrenic innervation and related diaphragmatic function. It allows easy access to the left chest and upper abdominal compartment through a single incision (Fig. 130A.12A,B).

The esophagus is mobilized from its bed, taking all its surrounding soft tissues and paraesophageal lymph nodes from the aortic arch, flush along the descending aorta and down to the hiatus (Fig. 130A.13). The pericardium can be resected en bloc if needed. The peritoneal fold behind the spleen is incised and the spleen, together with the tail of the pancreas, is mobilized. This exposes the left upper quadrant widely facilitating not only lymphadenectomy but also the clearing out of all surrounding fatty tissues and peritoneum as well as creating better exposure to safely and completely resect bulky tumors. The greater curvature is mobilized fully till the

level of the pylorus is reached. The gastrohepatic ligament is divided as well as the right gastric vessels. The left gastric vessels are divided as described above, and the gastric tube is fashioned.

In the abdomen the lymph node dissection starts at the splenic hilum going downward alongside the splenic artery till the left gastric artery stump is reached. To the right of the celiac trunk, the nodes and soft tissue surrounding the common hepatic artery are removed, the limit of the lymphadenectomy being the inferior vena cava and portal vein. Finally, the celiac axis nodes are removed completing the DII lymphadenectomy (Fig. 130A.14). When deemed necessary, a more extended lymph node dissection can be performed alongside the left side of the descending aorta and the left kidney hilum (Fig. 130A.15A,B).

Going back to the chest, a decision has to be made on the location of the anastomosis. It can be placed in the chest, usually between the inferior pulmonary vein and the aortic arch or in the neck. In the case of neck anastomosis, the esophagus has to be dissected more proximally and needs to be freed from the aorta. To do so the inferior bronchial artery and some arterial branches for the esophagus located near to the aortic arch need to be carefully identified and secured.

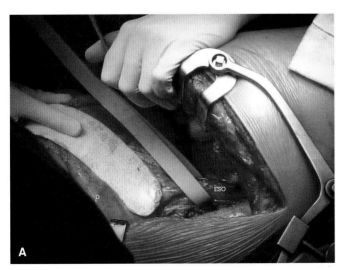

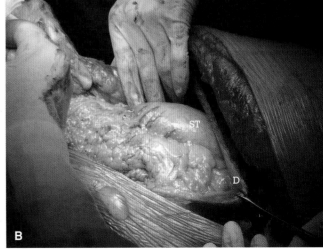

FIGURE 130A.12 Left thoracoabdominal incision: thoracic view (**A**) and abdominal view (**B**). ESO, esophagus; ST, stomach; D, diaphragm.

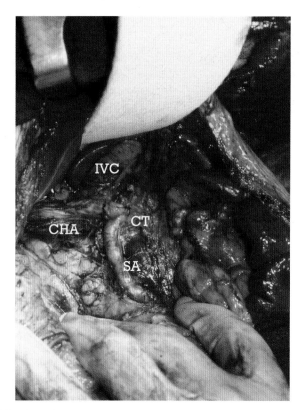

FIGURE 130A.14 Abdominal lymph node dissection. CT, celiac trunk with flush ligation of left gastric artery; SA, splenic artery; CHA, common hepatic artery; IVC, inferior vena cava; P, pancreas.

The thoracic esophagus is then freed behind the aortic arch using blunt dissection (decrossing of the aorta). The pleura is incised above the aortic arch and from there a blunt dissection of the esophagus is continued upward into the base of the neck. Great care is taken not to damage the recurrent nerve or the membranous part of the trachea in this blunt dissection.

Thoracic lymph node dissection is continued at the level of the subcarinal region and also includes the pulmonary hilar nodes,

para-aortic and aortopulmonary window nodes (Fig. 130A.16A,B). Left paratracheal nodes are normally removed from behind and above the aortic arch. Enlarged brachiocephalic nodes can be palpated from the left and when judged appropriate can be removed by performing a three-field lymphadenectomy.

The esophagus is transected at the top of the chest and the gastric tube is placed in the bed of the esophagus, brought up behind the aortic arch and fixed to the esophageal stump using two stay sutures for further extraction via the cervicotomy.

ANASTOMOSIS

Despite considerable improvements in surgical techniques and perioperative management, the anastomosis is still considered the Achilles' heel of esophagectomy. Indeed, anastomotic complications are still common (leakage rate varying from 3% to 53% and stricture occurrence rates of 14.7% to 56%) and their impact on morbidity, mortality, oral feeding initiation, hospital stay, and need for dilation should not be underestimated.[11,14–17]

The occurrence of anastomotic complications is associated with a wide range of predisposing factors. Some factors are specific to the gastroesophageal anastomosis itself, including absence of serosa of the esophagus, longitudinal orientation of its muscle fibers, ischemia of the gastric conduit with single vessel blood supply coming from the right gastroepiploic artery. But also systemic factors as inflammation, shock, hypoperfusion, steroid use, nutritional status, smoking, and alcohol consumption can play an important role in the development of such complications.

But above all surgical technique remains crucial and the quest for the perfect anastomosis has been going on for decades. The hand-sewn technique (HSA) represents the most traditional and economic method, but it takes longer to perform and requires more expertise compared to circular stapled anastomosis which are easier and faster to perform. Although no difference in leakage rates is seen between either technique, the stapled anastomosis seems more likely to cause stricture formation based on the results of a recent meta-analysis.[11]

In fact, both types of anastomosis are circular and limited in diameter size, making them prone to stricture formation anyway. Therefore, the more recent techniques, as developed by Collard et al.[18] and

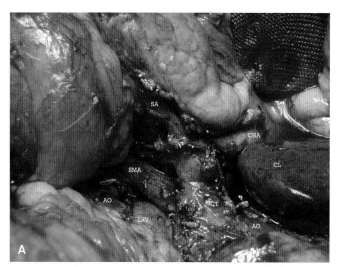
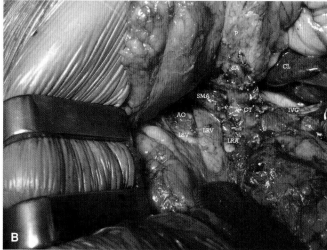

FIGURE 130A.15 **A, B:** View of a more extended lymph node dissection alongside the descending aorta on the left side. CL, caudate lobe of liver; CHA, common hepatic artery; AO, aorta; SA, splenic artery; P, pancreas tail, fully mobilized; SMA, superior mesenteric artery; LRV, left renal vein; LRA, left renal artery; SV, left spermatic vein; CT, celiac trunk; IVC, inferior vena cava.

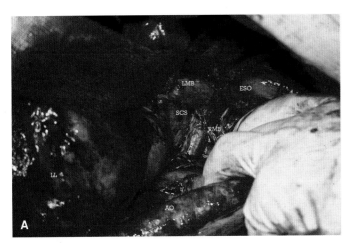 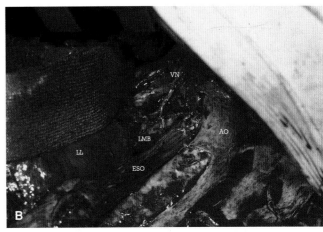

FIGURE 130A.16 **A, B:** Thoracic lymph node dissection. LMB, left main bronchus; RMB, right main bronchus; ESO, esophagus; AO, aorta; V, vagus nerve; SCS, subcarinal space; LL, left lung.

Orringer et al.[19] seem more promising. Indeed this partially stapled anastomosis, involving a side-to-side esophagogastric anastomosis, creates a larger triangular or droplet-shaped anastomosis with an almost doubling of the diameter and thus the potential to limit stricture formation without increasing the risk for leakage.[15,20]

In our institution, this semimechanical anastomosis, whenever possible, is the favored technique for a cervical anastomosis. Conversely, a circular stapled anastomosis is preferably for an intrathoracic anastomosis.

NECK ANASTOMOSIS

Since the patient is positioned and draped for laparotomy and cervicotomy, the surgical team can simultaneously proceed with a left-sided cervicotomy, over the medial border of the sternocleidomastoid muscle. After division of the platysma and omohyoid muscle and division of the inferior thyroid artery, access to the cervical esophagus is achieved. The esophagus, already mobilized up to the neck from within the chest cavity, can be hooked by the surgeon's finger and exteriorized into the cervical field. In the same movement the gastric conduit is carefully brought up through the diaphragmatic hiatus into the posterior mediastinum and eventually into the neck. Attention should be paid during this maneuver not to injure the left recurrent nerve. To prevent damage to the vascular pedicle, the conduit should nicely be guided by one hand of the surgeon through the hiatus to prevent detachment of the right gastroepiploic pedicle off the gastric tube in particular if a right-sided approach was used. Great care is taken to avoid axially twisting the gastric tube at the cervical level. Equally important is to have sufficient width (about three fingers) at the thoracic inlet to allow free passage into the cervical field without compressing the tube.

The specimen is brought out of the neck incision, with the proximal esophagus lying side by side to the gastric conduit. If the length of the conduit is sufficient (>5 cm overlap), we prefer to create a semimechanical modified Collard type end-to-side anastomosis.[19] To avoid leakage, the ischemic tip of the gastric conduit is to be resected with another linear stapler. When the conduit is considered not long enough for a semimechanical anastomosis, a two-layered hand-sewn anastomosis is preferred.

A. Hand-sewn anastomosis (Fig. 130A.17A–C):

The posterior seromuscular aspect of the anastomosis is performed using running nonabsorbable sutures, for example,

Ti-Cron 3/0. Esophagus and gastric tube are then incised alongside this suture line using the electrocoagulation on a 1 cm distance of the seromuscular layer. The posterior layer comprises full thickness of both the esophagus and gastric wall and this is sewn with a running absorbable suture, for example, Maxon 3/0 sutures. At this point, the nasogastric tube is advanced across the anastomosis The anterior part of the esophageal wall is transected and the anastomosis is finalized using a running absorbable suture, for example, Maxon 3/0 for the anterior layer and running nonabsorbable sutures, for example, Ti-Cron 3/0 for the outer seromuscular layer. Some authors prefer to use separated sutures, some authors prefer only a single layer anastomosis. Once the anastomosis is finished the esophagus and gastric tube are gently pushed back through the thoracic inlet in to the top of the chest.

B. Semimechanical anastomosis (Fig. 130A-18A–C)

A semimechanical anastomosis is started by putting five separate nonresorbable 3/0 stitches in the form of a pentagon between the muscular esophageal wall and the gastric serosal layer, with the tip being at the deepest point. Then, the gastric conduit is incised at the base of the pentagon, as well as the front wall of the esophagus. Next, a monofilament 3/0 resorbable suture is placed in the corners outward. Now, two 4/0 monofilament resorbable sutures are placed in the middle of the incision, bringing the base of the pentagon together and aligning gastric and esophageal walls. In between these sutures, a 45 mm linear stapler is fired over a distance of about 35 mm. This will create a V-shaped back wall, allowing a wider passage. It enlarges substantially the diameter and thus prevents narrowing down during the cicatrisation of the anastomosis. This results in less dysphagia for semi-solid and solid foods, consequently resulting in a lower need for repetitive anastomotic dilations and improving quality of life.[20]

The base of the back wall lateral to the stapler line is reinforced with separate 4/0 monofilament sutures. Now the nasogastric tube can be pushed down through the anastomosis into the proximal gastric conduit, in order to decompress the gastric conduit after surgery. The front wall of the anastomosis is then closed in a continuous two layer fashion with the earlier placed resorbable monofilament suture for the inner layer and the nonresorbable suture for the outer layer. To finish the anastomosis, the tip of the gastric tube is resected using a linear stapler leaving about 2 cm of healthy tissue away from the suture line of the anastomosis. Not resecting this redundant tip may result in the formation of a blind sac mimicking a diverticulum which can

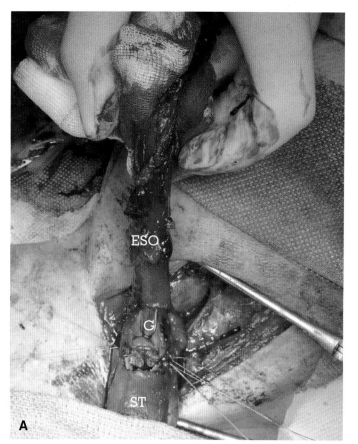

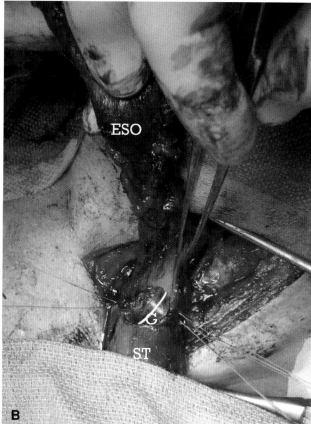

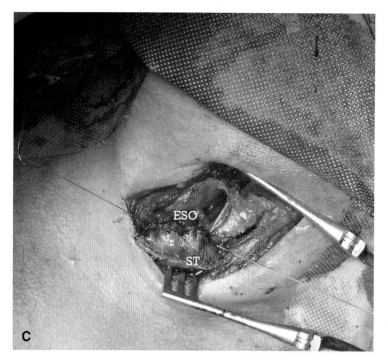

FIGURE 130A.17 Hand-sewn anastomosis: Posterior layers of the anastomosis, starting from corner to corner in a running fashion. The posterior seromuscular layer has just been performed. **A:** The next step will be a full thickness running suture also encompassing the mucosa. **B:** The nasogastric tube is then advanced in the tubulized esophagus. **C:** Finally, the anastomosis is completed by performing a double layer suture of the anterior part of the anastomosis. The redundant part of the tubulized stomach is then resected. ESO, esophagus; ST, tubulized stomach; G, nasogastric tube.

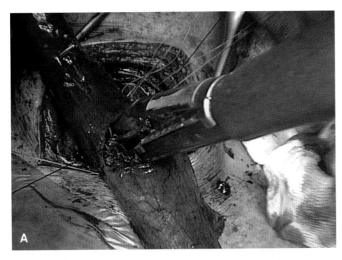

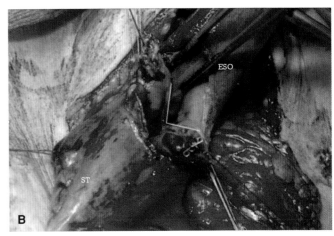

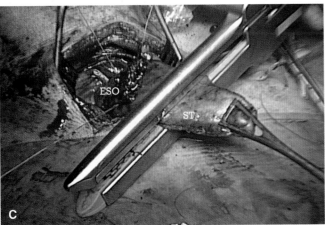

FIGURE 130A.18 A: The stapler has been fired on the sidewalls of the gastric tube and esophagus during the anastomosis to provide a wider passage. **B:** Demonstration of the V-shaped back wall of the esophagogastrostomy after firing of the linear stapler. **C:** Definitive shortening of the tip of the gastric tube by a linear stapler. ESO, esophagus; ST, tubulized stomach.

potentially impair the food passage further down the tube. In contrast, when resecting the gastric tip too close to the anastomotic area, necrosis might occur in between anastomosis and the transverse stapler line. This stapler line is then over sewn using a 3/0 nonresorbable suture. Again, as described above, the esophagus and conduit are gently pushed back in to the chest before closing the cervicotomy.

THORACIC ANASTOMOSIS

Anastomosis

The esophagogastrostomy can be performed in a variety of ways, including the use of a circular stapler or hand-sewn anastomosis.

A. Stapled anastomosis:

The esophagus is transected and a purse-string with a nonabsorbable suture, for example, prolene 4/0 running suture is placed through mucosa and the muscular layer. The anvil head of the circular stapler (size at least 25) is placed into the esophagus and the purse-string is tied snugly around the shaft of the anvil head. An incision is made at the top of the gastric tube to insert the gun of the circular stapler. The place where the gun will perforate the gastric wall is carefully chosen on the posterior aspect of the gastric tube, away from the longitudinal staple lines and from the greater curvature vessels. Of course one must also verify that once the anastomosis is performed, it will not be under tension. After perforating the gastric wall, the pointed

part in the shaft of the gun is detached and the gun is connected to the anvil head. The gun is then fired in the customary manner and the doughnuts inspected to ensure their integrity and completeness of anastomosis. Several nonabsorbable stitches may be placed between the muscular layer of the esophagus and the seromuscular lining of the stomach to strengthen and protect the anastomosis. The nasogastric tube is then advanced through the anastomosis into the gastric tube. The opening in the stomach and redundant part of the gastric tube is then transected with a linear stapler, the staple line is inverted with a running suture.

B. Hand-sewn anastomosis:

This anastomosis technique is comparable to the neck anastomosis. Usually a pleural flap is used to cover the anastomosis to protect the chest cavity from an anastomotic leakage.

REFERENCES

1. Torek F. The operative treatment of carcinoma of the oesophagus. *Ann Surg* 1915; 61:385–405.
2. Adams W, Phemister D. Carcinoma of the lower throacic esophagus: report of a successful resection and esophagogastrostomy. *J Thorac Surg* 1938;7:621.
3. Lewis I. The surgical treatment of carcinoma of the oesophagus; with special reference to a new operation for growths of the middle third. *Br J Surg* 1946;34:18–31.
4. Akiyama H, Tsurumaru M, Kawamura T, et al. Principles of surgical treatment for carcinoma of the esophagus: analysis of lymph node involvement. *Ann Surg* 1981;194:438–446.
5. Akiyama H, Tsurumaru M, Udagawa H, et al. Radical lymph node dissection for cancer of the thoracic esophagus. *Ann Surg* 1994;220:364–372; discussion 72–73.
6. McKeown KC. Total three-stage esophagectomy for cancer of esophagus. *Br J Surg* 1976;63:259–262.

7. Atkins BZ, Shah AS, Hutcheson KA, et al. Reducing hospital morbidity and mortality following esophagectomy. *Ann Thorac Surg* 2004;78:1170–1176; discussion 70–76.

8. Levy RM, Trivedi D, Luketich JD. Minimally invasive esophagectomy. *Surg Clin North Am* 2012;92:1265–1285.

9. Berger AC, Bloomenthal A, Weksler B, et al. Oncologic efficacy is not compromised, and may be improved with minimally invasive esophagectomy. *J Am Coll Surg* 2011;212:560–566; discussion 66–68.

10. Nafteux P, Durnez J, Moons J, et al. Assessing the relationships between health-related quality of life and postoperative length of hospital stay after oesophagectomy for cancer of the oesophagus and the gastro-oesophageal junction. *Eur J Cardiothorac Surg* 2013;44(3):525–533.

11. Honda M, Kuriyama A, Noma H, et al. Hand-sewn versus mechanical esophagogastric anastomosis after esophagectomy. A systematic review and meta-analysis. *Ann Surg* 2013;257;238–248.

12. Shah D, Martinez S, Canter R, et al. Comparative morbidity and mortality from cervical or thoracic esophageal anastomoses. *J Surg Oncol* 2013;108:472–476.

13. Arvaniti K, Lathyris D, Blot S, et al. Cumulative evidence of randomized controlled and observational studies on catheter-related infection risk of central venous catheter insertion site in ICU patients: a pairwise and network meta-analysis. *Crit Care Med* 2017;45(4):e437–e448.

14. Dewar L, Gelfand G, Finley RJ, et al. Factors affecting cervical anastomotic leak and stricture formation following esophagogastrectomy and gastric tube interposition. *Am J Surg* 1992;163:484–489.

15. Kondra J, Ong S, Clifton K, et al. A change in clinical practice: a partially stapled cervical esophagogastric anastomosis reduces morbidity and improves functional outcome after esophagectomy for cancer. *Dis Esoph* 2008;21:422–429.

16. Markar S, Arya S, Karthikesalingam A, et al. Technical factors that affect anastomotic integrity following esophagectomy: systematic review and meta-analysis. *Ann Surg Oncol* 2013;20:4274–4281.

17. Shah D, Martinez S, Canter R, et al. Comparative morbidity and mortality from cervical or thoracic esophageal anastomoses. *J Surg Oncol* 2013;108:472–476.

18. Collard JM, Tinton N, Malaise J, et al. Esophageal replacement: gastric tube or whole stomach? *Ann Thorac Surg* 1995;60:261–267.

19. Orringer M, Marshall M, Iannettoni M. Eliminating the cervical esophagogastric anastomotic leak with a side-to-side stapled anastomosis. *J Thorac Cardiovasc Surg* 2000;119:227–288.

20. Saluja S, Ray S, Pal S, et al. Randomized trial comparing side-to-side stapled and hand-sewn esophagogastric anastomosis in neck. *J Gastrointest Surg* 2012;16:1287–1295.

130B

Extended Resection for Esophageal Carcinoma

Jeffrey L. Port ▪ Mohamed K. Kamel ▪ Nasser K. Altorki

INTRODUCTION

Worldwide, esophageal carcinoma is the sixth most common cause of cancer deaths. In 2014, there were 18,170 cases of esophageal cancer in the United States.[1] This represents a 350% increase in incidence over the past two decades. For the majority of patients, treatment remains a formidable challenge and the overall survival is only 15%.[2–5] Despite advances in chemotherapy, radiotherapy, and molecularly targeted therapeutics; surgical resection remains an essential component of the treatment of localized esophageal carcinoma. However, there is ongoing controversy regarding the preferred surgical strategy in terms of the extent of lymph node dissection and the preferred surgical approach, namely open (transhiatal or transthoracic) or minimally invasive esophagectomy (MIE). Most surgeons regard esophageal cancer as a systemic disease at the time of diagnosis, with nodal clearance limited to easily accessible periesophageal and perigastric lymph nodes. In this paradigm, the surgical objective is essentially palliation with surgical cure being viewed as a chance phenomenon. Not surprisingly, overall, 5-year survival has remained in the 15% to 20% range with or without preoperative therapy.

A few surgical groups have advocated more extended resections for esophageal carcinoma. We have advocated the concept of an en bloc esophagectomy where resection of the esophagus is performed within a wide envelope of adjoining mediastinal tissue and accompanied by a thorough dissection of the mediastinal and upper abdominal retroperitoneal lymph nodes (two-field dissection). Further extension of the operation includes dissection of lymph nodes in the superior mediastinum and lower neck (three-field dissection) in an attempt to eliminate known or occult locoregional nodal disease. The objective of these extended resections is to improve disease control and thus possibly enhance survival. Although, the 5-year survival after these extended resections is encouraging, they remain controversial in most of Western Europe and the United States.[6]

PREOPERATIVE EVALUATION

Preoperative evaluation should be aimed at establishing the histologic diagnosis, determining the extent of local and distant disease and evaluating the patient's physiologic status. Radiologic evaluation should include a computed tomography (CT) scan of the chest and abdomen. A CT scan will establish the local extent of the tumor including mural penetration and infiltration into adjacent tissues, and may suggest nodal involvement or, more importantly, distant metastases. A barium swallow and/or an upper endoscopy preferably performed by the operating surgeon will document the location and length of the lesion and should include careful assessment of the stomach and duodenum for associated neoplastic lesions or ulcerative disease. During endoscopy, attention should be directed to identifying the relationship of the tumor to the cricopharyngeus, the squamocolumnar junction, and the diaphragmatic hiatus. It is also important to note the presence and extent of Barrett's esophagus and the presence of satellite lesions. This information is invaluable and may impact the decision on the extent and approach for esophagectomy. Most patients will also undergo both an endoscopic ultrasound (EUS) and positron emission tomography (PET) scan. EUS has been established as an invaluable tool in evaluating the depth of tumor penetration and involvement of regional lymph nodes and should be utilized in patients being considered for neoadjuvant therapy. Lightdale[7] reported that EUS has a diagnostic accuracy of 80% in predicting the T status and a 70% accuracy in predicting the N status. Also, transesophageal needle aspiration of periesophageal or perigastric nodes can often be performed with ultrasound guidance. PET scanning appears to add further sensitivity for the detection of distant visceral and skeletal metastases,[8] and may play a role in assessing response following induction therapy.[9]

Bronchoscopy is critical in evaluating tumors of the upper and middle third of the esophagus, to assess vocal cord function, and major airway involvement. Finally, thoracoscopy and laparoscopy have been suggested as staging modalities for esophageal cancer as they offer the potential to assess the extent of lymph node involvement, identify serosal and peritoneal implants, identify liver metastases, and perhaps most importantly detect T4 disease. While these minimally invasive procedures provide critical staging information beyond what is achievable by current staging modalities, their overall clinical benefit in patient management is unclear.[10]

Generally, patients are considered for primary surgical resection if preoperative evaluation reveals no evidence of distant visceral metastases or clear evidence of direct neoplastic invasion of the airway or major vascular structures. The presence of extensive nodal disease is not considered a contraindication to extended resection unless it clearly extends beyond the proposed fields of dissection.

All esophageal cancer patients must have a careful assessment of their pulmonary and cardiac status prior to resection. Patients who are current smokers must be counseled to abstain for at least 2 weeks prior to resection. Comorbidities, when present, must be optimally managed. Given the high incidence of pulmonary morbidity after esophagectomy, pulmonary function needs to be carefully evaluated.[11] Furthermore, patients with a significant history of cardiac disease will require thorough cardiac evaluation including cardiac stress testing.

ANESTHETIC MANAGEMENT

Patients undergoing a transthoracic esophagectomy should have an epidural catheter placed for postoperative pain control. In addition, a double-lumen endotracheal tube will allow for single lung ventilation and enhanced exposure. A radial artery catheter for continuous blood pressure monitoring is recommended. Two large-bore peripheral intravenous catheters should be inserted and urinary output monitored with a Foley catheter.

EN BLOC ESOPHAGECTOMY

The deep location of the esophagus within the narrow confines of the mediastinum and the lack of a well-defined mesentery have generally precluded the application of en bloc resection to patients with esophageal carcinoma. In 1963, Logan[12] reported on 250 patients with cancer of the cardia who underwent en bloc resection. While the operative mortality was high, the 5-year survival that was achieved was unparalleled at the time. Skinner[13] resurrected that approach in 1979 and extended its use to tumors of the middle and lower esophagus, publishing his first approach in 1983.

The basic principle underlying the operation is resection of the tumor-bearing esophagus within a wide envelope of adjoining periesophageal tissue that includes both pleural surfaces laterally and the pericardium anteriorly (Fig. 130B.1). The lymphatics between the esophagus and aorta, including the thoracic duct, are resected en bloc with the esophagus along with the surrounding mediastinal lymph nodes from the tracheal bifurcation to the hiatus. An upper abdominal lymphadenectomy is also performed including the

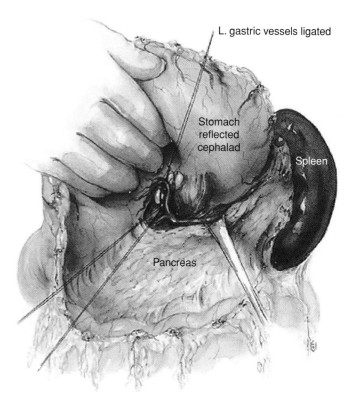

FIGURE 130B.2 Mediastinal and peritoneal nodal fields in the three-field dissection.

common hepatic, celiac, left gastric, lesser curvature, parahiatal, and retroperitoneal nodes (Fig. 130B.2). A "third-field" nodal dissection can be incorporated by extending the lymphadenectomy to include the superior mediastinal and cervical lymph nodes (Fig. 130B.3). Although the procedure has been historically carried out through three open incisions, a right thoracotomy followed by a laparotomy and collar neck incision, our current practice is to utilize a minimally invasive approach to accomplish the objectives of the en bloc dissection.

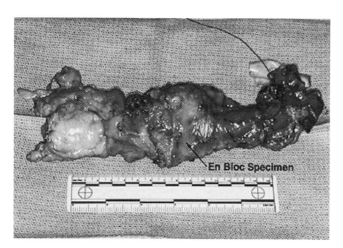

FIGURE 130B.1 En bloc specimen.

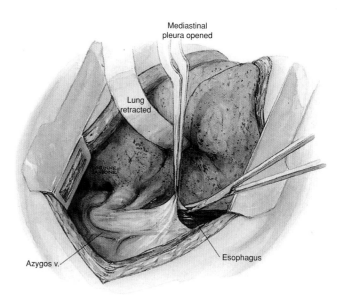

FIGURE 130B.3 Cervicothoracic nodal fields in the three-field dissection.

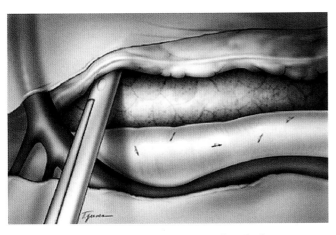

FIGURE 130B.4 Illustrated en bloc dissection in the right chest.

THE THORACIC PHASE

A right thoracotomy through the 5th interspace is performed. The "first field" comprises the middle and lower mediastinum and is bound superiorly by the tracheal bifurcation, inferiorly by the esophageal hiatus, anteriorly by the hilum of the lung and pericardium, and posteriorly by the descending thoracic aorta and the spine. The dissection begins by incising the pleura just anterior to the main trunk of the azygos vein throughout its course. The dissection proceeds leftward toward the aortic adventitia thus mobilizing the thoracic duct throughout its course in the lower and middle mediastinum (Figs. 130B.4 and 130B.5). The duct is ligated proximally at the aortic hiatus and distally as it crosses to the left side at the level of the aortic arch. The trunk of the azygos vein and the intercostal vessels are preserved. Dissection continues anterior to the aorta toward the left pleura, which is incised from the level of the left main bronchus to the diaphragm (Figs. 130B.6 and 130B.7). This completes the posterior mediastinectomy. The anterior dissection begins by division of the azygos vein at its caval junction. Dissection then proceeds along the back of the hilum of the right lung sweeping all lymphatic tissues including the subcarinal nodal chain toward the specimen. A patch of pericardium is excised en bloc with the specimen where the tumor-bearing esophagus abuts the pericardium. The right inferior pulmonary ligament is incised close to the lung and the esophagus is

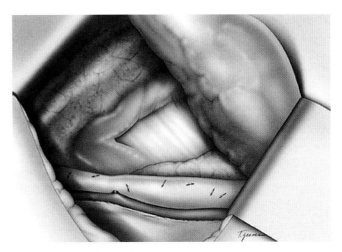

FIGURE 130B.6 Illustrated posterior mediastinectomy.

lifted out of its mediastinal bed exposing its attachment to the contralateral pulmonary ligament, which is divided, thus completing the esophageal mobilization. In tumors that transverse the hiatus, a cuff of diaphragm is circumferentially excised around the esophagus. Above the carina, the esophagus is separated from its prevertebral and retrotracheal attachments and dissected well into the neck. The completed dissection clears all nodal tissue in the middle and lower mediastinum including the right and left paraesophageal, parahiatal, para-aortic, subcarinal, bilateral hilar, and aortopulmonary lymph nodes. The specimen is left in situ and the chest is closed with pleural drainage.

THE ABDOMINAL PHASE

The patient is repositioned for a simultaneous laparotomy and cervical incision. An upper midline incision is created. Full abdominal exploration ensues with special attention paid to looking for evidence of tumor dissemination in the form of peritoneal and serosal implants and liver metastases. An abdominal self-retaining retractor such as the Omni is useful to maximize exposure. The omentum is dissected off of the transverse colon and transected several centimeters from the gastroepiploic arcade and the lesser sac is entered. Following division of the short gastric vessels, the retroperitoneum is incised along the superior border of the pancreas. The retroperitoneal lymphatic

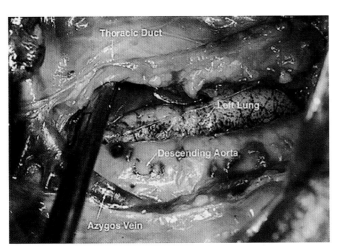

FIGURE 130B.5 Intraoperative photograph of the en bloc dissection in the right chest.

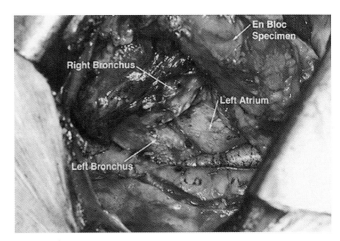

FIGURE 130B.7 Intraoperative photograph of posterior mediastinectomy.

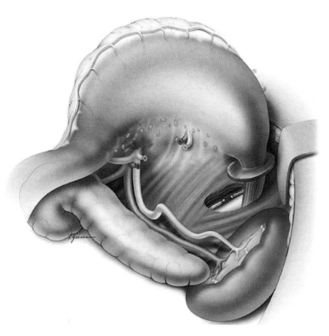

FIGURE 130B.8 Illustration of the intraperitoneal en bloc dissection.

and areolar tissues are swept superiorly toward the esophageal hiatus and medially along the splenic artery to the celiac trifurcation. The left gastric artery is divided flush with its celiac origin and the nodes along the common hepatic artery are dissected toward the specimen. This retroperitoneal dissection is bound by the dissected esophageal hiatus superiorly, the hilum of the spleen laterally, and the common hepatic artery and inferior vena cava medially (Fig. 130B.8). Finally, the lesser curvature and left gastric nodes are included with the specimen as the gastric tube is prepared.

THE CERVICAL PHASE

A low collar incision is performed and the subplatysmal flaps are raised inferiorly and superiorly (Fig. 130B.9). The prevertebral space is entered medial to the carotid sheath and the esophagus (previously fully mobilized from the thorax) is retrieved. The esophagus is divided and the specimen is retrieved in the abdomen. The stomach is transected from the fundus to the third or fourth branch of the left gastric artery. This preserves a full length of stomach for advancement into the neck. A pyloromyotomy is always performed. The gastric tube is advanced through the posterior mediastinum to the neck (Fig. 130B.10). The anastomosis is handsewn using a single layer running technique with a monofilament absorbable suture.

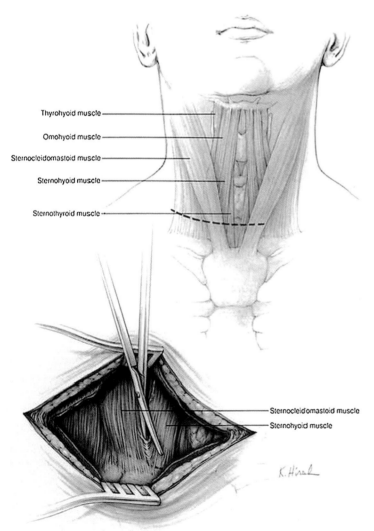

Thyrohyoid muscle
Omohyoid muscle
Sternocleidomastoid muscle
Sternohyoid muscle
Sternothyroid muscle

Sternocleidomastoid muscle
Sternohyoid muscle

K. Hirel

FIGURE 130B.9 Approach to the cervical esophagus. (Reprinted from Skinner DB. *Atlas of Esophageal Surgery.* New York: Churchill Livingstone; 1991:13. Copyright © 1991 Elsevier. With permission.)

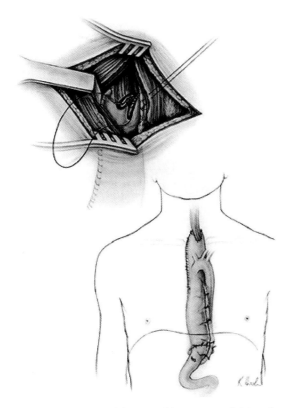

FIGURE 130B.10 Delivery of the apex of the gastric conduit into the cervical incision. The anastomosis is performed with a running suture technique. (Reprinted from Skinner DB. *Atlas of Esophageal Surgery*. New York: Churchill Livingstone; 1991:61. Copyright © 1991 Elsevier. With permission.)

More recently, we have performed a hybrid stapled anastomosis as described by Orringer et al.[14] Any redundant stomach is retracted into the abdomen and the gastric tube secured to the hiatus with care not to injure the gastroepiploic arcade. A feeding jejunostomy tube is routinely placed for early postoperative enteral feeding.

EN BLOC (TWO-FIELD) RESECTION VIA LEFT THORACOTOMY

A left thoracotomy is occasionally used for carcinomas of the gastroesophageal junction; 6th interspace thoracotomy is performed for carcinomas of the lower esophagus (Fig. 130B.11). This approach provides excellent exposure to the lower mediastinum, hiatal tunnel, and upper abdomen, particularly in obese patients. A thoracoabdominal incision is almost never necessary. Access to the abdomen is achieved through a peripherally placed semilunar incision of the left hemi-diaphragm. The diaphragmatic incision extends from the back of the sternum anteriorly to the spleen posteriorly. The thorax and abdomen are carefully assessed for visceral metastases and the tumor is assessed for mobility. The omentum is detached from the colon in the avascular plane, carefully preserving the gastroepiploic vessels. Dissection proceeds along the superior border of the pancreas sweeping all retroperitoneal lymphatics and areolar tissue toward the esophageal hiatus. The left gastric artery and vein are dissected at their origin and transected. Utilizing the cautery, a 1-in cuff of diaphragm is resected circumferentially around the esophagus. The thoracic duct is identified, ligated, and transected as it passes through the aortic hiatus. After completion of the abdominal portion of the operation, the posterior mediastinectomy begins by incising the mediastinal pleura overlying the aorta from the aortic

arch to the esophageal hiatus. Dissection proceeds along the aortic adventitia, dividing all esophageal and bronchoesophageal vessels. Further dissection proceeds dorsally and to the right to mobilize the thoracic duct toward the specimen. This dissection proceeds cephalad from the distal thoracic aorta to a point 10 cm proximal to the tumor. All lymphatics are carefully ligated. The thoracic duct is again ligated proximally and retained in the specimen. The right pleura is incised along the length of the entire dissection, thus entering the right pleural cavity. Anteriorly, the left pulmonary ligament is incised close to the lung and the dissection proceeds along the back of the hilus of the left lung. The pericardium is incised and entered and the incision carried distally along the pleuropericardial reflection to the diaphragm. The incision is carried to the right side behind the right inferior pulmonary vein and then caudally to the diaphragm (Fig. 130B.12). Dissection continues along the back of the hilum of the left lung to clear all lymphatics and areolar tissue toward the subcarinal space, which is thoroughly dissected. Dissection at this point is carried to the wall of the esophagus, which is visualized for the first time. The right and left vagus nerves are transected. The entire specimen is lifted out of the mediastinum to expose the right inferior pulmonary ligament, which is divided flush with the right lung to complete the dissection.

The digestive tract is divided 10 cm on either side of the tumor. Reconstruction can be performed in the subaortic position or alternatively, the esophagus is dissected underneath the aortic arch and into the neck. The conduit is then passed under the arch, and both the conduit and esophageal stump are gently placed into the prevertebral cervical space in preparation for a cervical anastomosis performed through a separate cervical incision. The diaphragm is

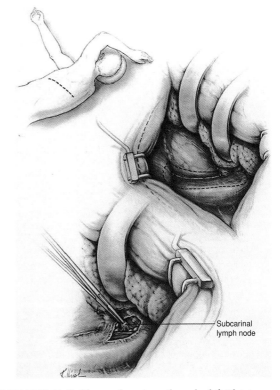

FIGURE 130B.11 En bloc esophagectomy through a left 6th interspace thoracotomy without division of the costal margin. The pulmonary ligament is divided. The *dotted lines* denote the extent of pleural, pericardial, and diaphragmatic incisions. The diaphragm will be detached from the chest wall in a semilunar fashion. (Reprinted from Skinner DB. *Atlas of Esophageal Surgery*. New York: Churchill Livingstone; 1991:23. Copyright © 1991 Elsevier. With permission.)

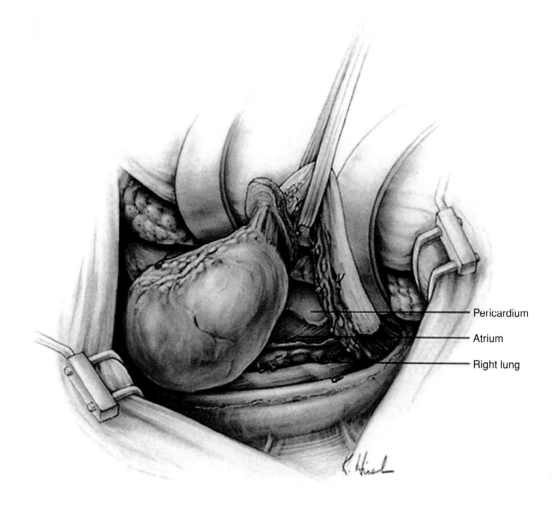

FIGURE 130B.12 En bloc mobilization of the esophagus. Note the right lung is visible in the depths of the field. (Reprinted from Skinner DB. *Atlas of Esophageal Surgery*. New York: Churchill Livingstone; 1991:31. Copyright © 1991 Elsevier. With permission.)

reattached with interrupted nonabsorbable sutures, and the conduit sutured to the hiatus. The chest incision is closed with bilateral pleural drainage.

A greater curvature gastric conduit is our preferred choice for esophageal reconstruction. When a gastric conduit is not feasible as for example, after prior gastrectomy, an isoperistaltic colon interposition may be utilized.

THREE-FIELD DISSECTION

The extension of the lymphadenectomy for carcinoma of the thoracic esophagus to include the superior mediastinal and cervical lymph nodes (three-field node dissection) was introduced by Japanese surgeons. This was prompted by large studies performed by Isono et al.[15] that demonstrated that up to 40% of patients resected by radical two-field esophagectomy developed isolated recurrences in the cervical nodes. A study reported by Isono et al.[16] on three-field lymph node dissection for carcinomas of the thoracic and abdominal esophagus demonstrated cervical nodal metastases in one-third of patients, and that up to 20% of patients with lower third lesions harbored cervical metastases. In addition, the frequency of nodal involvement increased with the depth of tumor penetration and up to 50% of patients with T1 lesions had nodal metastases. Although many studies have demonstrated an improvement in survival for patients who undergo

three-field dissection there has been considerable reluctance among Western surgeons to adopt the technique. This is related in part to the reported higher morbidity (which includes recurrent nerve injury) as well as to a general skepticism that esophageal cancer can be cured surgically once nodal disease is present.

Although the recurrent nodes are described as being cervical in location, the majority of this dissection can be accomplished through the chest. Dissection of the "third field" begins during the thoracic portion of the procedure and is later completed through a collar neck incision. Dissection of the nodes in the superior mediastinum includes the nodes along the right and left recurrent laryngeal nerves throughout their mediastinal course (Fig. 130B.3). The paratracheal retrocaval compartment is not disturbed. The left recurrent nerve is dissected using a "no-touch" technique and nodes along its anterior aspect are carefully excised. Notably, there is a paucity of nodal tissue along the left nerve in nearly all Caucasians. The right recurrent nerve is carefully exposed near its origin at the base of the right subclavian artery. The right vagus nerve serves as a good guide to locate the right recurrent nerve. The right recurrent nodal chain begins at that level and forms a continuous package that extends through the thoracic inlet to the neck. Through the cervical incision, the remainder of the recurrent nodes are dissected, as are the lower deep cervical nodes located posterior and lateral to the carotid sheath. Thus, the "third field" includes a continuous anatomically inseparable chain of nodes that extends from the superior mediastinum to the lower neck.

MINIMALLY INVASIVE/ROBOTIC ESOPHAGECTOMY

Recent advances in minimally invasive techniques have allowed for the application of laparoscopic, thoracoscopic, and even robotic approaches to an en bloc esophageal resection. They can be applied by themselves or in combination with their open counterparts, so called "hybrid" approaches. Most institutional reports with MIE in the non–en bloc setting have demonstrated safety with acceptable morbidity and mortality.[17–20] Oncologic endpoints such as lymph node yield also appear appropriate.[21] One of the largest series from the University of Pittsburgh with over 1,000 cases reported a mortality of 1.6% with declining operative time and morbidity with experience.[22] While all of the operative and perioperative complications seen in open approaches apply to MIE, there appears to be an increased incidence of airway injury in the earliest experience. The reported benefit of the MIE approach has been a decrease in postoperative pain, pulmonary complications, and a decrease in length of stay. To date most of the MIE experience had been in select center with extensive experience in minimally invasive techniques and esophageal surgery.

Our own experience with MIE for en bloc resection has mirrored our experience with the open approach in terms of lymph node yield and hospital mortality. An initial increase in pulmonary and anastomotic complications related mainly to unrecognized thermal airway injury and endoscopic "grasper" injury to the gastric fundus, has been remedied by appropriate technical modifications.

POSTOPERATIVE MANAGEMENT

In the past, mechanical ventilation was maintained until the following postoperative day. Currently, with improved pulmonary physiotherapy and epidural pain control, patients are extubated immediately following two-field en bloc resection. Patients who undergo the three-field dissection are often mechanically ventilated for 24 hours. Following radical resections (two- or three-field) patients demonstrate significant fluid sequestration as a result of the disruption of lymphatics and resection of the thoracic duct. A spontaneous diuresis will be evident by the third postoperative day. Patients are encouraged to be out of bed and ambulate. The nasogastric tube is often removed by the third day and jejunostomy feeding is begun by the fourth postoperative day. Chest tubes are left in place until drainage is less than 200 cc/day. A postoperative barium swallow is obtained on day 5 or 6 to verify anastomotic integrity and oral intake is subsequently begun. Patients are discharged often still requiring supplemental jejunostomy feeds at night. Eventually the j-tube is removed 4 weeks after operation.

MANAGEMENT OF COMPLICATIONS

ANASTOMOTIC LEAKS

A small anastomotic leak that is detected on a routine barium swallow and that appears to drain back into the esophageal lumen will usually heal without intervention. Larger uncontained leaks will require adequate drainage usually simply by opening the neck wound at the bedside. On rare occasion, a leak from a cervically placed anastomosis can track into the mediastinum and/or pleural space. In such instances drainage can usually be accomplished by tube thoracostomy. Thoracotomy is rarely necessary except in the face of persistent sepsis or multiloculated fluid collections. In complicated anastomotic leaks (large leaks or ongoing sepsis), esophagoscopy may be useful to determine viability of the conduit. Necrosis of the conduit should be treated by resection, cervical esophagostomy, and reconstruction at a later date.

ANASTOMOTIC STRICTURE

In many reports 30% to 50% of patients will develop a stricture at the anastomosis by 3 months after surgery. Dilatation of this stricture can be accomplished by several means. Our preference is for endoscopic balloon dilatation. Recalcitrant strictures may require monthly dilatation for several months postoperatively with occasional steroid injections into the stricture. To date, our anecdotal experience with temporary endoluminal stent placement has not been satisfactory, usually due to stent migration.

DELAYED GASTRIC EMPTYING

Clinically significant delayed gastric emptying is rare. Common causes of delayed gastric emptying include the lack of a pyloric drainage procedure, obstruction at a tight hiatus, or a redundant intrathoracic stomach. Balloon dilatation of the pylorus can be attempted along with the addition of promotility agents such as metoclopramide and erythromycin. Attention to the operative details, including performance of a pyloromyotomy, avoidance of intrathoracic redundancy of the conduit, and securing the conduit to the edges of the hiatus, greatly reduce the probability of clinically significant delayed gastric emptying.

REFLUX

Reflux is a common problem after gastric pullup. It appears that the severity of reflux will vary with the level of the anastomosis. Anastomoses above the azygos vein have a lower incidence of reflux than similarly constructed anastomoses below the vein. Reflux is particularly severe if the anastomosis is in the lower mediastinum. Conservative measures such as frequent smaller meals, avoidance of liquids with meals, and not reclining after meals may alleviate symptoms.

RESULTS

Although most patients with esophageal cancer will eventually develop metastatic disease, it is doubtful that a favorable long-term outcome could be achieved in the absence of adequate local control. A careful analysis of the patterns of failure after surgical resection suggests inadequate local control using the currently available treatment modalities. For example, the locoregional failure rate in randomized trials comparing surgery alone with various preoperative therapies followed by surgery is in the range of 30% to 40%.[23] In the large US trial comparing preoperative chemotherapy followed by surgery with surgery alone, locally recurrent or locally persistent disease was reported in 64% of patients.[24] More recently, locoregional recurrence was reported in 34% of patients in the surgery alone

TABLE 130B.1 Demographics, Clinical, Surgical, and Pathologic Characteristics of 465 Patients Undergoing En Bloc and Standard Esophageal Resection

	En Bloc	Standard	P-value
N	328	137	
Male	267 (81.4%)	103 (75.2%)	0.129
Age, year (median)	63	68	<0.001
Performance status			
PS 0	173 (52.7%)	70 (51.1%)	0.746
PS 1/2	155 (47.3%)	67 (48.9%)	
Clinical stage			
cStage 0[a]/I	33 (10.9%)	49 (41.2%)	<0.001
cStage II/III/IV	269 (89.1%)	70 (58.8%)	
Pathologic stage			
pStage 0[a]/I	71 (21.6%)	46 (33.6%)	0.007
pStage II/III/IV	257 (78.4%)	91 (66.4%)	
Adenocarcinoma	236 (72%)	105 (76.6%)	0.297
Location			
Proximal third	11 (3.4%)	3 (2%)	0.281
Middle third	55 (16.6%)	16 (12%)	
Lower third/GEJ	262 (80%)	118 (86%)	
Induction therapy	159 (48.5%)	20 (14.6%)	<0.001
Perioperative mortality	11 (3.4%)	5 (3.6%)	0.284

GEJ, gastroesophageal junction.
[a]Clinical stage 0 denotes Tis disease preoperatively and pathologic stage 0 denotes complete pathologic response after induction therapy.

arm of the CROSS trial where patients were randomized to either surgery alone or preoperative chemoradiation followed by surgery. These data suggest that current resection strategies are suboptimal in eradicating locoregional disease and that will most likely result in a negative impact on survival.

EN BLOC ESOPHAGECTOMY

We recently reported on our experience with 465 patients with completely resected esophageal cancer in the period from 1987 to 2009.[25] Of the whole cohort, 328 patients (70%) underwent en bloc resection (two-field in 199 patients and three-field in 129 patients). Although generally younger, the group with en bloc resection had clinically and pathologically more advanced disease and thus a higher incidence of induction therapy, when compared to the 137 patients that underwent standard esophagectomy (transthoracic in 49, transhiatal in 88), as shown in Table 130B.1. With a 30-day postoperative mortality of 3.4%, there were no difference between en bloc and standard resection in terms of perioperative morbidity and mortality, apart from a higher incidence of atrial arrhythmias after en bloc resection, possibly due to pericardial manipulation or resection. The number of dissected lymph nodes was significantly higher after en bloc resection (median 31 vs. 17, P <0.001). In patients with early pathologic stage (0/I), there was no statistically significant difference in freedom from recurrence (FFR) or disease-free survival (DFS) rates between those who underwent an en bloc resection and those who underwent a standard surgical resection. However, patients with advanced pathologic stages (II/III/IV) that underwent en bloc resection, exhibited significant improvement in DFS (5-yr DFS: 30.8% vs. 18.5%, p = 0.004), compared to those with standard resection (Fig. 130B.13). Similarly, en bloc resection was associated with a 30% reduction in the hazard for recurrence and an increase of almost 12 months in FFR (median of 32.4 vs. 20.7 months, HR, 0.64; CI, 0.43–0.96; P = 0.028), when compared to standard surgical resection in patients with advanced pathologic stages (II/III/IV) and upfront surgery. Multivariable analyses showed that en bloc resection was an independent predictor of FFR when adjusted for clinical stage (HR: 0.61, 95% CI: 43–0.88, p = 0.007) or pathologic stage (HR: 0.60, 95% CI: 0.40–0.90, p = 0.014). Similarly, en bloc resection was found to be an independent predictor of DFS in the whole cohort (HR: 0.63, 95% CI: 0.47–0.84, p = 0.002) (Table 130B.2), and

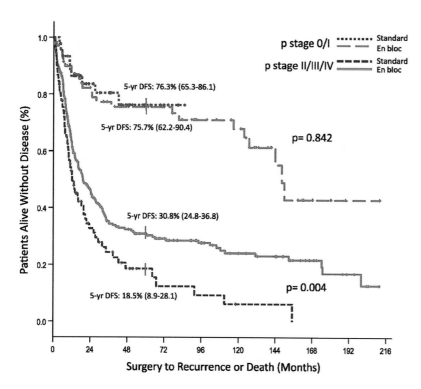

FIGURE 130B.13 DFS of patients undergoing en bloc versus the standard procedure, stratified by the pathologic stage.

TABLE 130B.2 Cox-Regression Multivariable Predictors of DFS of 465 Patients Following R0 Esophageal Resection

Independent Variables	HR (95% CI)	P Value
Age	1.00 (0.99–1.01)	0.575
Male gender	1.16 (0.85–1.58)	0.360
Performance status > 0	1.73 (1.34–2.23)	<0.001
Poor differentiation	1.25 (0.98–1.60)	0.069
Squamous cell type	1.25 (0.94–1.67)	0.120
Induction	1.34 (1.02–1.76)	0.033
En bloc resection	0.63 (0.47–0.84)	0.002
Advanced pathologic stage	3.16 (2.15–4.65)	<0.001

TABLE 130B.3 Logistic-Regression Multivariable Clinical Predictors of Cervical and Recurrent Laryngeal Nodal Metastases in Patients With Middle/Lower Third Esophageal Cancer

Independent Variables	OR (95% CI)	P Value
Squamous cell type	2.20 (0.90–5.38)	0.08
Middle third	1.70 (0.62–4.7)	0.31
cT3 to 4 or cN1 to 3, or both	2.56 (0.91–7.16)	0.07

the survival benefit increased when we limited the multivariable model to patients with advanced pathologic stages (HR: 0.56, 95% CI: 0.41–0.76, p <0.001).

EXTENT OF LYMPH NODE DISSECTION

Despite a growing interest in performing more radical lymph node dissections, limited lymph node resection remains the most commonly practiced procedure nationwide. A recent SEER review of more than 5,600 patients, who underwent esophagectomy for cancer, showed that the median number of total nodes resected was only eight lymph nodes.[26] It also demonstrated that resection of more than 30 nodes was associated with improved overall survival. We retrospectively reviewed 264 patients that underwent esophagectomy as the primary treatment modality and found that in node-negative patients with more than 25 nodes resected, the death hazard was reduced by almost 50% compared to patients with ≤16 nodes resected. This survival benefit was also seen in patients with positive nodal disease.[27] Rizk et al.[28] used the Worldwide Esophageal Cancer Collaboration data to identify the optimum number of nodes that should be resected to maximize survival. The minimum number of nodes that should be resected in node-negative disease was: 10 to 12 nodes for pT1, 15 to 22 nodes for pT2, and 31 to 42 nodes for pT3/T4. For node-positive patients, they recommended resection of 10 nodes for pT1, 15 for pT2, and 29 to 50 for pT3/T4.

THREE-FIELD DISSECTION

Despite the currently available data demonstrating a high incidence of metastasis in cervical and recurrent laryngeal (CRL) nodes, the addition of a third-field (cervical) dissection is rarely performed in the West. We retrospectively reviewed 185 patients, with middle or lower third esophageal tumors, that underwent three-field LN dissection to explore factors associated with CRL node positivity, thus identifying appropriate indications for cervical nodal dissection during esophagectomy for cancer.[29] Overall, 46 patients (24.9%) had positive CRL nodes. Interestingly, over 80% of these patients had no preoperative clinical evidence of cervical nodal involvement. The vast majority of patients with CRL nodal disease were found to be pT3/T4 (76%). Of note, CRL involvement was the only site of nodal involvement in nine patients (19.6%), all of whom had squamous cell carcinoma. On multivariate analysis, the factors prognostic for CRL nodal involvement were: squamous histology (adjusted OR 6.04, 95% CI: 2.21 to 16.56; p <0.0001), and higher pN classification (adjusted

OR 16.25, 95% CI: 5.40 to 48.87; p <0.0001). Moreover, in order to explore possible preoperative factors that may indicate CRL node involvement, a clinical multivariate model was constructed (excluding postoperative pathologic variables). Again, squamous cell histology predicted CRL nodal metastases (adjusted OR 2.20, 95% CI: 0.90 to 5.38; p = 0.083), and advanced clinical staging (cT3/T4 or cN1–3, or both) showed more than a two-fold increased risk of CRL nodal involvement (adjusted OR 2.56, 95% CI: 0.91 to 7.16; p = 0.074) (Table 130B.3). Although the study was not designed to explore the therapeutic value of the addition of a third field to the nodal dissection, we found that patients with CRL nodal metastases had a 5-year survival of 25% in the setting of a three-field lymph node dissection. The results were even more favorable for patients with squamous cell cancer as compared to those with adenocarcinoma (44% vs. 14%). Based on these results, CRL nodal dissection appears appropriate in some patients with locally advanced adenocarcinoma, and in most patients with squamous cell carcinoma.

EXTENDED RESECTION FOLLOWING INDUCTION THERAPY

The recent positive results favoring induction chemoradiotherapy have led some to question the benefit of a more extended resection. However, despite the significant reduction in the locoregional failure rate observed with the addition of preoperative chemoradiation compared to surgery alone, in the CROSS trial (14% vs. 27%; HR: 0.50, 95% CI: 0.29–0.86), there is little to suggest that patients may not benefit from an en bloc resection. Many patients in the trial underwent only transhiatal resection without an extended two-field dissection.[30] In contrast, Rizzetto et al. analyzed patients that underwent neoadjuvant therapy followed by an en bloc (n = 40) or transhiatal (n = 18) esophagectomy. Both groups had undergone neoadjuvant treatment. The results demonstrated that an en bloc resection was associated with a significantly lower locoregional recurrence rate (0% vs. 16.6%, p = 0.02), and an improved overall survival (5-year survival; 51% vs. 22%, p = 0.04).[31] Despite the nonrandomized nature and the small number of patients included in that study, there is a suggestion that patients do benefit from an en bloc approach even after induction chemoradiotherapy.

We reviewed our own experience with 156 patients that underwent esophagectomy following induction chemotherapy.[32] Ninety-six patients (63%) were noted to have persistent nodal disease, the majority underwent en bloc resection (n = 87, 91%). Metastatic disease in the recurrent laryngeal nodal basin was noted in 24 patients (25%), and celiac nodal involvement was noted in five patients (5%). The number of positive nodes was an independent predictor of overall survival (HR: 1.03 per node, P = 0.09) (Fig. 130B.14). Given the high incidence of persistent regional and nonregional nodal disease following induction chemotherapy or chemoradiotherapy, and the low perioperative morbidity associated with an en bloc resection in

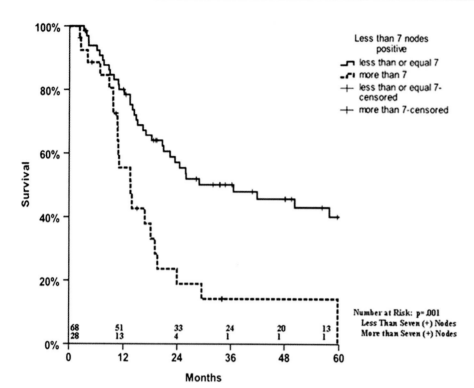

FIGURE 130B.14 Overall survival of patients with persistent nodal metastasis after induction chemotherapy stratified by the total number of positive lymph nodes resected.

experienced hands, we continue to encourage dedicated esophageal centers to perform an en bloc resection regardless of the preoperative treatment status.

RANDOMIZED TRIALS COMPARING EN BLOC AND CONVENTIONAL ESOPHAGECTOMY

A single randomized trial has been reported by Hulscher and colleagues[33] comparing transthoracic en bloc esophagectomy with conventional (transhiatal) resection. Although there was no statistically significant difference in survival between the two groups, there was a trend toward improved survival in the en bloc arm of the study. Overall and disease-free 5-year survival were 39% in the en bloc group compared to 29% and 27%, respectively, in the transhiatal group. Morbidity, but not mortality, was significantly higher in the en bloc group, consistent with the learning curve usually necessary with more complex procedures. Recently, an update has been published which demonstrates no significant overall survival benefit for the en bloc group. However, patients with adenocarcinoma of the distal esophagus as well as patients with a limited number of positive nodes did appear to benefit from the en bloc resection.[34]

CONCLUSION

En bloc resection with a three-field lymph node dissection continues to remain our procedure of choice for all patients with carcinoma of the esophagus who are surgical candidates. The operation can be performed with a low mortality and a reasonable morbidity. Radical resection improves tumor staging and may improve survival. The improvement in survival is attributed to resection of nodal metastases and a reduction in the rate of local recurrence. Nonetheless, most patients with node-positive disease will succumb to recurrent systemic disease despite aggressive surgical resection. Thus, there is

a dire need for the development of new and more effective systemic therapy for this dreaded disease.

REFERENCES

1. Rubenstein JH, Shaheen NJ. Epidemiology, diagnosis, and management of esophageal adenocarcinoma. *Gastroenterology* 2015;149(2):302–317.e1.
2. Jemal A, Siegel R, Ward E, et al. Cancer statistics. *CA Cancer J Clin* 2007;57(1):43–66.
3. Devesa SS, Blot WJ, Fraumeni JF. Changing patterns in the incidence of esophageal and gastric carcinoma in the United States. *Cancer* 1998;83(10):2049–2053.
4. Urba SG, Orringer MB, Turrisi A, et al. Randomized trial of pre-operative chemoradiation versus surgery alone in patients with locoregional esophageal carcinoma. *J Clin Oncol* 2001;19(2):305–313.
5. Walsh TN, Noonan N, Hollywood D, et al. A comparison of multimodal therapy and surgery for esophageal adenocarcinoma. *N Engl J Med* 1996;335(7):462–467.
6. Blot WJ, Mclaughlin JK. The changing epidemiology of esophageal cancer. *Semin Oncol* 1999;26(5 Suppl 15):2–8.
7. Lightdale CJ. Staging of esophageal cancer. Endoscopic ultrasonography. *Semin Oncol* 1994;21:438.
8. Meyers BF, Downey RJ, Decker PA, et al. The utility of positron emission tomography in staging of potentially operable carcinoma of the thoracic esophagus: results of the American College of Surgeons Oncology Group Z0060 trial. *J Thorac Cardiovasc Surg* 2007;133(3):738–745.
9. Port JL, Lee PC, Korst RJ, et al. Positron emission tomographic scanning predicts survival after induction chemotherapy for esophageal carcinoma. *Ann Thorac Surg* 2007;84(2):393–400.
10. Krasna MJ. Role of thoracoscopic lymph node staging for lung and esophageal cancer. *Oncology* 1996;10(6):793–802.
11. Marmuse JP, Maillochaud JH. Respiratory morbidity and mortality following transhiatal esophagectomy in patients with severe chronic obstructive pulmonary disease. *Ann Chir* 1999;53(1):23–28.
12. Logan A. The surgical treatment of carcinoma of the esophagus and cardia. *J Thorac Cardiovasc Surg* 1963;46:150–161.
13. Skinner DB. En bloc resection for neoplasms of the esophagus and cardia. *J Thorac Cardiovasc Surg* 1983;85(1):59–71.
14. Orringer MB, Marshall B, Iannettoni MD. Transhiatal esophagectomy: clinical experience and refinements. *Ann Surg* 1999;230(3):392–400.
15. Isono K, Onoda S, Okuyama K, et al. Recurrence of intrathoracic esophageal cancer. *Jpn J Clin Oncol* 1985;15(1):49–60.
16. Isono K, Sato H, Nakayama K. Results of a nationwide study on the three-field lymph node dissection of esophageal cancer. *Oncology* 1991;48(5):411–420.
17. Luketich JD, Pennathur A, Franchetti Y, et al. Minimally invasive esophagectomy: results of a prospective phase II multicenter trial—the eastern cooperative oncology group (E2202) study. *Ann Surg* 2015;261(4):702–707.
18. Van der sluis PC, Ruurda JP, Verhage RJ, et al. Oncologic long-term results of robot-assisted minimally invasive thoraco-laparoscopic esophagectomy with

two-field lymphadenectomy for esophageal cancer. *Ann Surg Oncol* 2015;22: 1350–1356.

19. Huang L, Onaitis M. Minimally invasive and robotic Ivor Lewis esophagectomy. *J Thorac Dis* 2014;6 Suppl 3:S314–S321.
20. Van der sluis PC, Ruurda JP, Van der horst S, et al. Robot-assisted minimally invasive thoraco-laparoscopic esophagectomy versus open transthoracic esophagectomy for resectable esophageal cancer, a randomized controlled trial (ROBOT trial). *Trials* 2012;13:230.
21. Shen Y, Zhang Y, Tan L, et al. Extensive mediastinal lymphadenectomy during minimally invasive esophagectomy: optimal results from a single center. *J Gastrointest Surg* 2012;16(4):715–721.
22. Luketich JD, Pennathur A, Awais O, et al. Outcomes after minimally invasive esophagectomy: review of over 1000 patients. *Ann Surg* 2012;256(1):95–103.
23. Nygaard K, Hagen S, Hansen HS, et al. Pre-operative radiotherapy prolongs survival in operable esophageal carcinoma: a randomized, multicenter study of pre-operative radiotherapy and chemotherapy. The second Scandinavian trial in esophageal cancer. *World J Surg* 1992;16(6):1104–1109.
24. Kelsen DP, Ginsberg R, Pajak TF, et al. Chemotherapy followed by surgery compared with surgery alone for localized esophageal cancer. *N Engl J Med* 1998;339(27):1979–1984.
25. Lee PC, Mirza FM, Port JL, et al. Predictors of recurrence and disease-free survival in patients with completely resected esophageal carcinoma. *J Thorac Cardiovasc Surg* 2011;141(5):1196–1206.
26. Schwarz RE, Smith DD. Clinical impact of lymphadenectomy extent in resectable esophageal cancer. *J Gastrointest Surg* 2007;11:1384–1393.
27. Altorki NK, Zhou X, Stiles B, et al. Total number of resected lymph nodes predicts survival in esophageal cancer. *Ann Surg* 2008;248:221–226.
28. Rizk NP, Ishwaran H, Rice TW, et al. Optimum lymphadenectomy for esophageal cancer. *Ann Surg* 2010;251:46–50.
29. Stiles BM, Mirza F, Port JL, et al. Predictors of cervical and recurrent laryngeal lymph node metastases from esophageal cancer. *Ann Thorac Surg* 2010;90(6): 1805–1811.
30. Oppedijk V, Van der gaast A, Van lanschot JJ, et al. Patterns of recurrence after surgery alone versus pre-operative chemoradiotherapy and surgery in the CROSS trials. *J Clin Oncol* 2014;32(5):385–391.
31. Rizzetto C, Demeester SR, Hagen JA, et al. En bloc esophagectomy reduces local recurrence and improves survival compared with transhiatal resection after neoadjuvant therapy for esophageal adenocarcinoma. *J Thorac Cardiovasc Surg* 2008;135(6):1228–1236.
32. Stiles BM, Christos P, Port JL, et al. Predictors of survival in patients with persistent nodal metastases after pre-operative chemotherapy for esophageal cancer. *J Thorac Cardiovasc Surg* 2010;139(2):387–394.
33. Hulscher JB, Van sandick JW, De boer AG, et al. Extended transthoracic resection compared with limited transhiatal resection for adenocarcinoma of the esophagus. *N Engl J Med* 2002;347(21):1662–1669.
34. Omloo JM, Lagarde SM, Hulscher JB, et al. extended transthoracic resection compared with limited transhiatal resection for adenocarcinoma of the mid/distal esophagus: five-year survival of a randomized clinical trial. *Ann Surg* 2007;246(6):992–1001.

Transhiatal Esophagectomy Without Thoracotomy

James E. Speicher ■ Mark D. Iannettoni

HISTORY OF TRANSHIATAL ESOPHAGECTOMY[1]

Historically, in 1913 Denk[2] performed the first reported blunt trans-mediastinal esophageal resection, without thoracotomy, using a vein stripper in cadavers. In 1933, the British surgeon Turner[3] reported the first successful transhiatal blunt esophagectomy for carcinoma and used an antethoracic skin tube to re-establish alimentary continuity at a second stage. With the advent of endotracheal anesthesia, however, esophageal resection under direct vision became possible, and transhiatal esophagectomy (THE) without thoracotomy became a seldom-used procedure reserved primarily for the patient undergoing a laryngopharyngectomy for carcinoma and restoration of alimentary continuity with the stomach.[4,5] As transthoracic operations became a reality, reports of resection of the thoracic esophagus—including those by Rehn (1898),[6] Llobet (1900),[7] and Torek (1915)[8]—began to appear.

The earliest reports of successful transthoracic esophagectomy and intrathoracic esophagogastric anastomosis for carcinoma were by Ohsawa in 1933,[9] Marshall in 1938,[10] Adams and Phemister in 1938,[11] and Churchill and Sweet in 1942.[12] Garlock in 1946[13] and Carter in 1947[14] popularized the combined left thoracoabdominal incision for carcinoma of the lower third of the esophagus, which had been used by Ohsawa.[9] In 1946, Ivor Lewis[15] described a right combined thoracic and abdominal approach for esophageal resection and reconstruction, citing the advantages over a left-sided approach of improved access to the upper two-thirds of the esophagus, exposure of the entire course of the esophagus after division of the azygos vein, and protection of the opposite pleural cavity provided by the descending thoracic aorta. Ong[16] used a right thoracotomy for resection of middle-third esophageal tumors but advocated a cervical esophagogastric anastomosis. McKeown[17,18] also preferred a cervical esophagogastric anastomosis and described his use of three incisions (i.e., laparotomy, right thoracotomy, and cervical) for resection of esophageal carcinoma and esophageal reconstruction with stomach. But some variation of a thoracoabdominal esophageal resection and reconstruction with an intrathoracic esophagogastric anastomosis was the most popular approach into the 1980s.

With the exception of a few reported series of transthoracic esophageal resection and reconstruction for carcinoma performed with a hospital mortality <5% by Akiyama and colleagues,[19] Mitchell,[20] and Mathisen and colleagues,[21] this operation remained a formidable one in the hands of surgeons worldwide, with mortality rates ranging from 15% to 40% in series reported through the 1970s and early 1980s,[22,23] and averaging 33%.[24,25] In reports published between 1980 and 1990, the mean mortality rate for resection of esophageal carcinoma, although significantly decreased compared with the previous decade, was still 13%.[26] Pulmonary complications in a debilitated patient caused by splinting and the resultant atelectasis associated with a combined thoracic and abdominal operation, and mediastinitis and sepsis after an intrathoracic esophageal anastomotic leak, remained the leading causes of death after esophageal resection in virtually every reported series.

Against this backdrop of more than 40 years of experience with transthoracic esophageal resection, Orringer and Sloan,[27] in 1978 reawakened interest in the technique of THE without thoracotomy as an alternative approach with potentially less risk and morbidity than the more traditional transthoracic resection. By avoiding a thoracotomy, it was argued that this approach lessens the physiologic impact of a combined thoracic and abdominal operation. Furthermore, mediastinitis from an anastomotic leak is virtually eliminated, since the cervical esophageal anastomosis results in a transient, easily drained salivary fistula if a leak occurs. The THE technique was criticized by some as being an unsafe operation that violates basic surgical principles of adequate exposure and hemostasis and denies the patient with carcinoma a complete mediastinal lymph node dissection. After 1978, a number of published reports described several surgeons' early experience with THE and discussed the indications and relative morbidity and mortality of transhiatal versus transthoracic esophagectomy. Many of these THE series represented the authors' early results with this procedure, and they were not reflective of the true morbidity and mortality of the operation performed after greater experience and facility with it were gained. Katariya and colleagues[28] (1994) reviewed 1,353 patients undergoing THE who were reported in the surgical literature between 1981 and 1992. Sixteen of the papers referenced (69.5%) were a series of 50 patients or less and as such were not a true reflection of the types of results that can be achieved by more experienced surgical teams. All but 12 of the operations were for cancer. Eighteen (1.3%) were converted to open thoracotomies for control of hemorrhage. Tracheal injuries occurred in nine (0.67%). The most common postoperative complications were "thoracic or pulmonary," which these authors grouped together as including pneumothoraces, pleural effusions, pneumonias, empyemas, and respiratory failure, and which occurred in nearly 50% of the patients. Inclusion of such diverse complications in a single category is difficult to analyze. The need for a chest tube because of entry into a pleural cavity is much less of a complication than pneumonia, empyema, or respiratory failure, which prolong hospitalization. Additional complications included anastomotic leak (15.1%), clinically detected recurrent laryngeal nerve injury (11.3%), cardiac arrhythmias, myocardial infarction or tamponade (11.9%), incidental splenectomy (2.6%), and chylothorax (0.7%).

In the next decade, there were at least nine different reports on THE and 37 series comparing transthoracic esophagectomy and THE. Table 130C.1 lists the series, totaling more than 6,300 patients.

In a more recent meta-analysis of transthoracic versus transhiatal resection for carcinoma of the esophagus by Hulscher and colleagues[66] (2001), perioperative blood loss was significantly higher after transthoracic resection (mean 1,001 mL vs. 728 mL), and transthoracic resection carried a higher risk for pulmonary complications, chylothorax, and wound infection. The length of postoperative intensive care after transthoracic resection was significantly longer (11.2 days vs. 9.1 days), the hospital stay significantly prolonged (21 days vs. 17.8 days), and the overall hospital mortality rate was significantly higher after transthoracic resections (9.2% vs. 5.7%). However, overall mean anastomotic leak rate was greater with transhiatal resection (13.6% vs. 7.2%), as was the rate of vocal cord paralysis (9.5% vs. 3.5%). There was no significant difference in survival at 3 or 5 years postoperatively between those undergoing transthoracic and transhiatal esophagectomies. Orringer and colleagues[67] reported the largest THE series in 2007 and described a 30-year retrospective experience with this operation in 2,007 patients undergoing esophageal resection for diseases of the intrathoracic esophagus (482 [24%] with benign disease and 1,525 [76%] with carcinoma); the total hospital mortality rate for the procedure was 3% and was only 1% in the last 1,000 patients. Hemorrhage requiring thoracotomy was reported in <1%, incidental splenectomy in 2%, tracheobronchial injury in <1%, chylothorax in 1%, and recurrent nerve injury in 5%, but only 2% in the last 1,000 patients. Anastomotic leak rate was 12% overall, and 9% in the last 1,000 patients.

PREOPERATIVE CONSIDERATIONS

THE has been completed in almost all patients requiring an esophagectomy for either benign or malignant disease at the author's institution. In patients with esophageal carcinoma, the operation is contraindicated if there is bronchoscopic evidence of tracheobronchial invasion, not contiguity, by the tumor. Significant cirrhosis with portal hypertension is also a contraindication to THE, due to the potential for major complications, poor healing, and massive hemorrhage. Histologic documentation of distant metastatic disease (i.e., biopsy-proven liver or supraclavicular, or distant lymph node metastasis) associated with an intrathoracic esophageal carcinoma should be a contraindication to esophagectomy by either approach, because patients with stage IV carcinomas have an average survival of only approximately 6 months and the risks of esophagectomy generally outweigh the short-term benefits in this population. Salvage esophagectomy is rarely offered in patients with advanced disease for the same reasons. Rarely, optimized patients with distant disease complicated by perforation, complete obstruction, or recurrent local disease may be considered for salvage esophagectomy; however, this indication has become even more infrequent as advances in endoscopic techniques are now capable of palliating many of these

TABLE 130C.1 Report on Transhiatal Esophagectomies, 1993–2003

Year	Investigators	No. of Patients (% Operative Mortality)	
		THE vs.	TTE
1993	Goldminc et al.[29]	32 (6.2)	35 (8.6)
1993	Hagen et al.[30]	30 (NS)	39 (NS)
1993	Naunheim et al.[31a]	11 (18)	27 (18)
1993	Pac et al.[32]	118 (6.7)	120 (11)
1993	Tilanus et al.[33]	141 (5)	152 (9)
1993	Gertsch et al.[34]	100 (3)	
1993	Vigneswaram et al.[35]	131 (2.3)	
1994	Bolton et al.[36]	48 (NS)	31 (NS)
1994	Putnam et al.[37]	134 (6.8)	221 (6.8)
1995	Berdejo[38]	21 (4.7)	20 (20)
1995	Bonavina[39]	85 (6)	168 (10.7)
1995	Horstmann et al.[40]	46 (15)	41 (10)
1995	Millikan et al.[41]	67 (4.5)	71 (12.7)
1995	Svanes et al.[42]	51 (0)	32 (4)
1996	Junginger and Dutkowski[43]	49 (6)	124 (8)
1996	Stark et al.[44]	32 (3.1)	16 (0)
1996	Beik et al.[45]	68 (8.8)	
1996	Gupta[46]	250 (6)	
1997	Chu et al.[47]	20 (10)	19 (5)
1997	Jacobi et al.[48]	16 (0)	16 (0)
1997	Thomas et al.[49]	49 (4)	103 (7)
1998	Pommier et al.[50]	38 (5)	40 (3)
1998	Dudhat and Shinde[51]	80 (7.5)	
1998	Gillinov and Heitmiller[52]	101 (3)	
1999	Gluch et al.[53]	65 (7)	33 (7)
1999	Torres et al.[54]	29 (17.2)	28 (7)
1999	Boyle et al.[55]	38 (8)	27 (19)
2000	van Sandick et al.[56]	115 (3.5)	
2001	Orringer et al.[57]	1,085 (4)	
2002	Uravic et al.[58]	29 (20.7)	
2002	Hulscher et al.[59]	106 (2)	114 (4)
2002	Rao et al.[60]	411 (11)	
2002	Averbach et al.[61]	14 (NS)	16 (NS)
2002	Doty et al.[62]	91 (0)	4 (0)
2002	de Boer et al.[63]	26 (NS)	22 (NS)
2002	Bousamra et al.[64]	43 (NS)	47 (NS)
2003	Rentz et al.[65]	383 (9.9)	562 (10)
	Total	**4,253**	**2,128**

[a]Series of septuagenarians.
THE, transhiatal esophagectomy; TTE, transthoracic esophagectomy; NS, not stated.

problems. In patients with benign esophageal disease, particularly those who have had previous esophageal operations and especially an esophagomyotomy, which may produce adhesions between the esophageal submucosa and adjacent aorta, the surgeon must be prepared to convert to a transthoracic esophagectomy if, on palpation of the esophagus through the diaphragmatic hiatus, periesophageal adhesions are found that would prevent a safe transhiatal resection.

Patients are seen and evaluated in a preoperative clinic, both at initial consultation and during the restaging process if a patient is receiving trimodality therapy with neoadjuvant chemoradiation. Pulmonary function tests are performed if the patient is a heavy smoker, and cardiac evaluation is requested if there is a prior history of cardiac disease or significant risk factors. Standard laboratory studies are obtained along with the staging workup as directed below if the indication for resection is esophageal cancer. A barium enema is obtained if the patient has had previous gastrointestinal surgery and there is concern for the need to use colon as a conduit. A multidisciplinary approach is used and all patients are presented at a multidisciplinary thoracic cancer conference. Of note, patients are required to quit smoking prior to the operation and a Cotinine blood test is used to confirm this on the day of surgery. If a patient has not stopped smoking, their surgery is postponed until smoking cessation is confirmed.

The preoperative staging of esophageal carcinoma has been greatly improved and refined with the availability of computed tomography (CT), endoscopic ultrasonography (EUS), and positron emission tomography (PET), all of which are now regarded as basic in the preoperative assessment of these patients.[68,69] CT scanning of the chest and upper abdomen in the preoperative assessment of these patients is helpful in defining the local extent of the tumor and the presence of distant metastatic disease, but this diagnostic modality is not a reliable indicator of resectability.[70,71] CT demonstration of contiguity of an esophageal tumor with adjacent organs does not prove that invasion is present or that the tumor is unresectable.[72] PET scanning is an integral part of the assessment of patients with esophageal carcinoma and should be performed in all patients during their initial staging evaluation as occult metastatic disease is often detected that is otherwise not evident.[73,74] EUS, which defines the five layers of alternating echogenicity of the esophageal wall, allows precise determination of the depth of tumor invasion ("T status"). EUS provides what is perhaps the best assessment of the depth of tumor invasion of the wall of the esophagus and adjacent organs and the presence of lymph node metastases that may preclude resection. The addition of fine-needle aspiration (FNA) biopsy of suspicious paraesophageal and celiac axis lymph nodes at the time of EUS greatly enhances the accuracy of staging. Currently, the majority of patients with esophageal carcinoma undergo neoadjuvant chemotherapy and radiation prior to resection. This is the case for any patient able to tolerate the trimodality approach that has a T3 or greater tumor (or in some cases, T2 and above), or any suspicious lymph nodes seen on staging studies. After receiving neoadjuvant therapies, patients are typically restaged with both a repeat PET scan as well as a repeat EUS procedure, to assess adequacy of response and to document that there has been no progression of disease or appearance of new metastatic disease. Although the addition of a contrast-enhanced CT scan to the restaging workup did not show any cost benefit in a recent study,[75] it identified several massive, asymptomatic pulmonary emboli that could have potentially impacted survival and outcome of the operation, had the operation proceeded without obtaining the scan first. The tangible diagnostic benefits of an additional contrast CT scan should be considered by providers during any restaging workup.

Preoperative epidural catheters are placed in all patients unless there is a contraindication. This allows for improved postoperative pain control and, in turn, improved respiratory dynamics, increased mobility, and decreased postoperative complications.[76] Intra-arterial blood pressure is monitored with a radial artery catheter in all patients undergoing THE, so that prolonged hypotension resulting from cardiac displacement by the surgeon's hand inserted into the posterior mediastinum during the transhiatal dissection can be avoided. Two large-bore intravenous catheters, generally placed in peripheral arm veins, should be available for rapid volume replacement if required, and the arms are padded and tucked at the patient's sides during the operation so that the surgeon has unimpeded access to the neck, chest, and abdomen. If central venous pressure is to be monitored intraoperatively, and this is not routine, a right-sided vein should be used to keep the left neck free for the operation. An unshortened standard endotracheal tube is used rather than a larger, more bulky double-lumen tube. If a posterior membranous tracheal tear occurs during the transhiatal dissection, the tube can be advanced into the left mainstem bronchus and one-lung anesthesia maintained while the tracheal injury is dealt with. If the tumor is adhered to the membranous trachea or left mainstem bronchus so much so as to prevent safe transhiatal dissection and a thoracotomy becomes necessary, the endotracheal tube can be exchanged for a double-lumen tube prior to repositioning for the thoracotomy. Because transient hypotension caused by cardiac displacement can occur during a transhiatal dissection, inhalation agents are decreased and inspired oxygen concentration increased during this phase of the operation. THE requires a close working relationship between the anesthetist and the surgeon. Intraoperative hypotension does not signal the need for pressor agents but rather for notifying the surgeon so that the hand can be temporarily removed from the mediastinum.

The patient is taken to the operating room and placed in the supine position. After intubation and placement of any lines, a Foley catheter is inserted to monitor urine output and the arms are tucked at the patient's sides. A shoulder roll is placed posterior to the scapula and the neck is extended and turned to the right. The skin is sterilely prepared and draped to expose the upper midline, the entire chest, and the left side of the neck up to the lobe of the ear. An iodophor-impregnated antimicrobial drape is used to cover the abdomen and chest, but not the neck. A multiarm retractor system is placed caudally on the table to facilitate the abdominal operation. Two suction lines, one at the head of the table and one from below, are used routinely. THE is executed in three phases: abdominal, mediastinal, and cervical.

ABDOMINAL PHASE

The supraumbilical midline incision extends from the xiphoid to several centimeters superior to the umbilicus (Fig. 130C.1). After exploring the abdominal cavity to rule out metastatic disease, the xiphoid process is usually removed for exposure. The triangular ligament of the liver is divided to visualize the esophageal hiatus and the left lobe of the liver retracted to the right with a splanchnic blade. The stomach is inspected to be certain that scarring or shortening from prior disease, or involvement of a significant portion of the upper

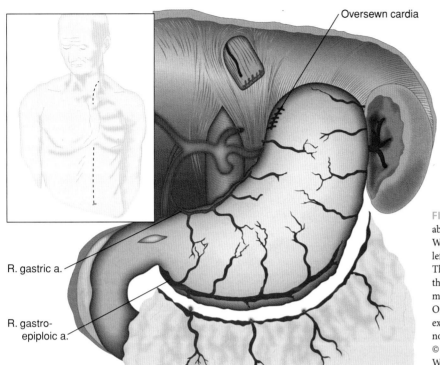

Oversewn cardia

R. gastric a.

R. gastro-
epiploic a.

FIGURE 130C.1 Cervical and supraumbilical midline abdominal incisions used for transhiatal esophagectomy. When the stomach is used to replace the esophagus, the left gastric and left gastroepiploic vessels are divided. The right gastric and right gastroepiploic arteries supply the mobilized stomach. A pyloromyotomy and Kocher maneuver are routinely performed. (Reprinted from Orringer MB, Sloan H. Substernal gastric bypass of the excluded esophagus for palliation of esophageal carcinoma. *J Thorac Cardiovasc Surg* 1975;70:836. Copyright © 1975 The American Association for Thoracic Surgery. With permission.)

stomach by tumor, does not preclude its use for a cervical esophagogastric anastomosis.

The right gastroepiploic artery is identified and evaluated to ensure it is adequate for conduit perfusion, and is carefully protected throughout the operation. Separation of the greater omentum from the stomach is begun high along the greater curvature at an avascular site where the right gastroepiploic artery terminates as it enters the stomach or anastomoses with small branches of the left gastroepiploic artery. The lesser sac behind the greater omentum is entered at this point, and—working progressively upward along the greater curvature of the stomach—the left gastroepiploic and short gastric vessels are sequentially ligated with an energy device, avoiding both injury to the gastric wall, which may result in later necrosis, and damage to the adjacent spleen. After the high greater curvature of the stomach has been mobilized away from the omentum and spleen, the dissection is continued anterior to the esophagus by dividing the phrenoesophageal membrane to expose the gastroesophageal junction. A finger is placed through the esophageal hiatus into the posterior mediastinum to evaluate mobility of the esophagus and tumor burden. Assuming no contraindications toward continuing with the transhiatal approach, attention is then turned back to the greater curvature.

Dissection is continued distally along the curvature, taking the greater omentum off the stomach while protecting the right gastroepiploic artery with the same hand used to elevate the stomach for retraction. Care is taken to palpate the pulse in the artery during each step in the dissection and to work at least 1.5 to 2.0 cm inferior to the vessel to avoid inadvertent injury to it. We attempt to visualize the gastroepiploic vein during this dissection as well, in order to avoid damage and the resultant venous congestion and conduit failure that would follow. The dissection is continued distally until the branching point of the artery is reached, where the gastroduodenal artery bifurcates into the right gastroepiploic and superior pancreaticoduodenal arteries. This dissection is aided if the assistant to the patient's right directs a headlight onto the field so that the surgeon on the patient's

left can easily see the vessels coursing through the mesentery. Any posterior adhesions to the stomach are then taken down and a finger is placed posterior to the antrum, through to the lesser curvature, and used to retract the stomach gently to spread out and expose the gastrohepatic ligament. The filmy portion of the gastrohepatic ligament is incised, and dissection is carried superiorly toward the esophageal hiatus, eventually connecting with the previous dissection from the side of the greater curvature. This exposes the fat pad containing the left gastric artery and vein, as well as any perigastric nodal tissue. The lymph node packet is swept off the celiac plexus toward the stomach and the left gastric vessels stapled with a vascular load below the nodes. The presence of a replaced or accessory left hepatic artery arising from the left gastric artery should always be assessed. If an aberrant left hepatic artery is found, the left gastric artery is dissected and divided at a point that will preserve the hepatic circulation. The right gastric artery is protected throughout the gastric mobilization. A generous Kocher maneuver is performed to ensure maximum mobility of the stomach. A pyloromyotomy extending from 2 cm proximal on the stomach through the pylorus and onto the duodenum is performed. The cutting current of a needle-tipped electrocautery is used, along with a fine-tipped mosquito clamp for dissection of the gastric and duodenal muscle away from the underlying submucosa. If the pyloric or duodenal mucosa is violated, the tear is repaired with 5-0 Prolene (Ethicon, Inc., Somerville, NJ) sutures and reinforced with adjacent omentum. Two metallic hemostatic clips are placed adjacent to the pylorus to facilitate its identification on subsequent radiographic examinations. Attention is then turned to the neck.

CERVICAL PHASE

A left-sided neck incision is made along the anterior border of the sternocleidomastoid muscle distally to just below the cricoid cartilage. The platysma is divided. The sternocleidomastoid muscle and carotid sheath are retracted laterally and the larynx and thyroid lobe

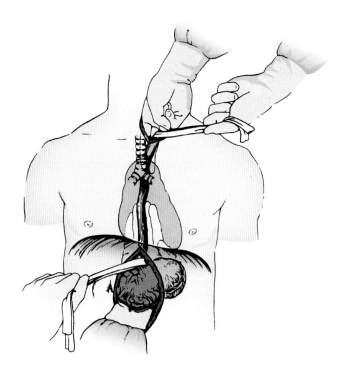

FIGURE 130C.2 Transhiatal esophagectomy is initiated as a midline dissection with the volar aspects of the fingers against the esophagus. Traction on rubber drains encircling either end of the esophagus can facilitate the dissection. (From Orringer MB. Surgical options for esophageal resection and reconstruction with stomach. In Baue AE et al., eds. *Glenn's Thoracic and Cardiovascular Surgery*, 5th ed. Norwalk, CT: Appleton & Lange; 1991:787, with permission.)

are retracted medially. A metal retractor should not be placed against the tracheoesophageal groove so as to avoid injury to the recurrent laryngeal nerve. The omohyoid is divided and the esophagus is identified by palpating the nasogastric tube. The inferior thyroid artery and occasionally the middle thyroid vein are ligated during this dissection.

The dissection is carried posteriorly to the prevertebral fascia medial to the carotid sheath. The prevertebral space behind the cervical esophagus is developed by blunt finger dissection, constantly keeping the fingers against the esophagus. The tracheoesophageal groove is developed by dissecting the plane between the trachea and cervical esophagus with a right-angled clamp, being careful to stay directly on the esophagus to avoid injury to the recurrent laryngeal nerve. The nerve is not routinely identified. The right-angled clamp is then placed up against the spine, medial to the esophagus, and passed back posteriorly to the esophagus and a Penrose drain grasped to encircle the esophagus. The drain is used to retract the esophagus superiorly as blunt dissection of the upper thoracic esophagus into the superior mediastinum is performed (Fig. 130C.2). The esophagus is mobilized in this fashion as far distally into the mediastinum as possible, preferably down to the level of the carina. Attention is then turned to the mediastinal dissection.

TRANSHIATAL DISSECTION

The transhiatal portion of the operation is begun by again evaluating the tumor. If the tumor-containing portion of the esophagus feels mobile and separable from adjacent structures as assessed by grasping the mass through the diaphragmatic hiatus and rocking it, THE is likely possible. The plane posterior to the esophagus is dissected

first. A hand is placed through the hiatus and advanced along the prevertebral fascia superiorly. The other hand is placed into the cervical incision and advanced inferiorly along the prevertebral fascia until the two hands meet. A half-sponge on a stick is occasionally advanced along the prevertebral fascia from the cervical incision until it can be palpated by the hand advancing through the diaphragmatic hiatus and used for traction and stability while dissecting the most superior mediastinal attachments (Fig. 130C.3). Once the posterior mediastinal plane is established, a 28-Fr Argyle Saratoga sump drain is inserted through the cervical incision and advanced through the posterior mediastinum into the upper abdominal cavity and connected to suction. This helps to maintain a dry field during the subsequent mediastinal dissection and facilitates identification and division of the lateral esophageal attachments under direct vision through the diaphragmatic hiatus.

The anterior mediastinal dissection is performed in a similar fashion as the posterior mobilization, again dissecting with the volar aspect of the fingers against the anterior esophagus until the hands placed through each incision can connect (Fig. 130C.4). As the esophagus is mobilized away from the pericardium and carina, care must be taken to avoid injury to the posterior membranous

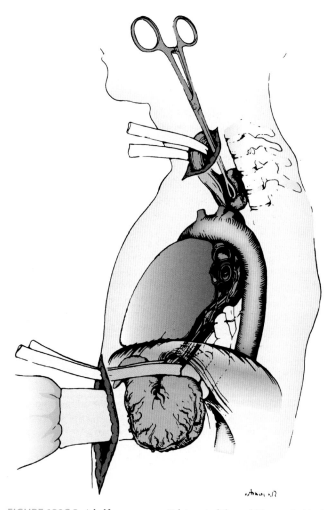

FIGURE 130C.3 A half sponge on a stick inserted through the cervical incision is advanced until it meets the hand inserted through the diaphragmatic hiatus posterior to the esophagus. (From Orringer MB. Surgical options for esophageal resection and reconstruction with stomach. In Baue AE et al., eds. *Glenn's Thoracic and Cardiovascular Surgery*, 5th ed. Norwalk, CT: Appleton & Lange; 1991:787, with permission.)

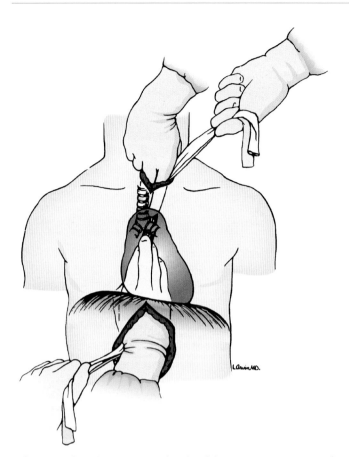

FIGURE 130C.4 The anterior transhiatal mobilization is a mirror image of the posterior dissection, again performed with the volar aspects of the fingers against the esophagus and using traction applied to drains around either end of the esophagus. Care must be taken to avoid injury to the posterior membranous trachea. (From Orringer MB. Surgical options for esophageal resection and reconstruction with stomach. In Baue AE, et al., eds. *Glenn's Thoracic and Cardiovascular Surgery*, 5th ed. Norwalk, CT: Appleton & Lange; 1991:787, with permission.)

trachea (Fig. 130C.5). As with the posterior dissection, a half-sponge on a stick can be used through the cervical incision to facilitate the dissection until the anterior plane is complete. At times during the anterior and posterior dissections, dense subcarinal or subaortic tissue requires fracture by firm pressure between the index finger and thumb, but this is where judgment must be exercised regarding the need to convert to a transthoracic mobilization of the esophagus under direct vision.

A deep Deaver retractor is then placed into the mediastinum, and used for retraction to visualize the remaining lateral attachments to the esophagus. Wherever possible, these are taken down sharply with an energy device. Any visualized paraesophageal and subcarinal lymph nodes are removed during this portion of the dissection. If any lateral attachments remain that are unreachable with the energy device or unable to be visualized even with the deep Deaver retractor in the mediastinum, a blunt technique can be used to complete the dissection. The right hand is inserted through the diaphragmatic hiatus anterior to the esophagus, which is retracted downward. The hand is advanced upward into the superior mediastinum until the transition from the circumferentially mobilized upper esophagus to the adjacent segment with its intact lateral attachments can be identified (Fig. 130C.6). The esophagus is trapped against the prevertebral fascia between the index and middle fingers, and with a downward raking motion of the hand, the remaining lateral periesophageal

attachments are avulsed (Fig. 130C.7). During this lateral dissection, vagal fibers passing from the hilum of the lungs onto the esophagus may be hooked by the index finger, identified through the diaphragmatic hiatus, and divided.

As an alternative to the blunt technique described above for dissection of the final lateral attachments, we often perform this portion of the dissection in a retrograde fashion. Once the esophagus has been mobilized as much as possible under direct vision, several inches of esophagus are gently pulled into the cervical wound, and the esophagus is divided obliquely in the neck with the GIA surgical stapler (Fig. 130C.8). The esophagus is divided as far distally as possible, within the anatomic constraints of the sternal notch, while insuring an adequate margin, intentionally leaving redundancy in the length of remaining cervical esophagus that will facilitate later construction of the cervical esophagogastric anastomosis. The distal end of the stapled esophagus can be delivered into the mediastinum and grasped with the hand through the diaphragmatic hiatus. Gentle traction is then placed on this section of esophagus, along with the distal portion of the intrathoracic esophagus to expose the final

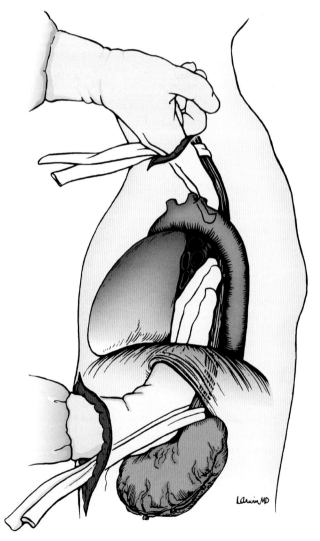

FIGURE 130C.5 In the process of dissecting the anterior esophagus, the hand should be pressed posteriorly against the esophagus to minimize cardiac displacement. (From Orringer MB. Surgical options for esophageal resection and reconstruction with stomach. In Baue AE, et al., eds. *Glenn's Thoracic and Cardiovascular Surgery*, 5th ed. Norwalk, CT: Appleton & Lange; 1991:787, with permission.)

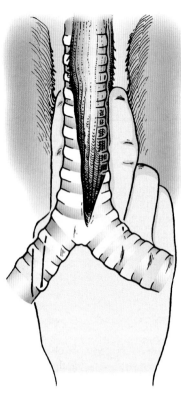

FIGURE 130C.6 After circumferential mobilization of the upper thoracic esophagus has been achieved through the cervical incision, the right hand is inserted through the diaphragmatic hiatus and advanced upward into the superior mediastinum until the undivided lateral esophageal attachments can be felt. (Reprinted from Orringer MB. Transhiatal esophagectomy. In: Dudley H, Pories WJ, Carter D, eds. *Rob and Smith's Operative Surgery*, 4th ed. London: Butterworth–Heinemann, 1983:192. Copyright © 1983 Elsevier. With permission.)

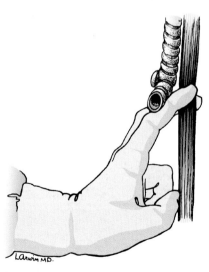

FIGURE 130C.7 Avulsion of filmy lateral esophageal attachments is achieved by a downward raking motion of the index and middle fingers, which have trapped the esophagus against the spine. Tougher vagal fibers that course along the esophagus may be delivered downward until they are visible through the hiatus and then divided under direct vision. (Republished with permission of John Wiley & Sons, Inc. from Orringer MB. Transhiatal blunt esophagectomy without thoracotomy. In: Cohn LH, ed. *Modern Technics in Surgery—Cardiothoracic Surgery*. Armonk, NY: Futura; 1983:62; permission conveyed through Copyright Clearance Center, Inc.)

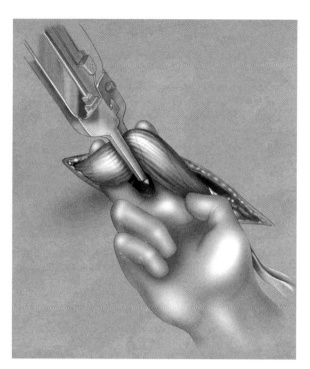

FIGURE 130C.8 The cervical esophagus is divided obliquely with the GIA stapler. (Reprinted from Orringer MB. Transhiatal esophagectomy without thoracotomy. *Oper Tech Thorac Cardiovasc Surg* 2005;10:63. Copyright © 2005 Elsevier. With permission.)

lateral and superior mediastinal attachments. These attachments can then be divided under direct vision and the specimen delivered into the abdominal cavity. Immediately after delivering the esophagus into the abdominal cavity, the posterior mediastinum is inspected for bleeding from the esophageal bed and any major hemorrhage controlled. A large abdominal gauze pack is inserted through the diaphragmatic hiatus into the posterior mediastinum and left in place to tamponade any minor bleeding as the stomach is prepared for its relocation into the chest. Similarly, narrow-gauge packs are gently inserted through the cervical incision into the upper mediastinum while continually protecting the recurrent laryngeal nerve from direct injury.

The stomach is then tubularized to create the conduit for reconstruction. The mobilized stomach and esophagus are lifted out of the abdominal cavity, and the gastric fundus is grasped and retracted superiorly. An area along the lesser curvature at the level of the second vascular arcade from the esophagus is cleared and the vascularized tissue is stapled with a vascular load. The gastric fundus is then retracted superiorly, and the lesser curvature of the stomach is progressively divided with sequential applications of a GIA stapler with a thick tissue load, approximately 4 to 6 cm distal to the palpable tumor (Fig. 130C.9). After each application of the stapler, the stomach is progressively stretched cephalad, thereby straightening the natural bend of the lesser curvature to the right and maximizing the upward reach of the stomach. For tumors of the upper and middle esophagus and in cases of benign disease requiring esophagectomy, as little stomach as possible is sacrificed to preserve gastric submucosal collateral circulation to the fundus. Care is taken during this portion of the operation to ensure that all perigastric lymph nodes are included with the specimen. After removal of the specimen, lymph node packets are often dissected off on the back table and sent as separate specimens, in order to ensure the highest yield of nodal tissue for staging. The staple line on the conduit is then

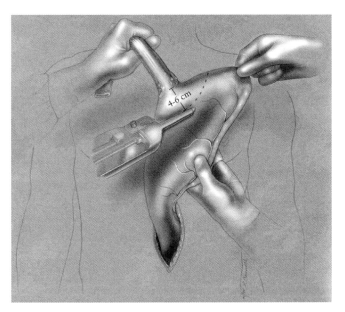

FIGURE 130C.9 After transhiatal mobilization of the esophagus has been completed, along with division of the cervical esophagus and mobilization of the stomach with the attached esophagus out of the abdomen and onto the anterior chest, traction is applied to the gastric fundus at the point that reaches most superior to the neck. For tumors of the distal esophagus and esophagogastric junction, the GIA surgical stapler is applied to the stomach 4 to 6 cm distal to the esophagogastric junction. For upper- and middle-third esophageal tumors and benign disease requiring an esophagectomy, as little stomach as possible is resected in order to maximize gastric submucosal collateral flow to the fundus. (Reprinted from Orringer MB. Transhiatal esophagectomy without thoracotomy. *Oper Tech Thorac Cardiovasc Surg* 2005;10:63. Copyright © 2005 Elsevier. With permission.)

oversewn with running 4-0 Prolene sutures. Traction on the stomach should be maintained as the staple line is oversewn, and two sutures are used: one for the first half and one for the second, to avoid "purse stringing" the staple line and interference with the upward reach of the stomach.

The abdominal pack that was placed into the mediastinum through the diaphragmatic hiatus and those in the superior mediastinum through the cervical incision are now removed. A long Penrose drain is suctioned to the Salem Sump drain and delivered through the cervical incision and into the abdominal cavity. Suction is turned off and the Penrose removed from the drain so that one end is in the abdominal cavity and the other end protruding from the cervical incision. The conduit is oriented appropriately and sutured to the Penrose in two places, taking care to maintain orientation. The gastric fundus is then grasped gently by the fingertips of one hand, which guide the stomach through the diaphragmatic hiatus and upward anterior to the spine, beneath the aortic arch, and into the superior mediastinum (Fig. 130C.10). Gentle traction is placed on the Penrose during this maneuver to assist in delivery of the conduit without twisting or kinking; however, it is important to avoid putting any actual tension on the conduit to avoid injury—the Penrose should only be used to facilitate a smooth transfer of the conduit without twisting of the gastric tip. A Babcock clamp inserted into the superior mediastinum through the cervical incision is used to deliver the gastric fundus into the neck wound until the stomach can be grasped with the fingers and gently pulled upward (Fig. 130C.11). Great care is taken to avoid traumatizing the stomach in this process. The Babcock clamp is not completely closed, and the stom-

ach is delivered into the neck more by pushing from below than traction from above. A healthy pink, correctly oriented gastric fundus tip in the neck wound is the goal of this repositioning of the stomach. A moistened thoracic gauze pack is inserted into the thoracic inlet posterior to the stomach to prevent the stomach from slipping back into the posterior mediastinum. The anterior surface of the stomach is carefully palpated through the hiatus and the neck incision to be certain that it has not become twisted within the posterior mediastinum during its positioning in the chest. In the rare situation in which mediastinal fibrosis from prior inflammation or irradiation results in posterior mediastinal narrowing that does not accommodate the stomach, it may be necessary to develop a retrosternal tunnel, resect the sternoclavicular joint, and place the stomach retrosternally.

The cervical esophagogastric side to side anastomosis is then performed using the 3-cm long, 3.5-mm Endo GIA stapler, as reported by Orringer and colleagues.[77] A 1.5-cm gastrotomy is made with the cutting current of the needle-tipped cautery device several centimeters proximal to the edge of the conduit (Fig. 130C.12). The location of the gastrotomy is chosen keeping in mind the length of the esophagus available and the size of the stapler cartridge to be used for the posterior portion of the anastomosis. The proximal esophagus is grasped with an atraumatic forceps and the staple line is amputated sharply with a fresh no. 10 blade in an oblique fashion so that the anterior portion of the esophagus is slightly longer than the posterior portion, which facilitates the shape of the anastomosis (Fig. 130C.13). The amputated staple line is sent to pathology as a proximal margin. Two full thickness 4-0 Vicryl stay sutures are placed for traction:

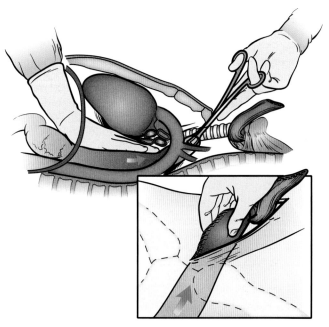

FIGURE 130C.10 The mobilized stomach is gently manipulated by one hand through the diaphragmatic hiatus upward beneath the aortic arch into the superior mediastinum until the tip of the gastric fundus can be grasped with a Babcock clamp inserted through the cervical incision. The clamp is applied gently, not completely ratcheting the handle, and is used to deliver the gastric fundus into the neck wound until it can be grasped with the fingertips (**inset**). Then, 4 to 6 cm of the stomach is brought into the neck wound more by pushing upward from below in the chest than by pulling from above in the neck. (Reprinted from Orringer MB, Marshall B, Iannettoni MD. Eliminating the cervical esophagogastric anastomotic leak with a side-to-side stapled anastomosis. *J Thorac Cardiovasc Surg* 2000;119:277. Copyright © 2000 The American Association for Thoracic Surgery. With permission.)

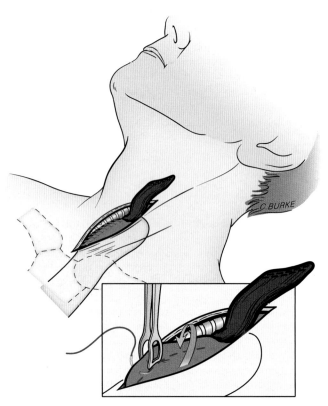

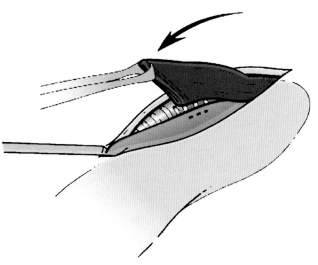

FIGURE 130C.11 When the stomach has been mobilized properly, 4 to 5 cm rests comfortably above the level of the clavicles along the cervical prevertebral fascia, well behind the end of the divided esophagus, which is retracted superiorly with an Allis clamp. The oversewn gastric staple line along the lesser curvature side of the stomach is toward the patient's right. A Babcock clamp (**inset**) grasps the anterior wall of the stomach low in the neck wound, where it emerges from the posterior mediastinum at the thoracic inlet, and the gastric staple line (*dotted line*) is rotated more medially. The stomach is elevated several more centimeters into the wound, and a seromuscular 3-0 cardiovascular silk traction suture is placed distal to the clamp. (Reprinted from Orringer MB, Marshall B, Iannettoni MD. Eliminating the cervical esophagogastric anastomotic leak with a side-to-side stapled anastomosis. *J Thorac Cardiovasc Surg* 2000;119:277. Copyright © 2000 The American Association for Thoracic Surgery. With permission.)

FIGURE 130C.12 The traction suture elevates the anterior gastric wall into the field and is fixed to the drapes with a hemostat. A point on the anterior gastric wall is selected for a 1.5-cm vertical gastrotomy (*dotted line*), which is performed with the cutting current of a needle-tipped electrocautery device. The gastrotomy must be located far enough inferior to the tip of the gastric fundus to allow subsequent full insertion of the 3-cm-long staple cartridge. Placement of the gastrotomy must also take into consideration the remaining length of cervical esophagus and should be performed with the realization that when the traction suture on the stomach is eventually removed, the stomach will partially retract downward into the thoracic inlet. Therefore, some redundancy in the length of the cervical esophagus should be allowed as the anastomosis is constructed. (Reprinted from Orringer MB, Marshall B, Iannettoni MD. Eliminating the cervical esophagogastric anastomotic leak with a side-to-side stapled anastomosis. *J Thorac Cardiovasc Surg* 2000;119:277. Copyright © 2000 The American Association for Thoracic Surgery. With permission.)

one through the anterior edge of the cut cervical esophagus and the other from the superior aspect of the gastrotomy through the posterior edge of the esophagus (Fig. 130C.14). The Endo GIA stapler is then positioned so that the anvil portion of the stapler is placed into the gastric conduit and the stapler cartridge is placed into the esophagus. With gentle downward traction on the stay sutures, the stapler is advanced, insuring correct alignment of the posterior wall of the esophagus and the anterior wall of the stomach (Fig. 130C.15). Once it is positioned appropriately, the stapler is closed. Two interrupted 4-0 Vicryl "suspension sutures" are placed on each side of the stapler, from the esophagus to the stomach. The stapler is then fired, creating the posterior portion of the esophagogastric anastomosis (Fig. 130C.16). After the stapler is fired, a 16-Fr nasogastric tube is inserted across the anastomosis and into the intrathoracic stomach for postoperative gastric decompression. The anterior portion of the anastomosis is completed in two layers (Fig. 130C.17). The first layer is a full-thickness layer performed with a running 4-0 PDS suture; one stitch is started from each corner of the anastomosis and ran toward the center where the two stitches are tied together. Care is taken to dunk the mucosa on each side into the anastomosis for adequate mucosal approximation. The second layer consists of interrupted 4-0

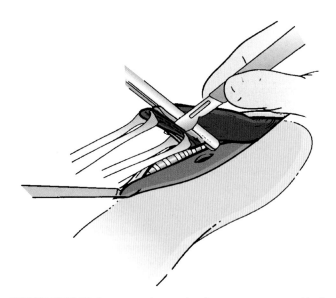

FIGURE 130C.13 An atraumatic vascular forceps serves as a guide for amputation of the cervical esophageal staple suture line, which is sent to the pathology department as the proximal esophageal margin. The original oblique placement of the stapler used to divide the cervical esophagus was purposeful, because the anterior tip of the esophagus should be longer than the posterior corner in construction of the anastomosis. (Reprinted from Orringer MB, Marshall B, Iannettoni MD. Eliminating the cervical esophagogastric anastomotic leak with a side-to-side stapled anastomosis. *J Thorac Cardiovasc Surg* 2000;119:277. Copyright © 2000 The American Association for Thoracic Surgery. With permission.)

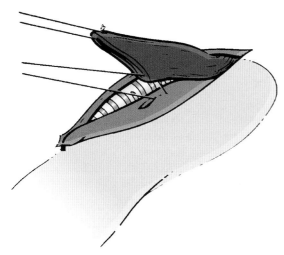

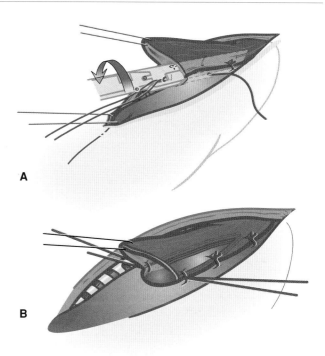

FIGURE 130C.14 Two full-thickness anastomotic stay sutures (4-0 Vicryl) are placed, one from the anterior tip of the cut cervical esophagus, and one at the midpoint of the upper edge of the transverse gastrotomy and the posterior corner of the esophagus. (Reprinted from Orringer MB, Marshall B, Iannettoni MD. Eliminating the cervical esophagogastric anastomotic leak with a side-to-side stapled anastomosis. *J Thorac Cardiovasc Surg* 2000;119:277. Copyright © 2000 The American Association for Thoracic Surgery. With permission.)

FIGURE 130C.16 **A:** The stapler is closed, thereby approximating the jaws, but before it is fired, two "suspension" sutures between the anterior stomach and the adjacent esophagus are placed on either side. **B:** When the knife assembly of the stapler is advanced, the "common wall" between the esophagus and stomach is cut and a 3-cm-long side-to-side anastomosis created. Corner sutures are then placed at either side of the gastrotomy. (Reprinted from Orringer MB, Marshall B, Iannettoni MD. Eliminating the cervical esophagogastric anastomotic leak with a side-to-side stapled anastomosis. *J Thorac Cardiovasc Surg* 2000;119:277. Copyright © 2000 The American Association for Thoracic Surgery. With permission.)

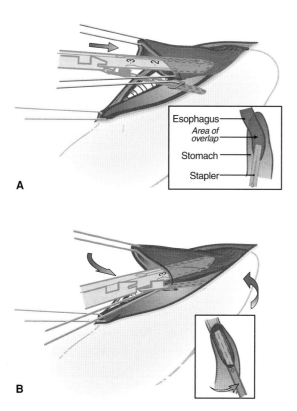

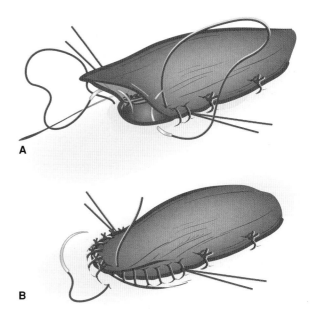

FIGURE 130C.15 **A:** With downward traction on the anastomotic stay sutures, the 3-cm-long EndoGIA staple cartridge is inserted: the thinner "anvil" portion into the stomach and the thicker staple-bearing portion into the esophagus. **B:** The staple cartridge is advanced into the esophagus and stomach. To achieve alignment of the posterior wall of the cervical esophagus and the anterior wall of the stomach, the stapler is rotated so that it is pointing toward the patient's right ear (**insets**) as it is inserted and advanced into the esophagus and stomach. (Reprinted from Orringer MB, Marshall B, Iannettoni MD. Eliminating the cervical esophagogastric anastomotic leak with a side-to-side stapled anastomosis. *J Thorac Cardiovasc Surg* 2000;119:277. Copyright © 2000 The American Association for Thoracic Surgery. With permission.)

FIGURE 130C.17 The gastrotomy and remaining open esophagus are approximated in two layers: a running inner layer of 4-0 monofilament absorbable suture (**A**) and an outer interrupted layer (**B**), which incorporates the anterior wall of the upper esophagus. (Reprinted from Orringer MB, Marshall B, Iannettoni MD. Eliminating the cervical esophagogastric anastomotic leak with a side-to-side stapled anastomosis. *J Thorac Cardiovasc Surg* 2000;119:277. Copyright © 2000 The American Association for Thoracic Surgery. With permission.)

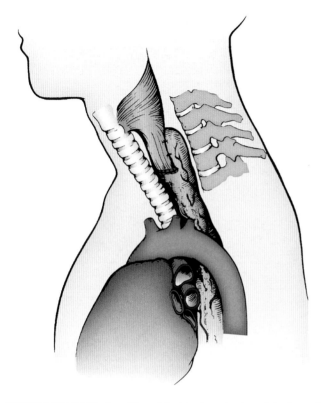

FIGURE 130C.18 Final position of the intrathoracic stomach in the neck after transhiatal esophagectomy and cervical esophagogastrostomy. The two sutures on either side of the anastomosis placed between the back of the cervical esophagus and the adjacent stomach limit tension on the anastomosis. These anterior "suspension" sutures are safer and preferable to tacking sutures between the stomach and the prevertebral fascia, which carry the risk of needle inoculation of the spine. (From Iannettoni MD, Whyte RI, Orringer MB. Catastrophic complications of the cervical esophagogastric anastomosis. *J Thorac Cardiovasc Surg* 1995;110:1493, with permission.)

PDS stitches placed in Lembert fashion. When the anastomosis is completed, metallic hemostatic clips are placed on either side of the anastomosis for future radiographic localization of the anastomosis. At the conclusion of the operation, the cervical anastomosis is located approximately 19 to 20 cm from the upper incisors or 4 to 5 cm distal to the upper esophageal sphincter (Fig. 130C.18), and the pyloromyotomy site rests 2 to 3 cm below the diaphragmatic hiatus. A small caliber Penrose drain is cut down the middle for several centimeters and draped over the anastomosis. The drain is brought out through the cervical incision and the incision is closed loosely with absorbable suture and two deep layers. The skin is closed with a running nylon suture that can easily be removed in the event of a leak.

The abdominal cavity is reinspected and hemostasis is ensured. The diaphragmatic hiatus is inspected and narrowed with 3-0 silk crural sutures as needed so that it loosely accommodates three fingers of the surgeon's hand alongside the stomach. The anterior gastric wall is sutured at one or two points to the edge of the diaphragmatic hiatus with interrupted 3-0 silk sutures to prevent subsequent intrathoracic herniation of abdominal viscera alongside the intrathoracic stomach.[78,79] A 14F feeding jejunostomy tube is placed in all patients, approximately 30 cm distal to the ligament of Treitz. A Witzel maneuver is performed and the tube brought out through a stab incision in the left lateral abdominal wall. The bowel is tacked to the abdominal wall in several places around the tube. The abdominal incision is closed in layers. Bilateral chest tubes are placed at the nipple level in the midaxillary line. The nasogastric tube is routinely

sewn to the nasal septum to prevent accidental dislodgement. The patient is extubated in the operating room and taken to the postanesthesia care unit (PACU).

A portable chest radiograph is obtained in the PACU to ensure that no unrecognized pneumothorax or hemothorax exists, and the tip of the nasogastric tube is in good position above the level of the diaphragmatic hiatus. With meticulous attention to preoperative pulmonary physiotherapy, including complete abstinence from cigarette smoking for at least 3 weeks and regular use of an incentive inspirometer, as well as postoperative epidural anesthesia to improve respiratory dynamics, neither postoperative mechanical ventilation nor intensive care unit stay is routinely required.

TRANSHIATAL ESOPHAGECTOMY FOR CARCINOMA OF THE ESOPHAGOGASTRIC JUNCTION

The technique of THE and proximal partial gastrectomy is applicable in most patients with carcinoma limited to the cardia and proximal stomach. It is generally possible to resect the proximal stomach in such a way that a 4 to 6 cm gastric margin still exists beyond the tumor (Fig. 130C.19). So long as the entire greater curvature of the

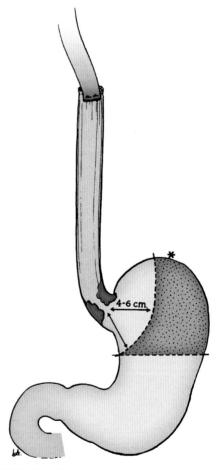

FIGURE 130C.19 Transhiatal esophagectomy for carcinoma of the cardia. Transection of the stomach along the lesser curvature 4 to 6 cm distal to palpable tumor preserves the point (*asterisk*) that reaches most cephalad and stomach that was formerly removed with a standard hemigastrectomy (*stippled area*). (Reprinted from Orringer MB, Sloan H. Esophagectomy without thoracotomy. *J Thorac Cardiovasc Surg* 1978;76:643. Copyright © 1978 The American Association for Thoracic Surgery. With permission.)

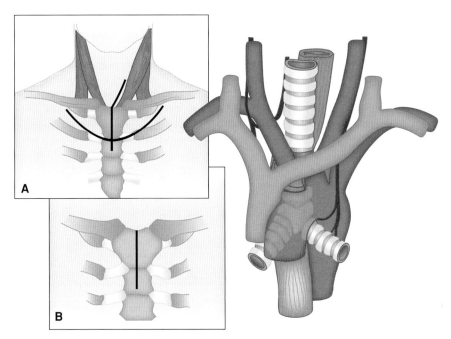

FIGURE 130C.20 Exposure of the upper mediastinum through a partial upper median sternotomy (**main drawing**). **A:** The usual left cervical skin incision used for transhiatal esophagectomy extends onto the anterior chest wall in the midline for a partial sternal split. Occasionally, a curved anterior thoracic skin incision with elevation of a skin flap can be used to avoid a scar in the low anterior neck. **B:** The sternotomy incision extending from the suprasternal notch through the manubrium. A small rib spreader inserted between the divided sternal edges provides the needed exposure to the cervicothoracic esophagus. (Reprinted from Orringer MB. Partial median sternotomy: anterior approach to the upper thoracic esophagus. *J Thorac Cardiovasc Surg* 1984;87:124. Copyright © 1984 The American Association for Thoracic Surgery. With permission.)

gastric fundus can be preserved, the point that reaches most cephalad to the neck is available for construction of the cervical anastomosis. Carcinomas of the cardia have a greater tendency to metastasize superiorly in the submucosal lymphatics of the esophagus rather than distally into the stomach, and recurrent carcinoma within the gastric remnant is uncommon and seldom produces recurrent dysphagia before the patient succumbs to metastatic disease. For all practical purposes, the traditional proximal hemigastrectomy, which has long been performed for carcinoma of the cardia, provides no better a cancer operation and wastes valuable stomach that can be used for esophageal replacement and a cervical esophagogastric anastomosis. It further commits the surgeon to an intrathoracic esophagogastric anastomosis with its potential attendant complications and postoperative challenges. DiMusto and Orringer[80] reported on 1,044 patients undergoing a THE, proximal partial gastrectomy (dividing the stomach 4 to 6 cm from palpable tumor), and cervical esophagogastric anastomosis for adenocarcinoma of the distal esophagus or cardia. Of these, only 20 (1.9%) were found to have a positive gastric margin on final pathologic evaluation. Eighty percent of these 20 patients died with distant metastases for which a more extensive gastric resection would have been futile. Local tumor recurrence in the intrathoracic stomach was documented in 20% and seldom caused dysphagia. Neither survival nor the incidence of local tumor recurrence was improved by adjuvant therapy in the nine patients who received it for their positive gastric margin. In summary, oncologic outcome was not diminished and the patients avoided a more extensive resection with its resultant morbidities.

TRANSSTERNAL APPROACH TO THE CERVICOTHORACIC ESOPHAGUS

Under certain circumstances, exposure of the esophagus distal to the point allowed via the standard cervical incision becomes necessary. Most commonly this occurs in patients with a short, thick neck in which adequate exposure for completion of the anastomosis cannot be obtained. Other situations that call for more distal exposure

include when patients have severe osteoarthritis of the neck or even torticollis, which limits neck extension and rotation, or when there is concern for adherence but not invasion of a mid- or upper-esophageal tumor to the membranous trachea. Anterior exposure of the low cervical and upper intrathoracic esophagus to the level of the carina is facilitated by performance of a partial upper median sternotomy (Fig. 130C.20).[81,82] The standard cervical incision is extended down the midline over the manubrium. The sternal notch is dissected out and the manubrium is split with a sternal saw. A small rib spreader is used to spread the manubrium after bluntly separating the sternomanubrial joint.

If transcervical and transhiatal mobilization of the esophagus suggests that there may be adherence of the tumor to the trachea, a partial upper sternotomy may allow direct visualization and sharp dissection of the esophagus from the posterior membranous trachea. After mobilizing the tumor away from the airway, the THE can then be performed as described previously.

MINIMALLY INVASIVE TRANSHIATAL ESOPHAGECTOMY

Recently, the authors have begun performing a minimally invasive hybrid approach to the THE, using a laparoscopic approach for the abdominal and transhiatal dissection, shaping the conduit extracorporeally, and a standard cervical incision and anastomosis. The goal is to minimize postoperative pain and complications while decreasing length of stay and maintaining oncologic outcomes.

The patient is placed in a low lithotomy position, but otherwise similar to standard positioning, with arms tucked, shoulder roll placed, and neck extended and rotated to the right. The patient is placed on a beanbag, to facilitate placement in reverse Trendelenburg position for the laparoscopic portion of the abdominal dissection. Ports are placed in similar position to a standard laparoscopic approach for a paraesophageal hernia, with the camera in a supraumbilical position. A 5-mm port is placed 2 cm under the right costal margin for the liver retractor. The main 12-mm dissecting ports are placed in the upper abdomen on the left and right sides and left lateral and right mid-abdominal 5-mm assistant ports are placed as well. The abdomen is insufflated with CO_2 gas to a pressure of 15 mm Hg. We attempt to maintain this pressure during the entire dissection, which can be a challenge during the mediastinal portion of the dissection as the abdominal cavity is connected with the open cervical incision. A laparoscopic liver retractor is used to elevate the left lobe of the liver and expose the diaphragmatic hiatus. The dissection begins in similar fashion to the standard open operation, using an energy device and starting just above the termination of the right gastroepiploic artery on the greater curvature and continuing to the left crus and then anterior through the phrenoesophageal membrane. Dissection is then continued distally along the greater curvature, making sure to visualize the gastroepiploic artery and vein during this dissection to avoid injury. The most complicated part of this portion of the operation, when done laparoscopically, is making sure to get as close to the bifurcation of the gastroduodenal artery as possible, without damaging the gastroepiploic vessels. Visualization of this area is much more difficult when done laparoscopically, especially if the patient has a large amount of intra-abdominal fat. The tendency is to terminate the dissection further away from the bifurcation than normal, in order to avoid injury; however, it is important to dissect as close as safely possible in order to preserve length for the conduit. The dissection is then continued through the gastrohepatic ligament to the right crus and the left gastric artery is stapled with an endovascular load, again taking care to sweep all perigastric lymph nodes to the specimen side of the stapler. A laparoscopic Kocher maneuver is completed to ensure maximum length on the conduit. Instead of a pyloromyotomy, botulinum toxin is routinely injected into the pylorus during the minimally invasive version of the THE. The pylorus is identified and grasped with a laparoscopic Babcock clamp and the injection is performed in three quadrants with a solution of 200u Botox in 5 mL normal saline. Intrapyloric botox has been shown to be an effective method of preventing delayed gastric emptying after esophagectomy in multiple studies, and appears to be a good alternative to pyloromyotomy.[83,84]

The mediastinal dissection is performed with an energy device, circumferential to the esophagus and progressing superiorly into the mediastinum. One advantage of performing this dissection in this manner is that visualization is often better than with the standard open operation. Lymph nodes can easily be seen and removed separately or with the specimen. Vessels are easily ligated with the energy device to decrease incidence of hemorrhage. As dissection progresses further into the mediastinum, the pleura can be violated. This can create hemodynamic instability, especially in the presence of CO_2 insufflation. If any hemodynamic instability or respiratory compromise is noted, bilateral chest tubes are placed immediately. Once chest tubes are in place, maintaining insufflation is more difficult and large volumes of CO_2 gas can be necessary to maintain the insufflation pressure at a level necessary for adequate visualization into the mediastinum. If necessary, the chest tubes are intermediately clamped and opened, to balance insufflation with hemodynamic stability. Alternatively, if available, a high-pressure trocar system, such as the AirSeal System (SurgiQuest, Milford, CT) is used to provide relatively stable pneumoperitoneum during this portion of the case. As dissection continues cephalad, the anterior portion of the dissection is completed using blunt dissection whenever possible, in order to avoid energy damage to the membranous trachea and aortic arch. Dissection is carried out as far into the mediastinum as can be visualized, circumferentially to the esophagus. A laparoscopic fan retractor is used anteriorly through the hiatus to facilitate visualization.

Once the mediastinal dissection has been completed as much as possible, the standard cervical incision is made and the esophagus identified and bluntly mobilized as directed above. A hand is placed into the cervical incision and the volar aspect of the fingers used to dissect bluntly down as far as possible into the mediastinum. At this point the camera is placed back into the mediastinum and the amount of tissue remaining between the two spaces evaluated. The laparoscopic mediastinal dissection is continued superiorly and cervical dissection continued inferiorly, often with assistance of a sponge on a stick until the two spaces can be connected posterior to the esophagus. The Salem Sump drain is again brought into the posterior mediastinum and grasped and pulled down into the abdominal cavity to help create a dry field. Once the two spaces are connected, the esophagus is stapled through the cervical incision in standard fashion. The distal stapled end is inverted down into the mediastinum and grasped from below. The two ends of the esophagus in the mediastinum can then be retracted for further exposure of the uppermost mediastinal attachments, which are then taken down bluntly and sharply to separate the specimen from the mediastinum. During this part of the dissection, the cervical wound is packed with a standard gauze pack to prevent loss of insufflation through the cervical wound. The esophagus and stomach are delivered down into the abdominal cavity. A laparoscopic jejunostomy tube is then placed 30 cm distal to the ligament of Treitz and secured to the abdominal wall with t-fasteners.

A 3 cm supraumbilical incision is then made and the specimen is brought out onto the field. The specimen is resected and the conduit shaped in the same manner as in the open operation. This portion is performed extracorporeally for two reasons: first, the incision must be made to remove the specimen from the field, and second, the aspect of shaping the conduit appropriately without compromising length is critical in order to have enough length to reach the cervical esophagus. When the conduit is shaped intracorporeally, it is difficult to straighten the stomach out enough to staple without curving and shortening the conduit. Once the conduit is created and oversewn, it is placed back into the abdominal cavity and the supraumbilical incision is closed with a Hassan trochar in place for the camera, and the abdomen is reinsufflated. The conduit is grasped and placed back through the mediastinum under direct vision, and oriented appropriately. It is directed superiorly until it can be grasped and brought out through the cervical incision. The rest of the operation is then completed in a similar manner as the standard open procedure described above. The authors only performed this minimally invasive technique for THE on carefully selected patients with low levels of intra-abdominal fat, no previous major intra-abdominal operations, and clearly resectable tumors. Neoadjuvant chemoradiotherapy has not been a contraindication for this technique. Results have been quite good. Operative blood loss and postoperative complications have been similar to that of patients undergoing the standard operation. Operative time is increased to approximately 5 hours, compared to around two and a half hours for open THE; however, this should improve along with the learning curve. No anastomotic leaks have occurred and average length of stay has been 4 days. More data must be accumulated, but minimally invasive THE appears to be a viable approach for selected patients.

POSTOPERATIVE CARE PROTOCOLS

Standardized postoperative care pathways have been shown to improve outcomes in surgical treatment of patients with esophageal cancer and this principle has been applied to the postoperative care of all patients undergoing THE.[85,86] In general, the patients are extubated in the operating room and do not go to the ICU, but rather to a specialized thoracic unit with telemetry and an experienced group of nursing staff who is familiar with the pathway and the standard care of postoperative THE patients. All patients receive a preoperative epidural catheter with a patient-controlled narcotic adjunct for optimal pain control, which is monitored daily by an experienced anesthesia team. This allows for early mobilization, as ambulation at the bedside is expected the day of surgery, followed by ambulation at least four times per day in the hallway starting on postoperative day 1. Chest tubes are removed when the output is serous and less than 200 cc per 8-hour shift, no air leak is present and the lung is completely inflated with no effusion or other concern on chest x-ray. This occurs on postoperative day 1 or 2 in the vast majority of patients. If there is concern for potential thoracic duct injury, the chest tubes are left in until patient is tolerating J-tube feeds. Jejunostomy tube feedings are started at 30 cc/hr on postoperative day 3 and advanced steadily toward goal. The epidural is usually removed on postoperative day 4, after all chest tubes are out and the patient is tolerating jejunostomy tube feedings at goal and able to take pain medicine via j-tube. The nasogastric tube is removed on postoperative day 4 and the patient undergoes an upper GI swallow study on day 5 to assess for leak or stricture (Fig. 130C.21). If the swallow study looks ok, the Penrose drain in the neck is removed and the patient is discharged home, on postoperative day 5. Patients are kept NPO until at least postoperative day 15, which has been shown in several retrospective studies, including one by the author, to be associated with a significant decrease in anastomotic leak rate.[87–89] Follow-up is arranged

approximately 3 weeks postoperatively, unless situations arise to necessitate an earlier evaluation.

DELAYED ORAL INTAKE AND ANASTOMOTIC LEAK RATE

In 2008, a prospective change in the postoperative pathway of the author's patients was undertaken, to eliminate all voluntary oral intake until at least postoperative day 15.[87] This change was applied to all patients undergoing THE for any reason. All patients underwent placement of a jejunostomy tube and tube feedings were initiated on postoperative day 3, if appropriate. This change was put in place based on the theory that increased tension from a food bolus or stress from gastric distension could contribute to anastomotic leaks, and by avoiding any unnecessary oral intake while the anastomosis heals, the leak rate can be reduced. A retrospective chart review of all patients undergoing THE by the author between February 2004 and November 2013 was performed to evaluate the effect of this prospective change. Ninety-four patients were included in the early oral intake group and 129 were included in the delayed oral intake group. All other postoperative variables were the same in both groups, and all operations were performed by the same senior surgeon, using the same technique, at the same institution. Of note, a significantly higher number of patients in the delayed oral intake group underwent THE for adenocarcinoma and had received neoadjuvant chemoradiation. In the past, neoadjuvant therapy has been considered to lead to higher anastomotic leak rate; however, recent studies have called this into question.[90–92] The delayed oral intake group could potentially be considered a higher risk group, however, because of the increased incidence of neoadjuvant therapy. The population profiles of the study groups were otherwise similar, and all leaks were reported, regardless of the timing of the leak.

Postoperative outcomes are shown in Table 130C.2. There was a statistically significant decrease in the rate of anastomotic leak between the delayed oral intake and early oral intake groups, which was 3.9% in the delayed oral intake group and 14.8% in the early oral intake group, respectively (P <0.01). The rate of esophageal stricture (known to be an associated sequelae of anastomotic leak)[77] in the delayed oral intake group was 12.4%, which was significantly less than the 27.6% present in the oral feeding group (p <0.01). One patient with a leak had a positive margin at a high cervical anastomosis and one had a stent in place during neoadjuvant chemoradiation that was difficult to remove resulting in significant gastric damage

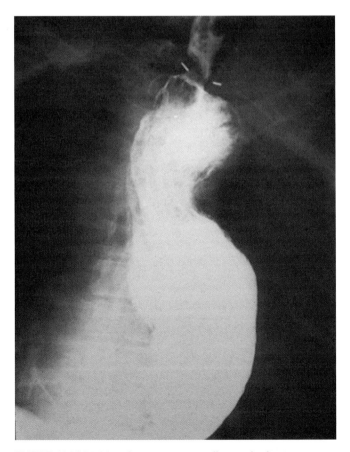

FIGURE 130C.21 Typical postoperative swallow study showing contrast passing through into the esophagus and filling the gastric conduit with no anastomotic leak. Metallic clips are seen at the anastomosis.

TABLE 130C.2 Postoperative Patient Outcomes: Early Oral Intake (POD 3) Versus Delayed Oral Intake (POD 15)

Variable[a]	POD 3 (n = 94)	POD 15 (n = 129)	P-value
Average blood loss (mL)	310 (200–300)	276 (200–300)	0.415
Operative mortality	3.0%	2.3%	0.693
Length of stay (days)	10.4 (6–11)	6.9 (5–6)	<0.001
Any ICU stay	20.8%	9.3%	0.004
Esophageal stricture	27.6%	12.4%	0.004
Anastomotic leak	14.8%	3.9%	0.004

[a]Continuous data are shown as mean (25 to 75th percentile) and categoric data are shown as a percent.

during removal. The leak rate in patients without positive margins and without a foreign body in place was 2.3%. Mean hospital length of stay was 6.9 days in the delayed intake group and 10.4 days in the early oral intake group (p <0.01). There was also a significant decrease seen in the percentage of patients who required any length of stay in the ICU (9.3% vs. 20.8%; p <0.01). Mortality and blood loss were similar among the groups. The decrease in rate of stricture formation appears to be directly correlated to the decrease in anastomotic leak rate, and results in the decrease in chronic morbidity following esophagectomy. This leads to earlier return to work and other normal activity and improved patient satisfaction. By analyzing the cost of serial dilations, along with the average number of dilations that a patient with a stricture receives (7.7 per stricture in our patient population), we calculate a cost savings of $3,233 per patient by eliminating the need for serial dilations alone, when a leak is avoided.

The data in this study are supported by two other recent studies.[88,89] Because of this data, the standard postoperative pathway has been permanently changed to delaying oral intake in all postesophagectomy patients under the author's care.

INTRAOPERATIVE COMPLICATIONS

Mediastinal hemorrhage is uncommon, but can occur from multiple sources. Splenic injury or splenic vascular injury is the most common intra-abdominal source of major hemorrhage during THE. During the mediastinal dissection, tearing of the azygos vein can lead to significant hemorrhage and the need for thoracotomy. Much more uncommon, but potentially devastating are injuries to the aorta and heart during mediastinal dissection, which carry a high mortality rate. In the largest reported series of THE, Orringer and colleagues[67] reported intraoperative death in 4/2007 (0.2%) THE patients from uncontrollable mediastinal hemorrhage, and another 8/2007 (0.4%) patients with inordinate massive blood loss (>4,000 mL), most commonly from a torn azygos vein. In the author's[87] series, evaluated as part of the delayed oral intake study above, the average reported operative blood loss was approximately 300 mL per case.

Left recurrent nerve injury during the cervical dissection is a known and preventable complication. It is important to avoid placement of a retractor against the tracheoesophageal groove during this dissection, and to ensure that the dissection occurs well posterolateral to the groove. The nerve is not routinely identified during the dissection, in order to avoid inadvertent injury while trying to visualize it. There is correlation between surgeon experience and incidence of recurrent nerve injury, and incidence is reported as 2% to 22% in various series.[67,93,94] In general, injury to the nerve is identified by the presence of postoperative hoarseness, which resolves in 3 to 6 months in the majority of cases.[67,94] If hoarseness is persistent, or if more serious complications occur, such as recurrent aspiration and respiratory distress, treatment involves a vocal cord medialization procedure.

Injury to the membranous trachea, which occurs in approximately 1% of cases, is a potentially significant complication that can occur during mediastinal dissection, especially in patients with mid- and upper-esophageal tumors and in those with significant adhesions in the upper mediastinum.[67,95] It is important to evaluate these patients preoperatively with a bronchoscopy to identify those with invasion of the membranous trachea, and even without invasion, to take extra care during the mediastinal dissection to avoid tracheal injury. If membranous tracheobronchial injury occurs, it must be repaired, either via thoracotomy or partial sternal split. Other potential intraoperative complications include injury to the spleen,

which occasionally leads to the need for splenectomy; mucosal injury during pyloromyotomy, which must be recognized, repaired, and reinforced with omentum; and damage to the gastric conduit itself or to the gastroepiploic vessels, which can necessitate abandonment of the stomach as the conduit and the need for a temporary esophageal diversion while preparing for reconstruction.

POSTOPERATIVE COMPLICATIONS

The incidence of anastomotic leak and anastomotic stricture is described above. Using the side-to-side stapled cervical anastomosis described by Orringer et al.[77] and delaying oral intake in patients until at least 15 days postoperatively has led to a reduction in the anastomotic leak rate to 2% to 3%. Anastomotic leaks typically present themselves with either increasing purulent drainage from the cervical drain, erythema and swelling or drainage from the cervical incision, or less commonly, as an occult leak on the swallow study. While some occult leaks can be treated with observation or endoscopic stenting, when purulence and subcutaneous inflammation occur, the standard treatment is opening of the cervical incision and drainage of the purulence. The vast majority of cervical anastomotic leaks can be treated this way, and rare is the case when immediate operative intervention is warranted. In the infrequent case of gastric tip necrosis, the conduit must be taken down and a cervical esophagostomy created. Gastric tip necrosis can be prevented by adhering strictly to conduit preservation and dissection techniques previously described, by taking care to preserve the entire length of the right gastroepiploic artery and vein, and by closely evaluating the gastric tip once it is positioned in the neck to make sure it remains pink and viable. If there is any question as to conduit viability, the anastomosis is often delayed and an esophagostomy is created.[96,97] The conduit is left in place and the patient is returned to the operating room in 8 to 12 weeks for re-evaluation of the conduit and anastomosis at that time. In 15 patients in the author's series who have undergone this management strategy, all have had complete healing with no anastomotic leak, and excellent functional results in all but one patient who required several elective dilations.[96]

While a cervical anastomotic leak rarely leads to mediastinitis or sepsis, a much more common problem is the long term sequela of the leak-anastomotic stricture. Chronic strictures and long-term dysphagia are seen in up to 60% of patients after a cervical anastomotic leak.[77] Serial dilations are often required in these patients, and complications of dilation, including conduit perforation and trachea-conduit fistulas, are not uncommon. Patients who develop an anastomotic stricture are serially dilated with 36-, 40-, and 46-Fr and larger Maloney dilators. The need for repeat dilation is determined by the reappearance of cervical dysphagia, and patients are encouraged to return for repeat dilation as soon as their dysphagia returns. Early intervention is critical to avoid worsening stenosis and scarring to the point where perforation and trachea-conduit fistulas are likely. In cases where multiple recurrent dilations are likely, motivated patients can be taught the technique of self-dilation.[98] In general, balloon dilatation of a cervical esophagogastric anastomotic stricture is not nearly as effective as the use of Maloney dilators.

Incidence of chylothorax is rare after THE (1% to 3%),[67,99,100] and in most cases aggressive treatment with ligation of the thoracic duct near the diaphragm is recommended. Some cases can be managed more conservatively, with nutritional adjustments, and thoracic duct embolization can be considered if available. Other potential postoperative complications include intra-abdominal and wound infections, and respiratory complications. While mortality is still reported as high as 9% in some low volume centers, much more acceptable mortality rates of 0.3% to 3% are typically reported in high volume centers with experienced surgeons and standardized postoperative pathways.[67,87,96] Randomized trials and meta-analyses have shown that the transhiatal approach has a reduced incidence of pulmonary complications, decreased pain, shorter length of stay, and lower perioperative mortality, when compared with a transthoracic approach.[90,101–103]

PATIENT SATISFACTION

In Orringer's large series of 2007 THEs, 89% of patients with either cancer or benign disease indicated that they were generally pleased with their ability to eat, 87% stated that they were better off than before their THE, and 96% stated that they would have the same operation again if faced with the same circumstances.[67] Patients undergoing a cervical anastomosis, when compared with those who have undergone transthoracic anastomosis, consistently have higher quality of life data, along with higher social and physical functioning scores. This is largely due to less frequent reflux-related symptoms in patients with a cervical anastomosis.[104]

SUMMARY

THE without thoracotomy is a reliable and effective method of esophageal resection when performed in accordance with a strict set of principles. Using recent advances in technique and postoperative care, complications are becoming less and less frequent and the leak rate can be reduced to minimal levels. A large majority of patients can be safely resected using this technique, with excellent outcomes and long-term survival for cancer that is equivalent to other resection techniques.

REFERENCES

1. Orringer MB. Transhiatal esophagectomy without thoracotomy In: Shields TW ed., *Thoracic Surgery*. Riverwoods, IL: LWW; 2009:1771–1794.
2. Denk W. Zur Radikaloperation des Oesophaguskarfzentralbl. *Chirurgie* 1913; 40:1065–1068.
3. Turner GG. Excision of the thoracic oesophagus for carcinoma with construction of extrathoracic gullet. *Lancet* 1933;2:1315–1316.
4. LeQuesne LP, Ranger D. Pharyngogastrectomy with immediate pharyngogastric anastomosis. *Br J Surg* 1966;53:105–109.
5. Ong GB, Lee TC. Pharyngogastric anastomosis after oesophagopharyngectomy for carcinoma of the hypopharynx and cervical oesophagus. *Br J Surg* 1960;48:193–200.
6. Rehn L. Operationen an dem Brustabschnitt der Speiserohre. (Operations on the Esophagus in the Region of the Chest.) *Verh Deutsch Ges Chir* 1898;27:448.
7. Llobet AF. L'operation de Nassilov: la premiére intervention á Buenos Aires. (Nassilous operation: first in Buenos Aires.) *Rev Chir Paris* 1900;21:647.
8. Torek F. The operative treatment of carcinoma of the oesophagus. *Ann Surg* 1915;61:385–405.
9. Ohsawa T. The surgery of the esophagus. *Arch Jpn Chir* 1933;10:605.
10. Marshall SF. Carcinoma of the esophagus. *Surg Clin North Am* 1938;18:643.
11. Adams WE, Phemister DB. Carcinoma of the lower thoracic esophagus: report of a successful resection and esophagogastrostomy. *J Thorac Surg* 1938;7:621.
12. Churchill ED, Sweet RH. Transthoracic resection of tumors of the stomach and esophagus. *Ann Surg* 1942;115:897–920.
13. Garlock JH. Combined abdominothoracic approach for carcinoma of cardia and lower esophagus. *Surg Gynecol Obstet* 1946;83:737–741.
14. Carter BN. The combined thoraco-abdominal approach with particular reference to its employment in splenectomy. *Surg Gynecol Obstet* 1947;84:1019–1028.
15. Lewis I. The surgical treatment of carcinoma of the esophagus with special reference to a new operation for growths of the middle third. *Br J Surg* 1946;34:18–31.
16. Ong GB. Resection and reconstruction of the esophagus. *Curr Probl Surg* 1971;8:3–56.
17. McKeown KC. Trends in oesophageal resection for carcinoma, with special reference to total oesophagectomy. *Ann R Coll Surg Engl* 1972;51:213–239.
18. McKeown KC. Total three-stage oesophagectomy for cancer of the esophagus. *Br J Surg* 1976;63:259–262.
19. Akiyama H, Tsurumaru M, Kawamura T, et al. Principles of surgical treatment for carcinoma of the esophagus: analysis of lymph node involvement. *Ann Surg* 1981;194:438–446.
20. Mitchell RL. Abdominal and right thoracotomy approach as standard procedure for esophagogastrectomy with low morbidity. *J Thorac Cardiovasc Surg* 1987; 93:205–211.
21. Mathisen DJ, Grillo HC, Wilkins EW, et al. Transthoracic esophagectomy: a safe approach to carcinoma of the esophagus. *Ann Thorac Surg* 1988;45:137–143.
22. Ellis FH Jr. Carcinoma of the esophagus. *CA Cancer J Clin* 1983;33:264–281.
23. Posthlethwait RW. Complications and deaths after operations for esophageal carcinoma. *J Thorac Cardiovasc Surg* 1983;85:827–831.
24. Earlam R, Cunha-Melo JR. Oesophageal squamous cell carcinoma. I. A critical review of surgery. *Br J Surg* 1980;67:381–390.
25. Giuli R, Gignoux M. Treatment of carcinoma of the esophagus. Retrospective study of 2400 patients. *Ann Surg* 1980;192:44–52.
26. Muller JM, Erasmi H, Stelzner M, et al. Surgical therapy of oesophageal carcinoma. *Br J Surg* 1990;77:845–857.
27. Orringer MB, Sloan H. Esophagectomy without thoracotomy. *J Thorac Cardiovasc Surg* 1978;76:643–654.
28. Katariya K, Harvey JC, Pina E, et al. Complications of transhiatal esophagectomy. *J Surg Oncol* 1994;57:157–163.
29. Goldminc M, Maddern G, LePrise E, et al. Oesophagectomy by transhiatal approach or thoracotomy: a prospective randomized trial. *Br J Surg* 1993;80:367–370.
30. Hagen JA, Peters JH, DeMeester TR. Superiority of extended en bloc esophagectomy for carcinoma of the lower esophagus and cardia. *J Thorac Cardiovasc Surg* 1993;106:850–859.
31. Naunheim KS, Hanosh J, Zwischenberger J, et al. Esophagectomy in the septuagenarian. *Ann Thorac Surg* 1993;56:880–883.
32. Pac M, Basoglu A, Kocak H, et al. Transhiatal versus transthoracic esophagectomy for esophageal cancer. *J Thorac Cardiovasc Surg* 1993;106:205–209.
33. Tilanus HW, Hop WC, Langenhorst BL, et al. Esophagectomy with or without thoracotomy. Is there any difference? *J Thorac Cardiovasc Surg* 1993;105:898–903.
34. Gertsch P, Vauthey JN, Lustenberger AA, et al. Long-term results of transhiatal esophagectomy for esophageal carcinoma. A multivariate analysis of prognostic factors. *Cancer* 1993;72:2312–2319.
35. Vigneswaran WT, Trastek VF, Pairolero PC, et al. Transhiatal esophagectomy for carcinoma of the esophagus. *Ann Thorac Surg* 1993;56:838–844; discussion 844–846.
36. Bolton JS, Ochsner JL, Abdoh A. Surgical management of esophageal cancer: a decade of change. *Ann Surg* 1994;219:475–480.
37. Putnam JB Jr, Suell DM, McMurtrey MJ, et al. Comparison of three techniques of esophagectomy within a residency training program. *Ann Thorac Surg* 1994;57:319–325.
38. Berdejo L. Transhiatal versus transthoracic esophagectomy for clinical stage I esophageal carcinoma. *Hepatogastroenterology* 1995;42:789–791.
39. Bonavina L. Early oesophageal cancer: results of a European multicentre survey. *Br J Surg* 1995;82:98–101.
40. Horstmann O, Verreet PR, Becker H, et al. Transhiatal oesophagectomy compared with transthoracic resection and systematic lymphadenectomy for the treatment of oesophageal cancer. *Eur J Surg* 1995;161:557–567.
41. Millikan KW, Silverstein J, Hart V, et al. A 15-year review of esophagectomy for carcinoma of thc csophagus and cardia. *Arch Surg* 1995;130:617–624.
42. Svanes K, Stangeland L, Viste A, et al. Morbidity, ability to swallow, and survival after oesophagectomy for cancer of the oesophagus and cardia. *Eur J Surg* 1995;161:669–675.
43. Junginger T, Dutkowski P. Selective approach to the treatment of oesophageal cancer. *Br J Surg* 1996;83:1473–1477.
44. Stark SP, Romberg MS, Pierce GE, et al. Transhiatal versus transthoracic esophagectomy for adenocarcinoma of the distal esophagus and cardia. *Am J Surg* 1996;172:478–481.
45. Beik AI, Jaffray B, Anderson JR. Transhiatal oesophagectomy: a comparison of alternative techniques in 68 patients. *J R Coll Surg Edinb* 1996;25:25–29.
46. Gupta NM. Oesophagectomy without thoracotomy: first 250 patients. *Eur J Surg* 1996;162:455–461.
47. Chu KM, Law SY, Fok M, et al. A prospective randomized comparison of transhiatal and transthoracic resection for lower-third esophageal carcinoma. *Am J Surg* 1997;174:320–324.
48. Jacobi CA, Zieren HU, Muller JM, et al. Surgical therapy of esophageal carcinoma: the influence of surgical approach and esophageal resection on cardiopulmonary function. *Eur J Cardiothorac Surg* 1997;11:32–37.
49. Thomas P, Doddoli C, Lienne P, et al. Changing patterns and surgical results in adenocarcinoma of the oesophagus. *Br J Surg* 1997;84:119–125.
50. Pommier RF, Vetto JT, Ferris BL, et al. Relationships between operative approaches and outcomes in esophageal cancer. *Am J Surg* 1998;175:422–425.
51. Dudhat SB, Shinde SR. Transhiatal esophagectomy for squamous cell carcinoma of the esophagus. *Dis Esophagus* 1998;11:226–230.
52. Gillinov AM, Heitmiller RF. Strategies to reduce pulmonary complications after transhiatal esophagectomy. *Dis Esophagus* 1998;11:43–47.
53. Gluch L, Smith RC, Bambach CP, et al. Comparison of outcomes following transhiatal or Ivor Lewis esophageactomy for esophageal carcinoma. *World J Surg* 1999;23:271–275.
54. Torres AJ, Sanchez-Pernaute A, Hernando F, et al. Two-field radical lymphadenectomy in the treatment of esophageal carcinoma. *Dis Esophagus* 1999;12:137–143.
55. Boyle MJ, Franceschi D, Livingstone AS. Transhiatal versus transthoracic esophagectomy: complication and survival rates. *Am Surg* 1999;65:1137–1141.

56. van Sandick JW, Obertop H, Fockens P, et al. Transhiatal esophagus resection without thoracotomy for carcinoma: complications, hospital mortality and prognosis in 115 patients. *Ned Tijdschr Geneeskd* 2000;144:2061–2066.

57. Orringer MB, Marshall B, Iannettoni MD. Transhiatal esophagectomy for treatment of benign and malignant esophageal disease. *World J Surg* 2001;25:196–203.

58. Uravic M, Petrosic N, Depolo A, et al. Transhiatal esophagectomy for carcinoma of the esophagus—our ten years experience. *Zentralbl Chir* 2002;127:956–959.

59. Hulscher JB, VanSandick JW, deBoer AG, et al. Extended transthoracic resection compared with limited transhiatal resection for adenocarcinoma of the esophagus. *N Engl J Med* 2002;347:1662–1669.

60. Rao YG, Pal S, Pande GK. Transhiatal esophagectomy for benign and malignant conditions. *Am J Surg* 2002;184:136–142.

61. Averbach A, Akbarov A, Sidel T, et al. Results of curative therapy for esophageal cancer in a community training hospital. *Int Surg* 2002;87:31–37.

62. Doty JR, Salazar JD, Forastiere AA, et al. Postesophagectomy morbidity, mortality, and length of hospital stay after preoperative chemoradiation therapy. *Ann Thorac Surg* 2002;74:227–231.

63. de Boer AG, Stalmeier PF, Sprangers MA, et al. Transhiatal versus extended transthoracic resection in oesophageal carcinoma: patients' utilities and treatment preferences. *Br J Cancer* 2002;86:851–857.

64. Bousamra M 2nd, Haasler GB, Parviz M. A decade of experience with transthoracic and transhiatal esophagectomy. *Am J Surg* 2002;183:162–167.

65. Rentz J, Bull D, Harpole D, et al. Transthoracic versus transhiatal esophagectomy: a prospective study of 945 patients. *J Thorac Cardiovasc Surg* 2003;125:1114–1120.

66. Hulscher JBF, Tijssen JG, Obertop H, et al. Transthoracic versus transhiatal resection for carcinoma of the esophagus: a meta-analysis. *Ann Thorac Surg* 2001;72:306–313.

67. Orringer MB, Marshall B, Chang AC, et al. Two thousand transhiatal esophagectomies: changing trends, lessons learned. *Ann Surg* 2007;246:363–374.

68. Korst RJ, Altorki NK. Imaging for esophageal tumors. *Thorac Surg Clin* 2004;14:61–69.

69. Rice TW. Clinical staging of esophageal carcinoma: CT, EUS, and PET. *Surg Clin North Am* 2000;10:471–485.

70. Quint LE, Hepburn LN, Francis IR, et al. Incidence and distribution of distant metastases in new diagnosed esophageal carcinoma. *Cancer* 1995;76:1120–1125.

71. vanOvehagen H, Becker CD. Diagnosis and staging of carcinomas of the esophagus and gastroesophageal junction, and detection of postoperative recurrence by computed tomography. In: Meyers MA, ed. *Neoplasms of the Digestive Tract. Imaging, Staging and Management.* Philadelphia, PA: Lippincott–Raven; 1998:31–48.

72. Quint LE, Glazer GM, Orringer MB, et al. Esophageal carcinoma: CT findings. *Radiology* 1985;155:171–175.

73. Block MI, Patterson GA, Sundaresan RS, et al. Improvement in staging of esophageal cancer with the addition of positron emission tomography. *Ann Thorac Surg* 1997;64:770–776.

74. Luketich JD, Schauer PR, Meltzer CC, et al. Role of positron emission tomography in staging esophageal cancer. *Ann Thorac Surg* 1997;64:765–769.

75. Gunn T, Speicher JE, Parekh K, et al. Benefit of computerized tomography scan with intravenous contrast prior to esophagectomy in patients with esophageal cancer. *Presented at 23rd European Conference on General Thoracic Surgery*, 31 May–3 June; Lisbon, Portugal; 2015.

76. Saeki H, Ishimura H, Jigashi J, et al. Postoperative management using intensive patient-controlled epidural analgesia and early rehabilitation after an esophagectomy. *Surg Today* 2009;39(6):476–480.

77. Orringer MB, Marshall B, Iannettoni MD. Eliminating the cervical esophagogastric anastomotic leak with a side-to-side stapled anastomosis. *J Thorac Cardiovasc Surg* 2000;119:277–288.

78. Heitmiller RF, Gillinov AM, Jones B. Transhiatal herniation of colon after esophagectomy and gastric pull-up. *Ann Thorac Surg* 1997;63:554–556.

79. Reich H, Lo AY, Harvey JC. Diaphragmatic herniation following transhiatal esophagectomy. *Scand J Thorac Cardiovasc Surg* 1996;30:101–103.

80. DiMusto P, Orringer MB. Transhiatal esophagectomy for distal and cardia cancers: implications of a positive gastric margin. *Ann Thorac Surg* 2007;83:1993–1998.

81. Orringer MB. Partial median sternotomy: anterior approach to the upper thoracic esophagus. *J Thorac Cardiovasc Surg* 1984;87:124–129.

82. Waddell WR, Scannell JG. Anterior approach to carcinoma of the superior mediastinal and cervical segments of the esophagus. *J Thorac Surg* 1957;33:663–669.

83. Kent MS, Pennathur A, Fabian T, et al. A pilot study of botulinum toxin injection for the treatment of delayed gastric emptying following esophagectomy. *Surg Endosc* 2007;21(5):754–757.

84. Bagheri R, Fattahi SH, Haghi SZ, et al. Botulinum toxin for prevention of delayed gastric emptying after esophagectomy. *Asian Cardiovasc Thorac Ann* 2013;21(6):689–692.

85. Markar SR, Schmidt H, Kunz S, et al. Evolution of standardized clinical pathways: refining multidisciplinary care and process to improve outcomes of the surgical treatment of esophageal cancer. *J Gastrointest Surg* 2014;18(7):1238–1246.

86. Speicher JE, Gunn TM, Rossi NP, et al. Eliminating the cervical anastomotic leak, while reducing costs and improving outcomes. *22nd European Conference on General Thoracic Surgery, European Society of Thoracic Surgeons; June 15–18,* Copenhagen, Denmark: 2014.

87. Low DE, Kunz S, Schembre D, et al. Esophagectomy—it's not just about mortality anymore: standardized perioperative clinical pathways improve outcomes in patients with esophageal cancer. *J Gastrointest Surg* 2007;11(11):1395–1402.

88. Bolton JS, Conway WC, Abbas AE. Planned delay of oral intake after esophagectomy reduces the cervical anastomotic leak rate and hospital length of stay. *J Gastrointest Surg* 2014;18:304–309.

89. Tomaszek SC, Cassivi SD, Allen MS, et al. An alternative postoperative pathway reduces length of hospitalisation following oesophagectomy. *Eur J Cardiothorac Surg* 2010;37:807–813.

90. Kassis ES, Kosinski AS, Ross P Jr, et al. Predictors of anastomotic leak after esophagectomy: an analysis of the society of thoracic surgeons general thoracic database. *Ann Thorac Surg* 2013;96:1919–1926.

91. Kelley ST, Coppola D, Karl RC. Neoadjuvant chemoradiotherapy is not associated with a higher complication rate vs. surgery alone in patients undergoing esophagectomy. *J Gastrointest Surg* 2004;8:227–231; discussion 231–232.

92. Bosset JF, Gignoux M, Triboulet JP, et al. Chemoradiotherapy followed by surgery compared with surgery alone in squamous-cell cancer of the esophagus. *N Engl J Med* 1997;337:161–167.

93. Gockel I, Kneist W, Keilmann A, et al. Recurrent laryngeal nerve paralysis (RLNP) following esophagectomy for carcinoma. *Eur J Surg Oncol* 2005;31(3):277–281.

94. Hulscher JB, van Sandick JW, Devriese PP, et al. Vocal cord paralysis after subtotal oesophagectomy. *Br J Surg* 1999;86(12):1583–1587.

95. Gupta V, Gupta R, Thingnam SK, et al. Major airway injury during esophagectomy: experience at a tertiary care center. *J Gastrointest Surg* 2009;13(3):438–441.

96. Iannettoni MD, Parekh KR, Lynch WR, et al. Delayed Reconstruction of the Compromised Esophageal Conduit. *19th European Conference on General Thoracic Surgery, European Society of Thoracic Surgeons; June 5-8, Parc Chanot, Marseille, France: 2011.*

97. Lanzarini E, Ramon JM, Grande L, et al. Delayed cervical esophagogastrostomy: a surgical alternative for patients with ischemia of the gastric conduit at time of esophagectomy. *Cir Esp* 2014;92(6):429–431.

98. Chang A, Orringer MB. Management of the cervical esophagogastric anastomotic stricture. *Semin Thorac Cardiovasc Surg* 2007;19:66–71.

99. Kranzfelder M, Gertler R, Hapfelmeier A, et al. Chylothorax after esophagectomy for cancer: impact of the surgical approach and neoadjuvant treatment: systematic review and institutional analysis. *Surg Endosc* 2013;27(10):3530–3538.

100. Rao DV, Chava SP, Sahni P, et al. Thoracic duct injury during esophagectomy: 20 years experience at a tertiary care center in a developing country. *Dis Esophagus* 2004;17(2):141–145.

101. Pennathur A, Zhang J, Chen H, et al. The "best operation" for esophageal cancer? *Ann Thorac Surg* 2010;89(6):S2163–S2167.

102. Rindani R, Martin CJ, Cox MR. Transhiatal versus Ivor-Lewis oesophagectomy: is there a difference? *Aust N Z J Surg* 1999;69:187–194.

103. Omloo JM, Lagarde SM, Hulscher JB, et al. Extended transthoracic resection compared with limited transhiatal resection for adenocarcinoma of the mid/distal esophagus: five-year survival of a randomized clinical trial. *Ann Surg* 2007;246:992–1000; discussion 1000–1001.

104. Schmidt CE, Bestmann B, Kuchler T, et al. Quality of life associated with surgery for esophageal cancer: differences between collar and intrathoracic anastomoses. *World J Surg* 2004;28:355–360.

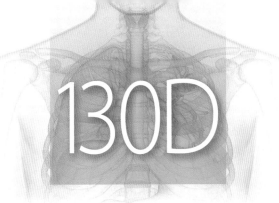

130D

Vagal-Sparing Esophagectomy

Steven R. DeMeester

WHY A VAGAL-SPARING ESOPHAGECTOMY?

An esophagectomy is a major operation associated with significant perioperative and long-term physiologic alterations. During the procedure, the dissection, typically involving the mediastinum and the abdomen, leads to extensive third-spacing and volume shifts in the perioperative period. These volume shifts frequently produce hemodynamic alterations and in some patients cardiopulmonary compromise. Later, the gastrointestinal alterations associated with esophagectomy and reconstruction often include dumping, diarrhea, early satiety, and gastroesophageal reflux symptoms. A laparoscopic vagal-sparing esophagectomy minimizes the dissection associated with an esophagectomy since the esophagus is stripped out of the mediastinum without formal dissection. In addition, many of the gastrointestinal alterations associated with an esophagectomy are secondary to division of the vagus nerves, and vagal preservation minimizes dumping, diarrhea and, depending on the type of reconstruction, early satiety and reflux symptoms. Finally, the technique for a vagal-sparing esophagectomy with gastric pull-up allows preservation of the left gastric arterial trunk and branches to the pylorus. This improves the perfusion of the proximal portion of the graft and may reduce the frequency of anastomotic leaks and strictures.

CANDIDATES FOR A VAGAL-SPARING ESOPHAGECTOMY

Candidates for a vagal-sparing esophagectomy are patients with benign disease or high-grade dysplasia or intramucosal esophageal cancer who require an esophagectomy. Over the past decade, there has been a paradigm shift in the management of patients with high-grade dysplasia or a superficial esophageal cancer. Most of these patients are now treated with organ preservation using endoscopic resection and ablation techniques. However, in some patients the esophageal function is so damaged by chronic reflux, or the disease is refractory or multifocal, and these patients are excellent candidates for a vagal-sparing esophagectomy. Importantly, there is no lymphadenectomy with a vagal-sparing esophagectomy, so only patients with no or only a very low risk of nodal metastases should be considered for the procedure. Thus, any lesion in the esophagus that may represent an early cancer must be endoscopically resected to confirm that, if malignant, the invasion is limited to the mucosa. Invasion into the submucosa is associated with an increased risk for nodal metastases and therefore, an esophagectomy should include a lymph node dissection in such cases.[1,2] Prior esophageal or gastric surgery will increase the complexity and may make vagal preservation impractical or impossible. However, even if the vagus nerves cannot be preserved there are still perioperative physiologic advantages to stripping the esophagus out and avoiding formal mediastinal dissection.

TYPES OF VAGAL-SPARING ESOPHAGECTOMIES

There are two types of vagal-sparing esophagectomies and two types of reconstruction. The options for removing the esophagus while preserving the vagus nerves include a mucosal stripping esophagectomy where only the mucosa is removed and the muscular portion of the esophagus remains in situ. Alternatively, the entire esophagus can be stripped out including all of the layers (mucosa, submucosa, and muscularis propria). The mucosal stripping vagal-sparing esophagectomy is reserved for patients with achalasia where the dilated muscular tube can accommodate the graft within it. In contrast, in patients with high-grade dysplasia or intramucosal cancer of the esophagus it is critical to strip out all the esophageal layers to avoid leaving any diseased mucosa behind. While acceptable, it is unlikely that mucosal stripping would be feasible in patients with end-stage reflux disease without Barrett's, secondary to chronic reflux-induced mucosal injury.

Reconstruction after a vagal-sparing esophagectomy can be either with a tubularized gastric pull-up or less commonly a colon interposition to the intact, innervated stomach. The gastric pull-up is preferred for simplicity and reliability but the colon may offer alimentary and quality of life advantages in the long-term.[3] With either reconstruction, the vagal innervation of the pylorus is preserved so a pyloroplasty is unnecessary, and preservation of the vagal innervation to the gastrointestinal tract minimizes dumping and diarrhea symptoms.[4]

VAGAL-SPARING ESOPHAGECTOMY TECHNIQUE

The technique for a vagal-sparing esophagectomy was described in the 1980s by Professor Akiyama from Japan.[5] We adopted his technique and over 150 patients with high-grade dysplasia, intramucosal cancer, or benign conditions including end-stage achalasia and reflux disease have undergone an open or laparoscopic vagal-sparing procedure at our center. Early in our experience we confirmed vagal integrity after the procedure using sham feeds, pancreatic polypeptide, Congo-red staining, and nuclear medicine gastric emptying studies. Further, we confirmed that esophagectomy with vagal preservation led to a significant reduction in the prevalence of dumping and diarrhea compared to patients that had a standard esophagectomy with vagotomy.[4,6]

Vagal-sparing procedures are done in a similar fashion to a transhiatal operation except the esophagus is stripped from the mediastinum without mediastinal or transhiatal dissection. The operation commences in the abdomen, and with a minimum of dissection the hiatus is opened and the anterior and posterior vagal trunks encircled with a vessel-loop. The vagus nerves are retracted gently toward the patient's right, and the gastroesophageal fat pad is dissected beginning on the left of the esophagus and stomach such that it allows the anterior vagus nerve to be brought well over to the right of the esophagus. Failure to do this step will lead in most cases to inadvertent injury of the anterior vagus nerve during the subsequent steps of the procedure. Once the anterior vagus is safely over to the right of the esophagus, a highly selective vagotomy is performed starting just above the crow's foot near the antrum of the stomach. This is necessary if the stomach is to be used as the esophageal replacement, and is beneficial with a colon interposition to reduce gastric acidity and the potential for ulceration in the colon graft. The highly selective vagotomy precisely follows the lesser curve of the stomach up to the point where the distal esophagus is reached and the vagus nerve trunks are separated from the esophagus. This dissection is facilitated by sequential grasping of the stomach with Babcock clamps along the lesser curve, and by using the Harmonic scalpel for division of the very vascular tissue in this area. Avoidance of a hematoma or bleeding in this area is critical to prevent unintended injury to the distal vagal braches.

At this point, the gastroesophageal junction should be completely exposed and the lesser curve above the crow's foot skeletonized. If the stomach is to be used for esophageal replacement then the greater curve is mobilized in the same fashion as for a standard gastric pull-up. However, if the colon is to be used then there is no need to mobilize the greater curve completely. Instead, the omentum is detached from the transverse colon and a window created near the left crus by dividing the most proximal one or two short gastric and posterior pancreaticogastric vessels. This creates a passage from the lesser sac to the hiatus for the colon graft. The colon is mobilized in the standard fashion based on the ascending branch of the left colic artery whenever possible.[7] The necessary length of colon is marked out by measuring the distance from the tip of the left ear to the xiphoid anteriorly with an umbilical tape and then marking a similar distance on the colon starting from the point where the left colic vessels tether the graft and going proximally on the colon from that site. The colon can then be divided and placed in the pelvis for later use.

Next, attention is directed to the left neck. The esophagus is exposed and, after placing a penrose drain around the esophagus to facilitate traction, blunt dissection is accomplished with a finger to free the upper mediastinal portion of the esophagus. A nasogastric tube is inserted and the esophagus is irrigated with a dilute Betadyne solution to reduce mediastinal contamination during the subsequent stripping procedure. The nasogastric tube is then removed. Next, a gastrotomy is made near the gastroesophageal junction, or alternatively the cardia is divided with a stapler and a small portion of the staple line is opened to provide access to the esophageal lumen. A standard vein stripper is then passed retrograde up the esophagus and brought out the anterior wall of the cervical esophagus as distally as possible. The esophagus is ligated distal to the exit site of the vein stripper in the neck using a heavy suture, and the cervical esophagus divided at the site where the vein stripper comes out. The divided distal end of the esophagus is then suture ligated and tied securely. I find that several endoloops facilitate secure ligation. This is a critical step since if the ligatures slip then the

vein stripper will merely pull out, leaving the partially stripped esophagus somewhere in the mediastinum. After changing the vein stripper to the large head, the esophagus is inverted on itself by pulling the vein stripper from below. It is useful to leave a long umbilical tape tied to the distal end of the cervical esophagus to provide access to the tract in the posterior mediastinum after the esophagus has been removed. The esophagus comes out inverted with the mucosa external to the muscular wall similar to taking off a sock inside-out. Generally bleeding is minimal and very little force is required to pull the esophagus out. Resistance should raise concern, and excessive resistance should prompt conversion to a transhiatal procedure.

Importantly, in patients with Barrett's and high-grade dysplasia or intramucosal cancer, all layers of the esophagus are stripped out so as not to inadvertently leave any Barrett's or tumor behind. However, in patients with benign conditions, such as achalasia, only the mucosa needs be stripped out. This is accomplished in similar fashion except a cervical esophageal myotomy is made and only the mucosa is encircled with a heavy tie, leaving the remaining muscular wall of the esophagus intact. After carefully securing the mucosal tie around the vein stripper, the mucosa can stripped out from below leaving the muscular wall of the esophagus in place. This works nicely through a gastrotomy high on the anterior fundus of the stomach. The mucosa is stapled off just distal to the squamocolumnar junction and the anterior gastrotomy closed.

The next step is to dilate the mediastinal tract to prevent constriction of the graft. We sequentially dilate the tract using a 90 cc balloon Foley catheter progressively filled with saline and pulled up through the mediastinum. Typically, 2 to 3 passes are made to ensure an adequate tract is created. This is particularly important in patients that have a normal caliber esophagus at the time of stripping. The graft can then be brought up through the posterior mediastinal tract.

When a gastric pull-up is being used, the stomach is tubularized in standard fashion leaving the crow's foot intact. The vascular supply of the gastric tube is typically excellent since the left gastric artery has been preserved and only the branches to the skeletonized lesser curve region were divided. This usually leaves several branches intact to the antrum, and in combination with preserved right gastric and gastroepiploic arteries, leads to excellent graft perfusion in most patients. We confirm the perfusion of the graft using SPY technology, and in this way ensure the anastomosis is done to a well-perfused area of the graft.[8] The gastric tube is then pulled up through the posterior mediastinum and an esophagogastric anastomosis constructed in standard fashion. After completing the cervical anastomosis, the graft is gently pulled into the abdomen to eliminate redundancy and sutured to the crura to prevent herniation of abdominal organs into the mediastinum. At this point, the operation is complete with the exception of passing a nasogastric tube and placing a feeding jejunostomy tube. Since the antral innervation has been preserved, no pyloroplasty is performed.

When a colon graft is used with vagal preservation of the stomach there are several important technical considerations. First, nearly the entire, innervated stomach is left intact and only the cardia immediately below the gastroesophageal junction is excised. A highly selective vagotomy is performed along the lesser curvature to reduce acid secretion and provide protection from the development of cologastric anastomotic ulcers. There is no need to do an extensive mobilization of the greater curvature. Instead, only the most proximal 1 to 2 short gastric vessels along with the posterior pancreaticoduodenal vessels are divided so that there is an approximately 10-cm window created near the left crus of the diaphragm. Importantly, the colon graft is passed up *posterior* to the stomach through this window, into the hiatus, and then up through the posterior mediastinum. In patients with achalasia where only the mucosa was stripped out through an anterior gastrotomy, the entire muscular tube of the native esophagus remains intact, and a sufficient-sized hole must be cut into the muscular tube along the left lateral aspect near the hiatus to allow the colon graft to be pulled up inside and passed to the neck. If all layers of the esophagus have been stripped out as in patients with high-grade dysplasia or intramucosal adenocarcinoma, then that issue does not exist, since the muscular wall of the esophagus is gone and only the mediastinal tract is present. The esophagocolonic anastomosis is done either with a stapled or hand-sewn technique in an end-to-end fashion. If the muscular tube of the esophagus has been preserved, it can be pulled up like a sheath to cover the anastomosis. The colon is then pulled firmly back into the abdomen to reduce any redundancy, and sutured to the left crus of the diaphragm to prevent twisting of the graft or herniation of abdominal contents into the mediastinum. In particular, sutures should be placed between the colon graft and the posterior aspect of the hiatus near the point where the left and right crus meet, since herniation can occur underneath the colon graft if these sutures are omitted.

The colon is divided approximately 10 to 15 cm distal to the hiatus taking care not to injure the vascular arcade. A stapled cologastric anastomosis is then done to the proximal posterior fundus using a 75-mm GIA stapler, and a nasogastric tube is guided into the stomach. Finally, the colocolostomy is accomplished in standard fashion with care taken to avoid traction on the left colic vessels or the marginal artery supplying the graft. Typically this requires that the right colon be brought up into the left upper quadrant. Finally, the mesenteric defects are closed and a feeding jejunostomy placed.

When a gastric pull-up is planned, the vagal-sparing procedure is readily adapted to a fully laparoscopic approach. The gastric mobilization as well as the highly selective vagotomy are straightforward laparoscopic procedures. I have found that the use of a 4-cm incision in the midline with placement of a hand port facilitates stripping the esophagus out (via the hand port) and subsequent dilatation of the mediastinal tract. The graft is pulled up attached to a chest tube and the cervical esophagogastric anastomosis accomplished in standard fashion. Similar to an open procedure, the gastric tube should be sutured to the left crus to prevent torsion of the graft or herniation of abdominal organs into the posterior mediastinum.

OUTCOME AFTER VAGAL-SPARING ESOPHAGECTOMY

Since nearly all patients that have a vagal-sparing esophagectomy have their operation for benign disease or curable stages of esophageal cancer, many of these patients live long lives with their replaced esophagus. In a study of patients 10 or more years after esophagectomy with colon interposition, we reported that 30 of the 63 patients (48%) had a vagal-sparing operation.[3] Compared to patients that had a standard esophagectomy with vagal division, those that had a vagal-sparing procedure had higher satisfaction with their alimentary comfort and less early satiety. There was no difference in quality of life scores between groups or in the frequency of dumping or diarrhea symptoms. This is likely due to the fact that after several years, most patients had learned how to control or minimize dumping and diarrhea if it had been present in the early postoperative period. Previously we showed that early after esophagectomy, perioperative weight loss and the frequency of dumping and diarrhea were reduced with vagal preservation.[4]

CONCLUSIONS

Barrett's surveillance programs and more liberal use of upper endoscopy are leading to the identification of an increasing number of patients with high-grade dysplasia or early-stage esophageal adenocarcinoma. Endoscopic resection and ablation are typically preferred in these patients, but in some of these patients, esophagectomy is a better option. In these patients as well as those with benign conditions that have reached the stage where esophagectomy is appropriate, a vagal-sparing operation provides the benefit of complete esophageal resection while minimizing the morbidity associated with a traditional esophagectomy that includes a vagotomy. The ease of the procedure, as well as its applicability to a fully laparoscopic approach, are additional factors that should encourage physician and patient acceptance.

REFERENCES

1. DeMeester SR. Evaluation and treatment of superficial esophageal cancer. *J Gastrointest Surg* 2010;14(suppl 1):S94–S100.
2. Leers JM, DeMeester SR, Oezcelik A, et al. The prevalence of lymph node metastases in patients with T1 esophageal adenocarcinoma a retrospective review of esophagectomy specimens. *Ann Surg* 2011;253:271–278.
3. Greene CL, DeMeester SR, Augustin F, et al. Long-term quality of life and alimentary satisfaction after esophagectomy with colon interposition. *Ann Thorac Surg* 2014;98:1713–1719; discussion 1719–1720.
4. Peyre C, DeMeester SR, Rizzetto C, et al. Vagal-sparing esophagectomy: the ideal operation for intramucosal adenocarcinoma and Barrett with high-grade dysplasia. *Ann Surg* 2007;246:665–674.
5. Akiyama H, Tsurumaru M, Kawamura T, et al. Esophageal stripping with preservation of the vagus nerve. *Int Surg* 1982;67:125–128.
6. Banki F, Mason RJ, DeMeester SR, et al. Vagal-sparing esophagectomy: a more physiologic alternative. *Ann Surg* 2002;236:324–335; discussion 335–336.
7. DeMeester SR. Colon interposition following esophagectomy. *Dis Esophagus* 2001;14:169–172.
8. Zehetner J, DeMeester SR, Alicuben ET, et al. Intraoperative assessment of perfusion of the gastric graft and correlation with anastomotic leaks after esophagectomy. *Ann Surg* 2015;262:74–78.

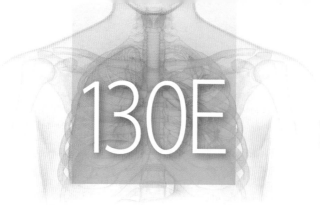

Video-Assisted and Robotic Esophagectomy

Inderpal S. Sarkaria ■ Lara Schaheen ■ James D. Luketich

INTRODUCTION

Minimally invasive esophagectomy (MIE) has become an increasingly accepted surgical approach for patients requiring esophageal resection for both malignant and benign conditions. When performed at high-volume centers, morbidity, mortality, and oncologic outcomes with MIE are comparable to, or improved, over open approaches. Several total and hybrid MIE techniques have evolved and been described, ranging from total thoracoscopic and laparoscopic approaches, to varying combinations of open and minimally invasive abdominal and/or thoracic approaches. The advent of robotics in surgery has brought an even more varied scope of procedures, including total robotic-assisted minimally invasive esophagectomy (RAMIE), and a host of procedures combining robotic-assisted and standard thoracoscopic and laparoscopic techniques, as well as laparotomy and thoracotomy. In this chapter, we will focus primarily on total thoracoscopic and laparoscopic MIE and RAMIE.

MIE

Current MIE approaches primarily include laparoscopic transhiatal, laparoscopic-thoracoscopic three-hole (McKeown), and laparoscopic-thoracoscopic Ivor Lewis esophagectomy. The choice of operation is largely influenced by surgeon preference, particularly the choice between a transthoracic versus transhiatal approach. Other factors influencing the operative approach include location of tumor, patient fitness, and morbidity profiles of specific operations. While a proximal tumor may require a three-hole McKeown approach, the creation of a cervical anastomosis has a higher incidence of recurrent laryngeal nerve injury and is more prone to anastomotic leak, stricture, and pharyngoesophageal swallowing dysfunction. By comparison, the Ivor Lewis approach, which we consider more suitable for mid- and lower thoracic tumors, may predisopse to greater morbidity in the event of an anastomotic leak.[1]

Our institutional approach at the University of Pittsburgh Medical Center has evolved over time, initially developed as a modified McKeown (three-hole) technique with a cervical anastomosis, and transitioned to a primarily Ivor Lewis approach with intrathoracic anastomosis.[1-3] In an initial series of 222 patients, 8 initial cases were performed as laparoscopic transhiatal operations, with quick adaptation thereafter to a modified McKeown approach with thoracoscopic

mobilization and cervical anastomosis. Results from this early experience yielded a median hospital stay of 7 days and an operative mortality of 1.4%, equivalent or better to the majority of open series. An anastomotic leak rate of 11.7% and stage specific survival were similar to open series. In a follow-up institutional series of 1,011 patients undergoing elective MIE, including 530 patients operated via the currently preferred Ivor Lewis MIE approach, operative mortality in this cohort was 0.9% and median length of hospital stay 8 days.[1]

Based on these single institution experiences and concern this operation might not be feasible at other institutions, we implemented the prospective multicenter intergroup Eastern Cooperative Oncology Group Phase II trial (E2202). Of the 106 patients enrolled, 95 patients from 17 credentialed institutions underwent a three-hole or Ivor Lewis MIE successfully.[4] Perioperative mortality was 2.9% with a median ICU and hospital stay of 2 and 9 days, respectively. Major anastomotic leak rate was 8.6% with morbidity profiles similar to open operations. The median lymph node count was 19 and 96% of patients received an R0 resection. Three-year survival was 58.4%, with local-regional recurrence occurring in only 6.7% of patients, suggesting equivalent survival and recurrence outcomes to open procedures. This landmark study demonstrated that MIE was feasible in the hands of experienced esophageal surgeons with good technical and oncologic outcomes in a variety of hospital settings.

A multicenter, randomized, controlled European study comparing open and minimally invasive esophagectomy primarily focused on the incidence of pulmonary complications. In this study of 56 patients undergoing open operations compared to 59 undergoing MIE, the incidence of respiratory complications in-house (34% vs. 12%, $p = 0.005$) and at 2 weeks (29% vs. 9%, $p = 0.005$) were more than threefold greater in the open esophagectomy group versus MIE. Mortality (3% vs. 2%) and anastomotic leak rates (12% vs. 7%) were similar between the two groups. This trial, although limited by a small patient population, provides the strongest level of evidence suggesting a significant decrease in morbidity with the MIE approach compared to open transthoracic operations, while maintaining similar oncologic outcomes.

Our current preferred approach is a completely laparoscopic-thoracoscopic (Ivor Lewis) esophagectomy with complete en bloc abdominal (celiac, left gastric, splenic) and mediastinal (paraesophageal and subcarinal) lymphadenectomy.[5] This approach is ideal for the majority of middle and distal esophageal cancers, gastroesophageal junction tumors with gastric cardia extension, short-to-moderate length Barrett esophagus with high-grade dysplasia, and in cases where there is concern regarding the available length of conduit.[6,7] In cases of primary gastric tumors with significant lesser curve extension that involve the incisura, we prefer a total gastrectomy with Roux-en-Y reconstruction. Total laparoscopic and thoracoscopic Ivor Lewis resections are not ideal for upper third or midesophageal cancers with significant proximal extension where the probability of achieving an adequate proximal margin may be compromised. The following describes our current technique for laparoscopic-thoracoscopic Ivor Lewis MIE.

MIE TECHNIQUE

Patients considered for esophagectomy are carefully evaluated and staged by upper endoscopy with biopsy, endoscopic ultrasound to assess depth of invasion and lymph node status, and positron emission tomography scanning in combination with computed tomography (PET-CT) to assess for metastatic disease as well as response to induction therapy. For patients with gastroesophageal junction carcinomas, initial staging laparoscopy is often performed to allow us to further characterize the extent of disease, determine the ideal operative timing and most appropriate surgical approach. If upon inspection it is decided that the disease warrants neoadjuvant therapy, an infusaport is placed, and consideration is given to performing a careful dilation of any existing malignant obstruction. In patients with a marginal nutritional status and a bulky obstructing tumor, we may elect to place a laparoscopic feeding tube at the time of staging; this is done in less than 10% of patients. For patients with T3 tumors, bulky local disease, or clinically evident malignant adenopathy, consideration is given to neoadjuvant chemotherapy with or without radiation.

MIE LAPAROSCOPIC APPROACH

On the day of operation, upper endoscopy is performed by the surgeon to assess the proximal and distal extent of tumor. A double-lumen tube is placed by the anesthesia team and appropriate intravenous access and monitoring lines obtained. The patient is placed supine on the operative table with the legs together, the arms at 45 degrees, and in steep reverse Trendelenburg position. The surgeon stands on the right and first assistant on the left.

Port placement is designed to allow ease of dissection and optimal visualization of the hiatus, gastroepiploic arcade, left gastric vascular pedicle, and retrogastric space, pylorus, and for placement of a feeding jejunostomy (Fig. 130E.1). A right paramedian 10- or 12-mm port is initially placed into the peritoneal cavity under direct vision via a direct Hasson cut-down technique, at approximately 2/3 the distance from the xiphoid process to the umbilicus. Subcostal 5-mm trocars are placed bilaterally, and an additional 5-mm trocar placed in the right lateral abdomen, near the posterior costal margin, for insertion of the liver retractor. A left paramedian camera port is placed. Depending on surgeon preference, a 5-mm or 10-mm camera may be used, and dictates the size of the port placed. An additional port may be placed in the right paramedian infraumbilical area as necessary for additional retraction during the procedure. This port also aids in placement of the feeding jejunostomy. This may be a 5-mm port if the surgeon is comfortable with intracorporeal freehand suturing. If an endoscopic suturing device is to be used, a 10-mm port may be necessary. Of note, patients with a large, protuberant abdomen or prior abdominal operations often require considerable judgment with regards to selecting port location and even in the decision to

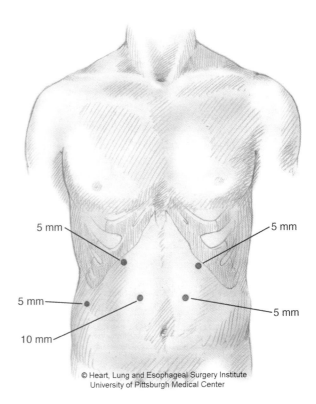

FIGURE 130E.1 Laparoscopic port placement. The 10-mm port is placed first in the right midabdomen using open Hasson trocar insertion technique. An additional 5/11-mm port (not shown) is placed in the right lower quadrant that is helpful for retraction during pyloroplasty and gastric tube creation. (No permission needed.)

proceed with a minimally invasive approach. In patient with an extensive prior abdominal surgical history, we often place exploratory ports to assist with adhesiolysis.

Ultrasonic coagulating shears are employed for the majority of the dissection. The lesser sac is visualized through the gastrohepatic omentum. The surgeon should take care to identify the presence of a replaced left hepatic artery in this space. Placement of a temporary clip on larger vessels and observation of the left hepatic lobe for ischemia may help determine the feasibility of dividing this artery. In the majority of cases, this vessel can be divided without clinical consequence, but on occasion, this is a dominant vessel and deserves consideration to changing the operative plan. Hiatal dissection and mobilization are performed to assess involvement of the crura and perihiatal structures, including the pleura and aorta. Division of the left gastric vascular pedicle is accomplished by lifting the lesser curve of the stomach anteriorly, thus exposing the retrogastric space (Fig. 130E.2). A full celiac and retrogastric lymphadenectomy is performed with dissection continued along the common hepatic and splenic arteries, and toward the hiatus, thus mobilizing and lifting all nodal-bearing tissue up with the left gastric vascular pedicle. The pedicle is divided with the use of an endovascular stapler through the right paramedian 12-mm trocar. Early division of the left gastric pedicle facilitates mobilization of the esophagus at the hiatus, particularly along the posterior aspect.

The greater curvature of the stomach is then mobilized by entering the lesser sac through the greater omentum. The ultrasonic shears are used to divide the omental perforating arteries, and great care is taken to identify, visualize, and preserve the right gastroepiploic arcade (Fig. 130E.2). For use as an anastomotic buttress, strong consideration is given to creation of an omental flap incorporating two

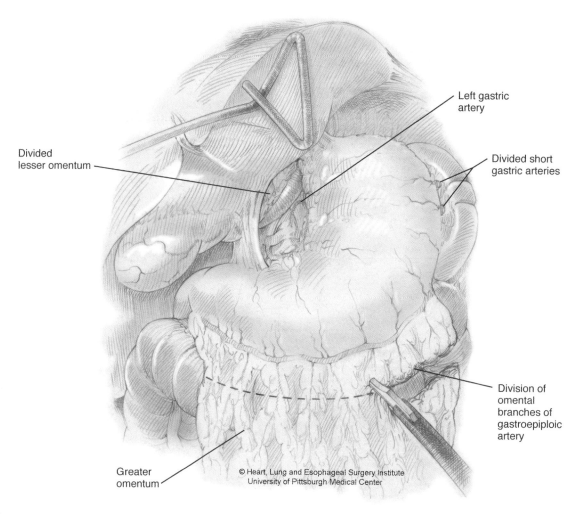

Divided
lesser omentum

Left gastric
artery

Divided short
gastric arteries

Division of
omental
branches of
gastroepiploic
artery

Greater
omentum

© Heart, Lung and Esophageal Surgery Institute
University of Pittsburgh Medical Center

FIGURE 130E.2 Lesser curve/retrogastric exposure and gastric mobilization. (No permission needed.)

to three omental arteries from the right gastroepiploic artery, particularly in patients receiving induction radiation. The dissection is continued along the fundus of the stomach with division of the short gastric arteries, if not previously divided during the crural dissection. The stomach is lifted and all retrogastric attachments and adhesions divided. Throughout the conduct of the entire operation and in particular during creation of the tubularized conduit, we employ a "no touch" technique which includes avoidance of unnecessary gastric conduit manipulation and only grasping the stomach in areas that will ultimately be resected, this is easily accomplished. Gastric mobilization is continued to the level of the pylorus. We mobilize the pyloroantral area until it easily reaches the caudate lobe of the liver and/or right crus without tension. We consider these pyloroantral mobilization maneuvers to be part of a modified Kocher maneuver, as full Kocherization is generally not necessary to gain the degree of pyloric mobility needed. In cases for which we anticipate the need for a longer conduit, such as those with a high esophageal tumor and/or Barrett's proximal extension, we spend additional time completely Kocherizing the pyloroantral duodenal areas in order to gain adequate mobilization.

We perform a pyloroplasty in virtually all patients. With experience a laparoscopic pyloroplasty can be performed safely, and with excellent technique, in less than 10 minutes. At the end of a 2-month rotation, most senior level residents are capable of performing a laparoscopic pyloroplasty if supervised by an experienced MIE surgeon. Initially, stay sutures are placed laterally on each side of the

pylorus to aid in retraction, in many cases this seems to decrease bleeding as these stay sutures frequently ligate branches of the vein of Mayo. A Heineke–Mikulicz pyloroplasty is then performed using the ultrasonic shear to enter the duodenum adjacent to the pylorus, and to divide the pyloric muscle in the axis of the lumen, continuing onto the thinner gastric antrum. We employ an endoscopic suturing device (Endo Stitch 2.0, US surgical, Norwalk, Connecticut) to close the pylorus transversely with interrupted sutures (Fig. 130E.3). Closure frequently requires 4-6 interrupted sutures. At the completion of the laparoscopic portion of the operation, we reinforce the pyloroplasty with a buttress of omentum.

A gastric conduit approximately 4 cm in width is fashioned (Fig. 130E.4). If a nasogastric tube has been placed, it is imperative the surgeon remember to have it withdrawn into the proximal esophagus at this time. Alignment of the stomach with gentle retraction of the fundus superiorly and the antrum inferiorly facilitates maximal "straightening" of the greater curvature of the stomach. The first staple load is applied at a near right angle to the lesser curve fat after careful consideration of the following: (1) the presence and extent of tumor extension onto the lesser curve; (2) "optimal" tube diameter, if narrow, you may want to start closer to the pylorus; and (3) history of neoadjuvant radiation therapy with concern for radiation damage to the stomach. An endovascular staple load is chosen to divide the lesser curve fat and vessels in order to minimize bleeding. As the subsequent loads divide the thicker muscle of the gastric antrum, a larger

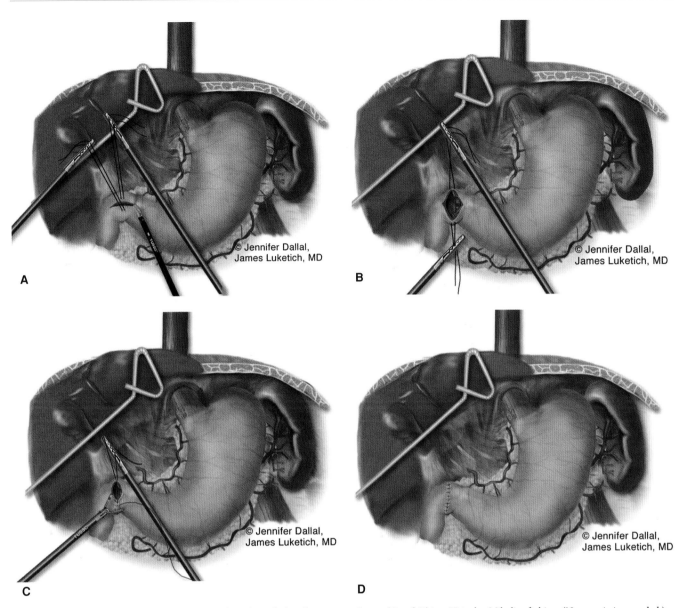

FIGURE 130E.3 Creation of longitudinal pyloroplasty (**A** and **B**) and transverse closure (**C** and **D**) in a Heineke–Mikulicz fashion. (No permission needed.)

staple height of 4 to 5 mm may be needed. As the staple line continues onto the body of the stomach wall, the wall thickness generally allows for an intermediate staple height of 4 mm. There are several important points to consider during the creation of the gastric conduit. The staple height chosen, as always should not be dogmatic, but in direct correlation to the thickness of the tissue being divided. Larger patients may require a 5 mm staple height for nearly all of the gastric stapling, due to the thickness of the tissue and the desire to obtain full staple closure. It is worth noting that we are attempting to make a straight conduit from the greater curvature, thus excessive lengths of the straight staple cartridges, 60 mm for example, may initially sound attractive, but can work against our goal from a geometrical consideration. For this reason, we prefer the shorter 45 mm lengths, and sometimes a 30 mm, as we are essentially trying to follow a curve with successive small straight lines. The gastric conduit is divided from the specimen, and the proximal tip fixed by suture to the specimen. It is important to be consistent in choosing a suture location that will allow you to properly orient the conduit in the chest with the staple line facing the surgeon during the right VATS and the greater curve

arcade and fat, facing toward the spleen. Appropriate orientation will help facilitate a safe and properly oriented transit into the thorax and avoid spiraling of the conduit. Our preference is to suture the greater curvature of the newly constructed conduit to the lesser curve staple line of the specimen. Prior to exiting the abdomen, we perform a 360-degree dissection around the esophagus, for a distance of 6 to 10 cm into the chest. This work, will facilitate delivery of the specimen into the chest, and will make the subsequent delivery of the conduit much easier during the VATS mobilization. If it is noted to be adherent to crus, or pleura, at this point we would attempt to keep a negative margin and include these areas in the specimen. Judgment is required here, and hopefully this was anticipated and planned for based on preoperative and/or laparoscopic staging. A stitch is then placed at the distal portion of the tubular conduit as it widens to form the gastric reservoir. This stitch will be used to mark the transition between the intra-abdominal and intrathoracic gastric conduit in order to minimize conduit redundancy in the chest.

A laparoscopic feeding jejunostomy is placed to complete the abdominal phase of the operation.

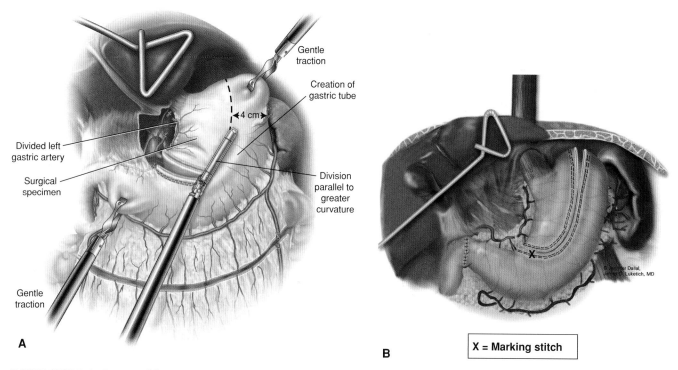

FIGURE 130E.4 A: Creation of the gastric conduit. The first stapler along the lesser curve is a vascular Endo GIA stapler after which the thick antrum is divided as described in the text. The antrum and the fundus are pulled in opposite directions to provide adequate tension during the gastric conduit creation. **B:** Completed gastric conduit with an intact right gastroepiploic arcade and an intact right gastric artery. A marking stitch is placed at the distal end of the gastric tube.

MIE THORACOSCOPIC APPROACH

The patient is turned into the standard left lateral decubitus position and single-lung ventilation instituted. An initial 10-mm port is placed in the eighth intercostal space in the midaxillary line and the thoracoscope introduced into the chest. Remaining ports are placed under direct vision (Fig. 130E.5). A 10-mm port is placed in approximately the eighth or ninth intercostal space in line with or just posterior to the scapular tip. This is the primary port used for introduction of the ultrasonic shears. An additional 5-mm port is placed inferior to the scapular tip for instrumentation and retraction in the operating surgeon's left hand. An additional 10-mm port is placed in the anterior axillary line at the third or fourth intercostal space for introduction of a fan-shaped lung retractor, as well as a 5-mm assist port in the fifth intercostal space in the anterior axillary line, primarily for

suction. A retraction stitch is placed on the diaphragm and brought out through a separate inferior stab incision.

The inferior pulmonary ligament is mobilized to the level of the inferior pulmonary vein. The lung is retracted anteriorly exposing the posterior mediastinal reflection. A dissection plane is begun inferiorly over the posterolateral aspect of the pericardium. In the absence of bulky tumor or significant inflammation, dissection of this plane can generally be accomplished swiftly with a combination of sharp and blunt dissection. Close adherence to the pericardium serves as a guide to complete the anterior-medial en-bloc dissection. Identification of the airway as the surgeon moves superiorly is critical to avoid injury, and allows successful completion of the subcarinal lymphadenectomy. The mediastinal pleura is opened above the azygous vein, which is divided with an endovascular stapler.

The posterior mediastinal pleura is incised along the length of the esophagus down to the level of the hiatus. We do not routinely resect

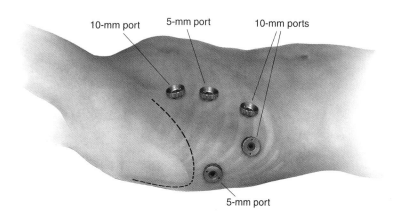

FIGURE 130E.5 Thoracoscopic port placement. (Reprinted from Tsai WS, Levy RM, Luketich JD. Technique of minimally invasive Ivor Lewis esophagectomy. *Oper Tech Thorac Cardiovasc Surg* 2009;14:176–192. Copyright © 2009 Elsevier. With permission.)

the thoracic duct, and care should be taken to identify it and leave it posterior to the dissection plane. The posterior esophageal dissection is carried out with the ultrasonic shears, with perforating lymphatics and aortoesophageal arteries also clipped prior to ligation.

The vagus nerve is divided at the level of the azygous vein to minimize risk of traction injury to the recurrent laryngeal nerve. Close approximation to the esophagus during mobilization above the azygous vein provides additional protection against recurrent laryngeal nerve injury.

Hiatal dissection is completed with careful attention to include all nodal tissue. Gentle cranial traction on the specimen is performed to introduce the conduit into the chest with proper orientation. The conduit is temporarily secured to the diaphragm and the distal specimen retracted laterally to complete the deep medial dissection along

the contralateral pleura and airway. Care should be taken to identify and safely dissect away the left mainstem bronchus and trachea.

The esophagus is sharply divided 2 to 3 cm above the azygous vein, and the posterior-inferior 10-mm port site increased in size by 3 to 4 cm to allow removal of the specimen after placement of a wound protection device. Margins are routinely assessed by frozen section.

A stapled anastomosis is created using an end-to-end anastomotic (EEA) stapler. The EEA anvil is placed within the proximal esophagus and a purse-string suture thoracoscopically placed. The gastric conduit is carefully brought into the chest and a gastrotomy performed in the proximal tip. The head of the EEA stapler is introduced through the posterior-inferior incision and into the proximal gastrotomy (Fig. 130E.6). The spike is brought out at a point above

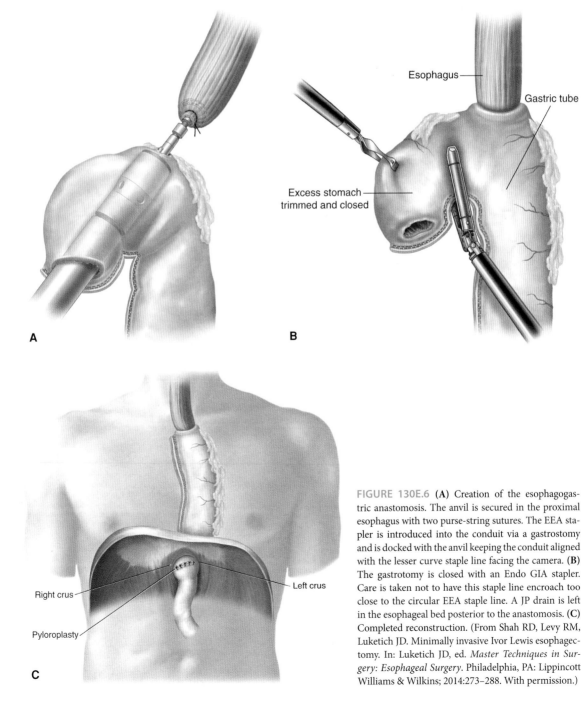

FIGURE 130E.6 **(A)** Creation of the esophagogastric anastomosis. The anvil is secured in the proximal esophagus with two purse-string sutures. The EEA stapler is introduced into the conduit via a gastrostomy and is docked with the anvil keeping the conduit aligned with the lesser curve staple line facing the camera. **(B)** The gastrotomy is closed with an Endo GIA stapler. Care is taken not to have this staple line encroach too close to the circular EEA staple line. A JP drain is left in the esophageal bed posterior to the anastomosis. **(C)** Completed reconstruction. (From Shah RD, Levy RM, Luketich JD. Minimally invasive Ivor Lewis esophagectomy. In: Luketich JD, ed. *Master Techniques in Surgery: Esophageal Surgery*. Philadelphia, PA: Lippincott Williams & Wilkins; 2014:273–288. With permission.)

the gastroepiploic arcade and docked to the anvil, with careful attention to advance the gastric conduit and stapler in concert and in proper orientation, with confirmation of intact anastomotic "donut" upon removal of EEA stapler. The stapler is fired and the anastomosis completed. The nasogastric tube is advanced past the anastomosis and into the proximal conduit under direct vision, and the proximal redundant gastric conduit resected with additional applications of the endogastrointestinal stapler. A standard posterior-apical chest tube and an additional small perianastomotic drain (No. 10 Jackson–Pratt drain) are placed, and the thoracoscopic phase completed.

MIE POSTOPERATIVE CARE

A routine esophagram is performed to assess the anastomosis between days 5 and 7 postoperatively. If there is no evidence of leak, the patient is started on oral intake. The patient is discharged on cycled tube feeding and with the perianastomotic drain in place. If the patient has advanced oral intake appropriately with no evidence of delayed leak, this drain is removed at the first postoperative visit, along with the feeding tube.

ROBOTIC-ASSISTED MINIMALLY INVASIVE ESOPHAGECTOMY

Although increasing, experience with RAMIE remains relatively limited to case reports and early institutional case series. Operative approaches are widely variable, with several combinations of abdominal and thoracic open, standard minimally invasive, and robotic-assisted approaches described, with robotics utilized most commonly for thoracic mobilization alone. The first detailed description of a total robotic-assisted laparoscopic and thoracoscopic procedure was in a patient undergoing a three-hole McKeown operation. Operative time was 660 minutes, although more than half the operating room time was nonsurgical in nature, highlighting the need to develop an experienced team.[8]

The same authors documented the first case series of completely robotic three-hole esophagectomy in a subset of eight patients.[9] An intraoperative injury to the left mainstem bronchus was recognized and repaired robotically. Median operative time was 672 minutes, and a median 18 lymph nodes were harvested. One patient died from pneumonia, and one patient required tracheostomy secondary to bilateral vocal cord paralysis. A subsequent report from the same institution reported an additional 22 cases undergoing total robotic three-hole esophagectomy, with a decrease in operative time to a median of 480 minutes and with 0% operative mortality.[10]

The first case series with an intrathoracic anastomosis was reported in 22 Ivor Lewis operations undergoing robotic-assisted thoracic mobilization and standard laparoscopy.[11] The authors switched to a two-layer hand-sewn technique after significant anastomotic complications, including five of six patients requiring reoperation in the initial patients undergoing a "hybrid" posterior stapled and anterior robotically hand-sewn anastomosis. Among the remaining 16 patients, there was a significant decrease in morbidity, thus leading the authors to advocate this anastomotic technique for intrathoracic robotic approaches.

In a subset of 17 of 21 patients undergoing RAMIE at Memorial Sloan Kettering Cancer Center, the current author described the first total robotic Ivor Lewis RAMIE procedure with robotic assistance in both the chest and abdomen with an EEA stapled intrathoracic anastomosis.[12] Median operative time was 556 minutes, and median lymph node harvest was 20. Anastomotic leaks occurred in

three patients. Of concern, three patients developed airway fistulas. While one small 1-mm fistula presented over 30 days after surgery and resolved quickly with stent therapy, two presented early in the postoperative course, with one resulting in mortality within 90 days of surgery. These complications are likely due to lateral spread of heat during airway dissection with rigid thermal devices resulting in unrecognized injury to the membranous airway. Although these complications have been largely unreported, they are not unique to RAMIE, and care must be taken to avoid airway contact with these devices during intrathoracic esophageal mobilization with all MIE operations, robotic assisted or otherwise. We have since tailored our approach to use available wristed bipolar energy sources (Maryland Bipolar, Intuitive Surgical Inc., Sunnyvale, CA) during the subcarinal dissection. In a follow-up experience with 100 RAMIE operations, we have had no further such complications, and operative outcomes have been excellent, with no additional 90-day mortality.[13] In an interim analysis of 45 patients undergoing RAMIE, intertertile comparisons between successive cohorts of 15 patients demonstrated significant improvement in rates of major complications, lymph node retrieval, conversions to open procedures, and operative time (from approximately 600 minutes to 370 minutes, with a median operative time for the last five patients of less than 300 minutes [unpublished data]).

Two reports from the same institution utilizing a similar RAMIE approach are largely in concordance with these findings.[14,15] In a series of 50 patients, approximately half of which underwent total robotic Ivor Lewis RAMIE procedures with EEA intrathoracic anastomoses and the remainder were hybrid procedures, operative outcomes were excellent, with no mortality, one anastomotic leak, and a median harvest of 19 lymph nodes.[15] Mean operative time decreased from 514 minutes to 397 minutes after the completion of 20 cases.[14]

Currently, no prospective data comparing RAMIE to standard laparoscopic or open procedures have been published. A prospective quality of life and outcomes trial comparing 65 RAMIE to 108 open esophagectomy patients at Memorial Sloan Kettering Cancer Center (ClinicalTrials.gov: NCT01558648) has completed accrual and short-term results have been analyzed identifying significantly improved short-term patient reported pain scores in the RAMIE cohort ($p = 0.007$) (Sarkaria et al., reported in abstract form, European Society of Thoracic Surgeons, Lisbon, Portugal, 2015). Blood loss ($p = 0.001$), hospital days ($p < 0.0001$), and median lymph node retrieval ($p < 0.0001$) was also superior in the RAMIE group. There was a trend toward decreased pulmonary complications (15% RAMIE vs. 32% open esophagectomy) and 90-day mortality was similar (1.5% RAMIE vs. 3.7% open esophagectomy).

These data suggest RAMIE appears to be an equivalent alternative to standard MIE and open esophageal resections. However, the level of evidence remains preliminary, with only a single meta-analysis by Clark et al., which indicated a 30% complication rate, 2.4% operative mortality, and 18% anastomotic leak rate in 60 patients undergoing RAMIE by various approaches.[16] A prospective, randomized, controlled trial comparing complications and outcomes in RAMIE versus open transthoracic esophagectomy (a.k.a. ROBOT trial) is under way in the Netherlands (ClinicalTrials.gov: NCT01544790).

RAMIE PROCEDURE

The current RAMIE procedure is largely adapted from the MIE operation as developed at the University of Pittsburgh Medical Center and as described above.[12,17] Selected procedural differences or adaptations are highlighted below.

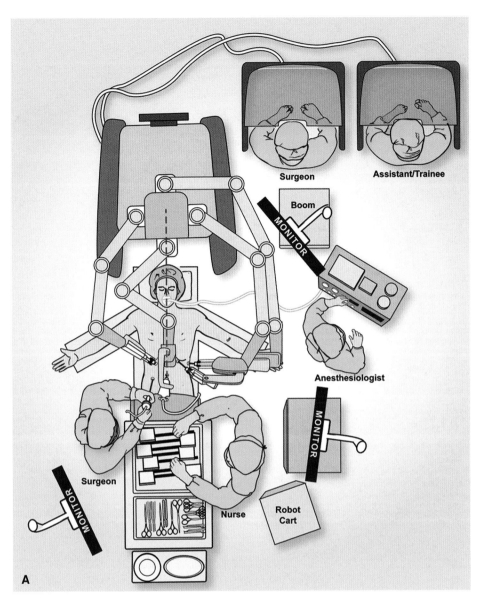

FIGURE 130E.7 RAMIE patient positioning. The operative setup for the abdominal (**A**) and thoracic (**B**) phases of the operation. (© 2014, Memorial Sloan Kettering Cancer Center.) (*continued*)

RAMIE PATIENT POSITIONING

The operative setup for the abdominal and thoracic phases of the operation is depicted in Figure 130E.7. The robotic instrumentation cart is set up on the patient's right side, and the tower is set up on the left. A four-arm robotic platform with two operating consoles is utilized, with the operating surgeon and surgical trainee at the robotic consoles, and an assistant at the bedside. Patient positioning is essentially identical to the MIE procedure, although the left arm may be tucked to avoid interaction with the robotic arms.

RAMIE SURGICAL APPROACH AND PORT PLACEMENT

A combined sequential laparoscopic and thoracoscopic approach is used, as previously described.[12] For the abdominal approach, the operative table is turned to allow easy entry of the robotic cart and arms (Da Vinci Surgical Robot, Intuitive Surgical Inc.) directly over the midline of the patient. A midline camera incision is marked preferably just above the umbilicus but no more than 23 cm from the supraxiphoid reference point. A left lateral subcostal 5-mm incision is marked for use by the robotic atraumatic grasper. A midclavicular 8-mm incision is marked in the left midabdomen. This port is for use with the ultrasonic shears (Harmonic Scalpel, Ethicon Incorporated, Somerville, NJ). An additional right lateral 5-mm subcostal port for placement of the liver retractor is marked, as well as an additional 8-mm midclavicular right midabdominal port for use with the bipolar atraumatic grasper. A 12-mm port is placed between the umbilical and the right midclavicular ports and is used by the assistant for both suctioning and additional retraction. This port may also be used as an alternative camera entry site to improve visualization along the greater curve of the stomach during mobilization of the omentum and gastroepiploic arcade. Port placement is outlined in Figure 130E.8. To minimize arm collisions, it is important to maintain a distance of at least 9 to 10 cm between robotic ports.

For the thoracic phase, the camera port is introduced into the chest in the eighth intercostal space in the mid to posterior axillary line under direct video guidance. Carbon dioxide insufflation is

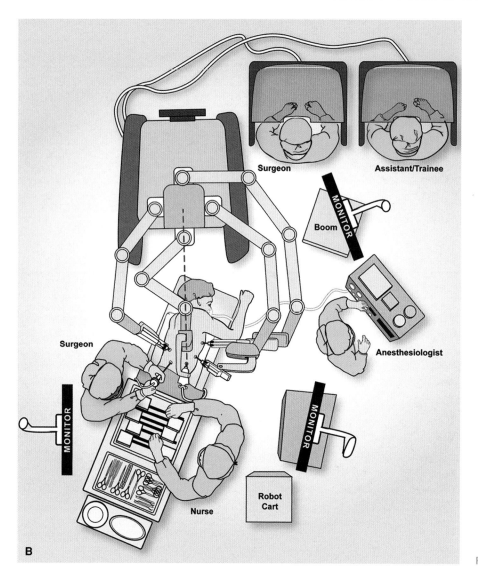

B

FIGURE 130E.7 (*Continued*)

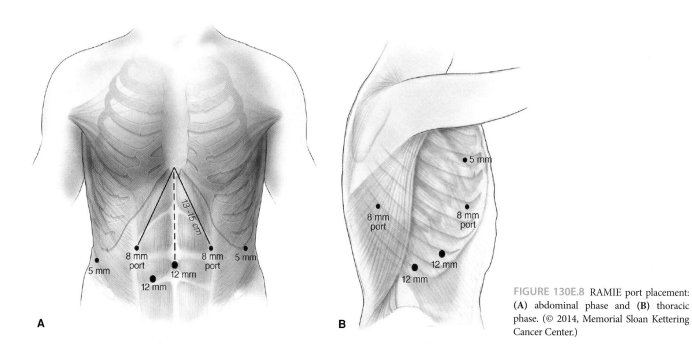

A

B

FIGURE 130E.8 RAMIE port placement: (**A**) abdominal phase and (**B**) thoracic phase. (© 2014, Memorial Sloan Kettering Cancer Center.)

employed, largely negating the need for a diaphragmatic retraction suture. A 5-mm robotic port is placed in the third intercostal space in the mid to posterior axillary line, and an 8-mm robotic port is placed in the fifth intercostal space. An additional 8-mm port is placed laterally in approximately the eighth or ninth interspace. A 12-mm assistant port is placed under direct vision at the diaphragmatic insertion midway between the camera port and the lateral 8-mm robotic port. The robot is docked to the ports, and the robotic camera is placed within the chest at a 30-degree downward orientation.

Basic procedural elements remain the same as MIE. The primary difference between the RAMIE and MIE procedures is the use of the additional robotic arm to allow self-assist by the surgeon, thus replacing the need for the bedside assist during the majority of exposures during the abdominal and thoracic phases of the operation (Fig. 130E.9). Visualization and control over the conduct of operation is also greatly enhanced, with the operative view under direct control of the surgeon at all times. Use of the wristed instruments allows for greater precision in suturing during closure of the pyloroplasty, and placement of the purse-string sutures during anastomotic creation (Fig. 130E.10). We have also found advanced indocyanine green based near infrared fluorescence imaging modalities available on the robotic platform to be of use in visualization of vital vascular structures, such as the gastroepiploic vessels, and potentially in assessment of conduit perfusion.[18] Potential disadvantages of the RAMIE approach

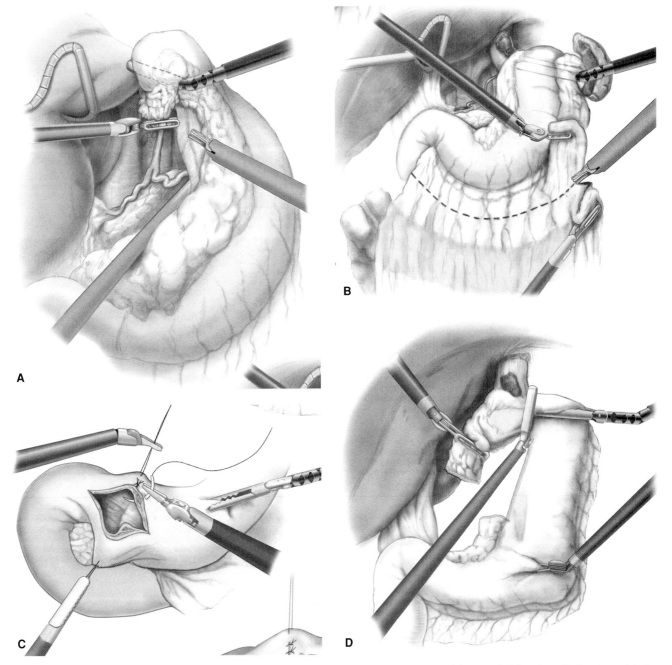

FIGURE 130E.9 Robotic-assisted exposures. **A:** Retrograde/celiac dissection. **B:** Greater gastric curve mobilization. **C:** Pyloroplasty. **D:** Gastric conduit formation. (From Sarkaria IS, Rizk NP, Finley DJ, et al. Combined thoracoscopic and laparoscopic robotic-assisted minimally invasive esophagectomy using a four-arm platform: experience, technique and cautions during early procedure development. *Eur J Cardiothorac Surg* 2013;43(5):e107–e115. Reproduced by permission of European Association for Cardiothoracic Surgery.)

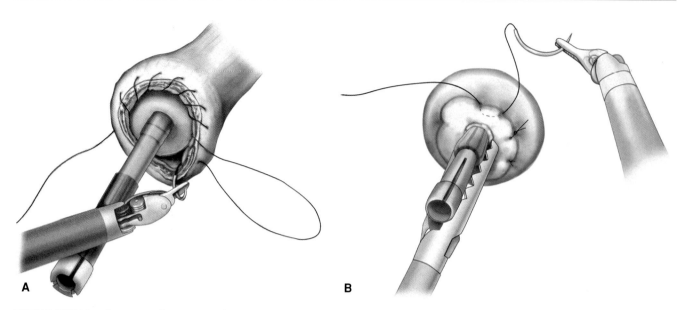

FIGURE 130E.10 Robotic-assisted purse-string placement during anastomotic creation. **A:** Placement of initial suture to secure the stapler anvil. **B:** Placement of second purse-string suture to gather in tissue folds. (From Sarkaria IS, Rizk NP, Finley DJ, et al. Combined thoracoscopic and laparoscopic robotic-assisted minimally invasive esophagectomy using a four-arm platform: experience, technique and cautions during early procedure development. *Eur J Cardiothorac Surg* 2013;43(5):e107–e115. Reproduced by permission of European Association for Cardiothoracic Surgery.)

include the reduced versatility and range in multifield visualization, as well as arm collisions, particularly within the thorax requiring a wide operative field from the hiatus to the thoracic inlet. It is also important to note that, once the ports are docked to the robotic arms, further positioning of the patient cannot occur without first undocking the arms. While these disadvantages will likely improve with future iterations of the technology, they may remain significant impediments to robotic adoption for esophagectomy.

SUMMARY

MIE is gaining wider acceptance, with an increasingly growing body of evidence suggesting improved quality of life and perioperative outcomes compared to open approaches, while maintaining oncologic equivalence. Although less established, RAMIE is also increasing in utilization, with early experiences suggesting equivalent outcomes to standard MIE approaches. Larger, prospective experiences are needed to clarify if the clear improvements in visualization, advanced imaging, surgeon control, and instrument dexterity afforded by these technologies translate into significant improvements in clinical outcomes.

REFERENCES

1. Luketich JD, Pennathur A, Awais O, et al. Outcomes after minimally invasive esophagectomy: review of over 1000 patients. *Ann Surg* 2012;256:95–103.
2. Luketich JD, Alvelo-Rivera M, Buenaventura PO, et al. Minimally invasive esophagectomy: outcomes in 222 patients. *Ann Surg* 2003;238:486–494; discussion 494–495.
3. Zhang J, Wang R, Liu S, et al. Refinement of minimally invasive esophagectomy techniques after 15 years of experience. *J Gastrointest Surg* 2012;16:1768–1774.
4. Luketich JD, Pennathur A, Franchetti Y, et al. Minimally invasive esophagectomy: results of a prospective phase II multicenter trial-the eastern cooperative oncology group (E2202) study. *Ann Surg* 2015;261:702–707.
5. Levy RM, Trivedi D, Luketich JD. Minimally invasive esophagectomy. *Surg Clin North Am* 2012;92:1265–1285.
6. Pennathur A, Awais O, Luketich JD. Minimally invasive esophagectomy for Barrett's with high-grade dysplasia and early adenocarcinoma of the esophagus. *J Gastrointest Surg* 2010;14:948–950.
7. Pennathur A, Awais O, Luketich JD. Technique of minimally invasive Ivor Lewis esophagectomy. *Ann Thorac Surg* 2010;89:S2159–S2162.
8. Kernstine KH, DeArmond DT, Karimi M, et al. The robotic, 2-stage, 3-field esophagolymphadenectomy. *J Thorac Cardiovasc Surg* 2004;127:1847–1849.
9. Kernstine KH, DeArmond DT, Shamoun DM, et al. The first series of completely robotic esophagectomies with three-field lymphadenectomy: initial experience. *Surg Endosc* 2007;21:2285–2292.
10. Anderson C, Hellan M, Kernstine K, et al. Robotic surgery for gastrointestinal malignancies. *Int J Med Robot* 2007;3:297–300.
11. Cerfolio RJ, Bryant AS, Hawn MT. Technical aspects and early results of robotic esophagectomy with chest anastomosis. *J Thorac Cardiovasc Surg* 2013;145:90–96.
12. Sarkaria IS, Rizk NP, Finley DJ, et al. Combined thoracoscopic and laparoscopic robotic-assisted minimally invasive esophagectomy using a four-arm platform: experience, technique and cautions during early procedure development. *Eur J Cardiothorac Surg* 2013;43:e107–e115.
13. Sarkaria IS, Rizk NP, Grosser R, et al. Attaining proficiency in robotic-assisted minimally invasive esophagectomy while maximizing safety during procedure development. *Innovations (Phila).* 2016;11(4):268–273.
14. Hernandez JM, Dimou F, Weber J, et al. Defining the learning curve for robotic-assisted esophagogastrectomy. *J Gastrointest Surg* 2013;17:1346–1351.
15. de la Fuente SG, Weber J, Hoffe SE, et al. Initial experience from a large referral center with robotic-assisted Ivor Lewis esophagogastrectomy for oncologic purposes. *Surg Endosc* 2013;27:3339–3347.
16. Clark J, Sodergren MH, Purkayastha S, et al. The role of robotic assisted laparoscopy for oesophagogastric oncological resection; an appraisal of the literature. *Dis Esophagus* 2011;24:240–250.
17. Sarkaria IS, Rizk NP. Robotic-assisted minimally invasive esophagectomy: the Ivor Lewis approach. *Thorac Surg Clin* 2014;24:211–222.
18. Sarkaria IS, Bains MS, Finley DJ, et al. Intraoperative near-infrared fluorescence imaging as an adjunct to robotic-assisted minimally invasive esophagectomy. *Innovations* 2014;9:391–393.

131

Alternative Conduits for Replacement of the Esophagus

Hugh G. Auchincloss ▪ Douglas J. Mathisen

INTRODUCTION

The stomach is the preferred conduit for reconstruction following resection of the esophagus for benign or malignant disease. However, situations arise in which the stomach cannot be used, mandating that thoracic surgeons be comfortable with alternative conduits to restore alimentary continuity. These conduits include colon, pedicled jejunum, and supercharged jejunum. Rarely, no intestinal conduit is available and a myocutaneous flap or skin tube is required. Alternative conduits may have the advantage of longer length, decreased postoperative acid reflux, and lower morbidity from anastomotic leak. Specific clinical situations are better suited to one conduit versus another and the techniques involved in their construction differ substantially. Thoracic surgeons must therefore be well versed in a broad variety of operative approaches. Short- and long-term outcomes following esophageal reconstruction with an alternative conduit are roughly comparable to those seen following traditional gastric pull-up, when one factors in the circumstances that led to an alternative conduit being required.

INDICATIONS

Rarely is an alternative conduit used for reconstruction following esophagectomy when the stomach is otherwise available. Some authors advocate for the use a colon or jejunum interposition graft as a primary option when long-term survival is expected, as with benign disease or in the pediatric population. Benign disease includes a wide range of pathology, including distal peptic stricture, long-segment caustic stricture, functional motility disorder, or failed antireflux procedure. For the majority of patients, though, an alternative conduit is used because the stomach is unsuitable. This may be because of prior abdominal surgery, pre-existing gastric pathology, or nonviability of the stomach (i.e., strangulated paraesophageal hernia). Alternatively, the patient may have previously undergone esophagectomy with gastric pull-up complicated by gastric necrosis or intractable stricture. Historically, alternative conduits were also used to bypass the esophagus in cases of unresectable malignant obstruction, with the obstructed esophagus left in situ and the conduit placed in an extra-anatomic location. However, the widespread availability of esophageal stents has rendered the need for esophageal bypass less common.

Our experience with colon and short-segment jejunum interposition for reconstruction following esophagectomy was published by Wain[1] and Gaissert[2] (Table 131.1), respectively. The indication for use of short-segment jejunum was related to gastroesophageal reflux disease in over 80% of patients, with the majority having undergone a failed antireflux procedure prior to surgery. Benign disease was also the most common indication for use of colon interposition, with special emphasis on long-segment caustic stricture.

CHOICE OF ALTERNATIVE CONDUIT

When an alternative conduit is required several factors must be considered. The conduit must be of suitable length, provide some mechanism of protection from reflux, have a reliable vascular supply, and be free of intrinsic pathology. When an anastomosis to the cervical esophagus is anticipated the options are limited to colon or supercharged jejunum. Pedicled jejunum is seldom long enough to reach into the adult neck for a tension-free esophagojejunostomy. Colon

TABLE 131.1 Indications for Jejunal Interposition

Indications for Short-Segment Interposition at Massachusetts General Hospital

Diagnosis	Percentage of 41 Patients
Gastroesophageal reflux disease	82.5
Failed antireflux procedure	50.5
Nondilatable stricture	21.5
Complication of treatment for achalasia	5.0
Complication of myotomy for motility disorder	2.5
Complication of intrathoracic esophagogastrostomy	2.5
Esophageal moniliasis with stricture	5.0
Barrett esophagus with carcinoma in situ	5.0
Leak from esophagotomy	2.5
Carcinoma of the esophagus	2.5
Leiomyosarcoma of the esophagus	2.5

interposition is less technically demanding than supercharged jejunum and provides good long-term functional result. However, colon pathology, including diverticular disease, functional motility disorders, and atherosclerotic vascular disease, is common and may limit its use. In contrast, intrinsic small bowel disease is uncommon and the jejunum has a rich albeit variable vascular arcade. The primary disadvantage of supercharged jejunal interposition is that considerable operative time and complexity must be devoted to performing multiple microvascular anastomoses. This critique does not apply to pedicled jejunum, though, which remains an excellent conduit for replacement of a short segment of distal esophagus. When the need for an alternative conduit was unanticipated but immediate reconstruction is desired, jejunum is preferred over colon because preoperative bowel prep and angiography are not required.

PREOPERATIVE PREPARATION

Ideally the potential for use of an alternative conduit is anticipated prior to esophageal resection. All patients should undergo a complete history and physical examination with special attention paid to vascular and gastrointestinal disease. Patients with a history of gastrointestinal bleeding, unexplained abdominal pain, colon polyps, or diverticular disease should be evaluated further with colonoscopy. A contrast enema is a reasonable and less invasive alternative. A history of constipation or other functional disorders may prompt formal motility studies; however, there is no evidence that peristalsis of the conduit directly impacts overall function after replacement.

A thorough assessment of nutritional status is crucial. This is especially true of patients who have undergone previous esophageal surgery with a failed conduit. Low levels of serum albumin and iron stores as well as physical signs of weight loss and muscle wasting indicate the need for a preoperative nutritional program. When possible, oral feeding with caloric supplementation is preferred. Some patients benefit from preoperative placement of an enteric feeding tube. Rarely, parenteral nutrition is required.

All patients in whom colon interposition is planned should undergo routine mesenteric angiography. Debate about this practice persists in the literature, with opponents arguing that intraoperative assessment of mesenteric vasculature is more reliable and cost effective than radiologic evaluation. Our perspective is that preoperative angiography aids immeasurably with surgical planning. In contrast to the richly vascularized stomach, the blood supply to the colon is highly variable and frequently tenuous.[3] Mesenteric angiography may demonstrate stenosis of the inferior mesenteric artery or the origin of the left colic artery, a bifid middle colic artery, or an incomplete marginal artery between the left branch of the middle colic artery and the ascending branch of the left colic artery. These findings may lead the surgeon to supercharge the conduit, select the right colon as an alternative conduit, or abandon the colon entirely in favor of jejunum. Having this information in advance saves valuable time in the operating room and prevents a tedious dissection of the mesentery guided by palpation. Patients undergoing planned jejunal interposition do not require preoperative angiography. Atherosclerotic disease involving the small bowel is uncommon, and despite the variability of jejunal blood supply,[4] angiography adds little to operative planning.

Mechanical bowel prep is appropriate when colon interposition is planned to avoid gross contamination of the chest. Antibiotic bowel preps are not indicated and may cause enteritis. Perioperative intravenous antibiotics targeted to skin and intestinal flora are given during both colon and jejunum interposition.

OPERATIVE TECHNIQUE

Replacement of the esophagus with colon or jejunum is a complex surgical procedure and, owing to its relative infrequency, one with which few thoracic surgeons can boast an extensive experience. Generally speaking, these operations should not be performed outside of centers familiar with complex esophageal surgery.

The principles of alternative-conduit esophageal replacement are consistent regardless of the indication: (1) meticulous attention to the vascular pedicle—both arterial and venous—of the conduit, (2) restoration of swallowing by placement of an isoperistaltic conduit with minimal intrathoracic redundancy, (3) positioning of the conduit in a location that provides for tension-free proximal and distal anastomoses, and (4) prevention of reflux. All esophageal surgery should begin with an endoscopic evaluation by the surgeon to confirm the location of pathology and the absence of other disease.

ANESTHESIA

Most patients benefit from placement of an epidural catheter prior to surgery with the caveat that an epidural placed to cover a thoracotomy incision will not cover pain related to the cervical incision and may not adequately cover a laparotomy incision. Intraoperative use of the epidural tends to result in intestinal peristalsis and distention and should be avoided. Placement of an arterial catheter for continuous blood pressure monitoring is essential given the need for accurate measurement when assessing the vasculature of the conduit and because of the potential for significant hemodynamic shifts associated with retraction of the heart during esophageal dissection. Single lung ventilation is required for the majority of esophageal resection and can be achieved with a double lumen endotracheal tube or Univent tube and bronchial blocker. Transhiatal esophagectomy with long-segment intestinal interposition can be accomplished without lung isolation; however, the patient should be physiologically able to tolerate lung isolation, should it be required.

POSITION OF CONDUIT

Four options exist for positioning a long-segment alternative conduit: posterior mediastinal, substernal, transpleural, or subcutaneous. A short-segment interposition with intrathoracic anastomosis by necessity lies in the posterior mediastinum with the mediastinal pleura opened into the left or right chest, depending on surgical approach. Placing the conduit in a sealed camera bag with suction applied eases the process of maneuvering it undamaged and with proper orientation into its chosen position.

POSTERIOR MEDIASTINAL

The posterior mediastinum in the bed of the resected esophagus is the preferred position of the conduit when the anastomosis is to the thoracic esophagus. It is also the shortest and most direct route to the cervical esophagus and should be used when there is limited length of the conduit. The posterior mediastinum is unavailable if the native esophagus is bypassed rather than resected, or if necrosis of a prior gastric pull-up has resulted in significant fibrosis and adhesions. An alternative route should also be considered when there is concern for an incomplete oncologic resection. This allows for additional radiation to be delivered to the esophageal resection

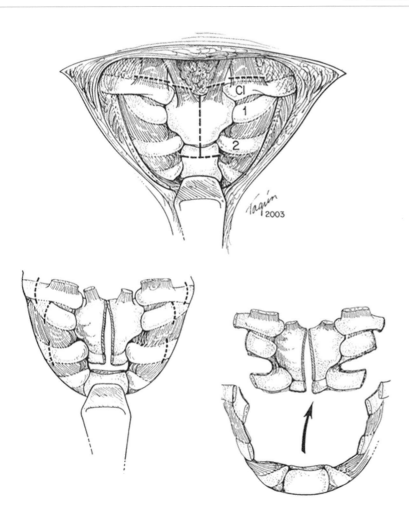

FIGURE 131.1 Enlargement of the thoracic inlet. (From Grillo HC. Surgery of the trachea and bronchi. PMPH-USA, 2004. With permission.)

bed without damage to the conduit, and avoids the potential for future obstruction of the conduit from local or regional nodal recurrence.

SUBSTERNAL

The substernal route is generally considered the primary option for reconstruction to the cervical esophagus. The course is between 5 and 10 cm longer than the posterior mediastinal route and comparatively more tortuous, with sharp angles at the manubrium and again at the xiphoid. Resection of the head of the clavicle, 1st rib, and part of the manubrium serves to enlarge the thoracic inlet and straighten the course (Fig. 131.1). We perform this maneuver routinely. A prior sternotomy usually prohibits use of the substernal route. Likewise, the presence of a substernal conduit complicates future sternotomy attempts; however, cautious sternotomy can be performed and may be the optimal incision if revision of the conduit is required.

TRANSPLEURAL

Either pleural space may be used in the lieu of the posterior mediastinal or substernal routes. Though shorter than the substernal route, a transpleural position risks comprising lung function and can cause poor emptying of the conduit. As with the substernal route, enlargement of the thoracic inlet to prevent compression of the conduit is typically required. In the pediatric population the transpleural route may be preferred.

SUBCUTANEOUS

Subcutaneous positioning of the conduit is undesirable from a cosmetic and functional perspective. It is reserved for the rare situation in which no other route is possible. Often the food bolus must be propelled manually through the resulting conduit.

EXPOSURE

Surgical approach depends on the indication for surgery, planned conduit, and surgeon preference. Resection of the distal esophagus followed by short-segment reconstruction with either colon or jejunum can be accomplished using a left thoracoabdominal incision through the 6th or 7th intercostal space with division of the costal arch. This provides excellent exposure to the distal esophagus, stomach, small bowel mesentery, and splenic flexure of the colon along with the middle and left colic arteries. It does not, however, permit mobilization of the right colon. The thoracoabdominal approach has the advantage of providing superior exposure to the esophageal hiatus, and requires only a single incision without the need for intraoperative repositioning. Its usefulness, however, is limited by poor access to the esophagus superior to the level of the aortic arch.

Long-segment colon or supercharged jejunum interposition requires access to both the abdomen and the cervical esophagus. Esophagectomy performed for benign disease may be done with a laparotomy and a left neck incision, with the esophagus resected in transhiatal fashion. Great care must be exercised when blindly passing the conduit into the esophageal bed to avoid injury to the conduit or blood supply. This approach avoids the morbidity of a thoracotomy and the need for single-lung ventilation. Esophageal carcinoma may also be resected using a transhiatal approach; however, many surgeons would advocate the addition of a right thoracotomy (i.e., three-field or McKeown esophagectomy) to ensure complete thoracic lymphadenectomy. Finally, the use of an alternative conduit to salvage a patient who has undergone prior esophagectomy complicated by gastric conduit necrosis requires a right thoracotomy to allow for resection of the failed conduit. This may be performed as a staged procedure: the alternative conduit is placed in a substernal position at the initial operation and the failed gastric conduit can be resected via thoracotomy at a later date.

PREPARATION AND PLACEMENT OF THE CONDUIT

COLON

Either the left or right colon may serve as an alternative conduit; however, the left colon is preferred over the right due to the relative constancy of the marginal artery. Wilkins[5] noted in his series from 1980 that conduit necrosis occurred in five out 32 patients reconstructed with right colon grafts and only two out of 68 patients with left colon grafts, an observation that is supported by current experience. The ideal colon conduit includes transverse colon and extends to a point distal to the splenic flexure. Extended length requires mobilization of the hepatic flexure as well. The vascular supply of a left colon graft arises from the left colic artery with the proximal conduit perfused via the marginal artery (Fig. 131.2). When

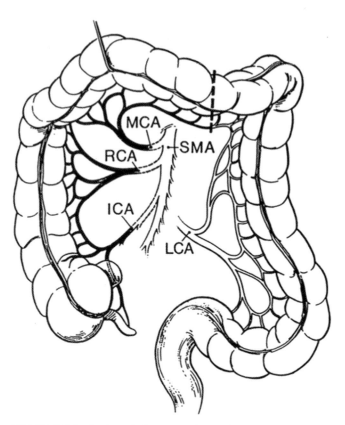

FIGURE 131.3 Blood supply for a right colon conduit.

the right colon is used the graft includes ascending and transverse colon, with or without terminal ileum depending on adequacy of the marginal artery (Fig. 131.3). The vascular pedicle becomes the middle colic artery.

Preparation of the colon for use as a conduit begins with mobilization of the avascular attachments to the greater omentum and retroperitoneum. The mesentery is then transilluminated to identify the middle and left colic pedicles. The middle colic artery and vein must be identified at their respective origins from the superior mesenteric artery and vein, a step that is made easier by careful review of preoperative angiography. Ultimately the middle colic artery is divided proximal to its bifurcation into middle and left branches, thereby creating an arcade to perfuse the proximal conduit. An early-branching middle colic artery should be approached cautiously, and a true bifid artery should prompt the surgeon to consider either performing a right colon graft or supercharging the left colon graft using the middle colic vessels.

The vasculature of the conduit is then isolated with the application of vascular clamps to the proximal middle colic artery and the collateral vessels of right colic artery. The conduit is now fed entirely by the left colic artery and an assessment can be made about the adequacy of this blood supply. Ideally, pulses are palpable in the mesentery of the proximal conduit. At minimum, Doppler signals should be present before proceeding with division of the middle colic artery. It is useful to perform this vascular isolation early in the course of the operation and then turn attention to mobilizing the stomach and preparing the cervical esophagus for anastomosis. If the proximal colon remains well perfused during this period, it can be divided with confidence.

Exposure of the cervical esophagus is performed through a left neck incision along the anterior border of the sternocleidomastoid

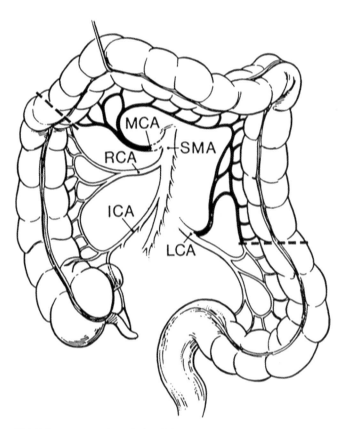

FIGURE 131.2 Blood supply for a left colon conduit.

muscle. The cervical esophagus is identified and encircled with a Penrose drain. Care must be taken to avoid injury to the recurrent laryngeal nerves that run in the tracheoesophageal groove. Complete mobilization of the thoracic esophagus facilitates delivery of the cervical esophagus into the incision where it can be prepared for anastomosis. The divided colon is drawn into the chest to lie in its chosen position. If a posterior mediastinal route is selected the conduit passes posterior to the stomach. A substernal route is better suited to an antegastric position. Multiple techniques have been described for cervical esophagocolostomy. The decision about whether to perform the anastomosis end-to-end versus end-to-side, and in handsewn fashion or with a circular stapler, is ultimately that of the surgeon. We prefer a two-layer interrupted suture technique. The most crucial aspect of the anastomosis is continued inspection for adequacy of blood supply. If there is concern for compression of the anastomosis, enlargement of the thoracic inlet should be performed using the previously described technique. After the anastomosis is complete the cervical incision is closed and attention returns to the abdomen. A closed suction drain may be left in the neck but should not be placed directly adjacent to the anastomosis as this may promote leak.

In the abdomen the distal colon is now divided at the previously designated site beyond the left colic pedicle. A handsewn or stapled colocolic anastomosis is performed with closure of the mesenteric defect. The gastrocolic anastomosis is performed with several factors in mind. Allowing 10 to 12 cm of intra-abdominal redundancy of the graft provides protection against reflux. Intrathoracic redundancy of the graft is poorly tolerated and should be managed by either resecting the distal graft or using a boxcar resection technique (Fig. 131.4). The

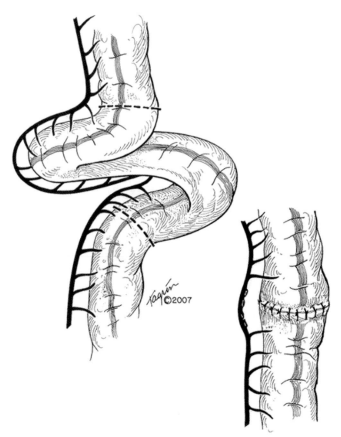

FIGURE 131.4 Boxcar resection of a colon conduit. (From de Delva PE, Morse CR, Austen Jr. WG, et al. Surgical management of failed colon interposition. *Eur J Cardiothorac Surg* 2008;34(2):432–437. Reproduced by permission of European Association for Cardiothoracic Surgery.)

conduit should be secured to the hiatus to prevent herniation. When a short-segment interposition is placed in the posterior mediastinal position, Wain[1] and colleagues perform the esophagocolic anastomosis to the midportion of the posterior stomach. For long-segment interposition in the substernal position an anterior anastomosis is preferred. Demeester[6] suggests performing a proximal gastrectomy with anastomosis to the gastric antrum except when a vagus-sparing esophagectomy has been performed. Regardless of site or technique, the resulting anastomosis should leave the graft with its pedicle free from torsion or kinking. When the stomach is unavailable the distal colon may be anastomosed to the duodenum or, preferably, to a Roux limb of jejunum.

Technique for right colon interposition is similar. The right colon and terminal ileum are mobilized from their retroperitoneal attachments and the ileocolic and right colic vessels are clamped. If adequate flow through the middle colic vessels is observed, the terminal ileum may be divided and brought into the neck for anastomosis. Alternatively the cecum and terminal ileum may be resected and the cervical anastomosis performed to the ascending colon. This shortens the graft but avoid the size discrepancy sometimes encountered when the cecum is involved in the anastomosis. The distal anastomosis is performed in the same fashion as described above.

PEDICLED JEJUNUM

Pedicled jejunum is an excellent conduit for replacement of the distal esophagus, particularly for benign disease; it may be used as an interposition graft with a distal anastomosis to the remaining stomach or in a Roux-en-Y configuration to replace both esophagus and stomach.

A left thoracoabdominal incision provides ideal exposure to the distal esophagus, hiatus, and abdominal contents. The esophagus is first mobilized circumferentially distal to the intended resection margin. When prior antireflux surgery has been performed there may be extensive scarring in the area of the esophageal hiatus. The short gastric vessels are ligated to provide exposure to the posterior stomach. The stomach may then be divided at the cardia using a linear stapler. An existing fundic wrap should be included in the resection. For benign disease the left gastric artery and the vagus nerves may be left intact. Complete lymphadenectomy is performed for malignant disease, and cancers of the esophagogastric junction may mandate more extensive gastrectomy.

The interposition graft is now fashioned. A suitable length of jejunum is selected and the vascular supply is inspected and palpated. The typical pedicled jejunal graft is based on a single jejunal branch of the superior mesenteric artery. The 1st, 2nd, and sometimes 3rd jejunal branches are short and provide collateral flow to the 4th portion of the duodenum (Fig. 131.5). Basing the conduit off these is unwise. More distally the vascular arcades of the jejunum produce increasing curvature and the geometry of the resulting conduit is difficult to negotiate. Proximal mid-jejunum is the preferred site, particularly when a Roux-en-Y reconstruction is to be used and total alimentary tract length must be factored in Figure 131.6.

With the site of the interposition graft now selected, vascular clamps are placed on all the collateral vessels and the conduit is observed for 10 minutes. If perfusion remains intact the segment may be divided proximally and distally. Jejunal continuity is restored using stapled or handsewn technique. The peritoneum overlying the mesentery to the conduit is divided to straighten it. If distal arcades are present a more proximal arcade may also be divided to achieve additional straightening, but care must be taken not compromise blood supply.

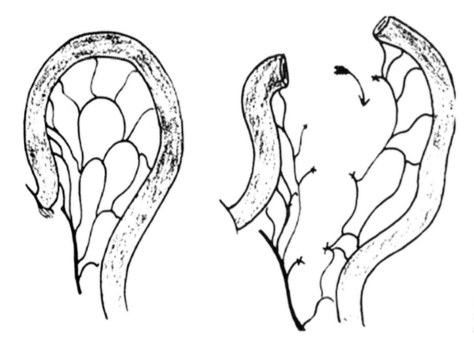

FIGURE 131.5 Blood supply for a pedicled jejunal interposition. The first several jejunal branches are left intact to supply the distal duodenum.

The conduit is transposed into the chest in retrocolic fashion by creating a small window in the transverse mesocolon. The graft is passed posterior to the stomach and through the esophageal hiatus into the posterior mediastinum. Isoperistaltic orientation is desirable. Meticulous attention must be paid the vascular pedicle to avoid kinking, torsion, or compression.

A two-layered handsewn end-to-side esophagojejunostomy is our preferred technique for the proximal anastomosis. The anastomosis should be performed to the antimesenteric border as close to the end of the graft as possible to avoid redundancy (i.e., "candy cane" defect) that results in stasis and regurgitation (Fig. 131.7). Others have described an end-to-end technique.

The gastrojejunal anastomosis is performed to the posterior wall of the stomach along the greater curve and a few centimeters away from the gastric staple line. This provides the most direct route from the posterior mediastinum and allows for several centimeters of intra-abdominal conduit, which in turn helps diminish reflux. Minimal intrathoracic redundancy should be tolerated. Redundancy may be dealt with by resecting distal jejunum leaving the mesentery intact, or by performing a boxcar resection at the midportion of

the graft (Fig. 131.8). If the latter method is employed the resection should stay immediately apposed to the bowel wall to prevent disruption of the vascular arcade. Finally, the conduit should be secured to the esophageal hiatus to prevent herniation.

Short-segment reconstruction using a Roux-en-Y configuration proceeds in much the same way as for a jejunal interposition graft. A point approximately 40 cm distal to the ligament of Treitz is selected and divided. The Roux limb is brought through the transverse mesocolon and into the chest through the esophageal hiatus. If the stomach is not surgically absent the Roux limb is typically brought posterior to it. The Roux limb can be straightened by dividing the peritoneal covering of the mesentery. The esophagojejunostomy is performed in the same fashion as described above. A jejunojejunostomy is

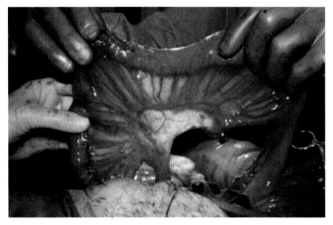

FIGURE 131.6 Preparing the jejunal interposition graft.

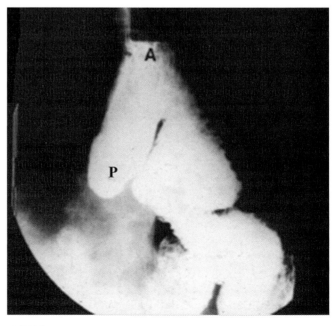

FIGURE 131.7 Barium swallow demonstrating a pouch at the esophagojejunal anastomosis.

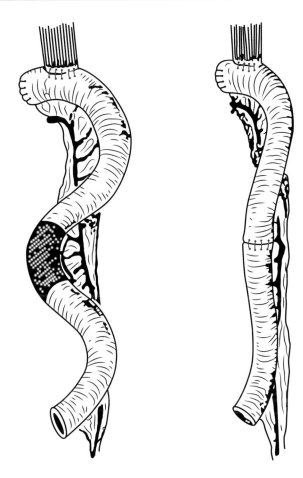

FIGURE 131.8 Boxcar resection of a jejunal interposition graft.

performed leaving at least an 80 cm Roux limb to prevent bile reflux. Mesenteric defects should be closed to prevent internal hernias and the Roux limb should be fixed to the esophageal hiatus.

SUPERCHARGED JEJUNUM

Supercharging refers to a technique in which the blood supply to the proximal conduit is augmented using microvascular anastomoses between the mesenteric vessels and vessels in the neck. While any conduit may be supercharged in the manner described below, the practice is commonly performed only for long-segment jejunal interposition. Ascioti[7] and colleagues describe performing microvascular anastomoses to the internal mammary and vein, occasionally using saphenous vein graft, as well as to branches of the carotid artery and jugular vein.

The mobilization of the jejunum is similar to that performed for short-segment interposition. However, a longer segment of jejunum is selected. This segment should be based on three jejunal branches: the most distal remains intact as a pedicle from the superior mesenteric artery, the middle is ligated, and the proximal is supercharged to the neck vessels. This conduit is then passed retrocolic and into its chosen position in the chest. If the posterior mediastinum is available the conduit passes retrogastric such that a posterior gastrojejunostomy can be performed. A substernal route is usually better suited to an anterior gastrojejunostomy. The distal anastomosis is performed after completion of the cervical esophagojejunostomy and in the same fashion as described earlier. Alternatively, if the

stomach is unavailable the conduit may be brought into the neck as a Roux limb.

Exposure to the cervical esophagus and neck vessels is performed via a left neck incision with resection of the head of the left clavicle, 1st rib, and part of the manubrium. The esophagojejunostomy is performed in the end-to-side or end-to-end fashion. The vein-to-vein and artery-to-artery anastomoses are performed under the operating microscope by a surgeon with microvascular training. Many methods of anastomosis have been described and are beyond the scope of this chapter. Blackmon[8] and others have adopted the use of a monitoring flap. This is a segment of proximal jejunum detached from the rest of the conduit but perfused by the microvascular anastomosis that is then externalized. Observed ischemia of the monitoring flap in the postoperative prompts re-exploration. If recovery is uncomplicated the flap can be excised at bedside after several days. Others have questioned the utility of the monitoring flap, noting that once the flap becomes ischemic the conduit is seldom salvageable.

OTHER CONSIDERATIONS

PYLORIC DRAINAGE

Once a mainstay of esophageal surgery, pyloric drainage procedures have not been shown to affect the rates of delayed conduit emptying. This is true for alternative conduit reconstruction as well.[9,10] We have moved away from routine pyloroplasty or pyloromyotomy in favor of selective postoperative pneumatic dilation of the pylorus for patients in whom conduit dysfunction occurs.

FEEDING JEJUNOSTOMY TUBES

Jejunostomy tubes allow for early enteral nutrition but come with their own set of complications, including local wound complications, intussusception, and small bowel obstruction. We feel that the benefits of jejunostomy tubes continue to outweigh these risks, especially in the context of alternative conduit reconstruction.

POSTOPERATIVE CARE

The majority of patients undergoing alternative conduit reconstruction following esophagectomy will require immediate monitoring in an intensive care setting. Initially, management is a balancing act between judicious fluid administration to avoid pulmonary complications and avoidance of high vasopressor requirements that may compromise vascular supply to the conduit. The patient remains strictly nil per os for at least a week. A nasoenteric drainage tube is placed in the operating room and used for decompression of the conduit during this period. Accidental dislodgement of this tube should prompt replacement only by a skilled practitioner. Placement of a feeding jejunostomy tube at the time of operation facilitates early enteric nutrition; however, small bowel and colonic ileus are common after both jejunum and colon interposition. A safe practice is to initiate tube feeds at a low, trophic rate and avoid advancement until bowel activity has been confirmed by passage of flatus. Drainage of the pleural space should continue until enteral nutrition has begun, given the propensity for thoracic duct leaks to present in delayed fashion. It is our practice to study all patients with a barium swallow after a week or so of uncomplicated recovery. If this study confirms adequate emptying of the conduit and the absence of leak or stricture, we initiate a clear liquid diet. This is advanced over a period of weeks to an appropriate esophageal diet. Alternatively, some surgeons forego a swallowing study and instead initiate oral feeding as an outpatient after several weeks have passed.

COMPLICATIONS

Early and late complications occur frequently following alternative conduit replacement of the esophagus. Pneumonia, arrhythmia, recurrent laryngeal nerve injury, wound infection, and small bowel obstruction may occur in as many as half of patients undergoing these complex procedures. Despite this, mortality in most major series is less than 10%, and serious procedure-specific complications requiring reoperation—including conduit necrosis, persistent anastomotic fistula, intractable stricture, conduit redundancy, and severe reflux—occur in less than 20% of patients Tables 131.2 and 131.3.[2,11]

CONDUIT NECROSIS

Necrosis of the conduit occurs rarely but failure to recognize and aggressively manage this complication results in significant disability or death. The cause is almost always vascular in origin. Arterial insufficiency is typically recognized and corrected intraoperatively; delayed ischemia is therefore often the result of venous compromise. Unexplained sepsis in the postoperative period should raise concern for conduit necrosis and prompt immediate return to the operating room. Endoscopic evaluation is a reasonable interim step when ambiguity exists; however, re-exploration with resection of the conduit and staged reconstruction is the safest option.

ANASTOMOTIC LEAK

Anastomotic leak most commonly occurs at the proximal anastomosis as a product of excessive tension, mild vascular compromise, or technical error. It presents as wound drainage or local swelling coupled with mild fever and pain. Importantly, in contrast to esophagogastric anastomotic leak, leak after colon or jejunum interposition tends to follow a more benign course. Frequently it can be managed with local drainage, antibiotics, and delayed feeding. As such, the use of covered stents—now commonplace in the management of esophagogastric anastomotic leak—has not been carried over to alternative conduit anastomotic leak.

TABLE 131.2 Complications Following Jejunal Interposition

Complications of Short-Segment Interposition at Massachusetts General Hospital

Mortality: 10.5%	
Graft necrosis	1
Myocardial infarction	1
Major complications: 31%	
Pneumonia	3
Gastric perforation	1
Paraparesis, aortoenteric erosion	1
Transient recurrent nerve injury	1

N = 41 patients.
Reprinted from Gaissert HA, Mathisen DJ, Grillo HC, et al. Short-segment intestinal interposition of the distal esophagus. *J Thorac Cardiovasc Surg* 1993;106(5):860–866. Copyright © 1993 The American Association for Thoracic Surgery. With permission.

TABLE 131.3 Complications Following Gastric Conduit Versus Supercharged Pedicled Jejunum[11]

Variable	Gastric Conduit (n = 31,69%)	SPJ (n = 14,31%)	p Value
Surgical complications:	15 (48%)	7 (50%)	NS
Pneumonia	7 (23%)	3 (21%)	
Afib	4 (13%)	1 (7%)	
Renal failure	1 (3%)	1 (7%)	
Respiratory failure	1 (10%)	1 (7%)	
UTI	1 (3%)	0 (0%)	
DVT	1 (3%)	1 (7%)	
1 year postop weight (lbs)	156.8 ± 35.6	144.7 ± 26.5	NS
1 year postop BMI	23.6 ± 5.5	22.6 ± 3.0	NS
1 year postop % weight loss	21.1 ± 22.4	22.5 ± 20.0	NS
1 year weight loss (lbs)	20.0 ± 20.3	20.9 ± 18.4	NS
Length of stay (days)	10 ± 4 (9)	17 ± 15 (12.5)	0.04
Leak within 60 days	7 (23%)	4 (29%)	NS
Reoperation	3 (10%)	1 (7%)	NS

Afib = atrial fibrillation; BMI = body mass index; DVT = deep vein thrombosis; NS = not statistically significant; postop = post-operative; SPJ = super-charged pedicled jejunal; LTI = urinary tract infection.
The number of patients of listed for each parameter followed by % of patients who answered that particular question is given in parenthesis. Mean ± standard deviation listed where appropriate with median in parenthesis.

STRICTURE

A late consequence of an anastomotic leak may be the formation of a stricture. Stricture may also form secondary to technical issues with the anastomosis or as a product of chronic venous stasis. Most strictures are amenable to endoscopic dilation, though improvement is seldom durable and serial dilations are required. Occasionally the severity of a stricture requires operative revision. This may take the form of a stricturoplasty (Fig. 131.9) or complete revision of the conduit.

REDUNDANCY

Excessive length of the intrathoracic conduit leads to poor emptying and mechanical obstruction. Redundancy is the most common indication for revision after long- and short-segment colon interposition (Table 131.4).[12] The same is not true for jejunal interposition because colon, unlike jejunum, tends to dilate and elongate over time. Redundancy is addressed surgically by removing excess conduit, either by revising the cologastric anastomosis or by performing a boxcar resection in the manner previously described.

LONG-TERM OUTCOME

Return to normal alimentation is the most important measure of the long-term success of reconstruction following esophagectomy. In this regard alternative conduits perform well. Blackmon[11] reported that over 80% of patients were able to return to a regular diet after supercharged jejunal interposition. Gaissert[2] found that 13 of 19 patients followed after short-segment jejunal interposition had excellent or good results, and three patients were able to eat but reported moderate dysphagia or regurgitation. On extended follow-up after colon

TABLE 131.4 Indications for Revision of Colon Interposition

Etiology of Colon Interposition Dysfunction in Patients Undergoing Revisional Surgery

Etiology	Number of Operations
Redundancy	13
Intractable stricture	11
Loss of intestinal continuity	8
Chronic fistula	6
Obstruction	6
Reflux esophagitis/colitis	4
Total	48

From de Delva PE, Morse CR, Austen WG Jr, et al. Surgical management of failed colon interposition. *Eur J Cardiothorac Surg* 2008;34(2):432–437; discussion 437. Reproduced by permission of European Association for Cardiothoracic Surgery.

interposition, Wain[1] noted that 11 of 50 patients had a completely unrestricted diet and 33 patients required some adjustment for aspiration but were free from supplemental nutrition. These results are consistent with the literature. There is general consensus that the function of an alternative conduit improves with time.

The ability of alternative conduits to participate in peristalsis and active food bolus propulsion remains a controversial subject. Studies using barium swallow, neoesophageal manometry, nuclear imaging, and endoscopy have been performed and yielded mixed results. These results may be summarized in the following terms: alternative conduits empty in delayed fashion, muscular contraction may be present but may also be disorganized, and there is little correlation between these findings and clinical results. It is our belief that most conduits function passively.

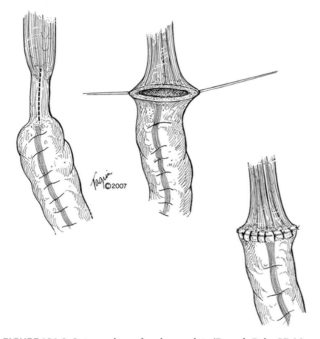

FIGURE 131.9 Stricturoplasty of a colon conduit. (From de Delva PE, Morse CR, Austen Jr. WG, et al. Surgical management of failed colon interposition. *Eur J Cardiothorac Surg* 2008;34(2):432–437. Reproduced by permission of European Association for Cardiothoracic Surgery.)

SKIN TUBES

In rare instances no intestinal conduit is available to bridge an esophageal defect. This usually occurs as a result of multiple failed attempts to restore alimentary continuity using the above alternative conduits, leaving the patient with cervical esophagostomy and a poor quality of life. In such cases we have had success using a myocutaneous pectoralis major flap fashioned into a tube fed by perforating vessels from the internal mammary artery. The inner layer of this tube is grafted with skin from a distant site to provide an epithelial border. The tube is connected in stages to the cervical esophagus proximally and a Roux limb distally.[13] Similar techniques using radial forearm and anterolateral thigh are well described for repairing defects in the pharynx and cervical esophagus. Though functionally immotile and cosmetically unappealing, these grafts can be successful in allowing patients to return to full oral nutrition.

CONCLUSION

Techniques for reconstruction of the esophagus using conduits other than the stomach are a valuable component of the thoracic surgeon's armamentarium. Because different clinical situations and patient factors may call for the use of colon, pedicled jejunum, supercharged jejunal interposition, or construction of a skin tube, familiarity with these operations is a requirement for practice of esophageal surgery. These reconstructive options may be performed with reasonable morbidity and yield functional results that approach those seen with a standard gastric conduit.

REFERENCES

1. Wain JC, Wright CD, Kuo EY, et al. Long-segment colon interposition for acquired esophageal disease. *Ann Thorac Surg* 1999;67(2):313–317; discussion 317–318.
2. Gaissert HA, Mathisen DJ, Grillo HC, et al. Short-segment intestinal interposition of the distal esophagus. *J Thorac Cardiovasc Surg* 1993;106(5):860–866; discussion 866–867.
3. Sonneland J, Anson BJ, Beaton LE. Surgical anatomy of the arterial supply to the colon from the superior mesenteric artery based upon a study of 600 specimens. *Surg Gynecol Obstet* 1958;106(4):385–398.
4. Barlow TE. Variations in the blood-supply of the upper jejunum. *Br J Surg* 1956;43(181):473–475.
5. Wilkins EW Jr. Long-segment colon substitution for the esophagus. *Ann Surg* 1980;192(6):722–725.
6. DeMeester TR, Johansson KE, Franze I, et al. Indications, surgical technique, and long-term functional results of colon interposition or bypass. *Ann Surg* 1988;208(4):460–474.
7. Ascioti AJ, Hofstetter WL, Miller MJ, et al. Long-segment, supercharged, pedicled jejunal flap for total esophageal reconstruction. *J Thorac Cardiovasc Surg* 2005;130(5):1391–1398.
8. Blackmon SH, Correa AM, Skoracki R, et al. Supercharged pedicled jejunal interposition for esophageal replacement: a 10-year experience. *Ann Thorac Surg* 2012;94(4):1104–1111; discussion 1111–1113.
9. Gaur P, Swanson SJ. Should we continue to drain the pylorus in patients undergoing an esophagectomy? *Dis Esophagus* 2014;27(6):568–573.
10. Antonoff MB, Puri V, Meyers BF, et al. Comparison of pyloric intervention strategies at the time of esophagectomy: is more better? *Ann Thorac Surg* 2014;97(6):1950–1957; discussion 1657–1658.
11. Stephens EH, Gaur P, Hotze KO, et al. Super-charged pedicled jejunal interposition performance compares favorably with a gastric conduit after esophagectomy. *Ann Thorac Surg* 2015;100(2):407–413.
12. de Delva PE, Morse CR, Austen WG Jr, et al. Surgical management of failed colon interposition. *Eur J Cardiothorac Surg* 2008;34(2):432–437; discussion 437.
13. Shen KR, Austen WG Jr, Mathisen DJ. Use of a prefabricated pectoralis major muscle flap and pedicled jejunal interposition graft for salvage esophageal reconstruction after failed gastric pull-up and colon interposition. *J Thorac Cardiovasc Surg* 2008;135(5):1186–1187.

132

Per-Oral Esophageal Procedures

Ezra N. Teitelbaum ▪ Nathaniel J. Soper

INTRODUCTION

Since the introduction of laparoscopic, and subsequently thoracoscopic, surgery in the late 1980s and early 1990s, options for operative interventions in the abdomen and chest have steadily evolved to become less invasive. These minimally invasive approaches have in turn resulted in superior patient outcomes in terms of reduced postoperative pain, narcotic requirements, length of stay, and wound complications. Interventions performed with a flexible endoscope inserted orally represent an endpoint in this progression toward making surgery as minimally invasive as possible. Currently, conditions as varied as gastroesophageal reflux disease (GERD), achalasia, and esophageal cancer, that formerly required open operations via laparotomy or thoracotomy, can often be treated using a flexible endoscope without incisions. This approach offers the potential to even further reduce pain and convalescence after surgery. However, as such new procedures are introduced they must be carefully evaluated and only considered for widespread adoption if they are proven to be as safe and as effective as their traditional predecessors in achieving the intended functional or oncologic goals of the operation. This chapter will discuss a variety of peroral endoscopic procedures that are currently available to treat diseases of the esophagus and esophagogastric junction (EGJ). It will examine their technical aspects, as well as the available outcomes data and any important limitations and contraindications to their use. In general, these endoscopic operations should not be thought of as replacements for open or videoscopic surgery, but rather as new tools in an increasingly varied armamentarium available to the surgeon treating esophageal disease. Only by becoming experienced and skilled in these novel endoscopic techniques can surgeons most effectively counsel patients regarding the advantages and drawbacks of each approach, and guide them toward making an informed decision regarding which treatment option best suits their individual condition.

PERCUTANEOUS ENDOSCOPIC GASTROSTOMY TUBE

While seemingly a simple operation, placement of a gastrostomy tube via either an open or laparoscopic technique is fraught with major complications and high rates of short- and long-term mortality. This is in a large part due to the underlying illnesses that necessitate long-term enteral access for feeding or decompression. These include oropharyngeal cancers, stoke, advanced dementia, debilitation from prolonged mechanical ventilation, and metastatic cancers in general.

Percutaneous endoscopic gastrostomy (PEG) tube insertion was first introduced in 1980[1] as a flexible endoscopic technique for creating enteral access without the need for laparotomy. PEG has evolved to become the most common procedure for placing an enteral feeding tube, with over 200,000 cases performed each year in the United States alone.[2] PEG has been shown to reduce operative times and health care costs when compared with traditional gastrostomy, but it still carries a significant burden of complications and postoperative mortality. While much of this morbidity is due to the frailty of the patients upon which the procedure is performed, the incidence of complications directly related to the operation is likely under appreciated. Because of this, an in-depth discussion with the patient and their family regarding their disease prognosis, goals of care, and procedural risks and benefits is mandatory prior to proceeding with PEG tube insertion.

PREOPERATIVE EVALUATION AND INDICATIONS

The indication for PEG tube placement is any condition requiring the need for long-term enteral access for feeding, medication administration, or gastric decompression. These include conditions causing obstruction of the oropharynx, such as malignancy or functional dysphagia, most commonly due to stroke or dementia. Debilitation and prolonged mechanical ventilation due to critical illness or trauma are also common indications for PEG. Contraindications include a complete luminal obstruction that precludes endoscope passage into the stomach and any condition that would interfere with percutaneous insertion of the feeding tube through the abdominal wall and into the stomach, or impede formation of a stable gastrostomy tract. These include prior gastric surgery, gastric varices, and abdominal ascites. Prior upper abdominal surgery in general should be considered as a relative contraindication to PEG placement, as the resulting adhesions can prevent direct apposition of the anterior stomach with the abdominal wall and increase the risk for injury of other organs such as the transverse colon.

OPERATIVE TECHNIQUE

PEG tube insertion can be performed under either sedation or general anesthesia, and in a monitored hospital bed setting, the operating room, or an endoscopy suite, depending on the overall condition of the patient and their ability to maintain a protected airway. Two proceduralists are typically required, one to operate the flexible endoscope and the other to pass instruments and the feeding tube through the abdominal wall. The procedure begins with a diagnostic upper endoscopy and the stomach is insufflated. The next, and possibly most critical, step in the procedure is to determine whether the anterior aspect of the stomach is in direct contact with the abdominal wall, and therefore whether the PEG tube can safely be passed between them. A number of techniques can be used to determine this, including one-to-one palpation, transillumination, and the use of a finder needle.[3] In the one-to-one palpation technique, the surgeon in the abdominal field presses posteriorly on the abdominal wall with a single finger while the endoscopist observes the anterior stomach. A clear impression of the finger should be seen indenting the stomach. If a wider area of stomach is depressed with finger palpation, another organ such as the transverse colon may be interposed between the abdominal and gastric walls. With the transillumination technique, the room lights are dimmed and with the endoscope pointed at the anterior stomach wall, the endoscope light is observed shining through the abdominal wall. Most flexible gastroscopes have a transillumination button on their light-source, which increases the intensity of the light for purposes of this test. Failure of the endoscope light to transilluminate through the abdominal wall can again be an indicator that there is not direct contact between the stomach and abdominal wall. Finally, a small-gauge finder needle can be passed as a test through the abdominal wall and into the stomach and observed endoscopically. This technique is used more as an anatomic guide before passage of a larger needle, rather than to determine whether such passage is safe. It should be noted that all three of these techniques are made significantly more difficult and their results more ambiguous in obese patients with thicker abdominal walls. If the surgeon is not convinced that the stomach and anterior abdominal wall are in direct contact after application of these techniques, the safest course of action is to convert the procedure to either a laparoscopic or open approach.

Next, a larger gauge needle is inserted through the abdominal wall and into the stomach under direct endoscopic observation. A long guide wire is then fed through the needle and captured endoscopically using a snare inserted through the endoscope's working channel. The endoscope is then withdrawn orally, so that one end of the wire now exits the patient's mouth and the other end still transverses the abdominal wall. There are then two primary methods for inserting the PEG tube: "pull" (i.e., Ponsky technique) and "push" (i.e., Sachs–Vine technique). A number of PEG kits are commercially available and each is designed to use one or the other of these methods. In the original "pull" technique, the PEG tube is secured to the wire (which has a loop on its end) outside the mouth and then pulled via the wire through the esophagus and stomach and across the abdominal wall into position. With the push technique, the PEG tube is fed over the wire and pushed forward until the end exits through the abdominal wall, at which point it is grasped and pulled into final position. In an early randomized trial, there was no difference in complications or outcomes following the two techniques[4]; however, a more recent nonrandomized study suggested that the push method may result in higher rates of complications, including dislocation and occlusion.[5] Ultimately, surgeons should be familiar with both and utilize whichever technique they are most comfortable with, depending on which kits are available.

OUTCOMES

Despite the fact that PEG placement is performed endoscopically without entry into the abdomen, it should be considered a high-risk procedure, carrying a considerable burden of complications and mortality. A recent meta-analysis found a pooled 5.5% 30-day mortality after PEG insertion.[6] While it is unclear whether the PEG

procedure itself contributed to these deaths or they were simply the consequence of the patients' debilitated condition and advanced illness, many complications can occur directly as a result of the procedure, including bleeding, local wound complications, injury to other intra-abdominal organs, and tube dislodgement from the stomach resulting in peritonitis. As a result, care must be taken in deciding which patients are appropriate for PEG placement and whether such a procedure fits within each patient's long-term goals of care.

ENDOSCOPIC INTERVENTIONS FOR ESOPHAGEAL VARICES

Esophageal varices are common in patients with cirrhosis and up to one-third of patients with varices will experience an acute bleeding episode at some point. Variceal bleeding is an extremely serious condition that carries a 30-day mortality of 15% to 20%.[7] In addition to resuscitation and correction of coagulopathy, endoscopic intervention to control the hemorrhage is the mainstay of treatment. The importance of swift and effective endoscopic control of variceal bleeding cannot be overemphasized, because if it is unsuccessful, the only available salvage therapies are transjugular intrahepatic portosystemic shunt (TIPS) or liver transplantation.

PREOPERATIVE EVALUATION AND INDICATIONS

As in any emergency situation, patients with massive gastrointestinal (GI) bleeding should be evaluated and treated in a systematic fashion that begins with addressing their airway, breathing, and circulation. If the patient has a significantly altered level of consciousness or ongoing hematemesis, they should undergo endotracheal intubation to protect their airway. Large bore intravenous access should be obtained and volume resuscitation initiated. In patients with hematemesis or melena, an upper GI bleed is the most likely source; however, hematochezia can also result from a brisk upper GI bleed. Nasogastric tube lavage can be used as a first step to help localize such bleeds and is safe even in patients with known varices. In patients with cirrhosis, variceal bleeding should be assumed to be the source of GI hemorrhage and once stabilized, they should proceed to upper endoscopy as quickly as possible. If variceal bleeding is suspected, intravenous octreotide and antibiotics should also be administered.

OPERATIVE TECHNIQUE

There are two main techniques for endoscopic control of variceal bleeding: rubber band ligation and sclerotherapy. The techniques are similarly effective in controlling hemorrhage; however, band ligation results in fewer complications so is typically used as the initial therapy. If band ligation fails to control the bleeding, sclerotherapy can then be attempted. Both techniques begin with an initial diagnostic upper endoscopy. Once varices are identified as the source of bleeding, the endoscope is removed and the band ligating device is placed over the tip of the scope. The original ligation devices could only be loaded with one band at a time, requiring endoscope removal for reloading after each firing. This necessitated placement of an esophageal overtube to facilitate multiple scope reinsertions. However, newer models of banding devices now allow for the application of up to 10 bands without scope reloading.[8]

Application of the ligating bands should start from the distal-most varix and proceed proximally, so that the applied bands do not obscure the endoscopic view once they are placed. To do this, individual varices are isolated and suctioned within the band applicator. It is important to fully suction each varix within the applicator before firing the band to ensure placement at the base of the varix. At the beginning of this process, bleeding may obscure the endoscopic field requiring the placement of bands semiblindly at the level of the EGJ. This is generally safe and can be continued until bleeding is temporized and visualization improves.

If band ligation fails to adequately control the hemorrhage, endoscopic sclerotherapy can be attempted before moving on to more morbid interventions such as TIPS. Sclerotherapy is performed by injecting a chemical sclerosing agent, such as sodium morrhuate or ethanolamine, directly into the varices using an endoscopic needle. It is important to inject these agents into only the varices, rather than the surrounding esophageal tissue, in order to limit local and systemic complications. This can obviously be difficult when treating acute hemorrhage given the limited visibility, and this is one of the main reasons why band ligation has largely replaced this technique as first-line therapy in this setting.

OUTCOMES

A randomized trial comparing band ligation and sclerotherapy found that ligation resulted in a lower rate of therapeutic failure (10% vs. 24%), as well as lower rates of complications.[9] For this reason, band ligation has become the preferred initial endoscopic therapy for acute variceal bleeding. However, despite the initial effectiveness of band ligation in controlling hemorrhage, patients who survive the 2-week period after a variceal bleed still have a 14% to 39% mortality rate over the following year depending on what aggressive prophylactic measures, such as TIPS, are taken to prevent re-bleeding.[10] This is likely due to a combination of re-bleeding episodes and the fact that a variceal bleed is an indicator of worsening liver function and cirrhosis overall.

ENDOSCOPIC RESECTION FOR ESOPHAGEAL MALIGNANCY

Recent advances in the understanding of the pathogenesis of esophageal adenocarcinoma as a progression from GERD-related esophageal acid exposure to metaplasia (i.e., Barrett esophagus) to dysplasia and finally to cancer, have prompted more active surveillance of patients who lie along this pathway. This in turn has created opportunities for early endoscopic intervention before patients progress to more advanced stages of esophageal cancer. While its use is still somewhat controversial and further long-term outcomes data are needed, endoscopic resection for early stage esophageal cancer is becoming increasingly utilized and offers a considerable reduction in postprocedure morbidity and mortality for patients who until recently had no treatment options other than esophagectomy.

PREOPERATIVE EVALUATION AND INDICATIONS

Upper endoscopy is the primary means for the initial diagnosis of esophageal cancer. Patients with GERD who have atypical or "alarm" symptoms (dysphagia, odynophagia, GI bleeding, unintentional weight loss) or those who are not responsive to initial proton-pump inhibitor (PPI) therapy should undergo upper endoscopy. During endoscopy, any suspicious lesions and mucosal irregularities should be biopsied to allow for histologic evaluation. The squamocolumnar

TABLE 132.1 TNM Classification for Esophageal Cancer

TNM staging for esophageal adenocarcinoma

Primary Tumor (T)	
Tx	Primary tumors cannot be assessed
T0	No evidence of primary tumor
Tis	High-grade dysplasia
T1	Tumor invades lamina propria, muscularis mucosae, or submucosa
T1a	Tumor invades lamina propria or muscularis mucosae
T1b	Tumor invades submucosa
T2	Tumor invades muscularis propria
T3	Tumor invades adventitia
T4	Tumor invades adjacent structures
Regional Lymph Nodes (N)	
Nx	Regional lymph node(s) cannot be assessed
N0	No regional lymph node metastasis
N1	Metastasis in 1–2 regional lymph nodes
N2	Metastasis in 3–6 regional lymph nodes
N3	Metastasis in seven or more regional lymph nodes
Distant Metastasis (M)	
M0	No distant metastasis
M1	Distant metastasis

junction (SCJ), or "z-line," is examined and any irregularity or migration of the SCJ proximal to the EGJ should be biopsied to evaluate for Barrett esophagus and dysplasia. Patients who are found to have esophageal adenocarcinoma on biopsies then require accurate cancer staging in order to determine the most effective treatment strategy. Staging for esophageal cancer is accomplished using endoscopic ultrasound (EUS) to assess depth of invasion and lymph node size, and computed tomography (CT) combined with positron-emission tomography (PET) to evaluate for distant metastases. Patients without evidence of metastatic disease or nodal spread on imaging are candidates for either endoscopic resection or esophagectomy based on the depth of invasion, or T-classification, of their tumor (Table 132.1). Patients with T1b tumors have a much higher rate of nodal metastases than those with T1a (16.6% vs. 5%),[11] therefore endoscopic resection is generally reserved for T1a tumors. Patients with T1a tumors but histologic lymphovascular invasion, tumor ulceration, and lesion size greater than 2 cm should also proceed to esophagectomy, as all of these are risk factors for lymph node involvement.

OPERATIVE TECHNIQUE

Endoscopic resection of esophageal tumors is performed using one of two techniques: endoscopic mucosal resection (EMR) or endoscopic submucosal dissection (ESD). EMR is essentially a large mucosal snare biopsy. A submucosal saline lift beneath the lesion is first performed using an endoscopic injection needle. This creates a plane between the tumor and underlying muscularis propria, allowing for complete tumor resection while decreasing the risk of full-thickness esophageal perforation. An endoscopic snare is then used to encircle the tumor. The endoscope is fitted with a transparent cap that allows the tumor to be suctioned into it while the snare is tightened. This facilitates encircling of an area of mucosa that includes the entire tumor area. Once tightened, electrocautery is

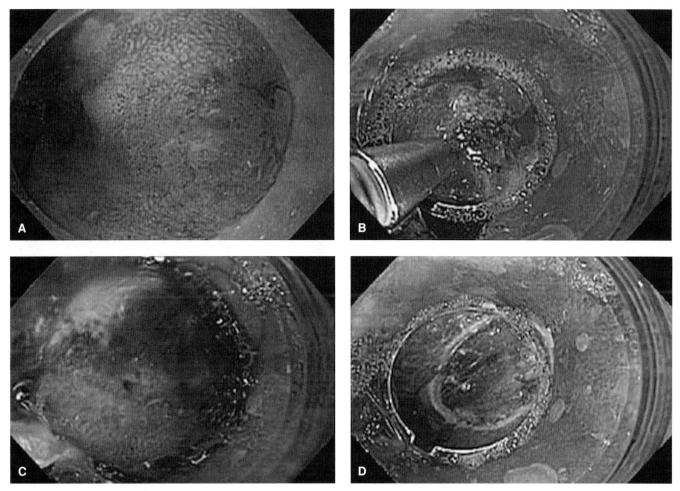

FIGURE 132.1 Endoscopic mucosal resection (EMR) is performed on an esophageal lesion. **(A)** The lesion is first identified. **(B)** A saline injection is performed to elevate the lesion. **(C)** A snare cautery is used to excise the lesion. **(D)** The resection bed is inspected for hemostasis. (Reprinted by permission from Macmillan Publishers Ltd: Waxman I, Konda VJ. Mucosal ablation of Barrett esophagus. *Nat Rev Gastroenterol Hepatol* 2009;6:393–401. Copyright © 2009.)

used to divide the specimen from the underlying layers and suction is maintained to capture the specimen against the face of the endoscope while it is removed (Fig. 132.1).

ESD is a more complicated technique that involves direct dissection of the submucosa in order to perform an en bloc resection of tumors of the mucosa, submucosa, and even muscularis propria of the esophagus. Because endoscopic resection of esophageal cancers that have invaded further than the mucosa is contraindicated due to high rates of lymph node involvement, the role of ESD for treatment of esophageal cancer has not been well defined. It may be best suited for en bloc resection of mucosally based tumors that are larger than 2 cm in diameter for which EMR is technically difficult to perform, although the use of endoscopic resection as primary therapy for these larger cancers is controversial.

The first step in ESD is marking the intended resection margin circumferentially with dots of electrocautery burn. A submucosal saline injection is then performed to create a potential space within this layer. The mucosa is then incised using an endoscopic electrocautery knife at the most proximal portion of the resection margin. The endoscope is fitted with a transparent dissecting cap, and this cap is used to bluntly maneuver the scope into the submucosal space through the previously created mucosal incision. A submucosal dissection is then performed deep to the tumor using electrocautery in order to completely separate the mucosa from the muscularis propria.

After this submucosal dissection is completed, the lateral and distal mucosal edges of the resection margin are incised to separate the en bloc specimen from the surrounding tissues (Fig. 132.2).

OUTCOMES

Procedural morbidity for both EMR and ESD is considerably lower than esophagectomy, with stricture rates of approximately 5% and perforation rates of less than 1%. Oncologic outcomes following endoscopic resection are also excellent, as long as the previously discussed inclusion criteria are followed. A comparison of endoscopic resections and esophagectomies performed for T1a esophageal cancers at two high-volume centers resulted in similar complete remission rates of 98.7% and 100%, respectively.[12] During a mean follow-up period of 4 years, 6.6% of patients in the endoscopic resection group had a local recurrence, but all of these patients underwent successful endoscopic re-resection. The importance of careful patient selection is highlighted by a study from the National Cancer Data Base, which showed lower 30-day mortality (hazard ratio 0.33) but higher 5-year mortality (hazard ratio 1.63) with endoscopic resection when compared with surgical esophagectomy.[11] However, 46% of the patients treated endoscopically had T1b tumors, a current contraindication to this approach, and this may have accounted for the poorer long-term survival seen in these patients.

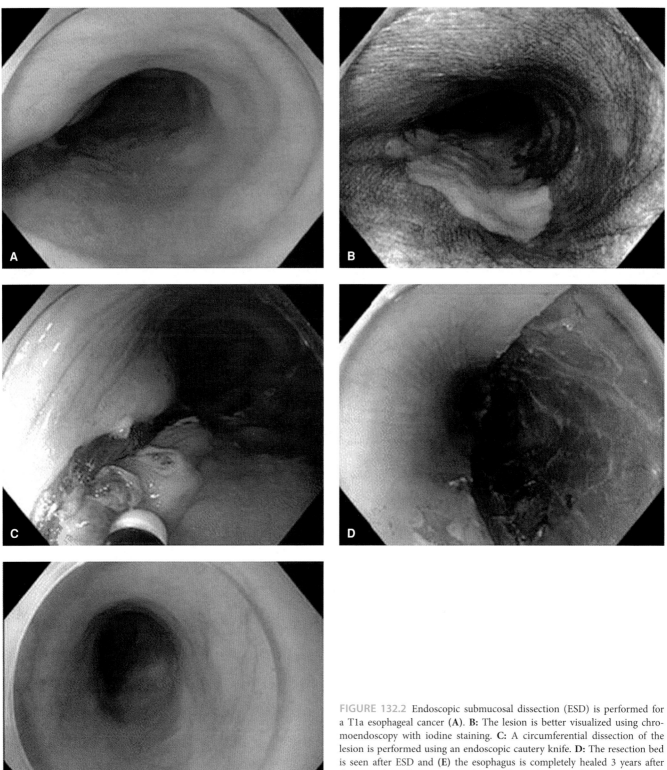

FIGURE 132.2 Endoscopic submucosal dissection (ESD) is performed for a T1a esophageal cancer (**A**). **B:** The lesion is better visualized using chromoendoscopy with iodine staining. **C:** A circumferential dissection of the lesion is performed using an endoscopic cautery knife. **D:** The resection bed is seen after ESD and (**E**) the esophagus is completely healed 3 years after the procedure. (From Hammad H, Kaltenbach T, Soetikno R. Endoscopic submucosal dissection for malignant esophageal lesions. *Curr Gastroenterol Rep* 2014;16:386. Copyright © 2014 Springer Science+Business Media. With permission of Springer.)

PERORAL ENDOSCOPIC MYOTOMY

Peroral endoscopic myotomy (POEM) is a novel endoscopic operation for the treatment of achalasia that draws from techniques of both traditional surgical myotomy and more recent advanced endoscopic procedures such as ESD. POEM creates a controlled surgical myotomy across the EGJ without skin incisions, using a standard flexible gastroscope and commercially available endoscopic instruments. The feasibility of an endoscopic myotomy using a submucosal tunnel technique was first demonstrated in an animal model by Pasricha and colleagues,[13] and POEM was first performed clinically in humans in 2008 by Inoue and colleagues.[14] Since that time, POEM has been performed at centers around the world, with over 1,000 cases reported in the literature thus far.[15] While initial outcomes after the procedure appear promising in terms of operative safety and short-term relief of dysphagia, further data are needed regarding long-term outcomes and the incidence of postoperative iatrogenic gastroesophageal reflux before POEM can be considered a standard-of-care treatment option for achalasia.

PREOPERATIVE EVALUATION AND INDICATIONS

Achalasia is the main indication for POEM, although the procedure has also been performed for other esophageal motility disorders that are refractory to medical management, such as jackhammer esophagus. Prior to surgery, patients should undergo a thorough work-up that includes upper endoscopy, contrast esophagram, and high-resolution manometry, in order to both establish a firm diagnosis and rule out any other causes of their symptoms, such as a malignancy at the EGJ causing pseudoachalasia. Although it has been described, performing POEM in patients with sigmoid esophagus is considerably technically more challenging, and should only be attempted by surgeons with substantial experience with the procedure in patients with more normal esophageal anatomy.

OPERATIVE TECHNIQUE

POEM begins with a diagnostic upper endoscopy and the esophagus should be irrigated to clear any remaining food particles. The endoscope is fitted with a transparent dissecting cap and a special insufflator is used so that only CO_2, and not room air, is transmitted through the scope. A saline solution containing blue dye is then injected into the anterior esophageal wall using an endoscopic needle, in order to form a submucosal fluid bleb and separate the mucosa from the muscularis propria of the esophagus. An endoscopic cautery knife (typically a triangle-tip knife), is then used to create a longitudinal opening in the mucosa overlying the fluid bleb and allow for access to the submucosa. Once this mucosotomy has been created, the endoscope is then guided through it and into the submucosal space.

The surgeon then creates a longitudinal submucosal tunnel down the length of the esophagus and onto the stomach, using a combination of blunt dissection with the scope cap and electrocautery with the triangle knife to clear away the fibrous submucosal fibers. Additional saline solution with blue dye is sequentially injected during this process to aid in hydrodissection. When completed, the tunnel must extend at least 3 cm onto the wall of the stomach, and this distance is checked by removing the scope from the tunnel and retroflexing in the stomach. In this position, progression of the tunnel is marked by the appearance of blue dye in the submucosa. Once the tunnel is complete, the myotomy is performed. Typically, this is begun 2 to 3 cm distal to the mucosotomy, 6 to 8 cm above the EGJ and extends 3 cm beyond the EGJ. During

POEM, as opposed to laparoscopic Heller myotomy, most surgeons perform a selective myotomy of only the inner, circular muscle layer. After the myotomy is complete, the scope is withdrawn from the tunnel and the mucosotomy is closed with endoscopic clips (Fig. 132.3).

OUTCOMES

Thus far, the published outcomes data after POEM have been excellent in terms of both symptomatic relief and improvement in EGJ physiology, although most of these series are relatively small and without long-term follow-up. POEM seems to have a perioperative safety profile similar to laparoscopic Heller myotomy.[16] Serious complications such as esophageal leak and clinically significant pneumothorax can occur, but are extremely rare (<1%). Clinical success after POEM, defined as significant relief of dysphagia, regurgitation, and chest pain symptoms (typically an Eckardt symptom score <4) has been shown to occur in >90% of patients at 3- to 12-month follow-up.[17–19] These outcomes also parallel results after both laparoscopic Heller myotomy and endoscopic pneumatic dilation. Multiple studies have demonstrated that POEM results in a marked reduction in EGJ relaxation pressures, as measured by manometry, and reductions in contrast column heights on esophagram.[17,18] Additionally, our group has shown that POEM results in a dramatic improvement in EGJ compliance, as measured by a functional lumen imaging probe (FLIP), an increase that appears to be larger than the effect produced by laparoscopic Heller myotomy.[20]

An early concern regarding POEM was that it would result in a high incidence of postoperative GER because it does not include an antireflux procedure, as opposed to laparoscopic Heller myotomy during which a partial fundoplication is typically performed. However, the outcomes data thus far have not reflected this. In our own POEM series, 31% of patients tested had pathologic esophageal acid exposure on 24-hour pH monitoring,[17] which is similar to recent studies of patients after Heller myotomy and partial fundoplication.[21] Bhayani and colleagues[18] compared their series of POEM and Heller patients and found similar rates of GER in the two groups (39% and 32% respectively). This result may be due to the fact that POEM does not involve dissection of the angle of His or opening of the diaphragmatic hiatus, and therefore it may preserve the natural antireflux valve intrinsic in the EGJ to a greater extent than Heller myotomy. While long-term outcomes after POEM still need to be carefully examined, thus far the procedure seems to be living up to its theoretical appeal of combining the durability of a controlled surgical myotomy with the minimally invasive nature of a purely endoscopic intervention.

ENDOSCOPIC PROCEDURES FOR GASTROESOPHAGEAL REFLUX DISEASE

GERD is one of the most common medical conditions in the United States, affecting 30% to 40% of the population, with 20% experiencing weekly symptoms. Given that the most effective medical therapy is indefinite acid suppression with a PPI, GERD represents an enormous societal burden in terms of health care costs.[22] Up to 50% of patients have symptoms that are refractory to PPI therapy and would possibly derive a quality-of-life benefit from undergoing antireflux surgery.[23] Despite this, less than 10% of such patients pursue surgical treatment for reflux, possibly due to concerns regarding the invasive nature and complications or side effects of such operations.[24] It is in this context that several endoscopic procedures for the treatment

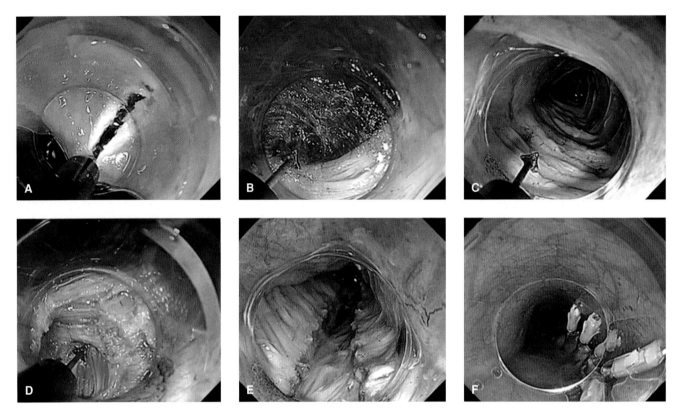

FIGURE 132.3 The steps of a peroral esophageal myotomy (POEM) procedure, starting with **(A)** creation of a mucosotomy in the anterior esophageal wall. **B:** The scope is advanced through the mucosotomy into the submucosal space and **(C)** a long submucosal tunnel is created. **D:** A longitudinal myotomy of the circular muscle fibers is performed and **(E)** shown after completion. **F:** The mucosotomy is closed with endoscopic clips to complete the procedure. (Reprinted by permission from Macmillan Publishers Ltd: Bechara R, Ikeda H, Inoue H. Peroral endoscopic myotomy: an evolving treatment for achalasia. *Nat Rev Gastroenterol Hepatol* 2015;12:410–426. Copyright © 2015.)

of GERD have been developed. While none of these has yet gained widespread acceptance or utilization, several have shown promising outcomes data, and such procedures likely represent a prime area for further research and clinical growth in the future. This section will focus on the two endoscopic procedures for GERD with the most robust outcomes data to support their use: EGJ radiofrequency therapy (RFT) using the Stretta device (Mederi Therapeutics, Greenwich, CT) and transoral incisionless fundoplication (TIF) using the EsophyX device (Endogastric Solutions, Redmond, WA).

PREOPERATIVE EVALUATION AND INDICATIONS

Evaluation of patients with suspected GERD begins with taking a thorough and careful history. Typical symptoms include pain that is retrosternal, ascending, and burning in nature, and also usually occurs after meals. Regurgitation of gastric acid and water brash hypersecretion of saliva are also common. Atypical symptoms include nonburning chest pain, dyspepsia, upper abdominal pain, and respiratory symptoms, such as wheezing, cough, and aspiration. So-called "warning symptoms" that should raise concern for the presence of malignancy include dysphagia, odynophagia, and unintentional weight loss. We encourage the use of a validated symptom score in the standard evaluation of all GERD patients, so that changes in symptoms after surgery can be more objectively measured and evaluated.

All patients being considered for any procedural intervention for GERD should undergo a preoperative endoscopy in order to rule out the presence of malignancy and evaluate for any other pathology that could be causing their symptoms. The entire esophagus should be evaluated for esophagitis, mucosal and submucosally based tumors,

dysplasia, and stricture. Any abnormal lesions should be biopsied in order to obtain a tissue diagnosis. The stomach and duodenum should likewise be evaluated for masses, gastritis, and ulcers. In patients with gastric and duodenal ulcers, biopsies should be taken of those lesions to evaluate for malignancy, and biopsies of normal gastric mucosa should be obtained to examine for *Helicobacter pylori* bacteria. Using a retroflexed position in the stomach, the EGJ should be evaluated for the presence of a hiatal hernia.

Patients with typical symptoms and the presence of reflux esophagitis on upper endoscopy have enough objective evidence of GERD to proceed with standard surgical intervention in the form of laparoscopic fundoplication. However, for patients with atypical symptoms, those without esophagitis, and those being considered for novel endoscopic interventions such as RFT or TIF, the presence of pathologic esophageal reflux should be confirmed using esophageal pH monitoring. This can be done using a transnasal catheter system that measures esophageal pH (at a position 5 cm above the EGJ over the course of 24 hours) or a wireless capsule system (Bravo pH Monitoring, Given Imaging, Yokneam, Israel) that can record esophageal pH over 48 or 72 hours. These studies are typically performed with the patient off acid suppression therapy, and the percentage of time esophageal pH below 4 is the main outcome measure for determining the presence of pathologic acid reflux.

While somewhat controversial, we recommend the routine use of high-resolution manometry in all patients being considered for surgical interventions for GERD. Manometry can reveal the presence of esophageal dysmotility that can adversely affect outcomes after surgery, and having a baseline manometry is useful for comparison purposes in the evaluation of patients who complain of dysphagia or

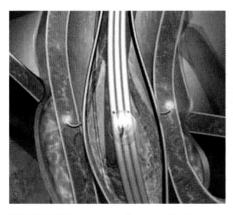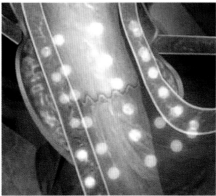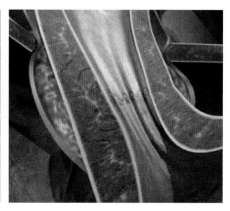

FIGURE 132.4 A cartoon depicting the Stretta procedure for treatment of gastroesophageal reflux disease. In the left image, the Stretta device is shown with electrodes deployed into the wall of the esophagogastric junction (EGJ) to deliver radiofrequency (RF) energy. The center image shows the locations of administration of RF treatment, and the right image shows the remodeling of the EGJ that results from the procedure. (From Auyang ED, Carter P, Rauth T, et al. SAGES clinical spotlight review: endoluminal treatments for gastroesophageal reflux disease (GERD). *Surg Endosc* 2013;27:2658–2672. Copyright © 2013 Springer Science+Business Media. With permission of Springer.)

other symptoms postoperatively. Contrast radiography of the esophagus and stomach (i.e., barium esophagram, "UGI series") can also be used preoperatively, primarily to evaluate esophageal and gastric anatomy for the presence of a hiatal hernia. This is important prior to the use of endoscopic therapies, as hiatal hernia is an important contraindication for these procedures. Finally, patients who complain of significant postprandial abdominal bloating or nausea should be evaluated for gastroparesis using gastric emptying scintigraphy.

The indications for peroral endoscopic procedures for GERD are similar to those for traditional laparoscopic fundoplication: objective evidence of pathologic reflux and symptoms that are poorly controlled with antisecretory medications or patients who wish to be weaned off such medications. All patients should undergo a trial of PPI therapy before being considered for an endoscopic intervention. The main contraindication for both RFT and TIF that differs from traditional surgery is the presence of a hiatal hernia that is >2 cm in axial length.

RADIOFREQUENCY THERAPY (STRETTA PROCEDURE)

OPERATIVE TECHNIQUE

The Stretta procedure can be performed under either sedation or general anesthesia. An upper endoscopy is first performed to measure the distance to the SCJ. The endoscope is then removed, and the Stretta device is inserted to the level of the SCJ. The device is a catheter-based system that consists of an inflatable balloon which deploys needle electrodes that extend 1 to 2 mm into the muscle of the esophageal and stomach wall (Fig. 132.4). These electrodes are connected to a radiofrequency generator and deliver low-power RF energy that elevates tissue temperature to 65° to 85°C during a series of treatment cycles. Energy is applied in this manner at four levels in the esophagus and two in the gastric cardia, while continuous intraluminal irrigation from the catheter prevents mucosal injury during this process.[25,26] After the ablation portion of the procedure is completed, a second upper endoscopy is performed to examine for mucosal injury. The RF energy application causes remodeling and thickening of the musculature of the EGJ. This results in decreased compliance at the EGJ and reductions in the number of transient LES relaxations, both of which contribute to reducing pathologic reflux.

OUTCOMES

Of the peroral procedures for GERD, the Stretta procedure has the most robust efficacy data in terms of both reducing esophageal acid exposure and improving patient symptoms. A recent meta-analysis by Perry and colleagues[27] pooled outcomes from 18 studies, which showed the procedure to be effective in both decreasing GERD-related symptoms and improving quality of life, while also reducing patient dependence on antisecretory medications. Most of these data are from follow-up periods of 12 to 48 months. Pooled results from studies that included pH monitoring showed a decrease in pathologic esophageal acid exposure from 10.3% to 6.5% after the procedure; however, it should be noted that the postprocedure mean of 6.5% still represents an abnormally elevated level of acid exposure, and that multiple studies examining laparoscopic Nissen fundoplication for the treatment of GERD have shown greater reductions in gastroesophageal reflux. Four randomized trials have evaluated the Stretta procedure in comparison to medical therapy for GERD, and one of these performed a double-blind comparison with a sham procedure.[28] At 6 months postprocedure, 61% of patients in the Stretta group had resolution of daily GERD symptoms, as compared with 33% in the sham control group.

TRANSORAL INCISIONLESS FUNDOPLICATION (ESOPHYX DEVICE)

OPERATIVE TECHNIQUE

As opposed to Stretta, the TIF procedure using the EsophyX device is more analogous to traditional surgery for GERD, as it forms a fundoplication that recreates the natural valve mechanism of the EGJ. TIF is performed under general anesthesia with endotracheal intubation and complete muscle paralysis. At the onset of the procedure, an upper endoscopy is performed to inspect the esophageal and gastric mucosa and to measure the distance to the SCJ. The endoscope is then removed and the EsophyX device is mounted over the endoscope. The device functions by inserting polypropylene fasteners (H-fasteners) in full-thickness bites between the gastric fundus and esophagus in order to create an approximately 270-degree fundoplication. At least 18 fasteners are placed in multiple rows under endoscopic visualization in a retroflexed scope position (Fig. 132.5). After

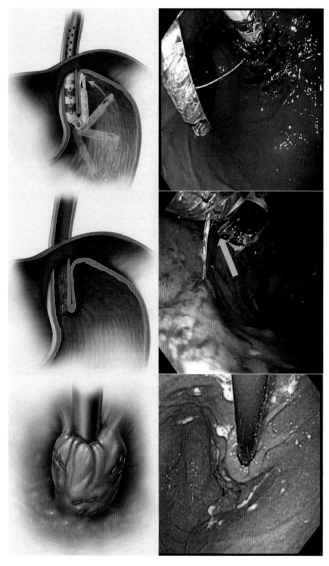

FIGURE 132.5 During a transoral incisionless fundoplication (TIF), the EsophyX device is used to apply polypropylene fasteners between the gastric fundus and esophagus in order to create a fundoplication endoscopically. (Reprinted from Hunter JG, Kahrilas PJ, Bell RC, et al. Efficacy of transoral fundoplication vs omeprazole for treatment of regurgitation in a randomized controlled trial. *Gastroenterology* 2015;148:324–333 e5. Copyright © 2015 AGA Institute. With permission.)

fastener deployment, the device is removed and a final endoscopy is performed to check fundoplication anatomy and ensure adequate hemostasis. Patients are typically admitted for overnight observation and pain control and some surgeons perform a routine postoperative contrast esophagram to check for leak. After discharge, patients are kept on a liquid diet and PPI for 2 weeks to allow for optimal healing and prevent ulceration and bleeding.

OUTCOMES

A number of single-center series of TIF procedures using the EsophyX device have shown improvements in symptoms and esophageal acid exposure with 6 to 24 months of follow-up. The best data available regarding the efficacy of the procedure comes from a recent randomized controlled trial.[29] This study compared 87 patients undergoing the TIF procedure followed by 6 months of placebo medication

to 42 patients who underwent a sham endoscopy followed by 6 months of PPI therapy. The primary outcome measure of troublesome regurgitation symptoms was eliminated in a higher percentage of the TIF patients than those in the sham plus PPI group (67% vs. 45%, p <0.05). There was also a significant reduction in esophageal acid exposure on pH monitoring after TIF (pre 9.3% vs. post 6.3%, p <.001), whereas the sham group had no change in esophageal acid exposure when tested off PPIs. Again, it should be noted that although the TIF procedure did result in a decrease in acid exposure, the mean post-TIF value of 6.3% is still above the cutoff for pathologic GERD (>4.5%).

CONCLUSIONS

As shown here, the applications of flexible upper endoscopy for both diagnostic and therapeutic purposes have undergone tremendous growth in recent years. As interventional medicine and surgery trend toward minimally invasive techniques, this expansion of peroral luminal interventions will certainly continue. It is therefore incumbent on surgeons to be at the forefront of learning and critically evaluating these techniques. It is only by being part of this process of innovation and having an array of procedures at our disposal, that we can choose the approach that best suits each individual patient.

REFERENCES

1. Gauderer MW, Ponsky JL, Izant RJ, Jr. Gastrostomy without laparotomy: a percutaneous endoscopic technique. *J Pediatr Surg* 1980;15:872–875.
2. Gauderer MW. Percutaneous endoscopic gastrostomy—20 years later: a historical perspective. *J Pediatr Surg* 2001;36:217–219.
3. Rahnemai-Azar AA, Rahnemaiazar AA, Naghshizadian R, et al. Percutaneous endoscopic gastrostomy: indications, technique, complications and management. *World J Gastroenterol* 2014;20:7739–7751.
4. Hogan RB, DeMarco DC, Hamilton JK, et al. Percutaneous endoscopic gastrostomy—to push or pull. A prospective randomized trial. *Gastrointest Endosc* 1986;32:253–258.
5. Kohler G, Kalcher V, Koch OO, et al. Comparison of 231 patients receiving either "pull-through" or "push" percutaneous endoscopic gastrostomy. *Surg Endosc* 2015;29:170–175.
6. Lim JH, Choi SH, Lee C, et al. Thirty-day mortality after percutaneous gastrostomy by endoscopic versus radiologic placement: a systematic review and meta-analysis. *Intest Res* 2016;14:333–342.
7. D'Amico G, De Franchis R, Cooperative Study Group. Upper digestive bleeding in cirrhosis. Post-therapeutic outcome and prognostic indicators. *Hepatology* 2003;38:599–612.
8. Committee AT, Liu J, Petersen BT, et al. Endoscopic banding devices. *Gastrointest Endosc* 2008;68:217–221.
9. Villanueva C, Piqueras M, Aracil C, et al. A randomized controlled trial comparing ligation and sclerotherapy as emergency endoscopic treatment added to somatostatin in acute variceal bleeding. *J Hepatol* 2006;45:560–567.
10. Garcia-Pagan JC, Caca K, Bureau C, et al. Early use of TIPS in patients with cirrhosis and variceal bleeding. *N Engl J Med* 2010;362:2370–2379.
11. Merkow RP, Bilimoria KY, Keswani RN, et al. Treatment trends, risk of lymph node metastasis, and outcomes for localized esophageal cancer. *J Natl Cancer Inst* 2014;106(7).
12. Pech O, Bollschweiler E, Manner H, et al. Comparison between endoscopic and surgical resection of mucosal esophageal adenocarcinoma in Barrett's esophagus at two high-volume centers. *Ann Surg* 2011;254:67–72.
13. Pasricha PJ, Hawari R, Ahmed I, et al. Submucosal endoscopic esophageal myotomy: a novel experimental approach for the treatment of achalasia. *Endoscopy* 2007;39:761–764.
14. Inoue H, Minami H, Kobayashi Y, et al. Peroral endoscopic myotomy (POEM) for esophageal achalasia. *Endoscopy* 2010;42:265–271.
15. Talukdar R, Inoue H, Reddy DN. Efficacy of peroral endoscopic myotomy (POEM) in the treatment of achalasia: a systematic review and meta-analysis. *Surg Endosc* 2015;29(11):3030–3046.
16. Hungness ES, Teitelbaum EN, Santos BF, et al. Comparison of Perioperative Outcomes Between Peroral Esophageal Myotomy (POEM) and Laparoscopic Heller Myotomy. *J Gastrointest Surg* 2013;17:228–235.
17. Teitelbaum EN, Soper NJ, Santos BF, et al. Symptomatic and physiologic outcomes one year after peroral esophageal myotomy (POEM) for treatment of achalasia. *Surg Endosc* 2014;28:3359–3365.
18. Bhayani NH, Kurian AA, Dunst CM, et al. A comparative study on comprehensive, objective outcomes of laparoscopic Heller myotomy with per-oral endoscopic myotomy (POEM) for achalasia. *Ann Surg* 2014;259:1098–1103.

19. von Renteln D, Inoue H, Minami H, et al. Peroral endoscopic myotomy for the treatment of achalasia: a prospective single center study. *Am J Gastroenterol* 2012;107:411–417.
20. Teitelbaum EN, Soper NJ, Pandolfino JE, et al. Esophagogastric junction distensibility measurements during Heller myotomy and POEM for achalasia predict postoperative symptomatic outcomes. *Surg Endosc* 2015;29:522–528.
21. Boeckxstaens GE, Annese V, des Varannes SB, et al. Pneumatic dilation versus laparoscopic Heller's myotomy for idiopathic achalasia. *N Engl J Med* 2011;364: 1807–1816.
22. Brook RA, Wahlqvist P, Kleinman NL, et al. Cost of gastro-oesophageal reflux disease to the employer: a perspective from the United States. *Aliment Pharmacol Ther* 2007;26: 889–898.
23. Liu JY, Finlayson SR, Laycock WS, et al. Determining an appropriate threshold for referral to surgery for gastroesophageal reflux disease. *Surgery* 2003;133:5–12.
24. Finks JF, Wei Y, Birkmeyer JD. The rise and fall of antireflux surgery in the United States. *Surg Endosc* 2006;20:1698–1701.

25. Utley DS. The Stretta procedure: device, technique, and pre-clinical study data. *Gastrointest Endosc Clin N Am* 2003;13:135–145.
26. Noar MD, Lotfi-Emran S. Sustained improvement in symptoms of GERD and antisecretory drug use: 4-year follow-up of the Stretta procedure. *Gastrointest Endosc* 2007;65:367–372.
27. Perry KA, Banerjee A, Melvin WS. Radiofrequency energy delivery to the lower esophageal sphincter reduces esophageal acid exposure and improves GERD symptoms: a systematic review and meta-analysis. *Surg Laparosc Endosc Percutan Tech* 2012;22:283–288.
28. Corley DA, Katz P, Wo JM, et al. Improvement of gastroesophageal reflux symptoms after radiofrequency energy: a randomized, sham-controlled trial. *Gastroenterology* 2003;125:668–676.
29. Hunter JG, Kahrilas PJ, Bell RC, et al. Efficacy of transoral fundoplication vs omeprazole for treatment of regurgitation in a randomized controlled trial. *Gastroenterology* 2015;148:324–33 e5.

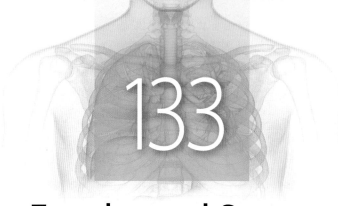

133

Esophageal Stents

Ory Wiesel ▪ Jon O. Wee

INTRODUCTION

Esophageal cancer is the sixth most common cause of cancer-related deaths throughout the world. In the past three decades there has been a persistent increase in the incidence of esophageal cancer attributed to the GERD and obesity epidemics. It is estimated that in 2015, 16,980 people in the United States will be diagnosed with esophageal cancer and 15,590 people will die of their disease.[1]

The tendency of esophageal cancer, to infiltrate early through lymphovascular channels and to grow intraluminally, makes early diagnosis difficult. In fact, in up to 50% of patients, surgical treatment is not indicated given the extent of the disease. Furthermore, patients usually seek medical attention when they are already experiencing some degree of dysphagia and thus already have some degree of luminal obstruction.

Palliation of dysphagia due to obstructing esophageal cancer is the main indication for which esophageal stents were developed. Stents are regarded as the best palliation for unresectable obstructing esophageal tumors.

Although the first description of an endoluminal esophageal prosthesis to treat malignant esophageal stricture dates back 120 years ago and is attributed to Sir Charter Symonds, it took half a century until Celestin described insertion of a plastic tube during laparotomy to bridge a malignant stricture in 1959.[2–4]

During the second half of the twentieth century, improvement in technology and endoscopy enabled physicians to diagnose and better treat endoluminal disease. Endoluminal stents were introduced for all parts of the gastrointestinal and hepatobiliary systems and the indications for endoluminal stenting expanded significantly as technology advanced. Newer and varied stents were introduced to the market, and more indications evolved as esophageal stents became more popular and easier to place.

In this chapter we will review the history of esophageal stent development, types of esophageal stents available, their application in both malignant and benign disease, and details about patient selection and method of stent deployment. Further discussion will be presented about the differences between stent types, common complications following stent placement, and finally, the future of stent technology.

HISTORY OF ESOPHAGEAL STENT DEVELOPMENT

Esophageal malignant strictures and the associated dysphagia were the driving force for development of novel techniques to bypass the stricture. The word "stent" is derived from Charles Stent, a nineteenth-century English dentist, who invented the material used to maintain skin graft patency. In 1845, the French innovator and scientist Leroy d'Etoilles unsuccessfully tried to use ivory tubes to traverse esophageal stenosis.[5] In 1856, Sir Charles Symmonds successfully introduced a 6-in. tube of boxwood into the esophagus of a patient. He attached a silk thread to the proximal end of the boxwood and wrapped it around the patient's ear to prevent further distal migration. Several prostheses were made through the subsequent years, and the first plastic prosthesis was described by Coyas in 1955.[6] Celestin subsequently described placement of an esophageal plastic endoprosthesis during laparotomy. Unfortunately these prosthetic insertions were associated with significant rate of morbidity and mortality. The first endoscopically inserted stent is attributed to Atkinson in 1970 who inserted a small (10 to 12 mm) plastic tube.[7,8] As technology developed, expanding spiral prostheses were developed. In the early 1980s, a Swedish engineer, Hans Wallstén, designed a braided cylindrical endoprosthesis ("wallstent") for vascular use; Frimberger reported his experience with expanding metal prosthesis introduced for the treatment of malignant esophageal stenosis in 1983; and in 1990, an expanding metal stent planned initially for vascular use was introduced through an endoscope for an esophageal stricture.[9] During the following two decades, expandable prostheses have been developed utilizing various metals and coverings to provide a range of characteristics such as self-expandable metallic stents (SEMS) and self-expandable plastic stents (SEPS).[10]

A working knowledge of the various stent types and their characteristics is essential for the practicing surgeon, and is reviewed below.

PRINCIPLES AND TYPES OF ESOPHAGEAL STENTS

Rigid stents are used in rare instances today, with the vast majority of stents utilized being expandable stents. These stents, which were originally designed for intravascular use, were shown to be very efficient for use in the GI and biliary tracts. Their ease of use and safety profile allow them to be placed with relatively low morbidity and mortality compared to the previous rigid esophageal stents.

In order to choose the correct stent, three factors should be considered: (1) the indication for which the stent is deployed; (2) patient characteristics (life expectancy, tumor biology, location of stricture, shape of the esophagus, etc.), and (3) stent characteristics. Stents characteristics depend on the stent design as well as the tissue response to the stent. Understanding the mechanics and characteristics behind

TABLE 133.1 Types of Esophageal Stents

1. Rigid tubes (Celestin tube)—historical
2. Expandable metal stents
3. Expandable plastic stents
4. Antireflux stents
5. Double-type stents
6. Biodegradable stents
7. Experimental (the future):
   a. Drug eluting stents
   b. Radiation emitting stents
   c. Allogenic grafts

the design of a stent will allow the clinician to choose the best stent for the proper indication. The various types of stents are listed in Table 133.1.

SELF-EXPANDABLE METALLIC STENTS

SEMS were the first expandable stents designed, and are divided into three types: uncovered stents, partially covered (PC) stents, and fully covered (FC) stents (Fig. 133.1).

Uncovered stents consist of bare metal mesh that is introduced with an introducer and expanded into the stenosis. A classic example is the Ultraflex (Boston Scientific). These stents often get tissue ingrained into the openings within the mesh, making its placement permanent. Attempts to remove the stent can create a challenge and lead to significant morbidity.

A completely covered stent is composed of a mesh membrane that covers the stent throughout its length. These are usually double funnel shaped and have a purse-string suture attached to the ends of the stent that can be grasped with forceps and withdrawn using a standard endoscope. The covering is usually made of silicone or a polymer which prevents tissue ingrowth. The benefit of using an FC stent is that it rarely gets imbedded in tissue, making its future removal much easier. It can also cover defects such as a perforation, enabling exclusion of injured sites. Commercially used FC stents are FC-Wallflex Stent (Boston Scientific), FC-Evolution Stent (Cook Endoscopy), Niti-S Stent (Taewoong Medical), AlimaXX-ES Stent (Merit Medical), FerX-Ella (Elia-CS), Bonastent (EndoChoice), and Dostent (MI Tech).

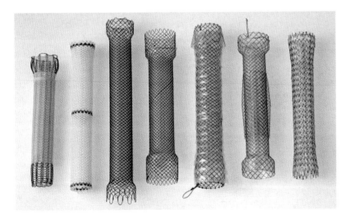

FIGURE 133.1 Spectrum of expandable esophageal stents. From *left* to *right*: partially covered Ultraflex stent, Polyflex stent, partially covered Wallflex stent, partially covered Evolution stent, fully covered SX-Ella stent, fully covered Niti-S antimigration stent, and fully covered Alimaxx-E stent. (Adapted from Vleggaar FP. Expandable stents for malignant esophageal disease. *Gastrointest Endosc Clin N Am* 2011;21(3):377–388. Copyright © 2011 Elsevier. With permission.)

PC stents consist of a membrane-covered stent body with the proximal and distal ends of the stent uncovered. Commercially available PC SEMS are PC Wallflex Stent (Boston Scientific), Evolution Stent (Cook Endoscopy), Flamingo Wallstent (Boston scientific), and Esophageal Z and Gianturco Z (Cook Endoscopy).[11,12]

Bethge and Vakil studied the tissue response to expandable stents placed in malignant esophageal stenosis.[13,14] Based on histologic examination of esophageal stents which were removed either during surgery or at the time of autopsy, they were able to propose a sequence of events following stent placement. When an uncovered metal stent expands, the wire of the stent expands and abuts against the tissue of both the malignant tumor and the normal esophageal wall. The radial forces of the stent cause initial mucosal necrosis followed by submucosal inflammation as the stent erodes into the submucosa of the esophageal wall. An inflammatory exudate covers the luminal aspect of the stent and few inflammatory cells are seen around the struts of the stent. In the tumor mass, the stent erodes into the tumor, and tumor tissue and cells are seen over the struts. As a result of the pressure necrosis exerted by the radial forces of an uncovered stent, fibrosis starts to develop. One month after stents placement, the fibrosis covers the stents, thus integrating it into the esophageal wall. Months later, the entire stent may no longer be visible as a result of the fibrosis and tumor ingrowth into the struts of the stent (Fig. 133.2).

FC stents also exert radial forces on both the tumor and the normal mucosa, but inflammatory exudate infiltration and tumor growth into the stent are prevented by the membrane bonded to the stent. This prevents imbedding the stent into the esophageal wall (Fig. 133.3).

PC stents have properties of both FC and uncovered stent types. The flared ends of a PC stent is usually uncovered in its proximal and distal ends, and thus PC stent behaves like any other uncovered stent, while the middle body of the stent is covered with a membrane preventing ingrowth of tissue into the stent itself (Fig. 133.4).

The tissue response to the stent can predict the clinical behavior of the specific stent being used. Tissue and tumor ingrowth into the struts of an uncovered stent make it difficult to remove but also decrease the rate of migration. Reintervention may be needed, however, if the stent becomes obstructed from tumor ingrowth. In

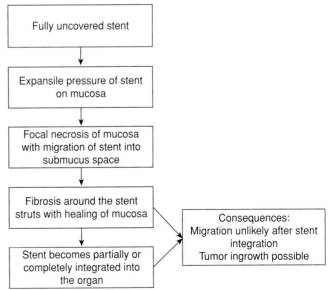

FIGURE 133.2 Sequence of events following uncovered esophageal stent deployment. (Adapted from Vakil N. Expandable metal stents: principles and tissue responses. *Gastrointest Endosc Clin N Am* 21(3):351–357. Copyright © 2011 Elsevier. With permission.)

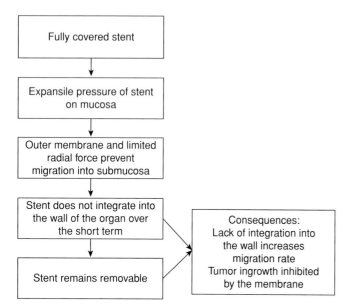

FIGURE 133.3 Sequence of events following fully covered esophageal stent deployment. (Adapted from Vakil N. Expandable metal stents: principles and tissue responses. *Gastrointest Endosc Clin N Am* 21(3):351–357. Copyright © 2011 Elsevier. With permission.)

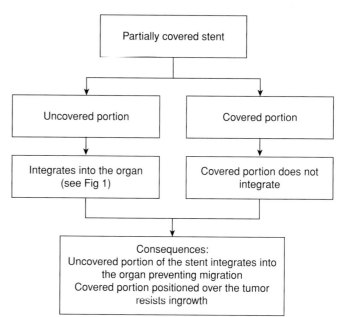

FIGURE 133.4 Sequence of events following partially covered esophageal stent deployment. (Adapted from Vakil N. Expandable metal stents: principles and tissue responses. *Gastrointest Endosc Clin N Am* 21(3):351–357. Copyright © 2011 Elsevier. With permission.)

contrast, FC stents are easier to remove and have a low risk of tissue ingrowth; however, reintervention can be needed as migration risk increases.[15]

The broad array of expandable stent types and designs available for use today attest that there is no "perfect" stent to date. Further, the fact that there is no stent that is superior in all aspects or fits to all patients and indications is important when discussing the advantage and disadvantage of a particular stent for a particular patient (Table 133.2).

SELF-EXPANDABLE PLASTIC STENTS

SEPS have been shown to be safe and effective for palliation of malignant dysphagia. Currently the only available SEPS is the Polyflex stent (Boston Scientific). It is made from a polyester mesh with an inner silicone lining designed to decrease the tissue reaction to the stent. The top of the stent is flared in order to decrease stent migration while the middle and lower portions of the stent are the same caliber. The stent is loaded on to the delivery system by the surgeon prior to deployment. This delivery system is fairly bulky (12 to 14 mm) and mandates stricture dilatation prior to stent placement in tight strictures. The same stent can be used after migration, by retrieval of the stent and reloading it onto the delivery device.

Several studies comparing SEPS to PC SEMS showed comparable technical success and dysphagia relief but SEPS has a higher migration

rate than PC SEMS.[11,16] Multiple studies have demonstrated the effectiveness of SEPS in benign esophageal disease (strictures, perforations fistulas, and anastomotic leaks) with success rates up to 95% in different studies, although most of these studies did not report long-term follow-up. When migration rate, long-term recurrence, and persistence of symptoms were examined over time, however, a high percentage of patients experienced recurrent symptoms (81.9%) with a high rate of stent migration (62% to 81%).[17,18]

According to these studies, SEPS can be safely used today but are mainly used in benign esophageal disease, with fare dysphagia relief scores, due to the high migration rate and poor long-term outcome compared to SEMS.

BIODEGRADABLE STENTS

Biodegradable esophageal stents are the latest development in stent technology in the past decade. The rationale of their design is to avoid the complications of tissue ingrowth and migration and to decrease the rate of reinterventions for stent removal. These are braided stents made of magnesium alloys, polymers of polylactic or polyglycolic acid, and polydiaxanon (ELLA-CS, Hradec Kralove, Czech Republic). Stent integrity is maintained for 6 to 8 weeks with complete disintegration after 12 weeks. Polydiaxanon is a semicrystalline polymer which degrades by

TABLE 133.2 Advantage and Disadvantage of Expandable Esophageal Stents		
Stent Type	Advantage	Disadvantage
Uncovered SEMS	Very low migration risk	Stent occlusion due to tumor ingrowth Difficult removal
Partially covered SEMS	Low migration risk	Stent occlusion if not removed
Fully covered SEMS	Easy removal Low risk of tissue ingrowth	High risk of stent migration
Self- expandable plastic stents (SEPS)	Low risk of tissue ingrowth Easy to remove Can reposition in same patient	High risk of stent migration Rigid introducer device

hydrolysis. The amorphous region of the matrix deteriorates first and the crystalline portion deteriorates later. The radial force of the stent is dependent on the crystalline portion of the stent and decreases by 50% at 9 weeks. Local tissue environment (low pH) may induce quicker disintegration. Biodegradable stents are still associated with complications such as migration, stricture recurrence, and obstruction; however, they may be a valuable alternative to SEMS and SEPS and may decrease the rate for repeated esophageal dilatations. Further studies and improved designs are needed to overcome the new challenges presented by these stents.[12,19–25]

ANTIREFLUX STENTS

Stents bridging the gastroesophageal junction keep the lower esophageal sphincter open and thus eliminate the major barrier against acid reflux. This can lead to significant acid reflux with its associated symptoms and complications. Patients who have stents across the GEJ should be placed on high-dose acid suppression. Potential aspiration risks should be addressed and preventive measures should be utilized (i.e., maintenance of an upright position and head-of-bed elevated to 30 degrees at all times).

Stents with an antireflux valve mechanism were developed with the intent to reduce acid reflux. The valve is an extension of the existing stent lining (mostly silicone or polyurethane), which is designed as a unidirectional flap valve on the gastric side of the stent that prevents reflux of the stomach acid content back through the stent into the esophagus. In a recent Cochrane-based meta-analysis, Dai and colleagues compared antireflux stents with conventional SEMS and demonstrated that these stents were similar in regard to adverse event rates and quality of life. Some of these stents were able to reduce gastroesophageal reflux, however, and were effective in rapidly palliating dysphagia.[26,27]

DOUBLE-TYPE STENTS

Recently, double-type stents have become available in the United States. These specially designed stents resist migration and tumor ingrowth with a stent-in-stent design. An inner nitinol FC stent prevents tumor ingrowth and an outer uncovered nitinol sleeve in the mid-portion of the covered internal stent prevents migration. Gonzales and colleagues used these double-type stents to manage postoperative fistulas, as well as leaks and perforation of the upper gastrointestinal tract around the GEJ. Overall success rate was 66% with 16% migration rate. All stents were removed in spite of the uncovered part of the stent. Other studies demonstrated similar results for malignant esophageal and cardia strictures.[28–30]

IMPORTANT FEATURES WHEN CHOOSING A STENT

To date, no ideal stent has been designed; however, several generalized rules can be made based on stent designs and patient characteristics.

1. *Stent indication*: The clinician should optimize the stent being used to the specific patient and disease characteristics. For example:
   a. Given the poor prognosis of malignant strictures and the tendency for occlusion, uncovered stents should be carefully considered for malignant esophageal obstruction.
   b. Covered stents and plastic stents can and should be used especially for benign esophageal strictures.

2. *Stricture dilatation*: This may be necessary before stent placement, especially in tight strictures. Esophageal dilatation can be achieved with mercury or tungsten-weighted bougies (Maloney bougie, Medovations) which are inserted blindly, polyvinyl dilators (Savary-Gilliard, Cook Medical) which are inserted over a guide wire passed through the scope, or balloon dilators (CRE, Boston Scientific).

3. *Stent length*: For tumor strictures, the stent should be long enough to bridge the whole length of the tumor to prevent tumor ingrowth along the length of the stent. Most stent manufacturers recommend placing the stent with a 2- to 4-cm margin proximal and distal to the tumor.

4. *Location of stent*:
   a. *Distal esophageal obstructions* (including gastroesophageal junction): Excessive stent length across the GEJ and into the stomach increases the risk for stent migration, impaction against the greater gastric curvature, and symptomatic reflux of gastric acid across the stented GEJ. Antireflux stents were designed to overcome this issue.
   b. *Proximal esophageal obstructions* (including high cervical strictures): Stenting the upper esophageal sphincter (UES) can be highly morbid for the patient (symptomatic reflux, pain, etc.) and may result in stent intolerance. It is recommended that a 1.5- to 2-cm free zone exist between the UES and the proximal end of the stent.

5. *Radial force of a stent*: Stents vary in their diameter and degree of radial force exerted on the tissue. Stents placed following chemoradiation can cause esophageal wall necrosis with perforation due to the high radial force on the wall if chosen incorrectly. Eroded stents into the esophageal wall and beyond have been reported to cause fatal aortic hemorrhage and paraspinal abscess.[31] In addition, stents placed at the proximal esophagus can cause tracheal compression and collapse with resultant stridor or respiratory distress if chosen incorrectly, and thus the surgeon must also evaluate the trachea and stent indications prior to placement of a proximal esophageal stent.

   Stent shape and tissue response: Some stents have proximal and distal uncovered flares that help to decrease the degree of migration. Stent designs might cause excessive tissue hyperplasia, and sharp wires at the end of the stent can cause tissue reaction. Modern stents have smoother ends that decrease the degree of tissue reaction and hyperplasia.

   Some stents tend to bend when inserted into a torturous esophagus and stricture, and as a result, FC stents are preferred if possible when planning procedure in such an esophagus.[32]

6. *Antimigration stent modifications*: Several methods have been developed to decrease the rate of migration (reported to be as high as 50% in some types of stents). The initial reports of passing a thread through the patient's nostril and tying it around the ear or in the nostril have been replaced with special stent designs and modification such as Struts design, antimigration collar, outer uncovered mesh, and large diameter flares, with some success.[33] Unfortunately, reports of hemorrhage, fistula, and esophageal perforation limit the use of these methods in some modern stents. Endoscopic clips at the proximal end of the stent are the latest attempt to fix the stent to the wall, though their efficacy remains unproven.[32]

TECHNIQUE

Prior to the procedure, all preoperative imaging should be available for the surgeon and fluoroscopy should be ordered in advance. Proper instrumentation (both adult and pediatric endoscopes, bronchoscope, esophageal dilators, guide wires, rat-toothed forceps, etc.) should be present in the operating room. Prior knowledge of the type of stent being used by both the operating surgeon and nursing personnel is imperative, and several sizes and types of stents should be available for the surgeon in the operating room as well. This is best done with stents in a dedicated cart. The surgeon should be trained to recognize and cope with unexpected complications such as perforations, airway compression, stent malpositioning, and incomplete stent deployment.

Proper anesthesia, either conscious sedation or preferably general anesthesia, should be administered. The patient is placed supine with arms tucked, and flexible endoscopy is performed to evaluate the lesion and to assess if the preoperative plan is feasible. In case of a high-grade stricture, dilation should be done under fluoroscopy and the decision to proceed with stent placement should be made at that time. The length of the area to be stented is mapped under fluoroscopy, and external radiopaque markers are placed over the patient's chest to mark the proximal and distal extent of the lesion. Next, a flexible guide wire is passed through the endoscope past the obstruction and the endoscope is withdrawn while the wire is kept in place.

Proper stent placement should be chosen to bridge the length of the proximal and distal margins marked by the radiopaque markers with an additional 2- to 3-cm margin proximal and distal beyond the lesion. In case of proximal or cervical lesions in proximity to the upper sphincter, a 1- to 1.5-cm proximal margin is shown to be sufficient. In case of distal obstruction, stenting the gastroesophageal junction is accompanied with both a high rate of stent migration and symptomatic reflux and thus should be kept to a minimum.

The stent and the delivery system should then be passed over the guide wire and, under continuous fluoroscopic guidance, carefully introduced until the distal external marker is aligned to match the distal stent marker. The stent is slowly deployed to bridge across both the proximal and distal skin markers. It is important to choose the correct size of stent to avoid excessive pressure on the wall which increases the risk of esophageal wall necrosis and perforation or choosing too narrow a stent which may migrate quickly.

After completion of stent deployment, stent position is confirmed by repeat endoscopy and confirmatory fluoroscopy. If malposition is detected, it is possible to pull the stent to the correct position with a rat-toothed forceps under fluoroscopy. If the stent is placed proximal to the stricture or released with its distal end inside the stricture, it should be removed and placed again and not pushed into the stricture.

The patient is allowed to wake up, and allowed to drink liquids initially, and further advanced to soft diet unless other contraindications exist. A PA and lateral chest x-ray is done following the procedure to record the stent position. Some authors recommend performing a gastrografin study on postoperative day 1 to assess patency before advancing the diet.[34]

STENT EFFICACY

Stent efficacy is measured by technical success and clinical factors such as improvement in the dysphagia score (Table 133.3), complication rate, and survival post-stent placement.

TABLE 133.3 Dysphagia Scoring Scale

0	Able to consume a normal diet
1	Dysphagia with certain solid foods
2	Able to swallow semi-solid foods
3	Able to swallow liquids only
4	Unable to swallow saliva (complete dysphagia)

Conio et al. summarized all prospective randomized trials which were published between 1993 and 2010 for stents placed for malignant esophageal disease.[16] The technical success rate for SEMS placement was close to 100% in all studies. The dysphagia score improved in 83% to 100% of patients.[15,35] The degree of improvement did not differ among studies as a function of stent type (covered SEMS, covered vs. uncovered SEMS, or SEMS vs. SEPS), although more interventions were needed for uncovered SEMS to treat recurrent dysphagia.[28,16,36–46] The degree of improvement did correlate with improvement in quality of life following SEMS placement, however.[47,48] Tumor ingrowth and/or overgrowth were common in cases of cancer progression. In the case of dysphagia secondary to a tracheoesophageal fistula (TEF), successful closure of the fistula has been reported in 70% to 100% of patients.[49–51] Up to 50% of patients will require additional interventions for recurrent dysphagia following stent placement.[52] Im et al. found that in patients with malignant esophageal and GEJ obstruction, stent patency rates at 30, 90, and 180 days were 94%, 78%, and 67%, respectively.[53]

INDICATION FOR STENT USE

Current indications for esophageal stent placement are centered around treating three conditions: (1) malignant esophageal disease, (2) extrinsic esophageal compression, and (3) benign esophageal disease.[54]

ESOPHAGEAL STENTS FOR MALIGNANT ESOPHAGEAL DISEASE

Surgical resection is the primary treatment for operable esophageal cancer. However, it is well recognized that up to 50% of patients are diagnosed with inoperable disease at the time of presentation. As a consequence, these patients are frequently sent for nonoperative modalities to palliate dysphagia due to malignant obstruction. In selected patients, stenting can be a bridge to surgical resection while neoadjuvant chemoradiation is given, whereas patients with incurable esophageal and other nonluminal malignancies of the head and neck often require longer-term palliation for dysphagia and/or a TEF.[55]

MALIGNANT ESOPHAGEAL STRICTURE

Endoluminal esophageal malignant stricture is the main indication for esophageal stent placement. Although many other modalities are being used to alleviate malignant esophageal obstruction (radiotherapy, laser, argon plasma coagulation, photodynamic therapy, local injection of ethanol or direct injection of chemotherapeutic agents), SEMS insertion is the most common intervention for palliation of dysphagia in inoperable esophageal cancer.[56] A published meta-analysis examined the efficacy of various treatments for dysphagia in 3,684 patients with inoperable or unresectable esophageal cancer in 53 studies.[26] Compared to plastic tube insertion, SEMS insertion was safer and more effective. Thermal and chemical ablative techniques including laser, photodynamic therapy, and ethanol injection had a greater incidence of reintervention and required greater expertise than SEMS placement.

Although SEMS provided faster relief of dysphagia, brachytherapy demonstrated better improvement in dysphagia and a decreased complication rate when compared to SEMS.[57–61] The combination of brachytherapy and SEMS placement is preferable due to a

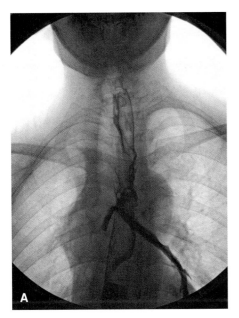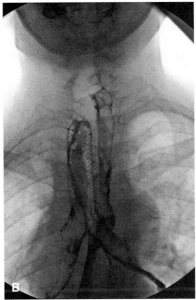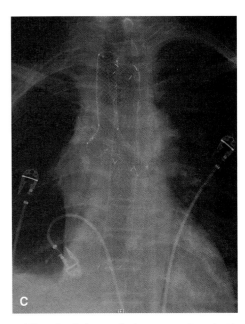

FIGURE 133.5 A 45-year-old lady with stage IIIA lung adenocarcinoma S/P VATS right upper lobectomy followed with chemoradiotherapy, complicated with proximal trachea-esophageal fistula, treated first with airway stent followed by esophageal stent placement and finally removal of the airway stent. **A:** Barium swallow study showing immediate contrast enhancement of the trachea and proximal bronchi. **B:** Trachea-bi-bronchial stent to bridge the TE fistula. **C:** Trachea-bi-bronchial stent and esophageal stent bridging the fistula.

reduced requirement for reinterventions. The authors concluded that brachytherapy might be a suitable alternative to SEMS in providing a survival advantage and possibly a better quality of life, and might provide better results when combined with argon plasma coagulation or external beam radiation therapy. Unfortunately brachytherapy is not widely available as only 6% of hospitals examined by Suntharalingam et al. had access to brachytherapy.[62]

MALIGNANT TRACHEA-ESOPHAGEAL FISTULA

Esophago-airway fistulas are complications secondary to growth of primary or recurrent esophageal or lung tumors or may result from radiation therapy or chemotherapy that leads to tumor necrosis. It is reported in 5% to 10% of patients and can recur after SEMS placement for malignant fistula in up to 35% of patients.

The consequence of an esophageal airway fistula (or TEF) is devastating as it predisposes the patient to recurrent respiratory tract infections and eventually limits the oral nutrition of the patient. The mean survival of a patient with an esophago-airway fistula is less than 6 weeks with supportive care alone.[63] Stent placement can be a good solution given the significant morbidity and mortality associated with surgical treatment of a TEF. Several reports show an 87% to 91% success rate of malignant fistula closure.[48,49,64] Retrospective evaluation of stents placed for closure of 264 TEFs over a period of 20 years showed that SEMS were associated with longer survival (13 weeks) compared to enteral feeding (4.5 weeks) or supportive care (5 weeks).[65]

Combined airway and esophageal stent placement should be considered only if the esophageal stent does not seal the fistula completely or risk of airway compression is anticipated from the esophageal stent since "kissing stents" can further erode the esophagus wall and enlarge the fistula. Herth et al. studied the difference between airway alone, esophagus alone, and combined airway and esophageal stents in 112 patients with malignant fistulas. Closure of the fistula

was initially achieved in 100% of patients. Survival was superior in the groups treated with the esophageal stent alone or the combined stents as compared to the airway stent only group (Fig. 133.5).[66]

RECURRENT LOCAL TUMOR GROWTH AFTER ESOPHAGECTOMY

Majority (~90%) of tumor recurrence after esophagectomy occurs within the first 2 years after completion of treatment. Late recurrence has been recognized more than 5 years after treatment as well. Loco-regional recurrence is usually at the level of the anastomosis, at gastric conduit, or in the mediastinum. SEMS have shown to provide good palliation for this group of patients, establishing luminal patency in nearly 100% of patients with good dysphagia score improvement and safety profile.[67,68]

ESOPHAGEAL STENTS AND CHEMORADIOTHERAPY

Increasing numbers of patients with esophageal cancer are getting either neoadjuvant or definitive chemoradiation. Some of these patients have malignant stricture and significant dysphagia leading to significant weight loss and/or malnutrition.

Temporary SEMS/SEPS are being used to either "bridge to surgery" in the patients who are surgical candidates or as a palliative measure in those who are non-operable in order to improve oral feeding and thus avoid placing a nasoenteric feeding tube, percutaneous endoscopic gastrostomy, or feeding jejunostomy.

Multiple studies have demonstrated that stents are highly effective in improving dysphagia scores and the quality of life in this specific group of patients. Stent migration as a result of tumor shrinkage following chemoradiation occurred in 15% to 60% of patients with SEPS and 2% to 40% of patients with SEMS.[46,69–72]

There is conflicting data regarding the contribution of radiation therapy to an increased risk of adverse events following stent placement. While several studies have shown increased rates of life-threatening complications and SEMS-related mortality with radiation therapy,[12,73–75] other studies and recent meta-analysis demonstrated that radiation therapy with or without chemotherapy had no relationship with the onset of complications, procedural death, or overall patient survival.[16,30,37,76–78]

EXTRINSIC MALIGNANT COMPRESSION ON THE ESOPHAGUS

Malignant compression on the esophagus either from bulky mediastinal tumor or lymphadenopathy is another indication for palliative stent placement.

A published study comparing SEMS for intrinsic and extrinsic compression showed 100% technical and 91% clinical success rate without significant differences between the groups and without immediate complications. Stents in the extrinsic compression group remained patent until death of the patient, with a median duration of patency time of 54.6 ± 45.1 days. The authors concluded that SEMS for extrinsic compression is not inferior to SEMS for intrinsic stenosis and has a comparable safety profile with good palliation of dysphagia. Both partially as well as FC stents have been used in this group of patients with good result.[79]

It is always important to remember to assess tracheal patency and potential tracheal compression following esophageal stent placement. If needed, it is safe to place a tracheal stent prior to esophageal stenting.

ESOPHAGEAL STENTS FOR BENIGN ESOPHAGEAL DISEASE

Following the experience gained in the past 20 years with the placement of esophageal stents for malignant stricture, several uses for expandable stents in nonmalignant (benign) esophageal conditions have also been described.

Benign esophageal diseases are a group of diseases that include

1. Nonmalignant refractory esophageal strictures
2. Nonmalignant esophageal rupture, perforation, fistula, leaks
3. Other nonmalignant conditions (achalasia, variceal bleeding)

REFRACTORY BENIGN ESOPHAGEAL STRICTURE

Benign esophageal strictures can result from esophageal mucosal injury as a part of the process of healing and scaring. Injuries from caustic injury, refractory peptic disease, radiation, and complication from endoscopic mucosal resection, photodynamic therapy, or other ablative therapies can result in benign esophageal stricture that might cause devastating dysphagia. Repeat endoscopic or self-bougienage, dilatation with or without steroid injection, and even esophagectomy have been used as treatments for benign stricture with variable rates of sustained success and improvement.

Before determining that a stricture is "benign," it is critical to rule out malignancy and to address the primary cause of the injury. Multiple biopsies are mandatory as part of the diagnostic endoscopy performed prior to stent placement. Reversible conditions should be treated prior to stent placement. For example, peptic strictures should be treated aggressively with PPIs before being labeled refractory.

Benign strictures are classified as simple or complex. Simple strictures are composed of a short straight esophageal segment (<2 cm) which is wide enough to allow a 9.5 mm standard endoscope to pass. Complex strictures are usually longer (>2 cm), tortuous, multiple, and often too narrow to allow passage of a standard adult endoscope. These strictures tend to become refractory to treatment over time.[32]

Simple strictures usually respond to simple dilatation; however, up to 40% may recur and require multiple periodic dilatations.[80] Complex strictures are difficult to treat, require multiple dilatations, and over time have higher risk of procedural complications. Kochman et al. defined a refractory benign esophageal stricture as an anatomic restriction due to critical luminal compromise or fibrosis that results in the clinical symptom of dysphagia in the absence of endoscopic evidence of inflammation. This may occur as the result of either an inability to successfully remediate the anatomic problem to a diameter of 14 mm over five sessions at 2-week intervals (refractory) or as a result of an inability to maintain a satisfactory luminal diameter for 4 weeks once the target diameter of 14 mm has been achieved (i.e., recurrent).[81]

Dilatation of a simple stricture stretching with a dilator allows momentary disruption of fibrous tissue with subsequent unopposed healing after the dilator is removed, thus maintaining temporary luminal patency. The benefit of using an expandable stent rather than simple dilatation is to allow the disrupted fibers to heal continuously and remodel over a fixed stent platform. Unlike malignant strictures, expandable stents for benign indication should be removed once healing has occurred. Tissue growth into the stent should be minimized to allow for stent removal. PC or FC SEMS and SEPS, and recently biodegradable stents, have been used with variable success rates for benign refractory strictures. Long-term stent-related complications occurred when stents were placed for a prolonged duration and included erosion into the esophageal wall (ulceration, bleeding, fistula formation), migration, granulation tissue formation with new stricture formation, and fatal bleeding following erosion into mediastinal structures including the aorta.

As the result of an unacceptably high rate of complications identified in multiple series due to the ingrowth of stents into the surrounding tissues, PC SEMS are not approved by the FDA for treatment of benign stricture.[11,13,82–86] FC SEMS are designed to overcome this problem of tissue ingrowth. Small case series and retrospective studies have demonstrated minimal tissue reaction and successful stent removal. The acceptable duration prior to stent removal has yet to be determined, but results with FC SEMS for benign strictures are encouraging. Certain FC SEMS are being used off label for benign strictures, although the high migration rate in some stents remains a significant issue. Further data are needed to determine the safety profile of SEMS for benign strictures.[87–90]

SEPS have replaced the PC SEMS in treating resistant esophageal strictures. The Polyflex stent is a SEPS that can be removed and is FDA approved for treating benign esophageal strictures. It is constructed of a polyester mesh completely covered with silicone membrane and has a flared proximal end to reduce the migration rate. Because it is a FC stent, tissue ingrowth is minimal, and the silicone and polyester provoke a less granulation reaction than metal. SEPS are available in various diameters and lengths, and unlike SEMS which are not preloaded, they need to be loaded at the time of placement. This has the advantage of being able to remove, reload, and redeploy the same stent if placement is not correct. As a result of the delivery system, SEPS deployment is more challenging and a pre-insertion dilatation can be required since the delivery system is large (12 to 21 mm). Stent migration is the most common complication and occurs in more than 50% of cases.[10,32,91] Multiple retrospective studies and one prospective trial showed an acceptable rate of technical success along with good dysphagia relief.[18,39–41,91,92]

There has been some interest in the use of biodegradable stents in the treatment of benign esophageal conditions, which would potentially decrease the need for reinterventions to remove the stent. Few case series with small patient cohort have been published, but further long-term prospective data obtained from controlled trials are awaited before biodegradable stents can be recommended for the management of benign esophageal lesions.[11]

ESOPHAGEAL STENTS FOR NONMALIGNANT ESOPHAGEAL RUPTURE, PERFORATION, FISTULA, OR LEAKS

Early recognition and diagnosis of esophageal rupture, perforation, and leaks is important and can significantly reduce the morbidity and mortality. The clinical context of these scenarios varies depending on the setting in which the rupture/perforation occurred (iatrogenic during endoscopy vs. spontaneous or traumatic), timing from the event (early vs. delayed diagnosis), condition of the patient (stable vs. unstable), location of the injury, and expertise of the clinician treating the patient.

Esophageal rupture is classified into iatrogenic or spontaneous:

1. Iatrogenic—instrumentation, esophageal dilatation, endoscopic mucosal resection/dissection, surgical myotomy, penetrating trauma, biopsies, and so on
2. Spontaneous—forceful vomiting (Boerhaave syndrome), forceful coughing, high-velocity MVA.

Leaks at the site of a surgical anastomosis have a tendency to evolve into a fistula. Fistulae can be a sequela of a long-standing chronic inflammation or as a consequence of a luminal or extra luminal process. Surgery is considered the gold standard for treatment of

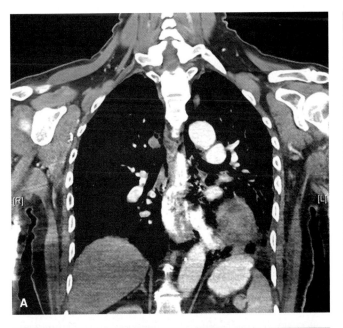

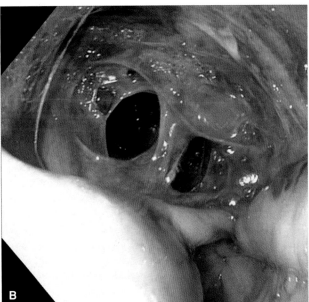

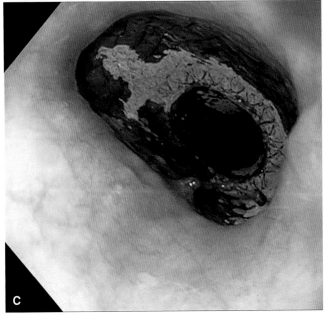

FIGURE 133.6 A 65-year-old male admitted with distal esophageal perforation following EGD biopsy and dilatation. **A:** Preoperative coronal view showing contrast extravasation from distal esophagus perforation (*arrow*). **B:** Intraoperative EGD showing large left-sided perforation with a direct view of the mediastinum (*), gastroesophageal junction (*arrow*). **C:** EGD view following stent deployment.

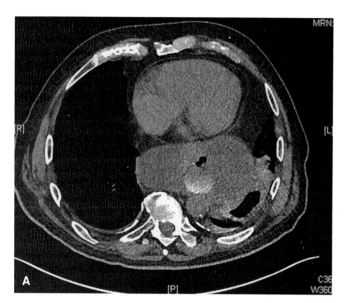
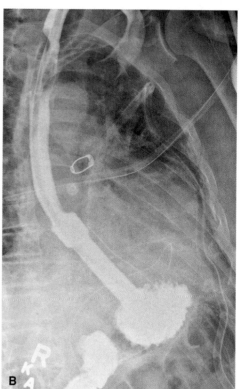

FIGURE 133.7 A 74-year-old male, 10 days S/P giant paraesophageal hernia repair with Nissen fundoplication and Collis gastroplasty, presented with fever. Computed tomography scan showed contrast extravasation into contained mediastinal collection. The patient was taken to the operating room for collection drainage followed by esophageal stent placement. **A:** Preoperative axial image showing contrast extravasation into large mediastinal fluid collection. **B:** Contrast traversing the stent into the stomach without evidence of extraluminal contrast extravasation.

an esophageal perforation/rupture or leak, although this is known to be associated with significant morbidity. Other nonsurgical alternatives have been developed and applied mainly on moribund patients such as elderly patients with multiple comorbidities where mortality rates are 20% to 45% if the perforation is left untreated.[93,94]

These nonsurgical or endoscopic options included placement of stents, sutures, and clips, application of tissue (fibrin) glue, or a combination of several methods. They can be used immediately after the perforation has been recognized during or immediately after the endoscopic procedure.

Primary endoscopic repair is usually reserved for acute small perforation of a few millimeters. Larger defects usually require surgical diversion and/or repair combined with mediastinal debridement and drainage. Occlusive stents can bridge the defect in select cases. As long as the seal is complete and the surrounding area remains well drained, complete healing is possible. At present, placement of a removable stent has become the first-line treatment for perforations and fistulas in many centers in the United States (Figs. 133.6 and 133.7).[95,96]

Stents including SEPS, FC metal stents, and biodegradable stents have been used for these indications and small series have reported on feasibility, efficacy, and complications with successful leak occlusion in 89% to 100% of patients and 23% to 50% stent migration rates.[17,25,41,86,97–105]

COMPLICATIONS OF STENT USE

Many factors contribute to stent-related complications. These include the nature of the disease (benign vs. malignant disease), the location

of the disease (proximal vs. distal esophagus), prior chemoradiotherapy, tumor vascularity, and consistency, and most importantly—stent design and diameter. Complications are usually highest (30% to 35%) for malignant strictures, SEPS, stents traversing the GEJ, and stents placed following chemoradiation, although as a general rule, the rate of serious adverse events is low, with only 0.5% to 2% stent-related mortality (oversedation, stent malposition, aspiration, perforation, etc.) being reported.[11] The timing of adverse events following stent placement is divided into immediate, early, and late as is shown in Table 133.4.

TABLE 133.4 Common Complications Related to Esophageal Stents

Immediate Complications (Intra-procedural)	Early Complications (<1 Week)	Late Complications (>1 Week)
Technical failure/ injury	Chest pain	Stent migration
Aspiration	Foreign body sensation	Tumor ingrowth/ occlusion
Airway compromise	Bleeding	Fistulization
Mortality	Nausea Tracheal compression Respiratory compromise	Perforation Bleeding GERD Aspiration

IMMEDIATE COMPLICATIONS

Hemorrhage

Stent-related bleeding is usually self-limited and is rarely life-threatening. It is usually secondary to mucosal and/or tumor erosion as a result of stent compression following deployment.

Mortality

Stent-related mortality is low (<1.4%) and is often procedure-related mortality secondary to oversedation, aspiration, or rarely perforation.

Technical Failure

In a US national survey, which included 212 endoscopists who had placed a total of 434 SEMS, the rate of overall technical adverse events was 5.4%. These included misplacement (0.3%), failed expansion or deployment (4.7%), and early migration (0.3%).[37]

EARLY COMPLICATIONS

Esophagorespiratory Fistula

Esophagorespiratory fistula (ERF) is one of the most severe complications (excluding perforation) resulting from stent placement and is associated with increased mortality. It leads to repeated respiratory aspirations and infections and inability to maintain adequate nutrition. The rate of ERF is 5% to 10% in different studies. In a study of 397 patients receiving stents for both malignant and benign indications, the overall rate of stent-related ERF was 4% after a median of 5 months, 6% in patients with proximal esophageal stents, and 14% in patients with midesophageal stents. None of the patients with distal esophageal stents developed a fistula. Radiation therapy also increased the risk for ERF.[106] In a study of 208 patients with stents for malignant stricture, the rate of TE fistula was 9%, with 94% of patients who developed a fistula having the associated risk factor of radiation therapy either before or after stent placement.[107]

Stent Migration

Stent migration occurs in 10% to 50% of patients, depending on stent type, stent location, and patient-related factors. If identified early, migrated stents can be repositioned. If already migrated into stomach, they can be either repositioned back to the esophagus, removed totally, or in event of a short prognosis, can be left in the stomach. Case reports of passing migrated stents per rectum have been described[108] but so has intestinal obstruction and thus removal is the treatment of choice.[31,109,110] In general, migration rates of FC stents, either SEMS or SEPS, are higher at 36% than those of PC stents which are reported at 4% to 23%.[111]

Food Obstruction

Food obstruction is a cause for recurrent dysphagia following stent placement. The rate of food obstruction is 5% to 7%.[112,113] This low frequency is attributed mainly to the silicone covering on the inner side of the newer stents. Patients should be advised to chew thoroughly, eat multiple small meals, and drink preferably non-carbonated beverages following meals.

Pain

Retrosternal pain can be related to tumor, radiation therapy, or the stent. Most of the time, it is multifactorial. A relatively high rate of retrosternal pain was observed after placement of the Wallflex partially covered stent (31%) and the Aliamaxx-E (22%) stent, and pain was significantly lower for other stent types such as Niti-S stents (10% to 12%), Ultraflex stents (6% to 7%), and Evolution stent (9%).[28,29,111,112–114] Retrosternal pain following stent placement is thought to be related to increased expansion force and decreased flexibility of some stent types over others. Occasionally the pain may be so severe and so persistent as to require removal.

DELAYED COMPLICATIONS

Tumor or Non-Tumoral Ingrowth and Overgrowth

Stent ingrowth (tissue growing through the stent mesh) or overgrowth (tissue growing into the lumen of the proximal or distal ends of the stent) can be caused by tumor or by a granulomatous tissue reaction. It can cause recurrent dysphagia or even stent occlusion. The incidence varies from 3% to 31% depending on the stent type.[29,30] The risk of stent occlusion due to tissue growth increases the longer the stent stays in place. Radial force and stent diameter, as well as the presence of nitinol or metal struts, increase the risk of reactive tissue growth. The risk of developing tissue growth can be reduced by using stents that are significantly longer than the malignant obstruction and by using FC stents. Thermal ablation or placement of a second stent (stent within a stent) can be used to treat stent occlusion as a result of tissue growth. Photodynamic therapy and thermal ablation are less durable and require frequent reintervention. Deployment of smaller SEPS/SEMS into previously placed SEMS is safe and effective and can palliate recurrent dysphagia caused by tissue growth.[115,116]

GERD/Aspiration

Stents placed across the GEJ and the lower esophageal sphincter can allow free reflux of gastric contents into the esophagus with the consequent regurgitation and aspiration risk. These patients are best treated with high-dose proton pump inhibitors and should be instructed to keep their head of bed elevated to 30 degrees or more. Antireflux stents (described earlier in the text) were developed to decrease the extent of acid reflux.

Aortoesophageal Fistula and Hemorrhage

Aortoesophageal fistula is a rare complication of SEMS with only a few cases reported. Prior thoracic aortic aneurysms, endovascular stent repair, and prior esophageal surgery predispose to fistula formation. Modern management utilizes endovascular aortic repair in the acute settings or more definitively endovascular repair and esophagectomy subsequently followed by gastroesophageal reconstruction. Given the extent of bleeding, morbidity and mortality are very high reaching up to 40%.[117,118]

SUMMARY/CONCLUSION

Esophageal stents have revolutionized the treatment of multiple esophageal pathologies. They have been shown to improve quality of life with reasonable safety and efficacy profiles and have decreased the morbidity of these severe clinical conditions. Esophageal stents have enabled the clinicians to treat moribund patients with esophageal perforation or leaks, ensure adequate enteral nutrition in cases of benign or malignant strictures, and improve the well-being of the patient with other esophageal pathologies.

Although significant research has been performed and intense industry competition exists, the ideal stent has yet to be designed. The variation between each individual patient's anatomy and the nature of the various diseases for which these stents are being used makes it difficult to have a perfect stent for all situations. However, some generalizations can be made on what is the "ideal stent":

1. Easy to deploy
2. Easy to remove
3. Reusable and able to be repositioned
4. Does not migrate
5. Reduces/prevents tumor ingrowth
6. "inert" (i.e., cause minimal tissue–stent interaction)
7. No discomfort
8. Inexpensive
9. Versatile so can be used for multiple indications

THE FUTURE

Besides revolutionizing the treatment of multiple esophageal diseases, expandable stents also created a new industry with new prototypes being tested frequently. Intense research to improve existing stents and to improve stent design for even better patient care is actively ongoing.

Drug Eluting Stents

Although widely used for endovascular applications, use of drug eluting stents for esophageal stenosis is still being investigated. In an animal model using 5-fluorouracil containing SEMS in rabbits, Guo et al., demonstrated high drug concentrations in the esophageal tissue whereas the 5-fluorouracil levels in the liver and the serum remained low even after 45 days.[119] Similarly, Jeon et al. showed that paclitaxel-covered stents exhibit little tissue reaction to the drug compared to the controls.[120] No human trials have been reported to date.

Radiation Emitting Stents

Synthetic radioactive holmium isotope [^{166}Ho] impregnated into the polyurethane membrane covering the outer surface of an esophageal stent has been studied in dogs. Histologic examination demonstrated radiation effect on the esophageal wall which was in direct contact with the SEMS.[121] Radiation seeds implanted into esophageal SEMS in rabbits demonstrated the desired local effect without serious complications.[122]

Allogenic Stent/Esophageal Replacement

The idea of using an allogenic aorta graft as a "stent" is best known in tracheal surgery; however, preliminary animal studies have shown success as a segmental esophageal replacement when tested in pigs. Gaujoux et al. replaced a 2 cm length of esophagus with 4 cm allogenic aortic graft bridged by a Polyflex stent placed within the aortic lumen. Six months following the replacement the stented "neo-esophagus" remained patent.[123] Unfortunately, when tested in rabbits, early postoperative aortic graft necrosis was observed.[124]

Although the data from the studies of these unique stents look promising, further validation and human studies will be needed before these stents can be used for patient care.

REFERENCES

1. Siegel RL, Miller KD, Jemal A. Cancer statistics, 2015. *CA Cancer J Clin* 2015; 65(1):5–29.
2. Irani S, Kozarek R. Esophageal stents: past, present, and future. *Tech Gastrointest Endosc* 2010;12(4):178–190.
3. Celestin LR. Permanent intubation in inoperable cancer of the oesophagus and cardia: a new tube. *Ann R Coll Surg Engl* 1959;25:165–170.
4. Symonds CJ. The treatment of malignant stricture of the oesophagus by tubage or permanent catheterism. *Br Med J* 1887;1:870–873.
5. Irani S, Kozarek R. History of GI stenting: rigid prostheses in the esophagus. In: Kozarek R, Baron T, Song HY, eds. *Self-Expandable Stents in the Gastrointestinal Tract*. New York: Springer; 2013:3–13.
6. Coyas A. Palliative intubation in carcinoma of oesophagus. *Lancet* 1955; 269(6891):647–649.
7. Atkinson M, Ferguson R, Ogilvie AL. Management of malignant dysphagia by intubation at endoscopy. *J R Soc Med* 1979;72(12):894–897.
8. Tytgat GN, den Hartog Jager FC, Haverkamp HJ. Positioning of a plastic prosthesis under fiberendoscopic control in the palliative treatment of cardio-esophageal cancer. *Endoscopy* 1976;8(4):180–185.
9. Mergener K, Kozarek RA. Stenting of the gastrointestinal tract. *Dig Dis* 2002;20(2): 173–181.
10. Siersema PD. Endoscopic therapeutic esophageal interventions: what is new? What needs further study? What can we forget? *Curr Opin Gastroenterol* 2005;21(4): 490–497.
11. Sharma P, Kozarek R, Practice Parameters Committee of American College of Gastroenterology. Role of esophageal stents in benign and malignant diseases. *Am J Gastroenterol* 2010;105(2):258–273; quiz 274.
12. Hindy P, Hong J, Lam-Tsai Y, et al. A comprehensive review of esophageal stents. *Gastroenterol Hepatol (N Y)* 2012;8(8):526–534.
13. Bethge N, Sommer A, Gross U, et al. Human tissue responses to metal stents implanted in vivo for the palliation of malignant stenoses. *Gastrointest Endosc* 1996;43(6):596–602.
14. Bethge N, Sommer A, von Kleist D, et al. A prospective trial of self-expanding metal stents in the palliation of malignant esophageal obstruction after failure of primary curative therapy. *Gastrointest Endosc* 1996;44(3):283–286.
15. Vakil N, Morris AI, Marcon N, et al. A prospective, randomized, controlled trial of covered expandable metal stents in the palliation of malignant esophageal obstruction at the gastroesophageal junction. *Am J Gastroenterol* 2001;96(6):1791–1796.
16. Conio M, Repici A, Battaglia G, et al. A randomized prospective comparison of self-expandable plastic stents and partially covered self-expandable metal stents in the palliation of malignant esophageal dysphagia. *Am J Gastroenterol* 2007;102(12):2667–2677.
17. Ott C, Ratiu N, Endlicher N, et al. Self-expanding Polyflex plastic stents in esophageal disease: various indications, complications, and outcomes. *Surg Endosc* 2007; 21(6):889–896.
18. Holm AN, de la Mora Levy JG, Gostout CJ, et al. Self-expanding plastic stents in treatment of benign esophageal conditions. *Gastrointest Endosc* 2008;67(1):20–25.
19. Mochizuki Y, Saito Y, Tanaka T, et al. Endoscopic submucosal dissection combined with the placement of biodegradable stents for recurrent esophageal cancer after chemoradiotherapy. *J Gastrointest Cancer* 2012;43(2):324–328.
20. van Boeckel PG, Vleggaar FP, Siersema PD. A comparison of temporary self-expanding plastic and biodegradable stents for refractory benign esophageal strictures. *Clin Gastroenterol Hepatol* 2011;9(8):653–659.
21. Cerna M, Kócher M, Válek V, et al. Covered biodegradable stent: new therapeutic option for the management of esophageal perforation or anastomotic leak. *Cardiovasc Intervent Radiol* 2011;34(6):1267–1271.
22. Repici A, Vleggaar FP, Hassan C, et al. Efficacy and safety of biodegradable stents for refractory benign esophageal strictures: the BEST (Biodegradable Esophageal Stent) study. *Gastrointest Endosc* 2010;72(5):927–934.
23. Jung GE, Sauer P, Schaible A. Tracheoesophageal fistula following implantation of a biodegradable stent for a refractory benign esophageal stricture. *Endoscopy* 2010;42(suppl 2):E338–E339.
24. Nogales Rincon O, Huerta Madrigal A, Merino Rodriguez B, et al. Esophageal obstruction due to a collapsed biodegradable esophageal stent. *Endoscopy* 2011; 43(suppl 2 UCTN):E189–E190.
25. Saito Y, Tanaka T, Andoh A, et al. Usefulness of biodegradable stents constructed of poly-l-lactic acid monofilaments in patients with benign esophageal stenosis. *World J Gastroenterol* 2007;13(29):3977–3980.
26. Dai Y, Li C, Xie Y, et al. Interventions for dysphagia in oesophageal cancer. *Cochrane Database Syst Rev* 2014;10:CD005048.
27. Laasch H-U, Martin DF. Antireflux stents. *Techn Gastrointest Endosc* 2010;12(4): 216–224.
28. Verschuur EM, Repici A, Kuipers EJ, et al. New design esophageal stents for the palliation of dysphagia from esophageal or gastric cardia cancer: a randomized trial. *Am J Gastroenterol* 2008;103(2):304–312.
29. Verschuur EM, Homs MY, Steyerberg EW, et al. A new esophageal stent design (Niti-S stent) for the prevention of migration: a prospective study in 42 patients. *Gastrointest Endosc* 2006;63(1):134–140.
30. Kim ES, Jeon SW, Park SY, et al. Comparison of double-layered and covered Niti-S stents for palliation of malignant dysphagia. *J Gastroenterol Hepatol* 2009; 24(1):114–119.
31. Dirks K, Schulz T, Schellmann B, et al. Fatal hemorrhage following perforation of the aorta by a barb of the Gianturco-Rosch esophageal stent. *Z Gastroenterol* 2002;40(2):81–84.
32. Dua KS. Expandable stents for benign esophageal disease. *Gastrointest Endosc Clin N Am* 2011;21(3):359–376.
33. Shim CS, Cho YD, Moon JH, et al. Fixation of a modified covered esophageal stent: its clinical usefulness for preventing stent migration. *Endoscopy* 2001;33(10):843–848.

34. Conio M, De Ceglie A, Blanchi S, et al. Esophageal strictures, tumors, and fistulae: stents for primary esophageal cancer. *Tech Gastrointest Endosc* 2010;12(4):191–202.
35. Sabharwal T, Morales JP, Irani FG, et al. Quality improvement guidelines for placement of esophageal stents. *Cardiovasc Intervent Radiol* 2005;28(3):284–288.
36. Siersema PD, Hop WC, van Blankenstein M, et al. A comparison of 3 types of covered metal stents for the palliation of patients with dysphagia caused by esophagogastric carcinoma: a prospective, randomized study. *Gastrointest Endosc* 2001;54(2):145–153.
37. Ramirez FC, Dennert B, Zierer ST, et al. Esophageal self-expandable metallic stents—indications, practice, techniques, and complications: results of a national survey. *Gastrointest Endosc* 1997;45(5):360–364.
38. Yakoub D, Fahmy R, Athanasiou T, et al. Evidence-based choice of esophageal stent for the palliative management of malignant dysphagia. *World J Surg* 2008;32(9):1996–2009.
39. Repici A, Conio M, De Angelis C, et al. Temporary placement of an expandable polyester silicone-covered stent for treatment of refractory benign esophageal strictures. *Gastrointest Endosc* 2004;60(4):513–519.
40. Evrard S, Le Moine O, Lazaraki G, et al. Self-expanding plastic stents for benign esophageal lesions. *Gastrointest Endosc* 2004;60(6):894–900.
41. Karbowski M, Schembre D, Kozarek R, et al. Polyflex self-expanding, removable plastic stents: assessment of treatment efficacy and safety in a variety of benign and malignant conditions of the esophagus. *Surg Endosc* 2008;22(5):1326–1333.
42. Siersema PD, Dees J, van Blankenstein M. Palliation of malignant dysphagia from oesophageal cancer. Rotterdam Oesophageal Tumor Study Group. *Scand J Gastroenterol Suppl* 1998;225:75–84.
43. Wilkes EA, Jackson LM, Cole AT, et al. Insertion of expandable metallic stents in esophageal cancer without fluoroscopy is safe and effective: a 5-year experience. *Gastrointest Endosc* 2007;65(6):923–929.
44. Lazaraki G, Katsinelos P, Nakos A, et al. Malignant esophageal dysphagia palliation using insertion of a covered Ultraflex stent without fluoroscopy: a prospective observational study. *Surg Endosc* 2011;25(2):628–635.
45. Siersema PD, Schrauwen SL, van Blankenstein M, et al. Self-expanding metal stents for complicated and recurrent esophagogastric cancer. *Gastrointest Endosc* 2001;54(5):579–586.
46. Adler DG, Fang J, Wong R, et al. Placement of Polyflex stents in patients with locally advanced esophageal cancer is safe and improves dysphagia during neoadjuvant therapy. *Gastrointest Endosc* 2009;70(4):614–619.
47. Ross WA, Alkassab F, Lynch PM, et al. Evolving role of self-expanding metal stents in the treatment of malignant dysphagia and fistulas. *Gastrointest Endosc* 2007;65(1):70–76.
48. Maroju NK, Anbalagan P, Kate V, et al. Improvement in dysphagia and quality of life with self-expanding metallic stents in malignant esophageal strictures. *Indian J Gastroenterol* 2006;25(2):62–65.
49. Raijman I, Siddique I, Ajani J, et al. Palliation of malignant dysphagia and fistulae with coated expandable metal stents: experience with 101 patients. *Gastrointest Endosc* 1998;48(2):172–179.
50. Morgan RA, Ellul JP, Denton ER, et al. Malignant esophageal fistulas and perforations: management with plastic-covered metallic endoprostheses. *Radiology* 1997;204(2):527–532.
51. Verschuur EM, Kuipers EJ, Siersema PD. Esophageal stents for malignant strictures close to the upper esophageal sphincter. *Gastrointest Endosc* 2007;66(6):1082–1090.
52. Rozanes I, Poyanli A, Acunas B. Palliative treatment of inoperable malignant esophageal strictures with metal stents: one center's experience with four different stents. *Eur J Radiol* 2002;43(3):196–203.
53. Im JP, Kang JM, Kim SG, et al. Clinical outcomes and patency of self-expanding metal stents in patients with malignant upper gastrointestinal obstruction. *Dig Dis Sci* 2008;53(4):938–945.
54. Schembre DB. Recent advances in the use of stents for esophageal disease. *Gastrointest Endosc Clin* 2010;20(1):103–121.
55. Petruzziello L, Costamagna G. Stenting in esophageal strictures. *Dig Dis* 2002;20(2):154–166.
56. Baerlocher MO, Asch MR, Dixon P, et al. Interdisciplinary Canadian guidelines on the use of metal stents in the gastrointestinal tract for oncological indications. *Can Assoc Radiol J* 2008;59(3):107–122.
57. Rosenblatt E, Jones G, Sur RK, et al. Adding external beam to intra-luminal brachytherapy improves palliation in obstructive squamous cell oesophageal cancer: a prospective multi-centre randomized trial of the International Atomic Energy Agency. *Radiother Oncol* 2010;97(3):488–94.
58. Rupinski M, Zagorowicz E, Regula J, et al. Randomized comparison of three palliative regimens including brachytherapy, photodynamic therapy, and APC in patients with malignant dysphagia (CONSORT 1a) (Revised II). *Am J Gastroenterol* 2011;106(9):1612–1620.
59. Sur R, Donde B, Falkson C, et al. Randomized prospective study comparing high-dose-rate intraluminal brachytherapy (HDRILBT) alone with HDRILBT and external beam radiotherapy in the palliation of advanced esophageal cancer. *Brachytherapy* 2004;3(4):191–195.
60. Bergquist H, Wenger U, Johnsson E, et al. Stent insertion or endoluminal brachytherapy as palliation of patients with advanced cancer of the esophagus and gastroesophageal junction. Results of a randomized, controlled clinical trial. *Dis Esophagus* 2005;18(3):131–139.
61. Homs MY, Steyerberg EW, Eijkenboom WM, et al. Single-dose brachytherapy versus metal stent placement for the palliation of dysphagia from oesophageal cancer: multicentre randomised trial. *Lancet* 2004;364(9444):1497–1504.
62. Suntharalingam M, Moughan J, Coia LR, et al. The national practice for patients receiving radiation therapy for carcinoma of the esophagus: results of the 1996–1999 Patterns of Care Study. *Int J Radiat Oncol Biol Phys* 2003;56(4):981–987.

63. Reed MF, Mathisen DJ. Tracheoesophageal fistula. *Chest Surg Clin N Am* 2003;13(2):271–289.
64. May A, Ell C. Palliative treatment of malignant esophagorespiratory fistulas with Gianturco-Z stents. A prospective clinical trial and review of the literature on covered metal stents. *Am J Gastroenterol* 1998;93(4):532–535.
65. Balazs A, Kupcsulik PK, Galambos Z. Esophagorespiratory fistulas of tumorous origin. Non-operative management of 264 cases in a 20-year period. *Eur J Cardiothorac Surg* 2008;34(5):1103–1107.
66. Herth FJ, Peter S, Baty F, et al. Combined airway and oesophageal stenting in malignant airway-oesophageal fistulas: a prospective study. *Eur Respir J* 2010;36(6):1370–1374.
67. Tong DK, Law S, Wong KH. The use of self-expanding metallic stents (SEMS) is effective in symptom palliation from recurrent tumor after esophagogastrectomy for cancer. *Dis Esophagus* 2010;23(8):660–665.
68. Van Heel NC, Haringsma J, Spaander MC, et al. Esophageal stents for the palliation of malignant dysphagia and fistula recurrence after esophagectomy. *Gastrointest Endosc* 2010;72(2):249–254.
69. Bower M, Jones W, Vessels B, et al. Nutritional support with endoluminal stenting during neoadjuvant therapy for esophageal malignancy. *Ann Surg Oncol* 2009;16(11):3161–3168.
70. Siddiqui AA, Glynn C, Loren D, et al. Self-expanding plastic esophageal stents versus jejunostomy tubes for the maintenance of nutrition during neoadjuvant chemoradiation therapy in patients with esophageal cancer: a retrospective study. *Dis Esophagus* 2009;22(3):216–222.
71. Vleggaar FP, Siersema PD. Expandable stents for malignant esophageal disease. *Gastrointest Endosc Clin N Am* 2011;21(3):377–388.
72. Langer FB, Schoppmann SF, Prager G, et al. Temporary placement of self-expanding oesophageal stents as bridging for neo-adjuvant therapy. *Ann Surg Oncol* 2010;17(2):470–475.
73. Siersema PD, Hop WC, Dees J, et al. Coated self-expanding metal stents versus latex prostheses for esophagogastric cancer with special reference to prior radiation and chemotherapy: a controlled, prospective study. *Gastrointest Endosc* 1998;47(2):113–120.
74. Kinsman KJ, DeGregorio BT, Katon RM, et al. Prior radiation and chemotherapy increase the risk of life-threatening complications after insertion of metallic stents for esophagogastric malignancy. *Gastrointest Endosc* 1996;43(3):196–203.
75. Lecleire S, Di Fiore F, Ben-Soussan E, et al. Prior chemoradiotherapy is associated with a higher life-threatening complication rate after palliative insertion of metal stents in patients with oesophageal cancer. *Aliment Pharmacol Ther* 2006;23(12):1693–1702.
76. Sgourakis G, Gockel I, Radtke A, et al. The use of self-expanding stents in esophageal and gastroesophageal junction cancer palliation: a meta-analysis and meta-regression analysis of outcomes. *Dig Dis Sci* 2010;55(11):3018–3030.
77. Raijman I, Siddique I, Lynch P. Does chemoradiation therapy increase the incidence of complications with self-expanding coated stents in the management of malignant esophageal strictures? *Am J Gastroenterol* 1997;92(12):2192–2196.
78. Homs MY, Hansen BE, van Blankenstein M, et al. Prior radiation and/or chemotherapy has no effect on the outcome of metal stent placement for oesophagogastric carcinoma. *Eur J Gastroenterol Hepatol* 2004;16(2):163–170.
79. Rhee K, Kim JH, Jung DH, et al. Self-expandable metal stents for malignant esophageal obstruction: a comparative study between extrinsic and intrinsic compression. *Dis Esophagus* 2016;29(3):224–228.
80. Spechler SJ. American Gastroenterological Association medical position statement on treatment of patients with dysphagia caused by benign disorders of the distal esophagus. *Gastroenterology* 1999;117(1):229–233.
81. Kochman ML, McClave SA, Boyce HW. The refractory and the recurrent esophageal stricture: a definition. *Gastrointest Endosc* 2005;62(3):474–475.
82. Wadhwa RP, Kozarek RA, France RE, et al. Use of self-expandable metallic stents in benign GI diseases. *Gastrointest Endosc* 2003;58(2):207–212.
83. Ackroyd R, Watson DI, Devitt PG, et al. Expandable metallic stents should not be used in the treatment of benign esophageal strictures. *J Gastroenterol Hepatol* 2001;16(4):484–487.
84. Fiorini A, Fleischer D, Valero J, et al. Self-expandable metal coil stents in the treatment of benign esophageal strictures refractory to conventional therapy: a case series. *Gastrointest Endosc* 2000;52(2):259–262.
85. Song HY, Park SI, Do YS, et al. Expandable metallic stent placement in patients with benign esophageal strictures: results of long-term follow-up. *Radiology* 1997;203(1):131–136.
86. Repici A, Rando G. Stent for nonmalignant leaks, perforations, and ruptures. *Tech Gastrointest Endosc* 2010; 12(4):237–245.
87. Song HY, Park SI, Jung HY, et al. Benign and malignant esophageal strictures: treatment with a polyurethane-covered retrievable expandable metallic stent. *Radiology* 1997;203(3):747–752.
88. Song HY, Jung HY, Park SI, et al. Covered retrievable expandable nitinol stents in patients with benign esophageal strictures: initial experience. *Radiology* 2000;217(2):551–557.
89. Eloubeidi MA, Lopes TL. Novel removable internally fully covered self-expanding metal esophageal stent: feasibility, technique of removal, and tissue response in humans. *Am J Gastroenterol* 2009;104(6):1374–1381.
90. Bakken JC, Wong Kee Song LM, de Groen PC, et al. Use of a fully covered self-expandable metal stent for the treatment of benign esophageal diseases. *Gastrointest Endosc* 2010;72(4):712–720.
91. Vleggaar FP, Siersema PD. Stents for benign esophageal strictures. *Tech Gastrointest Endosc* 2010;12(4):231–236.

92. Radecke K, Gerken G, Treichel U. Impact of a self-expanding, plastic esophageal stent on various esophageal stenoses, fistulas, and leakages: a single-center experience in 39 patients. *Gastrointest Endosc* 2005;61(7):812–818.

93. Brinster CJ, Singhal S, Lee L, et al. Evolving options in the management of esophageal perforation. *Ann Thorac Surg* 2004;77(4):1475–1483.

94. Brinster CJ, Kucharczuk JC. Evolving options in the management of esophageal perforation. *Ann Thorac Surg* 2004;77(4):1475–1483. Review.

95. Zumbro GL, Anstadt MP, Mawulawde K, et al. Surgical management of esophageal perforation: role of esophageal conservation in delayed perforation. *Am Surg* 2002; 68(1):36–40.

96. Jougon J, Mc Bride T, Delcambre F, et al. Primary esophageal repair for Boerhaave's syndrome whatever the free interval between perforation and treatment. *Eur J Cardiothorac Surg* 2004;25(4):475–479.

97. Fry SW, Fleischer DE. Management of a refractory benign esophageal stricture with a new biodegradable stent. *Gastrointest Endosc* 1997;45(2):179–182.

98. Fischer A, Thomusch O, Benz S, et al. Nonoperative treatment of 15 benign esophageal perforations with self-expandable covered metal stents. *Ann Thorac Surg* 2006; 81(2):467–472.

99. Pennathur A, Chang AC, McGrath KM, et al. Polyflex expandable stents in the treatment of esophageal disease: initial experience. *Ann Thorac Surg*; 2008;85(6): 1968–1972; discussion 1973.

100. Doniec JM, Schniewind B, Kahlke V, et al. Therapy of anastomotic leaks by means of covered self-expanding metallic stents after esophagogastrectomy. *Endoscopy* 2003;35(8):652–658.

101. Freeman RK, Van Woerkom JM, Ascioti AJ. Esophageal stent placement for the treatment of iatrogenic intrathoracic esophageal perforation. *Ann Thorac Surg.* 2007;83(6):2003–2007; discussion 2007–2008.

102. Siersema PD, Homs MY, Haringsma J, et al. Use of large-diameter metallic stents to seal traumatic nonmalignant perforations of the esophagus. *Gastrointest Endosc* 2003; 58(3):356–361.

103. van Heel NC, Haringsma J, Spaander MC, et al. Short-term esophageal stenting in the management of benign perforations. *Am J Gastroenterol* 2010;105(7): 1515–1520.

104. Johnsson E, Lundell L, Liedman B. Sealing of esophageal perforation or ruptures with expandable metallic stents: a prospective controlled study on treatment efficacy and limitations. *Dis Esophagus* 2005;18(4):262–266.

105. Petruzziello L, Tringali A, Riccioni ME, et al. Successful early treatment of Boerhaave's syndrome by endoscopic placement of a temporary self-expandable plastic stent without fluoroscopy. *Gastrointest Endosc* 2003;58(4):608–612.

106. Bick BL, Song LM, Buttar NS, et al. Stent-associated esophagorespiratory fistulas: incidence and risk factors. *Gastrointest Endosc* 2013;77(2):181–189.

107. Park JY, Shin JH, Song HY, et al. Airway complications after covered stent placement for malignant esophageal stricture: special reference to radiation therapy. *Am J Roentgenol* 2012;198(2):453–459.

108. Oh YS, Kochman ML. Polyflex esophageal stent migration with elimination per rectum. *Gastrointest Endosc* 2007;66(3):633.

109. Wang MQ, Sze DY, Wang ZP, et al. Delayed complications after esophageal stent placement for treatment of malignant esophageal obstructions and esophagorespiratory fistulas. *J Vasc Interv Radiol* 2001;12(4):465–474.

110. Baron TH. A practical guide for choosing an expandable metal stent for GI malignancies: is a stent by any other name still a stent? *Gastrointest Endosc* 2001; 54(2):269–272.

111. Uitdehaag MJ, van Hooft JE, Verschuur EM, et al. A fully-covered stent (Alimaxx-E) for the palliation of malignant dysphagia: a prospective follow-up study. *Gastrointest Endosc* 2009;70(6):1082–1089.

112. van Boeckel PG, Repici A, Vleggaar FP, et al. A new metal stent with a controlled-release system for palliation of malignant dysphagia: a prospective, multicenter study. *Gastrointest Endosc* 2010;71(3):455–460.

113. van Boeckel PG, Siersema PD, Sturgess R, et al. A new partially covered metal stent for palliation of malignant dysphagia: a prospective follow-up study. *Gastrointest Endosc* 2010;72(6):1269–1273.

114. Bona D, Laface L, Bonavina L, et al. Covered nitinol stents for the treatment of esophageal strictures and leaks. *World J Gastroenterol* 2010;16(18):2260–2264.

115. Conio M, Blanchi S, Filiberti R, et al. Self-expanding plastic stent to palliate symptomatic tissue in/overgrowth after self-expanding metal stent placement for esophageal cancer. *Dis Esophagus* 2010;23(7):590–596.

116. Langer FB, Zacherl J. Palliative endoscopic interventions in esophageal cancer. *Eur Surg* 2007;39(5):288–294.

117. Unosawa S, Hata M, Sezai A, et al. Surgical treatment of an aortoesophageal fistula caused by stent implantation for esophageal stenosis: report of a case. *Surg Today* 2008;38(1):62–64.

118. Allgaier HP, Schwacha H, Technau K, et al. Fatal esophagoaortic fistula after placement of a self-expanding metal stent in a patient with esophageal carcinoma. *N Engl J Med* 1997;337(24):1778.

119. Guo SR, Wang ZM, Zhang YQ, et al. In vivo evaluation of 5-fluorouracil-containing self-expandable nitinol stent in rabbits: efficiency in long-term local drug delivery. *J Pharm Sci* 2010;99(7):3009–3018.

120. Jeon SR, Jin SY. Effect of drug-eluting metal stents in benign esophageal stricture: an in vivo animal study. *Endoscopy* 2009;41(5):449–456.

121. Won JH, Lee JD, Wang HJ, et al. Self-expandable covered metallic esophageal stent impregnated with beta-emitting radionuclide: an experimental study in canine esophagus. *Int J Radiat Oncol Biol Phys* 2002;53(4):1005–1013.

122. Guo JH, Lee JD, Wang HJ, et al. Self-expandable stent loaded with 125I seeds: feasibility and safety in a rabbit model. *Eur J Radiol* 2007;61(2):356–361.

123. Gaujoux S, Le Balleur Y, Bruneval P, et al. Esophageal replacement by allogenic aorta in a porcine model. *Surgery* 2010;148(1):39–47.

124. Tessier W, Mariette C, Copin MC, et al. Replacement of the esophagus with fascial flap-wrapped allogenic aorta. *J Surg Res* 2015; 193(1):176–183.

CONGENITAL, STRUCTURAL, AND INFLAMMATORY DISEASES OF THE ESOPHAGUS

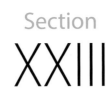

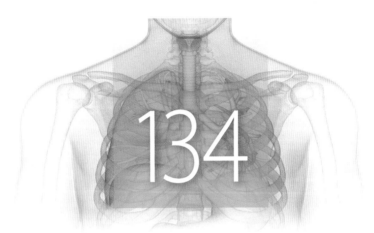

Congenital Anomalies of the Esophagus

David M. Notrica ▪ Dawn E. Jaroszewski

ESOPHAGEAL ATRESIA AND TRACHEOESOPHAGEAL FISTULA

DEFINITIONS

Esophageal atresia (EA) is a congenital anomaly in which the esophageal lumen is not in patent continuity with the stomach. Since more than 90% of cases of EA are associated with tracheoesophageal fistula (TEF), the anomalies are addressed together in this chapter, as is TEF without EA. The etiology of EA is unknown, but research continues into the understanding of the etiology.[1,2]

Embryology

Earlier descriptions regarding "division" of the trachea and esophagus have come into question.[3] Recent work using electron microscopy by Metzger et al.[4] found no evidence of lateral foregut ridges nor evidence of fusion to form a tracheoesophageal separation in embryonic development (Fig. 134.1). At the fourth week of gestation, the future trachea and lung begins as a ventral diverticulum off the foregut, just below the pharynx.[5] The future lungs are at the caudal end of this outpouching. The trachea initially grows as part of an "undivided foregut" and then becomes a separate structure as a result of a craniocaudal elongation, not a pinching between the esophagus and trachea as previous theories postulated.[4,6] In many ways, an undivided foregut separating by elongation offers a more satisfactory explanation of the EA/TEF spectrum than prior theories. Genetic research suggests this process is controlled by the developmental gene Sonic hedgehog (Shh) and members of its signaling cascade.[7,8]

History

Despite an initial attempt at repair by Charles Steele (reported in Lancet in 1888), repair of EA was unsuccessful until 1939 when multistage repairs where successfully done by Logan Leven and William Ladd, independently.[9] Haight's single-stage repair at the University of Michigan in 1941 on an ill 12-day-old baby girl[9] was the birth of the modern form of the operation. In 1999, the first thoracoscopic repair of EA was reported by Lobe et al.[10]

INCIDENCE

The incidence of EA is 1 in 4,100 to 4,500 pregnancies,[11] but only 1 in 5,500 live births.[12] In Europe, a 2.8% stillbirth rate and 3.0% elective termination rate was noted.[11] Only 18% to 20% of EA live births are diagnosed prenatally.[13] EA without TEF is more likely to be diagnosed prenatally than cases with a TEF.[12,13] A 1.3:1 male

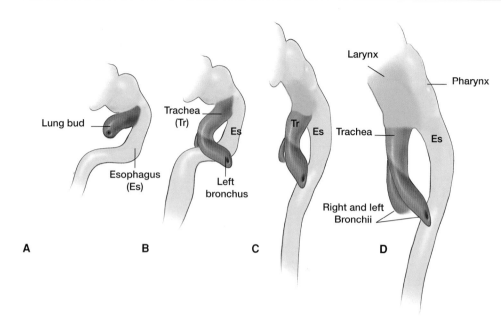

FIGURE 134.1 Current understanding of foregut development. The lungs and bronchi appear directly off the esophagus, initially with a shared foregut (oval). Next, the trachea develops and separates from the esophagus by caudal elongation. Panels by increasing Hamburger/Hamilton stage of development **A:** 19/20; **B:** 20/21; **C:** 22/23; **D:** 25/25. (Re-drawn from electron photomicrographs Metzger R, Wachowiak R, Kluth D. Embryology of the early foregut. *Semin Pediatr Surg* 2011;20(3):136–144.)

predominance is noted.[12] There does not appear to be any change in the overall world incidence over the last few decades, with the possible exception of Japan.[11,14]

Several classification schemes for EA and TEF exist. The preferred nomenclature is descriptive. Table 134.1 compares the current and historical classifications and incidence, while Figure 134.2 illustrates the common varieties.

Risk Classification

The earliest attempt at risk classification was the Waterston et al.[17] classification in 1962. The scheme identified risk factors for survival. With improved anesthetic and perioperative care, survival has increased considerably, but the concept of risk is still useful.[18] The Spitz classification looks at weight <1,500 g or major congenital heart disease to identify high-risk infants which allows comparison of outcomes between reported series (Table 134.4). The addition of preoperative respiratory distress to the classification may also prove to have prognostic merit,[19] but risk classification does not guide therapy in EA.

Associated Anomalies

Approximately 4% of patients with EA have definable genetic syndrome, including single gene disorders such as Feingold syndrome; CHARGE syndrome; Pallister–Hall syndrome; Opitz G syndrome; Fanconi anemia; trisomies 13, 18, and 21; gene deletions such as 22q11

deletion (DiGeorge) syndrome; Opitz syndrome; 13q deletion, 17q deletion,16q24 deletion; Oculo-Auriculo-Vertebral Spectrum (OAVS)/ Goldenhar syndrome; and Martinez-Frias syndrome.[20]

VACTERL

An additional 45% to 53% have a nongenetic associated anomaly.[21] These nonsyndromic associations are characterized by the acronym "VACTERL" for Vertebral, Anorectal, Cardiac, Tracheal, Esophageal, Renal, and Limb. Quan and Smith (1973) originally coined the acronym VATER to describe the association, but the terminology was later changed to include cardiac,[22] and the acronym was changed to VACTERL.[23] VACTERL is not a syndrome, but a nonrandom association of anomalies. The relative risks of the associated anomalies in patients with known EA or TEF are shown (Table 134.2).[27–29] "VACTERL + hydrocephalus" has also been well described.[24,25] The etiology of the VACTERL association is unknown, although research into the pathogenesis is ongoing.[26]

Cardiac disease occurs in approximately 25% to 60% of patients, and accounts for the majority of associated morbidity and mortality in patients without genetic syndromes. Major cardiac disease is defined by Spitz as "cyanotic congenital heart disease that required palliative or corrective surgery or noncyanotic heart anomaly that required medical or surgical treatment for cardiac failure." The relative frequencies of cardiac anomalies are listed in Table 134.3.

Duodenal atresia is occasionally seen in EA and requires special attention (Fig. 134.3).[31] If the duodenal obstruction is left unaddressed,

TABLE 134.1 Descriptive and Historical Classifications of EA and TEF

Descriptive Classification	Gross	Ladd	Incidence (%)[15]
EA, no TEF	A	I	7.5
EA, proximal TEF	B	II	1.1
EA, distal TEF	C	III, IV	86.6
EA, proximal and distal TEFs	D	V	1.0
TEF without EA (H-Type)	E		3.8
Esophageal stenosis	F		NR 3.6[16]

EA, Esophageal atresia; TEF, Tracheoesophageal fistula; NR, not reported.

TABLE 134.2 Frequency of VACTERL Associations in Patients in Either EA or TEF[27–29]

Vertebral	4–24%
Anorectal	9–14%
Cardiac	24–61%
Tracheal	92.5%
Esophageal	96.2%
Renal anomalies	9–21%
Limb anomalies	3–16%

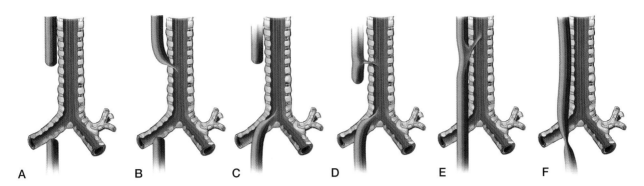

FIGURE 134.2 **A:** Esophageal atresia with distal tracheoesophageal fistula. **B:** Esophageal atresia without tracheoesophageal fistula. **C:** Tracheo-esophageal fistula without esophageal atresia. **D:** Esophageal atresia with proximal tracheoesophageal fistula. **E:** Esophageal atresia with both proximal and distal tracheoesophageal fistulas. **F:** Esophageal stenosis.

the duodenal atresia may lead to disruption of the esophageal anastomosis and tension pneumothorax. Options include decompressive gastrostomy with delayed repair of the duodenal atresia within a week, or immediate repair of the atresia after ligating the TEF. Both have been reported with good results.[32–35]

Malrotation is identified in approximately 3% of cases.[36] Unilateral pulmonary agenesis, hypothyroidism, and phenylketonuria have also been reported.[37,38] Communicating bronchopulmonary foregut malformations (CBFMs) are discussed at the end of the chapter, and may present important anatomic problems during repair.

CLINICAL PRESENTATION

Fetal diagnosis of EA is made on fetal ultrasound examination in approximately 20% of cases, more commonly in EA without TEF.[13] Typical findings include absent or small gastric bubble in conjunction with maternal polyhydramnios. Fetal magnetic resonance imaging (MRI) was only able to definitively diagnose 78% of cases presenting with clinical suspicion of EA.[39] Thus, the clinical presentation of drooling, choking, or cyanosis with feeds remain most common.

In a distal TEF, the abdomen quickly fills with air.[40] Bile and gastric secretions may enter the trachea through the fistula leading to chemical pneumonitis. The combination of aspiration and limitations of diaphragmatic breathing due to abdominal distention may lead to significant respiratory distress. In some cases, the respiratory status may worsen upon positive pressure ventilation as more air is driven into the abdomen through the fistula.[35] The fistula forms a one-way

TABLE 134.3 Description of Cardiac Disease Found in Association With EA

Cardiac Disease	Isolated Defect (%)	In Combination (%)
Ventricular septal defect (VSD)	16	42
Patent ductus arteriosus (PDA)	11	44
Tetralogy of Fallot	11	13
Right-sided aortic arch	7	9
Pulmonary stenosis	5	32
Atrial septal defect (ASD)	5	19
Total anomalous venous drainage	3	3
Double aortic arch	3	3
Coarctation of the aorta	2	6
Transposition of great vessels	2	2
Hypoplastic heart	2	2
Atrioventricular canal		7
Double outlet right ventricle		3
Aortopulmonary window		3
Aortic stenosis		3
Single ventricle		2

Data modified from Chittmittrapap S, Spitz L, Kiely EM, et al. Oesophageal atresia and associated anomalies. *Arch Dis Child* 1989;64(3):364–368.

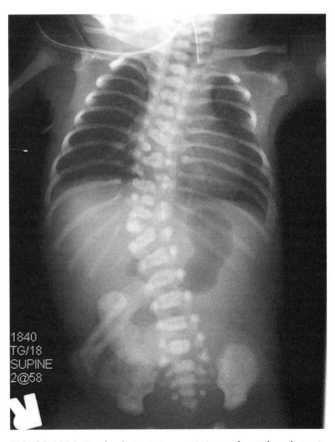

FIGURE 134.3 Duodenal atresia in association with esophageal atresia. Note the normal to small size of the stomach and duodenum as compared to typical duodenal atresia. Incidentally noted are numerous vertebral and rib anomalies.

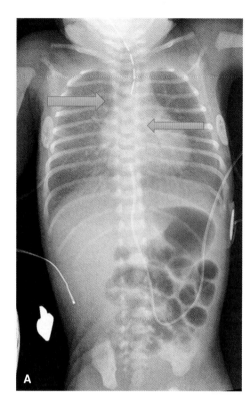
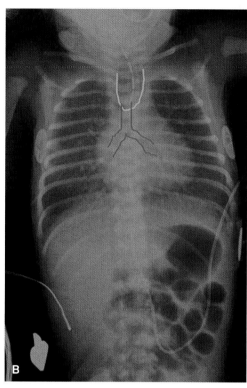

FIGURE 134.4 Chest (**A**) abdomen (**B**) plain film. Note the Replogle OGT stops at T3. The distance between the end of the esophagus and the carina is less than two vertebral bodies suggesting this is a short gap. The air in the stomach and small bowel indicated the presence of a TEF.

valve with subsequent massive abdominal distention. In rare cases, an emergent decompressive gastrostomy is necessary to restore ventilation following intubation. Gastric perforation in EA/TEF occurs in a small subset of patients.[41,42] Treatment generally consists of emergent aspiration of the tense pneumoperitoneum, urgent laparotomy, and repair of the stomach with or without a gastrostomy.

DIAGNOSIS

The initial diagnosis of EA is made by inability to pass an orogastric tube (OGT). As a general rule, the OGT in children with EA stops at approximately 10 cm,[43] although the length may vary with the length of the proximal esophageal pouch. A combined chest/abdomen radiograph is useful for multiple reasons. The study allows the clinician to confirm the position of the catheter; confirm the presence of a distal TEF (by presence of air below the diaphragm); evaluate for cardiac, intestinal, and vertebral anomalies; and allows the clinician to estimate the length of the gap between the proximal and distal fistula. Presence of air in the jejunum decreases the likelihood for duodenal atresia. While the distal esophagus is rarely seen, most fistula are near the carina, and an estimation of the gap may be calculated in terms of vertebral body heights between the carina and the end of the OGT. Greater than three vertebral bodies between the proximal esophagus and carina suggests the possibility of a long gap EA.

The differential diagnosis for EA includes iatrogenic esophageal perforation by OGT placement,[44–47] neonatal esophageal foreign body obstruction,[48] congenital esophageal stenosis,[49] or membranous diaphragm obstruction.[50] Other misdiagnoses have been reported due to malposition of the OGT into the trachea, through the TEF, and then into the stomach[51,52] or passing through proximal and distal TEFs into the stomach.[53] EA with TEF may rarely be misdiagnosed as EA without fistula in cases where the fistula is partially obstructed,[5] and concurrent distal esophageal stenosis (2% to 8%) may be difficult to identify preoperatively.[54] Missed proximal TEF is probably more common than

reported, particularly if preoperative laryngotracheobronchoscopy is not performed routinely.[15] Type IA and IB CBFMs are associated with EA but are often not diagnosed before or at the initial surgery.[55,56]

INITIAL MANAGEMENT AND EVALUATION

A prenatal history should be obtained and thorough physical examination for risk stratification and detection of other congenital anomalies should be performed. Prior to planning surgery, particular attention should be placed on confirming failure to pass an OGT, evaluating the degree of respiratory distress, and confirming the patency of the anus. A combined chest/abdomen radiograph should be performed with gentle pressure on the OGT (Fig. 134.4A). Occasionally, instillation of the Replogle tube with air may help define the proximal pouch, as well. Barium instillation is not recommended.[43] The presence of air in the stomach confirms the presence of a TEF. Air in the distal small bowel exclude an associated duodenal atresia. The gap length is estimated by counting vertebral bodies between the end of the proximal esophagus and the carina (Fig. 134.4B). Re-estimation of the gap length can be made at preoperative bronchoscopy using the technique described by Bagolan (Fig. 134.5).

An echocardiogram is required prior to surgery. This study allows the identification of potentially problematic cardiac anomalies, and allows identification of a right-sided aortic arch that occurs in approximately 2.5% to 9% of cases.[30,57] In cases of a right-sided aortic arch, a left sided approach may be advised. In cases where the right-sided arch was not identified preoperatively, it is possible to repair the EA on the same side of the aortic arch, but consideration should be given to closing and pursuing a left-sided approach.[21] If a right-sided arch is identified preoperatively, chest MRI may be helpful to exclude a vascular ring. In the presence of a vascular ring, the left-sided approach to the esophageal repair is difficult (or more difficult) than a right-sided approach.[57,58] Renal ultrasonography is done prior to surgery to identify renal anomalies requiring attention at the initial operation.

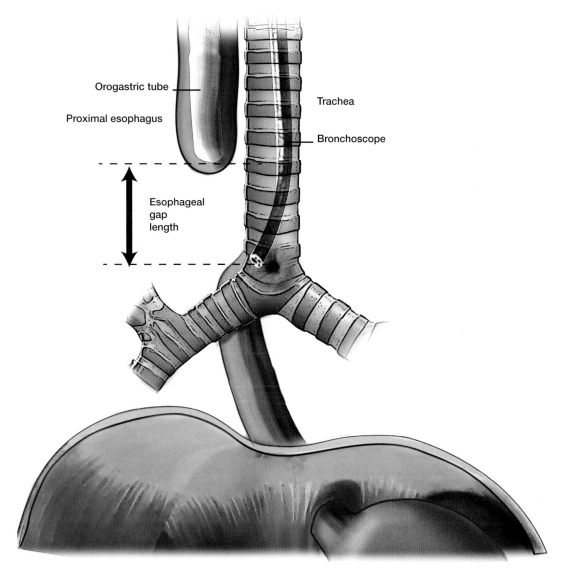

Orogastric tube

Proximal esophagus

Trachea

Bronchoscope

Esophageal
gap
length

FIGURE 134.5 Intraoperative measurement of esophageal gap length using the method described by Bagolan et al. An OGT or other radio-opaque object is placed in the proximal esophagus while flexible bronchoscopy is performed. The bronchoscope is at the tip of the fistula. Fluoroscopy then reveals the linear distance between the tips of the radio-opaque objects, thus providing an estimate of the esophageal gap length. The *double arrow* shows the distance between the proximal esophagus and the distal esophagus (at the fistula).

Modern management is guided by the patient's clinical stability. An algorithm is provided in Figure 134.6.

Unstable Infants

In patients who are unstable, the etiology needs to be determined. For patients with poor lung compliance and excessive venting through the fistula, options for management include intubation with a cuffed endotracheal tube to occlude the fistula, rigid bronchoscopic ventilation, transtracheal or transgastric occlusion of the fistula with a Fogarty catheter, passing the endotracheal tube beyond the fistula, gastric division, silastic gastric banding, high-frequency oscillators, or urgent thoracotomy.[35,59–62] In those cases where inability to ventilate is caused by a tense abdomen, consideration is given to urgent gastrostomy, occasionally at the bedside. For cases of gastric perforation, the preferred management as described by Maoate is: (1) needle decompression of the abdomen; (2) laparotomy and retrograde occlusion of the fistula through the gastric perforation; (3) thoracotomy, ligation, and division of TEF; (4) esophageal repair

if possible; and (5) repair of gastric perforation with or without gastrostomy.[40]

A staged repair, which consists of ligation and division of the fistula without repair of the EA is done in selected cases. These include the rare infant with highly unstable cardiac disease requiring urgent surgery, and those patients who develop worsening instability intraoperatively and fail to improve with control of the TEF. Note that most patients with cardiac anomalies will have their EA/TEF definitively addressed prior to their heart disease. Ligation alone (without division) only keeps the fistula closed for 7 to 14 days prior to recanalization, so this must be viewed as a temporizing measure.

Stable Infants

As shown in the algorithm, stable infants should undergo surgery within 24 to 48 hours, and bronchoscopy should be done if feasible. An initial ligation and division of the TEF should be performed for all stable infants. Even in small infants, a primary repair of the EA should be done if the tissues are adequate and ends can be brought

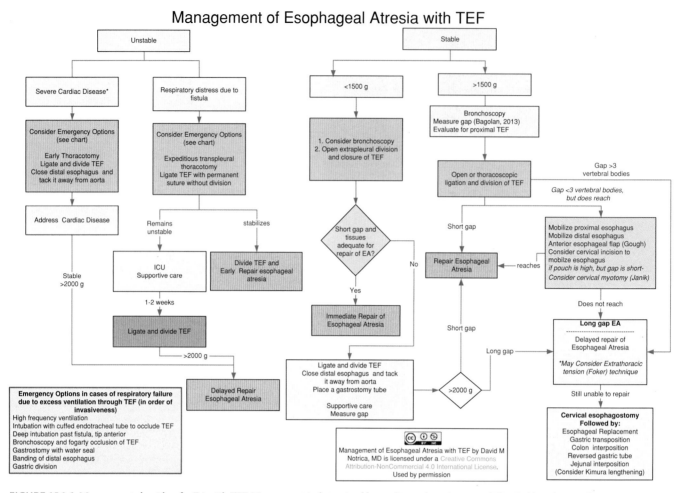

Management of Esophageal Atresia with TEF

FIGURE 134.6 Management algorithm for EA with TEF. Management is determined by cardiac and respiratory stability. Stable infants undergo repair at 24 to 48 hours after birth. EA, esophageal atresia; TEF, tracheoesophageal fistula; ICU, intensive care unit. (Used by permission.)

together.[63,64] For infants <1,500 g, repair may not be possible, and the distal esophagus may be ligated and tacked to the chest wall away from the aorta for later EA repair. Adjuncts to facilitate repair of the EA are listed in the algorithm and discussed below in the long gap EA section.

OPERATIVE CARE

Anesthetic Considerations

For patients with a distal TEF, classic management involves avoidance of muscle relaxation and avoidance of positive-pressure ventilation until after bronchoscopic evaluation of the fistula location, and prior to ligation of the fistula if the TEF is low or the fistula patulous. In stable infants, some series report inhalational or intravenous induction and muscle paralysis use.[65,66] Rothenberg's series of thoracoscopic TEFs reported use of pressure-control ventilation and tracheal intubation (regardless of the position of the fistula) even in patients with widely patent pericarinal fistulas,[65] although most of his patients were quite stable.

If planned, laryngotracheobronchoscopy is done prior to intubation to confirm the diagnosis and identify additional pathology as described below. Neither mainstem intubation nor left bronchial blockers are generally employed. Intubation beyond the fistula or occluding the TEF with a cuffed endotracheal tube may be possible in a very small subset of patients, but is not without risk.[62,67]

Laryngotracheobronchoscopy

Many surgeons advocate for routine endoscopy in the operating room to confirm the diagnosis prior to surgery (Fig. 134.7).[68–70] Recently a study found 20% of patients had unexpected, important findings identified at preoperative laryngotracheobronchoscopy. The additional findings included fistula at unusual sites, laryngotracheal clefts, vallecular cyst, EA/TEF in cases thought to be EA only, unusual fistula sites, upper pouch fistulae, double fistula, and fistula from main bronchus.[70] While a minority of UK centers do preoperative endoscopy, the benefits for diagnosis, planning, and treatment are significant enough to advocate for endoscopy immediately prior to repair in all cases where it is technically feasible and can be done safely.[71] Even in UK centers where they do not advocate for routine endoscopy, it is generally performed for EA without fistula.[21] In unstable patients, bronchoscopy allows a Fogarty catheter to be passed to occlude the fistula and to prevent continued loss of ventilation through the fistula in patients who are unstable or difficult to ventilate.[72] Simultaneous bronchoscopy and fluoroscopy allows an accurate preoperative assessment of the esophageal gap (Fig. 134.4).[35]

OPERATIVE REPAIR

Currently, operative repair is done through either open thoracotomy or thoracoscopic approach. As of this writing, approximately 94% of EA repairs in Europe are still done open, and the minority

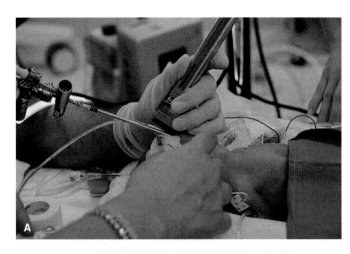

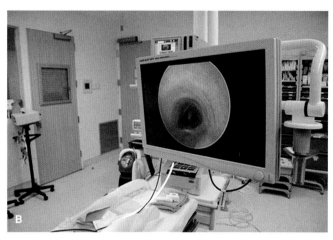

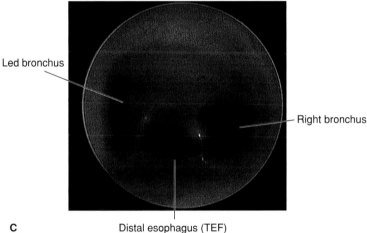

Led bronchus

Right bronchus

C   Distal esophagus (TEF)

FIGURE 134.7 Preoperative bronchoscopy may be done in stable infants. Ventilation through the bronchoscope is facilitated by use of small caliber lens. **A:** Stable 1,300 g infant undergoing a preoperative rigid bronchoscopy. **B:** Panel monitor showing the TEF in the midtrachea making chances for an anastomosis favorable, even in this small infant. **C:** Video of a patient with distal TEF at the carina, suggesting the possibility of a longer gap.

of repairs in the United States and Japan are thoracoscopic, even in centers doing minimally invasive surgery.[71,73,74] Both procedures are described below, as both techniques currently play a role.

OPEN REPAIR

PREPARATION AND POSITIONING

In cases with a confirmed left-sided aortic arch, the patient is positioned for right posterolateral thoracotomy (Fig. 134.8A). A left approach may be done for patients with a right-sided aortic arch if identified preoperatively, but if found intraoperatively, completion through right chest may be attempted if possible. A muscle-sparing extrapleural approach through the 4th interspace is achieved by gently pushing the intact pleura away from the chest wall. Moist cotton-tipped applicators are helpful (Figs. 134.9 and 134.10), as is moist gauze. The extrapleural dissection is begun mid-incision where a small tear in the pleura would be well away from the esophageal anastomosis. After an extensive extrapleural dissection is completed, the pleura and lung are retracted medially and the azygos vein identified, ligated, and divided (Fig. 134.8B). The TEF is often found under

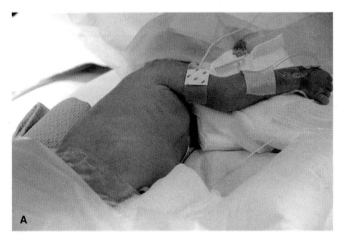

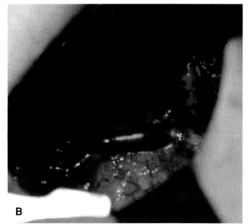

FIGURE 134.8 **A:** Positioning for open repair of EA/TEF. **B:** View of azygos vein crossing the TEF after extrapleural dissection.

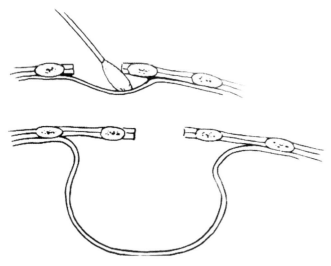

FIGURE 134.9 Drawing showing the extrapleural dissection. Prior to entering the chest, the pleura is pushed away and kept intact. The lung and pleura are then retracted as a unit to expose the esophagus and TEF. (Reprinted from Coran AG, Harmon CM. *Pediatric Surgery*. 7th ed. Philadelphia, PA: WB Saunders; 2012. Copyright © 2012 Elsevier. With permission.)

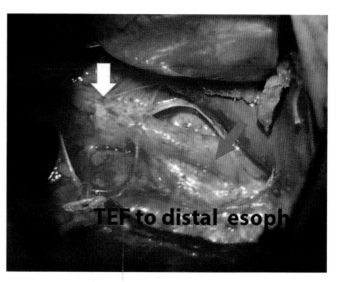

FIGURE 134.11 View of distal tracheoesophageal fistula. Head is toward left. Lung and pleura are retracted anteriorly. Junction with trachea is marked with *white arrow*. The *blue arrow* designates the distal esophagus.

the azygos (Fig. 134.11). The aorta is also often seen posterior to the TEF during the dissection and must not be confused for the TEF by the novice surgeon. The TEF is exposed and controlled with a vessel loop. The dissection of the TEF is continued to the trachea. Closure of the TEF may be handled in a variety of ways. Most commonly, fine polydioxanone (PDS) sutures are placed at the proximal fistula and the fistula divided. The fistula is then closed with interrupted PDS suture. Enough warm saline is placed in the chest to cover the fistula, and an airtight closure is confirmed to a pressure of 40 mm Hg generated via the endotracheal tube.

Next, the proximal esophagus is identified (Fig. 134.12). The extrapleural dissection should have been completed to the apex by this point. The lung within the pleural sac is retracted anteriorly. Gentle downward pressure on the untaped 10F Replogle tube by the anesthesiologist assists in identification (Fig. 134.12) (Video 134.1). In rare cases where the proximal esophagus does not extend into the chest, cervical

mobilization with or without myotomy and passage into the chest using a clamp may yield enough length to complete the repair in the chest (Fig. 134.13). The proximal atretic end of the esophagus is mobilized from the surrounding tissue. Use of a freer elevator may facilitate dissection laterally, while others prefer sharp dissection with tenotomy scissors. A traction suture may also be placed through the distal esophagus to facilitate dissection. The esophagus and trachea often share a common wall. The two structures must be adequately separated to allow mobilization for anastomosis. Once adequate esophageal length is confirmed, the proximal esophagus is opened. Several technical variations have been described to open the upper esophagus including as shown in the Figures 134.14 to 134.16[75–80] and an end-to-side technique has also been described.[81] The anterior esophageal flap (Fig. 134.14) is an

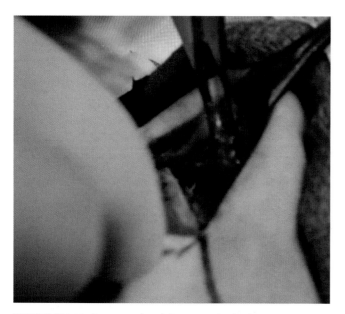

FIGURE 134.10 Open extrapleural dissection of right chest.

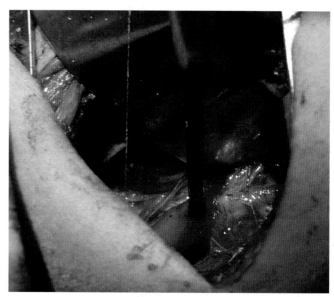

FIGURE 134.12 Operative exposure of the proximal esophagus. The forceps hold the proximal esophagus. (Video) This video shows the distal esophagus after division of the TEF and identification of the proximal esophagus aided by the OGT.

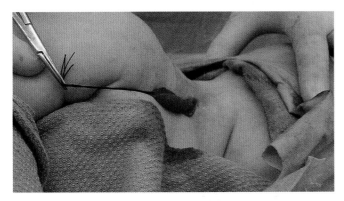

FIGURE 134.13 Cervical exposure of the esophagus without esophagostomy is an effective technique to achieve primary repair in EA when there is adequate distal esophagus, but the proximal esophagus does not reach into the chest.

important modification in moderately long gap cases as shown in the algorithm, while the others have not yet gained wide adoption.

The type of absorbable suture for the esophageal anastomosis is controversial, but probably is not an important determinant of stricture or leak. One randomized study has reported use of fibrin glue as an adjunct to decrease leakage and stricture.[82] Several nonanastomotic techniques have been reported, one with suture and another with magnets, but are not in clinical use at this time.[83–85] The authors currently prefer absorbable monofilament suture, such as 5-0 PDS with knots on the outside, which is a common choice, but previously used absorbable braided suture for many years without difficulty (Fig. 134.17).[86] The back wall stitches are placed sequentially by equally dividing the distance. The assistant brings together the ends of the esophagus together to decrease tension while the surgeon ties down the sutures in order. The OGT or a feeding tube is then passed into the stomach during the anastomosis and later removed. The front wall sutures are then placed prior to tying them sequentially. Due to the size mismatch, gaps in the proximal esophagus may require a vertical stitch to prevent leakage. The OGT is generally removed at completion of the anastomosis.

Placement of a chest tube has been questioned, and many experienced surgeons advocate for omitting chest drains.[21,87] Currently, the practice is still to use soft Blake extrapleural drains in small infants, cases with significant tension or friable esophageal tissue.

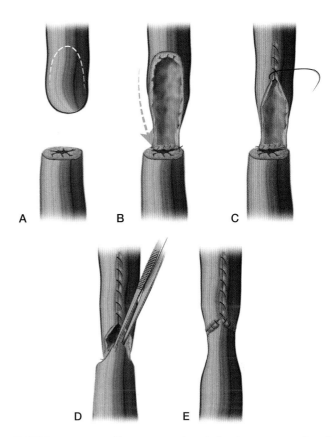

FIGURE 134.14 Gough's anterior esophageal flap for gaining esophageal length and tapering the proximal esophagus. This is an important technique when gap length is inadequate. **A:** Dotted lines indicate cut lines for flap. **B:** Flap is rotated down to reach the backwall. **C:** Proximal esophagus is closed longitudinally to taper the esophagus. **D:** Checking the ability of the distal esophagus to reach the proximal esophagus. **E:** Completed esophago-esophagostomy.

THORACOSCOPIC REPAIR

The first thoracoscopic repair of EA/TEF was performed in 2000, and more than 100 cases have been reported since that time.[73,88] Unlike other thoracoscopic procedures, adoption has been much slower for

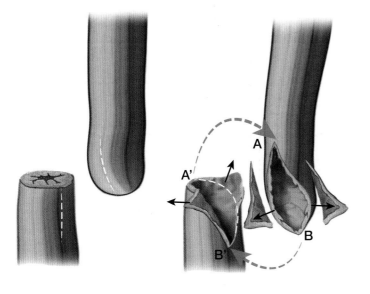

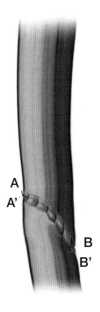

FIGURE 134.15 Spatulated anastomosis to reduce stricture formation when gap length is not a problem.

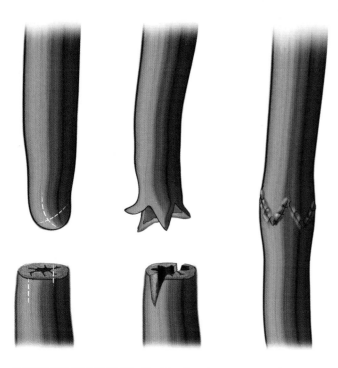

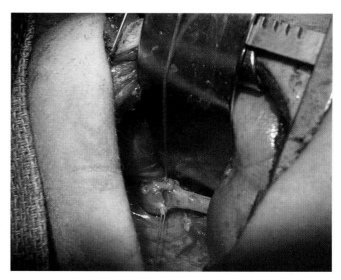

FIGURE 134.17 Intraoperative photo of primary repair of the esophagus. The back wall has been completed and the front wall is ready for closure after passage of an OGT.

FIGURE 134.16 Melak's "Plus" incision for primary anastomosis.

a variety of reasons.[73,89–91] As said so eloquently by Lee et al.[92] "when the initial learning curve was endured, surgical outcomes of thoracoscopic repair of EA/TEF were…comparable to past experiences with open thoracotomy." A definite learning curve exists in thoracoscopic repair of EA.[92] At the current time, ideal candidates appear to have a birth weight >2,000 g without severe cardiac malformations or chromosomal aberrations.[93] With experience, these criteria will most likely widen.[65,94] Simulation aimed specifically at EA/TEF repair is being developed to address the current slow adoption.[90,95]

POSITIONING AND PORT PLACEMENT

A right-sided approach is used. Patients with a known right-sided aorta may not be ideal candidates for less-experienced surgeons. A modified prone position with the right side elevated by 30 to 45 degrees, as described by Rothenberg is ideal to allow gravity to retract the lung anteriorly and exposure to the posterior mediastinum (Fig. 134.18).

No lung retractors are required. Three trocars are placed, generally two 5-mm ports, and one 3-mm port, (although some prefer to use a 3-mm scope and port in lieu of two 5-mm ports). The 3- or 5-mm 30-degree scope is placed just below the posteriorly tip of the scapula as shown in Figure 134.18. The surgeon works through two operative ports: a 5-mm port for the right hand in midaxillary line, and a 3-mm port placed posterior to the posterior axillary line for the left hand. Low flow carbon dioxide insufflation (1 L/min) and pressure of 4 to 5 mm Hg are used (as tolerated) to facilitate exposure.

TECHNIQUE

A transpleural approach is generally used, although an extrapleural approach has been described by Tsao et al.[96] After establishing exposure, the distal TEF is identified and dissected to its connection with the trachea using the 3-mm monopolar cautery. The distal TEF may be clipped or ligated, and then divided. Next, the proximal esophageal pouch is dissected. Separation of the proximal esophagus from the membranous trachea may also be done with hook cautery, or 3-mm

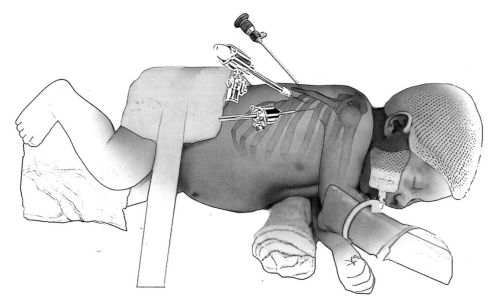

FIGURE 134.18 The drawing shows the modified prone position with port placement for thoracoscopic repair of EA/TEF. The camera is placed in the middle port below the scapula. The 5-mm port is used for clipping the fistula and passing suture.

scissors if preferred. The dissection is carried into the neck. Often the proximal esophagus will not mobilize until the congenitally fused portions in the upper chest have been separated from the trachea. The proximal esophagus is opened, and an end-to-end esophageal anastomosis is then performed. This may be done with either braided or monofilament absorbable suture, typically 4-0 or 5-0. Once the back wall has been sewn, the OGT is passed into the stomach prior to sewing the front wall. Techniques to facilitate the anastomosis have been described, including placing a stitch between the Replogle tube and the distal esophagus to pull up the distal esophagus and take tension off the anastomosis, or passing a Foley into the stomach to pull up on the gastroesophageal junction.[97,98] Clearly, other innovations will be developed.

POSTOPERATIVE CARE

Stable infants are extubated following the procedure. The child is kept NPO for a variable amount of time. Intubation, paralysis, and neck flexion has been advocated for some high-tension anastomosis.[99] Wide variability exists in initiation of feeding, use of transanastomotic feeding tubes, esophagram and timing of study, use of chest tubes, postoperative GER treatment, and antibiotic usage, often without any clear difference in outcome.[71] The authors study the esophagus on postoperative day 5, and initiate transanastomotic tube feeds if the esophagram shows no leak.

ESOPHAGEAL ATRESIA WITHOUT TRACHEOESOPHAGEAL FISTULA

PRESENTATION

Isolated EA often presents with symptoms of excessive drooling, coughing, and choking. In contrast to EA with TEF, radiographs show no air in the stomach.

MANAGEMENT

Figure 134.19 shows the treatment algorithm for EA without TEF. Most surgeons agree that endoscopic evaluation is mandatory in

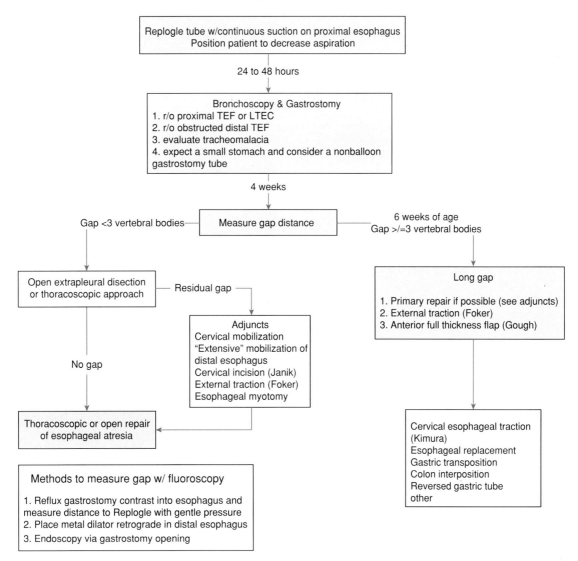

FIGURE 134.19 Management of EA without TEF. EA, esophageal atresia; TEF, tracheoesophageal fistula; LTEC, laryngotracheo-esophageal cleft; r/o, rule out.

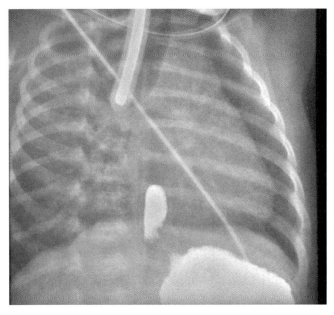

FIGURE 134.20 Intraoperative measurement of the esophageal gap in EA without TEF. A bougie is in the proximal esophagus and gastrostomy contrast refluxes into the distal esophagus under fluoroscopic guidance.

these infants.[21] The study confirms the diagnosis, evaluates for proximal TEF, allows assessment of tracheomalacia, and allows diagnosis of an occluded distal TEF that might be amenable to immediate repair.[68,70] Unlike children with a TEF, newborns with isolated EA undergo gastrostomy tube placement once the diagnosis is confirmed.[100] Often the stomach is quite small, and a small, nonballoon tube such as a Malecot catheter is required. Since duodenal atresia is sometimes associated with EA, a contrast study through the new gastrostomy is worthwhile in the operating room to exclude an atresia hidden by the EA.

A Replogle tube is kept on continuous suction in the proximal pouch to prevent aspiration of saliva. The majority of children are hospitalized during this period, although a few centers have been successful in allowing discharge in highly motivated families.[101] Feeds are initiated through the gastrostomy tube. Bolus feeds encourage enlargement of the tiny stomach, but caution must be exercised to avoid gastric rupture. After 4 weeks, the distance between the proximal and distal esophagus is measured. A variety of techniques have been described for doing this including contrast injection through the gastrostomy or retrograde passage of a dilator (Fig. 134.20).[102] Contrast may underestimate the distal esophagus, or it may not visualize at all if there is no reflux. Blind passage of the bougie does not guarantee correct placement within the esophagus. Endoscopy through the gastrostomy is the most reliable method, and fluoroscopy allows the gap to be measured in terms of vertebral bodies (Figs. 134.21 and 134.22).[103,104] If the surgeon determines that the distance between the two ends of the esophagus will not allow an anastomosis, several options are available and are discussed below.[105–116]

LONG GAP ESOPHAGEAL ATRESIA, WITH AND WITHOUT TEF

Long gap atresia has been variously defined, ranging from >two vertebral bodies to "when the distance between the upper and lower atretic segments is too far for primary anastomosis" (Fig. 134.22).[115,117,118]

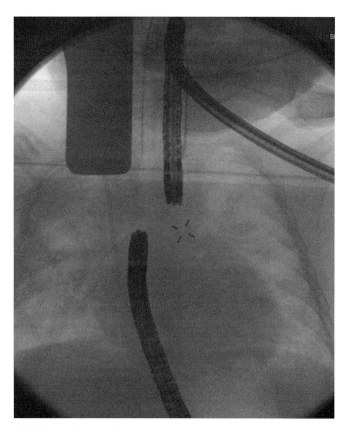

FIGURE 134.21 Double endoscopy (through the gastrostomy and orally) allows accurate assessment of the gap distance in esophageal atresia. The residual distance is less than one vertebral body. (Photo courtesy of K Graziano and author [David M. Notrica].)

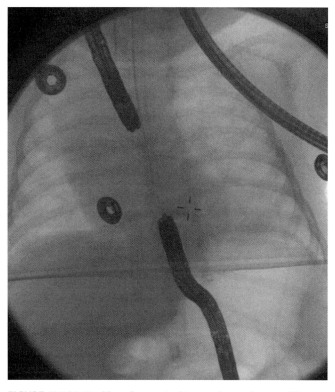

FIGURE 134.22 Double endoscopy in this case shows a long gap EA, measuring four vertebral bodies.

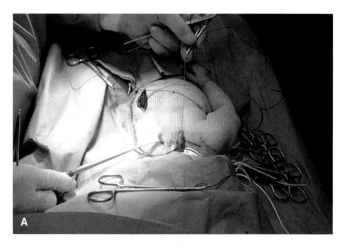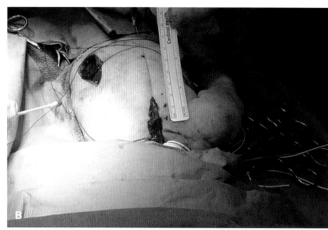

FIGURE 134.23 **A:** Cervical myotomy for esophageal atresia with short proximal esophagus. **B:** At the definitive esophageal repair operation, the esophagus did not extend into the chest at all, so a cervical incision was performed to mobilize the proximal esophagus. The first dot shows the esophagus prior to the myotomy. Each of the circular myotomies gained 1 cm in length as shown by the three purple dots.

Some describe it only in EA without fistula.[21] A nice series of long gap EA, however, showed that almost half of long gap EA also had distal a TEF.[35,119] In rare cases where the proximal esophagus is very short and inaccessible, but the fistula comes off high in the trachea, consideration should be given to cervical exteriorization of the esophagus, circular myotomy, and passage of the esophagus back into the chest with anastomosis as originally described by Janik et al.[120] (Fig. 134.23). A short proximal esophagus does not necessarily mean the child has a long gap, nor is there a guarantee the ultrashort esophagus will grow with time.

For true long gaps a variety of innovative techniques have been described. Allowing the proximal esophagus to grow is the oldest and most common. Bougie of the upper pouch is now infrequent, and of limited value.[58,102] Adjuncts to gain length include mobilization of the cervical esophagus, circular (Livaditis) myotomies (Fig. 134.24A),[121] spiral myotomies (Fig. 134.24B),[122,123] "excessive" mobilization of the distal esophagus,[105] anterior esophageal flap (Fig. 134.10),[75] Foker procedure (external esophageal traction (Fig. 134.25)),[106–108] or modifications of the Foker technique.[109–113] In a recent survey, approximately 47% of surgeons reported using the

Foker technique. Some authors now believe almost all long gaps can be repaired, although this may be premature.[21,124] Cervical esophagostomy ("spit fistula") is reserved for failure of other methods. Salvage after cervical esophagostomy has been reported using Kimura's lengthening technique,[125] with or without Foker-type traction on the lower pouch.[112,114,115,126] Lateral cervical esophagostomy has been reported, but has not gained wide acceptance.[116]

ESOPHAGEAL REPLACEMENT

Esophageal substitution is used for failed attempts at esophageal repair and is discussed in Chapter 131. The incidence of esophageal replacement has decreased for EA and ranges from 0.4% to 9%.[127,128] There is no consensus on the best operation for esophageal replacement,[129] but the most common replacement procedures after EA are gastric transposition and colon interposition.[86,130,131] With gastric transposition, Spitz reported a mortality of 2.5%, leak rate of 12%, and stricture of 20%. The follow-up satisfaction was 90%.[128] Colon interposition has been reported to have good results, but

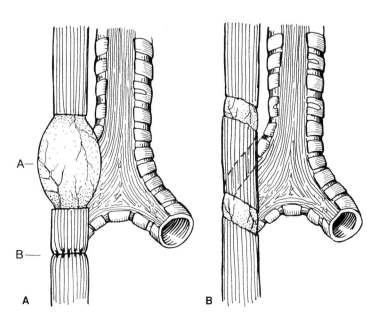

FIGURE 134.24 **A, B:** Circular and spiral myotomies for esophageal lengthening.

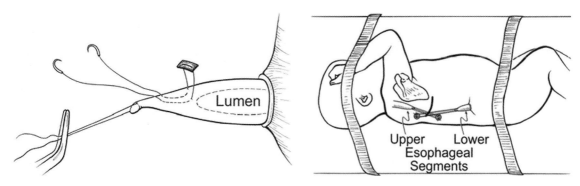

FIGURE 134.25 Foker traction procedure. A double-needle, pledgeted traction suture is placed through the muscular layer of the unopened upper and lower pouch. External traction is applied by threading the sutures through silastic buttons on the skin surface as shown. Over time, traction lengthens the segments allowing for primary anastomosis. Metal clips may be added to the esophageal ends to monitor progress radiographically. (Reprinted from Canty TG, Boyle EM, Linden B, et al. Aortic arch anomalies associated with long gap esophageal atresia and tracheoesophageal fistula. *J Pediatr Surg* 1997;32(11):1587–1591. Copyright © 1997 Elsevier. With permission.)

complication rates of leakage (5% to 60%), redundancy (2% to 28%), and stenosis (3% to 50%) vary significantly.[132–134] Other options include reversed gastric tube,[135] and various gastroplasties,[136–138] including the Scharli procedure, where the superior aspect of the stomach at the LES is divided in the transverse direction along the lesser curvature with ligation of the left gastric artery.[139] This procedure is sometimes described as similar to a Collis fundoplasty, but on the lesser curve.[140]

OUTCOMES

The original risk factors identified by Waterson et al.[17] in 1962 remain important, but other factors have also been identified.[141] Modifications by Spitz have gained wide acceptance, and updated survival numbers are shown in Table 134.4.[21] Overall survival after EA repair is now 95%, and considerably higher than just a few decades ago.[142] Current predictors and their relative importance of in-hospital mortality are nicely summarized by Sulkowski et al.[142] (Table 134.5). The average length of hospitalization is 27 days, with over half readmitted during the first 2 years of life (most commonly for pneumonia). Repeat esophageal reconstruction (without replacement) is required in 11% of cases, typically for leak or recalcitrant stricture.

COMPLICATIONS

Anastomotic Leak

Anastomotic leaks are common ranging between 2% and 21%.[144–146] Small leaks which are clinically insignificant will seal without inter-

vention, especially after an extrapleural approach.[147] Major disruption of the anastomosis results in pneumothorax, pleural effusion, or saliva or gastric contents draining from the chest drain. Some major leaks require reoperation, although many close spontaneously.[146] Recently, van der Zee et al.[148] reported that patients with a short proximal esophagus (<7 mm) and a distance from the carina to the proximal esophagus of >13.5 mm have an increased risk of leakage (Fig. 134.26).

Esophageal Anastomotic Strictures

Esophageal strictures after EA repair are very common. Typically, 35% to 40% of patients require dilation, with a median of four dilations in those developing symptomatic stricture. A short proximal esophagus or long gap between segments may be associated with an increased risk of postoperative stricture.[148] Signs and symptoms in infants with stricture include double swallowing (often manifest as a second, forceful attempt at swallowing a bolus of milk or formula), longer times to complete feeding, choking, gagging, refusal of milk, excessive drooling, regurgitation of food substance, or decreasing tolerance of the caliber of food.[149] In older children, they frequently complain of food "getting stuck" in their throats or epigastric region.

TABLE 134.4 The Spitz Risk Groupings With Updated Survival Numbers. Major Cardiac Disease Is Defined as "Cyanotic Congenital Heart Disease That Required Palliative or Corrective Surgery or Noncyanotic Heart Anomaly That Required Medical or Surgical Treatment for Cardiac Failure"[143]

Spitz Risk Groupings	Survival (%)
Group 1: Birth weight >1,500 g without major cardiac anomaly	98
Group 2: Birth weight <1,500 g or major cardiac	82
Group 3: Birth weight <1,500 g and major cardiac anomaly	50

TABLE 134.5 Independent Predictors of In-Hospital Mortality During the Initial Admission for Patients With EA. Odds Ratios Are Shown After Sensitivity Analysis in 3,479 Patients

Risk Factor	OR	(95% CI)	P Value
Genetic anomaly	2.04	(1.31–3.07)	<0.0001
Congenital heart disease	1.74	(1.19–2.57)	<0.0001
Respiratory anomaly	1.61	(1.09–2.33)	0.0008
Musculoskeletal anomaly	1.47	(1.03–2.06)	0.004
Preoperative mechanical ventilation	1.47	(1.03–2.08)	0.001
Eye anomaly	1.43	(0.79–2.35)	0.01
Preoperative ECMO	1.12	(0.43–2.25)	0.01
Birth weight (per 100 g increase)	0.88	(0.65–1.19)	<0.0001
Preoperative TPN	0.84	(0.58–1.19)	0.001

Data from Sulkowski JP, Cooper JN, Lopez JJ, et al. Morbidity and mortality in patients with esophageal atresia. *Surgery* 2014;156(2):483–491.

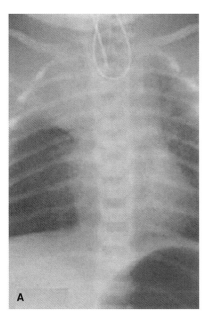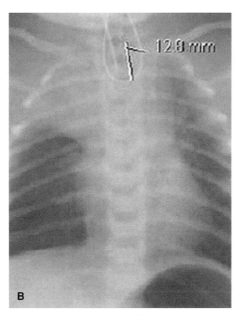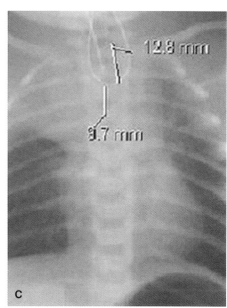

FIGURE 134.26 Estimation of the risk of leak may be done by evaluating the gap distance as well as the shortness of the proximal esophagus. A short proximal esophagus and a long gap are associated with increased risk of postoperative leak. (From van der Zee DC, Vieirra-Travassos D, de Jong JR, et al. A novel technique for risk calculation of anastomotic leakage after thoracoscopic repair for esophageal atresia with distal fistula. *World J Surg* 2008;32(7):1396–1399. Reproduced with permission of Springer New York LLC in the format Book via Copyright Clearance Center.)

An esophagram can identify the degree and length of stricture (Fig. 134.27). Esophageal dilation using balloon dilation is now the standard for the treatment of anastomotic strictures,[149–152] although bougie dilation is still in common usage.[153] Temporary use of self-expandable plastic stents and fully covered self-expandable metal stents has been reported in small infants and children with a history

of EA repair. They appear to be safe and beneficial in closing esophageal perforations, especially postdilation. However, the series from Boston noted a high stricture recurrence rate after stent removal, and suggested this may limit their usefulness in treating recalcitrant esophageal anastomotic strictures.[154] A comparative study done in the Netherlands looked at routine esophageal dilation versus dilation based on symptoms.[155] While there were slight differences in surgical techniques between the two centers, there appears to be no benefit to prophylactic dilation.

Recurrent TEF

Recurrent TEF is identified in 3% to 5% of patients.[144,146] Symptoms include coughing, choking, gagging, cyanosis, apnea, dying spells, wheezing, and recurrent chest infections.[156] Diagnosis is often difficult with multiple false-negative swallowing studies.[156] Treatment typically requires reoperation, closure, and interposition of tissue or biosynthetic mesh between the trachea and esophagus.[157] Endoscopic obliteration of the recurrent TEF has been reported using an electrocautery.[158,159] We prefer the 5F, ball-tipped, flexible urologic cautery (Bugbee, ACMI Corp) in this situation.[160]

Missed Proximal TEF

More common than recurrent TEF is a proximal TEF missed at the initial surgery (Fig. 134.28). Routine preoperative endoscopy will identify a proximal fistula in 4.9% of cases.[15] A missed proximal fistula is often correctable using a neck incision, unlike the recurrent fistula, which is typically lower in the chest.

Tracheomalacia and Bronchomalacia

Tracheomalacia refers to a flaccid trachea in which the trachea collapses during inspiration. Bronchomalacia is a similar problem effecting the major bronchi. When associated with EA, malacia typically results from inadequate cartilage support in a semicircular trachea (Fig. 134.29) (Video 134.2). Similarly, a bronchus may collapse with inspiration as well resulting in lobar atelectasis (Fig. 134.30).

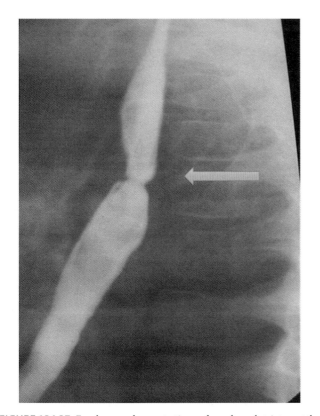

FIGURE 134.27 Esophagram demonstrating and esophageal stricture at the anastomosis. The *arrow* denotes the anastomotic stricture.

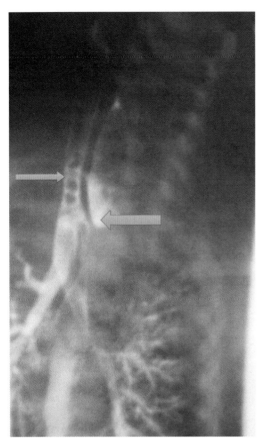

FIGURE 134.28 A dye study demonstrates a proximal as well as distal TEF. Contrast studies are no longer routinely done in EA and bronchoscopy is preferred.

A characteristic barking cough (often termed the "TOF Cough" in UK literature) is indicative of a degree of tracheomalacia, and it is important to let the family know prior to discharge that the barking cough is not unexpected. In some infants, the tracheomalacia may only become symptomatic when the infant swallows a large bolus of food resulting in posterior compression of a weak tracheal wall compressing the airway. The incidence of severe tracheomalacia (cyanotic spells, the requirement of an aortopexy or tracheostomy) is about 15%.[161]

In severe cases, the airway collapse may cause respiratory distress and require reintubation. Typically, these children require very little ventilator support, but fail extubation. Continuous positive airway pressure (CPAP) is helpful in these children.[162,163] Long-term options include aortopexy in which the aorta is sutured to the sternum to pull the front wall of the trachea anteriorly, away from the back wall. Since the aorta and trachea share connective tissue, the anterior displacement of the trachea will often prevent the posterior trachea wall from occluding the airway during respiration, thereby allowing extubation of patients with significant tracheomalacia. Thoracoscopic aortopexy was first reported in 2001[164] and has been demonstrated as a safe and effective treatment strategy for tracheomalacia associated with EA.[164–166] Stenting of the trachea and bronchi in tracheobronchomalacia has been reported, although some authors have reported unsatisfactory results in neonates.[166,167] Tracheostomy with or without CPAP is an option when other methods fail.

Recurrent Laryngeal Nerve Injury

The recurrent laryngeal nerves (RLNs) are typically found laterally in the groove between the trachea and esophagus. Symptomatic RLN injury after EA repair has been reported in 4% of cases, but largely ignored in other series.[161,168] Symptoms include persistent

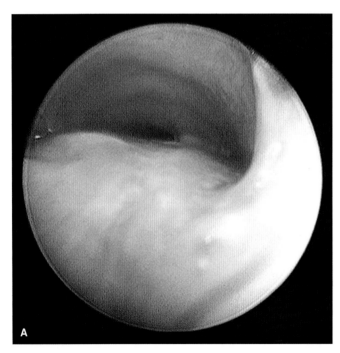
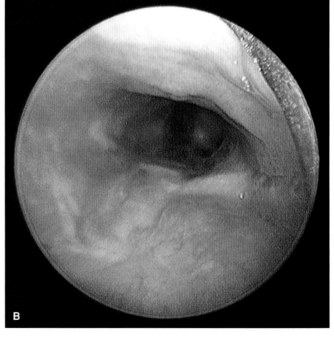

FIGURE 134.29 (Video): Tracheomalacia before (**A**) and after (**B**) aortopexy. Note the complete occlusion of the tracheal lumen by the posterior wall of the trachea in the panel on the left. The panel on the right shows a marked improvement of the lumen following aortopexy. The associated video shows the dynamic occlusion with inspiration.

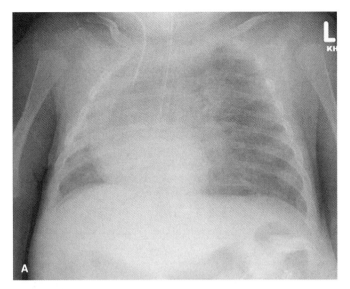

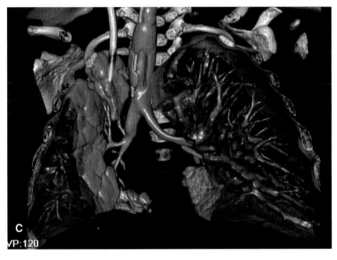

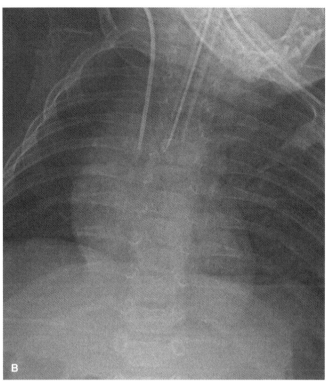

FIGURE 134.30 **A:** Repeated attempts at extubation failed after uneventful repair of EA/TEF. Bronchoscopy showed severe tracheomalacia as well as bronchomalaica. **B:** Following aortopexy, the patient extubated and the prior right upper lobe collapse and mediastinal shift are gone. **C:** Preoperative CT showing 3D reconstruction. Anterior view with right lung on the right. Note the collapsed right upper lobe.

stridor, dyspnea, and/or weak cry (dysphonia).[168] Diagnosis is made by endoscopic evaluation with the patient breathing spontaneously. Vocal cord paresis occurs with the finding of incomplete abduction or adduction of the vocal cord, while paralysis is the complete immobility of the vocal cord. Factors associated with RLN injury include anastomotic leak, cervical esophagostomy, and long gap EA.[168]

Gastroesophageal Reflux

GER in children with EA is very common, generally 50%. For EA without TEF, GER is even higher, almost 100% in some studies.[169] A survey done at the Canadian Association of Pediatric Surgeons found three-quarters of attendees advocate for prophylactic use of pump inhibitors or H2-receptor antagonists in children with EA. Patients were typically kept on antireflux medication for 3 to 12 months after repair.[170] The esophagus of EA/TEF often has dysmotility, abnormal innervation, and deficient sphincter function.[169] In the nicely done study by van Wijk et al.,[171] transient lower esophageal relaxation was shown to be the main mechanism underlying GER in infant and adult patients with EA. Adults born with EA continue to have impaired motility, delayed bolus clearance, and delayed gastric emptying. In one systematic review, overall antireflux surgery was performed in 26% of over 1,600 patients, suggesting many of the cases

are refractory to conservative therapy, although many series report lower rates (12%).[142,144,172] Risk factors for needing surgical fundoplication include pure EA, long gap EA, and associated duodenal atresia.[169] Fundoplication is often anatomically difficult after EA with failure rates of 30%.[169]

Eosinophilic Esophagitis

EoE was seen in 17% of children with EA in one study from Australia. Proton pump inhibitors, alone or with steroids, may provide symptomatic relief by reducing eosinophilic inflammation in esophageal strictures or the GERD associated with EA, particularly for patients with increasing dysphagia, and recurrent strictures.[173,174]

Chylothorax

Chylothorax occurs in as many as 5% of patient with EA.[161] Initial is generally conservative with total parenteral nutrition and adequate chest drainage.[175] If an injury to the duct is identified at surgery, ligation is indicated (Fig. 134.31) (Video134.3).

Late Complications

Barrett esophagus (5% to 20%), adenocarcinoma of the esophagus (as young as age 20, 50-fold increased risk), late onset achalasia (age

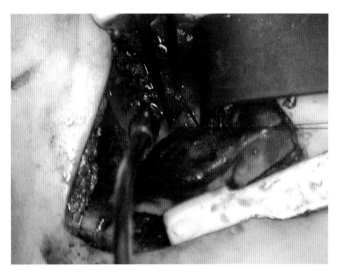

FIGURE 134.31 (Video) During the second surgery for repair of EA with TEF in a very small infant, a major chyle leak was noticed. The thoracic duct was identified, and the proximal duct ligated with permanent suture which ended the chyle leak.

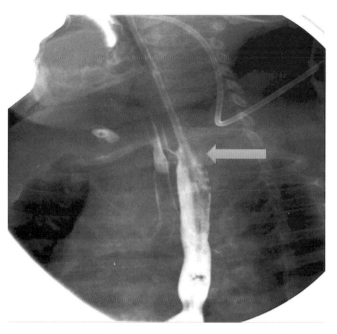

FIGURE 134.32 Pullback esophagram demonstrating a TEF without EA. *Blue arrow* at the level of the connection.

30 year), and spontaneous esophageal perforation (age 37) have all been reported.[169,176–180]

TRACHEOESOPHAGEAL FISTULA WITHOUT ESOPHAGEAL ATRESIA

DIAGNOSIS

TEF without EA occurs in approximately 1 in 75,000 births, making it very uncommon. The opening on the tracheal side is higher than the opening in the esophagus, giving the TEF an "N-shape." Despite this, the term "H-Type" TEF has become the accepted terminology of TEF without EA. Most H-type TEFs are located at or above the T2 level, and are generally repaired through a right cervical approach.[181–183]

Unlike TEF with EA, the diagnosis of H-type TEFs is often made late, despite the presence of significant symptomatology.[184] Typical symptoms include persistent coughing, choking, emesis, recurrent pneumonias, and rarely aerophagia.[185,186] Failure to diagnose on multiple esophagrams is common, as a single test has very limited sensitivity for H-type TEFs.[183,184,187] The pull-back tube esophagram[188] has been the study of choice for decades, although this has recently been challenged in the radiology literature (Fig. 134.32).[184,189] Rigid bronchoscopy of the proximal trachea may also be helpful in making the diagnosis, and often considered the single best test to make or exclude the diagnosis (Fig. 134.33).[186]

OPERATIVE APPROACH

After general anesthesia, a rigid bronchoscopy is performed. A hydrophilic wire (Glidewire®) or small Fogarty is then passed through the TEF into the esophagus (Fig. 134.33) (Video 134.4).

The wire or Fogarty is then retrieved from the esophagus and pulled out of the mouth to aid in identification of the fistula. The patient is then positioned supine with a roll under the neck, and the neck is placed in gentle extension. A right cervical incision is made and the neck, and the sternocleidomastoid muscle is encircled with a silastic loop to provide exposure (Fig. 134.34). The esophagus is

identified while the trachea is retracted anteriorly. The RLN is carefully identified in the tracheoesophageal groove and spared. Identification of the fistula can be facilitated by gentle traction on the wire or Fogarty catheter. Since the contralateral RLN is difficult to see, the fistula should be carefully dissected prior to division to avoid injury. Once the fistula is located, stitches are placed on either side, the fistula is opened, and the wire is removed. The esophageal and tracheal ends are closed with absorbable suture, and the two structures are separated using local muscle or soft tissue to help prevent recurrent TEF.

COMPLICATIONS

Recurrent TEF

As noted by Reynolds in the prior edition of this chapter, recurrent TEF can be a "challenging and disappointing experience." Fortunately,

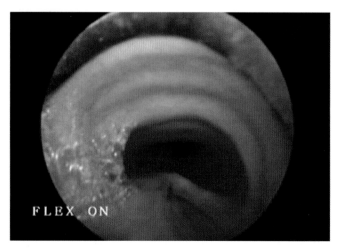

FIGURE 134.33 Video showing the H-type TEF as well as Fogarty catheter placement to aid in operative identification of the fistula. The identical technique is used as an emergency measure to occlude the fistula in cases where the patient cannot be effectively ventilated.

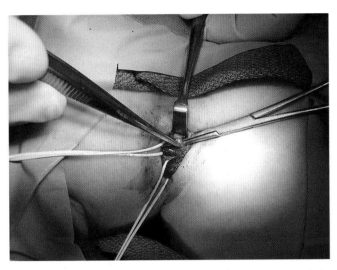

FIGURE 134.34 Operative view of the H-type TEF as shown through the right neck. The patient's head is on the left side of the photo. The fistula is elevated under the angled clamp. The sternocleidomastoid muscle is looped and retracted inferiorly. The other loop is around the proximal esophagus.

recurrences are uncommon, with a reported incidence of 0% to 14%.[183,190] Recurrences may be treated conservatively by nasogastric tube feedings for 4 to 6 weeks.[190] Endoscopic management using electrocautery fulgaration of the fistula or sealants have been reported. Reoperation should be undertaken at experienced centers.

Recurrent Laryngeal Nerve Injury

RLN injury can occur either through traction injury or transection.[191] Since the H-type TEF is generally in the proximal trachea,

the nerve is at higher risk than in other forms of TEF, generally 15% to 50%.[183] In cases of bilateral injury, the median position of the vocal chords may cause respiratory distress requiring tracheostomy. Over time, the vocal cords move away from the midline allowing decannulation. Successful microsurgical repair of the RLN has been reported.[191]

CONGENITAL LARYNGOTRACHEOESOPHAGEAL CLEFT

Laryngotracheoesophageal cleft (LTEC) is a congenital malformation of the posterior aspect of the larynx which can extend down variable lengths between the trachea and the esophagus.[192–199] Symptoms generally correlate with the severity of the defect. The most frequent clinical presentations include aspiration and cyanosis during feeding (53% to 80%), stridor (10% to 60%), and recurrent pneumonias (16% to 54%).[193,195–198,200–202] The incidence is low being estimated at about 1/10,000 to 20,0000 births.[194,201,203] LTEC is associated with a number of other congenital abnormalities (16% to 68%). These are most commonly malformations of the digestive tract.[197,198]

Benjamin and Inglis[192] typing is commonly used for describing the types based on the level of involvement (Fig. 134.35). Types I to IV are described as follows[192–198,200,202,204–209]:

Type I: Cleft involves the supraglottic larynx above the vocal fold level; usually presenting with mild to moderate symptoms, including stridor, a toneless or hoarse cry, and swallowing disorders. Diagnosis generally occurs before 6 months of age.
Type II: Cleft extending through the cricoid cartilages but not into the trachea; will generally have more swallowing issues, aspiration, and pneumonia. Diagnosis is usually made by 2 months of age.

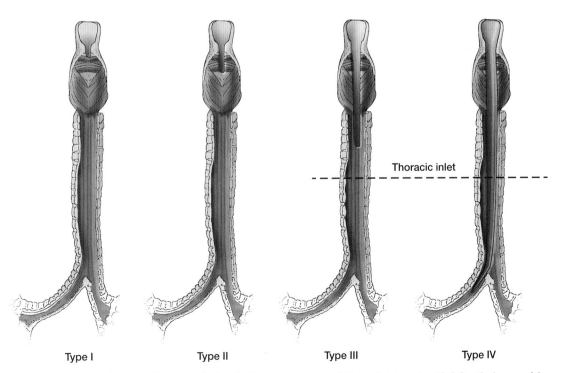

FIGURE 134.35 Classification of laryngotracheal clefts: Type 0, submucosal cleft; type I, interarytenoid cleft with absence of the interarytenoid muscle; type II, posterior cleft extending partially through the cricoid plate; type IIIa, posterior cleft extending down to the inferior border of the cricoid plate; type IIIb, posterior cleft extending into the cervical trachea, but not further down than the level of the sternal notch; type IVa, laryngotracheal cleft extending into the intrathoracic trachea to the carina; and type IVb, intrathoracic extension of the cleft involving one main bronchus.

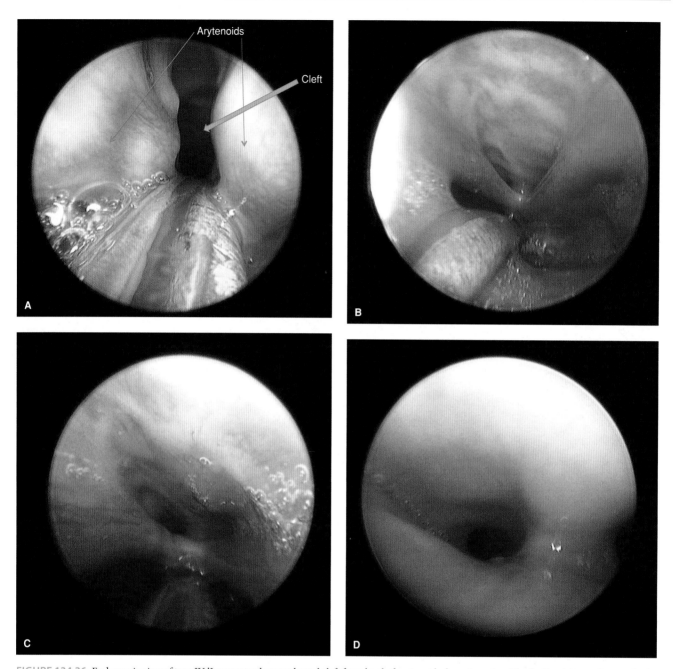

FIGURE 134.36 Endoscopic view of type IV lLaryngotracheoesophageal cleft from level of arytenoids down to carina. The feeding tube can be seen in the esophagus and the trachea anterior (**A**). Proximal view of the cleft (**B**). Widely open cleft. Note the view of the anterior tracheal rings through the opening and flattening of the trachea (**C**). The cleft ends just above the carina (**D**). The back wall of the trachea is intact above the carina. There is no extension into the bronchus, which is sometimes termed.

Type III: Cleft extending through the cricoid cartilage and into the cervical trachea; more severe swallowing and aspiration issues occur and diagnosis is first few months of life.

Type IV: Cleft extending into the thoracic trachea, potentially down to the carina or main stem bronchi. The most severe form with high mortality rate up to 50% is due to associated microgastria and reflux causing severe aspiration and pulmonary issues.[199,209–211]

DIAGNOSIS

A barium swallow can be used to identify the presence of a fistula with barium entering into the airway; however, definitive diagnosis requires endoscopic assessment.[193,195] Both fiberoptic and rigid bronchoscopy are recommended to fully assess the length and extent of the fistula (Fig. 134.36A–D).[193,208,212,213]

TREATMENT

Surgical repair should be undertaken as soon as possible to avoid aspiration complications and increased morbidity and mortality.[193–197,199,202,203,205,206,209] The type of cleft directs operative approach. Both endoscopic and external approaches are options.[193,194,197–199,203,205,206,211–219] External approaches including lateral pharyngotomy and anterior laryngotracheal open

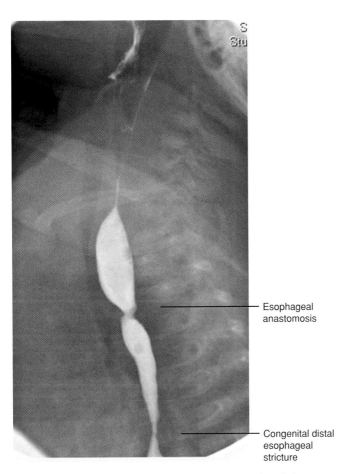

FIGURE 134.37 Congenital distal esophageal stricture identified on post-operative esophagram.

techniques.[193,203,216] The advantage of the anterior approach is the decreased risk of nerve injury due to minimal neck dissection.[202,216] Most Type I and II clefts, as well as some Type III, can be repaired endoscopically with 80% to 100% success.[194,197,204,214,215,217,219] The cleft closure is performed under suspension laryngoscopy using a microscope and microlaryngeal instruments. Combined cervical and thoracic approaches are often utilized for type IV clefts. Cardiopulmonary bypass or extracorporeal membrane oxygenation may also be necessary for successful repair.[199,209–211] Irrespective of closure method, reopening of the cleft is not uncommon (reported in 11% to 50%) with reoperation necessary.[193,197,203,207,210,214,217]

CONGENITAL ESOPHAGEAL STENOSIS

Congenital esophageal stenosis is quite rare.[220–222] These can be described histologically as three types: (a) fibromuscular stenosis (66%), (b) tracheobronchial remnants (26%), and membranous stenosis (8%).[222,223] Michaud reported on 61 patients with congenital esophageal stenosis, of which 47% also had EA.[222] Conversely, approximately 1% to 8% of EA also have a separate congenital esophageal stenosis (Fig. 134.37).[16] This entity has also been reported in TEF with and without EA.[221,224]

The mean age at diagnosis was 7 months for children with associated EA, and 10 years for those without. Over one-third of patients had no clinical symptoms. In the patients with symptoms, 50% presented with dysphasia, 40% with vomiting, 50% with food impaction, and 42% with respiratory symptoms. Among the asymptomatic patients, congenital stenosis was missed at surgery for EA in 38% of the cases. The definitive diagnosis is by esophagram with or without esophagoscopy.

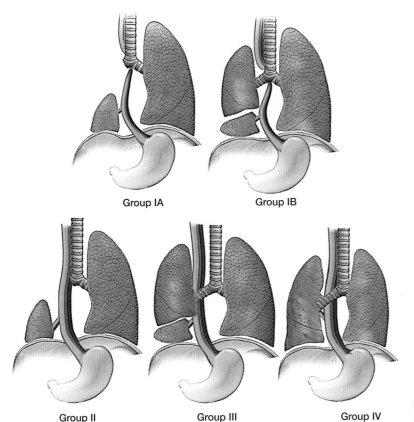

Group IA   Group IB

Group II   Group III   Group IV

FIGURE 134.38 Type IA and IB CBFMs are associated with EA.

Once diagnosed, initial treatment is by esophageal dilation. Dilation may be complicated by perforation in a small number of patients, and failure is not uncommon (44%). Dilation appears to be more effective for treating patients with fibromuscular stenosis and membranous stenosis as surgical repair is often required for those with tracheobronchial remnants. After treatment, dysphagia is common (36%) among children with esophageal stenosis, both with and without EA.[222]

COMMUNICATING BRONCHOPULMONARY FOREGUT MALFORMATIONS

CBFM are extremely rare anomalies in which the lung communicates with the esophagus or stomach.[225] Srikanth et al.,[226] classified CBFM as shown in Figure 134.38. Type I is associated with EA (Fig. 134.39), and is subdivided based on complete or partial lung communication. Communication with the lower esophagus is most common (66%), while communication with stomach is less common (16%). Most of the cases reported by Srikanth et al.[226] were associated with communications to pulmonary sequestrations with systemic arterial supply.

Treatment options in cases include resection of the esophageal bronchus and reimplantation into the trachea.[227] Imaging of the airway with CT and 3D reconstruction should be considered prior to surgery, as the trachea may be too small for reimplantation in those cases. In addition, the lung tissue may be pulmonary sequestration or otherwise not be salvageable. Consideration may be given to pneumonectomy in type IA, as attempts at reimplantation into an elongated left bronchus may cause kinking of the contralateral airway and death; pneumonectomy in the newborn, however, is not without its own risks.[228,229]

DIVERTICULUM OF THE ESOPHAGUS

True congenital esophageal diverticulum is extremely rare. More common presentations of diverticulum in infants and children are secondary to pulsion including Zenker and epiphrenic diverticula.[230–232] Symptoms are generally related to regurgitation of feeds and include vomiting, coughing, and aspiration. Barium swallow

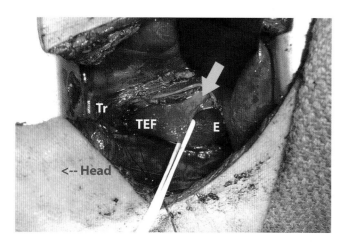

FIGURE 134.39 Right thoracotomy showing CBFM associated with EA, Type IA. *Blue arrow* denotes the right main bronchus coming off the esophagus. The CBFM had not been recognized prior to dividing the TEF at the initial operation. When the CBFM was discovered, the TEF was reattached to the trachea and the surgery terminated. Ultimately, attempts at reconstruction failed. Tr, trachea; TEF, tracheoesophageal fistula; E, distal esophagus.

and endoscopy can both be utilized for diagnosis. A number of surgical approaches have been described for repair and are similar to those described for adult diverticulum management. These include surgical extirpation, myotomy, and endoscopic stapling of the pouch.[231,233,234]

REFERENCES

1. Yang L, Shen C, Mei M, et al. De novo GLI3 mutation in esophageal atresia: reproducing the phenotypic spectrum of Gli3 defects in murine models. *Biochim Biophys Acta* 2014;1842(9):1755–1761.
2. Fragoso AC, Martinez L, Estevão-Costa J, et al. Abnormal Sonic hedgehog signaling in the lung of rats with esophageal atresia induced by adriamycin. *Pediatr Res* 2014;76(4):355–362.
3. Pinheiro PF, Simoes e Silva AC, Pereira RM. Current knowledge on esophageal atresia. *World J Gastroenterol* 2012;18(28):3662–3672.
4. Metzger R, Wachowiak R, Kluth D. Embryology of the early foregut. *Semin Pediatr Surg* 2011;20(3):136–144.
5. Spitz L. Oesophageal atresia. *Orphanet J Rare Dis* 2007;2:24.
6. Carlson BM. *Human Embryology and Developmental Biology*. Elsevier Health Sciences; 2013.
7. Faure S, de Santa Barbara P. Molecular embryology of the foregut. *J Pediatr Gastroenterol Nutr* 2011;52(suppl 1):S2–S3.
8. Litingtung Y, Lei L, Westphal H, et al. Sonic hedgehog is essential to foregut development. *Nat Genet* 1998;20(1):58–61.
9. Bae JO, Widmann WD, Hardy MA. Cameron Haight: pioneer in the treatment of esophageal atresia. *Curr Surg* 2005;62(3):327–329.
10. Lobe TE, Rothenberg S, Waldschmidt J, et al. Thoracoscopic repair of esophageal atresia in an infant: a surgical first. *Pediatric Endosurgery & Innovative Techniques* 1999;3(3):141–148.
11. Nassar N, Leoncini E, Amar E, et al. Prevalence of esophageal atresia among 18 international birth defects surveillance programs. *Birth Defects Res A Clin Mol Teratol* 2012;94(11):893–899.
12. Sfeir R, Bonnard A, Khen-Dunlop N, et al. Esophageal atresia: data from a national cohort. *J Pediatr Surg* 2013;48(8):1664–1669.
13. Fallon SC, Ethun CG, Olutoye OO, et al. Comparing characteristics and outcomes in infants with prenatal and postnatal diagnosis of esophageal atresia. *J Surg Res* 2014;190(1):242–245.
14. Takahashi D, Hiroma T, Takamizawa S, et al. Population-based study of esophageal and small intestinal atresia/stenosis. *Pediatr Int* 2014;56(6):838–844.
15. Parolini F, Morandi A, Macchini F, et al. Esophageal atresia with proximal tracheoesophageal fistula: a missed diagnosis. *J Pediatr Surg* 2013;48(6):E13–E17.
16. McCann F, Michaud L, Aspirot A, et al. Congenital esophageal stenosis associated with esophageal atresia. *Dis Esophagus* 2014;28(3):211–215.
17. Waterston DJ, Carter RB, Aberdeen E. Oesophageal atresia: tracheo-oesophageal fistula: a study of survival in 218 infants. *The Lancet* 1962;279(7234):819–822.
18. Konkin DE, O'hali WA, Webber EM, et al. Outcomes in esophageal atresia and tracheoesophageal fistula. *J Pediatr Surg* 2003;38(12):1726–1729.
19. Yagyu M, Gitter H, Richter B, et al. Esophageal atresia in Bremen, Germany–evaluation of preoperative risk classification in esophageal atresia. *J Pediatr Surg* 2000;35(4):584–587.
20. de Jong EM, Felix JF, de Klein A, et al. Etiology of esophageal atresia and tracheoesophageal fistula: "mind the gap". *Curr Gastroenterol Rep* 2010;12(3):215–222.
21. Spitz L. Esophageal atresia. Lessons I have learned in a 40-year experience. *J Pediatr Surg* 2006;41(10):1635–1640.
22. Temtamy SA, Miller JD. Extending the scope of the VATER association: definition of the VATER syndrome. *J Pediatr* 1974;85(3):345–349.
23. Nora JJ, Nora AH. Birth defects and oral contraceptives. *Lancet* 1973;1(7809):941–942.
24. McCauley J, Masand N, McGowan R, et al. X-linked VACTERL with hydrocephalus syndrome: further delineation of the phenotype caused by FANCB mutations. *Am J Med Genet A* 2011;155A(10):2370–2380.
25. Evans JA, Stranc LC, Kaplan P, et al. VACTERL with hydrocephalus: further delineation of the syndrome(s). *Am J Med Genet* 1989;34(2):177–182.
26. Kim JH, Kim P, Hui CC. The VACTERL association: lessons from the Sonic hedgehog pathway. *Clin Genet* 2001;59(5):306–315.
27. Stoll C, Alembik Y, Dott B, et al. Associated malformations in patients with esophageal atresia. *Eur J Med Genet* 2009;52(5):287–290.
28. Seo J, Kim DY, Kim AR, et al. An 18-year experience of tracheoesophageal fistula and esophageal atresia. *Korean J Pediatr* 2010;53(6):705–710.
29. Keckler SJ, St Peter SD, Valusek PA, et al. VACTERL anomalies in patients with esophageal atresia: an updated delineation of the spectrum and review of the literature. *Pediatr Surg Int* 2007;23(4):309–313.
30. Chittmittrapap S, Spitz L, Kiely EM, et al. Oesophageal atresia and associated anomalies. *Arch Dis Child* 1989;64(3):364–368.
31. Spitz L, Ali M, Brereton RJ. Combined esophageal and duodenal atresia: experience of 18 patients. *J Pediatr Surg* 1981;16(1):4–7.
32. Nabzdyk CS, Chiu B, Jackson CC, et al. Management of patients with combined tracheoesophageal fistula, esophageal atresia, and duodenal atresia. *Int J Surg Case Rep* 2014;5(12):1288–1291.
33. Holder TM, Ashcraft KW, Sharp RJ, et al. Care of infants with esophageal atresia, tracheoesophageal fistula, and associated anomalies. *J Thorac Cardiovasc Surg* 1987;94(6):828–835.

34. Ein SH, Palder SB, Filler RM. Babies with esophageal and duodenal atresia: a 30-year review of a multifaceted problem. *J Pediatr Surg* 2006;41(3):530–532.

35. Conforti A, Morini F, Bagolan P. Difficult esophageal atresia: trick and treat. *Semin Pediatr Surg* 2014;23(5):261–269.

36. Pachl M, Eaton S, Kiely EM, et al. Esophageal atresia and malrotation: what association? *Pediatr Surg Int* 2015;31(2):181–185.

37. Peker E, Tuncer O, Cagan E, et al. Esophageal atresia concomitant with congenital hypothyroidism and phenylketonuria in a newborn. *J Pediatr Endocrinol Metab* 2010;23(1–2):203–204.

38. Steadland KM, Langham MR, Greene MA, et al. Unilateral pulmonary agenesis, esophageal atresia, and distal tracheoesophageal fistula. *Ann Thorac Surg* 1995;59(2):511–513.

39. Ethun CG, Fallon SC, Cassady CI, et al. Fetal MRI improves diagnostic accuracy in patients referred to a fetal center for suspected esophageal atresia. *J Pediatr Surg* 2014;49(5):712–715.

40. Maoate K, Myers NA, Beasley SW. Gastric perforation in infants with oesophageal atresia and distal tracheo-oesophageal fistula. *Pediatr Surg Int* 1999;15(1):24–27.

41. Rathod KK, Bawa M, Mahajan JK, et al. Management of esophageal atresia with a tracheoesophageal fistula complicated by gastric perforation. *Surg Today* 2011;41(10):1391–1394.

42. Jones TB, Kirchner SG, Lee FA, et al. Stomach rupture associated with esophageal atresia, tracheoesophageal fistula, and ventilatory assistance. *AJR Am J Roentgenol* 1980;134(4):675–677.

43. Gopal M, Woodward M. Potential hazards of contrast study diagnosis of esophageal atresia. *J Pediatr Surg* 2007;42(6):e9–e10.

44. Vandenplas Y, Delree M, Bougatef A, et al. Cervical esophageal perforation diagnosed by endoscopy in a premature infant: review of recent literature. *J Pediatr Gastroenterol Nutr* 1989;8(3):390–393.

45. Mahomed A. Iatrogenic esophageal perforation that may sometimes masquerade as esophageal atresia. *J Pediatr Surg* 2005;40(4):751–752.

46. Knight RB, Webb DE, Coppola CP. Pharyngeal perforation masquerading as esophageal atresia. *J Pediatr Surg* 2009;44(11):2216–2218.

47. Meeralebbae SM, Zain SM, Basir AO, et al. Misdiagnosing esophageal perforation as esophageal atresia. *Saudi Med J* 2002;23(10):1287–1290.

48. Aggarwal SK, Gupta R. Esophageal foreign body mimicking esophageal atresia. *Indian Pediatr* 2005;42(4):392–393.

49. Nagae I, Tsuchida A, Tanabe Y, et al. High-grade congenital esophageal stenosis owing to a membranous diaphragm with tracheoesophageal fistula. *J Pediatr Surg* 2005;40(10):e11–e13.

50. Islam S, Shanbhogue LK. Membranous diaphragm presenting as esophageal atresia in a neonate. *Saudi Med J* 2007;28(11):1737–1738.

51. Celayir AC, Erdogan E. An infrequent cause of misdiagnosis in esophageal atresia. *J Pediatr Surg* 2003;38(9):1389.

52. Hombalkar N, Dhanawade S, Hombalkar B, et al. Esophageal atresia with tracheo-esophageal fistula: Accidental transtracheal gastric intubation. *J Indian Assoc Pediatr Surg* 2009;14(4):224–225.

53. Kane TD, Atri P, Potoka DA. Triple fistula: management of a double tracheoesophageal fistula with a third H-type proximal fistula. *J Pediatr Surg* 2007;42(6):E1–E3.

54. Spitz L. Congenital esophageal stenosis distal to associated esophageal atresia. *J Pediatr Surg* 1973;8(6):973–974.

55. Toyama WM. Esophageal atresia and tracheoesophageal fistula in association with bronchial and pulmonary anomalies. *J Pediatr Surg* 1972;7(3):302–307.

56. Usui N, Kamata S, Ishikawa S, et al. Bronchial reconstruction for bronchopulmonary foregut malformation: a case report. *J Pediatr Surg* 1995;30(10):1495–1497.

57. Babu R, Pierro A, Spitz L, et al. The management of oesophageal atresia in neonates with right-sided aortic arch. *J Pediatr Surg* 2000;35(1):56–58.

58. Canty TG, Boyle EM, Linden B, et al. Aortic arch anomalies associated with long gap esophageal atresia and tracheoesophageal fistula. *J Pediatr Surg* 1997;32(11):1587–1591.

59. Laeven NF, Derikx JP, van Hoorn JH, et al. Temporary gastric banding in a premature infant with esophageal atresia and severe respiratory distress syndrome. *Pediatr Surg Int* 2015;31(4):413–415.

60. Ratan SK, Rattan KN, Ratan J, et al. Temporary transgastric fistula occlusion as salvage procedure in neonates with esophageal atresia with wide distal fistula and moderate to severe pneumonia. *Pediatr Surg Int* 2005;21(7):527–531. DOI: 10.1007/s00383-005-1407-8.

61. Spitz L. Esophageal atresia: past, present, and future. *J Pediatr Surg* 1996;31(1):19–25.

62. Ehlen M, Bachour H, Wiebe B, et al. Esophageal atresia and severe respiratory failure–cuffed pediatric tracheal tubes as an additional therapeutic option? *J Pediatr Surg* 2005;40(6):e25–e27.

63. Seitz G, Warmann SW, Schaefer J, et al. Primary repair of esophageal atresia in extremely low birth weight infants: a single-center experience and review of the literature. *Biol Neonate* 2006;90(4):247–251.

64. Ito K, Ashizuka S, Kurobe M, et al. Delayed primary reconstruction of esophageal atresia and distal tracheoesophageal fistula in a 471-g infant. *Int J Surg Case Rep* 2013;4(2):167–169.

65. Ma L, Liu YZ, Ma YQ, et al. Comparison of neonatal tolerance to thoracoscopic and open repair of esophageal atresia with tracheoesophageal fistula. *Chin Med J (Engl)* 2012;125(19):3492–3495.

66. Krosnar S, Baxter A. Thoracoscopic repair of esophageal atresia with tracheoesophageal fistula: anesthetic and intensive care management of a series of eight neonates. *Pediatr Anesth* 2005;15(7):541–546.

67. Alabbad SI, Shaw K, Puligandla PS, et al. The pitfalls of endotracheal intubation beyond the fistula in babies with type C esophageal atresia. *Semin Pediatr Surg* 2009;18(2):116–118.

68. Pigna A, Gentili A, Landuzzi V, et al. Bronchoscopy in newborns with esophageal atresia. *Pediatr Med Chir* 2002;24(4):297–301.

69. Atzori P, Iacobelli BD, Bottero S, et al. Preoperative tracheobronchoscopy in newborns with esophageal atresia: does it matter? *J Pediatr Surg* 2006;41(6):1054–1057.

70. Sharma N, Srinivas M. Laryngotracheobronchoscopy prior to esophageal atresia and tracheoesophageal fistula repair–its use and importance. *J Pediatr Surg* 2014;49(2):367–369.

71. Zani A, , Hoellwarth ME, et al. International survey on the management of esophageal atresia. *Eur J Pediatr Surg* 2014;24(1):3–8.

72. Filston HC, Chitwood WR, Schkolne B, et al. The Fogarty balloon catheter as an aid to management of the infant with esophageal atresia and tracheoesophageal fistula complicated by severe RDS or pneumonia. *J Pediatr Surg* 1982;17(2):149–151.

73. Davenport M, Rothenberg SS, Crabbe DC, et al. The great debate: open or thoracoscopic repair for oesophageal atresia or diaphragmatic hernia. *J Pediatr Surg* 2015;50(2):240–246.

74. Okuyama H, Koga H, Ishimaru T, et al. Current practice and outcomes of thoracoscopic esophageal atresia and tracheoesophageal fistula repair: a multi-institutional analysis in Japan. *J Laparoendosc Adv Surg Tech A* 2015;25(5):441–444.

75. Gough MH. Esophageal atresia–use of an anterior flap in the difficult anastomosis. *J Pediatr Surg* 1980;15(3):310–311.

76. Brown AK, Gough MK, Nicholls G, et al. Anterior flap repair of oesophageal atresia: a 16-year evaluation. *Pediatr Surg Int* 1995;10(8):525–528.

77. Singh SJ, Shun A. A new technique of anastomosis to avoid stricture formation in oesophageal atresia. *Pediatr Surg Int* 2001;17(7):575–577.

78. Catalano P, Di Pace MR, Caruso AM, et al. A simple technique of oblique anastomosis can prevent stricture formation in primary repair of esophageal atresia. *J Pediatr Surg* 2012;47(9):1767–1771.

79. Tandon RK, Khan TR, Maletha M, et al. Modified method of primary esophageal anastomosis with improved outcome in cases of esophageal atresia with tracheoesophageal fistula. *Pediatr Surg Int* 2009;25(4):369–372.

80. Melek M, Cobanoglu U. A new technique in primary repair of congenital esophageal atresia preventing anastomotic stricture formation and describing the opening condition of blind pouch: plus ("+") incision. *Gastroenterol Res Pract* 2011;2011:527323.

81. Touloukian RJ, Seashore JH. Thirty-five-year institutional experience with end-to-side repair for esophageal atresia. *Arch Surg* 2004;139(4):371–374; discussion 374.

82. Upadhyaya VD, Gopal SC, Gangopadhyaya AN, et al. Role of fibrin glue as a sealant to esophageal anastomosis in cases of congenital esophageal atresia with tracheoesophageal fistula. *World J Surg* 2007;31(12):2412–2415.

83. Zaritzky M, Ben R, Zylberg GI, et al. Magnetic compression anastomosis as a nonsurgical treatment for esophageal atresia. *Pediatr Radiol* 2009;39(9):945–949.

84. Stringel G, Lawrence C, McBride W. Repair of long gap esophageal atresia without anastomosis. *J Pediatr Surg* 2010;45(5):872–875.

85. Garcia AV, Thirumoorthi AS, Traina JM, et al. Image-guided esophageal anastomosis in esophageal atresia. *J Pediatr Surg* 2012;47(10):1959–1961.

86. Lal D, Miyano G, Juang D, et al. Current patterns of practice and technique in the repair of esophageal atresia and tracheoesophageal fistula: an IPEG survey. *J Laparoendosc Adv Surg Tech A* 2013;23(7):635–638.

87. Paramalingam S, Burge DM, Stanton MP. Operative intercostal chest drain is not required following extrapleural or transpleural esophageal atresia repair. *Eur J Pediatr Surg* 2013;23(4):273–275.

88. Rothenberg SS. Thoracoscopic repair of a tracheoesophageal fistula in a newborn infant. *Pediatric Endosurgery & Innovative Techniques* 2000;4(4):289–294.

89. Laberge JM, Blair GK. Thoracotomy for repair of esophageal atresia: not as bad as they want you to think! *Dis Esophagus* 2013;26(4):365–371.

90. Barsness KA, Rooney DM, Davis LM, et al. Validation of measures from a thoracoscopic esophageal atresia/tracheoesophageal fistula repair simulator. *J Pediatr Surg* 2014;49(1):29–32; discussion 32–33.

91. Ron O, De Coppi P, Pierro A. The surgical approach to esophageal atresia repair and the management of long-gap atresia: results of a survey. *Semin Pediatr Surg* 2009;18(1):44–49.

92. Lee S, Lee SK, Seo JM. Thoracoscopic repair of esophageal atresia with tracheoesophageal fistula: overcoming the learning curve. *J Pediatr Surg* 2014;49(11):1570–1572.

93. Yamoto M, Urusihara N, Fukumoto K, et al. Thoracoscopic versus open repair of esophageal atresia with tracheoesophageal fistula at a single institution. *Pediatr Surg Int* 2014;30(9):883–887.

94. Rothenberg SS. Thoracoscopic repair of esophageal atresia and tracheo-esophageal fistula in neonates: evolution of a technique. *J Laparoendosc Adv Surg Tech A* 2012;22(2):195–199.

95. Barsness KA, Rooney DM, Davis LM, et al. Evaluation of three sources of validity evidence for a synthetic thoracoscopic esophageal atresia/tracheoesophageal fistula repair simulator. *J Laparoendosc Adv Surg Tech A* 2015;25(7):599–604.

96. Tsao K, Lee H. Extrapleural thoracoscopic repair of esophageal atresia with tracheoesophageal fistula. *Pediatr Surg Int* 2005;21(4):308–310.

97. Hiradfar M, Shojaeian R, Gharavi Fard M, et al. Thoracoscopic esophageal atresia repair made easy. An applicable trick. *J Pediatr Surg* 2013;48(3):685–688.

98. Boia ES, Nicodin A, Popoiu MC, et al. An effective method to release anastomotic tension after repair of esophageal atresia using a Foley catheter. *Chirurgia (Bucur)* 2013;108(2):189–192.

99. Uchida K, Inoue M, Otake K, et al. Efficacy of postoperative elective ventilatory support for leakage protection in primary anastomosis of congenital esophageal atresia. *Pediatr Surg Int* 2006;22(6):496–499.

100. Seguier-Lipszyc E, Bonnard A, Aizenfisz S, et al. The management of long gap esophageal atresia. *J Pediatr Surg* 2005;40(10):1542–1546.

101. Aziz D, Schiller D, Gerstle JT, et al. Can "long-gap" esophageal atresia be safely managed at home while awaiting anastomosis? *J Pediatr Surg* 2003;38(5):705–708.
102. Bagolan P, Iacobelli BD, De Angelis P, et al. Long gap esophageal atresia and esophageal replacement: moving toward a separation? *J Pediatr Surg* 2004;39(7): 1084–1090.
103. Gross ER, Reichstein A, Gander JW, et al. The role of fiberoptic endoscopy in the evaluation and management of long gap isolated esophageal atresia. *Pediatr Surg Int* 2010;26(12):1223–1227.
104. Kim S. Gas insufflation of stomach and laparoscope intubation of distal esophagus for measurement of gap in esophageal atresia without distal fistula. *Pediatr Surg Int* 2013;29(4):347–348.
105. Farkash U, Lazar L, Erez I, et al. The distal pouch in esophageal atresia – to dissect or not to dissect, that is the question. *Eur J Pediatr Surg* 2002;12(1):19–23.
106. Al-Qahtani AR, Yazbeck S, Rosen NG, et al. Lengthening technique for long gap esophageal atresia and early anastomosis. *J Pediatr Surg* 2003;38(5):737–739.
107. Foker JE, Kendall TC, Catton K, et al. A flexible approach to achieve a true primary repair for all infants with esophageal atresia. *Semin Pediatr Surg* 2005;14(1):8–15.
108. Nasr A, Langer JC. Mechanical traction techniques for long-gap esophageal atresia: a critical appraisal. *Eur J Pediatr Surg* 2013;23(3):191–197.
109. Sroka M, Wachowiak R, Losin M, et al. The Foker technique (FT) and Kimura advancement (KA) for the treatment of children with long-gap esophageal atresia (LGEA): lessons learned at two European centers. *Eur J Pediatr Surg* 2013;23(1): 3–7.
110. Tamburri N, Laje P, Boglione M, et al. Extrathoracic esophageal elongation (Kimura's technique): a feasible option for the treatment of patients with complex esophageal atresia. *J Pediatr Surg* 2009;44(12):2420–2425.
111. Till H, Rolle U, Siekmeyer W, et al. Combination of spit fistula advancement and external traction for primary repair of long-gap esophageal atresia. *Ann Thorac Surg* 2008;86(6):1969–1971.
112. Miyano G, Okuyama H, Koga H, et al. Type-A long-gap esophageal atresia treated by thoracoscopic esophagoesophagostomy after sequential extrathoracic esophageal elongation (Kimura's technique). *Pediatr Surg Int* 2013;29(11):1171–1175.
113. Mochizuki K, Obatake M, Taura Y, et al. A modified Foker's technique for long gap esophageal atresia. *Pediatr Surg Int* 2012;28(8):851–854.
114. Takamizawa S, Nishijima E, Tsugawa C, et al. Multistaged esophageal elongation technique for long gap esophageal atresia: experience with 7 cases at a single institution. *J Pediatr Surg* 2005;40(5):781–784.
115. Kimura K, Nishijima E, Tsugawa C, et al. Multistaged extrathoracic esophageal elongation procedure for long gap esophageal atresia: experience with 12 patients. *J Pediatr Surg* 2001;36(11):1725–1727.
116. Aloisi AS, de Freitas S, Colombo AC, et al. Lateral esophagostomy: an alternative in the initial management of long gap esophageal atresia without fistula. *J Pediatr Surg* 2000;35(12):1827–1829.
117. Liszewski MC, Bairdain S, Buonomo C, et al. Imaging of long gap esophageal atresia and the Foker process: expected findings and complications. *Pediatr Radiol* 2014;44(4):467–475.
118. van der Zee DC, Gallo G, Tytgat SH. Thoracoscopic traction technique in long gap esophageal atresia: entering a new era. *Surg Endosc* 2015;29(11):3324–3330.
119. Friedmacher F, Puri P. Delayed primary anastomosis for management of long-gap esophageal atresia: a meta-analysis of complications and long-term outcome. *Pediatr Surg Int* 2012;28(9):899–906.
120. Janik JS, Simpson JS, Filler RM. Wide gap esophageal atresia with inaccessible upper pouch. *J Thorac Cardiovasc Surg* 1981;82(2):198–202.
121. Livaditis A, Radberg L, Odensjo G. Esophageal end-to-end anastomosis. Reduction of anastomotic tension by circular myotomy. *Scand J Thorac Cardiovasc Surg* 1972;6(2):206–214.
122. Rossello PJ, Lebron H, Franco AA. The technique of myotomy in esophageal reconstruction: an experimental study. *J Pediatr Surg* 1980;15(4):430–432.
123. Kimura K, Nishijima E, Tsugawa C, et al. A new approach for the salvage of unsuccessful esophageal atresia repair: a spiral myotomy and delayed definitive operation. *J Pediatr Surg* 1987;22(11):981–983.
124. Bagolan P, Valfrè L, Morini F, et al. Long-gap esophageal atresia: traction-growth and anastomosis - before and beyond. *Dis Esophagus* 2013;26(4):372–379.
125. Kimura K, Soper RT. Multistaged extrathoracic esophageal elongation for long gap esophageal atresia. *J Pediatr Surg* 1994;29(4):566–568.
126. Kimura K, Hashimoto S, Nishijima E, et al. Percutaneous transhepatic cholangiodrainage after hepatic portoenterostomy for biliary atresia. *J Pediatr Surg* 1980;15(6):811–816.
127. Koivusalo AI, Pakarinen MP, Lindahl HG, et al. Revisional surgery for recurrent tracheoesophageal fistula and anastomotic complications after repair of esophageal atresia in 258 infants. *J Pediatr Surg* 2015;50(2):250–254.
128. Spitz L. Esophageal replacement: overcoming the need. *J Pediatr Surg* 2014;49(6):849–852.
129. Loukogeorgakis SP, Pierro A. Replacement surgery for esophageal atresia. *Eur J Pediatr Surg* 2013;23(3):182–190.
130. Ure BM, Jesch NK, Sümpelmann R, et al. Laparoscopically assisted gastric pull-up for long gap esophageal atresia. *J Pediatr Surg* 2003;38(11):1661–1662.
131. Iwanaka T, Kawashima H, Tanabe Y, et al. Laparoscopic gastric pull-up and thoracoscopic esophago-esophagostomy combined with intrathoracic fundoplication for long-gap pure esophageal atresia. *J Laparoendosc Adv Surg Tech A* 2011;21(10): 973–978.
132. Hamza AF. Colonic replacement in cases of esophageal atresia. *Semin Pediatr Surg* 2009;18(1):40–43.
133. Erdoğan E, Emir H, Eroğlu E, et al. Esophageal replacement using the colon: a 15-year review. *Pediatr Surg Int* 2000;16(8):546–549.
134. Freeman NV, Cass DT. Colon interposition: a modification of the Waterston technique using the normal esophageal route. *J Pediatr Surg* 17(1):17–21.
135. McCollum MO, Rangel SJ, Blair GK, et al. Primary reversed gastric tube reconstruction in long gap esophageal atresia. *J Pediatr Surg* 2003;38(6):957–962.
136. Rao KL, Menon P, Samujh R, et al. Fundal tube esophagoplasty for esophageal reconstruction in atresia. *J Pediatr Surg* 2003;38(12):1723–1725.
137. Schneider A, Ferreira CG, Kauffmann I, et al. Modified Spitz procedure using a Collis gastroplasty for the repair of long-gap esophageal atresia. *Eur J Pediatr Surg* 2011;21(3):178–182.
138. Nakahara Y, Aoyama K, Goto T, et al. Modified Collis-Nissen procedure for long gap pure esophageal atresia. *J Pediatr Surg* 2012;47(3):462–466.
139. Beasley SW, Skinner AM. Modified Scharli technique for the very long gap esophageal atresia. *J Pediatr Surg* 2013;48(11):2351–2353.
140. Mulholland MW, Doherty GM. *Complications in Surgery*. Lippincott Williams & Wilkins; 2011.
141. Gupta DK, Sharma S. Esophageal atresia: the total care in a high-risk population. *Semin Pediatr Surg* 2008;17(4):236–243.
142. Sulkowski JP, Cooper JN, Lopez JJ, et al. Morbidity and mortality in patients with esophageal atresia. *Surgery* 2014;156(2):483–491.
143. Koivusalo A, Pakarinen MP, Rintala RJ. Anastomotic dilatation after repair of esophageal atresia with distal fistula. Comparison of results after routine versus selective dilatation. *Dis Esophagus* 2009;22(2):190–194.
144. Schneider A, Blanc S, Bonnard A, et al. Results from the French National Esophageal Atresia register: one-year outcome. *Orphanet J Rare Dis* 2014;9:206.
145. Burford JM, Dassinger MS, Copeland DR, et al. Repair of esophageal atresia with tracheoesophageal fistula via thoracotomy: a contemporary series. *Am J Surg* 2011;202(2):203–206.
146. Engum SA, Grosfeld JL, West KW, et al. Analysis of morbidity and mortality in 227 cases of esophageal atresia and/or tracheoesophageal fistula over two decades. *Arch Surg* 1995;130(5):502–508; discussion 508–509.
147. Zhao R, Li K, Shen C, et al. The outcome of conservative treatment for anastomotic leakage after surgical repair of esophageal atresia. *J Pediatr Surg* 2011;46(12):2274–2278.
148. van der Zee DC, Vieirra-Travassos D, de Jong JR, et al. A novel technique for risk calculation of anastomotic leakage after thoracoscopic repair for esophageal atresia with distal fistula. *World J Surg* 2008;32(7):1396–1399.
149. Lan LC, Wong KK, Lin SC, et al. Endoscopic balloon dilatation of esophageal strictures in infants and children: 17 years' experience and a literature review. *J Pediatr Surg* 2003;38(12):1712–1715.
150. Ko HK, Shin JH, Song HY, et al. Balloon dilation of anastomotic strictures secondary to surgical repair of esophageal atresia in a pediatric population: long-term results. *J Vasc Interv Radiol* 2006;17(8):1327–1333.
151. Antoniou D, Soutis M, Christopoulos-Geroulanos G. Anastomotic strictures following esophageal atresia repair: a 20-year experience with endoscopic balloon dilatation. *J Pediatr Gastroenterol Nutr* 2010;51(4):464–467.
152. Lang T, Hummer HP, Behrens R. Balloon dilation is preferable to bougienage in children with esophageal atresia. *Endoscopy* 2001;33(4):329–335.
153. Serhal L, Gottrand F, Sfeir R, et al. Anastomotic stricture after surgical repair of esophageal atresia: frequency, risk factors, and efficacy of esophageal bougie dilatations. *J Pediatr Surg* 2010;45(7):1459–1462.
154. Manfredi MA, Jennings RW, Anjum MW, et al. Externally removable stents in the treatment of benign recalcitrant strictures and esophageal perforations in pediatric patients with esophageal atresia. *Gastrointest Endosc* 2014;80(2):246–252.
155. Koivusalo A, Turunen P, Rintala RJ, et al. Is routine dilatation after repair of esophageal atresia with distal fistula better than dilatation when symptoms arise? Comparison of results of two European pediatric surgical centers. *J Pediatr Surg* 2004;39(11):1643–1647.
156. Ein SH, et al. Recurrent tracheoesophageal fistulas seventeen-year review. *J Pediatr Surg* 1983;18(4):436–441.
157. St Peter SD, Calkins CM, Holcomb GW. The use of biosynthetic mesh to separate the anastomoses during the thoracoscopic repair of esophageal atresia and tracheoesophageal fistula. *J Laparoendosc Adv Surg Tech A* 2007;17(3):380–382.
158. Tzifa KT, Maxwell EL, Chait P, et al. Endoscopic treatment of congenital H-Type and recurrent tracheoesophageal fistula with electrocautery and histoacryl glue. *Int J Pediatr Otorhinolaryngol* 2006;70(5):925–930.
159. Rangecroft L, Bush GH, Lister J, et al. Endoscopic diathermy obliteration of recurrent tracheoesophageal fistulae. *J Pediatr Surg* 1984;19(1):41–43.
160. Richter GT, Ryckman F, Brown RL, et al. Endoscopic management of recurrent tracheoesophageal fistula. *J Pediatr Surg* 2008;43(1):238–245.
161. Castilloux J, Noble AJ, Faure C. Risk factors for short- and long-term morbidity in children with esophageal atresia. *J Pediatr* 2010;156(5):755–760.
162. Davis S, Jones M, Kisling J, et al. Effect of continuous positive airway pressure on forced expiratory flows in infants with tracheomalacia. *Am J Respir Crit Care Med* 1998;158(1):148–152.
163. Wiseman NE, Duncan PG, Cameron CB. Management of tracheobronchomalacia with continuous positive airway pressure. *J Pediatr Surg* 1985;20(5):489–493.
164. Decou JM, Parsons DS, Gauderer MW. Thoracoscopic aortopexy for severe tracheomalacia. *Pediatric Endosurgery & Innovative Techniques* 2001;5(2):205–208.
165. Dave S, Currie BG. The role of aortopexy in severe tracheomalacia. *J Pediatr Surg* 2006;41(3):533–537.
166. Schaarschmidt K, Kolberg-Schwerdt A, Pietsch L, et al. Thoracoscopic aortopericardiosternopexy for severe tracheomalacia in toddlers. *J Pediatr Surg* 2002;37(10):1476–1478.
167. Valerie EP, Durrant AC, Forte V, et al. A decade of using intraluminal tracheal/bronchial stents in the management of tracheomalacia and/or bronchomalacia: is it better than aortopexy? *J Pediatr Surg* 2005;40(6):904–907.

168. Morini F, Iacobelli BD, Crocoli A, et al. Symptomatic vocal cord paresis/paralysis in infants operated on for esophageal atresia and/or tracheo-esophageal fistula. *J Pediatr* 2011;158(6):973–976.

169. Tovar JA, Fragoso AC. Anti-reflux surgery for patients with esophageal atresia. *Dis Esophagus* 2013;26(4):401–404.

170. Shawyer AC, Pemberton J, Flageole H. Post-operative management of esophageal atresia-tracheoesophageal fistula and gastroesophageal reflux: a Canadian Association of Pediatric Surgeons annual meeting survey. *J Pediatr Surg* 2014;49(5):716–719.

171. van Wijk M, Knüppe F, Omari T, et al. Evaluation of gastroesophageal function and mechanisms underlying gastroesophageal reflux in infants and adults born with esophageal atresia. *J Pediatr Surg* 2013;48(12):2496–2505.

172. Shawyer AC, D'Souza J, Pemberton J, et al. The management of postoperative reflux in congenital esophageal atresia-tracheoesophageal fistula: a systematic review. *Pediatr Surg Int* 2014;30(10):987–996.

173. Dhaliwal J, Tobias V, Sugo E, et al. Eosinophilic esophagitis in children with esophageal atresia. *Dis Esophagus* 2014;27(4):340–347.

174. Yamada Y, Nishi A, Kato M, et al. Esophagitis with eosinophil infiltration associated with congenital esophageal atresia and stenosis. *Int Arch Allergy Immunol* 2013;161(suppl 2):159–163.

175. Panthongviriyakul C, Bines JE, Post-operative chylothorax in children: an evidence-based management algorithm. *J Paediatr Child Health* 2008;44(12):716–721.

176. Marinello FG, Targarona EM, Poca M, et al. Late-onset achalasia after esophageal atresia repair. *Dis Esophagus* 2013;26(3):311–313.

177. Merei J, Smith G. Spontaneous esophageal perforation 37 years after primary repair of esophageal atresia. *Eur J Pediatr Surg* 2009;19(4):267–268.

178. Ryckman FC, Warner BW. Barrett's esophagus after repair of esophageal atresia with tracheoesophageal fistula: yet another morbidity. *Gastroenterology* 2004;126(7):1913–1915; discussion 1915.

179. Krug E, Bergmeijer JH, Dees J, et al. Gastroesophageal reflux and Barrett's esophagus in adults born with esophageal atresia. *Am J Gastroenterol* 1999;94(10):2825–2828.

180. Adzick NS, Fisher JH, Winter HS, et al. Esophageal adenocarcinoma 20 years after esophageal atresia repair. *J Pediatr Surg* 1989;24(8):741–744.

181. Garcia NM, Thompson JW, Shaul DB. Definitive localization of isolated tracheoesophageal fistula using bronchoscopy and esophagoscopy for guide wire placement. *J Pediatr Surg* 1998;33(11):1645–1647.

182. Parolini F, Morandi A, Macchini F, et al. Cervical/thoracotomic/thoracoscopic approaches for H-type congenital tracheo-esophageal fistula: a systematic review. *Int J Pediatr Otorhinolaryngol* 2014;78(7):985–989.

183. Brookes JT, Smith MC, Smith RJ, et al. H-type congenital tracheoesophageal fistula: University of Iowa experience 1985 to 2005. *Ann Otol Rhinol Laryngol* 2007;116(5):363–368.

184. Kirk JM, Dicks-Mireaux C. Difficulties in diagnosis of congenital H-type tracheo-oesophageal fistulae. *Clin Radiol* 1989;40(2):150–153.

185. Ko BA, Frederic R, DiTirro PA, et al. Simplified access for division of the low cervical/high thoracic H-type tracheoesophageal fistula. *J Pediatr Surg* 2000;35(11):1621–1622.

186. Karnak I, Senocak ME, Hiçsönmez A, et al. The diagnosis and treatment of H-type tracheoesophageal fistula. *J Pediatr Surg* 1997;32(12):1670–1674.

187. Sundar B, Guiney EJ, O'Donnell B. Congential H-type tracheo-oesophageal fistula. *Arch Dis Child* 1975;50(11):862–863.

188. Stringer DA, Ein SH. Recurrent tracheo-esophageal fistula: a protocol for investigation. *Radiology* 1984;151(3):637–641.

189. Laffan EE, Daneman A, Ein SH, et al. Tracheoesophageal fistula without esophageal atresia: are pull-back tube esophagograms needed for diagnosis? *Pediatr Radiol* 2006;36(11):1141–1147.

190. Crabbe DC, Kiely EM, Drake DP, et al. Management of the isolated congenital tracheo-oesophageal fistula. *Eur J Pediatr Surg* 1996;6(2):67–69.

191. Olsen L, Meurling S, Grotte G. H-type tracheo-oesophageal fistula in children with special reference to surgical management and to repair of recurrent nerve injury. *Z Kinderchir* 1982;36(1):27–29.

192. Benjamin B, Inglis A. Minor congenital laryngeal clefts: diagnosis and classification. *Ann Otol Rhinol Laryngol* 1989;98(6):417–420.

193. Eriksen C, Zwillenberg D, Robinson N. Diagnosis and management of cleft larynx. Literature review and case report. *Ann Otol Rhinol Laryngol* 1990;99(9 Pt 1):703–708.

194. Evans JN. Management of the cleft larynx and tracheoesophageal clefts. *Ann Otol Rhinol Laryngol* 1985;94(6 Pt 1):627–630.

195. Leboulanger N, Garabedian EN. Laryngo-tracheo-oesophageal clefts. *Orphanet J Rare Dis* 2011;6:81.

196. Moungthong G, Holinger LD. Laryngotracheoesophageal clefts. *Ann Otol Rhinol Laryngol* 1997;106(12):1002–1011.

197. Rahbar R, Rouillon I, Roger G, et al. The presentation and management of laryngeal cleft: a 10-year experience. *Arch Otolaryngol Head Neck Surg* 2006;132(12):1335–1341.

198. Roth B, Rose KG, Benz-Bohm G, et al. Laryngo-tracheo-oesophageal cleft. Clinical features, diagnosis and therapy. *Eur J Pediatr* 1983;140(1):41–46.

199. Mathur NN, Peek GJ, Bailey CM, et al. Strategies for managing Type IV laryngotracheoesophageal clefts at Great Ormond Street Hospital for Children. *Int J Pediatr Otorhinolaryngol* 2006;70(11):1901–1910.

200. Andrieu-Guitrancourt J, Narcy P, Desnos J, et al. [Diastema or laryngeal or posterior laryngotracheal cleft. Analysis of 16 cases]. *Chir Pediatr* 1984;25(4–5):219–227.

201. Mitchell DB, Koltai P, Matthew D, et al. Severe tracheobronchomalacia associated with laryngeal cleft. *Int J Pediatr Otorhinolaryngol* 1989;18(2):181–185.

202. Myer CM, Cotton RT, Holmes DK, et al. Laryngeal and laryngotracheoesophageal clefts: role of early surgical repair. *Ann Otol Rhinol Laryngol* 1990;99(2 Pt 1):98–104.

203. Evans KL, Courteney-Harris R, Bailey CM, et al. Management of posterior laryngeal and laryngotracheoesophageal clefts. *Arch Otolaryngol Head Neck Surg* 1995;121(12):1380–1385.

204. Chien W, Ashland J, Haver K, et al. Type 1 laryngeal cleft: establishing a functional diagnostic and management algorithm. *Int J Pediatr Otorhinolaryngol* 2006;70(12):2073–2079.

205. Cotton RT, Schreiber JT. Management of laryngotracheoesophageal cleft. *Ann Otol Rhinol Laryngol* 1981;90(4 Pt 1):401–405.

206. Donahoe PK, Gee PE. Complete laryngotracheoesophageal cleft: management and repair. *J Pediatr Surg* 1984;19(2):143–148.

207. Kawaguchi AL, Donahoe PK, Ryan DP. Management and long-term follow-up of patients with types III and IV laryngotracheoesophageal clefts. *J Pediatr Surg* 2005;40(1):158–164; discussion 164–165.

208. Parsons DS, Herr T. Delayed diagnosis of a laryngotracheoesophageal cleft. *Int J Pediatr Otorhinolaryngol* 1997;39(2):169–173.

209. Shehab ZP, Bailey CM. Type IV laryngotracheoesophageal clefts–recent 5 year experience at Great Ormond Street Hospital for Children. *Int J Pediatr Otorhinolaryngol* 2001;60(1):1–9.

210. Simpson BB, Ryan DP, Donahoe PK, et al. Type IV laryngotracheoesophageal clefts: surgical management for long-term survival. *J Pediatr Surg* 1996;31(8):1128–1133.

211. Ryan DP, Muehrcke DD, Doody DP, et al. Laryngotracheoesophageal cleft (type IV): management and repair of lesions beyond the carina. *J Pediatr Surg* 1991;26(8):962–969; discussion 969–970.

212. Garabedian EN, Ducroz V, Roger G, et al. Posterior laryngeal clefts: preliminary report of a new surgical procedure using tibial periosteum as an interposition graft. *Laryngoscope* 1998;108(6):899–902.

213. Bell DW, Christiansen TA, Smith TE, et al. Laryngotracheoesophageal cleft: the anterior approach. *Ann Otol Rhinol Laryngol* 1977;86(5 Pt 1):616–622.

214. Garabedian EN, Pezzettigotta S, Leboulanger N, et al. Endoscopic surgical treatment of laryngotracheal clefts: indications and limitations. *Arch Otolaryngol Head Neck Surg* 2010;136(1):70–74.

215. Koltai PJ, Morgan D, Evans JN. Endoscopic repair of supraglottic laryngeal clefts. *Arch Otolaryngol Head Neck Surg* 1991;117(3):273–278.

216. Lipshutz GS, Albanese CT, Harrison MR, et al. Anterior cervical approach for repair of laryngotracheoesophageal cleft. *J Pediatr Surg* 1998;33(2):400–402.

217. Rahbar R, Chen JL, Rosen RL, et al. Endoscopic repair of laryngeal cleft type I and type II: when and why? *Laryngoscope* 2009;119(9):1797–1802.

218. Robie DK, Pearl RH, Gonsales C, et al. Operative strategy for recurrent laryngeal cleft: a case report and review of the literature. *J Pediatr Surg* 1991;26(8):971–973; discussion 973–974.

219. Sandu K, Monnier P. Endoscopic laryngotracheal cleft repair without tracheotomy or intubation. *Laryngoscope* 2006;116(4):630–634.

220. Vasudevan SA, Kerendi F, Lee H, et al. Management of congenital esophageal stenosis. *J Pediatr Surg* 2002;37(7):1024–1026.

221. van Poll D, van der Zee DC. Thoracoscopic treatment of congenital esophageal stenosis in combination with H-type tracheoesophageal fistula. *J Pediatr Surg* 2012;47(8):1611–1613.

222. Michaud L, Coutenier F, Podevin G, et al. Characteristics and management of congenital esophageal stenosis: findings from a multicenter study. *Orphanet J Rare Dis* 2013;8:186.

223. Ramesh JC, Ramanujam TM, Jayaram G. Congenital esophageal stenosis: report of three cases, literature review, and a proposed classification. *Pediatr Surg Int* 2001;17(2–3):188–192.

224. Homnick DN. H-type tracheoesophageal fistula and congenital esophageal stenosis. *Chest* 1993;103(1):308–309.

225. Leithiser RE, Capitanio MA, Macpherson RI, et al. "Communicating" bronchopulmonary foregut malformations. *AJR Am J Roentgenol* 1986;146(2):227–231.

226. Srikanth MS, Ford EG, Stanley P, et al. Communicating bronchopulmonary foregut malformations: classification and embryogenesis. *J Pediatr Surg* 1992;27(6):732–736.

227. Michel JL, Revillon Y, Salakos C, et al. Successful bronchotracheal reconstruction in esophageal bronchus: two case reports. *J Pediatr Surg* 1997;32(5):739–742.

228. Stolar C, Berdon W, Reyes C, et al. Right pneumonectomy syndrome: a lethal complication of lung resection in a newborn with cystic adenomatoid malformation. *J Pediatr Surg* 1988;23(12):1180–1183.

229. Szarnicki R, Maurseth K, de Leval M, et al., Tracheal compression by the aortic arch following right pneumonectomy in infancy. *Ann Thorac Surg* 1978;25(3):231–235.

230. Jackson C, Shallow TA. Diverticula of the oesophagus, pulsion, traction, malignant and congenital. *Ann Surg* 1926;83(1):1–19.

231. Lindholm EB, Hansbourgh F, Upp JR, et al. Congenital esophageal diverticulum – a case report and review of literature. *J Pediatr Surg* 2013;48(3):665–668.

232. Nelson AR. Congenital true esophageal diverticulum; report of a case unassociated with other esophagotracheal abnormality. *Ann Surg* 1957;145(2):258–264.

233. De BM, Creech O. Surgical treatment of epiphrenic diverticulum of the esophagus; review of literature and report of case treated by resection and esophagogastrostomy. *J Thorac Surg* 1952;23(5):486–494.

234. Patron V, Godey B, Aubry K, et al. Endoscopic treatment of pharyngo-esophageal diverticulum in child. *Int J Pediatr Otorhinolaryngol* 2010;74(6):694–697.

135

Inflammatory Diseases of the Esophagus

Joseph D. Phillips ■ Andrew C. Chang

Nonreflux inflammatory disorders of the esophagus were a relatively rare entity to encounter in clinical practice prior to the early 2000s. This is, in part, due to the recent expansion of the diagnosis and understanding of eosinophilic esophagitis (EoE). In the immunocompetent host, most benign diseases of the esophagus are related to disruption of host defense, the use of antibiotics, or a structural abnormality of the esophagus, such as a stricture. Many of these pathologies are more prevalent in the immunocompromised patient. Clinically significant infections with herpes simplex virus (HSV) and *Candida* species occur rarely in the immunocompetent individual. Acquired immunodeficiency syndrome (AIDS), immunosuppression for transplantation, and immune-suppressing therapies for malignant disease are underlying etiologies that predispose to benign inflammatory diseases of the esophagus. Common and uncommon opportunistic infections of the esophagus in immunocompromised patients are outlined in Table 135.1. The aggressive implementation of antiretroviral therapy to suppress the human immunodeficiency virus (HIV) and the routine use of antiviral and antibiotic prophylaxis in transplant recipients has resulted in an overall reduction in opportunistic infections of the esophagus in recent decades. This chapter will focus on benign inflammatory diseases of the esophagus related to infections and nonmalignant systemic disease. Esophagitis related to gastroesophageal reflux, radiation, caustic ingestion, and medication-induced damage to the esophagus are discussed in the other chapters of this text.

TABLE 135.1 Opportunistic Pathogens of the Esophagus in Immunocompromised Patients

Common
  Herpes simplex virus (HSV)
  Cytomegalovirus (CMV)
  Candida species

Uncommon
  Varicella-zoster virus (VZV)
  Enterovirus
  Adenovirus
  Cryptococcus species
  Aspergillus species
  Mucormycosis species
  Mycobacterium tuberculosis
  Histoplasmosis species
  Leishmania species

EOSINOPHILIC ESOPHAGITIS

Eosinophilic esophagitis (EoE) is a chronic inflammatory disorder characterized by symptomatic esophageal dysfunction and intraepithelial eosinophilic infiltration, which is thought to be an allergic etiology.[1] While it was first described in a handful of case reports in the 1970s and 80s, it was recognized as a distinct clinicopathologic entity only in 1993.[2] Common presenting symptoms in adults include dysphagia (93%), food impaction (62%), and heartburn unresponsive to proton pump inhibitor (PPI) therapy (24%). A history of allergy is found in 52% of patients and peripheral eosinophilia in 31%.[3] Other associated disorders include asthma, in approximately 50% of patients, allergic rhinitis (50%), or atopic dermatitis (20%).[4] Children typically exhibit heartburn, and/or regurgitation, abdominal pain, emesis, and food impaction, but only rarely report dysphagia. There is a 3 to 4:1 male to female predominance. In recent years there has been an increased incidence with an estimated 1.9% of patients undergoing biopsy for symptoms of dysphagia demonstrating findings of EoE.[5] The prevalence of EoE in children is estimated to be between 8.9 and 12.8 per 100,000.[6,7] A population-based study from the Mayo Clinic demonstrated that the incidence in the adult population has been increasing over the last 30 years from 0.35 per 100,000 before 1995 to 9.45 per 100,000 in 2005, although this increase paralleled an increase in endoscopy volume.[8]

The symptoms of dysphagia and food impaction are directly related to the phases of the disease process. Initially, acute inflammation and edema result in luminal narrowing. Remodeling of the esophageal lumen then leads to fixed narrowing and impaired distensibility. In addition, there is dynamic and variable narrowing caused by muscular contraction and spasm. While the relative contributions of these processes remain undetermined, the majority of research focuses on remodeling, which refers to acute and chronic inflammatory infiltration resulting in structural changes including epithelial hyperplasia, muscular hypertrophy, and fibrosis of the lamina propria.[9] While EoE is an antigen driven disease, the exact mechanism of activation of the immune system remains incompletely elucidated. One hypothesis suggests that direct contact of antigen with the esophageal epithelium leads to antigen presentation and resultant acute inflammation. Another theory is that antigen presentation to residing lymphoid tissue in the small bowel or respiratory mucosa leads to eosinophil activation and migration. While the normal esophagus does not contain eosinophils, their mere presence is not specific for EoE. Eosinophils are derived from myeloid precursors

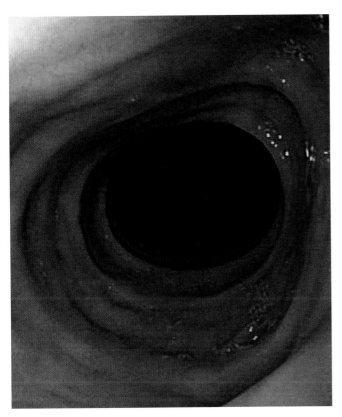

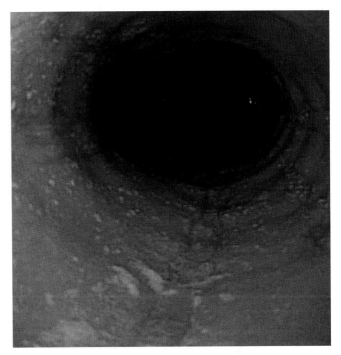

FIGURE 135.2 Endoscopic photograph demonstrating white exudates, longitudinal furrows, and mild rings in a patient with eosinophilic esophagitis. (Courtesy of Dr. Joel H. Rubenstein, Ann Arbor, MI.)

FIGURE 135.1 Endoscopic photograph demonstrating pronounced rings in the upper esophagus in a patient with eosinophilic esophagitis. (Courtesy of Dr. Joel H. Rubenstein, Ann Arbor, MI.)

in the bone marrow and mature in response to IL-5. Once activated they may reside in tissues for 2 to 14 days. They are attracted to target tissues by a variety of cytokines (IL-5, IL-9, IL-13) and chemokines (eotaxins 1, 2, and 3). Once in tissue, eosinophils release a variety of mediators that cause local tissue damage and recruit other inflammatory cells, such as mast cells, B- and T-lymphocytes, and basophils.[9] This inflammation can then lead to the long-term complications of stricture formation and chronic scarring.

Endoscopy reveals friable mucosa and edema (59%); single or multiple concentric rings, known as "trachealization" or "feline esophagus" (49%); strictures (40%); whitish papules (16%); or narrowing of the esophageal lumen (5%) (Figs. 135.1 and 135.2). However, 9% of endoscopies are normal.[3,5] Esophageal rings appear to be more common to EoE, occurring in 27% to 72% of patients.[10,11] Furthermore, rings were noted twice as often on endoscopy in patients with EoE compared to reflux esophagitis, possibly helping to distinguish the two processes, which can have considerable symptom and histologic overlap. The endoscopic finding of esophageal rings is thought to be secondary to the release of histamine from activated mast cells in the mucosa with resultant acetylcholine release and contraction of the muscularis mucosa.[4] In general, endoscopic findings correlate poorly with histologic severity and are not diagnostic.[12]

Histologically, EoE diagnosis in part rests on the number of eosinophils present in the squamous epithelium (Fig. 135.3). Normal biopsies of the esophagus of children show less than 1 eosinophil per HPF and 95% of healthy adults have no eosinophils on random biopsy.[13,14] Previously, a finding of 15 to 30 eosinophils per HPF had been used as diagnostic criteria. Standardized criteria were created by the American Gastroenterological Association Institute and the North American Society of Pediatric Gastroenterology, Hepatology,

and Nutrition in 2007[15] and updated in 2011.[1] A threshold of 15 to 20 eosinophils per HPF is now the accepted minimum for diagnosis in the appropriate clinical context, although biopsy specimens frequently contained >250 eosinophils per HPF.[16] This finding is not definitive, as multiple other disease processes can cause increased intraepithelial eosinophils, including GERD, parasitic infection, and drug-associated esophageal injury. Thus, eosinophil counts alone cannot be used to diagnosis the disease. Systematic biopsies along the length of the esophagus must also be taken, as eosinophilic infiltration may occur in a patchy distribution. In one study, diagnostic levels of eosinophils were present in fewer than 50% of biopsy specimens in 34% of patients with EoE.[11] In an affected individual, the sensitivity of one biopsy is 55%, rising to 100% with five biopsies.[17] The average

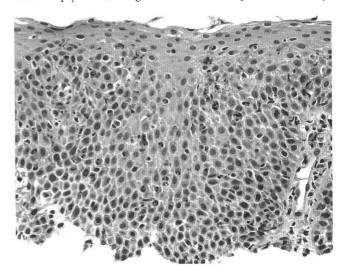

FIGURE 135.3 High power photomicrograph demonstrating eosinophil infiltration of the esophageal mucosa in a biopsy specimen from a patient with EoE. (Courtesy of Dr. Joel K. Greenson, Ann Arbor, MI.)

eosinophil density of patients diagnosed with EoE is >40 per HPF. In addition, biopsy location may aide in differentiation, with samples taken from the upper and mid-portions of the esophagus more likely to contain higher levels of eosinophils in patients with EoE than those with reflux esophagitis. Qualitative aspects of eosinophil infiltration also support the diagnosis of EoE. These include superficial layering of eosinophils, eosinophil microabscesses (superficial aggregates of 4 or more eosinophils), and eosinophil degranulation, all resulting in a "moth eaten" appearance to the squamous epithelium due to associated intercellular edema and acantholysis.[5] While these findings are more common in EoE, they can also occur in reflux esophagitis, and thus also are not pathognomonic for EoE. One study found that while biopsy specimens of EoE contained five times greater mean eosinophil counts per HPF, 17% of samples of gastroesophageal reflux disease patients contained >15 eosinophils per HPF.[18]

Esophageal pH probe testing and response to acid suppression can also be used to help differentiate EoE and reflux esophagitis. Up to one-third of patients with biopsies showing >15 eosinophils per HPF will demonstrate clinical and histologic improvement with PPI therapy.[19] Manometry may demonstrate nonspecific dysmotility and lower esophageal sphincter dysfunction. While manometry is essential to rule out other esophageal disorders, there are no distinct findings diagnostic of EoE. Esophageal pH monitoring is usually within the normal range, but 10% to 20% of patients will have coexisting reflux disease, which further complicates accurate diagnosis.[4]

The diagnostic value of additional ancillary studies has been studied extensively. To date no single marker has proven superior to correlation of clinical and histologic findings. Immunohistochemical staining for eosinophil peroxidase and eosinophilic major basic protein, as well as chemokine gene expression analysis are being studied. But currently these analyses remain either clinically unproven or not widely available.[5] Several noninvasive biomarkers of inflammation have been studied in an attempt to improve diagnostic accuracy for EoE. Plasma levels of eotaxin-3, an eosinophil-specific chemokine, have been shown to be elevated in children diagnosed with EoE; increased levels are correlated with mucosal eosinophilia and severity of disease.[20] Eotaxin-3 gene microarray, mRNA level, and protein level have also been demonstrated to be elevated in patients with EoE. Interestingly, mice deficient in eotaxin-3 receptors are unable to develop an experimental form of the disease.[21] Interferon-c, IL-5, and eotaxin-1 were all overexpressed in biopsy specimens of patients with EoE compared to normal controls, while eotaxin-2 was overexpressed in controls. Collectively, these findings suggest a Th2 type response that may be implicated in the pathogenesis of the disease.[22] Increased numbers of activated mast cells in the mucosa of patients with EoE have also been reported.[23] In addition, elevated levels of TGF-β, SMAD 2–3, and VCAM-1 have all been demonstrated to be elevated in EoE patients and may be related to stricture formation.[24] The clinical significance of these findings remains to be elucidated, but they may offer new ways to aid in diagnosis or the stratification of disease severity.

While elimination diets may offer symptomatic relief, management of EoE often includes systemic or parenteral administration of corticosteroids. Diet modification may consist of a completely liquid elemental formulation of crystalline amino acids, skin allergy testing-directed food elimination, or empiric elimination diets. A study from Northwestern University demonstrated that in pediatric patients 88% of those placed on an elemental diet and 74% of those placed on a six-food elimination diet (SFED)—(exclusion of milk protein, soy, egg, wheat, peanut/tree nuts, and seafood)—demonstrated improvement in esophageal inflammation as evidenced by significantly lower esophageal eosinophil counts. The vast majority of children in both groups demonstrated symptom resolution or improvement.[25] A

recent meta-analysis found that up to 67% of patients treated with diet modification had evidence of remission as evidenced by a peak eosinophil count of <15 per HPF.[26] The response rates of elemental diet, SFED, and allergy test-directed therapies were 90.8%, 72.1%, and 45.5%, respectively. There were no differences in overall response rates between adult and pediatric patients.

Although an elemental diet is the most effective treatment, its cost and often unpalatable taste with subsequent need for tube feedings can limit its efficacy. For those patients unresponsive or unwilling to undergo diet modification, steroids are the mainstay of treatment. Symptom improvement was achieved in up to 67% of pediatric patients with corticosteroids and 50% showed complete histologic remission in a double-blind placebo controlled trial of 3 months of fluticasone versus 3% in the placebo group.[20] Prior normal skin tests to foods and aeroallergens seemed to predict response to steroids. It may be that repeated exposure to allergens resulting in persistent inflammation leads to resistance to therapy.[27] In adults, symptoms usually regress following a 6-week course of topical therapy, although recurrence is common. Usually a combination of systemic steroids and other therapies, such as esophageal dilation and Montelukast, are necessary.[4] Long-term treatment with corticosteroids may lead to oral candidiasis and hoarseness in up to 25% of patients. Suppression of the hypothalamopituitary axis and decreased bone density are other complicating issues.[28] It should be noted that given the patchy distribution of eosinophils and the lack of correlation with number and symptom severity, eosinophil counts alone should not be used to gauge treatment response on follow-up biopsies. Therefore, a combination of clinical response and eosinophil counts in comparison to prior biopsies is the best assessment of treatment.[5]

CANDIDA ESOPHAGITIS

Approximately 20% of healthy adults will have colonization of the esophagus with *Candida* species. Often these organisms are innocuous. However, *Candida* esophagitis (CE) is the most common fungal infection of the esophagus, and *Candida albicans* is the most virulent and common organism. While this fungal infection predominantly affects immunocompromised individuals, numerous conditions may predispose a patient to its development including malignancy, malnutrition, alcohol abuse, corticosteroids, diabetes mellitus, pregnancy, HIV infection, organ transplantation, esophageal dysmotility, acid suppression, gastric surgery, and antibiotic use. Symptoms typically include dysphagia and odynophagia; concomitant oral thrush may be present.[5] Frick[29] and Winston[30] and their colleagues noted that whereas CE is quite common in patients with AIDS, it occurs less commonly in patients who undergo transplantation and immunosuppression, and the risk is less than 5% in transplant recipients given prophylactic antifungal therapy. CE is the most common esophageal disorder observed in HIV patients,[31] with a prevalence of 43% to 53% in the pre-HAART era that has decreased to 17% to 24% since the introduction of HAART.[32–34]

The diagnosis of CE is established by upper endoscopy with cytologic and tissue analysis. Endoscopy is the diagnostic procedure of choice, although antifungal empiric therapy when oral thrush is present is acceptable. Endoscopy should be considered if symptoms do not improve rapidly, for example, within 7 to 10 days. In addition, Brandt and colleagues[35] described a technique involving the blind passage of a cytology brush transnasally. This technique is quite sensitive for the diagnosis. Radiographically, patients with CE have large intramural defects owing to the pseudomembranous process and intramural pseudodiverticulosis sometimes is evident (Fig. 135.4). These findings can mimic viral esophagitis, thus cytologic or tissue diagnosis for confirmation is

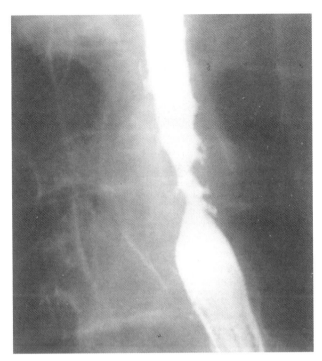

FIGURE 135.4 Esophagram showing pseudodiverticulosis in a patient with *Candida* esophagitis.

essential. The distribution and extent of involvement is variable. Findings on endoscopy are graded on a scale from 1 to 4 and range from tiny white or yellow plaques (<2 mm in diameter) to confluent pseudomembranes that constrict the lumen.[4] Most infections are isolated, superficial plaques. However, tissue invasion, ulcerations, and erosions can occur. More severe forms are encountered almost exclusively in immunocompromised patients.[5] *C. albicans* is the most common causative organism, though *C. glabrata, C. tropicalis, C. krusei,* and *C. stellatoidea* have also been identified.[36] Severe cases may be associated with complications such as hemorrhage, stenosis, and esophagotracheal fistula.[37,38] In a recent study, 62 of 733 patients (8.5%) with known HIV, including asymptomatic patients, had biopsy-proven CE on endoscopy.[39] Fifty-six percent of those found to have CE had no gastrointestinal symptoms, and 55% of those with severe CE were asymptomatic. HIV factors associated with CE were low CD4 count (<100) and higher viral load RNA levels. Severity of disease did not correlate with symptoms, but a lower CD4 count was more likely in patients found to have severe disease based on endoscopy findings.

Most immunocompetent patients with CE respond to the elimination of a predisposing antibiotic or corticosteroid. Agents such as clotrimazole and nystatin mouthwash are effective for oral candidiasis and as prophylaxis against esophageal infection but are generally less effective than oral azoles. Azoles (ketoconazole, fluconazole, and itraconazole) are first-line agents in treating CE. A dose of fluconazole of 100 to 200 mg daily typically is effective therapy. Fluconazole has been demonstrated to be superior to ketoconazole in patients with AIDS in a randomized controlled trial.[40] In severe cases the entire esophagus can be filled with a pseudomembranous exudative infiltrate. The infection can invade the esophageal wall and produce systemic candidiasis. In this setting, patients should receive intravenous amphotericin B if there is no rapid clinical response to fluconazole. In these severe cases, hospitalization is likely to be required. Amphotericin B is an effective agent but has potential renal toxicity. Lipid-based formulations of amphotericin B are available and decrease the risk of nephrotoxicity while maintaining effective antifungal coverage.

While the main choice for treatment remains fluconazole, increasing reports of clinical failures, particularly in patients who suffer repeated exposures, reveal opportunities for new therapies. The relatively recent development of the class of drugs known as echinocandins offers additional antifungal drug choices and are less toxic than amphotericin B.[27] Examples of these drugs are caspofungin, micafungin, and anidulafungin. Reports of similar efficacy between the echinocandins and fluconazole show promise for initial therapy.[41,42] However, similar or slightly higher rates of relapse have been noted in direct comparison trials of caspofungin and anidulafungin to fluconazole. While the echinocandins offer an effective option for azole-resistant fungal species, their extensive use has been associated with the development of organisms with reduced susceptibility or complete cross-resistance to these agents.[43]

OTHER FUNGAL DISEASES

Rarely, other fungal diseases can affect the esophagus, especially in patients with AIDS. Fungi typically involve the esophagus by contiguous spread from lymph nodes in the mediastinum or by vascular dissemination, although primary esophageal infection can occur. The presentations mimic other opportunistic esophageal infections, with odynophagia as the primary symptom. Long fibrosing esophageal strictures or fistulas should raise clinical suspicion of an atypical fungal infection. *C. glabrata* (formerly *Torulopsis glabrata*) is becoming an increasingly recognized pathogen for esophagitis. *C. glabrata* is a common cause of superficial fungal infections of the oral, urinary, and vaginal mucosa, but is a rare cause of esophagitis.[36] These organisms can be resistant to the typical azole therapy used to treat other *Candida* infections, but remain responsive to amphotericin B. Other species of *Candida*, including *C. tropicalis, C. krusei,* and *C. stellatoidea* have also been reported causes of esophagitis. In addition, aspergillosis, blastomycosis, mucormycosis, and histoplasmosis infections of the esophagus have been described.

VIRAL ESOPHAGITIS

Viral infections of the esophagus are common opportunistic infections in patients with HIV, malignancy, severe burns, transplant recipients, or patients on immunosuppressants or corticosteroid therapy. Clinically significant symptoms are often the result of reactivation of the pathogenic virus, although they can arise from primary infections. Cases of healthy subjects experiencing symptoms have been described.[44] As protease inhibitors have decreased viral replication in patients with AIDS and prophylaxis against HSV infection, the use of cytomegalovirus (CMV)-negative blood products and organs and preemptive ganciclovir has become standard in transplant recipients, the rates of these infections are decreasing. Viral infections of the esophagus are more common in bone marrow transplant recipients than in solid organ recipients because of the more profound immunosuppression.

In general, the incidence of CMV and HSV esophagitis is similar after organ transplantation, and coinfections have been described. HSV type 1 and type 2 may both result in esophagitis, although type 1 is more common. These patients usually present with odynophagia and dysphagia and involvement is typically in the mid- to lower esophagus.[5] Extraesophageal signs of herpes infection may or may not be seen concomitantly. Rattner and colleagues[45] reported that in rare circumstances, HSV esophagitis has presented with massive gastrointestinal hemorrhage. Endoscopically there are usually multiple separate 1- to 3-mm vesicles or coalescent ulcerations that have a "punched out" or "volcano-like" appearance with discreet edges. Biopsies should be taken from the rim of these lesions, as the virus infects intact or denuded squamous epithelial cells. Histology reveals giant cells with eosinophilic intranuclear inclusion bodies (Cowdry type A or B).[4] HSV generally responds to oral acyclovir therapy. Often, higher doses must be used in patients with AIDS, but the drug is generally well tolerated. Like CE, HSV esophagitis in the AIDS patient is usually not eradicated but rather only suppressed with acyclovir. Prophylaxis may be needed in some patients on a long-term basis. Valacyclovir, a prodrug of acyclovir, and famciclovir are available alternatives. These drugs can be administered at less frequent, daily doses with equal efficacy to acyclovir. Reports of resistant forms of HSV have been described in patients with AIDS[46] which may make therapy problematic.

CMV esophagitis is very unusual in the normal host. In HIV/AIDS patients, isolated HSV esophagitis is nine times less likely than CMV esophagitis, although the two may be seen as a coinfection.[4] Deep or longitudinal ulcers (>1 cm) should suggest CMV esophagitis. CMV can affect the esophagus alone, but it is more commonly associated with disseminated infection involving the lung, liver, eye, and small and large bowels. Presenting symptoms are dysphagia, odynophagia, nausea, vomiting, and abdominal pain. Aside from HIV/AIDS, it is seen in posttransplant patients, as well as end-stage renal disease patients on dialysis. Endoscopy reveals segmental erosions or frank ulcerations that can be several centimeters in length. The bed of the ulcer should be biopsied instead of the rim (as in HSV) because the virus infects endothelial and glandular cells instead of the squamous epithelium.[5] Viral antigen or DNA can be found on biopsy specimens by staining with antibodies or performing PCR, respectively. Classic histologic findings include giant cells with large pleomorphic nuclei and basophilic inclusions in the setting of acute or chronic inflammation and ulceration.[4] Effective suppressive treatment consists of ganciclovir, acyclovir, foscarnet, or immunoglobulin therapy. Since therapies are virostatic and not virocidal, relapse rates may approach 50% in patients with AIDS.[47] CMV retinitis may accompany CMV esophagitis. Thus, ophthalmologic evaluation is appropriate. Prophylactic ganciclovir has been effective in many high-risk transplant recipients who are CMV-seropositive or CMV-seronegative and receive a CMV-seropositive organ or blood product.

Idiopathic ulceration in patients with HIV/AIDS without an additional underlying etiology has been described, but is a rare condition, particularly in the current era of effective antiretroviral therapy. Some patients negative for CMV, HSV, and *Candida* have been shown to have severe esophagitis with deep, discrete esophageal ulcers. These idiopathic esophageal ulcers may be seen in up to 15% of patients with AIDS, typically in later stages of the disease.[48] The mechanism of injury is unknown, but direct viral infection of the squamous epithelium in unlikely to be the primary abnormality.[49] Early infection can lead to multiple small shallow ulcers that can progress to larger ulcers that extend several centimeters. These can lead to secondary infection, hemorrhage, fistula formation, or even perforation.[4] Diagnosis involves eliminating other infectious etiologies, particularly CMV or HSV, on biopsy and culture. Initiation of retroviral therapy is the mainstay of treatment. Systemic or local corticosteroids may be used once CMV and HSV have been eliminated as an underlying cause. Thalidomide has also been used to treat these lesions.

Other viruses have been associated with esophageal infection. Human papillomavirus (HPV) may infect the normal and immunocompromised host. HPV has been described in a series of patients with nodular squamous papillomas of the esophagus.[50] HPV DNA detected by PCR has also been found in cases of esophagitis.[51] Cases of Epstein–Barr viral esophagitis have been described in both immunocompetent and immunocompetent hosts.[52,53] Herpes zoster can sometimes affect the esophagus as part of a more generalized infection. Often, the esophagitis is mild. Rarely such inflammation can progress to necrotizing esophagitis and fistula formation in severely immunocompromised hosts.[54] Acyclovir is effective therapy, typically.

BACTERIAL INFECTIONS

Bacterial infections of the esophagus occur rarely. Bacterial colonization of the gastrointestinal tract is well known and it was previously thought that bacteria simply passed from the oral mucosa through the esophagus and into the stomach. However, culture studies in healthy subjects have revealed a microbiome similar to that of the oral mucosa, with viridans streptococci species present in greater than 96% of samples.[55] In healthy subjects these bacteria have close association with the distal esophageal epithelium, indicating colonization and not simply transit through to the stomach. It appears that the normal microbiome of the esophagus can also be influenced by disease states, such as reflux and Barrett metaplasia, that lead to a shift from mostly gram-positive organisms to a higher proportion of gram-negative anaerobic and microaerophilic bacteria.[56]

Mycobacterium tuberculosis esophagitis has been associated with either primary or secondary tuberculosis and is rare. Increased incidence, particularly with *Mycobacterium avium–intracellulare*, was noted in patients with HIV/AIDS. While these infections are often in immunocompromised hosts, infections in seemingly otherwise healthy patients have been reported.[57] Tuberculous esophagitis is typically due to extension from mediastinal disease or the organisms may be swallowed from a laryngeal focus. Primary TB can manifest with an exophytic process within the esophagus, suggesting ulceration or tumor, and it is one of the causes of pseudotumor. It may also cause obstructive esophageal stenosis and fistulization into the tracheobronchial tree or perforation. The diagnosis should be considered in any immunocompromised patient with multiple esophageal sinuses or fistulae. Diagnosis involves bronchoscopy, endoscopy, and CT scanning to evaluate for extra-esophageal sites of disease. Biopsy and culture are crucial to rule out other etiologies, such as Crohn disease and malignancy. Generally, primary or secondary tuberculosis responds to usual antimycobacterial therapy, including isoniazid, rifampin, and ethambutol.

Polymicrobial infection of the esophagus with multiple gram-positive organisms have been described. *Streptococcus viridans, Staphylococcus aureus, Staphylococcus epidermidis,* and beta-hemolytic streptococci are the most commonly found organisms.[5] These infections occur almost exclusively in the immunocompromised patient, particularly those with underlying hematologic malignancy and severe neutropenia. Secondary colonization of the previously injured esophagus is a common underlying etiology. Walsh and colleagues[58] established strict diagnostic criteria for the diagnosis of bacterial esophagitis: bacterial aggregates with invasion into deeper layers without evidence of fungal, viral, or neoplastic disease or previous esophageal surgery. Sheets of bacteria are typically present with associated necrosis and mucosal erosion. Neutropenic patients may have a varying degree of associated inflammation, which may be completely absent. In some patients, the development of bacteremia with no identifiable extra-esophageal source has occurred.[5] Treatment consists of appropriate antibiotic therapy. Depending on the clinical status of the patient, surgical intervention including debridement and drainage, esophageal stent placement, esophagectomy, and salivary diversion may be required.[59]

Actinomycosis is a relatively rare cause of esophagitis, but has been reported in both immunosuppressed and immunocompetent patients.[60] *Actinomyces* species are facultative anaerobic gram-positive bacilli that are present as normal flora in the oral and vaginal mucosa and in the gastrointestinal tract.[61] Disruption of the mucosal barrier appears to be a crucial step in the pathogenesis of actinomycosis. Once established in an anaerobic environment, the organism may spread without respect to fascial planes and create abscesses, sinus tracts, and fistulae. Diagnosis is typically via EGD demonstrating ulceration or eschar with tissue biopsy or culture showing gram-positive filamentous bacilli with sulfur granules and positive Gomori methenamine silver (GMS). A high index of suspicion is needed. Treatment is high-dose oral penicillin or doxycycline; prolonged therapy (4 to 52 weeks) may be needed for adequate treatment.[60,62]

UNCOMMON INFECTIONS AND INFLAMMATORY DISORDERS

Protozoal diseases can present with primary esophageal involvement. Patients with AIDS and primary cryptosporidiosis or *Pneumocystis carinii* of the esophagus have been reported, although these presentations are rare.

The esophagus can be involved with systemic diseases. Sarcoidosis rarely is associated with primary esophageal involvement but may result in an ulcerating or nodular esophagitis. Primary dermatologic conditions such as epidermolysis bullosa, pemphigus, pemphigoid, and erythema multiforme may involve the esophagus. Pemphigus vulgaris is the most common. Interestingly, more than 50% of patients with various bullous dermatitides will have esophageal involvement resulting in symptoms and notable endoscopic abnormalities. Identification of esophageal involvement may be the first step toward diagnosis of dermatologically asymptomatic pemphigus vulgaris.[5] Vesicle and blister formation is seen, and occasionally mucosal sloughing is observed. Biopsy specimens demonstrate suprabasilar clefting of the squamous epithelium with acantholysis and absence of substantial inflammation. Infiltrating inflammatory cells consist of lymphocytes and eosinophils. Direct immunofluorescence nearly always demonstrates intercellular deposition of IgG and C3 in the squamous epithelium. In contrast to pemphigus vulgaris, esophageal involvement in bullous pemphigoid is rare. The two can be distinguished histologically by the subepithelial clefting with associated eosinophilic infiltration and linear IgG and C3 deposition observed in bullous pemphigoid.[5] Often, the esophageal and pharyngeal involvement with erythema multiforme and epidermolysis bullosa is severe and is the most serious manifestation of the generalized process. Behçet disease also rarely involves the esophagus.

LICHEN PLANUS

Lichen planus is a chronic idiopathic disorder affecting less than 1% of the population and involves the skin, nails, and mucosal surfaces of the mouth, pharynx, and perineum. The pathogenesis of the disease is poorly understood, but seems to be related to T-cell (both CD4 and CD8) mediated inflammation.[63] Exogenous or endogenous antigen present in the basal layer of squamous epithelium seems to stimulate the immune response resulting in epithelial damage. The cutaneous form presents with violaceous, scaling, pruritic plaques. The oral form results in erosions and lace-like plaques. Esophageal involvement is thought to be rare, present in less than 1% of patients with the oral form of the disease.[64] When esophagitis is present, other sites of disease are commonly active. Patients may be asymptomatic or have dysphagia or odynophagia. Although the upper half of the esophagus is usually involved, the entire length may be affected, with sparing of the gastroesophageal junction. Most cases show a superficial peeling of the mucosa away from the underlying layers, leaving a friable surface

that is prone to bleed. Strictures and ulceration may also be seen. Histologically, there is a lichenoid or band-like lymphocytic infiltrate involving the superficial lamina propria and basal epithelial layer. This is usually composed of mature T-cells. Usual treatment includes systemic or topical steroid administration and is effective; however, recurrence is common following withdrawal of therapy. Oral lichen planus has an associated transformation to squamous cell carcinoma of 1% to 3%.[65] Currently, the implications of esophageal lichen planus as a premalignant condition are unknown, but cases of associated carcinoma have been reported. Thus, some would argue that patients diagnosed with esophageal lichen planus be followed closely.[63]

SCLERODERMA/CREST SYNDROME

Systemic sclerosis is an inflammatory connective tissue disorder characterized by fibrosis of the skin, vasculature, and internal organs. Scleroderma refers to the skin thickening that is characteristic of the disease and currently is used to describe both systemic sclerosis and a group of scleroderma variants that involve dermal fibrosis with rare internal organ involvement. Nearly all patients have peripheral vascular involvement in the form of Raynaud syndrome, and 80% have some gastrointestinal manifestations, although many may be asymptomatic.[66] Ten percent of patients present with gastrointestinal symptoms. Severe GI involvement affects only 8% of scleroderma patients, but only 15% of these patients survive 9 years.[67] Typical symptoms include heartburn, regurgitation, and dysphagia, but GI manifestations may not correlate with the severity of skin involvement. A retrospective analysis of asymptomatic patients with early scleroderma and mixed connective tissue disorders who underwent EGD revealed 77% had esophagitis, 85% had distal esophageal dysmotility, and 92% had gastritis.[68]

Women are affected three times more commonly than men. The incidence of systemic sclerosis is approximately 1 per 100,000 adults per year.[69] The disease is autoimmune mediated with 95% of patients testing positive for antinuclear antibodies (ANA); however, this is not specific to scleroderma.[66] Other clinically available antibody tests (anti-Scl 70, anti-RNA Polymerase III, and anticentromere) can be used to help group patients and predict clinical symptoms and organ involvement. While the pathogenesis is yet to be fully elucidated, the process seems to involve immune activation, endothelial cell injury, and fibroblast activation with resultant matrix deposition. The classic finding associated with systemic sclerosis is an aperistaltic tubular esophagus with an impaired lower esophageal sphincter. Esophageal manometry is used to document dysmotility. Features include low amplitude contractions in the distal two-thirds of the esophagus and slow transit time once a critically low pressure (<30 mm Hg) is reached.[69] As the disease progresses, the lower esophageal sphincter pressure diminishes and reflux occurs. Radiographically, the esophagus appears dilated and shortened. Air may be present as the esophagus becomes more fibrotic and loses the ability to collapse, particularly when reflux is present. A majority of patients will have abnormal 24-hour pH monitoring, but this also correlates poorly with the presence of symptoms.[69] Complications of reflux are common in these patients with up to one-third developing strictures prior to the advent of PPIs. Long-standing reflux can lead to Barrett metaplasia, which is a risk factor for developing esophageal cancer. Management of the esophageal symptoms include lifestyle modification (avoidance of nicotine, alcohol, and NSAIDs) and early initiation of high-dose PPI therapy. Evidence regarding the benefit of prokinetic agents is lacking. The performance and timing of antireflux surgery is controversial.[66] Unfortunately, there is no cure for systemic sclerosis and current treatments only slow the progression of disease. These patients often suffer from malnutrition, and coordination of care with a multidisciplinary team is critical.[67]

GRAFT-VERSUS-HOST DISEASE

In patients who have undergone bone marrow transplantation, graft-versus-host disease (GVHD) can affect the esophagus, although less commonly than other portions of the gastrointestinal tract. When involved, ulceration or vesicle formation in the esophagus similar to that found in other diseases is seen. These are typically present in the upper esophagus. Symptoms consist of dysphagia and noncardiac chest pain. In the acute setting, erosions and rarely mucosal sloughing may be seen. The histologic features of GVHD include necrotic and/or apoptotic basal squamous cells with lichenoid interface inflammation with lymphocyte infiltration predominantly in the basal layer and scattered dyskeratotic squamous cells.[5] The chronic form of GVHD (>100 days posttransplant) results in less inflammation. Fibrosis of the lamina propria can be difficult to discern; treatment is with corticosteroids. Potentially complicating the accuracy of diagnosis is the fact that mycophenolic acid, a common solid organ immunosuppressive medication, can cause mild changes in the esophagus that mimic GVHD. Correlation of the patient's clinical history, symptoms, and endoscopic findings are crucial to differentiate the underlying etiology.

CROHN DISEASE

Crohn disease can affect any portion of the gastrointestinal tract. When it is the causative etiology of esophagitis, there is usually coexistent active disease in other areas. Isolated Crohn esophagitis is extremely rare, especially in adults. The incidence of Crohn disease of the esophagus is less than 2% in adults. A higher incidence of upper gastrointestinal tract disease, including esophageal involvement has been reported in the pediatric population.[70] When the esophagus is involved, it is typically in the distal two-thirds with fissuring ulcers and fibrosis. The most common presenting symptom is dysphagia. Endoscopic features of Crohn esophagitis include strictures, fistulae, sinus tracts, and ulcers. Inflammation and cobblestoning similar to that seen in the lower portions of the GI tract can also be seen. Aphthous ulcers of the oral mucosa may indicate the diagnosis.[4] Histologically, there is a predominant transmural lymphocytic and neutrophilic infiltration, and nonnecrotizing granulomas are observed in approximately 60% of cases.[5] As discussed below, intraepithelial lymphocyte infiltration is a nonspecific finding in adults. However, there appears to be a more significant association with Crohn disease in children. Therapy involves immunomodulating agents, dilation for strictures, and surgery when indicated.

LYMPHOCYTIC ESOPHAGITIS

Lymphocytic esophagitis is a poorly characterized pattern of lymphocyte infiltration that likely results from a variety of causes including medications, motility disorders, and immune-mediated diseases. Biopsies show increased numbers of intraepithelial lymphocytes and edema, both around and distant from papillae, without associated neutrophil or eosinophil infiltration. Currently, there is no standardized criteria for diagnosis, but a cutoff of >55 lymphocytes per HPF has been proposed.[71] While lymphocytic infiltration of the esophagus may be a marker for Crohn disease, particularly in children, it has also been observed in achalasia, celiac disease, GERD, scleroderma, and other immune-mediated disorders. Thus, lymphocytic esophagitis may not represent a distinct entity, but rather might be a marker of injury resulting from a variety of disease processes or medications.[5]

ESOPHAGITIS DISSECANS SUPERFICIALIS (SLOUGHING ESOPHAGITIS)

Esophagitis dissecans superficialis is a poorly understood disease process that tends to affect the mid and distal portions of the esophagus in adults over the age of 50 and presents with reflux type symptoms or dysphagia. Nearly all patients have multiple comorbidities, are chronically debilitated, or taking multiple medications. Endoscopy reveals white plaques, membranes, or sloughed epithelium that forms a cast of the esophageal lumen. Histologically, there is a sharply demarcated superficial layer of necrotic squamous epithelium covering a viable, mature, uninflamed squamous layer. The necrotic layer is more eosinophilic than the underlying intact basal layer, which creates a "two-toned" appearance on microscopic examination. A variable amount of neutrophils and edema may be seen between the two layers, but inflammation is often mild.[5] Differentiation between sloughing esophagitis and other endoscopically similar etiologies with white plaques (chemical ingestion, medication-induced mucosal injury, fungal esophagitis, and pemphigus) can usually be made by the clinical history, degree of inflammation, and divergent histologic features. No standardized criteria for diagnosis exist, but proposed criteria are sloughed mucosal strips >2 cm that occur over normal underlying mucosa in the absence of nearby ulcerations or friable areas.[72] The natural history appears to be benign with endoscopic resolution occurring commonly. Treatment involves symptom control and most patients have no lasting sequelae.

SUMMARY

The esophagus can be involved in a wide variety of benign inflammatory disease processes. These range from immune-mediated inflammation primarily of the esophagus to opportunistic infections to systemic diseases that concomitantly affect the esophagus. Accurate diagnosis often hinges on an astute history and physical examination, a high index of suspicion, and correlation of endoscopy findings with appropriate microbiologic and pathologic results. Occasionally, additional ancillary testing may lead to the correct diagnosis. While some of these diseases can be easily treated or self-limiting, others have broad implications for patients. Esophageal symptoms may be the first signs of a serious systemic disease and prompt diagnosis and treatment is essential. Depending on the underlying etiology, involvement and coordination of a multidisciplinary team may be necessary to ensure appropriate care.

ACKNOWLEDGMENT

The authors wish to thank Joel H. Rubenstein, M.D. and Joel K. Greenson, M.D. from the University of Michigan Health System for supplying endoscopic and pathologic photographs, respectively.

REFERENCES

1. Liacouras CA, Furuta GT, Hirano I, et al. Eosinophilic esophagitis: updated consensus recommendations for children and adults. *J Allergy Clin Immunol* 2011;128(1):3–20, e6; quiz 21–22.
2. Attwood SE, Smyrk TC, Demeester TR, et al. Esophageal eosinophilia with dysphagia. A distinct clinicopathologic syndrome. *Dig Dis Sci* 1993;38(1):109–116.
3. Sgouros SN, Bergele C, Mantides A. Eosinophilic esophagitis in adults: a systematic review. *Eur J Gastroenterol Hepatol* 2006;18(2):211–217.
4. Attwood SE, Lamb CA. Eosinophilic oesophagitis and other non-reflux inflammatory conditions of the oesophagus: diagnostic imaging and management. *Best Pract Res Clin Gastroenterol* 2008;22(4):639–660.
5. Almashat SJ, Duan L, Goldsmith JD. Non-reflux esophagitis: a review of inflammatory diseases of the esophagus exclusive of reflux esophagitis. *Semin Diagn Pathol* 2014; 31(2):89–99.

6. Cherian S, Smith NM, Forbes DA. Rapidly increasing prevalence of eosinophilic oesophagitis in Western Australia. *Arch Dis Child* 2006;91(12):1000–1004.

7. Noel RJ, Putnam PE, Rothenberg ME. Eosinophilic esophagitis. *N Engl J Med* 2004; 351(9):940–941.

8. Prasad GA, Alexander JA, Schleck CD, et al. Epidemiology of eosinophilic esophagitis over three decades in Olmsted County, Minnesota. *Clin Gastroenterol Hepatol* 2009;7(10):1055–1061.

9. Philpott H, Nandurkar S, Thien F, et al. Eosinophilic esophagitis: a clinicopathological review. *Pharmacol Ther* 2015;146:12–22.

10. Potter JW, Saeian K, Staff D, et al. Eosinophilic esophagitis in adults: an emerging problem with unique esophageal features. *Gastrointest Endosc* 2004;59(3):355–361.

11. Parfitt JR, Gregor JC, Suskin NG, et al. Eosinophilic esophagitis in adults: distinguishing features from gastroesophageal reflux disease: a study of 41 patients. *Mod Pathol* 2006;19(1):90–96.

12. Genevay M, Rubbia-Brandt L, Rougemont AL. Do eosinophil numbers differentiate eosinophilic esophagitis from gastroesophageal reflux disease? *Arch Pathol Lab Med* 2010;134(6):815–825.

13. DeBrosse CW, Case JW, Putnam PE, et al. Quantity and distribution of eosinophils in the gastrointestinal tract of children. *Pediatr Dev Pathol* 2006;9(3):210–218.

14. Ronkainen J, Talley NJ, Aro P, et al. Prevalence of oesophageal eosinophils and eosinophilic oesophagitis in adults: the population-based kalixanda study. *Gut* 2007;56(5):615–620.

15. Furuta GT, Liacouras CA, Collins MH, et al. Eosinophilic esophagitis in children and adults: a systematic review and consensus recommendations for diagnosis and treatment. *Gastroenterology* 2007;133(4):1342–1363.

16. Shah A, Kagalwalla AF, Gonsalves N, et al. Histopathologic variability in children with eosinophilic esophagitis. *Am J Gastroenterol* 2009;104(3):716–721.

17. Gonsalves N, Policarpio-Nicolas M, Zhang Q, et al. Histopathologic variability and endoscopic correlates in adults with eosinophilic esophagitis. *Gastrointest Endosc* 2006;64(3):313–319.

18. Mueller S, Neureiter D, Aigner T, et al. Comparison of histological parameters for the diagnosis of eosinophilic oesophagitis versus gastro-oesophageal reflux disease on oesophageal biopsy material. *Histopathology* 2008;53(6):676–684.

19. Dellon ES, Speck O, Woodward K, et al. Clinical and endoscopic characteristics do not reliably differentiate PPI-responsive esophageal eosinophilia and eosinophilic esophagitis in patients undergoing upper endoscopy: a prospective cohort study. *Am J Gastroenterol* 2013;108(12):1854–1860.

20. Konikoff MR, Blanchard C, Kirby C, et al. Potential of blood eosinophils, eosinophil-derived neurotoxin, and eotaxin-3 as biomarkers of eosinophilic esophagitis. *Clin Gastroenterol Hepatol* 2006;4(11):1328–1336.

21. Blanchard C, Wang N, Stringer KF, et al. Eotaxin-3 and a uniquely conserved gene-expression profile in eosinophilic esophagitis. *J Clin Invest* 2006;116(2):536–547.

22. Gupta SK, Fitzgerald JF, Kondratyuk T, et al. Cytokine expression in normal and inflamed esophageal mucosa: a study into the pathogenesis of allergic eosinophilic esophagitis. *J Pediatr Gastroenterol Nutr* 2006;42(1):22–26.

23. Kirsch R, Bokhary R, Marcon MA, et al. Activated mucosal mast cells differentiate eosinophilic (allergic) esophagitis from gastroesophageal reflux disease. *J Pediatr Gastroenterol Nutr* 2007;44(1):20–26.

24. Aceves SS, Newbury RO, Dohil R, et al. Esophageal remodeling in pediatric eosinophilic esophagitis. *J Allergy Clin Immunol* 2007;119(1):206–212.

25. Kagalwalla AF, Sentongo TA, Ritz S, et al. Effect of six-food elimination diet on clinical and histologic outcomes in eosinophilic esophagitis. *Clin Gastroenterol Hepatol* 2006;4(9):1097–1102.

26. Arias A, González-Cervera J, Tenias JM, et al. Efficacy of dietary interventions for inducing histologic remission in patients with eosinophilic esophagitis: a systematic review and meta-analysis. *Gastroenterology* 2014;146(7):1639–1648.

27. Pace F, Pallotta S, Antinori S. Nongastroesophageal reflux disease-related infectious, inflammatory and injurious disorders of the esophagus. *Curr Opin Gastroenterol* 2007;23(4):446–451.

28. Lipworth BJ. Systemic adverse effects of inhaled corticosteroid therapy: a systematic review and meta-analysis. *Arch Intern Med* 1999;159(9):941–955.

29. Frick T, Fryd DS, Goodale RL, et al. Incidence and treatment of candida esophagitis in patients undergoing renal transplantation. Data from the Minnesota prospective randomized trial of cyclosporine versus antilymphocyte globulin-azathioprine. *Am J Surg* 1988;155(2):311–313.

30. Winston DJ, Gale RP, Meyer DV, et al. Infectious complications of human bone marrow transplantation. *Medicine (Baltimore)* 1979;58(1):1–31.

31. Werneck-Silva AL, Prado IB. Role of upper endoscopy in diagnosing opportunistic infections in human immunodeficiency virus-infected patients. *World J Gastroenterol* 2009;15(9):1050–1056.

32. Nkuize M, De Wit S, Muls V, et al. Upper gastrointestinal endoscopic findings in the era of highly active antiretroviral therapy. *HIV Med* 2010;11(6):412–417.

33. Bonacini M, Young T, Laine L. The causes of esophageal symptoms in human immunodeficiency virus infection. A prospective study of 110 patients. *Arch Intern Med* 1991;151(8):1567–1572.

34. Rolston KV, Rodriguez S. Upper gastrointestinal disease in human immunodeficiency virus-infected individuals. *Arch Intern Med* 1992;152(4):881–882.

35. Brandt LJ, Coman E, Schwartz E, et al. Use of a new cytology balloon for diagnosis of symptomatic esophageal disease in acquired immunodeficiency syndrome. *Gastrointest Endosc* 1993;39(4):559–561.

36. Macedo DP, da Silva VK, de Almeida Farias AM, et al. Candida glabrata esophagitis: new case reports and management. *Braz J Microbiol* 2008;39(2):279–281.

37. Gaissert HA, Breuer CK, Weissburg A, et al. Surgical management of necrotizing candida esophagitis. *Ann Thorac Surg* 1999;67(1):231–233.

38. Kanzaki R, Yano M, Takachi K, et al. Candida esophagitis complicated by an esophago-airway fistula: report of a case. *Surg Today* 2009;39(11):972–978.

39. Nishimura S, Nagata N, Shimbo T, et al. Factors associated with esophageal candidiasis and its endoscopic severity in the era of antiretroviral therapy. *PLoS One* 2013; 8(3):e58217.

40. Barbaro G, Barbarini G, Calderon W, et al. Fluconazole versus itraconazole for candida esophagitis in acquired immunodeficiency syndrome. Candida esophagitis. *Gastroenterology* 1996;111(5):1169–1177.

41. Krause DS, Simjee AE, van Rensburg C, et al. A randomized, double-blind trial of anidulafungin versus fluconazole for the treatment of esophageal candidiasis. *Clin Infect Dis* 2004;39(6):770–775.

42. de Wet NT, Bester AJ, Viljoen JJ, et al. A randomized, double blind, comparative trial of micafungin (FK463) vs. fluconazole for the treatment of oesophageal candidiasis. *Aliment Pharmacol Ther* 2005;21(7):899–907.

43. Laverdiere M, Lalonde RG, Baril JG, et al. Progressive loss of echinocandin activity following prolonged use for treatment of candida albicans oesophagitis. *J Antimicrob Chemother* 2006;57(4):705–708.

44. Castrillero C, García Durán F, Cabello N, et al. Herpes esophagitis in healthy adults and adolescents: report of 3 cases and review of the literature. *Medicine (Baltimore)* 2010;89(4):204–210.

45. Rattner HM, Cooper DJ, Zaman MB. Severe bleeding from herpes esophagitis. *Am J Gastroenterol* 1985;80(7):523–525.

46. Erlich KS, Mills J, Chatis P, et al. Acyclovir-resistant herpes simplex virus infections in patients with the acquired immunodeficiency syndrome. *N Engl J Med* 1989;320(5): 293–296.

47. Wilcox CM, Straub RF, Schwartz DA. Prospective evaluation of biopsy number for the diagnosis of viral esophagitis in patients with HIV infection and esophageal ulcer. *Gastrointest Endosc* 1996;44(5):587–593.

48. Wilcox CM, Schwartz DA. Endoscopic characterization of idiopathic esophageal ulceration associated with human immunodeficiency virus infection. *J Clin Gastroenterol* 1993;16(3):251–256.

49. Wilcox CM, Zaki SR, Coffield LM, et al. Evaluation of idiopathic esophageal ulceration for human immunodeficiency virus. *Mod Pathol* 1995;8(5):568–572.

50. Orlowska J, Jarosz D, Gugulski A, et al. Squamous cell papillomas of the esophagus: report of 20 cases and literature review. *Am J Gastroenterol* 1994;89(3):434–437.

51. Tornesello ML, Monaco R, Nappi O, et al. Detection of mucosal and cutaneous human papillomaviruses in oesophagitis, squamous cell carcinoma and adenocarcinoma of the oesophagus. *J Clin Virol* 2009;45(1):28–33.

52. Annahazi A, Terhes G, Deák J, et al. Fulminant Epstein-Barr virus esophagitis in an immunocompetent patient. *Endoscopy* 2011;43(Suppl 2):E348–E349.

53. Kitchen VS, Helbert M, Francis ND, et al. Epstein-Barr virus associated oesophageal ulcers in AIDS. *Gut* 1990;31(11):1223–1225.

54. Moretti F, Uberti-Foppa C, Quiros-Roldan E, et al. Oesophagobronchial fistula caused by varicella zoster virus in a patient with AIDS: a unique case. *J Clin Pathol* 2002;55(5):397–398.

55. Grusell N, Dahlén G, Ruth M, et al. Bacterial flora of the human oral cavity, and the upper and lower esophagus. *Dis Esophagus* 2013;26(1):84–90.

56. Walker MM, Talley NJ. Review article: bacteria and pathogenesis of disease in the upper gastrointestinal tract—beyond the era of Helicobacter pylori. *Aliment Pharmacol Ther* 2014;39(8):767–779.

57. Mou Y, Zeng H, Wang QM, et al. Esophageal tuberculosis initially misdiagnosed by endoscopy as a submucosal tumor. *Endoscopy* 2015;47(Suppl 1):E30–E31.

58. Walsh TJ, Belitsos NJ, Hamilton SR. Bacterial esophagitis in immunocompromised patients. *Arch Intern Med* 1986;146(7):1345–1348.

59. Gaissert HA, Roper CL, Patterson GA, et al. Infectious necrotizing esophagitis: outcome after medical and surgical intervention. *Ann Thorac Surg* 2003;75(2):342–347.

60. Murchan EM, Redelman-Sidi G, Patel M, et al. Esophageal actinomycosis in a fifty-three-year-old man with HIV: case report and review of the literature. *AIDS Patient Care STDS* 2010;24(2):73–78.

61. Abdalla J, Myers J, Moorman J. Actinomycotic infection of the oesophagus. *J Infect* 2005;51(2):E39–E43.

62. Chandrasekhara V, Zhang L, Floyd BN, et al. A rare cause of esophageal strictures: actinomyces. *Gastrointest Endosc* 2012;75(5):1111–1112.

63. Ynson ML, Forouhar F, Vaziri H. Case report and review of esophageal lichen planus treated with fluticasone. *World J Gastroenterol* 2013;19(10):1652–1656.

64. Eisen D. The evaluation of cutaneous, genital, scalp, nail, esophageal, and ocular involvement in patients with oral lichen planus. *Oral Surg Oral Med Oral Pathol Oral Radiol Endod* 1999;88(4):431–436.

65. Dickens CM, Heseltine D, Walton S, et al. The oesophagus in lichen planus: an endoscopic study. *BMJ* 1990;300(6717):84.

66. Domsic R, Fasanella K, Bielefeldt K. Gastrointestinal manifestations of systemic sclerosis. *Dig Dis Sci* 2008;53(5):1163–1174.

67. Gyger G, Baron M. Gastrointestinal manifestations of scleroderma: recent progress in evaluation, pathogenesis, and management. *Curr Rheumatol Rep* 2012;14(1):22–29.

68. Thonhofer R, Siegel C, Trummer M, et al. Early endoscopy in systemic sclerosis without gastrointestinal symptoms. *Rheumatol Int* 2012;32(1):165–168.

69. Ebert EC. Esophageal disease in progressive systemic sclerosis. *Curr Treat Options Gastroenterol* 2008;11(1):64–69.

70. De Felice KM, Katzka DA, Raffals LE. Crohn's disease of the esophagus: clinical features and treatment outcomes in the biologic era. *Inflamm Bowel Dis* 2015;21(9):2106–2113.

71. Rubio CA, Sjodahl K, Lagergren J. Lymphocytic esophagitis: a histologic subset of chronic esophagitis. *Am J Clin Pathol* 2006;125(3):432–437.

72. Hart PA, Romano RC, Moreira RK, et al. Esophagitis dissecans superficialis: clinical, endoscopic, and histologic features. *Dig Dis Sci* 2015;60(7):2049–2057.

136

Esophageal Motility Disorders

Janani S. Reisenauer ▪ Karthik Ravi ▪ Shanda H. Blackmon

Esophageal motility disorders are uncommon and usually present with dysphagia, its sequelae (regurgitation and aspiration), or atypical noncardiac chest pain. Diagnosis of these disorders typically utilizes multiple modalities, including upper endoscopy, esophagram, and esophageal manometry. However, esophageal manometry constitutes the gold standard for the evaluation of esophageal dysmotility. Esophageal manometry assesses lower esophageal sphincter (LES) pressure and relaxation. It also assesses the nature of esophageal contraction waves, including amplitude, duration, repetitive nature, the presence of nontransmitted or partially transmitted waves, and the presence of peristalsis in the body of the esophagus. Esophageal motility disorders are classified as primary when not related to a systemic disease, and secondary, if they are associated with a systemic disease. In a series published by Patti et al.[1] of the 3,471 patients referred to their swallowing center for evaluation, 11.4% were diagnosed with a primary esophageal motility disorder. Table 136.1 lists the primary motility disorders with their manometric profiles.[2,3] Reviews emphasizing the manometric diagnosis and medical management of the primary esophageal motility disorders have been published by Spechler and Castell[4] and Richter.[5]

ACHALASIA

Achalasia, a term of Greek origin, means failure to relax. Achalasia was first described and effectively treated (by dilation with whalebone) by Thomas Willis in 1672. The classic findings on manometry are failure of the LES to relax in response to a swallow and absent peristalsis in the smooth muscle of the distal esophagus. The etiology of achalasia is unknown. Possible causes include hereditary, degenerative, autoimmune, and infectious etiologies. Achalasia is rare, with

an incidence of only about 0.5 per 100,000 people and prevalence of 1 per 10,000 people. Although described in both the very young and elderly people, it occurs most commonly between the ages of 20 and 50 years. The gender distribution is equal.

HISTORY

Payne[7] reviewed the history of the surgical treatment of achalasia with an emphasis on Heller's contribution. Surgical treatment before the acceptance of Heller's technique was by a variety of anastomotic cardioplasties that relieved obstruction but led to severe esophagitis, with its attendant complications. In 1914, Heller reported a successful result in a patient treated with a transabdominal double (anterior and posterior) esophagomyotomy. His operation did not become standard until the devastating late effects of severe reflux disease were reported by Barrett and Franklin in 1949. Heller's operation was modified to a single anterior esophagomyotomy by Groeneveldt in 1918 and further popularized by Zaaijer in 1923.

PATHOPHYSIOLOGY

Pathologic studies have shown abnormalities in the esophageal myenteric (Auerbach's) plexus, which include inflammation, loss of ganglion cells, and fibrosis. Degenerative changes of the vagus nerve and changes of the dorsal motor nucleus of the vagus have also been described. Central vagal dysfunction and destruction of the peripheral myenteric plexus are the two hypotheses that could explain achalasia; it is unclear which is correct. The end result of the destruction of the myenteric plexus is a loss of postganglionic inhibitory neurons containing nitric oxide and vasoactive intestinal polypeptide. The result is relatively unopposed cholinergic stimulation, resulting

TABLE 136.1 Classification of Primary Esophageal Motility Disorders and Their Manometric Features

Disorder	Lower Esophageal Sphincter Pressure	Lower Esophageal Sphincter Relaxation	Wave Progression	Wave Amplitude
Achalasia, type I	High	Incomplete	Aperistalsis	Usually low
Achalasia, type II	High	Incomplete	Pressurization >30 mm Hg	Low
Achalasia type III	High, DLI <4.5 s	Incomplete	Spastic >20% swallows	Low
Diffuse esophageal spasm	Usually normal	Normal	Simultaneous, >20% swallows	Usually normal
Nutcracker esophagus	Usually normal	Normal	Normal	High
Hypertensive low esophageal sphincter[6]	High	Normal	Normal	Normal
Ineffective esophageal motility	Usually normal	Normal	Usually disordered	Low, >30% swallows

in loss of the normal progressive increased proportion of inhibitory input distally in the esophagus responsible for peristalsis as well as impaired LES relaxation.

DIAGNOSIS

Clinical Features

Patients with achalasia usually have dysphagia to solids and liquids (76%), as reported by Blam and colleagues.[8] Regurgitation is frequent (79%) and may contain food or saliva. Regurgitation is especially frequent at night during recumbency and may cause coughing or choking spells. Most patients (79%) learn to eat slowly and may have adaptive mechanisms such as repetitive swallows with the neck extended and using liquids to lubricate solid food. Chest pain occurs in some patients, especially those with early disease. Weight loss is common, but not universal and typically gradual. Obesity does not eliminate the possibility of achalasia. A history of food bolus impaction may be present. Heartburn is often present as a symptom (40% to 50%),[9–11] sometimes providing a diagnostic challenge. The etiology of heartburn in achalasia is not related to gastroesophageal reflux given the impairment of LES relaxation. Instead, it may result from the lactic acid from the fermented retained food. Additionally, distention of the esophageal body itself, as seen in achalasia, has been demonstrated to induce heartburn. Pulmonary symptoms may predominate, with occasional patients diagnosed after hospitalization for aspiration pneumonia. Most patients live with their symptoms for years, and misdiagnosis of early cases is frequent.

Radiographic Evaluation

Chest radiographs may show subtle findings such as an esophageal air–fluid level, absent gastric air bubble, abnormal mediastinal contour, or even evidence of aspiration pneumonia. Barium swallow may show the characteristic findings of a dilated esophagus and a smooth, tapered distal narrowing at the gastroesophageal junction (GEJ) ("bird's beak" appearance). However, in some cases an esophagram may fail to demonstrate typical findings of achalasia. See Chapter 133 for a more detailed discussion of contrast study and fluoroscopic findings in achalasia.

Endoscopy

An upper gastrointestinal endoscopy is necessary in the diagnostic evaluation. In achalasia, the body of the esophagus is usually dilated and often has retained food and liquid. Retention esophagitis may be present, with a cobblestone appearance to the mucosa. The LES is usually tonically closed, but it is possible to pass the endoscope with gentle pressure through the esophagogastric junction. Cameron and colleagues[12] have reported on the accuracy of video endoscopy to diagnose achalasia by noting the response of the visualized esophagus to a swallow. In almost all patients, there was an absence of lumen-occluding contractions with failure of the LES to open. However, it is estimated that upper endoscopy is normal in nearly 50% of patients with achalasia. Therefore, the primary role of EGD is to rule out pseudoachalasia, most often secondary to GEJ malignancy, which is present in up to 5% of patients meeting manometric criteria for achalasia.[13] If pseudoachalasia is suspected, a computed tomography (CT) scan or endoscopic ultrasound should also be performed to look for a mass at the esophagogastric junction.

Manometry

Manometry is the key diagnostic test because endoscopic and radiographic exams are less reliably diagnostic of achalasia.[14,15] The two

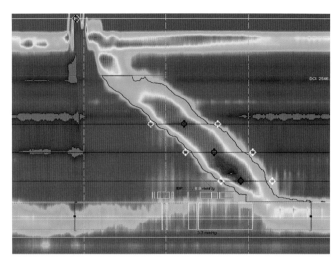

FIGURE 136.1 Normal image of high-resolution manometry demonstrating the findings of DCI, IRP, and DL (described in the text).

manometric features required to make a diagnosis of achalasia are (a) incomplete relaxation of the LES and (b) aperistalsis in the body of the esophagus (Table 136.1). The LES pressure is usually high (never low) but can be normal (10 to 45 mm Hg).

The recent advent of high-resolution esophageal manometry (HRM) has further refined our diagnosis of achalasia. Traditional esophageal manometry utilized a water perfusion catheter with sensors spaced 3 to 5 cm apart. This required multiple catheter manipulations to evaluate the entire esophageal body and LES. In comparison HRM utilizes circumferential solid state sensors which are placed 1 cm apart. This allows intraluminal manometry to be measured as a continuum along the entire length of the esophagus. This in turn allows for results to be displayed in an easy to interpret color-coded esophageal pressure topographic map, with high pressures demonstrated in red and orange and low pressures in blue and green (Fig. 136.1). The advent of HRM and the increased information gathered have necessitated a new classification system to interpret studies. The Chicago Classification has emerged to fill this niche.[16–18] This classification system utilizes several metrics involved with high-resolution manometry that are of vital importance to understanding the classification of motility disorders. Integrated relaxation pressure (IRP) is a measure of the GEJ relaxation during swallowing, defined by an average of the four noncontinuous seconds of lowest pressure during the deglutitive window of a swallow. Incomplete GEJ relaxation is defined by an IRP of 15 mm Hg or greater. The distal latency (DL) is a measure of peristaltic timing with normal defined as less than 4.5 seconds from the initiation of swallow to the conclusion of the distal peristaltic wave. The distal contractile integral is a measure of the vigor of the contraction and is the product of the amplitude, length of the esophagus, and the duration of the contraction.

Utilizing HRM, Pandolfino et al. were the first to identify three distinct types of achalasia.[18] In type I achalasia (Fig. 136.2) there is minimal esophageal pressurization while in type II (Fig. 136.3) there is panesophageal pressurization greater than 30 mm Hg in at least 20% of swallows. It is thought that types I and II achalasia exist along a continuum, with type II representing early achalasia in which the esophagus has minimal dilation while type I is late achalasia in which there is significant esophageal dilation and loss of elasticity. In contrast, type III achalasia (Fig. 136.4) is defined by nonperistaltic rapid and vigorous or spastic contractions within the distal esophageal body. Type III achalasia, formerly known as vigorous achalasia, was first reported by Sanderson and colleagues.[19] Some investigators have

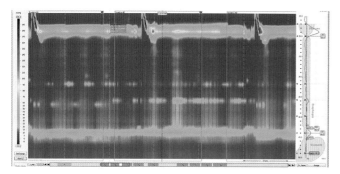

FIGURE 136.2 High-resolution manometry in a patient with type I achalasia. Type I achalasia is classically defined as aperistalsis with an elevated integrated relaxation pressure and incomplete lower esophageal sphincter relaxation with an elevated lower esophageal sphincter pressure.

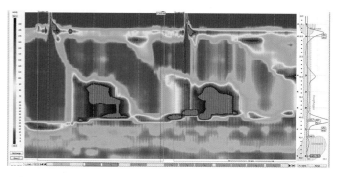

FIGURE 136.4 High-resolution manometry in a patient with type III achalasia. Classic findings include the detection of at least two spastic high-amplitude waves in the setting of aperistalsis and elevated integrated relaxation pressures (IRP).

proposed that atypical chest pain is more common in these patients, whereas others, such as Goldenberg and colleagues,[20] suggest that such patients cannot be distinguished from those with classic achalasia. Pasricha and colleagues[21] have reported that botulinum toxin injection is more effective in patients with vigorous as opposed to classic achalasia, whereas Cuilliere and colleagues[22] found no difference in response between the patients. Recent studies have suggested that per oral endoscopic myotomy (POEM), which will be discussed later in this chapter is an appealing solution for patients with type III achalasia.[23]

Several studies have evaluated the prognostic value of this scoring system.[24,25] Both a retrospective trial by Pandolfino et al.[26] conducted in 2008 and a recent randomized trial found that type II patients were more likely to respond to therapy regardless of pneumatic dilation or Heller myotomy compared to those patients with type I or type III (100% excellent results vs. 81% and 86%, respectively). Type I did, however, appear to have improved outcomes when comparing myotomy as initial treatment to dilation or botox.

TREATMENT

There is no curative treatment for achalasia because it is impossible to restore peristaltic function to the denervated esophagus. Current treatment is directed at reducing the pressure gradient across the LES, thus reducing outflow obstruction and allowing gravity to empty the esophagus. The two most effective treatments are mechanical: balloon dilation and surgical myotomy. Pharmacologic treatment is less effective and includes injection of botulinum toxin into the LES

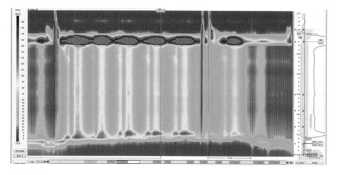

FIGURE 136.3 High-resolution manometry in a patient with type II achalasia. Patients once again have an elevated integrated relaxation pressure (IRP) with lack of normal peristalsis. However, there is pressurization of the esophagus demonstrated in greater than 20% of the swallows.

and orally administered drugs that reduce LES pressure. Esophageal resection is rarely needed for failure of primary therapy.

Medical Therapy

Several types of drugs are effective at reducing LES pressure. These include beta agonists, anticholinergics, nitrates, and calcium channel blockers. The effects of sildenafil (Viagra), a phosphodiesterase inhibitor, on the esophagus were reported by Eherer et al.[27] All of these medications have been used in achalasia, but all are of limited use because of either poor efficacy or adverse side effects.

Botulinum Toxin Injection

Pasricha and colleagues[21] reported favorable results of the first trial of botulinum toxin injection in patients with achalasia in 1994. Botulinum toxin inhibits acetylcholine release from nerve endings, thereby reducing the cholinergic drive to the LES, with resultant sphincter relaxation. Over time, neurotransmission and muscle activity recover after new nerve endings are sprouted and new synapses to adjacent muscle fibers are formed. Botulinum toxin is administered on an outpatient basis via an endoscope through a sclerotherapy needle (Fig. 136.5). Usually, 25 IU is delivered into each of the four quadrants of the cardia in 1-mL aliquots. The initial success rate is about 70% to 90%[28]; however, efficacy is transient with recurrent symptoms within 1 year in the majority of patients. Common side effects are transient chest pain after the procedure and reflux symptoms. A relatively rare but important complication is mediastinitis, related to injection of botox through the relatively thin-walled esophagus. Neubrand and colleagues[29,30] reported on medium-term results and prognostic factors with botulinum toxin injection. The LES pressure was significantly reduced from 62 to 43 mm Hg after treatment. Thirty-six patients had symptomatic relief a mean of 2.5 years after treatment, whereas 64% had a good initial result. Retreatment was of no benefit if results were assessed at 6 months. Patients with high LES pressures (mean 73 mm Hg) and younger patients (mean 46 years) had poor results. In a randomized controlled trial comparing 40 patients assigned to a set of two botulinum toxin injections 1 month apart with another 40 patients assigned to laparoscopic Heller myotomy, Zaninotto et al.[31] found that initial response to treatment was excellent and similar in both groups. Symptoms recurred in the botulinum group, however, for 40% of patients by 1 year and 66% by 2 years.

Botulinum toxin injection is likely best suited for high-risk elderly patients with comorbidities limiting their candidacy for more definitive therapy. Retreatment is of some value if there was an initial good response to injection but is of little benefit if the initial response was

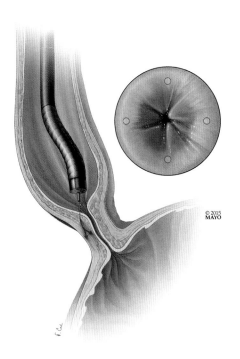

FIGURE 136.5 Method of botox injection is demonstrated in a patient with achalasia. An endoscope is inserted into the esophagus and under direct visualization; the lower esophageal sphincter is injected in four quadrants through the mucosa of the esophagus. Used with permission of Mayo Foundation for Medical Education and Research, all rights reserved.

poor. Increasing the dose of botulinum toxin has been of no benefit in improving the response.

Many believe that botulinum toxin injection may complicate the results of later myotomy, although studies have not shown a clear relationship. Raftopoulos and colleagues[32] found that myotomy patients who had undergone prior botulinum toxin injection did not have significant improvement in symptoms of heartburn, regurgitation, chest pain, or sense of well-being, while those without prior nonoperative treatment did improve in all of these areas. Nevertheless, the group that had undergone prior botulinum toxin injection did have significantly improved dysphagia scores, and the same study showed no significant effect of prior nonoperative treatment on surgical outcome. Patti et al.[33] attributed two of their myotomy failures (and intraoperative perforations) to transmural fibrosis from prior botulinum toxin injection. In contrast, Deb and colleagues[34] found that prior botulinum toxin injection was not associated with intraoperative perforation or poor functional outcome. Similarly, in comparing myotomy patients who had undergone prior endoscopic treatment for achalasia (including 34 patients who had undergone prior botulinum injection) with those who had not, Perrone et al.[35] found no significant difference in the rate of intraoperative perforation, myotomy failure, postoperative solid dysphagia score, or overall patient satisfaction. The degree to which botulinum therapy interferes with later myotomy remains a controversial issue.

Pneumatic Dilation

Forceful dilation of the LES is a noninvasive, time-tested treatment option in achalasia. Originally a large, relatively compliant bag dilator (Mosher bag) was swallowed and positioned across the cardia and inflated with contrast material under fluoroscopic control until the "waist" of the LES impression disappeared. The aim of pneumatic

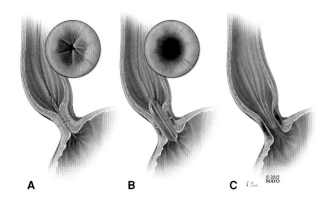

FIGURE 136.6 Balloon dilation demonstrated as a treatment modality for achalasia. The endoscope is inserted to view the lower esophageal sphincter. **A:** The non-dilated balloon is passed through the contracted lower esophageal sphincter. **B:** The balloon is dilated. **C:** Post-dilation view of the lower esophageal sphincter, demonstrating tearing of the esophageal muscle layer. Used with permission of Mayo Foundation for Medical Education and Research, all rights reserved.

dilation is rupture of the muscle fibers of the LES with maintenance of an intact esophageal mucosa (Fig. 136.6). The reason this seemingly contradictory result can occur is the different compliances of the esophageal sphincter (less compliant) and the mucosa (more compliant). Good results were obtained initially in about 70% of patients, with a perforation rate of 2% to 5%. More recently, balloon dilation has been performed with polyethylene noncompliant-sized balloons that can be passed through the working channel of an endoscope or over a guidewire. The most commonly used balloons are the Rigeflex balloons (Microinvasive, Watertown, MA). Utilizing nondeformable pneumatic pressure, the balloons are available in 30 and 35 mm Hg, and the procedure is usually done on an outpatient basis with sedation.[36] Patients have significant chest pain during the dilation, which rapidly improves. If the pain continues, the patient should be evaluated for perforation. Most gastroenterologists do the dilation under endoscopic but not radiographic control. Results are then judged by relief of dysphagia in follow-up. If there is inadequate relief, the next size of balloon dilator is used. A more precise technique is to use radiographic control with inflation of the balloon with dilute contrast; dilation is continued until the waist of the LES disappears. Kadakia and Wong[17] reviewed the results of modern balloon dilation. The symptomatic response rate was 74% to the 30 mm Hg balloon, 33% to the 35 mm Hg balloon, and 5% to the 40 mm Hg balloon. The perforation rate increased as balloon size increased: 1% with the 30 mm Hg and 15% with the 40 mm Hg balloon. In the short term, relapse occurs at about 6% per year. Troublesome heartburn occurred in only 5% of patients. Sabharwal and colleagues[37] reported results in 76 patients using radiographic control of balloon dilation. There were no perforations, and 89% of patients reported satisfactory improvement of their swallowing. Fifty-two patients required a single dilation, 22 patients between two and four dilations, and 2 patients needed five dilations. There is very little information on the long-term results of dilation. West and colleagues[38] recently reported long-term results in patients after dilation. At 5 years, the success rate was only 50%, and at 15 years, the success rate dropped to only 40%. Of the 32 patients who died during the study, 6 (19%) died of esophageal cancer. Sabharwal and colleagues[37] reported safe, effective balloon dilation after failed surgical myotomy. Alternatively, Ferguson and colleagues[39] and Dolan and colleagues[40] reported good results with surgical myotomy after failed balloon dilation. Balloon dilation remains an option for gastroenterologists, particularly due to its minimally invasive nature and seemingly more effective response in older women compared to younger men.[41] The esophageal perforation rate for balloon dilation is estimated as 2% to 5%.[42,43]

Esophagomyotomy

Esophageal myotomy is the definitive treatment for achalasia. The goals of the procedure are to reduce the LES pressure enough to allow gravity drainage of the esophagus and paradoxically maintain (or augment) control of gastroesophageal reflux. Heller's original technique was a two-sided myotomy through a laparotomy. This was abandoned because of late severe reflux complications. A single myotomy is now accepted by all as allowing enough reduction in LES pressure to relieve outflow obstruction (Fig. 136.7). Many South American and most European surgeons continued with the laparotomy approach because, in those areas historically, visceral surgeons usually operated on the esophagus. American thoracic surgeons who have historically operated on the esophagus, naturally approached a myotomy through the chest. With the advent of minimally invasive surgery in the early 1990s, esophageal myotomy was performed with video-assisted thoracic surgery (VATS) techniques. This approach had several disadvantages: the myotomy must be approached perpendicularly, single-lung ventilation is required intraoperatively, and chest drainage is required postoperatively.[44] Ramacciato and colleagues[45] compared the VATS and the laparoscopic approaches to myotomy within their own unit. Laparoscopic myotomy (Fig. 136.8) was found to be superior in several areas: shorter length of surgery, shorter length of stay, better dysphagia relief, less postoperative heartburn, and less incisional discomfort. Table 136.2 summarizes the recent study outcomes from laparoscopic Heller myotomy and POEM.

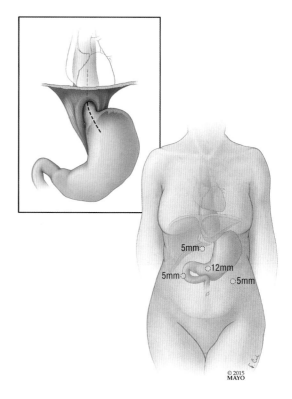

FIGURE 136.8 Technique for laparoscopic modified Heller myotomy. Laparoscopic access is gained via a supraumbilical camera port, placement of two 5 mm working ports in the right and left lower quadrant, and a subxiphoid 5 mm working port. Used with permission of Mayo Foundation for Medical Education and Research, all rights reserved.

Conversion to an open procedure is very rare. Intraoperative mucosal injury occurs in about 5% of patients and can almost always be handled with laparoscopic suturing and buttressing with an anterior Dor wrap. There are various techniques to perform the myotomy; it is not clear which is best.[46–48] Myotomy can be performed with scissors, hook, and cautery division, or by tearing muscle fibers between two forceps. It is very important not to injure the mucosa with the cautery, which could present as a delayed perforation. We prefer the scissors. Almost all bleeding from muscular vessels will stop with time and pressure during the myotomy, which helps to avoid the need for cauterization. Many surgeons obtain a control barium swallow the following morning to document the relief of LES obstruction and the absence of a leak. But authors of several large series report abandoning the routine use of postoperative barium swallow, citing extremely low yield and no effect on postoperative management. Liquids are allowed the first day and rapidly advanced to a soft diet. The average length of stay is 1 to 2 days. Most series report good results in 90% to 95% and heartburn in 5% to 25%. Well into the second decade of this technique, there are now long-term data demonstrating continued successful outcome. Wright and colleagues[49] followed, for a median of 63 months, 30 of their patients who underwent laparoscopic Heller myotomy and found no significant worsening of patient dysphagia during that period. After a mean follow-up of 95 months, Costantini and colleagues[47] found that although symptom scores with regard to dysphagia, regurgitation, and chest pain worsened over time, they were all still significantly improved from preoperative values. Furthermore, they found that more than half of the episodes of symptom recurrence appeared within the first year postoperatively. Although most surgeons consider laparoscopic Heller myotomy the surgical treatment of choice for achalasia, controversy still exists regarding

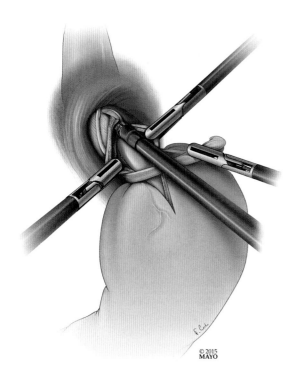

FIGURE 136.7 With a single myotomy, the esophagus is circumferentially dissected and a Penrose drain is placed around the esophagus to aid in retraction. Sharp dissection is then used to dissect the muscular layer along the anterior aspect of the esophagus. Dissection is carried proximally to the level of the inferior pulmonary ligament and distally 2 to 3 cm onto the gastric cardia, avoiding the left anterior vagal nerve. Used with permission of Mayo Foundation for Medical Education and Research, all rights reserved.

TABLE 136.2 Recent Studies on Laparoscopic Heller and Perioral Endoscopic Myotomy

Reference, Study	Type of Patients	No. of Fundoplications	Type of Fundoplication if Any (No. of Pts if Multiple Types Available)	Median/Mean Follow-up (Range)	Length of Gastric Cardiomyotomy	Intraoperative Endoscopy	Postoperative Outcomes Measured	Rate of Postoperative Dysphagia	Rate of Postoperative Gastroesophageal Reflux
Bessell et al.,[50] 2006	Retrospective	167	Dor	49 months	0.5–1 cm	Yes	Symptom score	18%, 27%, 23% at 1, 3, 5 years	By symptoms: 29%, 34%, 34% at 1, 3, 5 years (based on frequency daily or several times per week)
Bonatti et al.,[46] 2005	Retrospective	75 (includes 3 VATS)	Dor (8), Toupet (64), VATS none (3)	63.6 months (10–131)	1–2 cm	Yes	Symptom score	16%	By symptoms: 11%
Costan-tini M, et al.,[47] 2005	Retrospective	71	Dor	95 months (75–134)	1–1.5 cm	No	Symptom score, manometry, barium swallow, endoscopy	18.3%	By symptoms or pH probe: 12.7% (but no severe esophagitis on endoscopy)
Deb et al.,[34] 2005	Retrospective	211 (79% follow-up data available)	Dor (63), Toupet (135), none (13)	5.3 months (1–71)	2 cm	No	Symptom score, barium swallow	11%	By symptoms: 25%
Finley et al.,[51] 2007	Retrospective	95	Dor (71), none (24)	6.9 months	2 cm	Yes	Symptom score, esophageal clearance	6% Dor, 0% none	By symptoms: 6% Dor, 4% no wrap
Inoue et al.,[52] 2015	Prospective	500	POEM	36 months	3 cm	Yes	Symptom score, manometry	NR (median ES-1 @ 1 yr and 1 @ 3 yrs)	16.8% 2 months 21.3% at 3 yrs
Khasab et al.,[53] 2015	Retrospective	73	POEM	234 days	2 cm	Yes	Symptom score, pH probe	NR (75% ES 0–1 @ 118 days)	Symptoms 10% at 6–8 weeks
Khajanchee et al.,[23] 2005	Retrospective	121	Toupet	9 months (6–48)	2 cm	No	Symptom score, manometry, pH probe	9%	By pH probe: 33.3%
Rice et al.,[54] 2005	Retrospective	149	Dor (88), none (61)	64–69 days	>2 cm	No	Manometry, timed barium swallow, pH probe	Not reported	See discussion
Rossetti et al.,[55] 2005	Retrospective	195	Nissen	83.2 months (3–141)	>2 cm	Yes	Symptom score, 38% had manometry, pH probe, and barium swallow	8.2%	By pH probe: 0
Wright et al.,[49] 2007	Retrospective	115	Dor (52), Toupet (63)	46 months	1–2 cm (Dor group), >3 cm (Toupet group)	No	Symptom score, 33% had pH probe and manometry	17% Dor (short myotomy), 5% Toupet	By pH probe: 31.3% Toupet (long myotomy), 13.5% Dor

ES = Eckhardt Score.

the length of the gastric portion of the myotomy,[56] and which, if any, antireflux repair should be performed.

Whether to include an antireflux procedure is a highly debated issue. In a meta analysis of 21 studies from 1995 to 2000, Lyass et al.[57] compared 532 patients who underwent laparoscopic Heller with fundoplication to 69 patients without fundoplication. There was no significant difference in the severity of gastroesophageal reflux symptoms or the rate of reflux detected by pH monitor between the two groups, although there was a trend toward a lower rate of reflux on pH probe studies in the group with fundoplication. Recurrent postoperative dysphagia occurred in 1.5% of the nonfundoplication patients, with one patient requiring reoperation, and in 3.2% of the fundoplication patients, with three requiring takedown of the fundoplication, two requiring myotomy revision, and one ultimately requiring esophagectomy. In a recent study with short-term follow-up by Finley and colleagues,[51] 24 patients who underwent laparoscopic Heller without fundoplication had greater improvement in esophageal clearance time (by nuclear study) than did 71 patients whose procedure included a Dor fundoplication. The authors noted, however, that there was significantly worse esophageal clearance in the no-wrap group compared with the Dor group preoperatively, perhaps allowing more "room for improvement." Nevertheless, there were no significant differences in the symptom scores for dysphagia, regurgitation, or heartburn between the two groups postoperatively. Bloomston and Rosemurgy[58] reported their experience using fundoplication only for specific indications: to buttress an esophageal repair or to manage a patulous hiatus or hiatal hernia. They found no significant difference in postoperative dysphagia scores between patients who had fundoplication and those who did not. Rice et al.[54] found that patients with fundoplication (N = 88) had higher resting and residual LES pressures postoperatively than those without fundoplication (N = 61). The investigators did not report patients' symptoms to corroborate the clinical impact of these data. The no-wrap group had more time of pathologic reflux (percentage of time with pH <4 on 24-hour pH probe) while supine postoperatively than the wrap group, although there was no significant difference in percentage of time with pathologic reflux while upright.

In a landmark prospective study, Richards and colleagues[59] randomized patients to laparoscopic myotomy with (N = 22) and without (N = 21) Dor fundoplication and followed their symptoms as well as manometric and 24-hour pH probe results postoperatively. There was no significant difference in postoperative dysphagia between the groups. The non-fundoplication patients had higher median acid exposure time, higher number of episodes of acid exposure, and higher percentage time of acid exposure both supine and upright. Although these are impressive data, their clinical impact, for example, on the incidence of peptic stricture or Barrett's transition, is unknown. Moreover, the incidence of pathologic gastroesophageal reflux disease (GERD) (as defined by >4.2% of a 24-hour period with pH <4) in non-fundoplication patients in this study (47.6%) was markedly higher than that in other series, including one by the same group.[60] The authors attribute this difference to the more recent study involving a younger patient population with lower LES pressures; they had found these two risk factors to be associated with the development of pathologic GERD after Heller myotomy. In an interesting report, the same group performed a cost-utility analysis based on 1-year follow-up data from their randomized trial.[61] They used the Markov simulation model to project cost and adjust quality of life for postoperative GERD and dysphagia. Although the operative cost of the Dor group was higher owing to longer operating room time, projected costs at 10 years showed Dor to be cost-effective when the cost of proton-pump inhibitor therapy was taken into account ($6,800 vs. $9,500 per patient over 10 years).

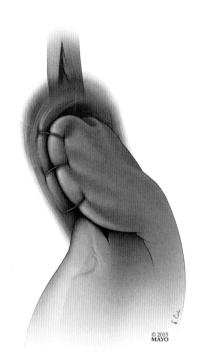

FIGURE 136.9 Demonstration of a Dor fundoplication. An anterior 180-degree Dor fundoplication can be performed where the cardia of the stomach is sewn to the muscular fibers of the left side of the myotomy, then the right side of the myotomy, and finally to the right crus of the diaphragm. Used with permission of Mayo Foundation for Medical Education and Research, all rights reserved.

Even among those who agree that routine partial fundoplication should be added to a laparoscopic myotomy, the type of wrap has varied. Although nearly all surgeons agree that a Nissen total fundoplication results in excessive obstruction in the face of an aperistaltic esophagus, Rossetti and colleagues[55] reported 92% excellent or good outcomes and no postoperative reflux using a modified Nissen, in which they did not take down the short gastric vessels and their sutures did not include the esophagus or the diaphragmatic crura. Also, they calibrated the high-pressure zone using intraoperative manometry and reconstructed the wrap if it was not within a 20 to 40 mm Hg range. The Dor anterior wrap (Fig. 136.9) is favored by many because it can buttress small perforations and does not require taking down the posterior esophageal attachments. On the other hand, many feel the Toupet wrap (Fig. 136.10) keeps the myotomy edges distracted, decreasing the chance of sclerosis between the edges, which can cause delayed and recurrent postoperative dysphagia. In two papers, Oelschlager and Pellegrini's group[49,62] compared their patients who had undergone laparoscopic Heller with Dor to those with Toupet as they modified their technique in 1998. The Toupet group had significantly less severe and less frequent dysphagia than their Dor counterparts in the short and long term, with no difference in the frequency of heartburn or percentage of pathologic reflux on pH probe. Over time, the Toupet group had a significantly higher percentage of patients requiring proton-pump inhibitor therapy. The results of these two studies are difficult to interpret, however, because two variables were changed in the authors' technique: both the type of fundoplication and the length of gastric cardiomyotomy, with the Dor patients undergoing a short myotomy (1 to 2 cm) and the Toupet patients undergoing a longer myotomy (3 cm) onto the cardia. In reviewing their experience with laparoscopic myotomy, Deb and colleagues[34]

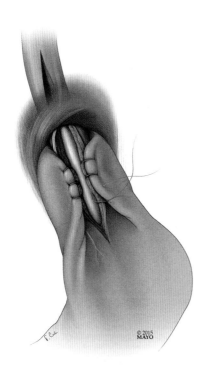

found no significant difference in functional outcome between 63 patients who underwent Heller with Dor and 135 patients with Toupet. To date, there have been no randomized prospective trials comparing types of fundoplication, and although it seems that a partial wrap should be added to the laparoscopic Heller myotomy, there is no consensus on the type that should be performed.

There has been some disagreement over the length of the gastric portion of the myotomy. While laparoscopy allows access for a longer gastric cardiomyotomy, some surgeons historically prefer a shorter myotomy (0.5 cm) to preserve the sling fibers of Willis, hoping to minimize postoperative reflux. The only major reports comparing shorter with longer myotomy have been published by Oelschlager[62] and Wright[49] from the same series of patients. The authors modified their technique over time when they noticed that dysphagia improved profoundly after the myotomy was extended well below the GEJ in patients who required reoperation after thoracoscopic myotomy. The studies compared a group of patients who had shorter gastric myotomies (1 to 2 cm) with Dor fundoplication to a group that had a 3-cm "extended" gastric myotomy with Toupet. Again, the authors found that the extended myotomy group had less postoperative dysphagia and required fewer interventional procedures for recurrent dysphagia, but there were two major variables that differed between the groups (myotomy length and antireflux procedure). Although there are no randomized trials supporting a specific length, most current studies report using a 1- to 2-cm gastric cardiomyotomy.

Most surgeons have found intraoperative endoscopy to be helpful, especially early in their experience, to locate the squamocolumnar junction and gauge the adequacy of the distal extent of the myotomy (the LES is seen, and one can readily see into the stomach from the distal esophagus when the last few gastric fibers are cut). Alves et al.[29] evaluated the benefit of intraoperative endoscopy in a retrospective series using laparoscopic and endoscopic criteria to identify the location of the cardia in 19 patients. By laparoscopy, the cardia was identified by its vessels, the change in muscle fiber direction and thickness, and adherence of the muscular layer to the mucosa. The endoscopic criteria were change in the color and appearance of mucosal folds with transillumination to identify this area for myotomy. There was discordance in cardia location in 58% of cases, with the endoscopic criteria pointing to a more distal location each time. These patients were compared with the 16 patients who underwent laparoscopic Heller in the practice of Alves and colleagues[29] before the introduction of intraoperative endoscopy. The authors attributed delayed complications to suboptimal myotomy in 11% of their intraoperative endoscopy patients and in 44% of their nonendoscopy patients. Given the learning curve involved in laparoscopic myotomy, this difference may be related to evolution of the surgeons' skills, as the nonendoscopy patients were earlier cases in their experience. Overall, while many surgeons favor intraoperative endoscopy to guide myotomy and help evaluate for perforation, there are no convincing series to support its routine use.

The selection of therapy for an individual patient remains controversial. A randomized trial from 2011 does demonstrate similar rates of therapeutic success between pneumatic dilation and laparoscopic Heller myotomy; however, it should be noted that this trial had limited follow-up at 2 years.[36] It is not surprising that the technical procedural results are better with surgical myotomy because it is done under direct vision and is quite precise. In the end, the patient must be presented with the management options and have a thorough discussion of the risks and benefits of each technique to help make an individual decision.

POEM (PER ORAL ENDOSCOPIC MYOTOMY)

Per oral endoscopic myotomy is an endoscopic treatment modality utilized in the treatment of achalasia that was first described in the 1980s. Pasricha,[63] first described the technique in a human in 2007 and was the first to demonstrate outcomes in a series of patients.

All patients with primary symptoms and manometric findings of achalasia can be considered for the POEM procedure. Initially sigmoid esophagus and prior gastric bypass surgery were thought to be relative contraindications; however, recent data have demonstrated feasibility in these patients.

The technique is described by placing a forward viewing endoscope with the patient under general anesthesia (Fig. 136.11). A submucosal tunnel is created proximal to the LES with a mixture of saline and 0.3% indigo carmine and carried down 2 to 3 cm onto the proximal stomach (Figs. 136.12 to 136.15). The circular muscle layer is then cut with a triangle-tip knife and spray coagulation current (Fig. 136.16). Initially, only the circular layer was divided, but as techniques have evolved, many endoscopists are now performing a full thickness myotomy. The mucosal entry site is then closed with endoscopic clips (Fig. 136.17). Patients are typically admitted overnight for observation and discharged the following day on a soft solid diet.

Current literature supports the feasibility and safety of POEM.[64] Inoue[37] reported a statistically significant decrease in the symptoms of dysphagia within his patient population and a decrease in LES pressure. Outcomes from further studies appear to corroborate this data, with a multicenter study of 804 patients[66] demonstrating clinical success in 82% to 100% of patients. A systematic review with meta-analysis conducted in 2015 further demonstrated technical success of 97% and clinical success of 93%.[67] More recently, intraoperative technology titled Endolumenal Functional Lumen Imaging Probe (EndoFLIP) involves using a balloon catheter to quantitatively

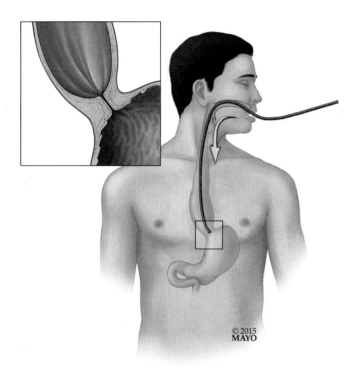

FIGURE 136.11 Peroral endoscopic myotomy (POEM). The upper endoscope is inserted into the patient while under general anesthesia. The lower esophageal sphincter is visualized. Used with permission of Mayo Foundation for Medical Education and Research, all rights reserved.

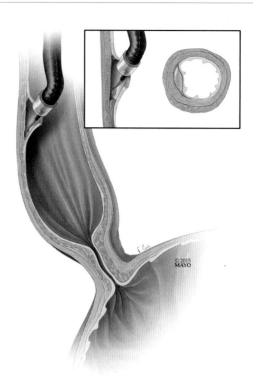

FIGURE 136.13 Submucosal fluid is injected to dissect the submucosa away from the muscle layers, facilitating the mucosotomy. Used with permission of Mayo Foundation for Medical Education and Research, all rights reserved.

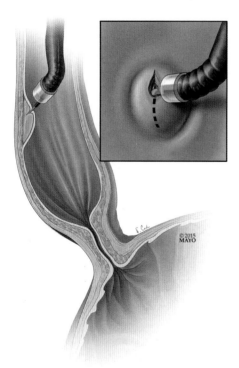

FIGURE 136.12 A mucosotomy is performed 25 to 30 cm from the incisors. Used with permission of Mayo Foundation for Medical Education and Research, all rights reserved.

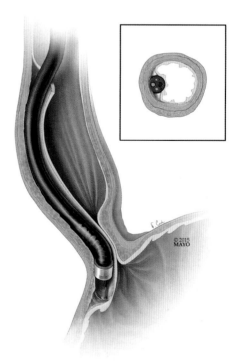

FIGURE 136.14 The mucosotomy allows the creation of a submucosal tunnel along the posterior wall of the esophagus. The ERBE hybrid-T knife is used to extend the submucosal tunnel. Used with permission of Mayo Foundation for Medical Education and Research, all rights reserved.

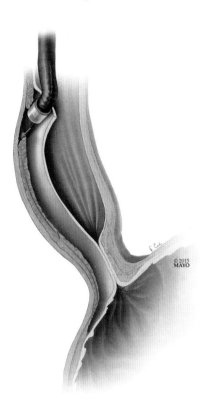

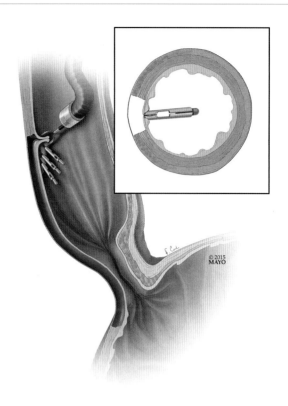

FIGURE 136.15 A posterior myotomy is typically initially performed. Used with permission of Mayo Foundation for Medical Education and Research, all rights reserved.

FIGURE 136.17 Following myotomy, resolution clips are placed on the mucosotomy site in a zipper fashion to facilitate closure. Used with permission of Mayo Foundation for Medical Education and Research, all rights reserved.

measure the luminal diameter to estimate gastroesophageal sphincter distention as a predictor of postoperative resolution of symptoms.

Barbieri's group[67] reported no mortality events with an adverse event incidence of 14%, mostly related to pneumoperitoneum, perforation, or bleeding. The rate of post-POEM esophagitis was 13%, which is comparable to the 21% which is reported in some larger series of patients undergoing laparoscopic myotomy.

Inoue[52] recently published a single-center prospective review of 500 consecutive patients treated with POEM for achalasia. The results are encouraging, demonstrating a reduction in LES pressure from 25.4 to 13.4 mg Hg at 2 months post-procedure with a 21% incidence of GERD reported at 3 years. Adverse events were also low, reported at 3.2%. Although there has yet to be a direct randomized comparison between Heller myotomy and POEM, the current data would suggest that POEM is a successful treatment option in patients.

ACHALASIA ASSOCIATED WITH EPIPHRENIC DIVERTICULUM

Epiphrenic diverticulum is almost always associated with an esophageal motility disorder, with about half the cases characterized as achalasia. Nehra and colleagues[68] reported 21 patients with diverticula and reviewed the recent literature. All of their patients had a motility disorder, and a consistent finding on ambulatory motility studies was a high percentage of simultaneous waveforms with esophageal body contractions of increased amplitude and duration. Pneumatic dilation is not appropriate because the torn esophageal muscle will not extend to the base of the diverticulum, and the diverticulum is left in place. The standard procedure is a left transthoracic myotomy to the base of the diverticulum and a diverticulectomy. There are numerous reports, including that of Rosati and colleagues,[69] of laparoscopic myotomy

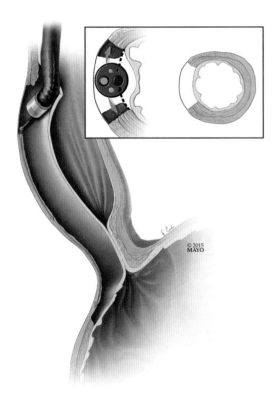

FIGURE 136.16 A full thickness myotomy is performed in the distal esophagus, lower esophageal sphincter, and cardia. A resolution clip is placed on the anterior wall of the gastroesophageal junction and the endoscope advanced to distal end of the myotomy. Fluoroscopy is used to confirm the tip of the endoscope distal to this clip and well into the cardia. Used with permission of Mayo Foundation for Medical Education and Research, all rights reserved.

and diverticulectomy. For a laparoscopic approach to be feasible, the diverticulum has to be very close to the cardia (as it usually is) for sufficient access through the hiatus. Details of the management of epiphrenic diverticula are presented in Chapter 156.

ESOPHAGECTOMY FOR ACHALASIA

Esophagectomy is rarely appropriate as primary therapy for achalasia and occasionally appropriate as a salvage treatment for late complications. Absolute indications for esophagectomy include resectable cancer, multiple failed previous treatments, reflux strictures, intractable esophagitis, obstruction associated with an overly competent fundoplication, and perforation of an end-stage dilated esophagus. Relative indications include a single failed myotomy in an end-stage dilated esophagus and initial treatment of an end-stage sigmoid-shaped esophagus. Most surgeons suggest that the results of dilation or myotomy with a sigmoid esophagus are so poor that the additional risk for esophagectomy is warranted. The massively dilated sigmoid-shaped esophagus (Fig. 136.18) empties so poorly that an aperistaltic narrow gastric conduit empties better. Banbury,[70] Miller,[71] Peters,[72] and Devaney[73] have reported large series of esophagectomies for achalasia. In Devaney's[73] report on 93 patients, the indications for resection were sigmoid esophagus (64%), failed previous procedures (29%), and reflux stricture (7%). Transhiatal resection was possible in 94% of patients. The stomach was used in all but two patients. There were two postoperative deaths. The average hospital stay was 12.5 days. Ninety-five percent of the patients are able to eat a regular diet, 71% had a good or excellent result, and 88% were pleased they had an operation. The authors made several

technical points: (a) the esophagus is usually very deviated into the right chest, which complicates resection; (b) the direct esophageal aortic arteries are often quite enlarged and must be carefully controlled; (c) the dilated esophagus makes the cervical esophagus difficult to encircle, so that caution must be used to avoid recurrent nerve injuries; and (d) the exposed esophageal submucosa after prior myotomy is often very adherent to the aorta and lung that complicates resection. Peters[72] and DeMeester have long advocated the use of colon as a better conduit for esophageal replacement in achalasia. He emphasizes that the stomach regains its acid-secreting ability despite the vagotomy, which can lead to late esophagitis and strictures of the proximal esophagus. His group reported excellent results with the use of a colon interposition, with no deaths in 19 patients. Most groups, however, report more early complications with the use of the colon rather than the stomach, especially the occasional devastating ischemic colon graft.

ACHALASIA AND ESOPHAGEAL CANCER

The end result of years of chronic esophageal mucosal irritation from saliva, undigested food, bacteria, and refluxate in the end stage of achalasia esophagus is cancer. Streitz and colleagues[74] reported on 241 collected patients who developed squamous cell cancer of the esophagus in association with achalasia. The patients uniformly presented with advanced disease and accordingly had a dismal prognosis. They made the point that in the dilated obstructed achalasia esophagus a cancer has to grow to a large size and cause severe dysphagia before the patient can recognize this as a new problem. The risk was estimated to be 14.5 times that of the normal population. Reflux esophagitis is also a late chronic complication of achalasia. It is therefore not surprising that Barrett's mucosa and adenocarcinoma have also been reported by Di Simone and colleagues.[75]

GE JUNCTION OUTFLOW OBSTRUCTION OUTFLOW

GEJ outflow (Fig. 136.19) is a unique entity that is defined as a failure of LES relaxation, evidenced on HRM as an elevated IRP >15 mm Hg. It is differentiated from achalasia by a preservation of peristalsis. Diagnostic evaluation consists of barium esophagram, EGD, and potentially EUS, as many causes of GEJ outflow obstruction may be related to mechanical causes, such as neoplasm.

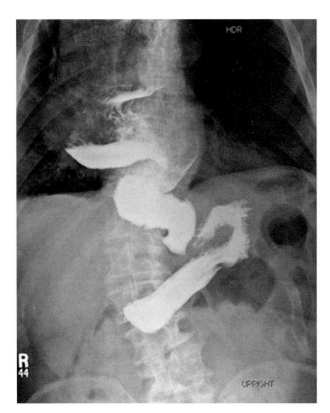

FIGURE 136.18 Upright abdominal barium swallow esophagram depicting sigmoidization of the esophagus as end-stage achalasia, with a "bird-beak" esophagogastric junction, with an increased transverse diameter of the thoracic esophagus at greater than 8 cm.

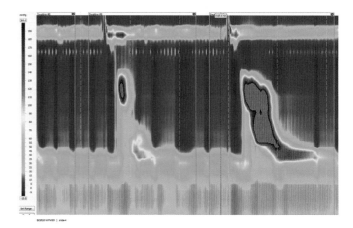

FIGURE 136.19 High-resolution manometry in a patient with gastroesophageal outflow obstruction. Pertinent findings include preserved peristalsis with an IRP greater than 15.

If radiographic studies fail to demonstrate a mechanical cause and functional GEJ outflow obstruction is diagnosed, medical therapy comparable to the treatment of achalasia can be considered. However, treatment should be tailored to meet symptomatology.

DIFFUSE ESOPHAGEAL SPASM

Diffuse esophageal spasm (DES) (Fig. 136.20) is a rare motility disorder characterized by intermittent dysphagia and chest pain with normal peristalsis intermittently interrupted by simultaneous contractions. DES is rare and is seen in <5% of patients with motility disorders. The mean age of affected patients is about 50 years, and more women are affected than men.

HISTORY

Osgood[76] reported the first cases of esophageal spasm with dysphagia. Creamer and colleagues[77] were the first to report the manometric feature of simultaneous contractions in DES. Richter and Castell[5] clarified the manometric definition for DES: simultaneous contractions associated with >20% of wet swallows (but <100%) and mean simultaneous contraction amplitude >30 mm Hg.

PATHOPHYSIOLOGY

The etiology of DES is unknown. Most reports, including those of Friesen[78] and Eypasch[79] and their colleagues, demonstrate no changes in the esophageal muscle and myenteric plexus. Patients with DES are hypersensitive to cholinergic and hormonal (pentagastrin) stimulation. Recent studies implicate decreased available nitric oxide in the etiology of DES, as reported by Behr and Biancani[80] and Konturek and colleagues.[81]

DIAGNOSIS

Clinical Features

Intermittent chest pain and dysphagia are the common presenting symptoms. The chest pain can be indistinguishable from ischemic cardiac pain and can also respond to nitroglycerin. The pain can vary in intensity, location, and frequency. It is not related to exertion and may relate to meals. The pain is usually substernal but may be epigastric and can radiate to the neck and arm like ischemic pain. The dysphagia is intermittent, is nonprogressive, and can occur with both solids and liquids. Dysphagia may be precipitated by stress, very hot or cold liquids, or rapid eating. Some patients also have other intestinal dysmotility syndromes, such as irritable bowel syndrome.

Radiographic Evaluation

Contrast esophagograms can be normal but classically show segmental spasm of the distal esophagus, which has been described as corkscrew esophagus or pseudodiverticulosis of the esophagus. Diffuse spasm can be suggested by the barium swallow appearance but is not diagnostic, as reported by Fuller and colleagues.[82] CT of the esophagus invariably demonstrates a markedly thickened esophageal wall.

Manometry

DES is defined as >20% simultaneous contractions intermixed with normal peristalsis (Fig. 136.2). If all contractions are simultaneous,

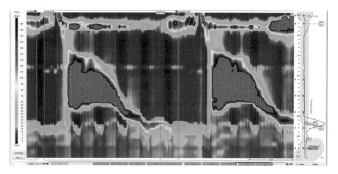

FIGURE 136.20 High-resolution manometry in a patient with diffuse esophageal spasm. Characteristic findings include normal lower esophageal pressure with normal LES relaxation. Wave progression is simultaneous and should be visualized in greater than 20% of the swallows with normal wave amplitude.

the diagnosis is achalasia. Patients with pain tend to have high contraction pressures, whereas those without pain have lower pressures. The simultaneous contractions are often >30 mm Hg. Other findings include long-duration contractions, spontaneous non-swallow–induced contractions, repetitive waves (three peaks or more), and occasionally incomplete LES relaxation, as reported by Richter.[5] Ambulatory 24-hour manometry is more sensitive for the diagnosis of DES, and meal-induced swallows are especially disordered, as reported by Eypasch and colleagues.[79]

Based on high-resolution manometry, a patient would be considered to have DES if 20% or greater of the swallows had a DL of less than 4.5 seconds, suggesting a premature contraction. According to the Chicago Classification, normal LES relaxation would be expected.

TREATMENT

There is no definitive treatment for DES. It is critical to eliminate ischemic cardiac disease as the cause of the patient's symptoms. Some patients with mild DES improve with simple reassurance. More symptomatic patients require medical treatment. Patients who fail a prolonged trial of all medical therapies and who have a persistently poor quality of life are candidates for extended myotomy.

Medical Therapy

Patients should be evaluated for gastroesophageal reflux by 24-hour pH probe testing and treated, if reflux is found, with proton-pump inhibitors. The same drugs that can be used in achalasia have some degree of efficacy in DES. These include nitrates, anticholinergics, and calcium channel blockers. The frequent presence of anxiety and affective disorders in these patients has led to the use of anxiolytics and antidepressants. Clouse and colleagues[83] have reported a randomized trial of trazodone (an antidepressant) to treat the chest pain. The drug was effective in relieving pain perception but did not alter manometric findings.

Dilation

Simple dilation has been described for patients with dysphagia but has no physiologic basis; any response is likely to be the placebo effect only. Forceful dilation has no role in most patients because the entire distal esophagus is affected. The rare patient with impaired LES relaxation and dysphagia may benefit from pneumatic dilation.

Botulinum Toxin Injection

Numerous reports suggest some efficacy for the treatment of both dysphagia and chest pain in patients with DES, including those of Miller[84] and Storr[85] and their colleagues. Storr treated nine patients by multiple injections of botulinum toxin from the LES and along the body of the esophagus. At 1 month, eight of nine patients were markedly improved, with reduction in symptom scores from 8 to 2 after treatment. At 6 months, all eight responders were still improved. Four patients needed repeat injections at a mean of 15 months, with similar good results.

Extended Esophagomyotomy

Surgical treatment is reserved for true medical failures because the surgical results are not as good or as predictable as those for achalasia. Patients should be cautioned that the procedure is palliative and is intended to reduce symptoms rather than eliminate them altogether. The extent of myotomy is determined by preoperative manometry. The myotomy can be extended under the aortic arch through the left chest to the thoracic inlet if needed. The LES does not need to be divided if it is normal on manometry. Most surgeons approach an extended myotomy through the left chest. The extent of myotomy (proximal and distal) and the need for an antireflux repair are areas of controversy. Leonardi and colleagues[86] reported the results of extended myotomy (sparing the LES and avoiding an antireflux procedure) in 11 patients; 10 patients improved, and reflux was a problem in only 1 patient. Eypasch and colleagues[79] reported the results of extended myotomy (dividing the LES and adding a Dor fundoplication) in 15 patients. There was improvement in chest pain in 12 patients and dysphagia in 14. Twelve of 14 patients stated they would have the operation again. Patti and colleagues[15] reported a thoracoscopic approach to extended myotomy for DES.

HYPERCONTRACTILE/JACKHAMMER ESOPHAGUS (FORMERLY NUTCRACKER ESOPHAGUS)

Hypercontracting (or nutcracker) esophagus is a motility disorder with high-amplitude esophageal contractions and chest pain. With advent of high-resolution manometry this clinical entity has been redefined as jackhammer esophagus and was first described by Roman and colleagues.[87]

PATHOPHYSIOLOGY

The etiology of jackhammer esophagus is unknown. No pathologic changes are seen in the muscle or myenteric plexus. Some high-pressure contractions are related to either reflux or stress. The correlation between the high-amplitude contractions and pain is unclear because most patients can be asymptomatic while undergoing manometry. Relief of chest pain does not reliably correlate with reduction of contraction amplitude following medical or surgical therapy. The

abnormal contractions may represent an epiphenomenon rather than a true motility disorder. Richter[88] and Mujica[89] and their colleagues reproduced chest pain in these patients with balloon distention of the esophagus.

DIAGNOSIS

Clinical Features

The average age of the patients is the fifth decade, and most are women. Almost all patients complain of dysphagia as the primary symptom, with reflux or chest pain as secondary complaints. Cardiac ischemia must be eliminated as a possible cause of pain in these patients, just as in those with DES.

Radiographic Evaluation

Peristalsis is normal in these patients; thus contrast esophagrams are usually normal.

Manometry

Primary manometric findings (Fig. 136.21) include normal gastroesophageal relaxation pressure (IRP <15), with a hypercontractile esophageal body peristalsis. DCI is elevated in greater than 20% of swallows.

TREATMENT

As with DES, the treatment of hypercontracting esophagus has unpredictable results. In a double-blind crossover study, Richter and colleagues[5,90] showed no difference between nifedipine and placebo in relieving patients' chest pain. In contrast, Cattau and colleagues[91] showed reduced chest pain and lower contraction amplitudes with diltiazem. Trazodone, imipramine, tricyclic antidepressants, and theophylline[92] have been suggested as beneficial. Winters and colleagues[93] reported an interesting trial of placebo dilation with a 24-Fr dilator versus a therapeutic 54-Fr dilator. Neither would be expected to provide any benefit, given the pathophysiology of hypercontracting esophagus. Both groups of patients reported reduced chest pain, with no difference between the two. As esophageal contractions do not reliably correlate with chest pain and symptoms, extended myotomy may not help these patients. Traube[94] and Shimi[95] and their colleagues have reported mixed success with surgical myotomy.

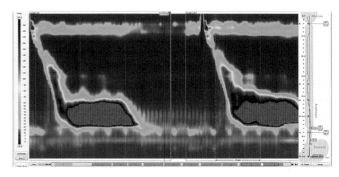

FIGURE 136.21 High-resolution manometry in a patient with Jackhammer esophagus. This disorder is characteristically defined by high-amplitude repetitive contractions in the setting of elevated digital contractile intervals (DCI) in the presence of normal lower esophageal sphincter relaxation.

HYPOCONTRACTING ESOPHAGUS (INEFFECTIVE ESOPHAGEAL MOTILITY)

Most patients who were previously diagnosed with a nonspecific motility disorder have motility tracings with low-amplitude (<30 mm Hg) peristaltic waves, simultaneous contractions in the distal esophagus, or failed peristalsis (Fig. 136.4). These abnormalities have been renamed *ineffective esophageal motility* by Leite and colleagues.[4] Patients often have low LES pressure, but it may be normal. Low-amplitude (<30 mm Hg) waves have been demonstrated by Kahrilas and colleagues,[96] using simultaneous manometry and barium video radiography, to be ineffective at esophageal clearance. Most patients with ineffective esophageal motility have GERD with heartburn and regurgitation. The abnormal acid exposure in these patients correlates more with poor esophageal clearance than does resting LES pressure. Dysphagia is usually absent or mild in these patients. Severe dysphagia implies that there is an anatomic lesion such as severe esophagitis, stricture, or cancer. It is unclear whether gastroesophageal reflux leads to the development of ineffective esophageal motility by repeated esophageal acid exposure or whether the presence of preexisting poor esophageal peristalsis leads to ineffective esophageal clearance mechanisms, producing abnormal gastroesophageal reflux. Scleroderma is the classic example of severe esophageal hypocontraction. Patients with scleroderma have vascular obliteration and secondary fibrosis of the nerves and muscle, which weaken contractions and result in loss of normal peristalsis. It is defined on HRM as aperistalsis with low or absent LES pressure <10 mm Hg. Similar manometric findings can be seen in other connective tissue diseases as well as a variety of systemic diseases such as alcoholism, diabetes, amyloidosis, and myxedema. Treatment is directed at controlling gastroesophageal reflux with proton-pump inhibitors. There is no effective drug to increase esophageal motility. Cisapride was used in the past, but it has been withdrawn from the market because of its rare association with cardiac arrhythmias.

SECONDARY ESOPHAGEAL MOTILITY DISORDERS

Patients with secondary disorders of esophageal motility have motility disorders from another systemic disease, such as scleroderma (Fig. 136.22). Table 136.3 lists the most common diseases that affect esophageal motility. Treatment is usually directed at the underlying disease, and reflux symptoms are treated with proton-pump inhibitors. Chagas' disease is a special case and is discussed in detail in Chapter 150.

TABLE 136.3 Secondary Esophageal Motility Disorders

Secondary achalasia
  Pseudoachalasia (cancer)
  Chagas' disease
  Infiltrating diseases
  Amyloidosis
  Sarcoidosis
  Systemic diseases
  Diabetes mellitus
  Generalized intestinal dysmotility
  Neuromuscular diseases
  Parkinson's disease

Secondary dysmotility disorders
  Scleroderma
  Diabetes mellitus
  Amyloidosis
  Connective tissue disorders
  Parkinson's disease
  Myxedema
  Crohn's disease
  Presbyesophagus
  Neuromuscular disorders
  Intestinal dysmotility
  Alcoholism

PSEUDOACHALASIA (SECONDARY ACHALASIA)

The radiologic and manometric diagnosis of primary achalasia is not absolute, because approximately 4% of patients who present with "classic" achalasia actually have pseudoachalasia. This entity is an achalasia-like syndrome most often due to a cancer of the esophagogastric junction infiltrating the myenteric plexus, as noted by DiBaise and Quigley.[97] All patients with newly suspected achalasia must have endoscopic evaluation of the upper gastrointestinal tract (Fig. 136.23). If there is significant resistance to passage of the scope through the esophagogastric junction, a cancer should be suspected, even in the absence of a mucosal abnormality. An endoscopic ultrasound exam and a CT scan should be done to evaluate this area thoroughly. Kahrilas and colleagues[2,98,99] compared the clinical features of the two types of achalasia. Clinical features that suggest carcinoma-induced achalasia include older age, rapid symptom development, significant weight loss, progressive dysphagia, and difficulty passing the manometry catheter through the LES. Liu and colleagues[100] reported 13 cases of pseudoachalasia and found neoplastic infiltration of the myenteric plexus in 11 patients. A paraneoplastic syndrome was thought to be the cause in the other two patients. The neoplasms included adenocarcinoma of the esophagogastric junction (7), esophageal cancer (1), metastatic renal cell cancer to the esophagogastric junction (1), breast cancer (1), small-cell lung cancer (1), mesothelioma (1), and mediastinal fibrosis

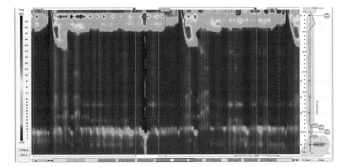

FIGURE 136.22 Esophageal manometry tracing from a patient with aperistalsis (such as scleroderma). Aperistalsis is visualized with low or absent LES pressure <10 mm Hg and low wave amplitudes.

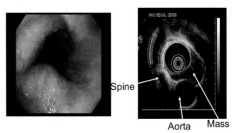

FIGURE 136.23 Endoscopic and EUS findings in a patient with pseudoachalasia.

(1). The treatment of pseudoachalasia is the treatment of the underlying cancer.

INEFFECTIVE ESOPHAGEAL MOTILITY

Ineffective esophageal motility is a very commonly identified manometric abnormality defined by weak peristaltic contractions in more than 50% of swallows.[4] Patients present with GERD, with dysphagia being a less common complaint. Although the disorder has been identified on imaging studies and has been associated with failure of bolus clearance, the clinical significance of this entity remains unknown.

REFERENCES

1. Patti MG, Molena D, Fisichella PM, et al. Laparoscopic Heller myotomy and Dor fundoplication for achalasia: analysis of successes and failures. *Arch Surg* 2001;136:870–877.
2. Kahrilas PJ, Bredenoord AJ, Fox M, et al. The Chicago Classification of esophageal motility disorders v. 3.0. International High Resolution Manometry Working Group. *Neurogastroenterol Motil* 2015;27(2):160–174.
3. Leite LP, Johnston BT, Barrett J, et al. Ineffective esophageal motility (IEM): the primary finding in patients with non-specific motility disorder. *Dig Dis Sci* 1997;42:1859–1865.
4. Spechler SJ, Castell DO. Classification of oesophageal motility abnormalities. *Gut* 2001;49:145–151.
5. Richter JE, Castell DO. Diffuse esophageal spasm: a reappraisal. *Ann Intern Med* 1984;100:242–245.
6. Bassotti G, Alunni G, Cocchieri M, et al. Isolated hypertensive lower esophageal sphincter. Clinical and manometric aspects of an uncommon esophageal motor disorder. *J Clin Gastroenterol* 1992;14:285–287.
7. Payne WS. Heller's contribution to the surgical treatment of achalasia of the esophagus. *Ann Thorac Surg* 1989;48:876–881.
8. Blam ME, Delfyett W, Levine MS, et al. Achalasia: a disease of varied and subtle symptoms that do not correlate with radiographic findings. *Am J Gastroenterol* 2002;97:1916–1923.
9. Abid S, Champion G, Richter JE. Treatment of achalasia: the best of both worlds. *Am J Gastroenterol* 1994;89(7):979–985.
10. Fisichella PM, Raz D, Palazzo F, et al. Clinical, radiological, and manometric profile in 145 patients with untreated achalasia. *World J Surg* 2008;32:1974–1979.
11. Katzka DA, Farrugia G, Arora AS. Achalasia secondary to neoplasia: a disease with a changing differential diagnosis. *Dis Esophagus* 2012;25(4):331–336.
12. Cameron, AJ, Malcom A, Prather CM, et al. Videoendoscopic diagnosis of esophageal motility disorders. *Gastrointest Endosc* 1999;49:62–69.
13. Katzka DA, Castell DO. Review article: an analysis of the efficacy, perforation rates and methods used in pneumatic dilation for achalasia. *Aliment Pharmacol Ther* 2011;34(8):832–839.
14. Kessing BF, Bredenoord AJ, Smout AJ. Erroneous diagnosis of gastroesophageal reflux disease in achalasia. *Clin Gastroenterol Hepatol* 2011;9:1020–1024.
15. Patti MG, Gorodner MV, Galvani C, et al. Spectrum of esophageal motility disorders: implications for diagnosis and treatment. *Arch Surg* 2005;140:442–449.
16. Bowers S. Esophageal motility disorders. *Surg Clin N Am* 2015;95:467–482.
17. Kadakia SC, Wong RK. Pneumatic balloon dilation for esophageal achalasia. *Gastrointest Endosc Clin North Am* 2001;11:325–346.
18. Roman S, Gyawali P, Xiao Y, et al. The Chicago Classification of motility disorders. *Gastrointest Endosc Clin N Am* 2014;24:545–561.
19. Sanderson DR, Ellis FH Jr, Schlegel JF, et al. Syndrome of vigorous achalasia: clinical and physiologic observations. *Dis Chest* 1967;52:508–517.
20. Goldenberg SP, Burrell M, Fette GG, et al. Classic and vigorous achalasia: a comparison of manometric, radiographic, and clinical findings. *Gastroenterology* 1991;101:743–748.
21. Pasricha PJ, Rai R, Ravich WJ, et al. Botulinum toxin for achalasia: long-term outcome and predictors of response. *Gastroenterology* 1996;110:1410–1415.
22. Cuilliere C, Ducrotte P, Zerbib F, et al. Achalasia: outcome of patients treated with intrasphincteric injection of botulinum toxin. *Gut* 1997;41:87–92.
23. Khajanchee Y, Kanneganti S, Leatherwood AEB, et al. Laparoscopic Heller myotomy with Toupet fundoplication: outcomes predictors in 121 consecutive patients. *Arch Surg* 2005;140:827–834.
24. Fisichella PM, Jalilvand A, Lebenthal A. Diagnostic evaluation of achalasia: from the whalebone to the Chicago Classification. *World J Surg* 2015;39:1593–1597.
25. Rohof WO, Salvador R, Annese V, et al. Outcomes of treatment for achalasia depend on manometric subtype. *Gastroenterology* 2013;144:718–725.
26. Pandolfino JE, Gawron AJ. Achalasia: a systematic review. *JAMA* 2015;313(18):1841–1852.
27. Eherer AJ, Schwetz I, Hammer HF, et al. Effect of sildenafil on oesophageal motor function in healthy subjects and patients with oesophageal motor disorders. *Gut* 2002;50:758.
28. Pasricha PJ, Hawari R, Ahmed I. Submucosal endoscopic esophageal myotomy: a novel experimental approach for the treatment of achalasia. *Endoscopy* 2007;39:761–764.
29. Alves A, Perniceni P, Godeberge P, et al. Laparoscopic Heller's cardiomyotomy in achalasia: Is intraoperative endoscopy useful, and why? *Surg Endosc* 1999;13;600–603.
30. Neubrand M, Scheurlen C, Schepke M, et al. Long-term results and prognostic factors in the treatment of achalasia with botulinum toxin. *Endoscopy* 2002;34.519–523.
31. Zaninotto ZG, Annese V, Costantini M, et al. Randomized controlled trial of botulinum toxin versus laparoscopic Heller myotomy for esophageal achalasia. *Ann Surg* 2004;239:364–370.
32. Raftopoulos Y, Landreneau RJ, Hayetian F, et al. Factors affecting quality of life after minimally invasive Heller myotomy for achalasia. *J Gastrointest Surg* 2004;8:233–239.
33. Patti MG, Pellegrini CA, Arcerito M, et al. Comparison of medical and minimally invasive surgical therapy for esophageal motility disorders. *Arch Surg* 1995;130:609–616.
34. Deb S, Deschamps C, Allen MS, et al. Laparoscopic esophageal myotomy for achalasia: factors affecting functional results. *Ann Thorac Surg* 2005;80:1191–1195.
35. Perrone JM, Frisella MM, Desai KM, et al. Results of laparoscopic Heller–Toupet operation for achalasia. *Surg Endosc* 2004;18:1565–1571.
36. Boeckxstaens GE, Annese V, des Varannes SB, et al. Pneumatic dilation versus laparoscopic Heller's myotomy for idiopathic achalasia. *N Engl J Med* 2011;364(19):1807–1816.
37. Sabharwal T, Cowling M, Dussek J, et al. Balloon dilation for achalasia of the cardia: experience in 76 patients. *Radiology* 2002;224:719–724.
38. West RL, Hirsch DP, Bartelsman JF, et al. Long term results of pneumatic dilation in achalasia followed for more than 5 years. *Am J Gastroenterol* 2002;97:1346–1351.
39. Ferguson MK, Reeder LB, Olak J. Results of myotomy and partial fundoplication after pneumatic dilation for achalasia. *Ann Thorac Surg* 1996;62:327–330.
40. Dolan K, Zafirellis K, Fountoulakis A, et al. Does pneumatic dilatation affect outcome of laparoscopic cardiomyotomy? *Surg Endosc* 2002;16:84–87.
41. Alderliesten J, Conchillo JM, Leeuwenburgh I. Predictors for outcome of failure of balloon dilatation in patients with achalasia. *Gut* 2011;60:10–16.
42. Hunt DR, Wills VL, Weis B, et al. Management of esophageal perforation after pneumatic dilation. *J Gastrointest Surg* 2000;4:411–415.
43. Vanuytsel T, Lerut T, Coosemans W, et al. Conservative management of esophageal perforations during pneumatic dilation for idiopathic esophageal achalasia. *Clin Gastroenterol Hepatol* 2012;10:142–149.
44. Hunter J, Trus TL, Branum GD, et al. Laparoscopic Heller myotomy and fundoplication for achalasia. *Ann Surg* 1997;225:655–665.
45. Ramacciato G, Mercantini P, Amodio PM, et al. The laparoscopic approach with antireflux surgery is superior to the thoracoscopic approach for the treatment of esophageal achalasia. Experience of a single surgical unit. *Surg Endosc* 2002;16:1431–1437.
46. Bonatti H, Hinder RA, Klocker J, et al. Long-term results of laparoscopic Heller myotomy with partial fundoplication for treatment of achalasia. *Am J Surg* 2005;190:883–887.
47. Costantini M, Zaninotto G, Guirroli E, et al. The laparoscopic Heller–Dor operation remains an effective treatment for esophageal achalasia at a minimum 6-year follow-up. *Surg Endosc* 2005;19:345–351.
48. Donahue PE, Horgan S, Liu K, et al. Floppy Dor fundoplication after esophagocardiomyotomy for achalasia. *Surgery* 2002;132:716–723.
49. Wright AS, Williams CW, Pellegrini CA, et al. Long-term outcomes confirm the superior efficacy of extended Heller myotomy with Toupet fundoplication for achalasia. *Surg Endosc* 2007;21:713–718.
50. Bessell JR, Lally CJ, Schloithe A, et al. Laparoscopic cardiomyotomy for achalasia: long-term outcomes. *Aust NZ J Surg* 2006;76:558–562.
51. Finley C, Clifton J, Yee J, et al. Anterior fundoplication decreases esophageal clearance in patients undergoing Heller myotomy for achalasia. *Surg Endsc* 2007;12:2178–2182.
52. Inoue H, Sato H, Ikeda H, et al. Per-oral endoscopic myotomy: a series of 500 patients. *J Am Coll Surg* 2015;221(2):256–256.
53. Khasab MA. International multicenter experience with peroral endoscopic myotomy for the treatment of spastic esophageal disorders refractory to medical (with video). *Gastrointest Endosc* 2015;81:1170–1177.
54. Rice TW, McKelvey AA, Richter JE, et al. A physiologic clinical study of achalasia: Should Dor fundoplication be added to Heller myotomy? *J Thorac Cardiovasc Surg* 2005;130:1593–1600.
55. Rossetti G, Brusciano L, Amato G, et al. A total fundoplication is not an obstacle to esophageal emptying after Heller myotomy for achalasia: results of a long-term follow up. *Ann Surg* 2005;241:614–621.
56. Zaninotto ZG, Costantini M, Portale G, et al. Etiology, diagnosis and treatment of failures after laparoscopic Heller myotomy for achalasia. *Ann Surg* 2002;235:186–192.
57. Lyass S, Thoman D, Steiner JP, et al. Current status of an antireflux procedure in laparoscopic Heller myotomy. *Surg Endosc* 2003;17:554–558.
58. Bloomston M, Rosemurgy A. Selective application of fundoplication during laparoscopic Heller myotomy ensures favorable outcomes. *Surg Laparosc Endosc Percutan Techn* 2002;5:309–315.
59. Richards W, Torquati A, Holzman MD, et al. Heller myotomy versus Heller myotomy with Dor fundoplication for achalasia: a prospective randomized double-blind clinical trial. *Ann Surg* 2004;240:405–415.
60. Richards WO, Clements RH, Wang PC, et al. Prevalence of gastroesophageal reflux after laparoscopic Heller myotomy. *Surg Endosc* 1999;13:1010–1014.
61. Torquati A, Lutfi R, Khaitan L, et al. Heller myotomy vs. Heller myotomy plus Dor fundoplication: cost–utility analysis of a randomized trial. *Surg Endosc* 2006;20:389–393.

62. Oelschlager BK, Chang L, Pellegrini CA. Improved outcome after extended gastric myotomy for achalasia. *Arch Surg* 2003;138:490–497.

63. Pasricha PJ, Ravich WJ, Hendrix TR, et al. Treatment of achalasia with intrasphincteric injection of botulinum toxin: a pilot trial. *Ann Intern Med* 1994;121: 590–591.

64. Kumbhari V, Khashab MA. Peroral endoscopic myotomy. *World J Gastrointest Endosc* 2015;7(5):496–509.

65. Inoue H, Minami H, Kobayashi Y, et al. Peroral endoscopic myotomy (POEM) for esophageal achalasia. *Endoscopy* 2010;42:265–271.

66. Stavropoulos SN, Desilets DJ, Fuchs KH, et al. Per-oral endoscopic myotomy white paper summary. *Gastrointest Endosc* 2014;80:1–15.

67. Barbieri LA, Hassan C, Rosati R, et al. Systematic review and meta-analysis: efficacy and safety of POEM for achalasia. *United European Gastroenterol J* 2015; 3(4):325–334.

68. Nehra D, Lord RV, DeMeester TR, et al. Physiologic basis for the treatment of epiphrenic diverticulum. *Ann Surg* 2002;235:346–354.

69. Rosati R, Fumagalli U, Bona S, et al. Diverticulectomy, myotomy and fundoplication through laparoscopy: a new option to treat epiphrenic diverticula? *Ann Surg* 1998;227:174.

70. Banbury MK, Rice TW, Goldblum JR, et al. Esophagectomy with gastric reconstruction for achalasia. *J Thorac Cardiovasc Surg* 1999;117:1077–1085.

71. Miller DL, Allen MS, Trastek VF, et al. Esophageal resection for recurrent achalasia. *Ann Thorac Surg* 1995;60:922–926.

72. Peters JH, Kauer WK, Crookes PF, et al. Esophageal resection with colon interposition for end-stage achalasia. *Arch Surg* 1995;130:632–637.

73. Devaney EJ, Lannettoni MD, Orringer MB, et al. Esophagectomy for achalasia: patient selection and clinical experience. *Ann Thorac Surg* 2001;72:854–858.

74. Streitz JM Jr, Ellis FH Jr, Gibb SP, et al. Achalasia and squamous cell carcinoma of the esophagus: analysis of 241 patients. *Ann Thorac Surg* 1995;59:1604–1609.

75. Di Simone MP, Felice V, D'Errico A, et al. Onset timing of delayed complications and criteria of follow-up after operation for esophageal achalasia. *Ann Thorac Surg* 1996;61:1106–1111.

76. Osgood H. A peculiar form of esophagismus. *Boston Med Surg J* 1889;120:140.

77. Creamer B, Donoghue FE, Code CF. Pattern of esophageal motility in diffuse spasm. *Gastroenterology* 1958;34:782–796.

78. Friesen DL, Henderson RD, Hanna W. Ultrastructure of the esophageal muscle in achalasia and diffuse esophageal spasm. *Am J Clin Pathol* 1983;79:319–325.

79. Eypasch EP, DeMeester TR, Klingman RR, et al. Physiologic assessment and surgical management of diffuse esophageal spasm. *J Thorac Surg* 1992;104:859–868.

80. Behr J, Biancani P. Pathogenesis of simultaneous esophageal contractions in patients with motility disorders. *Gastroenterology* 1993;105:111–118.

81. Konturek JW, Gillessen A, Domschke W. Diffuse esophageal spasm: a malfunction that involves nitric oxide? *Scand J Gastroenterol* 1995;30:1041–1045.

82. Fuller L, Huprich JE, Theisen J, et al. Abnormal esophageal body function: radiographic–manometric correlation. *Am Surg* 1999;65:911.

83. Clouse RE, Lustman PJ, Eckert TC, et al. Low-dose trazodone for symptomatic patients with esophageal contraction abnormalities. A double-blind, placebo-controlled trial. *Gastroenterology* 1987;92:1027–1036.

84. Miller LS, Pullela SV, Parkman HP, et al. Treatment chest pain in patients with noncardiac, nonreflux, nonachalasia spastic esophageal motor disorders using botulinum toxin injection into the gastroesophageal junction. *Am J Gastroenterol* 2002;97:1640–1646.

85. Storr M, Allescher HD, Rosch T, et al. Treatment of symptomatic diffuse esophageal spasm by endoscopic injections of botulinum toxin: a prospective study with long-term follow-up. *Gastrointest Endosc* 2001;54:754–759.

86. Leonardi HK, Shea JA, Crozier RE, et al. Diffuse spasm of the esophagus. Clinical, manometric, and surgical considerations. *J Thorac Cardiovasc Surg* 1997;74:736–743.

87. Roman S, Pandolfindo JE, Chen J, et al. Phenotypes and clinical context of hypercontractility in high-resolution esophageal pressure topography (EPT). *Am J Gastroenterol* 2011;107(1):37–45.

88. Richter JE, Barish CF, Castell DO. Abnormal sensory perception in patients with esophageal pain. *Gastroenterology* 1986;91:845–852.

89. Mujica VR, Mudipalli RS, Rao SS. Pathophysiology of chest pain in patients with nutcracker esophagus. *Am J Gastroenterol* 2001;96:1371–1377.

90. Richter JE. Oesophageal motility disorders. *Lancet* 2001;358:823–828.

91. Cattau EL Jr, Castell DO, Johnson DA, et al. Diltiazem therapy for symptoms associated with nutcracker esophagus. *Am J Gastroenterol* 1991;86:272–276.

92. Rao SSC, Mudipalli RS, Remes-Troche JM. Theophylline improves esophageal chest pain—a randomized, placebo-controlled study. *Am J Gastroenterol* 2007; 102(5):930–938.

93. Winters C, Artnak EJ, Benjamin SB, et al. Esophageal bougienage in symptomatic patients with the nutcracker esophagus. *JAMA* 1984;252:363.

94. Traube M, Tummala V, Baue AE, et al. Surgical myotomy in patients with high-amplitude peristaltic contractions: manometric and clinical effects. *Dig Dis Sci* 1987;32:16–21.

95. Shimi SN, Nathanson LK, Cuscheri A. Thoracoscopic long oesophageal myotomy for nutcracker oesophagus: initial experience of a new surgical approach. *Br J Surg* 1992;79:533–536.

96. Kahrilas PJ, Dodds WJ, Hogan WJ. Effect of peristaltic dysfunction on esophageal volume clearance. *Gastroenterology* 1988;94:73–80.

97. DiBaise JK, Quigley EMM. Tumor-related dysmotility: gastrointestinal dysmotility syndromes associated with tumors. *Dig Dis Sci* 1998;43:1369–1401.

98. Kahrilas PJ, Ghosh SK, Pandolfino JE. Esophageal motility disorders in terms of pressure topography: the Chicago Classification. *J Clin Gastroenterol* 2008;42(5): 627–635.

99. Kahrilas PJ, Kishk SM, Helm JF, et al. Comparison of pseudoachalasia and achalasia. *Am J Med* 1987;82:439–446.

100. Liu W, Fackler W, Rice TW, et al. The pathogenesis of pseudoachalasia: a clinicopathologic study of 13 cases of a rare disorder. *Am J Surg Pathol* 2002;26:784–788.

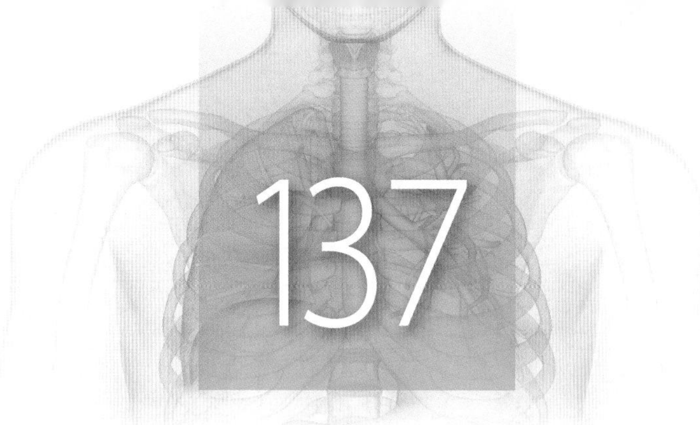

137

Gastroesophageal Reflux Disease

Thomas J. Watson

INTRODUCTION

Gastroesophageal reflux disease (GERD) is the most common disorder affecting the foregut. Epidemiologic studies have determined that approximately 7% of adults in the United States suffer from heartburn on a daily basis, nearly 20% have weekly symptoms, and up to a third experience at least one episode per month.[1,2] Importantly, those patients complaining of "typical" reflux symptoms of heartburn, regurgitation, or dysphagia represent only a fraction of the overall population suffering from GERD, with many individuals experiencing "atypical" or occult manifestations and others presenting with complications such as Barrett esophagus (BE) or esophageal stricture (Fig. 137.1).

The prevalence of GERD varies considerably by geography, with the highest rates in North America, western Europe, and Australia, and the lowest rates in Africa and Asia.[3] In addition, both the prevalence and severity of GERD appear to be increasing over the past few decades in certain locations, including the United States, Singapore, and China.[4] The diagnosis of BE, a GERD-related condition, is also increasing[5-7] as are deaths from benign esophageal diseases,[8] both

suggesting that current therapies for GERD are inadequate. These increases are a stark contrast to the prevalence of peptic ulcer disease, which has decreased markedly over the same time period.[9] While surgery for complications of peptic ulcer disease occupied a predominant place in the practice of foregut surgeons a generation ago, operations for GERD and obesity are now the most common.

Two factors have been identified as contributors to the increase in prevalence and severity of GERD. Population-based analyses have found that GERD is associated with obesity and negatively correlated to gastric colonization with *Helicobacter pylori*.[10-12] Over the past few decades, the former has increased markedly, while the latter has decreased, in the United States and most Western countries.

Given the diversity of its presentations, GERD is difficult to define. A panel of experts convened in Montreal in 2004 to provide a consensus opinion and concluded that GERD is defined best as a condition "which develops when the reflux of stomach contents causes troublesome symptoms and/or complications."[13] Symptoms are considered to be troublesome if they occur at least two times per week and adversely affect the individual's well-being. Patients with GERD may experience increased time off work, diminished work productivity, low sleep scores, and a decrease in physical functioning.[14] As there is no single objective study that is completely reliable, and as associated signs and symptoms may be occult, subtle, or attributable to other causes, the diagnosis of GERD may be challenging in some cases.

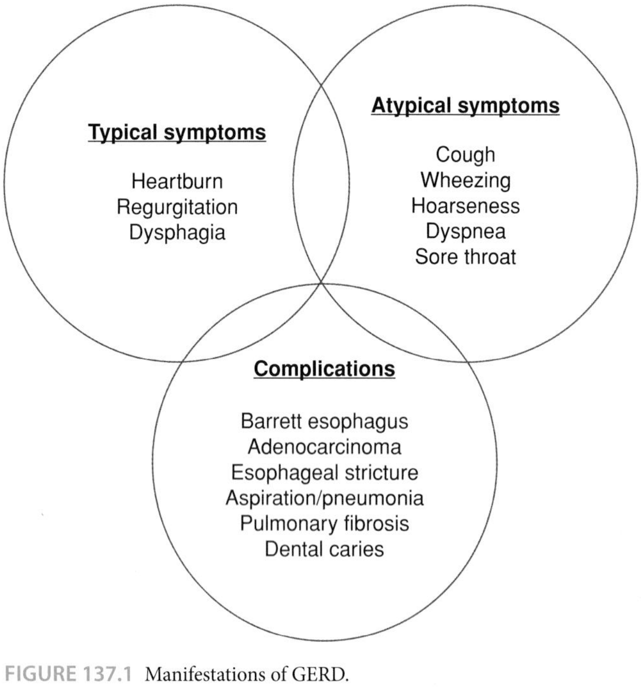

PATHOPHYSIOLOGY OF GERD

"PUMP–VALVE–RESERVOIR" SYSTEMS

Anatomic or physiologic models may be used to describe the foregut. To the classical anatomist, the esophagus is discrete from the pharynx, more cephalad, and the stomach, more caudad. Similarly, the small intestines are a discrete organ caudal to the stomach. To the physiologist, the pharynx, esophagus, stomach, and duodenum function as three "pump–valve–reservoir" systems (Fig. 137.2). The system most studied and best understood is the esophageal muscular pump consisting of the smooth muscle portion of the esophagus, the lower esophageal sphincter (LES) valve, and the gastric fundic reservoir. In this model, the esophageal pump functions as a piston, propagating food and saliva from the pharynx toward the stomach. The LES functions as a one-way valve, permitting distal passage of esophageal contents while preventing proximal reflux of gastric juice. The fundic reservoir holds food, liquid, and gas for storage until the antral pump propels the gastric contents toward the duodenum.

Typical symptoms

Heartburn
Regurgitation
Dysphagia

Atypical symptoms

Cough
Wheezing
Hoarseness
Dyspnea
Sore throat

Complications

Barrett esophagus
Adenocarcinoma
Esophageal stricture
Aspiration/pneumonia
Pulmonary fibrosis
Dental caries

FIGURE 137.1 Manifestations of GERD.

Pump	Valve	Reservoir
Pharynx	UES	Proximal esophagus (striated muscle)
Esophageal body (smooth muscle)	LES	Gastric fundus
Gastric antrum	Pylorus	Duodenum

UES = upper esophageal sphincter
LES = lower esophageal sphincter

FIGURE 137.2 "Pump–valve–reservoir" systems of the foregut.

The second "pump–valve–reservoir" system consists of the gastric antral pump, the pyloric valve, and the duodenal reservoir. The third system is the pharyngeal pump, the upper esophageal sphincter (UES) valve, and the proximal esophageal reservoir consisting of the striated muscular segment. Each of these systems plays an important role in normal foregut function. Likewise, derangements in any can lead to symptoms or associated pathology.

Starting from the most distal level, dysfunction of the antro-pyloro-duodenal system may lead to retrograde passage of chyme and the manifestations of delayed gastric emptying, such as nausea, vomiting, early satiety, or epigastric pain. Duodenogastric reflux may also result, bringing bile and pancreatic enzymes into the gastric lumen and exposing the gastric mucosa to these agents. As duodenogastric reflux may coexist with gastroesophageal reflux, gastric contents crossing the LES into the esophagus may consist not only of acid but also of the components of the duodenal refluxate. Thus, "acid reflux" commonly is more appropriately considered "duodenogastroesophageal reflux."

Dysmotility of the esophageal pump, as well as hypertension or poor relaxation of the LES such as that occurring with achalasia, can lead to dysphagia. Similarly, discoordination of the pharyngeal pump and UES can cause cervical dysphagia or aspiration. Reflux may occur from the esophagus across the UES into the pharynx, leading to regurgitation, sore throat, or water brash. If such reflux occurs together with gastroesophageal reflux, duodenal, pancreatic, and gastric contents may be delivered into the throat.

Once the refluxate reaches the pharynx, its course may continue into the mouth, nasal passages, or airway. Each of these routes is associated with potential symptoms or complications. Transoral flow can cause oral regurgitation, dental caries, tongue pain, or halitosis. With nasal passage comes the potential for nasal regurgitation or sinus infections. Laryngeal contact or frank aspiration into the tracheobronchial tree can trigger cough, wheezing, hoarseness, pneumonia/pneumonitis, or the more insidious onset of bronchiectasis or pulmonary fibrosis.

ESOPHAGOGASTRIC HIGH-PRESSURE ZONE

Much attention has been paid to the role of the esophagogastric high-pressure zone (HPZ) in the prevention of reflux from the high-pressure environment of the stomach to the lower pressure environment of the esophagus. The HPZ consists of both anatomic (flap valve and crural diaphragm) and physiologic (LES) components. The main determinants of competency of the HPZ include:

1. The presence or absence of a hiatal hernia, which alters the juxtaposition of the LES to the crural diaphragm and affects the geometry of the gastroesophageal flap valve created by the angle of His;
2. The intrinsic contractility of the LES;

3. The frequency of swallow- and nonswallow-induced transient LES relaxations (TLESRs).

Factors other than the loss of the HPZ barrier, such as gastric hypersecretion, delayed gastric emptying, decreased salivation (i.e., xerostomia), or poor esophageal clearance, also can contribute to excessive esophageal acid exposure but are less commonly the main culprits.

THE ESOPHAGOGASTRIC JUNCTION FLAP VALVE

Hill and colleagues[15] emphasized the importance of the physiologic flap valve created by the angle of His as a barrier against gastroesophageal reflux. Esophageal acid exposure has been correlated to the endoscopic appearance of the flap valve, highlighting the importance of geometry and anatomy at the esophagogastric junction in the prevention of GERD.[16] A hiatal hernia alters the anatomy in this region, rendering the flap valve less competent. In addition, gastric distention affects the flap valve by shortening of the LES and lessening the acuity of the angle of His, also leading to sphincter incompetence.[17]

INTEGRITY OF THE LES

An HPZ can be identified at the esophagogastric junction during the course of manometric assessment. This "sphincter" has no anatomic landmarks, but typically is comprised of contributions from the crural diaphragm and the intrinsic LES. The presence of a hiatal hernia alters the anatomic relationship between the diaphragm and the LES, negatively impacting the physiology of the reflux barrier. Three components of the LES have been shown to contribute to its efficacy at preventing reflux: its pressure (best measured at end-expiration), its overall length, and the length exposed to the positive pressure environment of the abdomen.[18]

The resting resistance imposed by the LES is a function of both its intrinsic tone and the length over which that tone is applied.[19] The shorter the overall or abdominal length of the sphincter, the higher the pressure must be to maintain sphincter competence. An important principle is that a short length can render an LES incompetent despite an adequate intrinsic tone. With gastric distention, the LES can be foreshortened, similar to the shortening of the neck of a balloon as it is inflated, making an LES of marginal resting length incompetent despite an adequate pressure and length in the nondistended state. This mechanism explains why GERD can be induced with overeating.

The intra-abdominal sphincter length aids in the prevention of reflux during periods of increased abdominal pressure. If pressure applied externally to the stomach is not countered with an equal pressure applied to the LES, reflux of gastric contents can result. A hiatal hernia contributes to the loss of intra-abdominal sphincter length. This fact, along with diminution of the crural contribution to the HPZ and the loss of the flap valve, are the proposed mechanisms by which a hiatal hernia contributes to GERD.

If the HPZ is characterized by a low LES resting pressure, a short overall length, or decreased exposure to the intra-abdominal pressure environment, then permanent loss of barrier function has occurred and significant gastroesophageal reflux can be anticipated. A mechanically defective HPZ is characterized by a mean LES pressure less than 6 mm Hg, an overall length of 2 cm or less, or an abdominal length of 1 cm or less.[18] These cut-off values are below the 2.5 percentile for normal subjects for each parameter. The most common cause of a mechanically defective LES is a shortened intra-abdominal length resulting from a hiatal hernia.

A permanently defective LES can lead to several consequences. Patients may have symptoms that are difficult to eradicate with acid suppression therapy, given the propensity for reflux to occur despite the neutralization of acid gastric content. In addition, esophageal mucosal injury typically occurs in the setting of frequent and repetitive reflux, such as occurs when the LES has failed. Deficits in LES function are not reversible with medical therapy, even when esophagitis is healed. In addition, longstanding reflux can lead to a progressive loss of esophageal body function, impairing esophageal clearance and leading to increased esophageal acidification from stasis after reflux events. Cases of HPZ failure can only be corrected with interventions aimed at augmenting the LES and repairing a hiatal hernia.

TRANSIENT LOWER ESOPHAGEAL SPHINCTER RELAXATIONS

The esophagogastric HPZ is normally present in the resting state. This HPZ is temporarily lost in two situations: (1) following a swallow, to allow passage of a food or fluid bolus into the stomach, and (2) when the fundus is distended with air or gas, to allow venting (a belch). These nonswallow-induced TLESRs are a proposed mechanism for gastroesophageal reflux episodes in normal individuals and those with symptomatic GERD.[20] Such TLESRs may occur without an antecedent pharyngeal contraction, may be prolonged (>10 seconds), and when reflux occurs, may be associated with relaxation of the crural diaphragm. As evidence of the importance of the crural diaphragm contribution to LES competence, experiments whereby the intrinsic tone of the LES is reduced pharmacologically to zero have shown that reflux does not occur unless crural diaphragmatic contraction also is absent.[21]

A prevailing theory is that TLESRs are vagally mediated reflex phenomena triggered by gastric distention. Mechanoreceptors in the proximal stomach communicate with the brainstem via vagal afferent pathways, and vagal efferent pathways communicate with inhibitory neurons in the LES. Gamma-aminobutyric acid B-class (GABA$_B$) receptors inhibit signaling from the vagal afferent endings located in the stomach and esophagus, reducing mechanosensitivity, and also inhibit both central nervous system pathways in the brainstem as well as vagal efferent pathways.[22] Selective agonists of GABA$_B$ receptors, such as baclofen, have been utilized to inhibit this vagovagal reflex, and thus inhibit TLESRs.

Obesity, gastric distention, an upright posture, and a high fat content in meals all have been shown to increase the frequency of TLESRs.[21-23] Given these observations, an alternate theory is that TLESRs may be the result of unfolding of the LES rather than a reflexively induced phenomenon. When the stomach is distended, the forces exerted at the esophagogastric junction vary depending upon the geometry at the cardia. When a hiatal hernia is present and the angle of His is compromised, intragastric pressure is transmitted to the distal esophagus, leading to a reduction in the length of the HPZ. Once a critical shortening has occurred, the sphincter can be overcome, leading to a sudden drop in LES tone and a reflux event. This mechanism conceptualizes a TLESR as a mechanical event resulting from gastric distention and LES unfolding rather than a neuromuscular reflex. These transient LES "shortenings" rather than "relaxations" likely explain the early stages of GERD, especially in the postprandial period. After the stomach is vented, the length of the HPZ is returned toward normal, re-establishing sphincter competence until further distention occurs, leading to additional venting and reflux. A normal response to reflux events is to swallow, as saliva acts to neutralize acid within the esophageal lumen. The sequence of reflux and swallowing

can lead to the common complaints of belching and bloating resulting from aerophagia in patients with GERD.

Since the concept of TLESRs was first introduced, they have been implicated as the major reason for GERD regardless of severity. This theory contradicts the fact that over 80% of patients with symptomatic GERD have an associated hiatal hernia, which is responsible for a mechanically defective LES. In addition, most patients with erosive esophagitis or BE also have an incompetent LES. In light of these facts, TLESRs likely are not the mechanism for the development of GERD in most cases, but rather: (1) result from gastric distention, allowing a belch, and (2) are responsible for physiologic reflux, or mild cases of pathologic reflux, in individuals with normal hiatal anatomy and LES tone.

THE "ACID POCKET"

A recognized phenomenon is that combined pH monitoring of the esophagus and stomach can reveal postprandial esophageal acidification simultaneous with gastric alkalinization. As the presence of acid in the esophagus presumes that reflux of gastric content has occurred, this contradiction is difficult to explain. To test whether an "acid pocket" exists in the proximal stomach, cephalad to gastric content buffered by a meal, luminal pH was measured at 1 cm increments distal and proximal to the LES in healthy volunteers before and after a meal.[24] Such a pocket was identified, extending on average 1.8 cm into the lumen of the esophagus. This distal esophageal reflux could occur despite a normal esophageal pH study, as assessed by a probe positioned 5 cm proximal to the upper border of the LES, and in the absence of endoscopic esophagitis.[25] These findings provide an explanation for the observations of inflammation and metaplasia that can occur at the esophagogastric junction even in the absence of overt GERD symptoms.

IMPLICATIONS OF GERD PATHOPHYSIOLOGY FOR ITS MANAGEMENT

The vast body of literature outlining the pathophysiology of GERD supports the concept that it begins in the stomach. Gastric distention from overeating and delayed gastric emptying secondary to a high-fat Western diet leads to a loss of the angle of His, compromise of the cardia flap valve, and shortening of the HPZ. The barrier against reflux can be overcome, leading to reflux events, and exposing the distal esophagus to the contents of gastric juice including pepsin, as well as possible bile and pancreatic enzymes. Repetitive exposure of the esophageal mucosa to gastric refluxate leads to inflammation, carditis, and the potential for metaplasia. In the early stages, symptoms are mild, intermittent, and easily controllable with dietary or lifestyle modifications and intermittent acid suppressive therapy. Esophagitis is generally mild and limited to the distal esophagus. A "Schatzki ring" consisting of fibrotic mucosa at the squamocolumnar junction can result. Patients learn to compensate by swallowing saliva to buffer esophageal acid, though aerophagia may be troublesome, leading to a sequence of repetitive belching and bloating.

As the disease progresses, the reflux barrier is compromised in a distal to proximal direction until a permanently defective HPZ results. At this point, symptoms become more difficult to control and severe esophagitis can occur. Esophageal acid exposure increases as the severity of esophagitis worsens, and is highest for patients with BE.[26] Although acid suppression medications may help to alleviate heartburn, reflux of gastric content continues and can lead to ongoing esophageal injury, including mucosal complications such as esophagitis, metaplasia, or neoplasia, as well as transmural damage causing esophageal stricturing or loss of peristaltic function. In addition, any of variety of extraesophageal manifestations of GERD can continue, including the potential for end-stage pulmonary disease from repetitive aspiration. Therapy aimed at restoring competency of the LES and repairing an associated hiatal hernia is the only durable solution in such cases.

MECHANISMS OF SYMPTOM DEVELOPMENT

The clinical manifestations of esophageal pathophysiology are diverse in their presentation and causation. Noxious luminal contents and distention drive esophageal symptom development. Symptoms of esophageal origin, however, easily may be confused with those attributable to other sites or organs. Studies of embryologic foregut development, as well as anatomic dissections in adults, reveal that the visceroneural pathways of the esophagus are intertwined with those of the respiratory tract and heart. This fact explains the common overlap in clinical presentations of disease processes involving the upper gastrointestinal, pulmonary, and cardiac systems and the frequent inability to localize the source of symptoms to one organ system or another.

Early studies on the pathophysiology of esophageal symptomatology focused on intraluminal balloon distention or acid perfusion. A classic study from 1931 assessed the location of symptoms after serial balloon inflations at 5 cm increments along the length of the esophageal body.[27] Pain was poorly localized, consistent with visceral nociception in other parts of the alimentary tract, and was identified at diverse sites including the base of the neck, between the shoulder blades, or even in the retrobulbar region. In addition, symptoms were reported with a variety of descriptors including heartburn, chest pain, or nausea.

Esophageal perfusion with either acid or bile salts can induce heartburn or angina-like chest pain. Symptom severity is dependent upon concentration and contact time, though is quite variable between individuals. Discomfort tends to be reproducible below a pH of 4, a fact appreciated in the early years of esophageal pH monitoring. This threshold is a factor in the selection of pH 4 as the value below which acid reflux into the esophagus is defined on ambulatory pH studies. The Bernstein test, now mainly of historic interest, utilized the instillation of acid into the esophagus to induce reflux symptoms as a way to diagnose the presence of GERD. The test, however, lacked both sensitivity and specificity. Studies assessing bile salt infusion in the esophagus have shown the ability to invoke symptoms in a similar manner.

CLINICAL PRESENTATION AND SYMPTOM ASSESSMENT

The classic or "typical" symptoms associated with GERD are heartburn, regurgitation, and dysphagia. The term "heartburn" is not consistently interpreted by patients, and may be described more reliably as a "burning feeling rising from the stomach or lower chest up toward the neck."[28] Given the nonspecificity of this complaint, multiple other diagnoses can masquerade as GERD (Table 137.1). Although none of the typical reflux symptoms is specific to the diagnosis of GERD, dysphagia is often the most concerning in that it can signify a more serious condition, such as esophageal cancer. Any

TABLE 137.1 Medical Conditions That May Present With Symptoms Similar to GERD

- Coronary artery disease
- Esophageal motility disorders
- Pill-induced esophagitis
- Eosinophilic esophagitis
- Functional foregut disorders
- Esophagogastric carcinoma
- Peptic ulcer disease
- Cholelithiasis

complaint of dysphagia of recent onset necessitates a prompt and through evaluation to rule out this possibility.

Most patients with infrequent or mild GERD symptoms self-medicate with antacids or antisecretory medications. With the introduction and subsequent extensive market penetration of inexpensive, generic, and over-the-counter histamine 2-receptor antagonists (H2RAs) and proton pump inhibitors (PPIs), the accessibility of effective GERD therapies has increased. Acid suppression therapy, however, only addresses the acid component of the gastric refluxate and does not prevent injury from refluxed pepsin, bile, or pancreatic enzymes that may be proinflammatory or carcinogenic. As patients commonly present to a physician only when symptoms are severe or persist despite therapy, delays in seeking evaluation may have deleterious consequences.

The art of accurate symptom assessment in the evaluation of GERD is critical to successful management and has been underemphasized in the literature. As the clinical manifestations of GERD can be quite variable and its presence is not always obvious, insight and perseverance may be necessary on the part of the evaluating clinician. The decision to proceed with antireflux surgery is generally made on the basis of both subjective and objective findings, anticipating how symptoms will be impacted. Symptoms should be prioritized in order of severity, and the probability of relief of each with treatment estimated. Given the importance of an accurate and reliable assessment, an experienced provider should obtain the clinical history; the task should not be relegated solely to the inexperienced house officer, nurse practitioner, or physician assistant.

The presence of "typical" reflux symptoms, such as heartburn, regurgitation, or dysphagia, as well as "atypical" symptoms that might be due to GERD, such as cough, wheezing, hoarseness, shortness of breath, or sore throat should be noted. Atypical symptoms are the primary complaint in approximately 20% to 25% of patients with GERD and are associated with typical symptoms in even more.[29] As there are fewer potential mechanisms for their generation, typical symptoms are more likely to be secondary to refluxed gastric contents than are atypical symptoms. Other common contributors to respiratory symptoms should be investigated, such as smoking, postnasal drip, asthma, or the use of angiotensin converting enzyme (ACE) inhibitors. A chest radiograph should be considered to detect associated lung parenchymal abnormalities. The patient should be counseled about the decreased probability of success of antireflux surgery when atypical symptoms are the primary factors driving intervention, in that other contributors may remain. Of significance is the relatively long time necessary for respiratory symptoms to improve after surgery compared to typical symptoms.

Symptomatic response to acid suppression medications is of importance as it can predict relief following surgery.[30] A paradox of patient referral for antireflux surgery is that patients well controlled on medical therapy, who may be among the best candidates for surgery, often are not considered, while those who do not respond to medical therapy and, therefore, may not respond well to surgery, may seek surgical intervention. A detailed objective evaluation for the presence of pathologic esophageal acid exposure is particularly important in the latter group, as well as a careful consideration of whether the patient's main complaints are reflux-related. The surgeon needs to be alert to primary symptoms such as nausea, early satiety, epigastric pain, or bloating, which may be attributable to foregut pathology but may not be caused by GERD. Additional historical factors to note include asthma and other pulmonary disorders (e.g., recurrent aspiration/pneumonia, "idiopathic" pulmonary fibrosis or interstitial lung disease).

As symptoms generally are not pathognomonic for GERD, are varied in their presentation, and can be unreliable in determining etiology, using symptoms alone to guide therapy can be misleading. In fact, the diagnosis of GERD using symptoms alone has been shown to be accurate in only approximately two-thirds of patients.[31] In addition, each of the available esophageal diagnostic studies has strengths and limitations that must be understood to determine their place in the assessment of GERD. Only through consideration and consolidation of both subjective and objective findings can the optimal treatment course be determined.

COMPLICATIONS OF GERD

The reflux of gastric contents has the potential to damage the esophagus, pharynx, larynx, and respiratory tract. Injury from exposure to gastric juice can be categorized into esophageal mucosal and mural complications, such as esophagitis or stricture; extraesophageal or pulmonary manifestations such as cough, asthma, or pulmonary fibrosis; and metaplastic or neoplastic transformation of the esophageal mucosa, which will be addressed in a separate chapter.

ESOPHAGEAL MUCOSAL COMPLICATIONS

Symptoms of GERD do not predict the presence of erosive esophagitis. Gastric refluxate contains multiple potentially noxious agents, including those secreted by the stomach (acid and pepsin), as well as those refluxed into the stomach from the duodenum (bile and pancreatic enzymes, including trypsin). In addition, toxic compounds can be generated in the mouth, esophagus, and stomach by the action of bacteria on dietary substrates.

Landmark animal studies by Lillemoe and others[32,33] demonstrated that acid alone inflicts minimal damage to the esophageal mucosa, though the combination of acid and pepsin is highly inflammatory. Hydrogen ions injure the squamous esophageal mucosa only at a pH below 2. With acid reflux, pepsin appears to be the main culprit underlying esophagitis. Similarly, the reflux of duodenal juice alone does little damage to the esophageal lining, though the combination of bile, pancreatic enzymes, and gastric secretions may be either noxious or protective. For example, in an acid environment trypsin is inactivated while bile salts precipitate and attenuate the injurious effects of pepsin. In this scenario, duodenogastric refluxate injures the esophageal mucosa less than pure gastric juice. In an alkaline environment, on the other hand, trypsin activity is maximized while bile salts with a high pk_a are ionized and solubilized, preventing interference with pepsin. In this setting, duodenogastric refluxate is more damaging to the esophagus than gastric juice alone. Given the complexity of these interactions and the chemistry of bile salts, the poor correlation between the presence of heartburn and the finding of endoscopic esophagitis can be understood.

RESPIRATORY COMPLICATIONS

Many individuals suffering from GERD will experience respiratory symptoms either as their primary complaints or in association with more troublesome heartburn and regurgitation. In the absence of typical symptoms, establishing the diagnosis of GERD may be difficult, yet is critical to appropriate management. Reflux may cause asthma, may underlie "idiopathic" pulmonary fibrosis, and may complicate chronic obstructive pulmonary disease (COPD). In fact, patients with COPD and GERD are twice as likely to have significant COPD exacerbations as patients with COPD alone.[34] Studies have found that 35% to 50% of asthmatics have excessive esophageal acid exposure, esophagitis, or a hiatal hernia.[35] Bronchospasm may be induced by "reflex" or "reflux" mechanisms, the former due to vagally mediated airway reactivity from acidification of the esophagus[36,37] and the latter due to the direct effect of aspirated gastric contents on the respiratory epithelium.

NONRESPIRATORY EXTRAESOPHAGEAL COMPLICATIONS

A spectrum of extraesophageal manifestations of GERD other than pulmonary complications exists, including hoarseness from laryngitis, sore throat associated with pharyngitis, sinusitis, dental caries, halitosis, and sleep disturbances. Nearly half of individuals referred for antireflux surgery may exhibit one or more nonesophageal complaints. The term laryngopharyngeal reflux (LPR) has been used to explain these various pulmonary and nonpulmonary extraesophageal symptoms. Unfortunately, diagnostic testing for the presence of LPR remains imprecise, making proof of causality a challenge in many cases.

MEDICAL THERAPY FOR GERD

GERD is one of the most common conditions encountered in general medical practices. It is the most frequent outpatient diagnosis in the United States, the most common indication for flexible upper endoscopy, and the most prevalent gastrointestinal-related diagnosis encountered by primary care physicians.[38] As a result, medications for control of GERD comprise one of the largest pharmaceutical markets in the United States and abroad. Since PPIs were introduced in the United States in 1989, a number of different medications have emerged in this class, each with substantial penetration into the marketplace. In 2015, sales of the PPI esomeprazole accounted for over $5.5 billion in expenditures in the United States alone, although this figure represents a 23% decrease from the prior year due to the introduction of generic versions.[39] On a yearly basis in the United States, direct and indirect costs associated with the management of GERD and its complications exceed $10 billion.[38]

With the widespread availability of over-the-counter acid neutralizing and suppressive medications, including H2RAs as well as PPIs, self-medication of the patient with mild GERD symptoms has become a frequent occurrence. PPIs are generally effective at improving symptoms and quality of life, healing esophagitis, and preventing complications. They are also well tolerated with a once or twice per day dosing schedule.

Initial therapy for heartburn and regurgitation in the absence of obvious complications consists of PPI therapy, once or twice daily, for 2 to 4 weeks. Many patients will experience symptom resolution and, in such cases, an extensive objective evaluation is not necessary.

TABLE 137.2 Arguments for the Use of Acid Suppression Medications for Control of GERD

- No particular expertise necessary to prescribe
- No detailed work-up necessary in the absence of "alarm" symptoms
- Low morbidity and side effects
- Rare mortality
- No irreversible consequences
- Efficacious in many

TABLE 137.3 Arguments Against the Use of Acid Suppression Medications for Control of GERD

- May require life-long daily therapy, even in multiple doses
- Compliance
- Cost
- Desire not to take medications
- Long-term risks
- Does not address the mechanically defective LES
- Does not prevent reflux of nonacid gastric contents

The dose and duration of such a "PPI test," as well as the definition of a satisfactory response, are not standardized. Consequently, the results of a therapeutic trial have a low sensitivity and specificity for the diagnosis of GERD. Additional recommendations include the avoidance of triggering foods and liquids, such as fatty, fried, spicy, or greasy foods; citrus; peppermint; chocolate; alcohol; and coffee. Patients are advised to elevate the head of the bed at night, avoid tight clothing, eat small meals, not eat immediately prior to bedtime, quit smoking and, if obese, lose weight. Flexible upper endoscopy is indicated for so-called "alarm symptoms" of dysphagia, upper gastrointestinal bleeding, or weight loss.

Mild esophagitis will usually heal with a short course of therapy; the available data show healing of mild esophagitis in 88% to 96% of patients after 8 weeks of treatment.[40] The efficacy of PPIs in relieving symptoms is less, with a response rate of only 36.7% in patients with nonerosive reflux disease (NERD) and 55.5% in patients with erosive esophagitis, after 4 weeks of standard dose therapy.[41] In patients with mixed acid and bile reflux, esophageal mucosal damage may continue despite symptom relief.

Studies have shown that the majority of patients, unfortunately, will experience recurrence of symptoms within 6 months of discontinuation of therapy.[42] Thus, long-term treatment will be necessary for many individuals, requiring compliance not only with a medical regimen but also with a multitude of dietary and lifestyle modifications. For patients on long-term PPI therapy, 59% of patients with erosive GERD, 40% of patients with NERD, and 40% of patients complaining of the extraesophageal manifestations of GERD will have persistent symptoms on a once-a-day PPI dosing schedule.[43]

Much work has revolved around understanding the reasons underlying medical treatment failures for GERD. Esophageal acid exposure is decreased up to 80% with H2RAs and up to 95% with PPIs. Despite these high degrees of acid suppression, the clinical response may not be sustained and breakthrough reflux episodes may occur, particularly at night. Split PPI dosing regimens and the use of H2RAs prior to bedtime have been advocated to help prevent nocturnal reflux events. Other potential reasons underlying an incomplete symptomatic response to medications include poor compliance, low bioavailability, inappropriate timing of medication administration relative to meals, diagnostic errors, the presence of duodenogastroesophageal reflux, delayed gastric emptying, and visceral hypersensitivity to physiologic amounts of esophageal acid exposure. When the esophagogastric HPZ has failed, such as occurs with a hiatal hernia, sustained symptom relief may be a challenge despite optimal use of medications.

A significant body of literature has accumulated and reached the lay press regarding potential adverse consequences of long-term acid suppressive therapies. Various studies have shown higher rates of community-acquired pneumonia,[44] osteoporosis-related fractures due to impaired calcium absorption,[45,46] hypomagnesemia,[47] and *Clostridium difficile* pseudomembranous colitis[48] in patients taking PPIs compared to appropriately matched control subjects. Of course, the relatively small magnitude of these risks needs to be considered

and weighed against the benefits of therapy, as well as the risks and benefits of alternative treatments, in deciding upon optimal management for the individual (Tables 137.2 and 137.3).

SURGERY FOR GERD

The nature of medical therapy for GERD is that symptom relief is attempted by means of acid suppression. The factors responsible for the disease, especially the defective esophagogastric HPZ as well as TLESRs, are not corrected by acid suppressive medications. The importance of this fact is underscored by a continued interest within the medical community to develop endoscopic or other minimally invasive techniques to restore LES competence in GERD patients, despite a recent history of failures of some devices created for this purpose (Fig. 137.3).

Over 60 years have passed since Rudolph Nissen[49] first reported the use of fundoplication for the treatment of GERD. Surgical therapy for GERD was revolutionized by the introduction of laparoscopic techniques in the early 1990s.[50] The indications for surgery, preoperative evaluation, and techniques of fundoplication have been refined, leading to favorable outcomes in the vast majority of cases as assessed by both subjective and objective parameters. The introduction of a minimally invasive approach to fundoplication, coupled with the excellent long-term control of symptoms afforded by such procedures, has made antireflux surgery an attractive alternative. Today, laparoscopic Nissen fundoplication remains the most commonly performed antireflux operation and is the gold standard against which other types of surgical or endoscopic therapies are judged (Fig. 137.4).

On the other hand, the potential morbidity and cost of surgery, as well as suboptimal short- or long-term symptomatic and functional outcomes resulting in some patients undergoing antireflux

- Endoluminal suturing technologies
  - Endocinch (C.R. Bard, Murray Hill, New Jersey)
  - ESD (Wilson-Cook, Winston-Salem, North Carolina)

- Endoluminal injection therapies
  - Enteryx (Boston Scientific, Natick, Massachusetts)
    - *no longer available*
  - Gatekeeper (Medtronic, Minneapolis, Minnesota)
    - *no longer available*

- Endoluminal plication
  - EsophyX (EndoGastric Solutions, Redmond, Washington)
  - Medigus MUSE™ System (Medigus USA, Danville, California)
  - NDO plicator (NDO Medical, Mansfield, Massachusetts)
    - *no longer available*

- Endoluminal radiofrequency application to LES
  - Stretta procedure (Mederi Therapeutics, Norwalk, Connecticut)

FIGURE 137.3 Recent endoscopic technologies for control of GERD.

- Fundoplication
  - Laparoscopic
  - Open transabdominal
  - Open transthoracic
  - Complete (Nissen)
  - Partial (Toupet, Dor)

- Posterior gastropexy (Hill repair)
  - Laparoscopic
  - Open transabdominal

- Magnetic sphincter augmentation

- LES electrostimulation

- Other:
  - Roux-en-Y gastric bypass
  - Gastrectomy (total or partial)

FIGURE 137.4 Surgical options for GERD.

TABLE 137.4 Arguments for the Use of Fundoplication for Control of GERD

- Effective at controlling typical symptoms
- Safe in experienced hands
- Generally durable
- Low incidence of severe side effects
- Generally good postoperative quality of life

TABLE 137.5 Arguments Against the Use of Fundoplication for Control of GERD

- Perioperative morbidity/mortality
- Potential for breakdown and need for reoperation
- Side effects (especially dysphagia or gas-bloat)

procedures, has led to criticism regarding the use of fundoplication and has fostered the development of novel medical, endoscopic, or surgical treatments for GERD (Tables 137.4 and 137.5). Given the various strategies for managing GERD, each with its potential advantages and shortcomings, accurate and current data regarding outcomes after antireflux surgery are necessary as a basis against which other established and evolving therapies must be judged. The various techniques of fundoplication and other antireflux operations, as well as the data documenting subjective and objective outcomes, will be reviewed in a separate chapter.

SUMMARY

Much has been learned about the mechanisms underlying GERD and its diverse manifestations. Despite an extensive literature detailing its pathogenesis and treatment, GERD remains an extremely common malady occupying a prominent place in medical practice and consuming vast resources. While improvements in the medical, endoscopic, and surgical therapy for GERD have taken shape in recent decades, its prevalence and severity remain on the increase, possibly related to the impact of a Western diet and resultant obesity. Acid suppression therapy, the mainstay of medical management of GERD, improves symptoms and heals esophagitis in the majority of cases of mild disease. In more advanced cases, when the competence of the reflux barrier has been compromised, therapy targeted at augmenting the esophagogastric HPZ and correcting a hiatal hernia is necessary

for sustained relief. While laparoscopic fundoplication has been the standard surgical treatment, novel pharmacologic, endoscopic, and surgical therapies may supplant traditional operative approaches in the years to come. Much remains to be learned about GERD and its management, making the pursuit of GERD relief a worthy endeavor for the clinician and academician.

REFERENCES

1. Locke GR, Talley NY, Fett SL, et al. Prevalence and clinical spectrum of gastroesophageal reflux; a population-based study in Olmsted County Minnesota. *Gastroenterology* 1997;112:1448.
2. Isolauri J, Laippala P. Prevalence of symptoms suggestive of gastroesophageal reflux disease in an adult population. *Ann Med* 1995;27:67.
3. Sharma P, Wani S, Romero Y, et al. Racial and geographic issues in gastroesophageal reflux disease. *Am J Gastroenterol* 2008;103:2669–2680.
4. El-Serag H. Time trends in gastroesophageal reflux disease: a systematic review. *Clin Gastroenterol Hepatol* 2007;5:17–26.
5. Conio M, Cameron AJ, Romero Y, et al. Secular trends in the epidemiology and outcome of Barrett's oesophagus in Olmsted County, Minnesota. *Gut* 2001;48:304–309.
6. Coleman HG, Bhat S, Murray LJ, et al. Increasing incidence of Barrett's oesophagus: a population-based study. *Eur J Epidemiol* 2011;26:739–745.
7. Van Soest EM, Dieleman JP, Siersema PD, et al. Increasing incidence of Barrett's oesophagus in the general population. *Gut* 2005;54:1062–1066.
8. Panos MZ, Walt RP, Stevenson C, et al. Rising death rate from non-malignant disease of the oesophagus (NMOD) in England and Wales. *Gut* 1995;36:488.
9. El-Serag HB, Sonnenberg A. Opposing time trends of peptic ulcer and reflux disease. *Gut* 1998;434:427.
10. Jacobson BC, Somers SC, Fuchs CS, et al. Body-mass index and symptoms of gastroesophageal reflux in women. *N Engl J Med* 2006;354:2340–2348.
11. Corely DA, Kubo A. Body mass index and gastroesophageal reflux disease: a systematic review and meta-analysis. *Am J Gastroenterol* 2006;108:2619–2628.
12. Bowrey DJ, Williams GT, Clark GW. Interactions between Helicobacter pylori and gastroesophageal reflux disease. *Dis Esophagus* 1998;11:203–209.
13. Vakil N, van Zanten SV, Kahrilas P, et al. The Montreal definition and classification of gastroesophageal reflux disease; a global evidence-based consensus. *Am J Gastroenterol* 2006;101:1900–1920.
14. Becher A, El-Serag H. Systematic review: the association between symptomatic response to proton pump inhibitors and health-related quality of life in patients with gastro-oesophageal reflux disease. *Aliment Pharmacol Ther* 2011;34:618–627.
15. Hill JD, Kozarek RA, Kraemer SJM, et al. The gastroesophageal flap valve: in vitro and in vivo observations. *Gastrointest Endosc* 1996;44:541–547.
16. Oberg S, Peters JH, DeMeester TR, et al. Endoscopic grading of the gastroesophageal valve in patients with symptoms of gastroesophageal reflux disease (GERD). *Surg Endosc* 1999;13:1184–1188.
17. Ismail T, Bancewicz J, Barlow J. Yield pressure, anatomy of the cardia and gastro-esophageal reflux. *Br J Surg* 1995;82:943.
18. Zaninotto G, DeMeester TR, Schwizer W, et al. The lower esophageal sphincter in health and disease. *Am J Surg* 1988;155:104.
19. O'Sullivan GC, DeMeester TR, Joelsson BE, et al. The interaction of the lower esophageal sphincter pressure and length of sphincter in the abdomen as determinants of gastroesophageal competence. *Am J Surg* 1982;143:40.
20. Dodds WJ, Dent J, Hogan WJ, et al. Mechanisms of gastroesophageal reflux disease in patients with reflux esophagitis. *N Engl J Med* 1982;307:1547–1552.
21. Mittal RK, Holloway R, Dent J. Effect of atropine on the frequency of reflux and and transient lower esophageal sphincter relaxation in normal subjects. *Gastroenterology* 1995;109:1547–1554.
22. Falk GW. Inhibition of transient lower esophageal sphincter relaxation in GERD: will Lesogaberan advance the field? *Gastroenterology* 2010;139:377–386.
23. Mittal RK, Holloway RH, Penagini R, et al. Transient lower esophageal sphincter relaxation. *Gastroenterology* 1995;109:601–610.
24. Fletcher J, Wirz A, Young J, et al. Unbuffered highly acidic gastric juice exists at the gastroesophageal junction after a meal. *Gastroenterology* 2001;1221:775.
25. Fletcher J, Wirz A, Henry E, et al. Studies of acid exposure immediately above the gastroesophageal squamocolumnar junction: evidence of short segment reflux. *Gut* 2004;53:168.
26. Bredenoord AJ, Hemmink GJ, Smout AJ. Relationship between gastro-oesophageal reflux pattern and severity of mucosal damage. *Neurogastroenterol Motil* 2009;21:807–812.
27. Polland WS, Bloomfield AL. Experimental referred pain from the gastrointestinal tract: I. The esophagus. *J Clin Invest* 1931;10:435–452.
28. Carlsson R, Dent J, Bolling-Sternevald E, et al. The usefulness of a structured questionnaire in the assessment of symptomatic gastroesophageal reflux disease. *Scand J Gastroenterol* 1998;33:1023–1029.
29. Sontag SJ. In: Stein M, ed. *Gastroesophageal Reflux Disease and Airway Disease*. New York: Marcel Dekker; 1999:115–138.
30. Campos GM, Peters JH, DeMeester TR, et al. Multivariate analysis of factors predicting outcome after laparoscopic Nissen fundoplication. *J Gastrointest Surg* 1999;3:292–300.
31. Costantini M, Crookes PF, Bremner RM, et al. The value of physiologic assessment of foregut symptoms in a surgical practice. *Surgery* 1993;114:780.

32. Lillemoe KD, Johnson LF, Harmon JW. Role of the components of the gastroduodenal contents in experimental acid esophagitis. *Surgery* 1982;92:276–284.

33. Lillemoe KD, Johnson LF, Harmon JW. Alkaline esophagitis: a comparison of the ability of components of gastroduodenal contents to injure the rabbit esophagus. *Gastroenterology* 1983;85:621–628.

34. Rascon-Aguilar IE, Pamer M, Wludyka P, et al. Role of gastroesophageal reflux symptoms in exacerbations of COPD. *Chest* 2006;130:1096–1101.

35. Havemann BD, Henderson CA, El-Serag HB. The association between gastro-oesophageal reflux disease and asthma: a systematic review. *Gut* 2007;56: 1654–1664.

36. Mansfield LE, Hameister HH, Spaulding HS, et al. The role of the vagus nerve in airway narrowing caused by intraesophageal hydrochloric acid provocation and esophageal distention. *Ann Allergy* 1981;47:431–434.

37. Wright RA, Miller SA, Corsello BF. Acid-induced esophagobronchial-cardiac reflexes in humans. *Gastroenterology* 1990;99:71–73.

38. Peery AF, Dellon ES, Lund J, et al. Burden of gastrointestinal disease in the United States: 2012 update. *Gastroenterology* 2012;143:1179–1187.

39. Schumock GT, Li EC, Suda KT, et al. National trends in prescription drug expenditures and projections for 2016. *Am J Health Syst Pharm* 2016;73:1058–1075.

40. Kahrilas PJ, Shaheen NJ, Vaezi MF. American gastroenterological association institute technical review on the management of gastroesophageal reflux disease. *Gastroenterology* 2008;135:1392–1413.

41. Fass R, Shapiro M, Dekel R, et al. Systematic review: proton-pump inhibitor failure in gastro-esophageal reflux disease—where next? *Aliment Pharmacol Ther* 2005;22:79–84.

42. Sandmark S, Carlsson R, Fausa O, et al. Omeprazole or ranitidine in the treatment of reflux esophagitis. *Scand J Gastroenterol* 1988;23:625.

43. Raghunath AS, Hungin AP, Mason J, et al. Symptoms in patients on long-term proton pump inhibitors: prevalence and predictors. *Aliment Pharmacol Ther* 2009;29:431–439.

44. Laheij RJF, Sturkenboom MCJM, Hassing RJ, et al. Risk of community-acquired pneumonia and use of gastric acid-suppressive drugs. *JAMA* 2004;292:1955–1960.

45. Yang Y-X, Lewis JD, Epstein S, et al. Long-term proton pump inhibitor therapy and the risk of hip fracture. *JAMA* 2006;296:2947–2953.

46. Targownik LE, Lix LM, Metge CJ, et al. Use of proton pump inhibitors and risk of osteoporosis-related fractures. *CMAJ* 2008;179:319–326.

47. Cheungpasitporn W, Thongprayoon C, Kittanmongkolchai W, et al. Proton pump inhibitors linked to hypomagnesemia: a systematic review and meta-analysis of observational studies. *Ren Fail* 2015;37:1237–1241.

48. Lewis PO, Litchfield JM, Tharp JL, et al. Risk and severity of hospital-acquired clostridium difficile infection in patients taking proton pump inhibitors. *Pharmacotherapy* 2016;36:986–993.

49. Nissen R. A simple operation for control of reflux esophagitis. *Schweiz Med Wochenschr* 1956;86:590–592.

50. Dallemagne B, Weerts JM, Jehaes C. Laparoscopic Nissen fundoplication: preliminary report. *Surg Laparosc Endosc* 1991;1:138–143.

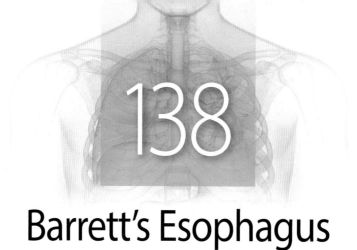

138

Barrett's Esophagus

Kamran Mohiuddin ▪ Donald E. Low

INTRODUCTION AND EPIDEMIOLOGY

Barrett's is an acquired and premalignant condition which has been associated with many etiologic factors but most specifically with chronic gastroesophageal reflux disease (GERD). Barrett's esophagus demonstrates significant variation in incidence among different populations around the world associated with marked variability in incidence rates according to geography, race, and gender.[1,2] Therefore, an insight into its pathogenetic mechanisms may help to better understand its epidemiologic patterns around the world.[1,3-5]

Risk factors for the development of Barrett's esophagus include demographics (Caucasian), obesity (↑risk of GERD), behavior and lifestyle (smoking), diet (omega-3 fatty acids), socioeconomic status (high income), GERD, male gender, and increasing age. Smoking might increase the risk of Barrett's, whereas *Helicobacter pylori* infection and specific "healthy" dietary factors may lower the risk.[6]

Barrett's esophagus is accepted as the major precursor of esophageal adenocarcinoma (EAC). The conversion of Barrett's epithelium into adenocarcinoma is believed to be associated with an evolution over time. It likely follows a sequence of events from non-dysplastic metaplasia through low-grade dysplasia (LGD), high-grade dysplasia (HGD) to early cancer. With HGD there is an increased risk of conversion to malignancy. There is ample evidence that Barrett's esophagus and EAC predominantly affect Caucasian males, less commonly in African-American males, and least likely to affect African-American females.[6-9] Thrift et al. analyzed data of 999 patients with EAC, 2,061 patients with Barrett's, and 2,169 population controls and performed genetic risk score derived from 29 genetic variants shown to be associated with BMI. They reported that people with high genetic propensity to obesity have higher risk of esophageal metaplasia and neoplasia.[10] The annual incidence in Caucasian men is 3.6/100,000 compared to 0.8 in African-American men and 0.3 in Caucasian women.[11] Prevalence of Barrett's esophagus in Hispanics is similar to Caucasians in the United States.[11]

In Europe, the prevalence of Barrett's esophagus among patients undergoing upper endoscopy for GERD symptoms is similar to the United States. Barrett's esophagus is relatively uncommon among Asian populations (Japan or Singapore) but more prevalent among Chinese population in Taiwan.[13] Also, Africa and the Middle East represent geographical regions with low prevalence of both Barrett's

esophagus and adenocarcinoma, although these regions demonstrate high incidence of squamous cell esophageal cancer.[6,8,9] Barrett's is rare in children and tends to become more prevalent with age.[12] The incidence of EAC has increased rapidly over the past four decades in the United States and other western countries. In the United States, the incidence rates rose from 1975 through 2004 among white men (463%) and women (335%).[13] In 2014 approximately 18,170 people were newly diagnosed with EAC accompanied by an estimated 15,450 EAC-related cancer deaths in the United States.[14] Despite substantial improvements in survival over the past three decades 5-year overall survival in all patients presenting with EAC remains approximately 17.5%. Patients with early-stage disease demonstrate better outcomes with the majority of studies describing 5-year survival rates in stage I patients exceeding 80%.[15]

AGA current recommendations for treatment of Barrett's include medical therapy with proton pump inhibitors (PPIs).[16] There is some evidence that successful surgical anti-reflux therapy may help to prevent the development of cancer in Barrett's and that the risk of progression of Barrett's to dysplasia and cancer may decrease[17]; however, this protective effect of anti-reflux surgery has not been definitely proven.

PRESENTATION, ASSESSMENT, AND SCREENING FOR BARRETT'S

It is difficult to accurately document the actual incidence and prevalence of Barrett's esophagus. This is due to the fact that the majority of individuals with Barrett's are asymptomatic. However, in a study from Sweden with the objective of validating the Gastrointestinal Symptom Rating Scale, a random selection of 1,000 individuals underwent endoscopy. Patients with symptoms of reflux had an overall prevalence of Barrett's esophagus of 2.3%, whereas the prevalence in asymptomatic individuals was 1.4%.[18] In another study Westhoff et al. demonstrates that 13.2% of patients with chronic GERD symptoms have Barrett's metaplasia. Paradoxically, patients with short-segment Barrett's esophagus had more frequent and intense symptoms than did those with long-segment Barrett's esophagus suggesting that patients with long-segment Barrett's may be less likely to manifest classic symptoms of GERD.[19]

Barrett's esophagus can be diagnosed easily by endoscopic visualization of columnar mucosa in the distal esophagus (Fig. 138.1A,B)

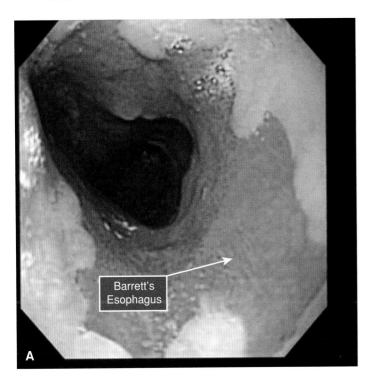

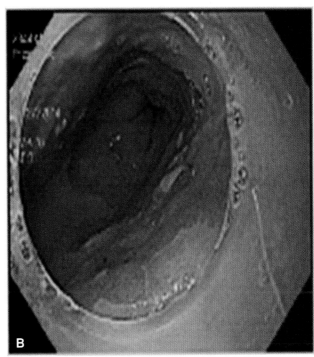

FIGURE 138.1 **A:** Endoscopic view of Barrett's esophagus. **B:** Pre-EMR view of LGD and foci of HGD.

and can be confirmed by biopsy demonstrating intestinal metaplasia (Fig. 138.2). Patients with the diagnosis of Barrett's who then undergo routine surveillance will hypothetically have progression to dysplasia or cancer diagnosed at an earlier stage. In spite of this there have historically been no generally accepted recommendations for Barrett's screening of the general population due mostly to concerns for cost-effectiveness.

The biopsy specimens of columnar mucosa show specialized intestinal metaplasia with its characteristic goblet cells (Fig. 138.2). The distance between the gastroesophageal junction and the most proximal extent of Barrett's metaplasia establishes whether there is long-segment (>3 cm) or short-segment (<3 cm) Barrett's.[20,21] Long-segment Barrett's is strongly associated with chronic heartburn,

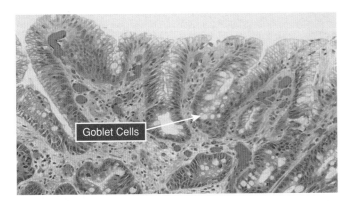

FIGURE 138.2 Barrett's histology showing negative for dysplasia and importance of seeing goblet cells in differentiating "intestinal metaplasia." The metaplastic glands consistently show nuclear atypism when contrasted with normal columnar epithelium. The atypism comprises nuclear enlargement, crowding, hyperchromatism, prominence of nucleoli, and occasional mild stratification.

hiatal hernia, and severe reflux esophagitis. Barrett's metaplasia itself typically causes no symptoms.

In spite of the historic controversy, new data on risk stratification increasingly favor selective screening. Patients can be stratified based on known risk factors for Barrett's esophagus, including age >40, chronic heartburn, smoking, obesity (body mass index greater than 30 kg per m^2), and longer duration of GERD symptoms.[22] The patients with highest yield for Barrett's are older Caucasian males with long-standing heartburn. These data are strengthened by nationwide retrospective cohort studies confirming that male sex, older age, and LGD at initial diagnosis are independent predictors of malignant progression in Barrett's esophagus.[23] The American Gastroenterological Association (AGA) and the American College of Physicians (ACP) clinical guidelines[16,24] have been published. Two additional guidelines are yet to be published from the BOB CAT consensus[25] and the Society of Thoracic Surgeons.[26] The former is an international, multidisciplinary, systematic search and evidence-based review of Barrett's esophagus and provided consensus recommendations for clinical use in patients with non-dysplastic, indefinite, and LGD; the latter comes from the STS General Thoracic Surgery Esophageal Cancer Taskforce. They all suggest that EGD screening for Barrett's can be considered for men over 50 with long-standing heartburn (GERD) symptoms (typically more than 5 years) especially those with additional risk factors such as nocturnal reflux, hiatal hernia, smoking history, and elevated BMI especially those with high proportions of intra-abdominal fat or visceral obesity (see Table 138.1).

Cancer Research UK is currently conducting a multicenter clinical trial, in which the researchers are reviewing a new screening tool called the cytosponge (Fig. 138.3) (non-endoscopic immuno-cytologic device) for screening Barrett's in the primary care setting. High-risk patients swallow a pill with an attached string. Once in the stomach the pill dissolves releasing a cytosponge and the string

TABLE 138.1 Current Recommendations for Screening Guidelines on the Management of Barrett's Esophagus

AGA, 2014	ASGE, 2014	ACG, 2008	STS, 2015	SSAT, 2005	ACP, 2012	BOB CAT, 2015
Patients with additional risk factors for esophageal adenocarcinoma*	Long-standing reflux, additional risk factors for esophageal adenocarcinoma*	Age >50 yrs, Caucasian, male with long-standing heartburn	NA	Patients who require long-term medical therapy for GERD	Men, age >50 yrs with chronic GERD symptoms (>5 yrs) and additional risk factors for EA*	Men, age >50 yrs, Uncontrolled GERD White race, Central Obesity

ACG, American College of Gastroenterology; ACP, American College of Physicians; ASGE, American Society for Gastrointestinal Endoscopy; SSAT, Society for Surgery of the Alimentary Tract; AGA, American Gastroenterological Association; STS, Society of Thoracic Surgeons; BOB CAT, Benign Barrett's and Cancer Taskforce.
*Additional Risk Factors: Age >50 years, male, white, chronic GERD, hiatal hernia, elevated body mass index, tobacco use, intra-abdominal body fat distribution, nocturnal reflux symptoms

is used to retrieve the sponge up the esophagus collecting mucosal cells. Cytologic assessment allows for the detection of Barrett's or cancer while additional studies are assessing cellular markers that may identify patients at higher risk of Barrett's esophagus progressing to cancer. This system may ultimately provide a suitable, low-cost alternative to endoscopy screening and potentially can be applied in the office of a primary caregiver.

Recently, a consortium of international scientists from the University of Cambridge (UK) and the University of Southampton (UK) sequenced the DNA of patients with Barrett's esophagus and patients with esophageal cancer and mapped out their genetic similarities and differences. They found mutations in the gene's tumor protein 53 (TP53) and SMAD family member 4 (SMAD4) that may offer a way of identifying which Barrett's patients will progress into cancer. There is increasing optimism that at some point in the future genetic mapping will allow Barrett's patients with high risk for progression to be identified at the time of initial diagnosis.[27]

The risk of adenocarcinoma appears to vary with the length of esophagus lined by Barrett's. Short-segment Barrett's is more common than long-segment. However, patients with long-segment are at higher risk of developing adenocarcinoma.[28] The current recommendations for screening programs for Barrett's will not identify the 50% of patients with short-segment disease who have no GERD symptoms.

SURVEILLANCE

In patients with Barrett's esophagus and/or LGD, treatment with acid suppression therapy remains the standard of care, with evidence

assessing survival data supporting routine surveillance in patients with Barrett's esophagus. All patients with non-dysplastic Barrett's esophagus should be treated with PPIs because there is a 37 percent absolute risk reduction for developing dysplasia based on a 20-year prospective cohort.[29] According to the American College of Gastroenterology (ACG)'s Practice Guidelines, patients diagnosed with Barrett's esophagus (without dysplasia) should receive two upper endoscopies within 1 year and then every 3 years thereafter. More frequent intervals are recommended if dysplasia is present.[30] Similarly the ACP recommend that upper endoscopy should be performed at intervals no more frequent than 3 to 5 years in men and women with Barrett's esophagus and no dysplasia and more frequently in patients with dysplasia.[24] The current guidelines to determine surveillance intervals are based on the degree of dysplasia.

Biopsies showing any grade of dysplasia should be reassessed by an expert gastrointestinal pathologist. In patients with known LGD endoscopic surveillance is justified and has been shown to be cost-effective.[31] However, important developments in the area of endoscopic ablation therapies for Barrett's have provided effective therapeutic alternative in patients with Barrett's and dysplasia.

Crockett et al. investigated the association of endoscopic surveillance in non-dysplastic Barrett's. They conducted a multicenter study and found that most patients (65%) had more endoscopic surveillance than recommended within current guidelines.[32] Das et al. performed an economic analysis evaluating the cost-effectiveness of endoscopic ablation versus endoscopic surveillance in non-dysplastic Barrett's and reported that endoscopic ablation is more cost-effective. Adhering to current endoscopic surveillance recommendations by ACG and ACP is expensive and costs approximately $290 million every year in the United States alone.[33] Current recommendations are based on the assumptions that Barrett's adversely influences survival. Surveillance has the potential to detect progression of dysplasia into cancer, and early detection will reduce mortality and improve the survival in these patients. However, several randomized prospective trials did not demonstrate survival benefits in non-dysplastic Barrett's patients undergoing surveillance.[30]

In HGD, Barrett's is associated with a 6% per year incidence of cancer[34] justifying intervention.[18] In patients with HGD current recommendations do not recommend surveillance as these patients should be considered for ablation. Two important areas for future assessment are to formalize recommendations for surveillance in patients following successful endoscopic ablation and design clinical trials to establish the clinical and cost-effectiveness of surveillance and ablation in non-dysplastic Barrett's esophagus. The AGA and the American Society for Gastrointestinal Endoscopy (ASGE) now recommend endoscopic eradication therapy rather than surveillance for patients with confirmed HGD in Barrett's.[16,35]

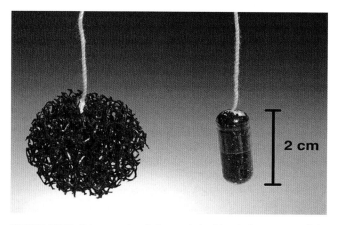

FIGURE 138.3 Cytosponge in gelatin capsule (*right*) and after expansion (*left*).

PATHOLOGIC ASSESSMENT OF BARRETT'S ESOPHAGUS

Due to the significance of recognizing Barrett's metaplasia and of identifying dysplasia, much work has gone into clarifying and refining the criteria used to interpret biopsies.[36–38] Multiple previous assessments have demonstrated marked inter-observer variation in pathologic interpretation of standard biopsy specimens of columnar lined esophagus especially in the presence of dysplasia. Accurate pathologic interpretation is essential for recommending subsequent endoscopic surveillance or surgical or endoscopic intervention. The degree of dysplasia is determined by evaluating the cytology (nuclear and cytoplasmic features), architecture (relationship of glands and lamina propria), and degree of surface maturation (comparison of nuclear size within crypts to nuclear size at the mucosal surface) and interpreting these findings in conjunction with the amount of background inflammation. There are standardized categories for grading dysplastic change based on histology: (1) negative for dysplasia (Fig. 138.2), (2) indefinite for dysplasia, (3) LGD (Fig. 138.4), and (4) HGD (Fig. 138.5).

LGD carries a higher risk of progression to esophageal cancer compared to negative and indefinite for dysplasia. The diagnosis of LGD should be confirmed by an expert GI pathologist because previous studies have shown significant inaccuracy in the initial interpretation of LGD. Curvers et al. reviewed the histopathology reports of all patients diagnosed with LGD between 2000 and 2006 in six community-based hospitals and found that 85% of the patients were downstaged to non-dysplastic or to indefinite for dysplasia.[39] Accurate initial interpretation is clinically relevant because a large Dutch cohort study demonstrated an increased rate of progression from LGD to cancer of 0.77% per year and many centers are now recommending endoscopic ablation in patients with LGD.[23] Thomas et al. performed a meta-analysis to determine the incidence of esophageal cancer in Barrett's and found similar rates of progression in studies of patients in surveillance programs: 0.7% per year in the United Kingdom, 0.7% per year in the United States, and 0.8% per year in Europe.[40] For patients with a consensus diagnosis of LGD, the cumulative risk of progressing to HGD or carcinoma was 85.0% in 9.1 years compared with 4.6% in 9 years for patients histologically confirmed to have non-dysplastic Barrett's (p <0.0001).[41]

HGD also requires confirmation by an expert pathologist and routinely represents a threshold for intervention. Two major issues in producing accurate pathologic interpretation are sampling error at the time of endoscopy and observer variability among pathologists in interpreting the severity of dysplasia. Kelly et al. studied the inter-observer reproducibility among a group of seven gastrointestinal

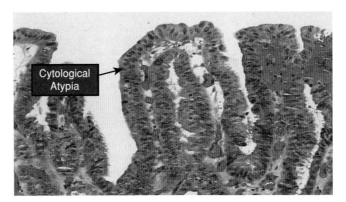

FIGURE 138.5 Barrett's histology showing high-grade dysplasia. The distortion of glandular architecture is present and marked; branching and lateral budding of crypts, a villiform configuration of the mucosal surface, intraglandular bridging of epithelium to form a cribriform pattern of "back-to-back" glands, with loss of nuclear polarity, characterized by "rounding up" of the nuclei, and absence of a consistent relationship of nuclei.

pathologists in the interpretation of 163 consecutive pre-resection biopsies with at least HGD who ultimately underwent esophagectomy. There was 100% agreement among all seven pathologists in only 7.4% of the cases.[41] More recently Sangle et al. studied 485 biopsies from patients with an initial diagnosis of HGD who were rescreened pathologically in preparation for being included in an endoscopic ablation trial. Only 51% were confirmed to have HDG. The remainder demonstrated inflamed gastric mucosa (no Barrett's) 7%, Barrett's no dysplasia 15%, indefinite for dysplasia 26%, LGD 33%, and adenocarcinoma 18%. However, the specialized GI pathologists involved demonstrated a 90% rate of agreement with respect to the pathologic review.[42]

For this reason, all patients with biopsies showing HGD should have a secondary pathologic review, preferably by a gastrointestinal pathologist. A review of the current literature indicates that the percentage of patients with HGD who progress to cancer ranges from 16% to 59%.[43–46] Studies have suggested that for HGD the spacing of four-quadrant biopsies should be every 1 cm because larger intervals (2 cm) lead to a 50% greater miss rates of cancer.[47]

Any mucosal irregularity, such as nodularity or ulcer (Fig. 138.6A), is best assessed with endoscopic mucosal resection (EMR) to provide a more extensive histologic evaluation (Fig. 138.6B). Nodularity has been demonstrated to be associated with a much higher frequency of malignancy and increased potential for spread to regional lymph nodes.[45] At the present time endoscopic ultrasound does not add any useful information to the assessment of HGD.[48]

MANAGEMENT OF NON-DYSPLASTIC BARRETT'S

The current literature provides limited evidence that anti-secretory agents or anti-reflux surgery definitively decreases the occurrence of adenocarcinoma or leads to regression of Barrett's esophagus.[49] In the mid-1980s, histamine 2 (H2) receptor antagonists were the most commonly prescribed agents for treatment of GERD. However, a number of studies were conducted with either cimetidine or ranitidine, and none documented regression of Barrett's. The introduction of PPIs in the late 1980s proved to be much more efficacious at reducing gastric acid secretion.

The goals of treatment of Barrett's in the absence of dysplasia are essentially the same as for uncomplicated GERD. Therapeutic

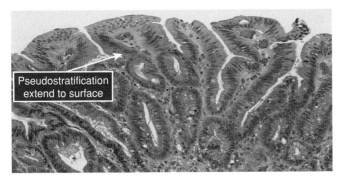

FIGURE 138.4 Barrett's histology showing low-grade dysplasia. The slide shows glands lined by cells with crowded, stratified, hyperchromatic nuclei that extend onto the mucosal surface.

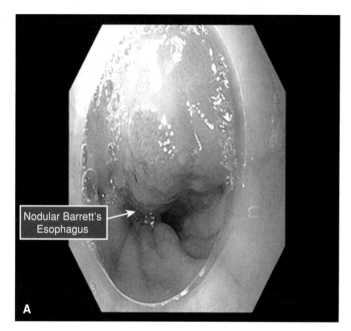
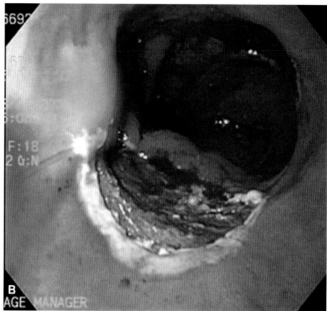

FIGURE 138.6 **A:** Endoscopic view of nodular Barrett's esophagus. **B:** Area of nodular mucosa after EMR.

options include medical therapy with PPIs, H2 receptor antagonists, and/or prokinetic agents or a surgical anti-reflux procedure. There are advantages and disadvantages of each. Medical therapy is noninvasive, is directed at acid suppression, and is effective at controlling reflux symptoms and maintaining the healing of esophagitis in the majority of patients. However, a proportion of patients treated medically will continue to demonstrate reflux, which may contribute to the development of dysplasia and adenocarcinoma. There are also concerns for side effects of long-term PPI therapy especially with respect to their effect on calcium and magnesium metabolism with increasing incidence of osteoporosis and hip fracture especially in women.[50] There is also documented increase in certain GI infections and recognized interactions with other medications, particularly antiplatelet agents. Historical evidence exists supporting the concern that bile reflux (not just acid reflux) plays an important part in the pathogenesis of Barrett's. Bile injury to the esophageal mucosa results in a "chemical" esophagitis and can contribute to the development of metaplasia.[51]

In several prospective studies for the treatment of GERD, surgical anti-reflux therapy has been shown to be superior to medical therapy in effectively controlling the symptoms of reflux, preventing both acid and nonacid reflux. There is some evidence that surgery may delay the progression of Barrett's to dysplasia and adenocarcinoma more effectively than medical therapy.[52] Low et al. examined the effect of anti-reflux surgery in 14 patients who had histologically proven Barrett's and underwent anti-reflux surgery. They were followed by careful endoscopic, histologic, and symptomatic follow-up beginning at 2 to 4 weeks after surgery with the mean follow-up of 25.1 months (range 12 to 36 months) and found that 72% had squamous re-epithelialization and 28% had stabilization or improvement in dysplasia without the need for long-term medications.[53] Similarly Morrow et al. studied the impact of laparoscopic anti-reflux surgery on 82 patients who had postoperative esophageal biopsies and found regression of Barrett's in 22% and progression in only 7%.[54]

Nonsteroidal anti-inflammatory drugs (NSAIDs) can exert anti-tumor effects through the inhibition of cyclooxygenase 2 and through actions independent of cyclooxygenase inhibition. Indirect evidence suggests that NSAID use might decrease the risk of EAC. However, NSAIDs can have severe adverse effects, and presently, the use of NSAIDs solely for chemoprevention in Barrett's is discouraged.[55]

TREATMENT OF LOW-GRADE AND HIGH-GRADE DYSPLASIA

ROLE OF ABLATION THERAPY

Ablation therapy is an endoscopic technique in which Barrett's epithelium is exposed to heat energy and destroyed. The goal is to destroy the epithelium to a sufficient depth to eliminate the intestinal metaplasia and allow regrowth of normal squamous epithelium. There are a number of endoscopic ablative modalities including radiofrequency ablation (RFA), photodynamic therapy (PDT), argon plasma coagulation (APC), multipolar electrocoagulation (MPEC), heater probes, various forms of lasers, and cryotherapy which have been utilized, typically in combination with medical therapy. For ablation to be successful an antacid environment is recommended.

Although esophagectomy remains an acceptable option in patients with HGD, the American Gastroenterology Association and the Guidelines of the Society of Thoracic Surgeons recommend endoscopic eradication therapy (RFA, PDT, or EMR) rather than surveillance for patients with HGD and identify endoscopic ablation as an acceptable therapeutic option for patients with LGD.[16,56] For the general population of patients with Barrett's in the absence of dysplasia, endoscopic eradication therapy is not currently generally recommended. Although, in selected individuals with non-dysplastic Barrett's who are judged to be at increased risk for progression to HGD or with a family history of EAC RFA (Fig. 138.7) with or without EMR (Fig. 138.8) can be a therapeutic option.[16]

Shaheen et al. in a multicenter, randomized, sham-controlled trial assessed whether endoscopic RFA can eradicate dysplastic Barrett's and decrease the rate of neoplastic progression in 127 patients. In LGD, complete eradication of dysplasia occurs in 91% in the ablation group and 23% in the sham group (p = 0.001), whereas in HGD,

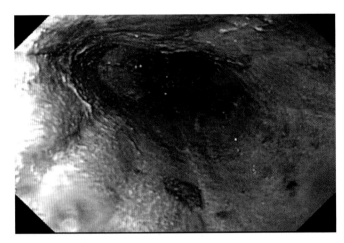

FIGURE 138.7 Endoscopic picture after RFA of patient shown in Figure 138.1B. RFA produces a superficial continuous burn of metaplastic and dysplastic Barrett's epithelium to allow regrowth of normal squamous mucosa.

complete eradication was achieved in 81% compared with 19% in sham group (p = 0.001).[57] Similarly, Phoa et al. recently conducted a multicenter, randomized trial at nine Barrett's centers in Europe, enrolling 136 patients to investigate whether endoscopic RFA could decrease the rate of neoplastic progression in patients with LGD. They concluded that RFA substantially reduced the rate of neoplastic progression to HGD and adenocarcinoma over 3 years of follow-up and recommended that patients with a pathologically confirmed diagnosis of LGD should be considered for ablation therapy.[58] Orman et al. performed a systemic review and meta-analysis of 18 studies to determine the efficacy and durability of RFA in patients with dysplastic and non-dysplastic Barrett's and reported that complete eradication of dysplasia was achieved in 91% whereas complete eradication of intestinal metaplasia occurred in 78%. Progression to cancer was seen in only 0.2% during treatment. Esophageal stricture (Fig. 138.9) was the most common adverse event reported in 5% of patients.[59] Spechler et al. reported complete neoplasia eradication in 97% of 349 patients undergoing endoscopic therapies for mucosal cancer in Barrett's.[16] During a mean follow-up of 64 months, metachronous neoplasms were discovered in 21%. A retrospectively identified major risk factor for these metachronous lesions was failure to eradicate the residual, non-neoplastic Barrett's. Thus, it is now recommended that all of the Barrett's, not just the apparent neoplastic foci, be eradicated during endoscopic treatment.[2,18]

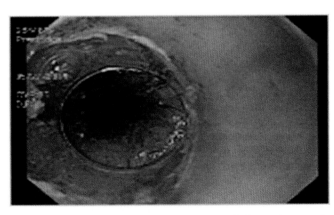

FIGURE 138.8 EMR can be applied circumferentially but is also typically recommended due to risk of stricture (see Fig. 138.9). Generally EMR should be limited to 50% of the circumference during any single treatment.

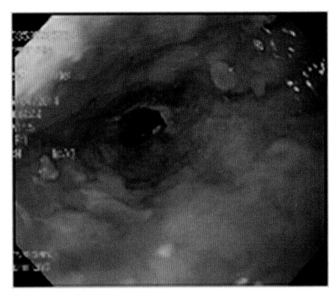

FIGURE 138.9 Post circumferential EMR stricture.

The recent ASGE guidelines recommend endoscopic ablation for Barrett's with HGD; RFA should also be considered and discussed with patients with LGD. Due to the safety, apparent efficacy, and minimal morbidity of RFA (Fig. 138.10A,B), however, some authors feel that these guidelines are too restrictive and argue that virtually all patients with Barrett's, irrespective of dysplasia, should be treated with RFA.[60] There is currently no consensus regarding ablation of non-dysplastic Barrett's.

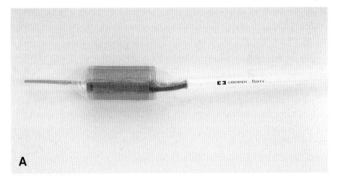

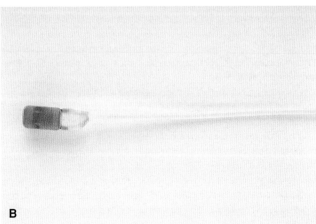

FIGURE 138.10 **A:** The Barrx™ circumferential ablation system facilitates a 360-degree, 3-cm long ablation for treating short and long segments of Barrett's epithelium. **B:** Barrx™ 90 RFA focal catheter.

EMR (Fig. 138.6B) and endoscopic submucosal dissection are alternative approaches to ablation which involve the removal of larger areas of mucosa and submucosa than can be sampled by standard biopsies. These approaches provide much improved samples for pathologic interpretation and can be used as definitive treatment in selected patients with Barrett's. EMR should be considered for the primary sampling of any mucosal lesions seen in Barrett's and circumferential EMR or ESD can be done but should be done in multiple sessions to minimize the risk of significant stricture (Fig. 138.9).

Bennett et al. analyzed data from the current literature to examine the effectiveness of endotherapies compared with surgery in people with Barrett's and concluded that there is currently no randomized control trial to compare management options. They also recommended that in patients with early cancer or HGD use of endotherapies should be done in association with a recommendation from a multidisciplinary team. There is an excellent correlation between preoperative EMR T staging of early Barrett's cancers and postoperative T staging from examination of esophagectomy specimens.[61]

Management of patients with HGD is dependent on local expertise, as well as taking into account the patient's age, comorbidity, and preferences. The current recommendation suggests that if HGD is detected and confirmed, such patients should be referred to a center with expertise in interventional endoscopy techniques and esophageal resection, since there is a high likelihood of occult cancers in these patients.

MANAGEMENT OF T1A AND T1B

In the United States, 20% of all esophageal cancers are currently detected in the early stage (T1) with disease confined to the mucosa or submucosa.[62,63] Historically, the treatment of mucosal cancer has been surgery. However, there remains a potential for substantial morbidity (30% to 50%) associated with esophagectomies.[64,65] In addition in-hospital mortality rates can be as high as 8% in low-volume hospitals compared to 2% to 3% in high-volume institutions.[66] A less invasive alternative to surgery for early-stage mucosal malignancy (T1a) is endoscopic resection and ablation. Depth of invasion is one of the most important prognostic indicators in esophageal cancer. T1a cancers are categorized as intra-mucosal carcinomas because they involve the epithelium, basement membrane, and lamina propria, but do not invade farther than the muscularis mucosae. T1a cancers are rarely associated with lymph node metastasis.[67] T1b lesions extend into the submucosa, and the American Joint Committee on Cancer (AJCC) TNM classification of carcinoma of the esophagus and the esophageal-gastric junction adenocarcinoma (7th edition, 2010)[68,69] highlights that distinguishing between the T1a and T1b stages of esophageal carcinoma is critical for appropriate disease management (Fig. 138.11).

Duplication of muscularis mucosae frequently develops in esophageal metaplasia, and this is not only under-recognized but creates problems for appropriate staging.[70] The muscularis mucosae of the esophagus is the thickest layer and becomes even thicker in response to repeated ulcerations due to acid reflux and therefore it can be easily misidentified on EMR specimens as being the much deeper and typically much larger muscularis propria. Furthermore, when the muscularis mucosae "splits" into superficial and deep layers, the space in between often is misjudged as submucosa. Cancers invading muscularis mucosa actually behave as intra-mucosal cancer. A large study of 99 early Barrett's adenocarcinomas suggested that up to 60% of intra-mucosal lesions are overstaged by EUS and EMR as submucosal cancers.[71]

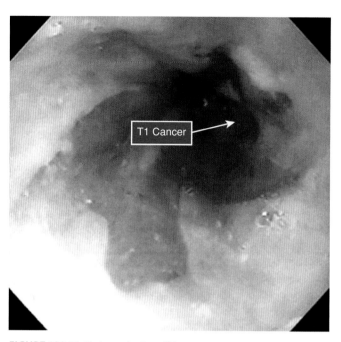

FIGURE 138.11 Endoscopic view of T1 cancer.

Lymph node metastases occur in approximately 3% to 6% of T1a cases, and current guidelines[72–75] recommend the routine application of EMR or ESD for the initial assessment of any mucosal lesions or whenever routine biopsies show malignancy. EMR is well tolerated and is the most appropriate assessment to discriminate between T1a versus T1b tumors.[73–75] In contrast, lymph node metastases occur in 21% to 24% of those with T1b stage of esophageal cancer, and these patients are generally considered not suitable for endoscopic treatment and require surgical resection.[76–80] Selected high-volume endoscopic centers have suggested that "low-risk" T1b cancers can be considered for endoscopic management. These patients must have invasion only into the most superficial submucosal layer (sm1), be confirmed as well-differentiated tumors, and have no lymphovascular invasion on pathologic assessment of EMR specimen.[81] However, most centers recommend that physiologically fit patients with T1b cancer be offered esophageal resection.

Surgery remains an appropriate option in patients with HGD, especially in patients with long-segment Barrett's, in patients with multifocal HGD, and in whom follow-up cannot be guaranteed. In high-volume esophagectomy centers mortality should be 0% to 2% and postoperative quality of life can be comparable to the general population.[82]

REFERENCES

1. Hughes WS. Esophageal cancer. In: Everhart JE, ed. *Digestive Diseases in the United States: Epidemiology and Impact*. Bethesda, MD: NIH; 1994:159–180.
2. Sonnenberg A. Esophageal diseases. In: Everhart JE, ed. *Digestive Diseases in the United States: Epidemiology and Impact*. Bethesda, MD: NIH; 1994:301–355.
3. Bersentes K, Fass R, Sukhdeep P, et al. Prevalence of Barrett's esophagus in Hispanics is similar to Caucasians. *Dig Dis Sci* 1998;43:1038–1041.
4. Cameron AJ, Lomboy CT. Barrett's esophagus: age, prevalence, and extent of columnar epithelium. *Gastroenterology* 1992;103:1241–1245.
5. Yeh C, Hsu CT, Ho AS, et al. Erosive esophagitis and Barrett's esophagus in Taiwan. *Dig Dis Sci* 1997;42:702–706.
6. Spechler SJ, Goyal RK. Barrett's esophagus. *N Engl J Med* 1986;315:362–371.
7. Wong AI, Fitzgerald RC. Epidemiologic risk factors for Barrett's esophagus and associated adenocarcinoma. *Clin Gastroenterol Hepatol* 2005;3(1):1–10.
8. Blot WJ, Devesa SS, Kneller RW, et al. Rising incidence of adenocarcinoma of the esophagus and gastric cardia. *JAMA* 1991;265:1287–1289.
9. Blot WJ, Devesa SS, Fraumeni JF. Continuing climb rates of esophageal adenocarcinoma. *JAMA* 1993;270:1320–1221.

10. Thrift AP, Risch HA, Onstad L, et al. Risk of esophageal adenocarcinoma decreases with height based on consortium analysis and confirmed by Mendelian randomization. *Clin Gastroenterol Hepatol* 2014;12(10):1667–1676.e1.

11. Brown LM, Devesa SS. Epidemiologic trends in esophageal and gastric cancer in the United States. *Surg Oncol Clin N Am* 2002;11:235–256.

12. Hassall E. Columnar-lined esophagus in children. *Gastroenterol Clin North Am* 1997;26(3):533–548.

13. Brown LM, Devesa SS, Chow WH. Incidence of adenocarcinoma of the esophagus among white Americans by sex, stage, and age. *J Natl Cancer Inst* 2008;100(16):1184–1187.

14. Hur C, Miller M, Kong CY, et al. Trends in esophageal adenocarcinoma incidence and mortality. *Cancer* 2013;119:1149–1159.

15. Howlader N, Noone AM, Krapcho M, et al. *SEER Cancer Statistics Review.* Bethesda, MD: National Cancer Institute; 1975–2011. http://seer.cancer.gov/csr/1975_2011/, based on November 2013 SEER data submission, posted to the SEER web site, April 2014.

16. Spechler SJ, Sharma P, Souza RF, et al; American Gastroenterological Association. American Gastroenterological Association medical position statement on the management of Barrett's esophagus. *Gastroenterology* 2011;140(3):1084–1091.

17. Wayne L. Hofstetter, MD, Jeffrey H. et al. Long-term outcome of antireflux surgery in patients with Barrett's esophagus. *Ann Surg* 2001;234(4):532–539.

18. Ronkainen J, Aro P, Storskrubb T, et al. Prevalence of Barrett's esophagus in the general population: an endoscopic study. *Gastroenterology* 2005;129(6):1825–1831.

19. Westhoff B, Brotze S, Weston A, et al. The frequency of Barrett's esophagus in high-risk patients with chronic GERD. *Gastrointest Endosc* 2005;61:226–231.

20. Sharma P, Morales TG, Sampliner RE. Short segment Barrett's esophagus: the need for standardization of the definition and of endoscopic criteria. *Am J Gastroenterol* 1998;93:1033–1036.

21. Sampliner RE. Updated guidelines for the diagnosis, surveillance, and therapy of Barrett's esophagus. *Am J Gastroenterol* 2002;97:1888–1895.

22. Whiteman DC, Sadeghi S, Pandeya N, et al.; Australian Cancer Study. Combined effects of obesity, acid reflux and smoking on the risk of adenocarcinomas of the oesophagus. *Gut* 2008;57(2):173–180.

23. de Jonge PJ, van Blankenstein M, Looman CW, et al. Risk of malignant progression in patients with Barrett's oesophagus: a Dutch nationwide cohort study. *Gut* 2010; 59(8):1030–1036.

24. Shaheen NJ, Weinberg DS, Denberg TD, et al.; Clinical Guidelines Committee of the American College of Physicians. Upper endoscopy for gastro esophageal reflux disease: best practice advice from the Clinical Guidelines Committee of the American College of Physicians. *Ann Intern Med* 2012;157(11):808–816.

25. Kadri S, Lao-Sirieix P, Fitzgerald RC. Developing a nonendoscopic screening test for Barrett's esophagus. *Biomark Med* 2011;5(3):397–404.

26. Bennett C, Moayyedi P, Corley AD, et.al. BOB-CAT: a large-scale review and Delphi consensus for management of Barrett's esophagus with no dysplasia, indefinite for, or low-grade dysplasia. *Am J Gastroenterol* 2015;110(5):662–682; quiz 683.

27. Weaver JMJ, Ross-Innes CS, Shannon N, et al.; OCCAMS consortium. Ordering of mutations in pre-invasive disease stages of esophageal carcinogenesis. *Nat Genet* 2014;46(8):837–843.

28. Weston AP, Sharma P, Mathur S, et al. Risk stratification of Barrett's esophagus: updated prospective multivariate analysis. *Am J Gastroenterol* 2004;99:1657–1666.

29. El-Serag HB, Aguirre TV, Davis S, et al. Proton pump inhibitors are associated with reduced incidence of dysplasia in Barrett's esophagus. *Am J Gastroenterol* 2004; 99(10):1877–1883.

30. Wang KK, Sampliner RE; Practice Parameters Committee of the American College of Gastroenterology. Updated guidelines 2008 for the diagnosis, surveillance and therapy of Barrett's esophagus. *Am J Gastroenterol* 2008;103(3):788–797.

31. Hirota WK, Zuckerman MJ, Adler DG, et al; Standards of Practice Committee, American Society for Gastrointestinal Endoscopy. ASGE guideline: the role of endoscopy in the surveillance of premalignant conditions of the upper GI tract. *Gastrointest Endosc* 2006;63(4):570–580.

32. Crockett SD, Lipkus IM, Bright SD, et al. Overutilization of endoscopic surveillance in nondysplastic Barrett's esophagus: a multicenter study. *Gastrointest Endosc* 2012; 75(1):23–31.e2.

33. Das A, Wells C, Kim HJ, et al. An economic analysis of endoscopic ablative therapy for management of non-dysplastic Barrett's esophagus. *Endoscopy* 2009; 41(5):400–408.

34. Kuipers EJ. Barrett esophagus and life expectancy: implications for screening? *Gastroenterol Hepatol (N Y)* 2011;7(10):689–691.

35. Evans JA, Early DS, Fukami N, et al.; Standards of Practice Committee of the American Society for Gastrointestinal Endoscopy. The role of endoscopy in Barrett's esophagus and other premalignant conditions of the esophagus. *Gastrointest Endosc* 2012;76(6):1087–1094.

36. Montgomery E, Bronner MP, Goldblum JR, et al. Reproducibility of the diagnosis of dysplasia in Barrett esophagus: a reaffirmation. *Hum Pathol* 2001;32:368–378.

37. Theisen J, Nigro JJ, DeMeester TR, et al. Chronology of the Barrett's metaplasia-dysplasia-carcinoma sequence. *Dis Esophagus* 2004;17:67–70.

38. Zhu W, Appelman HD, Greenson JK, et al. A histologically defined subset of high-grade dysplasia in Barrett mucosa is predictive of associated carcinoma. *Am J Clin Pathol* 2009;132:94–100.

39. Curvers WL, ten Kate FJ, Krishnadath KK, et al. Low-grade dysplasia in Barrett's esophagus: over diagnosed and underestimated. *Am J Gastroenterol* 2010;105(7): 1523–1530.

40. Thomas T, Abrams KR, De Caestecker JS, et al. Meta-analysis: cancer risk in Barrett's oesophagus. *Aliment Pharmacol Ther* 2007;26(11–12):1465–1477.

41. Downs-Kelly E, Mendelin JE, Bennett AE, et al. Poor interobserver agreement in the distinction of high-grade dysplasia and adenocarcinoma in pretreatment Barrett's esophagus biopsies. *Am J Gastroenterol* 2008;103(9):2333–2340; quiz 2341.

42. Sangle NA, Taylor SL, Emond MJ, et al. Over diagnosis of high-grade dysplasia in Barrett's esophagus: a multicenter, international study. *Mod Pathol* 2015;28:758.

43. Schnell TG, Sontag SJ, Chejfec G, et al. Long-term nonsurgical management of Barrett's esophagus with high-grade dysplasia. *Gastroenterology* 2001;120: 1607–1619.

44. Buttar NS, Wang KK, Sebo TJ, et al. Extent of high-grade dysplasia in Barrett's esophagus correlates with risk of adenocarcinoma. *Gastroenterology* 2001;120: 1630–1639.

45. Reid BJ, Levine DS, Longton G, et al. Predictors of progression to cancer in Barrett's esophagus: baseline histology and flow cytometry identify low- and high-risk patient subsets. *Am J Gastroenterol* 2000;95:1669–1676.

46. Overholt BF, Lightdale CJ, Wang KK, et al. Photodynamic therapy with porfimer sodium for ablation of high-grade dysplasia in Barrett's esophagus: international, partially blinded, randomized phase III trial. *Gastrointest Endosc* 2005;62:488–498.

47. Reid BJ, Blount P, Feng Z, et al. Optimizing endoscopic biopsy detection of early cancers in Barrett's high-grade dysplasia. *Am J Gastroenterol* 2000;95: 3089–3096.

48. Fernández-Sordo JO, Konda VJ, Chennat J, et al. Is endoscopic ultrasound (EUS) necessary in the pre-therapeutic assessment of Barrett's esophagus with early neoplasia? *J Gastrointest Oncol* 2012;3(4):314–321.

49. Haag S, Nandurkar S, Talley NJ. Regression of Barrett's esophagus: the role of acid suppression, surgery, and ablative methods. *Gastrointest Endosc* 1999;50(2): 229–240.

50. Khalili H, Huang ES, Jacobson BC, et al. Use of proton pump inhibitors and risk of hip fracture in relation to dietary and lifestyle factors: a prospective cohort study. *BMJ* 2012;344:e372.

51. Souza RF. The role of acid and bile reflux in oesophagitis and Barrett's metaplasia. *Biochem Soc Trans* 2010;38(2):348–352.

52. DeMeester TR. Antireflux surgery in the management of Barrett's esophagus. *J Gastrointest Surg* 2000;4:124–128.

53. Low DE, Levine DS, Dail DH, et al. Histological and anatomic changes in Barrett's esophagus after antireflux surgery. *Am J Gastroenterol* 1999;94:80–85.

54. Morrow E, Bushyhead D, Wassenaar E, et al. The impact of laparoscopic anti-reflux surgery in patients with Barrett's esophagus. *Surg Endosc* 2014;28(12):3279–3284.

55. Kastelein F, Spaander MC, Biermann K, et al.; Probar Study Group. Nonsteroidal anti-inflammatory drugs and statins have chemopreventative effects in patients with Barrett's esophagus. *Gastroenterology* 2011;141(6):2000–2008; quiz e13–e14.

56. Fernando HC, Murthy SC, Hofstetter W, et al.; Society of Thoracic Surgeons. The Society of Thoracic Surgeons practice guideline series: guidelines for the management of Barrett's esophagus with high-grade dysplasia. *Ann Thorac Surg* 2009; 87(6):1993–2002.

57. Shaheen NJ, Sharma P, Overholt BF, et al. Radiofrequency ablation in Barrett's esophagus with dysplasia. *N Engl J Med* 2009;360:2277–2288.

58. Phoa KN, Pouw RE, Bisschops R, et al. Multimodality endoscopic eradication for neoplastic Barrett esophagus: results of an European multicentre study (EURO-II). *Gut* 2016;65(4):555–562.

59. Orman ES, Li N, Shaheen NJ. Efficacy and durability of radiofrequency ablation for Barrett's esophagus: systematic review and meta-analysis. *Clin Gastroenterol Hepatol* 2013;11(10):1245–1255.

60. Fleischer DE, Odze R, Overholt BF, et al. The case for endoscopic treatment of non-dysplastic and low-grade dysplastic Barrett's esophagus. *Dig Dis Sci* 2010;55: 1918–1931.

61. Bennett C, Green S, Decaestecker J, et al. Surgery versus radical endotherapies for early cancer and high-grade dysplasia in Barrett's oesophagus. *Cochrane Database Syst Rev* 2012;11:CD007334.

62. Enzinger PC, Mayer RJ. Esophageal cancer. *N Engl J Med* 2003;349:2241–2252.

63. Das A, Singh V, Fleischer DE, et al. A comparison of endoscopic treatment and surgery in early esophageal cancer: an analysis of surveillance epidemiology and end results data. *Am J Gastroenterol* 2008;103:1340–1345.

64. Lagarde SM, Vrouenraets BC, Stassen LP, et al. Evidence-based surgical treatment of esophageal cancer: overview of high-quality studies. *Ann Thorac Surg* 2010;89: 1319–1326.

65. Chang AC, Ji H, Birkmeyer NJ, et al. Outcomes after transhiatal and transthoracic esophagectomy for cancer. *Ann Thorac Surg* 2008;85:424–429.

66. Markar SR, Karthikesalingam A, Thrumurthy S, et al. Volume-outcome relationship in surgery for esophageal malignancy: systematic review and meta-analysis 2000–2011. *J Gastrointest Surg* 2012;16:1055–1063.

67. Merkow RP, Bilimoria KY, Keswani RN, et al. Treatment trends, risk of lymph node metastasis, and outcomes for localized esophageal cancer. *J Natl Cancer Inst* 2014; 106(7):pii: dju133.

68. Sobin L, Gospodarowicz M, Wittekind C. International Union Against Cancer. TNM Classification of Malignant Tumours. 7th ed. Oxford, UK: Wiley-Blackwell; 2009, pp 15–18.

69. National Comprehensive Cancer Network (NCCN). NCCN practice guideline for oncology (esophageal and esophagogastric junction cancer) version 2. http://www.nccn.org/professionals/physician_gls/f_guidelines.asp#site. 2011

70. Abraham SC, Krasinskas AM, Correa AM, et al. Duplication of the muscularis mucosae in Barrett esophagus: an under recognized feature and its implication for staging of adenocarcinoma. *Am J Surg Pathol* 2007;31(11):1719–1725.

71. Estrella JS, Hofstetter WL, Correa AM, et al. Duplicated muscularis mucosae invasion has similar risk of lymph node metastasis and recurrence-free survival as intramucosal esophageal adenocarcinoma. *Am J Surg Pathol* 2011;35(7): 1045–1053.

72. Ell C, May A, Pech O, et al. Curative endoscopic resection of early esophageal adenocarcinomas (Barrett's cancer) *Gastrointest Endosc* 2007;65:3–10.

73. Pech O, Behrens A, May A, et al. Long-term results and risk factor analysis for recurrence after curative endoscopic therapy in 349 patients with high-grade intraepithelial neoplasia and mucosal adenocarcinoma in Barrett's oesophagus. *Gut* 2008;57:1200–1206.

74. Pech O, Gossner L, May A, et al. Endoscopic resection of superficial esophageal squamous-cell carcinomas: western experience. *Am J Gastroenterol* 2004;99:1226–1232.

75. Stahl M, Budach W, Meyer HJ, et al. Esophageal cancer: clinical practice guidelines for diagnosis, treatment and follow-up. *Ann Oncol* 2010;21(Suppl 5):v46–v49.

76. Nealis TB, Washington K, Keswani RN. Endoscopic therapy of esophageal premalignancy and early malignancy. *J Natl Compr Canc Netw* 2011;9:890–899.

77. Lee JH, Hong SJ, Jang JY, et al. Outcome after endoscopic submucosal dissection for early gastric cancer in Korea. *World J Gastroenterol* 2011;17:3591–3595.

78. Saito Y, Takisawa H, Suzuki H, et al. Endoscopic submucosal dissection of recurrent or residual superficial esophageal cancer after chemoradiotherapy. *Gastrointest Endosc* 2008;67:355–359.

79. Othman MO, Wallace MB. Endoscopic mucosal resection (EMR) and endoscopic submucosal dissection (ESD) in 2011, a Western perspective. *Clin Res Hepatol Gastroenterol* 2011;35:288–294.

80. Kwee RM, Kwee TC. Imaging in local staging of gastric cancer: a systematic review. *J Clin Oncol* 2007;25:2107–2116.

81. Lin JL. T1 esophageal cancer, request an endoscopic mucosal resection (EMR) for in-depth review. *J Thorac Dis* 2013;5(3):353–356.

82. Porteous GH, Neal JM, Slee A, et al. A standardized anesthetic and surgical clinical pathway for esophageal resection: impact on length of stay and major outcomes. *Reg Anesth Pain Med* 2015;40(2):139–149.

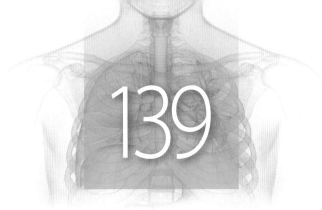

139

Paraesophageal Hiatal Hernia

Janet Edwards ▪ Colin Schieman ▪ Sean C. Grondin

CLASSIFICATION OF HIATAL HERNIA

Hiatal hernias are generally classified into four types, the most common of which is the sliding or type I hiatal hernia. Types II through IV hiatal hernias are paraesophageal hernias (PEHs) which vary with regard to the degree of intrathoracic migration, as well as, the contents of the hernial sac (see Fig. 139.1).

In order to appreciate the differences between the types of hernias, it is important to understand the anatomy of the hiatus and the gastroesophageal (GE) junction. The esophageal hiatus is formed by

muscle fibers of the right crus of the diaphragm, with little or no contribution from the left crus. These fibers overlap inferiorly where they attach over and along the right side of the median arcuate ligament, which is attached to the lateral aspects of vertebral bodies. The orifice is therefore teardrop-shaped, with the point to the right of the aorta and the ventral rounded portion in the midline close to the connecting portion of the central tendon of the diaphragm. The crural fibers form a tunnel that encloses the esophagus. The phrenicoesophageal ligament is formed by fusion of the endothoracic and endoabdominal fascia at the diaphragmatic hiatus. This ligament inserts onto the

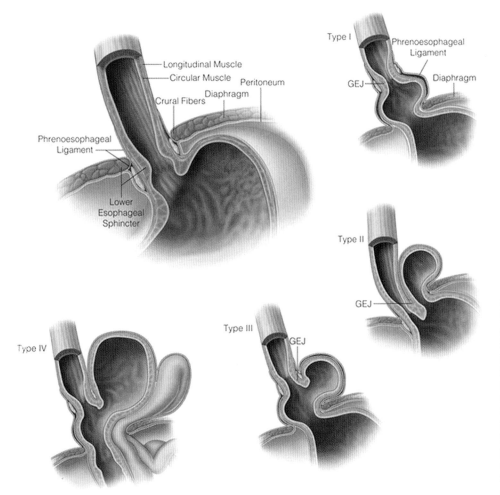

FIGURE 139.1 Types of hiatal hernia. Type I is a sliding hernia. Types II, III and IV are paraesophageal hernias (PEHs). In type II PEHs, the gastroesophageal (GE) junction remains below the diaphragm whereas in type I PEHs the GE junction is above the diaphragm. Type IV PEHs include herniation of the stomach as well as other abdominal organs into the chest cavity. (Used with kind permission from Wiener DC, Wee JO. Thorax. Minimally invasive esophageal procedures. In: Ashley SW, ed. *Scientific American Surgery [online]*. Hamilton, ON: Decker Intellectual Properties; 2012. Available at: http://www.sciamsurgery.com.[1])

esophagus just above the GE junction circumferentially and holds the distal esophagus in place, with the most caudal 2 to 3 cm residing within the abdomen.

TYPE I

In this sliding type of hiatal hernia the GE junction moves upward through the diaphragmatic hiatus into the posterior mediastinum so that it occupies an intrathoracic position and the proximal cardia resides within the chest. This process occurs because of circumferential weakening of the phrenicoesophageal ligament (see Fig. 139.1). Factors that may contribute to the development of this hernia include increased abdominal pressure (e.g., with pregnancy, obesity, or vomiting) and vigorous esophageal contraction, both of which may pull the GE junction up into the mediastinum. This type of hiatal hernia is frequently accompanied by low resting pressure or inappropriate relaxation of the lower esophageal sphincter (LES), which may result in GE reflux and esophagitis. The LES effects may be related to the loss of mechanical advantage at the GE junction when it is displaced into the chest. The diagnosis and treatment of reflux esophagitis and type I hiatal hernia is reviewed elsewhere in this text.

TYPE II

Type II PEH is an uncommon disorder that is distinct from the sliding hiatal hernia. In type II hernias, the phrenicoesophageal membrane is not weakened diffusely but rather focally, anterior and lateral to the esophagus. The gastric cardia and lower esophagus remain at or below the diaphragm, while the gastric fundus and/or greater curvature protrudes through the defect into the mediastinum (see Fig. 139.1). The protruding organs are covered circumferentially by a layer of peritoneum that forms a true hernial sac.

This intrathoracic migration of the stomach evolves by so-called organo-axial rotation (see Fig. 139.2). The lesser curve of the stomach is anchored in the abdomen by the posterior attachments of the lower esophagus, the left gastric artery, and the retroperitoneal fixation of the pylorus and duodenum. These three points define the long axis of the stomach and remain relatively fixed within the abdomen in a type II hiatal hernia. The greater curve of the stomach, however, is relatively mobile and rotates about the "long axis" by moving first anteriorly and then upward as the hernia evolves. The fundus is the first part of the stomach to protrude upward through the anterior hernial sac. As the hiatal defect enlarges, the body and antrum continue the axial rotation and migrate into the thorax, leaving the cardia and pylorus in the abdomen. The stomach then resides "upside down" in the chest, with the remaining greater curve pointing cephalad and the cardia remaining at or below the diaphragm (see Fig. 139.2). The stomach initially may occupy a retrocardiac position, but as the hernia enlarges rotation occurs, usually into the right chest. With huge hernias, most of the stomach lies within the right hemithorax and the greater curvature of the stomach points toward the right shoulder. The organo-axial rotation of the stomach is most commonly upward into the chest and toward the right. This is the path of least resistance because of the aorta to the left and the heart anterior into the left chest. Occasionally, however, the stomach may rotate directly in a superior direction without a rightward deviation so that the greater curvature lies transversely behind the heart.

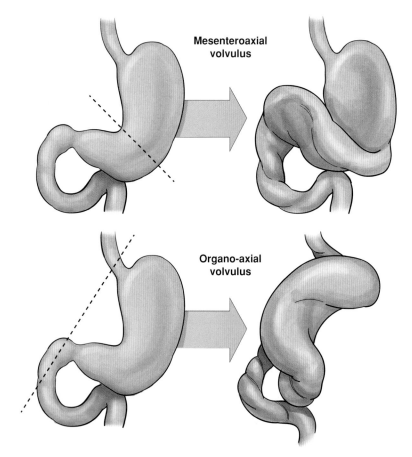

Mesenteroaxial volvulus

Organo-axial volvulus

FIGURE 139.2 Mechanism of incarceration and strangulation with paraesophageal hiatal hernia. In organo-axial volvulus, the stomach rotates around an axis which runs from the pylorus to the gastroesophageal junction thereby causing a closed-loop foregut obstruction. The resulting occlusion of the gastric vessels may lead to ischemia, necrosis, and perforation. In a meso-axial volvulus, the axis bisects the lesser and greater curvatures. The antrum rotates anteriorly and superiorly so that the posterior surface of the stomach lies anteriorly. The rotation is usually incomplete and occurs intermittently. Vascular compromise is uncommon.

The term "parahiatal hernia" has been used in the past, but this type of defect may not actually exist. Aside from post-traumatic diaphragmatic injury, the authors have never encountered a defect in the diaphragm along the side of the esophageal hiatus with protrusion of the stomach into the chest and identifiable crural or diaphragmatic fibers separating the hernial orifice from the true hiatus.

TYPE III

The type III or mixed hiatal hernia is a combination of types I and II in that it includes both sliding and rolling components (see Fig. 139.1). If a type I hiatal hernia enlarges, the attenuated phrenicoesophageal membrane may also weaken focally in its anterior aspect and thus allow protrusion of the gastric fundus into the chest. Rotation of the stomach may result in the body or fundus obtaining a higher position within the chest than the cardia. But, unlike the type II hiatal hernia, in this situation the cardia itself is above the level of the hiatus. The term "giant PEH" typically refers to a hernia where more than a third of the stomach has migrated into the chest cavity above the diaphragm.[2]

It has also been suggested that a type III defect may very well be just progression or evolution over time of a type II defect. Presumably, with ongoing negative intrathoracic pressure and positive intra-abdominal pressure the severity of the gastric herniation may advance over the years until the cardia is drawn up above the level of the diaphragm, thus resulting in a type III defect. In this case, attachments of the GE junction would remain intact posteriorly.

TYPE IV

Progressive enlargement of the diaphragmatic opening can eventually lead to herniation of organs other than the stomach into the chest (see Fig. 139.1). The transverse colon and omentum are most commonly involved, but the spleen and small bowel may also herniate into the chest. However, it is uncommon for patients to demonstrate obstructive symptoms from herniation of either large or small intestine into the chest in this setting.

EPIDEMIOLOGY

PEHs account for approximately 5% to 15% of all hiatal hernias and are thus far less common than the typical sliding hiatal hernia.[3–5] Hill and Tobias,[6] Ozdemir,[7] and Sanderug[8] have reported that this condition accounted for only 3% to 6% of all patients undergoing surgical repair of hiatal hernias. Allen and colleagues[9] reviewed the records of over 46,000 patients diagnosed with a hiatal hernia at the Mayo Clinic from 1980 to 1990. These investigators found that only 147 patients (0.32%) had PEHs with 75% or more of the stomach within the chest. Of the 124 patients who underwent operation, 51 (41%) had a type II hiatal hernia, 52 (43%) had a type III (mixed sliding and paraesophageal) hiatal hernia, and 21 (17%) had a type IV hiatal hernia with other organs identified within the intrathoracic hernial sac.

Little data are available on the risk of progression from asymptomatic to symptomatic PEH but estimates suggest the rate is approximately 14% per year.[10] In the Allen study,[9] only 4 of the 23 patients (17%) who initially refused surgery developed significant symptoms requiring surgery. It is estimated that the risk of developing acute symptoms requiring urgent surgery is 1% to 2%.[5,11]

In terms of risk factors, elderly female patients are most commonly affected.[12,13] Obesity is also a clear risk factor for developing a hiatal hernia with one meta-analysis demonstrating an odds ratio of 1.93 for patients with a body mass index greater than 25 with risk increasing in parallel with body mass index.[14] PEHs are also associated with previous GE surgery such as esophagomyotomy, antireflux surgery, and thoracoabdominal trauma. The presence of skeletal deformities such as kyphosis or scoliosis may also lead to the development of PEH due to distortion of the anatomy of the diaphragm.[15] In children, congenital defects are the most common cause of PEH and are often associated with other congenital anomalies such as intestinal malformation.[5]

SYMPTOMS

Some PEHs cause few or no symptoms and remain undiagnosed for years until they are recognized on a routine chest radiograph or computed tomography (CT) scan, often performed for another reason. In those patients with a supradiaphragmatic cardia, the LES may be incompetent; such patients can present with symptoms of GE reflux, such as substernal burning and water brash. However, the most common symptoms result from the mechanical consequences of an intrathoracic stomach. As with any true anatomic hernia, potential complications include bleeding, incarceration, volvulus, obstruction, strangulation, and perforation. The most common symptoms overall are related to the obstructive nature of the PEH, with early satiety, postprandial pain, vomiting, and dysphagia being common complaints. In some patients, these symptoms may be insidious and not immediately apparent when a history is first taken. As a result of their symptoms, patients may gradually alter the pattern of their food intake to minimize or prevent postprandial discomfort. Thus decreased quantities of food are taken at increasingly longer intervals to minimize those symptoms that occur routinely during eating. Many patients who have been symptomatic for years or even decades will initially deny eating difficulties; it is only upon focused, persistent questioning of the patients and their family members that one finds that their oral intake has changed both in frequency and amount over a period of years, often with a concomitant weight loss.

Allen and colleagues[9] documented the symptoms in the 147 patients undergoing a repair of PEH and found that only 5% of their patients were asymptomatic. Postprandial pain occurred in 87 (59%), vomiting in 46 (31%), and dysphagia in 44 (30%). GE reflux was a complaint in only 23 patients (16%).

Bleeding is also a complication of PEH and most commonly occurs from "saddle or Cameron lesions" found within the gastric wall at the level of the hiatus.[16,17] It has been suggested that these lesions may be purely a consequence of mechanical abrasion on the mucosa. Often patients will present not with acute bleeding but rather with chronic fatigue, and they may then be found to have anemia. This was the case for 21% of patients in the previously mentioned study of Allen et al.[9] Bleeding is rarely rapid enough to result in melena, which the above authors found in three patients (2%). Irritation of mucosa leading to esophagitis and/or gastritis may also lead to bleeding.

Large type III (i.e., giant PEH) or IV hiatal hernias may occupy a large portion of the thoracic cavity and result in postprandial respiratory symptoms of breathlessness with a sense of suffocation. Such symptoms, however, can also be mild despite the presence of a huge hernia. Many patients have become accustomed to these symptoms and tolerate them well. They will sometimes describe this as a sensation of substernal fullness or pressure, and it can on occasion be mistaken for angina. This discomfort is frequently accompanied by nausea and may be somewhat relieved by belching or regurgitation.

The most serious complication of giant PEH is incarceration and/or strangulation. After a meal, with gastric distention, the stomach may twist in its midportion just proximal to the antrum, resulting in partial or complete obstruction (see Fig. 139.2). Progressive distention of the intrathoracic stomach and further rotation of the fundus may result in obstruction at the GE junction. Still further twisting may lead to pyloric obstruction, which results in an incarcerated gastric segment and a closed-loop obstructive physiology. If unchecked, this process ultimately leads to strangulation, necrosis, and perforation. Unless it is recognized and corrected, the resulting mediastinitis and shock could prove fatal. Such patients usually present in extreme distress and when prompted will often give a long history of complaints for which they may never have sought medical advice. The chief complaints at the time of presentation are severe pain and pressure in the chest or the epigastric region. The discomfort is usually accompanied by nausea and may be misdiagnosed as an acute myocardial infarction. Vomiting may occur, but more frequently the patient complains of retching and an inability to regurgitate. The patient may also complain of an inability to swallow saliva. If the volvulus is allowed to progress, strangulation of the intrathoracic portion of the stomach occurs, resulting in a toxic clinical picture including fever, third-spacing of a fluid, and hypovolemic shock. Borchardt[18] originally described the constellation of substernal chest pain, retching with an inability to vomit, and the inability to pass a nasogastric tube. This triad of symptoms essentially is pathognomic for an intrathoracic gastric volvulus.

Fortunately, this life-threatening complication occurs relatively infrequently today. In the past, it has been reported to occur more often. Hill and Tobias,[6] Ozdemir,[7] and Wichterman[19] and their colleagues have reported that approximately 30% of their patients with PEHs presented with gastric volvulus. However, Allen and colleagues[9] reported only five such patients requiring emergency operations for suspected strangulation, an incidence of 3%. In a pooled analysis by Stylopoulos,[11] it was estimated that only 1.16% of patients diagnosed with PEH will develop acute symptoms requiring emergent surgery. The reason for this may be that PEHs are now recognized more frequently at an earlier stage. With the performance of routine chest X-rays and the wide dissemination of advanced radiologic testing such as CT and magnetic resonance imaging (MRI), the identification of asymptomatic or minimally symptomatic PEHs has become a relatively frequent occurrence. Thus, patients who carry that diagnosis can undergo earlier surgical intervention, before obstructive symptomatology becomes severe.

DIAGNOSIS

The diagnosis of PEH is often first suspected because of an abnormal chest radiograph. The most frequent finding is a retrocardiac air bubble with or without an air-fluid level noted on the lateral view of a standard chest x-ray (see Fig. 139.3). In a giant PEH, the hernial sac and its contents occasionally protrude into the right thoracic cavity. The differential diagnosis includes mediastinal cyst or abscess and dilated obstructive esophagus, as one would see with megaesophagus in a patient with end-stage achalasia. A barium study of the upper gastrointestinal tract is usually diagnostic, with a pathognomonic finding being that of the upside-down stomach in the chest (see Fig. 139.4). The radiologist should pay careful attention to the position of the cardia relative to the hiatus; this often requires lateral and/or oblique views during the performance of the swallow. This helps to differentiate between type II and type III hiatal hernias. A barium enema or CT of the chest can help to determine whether

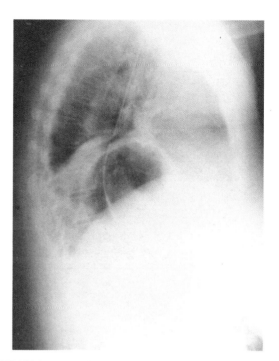

FIGURE 139.3 Retrocardiac air bubble. Note the wedge of atelectatic lung compressed by a large hernial sac.

any portion of the colon is involved; however, this is not strictly indicated in all patients as it adds little or nothing to the decision-making process. An MRI of the chest can suggest the diagnosis of PEH, but there is a little or no role for the routine utilization of such testing in the standard diagnostic workup.

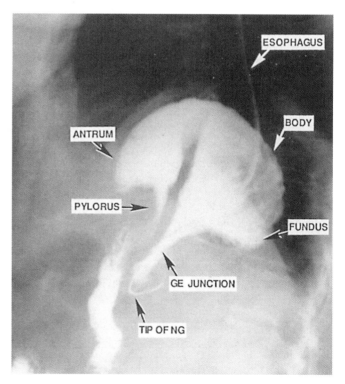

FIGURE 139.4 Barium study of the stomach that demonstrates the "upside-down" appearance of the stomach in the thoracic cavity. Note the nasogastric tube (NG) extending through the length of the esophagus with the tip at the gastroesophageal junction (GE) below the esophageal hiatus. The fundus, body, and antrum of the stomach are above the diaphragm.

Esophagogastroduodenoscopy (EGD) is now routinely performed in all patients in whom consideration of operative repair is entertained. The EGD allows for identification of the presence or absence of esophagitis, which may confirm a diagnosis of GE reflux concomitant to the mechanical perturbations resulting from a PEH. This also allows for the identification of the potential presence of Barrett's esophagus, a finding that not only indicates the presence of GE reflux but also mandates long-term surveillance with follow-up EGD procedures. Finally, it is important to rule out unsuspected endoluminal causes of obstructive symptomatology, such as fibrotic stricture, esophageal neoplasm, or concomitant epiphrenic diverticulum. The typical endoscopic findings in an uncomplicated PEH are a somewhat serpiginous distal esophagus with a GE junction at or above the level of a hiatus. That portion of the stomach which is supradiaphragmatic is twisted, and it may be difficult to traverse the entire length of the stomach into the pylorus due to this tortuosity. The EGD also allows for identification of intragastric ulcers, which may be the cause of the chronic anemia that many paraesophageal hiatal hernia patients have at presentation. Notably, major complications such as aspiration or perforation which may occur when performing an EGD on a patient diagnosed with PEH are rare (less than 1 in 1,000 procedures).[5]

Controversy exists as to the role of preoperative esophageal function testing. Many surgeons routinely perform a preoperative esophageal manometry and 24-hour pH testing in order to help them decide whether or not a concomitant fundoplication at the time of hernia repair is indicated or contraindicated. Esophageal manometry tests, which can demonstrate severe esophageal dysmotility, can help the surgeon make an appropriate decision regarding whether to perform a fundoplication and if so what type of fundoplication (total or partial) would prove optimal. Manometry can also rule out concomitant esophageal dysmotility disorders, which can themselves result in dysphagia. Importantly, experience in interpreting manometry in this setting is required as it can be difficult and sometimes not possible to place the manometry probe as a result of the PEH. Additionally, typical pressure differentials seen between the thorax and abdominal cavities are often not present. Although ambulatory 24-hour pH is not useful in diagnosing a PEH, it may be useful in identifying GE reflux, which is certainly best treated by a concomitant fundoplication at the time of surgical correction.[5] Not all patients with PEH actually have GE reflux, although it can be a common finding. Walther and colleagues[20] found pH testing consistent with pathologic reflux in 9 of 15 patients (60%) with type II hiatal hernias. Fuller and colleagues[21] found similar evidence of reflux in 69% of their patients.

At our institution, patients referred with PEH routinely undergo EGD, barium study of the upper gastrointestinal tract, and esophageal manometry to fully characterize the anatomy and physiology as well as rule out any possible concomitant conditions. In this way, the surgeon can tailor the operative approach appropriately for each patient. Ambulatory reflux monitoring is not routinely performed in our patients with giant PEH since all patients at our institution undergo the addition of a partial or full fundoplication with their PEH repair.

DECISION FOR SURGERY

For many decades the mere presence of a PEH was felt to be a strong indication for definitive repair. This belief stemmed from a report by Skinner and Belsey[22] who found a 29% mortality rate in 21 patients followed with nonoperative treatment. Similarly, Hill[23] reported the outcomes of 29 patients with PEH, 10 of whom developed

incarceration. Two of the four patients operated on emergently died. The 50% operative mortality rate for emergent repair of incarcerated PEH has since been widely disseminated. Many surgeons have based their practice of immediate repair for PEH on these alarming mortality figures and this has been surgical dogma for nearly 40 years.

However, it is highly likely that few, if any, of the patients in the aforementioned series above were truly asymptomatic. Medical practice has advanced significantly over the past five decades, and the identification of asymptomatic PEH is not uncommon. With the widespread dissemination of the use of barium swallows, CT, or MRI scans, and esophagoscopy for patients with even mild upper abdominal complaints, practitioners are now identifying PEH with little or no associated symptomatology.

The first investigators to suggest that such patients might be safely followed were Treacy and Jamieson.[24] In their series, 29 of 71 patients were managed conservatively with a mean follow-up of 6 years. Thirteen of the conservatively managed patients developed progression of symptoms and eventually underwent surgical repair, although none required emergency intervention. Similar experience was reported from the Mayo Clinic by Allen and colleagues.[9] Of the 147 patients with PEH identified, 23 were followed nonoperatively and 19 of these were successfully managed in this fashion. Only four patients were noted to have progressive symptoms. These four eventually underwent repair and one died of complications related to the hernia.

More recently, Stylopoulos and colleagues[11] utilized a Markov Monte Carlo decision analytic model to determine the advisability of elective laparoscopic repair of PEH in patients with minimal or no symptoms. In their pooled analysis from five published studies, it was estimated that the incidence of acute complication was 0.7% to 7% per patient per year resulting in a weighted value of 1.16% per patient per year. Using mean life expectancy tables, the risk of developing acute symptoms requiring emergency surgery decreases with age and was calculated to be 18% for a patient diagnosed with PEH at age 65, 12% at the age of 75, and less than 8% by the age of 85. Based on these results, the authors concluded that patients with a PEH at age 65 should undergo elective surgical repair, whether symptomatic or not, because of a 20% benefit from surgical intervention. A benefit of only 10% was observed in patients beyond the age of 80; therefore, surgical repair should be reserved for symptomatic patients in this age range.[11,25]

Thus, many experts in this field have now come to recognize that all patients must be considered individually and that it is not appropriate to automatically recommend surgery for any and all patients presenting with PEH especially if symptoms are mild or nonexistent. Many such patients are septuagenarians or octogenarians with multiple comorbidities and relatively minor symptomatology. Given that fragile patients are subject to relatively high rates of perioperative morbidity, strong consideration should be given to expectant management, as most will live out their lives without serious incident due to their hiatal hernia.

However, in those patients with predominantly obstructive symptoms, there is no effective medical treatment that can adequately resolve most complaints. Although symptoms of reflux alone can often be effectively treated with proton pump inhibitors, most postprandial symptoms of pain and early satiety will remain. In such patients operative therapy is indeed indicated.

OPERATIVE PRINCIPLES

There is controversy regarding both the optimal procedure to be performed and the best operative approach to be employed. However, there are certain tenets of operative management that are agreed upon by virtually all experts in the field. These principles include reduction of the hernial sac's contents, removal of the hernial sac from the chest, assessment of esophageal shortening, crural closure, and fixation of the stomach within the abdomen. Despite almost universal acceptance of these principles, there are some variations in the techniques utilized to achieve each of these goals.

REDUCTION OF THE HERNIAL SAC'S CONTENTS

Although this is relatively easy to accomplish in the majority of patients, it can occasionally be difficult in those with a tight hiatal ring or with volvulus who have developed gastric distention with mural edema. In patients whose sac contents are difficult to extricate, excessive force should be avoided lest serosal or full-thickness tears of the stomach occur. Such tears, if unrecognized, can lead to perioperative leaks and the need for reoperation. It is important to achieve gastric decompression, as effectively as possible with a nasogastric tube, so as to maximize the chance of reducing the stomach into the abdomen without adjunctive maneuvers. It has been suggested that insertion of a soft red rubber catheter into the hernial sac with insufflation of a small amount of air may help facilitate reduction of the hernia contents by breaking a vacuum within the sac. For those patients in whom gentle traction and the above-mentioned maneuvers are not effective, a small (1 to 2 cm) incision of the hiatal ring will usually make it possible to accomplish reduction.

MOBILIZATION AND RESECTION OF THE HERNIAL SAC

The vast majority of experts suggest that the intrathoracic hernial sac should be dissected completely from its mediastinal location and delivered into the abdomen. It is thought that resection of the hernial sac results in a significant reduction in the recurrence rate.[26,27] The rationale is that this minimizes the chance for intrathoracic recurrence for two reasons. First, it allows obliteration of the large mediastinal potential space occupied by the sac. Second, it results in more effective healing of the hiatal repair because the mediastinal tissues and crural pillars will no longer be lined by mesothelial tissue which would prevent healing and scar formation following suture apposition of the crura. There is a controversy as to whether or not the hernial sac, once mobilized from its intrathoracic position, has to be resected. Some surgeons do not resect the sac off the cardia as they feel it will increase the chance for vagal nerve damage during sac dissection. Others suggest that leaving a portion of the hernial sac in place, especially in continuum with the peritoneum, may create a path that will lead to a recurrent herniation.[28] Our own practice is to resect the sac as completely as possible beginning at the GE junction where the lesser curve begins. We believe that resecting the hernial sac allows for precise visualization of the GE junction location and thus a better assessment of the necessity for an esophageal lengthening procedure. Further, resection of the sac forces the surgeon to perform complete mediastinal dissection of the esophagus, which in turn maximizes esophageal length. Lastly, sac resection usually results in removal of the GE junction fat pad which may allow for more effective sizing and suture placement during construction of the gastric wrap. Once the hernial sac has been removed from its intrathoracic position, the dead space in the mediastinum will disappear as the lungs expand. No drainage of this space is necessary.

CRURAL CLOSURE

The crural closure at the esophageal hiatus at the time of PEH repair is often complicated by attenuated crura with poor tissue quality and excessive tension of the hiatal closure. These factors, along with unrecognized esophageal shortening, predispose the crural repair to disruption leading to reherniation of the stomach into the thorax. Understanding and recognizing the anatomy of the esophageal diaphragmatic hiatus at the time of dissection during surgery is critical for effective crural closure.

Once the hernial sac has been mobilized into the abdomen, a large diaphragmatic defect is noted to be anterior to the lower esophagus. It must be remembered that the distal esophagus makes up the posterior wall of the intrathoracic hernia, with the gastric fundus residing anterior to it. Once the fundus has been mobilized, the esophagus usually sits in a posterior mediastinal position immediately anterior to the aorta. Although some surgeons then perform an anterior crural closure, the authors feel it is important to dissect the esophagus circumferentially and raise it up off the aorta. With intramediastinal dissection the distal esophagus can routinely be mobilized for a length of approximately 8 to 10 cm, about to the level of the carina anteriorly. This intrathoracic dissection allows for the maximum intra-abdominal length of the esophagus and also moves the esophagus in an anterior direction in the hiatus up to the 12 o'clock position immediately behind the ventral midpoint of the hiatus. A posterior crural closure can then be performed, thereby re-establishing normal anatomic relationships. It is critical to dissect out the crural pillars carefully and maintain the crural integrity.[29] Stripping the endoabdominal or endothoracic fascia from the crura results in exposed and macerated muscle fibers, which do not hold sutures well. Closure of this posterior crural defect is accomplished with the placement of nonabsorbable sutures, with the stitches placed 8 to 10 mm apart and encompassing stout bites of the crura along with its peritoneal covering. The use of some sort of reinforcement for these sutures is a topic of controversy. Some surgeons have suggested using Teflon or felt pledgets to reinforce the crural stitches, but there is limited objective evidence to suggest that such a practice decreases the incidence of recurrence.[30]

To improve the strength of the crural repair, and to minimize tissue tension, surgeons have used prosthetic mesh much like it has been applied for inguinal and incisional hernias.[31–33] The mesh is thought to cause fibrosis and tissue in-growth thereby reducing the rate of recurrence. For PEH repairs, a variety of meshes with different compositions have been used to buttress the crural closure. Each type of mesh has advantages and disadvantages based on its component material (e.g., polypropylene, polytetrafluoroethylene [PTFE], polyvinyl, porcine small intestine submucosa, acellular dermal matrix).[26,34]

A variety of techniques have been used to position mesh at the hiatus to reinforce the crural closure. The most common approaches described by surgeons include primary closure of the crura followed by prosthetic onlay (either anterior or posterior placement),[35] the keyhole technique with an onlay piece of mesh with a hole facilitating the passage of the esophagus,[36] and the "tension-free" repair whereby the hiatal defect is not closed with sutures rather the mesh is used to bridge the gap between the crura.[37,38] Figure 139.5 illustrates examples of approaches for mesh placement.

There have been three randomized clinical trials published comparing simple cruroplasty versus mesh repair. In 1999, Carlson and colleagues[39] reported a randomized trial of 31 patients suggesting that the rate of hernial recurrence was significantly decreased utilizing mesh to reinforce the crural closure. In 2002, Frantzides and

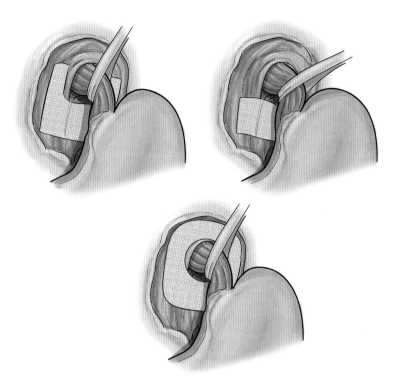

colleagues[36] reported a study of a total of 72 patients with giant hiatal hernias greater than 8 cm that were equally randomized to simple crural repair with interrupted sutures versus 36 patients with mesh repair using PTFE. A statistically significant increased recurrence rate was observed in the cruroplasty group (22%) versus no recurrences in the mesh group (p <0.006). In this study with a median follow-up of 30 months, no increase in incidence of erosions, strictures, or dysphagia was reported in the mesh group. Interestingly, a subsequent prospective randomized trial by Granderath et al.[35] demonstrated that the utilization of polypropylene mesh to reinforce the crural repair did increase postoperative dysphagia rates for short-term and mid-term follow-up. Other surgeons have noted similar problems and there are case reports describing significant periesophageal inflammation, erosion, stricture, and fistula formation.[40] Given the substantial morbidity of mesh complications when compared to recurrence, surgeons who are expert in this area generally avoid using mesh if at all possible.

There has been one prospective randomized trial reporting the utilization of an absorbable biologic prosthesis to reinforce the crural repair following PEH procedures.[41] First reported in 2006, this multi-institutional study included only surgeons with extensive experience in laparoscopic esophageal surgery. There were 108 patients randomized to either simple suture closure of the hiatus versus closure with reinforcement utilizing a porcine subintestinal submucosal allograft patch. Routine upper intestinal radiography was performed at 6 months and the investigators documented a significantly decreased incidence of radiologic recurrence when the allograft patch was used compared with primary repair alone (9% versus 24%, p = 0.04). Those patients who did develop recurrent hernia reported slightly higher levels of postprandial chest pain and early satiety but there was no difference in dysphagia. None of the postoperative symptoms was severe enough to warrant reoperation. The conclusion of this study after short-term follow-up was that the use of biologic mesh may be warranted in giant PEH. A follow-up report of this study cohort in 2011 by Oelschlager and colleagues[42] reported

that laparoscopic repair of PEH resulted in long and durable relief of symptoms and improvement in quality of life with either primary suture repair or buttressed repair with a biologic mesh. Importantly, long-term recurrence rates were similar in both groups, reported to be 54% to 59%. Interestingly, in a recent survey by the Society of American Gastrointestinal and Endoscopic Surgery (SAGES), a higher recurrence rate using bioprosthetic versus synthetic mesh was reported by members.[43]

Table 139.1 outlines the results of the mesh versus non-mesh repair for both the open and laparoscopic approaches. Recently, two literature reviews on the controversial subject of selective use of prosthetic material have been reported. In the first study, a meta-analysis of three randomized trials reported that prosthetic reinforcement of the crural repair decreased the 1-year risk of recurrence fourfold.[47] The second study used a decision analysis model based on retrospective studies with a much longer follow-up period of 15 to 50 months.[48] In this study minimal differences between repairs with or without mesh were reported. These discordant results highlight the low quality of overall published evidence and reporting variability suggesting that a firm recommendation to proceed with mesh reinforcement must await long-term follow-up and confirmatory studies.[30]

INTRA-ABDOMINAL FIXATION

Key among the factors contributing to recurrence and reherniation is the negative intrathoracic pressure creating a cephalad force that favors displacement of the stomach into the chest cavity. It is generally accepted that some form of intra-abdominal gastric fixation is warranted as a component of repairing PEH. It is thought that anchoring the stomach below the diaphragm by anterior gastropexy, tube gastrostomy, or a partial or complete fundoplication prevents migration of the stomach into the chest.[49]

Surgeons who favor gastropexy for fixation emphasize that this technique is fast and simple to perform; however, high rates of recurrence have been reported.[50,51] Those surgeons who favor fixation of

TABLE 139.1 Studies Investigating Laparoscopic Operative Approach With and Without Mesh Repair for Giant Paraesophageal Hernia (Percentages Are Overall Unless Specified)

First Author	Year	No. Pts.	Mesh (n)	No Mesh (n)	Intraoperative Complications (%)	Postoperative Complications (%)	Recurrence (%)	Reoperation (%)
Carlson[39]	1999	35	15	16	Mesh: 13 No mesh: 6	NS	Mesh: 0 No mesh: 19	Mesh: 0 No mesh: 12
Frantzides[36]	2002	72	36	36	NS	Mesh: 6 No mesh: 3	Mesh: 0 No mesh: 22	Mesh: 0 No mesh: 14
Morino[44]	2006	51	37	14	0	NS	Mesh: 35 No mesh: 77	Mesh: 14 No mesh 36
Muller-Stitch[45]	2006	56	16	40	Mesh: 19 No mesh: 5	Mesh: 13 No mesh: 15	Mesh: 0 No mesh: 19	Mesh: 0 No mesh: 5
Zaninotto[46]	2007	54	35	19	NS	NS	Mesh: 9 No mesh: 42	NS
Oelschlager[42]	2011	108	57	51	NS	NS	Mesh: 54 No mesh: 59	Mesh: 0 No mesh: 4

NS, not stated.

the stomach intra-abdominally with a gastrostomy tube argue that this technique decompresses the stomach thus eliminating the need for nasogastric drainage postoperatively and also provides a solid anchoring point to prevent intra-abdominal volvulus and rehemiation into the thorax.[52] This has been described utilizing a purse-string technique or a commercially prepared percutaneous enterostomy technique. Those surgeons who oppose the use of a gastrostomy tube report that rehemiation is not prevented because the stomach is pliable and stretches back into the chest in response to the cephalad force. To date, no randomized trials have proven that the use of gastropexy or tube gastrostomy reduces the rate of recurrence of PEH.[53]

Many surgeons support the routine performance of a fundoplication at the time of PEH repair regardless of the presence or absence of GE reflux symptomatology or esophagitis.[9,54] These surgeons report that the fundoplication not only helps anchor the stomach in the abdomen but also decreases the incidence of postoperative reflux. These results have been disputed by some authors who argue that significant postoperative GE reflux can be adequately managed with medical therapy.[50,55] These surgeons support the notion that fundoplication should only be performed selectively in patients with GE reflux diagnosed on preoperative testing. Williamson and colleagues[55] reviewed 119 patients with PEH, of whom only 19 underwent an antireflux procedure in addition to anatomic repair of the hernia. The antireflux procedures were performed for those patients with reflux as diagnosed by symptoms, endoscopic findings, and manometric or pH findings. Postoperatively, two of these patients (2%) developed severe symptoms of GE reflux, while 17 others (15%) developed mild and easily controllable symptoms. These authors reported the development of recurrent hernia in 12 of 117 patients, with good to excellent result in 86% of patients. It is thought that this selective approach may decrease the incidence of postoperative dysphagia and other complications simplifying the dissection and potentially shortening the operative time for patients, many of whom are elderly and have significant medical comorbidities. Although limited data exist to confirm the need for fundoplication, most surgeons perform an antireflux procedure when repairing a PEH to limit reflux and to fix the stomach below the diaphragm.

The predominant approach to anchor the stomach below the diaphragm at present appears to be a partial or full circumferential fundoplication, such as a Belsey or Nissen procedure. The Belsey Mark IV (BMIV) is a classic operation performed transthoracically which has

demonstrated good to excellent results in most patients.[56] The BMIV provides an incomplete 240-degree anterior fundal wrap as opposed to the 360-degree Nissen fundoplication. This partial wrap appears useful in decreasing the potential for dysphagia and gas bloating in patients with decreased esophageal motility.[57] In addition to reapproximating the crura and performing the anterior 240-degree fundoplication, the BMIV also helps recreate the high-pressure zone of the LES by securing the fundoplication in the infradiaphragmatic position (see Fig. 139.6[57]). Attempts to reproduce the Belsey approach using thoracoscopic minimally invasive techniques have been largely abandoned due to the complexity of the procedure.[58] With recent advances in laparoscopic surgery techniques, the 180-degree anterior Dor and 270-degree posterior Toupet fundoplication have gained popularity for patients with significant esophageal dysmotility.

The authors' own practice is to routinely perform a Nissen fundoplication procedure to minimize the risk of recurrence. A partial fundoplication is performed in patients with significant esophageal dysmotility documented on preoperative manometric testing. If lengthening is necessary, we perform a Collis gastroplasty with a 50 to 54 Fr dilator placed along the lesser gastric curve. The size of the bougie is adjusted based on the patient's body habitus and preoperative manometry results. We will occasionally and selectively use gastropexy and/or a tube gastrostomy as abdominal fixation in those rare patients who have markedly decreased esophageal motility (as determined by manometry) or in very elderly, fragile patients for whom we wish to minimize the length of the operative procedure. In such cases we use a combined operative approach using laparoscopy to reduce the hernia allowing the insertion of a percutaneous gastrostomy (PEG) tube. The gastrostomy can provide adequate intra-abdominal gastric fixation as well as an alternative method for alimentation should the patient's oral intake be inadequate. If GE reflux is encountered in such a patient it can usually be managed adequately with proton pump inhibitors.

ESOPHAGEAL SHORTENING

Although first described in 1957, controversy remains regarding the true incidence and management of esophageal shortening.[59–62] Those who do not believe that esophageal shortening exists argue that the esophagus appears shortened because of the cephalad displacement of the stomach into the chest. Correction of the anatomic defect and

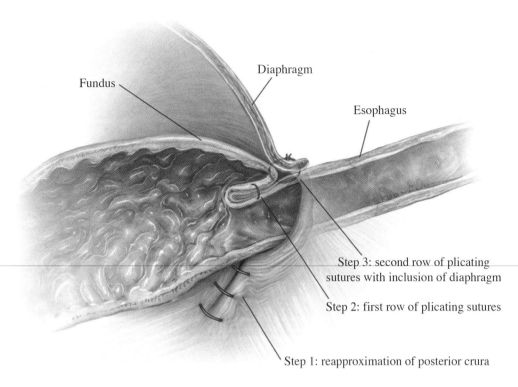

Fundus

Diaphragm

Esophagus

Step 3: second row of plicating
sutures with inclusion of diaphragm

Step 2: first row of plicating sutures

Step 1: reapproximation of posterior crura

FIGURE 139.6 A sagittal view of the Belsey Mark IV repair demonstrating the three steps in the repair. (Adapted from Cooke DT. Belsey Mark IV repair. *Op Tech Thorac Cardiovasc Surg* 2013;18(3):215–229.[57] Copyright © 2013 Elsevier. With permission.)

reduction of the stomach back into the abdomen avoids the need for a lengthening procedure. The more commonly held view is that esophageal shortening does exists and results from periesophageal inflammation and irritation due to long-standing GE reflux which in turn leads to healing and subsequent fibrosis and shortening. This shortening, although uncommon, is thought to contribute to wrap herniation resulting in anatomic recurrence due to the inability of the surgeon to place the GE junction below the diaphragm without undue tension.

Identifying patients with esophageal shortening may be challenging. Preoperative testing with radiologic or endoscopic measurements has not been reliable at predicting esophageal shortening intraoperatively.[63] A short esophagus is usually identified at the time of surgery by assessing the position of the GE junction below the diaphragmatic hiatus after maximal distal esophageal mobilization. If the GE junction cannot be reduced to the requisite 2 to 3 cm below the hiatus necessary for a tension-free intra-abdominal fundoplication to be performed, the classic solution is to perform an esophageal lengthening procedure known as a Collis gastroplasty. The technique consists of a vertical gastric incision usually made with a stapler placed flush alongside an intraesophageal dilator advanced into the stomach (see Fig. 139.7). This creates a "neoesophagus" out of the lesser curvature of the stomach. This neoesophagus resides within the abdomen and allows a circumferential intra-abdominal fundoplication to be performed without undue tension. Collis[59] first described this technique without fundoplication; however, fundoplication such as Nissen was later added (e.g., Collis–Nissen fundoplication) to minimize reflux.[64]

While the classic Collis gastroplasty was performed utilizing a stapler from an intrathoracic approach, Luketich and colleagues[65] have described a modified Collis gastroplasty, which can be performed during laparoscopy. This is achieved utilizing circular and linear staplers to form the neoesophagus with a dilator residing in the esophagus to prevent excessive narrowing (see Fig. 139.7). More recently, a

wedge gastroplasty has been utilized by sequentially firing an articulating linear stapler to resect a wedge of the stomach, thus effecting the creation of a neoesophagus similar to that resulting from the other techniques (see Fig. 139.7). Whitson et al.[66] has recently reported a large series of PEH repairs using this technique with excellent results. Interestingly, the presence of esophageal shortening is less frequent with the laparoscopic repair.[52] This observation may be related to the challenges in accurately identifying the position of the GE junction at the hiatus due to elevation of the diaphragm from insufflation of carbon dioxide, failure to accurately visualize the GE junction due to the esophageal fat pad, or improved distal esophageal mobilization. Some surgeons may also be reluctant to perform a lengthening procedure due to the technical challenges using laparoscopic techniques.

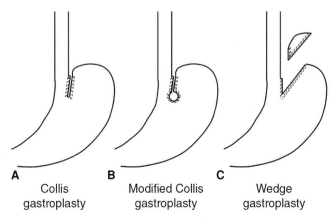

A   Collis gastroplasty

B   Modified Collis gastroplasty

C   Wedge gastroplasty

FIGURE 139.7 Surgical options for lengthening a foreshortened esophagus by creation of a neoesophagus. **A:** Classic stapled Collis gastroplasty. **B:** Modified laparoscopic stapled Collis gastroplasty. **C:** Wedge gastroplasty.

TABLE 139.2 Reports with ≥50 Open Paraesophageal Hiatal Hernia Repairs

First Author	Year	No. Pts.	Approach	Median LOS (Days)	Morbidity (%)	Mortality (%)	Median F/U (Months)	Known Recurrences (%)
Ellis[50]	1986	55	Abdominal	9.5[a]	24	2	52[a]	9
Allen[9]	1993	124	Thoracic	9	26	0	42	1
Williamson[55]	1993	119	Abdominal	NS	12	2	61	10
Martin[70]	1997	51	Thoracic/abdominal	9.1[a]	29	0	27[a]	NS
Maziak[71]	1998	94	Thoracic	NS	19	2	72	2
Geha[72]	2000	100	Thoracic/abdominal	NS	6	2	NS	0
Rogers[73]	2001	60	Thoracic	9	8	2	19	2
Patel[74]	2004	240	Thoracic	7	24	1	42	8
Low[75]	2005	72	Abdominal	4.5	15	0	30[a]	18

LOS, length of stay; F/U, follow-up in months.
[a]Mean, not median.

OPERATIVE APPROACH

Controversy continues regarding the optimal approach to the repair of a PEH. Options include the open approaches (thoracotomy, laparotomy) as well as the laparoscopic approach. Both the open and the minimally invasive approaches are championed by supporters who emphasize the advantages and disadvantages of one approach over the other. The proponents of an open approach tout the ease of decompression of the herniated viscera, the ability to palpate and thereby protect the vagus nerves intraoperatively, as well as the ability to place stout stitches for the crural repair. Those who prefer the thoracotomy approach note the ease with which complete esophageal mobilization can be undertaken all the way up to the inferior aspect of the aortic arch as well as the excellent view of the crura. The thoracotomy proponents also note the ease of performing a Collis gastroplasty from a supradiaphragmatic approach. Rarely do these same experts note the difficulty of achieving short gastric artery division through this approach, nor do they note the painful nature of the thoracotomy incision with the resultant prolonged hospital stay and the risk of chronic thoracotomy pain. Finally, proponents of the open approaches routinely cite the steep learning curve for the laparoscopic repair of PEH. Interestingly, they never mention the similar steep learning curve for achieving a successful open repair.

Those experts who advise a laparoscopic approach emphasize the minimally invasive nature of the procedure. They can appropriately point to less postoperative pain with shorter length of hospital stay as well as a faster return to work.[67–69] In addition, they note that crural visualization is likely even better with a laparoscopic approach than with either the open abdominal or thoracic approach. Extensive laparoscopic mobilization of the intrathoracic esophagus is now routinely achievable and esophageal lengthening can be accomplished with minimally invasive techniques, as reported by Luketich[65] and Whitson.[66] The technique of wedge gastroplasty reported by the latter author has become widely utilized because of its relative technical ease of execution.

Table 139.2 lists the results of studies with ≥50 open (thoracotomy or laparotomy) paraesophageal hiatal hernia repairs. In most series, both approaches result in durable repairs with a slight improved result with the transthoracic approach. Table 139.3 outlines the results of studies with >100 laparoscopic repairs of giant PEH. Reported morbidity is generally lower with the minimally invasive approach and this correlates with a much shorter length of hospital stay. There does not appear to be a great difference with regard to overall operative mortality.[68,84–86]

Perhaps the strongest argument against a minimally invasive approach has to do with the risk of recurrence of the hiatal hernia with long-term follow-up. Proponents of the open approach suggest

TABLE 139.3 Reports With ≥100 Laparoscopic Paraesophageal Hiatal Hernia Repairs

First Author	Year	No. Pts.	Conversion (%)	Mean LOS (Days)	Mortality (%)	Mean F/U (Months)	Known Recurrences (%)
Mattar[76]	2002	125	2.4	3.9	3	40	33
Pierre[77]	2002	203	1.5	3	1	18	3
Diaz[78]	2003	116	2.5	2[a]	2	30	22
Andujar[79]	2004	166	1.2	3.9	NS	15	20
Aly[80]	2005	100	1.0	3.6	0	47	14
Nason[81]	2008	187	1.1	NS	NS	77[a]	15
Luketich[82]	2010	662	1.5	3[a]	2	NS	16
Latzko[83]	2014	126	4.8	4.0	2	23	21

[a]median, not mean.
LOS, length of stay; F/U, follow-up in months; NS, not stated.

TABLE 139.4 Educational Video Links Related to Laparoscopic Paraesophageal Hernia Repair

Type of Hernia Repair	Strengths/Unique Features	Type	Author(s)	Link or Reference
Laparoscopic	Excellent, brief video of laparoscopic technique, demonstrates mesh repair of crura	Online video	Dr. Robert Sewel	https://www.youtube.com/watch?v=cAkETBbo1jk
Laparoscopic	Demonstrates repair of large hiatal defect. Demonstrates Endostitch Autosure device, mesh repair of crura	Online video	Dr. Ehab Akkary	https://www.youtube.com/watch?v=WwRMUCH4NU8
Laparoscopic	Demonstrates repair of large hiatal defect, illustrates felt pledgeted suturing and anterior gastropexy	Online video	Dr. Daniel Rosen	https://www.youtube.com/watch?v=MjQuUi1bPOY
Laparoscopic	Demonstrates Toupet partial fundoplication	Online video	Dr. Bernard Dallemagne	http://www.websurg.com/doi-vd01en2101.htm
Laparoscopic	Excellent summary video of principles and techniques	Online video	Dr. Nathaniel Soper	http://www.websurg.com/doi-lt03ensoper005.htm
Laparoscopic	Excellent summary of controversies and challenges	Online video	Dr. Lee L. Swanstrom	http://www.websurg.com/doi-lt03enswanstrom014.htm

that it allows for much more thorough esophageal mobilization and more accurate crural closure, two factors that help to prevent recurrent intrathoracic herniation of the stomach. While laparoscopy enthusiasts point out that the vast majority of these recurrences are asymptomatic, proponents of the open approach suggest that the incidence of recurrent herniation, symptomatic or not, is simply too high and thus supports their method of open repair.

The weakness of the prior arguments is related to the fact that the information on the recurrence rate following laparoscopic repair comes from authors who performed routine radiologic follow-up. Many investigators now routinely obtain a contrast esophagogram not just in the immediate postoperative period but also during long-term follow-up. This identifies even small asymptomatic recurrent hernias that would otherwise go undetected. Such follow-up had not been a routine practice for investigators performing open repair; thus only symptomatic patients were felt to warrant an investigation that would identify recurrent hernias. There is only one reported series in which routine radiographic follow-up was sought following open repair. Low and Unger[75] performed routine radiologic follow-up in the patients they had repaired through an open abdominal approach and found recurrent hiatal hernia in 11 of 61 patients (18%) who returned for routine radiologic follow-up. One direct comparison of long-term results has recently been reported by Ferri et al.[87] His group compared recurrence rates in 25 open transabdominal and 35 laparoscopic repairs. There was no significant difference between the groups, although the open cohort did have a higher recurrence rate than the laparoscopic cohort (44% vs. 23%, $p = 0.11$).

Thus, the reported superiority of the open approach with regard to prevention of long-term recurrence may be based largely on the clinical picture of patients returning with symptomatic recurrence, whereas the recurrence rate for the laparoscopic approach is based on routine radiologic follow-up. This comparison of "apples and oranges" makes it difficult to determine whether an approach is indeed superior with regard to long-term results. Nonetheless, in order to respond to the reported increase in number of recurrences with the laparoscopic approach, many surgeons have employed the use of prosthetic mesh to reinforce the crural repair. In a self-reported survey of surgeons by SAGES in 2012, 25% of surgeons use mesh regularly, while 23% did not use mesh at all.[88]

Nationally, the trend appears to be favoring the laparoscopic approach for the repair of PEHs. While thoracic surgeons who are untrained in laparoscopic techniques will continue to perform open procedures, it seems probable that patients will increasingly be referred to those surgeons who use a less invasive approach. While this shift in referral pattern may not be based on hard data, it follows the trend for other procedures that can be accomplished laparoscopically and it seems likely to continue. This is not to say, however, that the open approach is without its advantages. Especially in those patients who have concomitant intrathoracic pathology, a transthoracic approach can be advantageous in that it allows all procedures to be performed with a single incision. The open thoracic approach can also be useful in patients who have had multiple upper abdominal surgical procedures that render an abdominal approach problematic, whether in an open or laparoscopic fashion. Finally, in those patients who have recurrent herniation following a laparoscopic approach, a transthoracic approach may prove to be somewhat easier and allow for complete esophageal mobilization.

ADDITIONAL LEARNING AIDS

For additional information, Table 139.4 lists several links to videos that detail the various laparoscopic techniques for the repair of PEH with and without mesh. Additionally, contributions by Cooke, Ellis, and Soper help illustrate the operative techniques for open Nissen fundoplication, BMIV repair, and laparoscopic PEH repair.[57,89,90]

REFERENCES

1. Wiener DC, Wee JO. Thorax. Minimally invasive esophageal procedures. In: Ashley SW, ed. *Scientific American Surgery [online]*. Hamilton, ON: Decker Intellectual Properties; 2012. Available at: http://www.sciamsurgery.com.
2. Mitiek MO, Andrade RS. Giant hiatal hernia. *Ann Thorac Surg* 2010;89(6):S2168–S2173.
3. Herwaarden MA, Samson M, Smout AJ, et al. The role of hiatus hernia in gastro-oesophageal reflux disease. *Eur J Gastroenterol Hepatol* 2004;16(9):831–835.
4. Dahlberg PS, Deschamps C, Miller DL, et al. Laparoscopic repair of large paraesophageal hiatal hernia. *Ann Thorac Surg* 2001;72(4):1125–1129.
5. Roman S, Kahrilas PJ. The diagnosis and management of hiatal hernia. *BMJ* 2014;349:g6154.
6. Hill LD, Tobias JA. Paraesophageal hernia. *Arch Surg* 1968;96(5):735–744.

7. Ozdemir IA, Burke WA, Ikins PM. Paraesophageal hernia. A life-threatening disease. *Ann Thorac Surg* 1973;16(6):547–554.

8. Sanderud A. Surgical treatment for the complications of hiatal hernia. *Acta Chir Scand* 1967;133(3):223–227.

9. Allen MS, Trastek VF, Deschamps C, et al. Intrathoracic stomach. Presentation and results of operation. *J Thorac Cardiovasc Surg* 1993;105(2):253–258.

10. Poulose BK, Gosen C, Marks JM, et al. Inpatient mortality analysis of paraesophageal hernia repair in octogenarians. *J Gastrointest Surg* 2008;12(11):1888–1892.

11. Stylopoulos N, Gazelle GS, Rattner DW. Paraesophageal hernias: operation or observation? *Ann Surg* 2002;236(4):492–500.

12. Thukkani N, Sonnenberg A. The influence of environmental risk factors in hospitalization for gastro-esophageal reflux disease-related diagnoses in the United States. *Aliment Pharmacol Ther* 2013;31(8):852–861.

13. Hennessey D, Convie L, Barry M, et al. Paraoesophageal hernia: an overview. *Br J Hosp Med (Lond)* 2012;73(8):437–440.

14. Menon S, Trughill N. Risk factors for the aetiology of hiatus hernia: a meta-analysis. *Eur J Gastroenterol Hepatol* 2011;23(2):133–138.

15. Schubert MJ, Adusumilli PS, Cook CC, et al. The impact of scoliosis among patients with giant paraesophageal hernia. *J Gastrointest Surg* 2011;15(1):23–28.

16. Annibale B, Capurso G, Chistolini A, et al. Gastrointestinal causes of refractory iron deficiency anemia in patients without gastrointestinal symptoms. *Am J Med* 2001;111(6):439–445.

17. Meganty K, Smith RL. Cameron lesions: unusual cause of gastrointestinal bleeding and anemia. *Digestion* 2008;77(3–4):214–217.

18. Borchardt M. Zur pathologie und therapie des magen volvulus. *Arch Klin Chir* 1904;74:243.

19. Wichterman K, Geha AS, Cahow CE, et al. Giant paraesophageal hiatus hernia with intrathoracic stomach and colon: the case for early repair. *Surgery* 1979;86(3):497–506.

20. Walther B, DeMeester TR, Lafontaine E, et al. Effect of paraesophageal hernia on sphincter function and its implication on surgical therapy. *Am J Surg* 1984;147(1):111–116.

21. Fuller CB, Hagen JA, DeMeester TR, et al. The role of fundoplication in the treatment of type II paraesophageal hernia. *J Thorac Cardiovasc Surg* 1996;111(3):655–661.

22. Skinner DB, Belsey RH. Surgical management of esophageal reflux and hiatus hernia. Long-term results with 1,030 patients. *J Thorac Cardiovasc Surg* 1967;53(1):33–54.

23. Hill LD. Incarcerated paraesophageal hernia. A surgical emergency. *Am J Surg* 1973;126(2):286–291.

24. Treacy PJ, Jamieson GG. An approach to the management of para-oesophageal hiatus hernias. *Aust N Z J Surg* 1987;57(11):813–817.

25. Collet D, Luc G, Chiche L. Management of large para-esophageal hiatal hernias. *J Visc Surg* 2013;150(6):395–402.

26. Mori T, Nagao G, Sugiyama M. Paraesophageal hernia repair. *Ann Thorac Cadiovasc Surg* 2012;18(4):297–305.

27. Edye M, Salky B, Posner A, et al. Sac excision is essential to adequate laparoscopic repair of paraesophageal hernia. *Surg Endosc* 1998;12(10):1259–1263.

28. Oddsdottir M. Paraesophageal hernia. *Surg Clin N Am* 2000;80(4):1243–1252.

29. Antonoff MB, D'Cunha J, Andrade RS, et al. Giant paraesophageal hernia repair: technical pearls. *J Thorac Cardiovasc Surg* 2012;144(3):567–570.

30. Nason KS. Synthetic reinforcement of diaphragm closure for large hiatal hernia repair. In: Ferguson MK, ed. *Difficult Decisions in Thoracic Surgery: An Evidence-Based Approach*, 3rd ed. London: Springer-Verlag; 2014: 473–496.

31. Lichtenstein IL, Shulman AG, Amid PK, et al. The tension-free hernioplasty. *Am J Surg* 1989;157(2):188–193.

32. Hinson EL. Early results with Lichtenstein tension-free hernia repair. *Br J Surg* 1995;82(3):418–419.

33. Utrera Gonzalez A, de la Portilla de Juan F, Carranza Albarran G. Large incisional hernia repair using intraperitoneal placement of expanded polytetrafluoroethylene. *Am J Surg* 1999;177(4):291–293.

34. Herbella FA, Patti MG, Del Grande JC. Hiatal mesh repair—current status. *Surg Laparosc Endosc Percutan Tech* 2011;21(2):61–66.

35. Granderath FA, Kamolz T, Schweiger UM, et al. Impact of laparoscopic Nissen fundoplication with prosthetic hiatal closure on esophageal body motility: results of a prospective randomized trial. *Arch Surg* 2006;141(7):625–632.

36. Frantzides CT, Madan AK, Carlson MA, et al. A prospective, randomized trial of laparoscopic polytetrafluoroethylene (PTFE) patch repair vs simple cruroplasty for large hiatal hernia. *Arch Surg* 2002;137(6):649–652.

37. Basso N, De Leo A, Genco A, et al. 360 degrees laparoscopic fundoplication with tension-free hiatoplasty in the treatment of symptomatic gastrointestinal reflux disease. *Surg Endosc* 2000;14(2):164–169.

38. Targarona EM, Bendahan G, Balague C, et al. Mesh in the hiatus: a controversial issue. *Arch Surg* 2004;139(12):1286–1296.

39. Carlson MA, Richards GG, Frantzides CT. Laparoscopic prosthetic reinforcement of hiatal herniorrhaphy. *Dig Surg* 1999;16(5):407–410.

40. Zugel N, Lang RA, Kox M, et al. Severe complications of laparoscopic mesh hernioplasty for paraesophageal hernia. *Surg Endosc* 2009;23(11):2563–2567.

41. Oelschlager BK, Pellegrini CA, Hunter J, et al. Biologic prosthesis reduces recurrence after laparoscopic paraesophageal hernia repair: a multicenter, prospective, randomized trial. *Ann Surg* 2006;244(4):481–490.

42. Oelschlager BK, Pellegrini CA, Hunter J, et al. Biologic prosthesis to prevent recurrence after laparoscopic paraesophageal hernia repair: long-term follow-up from a multicenter, prospective randomized trial. *J Am Coll Surg* 2011;213(4):461–468.

43. Frantzides CT, Carlson MA, Loizides S, et al. Hiatal hernia repair with mesh: a survey of SAGES members. *Surg Endosc* 2010;24(5):1017–1024.

44. Morino M, Giaccone C, Pellegrino L, et al. Laparoscopic management of giant hiatal hernia: factors influencing long-term outcome. *Surg Endosc* 2006;20(7):1011–1016. Epub 2006 Jun 8.

45. Muller-Stitch BP, Holzinger F, Kapp T, et al. Laparoscopic hiatal hernia repair: long-term outcome with the focus on the influence of mesh reinforcement. *Surg Endosc* 2006;20(3):380–384. Epub 2006 Jan 21.

46. Zaninotto G, Portale G, Costantini M, et al. Objective follow-up after laparoscopic repair of large type III hiatal hernia. Assessment of safety and durability. *World J Surg* 2007;31(11):2177–2183. Epub 2007 Aug 29.

47. Antoniou SA, Antoniou GA, Koch OO, et al. Lower recurrence rates after mesh-reinforced versus simple hiatal hernia repair: a meta-analysis of randomized trials. *Surg Laparosc Endosc Percutan Tech* 2012;22(6):498–502.

48. Obeid NM, Velanovich V. The choice of primary repair or mesh repair for paraesophageal hernia: a decision analysis based on utility scores. *Ann Surg* 2013;257(4):655–664.

49. Ponsky J, Rosen M, Fanning A, et al. Anterior gastropexy may reduce the recurrence rate after laparoscopic paraesophageal hernia repair. *Surg Endosc* 2003;17(7):1036–1041.

50. Ellis FH, Crozier RE, Shea JA. Paraesophageal hiatus hernia. *Arch Surg* 1986;121(4):416–420.

51. Braslow L. Transverse gastropexy vs. Stamm gastrostomy in hiatal hernia. *Arch Surg* 1987;122(7):851.

52. Wolf PS, Oelschlager BK. Laparoscopic paraesophageal hernia repair. *Adv Surg* 2007;41:199–210.

53. Schieman C, Grondin SC. Paraesophageal hernia: clinical presentation, evaluation, and management controversies. *Thorac Surg Clin* 2009;19(4):473–484.

54. Pearson FG, Cooper JD, Ilves R, et al. Massive hiatal hernia with incarceration: a report of 53 cases. *Ann Thorac Surg* 1983;35(1):45–51.

55. Williamson WA, Ellis FH Jr, Streitz JM Jr, et al. Paraesophageal hiatal hernia: is an antireflux procedure necessary? *Ann Thorac Surg* 1993;56(3):447–451.

56. Orringer MB, Skinner DB, Belsey RH. Long term results of the Mark IV operation for hiatal hernia and analyses of recurrences and their treatment. *J Thorac Cardiovasc Surg* 1972;63(1):25–33.

57. Cooke DT. Belsey Mark IV repair. *Op Tech Thorac Cardiovasc Surg* 2013;18(3):215–229.

58. Nguyen NT, Schauer PR, Hutson W, et al. Preliminary results of thoracoscopic Belsey Mark IV antireflux procedure. *Surg Laparosc Endosc* 1998;8(3):185–188.

59. Collis JL. An operation for hiatus hernia with short esophagus. *Thorax* 1957;12(3):181–188.

60. Hill LD, Gelfand M, Bauermeister D. Simplified management of reflux esophagitis with stricture. *Ann Surg* 1970;172(4):638–651.

61. Pearson FG, Cooper JD, Patterson GA, et al. Gastroplasty and fundoplication for complex reflux problems: long-term results. *Ann Surg* 1987;206(4):473–481.

62. Herbella FA, Del Grande JC, Colleoni R. Short esophagus: literature incidence. *Dis Esophagus* 2002;15(2):125–131.

63. Urbach DR, Khajanchee YS, Glascow RE, et al. Preoperative determinants of an esophageal lengthening procedure in laparoscopic antireflux surgery. *Surg Endosc* 2001;15(12):1408–1412.

64. Orringer MB, Orringer JS. The combined Collis-Nissen operation: early assessment of reflux control. *Ann Thorac Surg* 1982;33(6):534–539.

65. Luketich JD, Raja S, Fernando HC, et al. Laparoscopic repair of giant paraesophageal hernia: 100 consecutive cases. *Ann Surg* 2000;232(4):608–618.

66. Whitson BA, Hoang CD, Boettcher AK, et al. Wedge gastroplasty and reinforced crural repair: important components of laparoscopic giant or recurrent hiatal hernia repair. *J Thorac Cardiovasc Surg* 2006;132(5):1196–1202.

67. Draainsma WA, Gooszen HG, Tournoij E, et al. Controversies in paraesophageal hernia repair: a review of literature. *Surg Endosc* 2005;19(10):1300–1308. Epub 2005 Aug 4.

68. Karmali S, McFadden S, Mitchell P, et al. Primary laparoscopic and open repair of paraesophageal hernias: a comparison of short-term outcomes. *Dis Esophagus* 2008;21(1):63–68.

69. Rathore MA, Andrabi SI, Bhatti MI, et al. Metaanalysis of recurrence after laparoscopic repair of paraesophageal hernia. *JSLS* 2007;11(4):456–460.

70. Martin TR, Ferguson MK, Naunheim KS. Management of giant paraesophageal hernia. *Dis Esophagus* 1997;10(1):47–50.

71. Maziak DE, Todd TR, Pearson FG. Massive hiatus hernia: evaluation and surgical management. *J Thorac Cardiovasc Surg* 1998;115(1):53–62.

72. Geha AS, Massad MG, Snow NJ, et al. A 32-year experience in 100 patients with giant paraesophageal hernia: the case for abdominal approach and selective antireflux repair. *Surgery* 2000;128(4):623–630.

73. Rogers ML, Duffy JP, Beggs FD, et al. Surgical treatment of para-oesophageal hiatal hernia. *Ann R Coll Surg Engl* 2001;83(6):394–398.

74. Patel HJ, Tan BB, Yee J, et al. A 25-year experience with open primary transthoracic repair of paraesophageal hiatal hernia. *J Thorac Cardiovasc Surg* 2004;127(3):843–849.

75. Low DE, Unger T. Open repair of paraesophageal hernia: reassessment of subjective and objective outcomes. *Ann Thorac Surg* 2005;80(1):287–294.

76. Mattar SG, Bowers SP, Galloway KD, et al. Long-term outcome of laparoscopic repair of paraesophageal hernia. *Surg Endosc* 2002;16(5):745–749. Epub 2002 Feb 8.

77. Pierre AF, Luketich JD, Fernando HC, et al. Results of laparoscopic repair of giant paraesophageal hernias: 200 consecutive patients. *Ann Thorac Surg* 2002;74(6):1909–1915.

78. Diaz S, Brunt LM, Klingensmith ME, et al. Laparoscopic paraesophageal hernia repair, a challenging operation: medium-term outcome of 116 patients. *J Gastrointest Surg* 2003;7(1):59–66.

79. Andujar JJ, Papasavas PK, Birdas T, et al. Laparoscopic repair of large paraesophageal hernia is associated with a low incidence of recurrence and reoperation. *Surg Endosc* 2004;18(3):444–447. Epub 2004 Feb 2.

80. Aly A, Munt J, Jamieson GG, et al. Laparoscopic repair of large hiatal hernias. *Br J Surg* 2005;92(5):648–653.
81. Nason KS, Luketich JD, Qureshi I, et al. Laparoscopic repair of giant paraesophageal hernia results in long-term patient satisfaction and a durable repair. *J Gastrointest Surg* 2008;12(12):2066–2077. Epub 2008 Oct 8.
82. Luketich JD, Nason KS, Christie NA, et al. Outcomes after a decade of laparoscopic giant paraesophageal hernia repair. *J Thorac Cardiovasc Surg* 2010;139(2):395–404. Epub 2009 Dec 11.
83. Latzko M, Borao F, Squillaro A, et al. Laparoscopic repair of paraesophageal hernias. *JSLS* 2014;18(3):pii: e2014.00009.
84. Edwards JP, Grondin SC. Minimally invasive versus open repair of giant paraesophageal hernia. In: Ferguson MK, ed. *Difficult Decisions in Thoracic Surgery: An Evidence-Based Approach,* 3rd ed. London: Springer-Verlag; 2014: 461–472.
85. Schauer PR, Ikramuddin S, McLaughlin RH, et al. Comparison of laparoscopic versus open repair of paraesophageal hernia. *Am J Surg* 1998;176(6):659–665.
86. Zehetner J, DeMeester SR, Ayazi S, et al. Laparoscopic versus open repair of paraesophageal hernia: the second decade. *J Am Coll Surg* 2011;212(5):813–820. Epub 2011 Mar 23.
87. Ferri LE, Feldman LS, Stanbridge D, et al. Should laparoscopic paraesophageal hernia repair be abandoned in favour of the open approach? *Surg Endosc* 2005;19(1):4–8. Epub 2004 Nov 11.
88. Pfluke JM, Parker M, Bowers SP, et al. Use of mesh for hiatal hernia repair: a survey of SAGES members. *Surg Endosc* 2012;26(7):1843–1848. Epub 2012 Jan 25.
89. Ellis Henry F Jr. Open Nissen Fundoplication. In: *Pearson's Thoracic and Esophageal Surgery.* 3rd ed. Philadelphia, PA: Churchill Livingston Elsevier; 2008:261–268.
90. Soper NJ, Teitelbaum EN. Laparoscopic paraesophageal repair: current controversies. *Surg Laparosc Endosc Percutan Tech* 2013;23(5):442–445.

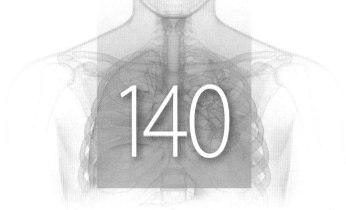

140

Esophageal Diverticula

Pamela Samson ▪ Varun Puri

Esophageal diverticula are acquired conditions of the esophagus occurring almost exclusively in adults. There are two major categories: pulsion diverticula and traction diverticula. Pulsion diverticula result from herniation of the mucosa through a weak point in the muscle layer (pseudodiverticulum) and consist of mucosa and submucosa only. Two types of pulsion diverticula are clinically recognized: pharyngoesophageal (Zenker's) and epiphrenic. The second category, traction diverticulum, results from inflammation and fibrosis in adjacent lymph nodes and is composed of all layers of the esophageal wall (true diverticulum). There is also a very rare entity called diffuse intramural esophageal diverticulosis.

PHARYNGOESOPHAGEAL (ZENKER'S) DIVERTICULUM

The pharyngoesophageal diverticulum, the most common diverticulum of the esophagus, is situated posteriorly and immediately superior to the physiologic and anatomic area of the upper esophageal sphincter (UES). It is most prevalent in the fifth to eighth decades of life. Prevalence is believed to be less than 1% of the general population.[1] Although first described in 1769 by the English surgeon Ludlow, it was as a consequence of the classic review written by the German pathologists Zenker and von Ziemssen in 1874 that the eponym Zenker's diverticulum arose.[2,3]

PATHOPHYSIOLOGY

Because Zenker's diverticulum is usually seen in patients >50 years of age (peaking in older adults during the seventh and eight decades of life), it is considered an acquired condition. In the 1950s Negus[4] described the constant site of origin just above the cricopharyngeus muscle and suggested the possibility of an anatomic weak point in the muscular layers. This area of the cervical esophagus, known as Killian's triangle, is bordered by the oblique fibers of the inferior constrictor muscle of the pharynx superiorly, and by the transverse fibers of the cricopharyngeus muscle inferiorly. This is the most common site for a pharyngoesophageal diverticulum. Less commonly, a pharyngoesophageal diverticulum may occur in Lamier's triangle (inferior to the cricopharyngeus and superior to the longitudinal fibers of the esophagus) or in the Killian–Jamieson triangles (inferior to the cricopharyngeus on either side of the muscle's insertion into the cricoid cartilage). These diverticula are referred to as Lamier's diverticulum and Killian's diverticulum, respectively. Manometric studies conducted by Ellis[5] did not confirm the presence of either

achalasia or hypertension of the cricopharyngeus in patients with a pharyngoesophageal diverticulum.

An evaluation by Lerut[6] of the characteristics of the muscles making up the UES area suggests that myogenic degeneration and neurogenic disease are not limited to just the cricopharyngeus muscle but affect the striated muscles as well. Therefore incoordination of the cricopharyngeus muscle could be considered only one aspect of a more complex functional problem rather than a disease on its own, and a pharyngoesophageal diverticulum could be just one expression of this process. Venturi and colleagues[7] also demonstrated a higher collagen-to-elastin ratio in the cricopharyngeus muscle, as well as the upper esophageal muscularis propria in patients with a Zenker's diverticulum as compared with controls. This suggests a primary difference in the biochemical composition of the muscles of the UES area.

Cook and colleagues[8] studied patients with Zenker's diverticula and controls using simultaneous videoradiography and manometry. They were able to document significantly reduced sphincter opening and greater intrabolus pressure in patients with Zenker's diverticulum. They concluded that the primary abnormality in patients with Zenker's diverticulum is one of incomplete UES opening rather than abnormal coordination between pharyngeal contraction and UES relaxation or opening. Thus, the act of swallowing in the presence of cricopharyngeal dysfunction, combined with the usual pressure phenomena during deglutition, is believed to generate sufficient transmural pressure to allow mucosal herniation through an anatomically weak point in the posterior pharynx above the cricopharyngeus muscle. Owing to the recurrent nature of the pressures involved and the constant distention of the sac with ingested material, the established diverticulum enlarges progressively and descends dependently. The neck of the diverticulum hangs over the cricopharyngeus, and the sac becomes interposed between the esophagus and the vertebrae. Indeed, an advanced diverticulum may come to lie in the same vertical axis as the pharynx, permitting selective filling of the sac, which may compress and cause the adjacent esophagus to angle anteriorly. These anatomic changes further obstruct swallowing. Moreover, because the mouth of the diverticulum is above the cricopharyngeus, spontaneous emptying of the diverticulum is unimpeded and is often associated with laryngotracheal aspiration as well as regurgitation into the mouth.

SYMPTOMS AND DIAGNOSIS

Although a Zenker's diverticulum may be asymptomatic, most patients develop symptoms early in the course of the disease. Once the condition is established, it progresses both in size and in the

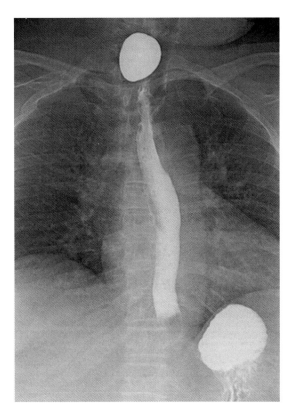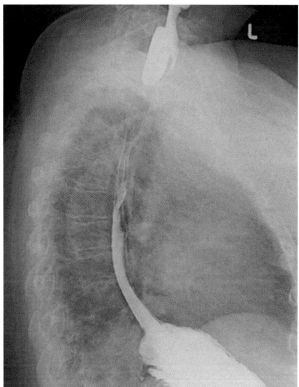

FIGURE 140.1 Anterior–posterior (AP) and lateral view of a Zenker's diverticulum in a patient presenting with regurgitation.

frequency and severity of symptoms and complications. Characteristically, the symptoms consist of high cervical esophageal dysphagia, halitosis, noisy deglutition, and spontaneous regurgitation with or without coughing or choking episodes. The regurgitated food is characteristically undigested; it is not bitter (bilious), sour (acidic), or contaminated by gastroduodenal secretions, and can occur up to a few hours after eating. The chief complications of a pharyngoesophageal diverticulum are nutritional and respiratory. If the condition is neglected, weight loss, hoarseness, asthma, respiratory insufficiency, and pulmonary sepsis leading to abscess are all potential complications. A palpable cervical mass is rarely noted. Carcinoma arising in a pharyngoesophageal diverticulum has been described in the literature to range from 0.3% to 7% and is of the squamous cell type.[9–11] Iatrogenic diverticular perforation may occur with esophageal intubation, instrumentation, or the accidental ingestion of a foreign body.

The diagnosis is confirmed by a barium swallow, which demonstrates the diverticulum (Fig. 140.1). Though an endoscopy is not specifically indicated for diagnosis of Zenker's diverticulum, if the patient is undergoing endoscopy as indicated for other esophageal symptoms, the endoscopist should be warned of the possibility of a pharyngoesophageal diverticulum because of the risk of perforation with the endoscope. Once the diagnosis of Zenker's diverticulum is made with a barium swallow, manometry is not typically indicated.

TREATMENT

The treatment of a pharyngoesophageal diverticulum is surgical. There is no medical therapy for this condition, and all patients with such diverticula should be considered candidates for surgical treatment irrespective of the size of the diverticulum.[11] Advanced age is not a contraindication to treatment. Indeed, it is highly recommended

as it will protect a vulnerable population from aspiration pneumonia and progressive malnutrition. A review from the Mayo Clinic demonstrated improvement in 94% of patients treated surgically with no operative deaths.[12] In a similar modern series, 99% of patients treated with cricopharyngeal myotomy had excellent results.[13] Treatment is best performed on an elective basis while the pouch is of small or moderate size and before complications have occurred. When nutritional or respiratory complications are present or when neoplasia is suspected, surgical intervention is still warranted. In a retrospective review of patients receiving surgery for Zenker's diverticulum, the complication rates for malnourished patients (defined as weight loss ≥10% in 6 months, albuminemia <35 g/L, and/or BMI <21) and non-malnourished patients were similar, but malnourished patients had a longer length of inpatient stay (3.8 vs. 1.9 days, respectively).[14]

The most common surgical procedure for a Zenker's diverticulum is either diverticulectomy or diverticulopexy combined with myotomy.[15–17] A comparison of techniques found that diverticulectomy without myotomy predisposed the patient to developing postoperative fistulas and diverticular recurrences, thus emphasizing the importance of myotomy in the treatment of this disorder.[17] Other approaches have also been used successfully. Dohlman and Mattsson first described peroral endoscopic diathermic division of the septum or common wall between the diverticulum and the esophagus.[18] Additionally, van Overbeek[19] has described the use of a carbon dioxide laser to divide the common wall. Collard[20] and Peracchia[21] later developed an endoluminal stapler technique to perform an endoscopic cricopharyngeal myotomy. In particular, the transoral endoluminal stapler myotomy and carbon dioxide laser techniques have emerged as the most frequently performed nonopen surgical approaches. Retrospective series have shown that an open approach (including cricopharyngeal myotomy and diverticulectomy or diverticulopexy) offers improved long-term results (persistent symptoms, recurrent symptoms, need for a repeat procedure) when compared to transoral endoscopic diverticulostomy with myotomy.[17,22] Of note, this is even more pronounced in diverticula ≤3 cm (where recurrence rates with peroral endoscopic stapling may be as high as 36%), likely because the anvil of the stapler (which is not able to staple or divide the tissue) can constitute one-third to one-half the length of these smaller diverticula.[22,23] Some authors have recommended that endoscopic diverticulostomy is best suited for patients with medium sized diverticula (3–5 cm), while open surgical myotomy, with or without diverticulectomy, should be the treatment of choice for smaller diverticula to lower the risk of incomplete myotomy.[22,23] Furthermore, transoral endoscopic approaches may also be prohibited in patients with a history of cervical disk fusion, limited neck extension, a short neck length, and in patients with kyphosis. Compared to transoral endoscopic approaches, the carbon dioxide laser technique has been reported to show a greater improvement in dysphagia and regurgitation symptoms, and a lower revision rate, but a higher rate of overall complications.[24]

Most patients undergoing surgical treatment require minimal preoperative preparation. A few patients (<10%) may have nutritional deficiencies severe enough to require preoperative parenteral hyperalimentation or gastrostomy.[14] Prompt repair of the diverticulum provides the best means of correcting most deficiencies and preventing further sequelae. Suppurative lung diseases also often require definitive resolution of the diverticular problem before they can be managed effectively.

SURGICAL TECHNIQUE

Open Cricopharyngeal Myotomy with Diverticulectomy or Diverticulopexy

The surgical procedure of choice among the authors' thoracic group at Washington University is an open cricopharyngeal myotomy with either diverticulectomy or diverticulopexy. At this time, an open approach facilitates the best chance for a complete myotomy of the cricopharyngeus. Diverticulectomy offers the theoretical benefit of a pathologic evaluation to rule out the small risk of esophageal cancer. Diverticulopexy avoids a suture line, and the small risk of complications associated with a diverticulectomy (fistula).

Patients first receive general anesthesia with a cuffed endotracheal tube. This technique controls ventilation and helps prevent intraoperative aspiration. The neck should be extended with a shoulder roll, and the head rotated to the right, approximately 45 degrees. The patient may undergo endoscopy at this time to ensure the diverticulum is adequately clear of food material (even if the patient has been appropriately n.p.o.) and document its appearance. Most commonly, a left cervical approach provides the best exposure. An oblique incision paralleling the anterior border of the sternocleidomastoid muscle and extending from the level of the hyoid bone to a point 1 cm above the clavicle is utilized. The platysma and omohyoid muscles are divided. By retracting the sternocleidomastoid muscle and carotid sheath laterally and the thyroid gland and larynx medially,

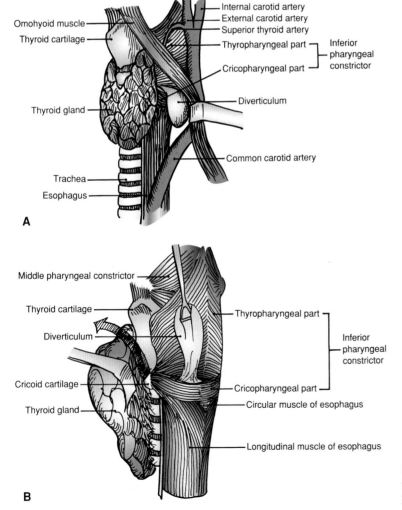

FIGURE 140.2 Cricopharyngeal myotomy. **A:** Exposure of diverticulum. **B:** Cephalad traction on diverticulum to expose cricopharyngeal part of inferior pharyngeal constrictors. (*continued*)

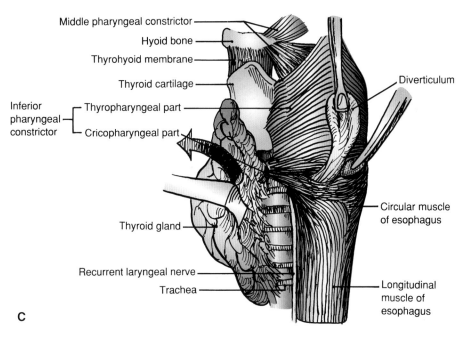

Middle pharyngeal constrictor
Hyoid bone
Thyrohyoid membrane
Thyroid cartilage
Inferior pharyngeal constrictor
Thyropharyngeal part
Cricopharyngeal part
Thyroid gland
Recurrent laryngeal nerve
Trachea

Diverticulum
Circular muscle of esophagus
Longitudinal muscle of esophagus

C

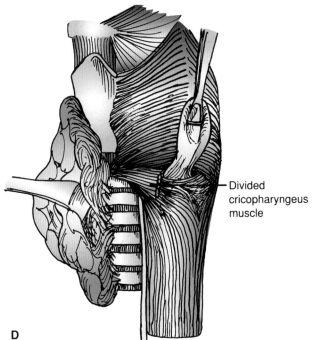

Divided cricopharyngeus muscle

D

FIGURE 140.2 (*Continued*) **C:** Dissection to delineate neck of diverticulum. **D:** Myotomy. (From Carol E Scott-Conner. *Scott-Conner & Dawson: Essential Operative Techniques and Anatomy.* 4th ed. Philadelphia, PA: Lippincott Williams & Wilkins; 2013.)

the retropharyngeal space and diverticulum are exposed. During this dissection, it may be necessary to divide the middle thyroid vein. Electrocautery should be avoided or used with extreme caution to prevent injury to the left recurrent laryngeal nerve. The diverticulum can promptly be recognized as arising from the posterior wall of the pharynx.

Once the diverticulum is identified, it is mobilized and elevated with a clamp (Fig. 140.2). At this point, a bougie (typically 40 to 50 Fr) may be introduced into the esophagus to facilitate the dissection. The area of the neck of the diverticulum is freed from surrounding fibrofatty tissue. The surgeon must thoroughly dissect out the diverticulum, identifying the margins of the pharyngeal muscular defect through which the mucosal sac protrudes. The decision to perform myotomy before diverticulectomy or diverticulopexy is an individual

one. We feel that when the choice between diverticulectomy and diverticulopexy is not clear, it is beneficial to perform the myotomy first and that can make medium-sized diverticula appear smaller and thus less likely to need a diverticulectomy.

The myotomy is performed beginning at the inferior aspect of the diverticulum and extending at least 3 to 4 cm inferiorly until the characteristic horizontal fibers of the cricopharyngeus have been adequately divided. We prefer using myotomy scissors, rather than low-intensity electrocautery, to avoid the risk of thermal injury. Simultaneously, a Kittner dissector is used to retract the divided muscle layer laterally. The myotomy is placed roughly at 135 degrees laterally from the anterior aspect of the esophagus. Of note, most sacs <2 cm simply disappear after the myotomy. Some surgeons prefer to have a 40- to 50-Fr esophageal bougie in place while performing the myotomy.

At this point, the size of the diverticulum is assessed. If a diverticulectomy is deemed necessary, a linear cutting stapler (white cartridge, 2.5 mm staples) is utilized with an esophageal bougie in place. It is easy to excise too much mucosa and create an iatrogenic esophageal stenosis if a bougie is not used during the diverticulectomy. The staple line is not typically reinforced. Alternatively, a diverticulopexy can be performed by inverting the diverticulum, and using absorbable suture to fix the superior portion of the diverticulum to either the left lateral wall of the hypopharynx or the anterior longitudinal ligament.[15]

A small suction drain (Jackson–Pratt) is placed in the retropharyngeal space. After the operation, the patient is managed routinely. A radiographic examination of the esophagus using contrast may be done the next day; if this is satisfactory, a soft diet is started. The drain is then removed and the patient may be discharged on the second postoperative day. A normal diet is resumed, 2 to 3 weeks later, as tolerated.

Transoral Endoscopic Stapled Diverticulotomy

Patients considered for this technique usually are those with a diverticulum of ≥3 cm in size in order to allow for introduction of the endoscopic stapling device and effectively transect the cricopharyngeus muscle. Contraindications to this approach were listed previously in the treatment selection section.

Under general anesthesia, the posterior oropharynx and upper esophagus is visualized using a Weerda laryngoscope. The laryngoscope is positioned with the anterior jaw in the esophagus and the posterior jaw in diverticulum. The common septum, located at the level of the neck of the diverticulum and formed by the cricopharyngeus muscle, is visualized by opening the jaws of the laryngoscope. An endoscopic suturing device is then used to place a suture across the septum, allowing it to be retracted cephalad.

A modified endoscopic stapling device (Endo-GIA 30) with a non-tapered anvil tip has been used to allow stapling and cutting to be performed to the very tip of the device to improve the myotomy completeness.[25] The modified anvil is positioned in the diverticulum, whereas the side of the stapling cartridge is positioned within the esophageal lumen. One or more applications of the stapling device may be required to allow for complete division of the common septum up to the apex of the diverticulum. By dividing the entire common septum, the required cricopharyngeal myotomy is performed. Effectively, the stapler creates a common cloaca between the true esophageal lumen and the diverticulum, simultaneously dividing the cricopharyngeus muscle. Similar postoperative care is employed as in the open technique, although no drain is placed in the endoscopic technique. In some centers, this procedure is performed on an outpatient basis.[26]

RESULTS

A retrospective review of elderly patients receiving an open surgical approach for their Zenker's diverticulum over two decades showed that the majority received diverticulectomy and myotomy (76%), while a minority received diverticulopexy and myotomy (7%) or diverticulopexy alone (5%).[12] The median age was 79 years, with the range being 75 to 91 years. Complications occurred in eight patients (11%) and included esophagocutaneous fistula in four, pneumonia and urinary tract infection in one, and wound infection, myocardial infarction, and persistent diverticulum in one patient each. At follow-up, 64 patients (88%) were completely asymptomatic and 4 (6%) were improved with minimal symptoms. Lerut reported similar results: no postoperative mortality, minimal morbidity, and very good to excellent results in 96% of patients.[27]

With regard to the endoscopic stapled diverticulotomy technique, several groups have reported very good results with minimal complications.[25,28,29] In a review of the long-term outcomes and quality of life after transoral stapling of Zenker's diverticulum from 2001 to 2013, the overall complication rate was found to be 4%, with no mortality. There was an overall success rate (no or minimal symptoms) of 76% over a median follow-up period of 63 months.[29] Of note, patients that were older (>70 years), had larger diverticula (>3 cm), and had an endostitch placed in the septum for traction prior to stapling,[29] all had significantly improved symptom resolution compared to those that were younger, had smaller diverticula, and did not have an endostitch placed.

Reoperation for recurrent pharyngoesophageal diverticulum is difficult and carries an increased risk of early postoperative morbidity.[30,31] Patients who have had previous surgery for Zenker's diverticulum should be considered for reoperation only if they have definite evidence of a diverticulum on barium swallow and progressively disabling or life-threatening symptoms. Reoperation on the UES can be a technical challenge. Previous surgery causes obliterated tissue planes and friable esophageal mucosa. Payne[32] reported that the use of an indwelling bougie is particularly helpful both as a landmark for the esophagus and as a mandrel over which esophageal repair can be accomplished without fear of luminal compromise. Revision endoscopic staple diverticulostomy has been recently reported by two groups (in patients that had an initial endoscopic staple diverticulostomy), and while one demonstrated a 95% partial or complete resolution of symptoms with no major complications, another has described perforation and mediastinitis occurring in 11% of their small series, to which they cited concern for a "staple over staple" effect.[28,33]

Cancer arising in a Zenker's diverticulum is rare and is usually of the squamous cell type.[9–11] It appears to occur in chronically neglected or retained diverticula. In a report of two patients with cancer totally confined to the sac, simple diverticulectomy provided long-term survival.[34] More aggressive management is indicated if the malignancy extends beyond the sac.[11]

EPIPHRENIC DIVERTICULUM

Epiphrenic diverticula are quite uncommon and are outnumbered by Zenker's diverticulum by a ratio of 1:6. They usually arise in the lower 10 cm of the thoracic esophagus. Most of these diverticula are found in middle-aged or elderly patients, and there is a slight predominance in men.

PATHOPHYSIOLOGY

With the advent of manometric studies, it became increasingly evident that functional obstruction of the distal esophagus may not only be the cause of the diverticulum but also a major cause of symptoms.[35,36] Achalasia, diffuse esophageal spasm, hypertensive lower esophageal sphincter, and nonspecific motor abnormalities have all been seen in conjunction with epiphrenic diverticula.[37,38] Achalasia and diffuse esophageal spasm are the esophageal motility disorders most commonly documented when an epiphrenic diverticulum is diagnosed.[38] However, when such conditions have been present, both the type of manometric disturbance and the severity of symptoms have varied.[39,40] Nehra and colleagues,[41] using 24-hour ambulatory manometry, prospectively studied patients with epiphrenic diverticula cases and found that the prevalence of abnormal esophageal motility was 100%.

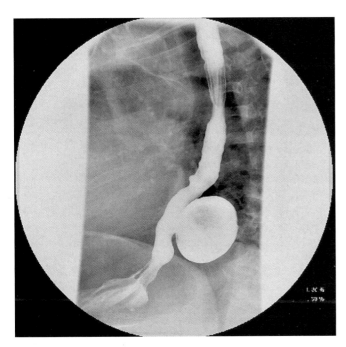

FIGURE 140.3 Barium esophagram of patient with a large epiphrenic diverticulum (8.4 by 6.9 cm, with a 2.5 cm opening) before surgical resection. This patient received a diagnostic fiberoptic esophagogastroduodenoscopy, left posterolateral thoracotomy, excision of the ephiphrenic diverticulum, esophagogastric myotomy, and partial fundoplication.

SYMPTOMS AND DIAGNOSIS

Symptoms in patients with epiphrenic diverticula are variable and are likely to be caused by the condition causing esophageal dysmotility rather than the diverticulum itself. Some patients may have only mild dysphagia that is readily managed with conservative methods, such as thorough mastication and adequate fluids at mealtime. The epiphrenic diverticulum is often diagnosed as an incidental finding on barium swallow done as part of a dysphagia evaluation. A small number of patients have progressive and incapacitating symptoms, including severe dysphagia, chest pain, food retention, regurgitation, and aspiration. The last two of these symptoms may become life-threatening, since repeated episodes of pneumonia may result in progressive destruction of lung parenchyma.

All patients with a suspected epiphrenic diverticulum should have a barium contrast upper gastrointestinal radiograph. A barium swallow provides proof of diagnosis (Fig. 140.3), serves as a baseline if the patient is asymptomatic, may provide clues to any associated motility disorder, and may detect other lesions, such as cancer, stricture, or hiatal hernia. Patients with symptoms of dysphagia and weight loss should have further evaluation with esophagoscopy and esophageal manometry. Esophagoscopy allows evaluation for esophagitis and the rare presence of cancer. Manometry is mandatory to characterize any associated motility disorders. However, the manometry catheter may coil within the epiphrenic diverticulum, and guidance under either endoscopy or fluoroscopy may be needed to ensure an appropriate and accurate study.[38] Primary carcinoma has rarely been reported noted with epiphrenic diverticula.[42,43]

TREATMENT

Patients with an epiphrenic diverticulum that is found incidentally with no or minimal symptoms can be managed conservatively and followed at regular intervals. If symptoms are present and the patient is otherwise in good health, an operation should be advised. Additionally, even when symptoms cannot be definitely attributed to the diverticulum, diverticulectomy should be considered when an operation is planned for the management of associated esophageal conditions.

SURGICAL TECHNIQUE

Two techniques are currently employed: a left transthoracic diverticulectomy, usually with a long esophagomyotomy or a laparoscopic approach. A double lumen cuffed endotracheal tube is placed to provide single lung ventilation. The diverticulum is mobilized from adjacent tissues until it is mobilized to the neck and proximal origin. Care should be taken not to injure the vagus nerve. With a bougie in place (usually 48 Fr or larger), a linear surgical stapler is applied parallel to the vertical axis of the esophagus to resect the diverticulum.[44] The staple line is then covered with the esophageal muscle and/or overlying mediastinal tissues. Though it is often recommended that a myotomy be performed on the opposite side of the esophagus (180 degrees from the epiphrenic diverticulum), we find that as long as there is 90 degrees or more axial separation between the diverticulectomy and the myotomy, there should be no risk of compromising the diverticulectomy and the exposure of the myotomy site is much easier. A long esophagomyotomy is performed from as high as the level of the pulmonary veins onto the proximal 1 to 2 cm of the gastric cardia. Testing may be performed with insufflation of air from an endoscope or nasogastric tube while the esophagus is submerged under saline, while observing for the leakage of any bubbles. Finally, if the transthoracic approach is utilized, a modified Belsey Mark IV repair (240 degrees) is commonly performed as an antireflux procedure.[44] A chest tube should be placed before closure.

A laparoscopic approach is typically used if the diverticulum is within 4 to 5 cm of the hiatus. For this operation, the patient is intubated and placed in the lithotomy position in reverse Trendelenburg. After entry into the abdomen and placement of 5-mm trocars in a manner consistent with a Heller myotomy, the transhiatal dissection is begun. Once the esophagus is mobilized from the left and right crus, the esophagus may be encircled with a tape for traction. The diverticulum is identified with careful blunt mediastinal dissection. Once the diverticulum is identified, it must be dissected from all adherent tissues. Again, care should be taken not to injure the vagus nerve. Once the diverticulum is completely mobilized to the neck, a linear endoscopic stapler is brought in through the left upper quadrant trocar to obtain appropriate apposition.[45] A bougie and/or endoscope should be placed in the esophagus, distal to the diverticulum, to prevent luminal compromise. It is again recommended to oversew the staple line with a muscular layer, in a laparoscopic interrupted manner with absorbable suture.[45] The myotomy is again carried out past the upper limit of the diverticulum excision, and down onto the cardia for 1 to 2 cm. Patients should receive a concomitant partial fundoplication.

RESULTS

A series from the University of Michigan included 35 patients over a 30-year period who underwent surgery via the open transthoracic approach.[44] The operative mortality was 2.8% and the leak rate 5.6%. With a median follow-up of 33.4 months, 74% of patients were symptom-free. Periodic esophageal dilatation was required in 20% of the cohort to treat postoperative dysphagia. In review of 20 patients undergoing a laparoscopic operation, esophageal leak was reported in 1 patient (5%), with recurrence of symptoms in 3 patients (15%) over a median follow-up period of 52 months.[46]

The need for meticulous surgical technique in these patients has been stressed in a prior report by Orringer,[47] and this cannot be overemphasized. Paramount to achieving a good result is careful reapproximation of tissue and relief of distal obstruction. Failure to perform esophagomyotomy in conjunction with diverticulectomy may be associated with recurrence or suture line complications and postoperative death. Early radiographic examination of the esophagus using a water-soluble contrast medium prior to starting an oral diet is usually advised. This examination permits an assessment of the staple line at the diverticulectomy site as well as evaluation of the esophagogastric lumen and esophageal emptying. Patients are generally asymptomatic postoperatively if associated esophageal conditions have been adequately dealt with during the operation.

TRACTION DIVERTICULUM

The incidence of traction diverticula appears to parallel that of specific granulomatous diseases, especially tuberculosis and histoplasmosis. Esophageal involvement by mediastinal granuloma is uncommon but may manifest as esophageal compression, stricture, diverticulum, sinus tract, or airway-esophageal fistula.[48,49] Because of the configuration and size of these diverticula, symptoms are rare. Occasionally, dysphagia or odynophagia occurs, presumably due to compression, stricture, or inflammation in the diverticulum. Local esophagitis may occur, suggesting that the caseous material may irritate the esophageal mucosa. Fistulization to the tracheobronchial tree occasionally results from inflammatory necrosis of the originating granuloma.[49] Similar but rarer communications have been found between the esophagus and great vessels.[50] Most hemorrhagic manifestations, however, probably result from friable granulation tissue or erosion of small bronchial or esophageal vessels by calcific debris.

When the condition is symptomatic, surgical treatment is indicated. Local excision of the diverticulum and adjacent inflammatory mass, with layered closure of the esophagus over an indwelling 40- to 50-Fr bougie, may be performed for the symptomatic uncomplicated traction diverticulum. Medical management of the underlying condition causing the granulomatous disease is also recommended.

The possibility of a tracheoesophageal fistula should be considered in a patient with esophageal diverticulum and chronic suppurative lung disease or in one with symptoms of cough after swallowing. In evaluating such patients, radiographic examination of the esophagus should be performed. Cinefluoroscopy during the ingestion of contrast medium usually defines the site and size of the communication and aids in screening patients suspected of having a fistula. Patients actually aspirating ingested material through the larynx because of some mechanism other than a fistula should be identified. This is important as in a debilitated patient with pulmonary symptoms and a traction esophageal diverticulum identified on esophagram, oropharyngeal aspiration is just as likely to be the cause of cough as the esophageal diverticulum.

Endoscopic examination of both the esophagus and the tracheobronchial tree is indicated, and the orifices of the fistula can usually be visualized. The introduction of methylene blue or other dye into the esophagus during bronchoscopy may facilitate this identification but is usually unnecessary. Appropriate biopsy material should be

obtained for histopathologic and microbiologic study, although viable organisms are rarely identified. If symptoms suggest chronic pulmonary suppuration, computed tomographic scanning of the lungs is indicated. This will delineate the extent of infection, which might require surgical management at the time of fistula repair. Recurrence of fistula is minimized by the interposition of healthy mediastinal tissue or muscle flap between the airway and the esophagus. In addition to division of the fistula and repair of the esophagus and airway, attention must be paid to correction of any distal esophageal obstruction, whether it is organic or one of the defined esophageal motility disturbances.

Esophagovascular fistulas are rare complications of traction diverticula. Impressive hemorrhage may occur without communication with a major vessel as mediastinal and bronchial vessels are often hypertrophied due to inflammation; fortunately, communication with a small unnamed vessel may provide additional time for orderly study and treatment. Unfortunately, initial bleeding is sudden, massive, and fatal when major vessels are involved. In addition to standard endoscopic and radiographic studies, selective arteriography during active bleeding can help define the site of hemorrhage.

KILLIAN–JAMIESON "DIVERTICULUM"

Radiologically identified outpouchings in the lateral wall of the upper esophagus below the level of the cricopharyngeus muscle occur in an area of weakness in the anterolateral aspect of the pharyngoesophageal junction (Fig. 140.4), which was described by Killian in 1908 and Jamieson in 1934.[51,52] The pathophysiology of this entity is unknown, since no specific motility disorder has been identified in association

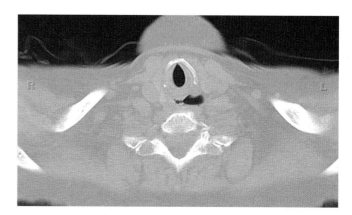

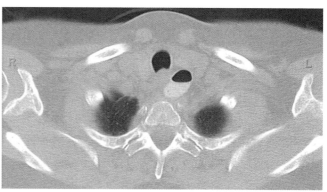

FIGURE 140.4 Sequential images of a Killian–Jamieson diverticulum on CT imaging with oral contrast. During surgical resection of this diverticulum, extreme caution must be taken to protect the recurrent laryngeal nerve.

with these radiologic findings. These cases usually represent radiologic demonstrations of local esophageal mural weakness rather than actual diverticula. These so-called Killian–Jamieson "diverticula" should not be confused with Zenker's diverticula, which originate in the posterior midline above the cricopharyngeus and can be effectively treated by cricopharyngeal myotomy, as described earlier in this chapter. For patients with symptoms of dysphagia, regurgitation, or aspiration from this diverticulum, an open transcervical approach similar to that for a Zenker's diverticulum may be used (diverticulopexy or diverticulectomy with distal myotomy). Extreme caution must be used during dissection of the diverticulum to not injure the recurrent laryngeal nerve, as this will be lying immediately posterior to the Killian–Jamieson diverticulum. In fact, due to the proximity of the recurrent laryngeal nerve to this diverticulum, a transoral endoscopic stapler approach should be avoided, as the likelihood of stapling and dividing the nerve is too high.[53]

DIFFUSE INTRAMURAL ESOPHAGEAL DIVERTICULOSIS

Diffuse intramural esophageal diverticulosis is a rare disease that usually presents as dysphagia. These patients are found to have multiple diverticula and esophageal strictures secondary to chronic inflammation and fibrosis (Fig. 140.5). The pathologic basis of this disease is thought to involve dilatation of the deep esophageal glands within the wall of the esophagus, forming pseudodiverticula.[54] A clear association with a distinct motility disorder has not been found. While there is no specific treatment for diffuse intramural esophageal diverticulosis, the strictures involved in this disease can sometimes

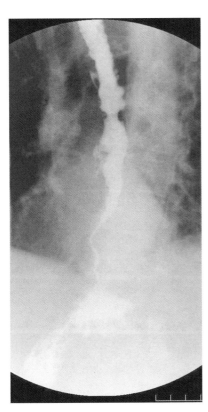

FIGURE 140.5 Contrast esophagram of patient with diffuse intramural esophageal diverticulosis demonstrating multiple esophageal diverticula and fibrotic strictures at various levels.

be treated by bougie dilatation for symptomatic relief.[55] Esophagectomy may be required for definitive treatment, with the caveat of increased hazard due to the significant periesophageal inflammation and fibrosis.

REFERENCES

1. Ferreira LE, Simmons DT, Baron TH. Zenker's diverticula: pathophysiology, clinical presentation, and flexible endoscopic management. *Dis Esophagus* 2008; 21(1):1–8.
2. Ludlow A. A case of obstructed deglutition, from a preternatural dilation of, and bag formed in the pharynx. *Med Observ Inquiries* 1769;3:85–101.
3. Zenker FA, von Ziemssen H. Krankheiten des oesophagus. In: von Ziemssen H, ed. *Handbuch der speziellen Pathologie und Therapie. Vol. 7, Part 1.* Leipzig: FCW Vogel; 1874.
4. Negus VE. Pharyngeal diverticula: observations on their evolution and treatment. *Br J Surg* 1950;38:129–146.
5. Ellis FH Jr., Schlegel JF, Lynch VP, et al. Cricopharyngeal myotomy for pharyngoesophageal diverticulum. *Ann Surg* 1969;170:340–349.
6. Lerut T, Guelinckx P, Dom R, et al. Does the musculus cricopharyngeus play a role in the genesis of Zenker's diverticulum? Enzyme histochemical and contractility properties. In: Siewert JR, Holscher AM, eds. *Diseases of the Esophagus.* New York: Springer, 1988.
7. Venturi M, Bonavina L, Colombo L, et al. Biochemical markers of upper esophageal sphincter compliance in patients with Zenker's diverticulum. *J Surg Res* 1997;70:46–48.
8. Cook IJ, Gabb M, Panagopoulos V, et al. Pharyngeal (Zenker's) diverticulum is a disorder of upper esophageal sphincter opening. *Gastroenterology* 1992;103:1229–1235.
9. Brucher BL, Sarbia M, Oestreicher E, et al. Squamous cell carcinoma and Zenker diverticulum. *Dis Esophagus* 2007;20:75–78.
10. Sauvanet A, Gayet B, Lemee J, et al. Cancer on an esophageal diverticulum. *Presse Med* 1992;21:305–308.
11. Herbella FA, Dubecz A, Patti MG. Esophageal diverticula and cancer. *Dis Esophagus* 2012;25(2):153–158.
12. Crescenzo DG, Trastek VF, Allen MS, et al. Zenker's diverticulum in the elderly: Is operation justified? *Ann Thorac Surg* 1998;66:347–350.
13. Jougon J, Le Taillandier-de-Gabory L, Raux F, et al. Plea in favour of external approach of Zenker's diverticulum: 73 cases reported. *Ann Chir* 2003;128:167–172.
14. Boucher S, Breheret R, Laccourreye L. Importance of malnutrition and associated diseases in the management of Zenker's diverticulum. *Eur Ann Otorhinolaryngol Head Neck Dis* 2015;132(3):125–128.
15. Mariette C. Zenker's pharyngoesophageal diverticulum: diverticulectomy and diverticulopexy. *J Vasc Surg* 2014 151(2):145–149.
16. Yuan Y, Zhao YF, Hu Y, et al. Surgical treatment of Zenker's diverticulum. *Dig Surg* 2013;30(3):207–218.
17. Gutschow CA, Hamoir M, Rambaux P, et al. Management of pharyngoesophageal (Zenker's) diverticulum: Which technique? *Ann Thorac Surg* 2002;74:1677–1682.
18. Dohlman G, Mattsson O. The endoscopic operation for hypopharyngeal diverticula: a roentgencinematographic study. *AMA Arch Otolaryngol* 1960;71:744–752.
19. van Overbeek JJ. Microendoscopic CO_2 laser surgery of the hypopharyngeal (Zenker's) diverticulum. *Adv Otorhinolaryngol* 1995;49:140–143.
20. Collard JM, Otte JB, Kestens PJ. Endoscopic stapling technique of esophagodiverticulostomy for Zenker's diverticulum. *Ann Thorac Surg* 1993;56:573–576.
21. Peracchia A, Bonavina L, Narne S, et al. Minimally invasive surgery for Zenker diverticulum: analysis of results in 95 consecutive patients. *Arch Surg* 1998;133:695–700.
22. Rizzetto C, Zaninotto G, Costantini M, et al. Zenker's diverticula: feasibility of a tailored approach based on diverticulum size. *J Gastrointest Surg* 2008;12(12):2057–2064.
23. Kannabiran VR, Gooey J, Fisichella PM. A tailored approach to the surgical treatment of Zenker's Diverticula. *J Gastrointest Surg* 2015;19(5):949–954.
24. Parker NP, Misono S. Carbon dioxide laser versus stapler-assisted endoscopic Zenker's diverticulotomy: a systematic review and meta-analysis. *Otolaryngol Head Neck Surg* 2014;150(5):750–753.
25. Morse CR, Fernando HC, Ferson PF, et al. Preliminary experience by a thoracic service with endoscopic transoral stapling of cervical (Zenker's) diverticulum. *J Gastrointest Surg* 2007;11:1091–1094.
26. Saetti R, Silvestrini M, Peracchia A, et al. Endoscopic stapler-assisted Zenker's diverticulotomy: Which is the best operative facility? *Head Neck* 2006;28:1084–1089.
27. Lerut T, van Raemdonck D, Guelinckx P, et al. Pharyngo-oesophageal diverticulum (Zenker's): clinical, therapeutic, and morphological aspects. *Acta Gastroenterol Belg* 1990;53:330–337.
28. Wiklen R, Whited C, Scher RL. Endoscopic staple diverticulostomy for Zenker's diverticulum: review of experience in 337 cases. *Ann Otol Rhinol Laryngol* 2015; 214(1):21–29.
29. Bonavina L, Aiolfi A, Scolari F, et al. Long-term outcome and quality of life after transoral stapling for Zenker diverticulum. *World J Gastroenterol* 2015;21(4);1167–1172.
30. Huang B, Payne WS, Cameron AJ. Surgical management for recurrent pharyngoesophageal (Zenker's) diverticulum. *Ann Thorac Surg* 1984;37:189–191.
31. Rocco G, Deschamps C, Martel E, et al. Results of reoperation on the upper esophageal sphincter. *J Thorac Cardiovasc Surg* 1999;117:28–30.
32. Payne WS. The treatment of pharyngoesophageal diverticulum: the simple and complex. *Hepatogastroenterology* 1992;39:109–114.

33. Buchanan MA, Riffat F, Mahrous AK, et al. Endoscopic or external approach revision surgery for pharyngeal pouch following primary endoscopic stapling: Which is the favored approach? *Eur Arch Otorhinolaryngol* 2013;270:1707–1710.

34. Huang B, Unni KK, Payne WS. Long-term survival following diverticulectomy for cancer in pharyngoesophageal (Zenker's) diverticulum. *Ann Thorac Surg* 1984;38:207–210.

35. Habein HC, Kirklin JW, Clagett OT, et al. Surgical treatment of lower esophageal pulsion diverticula. *Arch Surg* 1956;72:1018–1024.

36. Habein HC, Moersch HJ, Kirklin JW. Diverticula of the lower part of the esophagus: a clinical study of one hundred forty-nine nonsurgical cases. *Arch Intern Med* 1956;97:768–777.

37. Fisichella PM, Jalilvand A, Dobrowolsky A. Achalasia and epiphrenic diverticulum. *World J Surg* 2015;39(7):1614–1619.

38. Soares R, Herbella FA, Prachand VN, et al. Epiphrenic diverticulum of the esophagus: from pathophysiology to treatment. *J Gastrointest Surg* 2010;14(12):2009–2015.

39. Bontempo L, Corazziari E, Mineo TC, et al. Esophageal motor activity in patients with esophageal diverticula. In: DeMeester TR, Skinner DB, eds. *Esophageal Disorders, Pathophysiology and Therapy*. New York: Raven Press, 1985:427.

40. Debas HT, Payne WS, Cameron AJ, et al. Physiopathology of lower esophageal diverticulum and its implications for treatment. *Surg Gynecol Obstet* 1980;151:593–600.

41. Nehra D, Lord RV, DeMeester TR, et al. Physiologic basis for the treatment of epiphrenic diverticulum. *Ann Surg* 2002;235:346–354.

42. Lai ST, Hsu CP. Carcinoma arising from an epiphrenic diverticulum: a frequently misdiagnosed disease. *Ann Thorac Cardiovasc Surg* 2007;13(2):110–113.

43. Avisar E, Luketich JD. Adenocarcinoma in a mid-esophageal diverticulum. *Ann Thorac Surg* 2000;69(1):288–289.

44. Varghese TK Jr., Marshall B, Chang AC, et al. Surgical treatment of epiphrenic diverticula: a 30-year experience. *Ann Thorac Surg* 2007;84(6):1801–1809.

45. Romario U, Ceolin M, Porta M, et al. Laparoscopic repair of epiphrenic diverticulum. *Semin Thoracic Surg* 2012;24:213–217.

46. Rosati R, Fumagalli U, Elmore U, et al. Long-term results of minimally invasive surgery for symptomatic epiphrenic diverticulum. *Am J Surg* 2011;201(1):132–135.

47. Orringer MB. Epiphrenic diverticula: fact and fable. *Ann Thorac Surg* 1993;55:1067–1068.

48. Rastogi A, Sarda D, Kothari P, et al. Mediastinal tuberculosis presenting as traction diverticulum of the esophagus. *Ann Thorac Med* 2007;2(3):126–127.

49. Lopez A, Rodriquez P, Santana N, et al. Esophagobronchial fistula caused by traction esophageal diverticulum. *Eur J Cardiothorac Surg* 2003;23(1):128–130.

50. Ballehaninna UK, Shaw JP, Brichkov I. Traction esophageal diverticulum: a rare cause of gastrointestinal bleeding. *SpringerPlus* 2012;1(1):50.

51. Killian G. Uber den mund der speiserohre. *Zeitschr Ohrenheilk* 1908;55:1–44.

52. Jamieson EB. *Illustrations of Regional Anatomy*. Edinburgh: E & S Livingstone; 1934.

53. Undavia S, Anand SM, Jacobson AS. Killian-Jamieson diverticulum: a case for open transcervical excision. *Laryngoscope* 2013;123(2):414–417.

54. Medeiros LJ, Doos WG, Balogh K. Esophageal intramural pseudodiverticulosis: a report of two cases with analysis of similar, less extensive changes in normal autopsy esophagi. *Hum Pathol* 1988;19:928–931.

55. Teraishi F, Fujiwara T, Jikuhara A, et al. Esophageal intramural pseudodiverticulosis with esophageal strictures successfully treated with dilation therapy. *Ann Thorac Surg* 2006;82:1119–1121.

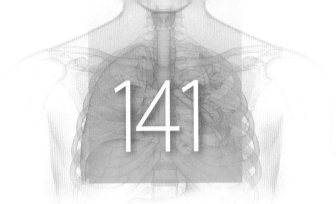

141

Benign Tumors, Cysts, and Duplications of the Esophagus

Kiran Lagisetty ■ Rishindra M. Reddy

Benign esophageal lesions are uncommon tumors with uncertain long-term sequelae and controversial indications regarding how and when to intervene operatively. The incidence of these lesions is quiet low, with autopsy reports suggesting prevalence rates of 0.17% to 0.59%,[1] and malignant esophageal tumors being found up to 5 to 10 times more often.[1,2] Esophageal leiomyomas are the most common lesions based on autopsy studies, but in retrospect, some tumors classified in those series may have been gastrointestinal stromal tumors (GISTs), incorrectly classified as leiomyomas. Esophageal cysts are the next most common, followed by granular cell tumors (GCTs), fibrovascular polyps, and squamous papillomas. Most of these lesions in the large incidence studies were found after endoscopy performed for symptoms of dysphagia, but more recently, an increasing number of lesions have been found incidentally as a result of the increased use of endoscopy and endoscopic ultrasound (EUS). The indications for surgery are changing, as some lesions are being seen as safe to be observed long term without resection.

This chapter describes the incidence, pathology, diagnosis, and treatment for benign esophageal tumors and cysts. Surgical approaches will be briefly reviewed and a proposed treatment algorithm is provided at the end of the chapter.

OVERVIEW

The first report of a benign esophageal tumor was recorded as early as 1559 by Sussius; however, there is no pathologic record to confirm his findings.[3] The first pathologically confirmed benign esophageal tumor may have been described by Virchow in 1867.[4] Sauerbruch is credited with the first reported resection of a benign esophageal tumor by performing a partial esophagectomy with esophagogastrostomy in 1932.[4] This was followed by a report of an esophageal tumor enucleation by Ohsawa 1 year later.[5] Following the advent of video-assisted thoracoscopic surgery (VATS), 1992 was marked by the first two reports of minimally invasive resection of leiomyomas.[6,7] Advances in endoscopic treatments have now led to descriptions of trans-oral endoscopic resections of smaller tumors.[8] Currently, benign esophageal tumors are relatively rare and comprise less than 1% of all clinically detected esophageal tumors.

The true incidence of benign esophageal tumors is impossible to characterize as most are diagnosed only when symptomatic or otherwise discovered incidentally on autopsy. There have been several autopsy series published demonstrating an overall incidence of less than 1%. Patterson reported 62 benign esophageal tumors described in the ancient literature over a 215-year period between 1717 and 1932.[9] Subsequent autopsy series by Moersch, Plachta, and Attah have all yielded a prevalence estimate of less than 1%.[1,10,11] Benign esophageal tumors typically present between the third and fifth decades of life with a male to female predominance of 2:1.[4]

Benign tumors of the esophagus are rare entities, even at high-volume thoracic surgery centers with vast experience in esophageal cancer and benign functional conditions. Several basic tenets of management will help guide the decision-making process in the workup and management of these tumors. Evaluating patients for symptoms such as dysphagia, odynophagia, chest pain, obstruction, or bleeding is important as the lesions causing these symptoms should generally be removed. Cystic lesions of the esophagus are often removed in order to "prevent possible infection" but the data supporting such a stance are not well established. In order to differentiate these lesions from malignant lesions, a standard endoscopic evaluation with EUS should be undertaken. One goal of such an assessment would be to avoid unnecessary biopsy for clearly benign lesions. Surgical resection can be approached in a minimally invasive manner when feasible with the choice of operation based on adequate exposure, myotomy of the muscularis propria, and full enucleation of the mass with avoidance of mucosal injury.

Benign esophageal masses can typically be classified as either solid or cystic masses and can be characterized by the specific layer of the esophageal wall from which they arise. Figure 141.1 displays a list of the variety of subtypes of benign esophageal lesions with regard to the EUS layer from which they originate. These tumors tend to be slow growing and approximately 50% are asymptomatic.[11] The most common presenting symptom is dysphagia secondary to increasing size and luminal obstruction. Most tumors greater than 5 cm will cause dysphagia secondary to luminal narrowing. Less frequent symptoms include retrosternal or epigastric pain, bleeding, ulceration, or regurgitation.[4,12] Most patients present with long-standing symptoms and, according to Seremetis and colleagues, 30% will have experienced symptoms for 5 years or greater, while 30% will have 2 to 5 years of symptoms and the remaining minority will describe an average of 11 months of symptoms.[2] Malignant transformation of benign esophageal lesions is extremely rare and malignant lesions other than squamous cell or adenocarcinoma are exceedingly rare themselves. The distinction between benign and malignant tumors can typically be made based on endoscopy and EUS.

Esophageal 1st/2nd layers
(Mucosa)
Granular Cell Tumor
Fibrovascular Polyp
Squamous Papilloma
Retention Cyst

Esophageal 4th layer
(Muscularis propria)
Leiomyoma
GIST
Leiomyosarcoma

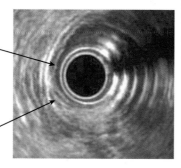

Esophageal 3rd layer
(Submucosa)
Lipoma
Hemangioma
Fibroma
Neurofibroma

Esophageal 5th layer
(Paraesophageal tissue)
Cysts

FIGURE 141.1 Benign esophageal lesion subtype by location within the esophageal wall. (EUS picture courtesy of Dr. Erik Wamsteker, University of Michigan, Ann Arbor, MI.)

IMAGING AND ENDOSCOPY

Most benign lesions of the esophagus are discovered incidentally during workup for other lesions; however, when these lesions become large enough, the patient will present with dysphagia. Chest radiographs have low value in the diagnosis of benign esophageal lesions; however, such studies occasionally demonstrate posterior or middle mediastinal masses. The most commonly performed diagnostic tests include barium esophagram, computed tomography (CT), esophagogastroduodenoscopy (EGD), and EUS. These tests require a firm understanding of the anatomy of the esophagus and the composition of the esophageal wall. Other chapters in this book provide detailed descriptions of esophageal wall anatomy, imaging studies, and endoscopy.

During workup of benign esophageal lesions, special attention must be made to clearly identify the mucosa, submucosa, and muscularis propria. The mucosa is made up of the innermost layer of epithelium followed by the basement membrane, lamina propria, and muscularis mucosa. The next deeper layer is the submucosa, containing the elastic fibers, collagen, and glands of the esophageal wall. The outermost layer is the muscularis propria, composed of the inner circular muscle and the outer longitudinal muscle. These muscles are initially striated muscle in the cervical esophagus and transition to becoming smooth muscle in the mid- to lower esophagus. It is commonly pointed out that the esophagus has no serosal layer; therefore, the outermost wall is made of the longitudinal muscle.

A barium esophagram is typically the first diagnostic test ordered for a patient presenting with dysphagia. This test is typically performed in a biphasic manner with an upright double-contrast view with high-density barium allowing for the evaluation of the mucosa and a prone single-contrast view with low-density barium allowing for evaluation of luminal narrowing. Most benign lesions will be seen as mobile masses with smooth contours. Barium esophagrams will occasionally demonstrate altered peristalsis.[13]

CT imaging is useful when evaluating for extra-esophageal tumors or to exclude the possibility of other mediastinal tumors that may present in a similar fashion. CT cannot differentiate between the several layers of the esophageal wall; however, it does give important anastomotic relationships to nearby structures, especially important information during surgical planning.

EGD and EUS are extremely helpful for the evaluation of esophageal lesions and provide the most direct evaluation of the esophageal mucosa and the relationship of the mass to the layers of the esophageal wall. On EUS, the layers of the esophageal wall are seen

as concentric hyperechoic (white) and hypoechoic (black) rings. The innermost ring represents the superficial mucosa (white) followed by the lamina propria/basement membrane (black). Moving outward, one encounters the submucosa (white), muscularis propria (black), and finally the peri-esophageal tissue (white). There are a total of five rings seen on typical EUS imaging. EGD and EUS allow for evaluation of the mass size and the depth of invasion while allowing for potential biopsy of the mass or adjacent lymph nodes if malignancy is suspected. Although EGD can only see the mucosa, it is important to ensure that the overlying mucosa is intact if an intramural tumor is suspected. Features favoring a benign lesion on EUS include small size, smooth borders, homogenous echo pattern, and lack of surrounding enlarged lymph nodes. Lesions that appear heterogeneous and greater than 3 cm in diameter should raise the suspicion for malignancy and warrant fine-needle aspiration (FNA) for diagnosis.[14,15] EUS has the added benefit of differentiating between solid and cystic masses; however, the viscous nature of typical esophageal cysts may make differentiating cystic from solid a difficult task.

FNA of esophageal lesions should be carried out with caution and is generally not favored in the workup of benign lesions. There is an inherent risk of causing an infection within a cystic lesion secondary to the transmucosal nature of the needle aspiration procedure. FNA may also create inflammatory adhesions between the mucosa and mass, an event which may make subsequent resection more difficult and increase the chance of mucosal injury. Given the indolent nature of most benign esophageal lesions, if an asymptomatic lesion appears solid and benign on EUS, the typical treatment is observation alone.

BENIGN TUMORS OF THE MUCOSA

Benign tumors of the esophageal mucosa are typically seen on endoscopy during workup for a symptomatic patient. Secondary to their location these lesions are easily biopsied with endoscopic pinch forceps during endoscopy. EUS should also be undertaken to examine the size and depth of invasion.

GRANULAR CELL TUMORS

Abrikossoff first described GCTs in the 1920s. These tumors were historically known as granular cell myoblastomas. GCTs are the third most common benign esophageal tumors after leiomyomas and cysts. These tumors can be found in multiple locations with approximately 1% to 8% seen in the gastrointestinal tract and of those, one-third in the esophagus. Other less common locations include the respiratory tract and breast.[16–18] Within the esophagus the most common location is the distal third and these tumors are thought to originate from Schwann cell because of their staining patterns. GCTs tend to be asymptomatic and are typically discovered on endoscopy for other reasons or autopsy. Patients with larger lesions can present with dysphagia, chest pain, cough, nausea, or reflux.[19] GCTs can be seen on barium studies or on endoscopy. Endoscopically, these tumors appear pale-yellow, wide-based, and firm with intact overlying mucosa. EUS demonstrates a hypoechoic mass surrounded by a hypoechoic mucosa found in the inner two layers.[15] Definitive diagnosis of GCTs based on EGD and EUS can sometimes be difficult; therefore, direct biopsy using endoscopic forceps is sometimes required. There is no current consensus on the treatment of GCTs. If the tumor is benign on biopsy, there have been no reported cases of subsequent malignant transformation. There is however a 1% to 3% malignancy rate and tumors which are symptomatic, larger than 10 mm, rapidly growing, or harbor malignancy should be resected.[19,20] The remainder of tumors may be biopsied and clinically followed.

FIBROVASCULAR POLYPS

Benign fibrovascular polyps are typically found in the upper third of the esophagus, typically located in the posterior midline above the confluence of the longitudinal layer of muscle known as the Lamier triangle. These tumors are caused by submucosal thickening and are often based on a long pedicle secondary to the effects of peristalsis.[21] Large fibrovascular polyps can present with dysphagia and/or obstruction and rarely with regurgitation with asphyxiation and sudden death.[22,23] Histologically these tumors have variable makeup including fibrous, vascular, adipose, and neural tissues. Contrast imaging demonstrates a sausage-shaped lesion and endoscopy will show the same, typically located in the upper esophagus (Fig. 141.2).[12] Resection is recommended secondary to the risk of airway compromise. EUS is beneficial in determining the vascularity of the stalk, the location, and the size: all of which are helpful in planning resection.[8] Smaller lesions can be removed endoscopically with direct snare or EMR techniques. Larger lesions or lesions with a highly vascular stalk should be resected via a longitudinal esophagotomy on the side opposite the tumor stalk followed by ligation and resection of the tumor and two-layer closure of the esophagotomy.[24]

SQUAMOUS PAPILLOMAS

Esophageal papillomas are exceedingly rare with an incidence of 0.01% on autopsy series and 0.07% on endoscopy series.[25,26] Patients are typically older and these lesions are thought to be secondary to infection with papillomavirus or the result of chronic inflammation from gastroesophageal reflux; however, this remains an area of controversy.[15,27–29] Lesions are small and solitary and typically found in the distal esophagus.[25] Multiple lesions can be found throughout the esophagus in a rare condition referred to as esophageal papillomatosis.[30] These sessile lesions are usually discovered incidentally on endoscopy where they appear as small, pink, and fleshy and are typically less than 1 cm. Biopsies are typically taken in order to distinguish these mucosal lesions from squamous cell carcinoma. Resection via endoscopic mucosal resection or open surgical techniques is recommended when patients are symptomatic due to obstruction, or

when a biopsy demonstrates atypical features and malignancy cannot be ruled out. There has been only one case report of malignant transformation of an esophageal papilloma, and cases where cancer is still a concern after EMR should be treated with additional EMR or, possibly, esophagotomy and local resection.[31]

BENIGN TUMORS OF THE SUBMUCOSA

Benign esophageal tumors of the submucosa include lipomas, fibromas, neurofibromas, and hemangiomas. Tumors of this variety have similar diagnostic workup and are most commonly clinically followed or resected based on symptomatology and EUS findings.

LIPOMAS

Lipomas of the esophagus are very rare, accounting for only 0.4% of benign digestive tract tumors. They are asymptomatic; however, they can become symptomatic with dysphagia if they grow large.[32] These tumors tend to be soft, yellow tumors that bulge into the esophageal lumen with an intact mucosa (Fig. 141.3). Lipomas have presented in patients ranging from ages of 4 to 80 years with an average age of 50 years. These tumors are most commonly found in the cervical and upper thoracic esophagus.[33] Radiographically, lipomas appear as filling defects and will change contour and configuration as a result of peristalsis.[34] Endoscopically, these lesions have yellow hue and highly experienced endoscopists may notice a "soft texture" with probing of the mass. EUS demonstrates hyperechoic, homogenous, submucosal lesions. Biopsy is rarely helpful and should only be done if there is concern for liposarcoma or other malignancy. Lipomas are generally clinically observed; however, when symptomatic, they can be resected via an endoscopic or minimally invasive surgical approach.[35]

HEMANGIOMAS

Esophageal hemangiomas are benign vascular tumors that arise from the hypertrophy of blood vessels within the submucosa of the esophagus. These tumors appear as dark purplish-red nodules and account for 3% of all benign tumors of the esophagus.[11] Hemangiomas can present as a solitary lesion or as multiple lesions in cases of the Rendu–Osler–Weber syndrome. Most are asymptomatic. Symptomatic lesions may present with dysphagia and retrosternal pain but afflicted patients rarely describe hematemesis, which may be secondary to mucosal ulceration. EGD is helpful in diagnosing these tumors given their characteristic appearance and EUS will show a hypoechoic, submucosal mass arising from the second or third layer with sharp margins.[36] CT with contrast and MRI are useful in confirming the diagnosis and further delineating these tumors. Asymptomatic tumors are followed clinically and symptomatic lesions can be treated with endoscopic resection, sclerotherapy, radiation, laser fulguration, or minimally invasive surgical resection.[15,37–40]

FIBROMAS AND NEUROFIBROMAS

With fewer than 30 case reports, fibromas and neurofibromas are the least common of the benign esophageal mesenchymal tumors, accounting for approximately 0.9% of esophageal submucosal tumors.[11] Neurofibromas are typically associated with von Recklinghausen disease and are most commonly seen in the stomach or colon. These tumors are found in the submucosa and arise from Schwann cells and are classified into three types: localized, diffuse,

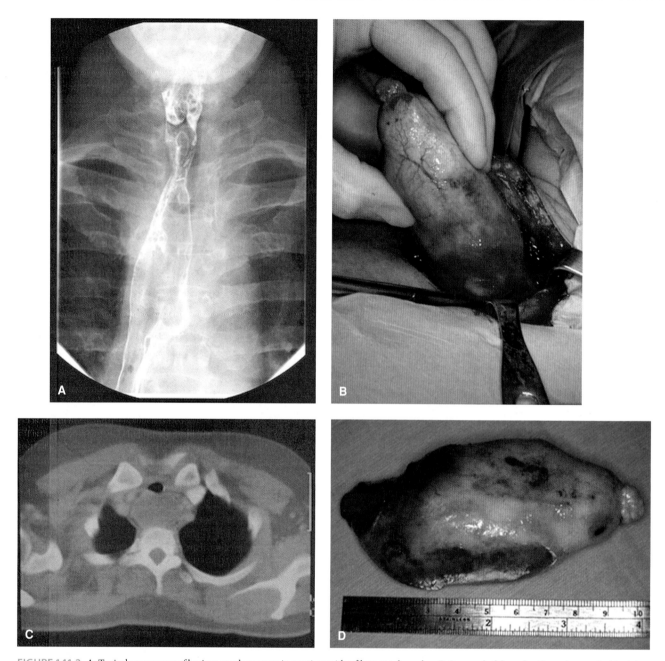

FIGURE 141.2 **A:** Typical appearance of barium esophagogram in a patient with a fibrovascular polyp. **B:** Removal of the polyp through a cervical incision. **C:** CT scan of the chest demonstrating the polyp in the chest. **D:** Typical picture of a fibrovascular polyp. (Photos courtesy of Dr. Mark B. Orringer, University of Michigan, Ann Arbor, MI.)

and plexiform. Tumors most commonly present between age 50 and 60 with a range of 10 to 79 years and a slight female to male predominance.[41] Tumors are typically found in the cervical or upper esophagus and can range in size from 0.5 to 16 cm.[42] Most tumors are asymptomatic and are discovered incidentally on endoscopy; however, when symptomatic, they will present with dysphagia and chest discomfort.[42]

The diagnostic workup for suspected esophageal fibromas is similar to that of the previously described esophageal lesions, namely, barium esophagram, EGD, and EUS. Given the rarity of these tumors, they often have to be differentiated from leiomyomas, leiomyosarcomas, or GISTs. Grossly these tumors appear as yellow-white colored, rubbery masses with smooth surfaces. Histologically, these tumors feature peripheral lymphoid cuffs composed of lymphoid

follicles, moderate cellularity, broad bundles, interlacing fascicles or whorls, or elongating cells.[43] Immunohistochemical analysis will demonstrate positive staining for S-100 and will stain negative for CK117, CD34, desmin, and SMA, thus distinguishing these tumors from GISTs and leiomyomas.

Management of these tumors is similar to that of leiomyomas and is typically based on size and presence of symptoms. Tumors smaller than 2 cm in diameter can be observed and resection is reserved for larger tumors, the presence of symptoms, or increasing size on surveillance endoscopy.[44] As with leiomyomas, small lesions can be safely resected endoscopically, but larger tumors (>2 cm) typically require resection via thoracotomy or thoracoscopy.[41,45,46] In rare occasions, an esophagectomy may be required if the lesions are extremely large.[47]

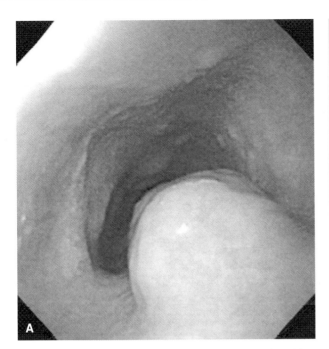
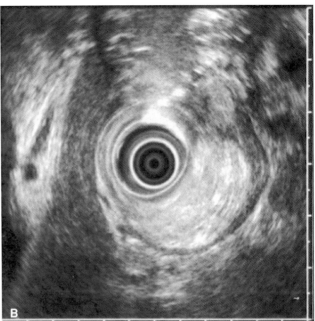

FIGURE 141.3 **A:** Typical endoscopic appearance of an esophageal lipoma. **B:** Typical homogeneous and hyperechoic esophageal ultrasound appearance of an esophageal lipoma within the third ultrasound layer (submucosa). (Photos courtesy of Dr. David Diehl, Geisinger Medical Center, Danville, PA.)

BENIGN TUMORS OF THE MUSCULARIS PROPRIA

Leiomyomas and esophageal cysts are the two most common tumors of the muscularis propria.

LEIOMYOMAS

The first description of an esophageal leiomyoma was by Morgagni in 1761.[48] Leiomyomas are the most common benign tumor of the esophagus accounting for over 70% of benign tumors; however, only 10% of gastrointestinal leiomyomas occur in the esophagus.[49] The overall prevalence of these tumors ranges from 0.006% to 0.1%; however, the presentation of clinically significant leiomyomas is much more rare.[49] Leiomyomas arise from the muscularis propria, specifically from the smooth muscle. Approximately 80% of these tumors are found intramurally and 7% are extra-esophageal. Most are localized and solitary; however, 2.4% occur in multiple sites within the esophagus and 10% to 13% will be circumferential at the time of presentation.[50] Leiomyomas are usually found in the middle to distal third of the esophagus arising from the inner circular layer. A review of 838 cases by Seremetis et al. found that 57% of tumors were in the distal third of the esophagus, 32% in the middle third, and 11% in the upper third.[2] There is a 2:1 male to female predominance and these tumors are overwhelmingly benign tumors with only four documented cases of malignant degeneration.[2] These tumors have been associated with other benign esophageal conditions such as gastrointestinal reflux, esophageal diverticuli, achalasia, and other esophageal dysmotility disorders.

Grossly, leiomyomas are tan-yellow, firm, rubbery, well-encapsulated, and smooth-bordered masses (Fig. 141.4). Approximately 50% of these masses are less than 5 cm, with 93% less than 15 cm.[50] Histologically,

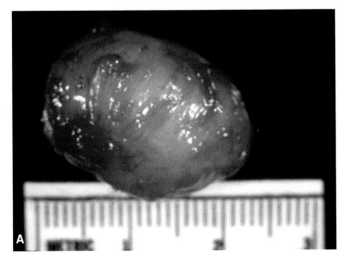
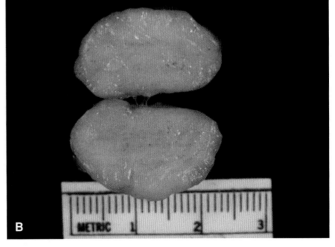

FIGURE 141.4 **A:** Sample picture of 2.2 cm esophageal leiomyoma. **B:** Transected leiomyoma showing the rubbery inner appearance. (Photos courtesy of Dr. Mark B. Orringer, University of Michigan, Ann Arbor, MI.)

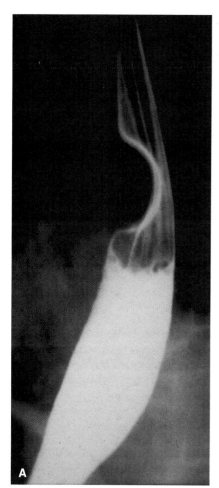

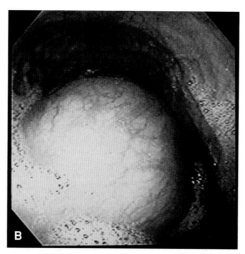

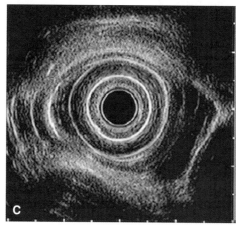

FIGURE 141.5 **A:** Barium esophagram demonstrating smooth-lined filling defect in the midesophagus caused by a leiomyoma. **B:** Typical endoscopic appearance of a midesophageal leiomyoma. **C:** Typical hypoechoic esophageal ultrasound appearance of an esophageal leiomyoma arising in the fourth ultrasound layer (muscularis propria). (Photo courtesy of Dr. David Diehl, Geisinger Medical Center, Danville, PA.)

these tumors are hypocellular with minimal to no atypia, uniform spindle cells arranged in whorls or fascicles, few mitotic figures, and eosinophilic cytoplasm. Leiomyomas must be distinguished from GISTs which are a separate entity of esophageal mesenchymal tumors. Leiomyomas will stain positive for smooth muscle antigen (SMA) and desmin while staining negative for CK117 and CD34. GISTs will uniformly stain positive for CK117 and CD34 while staining negative for SMA and desmin. Histologically, GISTs are very cellular tumors with increased cellular atypia and mitotic figures.[51] Diffuse leiomyomatosis is a rare benign condition of the esophagus that must be differentiated from discrete leiomyoma tumors. The tumors of diffuse leiomyomatosis involve the muscularis propria and muscularis mucosa along the entire length of the esophagus. Leiomyomatosis patients are typically asymptomatic and this condition may be found in conjunction with Alport syndrome.[52]

Clinically, leiomyoma tumors are asymptomatic in 50% of patients with clinical findings such as dysphagia and chest pain being limited to patients with tumors that are greater than 5 cm in size.[4] Other symptoms that have been reported with leiomyomas include epigastric/retrosternal chest pain, heartburn, weight loss, dyspnea, or cough. Other less frequent symptoms include ulceration and hemorrhage which constitute strong reasons for tumor resection.[53]

Diagnostically, leiomyomas are typically found on barium swallow or endoscopy; however, a variety of imaging modalities can help diagnose leiomyomas. Plain chest radiographs have been able to suggest the presence of leiomyomas by demonstrating a smooth, round hyperdense mass in the posterior mediastinum.[3]

CT imaging is typically low yield; however, it may be useful in evaluating for anatomic relationship to nearby structures and for presence of extrinsic compression.[50] Barium esophagrams are typically the first diagnostic test obtained and will demonstrate a smooth, convex filling defect within the esophagus (Fig. 141.5A). These masses tend not to be obstructing and will usually not have proximal esophageal dilation.

Masses discovered on barium swallow should be further evaluated by endoscopy. Endoscopy allows for direct visualization and will demonstrate a bulging mass with an intact overlying mucosa (Fig. 141.5B). Postlethwait et al. described four characteristic endoscopic findings for leiomyomas which include intact overlying mucosa, projection of the tumor into the esophagus at varying degrees, tumor mobility allowing for the overlying mucosa to slide over it, and possible narrowing of the esophageal lumen but no findings of obstruction or stenosis.[54] Blind biopsies of these lesions are not typically recommended as these are typically nondiagnostic since the sample is not usually deep enough to be from the muscularis propria.[55,56] Biopsies also add the additional complication of mucosal adhesions making subsequent enucleation of the tumor more difficult by risking mucosal perforation.[15,49]

Further characterization of esophageal leiomyomas can be made with EUS. EUS allows for the visualization of all the esophageal layers and allows for determination of which exact layer the mass is arising from. EUS also allows for the determination of size, borders and depth, and extent of local invasion. On EUS, leiomyomas arise from the third submucosal layer (Fig. 141.5C). Biopsies with

EUS-FNA should be undertaken if there are features concerning for malignancy such as irregular borders, invasion in adjacent layers, or regional lymphadenopathy.[5] EUS-FNA should, however, be used with caution since it is difficult to obtain enough cellular architecture on biopsy to differentiate between benign leiomyoma and malignant leiomyosarcoma.[15] One case series reported that FNA used in the evaluation of leiomyomas provided no important clinical information.[49] Small and asymptomatic lesions can be followed clinically using EUS surveillance.[15]

ESOPHAGEAL CYSTS

Esophageal cysts are the second most common benign tumor of the esophagus accounting for 20% of lesions. These lesions are not neoplasms and are classified as malformations of the esophagus. They typically occur within an intramural location; however, they can also occur adjacent to the esophagus. Congenital cysts (covered in depth elsewhere) also include bronchogenic, gastric, and inclusion cysts.

The diagnosis of esophageal cysts is typically based on the following criteria: cyst is contained within the esophageal wall, it is covered by two muscle layers, and it contains squamous epithelium or a lining compatible with that found in the embryonic esophagus (i.e., columnar, cuboid, pseudostratified, or ciliated). True esophageal duplications consist of persistent isolated embryonic vacuoles which normally coalesce with others to form the esophageal lumen.[57] Esophageal cysts are usually asymptomatic in adults and are often discovered incidentally on chest radiograph.[4] Those patients who are symptomatic will present most commonly with dysphagia; however, some can present with obstruction, hemorrhage, rupture, or infection.[58] The majority of these cysts arise in the middle or lower third of the esophagus and are typically found on the right side of the distal esophagus.

Acquired esophageal cysts are known as retention cysts and are generally assumed to arise in the lamina propria and exist as a result of chronic inflammation within submucosal glands. These lesions may be single or multiple, and the term *esophagitis cystica* describes the presence of multiple retention cysts. The majority are located within the upper esophagus, and only a minority cause any symptoms.

Diagnostic evaluation of esophageal cysts typically starts with barium esophagram followed by endoscopy, EUS and CT (Fig. 141.6A) or MRI (Fig. 141.6B) imaging. Barium esophagram will demonstrate a smooth surfaced filling defect, similar to that of a leiomyoma. However, this defect is caused secondary to extrinsic compression of the esophagus by the cyst (Fig. 141.6). On CT imaging, a fluid filled structure is typically seen, although the thick mucoid content may be difficult to differentiate from solid leiomyoma or posterior mediastinal lymphadenopathy using routine imaging.

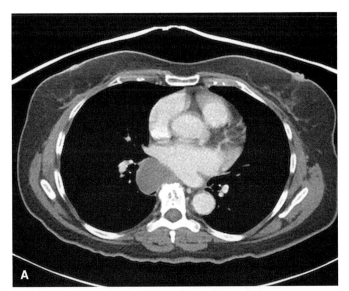

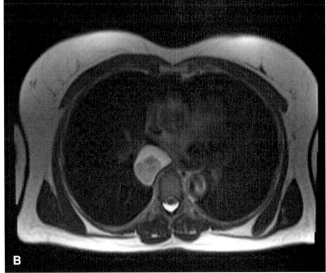

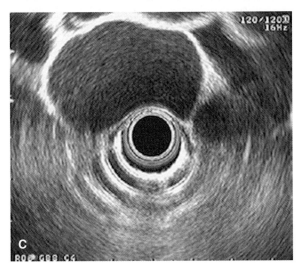

FIGURE 141.6 **A:** Typical appearance of esophageal cyst on CT scan. **B:** Typical appearance of esophageal cyst from the same patient (A) shown on MRI. **C:** Typical anechoic esophageal ultrasound appearance of an esophageal cyst arising from the fifth ultrasound layer (paraesophageal tissue). (Photo courtesy of Dr. David Diehl, Geisinger Medical Center, Danville, PA.)

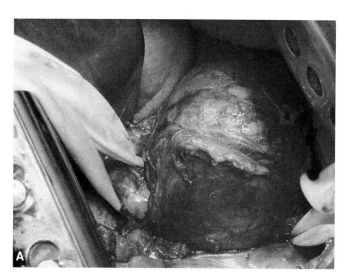
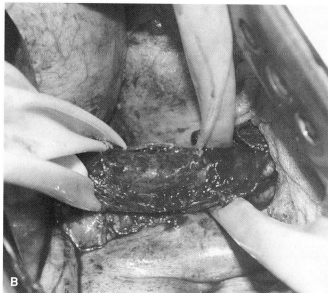

FIGURE 141.7 **A:** Left thoracotomy exposure of large, infected esophageal cyst (patient's head is toward the right of the photo). **B:** Appearance of the esophagus after myotomy and removal of the infected cyst.

Endoscopy will allow for direct visualization of the esophagus and the mucosa which will demonstrate a bulging lesion with normal overlying mucosa. Endoscopic biopsy or cyst aspiration is not recommended! There is a real risk of seeding the cyst with bacteria leading to infection or scar formation that makes subsequent resection more difficult. EUS has developed into a useful adjunct to confirm and characterize these benign lesions. EUS will reveal an anechoic lesion with distinct borders seen between the fourth and fifth ultrasound layers (Fig. 141.6C) corresponding to the muscularis propria and paraesophageal tissue, respectively.[15] Transesophageal cyst drainage has been attempted; however, recurrence is common secondary to the persistence of the epithelial lined cavity.[59] Cyst drainage could result in infection of the cyst and even in mediastinitis. Mediastinitis in these situations can be potentially life-threatening and will require an emergent debridement procedure exposing the patient to potential risk of esophageal perforation, increased morbidity, and possible mortality if not cared for promptly. Esophageal cysts, although benign, are commonly recommended by most authors to be surgically resected. This appeal for resection is based on the claim that most will become symptomatic at some point in adult life, though the quality of evidence for this recommendation is low (Fig. 141.7).

RESECTION OF BENIGN ESOPHAGEAL TUMORS

Open thoracotomy with limited myotomy and simple enucleation is the classic description for the removal of benign esophageal tumors (Figs. 141.7 and 141.8). With the evolution of minimally invasive techniques, this type of surgery is commonly approached with thoracoscopic, robotic, or endoscopic techniques. The key surgical principles include a longitudinal myotomy over the mass, blunt dissection of the tumor away from the mucosa, avoidance of injury to the adjacent mucosa, and closure of the overlying muscular wall.[5] The right or left chest may be entered, based on the location of the lesion. Tumors in the mid to upper esophagus are best approached from the right chest and tumors located closer to the gastroesophageal junction are ideally approached from the left chest. Mobilization and

exposure of an esophageal leiomyoma is shown (Fig. 141.8). Other exposures include transcervical, thoracoabdominal, or transabdominal and are selected based on the tumor location. Most authors agree that closure of the overlying muscular wall should be performed and the muscle may be somewhat redundant secondary to chronic stretch from the tumor. Closure of the wall is also thought to help minimize the occurrence of a future diverticulum. Endoscopy should be performed at the completion of the case to ensure that there is no mucosal injury. A case series from Mutrie et al. reported no perioperative morbidity or mortality over 40 years of experience using the above surgical principles.[49]

Minimally invasive techniques have been widely reported and are now frequently used to resect benign esophageal lesions.[60,61] Minimally invasive techniques include VATS, robotic-assisted thoracoscopic or laparoscopic surgery, and advanced endoscopy. Robotic-assisted resection allows for enhanced magnification, three-dimensional views, and excellent dexterity when compared with VATS.[62] Endoscopic resection of small tumors such as leiomyomas has recently been described using EMR; however, that approach is typically limited to small lesions with pedunculated, intraluminal or polypoid growth patterns. Ethanol injection has been described to facilitate lesion necrosis; however, this strategy has had limited use in the United States.[49,50]

Esophagectomy may be required in up to 10% of leiomyoma patients. Indications for esophagectomy include size of tumor greater than 8 cm, annular morphology, multiple tumors or diffuse esophageal involvement, extensive damage/ulceration to the mucosa, or the presence or high suspicion of malignancy.[2] Mortality from esophagectomy would be expected to be higher than that seen with open enucleation.[5] It is not clear that morbidity or mortality of esophagectomy in this setting would be any different than what is seen for patients with esophageal cancer.

Enucleation of benign esophageal tumors typically results in complete resolution of symptoms. Recurrence of lesions after enucleation is rare and there have been no reported cases of recurrence of leiomyomas after esophageal resection. Postoperative complications include esophageal leak from mucosal injury and GERD in those patients with lesions close to the gastroesophageal junction.

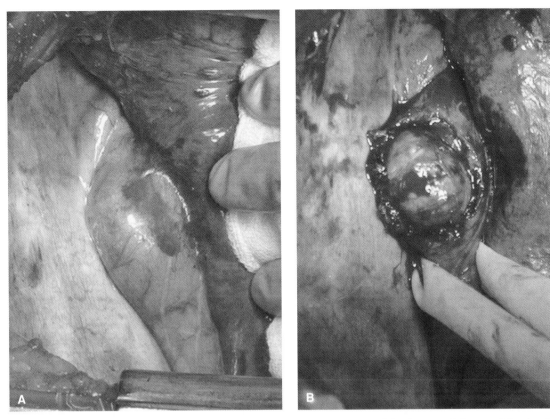

FIGURE 141.8 **A:** Classic right thoracotomy exposure of the midesophagus (patient's head is toward the top of the photo), revealing the typical bulge of an esophageal leiomyoma. **B:** Same patient, but with the tumor now exposed by classic myotomy.

RECOMMENDATIONS

Benign esophageal tumors constitute a small portion of esophageal masses. Benign tumors are often discovered incidentally but can also present with symptoms. Testing includes barium esophagography, endoscopy, EUS, and CT imaging. Symptomatic lesions should be referred for elective enucleation or resection upon diagnosis to prevent future symptoms or complications. Benign, asymptomatic lesions and smaller lesions can be followed by serial EUS or endoscopic examinations. Biopsies of these lesions should be avoided if they do not change management; however, lesions highly suspicious for malignancy should be biopsied. An algorithm on diagnosis and treatment of benign esophageal tumors is presented in Figure 141.9. Resection

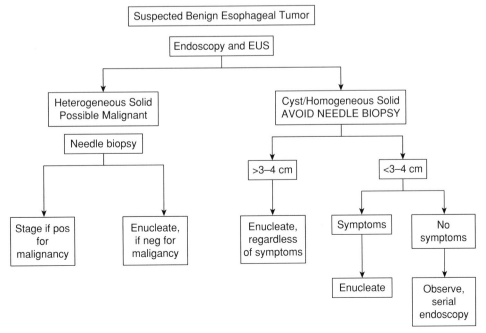

FIGURE 141.9 Suggested management algorithm for benign esophageal tumors.

techniques are dependant on the comfort level of the surgeon and include resection via open thoracotomy, VATS, robotic-assisted, and advanced endoscopic techniques. Adhering to key principles of resection allows for a safe operation with limited morbidity/mortality and provides excellent patient outcomes.

REFERENCES

1. Attah EB, Hajdu SI. Benign and malignant tumors of the esophagus at autopsy. *J Thorac Cardiovasc Surg* 1968;55(3):396–404.
2. Seremetis MG, Lyons WS, deGuzman VC, et al. Leiomyomata of the esophagus. An analysis of 838 cases. *Cancer* 1976;38(5):2166–2177.
3. Watson RR, O'Connor TM, Weisel W. Solid benign tumors of the esophagus. *Ann Thorac Surg* 1967;4(1):80–91.
4. Choong CK, Meyers BF. Benign esophageal tumors: introduction, incidence, classification, and clinical features. *Semin Thorac Cardiovasc Surg* 2003;15(1):3–8.
5. Samphire J, Nafteux P, Luketich J. Minimally invasive techniques for resection of benign esophageal tumors. *Semin Thorac Cardiovasc Surg* 2003;15(1):35–43.
6. Bardini R, Segalin A, Ruol A, et al. Videothoracoscopic enucleation of esophageal leiomyoma. *Ann Thorac Surg* 1992;54(3):576–577.
7. Everitt NJ, Glinatsis M, McMahon MJ. Thoracoscopic enucleation of leiomyoma of the oesophagus. *Br J Surg* 1992;79(7):643.
8. Kinney T, Waxman I. Treatment of benign esophageal tumors by endoscopic techniques. *Semin Thorac Cardiovasc Surg* 2003;15(1):27–34.
9. Patterson EJ. Benign neoplasms of the esophagus: report of a case of myxofibroma. *Ann Otol Rhinol Laryngol* 1932;41:942–950.
10. Moersch JH, Harrington SW. Benign tumor of the esophagus. *Ann Otol Rhinol Laryngol* 1944;53:800–817.
11. Plachta A. Benign tumors of the esophagus. Review of literature and report of 99 cases. *Am J Gastroenterol* 1962;38:639–652.
12. Levine MS, Buck JL, Pantongrag-Brown L, et al. Fibrovascular polyps of the esophagus: clinical, radiographic, and pathologic findings in 16 patients. *Am J Roentgenol* 1996;166(4):781–787.
13. Levine MS. Benign tumors of the esophagus: radiologic evaluation. *Semin Thorac Cardiovasc Surg* 2003;15(1):9–19.
14. Lennon AM, Penman ID. Endoscopic ultrasound in cancer staging. *Br Med Bull* 2007;84:81–98.
15. Rice TW. Benign esophageal tumors: esophagoscopy and endoscopic esophageal ultrasound. *Semin Thorac Cardiovasc Surg* 2003;15(1):20–26.
16. Lack EE, Worsham GF, Callihan MD, et al. Granular cell tumor: a clinicopathologic study of 110 patients. *J Surg Oncol* 1980;13(4):301–316.
17. McSwain GR, Colpitts R, Kreutner A, et al. Granular cell myoblastoma. *Surg Gynecol Obstet* 1980;150(5):703–710.
18. Johnston J, Helwig EB. Granular cell tumors of the gastrointestinal tract and perianal region: a study of 74 cases. *Dig Dis Sci* 1981;26(9):807–816.
19. Coutinho DS, Soga J, Yoshikawa T, et al. Granular cell tumors of the esophagus: a report of two cases and review of the literature. *Am J Gastroenterol* 1985;80(10):758–762.
20. De Rezende L, Lucendo AJ, Alvarez-Arguelles H. Granular cell tumors of the esophagus: report of five cases and review of diagnostic and therapeutic techniques. *Dis Esophagus* 2007;20(5):436–443.
21. Pitichote H, Ferguson MK. Minimally invasive treatment of benign esophageal tumors. *Surgical Management of Benign Esophageal Disorders.* Springer; 2014:181–199.
22. Allen MS, Jr., Talbot WH. Sudden death due to regurgitation of a pedunculated esophageal lipoma. *J Thorac Cardiovasc Surg* 1967;54(5):756–758.
23. Cochet B, Hohl P, Sans M, et al. Asphyxia caused by laryngeal impaction of an esophageal polyp. *Arch Otolaryngol* 1980;106(3):176–178.
24. Solerio D, Gasparri G, Ruffini E, et al. Giant fibrovascular polyp of the esophagus. *Dis Esophagus* 2005;18(6):410–412.
25. Weitzner S, Hentel W. Squamous papilloma of esophagus. Case report and review of the literature. *Am J Gastroenterol* 1968;50(5):391–396.
26. Mosca S, Manes G, Monaco R, et al. Squamous papilloma of the esophagus: long-term follow up. *J Gastroenterol Hepatol* 2001;16(8):857–861.
27. Politoske EJ. Squamous papilloma of the esophagus associated with the human papillomavirus. *Gastroenterology* 1992;102(2):668–673.
28. Poljak M, Orlowska J, Cerar A. Human papillomavirus infection in esophageal squamous cell papillomas: a study of 29 lesions. *Anticancer Res* 1995;15(3):965–969.
29. Winkler B, Capo V, Reumann W, et al. Human papillomavirus infection of the esophagus. A clinicopathologic study with demonstration of papillomavirus antigen by the immunoperoxidase technique. *Cancer* 1985;55(1):149–155.
30. Sandvik AK, Aase S, Kveberg KH, et al. Papillomatosis of the esophagus. *J Clin Gastroenterol* 1996;22(1):35–37.
31. Van Cutsem E, Geboes K, Vantrappen G. Malignant degeneration of esophageal squamous papilloma associated with the human papillomavirus. *Gastroenterology* 1992;103(3):1119–1120.
32. Mayo CW, Pagtalunan RJ, Brown DJ. Lipoma of the alimentary tract. *Surgery* 1963;53:598–603.
33. Wang CY, Hsu HS, Wu YC, et al. Intramural lipoma of the esophagus. *J Chin Med Assoc* 2005;68(5):240–243.
34. Hurwitz MM, Redleaf PD, Williams HJ, et al. Lipomas of the gastrointestinal tract. An analysis of seventy-two tumors. *Am J Roentgenol Radium Ther Nucl Med* 1967;99(1):84–89.
35. Cheriyan D, Guy C, Burbridge R. Giant esophageal lipoma: endoscopic resection. *Gastrointest Endosc* 2015;82(4):742.
36. Araki K, Ohno S, Egashira A, et al. Esophageal hemangioma: a case report and review of the literature. *Hepatogastroenterology* 1999;46(30):3148–3154.
37. Yoshikane H, Suzuki T, Yoshioka N, et al. Hemangioma of the esophagus: endosonographic imaging and endoscopic resection. *Endoscopy* 1995;27(3):267–269.
38. Shigemitsu K, Naomoto Y, Yamatsuji T, et al. Esophageal hemangioma successfully treated by fulguration using potassium titanyl phosphate/yttrium aluminum garnet (KTP/YAG) laser: a case report. *Dis Esophagus* 2000;13(2):161–164.
39. Aoki T, Okagawa K, Uemura Y, et al. Successful treatment of an esophageal hemangioma by endoscopic injection sclerotherapy: report of a case. *Surg Today* 1997;27(5):450–452.
40. Ramo OJ, Salo JA, Bardini R, et al. Treatment of a submucosal hemangioma of the esophagus using simultaneous video-assisted thoracoscopy and esophagoscopy: description of a new minimally invasive technique. *Endoscopy* 1997;29(5):S27–S28.
41. Yoon HY, Kim CB, Lee YH, et al. An obstructing large schwannoma in the esophagus. *J Gastrointest Surg* 2008;12(4):761–763.
42. Kobayashi N, Kikuchi S, Shimao H, et al. Benign esophageal schwannoma: report of a case. *Surg Today* 2000;30(6):526–529.
43. Murase K, Hino A, Ozeki Y, et al. Malignant schwannoma of the esophagus with lymph node metastasis: literature review of schwannoma of the esophagus. *J Gastroenterol* 2001;36(11):772–777.
44. Iwata H, Kataoka M, Yamakawa Y, et al. Esophageal schwannoma. *Ann Thorac Surg* 1993;56(2):376–377.
45. Kwon MS, Lee SS, Ahn GH. Schwannomas of the gastrointestinal tract: clinicopathological features of 12 cases including a case of esophageal tumor compared with those of gastrointestinal stromal tumors and leiomyomas of the gastrointestinal tract. *Pathol Res Pract* 2002;198(9):605–613.
46. Nishikawa K, Omura N, Yuda M, et al. Video-assisted thoracoscopic surgery for localized neurofibroma of the esophagus: case report and review of the literature. *Int Surg* 2013;98(4):461–465.
47. Park BJ, Carrasquillo J, Bains MS, et al. Giant benign esophageal schwannoma requiring esophagectomy. *Ann Thorac Surg* 2006;82(1):340–342.
48. Storey CF, Adams WC, Jr. Leiomyoma of the esophagus; a report of four cases and review of the surgical literature. *Am J Surg* 1956;91(1):3–23.
49. Mutrie CJ, Donahue DM, Wain JC, et al. Esophageal leiomyoma: a 40-year experience. *Ann Thorac Surg* 2005;79(4):1122–1125.
50. Lee LS, Singhal S, Brinster CJ, et al. Current management of esophageal leiomyoma. *J Am Coll Surg* 2004;198(1):136–146.
51. Miettinen M, Sarlomo-Rikala M, Sobin LH, et al. Esophageal stromal tumors: a clinicopathologic, immunohistochemical, and molecular genetic study of 17 cases and comparison with esophageal leiomyomas and leiomyosarcomas. *Am J Surg Pathol* 2000;24(2):211–222.
52. Calabrese C, Fabbri A, Fusaroli P, et al. Diffuse esophageal leiomyomatosis: case report and review. *Gastrointest Endosc* 2002;55(4):590–593.
53. Hatch GF, 3rd, Wertheimer-Hatch L, Hatch KF, et al. Tumors of the esophagus. *World J Surg* 2000;24(4):401–411.
54. Postlethwait RW. Benign tumors and cysts of the esophagus. *Surg Clin North Am* 1983;63(4):925–931.
55. Schafer TW, Hollis-Perry KM, Mondragon RM, et al. An observer-blinded, prospective, randomized comparison of forceps for endoscopic esophageal biopsy. *Gastrointest Endosc* 2002;55(2):192–196.
56. Woods KL, Anand BS, Cole RA, et al. Influence of endoscopic biopsy forceps characteristics on tissue specimens: results of a prospective randomized study. *Gastrointest Endosc* 1999;49(2):177–183.
57. Kirwan WO, Walbaum PR, McCormack RJ. Cystic intrathoracic derivatives of the foregut and their complications. *Thorax* 1973;28(4):424–428.
58. Cioffi U, Bonavina L, De Simone M, et al. Presentation and surgical management of bronchogenic and esophageal duplication cysts in adults. *Chest* 1998;113(6):1492–1496.
59. Van Dam J, Rice TW, Sivak MV, Jr. Endoscopic ultrasonography and endoscopically guided needle aspiration for the diagnosis of upper gastrointestinal tract foregut cysts. *Am J Gastroenterol* 1992;87(6):762–765.
60. Demmy TL, Krasna MJ, Detterbeck FC, et al. Multicenter VATS experience with mediastinal tumors. *Ann Thorac Surg* 1998;66(1):187–192.
61. Kent M, d'Amato T, Nordman C, et al. Minimally invasive resection of benign esophageal tumors. *J Thorac Cardiovasc Surg* 2007;134(1):176–181.
62. Bodner JC, Zitt M, Ott H, et al. Robotic-assisted thoracoscopic surgery (RATS) for benign and malignant esophageal tumors. *Ann Thorac Surg* 2005;80(4):1202–1206.

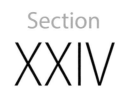

MALIGNANT LESIONS OF THE ESOPHAGUS

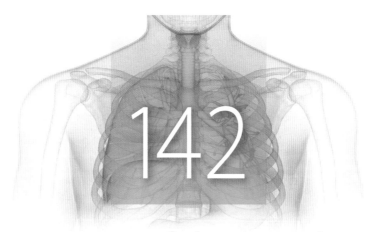

142

Carcinoma of the Esophagus

Biniam Kidane ▪ Mathieu Derouet ▪ Gail E. Darling

Esophageal cancer is the 8th most common cancer worldwide and 18th most common in the United States.[1,2] It is second to pancreatic cancer in case fatality rate. There are two dominant histologies: squamous cell carcinoma and adenocarcinoma. Rare histologies include adenosquamous, small cell cancer, melanoma, lymphoma, malignant granular cell tumor, and leiomyosarcoma. The aim of this chapter is to provide an overview of squamous cell carcinoma and adenocarcinoma. Adenocarcinoma was previously rare but since the 1970s has become the fastest growing solid tumor **and** now is the dominant histology in the Western world, particularly North America and Europe.[3] See Figure 142.1. The rapid growth in the incidence of adenocarcinoma suggests that genetic factors are not the major driver of this change.

The presenting features of esophageal neoplasms have remained constant for decades: dysphagia and weight loss (see Table 142.1). The overwhelming majority of tumors are malignant, and most patients present with locally advanced disease.

EPIDEMIOLOGY

Using data from the WHO International Agency of Research on Cancer's (IARC) GLOBOCAN project, 455,774 new cases of esophageal cancer were estimated to have been diagnosed worldwide in 2012.[2,4] The world age-standardized incidence rate is estimated at 9 males per 100,000 males and 3.1 females per 100,000 females.[2]

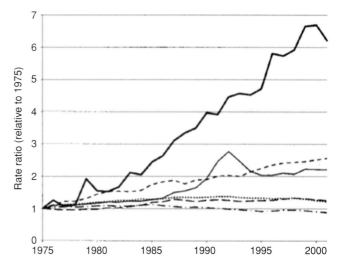

FIGURE 142.1 Relative change in incidence of esophageal adenocarcinoma and other malignancies (1975–2001). Data for the National Cancer Institue's Surveillance Epidemiology and End Results program with age-adjustment between 1973 and 1975. **Solid black line:** esophageal adenocarcinoma; **short dashed line:** melanoma; **line:** prostate cancer; **dashed line:** breast cancer; **dotted line:** lung cancer; **dashes and dotted line:** colorectal cancer. (From Pohl H, Welch HG. The role of overdiagnosis and reclassification in the marked increase of esophageal adenocarcinoma incidence. *J Natl Cancer Inst* 2005;97(2):142–146. Reproduced by permission of Oxford University Press.)

TABLE 142.1 Signs and Symptoms Produced by Advanced Esophageal Carcinoma

Dysphagia
Weight loss
Hoarseness from recurrent laryngeal nerve paralysis
Dyspnea from diaphragm paralysis (phrenic nerve)
Cough (tracheoesophageal fistula)
Superior vena cava syndrome
Palpable supraclavicular lymphadenopathy
Malignant effusion (pleural or peritoneal)

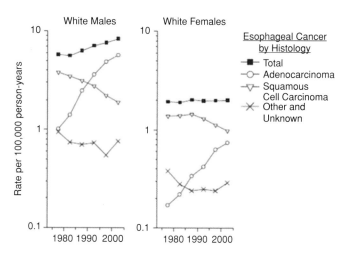

FIGURE 142.2 Incidence of adenocarcinoma of the esophagus among white Americans by sex. (From Brown LM, Devesa SS, Chow WH; Incidence of Adenocarcinoma of the Esophagus Among White Americans by Sex, Stage, and Age. *J Natl Cancer Inst* 2008;100(16):1184–1187. Reproduced by permission of Oxford University Press.)

Among nations with high-quality data capture, there is wide range of age-standardized incidence ranging from 1.6 males and 0.5 females per 100,000 in Cyprus to 10 males and 3.5 females per 100,000 in the United Kingdom. In general, the highest incidence rates globally are found in Brazil, UK, Netherlands, Eastern Sub-Saharan Africa, and particularly in the "esophageal cancer belt" starting from Iran and extending across the central Asian republics to China.[5] The world age-standardized mortality rate is estimated at 7.7 males per 100,000 males and 2.7 females per 100,000 females. Among nations with high-quality mortality data, the age-standardized mortality rate ranges from 1.8 males and 0.3 females per 100,000 in Georgia to 22.7 males and 15.2 females per 100,000 in Turkmenistan.[2]

In the United States, using data from the National Cancer Institute's SEER program (Surveillance, Epidemiology, and End Results), the age-standardized incidence rate is estimated at 7.7 males per 100,000 males and 1.8 females per 100,000 females. Interestingly, when stratified by race, the age-standardized incidence rate appears considerably lower among men with Asian, First Nations, and Hispanic ethnicities. It is estimated that 18,170 new cases of esophageal cancer were diagnosed in 2014, accounting for approximately 1.1% of all new cancers diagnosed. Esophageal cancer was estimated to account for 2.6% of all cancer deaths in 2014, making it the sixth most common cause of cancer death. The median age is 67 at diagnosis and 69 at death, with the highest proportion of people being diagnosed and dying from esophageal cancer in the 65 to 74 age group.[1]

The lower incidence of esophageal cancer in women is thought to be related to other confounding risk factors that are more commonly found in men than women but there is some evidence that estrogen may be protective.[6] The risk of esophageal cancer is significantly higher in postmenopausal women (RR 1.46 95% confidence interval [CI] = 1.07–2.00) and is increased further for women who were younger at menopause.[6] Further, oral contraceptive use (OR = 0.76; 95% CI = 0.57–1.00) and hormone replacement therapy (OR = 0.75; 95% CI = 0.58–0.98) also appear to reduce the risk of adenocarcinoma.[7]

Other potentially protective factors include the use of statins, aspirin, NSAIDs, and increased consumption of fruits and raw vegetables as well as decreased consumption of red meat.[8–10]

In the United States, both the incidence and mortality rates associated with esophageal cancer have been decreasing by approximately 1% per year over the past 10 years.[1] However, the incidence of **adenocarcinoma** has been increasing in developed countries including the United States. In contrast, squamous cell cancer has been decreasing in incidence in developed countries as well as developing nations. Previously rapidly rising, the incidence rates of adenocarcinoma have started to slow in the United States and appeared to have leveled off in the Netherlands and United Kingdom (Fig. 142.2).[11,12]

CLINICAL PRESENTATION

Dysphagia is the most common initial symptom gradually progressing from occasional dysphagia for solid foods to continuous dysphagia for solids, then soft foods and ultimately liquids, over a period of weeks to months. Weight loss is the inevitable result. Untreated patients end up spitting up their own saliva. The symptoms of esophageal cancer are similar regardless of the histology. Odynophagia may occur and may be caused by an ulcerated lesion or invasion of surrounding mediastinal structures. Constant pain in the midback or midchest suggests mediastinal invasion. Regurgitation of food immediately after swallowing may occur as the growing neoplasm narrows the esophageal lumen. Hoarseness may also occur with proximal tumors and indicates involvement of the recurrent laryngeal nerve.

Patients with EAC often have a history of reflux symptoms, although clinical features do not distinguish patients with and without Barrett mucosa, which itself is asymptomatic. Patients in a Barrett's surveillance program may be identified at an early stage when the disease is asymptomatic. The signs and symptoms of advanced esophageal carcinoma are shown in Table 142.1.[12] In a series of 115 patients, van Sandick reported dysphagia, retrosternal/epigastric pain, and hematemesis/melena in approximately 70%, 10%, and 5% of patients, respectively. While 7% of cases were asymptomatic and discovered during surveillance, approximately 50% of patients presented with weight loss of greater than 5%.[13]

Physical examination may reveal entirely normal findings and generally does not aid in the diagnosis. Temporal wasting, weight loss, and dehydration can be seen. It is not clear whether this is simply malnutrition resulting from an obstructed esophageal lumen or whether the tumor is secreting factors that promote cachexia. The ability of patients to gain weight after successful palliation of dysphagia suggests the former. It is important to look for physical findings that may alter the therapeutic approach, including supraclavicular or cervical adenopathy, or an abdominal mass.

Laboratory examinations may reveal anemia from chronic blood loss, hypoproteinemia from malnutrition, and hypercalcemia and abnormal liver function tests from distant metastases. Hypercalcemia is more common than previously appreciated and was seen in about 15% of patients with esophageal squamous cell carcinoma.[14,15]

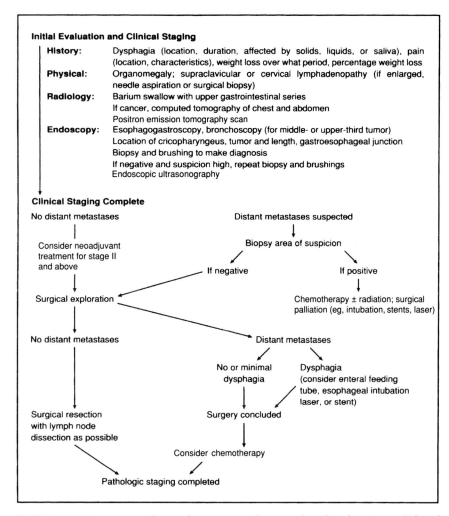

Initial Evaluation and Clinical Staging

History:	Dysphagia (location, duration, affected by solids, liquids, or saliva), pain (location, characteristics), weight loss over what period, percentage weight loss
Physical:	Organomegaly; supraclavicular or cervical lymphadenopathy (if enlarged, needle aspiration or surgical biopsy)
Radiology:	Barium swallow with upper gastrointestinal series
	If cancer, computed tomography of chest and abdomen
	Positron emission tomography scan
Endoscopy:	Esophagogastroscopy, bronchoscopy (for middle- or upper-third tumor)
	Location of cricopharyngeus, tumor and length, gastroesophageal junction
	Biopsy and brushing to make diagnosis
	If negative and suspicion high, repeat biopsy and brushings
	Endoscopic ultrasonography

Clinical Staging Complete

No distant metastases — Consider neoadjuvant treatment for stage II and above — Surgical exploration — No distant metastases — Surgical resection with lymph node dissection as possible — Pathologic staging completed

Distant metastases suspected — Biopsy area of suspicion — If negative / If positive — Chemotherapy ± radiation; surgical palliation (eg, intubation, stents, laser)

Distant metastases — No or minimal dysphagia / Dysphagia (consider enteral feeding tube, esophageal intubation laser, or stent) — Surgery concluded — Consider chemotherapy — Pathologic staging completed

FIGURE 142.3 Diagnostic evaluation for a patient with suspected esophageal carcinoma. (Adapted from Putnam JB Jr, et al. Neoplasms of the esophagus. In: Bell RH Jr, et al., eds. *Digestive Tract Surgery. A Text and Atlas.* Philadelphia, PA: Lippincott-Raven; 1996:50. With permission.)

INVESTIGATIONS

The evaluation of a patient with a suspected esophageal carcinoma is depicted in Figure 142.3 and more in detail elsewhere in this book.[16]

ENDOSCOPY

Esophagoscopy

Endoscopic evaluation is essential in all patients suspected of having a carcinoma of the esophagus. Endoscopy is usually diagnostic and therefore the first choice for investigation of dysphagia. Barium swallow is an alternative first test but findings suspicious for cancer require endoscopic confirmation. Barium swallow may offer an advantage as a first test over endoscopy if the etiology of dysphagia is potentially not malignant. The location of the lesion, degree of obstruction, and longitudinal as well as circumferential extent of the lesion should be determined in all patients. The endoscopic features of late carcinoma are generally easily recognized, although the associated stenosis by submucosal infiltration of the tumor can prevent actual identification of the tumor in some cases. Biopsy and cytologic smears should be performed routinely for all visible lesions.

The biopsy specimen should be taken from the edge of the lesion and not from the necrotic center. With multiple biopsy specimens, a positive tissue diagnosis is obtained in 95% of tumors.[17]

In patients with early carcinoma identified by surveillance, the endoscopic changes are subtle and may be difficult to recognize. Changes include mucosal erosion, focal congestion, and roughness of the mucosa. A small nodule, ulcer, or even a small tumor mass may be seen.

Bronchoscopy

Bronchoscopy is important in the evaluation of possible tracheal or bronchial invasion by a carcinoma in the cervical and the upper or middle thirds of the thoracic esophagus. Postlethwait,[18] noted tracheobronchial invasion in 26 of 153 patients with carcinoma of the cervical esophagus, in 82 of 487 patients with carcinoma located in the upper thoracic esophagus, and in 6 of 268 patients with tumor in the distal thoracic esophagus. Of the 114 patients with tracheobronchial invasion, 60 had tracheal involvement and 54 had bronchial invasion. Thirty-seven patients developed a tracheoesophageal or bronchoesophageal fistula. Angorn noted tracheobronchial invasion in 184 of 1,045 patients with carcinoma of the upper thoracic esophagus with a fistula present in 75 patients of which tracheal invasion

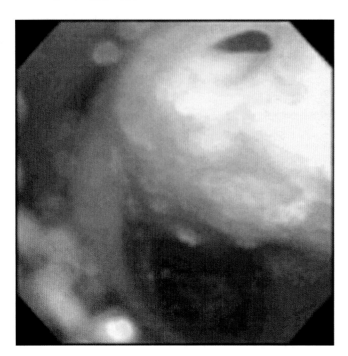

FIGURE 142.4 Bronchoscopy with tracheoesophageal fistula.

was present in 57%, bronchial invasion in 40%, and direct involvement of the lung parenchyma in 3%.[19]

Patients with infracarinal bulky tumors or subcarinal lymphadenopathy on CT should undergo bronchoscopy to evaluate for carinal involvement. Bronchoscopic findings may range from simple bulging, loss of striations, bulging with fixation of the posterior wall of the trachea or the main bronchi (most commonly the left main bronchus), frank tumor invasion, or the presence of a fistula. The carina may also appear widened owing to metastatic disease to the subcarinal nodes. However, bulging does not necessarily indicate invasion. A cytologic or histologic diagnosis obtained by bronchial brushings or biopsies is helpful in confirming invasion (Figs. 142.4 and 142.5).

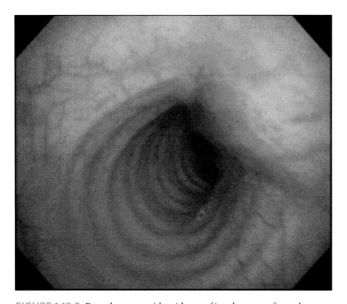

FIGURE 142.5 Bronchoscopy with evidence of involvement of membranous trachea.

RADIOGRAPHIC STUDIES

Investigations are addressed in detail in subsequent chapters. A brief overview follows here.

CHEST RADIOGRAPHS

Standard chest radiographs are generally not helpful but in advanced esophageal cancer 48% of patients will have an abnormal finding albeit subtle and nondiagnostic.[20] These include an abnormal azygoesophageal line, widened mediastinum, posterior tracheal indentation or mass, widened retrotracheal stripe, and compression, displacement, or irregularity of the tracheal air column.

Contrast Studies

The barium swallow has been an important diagnostic study for the evaluation of dysphagia, as it is a low-risk, expedient study of the esophageal mucosa, luminal distensibility, motility, and any anatomic pathology, as shown in Figure 142.6. It has largely been replaced by endoscopy however still has value if when the diagnosis of dysphagia includes nonmalignant etiologies. Double contrast studies provide optimum visualization. The positive predictive value for detection of esophageal cancer is 42%.[21] Benign strictures typically have symmetric areas of narrowing with smooth contours and tapered proximal and distal margins whereas malignant strictures typically have asymmetric narrowing with abrupt, shelf-like margins, and irregular contours with nodular or ulcerated mucosal surfaces. Barium is also a safe contrast agent to use when a tracheoesophageal fistula is suspected. See Figures 142.6 and 142.7.

Computed Tomography

Computed tomography (CT) scans of the chest and abdomen are important studies in the initial evaluation of esophageal carcinoma to determine the local extent of the tumor, the relationship to adjacent structures, and distant metastases, as shown in Figure 142.8. CT is generally not useful for determining T status, although preservation of fat planes suggests that the tumor is limited to the esophagus without invasion of adjacent structures. Compression of the trachea or of a mainstem bronchus raises suspicion of airway involvement, as shown in Figure 142.8D. Compression or thickening of the wall of the tracheobronchial tree abutting the tumor or loss of fat planes in that region mandates bronchoscopic evaluation. Involvement of the aorta is uncommon and in an autopsy study was present in only 2% of 2,440 patients.[22] Aortic invasion is suggested by >90 degrees of contact but this is not definitive. Invasion of the pericardium is difficult to detect although obliteration of the intervening fat planes is suggestive. The accuracy of CT in diagnosing mediastinal invasion has been reported in the range of 59% to 82%.[23]

Sensitivity for detecting abnormal lymph nodes (>1 cm) is 34% to 61% in the mediastinum and 50% to 76% in the abdomen, although false-positive rate may be as high as 25%.[24] CT may not be as sensitive for detecting disease in the celiac region.[25] For metastatic disease, CT has a sensitivity of 70% to 80% for identifying metastases >2 cm.[26]

Magnetic Resonance Imaging

Magnetic resonance imaging (MRI) is useful in evaluation of airway, pericardial, or aortic invasion particularly in coronal or sagittal views.

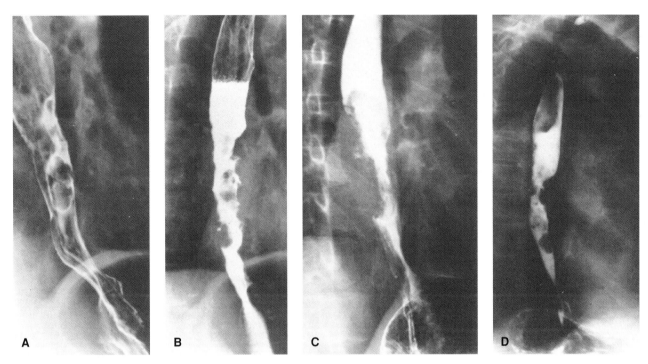

FIGURE 142.6 Barium esophagogram demonstrating late esophageal squamous cell carcinoma. **A:** Polypoid lesion. **B:** Multiple polypoid tumors. **C:** Long ulcerative tumor. **D:** Stenotic, infiltrative tumor.

Positron Emission Tomography

^{18}F-FDG positron emission tomography (PET) is very sensitive for identification of primary esophageal cancer in 97% of cases compared to 81% with CT.[27,28] Current guidelines recommend PET for

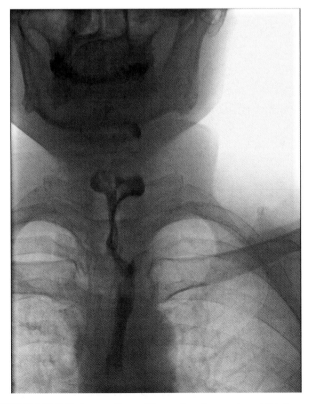

FIGURE 142.7 Barium swallow evidence of tracheoesophageal fistula.

staging of esophageal cancer, however, early-stage tumors may not be identified on PET.[29] Although current guidelines recommend PET for locally advanced esophageal cancer, PET is optional in early-stage esophageal cancer.[30] PET cannot distinguish the layers of the esophageal wall so cannot be used to determine T stage but PET-CT is useful for detection of nodal metastases, particularly nodes distant from the primary tumor. Meta-analysis report that PET-CT demonstrates sensitivities and specificities ranging from 55% to 62% and 76% to 96%, respectively in the detection of nodal disease (Fig. 142.9).[27] More importantly, PET-CT is able to identify nodal disease that is missed by CT alone. Meta-analysis has shown that the pooled sensitivity and specificity for nodal disease of PET-CT is 0.57 and 0.85 compared to 0.50 and 0.83 for CT alone.[28]

PET-CT is even more useful in identifying occult metastatic disease not identified by CT alone; the pooled sensitivity and specificity of PET-CT is 0.71 and 0.93 compared to 0.52 and 0.91 for CT alone.[28] PET-CT can detect 15% to 20% additional metastases compared with CT scan.[28,31–33] The diagnostic accuracy of CT in determining resectability was 65%, compared with 92% for PET-CT.[34] PET also has the advantage of assessing the whole body as compared with conventional imaging allowing for identification of distant metastatic disease at initial evaluation. In addition, PET may have a role in selecting therapy. Responses to induction chemotherapy on PET scans were predictive of a complete surgical resection and longer survival but unfortunately not accurate enough to allow patients to avoid surgery.[35,36] Some literature suggests that PET-CT may serve as a clinical predictor of pathologic response to neoadjuvant therapy. These studies suggest a diagnostic accuracy ranging from 68% to 86% of predicting pathologic response.[37–40] Moreover, PET-CT response to treatment has been shown to predict longer-term outcomes such as overall survival.[38–42] In the largest report of patients assessed with PET-CT postneoadjuvant chemoradiation therapy, Kukar et al. found that 29% of patients had complete pathologic

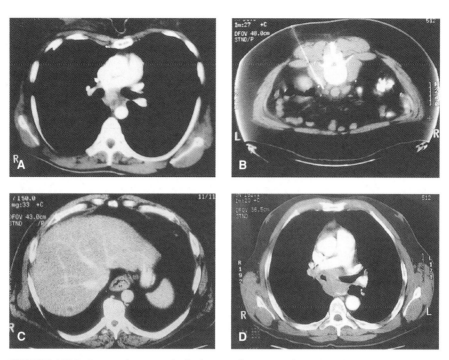

FIRGURE 142.8 Computed tomography (CT) scans of patients with esophageal carcinoma. **A:** Tumor in contact with the thoracic aorta. **B:** CT- guided biopsy of nodal disease. **C:** Metastatic hepatic nodules. **D:** Local invasion of the right mainstem bronchus.

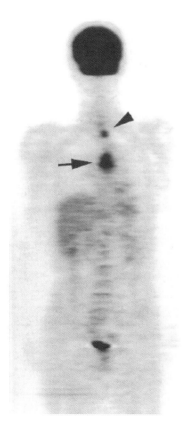

FIGURE 142.9 Positron emission tomography (PET) scan reveals a middle esophageal primary tumor (*arrow*) and a positive upper mediastinal lymph node (*arrowhead*). (From Kato H, Kuwano H, Nakajima M, et al. Comparison between positron emission tomography and computed tomography in the use of the assessment of esophageal carcinoma. *Cancer* 2002;94:921.)

response and that a decrease in SUV of greater than 45% was significantly predictive of complete pathologic response.[43] However, the negative predictive value of PET-CT following chemoradiation is not sufficiently high to recommend it for routine clinical use in avoiding surgery.[30,43]

Endoscopic Ultrasound

Endoscopic ultrasound (EUS) is the modality of choice for T staging; EUS can assess the depth of penetration of the primary tumor and is able to detect local, perigastric, and celiac lymph nodes.[44] EUS can identify five distinct layers in the esophageal wall, permitting assessment of the depth of tumor invasion, as depicted in Figure 142.10. The significance of determining the depth of invasion relates to the likelihood of lymph node metastases with deeper invasion. T1a lesions are confined to the mucosa and rarely spread to lymph nodes, while T1b lesions involve the submucosa and may have lymph node metastases in 15% to 30% of cases.[44] In resected patients, 5% of T1a tumors were found to have lymph node metastases but this increased to 16.6% for T1b lesions. Nodal metastases were associated with tumor size greater than 2 cm and intermediate/high-grade lesions.[45] Although the overall accuracy of T staging is reported to range from 72% to 84%, it is not reliable enough to distinguish T1a from T1b tumors and thus identify tumors that can be safely resected endoscopically.[28,46] However, a recent meta-analysis has reported pooled sensitivity and specificity of 0.86 and 0.86 for distinguishing T1 tumors from higher T stages.[47] With respect to nodal staging, another meta-analysis has shown that EUS has the highest sensitivity with pooled sensitivity of 80% as compared to 57% and 50% for PET-CT and CT, respectively.[28] Accuracy was most notable in the staging of early carcinoma and in evaluating the extent of periesophageal invasion.

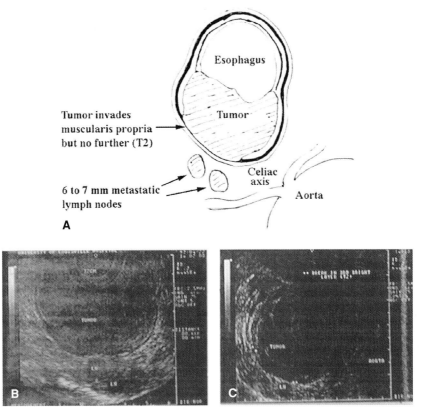

FIGURE 142.10 **A:** Illustration of the endoscopy sonographic (EUS) views shown in **B** and **C**, of a T2 esophageal adenocarcinoma with metastatic celiac nodes.

In up to one-third of patients, the 13-mm endoscope cannot be passed because of esophageal stenosis, although a narrow-caliber EUS can be used.[48] This has been noted to be one of the limitations of EUS. If the probe cannot be passed beyond the stenosis or tumor, the tumor may be understaged. However, this finding in itself is consistent with T2 or T3 tumors and thus the EUS in this circumstance likely adds very little to clinical decision making.[49] Miniprobes that can be passed in nearly all patients are now available in 12-, 15-, and 20-MHz frequencies. Unlike dedicated EUS, a probe can be passed through the biopsy channel, and endoscopic evaluation can be performed while the tumor is being visualized, thus obviating the need to exchange instruments. Higher-frequency probes can provide greater detail of a superficial lesion, but deeper structures such as regional lymph nodes may not be visualized.[50,51]

Endoscopic Mucosal Resection

Endoscopic mucosal resection (EMR) or endoscopic submucosal dissection (ESD) can be considered as an adjunct to diagnosis/staging if EUS suggests a potential for T1a disease and endoscopic, organ-sparing resection is being considered. EMR allows for pathologic assessment of depth of invasion.[30,52] Precise protocols for en-bloc endoscopic dissection and preparation of the specimen should be followed; these have been outlined in the Guidelines for Diagnosis and Treatment of Carcinoma of the Esophagus published by the Japan Esophageal Society.[52] In circumstances wherein EMR confirms true pT1a disease on pathologic examination, it may also serve as definitive therapy.[52]

THORACOSCOPY AND LAPAROSCOPY

Thoracoscopy and laparoscopy have been used as staging tools in esophageal cancer and are potentially more accurate in determining nodal status than noninvasive techniques as well as in evaluating the extent of local invasion but have not been widely adopted. Krasna reported a 93% and 94% accuracy in detecting metastatic disease for thoracoscopy and laparoscopy, respectively.[53] Six cases of unsuspected celiac nodal disease were identified in 19 patients despite preoperative CT and EUS. A prospective multi-institutional study of 107 patients found that CT, EUS, and MRI failed to detect positive nodal disease identified in 25% of patients using thoracoscopy and laparoscopy.[54] Minimally invasive techniques changed the staging in 32% of patients.[55] However, these studies were all completed prior to the routine use of PET-CT.

Laparoscopy is useful for identifying peritoneal metastases with 96% sensitivity and is recommended for gastric and gastroesophageal junction cancers and is more useful in patients with adenocarcinoma than with squamous cell carcinoma of the esophagus. Stein found a 22% incidence of previously unidentified hepatic metastases and a 25% incidence of positive fluid cytology in patients with EAC, whereas laparoscopy provided minimal additional information in the evaluation of patients with ESCC.[56] Thoracoscopy through the right hemithorax, particularly in combination with laparoscopy, is of value in patients with both types of carcinoma.

Laparoscopic Ultrasound

Laparoscopic ultrasound (LUS) is also being investigated as a staging modality and may provide improved accuracy in T and N staging however, has not been widely adopted. In one study, LUS improved staging accuracy of celiac nodal disease to 92%, compared with final pathology in 44 patients.[57] There was a significant difference in disease-free survival between node-positive and node-negative patients identified by LUS.

With increased cost and invasiveness, the role of these techniques will require further assessment. In a comparison of health care costs, CT scan, followed by EUS-FNA when necessary, was the most inexpensive evaluation and provided the most quality-adjusted years of life except for PET with EUS-FNA, which was slightly more effective but more expensive.[58] At present, EUS and CT should be the initial staging examination, followed by PET-CT.[30]

MOLECULAR MARKERS

The identification of molecular markers may offer earlier diagnosis than currently available through radiology or pathology and may provide prognostic information on tumors that are more advanced and likely to metastasize. Molecular markers could also be useful in identifying micrometastases. To date there are no molecular markers that have proven to be robust enough for clinical practice.

A number of potential markers have been identified in the literature. In Barrett esophagus, assessment of sucrase–isomaltase might improve the ability to detect Barrett metaplasia and dysplasia.[59] Several studies have found associations between aneuploid or increased tetraploid fractions and metastases, advanced disease, and poor survival, with reports that 70% of patients with such findings develop high-grade dysplasia or adenocarcinoma.[60,61] Although p53 mutations have been reported by Altorki and colleagues[62] in more than 50% of esophageal adenocarcinomas (EACs) while Casson and colleagues[63] reported decreased patient survival, a p53 mutation is not sufficient by itself to predict progression to adenocarcinoma.

Of the molecular markers studied a number have been found to be possible predictive or prognostic markers (e.g., growth factor receptors, angiogenesis factors, tumor suppressor genes, apoptotic factors, matrix metalloproteinases, and cell cycle regulators) for esophageal cancer.[64,65] Low intratumoral expression levels of HER2/neu were associated with better histopathologic response to neoadjuvant therapy as compared to higher levels.[66] Angiogenetic factors have also been found to play a role in predicting response to neoadjuvant therapy. Kulke and colleagues determined that in patients with SCC, low Cox-2 expression correlated with pathologic response.[67]

Several groups have been focusing on micro-RNA (miRNA) as potential new biomarkers. These 21 nucleotide RNAs have the ability to regulate gene expression and have been shown to play an important role in carcinogenesis, angiogenesis, and metastasis.[68,69] miRNA profiling has been used to identify the Healthy-BE-EAC sequence[70] and predicts the response to neoadjuvant therapy.[71]

Currently, a reliable biomarker is not available, and the prevalence of most markers is low. Because of the diverse genetic changes seen in EAC, a panel of biomarkers may be most useful.

PROGNOSIS

Esophageal cancer is one of the poorest prognosis cancers. Despite being the 18th most common cause of cancer in the United States, it is the 6th most common cause of cancer death. The estimated 5-year relative survival of people with esophageal cancer in the United States is 17.5% but has been increasing from 4% for those diagnosed in 1975 to 20% for those diagnosed in 2006.[1] Although part of this improvement in relative survival may be due to improvements in therapy and changing trends over the decades in histology and risk factors, much of it is due to earlier diagnosis and thus earlier treatment.[72,73] SEER data from 2004 to 2010 showed that 21% of people with esophageal cancer were diagnosed with localized disease compared to 37% with metastatic disease. The 5-year survival for those with localized disease was 39.5% compared to 3.8% in those with metastatic disease.[1] Positive nodal disease is an important prognostic factor. As can be seen in Figure 142.11, there are significant drop-offs in survival in those with 1 to 5 and greater than 5 positive lymph nodes.[74] This has also been replicated in more recent series using 0, 1–2, 3–6, and ≥7 lymph nodes as cut-offs.[75] In addition to the prognostic impact of having positive nodal disease, having a higher ratio of positive to harvested lymph nodes has been reported to predict poorer prognosis (Fig. 142.12).[76–80]

In the last 5 years, the staging system was revised based on data derived from the Worldwide Esophageal Cancer Collaboration. Data on 4,627 patients from 13 countries in 3 different continents were used to define new stage groupings and associated survival curves. Staging and prognosis were different for adenocarcinoma and squamous cell cancer.[81] See Figure 142.13.

SQUAMOUS CELL CARCINOMA OF THE ESOPHAGUS

RISK FACTORS

Demographic and Geographic Factors

Regardless of ethnicity and country, men are affected by ESCC three to four times as often as women.[2,82,83] This conserved epidemiologic finding is likely related to other confounding risk factors that are more commonly found in men compared to women rather than a unique genetic risk related to male sex although as noted above estrogen may be protective. There is geographic variation in the incidence of ESCC, suggesting that environmental exposure and socioeconomic factors are causally important.[84] Regions with a high incidence are generally located in poorer parts of the world, often associated with nutritional deficiencies. In China, where the majority of the world's cases occur annually, the incidence is clustered into sharply demarcated geographic areas. Areas located in the southern parts of the Taihang Mountains on the borders of Henan, Shansi, and Hopei provinces in China have some of the highest incidence and mortality rates of ESCC in the world.[2,85] In Central Asia, an esophageal cancer belt extending from northern Sinkiang through the former Soviet central Asian republics of Kazakhstan, Uzbekistan, and Turkmenistan and including northern Afghanistan and northeastern Iran has been described.[5]

High rates have also been noted in the Indian subcontinent, and intermediate to high rates exist in the Caribbean and portions of Latin America.[86] In the United States, where ESCC is less common, urban African-American men seem particularly affected, especially in Washington, DC, and coastal South Carolina.[87] Low income and education have also been shown to be associated with increased ESCC, although it is unclear whether these risk factors operate independently of factors such as alcohol and tobacco consumption and nutritional deficiencies.[88]

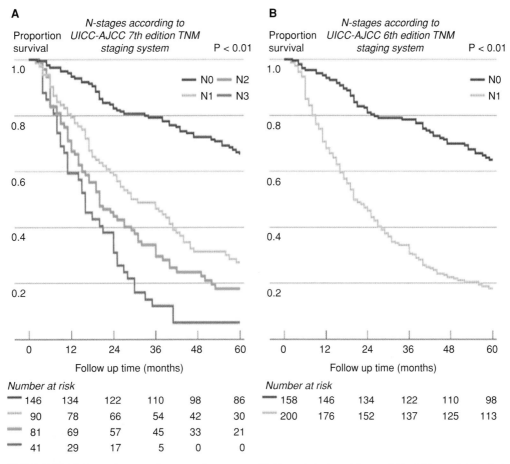

FIGURE 142.11 Survival curves of patients subgroups stratified by pathologic nodal status (N0 = 0, N1 = 1–2, N2 = 3–6, N3 ≥7 lymph nodes). (Talsma K, van Hagen P, Grotenhuis BA, et al. Comparison of the 6th and 7th editions of UICC-AJCC TNM classification for esophageal cancer. *Ann Surg Oncol* 2012;19:2142–2148.)

NUTRITION AND FOOD PRACTICES

High consumption of foods containing N-nitrosamines, have been associated with increasing risk of ESCC.[89,90] For example, pickled vegetables contain high levels of N-nitrosamines and high consump-

tion of these has been associated with increased risk of ESCC.[91] Nitrates and nitrites can be converted within the body to carcinogenic N-nitrosamines and are suspected etiologic factors in the development of ESCC. The mechanism of increased carcinogenesis is thought to be via alkylation of DNA by N-nitrosamines.[89,90] Diets low in fruits, particularly citrus, and low vitamin C intake have been

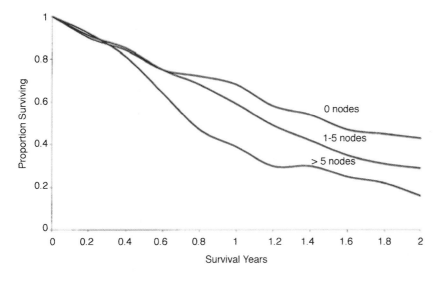

FIGURE 142.12 Kaplan–Meier survival plots for 1,340 patients stratified by the number of positive lymph nodes. (From Eloubedi MA, Desmond R, Arguedas MR, et al. Prognostic factors for the survival of patients with esophageal carcinoma in the U.S.: the important of tumour length and lymph node status. *Cancer* 2002;95:1437–1440. Copyright © 2002 by John Wiley Sons, Inc. Reprinted by permission of John Wiley & Sons, Inc.)

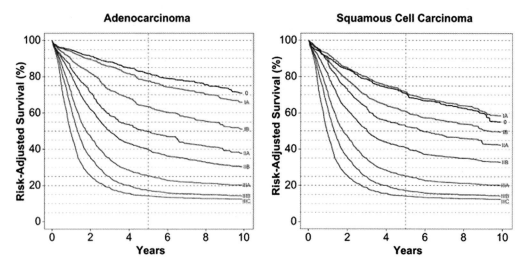

FIGURE 142.13 WECC figures. Risk-adjusted survival curves for adenocarcinoma and squamous cell carcinoma. (From Rice TW, Rusch VW, Ishwaran H, et al.; Worldwide Esophageal Cancer Collaboration. Cancer of the esophagus and esophagogastric junction: data-driven staging for the seventh edition of the American Joint Committee on Cancer/International Union Against Cancer Cancer Staging Manuals. *Cancer* 2010;116(16):3763–3773. Copyright © 2010 by John Wiley Sons, Inc. Reprinted by permission of John Wiley & Sons, Inc.)

associated with an increased risk for ESCC.[92] Citrus fruits and vitamin C may inhibit endogenous nitrosation and reduce the risk for ESCC.[93]

Nutritional deficiencies have been implicated in the pathogenesis of ESCC, along with a number of other etiologic factors listed in Table 142.2. Low levels of retinol, riboflavin, vitamin C, folate, vitamin D, beta-carotene, and alpha-tocopherol are prevalent among the people in high-incidence regions of China.[94]

TABLE 142.2 Etiologic Factors in Squamous Cell Carcinoma of the Esophagus

Carcinogens
  Tobacco
    Smoking cigarettes, cigars, and pipes
    Chewing tobacco alone or with quid or betel nut
  Alcohol
    Locally brewed
    Apple brandy
    Maize beer
  Nitrosamines
  Furacin c
  Opiates; combustible residue
  Fungal toxins
  Spices
Nutritional deficiencies
  Vitamins A, C, riboflavin
  Trace elements: molybdenum, zinc
Physical factors
  Thermal trauma
  Hot food or drinks
  Abrasive material (soil) and food
  Lye
Predisposing factors
  Tylosis
  Plummer–Vinson syndrome
  Achalasia
  Celiac sprue
Human papilloma virus

Deficiencies in various mineral elements, such as selenium, zinc, and molybdenum, have also been associated with increased risk of ESCC.[36,95–99] These deficiencies are believed to make one more susceptible to the carcinogenic effects of exogenous factors such as carcinogenic N-nitrosamines.

In addition to geographic variations in diet and nutrition, geographic variation in food practices also appears to increase risk of ESCC. Certain regions and cultures (e.g., northern Iran) engage in consumption of very hot foods and beverages (e.g., tea) and this has been associated with an increased risk of ESCC. In addition to hot beverages, consuming very hot foods such as boiled, roasted, or fried meat also appears associated with ESCC. A recent meta-analysis suggests that high red meat consumption and low poultry consumption are associated with higher risk for ESCC whereas high consumption of any kind of processed meats was associated with higher risk of EAC. It is hypothesized that hot food or drinks may cause the development of cancer through repeated thermal injury and the consequent inflammatory process. Daily consumption of roasted meats also is associated with increased risk of ESCC likely through the methylation of the p16 promoter. Salted meat also increases the risk of ESCC and appears to also have a synergistic effect with alcohol and smoking, such that ESCC risk increases with a combination of high-salted meat diet and smoking or alcohol history.[95,100–103]

Environmental Carcinogens

Low molybdenum levels in the soil may cause higher nitrate and nitrite levels in plants and thus increase N-nitrosamine levels when consumed. Molybdenum functions as a cofactor for the plant enzyme nitrate reductase and thus would be expected to reduce the nitrate and nitrite levels in plants.[95] Contamination of water by impurities such as petroleum has been associated with a higher prevalence of ESCC in the Gassim region of Saudi Arabia.[104]

Alcohol and Smoking

Alcohol and tobacco are the primary etiologic factors for ESCC.[105–107] Ethanol is associated with nearly 80% of the neoplasms among esophageal cancer patients, and the relative risk increases with the amount of alcohol consumed with a 20% to 30% increased risk overall.[107] There is also an association between increasing alcohol consumption and poor nutrition. The risks associated with tobacco use appear to increase with the number of cigarettes smoked per day, duration of smoking, and tar content with an overall increased risk of 20% to 30%. Ex-smokers have a reduced risk, and after 10 years, their risk returns to baseline. A synergistic effect of alcohol consumption and tobacco use has been reported with a threefold increased risk and an adjusted odds ratio of 3.28 (95% CI = 2.11–508).[105,108]

In addition to consumption, genetic variations in alcohol metabolism have recently been shown to be risk factors for ESCC.[109] Alcohol dehydrogenase, an important enzyme in alcohol metabolism, has been shown to have genetic variants which increase the risk for ESCC, predominantly in Asian populations.[109–111] Moreover, some studies have shown evidence of complex gene–environment interactions; for example, risk of ESCC was shown to be higher in Asian men with specific aldehyde dehydrogenase gene variants who drank heavily than those heavy drinkers without those gene variants.[110,111]

Achalasia

Achalasia is recognized as a risk factor for the development of ESCC with an estimated 16- to 30-fold greater likelihood of developing ESCC compared to the normal population.[112–114] The average duration between symptoms and detection of esophageal carcinoma is 11 to 17 years, with cancer developing at an earlier age in patients with achalasia.[113–115] In patients treated with dilation or esophagomyotomy, esophageal cancer developed at a rate only slightly higher than that for the general population.[116] Thus, the increased risk of ESCC may be related to the stasis of food and saliva in the esophagus and the consequent inflammatory microenvironment.[117] Current clinical guidelines of the American Society for Gastrointestinal Endoscopy (ASGE) do not recommend for or against endoscopic surveillance; however, in those considering surveillance, the ASGE recommends starting 15 years after the onset of achalasia symptoms.[118]

Caustic Injury

The incidence of esophageal cancer among patients with a history of caustic ingestion has been estimated to be 1,000-fold greater than that of the general population.[119] ESCC is the most common subtype and typically occurs in the middle third of the esophagus at the level of the tracheal bifurcation. Most cases present four to five decades after the initial injury and 10 to 20 years earlier than in the general population.[120] Carcinoma should be suspected with any change in the ability to dilate a chronic stricture or in the presence of increasing dysphagia.

Scarring of the esophagus may actually alter the natural history of the esophageal cancer. Because the lumen is less distensible, dysphagia is more likely to present earlier in the course of the disease. In addition, damage to submucosal lymphatics and the presence of dense scar tissue within the esophageal wall may limit lymphatic spread.[121] Current ASGE guidelines suggest endoscopic surveillance patients starting 15 to 20 years after caustic ingestion, with a frequency of every 1 to 3 years.[118]

Tylosis, an autosomal dominant disorder characterized by hyperkeratosis of the palms and soles, is the only well-documented genetic disorder associated with esophageal cancer.[121] Patients with tylosis (also known as nonepidermolytic palmoplantar keratoderma) have up to 95% chance of developing ESCC during

their lifetimes.[122] The culprit TEC (tylosis with esophageal cancer) gene has been mapped to chromosome 17q25.[123] There is some evidence supporting gene–environment interactions; in smokers, gene polymorphisms of the CYP2A6 gene have been noted play a role in the formation of carcinogenic nitrosamines.[124] Those with known family history of tylosis are recommended to begin upper gastrointestinal endoscopic surveillance after age 20.[125] Other hereditary syndromes associated with an increased risk of ESCC are Fanconi Anemia and Bloom syndrome. These are both autosomal recessive syndromes in which screening with upper gastrointestinal endoscopy may be considered although there are no guidelines to support this approach.[126,127]

Other Risk Factors

Esophageal cancer has also been associated with several other risk factors. Patients with a history of exposure to ionizing radiation, head and neck cancer, Plummer–Vinson syndrome, celiac disease, and thyroid disease have been reported to be at increased risk for developing ESCC.[128–131] Women who receive radiation for breast cancer were found to have an increased risk for esophageal cancer.[132] Human papilloma virus (HPV) infection has been shown to be significantly associated with increased risk of ESCC; however, there is wide heterogeneity in the evidence with data both supporting and refuting HPV as a risk factor for ESCC.[99] Close contact with ruminants may also increase the risk of ESCC but it is unknown whether this is an independent risk factor.[133] Poor oral hygiene has been shown to be associated with increased risk of ESCC, even when controlling for the effect of tobacco-use.[134–136]

Genetic Factors

Much research has centered around p53, a tumor suppressor gene important in cell cycle control, DNA repair and synthesis, genomic stability, and apoptosis. p53 mutations and allelic losses are common abnormalities in many human neoplasms. Mutations in p53 as independent somatic mutations in different regions of the esophagus have been postulated to be key molecular events in multifocal esophageal carcinogenesis.[137] Elevated levels of p53 mutations have been described in both esophageal cancer patients as well as patients with dysplasia.[138,139] Mutant p53 protein expression was also increased in the nonmalignant mucosa of patients after gastrectomy (68%) and in patients with advanced achalasia (44%), two conditions considered to be risk factors for ESCC. Mutant p53 overexpression has been shown to correlated with poorer patient survival.[140] Mutations of the TP53 gene appear to link chronic inflammation with cancer; mutations such as G:C and A:T transitions at CpG dinucleotides were highly prevalent in SCC in high-risk parts of Asia.[141] These particular codon regions appear to code for moieties responsible for interacting with benzopyrene metabolites as are found in tobacco.[142,143] Thus, mutation of p53 at these loci may be induced by repeated exposure to environmental factors such as benzopyrene in tobacco.[142,143] Other mutated genes identified in ESCC include PIK3CA, NOTCH1, FAT1, FAT2, ZNF750, and KMT2D.[144]

Potential Biomarkers

Periostin protein expression is reported to be an independent prognostic factor in ESCC. Overexpression is prevalent in ESCC and is significantly associated with lymphatic metastasis ($p = 0.008$), tumor differentiation ($p = 0.04$), venous invasion ($p = 0.014$), and TNM stage ($p = 0.001$).[145] Osteopontin may also be a useful biomarker as it is expressed in 30 of 63 cancer lesions (48%) and significantly associated with pathologic T stage ($p = 0.038$) and overall stage

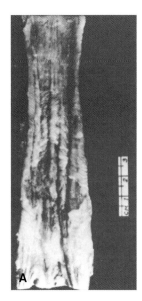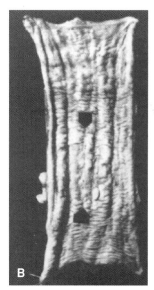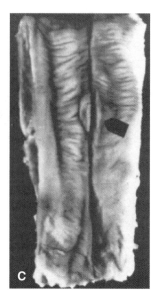

FIGURE 142.14 Early esophageal carcinoma. **A:** Erosive type. **B:** Plaquelike type. **C:** Papillary type. (From Liu FS, Zhou CN. Pathology of carcinoma of the esophagus. In Huang GJ, Wu YK, eds. *Carcinoma of the Esophagus and Gastric Cardia*. Berlin: Springer; 1984:80, 82. Copyright © 1984 Springer-Verlag Berlin Heidelberg. With permission of Springer.)

(p = 0.023).[146] MicroRNAs may also be useful as biomarkers. For example, mir-25 and mir-100 can predict poor survival in ESCC.[147]

PATHOLOGY

MACROSCOPIC FEATURES

ESCC is most commonly located in the middle third of the thoracic esophagus; with approximately 50% ESCC found there.[22] This region of the esophagus extends from the level of the carina to the inferior

pulmonary veins. Thirty to 40% of lesions arise in the lower third of the esophagus whereas only 10% to 20% of squamous cell carcinomas occur in the upper esophagus.

Early-stage ESCC is infrequently encountered in North America and Europe but are seen more commonly in China and other endemic areas where routine screening is practiced. Early lesions are generally small or even occult but may involve the entire circumference of the mucosa and appear as plaque-like, erosive, or papillary lesions (Fig. 142.14). More advanced lesions have been described as fungating, ulcerative, or infiltrative tumors (Fig. 142.15). Ulcerated lesions have regular or irregular everted edges with a deep base and

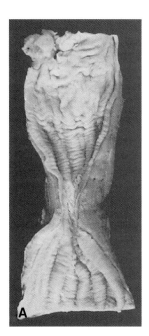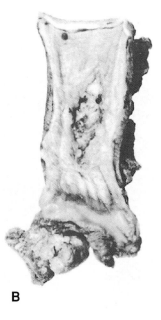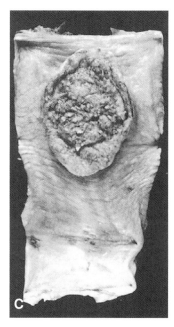

FIGURE 142.15 Late esophageal carcinoma. **A:** Scirrhous type. **B:** Medullary type. **C:** Fungating type. (From Liu FS, Zhou CN. Pathology of carcinoma of the esophagus. In Huang GJ, Wu YK, eds. *Carcinoma of the Esophagus and Gastric Cardia*. Berlin: Springer; 1984:83–85. With permission.)

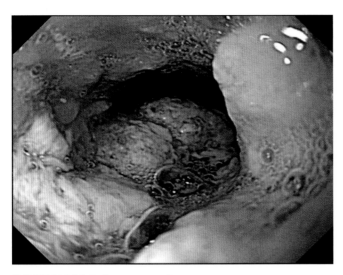

FIGURE 142.16 Endoscopic view of verrucous carcinoma.

associated infiltration of the esophageal wall. Infiltrative tumors are characterized by extensive intramural spread and desmoplastic response producing a tight esophageal stricture without obvious tumor. A variant of ESCC is verrucous carcinoma which appears as an exophytic mass, biopsies of which often show squamous hyperplasia, atypical or dysplasia but not invasive carcinoma (Fig. 142.16).

There exist a variety of gross classification schemes. Descriptions of the different types overlap, but the extent of invasion and the presence of nodal metastases are the critical features that determine patient prognosis.

Microscopic Features

Early squamous cell carcinomas can be divided into intraepithelial, intramucosal, and submucosal tumors. Intraepithelial lesions are carcinoma in situ with an intact basement membrane (Fig. 142.17). This intraepithelial neoplasia has been graded according to the degree of epithelial involvement into low-grade (superficial third of the epithelium), moderate-grade (middle third of the epithelium), and high-grade (deep third of the epithelium) intraepithelial

neoplasia.[148–150] The risk of progression to ESCC has been estimated at 24%, 50%, and 75% at 14 years from diagnosis for low-, moderate-, and high-grade intraepithelial neoplasia, respectively.[148,149] In intramucosal carcinomas, the tumor cells penetrate the basement membrane and infiltrate the lamina propria or part of the muscularis mucosa. Once the cells have penetrated the muscularis mucosa, the lesions are classified as submucosal carcinomas, as depicted in Figure 142.18. In the more advanced stages of squamous cell carcinoma, there is invasion into or through the muscular layers of the esophagus and into the adventitia. The degree of tumor differentiation varies from well to poorly differentiated, with 60% of tumors being moderately differentiated.

Recently, there has been more interest in the extent of mucosal and submucosal infiltration of tumor in both ESCC and EAC. The mucosal and submucosal layers have each been divided into thirds (m1, m2, m3 and sm1, sm2, sm3) and studies have reported differences in oncologic outcomes according to tumor invasion of these layers.[151,152] Tumors in the m1 and m2 layers are reported to have 0% to 3.3% risk of nodal disease whereas tumors in the m3 and sm1 layers have risks of nodal disease ranging from 12% to 27%. Tumors in the sm2 and sm3 layers have been reported to carry risks of 36% to 46% of harboring nodal disease. In addition to having implications on prognosis, these studies suggest that selection of patients for endoscopic, organ-sparing treatment should not only be limited to T1a disease but also perhaps to those without m3 infiltration.[151,152]

Metastases

In the advanced pathologic stages of the disease, direct extension through the wall of the esophagus is common, as are lymphatic metastases. Lymphatic metastases were found in about 60% of patients undergoing esophagectomy.[153] In an autopsy series, lymphatic metastasis were seen in 75%.[154] Hematogenous spread was also common in autopsy specimens, with an incidence ranging from 50% to 63%.[128,154]

Intraesophageal Spread

Microscopically, most tumors have spread more extensively than their gross appearance would indicate. Wong[155] noted the correlation between the proximal resection margin and the incidence of

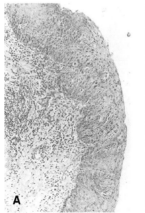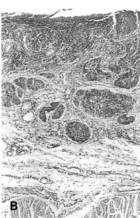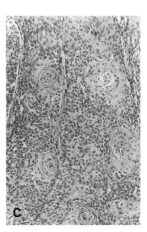

FIGURE 142.17 Esophageal squamous carcinoma. **A:** In situ with an intact basement membrane. **B:** Submucosal carcinoma. **C:** Well-differentiated carcinoma with pearl formations. (From Liu FS, Zhou CN. Pathology of carcinoma of the esophagus. In Huang GJ, Wu YK, eds. *Carcinoma of the Esophagus and Gastric Cardia.* Berlin: Springer; 1984:88, 90, 91. Copyright © 1984 Springer-Verlag Berlin Heidelberg. With permission of Springer.)

Tumor extent and lymph node metastatic rate of Clinical Stage I esophageal cancer

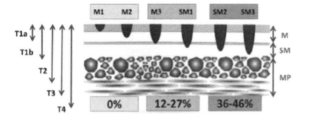

FIGURE 142.18 Tumor infiltration and lymph node metastases of T1 cancer. Early cancers are in situ lesion (Tis) or T1 tumors. T1 tumors are split into T1a and T1b subcategories depending of the depth of invasion. T1a (m1 or SSM, intraepithelial cancer; m2 or LPM, cancer with invasion into the lamina propria mucosae; m3 or DMM, cancer reaching to the muscularis mucosae), T1b (m1, cancer with invasion into **one-third** of the submucosa; sm2, cancer with invasion into the middle third of the submucosa; sm3, cancer with invasion into the lower third of submucosa). The incidence of lymph nodes metastasis in M1, M2, and M3 was 0%, 3.3%, and 12.2%, respectively. In submucosal cancer, nodal metastasis was found in 26.5% of SM1, 35.8% of SM2, and 45.9% of SM3. (From Tangoku A, Yamamoto Y, Furukita Y, Goto M, Morimoto M. The New Era of Staging as a Key for an Appropriate Treatment for Esophageal Cancer. *Ann Thorac Cardiovasc Surg* 2012;18(3):190–199. Copyright © The Editorial Committee of Annals of Thoracic and Cardiovascular Surgery (ATCS). All Rights Reserved.)

anastomotic recurrence as shown in Table 142.3. Microscopic spread distal to the gross tumor, for reasons that are unclear, extends for a shorter distance of approximately 4 cm from the tumor.[156] Submucosal lymphatic spread occurs often and may result in tumor emboli producing satellite nodules with significant adverse prognostic implications.

Direct Extension

After penetration of the adventitial layers covering the esophagus, the tumor may invade adjacent structures, including the pleura, trachea, left mainstem bronchus, pericardium, great vessels, thoracic duct, and the anterior ligaments of the vertebral column. In the upper esophagus, the recurrent laryngeal nerves may also be involved, whereas in the lower esophagus, tumors may invade the diaphragm, stomach, and liver. However, it has been noted at postmortem examination that the extent of invasion in one-third of the tumors was restricted to the periesophageal tissues.[157]

TABLE 142.3 Proximal Resection Margin and Anastomotic Recurrence

Length of Margin (cm)	Number of Patients	Percentage of Patients
0–2	1/4	25
2–4	2/11	18
4–6	2/13	15
6–8	2/26	8
8–10	1/15	7
10	0/26	0

Reprinted from Wong J. Esophageal resection for cancer: the rationale of current practice. *Am J Surg* 1987;153:8.

TABLE 142.4 Degree of Invasion and Lymph Node Status of 504 Resected Specimens of Esophageal Cancer

Degree of Invasion	Number of Specimens	Resected Lymph Node Metastasis	Percentage of Invasion Specimens
Submucosa	1	0	0
Muscularis	175	52	29.7[a]
Full thickness	273	118	42.2[a]
Adjacent tissue	55	38	69.1[a]
Totals	**504**	**208**	**41.3**

[a]Proportion is significantly different at $p < 0.05$.
From Lu YK, Li YM, Gu YZ. Cancer of esophagus and esophagogastric junction: analysis of results of 1,025 resections after 5 to 20 years. *Ann Thorac Surg* 1987;43:176. Copyright © 1987 Elsevier. With permission.

Lymphatic Spread

The direction of flow in the extensive lymphatic network of the esophagus is primarily longitudinal. Using lymphoscintigraphy, Tanabe[158] demonstrated that lymph from the upper third of the esophagus drains primarily to the upper mediastinum and neck, whereas lymph from the lower esophagus flows to the abdomen. However, despite this predominantly unidirectional flow, cervical, supraclavicular, and abdominal lymphadenopathy are seen in both upper and lower esophageal cancers.

As shown in Table 142.4, the incidence of lymphatic metastases in surgical specimens ranges from 30% to 70% and is related to the depth of invasion of the primary tumor.[159] Even in early esophageal cancer, ESCC is more likely to result in lymphatic spread with mucosal and submucosal tumors than EAC.[160] Stein et al. showed that ESCC and EAC limited to the mucosa had 7.7% and 0% rate of positive nodal disease, respectively. In the same study, they also reported that ESCC and EAC limited to the submucosa had 36.4% and 20.7% rate of positive nodal disease, respectively.[160] Postlethwait found supraclavicular nodal involvement in 6.9% based on a series of autopsy studies.[22] In two smaller surgical series, supraclavicular and cervical nodal involvement were seen in about 19% to 26%.[161–163] In contrast, spread below the diaphragm is more common. Akiyama et al.[153] reported nodal metastases in the superior epigastrium in 31.8% of patients with tumors located in the cervical esophagus, 32.8% with tumors in the middle third, and 61.5% with tumors in the lower third of the esophagus (Fig. 142.19).

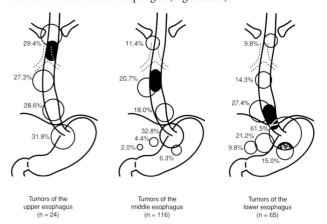

FIGURE 142.19 Sites of lymph node metastases from esophageal squamous carcinoma. (From Akiyama H, Tsurumaru M, Kawamura T, et al. Principles of surgical treatment for carcinoma of the esophagus: analysis of lymph node involvement. *Ann Surg* 1981;194:438. With permission.)

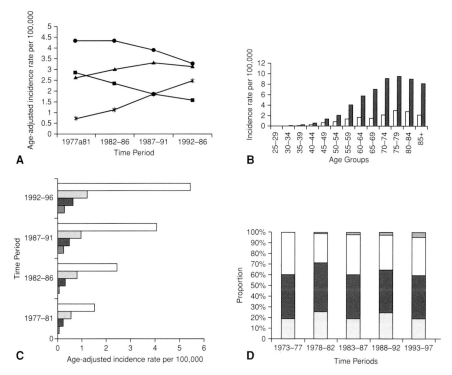

FIGURE 142.20 **A:** Age-adjusted incidence rates per 100,000 population in the United States from the Surveillance, Epidemiology, and End Results Program of the National Cancer Institute between 1977 and 1996 for esophageal squamous cell carcinoma (*circles*), carcinoma of the gastric cardia (*triangles*), gastric cancer (*squares*), and esophageal adenocarcinoma (*stars*). **B:** Age distribution of patients diagnosed with esophageal adenocarcinoma between 1977 and 1981 (*white bars*) and 1992 and 1996 (*black bars*) in the United States. **C:** Age-adjusted incidence of esophageal adenocarcinoma by gender and ethnicity for Caucasian men (*white bars*) and women (*black bars*) and African-American men (*light gray bars*) and women (*dark gray bars*). **D:** Trends in the stage of esophageal adenocarcinoma. (Light gray, unstaged; black, distant; white, regional; dark gray, in situ). (Reprinted from El-Serag HB. The epidemic of esophageal adenocarcinoma. *Gastroenterol Clin North Am* 2002;31:422. Copyright © 2002 Elsevier. With permission.)

Distant Metastatic Disease

Visceral metastases may be present in up to 30% of patients at the time of diagnosis and are manifestations of advanced disease. In an autopsy series, 40% of patients with well-differentiated ESCC had visceral metastases while 87% of those with undifferentiated ESCC had widespread disease. Metastases were found in the lungs, liver, pleura, bone, kidneys, and adrenal glands, in order of decreasing frequency.[154] The nervous system was involved in 2.7% of specimens, with 1% incidence of metastases to the brain.[164]

ESOPHAGEAL ADENOCARCINOMA

EAC is the most rapidly increasing solid malignancy in the United States. It is estimated 15,690 deaths from esophageal carcinoma will occur in 2017. In the mid-1990s, adenocarcinoma overtook squamous cell carcinoma as the most common cancer of the esophagus in America.[165] Surgical resection remains the only chance for cure, and approximately 90% of those diagnosed ultimately die of their disease. Although there have been significant improvements in surgical technique and perioperative care, the prognosis remains poor, with an overall 5-year survival rate of only approximately 19%. However, with improvements in staging, detection and multimodality treat-

ments, estimated 5-year survival for those with localized disease is over 40%.[166]

The incidence of EAC has increased progressively since the 1970s. SEER data indicate that the incidence has increased from 0.7 per 100,000 in 1974 to 1976 to 2.58 per 100,000 in 2009 (see Fig. 142.20).[167] More recent SEER data have estimated that incidence has increased dramatically between 1975 and 1997 with an annual percentage change of 8.4 per 100,000 but the rate of increase subsequently decreased with an annual percentage change of 1.6 per 100,000 between 1997 and 2009 (Fig. 142.21).[167,168] The reason for the increase in incidence of EAC is unclear. Although the use of diagnostic techniques such as endoscopy has increased, it is believed that there has been a true increase in incidence. Recently, a modeling study utilizing 16 cancer registries from 8 countries presented compelling data that suggests that the global EAC epidemic appears to have started due to some as-yet-undetermined exposure introduced within a short time period between 1950s and 1970s.[3] The complex and rigorous statistical modeling suggests that this exposure likely originated in the United Kingdom in the 1950s and over a 30-year time period spread to North America, Australia, and Western Europe. This exposure, which might be discrete or multi-factorial, is not explained solely by gastroesophageal reflux disease (GERD) or obesity as the epidemiologic trends of these risk factors over those periods do not fit the trends observed for the EAC epidemic.[3]

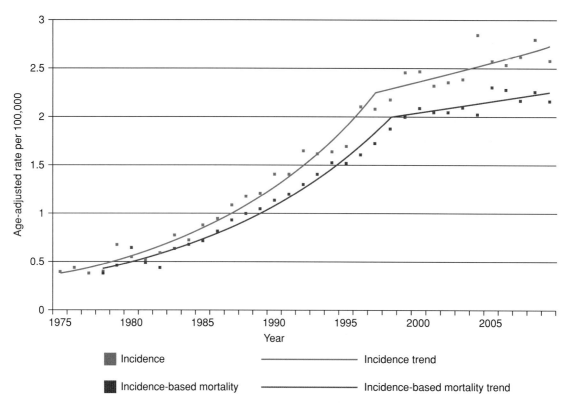

FIGURE 142.21 Graph shows SEER 9 esophageal adenocarcinoma incidence and incidence-based mortality, 1975 to 2009. From 1975 to 1997, EAC incidence increased at an annual percentage change (APC) of 8.4 (95% confidence interval [CI] = 7.7–9.1), whereas the APC was 1.6 (95% CI = 0.0–3.3) from 1997 to 2009. For incidence-based mortality, the APC was 8.0 from 1978 to 1998 (95% CI = 7.2–8.8) and 1.1 from 1998 to 2009 (95% CI = –0.7 to 2.9). All rates were age adjusted to the 2000 Standard population using 19 age groups. (From Hur C, Miller M, Kong CY, et al. Trends in esophageal adenocarcinoma incidence and mortality. *Cancer* 2013;119(6):1149–1158.)

Between 1994 and 2008, in Australia and the United States the *rate* of increase in incidence of adenocarcinoma has decreased, although the incidence is still increasing by 2.2% for men in Australia and 1.5% in the United States. The prevalence of gastroesophageal reflux symptoms appears to have plateaued in the 1990s in the United States and this may be a factor in the slower rate of increase in incidence of adenocarcinoma.[169] In Sweden, EAC incidence among men is stabilizing.[170] Elsewhere in Europe, the incidence of adenocarcinoma appears to have stabilized in the United Kingdom and the Netherlands since 2003.[171]

RISK FACTORS

Studies focusing on population attributable risk for EAC have shown that GERD, obesity, smoking, and a low-fruit/vegetable diet accounted for nearly 80% of EACs in the United States.[172] Alcohol use, in contrast to ESCC is not a risk factor for EAC or for Barrett esophagus.[173] Moreover, interactions between these risk factors and genetic polymorphisms may further drive risk.[174] Furthermore, genetic mutations appear to occur early in the evolution of EAC.[175]

DEMOGRAPHIC AND GEOGRAPHIC FACTORS

As for most cancers, increasing age is risk factor for EAC. Although the median age at diagnosis was 68 years among patients entered into the SEER database after 1988, there has been a considerable increase

in the proportion of patients diagnosed between the ages of 45 and 65.[176] As with ESCC, sex is a significant and important risk factor with men affected six to eight times more often than women. Race is also a risk factor with Caucasians being affected five times as often as African Americans.[176] Incidence rates are higher in developed countries, and there are geographic variations including within nations themselves; for example, SEER data from 1973 to 1998 show that the incidence in Seattle was twice as high as in Utah.[3,177]

Reflux Disease and Barrett Esophagus

Nearly all EAC arises from areas of Barrett metaplasia, which itself is an acquired condition resulting from chronic inflammation due to gastroesophageal reflux.

Barrett mucosa is the precursor lesion to EAC (Fig. 142.22) and the risk is increased 30 to 125 times the risk of the age-matched population with an incidence of 1 to 2 cancers per 100 patient-years.[178,179] It is more common in males, with a 2:1 ratio and a mean age of diagnosis of 62 years in males and 67 years in females. EAC develops in about 7% to 20% of patients with Barrett metaplasia.[1] Although Barrett epithelium is seen in 24% to 64% of surgical specimens, its absence in the remaining specimens may be due to overgrowth of the Barrett mucosa by tumor or sampling errors.[180,181] In an autopsy study in 1990, Barrett metaplasia was found in 0.4% or 376 per 100,000 Caucasians, which is significantly higher than the clinically diagnosed prevalence of only 80 per 100,000.[182] This suggests that most cases of Barrett esophagus have not been diagnosed. Simulation studies using SEER data estimate

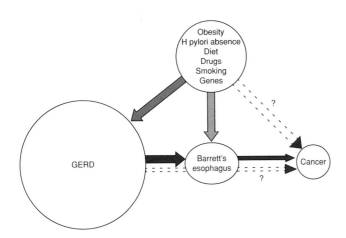

that the incidence of Barrett esophagus is approximately 5.6% of the US population.[183]

On endoscopy, these lesions appear as red, velvety areas. In the past, Barrett mucosa has been described as columnar epithelium extending >3 cm above the gastroesophageal junction and was originally believed to be congenital. However, short-segment Barrett's <3 cm above the gastroesophageal junction has been increasingly recognized as a risk factor for EAC, and 35% of such tumors arise in short-segment Barrett's.[184] Although there are three types of columnar epithelium—including the gastric fundic, gastric junctional, and intestinal type—only the intestinal type is associated with an increased risk of EAC. See Figure 142.23. Indeed, only columnar epithelium with goblet cells shares genetic mutations found in adenocarcinoma.[185,186]

It has been reported that 18% of the US population experiences heartburn once per week and that 7% have daily symptoms.[187,188] At endoscopy for reflux, Barrett mucosa was found in 12% to 18% of patients.[189,190] Nevertheless, studies have also shown an increased risk of EAC with reflux without necessarily pointing to Barrett's as the mediating factor. A large population study in Sweden revealed that the odds of developing EAC are 7.7 times if one has recurrent reflux and 44 times higher if one has long-standing reflux.[191] Further studies replicated the finding of increased risk of EAC with reflux disease; however, current evidence suggests that antireflux surgery does not reduce the risk of EAC associated with reflux disease.[192]

Obesity

Associations have also been found between obesity and EAC. EAC was 7.6 times more common in the heaviest quartile of the population in a Swedish study.[193] A recent meta-analysis of 22 studies demonstrated an increased risk of EAC with overweight and obese status.[194] This study also demonstrated a dose-dependent effect with incremental higher odds of developing EAC with incremental increases of BMI of 5 kg/m². [194] Although the question whether obesity increases the risk of EAC by increasing the risk of GERD remains unanswered, recent work using genome-wide association studies have shown that obesity is associated with increased risk of EAC even when one controls for GERD. Using a genetic risk score, derived from 29 genetic variants shown to be associated with BMI with a higher score indicating a propensity to obesity, EAC risk increased by 16% (OR = 1.16, 95% CI = 1.01–1.33) and BE risk increased by 12% (OR = 1.12, 95% CI = 1.00 to 1.25) per kg/m² increase in BMI. The genetic risk score was not associated with poten-

tial confounders, including gastroesophageal reflux symptoms and smoking.[195] Further, it appears that visceral obesity is more important than subcutaneous fat or BMI overall. While body mass index was similar in EAC patients (26.1 kg/m²) and controls (26.2 kg/m²), visceral adipose tissue was significantly higher in EAC patients in controls (276 vs. 231 cm²; $p = 0.015$) but there was no difference in subcutaneous adipose tissue.[196] Thus, this suggests that even though GERD may mediate some of the EAC risk, it is not the sole mediator explaining the increased risk of EAC seen with obesity.

Physical activity may reduce the risk of EAC (RR = 0.79; 95% CI = 0.66–0.94); however, it is unclear how much of this risk reduction is mediated by weight loss itself.[197,198]

H. pylori Infection Eradication

Evidence exists suggesting that eradication of *Helicobacter pylori* is associated with increased EAC.[199–202] Erosive esophagitis has been found in 26% of patients who were cleared of *H. pylori* compared with 13% of those with persistent infections.[201] Furthermore, a population-based case-control study in Australia reported a decreased risk of EAC and Barrett esophagus with *H. pylori* infection.[201] This risk was independent of the severity of GERD.[201] Although this might lead some to hypothesize that *H. pylori* infection somehow be protective against EAC, it may also reflect some degree of detection bias. It may be that the apparent protective effect relates to reduced stomach acid associated with *H. pylori* infection or that improved sanitation and affluence are associated with reduced *H. pylori* but more GERD and obesity.

Smoking

A few studies have reported approximately twofold higher risk for EAC among smokers.[203,204] There is a dose–response relationship with higher tobacco use being associated with higher risk of EAC.[203] Although the risk of EAC was reduced with smoking cessation, it was not fully nullified and persisted for up to 30 years after quitting.[88,204]

Other Risk Factors

Low-level evidence suggests that use of medications that decrease LES tone (and thus promote reflux) is associated with higher risk of EAC.[191,205] These medications include nitroglycerin, anticholinergics, beta-adrenergic agonists, aminophyllines, and benzodiazepines.[205] Bisphosphonates have also been investigated but results are conflicting.[206–208]

Swedish population-based study showed that having a cholecystectomy was associated with a higher risk of EAC.[209] They hypothesized that this might be due to increased bile acid reflux after cholecystectomy. Reflux of both acid and bile has a major role in the development of Barrett esophagus. Although esophageal mucosa appears to be relatively resistant to acid, mixed reflux with bile acids, pepsin, trypsin, gastric acid, and lysolecithin appears to be more harmful and has been implicated in mucosal injury, as depicted in Figure 142.23.[210] Although primary bile acids are not carcinogenic, it has been noted that secondary bile acids are potential carcinogens, depending on the pH and conjugation status.[210] One study showed that 67% of patients with Barrett metaplasia have duodenogastric reflux.[202]

There is a question whether a history of tracheoesophageal fistula or esophageal atresia as a child is a risk factor for developing esophageal cancer as an adult. Some limited data suggest that patients may be at increased risk of both ESCC and EAC.[210–212] Patients with a history of tracheoesophageal fistula or esophageal atresia have been

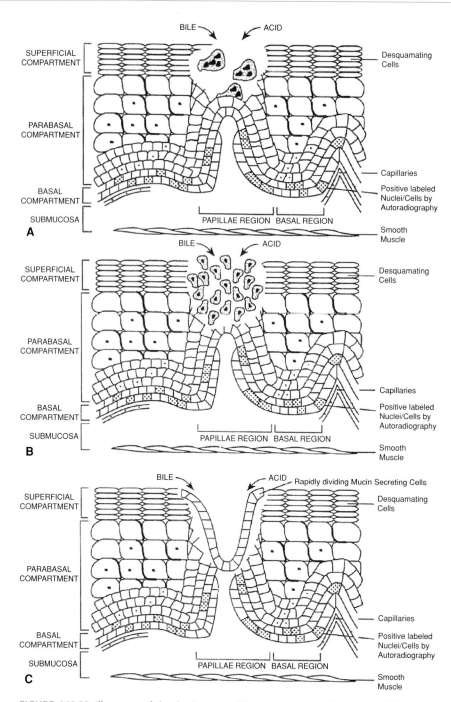

FIGURE 142.23 Illustration of the development of Barrett mucosa. **A:** Damage to differentiated esophageal cells in the superficial and parabasal compartments. **B:** Damage in the basal compartment involving the epithelial stem cells (speckled nuclei). **C:** Generation of mucin-secreting acid-bile-resistant clones. (Reprinted from Jankowski JA, Wright NA, Meltzer SJ, et al. Molecular evolution of the metaplasia-dysplasia-adenocarcinoma sequence in the esophagus. *Am J Pathol* 1999;154:968. Copyright © 1999 American Society for Investigative Pathology. With permission.)

reported to have increased rates of GERD and esophagitis and this may be the mechanism through which an increased risk of EAC may exist.[212,213]

Nutrition

A Swedish population-based study demonstrated that increased cereal fiber intake was associated with decreased risk of EAC.[214] The inference drawn from this observation was that the wheat fibers may be acting to neutralize the mutagenic properties of nitrosamines. However, the same study did not show a concomitant decrease in ESCC (in which nitrosamines are a well-described risk factor) and thus this calls into question that hypothesized mechanism of action. There is, nevertheless, some evidence suggesting that nitrosamines may increase the risk of EAC.[215]

In addition to high-fiber diets, diets with increased intake of fruits, vegetables, folate, beta-carotene, vitamins B6 and C were associated with decreased risk of EAC.[8,216–218]

Protective Effect of NSAIDs and Other Drugs

There is mixed evidence about the potential protective effect of aspirin and NSAIDs. Aspirin and NSAIDs inhibit cyclooxygenase (COX). COX-2 has been found to be upregulated in Barrett metaplasia and continues to increase in the progression to dysplasia and adenocarcinoma.[219] Bile acids may activate COX-2 through the protein kinase C pathway.[220] These changes may result in decreased cell–cell adhesion, increased angiogenesis, or inhibited apoptosis which in turn facilitate multiple features of malignancy. Aspirin and specific COX-2 inhibitors have been shown to suppress growth and induce apoptosis.[221] COX-2–mediated inflammatory changes may be important in facilitating a microenvironment that promotes carcinogenesis.[222] Thus, this mechanistic-level data support a potential protective effect of NSAID-induced COX-2 inhibition for prevention of EAC. Some have postulated that the effect of NSAIDs might also be through COX-independent pathways.[223]

At the epidemiologic level, a large individual-patient meta-analysis of observational studies demonstrated reduced risk of EAC with NSAID usage in both GERD and non-GERD populations.[224] Aspirin alone appears protective (OR 0.67; 95% CI = 0.526–0.856, $p = 0.001$).[225–227] However, a small randomized study failed to show any significant decrease in progression from Barrett esophagus to EAC or changes in biomarkers with use of twice-daily celecoxib (COX-2 inhibitor).[228]

Statin use is associated with reduced risk of development of EAC (odds ratio = 0.58; 95% CI = 0.39–0.87), esophagogastric junctional adenocarcinoma (odds ratio = 0.29; 95% CI = 0.09–0.92) and ESCC (odds ratio = 0.51; 95% CI = 0.27–0.98).[229] However, the number needed to treat to prevent one case of esophageal cancer was more than 1,000.

Although metformin use was hypothesized to potentially modulate the risk of EAC in Barrett esophagus, metformin use was not found to be protective against the development of EAC.[230]

PATHOGENESIS

After the squamous epithelium is injured by reflux, there is an inflammation-stimulated hyperplasia and metaplastic change to a columnar epithelium. One hypothesis is that pluripotent stem cells in the basal layers undergo metaplasia after repeated stimulation from reflux. Other possible origins of columnar cells are the gastric cardia and propagation of columnar cells from the esophageal gland ducts.

Replacement by long-segment Barrett's is believed to occur rapidly and reaches its maximal proximal extent within 3 years.[231] With further injury and multiple genetic changes, further progression occurs in a stepwise fashion in a metaplasia–dysplasia–adenocarcinoma sequence.[232]

Recent studies have evaluated the role of intraluminal nitric oxide and the change in the esophageal biome as risk factors for the development of EAC. Ingested dietary nitrate can lead to intraluminal nitric oxide through enterosalivary re-circulation. Nitric oxide can disrupt epithelial barrier function and lead to increased inflammation and increased transformation of squamous epithelium to columnar epithelium.[233] Changes in the esophageal microbiome from predominantly gram-positive bacilli in GERD and Barrett's to predominantly gram-negative bacteria in EAC suggest that dysbiosis may play a role in the pathogenesis of EAC.[234]

MOLECULAR BASIS

Carcinoma that arises in the setting of Barrett metaplasia is thought to develop as part of the metaplasia–dysplasia–carcinoma sequence. It seems that the accumulation of several changes in gene and protein rather than the sequence of events is more essential.[235] Some of these changes are depicted in Figure 142.24.[61]

Various growth factors and receptors are increased in the progression to EAC including epidermal growth factor (EGF), EGF receptor, and fibroblast growth factor (FGF).[236,237] EGFR gene amplification is correlated with lymph node invasion, and its overexpression with decreased postoperative survival in patients with locally advanced cancer treated with preoperative chemo and radiotherapy.[238] C-erb B2 (Her2/neu) protein overexpression was found in 10% to 70% of EAC; however, it was not demonstrated in metaplastic or low-grade dysplastic Barrett's suggesting that it is a late event.[239,240] Furthermore, C-erb B2 amplification independently predicted poor outcome and short survival in patients with Barrett-associated adenocarcinoma.[241] C-myc upregulation was found in 50% of metaplasia and 90% of adenocarcinoma with a role for acidified bile as an agent responsible for inducing this oncogene.[242]

Tumor suppressors—including p16, Rb, VHL, CDKN2, and DCC—are decreased in adenocarcinomas.[183,243,244] APC, another tumor suppressor, accumulates in the nucleus in its mutated form.[245] Changes have also been seen in cell–cell adhesion, facilitating tumor invasion; decreased expression of E-cadherin and β-catenin have been correlated with a poor prognosis.[246]

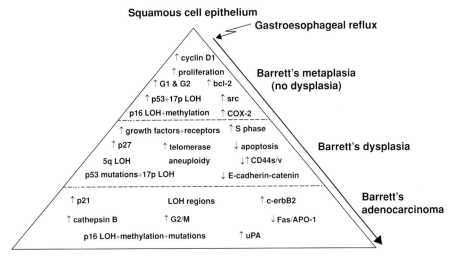

FIGURE 142.24 Genetic changes involved in the progression from Barrett metaplasia to esophageal adenocarcinoma. (From Wijnhoven BP, Tilanus HW, Dinjens WN. Molecular biology of esophageal adenocarcinoma. *Ann Surg* 2001;233:331. With permission.)

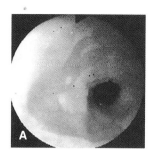
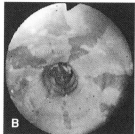
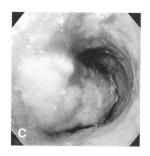

FIGURE 142.25 Endoscopic view of Barrett metaplasia (**A,B**) and an esophageal adenocarcinoma (**C**).

Inhibition of apoptosis is also seen in dysplastic cells as well as an increase in apoptotic rate with increasing histologic severity. Decreased expression of Fas receptor at the cell surface in dysplasia and adenocarcinoma, leads to a decrease in apoptosis.[247] Bcl-2, an antiapoptotic protein, was found to be overexpressed in 72% of Barrett metaplasia and 100% of low-grade dysplasia, although only 20% to 40% of high-grade dysplasia or adenocarcinoma showed overexpression.[248] Bcl-2 may be important early in the dysplasia–carcinoma sequence in allowing dysplastic cells to proliferate. The p53 gene is one of the most commonly mutated genes in cancer. Accumulation of mutated p53 increases with progression to dysplasia and adenocarcinoma, and loss of heterozygosity is found in more than 50% of adenocarcinomas.[249] Gene alterations of p53 appear to be early and frequent events in EAC and are associated with the malignant transformation of Barrett esophagus.

There are likely multiple genetic routes to cancer from Barrett metaplasia, an inference derived from studies using clonal ordering of neoplastic lineages.[250] Other chromosomal changes seen in EAC include genomic amplifications, deletions, and microsatellite instability.[251–253] Some have suggested that nuclear DNA ploidy analysis on flow cytometry might provide a more objective and reliable biomarker of progression from metaplasia to carcinoma than the histologic diagnosis of high-grade dysplasia.[254,255] Loss of chromosome Y is found in 31% to 93% of tumors.[61] In addition, repression of gene expression through promoter hypermethylation is frequently seen. Hypermethylation of the APC promoter has been found in 94% of EACs and has also been associated with advanced stage and reduced survival.[256]

PATHOLOGY

Barrett Esophagus

On endoscopy, these lesions appear as red, velvety areas between smooth, pale esophageal squamous mucosa, as shown in Figure 142.25A

and B. Microscopically, columnar epithelium is seen with mucosal glands that often contain intestinal goblet cells, as shown in Figure 142.26A. Barrett metaplasia is the precursor to EAC, and high-grade dysplasia seen on histopathology remains the best predictor of progression to adenocarcinoma.[255] Dysplasia is defined as cytologic and structural abnormalities that are distinguishable from reactive changes and extend to the luminal surface, as shown in Figure 142.26B.[257] Lesions are classified as low- or high-grade dysplasia and are distinguished by the nuclear orientation along the base of the epithelium as well as other characteristics, as illustrated in Table 142.5. Lesions are often a mosaic of low- and high-grade dysplasia adjacent to nondysplastic mucosa. It is important to remember there can be inter- and intraobserver variability.

Esophageal Adenocarcinoma

EACs usually arise in the distal esophagus. Based on SEER data, 79.3% of adenocarcinomas arise from the lower esophagus, 17.9% from the middle, and 2.8% from the upper third.[83] Lesions are initially flat or raised patches of mucosa that may become infiltrative or deeply ulcerated lesions. Microscopically, most tumors are composed of mucin-producing intestinal-type glands, as shown in Figure 142.25C. Diffusely infiltrating gastric-type signet-ring cells can be seen but are less common.

Metastases

The number of EACs detected at an early stage is small. However, this proportion is increasing due to screening programs of patients with Barrett esophagus.[258] Using SEER data, the proportion of esophageal cancer presenting as carcinoma in situ increased from 0.4% in the 1970s to 2% of patients in the 2000s.[259] In a cohort study of 295 patients published in 1999, Rice et al. found nodal disease in 10% of patients with T1 lesions, 46% of those with T2, and 83% of those

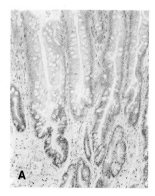
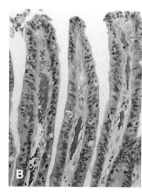
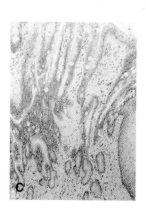

FIGURE 142.26 Microscopic view of Barrett metaplasia (**A**), high-grade dysplasia (**B**), and invasive adenocarcinoma (**C**).

TABLE 142.5 Grading Dysplasia in Barrett Esophagus

Feature	Negative	IND	LGD	HGD
Surface maturation	+	+	–	–
Architecture	Normal	Normal or mild alteration	Mild alteration	Marked alteration
Cytology	Normal or reactive	Mild alterations or focal marked atypia with inflammation	Mild alterations, diffuse or marked alterations, focal; maintained polarity	Marked alterations; loss of polarity

IND, indeterminate; LGD, low-grade dysplasia; HGD, high-grade dysplasia.
Reprinted from Montgomery E, Bronner MP, Goldblum JR, et al. Reproducibility of the diagnosis of dysplasia in Barrett's esophagus: a reaffirmation. *Hum Pathol* 2001;32:376. Copyright © 2001 Elsevier. With permission.

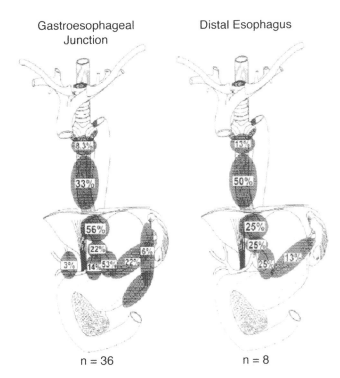

Gastroesophageal Junction   Distal Esophagus

n = 36   n = 8

FIGURE 142.27 Sites of lymph node metastases in patients with transmural esophageal adenocarcinoma. (Reprinted from Nigro JJ, DeMeester SR, Hagen JA, et al. Node status in transmural esophageal adenocarcinoma and outcome after en bloc esophagectomy. *J Thorac Cardiovasc Surg* 1999;117:962. Copyright © 1999 The American Association for Thoracic Surgery. With permission.)

TABLE 142.6 Occurrence of Metastases in Patients with Esophageal Cancer

Sites	Occurrence (%)
Liver	35
Lung	20
Bone	9
Adrenal glands	2
Brain	2
Pericardium	1
Pleura	1
Stomach	1
Pancreas	1
Spleen	1

From Quint LE, Hepburn LM, Francis IR, et al. Incidence and distribution of distant metastases in newly diagnosed esophageal carcinoma. *Cancer* 1995;76:1120. Copyright © 1995 by John Wiley Sons, Inc. Reprinted by permission of John Wiley & Sons, Inc.

with T3.[260] More recent data, however, have shown that even when tumors are confined to the muscularis mucosa and submucosa, up to 12% and 46% have nodal disease, respectively.[151,261,262] As previously discussed, EAC is less likely to demonstrate nodal disease in T1 stages than ESCC.[262,263] Nodal status is a major prognostic factor and influences survival (Figs. 142.11 and 142.13).

Lymphatic channels begin in the mucosa and drain into the submucosa, forming long collecting channels. Numerous valves direct the lymphatic flow longitudinally. Although in normal conditions lymph above the carina flows into the thoracic duct or subclavian lymphatic trunks and lymph below the carina drains into the cisterna chyli in the abdomen, reversal of flow can occur when nodes are blocked by tumor. Because of this extensive lymphatic network, most patients with symptomatic EAC and ESCC have lymph node metastases at the time of diagnosis (see Fig. 142.27).[45,261–263]

Distant metastases are also common at the time of diagnosis.[25,91,264] The most common sites of distant metastases include the liver (35%), lungs (20%), bone (9%), brain or adrenal glands (2%), and pericardium, pancreas, spleen, or stomach (1%) (Table 142.6).[265]

REFERENCES

1. American Cancer Society. *Cancer Facts and Figures 2015*. Atlanta: American Cancer Society; 2015.
2. Ferlay J, Soerjomataram I, Ervik M, et al. Globocan 2012 v1.0, *Cancer Incidence and Mortality Worldwide: IARC Cancerbase No. 11*(Internet). Lyon, France: International Agency for Research on Cancer: 2013. Available at: http://globocan.iarc.fr. Accessed June 23, 2015.
3. Edgren G, Adami HO, Weiderpass I, et al. A global assessment of the oesophageal adenocarcinoma epidemic. *Gut* 2005;54:187–192.
4. Arnold M, Soerjomataram I, Ferlay J, et al. Global incidence of oesophageal cancer by histological susbtype in 2012. *Gut* 2015;64(3) 381–387.
5. Day NE. The geographic pathology of cancer of the oesophagus. *Br Med Bull* 1984;40(4):329–334.
6. Green J, Roddam A, Pirie K et al; Million Women Study collaborators. Reproductive factors and risk of oesophageal and gastric cancer in the Million Women Study cohort. *Br J Cancer* 2012;106(1) 210–206.
7. Lagergren K, Lagergren J, Brusselaers N. Hormone replacement therapy and oral contraceptives and risk of oesophageal adenocarcinoma: a systematic review and meta-analysis. *Int J Cancer* 2014;135 (9):2183–2190.
8. Steevens J, Schouten LJ, Goldbohm RA, et al. Vegetables and fruits consumption and risk of esophageal and gastric cancer subtypes in the Netherlands Cohort Study *Int J Cancer* 2011;129(11):2681–2693.
9. Daniel CR, Cross AJ, Graubard BI, et al. Sinha R Prospective investigation of poultry and fish intake in relation to cancer risk. *Cancer Prev Res (Phila)* 2011;4(11):1903–1911.
10. Hippisley-Cox J, Coupland C. Unintended effects of statins in men and women in England and Wales: population based cohort study using the QResearch database. *BMJ* 2010;340:c2197.
11. Pohl H, Welch HG. The role of overdiagnosis and reclassification in the marked increase of esophageal adenocarcinoma incidence. *J Natl Cancer Inst* 2005;97:142–146.
12. Brown LM, Devesa SS, Chow WH. Incidence of adenocarcinoma of the esophagus among white Americans by sex, stage, and age. *J Natl Cancer Inst* 2008;100:1184–1187.
13. Putnam JB Jr, et al. Neoplasms of the esophagus. In Bell RH Jr, et al, eds. *Digestive Tract Surgery. A Text and Atlas*. Philadelphia, PA: Lippincott-Raven; 1996:45, 50.
14. Chandrasekhara R, Pilz CG, Levitan R. Hypercalcemia associated with esophageal carcinoma in the absence of bone metastasis. *Am J Dig Dis* 1975;20:173–175.
15. van Sandick JW, van Lanschot JJ, ten Kate FJ, et al. Indicators of prognosis after transhiatal esophageal resection without thoracotomy for cancer. *J Am Coll Surg* 2002;194:28–36.

16. Stephens RL, Hansen HH, Muggia FM. Hypercalcemia in epidermoid tumors of the head and neck and esophagus. *Cancer* 1973;31:1487–1491.

17. Orringer MB. Esophageal tumors. In Cameron JL, ed. *Current Surgical Therapy*. 7th ed. St. Louis, MO: Mosby; 2001:58.

18. Postlethwait RW. Tracheobronchial invasion by carcinoma of the esophagus. In DeMeester NR, Skinner DB, eds. *Esophageal Disorders. Pathophysiology and Therapy*. New York: Raven Press; 1985:389.

19. Angorn IB. Intubation in the treatment of carcinoma of the esophagus. *World J Surg* 1981;5:535–541.

20. Lindell MM Jr, Hill CA, Libshitz HI. Esophageal cancer. radiographic chest findings and their prognostic significance. *AJR Am J Roentgenol* 1979;133:461–465.

21. Levine MS, Chu P, Furth EE, et al. Carcinoma of the esophagus and esophagogastric junction: sensitivity of radiographic diagnosis. *AJR Am J Roentgenol* 1997;168:1423–1426.

22. Postlethwait RW. *Surgery of the Esophagus*. 2nd ed. East Norwalk, CT: Appleton-Century-Crofts; 1986.

23. Iyer R, DuBrow R. Imaging of esophageal cancer. *Cancer Imaging* 2004;4:125.

24. Saunders HS, Wolfman NT, Ott DJ. Esophageal cancer: radiologic staging. *Radiol Clin North Am* 1997;35:281–294.

25. Reed CE, Mishra G, Sahai AV, et al. Esophageal cancer staging: improved accuracy by endoscopic ultrasound of celiac lymph nodes. *Ann Thorac Surg* 1999;67: 319–321.

26. Rice TW. Clinical staging of esophageal carcinoma. CT, EUS, and PET. *Chest Surg Clin North Am* 2000;10:471–485.

27. Shi W, Wang W, Wang J, et al. Meta-analysis of 18FDG PET-CT for nodal staging in patients with esophageal cancer. *Surg Oncol* 2013;22(2):112–116.

28. Van Vliet EP, Heijenbrok-Kal MH, Hunink MG, et al. Staging investigations for oesophageal cancer. a meta-analysis. *Br J Cancer* 2008;98:547–557.

29. Block MI, Patterson GA, Sundaresan RS, et al. Improvement in staging of esophageal cancer with the addition of positron emission tomography. *Ann Thorac Surg* 1997;64:770–776.

30. Varghese Jr TK, Hofstetter WL, Rizk NP et al. The Society of thoracic surgeons guidelines on the diagnosis and staging of patients with esophageal cancer. *Ann Thor Surg* 2103;96:346–356.

31. Luketich JD, Schauer PR, Meltzer CC, et al. Role of positron emission tomography in staging esophageal cancer. *Ann Thorac Surg* 1997;64:765–769.

32. Kole AC, Plukker JT, Nieweg OE, et al. Positron emission tomography for staging of oesophageal and gastroesophageal malignancy. *Br J Cancer* 1998;78:521–527.

33. Kumar P, Damle NA, Bal C. Role of F18-FDG PET/CT in the Staging and Restaging of Esophageal Cancer: A Comparison with CT. *Indian J Surg Oncol* 2011;2(4):343–350.

34. Luketich JD, Friedman DM, Weigel TL, et al. Evaluation of distant metastases in esophageal cancer: 100 consecutive positron emission tomography scans. *Ann Thorac Surg* 1999;68:1133–1136.

35. Stiles BM, Salzler G, Jorgensen A, et al. Complete metabolic response is not uniformly predictive of complete pathologic response after induction therapy for esophageal cancer. *Ann Thorac Surg* 2013;96(5):1820–1825.

36. Weber WA, Ott K, Becker K, et al. Prediction of response to preoperative chemotherapy in adenocarcinomas of the esophagogastric junction by metabolic imaging. *J Clin Oncol* 2001;19:3058–3065.

37. Duong CP, Hicks RJ, Weih L, et al. FDG-PET status following chemoradiotherapy provides high management impact and powerful prognostic stratification in oesophageal cancer. *Eur J Nucl Med Mol Imaging* 2006;33(7):770–778.

38. Kim MK, Ryu JS, Kim SB, et al. Value of complete metabolic response by (18)F-fluorodeoxyglucose-positron emission tomography in oesophageal cancer for prediction of pathologic response and survival after preoperative chemoradiotherapy. *Eur J Cancer* 2007;43:1385–1391.

39. Wieder HA, Ott K, Lordick F, et al. Prediction of tumor response by FDG-PET: comparison of the accuracy of single and sequential studies in patients with adenocarcinomas of the esophagogastric junction. *Eur J Nucl Med Mol Imaging* 2007;34(12):1925–1932.

40. Smithers BM, Couper GC, Thomas JM, et al. Positron emission tomography and pathological evidence of response to neoadjuvant therapy in adenocarcinoma of the esophagus. *Dis Esophagus* 2008;21(2):151–e158.

41. Klaeser B, Nitzsche E, Schuller JC, et al. Limited predictive value of FDG-PET for response assessment in the preoperative treatment of esophageal cancer: results of a prospective multi-center trial (SAKK 75/02). *Onkologie* 2009;32(12): 724–730.

42. Shenfine J, Barbour AP, Wong D, et al. Prognostic value of maximum standardized uptake values from preoperative positron emission tomography in resectable adenocarcinoma of the esophagus treated by surgery alone. *Dis Esophagus* 2009;22(8):668–675.

43. Kukar M, Alnaji RM, Jabi F, et al. Role of repeat 18F-Fluorodeoxyglucose positron emission tomography examination in predicting pathologic response following neoadjuvant chemoradiotherapy for esophageal adenocarcinoma. *JAMA Surg* 2015;150(6):555–562.

44. Reed CE, Eloubeidi MA. New techniques for staging esophageal cancer. *Surg Clin North Am* 2002;82:697–710.

45. Merkow RP, Bilimoria KY, Keswani RN, et al. Treatment trends, risk of lymph node metastasis and outcomes for localized esophageal cancer. *J Natl Cancer Inst* 2014;106(7):pii: dju133

46. Bergeron EJ, Lin J, Chang AC, et al. Endoscopic ultrasound is inadequate to determine which T1/T2 esophageal tumors are candidates for endoluminal therapies. *J Thorac Cardiovasc Surg* 2014;147(2):765–771.

47. Thosani N, Singh H, Kapadia A, et al. Diagnostic accuracy of EUS in differentiating mucosal versus submucosal invasion of superficial esophageal cancers: a systematic review and meta-analysis. *Gastrointest Endosc* 2012;75:242–253.

48. Eloubeidi MA, Wallace MB, Hoffman BJ, et al. Predictors of survival for esophageal cancer patients with and without celiac axis lymphadenopathy. impact of staging endosonography. *Ann Thorac Surg* 2001;72:212–219.

49. Worrell SG, Oh DS, Greene CL, et al. Endoscopic ultrasound staging of stenotic esophageal cancers may be unnecessary to determine the need for neoadjuvant therapy. *J Gastrointest Surg* 2014;18(2):318–320.

50. Hunerbein M, Ghadimi BM, Haensch W, et al. Transendoscopic ultrasound of esophageal and gastric cancer using miniaturized ultrasound catheter probes. *Gastrointest Endosc* 1998;48:371–375.

51. Waxman I. Clinical impact of high-frequency ultrasound probe sonography during diagnostic endoscopy—a prospective study. *Endoscopy* 1998;30(Suppl 1): A166–A168.

52. Kuwano H, Nishimura Y, Oyama T, et al. Guidelines for diagnosis and treatment of carcinoma of the esophagus April 2012 edited by the Japan esophageal Society. *Esophagus* 2015;12(1):1–30.

53. Krasna MJ, Flowers JL, Attar S et al. Combined thoracoscopic/laparoscopic staging of esophageal cancer. *J Thorac Cardiovasc Surg* 1996;111:800–806.

54. Krasna MJ, Reed CE, Nedzwiecki D et al. CALGB 9380. A prospective trial of the feasibility of thoracoscopy/laparoscopy in staging esophageal cancer. *Ann Thorac Surg* 2001;71:1073–1079.

55. Luketich JD, Meehan M, Nguyen NT, et al. Minimally invasive surgical staging for esophageal cancer. *Surg Endosc* 2000;14:700–702.

56. Stein HJ, Kraemer SJ, Feussner H, et al. Clinical value of diagnostic laparoscopy with laparoscopic ultrasound in patients with cancer of the esophagus or cardia. *J Gastrointest Surg* 1997;1:167–172.

57. Flett ME, Lim MN, Bruce D, et al. Prognostic value of laparoscopic ultrasound in patients with gastro-esophageal cancer. *Dis Esophagus* 2001;14:223–226.

58. Wallace MB, Nietert PJ, Earle C, et al. An analysis of multiple staging management strategies for carcinoma of the esophagus: computed tomography, endoscopic ultrasound, positron emission tomography, and thoracoscopy/laparoscopy. *Ann Thorac Surg* 2002;4:1026–1032.

59. Iannettoni MD, Lee SS, Bennell MR, et al. Detection of Barrett's adenocarcinoma of the gastric cardia with sucrase isomaltase and p53. *Ann Thorac Surg* 1996;62:1460–1466.

60. Reid BJ, Bount PL, Rubin CE, et al. Flow-cytometric and histological progression to malignancy in Barrett's esophagus: prospective endoscopic surveillance of a cohort. *Gastroenterology* 1992;102:1212–1219.

61. Wijnhoven BP, Tilanus HW, Dinjens WN. Molecular biology of Barrett's adenocarcinoma. *Ann Surg* 2001;233:322–337.

62. Altorki NK, Oliveria S, Schrump DS. Epidemiology and molecular biology of Barrett's adenocarcinoma. *Semin Surg Oncol* 1997;13:270–280.

63. Casson AG, Tammemagi M, Eskandarian S, et al. p53 Alterations in oesophageal cancer: association with clinicopathological features, risk factors, and survival. *Mol Pathol* 1998;51:71–79.

64. Lagarde SM, ten Kate FJ, Richel DJ, et al. Molecular prognostic factors in adenocarcinoma of the esophagus and gastroesophageal junction. *Ann Surg Oncol* 2007;14:977–991.

65. Vallbohmer D, Lenz HJ. Predictive and prognostic molecular markers in outcome of esophageal cancer. *Dis Esophagus* 2006;19:425–432.

66. Miyazono F, Metzger R, Warnecke-Eberz U, et al. Quantitative c-erbB-2 but not c-erbBo-1 mRAN expression is a promising marker to predict minor histopathologic response to neoadjuvant radiochemotherapy in oesophageal cancer. *Br J Cancer* 2004;91:666–672.

67. Kulke MH, Odze RD, Mueller JD, et al. Prognostic significance of vascular endothelial growth factor and cyclooxygenase 2 expression in patients receiving preoperative chemoradiation for esophageal cancer. *J Thorac Cardiovasc Surg* 2004;127:1579–1586.

68. Metias SM, Lianidou E, Yousef GM. MicroRNAs in clinical oncology: at the crossroads between promises and problems. *J Clin Pathol* 2009;62(9):771–776.

69. Esquela-Kerscher A, Slack FJ. Oncomirs—microRNAs with a role in cancer. *Nat Rev Cancer* 2006;6(4):259–269.

70. Feber A, Xi L, Luketich JD, Pennathur A, et al. MicroRNA expression profiles of esophageal cancer. *J Thorac Cardiovasc Surg* 2008;135(2):255–260.

71. Ko MA, Zehong G, Virtanen C, et al. MicroRNA expression profiling of esophageal cancer before and after induction chemoradiotherapy. *Ann Thorac Surg* 2012;94(4):1094–1102.

72. Ronellenfitsch U, Schwarzbach M, Hofheinz R, et al; GE Adenocarcinoma Meta-analysis Group. Perioperative chemo(radio)therapy versus primary surgery for resectable adenocarcinoma of the stomach, gastroesophageal junction, and lower esophagus. *Cochrane Database Syst Rev* 2013;5:CD008107.

73. Kidane B, Coughlin S, Vogt K, Malthaner R. Preoperative chemotherapy for resectable thoracic esophageal cancer. *Cochrane Database Syst Rev* 2015;5:CD001556.

74. Eloubeidi MA, Desmond R, Arguedas MR, et al. Prognostic factors for the survival of patients with esophageal carcinoma in the U.S.: the importance of tumor length and lymph node status. *Cancer* 2002;95:1434–1443.

75. Wang J, Wu N, Zheng QF, et al. Evaluation of the 7th edition of the TNM classification in patients with resected esophageal squamous cell carcinoma. *World J Gastroenterol* 2014;20(48):18397–18403.

76. Talsma K, van Hagen P, Grotenhuis BA, et al. Comparison of the 6th and 7th Editions of the UICC-AJCC TNM classification for esophageal cancer. *Ann Surg Oncol* 2012;19(7):2142–2148

77. Liu YP, Ma L, Wang SJ, et al. Prognostic value of lymph node metastases and lymph node ratio in esophageal squamous cell carcinoma. *Eur J Surg Oncol* 2010; 36(2):155–159.

78. Greenstein AJ, Litle VR, Swanson SJ, et al. Effect of the number of lymph nodes sampled on postoperative survival of lymph node-negative esophageal cancer. *Cancer* 2008;112(6):1239–1246.

79. Greenstein AJ, Litle VR, Swanson SJ, et al. Prognostic significance of the number of lymph node metastases in esophageal cancer. *J Am Coll Surg* 2008;206(2):239–246.

80. Xu XL, Zheng WH, Zhu SM, et al. The prognostic impact of lymph node involvement in large scale operable node-positive esophageal squamous cell carcinoma patients: A 10-year experience. *PLoS One* 2015;10(7):e0133076.

81. Rice TW, Rusch VW, Ishwaran H, et al; Worldwide Esophageal Cancer Collaboration. Cancer of the esophagus and esophagogastric junction: data-driven staging for the seventh edition of the American Joint Committee on Cancer/International Union Against Cancer Cancer Staging Manuals. *Cancer* 2010;116(16): 3763–3773.

82. Chalasani N, Wo JM, Waring JP. Racial differences in the histology, location, and risk factors of esophageal cancer. *J Clin Gastroenterol* 1998;26:11–13.

83. Yang PC, Davis S. Incidence of cancer of the esophagus in the US by histologic type. *Cancer* 1988;61:612–617.

84. Ribeiro U Jr, Posner MC, Safatle-Ribeiro AV, et al. Risk factors for squamous cell carcinoma of the oesophagus. *Br J Surg* 1996;83:1174–1185.

85. Stoner GD, Gupta A. Etiology and chemoprevention of esophageal squamous cell carcinoma. *Carcinogenesis* 2001;22:1737–1746.

86. Vassallo A, Correa P, De Stefani E, et al. Esophageal cancer in Uruguay: a case-control study. *J Natl Cancer Inst* 1985;75:1005–1009.

87. Fraumeni JF Jr, Blot WJ. Geographic variation in esophageal cancer mortality in the United States. *J Chronic Dis* 1977;30:759–767.

88. Gammon MD, Schoenberg JB, Ahsan H, et al. Tobacco, alcohol, and socioeconomic status and adenocarcinomas of the esophagus and gastric cardia. *J Natl Cancer Inst* 1997;89(17):1277–1284.

89. Lu SH, Montesano R, Zhang MS, et al. Relevance of N-nitrosamines to esophageal cancer in China. *J Cell Physiol Suppl* 1986;4:51–58.

90. Wang L, Zhu D, Zhang C, et al. Mutations of O6-methylguanine-DNA methyltransferase gene in esophageal cancer tissues from Northern China. *Int J Cancer* 1997;71(5):719–723.

91. Islami F, Ren JS, Taylor PR, et al. Pickled vegetables and the risk of oesophageal cancer: a meta-analysis. *Br J Cancer* 2009;101(9):1641–1647.

92. Liu J, Wang J, Leng Y, et al. Intake of fruit and vegetables and risk of esophageal squamous cell carcinoma: a meta-analysis of observational studies. *Int J Cancer* 2013;133(2):473–485.

93. Lu SH, Ohshima H, Fu HM, et al. Urinary excretion of N-nitrosamino acids and nitrate by inhabitants of high- and low-risk areas for esophageal cancer in Northern China: endogenous formation of nitrosoproline and its inhibition by vitamin C. *Cancer Res* 1986;46:1485–1491.

94. Huang GL, Yang L, Su M, et al. Vitamin D3 and beta-carotene deficiency is associated with risk of esophageal squamous cell carcinoma—results of a case-control study in China. *Asian Pac J Cancer Prev* 2014;15(2):819–823.

95. Burrell RJ, Roach WA, Shadwell A. Esophageal cancer in the Bantu of the Transkei associated with mineral deficiency in garden plants, *J Natl Cancer Inst* 1966;36:201–209.

96. Jaskiewicz K, Marasas WF, Rossouw JE, et al. Selenium and other mineral elements in populations at risk for esophageal cancer. *Cancer*1988;62:2635–2639.

97. Steevens J, van den Brandt PA, Goldbohm RA, et al. Selenium status and the risk of esophageal and gastric cancer subtypes: the Netherlands cohort study. *Gastroenterology* 2010;138(5):1704–1713.

98. Xiao Q, Freedman ND, Ren J, et al. Intakes of folate, methionine, vitamin B6 and vitamin B12 with risk of esophageal and gastric cancer in a large cohort study. *Br J Cancer* 2014;110:1328–1333.

99. Li X, Gao C, Yang Y, et al. Systematic review with meta-analysis: the association between human papillomavirus infection and oesophageal cancer. *Aliment Pharmacol Ther* 2014;39(3):270–281.

100. Tang L, Xu F, Zhang T, et al. High temperature of food and beverage intake increase the risk of oesophageal cancer in Xinjiang, China. *Asian Pac J Cancer Prev* 2013;14:5085–5088.

101. Chen W, Yang C, Yang L, et al. Zheng Association of roasting meat intake with the risk of esophageal squamous cell carcinoma of Kazakh Chinese via affecting promoter methylation of p16 gene. *Y Asia Pac J Clin Nutr* 2014;23(3):488–497.

102. Hakami R, Etemadi A, Kamangar F, et al. Cooking methods and esophageal squamous cell carcinoma in high-risk areas of Iran. *Nutr Cancer* 2014;66(3):500–505.

103. Lin S, Wang X, Huang C, et al. Consumption of salted meat and its interactions with alcohol drinking and tobacco smoking on esophageal squamous-cell carcinoma. *Int J Cancer* 2015;137(3):582–589.

104. Amer MH, El-Yazigi A, Hannan MA, et al. Water contamination and esophageal cancer at Gassim Region, Saudi Arabia. *Gastroenterology* 1990;98:1141–1147.

105. Notani PN. Role of alcohol in cancers of the upper alimentary tract. Use of models in risk assessment. *J Epidemiol Community Health* 1988;42:187–192.

106. Yu MC, Garabrant DH, Peters JM, et al. Tobacco, alcohol, diet, occupation, and carcinoma of the esophagus. *Cancer Res* 1988;48:3843–3848.

107. Ziegler RG. Alcohol-nutrient interactions in cancer etiology. *Cancer* 1986;58:1942–1948.

108. Prabhu A, Obi KO, Rubenstein JH. The synergistic effects of alcohol and tobacco consumption on the risk of esophageal squamous cell carcinoma: a meta-analysis. *Am J Gastroenterol* 2014;109(6):822–827.

109. Hashibe M, McKay JD, Curado MP, et al. Multiple ADH genes are associated with upper aerodigestive cancers. *Nat Genet* 2008;40(6):707–709.

110. Wang H, Tong L, Wei J, et al. The ALDH7A1 genetic polymorphisms contribute to development of esophageal squamous cell carcinoma. *Tumour Biol* 2014;35(12):12665–12670.

111. Zhang L, Jiang Y, Wu Q, et al. Gene-environment interactions on the risk of esophageal cancer among Asian populations with the G48A polymorphism in the alcohol dehydrogenase-2 gene: a meta-analysis. *Tumour Biol* 2014;35(5): 4705–4717.

112. Meijssen MA, Tilanus HW, van Blankenstein M, et al. Achalasia complicated by esophageal squamous cell carcinoma: a prospective study in 195 patients. *Gut* 1992;33:155–158.

113. Sandler RS, Nyrén O, Ekbom A, et al. The risk of esophageal cancer in patients with achalasia. A population-based study. *JAMA* 1995;274(17):1359–1362.

114. Leeuwenburgh I, Scholten P, Alderliesten J, et al. Long-term esophageal cancer risk in patients with primary achalasia: a prospective study. *Am J Gastroenterol* 2010;105(10):2144–2149.

115. Carter R, Brewer LA III. Achalasia and esophageal carcinoma. Studies in early diagnosis for improved surgical management. *Am J Surg* 1975;130:114–120.

116. Wychulis AR, Woolam GL, Andersin HA, et al. Achalasia and carcinoma of the esophagus. *JAMA* 1971;215:1638–1641.

117. O'Sullivan KE, Phelan JJ, O'Hanlon C, et al. The role of inflammation in cancer of the esophagus. *Expert Rev Gastroenterol Hepatol* 2014;8(7):749–760.

118. American Gastroenterological Association Guidelines. Endoscopic Surveillance of premalignant conditions of the upper gastrointestinal tract. Available at www. gastro.org/guidelines. Accessed November 3, 2017.

119. Isolauri J, Markkula H. Lye ingestion and carcinoma of the esophagus. *Acta Chir Scand* 1989;155:269–271.

120. Appelqvist P, Salmo M. Lye corrosion carcinoma of the esophagus: a review of 63 cases. *Cancer* 1980;45:2655–2658.

121. Schwindt WD, Bernhardt LC, Johnson AM. Tylosis and intrathoracic neoplasms. *Chest* 1970;57:590–591.

122. Howel-Evans W, McConnell RB, Clarke CA, et al. Carcinoma of the oesophagus with keratosis palmaris et plantaris (tylosis). *Q J Med* 1958;27:413–429.

123. Risk JM, Evans KE, Jones J, et al. Characterization of a 500 kb region on 17q25 and the exclusion of candidate genes as the familial Tylosis Oesophageal Cancer (TOC) locus. *Oncogene* 2002;21(41):6395–6402.

124. Lambert R, Hainaut P. Esophageal cancer II: The precursors. *Endoscopy* 2007;39:659–664.

125. Lindor NM, McMaster ML, Lindor CJ, et al. Concise handbook of familial cancer susceptibility syndromes. 2nd ed. *J Natl Cancer Inst Monogr* 2008:1–93.

126. Trivers KF, Sabatino SA, Stewart SL. Trends in esophageal cancer incidence by histology, United States, 198–2003. *Int J Cancer* 2008;123:1422–1428.

127. Jemal A, Bray F, Center MM, et al. Global cancer statistics. *CA Cancer J Clin* 2011;61:69–90.

128. Arnott SJ, Pearson JG, Finlayson ND et al. et al. The association of squamous oesophageal cancer and thyroid disease. *Br J Cancer* 1971;25:33–36.

129. Atabek U, Mohit-Tabatabai MA, Rush BF, et al.et al. Impact of esophageal screening in patients with head and neck cancer. *Am Surg* 1990;56:289–292.

130. Selby WS, Gallagher ND. Malignancy in a 19-year experience of adult celiac disease. *Dig Dis Sci* 1979;24:684–688.

131. Shimizu T, Matsui T, Kimura O, et al. Radiation-induced esophageal cancer. A case report and a review of the literature. *Jpn J Surg* 1990;20:97–100.

132. Ahsan H, Neugut AI. Radiation therapy for breast cancer and increased risk for esophageal carcinoma. *Ann Intern Med* 1998;128:114–117.

133. Nasrollahzadeh D, Ye W, Shakeri R, et al. Contact with ruminants is associated with esophageal squamous cell carcinoma risk. *Int J Cancer* 2015;136(6): 1468–1474.

134. Abnet CC, Kamangar F, Islami F, et al. Tooth loss and lack of regular oral hygiene are associated with higher risk of esophageal squamous cell carcinoma. *Cancer Epidemiol Biomarkers Prev* 2008;187(11):3062–3068.

135. Guha N, Boffetta P, Wünsch Filho V, et al. Oral health and risk of squamous cell carcinoma of the head and neck and esophagus: results of two multicentric case-control studies. *Am J Epidemiol* 2007;166(10):1159–1173.

136. Ahrens W, Pohlabeln H, Foraita R, et al. Oral health, dental care and mouthwash associated with upper aerodigestive tract cancer risk in Europe: the ARCAGE study. *Oral Oncol* 2014;50(6):616–625.

137. Wang LD, Zhou Q, Hong JY, et al. p53 Protein accumulation and gene mutations in multifocal esophageal precancerous lesions from symptom free subjects in a high incidence area for esophageal carcinoma in Henan, China. *Cancer* 1996;77:1244–1249.

138. Chaves P, Periera AD, Pinto A, et al. p53 Protein immunoexpression in esophageal squamous cell carcinoma and adjacent epithelium. *J Surg Oncol* 1997;65: 3–9.

139. Safatle-Ribeiro AV, Riveira U Jr, Sakai P, et al. Integrated p53 histopathologic/genetic analysis of premalignant lesions of the esophagus. *Cancer Detect Prev* 2000;24:13–23.

140. Uchino S, Saito T, Inomata M, et al. Prognostic significance of the p53 mutation in esophageal cancer. *Jpn J Clin Oncol* 1996;26:287–292.

141. Lambert R, Hainaut P. Esophageal cancer I: Cases and causes. *Endoscopy* 2007;39:233–238.

142. Saeki H, Kitao H, Yoshinaga K, et al. Copy-neutral loss of heterozygosity at the p53 locus in carcinogenesis of esophageal squamous cell carcinomas associated with p53 mutations. *Clin Cancer Res* 2011;17(7):1731–1740.

143. Abedi-Ardekani B, Kamangar F, Sotoudeh M et al. Extremely high TP53 mutation load in esophageal squamous cell carcinoma in Golestan Province, Iran. *PLoS ONE* 2011;6(12): e29488.

144. Lin DC, Hao JJ, Nagata Y, et al. Genomic and molecular characterization of esophageal squamous cell carcinoma. *Nat Genet* 2014;46(5):467–473.

145. Wang W, Sun QK, He YF, et al. Overexpression of periostin is significantly correlated to the tumor angiogenesis and poor prognosis in patients with esophageal squamous cell carcinoma. *Int J Clin Exp Pathol* 2014;7:593–601.

146. Zhang MX, Xu YJ, Zhu MC, et al. Overexpressed ostepontin-c as a potential biomarker for esophageal squamous cell carcinoma. *Asian Pac J Cancer Prev* 2013;14(12):7315–7319.

147. Wu C, Wang C, Guan X, et al. Diagnostic and prognostic implications of a serum miRNA panel in oesophageal squamous cell carcinoma. *Plos One* 2014;9(3):e92292.

148. Dawsey SM, Lewin KJ, Liu FS et al. Esophageal morphology from Linxian, China. Squamous histologic findings in 754 patients. *Cancer* 1994;73:2027–2037.

149. Dawsey SM, Lewin KJ, Wang GQ et al. Squamous esophageal histology and subsequent risk of squamous cell carcinoma of the esophagus. A prospective follow-up study from Linxian, China. *Cancer* 1994;74:1686–1692.

150. Taylor PR, Abnet CC, Dawsey SM. Squamous dysplasia—the precursor lesion for esophageal squamous cell carcinoma. *Cancer Epidemiol Biomarkers Prev* 2013;22(4):540–552.

151. Yoshida M. Recent development of studies on superficial cancer in Japan. *Esophagus* 2007;4:91–92.

152. Hölscher AH, Bollschweiler E, Schröder W, et al. Prognostic impact of upper, middle, and lower third mucosal or submucosal infiltration in early esophageal cancer. *Ann Surg* 2011;254(5):802–807.

153. Akiyama H, Tsurumaru M, Kawamura T, et al. Principles of surgical treatment for carcinoma of the esophagus. analysis of lymph node involvement. *Ann Surg* 1981;194:438–446.

154. Mandard AM, Chasle J, Marnay J, et al. Autopsy findings in 111 cases of esophageal cancer. *Cancer* 1981;48:329–325.

155. Wong J. Esophageal resection for cancer: the rationale of current practice. *Am J Surg* 1987;153:18–24.

156. Casson AG, Darnton SJ, Subrmanian S, et al. What is the optimal distal resection margin for esophageal carcinoma? *Ann Thorac Surg* 2000;69:205–209.

157. Roberts JG. Cancer of the oesophagus—how should tumour biology affect treatment? *Br J Surg* 1980;67:791–797.

158. Tanabe G, Baba M, Kuroshima K, et al. [Clinical evaluation of the esophageal lymph flow system based on RI uptake of dissected regional lymph nodes following lymphoscintigraphy]. *Nippon Geka Gakkai Zasshi* 1986;87:315–323.

159. Lu YK, Li YM, Gu YZ. Cancer of esophagus and esophagogastric junction. analysis of results of 1,025 resections after 5 to 20 years. *Ann Thorac Surg* 1987;43:176–181.

160. Stein HJ, Feith M, Bruecher BL, et al. Early esophageal cancer: pattern of lymphatic spread and prognostic factors for long-term survival after surgical resection. *Ann Surg* 2005;242(4):566–573.

161. Ide H. Extended lymph node dissection for thoracic esophageal cancer: efficacy of three field dissection based on preoperative staging. *Jpn J Gastroenterol Surg* 1995;37:382.

162. Kato H, Watanabe H, Tachimori Y, et al. Evaluation of neck lymph node dissection for thoracic esophageal carcinoma. *Ann Thorac Surg* 1991;51:931–935.

163. Sannohe Y, Hiratsuka R, Doki K. Lymph node metastases in cancer of the thoracic esophagus. *Am J Surg* 1981;141:216–218.

164. Anderson LL, Lad TE. Autopsy findings in squamous-cell carcinoma of the esophagus. *Cancer* 1982;50:1587–1590.

165. Devesa SS, Blot WJ, Fraumeni JF Jr. Changing patterns in the incidence of esophageal and gastric carcinoma in the United States. *Cancer* 1998;83:2049–2053.

166. Howlader N, Noone AM, Krapcho M, et al. *SEER Cancer Statistics Review, 1975–2014.* Bethesda, MD: National Cancer Institute. Available at: http://seer.cancer.gov/csr/1975_2014/, based on November 2016 SEER data submission, posted to the SEER web site, April 2017. Accessed November 3, 2017.

167. Hur C, Miller M, Kong CY, et al. Trends in esophageal adenocarcinoma incidence and mortality. *Cancer* 2013;119(6):1149–1158.

168. El-Serag HB. The epidemic of esophageal adenocarcinoma. *Gastroenterol Clin North Am* 2002;31:421–440.

169. Rubenstein JH, Chen JW. Epidemiology of gastroesophageal reflux disease. *Gastroenterol Clin North Am* 2014;43(1):1–14.

170. Thrift AP, Whiteman DC. The incidence of esophageal adenocarcinoma continues to rise: analysis of period and birth cohort effects on recent trends. *Ann Oncol* 2012;23(12):3155–3162.

171. Masclee GM, Coloma PM, de Wilde M, et al. The incidence of Barrett's oesophagus and oesophageal adenocarcinoma in the United Kingdom and The Netherlands is levelling off. *Aliment Pharmacol Ther* 2014;39(11):1321–1330.

172. Engel LS, Chow WH, Vaughan TL, et al. Population attributable risks of esophageal and gastric cancers. *J Natl Cancer Inst* 2003;95(18):1404.

173. Steyerberg EW, Looman CW, Kuipers EJ. Alcohol and the risk of Barrett's esophagus: a pooled analysis from the International BEACON Consortium. *Am J Gastroenterol* 2014;109(10):1586–1594.

174. Zhai R, Chen F, Liu G, et al. Interactions among genetic variants in apoptosis pathway genes, reflux symptoms, body mass index, and smoking indicate two distinct etiologic patterns of esophageal adenocarcinoma. *J Clin Oncol* 2010;28(14):2445–2451.

175. Weaver JM, Ross-Innes CS, Shannon N, et al.; OCCAMS Consortium. Ordering of mutations in preinvasive disease stages of esophageal carcinogenesis. *Nat Genet* 2014;46(8):837–843.

176. El-Serag HB, Mason AC, Petersen N, et al. Epidemiological differences between adenocarcinoma of the oesophagus and adenocarcinoma of the gastric cardia in the USA. *Gut* 2002;50:368–372.

177. Kubo A, Corley DA. Marked regional variation in adenocarcinomas of the esophagus and the gastric cardia in the United States. *Cancer* 2002;95:2096–2102.

178. Cameron AJ. Epidemiology of columnar-lined esophagus and adenocarcinoma. *Gastroenterol Clin North Am* 1997;26:487–494.

179. O'Connor JB, Falk GW, Richter JE. The incidence of adenocarcinoma and dysplasia in Barrett's esophagus: report on the Cleveland Clinic Barrett's Esophagus Registry. *Am J Gastroenterol* 1999;94:2037–2042.

180. Hamilton SR, Smith RR, Cameron JL. Prevalence and characteristics of Barrett's esophagus in patients with adenocarcinoma of the esophagus or esophagogastric junction. *Hum Pathol* 1988;19:942–948.

181. Sarr MG, Hamilton SR, Marrone GC, et al. Barrett's esophagus: its prevalence and association with adenocarcinoma in patients with symptoms of gastroesophageal reflux. *Am J Surg* 1985;149:187–193.

182. Cameron AJ, Ott BJ, Payne WS. The incidence of adenocarcinoma in columnar-line (Barrett's) esophagus. *N Eng J Med* 1985;313:857–859.

183. Hayeck TJ, Kong CY, Spechler SJ, et al. The prevalence of Barrett's esophagus in the US: estimates from a simulation model confirmed by SEER data. *Dis Esophagus* 2010;23(6):451–457.

184. Jankowski JA, Wright NA, Meltzer SJ. et al. Molecular evolution of the metaplasia-dysplasia-adenocarcinoma sequence in the esophagus. *Am J Pathol* 1999;154: 965–973.

185. Bandla S, Peters JH, Ruff D, et al. Comparison of cancer-associated genetic abnormalities in columnar-lined esophagus tissues with and without goblet cells. *Ann Surg* 2014;260:72–80.

186. Buas MF, Levine DM, Makar KW, et al. Integrative post-genome-wide association analysis of CDKN2A and TP53 SNPs and risk of esophageal adenocarcinoma. *Carcinogenesis* 2014;35(12):2740–2747.

187. Locke GR III, Talley NJ, Fett SL, et al. Prevalence and clinical spectrum of gastroesophageal reflux: a population based study in Olmsted County, Minnesota. *Gastroenterology* 1997;112:1448–1456.

188. Nebel OT, Fornes MF, Castell DO. Symptomatic gastroesophageal reflux: incidence and precipitating factors. *Am J Dig Dis* 1976;21:953–956.

189. Spechler SJ, Zeroogian JM, Antonioli DA et al. Prevalence of metaplasia at the gastro-oesophageal junction. *Lancet* 1994;344:1533–1536.

190. Winters C Jr, Spurling TJ, Chobanian SJ, et al. Barrett's esophagus. A prevalent, occult complication of gastroesophageal reflux disease. *Gastroenterology* 1987;92:118–124.

191. Lagergren J, Bergström R, Lindgren A, et al. Symptomatic gastroesophageal reflux as a risk factor for esophageal adenocarcinoma. *N Engl J Med* 1999;340: 825–831.

192. Lagergren J, Ye W, Lagergren P, et al. The risk of esophageal adenocarcinoma after antireflux surgery. *Gastroenterology* 2010;138(4):1297–1301.

193. Lagergren J, Bergstrom R, Nyren O. Association between body mass and adenocarcinoma of the esophagus and gastric cardia. *Ann Intern Med* 1999;130: 883–890.

194. Turati F, Tramacere I, La Vecchia C, et al. A meta-analysis of body mass index and esophageal and gastric cardia adenocarcinoma. *Ann Oncol* 2013;24(3): 609–617.

195. Thrift AP, Shaheen NJ, Gammon MD, et al. Obesity and risk of esophageal adenocarcinoma and Barrett's esophagus: a Mendelian randomization study. *J Natl Cancer Inst* 2014;106(11). Pii: dju252

196. Massl R, van Blankenstein M, Jeurnink S, et al. Visceral adipose tissue: the link with esophageal adenocarcinoma. *Scand J Gastroenterol* 2014;49(4):449–457.

197. Singh S, Devanna S, Edakkanambeth Varayil J, et al. Physical activity is associated with reduced risk of esophageal cancer, particularly esophageal adenocarcinoma: a systematic review and meta-analysis. *BMC Gastroenterol* 2014;14:101.

198. Behrens G, Jochem C, Keimling M, et al. The association between physical activity and gastroesophageal cancer: systematic review and meta-analysis. *Eur J Epidemiol* 2014;29(3):151–170.

199. Chow WH, Blaser MJ, Blot WJ, et al. An inverse relation between cagA+ strains of Helicobacter pylori infection and risk of esophageal and gastric cardia adenocarcinoma. *Cancer Res* 1998;58:588–590.

200. Ye W, Held M, Lagergren J, et al. Helicobacter pylori infection and gastric atrophy: risk of adenocarcinoma and squamous-cell carcinoma of the esophagus and adenocarcinoma of the gastric cardia. *J Natl Cancer Inst* 2004;96(5):388–396.

201. Whiteman DC, Parmar P, Fahey P, et al. Australian Cancer Study. Association of Helicobacter pylori infection with reduced risk for esophageal cancer is independent of environmental and genetic modifiers. *Gastroenterology* 2010;139(1): 73–83.

202. Labenz J, Blum Al, Bayerdörffer E, et al. Curing Helicobacter pylori infection in patients with duodenal ulcer may provoke reflux esophagitis. *Gastroenterology* 1997;112:1442–1447.

203. Cook MB, Kamangar F, Whiteman DC, et al. Cigarette smoking and adenocarcinomas of the esophagus and esophagogastric junction: a pooled analysis from the international BEACON consortium. *J Natl Cancer Inst* 2010;102(17): 1344–1353.

204. Tramacere I, La Vecchia C, Negri E. Tobacco smoking and esophageal and gastric cardia adenocarcinoma: a meta-analysis. *Epidemiology* 2011;22:344–349.

205. Lagergren J, Bergström R, Adami HO, et al. Association between medications that relax the lower esophageal sphincter and risk for esophageal adenocarcinoma. *Ann Intern Med* 2000;133:165–175.

206. Green J, Czanner G, Reeves G, et al. Oral bisphosphonates and risk of cancer of oesophagus, stomach, and colorectum: case-control analysis within a UK primary care cohort. *BMJ* 2010;341:c4444.

207. Cardwell CR, Abnet CC, Cantwell MM, et al. Exposure to oral bisphosphonates and risk of esophageal cancer. *JAMA* 2010;304:657–663.

208. Vinogradova Y, Coupland C, Hippisley-Cox J. Exposure to bisphosphonates and risk of gastrointestinal cancers: series of nested case-control studies with QResearch and CPRD data. *BMJ* 2013;346:f114.

209. Freedman J, Ye W, Näslund E, et al. Association between cholecystectomy and adenocarcinoma of the esophagus. *Gastroenterology* 2001;121(3):548–553.

210. Kauer WK, Peters JH, DeMeester TR, et al. Mixed reflux of gastric and duodenal juices is more harmful to the esophagus than gastric juice alone. The need for surgical therapy re-emphasized. *Ann Surg* 1995;222:525–531.

211. Deurloo JA, van Lanschot JJ, Drillenburg P, et al. Esophageal squamous cell carcinoma 38 years after primary repair of esophageal atresia. *J Pediatr Surg* 2001;36:629–630.

212. Alfaro L, Bermas H, Fenoglio M, et al. Are patients who have had a tracheoesophageal fistula repair during infancy at risk for esophageal adenocarcinoma during adulthood? *J Pediatr Surg* 2005;40:719–720.

213. Deurloo JA, Ekkelkamp S, Bartelsman JF, et al. Gastroesophageal reflux: prevalence in adults older than 28 years after correction of esophageal atresia. *Ann Surg* 2003;238(5):686–689.

214. Terry P, Lagergren J, Ye W, et al. Inverse association between intake of cereal fiber and risk of gastric cardia cancer. *Gastroenterology* 2001;120:387–391.

215. Iijima K, Grant J, McElroy K, et al. Novel mechanism of nitrosative stress from dietary nitrate with relevance to gastro-oesophageal junction cancers. *Carcinogenesis* 2003;24:1951–1960.

216. Mayne ST, Risch HA, Dubrow R, et al. Nutrient intake and risk of subtypes of esophageal and gastric cancer. *Cancer Epidemiol Biomarkers Prev* 2001;10(10):1055–1062.

217. Larsson SC, Giovannucci E, Wolk A. Folate intake, MTHFR polymorphisms, and risk of esophageal, gastric, and pancreatic cancer: a meta-analysis. *Gastroenterology* 2006;131:1271–1283.

218. Keszei AP, Goldbohm RA, Schouten LJ, et al. Dietary N-nitroso compounds, endogenous nitrosation, and the risk of esophageal and gastric cancer subtypes in the Netherlands Cohort Study. *Am J Clin Nutr* 2013;97:135–146.

219. Wilson KT, Fu S, Ramanujam KS et al. Increased expression of inducible nitric oxide synthase and cyclooxygenase-2 in Barrett's esophagus and associated adenocarcinomas. *Cancer Res* 1998;58:2929–2934.

220. Zhang F, Subbaramaiah K, Altorki N, et al. Dihydroxy bile acids activate the transcription of cyclooxygenase-2. *J Biol Chem* 1998;273:2424–2428.

221. Souza RF, Shewmake K, Beer DG, et al. Selective inhibition of cyclooxygenase-2 suppresses growth and induces apoptosis in human esophageal adenocarcinoma cells. *Cancer Res* 2000;60:5767–5772.

222. Moons LMG, Kuipers EJ, Rygiel AM, et al. COX-2 CA-haplotype is a risk factor for the development of esophageal adenocarcinoma. *Am J Gastroenterol* 2007;102:2373–2379.

223. Mehta S, Boddy A, Johnson IT, et al. Systematic review: cyclo-oxygenase-2 in human esophageal adenocarcinogenesis. *Aliment Pharmacol Ther* 24:1321–1331.

224. Liao LM, Vaughan TL, Corley DA, et al. Nonsteroidal anti-inflammatory drug use reduces risk of adenocarcinomas of the esophagus and esophagogastric junction in a pooled analysis. *Gastroenterology* 2012;142:442–452.

225. Macfarlane TV, Lefevre K, Watson MC. Aspirin and non-steroidal anti-inflammatory drug use and the risk of upper aerodigestive tract cancer. *Br J Cancer* 2014;111:1852–1859.

226. Sivarasan N, Smith G. Role of aspirin in chemoprevention of esophageal adenocarcinoma: a meta-analysis. *J Dig Dis* 2014;14:222–230.

227. Bosetti C, Rosato V, Gallus S, et al. Aspirin and cancer risk: a quantitative review to 2011. *Ann Oncol* 2012;23:1403–1415.

228. Heath EI, Canto MI, Piantadosi S, et al. Chemoprevention for Barrett's Esophagus Trial Research Group. Secondary chemoprevention of Barrett's esophagus with celecoxib: results of a randomized trial. *J Natl Cancer Inst* 2007;99(7):545–557.

229. Alexandre L, Clark AB, Bhutta HY, et al. Statin use is associated with reduced risk of histologic subtypes of esophageal cancer: a nested case-control analysis. *Gastroenterology* 2014;146:661–668.

230. Agrawal S, Patel P, Agrawal A, et al. Metformin use and the risk of esophageal cancer in Barrett esophagus. *South Med J* 2014;17:774–779.

231. Morales TG, Bhattacharyya A, Johnson C, et al. Is Barrett's esophagus associated with intestinal metaplasia of the gastric cardia? *Am J Gastroenterol* 1997;92:1818–1822.

232. Geboes K. Barrett's esophagus: the metaplasia-dysplasia-carcinoma sequence: morphological aspects. *Acta Gastroenterol Belg* 2000;63:13–17.

233. Iijima K, Shimosegawa T. Involvement of luminal nitric oxide in the pathogenesis of the gastroesophageal reflux disease spectrum. *J Gastroenterol Hepatol* 2014;29:898–905.

234. Sheflin AM, Whitney AK, Weir TL. Cancer-promoting effects of microbial dysbiosis. *Curr Oncol Rep* 2014;16:406.

235. Koppert LB, Wijnhoven BP, van Dekken H, et al. The molecular biology of esophageal adenocarcinoma. *J Surg Oncol* 2005;92:169–190.

236. Brito MJ, Filipe MI, Linehan J, et al. Association of transforming growth factor alpha (TGFA) and its precursors with malignant change in Barrett's epithelium: biological and clinical variables. *Int J Cancer* 1995;60:27–32.

237. Soslow RA, Nabeya Y, Ying L, et al. Acidic fibroblast growth factor is progressively increased in the development of oesophageal glandular dysplasia and adenocarcinoma. *Histopathology* 1999;35:31–37.

238. Gibson MK, Abraham SC, Wu TT, et al. Epidermal growth factor receptor, P53 mutation, and pathological response predict survival in patients with locally advanced esophageal cancer treated with preoperative chemoradiotherapy. *Clin Cancer Res* 2003;9;6461–6438.

239. Hardwick RH, Shepherd NA, Moorghen M, et al. C-erbB-2 overexpression in the dysplasia/carcinoma sequence of Barrett's esophagus. *J Clin Pathol* 1995;48:129–132.

240. Walch A, Specht K, Braselmann H, et al. Coamplification and coexpression of GRB7 and ERBB2 is found in high grade intraepithelial neoplasia and in invasive Barrett's carcinoma. *Int J Cancer* 2004;112:747–753.

241. Brien TP, Odze RD, Sheehan CE, et al. HER-2/neu gene amplification by FISH predicts poor survival in Barrett's esophagus-associated adenocarcinoma. *Hum Pathol* 2000;31:35–39.

242. Tselepis C, Morris CD, Wakelin D, et al. Upregulation of the oncogene c-myc in Barrett's adenocarcinoma: Induction of c-myc by acidified bile acid in vitro. *Gut* 2003;52:174–180.

243. Barrett MT, Sanchez CA, Galipeau PC, et al. Allelic loss of 9p21 and mutation of the CDKN2/p16 gene develop as early lesions during neoplastic progression in Barrett's esophagus. *Oncogene* 1996;13:1867–1873.

244. Coppola D, Schreiber RH, Mora L, et al. Significance of Fas and retinoblastoma protein expression during the progression of Barrett's metaplasia to adenocarcinoma. *Ann Surg Oncol* 1999;6:298–304.

245. Bektas N, Donner A, Wirtz C, et al. Allelic loss involving the tumor suppressor genes APC and MCC and expression of the APC protein in the development of dysplasia and carcinoma in Barrett's esophagus. *Am J Clin Pathol* 2000;114:890–895.

246. Bailey T, Biddlestone L, Shepherd N, et al. Altered cadherin and catenin complexes in the Barrett's esophagus-dysplasia-adenocarcinoma sequence: correlation with disease progression and dedifferentiation. *Am J Pathol* 1998;152:135–144.

247. Hughes SJ, Nambu Y, Soldes OS, et al. Fas/APO-1 (CD95) is not translocated to the cell membrane in esophageal adenocarcinoma. *Cancer Res* 1997;57:5571.

248. Katada N, Hinder RA, Smyrk TC, et al. Apoptosis is inhibited early in the dysplasia-carcinoma sequence of Barrett esophagus. *Arch Surg* 1997;132:728–733.

249. Gimenez A, Minguela A, Parrilla P, et al. Flow cytometric DNA analysis and p53 protein expression show a good correlation with histologic findings in patients with Barrett's esophagus. *Cancer* 1998;83:641–651.

250. Barrett MT, Sanchez CA, Prevo LJ, et al. Evolution of neoplastic cell lineages in Barrett's oesophagus. *Nat Genet* 1999;22:106–109.

251. al-Kasspooles M, Moore JH, Orringer MB et al. Amplification and over-expression of the EGFR and erbB-2 genes in human esophageal adenocarcinomas. *Int J Cancer* 1993;54:213–219.

252. Lin L, Aggarwal S, Glover TW, et al. A minimal critical region of the 8p22–23 amplicon in esophageal adenocarcinomas defined using sequence tagged site-amplification mapping and quantitative polymerase chain reaction includes the GATA-4 gene. *Cancer Res* 2000;60:1341–1347.

253. Lin L, Prescott MS, Zhu Z, et al. Identification and characterization of a 19q12 amplicon in esophageal adenocarcinomas reveals cyclin E as the best candidate gene for this amplicon. *Cancer Res* 2000;60:7021–7027.

254. Fang M, Lew E, Klein M, et al. DNA abnormalities as marker of risk for progression of Barrett's esophagus to adenocarcinoma: Image cytometric DNA analysis in formalin-fixed tissues. *Am J Gastroenterol* 2004;99:1887–1894.

255. Reid BJ, Levine DS, Longton G, et al. Predictors of progression to cancer in Barrett's esophagus: baseline histology and flow cytometry identify low- and high-risk patient subsets. *Am J Gastroenterol* 2000;95:1669–1676.

256. Kawakami K, Brabender J, Lord RV, et al. Hypermethylated APC DNA in plasma and prognosis of patients with esophageal adenocarcinoma. *J Natl Cancer Inst* 2000;92:1805–1811.

257. Reid BJ, Haggitt RC, Rubin CE, et al. Observer variation in the diagnosis of dysplasia in Barrett's esophagus. *Hum Pathol* 1988;19:166–178.

258. Pohl H, Sirovich B, Welch HG. Esophageal adenocarcinoma incidence: are we reaching the peak? *Cancer Epidemiol Biomarkers Prev* 2010;19:1468–1470.

259. Dubecz A, Gall I, Solymosi N, et al.Temporal trends in long-term survival and cure rates in esophageal cancer: a SEER database analysis. *J Thorac Oncol* 2012;7(2):443–447.

260. Rice TW, Zuccaro G Jr, Adelstein DJ, et al. Esophageal carcinoma: depth of tumor invasion is predictive of regional lymph node status. *Ann Thorac Surg* 1998;65:787–792.

261. Dubecz A, Kern M, Solymosi N, et al. Predictors of lymph node metastasis in surgically resected T1 esophageal cancer. *Ann Thorac Surg* 2015;99(6):1879–1886.

262. Wang GQ, Jiao GG, Chang FB, et al. Long-term results of operation for 420 patients with early squamous cell esophageal carcinoma discovered by screening. *Ann Thorac Surg* 2004;7 7:1740–1744.

263. Lorenz D, Origer J, Pauthner M, et al. Prognostic risk factors of early esophageal adenocarcinomas. *Ann Surg* 2014;259:469–476.

264. Cen P, Banki F, Cheng L, et al. Changes in age, stage distribution, and survival of patients with esophageal adenocarcinoma over three decades in the United States. *Ann Surg Oncol* 2012;19(5):1685–1691.

265. Quint LE, Hepburn LM, Francis IR, et al. Incidence and distribution of distant metastases from newly diagnosed esophageal carcinoma. *Cancer* 1995;76:1120–1125.

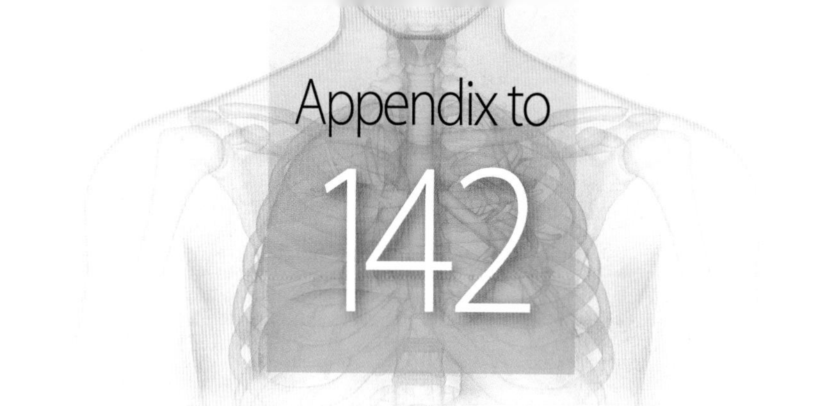

2009 AJCC/UICC Staging of Esophageal Cancer

Thomas W. Rice ▪ Valerie W. Rusch ▪ Eugene H. Blackstone

TABLE 142A.1 Summary of Changes in Anatomic Classifications and Additions of Nonanatomic Cancer Characteristics

Changes in Anatomic Classifications

T classification
  Tis is redefined and T4 is subclassified
  Tis   High-grade dysplasia
    T4a   Resectable cancer invades adjacent structures such as pleura, pericardium, diaphragm, etc.
    T4b   Unresectable cancer invades adjacent structures such as aorta, vertebral body, trachea, etc.

N classification
  Regional lymph node is redefined
  Any periesophageal lymph node from cervical lymph nodes
  N is subclassified
    N0   No regional lymph node metastases
    N1   1–2 positive regional lymph nodes
    N2   3–6 positive regional lymph nodes
    N3   ≥7 positive regional lymph nodes

M classification
  M is redefined
    M0   No distant metastases
    M1   Distant metastases

Additions of Nonanatomic Cancer Characteristics

Histopathologic cell type
  Adenocarcinoma
  Squamous cell carcinoma

Histologic grade
  G1   Well differentiated
  G2   Moderately differentiated
  G3   Poorly differentiated
  G4   Undifferentiated

Cancer location
  Upper thoracic   20–25 cm from incisors
  Middle thoracic   >25–30 cm from incisors
  Lower thoracic   >30–40 cm from incisors
  Esophagogastric junction   Includes cancers whose epicenter is in the distal thoracic esophagus, esophagogastric junction, or within the proximal 5 cm of the stomach (cardia) that extends into the esophagogastric junction or esophagus

Previous stage groupings of esophageal cancer were based on a simple, orderly arrangement of increasing anatomic T, then N, then M classifications.[1] These previous groupings are inconsistent with both the data and cancer biology.[2-7] Some explanations for the discrepancies relate to the interplay among TNM classifications, histopathologic type, biologic activity of the tumor (histologic grade, G), and cancer location. In contrast, the 2009 AJCC/UICC staging system is data-driven, based on a risk-adjusted random-survival forest analysis of worldwide data.[8,9] It accounts for interactions of anatomic and nonanatomic cancer characteristics.

In addition to creating a data-driven staging system, the AJCC Lung and Esophageal Task Force was charged with harmonizing the staging of cancer across the esophagogastric junction. The previous staging system produced different stage groupings for these cancers, depending on the use of either esophageal or gastric stage groupings. The 2009 AJCC/UICC staging system is for cancers of the esophagus and esophagogastric junction and includes cancer within the first 5 cm of the stomach that invade the esophagogastric junction (Siewert III).

TABLE 142A.2 Stage Groupings: Adenocarcinoma

Stage	T	N	M	G
0	is (HGD)	0	0	1
IA	1	0	0	1–2
IB	1	0	0	3
	2	0	0	1–2
IIA	2	0	0	3
IIB	3	0	0	Any
	1–2	1	0	Any
IIIA	1–2	2	0	Any
	3	1	0	Any
	4a	0	0	Any
IIIB	3	2	0	Any
IIIC	4a	1–2	0	Any
	4b	Any	0	Any
	Any	N3	0	Any
IV	Any	Any	1	Any

HGD, high-grade dysplasia.

TABLE 142A.3 Stage Groupings: Squamous Cell Carcinoma

Stage	T	N	M	G	Location
0	is (HGD)	0	0	1	Any
IA	1	0	0	1	Any
IB	1	0	0	2–3	Any
	2–3	0	0	1	Lower
IIA	2–3	0	0	1	Upper, middle
	2–3	0	0	2–3	Lower
IIB	2–3	0	0	2–3	Upper, middle
	1–2	1	0	Any	Any
IIIA	1–2	2	0	Any	Any
	3	1	0	Any	Any
	4a	0	0	Any	Any
IIIB	3	2	0	Any	Any
IIIC	4a	1–2	0	Any	Any
	4b	Any	0	Any	Any
	Any	N3	0	Any	Any
IV	Any	Any	1	Any	Any

HGD, high-grade dysplasia.

The analysis produced separate stage groupings for squamous cell carcinoma and adenocarcinoma. Histologic grade (G) was found to be an important nonanatomic cancer characteristic for early-stage grouping of both adenocarcinoma and squamous cell carcinoma.

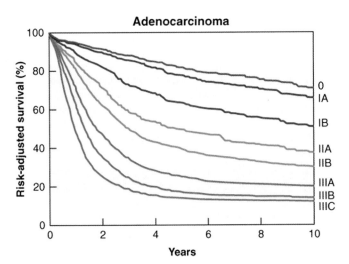

FIGURE 142A.1 Risk-adjusted survival for adenocarcinoma according to 2009 AJCC/UICC stage groups. (From DeVita VT Jr., Lawrence TS, Rosenberg SA. DeVita, Hellman, and Rosenberg's *Cancer: Principles & Practice of Oncology*. 10th ed. Philadelphia, PA: Wolters Kluwer Health; 2015.)

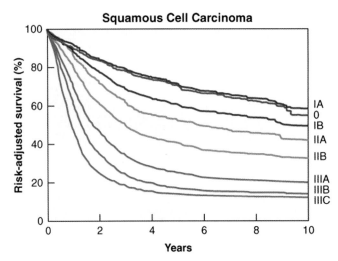

FIGURE 142A.2 Risk-adjusted survival for squamous cell carcinoma according to 2009 AJCC/UICC stage groups. (From DeVita VT Jr., Lawrence TS, Rosenberg SA. DeVita, Hellman, and Rosenberg's *Cancer: Principles & Practice of Oncology*. 10th ed. Philadelphia, PA: Wolters Kluwer Health; 2015.)

Cancer location, defined as the proximal tumor margin measured at esophagoscopy, was found to be a critical nonanatomic characteristic for squamous cell cancers. A summary of the changes in anatomic classifications and nonanatomic cancer characteristics is given in Table 142A.1. Stage groupings and corresponding risk-adjusted survival curves are presented in Tables 142A.2 and 142A.3 and Figures 142A.1 and 142A.2, respectively.

REFERENCES

1. *AJCC Cancer Staging Handbook*. 6th ed. Philadelphia, PA: Lippincott-Raven; 2002;3–8:91–103.
2. Bollschweiler E, Baldus SE, Schroder PM, et al. Staging of esophageal carcinoma: length of tumor and number of involved nodes. Are these independent prognostic factors? *J Surg Oncol* 2006;94(5):355–363.
3. Dickson GH, Singh KK, Escofet X, et al. Validation of a modified GTNM classification in peri-junctional oesophago-gastric carcinoma and its use as a prognostic indicator. *Eur J Surg Oncol* 2001;27(7):641–644.
4. Hofstetter W, Correa AM, Bekele N, et al. Proposed modification of nodal status in AJCC esophageal cancer staging system. *Ann Thor Surg* 2007;84(2):365–375.
5. Rice TW, Blackstone EH, Rybicki LA, et al. Refining esophageal cancer staging. *J Thorac Cardiovasc Surg* 2003;125(5):1103–1113.
6. Rizk N, Venkataraman E, Park B, et al. The prognostic importance of the number of involved lymph nodes in esophageal cancer: implications for revisions of the American Joint Committee on cancer staging system. *J Thorac Cardiovasc Surg* 2006;132(6):1374–1381.
7. Rusch VW. Should the esophageal cancer staging system be revised? *J Thorac Cardiovasc Surg* 2003;125(5):992–993.
8. *AJCC Cancer Staging Handbook*. 7th ed. New York: Elsevier (2014).
9. Rice TW, Rusch VW, Apperson-Hansen C, et al. Worldwide Esophageal Cancer Collaboration. *Dis Esophagus* 2009;22(1):1–8.

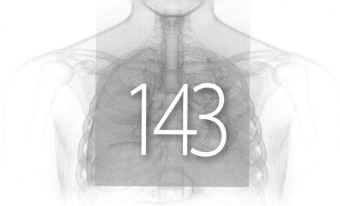

143

Staging of Esophageal Cancer

Mark Onaitis

MALIGNANT LESIONS OF THE ESOPHAGUS

The incidence of esophageal cancer is increasing, with an estimated 17,460 new cases in the United States in 2012.[1] Overall 5-year survival for patients with esophageal cancer remains poor, although some improvement has been achieved with an increase of 5-year survival from 5% to 17%–19% over the past four decades.[1-6] Because approximately 50% to 60% of patients with esophageal cancer present with incurable locally advanced or metastatic disease, prolonged progression-free survival is possible in only a few patients. Recent evidence suggests that induction chemoradiation treatment (CRT) followed by surgical resection is the optimal treatment for patients with locally advanced disease.[7-13] However, obtaining accurate pretreatment staging and then subsequently providing stage-appropriate treatment is crucial in optimizing esophageal cancer outcomes to avoid both inadequate and unnecessary treatment. The TNM staging system provided by the American Joint Committee on Cancer (AJCC) and the International Union Against Cancer (UICC) for esophageal cancer is an important guide for the grouping and subsequent treatment of esophageal cancer patients and is used throughout the world.

7TH EDITION OF THE AJCC/UICC TNM ESOPHAGEAL CANCER STAGING SYSTEM

The 7th and latest edition of the AJCC and the UICC TNM system was created in 2010. It is a data-driven system that was based on a risk-adjusted random-survival forest analysis of worldwide data. During this 7th edition, the writers analyzed the outcomes of 4,627 patients who underwent esophagectomy as sole treatment and found that in node-negative patients, prognosis was dependent on T status, histology, grade, and tumor location.[6,14,15] These findings led to the separation of the stage groupings according to esophageal cancer histology for the first time. It also led to the integration of grade into the adenocarcinoma and squamous cell cancer stage groupings while location was integrated into the squamous cell cancer stage grouping.

The new 7th edition bases nodal status on the number of positive lymph nodes which is a change from the prior edition which based nodal status on the location of these nodes. Several studies have revealed that the number of regional lymph nodes containing metastases is the most important prognostic factor in patients undergoing resection for esophageal cancer.[14-18] The change in nodal status definition will hopefully lead to more precise staging that is more closely associated with prognosis. The task force charged with updating the edition was also asked to work on harmonization of the esophageal and gastric cancer staging and thus in the 7th edition, tumors of the esophagogastric junction and proximal 5 cm of the stomach that extends into the GEJ or esophagus are classified and staged as esophageal cancers. All other tumors with an epicenter in the stomach >5 cm from the GEJ, or those within 5 cm of the GEJ without extension into the esophagus are staged as gastric cancers.

In the 7th edition, Tis (carcinoma in situ) was redefined as high-grade dysplasia and T4 was reclassified based on resectability of the involved structure(s), that is, T4a involves invasion of pleura, pericardium, diaphragm, etc., while T4b involves invasion of aorta, trachea, or vertebral body, etc. With all of the above changes, the 7th edition TNM system accounted for interactions of anatomic and nonanatomic cancer characteristics. It is hoped that these changes will lead to a better separation of prognostic groups for both histologies as determined by the T, N, and M categories at the time of initial diagnosis,[19] thus making clinical staging more impactful as it correlates more closely with prognosis. The tables depicting the TNM classification (Table 143.1), stage groupings for adenocarcinoma (Table 143.2), and stage groupings for squamous cell cancer (Table 143.3) are shown.[20]

PREOPERATIVE STAGING EVALUATION

The steps of staging in patients with esophageal cancer will be described in this text. Staging typically begins at the time of diagnosis of esophageal cancer and with evaluation by CT scan (CT) of the chest and abdomen.

CT SCAN

CTs of the chest and abdomen are obtained to evaluate the extent of the primary tumor and presence of distant metastatic disease. The extent of the tumor is determined by the preservation of the surrounding fat planes. Obliteration of these planes near the tumor suggests local invasion. In one study, when the nutritional status of a patient was adequate and the fat plane obliterated, the tumor extended to the adjacent structures in at least 90% of patients.[21] Only 21% of patients in whom fat planes were preserved had tumor extension beyond the esophageal wall. Although this observation suggests that CT is helpful in distinguishing T3 and T4 disease, Iyer and DuBrow[22] found that CT has an accuracy of only 59% to 82% in diagnosing mediastinal invasion.

TABLE 143.1 Summary of Changes in Anatomic Classifications and Additions of Nonanatomic Cancer Characteristics

Changes in Anatomic Classifications

T Classification

Tis is redefined and T4 is subclassified

Tis	High-grade dysplasia
T4a	Resectable cancer invades adjacent structures such as pleura, pericardium, diaphragm
T4b	Unresectable cancer invades adjacent structures such as aorta, vertebral body, trachea

N Classification

Regional lymph node is redefined
Any periesophageal lymph node from cervical nodes to celiac nodes

N is subclassified

N0	No regional lymph node metastases
N1	1 to 2 positive regional lymph nodes
N2	3 to 6 positive regional lymph nodes
N3	≥7 positive regional lymph nodes

M Classification

M is redefined

M0	No distant metastases
M1	Distant metastases

Additions of nonanatomic cancer characteristics

Histopathologic cell type
  Adenocarcinoma
  Squamous-cell carcinoma

Histologic grade

G1	Well differentiated
G2	Moderately differentiated
G3	Poorly differentiated
G4	Undifferentiated

Cancer location

Upper thoracic	20–25 cm from incisors
Middle thoracic	>25 to 30 cm from incisors
Lower thoracic	>30 to 40 cm from incisors
Esophagogastric junction	Includes cancers whose epicenter is in the distal thoracic esophagus, esophagogastric junction, or within the proximal 5 cm of the stomach (cardia) that extends into the esophagogastric junction or distal thoracic esophagus (Siewert III). These stomach cancers are stage grouped similarly to adenocarcinoma of the esophagus.

Sensitivity of CT for detecting abnormal lymph nodes (>1 cm) is 34% to 61% in the mediastinum and 50% to 76% in the abdomen.[23] Thompson and colleagues found that CT identified 69% of patients with positive subdiaphragmatic lymph node involvement. However, there was a 23% false-negative rate.[21] Reed and colleagues[24] suggested that CT may not be a sensitive imaging choice for evaluation of celiac nodes. Lowe and colleagues[25] found that local tumor staging was correctly predicted by CT in only 42% of patients.

CTs are also used to evaluate the presence of distant metastatic disease. In the detection of distant metastases, the sensitivity and specificity for CT were 52% and 91%, and for FDG-PET 71% and 93%, respectively.[26] The authors concluded that for the evaluation of distant metastases, FDG-PET has a higher sensitivity than CT.[26] Although CT is frequently the first modality used in staging patients,

TABLE 143.2 Adenocarcinoma Stage Groupings

Stage	T	N	M	G
0	is (HGD)	0	0	1
IA	1	0	0	1–2
IB	1	0	0	3
	2	0	0	1–2
IIA	2	0	0	3
IIB	3	0	0	Any
	1–2	1	0	Any
IIIA	1–2	2	0	Any
	3	1	0	Any
	4a	0	0	Any
IIIB	3	2	0	Any
IIIC	4a	1–2	0	Any
	4b	Any	0	Any
	Any	N3	0	Any
IV	Any	Any	1	Any

it has not been shown to be the best at determining either component of the TNM system. As above, PET is more sensitive in determining the M status and neither the depth of wall invasion nor the number of lymph nodes involved is well-evaluated on CT. Endoscopic ultrasound (EUS) is considered first-line for determining the T and N status in esophageal cancer patients.

ENDOSCOPIC ULTRASOUND

If the chest/abdomen CT has not shown metastatic disease then EUS should be performed to evaluate the depth of invasion and regional

TABLE 143.3 Squamous-Cell Carcinoma Stage Groupings

Stage	T	N	M	G	Location
0	is (HGD)	0	0	1	Any
IA	1	0	0	1	Any
IB	1	0	0	2–3	Any
	2–3	0	0	1	Lower
IIA	2–3	0	0	1	Upper, middle
	2–3	0	0	2–3	Lower
IIB	2–3	0	0	2–3	Upper, middle
	1–2	1	0	Any	Any
IIIA	1–2	2	0	Any	Any
	3	1	0	Any	Any
	4a	0	0	Any	Any
IIIB	3	2	0	Any	Any
IIIC	4a	1–2	0	Any	Any
	4b	Any	0	Any	Any
	Any	N3	0	Any	Any
IV	Any	Any	1	Any	Any

nodal status of patients with esophageal cancer. It is the most accurate technique for locoregional staging with an accuracy of 80% to 90% in T (tumor) and N (nodes) staging.[27,28] One study suggested that with less invasive disease, the accuracy can fall as low as 67%,[29] whereas a larger meta-analysis found that EUS was accurate for staging T1a and T1b tumors.[30] The authors found the sensitivity and specificity of EUS in the diagnosis of T1a tumors to be 85% and 87%, respectively. For T1b tumors, the sensitivity and specificity were both 86%. The overall accuracy of EUS was 81% for squamous cell carcinoma and 84% for adenocarcinoma.[30]

The EUS probe may be unable to traverse an area of stenosis or occlusion due to tumor, thus preventing the accurate assessment of the depth of tumor invasion and staging. Several options are available in this setting. Firstly, the area can be dilated with either Savary or pneumatic balloon dilation, however the perforation rate with this technique can be up to 24%.[31] Secondly, an ultrasound catheter that is 3 mm or less in diameter can be introduced through the biopsy channel to traverse the stricture. This option is limited by the depth of penetration that these small caliber catheters can visualize. Finally, wire-guided echoendoscopes are available and have increased the ability to stage stenotic lesions.[32]

When compared with CT, MRI, or PET, EUS consistently provides better tumor staging. van Vliet and colleagues[26] performed a meta-analysis determining the diagnostic performance of EUS, CT, and PET in the staging of esophageal cancer. For detection of celiac lymph node metastases by EUS, sensitivity and specificity were 85% and 96%, respectively and the sensitivity and specificity of EUS for other regional node metastases were 80% and 70%, respectively. For abdominal lymph node metastases detection by CT, these values were 42% and 93%, respectively, but was 50% and 83% for regional lymph nodes. The sensitivity and specificity for regional lymph node metastases were 57% and 85%, respectively for FDG-PET scanning. The authors concluded that EUS is most sensitive for the detection of regional lymph node metastases, whereas CT and FDG-PET are more specific tests.[26]

EUS FNA biopsy increases the accuracy of lymph node diagnosis beyond just EUS alone. The sensitivity, specificity, and accuracy of EUS FNA for locoregional lymph nodes are all over 85% compared to the gold standard of the surgical resection specimen or cytology results.[33–35] The sensitivity of EUS FNA for celiac lymph nodes was 88% to 100%.[24,34,36] FNA biopsy should be used in patients undergoing EUS who have suspicious nodes (>10 mm, hypoechoic, smooth border, or round) if the actual tumor will not be traversed during aspiration of the node.

ENDOSCOPIC RESECTION

As noted above, the accuracy in distinguishing T1a from T1b lesions by EUS is not 100%. The distinction between the two is critical, however, as T1a and T1b lesions are treated quite differently. Endoscopic resection (ER) is frequently definitive therapy for patients with T1a disease. The elevated risk of lymph node spread in patients with T1b disease limits the utility of ER as treatment in this cohort and surgical resection is typically recommended in those who are good operative candidates. Because treatment is very different based on whether the muscularis mucosa is invaded, ER can be considered to remove the tumor and precisely define the depth of invasion. The pathology result from the ER (particularly the presence or absence of lymphovascular invasion) can then be used to guide the final decision as to whether endoscopic therapy alone is sufficient or if surgery should be recommended.

POSTINDUCTION EUS STAGING

Many studies have shown that EUS is not an accurate means of determining response after chemotherapy or chemoradiation.[38,39] Zuccaro and colleagues[38] found that EUS correctly predicted a complete response to chemoradiotherapy in only 17% of patients. Another study by Sankaria and colleagues found that, in 118 patients no tumor was found on endoscopic biopsy after receiving cisplatin-based chemotherapy and 5,040 cGy of radiation. However, 69% of these patients were found to have local disease at esophagectomy, leading the authors to conclude that a negative endoscopic biopsy is not a useful predictor of a pathologic complete response after chemoradiation.[39] At this time, postinduction EUS staging is not standard practice.

PET

Positron emission tomography (PET) scans identify increased glycolysis using ^{18}F-fluorodeoxyglucose (^{18}F-FDG), which accumulates in 97% of esophageal adenocarcinomas.[40] However, like CT, PET cannot define the layers of the esophagus. This modality has been found to be 69% sensitive and 93% specific in identifying distant metastases, compared with CT, which was 46% sensitive and 74% specific.[41] PET can detect 15% to 20% additional metastases compared with CT scan.[42] Liberale and colleagues[43] found that the sensitivity, specificity, and accuracy of (PET) scanning was 38%, 81%, and 67%, respectively, for lymph node involvement detection and 88%, 88%, and 88%, respectively, for distant metastasis detection in patients with esophageal cancer. van Vliet and colleagues found similar results in a meta-analysis that looked at imaging techniques used to evaluate esophageal cancer.[26] The diagnostic accuracy of CT in determining resectability was 65%, compared with 88% with PET and 92% when both modalities were utilized.[42] PET also has the advantage of assessing the whole body as compared with conventional imaging, thus allowing for identification of distant metastatic disease at the initial evaluation.

It is important to note that Malik and colleagues[44] found that PET imaging had a high false-positive rate in regard to detection of metastatic disease in patients with esophageal cancer. Myers and colleagues of the American College of Surgeons Oncology Group (ACOSOG) Z0060 trial evaluated 189 patients with resectable esophageal cancer and studied the impact that PET had on these patients. In this study, patients with nonmetastatic potentially resectable esophageal cancer evident on CT of the chest and abdomen were randomly assigned to PET or no PET. The authors found that although 22% of eligible patients did not undergo esophagectomy, FDG-PET after standard clinical staging for esophageal carcinoma identified subsequently confirmed M1b disease in at least 4.8% of patients. Unconfirmed PET evidence of M1 disease and regional adenopathy (N1 disease) led to definitive nonsurgical or induction therapy in additional patients.[45] Overall, the authors found that PET usage was clearly favorable but that of the 35 lesions found to be suspicious for metastatic disease on PET (2 M1a, 33 M1b), 7 (20%) were found to be falsely positive by biopsy. The authors wrote that the risks and costs that characterize the burden of false positive results are likely underestimated.[45] Although imperfect, the addition of preoperative PET to the staging evaluation results in a change in management in up to 20% of patients with esophageal cancer.[19]

POSTINDUCTION PET STAGING

PET use for restaging after induction therapy is increasing in patients with locally advanced disease. A study suggests that whole-body PET/CT imaging detects distant metastases in approximately 8% of patients following induction chemoradiotherapy.[46] In addition to detecting otherwise occult metastatic disease, other data suggests that responses observed on PET scan during induction chemotherapy have significant predictive and prognostic benefit. PET-directed therapy for esophageal or GEJ cancer cannot be considered a standard approach as data is awaiting an upcoming US cooperative group trial (CALGB 80803) that will use the results of postinduction chemotherapy PET scan to determine the choice of the chemotherapy regimen during subsequent chemoradiotherapy, followed by surgery.

LAPAROSCOPY

As noted above, the staging of esophageal cancer is imprecise. In CALGB 9380, a prospective, multi-institutional study, Krasna and colleagues evaluated the feasibility and accuracy of thoracoscopic and laparoscopic staging in patients with esophageal cancer. They found that noninvasive tests (CT, MRI, and EUS) each incorrectly identified the stage as noted by missed positive or false-negative lymph nodes or metastatic disease found at thoracoscopic and laparoscopic staging in 50%, 40%, and 30% of patients, respectively. Median operating time was 210 minutes. Median postoperative hospital stay was 3 days. There were no deaths or major complications.[47] Krasna and colleagues[48] found thoracoscopy to be accurate in 93% and laparoscopy in 94% of patients in identifying metastatic disease. Six cases of unsuspected celiac nodal disease were identified in 19 patients despite preoperative CT and EUS. Similar results were confirmed by Luketich and colleagues[49] in 26 patients. Minimally invasive techniques changed the staging in 32% of patients.[50] Laparoscopy is also useful for identifying peritoneal metastases and was found to be 96% sensitive.

Laparoscopy alone is more effective in patients with adenocarcinoma than with squamous cell carcinoma of the esophagus. Stein and colleagues[51] found a 22% incidence of previously unidentified hepatic metastases and a 25% incidence of positive fluid cytology in patients with adenocarcinomas, whereas laparoscopy provided minimal additional information in the evaluation of patients with squamous cell tumors. Thoracoscopy through the right hemithorax, particularly in combination with laparoscopy, is of value in patients with both types of carcinoma.[42]

The need for diagnostic laparoscopy for patients who appear to have resectable adenocarcinoma of the distal esophagus is controversial and there is currently no consensus. Most patients will not have abnormalities found on laparoscopy that will change their course of treatment. The use of this more invasive staging technique will need to be considered on a case-by-case basis in patients with suspicion for peritoneal metastases.

CONCLUSIONS

Survival in patients with esophageal cancer remains quite low. Stage is the most important prognostic factor and therefore, appropriate staging is paramount for treatment selection and prognosis. The current 7th edition of the AJCC/UICC esophageal cancer staging manual is data-driven and will better help align stage with survival. EUS is the gold standard for T and N staging while PET provides the most accurate M staging. Surgical staging is becoming more useful, especially in those with suspected intraperitoneal metastases. The indications and limitations of both noninvasive and invasive staging techniques should be understood by clinicians caring for patients with esophageal cancer.

REFERENCES

1. Seigel R, Naishadham D, Jemal A. Cancer Statistics, 2013. *CA Journal Clin* 2013;63(1):11–30.
2. Dubecz A, Gall I, Solymosi N, et al. Temporal trends in long-term survival and cure rates in esophageal cancer: a SEER database analysis. *J Thorac Oncol* 2012;7:443–447.
3. Horner M, Ries L, Krapcho M, et al. *SEER Cancer Statistics Review, 1975–2006.* Bethesda, MD: National Cancer Institute; 2009. http://seer.cancer.gov/csr/1975_2006/ [based on November 2008 SEER data submission, posted to the SEER website].
4. Howlader N, Noone AM, Krapcho M, et al. *SEER Cancer Statistics Review, 1975–2008.* Bethesda, MD: National Cancer Institute; 2011. http://seer.cancer.gov/csr/1975_2008/ [based on November 2010 SEER data submission, posted to the SEER website].
5. Enzinger PC, Mayer RJ. Esophageal cancer. *N Engl J Med* 2003;349:2241–2252.
6. Rice TW, Rusch VW, Ishwaran H, et al. Cancer of the esophagus and esophago-gastric junction: Data-driven staging for the seventh edition of the American joint committee on cancer/international union against cancer staging manuals. *Cancer* 2010;116:3763–3773.
7. Worni M, Castleberry AW, Gloor B, et al. Trends and outcomes in the use of surgery and radiation for the treatment of locally advanced esophageal cancer: a propensity score adjusted analysis of the surveillance, epidemiology, and end results registry from 1998 to 2008. *Dis Esophagus* 2014;27:662–669.
8. Burmeister BH, Smithers BM, Gebski V, et al. Surgery alone versus chemoradiotherapy followed by surgery for resectable cancer of the oesophagus: a randomised controlled phase III trial. *Lancet Oncol* 2005;6:659–668.
9. Tepper J, Krasna MJ, Niedzwiecki D, et al. Phase III trial of trimodality therapy with cisplatin, fluorouracil, radiotherapy, and surgery compared with surgery alone for esophageal cancer: CALGB 9781. *J Clin Oncol* 2008;26:1086–1092.
10. Sjoquist KM, Burmeister BH, Smithers BM, et al. Survival after neoadjuvant chemotherapy or chemoradiotherapy for resectable oesophageal carcinoma: an updated meta-analysis. *Lancet Oncol* 2011;12:681–692.
11. Schwer AL, Ballonoff A, McCammon R, et al. Survival effect of neoadjuvant radiotherapy before esophagectomy for patients with esophageal cancer: a surveillance, epidemiology, and end-results study. *Int J Radiat Oncol Biol Phys* 2009;73:449–455.
12. Solomon N, Zhuge Y, Cheung M, et al. The roles of neoadjuvant radiotherapy and lymphadenectomy in the treatment of esophageal adenocarcinoma. *Ann Surg Oncol* 2010;17:791–803.
13. van Hagen P, Hulshof MC, van Lanschot JJ, et al. Preoperative chemoradiotherapy for esophageal or junctional cancer. *N Engl J Med* 2012;366:2074–2084.
14. Edge SB, Byrd DR, Compton CC, et al., eds. *American Joint Committee on Cancer Staging Manual.* 7th ed. New York: Springer; 2010:103.
15. Rice TW, Rusch VW, Ishwaran H, et al.; Worldwide Esophageal Cancer Collaboration. Cancer of the esophagus and esophagogastric junction: data-driven staging for the seventh edition of the American Joint Committee on Cancer/International Union Against Cancer cancer staging manuals. *Cancer* 2010;116(16):3763–3773.
16. Rizk NP, Venkatraman E, Park B, et al.; American Joint Committee on Cancer staging system. The prognostic importance of the number of involved lymph nodes in esophageal cancer: implications for revisions of the American Joint Committee on Cancer staging system. *J Thorac Cardiovasc Surg* 2006;132:1374–1381.
17. Mariette C, Piessen G, Briez N, et al. The number of metastatic lymph nodes and the ratio between metastatic and examined lymph nodes are independent prognostic factors in the esophageal cancer regardless of neoadjuvant chemoradiation or lymphadenectomy extent. *Ann Surg* 2008;247:365–371.
18. Hofstetter W, Correa AM, Bekele N, et al. Proposed modification of nodal status in AJCC esophageal cancer staging system. *Ann Thorac Surg* 2007;84:365–375.
19. Saltzman JR, Gibson MK. Diagnosis and staging of esophageal cancer. www.uptodate.com. Last visited 4/27/15.
20. Rice TW, Blackstone EH, Rusch VW. 7th edition of the AJCC cancer staging manual: Esophagus and esophagogastric junction. *Ann Surg Oncol* 2010;17:1721–1724.
21. Thompson WM, Halvorsen RA, Foster WL Jr, et al. Computed tomography for staging esophageal and gastroesophageal cancer: reevaluation. *AJR Am J Roentgenol* 1983;141:951–958.
22. Iyer R, DuBrow R. Imaging of esophageal cancer. *Cancer Imaging* 2004;4:125–132.
23. Saunders HS, Wolfman NT, Ott DJ. Esophageal cancer: radiologic staging. *Radiol Clin North Am* 1997;35:281–294.
24. Reed CE, Mishra G, Sahai AV, et al. Esophageal cancer staging: improved accuracy by endoscopic ultrasound of celiac lymph nodes. *Ann Thorac Surg* 1999;67:319–321; discussion 322.
25. Lowe VJ, Booya F, Fletcher JG, et al. Comparison of positron emission tomography, computed tomography, and endoscopic ultrasound in the initial staging of patients with esophageal cancer. *Mol Imaging Biol* 2005;7:422–430.

26. van Vliet EP, Jeijenbrok-Kal MJ, Hunink MG, et al. Staging investigations for oesophageal cancer: a meta-analysis. *Br J Cancer* 2008;98(3):547–557.

27. Rosch T. Endosonographic staging of esophageal cancer: a review of literature results. *Gastrointest Endosc Clin N Am* 1995;5:537–547.

28. Chandawarkar RY, Kakegawa T, Fujita H, et al. Endosonography for preoperative staging of specific nodal groups associated with esophageal cancer. *World J Surg* 1996;20:700–702.

29. Young PE, Gentry AB, Acosta RD, et al. Endoscopic ultrasound does not accurately stage early adenocarcinoma or high-grade dysplasia of the esophagus. *Clin Gastroenterol Hepatol* 2010;8:1037–1041.

30. Thosani N, Singh H, Kapadia A, et al. Diagnostic accuracy of EUS in differentiating mucosal versus submucosal invasion of superficial esophageal cancers: a systematic review and meta-analysis. *Gastrointest Endosc* 2012;75(2):242–253.

31. Van Dam J, Rice TW, Catalano MF, et al. High-grade malignant stricture is predictive of esophageal tumor stage. Risks of endosonographic evaluation. *Cancer* 1993;71:2910–2917.

32. Mallery S, Van Dam J. Increase rate of complete EUS staging of patients with esophageal cancer using the nonoptical, wire-guided echoendoscope. *Gastrointest Endosc* 1999;50:53–57.

33. Wiersema MJ, Vilmann P, Giovannini M, et al. Endosonography-guided fine-needle aspiration biopsy: diagnostic accuracy and complication assessment. *Gastroenterology* 1997;112:1087–1095.

34. Giovannini M, Seitz JF, Monges G, et al. Fine-needle aspiration cytology guided by endoscopic ultrasonography: results in 141 patients. *Endoscopy* 1995;27:171–177.

35. Eloubeidi MA, Wallace MB, Reed CE, et al. The utility of EUS and EUS-guided fine needle aspiration in detecting celiac lymph node metastasis in patients with esophageal cancer: a single-center experience. *Gastrointest Endosc* 2001;54:714–719.

36. Catalano MF, Alcocer E, Chak A, et al. Evaluation of metastatic celiac axis lymph nodes in patients with esophageal carcinoma: accuracy of EUS. *Gastrointest Endosc* 1999;50:352–356.

37. Wiersema MJ, Howell DA, Travis AC, eds. *Endoscopic ultrasound in esophageal carcinoma.* www.uptodate.com. Last visited April 29, 2015.

38. Zuccaro G Jr, Rice TW, Goldblum J, et al. Endoscopic ultrasound cannot determine suitability for esophagectomy after aggressive chemoradiotherapy for esophageal cancer. *Am J Gastroenterol* 1999;94:906–912.

39. Sankaria IS, Rizk NP, Bains MS, et al. Post-treatment endoscopic biopsy is a poor-predictor of pathologic response in patients undergoing chemoradiation therapy for esophageal cancer. *Ann Surg* 2009;249:764–767.

40. Luketich JD, Schauer PR, Meltzer CC, et al. Role of positron emission tomography in staging esophageal cancer. *Ann Thorac Surg* 1997;64:765–769.

41. Luketich JD, Friedman DM, Weigel TL, et al. Evaluation of distant metastases in esophageal cancer: 100 consecutive positron emission tomography scans. *Ann Thorac Surg* 1999;68:1133–1136.

42. Jasmine H, Mohammad B, Iannettoni MD. Carcinoma of the esophagus. In: Shields TW, ed. *General Thoracic Surgery.* 6th ed. Philadelphia, PA: Wolters Kluwer; 2009:1983–2015.

43. Liberale G, Van Laethem JL, Gay F, et al. The role of PET scan in the preoperative management of oesophageal cancer. *Eur J Surg Oncol* 2004;30:942–947.

44. Malik V, Keogan M, Gilham C, et al. FDG-PET Scanning in the management of cancer of the oesophagus and oesophagogastric junction: early experience with 100 consecutive cases. *Ir J Med Sci* 2006;174(4):48–54.

45. Myers BF, Downey RJ, Decker PA, et al. The utility of positron emission tomography in staging of potentially operable carcinoma of the thoracic esophagus: results of the American College of Surgeons Oncology Group Z0060 trial. *The J Thorac Card* 2007;133:738–745.

46. Bruzzi JF, Swisher SG, Truong MT, et al. Detection of interval distant metastases: clinical utility of integrated CT-PET imaging in patients with esophageal carcinoma after neoadjuvant therapy. *Cancer* 2007;109:125–134.

47. Krasna MJ, Reed CE, Nedzwiecki D, et al. CALGB 9380. A prospective trial of the feasibility of thoracoscopy/laparoscopy in staging esophageal cancer. *Ann Thorac Surg* 2001;71:1073–1079.

48. Krasna MJ, Flowers JL, Attar S, et al. Combined thoracoscopic/laparoscopic staging of esophageal cancer. *J Thorac Cardiovasc Surg* 1996;111:800–806.

49. Luketich JD, Schauer P, Landreneau R, et al. Minimally invasive surgical staging is superior to endoscopic ultrasound in detecting lymph node metastases in esophageal cancer. *J Thorac Cardiovasc Surg* 1997;114:817–821.

50. Luketich JD, Meehan M, Nguyen NT, et al. Minimally invasive surgical staging for esophageal cancer. *Surg Endosc* 2000;14:700–702.

51. Stein HJ, Kraemer SJ, Feussner H, et al. Clinical value of diagnostic laparoscopy with laparoscopic ultrasound in patients with cancer of the esophagus or card. *J Gastrointest Surg* 1997;1:167.

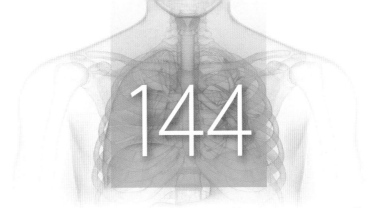

144

Multimodality Therapy for Esophageal Cancer

Abby White ▪ Scott J. Swanson

Radical resection has been part of the standard of care for esophageal cancer for decades; yet the incidence of local and distant treatment failures have propelled vast amounts of research in complimentary therapies. Because of the tendency to spread systemically early in the disease course, chemotherapeutic agents have been the focus of many studies, while radiotherapy approaches have been employed to decrease tumor bulk and burden. Although overall survival rates remain below 20%, long-term survival is improving for those with early or locally advanced disease, in the era of multimodality therapy.[1]

Until 2000, the only U.S. Food and Drug Administration (FDA)-approved agents for the treatment of gastrointestinal (GI) cancers included platinums (cisplatin, carboplatin), anthracyclines (doxorubicin, epirubicin), and pyrimidine analogs (5-fluorouracil [5-FU]). In the early 2000s, oxaliplatin, which is a third-generation platinum, and capecitabine, a newer version of 5-FU, emerged with similar efficacy and improved toxicity profiles. Taxanes (docetaxel, paclitaxel), so named for their derivation from plants of the genus Taxus (yews), first became FDA approved in 2007 for the treatment of upper GI tumors. This came after the success of taxanes in advanced breast, lung, and prostate cancer.[2]

Advances in radiotherapy have made neoadjuvant and adjuvant treatment of upper GI tumors more tolerable as well. Intensity-modulated radiation therapy (IMRT) is a newer, more precise method of delivery for radiation that uses computerized linear accelerators to deliver the dose in a manner such that the dose is conformed (or modulated) to the three-dimensional (3D) aspects of the tumor. This allows higher radiation doses to be focused to regions within the tumor while minimizing the dose to surrounding vital structures, as is particularly important with the thoracic esophagus and its proximity to mediastinal structures and the lungs.

Minimally invasive approaches to esophageal resection, as described in prior chapters, have increased the spectrum of patients able to undergo surgical treatment of esophageal cancers. While maintaining oncologic principles, many centers have been able to minimize pain, improve early mobility, and shorten hospital stay with laparoscopic and thoracoscopic approaches to resection.

Without a doubt, lessons learned from decades of care and research have informed current strategies in management and made esophageal cancer treatment an excellent example of evidence-based multidisciplinary care. What follows is a review of the data that brought us here.

STAGING

The revised 2010 AJCC[3] staging classification is based on data provided by the Worldwide Esophageal Cancer Collaboration (WECC), which contains data for 4,627 patients who were treated with surgery alone without pre- or postoperative therapy. It is discussed in greater detail in the preceding chapter; however, the authors wish to emphasize that outcomes may correlate with the clinical stage at the time of diagnosis, but the clearest correlation with survival is associated with surgical pathologic staging.

APPROACHES TO TREATMENT

EARLY STAGE ESOPHAGEAL CANCER

Although a detailed review of Barrett esophagus with and without dysplasia and mucosal-based cancers is beyond the scope of this chapter, the authors wish to note major advances in the treatment of early stage esophageal cancer in the last decade. Endomucosal resection (EMR) and endoscopic ablation are recommended as effective therapies for tumors invading the lamina propria and muscularis mucosa.[4] Successful endoscopic treatment programs for early esophageal cancer must involve meticulous pathologic review, in-depth patient education and commitment to surveillance endoscopies, and further therapies. No randomized studies have compared EMR and endoscopic ablative therapies to surgery, but a large retrospective analysis of the Surveillance, Epidemiology, and End Results (SEER) database reviewed all patients who underwent surgery or endoscopic therapy for T1N0 esophageal cancer.[5] Patients treated with endoscopic therapy had better cancer-specific survival and overall survival was equivalent. Endoscopic therapy is recommended for patients with early stage cancer because the risk of lymph node involvement, local recurrence, and cancer-related death is low following treatment. Patients with any involvement of the submucosa (T1b), tumor size >2 cm, or poor differentiation should be considered for esophagectomy.[4,6]

Clinical staging of esophageal cancer has improved with positron-emission tomography/computed tomography (PET/CT) and endoscopic ultrasound imaging (EUS). Yet, small single-center studies have questioned the reliability of clinical staging of T2N0 esophageal cancer, and management controversies abound. In studies specifically examining cT2N0M0 tumors, Rice et al.[7] and Zhang et al.[8] observed 13% and 28% accuracy for EUS, respectively. A broader review of the Society of Thoracic Surgeons, General Thoracic Database, was published in 2012.[9] Of 482 clinically staged T2N0 patients who went directly to surgical intervention, only 27% were confirmed as pathologic T2N0, 26% were downstaged and 47% were upstaged on pathologic review. The majority of patients upstaged were due to the identification of occult nodal disease, with exclusive tumor upstaging (T status) being in the minority. Given the high incidence of occult nodal disease and the unreliability of clinical staging of T2N0 disease, some authors have advocated for routine administration of induction therapy in this population and in fact, there is an increasing trend of patients with clinical T2N0 esophageal cancer receiving neoadjuvant therapy. Such a broad application of induction therapy will inevitably result in a percentage of patients being "overtreated" with induction therapy, and future studies will help to delineate whether the consequences of induction therapy in this subset outweigh the associated morbidity and cost.

LOCALLY ADVANCED ESOPHAGEAL CANCER: NEOADJUVANT THERAPIES

Neoadjuvant Radiation

A meta-analysis published from the Cochrane Library in 2005 reviewed five randomized controlled trials, including a total of 1,147 patients and providing the most comprehensive evaluation of preoperative radiotherapy to date.[10] The majority of the patients included in these studies had squamous cell carcinoma. Each of the trials compared neoadjuvant radiotherapy followed by surgery to surgery alone. The overall hazard ratio (HR) was 0.89 and the authors concluded that neoadjuvant radiotherapy confers a modest survival

benefit, reducing the mortality rate by 11% and improving the absolute survival at 2 years from 30% to 34%. It should be noted that the majority of these studies were enrolled more than 20 years prior to the meta-analysis, and though careful review and updating of survival data was accomplished, these patients were staged in the era prior to EUS and PET CT. In addition, the timing to surgery was inconsistent among the various trials and the anticipated improvement in resectability was not seen. Currently, neoadjuvant radiation alone prior to surgery is not recommended outside the context of a clinical trial, or clinical circumstances that make individual patients poor candidates for combined chemoradiation (e.g., prior chemotherapy).

Neoadjuvant Chemotherapy

Early controversy surrounding the efficacy of radiation therapy in esophageal and gastric cancers ignited numerous investigations into the efficacy of preoperative chemotherapy as an adjunct to surgery.[11–20] Several randomized controlled trials examined this treatment approach, and are summarized in Table 144.1. Four trials demonstrated survival benefit for patients undergoing combined preoperative chemotherapy followed by surgery versus surgery alone.[15–17,19] The largest enrolled study was from the United Kingdom and involved 802 patients, with mixed adenocarcinoma and squamous cell histology. Survival at 5 years in the combined-modality arm was 23% versus 17% in the surgery-alone cohort.[15] The more recent, and widely cited, MAGIC study was published in 2006, but included only patients with adenocarcinoma, of which only 25% were distal esophageal or GE junction cancers.[16] A total of 502 patients were randomized and significant downstaging was noted in patients following chemotherapy. Combined-modality therapy in the MAGIC study involved preoperative *and* postoperative chemotherapy; yet only 50% of patients were able to complete the prescribed

TABLE 144.1 Randomized Trials Comparing Preoperative Chemotherapy to Surgery Alone

Study	n	Publication Year	Histology	Treatment Mortality (Preop Chemo/Surgery Alone) (%)	Chemo Response Rate (%)	Survival of Responders	p Value	Notes
Schlag et al.[11]	46	1992	SCC	19/10	50	13 mo vs. 5 mo	ns	
Maipang et al.[12]	46	1994	SCC	20/NR	53	NR	ns	
Law et al.[13]	147	1997	SCC	8/8	58	42 mo vs. 8 mo	ns	
Ancona et al.[14]	96	2001	SCC	4/4	40	53 mo vs. 19 mo	ns	
Allum et al.[15]	**802**	**2002**	**67% AC**	**10/10**	**NR**	**NR**	**0.03**	**Follow-up data published in 2009**
Cunningham et al.[16] (MAGIC)	**503**	**2006**	**AC**	**14/15**	**NR**	**NR**	**0.009**	**Only 25% distal esophagus and GEJ tumors**
Ychou et al.[17]	**224**	**2006**	**AC**	**NR**	**NR**	**NR**	**0.02**	**75% of tumors were distal esophagus and GEJ**
Kelsen et al.[18] (RTOG)	216	2007	52% AC	NR	19	3.3 yrs vs. 1.1 yrs	ns	
Boonstra et al.[19] (MRC)	**169**	**2011**	**SCC**	**5/4**	**38**	**NR**	**0.03**	

adjuvant therapy. Five-year overall survival was significantly higher in the chemotherapy arm compared to surgery alone (36% vs. 23%).[16] A similar study, published by Ychou et al., was published the same year and included 224 patients with adenocarcinoma, 75% of which were distal esophageal or GE junction tumors. In this study, preoperative chemotherapy followed by surgery conferred a 38% versus 24% 5-year survival advantage. Similarly, only 50% of patients completed adjuvant treatment.[17] While many of the early studies examining preoperative chemotherapy did not reach statistical significance, these trials mainly included patients with squamous cell histology only. Though many of the investigations which included subgroup analyses of responders to chemotherapy defined "responders" differently, undeniably the results indicated that patients with some measurable response to the therapy had significantly improved survival (Table 144.1).

Three meta-analyses were published between 2007 and 2011 to determine the survival benefit of neoadjuvant chemotherapy for esophageal cancer.[20–22] Gebski et al. reviewed eight trials, which included 1,724 patients and showed a significant reduction in mortality for neoadjuvant chemotherapy (HR 0.90, $p = 0.01$). While the analysis included patients with both squamous cell and adenocarcinoma, the survival benefit was exclusive to adenocarcinoma.[20] The meta-analysis by Kranzfelder et al.[21] included only patients with squamous cell carcinoma from eight randomized trials and did not demonstrate any benefit to preoperative chemotherapy. Sjoquist et al.[22] reviewed nine randomized trials, including 1,981 patients and showed an absolute 2-year survival benefit of 7% with neoadjuvant chemotherapy (HR 0.87, $p = 0.01$), but again, only for patients with adenocarcinoma.

Neoadjuvant Chemoradiotherapy

Citing the synergistic effects of chemotherapy and radiation, and noting the challenges of completing adjuvant therapy as evidenced in the MAGIC[16] and other trials like it,[23] preoperative combined chemoradiation has been extensively studied.

Numerous phase III trials have compared preoperative concurrent chemoradiation therapy to surgery alone for patients with esophageal cancer. An Irish study, published in 1996, examined patients treated with induction chemoradiation therapy consisting of 5-FU, cisplatin, and 40 Gy plus surgery over resection alone. A modest survival benefit was found for multimodal treatment, although the survival in the surgery-alone group was very low and bring into question the reliability of the overall conclusion. A French multicenter prospective randomized trial, published in 1997, in which preoperative combined chemotherapy (i.e., cisplatin)

and radiation therapy (37 Gy) followed by surgery was compared to surgery alone in patients with squamous cell carcinoma, showed no improvement in OS and a significantly higher postoperative mortality (12% vs. 4%) in the combined-modality arm.[24] Dr. Orringer's group at the University of Michigan randomized 100 patients (75% of which had adenocarcinoma) to surgery alone or preoperative 5-FU, cisplatin, vinblastine, and radiation therapy to a total of 45 Gy. Their results were published in 2001 and with a median follow-up of more than 8 years, there was no significant difference between the surgery-alone and combined-modality therapy with respect to median survival (17.6 vs. 16.9 months), overall survival (16% vs. 30% at 3 years), or disease-free survival (16% vs. 28% at 3 years); however, the study was powered only to detect a substantial survival benefit (1 year) over surgery alone.[25] The CALGB led an Intergroup trial which compared surgery alone to preoperative cisplatin, 5-FU, and 50.4 Gy followed by resection.[26] Resection via left chest or Ivor-Lewis (right chest and abdomen) was recommended for midesophageal and GE junction cancers. The study was slated for 475 patients, but after 3 years (1997–2000), only 56 patients had been accrued and the trial was closed, citing physician biases and patient preferences as the reasons for difficulty in accrual. Nonetheless, the group published. The results of the 56 randomized patients were published in 2008 following a median 6-year follow-up and demonstrated a benefit in overall survival (39% vs. 16%) and progression-free survival with trimodality therapy. There was no indication that operative mortality was increased by the use of trimodality therapy, and the preoperative treatment was accomplished with reasonable toxicity.[26]

Several meta-analyses were published between 2003 and 2011 to determine the survival benefit of neoadjuvant chemotherapy or chemoradiotherapy prior to resection over surgery alone, summarized in Table 144.2. The largest and most quoted of those studies were published by Gebski et al.[20] in 2007 and Sjoquist et al.[22] in 2011. Gebski et al. reviewed 10 chemoradiation studies and 8 chemotherapy studies and found a survival benefit for both chemoradiation and chemotherapy as neoadjuvant treatment strategies. Sjoquist reviewed 12 chemoradiotherapy studies and 9 chemotherapy-only studies and published statistically significant HRs favoring multimodality treatment as well.

Published in 2012, the Dutch CROSS[27] trial has shaped the way many are treating esophageal cancer at centers worldwide. The study randomly assigned 366 patients with resectable esophageal or junctional cancers to receive either surgery-alone or weekly administration of carboplatin and paclitaxel with concurrent radiation therapy (41.4 Gy in 23 fractions) administered over 5 weeks, followed by resection. Seventy-five percent of patients enrolled had adenocarcinoma,

TABLE 144.2 Meta-analyses of Preoperative Chemotherapy or Chemoradiation Versus Surgery Alone

Study	n	Publication Year	Therapy	Number of Studies	HR	p Value
Urschel and Vasan[28]	1,116	2003	CRT	9	0.66	0.016
Fiorica et al.[29]	764	2004	CRT	6	0.53	0.03
Greer et al.[30]	738	2005	CRT	6	0.86	0.07
Gebski et al.[20]	CRT 1,209/ Chemo 1,724	2007	CRT/Chemo	CRT 10/Chemo 8	CRT 0.81/ Chemo 0.90	CRT 0.002/ Chemo 0.05
Jin et al.[31]	1,308	2009	CRT	11	1.46	0.02
Kranzfelder et al.[21] (100% SCC)	CRT 1,099/ Chemo 1,707	2011	CRT/Chemo	CRT 9/Chemo 8	CRT 0.81/ Chemo 0.93	CRT 0.008/ Chemo 0.368
Sjoquist et al.[22]	CRT 1,854/ Chemo 1,981	2011	CRT/Chemo	CRT 12/Chemo 9	CRT 0.78/ Chemo 0.87	CRT <0.0001/ Chemo 0.005

and the majority of tumors were in the distal esophagus and GE junction. With a median follow-up of 45 months, preoperative chemoradiation was found to improve median overall survival from 24 months in the surgery-alone group to 49.4 months (HR = 0.657, p = 0.03). Of particular interest to surgeons, preoperative chemoradiation improved the rate of R0 resections (defined as no tumor within 1 mm of resection margins) and a pathologic complete response (pCR) was noted in 29% of chemoradiation patients. Of note, 91% of patients completed the prescribed chemotherapy and 92% of patients completed the prescribed radiation therapy, with few serious side effects.[27]

Patients in the chemoradiotherapy followed by surgery group underwent surgery as soon as possible after completion of chemoradiotherapy (preferably, within 4 to 6 weeks), whereas the surgery-alone group underwent resection immediately following randomization. The median time to resection from chemoradiation was 6.6 weeks. A transthoracic approach with two-field lymph node dissection was performed for tumors extending proximal to the carina. A transhiatal esophagectomy was performed for tumors at the GE junction, though there was some flexibility in the approach across centers, based on surgeon experience and preference. The preferred method of restoring continuity was a cervical anastomosis. Postoperative complications and mortality were equivalent between the two treatment arms. Complete remission in both the primary tumor and the lymph nodes (ypT0N0) was the best possible pathologic outcome of chemoradiotherapy. The observed percentage of patients with a pathologic complete response (29%) is in line with the reported percentages in other phase III studies. An R0 resection was achieved in 148 of 161 patients (92%) in the chemoradiotherapy–surgery group, as compared with 111 of 161 (69%) in the surgery group (P < 0.001).[27] While results of earlier randomized trials and meta-analyses conflicted, those employing updated staging techniques and newer, less toxic chemotherapy and radiotherapy strategies have demonstrated a survival benefit. Chemoradiation followed by surgery is the standard treatment option for patients with locally advanced esophageal cancer.

LOCALLY ADVANCED ESOPHAGEAL CANCER: ADJUVANT THERAPIES

Adjuvant Chemotherapy

Adjuvant chemotherapy is traditionally recommended only for patients with positive lymph nodes. Studies that have included adjuvant chemotherapy after neoadjuvant chemotherapy and/or surgery, such as the MAGIC trial,[16] have noted that only 50% complete their intended postoperative therapy.

A few trials have evaluated adjuvant chemotherapy only. Published in 1996, a Japanese Oncology Group (JCOG) study by Ando randomized 205 patients with squamous cell cancer to surgery alone or surgery followed by cisplatin and vindesine. There was no statistical significance in 5-year survival rates between the two groups.[32] A follow-up study by the same group in 2003 evaluated postoperative cisplatin and 5-FU, again in patients with squamous cell cancer only, and found a modest improvement in survival with the adjuvant therapy group (61% vs. 52%) that did not reach statistical significance.[33]

A more recent JCOG study, published in 2012, compared neoadjuvant to adjuvant chemotherapy in patients with esophageal squamous cancer and found a significant survival benefit to adjuvant chemotherapy, albeit less than the benefit accrued by the preoperative group. Overall 5-year survival rates were 55% in the preoperative group and 43% in the postoperative therapy group.[34]

The use of adjuvant therapy after esophagectomy for adenocarcinoma is less well characterized, and the National Comprehensive

Care Network (NCCN) guideline recommendations are based on trials which predominately included patients with gastric and not esophageal and GE junction cancers.[4] For instance, the Southwest Oncology Group (SWOG)-led Intergroup trial, published in 2001, included 556 patients, of which only 20% had proximal stomach or GE junction tumors. Postoperative chemoradiation was offered to patients with tumors T1 or higher, regardless of nodal stage. In this study, patients given adjuvant treatment with 5-FU and leucovorin plus 45 Gy radiotherapy, experienced a statistically significant 5-year survival benefit compared to those who underwent surgery alone (50% vs. 41%). There were less local failures in the multimodality group, even though only 64% of patients prescribed adjuvant chemoradiation were able to complete the therapy and hematologic and GI toxicities were common.[35] Retrospective analyses of the data have yielded survival benefits in patients with node-positive gastroesophageal cancer. Median survival was improved by 10 months in the subset of patients who received adjuvant chemoradiation, and 3-year disease-free survival was improved in node-positive patients who underwent adjuvant treatment versus surgery alone (37% vs. 24%).[35] The results of the SWOG trial have set the standard of care in patients with completely resected gastric or GE junction who did not receive neoadjuvant therapy.

Extrapolating data from adjuvant studies of gastric adenocarcinoma is likely valid when considering the biology of disease relative to GE junction and gastric adenocarcinomas. However, the ability to tolerate adjuvant therapy following esophageal reconstruction versus gastric resection and reconstruction may differ significantly. A retrospective database review was recently published which attempts to specifically address those concerns. Speicher et al.[36] reviewed the National Cancer Database to evaluate adjuvant chemotherapy following esophagectomy for adenocarcinoma in node-positive patients who did not receive preoperative treatment. The study included 1,694 patients, 51.6% of which received adjuvant chemotherapy. Patients given adjuvant chemotherapy exhibited improved 5-year survival (24.2 vs. 14.9%, p = <0.001), although adjuvant radiation (70.7% of patients) did not improve survival. Older age, longer travel distance to a cancer center, and complications related to surgery (length of stay greater than 20 days or unplanned readmission with 30 days), correlated with the failure to receive adjuvant chemotherapy. Although complications related to surgery were associated with worse survival and lower chance of receiving adjuvant chemotherapy, those that ultimately recovered and went on to postoperative treatment, experienced improved survival.[36] This study suggests that even those patients who do not experience a straightforward postoperative course will benefit from adjuvant chemotherapy once they have recovered.

The efficacy of adjuvant chemotherapy for node-positive esophageal adenocarcinoma has not been proven in randomized controlled trials, but continues to be recommended as the standard of care in the NCCN guidelines.[4] In contrast, patients with esophageal squamous cell cancer who undergo R0 resection, regardless of nodal status, are designated for surveillance only. Postoperative therapies for patients with squamous cell carcinoma are considered only for positive resection margins (R1 or higher). Future studies may help delineate the survival benefits of adjuvant chemotherapy and/or chemoradiotherapy.

LOCALLY ADVANCED ESOPHAGEAL CANCER: ROLE OF SURGERY

Esophageal resection was one of the operations identified in a 2002 study published in the *New England Journal of Medicine*, which demonstrated a correlation between hospital volume and surgical mortality by analyzing Medicare databases.[37] Mortality ranged from the single digits at high-volume centers to above 20% at low volume centers, drawing attention to regionalized care by experienced surgeons for what was traditionally considered a quite morbid procedure. Since then, other surgeons have published data which clearly delineates reduced morbidity and mortality associated with less invasive approaches.[38–40] Most recently, a prospective randomized trial supported by the Eastern Cooperative Oncology Group (ECOG) demonstrated 2.1% mortality with reasonable morbidity in 104 patients undergoing minimally invasive esophagectomy. The trial authors conducted site and surgeon credentialing to ensure quality and consistency in the surgical approach and that oncologic outcomes were acceptable at a median follow-up of 36 months.[41] Analysis of Medicare databases reviewed national trends in esophagectomy in the era after the *New England Journal of Medicine* article was published and found that just over 30% of esophagectomies had moved to high-volume centers with an associated 11% decrease in surgical mortality.[42]

The extent of lymphadenectomy during esophagectomy has significant prognostic implications, as both the absolute number and the ratio of positive lymph nodes in a given specimen correlate with survival. As pointed out by a query of the National Cancer Database, the absolute number of lymph nodes examined is confounded by the total number of lymph nodes removed, and fewer than one-third of hospitals in the United States were meeting national standards as of 2012.[43] Greenstein and Swanson published an analysis of over 800 esophagectomy patients from the SEER database. Patients were classified into three groups by the ratio of positive-to-total number of lymph nodes removed and esophageal cancer-specific survival was compared among these groups. Higher lymph node ratio among patients with node-positive esophageal cancer was demonstrated to be associated with significantly worse survival ($p <0.001$).[44] The total number of lymph nodes needed to assure accurate staging and prognosticating is not known, but evidence continues to suggest that more is better, and current NCCN guidelines suggest at least 15 lymph nodes be evaluated.[4] However, a second SEER analysis by Greenstein and Swanson suggested that even in patients with node-negative disease, the number of negative lymph nodes correlated with survival. In their analysis, node-negative esophageal cancer patients with 18 or more lymph nodes demonstrated a 20% improvement in 5-year disease-specific survival compared to node-negative patients with 10 or less lymph nodes evaluated (75% vs. 55%, respectively).[45] Thus, since a higher number of negative lymph nodes is independently associated with higher disease-specific survival, more really is better when it comes to lymphadenectomy during esophagectomy for esophageal cancer.

LOCALLY ADVANCED ESOPHAGEAL CANCER: DEFINITIVE CHEMORADIATION

In addition to controlling micrometastatic disease, chemotherapy is thought to sensitize tumor cells to radiation. Therefore, patients ineligible for surgery have been studied in the context of combined chemoradiotherapy as definitive treatment for esophageal cancer. A Cochrane Database review of 19 randomized trials, comparing chemoradiation to radiation alone, was published in 2006 by Wong and Malthaner.[46] There was a reduction in mortality and in local recurrence rates, but these came at the cost of significant toxicities. An ECOG trial evaluated mitomycin-C and 5-FU with radiation compared to radiation alone and noted a median survival of 14.5 months compared to 9.2 months in the radiation-alone group.

Given the success of an earlier ECOG trial for squamous cell cancer of the anus using the same regimen, all patients in this study had squamous cell cancer. The results of this trial were replicated by the Radiation Therapy Oncology Group (RTOG) using cisplatin and 5-FU, without the mitomycin-C. Yet despite the overall survival benefit, a local failure rate of 47% was noted leading to the RTOG INT 0123 trial, designed to evaluate whether increased radiation doses would affect local control. The phase III study compared 50.4 Gy versus 64.8 Gy radiation doses along with the aforementioned chemotherapy regimen. There was no significant difference in median survival, 2-year survival, or local/regional failure between the high-dose and standard-dose arms. As such, 50.4 Gy continues to be the standard delivered dose of radiation.

Analyzed in the context of today's standards, the above trials have several limitations. The majority of the patients had squamous cell carcinoma. The patients were enrolled in the era prior to EUS or PET and were treated using two-dimensional (2D) treatment planning with simple esophograms and chest x-rays, significantly different from 3D and four-dimensional (4D) image-guided techniques, fiducial placement for live tumor marking, and tumor volume calculations employed more commonly today. Without PET scans, it is unclear how many patients may have had metastatic disease and would likely be excluded from current studies. There may be a role for an updated look at dose escalation studies in the era of PET, EUS, and advanced radiation techniques. At present, the RTOG data provides the foundation for the dosages used in practice today.

LOCALLY ADVANCED ESOPHAGEAL CANCER: ROLE OF TARGETED THERAPIES

Human epidermal growth factor-2 (HER2) is a well-known molecular target in breast cancer and there is a significant body of evidence that HER2 is an important biomarker and key driver of tumorigenesis. As such, HER2 has been extensively studied in gastric and GE junction adenocarcinoma. Trastuzumab, a monoclonal antibody that targets HER2, has shown a survival advantage in early and metastatic breast cancer and is now the standard of care. The ToGA trial,[47] published in 2010, is the first randomized phase III trial to evaluate the efficacy of trastuzumab in HER2 positive gastric and GE junction adenocarcinoma. The study included 594 patients with HER2 positivity and locally advanced, recurrent, or metastatic gastric or GE junction adenocarcinoma. The patients in the study were randomized to standard chemotherapy alone or chemotherapy plus trastuzumab. The majority of patients had gastric cancer (80%); the results demonstrated a significant improvement in median overall survival with the addition of trastuzumab (13.8 vs. 11 months, $p = 0.046$). It is important to note that encouraging results are limited to patients with tumors who were fluorescence in situ hybridization (FISH) positive or had immunohistochemistry scores of 2 or 3+. Weakly HER2-positive patients did not derive benefit.

An additional monoclonal antibody targeting vascular endothelial growth factor receptor (VEGFR), ramucirumab, has also demonstrated some viability in patients with previously treated advanced or metastatic gastric and GE junction cancers. The REGARD international phase III trial[48] demonstrated a survival benefit for patients who failed first-line chemotherapy and thus ramucirumab is FDA approved for the treatment of patients with advanced GE junction adenocarcinoma refractory to first-line chemotherapy. Hypertension was an associated complication noted in the ramucirumab group. Other targets and agents are under investigation and results of ongoing trials will shed more light on the role of targeted therapy for esophageal cancer.

CONCLUSIONS

Improvements in the tolerance profiles of chemotherapeutic agents, adaptations to surgical technique, and modifications in the delivery of radiation therapy are making treatment increasingly tolerable to a wider range of patients with esophageal cancer and have set the standard of care for multimodality therapy worldwide. With careful patient selection, endoscopic therapies are effective for early-stage disease. Controversy surrounds clinical T2N0 esophageal cancer, but available data suggests neoadjuvant therapy improves survival and ongoing research will continue to inform current strategies. The best opportunity for cure in locally advanced esophageal cancer is offered by induction chemoradiotherapy followed by surgery. No specific surgical approach is supported by national guidelines; however, evidence clearly delineates reduced morbidity and mortality associated with less invasive approaches, and equivalent oncologic outcomes when compared to open procedures. Thorough lymphadenectomy is a crucial part of esophageal resection for malignancy with impact on disease-free survival. Though patient fitness and postoperative course are important, completing adjuvant chemotherapy provides a survival benefit to node-positive patients who did not receive preoperative therapy. Targeted therapy currently plays a role in locally advanced, recurrent, or metastatic GE junction adenocarcinoma and further research will provide valuable insight into the biology of the disease.

REFERENCES

1. Rustgi AK, El-Serag HB. Esophageal carcinoma. *N Engl J Med* 2014;371:2499–2509.
2. Jiminez P, Pathak A, Phan AT. The role of taxanes in the management of gastroesophageal cancer. *J Gastroint Oncol* 2011;2(4):240–249.
3. Edge SB, Byrd DR, Compton CC, et al. *AJCC Cancer Staging Manual.* 7th ed. New York: Springer; 2010.
4. Ajani JA, D'Amico TA, Almhanna K, et al.; National Comprehensive Cancer Network. Esophageal and Esophagogastric Junction Cancers (Version 1.2015). http://www.nccn.org/professionals/physician_gls/pdf/esophageal.pdf. Accessed February 6, 2015.
5. Berry MF, Brunner JZ, Castleberry AW, et al. Treatment modalities for T1N0 esophageal cancers: a comparative analysis of local therapy versus surgical resection. *J Thorac Oncol* 2013;8(6):796–802.
6. Leers JM, DeMeester SR, Oezcelik A, et al. The prevalence of lymph node metastases in patients with T1 esophageal adenocarcinoma a retrospective review of esophagectomy specimens. *Ann Surg* 2011;253(2):271–278.
7. Rice TW, Mason DP, Murthy SC, et al. T2N0M0 esophageal cancer. *J Thorac Cardiovasc Surg* 2007;133:317–324.
8. Zhang JQ, Hooker CM, Brock MV, et al. Neoadjuvant chemoradiation therapy is beneficial for clinical stage T2 N0 esophageal cancer patients due to inaccurate preoperative staging. *Ann Thorac Surg* 2012;93:429–435.
9. Crabtree TD, Kosinski AS, Puri V, et al. Evaluation of the reliability of clinical staging of T2 N0 esophageal cancer: a review of the Society of Thoracic Surgeons database. *Ann Thorac Surg* 2013;96:382–390.
10. Arnott SJ, Duncan W, Gignoux M, et al.; Oesophageal Cancer Collaborative Group. Preoperative radiotherapy for esophageal carcinoma. *Cochrane Database Syst Rev* 2005;(4):CD001799.
11. Schlag PM. Randomized trial of preoperative chemotherapy for squamous cell cancer of the esophagus. The Chirurgische Arbeitsgemeinschaft Fuer Onkologie der Deutschen Gesellschaft Fuer Chirurgie Study Group. *Arch Surg* 1992;127(12):1446–1450.
12. Maipang T, Vasinanukorn P, Petpichetchian C, et al. Induction chemotherapy in the treatment of patients with carcinoma of the esophagus. *J Surg Oncol* 1994;56(3):191–197.
13. Law S, Fok M, Chow S, et al. Preoperative chemotherapy versus surgical therapy alone for squamous cell carcinoma of the esophagus: a prospective randomized trial. *J Thorac Cardiovasc Surg* 1997;114(2):210–217.
14. Ancona E, Ruol A, Santi S, et al. Only pathologic complete response to neoadjuvant chemotherapy improves significantly the long term survival of patients with resectable esophageal squamous cell carcinoma: final report of a randomized, controlled trial of preoperative chemotherapy versus surgery alone. *Cancer* 2001;91(11):2165–2174.
15. Allum WH, Stenning SP, Bancewicz J, et al. Long-term results of a randomized trial of surgery with or without preoperative chemotherapy in esophageal cancer. *J Clin Oncol* 2009;27(30):5062–5067.
16. Cunningham D, Allum WH, Stenning SP, et al. Perioperative chemotherapy versus surgery alone for resectable gastroesophageal cancer. *N Engl J Med* 2006;355(1):11–20.
17. Ychou M, Boige V, Pignon JP, et al. Perioperative chemotherapy compared with surgery alone for resectable gastroesophageal adenocarcinoma: an FNCLCC and FFCD multicenter phase III trial. *J Clin Oncol* 2011;29(13):1715–1721.
18. Kelsen DP, Winter KA, Gunderson LL, et al. Long-term results of RTOG trial 8911 (USA Intergroup 113): a random assignment trial comparison of chemotherapy followed by surgery compared with surgery alone for esophageal cancer. *J Clin Oncol* 2007;25(24):3719–3725.
19. Boonstra JJ, Kok TC, Wijnhoven BP, et al. Chemotherapy followed by surgery versus surgery alone in patients with resectable oesophageal squamous cell carcinoma: long-term results of a randomized controlled trial. *BMC Cancer* 2011;11:181.
20. Gebski V, Burmeister B, Smithers BM, et al. Survival benefits from neoadjuvant chemoradiotherapy or chemotherapy in oesophageal carcinoma: a meta-analysis. *Lancet Oncol* 2007;8:226–234.
21. Kranzfelder M, Schuster T, Geinitz H, et al. Meta-analysis of neoadjuvant treatment modalities and definitive non-surgical therapy for oesophageal squamous cell cancer. *Br J Surg* 2011;98(6):768–783.
22. Sjoquist KM, Burmeister BH, Smithers BM, et al. Survival after neoadjuvant chemotherapy or chemoradiotherapy for resectable oesophageal carcinoma: an updated meta-analysis. *Lancet Oncol* 2011;12(7):681–692.
23. Walsh TN, Noonan N, Hollywood D, et al. A comparison of multimodal therapy and surgery for esophageal adenocarcinoma. *N Engl J Med* 1996;335(7):462–467.
24. Bosset JF, Gignoux M, Triboulet JP, et al. Chemoradiotherapy followed by surgery compared with surgery alone in squamous cell cancer of the esophagus. *N Engl J Med* 1997;337(3):161–167.
25. Urba SG, Orringer MB, Turrisi A, et al. Randomized trial of preoperative chemoradiation versus surgery alone in patients with locoregional esophageal carcinoma. *J Clin Oncol* 2001;19(2):305–313.
26. Tepper J, Krasna MJ, Niedzwiecki D, et al. Phase III trial of trimodality therapy with cisplatin and fluorouracil, radiotherapy and surgery compared with surgery alone for esophageal cancer: CALGB 9781. *J Clin Oncol* 2008;26(7):1086–1092.
27. van Hagen P, Hulshof MC, van Lanschot JJ, et al. Preoperative chemoradiotherapy for esophageal or junctional cancer. *N Engl J Med* 2012;366(22):2074–2084.
28. Urschel JD, Vasan H. A meta-analysis of randomized controlled trials that compared neoadjuvant chemoradiation and surgery to surgery alone for resectable esophageal cancer. *Am J Surg* 2003;185(6):538–543.
29. Fiorica F, Di Bona D, Licate A, et al. Preoperative chemoradiotherapy for oesophageal cancer: a systematic review and meta-analysis. *Gut* 2004;53(7):925–930.
30. Greer SE, Goodney PP, Sutton JE, et al. Neoadjuvant chemoradiotherapy for esophageal carcinoma: A meta-analysis. *Surgery* 2005;137(2):172–177.
31. Jin HL, Zhu H, Ling TS, et al. Neoadjuvant chemoradiotherapy for resectable esophageal carcinoma: A meta-analysis. *World J Gastroenterol* 2009;15(47):5983–5991.
32. Ando N, Iizuka T, Kakegawa T, et al. A randomized trial of surgery with and without chemotherapy for localized squamous carcinoma of the thoracic esophagus: the Japan Clinical Oncology Group study. *J Thorac Cardiovasc Surg* 1997;114(2):205–209.
33. Ando N, Iizuka T, Ide H, et al. Surgery plus chemotherapy compared to surgery alone for localized squamous cell carcinoma of the thoracic esophagus: A JCOG group study—JCOG9204. *J Clin Oncol* 2003;21(24):4592–4596.
34. Ando N, Kato H, Igaki H, et al. A randomized trial comparing postoperative adjuvant chemotherapy with cisplatin and 5-fluorouracil versus preoperative chemotherapy for localized advanced squamous cell carcinoma of the thoracic esophagus (JCOG9907). *Ann Surg Oncol* 2012;19(1):68–74.
35. Smalley SR, Benedetti JK, Haller DG, et al. Updated analysis of SWOG-directed intergroup study 0116: a phase III trial of adjuvant radiochemotherapy versus observation after curative gastric cancer resection. *J Clin Oncol* 2012;30:2327–2333.
36. Speicher PJ, Englum BR, Ganapathi AM, et al. Adjuvant chemotherapy is associated with improved survival after esophagectomy without induction therapy for node-positive adenocarcinoma. *J Thorac Oncol* 2015;10(1):181–188.
37. Birkmeyer JD, Siewers AE, Finlayson EV, et al. Hospital volume and surgical mortality in the United States. *New Engl J Med* 2002;346(15):1128–1137.
38. Palazzo F, Rosato E, Chaudhary A, et al. Minimally invasive esophagectomy provides significant survival advantage compared with open or hybrid esophagectomy for patients with cancers of the esophagus and gastroesophageal junction. 2014. Presented at the Southern Surgical Association 126th Annual Meeting.
39. Luketich JD, Pennathur A, Awais O, et al. Outcomes after minimally invasive esophagectomy: review of over 1000 patients. *Ann Surg* 2012;256(1):95–103.
40. Warner S, Chang YH, Paripati H, et al. Outcomes of minimally invasive esophagectomy in esophageal cancer after neoadjuvant chemoradiotherapy. *Ann Thorac Surg* 2014;97(2):439–445.
41. Luketich JD, Pennathur A, Franchetti Y, et al. Minimally invasive esophagectomy: results of a prospective phase II multicenter trial—the Eastern Cooperative Oncology Group (E2202) study. *Ann Surg* 2015;261(4):702–707.
42. Finks JF, Osborne NH, Birkmeyer JD. Trends in hospital volume and operative mortality for high-risk surgery. *New Engl J Med* 2011;364(22):2128–2137.
43. Merkow RP, Bilimoria KY, Chow WB, et al. Variation in lymph node examination after esophagectomy for cancer in the United States. *Arch Surg* 2012;147(6):505–511.
44. Greenstein AJ, Litle VR, Swanson SJ, et al. Prognostic significance of the number of lymph node metastases in esophageal cancer. *J Am Coll Surg* 2008;206(2):239–246.
45. Greenstein AJ, Litle VR, Swanson SJ, et al. Effect of the number of lymph nodes sampled on postoperative survival of lymph node-negative esophageal cancer. *Cancer* 2008; 112(6):1239–1246.
46. Wong R, Malthaner R. Combined chemotherapy and radiotherapy (without surgery) compared with radiotherapy alone in localized carcinoma of the esophagus. *Cochrane Database Syst Rev* 2006;(1):CD002092.
47. Bang Y, Van Cutsem E, Feyereislova A, et al. Trastuzumab in combination with chemotherapy versus chemotherapy alone for the treatment of HER2-positive advanced gastro-oesophageal junction cancer (ToGA): a phase 3, open-label, randomised controlled trial. *Lancet* 2010;376(9742):687–697.
48. Liquiqli W, Tomasello G, Toppo L, et al. Remucirumab for metastatic gastric or gastroesophageal junction cancer: results and implications of the REGARD trial. *Future Oncol* 2014;10(9):1549–1557.

145

Less Common Malignant Tumors of the Esophagus

Kiran Lagisetty ▪ Andrew C. Chang

The less common malignant tumors of the esophagus include a variety of rare tumors. Table 145.1 provides a list of malignant esophageal tumors outside the more common epidermoid and adenocarcinomas. These tumors oftentimes share many of the same clinical and pathologic behavior as their more typical and adenocarcinoma counterparts. Given their similarity to squamous cell and adenocarcinoma of the esophagus, the less common malignant tumors of the esophagus also have poor survival rates despite advances in surgery and adjuvant therapies.

Although there are wide varieties of tumor cell types and degrees of differentiation, these have limited prognostic capacity due to the poor response of such tumors to conventional treatment. Some tumors such as the uncommon polypoid carcinoma and sarcomas of the esophagus may allow for improved survival when discovered in their early stages; however, spread beyond the esophagus is typically fatal. Other tumors include glandular carcinomas such as cylindroma, mucoepidermoid carcinoma, and adenoacanthoma, whereas rare epitheliomatous lesions include verrucous carcinoma and polypoid carcinoma. Tumors found more commonly in other locations such as neuroendocrine carcinoma, melanoma, and sarcomas can also occasionally be found as a primary lesion of the esophagus. Metastatic lesions to the esophagus from other primary lesions are a rare occurrence.

TABLE 145.1 Less Common Malignant Tumors of the Esophagus

Malignant epithelial tumors
  Adenocarcinoma variants
    Type "ordinaire"
    Adenoid cystic carcinoma (cylindroma)
    Mucoepidermoid carcinoma
    Adenoacanthoma
    Choriocarcinoma
  Squamous cell carcinoma variants
    Verrucous carcinoma
    Polypoid carcinoma
      Carcinosarcoma
      Pseudosarcoma
  Neuroendocrine tumors
    Small cell carcinoma
    Carcinoid tumor
    Atypical carcinoid tumor
  Melanoma
Malignant mesenchymal tumors
  Leiomyosarcoma
  Rhabdomyosarcoma
  Fibrosarcoma
  Chondrosarcoma
  Osteosarcoma
  Liposarcoma
  Kaposi sarcoma
  Malignant schwannoma
Lymphoma
  Histiocytic lymphosarcoma
  Reticulum cell sarcoma
  Hodgkin lymphoma
  Plasmacytoma
Metastatic tumors to the esophagus

EPITHELIAL TUMORS

Adenocarcinoma of the esophagus, once a rare form of esophageal cancer, is now one of the fastest growing solid organ cancers in America. In 2015, it is estimated that 16,980 patients will be diagnosed with esophageal cancer with 15,590 deaths. These tumors still only make up less than 1% of new cancer diagnoses overall. Of the over 16,000 cases of esophageal cancer diagnosed in the United States, approximately 60% of these tumors are of adenocarcinoma histology.[1] Worldwide, squamous cell carcinoma is still the most prevalent histology of esophageal cancer with 398,000 cases compared to 52,000 cases of adenocarcinoma in 2012.[2] The percentage of patients surviving at 5 years is poor at 17.9%, which has not changed significantly over the past decade despite advances in cancer therapy. Adenocarcinoma of the esophagus and gastroesophageal junction is discussed in more detail in Chapter 142.

A review of glandular epithelial structures that may be found within the esophagus is essential for understanding the development of esophageal adenocarcinoma. Only a few sources of columnar epithelium in the esophagus have been recognized (Fig. 145.1). Superficial and deep submucosal glands constitute part of the normal anatomy of the esophagus. Heterotopic islands of aberrant gastric mucosa occur in many organs of the body, including the esophagus. Columnar epithelium-lined lower esophagus (Barrett's metaplasia) is now thought to be the most common underlying pathologic process that may progress to frank, typical adenocarcinoma of the esophagus. The columnar epithelium in all these locations may become a site for malignant transformation. In Barrett's metaplasia, only the

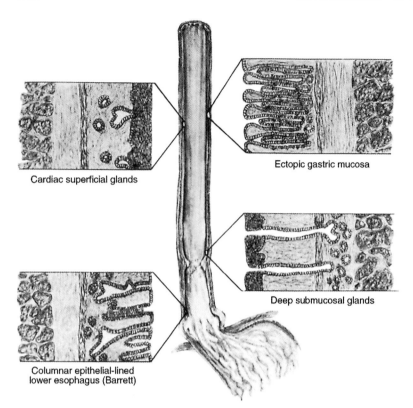

Ectopic gastric mucosa

Cardiac superficial glands

Deep submucosal glands

Columnar epithelial-lined
lower esophagus (Barrett)

FIGURE 145.1 Sources of columnar epithelium in the esophagus recognized in the origin of primary esophageal adenocarcinoma.

intestinal type of columnar epithelial cells is believed to be premalignant. Detailed discussions of Barrett's metaplasia are presented in Chapter 138.

UNUSUAL VARIANTS OF ADENOCARCINOMA

Embryologic development of the superficial esophageal glands arises from the tall columnar epithelium which subsequently localizes to the upper and lower ends of the esophagus. These mucous-secreting glandular cells are found in the lamina propria and cannot be distinguished from the cardiac glands of the stomach. Although these glands may give rise to adenocarcinoma the described incidence of adenocarcinoma is limited to case reports.[2,3] In one such case report, Goldfarb et al. describe the malignant transformation arising from the cardiac submucosal glands.[4]

The deeper esophageal submucosal glands, which develop during the postnatal period, are found throughout the esophagus. These cells can sometimes secrete serous fluid making them indistinguishable from minor salivary glands. Adenoid cystic carcinoma or cylindroma (Fig. 145.2) is a common tumor found in the salivary glands; however, it is extremely rare in the esophagus with no known counterpart in the stomach. Histologically, these tumors typically exhibit three distinct growth patterns: cribriform, tubular, and solid. The cribriform pattern demonstrates nest of cells with cylindromatous microcystic spaces. The tubular form has well-formed ducts and tubules lined with inner epithelial cells and outer myoepithelial cells. The solid form is characterized by uniform sheets of basaloid cells lacking tubular or microcystic formation.[3] Patients typically present with progressive dysphagia with the average age of patients being 65 years with a 3.4:1 male to female ratio. These tumors are most commonly found in the middle third of the esophagus (63%) with 30% in the lower third and 7% in the upper third.[4,5]

True mucoepidermoid tumors of the esophagus are extremely rare and typically have a histologic resemblance to tumors found in major salivary glands.[6] These tumors have mucous-secreting properties and have distinct epidermoid features. These tumors originate in the submucosa and typically present as intramural masses. Adenosquamous carcinoma is also another rare variant which is similar to mucoepidermoid carcinoma because of its epidermoid and glandular components.[7] Similar to Paget's disease of the breast, mucoepidermoid carcinomas may sometimes demonstrate both in situ and infiltrative components along with pagetoid spread to the surface epithelium.

Heterotopic islands of gastric mucosa replacing portions of the squamous lining of the esophagus have been reported (Fig. 145.3). These islands typically consist of cardiac glands, but also can contain parietal cells. These islands are often seen in the upper third of the esophagus and are present in up to 7.8% of 1,000 consecutive pediatric autopsies. Carrie reported the first case of adenocarcinoma arising from one of these heterotopic islands of gastric tissue.[8] In situ malignant changes seen in these islands are morphologically indistinguishable from gastric carcinoma.

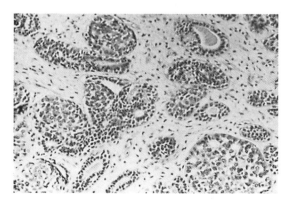

FIGURE 145.2 Adenoid cystic carcinoma of the esophagus. (From Sobin LH, Oota K, Ōta K. Histologic Typing of Gastric and Oesophageal Tumours. Geneva: World Health Organization, 1977. With permission.)

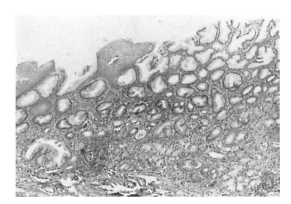

FIGURE 145.3 Gastric heterotopia, upper esophagus. (From Sobin LH, Oota K, Ôta K. Histologic Typing of Gastric and Oesophageal Tumours. Geneva: World Health Organization, 1977. With permission.)

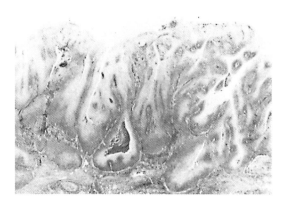

FIGURE 145.4 Verrucous squamous cell carcinoma of the esophagus with typical blunt contours of deep margin. (From Sobin LH, Oota K, Ôta K. Histologic Typing of Gastric and Oesophageal Tumours. Geneva: World Health Organization, 1977. With permission.)

Adenocanthoma is another variant of adenocarcinoma which displays concomitant squamous metaplastic elements. Histologically this is a well-differentiated adenocarcinoma with islands of squamous cells surrounded by glandular tumor. Distinct from these tumors is the squamous cell carcinoma with pseudoglandular degeneration characterized by lack of mucus secretion and the rare composite adenosquamous malignancy with aggressive glandular and epidermoid elements. It has been suggested that metaplasia of esophageal adenocarcinoma forms hormonally active choriocarcinoma.[9] This tumor is rare; it may be a giant cell variant of adenocarcinoma that is attempting trophoblastic differentiation.

Treatment

The mainstay of treatment of unusual variants for adenocarcinoma of the esophagus is resection. During resection, frozen sections are typically obtained given the extensive infiltration in the wall and lymphatic spread. As is the standard of care for typical adenocarcinoma of the esophagus some patients derive benefit from the use of radiation and chemotherapy. Survival is typically dependent on completeness of resection and is the only modality achieving survival of 5 years or more. Histologic subtype has not been shown to be an independent predictor of survival in patients undergoing resection.[7] TNM staging continues to be the best predictor in the outcome of the disease.

Prognosis

Prognosis in unusual variants of adenocarcinoma is uniformly poor with most patients presenting with extensive invasion and often metastases. Adenocystic lesions found in other areas are relatively benign and are applicable to esophageal lesions. These tumors typically have extensive intramural spread with distant metastases. Treatment of these lesions is similar to that of squamous cell carcinoma utilizing multimodality therapy including chemotherapy, radiation, and surgical resection.

UNUSUAL VARIANTS OF SQUAMOUS CELL CARCINOMA

Verrucous Carcinoma

Verrucous carcinoma is a rare form of esophageal cancer that is a variant of squamous cell carcinoma. This unique tumor was first described by Minelly in 1967 and there have only been 30 cases reported in the literature. Verrucous cell carcinomas are associated with human papillomavirus infection and are slow growing tumors

which are most commonly found in the oral cavity but can also be found in the larynx, glans penis, vulva, endometrium, bladder, anorectum, and the soles of the feet.[6,10] These lesions demonstrate papillary or warty, cauliflower-like epidermoid growths that are well differentiated histologically and show acanthosis and hyperkeratosis (Fig. 145.4). Although there is no clear etiology reported in the literature, chronic retention of esophageal contents may contribute to the development of these verrucous lesions. Verrucous cell carcinoma may also be associated with smoking, alcohol abuse, hiatal hernia, esophagitis, caustic injury from lye, battery or kerosene ingestion, or nutcracker esophagus. Although leukoplakia is commonly associated with verrucous squamous carcinoma in other sites, such as the oral cavity or penis, it is rarely encountered in the esophagus except in association with achalasia or esophageal diverticulum.

The incidence of verrucous cell carcinomas is higher in males versus females and the average age at diagnosis is 61.[7,11] The most common presenting symptoms are dysphagia and weight loss, although there are also reports of hematemesis, coughing, and odynophagia.[10] Tumors are most often found in the lower esophagus but can be located in the middle and upper esophagus.

Diagnosis of verrucous cell carcinoma is typically made by endoscopic biopsy or endoscopic ultrasound (EUS). Lesions can appear as shaggy, white, exophytic, wart-like, velvety, papillary, spiked, cauliflower-like masses. The typical progression of verrucous cell tumors is stepwise progression from acanthosis, hyperkeratosis, parakeratosis, leukoplakia, verrucous lesions, and papillary hyperplasia to verrucous carcinoma.[10] Superficial biopsies may only reveal nonspecific acanthosis, parakeratosis, or hyperkeratosis which can make diagnosis difficult. EUS has the added benefit of allowing for accurate evaluation of depth of invasion, ability to secure accurate biopsies, and evaluation of lymph nodes.

Although verrucous cell carcinomas are slow growing and well differentiated, these tumors have a poor prognosis. There often is a considerable delay in the time between symptom onset and diagnosis; therefore, the majority of these cases are locally advanced. Morbidity and mortality are typically related to local invasion or surgical complications. These tumors can invade the lungs, pleura, bronchi, or pericardium.[7,10,12] When diagnosed at an early stage these tumors can be treated by esophagectomy, polypectomy, or endomucosal resection. There is a recent case report of treatment of a locally advanced verrucous cell tumor with an esophageal stent.[12] Given the lack of cases in the literature there are limited data demonstrating the benefit of chemotherapy or radiation. Post-surgical survival has ranged from 9 months to 3 years.[10,11]

Polypoid Carcinoma

Polypoid carcinoma was first described by Virchow in 1865. Polypoid carcinoma with spindle cell sarcomatous features or carcinosarcoma is another rare variant of squamous carcinoma. It has a reported incidence of 2% of all esophageal neoplasms.[13] Tumors often present with symptoms of dysphagia, odynophagia, and weight loss and are typically found in the middle third of the esophagus. Patients will typically present at an early stage because of the relatively large size and obstructive symptoms. These tumors are most frequently seen in the upper aerodigestive tract and mouth and can often arise in response to radiation given for treatment of other conditions (benign or malignant). However, this association has not been shown for the esophageal lesions. Carcinosarcoma typically spreads via direct invasion, hematogenously or through the lymphatic circulation. Doubling time of 2.2 months has been described.[14]

Grossly these tumors can be as large as 15 cm and are most commonly attached to the esophageal wall via a pedicle but can also be seen attached via a broad base. The surface of these tumors can be smooth, intact, or ulcerated.[15] On microscopic evaluation there is a mixture of carcinoma mixed with malignant sarcomatoid elements. The epithelial component is typically an in situ or minimally invasive squamous cell. Adenocarcinoma can also be found but has been rarely described.[15,16] Metastatic potential is typically assigned to either the epithelial or sarcomatous component or both. By contrast, in pseudosarcoma, the carcinomatous element, in situ or invasive, is confined to the surface epithelium near the base of the polyp (Fig. 145.5). Only the carcinomatous component of polypoid pseudosarcoma has been considered to have metastatic potential, but also described are the polypoid esophageal malignancies with all the morphologic features of pseudosarcoma and definite evidence of metastasis of the spindle cell element (Fig. 145.6).[17,18] There is no significant differences in the clinicopathologic features of carcinosarcoma and pseudosarcoma and no important distinction can be made between the two tumors; therefore, the unifying term *polypoid carcinoma* was suggested by Osamura et al.[18]

The idea that the sarcomatous elements of polypoid carcinoma arise from transformation of squamous cells was proposed at the turn of the century, and this viewpoint represents the current consensus. Electron microscopic studies supporting the squamous origin of the sarcomatous cells resolved the controversy. In 1972, the first reported electron microscopic study of a polypoid carcinoma of the esophagus (Fig. 145.7) was described, where many cells exhibited desmosomal

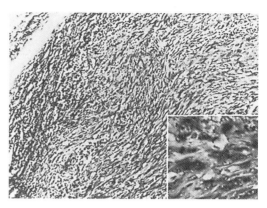

FIGURE 145.6 Metastatic sarcoma in lymph node. (*Inset*) Detail of spindle cells and several mitoses, including abnormal forms (H&E stain, original magnification ×125; inset, original magnification ×320). (From Martin MR, Kahn LB. So-called pseudosarcoma of the esophagus. *Arch Pathol Lab Med* 1977;101:607. With permission.)

attachment to neighboring cells with well-developed junctional complexes including tonofilaments (Fig. 145.8).[19] Numerous typical branching tonofibrils were seen in a few cells (Fig. 145.9). Tonofibrils are found only in epithelial cells, predominantly squamous types, and are thought to be related to the process of keratinization. Well-developed, tonofilament-associated desmosomes are also common in epithelial tumors, especially in those of squamous cell origin; thus, it was concluded that the spindle-shaped cells in the polypoid tumor originated from squamous cells.[19] Indeed, ultrastructural evidence of the squamous origin of the spindle cell element of polypoid esophageal carcinoma was later found.[19] From these findings, it was suggested that the sarcomatous component of the tumor originates from mesenchymal metaplasia of squamous cells and that these metaplastic cells produce collagen. On the basis of immunohistochemical analysis, however, Kimura et al. suggested that the anaplastic cells have a myogenic origin.[20]

Esophagectomy with adequate lymph node dissection is the mainstay of treatment of polypoid carcinoma and will effectively palliate the symptomatic patient. The extent of resection and requisite restoration of gastrointestinal continuity depends on the level of the lesion rather than the estimated degree of malignancy. Local resection is avoided given the high incidence of recurrence. Survival after resection has generated a 5-year survival rate of 71% and many long-term survivors have been reported.[14] Other modalities such as radiation have only been met with limited success. Polypoid carcinoma

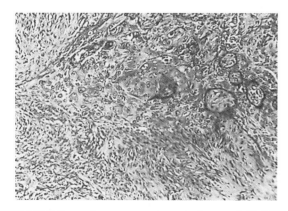

FIGURE 145.5 Focus of squamous carcinoma in the upper half of this photomicrograph adjacent to sarcoma in the lower half of a section from the base of a polyp (H&E stain, original magnification ×125). (From Martin MR, Kahn LB. So-called pseudosarcoma of the esophagus. *Arch Pathol Lab Med* 1977;101:607. With permission.)

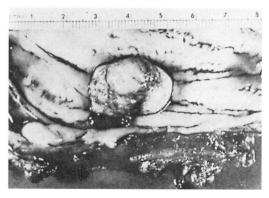

FIGURE 145.7 Polypoid pseudosarcoma of the esophagus. (Reproduced from Shields TW, Eilert JB, Battifora H. Pseudosarcoma of the oesophagus. *Thorax* 1972;27:474, with permission from BMJ Publishing Group Ltd.)

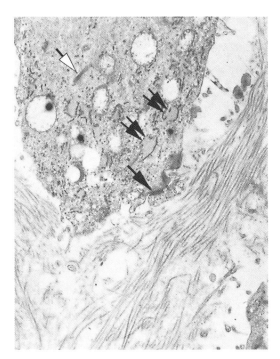

FIGURE 145.8 Electron micrograph of pseudosarcoma of the esophagus showing part of a spindle cell and a small segment from another cell. At point of contact, a well-developed desmosome is present (*solid arrow*). The cytoplasm is rich in tonofilaments that form bundles in some places (*hollow arrow*). Several distended cisternae of rough endoplasmic reticulum are visible (*double arrows*). Collagen fibers abound in the vicinity of the cell (original magnification ×22,000).

typically carries a better prognosis than typical squamous cell carcinoma given its limited extent of penetration into the esophageal wall. There has been no clear correlation between gross appearance and biologic behavior.

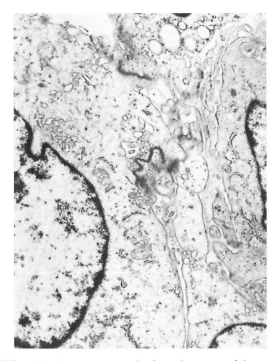

FIGURE 145.9 Electron micrograph of pseudosarcoma of the esophagus shows the contact site of four tumor cells. Well-developed desmosomes are prominent and numerous (original magnification ×22,000).

NEUROENDOCRINE TUMORS OF THE ESOPHAGUS

Small Cell Carcinoma

Small cell carcinoma (SCC) of the esophagus was initially described in 1952 by McKeown.[21] These tumors are also referred to as oat cell, anaplastic carcinoma or APUDomas. SCC of the esophagus makes up 0.3% to 2.4% of primary esophageal cancers with fewer than 300 case reports in the literature. These tumors are highly malignant with early metastases and limited overall survival. The median age at diagnosis is 60 years and occurs more commonly in males.[22] Histologically these tumors are similar to small cell lung cancer with similar aggressive biology. Approximately 40% to 60% of SCC patients have metastatic disease at presentation.[23] About 5% of small cell tumors have an extrapulmonary origin including nasal cavity, salivary gland, paranasal sinus, larynx, hypopharynx, esophagus, thymus, pancreas, small and large intestines, and stomach.

The most common presenting symptoms are dysphagia, pain, and weight loss. Endoscopy with biopsy is the mainstay of diagnosis. Lesions are typically located in the mid to distal third of the esophagus and appear as fungating, polypoid lesions. On histologic examination these tumors appear small, round, ovoid or spindle-shaped cells with scant cytoplasm, ill-defined cell borders, finely granular nuclear chromatin, and absent or inconspicuous nucleoli. Cells are arranged in sheets or ribbons with streaming patterns (Fig. 145.10). Immunohistochemical analysis of SCC tumors will also indicate expression of markers including synaptophysin, chromogranin A, CD56, TTF-1, and neuron-specific enolase. Staging consists of imaging to evaluate for regional and distal spread. Distal spread is typically found in the liver, bone, and distant lymph nodes. According to the largest retrospective review of SCC of the esophagus 49% of patients presented with metastatic disease at the time of diagnosis.[24]

Treatment of SCC of the esophagus is controversial since there are limited data to suggest a benefit for one treatment type over another. Options for therapy include resection with or without chemotherapy or chemotherapy with or without radiotherapy. Because of its close relationship to SCC of the lung, many investigators have advocated for a similar treatment approach.[22,24] Chemotherapy treatment consists of a platinum agent combined with etoposide. Recent studies have shown superiority in SCC of the lung using a regimen consisting of cisplatin and irinotecan; this has not been studied in SCC of the esophagus in any large series.[25] Patients with limited disease and no evidence of distant metastasis may benefit from resection. In a retrospective review of esophageal small cell cancer at the MD

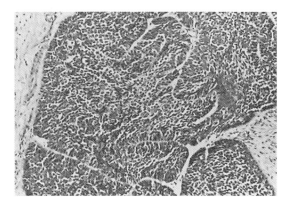

FIGURE 145.10 Undifferentiated carcinoma of the esophagus. A distinct form referred to as small-cell carcinoma is described in the text. (From Sobin LH, Oota K, Ōta K. Histologic Typing of Gastric and Oesophageal Tumours. Geneva: World Health Organization, 1977. With permission.)

Anderson Cancer Center two patients treated with esophagectomy had overall survival of more than 10 and 57 months.[26]

Overall survival is typically measured in months, and in a review from Ku et al. patients had a median survival of 8 months among those with limited disease and 3 months among those with extended disease.[22] In a recent review of the SEER database of over 300 patients with SCC of the esophagus, risk factors associated with poor overall survival included age, female sex, black race, and stage.[14] In this study, resection with removal of greater than 10 lymph nodes and pre- or postoperative radiotherapy were all associated with improved survival.

CARCINOID TUMORS OF THE ESOPHAGUS

Carcinoid tumors are neuroendocrine tumors often found in the gastrointestinal tract with the most common sites being the stomach, small bowel, appendix, and rectum. Carcinoid tumors of the esophagus are a rare entity first described by Brenner in 1969.[26] Since its first description, multiphasic clinical and pathologic features of 100 cases reported in the world literature of carcinoid tumors of the esophagus have been reviewed; 28 cases were of the typical variety and 72 were of the atypical type.[28] Lesions are typically found in males in a 6:1 ratio compared to females and the typical age at diagnosis is 60.[29] The most common presenting symptoms are weight loss and dysphagia. Carcinoid syndrome is a rare clinical finding. Tumors are typically located in submucosa and most commonly occur in the lower esophagus. Histologically, esophageal carcinoids consist of fair to well-differentiated argyrophilic cells organized as solid nests or as acinar or tubular structures. As with neuroendocrine tumors elsewhere in the body, esophageal carcinoids will stain positive for chromogranin A and synaptophysin. In 2010 the World Health Organization began classifying neuroendocrine tumors based on mitotic count and Ki67 index and graded these tumors as G1 (low grade, well differentiated) <2 mitoses/10 hpf and/or ≤2% Ki67 index; G2 (intermediate grade, moderate differentiated) 2 to 20 mitoses/10 hpf and/or 3 to 20% Ki67 index; and G3 neuroendocrine carcinomas (high grade, poorly differentiated) >20 mitoses/10 hpf and/or >20% Ki67 index. The majority of esophageal carcinoids are classified as G3.

Treatment strategies vary for typical versus atypical carcinoids. Typical carcinoids are as a rule smaller in size, confined to the lamina propria, and have a low incidence of metastasis. Surgical resection is the primary method of treatment and is typically curative for typical carcinoids. Recently there have been increasing reports of endoscopic resection and endomucosal resection yielding similar results to more standard approaches to surgical resection.[30]

Compared to typical carcinoids, atypical carcinoids are more aggressive in nature, although optimal management of atypical esophageal carcinoid is difficult to ascertain given the limited literature. There have been reports of esophagectomy with and without chemoradiotherapy.[31–33] Survival rates even with resection for atypical carcinoid typically range from 6 to 12 months.

MELANOMA

Primary malignant melanoma of the esophagus (PMME) is a rare form of esophageal cancer and makes up approximately 0.1% to 0.2% of primary esophageal cancers (Fig. 145.11).[34] Most of what is described about the pathogenesis and natural history of PMME is based on single-incident case reports. PMME is highly aggressive with widespread disease occurring rapidly and typically has a poor prognosis. Most patients present in the sixth and seventh decades of life with a 2:1 male to female ratio.

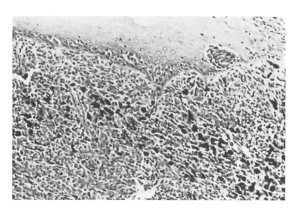

FIGURE 145.11 Malignant melanoma of the esophagus. The primary tumor is heavily pigmented. (From Sobin LH, Oota K, Ōta K. Histologic Typing of Gastric and Oesophageal Tumours. Geneva: World Health Organization, 1977. With permission.)

No specific risk factors have been identified for PMME; however, some have suggested that the presence of melanoblasts with melanin granules and dendrites in the basal layer of the esophageal epithelium could be a potential source.[35] Tumors are typically found as pigmented lesions in the middle to lower third of the esophagus; up to one-quarter of these lesions can be amelanotic making diagnosis based on gross appearance difficult.[36,37] Absence of melanosis in most melanomas of the esophagus indicates a potential different progenitor such as normally occurring melanoblasts, metaplasia of normal basal epithelial cells of esophagus, or ectopic melanoblast-containing epithelium rising within the esophagus during development.

Immunohistochemical analysis of these tumors indicates vimentin, S-100, HB-45, Melan-A, and tyrosinase. Presence of junctional changes in the overlying adjacent epithelium is considered evidence of primary cutaneous malignant melanoma. Diagnosis of PMME should be based on the following criteria: (a) the tumor should have the characteristic histology of melanoma and should contain melanin; (b) the tumor should arise from an area of junctional change in squamous epithelium; (c) the adjacent epithelium should demonstrate junctional change with the presence of melanin-containing cells; (d) careful evaluation must exclude skin, ocular, or anal mucosal primary melanomatous malignancy; and (e) a positive reaction to the monoclonal antigen HMB-45 should be present.[38]

The most common presenting symptom in PMME is dysphagia. By the time of symptom onset such tumors will have significant bulk and often will have already metastasized.[34,36] The radial growth pattern of PMME is similar to that of lentigo maligna melanoma although its biologic behavior is more aggressive. Staging of tumors typically consists of esophagograms, CT imaging, endoscopy, and EUS. PET imaging is useful for detecting lymph node and distant metastasis. Endoscopic findings typically include lobulated tumor situated on a wide pedicle in the lower or middle esophagus with ulceration and friable tissue. Although the initial diagnosis usually is established by identification of a solitary lesion, there should be a high suspicion for satellite lesions. Metastatic lesions are found in approximately 40% to 66% of cases. Metastatic spread is typically lymphatic and vascular. The most common sites of metastasis include paraesophageal and supraclavicular lymph nodes, liver, kidney, and bone.[36,37]

The mainstay of therapy of localized PMME is esophagectomy with wide margins given its aggressive nature. The survival benefit from resection is difficult to measure since only case reports are available with up to 77% of patients succumbing to disease within the first postoperative year.[34] Adjuvant therapies with dacarbazine, immunotherapy, radiotherapy, or biologic agents such IL2 and interferon-alpha are typically ineffective. These treatments are most often given in a palliative setting; response is variable and poor.[39–41] Overall survival is typically 10 to 14 months with a 5-year survival rate of 4%.[36,42]

MALIGNANT MESENCHYMAL TUMORS

Esophageal sarcomas are extremely rare tumors. The median age of diagnosis is 58 years and patients typically will present with dysphagia. These tumors are diagnosed using a combination of esophagograms, endoscopy, EUS, CT, and PET imaging. Leiomyosarcoma is the most commonly occurring esophageal sarcoma with leiomyoma being the most common benign tumor. Rhabdomyosarcoma and fibrosarcoma are infrequent with only several case reports in the literature. These tumors are difficult to distinguish from their nonmalignant counterparts given the polypoid and pedunculated gross appearance. Tumors are identified superficially within the wall of the esophagus and seldom metastasize to regional lymphatics or distant sites. The mainstay of treatment is surgical resection and with early detection has a more favorable prognosis when compared to squamous cell or adenocarcinoma of the esophagus. The role of chemotherapy and radiotherapy is controversial with conflicting results. The most common factors affecting survival are completeness of surgical resection, tumor size, grade, location, and growth pattern.

LEIOMYOSARCOMA

Leiomyosarcoma is the most common sarcoma of the esophagus, first described by Howard in 1902. Since then there have been more than 100 case reports in the literature.[43] These tumors typically occur in the fifth and sixth decades of life, have a 2:1 male to female ratio, are slow growing, and have late metastases. These tumors can be found throughout the esophagus (Fig. 145.12A) but most frequently occur in the middle and distal thirds, given their smooth muscle origin. These tumors are classified as polypoid (60%) or infiltrative.[44]

Although difficult to distinguish from leiomyoma, leiomyosarcoma tends to be larger and more commonly ulcerated at presentation (Fig. 145.12A). Leiomyomas occur in the younger population with a mean age of 35. In both cases patient will typically present with dysphagia once these tumors have grown sufficiently to cause luminal narrowing. Leiomyosarcomas can also infiltrate adjacent structures, in contrast to leiomyomas which typically have only a mass effect on

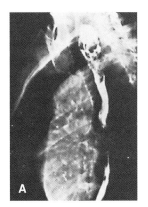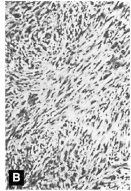

FIGURE 145.12 Leiomyosarcoma. **A:** Barium swallow shows a polypoid mass in the upper thoracic and cervical esophagus. **B:** Photomicrograph of the polyp demonstrates large spindle-shaped cells with numerous mitoses (H&E stain, original magnification ×150). (Reprinted from DeMeester TR, Skinner DB. Polypoid sarcomas of the esophagus. *Ann Thorac Surg* 1975;20:405. Copyright © 1975 The Society of Thoracic Surgeons. With permission.)

adjacent structures. Grossly, leiomyomas are firm tumors in contrast to the soft, fleshy sarcomatous counterpart. CT and EUS can sometimes distinguish leiomyosarcomas secondary to the presence of intraluminal and exophytic growth.[45] EUS yields the added benefit of facilitating ultrasound-guided biopsies. Microscopically, the findings of interlacing spindle-shaped pleomorphic cells with numerous mitotic figures are characteristic of leiomyosarcoma (Figs. 145.12B and 145.13). Histologically, leiomyosarcomas stain positive for CD34 and CD117 and negative for desmin. Malignant potential can be determined by abnormal nucleoli and the absence or scarcity of organelles in the smooth muscle cells.[46] PET CT is an emerging diagnostic tool for the detection of leiomyosarcomas, although there have been reports of false-positive results for patients found to have leiomyomas.[47]

Patients will typically present with dysphagia but can also present with retrosternal/back pain, weight loss, emesis, and, in rare cases, bleeding from tumor ulceration.[48] The treatment of choice for leiomyosarcoma is surgical resection and can lead to 3-, 5-, and 10-year survivals of 80%, 58%, and 31%, respectively.[49] Preoperative radiotherapy has demonstrated regression in some patients and may be used for palliative relief in unresectable cases. There are conflicting reports regarding the response rate and survival benefits of salvage chemoradiotherapy for recurrent disease with some demonstrating improvement in survival but others showing no improvement in size or survival.[50,51]

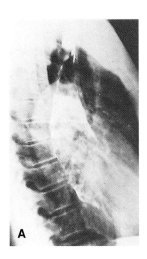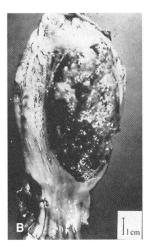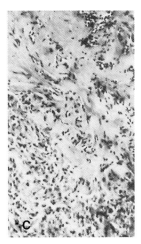

FIGURE 145.13 Leiomyoblastoma. **A:** Barium swallow reveals a large polypoid mass within the middle third of the esophagus. **B:** Surgical specimen shows a 9-cm polypoid tumor within the esophagus with necrotic and hemorrhagic changes on its surface. **C:** Photomicrograph of the pedicle portion of the polyp demonstrates cells containing eccentric nuclei with cytoplasmic vacuolization (H&E stain, original magnification ×150). (Reprinted from DeMeester TR, Skinner DB. Polypoid sarcomas of the esophagus. *Ann Thorac Surg* 1975;20:405. Copyright © 1975 The Society of Thoracic Surgeons. With permission.)

RHABDOMYOSARCOMA

There are only 16 reported cases of rhabdomyosarcoma in the literature. Debate exists over whether such tumors represent a poorly differentiated leiomyosarcoma especially in the distal esophagus given the lack of striated muscle. Microscopic diagnosis is difficult and is typically based on the presence of cells shaped like a tennis racket, with one long protoplasmic projection. Diagnosis is typically made after resection and there are only two case reports of preoperative diagnosis.[52] Tissue staining via the May–Grünwald–Giemsa method will demonstrate abundant, pleomorphic, malignant cells with basophilic cytoplasm and intracytoplasmic cross-striations. Unlike rhabdomyosarcoma elsewhere, primary esophageal tumors will often metastasize regionally to lymphatics.

The mainstay of treatment for esophageal rhabdomyosarcoma is the same as other esophageal sarcoma variants with surgical resection being the preferred treatment. There have been no reports of long-term survivors after resection. As with rhabdomyosarcomas located elsewhere in the body, tumors in the esophagus are not radiosensitive and radiation therapy is rarely effective.

FIBROSARCOMA

Fibrosarcoma of the esophagus has been described only once in the literature.[53] These tumors are typically low-grade, indolent tumors with low metastatic potential. Tumors cause narrowing within the esophagus and patients typically present with dysphagia. Treatment of these tumors has required local resection; however, with cases of high-grade histology or recurrence the treatment of choice would be "standard" esophagectomy.

CHONDROSARCOMA

Chondrosarcoma of the esophagus was first described in 1976 by Yaghmai et al.[54] Chrondrosarcomas of the esophagus are unique as they arise from tissues that are devoid of cartilage forming cells. A proposed mechanism of formation is that separation of the embryonic respiratory tract from the primitive foregut leaves behind clusters of tracheobronchial precursor cells with resultant formation of cartilaginous rings and nodules. Metaplasia of the mesenchymal cell has also been suggested as the mechanism of action. These tumors are polypoid in nature and result in narrowing of the esophagus typically seen in the mid to distal third of the esophagus. Treatment consists of en bloc resection with possible postoperative radiation.

OTHER SARCOMAS

Liposarcoma of the esophagus occurs mostly in males with a median age of 62 and typically present with dysphagia.[55] Preoperative biopsies are typically non-diagnostic. Tumors tend to be located in the upper esophagus and are pedunculated, well circumscribed, and well differentiated. There are five subtypes of liposarcomas which include well differentiated, myxoid, round cell, dedifferentiated, and pleomorphic. Local resection is the most often described treatment with excellent long-term outcomes. Other reports include endoscopic resection and debulking using CO_2 laser.[56] Long-term follow-up is recommended since up to 10% can recur.[55]

Myxofibrosarcoma and osteosarcoma each have been reported only once in the literature.[53,57] In the myxofibrosarcoma case report a 40-year-old woman presented with dysphagia and was found to have a 5 cm by 3 cm mass, located 8 cm proximal to the esophagogastric junction. The patient was treated with surgical resection. Low-grade tumors have a favorable prognosis, but given their indolent course patients should have regular oncologic surveillance.

Kaposi sarcoma is commonly seen in patients with HIV infection or other immunosuppressive states including history of prior transplantation. Gastrointestinal lesions are most commonly seen in the small bowel followed by the stomach, esophagus, and colon. The first case of esophageal Kaposi sarcoma was reported in 1980 by Umerah in a 23-year-old patient with Kaposi lesions of the foot and polypoid lesions in the lower half of the esophagus. Autopsy demonstrated Kaposi sarcoma of the esophagus.[57] Kaposi sarcoma of the upper gastrointestinal tract is typically asymptomatic and rare without extensive cutaneous disease. There have been cases describing anemia and gastrointestinal bleeding, which can be treated with injection therapy, heat coagulation, H_2 blockers, and sucralfate.[59] Diagnosis via endoscopic biopsy is usually difficult secondary to the submucosal location of the tumor. Kaposi sarcoma typically regresses with reduction of immunosuppressive agents in transplant patients and improved survival can be achieved with antiretroviral therapy for HIV-infected patients.[60]

There are scant reports of synovial cell sarcoma of the esophagus in the literature. Patients presented between the ages of 14 and 75, with equal sex distribution. Tumors were found mostly in the cervical and upper esophagus. Histologic findings included biphasic patterns including spindle cell and epithelial components. Synovial cell sarcomas are highly malignant and therapy is based on the aggressiveness of the tumor. Treatments have ranged from local resection with adjuvant chemotherapy to esophagectomy.[61,62]

In a review of the literature on malignant esophageal schwannomas there are only four reported cases.[63–66] Diagnosis of malignant schwannomas are typically based on histologic review and consists of the presence of 5 or more mitotic figures in 50 high power fields, increased cellularity, nuclear atypia, and tumor necrosis. Treatment typically consists of surgical resection when possible with adjuvant radiation therapy. Patients with a "triton" tumor, i.e., a malignant peripheral nerve sheath tumor with rhabdomyosarcomatous differentiation, may be given additional chemotherapy.

Malignant granular cell tumor of the esophagus comprises only 2% to 4% of esophageal granular cell tumors.[67] While benign tumors can be treated with endoscopic endomucosal resection, malignant lesions should be excised surgically.[68,69] Malignant fibrous histiocytomas of the esophagus have been reported several times and have been treated with surgical resection.[70]

LYMPHOMA

Esophageal lymphoma is an exceedingly rare occurrence and makes up less than 1% of patients with gastrointestinal lymphoma. There are fewer than 25 case reports of primary esophageal lymphoma in the literature, with the diagnosis typically established at autopsy. When identified, esophageal lymphoma usually is widespread, extensive, and not evident clinically. The stomach is the most common site of gastrointestinal lymphoma followed by small bowel, ileocecal region, and esophagus. Esophageal lymphoma is typically the result of direct extension from the stomach, mediastinal, or cervical lymph nodes. Primary gastrointestinal lymphoma is diagnosed based on having the predominant lesion within the gastrointestinal tract with lymph node involvement confined to the lymph node chain draining the specific organ of involvement.

Most patients are asymptomatic but can present with symptoms from hemorrhage, perforation, stricture, obstruction, vocal cord paralysis, or tracheoesophageal fistula formation. Invasion into the distal esophagus along the myenteric plexus may simulate achalasia. The exact etiology of gastrointestinal lymphoma is unknown although risk factors for its development include HIV/AIDS, Epstein–Barr infection, and oncogene overexpression such as c-Myc. The most common histologic variant is B-cell lymphoma but other subtypes such as Hodgkin, non-Hodgkin, and Burkitt lymphoma can be identified. There have been increasing reports of mucosa-associated lymphoid tissue (MALT) which unlike gastric lymphoma is not associated with *H. pylori* infections.[71] Initial staging studies include a complete blood count, bone marrow biopsy, and CT scan of the chest, abdomen, and pelvis.

Treatment of esophageal lymphoma is based on the underlying histology and the extent of involvement. Therapy ranges from surgical resection to chemotherapy and/or radiation, or combinations of any or all three modalities. Recent reports have even suggested the use of endomucosal resection for the treatment of MALT lymphomas.[72] The standard chemotherapy regimen consists of cyclophosphamide, doxorubicin, vincristine, and prednisone (commonly referred to as CHOP). In addition to the CHOP regimen, addition of a chimeric anti-CD20 monoclonal antibody, rituximab, has been shown to improve survival. Radiotherapy is often used in combination with chemotherapy but has also been used as a single agent. Complications from radiotherapy include esophagotracheal or esophago-aortic fistulae.

METASTATIC TUMORS TO THE ESOPHAGUS

Most metastatic tumors to the esophagus are the result of direct extension from adjacent organs. Tumor invasion into the esophagus can be seen from the stomach, lungs, pharynx, larynx, bronchus, mediastinal lymph nodes, and thyroid but they can occur via metastasis from lymphatic and hematogenous spread from other malignancies. Metastatic cancer to the esophagus makes up 8% of gastrointestinal malignancies. Esophageal metastases from remote organs include prostate, pancreas, testis, eye, tongue, tibia, liver, uterus, breast, skin, lung, and wrist synovium. Remote sites of metastases that are exceedingly rare, however, have been described. Metastases from breast cancer are the most commonly described and are hypothesized to be the result of spread along the internal mammary lymph nodes. Some autopsy series have reported that 6% of breast cancer patients will have esophageal metastases.[73]

Dysphagia is a common presenting symptom in patients with metastatic spread to the esophagus and occurs in up to one-third of patients. Additional testing includes esophagogram, which demonstrates a smooth, concentric stricture or indentation with overlying intact mucosa (Fig. 145.14). Esophagoscopy typically reveals a smooth or nodular mucosal surface with luminal narrowing. Endoscopic ultrasound can better characterize these lesions as this modality can localize the lesion, yield information regarding size and depth of invasion, and permit biopsy.[74] Other diagnostic and imaging modalities include CT imaging and PET imaging.

Treatment of esophageal metastases is typically centered around palliation of symptoms. Surgical therapy consisting of esophagectomy is reserved for patients with isolated metastatic disease and has been described in metastatic lesions from ovary, lung, and breast cancer.[73] Esophageal dilation of a malignant stricture is an area of controversy. Many will argue that bougie dilation exposes the patient to potential catastrophic perforation given the friable nature of the esophageal mucosa. However, there are recent reports that dilation as well as endoscopy with stent placement is a safe and reliable procedure.[75] Other treatment strategies for metastatic lesions include adjuvant

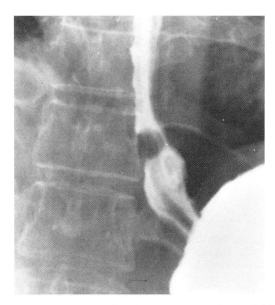

FIGURE 145.14 Barium swallow demonstrates typical smooth filling of metastatic breast carcinoma in the distal esophagus.

therapy directed toward the primary malignancy such as for melanoma or chemotherapy and radiation depending on the histology of the tumor.

REFERENCES

1. Anonymous (Surveillance, Epidemiology, and End Results (SEER) Program) (www.seer.cancer.gov). Research Data (1973–2012). National Cancer Institute, DCCPS, Surveillance Research Program, Surveillance Systems Branch, released April 2015, based on the November 2014 submission.
2. Arnold M, Soerjomataram I, Ferlay J, et al. Global incidence of oesophageal cancer by histological subtype in 2012. *Gut* 2015;64(3):381–387.
3. Nascimento AG, Amaral AL, Prado LA, et al. Adenoid cystic carcinoma of salivary glands. A study of 61 cases with clinicopathologic correlation. *Cancer* 1986;57(2):312–319.
4. Petursson SR. Adenoid cystic carcinoma of the esophagus. Complete response to combination chemotherapy. *Cancer* 1986;57(8):1464–1467.
5. Sweeney EC, Cooney T. Adenoid cystic carcinoma of the esophagus: A light and electron microscopic study. *Cancer* 1980;45(6):1516–1525.
6. Tonna J, Palefsky JM, Rabban J, et al. Esophageal verrucous carcinoma arising from hyperkeratotic plaques associated with human papilloma virus type 51. *Dis Esophagus* 2010;23(5):E17–E20.
7. Malik AB, Bidani JA, Rich HG, et al. Long-term survival in a patient with verrucous carcinoma of the esophagus. *Am J Gastroenterol* 1996;91(5):1031–1033.
8. Carrie A. Adenocarcinoma of the upper end of the oesophagus arising from ectopic gastric epithelium. *Br J Surg* 1950;37:474.
9. McKechnie JC, Fechner RE. Choriocarcinoma and adenocarcinoma of the esophagus with gonadotropin secretion. *Cancer* 1971;27(3):694–702.
10. Osborn NK, Keate RF, Trastek VF, et al. Verrucous carcinoma of the esophagus: Clinicopathophysiologic features and treatment of a rare entity. *Dig Dis Sci* 2003; 48(3):465–474.
11. Devlin S, Falck V, Urbanski SJ, et al. Verrucous carcinoma of the esophagus eluding multiple sets of endoscopic biopsies and endoscopic ultrasound: A case report and review of the literature. *Can J Gastroenterol* 2004;18(7):459–462.
12. Ramani C, Shah N, Nathan RS. Verrucous carcinoma of the esophagus: A case report and literature review. *World J Clin Cases* 2014;2(7):284–288.
13. Iyomasa S, Kato H, Tachimori Y, et al. Carcinosarcoma of the esophagus: A twenty-case study. *Jpn J Clin Oncol* 1990;20(1):99–106.
14. Kukar M, Groman A, Malhotra U, et al. Small cell carcinoma of the esophagus: A SEER database analysis. *Ann Surg Oncol* 2013;20(13):4239–4244.
15. Raza MA, Mazzara PF. Sarcomatoid carcinoma of esophagus. *Arch Pathol Lab Med* 2011;135(7):945–948.
16. Orsatti G, Corvalan AH, Sakurai H, et al. Polypoid adenosquamous carcinoma of the esophagus with prominent spindle cells. Report of a case with immunohistochemical and ultrastructural studies. *Arch Pathol Lab Med* 1993;117(5):544–547.
17. Martin MR, Kahn LB. So-called pseudosarcoma of the esophagus: Nodal metastases of the spindle cell element. *Arch Pathol Lab Med* 1977;101(11):604–609.
18. Osamura RY, Shimamura K, Hata JI, et al. Polypoid carcinoma of the esophagus. A unifying term for "carcinosarcoma" and "pseudosarcoma." *Am J Surg Pathol* 1978; 2(2):201–208.
19. Shields TW, Eilert JB, Battifora H. Pseudosarcoma of the oesophagus. *Thorax* 1972; 27(4):472–479.
20. Kimura N, Tezuka F, Ono I, et al. Myogenic expression in esophageal polypoid tumors. *Arch Pathol Lab Med* 1989;113(10):1159–1165.

21. McKeown F. Oat-cell carcinoma of the oesophagus. *J Pathol Bacteriol* 1952;64(4): 889–891.
22. Ku GY, Minsky BD, Rusch VW, et al. Small-cell carcinoma of the esophagus and gastroesophageal junction: Review of the Memorial Sloan-Kettering experience. *Ann Oncol* 2008;19(3):533–537.
23. Lv J, Liang J, Wang J, et al. Primary small cell carcinoma of the esophagus. *J Thorac Oncol* 2008;3(12):1460–1465.
24. Casas F, Ferrer F, Farrus B, et al. Primary small cell carcinoma of the esophagus: A review of the literature with emphasis on therapy and prognosis. *Cancer* 1997;80(8):1366–1372.
25. Noda K, Nishiwaki Y, Kawahara M, et al. Irinotecan plus cisplatin compared with etoposide plus cisplatin for extensive small-cell lung cancer. *N Engl J Med* 2002;346(2):85–91.
26. Medgyesy CD, Wolff RA, Putnam JB, Jr., et al. Small cell carcinoma of the esophagus: The University of Texas M.D. Anderson Cancer Center experience and literature review. *Cancer* 2000;88(2):262–267.
27. Brenner S, Heimlich H, Widman M. Carcinoid of esophagus. *N Y State J Med* 1969; 69(10):1337–1339.
28. Soga J. Esophageal endocrinomas, an extremely rare tumor: A statistical comparative evaluation of 28 ordinary carcinoids and 72 atypical variants. *J Exp Clin Cancer Res* 1998;17(1):47–57.
29. Lindberg GM, Molberg KH, Vuitch MF, et al. Atypical carcinoid of the esophagus: A case report and review of the literature. *Cancer* 1997;79(8):1476–1481.
30. Yagi M, Abe Y, Sasaki Y, et al. Esophageal carcinoid tumor treated by endoscopic resection. *Dig Endosc* 2015;27(4):527–530.
31. Xiaogang Z, Xingtao J, Huasheng W, et al. Atypical carcinoid of the esophagus: Report of a case. *Ann Thorac Cardiovasc Surg* 2002;8(5):302–305.
32. Oz MC, Ashley PF, Oz M. Atypical gastroesophageal carcinoid: A case report and review of the literature. *Del Med J* 1987;59(12):785–788.
33. Shah MJ, Birwa SB, Samanta ST, et al. Atypical carcinoid of the esophagus. *Indian J Pathol Microbiol* 2015;58(2):223–225.
34. Volpin E, Sauvanet A, Couvelard A, et al. Primary malignant melanoma of the esophagus: A case report and review of the literature. *Dis Esophagus* 2002;15(3):244–249.
35. De La Pava S, Nigogosyan G, Pickren JW, et al. Melanosis of the esophagus. *Cancer* 1963;16:48–50.
36. Sabanathan S, Eng J, Pradhan GN. Primary malignant melanoma of the esophagus. *Am J Gastroenterol* 1989;84(12):1475–1481.
37. Stringa O, Valdez R, Ruiz Beguerie J, et al. Primary amelanotic melanoma of the esophagus. *Int J Dermatol* 2006;45(10):1207–1210.
38. Allen AC, Spitz S. Malignant melanoma. A clinicopathological analysis of the criteria for diagnosis and prognosis. *Cancer* 1953;6(1):1–45.
39. Yano M, Shiozaki H, Murata A, et al. Primary malignant melanoma of the esophagus associated with adenocarcinoma of the lung. *Surg Today* 1998;28(4):405–408.
40. Naomoto Y, Perdomo JA, Kamikawa Y, et al. Primary malignant melanoma of the esophagus: Report of a case successfully treated with pre- and post-operative adjuvant hormone-chemotherapy. *Jpn J Clin Oncol* 1998;28(12):758–761.
41. Kato H, Watanabe H, Tachimori Y, et al. Primary malignant melanoma of the esophagus: Report of four cases. *Jpn J Clin Oncol* 1991;21(4):306–313.
42. Chalkiadakis G, Wihlm JM, Morand G, et al. Primary malignant melanoma of the esophagus. *Ann Thorac Surg* 1985;39(5):472–475.
43. Howard WT. Primary sarcoma of the esophagus and stomach. *JAMA* 1902;38(6): 392–394.
44. Patel SR, Anandarao N. Leiomyosarcoma of the esophagus. *N Y State J Med* 1990; 90(7):371–373.
45. Aimoto T, Sasajima K, Kyono S, et al. Leiomyosarcoma of the esophagus: Report of a case and preoperative evaluation by CT scan, endoscopic ultrasonography and angiography. *Gastroenterol Jpn* 1992;27(6):773–779.
46. Gaede JT, Postlethwait RW, Shelburne JD, et al. Leiomyosarcoma of the esophagus. Report of two cases, one with associated squamous cell carcinoma. *J Thorac Cardiovasc Surg* 1978;75(5):740–746.
47. Grover RS, Kernstine K, Krishnan A. A case of diffuse large B-cell lymphoma in association with paraesophageal leiomyoma: Highlighting false-positivity of PET scan and importance of tissue diagnosis. *J Natl Compr Canc Netw* 2012;10(5):577–581.
48. Levine MS, Buck JL, Pantongrag-Brown L, et al. Leiomyosarcoma of the esophagus: Radiographic findings in 10 patients. *AJR Am J Roentgenol* 1996;167(1):27–32.
49. Zhang BH, Zhang HT, Wang YG. Esophageal leiomyosarcoma: Clinical analysis and surgical treatment of 12 cases. *Dis Esophagus* 2014;27(6):547–551.
50. Shiraishi M, Takahashi T, Yamashiro M, et al. [A report of leiomyosarcoma of the esophagus]. *Nihon Ronen Igakkai Zasshi* 1995;32(4):286–291.
51. Perch SJ, Soffen EM, Whittington R, et al. Esophageal sarcomas. *J Surg Oncol* 1991; 48(3):194–198.
52. Batoroev YK, Nguyen GK. Esophageal rhabdomyosarcoma: Report of a case diagnosed by imprint cytology. *Acta Cytol* 2006;50(2):213–216.
53. Song HK, Miller JI. Primary myxofibrosarcoma of the esophagus. *J Thorac Cardiovasc Surg* 2002;124(1):196–197.
54. Yaghmai I, Ghahremani GG. Chondrosarcoma of the esophagus. *AJR Am J Roentgenol* 1976;126(6):1175–1177.
55. Dowli A, Mattar A, Mashimo H, et al. A pedunculated giant esophageal liposarcoma: A case report and literature review. *J Gastrointest Surg* 2014;18(12):2208–2213.
56. Ginai AZ, Halfhide BC, Dees J, et al. Giant esophageal polyp: A clinical and radiological entity with variable histology. *Eur Radiol* 1998;8(2):264–269.
57. McIntyre M, Webb JN, Browning GC. Osteosarcoma of the esophagus. *Hum Pathol* 1982;13(7):680–682.
58. Umerah BC. Kaposi sarcoma of the oesophagus. *Br J Radiol* 1980;53(632):807–808.
59. Lin CH, Hsu CW, Chiang YJ, et al. Esophageal and gastric Kaposi's sarcomas presenting as upper gastrointestinal bleeding. *Chang Gung Med J* 2002;25(5):329–333.
60. Tam HK, Zhang ZF, Jacobson LP, et al. Effect of highly active antiretroviral therapy on survival among HIV-infected men with Kaposi sarcoma or non-Hodgkin lymphoma. *Int J Cancer* 2002;98(6):916–922.
61. Habu S, Okamoto E, Toyosaka A, et al. Synovial sarcoma of the esophagus: Report of a case. *Surg Today* 1998;28(4):401–404.
62. Amr SS, Shihabi NK, Al Hajj H. Synovial sarcoma of the esophagus. *Am J Otolaryngol* 1984;5(4):266–269.
63. Wang S, Zheng J, Ruan Z, et al. Long-term survival in a rare case of malignant esophageal schwannoma cured by surgical excision. *Ann Thorac Surg* 2011;92(1): 357–358.
64. Manger T, Pross M, Haeckel C, et al. Malignant peripheral nerve sheath tumor of the esophagus. *Dig Surg* 2000;17(6):627–631.
65. Murase K, Hino A, Ozeki Y, et al. Malignant schwannoma of the esophagus with lymph node metastasis: Literature review of schwannoma of the esophagus. *J Gastroenterol* 2001;36(11):772–777.
66. Basoglu A, Celik B, Sengul TA, et al. Esophageal schwannoma. *J Thorac Cardiovasc Surg* 2006;131(2):492–493.
67. Voskuil JH, Van Dijk MM, Wagenaar SS, et al. Occurrence of esophageal granular cell tumors in The Netherlands between 1988 and 1994. *Dig Dis Sci* 2001;46(8): 1610–1614.
68. Lu W, Xu MD, Zhou PH, et al. Endoscopic submucosal dissection of esophageal granular cell tumor. *World J Surg Oncol* 2014;12:221.
69. Loo CK, Santos LD, Killingsworth MC. Malignant oesophageal granular cell tumour: A case report. *Pathology* 2004;36(5):506–508.
70. Geboes K, De Vos R, Lomami-Luakabanga B, et al. Primary malignant fibrous histiocytoma of the esophagus. *J Surg Oncol* 1989;40(1):49–57.
71. Hosaka S, Nakamura N, Akamatsu T, et al. A case of primary low grade mucosa associated lymphoid tissue (MALT) lymphoma of the oesophagus. *Gut* 2002;51(2): 281–284.
72. Kudo K, Ota M, Narumiya K, et al. Primary esophageal mucosa-associated lymphoid tissue lymphoma treated by endoscopic submucosal dissection. *Dig Endosc* 2014;26(3):478–481.
73. Mizobuchi S, Tachimori Y, Kato H, et al. Metastatic esophageal tumors from distant primary lesions: Report of three esophagectomies and study of 1835 autopsy cases. *Jpn J Clin Oncol* 1997;27(6):410–414.
74. Matsumoto Y, Matsukawa H, Seno H, et al. Education and imaging. Gastrointestinal: Breast cancer metastasis to the esophagus diagnosed using endoscopic ultrasound-guided fine-needle aspiration. *J Gastroenterol Hepatol* 2015;30(2):233.
75. Simchuk EJ, Low DE. Direct esophageal metastasis from a distant primary tumor is a submucosal process: A review of six cases. *Dis Esophagus* 2001;14(3–4):247–250.

146

Palliative Approaches to Inoperable Esophageal Cancer

Jonathan D. Spicer ▪ Garrett L. Walsh

INTRODUCTION

Inoperable esophageal cancer can be defined according to several clinical findings. Some esophageal neoplasms present with no evidence of systemic spread and are technically resectable; however, the patient's condition may prohibit surgical management based on poor performance status. Alternatively, a patient may be fit for surgery, but presents with a technically unresectable lesion or evidence of systemic spread. Regardless of the situation, dysphagia is the primary symptom for which the thoracic surgeon will be called upon to provide palliation in patients with inoperable esophageal cancer. Hence, this chapter will focus on the currently available techniques for palliation of dysphagia caused by locally advanced esophageal cancer.

Dysphagia is defined as a difficulty encountered when attempting to swallow solids or liquids. The problem can originate from oropharyngeal dyscoordination, from neurological impairment of normal esophageal peristalsis and in the case of esophageal cancer, most commonly from mechanical obstruction caused by the primary tumor. The impact of dysphagia for the esophageal cancer patient can be dramatic leading to severe weight loss and significant nutritional deficits, and can also cause recurrent aspiration. Needless to say, the ability to eat is one of the most basic aspects of our daily lives and the impairment caused by esophageal cancer has a profound impact on the quality of life and general psychological status of these patients, beyond the obvious physiologic consequences. As a result, our ability to improve our patients' ability to eat after a diagnosis of inoperable esophageal cancer is of paramount importance to improving their end-of-life experience and minimizing the suffering caused by this fatal disease.

CLINICAL ASSESSMENT

Squamous cell carcinoma and adenocarcinoma of the esophagus account for approximately 95% of esophageal malignancies.[1] Typically, squamous cell carcinoma has a predilection for the upper and middle thirds of the esophagus and is more prevalent in Asia where smoking and alcohol abuse are the predominant risk factors. The incidence of esophageal adenocarcinoma is rising faster than almost any other malignancy in North America and is certainly the predominant type in the Western hemisphere.[2] They are generally located in the middle and distal thirds (including the esophagogastric junction or EGJ). Again, with both, the most common presenting symptom is dysphagia. An essential part of the work up of any esophageal cancer patient is a symptomatic assessment of their dysphagia for it is both predictive of their clinical T stage and a critical consideration when choosing the best approach to manage their condition. While several dysphagia scoring systems exist, we favor the one published by Bergquist et al.[3] where dysphagia is graded on a 5-point Likert scale: 0, no dysphagia; 1, dysphagia to solids; 2, dysphagia to semi-solids; 3, dysphagia to liquids; 4, dysphagia to own saliva. In addition, patients will frequently be able to locate the level at which they notice bolus impaction which frequently correlates with the level of the lesion.

The remainder of the history and physical exam is fairly standard and focuses on the extent of the local and systemic impacts of the cancer. Anorexia, weight loss, chest pain, odynophagia, stridor, and bone pain are all ominous signs of an advanced stage. Hoarseness is an important finding to elicit since it may signal recurrent laryngeal nerve involvement by the tumor or invaded lymph nodes and is associated with a much higher risk of aspiration. The physical exam is geared toward further evaluating aspects of esophageal cancer progression that may further impact their ability to swallow and eat. A cervical and supraclavicular nodal exam is critical, along with a thorough cranial nerve examination. A quick and inexpensive bedside swallowing assessment can be performed using 10 cc of fluid ingestion and monitoring for cough or desaturation.[4] Such a screening tool will help guide the need for more involved radiographically assisted swallowing assessments by a speech and language therapist.

The work-up of such patients will often already have been performed to determine that they have inoperable esophageal cancer, nevertheless, an upper endoscopy is essential to obtain a tissue diagnosis and gain an appreciation for the level at which the tumor is located and the degree to which it obstructs the lumen. Thus, even when such exams have been previously performed for the sake of diagnosis and staging, a patient with progressive esophageal cancer may require reinvestigation either by CT scan or endoscopy to determine the optimal palliative approach. The location of the lesion is an essential consideration due to potential involvement of the airway when dealing with lesions of the upper and middle thirds of the esophagus. Similarly, lower third and EGJ tumors can present challenges due to the massive reflux that can occur when such lesions are stented.

ASSESSING OPERABILITY

Standard criteria to determining whether a patient is operable do not universally exist. Certainly, patients with evidence of systemic spread do not benefit from surgical resection. However, practice patterns vary significantly amongst surgeons and institutions for patients with locally advanced disease (T4 lesions) or evidence of regional and nonregional lymph node spread (Fig. 146.1). Many would consider clinically evident T4 lesions or N3 disease to be contraindications to surgery while others have tackled such cases in the context of multimodality therapy with some success.[5] Hence, determining resectability from a tumor standpoint is fairly variable and will depend on response to induction treatments and surgical expertise. Clearly, the goal of any surgical interventions ought to be geared toward achieving an R0 resection.

Physiologic factors are of utmost importance when assessing operability. Esophagectomy is a major surgical undertaking regardless of the mode of approach, Ivor-Lewis, transhiatal, minimally invasive or other. Consequently, surgeons must evaluate both modifiable and nonmodifiable factors that are predictive of surgical outcome. In patients eligible for surgery, nutritional status may initially be prohibitive, but with neoadjuvant therapy and nutritional supportive measures can be rehabilitated to become good surgical candidates. However, advanced age is a nonmodifiable factor that is associated with higher rates of pulmonary complications, which requires careful cardiopulmonary evaluation prior to choosing the ideal treatment modality and whether surgery is advisable. Generally speaking, the surgeon must carefully evaluate the patient's desire to proceed with surgery and take all comorbidities into consideration to determine whether the operative risk is prohibitive.[6,7] Finally, each case must be discussed

in the context of a multidisciplinary tumor board to establish a consensus-based approach to each individual patient.

MANAGEMENT

Once a patient has been deemed inoperable, the treatment team must determine whether the patient remains eligible for curative intent treatment utilizing bimodality chemoradiation therapy (CRT). In such cases, excellent palliation of dysphagia can be achieved within 2 to 4 weeks after initiation of treatment (Fig. 146.2). It should be noted that CRT can cause initial swelling that converts a patient with partial dysphagia to a patient with a complete inability to eat and drink. As a result, due to the excellent partial response rates with induction chemotherapy using Docetaxel, Cisplatin and Fluorouracil (DCF),[8] many centres have adopted such an approach even in unresectable patients prior to definitive CRT.[9] Hence, some patients will require some form of invasive tube feeding. For short-term bridging, nasogastric feeding tubes are used, given their safety profile and the fact that they are relatively inexpensive. While these can often be placed at the bedside for patients with smaller lesions, they occasionally require endoscopic or radiographic guidance to achieve proper placement beyond the obstructing lesion. Percutaneous gastrostomy tubes can be placed endoscopically or radiographically as an outpatient procedure and are useful in cases where the lesion causes a complete obstruction. Feeding jejunostomies are not usually necessary in the palliative or nonoperative setting. Depending on the histology of the lesion, results with bimodality definitive therapy vary with squamous cell carcinoma showing the best outcomes.[10,11] Overall survival in this cohort, all histologies combined, is in the range of 25% at 5 years, though outcomes are likely to continue to improve with the advent of such technologies as proton-based radiotherapy and increasingly effective systemic agents.

When curative intent therapy is not an option, the clinician must determine the importance and feasibility of restoring normal

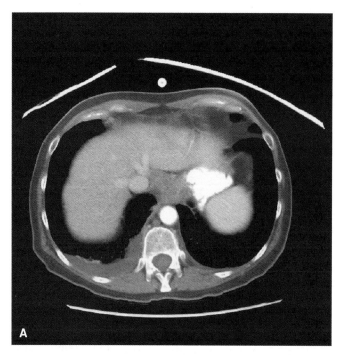

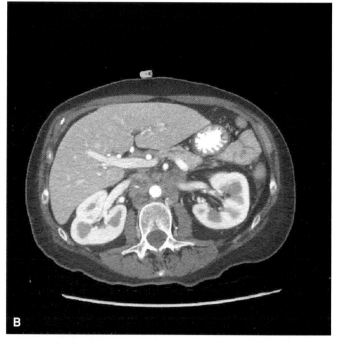

FIGURE 146.1 Unresectable T4 esophageal adenocarcinoma. **A:** Completely obstructing esophageal mass. **B:** Bulky circumferential periaortic adenopathy.

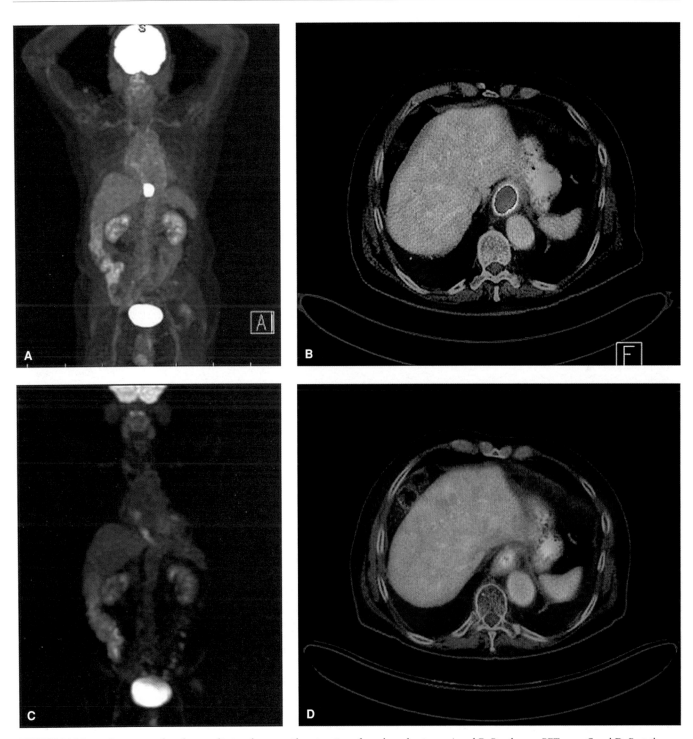

FIGURE 146.2 Local response after chemoradiation therapy with restoration of esophageal patency. **A** and **B**: Pre-therapy PET scan. **C** and **D**: Post-therapy PET scan.

oral nutrition. A helpful guide is whether the patient's appetite has been maintained. If it has, relief of the obstruction can provide good palliation. This is not the case if the tumor burden has produced nausea and pain from eating or even a total loss of appetite. For patients with a very short prognosis on the order of days, invasive therapies are not beneficial. Indeed, dehydration and inability to eat do not contribute to patient distress in the final moments of life.[12] This may be difficult for the patient's family to understand, which highlights the importance of careful discussion with family members and loved ones.

However, for patients with a longer prognosis who are contemplating palliative chemotherapy or who have a lower burden of disease, a number of options exist to provide durable relief from dysphagia.

ESOPHAGEAL STENTS

Self-expanding metallic stents (SEMS) have become one of the most commonly utilized strategies to manage malignant esophageal strictures. They are available in a variety of lengths and diameters, and can be partially or fully covered. Fully covered stents are more prone

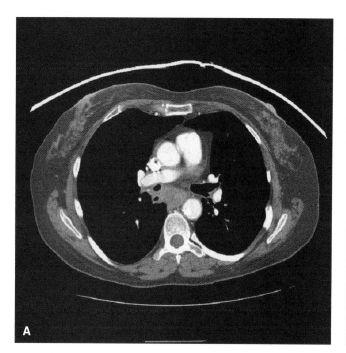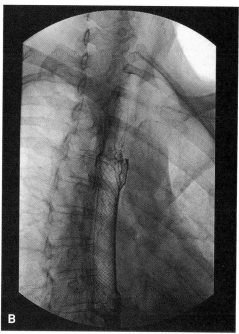

FIGURE 146.3 Patient with complete dysphagia pre (**A**) and post (**B**) placement of SEMS.

to migration but less susceptible to tumor ingrowth.[13] Because stent migration is a particularly vexing problem for patients, the use of partially covered stents is preferred for the purposes of palliation. The uncovered ends offer good grip along the esophageal wall and the covered central portion provides resistance to tumor ingrowth and therefore a more prolonged patency as compared to an uncovered stent.

Relief of dysphagia using such stents can be almost immediate depending on the bulk and rigidity of the area being bridged (Fig. 146.3). They are effective in 85% to 100% of cases and have been associated with increased appetite and overall well-being.[14] On the down side, relief of dysphagia is not permanent with recurrence frequently occurring at 5 to 6 months.[15] Other potential complications include migration in approximately 30% of cases, bleeding, perforation, and aspiration. Some limitations to stent use include lesions located in the high cervical regions of the esophagus. The mucosal sensitivity of the oropharynx precludes stent placement due to the significant pain and constant triggering of the gag reflex when the proximal portion of the stent is deployed in this area. Placement across the EGJ may also be problematic due to the stent assuming a transverse orientation such that its distal portion can abut the greater curvature of the stomach leading to mechanical obstruction. Such placement can also result in massive and uncontrollable reflux, the symptoms of which may be impossible for the patient to tolerate. While valved stents do exist, they have yet to show promising results for this application. Stents can sometimes produce substernal pain. While most often lasting only 1 to 2 days, occasionally the pain persists necessitating stent removal. A more detailed discussion of esophageal stents is presented in Chapter 131.

OTHER ENDOSCOPIC TECHNIQUES

A number of endoscopic techniques have been developed over the years to manage local tumor growth. None of these has surpassed the effectiveness of modern stents and for this reason most have fallen out of favor. Photodynamic therapy (PDT) has been utilized in this context although it is better recognized for its use in the management of Barrett's esophagus.[16] The technique requires injection of a photosensitizing agent followed by endoscopy 48 hours later, at which time, the esophageal mucosa/tumor is exposed to laser light. This exposure results in ablation of the surrounding tissue. Repeat endoscopy at a later date is required to debride the necrotic tissue and this technique has been associated with such complications as perforation and significant chest pain resulting from the inflammation caused by the local tissue destruction. Furthermore, patients undergoing PDT must avoid sunlight for 1 month after therapy to avoid cutaneous burns.

Several other endoscopic ablative techniques exist. Neodymium-yttrium-aluminum-garnet (Nd:YAG) laser is an effective technique to debulk a lesion endoscopically. It is effective in up to 70% of patients for relief of dysphagia and it is most useful for exophytic tumors that are less than 5 cm in length and in a nontortuous portion of the esophagus.[17] Complications, such as perforation or tracheoesophageal fistula, have been reported in as many as 5% of patients. Similarly, argon plasma coagulation has been used, however, tissue penetration is less than with an Nd-YAG laser and therefore the ability to debulk is reduced.[18] It has, therefore, been used frequently in combination with other modalities such as PDT. Similarly to Nd-YAG, the risk of perforation remains high and can reach up to 8%. Absolute alcohol injection has also been used as a local ablative therapy. While it is cheap and effective on the short term, its use is limited by early recurrence and the need for multiple treatments.[19]

RADIATION THERAPY

While radiation therapy alone has not demonstrated any efficacy to achieve cure for locally advanced esophageal cancer, it can be a very effective form of palliation. As mentioned, radiation is preferably used in combination with chemotherapy due to the increased efficacy and potential chance of achieving complete response for patients without evidence of systemic spread. However, because it is very well tolerated when used alone, it provides effective results for patients who are unable to tolerate systemic chemotherapy. The mode of delivery can be either via multifractionated external beam radiotherapy or by endoluminal brachytherapy. Although external beam radiotherapy can provide good results with relief of dysphagia in as many as 69% of patients,[20] several fractions (between 2 and 10) are required to achieve good results, which can be problematic for palliative patients who lack the energy or resources to have the treatments delivered several times per week. As an alternative, brachytherapy delivered via an endoscopic route provides a convenient approach for the patient. High doses can be achieved with one or two endoscopic interventions. The primary drawback to brachytherapy is the time required to achieve results which do not compare favorably to SEMS.[21] Nevertheless, with time, brachytherapy achieves equal effectiveness as compared to SEMS one month after institution of treatment. A recent trial has investigated the effectiveness of SEMS loaded with brachytherapy beads and found that this technique actually prolonged survival in inoperable esophageal cancer patients. Such technology is likely the ideal approach at this time given the early effectiveness of the SEMS with the long-term durability of brachytherapy and the convenience of avoiding multiple visits to undergo external beam therapy.[22]

MEDICAL INTERVENTIONS

One of the most common problems that arises with malignant dysphagia is oral and esophageal candidiasis. Due to the stasis of organic matter within the esophagus proximal to the obstructing lesion, fungal overgrowth is a common problem leading to significant discomfort. Hence, while the obstruction may be relieved by the placement of a SEMS or by application of radiation therapy, dysphagia may persist as a result of untreated candidiasis. Excellent results can be achieved by treating oral and esophageal candidiasis with nystatin swish and swallow at 400,000 to 600,000 units four times a day. If symptoms persist, oral fluconazole provides 90% effectiveness.[23] To deal with the mucositis caused by chemotherapy and/or radiation therapy, we recommend careful oral hygiene and an orally available cocktail of drugs such as lidocaine, diphenhydramine, antacid, and dexamethasone. Such medication is focused on managing the persistent odynophagia that can plague these frail patients.[24]

MANAGEMENT OF MALIGNANT ESOPHAGEAL FISTULAE

Fortunately, esophageal fistula resulting from primary esophageal carcinoma is relatively rare. However, when it occurs, the consequences can be fairly dramatic with aspiration of stagnant polymicrobial foodstuff into the airway or major bleeding from the heart or great vessels. In the case of a fistula with the airway, most patients can be palliated with an esophageal SEMS.[25] However, in some cases, adequate exclusion of the airway cannot be achieved in this manner and double airway and esophageal stenting is required (Fig. 146.4).[26,27] Naturally, such a situation can aggravate the size of the fistula. In the inoperable patient with a relatively limited lifespan, providing temporary relief from aspiration and the ability to ingest food are worthy goals, yet such events generally portend a dismal prognosis and major emphasis ought to be placed on adequate palliation of the patient's symptoms by noninterventional means. With regards to bleeding, such events are most often fatal due to the nature of the structures with which the esophagus may communicate. Nevertheless, rare reports utilizing aortic stents have demonstrated temporary success to prevent massive exsanguination.[28]

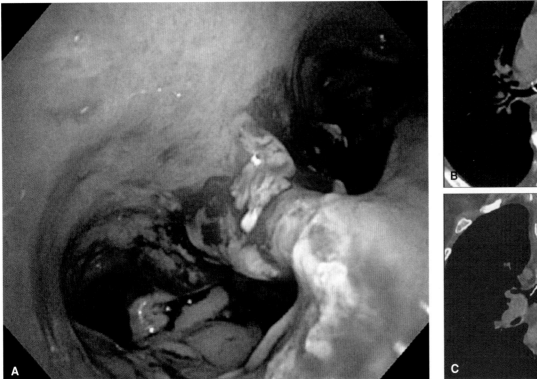
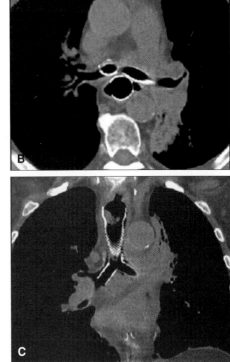

FIGURE 146.4 Use of double esophageal and bronchial stent to exclude a malignant esophagobronchial fistula. **A:** Endoscopic view of large malignant bronchoesophageal fistula. **B** and **C:** Axial and coronal views of patient post double trachea-bronchial Y stent and esophageal stent placement. (Images courtesy of Dr. Moishe Liberman.)

SUMMARY

Patients with inoperable esophageal cancer can still achieve cure when definitive bimodality CRT therapy is feasible as determined by tumor factors and the patient's ability to tolerate this therapeutic course. Systemic chemotherapy is an effective means of achieving rapid relief of dysphagia prior to definitive CRT. SEMS provide the most effective immediate relief of dysphagia when chemotherapy is not feasible or if the degree of dysphagia is prohibitive. SEMS are ideal for inoperable patients who cannot tolerate any form of curative intent therapy and, when combined with brachytherapy, durability and overall survival are improved. Finally, SEMS are an effective means of palliating the rare instances where disease progression and/or complications of therapy have led to fistulization with the airway or neighboring great vessels. Overall, the primary objective is respecting patient wishes and providing optimal relief of symptoms in a multidisciplinary fashion.

REFERENCES

1. Daly JM, Karnell LH, Menck HR. National Cancer Data Base report on esophageal carcinoma. *Cancer* 1996;78:1820–1828.
2. Siegel R, Naishadham D, Jemal A. Cancer statistics, 2013. *CA Cancer J Clin* 2013; 63(1):11–30.
3. Bergquist H, Wenger U, Johnsson E, et al. Stent insertion or endoluminal brachytherapy as palliation of patients with advanced cancer of the esophagus and gastroesophageal junction. Results of a randomized controlled clinical trial. *Dis Esophagus* 2005; 18:131–139.
4. Smith HA, Lee SH, O'Neill PA, et al. The combination of bedside swallowing assessment and oxygen saturation monitoring of swallowing in acute stroke: a safe and humane screening tool. *Age Ageing* 2000;29:495–499.
5. Pimiento JM, Weber J, Hoffe S, et al. Outcomes associated with surgery for T4 esophageal cancer. *Ann Surg Oncol* 2013;20:2706–2712.
6. Backemar L, Lagergen P, Djärv T, et al. Comorbidities and risk of complications after surgery for esophageal cancer: a nationwide cohort study in Sweden. *World J Surg* 2015;39(9):2282–2288.
7. O'Grady G, Hameed AM, Pang TC, et al. Patient selection for oesophagectomy: impact of age and comorbidities on outcome. *World J Surg* 2015;39(8):1994–1999.
8. Cools-Lartigue J, Jones D, Spicer J, et al. Management of dysphagia in esophageal adenocarcinoma patients undergoing neoadjuvant chemotherapy: can invasive tube feeding be avoided? *Ann Surg Oncol* 2015;22(6):1858–1865.
9. Satake H, Tahara M, Mochizuki S, et al. A prospective, multicenter phase I/II study of induction chemotherapy with docetaxel, cisplatin and fluorouracil (DCF) followed by chemoradiotherapy in patients with unresectable locally advanced esophageal carcinoma. *Cancer Chemother Pharmacol* 2016;78(1):91–99.
10. Cooper JS, Guo MD, Herskovic A, et al. Chemoradiotherapy of locally advanced esophageal cancer: long-term follow-up of a prospective randomized trial (RTOG 85-01). Radiation Therapy Oncology Group. *JAMA* 1999;281(17):1623–1627.
11. Suzuki A, Xiao L, Hayashi Y, et al. Nomograms for prognostication of outcome in patients with esophageal and gastroesophageal carcinoma undergoing definitive chemoradiotherapy. *Oncology* 2012;82(2):108–113.
12. McCann RM, Hall WJ, Groth-Juncker A. Comfort care for terminally ill patients. The appropriate use of nutrition and hydration. *JAMA* 1994;272:1263–1266.
13. Kim SG, Yang CH. Upper gastrointestinal stent. *Clin Endosc* 2012;45:386–391.
14. Madhusudhan C, Saluja SS, Pal S, et al. Palliative stenting for relief of dysphagia in patients with inoperable esophageal cancer: impact on quality of life. *Dis Esophagus* 2009;22:331–336.
15. Hanna WC, Sudarshan M, Roberge D, et al. What is the optimal management of dysphagia in metastatic esophageal cancer? *Curr Oncol* 2012;19:e60–e66.
16. Lightdale CJ, Heier SK, Marcon NE, et al. Photodynamic therapy with porfimer sodium versus thermal ablation therapy with Nd:YAG laser for palliation of esophageal cancer: a multicenter randomized trial. *Gastrointest Endosc* 1995;42: 507–512.
17. Haddad NG, Fleischer DE. Endoscopic laser therapy for esophageal cancer. *Surg Clin North Am* 1994;4:863–874.
18. Heindorff H, Wøjdemann M, Bisgaard T, et al. Endoscopic palliation of inoperable cancer of the oesophagus or cardia by argon electrocoagulation. *Scand J Gastroenterol* 1998;33:21–23.
19. Ozdil B, Kece C, Akkiz H, et al. Management of an esophageal metallic stent obstructed by tumor progression: endoscopic alcohol injection therapy instead of restenting. *Endoscopy* 2010;42(suppl 2):E91.
20. Kassam Z, Wong RK, Ringash J, et al. A phase I/II study to evaluate the toxicity and efficacy of accelerated fractionation radiotherapy for the palliation of dysphagia from carcinoma of the oesophagus. *Clin Oncol (R Coll Radiol)* 2008;20(1):53–60.
21. Amdal CD, Jacobsen AB, Sandstad B, et al. Palliative brachytherapy with or without primary stent placement in patients with oesophageal cancer, a randomised phase III trial. *Radiother Oncol* 2013;107(3):428–433.
22. Zhu HD, Guo JH, Mao AW, et al. Conventional stents versus stents loaded with (125) iodine seeds for the treatment of unresectable oesophageal cancer: a multicentre, randomised phase 3 trial. *Lancet Oncol* 2014;15(6):612–619.
23. Finlay PM, Richardson MD, Robertson AG. A comparative study of the efficacy of fluconazole and amphotericin B in the treatment of oropharyngeal candidiasis in patients undergoing radiotherapy for head and neck tumours. *Br J Oral Maxillofac Surg* 1996;34:23–25.
24. Galloway T, Robert JA. Management and prevention of complications during initial treatment of head and neck cancer. In: Posner M, Brockstein B, Brizel D, et al. eds. Waltham, MA: UpToDate; 2012.
25. Schweigert M, Dubecz A, Beron M, et al. Management of anastomotic leakage-induced tracheobronchial fistula following oesophagectomy: the role of endoscopic stent insertion. *Eur J Cardiothorac Surg* 2012;41(5):e74–e80.
26. Schweigert M, Posada-González M, Dubecz A, et al. Recurrent oesophageal cancer complicated by tracheo-oesophageal fistula: improved palliation by means of parallel tracheal and oesophageal stenting. *Interact Cardiovasc Thorac Surg* 2014; 18(2):190–196.
27. Hamai Y, Hihara J, Emi M, et al. Airway stenting for malignant respiratory complications in esophageal cancer. *Anticancer Res* 2012;32(5):1785–1790.
28. Uchida N, Katayama K, Sueda T. Endovascular stent graft for aortoesophageal fistula caused by esophageal stent. *Asian Cardiovasc Thorac Ann* 2014;22(3):368.

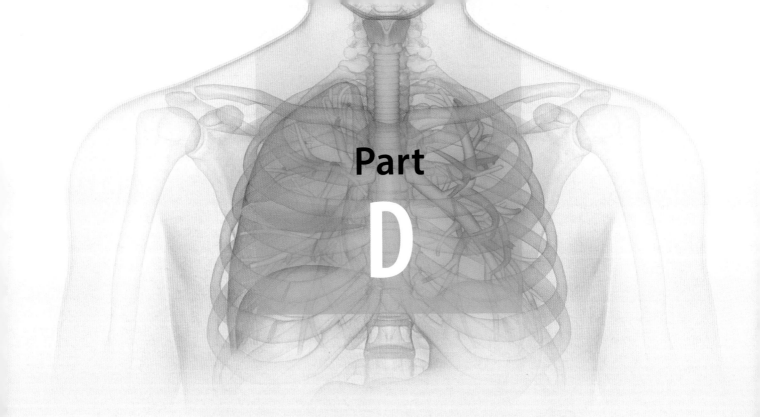

THE MEDIASTINUM

STRUCTURE AND FUNCTION OF THE MEDIASTINAL CONTENTS

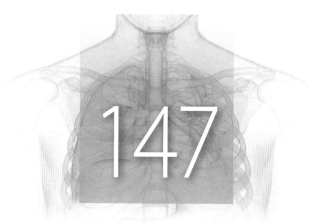

147

The Mediastinum, Its Compartments, and the Mediastinal Lymph Nodes

Hisao Asamura ▪ Masaya Yotsukura

DEFINITION OF THE MEDIASTINUM

The mediastinum is defined as the thoracic space located between the two pleural cavities. It originates at the thoracic inlet and extends inferiorly to the superior surface of the diaphragm. It is anteriorly bounded by the undersurface of the sternum and posteriorly by the thoracic vertebral column. Several organs and structures, such as heart and great vessels, trachea and main bronchi, esophagus, thymus, and lymphatic vessels, are contained in the mediastinum.[1]

SUBDIVISIONS OF THE MEDIASTINUM

Different radiographical and surgical subdivisions of the mediastinum have been proposed in the literature.[1-4] Generally, the mediastinum can be divided into four or three compartments, depending on whether the superior mediastinal compartment is considered as a separate anatomical entity.

FOUR-COMPARTMENT MODEL

The most common type of anatomical subdivision is the four-compartment model, which was described in Gray's anatomy.[5] It divides the mediastinum into the superior, anterior, middle, and posterior compartments (Fig. 147.1). The superior mediastinum originates at the thoracic inlet and extends inferiorly to a horizontal line connecting the sternomanubrial junction (angle of Louis) and the lower part of the fourth thoracic vertebra. The major components of the superior mediastinum are the aorta and great vessels, trachea, upper third of the esophagus, upper thymus, vagus and phrenic nerves, lymphatic tissues, and upper thoracic duct. The anterior mediastinum is located between the body of the sternum and the anterior pericardium. It contains mediastinal fat, lymph nodes, and the thymus. The middle mediastinum is anteriorly bounded by the pericardium. It is posteriorly bounded by the bifurcation of the trachea, pulmonary vessels, and pericardium. It encompasses the pericardium and its contents, carina, lymphatic tissues, and proximal portions of the main bronchi. The posterior mediastinum extends from the dorsal surface of the pericardium, bifurcation of the trachea, pulmonary vessels, and the posterior part of the upper surface of the diaphragm to the ventral surface of the lower eight thoracic vertebrae (T5-12). It contains the esophagus, descending thoracic aorta, azygos vein, sympathetic trunk, lymphatic tissues, and thoracic duct.[4,6]

A major problem with this classification is the fact that some of the organs or structures are included into multiple compartments. Therefore, the location of the organs or structures in the mediastinum cannot be simply described with one specific mediastinal site.

In 2013, a new method for a classification of mediastinal compartment was proposed by the Japanese Association for Research on the

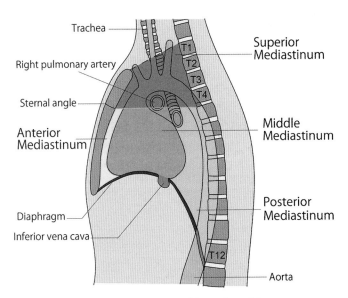

FIGURE 147.1 Schematic illustration of the traditional four-compartment subdivision of the mediastinum.

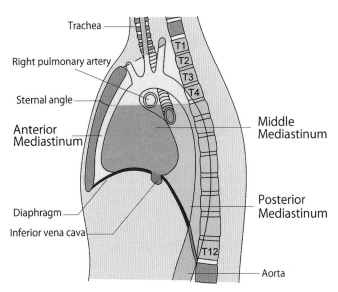

FIGURE 147.2 An example of the schematic illustration of the traditional three-compartment subdivision of the mediastinum.

Thymus (JART).[2] This method divides the mediastinum into four compartments based on anatomical boundary, using transverse computed tomography (CT) images. In this model, the superior and the anterior mediastinum is separated by the anatomical line defined by the intersection of caudal margin of left innominate vein with the trachea. This boundary is linked with the definition of the paratracheal lymph nodes proposed by the International Association for the Study of Lung Cancer (IASLC).[7] The esophagus, trachea, and bronchi, all of which share the same embryological origin, are included in the middle mediastinum compartment. This classification aims to categorize mediastinal lesions in a simple way, and to make differential diagnosis easier.

THREE-COMPARTMENT MODEL

There are several different types of three-compartment models, which subdivide the mediastinum into anterior, middle, and posterior compartments. In this article, we describe three common types of classifications.

Traditional Model

In the traditional three-compartment model, the anterior mediastinum includes the superior mediastinum as outlined in the traditional four-compartment model (Fig. 147.2).[4,6] The middle mediastinum is the area located between the anterior and posterior mediastinum, which is the same definition used in the traditional four-compartment model. The posterior mediastinum extends from the superior aspect of the first thoracic vertebra to the diaphragm inferiorly, containing the area where the traditional four-compartment model defined as the posterior compartment.[4] This model ignores anatomical boundaries, similar to the traditional four-compartment model.

As another traditional three-compartment model, a mediastinal classification based on lateral chest radiographs was defined in the Felson's textbook (Fig. 147.3).[3] Precisely, this was not intended to subdivide the mediastinum, but to show a method for indicating the location of a mass on radiography. A line drawn along the tracheal anterior and cardiac posterior edges is assumed to be the boundary between the anterior and middle mediastinum. The boundary of the middle and posterior mediastinum is drawn by a line that connects a point located 1 cm behind the anterior margin of each thoracic

vertebral body.[2] This method is purely dependent on lateral profiles of two-dimensional chest radiography. Therefore, exact location of a mass cannot be correctly determined when compared with three-dimensional findings detected by CT or surgical procedure.

Shields' Classification

Shields suggested an original method for dividing the mediastinum in 1972 (Fig. 147.4).[8] He classified the mediastinum into the anterior compartment, middle compartment (also referred to as the visceral compartment), and bilateral paravertebral sulci. The anterior compartment is bounded anteriorly by the undersurface of the sternum, superiorly by the innominate veins, and posteriorly by an imaginary line formed by the anterior surfaces of the great vessels and pericardium. The middle compartment extends from the posterior surface of the superior portion of the sternum above the innominate veins, and the posterior limit of the anterior compartment below these

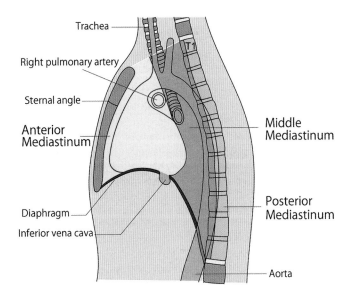

FIGURE 147.3 Schematic illustration of Felson's classification of the mediastinum compartment. Felson's classification is based on the chest roentgenology, therefore the boundary line could be vague.

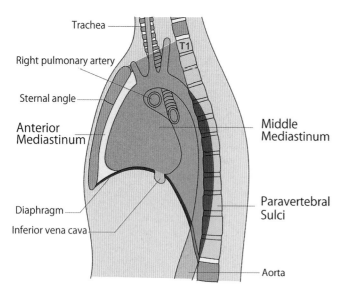

FIGURE 147.4 Schematic illustration of the Shields' mediastinal subdivision.

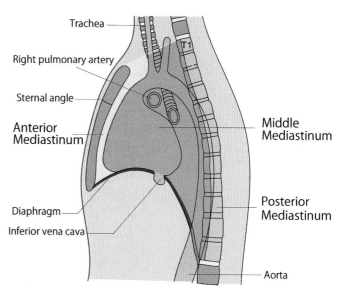

FIGURE 147.5 A schematic illustration of subdivisions of the mediastinum proposed by the International Thymic Malignancy Interest Group. This is an example of an illustration which shows a sagittal reformatted image of computed tomography. It should be noted that the anterior mediastinum wraps around the heart and pericardium.

veins, to the ventral surface of the vertebral column. The paravertebral sulci are not truly mediastinal compartments, but are spaces along each side of the vertebral column just adjacent to the proximal portions of the ribs. The thoracic inlet space is occupied with the middle compartment and two paravertebral sulci. The anterior compartment does not directly communicate with the thoracic inlet.

Shields described that the anterior compartment generally contains the thymus, internal mammary vessels, lymph nodes, and fat. He also indicated that displaced parathyroid glands and true ectopic thyroid tissues may also be present in this compartment.

The middle compartment contains the pericardium, heart, and great vessels, and the major visceral structures including the trachea, proximal portions of the main bronchi, and esophagus. This compartment also contains extensive lymphatic tissues, the vagus and phrenic nerves, the supraaortic and paraaortic bodies, multiple nerve plexuses and fibers, thoracic duct, proximal portion of the azygos venous system, connective tissue, and fat.

The paravertebral sulci primarily contain the proximal portions of the intercostal arteries, veins, and nerves, thoracic spinal ganglions, sympathetic trunk and its major branches, connective and lymphatic tissues, as well as the distal azygos vein.

International Thymic Malignancy Interest Group Classification

In 2014, the International Thymic Malignancy Interest Group (ITMIG) described a new method of CT-based mediastinal subdivision, based on the aforementioned JART model.[1] However, unlike the JART model, the ITMIG model does not define the superior mediastinum, because the superior segment is not inevitable to obtain useful information for making diagnosis. In this new classification, the anterior compartment is defined anteriorly by the sternum and posteriorly by the anterior aspect of the pericardium (Fig. 147.5). The middle compartment is bounded anteriorly by the anterior aspect of the pericardium and posteriorly by a vertical line connecting the points that are located 1 cm posterior to the anterior margin of the vertebral columns. The posterior compartment is bounded anteriorly by the visceral compartment and posteriorly by a vertical line along the posterior margin of the chest wall on the lateral aspect of the transverse processes. Each compartment is bound superiorly by the thoracic inlet and inferiorly by the diaphragm.

The ITMIG indicated that the major components of the anterior compartment include the thymus, fat, and left brachiocephalic vein. The

components of the middle compartment are classified into two categories. The one is a vascular category, which contains the heart, superior vena cava, ascending thoracic aorta, aortic arch, descending thoracic aorta, intrapericardial pulmonary arteries, and thoracic duct. The other category contains the trachea, carina, and esophagus, all of which share the same embryological origin. The major components of the posterior compartment include the thoracic spine and paravertebral soft tissues.

MEDIASTINAL LYMPH NODES

The mediastinum is rich in the lymphatic vessels and lymph nodes. It is essential for thoracic surgeons to understand the route of the

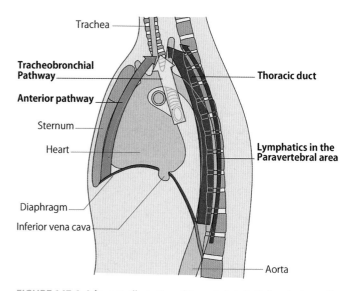

FIGURE 147.6 Schematic illustration of the main lymphatic flow in the mediastinum. The anterior pathway (*green arrow*), tracheobronchial pathway (*yellow arrow*), thoracic duct (*red arrow*), and the lymphatics in the paravertebral area (*blue arrow*) are shown.

lymphatic pathways and location of lymph nodes in order to perform safe surgeries with high-curability, since it has been well recognized that, together with venous route, the lymphatic channel is one of the most important route of the spread of cancer cells.

We classify the major lymphatic pathways of the mediastinum into four categories: the anterior pathway, tracheobronchial pathway, thoracic duct, and pathway in paravertebral area (Fig. 147.6). It has been clinically well recognized that malignant tumors, especially carcinomas, tend to spread through regional lymphatics and lymph nodes, and therefore, in the surgical treatment of the malignant tumors in the chest,

the clearance of the lymphatic route is an important part of the radical procedures termed as "lymph node dissection" or "lymphadenectomy" together with removal of the primary tumor. In performing this, surgeons are required to adequately perform the dissection based upon the anatomy of the regional lymphatics and lymph nodes.

ANTERIOR PATHWAY

Regarding the anterior pathway of lymphatics in the mediastinum, the internal mammary chain, which is located along the bilateral

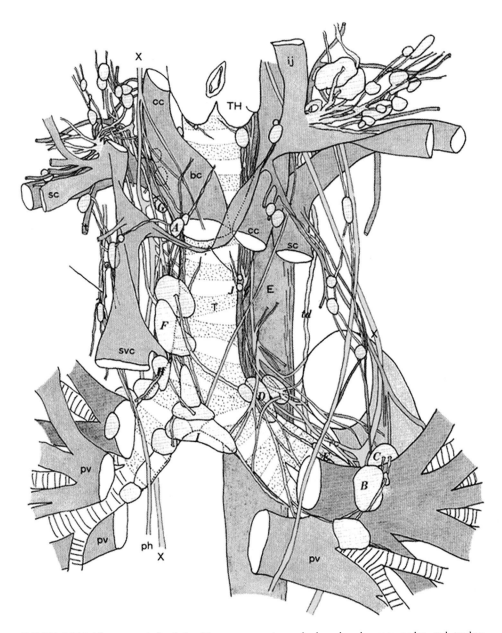

FIGURE 147.7 The anatomical relationship among great vessels, bronchopulmonary nodes, and tracheobronchial nodes. Arteries, veins, and nerves are shown in red, blue, and yellow, respectively. TH, thyroid gland; T, trachea; cc, common carotid artery; bc, brachiocephalic artery; sc, subclavian artery/vein; it, internal thoracic artery; ij, internal jugular vein; svc, superior vena cava; pv, pulmonary vein; ph, phrenic nerve; X, vagus nerve; E, esophagus; A, venous angle lymph node; B, lymph node anterior to pulmonary artery; C, lymph node of ligamentum arteriosum; D, left paratracheal or parabronchial lymph node; E, lymph node nearby the ligamentum arteriosum; F, right paratracheal lymph node; G, lymph node of right recurrent nerve; H, right paratracheal or parabronchial lymph node, I, subcarinal lymph node; J, left paratracheal lymph node; td, thoracic duct. (From Sato T. *Color Atlas of Applied Anatomy of Lymphatics.* Tokyo: Nanko-Do; 1997:149. Copyright © Gen Murakami. With permission.)

internal thoracic arteries drains the upper anterior abdominal wall, anterior chest wall, anterior portion of the diaphragm, and medial portions of the breast.[8] This lymphatic flow ascends along the bilateral internal thoracic arteries, and finally merges with the systemic venous flow at the venous angles.

The internal mammary chain also collects some of the lymphatic flow which comes from the area anterior to superior vena cava, left brachiocephalic vein, and ascending aorta. The lymph nodes in this area are named "prevascular nodes" in the IASLC map (Table 147.1). The internal mammary chain is associated with metastasization from breast, lung, and esophageal cancers. Among these, breast cancer uses this route as the prominent lymphatic pathway.

TRACHEOBRONCHIAL PATHWAY

Generally, the tracheobronchial pathway originates from pulmonary hilum and ascends along with main bronchi and trachea. Finally, it merges with subclavian veins at venous angles in both sides. It communicates with the lymphatic vessels originating from the esophagus, forming a complicated lymphatic network.

Usually, the lymphatics originating from the hilum ascend along with trachea in ipsilateral side. However, it should be noted that there may be other pathways that communicate with lymphatics in contralateral side (Figs. 147.7 and 147.8).[9] Since the left paratracheal channels are not as well developed as the right paratracheal ones, several sections of lymphatic vessels from the left side merge with

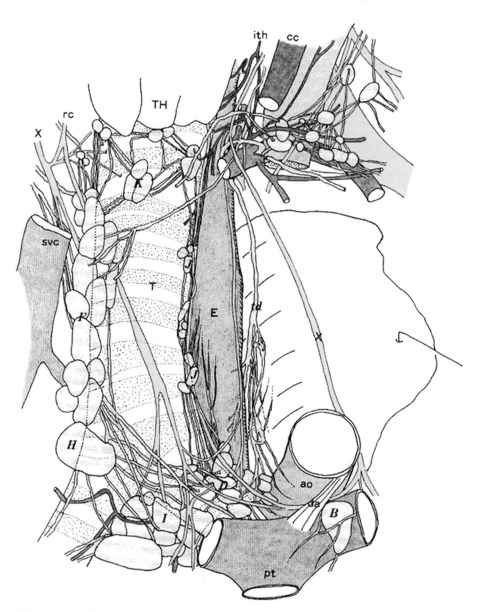

FIGURE 147.8 Schematic illustration of the paratracheal and left parabronchial lymphatic vessels. Arteries, veins, and nerves are shown in red, blue, and yellow, respectively. It is important to note that several branches of lymphatic vessels from the left side merge with the right paratracheal branches. TH, thyroid gland; T, trachea; cc, common carotid artery; da, ligamentum arteriosum; ith, inferior thyroid artery; ao, aorta; pt, pulmonary trunk; svc, superior vena cava; rc, recurrent nerve; X, vagus nerve; E, esophagus; B, lymph node anterior to pulmonary artery; F, right paratracheal lymph node; H, right paratracheal or parabronchial lymph node; I, subcarinal lymph node; K, cervical lymph node anterior to the trachea; td, thoracic duct. (From Sato T. *Color Atlas of Applied Anatomy of Lymphatics.* Tokyo: Nanko-Do; 1997:152. Copyright © Gen Murakami. With permission.)

TABLE 147.1 The Anatomical Definitions for Each Lymph Node Station According to the IASLC Classification Used in the 7th Edition of the TNM Classification for Lung Cancer

#1 Low Cervical, Supraclavicular, and Sternal Notch Nodes
    Upper border: lower margin of cricoid cartilage
    Lower border: clavicles bilaterally and, in the midline, the upper
        border of the manubrium, 1R designates right-sided nodes, 1L,
        left-sided nodes in this region
    For lymph node station 1, the midline of the trachea serves as the
        border between 1R and 1L

#2 Upper Paratracheal Nodes
    2R Upper border: apex of the right lung and pleural space, and in
            the midline, the upper border of the manubrium
        Lower border: intersection of caudal margin of innominate vein
            with the trachea
        As for lymph node station 4R, 2R includes nodes extending to
            the left lateral border of the trachea
    2L Upper border: apex of the left lung and pleural space, and in the
            midline, the upper border of the manubrium
        Lower border: superior border of the aortic arch

#3 Prevascular and Retrotracheal Nodes
    3a: Prevascular
        On the right:
            Upper border: apex of chest
            Lower border: level of carina
            Anterior border: posterior aspect of sternum
            Posterior border: anterior border of superior vena cava
        On the left:
            Upper border: apex of chest
            Lower border: level of carina
            Anterior border: posterior aspect of sternum
            Posterior border: left carotid artery
    3p: Retrotracheal
        Upper border: apex of chest
        Lower border: carina

#4 Lower Paratracheal Nodes
    4R: includes right paratracheal nodes, and pretracheal nodes
            extending to the left lateral border of trachea
        Upper border: intersection of caudal margin of innominate vein
            with the trachea
        Lower border: lower border of azygos vein
    4L: includes nodes to the left of the left lateral border of the trachea,
            medial to the ligamentum arteriosum
        Upper border: upper margin of the aortic arch
        Lower border: upper rim of the left main pulmonary artery

#5 Subaortic (Aortopulmonary Window)
    Subaortic lymph nodes lateral to the ligamentum arteriosum
    Upper border: the lower border of the aortic arch
    Lower border: upper rim of the left main pulmonary artery

#6 Paraaortic Nodes (Ascending Aorta or Phrenic)
    Lymph nodes anterior and lateral to the ascending aorta and aortic arch
    Upper border: a line tangential to the upper border of the aortic arch
    Lower border: the lower border of the aortic arch

#7 Subcarinal Nodes
    Upper border: the carina of the trachea
    Lower border: the upper border of the lower lobe bronchus on the
        left; the lower border of the bronchus intermedius on the right

#8 Paraesophageal Nodes (Below Carina)
    Nodes lying adjacent to the wall of the esophagus and to the right or
        left of the midline, excluding subcarinal nodes
    Upper border: the upper border of the lower lobe bronchus on the
        left; the lower border of the bronchus intermedius on the right
    Lower border: the diaphragm

#9 Pulmonary Ligament Nodes
    Nodes lying within the pulmonary ligament
    Upper border: the inferior pulmonary vein
    Lower border: the diaphragm

#10 Hilar Nodes
    Includes nodes immediately adjacent to the mainstem bronchus and
        hilar vessels including the proximal portions of the pulmonary
        veins and main pulmonary artery
    Upper border: the lower rim of the azygos vein on the right; upper
        rim of the pulmonary artery on the left
    Lower border: interlobar region bilaterally

#11 Interlobar Nodes
    Between the origin of the lobar bronchi
    11s: between the upper lobe bronchus and bronchus intermedius on
            the right
    11i: between the middle and lower lobe bronchi on the right

#12 Lobar Nodes
    Adjacent to the lobar bronchi

#13 Segmental Nodes
    Adjacent to the segmental bronchi

#14 Subsegmental Nodes
    Adjacent to the subsegmental bronchi

IASLC, International Association for the Study of Lung Cancer.

the right paratracheal chains. Also, a few lymphatics which come from right tracheobronchial channels merge with the left tracheo-bronchial ones. This cross communication of lymphatics plays an important role in determining the contralateral metastasization of lung cancer.

With regard to lung cancer, the common thoracic lymph nodes were defined in 2009 as a proposal by IASLC (Table 147.1).[7] At present, this definition is used internationally. There used to be discrepancies in the definition of lymph nodes between the Japanese–Naruke Map (1978)[10] and the Mountain and Dresler Map (1997).[11] The former was used mainly in Asian countries, and the latter was used in the Western countries. The IASLC proposal aimed to achieve international uniformity and provide precise anatomic definitions. In the proposal, lymph nodes potentially associated with lung cancer drainage were classified into 14 stations depending on the anatomical structure (Figs. 147.9 and 147.10). Stations no. 2 to no. 9 are located

within the mediastinal pleura and are thus assumed to be mediastinal lymph nodes. Stations no. 10 to 14 are hilar, interlobar, and intrapulmonary nodes. The lymphatic flows from no. 10 (hilar nodes) to no. 7 (subcarinal nodes), no. 4 (lower paratracheal nodes), and no. 2 (upper paratracheal nodes) represent the main stream of the tracheobronchial pathway.

In the staging of lung cancer, metastases to lymph nodes are classified into three categories, named N1, N2 and N3.[12] N1 means the metastasis in ipsilateral peribronchial, hilar, and/or intrapulmonary lymph nodes—namely nodes no. 10 to 14. N2 means the metastasis in ipsilateral mediastinal lymph nodes—namely nodes no. 2 to 9. N3 means the metastasis in contralateral mediastinal and/or hilar lymph nodes, and/or ipsilateral or contralateral supraclavicular nodes—namely nodes no. 1. The tumor usually spreads from N1 to N2 or N3 regions; therefore, the stage of cancer progresses in accordance with N status.

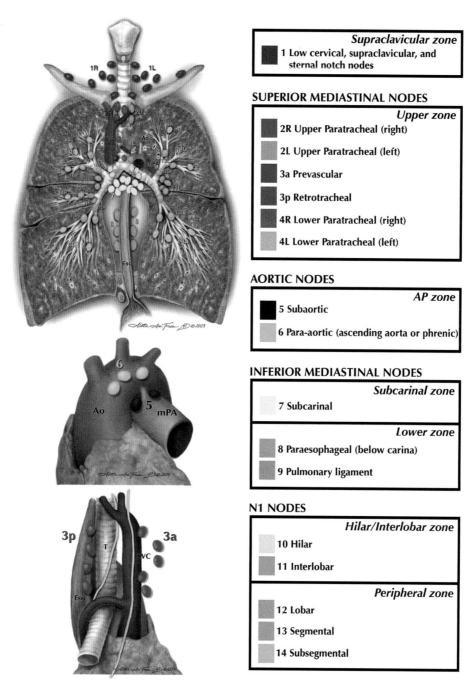

FIGURE 147.9 The International Association for the Study of Lung Cancer lymph node map. Ao, aorta; Eso, esophagus; mPA, main pulmonary artery; SVC, superior vena cava; T, trachea. (Reprinted from Rusch VW, Asamura H, Watanabe H, et al. The IASLC lung cancer staging project: a proposal for a new international lymph node map in the forthcoming seventh edition of the TNM classification for lung cancer. *J Thorac Oncol* 2009;4:568–577. Copyright © 2009 International Association for the Study of Lung Cancer. With permission.)

THORACIC DUCT

The thoracic duct is the largest lymphatic vessel in the body, which arises from the combination of bilateral lumber trunks and the intestinal trunk in the abdomen.[5] It enters the thoracic cavity via the aortic hiatus, and ascends between the azygos vein and the descending aorta. It crosses from the right to the left at the level of the 4th or 5th thoracic vertebrae. Finally, it flows into the left sub-clavian vein at the left venous angle. It collects the lymphatics from esophagus and chest wall, and furthermore, it communicates with tracheobronchial pathways. Just before flowing into the subcla-vian vein, it also merges with left subclavian trunk, and left jugular trunk.

LYMPHATICS IN THE PARAVERTEBRAL AREA

It has been described that the paravertebral area has lymphatic flow which originates from the chest wall including intercostal spaces, parietal pleura, and vertebral column.[8] The lymphatics in the para-vertebral area communicate with the thoracic duct, and they finally

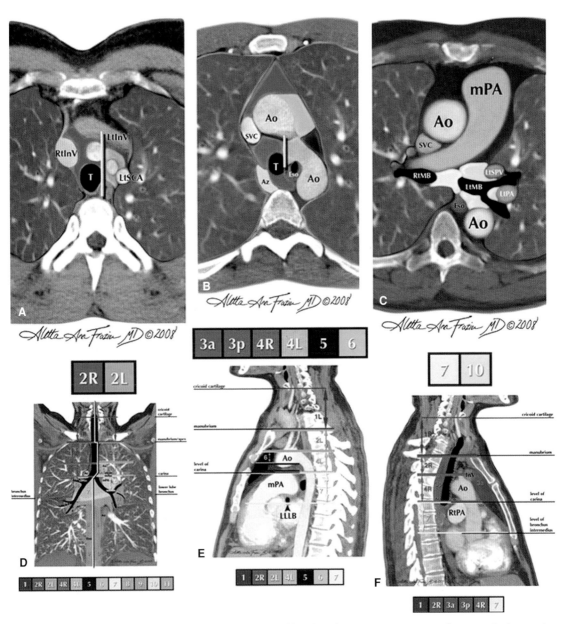

FIGURE 147.10 Illustrations of the locations of the mediastinal lymph nodes on transverse computed tomography images. Ao, aorta; Az, azygos vein; Br, bronchus; Eso, esophagus; InV, innominate vein; LLLB, left lower lobe bronchus; MB, main bronchus; mPA, main pulmonary artery; PA, pulmonary artery; PV, pulmonary vein; SCA, subclavian artery; SPV, superior pulmonary vein; SVC, superior vena cava; T, trachea. (Reprinted from Rusch VW, Asamura H, Watanabe H, et al. The IASLC lung cancer staging project: a proposal for a new international lymph node map in the forthcoming seventh edition of the TNM classification for lung cancer. *J Thorac Oncol* 2009;4:568–577. Copyright © 2009 International Association for the Study of Lung Cancer.)

merge in venous angles. However, the lymph nodes in the paravertebral area are rarely seen in the routine surgical procedure.

REFERENCES

1. Carter BW, Tomiyama N, Bhora F, et al. A modern definition of mediastinal compartments. *J Thorac Oncol* 2014;9:S97–S101.
2. Fujimoto K, Hara M, Tomiyama N, et al. Proposal for a new mediastinal compartment classification of transverse plane images according to the Japanese Association for Research on the Thymus (JART) General Rules for the Study of Mediastinal Tumors. *Oncol Rep* 2014;31:565–572.
3. Goodman LR. *Felson's Principles of Chest Roentgenology: A Programmed Text.* 4th ed. Philadelphia, PA: Saunders Elsevier; 2014:172–191.
4. Liu W, Deslauriers J. Mediastinal divisions and compartments. *Thorac Surg Clin* 2011;21:183–190.
5. Susan S. *Gray's Anatomy: the Anatomical Basis of Clinical Practice.* 41st ed. New York: Elsevier; 2016:976–980.
6. Kirschner PA. Anatomy and surgical access of the mediastinum. In: Pearson FG, ed. *Thoracic Surgery.* 2nd ed. New York: Churchill Livingstone; 2002:1563–1566.
7. Rusch VW, Asamura H, Watanabe H, et al. The IASLC lung cancer staging project: a proposal for a new international lymph node map in the forthcoming seventh edition of the TNM classification for lung cancer. *J Thorac Oncol* 2009;4:568–577.
8. Shields TW. The mediastinum, its compartments, and the mediastinal lymph nodes. In: Shields TW, ed. *General Thoracic Surgery.* 7th ed. Philadelphia, PA: Wolters Kluwer/Lippincott Williams & Wilkins; 2009:2055–2058.
9. Mountain CF, Dresler CM. Regional lymph node classification for lung cancer staging. *Chest* 1997;111:1718–1723.
10. Naruke T, Suemasu K, Ishikawa S. Lymph node mapping and curability at various levels of metastasis in resected lung cancer. *J Thorac Cardiovasc Surg* 1978;76:833–839.
11. Sato T. *Color Atlas of Applied Anatomy of Lymphatics.* Tokyo: Nanko-Do; 1997:145–155.
12. Goldstraw P, Crowley J, Chansky K, et al. The IASLC Lung Cancer Staging Project: proposals for the revision of the TNM stage groupings in the forthcoming (seventh) edition of the TNM Classification of malignant tumours. *J Thorac Oncol* 2007;2:706–714.

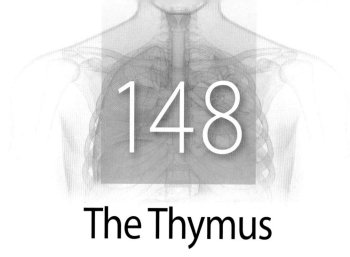

The Thymus

Michael S. Mulvihill ▪ Jacob A. Klapper ▪ Matthew G. Hartwig

EMBRYOLOGY

The thymus in humans primarily arises late in the sixth week of gestation as ventral outgrowths of the third pharyngeal pouches (thymus III). Occasionally, thymic tissue may arise from the fourth pharyngeal pouches (thymus IV). When present this thymic IV tissue most frequently becomes associated with the thyroid and may ultimately become embedded within its substance. The primordial cell mass is the result of fusion of the second, third, and fourth branchial clefts which furrow resulting in the ventral pharyngeal

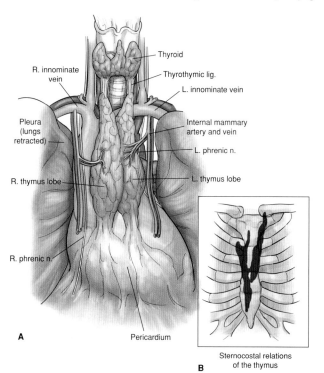

A   Pericardium

B   Sternocostal relations of the thymus

FIGURE 148.1 Anatomy of the thymus in the adult, emphasizing the form, visceral relations, and blood supply. In detailed drawing (**A**), showing a typical adult specimen, the thymus is elongated and finger-shaped; it consists of two parts and has the gross appearance of paired fatty lobes. The thymic arteries usually derive from the adjacent internal mammary arteries, and at least some of the veins terminate in the left innominate vein (thymic bodies are retracted to expose the chief veins). The lobes occupy the sulcus between the anterior borders of the lungs and may extend downward into the cardiac notch. Schematic drawing (**B**) shows the sternocostal relations of the thymus in the same specimen.

pouch III endoderm and the ectoderm. Ectodermal cells are thus the main origin of the epithelial cells of the cortex, while endodermal cells act as the source of the medullary epithelial cells.

The primordia of the thymus then elongates rapidly in the seventh week but retains its connection with the third pouch and remains associated with parathyroid tissue III. The right and left thymic tissue masses move toward the midline just caudal to the thyroid primordium and by the eighth week make contact with each other but do not fuse. They remain separate but connected lobes. The gland migrates caudad and slides under the sternum in front of the great vessels into the mediastinum to lie in contact with the superior portion of the ventral aspect of the pericardium (Fig. 148.1).

Thymic epithelial cells (TECs) are divided into cortical TECs (cTECs) located in the outer cortex region and medullary TECs (mTECs) located in the inner medulla area. These two groups of TECs play distinct roles in the positive and negative selection during thymocyte maturation. By way of immunohistochemistry and flow cytometry, these epithelial cells of the thymic cortex and the thymic medulla can be distinguished by the expression of distinctive surface antigens.[1–3] The localization of TEC markers in the newborn human thymus reflects different phenotypic origins of epithelial cells in the cortex and medulla.[4] The clinical relevance of differentiating between phenotypes is that these immunohistochemical and morphologic differences of the cortical and medullary epithelial cells can be used to classify epithelial thymic tumors (thymomas), most of which are of cortical epithelial cell origin (see Chapter 166).[5–7]

GROSS ANATOMY

In the newborn, the thymus gland reaches a mean weight of 15 g.[8] The gland continues to grow until puberty reaching a mean weight of 30 to 40 g. A representative specimen from a 5-kg patient is shown in Figure 148.2 both in situ and following subtotal resection. A gradual process of involution then occurs throughout adulthood, and the gland is reduced in weight by approximately 1% to 3% per year. In adults <85 years of age, the mean thymic weight varies between 20 and 28 g, with an average standard deviation of 12.5. Figure 148.3 shows the variations in size of the gland on computed tomography (CT) in an adolescent boy and an adult woman.

The thymus, although classically described as having a right and left lobe, may on occasion be a composite of three or more lobular structures. Nonetheless, the gland tends to maintain its original paired character. Grossly, the gland has a roughly H-shaped configuration, with extension of the upper poles of either side into the base of the neck, and with a greater or lesser attachment to the thyroid

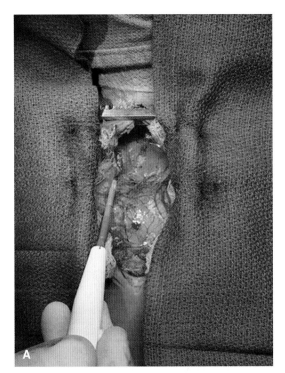
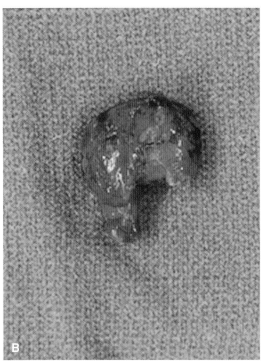

FIGURE 148.2 The thymus at sternotomy and following subtotal excision in a 5-kg patient. Subtotal thymectomy is frequently performed to facilitate exposure in operations for congential heart disease.

gland by the thyrothymic ligament. The lower poles of each side extend down over the pericardium.

In addition to the variations in size and configuration of the thymic gland, numerous collections of varying amounts of identifiable thymic tissue, both gross and microscopic, may be found as additional mediastinal lobes and islets of tissue outside the capsule of the "gland" extending from the neck to the diaphragm. Microscopic collections of thymic tissue in the mediastinal fatty tissues of the anterior compartment outside the thymic capsule have in some series occurred with an incidence of 40% to 72%.[9–11] The most common locations of extra thymic tissues are the anterior mediastinal fat, retrocarinal fat, the fat of the cardiophrenic angle, and the neck.[12] Unencapsulated thymic tissue can also be found in the region of the phrenic nerves, behind the innominate vein, in the aortopulmonary window, and in the aortocaval groove. Clinically, these anatomic variations form the basis for why a radical thymectomy must include all mediastinal fat, including the thymus, the diaphragm to the thoracic inlet, and out laterally to the phrenic nerves. The cervical and mediastinal variations in the location of these thymic tissue foci are schematically illustrated in Figure 148.4. Thymic tissue may be found in the neck in about 36% of patients, which is outside the "normal" cervical extensions of the thymic lobes. Most or all such tissue likely represents arrested descent of thymus III tissues. The presence of thymic tissue in these locations readily explains the occasional occurrence of epithelial thymic tumors (see Chapter 166) and true thymic cysts (see Chapters 173 and 174) in these areas. The significance of these variations in location in the management of myasthenia gravis is discussed in Chapters 162 and 163.

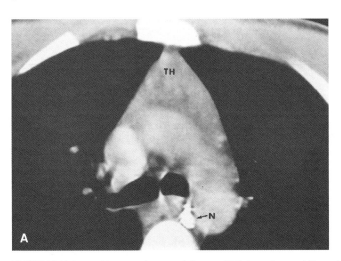
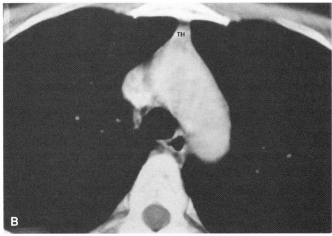

FIGURE 148.3 **A:** CT image of a normal thymus (TH) in a 17-year-old boy. A calcified subcarinal lymph node (N) is demonstrated. **B:** Normal residual thymic tissue (TH) in a 36-year-old woman is demonstrated.

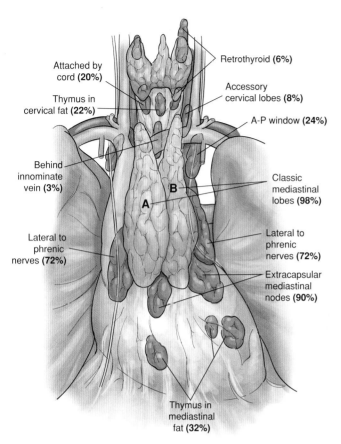

FIGURE 148.4 Composite anatomy of the thymus. The illustration is based on surgical–anatomic studies of 50 transcervical–transsternal maximal thymectomies for myasthenia gravis. Thymic tissue was found outside the classic cervical mediastinal lobes (**A,B**) in 32% of specimens in the neck and in 98% of specimens in the mediastinum.

In the adult, the upper portions of the gland normally lie on the anterior surface of the left innominate vein. In a small fraction of patients (2% to 4%), one or both lobes lie behind this vein instead of in front of it.[13] Other anomalies in position include partial or complete failure of descent of one or both thymic lobes and the presence of thymic tissue at the root of either lung or even within the pulmonary parenchyma.[14,15]

The arterial blood supply of the thymus is mainly from branches of the internal mammary arteries, but the gland may also receive small branches from the inferior thyroid arteries and the pericardiophrenic arteries. Venous drainage may be partially through small veins accompanying these arterial branches. The main drainage, however, is through a centrally located venous trunk on the posterior aspect of the gland that drains into the anterior aspect of the left innominate vein as a single vessel; occasionally a branch may enter the superior vena cava.

No afferent lymph channels enter the gland, although efferent channels have been identified. These are believed to drain only the capsule and fibrous septa of the gland. These efferent channels terminate at the anterior mediastinal, pulmonary hilar, and internal mammary lymph nodes. Both sympathetic and parasympathetic nerve fibers enter the gland.

HISTOLOGIC FEATURES

Each thymic lobe is covered by a fibrous capsule that extends into the parenchyma as fibrous connective tissue septa, which divide the

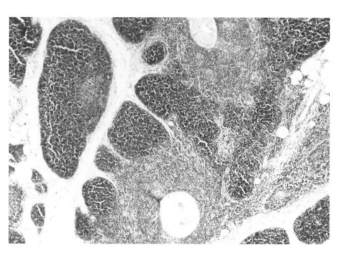

FIGURE 148.5 Photomicrograph of thymic lobule. Cortex and medullary area separated by septal connective tissue are well seen.

gland into various-sized lobules ranging from 0.5 to 2.0 mm in size. Each lobule is composed of a cortex and medulla. The medullary areas extend from one lobule into adjacent ones (Fig. 148.5).

THYMIC EPITHELIAL CELLS

The cortex is composed of densely packed lymphocytes (thymocytes), admixed with epithelial and mesenchymal cells. As introduced above, TECs can be differentiated broadly between cTECs and mTECs. These pools of cells share a common progenitor in bipotent TEC precursors (TEPCs) that differentiate into both cTECs and mTECs.[16–18] The medullary cells appear more electron dense than the peripheral (cortical) epithelial cells. However, similar darkly stained epithelial cells may also be seen in the inner cortex. The cell types in the two areas are heterogeneous, as noted by their antigenic determinants found in other various cells of the thymus.

Enzyme histochemical studies indicate a functional heterogeneity among TECs, showing different immunohistochemical phenotypes in the subcortical, inner cortex, and medullary areas, including those of the Hassall's corpuscles.[7] Subcapsular epithelial cells and medullary epithelial cells have similar but not identical antigen expression. Both have secretory function, and various thymic hormones have been identified immunohistochemically within cytoplasm of these cells. The inner cortical cells have a different antigenicity and are nonsecretory.

In the medullary portions of the gland, large epithelial cells with abundant tonofilaments with well-developed rough endoplasmic reticulum and numerous cytoplasmic vesicles are also present. These cells often are arranged in round, keratinized structures known as Hassall's corpuscles (Fig. 148.6). These complex tubular structures are composed of clumps of mature medullary epithelial cells forming concentric layers. Varying degrees of central keratinization, calcification, or both may be present. Occasionally, these structures may become cystic. Hassall's corpuscles react strongly to high-molecular-weight keratin—a feature of mature epithelial cells. So-called nurse cells are a subset of epithelial cells primarily located in the cortex.

THYMIC LYMPHOCYTES

Lymphocytes (thymocytes) dominate the histologic picture of the gland. Embryologically, by the 10th week, prothymocytes (small

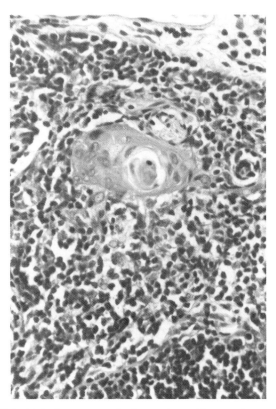

FIGURE 148.6 Photomicrograph of a typical Hassall's corpuscle.

Thymocyte selection proceeds by way of the affinity model, a process characterized by the interaction between the T-cell receptor and self-peptide-MHC complexes. Strong interactions lead to negative selection by apoptosis, while weak interactions protect thymocytes from death by neglect and promote positive selection. This process of maturation ensures self-tolerance and permits the recognition and elimination of foreign antigen that enters the body.[21] The process of maturation is also essential for the selection of T lymphocytes that do not recognize self antigens.[22] During this process, the thymocytes become initially CD3+ CD4+ CD8+. As maturation approaches completion, the T lymphocytes become either CD3+ CD4+ or CD3+ CD8+. This complex process of maturation to the mature T lymphocytes of either type is regulated by cytokines, cell adhesion molecules, thymic polypeptide hormones, and cell surface self-recognition antigens especially related to each individual human leukocyte type. The CD4+ T lymphocytes become "helper" cells and are the more common of the two. These cells also promote antibody formation by B lymphocytes. The CD8+ T lymphocytes become suppressor, cytotoxic "killer" cells. At maturity, the thymocytes located in the subcapsular region of the gland constitute 0.5% to 5% of the total, the cortically located thymocytes 60% to 80%, and the medullary located thymocytes 15% to 20%. Most of the thymic lymphocytes die within the thymic cortex by the process of programmed cell death (apoptosis), and only about 10% of the mature thymocytes reach the bloodstream (Fig. 148.7).

With aging, the involuting thymus shows a decrease in lymphocytes, Hassall's corpuscles, and other normal elements. Lipid-laden macrophages and adipose cells increase in number, but normal thymic tissue, although atrophic, persists throughout life. The epithelial stromal tissue, particularly the cortex, is replaced by fat.[23] The organohistologic features of the child's and adolescent's thymus and that of the involuted thymus of the adult are listed in Table 148.1. The T-cell compartment shows a reduction of CD4+ cells, and the aged thymus is impaired in its ability to repopulate the T cells when repletion is required.

OTHER CELL TYPES

B lymphocytes may be found grouped as lymphoid follicles or distributed as individual cells within the thymus. Of note, a proportion of

lymphoid cells) originating in the fetal liver (by the seventh week of gestation) and bone marrow (from the 22nd week onward) enter the thymus.[3,19] Initially, the cells migrate to the outer cortex and the corticomedullary junction.[20] At the time of entrance into the thymus, the prothymocytes (T-lymphocyte precursors) are immature, triple-negative T lymphocytes (CD3, CD4, CD8). The CD number refers to a cluster of differentiation of all surface markers that are negative in immature cells but become positive (immunocompetent) to various monoclonal antibodies during the process of thymic lymphocyte maturation.

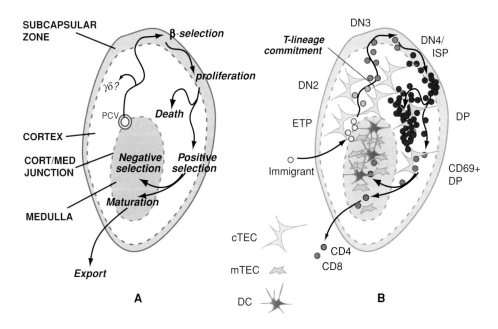

FIGURE 148.7 Anatomical compartments of the thymus and migration pathways of developing T-Cell precursors. **A:** Major compartments and migration pathways are depicted with key checkpoints in T-cell development indicated. **B:** Phenotypes of T-cell precursors (*pink, red, violet*) and stromal cell types in different compartments. For clarity, the "outbound" path from ETP to DN3 is separated from the "inbound" path from DN4 to CD4 or CD8 single positive maturation, but in vivo the "outbound" transit is surrounded with the "inbound" cells. Cort/med junction, cortical-medullary junction; PCV: postcapillary venule (immigration portal); cTEC, cortical thymic epithelial cells; DC, dendritic; mTEC, medullary thymic epithelial cells. (From William E Paul. Fundamental Immunology. 7th ed. Philadelphia, PA: Lippincott Williams & Wilkins; 2012.)

TABLE 148.1 Organotypical Features of Differentiation of the Normal Thymus of Children and Adolescents and of the Involuted Thymus of the Adult

Normal mature thymus of childhood and adolescents
Lobulation and encapsulation
Dual (epithelial/lymphoid) cell population with variable numbers of immature T lymphocytes
Perivascular spaces
Areas of medullary differentiation
Normal involuted thymus of the adult
Spindle-cell population devoid of cytologic atypia
Scant immature T lymphocytes
Rosette-like epithelial structures
Cystic and glandular structures

From Suster S, Moran CA. Thymoma classification. Current status and future trends. *Am J Clin Pathol* 2006;125:542–554. Reproduced by permission of American Society of Clinical Pathologists.

non-Hodgkin's lymphomas of the B-cell type, located in the anterior mediastinum, may arise from the B-cell population within the thymus. Neuroendocrine cells are few, but their presence has been postulated as the probable reservoir for the development of carcinoid tumors and other neuroendocrine neoplasms, including calcitonin-positive medullary carcinomas. Myoid cells are readily demonstrated in the gland and may play a role in the pathogenesis of myasthenia gravis.[13] These myoid cells are characterized by an acidophilic cytoplasm that contains cross striations. These striations react with antisera to give actin and myosin. These myoid cells also react to troponin and to acetylcholine receptor. Rare thymic neoplasms thought to be derived from the myoid cells have been described.[24,25] Nevus cell aggregates have also been identified in the thymus.[26] These cells react positively to S100 protein but show no reactivity to keratins, HMB-45, or p53. A low reactivity to Ki67 is observed in some of these aggregates of nevus cells. Occasionally, ectopic parathyroid tissue may be embedded in or adjacent to thymic tissue in the mediastinum (see Chapter 149).

THYMIC FUNCTION

The thymus is essential for the development of cellular immunity. The origin of thymic lymphocytes is, as noted, extrathymic from the bone marrow in the embryo. These prothymocyte lymphocytes enter the thymus, proliferate, gain their cellular immunocompetency, and mature into T lymphocytes, the majority of which are inducer cells (CD3+ CD4+) and a minority of which are suppressor cytotoxic cells (CD3+ CD8+).

The proper function of the immune system depends on the normal development of cellular and antibody-mediated components. The thymus-dependent system consists principally of the thymus and a circulating pool of T lymphocytes. These lymphocytes act as recognition agents capable of discerning self antigens from non–self antigens and producing cell-mediated immune reactions, as are seen in delayed hypersensitivity and allograft reactions. The antibody-mediated system is responsible for the production of immunoglobulins (IgA, IgG, and IgM) and specific antibodies. This stimulation of B cells to become plasma cells proceeds in an IL-4-dependent fashion. Any disturbance in the development of either system can be expected to lead to one of the various immunologic deficiency syndromes which have been associated with neoplasms of the thymus as well as with congenital thymic hypoplasias and agenesis. In addition, the thymus has been implicated in certain hematologic, endocrinologic, autoimmune, collagen, and neuromuscular defects.

Of particular interest to surgeons are the immunologic consequences of thymectomy, because extirpation is the only commonly used thymic operation. Although thymectomy in certain species, particularly neonatal thymectomy, is often associated with significant alterations in immunity, this relationship has not been observed in either adult or pediatric patients. Although lymphocyte count and tests of immunologic capacity may be diminished by thymectomy in humans, no particular clinical problems have developed to correlate with these laboratory observations.[27] With the exception of the management of thymic neoplasms and the empiric management of myasthenia gravis, no clear indications for thymectomy exist in clinical practice at present.

THYMIC HYPERPLASIA

Changes in the lymphatic content and structure of the thymus are seen to accompany many autoimmune states. Thymic hyperplasia is separated into two categories based on gross and histologic criteria. The first is lymphoid or follicular hyperplasia, characterized by the presence of lymphoid follicles with activated germinal centers (Fig. 148.8). The second is true hyperplasia, characterized by an increase in the size and weight of the thymus gland, which retains a normal or nearly normal morphology for the patient's age and is not accompanied by lymphoid follicles with activated germinal centers.

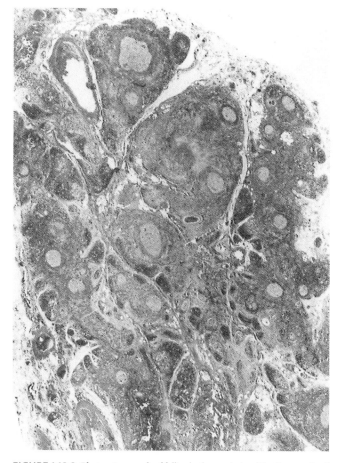

FIGURE 148.8 Photomicrograph of follicular hyperplasia of the thymus gland in a patient with myasthenia gravis. Note prominent activated germinal centers. (From Cove H. The mediastinum. In: Coulson SF, ed. *Surgical Pathology.* 2nd ed. Philadelphia, PA: Lippincott; 1988. With permission.)

LYMPHOID OR FOLLICULAR HYPERPLASIA

The thymus may be of normal or abnormal size and weight. Lymphoid or follicular hyperplasia is frequently associated with autoimmune diseases. It is estimated that 60% to 90% of myasthenic patients who do not have a thymoma have histologically demonstrable follicular hyperplasia of the thymus gland.

TRUE THYMIC HYPERPLASIA

Two types of true thymic hyperplasia are seen: (a) idiopathic or true hyperplasia with marked to massive enlargement of the gland of no apparent cause and (b) rebound thymic hyperplasia in children after treatment of various tumors. The second type occurs particularly after chemotherapy and is occasionally associated with other systemic disease states, especially Graves' disease, or after a period of physical stress (e.g., burns, operations, and other similar events).

Thymic Rebound Hyperplasia

There remains a paucity of literature into the pathogenesis of rebound hyperplasia. The extent to which the relationship between these disease states and thymus is one of cause and effect or only coincidental remains unclear. Nevertheless, thymic rebound enlargement has been observed after the treatment of Hodgkin's disease and other malignancies.[28–30] In terms of its association with non-neoplastic diseases, this condition has been identified after burn injuries and during the treatment of primary hypothyroidism and is a known common feature of Graves' disease.[31–33] Incidentally, rebound hyperplasia has also been described in a newborn with Beckwith–Wiedemann syndrome (exophthalmos, macroglossia, and gigantism, often associated with neonatal hypoglycemia).[33,34] The importance of recognizing the rebound nature of thymic hyperplasia is that once the diagnosis is established, no specific treatment is necessary. This is in marked contrast to the management of idiopathic true (massive) thymic hyperplasia, which, except in rare incidences, requires surgical excision.

Idiopathic True (Massive) Thymic Hyperplasia

True massive thymic hyperplasia is a very rare clinical entity, with approximately 50 cases reported.[35,36] The major feature is that there is no discernible cause; most cases occur between the ages of 1 and 15 years. The next common age group is less than 1 year of age or younger. Rarely does idiopathic massive hyperplasia occur after age 15 years. True massive thymic hyperplasia occurs twice as often in boys as in girls. About 85% of patients are symptomatic. Cough, shortness of breath, respiratory distress, and pulmonary infection are the more common symptoms, though more serious sequelae including mediastinal hemorrhage has been described. Lymphocytosis in the peripheral blood is seen in about one-fourth of patients. The radiographic findings are of a large anterior mass that extends into both hemithoraces, generally to a greater extent into one than into the other (Fig. 148.9). Axial imaging by way of CT and MRI has been utilized to assist in diagnosis, as has diagnostic fine-needle aspiration. A trial of steroids may be initiated as a conservative approach to therapy, but in patients with persistent symptoms surgical excision remains standard therapy. The surgical approach may be accomplished through a median sternotomy, a clamshell incision, or even a unilateral posterolateral thoracotomy. The operation is curative, and no subsequent difficulty has been recorded.

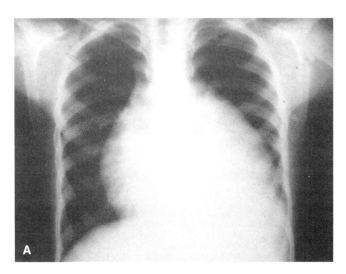

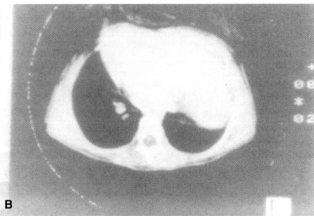

FIGURE 148.9 True thymic hyperplasia. **A:** Posteroanterior radiograph of a massive enlargement of the thymus obscuring the cardiac silhouette on the left in a 12-year-old boy presenting with mild dyspnea. **B:** Computed tomographic scan showing the presence of a large parenchymatous density adjacent to the heart, which has shifted to the right. (Reprinted from Ricci CM, Pescarmona E, Rendina EA, et al. True thymic hyperplasia: a clinicopathological study. *Ann Thorac Surg* 1989;47:741–745. Copyright © 1989 The Society of Thoracic Surgeons. With permission.)

REFERENCES

1. von Gaudecker B, Steinmann GG, Hansmann ML, et al. Immunohistochemical characterization of the thymic microenvironment. *Cell Tissue Res* 1986;244:403–412.
2. McFarland EJ, Scearce RM, Haynes BF. The human thymic microenvironment: cortical thymic epithelium is an antigenically distinct region of the thymic microenvironment. *J Immunol* 1984;133:1241–1249.
3. Haynes BF. The human thymic microenvironment. *Advances in Immunology.* Elsevier BV;1984:87–142.
4. Hirokawa K, Utsuyama M, Moriizumi E, et al. Immunohistochemical studies in human thymomas. Localization of thymosin and various cell marker. *Virchows Arch B Cell Pathol Incl Mol Pathol* 1988;55:371–380.
5. Suster S, Moran CA. Thymoma classification. *Am J Clin Pathol* 2006;125:542–554.
6. Marino M, Müller-Hermelink HK. Thymoma and thymic carcinoma. *Virchows Archiv A Pathol Anat* 1985;407:119–149.
7. Müller-Hermelink HK, Marino M, Palestio G. Pathology of thymic epithelial tumors. *Curr Top Pathol* 1986;75:206.
8. Boyd E. The weight of the thymus gland in health and disease. *Arch Pediatr Adolesc Med* 1932;43:1162.
9. Masaoka A, Nagaoka Y, Kotake Y. Distribution of thymic tissue at the anterior mediastinum. Current procedures in thymectomy. *J Thorac Cardiovasc Surg* 1975;70:747–754.
10. Fukai I, Funato Y, Mizuno T, et al. Distribution of thymic tissue in the mediastinal adipose tissue. *J Thorac Cardiovasc Surg* 1991;101:1099–1102.
11. Ashour M. Prevalence of ectopic thymic tissue in myasthenia gravis and its clinical significance. *J Thorac Cardiovasc Surg* 1995;109:632–635.

12. Lee Y, Moallem S, Clauss RH. Massive hyperplastic thymus in a 22-month-old infant. *Ann Thorac Surg* 1979;27:356–358.
13. Drenckhahn D, von Gaudecker B, Muller-Hermelink HK, et al. Myosin and actin containing cells in the human postnatal thymus. Ultrastructural and immunohisto-chemical findings in normal thymus and in myasthenia gravis. *Virchows Arch B Cell Pathol Incl Mol Pathol* 1980;32:33–45.
14. Jaretzki A. Thymectomy for myasthenia gravis: analysis of the controversies regarding technique and results. *Neurology* 1997;48:52S–63S.
15. Bell RH, Knapp BI, Anson BJ, et al. Form, size, blood-supply and relations of the adult thymus. *Q Bull Northwest Univ Med Sch* 1954;28:156–164.
16. Bleul CC, Corbeaux T, Reuter A, et al. Formation of a functional thymus initiated by a postnatal epithelial progenitor cell. *Nature* 2006;441:992–996.
17. Rossi SW, Jenkinson WE, Anderson G, et al. Clonal analysis reveals a common progenitor for thymic cortical and medullary epithelium. *Nature* 2006;441:988–991.
18. Suster S, Rosai J. Histology of the normal thymus. *Am J Surg Pathol* 1990;14:284–303.
19. Haynes BF, Hale LP. The human thymus. *Immunol Res* 1998;18:175–192.
20. Boyd RL, Hugo P. Towards an integrated view of thymopoiesis. *Immunol Today* 1991;12:71–79.
21. Klein L, Kyewski B, Allen PM, et al. Positive and negative selection of the T cell repertoire: what thymocytes see (and don't see). *Nat Rev Immunol* 2014;14:377–391.
22. Res P, Spits H. Developmental stages in the human thymus. *Semin Immunol* 1999;11:39–46.
23. George AJ, Ritter MA. Thymic involution with ageing: Obsolescence or good housekeeping? *Immunol Today* 1996;17:267–272.
24. Henry K. An unusual thymic tumour with a striated muscle (myoid) component (with a brief review of the literature on myoid cells). *Br J Dis Chest* 1972;66:291–299.
25. Murakami S, Shamoto M, Miura K, et al. A thymic tumor with massive proliferation of myoid cells. *Pathol Int* 1984;34:1375–1383.
26. Parker JR, Ro JY, Ordonez NG. Benign nevus cell aggregates in the thymus: a case report. *Mod Pathol* 1999;12:329–332.
27. Adner MM, Isé C, Schwab R, et al. Immunologic studies of thymectomized and nonthymectomized patients with myasthenia gravis. *Ann N Y Acad Sci* 1966;135:536–548.
28. Gelfand DW, Goldman AS, Law EJ, et al. Thymic hyperplasia in children recovering from thermal burns. *J Trauma* 1972;12:813–817.
29. Tartas NE. Diffuse thymic enlargement in Hodgkin's disease. *JAMA* 1985;254:406–406.
30. Cohen M, Hill CA, Cangir A, et al. Thymic rebound after treatment of childhood tumors. *Am J Roentgenol* 1980;135:151–156.
31. Judd R, Bueso-Ramos C. Combined true thymic hyperplasia and lymphoid hyperplasia in Graves' disease. *Pediatr Pathol* 1990;10:829–836.
32. Bergman TA, Mariash CN, Oppenheimer JH. Anterior mediastinal mass in a patient with Graves' disease. *J Clin Endocrinol Metab* 1982;55:587–588.
33. Nomori H. A case of massive true thymic hyperplasia with non-Hodgkin's lymphoma. *Chest* 1990;98:1304–1305.
34. Balcom RJ, Hakanson DO, Werner A, et al. Massive thymic hyperplasia in an infant with Beckwith-Wiedemann syndrome. *Arch Pathol Lab Med* 1985;109:153–155.
35. Ricci C, Pescarmona E, Rendina EA, et al. True thymic hyperplasia: a clinicopatho-logical study. *Ann Thorac Surg* 1989;47:741–745.
36. Linegar AG, Odell JA, Fennell WM, et al. Massive thymic hyperplasia. *Ann Thorac Surg* 1993;55:1197–1201.

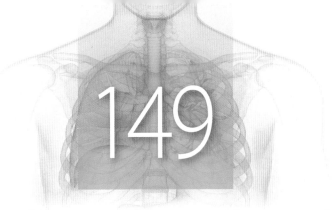

149

Mediastinal Parathyroids

Daniel J. Boffa

INTRODUCTION

Surgical removal of hyperfunctional parathyroid glands is a highly effective treatment of primary and secondary hyperparathyroidism. Approximately 15% of patients undergoing surgery for hyperparathyroidism (either primary or secondary) will have a hyperfunctional ectopic parathyroid gland.[1,2] The vast majority of ectopic glands (including those lying in the superior mediastinum) can be removed through a cervical incision. However, 1% to 3% of patients with hyperparathyroidism will require a thoracic surgical procedure to remove a hyperfunctional parathyroid gland from the mediastinum.[3–7] The clinical outcomes associated with transthoracic resection of hyperfunctional parathyroid glands in the mediastinum have been excellent, curing the vast majority of patients of hyperparathyroidism. However, the surgical approach and the overall success of the procedure are dependent upon the process used to localize the culprit gland(s) to the mediastinum. Therefore, it is important for thoracic surgeons to be aware of the anatomic aspects of hyperfunctional mediastinal parathyroids, as well as the strategies to localize and remove the abnormal glands.

EMBRYOLOGY/ANATOMY

The superior parathyroid glands arise from the fourth pharyngeal pouch. When a superior gland is ectopic, it is typically associated with the esophagus, airway, thyroid gland, carotid sheath, or great vessels. The inferior parathyroid glands arise from the third pharyngeal pouch. The inferior parathyroid glands travel a greater embryologic distance to reach their classic anatomic position, and are twice as likely to be ectopic.[2] Because the third pharyngeal pouch also gives rise to the thymus, ectopic inferior parathyroid glands are most commonly located within or around the thymus. Supernumerary glands appear to have a predilection for the mediastinum as 60% are located in the mediastinum (typically in the thymus).[8]

HYPERFUNCTIONAL PARATHYROID GLANDS IN THE MEDIASTINUM

Approximately 85% of primary hyperparathyroidism is the result of a solitary parathyroid adenoma. Although the majority of hyperfunctional glands are located in the neck, a solitary adenoma is also the most common scenario when hyperparathyroidism is driven by a hyperfunctional parathyroid gland in the mediastinum.[9–11]

For secondary hyperparathyroidism, the vast majority of patients will have hyperplasia (rather than adenoma). Hyperplasia may involve more than one mediastinal parathyroid gland.[12] Hyperplastic mediastinal parathyroid glands may also be associated with hyperplastic glands in the neck; therefore, the thoracic surgeon should be aware of patient's cervical parathyroid status with respect to prior exploration and imaging to counsel the patient regarding the likelihood that the thoracic procedure will eliminate all *hyperfunctional* glands (i.e., discuss the possibility that cervical glands may leave the patient hyperparathyroid after the removal of a pathologic mediastinal gland). On the other hand, if the patient has been left without functional glands in the neck (as a result of prior surgeries), the patient should be counseled on the possibility that the removal of the hyperfunctional mediastinal parathyroid could leave the patient without any functional parathyroid tissue.

THYMOMA AND HYPERPARATHYROIDISM

Thymomas have been identified in patients with primary hyperparathyroidism. The thymoma may be mistaken for an ectopic parathyroid gland, as it is not unusual for a thymoma be positive by parathyroid localization studies (see Tc-99m sestamibi scan below).[12,13] In addition, thymic carcinoids have been seen in patients with MEN I syndrome (which typically includes parathyroid adenomas). However, in the vast majority of patients with hyperparathyroidism and a thymoma, the hyperparathyroidism is related to parathyroid pathology (such as a coexisting adenoma)[14,15] and not the thymoma. On extremely rare occasions, the thymoma itself may produce parathyroid hormone (PTH).[16]

LOCATION OF ECTOPIC HYPERFUNCTIONAL PARATHYROID GLANDS IN THE MEDIASTINUM

Over the past 75 years, case reports and case series have described a seemingly endless list of possible locations of hyperfunctional parathyroid glands within the mediastinum.[3–5,7,9,12,17,18] Therefore, thoracic surgeons should be aware that a culprit parathyroid gland can exist virtually anywhere in the mediastinum. That being said, there are several mediastinal locations with a clear predilection for hyperfunctional parathyroid glands (Table 149.1). The inferior parathyroid glands (which are the most commonly ectopic) are most often located within or around the thymus (likely relating to shared

TABLE 149.1 Locations of Ectopic Hyperfunctioning Parathyroid Glands

Most Common Locations of Mediastinal Parathyroid Glands[a]	Rare Locations of Mediastinal Parathyroid Glands
Within or adjacent to the thymus	Wall of atrial appendage
Periaortic (ascending aorta, aortic arch)	Paraspinal[19]
Aortopulmonary window	Endotracheal[20]
Adjacent to thoracic esophagus	Pulmonary hilum[21]
Adjacent to SVC/innominate veins	
Overlying the pericardium	
Peritracheal (similar to mediastinal lymph node stations)	
Retrosternal (adherent to underside of sternum)	

[a]Since there is no consistent nomenclature to describe the anatomic location of mediastinal parathyroids, this table includes some estimated locations based on similar anatomic descriptions.[3–5,7,9,12,17,18]

embryologic origins mentioned above). Most ectopic parathyroid glands within the thymus are accessible through a traditional cervical parathyroidectomy incision (i.e., without using a transcervical thymectomy retractor). However, when a thoracic surgery approach is required, the thymus remains the most common location. On the other hand, the superior glands are more commonly located around the esophagus, trachea, or great vessels in the mediastinum.

LOCALIZING A HYPERFUNCTIONAL PARATHYROID GLAND

In the current era of endocrine surgery, the majority of hyperfunctional parathyroid glands are able to be localized prior to surgical exploration. Localization enables surgery to be done less invasively, and with fewer nontherapeutic explorations. More recently, tissue-specific metabolic imaging techniques and high-resolution anatomic imaging have been used to greatly increase the accuracy of identifying hyperfunctional parathyroid glands in the mediastinum (Table 149.2).[22] As a result, transthoracic exploration of the mediastinum for hyperparathyroidism is typically in pursuit of a localized

TABLE 149.2 Sensitivity of Diagnostic Modalities for Detecting Ectopic Parathyroids

Diagnostic Modality	Sensitivity
1. Neck ultrasound	1. 27–89%
2. ^{99m}Tc-sestamibi scan	2. 54–100% (mostly 80–90%)
3. Computerized tomography	3. 65%
4. Magnetic resonance imaging	4. 75–78%
5. Single photon emission CT (SPECT)	5. 95%
6. Dual-phase ^{99m}Tc sestamibi scan with SPECT	6. 96%

Reproduced and modified with permission from Noussios G, Anagnostis P, Natsis K. Ectopic parathyroid glands and their anatomical, clinical and surgical implications. *Exp Clin Endocrinol Diabetes* 2012;120(10):604–610. Copyright © Georg Thieme Verlag KG.

imaging abnormality. However, each of the localization techniques varies with respect to sensitivity and specificity in different clinical scenarios and it is important for the thoracic surgeon to understand the strengths and limitations of these studies.

4D-CT SCANNING

4D-CT scanning refers to the use of multiphase scanning from the mandible to the mediastinum to look for hyperfunctional parathyroid glands. The four "dimensions" refer to the 3 planes (axial, coronal, sagittal) and a "temporal" dimension referring to the multiple phases (or time points) relating to the injection of intravenous contrast. Similar to angiography, 4D-CT scanning uses multiphase imaging (noncontrast, early post-contrast and late post-contrast) to distinguish abnormal parathyroid tissue based on a characteristic blush and early washout with contrast injection. This technique has shown encouraging results among case series with accuracy of over 80%[23,24] and appears to be particularly useful in patients whose sestamibi scan is negative, as one series found 4D-CT to be 89% sensitive for locating the abnormal gland in this setting.[25] The extent to which 4D-CT scanning performs in the mediastinum is unclear, but there are case reports of successful localizations. A limitation of 4D-CT scanning is the radiation exposure. The multiple phases required (multiple runs before and after contrast) results in a significant radiation exposure (28 mSv for 4D-CT compared to a chest CT which is around 7 mSv). Some centers have lowered radiation dosing by limiting the areas scanned and eliminated the noncontrast imaging in an effort to bring the radiation exposure more in line with other localization techniques. 4D-CT also involves the use of iodinated contrast which may be an issue in patients with renal insufficiency of iodine allergies. Finally, there is a subjective component to the interpretation of 4D-CT by radiologists, and reactive lymph nodes may appear as false positives.

^{99m}Tc-SESTAMIBI (TECHNETIUM-99m METHOXYISOBUTYL ISONITRILE)

In the late 1980s it was noted that the ^{99m}Tc-sestamibi compound injected into patients to study cardiac perfusion also accumulates in the mitochondria of hyperfunctional parathyroid tissue.[26] Since that time, ^{99m}Tc-sestamibi has been increasingly used to localize parathyroid adenomas and hyperplastic glands. The radioactive signal is proportional to the size and activity of the abnormal parathyroid gland. Therefore, the sensitivity can be limited in the setting of small (<600 mg), or moderate to low functioning adenomas (<20% oxyphilic cells).[27] ^{99m}Tc-sestamibi is also taken up by the thyroid. As a result, in order to visualize parathyroid glands, a separate step must be taken to distinguish the two sources of uptake. The sestamibi compound is cleared from the thyroid more quickly than parathyroid tissue, so one strategy is to obtain early and delayed imaging to distinguish parathyroid tissue. Another strategy is to use a thyroid-specific imaging compound (such as ^{123}I scanning) to map (and then subtract) the thyroid contribution from the sestamibi.[28] The resolution of ^{99m}Tc-sestamibi scanning can be poor, particularly in the mediastinum. As a result, it may be challenging to pinpoint the location of the abnormal signal in the mediastinum (which typically contains lymph nodes of a size and shape similar to a parathyroid adenoma). Thymomas can also take up ^{99m}Tc-sestamibi, leading to false positives in the mediastinum.

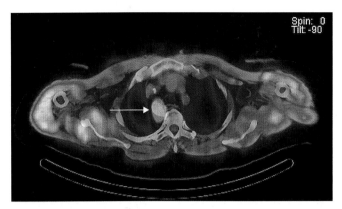

FIGURE 149.1 ^{99m}Tc-sestamibi SPECT scan. Axial image from a ^{99m}Tc-sestamibi SPECT scan demonstrating a hyperfunctional mediastinal parathyroid gland between the esophagus and trachea on the right (*arrow on bright oval structure*).

^{99m}Tc-SESTAMIBI SPECT

One of the principal limitations of the ^{99m}Tc-sestamibi has been poor resolution of anatomic detail. More recently, ^{99m}Tc-sestamibi has been combined with single photon emission computed tomography (SPECT). This has greatly increased the ability to precisely localize ectopic parathyroid glands, particularly in the mediastinum (Fig. 149.1). There is some indication that ^{99m}Tc-sestamibi SPECT is not as effective at identifying hyperplastic glands as it is adenomas.[28] The positive predictive value of ^{99m}Tc-sestamibi SPECT is 79% and the sensitivity around 90%.[29]

MAGNETIC RESONANCE IMAGING

Parathyroid adenomas enhance on T_1-weighted images, which can be used to localize adenomas in the mediastinum. Magnetic resonance imaging (MRI) performs well in patients with persistent hyperparathyroidism after treatment of cervical disease, with a sensitivity of 88% and an accuracy of 84%, but does not perform as well for hyperplasia.[30] There is some indication that combining MRI with another form of imaging may have synergistic localization results. MRI has appeal in patients that are unable to receive iodinated contrast material. MRI cannot be done in patients with certain metallic implants unless specifically certified to be MRI safe (pacemakers, internal defibrillators, intrauterine birth control devices).

SELECTIVE VENOUS SAMPLING

Selective venous sampling involves the measurement of PTH at multiple levels throughout the venous drainage system of the neck and mediastinum to localize the region of the source of elevated PTH. This technique has been most commonly advocated for patients with persistently elevated PTH after neck exploration and multiple negative noninvasive localization studies (or if there is disagreement between the studies).[31] The technique involves introducing a catheter into neck and mediastinum, typically through a transfemoral approach.[32] This requires sedation and local anesthesia. The catheter is maneuvered into various locations within the venous anatomy to create a venous map (Fig. 149.2). The PTH levels are then correlated

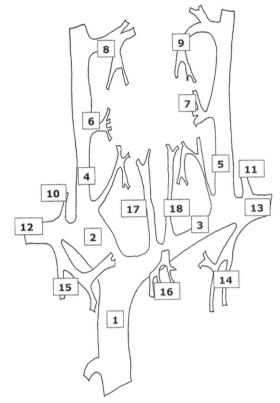

FIGURE 149.2 Selective venous sampling map. Cervical and mediastinal venous sites selected for blood sampling (*n* = 18). *1*, superior vena cava; *2*, right brachiocephalic vein; *3*, left brachiocephalic vein; *4*, right internal jugular vein; *5*, left internal jugular vein; *6*, right middle thyroid vein; *7*, left middle thyroid vein; *8*, right superior thyroid vein; *9*, left superior thyroid vein; *10*, right vertebral vein; *11*, left vertebral vein; *12*, right subclavian vein; *13*, left subclavian vein; *14*, left internal thoracic vein; *15*, right internal thoracic vein; *16*, superior thymic vein; *17*, right inferior thyroid vein; *18*, left inferior thyroid vein. (From Chaffanjon PC, Voirin D, Vasdev A, et al. Selective venous sampling in recurrent and persistent hyperparathyroidism: indication, technique, and results. *World J Surg* 2004;28(10):958–961. Copyright © 2004 Société Internationale de Chirurgie. With permission of Springer.)

with that of a peripheral vein and a twofold gradient is considered to be indicative of a positive localization. Selective venous sampling has been shown by two large series of reoperative hyperparathyroid patients who were not able to be localized with noninvasive imaging studies, to be specific (true positive rate 76%, false positive rate 4%) and reasonably sensitive (sensitivity 76%).[33,34]

Interestingly, false positives have been reported in this context. In one series of suspected mediastinal parathyroids, selective venous sampling was "falsely" positive in three of five cases where the venous sampling was the only study to localize the abnormal gland (and other imaging modalities such as CT and MIBI failed to localize).[5] Therefore, one should be cautious if selective venous sampling localizes the gland to an area that appears to be normal on other imaging exams (i.e., CT scanning). It is important to be cognizant of venous anatomy, as the sampling study can at times demonstrate counter intuitive findings. For example, in one of the author's cases, the gradient localized to the hemiazygos vein, which includes venous return from the pleura. CT imaging had identified two indeterminate peripheral subpleural pulmonary nodules that ultimately proved to be small pleural metastases from parathyroid carcinoma. Venous sampling typically involves intravenous contrast to map out the venous anatomy, so caution must be used in patients with renal insufficiency.

¹¹C-METHIONINE PET/CT

In patients with a negative ^{99m}Tc-sestamibi SPECT imaging, there may be value in performing a ¹¹C-methionine PET/CT.[35,36] It is not entirely clear why the methionine accumulates in parathyroid tissue (also accumulates in osteoblasts and gastrointestinal mucosa), but may relate to an interaction with the PTH1 receptor.[35] The sensitivity and specificity of this modality appears to be on par with other imaging modalities; however, the performance of ¹¹C-methionine PET/CT for mediastinal parathyroids has not been determined. Some recommend ¹¹C-methionine PET/CT in patients after a neck exploration has failed to normalize PTH and ^{99m}Tc-sestamibi SPECT imaging has not demonstrated the source.[37]

FALSE POSITIVES

Several structures in the mediastinum may resemble hyperfunctional ectopic parathyroid glands, which may lead to false positives on localization studies. For example, thymomas may concentrate sestamibi (false positive ^{99m}Tc-sestamibi SPECT imaging) and may enhance with intravenous contrasts (false positive 4D-CT). Mediastinal lymph nodes often are the shape and size of a hyperfunctional parathyroid gland and may enhance with intravenous contrast (falsely positive 4D-CT and MRI) (Fig. 149.3). Thymomas and other thymic lesions (hamartoma) can arterially enhance as an ectopic parathyroid gland (Fig. 149.4). At times, the portion of the right atrial appendage can be mistaken for a mediastinal parathyroid gland on ^{99m}Tc-sestamibi imaging. Overall, the false positive rates are generally low, and localization studies may be used to reduce the invasiveness, and the rate of nontherapeutic thoracic surgical procedures for hyperparathyroidism.

BIOPSY

It is currently not routine practice to biopsy target lesions in the mediastinum prior to resection. However, in the event that tissue confirmation would influence the patient's care, an FNA can be performed

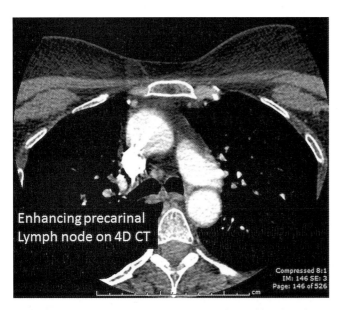

FIGURE 149.3 False positive 4D-CT scan. A mediastinal lymph node was read as a hyperfunctional mediastinal parathyroid gland.

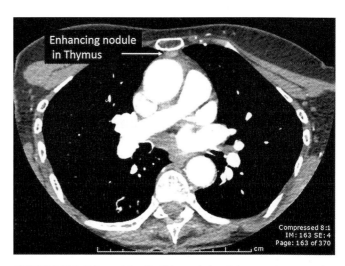

FIGURE 149.4 False positive 4D-CT scan. A thymic hamartoma was read as a hyperfunctional mediastinal parathyroid gland.

on accessible lesions to reveal the diagnosis. If information is needed in a more timely fashion, the aspirate can be run through the PTH assay and an "off the chart" reading be taken as confirmation of parathyroid tissue.[38]

PREOPERATIVE PLANNING

Prior to surgically removing a mediastinal parathyroid gland, the surgeon should attempt to understand the status of the patient's cervical parathyroid glands. This is particularly true in patients with multiple prior cervical explorations, because the cervical glands may have been removed or compromised (devascularized) during the prior surgeries. Leaving a patient without any functioning, parathyroid tissue can have profound clinical implications and should be avoided when possible. It may be necessary to perform an autografting of hyperfunctional parathyroid tissue. Therefore, the thoracic surgeon should be aware of this scenario and if necessary, engage an endocrine surgeon to participate in the care of the patient.

DE NOVO EXPLORATION OF THE MEDIASTINUM

The classic teaching has been for patients to undergo bilateral neck exploration prior to undergoing mediastinal exploration. However, with greater resolution of localization studies, more recent series have managed mediastinal disease without prior neck exploration.[39–41] The decision to proceed first with mediastinal exploration (and defer cervical exploration) would imply confidence of the clinical team that (A) the mediastinal lesion is the "culprit" lesion, (B) the mediastinal lesion is not reachable through a cervical incision, and (C) there is not a lesion is the neck (or at least the patient understands that he or she may require a second procedure).

MEDIASTINAL EXPLORATION WITHOUT A LOCALIZED TARGET

Exploration of the mediastinum through a thoracic approach is not generally advised for hyperparathyroidism without an imaging localized target. The yield of empiric exploration is presumed to be substantially lower than that of patients with a defined target. The mediastinum contains a number of tissues and structures of a similar size and shape of a hyperfunctional parathyroid gland (lymph nodes, fat, etc.) that could lead to extensive resection without impacting the patient's hyperparathyroidism. There are times in which refractory patients have no other option and are willing to embark down this pathway. An empiric thymectomy would be a reasonable step in this process. The surgeon should have intraoperative PTH monitoring capability for a real-time assessment of the impact that each resected structure has on the PTH level (to limit the extent of nontherapeutic tissue removal).

SURGICAL APPROACHES

The preferred surgical approach may vary based on the size and location of the gland within the mediastinum, as well as the experience and preferences of the involved thoracic surgeon. Historically, median sternotomy has been the most common approach for hyperfunctional mediastinal parathyroids, with thoracotomy being used more selectively. Through either of these open approaches, the majority of the mediastinum would be accessible, with a clear advantage of sternotomy being access to bilateral and central portions of the mediastinum. However, advances in localization techniques and greater experience with less invasive surgical approaches have led to increasing use of minimally invasive surgery for mediastinal parathyroid resection. In this regard, some surgeons have found success using immediate preoperative injection of Tc-99m sestamibi (MIBI) injection and intraoperative handheld gamma probe scanning to provide both localization of parathyroid adenoma and confirmation of completeness of resection.[52]

The transcervical thymectomy may be used for intrathoracic parathyroid glands. A partial sternotomy may be appropriate for lesions in the superior and anterior mediastinum. Video-assisted thoracic surgery has been used to resect mediastinal parathyroids from a wide array of locations (periesophageal, peritracheal, periaortic, overlying pericardium, etc.). There is some indication that the VATS approach is associated with fewer complications than sternotomy.[4] Video mediastinoscopy has also been used for glands around the trachea.[39,42] In this location, the author prefers the use of the two-bladed, expanding video mediastinoscope (as opposed to a rigid single barrel design). The expanding mediastinoscope allows the scope to progressively widen in the mediastinum (much like a speculum), providing a fixed retraction of mediastinal tissues and allows the surgeon to operate multiple instruments simultaneously. There are also several case reports of successful mediastinal parathyroidectomy using robot-assisted techniques.[43–45]

PARATHYROMATOSIS

Irrespective of the surgical approach, gentle tissue handling is critical. Seeding of tissues has occurred during parathyroidectomy in the neck (referred to as "parathyromatosis").[46,47] While it is likely the result of traumatic handling of the parathyroid tissue, it is worth noting that the majority of patients who experienced capsular disruption will not develop parathyromatosis.[48] That being said, every effort should be made to remove ectopic parathyroids intact.

INTRAOPERATIVE PTH MONITORING

The half-life of PTH in the circulation is short (3 to 5 minutes) and therefore serial PTH measurements can be used intraoperatively to assess whether or not the source of hyperparathyroidism has been eliminated.[27] A reduction in PTH 50% in 15 minutes corresponds to high surgical success rates, however, the value will often fall more dramatically (80% in 10 minutes). It is not uncommon for a patient's value to spike as a result of the manipulation of the gland, so this possibility should be considered as the perioperative values are interpreted. A return to a normal range is the most compelling indication that the source of hyperparathyroidism has been eliminated.[48] The same assay may be used on an aspirate of removed tissue with an "out of range" high reading (PTH >1000 pg/mL) being highly correlative with a hyperfunctional gland on histopathology.

PERIOPERATIVE MANAGEMENT

The surgical removal of a hyperfunctional mediastinal parathyroid gland is likely to significantly alter this hormonal axis of calcium regulation. The abrupt decline in circulating PTH may lead to a reduction in serum calcium that peaks between postoperative days 2 and 4. Patients are routinely supplemented with oral calcium (e.g., TUMS) and counseled for the signs and symptoms of hypocalcemia (numbness and tingling in fingers, toes, perioral areas).[49,50] An exaggerated form of rebound hypocalcemia is referred to as "hungry bone syndrome," and is thought to result from a loss of PTH-driven osteoclastic activity in the setting of chronically upregulated (compensatory) osteoblastic activity.[51]

CONCLUSION

Transthoracic resection of hyperfunctional mediastinal parathyroid glands can be a highly effective approach to a challenging problem. Preoperative localization is a very important component of the thoracic evaluation, because the ectopic glands can be located throughout the mediastinum and may be confused with other mediastinal structures (lymph nodes, thymic neoplasms, etc.). The management of hyperparathyroidism may be complex, particularly if the mediastinal gland represents the patient's only viable parathyroid tissue; therefore, it is critical to have some assessment of the patient's cervical parathyroid status. Thoracic surgeons should be aware of the potential for perioperative hypocalcemia, and engage clinicians with endocrine expertise to assist in the management of these patients.

REFERENCES

1. Gomes EM, Nunes RC, Lacativa PG, et al. Ectopic and extranumerary parathyroid glands location in patients with hyperparathyroidism secondary to end stage renal disease. Acta Cir Bras 2007;22(2):105–109.
2. Phitayakorn R, McHenry CR. Incidence and location of ectopic abnormal parathyroid glands. Am J Surg 2006;191(3):418–423.
3. Russell CF, Edis AJ, Scholz DA, et al. Mediastinal parathyroid tumors: experience with 38 tumors requiring mediastinotomy for removal. Ann Surg 1981;193(6):805–809.
4. Alesina PF, Moka D, Mahlstedt J, et al. Thoracoscopic removal of mediastinal hyperfunctioning parathyroid glands: personal experience and review of the literature. World J Surg 2008;32(2):224–231.
5. Cupisti K, Dotzenrath C, Simon D, et al. Therapy of suspected intrathoracic parathyroid adenomas. Langenbeck's Arch Surg 2002;386(7):488–493.
6. Conn JM, Goncalves MA, Mansour KA, et al. The mediastinal parathyroid. Am Surg 1991;57(1):62–66.
7. Randone B, Costi R, Scatton O, et al. Thoracoscopic removal of mediastinal parathyroid glands: a critical appraisal of an emerging technique. Ann Surg 2010;251(4):717–721.
8. Uludag M, Isgor A, Yetkin G, et al. Supernumerary ectopic parathyroid glands. Persistent hyperparathyroidism due to mediastinal parathyroid adenoma localized by preoperative single photon emission computed tomography and intraoperative gamma probe application. Hormones (Athens) 2009;8(2):144–149.
9. Cope O. Surgery of hyperparathyroidism: the occurrence of parathyroids in the anterior mediastinum and the division of the operation into two stages. Ann Surg 1941;114(4):706–733.

10. Chaffanjon PC, Voirin D, Vasdev A, et al. Selective venous sampling in recurrent and persistent hyperparathyroidism: indication, technique, and results. *World J Surg* 2004;28(10):958–961.

11. Kumar A, Kumar S, Aggarwal S, et al. Thoracoscopy: the preferred method for excision of mediastinal parathyroids. *Surg Laparosc Endosc Percutan Tech* 2002;12(4):295–300.

12. Iihara M, Suzuki R, Kawamata A, et al. Thoracoscopic removal of mediastinal parathyroid lesions: selection of surgical approach and pitfalls of preoperative and intraoperative localization. *World J Surg* 2012;36(6):1327–1334.

13. Fiorelli A, Vicidomini G, Laperuta P, et al. The role of Tc-99m-2-methoxy-isobutyl-isonitrile single photon emission computed tomography in visualizing anterior mediastinal tumor and differentiating histologic type of thymoma. *Eur J Cardiothorac Surg* 2011;40(1):136–142.

14. Park HS, Lee SW, Yun SU, et al. Atypical thymoma (World Health Organization Type B3) with neuroendocrine differentiation combined with hyperparathyroidism. *J Thorac Oncol* 2010;5(9):1490–1491.

15. Ceriani L, Giovanella L. Simultaneous imaging of pericardial thymoma and parathyroid adenoma by sestamibi scan. *Clin Nucl Med* 2008;33(8):542–544.

16. Cunningham LC, Yu JG, Shilo K, et al. Thymoma and parathyroid adenoma: false-positive imaging and intriguing laboratory test results. *JAMA Otolaryngol Head Neck Surg* 2014;140(4):369–373.

17. Said SM, Cassivi SD, Allen MS, et al. Minimally invasive resection for mediastinal ectopic parathyroid glands. *Ann Thorac Surg* 2013;96(4):1229–1233.

18. Arnault V, Beaulieu A, Lifante JC, et al. Multicenter study of 19 aortopulmonary window parathyroid tumors: the challenge of embryologic origin. *World J Surg* 2010;34(9):2211–2216.

19. Nakai K, Fujii H, Maeno K, et al. A case of parathyroid adenoma adjacent to the thoracic spine in a hemodialysis patient. *Clin Nephrol* 2014;81(1):52–57.

20. Özgül MA, Seyhan EC, Özgül G, et al. Endotracheal ectopic parathyroid adenoma mimicking asthma. *Respir Med Case Rep* 2014;13:28–31.

21. Panchani R, Varma T, Goyal A, et al. A challenging case of an ectopic parathyroid adenoma. *Indian J Endocrinol Metab* 2012;16(suppl 2):S408–S410.

22. Noussios G, Anagnostis P, Natsis K. Ectopic parathyroid glands and their anatomical, clinical and surgical implications. *Exp Clin Endocrinol Diabetes* 2012;120(10):604–610.

23. Kelly HR, Hamberg LM, Hunter GJ. 4D-CT for preoperative localization of abnormal parathyroid glands in patients with hyperparathyroidism: accuracy and ability to stratify patients by unilateral versus bilateral disease in surgery-naïve and re-exploration patients. *AJNR Am J Neuroradiol* 2014;35(1):176–181.

24. Starker LF, Mahajan A, Björklund P, et al. 4D parathyroid CT as the initial localization study for patients with de novo primary hyperparathyroidism. *Ann Surg Oncol* 2011;18(6):1723–1728.

25. Day KM, Elsayed M, Beland MD, et al. The utility of 4-dimensional computed tomography for preoperative localization of primary hyperparathyroidism in patients not localized by sestamibi or ultrasonography. *Surgery* 2015;157(3):534–539.

26. Coakley AJ, Kettle AG, Wells CP, et al. 99Tcm sestamibi—a new agent for parathyroid imaging. *Nucl Med Commun* 1989;10(11):791–794.

27. Van Udelsman B, Udelsman R. Surgery in primary hyperparathyroidism: extensive personal experience. *J Clin Densitom* 2013;16(1):54–59.

28. Mohebati A, Shaha AR. Imaging techniques in parathyroid surgery for primary hyperparathyroidism. *Am J Otolaryngol* 2012;33(4):457–468.

29. Cheung K, Wang TS, Farrokhyar F, et al. A meta-analysis of preoperative localization techniques for patients with primary hyperparathyroidism. *Ann Surg Oncol* 2012;19(2):577–583.

30. Numerow LM, Morita ET, Clark OH, et al. Persistent/recurrent hyperparathyroidism: a comparison of sestamibi scintigraphy, MRI, and ultrasonography. *J Magn Reson Imaging* 1995;5(6):702–708.

31. Lebastchi AH, Aruny JE, Donovan PI, et al. Real-time super selective venous sampling in remedial parathyroid surgery. *J Am Coll Surg* 2015;220(6):994–1000.

32. Lau JH, Drake W, Matson M. The current role of venous sampling in the localization of endocrine disease. *Cardiovasc Intervent Radiol* 2007;30(4):555–570.

33. Jaskowiak N, Norton JA, Alexander HR, et al. A prospective trial evaluating a standard approach to reoperation for missed parathyroid adenoma. *Ann Surg* 1996;224(3):308–320; discussion 320–321.

34. Jones JJ, Brunaud L, Dowd CF, et al. Accuracy of selective venous sampling for intact parathyroid hormone in difficult patients with recurrent or persistent hyperparathyroidism. *Surgery* 2002;132(6):944–950; discussion 950–951.

35. Traub-Weidinger T, Mayerhoefer ME, Koperek O, et al. 11C-methionine PET/CT imaging of 99mTc-MIBI-SPECT/CT-negative patients with primary hyperparathyroidism and previous neck surgery. *J Clin Endocrinol Metab* 2014;99(11):4199–4205.

36. Hellman P, Ahlström H, Bergström M, et al. Positron emission tomography with 11C-methionine in hyperparathyroidism. *Surgery* 1994;116(6):974–981.

37. Kettle AG, O'Doherty MJ. Parathyroid imaging: how good is it and how should it be done? *Semin Nucl Med* 2006;36(3):206–211.

38. Graff-Baker A, Roman SA, Boffa D, et al. Diagnosis of ectopic middle mediastinal parathyroid adenoma using endoscopic ultrasonography-guided fine-needle aspiration with real-time rapid parathyroid hormone assay. *J Am Coll Surg* 2009;209(3):e1–e4.

39. Wei B, Inabnet W, Lee JA, et al. Optimizing the minimally invasive approach to mediastinal parathyroid adenomas. *Ann Thorac Surg* 2011;92(3):1012–1017.

40. Amar L, Guignat L, Tissier F, et al. Video-assisted thoracoscopic surgery as a first-line treatment for mediastinal parathyroid adenomas: strategic value of imaging. *Eur J Endocrinol* 2004;150(2):141–147.

41. Liu RC, Hill ME, Ryan JA. One-gland exploration for mediastinal parathyroid adenomas: cervical and thoracoscopic approaches. *Am J Surg* 2005;189(5):601–604; discussion 605.

42. Tcherveniakov P, Menon A, Milton R, et al. Video-assisted mediastinoscopy (VAM) for surgical resection of ectopic parathyroid adenoma. *J Cardiothorac Surg* 2007;2:41.

43. Sridhar P, Steenkamp DW, Lee SL, et al. Mediastinal parathyroid adenoma with osteitis fibrosa cystica: robot-assisted thoracic surgical resection. *Innovations (Phila)* 2014;9(6):445–447.

44. Van Dessel E, Hendriks JM, Lauwers P, et al. Mediastinal parathyroidectomy with the da Vinci robot. *Innovations (Phila)* 2011;6(4):262–264.

45. Chan AP, Wan IY, Wong RH, et al. Robot-assisted excision of ectopic mediastinal parathyroid adenoma. *Asian Cardiovasc Thorac Ann* 2010;18(1):65–67.

46. Rattner DW, Marrone GC, Kasdon E, et al. Recurrent hyperparathyroidism due to implantation of parathyroid tissue. *Am J Surg* 1985;149(6):745–8.

47. Sokol MS, Kavolius J, Schaaf M, et al. Recurrent hyperparathyroidism from benign neoplastic seeding: a review with recommendations for management. *Surgery* 1993;113(4):456–461.

48. Callender GG, Udelsman R. Surgery for primary hyperparathyroidism. *Cancer* 2014;120(23):3602–3616.

49. De Sanctis V, Soliman A, Fiscina B. Hypoparathyroidism: from diagnosis to treatment. *Curr Opin Endocrinol Diabetes Obes* 2012;19(6):435–442.

50. Selberherr A, Scheuba C, Riss P, et al. Postoperative hypoparathyroidism after thyroidectomy: efficient and cost-effective diagnosis and treatment. *Surgery* 2015;157(2):349–353.

51. Witteveen JE, van Thiel SW, Romijn JA, et al. Therapy of endocrine disease: hungry bone syndrome: still a challenge in the post-operative management of primary hyperparathyroidism: a systematic review of the literature. *Eur J Endocrinol* 2013;168(3):R45–R53.

52. Mehrabibahar M, Mousavi Z, Sadeghi R, et al. Feasibility and safety of minimally invasive radioguided parathyroidectomy using very low intraoperative dose of Tc-99m MIBI. *Int J Surg* 2017;39:229–233.

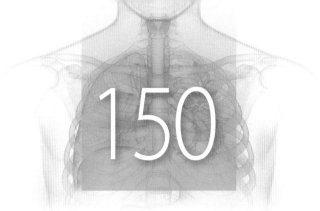

150

Neurogenic Structures of the Mediastinum

Ghulam Abbas ▪ Mark J. Krasna

A thorough knowledge of the normal anatomy and their variants of the neurogenic structures of the thorax is essential for surgeons to prevent intraoperative injuries that can be debilitating for the patients. The most important neurogenic structures in the mediastinum are the phrenic and vagus nerves, the thoracic spinal nerves, the sympathetic trunks and ganglia, and the autonomic plexus.

PHRENIC NERVE

The phrenic nerves arise from the nerve roots of C3, C4, and C5 in the neck at the border of anterior scalene muscles on each side (Figs. 150.1A,B and 150.2). It enters the thoracic cavity behind the first rib and is accompanied by the pericardiophrenic arteries and veins of the internal mammary vessels.[1]

The right phrenic nerve passes between the innominate artery and vein as it enters the thoracic cavity via the thoracic inlet. The nerve runs along with the pericardiophrenic vessels, passes over the pleural cupola, and descends caudally on the right side of the innominate vein and then on the anterolateral surface of the superior vena cava. In its caudal descent it passes ventrally to the hilar structures (Fig. 150.1A). The nerve lies deeper and has a more vertical course than the left nerve as it passes along the lateral aspect of the pericardium deeper to the mediastinal pleura. Finally, just above the diaphragm or at the diaphragmatic level it divides into its terminal branches.[2,3]

The left phrenic nerve is longer than the right and descends between the common carotid and subclavian arteries. It lies behind the left innominate vein, lateral to the vagus nerve and then crosses to lie medial and anterior to the vagus and descends anterior to the hilar structures along the pericardium in the similar fashion as the right (Fig. 150.1B).

Both phrenic nerves just above or at the diaphragmatic level usually divide into three terminal branches, anteromedial (sternal), anterolateral, and posterolateral branch (Fig. 150.3). These are relatively consistent branches which lie deep in the muscle, making it safe to incise diaphragmatic muscles radially or alternatively circumferencially a few centimeters from the costal attachment without damaging the nerve branches.[4]

VAGUS NERVE

The vagus nerves are the 10th cranial nerves which enter the neck via the jugular foramen, anterior to the jugular vein. They descend caudally in the carotid sheath behind the carotid artery and jugular vein. Each nerve enters the neck behind the sternoclavicular joint and the brachiocephalic vein (Fig. 150.4A).

At the thoracic inlet, the right vagus nerve crosses the first part of the subclavian artery and gives off the recurrent laryngeal nerve. This branch loops around the vessel and ascends to travel in the tracheoesophageal groove to the larynx. Caudally the main trunk lies on the right side of trachea and passes dorsal to the pulmonary hilum (Fig. 150.4B). The trunk then makes the dorsal pulmonary plexus and nerve plexus on the dorsal surface of the esophagus. After receiving a branch from the left vagus it becomes the posterior vagus nerve, running on the posterior surface of the esophagus as the posterior vagus nerve and enters the abdomen along with the esophagus through the hiatus.

The left vagus nerve enters the thorax between the left carotid and subclavian arteries deep to the left innominate vein. It passes over the aortic arch and then between the aorta and the left pulmonary artery just distal to the ligamentum arteriosum. At this level, it gives off the left recurrent laryngeal branch, which loops under the surface of the aortic arch to lie next to trachea and then ascend in the tracheoesophageal groove to the neck (Fig. 150.4C). The main vagal trunk passes dorsal to the pulmonary hilum and gives off the pulmonary plexus. Subsequently, it descends on the ventral surface of the esophagus, entering the abdomen through the hiatus as the left vagus nerve. It then lies in the gastroesophageal fat pad giving off small branches to the stomach along its lesser curvature. Filaments from these branches enter the lesser sac and join the hepatic plexus.

THORACIC SPINAL NERVES

Each nerve emerges from the vertebral canal through the intervertebral foramen below the corresponding vertebra and divides into an anterior (ventral) and a posterior (dorsal) ramus, ramus communicantes, through which it connects with the sympathetic trunk, and a smaller ramus meningeus that returns to the spinal canal (Fig. 150.5). The dorsal ramus runs posteriorly to supply the muscles, bone, and skin of the back and terminates by dividing into a medial cutaneous and a lateral muscular branch.

The ventral ramus, known as intercostal nerve, runs laterally and is joined by the respective intercostal artery and vein and lie in the groove at the inferior border of each rib.

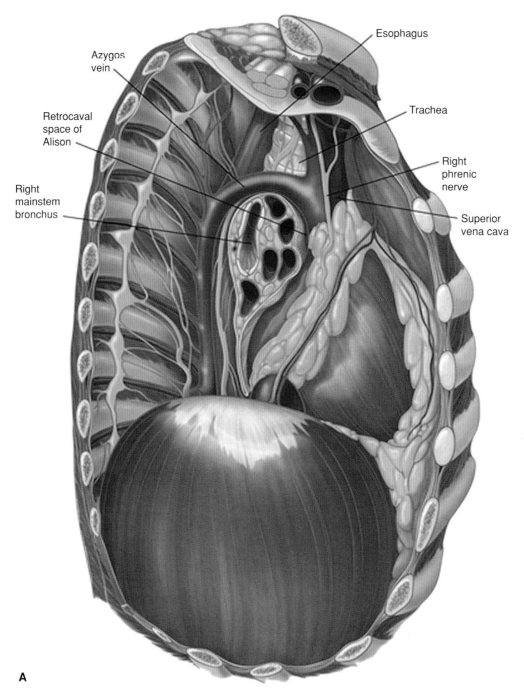

A

FIGURE 150.1 **A:** Right phrenic nerve and hilum of right lung. Phrenic nerve descends anterior to the right hilum. **B:** Left phrenic nerve and its relation to the hilum and the aortic arch. (Reprinted from Wang J, Li J, Liu G, et al. Nerves of the mediastinum. *Thorac Surg Clin* 2011; 21(2):239–249. Copyright © 2011 Elsevier. With permission.) (*continued*)

SYMPATHETIC TRUNKS AND GANGLIA

The thoracic sympathetic chain is made up of a variable number of ganglia connected by the sympathetic trunk, which lies ventral to the heads of the ribs, behind the endothoracic fascia and parietal pleura. These nerves enter the abdomen under the median arcuate ligaments and join the lumbar sympathetic trunks (Fig. 150.6).

The number of the thoracic ganglia is variable but is usually 10 or 11. The first ganglia is usually fused with the inferior cervical ganglion,

forming the "stellate ganglion" located anterior to the transverse process of the C7 and superior to the neck of the first rib. The remaining thoracic ganglia are situated at the level of the intervertebral discs and communicate with the corresponding spinal nerve with one or two rami communicantes.

The anatomy of the sympathetic chain, especially the origin and branching of the second thoracic nerve root—including the "nerve of Kuntz" is of interest to surgeons interested in performing VATS sympathectomy for palmar hyperhidrosis. The "nerve of Kuntz" is an inconsistent ramus described by Kuntz in 1927

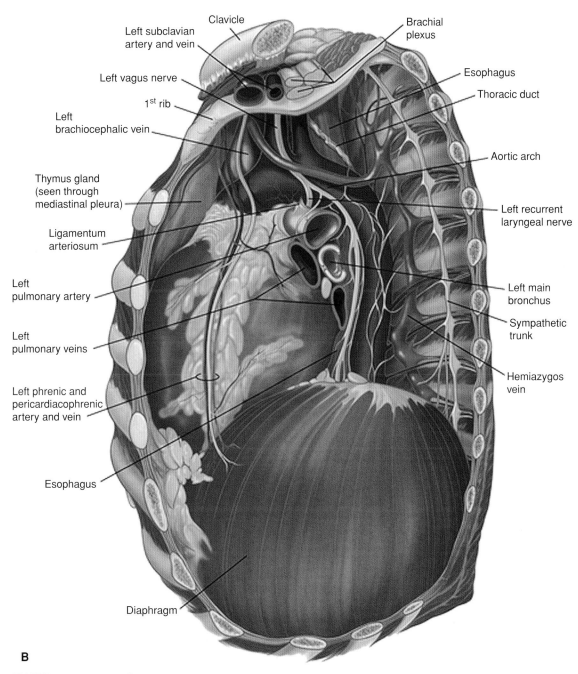

B

FIGURE 150.1 (*Continued*)

connecting the first and second thoracic nerves in a variable fashion.[5] It is present in 50% to 75% of patients. In the most common patterns the nerve of Kuntz connects from T2 to the T1 nerve, from the T2 to first intercostal nerve, from T2 to ramus communicates between the stellate ganglion and the T1 nerve, or the nerve branching to connecting from the T2 nerve to T1 nerve and the first intercostal nerve.[6] If present, its transection is important in order to achieve a successful sympathectomy and requires extending the dissection at least 1.5 cm to 2 cm laterally from the chain over the parietal pleura.[7,8] The position of the second ganglion can be variable. Most frequently it is present in the second intercostal space or the upper border of the third rib. It can also be elongated from the second rib to third rib or the second

intercostal space to the third intercostal space covering the entire width of the third rib.

SPLANCHNIC NERVES

The branches from the fifth to ninth ganglia make the greater splanchnic nerve at the level of the tenth thoracic vertebra. These nerves pass inferomedially through the ipsilateral diaphragmatic crus to join the celiac ganglia. The branches from the 10th to 12th thoracic ganglia make the lesser splanchnic nerves. They pass behind the greater splanchnic nerves, laterally to end in the renal plexus (Fig. 150.7).

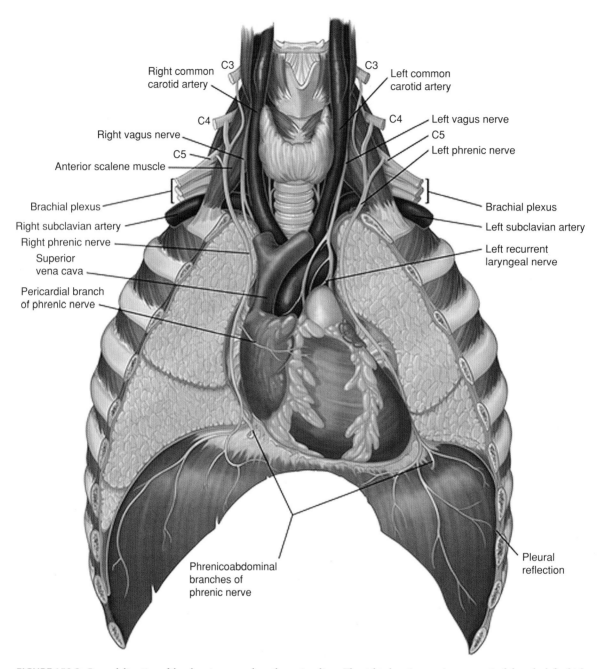

FIGURE 150.2 General direction of the phrenic nerves along the pericardium. The right phrenic nerve is more vertical than the left which has an oblique course. (From Wang J, Li J, Liu G, et al. Nerves of the mediastinum. *Thorac Surg Clin* 2011;21(2):239–249. Copyright © 2011 Elsevier. With permission.)

MAJOR THORACIC PLEXUSES

Following are the major nerve plexus in the thoracic cavity.[9]

PULMONARY PLEXUSES

The posterior pulmonary plexus is formed by the branches from vagus nerve as it passes dorsal to the hilum and branches from the upper thoracic ganglia. The anterior pulmonary plexus is less well developed and is formed by a branch of the vagus nerve and rami from cervical ganglion. Post plexus nerves pierce the pulmonary parenchyma and divide into periarterial and peribronchial plexus.

CARDIAC PLEXUSES

The branches from the lower cervical trunk and stellate ganglion make up the cardiac plexus. The parasympathetic cardiopulmonary nerves are formed by the branches of the recurrent laryngeal nerve and main vagus nerves. These nerves interconnect with sympathetic cardiopulmonary nerves anterior and posterior to the main pulmonary artery to form the ventral and dorsal cardiopulmonary plexuses which supply the heart.

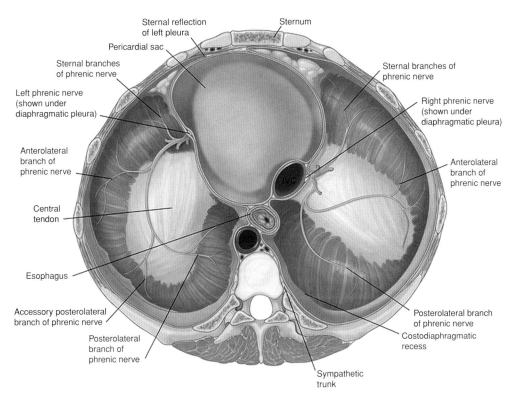

FIGURE 150.3 Main branches of the phrenic nerves at the diaphragmatic level. (Reprinted from Wang J, Li J, Liu G, et al. Nerves of the mediastinum. *Thorac Surg Clin* 2011;21(2):239–249. Copyright © 2011 Elsevier. With permission.)

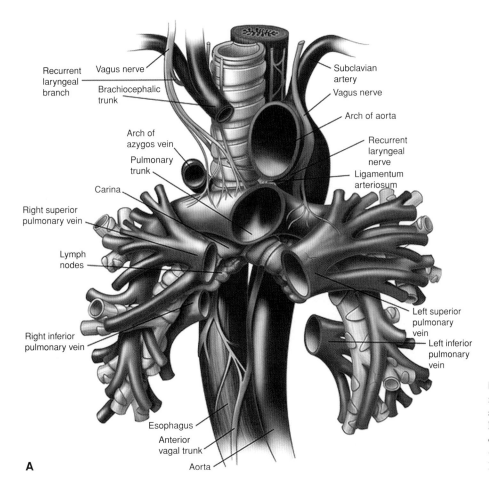

A

FIGURE 150.4 **A:** Course of the vagus and recurrent nerves and their relation to great vessels. **B:** Anatomy of right vagus. **C:** Anatomy of left vagus. (Reprinted from Wang J, Li J, Liu G, et al. Nerves of the mediastinum. *Thorac Surg Clin* 2011;21(2):239–249. Copyright © 2011 Elsevier. With permission.) (*continued*)

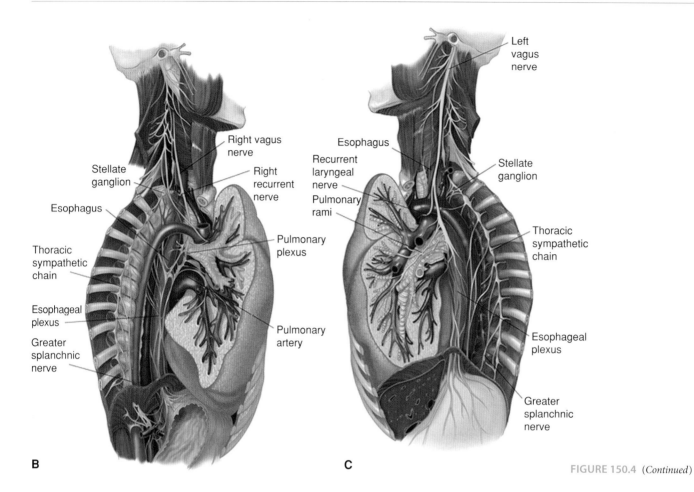

B

C

FIGURE 150.4 (*Continued*)

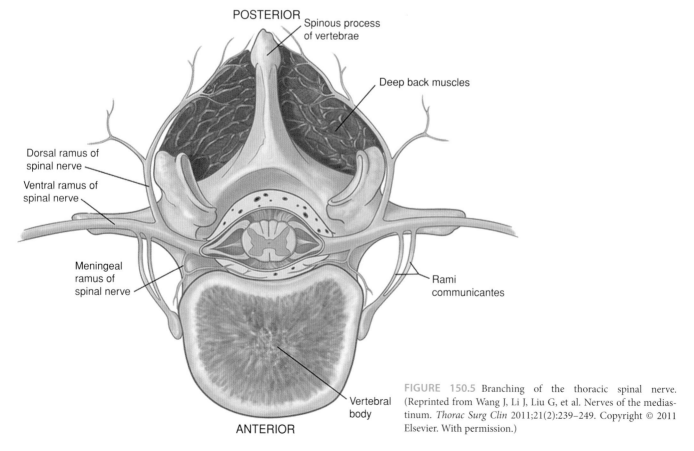

FIGURE 150.5 Branching of the thoracic spinal nerve. (Reprinted from Wang J, Li J, Liu G, et al. Nerves of the mediastinum. *Thorac Surg Clin* 2011;21(2):239–249. Copyright © 2011 Elsevier. With permission.)

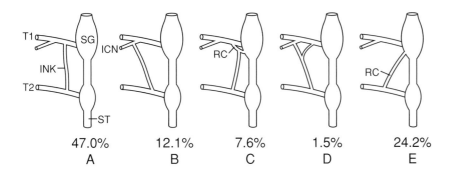

FIGURE 150.6 Four types of the intrathoracic nerves of Kuntz and ramus communicates from the T2 nerve to the stellate ganglion. Inc, intercostal nerve: ramus communicates; SG, stellate ganglion; ST, sympathetic trunk. (Reprinted from Chung IH, Oh CS, Koh KS, et al. Anatomic variations of the T2 nerve root (including the nerve of Kuntz) and their implications for sympathectomy. *J Thorac Cardiovsc Surg* 2002;123:498. Copyright © 2011 Elsevier. With permission.)

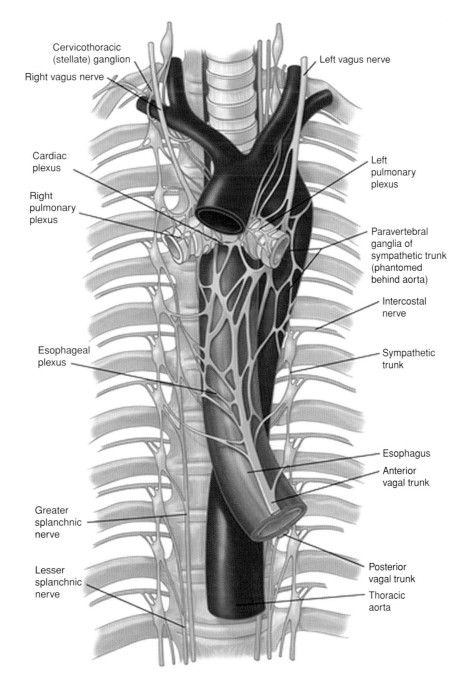

FIGURE 150.7 Pulmonary and esophageal plexus and splanchnic nerves. (Reprinted from Wang J, Li J, Liu G, et al. Nerves of the mediastinum. *Thorac Surg Clin* 2011;21(2):239–249. Copyright © 2011 Elsevier. With permission.)

ESOPHAGEAL PLEXUS

The esophageal plexus is formed by the left and right vagus nerves on the ventral and dorsal surface of the esophagus respectively. At the level of the lower third of the esophagus the ventral esophageal plexus collects into the anterior vagus nerve and the dorsal plexus collects into the posterior vagus nerve.

AORTIC BODIES AND PARAGANGLIA

The paraganglia are a collection of neural crest cells that are distributed throughout the body. They are composed of the adrenal medulla, the carotid and aortic bodies, the vagal body, and small groups of cells associated with the thoracic, intra-abdominal, and retroperitoneal ganglia.[10] In 2004 the World Health Organization defined a pheochromocytoma as an intra-adrenal paraganglioma, whereas closely related tumors of extra-adrenal sympathetic or parasympathetic paraganglia are classified as extra-adrenal paragangliomas.[11] The aortic and carotid bodies are chemoreceptors and react weakly with chromate solutions and thus are called nonchromaffin paragangliomas. The aortic body on the right lies between the angle of the right subclavian and carotid arteries. On the left, it is found above the aorta medial to the origin of the left subclavian artery (Fig. 150.8).

Beside aortic bodies, the connective tissue between the aorta and pulmonary artery on each side contains a collection of readily identifiable chromaffin cells. Most of the tumors arising from the aortic bodies and other paragangliomas of the visceral mediastinum are inactive.

The para-aortic sympathetic paraganglia are the collections of chromaffin cells in both paravertebral sulci in association with the connective tissues around the spinal ganglia bilaterally. They are the sites of the origin of the chromaffin tumors in the paravertebral sulci.[12] Surgical resection of mediastinal paragangliomas is an effective treatment with most cases being curative. However, the Mayo Clinic investigators[13] found that, even with complete resection of the mediastinal tumor, the majority of their patients (64%) remained hypertensive requiring antihypertensive treatment. There was no evidence of recurrent or residual tumors. These patients need life-long surveillance.

CLINICAL IMPLICATIONS

Injuries to the neurogenic structures of the mediastinum can lead to life-long, debilitating outcomes for the patients. For example, the recurrent laryngeal nerve is susceptible to injuries during routine cardiothoracic surgical procedures, more on the left in aortopulmonary window.[14] Aside from hoarseness of voice, it can lead to fatal aspiration events in the immediate postoperative period. Similarly, injury to vagus nerves can lead to delayed gastric emptying and digestive problems. Phrenic nerve injury during tumor resection or cardiovascular procedures can lead to diaphragmatic paralysis.[3] This leads to diaphragmatic elevation and paradoxical movement of diaphragm during respiration, significantly impairing patient's breathing capacity and in many instants leading to permanent oxygen requirement. During sympathectomy, injury to stellate ganglia leads to Horner syndrome with ptosis of eyelid, decrease in pupil size, and

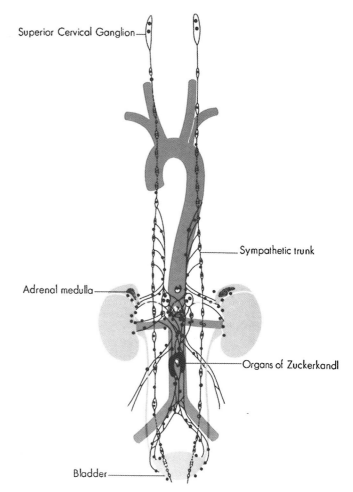

FIGURE 150.8 Sites of the aorticosympathetic paraganglia. Diagram of extramedullary chromaffin tissue in a newborn child. (From Gleener CG, Grimley PM. Tumors of the extra-adrenal paraganglion system (including chemoreceptors). In: *Atlas of Tumor Pathology*. Second Series, Fascicle 9. Washington, DC: Armed Forces Institute of Pathology; 1974.)

decreased sweating of the affected side of the face. The other important anatomical structure in thoracic sympathectomy is the "Nerve of Kuntz."[6] The surgeon must be familiar with the anatomic variations of this nerve in order to make sure that is transected for good outcome after sympathectomy.

REFERENCES

1. Agur MR, Dalley AF. *Grant's Atlas of Anatomy*. 13th ed. Lippincott Williams & Wilkins; 2012.
2. Fell SC. Surgical anatomy of the diaphragm and the phrenic nerve. *Chest Surg Clin N Am* 1998;8:281–294.
3. Owens WA, Gladstone DJ, Heylings DJ. Surgical anatomy of the phrenic nerve and internal mammary artery. *Ann Thorac Surg* 1994;58:843–844.
4. Downey R. Anatomy of the normal diaphragm. *Thorac Surg Clin* 2011;21(2): 273–279.
5. Kuntz A. Distribution of sympathetic rami to the brachial plexus: Its relation to sympathectomy affecting the upper extremity. *Arch Surg* 1927;15:871.
6. Chung IH, Oh CS, Koh KS, et al. Anatomic variations of the T2 nerve root (including the nerve of Kuntz) and their implications for sympathectomy. *J Thorac Cardiovasc Surg* 2002;123:498–501.
7. Marhold F, Izay B, Zacherl J, et al. Thoracoscopic and anatomic landmarks of Kuntz's nerve: Implications for sympathetic surgery. *Ann Thorac Surg* 2008;86(5): 1653–1658.

8. Ramsaroop L, Partab P, Singh B, et al. Thoracic Origin of a sympathetic supply to the upper limb: The 'nerve of Kuntz' revisited. *J Anat.* 2001;199(Pt 6):675–682.

9. Wang J, Li J, Liu G, et al. Nerves of the mediastinum. *Thorac Surg Clin* 2011;21(2):239–249.

10. Kimura N, Chetty R, Capella C, et al. Extra-adrenal paraganglioma: carotid body, jugulotympanic, vagal, laryngeal, aortico-pulmonary. In: Lloyd RV, Heitz PU, et al. eds. *Pathology and Genetics of Tumours of Endocrine Organs.* Lyon, France: IARC Press; 2004:159–161.

11. Chen J, Sippel RS, O'Dorisio MS, et al. The North American Neuroendocrine Tumor Society consensus guideline for the diagnosis and management of neuroendocrine tumors: Pheochromocytoma, paraganglioma and medullary thyroid cancer. *Pancreas* 2010;39(6):775–783.

12. Shields TW, Locicer J, Ponn RB, et al. *General Thoracic Surgery.* 7th ed. Philadelphia, PA: Lippincott Williams & Wilkins; 2005.

13. Brown ML, Zayas GE, Abel MD, et al. Mediastinal paragangliomas: The Mayo Clinic experience. *Ann Thorac Surg* 2008;86(3):946–951.

14. Myssiorek D. Recurrent Laryngeal nerve paralysis: anatomy and etiology. *Otolaryngol Clin North Am* 2004;37:25–44.

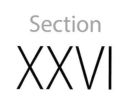

NONINVASIVE INVESTIGATIONS

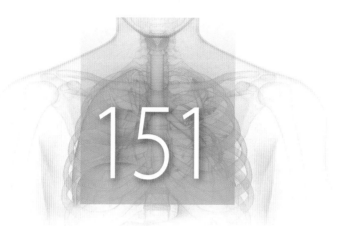

151

Radiographic, Computed Tomographic, and Magnetic Resonance Investigation of the Mediastinum

Nadeem Parkar ■ Sanjeev Bhalla

INTRODUCTION

The mediastinum is the designation given to the anatomical region of the thorax bounded laterally by the pleura, anteriorly by the sternum, posteriorly by the vertebrae, superiorly by the thoracic inlet, and inferiorly by the diaphragm.[1-3] The mediastinum is divided into compartments to aid in generating a differential diagnosis at initial presentation and to facilitate surgical treatment plan. However, there are no physical boundaries between compartments and several different classification systems have been developed in the past by anatomists, clinicians, and radiologists.

Anatomically the mediastinum is divided into superior and inferior compartments by an imaginary line traversing the manubriosternal joint and the lower margin of the fourth thoracic vertebra. The inferior compartment is further divided into three parts: the anterior, middle, and posterior compartments. The Felson method of division is based on findings at lateral radiography. A line that extends from the thoracic inlet to the diaphragm along the back of the heart (inferior vena cava) and anterior to the trachea separates the anterior from the middle mediastinal compartment. The middle and posterior compartments of the mediastinum are separated by a line that runs 1 cm behind the anterior margins of the vertebral bodies (Fig. 151.1). A popular modification divides the entire mediastinum into anterior, middle, and posterior compartments but does not have a separate superior compartment.[4] The Japanese Association for Research on the Thymus (JART) proposed four mediastinal compartments based on axial CT images: superior portion of the mediastinum, anterior mediastinum (prevascular), middle mediastinum (peritracheoesophageal), and posterior mediastinum (paravertebral).[5] The International Thymic Malignancy Group (ITMIG) proposed a new classification defining a prevascular (anterior), visceral (middle), and a paravertebral (posterior) compartment with anatomic boundaries clearly defined by computed tomography (CT).[6]

IMAGING TECHNIQUES

RADIOGRAPHY

Most mediastinal masses are detected incidentally on chest radiographs and a chest radiograph is the most frequent method used initially to localize a mass to the mediastinum. A mediastinal mass makes obtuse margins with the lungs and it does not have air bronchograms. Knowledge of the normal mediastinal reflections that can be appreciated on chest radiographs is very useful in identifying a mediastinal mass and subsequently to localize it in the anterior, middle, or posterior compartments of the mediastinum. Radiographs are limited in their ability to delineate the extent of mediastinal abnormality and the relationship of the mediastinal masses to specific mediastinal structures.

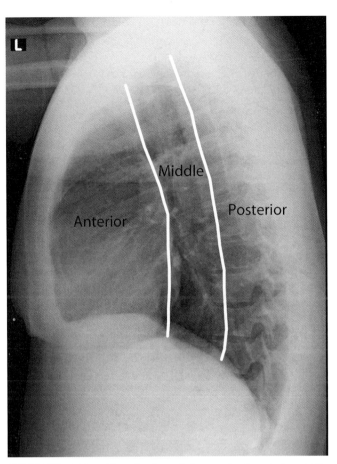

FIGURE 151.1 Normal lateral radiograph demarcating the anterior, middle, and posterior mediastinal compartments.

COMPUTED TOMOGRAPHY OF THE MEDIASTINUM

CT is the most useful cross-sectional imaging technique in localizing the origin of a mediastinal lesion to one of the mediastinal compartments and to evaluate the extent of the disease. CT is also useful in detecting calcium within the mediastinal lesion and helps in narrowing the differential diagnosis. Contrast-enhanced CT with multiplanar reformats in coronal and sagittal planes provides a very good assessment of the relationship of the vascular structures and other mediastinal structures to the mediastinal mass. Very large mediastinal lesions can extend from one compartment to another making it difficult to determine the site of origin. There are two tools to assist in deciphering the compartment where the mass originated while reviewing the cross-sectional CT images. One is to determine the center point of the lesion on the axial CT image showing the greatest size of the lesion and localizing to a specific compartment. The second is that large mediastinal masses can displace organs in other compartments that abut the compartment from which the tumor originated. In the JART study, this method resulted in classification of all 445 mediastinal masses to specific compartments.[5] CT can also be used to guide biopsy and to follow treatment response.

MAGNETIC RESONANCE IMAGING OF THE MEDIASTINUM

Magnetic resonance imaging (MRI) can provide better soft tissue characterization than CT and in some instances is helpful in delineating the composition of the mass. MRI can be useful in determining the extent of the cystic component of the mass. MR can demonstrate the extent of the intraspinal extension of a mediastinal mass or the relationship of the mediastinal mass to the heart and blood vessels. MRI is very useful in imaging neurogenic tumors. MR may have advantages over contrast-enhanced CT for distinguishing between solid tissue and adjacent vessels (fast flowing blood in vessels results in a signal void on spin-echo sequences). MRI is not as sensitive to the presence of calcification as CT. MRI is sensitive to motion artifacts related to respiratory motion and cardiac contractility.

NUCLEAR MEDICINE IMAGING OF THE MEDIASTINUM

Positron emission tomography (PET) and PET-CT using [F-18]2-deoxy-D-glucose (^{18}F-FDG) have been utilized in the evaluation of mediastinal lymph node involvement in lung cancer and lymphoma.[7,8] PET-CT is commonly used to evaluate treatment response in lymphoma and other malignancies. Radionuclide imaging with ^{123}I or ^{131}I demonstrates the presence of thyroid tissue within the mediastinum in almost all intrathoracic goiters. Radionuclide examination can play a role in imaging neuroendocrine tumors and pheochromocytomas.

ULTRASOUND IMAGING OF THE MEDIASTINUM

Echocardiography is useful in differentiating cardiac from paracardiac masses. Endoscopic ultrasound is used in guiding biopsy of mediastinal lymph nodes. Ultrasound can help in distinguishing cystic from solid masses in the mediastinum.

APPROACH TO MEDIASTINAL MASSES

Most mediastinal masses are (>60%)

- Thymomas
- Neurogenic tumors
- Benign cysts
- Lymphadenopathy

In children most common mediastinal masses are (>80%)

- Neurogenic tumors
- Germ-cell tumors
- Foregut duplication cysts

In adults the most common mediastinal masses are

- Lymphomas
- Lymphadenopathy
- Thymomas
- Thyroid masses

The approach to mediastinal masses is to

1. Localize the mass to the mediastinum
2. Localize the mass within the mediastinum
3. Characterize the mass on CT or MR

LOCALIZE TO THE MEDIASTINUM

As most mediastinal masses are initially detected on a chest radiograph, the following features can help localize a lesion to the mediastinum.

1. The margins of the lesion with the lungs will be obtuse whereas if the lesion is in the lung, the margins of the lesion with the lungs will be acute.
2. There will be disruption or alteration of the mediastinal lines (such as the anterior and posterior junction lines, right paratracheal stripe, paraspinal lines, and the azygo-esophageal recess).
3. A mediastinal mass will contain air bronchograms.
4. Associated abnormalities may be seen in the spine, sternum, and ribs.

LOCALIZE WITHIN THE MEDIASTINUM

Many mediastinal reflections can be appreciated at conventional radiography and their presence or distortion is the key to interpretation of mediastinal masses. The hilum overlay sign is present when the normal hilar structures project through a mass, such that the mass can be understood as being either anterior or posterior to the hilum. Anterior mediastinal masses can be identified when both the hilum overlay sign and preservation of the posterior mediastinal lines are present.

The azygo-esophageal recess reflection is a prevertebral structure and is, therefore, disrupted by prevertebral disease. It has an interface with the middle mediastinum; thus, the resulting line seen at radiography can be interrupted by abnormalities in both the middle and posterior compartments. A right paratracheal stripe 5 mm or more in width is considered widened. A convex border between the AP window and the lung is considered abnormal. The paraspinal lines are disrupted by paravertebral disease which commonly includes diseases originating in the intervertebral disks and vertebrae and by neurogenic tumors.[9] Posterior mediastinal masses above the level of the clavicles have sharp margins due to their interface with lung whereas anterior mediastinal masses do not have sharp margins extending above the level of the clavicles. Although there is no tissue plane separating the divisions of the mediastinum, attempting to more accurately localize an abnormality with reference to the local anatomy of the mediastinum helps in narrowing the differential diagnosis and determining appropriate further imaging.

IMAGING FEATURES ON CT OR MRI TO CHARACTERIZE THE MASS

In most cases of mediastinal masses detected on radiography, CT is performed to further analyze and characterize the anterior and middle mediastinal masses. MR is performed to analyze and characterize posterior mediastinal masses as majority of these are nerve sheath tumors. If evaluation of osseous structures is needed a CT scan is more useful. Mediastinal masses can be further characterized by CT or MR depending on whether they contain fat, fluid, or are vascular.

Anterior mediastinum:

a. Fluid containing lesions: thymoma, thymic carcinoma, pericardial cyst, germ-cell tumor, lymphoma
b. Fat containing lesions: germ-cell tumor, thymolipoma, fat pad, Morgagni hernia
c. Vascular lesions: thyroid, ascending aorta, cardiac or coronary

Middle mediastinal lesions:

a. Fluid containing lesions: duplication cyst, necrotic nodes, pericardial recess
b. Fat containing lesions: lipoma, esophageal fibrovascular polyp
c. Vascular lesions: arch anomaly, azygos vein, vascular nodes

Posterior mediastinal lesions:

a. Fluid containing lesions: neuroenteric cyst, schwannoma, meningocele
b. Fat containing lesions: extramedullary hematopoiesis
c. Vascular lesions: descending aorta

Mediastinal lesions that disregard compartments:

a. Fluid containing lesions: lymphangiomas, mediastinal abscess (mediastinitis)
b. Fat containing lesions: liposarcoma
c. Vascular lesions: hemangioma, hemorrhage
d. Other: lung cancer

THYROID MASSES

Approximately 3% and 17% of goiters extend inferiorly from the neck into the thorax.[10,11] Most thyroid masses in the mediastinum represent downward extensions of either a multinodular colloid goiter or, occasionally, an adenoma or carcinoma. Rounded or irregular, well-defined areas of calcification in the intrathoracic thyroids may be seen in benign areas, whereas amorphous cloud-like calcification is occasionally seen within carcinomas.

Intrathoracic thyroid masses may cause tracheal narrowing or deviation of the trachea depending on the location of the mass (Fig. 151.2). Thyroid masses are commonly anterior and lateral to the trachea but posteriorly the masses often separate the trachea and the esophagus, and such separation by a localized mass continuing into the neck is virtually diagnostic of a thyroid mass. CT imaging features of mediastinal thyroid goiters are

1. High attenuation on a non-contrast exam (higher than muscle), reflecting high iodine content of thyroid tissue
2. Intense and prolonged enhancement following intravenous contrast enhancement
3. Continuity of the mass with the cervical thyroid gland
4. Calcifications and cystic regions resulting in foci of heterogeneous attenuation

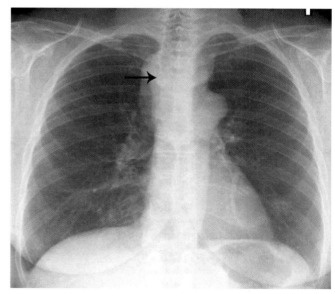

FIGURE 151.2 Intrathoracic thyroid goiter resulting in rightward deviation of the trachea (black arrow).

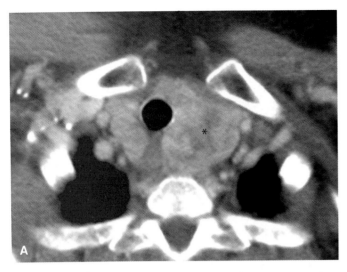

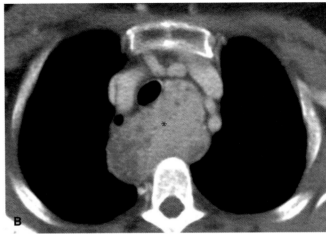

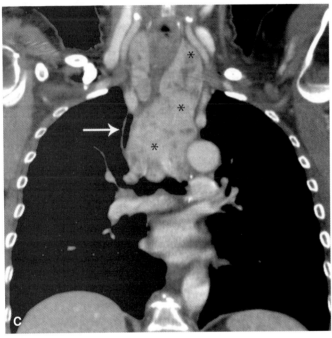

FIGURE 151.3 **A–C:** Large thyroid goiter (*asterisk*) arising from the left lobe of the thyroid extending into the thorax. The heterogeneous goiter demonstrates intense enhancement on post-contrast images with areas of low attenuation reflective of cystic change. There is resultant mass effect on the mediastinum causing rightward deviation of the trachea (*white arrow*, **C**).

Radionuclide imaging with ^{123}I or ^{131}I demonstrates the presence of thyroid tissue within the mediastinum in almost all intrathoracic goiters. Although radionuclide imaging is a sensitive and specific method of determining an intrathoracic thyroid mass, CT is more useful as the initial investigation because it provides more information if the mass is not a thyroid lesion. CT optimally demonstrates the shape, size, and position of the mass[12,13] (Fig. 151.3A–C).

The most important feature of CT is to demonstrate continuity of the mass with the cervical thyroid. It is not possible to distinguish between a benign and malignant mass on CT unless the tumor has clearly spread beyond the thyroid gland. Multiple masses are a feature of benign multinodular goiter, though carcinoma can develop in multinodular goiter. MRI of intrathoracic goiter, like CT, can identify cystic and solid components, and in addition can demonstrate hemorrhage.

Ultrasonography may be useful in demonstrating that a thyroid mass is a simple cyst and in guiding needle aspiration in patients with nonpalpable nodules. Simple cysts are seen in ultrasound imaging as sharply marginated, thin-walled, round or oval structures with no internal echoes and with through transmission.

THYMIC MASSES

The thymus is a bilobed, triangular-shaped organ in the anterior mediastinum occupying the retrosternal space and varies widely in size and shape depending on the age.[14] In young people, the attenuation value of the thymus is approximately 30 Hounsfield units. With age, the gland involutes and becomes replaced by fat and is no longer recognizable as a soft tissue structure in persons over 25 years but is seen as islands of soft tissue attenuation within a background of fat tissue. Although the thymus may still be seen as a discrete structure up to 40 years it usually involutes and is completely replaced by fat. Anterior mediastinal masses of thymic origin include thymomas, thymic carcinoma, thymolipoma, thymic lymphoma, thymic carcinoid, and thymic hyperplasia. Thymic cysts are another cause of a thymic mass. They may be simple cysts and occur in an otherwise normal gland, may lie within a thymoma, or may follow thymic irradiation for Hodgkin's disease.[15]

Thymomas

Thymoma is the most common neoplasm of the anterior mediastinum and the most common primary tumor of the anterior mediastinum in adults. They are benign or low-grade malignant tumors of thymic epithelium. A thymoma demonstrates an abnormal contour or widening of the mediastinum on PA radiographs and an opacity in the anterior clear space on the lateral radiograph (Fig. 151.4A,B). Thymomas can

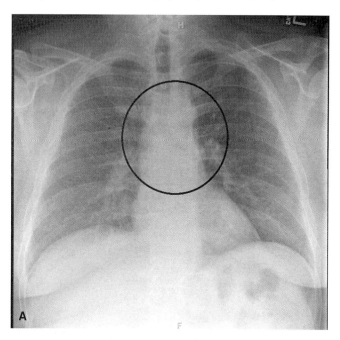

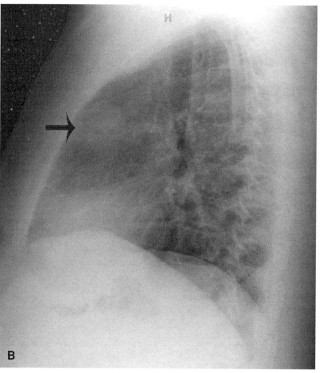

FIGURE 151.4 **A–B:** PA demonstrating enlargement of the mediastinum (*black circle*). Lateral radiograph showing a mass within the anterior clear space (*black arrow*).

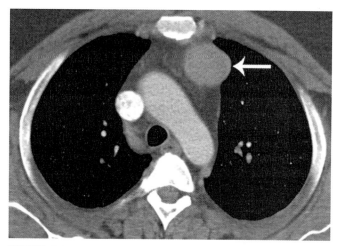

FIGURE 151.5 Contrast-enhanced CT images demonstrate a well-defined, homogeneously enhancing, spherical mass (*arrow*) located within the anterior mediastinum consistent with a thymoma.

be seen anywhere from the level of the thyroid gland to the cardiophrenic angles on either side of the heart. Most thymomas (90%) arise in the anterior mediastinum. The average age at diagnosis is approximately 50 years, earlier in those who present with myasthenia gravis. Thymomas are rare under 20 years of age and extremely unusual below the age of 15. Up to 50% of patients with thymoma have myasthenia gravis, and approximately 10% to 20% of patients with myasthenia gravis have a thymoma. A variety of other syndromes are seen in patients with thymoma, including hypogammaglobulinemia and red cell aplasia.[16,17] Thymomas can be encapsulated noninvasive type or the invasive type that has spread beyond the capsule. The terms "invasive" and "noninvasive" are commonly used instead of "benign" and "malignant" because invasive tumors may not show malignancy on pathology but they may be aggressive and difficult to treat.

Thymomas are usually spherical or oval in shape, may show lobulated borders, and may have cystic components. Thymomas usually show homogeneous density and uniform enhancement after contrast injection (Fig. 151.5). Calcification, punctate or curvilinear, may be seen. All of these features are best demonstrated using CT,[18,19] which is the most sensitive technique for the detection of thymoma in patients with myasthenia gravis.[20] Thymomas as small as 1.5 to 2.0 cm in diameter are readily identified over the age of 40, largely because the rest of the thymus is atrophic.

Invasion of the mediastinal fat and adjacent pleura may be identified with invasive thymomas and it can be seen insinuating between mediastinal structures. While CT can demonstrate such invasion, it cannot reliably diagnose invasive thymoma if the tumor is still confined to the thymus.[21] Pleural metastasis from transpleural spread is a characteristic feature of invasive thymomas, and therefore the entire pleura should be carefully examined.[21]

On MRI, the normal thymus in children and young adults characteristically demonstrates homogeneous and intermediate signal intensity on T1- and T2-weighted sequences which is less intense than mediastinal fat but greater than muscle. After puberty, the T1 and T2 signal intensity of the thymus increase with age since the thymus begins to involute and is replaced by fat.[22,23] Thymomas typically demonstrate low T1 signal intensity similar to muscle and relatively high T2 signal intensity. T2-weighted images occasionally show lobulated internal architecture and scattered areas of high intensity that correspond to fibrous septa and cystic areas.[24] MRI is superior to CT for defining the invasion of contiguous structures such as the pleura and pericardium in patients with invasive thymoma.[25] Complete preservation of the adjacent fat planes excludes extensive invasive disease but not minimal capsular invasion.[20]

Thymic Carcinomas

Thymic carcinomas are thymic epithelial tumors with a high degree of anaplasia, cell atypia, and increased proliferation.[26] They predominantly occur in adults and have a poor prognosis despite treatment with surgery and radiotherapy. Thymic carcinomas are typically large, heterogeneous masses, with areas of necrosis and calcification and evidence of invasion of adjacent structures, such as the mediastinum, pericardium, and pleura[27,28] (Fig. 151.6A–C). Thymic carcinomas are

aggressive locally invasive malignancies that have frequently metastasized to regional lymph nodes and distant sites at presentation. On MRI, thymic carcinoma demonstrates intermediate signal intensity slightly higher than muscle on T1-weighted sequence and high signal intensity on T2-weighted sequence.[29] Thymic carcinomas are more commonly associated with mediastinal node and extrathoracic metastasis but less commonly associated with pleural implants compared to invasive thymomas.[28]

Thymic Hyperplasia

Thymic hyperplasia is an increase in the size of the thymus with normal gross and histologic appearance and commonly occurs following

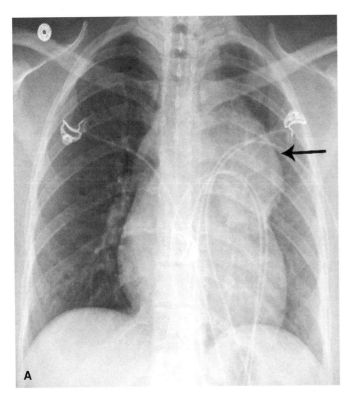

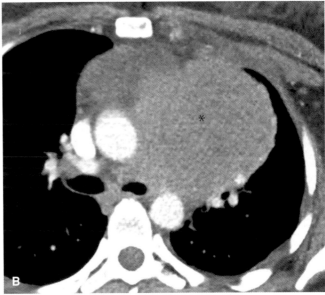

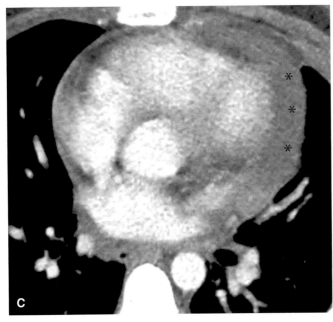

FIGURE 151.6 **A:** Radiographic images demonstrating a large mass (*arrow*) located within the anterior mediastinum which causes rightward displacement of the trachea. **B, C:** Subsequent contrast-enhanced CT images show a large, heterogeneous appearing anterior mediastinal mass (*black asterisk*, **B**) which invades the surrounding mediastinal soft tissue and exerts rightward mass effect on the mediastinum. Additionally, there is invasion of the pericardium (*black asterisk*, **C**).

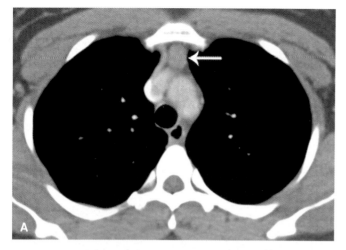

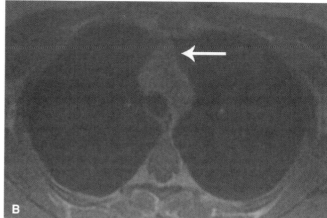

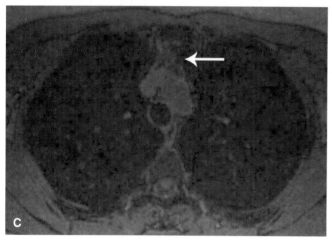

FIGURE 151.7 **A:** Axial CT image demonstrating a well-defined, homogeneous appearing mass within the anterior mediastinum suggestive of thymic hyperplasia (*arrow*). Subsequent axial MR images demonstrating chemical shift artifact of the anterior mediastinal mass with loss of signal intensity on the opposed-phase images (**C**) relative to the in-phase images (**B**).

atrophy due to stress, as a result of steroid therapy or chemotherapy.[30,31] The gland usually returns to its original size on recovery or cessation of treatment, but it may become larger than its previous normal size, a phenomenon known as rebound thymic hyperplasia.

It may then be difficult to distinguish between thymic rebound and thymic involvement by neoplasm. The diagnosis depends on a known reason for thymic rebound, the absence of clinical features to indicate tumor recurrence, and the presence of an enlarged, normally shaped thymus.[31,32] In patients older than 15 years with enlarged thymus, chemical shift MR can diagnose thymic hyperplasia by detecting fatty infiltration in the thymus and help differentiation from a neoplastic process. In thymic hyperplasia there is a drop in signal intensity at opposed-phase images when compared to in-phase images while in thymic tumors there is no drop in signal intensity on the opposed-phase images (Fig. 151.7A–C). It should be emphasized that chemical shift MR can depict physiologic fatty infiltration of the thymus in 50% of persons between ages 11 and 15 years and in 100% of those over 15 years but none of those under the age of 15 years.[33,34]

Thymic Cyst

Thymic cysts are uncommon, representing 1% of all mediastinal masses. Congenital thymic cysts are derived from a patent thymopharyngeal duct, are usually unilocular, and approximately 50% are discovered in the first two decades of life. Acquired thymic cysts are multilocular and occur in association with thymic tumors or in patients after radiation therapy for Hodgkin's disease. Occasionally, multiple cysts seen in the thymus may represent lymphoepithelial

cysts seen in HIV/AIDS or as a manifestation of Langerhans cell histiocytosis (in children). On chest radiographs, thymic cysts cannot be differentiated from other thymic masses. On CT, thymic cysts are seen as well-defined water attenuation masses with imperceptible walls (Fig. 151.8A). On MR, thymic cysts demonstrate typical characteristics of fluid with low T1 and high T2 signal intensity (Fig. 151.8B,C). In the presence of hemorrhage or infection, the cysts can demonstrate high signal on T1- and T2-weighted images.

Thymolipomas

Thymolipomas are rare tumors composed of a mixture of thymic stroma and mature fat. These tumors occur low in the anterior mediastinum, often in the cardiophrenic angle. The average age is 22 to 26 years and most patients are symptomatic.[35] Thymolipomas can grow to a very large size by the time they are detected and may mimic cardiomegaly or lobar collapse.[36] CT demonstrates fat, with islands of thymus and fibrous septa running through the lesion.[35,36] On MRI, fat within the tumor appears as high signal intensity and soft tissue appears as low signal intensity bands coursing through the mass.[37]

Thymic Neuroendocrine Tumors (Thymic Carcinoid)

Primary neuroendocrine tumors of the thymus are rare. Approximately 40% of patients have Cushing's syndrome due to adrenocorticotropic hormone secretion by the tumor and up to 20% have multiple endocrine neoplasia (MEN) syndromes I and II.[26] These tumors are aggressive and at least 20% of patients have distant metastasis at

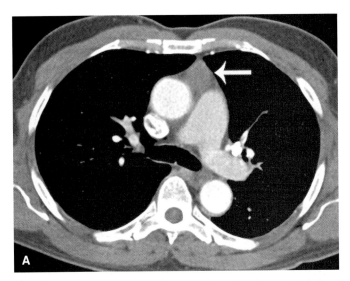

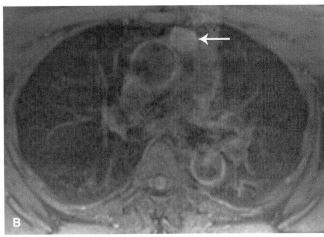

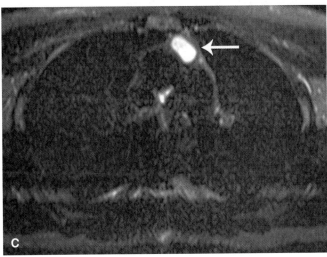

FIGURE 151.8 **A:** Axial CT image demonstrating a well-defined fluid atten-uation mass within the anterior mediastinum. MR images of the mass demon-strate a low signal intensity on T1-weighted imaging (**B**) and a high signal intensity on T2-weighted imaging (**C**). These findings are characteristic of a thymic cyst (*arrow*).

presentation to the liver, lung, bone, pleura, and pancreas.[38] Bone metastases are typically osteoblastic.

Thymic carcinoid is histologically distinct from thymoma. The imaging features of thymic carcinoid are indistinguishable from those of thymoma. On CT or MR, the tumors appear as lobulated thymic mass with heterogeneous enhancement and central areas of low attenuation secondary to necrosis or hemorrhage and may show local invasion.

PARATHYROID TUMORS

The parathyroid glands may migrate into the chest during develop-ment of the fetus. Parathyroid tumors are a rare cause of an ante-rior mediastinal mass. Most abnormal parathyroid glands contain an adenoma or are hyperplastic. Mediastinal parathyroid tumors causing hyperparathyroidism are most commonly located in or around the thymus but can be present anywhere from the base of the tongue to the surface of the pericardium. They are small and almost never visible on plain radiographs. Technetium-99m (^{99m}Tc)–sestamibi scintigraphy is the most sensitive imaging pro-cedure for parathyroid adenomas.[39,40] They can also be detected by ultrasound. On CT mediastinal adenomas manifest as small nod-ules that show minimal or no enhancement (Fig. 151.9). MRI may

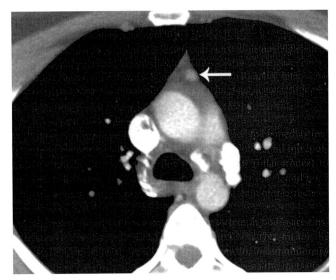

FIGURE 151.9 Axial CT image demonstrating a tiny minimally enhancing nodule within the anterior mediastinum (*arrow*) suggestive of a parathyroid adenoma in a patient with hyperparathyroidism.

also be useful for identifying mediastinal parathyroid adenomas in patients with unexplained hypercalcemia. They are isointense to muscle on T1-weighted images and hyperintense to muscle on T2-weighted images.

GERM-CELL TUMORS OF THE MEDIASTINUM

Germ-cell tumors of the mediastinum are derived from primitive germ-cell elements left behind after embryonal cell migration. Most germ-cell tumors present during the second to fourth decades of life with an average age of 24 years.[41] Mediastinal germ-cell tumors include teratoma, seminoma, and non-seminomatous germ-cell tumors such as embryonal carcinoma, choriocarcinoma, endodermal sinus tumor, and tumors with mixtures of these cell types.[42] The most common extragonadal site for these tumors is the mediastinum, 60% of which arise in the anterior mediastinum. These tumors account for 10% to 15% of anterior mediastinal masses in adults and approximately 25% in children. Malignant germ-cell tumors secrete human chorionic gonadotropin and α-fetoprotein.

TERATOMAS

All three germinal layers, ectoderm, mesoderm, and endoderm, are present in teratomas. Mature teratomas with predominantly ectodermal element and well-differentiated benign tissues are referred to as dermoid cyst. Mature teratomas are the most common mediastinal germ-cell tumor, predominantly cystic, usually have a benign course, and surgical resection is the treatment of choice. Malignant teratomas have a poor prognosis. Immature teratomas have a benign course in childhood and a more aggressive course in adults. Mature teratomas are found at all ages, particularly in adolescents and young adults, with women slightly outnumbering men.[41,43] They are usually asymptomatic and diagnosed incidentally on chest radiography or CT, but may be symptomatic if they compress the bronchial tree or superior vena cava, or if they rupture into the mediastinum or lung. They are usually stable, but hemorrhage or infection may lead to a rapid increase in size.

Teratomas present as a well-defined, rounded or lobulated mass, localized to the anterior mediastinum. Calcification may occasionally be identified on chest radiograph. On CT combinations of fat, fluid, soft tissue components, and calcification may be seen[25] (Fig. 151.10A,B). The presence of fat is a very helpful diagnostic feature favoring mature (benign) cystic teratoma over the other causes of anterior mediastinal mass. MRI can help in differentiating teratoma from thymoma and lymphoma. Soft tissue elements in the teratoma are isointense to muscle, cystic elements demonstrate low T1 intensity and high T2 intensity, and fat appears as high T1 intensity with signal loss on fat saturation sequence. Fat fluid levels are virtually diagnostic of teratomas.[44]

SEMINOMAS

Seminomas occur almost exclusively in males during the second through fourth decades. They are usually well-defined solid masses with small foci of degenerative changes representing hemorrhage and necrosis.[45] Symptoms are usually due to mass effect on adjacent structures. On CT and MR seminomas have homogenous attenuation and signal intensity and may have areas of hemorrhage and necrosis (Fig. 151.11).

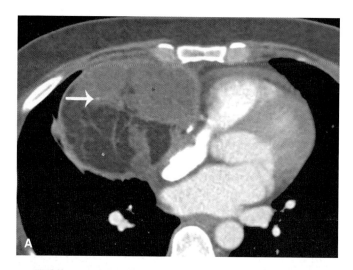

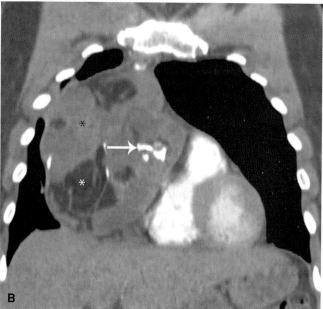

FIGURE 151.10 Axial (**A**) and coronal (**B**) CT images demonstrating a well-defined, large mass in the anterior mediastinum containing a combination of soft tissue (*black asterisk*), fat (*white asterisk*), and calcification (*white arrow*). The presence of these tissue components is highly suggestive of a teratoma.

NON-SEMINOMATOUS GERM-CELL TUMORS

Non-seminomatous germ-cell tumors include embryonal carcinoma, choriocarcinoma, endodermal sinus tumor, and tumors with mixtures of these cell types.[42] Malignant germ-cell tumors are usually seen in young adults and are much more common in men (>90%) than women. They are more commonly more symptomatic than mature teratoma, usually due to mass effect or invasion of adjacent structures.

On radiographs, the malignant tumors are more often lobular, and calcifications or fat density rarely seen. Malignant tumors grow rapidly and metastasize readily to the lungs, bones, or pleura. CT shows a lobular, asymmetrical mass. CT can demonstrate obliteration of mediastinal fat, multiple areas of contrast enhancement interspersed with areas of decreased attenuation due to necrosis and hemorrhage[46,47] (Fig. 151.12). On MRI these tumors demonstrate heterogeneous intensities with areas of high T2 signal intensity corresponding to degenerative cystic changes.

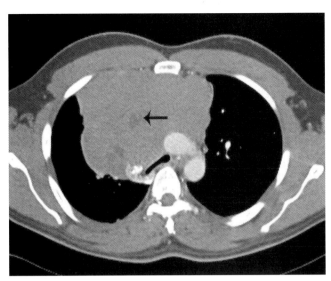

FIGURE 151.11 Axial CT image demonstrating a large, predominantly solid mass within the anterior mediastinum. Small areas of low attenuation (*black arrow*) are consistent with degenerative changes. Note the extensive mass effect exerted by the mass on the adjacent trachea and vascular structures.

MEDIASTINAL LYMPHADENOPATHY

Enlarged mediastinal lymph nodes may have a variety of causes, including metastatic tumor, lymphoma, sarcoidosis, and other granulomatous or inflammatory causes. CT is an excellent and accurate method for detecting the extent and distribution of mediastinal lymph node enlargement. It is usually easy to distinguish between the normal vascular structures and enlarged lymph nodes using contrast-enhanced CT. The short-axis measurement provides the most representative guide to true size, since long-axis measurements vary to a significant degree according to the orientation of the lymph node within the CT section. Detection of enlarged nodes on plain radiographs varies according to their location. Hilar lymph node

enlargement causes enlargement and/or lobulation of the outline of the hilar shadows. Nodes in the right paratracheal group are identified by widening of the right paratracheal stripe. Enlarged azygos nodes displace the azygos vein laterally and enlarge the shadow that normally represents just the azygos vein. If the lymph nodes beneath the aortic arch become large enough to project beyond the aortopulmonary window they cause a local bulge in the angle between the aortic arch and the main pulmonary artery. Subcarinal lymph node enlargement widens the carinal angle and displaces the azygo-esophageal line, so that the subcarinal portion of the azygo-esophageal line, which is normally concave toward the lung, flattens or becomes convex toward the lung (this can be confused with left atrial enlargement). Posterior mediastinal lymph node enlargement causes localized displacement of the paraspinal and paraesophageal lines. MRI provides essentially the same information as CT in evaluating lymph nodes, although its use is limited due to longer acquisition times and relatively limited spatial resolution (which may make measurement of individual nodes difficult). MR is not very helpful to detect calcification.

LYMPHOMA

Lymphoma is a common cause of mediastinal adenopathy and often involves the mediastinal and hilar lymph nodes, with multiple nodal groups usually being involved, particularly in Hodgkin's disease. Lymph node enlargement is seen in a higher proportion of patients with Hodgkin's than non-Hodgkin's lymphoma (Figs. 151.13 and 151.14). Any intrathoracic nodal group may be enlarged in lymphoma and the following generalizations regarding plain radiograph, CT, and MRI findings can be made.[48,49]

The prevascular and paratracheal nodes are the groups most frequently involved, the tracheobronchial and subcarinal nodes also being enlarged in many cases. In most cases, the lymphadenopathy is bilateral but asymmetrical. Hodgkin's disease, particularly the nodular sclerosing form, has a propensity to involve the prevascular and paratracheal nodes (Fig. 151.13). Hilar lymphadenopathy is usually seen along with mediastinal lymphadenopathy. Hilar lympadenopathy is rare without accompanying mediastinal lymph node enlargement, particularly in Hodgkin's disease.

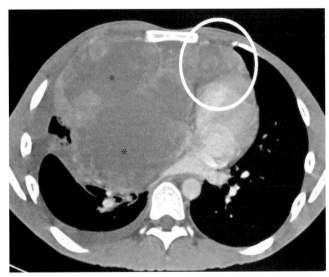

FIGURE 151.12 Axial CT image showing a lobulated large anterior mediastinal mass. There is obliteration of the normal anterior mediastinal fat (*white circle*) with extensive leftward mass effect exerted on the entire mediastinum. Extensive areas of low attenuation (*black asterisks*) are suggestive of hemorrhage and necrosis.

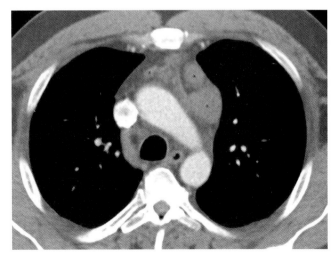

FIGURE 151.13 Axial CT image of the mediastinum in a patient with Hodgkin's lymphoma which shows enlarged lymph nodes in the prevascular location (*black asterisks*).

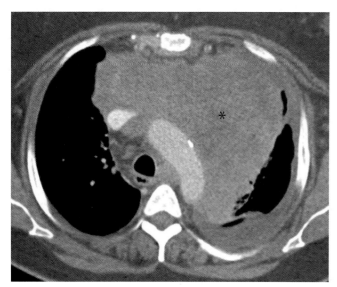

FIGURE 151.14 Axial CT image in a patient with diffuse large B-cell lymphoma demonstrating a slightly heterogeneous soft tissue mass (*black asterisk*) centered within the anterior mediastinum which encases the aorta and superior vena cava. The trachea is displaced leftward by the mass.

The posterior mediastinal nodes are infrequently involved—the enlarged nodes are often low down in the mediastinum and contiguous retroperitoneal disease is likely.

The cardiophrenic angle lymph nodes are rarely involved but become important as sites of recurrent disease because they may not be included in the initial radiation therapy fields.[50]

The lymph node enlargement in lymphoma may resolve remarkably rapidly with therapy.

METASTATIC LYMPHADENOPATHY

Mediastinal lymph node metastases can occur from primary bronchogenic carcinoma or from extrathoracic malignancy. Metastatic lung cancer is the most common cause of malignant adenopathy. The extrathoracic tumors likely to metastasize to the mediastinum are head and neck, breast, genitourinary, and melanoma. In one large series, half the cases of mediastinal lymph node enlargement from extrathoracic primary carcinomas arose from tumors of the genitourinary tract, particularly the kidney and testis.[51] Most metastatic tumors cause lymph node enlargement without distinguishing characteristics. However, enhancing lymph nodes are seen with melanoma, renal cell carcinoma, carcinoid, papillary thyroid cancer, and Kaposi's sarcoma.[52] Calcified lymph node metastases are typical of mucinous adenocarcinoma or thyroid carcinoma. Assessment of nodal size by CT is not sufficiently accurate for routine clinical staging, because significant numbers of small lymph nodes contain microscopic metastasis and some large lymph nodes are free of metastatic disease. PET/CT scanning, with its ability to distinguish between metabolically active and quiescent tissues, has proved increasingly beneficial in the noninvasive staging of the mediastinal lymphadenopathy (Fig. 151.15A–C).

SARCOIDOSIS

Sarcoidosis is the most common non-neoplastic cause of intrathoracic lymph node enlargement. Mediastinal lymph node enlargement occurs in a majority of the patients with sarcoidosis at some stage in their disease with the hilar nodes being enlarged in almost all cases.[53]

Additionally, tracheobronchial, aortopulmonary, and subcarinal nodes are enlarged in over half the patients.[54] The important diagnostic feature of lymphadenopathy in sarcoidosis is its symmetry. Lymph node calcification may have a stippled or egg shell appearance. Many patients have concurrent interstitial lung disease (Fig. 151.16A,B).

MYCOBACTERIAL AND FUNGAL INFECTIONS

Lymph node enlargement due to tuberculous or fungal infection may affect any of the nodal groups in the hila or mediastinum. One or more lymph nodes may be visibly enlarged and an associated area of pulmonary consolidation may or may not be present. Lymph node enlargement is usually seen on the side of the lung disease but involvement of the contralateral nodes may be present. Occasionally, widespread massive mediastinal and hilar node enlargement is seen. With healing, the nodes usually become smaller, often returning to normal size. Dense calcification is frequent both in nodes that stay enlarged and in those that shrink. The enlarged nodes, together with surrounding fibrosis, may compress the superior vena cava or pulmonary veins and cause obstruction. Rim enhancement with a low-density center may be seen with tuberculosis on contrast-enhanced CT examination[55] (Fig. 151.17A–C).

REACTIVE LYMPHADENOPATHY

Reactive hyperplasia in nodes draining infection/inflammation may cause mild enlargement of lymph nodes that is recognizable on CT but not on plain radiographs. Reactive lymphadenopathy can be seen in a wide variety of conditions including pneumonias, interstitial lung disease, and many other conditions. The clinician must be aware that in the setting of a known inflammatory process in the thorax, a few mildly enlarged lymph nodes may be present. Castleman's disease (also referred to as angiofollicular lymph node hyperplasia) is a specific type of lymph node hyperplasia of uncertain etiology which can cause substantial lymph node enlargement in many sites in the body. The lymph node mass is often localized to one area, can be huge, and may be very vascular. The nodes may calcify and may show striking contrast enhancement on both CT and MRI.[56,57] Histologically, there are two types: the hyaline vascular type and the plasma cell type.

LYMPH NODE CALCIFICATION

Extensive lymph node calcification is common following tuberculosis and fungal infection and may also be seen in sarcoidosis, silicosis, and amyloidosis. Lymph node calcification is not seen in untreated lymphoma though it is seen in nodes involved by Hodgkin's disease following therapy. Calcification may be seen in lymph node metastases from calcifying primary malignancies, such as osteosarcoma, chondrosarcoma, and mucinous colorectal and ovarian tumors, although it is not very common in metastatic disease (Fig. 151.18).

CT is more sensitive in detecting calcification in the lymph nodes compared to plain radiographic techniques. Calcification is not usually visible on MRI. Two common patterns of calcification are coarse, irregularly distributed clumps within the node and homogeneous calcification of the entire lymph node. A strikingly foamy appearance is seen with *Pneumocystis jiroveci* (previously *P. carinii*) infection in acquired deficiency syndrome (AIDS) patients[58] and in some cases of metastatic mucinous neoplasms. A ring of calcification at the periphery of the node—so-called "eggshell calcification"—is a particular feature of sarcoidosis and of prolonged dust exposure in coal and metal mines.

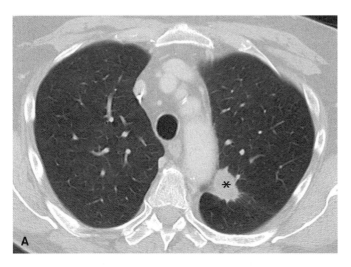

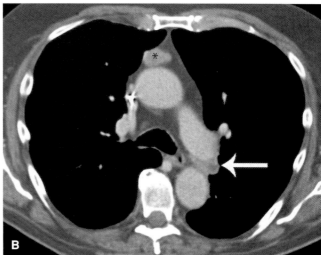

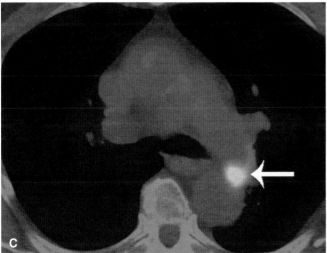

FIGURE 151.15 **A:** Axial CT image of a patient with spiculated mass within the left upper lobe (*black asterisk*) consistent with biopsy-proven primary lung cancer. **B:** A lymph node with central low attenuation suggestive of necrosis is seen within the aortopulmonary location (*white arrow*) and a mildly enhancing lymph node is seen within the anterior mediastinum (*black asterisk*). **C:** PET/CT imaging demonstrates increased radiotracer activity within the lymph node located within the aortopulmonary location (*white arrow*) indicating metabolically active metastatic lymphadenopathy.

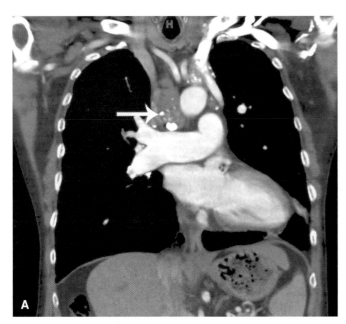

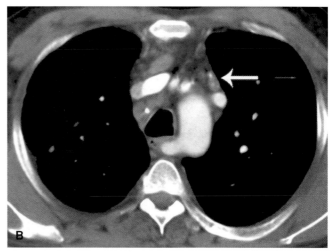

FIGURE 151.16 Coronal and axial CT images demonstrating stippled and egg shell calcifications within lymph nodes (*arrows*) located within the right para-tracheal (**A**) and prevascular (**B**) locations.

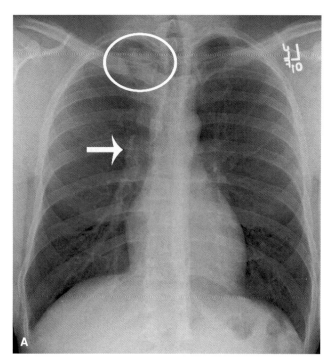

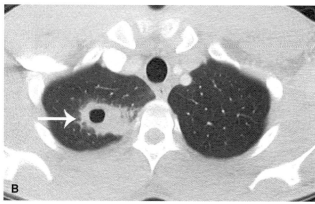

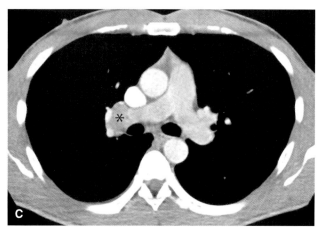

FIGURE 151.17 A: Radiograph demonstrating an opacity (*white circle*) within the right upper lobe suggestive of tuberculosis. There is right hilar enlargement (*white arrow*) which is suspicious for lymphadenopathy. **B, C:** Axial CT images of this patient with suspect tuberculosis confirm a cavitary right upper lobe opacity (*white arrow*, **B**). A rim enhancing right lymph node with central low attenuation (*black asterisk*, **C**) is seen within the right hilum.

LOW ATTENUATION NODES

Lymph nodes with central areas of low attenuation on CT representing necrosis may be seen in tuberculosis,[55] fungal infections,[59] infections in immunocompromised patients, metastatic disease (notably from testicular tumors[60]), and lymphoma[61] (Figs. 151.15B and 151.17C). Necrotic lymph nodes are common in patients with active tuberculosis. They demonstrate central areas of low attenuation with peripheral enhancement when intravenous contrast has been administered. Attenuation values below that of water are seen in fatty replacement of inflammatory nodes and have also been described in Whipple's disease.[62]

ENHANCING LYMPH NODES

Castleman's disease is a rare cause of strikingly uniform enhancing lymph nodes. In addition to Castleman's disease marked lymph node enhancement may occur in hypervascular metastases from melanoma, renal cell carcinoma, carcinoid, papillary thyroid cancer, and Kaposi's sarcoma[52] (Fig. 151.19).

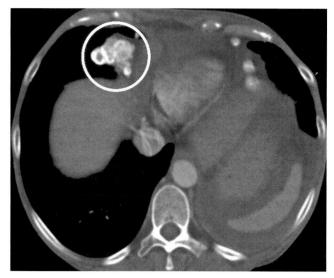

FIGURE 151.18 Peripherally calcified lymphadenopathy (*white circle*) in a patient with known metastatic mucinous ovarian carcinoma.

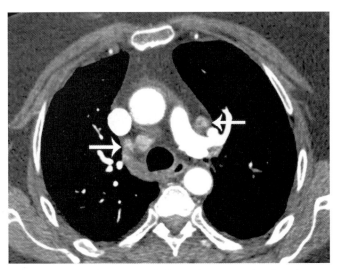

FIGURE 151.19 Enhancing lymphadenopathy is seen within the right paratracheal and prevascular locations (*white arrows*) in a patient with metastatic melanoma.

Contrast enhancement of enlarged nodes, when moderate in degree, is nonspecific, being seen with inflammatory disorders, particularly tuberculosis, fungal disease,[59] sarcoidosis, and neoplasm. Central low attenuation with rim enhancement of the enlarged node is a useful pointer toward the diagnosis of tuberculous infection[55] (Fig. 151.17C).

FOREGUT DUPLICATION CYSTS

"Foregut duplication cysts" are congenital cysts derived from the embryologic foregut. When a portion of this embryologic structure becomes isolated it results in a congenital epithelial cyst. These include bronchogenic cyst, enteric cyst, and neurenteric cyst.

BRONCHOGENIC CYSTS

Bronchogenic cysts occur as a result of abnormal budding of the developing tracheobronchial tree with separation of the buds from the normal airways.[63] Bronchogenic cysts are usually asymptomatic solitary mediastinal masses but they may compress surrounding structures and cause symptoms. The most common location is subcarinal but they are commonly adjacent to the trachea or main bronchi.[64] Typically they have a thin fibrous capsule, are lined with ciliated columnar epithelium, and may contain thick mucoid material. In rare cases they become infected or hemorrhage occurs into the cyst.

On chest radiography bronchogenic cysts present as round masses in the middle mediastinum abutting the carina or main bronchi (Fig. 151.20A). Foregut duplication cysts may displace the carina forward and the esophagus backward. CT is extremely good at demonstrating the size, shape, and location of a bronchogenic cyst and defining its extent and relation to key structures.[65] CT may show a thin-walled mass, with contents measuring simple fluid attenuation representing a fluid-filled cyst[66] or may demonstrate soft tissue attenuation confusing it with tumors (Fig. 151.20B). Occasionally, the cyst may show uniformly high density, probably due to a high protein content.

T1-weighted MR images show that the intrinsic signal intensity varies from low to high depending on the cyst contents. T2-weighted images demonstrate high signal intensity. Malignancy should be excluded when a solid component is seen in the cyst. Contrast-enhanced MRI examination can assess for subtle enhancement present in masses with cystic components but not in true cysts.

ESOPHAGEAL DUPLICATION CYSTS

Esophageal duplication cysts are distinguished from bronchogenic cysts pathologically by the presence of smooth muscle in the walls, absence of cartilage, and presence of mucosa resembling that of the esophagus, stomach, or small intestine.[67] They are incidentally found

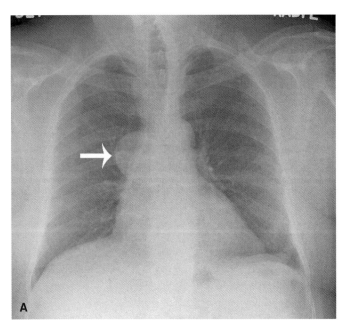

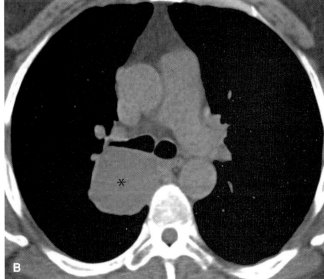

FIGURE 151.20 **A:** Frontal radiograph demonstrates a round, well-circumscribed mass projecting over the carina (*arrow*). **B:** CT demonstrates a well-circumscribed fluid attenuation cystic mass (*black asterisk*) within the middle mediastinum in the subcarinal location.

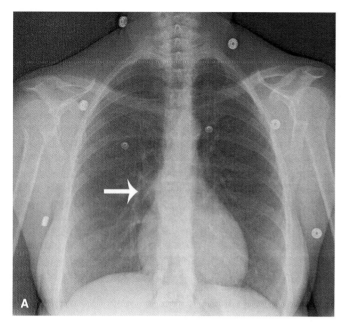

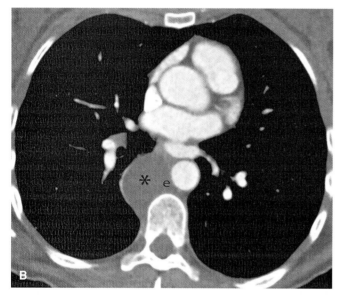

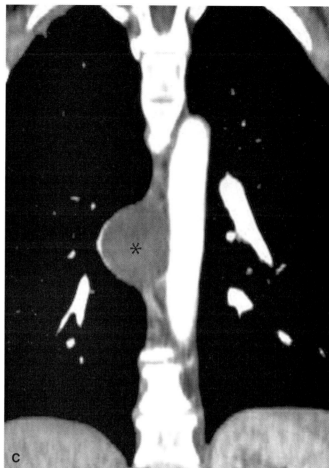

FIGURE 151.21 Frontal radiograph demonstrates a well-circumscribed mass projecting over the mediastinum (**A,** *white arrow*). Axial (**B**) and coronal (**C**) CT images demonstrate a well-circumscribed, fluid attenuation, thin-walled mass within the middle mediastinum (*black asterisk*). The mass is in intimate contact with the adjacent esophagus (*e*).

as an asymptomatic mass on an imaging of the chest, but they may cause dysphagia and pain. They usually present in childhood. A duplication cyst may become infected or there may be hemorrhage secondary to the ectopic gastric mucosa within the cyst. Extrinsic or intramural compression may be seen on esophagram due to their close proximity to the esophageal wall. The CT and MRI imaging features of esophageal duplication cysts are similar to those of bronchogenic cysts except that in the former the wall of the lesion may be thicker, the mass may assume a more tubular shape, and it may be in more intimate contact with the esophagus[64] (Fig. 151.21A–C).

PERICARDIAL CYSTS

Pericardial cysts are formed when a portion of the pericardium is pinched off during early development and are thought to be the result of persistence of blind-ending ventral parietal pericardial recesses. They almost invariably appear as a well-defined, oval or occasionally lobulated mass attached to the pericardium.[68] Most pericardial cysts occur in the right cardiophrenic angle (approximately 70%), with some

in the left cardiophrenic angle (approximately 20%), and some higher in the mediastinum. The cysts that communicate with the pericardial space are termed pericardial diverticula. With increase or decrease in pericardial fluid, diverticula can change in size. Pericardial cysts contain fluid and demonstrate imaging characteristics of water on echocardiography, CT, or MRI[69] (Fig. 151.22A,B). On MRI, they have low to intermediate T1 signal intensity and high T2 signal intensity and do not enhance following intravenous gadolinium administration.

NEUROENTERIC CYSTS

In early embryonic life, incomplete separation of the foregut from the notochord leads to the formation of neuroenteric cysts. A fibrous connection to the spine or an intraspinal component is usually present. The wall of the cyst has an enteric epithelial lining and contains neural and gastrointestinal elements. Associated vertebral body anomalies such as butterfly or hemivertebra are seen. Neuroenteric cysts frequently produce pain and are often found early in life. On radiographs, a neurenteric cyst is a well-defined, round, oval or lobulated

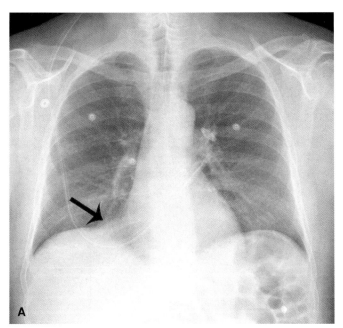

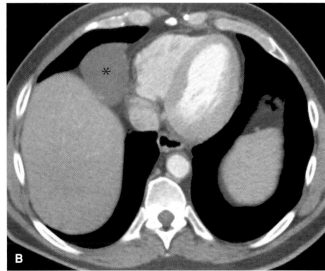

FIGURE 151.22 **A:** Frontal radiograph demonstrating a rounded mass (*black arrow*) centered at the right cardiophrenic angle. **B:** On the CT, there is a well-circumscribed water attenuation mass (*black asterisk*) abutting the right heart border and pericardium consistent with a pericardial cyst.

mass in the posterior mediastinum between the esophagus (which is usually displaced) and the spine. Imaging features on CT are similar to those of other foregut duplication cysts (Fig. 151.23A,B). MRI is the best imaging modality for evaluation of neuroenteric cysts as it demonstrates the extent of intraspinal involvement.[64]

NEUROGENIC TUMORS

Neurogenic tumors are the most common tumors to arise in the posterior mediastinum, and most neurogenic tumors occur in this location.[64] Neurogenic tumors represent 20% of all adult and 35% of all pediatric mediastinal neoplasms. Most neurogenic tumors in adults are benign and are discovered as asymptomatic masses on

chest radiographs. Neurogenic tumors are classified as tumors arising from peripheral nerves, such as neurofibroma, schwannoma, and malignant tumors of nerve sheath origin (neurogenic sarcomas), or as tumors arising from sympathetic ganglia such as neuroblastomas and ganglioneuroblastoma. Neurofibromas or schwannomas are more common in adults whereas neuroblastomas and ganglioneuroblastomas are more common in children. The best modality for imaging these tumors is MRI.[70]

PERIPHERAL NERVE SHEATH TUMORS

Peripheral nerve tumors are the most common posterior mediastinal neurogenic tumors. The nerve sheath tumors typically originate

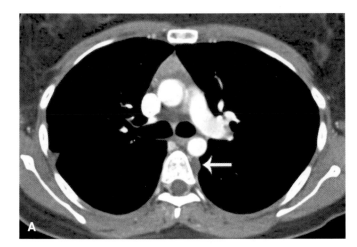

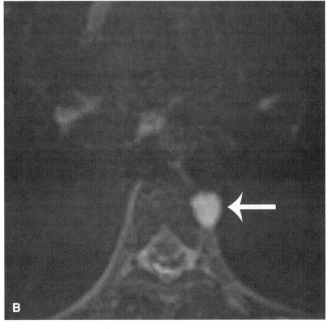

FIGURE 151.23 Axial CT image demonstrates a well-defined, oval mass (**A,** *white arrow*) located within the posterior mediastinum abutting the spine. T2-weighted MR image of the same lesion (**B,** *white arrow*) demonstrates increased signal intensity consistent with a cyst.

in an intercostal nerve in the paravertebral region. Radiologically, the benign tumors (neurofibromas and schwannomas) present as well-defined round or oval posterior mediastinal masses. Pressure deformity causing a smooth, scalloped indentation on the adjacent ribs, vertebral bodies, pedicles, or transverse processes is common, particularly with the larger tumors[64,71] with thickening of the scalloped cortex. The rib spaces and the intervertebral foramina may be widened by the tumor (Fig. 151.24A,B). These characteristic bone changes are diagnostic of a neurogenic tumor, the only differential diagnosis being that of a lateral thoracic meningocele. On CT the tumors may be homogeneous or heterogeneous in attenuation and foci of calcification may be seen. Neurogenic tumors usually enhance heterogeneously after intravenous contrast administration (Fig. 151.24C,D). On MRI neurofibromas and schwannomas have

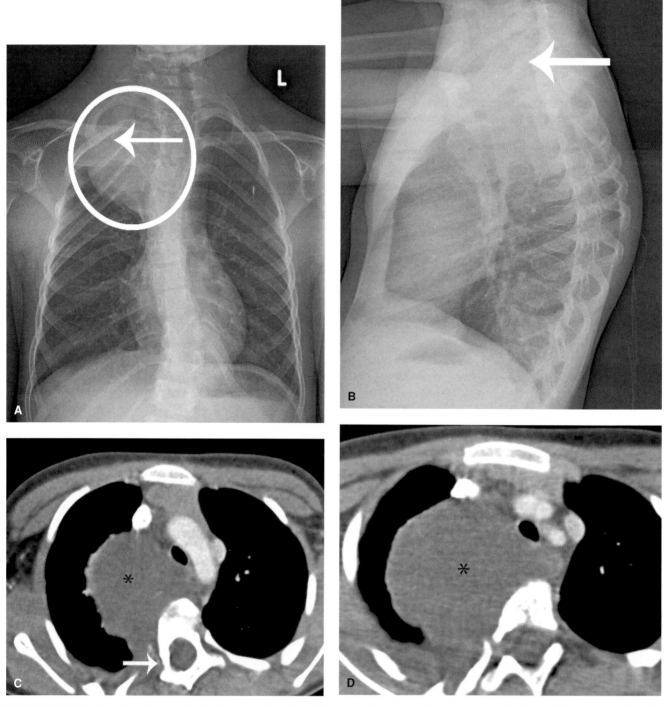

FIGURE 151.24 Frontal radiograph demonstrates a large mass (**A,** *white circle*) overlying the upper mediastinum. The lateral radiograph shows the mass (**B,** *white arrow*) is located within the posterior mediastinum. Widening of the rib spaces and scalloping of the cortex of the ribs (**A,** *white arrow*) are noted. **C, D:** CT images demonstrate a homogeneously enhancing mass (*black asterisk*) centered within the posterior mediastinum. There is rightward mass effect on the mediastinum, as well as scalloping of the pedicle of the adjacent vertebral body (*white arrow*). (*continued*)

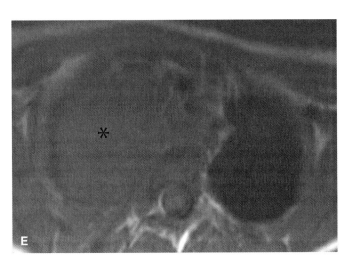

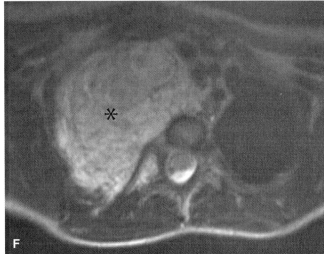

FIGURE 151.24 (*Continued*) **E, F:** T1 pre-contrast images (**E**) of the mass (*black asterisk*) within the posterior mediastinum demonstrate low to intermediate signal intensity. Post-contrast MRI images (**F**) demonstrate heterogeneous enhancement suggestive of a peripheral nerve sheath tumor.

low to intermediate signal intensity on T1-weighted images and may have characteristic high signal intensity peripherally and low signal intensity centrally (target sign) on T2-weighted images.[72] Neurogenic tumors enhance following the intravenous administration of gadolinium (Fig. 151.24E,F). Extension of the neurogenic tumor into the spinal canal may occur in as many as 10% of paravertebral neurofibromas giving a dumb-bell-shaped appearance with widening of the affected neural foramen.[73]

Malignant tumors of nerve sheath origin are spindle cell sarcomas, typically occurring in the third to fifth decades, although they may occur earlier in patients with neurofibromatosis type 1. On imaging, the masses are usually larger than 5 cm in diameter.[64] MRI is not helpful in distinguishing benign from malignant neurogenic tumors, but hemorrhage and necrosis resulting in a heterogeneous signal intensity, sudden interval increase in size of the mass, or invasion of adjacent structures are features of concern for malignant nerve sheath tumors.[74] Hematogenous metastases to the lung have been reported but lymph node metastases are rare.[64]

TUMORS OF SYMPATHETIC GANGLION

Tumors of the sympathetic ganglion arise from the nerve cells rather than the nerve sheaths. They are rare neoplasms ranging from benign ganglioneuroma to intermediate ganglioneuroblastoma and malignant neuroblastoma.[64] Ganglioneuromas are benign neoplasms usually occurring in children and young adults. Ganglioneuroblastomas exhibit variable degrees of malignancy and usually occur in children.[75] Ganglioneuromas and ganglioneuroblastomas usually arise from the sympathetic ganglia in the posterior mediastinum and therefore usually present radiologically as well-defined elliptical masses, with a vertical orientation, extending over the anterolateral aspect of three to five vertebral bodies.[64,76] Imaging features on CT are variable and calcification is seen in approximately 25%[64] (Fig. 151.25A,B). On MRI ganglioneuromas and ganglioneuroblastomas are usually of homogeneous intermediate signal intensity on T1- and T2-weighted images (Fig. 151.25C,D). Neuroblastomas are highly malignant tumors that typically occur in children younger than 5 years of age.[75] The most common extra abdominal location of a neuroblastoma is the posterior. Neuroblastomas are typically more heterogeneous on imaging due to areas of hemorrhage, necrosis,

cystic degeneration, and calcium; may be locally invasive; and have a tendency to cross the midline.[74]

PARAGANGLIOMAS

Intrathoracic paragangliomas are of two types: chemodectomas or pheochromocytomas (functioning paragangliomas), either of which may be benign or malignant. Less than 2% of pheochromocytomas occur in the thoracic cavity. Most intrathoracic pheochromocytomas are found in the posterior mediastinum or closely related to the heart, particularly in the wall of the left atrium or the interatrial septum. Approximately one-third of mediastinal pheochromocytomas are nonfunctioning and asymptomatic, the remaining present with symptoms, signs, and laboratory findings of excess catecholamines.

The various paragangliomas have similar imaging features on CT and MRI. They are round soft tissue masses, which are usually very vascular and therefore enhance intensely on CT[77] (Fig. 151.26A). On MRI, pheochromocytomas usually show a signal intensity similar to muscle on T1-weighted images and very high signal intensity on T2-weighted images.[78] MRI is particularly useful for demonstrating intracardiac pheochromocytomas. MIBG (meta-iodobenzylguanidine) and somatostatin receptor scintigraphy both show increased activity in paragangliomas and are extremely helpful in identifying extra-adrenal pheochromocytomas[78,79] (Fig. 151.26B).

LATERAL THORACIC MENINGOCELE

Lateral thoracic meningoceles are characterized by redundant meninges that protrude through the spinal foramen and are filled with cerebrospinal fluid. They are usually asymptomatic and commonly associated with neurofibromatosis.[80] CT and MRI can both indicate the correct diagnosis by showing the mass to be fluid filled rather than solid[64] and demonstrating continuity between the CSF in the meningocele and that contained in the thecal sac. If warranted, CT following the intrathecal injection of contrast will demonstrate flow into the lesion and help confirm the diagnosis (Fig. 151.27A–C).

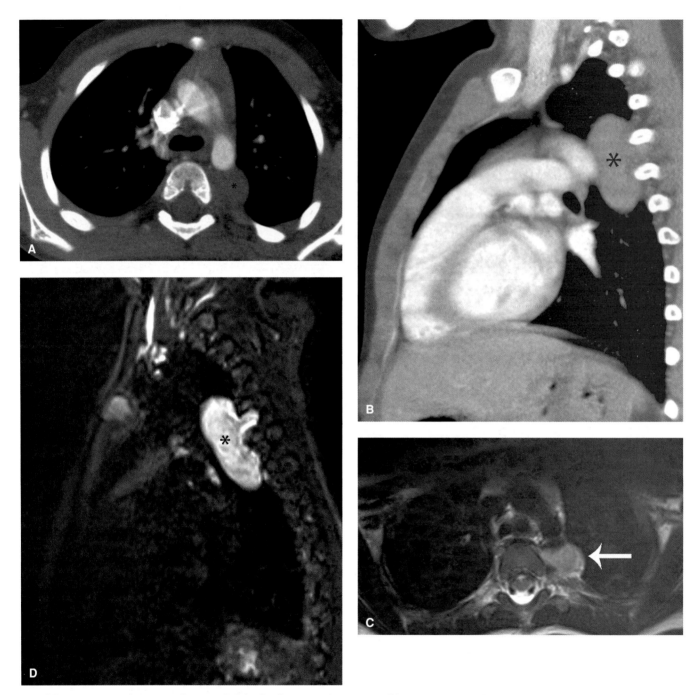

FIGURE 151.25 A: Axial CT image shows a well-defined, soft tissue attenuation mass (*black asterisk*) within the posterior mediastinum. **B:** Sagittal CT image showing the elliptical shape and vertical orientation of the ganglioneuroblastoma (*black asterisk*). **C:** Axial T2-weighted MR image of the mass (*white arrow*) within the posterior mediastinum shows increased signal intensity. **D:** Sagittal post-contrast MR image shows relatively homogeneous enhancement of the vertically orientated, elliptical mass (*black asterisk*) within the posterior mediastinum. Note the extension posteriorly through the neural foramen.

EXTRAMEDULLARY HEMATOPOIESIS

Severe anemia caused by inadequate production or excessive destruction of blood cells results in extramedullary hematopoiesis with compensatory expansion of bone marrow causing paravertebral masses. It can be seen in the presence of thalassemia, hereditary spherocytosis, and sickle cell anemia. Usually bilateral, multiple, and well-marginated lobulated paravertebral masses are seen in the lower thoracic vertebra on radiographs. The bones may be normal or may show an altered lacelike trabecular pattern due to marrow expansion. The masses are usually of homogeneous soft tissue attenuation on CT, although, occasionally, a fatty component may be visible[81] (Fig. 151.28).

CYSTIC HYGROMAS (LYMPHANGIOMAS)

Lymphangiomas or cystic hygromas are benign tumors of lymphatic system consisting of focal proliferations of well-differentiated lymphatic tissue comprising complex lymph channels or cystic spaces containing clear or straw-colored fluid.[82] They are classified histologically as simple (capillary), cavernous,

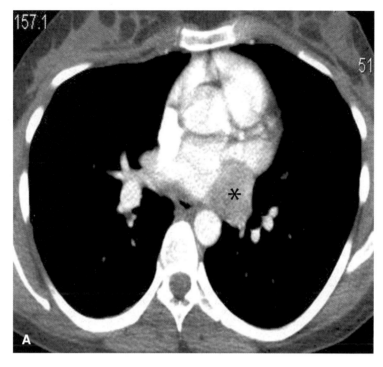

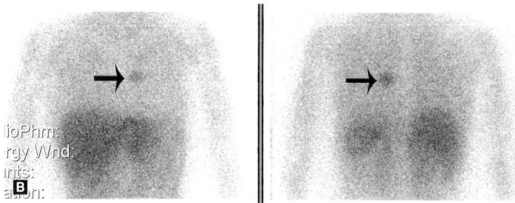

FIGURE 151.26 **A:** Axial CT image demonstrating a round, enhancing mediastinal mass (*black asterisk*). **B:** MIBG scintigraphic images show increased activity within the lesion (*black arrows*) suggestive of an extra-adrenal pheochromocytoma.

or cystic (hygroma) depending on the size of the lymphatic channels they contain. Cystic lymphangiomas are most common. They are usually present at birth and detected in the first 2 years of life. Lymphangiomas are most common in the neck and axilla and about 10% of lymphangiomas in the neck extend into the mediastinum,[82,83] most commonly in the anterior mediastinum. Most cervicomediastinal lymphangiomas present in early life as a neck mass, whereas the purely mediastinal lymphangiomas usually present in older children and adults as an asymptomatic mediastinal mass. Lymphangiomas are usually asymptomatic due to their soft consistency. However, compression of mediastinal structures can produce symptoms such as chest pain, cough, and dyspnea. Complications include airway compromise, infection, chylothorax, and chylopericardium.[84] CT demonstrates a lobulated smooth mass insinuating between the adjacent mediastinal structures rather than displacing them.[83] Lymphangiomas generally have fluid attenuation but may have a combination of fluid and soft tissue[85] (Fig. 151.29A–C). Lymphangiomas may demonstrate

thin septations within the mass.[83,85] On MR, the lesions may have heterogeneous T1 signal intensity but usually have high T2 signal intensity (Fig. 151.29D–F). Complete resection of lymphangiomas may be difficult because of their insinuating nature and follow-up may be helpful to exclude recurrence.[86]

HEMANGIOMAS

Hemangiomas are rare vascular tumors composed of interconnecting vascular channels with areas of thrombosis and fibrous stroma. Hemangiomas can be capillary, cavernous, or venous with cavernous hemangiomas accounting for approximately three quarters of the cases. Hemangiomas occur in young patients with half of the patients being asymptomatic. Symptoms are usually caused by compression of adjacent structures. Contrast-enhanced CT demonstrates dense, focal, or diffuse and peripheral or central enhancement. Phleboliths or punctate calcifications are seen in 10% to 20% of the cases.

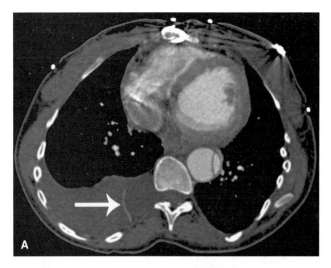

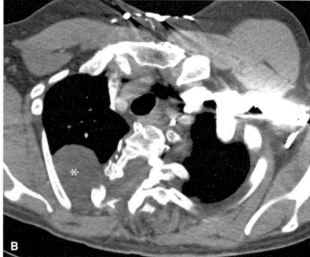

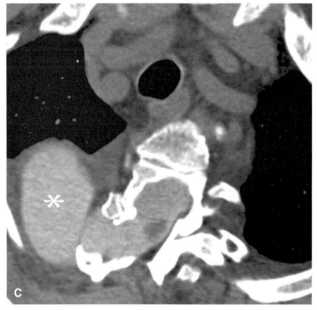

FIGURE 151.27 **A:** Axial CT image demonstrating a fluid-filled mass (*white arrow*) located within the posterior mediastinum which appears to protrude neural foramen. Pre- (**B**) and post-intrathecal injection (**C**) images show intrathecal contrast material flowing into the mass (*white asterisk*) which confirms the diagnosis of a lateral thoracic meningocele.

FAT CONTAINING LESIONS IN THE MEDIASTINUM

Fat is normally present in the mediastinum and the amount of fat in the mediastinum increases with age. Normal fat is equally distributed throughout the mediastinum and is not encapsulated. An abnormality of fat distribution in the mediastinum can be diffuse (mediastinal lipomatosis) or focal (fat containing diaphragmatic hernia or mediastinal lipoma). Relatively large amounts of fat may be seen in the cardiophrenic angles, particularly in obese subjects, resembling a mass on radiographs. In a majority of the cases, the presence of fat indicates benign nature of the mass.

MEDIASTINAL LIPOMATOSIS

Mediastinal lipomatosis is a benign accumulation of excessive amount of unencapsulated histologically normal fat in the mediastinum. Mediastinal lipomatosis is a phenomenon seen particularly in Cushing's disease, in patients on steroid therapy, and in obese subjects. When the fat deposits are extensive and symmetrical, the diagnosis is usually obvious. The excess fat deposition is most prominent in the upper mediastinum, resulting in

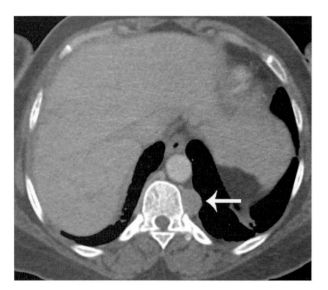

FIGURE 151.28 Axial CT image of a patient with sickle cell anemia shows a well-circumscribed soft tissue attenuation paravertebral mass (*white arrow*) consistent with extramedullary hematopoiesis.

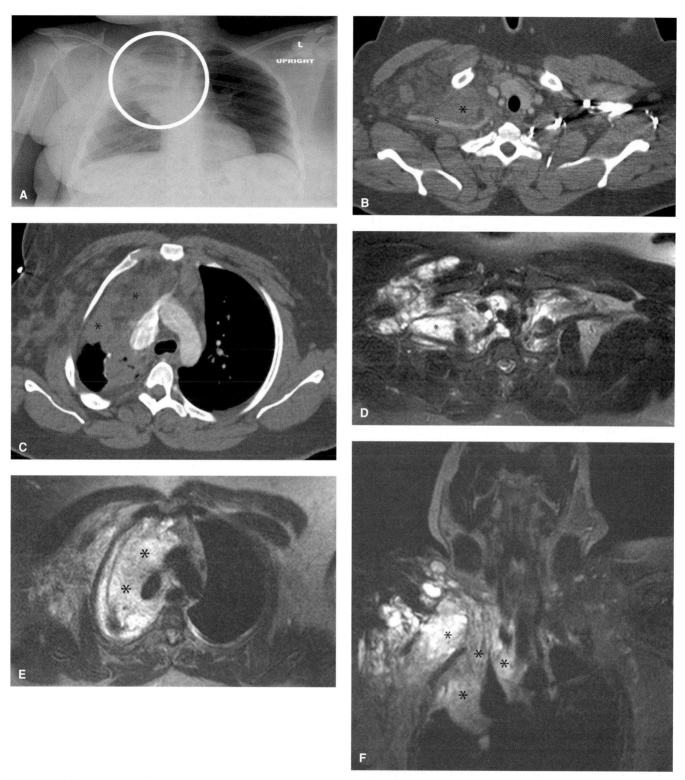

FIGURE 151.29 **A:** Frontal radiograph demonstrating a large mass (*white circle*) within the upper mediastinum which appears to displace the trachea to the left. **B, C:** CT images demonstrate a lobulated, fluid and soft tissue attenuation mass (*black asterisks*) located within the upper mediastinum. The mass insinuates between the mediastinal structures and surrounds but does not occlude the right subclavian vein (*S*). **D, E, F:** T2-weighted MR images show a multiseptated high signal intensity mass (*black asterisks*) extending from the neck into the upper mediastinum. The mass insinuates between mediastinal structures rather than displacing them.

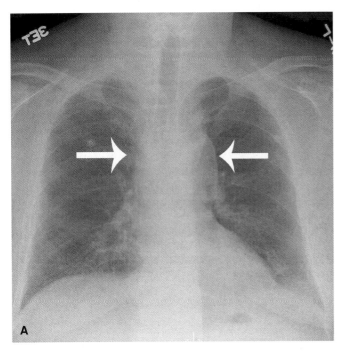
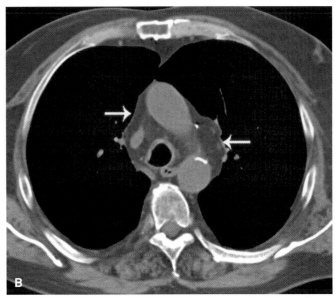

FIGURE 151.30 **A:** Frontal radiograph showing smooth mediastinal widening of the upper mediastinum (located between *white arrows*). **B:** Axial CT image of the same patient shows homogenous fat attenuation lobulations outlining the mediastinum (*white arrows*) corresponding to the widening seen on the radiograph and suggestive of mediastinal lipomatosis.

a smooth symmetrical mediastinal widening on the chest radiograph. On CT, the fat should appear homogenously low in attenuation, sharply outlining the mediastinal vessels and lymph nodes (Fig. 151.30A,B).

FATTY TUMORS OF THE MEDIASTINUM

Fatty tumors of the mediastinum are seen as well-defined round or oval mediastinal masses on chest radiography regardless of whether they are benign or malignant.

Mediastinal lipomas are most common in the prevascular space and constitute 2% of all mediastinal tumors. Benign lipomas are soft and do not compress surrounding structures unless they are

very large. On CT they show uniform fat attenuation with smooth boundaries and are sharply demarcated from adjacent structures in the mediastinum.[87]

Mediastinal liposarcomas are rare malignant fat containing tumors often seen in the anterior mediastinum. They usually contain large areas of soft tissue density unlike lipomas. Histologic differentiation between lipoma and liposarcoma depends on the presence of mitotic activity, cellular atypia, neovascularization, and tumor infiltration.

Imaging features on CT demonstrate inhomogeneous attenuation with significant soft tissue component in a mass with fat attenuation, poor demarcation of adjacent mediastinal structures, and infiltration/invasion of mediastinal structures (Fig. 151.31A,B).

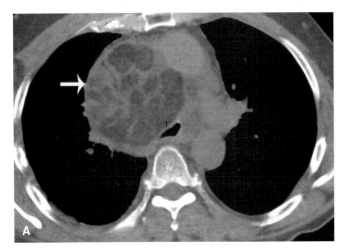
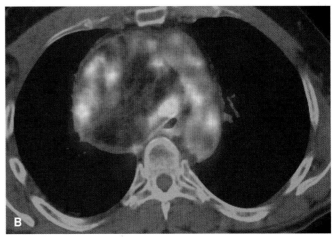

FIGURE 151.31 **A, B:** Axial CT image demonstrates a mediastinal mass (**A,** *white arrow*) containing fat and enhancing, thick, nodular septations. The lesion exerts mass effect on the trachea (**A,** *T*). PET/CT image of the mass shows increased metabolic activity within the mass, suggestive of a liposarcoma (**B**).

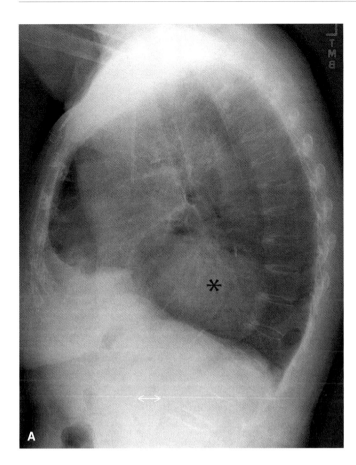

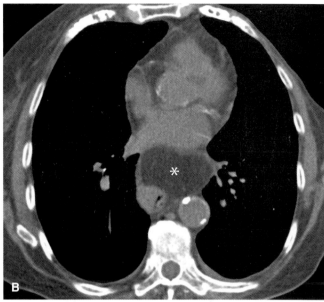

FIGURE 151.32 **A:** Lateral radiograph showing a mass (*black asterisk*) located within the posterior mediastinum. **B:** CT image of the same patient demonstrates that the mass seen on the lateral radiograph corresponds to herniated fat (*white asterisk*) through the esophageal hiatus.

FAT CONTAINING HERNIAS

Omental fat can herniate through the foramen of Morgagni and give the appearance of a cardiophrenic angle mass on the right. Fat herniation through the foramen of Bochdalek occurs most frequently on the left side posteriorly. The fat can also herniate through the esophageal hiatus (Fig. 151.32A,B). These fat herniations are easily diagnosed because of their characteristic locations. Fat attenuation on CT or fat intensity on MR along with the characteristic locations of these hernias is useful in differentiating these hernias from other mediastinal masses.[88]

MEDIASTINITIS

Acute Mediastinitis

The most common cause of acute mediastinitis is perforation of the esophagus during diagnostic or therapeutic endoscopic procedures. Forceful vomiting may result in esophageal perforation (Boerhaave's syndrome) and a leak into the mediastinum can result in acute mediastinitis. Such tears are usually just above the gastro-esophageal junction. Acute infection of the mediastinum is rare. Other causes of acute mediastinitis are perforation secondary to a necrotic tumor and extension of infection from the neck, retroperitoneum, or adjacent intrathoracic or chest wall structures into the mediastinum. Diffuse mediastinitis has a very poor prognosis and the mortality associated with acute mediastinitis from esophageal perforation is 5% to 30% even with appropriate treatment.[89]

The chest radiograph may show mediastinal widening. Streaks of air and even air–fluid levels may be seen within the mediastinum.

Air may also be seen in the soft tissues of the neck. Pleural effusions are frequent and are usually on the left. Radiologically, detection of esophageal perforation relies on the presence of indirect signs, including pneumomediastinum, left pleural effusion, and pneumothorax. An esophagram using water-soluble contrast medium may show the site of perforation, with extravasation into the mediastinum.

CT is the modality of choice in the evaluation of suspected mediastinitis and mediastinal abscess demonstrating obliteration of the normal mediastinal fat planes, esophageal thickening, and extraluminal gas bubbles within the mediastinum. In advanced cases there may be walled-off discrete fluid or air–fluid collections indicating abscess formation. Associated pleural effusion, empyema, sub-phrenic, or pericardial collection may be present. When acute mediastinitis is suspected following sternotomy, CT can demonstrate the extent of inflammation and any drainable mediastinal or pericardial fluid collections.[90] It should be remembered that substernal fluid collections and tiny pockets of air are normal in the first 20 days following sternotomy. Therefore, before gas-forming infections can be diagnosed, the air collections must appear de novo or must progressively increase in the absence of any other explanation.[91]

Fibrosing Mediastinitis

Fibrosing mediastinitis occurs due to proliferation of collagen and fibrous tissue in the mediastinum usually secondary to prior infection with histoplasmosis or tuberculosis.[92] Other etiologies include sarcoidosis, autoimmune diseases, retroperitoneal fibrosis radiation, and drugs such as methysergide.

The chest radiograph may show calcified mediastinal or hilar lymph nodes in cases of fibrosing mediastinitis secondary to prior histoplasmosis or tuberculosis infection. The chest radiograph otherwise often underestimates the extent of mediastinal disease. CT demonstrates an infiltrative, often calcified mediastinal process, which may be relatively focal when disease is due to previous histoplasmosis or tuberculosis, and more diffuse in the idiopathic form.[93] CT is an excellent modality for the evaluation of the extent of mediastinal soft tissue infiltration and identifying the degree of vascular encasement or obstruction and narrowing of other mediastinal structures.

Two patterns of fibrosing mediastinitis have been described: a focal pattern and a diffuse pattern.[93,94] The focal pattern caused by histoplasmosis, seen in 82% of cases, manifests as a mass of soft tissue attenuation that is frequently calcified (63% of cases) and is usually located in the right paratracheal or subcarinal regions or in the hila. The diffuse pattern not related to histoplasmosis, often occurs in the setting of retroperitoneal fibrosis seen in 18% of cases, manifests as a diffusely infiltrating, noncalcified mass that affects multiple mediastinal compartments.

MRI lacks sensitivity for detection of calcification, which is an important feature for differentiating fibrosing mediastinitis from other infiltrative disorders of the mediastinum, such as lymphoma and metastatic carcinoma. Fibrosing mediastinitis typically demonstrates a heterogeneous, infiltrative mass of intermediate signal intensity on T1-weighted MR images. On T2-weighted MR images it is more variable with areas of both increased and markedly decreased signal intensity seen in the same lesion.[94-96] Areas of decreased signal intensity represent calcification or fibrous tissue, and areas of increased signal intensity may indicate more active inflammation. Extensive regions of decreased signal intensity within the lesion, when present, help differentiate fibrosing mediastinitis from other infiltrative lesions of the mediastinum, such as metastatic carcinoma and lymphoma, that typically have increased T2 signal intensity. Heterogeneous enhancement of the mass may be seen after intravenous administration of a gadolinium contrast.

REFERENCES

1. Gatzoulis MA. Mediastinum. In: Standring S, ed. *Gray's Anatomy. The Anatomical Basis of Clinical Practice.* 40th ed. Philadelphia, PA: Churchill Livingstone (Elsevier); 2008:939–957.
2. Fraser RS, Müller NL, Colman N, et al. The mediastinum. In: *Fraser and Paré's Diagnosis of Diseases of the Chest.* 4th ed. Philadelphia, PA: WB Saunders; 1999:196–234.
3. Fraser RG, Paré JA. *The Normal Chest. Diagnosis of Diseases of the Chest.* 2nd ed. Philadelphia PA: WB Saunders; 1977:1–183.
4. Zylak CJ, Pallie W, Jackson R. Correlative anatomy and computed tomography: a module on the mediastinum. *RadioGraphics* 1982;2(4):555–592.
5. Fujimoto K, Hara M, Tomiyama N, et al. Proposal for a new mediastinal compartment classification of transverse plane images according to the Japanese Association for Research on the Thymus (JART) General Rules for the Study of Mediastinal Tumors. *Oncol Rep* 2014;31:565–572.
6. Carter BW, Tomiyama N, Bhora FY, et al. A modern definition of mediastinal compartments. *J Thorac Oncol* 2014;9(9 Suppl 2):S97–S101.
7. Friedberg JW, Chengazi V. PET scans in the staging of lymphoma: current status. *Oncologist* 2003;8: 438–447.
8. Verboom P, van Tinteren H, Hoekstra OS, et al. Cost-effectiveness of FDG-PET in staging non-small cell lung cancer: the PLUS study. *Eur J Nucl Med Mol Imaging* 2003;30:1444–1449.
9. Whitten CR, Khan S, Munneke GJ, et al. A diagnostic approach to mediastinal abnormalities. *RadioGraphics* 2007;27:657–671.
10. Mack E. Management of patients with substernal goiters. *Surg Clin N Am* 1995;75:377–394.
11. Buckley JA, Stark P. Intrathoracic mediastinal thyroid goiter: imaging manifestations. *Am J Roentgenol* 1999;173:471–475.
12. Glazer GM, Axel L, Moss A. CT diagnosis of mediastinal thyroid. *Am J Roentgenol* 1982;138:495–498.
13. Bashist B, Ellis K, Gold RP. Computed tomography of intrathoracic goiter. *Am J Roentgenol* 1983;140:455–460.
14. Baron RL, Lee JK, Sagel SS, et al. Computed tomography of the normal thymus. *Radiology* 1982;142:121–125.
15. Baron RL, Sagel S, Bagman RJ. Thymic cysts following radiation therapy for Hodgkin disease. *Radiology* 1981;141:593–597.
16. Souadjian JV, Enriquez P, Silverstein MN, et al. The spectrum of diseases associated with thymoma. Coincidence or syndrome? *Arch Intern Med* 1974;134:374–379.
17. Strollo DC, Rosado-de-Christenson ML. Tumors of the thymus. *J Thorac Imaging* 1999;14:152–171.
18. Brown LR, Muhm JR, Sheedy PF, et al. The value of computed tomography in myasthenia gravis. *Am J Roentgenol* 1983;140:31–35.
19. Ellis K, Austin JH, Jaretzki A III. Radiologic detection of thymoma in patients with myasthenia gravis. *Am J Roentgenol* 1988;151:873–881.
20. Chen JL, Weisbrod GL, Herman SJ. Computed tomography and pathologic correlations of thymic lesions. *J Thorac Imaging* 1988;3:61–65.
21. Rosado-de-Christenson ML, Galobardes J, Moran CA. Thymoma: radiologic–pathologic correlation. *RadioGraphics* 1992;12:151–168.
22. De Geer G, Webb WR, Gamsu G. Normal thymus: associated with MR and CT. *Radiology* 1986;158:313–317.
23. Boothroyd AE, Hall-Graggs MA, Dicks-Mireaux C, et al. The magnetic resonance appearances of the normal thymus in children. *Clin Radiol* 1992;45:378–381.
24. Sakai F, Sone S, Kiyono K, et al. MR imaging of thymoma: radiological-pathologic correlation. *Am J Roentgenol* 1991;158:751–756.
25. Fujimoto K, Nishihara H, Abe T, et al. MR imaging of thymoma—comparison with CT, operative, and pathological findings. *Nippon Igaku Hoshasen Gakkai Zasshi* 1992;52:1128–1138.
26. Takahashi K, Al-Janabi NJ. Computed tomography and magnetic resonance imaging of mediastinal masses. *J Magn Reson Imaging* 2010;32:1325–1339.
27. Lee JD, Choe KO, Kim SJ, et al. CT findings in primary thymic carcinoma. *J Comput Assist Tomogr* 1991;15:429–433.
28. Do YS, Im JG, Lee BH, et al. CT findings in malignant tumors of thymic epithelium. *J Comput Assist Tomogr* 1995;19:192–197.
29. Kushihashi T, Fujisawa H, Munechika H. Magnetic resonance imaging of thymic epithelial tumors. *Crit Rev Diagn Imaging* 1996;37:191–259.
30. Choyke PL, Zeman RK, Gootenberg JE, et al. Thymic atrophy and regrowth in response to chemotherapy: CT evaluation. *Am J Roentgenol* 1987;149:269–272.
31. Kissin CM, Husband JE, Nicholas D, et al. Benign thymic enlargement in adults after chemotherapy: CT demonstration. *Radiology* 1987;163:67–70.
32. Cohen M, Hill CA, Cangir A, et al. Thymic rebound after treatment of childhood tumors. *Am J Roentgenol* 1980;135:151–156.
33. Inaoka T, Takahashi K, Iwata K, et al. Evaluation of normal fatty replacement of the thymus with chemical-shift MR imaging for identification of the normal thymus. *J Magn Reson Imaging* 2005;22:341–346.
34. Inaoka T, Takahashi K, Mineta M, et al. Thymic hyperplasia and thymus gland tumors: differentiation with chemical shift MR imaging. *Radiology* 2007;243:869–876.
35. Rosado-de-Christenson ML, Pugatch RD, Moran CA, et al. Thymolipoma: analysis of 27 cases. *Radiology* 1994;193:121–126.
36. Chew FS, Weissleder R. Mediastinal thymolipoma. *Am J Roentgenol* 1991;157:468.
37. Shirkhoda A, Chasen MH, Eftekhari F, et al. MR imaging of mediastinal thymolipoma. *J Comput Assist Tomogr* 1987;11:364–365.
38. Chaer R, Massad MG, Evans A, et al. Primary neuroendocrine tumors of the thymus. *Ann Thorac Surg* 2002;74:1733–1740.
39. Lee VS, Spritzer CE, Coleman RE, et al. The complementary roles of fast spin-echo MR imaging and double-phase 99mTc-sestamibi scintigraphy for localization of hyperfunctioning parathyroid glands. *Am J Roentgenol* 1996;167:1555–1562.
40. Lee VS, Spritzer CE. MR imaging of abnormal parathyroid glands. *Am J Roentgenol* 1998;170:1097–1103.
41. Moeller KH, Rosado-de-Christenson ML, Templeton PA. Mediastinal mature teratoma: imaging features. *Am J Roentgenol* 1997;169:985.
42. Moran CA, Suster S. Primary germ cell tumors of the mediastinum: I. Analysis of 322 cases with special emphasis on teratomatous lesions and a proposal for histopathologic classification and clinical staging. *Cancer* 1997;80:681–690.
43. Strollo DC, Rosado de Christenson ML, Jett JR. Primary mediastinal tumors. Part 1: tumors of the anterior mediastinum. *Chest* 1997;112:511–522.
44. Fulcher AS, Proto AV, Jolles H. Cystic teratoma of the mediastinum: demonstration of fat/fluid level. *Am J Roentgenol* 1990;154:259–260.
45. Shimosato Y, Mukai K. Tumors of the thymus and related lesions. In: Rosai J, ed. *Tumors of the Mediastinum*, 3rd ed. Washington, DC: Armed Forces Institute of Pathology; 1997: 33.
46. Lee K, Im J, Han M, et al. Malignant primary germ cell tumors of the mediastinum: CT features. *Am J Roentgenol* 1989;153:947–951.
47. Rosado-de-Christenson ML, Templeton PA, Moran CA. From the archives of the AFIP. Mediastinal germ cell tumors: radiologic and pathologic correlation. *RadioGraphics* 1992;12:1013–1030.
48. Castellino RA, Hilton S, O'Brien JP, et al. Non-Hodgkin lymphoma: contribution of chest CT in the initial staging evaluation. *Radiology* 1996;199:129–132.
49. Castellino RA, Blank N, Hoppe RT, et al. Hodgkin disease: contributions of chest CT in the initial staging evaluation. *Radiology* 1986;160:603–605.
50. Jochelson MS, Balikian JP, Mauch P, et al. Peri- and paracardial involvement in lymphoma: a radiographic study of 11 cases. *Am J Roentgenol* 1983;140:483–488.
51. McLoud TC, Kalisher L, Stark P, et al. Intrathoracic lymph node metastases from extrathoracic neoplasms. *Am J Roentgenol* 1978;131:403–407.
52. Suwatanapongched T, Gierada DS. CT of thoracic lymph nodes. Part II: diseases and pitfalls. *Br J Radiol* 2006;79:999–1000.
53. Miller BH, Rosado-de-Christenson ML, McAdams HP, et al. Thoracic sarcoidosis: radiologic–pathologic correlation. *RadioGraphics* 1995;15:421–437.
54. Bein ME, Putman CE, McLoud TC, et al. A reevaluation of intrathoracic lymphadenopathy in sarcoidosis. *Am J Roentgenol* 1978;131:409–415.
55. Pombo F, Rodriguez E, Mato J, et al. Patterns of contrast enhancement of tuberculous lymph nodes demonstrated by computed tomography. *Clin Radiol* 1992;46:13–17.
56. McAdams HP, Rosado-de-Christenson M, Fishback NF, et al. Castleman disease of the thorax: radiologic features with clinical and histopathologic correlation. *Radiology* 1998;209:221–228.

57. Yamashita Y, Hirai T, Matsukawa T, et al. Radiological presentations of Castleman's disease. *Comput Med Imaging Graph* 1993;17:107–117.
58. Radin DR, Baker EL, Klatt EC, et al. Visceral and nodal calcification in patients with AIDS-related Pneumocystis carinii infection. *Am J Roentgenol* 1990;154:27–31.
59. Landay MJ, Rollins NK, Mediastinal histoplasmosis granuloma: evaluation with CT. *Radiology* 1989;172:657–659.
60. Yousem DM, Scatarige JC, Fishman EK, et al. Low-attenuation thoracic metastases in testicular malignancy. *Am J Roentgenol* 1986;146:291–293.
61. Hopper KD, Diehl LF, Cole BA, et al. The significance of necrotic mediastinal lymph nodes on CT in patients with newly diagnosed Hodgkin disease. *Am J Roentgenol* 1990;155:267–270.
62. Samuels T, Hamilton P, Shaw P. Whipple disease of the mediastinum. *Am J Roentgenol* 1990;154:1187–1188.
63. Zylak CJ, Eyler WR, Spizarny DL, et al. Developmental lung anomalies in the adult: radiologic-pathologic correlation. *RadioGraphics* 2002;22:S25–S43.
64. Strollo DC, Rosado-de-Christenson ML, Jett JR. Primary mediastinal tumors: part II. Tumors of the middle and posterior mediastinum. *Chest* 1997;112: 1344–1357.
65. Berrocal T, Madrid C, Novo S, et al. Congenital anomalies of the tracheobronchial tree, lung, and mediastinum: embryology, radiology, and pathology. *RadioGraphics* 2004;24:e17.
66. Nakata H, Nakayama C, Kimoto T, et al. Computed tomography of mediastinal bronchogenic cysts. *J Comput Assist Tomogr* 1982;6:733–738.
67. Jeung MY, Gasser B, Gangi A, et al. Imaging of cystic masses of the mediastinum; *RadioGraphics* 2002;22:S79–S93.
68. Feigin DS, Fenoglio J, McAllister HA, et al. Pericardial cysts. A radiologic-pathologic correlation and review. *Radiology* 1977;125:15–20.
69. Sechtem U, Tscholakoff D, Higgins CB. MRI of the abnormal pericardium. *Am J Roentgenol* 1986;147:245–252.
70. Kawashima A, Fishman EK, Kuhlman JE, et al. CT of posterior mediastinal masses. *RadioGraphics* 1991;11:1045–1067.
71. Reed JC, Hallet K, Feigin DS. Neural tumors of the thorax: subject review from the AFIP. *Radiology* 1978;126:9–17.
72. Baraga R, Parham DM, Lasater OE, et al. MR imaging differentiation of benign and malignant peripheral nerve sheath tumors: use of the target sign. *Pediatr Radiol* 1997;27:124–129.
73. Aughenbaugh GL. Thoracic manifestations of neurocutaneous diseases. *Radiol Clin North Am* 1984;22:741–756.
74. Erasmus JJ, McAdams HP, Donnelly LF, et al. MR imaging of mediastinal masses. *Magn Reson Imaging Clin N Am* 2000;8:59–89.
75. Adam A, Hochholzer L. Ganglioneuroblastoma of the posterior mediastinum: a clinicopathologic review of 80 cases. *Cancer* 1981;47:373–381.
76. Bar-Ziv J, Nogrady MB. Mediastinal neuroblastoma and ganglioneuroma. The differentiation between primary and secondary involvement on the chest roentgenogram. *Am J Roentgenol Radium Ther Nucl Med* 1975;125:380–390.
77. Spizarny DL, Rebner M, Gross BH. CT evaluation of enhancing mediastinal masses. *J Comput Assist Tomogr* 1987;11:990–993.
78. Van Gils AP, Falke TH, van Erkel AR, et al. MR imaging and MIBG scintigraphy of pheochromocytomas and extra adrenal functioning paragangliomas. *RadioGraphics* 1991;11:37–57.
79. Krenning EP, Kwekkeboom DJ, Bakker WH, et al. Somatostatin receptor scintigraphy with [111In-DTPA-D-Phe1]- and [123I-Tyr3]-octreotide: the Rotterdam experience with more than 1000 patients. *Eur J Nucl Med* 1993;20:716–731.
80. Miles J, Pennybacker J, Sheldon P. Intrathoracic meningocele. Its development and association with neurofibromatosis. *J Neurol Neurosurg Psychiatry* 1969;32:99–110.
81. Long JA Jr, Doppman JL, Nienhuis AW. Computed tomographic studies of thoracic extramedullary hematopoiesis. *J Comput Assist Tomogr* 1980;4:67–70.
82. Faul JL, Berry GJ, Colby TV, et al. Thoracic lymphangiomas, lymphangiectasis, lymphangiomatosis, and lymphatic dysplasia syndrome. *Am J Respir Crit Care Med* 2000;161:1037–1046.
83. Miyake H, Shiga M, Takaki H, et al. Mediastinal lymphangiomas in adults: CT findings. *J Thorac Imaging* 1996;11:83–85.
84. Tecce PM, Fishman EK, Kuhlman JE. CT evaluation of the anterior mediastinum: spectrum of disease. *RadioGraphics* 1994;14:973–990.
85. Shaffer K, Rosado-de-Christenson ML, Patz EF Jr, et al. Thoracic lymphangioma in adults: CT and MR imaging features. *Am J Roentgenol* 1994;162:283–289.
86. Brown LR, Reiman HM, Rosenow EC III, et al. Intrathoracic lymphangioma. *Mayo Clin Proc* 1986;61:882–892.
87. Glazer HS, Wick MR, Anderson DJ, et al. CT of fatty thoracic masses. *Am J Roentgenol* 1992;159:1181–1187.
88. Gaerte SC, Meyer CA, Winer-Muram HT, et al. Fat-containing lesions of the chest. *RadioGraphics* 2002;22:615–678.
89. Pasricha PJ, Fleischer DE. Endoscopic perforations of the upper digestive tract: a review of their pathogenesis, prevention and management. *Gastroenterology* 1994;106; 787–802.
90. Jolles H, Henry DA, Roberson JP, et al. Mediastinitis following median sternotomy: CT findings. *Radiology* 1996;201:463–466.
91. Carter AR, Sostman HD, Curtis AM, et al. Thoracic alterations after cardiac surgery. *Am J Roentgenol* 1983;140:475–481.
92. Goodwin RA, Nickell JA, Des Prez RM. Mediastinal fibrosis complicating healed primary histoplasmosis and tuberculosis. *Medicine Balt* 1972;51:227–246.
93. Sherrick AD, Brown LR, Harms GF, et al. The radiographic findings of fibrosing mediastinitis. *Chest* 1994;106:484–489.
94. Rossi SE, McAdams HP, Rosado-de-Christenson ML, et al. Fibrosing mediastinitis. *RadioGraphics* 2001;21:737–757.
95. Rodriguez E, Soler R, Pombo F, et al. Fibrosing mediastinitis: CT and MR findings. *Clin Radiol* 1998;53:907–910.
96. Rholl KS, Levitt RG, Glazer HS. Magnetic resonance imaging of fibrosing mediastinitis. *Am J Roentgenol* 1985;145:255–259.

Radionuclide Studies of the Mediastinum

Philip Maximilian Scherer ▪ Delphine L. Chen

Until recently, the role of radionuclide imaging in the chest was primarily related to evaluation of disorders of the heart and lungs, particularly the evaluation of myocardial perfusion and ventricular function, the use of ventilation/perfusion scintigraphy in the detection of pulmonary embolism, and the diagnosis of inflammatory and neoplastic disorders of the lungs and bony thorax using traditional single-photon radionuclides. In the course of pulmonary scintigraphy, findings may indirectly identify the presence of pathology in the mediastinum, such as obstructive airways disease on ventilation studies or the presence of mediastinal lesions producing secondary effects on pulmonary ventilation, perfusion, or both, including mass lesions and fibrosing mediastinitis.

A number of targeted nuclear medicine agents can be used to image specific lesions of the mediastinum that can lead to ventilation–perfusion scintigraphy abnormalities or directly assess the extent of mediastinal involvement of specific processes. These include In-111-labeled pentetreotide (^{111}In-Octreotide), I-123 labeled metaiodobenzylguanidine (^{123}I-MIBG), iodine itself (either ^{123}I or ^{131}I), and In-111-labeled white blood cells (WBCs). The distribution of these tracers has historically been assessed by planar imaging. However, with the increasing availability of combined SPECT and x-ray computed tomography (SPECT-CT) cameras, the ability to more precisely localize the uptake of these tracers anatomically is now tremendously improved. SPECT-CT also has the potential to increase the sensitivity of detecting abnormal uptake in the mediastinum. The current clinical applications for these targeted radiopharmaceuticals as well as the role of SPECT-CT will be discussed in this chapter.

Positron emission tomographic (PET) and CT imaging with the radiopharmaceutical fluorine-18 (^{18}F) 2-fluoro-2-deoxy-D-glucose (^{18}F-FDG) is now the primary imaging modality for the detection and staging of a number of common malignancies. ^{18}F-FDG PET/CT is approved for diagnosis, initial staging, treatment monitoring, and restaging of the most important malignancies of the chest and mediastinum, including non–small cell lung carcinoma (NSCLC), lymphoma, esophageal carcinoma, and non–iodine-avid thyroid carcinomas. The current clinical applications of ^{18}F-FDG PET/CT in these cancers will be discussed.

VENTILATION/PERFUSION SCINTIGRAPHY

Radionuclide imaging of the lungs remains one of the most commonly performed nuclear medicine procedures of the chest. Although spiral CT imaging of the chest has emerged as a viable alternative modality for the evaluation of patients with suspected pulmonary thromboembolism, ventilation/perfusion (V/Q) lung scintigraphy remains an important screening modality in the evaluation of these patients, and this application is by far the most important indication for this procedure. This subject is discussed in greater detail in Chapter 13. However, V/Q imaging can also provide useful information regarding certain types of mediastinal pathology. Ventilation imaging is performed using either radioactive gases, such as xenon-133 (^{133}Xe) or krypton 81m ([81m]Kr) or using fine, uniform aerosols labeled with ^{99m}Tc, which are inhaled by the patient. Alderson and colleagues[1–3] have shown that these studies are extremely sensitive for the detection of obstructive airways disease, nearly twice as sensitive as routine chest radiographs. The ^{133}Xe study is performed by having the patient rapidly inhale as a 10- to 20-mCi (370- to 740-mBq) dose of the radioactive gas is injected into a breathing apparatus, similar to a standard spirometer. The patient holds his or her breath as long as possible while a posterior "single-breath" image is acquired, which reflects regional ventilation. The patient then breathes a ^{133}Xe/air mixture in a closed system for 3 to 5 minutes to allow equilibration of the gas in the airways to occur. During or at the conclusion of this period, an "equilibrium washin" image or images are obtained, which reflect total ventilated lung volume. Finally, the patient exhales the radioactive gas and breathes room air while additional images are obtained every 30 to 60 seconds for an additional 5 minutes, constituting the "washout" phase. This latter phase is the most sensitive for detection of obstructive airways disease and cannot be obtained with either [81m]Kr or ^{99m}Tc aerosols. In ^{133}Xe imaging (unlike the other ventilation imaging agents), all images are acquired in the posterior projection, but posterior oblique views are often obtained during the washin and washout phases to improve the localization of abnormalities in the anteroposterior plane.

In addition to diffuse involvement in emphysema, asthma, or chronic bronchitis, the presence of endobronchial masses, foreign bodies, mucous plugging, or extrinsic airway obstruction from either masses or other processes can be detected by these studies, particularly using ^{133}Xe imaging. The most significant finding in such cases is the presence of decreased uptake of the gas on the single-breath study, with prolonged retention of the tracer in the affected lung during the washout phase, when the patient is breathing room air. Whole-lung hypoventilation is particularly suggestive of a central mass, foreign body, or mucous plug causing a ball–valve type of airway obstruction and often results in a secondary global decrease in perfusion to the affected lung via hypoxic vasoconstriction, as demonstrated by a bronchial obstructing carcinoid tumor shown in Figure 152.1. [133]Xe ventilation imaging can also be helpful for assessing the integrity of bronchial closures after pneumonectomy. With aerosol ventilation agents, areas of obstructive airways disease present as focal defects

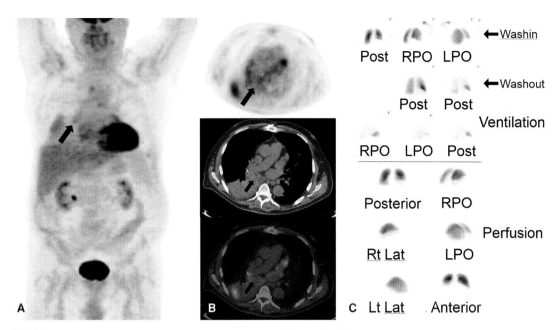

FIGURE 152.1 Airway obstruction due to obstructing carcinoid tumor with hypoxic vasoconstriction leading to a matched ventilation-perfusion defect. **A:** Maximum-intensity-projection image from an ^{18}F-FDG PET/CT scan. There is no increased activity in the obstructing carcinoid tumor in the bronchus intermedius (*arrow*). There is increased activity in the right lower lobe consolidation, most consistent with postobstructive pneumonia. **B:** Attenuation-corrected, noncontrast CT, and fused PET-CT images of the chest. These images confirm that there is no increased ^{18}F-FDG uptake in the known obstructing carcinoid tumor in the bronchus intermedius (*arrows*). **C:** Washin images in posterior (Post), right posterior oblique (RPO), and left posterior oblique (LPO) views and five serial 60-second washout images from a Xe-133 ventilation study. There is decreased perfusion in the right lower lobe with retention. There is mild retention at the left lung base. There is markedly decreased perfusion in the right middle and right lower lobes. These findings are most consistent with obstruction of the right lower lobe bronchus and hypoxic vasoconstriction of the right middle and lower lobar pulmonary arteries. Rt Lat, right lateral view; Lt Lat, left lateral view.

in ventilation.[4] In severe cases of chronic obstructive airways disease, clumping of the radioaerosol in the central airways may also be observed.

Pulmonary perfusion imaging is performed by intravenous injection of ^{99}Tc-labeled particles, such as macroaggregated albumin (MAA), which are trapped in the pulmonary capillary system in proportion to regional pulmonary blood flow. Although pulmonary embolism is again the most important cause of perfusion defects, perfusion abnormalities are also commonly associated with the presence of mediastinal lesions, which produce hypoperfusion as the result of compression or invasion of pulmonary arterial or venous branches. In combination with the ventilation study, it can be determined whether the perfusion defect is the primary abnormality (producing V/Q mismatch) or whether there is secondary hypoxic vasoconstriction and shunting of blood flow away from a site of ventilatory deficit (matching abnormalities). Important mediastinal lesions producing such changes in pulmonary blood flow include mediastinal masses due to lung carcinoma or other tumors and fibrosing mediastinitis (see Figs. 152.2 to 152.4). The finding of lobar or whole-lung V/Q mismatch is suggestive of these disorders, although these findings may also occur in other situations, as discussed by Datz,[5] including massive unilateral pulmonary embolism and other primary vascular lesions, such as arteritis or prior radiation therapy. Thus a mediastinal mass lesion, depending on its location, may produce either V/Q match or mismatch.

The radiopharmaceutical uptake in ventilation/perfusion imaging is easily quantified using commercially available nuclear medicine image processing software packages. White and colleagues[6] demonstrated perfusion defects associated with bronchial carcinoma and determined that the size of the perfusion defect correlated with the extent of the lesion. They found that if the perfusion to the ipsilat-

eral lung was less than 33% of total pulmonary perfusion, the lesion was nearly always unresectable. Quantitation of both perfusion and ventilation allows calculation of regional V/Q ratios. Comparison of these ratios with normal values can also help to predict resectability of tumors, although this analysis is not commonly performed because of relatively low sensitivity and the availability of more accurate staging of lung carcinoma by CT and, more recently, PET imaging. However, quantitative V/Q imaging is now performed to predict pulmonary function following contemplated pneumonectomy, as initially described by Kristersson,[7] Olsen,[8] and Boysen[9] and their colleagues. Assessment of postresection pulmonary reserve is an important aspect of the preoperative evaluation of patients considered for lung resection. Significant disability can result from chronic ventilatory insufficiency if the postoperative forced expiratory volume in 1 second (FEV_1) is less than 0.8 L, as reported by Olsen and colleagues[8] and by Williams and Brenowitz.[10] Quantitative V/Q scintigraphy can accurately predict the postoperative pulmonary function in these patients, as reported by Wernly and colleagues,[11] and surgery is usually not performed if the predicted FEV_1 is less than 0.8 L, as described by Block and Olsen.[12] This technique has also been used to monitor pulmonary function following pulmonary transplantation, as described by the Toronto Lung Transplant Group,[13] and to assess patients preoperatively prior to lung reduction surgery, as described by Wang and colleagues.[14]

SPECT-CT has added additional capabilities for functional quantification of ventilation and perfusion. Because of the tomographic representation of the images, SPECT-CT images have greater sensitivity for demonstrating ventilation and perfusion defects.[15] The CT images used for attenuation correction of the SPECT images potentially improve the precision of quantifying regional ventilation

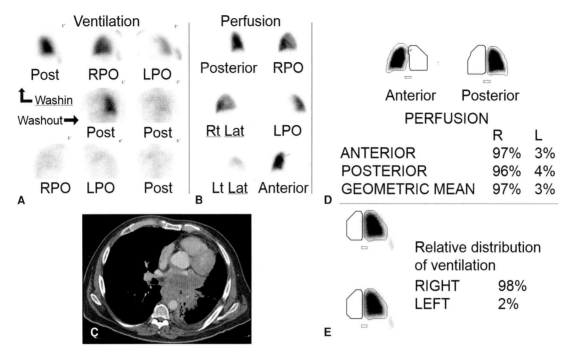

FIGURE 152.2 Whole-lung ventilation/perfusion match. The patient is a 52-year-old man with non–small cell lung cancer presenting with symptoms concerning for bronchial obstruction. **A:** Washin images in posterior (Post), right posterior oblique (RPO) and left posterior oblique (LPO) views and five serial 60-second washout images from a Xe-133 ventilation study. There is essentially absent ventilation of the left lung. **B:** Perfusion images in the posterior, left posterior oblique, right posterior oblique, right lateral (Rt Lat), left lateral (Lt Lat), and anterior projections. There is trace perfusion of the left upper lobe with absent perfusion throughout the remainder of the left lung. **C:** CT of the chest with Optiray-350 intravenous contrast. There is a large infiltrative soft tissue mass in the left hilum and subcarinal region. This mass compresses and nearly completely obstructs the left mainstem bronchus, invades the left atrium, occludes the left pulmonary veins, attenuates the left pulmonary artery, and encases the esophagus and aorta. **D:** Quantitative perfusion. The right lung receives 97% and the left lung receives 3% of total pulmonary perfusion. **E:** Quantitative ventilation. The right lung contributes 98% and the left lung contributes 2% of total pulmonary ventilation.

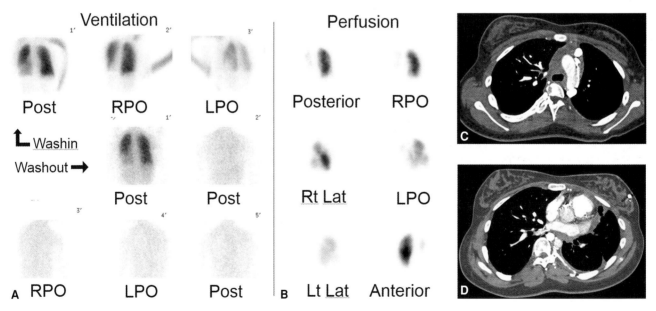

FIGURE 152.3 Decreased ventilation and perfusion secondary to fibrosing mediastinitis. The patient is an 18-year-old girl with pulmonary hypertension. **A:** Washin images in posterior, right posterior oblique and left posterior oblique views and five serial 60-second washout images from a Xe-133 ventilation study. There is decreased ventilation in the left lower lobe. There is no abnormal retention during the washout phase. **B:** Perfusion images in the posterior (Post), left posterior oblique (LPO), right posterior oblique (RPO), right lateral (Rt Lat), left lateral (Lt Lat), and anterior projections. There is nearly absent perfusion in the left lung. There is nearly absent perfusion in the right lower lobe and decreased perfusion in the right upper lobe. **C:** CT angiography (CTA) of the chest with Optiray-350 intravenous contrast. There is soft tissue thickening throughout the mediastinum with matted lymphadenopathy. There is complete obstruction of the superior vena cava with enlarged venous collaterals in the mediastinum. **D:** CTA of the chest with Optiray-350 intravenous contrast. There is focal stenosis in the right inferior pulmonary vein stent. There is complete occlusion of the left superior and inferior pulmonary veins.

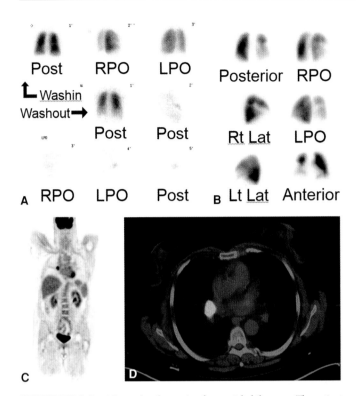

FIGURE 152.4 Partial vascular obstruction from a right hilar mass. The patient is a 63-year-old woman with non–small cell lung cancer. **A:** Washin images in posterior (Post), right posterior oblique (RPO) and left posterior oblique (LPO) views and five serial 60-second washout images from a Xe-133 ventilation study. There is decreased ventilation in the right middle lobe with retention during the washout phase. **B:** Perfusion images in the posterior, left posterior oblique, right posterior oblique, right lateral (Rt Lat), left lateral (Lt Lat), and anterior projections. There is markedly decreased perfusion to the right middle and lower lobes. **C:** Coronal MIP image from an ^18F-FDG PET/CT scan. There is a hypermetabolic mass in the right hilum. There is physiologic ^18F-FDG uptake in the brain and left ventricular myocardium and physiologic excretion in the kidneys and urinary bladder. **D:** Fused ^18F-FDG PET/CT image. There is a hypermetabolic mass in the right hilum.

and perfusion over SPECT alone. Right- and left whole-lung quantification of perfusion with SPECT-CT is essentially identical to that obtained from planar images.[16] However, SPECT-CT images yield greater differences than planar images in regional perfusion quantification,[16,17] most likely due to the reduction in overlap of segments on the tomographic images. The degree of improved accuracy in these measurements remains to be validated.

POSITRON EMISSION TOMOGRAPHY

PET/CT imaging is now a key imaging modality for the staging of most cancers. PET has long been available as a research tool in the evaluation of brain and cardiac metabolism, often using ultra–short-lived positron-emitting radionuclides such as carbon-11, nitrogen-13, and oxygen-15. Although these agents permit the labeling of biologically important molecules that serve as excellent tracers that can measure the activity of various metabolic functions their physical nature (half-lives in the range of 2 to 20 minutes) demands that they be prepared locally for immediate use. This preparation requires the availability of an on-site medical cyclotron and the equipment needed to radiolabel the necessary compounds with these isotopes, which involves complex and expensive instrumentation as well as dedicated,

highly trained personnel who operate the equipment. The use of such short-lived isotopes remains confined to medical centers with experience in handling these radionuclides, though the installation of smaller cyclotrons now also makes these short-lived isotopes more readily available at more centers. However, with widespread availability of PET/CT scanners, distribution networks are now set up across the United States to deliver radiopharmaceuticals with longer-lived isotopes, primarily ^18F-FDG, whose F-18 label has a longer half-life of 1.83 hours (~110 minutes) that enables shipping unit doses from centralized pharmacies.

^18F-FDG is an analog of glucose, with the F-18 label replacing a hydroxyl group at the 2-carbon position, and is the workhorse radiopharmaceutical for clinical PET/CT imaging. ^18F-FDG is taken up by the same mechanisms as glucose, namely the glucose transporters, and then trapped because the absence of the hydroxyl group prevents its phosphorylation by hexokinase-I and subsequent metabolism via entry into the Krebs cycle. Besides the ability of ^18F-FDG to image cardiac and brain glucose metabolism, the use of ^18F-FDG for cancer staging and treatment response assessment is now well-established. As a result of the Warburg effect, in which tumor cells exhibit increased glucose utilization compared to normal tissues, PET imaging with ^18F-FDG can clearly distinguish metabolically active malignant disease more readily than CT, particularly in lesions that may be normal by size criteria for CT and in previously treated disease that may have residual tissue by CT that is no longer metabolically active. As a result, ^18F-FDG PET/CT imaging is now the standard of care for initial staging of lung cancer and is being utilized for radiation treatment planning as well.[18] ^18F-FDG PET/CT is currently approved and reimbursed for the diagnosis, initial staging, and restaging of nearly all cancers as well as for monitoring for treatment responses and detecting suspected recurrences.

Because PET is an inherently quantitative imaging modality, multiple different methods of quantifying ^18F-FDG uptake have been proposed to determine what provides the most representative and clinical relevant information about the tumor to guide diagnosis, prognostication, and treatment response assessments. The standard uptake value (SUV) is the primary measurement used clinically to supplement visual assessment of the PET images and is calculated by dividing the activity in a region of interest (ROI) by the injected dose per kilogram of body weight. Because the average SUV within any given ROI depends on the size of the ROI, many studies have focused on using the maximum SUV, which gives the maximum value within the ROI. While this measurement is based on the single hottest pixel within the ROI and thus may be overly influenced by noise, it is the most frequently used as this value is the least observer dependent as its value does not depend on the size of the ROI drawn. Other measurements have been proposed, such as the total lesion glycolysis (TLG), which is the product of the average SUV within a tumor and the tumor volume, and peak SUV, which sums the SUV values of the voxels around the voxel containing the maximum SUV. These alternative approaches are still being investigated to assess what their clinical role will be in the reporting of ^18F-FDG uptake. However, the SUV can be influenced by a number of factors, as reviewed by Gámez-Cenzano and colleagues[19] and Tomasi and colleagues,[20] including the uptake time (the amount of time between the time of ^18F-FDG injection and PET/CT scan acquisition) and blood glucose levels (with high glucose levels, glucose will directly compete with ^18F-FDG for tumor uptake, leading to reduced ^18F-FDG uptake) as well as technical variables such as the scanner type and image acquisition and reconstruction parameters. These factors make accurate comparisons of absolute SUVs between centers difficult; however, within the same center using the same equipment, SUV comparisons can be reliably performed to assess for treatment responses.[20]

^{18}F-FDG PET/CT easily images the extent of involvement in many of the cancers that involve the mediastinum, including non–small cell lung cancer, small cell lung carcinoma (SCLC), lymphoma (both Hodgkin and non-Hodgkin as well as other subtypes) and esophageal cancer. Metastatic disease from melanoma, breast cancer, cervical cancer, and other genitourinary or gastrointestinal tumors are also easily identified. False-positive findings may occur in granulomas or in noninfectious inflammatory processes, such as sarcoidosis, however, which frequently involve the mediastinum. False-negative imaging results may occur with cell types that may be associated with lower levels of metabolic activity, such as bronchoalveolar carcinoma and carcinoid tumors (see Fig. 152.1) as well as tumors with mucinous features, which tend to have less tissue associated with the tumor because of the mucin content, thus reducing the amount of tissue available to take up the ^{18}F-FDG. False-negative imaging results or underestimation of the metabolic activity of lesions may also occur in the case of very small nodules less than 1 cm in diameter. Though the 1 cm cutoff remains in use, for PET/CT, the true spatial resolution limit has not been systematically studied in newer PET/CT scanners that have better spatial resolution and count rate handling capabilities compared to the original dedicated PET scanners which were originally used to establish the smallest detectable lung nodule by ^{18}F-FDG PET/CT. This chapter will focus on the existing evidence for using ^{18}F-FDG PET in staging the mediastinal involvement from non–small cell lung cancer, lymphoma, and esophageal cancer.

With regard to assessment of mediastinal involvement with NSCLC, prior reports have clearly demonstrated improved sensitivity, specificity, and accuracy using ^{18}F-FDG PET over CT alone. The overall sensitivity and specificity of CT in the staging of NSCLC has been reported to be only 52% and 69%, respectively, which is representative of the findings of most studies with CT alone.[21] By contrast, as reviewed by Al-Sugair and Coleman,[22] numerous studies have shown PET to have sensitivities and specificities for mediastinal lymph node staging in the range of 70% to 90% and 75% to 100%, respectively. ^{18}F-FDG uptake also positively correlates with histopathologic findings in mediastinal lymph nodes, and the results of the PET study led to in changes in staging in 62 of 102 patients, raising the stage in 42 and lowering it in 20. However, the potential for false-positive results secondary to infectious or noninfectious inflammatory processes, such as fungal infection, tuberculosis or sarcoidosis, significantly compromises the specificity of ^{18}F-FDG PET/CT for assessing mediastinal metastases. On the other hand, the very high negative predictive value of PET obviates the need for preoperative invasive procedures. This was confirmed in a recent meta-analysis that included 45 studies between 1946 and 2013.[23] The authors concluded that the accuracy of ^{18}F-FDG PET/CT alone is not sufficient to guide management appropriately, but could be used to guide biopsy procedures for additional staging when positive or, when negative with small nodes, allow patients to proceed straight to surgery. Finally, the ease with which the whole body can be imaged with PET also permits the detection of occult distant metastases, such as involvement of the adrenal glands, liver, or skeleton. PET imaging is also extremely valuable in the follow-up assessment of the response to therapy, again outperforming CT in detecting recurrences and differentiating between posttreatment fibrosis versus residual or recurrent tumor involvement. As reviewed by Skoura and colleagues,[24] seven published studies report that reductions in ^{18}F-FDG uptake by 20% to 50% after 1 to 3 cycles of standard chemotherapy, based on the mean SUV in the tumor or other quantification approaches, identify patients who will have longer progression-free or overall survival. While these results are promising, all were based on small clinical trials and thus still require prospective validation. See

Figure 152.4 for an example of a right hilar NSCLC. ^{18}F-FDG PET/CT is also sensitive for the detection of SCLC; but because of the typically extensive involvement encountered in SCLC at initial presentation and its usually poor prognosis, management is often similar for many patients. Additionally, ^{18}F-FDG PET/CT is not useful in assessing the presence of cranial disease, which occurs frequently with SCLC, due to the high normal brain uptake of ^{18}F-FDG. Therefore, although a recent limited meta-analysis demonstrated high sensitivity, specificity, and accuracy for ^{18}F-FDG PET/CT in staging SCLC,[25] its role in the clinical management of this disease remains to be defined.

^{18}F-FDG PET/CT is the primary diagnostic imaging modality for assessing lymphoma, including both Hodgkin's and non-Hodgkin's lymphoma, and has nearly completely replaced ^{67}Ga-citrate imaging for this purpose given its superior diagnostic performance. A review by Tirumani and colleagues of the current state of ^{18}F-FDG PET/CT succinctly summarizes its central role in the management of lymphoma.[26] Whole-body ^{18}F-FDG PET/CT imaging has been shown to be more accurate in the diagnosis and staging of both Hodgkin and non-Hodgkin's lymphoma than PET or CT alone.[27] More importantly, as in the case of NSCLC, PET has proven to be superior to CT in the evaluation of patients with lymphoma for assessing end-of-therapy response and detecting recurrences. ^{18}F-FDG PET/CT is now the primary basis for determining treatment responses in lymphoma using mediastinal blood pool or liver activity as the visual reference by which to determine ^{18}F-FDG positivity.[28] Nearly all studies have shown that ^{18}F-FDG-avid disease at the end of treatment predicts a poor prognosis, while negative end-of-treatment ^{18}F-FDG PET/CT scans predict improved outcomes.[26] Negative PET/CT studies demonstrating both functional and anatomic resolution of disease also predict improved survival compared to those with residual masses as minimal residual disease that is not detectable by ^{18}F-FDG PET/CT may still be present.[29] Multiple studies now also have demonstrated the prognostic value of ^{18}F-FDG PET/CT for assessing interim response after 2 to 3 cycles of chemotherapy.[30–32] The Deauville criteria are the most widely used criteria for assessing interim responses for aggressive lymphomas.[33,34] Ongoing trials are now testing whether risk-adaptive treatment strategies employing interim PET/CT imaging can improve outcomes for both Hodgkin and non-Hodgkin's lymphoma. An example of PET imaging in mediastinal lymphoma, as well as demonstrating treatment response, is shown in Figures 152.5 and 152.6. As in the case of lung carcinoma, false-negative imaging results may occur with small lesions and in certain cell types, for example, the mucosa-associated lymphoid tumor (MALT) variety, as reported by Hoffmann and colleagues.[35]

^{18}F-FDG PET/CT imaging can be useful in the initial staging of patients with esophageal carcinoma and in detecting suspected recurrences. In normal studies, faint uptake may be seen in the distal esophagus, which may represent a normal variant, or in some cases may reflect mild inflammatory changes secondary to gastroesophageal reflux. As reviewed by Kwee and colleagues,[36] ^{18}F-FDG PET/CT is sensitive for the detection of both squamous cell and adenocarcinoma of the esophagus but not useful for small tumors given the superior performance of endoscopic ultrasound for T staging and assessment of locoregional metastatic disease.[37] ^{18}F-FDG PET/CT is also useful in improving the accuracy of staging by detecting distant metastases or confirming nonmalignancy in suspected metastatic sites by conventional imaging, leading to a significant change in stage and management strategy in approximately one-third of patients.[38] ^{18}F-FDG PET/CT also detects second primary malignancies in a few percentage of patients undergoing initial staging for esophageal cancer, which can also significantly alter the initial treatment strategy.[39] Not surprisingly, given the advantages of ^{18}F-FDG PET/CT in

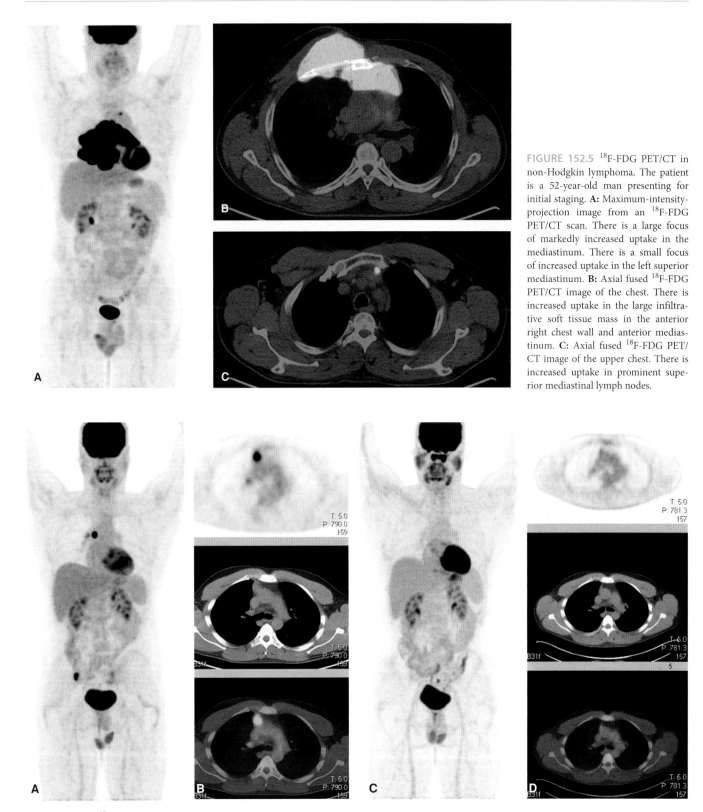

FIGURE 152.5 ^{18}F-FDG PET/CT in non-Hodgkin lymphoma. The patient is a 52-year-old man presenting for initial staging. **A:** Maximum-intensity-projection image from an ^{18}F-FDG PET/CT scan. There is a large focus of markedly increased uptake in the mediastinum. There is a small focus of increased uptake in the left superior mediastinum. **B:** Axial fused ^{18}F-FDG PET/CT image of the chest. There is increased uptake in the large infiltrative soft tissue mass in the anterior right chest wall and anterior mediastinum. **C:** Axial fused ^{18}F-FDG PET/CT image of the upper chest. There is increased uptake in prominent superior mediastinal lymph nodes.

FIGURE 152.6 ^{18}F-FDG PET/CT in Hodgkin lymphoma (pre- and posttherapy). The patient is a 29-year-old man with classical Hodgkin lymphoma post autologous stem cell transplant and chemotherapy presenting with enlarging mediastinal lymph nodes on a recent diagnostic CT. **A:** Maximum-intensity-projection image from an ^{18}F-FDG PET/CT scan. There is focally increased uptake in the right aspect of the anterior mediastinum and right iliac bone. There are foci of mildly increased uptake in the right hilum and left sacral ala. These findings are most consistent with recurrent disease. **B:** Attenuation-corrected ^{18}F-FDG PET, non-contrast-enhanced CT, and fused ^{18}F-FDG PET/CT images of the chest. There is increased uptake in the right anterior mediastinal mass and mildly increased uptake in a right hilar lymph node. **C:** Maximum-intensity-projection image from an ^{18}F-FDG PET/CT scan 6 weeks later following multiple cycles of chemotherapy. There has been interval resolution of abnormal uptake with no abnormal foci remaining, most consistent with a complete metabolic response. **D:** Attenuation-corrected ^{18}F-FDG PET, non-contrast-enhanced CT, and fused ^{18}F-FDG PET/CT images of the chest. There has been decrease in size of the anterior mediastinal mass with residual abnormal soft tissue density. The intensity of ^{18}F-FDG uptake is equal to blood pool, indicating complete metabolic response.

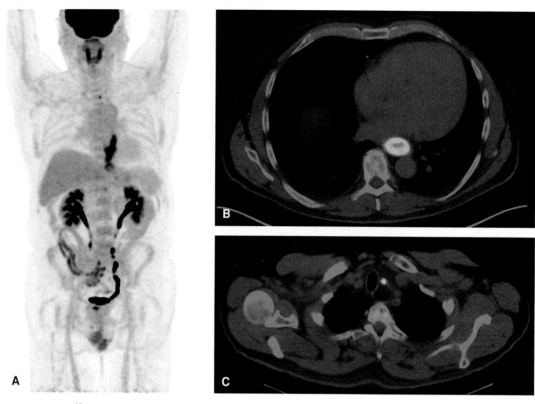

FIGURE 152.7 ^{18}F-FDG PET/CT in esophageal cancer. **A:** Maximum-intensity-projection image from an ^{18}F-FDG PET/CT scan in a 58-year-old man with recently diagnosed distal esophageal carcinoma. There is increased uptake in the lower third of the esophagus, corresponding to the primary lesion. There is focally increased uptake in the left superior paratracheal region, most consistent with mediastinal nodal metastasis. There is normal brain, kidney, urinary bladder, and bowel activity. **B:** Fused ^{18}F-FDG PET/CT image of the chest. There is increased uptake in the lower third of the esophagus, corresponding with circumferential esophageal wall thickening of the primary lesion. **C:** Fused ^{18}F-FDG PET/CT image of the thoracic inlet. There is abnormally increased uptake in the prominent left superior paratracheal lymph node.

detecting distant disease, the literature to date suggests that ^{18}F-FDG PET/CT may also be useful in the restaging of esophageal cancers after treatment and in detecting suspected recurrences, though the presence of inflammation or infection reduces the specificity of ^{18}F-FDG PET/CT for this purpose.[36] The prognostic significance of the SUV in the primary tumor remains to be established. Although multiple studies have demonstrated that high SUV predicts poor prognosis by univariate analysis, as analyzed in two meta-analyses of 11 and 15 studies,[40,41] only two of the studies reported SUV as an independent predictor of prognosis in multivariate analyses.[41] The results of studies investigating the utility of ^{18}F-FDG PET/CT for predicting response to neoadjuvant chemotherapy or chemoradiation therapy overall have demonstrated inadequate performance for this purpose.[36] Examples of primary and metastatic esophageal carcinoma are shown in Figures 152.7 and 152.8.

In the case of breast carcinoma, PET imaging has been used both in the characterization of benign versus malignant lesions as well as in the evaluation of the extent of tumor spread, especially with respect to axillary lymph node involvement, as recently reviewed by Lebron and colleagues.[42] ^{18}F-FDG PET/CT is highly specific but not sensitive for detecting axillary node disease; therefore, staging the axillae in breast carcinoma requires lymphoscintigraphy (see Fig. 152.9) with directed lymph node dissection and immunohistochemical analysis.[43] PET may also permit superior evaluation of the internal mammary nodes, which, as previously discussed, are difficult to evaluate using other existing modalities. The greatest value for ^{18}F-FDG PET/CT is in diagnosing distant metastases, which is more sensitive than bone scan for detecting osteolytic metastases.[42] High ^{18}F-FDG

uptake predicts a poorer prognosis, and changes in ^{18}F-FDG uptake can also be used to assess the response to therapy.[42] Research involving PET imaging using ^{18}F-labeled estrogen analogs holds promise in the assessment of the receptor function of breast tumors, which may also have a significant impact on therapeutic decisions.

OCTREOTIDE IMAGING

The somatostatin receptor agent octreotide is a peptide-based agent that has been labelled for imaging. Somatostatin is a naturally occurring peptide hormone first isolated from hypothalamic extracts, as reviewed by Olsen and colleagues.[44] Acting as an anti–growth-hormone factor, this peptide inhibits the synthesis and secretion of various peptide hormones—including insulin, gastrin, vasoactive intestinal peptide, and many others—by neuroendocrine tissue. Octreotide is a synthetic somatostatin analog possessing a longer serum half-life and higher potency than other similar agents. Early imaging studies used a ^{123}I-labeled octreotide. Disadvantages of this agent included the short 13-hour half-life of ^{123}I relative to the longer biological half-life of octreotide, a technically difficult labeling procedure, and interference by large amounts of intestinal activity secondary to its rapid hepatic and biliary clearance, as discussed by Krenning and colleagues.[45] The commercially available FDA-approved agent Octreoscan (Mallinckrodt Inc., Hazelwood, CO) is the ^{111}In-labeled octreotide derivative pentetreotide, which incorporates the compound diethylenetriaminepentaacetic acid (DTPA);

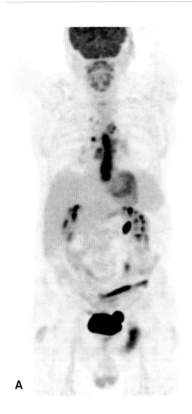
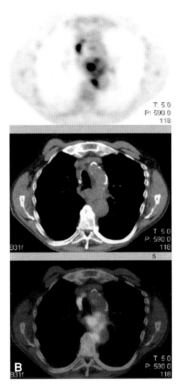

FIGURE 152.8 ^{18}F-FDG PET/CT in esophageal cancer. **A:** Maximum-intensity-projection image from an ^{18}F-FDG PET/CT scan in a 72-year-old man with newly diagnosed esophageal adenocarcinoma and suspicious mediastinal lymphadenopathy on a recent diagnostic CT. There is markedly increased uptake in the mid to distal esophagus in the primary lesion. There are multiple foci of increased uptake in the mediastinum, most consistent with mediastinal nodal metastasis. There is focally increased uptake in the left ischium, most consistent with distant osseous metastasis. **B:** Attenuation-corrected ^{18}F-FDG PET, noncontrast CT, and fused ^{18}F-FDG PET/ CT images of the chest. There is increased uptake in the mid to distal esophagus in the primary lesion. There is also increased uptake in the subcarinal and inferior paratracheal lymphadenopathy.

this compound is commonly used in radiopharmaceuticals, being a glomerular filtration imaging agent itself when labeled with ^{99m}Tc. This radiopharmaceutical localizes with high affinity in a number of neuroendocrine tumors (NETs), including carcinoid tumor, islet cell carcinoma of the pancreas, medullary carcinoma of the thyroid, pheochromocytoma, paragangliomas, pituitary tumors, SCLC, and some lymphomas. It has demonstrated sensitivity in the range of 80% to 100% for the detection of many NETs, with lower sensitivities reported for insulinomas and medullary carcinoma of the thyroid. An example of an abnormal pentetreotide scan is shown in Figure 152.10. As is the case for most new tumor imaging agents and even gallium scintigraphy, SPECT and SPECT/CT imaging has proven to be an essential element of octreotide imaging in order to maximize the sensitivity of the study. However, with the wide availability and improved sensitivity and spatial resolution of PET/CT scanners, a number of PET tracers for imaging somatostatin receptors are now

under evaluation for FDA approval, summarized by Johnbeck and colleagues.[46] The most commonly used tracers, ^{68}Ga-DOTANOC, ^{68}Ga-DOTATATE, and ^{68}Ga-DOTATOC, all identify more lesions than ^{111}In-pentetreotide SPECT/CT and are recommended for use in Europe whenever possible for the evaluation of NETs,[47–50] particularly for colonic NETs, insulinomas, and multiple endocrine neoplasia syndromes.[51,52] These tracers have the advantage of being labelled with Ga-68, which is a generator-produced isotope and thus does not require an on-site cyclotron for availability. However, the short half-life of Ga-68 (68 minutes) requires that the production of these tracers must be carefully timed with the patient's scheduled scan. More recently, PET/CT imaging with ^{64}Cu-DOTATATE was also shown to have significantly improved performance over ^{111}In-pentetreotide SPECT/CT.[53] Though Cu-64 is cyclotron produced, its longer half-life (12.7 hours) enables it shipment from central radiopharmacies and allows more flexibility in the production

20 min post injection

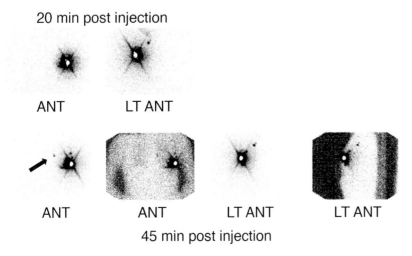

45 min post injection

FIGURE 152.9 Lymphoscintigraphy with sentinel lymph node mapping. Serial images from a lymphoscintigraphy study in a patient with recently diagnosed carcinoma of the left breast demonstrate markedly increased uptake in the region of the injection sites overlying the patient's breast mass. The "star" artifact emanating from the region of the injection sites is secondary to the phenomenon of septal penetration artifact, which occurs when high concentrations of activity exist in a small location, allowing some photons to penetrate between the holes of the gamma camera collimator. In addition, there is visualization of focal areas of lymph node uptake superior and posterior to the lesion and medial to the lesion, representing the sentinel left axillary and left internal mammary lymph nodes, respectively. Ant, anterior; Lt Ant, left anterior.

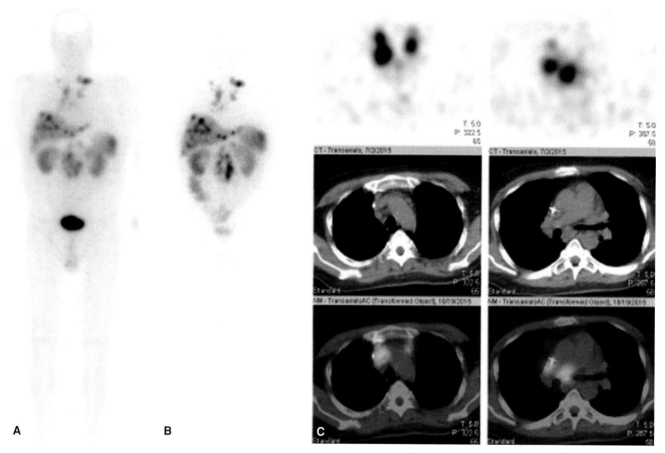

FIGURE 152.10 Abnormal Octreoscan study. The patient is a 45-year-old man with metastatic pancreatic neuroendocrine tumor presenting with intractable nausea and vomiting. Four-hour (**A**) and 24-hour (**B**) whole-body images. There are multiple foci of abnormal ^{111}In-pentetreotide activity in the left supraclavicular, mediastinal and retroperitoneal regions and in the liver. The uptake in the spleen, kidneys, bowel, and urinary bladder is normal. **C:** SPECT/CT images of the mediastinum demonstrate increased activity in multiple mediastinal lymph nodes in the right paratracheal, prevascular, and pre-aortic regions.

of the radiopharmaceutical relative to when patient scans are scheduled. FDA approval was recently granted for ^{68}Ga-DOTATATE, in the United States.

METAIODOBENZYLGUANIDINE IMAGING

Pheochromocytomas are tumors containing adrenal medullary tissue and are located in the adrenal glands in approximately 90% of patients. These tumors are initially detected by elevations of biochemical markers, including various catecholamine metabolites, such as vanillylmandelic acid (VMA) and metanephrines. The adrenal lesions are often localized on CT as large soft tissue masses, which may have necrotic centers. In the remaining 10% of cases, the lesion or lesions are extra-adrenal, often located along the paravertebral para-aortic or mediastinal regions. These lesions are detectable in some cases by CT or MRI, but only if extensive imaging of the entire chest, abdomen, and pelvis is performed. The radiopharmaceutical ^{123}I-MIBG localizes in these tumors as well as related neural tumors, including ganglioneuromas and neuroblastomas in children. Though ^{131}I-MIBG has been used in the past, ^{123}I-MIBG has a more favorable radiation dosimetry profile and superior imaging characteristics that give it higher sensitivity than ^{131}I-MIBG.[54] Since I-123 can dissociate from the MIBG and concentrate in the thyroid, iodine solution is routinely administered at the time of tracer injection to block the thyroid uptake and reduce the thyroid radiation exposure. Bleeker and colleagues[55] performed a meta-analysis of 11 studies

that reported sensitivities of ^{123}I-MIBG SPECT/CT for imaging neuroblastoma ranging from 67% to 100%; however, the currently available data were inadequate for determining the specificity of this imaging approach for this particular tumor. The same meta-analysis also assessed the data supporting the use of ^{18}F-FDG PET/CT in this setting but found only one study reporting a 100% sensitivity and no data to determine specificity of ^{18}F-FDG PET/CT for detecting neuroblastoma. ^{18}F-FDG PET/CT was considered a potentially reasonable study to assess ^{123}I-MIBG negative tumors, which occur in 10% of cases, but not enough data exist to support this as a firm recommendation. An example of a positive imaging result in a mediastinal neuroblastoma in a 3-year-old child is shown in Figure 152.11. The data for ^{123}I-MIBG imaging in pheochromocytomas and paragangliomas is more limited. In a total of 400 patients, Shapiro and colleagues[56] from the same group reported an overall sensitivity of 87.4% and a specificity of 98.9% for ^{131}I-MIBG, including patients with primary sporadic pheochromocytoma, malignant pheochromocytoma, and familial pheochromocytoma, with slightly poorer results in the former category. Small studies have demonstrated improved lesion detection with ^{123}I-MIBG over ^{131}I-MIBG SPECT/CT,[57] with sensitivity of 92% and specificity of 100% for pheochromocytoma detection.[58] A meta-analysis of five studies confirmed that the sensitivity and specificity of ^{123}I-MIBG imaging are high (96% and 100%).[58] However, for malignant pheochromocytomas, imaging after high-dose ^{131}I-MIBG demonstrates more lesions than diagnostic ^{123}I-MIBG scans.[59] An example of a mediastinal pheochromocytoma is shown in Figure 152.12.

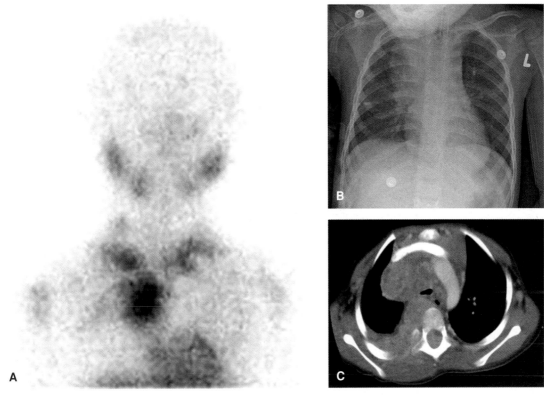

FIGURE 152.11 Posterior mediastinal neuroblastoma on a ^{123}I-MIBG study. The patient is a 3-year-old child presenting with cough and cervical lymphadenopathy. **A:** 24-hour image of the head, neck, and trunk from an anterior acquisition. There is abnormal ^{123}I-MIBG accumulation in the large right posterior mediastinal mass. There is abnormal ^{123}I-MIBG accumulation in the right cervical, bilateral supraclavicular, and superior mediastinal regions and in the proximal humeri. **B:** Frontal chest radiograph. There is a large right paraspinal and superior mediastinal mass. **C:** Contrast-enhanced CT image of the chest. There is a large necrotic right posterior mediastinal mass with neuroforaminal extension into the spinal canal. There is bulky mediastinal lymphadenopathy.

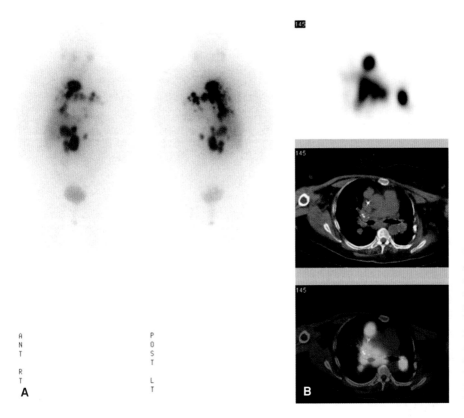

FIGURE 152.12 Metastatic pheochromocytoma diagnosed on a ^{123}I-MIBG study. The patient is a 69-year-old woman post right adrenalectomy and right nephrectomy presenting with suspected recurrence in the chest and abdomen. **A:** 24-hour whole-body images. There is intense uptake in multiple nodal masses in the mediastinum and upper abdomen, with less intense uptake in numerous masses and nodules in both lungs. **B:** SPECT/CT image of the chest. There is intense uptake in prevascular, inferior paratracheal, and hilar adenopathy. There is uptake in right perihilar lung nodules.

THYROID AND PARATHYROID IMAGING

Thyroid imaging using ^{99m}Tc pertechnetate or iodine radionuclides (^{123}I or ^{131}I) is primarily used for the evaluation of thyroid size and morphology, detection and assessment of the functional status of thyroid nodules, evaluation of patients with suspected abnormalities in thyroid function, and detection of metastatic disease in patients with well-differentiated thyroid carcinomas. Iodine radionuclides are trapped and organified by the gland. ^{99m}Tc pertechnetate is a monovalent anion similar in size to an iodide ion and is also trapped but not organified by the thyroid. Because of the high sensitivity of radionuclide thyroid imaging for the detection of functioning thyroid tissue, it is extremely valuable for the detection of ectopic functioning thyroid tissue. Specifically, thyroid imaging can be used to detect substernal extension of the thyroid presenting as a mediastinal mass or functioning metastases from well-differentiated thyroid carcinoma.

Substernal extension of the thyroid may be suggested by the incidental finding of a superior mediastinal mass with tracheal deviation on a routine chest radiograph. Evaluation of substernal extension of the thyroid is now most often performed using ^{123}I sodium iodide. ^{131}I was previously used for this purpose but has been largely replaced by ^{123}I because of the latter's much lower radiation dose to the patient and the relatively better spatial resolution of the ^{123}I images. The shortcomings of ^{131}I as a diagnostic imaging agent result from the long 8-day half-life and beta decay of ^{131}I (resulting in a high patient radiation dose and limiting the dose that may be administered) and high 364-keV energy gamma emission, which is not optimal for the nuclear medicine gamma camera, resulting in lower-resolution images. The previously discussed advantage of using ^{131}I rather than ^{99m}Tc pertechnetate because of the former's higher energy, allowing better penetration of photons through the sternum, is probably a minor factor that is far less significant than the aforementioned considerations. ^{123}I has a half-life of only 13 hours and a gamma photon energy of 159 keV, which is readily imaged with a gamma camera. ^{123}I offers some advantages over ^{99m}Tc pertechnetate in this application as well because it can be used in imaging anywhere from 4 to 24 hours after administration and is associated with less interfering background activity in the blood pool and soft tissues. Blood pool activity in the great vessels on pertechnetate images may interfere with the visualization of small foci of thyroid tissue or poorly functioning mediastinal goiters. In addition, ^{123}I may be given orally in

capsule form, typically in doses of 200 to 300 µCi (7.4 to 11.1 MBq), whereas ^{99m}Tc pertechnetate must be given intravenously, in doses of 8 to 10 mCi (296–370 MBq). Radionuclide thyroid imaging must be performed prior to CT imaging with iodinated contrast material or any other studies involving administration of contrast material. Even small amounts of nonradioactive iodine released into the bloodstream from iodinated contrast material can flood the extracellular iodide pool, resulting in competitive inhibition of tracer uptake by the thyroid and subsequent nonvisualization of thyroid tissue. If the patient has recently received iodinated contrast material or has ingested large amounts of iodine from food or other medications, then radionuclide thyroid imaging must be delayed for at least 4 weeks. An example of a substernal goiter is shown in Figure 152.13.

In the assessment of patients with well-differentiated thyroid carcinoma, whole-body imaging is performed using 2 to 10 mCi (74–370 MBq) of ^{131}I administered orally. The best dose to use for diagnostic ^{131}I whole-body imaging is controversial, as discussed by Reynolds and Robbins.[60] Higher doses of 5 to 10 mCi (185 to 370 MBq) are associated with higher sensitivity for the detection of metastatic disease, but the higher doses may also produce a "stunning" phenomenon, resulting in lower uptake by lesions after subsequent therapeutic administration of ^{131}I, creating the potential for less effective ablation of thyroid carcinoma metastases. Lower doses of 1 to 2 mCi (37 to 74 MBq) avoid the problem of stunning but also result in poorer image quality and decreased sensitivity for the detection of metastases. This study is appropriately performed only in patients who have already undergone subtotal or total thyroidectomy. Beierwaltes[61] and others have suggested that this study be performed 4 to 6 weeks after thyroidectomy without thyroid hormone supplementation or after withdrawal of thyroid supplements for approximately 6 weeks in order to obtain maximal endogenous thyroid-stimulating hormone (TSH) stimulation of uptake by functioning metastases. Previously, it was widespread practice to switch patients to the shorter-acting 3,5,5-triiodothyronine (Cytomel, Jones Pharma, St. Louis, MO) 6 weeks before imaging and to withdraw the hormone at 2 to 3 weeks before the study, permitting the patient to suffer a shorter period of symptomatic hypothyroidism. It is highly recommended to obtain serum TSH and thyroglobulin levels prior to imaging, with a TSH level of >30 µ IU/mL being indicative of adequate stimulation. The FDA has approved the use of a new form of recombinant human TSH (Thyrotropin alfa, Thyrogen, Genzyme Corporation, Cambridge, MA), which may be administered to patients

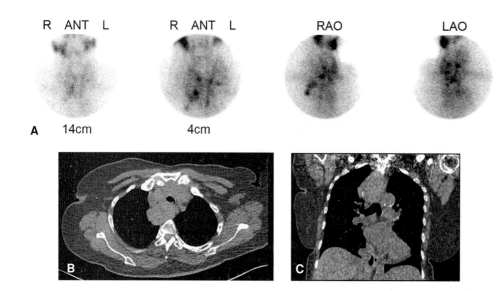

FIGURE 152.13 Substernal goiter. The patient is an 84-year-old woman with hyperthyroidism and multinodular goiter. I-131 uptake was normal at 19%. **A:** I-131 anterior pinhole image of the neck and upper mediastinum at 14 cm, with anterior, right anterior oblique, and left anterior oblique images of the neck and upper mediastinum at 4 cm. There is heterogeneous activity in the enlarged thyroid gland with substernal component, most consistent with a multinodular, substernal goiter. Axial (**B**) and coronal (**C**) CT images of the chest demonstrate enlargement of the thyroid gland with substernal extension into the upper mediastinum.

for 2 or 3 days prior to imaging without undergoing thyroid hormone withdrawal. This approach has been shown to be a less sensitive but acceptable alternative for diagnostic imaging in patients with low clinical risk for recurrent disease or those unable to tolerate hormone withdrawal, as described in the Thyrotropin alfa package insert.[62] It is best used in patients who have already undergone at least one negative hormone-withdrawal scan. The use of Thyrotropin alfa is probably not advisable for first postoperative evaluations or evaluation of patients at high risk for recurrence, since it has been shown to be less sensitive than hormone withdrawal for detecting lesions. Furthermore, the use of recombinant TSH is definitely not recommended for the preparation of patients for high-dose radioiodine therapy. In addition, serum pregnancy tests must be performed in women of childbearing age to preclude the possibility of administering the dose during pregnancy, which could have adverse effects on the fetus, especially if given after function of the fetal thyroid has begun. Women who are breast-feeding and even those still lactating after cessation of breast-feeding should not receive ^{131}I for evaluation of thyroid carcinoma because of unacceptably high radiation exposure to the fetus and maternal breasts, respectively. In selected cases, other radiopharmaceuticals may be used to evaluate specific patients, such as ^{18}F-FDG, thallium, ^{99m}Tc sestamibi, and, in the case of medullary carcinoma of the thyroid (which does not accumulate ^{131}I), ^{111}In octreotide, which was discussed earlier in this chapter.

Although metastases from thyroid carcinoma are most often found in cervical lymph nodes, the lungs, or skeleton, mediastinal metastases can also occur and can be detected by whole-body ^{131}I imaging, as demonstrated in Figure 152.14. Metastatic lesions and normal thyroid remnants, which may interfere with the future detection of recurrences, may be ablated with larger, therapeutic doses of ^{131}I, usually given in doses of 100 to 200 mCi (3,700 to 7,400 mBq) or even higher if dosimetry estimates are performed. Patients receiving therapeutic doses of >30 mCi (1,110 MBq) of ^{131}I generally do not need to be hospitalized according to the most recent Nuclear Regulatory Commission (NRC) regulations. All patients should undergo posttherapy whole-body ^{131}I scans, which are typically performed 3 to 7 days after the therapy. Because of the higher amount of radioactivity present, these posttherapy studies often demonstrate additional findings or better delineation of abnormalities than the diagnostic study, as described by Spies and colleagues.[63] Follow-up studies performed annually can be used to assess the response to therapy and detect and treat recurrences. In patients without evidence of recurrence, the follow-up interval may be increased to every 2 to 5 years. Suppressive doses of thyroid hormone are administered between studies, and serial thyroglobulin levels are also monitored. Recently, there has been growing support for ^{131}I treatment of patients with normal whole-body ^{131}I diagnostic studies but elevated serum thyroglobulin levels, as reviewed by Reynolds and Robbins.[60] In many such cases, functioning metastases may be visible on follow-up posttherapy scans. Alternatively, such patients may first undergo ^{18}F-FDG PET/CT imaging to assess for metastases without significant iodine uptake but with increased glucose metabolism, as reported by Chung,[64] Grunwald,[65] and Alnafisi[66] and their colleagues. An example of the utility of this approach is demonstrated in Figure 152.15. Lesions identified by this technique may be treated either with ^{131}I or surgically. In general, the better-differentiated lesions are more likely to be detected with ^{131}I imaging, whereas those that are less well-differentiated may be better detected with ^{18}F-FDG PET/CT.

Parathyroid imaging is useful in the preoperative evaluation of patients with biochemical evidence of primary or secondary

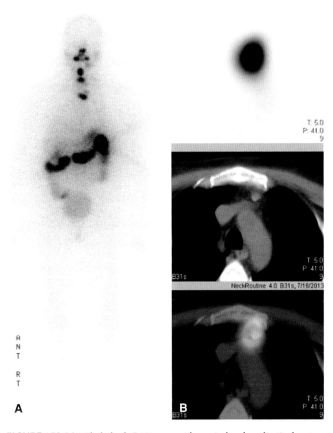

FIGURE 152.14 Whole-body I-131 scan with cervical and mediastinal metastases. The patient is a 44-year-old woman with papillary thyroid cancer post thyroidectomy 3 weeks earlier. **A:** Anterior whole-body I-131 image obtained 4 days after administration of a therapeutic dose of 150 mCi of I-131. There are foci of activity in the upper neck, lower neck, and upper mediastinum, most consistent with functioning thyroid tissue in the thyroidectomy bed and metastatic left level II and superior anterior mediastinal nodes. **B:** SPECT/CT image of the upper chest. There is increased activity in a partially-calcified, enlarged superior mediastinal lymph node, indicating that this is most likely a thyroid cancer metastasis.

hyperparathyroidism. Eighty-five percent of patients with primary hyperparathyroidism have a solitary parathyroid adenoma and 10% to 15% have hyperplasia of all four glands. While there is a 90% to 95% cure rate in experienced hands without any preoperative localization procedure, there remains a 5% to 10% recurrence rate, primarily due to ectopic lesions not located in the thyroid bed. Furthermore, reexploration is technically difficult and associated with higher morbidity and a poorer cure rate. The goals of preoperative localization include decreasing operative time, allowing unilateral neck dissection in some cases and minimizing the frequency of reexploration. Noninvasive parathyroid localization techniques include high-resolution ultrasonography, CT, MRI, and radionuclide imaging. Many authorities believe that ultrasonography and radionuclide imaging may be the best screening techniques for most patients at present, although both CT and MRI may play a role as well. Ultrasonography in particular is less likely to detect lesions in the upper mediastinum, where imaging is limited by absorption or reflection of the sound waves by air in lung tissue and the bones of the sternum.

Clinical studies for parathyroid imaging currently employ a single-isotope method using ^{99m}Tc sestamibi (methoxyisobutylisonitrile), a commonly used myocardial perfusion imaging agent. Sestamibi is taken up by thyroid and parathyroid tissue but demonstrates differential washout. Thus, immediate static images demonstrate

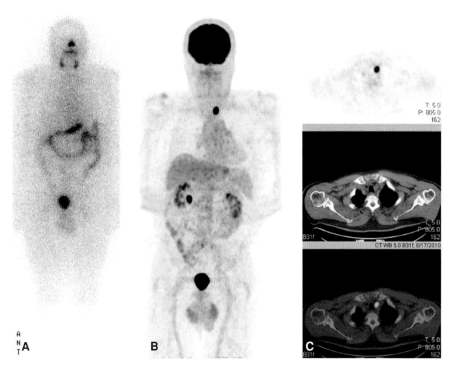

FIGURE 152.15 Whole-body I-131 scan and ^{18}F-FDG PET/CT scan in papillary thyroid carcinoma. This patient underwent total thyroidectomy 4 years earlier with multiple treatments with I-131. **A:** Follow-up I-131 whole-body scan. This study was normal, without functioning thyroid tissue. Serum thyroglobulin was <0.1 ng/mL with an elevated thyroglobulin antibody at 67 IU/mL. **B:** Maximum-intensity-projection image from an ^{18}F-FDG PET/CT scan. There is focally increased ^{18}F-FDG uptake in the left superior paratracheal region. **C:** Fused ^{18}F-FDG PET/CT image of the upper chest. There is focally increased ^{18}F-FDG uptake in an enlarged left superior paratracheal lymph node, most consistent with metastatic disease in a site not associated with significant I-131 uptake.

uptake in normal thyroid tissue and abnormal parathyroid tissue (i.e., adenomas or hyperplastic glands), but the normal thyroid activity washes out over time more rapidly than the parathyroid uptake. Three-hour delayed images demonstrate clear visualization of parathyroid adenomas without the need for subtraction, reregistration, or correction of dual-isotope cross talk (downscatter). In addition, the more favorable imaging characteristics of ^{99m}Tc compared with thallium also result in improved lesion visibility. Normal parathyroid glands are not usually visualized. Some authorities prefer to use ^{123}I subtraction even with sestamibi parathyroid imaging, but this step is often unnecessary. Multiple studies and two small meta-analyses have since shown that SPECT/CT imaging with ^{99m}Tc-sestamibi is superior to SPECT alone for diagnosis of parathyroid adenomas and preoperative planning and thus is the optimal imaging modality for this purpose.[67–72]

Using either technique, the presence of a parathyroid adenoma or diffuse parathyroid hyperplasia is indicated by a focal "hot" spot or spots. Although these lesions are most often found in the region of the thyroid bed, ectopic parathyroid tissue may occur in the neck or superior mediastinum, since the parathyroids embryologically descend into the neck and are variably located, especially the inferior parathyroids (see Fig. 152.16). As discussed, such mediastinal foci of tumor may be difficult to localize preoperatively using other modalities, particularly ultrasonography and especially in patients with recurrent hyperparathyroidism after a prior neck exploration. Radionuclide parathyroid scintigraphy has been reported to have a sensitivity in the range of 80% to 90%, with better results reported since the use of the single-isotope sestamibi method has become widespread. Sensitivity is related to the size of the lesion, with poorer sensitivity for lesions of <500 mg and for hyperplastic glands and with virtually 100% detection of lesions of >1,500 mg. Specificity is lower in patients without definite biochemical evidence of hyperparathyroidism. A common cause of false-positive imaging results is focal thyroid pathology, such as thyroid adenomas or, less often, carcinomas, which also accumulate thallium and ^{99m}Tc-sestamibi. Like all of the other methods, radionuclide parathyroid scintigraphy is also

less sensitive for detection of parathyroid hyperplasia, which is more common in secondary hyperparathyroidism, than it is for adenomas. Recently, the use of the intraoperative probe techniques developed for intraoperative lymphoscintigraphy studies, as discussed, has been applied to parathyroid scintigraphy as well, resulting in shorter, less invasive surgical procedures in these patients.

GALLIUM AND INDIUM LEUKOCYTE SCINTIGRAPHY

Gallium-67 (^{67}Ga) citrate and indium-111-labeled autologous WBCs (^{111}In-WBC) have been mainstays of imaging infections in the mediastinum. ^{67}Ga is a cyclotron-produced radionuclide with a physical half-life of 78 hours and several gamma photopeaks for imaging. ^{67}Ga is an iron analogue administered in the form of ^{67}Ga-citrate and has been used for evaluation of both inflammatory and neoplastic lesions; however, most neoplastic lesions assessed by ^{67}Ga-citrate are now routinely imaged with ^{18}F-FDG PET/CT. ^{111}In-WBC is generated by labelling leukocytes with ^{111}In-oxine ex vivo and then reinjecting them into the patient.

Currently, autologous leukocytes can be labeled with ^{111}In oxine and reinjected for imaging with SPECT/CT, as reviewed by Navalkissoor.[73] This radiopharmaceutical is more specific for infection than ^{67}Ga-citrate and is rarely taken up by neoplasms. Normal uptake is seen in the spleen, bone marrow, and liver. ^{111}In-WBC imaging may be preferred over gallium in certain clinical settings, but both are useful in evaluating suspected mediastinal infections. It should be noted that uptake in the lungs is normal early after injection of approximately 500 µCi (18.5 MBq) ^{111}In WBCs; imaging is therefore usually performed at 18 to 24 hours. Partly for this reason, Fineman and colleagues[74] and most other investigators favor the use of gallium over indium leukocytes when pulmonary parenchymal infections are suspected, as in AIDS patients. In indium leukocyte scintigraphy, unlike gallium, delayed imaging beyond 24 hours is rarely necessary. Gallium is probably also more useful in suspected chronic infections, since the

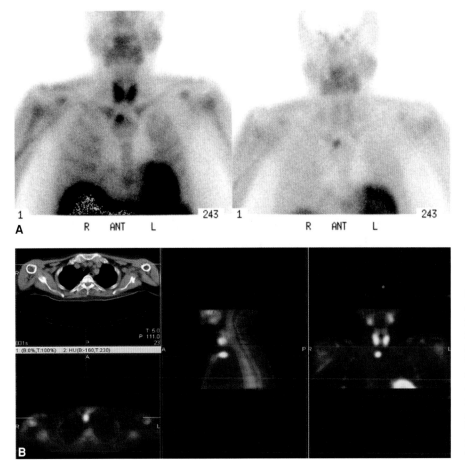

FIGURE 152.16 Ectopic parathyroid adenoma on a ^{99m}Tc-sestamibi study with SPECT/CT. **A:** Anterior immediate and delayed planar images of the entire neck and chest, obtained at 10 minutes and 2 hours, respectively, following intravenous administration of ^{99m}Tc-sestamibi. There is normal uptake in the thyroid and salivary glands and myocardium. There is a focus of persistent activity in the right aspect of the superior mediastinum. **B:** Non-contrast-enhanced CT image and SPECT/CT images of the chest. There is focal ^{99m}Tc-sestamibi uptake in the soft tissue nodule in the right aspect of the superior mediastinum, most consistent with an ectopic parathyroid adenoma.

majority of labeled leukocytes in ^{111}In-WBC imaging are neutrophils; thus the sensitivity of ^{111}In-WBC imaging for chronic infection is often lower. Other radiopharmaceuticals have also been developed for the detection of sites of infection—including ^{99m}Tc hexamethyl-propylene amine oxime (HMPAO)–labeled leukocytes, monoclonal antigranulocyte and polyclonal immunoglobulin G nonspecific antibodies, chemotactic peptide agents, liposomes, nanocolloids, and others—as reviewed by Peters[75] and by Becker,[76] Corstens,[77] and Fischman[78] and their colleagues. Of these, only the ^{99m}Tc-labeled leukocytes have achieved widespread clinical use to date.

^{18}F-FDG PET/CT imaging, as alluded to previously, can also easily detect infectious and inflammatory processes as the most common false-positive findings on PET imaging obtained for cancer staging are due to infection or inflammation-related increased glucose metabolism, including sarcoidosis, tuberculosis, abscesses, and other infections. As a result, ^{18}F-FDG PET/CT imaging may also play a potential role in the evaluation of suspected inflammatory processes, such as enterocolitis, musculoskeletal infections, cerebral infections and others, as described by Kresnik,[79] Temmerman,[80] DeWinter,[81] Stumpe,[82] Sugawara,[83] and Meyer[84] and their colleagues. This topic has also recently been reviewed by Hess and colleagues[85] and Vaidyanathan and colleagues.[86] However, this application of PET imaging is not currently approved or reimbursed for clinical use.

MONOCLONAL ANTIBODIES

Murine-produced monoclonal antibodies directed against a wide variety of human tumor antigens have been developed using hybrid-

oma techniques, as discussed by Halpern,[87] Oldham,[88] and Keenan[89] and their colleagues and by Larson.[90] Many of these antibodies have high affinity for human neoplasms, although there is often some overlap in specificity for related tumors. Currently, newer monoclonal antibodies with superior tumor uptake characteristics, including human and chimeric antibodies, are being developed. Monoclonal antibodies have been successfully radiolabeled with a variety of radionuclides, including ^{131}I, ^{111}In, yttrium-90 (^{90}Y), ^{99m}Tc, and others. These radiopharmaceuticals have been evaluated for use in the imaging of neoplasms such as lymphomas, melanoma, lung, colon, ovarian, prostatic, and breast carcinoma. At present, several monoclonal antibody radiopharmaceuticals have received FDA approval for clinical use as imaging agents, including agents directed against colorectal, ovarian, and prostate carcinoma and anticarcinoembryonic antigen antibodies, as reviewed by Abdel-Nabi and Doerr[91] as well as by Neal,[92] and Podoloff[93] and their colleagues. These studies have the potential advantage of more specific detection of tumor than standard anatomic imaging techniques. For example, it is possible to have enlarged but nonneoplastic lymph nodes detected by CT or, conversely, to have normal-sized but involved nodes, as often occurs in Hodgkin's lymphoma. Furthermore, monoclonal antibody imaging also allows for whole-body surveys, leading to the potential for detection of occult disease in clinically unsuspected sites. An example of a ProstaScint study is shown in Figure 152.17.

Labeling monoclonal antibodies with high-energy beta- or alpha-emitting radionuclides, such as ^{131}I and ^{90}Y, allows these agents to be used therapeutically, analogous to the use of free ^{131}I for treatment in well-differentiated thyroid carcinoma. Unlabeled monoclonal antibodies are also used for treatment of various neoplasms,

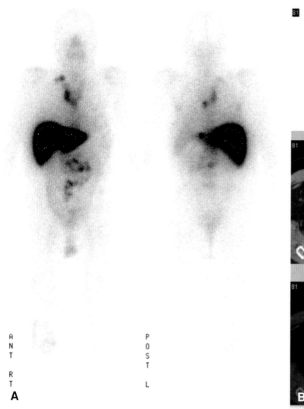

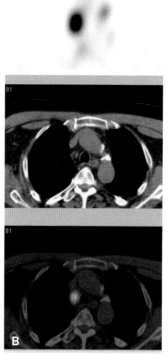

FIGURE 152.17 Abnormal ^{111}In-capromab pendetide (ProstaScint) monoclonal antibody study. The patient is a 70-year-old man presenting with increase in the serum prostate-specific antigen level approximately 3 years after radical prostatectomy for prostatic adenocarcinoma and adjuvant radiation therapy. He was placed on androgen blockade. **A:** Four-day whole-body planar images. There are numerous foci of increased activity in the right supraclavicular, mediastinal, retroperitoneal, and mesenteric regions, most consistent with widespread nodal metastases. The activity in the liver and faint activity in the spleen and blood pool represent normal findings. **B:** Attenuation-corrected ^{111}In-capromab pendetide, non-contrast-CT, and SPECT/CT images of the chest. There is focally increased activity in a right paratracheal lymph node, most consistent with nodal metastasis.

most commonly non-Hodgkin's lymphoma. The most commonly used agent of this type is the murine monoclonal antibody rituximab (Rituxan, Genentech, Inc., Vacaville, CA). The addition of radiolabeling with beta-emitting isotopes to the monoclonal antibody has been shown to enhance the tumoricidal effects of the agent. In general, radioimmunotherapy is associated with far fewer systemic side effects than standard chemotherapy or irradiation, although in some instances the high doses of radioactivity used may require hospitalization of patients for radiation safety considerations, particularly if the radionuclide used also has significant gamma emission, like [131]I. These therapeutic agents are associated with clinically significant bone marrow depression or, less often, other toxicity, but these adverse effects are usually self-limited and do not frequently require further intervention.

At present, most of the therapeutic monoclonal antibody agents being evaluated are directly against non-Hodgkin's lymphoma, as reviewed by Bischof Delaloye.[94] Previous agents of this type, such as the LYM-1 antibody (Oncolym, Peregrine Inc., Tustin, CA) were used with some success during the 1980s and 1990s, as reported by DeNardo and colleagues.[95] Newer agents are directed against the CD-20 cell surface antigen, which is found on over 90% of non-Hodgkin's lymphoma tumor cells. Studies to date have focused on the treatment of patients with refractory disease or those who have undergone transformation to more aggressive forms of non-Hodgkin's lymphoma. Studies demonstrating significant efficacy of these agents in this clinical setting, following standard therapy and even in patients refractory to unlabeled monoclonal antibody therapy, as reported by Witzig and colleagues,[96–98] have led to FDA approval of one ^{90}Y-labeled agent, ibritumomab tiuxetan (Zevalin, IDEC Pharmaceuticals Corporation, San Diego, CA). Overall response rates of approximately 70% have been reported, with complete response rates of up to 15%

to 30%, lasting for a mean of approximately 7 months. Another ^{131}I-labeled agent, tositumomab (Bexxar, Corixa Corporation, Seattle, WA), directed against the same antigen, has demonstrated similar efficacy and may soon receive approval as well. Hematologic toxicity is the primary form of toxicity noted in these patients, but as mentioned earlier, it is usually moderate in degree and is self-limited. Even patients with mild thrombocytopenia can safely be treated with reduced doses, as reported by Wiseman and colleagues.[99] Future developments in this field will focus on the wider application of radioimmunotherapy, the continued development of new antibodies having greater affinity and specificity for specific neoplasms, and perhaps the development of more human or humanized monoclonal antibodies, which could further reduce the problem of the development of human antimouse antibody (HAMA) responses, as described by De Jager and colleagues.[100] The development of a HAMA response, when it occurs, interferes with the repeated use of the antibody for imaging or therapy.

FUTURE DEVELOPMENTS

In this era of superb spatial resolution and three-dimensional digital image display provided by the various anatomic imaging modalities, such as CT and MRI, the thrust of nuclear medicine research has appropriately returned to the development of improved methods for the evaluation of human physiology and pathophysiology. Recent innovations in nuclear medicine techniques have largely involved the development of new radiopharmaceuticals that are better suited to specific clinical indications as well as improvements in instrumentation and data processing. The goals in developing new radiopharmaceuticals are to design agents that provide better image quality; more specific localization in various lesions and regions of interest; lower radiation

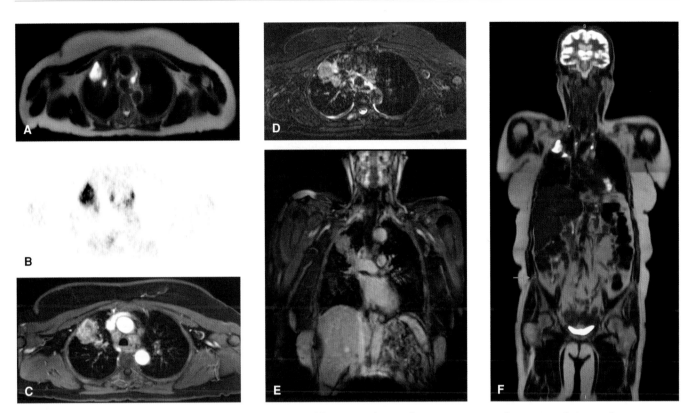

FIGURE 152.18 Abnormal PET MR study. The patient is a 60-year-old woman with cervical cancer presenting with extensive soft tissue and osseous metastases. **A:** Axial ^{18}F-FDG PET/MR image of the chest. There is markedly increased uptake in the right upper lobe mass and mediastinal lymphadenopathy. Axial non-attenuation–corrected ^{18}F-FDG PET/CT (**B**) and post-contrast T1 (**C**), pre-contrast fluid-sensitive (**D**), and coronal post-contrast T1 (**E**) MRI sequences demonstrate the large right upper lobe lung mass extending to the right hilum with paratracheal lymphadenopathy. The coronal ^{18}F-FDG PET/MR image (**F**) also demonstrates increased uptake in the right supraclavicular and superior mediastinal lymphadenopathy and in a right iliac crest lesion (*green arrow*).

exposure to patients, technologists, and physicians; easier preparation; lower cost; wider availability; and a minimum of side effects. Novel radiopharmaceuticals for PET imaging are being developed such as those discussed above for NETs, including new monoclonal antibodies and peptide receptor imaging agents, and the development of radioimmunotherapy and other forms of targeted radionuclide therapy using unsealed sources. In addition, the rapid growth of PET imaging in clinical oncology has spurred research aimed at developing newer PET radiopharmaceuticals directed against specific lesions not adequately addressed by ^{18}F-FDG. For example, ^{11}C-choline is now being used under an expanded access IND at several medical centers to image prostate cancer, which is not generally visualized with ^{18}F-FDG. Other PET radiopharmaceuticals labeled with ^{18}F and other radionuclides, such as ^{11}C, and agents consisting of radiolabeled compounds targeting other physiologic functions, such as protein synthesis, hormone receptors, and DNA synthesis, are also being developed and evaluated. Specifically, the clinical role of PET/CT imaging in the diagnosis, staging, and follow-up of primary and secondary tumors in the mediastinum with non-^{18}F-FDG radiopharmaceuticals is likely to be further expanded as additional data corroborating its use and increased reimbursement become available. PET/CT imaging is already now widely available at both academic and clinical imaging facilities, with both private and commercial ventures expanding the availability and affordability of ^{18}F-FDG as a routine clinical radiopharmaceutical. At present, the metabolic and pathophysiologic information provided by PET imaging is not obtainable by any other imaging modality, although research in whole-body diffusion-weighted MRI holds promise for imaging such processes.[101,102]

The major instrumentation development on the horizon is PET/MR imaging, with the number of scanners being installed in medical centers growing worldwide. An example of PET/MR images for a patient with metastatic cervical cancer involving the chest is shown in Figure 152.18. Early reports suggest that PET/MR performs similarly to PET/CT for most cancers, including non–small cell lung cancer.[103–105] The role of PET/MR remains to be investigated prospectively, however, as CT and MRI each have unique properties that make them suitable for specific indications (e.g., MRI provides better soft tissue contrast in the liver and pelvis than noncontrast CT). Further improvements in SPECT/CT and PET/CT image acquisition and reconstruction techniques also promise to improve the sensitivity and spatial resolution of images obtained with any radiopharmaceutical imaged with these modalities. Images from time-of-flight PET/CT scanners show improved lesion detectability, especially for larger patients, and are less susceptible to motion artifacts.[106] New ultrafast SPECT/CT cameras employing cadmium-zinc-telluride (CZT) solid-state detectors, developed for cardiac imaging, have improved count sensitivity and spatial resolution[107] when compared to the traditional NaI crystal-based Anger cameras that have been the cornerstone of nuclear medicine imaging for decades. Improvements in iterative reconstructive techniques for SPECT/CT can also reduce the acquisition time required while preserving or even improving spatial resolution.[107] Such improvements may also reduce the amount of radiopharmaceutical needed to obtain interpretable images, thus reducing radiation exposures for patients. These developments are likely to expand the imaging tools available to assess mediastinal pathology.

REFERENCES

1. Alderson PO, Line BR. Scintigraphic evaluation of regional pulmonary ventilation. *Semin Nucl Med* 1980;10(3):218–242.
2. Alderson PO, Rujanavech N, Sicker-Walker RH, et al. The role of 133Xe ventilation studies in the scintigraphic detection of pulmonary embolism. *Radiology* 1976;120(3):633–640.
3. Alderson PO, Secker-Walker RH, Forrest JV. Detection of obstructive pulmonary disease. Relative sensitivity of ventilation-perfusion studies and chest radiography. *Radiology* 1974;112(3):643–648.
4. Jogi J, Jonson B, Ekberg M, et al. Ventilation-perfusion SPECT with 99mTc-DTPA versus Technegas: a head-to-head study in obstructive and nonobstructive disease. *J Nucl Med* 2010;51(5):735–741.
5. Datz FL. Ventilation-perfusion mismatch: lung imaging. *Semin Nucl Med* 1980; 10(2):193–194.
6. White RI, James AE, Wagner HN. The significance of unilateral absence of pulmonary artery perfusion by lung scanning. *Am J Roentgenol Radium Ther Nucl Med* 1971;111(3):501–509.
7. Kristersson S, Lindell SE, Svanberg L. Prediction of pulmonary function loss due to pneumonectomy using 133 Xe-radiospirometry. *Chest* 1972;62(6):694–698.
8. Olsen GN, Block AJ, Swenson EW, et al. Pulmonary function evaluation of the lung resection candidate: a prospective study. *Am Rev Respir Dis* 1975;111(4):379–387.
9. Boysen PG, Block AJ, Olsen GN, et al. Prospective evaluation for pneumonectomy using the 99mtechnetium quantitative perfusion lung scan. *Chest* 1977; 72(4):422–425.
10. Williams CD, Brenowitz JB. "Prohibitive" lung function and major surgical procedures. *Am J Surg* 1976;132(6):763–766.
11. Wernly JA, DeMeester TR, Kirchner PT, et al. Clinical value of quantitative ventilation-perfusion lung scans in the surgical management of bronchogenic carcinoma. *J Thorac Cardiovasc Surg* 1980;80(4):535–543.
12. Block AJ, Olsen GN. Preoperative pulmonary function testing. *JAMA* 1976; 235(3):257–258.
13. Toronto Lung Transplant Group. Unilateral lung transplantation for pulmonary fibrosis. *N Engl J Med* 1986;314(18):1140–1145.
14. Wang SC, Fischer KC, Slone RM, et al. Perfusion scintigraphy in the evaluation for lung volume reduction surgery: correlation with clinical outcome. *Radiology* 1997; 205(1):243–248.
15. Leblanc M, Paul N. V/Q SPECT and computed tomographic pulmonary angiography. *Semin Nucl Med* 2010;40(6):426–441.
16. Toney LK, Wanner M, Miyaoka RS, et al. Improved prediction of lobar perfusion contribution using technetium-99m-labeled macroaggregate of albumin single photon emission computed tomography/computed tomography with attenuation correction. *J Thorac Cardiovasc Surg* 2014;148(5):2345–2352.
17. Knollmann D, Meyer A, Noack F, et al. Preoperative assessment of relative pulmonary lobar perfusion fraction in lung cancer patients. A rather simple three-dimensional CT-based vs. planar image-derived quantification. *Nuklearmedizin* 2015;54(4):178–182.
18. Chang AJ, Dehdashti F, Bradley JD. The role of positron emission tomography for non-small cell lung cancer. *Pract Radiat Oncol* 2011;1(4):282–288.
19. Gámez-Cenzano C, Pino-Sorroche F. Standardization and quantification in FDG-PET/CT imaging for staging and restaging of malignant disease. *PET Clin* 2014;9(2):117–127.
20. Tomasi G, Turkheimer F, Aboagye E. Importance of quantification for the analysis of PET data in oncology: review of current methods and trends for the future. *Mol Imaging Biol* 2012;14(2):131–146.
21. Webb WR, Gatsonis C, Zerhouni EA, et al. CT and MR imaging in staging non-small cell bronchogenic carcinoma: report of the Radiologic Diagnostic Oncology Group. *Radiology* 1991;178(3):705–713.
22. Al-Sugair A, Coleman RE. Applications of PET in lung cancer. *Semin Nucl Med* 1998;28(4):303–319.
23. Schmidt-Hansen M, Baldwin DR, Hasler E, et al. PET-CT for assessing mediastinal lymph node involvement in patients with suspected resectable non-small cell lung cancer. *Cochrane Database Syst Rev* 2014;11:CD009519.
24. Skoura E, Datseris IE, Platis I, et al. Role of positron emission tomography in the early prediction of response to chemotherapy in patients with non–small-cell lung cancer. *Clin Lung Cancer* 2012;13(3):181–187.
25. Lu YY, Chen JH, Liang JA, et al. 18F-FDG PET or PET/CT for detecting extensive disease in small-cell lung cancer: a systematic review and meta-analysis. *Nucl Med Commun* 2014;35(7):697–703.
26. Tirumani SH, LaCasce AS, Jacene HA. Role of 2-deoxy-2-[18F]-fluoro-d-glucose-PET/computed tomography in lymphoma. *PET Clin* 2015;10(2):207–225.
27. Rigacci L, Vitolo U, Nassi L, et al. Positron emission tomography in the staging of patients with Hodgkin's lymphoma. A prospective multicentric study by the Intergruppo Italiano Linfomi. *Ann Hematol* 2007;86(12):897–903.
28. Cheson BD, Fisher RI, Barrington SF, et al. Recommendations for initial evaluation, staging, and response assessment of Hodgkin and non-Hodgkin lymphoma: The Lugano classification. *J Clin Oncol* 2014;32(27):3059–3067.
29. Jerusalem G, Beguin Y, Fassotte MF, et al. Whole-body positron emission tomography using 18F-fluorodeoxyglucose for posttreatment evaluation in Hodgkin's disease and non-Hodgkin's lymphoma has higher diagnostic and prognostic value than classical computed tomography scan imaging. *Blood* 1999;94(2):429–433.
30. Markova J, Kahraman D, Kobe C, et al. Role of [18F]-fluoro-2-deoxy-D-glucose positron emission tomography in early and late therapy assessment of patients with advanced Hodgkin lymphoma treated with bleomycin, etoposide, adriamy-cin, cyclophosphamide, vincristine, procarbazine and prednisone. *Leuk Lymphoma* 2012;53(1):64–70.
31. Terasawa T, Lau J, Bardet S, et al. Fluorine-18-fluorodeoxyglucose positron emission tomography for interim response assessment of advanced-stage Hodgkin's lymphoma and diffuse large B-cell lymphoma: a systematic review. *J Clin Oncol* 2009;27(11):1906–1914.
32. Zinzani PL, Rigacci L, Stefoni V, et al. Early interim 18F-FDG PET in Hodgkin's lymphoma: evaluation on 304 patients. *Eur J Nucl Med Mol Imaging* 2012;39(1):4–12.
33. Meignan M, Gallamini A, Haioun C, et al. Report on the Second International Workshop on interim positron emission tomography in lymphoma held in Menton, France, 8-9 April 2010. *Leuk Lymphoma* 2010;51(12):2171–2180.
34. Meignan M, Gallamini A, Itti E, et al. Report on the Third International Workshop on interim positron emission tomography in lymphoma held in Menton, France, 26-27 September 2011 and Menton 2011 consensus. *Leuk Lymphoma* 2012;53(10):1876–1881.
35. Hoffmann M, Kletter K, Diemling M, et al. Positron emission tomography with fluorine-18-2-fluoro-2-deoxy-D-glucose (F18-FDG) does not visualize extranodal B-cell lymphoma of the mucosa-associated lymphoid tissue (MALT)-type. *Ann Oncol* 1999;10(10):1185–1189.
36. Kwee RM, Marcus C, Sheikhbahaei S, et al. PET with fluorodeoxyglucose F 18/computed tomography in the clinical management and patient outcomes of esophageal cancer. *PET Clin* 2015;10(2):197–205.
37. Walker AJ, Spier BJ, Perlman SB, et al. Integrated PET/CT fusion imaging and endoscopic ultrasound in the pre-operative staging and evaluation of esophageal cancer. *Mol Imaging Biol* 2011;13(1):166–71.
38. Barber TW, Duong CP, Leong T, et al. 18F-FDG PET/CT has a high impact on patient management and provides powerful prognostic stratification in the primary staging of esophageal cancer: a prospective study with mature survival data. *J Nucl Med* 2012;53(6):864–871.
39. Malik V, Johnston C, Donohoe C, et al. (18)F-FDG PET-detected synchronous primary neoplasms in the staging of esophageal cancer: incidence, cost, and impact on management. *Clin Nucl Med* 2012;37(12):1152–1158.
40. Pan L, Gu P, Huang G, et al. Prognostic significance of SUV on PET/CT in patients with esophageal cancer: a systematic review and meta-analysis. *Eur J Gastroenterol Hepatol* 2009;21(9):1008–1015.
41. Omloo JM, van Heijl M, Hoekstra OS, et al. FDG-PET parameters as prognostic factor in esophageal cancer patients: a review. *Ann Surg Oncol* 2011;18(12):3338–3352.
42. Lebron L, Greenspan D, Pandit-Taskar N. PET imaging of breast cancer: role in patient management. *PET Clin* 2015;10(2):159–195.
43. Veronesi U, De Cicco C, Galimberti VE, et al. A comparative study on the value of FDG-PET and sentinel node biopsy to identify occult axillary metastases. *Ann Oncol* 2007;18(3):473–478.
44. Olsen JO, Pozderac RV, Hinkle G, et al. Somatostatin receptor imaging of neuroendocrine tumors with indium-111 pentetreotide (Octreoscan). *Semin Nucl Med* 1995;25(3):251–261.
45. Krenning EP, Bakker WH, Kooij PP, et al. Somatostatin receptor scintigraphy with indium-111-DTPA-D-Phe-1-octreotide in man: metabolism, dosimetry and comparison with iodine-123-Tyr-3-octreotide. *J Nucl Med* 1992;33(5):652–658.
46. Johnbeck CB, Knigge U, Kjaer A. PET tracers for somatostatin receptor imaging of neuroendocrine tumors: current status and review of the literature. *Future Oncol* 2014;10(14):2259–2277.
47. Al-Nahhas A, Win Z, Szyszko T, et al. Gallium-68 PET: a new frontier in receptor cancer imaging. *Anticancer Res* 2007;27(6B):4087–4094.
48. Pavel M, Baudin E, Couvelard A, et al. ENETS Consensus Guidelines for the management of patients with liver and other distant metastases from neuroendocrine neoplasms of foregut, midgut, hindgut, and unknown primary. *Neuroendocrinology* 2012;95(2):157–176.
49. Pape UF, Perren A, Niederle B, et al. ENETS Consensus Guidelines for the management of patients with neuroendocrine neoplasms from the jejuno-ileum and the appendix including goblet cell carcinomas. *Neuroendocrinology* 2012;95(2):135–156.
50. Falconi M, Bartsch DK, Eriksson B, et al. ENETS Consensus Guidelines for the management of patients with digestive neuroendocrine neoplasms of the digestive system: well-differentiated pancreatic non-functioning tumors. *Neuroendocrinology* 2012;95(2):120–134.
51. Caplin M, Sundin A, Nillson O, et al. ENETS Consensus Guidelines for the management of patients with digestive neuroendocrine neoplasms: colorectal neuroendocrine neoplasms. *Neuroendocrinology* 2012;95(2):88–97.
52. Jensen RT, Cadiot G, Brandi ML, et al. ENETS Consensus Guidelines for the management of patients with digestive neuroendocrine neoplasms: functional pancreatic endocrine tumor syndromes. *Neuroendocrinology* 2012;95(2):98–119.
53. Pfeifer A, Knigge U, Binderup T, et al. 64Cu-DOTATATE PET for neuroendocrine tumors: a prospective head-to-head comparison with 111In-DTPA-octreotide in 112 patients. *J Nucl Med* 2015;56(6):847–854.
54. Lynn MD, Shapiro B, Sisson JC, et al. Pheochromocytoma and the normal adrenal medulla: improved visualization with I-123 MIBG scintigraphy. *Radiology* 1985; 155(3):789–792.
55. Bleeker G, Tytgat GA, Adam JA, et al. 123I-MIBG scintigraphy and 18F-FDG-PET imaging for diagnosing neuroblastoma. *Cochrane Database Syst Rev* 2015;9: CD009263.
56. Shapiro B, Copp JE, Sisson JC, et al. Iodine-131 metaiodobenzylguanidine for the locating of suspected pheochromocytoma: experience in 400 cases. *J Nucl Med* 1985;26(6):576–585.
57. Elgazzar AH, Gelfand MJ, Washburn LC, et al. I-123 MIBG scintigraphy in adults. A report of clinical experience. *Clin Nucl Med* 1995;20(2):147–152.

58. Van Der Horst-Schrivers AN, Jager PL, Boezen HM, et al. Iodine-123 metaiodo-benzylguanidine scintigraphy in localising phaeochromocytomas-experience and meta-analysis. *Anticancer Res* 2006;26(2B):1599–1604.
59. Fukuoka M, Taki J, Mochizuki T, et al. Comparison of diagnostic value of I-123 MIBG and high-dose I-131 MIBG scintigraphy including incremental value of SPECT/CT over planar image in patients with malignant pheochromocytoma/paraganglioma and neuroblastoma. *Clin Nucl Med* 2011;36(1):1–7.
60. Reynolds JC, Robbins J. The changing role of radioiodine in the management of differentiated thyroid cancer. *Semin Nucl Med* 1997;27(2):152–164.
61. Beierwaltes WH. The treatment of thyroid carcinoma with radioactive iodine. *Semin Nucl Med* 1978;8(1):79–94.
62. *Thyrogen Complete Prescribing Information.* Cambridge, Massachusetts: G.C. Genzyme Therapeutics, and Knoll Pharmaceutical Company; 1998.
63. Spies WG, Wojtowicz CH, Spies SM, et al. Value of post-therapy whole-body I-131 imaging in the evaluation of patients with thyroid carcinoma having undergone high-dose I-131 therapy. *Clin Nucl Med* 1989;14(11):793–800.
64. Chung JK, So Y, Lee JS, et al. Value of FDG PET in papillary thyroid carcinoma with negative 131I whole-body scan. *J Nucl Med* 1999;40(6):986–992.
65. Grunwald F, Kalicke T, Feine U, et al. Fluorine-18 fluorodeoxyglucose positron emission tomography in thyroid cancer: results of a multicentre study. *Eur J Nucl Med* 1999;26(12):1547–1552.
66. Alnafisi NS, Driedger AA, Coates G, et al. FDG PET of recurrent or metastatic 131I-negative papillary thyroid carcinoma. *J Nucl Med* 2000;41(6):1010–1015.
67. Lavely WC, Goetze S, Friedman KP, et al. Comparison of SPECT/CT, SPECT, and planar imaging with single- and dual-phase (99m)Tc-sestamibi parathyroid scintigraphy. *J Nucl Med* 2007;48(7):1084–1089.
68. Eslamy HK, Ziessman HA. Parathyroid scintigraphy in patients with primary hyperparathyroidism: 99mTc sestamibi SPECT and SPECT/CT. *Radiographics* 2008;28(5):1461–1476.
69. Shafiei B, Hoseinzadeh S, Fotouhi F, et al. Preoperative (9)(9)mTc-sestamibi scintigraphy in patients with primary hyperparathyroidism and concomitant nodular goiter: comparison of SPECT-CT, SPECT, and planar imaging. *Nucl Med Commun* 2012;33(10):1070–1076.
70. Kim YI, Jung YH, Hwang KT, et al. Efficacy of (9)(9)mTc-sestamibi SPECT/CT for minimally invasive parathyroidectomy: comparative study with (9)(9)mTc-sestamibi scintigraphy, SPECT, US and CT. *Ann Nucl Med* 2012;26(10):804–810.
71. Wong KK, Fig LM, Gross MD, et al. Parathyroid adenoma localization with 99mTc-sestamibi SPECT/CT: a meta-analysis. *Nucl Med Commun* 2015;36(4):363–375.
72. Wei WJ, Shen CT, Song HJ, et al. Comparison of SPET/CT, SPET and planar imaging using 99mTc-MIBI as independent techniques to support minimally invasive parathyroidectomy in primary hyperparathyroidism: a meta-analysis. *Hell J Nucl Med* 2015;18(2):127–135.
73. Navalkissoor S, Nowosinska E, Gnanasegaran G, et al. Single-photon emission computed tomography-computed tomography in imaging infection. *Nucl Med Commun* 2013;34(4):283–290.
74. Fineman DS, Palestro CJ, Kim CK, et al. Detection of abnormalities in febrile AIDS patients with In-111-labeled leukocyte and Ga-67 scintigraphy. *Radiology* 1989;170(3 Pt 1):677–680.
75. Peters AM. The utility of [99mTc]HMPAO-leukocytes for imaging infection. *Semin Nucl Med* 1994;24(2):110–127.
76. Becker W, Goldenberg DM, Wolf F. The use of monoclonal antibodies and antibody fragments in the imaging of infectious lesions. *Semin Nucl Med* 1994;24(2):142–153.
77. Corstens FH, Oyen WJ, Becker WS. Radioimmunoconjugates in the detection of infection and inflammation. *Semin Nucl Med* 1993;23(2):148–164.
78. Fischman AJ, Babich JW, Rubin RH. Infection imaging with technetium-99m-labeled chemotactic peptide analogs. *Semin Nucl Med* 1994;24(2):154–168.
79. Kresnik E, Gallowitsch HJ, Mikosch P, et al. (18)F-FDG positron emission tomography in the early diagnosis of enterocolitis: preliminary results. *Eur J Nucl Med Mol Imaging* 2002;29(10):1389–1392.
80. Temmerman OP, Heyligers IC, Hoekstra OS, et al. Detection of osteomyelitis using FDG and positron emission tomography. *J Arthroplasty* 2001;16(2):243–246.
81. de Winter F, van de Wiele C, Vogelaers D, et al. Fluorine-18 fluorodeoxyglucose-position emission tomography: a highly accurate imaging modality for the diagnosis of chronic musculoskeletal infections. *J Bone Joint Surg Am* 2001;83-A(5):651–660.
82. Stumpe KD, Dazzi H, Schaffner A, et al. Infection imaging using whole-body FDG-PET. *Eur J Nucl Med* 2000;27(7):822–832.
83. Sugawara Y, Braun DK, Kison PV, et al. Rapid detection of human infections with fluorine-18 fluorodeoxyglucose and positron emission tomography: preliminary results. *Eur J Nucl Med* 1998;25(9):1238–1243.
84. Meyer MA, Hubner KF, Raja S, et al. Sequential positron emission tomographic evaluations of brain metabolism in acute herpes encephalitis. *J Neuroimaging* 1994;4(2):104–105.
85. Hess S, Hansson SH, Pedersen KT, et al. FDG-PET/CT in infectious and inflammatory diseases. *PET Clin* 2014;9(4):497–519, vi–vii.
86. Vaidyanathan S, Patel CN, Scarsbrook AF, et al. FDG PET/CT in infection and inflammation—current and emerging clinical applications. *Clin Radiol* 2015;70(7):787–800.
87. Halpern SE, Dillman RO, Hagan PL. The problems and promise of monoclonal antitumor antibodies. *Diagn Imaging* 1983;5:40–47.
88. Oldham RK. Monoclonal antibodies in cancer therapy. *J Clin Oncol* 1983;1(9):582–590.
89. Keenan AM, Harbert JC, Larson SM, Monoclonal antibodies in nuclear medicine. *J Nucl Med* 1985;26(5):531–537.
90. Larson SM. Radiolabeled monoclonal anti-tumor antibodies in diagnosis and therapy. *J Nucl Med* 1985;26(5):538–545.
91. Abdel-Nabi H, Doerr RJ. Clinical applications of indium-111-labeled monoclonal antibody imaging in colorectal cancer patients. *Semin Nucl Med* 1993;23(2):99–113.
92. Neal CE, Swenson LC, Fanning J, et al. Monoclonal antibodies in ovarian and prostate cancer. *Semin Nucl Med* 1993;23(2):114–126.
93. Podoloff DA, Patt YZ, Curley SA, et al. Imaging of colorectal carcinoma with technetium-99m radiolabeled Fab' fragments. *Semin Nucl Med* 1993;23(2):89–98.
94. Bischof Delaloye A. Radioimmunoimaging and radioimmunotherapy: will these be routine procedures? *Semin Nucl Med* 2000;30(3):186–194.
95. DeNardo SJ, DeNardo GL, O'Grady LF, et al. Treatment of B cell malignancies with 131I Lym-1 monoclonal antibodies. *Int J Cancer Suppl* 1988;3:96–101.
96. Witzig TE, Flinn IW, Gordon LI, et al. Treatment with ibritumomab tiuxetan radioimmunotherapy in patients with rituximab-refractory follicular non-Hodgkin's lymphoma. *J Clin Oncol* 2002;20(15):3262–3269.
97. Witzig TE, Gordon LI, Cabanillas F, et al. Randomized controlled trial of yttrium-90-labeled ibritumomab tiuxetan radioimmunotherapy versus rituximab immunotherapy for patients with relapsed or refractory low-grade, follicular, or transformed B-cell non-Hodgkin's lymphoma. *J Clin Oncol* 2002;20(10):2453–2463.
98. Witzig TE, White CA, Wiseman GA, et al. Phase I/II trial of IDEC-Y2B8 radioimmunotherapy for treatment of relapsed or refractory CD20(+) B-cell non-Hodgkin's lymphoma. *J Clin Oncol* 1999;17(12):3793–3803.
99. Wiseman GA, Gordon LI, Multani PS, et al. Ibritumomab tiuxetan radioimmunotherapy for patients with relapsed or refractory non-Hodgkin lymphoma and mild thrombocytopenia: a phase II multicenter trial. *Blood* 2002;99(12):4336–4342.
100. De Jager R, Abdel-Nabi H, Serafini A, et al. Current status of cancer immunodetection with radiolabeled human monoclonal antibodies. *Semin Nucl Med* 1993;23(2):165–179.
101. Ohno Y, Koyama H, Onishi Y, et al. Non-small cell lung cancer: whole-body MR examination for M-stage assessment—utility for whole-body diffusion-weighted imaging compared with integrated FDG PET/CT. *Radiology* 2008;248(2):643–654.
102. Yi CA, Shin KM, Lee KS, et al. Non-small cell lung cancer staging: efficacy comparison of integrated PET/CT versus 3.0-T whole-body MR imaging. *Radiology* 2008;248(2):632–642.
103. Al-Nabhani KZ, Syed R, Michopoulou S, et al. Qualitative and quantitative comparison of PET/CT and PET/MR imaging in clinical practice. *J Nucl Med* 2014;55(1):88–94.
104. Heusch P, Buchbender C, Kohler J, et al. Thoracic staging in lung cancer: prospective comparison of 18F-FDG PET/MR imaging and 18F-FDG PET/CT. *J Nucl Med* 2014;55(3):373–378.
105. Drzezga A, Souvatzoglou M, Eiber M, et al. First clinical experience with integrated whole-body PET/MR: comparison to PET/CT in patients with oncologic diagnoses. *J Nucl Med* 2012;53(6):845–855.
106. Surti S. Update on time-of-flight PET imaging. *J Nucl Med* 2015;56(1):98–105.
107. Garcia EV, Faber TL, Esteves FP. Cardiac dedicated ultrafast SPECT cameras: new designs and clinical implications. *J Nucl Med* 2011;52(2):210–217.

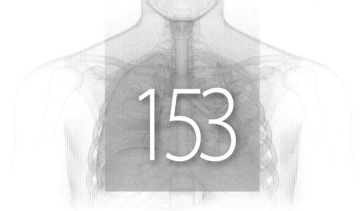

153

Mediastinal Tumor Markers

Mirella Marino ▪ Rossano Lattanzio ▪ Edoardo Pescarmona

TUMOR MARKERS: DEFINITION AND OVERVIEW

Tumor markers are indicators with diagnostic or prognostic or predictive relevance for each type of neoplasia. Tumor markers with high levels of specificity and/or sensitivity, however, are still not yet known. According to the NIH, a biomarker is defined as "a characteristic used to measure and evaluate objectively normal biological processes, pathogenic processes, or pharmacological responses to a therapeutic intervention."[1]

Biomarkers belong to different molecular classes of organic compounds, such as DNA, RNA, proteins, peptides, and metabolites. The most studied and used molecules are proteins, controlling most biological processes. Protein biomarkers are widely used in the diagnostic phase. A marker with prognostic relevance is a disease characteristic at the time of diagnosis providing information about the natural history of the disease, independent of therapy. On the other hand, a predictive biomarker predicts response to a therapeutic intervention compared to the effect of a different therapy or no treatment. Predictive biomarkers set the stage for the development of personalized medicine. Serum tumor markers include hormones, enzymes, intracellular proteins, or cell membrane antigens detectable or measured in serum, plasma, urine or other body fluids. Tissue tumor markers are differentiating or signaling antigens or cellular structural components/products, such as proteins or hormones, detectable by immunologic techniques in different cellular compartments (membrane, cytoplasm, or nucleus) in fresh, frozen, or in formalin-fixed, paraffin-embedded (FFPE) tissue sections. Here, the authors present and discuss serum markers of mediastinal tumors with a variety of sensitivity/specificity, to be used in the appropriate clinical and laboratory context for diagnostic purposes. None of these markers are really specific to a single tumor that can be used in a screening test, however, all contribute to the diagnosis. Some diagnostic biomarkers imply a prognostic relevance and have to be looked at for staging and follow-up (FU). Furthermore, the authors introduce and discuss immunity-related serum markers variably associated with mediastinal tumors/pseudotumors.

MEDIASTINAL TUMOR MARKERS

The broad spectrum of mediastinal tumors is reflected in the variety of markers they can elicit. Markers reflecting the genetic characteristics, the differentiation lineage, and endocrine or neuroendocrine production specificities of the tumor are of diagnostic value in the preliminary workup of a new case. Whereas markers of prognostic/predictive significance drive the patient's evaluation and treatment. Markers related to the most frequent and relevant diagnostic tumor categories are discussed according to the 2015 WHO classification.[2] Due to the variety of mediastinal tumors, among the less frequent neoplastic entities, only those associated with specific/characteristic serum or tissue markers or clinical syndromes will be discussed here. Moreover, a brief mention will be made in the Genetic markers section, for those tumors with an identified genetic trait. The reader must refer to specific treatises or reviews or to updated references for tumors not covered here. The mediastinum is a virtual space consisting of vital anatomical structures. Its complex embryological derivation and the difficulty in approaching deep-located masses for diagnostic purposes justify either marker's relevance in diagnostics or interest in developing this field. The surgeon and/or the neurosurgeon or the oncologist during the preliminary workup of patients with mediastinal masses should consider a variety of demographical characteristics, symptoms, imaging features, and serological findings in order to start/proceed with a diagnostic algorithm able to dissect among several diagnostic possibilities and to address adequate diagnostic procedures. The diagnostic algorithm should first take into consideration the age, sex, and location of the mass.[3,4] Contemporarily, a blood-based exam (blood cells and serum products) should be considered in order to exclude leukemic spread from the mass and/or tumor products/hormones increased levels.

Table 153.1 reports the distribution in the mediastinal tumors by their location and Table 153.2 according to their age and frequency distribution. Table 153.3 proposes a list of mediastinal tumors specifically associated with serum and laboratory markers and associated diseases. Whereas the most frequent tumors of the

TABLE 153.1 Diagnosis of Mediastinal Masses by Location

Superior mediastinum	Thymic epithelial tumors (TET); ectopic thyroid tissue
Anterior mediastinum	Teratoma Lymphoma Germ cell tumors (GCT) TET
Middle mediastinum	Pericardial–Bronchogenic–Enteric cysts Lymphoma
Posterior mediastinum	Neurogenic tumors Esophageal diseases

TABLE 153.2 Diagnosis of Mediastinal Masses by Age and Frequencies

Children	Adults
Neurogenic tumors 40%	Thymic epithelial tumors (TETs) 30%
Neuroblastoma 27%	Germinal cell tumors (GCT) 23%
Teratoma and non-Hodgkin lymphomas 14%	Lymphoma 19%
Enteric cysts and ganglio-neuroma 0.09%	Neurogenic tumors 12%

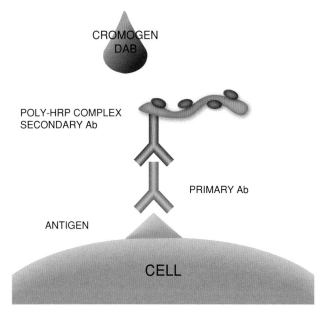

CROMOGEN DAB

POLY-HRP COMPLEX SECONDARY Ab

PRIMARY Ab

ANTIGEN

CELL

mediastinum occurring in adults, the thymic epithelial tumors (TETs) (Table 153.4) are not associated with a currently recognized and relevant hormonal/cell product increase in the serum, an important exception must be made. In fact, a vast percentage of TET is associated with autoimmune derangements/immune disorders and/or immunodeficiency leading to neuromuscular disorders or collagen/autoimmune diseases (ADs) (Table 153.5).[5] In ADs, autoantibody detection, alone or associated with already present symptoms, could constitute a "clue" in the detection of an underlining mediastinal tumor. Among the most relevant mediastinal tumors producing hormones or cell products are the germ cell tumors (GCTs), similar to their gonadal counterparts (Table 153.6). Therefore, a new tool for diagnostics arises, as an informed diagnostic algorithm considering the tumor-serum interplay has to be planned by the specialist who first deal with the mediastinal mass. As a further advance, immunohistochemistry (IHC) is nowadays a fundamental tool for pathologists, contributing to the diagnosis

FIGURE 153.1 Bond Polymer Refine Detection works as follows: The specimen is incubated with hydrogen peroxide to quench endogenous peroxidase activity. A user-supplied specific primary antibody is applied. Post primary IgG linker reagent localizes mouse antibodies. Poly-HRP IgG reagent localizes rabbit antibodies. The substrate chromogen, 3,3′-diaminobenzidine tetrahydrochloride (DAB), visualizes the complex via a brown precipitate. Hematoxylin (blue) counterstaining allows the visualization of cell nuclei. Using Bond Polymer Refine Detection in combination with the Bond automated system reduces the possibility of human error and inherent variability resulting from individual reagent dilution, manual pipetting, and reagent application.

TABLE 153.3 Tumors and Pseudotumors of the Mediastinum Associated to Their (Most Relevant) Serum Markers

Tumor (or Pseudotumor) Type	Hormones or Cellular Product Increase or Alterations in Normal Serum/Blood Components	Antibody Production	Associated Disease or Tumors
Germ cell tumors	alpha-fetoprotein β-HCG CEA PLAP[a] NSE[a] LDH[a]	–	Seminoma, embryonal carcinoma, yolk-sac tumor, choriocarcinoma, teratocarcinoma
Thymoma	Hypogammaglobulinemia Lymphopenia	Anti-AChr[b] Anti-MuSK[b] Anti-Titin[b] Anti-RyR[b] Other specific tissue auto-Ab	Myasthenia gravis (MG) Good syndrome Pure red cell aplasia Hashimoto thyroiditis Systemic Lupus Erythematosus (SLE) other collagen diseases
Thymic Neuroendocrine tumors	ACTH Parathyroid hormone increase		Cushing syndrome Hypercalcaemia and hypophosphatemia
Thymolipoma		Anti-AChR	MG
Pheochromocytomas, Neuroblastomas, Ganglioneuroblastomas	Catecholamine increase VIP increase ADH increase		Hypertension and headaches VIP and ADH production syndromes
Castleman disease	Hypergammaglobulinemia Thrombocytopenia	Anti-HHV8 Antibodies	Lymphoproliferative disorder
Sclerosing mediastinitis	IgG4 increase		IgG4-RD

[a]Not specific.
[b]Ball the antibodies are associated to myasthenia gravis.
AFP, α-fetoprotein; β-HCG, β-subunit of human chorionic gonadotropin; CEA, carcinoembryonic antigen; NSE, neuron-specific enolase; LDH, lactate dehydrogenase; SLE, systemic lupus erythematosus; MuSK, muscle-specific tyrosine kinase; anti-RyR, anti-ryanodine receptor; ACTH, adrenocorticotropic hormone; VIP, vasoactive intestinal peptide secretion; ADH, antidiuretic hormone; IgG4-RD, IgG4-related disease.

TABLE 153.4 WHO Classification 2015 of Thymic Epithelial Tumours

Epithelial tumors	Thymic neuroendocrine tumors
Thymoma	Carcinoid tumors
Type A Thymoma (including atypical variant)	Typical carcinoid
Type AB thymoma	Atypical carcinoid
Type B1 thymoma	Large cell neuroendocrine carcinoma
Type B2 thymoma	Combined large cell neuroendocrine carcinoma
Type B3 thymoma	Small cell carcinoma
Micronodular thymoma with lymphoid stroma	Combined small cell carcinoma
Metaplastic thymoma	
Other rare thymomas	
Microscopic thymoma	Combined thymic carcinomas
Sclerosing thymoma	
Lipofibroadenoma	
Thymic carcinoma	
Squamous cell carcinoma	
Basaloid carcinoma	
Mucoepidermoid carcinoma	
Lymphoepithelioma-like carcinoma	
Clear cell carcinoma	
Sarcomatoid carcinoma	
Adenocarcinomas	
Papillary adenocarcinoma	
Thymic carcinoma with adenoid cystic carcinoma-like features	
Mucinous adenocarcinoma	
Adenocarcinoma NOS	
NUT carcinoma	
Undifferentiated carcinoma	
Other rare thymic carcinomas	
Adenosquamous carcinoma	
Hepatoid carcinoma	
Thymic carcinoma, NOS	

Modified with permission from Travis WD, Brambilla E, Burke AP, Marx A, Nicholson AG. *World Health Organization Classification of Tumours of the Lung, Pleura, Thymus and Heart*. Vol. 7. 4th ed. Lyon: IARC Press, 2015.

TABLE 153.5 Autoimmune and Paraneoplastic Disorders Associated With Thymoma[a,b]

Neuromuscular Disorders	*Immune Deficiency Disorders*
Myasthenia gravis (MG)	Hypogammaglobulinemia (Good's syndrome)
Limbic encephalopathy	T-cell deficiency syndrome
Peripheral Neuropathy	
Neuromyotonia	Endocrine disorders
Stiff person syndrome	Autoimmune polyglandular syndrome
Polymyositis	Addison syndrome
	Thyroiditis
Hematological Disorders	
Red cell aplasia	Dermatological disorders
Pernicious anemia	Pemphigus
Pancytopenia	Lichen planus
Hemolytic anemia	Chronic mucocutaneous candidiasis
	Alopecia areata
Collagen and Autoimmune Disorders	
Systemic lupus erythematosus	Miscellaneous disorders
Rheumatoid arthritis	Giant cell myocarditis
Sjögren syndrome	Glomerulonephritis/nephritic syndrome
Scleroderma	Ulcerative colitis
Interstitial pneumonitis	Hypertrophic osteoarthropathy

[a]Klein R, Marx A, Ströbel P, et al. Autoimmune associations and autoantibody screening show focused recognition in patient subgroups with generalized myasthenia gravis. *Hum Immunol* 2013;74:1184–1193.
[b]Marx A, Willcox N, Leite MI, et al. Thymoma and paraneoplastic myasthenia gravis. *Autoimmunity* 2010;43:413–427.
Modified with permission from Travis WD, Brambilla E, Burke AP, Marx A, Nicholson AG. *World Health Organization Classification of Tumours of the Lung, Pleura, Thymus and Heart*. Vol. 7. 4th ed. Lyon: IARC Press, 2015.

on tumor tissue and cells derived from surgical approaches (Fig. 153.1). A further important point to consider is that most of mediastinal tumors are rare. It would be advisable to discuss and to share cases and diagnostic procedures and problems with a local institutional and/or regional/national tumor board.[6,7]

PRIMARY MEDIASTINAL GERM CELL TUMORS—SERUM AND IMMUNOHISTOCHEMICAL MARKERS

Primary mediastinal GCTs are rare neoplasms that account for only 10% to 20% of all mediastinal tumors.[8,9] GCTs are believed to arise from ectopic primordial germ cells (GC) that fail to migrate to the urogenital ridge during development, escaping from the influence of their primary organizer during embryonic development and which reside in the thymic gland, or in thymic cells that possess the potential to differentiate toward germ cells.[10] Another hypothesis

is that they represent metastatic testicular lesions where the primary lesion has regressed. GCTs maintain the same histological features, cytogenetic abnormalities (isochromosome 12p), and serum tumor marker expression of the gonadal counterpart.[11] Even if rare, approximately 54% of extragonadal GCTs are located in the anterior mediastinum. This is disproportionally high among the midline structures, presumably due to a favorable microenvironment for GCT development in the developing thymus.[12] GCTs pose diagnostic challenges due to their rarity and often there is limited tissue obtained for diagnosis.[13] The clinical course of GCTs should

TABLE 153.6 WHO Classification 2015 of Germ Cell Tumors of the Mediastinum

Seminoma
Embryonal carcinoma
Yolk sac tumor
Choriocarcinoma
Teratoma
Mature teratoma
Immature teratoma
Mixed germ cell tumors
Germ cell tumors with somatic-type malignancy
Germ cell tumors with associated
Hematologic malignancy

Modified with permission from Travis WD, Brambilla E, Burke AP, Marx A, Nicholson AG. *World Health Organization Classification of Tumours of the Lung, Pleura, Thymus and Heart*. Vol. 7. 4th ed. Lyon: IARC Press, 2015.

TABLE 153.7 Immunohistochemical Staining Markers of Germ Cell Tumors

Immunomarker	Seminoma	Yolk Sac Tumor	Embryonal Carcinoma	Choriocarcinoma
α-Fetoprotein (AFP)	–	+	+/–	–
β-HCG	–	–	–	++
PLAP	+	+/–	+/–	+/–
CD30	–	+/–	+	–
D2-40	++	+/–	+/–	
c-KIT (CD117)	++	+/–	+/–	
Cytokeratin	+/–	++	++	+
OCT4 and NANOG	++	–	++	–
SALL4	++	++	++	
SOX2	–	–	++	–
SOX17	+		–	
TCL1	+/–	–		
UTF1	++	–	++	–
Glypican-3	–	++	+/–	++
MAGEC2	+			

++, always positive; +, usually positive; +/–, positive or negative; –, negative; β-HCG, β-human chorionic gonadotropin; PLAP, placental alkaline phosphatase; MAGEC2, melanoma-associated antigen C2.
Reprinted from Iczkowski KA, Butler SL, Shanks JH, et al. Trials of new germ cell immunohistochemical stains in 93 extragonadal and metastatic germ cell tumors. *Hum Pathol* 2008;39:275–281. Copyright © 2008 Elsevier. With permission.

be differentiated according to the main histologic groups and the age of occurrence, as teratomas and yolk sac tumors occur only in prepubertal age.[14] Although pure seminomas did not demonstrate to be much more aggressive, primary mediastinal nonseminomas are characterized by poor prognosis, higher chemoresistance, and shorter survival.[15,16] However, improvement in the prognosis has been reported through using cisplatin-based neoadjuvant therapy.[17,18] Given the different treatment plan and prognosis between GCTs, correct diagnosis of these tumors is critical for clinical management.

GCTs were among the first tumors for which serum markers were applied. The first report dates back to 1930, when beta human chorionic gonadotropin (β-HCG) was detected in the urine of men with choriocarcinoma.[19] Since that time, serum protein markers such as α-fetoprotein (AFP), β-HCG, and lactate dehydrogenase (LDH) acquired increasing importance in the management of GCTs. In adults, preoperative tumor markers are part of the criteria for risk grouping (good, intermediate, poor) of GCT according to the International Germ Cell Cancer Collaborative Group (IGCCCG) system.[20] These markers provide critical information for diagnosis, prognosis, staging, monitoring response to therapy, and diagnosis recurrence. Moreover, the National Academy of Clinical Biochemistry (NACB) published a practice guideline on analytic methods for tumor markers in testicular GCTs and other cancers,[21] which could be of interest even in extragonadal GCTs. Moreover, guidelines regarding recommendations on appropriate uses for serum markers of GCTs in their normal sites, to be considered also for their mediastinal occurrences, were developed.[21,22] For extragonadal GCTs, anatomic site, morphology, and staging parameters are relevant to patient outcome.[23] Immunohistochemical characterization on bioptic/surgical material obtained is needed. In GCT characterization, the optimal IHC panel must include detection of AFP and β-HCG for identifying yolk sac

tumors and choriocarcinomas, respectively.[24] Other markers used for diagnosing GCTs include c-KIT (CD117), placental-like alkaline phosphatase (PLAP), and CD30. However, these markers lack adequate sensitivity and/or specificity.[25–29] Recently, stem cell markers (SCMs) (SALL4, OCT4, NANOG, UTF1, and TCL1) have been used as more sensitive markers for GCTs.[30–32] Applications of these and other immunohistochemical markers (LDH-1, glypican-3 [GPC3], M2A, melanoma-associated antigen C2 [MAGEC2]) in GCTs will be certainly further addressed (Table 153.7).

Overall, there is a strong and uniform consensus on the necessity of a close multidisciplinary collaboration in diagnosis and management of GCTs tumors by centralizing care at experienced centers, particularly for patients with intermediate and poor prognosis at diagnosis as well as for all relapsed germ cell cancer patients.[33]

Here a detailed report for GCT markers is given. Most serum markers are also detectable by IHC on FFPE slides (Table 153.8).

ALPHA-FETOPROTEIN (AFP)

AFP, which resembles albumin in many physicochemical properties, is a major fetal serum protein with a molecular weight of approximately 70 kDa. AFP is normally produced during gestation by fetal liver and gastrointestinal tract, and by the yolk sac. The detection of AFP is referred to cells of yolk sac origin present in embryonal carcinoma and in yolk sac tumors. These cells, however, are never present in pure seminomas or choriocarcinomas. Even when these cells cannot be histologically demonstrated in pure seminomas or choriocarcinomas, they must be assumed to be present when AFP shows elevated levels. In patients with mature teratomas, AFP is always negative in the serum. However, a case of metachronous

1978 XXVI Noninvasive Investigations

Germ Cell Tumor (GCT)	Serum Markers
SEMINOMA	β-HCG (occasionally); LDH
EMBRYONAL CARCINOMA	AFP; β-HCG
YOLK-SAC TUMOR (endodermal sinus tumor; YST)	AFP; CEA (occasionally)
CHORIOCARCINOMA	β-HCG; AFP; PLAP;
MATURE AND IMMATURE TERATOMA	—
MIXED GERM CELL TUMOR	AFP; β-HCG rarely
GERM CELL TUMOR WITH SOMATIC-TYPE SOLID MALIGNANCY	AFP and/or β-HCG; CEA; NSE

TABLE 153.8 Summary of Serological Markers in GCTs

AFP, α-fetoprotein; β-HCG, β-subunit of human chorionic gonadotropin; CEA, carcinoembryonic antigen; NSE, neuron-specific enolase; LDH, lactate dehydrogenase.

bilateral recurrent ovarian and mediastinal teratomas with elevated AFP has been recently described.[34]

BETA HUMAN CHORIONIC GONADOTROPIN (β-HCG)

β-HCG, the first pregnancy-specific protein to be described, is a 38-kDa glycoprotein secreted by placental syncytiotrophoblasts, whose function is to maintain the corpus luteum during the first few weeks of pregnancy. Elevated serum levels of β-HCG have been reported in patients with hepatic, pancreatic, gastric, pulmonary, breast, renal, and bladder tumors.[35] However, serum levels of β-HCG >10.000 U/L are seen only in pregnancy and in patients with GCTs, gestational trophoblastic disease, and (rarely) trophoblastic differentiation of lung or gastric primary tumors.[36] Choriocarcinoma is a highly aggressive GCT. Serum β-HCG is elevated in the majority of cases of choriocarcinoma and in up to 10% of patients with seminomas. By IHC in tumor tissue, choriocarcinoma β-HCG is positive in the syncytiotrophoblastic cells, while PLAP is positive in about half.[27] In tumor tissue, also one-third of embryonal carcinomas show β-HCG expression in scattered syncytiotrophoblastic cell.

PLACENTAL ALKALINE PHOSPHATASE (PLAP)

PLAP is a fetal isoenzyme of the ubiquitous adult alkaline phosphatase. It is normally expressed in placental syncytiotrophoblast cells and released into maternal circulation after the 12th week of pregnancy,[37] and is also detected in children less than 1 year old.

Although widely accepted as a reliable immunohistochemical marker for seminomas, its role as a serum tumor marker is uncertain. In seminomas, serum PLAP is elevated in 50% to 72% of patients, with elevated levels more frequently reported in patients with higher stage disease.[38,39] Thus, high serum levels of PLAP are considered to have the highest sensitivity for detecting metastasis.[40] Specificity, however, is poor. Elevated levels of PLAP can be found in both healthy smokers and in patients with other diseases, including lung, ovary, breast, and gastrointestinal malignancies.[41] Immunohistochemically, otherwise, the typical seminoma phenotype is that of a cytokeratin-negative tumor with uniform, cell membrane–based reactivity for PLAP.[26,27] Approximately 10% to

15% of such lesions, however, will indeed demonstrate labelling for cytokeratins.[26,27] On the other hand, mediastinal seminomas show strong dot-like positivity for CAM5.2, a low–molecular-weight cytokeratin, in 80% of cases as compared with only 20% positivity in testicular seminomas.[42] Amongst other GCTs, embryonal carcinomas are also immunohistochemically positive for PLAP as well as for low–molecular-weight cytokeratin, and about one-third are positive for AFP.[27]

LACTATE DEHYDROGENASE (LDH)

LDH is an enzyme of 134 kDa which is highly expressed in muscles as well as in the liver, kidney, and brain. It plays an important role in metabolism, through oxidation of lactic acid to pyruvic acid. Five isoenzymes of LDH have been described.

Serum levels of LDH are elevated in a wide spectrum of diseases, and its specificity for GCTs is extremely poor. In addition, it has not been shown to have strong predilection for specific histologies in GCTs. Therefore, LDH is not particularly useful in diagnosis. However, in GCTs, LDH (LDH-1 isoform) has an important role in monitoring response to treatment and recurrence, and has been shown to predict relapse-free survival, and overall survival.[43,44] Therefore, in patients with GCTs, the evaluation of LDH levels, together with levels of AFP and β-HCG, is strongly recommended.[45] LDH is only a serum marker.

TISSUE (ONLY) MARKERS FOR GCT

CD30

CD30 is a member of the tumor necrosis factor superfamily and has pleiotropic effects on cells carrying it. It was initially described as a diagnostic marker for Hodgkin lymphoma (HL)[46–48] so it is neither tumor specific nor lymphoma specific. Immunohistochemically, CD30 (Ki-1) is expressed in 85% to 100% of embryonal carcinoma,[49,50] while other GCTs, with the exception of rare cases of seminomas and yolk sac tumors,[25,51] and other nonhematopoietic tumors are CD30 negative.[50] AFP[25,42] and PLAP[42,52] can occur in scattered tumor cells or small foci in about 30% of cases.

M2A (D2-40)

Transcription factor M2A is a highly glycosylated monomeric sialoglycoprotein antigen of unknown origin, and is detected by the commercially available antibody D2-40. M2A is expressed in intratubular germ cell neoplasia of unclassified type (IGCNU), seminomas, and immature fetal germ cells.[53,54]

Lau and colleagues[55] used D2-40 monoclonal antibody as an immunohistochemical tumor marker to differentiate seminomas from embryonal carcinomas. They found that all of their seminomas stained for M2A, but about 30% of embryonal carcinomas also stained for it. Similar results were obtained by Iczkowski and colleagues.[56] Overall, therefore, D2-40 is not a useful tool to differentiate seminomas from embryonal carcinomas.

c-KIT (CD117)

CD117, the c-KIT proto-oncogene product, is a tyrosine growth factor receptor. It is expressed by interstitial cells of Cajal, which are involved in the regulation of gut motility (pacemaker cell). The interaction of CD117 with its natural ligand, stem cell factor (SCF), has been implicated in enhanced tumor growth. CD117 expression has been observed in a range of human malignancies, including mast cell leukemia, gastrointestinal stromal tumors (GISTs), melanomas, and seminomas.[57–60] Mediastinal seminomas were found to have c-KIT mutations in approximately 50% of cases, whereas no such mutation was identified in any of the testicular tumors.[28]

Immunohistochemically, CD117 has been found to be predominantly expressed by mediastinal seminomas, where immunoreactivity is commonly seen at the cell membrane or in the paranuclear region.[61,62]

Stem Cell Markers

Earlier markers used for diagnosing primary mediastinal GCTs like c-KIT, PLAP, AFP, and CD30 lack adequate sensitivity and/or specificity.[25,27–29,32] OCT4, a transcription factor expressed in embryonic stem cells and germ cells, has been found to be a useful marker in the identification of testicular seminomas and embryonal carcinomas,[62] as well as dysgerminomas and the germ cell component of ovary gonadoblastoma.[63] OCT4 has been used as a more sensitive marker for mediastinal seminomas.[30,32] However, OCT4 labels only seminomas and embryonal carcinomas whereas yolk sac tumors are negative for this marker.[30,32] The most commonly used markers for yolk sac tumors are AFP and PLAP, but they had relatively low sensitivity.[25,27,32,42] Therefore, more sensitive markers, especially for mediastinal yolk sac tumors, are needed.

SALL4 is an SCM involved in maintaining self-renewal and pluripotency of embryonic stem cells by forming a regulatory network with other SCMs: OCT4, SOX2, NANOG, UTF1, and TCL1.[64–66] In this network, SALL4 regulates OCT4,[67] which then regulates UTF1[68,69] and TCL1.[70] Recently, SALL4 has been identified as diagnostic marker for gonadal GCTs.[71,72] It showed 100% sensitivity for gonadal yolk sac tumors and seminomas/dysgerminomas and embryonal carcinomas.

Available data indicate that SCMs are relatively specific for GCTs. SALL4 showed the highest sensitivity as it stained not only seminomas and embryonal carcinomas but also yolk sac tumors. OCT4, NANOG, and UTF1 stained both seminomas and embryonal carcinomas whereas TCL1 stained only seminomas. SOX2 stained embryonal carcinomas and teratomas. Of these six markers, SALL4 is the only one to stain yolk sac tumors.[31] In addition, except for that some lymphomas may express strong SALL4[73] and TCL1[74,75] and some carcinomas express strong SOX2,[76,77] non-GCTs do not show strong staining for these SCMs. Overall, SCMs are highly specific for mediastinal GCTs. Their determination, however, has to be integrated with the other clinical and laboratory findings.

Glypican-3 (GPC3)

GPC3 belongs to the glypican family that is a group of heparan sulfate proteoglycans linked to the outer surface of cell membrane through a glycosylphosphatidylinositol anchor.[78] In mammals, six members of GPCs have been reported, GPC1 to GPC6. GPCs are released from the cell surface by a lipase called notum to regulate the signaling of Wnts of Hedgehogs,[79] of fibroblast growth factors (FGFs) and bone morphogenetic proteins (BMPs).[80–83] Depending on the cellular context, their function can be stimulatory or inhibitory, or of signaling. The expression of GPC3 is detected in placenta and fetal liver, but not in other normal organs. GPC3 has proven also useful for the diagnosis of nonseminomatous GCTs of the testis, in particular yolk sac tumors.[84] Recently, Weissferdt and colleagues[85] reported an absence of immunohistochemical expression of GPC3 in 32 mediastinal seminomas. This result encourages the use of this marker, as it could allow to separate seminomatous from nonseminomatous GCTs.

Melanoma-Associated Antigen C2 (MAGEC2)

In 2011, Bode and colleagues[86] studied the expression of MAGEC2, a cancer testis antigen present in normal germ cells and various human cancers, in a tissue microarray of 325 testicular GCTs including 254 seminomas. They found positive results in 94% of their cases, postulating that this marker is another sensitive tool in the differential diagnosis of seminomas. In 2015, Weissferdt and colleagues[85] reported staining for MAGEC2 in 28 (88%) out of 32 mediastinal seminomas. Similar to testicular seminomas, mediastinal seminomas show consistent expression of MAGEC2 making it a valuable marker in the context of an antibody panel.

THYMIC EPITHELIAL TUMORS (TET)

TETs include thymomas and thymic carcinomas (Table 153.4). Although rare,[87] they represent the most frequent primary mediastinal neoplasias in adults, whereas in pediatric ages they are even rarer. They derive from thymic epithelial cells (TECs), with thymoma representing "organotypic" tumors (Figs. 153.2, 153.3, and 153.4A,B), whereas thymic carcinoma subtypes resemble carcinomas occurring in other organs (Fig. 153.4C,D). It is important to note that the anterior mediastinum represents the most frequent site, but that they occur in several ectopic thoracic, and rarely, extrathoracic locations. Therefore, every tissue mass in the mediastinum, even in pleural or pericardial localization, should be preoperatively considered a TET until it is histologically verified. After recent re-evaluation, thymomas are now considered tumors with distinct even if low-malignant potential tumors.[88] The reader should refer to other chapters in this book (Chapter 166) regarding prognostic factors for thymomas, above all including staging. Here we deal primarily with diagnostic markers for routine tumor diagnostics. Serum markers specific for TET as neoplasms are still unknown. However, several serum markers are found in ADs (see section: Autoimmune Disorders Thymoma-Associated and Their Serum Markers) and in the thymoma-associated immunodeficiencies (see section: Immunodeficit in Thymoma and Related Markers) (Tables 153.3, 153.5, and 153.9).

Even though serum markers are not specific for TET themselves, a variety of tissue-specific markers are of help in characterizing the tissue removed for diagnosis, as reported in Table 153.10. In fact, the role of IHC in TET histological diagnosis appears to be relevant when dealing with specific subtypes and their variants/peculiarities, and crucial when considering fine needle biopsies or bioptic specimens. The reader should refer to recent publications that deal with diagnostic considerations on this subject.[89–91] Differential diagnostic features highlighted by immunohistochemical markers will be briefly discussed here.

TABLE 153.9 Striational Abs in MG Associated With Anti-AChR Abs

Antibody	MG Population	Thymoma MG	Late-onset MG	Early-onset MG
Anti-Titin	20–40%	80–90%	50–60%	10%
Anti-RyR	13–38%	50–70%	20–30%	—
Anti-Kv1.4	12–15%	40–70%[a]	18–20%	10%

[a]In Japanese patients, associated with myositis and myocarditis. (Courtesy of Prof. A. Evoli, Rome, Italy.)

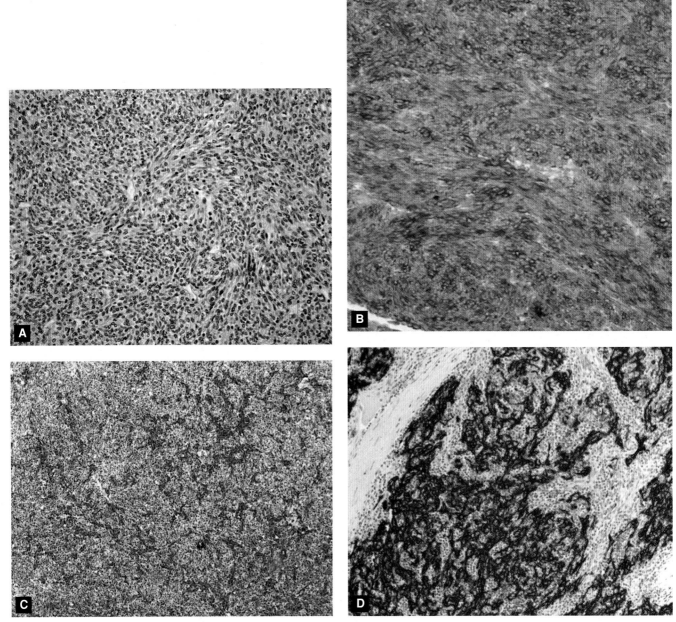

FIGURE 153.2 Type A thymoma: (**A**) H&E, 200×; (**B**) CKMNF116, 200×; Type AB thymoma: (**C**) AB thymoma H&E, 100×; (**D**) AB thymoma CD20 staining of epithelial cells, 200×.

The current classification of TET 2 (Table 153.4) represents the actual consensus of a long debate between pathologists to identify not only diagnostic criteria[89] but also to interpret the TEC spectrum and the patterns that TEC exhibit in tumors and their biological characteristics. In the authors opinion, the WHO classification, through its different editions[2,96,97] appears in some way related (or derived from) to the concept of corticomedullary differentiation in thymoma[98] and to the later developed concept of a well-differentiated thymic carcinoma (Fig. 153.4A,B).[99] However, it should be mentioned that other pathologists disagreed on recognizing distinct TEC subtypes and biological entities in thymic tumors, by describing the heterogeneity of thymomas as result of a continuous morphologic spectrum exhibited by epithelial cells. The reader could refer to some earlier references[100,101] and to recent reviews regarding this issue.[102]

IMMUNOHISTOCHEMICAL MARKERS OF TET

All TETs react with keratins, particularly with CK19, by showing, according to the subtypes and density of their growth, a network of TEC (Figs. 153.2B and 153.3B); other keratins and epithelial markers are listed in Table 153.4. Detailed studies of EC and lymphoid cell immunohistochemical findings were reported.[103–106] Terminal deoxynucleotidyl transferase (Tdt) in the cortical type thymocytes in AB and in B type tumors being the fundamental marker for lymphoid T cells (Fig. 153.3D). New TEC markers have also been described recently.[107–110] A TET immunohistochemical profile of diagnostic value in the differential diagnosis of mediastinal/pulmonary and pleural neoplasms was defined by surveying wide and complex literature.[111–113] Moreover, the density of TEC network in the B type thymoma represents a major

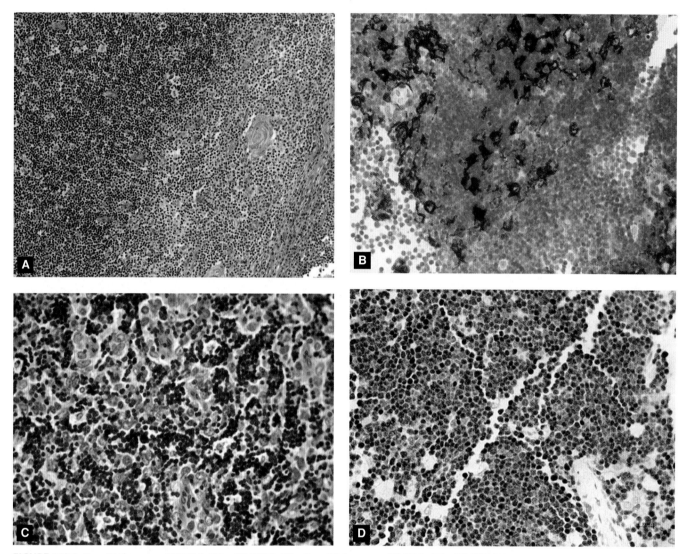

FIGURE 153.3 Type B1 thymoma: (**A**) H&E, 100×; (**B**) CK19, 400×; Type B2 thymoma: (**C**) H&E, 400×; (**D**) TdT, 400×.

criterium in order to distinguish, in case of doubt, the B1 from the B2 cases.[89,91]

Besides classical epithelial markers, some antibodies not originally designed for TEC are frequently applied in TET diagnostics: CD20, CD5, and CD117. Chilosi and colleagues[114] described the occurrence of CD20 as an aberrant marker in spindle TEC of "mixed" type thymomas (or AB). This marker was shown to stain "medullary" TEC type in A and AB type thymomas (Fig. 153.2D). This antibody is useful associated to epithelial markers pointing out a possible TEC derivation of the tumor, even if located in the pleura[111] or in ectopic localization.[115] A further diagnostic improvement was the identification of CD5 as a marker of thymic squamous cell carcinomas (TSCCs)[116–118] and of KIT (CD117) (Fig. 153.4D), which stains most thymic carcinomas at variance with most epithelial neoplasms.[119,120] The positivity for CD5 and CD117 together represent a diagnostic "key" in evaluating mediastinal carcinomas of uncertain origin. However, one must consider that some carcinoma metastases are CD5+.[4] Recently, a new antibody has been described, MUC1, with diagnostic and prognostic value in differentiating thymic carcinoma from B3 thymomas.[121] Furthermore, the concept of a histogenetic thymoma correlation with cortical and/or medullary TEC derivation was recently reinforced by the characterization of several

compartment-specific TEC markers in thymomas.[92] These observations derived from an early description of a proteasome β subunit expressed exclusively in thymic cortical epithelial cells in mice and humans.[93,94] This subunit, designated β5t, is a component of the thymoproteasome, a specialized type of proteasome implicated in thymic lymphocyte positive selection. A Japanese study[95] demonstrated that β5t, when used in a panel of diagnostic markers, could be a relevant marker in differentiating type B3 thymomas from thymic carcinomas, being expressed in most type B and in some type AB thymomas. These molecules also appear to play a central role in thymic immunologic function such as the generation of the MHC class-I–restricted CD8+ T cell repertoire.[93] In thymomas, the characterization by a panel of compartment-specific immunohistochemical markers allowed to hypothesize that thymomas arise from thymic precursors with cortical/medullary maturation defects (Fig. 153.5).[92]

Among differentiation-related antigens, it should be noted that positivity for antibodies useful in diagnostics could also be informative for predictive use. It is well known that overexpression of c-kit could correspond to a mutated gene. Ströbel and colleagues[122] described a c-kit–activating mutation in thymic carcinomas in a tumor hyperexpressing KIT. The patient harboring the c-kit mutation was responsive for 6 months to imatinib therapy, then the

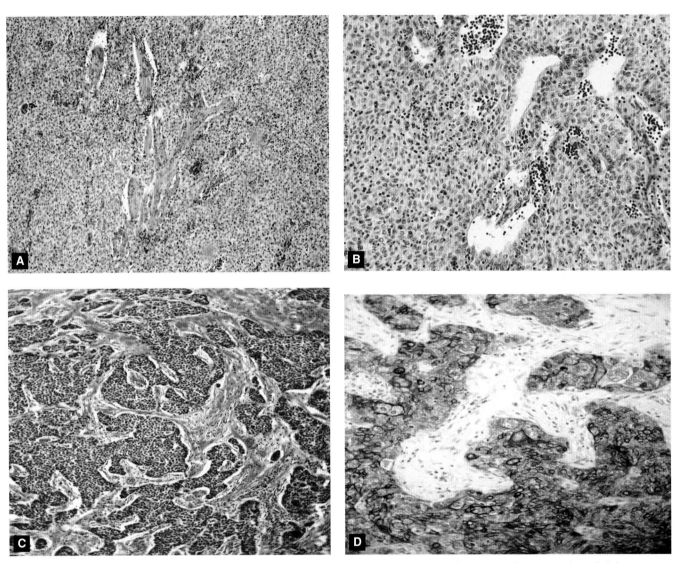

FIGURE 153.4 Type B3 thymoma: (**A**) H&E 100×; (**B**) H&E 200×; Thymic carcinoma, poorly differentiated squamous cell carcinoma (TSCC): (**C**) H&E, 100×; (**D**) CD117, 400×.

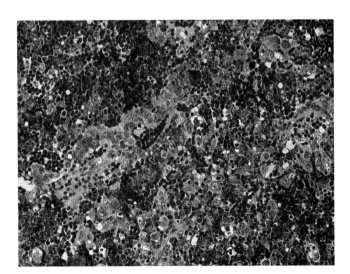

FIGURE 153.5 Thymus (cortex) staining of proteasome β5t, 400×. (Courtesy of Prof. A. Marx, Mannheim, Germany, and of Prof. P. Ströbel, Göttingen, Germany.)

disease progressed despite radiochemotherapy. KIT, corresponding to CD117, a transmembrane tyrosine kinase receptor protein encoded by a proto-oncogene c-kit, triggers intracellular signals controlling cell proliferation and apoptosis. By IHC on whole sections and on TMA, KIT was found to be consistently expressed (heterogeneous or diffuse cytoplasmic staining) by thymic carcinomas but not by thymomas.[120] However, no mutations were found in the tumors (exons 9, 11 and exons 13 and 17). Similar data were provided by other studies.[119,123,124] However, it appears that KIT mutations as well as EGFR mutations are rare.[125] However, nowadays, small tyrosine kinase inhibitors (TKIs) are widely used in clinics to treat advanced TET, both thymomas and thymic carcinomas.[126–128]

AUTOIMMUNE DISORDERS THYMOMA-ASSOCIATED AND THEIR SERUM MARKERS

The variety of thymoma-associated AD and immune dysfunctions is only briefly mentioned here. Table 153.5 reports the major AD thymomas associated with this. Most of them cause neurological symptoms and syndromes. The occurrence of myasthenia gravis (MG), which is by far the most frequent autoimmune thymoma–associated

TABLE 153.10 Immunohistochemical Markers Helpful in Distinguishing TET Subtypes and in the Differential Diagnosis of TET From Other Cancers

Marker	Reactivity
Cytokeratins	Cortical and medullary thymic epithelial cells
CK19	Cortical and medullary thymic epithelial cells
CK10	Terminally mature medullary thymic epithelial cells, Hassall corpuscles, and squamous epithelial cells Focally positive in type B thymoma and thymic squamous cell carcinoma Negative in type A and AB thymoma
CK20	Negative in normal and neoplastic thymic epithelial cells May be positive in rare thymic adenocarcinomas (differential diagnosis: in metastases to the mediastinum)
p63	Cortical and medullary thymic epithelial cells Cross-reacts with tumor cells of primary mediastinal large B-cell lymphoma [Chilosi, et al.,[293]]
CD5	T cells Epithelial cells in ~70% of thymic squamous cell carcinomas (TSCC) Variably positive in thymic (and other) adenocarcinomas
CD20	B cells Epithelial cells in ~50% of type A and AB thymomas [Chilosi, et al.,[114]]
CD117	Epithelial cells in ~80% of thymic squamous cell carcinomas (TSCC)
PAX8	Positive in thymomas and most thymic carcinomas [Weissferdt, et al.,[166]]
Terminal deoxynucleotidyl transferase (Tdt)	Immature T cells in thymus and thymoma T-cell lymphoblastic lymphoma
Desmin	Myoid cells of thymic medulla, type B1 thymoma, rare type B2 and B3 thymomas, and thymic carcinomas
Ki-67	Any proliferating cells (immature T cells in normal thymic cortex, most thymomas, T-cell lymphoblastic lymphoma, etc.)
Compartment-specific antibody targets[92–95]	
Beta5t	Thymic epithelial cells with cortical differentiation (thymus and thymoma)
PRSS16	Thymic epithelial cells with cortical differentiation (thymus and thymoma)
Cathepsin V	Thymic epithelial cells with cortical differentiation (thymus and thymoma)
Claudin 4	Subset of thymic epithelial cells with medullary differentiation
CD40	Subset of thymic epithelial cells with medullary differentiation
Autoimmune regulator	Subset of thymic epithelial cells with medullary differentiation
Autoimmune regulator	Subset of thymic epithelial cells with medullary differentiation
Involucrin	Like CK10, but focally positive in type AB thymoma

Modified with permission from Travis WD, Brambilla E, Burke AP, Marx A, Nicholson AG. *World Health Organization Classification of Tumours of the Lung, Pleura, Thymus and Heart.* Vol. 7. 4th ed. Lyon: IARC Press, 2015.

disease, is recorded in 24.5% to 40% of thymoma patients, whereas 15% to 20% of MG patients have a thymoma. More than 50% of MG patients have follicular thymic hyperplasia.

The chapter on MG (Chapter 164) in this book and specific review and papers[129,130] cover this subject in detail. In the diagnostic preoperative workup of patients with a mediastinal mass the detection of neurological, even subtle symptoms and appropriate serological investigations, appear to be very relevant. Table 153.9 reports on the major autoantibodies (Anti-AChR and antistriational autoantibodies) to be searched for in case of suspect MG and their frequencies in the different forms of MG, either paraneoplastic, or associated with thymic nonneoplastic changes. Awareness of an underlying paraneoplastic MG is of paramount relevance in the preoperative workup, as many patients undergo a myasthenic crisis following tumor removal.[131]

It is also important to note that autoimmune symptoms could arise as early signs of a TET, or could appear after the removal of the tumor or even several years later. In addition, symptoms and signs of neurological paraneoplastic disease could be associated with thymoma recurrence (Table 153.11).[129]

Pathogenic antibodies (Abs) in MG bind to extracellular epitopes of postsynaptic membrane proteins, causing molecular and functional

TABLE 153.11 Autoimmune Diseases Associated With Thymoma

Disease	Remission Post-thymectomy
MG	Reduction in anti-AChR antibodies
SLE	YES
SIADH	YES
ARCA	YES
BP	YES
Others	Unknown
Polymyositis, pernicious anemia, Hashimoto thyroiditis, hyperthyroidism, RA, UC, DM, scleroderma, Takayasu syndrome, Graves disease, encephalitis	

AChR, acetylcholine receptor; ARCA, acquired red cell aplasia; BP, bullous pemphigoid; DM, dermatomyositis; MG, myasthenia gravis; RA, rheumatoid arthritis; SIADH, syndrome of inappropriate antidiuretic hormone secretion; SLE, systemic lupus erythematosus; UC, ulcerative colitis.
Modified with permission from Macmillan Publishers Ltd: Shelly S, Agmon-Levin N, Altman A, et al. Thymoma and autoimmunity. *Cell Mol Immunol* 2011;8:199–202. Copyright © 2011.

alterations interfering with neuromuscular transmission (NMT). In thymoma patients, MG is nearly invariably associated with AChR-Abs, which can also occur in rare thymoma cases without neurological symptoms. Abs against the muscle giant protein *titin*, also called connectin, previously identified as "striational" muscle Abs, and antiryanodine receptor are also found in a high proportion of thymoma-MG cases (Table 153.9). These antibodies are also found in late-onset MG, although with a low frequency. Although of uncertain pathogenicity (as directed against intracellular antigens), these Abs are markers of thymomas, at least in patients younger than 50 years at MG onset; diagnosis is confirmed by Ab testing and electromyography.[130] In thymoma, frequent concurrent autoimmunity against seemingly unrelated autoantigens suggests that potentially cross-reacting proteins expressed by the tumor play a role in disease production.[132] Thymomas from MG patients are rich in auto-reactive T cells, consistent with this postulate.[133] It may also be hypothesized that these autoreactive T cells are positively selected (selected for survival) and exported to the periphery, where they are activated and provided help for autoantibody-producing B cells. Negative selection and regulation of potentially self-reactive T cells may also play a role in abnormal thymus tissue due to a deficiency in the expression of the autoimmune regulator (AIRE) gene and possibly the selective loss of regulatory T cells.[134–136]

Beside thymomas, other tumors in the mediastinum or elsewhere are eventually associated with MG. Among these, there is thymolipoma (see section: Thymolipoma, Table 153.3). Thymic carcinoma very rarely is associated with MG.[137] Moreover, MG has been exceptionally reported in a case of localized thymic amyloidosis[138] and in one case of Castleman disease (CD) of hyaline vascular type, associated with anti-AchR antibodies (see section on Immunity-related tumor-like conditions). The MG-CD association is reported to be more than occasional.[139]

IMMUNODEFICIT IN THYMOMA AND RELATED MARKERS

Among the variety of ADs and immunodeficiencies associated with thymoma (Table 153.5), a rare syndrome has been named Good's syndrome (GS), characterized by increased susceptibility to bacterial, viral, and fungal infections, as well as by autoimmunity. A wide spectrum of autoimmunity manifestations has been described in GS, comprising oral lichen planus, graft-versus-host disease-like colitis, and pure red cell aplasia. In fact, many patients have profound B-lymphopenia, until to absence of circulating B cells.[140] GS is associated with hypogammaglobulinemia which may be fatal. GS was also shown to be associated with a severe loss of CD4+, NK, and B cells, and with accumulation of CD8+CD45RA+ T lymphocytes. In GS, the immunological features and pathogenetic mechanisms are still poorly investigated and unclear.[141]

Table 153.5 lists other immunodeficiencies and autoimmune disorders (hematological, endocrine, dermatological) and collagen diseases associated with TETs.

THYMIC NEUROENDOCRINE TUMORS

THYMIC CARCINOIDS

Carcinoid tumors of the thymus gland account for only 0.4% of all neuroendocrine tumors.[142] Their morphological appearance histologically close mimic carcinoids of the other organ systems, with ultrastructural evidence of neuroendocrine granules and immunohistochemical expression of neuroendocrine markers. These tumors, alongside the atypical carcinoids, have been reported in the setting of type 1 multiple

neuroendocrine neoplasia (MEN1).[143] Evidence of neuroendocrine differentiation is revealed by reactivity with antibodies to neuroendocrine markers: synaptophysin, chromogranin A, and neuron-specific enolase (NSE). NSE is more sensitive (about >90%) than chromogranin A (70% to 90%)[144,145] and synaptophysin.[144] Carcinoid tumors are often associated with endocrine dysfunctions (Table 153.3).[146] Between 7% and 30% of adult and >50% of childhood carcinoids of the thymus are associated with Cushing syndrome due to adrenocorticotropic hormone (ACTH) production.[145,147,148] Although intracytoplasmic ACTH positive cells are detected in some carcinoids clinically associated with Cushing syndrome,[149] it is difficult to prove the presence of ACTH immunohistochemically in other cases. In such cases, radioimmunoassay of an extract of tumor tissue confirms the presence of the peptide. Of note, there is no close correlation between the hormones detected by IHC and the clinical symptoms.[150] The expression of ACTH is quite common, whereas the finding of serotonin, gastrin, and parathormone is uncommon.[145,151] Somatostatin, on the contrary, is frequently detected.[152] In addition to Cushing syndrome, parathyroid hormone production syndrome was reported in thymic carcinoids, causing hypercalcemia and hypophosphatemia.[153] More rarely, acromegaly and antidiuretic hormone (ADH) production have been reported.[154,155]

The survival rate for patients with thymic carcinoids has been reported as 50% at 5 years,[146] and it is significantly worse than for patients with other nonepithelial mediastinal neuroendocrine tumors (paraganglioma), and for patients with neuroendocrine tumors of the lung. Thus, the importance of correctly identifying thymic carcinoids is evident. This is particularly true considering that mediastinoscopic biopsies yield only little amounts of tissue.[146]

Carcinoid tumors are virtually all immunoreactive for low-molecular-weight cytokeratins, with tumor cells showing dot-like immunostaining with CAM5.2 or AE1/3 in the paranuclear region, as opposed to paraganglioma.[146,156–158]

Recently, Pax8, a transcription factor commonly expressed in epithelial tumors of the thyroid gland, parathyroid gland, kidneys, and Müllerian tract,[159–162] was found to label neoplastic epithelial cells of thymus gland.[163] On the other hand, primary pulmonary neuroendocrine tumors failed to stain this marker.[164,165] In thymic carcinoids, Pax8 was found to be positive in approximately one-third of the cases (8/25; 32%)[166] with a diffuse staining pattern, weak to strong in intensity.

Thyroid transcription factor-1 (TTF-1) has been reported to be expressed in lung and thyroid tumors.[159,167,168] Expression of TTF-1 was noted in 19 out of 25 (76%) of pulmonary neuroendocrine carcinoma cases,[166] while TTF-1 expression was absent in the vast majority of thymic carcinoids.[166,169] Among the criteria required for the diagnosis, absence of necrosis and a low mitotic count (<2 mitoses per 2 mm^2) have been included.[170] On the contrary, GATA-3, a zinc finger DNA-binding transcription factor involved in cell development and differentiation of multiple organs (see section Paraganglioma), was not found to be expressed in 24 thymic carcinoids evaluated.[171] Based on these results, not only the routine evaluation of conventional neuroendocrine markers and cytokeratins expression, but also novel markers such as Pax8, TTF-1, and GATA-3 could compose a relevant panel for the differential diagnosis of thoracic neuroendocrine tumors, and carcinoids in particular.

ATYPICAL CARCINOID

Atypical carcinoids (Fig. 153.6A) differ from carcinoids as they exhibit 2 to 10 mitoses per 2 mm^2 and show foci of necrosis. The clinical presentation includes extrathoracic lymph nodes and parenchymal metastases. The immunohistochemical features are similar to typical carcinoids (Fig. 153.6B–D).

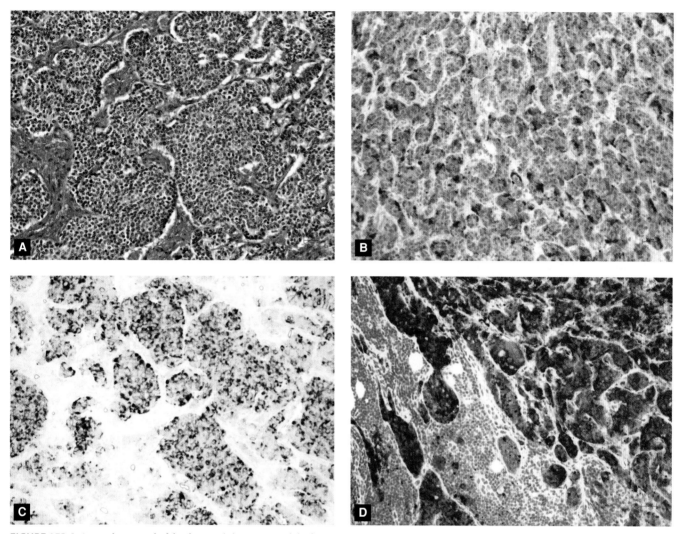

FIGURE 153.6 Atypical carcinoid of the thymus: (**A**) H&E 200×; (**B**) Chromogranin A, 200×; (**C**) Synaptophysin, 200×; (**D**) CK MNF116, 200×.

HIGH-GRADE NEUROENDOCRINE CARCINOMA

High-grade neuroendocrine carcinomas occur in the thymic region, composed either of large or of small cells. In the large cell variant (Large Cell Neuroendocrine Carcinoma, LCNC), mitoses overcome the threshold of 10 per 2 mm², and necrosis is prominent (Fig. 153.7A). Immunohistochemical expression of keratins[172] (Fig. 153.7B) and of NSE, synaptophysin (Fig. 153.7D) and CD56 has been reported. CD117 staining may occur (Fig. 153.7C). These tumors do not appear in the setting of MEN1.

In the small cell carcinoma (SCC) variant a Cushing syndrome has been exceptionally described.[173] Necrosis and hemorrhages are constant features. Immunohistochemical positivity of markers such as keratins and neuroendocrine markers have been reported as well as hormonal production.

NUT MIDLINE CARCINOMA

Nuclear protein in testis (NUT) midline carcinoma (NMC) is a rare form of poorly differentiated squamous cell carcinoma. NMC typically arises within the midline epithelial structures of the upper aerodigestive tract (50%) and the mediastinum (41%), and

occasionally outside the midline structures as the parotid gland, pancreas, adrenal gland, subcutis, orbit, lung, bladder, and iliac bone.[174] NMC is a lethal disease with a median overall survival of 6.7 months,[175] far more aggressive than typical noncutaneous squamous cell carcinomas.

NMC is associated with chromosomal rearrangements of the *NUT* gene (also known as *NUTM1*) on chromosome 15q14.[176–178] Molecular demonstration of the *NUT* rearrangement, with conventional karyotyping, reverse transcriptase polymerase chain reaction (RT-PCR), or fluorescence in situ hybridization (FISH) studies, is diagnostic of NMC.[179] In about two-thirds of cases, a reciprocal chromosomal translocation occurs between the *NUT* gene and the bromodomain-containing protein (*BRD*) 4 gene on chromosome 19, t(15;19),[176] resulting in an oncogenic fusion gene known as *BRD4-NUT*.[180] The remaining one-third of cases have varying *NUT* rearrangements involving *BRD3* or other unknown partners.[181–183] Initial reports of NMC harboring the *BRD4-NUT* translocation described the tumor in a pediatric population.[184] As more cases are recognized, tumors harboring the *BRD4-NUT* translocation are now understood to affect a broad demographic (range 0.1 to 78 years), with men and women equally affected. The BRD4-NUT oncoprotein acts by blocking the differentiation of NMC cells.[183] BRD4 bromodomain binds to acetylated chromatin and attaches the BRD4-NUT

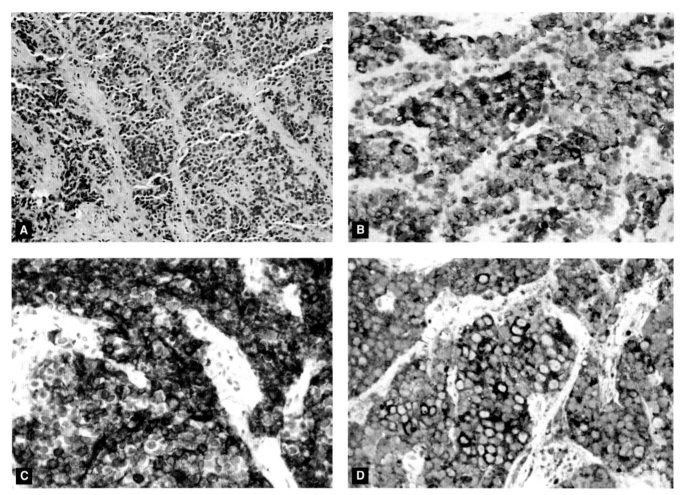

FIGURE 153.7 Large cell neuroendocrine carcinoma of the thymus: (**A**) H&E, 200×; (**B**) CK MNF116, 400×; (**C**) CD117, 400×; (**D**) Synaptophysin, 400×.

oncoprotein to (transcriptionally active) euchromatin.[183] This mechanism is essential to abrogate cellular differentiation in NMC tumors.

NMC tumors typically exhibit the histopathologic features of a poorly differentiated carcinoma, with varying degrees of abrupt, well-differentiated squamous cell islands[185] and an absence of glandular[186] and mesenchymal[187] differentiation, and are not morphologically distinguishable from other undifferentiated carcinomas.[176] The tumor can be diagnosed with virtually 100% specificity by immunohistochemical expression of the NUT protein.[188] In general, it is recommended that testing for the NUT expression by IHC be performed in all poorly differentiated carcinomas that lack glandular differentiation. Pancytokeratin is positive in the majority of NMC tumors, although rare cases are negative.[189,190] Variable results have been obtained with other epithelial markers, such as epithelial membrane antigen (EMA), while markers of squamous and basal cell carcinomas such as p63 have high positivity rates.[191] Variable positivity of NMC tumors has been noted for a variety of markers including CD99, FLI1, CD45 RO, NSE, CD34, vimentin, and focally, p16, CD56, CD138, TTF1, S-100, CD117, and PLAP.[163,176,191–197] Neuroendocrine markers such as chromogranin A and synaptophysin are mostly negative in NMC; however, a few cases of NMC have weak positivity to neuroendocrine markers.[187,198–200] No specific chemotherapeutic regimen has demonstrated efficacy in treating NMC. Traditional chemotherapeutic and radiotherapeutic regimens may be effective early in the disease, but patients frequently relapse later.[184,192,196] With the molecular basis of NMC being more

completely understood, more effective treatment options are under investigation[182] for this very aggressive neoplasm.

SOFT TISSUE TUMORS OF THE MEDIASTINUM

THYMOLIPOMA

Thymolipoma, already mentioned previously, represents a hamartomatous condition composed of adipose fat tissue associated with mature thymic tissue (Table 153.12). This condition occurring mostly in a mature age group (47.9 years in a recent series) was associated with MG occurring in a variety of grades, from grade I Osserman to grade III, most patients being in class IIb (50%).[201] Association with other ADs has been reported.[202,203]

NEUROGENIC TUMORS

Neurogenic tumors of the mediastinum comprise approximately 12% to 21% of all mediastinal masses,[204] most of them occurring in the posterior compartment.[205] Seventy percent to 80% of neurogenic tumors are benign, and nearly half are asymptomatic, however, they occasionally cause compressive or neurologic symptoms.[206,207] These neurogenic tumors include ependymomas, schwannomas,

TABLE 153.12 Soft Tissue Tumors of the Mediastinum

Thymolipoma
Lipoma
Liposarcoma
   Well-differentiated
   Dedifferentiated
   Myxoid
   Pleomorphic
Solitary fibrous tumor
   Malignant
Synovial sarcoma
   Synovial sarcoma, NOS
   Synovial sarcoma, spindle cell
   Synovial sarcoma, epithelioid cell
   Synovial sarcoma, biphasic
Vascular neoplasms
   Lymphangioma
   Hemangioma
   Epithelioid hemangioendothelioma
   Angiosarcoma
Tumors of peripheral nerves
   Ganglioneuroma
   Ganglioneuroblastoma
   Neuroblastoma
   Other rare mesenchymal tumors

Modified with permission from Travis WD, Brambilla E, Burke AP, Marx A, Nicholson AG. *World Health Organization Classification of Tumours of the Lung, Pleura, Thymus and Heart.* Vol. 7. 4th ed. Lyon: IARC Press, 2015.

neurofibromas, malignant peripheral nerve sheath tumors (MPNSTs), ganglioneuromas, ganglioneuroblastomas, neuroblastomas, infrequently pheochromocytomas, and paragangliomas.

Ependymoma

Ependymomas are tumors of neurogenic nature, derived from paravertebral ependymal rests. They are very rare and localized in the posterior mediastinum, entering in differential diagnosis (DD) with other rare posterior mediastinal tumors such as neuroendocrine carcinomas, schwannomas, and metastatic melanoma. GFAP is positive (cytoplasmic staining) in ependymomas, as well as in granular cell tumor, in neural parts of teratomas and in ganglioneuroblastomas. CK and S100 are occasionally weak positive. These neural neoplasms when in the mediastinum show intermediate malignant potential.[208]

Paraganglioma

Paragangliomas (PGL), also defined as extra-adrenal paraganglioma, are tumors with a characteristic morphological "Zellballen" growth pattern and marked cellular atypia.[208] Paragangliomas are probably derived from neuroendocrine tissue located on both side of the vertebral axis and from normal paraganglia. They may occur in the anterior and posterior mediastinum, part of them being part of the hereditary paraganglioma–pheochromocytoma (PGL/PCC) syndromes.[209,210] Extra-adrenal *parasympathetic* paragangliomas are located predominantly in the upper mediastinum; approximately 95% of such tumors are nonsecretory. In contrast, *sympathetic* extra-adrenal paragangliomas are generally confined to the lower mediastinum and typically hypersecrete catecholamines. Therefore, in addition to aspecific signs they may be therefore associated with hypertension and headaches. PGL are mostly benign with few of them showing aggressive metastatic behavior. The initial workup for suspicious PGL should include measurements of plasma free

or urinary fractionated metanephrines. Moreover, genetic testing in all patients by accredited laboratories is recommended. Patients with paragangliomas should be tested for SDHx mutations, and those with metastatic disease for SDHB mutations. It should also be considered that all patients with functional PGL should undergo preoperative blockade to prevent perioperative complications.[211] PGL are strongly positive for neuroendocrine markers but not for CKs. S100 is positive in sustentacular cells pointing to the paraganglionic origin. Moreover, the GATA-3 transcription factor was recently described as expressed. GATA-3, a zinc finger transcription factor, is involved in cell development and differentiation of multiple organs including the nervous system and the urogenital tract.[212,213] It is primarily expressed in urothelial carcinomas and breast cancer,[214,215] but has more recently also been shown to label paragangliomas. In a study of 32 cases of paragangliomas of the urinary bladder and nonurologic sites, So and Epstein[216] found that 78.7% of their cases were positive for GATA-3, irrespective of site. Weissferdt and colleagues[171] found 55% of GATA-3 positivity in their series of 22 paragangliomas.

Benign Schwannomas and Malignant Peripheral Nerve Sheath Tumors

These tumors are briefly mentioned here; they respectively represent the benign and malignant varieties of the Schwann cell tumors. The benign tumors are located mainly in the posterior mediastinum[217] commonly originating along intercostal nerves. Rarely are malignant tumors (MPNST) found in the anterior mediastinum.[218]

Ganglioneuromas, Ganglioneuroblastomas

Ganglioneuromas and ganglioneuroblastomas are respectively tumors of mature ganglion cells or primitive neuroblasts with a component of mature ganglion cells occurring mainly in children. They are rarely associated with hypertension, opsomyoclonus, vasoactive intestinal peptide secretion (VIP) production or with ADH secretion syndrome.[219]

OTHER RARE SOFT TUMORS OF THE MEDIASTINUM

The liposarcoma, the synovial sarcoma, the vascular infantile hemangioendothelioma, and the neuroblastoma are mentioned in the genetic markers section.

HEMATOLOGIC TUMORS OF THE MEDIASTINUM OTHER THAN LYMPHOMAS

Hematologic tumors of the mediastinum other than lymphomas include (a) histiocytic and dendritic cell neoplasms; and (b) myeloid (granulocytic) sarcomas and extramedullary acute myeloid leukemia.

HISTIOCYTIC AND DENDRITIC CELL NEOPLASMS

This group includes Langerhans cell histiocytosis and Langerhans cell sarcomas, histiocytic sarcomas, follicular dendritic cell sarcomas, and interdigitating dendritic cell sarcomas (Table 153.13). These entities are at present classified according to the WHO classification of tumors of hematopoietic and lymphoid tissues.[220] As far as the mediastinum is concerned, lymph nodes are the most frequently involved sites.

TABLE 153.13 Histiocytic and Dendritic Cell Neoplasms of the Mediastinum

Langerhans cell lesions
Langerhans cell histiocytosis
Langerhans cell sarcoma
Histiocytic sarcoma
Follicular dendritic cell sarcoma
Interdigitating dendritic cell sarcoma
Fibroblastic reticular cell tumor
Other dendritic cell tumors
Indeterminate dendritic cell tumor
Myeloid sarcoma and extramedullary acute
Myeloid leukaemia

Modified with permission from Travis WD, Brambilla E, Burke AP, Marx A, Nicholson AG. *World Health Organization Classification of Tumours of the Lung, Pleura, Thymus and Heart.* Vol. 7. 4th ed. Lyon: IARC Press, 2015.

Langerhans Cell Histiocytosis and Langerhans Cell Sarcomas

Langerhans cell histiocytosis and Langerhans cell sarcomas are neoplasms of Langerhans cells, and may involve the lymph nodes and, more rarely, the thymus.[221,222] The most characteristic and diagnostic markers are S-100 protein, CD1a, and the langerin protein (CD207) (overall positive in 100% of cases) and, at ultrastructural level, the presence of Birbeck granules. Notably, in Langerhans cell sarcomas which are the less differentiated and aggressive type of Langerhans cell neoplasms, one (or more) of these markers may not be expressed.[223] The histiocytic marker CD68 is also very frequently expressed (90% to 100% of cases), whereas dendritic cell markers such as CD21 and CD35 are usually negative.

Histiocytic Sarcomas

Histiocytic sarcomas are a rare, highly aggressive neoplastic proliferation of cells with morphologic and immunophenotypic features of histiocytes, which are considered their putative normal counterpart. Histiocytic sarcomas may involve the lymph nodes but also extranodal sites, and, in case of systemic involvement, the definition malignant histiocytosis seems to be appropriate. A single case was reported with predominant mediastinal involvement.[224] The histiocytic markers CD68 and lysozyme are expressed in 95% to 100% of cases. S-100 protein may be expressed in about 30% of cases, whereas CD1a, CD21, and CD35 are as a rule negative.

Follicular Dendritic Cell Sarcomas

Follicular dendritic cell sarcomas are rare neoplasms with evidence of follicular dendritic cell differentiation, which may involve both the lymph nodes and extranodal sites. The most distinctive and diagnostic markers are CD21 and/or CD35 (100% of cases), but also CD68 is frequently expressed (about 50% of cases). S-100 protein and CD1a are usually negative. Interestingly, some cases of follicular dendritic cell neoplasms were described in association with (and even as a transformation of) CD (which is not uncommon in the mediastinum), thus suggesting a pathogenetic link between these two entities.[225–227]

Interdigitating Dendritic Cell Sarcomas

Interdigitating dendritic cell sarcomas are rare neoplasms showing immunophenotypic features of interdigitating reticulum cells, that is, the dendritic nonphagocytic cells typically found in the T-dependent areas of lymphoid tissues (mainly lymph nodes). The involvement of mediastinal lymph nodes usually occurs in the setting of disseminated disease, and it is very rare.[228] The most distinctive immunophenotypic marker is S-100 protein (positive in 100% of cases). Histiocyte/macrophage markers such as CD68, lysozyme, and alpha-1-antichymotrpsin may be expressed at a lesser extent (25% to 50% of cases). CD21, CD35, CD1a are negative, and Birbeck granules are not detectable at ultrastructural level. The differential diagnosis is to be done with primary or metastatic malignant melanoma.[2]

MYELOID (GRANULOCYTIC) SARCOMA AND EXTRAMEDULLARY ACUTE MYELOID LEUKEMIA

Myeloid (or granulocytic) sarcoma is by definition an extramedullary neoplasm composed of immature myeloid cells. It is frequently associated with hematologic disorders such as acute myeloid and chronic myelogenous leukemia, and myelodysplastic syndrome. Notably, these hematologic diseases may be observed synchronously or, on the contrary, may develop subsequent to the detection of myeloid sarcoma. In the former case, myeloid sarcoma represents indeed an extramedullary involvement of an overt hematologic disorder, whereas in the latter case, the definition of myeloid sarcoma seems to be more appropriate. Myeloid sarcoma is mainly composed of immature myeloid cells, featured by the expression of myeloid and/or monocytic markers, such as myeloperoxidase, AS-D chloroacetate esterase, CD13, CD33 and lysozyme, and by variable expression of hematopoietic precursors markers, such as CD34 and TdT. Mediastinal involvement by myeloid sarcoma (Fig. 153.8) or by blastic crisis in chronic myeloid leukemia is a rare occurrence.[229] However, it should be pointed out that the hematopoietic precursor cells eventually present within a mediastinal GCT (and in particular the yolk sac tumor), and may give rise to secondary hematologic malignancies.[230]

LYMPHOMAS OF THE MEDIASTINUM

Lymphomas of the mediastinum (Table 153.14) are only briefly reported here, and the reader should refer to Chapter 168 in this book. Here mainly is a description of the relevant markers and the "clues" for the diagnosis are described with a particular relationship to their markers.

Lymphomas of the mediastinum may be primary (in which the mediastinum is the primary site of disease involvement) or, on the

TABLE 153.14 Lymphomas of the Mediastinum

Primary mediastinal large B-cell lymphoma
Extranodal marginal zone lymphoma of MALT type[a]
Other mature B-cell lymphomas
T-cell lymphoblastic lymphoma/leukemia
ALCL[b] and other rare mature T- and NK-cell lymphomas
ALCL, ALK-positive (ALK+)
ALCL, ALK-negative (ALK-)
Hodgkin lymphoma
B-cell lymphoma, unclassifiable, with features
  intermediate between diffuse large B-cell
  lymphoma and classical Hodgkin lymphoma

[a]MALT, Mucosa-associated lymphoid tissue.
[b]ALCL, Anaplastic large cell lymphoma.
Modified from Travis WD, Brambilla E, Burke AP, et al. *World Health Organization Classification of Tumours of the Lung, Pleura, Thymus and Heart.* Vol. 7. 4th ed. Lyon: IARC Press.

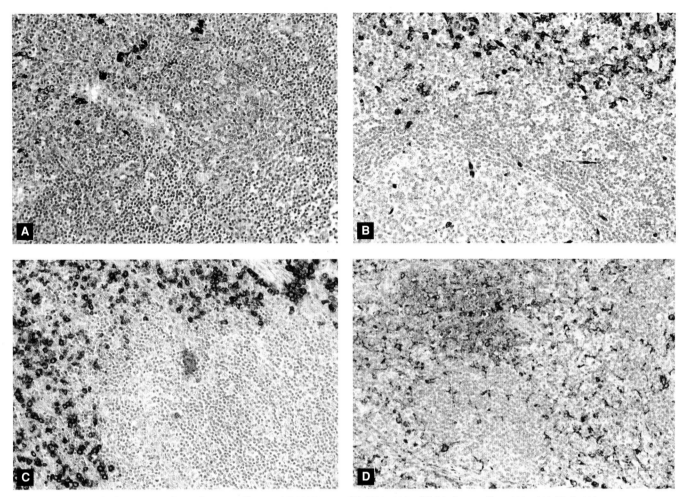

FIGURE 153.8 Myeloid sarcoma in the mediastinum/thymus: (**A**) H&E, 200×; (**B**) CD34, 200×; (**C**) Myeloperoxidase, 200×; (**D**) CD68, 200×.

contrary, secondary (to a more or less generalized lymphoproliferative disorders). The former definition basically refers to four entities, that is, primary mediastinal (thymic) large B-cell lymphomas, thymic extranodal marginal zone B-cell lymphomas, precursor T-lymphoblastic lymphomas, and Hodgkin lymphoma. In the latter case, virtually all types of lymphomas may be considered. Mediastinal lymphomas may arise in and involve both the thymus (most frequently in case of primary lymphomas) and/or the mediastinal lymph nodes (most frequently in case of secondary lymphomas). Primary mediastinal lymphoma usually occurs in the anterior mediastinum, without clinical and/or pathological evidence of other involved sites.

PRIMARY MEDIASTINAL LYMPHOMAS

B-Cell Lymphoma

Primary Mediastinal (Thymic) Large B-Cell Lymphoma
Primary mediastinal (thymic) large B-cell lymphoma (PMBL) is a mature B-cell lymphoma with large cell morphology, that involves (and most likely arises within) the thymus. PMBL expresses B-cell antigens (CD19, CD20, CD79a), but typically lacks immunoglobulins in spite of the expression of transcription factors such as BOB1, OCT2, and PU.1.[231,232] CD23 and CD30 are expressed in most cases of PMBL. However, the CD30 expression is rather weak and

not homogeneous.[233,234] On the contrary, Bcl2, germinal center cell (CD10 and Bcl6), and postgerminal center cell (MUM1/IRF4) markers are more variably expressed. Overall, the cytological diagnosis by fine needle aspiration is not recommended as differential diagnosis and subclassification is complex.[2]

Genetic markers in chromosome 9p24.1 and the transcriptional signature are rather specific for PMBL with comparison with DLBCL of other primary source,[235,236] but similar or related to classical Hodgkin lymphoma,[237] underlining the existing similarity and supporting a "gray zone" area.

Thymic Extranodal Marginal Zone B-Cell Lymphoma
Thymic extranodal marginal zone B-cell lymphoma is a very rare lymphoma that occurs in the setting of AD and therefore is eventually associated with the signs and markers of the autoimmunity (Sjögren disease, rheumatoid arthritis).[238] It should be considered that the Hassall bodies represent an epithelial boundary similar to glandular structures in the sites of the mucosa-associated lymphatic tissue (MALT)[239] and that the thymus develops as an endodermal derivative from branchial clefts moving to the thorax. Therefore, an antigenic entry may be postulated for these epithelial enigmatic structures. In addition, the occurrence of lymphoepithelial lesions is described also in thymic MALT-type lymphoma even if the epithelium usually is almost destroyed at the time of diagnosis. Only rarely early phases of this kind of lymphoma are observed, even though

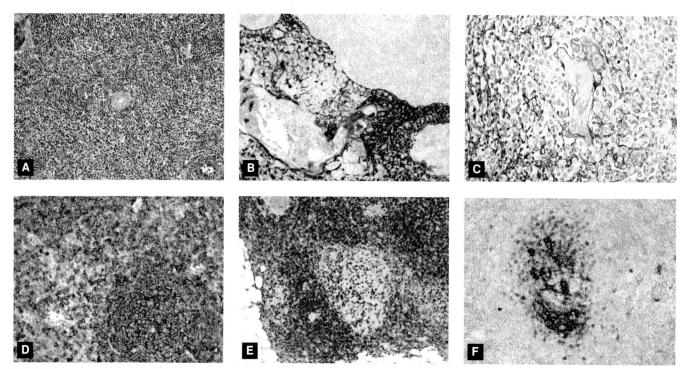

FIGURE 153.9 Thymic marginal lymphoma: (**A**) H&E, lymphoid proliferation substituting the normal thymic structure 100×; (**B**) CK19 residual but interrupted epithelial cell networks of the thymic medulla, 100×; (**C**) CK19, highlighting lymphoepithelial lesions in a Hassall body, 200×; (**D**) CD20+ cells invading the thymic medulla, 200×; (**E**) CD5, staining of small T-lymphocytes, 100×; (**F**) CD23, highlighting residual follicular dendritic cell networks in a germinal center, 100×. (Images courtesy of Prof. L Lauriola, Rome.)

they cause a mass developing in the anterior mediastinum in the thymic area (Fig. 153.9).

T-Cell Lymphoma

Precursor T-Lymphoblastic Lymphoma (T-Lb)

Precursor T-lymphoblastic lymphoma is usually observed in childhood and is associated with leukemic involvement. However, cases have been observed which show a mass-forming phase prior to leukemia development. These lymphoblastic proliferations have to be distinguished from B2 or B1 type thymomas, and the keratin staining is very useful in detecting the disordered EC network characterizing thymoma as opposed to lymphoblastic lymphoma, which is an early destructor of the TEC network/remnants. Whereas the immunophenotype of T-Lb lymphoma is similar to that of cortical type thymocytes in thymomas of the B group, the monotony and the atypia of the neoplastic proliferation distinguish the lymphoma from the thymoma (Fig. 153.10).[240] In these cases, an assiduous surveillance of peripheral blood cell count may disclose the sudden increase in the lymphocytic count following surgery.

Hodgkin Lymphoma

Hodgkin's Lymphoma of the Thymus B Cells

Hodgkin lymphoma arises in the thymus and lymph nodes. In the thymus, it possibly arises from B cells,[237] and is usually associated with thick sclerosis. Classical HL cells are CD30+ with a dot-like perinuclear and membranous staining. CD15 is only sometimes positive, while PAX5 and fascin are also positive.[220] Cases with overlapping aspects among PMBL and Hodgkin lymphoma are defined B-cell lymphoma, unclassifiable, with intermediate features among diffused large B-cell lymphoma and classical HL, also known as "gray zone lymphoma."[241-243]

SECONDARY MEDIASTINAL LYMPHOMAS

The mediastinum may be involved by virtually all types of systemic lymphomas, the most frequent ones being diffused large B-cell lymphomas, follicular lymphomas, and Hodgkin lymphoma. These cases are classified according to the WHO classification of lymphomas.[220]

IMMUNITY-RELATED TUMOR-LIKE CONDITIONS OF THE MEDIASTINUM

A heterogeneous group of immunity-related disorders and their serological signs/markers are associated with different pathogenetic mechanisms in mediastinal mass development. These disorders alter the overall immunoglobulin production by B cells and/or associate with autoantibody production. They are described here in a distinct section specifically devoted to immune disorders, reflecting either hypergammaglobulinemia or hypogammaglobulinemia, or autoantibody production (Table 153.3). All these disorders either affect the thymus itself, as a main lymphatic organ, or affect mediastinal lymph nodes and/or the mediastinal structures.

CASTLEMAN DISEASE OF THE MEDIASTINUM

CD is a heterogeneous group of nonneoplastic disorders of the lymphatic tissue, occasionally giving rise to neoplasms of the constituting cells (both lymphoid and "accessory").[225-227] It occurs either in the anterior mediastinum or in the middle or posterior mediastinum, constituting a large mass involving lymph nodes or lymph node groups. Usually it gives rise to a well-circumscribed round nodule

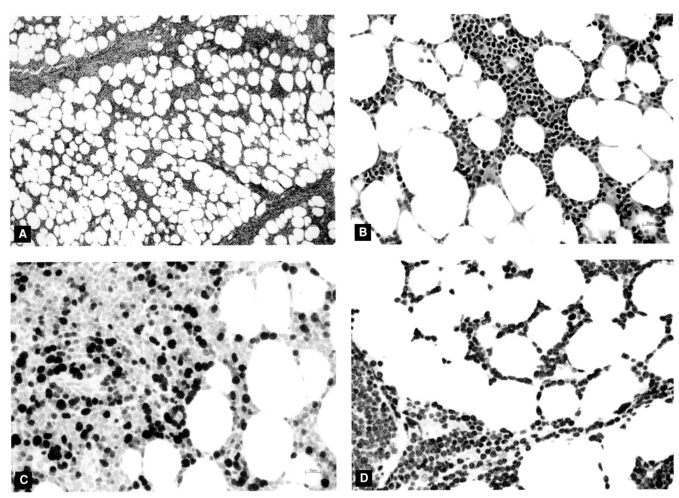

FIGURE 153.10 T-lymphoblastic lymphoma of the mediastinum/thymus: (**A**) H&E 100×; (**B**) H&E 400×; (**C**) Ki67, 400×; (**D**) TdT, 400×.

(Fig. 153.11) on one side of the midline.[244] In the mediastinum, the most frequent type is the hyaline-vascular type. It may be asymptomatic or it may give rise to compression symptoms. Most of the CD of multicentric types are associated with polyclonal hypergammaglobulinemia, elevated VES rate, increase in LDH or IL-6 or with thrombocytopenia. HHV-8 and HIV infections are often associated with the multicentric type of CD. Associated lymphomas may also develop. Single cases have been reported in association with MG.[139]

IGG4 DISEASE AND SCLEROSING MEDIASTINITIS

IgG4-related disease (IgG4-RD) is a recently recognized wide-spectrum, multiorgan idiopathic fibroinflammatory disorder, which is characterized by hypergammaglobulinemia and increased serum levels of IgG, particularly IgG4. Since the observation that many patients affected by autoimmune pancreatitis (AIP), a specific type of chronic pancreatitis, had elevated serum levels of IgG4, it was reported that these patients also had increased numbers of IgG4-positive plasma cells both in the inflamed pancreatic tissue and in extrapancreatic localizations, including sclerosing cholangitis, retroperitoneal fibrosis, sclerosing sialoadenitis (Küttner tumor), lymphadenopathy, nephritis, thyroiditis, interstitial pneumonia, and sclerosing mediastinitis, giving rise to inflammatory pseudotumors. Moreover, increased IgG4+ plasma cell infiltrate has been reported in the hypophysis and in IgG4-associated prostatitis.[245] Cellular and storiform fibrosis, lymphoplasmacytic infiltration,

increased numbers of IgG4-positive plasma cells, and obliterative phlebitis are the histological features in IgG4-RD. In the mediastinum, lymph node enlargement is associated with lung disease and it is very frequent in patients with AIP.[246] Sclerosing mediastinitis may develop as a rare aggressive syndrome characterized by the formation of invasive fibrous tissue in the mediastinum compromising the vital structures. IHC performed on the plasma cellular infiltrate may reveal high expression of IgG4 immunoglobulin in the fibrosing lesions. Recently published International Consensus Diagnostic Criteria for Autoimmune Pancreatitis include Guidelines by the International Association of Pancreatology, classifying AIP into types 1 and 2, using five cardinal features of AIP, namely, imaging of pancreatic parenchyma and duct, serology, other organ involvement, pancreatic histology, and an optional criterion of response to steroid therapy.[247]

PRIMARY LOCALIZED AMYLOIDOSIS

The thymus is very rarely involved by amyloidosis presenting a localized mediastinal mass. A case of primary (type A) amyloidosis was reported, associated with MG, thus simulating a thymoma. The mass showed birefringence under polarized light microscopy after Congo red staining and immunohistochemical analysis revealed polyclonal light chains. No alterations in serum and urine immunoglobulin protein electrophoresis were found, with no evidence of plasma cell dyscrasia on bone marrow aspirate, urine, or serum.[138]

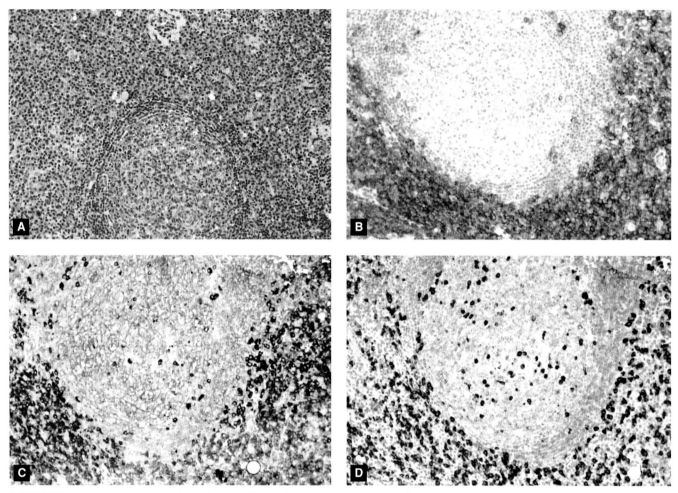

FIGURE 153.11 Castleman disease of the mediastinum/thymus: (**A**) H&E staining showing a large germinal center surrounded by sheets of plasmacells (pc), 200×; (**B**) CD138 underlying the pc sheet, 200×; (**C**) CAT K+ positive pc, outside and in the germinal center, 200×; (**D**) CAT λ+ pc outside and in the germinal center, 200× (the pc are polyclonal).

THE NEW SPECTRUM OF AIDS-RELATED MALIGNANCIES

The incidence of AIDS specifically related to (AIDS defining malignancies, namely Kaposi sarcoma and non-Hodgkin lymphoma) neoplasms has declined in the ART era. Conversely, the number of cases of non–AIDS-defining malignancies has increased,[248–250] reflecting the longer survival of HIV-infected patients. Among these diseases, Hodgkin lymphoma and human herpesvirus 8 (HHV8)-related diseases have changed their epidemiological profile. In these situations, HIV positivity appears to be an independent risk factor. Epstein virus (EBV)-associated Hodgkin lymphoma has increased its incidence several times in HIV-infected patients and ART-induced improvement in CD4 counts from severe to moderate immunosuppression resulting in this increased incidence of Hodgkin lymphoma.[251] The lymphadenopathy typically occurs in the mediastinum.[251] Among HHV8-related AIDS associated diseases, Kaposi sarcoma usually involves the lungs. HHV8-associated multicentric Castleman disease (MCD) is among the increasing pathologies. Hilar and mediastinal lymphadenopathies are common, and MCD of the plasma cellular type is the variant encountered, associated with laboratory abnormalities typical of MCD of plasma cellular type.[252–254] The occurrence also of multilocular thymic cysts (MTC), mostly in children, is among the mediastinal masses, associated with CD8+ lymphocytes in the blood.[255]

ECTOPIC TUMOR MARKERS

THYROID TISSUE

Thyroid tissue can also be found in remote structures associated with the thyroid anlage during development, including the esophagus, mediastinum, heart, aorta, adrenal, pancreas, gallbladder, and skin. Ectopic thyroid tissue can be subject to the same pathological processes as normal ectopic thyroid tissue such as inflammation, hyperplasia, and tumorigenesis. In the mediastinum, most of the ectopic tissue is found in continuity with a thyroid goiter, very rare cases of distinct thyroid tissue and tumors being detected elsewhere in the mediastinum.[256,257] Every kind of thyroid neoplasia can occur, but follicular adenomas and papillary carcinomas are the most frequent. Medullary carcinomas may occur, and may be associated with several hormonal secretion syndromes.[258]

PARATHYROID TISSUE

Parathyroid tissue may give rise to ectopic parathyroid tumors (both adenomas and carcinomas) in the mediastinum. About 20% of parathyroid neoplasms develop in the mediastinum, most of them (80%) occurring in the anterior mediastinum, near or within the thymus.[259] In fact, the thymus and parathyroid share a common embryologic origin from the third branchial cleft. Mediastinal parathyroid adenomas are an uncommon cause of persistent hyperparathyroidism and rarely cause a discernible mass. Among symptoms of hyperparathyroidism, kidney stones and bone pain can develop. Serum calcium and phosphorus levels (hypercalcemia and hypophosphatemia) could be altered, even symptomless, in relationship with hormonal secretion.[260,261]

METASTASES TO THE THYMUS OR MEDIASTINUM

When evaluating masses in the mediastinum, it is important to remember that most neoplasias in the mediastinum are indeed metastatic neoplasms from the lung. The lymphatic route is first utilized by pulmonary carcinomas, and therefore the mediastinal nodes, mostly in the middle compartment of the mediastinum, are interested first. Other frequent sources of thymic/anterior mediastinal metastases include thyroid, breast, and prostatic carcinomas.[2] Very rarely, metastases from other cancers may occur in a thymoma (Fig. 153.12). Immunohistochemical and genetic characterizations might provide data on the primary origin of these tumors.[113] The mediastinum was also recently indicated for the diagnosis and M1 staging of extrathoracic neoplasms.[262,263] A recent review illustrated the role of IHC in the differential diagnosis of tumor of the mediastinum.[264]

GENETIC MARKERS

The discovery of genetic markers of mediastinal tumors encompasses expanding fields that cannot be presented synthetically. Genomic alterations specific to diagnostic categories of mediastinal tumors could support the diagnosis and eventually give insight to the prognosis and to the predictive personalized medicine. Genetic markers are also applied to dissect the primary origin, although not applicable for routine cases. The most intriguing problem is the differential diagnosis of TSCC and lung squamous cell carcinoma.[265–267] However, only a synthetic overview of genetic markers will be presented here.

A SHORT SURVEY OF GENETIC MARKERS IN GCTS, IN TET, AND IN MEDIASTINAL LYMPHOMAS

As recurrent genomic alterations in malignant GCTs, the occurrence of the isochromosome i(12p) genotype has been described in most variants in postpubertal cases (irrespective of their primary site),[32,268,269] and even in somatic-type–associated malignancies arising in GCTs.[270] However, in these secondary components, complex and tissue specific, further abnormalities have been additionally found in both solid and hematological malignancies.[270]

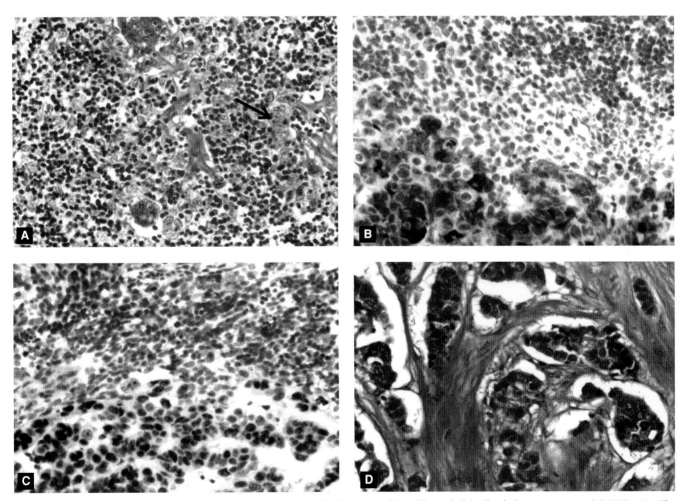

FIGURE 153.12 B2 thymoma with metastasis of breast carcinoma: (A–C) Thymoma infiltrated by epithelial cells of a breast carcinoma: (A) H&E, 400×. The *arrow* indicates nests of large epithelial cells in a B2 thymoma; (B) Mammoglobin staining of the same cells, 400×; (C) Estrogen receptor (ER) staining of metastatic epithelial cells, 400×; (D) Primary breast carcinoma, giving rise to lymphatic metastases in the thymoma showed in A–C: H&E, 400×.

In TET, the discovery of new genetic markers is increasing. The reader could refer to a recent review in such a field.[271] By cluster microRNA sequencing, a specific characteristic of WHO type A and AB thymomas has been reported in chromosome 19.[272] Mature microRNA in TET have just started to be explored in thymomas and thymic carcinomas.[273]

Primary mediastinal B-cell lymphoma (PMBCL) has been associated to gains in chromosomes 9p24.1 and 2p15.[235] Subsequent data confirmed this tumor's genomic uniqueness.[274] However, the study of the main lymphoma entities in the mediastinum is very complex due to the occurrence of cases with overlapping features among PMBCL and Hodgkin lymphoma, described as "mediastinal grey zone lymphomas"[258,275] and showing overlapping genetic features among the two entities,[276] as well as differences.[277]

GENETIC MARKERS IN MEDIASTINAL SOFT TISSUE TUMORS

Both differentiated and dedifferentiated liposarcomas show a complex 12q13-21 amplicon with constant MDM2 amplification.[2] The rare mediastinal synovial sarcoma is characterized by a specific translocation t(X;18)(p11;q11).[278] Neuroblastomas and ganglioneuroblastomas, both malignant tumors deriving from primitive neuroblastst the first, and from neuroblasts and mature ganglion cells the second, a recurrent genetic aberration, rarely shared with ganglioneuroblastomas, is MYCN amplification.[279] The rare epithelioid hemangioendothelioma recognizes translocation t(1;3)q36;q23-25) as specific genetic markers in all cases resulting in a fusion gene known as WWTR1 and CAMTA1.[280]

ROLE OF SURGEON IN MARKER VALIDATION AND BIOBANKING

Integration among specialty areas considers the role of surgeons in marker validation and biobanking as fundamental. In fact, the surgeon involved in mediastinal tumor treatment (in the thoracic surgery or neurosurgery) is the first able to plan the diagnostic procedure and to organize the necessary preliminary laboratory workup of the patient. Nowadays, the global concept of biobanking, in addition to cytological and tissue specimens, includes several other biospecimen types (e.g., matched blood, serum, plasma, buffy coat, saliva, urine),[281] that together contribute to the biorepository.[282–284] Baseline biological characteristics of tumors should be recorded similarly to demographic and clinical data. The biorepository is most useful for diagnosis and research. An integrated effort among specialties is mandatory. Biobanking is one of the tasks that the clinical pathologist carries out for blood, serum, plasma, and that pathology carries out both for tumor tissue and for normal tissue, when available. However, preoperative blood/serum and other body fluids collection and storage should become part of the routine surgical diagnostic workup. Postsurgical sampling and storage of tumor specimens should be immediately performed by the pathologists according to the standard operating procedure (SOP) of the existing local biobank.[285] Patient stored samples will be increasingly necessary to identify new biomarkers with biological meaning and statistical relevance. The markers showing significance will need prospective tissue banking and validation studies. Biopsies and blood/serum sampling at baseline, on treatment and at progression will become an integral part of future clinical trials.[286]

LIQUID BIOPSY, THE NEW FRONTIER

Liquid biopsy is a developing noninvasive practice in the detection and molecular characterization of circulating tumor cells (CTC) versus circulating tumor DNA (ctDNA) as a therapeutic strategy supporting personalized medicine. The information derived from CTC (cells or DNA shed from the tumor into the blood/serum) detection may provide diagnostic, monitoring, prognostic, and predictive elements. A variety of innovative technologies for the enrichment and detection of CTC are undergoing experimental validation, and the time and cost limitations are under evaluation.[287–289] The role of CTC and ctDNA detection as screening approaches in cancer diagnosis is still being debated.[290] The reader should refer to several recent reviews dealing with this topic and with the findings available in thoracopulmonary oncology.[291,292]

All these technological advances and the information they provide are still waiting to be translated into clinical practice. In the clinical practice and for research purposes, multidisciplinary teams are requested to improve detection, diagnosis, surveillance, and treatment in patients with mediastinal tumors.

ACKNOWLEDGMENTS

The Authors received no support for this work.

The authors are grateful to Prof. Francesco Facciolo (Rome, Italy) and his collaborators and to Prof. G. Palmieri (Naples, Italy) for their continuous support. Moreover, the authors thank Dr. Maria Teresa Ramieri and Dr. Enzo Gallo for their support in the photographical and editorial overview and to Mrs. Arianna Papadantonakis for her technical assistance. The authors are also grateful to Dr. T. Merlino for English language editing.

This chapter is dedicated to the late Prof. Dr. Piero Musiani (Rome and Chieti, Italy) for his enthusiastic encouragement on thymus gland study and research.

REFERENCES

1. Biomarkers Definitions Working Group. Biomarkers and surrogate endpoints: preferred definitions and conceptual framework. *Clin Pharmacol Ther* 2001;69:89–95.
2. Travis WD, Brambilla E, Burke AP, et al. *World Health Organization Classification of Tumours of the Lung, Pleura, Thymus and Heart*. Vol. 7. 4th ed. Lyon: IARC Press; 2015.
3. Carter BW, Marom EM, Detterbeck FC. Approaching the patient with an anterior mediastinal mass: a guide for clinicians. *J Thorac Oncol* 2014;9:S102–S109.
4. Marchevsky A, Marx A, Strobel P, et al. Policies and reporting guidelines for small biopsy specimens of mediastinal masses. *J Thorac Oncol* 2011;6:S1724–S1729.
5. Weksler B, Lu B. Alterations of the immune system in thymic malignancies. *J Thorac Oncol* 2014;9:S137–S142.
6. Chalabreysse L, Thomas De Montpreville V, De Muret A, et al. [Rythmic-pathology: the French national pathology network for thymic epithelial tumours]. *Ann Pathol* 2014;34:87–91.
7. Quint LE, Reddy RM, Lin J, et al. Imaging in thoracic oncology: case studies from Multidisciplinary Thoracic Tumor Board (part 1 of 2 part series). *Cancer Imaging* 2013;13:429–439.
8. le Roux BT, Kallichurum S, Shama DM. Mediastinal cysts and tumors. *Curr Probl Surg* 1984;21:1–77.
9. Mullen B, Richardson JD. Primary anterior mediastinal tumors in children and adults. *Ann Thorac Surg* 1986;42:338–345.
10. Chaganti RS, Rodriguez E, Mathew S. Origin of adult male mediastinal germ-cell tumours. *Lancet* 1994;343:1130–1132.
11. Albany C, Einhorn LH. Extragonadal germ cell tumors: clinical presentation and management. *Curr Opin Oncol* 2013;25:261–265.
12. Zhao GQ, Dowell JE. Hematologic malignancies associated with germ cell tumors. *Expert Rev Hematol* 2012;5:427–437.
13. Dominguez Malagon H, Perez Montiel D. Mediastinal germ cell tumors. *Semin Diagn Pathol* 2005;22:230–240.
14. Oosterhuis JW, Looijenga LH. Testicular germ-cell tumours in a broader perspective. *Nat Rev Cancer* 2005;5:210–222.
15. Baranzelli MC, Kramar A, Bouffet E, et al. Prognostic factors in children with localized malignant nonseminomatous germ cell tumors. *J Clin Oncol* 1999;17:1212.

16. Hartmann JT, Nichols CR, Droz JP, et al. Prognostic variables for response and outcome in patients with extragonadal germ-cell tumors. *Ann Oncol* 2002;13:1017–1028.

17. Bokemeyer C, Nichols CR, Droz JP, et al. Extragonadal germ cell tumors of the mediastinum and retroperitoneum: results from an international analysis. *J Clin Oncol* 2002;20:1864–1873.

18. Schneider DT, Calaminus G, Reinhard H, et al. Primary mediastinal germ cell tumors in children and adolescents: results of the German cooperative protocols MAKEI 83/86, 89, and 96. *J Clin Oncol* 2000;18:832–839.

19. Zondek B. Versuch einer biologischen (hormonalen) Diagnos- tik beim mailgnen Hodentumor. *Chirurg* 1930;2:1072–1080.

20. Mead GM, Stenning SP. International Germ Cell Consensus Classification: a prognostic factor-based staging system for metastatic germ cell cancers. International Germ Cell Cancer Collaborative Group. *J Clin Oncol* 1997;15:594–603.

21. Sturgeon CM, Duffy MJ, Stenman UH, et al. National Academy of Clinical Biochemistry laboratory medicine practice guidelines for use of tumor markers in testicular, prostate, colorectal, breast, and ovarian cancers. *Clin Chem* 2008;54:e11–e79.

22. Gilligan TD, Seidenfeld J, Basch EM, et al. American Society of Clinical Oncology Clinical Practice Guideline on uses of serum tumor markers in adult males with germ cell tumors. *J Clin Oncol* 2010;28:3388–3404.

23. McKenney JK, Heerema-McKenney A, Rouse RV. Extragonadal germ cell tumors: a review with emphasis on pathologic features, clinical prognostic variables, and differential diagnostic considerations. *Adv Anat Pathol* 2007;14:69–92.

24. van Casteren NJ, de Jong J, Stoop H, et al. Evaluation of testicular biopsies for carcinoma in situ: immunohistochemistry is mandatory. *Int J Androl* 2009;32:666–674.

25. Moran CA, Suster S, Koss MN. Primary germ cell tumors of the mediastinum: III. Yolk sac tumor, embryonal carcinoma, choriocarcinoma, and combined nonteratomatous germ cell tumors of the mediastinum—a clinicopathologic and immunohistochemical study of 64 cases. *Cancer* 1997;80:699–707.

26. Moran CA, Suster S, Przygodzki RM, et al. Primary germ cell tumors of the mediastinum: II. Mediastinal seminomas—a clinicopathologic and immunohistochemical study of 120 cases. *Cancer* 1997;80:691–698.

27. Niehans GA, Manivel JC, Copland GT, et al. Immunohistochemistry of germ cell and trophoblastic neoplasms. *Cancer* 1988;62:1113–1123.

28. Przygodzki RM, Hubbs AE, Zhao FQ, et al. Primary mediastinal seminomas: evidence of single and multiple KIT mutations. *Lab Invest* 2002;82:1369–1375.

29. Wick MR, Swanson PE, Manivel JC. Placental-like alkaline phosphatase reactivity in human tumors: an immunohistochemical study of 520 cases. *Hum Pathol* 1987;18:946–954.

30. Jung SM, Chu PH, Shiu TF, et al. Expression of OCT4 in the primary germ cell tumors and thymoma in the mediastinum. *Appl Immunohistochem Mol Morphol* 2006;14:273–275.

31. Liu A, Cheng L, Du J, et al. Diagnostic utility of novel stem cell markers SALL4, OCT4, NANOG, SOX2, UTF1, and TCL1 in primary mediastinal germ cell tumors. *Am J Surg Pathol* 2010;34:697–706.

32. Sung MT, Maclennan GT, Lopez-Beltran A, et al. Primary mediastinal seminoma: a comprehensive assessment integrated with histology, immunohistochemistry, and fluorescence in situ hybridization for chromosome 12p abnormalities in 23 cases. *Am J Surg Pathol* 2008;32:146–155.

33. Beyer J, Albers P, Altena R, et al. Maintaining success, reducing treatment burden, focusing on survivorship: highlights from the third European consensus conference on diagnosis and treatment of germ-cell cancer. *Ann Oncol* 2013;24:878–888.

34. Caposole MZ, Aruca-Bustillo V, Mitchell M, et al. Benign metachronous bilateral ovarian and mediastinal teratomas with an elevated alpha-fetoprotein. *Ann Thorac Surg* 2015;99:1073–1075.

35. Richie JP. *Neoplasm of the Testis*. 6th ed. Philadelphia, PA: W.B. Saunders; 1992.

36. Bower M. *Serum Tumor Markers*. 2nd ed. Philadelphia, PA: Lippincott Williams & Wilkins; 1999.

37. Fishman WH, Bardawil WA, Habib HG, et al. The placental isoenzymes of alkaline phosphatase in sera of normal pregnancy. *Am J Clin Pathol* 1972;57:65–74.

38. Koshida K, Nishino A, Yamamoto H, et al. The role of alkaline phosphatase isoenzymes as tumor markers for testicular germ cell tumors. *J Urol* 1991;146:57–60.

39. Lange PH, Millan JL, Stigbrand T, et al. Placental alkaline phosphatase as a tumor marker for seminoma. *Cancer Res* 1982;42:3244–3247.

40. Weissbach L, Bussar-Maatz R, Mann K. The value of tumor markers in testicular seminomas. Results of a prospective multicenter study. *Eur Urol* 1997;32:16–22.

41. Nielsen OS, Munro AJ, Duncan W, et al. Is placental alkaline phosphatase (PLAP) a useful marker for seminoma? *Eur J Cancer* 1990;26:1049–1054.

42. Suster S, Moran CA, Dominguez-Malagon H, et al. Germ cell tumors of the mediastinum and testis: a comparative immunohistochemical study of 120 cases. *Hum Pathol* 1998;29:737–742.

43. von Eyben FE, Blaabjerg O, Hyltoft-Petersen P, et al. Serum lactate dehydrogenase isoenzyme 1 and prediction of death in patients with metastatic testicular germ cell tumors. *Clin Chem Lab Med* 2001;39:38–44.

44. von Eyben FE, Blaabjerg O, Madsen EL, et al. Serum lactate dehydrogenase isoenzyme 1 and tumour volume are indicators of response to treatment and predictors of prognosis in metastatic testicular germ cell tumours. *Eur J Cancer* 1992;28:410–415.

45. Laguna MP, Pizzocaro G, Klepp O, et al. EAU guidelines on testicular cancer. *Eur Urol* 2001;40:102–110.

46. Durkop H, Latza U, Hummel M, et al. Molecular cloning and expression of a new member of the nerve growth factor receptor family that is characteristic for Hodgkin's disease. *Cell* 1992;68:421–427.

47. Smith CA, Gruss HJ, Davis T, et al. CD30 antigen, a marker for Hodgkin's lymphoma, is a receptor whose ligand defines an emerging family of cytokines with homology to TNF. *Cell* 1993;73:1349–1360.

48. Stein H, Mason DY, Gerdes J, et al. The expression of the Hodgkin's disease associated antigen Ki-1 in reactive and neoplastic lymphoid tissue: evidence that Reed-Sternberg cells and histiocytic malignancies are derived from activated lymphoid cells. *Blood* 1985;66:848–858.

49. Latza U, Foss HD, Durkop H, et al. CD30 antigen in embryonal carcinoma and embryogenesis and release of the soluble molecule. *Am J Pathol* 1995;146:463–471.

50. Pallesen G, Hamilton-Dutoit SJ. Ki-1 (CD30) antigen is regularly expressed by tumor cells of embryonal carcinoma. *Am J Pathol* 1988;133:446–450.

51. Hittmair A, Rogatsch H, Hobisch A, et al. CD30 expression in seminoma. *Hum Pathol* 1996;27:1166–1171.

52. Shimosato Y, Mukai K. *Tumors of the Mediastinum*. 3rd ed. Washington, DC: AFIP; 1997.

53. Franke FE, Pauls K, Rey R, et al. Differentiation markers of Sertoli cells and germ cells in fetal and early postnatal human testis. *Anat Embryol (Berl)* 2004;209:169–177.

54. Marks A, Sutherland DR, Bailey D, et al. Characterization and distribution of an oncofetal antigen (M2A antigen) expressed on testicular germ cell tumours. *Br J Cancer* 1999;80:569–578.

55. Lau SK, Weiss LM, Chu PG. D2-40 immunohistochemistry in the differential diagnosis of seminoma and embryonal carcinoma: a comparative immunohistochemical study with KIT (CD117) and CD30. *Mod Pathol* 2007;20:320–325.

56. Iczkowski KA, Butler SL, Shanks JH, et al. Trials of new germ cell immunohistochemical stains in 93 extragonadal and metastatic germ cell tumors. *Hum Pathol* 2008;39:275–281.

57. Bokemeyer C, Kuczyk MA, Dunn T, et al. Expression of stem-cell factor and its receptor c-kit protein in normal testicular tissue and malignant germ-cell tumours. *J Cancer Res Clin Oncol* 1996;122:301–306.

58. Hirota S, Isozaki K, Moriyama Y, et al. Gain-of-function mutations of c-kit in human gastrointestinal stromal tumors. *Science* 1998;279:577–580.

59. Sarlomo-Rikala M, Kovatich AJ, Barusevicius A, et al. CD117: a sensitive marker for gastrointestinal stromal tumors that is more specific than CD34. *Mod Pathol* 1998;11:728–734.

60. Tian Q, Frierson HF Jr, Krystal GW, et al. Activating c-kit gene mutations in human germ cell tumors. *Am J Pathol* 1999;154:1643–1647.

61. Leroy X, Augusto D, Leteurtre E, et al. CD30 and CD117 (c-kit) used in combination are useful for distinguishing embryonal carcinoma from seminoma. *J Histochem Cytochem* 2002;50:283–285.

62. Ulbright TM. Germ cell tumors of the gonads: a selective review emphasizing problems in differential diagnosis, newly appreciated, and controversial issues. *Mod Pathol* 2005;18(suppl 2):S61–S79.

63. Cheng L, Thomas A, Roth LM, et al. OCT4: a novel biomarker for dysgerminoma of the ovary. *Am J Surg Pathol* 2004;28:1341–1346.

64. Wang J, Rao S, Chu J, et al. A protein interaction network for pluripotency of embryonic stem cells. *Nature* 2006;444:364–368.

65. Wu Q, Chen X, Zhang J, et al. Sall4 interacts with Nanog and co-occupies Nanog genomic sites in embryonic stem cells. *J Biol Chem* 2006;281:24090–24094.

66. Zhou Q, Chipperfield H, Melton DA, et al. A gene regulatory network in mouse embryonic stem cells. *Proc Natl Acad Sci U S A* 2007;104:16438–16443.

67. Zhang J, Tam WL, Tong GQ, et al. Sall4 modulates embryonic stem cell pluripotency and early embryonic development by the transcriptional regulation of Pou5f1. *Nat Cell Biol* 2006;8:1114–1123.

68. Nishimoto M, Fukushima A, Okuda A, et al. The gene for the embryonic stem cell coactivator UTF1 carries a regulatory element which selectively interacts with a complex composed of Oct-3/4 and Sox-2. *Mol Cell Biol* 1999;19:5453–5465.

69. Nishimoto M, Miyagi S, Yamagishi T, et al. Oct-3/4 maintains the proliferative embryonic stem cell state via specific binding to a variant octamer sequence in the regulatory region of the UTF1 locus. *Mol Cell Biol* 2005;25:5084–5094.

70. Matoba R, Niwa H, Masui S, et al. Dissecting Oct3/4-regulated gene networks in embryonic stem cells by expression profiling. *PLoS One* 2006;1:e26.

71. Cao D, Guo S, Allan RW, et al. SALL4 is a novel sensitive and specific marker of ovarian primitive germ cell tumors and is particularly useful in distinguishing yolk sac tumor from clear cell carcinoma. *Am J Surg Pathol* 2009;33:894–904.

72. Cao D, Li J, Guo CC, et al. SALL4 is a novel diagnostic marker for testicular germ cell tumors. *Am J Surg Pathol* 2009;33:1065–1077.

73. Cui W, Kong NR, Ma Y, et al. Differential expression of the novel oncogene, SALL4, in lymphoma, plasma cell myeloma, and acute lymphoblastic leukemia. *Mod Pathol* 2006;19:1585–1592.

74. Herling M, Patel KA, Hsi ED, et al. TCL1 in B-cell tumors retains its normal b-cell pattern of regulation and is a marker of differentiation stage. *Am J Surg Pathol* 2007;31:1123–1129.

75. Narducci MG, Pescarmona E, Lazzeri C, et al. Regulation of TCL1 expression in B- and T-cell lymphomas and reactive lymphoid tissues. *Cancer Res* 2000;60:2095–2100.

76. Long KB, Hornick JL. SOX2 is highly expressed in squamous cell carcinomas of the gastrointestinal tract. *Hum Pathol* 2009;40:1768–1773.

77. Schoenhals M, Kassambara A, De Vos J, et al. Embryonic stem cell markers expression in cancers. *Biochem Biophys Res Commun* 2009;383:157–162.

78. Filmus J. The contribution of in vivo manipulation of gene expression to the understanding of the function of glypicans. *Glycoconj J* 2002;19:319–323.

79. Nusse R. Wnts and Hedgehogs: lipid-modified proteins and similarities in signaling mechanisms at the cell surface. *Development* 2003;130(22):5297–5305.

80. Capurro MI, Shi W, Sandal S, et al. Processing by convertases is not required for glypican-3-induced stimulation of hepatocellular carcinoma growth. *J Biol Chem* 2005;280:41201–41206.

81. Filmus J, Capurro M, Rast J. Glypicans. *Genome Biol* 2008;9:224.

82. Song HH, Shi W, Xiang YY, et al. The loss of glypican-3 induces alterations in Wnt signaling. *J Biol Chem* 2005;280:2116–2125.

83. Torisu Y, Watanabe A, Nonaka A, et al. Human homolog of NOTUM, overexpressed in hepatocellular carcinoma, is regulated transcriptionally by beta-catenin/TCF. *Cancer Sci* 2008;99:1139–1146.

84. Zynger DL, Dimov ND, Luan C, et al. Glypican 3: a novel marker in testicular germ cell tumors. *Am J Surg Pathol* 2006;30:1570–1575.

85. Weissferdt A, Rodriguez-Canales J, Liu H, et al. Primary mediastinal seminomas: a comprehensive immunohistochemical study with a focus on novel markers. *Hum Pathol* 2015;46:376–383.

86. Bode PK, Barghorn A, Fritzsche FR, et al. MAGEC2 is a sensitive and novel marker for seminoma: a tissue microarray analysis of 325 testicular germ cell tumors. *Mod Pathol* 2011;24:829–835.

87. Engels EA. Epidemiology of thymoma and associated malignancies. *J Thorac Oncol* 2010;5:S260–S265.

88. Kim E, Thomas CR Jr. Conditional survival of malignant thymoma using national population-based surveillance, epidemiology, and end results (SEER) registry (1973-2011). *J Thorac Oncol* 2015;10:701–707.

89. Marx A, Strobel P, Badve SS, et al. ITMIG consensus statement on the use of the WHO histological classification of thymoma and thymic carcinoma: refined definitions, histological criteria, and reporting. *J Thorac Oncol* 2014;9:596–611.

90. Weissferdt A, Moran CA. Immunohistochemistry in the diagnosis of thymic epithelial neoplasms. *Appl Immunohistochem Mol Morphol* 2014;22:479–487.

91. den Bakker MA, Roden AC, Marx A, et al. Histologic classification of thymoma: a practical guide for routine cases. *J Thorac Oncol* 2014;9:S125–S130.

92. Ströbel P, Hartmann E, Rosenwald A, et al. Corticomedullary differentiation and maturational arrest in thymomas. *Histopathology* 2014;64:557–566.

93. Murata S, Sasaki K, Kishimoto T, et al. Regulation of CD8+ T cell development by thymus-specific proteasomes. *Science* 2007;316:1349–1353.

94. Tomaru U, Ishizu A, Murata S, et al. Exclusive expression of proteasome subunit {beta}5t in the human thymic cortex. *Blood* 2009;113:5186–5191.

95. Yamada Y, Tomaru U, Ishizu A, et al. Expression of proteasome subunit beta5t in thymic epithelial tumors. *Am J Surg Pathol* 2011;35:1296–1304.

96. Rosai J, Sobin LH. *World Health Organization Classification of Tumors: Histological Typing of Tumours of the Thymus.* 2nd ed. Berlin-Heidelberg: Springer-Verlag; 1999.

97. Travis WD, Brambilla E, Muller-Hermelink HK, et al. *World Health Organization Classification of Tumors: Pathology and Genetics of Tumors of the Lung, Pleura, Thymus, and Heart.* 3rd ed. Lyon: IARC Press, 2004.

98. Marino M, Müller-Hermelink HK. Thymoma and thymic carcinoma. Relation of thymoma epithelial cells to the cortical and medullary differentiation of thymus. *Virchows Arch A Pathol Anat Histopathol* 1985;407:119–149.

99. Kirchner T, Schalke B, Buchwald J, et al. Well-differentiated thymic carcinoma. An organotypical low-grade carcinoma with relationship to cortical thymoma. *Am J Surg Pathol* 1992;16:1153–1169.

100. Suster S, Moran CA. Thymoma, atypical thymoma, and thymic carcinoma. A novel conceptual approach to the classification of thymic epithelial neoplasms. *Am J Clin Pathol* 1999;111:826–833.

101. Suster S, Moran CA. Primary thymic epithelial neoplasms: spectrum of differentiation and histological features. *Semin Diagn Pathol* 1999;16:2–17.

102. Kalhor N, Moran CA. Thymoma: current concepts. *Oncology (Williston Park)* 2012;26:975–981.

103. Kodama T, Watanabe S, Sato Y, et al. An immunohistochemical study of thymic epithelial tumors. I. Epithelial component. *Am J Surg Pathol* 1986;10:26–33.

104. Kuo T. Cytokeratin profiles of the thymus and thymomas: histogenetic correlations and proposal for a histological classification of thymomas. *Histopathology* 2000;36:403–414.

105. Kuo TT, Chan JK. Thymic carcinoma arising in thymoma is associated with alterations in immunohistochemical profile. *Am J Surg Pathol* 1998;22:1474–1481.

106. Sato Y, Watanabe S, Mukai K, et al. An immunohistochemical study of thymic epithelial tumors. II. Lymphoid component. *Am J Surg Pathol* 1986;10:862–870.

107. Kaira K, Oriuchi N, Imai H, et al. L-type amino acid transporter 1 (LAT1) is frequently expressed in thymic carcinomas but is absent in thymomas. *J Surg Oncol* 2009;99:433–438.

108. Nonaka D, Henley JD, Chiriboga L, et al. Diagnostic utility of thymic epithelial markers CD205 (DEC205) and Foxn1 in thymic epithelial neoplasms. *Am J Surg Pathol* 2007;31:1038–1044.

109. Raica M, Kondylis A, Mogoanta L, et al. Diagnostic and clinical significance of D2-40 expression in the normal human thymus and thymoma. *Rom J Morphol Embryol* 2010;51:229–234.

110. Sarafian VS, Marinova TT, Gulubova MV. Differential expression of LAMPs and ubiquitin in human thymus. *APMIS* 2009;117:248–252.

111. Attanoos RL, Galateau-Salle F, Gibbs AR, et al. Primary thymic epithelial tumours of the pleura mimicking malignant mesothelioma. *Histopathology* 2002;41:42–49.

112. Pan CC, Chen PC, Chou TY, et al. Expression of calretinin and other mesothelioma-related markers in thymic carcinoma and thymoma. *Hum Pathol* 2003;34:1155–1162.

113. Pomplun S, Wotherspoon AC, Shah G, et al. Immunohistochemical markers in the differentiation of thymic and pulmonary neoplasms. *Histopathology* 2002;40:152–158.

114. Chilosi M, Castelli P, Martignoni G, et al. Neoplastic epithelial cells in a subset of human thymomas express the B cell-associated CD20 antigen. *Am J Surg Pathol* 1992;16:988–997.

115. Marandino F, Zoccali C, Salducca N, et al. Ectopic primary type A thymoma located in two thoracic vertebras: a case report. *BMC Cancer* 2010;10:322.

116. Dorfman DM, Shahsafaei A, Chan JK. Thymic carcinomas, but not thymomas and carcinomas of other sites, show CD5 immunoreactivity. *Am J Surg Pathol* 1997;21:936–940.

117. Kornstein MJ, Rosai J. CD5 labeling of thymic carcinomas and other nonlymphoid neoplasms. *Am J Clin Pathol* 1998;109:722–726.

118. Tateyama H, Eimoto T, Tada T, et al. Immunoreactivity of a new CD5 antibody with normal epithelium and malignant tumors including thymic carcinoma. *Am J Clin Pathol* 1999;111:235–240.

119. Henley JD, Cummings OW, Loehrer PJ Sr. Tyrosine kinase receptor expression in thymomas. *J Cancer Res Clin Oncol* 2004;130:222–224.

120. Pan CC, Chen PC, Chiang H. KIT (CD117) is frequently overexpressed in thymic carcinomas but is absent in thymomas. *J Pathol* 2004;202:375–381.

121. Kaira K, Murakami H, Serizawa M, et al. MUC1 expression in thymic epithelial tumors: MUC1 may be useful marker as differential diagnosis between type B3 thymoma and thymic carcinoma. *Virchows Arch* 2011;458:615–620.

122. Ströbel P, Hartmann M, Jakob A, et al. Thymic carcinoma with overexpression of mutated KIT and the response to imatinib. *N Engl J Med* 2004;350:2625–2626.

123. Nakagawa K, Matsuno Y, Kunitoh H, et al. Immunohistochemical KIT (CD117) expression in thymic epithelial tumors. *Chest* 2005;128:140–144.

124. Palmieri G, Marino M, Buonerba C, et al. Imatinib mesylate in thymic epithelial malignancies. *Cancer Chemother Pharmacol* 2012;69:309–315.

125. Yoh K, Nishiwaki Y, Ishii G, et al. Mutational status of EGFR and KIT in thymoma and thymic carcinoma. *Lung Cancer* 2008;62:316–320.

126. Simonelli M, Zucali PA, Suter MB, et al. Targeted therapy for thymic epithelial tumors: a new horizon? Review of the literature and two cases reports. *Future Oncol* 2015;11:1223–1232.

127. Ströbel P, Hohenberger P, Marx A. Thymoma and thymic carcinoma: molecular pathology and targeted therapy. *J Thorac Oncol* 2010;5:S286–S290.

128. Thomas A, Rajan A, Berman A. Correction to Lancet Oncol 2015; 16: 181, 184. *Lancet Oncol* 2015;16:e105.

129. Evoli A, Lancaster E. Paraneoplastic disorders in thymoma patients. *J Thorac Oncol* 2014;9:S143–S147.

130. Meriggioli MN, Sanders DB. Muscle autoantibodies in myasthenia gravis: beyond diagnosis?. *Expert Rev Clin Immunol* 2012;8:427–438.

131. Fang W, Chen W, Chen G, et al. Surgical management of thymic epithelial tumors: a retrospective review of 204 cases. *Ann Thorac Surg* 2005;80:2002–2007.

132. Mygland A, Vincent A, Newsom-Davis J, et al. Autoantibodies in thymoma-associated myasthenia gravis with myositis or neuromyotonia. *Arch Neurol* 2000;57:527–531.

133. Kadota Y, Okumura M, Miyoshi S, et al. Altered T cell development in human thymoma is related to impairment of MHC class II transactivator expression induced by interferon-gamma (IFN-gamma). *Clin Exp Immunol* 2000;121:59–68.

134. Marx A, Hohenberger P, Hoffmann H, et al. The autoimmune regulator AIRE in thymoma biology: autoimmunity and beyond. *J Thorac Oncol* 2010;5:S266–S272.

135. Scarpino S, Di Napoli A, Stoppacciaro A, et al. Expression of autoimmune regulator gene (AIRE) and T regulatory cells in human thymomas. *Clin Exp Immunol* 2007;149:504–512.

136. Ströbel P, Rosenwald A, Beyersdorf N, et al. Selective loss of regulatory T cells in thymomas. *Ann Neurol* 2004;56:901–904.

137. Zhao Y, Zhao H, Hu D, et al. Surgical treatment and prognosis of thymic squamous cell carcinoma: a retrospective analysis of 105 cases. *Ann Thorac Surg* 2013;96:1019–1024.

138. Son SM, Lee YM, Kim SW, et al. Localized thymic amyloidosis presenting with myasthenia gravis: case report. *J Korean Med Sci* 2014;29:145–148.

139. Ishikawa K, Kato T, Aragaki M, et al. A case of Castleman's disease with myasthenia gravis. *Ann Thorac Cardiovasc Surg* 2014;20(suppl):585–588.

140. Malphettes M, Gerard L, Galicier L, et al. Good syndrome: an adult-onset immunodeficiency remarkable for its high incidence of invasive infections and autoimmune complications. *Clin Infect Dis* 2015;61:e13–e19.

141. Vitiello L, Masci AM, Montella L, et al. Thymoma-associated immunodeficiency: a syndrome characterized by severe alterations in NK, T and B-cells and progressive increase in naive CD8+ T Cells. *Int J Immunopathol Pharmacol* 2010;23:307–316.

142. Modlin IM, Lye KD, Kidd M. A 5-decade analysis of 13,715 carcinoid tumors. *Cancer* 2003;97:934–959.

143. Brandi ML, Gagel RF, Angeli A, et al. Guidelines for diagnosis and therapy of MEN type 1 and type 2. *J Clin Endocrinol Metab* 2001;86:5658–5671.

144. Moran CA, Suster S. Primary neuroendocrine carcinoma (thymic carcinoid) of the thymus with prominent oncocytic features: a clinicopathologic study of 22 cases. *Mod Pathol* 2000;13:489–494.

145. Soga J, Yakuwa Y, Osaka M. Evaluation of 342 cases of mediastinal/thymic carcinoids collected from literature: a comparative study between typical carcinoids and atypical varieties. *Ann Thorac Cardiovasc Surg* 1999;5:285–292.

146. Moran CA, Suster S. Neuroendocrine carcinomas (carcinoid tumor) of the thymus. A clinicopathologic analysis of 80 cases. *Am J Clin Pathol* 2000;114:100–110.

147. de Perrot M, Spiliopoulos A, Fischer S, et al. Neuroendocrine carcinoma (carcinoid) of the thymus associated with Cushing's syndrome. *Ann Thorac Surg* 2002;73:675–681.

148. Suster S, Moran CA. Neuroendocrine neoplasms of the mediastinum. *Am J Clin Pathol* 2001;115(suppl):S17–S27.

149. Huntrakoon M, Lin F, Heitz PU, et al. Thymic carcinoid tumor with Cushing's syndrome. Report of a case with electron microscopic and immunoperoxidase studies for neuron-specific enolase and corticotropin. *Arch Pathol Lab Med* 1984;108:551–554.

150. Herbst WM, Kummer W, Hofmann W, et al. Carcinoid tumors of the thymus. An immunohistochemical study. *Cancer* 1987;60:2465–2470.

151. Takayama T, Kameya T, Inagaki K, et al. MEN type 1 associated with mediastinal carcinoid producing parathyroid hormone, calcitonin and chorionic gonadotropin. *Pathol Res Pract* 1993;189:1090–1096; discussion 1096–1100.

152. Wick MR, Scheithauer BW. Thymic carcinoid. A histologic, immunohistochemical, and ultrastructural study of 12 cases. *Cancer* 1984;53:475–484.

153. Yoshikawa T, Noguchi Y, Matsukawa H, et al. Thymus carcinoid producing parathyroid hormone (PTH)-related protein: report of a case. *Surg Today* 1994;24:544–547.

154. Jansson JO, Svensson J, Bengtsson BA, et al. Acromegaly and Cushing's syndrome due to ectopic production of GHRH and ACTH by a thymic carcinoid tumour: in vitro responses to GHRH and GHRP-6. *Clin Endocrinol (Oxf)* 1998;48:243–250.

155. Okada S, Ohshima K, Mori M. The Cushing syndrome induced by atrial natriuretic peptide-producing thymic carcinoid. *Ann Intern Med* 1994;121:75–76.

156. Googe PB, Ferry JA, Bhan AK, et al. A comparison of paraganglioma, carcinoid tumor, and small-cell carcinoma of the larynx. *Arch Pathol Lab Med* 1988;112:809–815.

157. Martinez-Madrigal F, Bosq J, Micheau C, et al. Paragangliomas of the head and neck. Immunohistochemical analysis of 16 cases in comparison with neuro-endocrine carcinomas. *Pathol Res Pract* 1991;187:814–823.

158. Moran CA, Suster S, Fishback N, et al. Mediastinal paragangliomas. A clinicopathologic and immunohistochemical study of 16 cases. *Cancer* 1993;72:2358–2364.

159. Fabbro D, Di Loreto C, Beltrami CA, et al. Expression of thyroid-specific transcription factors TTF-1 and PAX-8 in human thyroid neoplasms. *Cancer Res* 1994;54:4744–4749.

160. Laury AR, Perets R, Piao H, et al. A comprehensive analysis of PAX8 expression in human epithelial tumors. *Am J Surg Pathol* 2011;35:816–826.

161. Ozcan A, Shen SS, Hamilton C, et al. PAX 8 expression in non-neoplastic tissues, primary tumors, and metastatic tumors: a comprehensive immunohistochemical study. *Mod Pathol* 2011;24:751–764.

162. Tacha D, Zhou D, Cheng L. Expression of PAX8 in normal and neoplastic tissues: a comprehensive immunohistochemical study. *Appl Immunohistochem Mol Morphol* 2011;19:293–299.

163. Weissferdt A, Moran CA. Pax8 expression in thymic epithelial neoplasms: an immunohistochemical analysis. *Am J Surg Pathol* 2011;35:1305–1310.

164. Long KB, Srivastava A, Hirsch MS, et al. PAX8 Expression in well-differentiated pancreatic endocrine tumors: correlation with clinicopathologic features and comparison with gastrointestinal and pulmonary carcinoid tumors. *Am J Surg Pathol* 2010;34:723–729.

165. Sangoi AR, Ohgami RS, Pai RK, et al. PAX8 expression reliably distinguishes pancreatic well-differentiated neuroendocrine tumors from ileal and pulmonary well-differentiated neuroendocrine tumors and pancreatic acinar cell carcinoma. *Mod Pathol* 2011;24:412–424.

166. Weissferdt A, Tang X, Wistuba, II, et al. Comparative immunohistochemical analysis of pulmonary and thymic neuroendocrine carcinomas using PAX8 and TTF-1. *Mod Pathol* 2013;26:1554–1560.

167. Du EZ, Goldstraw P, Zacharias J, et al. TTF-1 expression is specific for lung primary in typical and atypical carcinoids: TTF-1-positive carcinoids are predominantly in peripheral location. *Hum Pathol* 2004;35:825–831.

168. Saad RS, Liu YL, Han H, et al. Prognostic significance of thyroid transcription factor-1 expression in both early-stage conventional adenocarcinoma and bronchioloalveolar carcinoma of the lung. *Hum Pathol* 2004;35:3–7.

169. Oliveira AM, Tazelaar HD, Myers JL, et al. Thyroid transcription factor-1 distinguishes metastatic pulmonary from well-differentiated neuroendocrine tumors of other sites. *Am J Surg Pathol* 2001;25:815–819.

170. Travis WD, Rush W, Flieder DB, et al. Survival analysis of 200 pulmonary neuroendocrine tumors with clarification of criteria for atypical carcinoid and its separation from typical carcinoid. *Am J Surg Pathol* 1998;22:934–944.

171. Weissferdt A, Kalhor N, Liu H, et al. Thymic neuroendocrine tumors (paraganglioma and carcinoid tumors): a comparative immunohistochemical study of 46 cases. *Hum Pathol* 2014;45:2463–2470.

172. Chetty R, Batitang S, Govender D. Large cell neuroendocrine carcinoma of the thymus. *Histopathology* 1997;31:274–276.

173. Hekimgil M, Hamulu F, Cagirici U, et al. Small cell neuroendocrine carcinoma of the thymus complicated by Cushing's syndrome. Report of a 58-year-old woman with a 3-year history of hypertension. *Pathol Res Pract* 2001;197:129–133.

174. French CA. Pathogenesis of NUT midline carcinoma. *Annu Rev Pathol* 2012;7:247–265.

175. Bauer DE, Mitchell CM, Strait KM, et al. Clinicopathologic features and long-term outcomes of NUT midline carcinoma. *Clin Cancer Res* 2012;18:5773–5779.

176. French CA, Kutok JL, Faquin WC, et al. Midline carcinoma of children and young adults with NUT rearrangement. *J Clin Oncol* 2004;22:4135–4139.

177. Kees UR, Mulcahy MT, Willoughby ML. Intrathoracic carcinoma in an 11-year-old girl showing a translocation t(15;19). *Am J Pediatr Hematol Oncol* 1991;13:459–464.

178. Kubonishi I, Takehara N, Iwata J, et al. Novel t(15;19)(q15;p13) chromosome abnormality in a thymic carcinoma. *Cancer Res* 1991;51:3327–3328.

179. French CA. Demystified molecular pathology of NUT midline carcinomas. *J Clin Pathol* 2010;63:492–496.

180. French CA, Miyoshi I, Kubonishi I, et al. BRD4-NUT fusion oncogene: a novel mechanism in aggressive carcinoma. *Cancer Res* 2003;63:304–307.

181. French CA. NUT midline carcinoma. *Cancer Genet Cytogenet* 2010;203:16–20.

182. French CA. The importance of diagnosing NUT midline carcinoma. *Head Neck Pathol* 2013;7:11–16.

183. French CA, Ramirez CL, Kolmakova J, et al. BRD-NUT oncoproteins: a family of closely related nuclear proteins that block epithelial differentiation and maintain the growth of carcinoma cells. *Oncogene* 2008;27:2237–2242.

184. Vargas SO, French CA, Faul PN, et al. Upper respiratory tract carcinoma with chromosomal translocation 15;19: evidence for a distinct disease entity of young patients with a rapidly fatal course. *Cancer* 2001;92:1195–1203.

185. Stelow EB. A review of NUT midline carcinoma. *Head Neck Pathol* 2011;5:31–35.

186. Lee AC, Kwong YI, Fu KH, et al. Disseminated mediastinal carcinoma with chromosomal translocation (15;19). A distinctive clinicopathologic syndrome. *Cancer* 1993;72:2273–2276.

187. den Bakker MA, Beverloo BH, van den Heuvel-Eibrink MM, et al. NUT midline carcinoma of the parotid gland with mesenchymal differentiation. *Am J Surg Pathol* 2009;33:1253–1258.

188. Haack H, Johnson LA, Fry CJ, et al. Diagnosis of NUT midline carcinoma using a NUT-specific monoclonal antibody. *Am J Surg Pathol* 2009;33:984–991.

189. Evans AG, French CA, Cameron MJ, et al. Pathologic characteristics of NUT midline carcinoma arising in the mediastinum. *Am J Surg Pathol* 2012;36:1222–1227.

190. Zhu B, Laskin W, Chen Y, et al. NUT midline carcinoma: a neoplasm with diagnostic challenges in cytology. *Cytopathology* 2011;22:414–417.

191. Bellizzi AM, Bruzzi C, French CA, et al. The cytologic features of NUT midline carcinoma. *Cancer* 2009;117:508–515.

192. Davis BN, Karabakhtsian RG, Pettigrew AL, et al. Nuclear protein in testis midline carcinomas: a lethal and underrecognized entity. *Arch Pathol Lab Med* 2011;135:1494–1498.

193. Engleson J, Soller M, Panagopoulos I, et al. Midline carcinoma with t(15;19) and BRD4-NUT fusion oncogene in a 30-year-old female with response to docetaxel and radiotherapy. *BMC Cancer* 2006;6:69.

194. Nakamura H, Tsuta K, Tsuda H, et al. NUT midline carcinoma of the mediastinum showing two types of poorly differentiated tumor cells: a case report and a literature review. *Pathol Res Pract* 2015;211:92–98.

195. Parikh SA, French CA, Costello BA, et al. NUT midline carcinoma: an aggressive intrathoracic neoplasm. *J Thorac Oncol* 2013;8:1335–1338.

196. Teo O, Crotty P, O'Sullivan M, et al. NUT midline carcinoma in a young woman. *J Clin Oncol* 2011;29:e336–e339.

197. Ziai J, French CA, Zambrano E. NUT gene rearrangement in a poorly-differentiated carcinoma of the submandibular gland. *Head Neck Pathol* 2010;4:163–168.

198. Bishop JA, Westra WH. NUT midline carcinomas of the sinonasal tract. *Am J Surg Pathol* 2012;36:1216–1221.

199. Gokmen-Polar Y, Cano OD, Kesler KA, et al. NUT midline carcinomas in the thymic region. *Mod Pathol* 2014;27:1649–1656.

200. Gokmen-Polar Y, Kesler K, Loehrer PJ Sr, et al. NUT midline carcinoma masquerading as a thymic malignancy. *J Clin Oncol* 2016;34:e126–e129.

201. Huang CS, Li WY, Lee PC, et al. Analysis of outcomes following surgical treatment of thymolipomatous myasthenia gravis: comparison with thymomatous and non-thymomatous myasthenia gravis. *Interact Cardiovasc Thorac Surg* 2014;18:475–481.

202. McManus KG, Allen MS, Trastek VF, et al. Lipothymoma with red cell aplasia, hypogammaglobulinemia, and lichen planus. *Ann Thorac Surg* 1994;58:1534–1536.

203. Takahashi H, Harada M, Kimura M, et al. Thymolipoma combined with hyperthyroidism discovered by neurological symptoms. *Ann Thorac Cardiovasc Surg* 2007;13:114–117.

204. Duwe BV, Sterman DH, Musani AI. Tumors of the mediastinum. *Chest* 2005;128:2893–2909.

205. Reeder LB. Neurogenic tumors of the mediastinum. *Semin Thorac Cardiovasc Surg* 2000;12:261–267.

206. Kumar A, Kumar S, Aggarwal S, et al. Thoracoscopy: the preferred approach for the resection of selected posterior mediastinal tumors. *J Laparoendosc Adv Surg Tech A* 2002;12:345–353.

207. Saenz NC. Posterior mediastinal neurogenic tumors in infants and children. *Semin Pediatr Surg* 1999;8:78–84.

208. Suster S, Moran C. *Diagnostic Pathology: Thoracic*. 1st ed. Amirsys Publishing, Inc. Philadelphia, PA: Lippincott Williams & Wilkins; 2012.

209. Kirmani S, Young WF. Hereditary paraganglioma-pheochromocytoma syndromes. In: Adam MP, Ardinger HH, Pagon RA, et al., eds. GeneReviews® [Internet]. Seattle (WA): University of Washington, Seattle; 2008:1993–2017. [updated 2014 Nov 6]

210. Raygada M, Pasini B, Stratakis CA. Hereditary paragangliomas. *Adv Otorhinolaryngol* 2011;70:99–106.

211. Lenders JW, Duh QY, Eisenhofer G, et al. Pheochromocytoma and paraganglioma: an endocrine society clinical practice guideline. *J Clin Endocrinol Metab* 2014;99:1915–1942.

212. Grote D, Souabni A, Busslinger M, et al. Pax 2/8-regulated Gata 3 expression is necessary for morphogenesis and guidance of the nephric duct in the developing kidney. *Development* 2006;133:53–61.

213. Tsarovina K, Pattyn A, Stubbusch J, et al. Essential role of Gata transcription factors in sympathetic neuron development. *Development* 2004;131:4775–4786.

214. Liang Y, Heitzman J, Kamat AS, et al. Differential expression of GATA-3 in urothelial carcinoma variants. *Hum Pathol* 2014;45:1466–1472.

215. Liu H, Shi J, Prichard JW, et al. Immunohistochemical evaluation of GATA-3 expression in ER-negative breast carcinomas. *Am J Clin Pathol* 2014;141:648–655.

216. So JS, Epstein JI. GATA3 expression in paragangliomas: a pitfall potentially leading to misdiagnosis of urothelial carcinoma. *Mod Pathol* 2013;26:1365–1370.

217. Amin R, Waibel BH. An unusual presentation of a posterior mediastinal schwannoma associated with traumatic hemothorax. *Case Rep Surg* 2015;2015:175645.

218. Boland JM, Colby TV, Folpe AL. Intrathoracic peripheral nerve sheath tumors-a clinicopathological study of 75 cases. *Hum Pathol* 2015;46:419–425.

219. Husain K, Thomas E, Demerdash Z, et al. Mediastinal ganglioneuroblastoma-secreting vasoactive intestinal peptide causing secretory diarrhoea. *Arab J Gastroenterol* 2011;12:106–108.

220. Swerdlow SH, Campo E, Harris NL, et al. *WHO Classification of Tumours of Haematopoietic and Lymphoid Tissues*. Vol 2. 4th ed. Lyon: IARC Press; 2008.

221. Pescarmona E, Rendina EA, Ricci C, et al. Histiocytosis X and lymphoid follicular hyperplasia of the thymus in myasthenia gravis. *Histopathology* 1989;14:465–470.

222. Wakely P Jr, Suster S. Langerhans' cell histiocytosis of the thymus associated with multilocular thymic cyst. *Hum Pathol* 2000;31:1532–1535.

223. Pileri SA, Grogan TM, Harris NL, et al. Tumours of histiocytes and accessory dendritic cells: an immunohistochemical approach to classification from the International Lymphoma Study Group based on 61 cases. *Histopathology* 2002;41:1–29.

224. Kamel OW, Gocke CD, Kell DL, et al. True histiocytic lymphoma: a study of 12 cases based on current definition. *Leuk Lymphoma* 1995;18:81–86.

225. Chan AC, Chan KW, Chan JK, et al. Development of follicular dendritic cell sarcoma in hyaline-vascular Castleman's disease of the nasopharynx: tracing its evolution by sequential biopsies. *Histopathology* 2001;38:510–518.

226. Desai SB, Pradhan SA, Chinoy RF. Mediastinal Castleman's disease complicated by follicular dendritic cell tumour. *Indian J Cancer* 2000;37:129–132.

227. Perez-Ordonez B, Rosai J. Follicular dendritic cell tumor: review of the entity. *Semin Diagn Pathol* 1998;15:144–154.

228. Saygin C, Uzunaslan D, Ozguroglu M, et al. Dendritic cell sarcoma: a pooled analysis including 462 cases with presentation of our case series. *Crit Rev Oncol Hematol* 2013;88:253–271.

229. Ravandi-Kashani F, Cortes J, Giles FJ. Myelodysplasia presenting as granulocytic sarcoma of mediastinum causing superior vena cava syndrome. *Leuk Lymphoma* 2000;36:631–637.

230. Orazi A, Neiman RS, Ulbright TM, et al. Hematopoietic precursor cells within the yolk sac tumor component are the source of secondary hematopoietic malignancies in patients with mediastinal germ cell tumors. *Cancer* 1993;71:3873–3881.

231. Kanavaros P, Gaulard P, Charlotte F, et al. Discordant expression of immunoglobulin and its associated molecule mb-1/CD79a is frequently found in mediastinal large B cell lymphomas. *Am J Pathol* 1995;146:735–741.

232. Loddenkemper C, Anagnostopoulos I, Hummel M, et al. Differential Emu enhancer activity and expression of BOB.1/OBF.1, Oct2, PU.1, and immunoglobulin in reactive B-cell populations, B-cell non-Hodgkin lymphomas, and Hodgkin lymphomas. *J Pathol* 2004;202:60–69.

233. Higgins JP, Warnke RA. CD30 expression is common in mediastinal large B-cell lymphoma. *Am J Clin Pathol* 1999;112:241–247.

234. Pileri SA, Gaidano G, Zinzani PL, et al. Primary mediastinal B-cell lymphoma: high frequency of BCL-6 mutations and consistent expression of the transcription factors OCT-2, BOB.1, and PU.1 in the absence of immunoglobulins. *Am J Pathol* 2003;162:243–253.

235. Bentz M, Barth TF, Bruderlein S, et al. Gain of chromosome arm 9p is characteristic of primary mediastinal B-cell lymphoma (MBL): comprehensive molecular cytogenetic analysis and presentation of a novel MBL cell line. *Genes Chromosomes Cancer* 2001;30:393–401.

236. Joos S, Otano-Joos MI, Ziegler S, et al. Primary mediastinal (thymic) B-cell lymphoma is characterized by gains of chromosomal material including 9p and amplification of the REL gene. *Blood* 1996;87:1571–1578.

237. Rosenwald A, Wright G, Leroy K, et al. Molecular diagnosis of primary mediastinal B cell lymphoma identifies a clinically favorable subgroup of diffuse large B cell lymphoma related to Hodgkin lymphoma. *J Exp Med* 2003;198:851–862.

238. Inagaki H, Chan JK, Ng JW, et al. Primary thymic extranodal marginal-zone B-cell lymphoma of mucosa-associated lymphoid tissue type exhibits distinctive clinicopathological and molecular features. *Am J Pathol* 2002;160:1435–1443.

239. Isaacson PG, Chan JK, Tang C, et al. Low-grade B-cell lymphoma of mucosa-associated lymphoid tissue arising in the thymus. A thymic lymphoma mimicking myoepithelial sialadenitis. *Am J Surg Pathol* 1990;14:342–351.

240. den Bakker MA, Oosterhuis JW. Tumours and tumour-like conditions of the thymus other than thymoma; a practical approach. *Histopathology* 2009;54:69–89.

241. Eberle FC, Salaverria I, Steidl C, et al. Gray zone lymphoma: chromosomal aberrations with immunophenotypic and clinical correlations. *Mod Pathol* 2011;24:1586–1597.

242. Mani H, Jaffe ES. Hodgkin lymphoma: an update on its biology with new insights into classification. *Clin Lymphoma Myeloma* 2009;9:206–216.

243. Traverse-Glehen A, Pittaluga S, Gaulard P, et al. Mediastinal gray zone lymphoma: the missing link between classic Hodgkin's lymphoma and mediastinal large B-cell lymphoma. *Am J Surg Pathol* 2005;29:1411–1421.

244. Shimosato Y, Mukai K. *Tumors of the Mediastinum*. Vol. 11. 4th ed. Washington, DC: AFIP; 2010.

245. Detlefsen S. IgG4-related disease: a systemic condition with characteristic microscopic features. *Histol Histopathol* 2013;28:565–584.

246. Ishimoto H, Yatera K, Shimabukuro I, et al. Case of immunoglobulin G4 (IgG4)-related disease diagnosed by transbronchial lung biopsy and endobronchial ultrasound-guided transbronchial needle aspiration. *J UOEH* 2014;36:237–242.

247. Shimosegawa T, Chari ST, Frulloni L, et al. International consensus diagnostic criteria for autoimmune pancreatitis: guidelines of the International Association of Pancreatology. *Pancreas* 2011;40:352–358.

248. Engels EA, Biggar RJ, Hall HI, et al. Cancer risk in people infected with human immunodeficiency virus in the United States. *Int J Cancer* 2008;123:187–194.

249. Patel P, Hanson DL, Sullivan PS, et al. Incidence of types of cancer among HIV-infected persons compared with the general population in the United States, 1992–2003. *Ann Intern Med* 2008;148:728–736.

250. Shiels MS, Cole SR, Kirk GD, et al. A meta-analysis of the incidence of non-AIDS cancers in HIV-infected individuals. *J Acquir Immune Defic Syndr* 2009;52:611–622.

251. Biggar RJ, Jaffe ES, Goedert JJ, et al. Hodgkin lymphoma and immunodeficiency in persons with HIV/AIDS. *Blood* 2006;108:3786–3791.

252. Cesarman E. Gammaherpesvirus and lymphoproliferative disorders in immunocompromised patients. *Cancer Lett* 2011;305:163–174.

253. Chadburn A. Immunodeficiency-associated lymphoid proliferations (ALPS, HIV, and KSHV/HHV8). *Semin Diagn Pathol* 2013;30:113–129.

254. Chou SH, Prabhu SJ, Crothers K, et al. Thoracic diseases associated with HIV infection in the era of antiretroviral therapy: clinical and imaging findings. *Radiographics* 2014;34:895–911.

255. Shi X, Nasseri F, Berger DM, et al. Large multilocular thymic cyst: a rare finding in an HIV positive adult female. *J Clin Imaging Sci* 2012;2:55.

256. Noussios G, Anagnostis P, Goulis DG, et al. Ectopic thyroid tissue: anatomical, clinical, and surgical implications of a rare entity. *Eur J Endocrinol* 2011;165:375–382.

257. Triggiani V, Giagulli VA, Licchelli B, et al. Ectopic thyroid gland: description of a case and review of the literature. *Endocr Metab Immune Disord Drug Targets* 2013;13:275–281.

258. Wang XL, Mu YM, Dou JT, et al. Medullar thyroid carcinoma in mediastinum initially presenting as Ectopic ACTH syndrome. A case report. *Neuro Endocrinol Lett* 2011;32:421–424.

259. Clark OH. Mediastinal parathyroid tumors. *Arch Surg* 1988;123:1096–1100.

260. Janko O, Hubmann R, Zazgornik J, et al. Recurrent hyperparathyroidism after total parathyroidectomy due to multiple ectopic parathyroid glands in a patient with long-term haemodialysis. *Wien Med Wochenschr* 2001;151:288–290.

261. Noussios G, Anagnostis P, Natsis K. Ectopic parathyroid glands and their anatomical, clinical and surgical implications. *Exp Clin Endocrinol Diabetes* 2012;120:604–610.

262. Peric R, Schuurbiers OC, Veselic M, et al. Transesophageal endoscopic ultrasound-guided fine-needle aspiration for the mediastinal staging of extrathoracic tumors: a new perspective. *Ann Oncol* 2010;21:1468–1471.

263. Tournoy KG, Govaerts E, Malfait T, et al. Endobronchial ultrasound-guided transbronchial needle biopsy for M1 staging of extrathoracic malignancies. *Ann Oncol* 2011;22:127–131.

264. Zhang K, Deng H, Cagle PT. Utility of immunohistochemistry in the diagnosis of pleuropulmonary and mediastinal cancers: a review and update. *Arch Pathol Lab Med* 2014;138:1611–1628.

265. Bockmuhl U, Wolf G, Schmidt S, et al. Genomic alterations associated with malignancy in head and neck cancer. *Head Neck* 1998;20:145–151.

266. Squire JA, Bayani J, Luk C, et al. Molecular cytogenetic analysis of head and neck squamous cell carcinoma: By comparative genomic hybridization, spectral karyotyping, and expression array analysis. *Head Neck* 2002;24:874–887.

267. Zettl A, Strobel P, Wagner K, et al. Recurrent genetic aberrations in thymoma and thymic carcinoma. *Am J Pathol* 2000;157:257–266.

268. Bussey KJ, Lawce HJ, Olson SB, et al. Chromosome abnormalities of eighty-one pediatric germ cell tumors: sex-, age-, site-, and histopathology-related differences—a Children's Cancer Group study. *Genes Chromosomes Cancer* 1999;25:134–146.

269. Schneider DT, Schuster AE, Fritsch MK, et al. Genetic analysis of mediastinal non-seminomatous germ cell tumors in children and adolescents. *Genes Chromosomes Cancer* 2002;34:115–125.

270. Motzer RJ, Amsterdam A, Prieto V, et al. Teratoma with malignant transformation: diverse malignant histologies arising in men with germ cell tumors. *J Urol* 1998;159:133–138.

271. Rajan A, Carter CA, Berman A, et al. Cixutumumab for patients with recurrent or refractory advanced thymic epithelial tumours: a multicentre, open-label, phase 2 trial. *Lancet Oncol* 2014;15:191–200.

272. Radovich M, Solzak J, Conces M. A large microRNA cluster on chromosome 19 identified by RNA-sequencing is a transcriptional hallmark of WHO type A and AB thymomas. *J Thorac Oncol* 2013;8:46(suppl 1; P2.13).

273. Ganci F, Vico C, Korita E, et al. MicroRNA expression profiling of thymic epithelial tumors. *Lung Cancer* 2014;85:197–204.

274. Wessendorf S, Barth TF, Viardot A, et al. Further delineation of chromosomal consensus regions in primary mediastinal B-cell lymphomas: an analysis of 37 tumor samples using high-resolution genomic profiling (array-CGH). *Leukemia* 2007;21:2463–2469.

275. Hutchinson CB, Wang E. Primary mediastinal (thymic) large B-cell lymphoma: a short review with brief discussion of mediastinal gray zone lymphoma. *Arch Pathol Lab Med* 2011;135:394–398.

276. Steidl C, Gascoyne RD. The molecular pathogenesis of primary mediastinal large B-cell lymphoma. *Blood* 2011;118:2659–2669.

277. Vanhentenrijk V, Vanden Bempt I, Dierickx D, et al. Relationship between classic Hodgkin lymphoma and overlapping large cell lymphoma investigated by comparative expressed sequence hybridization expression profiling. *J Pathol* 2006;210:155–162.

278. Suurmeijer AJH. *WHO Classification of Tumours of Soft Tissue and Bone*. 4th ed. Lyon: IARC Press; 2013.

279. Owens C, Irwin M. Neuroblastoma: the impact of biology and cooperation leading to personalized treatments. *Crit Rev Clin Lab Sci* 2012;49:85–115.

280. Weiss SW. *WHO Classification of Tumours of Soft Tissue and Bone*. 4th ed. Lyon: IARC Press; 2013.

281. Mohamadkhani A, Poustchi H. Repository of human blood derivative biospecimens in biobank: technical implications. *Middle East J Dig Dis* 2015;7:61–68.

282. Grizzle WE, Bell WC, Sexton KC. Issues in collecting, processing and storing human tissues and associated information to support biomedical research. *Cancer Biomark* 2010;9:531–549.

283. Marko-Varga G, Baker MS, Boja ES, et al. Biorepository regulatory frameworks: building parallel resources that both promote scientific investigation and protect human subjects. *J Proteome Res* 2014;13:5319–5324.

284. Mee B, Gaffney E, Glynn SA, et al. Development and progress of Ireland's biobank network: ethical, legal, and social implications (ELSI), standardized documentation, sample and data release, and international perspective. *Biopreserv Biobank* 2013;11:3–11.
285. Bevilacqua G, Bosman F, Dassesse T, et al. The role of the pathologist in tissue banking: European Consensus Expert Group Report. *Virchows Arch* 2010;456:449–454.
286. Casson PR, Krawetz SA, Diamond MP, et al. Proactively establishing a biologic specimens repository for large clinical trials: an idea whose time has come. *Syst Biol Reprod Med* 2011;57:217–221.
287. Ilie M, Hofman V, Long E, et al. Current challenges for detection of circulating tumor cells and cell-free circulating nucleic acids, and their characterization in non-small cell lung carcinoma patients. What is the best blood substrate for personalized medicine? *Ann Transl Med* 2014;2:107.
288. Joosse SA, Gorges TM, Pantel K. Biology, detection, and clinical implications of circulating tumor cells. *EMBO Mol Med* 2014;7:1–11.

289. Millner LM, Linder MW, Valdes R Jr. Circulating tumor cells: a review of present methods and the need to identify heterogeneous phenotypes. *Ann Clin Lab Sci* 2013;43:295–304.
290. Schiffman JD, Fisher PG, Gibbs P. Early detection of cancer: past, present, and future. *Am Soc Clin Oncol Educ Book* 2015;35:57–65.
291. Marchetti A, Del Grammastro M, Felicioni L, et al. Assessment of EGFR mutations in circulating tumor cell preparations from NSCLC patients by next generation sequencing: toward a real-time liquid biopsy for treatment. *PLoS One* 2014;9:e103883.
292. Yu N, Zhou J, Cui F, et al. Circulating tumor cells in lung cancer: detection methods and clinical applications. *Lung* 2015;193:157–171.
293. Chilosi M, Zamò A, Brighenti A, et al. Constitutive expression of DeltaN-p63alpha isoform in human thymus and thymic epithelial tumours. *Virchows Arch* 2003; 443(2):175–183.

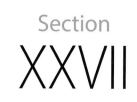

Section

XXVII

INVASIVE DIAGNOSTIC INVESTIGATIONS AND SURGICAL APPROACHES

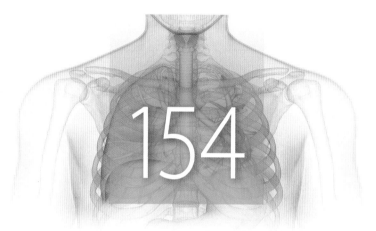

154

Sternotomy and Thoracotomy for Mediastinal Disease

Giulio Maurizi ▪ Federico Venuta ▪ Erino A. Rendina

INTRODUCTION

Surgical approaches for the diagnosis of mediastinal disease are anterior mediastinotomy, cervical mediastinoscopy, and video-assisted thoracic surgery (VATS). The parasternal anterior mediastinotomy was first described in 1966 by Chamberlain and McNeil.[1] This approach is most commonly indicated for large masses located in the anterior mediastinum, especially when they demonstrate direct contact with the posterior aspect of the sternum and the adjacent chest wall. Moreover, this technique has been proposed and largely employed for the histologic diagnosis of lymphadenopathies and masses located in the paraortic region and in the aorto-pulmonary window. This procedure is most frequently performed with the patient under general anesthesia.[2] Conventional cervical mediastinoscopy is useful for the diagnosis of lesions located in the superior-middle mediastinum at the level of paratracheal and pretracheal spaces and subcarinal lymph nodes. Therefore, the role of this technique in the histologic definition of anterior mediastinal masses is limited. The use of the latter approach in such cases is generally restricted to those tumors that extend outside the limits of the anterior mediastinum involving the peritracheal region. General anesthesia is required. In addition, VATS does not have wide application for the histologic definition of invasive tumors located in the anterior mediastinum. It may be indicated in case of large masses protruding in the pleural cavity, especially when separate lesions involving the pleura are associated.

However, for complete tumor removal, larger incisions must be used. The two most common incisions for exposure of the mediastinum are median sternotomy (full or partial) and thoracotomy. The most common thoracotomy incision for mediastinal exposure is bilateral inframmary thoracotomy with sternal transsection: clamshell incision. These approaches are better detailed in the following paragraphs.

STERNOTOMY

The mediastinal exposure for tumor removal was described for the first time in 1897[3]: the division of the whole sternum in a procedure termed "osteoplastic anterior mediastinotomy." A few years later, this approach was introduced for cardiac procedures.[4] Nowadays, median sternotomy and splitting sternotomy are the most commonly used anterior approaches to the mediastinum.[5] In addition, a sternal

2000

transverse transsection (in combination with a bilateral anterior thoracotomy) is carried out for the clamshell approach.

Median sternotomy provides the most complete exposure to the anterior mediastinum and most of the mediastinal structures with the exception of the esophagus. This approach allows the most effective removal of anterior mediastinal tumors, providing good exposure even in the presence of invasion of the adjacent structures such as the lung or the great vessels.[6,7] Full control of the entire anterior mediastinal compartment is provided by this approach. Furthermore, upper lobectomy, bilobectomy, or pneumonectomy (along with removal of the mediastinal mass), as well as pulmonary artery resection and repair, can be performed with this approach.[8] Simultaneously, exploration of both pleural cavities is feasible. This incision may be easily extended to the neck in case of cervicothoracic lesions. The full sternotomy also offers good exposure for tracheal resection and reconstruction. For thymectomy, a partial upper sternotomy may be indicated, in particular for benign and localized diseases, in order to provide better cosmetic results.

TECHNIQUE FOR FULL STERNOTOMY

The patient is positioned supine. The skin incision may differ for special approaches or for cosmesis. Two skin incisions are generally used: the most common midline incision and, as an alternative, the inframmary incision.

The standard midline incision is from the suprasternal notch to a point just below the xiphoid process. The incision can be made shorter at either or both ends for cosmetic purpose. Having the neck extended when the skin incision is made results in a lower location for the incision when the neck is returned to neutral at the conclusion of the procedure and results in a more cosmetically appealing incision. Subcutaneous tissue dissection, generally performed with the electrocautery, is carried out to the anterior sternal fascia. There is a space between the attachments of the pectoralis major muscles from

right and left, leaving a muscle-free area directly on the sternal surface. Superiorly, the subcutaneous tissue is swept bluntly away from the sternal notch, exposing the sternal ligament. There is usually a bridging anterior jugular vein, which may be swept bluntly superiorly or divided if necessary. The sternal ligament is a broad-based ligament beginning posteriorly at the manubrial notch. There is often a small vein in this area that can produce bothersome bleeding. The interclavicular ligament can be divided sharply or with cautery. Inferiorly, the incision is completed diving the linea alba 1 or 2 cm beyond the xiphoid. Blunt dissection is used to open superiorly and inferiorly the retrosternal space.

The alternative inframmary skin incision is generally reserved for cosmetic purposes but may be necessary to provide the best closure after extensive tumor resection. It may be indicated if the upper mediastinum has been irradiated or in case of tracheostomy, to avoid contamination of the wound. The incision is carried under both breasts and joined to a semicircular incision over the sternum. The subcutaneous incision is carried down to the prepectoral fascia creating large flaps bilaterally until the sternal notch is reached, since the necessary exposure of the sternum requires extensive mobilization bilaterally underneath the breasts.

Before splitting the sternum in the midline, it is necessary to identify the sternal notch and xiphoid. To find the exact midpoint of the sternum, two straight hemostats are usually placed next to the bone at the angle of Louis. This is a useful tip since the insertions of the pectoralis muscles do not always delineate the center of the sternum. The anterior surface of the sternum is marked by incising the periosteum with the electrocautery. The xiphoid is divided sharply with scissors. The sternum is divided by an oscillating sternal saw from top down or bottom up. This is performed with the lungs deflated (Fig. 154.1A, Video 154.1). Bone marrow bleeding can be controlled by judicious use of cautery and bone wax without increasing infectious complications. The sternum is generally divided straight, in the middle of the sternum; however, a lazy-S incision in the sternum, "the interlocking

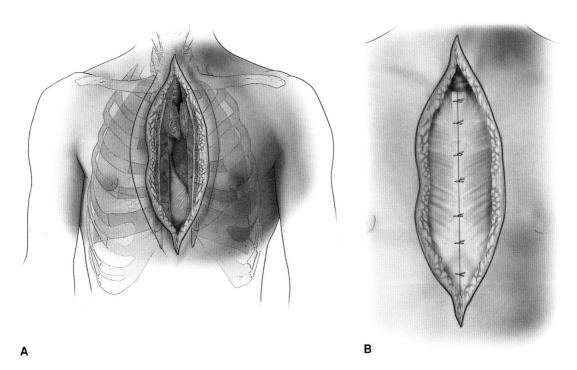

A   **B**

FIGURE 154.1 **A,B:** When a full median sternotomy is to be made, a long vertical incision is generally used. **A:** The mediastinum is exposed after complete median sternotomy. **B:** The sternum is reapproximated using interrupted stainless steel sutures.

incision," has been described by Joshi.[9] They reported no dehiscences and only a few cases of sternal instability.

At the end of sternotomy, two chest tubes are generally used to drain the mediastinum. If the pleura has been entered, one of the chest tubes is placed in that pleural space. If postoperative bleeding is anticipated in the open pleural space, it can be necessary to place a separate thoracostomy tube in a posterolateral position. The sternum is reapproximated using interrupted sutures around the sternum. Usually the suture used for this is a no. 5 or 6 wire (Fig. 154.1B, Video 154.2). No definitive guidelines for the optimal number of wires have been established; however, the usual criterion is to put 1 suture per 10 kg of bodyweight. Alternatively, no. 6 Mersilene or no. 5 Tycron suture can be used and have given excellent results. Different fastener systems have also been designed. The use of resorbable suture (vicryl) after median sternotomy in children allows stability of the sternum without complications, good wound healing, and very good compatibility. The subcutaneous tissue and fascia can be closed in layers. The fascia over the sternum should be approximated tightly to prevent outside contamination or collection of fluids, which could act as a culture medium for bacteria. If the incisions are inframammary, closed suction drains are placed in the subcutaneous plane before closing the subcutaneous tissue and the skin in layers.

TECHNIQUE FOR PARTIAL STERNOTOMY

The patient is positioned supine as for a standard sternotomy. In the partial sternotomy approach, only the upper sternum is split and a

short collar-type incision may be appropriate. The skin incision consists in a curved incision whose center is located at the angle of Louis. A compass, a goniometer, or an obstetric caliper could be useful to inscribe an arc, whose center is located at the cricoid cartilage and whose radius extends to the superior border of the third rib. A skin flap must be created from the area of the incision up to and above the sternal notch. The incision extends for a distance of 5 cm on either side of the midline. This is usually sufficient to allow development of the superior flap. An appropriate length is important before making the incision because distortion after development of the flap makes accurate lengthening difficult.

A thick flap is developed symmetrically cephalad. The flap extends in a triangular fashion, widest at its base and tighter at its end, 2 cm above the sternal notch. The incision is carried down through the subcutaneous tissue to the pectoralis and sternal fascia. As in the inframammary incision, a flap of skin and subcutaneous tissue is raised until the sternal notch is reached.

The upper sternum will be split down to the second interspace. The internal thoracic arteries must be exposed bilaterally at the level of the second intercostal space by incising the pectoralis and exposing the branches of the vessel. By blunt dissection, these incisions are connected through the midline under the sternum which is divided using an oscillating sternal saw. Placing the saw in the sternal notch, the surgeon divides the sternum in the midline down to this incision. The internal mammary pedicles need to be ligated bilaterally to open this incision for proper exposure (Fig. 154.2). A transverse incision with the sternal saw is frequently not necessary,

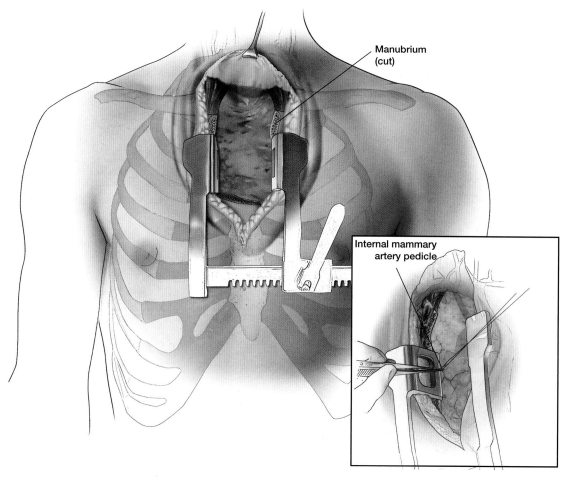

FIGURE 154.2 Partial sternotomy. The internal mammary artery pedicles are ligated bilaterally.

as the sternum will fracture at the appropriate interspace as the sternal retractor is opened.

In a partial sternotomy incision, closed suction drains are used for both the mediastinum and subcutaneous tissue. One drain is placed on either side of the sternum, with one going through the intercostal space and into the mediastinum and the other lying over the sternum. The manubrium is closed with stainless steel wire, with two additional sutures used to anchor the manubrium to the sternum in a criss-crossing X-type pattern. Soft tissue and skin are then closed in layers.

COMPLICATIONS

Complications of sternal incisions in general are rare and should occur in <3% of cases. The incidence of mediastinitis after sternotomy is reported around 1% to 2%. In addition to favorable patient factors, intraoperative hemostasis, proper sternal closure, and early extubation are the most significant factors preventing mediastinitis.[10] Delayed complications of median sternotomy include costochondral separation, occult rib fractures, chronic osteomyelitis of the sternum, rib cartilage necrosis, sternal nonunion, and sternal wire erosion.[11]

STRENGTHS AND LIMITATIONS

Advantages of sternotomy include the speed of opening and closing, the sparing of major thoracic muscles, and the relatively reduced postoperative pain. Main disadvantages are the limited exposure of the posterolateral compartment of the pleural cavities and of the pulmonary hili and the risk of sternal infection, which can carry significant morbidity.

THORACOTOMY

Thoracotomy (muscle sparing lateral or posterolateral) is the most common approach in general thoracic surgery, in particular for lung resections. Through this approach, excellent exposure can be achieved to the mediastinum laterally for both biopsy and resection. Furthermore, thoracotomy is the approach of choice for esophageal lesions and for posterior mediastinal and paravertebral sulcus tumors. On the opposite side, anterior mediastinum exposure is limited. Thoracotomy allows the exposure to different mediastinal structures depending on the side: The esophagus, superior vena cava, thoracic duct, trachea, and the carina can be adequately exposed through a right thoracotomy, while a left thoracotomy is necessary to expose the aorta, superior and inferior portions of the thoracic duct, and lower third of the esophagus.

TECHNIQUE

A high lateral thoracotomy is usually the best approach to the mediastinum except for operations on the lower third of the esophagus or for giant posterior mediastinal lesions. Sometimes, an axillary thoracotomy is most useful for high mediastinal lesions.

The patient is positioned in a lateral decubitus position. Performing a lateral thoracotomy, an incision is made just below the tip of the scapula. The incision is carried down with the electrocautery through the subcutaneous tissue to the fascia of the serratus anterior and beyond the border of the latissimus dorsi. A muscle-sparing incision can be advantageous to the patient, so the latissimus and

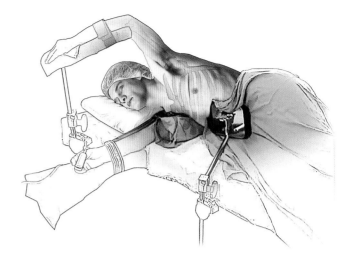

FIGURE 154.3 Usual skin incision for thoracotomy as approach for mediastinal diseases.

serratus muscles should be spared if possible. This is done by mobilizing the latissimus dorsi posteriorly, by splitting the serratus anterior in the direction of its fibers and retracting them away from the intercostal space to be entered. The fourth intercostal space is the usual entry point for exposure to the anterior mediastinum. If higher exposure is necessary, then an axillary thoracotomy is usually chosen (Fig. 154.3).

For an axillary thoracotomy, the patient is in the lateral thoracotomy position and the arm is flexed and abducted to 90 degrees. This delineates both the pectoralis and the latissimus muscles. The incision is performed between these two muscles and carried down through the subcutaneous tissue to the second or the third intercostal space. Long thoracic nerve injury must be avoided and it is important to be aware of the intercostobronchial vascular bundle. Once the muscles are dissected and retracted from the area of the incision, the intercostal space may be entered. Cerfolio in 2005[12] described an alternative method including the separation of the intercostal muscle so the retractor can lie directly on the rib, avoiding compression of the intercostal bundle. This technique has been validated by several randomized studies.

At the end of the procedure, anterior and posterior chest tubes are usually placed. The ribs are reapproximated using heavy pericostal absorbable sutures. In 2003 Cerfolio and colleagues described a technical modification in the closure of the intercostal space placing the suture through the rib transcostally or intracostally.[13] Muscles, the subcutaneous tissue, and skin are closed in layers.

COMPLICATIONS

The most frequent complication after a thoracotomy is bleeding that usually comes from the area of mediastinal resection or from an injured intercostal artery. No definitive guidelines for re-exploration have been established, but the usual criterion for bleeding revision is more than 250 mL per hour for 2 hours.

Acute post-thoracotomy pain occurs in most patients, but it must be carefully prevented and avoided with an adequate perioperative management including intraoperative intercostal nerve blocks and postoperative continuous intravenous infusion of analgesic drugs.[14]

Thoracotomy has been associated with long-term postoperative chronic pain. The literature shows a high rate of post-thoracotomy chronic pain; nevertheless, severe and disabling chronic pain rate is approximately 5%.

When closing the thoracotomy, large subcutaneous pockets must be avoided as it may lead to seroma formation. These are usually self-limited but may be aspirated for patient comfort.

Infections of thoracotomy incisions are rare and should occur in <1% of all thoracotomies. Because resectional therapy of the mediastinum is usually performed for indications other than infection, contamination of the thoracotomy wound should be less than for other indications. The infection usually occurs following inappropriate antisepsis management during a surgical procedure, and the organism is most often *Staphylococcus aureus*.

STRENGTHS AND LIMITATIONS

Advantages of thoracotomy for mediastinal diseases include speed of the procedure and the best exposure to esophageal lesions and to posterior mediastinal and paravertebral sulcus tumors. Main disadvantages are the limited exposure to the controlateral mediastinum and the associated high rates of acute and long-term chronic postoperative pain.

CLAMSHELL INCISION

As an alternative to the previously described incisions, a clamshell approach (bilateral anterior thoracotomy with transverse sternotomy)

has been proposed for the excision of giant masses extending into both pleural cavities, since it allows reasonably good exposure to both the right and left hilar structures.[6,15]

This incision has been described as a useful alternative to sternotomy also in patients with tracheostomy, because it allows avoiding the communication between the superior mediastinum and the lower cervical region.[16] It was the standard approach in the early years of open heart surgery, until it was replaced by the less invasive median sternotomy. Nevertheless, its usefulness was demonstrated for a variety of malignant diseases. Although usually done for bulky mediastinal tumors, it was employed for mediastinal infections.[17] However, currently it has gained most of its popularity as providing access for bilateral lung and heart–lung transplantation.

TECHNIQUE

A curvilinear bilateral submammary incision is performed, extending from one midaxillary line to the contralateral across the anterior aspect of the chest wall (Fig. 154.4A).

For cosmetic reasons, the incision generally follows the submammary folds located at the level of the sixth rib. The pectoralis major muscle is separated from its inferior and medial attachments and lifted with the overlying skin and soft tissues exposing the chest wall. Incision of the intercostal muscles at the level of the fourth space is conducted starting from the sternum bilaterally and extended more laterally and posteriorly than the skin incision to allow increased

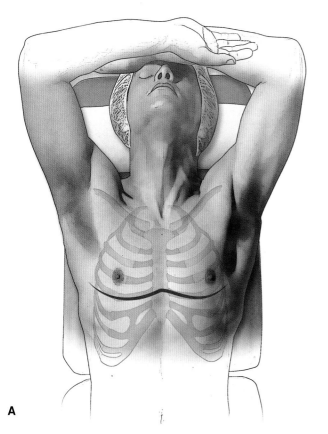 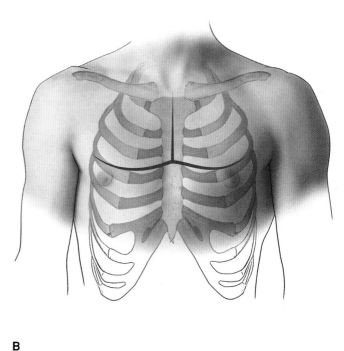

A **B**

FIGURE 154.4 **A,B:** The clamshell incision. **A:** The alternative approach to sternotomy for removal of giant mediastinal masses is an inframammary incision combined with a transverse sternotomy through the fourth interspace. **B:** The inverse-T incision is an extension of clamshell incision: a full clamshell combined with partial upper median sternotomy.

rib spreading. The internal mammary vessels are isolated, tied, and divided. The sternum is then sectioned transversally, usually with an oscillating saw.

Some authors recommend the placement of several Kirschner wires in the reapproximated sternum to reduce override and shifts of the sternal wedges, although complications due to migration of wires have been reported. Others suggest the offset of sternal tables by beveling the bone incision (tipping the saw at an angle of 45 degrees) to allow a more stable closure.[18] Recently,[19] a further extension of the clamshell approach has been described—the so-called inverse-T incision. This approach consists of a full clamshell incision together with a partial upper median sternotomy (Fig. 154.4B). This incision provides excellent access to the upper mediastinum and both the pulmonary hili. It thus allows an effective dissection of the entire upper third of the thorax. Moreover, this incision can be easily extended to the cervical region. Despite the magnitude of the incision, good results in terms of chest wall stability and preservation of the sternocostal arch functionality have been reported. These technical results have allowed fast recovery and rapid postoperative respiratory rehabilitation.

COMPLICATIONS

After clamshell incision, complications may include increased postoperative pain and the increased risk of sternal override or pseudoarthrosis.[20]

STRENGTHS AND LIMITATIONS

This incision provides an excellent exposure of both the pleural cavities and pulmonary hili and can be particularly useful for the treatment of giant tumors involving the lungs bilaterally. Main disadvantages include increased postoperative pain and the increased risk of sternal complications. Therefore, although the utility of this

approach has been emphasized in an oncologic setting by some investigators, its use in this field is still limited to very selected cases.

REFERENCES

1. McNeil TM, Chamberlain JM. Diagnostic anterior mediastinotomy. *Ann Thorac Surg* 1966;2:532–539.
2. Rendina EA, Venuta F, De Giacomo T, et al. Biopsy of anterior mediastinal masses under local anesthesia. *Ann Thorac Surg* 2002;74(5):1720–1722.
3. Milton H. Mediastinal surgery. *Lancet* 1897;1:872–875.
4. Julian OC, Lopez-Belio M, Dye WS, et al. The median sternal incision in intracardiac surgery with extracorporeal circulation: a general evaluation of its use in heart surgery. *Surgery* 1957;42:753.
5. Maurizi G, D'Andrilli A, Sommella L, et al. Transsternal thymectomy. *Thorac Cardiovasc Surg* 2015;63(3):178–186.
6. Bacha EA, Chapelier AR, Macchiarini P, et al. Surgery for invasive primary mediastinal tumors. *Ann Thorac Surg* 1998;66:234–249.
7. Chen KN, Xu SF, Gu ZD, et al. Surgical treatment of complex malignant anterior mediastinal tumors invading the superior vena cava. *World J Surg* 2006;30:162–170.
8. Venuta F, Rendina EA, Klepetko W, et al. Surgical management of stage III thymic tumors. *Thorac Surg Clin* 2011;21(1):85–91, vii.
9. Joshi R, Abraham S, Sampath Kumar A. Interlocking sternotomy: initial experience. *Asian Cardiovasc Thorac Ann* 2004;12:16–18.
10. Demmy TL, Park SB, Liebler GA, et al. Recent experience with major sternal wound complications. *Ann Thorac Surg* 1990;49:458–462.
11. Weber L, Peters RW. Delayed chest wall complications of sternotomy. *South Med J* 1986;79:723–727.
12. Cerfolio RJ, Bryant AS, Patel B, et al. Intercostal muscle flap reduces the pain of thoracotomy: a prospective randomized trial. *J Thorac Cardiovasc Surg* 2005;130:987–993.
13. Cerfolio RJ, Price TN, Bryant AS, et al. Intracostal sutures decrease the pain of thoracotomy. *Ann Thorac Surg* 2003;76:407–411.
14. D'Andrilli A, Ibrahim M, Ciccone AM, et al. Intrapleural intercostals nerve block associated with mini-thoracotomy improves pain control after major lung resection. *Eur J Cardiothorac Surg* 2006;29:790–794.
15. Bains MS, Ginsberg RJ, Jones WG 2nd, et al. The clamshell incision: an improved approach to bilateral pulmonary and mediastinal tumor. *Ann Thorac Surg* 1994;58:30–32.
16. Marshall WG Jr, Meng RL, Ehrenhaft JL. Coronary artery bypass grafting in patients with a tracheostoma: use of a bilateral thoracotomy incision. *Ann Thorac Surg* 1988;46:465–466.
17. Ris HB, Banic A, Furrer M, et al. Descending necrotizing mediastinitis: surgical treatment via clamshell approach. *Ann Thorac Surg* 1996;62:1650–1654.
18. Durrleman N, Massard G. Clamshell and hemiclamshell incisions. *Multimed Man Cardiothorac Surg* 2006;2006(810):mmcts.2006.001867.
19. Marta GM, Aigner C, Klepetko W. Inverse T incision provides improved accessibility to the upper mediastinum. *J Thorac Cardiovasc Surg* 2005;129:221–223.
20. Brown RP, Esmore DS, Lawson C. Improved sternal fixation in the transsternal bilateral thoracotomy incision. *J Thorac Cardiovasc Surg* 1996;112:137–141.

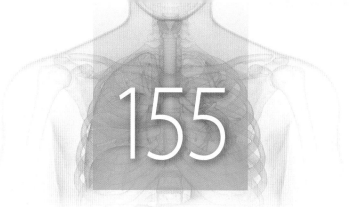

Video-Assisted Thoracic Surgery for Mediastinal Tumors and Cysts and Other Diseases Within the Mediastinum

Maxime Heyndrickx ▪ Amaia Ojanguren ▪ Agathe Seguin-Givelet ▪ Dominique Gossot

BACKGROUND

Even early in the development of video-assisted thoracic surgery (VATS), the feasibility of thoracoscopic resection of mediastinal tumors was reported. Now that advanced thoracoscopic techniques, such as major pulmonary resections, are gaining acceptance, surgical skills have improved, and new technologies have become available, facilitating accurate dissection in the mediastinum. Most benign mediastinal tumors and some malignant ones can now be approached by VATS.

As most large tumors should be removed en-bloc and not morcellated before retrieval, some surgeons may wonder if a thoracotomy would not be a better option, as a large incision will ultimately be needed for extraction of the specimen. Our answer is threefold:

- Dissecting and mobilizing a bulky mediastinal tumor requires a larger thoracotomy in order for the surgeon to introduce both hands into the chest and allow sufficient vision.
- Some young patients presenting with malignant tumors such as nonseminomatous germ cell tumors (NSGCTs) may potentially require reoperation. Avoiding a thoracotomy and performing a thoracoscopy that limits adhesions etc., may be helpful in these patients.
- Eventually, many benign lesions, even bulky ones, are incidentally discovered and the benefit of surgery is uncertain, as the evolution of these tumors is not predictable. Therefore, minimizing the consequences of the operation is important and a minimally invasive approach is an appealing alternate in these patients. On the other hand, thoracotomy or sternotomy must remain an option when there is concern for local invasion or if the dimensions of the tumor obscure visualization of vessels or nerves and make the procedure hazardous.

TECHNICAL CONSIDERATIONS

GENERAL POINTS

In this chapter, all techniques described are performed according to a full thoracoscopic technique, as we reported for major pulmonary

resections.[1] We will not deal with thymectomies which are described in another chapter (Chapter 156). We will also not describe the thoracoscopic approach to mediastinal lymph nodes for two reasons: (1) the indications may be decreasing with the availability of modern imaging modalities and endobronchial ultrasound (EBUS) biopsies and (2) the technique is similar to lymph node dissection performed for lobectomies (Chapter 147).

The procedure is performed under general anesthesia with split ventilation using a double-lumen endotracheal tube. Patients are positioned in lateral decubitus. The surgeon stands at the patient's anterior or posterior chest wall, depending on the tumor location. Three monitors are used, so that all members of the team have excellent vision during the procedure. The thorascope is placed on a mechanical scope holder. We use a deflectable videoscope connected to a high definition camera system (HDTV). Only dedicated thoracoscopic instruments are used. These are inserted through 3 to 4 trocars, depending on the operative need to achieve adequate exposure.

SPECIAL FEATURES OF THORACOSCOPIC SURGERY OF MEDIASTINAL TUMORS

- For small size benign tumors, especially in young patients with a small chest cavity, a 5-mm thoracoscope is sufficient.
- As it is important to have a view over and behind tumors, an oblique viewing scope, that is, 30 or 45 degrees, is often necessary. We prefer using a deflectable scope whose angulation ranges from 0 to 100 degrees allowing seeing *around the corner*.
- For tumors located in the posterior mediastinum, it may be preferable to face the lesion and stand at the patient's front (Fig. 155.1).
- For all tumors in close contact with a nerve, especially when the nerve must be preserved, for example, during the dissection of a teratoma close to the phrenic nerve, the use of monopolar cautery must be avoided. Conventional or electrothermal bipolar cautery is preferred. Ultrasonic dissectors are an alternative,[2] provided the tip of the instrument is always visible, to avoid direct trauma of vessels or nerve from the cavitation effect.[3]

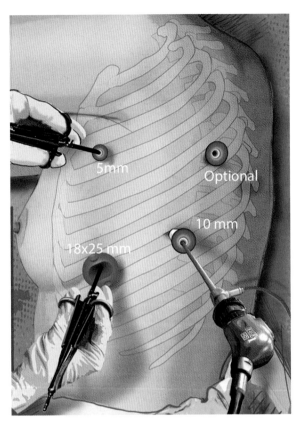

FIGURE 155.1 Port placement for thoracoscopic resection of a neurogenic tumor located in the posterior mediastinum.

- Most mediastinal tumors should be removed en-bloc. Avoiding breaking the tumor and spillage of its contents should be a constant concern. This means that dissection must progress slowly with gentle mobilization using blunt tip instruments. Direct grasping of the tumor must be avoided.
- Some tumors are bulky and dissection requires a perfect exposure. This can be achieved by the use of additional 3-mm forceps (Fig. 155.2) or throw-off instruments—instruments that can be released inside the chest cavity—as vascular clamp or lung retractors grasping forceps (Fig. 155.3) (Video 155.1).[4]

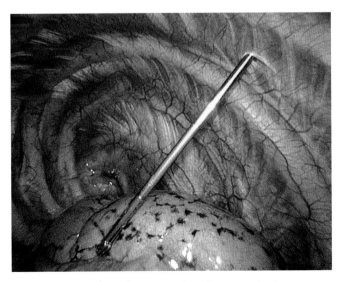

FIGURE 155.2 Mediastinal exposure using a 3-mm grasping forceps.

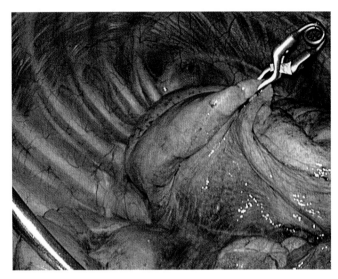

FIGURE 155.3 Mediastinal exposure using throw-off grasping forceps.

- The access incision through which the specimen is removed must be made in a location where it can easily be enlarged and where the intercostal space (ICS) is not too rigid, usually anteriorly and in the 7th or 8th ICS. Contrary to VATS lobectomy where the resected lobe is soft and is easily retrieved through a small incision, one must not hesitate to perform a sufficiently large incision in order to not crush the specimen during removal.

NEUROGENIC TUMORS

HISTOLOGIC CLASSIFICATION

Intrathoracic neurogenic tumors (NT) are neoplasms arising from any of the neurogenic structures of the mediastinum. They are divided into three groups:

- Autonomic ganglion tumors: neuroblastoma, ganglioblastoma (or ganglioneuroblastoma), and ganglioneuroma;
- Nerve sheath tumors: benign schwannoma (or neurilemomma), malignant schwannoma, and neurofibroma;
- Paraganglioma: primitive neuroectodermal tumors (PNET) or pheochromocytoma, which are rare conditions.

More than 90% of posterior mediastinum tumors are neurogenic and are concentrated in the paravertebral sulcus region (Fig. 155.4). They account for 12% to 21% of primary mediastinum tumors.[5] In adults, most NTs are benign while, in children, about 50% are malignant. Table 155.1 summarizes the pathologies according to age in two large series comprising more than 120 pediatric cases and 150 adult cases.[6,7] Dumbbell tumors, that is, with intraspinal component through the intervertebral foramen, account for 10% of all NTs of the mediastinum.[8]

TREATMENT

Principles

Most NTs are incidentally discovered. However, in order to establish a benign or malignant diagnosis, the tumor must be resected, at least in young patients. Treatment relies on achieving a complete surgical resection.[5] Benign NTs rarely recur and simple excision

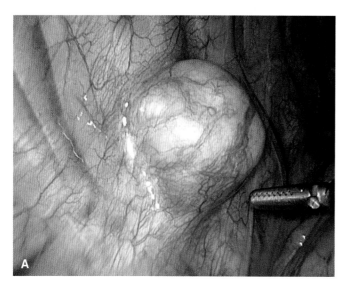 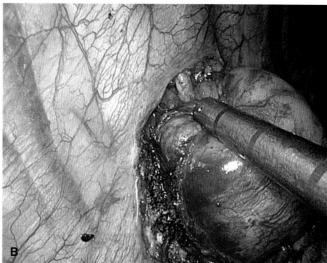

FIGURE 155.4 Typical benign neurogenic tumor (**A**). Once the pleura has been opened, the intercostal nerve is discovered (**B**).

is sufficient. When the tumor looks suspicious, for instance, when abnormal vascularization or an irregular tumor border is observed (Figs. 155.5 and 155.6), it is advisable to perform a larger resection with en-bloc excision of the tumor, adjacent pleural and muscular wall if involved.

Thoracotomy has been the traditional surgical approach. Video-assisted thoracoscopic surgery (VATS) is now documented as a safe and effective method for excising NTs and is the preferred approach.[9] In the early development of VATS, thoracoscopy was contraindicated for NT in the following situations: tumor over 6 cm, malignant tumors, tumors extending into the spinal cord, tumor located at the costophrenic angle, and tumors at the superior sulcus.[10] However recent publications demonstrate that these situations are only a relative contraindication to a VATS approach:

- Some bulky intrathoracic tumors (>5 cm) can be removed by VATS. Contraindication is more related to the location than to the diameter.
- Recurrence after VATS excision of NTs, even in pediatric patients with malignant tumors such as neuroblastoma, ganglioblastoma, seems to be very low.[7,11,12] However, port site recurrence has been reported.[13]

- Dumbbell tumors can be removed by a combined approach including laminectomy followed by VATS resection.[7,8,14,15]
- VATS resection of some benign NTs of the superior sulcus is also possible, although there is an increased incidence of brachial plexus injury (up to 21% in contrast to 2.3% by thoracotomy) and great caution must be exercised to avoid this injury.[16]

Technical Aspects

- An Adamkiewicz spinal artery must always been searched preoperatively when the NT is below T8. Although some authors have reported performing surgery with preservation of this artery[17] or with neurological monitoring,[18] it is safer to monitor these lesions except if there is a high suspicion of malignancy.
- Once the tumor has been identified, the pleura is incised circumferentially around the lesion, close to the tumor surface, using either an electrocautery hook or an ultrasonically activated (US) hook. The lesion is gently mobilized and lifted up with a blunt tip instrument in order to expose the vessels. Intercostal and vertebral vessels are coagulated with US scissors (the use of monopolar diathermy is avoided around the spinal foramen) (Fig. 155.4). In most cases, the nerve has to be sacrificed.

TABLE 155.1 Histological Results of Neurogenic Tumors According to Age[6,7]		Children (<15 years)	Adults (>15 years)	Total
Histologic Class				
Autonomic ganglion tumors	Neuroblastoma	46 (36.5%)	0 (0.0%)	**46 (16.3%)**
	Ganglioblastoma	14 (11.0%)	0 (0.0%)	**14 (5.0%)**
	Ganglioneuroma	51 (40.5%)	35 (22.4%)	**86 (30.5%)**
Paraganglioma[a]		3 (2.4%)	6 (3.8%)	**9 (3.2%)**
Nerve sheath tumors	Neurilemmoma (*benign schwannoma*)	7 (5.6%)	74 (47.4%)	**81 (28.7%)**
	Malignant schwannoma	2 (1.6%)	7 (4.5%)	**9 (3.2%)**
	Neurofibroma	3 (2.4%)	34 (21.8%)	**37 (13.1%)**
Benign diseases		61 (48.4%)	143 (91.7%)	**204 (72.3%)**
Malignant diseases		65 (51.6%)	13 (8.3%)	**78 (27.7%)**
Total		**126 (44.7%)**	**156 (55.3%)**	**282 (100.0%)**

[a]Paraganglioma include various histology such as chemodectoma, pheochromocytoma, primitive neuroectodermal tumors, Askin tumor.

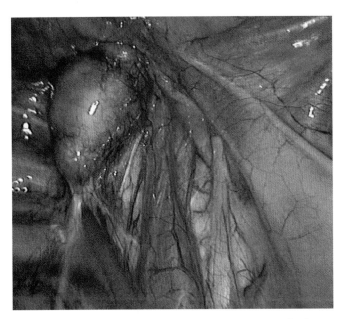

FIGURE 155.5 18-year-old male operated on for suspicion of a benign neurinoma of the right apex on the sympathetic chain. Note hypervascularization of the tumor wall. Final diagnosis: neurofibrosarcoma.

- When the tumor is bulky and stuck inside the thoracic inlet, mobilization and dissection are difficult (Fig. 155.7). Patients must be informed as to the risk of postoperative Horner syndrome. Traction on the tumor by mean of a stay stitch—as for esophageal leiomyomas—must be avoided since spreading of the tumor in the chest cavity can have serious consequences in the case of an unexpected malignancy. Gentle progressive mobilization of the tumor with blunt tip tools, such as endopeanuts, help expose the nerve and vessels. US scissors can usually not be used at the top of the thoracic inlet since the tip of the scissors cannot be visualized to assure safety.[3] Bipolar cautery is preferable.
- For patients with dumbbell tumors, a combined approach is used (Fig. 155.8).[8] The dissection of the intraspinal component must be performed first, in order to free the tumor from the cord. Thus, traction on the spinal cord is avoided during the thoracic dissection. This step is performed on a patient in prone position using a posterior approach. A unilateral laminectomy and complete facetectomy is performed. After dural opening, the intraspinal component is removed and the spinal nerve root is sacrificial. The dura is then sutured closed in a watertight manner. An associated fusion is necessary because of the instability related to the facetectomy (Fig. 155.8D). The patient is then placed in a lateral decubitus position for the thoracoscopic stage.

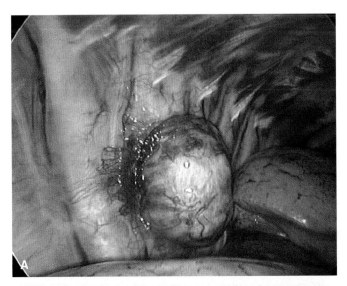

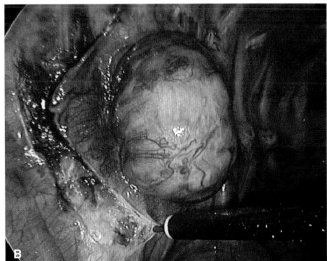

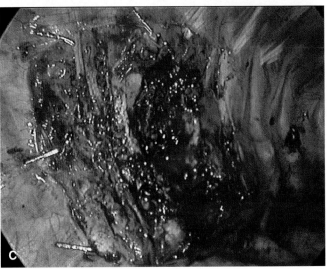

FIGURE 155.6 45-year-old male operated on for suspicion of a benign neurinoma of an intercostal nerve. Note hypervascularized tumor wall (**A**), leading to large en-bloc resection of the tumor, pleura (**B**), and adjacent muscular wall (**C**). Final diagnosis: benign schwannoma.

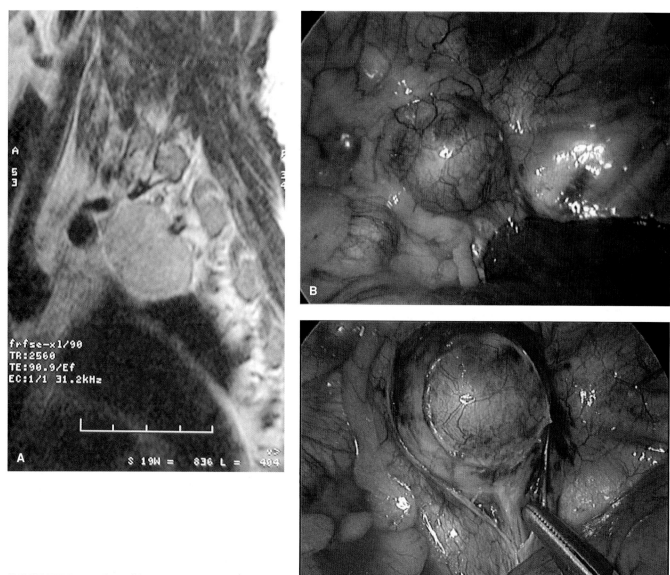

FIGURE 155.7 Typical NT of the apex involving the thoracic inlet. **A:** MRI. **B:** Thoracoscopic view. **C:** Thoracoscopic dissection after opening of the mediastinal pleura, showing the sympathetic nerve.

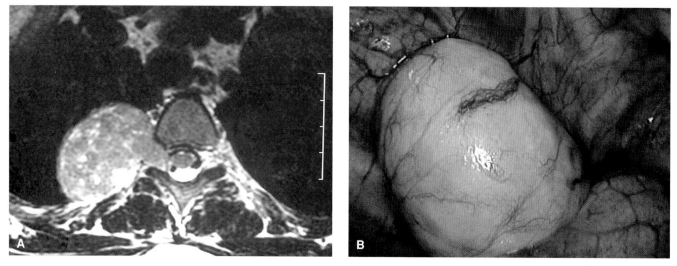

FIGURE 155.8 Typical dumbbell tumor. **A:** MRI showing the spinal component which is first severed after laminectomy. **B:** Thoracoscopic view. (*continued*)

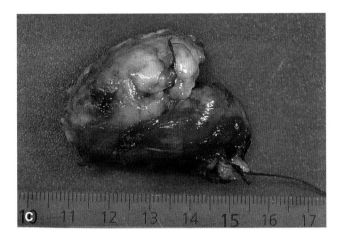

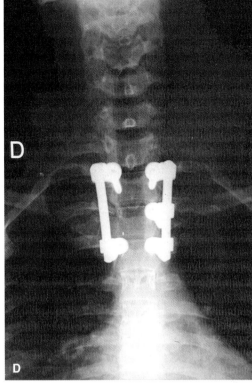

FIGURE 155.8 (*Continued*) **C:** Specimen with suture showing the spinal nerve root, **D:** X-ray showing the orthopedic spine stabilization.

Results

Table 155.2 demonstrates the results of published data for a VATS approach for the resection of NTs. Several findings have arisen from recent publications:

- Operative time is shorter by VATS when compared to open approach.[9,16,19]
- Duration of chest drainage and postoperative stay are shorter after VATS than after thoracotomy.[9,10,16,19]
- Only two studies[9,19] reported the results of postoperative pain assessment. Postoperative pain was less after VATS resection. However, patients must be aware that they may experience intense intercostal or posterior pain after removal of an intercostal NT regardless of approach.
- The most consistent complication seems to be Horner syndrome in NT of the superior sulcus. A higher rate of brachial plexus injury in neurogenic tumor of the apex in VATS approach (21% vs. 2%) has also been reported.[16] In these cases, a conventional transcervical-thoracic incision, as used for tumors of the thoracic inlet, may be preferred to VATS, to minimize the risk of neurological complications. However, no comparative study has been done and the larger incision is more invasive with significant cosmetic impact in patients who are commonly young and asymptomatic.
- Conversion rates are heterogeneous, ranging from 0% to 22.8% in the literature[9,15] with the most frequent reasons being bleeding, tumor size, or the presence of adhesions.[10,15,20]

BRONCHOGENIC CYSTS

INTRODUCTION

Bronchogenic cysts (BCs) are one type of foregut cyst (a closed epithelial-lined sac developing from both the upper gut and respiratory tracts). A BC develops as a diverticulum of the primitive foregut. Since most BCs form very early, usually at 4 to 8 weeks' gestation and before the development of distal airways, they rarely connect to a normal bronchus. The location of the cyst depends on the embryological stage of development at which the anomaly occurs.[21] When these abnormal buddings occur during early development, the cyst is located along the tracheobronchial tree. Cysts that arise later are more peripheral and may be located within the lung parenchyma. Most BCs are right sided and in close proximity to the tracheobronchial tree. On rare occasions, they can separate from the airway and migrate to the periphery, parahilar area, the neck, or below the diaphragm. Double BCs have also been reported.[22] BC can contain normal tracheal tissue including mucus glands, elastic tissue, smooth muscle, and cartilage. They are lined with ciliated epithelium, range from 2 to 10 cm in diameter, and may contain serous, blood, or proteinaceous fluid.[23] BC can be associated with other congenital malformations, such as congenital cystic adenoid malformation and pulmonary sequestration.[24] They are more frequently discovered during childhood than in adults.

PREOPERATIVE WORKUP

Bronchoscopy usually only reveals extrinsic bronchial compression. Rarely, it demonstrates a fistula between the cyst and the carina or main bronchus. Such a finding should probably lead to open surgery. Transbronchial biopsy is not only useless but contraindicated because of infectious risks. In addition, it can make surgery more difficult.

The diagnosis of BC relies on a CT scan, which shows a round, well-circumscribed, sometimes loculated mass with a density ranging from 10 to 80 Hounsfield units. Most common location for BC is subcarinal, therefore, in this typical location, (Fig. 155.9), the diagnosis is usually obvious and there is no need for any other imaging modality.

If the cyst is in the right paratracheal space, above the azygos arch, it can be mistaken for a mesenchymal cyst, which does not require

TABLE 155.2 Details of Largest Series of VATS Resection of Neurogenic Tumors

Author	Year	Details of the Study (Years)	No.	Pathology	Approach Type	Approach No.	Tumors Size (cm)	Operative Time (min)	Postoperative Pain	Postoperative Stay (Days)	Chest Tube (Days)	Conversion Rate	Conversion Details	Morbidity
Yang	2015	Retrospective single institution report of patient with neurogenic tumors of the apex (above 1st rib) (1992–2012). Exclusion of tumors >6cm, diabetes mellitus, coronary heart disease, hypertension, or other chronic disease	63	47 schwannoma, 5 neurofibroma, 11 ganglioneuroma	Open	44	4.9 ± 1	120 ± 43	NA	7 ± 2	NA	—	—	3 Horner syndrome, 1 Brachial plexus injury, 1 bleeding >1L from subclavian artery
					VATS	19	4.1 ± 1.2	93 ± 34	NA	4.8 ± 2	NA	None	—	1 Horner syndrome, 4 Brachial plexus injury
Li	2013	Retrospective single institution report of VATS approach for posterior mediastinal neurogenic tumors (2001–2011)	58	NA	VATS	58	4.9 (median)	127	NA	5.2	2.7	8.6% ($n = 5/58$)	Massive bleeding, dense adhesion, and bulky tumors	4 Horner syndrome
Cansever	2010	Retrospective single institution report of patients with posterior mediastinal neurogenic tumors (1996–2009)	20	NA	Open	13	NA	124 ± 16	VATS group required fewer analgesics that open group ($p < 0.001$)	3 ± 0.9	1.6 ± 0.5			NA
					VATS	7	NA	$84 +/-19$		1	1	NA	NA	NA
Cardillo	2008	Retrospective single institution report of patient with benign neurogenic tumors (1992–2007)	93	75 schwannoma, 7 neurofibroma, 12 ganglioneuroma	Open	36	5.2 ± 1.9	149 ± 77	Median postoperative pain was lower ($p < 0.001$) at day 1 and day 7 in VATS group	6	NA	22.8% ($n = 13/57$)	None	37.8% ($n = 14/37$)
					VATS	57	6.1 ± 2.4	111 ± 58		4	NA		3 pleuro-pulmonary adhesions, 5 huge tumors, 5 risk of injury (3 subclavian artery, 1 esophagus, 1 aorta)	7% ($n = 4/57$)

Author	Year	Description	n	Histology	Approach									
Ciriaco	2006	Retrospective single institution report of patients with benign neurogenic tumors of posterior mediastinum (1993–2005)	30	25 schwannoma 1 neurofibroma 4 ganglioneuroma	VATS in all cases	5.6 ± 1.4 (range 4–11)	140 ± 55 (range 95–230)	NA	4.55 (mean)	NA	13.3% (n = 4/30)	1 pleural adhesion, 3 bleeding	—	None
Venissac	2004	Retrospective single institution report of systematic VATS approach in all cases of mediastinal neurogenic tumors (1992–2002)	15	12 schwannoma 3 neurofibroma	VATS	15	NA	99 (range 60–180)	NA	5.5 (mean)	NA	None	—	2 Horner syndrome
Liu	2000	Retrospective three institution report of patients with neurogenic tumors (1992–1999). Exclusion of tumors >8 cm or obviously malignant	143	72 neurofibroma 33 schwannoma 7 paraganglioma 31 ganglioneuroma	VATS in all cases	3.5 (range 1.5–8)	40 (range 15–110)	NA	4.1 (range 1–11)	NA	None	9.8% (n = 14/143) need 6-cm "thoratomy utility incision"	1 Horner syndrome, 1 local empyema, 9 chest wall paresthesia	
Riquet	1995	Retrospective five institution report of patient with neurogenic tumors (1991–1994)	26	17 schwannoma 3 neurofibroma 2 ganglioneuroma	VATS	8	7.4 (range 3–14)	NA	NA	7.75 (range 5–14)	3 (range 2–5)			NA
					VATS	18	3.7 (range 1.5–6)	92 (range 40–120)	NA	5.3 (range 2–9)	2.5 (range 1–5)	16.7% (n = 3/18)	1 bleeding of internal mammary artery, 1 venous bleeding of spinal extension, 1 deformation of ribs	NA

N.A: Not Available.

2013

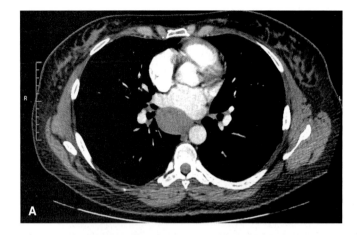

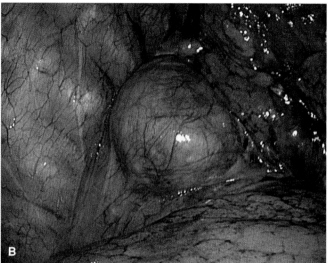

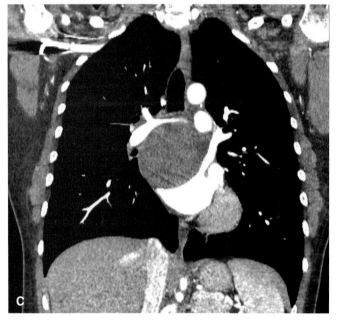

FIGURE 155.9 Typical subcarinal bronchogenic cyst. **A:** CT scan. **B:** Thoracoscopic aspect. **C:** Bulky bronchogenic cyst with compression of pulmonary artery and pulmonary vein.

surgical resection. Magnetic resonance imaging (MRI) can help by demonstrating a thin-walled, purely fluid-filled cyst (Figs. 155.10 and 155.11).

If the cyst is in the lower third of the posterior mediastinum, esophageal ultrasound (EUS) is indicated to check the integrity of the esophageal wall, in order to eliminate a duplication cyst (Fig. 155.12).[25] These have a layer of surrounding smooth muscle and are either attached to the esophagus in a paraesophageal or intramural location. On EUS, esophageal duplication cysts appear as a periesophageal homogenous hypoechoic mass with a multilayered wall and well-defined margins. Fine needle aspiration (FNA) should be avoided because of the risk of infecting the cyst. Special care is warranted during dissection of the esophageal wall.

Other unusual locations are illustrated on Figures 155.13 and 155.14).

TREATMENT

Principles

The majority of cases reported in the literature are in the pediatric population, as the main limitation for thoracoscopy in adults is that the BC is generally more advanced, with adhesions to bronchi,

esophagus, or even large vessels (pulmonary artery, pulmonary vein). Although often asymptomatic, BC can lead to infection and cause serious complications by compression of the tracheobronchial tree, heart, or both. Spontaneous ruptures and air embolism have also been reported. These rare, but life-threatening, complications favor removal, especially in young patients, even if asymptomatic.[26]

Except in very bulky and/or infected cysts, the standard approach for BC should be thoracoscopy. Conversion rates range from 0% to 35%.[26,27] In an early multi-institutional study, the conversion rate was 35%[28] while it is only 3.6% in a recent large single institution study,[26] suggesting that experience plays a role in the success of the thoracoscopic procedure. Although seen as a straightforward procedure, resection of BC can be tedious and hazardous due to close adhesions to the bronchial tree, esophagus, and even vessels. Vascular and bronchial injuries have been reported[26] so that conversion into thoracotomy should always be considered if needed.

Complete excision should always be the primary goal, as late recurrences have been described following incomplete resection, even 20 years later.[29] However, since most patients are asymptomatic, *primum non nocere* must remain the rule. Serious intraoperative complications, for example, bronchial or esophageal injuries must be

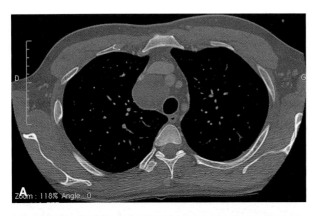

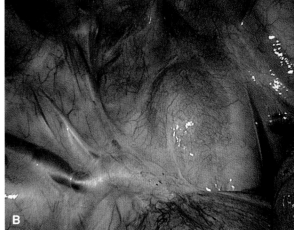

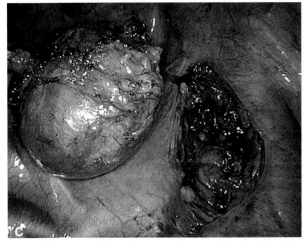

FIGURE 155.10 Paratracheal bronchogenic cyst. **A:** CT scan. **B:** Thoracoscopic aspect before resection. **C:** Thoracoscopic aspect after resection.

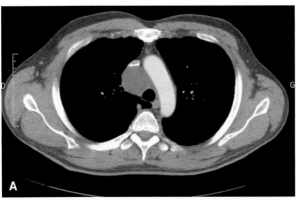

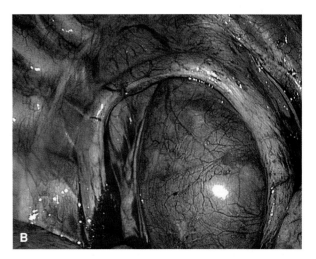

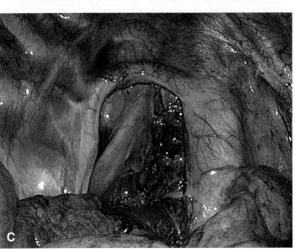

FIGURE 155.11 Paratracheal mesenchymal cyst, which can be confused with a bronchogenic cyst. **A:** CT scan. **B:** Thoracoscopic aspect before resection (note the thin wall). **C:** Thoracoscopic aspect after resection.

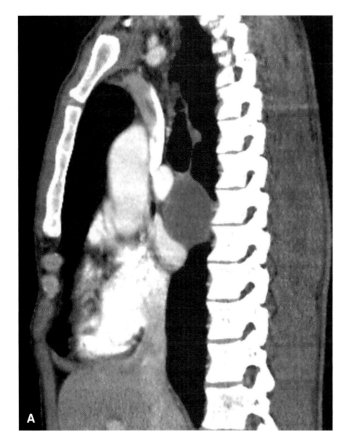

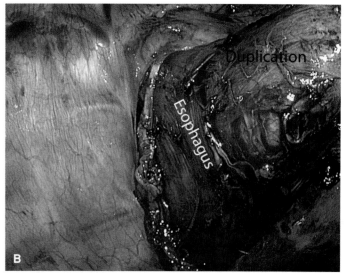

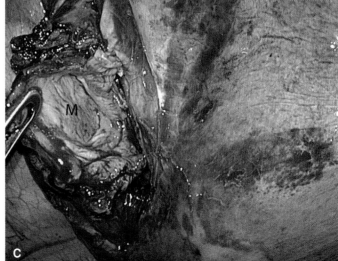

FIGURE 155.12 Esophageal duplication cyst. **A:** CT scan. **B:** Thoracoscopic aspect before resection (note continuity of the cyst with the esophageal muscular layer). **C:** Thoracoscopic aspect after resection (note that a mucosal patch (M) had to be left in place on the esophagus).

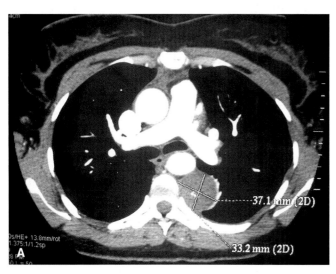

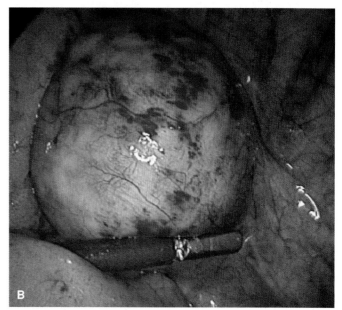

FIGURE 155.13 Left bronchogenic cyst in the lower mediastinum. **A:** CT scan. **B:** Thoracoscopic aspect. (*continued*)

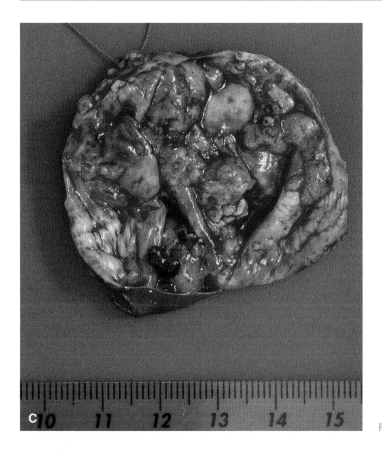

FIGURE 155.13 (*Continued*) **C:** Specimen.

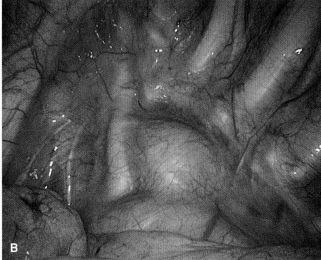

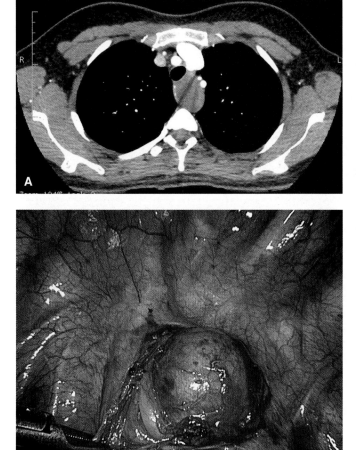

FIGURE 155.14 Left bronchogenic cyst in the upper mediastinum. **A:** CT scan. **B:** Thoracoscopic view before dissection. **C:** Thoracoscopic view after pleural incision.

avoided. Therefore, a compromise between long-term outcomes and immediate safety must be found.

Technical Aspects

- A high-quality imaging system is desirable, as the main challenge during these procedures is the identification of the correct dissection plane between the cyst and the bronchus or between the cyst and the esophagus.
- A nasogastric tube should be placed for better identification of the esophagus.
- Equipment for esophageal endoscopy should be available if needed. The endoscopist should be aware that the patient is in the lateral decubitus position with a double-lumen tube, a feature that can make intraoperative esophagoscopy difficult.
- Once the mediastinal pleura has been opened, the cyst wall should be kept intact—as far as possible—as this facilitates dissection. Once ruptured, the cyst shrinks and dissections planes are more difficult to identify as well as understanding of the anatomical landmarks.

- Bipolar is preferable to monopolar cautery, to avoid thermal injury and current spreading to the bronchial wall.
- In case of tight adhesion to the bronchial tree, one has to decide if digital palpation and digital handling would be helpful. If so, conversion to open thoracotomy should be entertained. In general, there are two scenarios: (1) either the cyst wall can be separated from the bronchus and careful dissection should be pursued or (2) there is no dissection plane, and one should consider leaving a patch of the cyst wall in situ. In those cases, destruction of mucosal lining by electrocautery may help prevent cyst recurrences.[30] The mucosa should be cauterized with caution and gentle application with a smooth-tip cautery device (Fig. 155.15).

Results

The largest series was reported by Jung et al.[26] in 2014 and included 113 cases over 8 years with a low complication and conversion rate. Results of large series are reported in Table 155.3.

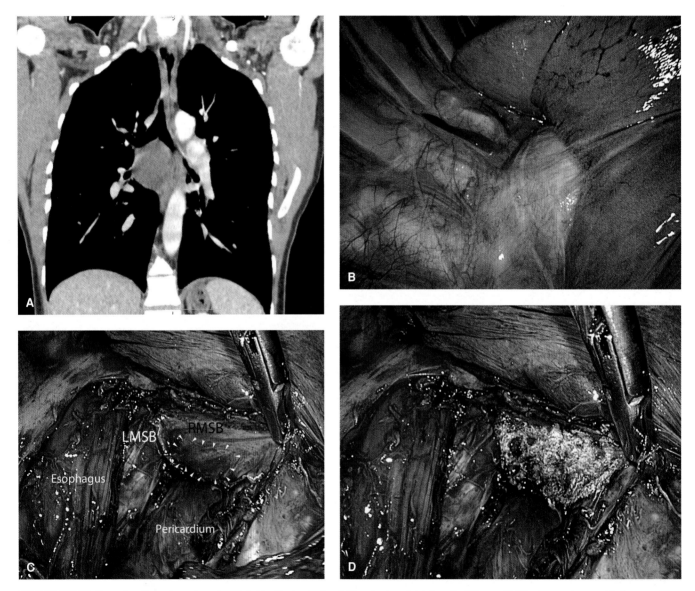

FIGURE 155.15 Example of bronchogenic cyst with tight adhesion to the right main stem bronchus. **A:** CT scan. **B:** Thoracoscopic aspect before resection. **C:** Thoracoscopic aspect after resection, with a mucosal patch left on the right main stem bronchus (*small arrows*). **D:** Cautery of the mucosal patch. RMSB, right main stem bronchus; LMSB, left main stem bronchus.

TABLE 155.3 Results of VATS Excision of Bronchogenic Cyst

Author	Year	Details of the Study (Years)	No.	Sex Ratio	Age (Range)	Approach Type	Approach No.	Tumors Size (Mean) in cm	Operative Time (min)	Length of Postoperative Stay (Days)	Length of Chest Tube (Days)	Conversion Rate	Conversion Details	Morbidity
Jung	2014	Retrospective single-institution report (1995–2013)	113	53M/60F	41.3 (4–78)	VATS in all cases		3.7 (range 1–10)	96.8 ± 48.7 (range 15–320)	3.7 ± 1.3 (range 1–23)	2.3 ± 1.6 (range 1–21)	n = 4/113 (3.6%)	2 majors adhesions of the bronchus, 1 left inominate venous injury, 1 repair of bronchial tear	2 prolonged air leak over 7 days 3 chylothorax
Kozu	2014	Retrospective single-institution report (1997–2012) of resection of mediastinal cyst	26	13M/13F	44 ± 17	VATS	17	3.6 ± 1.9	122 ± 47	7.0 ± 4.7	NA	None	—	2 atrial fibrillation 1 respiratory distress
						Open	9							
De Giacomo	2009	Retrospective multi-institution report (1995–2008)	30	19M/13F	39 (19–59)	VATS in all cases		5.2 (range 3–10.5)	80 (range 45–160)	3.7 (range 2–5)	NA	n = 2/30 (6.7%)	2 majors pleural adhesion	None
Weber	2004	Retrospective single-institution report (1995–2002)	12	6M/6F	43 (22–62)	VATS in all cases		4.5 (range 2–6.6)	75 (range 35–145)	5.5 (range 4–14)	NA	n = 1/12 (8.3%)	Massive pleural adhesion	1 postoperative diarrhea of unknown origin
Martinod	2000	Retrospective multi-institution report (1990–1993)	20	12M/8F	41.9 (22–73)	VATS in all cases		4,9 (range 2.5–0)	NA (range 60–300)	VATS: 5.2 / Open: 8.5	1.9	n = 7/20 (35%)	2 bleeding (azygos vein and left inferior pulmonary vein), 5 adhesions to vital structures	None

NA: Not Available.

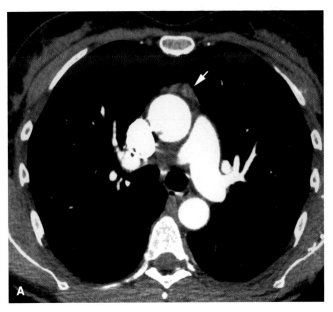
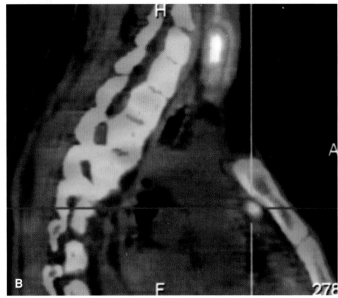

FIGURE 155.16 Parathyroid adenoma in the anterior mediastinum. **A:** CT scan. **B:** MIBI scintigraphy.

MEDIASTINAL PARATHYROID ADENOMA

INTRODUCTION

Primary hyperparathyroidism is usually caused by a parathyroid adenoma (PA). In the majority of patients with primary hyperparathyroidism, the responsible PA is located in the neck. However, parathyroid glands are ectopic in 20% of cases, and 2% are located deep within the mediastinum. Traditionally, sternotomy, mediastinotomy, and thoracotomy were required for complete surgical removal of ectopic mediastinal PA.

The embryologic origin of parathyroid glands is the endoderm of the third and fourth pharyngeal pouches.[31] From there, these glands migrate to their usual position, that is, behind the thyroid gland. If migration is too far, the parathyroids may be found in the cervical thymic horns but also inside or along the intrathoracic thymus or in the anterior mediastinum (Fig. 155.16). Other locations such as retrotracheal or paraesophageal are rare (Fig. 155.17). Although estimates of mediastinal parathyroid glands in primary hyperparathyroidism have been as high as 20%, only about 2% are not amenable to removal through a cervical incision.[32] However, a thoracic approach, regardless of the technique used, is noncontributive in 20% of cases.[33] This is mainly due to the fact that the adenoma, if small, is often not visible, especially in overweight patients. In addition, the surgeon is legitimately anxious about crushing a hidden adenoma with the inherent risk of spilling parathyroid tissue.

Localization of concealed parathyroid glands in the deep mediastinum can be achieved by a variety of imaging techniques, although no single study or combination of studies 100% sensitive because of false-negatives and false-positive results.

Parathyroid glands larger than 1 cm are typically seen on computed tomographic scans but smaller-sized glands can be difficult to identify. Strategies to localize parathyroid tissue include CT, MRI, [99]Tc Sestamibi scan, arteriography, selective venous sampling and FDG PET, and ^{11}C methionine PET. The [99]Tc Sestamibi scan may offer the highest success rate. In tumors greater than 1 g, the success is 86%, and it is 100% in tumors greater than 2 g. The sensitivity of MRI was greater than CT scan for detecting mediastinal lesions, but less than ^{99}Tc sestamibi alone.[34] The accuracy of ^{11}C methionine PET in successfully locating PAs was reported at 88%.[35]

TREATMENT

The options for treatment of an ectopic gland traditionally include sternotomy, thoracotomy, or thoracoscopy. A thoracoscopic approach is most likely the best compromise in terms of yield and safety.

Technical Features

- A thoracoscopic resection of a PA is possible only if supported by high-quality preoperative imaging, including CT scan and [99]Tc Sestamibi scan, so that the target is defined with optimal accuracy.
- If the adenoma is not rapidly discovered, tissue manipulation should be as gentle and as cautious as possible to prevent accidental injury to the adenoma with a high risk of parathyroid tissue spillage.
- Approximately 80% of all deep mediastinal PA are located in the anterior mediastinum and are usually situated within or in close contact with the thymus.[36] Thus, if the adenoma is not easily discovered, it is advisable to perform a hemithymectomy (Figs. 155.18 and 155.19).[37]
- Other minimally invasive surgical routes have been described including thoracoscopy via a small cervical incision[38] and sub-xiphoid thoracoscopic approach after preoperative localization by Tc sestamibi radionuclide scan.[39] However, with currently available instrumentation and high definition imaging systems, a standard thoracoscopy is probably a better option as it allows exploration of the whole mediastinum, if needed.

Intraoperative assays of parathormone levels is very helpful. A dramatic drop in levels after removal of tissue indicates the functioning PA has been removed.

Results

Minimally invasive techniques have been reported with increasing frequency in the past two decades but most of the cases are case

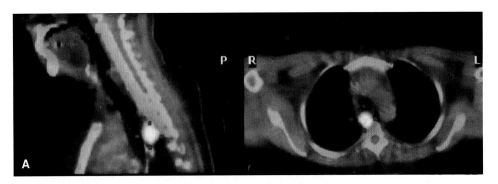

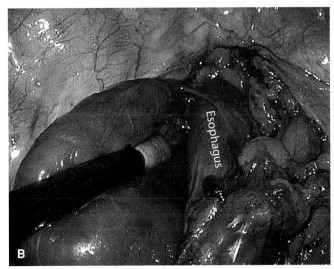

FIGURE 155.17 Parathyroid adenoma in the posterior mediastinum. **A:** MIBI scintigraphy. **B:** Thoracoscopic view of a large adenoma behind the esophagus.

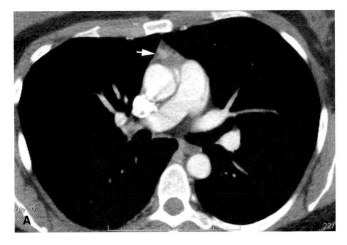

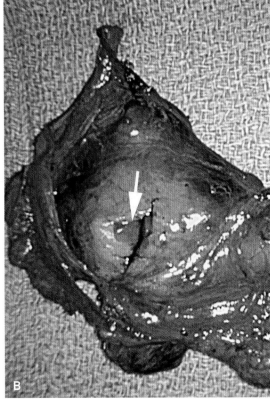

FIGURE 155.18 Small parathyroid adenoma (*arrow*) in the right thymus. **A:** CT scan. **B:** Open specimen revealing the adenoma.

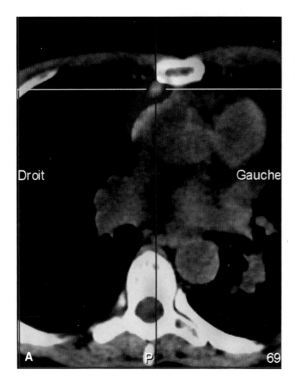

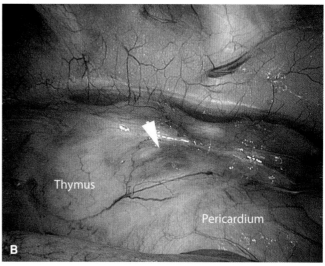

FIGURE 155.19 Parathyroid adenoma (*arrow*) in the right thymus. **A:** MIBI scintigraphy. **B:** Thoracoscopic view of the adenoma inside the thymus (*arrow*).

reports.[36,37,40–42] The largest series are shown in Table 155.4. Medrano and colleagues reported seven successful mediastinal parathyroid cases resected by a VATS approach. Resection was uneventful in all cases. In contrast to sternotomy, where up to 21% incidence of pulmonary complications has been reported,[43,44] this series only reported an intercostal neuralgia that resolved within 2 weeks.[36] Iihara et al.[42] succeeded in removing a mediastinal PA in 7 out of 14 patients, with the remaining seven cases with parathyroid lesions at the aortic arch or upper region, treated via a cervical approach. One patient required partial thymectomy because of a tumor embedded in the thymus. No significant postoperative complications were reported. Similar results were reported by Alesina and colleagues also in a series of seven patients.[40]

MEDIASTINAL GOITERS

INTRODUCTION

Intrathoracic goiter (ITG) is defined as a thyroid enlargement in which the majority of the mass is inferior to the thoracic inlet.[45] Reported incidences of ITGs range from less than 1% to more than 20%. Diagnosis of ITG is commonly made in the fifth or sixth decade of life, with a female:male ratio of 4:1. They are classified as either primary or secondary:

- Primary ITGs are rare. They arise from aberrant thyroid tissue located in the mediastinum, receive blood supply from mediastinal vessels, and are not connected to the cervical thyroid.
- Secondary ITGs arise from cervical thyroid tissue and grow downward through the thoracic inlet. Most ITG arise the from cervical thyroid gland and descend through a fascial plane into the superior mediastinum. They are usually situated in the anterior mediastinum and arise equally from the right or left lobes of the thyroid gland. However, 10% to 15% of ITGs grow retrotracheally into the posterior mediastinum. The attachment between the ITG and

the thyroid can be very thin and even absent, so that the intrathoracic portion of a goiter is frequently missed during a thyroidectomy. An anterior mediastinal mass discovered in a patient with a previous history of thyroidectomy is most often an ITG.

In over 30% of cases, ITGs are asymptomatic. The most commonly reported finding is a slowly growing cervical mass. There may be symptoms caused by compression of intrathoracic structures with predominance of respiratory disorders (dyspnea, stridor), and dysphagia may occur in up to one-third of patients. Conventional chest x-ray and CT scan provide the most important information related to location and extent of the lesion. The majority of patients with ITG are euthyroid.

TREATMENT

Resection of an ITG is indicated only in young patients or in the elderly that present with symptoms or with tracheal compression on CT. Surgical removal of ITG can be performed by cervicotomy in the majority of patients. Sternotomy or thoracotomy are necessary only in a minority of patients (<5%).[46] The most significant criteria for selecting patients requiring sternotomy or thoracotomy are CT scan features, that is, thyroid volume and extension below the carina or aortic arch.[47] There is little available information[48] about the best surgical approach for retrotracheal ITGs extending beyond the aortic arch into the posterior mediastinum. In such cases, sternotomy is not optimal as access to the posterior mediastinum is impaired by the heart and great vessels immediately anterior to the thyroid mass. Such exposure leads to blind dissection with the risk of uncontrolled hemorrhage, injury to the recurrent laryngeal nerve, and incomplete removal of the goiter. In these instances, high lateral muscle-sparing thoracotomy in combination with a cervical incision has been described and allows control and direct visualization of great vessels as well as the posterior mediastinum.[49] The feasibility of a VATS approach combined with a transverse cervical incision has also been reported[50] with less morbidity than open techniques and excellent exposure.

TABLE 155.4 Largest Series of Thoracoscopic Resections of Mediastinal Parathyroid Lesions

Author	Year	Type of Study (Years)	No.	Sex Ratio	Age (Range)	Approach	Nuclear Scan	CT	MRI	Previous Neck Operation	Gland Size (cm)	Blood Loss mL (Mean)	Operative Time min (Mean)	Length of Chest Tube (Days)	Length of Postoperative Stay	Histology	Conversion Rate
Iihara	2012	Retrospective single institution report of thoracoscopic removal of mediastinal parathyroid lesions (1997–2010)	8	1M/6F	57 (r:39–66)	VATS	8	8	1	2	—	19 (r:5–43)	144 (r:69–258)	—	—	Adenoma: 3 Hyperplasia: 4 Thymoma: 1	None
Alesina	2008	Retrospective single institution report of thoracoscopic removal of mediastinal hyperfunctioning parathyroid glands (2002–2007)	7	4M/3F	47 (r:28–67)	VATS	7	7	—	1	—	Minimal	90 (r:40–180)	No tube	3.8 (r:2–6)	Adenoma: 5 Hypoplasia: 2	None
Cupisti	2002	Retrospective single institution report using open transthoracic approach and VATS for suspected intrathoracic parathyroid adenomas (1986–2000)	19	8M/11F	50 (r:16–79)	Open: 14 VATS: 4 VAMS:1	9	9	6	13	1.82 (r:0.7–3.7)	—	—	—	Open: 14 (r:5–46) VATS: 7 (r:3–10) VAMS: 8	Adenoma: 14 Hyperplasia: 1 Unknown: 4	25% (n = 1/4)
Medrano	2000	Retrospective single institution report of thoracoscopic resection of ectopic parathyroid glands (1990–1999)	7	5M/2F	39 (r:22–57)	VATS	7	7	2	7	2.3	—	65 (r:40–92)	0,85 (r:0–2)	2.7 (r:2–3)	Adenoma: 6 Hyperplasia: 1	None
Prinz	1994	Retrospective two institutions report of thoracoscopic excision of enlarged mediastinal parathyroid glands (–)	4	2M/2F	52 (r:26–82)	VATS	4	4	1	4	—	—	195 (r:120–240)	1	3.25 (r:1–6)	Adenoma: 2 Hyperplasia: 2	None

NA, Not available; VAMS, video-assisted mediastinoscopic surgery; r, range.

In the combined approach, precise cervical dissection is mandatory to remove all attachments from the surrounding tissues to the thyroid. Digital dissection following the lower thyroid lobe as far as the thoracic inlet facilitates mobilization. Such a maneuver allows the goiter to be retracted and removed via VATS approach with previous dissection of the posterior mediastinum. Clips, ultrasonic or bipolar sealing device are useful for coagulation and ligation of small thyroid vessels in the mediastinum as well as lymphatic vessels between the superior cava vein and the trachea.

Reports on VATS approach for ITG removal are scarce and consist of case reports.[50–52] However these reports are convincing and VATS is most likely a valid option for ITG extending beyond the aortic arch into the posterior mediastinum.

MEDIASTINAL GERM CELLS TUMORS

INTRODUCTION

Germ cell tumors (GCTs) consist of a wide array of histologic subtypes ranging from benign mature teratoma to malignant embryonal carcinoma. The origin of these tumors is a primitive germ cell with multipotent capability for differentiation. Several theories have been proposed to explain the origin and location of these tumors. Some support the theory of aberrant migration of primitive germ cells originating in the embryonic yolk sac.[53] Others think that these tumors arise from totipotential cells originating in the primitive knot and primitive streak that invaginate between the layers of the bilaminar disc to form the mesoderm.[54]

GCTs are seen in childhood and adults up to the fourth decade, with different age peaks according the various anatomic sites. GCTs tend to occur in the midline of the body. The most common extragonadal locations in adults, in order of frequency, are the anterior mediastinum, retroperitoneum, and the pineal and suprasellar regions. In infants and young children, sacrococcygeal and intracranial GCTs are the most frequent.

Extragonadal GCTs include seminomas and NSGCTs. The NSGCTs tumors comprise yolk sac tumors, choriocarcinomas, embryonal carcinomas, teratomas, and mixed tumors that contain more than one cell line. Benign GCTs also have been referred to as epidermoid cysts, dermoids, benign teratomas, or simply teratomas. Differences in prognosis and treatment make the distinction of seminomas and NSGCTs essential.

PATHOLOGICAL AND CLINICAL FEATURES

GCTs account for approximately 15% of the anterior mediastinal tumors in adults and 25% in children.[55] Whether these tumors represent a malignant transformation of the thymus with germ cell potential is still not established. The close association of mediastinal GCT with the thymus and the presence of placental-like alkaline phosphatase (PLAP)-positive cell within the normal thymus support a potential thymic etiology.[56]

Mature Teratomas

Mature teratomas represent 60% to 70% of all mediastinal GCTs. Benign teratomas present equally in men and women, being found as early as the first month of life or as late as to the eighth decade of life. Tumors tend to be slow growing and many patients have no symptoms when the mass is discovered, often incidentally. Benign teratomas can be either cystic or solid or a combination of both,

measuring up to 21 cm (Fig. 155.20). They consist of all three primordial layers: ectoderm (skin and hair), mesoderm (bone, fat, and muscle), and endoderm (respiratory epithelium and gastrointestinal tract). Skin, pilosebaceous tissue, smooth muscle, fat, and respiratory epithelium are found in more than half of the tumors. The most common symptom is chest pain, and sometimes dyspnea, cough, and fever. Occasionally when the tumor erodes into an airway, patients may expectorate hair (trichoptysis) or sebum.[57] Hemoptysis also can occur, presumably from irritation of the bronchial mucosa by the tumor or from erosion into a vascular structure.[58] Benign teratomas, also can rupture and fistulize into the pleural or pericardium or to the skin. The cause of rupture is postulated to be from the tumor-secreting proteolytic enzymes with subsequent digestion of the tumor wall. Secretion of insulin, human chorionic gonadotropin, follicle-stimulating hormone, and androgenic substances resulting in sexual precocity has also been reported. Secretion of pancreatic enzymes can cause inflammation and necrosis. More recently, anti–N-methyl-D-aspartate (anti-NMDA) receptor antibody encephalitis has been reported in patients with mature mediastinal teratoma.[59,60]

Immature Teratomas

Teratomas of the mediastinum comprise a spectrum of purely mature to predominantly immature tissue from all three germinal layers mixed with embryonic immature tissue. Macroscopically, immature teratomas are made of cystic masses with areas of hemorrhage and necrosis. Although the majority of immature teratomas are limited to the mediastinum, those associated with malignant elements can invade surrounding structures or disseminate. Immature teratomas containing elements of other GCTs should be clinically considered to be mediastinal NSGCTs.

Mediastinal Seminomas

Primary mediastinal seminomas are the most common malignant mediastinal GCTs accounting for 40% to 50% of these tumors.[61] Such tumors predominantly occur in asymptomatic young males in their twenties to forties and have a good prognosis. Seminomas are slow-growing tumors that present as large mediastinal masses with a lobulated appearance, including areas of necrosis, hemorrhage, or both. Macroscopically, the tumor may present as a cystic structure in 8% to 20% of cases. They consist of multilocular thymic cyst with seminomatous tumor cells present in the wall of the cyst. The differential diagnosis includes thymoma and thymic cyst, nodular sclerosing Hodgkin lymphoma, reactive lymphoid hyperplasia, and nonspecific granulomatous inflammation. Symptoms are variable and can be vague, such as chest pain, cough, dyspnea, fever, and weight loss. Symptoms due to compression of adjacent structures, including hoarseness, dysphagia, or superior vena cava syndrome are seen in up to 10% of patients. More than 80% of patients are symptomatic at the time of presentation, and 60% to 70% have metastatic disease, with metastases to bone, lung, liver, spleen, spinal cord, or brain.[62] Although metastases from testicular seminoma to the mediastinum in the absence of retroperitoneal lymph node involvement are rare, all men with mediastinal seminoma should undergo testicular exploration to exclude gonadal origin. If testicular involvement is confirmed, orchiectomy is indicated. Immunohistochemical staining of mediastinal seminomas typically shows PLAP in 50% to 96% of the tumors. Serum β-HCG is elevated in one-third of patients. Seminomas do not produce alpha-fetoprotein (AFP), thus, an increased serum AFP is incompatible with the diagnosis of a pure seminoma and indicates that

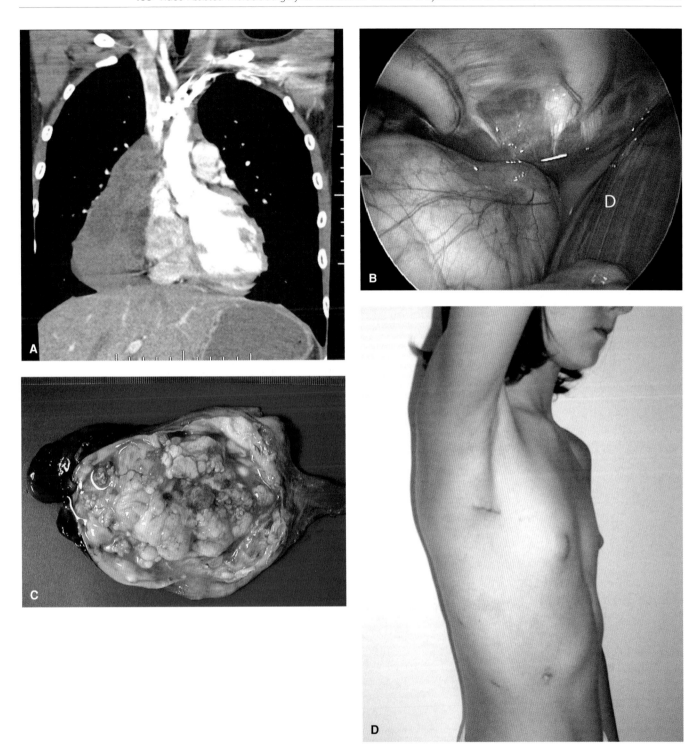

FIGURE 155.20 Bulky benign mature teratoma in a 13-year-old girl, removed via thoracoscopy. **A:** Preoperative CT scan. **B:** Intraoperative view (via 5-mm scope). **C:** Specimen. **D:** Scar at 1-month follow-up. *D, diaphragm.*

nonseminomatous elements are present. Currently, more sensitive and specific germ cell immunohistochemical stains are available for the diagnosis of seminomas as follows: D2-40 and AP-2gamma stains are positive in extragonadal seminomas, OCT3/4 shows nuclear staining and C-kit demonstrates membranous staining in the majority of seminomas.[63] Tumors consisting of a mixture of seminoma and other histologic types are defined as mixed GCTs and are classified as NSGCTs.

Nonseminomatous Germ Cell Tumors

Primary mediastinal NSGCTs are seen in children and young men, mainly in the second to fourth decade of life. These tumors are less frequent than seminomas or teratomas and have a markedly worse prognosis with reported 5-year overall survival ranging from 40% to 45%. Thus, although rare, the diagnosis should be considered in any young male patient presenting with an anterior mediastinal mass.

TABLE 155.5 Largest Series of Thoracoscopic Resections of Mediastinal Mature Teratoma

Author	Year	Type of Study (Years)	No.	Sex Ratio	Age Mean (Range)	Approach	Tumor Size cm (Range)	Blood Loss mL (Range)	Operative Time (mean) min	Length of Chest Tube (Days)	Length of Postoperative Stay	Conversion Rate
Tsubochi	2015	Retrospective single institution report of patients with complete thoracoscopic resection of mediastinal teratoma (1998–2013)	13	4M/9F	33 (17–54)	VATS	8 (range 5–13)	78 (10–300)	132 (range 95–184)	2 (range 1–6)	5 (range 4–7)	None
Shintani	2013	Retrospective single institution report of patients with thoracoscopic resection for mediastinal mature teratoma (2001–2012)	15	6M/9F	38 (21–62)	VATS	5.3 (range 3.2–8.5)	138 (10–450)	188 (range 78–430)	NA	NA	20% ($n = 3/15$)
Chang	2010	Retrospective single institution report of 18 years surgical experience with mediastinal mature teratoma (1988–2005)	57	18M/39F	28,8 (6–69)	Open: 43	10.4 ± 4.7	288.2 ± 406.6	205.4 ± 75.7	4.1 ± 2.1	8.1 ± 3.5	21% ($n = 3/14$)
						VATS: 14	8.5 ± 2.9	68.2 ± 152.1	106.4 ± 35.7	5.0 ± 3.4	6.0 ± 2.7	
Nakano	2008	Retrospective single institution report of patients who underwent video-assisted thoracoscopic removal for mediastinal mature teratoma following extraction of cystic components (1998–2008)	6	1M/5F	36,3 (24–54)	VATS	9 (range 5–11)	103	143	NA	NA	None

NA, Not Available.

NSGCTs represent up to 5% of anterior mediastinal masses in adults and 10% to 15% in children. Mediastinal origin of NSGCT is an independent predictor of poor prognosis compared with those of gonadal origin. There are several histological types including embryonal carcinoma, yolk sac carcinoma, choriocarcinoma, teratoma, and mixed types containing seminomatous components. Malignant mediastinal NSGCTs are characterized clinically by rapid local growth and early distal metastasis. At the time of diagnosis, most patients have symptoms caused by compression and/or invasion of local mediastinal structures. In addition, large series reported that 20% to 42% of these patients have at least one site of metastatic disease at diagnosis.[64–66] Common site of metastases are lung, pleura, lymph nodes, and liver with bone, brain, and kidneys less frequently involved. Gynecomastia is present in some patients who have high serum levels of β-HCG. Constitutional symptoms, such as weight loss, fever, and weakness, are more common in patients with nonseminomatous tumors than in those with pure seminoma. Serum AFP is increased in up to 80% of NSGCTs and β-HCG in up to 35%. This marker pattern differs slightly from that observed in nonseminomatous testicular tumors, where both markers are elevated with equal frequency. Elevation of AFP levels always indicates the presence of nonseminomatous elements within the tumor.

Association With Other Malignancies

Mediastinal NSGCTs, especially those with teratomatous elements can evolve into sarcomas and carcinomas that are extremely resistant to chemotherapy and radiotherapy.[67] NSGCTs may also be associated with a variety of hematologic malignancies: acute nonlymphocytic leukemia, acute lymphocytic leukemia, erythroleukemia, acute megakaryocytic leukemia, myelodysplastic syndrome, and malignant histiocytosis. NSGCTs are occasionally associated with Klinefelter syndrome.[68]

DIAGNOSIS

Imaging

In patients with a mediastinal lesion on standard chest radiograph, the differential diagnosis is determined based on the patient's age, location of the mass, clinical manifestations, and tumor markers. Once diagnosis of a mediastinal GCT is established, testicular exploration should be done, including gonadal palpation and testicular ultrasonography.

Currently, excellent depiction of the mediastinal lesions is possible with several imaging modalities: CT, MRI, and PET. Vascular contrast enhanced chest CT allows a reliable evaluation of the mediastinal anatomy and the involvement of surrounding structures and may help determine tissue composition. However, MRI is more accurate than CT in assessing tumor invasion of the great vessels or chest wall and in distinguishing a cyst from a solid tumor. PET is especially useful for the evaluation of residual disease from seminomas. Seminomas are extremely sensitive to chemotherapy and radiation and are initially treated nonsurgically. Therefore, identification and management of residual disease is critical. Traditionally, masses larger than 3 cm on CT have been considered to potentially contain residual disease and consequently offered additional treatment, usually surgery. In a series by De Santis and colleagues,[69] PET was superior to CT scan in detecting residual disease after chemotherapy in seminoma patients with a positive predictive value of 100% versus 37% and a negative predictive value of 96% versus 92%, respectively. Similarly, residual masses in NSGCTs may contain necrotic tissue, viable NSGCT, or teratoma. It has been demonstrated that a positive PET image after treatment was a strong predictor for the presence of viable carcinoma/teratoma.[70]

Biopsy

Several biopsy techniques have been described: ultrasound-guided endoscopic biopsy, CT-guided needle biopsy, parasternal anterior mediastinotomy, cervical mediastinoscopy, VATS, and open surgical procedures. The choice of technique depends on location of the lesion, clinical factors, and the availability of special techniques with the required expertise and the necessary equipment.

Transthoracic needle biopsy of suspected teratoma remains controversial. When imaging techniques show typical signs of mature teratoma, surgical resection is recommended without biopsy. In suspected seminomas, a biopsy is warranted. Core needle biopsy should be performed when possible. But there is a pathologic discrepancy of 6% between histology and fine-needle aspiration, and difficulty may arise in differentiating a GCT from poorly differentiated carcinoma. If the core needle biopsy is not conclusive, a surgical biopsy is usually the procedure of choice, preferably by VATS. In addition, if NSGCT is suspected, although prior histological diagnosis by means of surgical biopsy or large-bore needle is preferable, treatment may be started on the basis of increased tumor markers.

TREATMENT

Teratomas

The treatment of choice for benign GCTs is a total resection to definitively confirm the diagnosis and prevent development of local symptoms due to tumor growth. Small or medium size teratomas (Fig. 155.21) can be resected via thoracoscopy but when their size obscures visualization of anatomical landmarks, thoracotomy remains a reasonable option (Fig. 155.22).

Although mature teratomas are benign, they may pose difficult surgical problems because of the nearby structures involved such as pericardium, lung, vascular structures, and thymus. Nonetheless, complete surgical excision can usually be done. Some surgeons advocate that giant tumors can be removed through an open approach,[66] whereas others, including our team, have reported successful resection of giant teratomas up to 16 cm via a thoracoscopic approach.[71,72] Results of large series of thoracoscopic removal of mediastinal mature teratoma are shown in Table 155.5.

When a thoracoscopic approach is used for cystic tumors, puncturing the cyst and aspirating its fluid content facilitate mobilization, dissection, and specimen removal (Video 155.2).[71,73] In cystic teratoma, the mass can be only partially deflated as it also contains solid components. A similar technique has been described[74] using a cannula and a balloon cholangiography catheter connected to a syringe. This maneuver must not be done if a malignant component is suspected in order to avoid spillage of tumor contents into the thoracic cavity. Indeed, rapid tumor dissemination has been reported in a patient who underwent VATS resection of a teratoma with malignant transformation, in whom an intraoperative rupture of the cystic tumor occurred.[75]

Chang et al.[75] reported an 18-year surgical experience with mediastinal mature teratoma in a single institution. Forty-three patients received conventional open surgery whereas 14 received VATS. The patients in the thoracoscopic group had significantly decreased operative time (106 vs. 205 min), fewer ventilator days (0.2 vs. 0.5), and shorter stay in the intensive care unit (0.6 vs. 1.5 days) compared to thoracotomy group. Three patients underwent

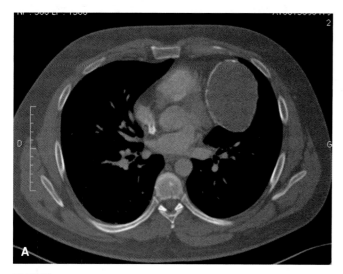

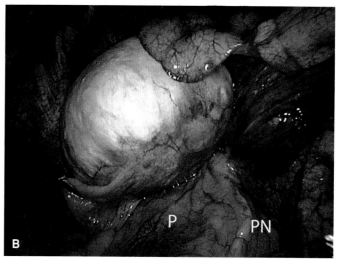

FIGURE 155.21 Teratoma resected via thoracoscopy. Note the adhesion to the phrenic nerve. **A:** preoperative CT scan. **B:** intraoperative view. *P, pericardium; PN, phrenic nerve.*

intraoperative conversion from VATS to anterolateral minithoracotomy because of dense adhesions to the surrounding structures. In a series of 15 patients who underwent thoracoscopic teratoma resection,[76] a higher incidence of complications was found in symptomatic patients. Whether the presence of symptoms should be considered as a relative contraindication for the thoracoscopic approach in mediastinal teratoma cases, is still not clear. The prognosis of benign teratoma after resection is excellent. Postoperative irradiation or other adjuvant treatments are not indicated.

Seminomas

The International Germ Cell Consensus Classification stratifies patients with mediastinal seminomas without evidence of nonpulmonary visceral metastases as good-risk GCTs. This group has

a 5-year survival rate of over 90%.[77] Seminomas are sensitive to both cisplatin-based chemotherapy and radiotherapy. Radiotherapy alone results in a long-term complete remission in only about 65% of patients,[78] whereas long-term disease-free survival is achieved in approximately 90% of patients treated with platinum-based chemotherapy.[62] Thus, the first line of treatment is chemotherapy in the majority of cases.

The role of surgical resection in the treatment of primary mediastinal seminoma is debated and is currently evolving. Some authors have suggested primary resection in good-risk surgical candidates with small, localized mediastinal tumors. In addition, surgical resection may be performed for an undiagnosed anterior mediastinal mass that is postoperatively found to be a seminoma. Surgical resection, however, is not recommended as the sole treatment modality.

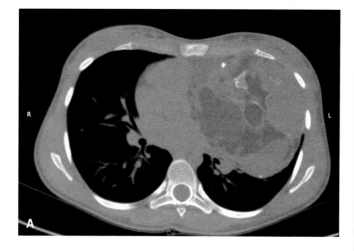

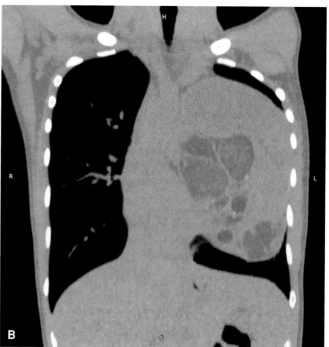

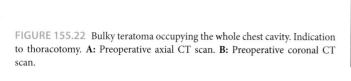

FIGURE 155.22 Bulky teratoma occupying the whole chest cavity. Indication to thoracotomy. **A:** Preoperative axial CT scan. **B:** Preoperative coronal CT scan.

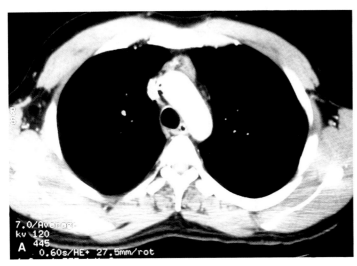 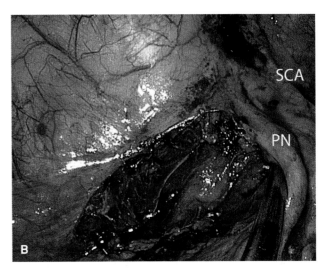

FIGURE 155.23 Residual mass after chemotherapy for a nonseminomatous germ cell tumor. **A:** CT scan. **B:** Intraoperative view. *PN, phrenic nerve; SCA, subclavian artery.*

Liu et al.[25] reported a series of 54 malignant primary mediastinal GCTs that contained 18 patients with seminoma. Among seminoma patients, eight cases were initially treated with surgery, eight had induction therapy followed by surgery, and two received chemoradiotherapy alone. The overall 5-year survival rate of the patients with mediastinal seminoma was 87.7%. Takeda and colleagues[7] in their series of 126 mediastinal GCTs, reported 13 seminoma patients. Among those 13 patients, 10 underwent surgery plus adjuvant or neoadjuvant therapy with long-term survival rates. All reported series performed an open approach either by sternotomy, thoracotomy, or clamshell incisions. No cases of thoracoscopic approach have been reported.

Likewise, consensus regarding the optimal postchemotherapy management has not been reached. It is reported that patients with a residual mass greater or equal to 3 cm after chemotherapy should undergo resection as those may contain residual malignancy in up to 30% of cases.[79] The role of resection for residual tumor is twofold in this situation. First, it is to document if there is residual disease as opposed to necrotic debris following treatment. Second, is to rule out the presence of a nonseminomatous component to the tumor that was previously unrecognized. Other authors recommend close follow-up for patients with a persistent radiographic mass after completion of induction chemotherapy and salvage treatment in case a relapse occurs. Recently, FDG-PET has been proposed to estimate viable residual lesions in seminoma patients after chemotherapy.[80]

Thoracoscopy has a place in the treatment of these lesions as the difficulty of the resection is not predictable, particularly for small lesions. It may be worth starting the procedure via thoracoscopy and determine if the lesion is easily resectable (Fig. 155.23).

NSGCTs

Mediastinal origin of NSGCTs is considered an independent predictor of poor prognosis compared with those of gonadal origin. Lack of durable response and resistance to first-line chemotherapy regimens, associated hematologic malignancies, and malignant transformation of the primary tumor to nongerm cell tumor elements have been cited as reasons for these poor outcomes.[68,78] Chemotherapy is the mainstay of initial treatment and surgery should be viewed as an adjuvant to chemotherapy. Bleomycin, etoposide and cisplatin (BEP) is the current standard regimen.[77] A rapid decline in tumor marker

levels with cisplatin-based chemotherapy is associated with improved response rates and overall survival. Postsurgical chemotherapy is indicated when viable tumor is present in the resected specimen. Despite multimodality treatment, outcomes are commonly poor, with 5-year survival rates reported between 30% and 48%.[66,77]

The most favorable candidates for surgical resection are patients with tumor marker normalization after initial treatment with chemotherapy. In the past, patients demonstrating a residual mass on CT and persistently elevated tumor markers have been treated with salvage chemotherapy in an effort to obtain normal tumor maker levels prior to surgery. This approach, however, has not improved outcome and currently postchemotherapy adjuvant surgery, regardless of persistently elevated tumor markers, has evolved as a mainstay of therapy in an attempt of achieving durable remission on these patients.[25,81] In rare circumstances, postchemotherapy patients will demonstrate normalized tumor marker levels but no residual mass on CT. Follow-up with serial computed tomography scans is recommended in these patients instead of surgery.

Preoperative and postoperative normalization of tumor markers, complete resection of any residual tumor, absence of extramediastinal disease, and absence of residual viable tumor in the resected specimen are factors predictive of better outcomes.[64,78] Predictors of worse survival included persistent malignancy in the postresection specimen, the need for extramediastinal resection, and increasing tumor markers following chemotherapy.[66] In a series of 158 patients, Kesler et al.[64] found persistent tumor in the resectioned specimen and increased markers postresection to be associated with worse survival on multivariate analysis.

Reported surgical approaches favor a hemiclamshell or clamshell incision to insure maximal exposure, especially when resection of involved lung and other mediastinal structures is planned.[82] Chemotherapy can cause the residual mass to be intimately adherent to surrounding structures. Thoracoscopic resection of mediastinal NSGCT is not reported in the literature.

REFERENCES

1. Gossot D. *Atlas of Endoscopic Major Pulmonary Resections.* Cham, Switzerland: Springer International Publishing AG; 2018.
2. Pons F, Lang-Lazdunski L, Bonnet P, et al. Videothoracoscopic resection of neurogenic tumors of the superior sulcus using the harmonic scalpel. *Ann Thorac Surg* 2003;75:602–604.

3. Gossot D. Ultrasonic dissectors for neurogenic tumors of the superior sulcus. *Ann Thorac Surg* 2004;77:2263–2264.
4. Gossot D, Pryschepau M, Martinez Berenys C, et al. Throw-off instruments for advanced thoracoscopic procedures. *Interact Cardiovasc Thorac Surg* 2009;10:159–160.
5. Reeder L. Neurogenic tumors of the mediastinum. *Semin Thorac Cardiovasc Surg* 2000;12:261–267.
6. Ribet M, Cardot G. Neurogenic tumors of the thorax. *Ann Thorac Surg* 1994;58:1091–1095.
7. Takeda S, Miyoshi S, Minami M, et al. Intrathoracic neurogenic tumors—50 years' experience in a Japanese institution. *Eur J Cardiothorac Surg* 2004;26:807–812.
8. Arapis C, Gossot D, Debrosse D, et al. Thoracoscopic removal of neurogenic mediastinal tumors: technical aspects. *Surg Endosc* 2004;18:1380–1383.
9. Cardillo G, Carleo F, Khalil M, et al. Surgical treatment of benign neurogenic tumours of the mediastinum: a single institution report. *Eur J Cardiothorac Surg* 2008;34:1210–1214.
10. Riquet M, Mouroux J, Pons F, et al. Videothoracoscopic excision of thoracic neurogenic tumors. *Ann Thorac Surg* 1995;60:943–946.
11. Fraga J, Aydogdu B, Aufieri R, et al. Surgical treatment for pediatric mediastinal neurogenic tumors. *Ann Thorac Surg* 2010;90:413–418.
12. Petty J, Bensard D, Partrick D, Hendrickson R, Albano E, Karrer F. Resection of neurogenic tumors in children: is thoracoscopy superior to thoracotomy? *J Am Coll Surg* 2006;203:699–703.
13. Anraku M, Nakahara R, Matsuguma H, et al. Port site recurrence after video-assisted thoracoscopic resection of chest wall schwannoma. *Interact Cardiovasc Thorac Surg* 2003;2:483–485.
14. Barrenechea I, Fukumoto R, Lesser J, et al. Endoscopic resection of thoracic paravertebral and dumbbell tumors. *Neurosurg* 2006;59:1195–1202.
15. Liu H, Yim A, Wan J, et al. Thoracoscopic removal of intrathoracic neurogenic tumors: a combined Chinese experience. *Ann Surg* 2000;232:187–190.
16. Yang C, Zhao D, Zhou X, et al. A comparative study of video-assisted thoracoscopic resection versus thoracotomy for neurogenic tumours arising at the thoracic apex. *Interact Cardiovasc Thorac Surg* 2015;20:35–39.
17. Shiiya H, Tanaka A, Sakuraba M, et al. Complete resection of a posterior mediastinal tumor after preoperative identification of artery of Adamkiewicz. *Kyobu Geka* 2014;67:371–374.
18. Smail H, Baste JM, Melki J, et al. Challenging posterior mediastinal mass resection via a minimally invasive approach with neurological monitoring. *Eur J Cardiothorac Surg* 2013;43:e44–e46.
19. Cansever L, Kocaturk C, Cinar H, et al. Benign posterior mediastinal neurogenic tumors: results of a comparative study into video-assisted thoracic surgery and thoracotomy (13 years' experience). *Thorac Cardiovasc Surg* 2010;58:473–475.
20. Li Y, Wang J. Experience of video-assisted thoracoscopic resection for posterior mediastinal neurogenic tumours: a retrospective analysis of 58 patients. *ANZ J Surg* 2013;83:664–668.
21. Ronson R, Duarte I, Miller J. Embryology and surgical anatomy of the mediastinum with clinical implications. *Surg Clin North Am* 2000;80:157–169.
22. Zaimi R, Fournel L, Chambon E, et al. Double bronchogenic cyst. *Rev Mal Resp* 2014;31:864–866.
23. Lev S, Lev M. Imaging of cystic lesions. *Radiol Clin North Am* 2000;38:1013–1027.
24. Traibi A, Strauss C, Validire P, et al. Intralobar pulmonary sequestration associated with bronchogenic cyst in adult. *Asian Cardiovasc Thorac Ann* 2012;5:597–599.
25. Liu R, Adler D. Duplication cysts: Diagnosis, management, and the role of endoscopic ultrasound. *Endosc Ultrasound* 2014;3:152–160.
26. Jung H, Kim D, Lee G, et al. Video-assisted thoracic surgery for bronchogenic cysts: is this the surgical approach of choice? *Interact Cardiovasc Thorac Surg* 2014;19:824–829.
27. Kozu Y, Suzuki K, Oh S, et al. Single institutional experience with primary mediastinal cysts: clinicopathological study of 108 resected cases. *Ann Thorac Cardiovasc Surg* 2014;5:365–369.
28. Martinod E, Pons F, Azorin J, et al. Thoracoscopic excision of mediastinal bronchogenic cysts: results in 20 cases. *Ann Thorac Surg* 2000;69:1525–1528.
29. Gharagozloo F, Dausmann M, McReynolds S, et al. Recurrent bronchogenic pseudocyst 24 years after incomplete excision. *Chest* 1995;108:880.
30. Weber T, Roth T, Beshay M, et al. Video-assisted thoracoscopic surgery of mediastinal bronchogenic cysts in adults: a single-center experience. *Ann Thorac Surg* 2004;78:987–991.
31. Kurtay M, Crile G. Aberrant parathyroid glands in relationship to the thymus. *Am J Surg* 1969;117:705.
32. Ipponsugi S, Takamori S, Suga K, et al. Mediastinal parathyroid adenoma detected by 99mTc-methoxyisobutylisonitrile: report of a case. *Surg Today* 1997;27:80–83.
33. Randone B, Costi R, Scatton O, et al. Thoracoscopic removal of mediastinal parathyroid glands: a critical appraisal of an emerging technique. *Ann Surg* 2010;251:717–721.
34. Ishibashi M, Nishida H, Hiromatsu Y, et al. Localization of ectopic parathyroid glands using technetium-99m sestamibi imaging: comparison with magnetic resonance and computed tomographic imaging. *Eur J Nucl Med* 1997;24:197–201.
35. Beggs A, Hain S. Localization of parathyroid adenomas using 11C-methionine positron emission tomography. *Nucl Med Commun* 2005;26:133–136.
36. Medrano C, Hazelrigg S, Landreneau R, et al. Thoracoscopic resection of ectopic parathyroid glands. *Ann Thorac Surg* 2000;69:221–223.
37. Hentati A, Gossot D. Thoracoscopic partial thymectomy for untraceable mediastinal parathyroid adenomas. *Interac Cardiovasc Surg* 2011;13:542–544.
38. Komanapalli C, Cohen J, Sukumar M. Extended transcervical video-assisted thymectomy. *Thorac Surg Clin* 2010;20:235–243.
39. Wei J, Gadacz T, Weisner L, et al. The subxiphoid laparoscopic approach for resection of mediastinal parathyroid adenoma after successful localization with Tc-99m-sestamibi radionuclide scan. *Surg Laparosc Endosc* 1995;5:402–406.
40. Alesina P, Moka D, Mahlstedt J, et al. Thoracoscopic removal of mediastinal hyperfunctioning parathyroid glands: personal experience and review of literature. *World J Surg* 2008;32:224–231.
41. Cupisti K, Dotzenrath C, Simon D, et al. Therapy of suspected intrathoracic parathyroid adenomas. Experiences using open transthoracic approach and video-assisted thoracoscopic surgery. *Langenbecks Arch Surg* 2002;386:488–493.
42. Iihara M, Suzuki R, Kawamata A, et al. Thoracoscopic removal of mediastinal parathyroid lesions: selection of surgical approach and pitfalls of preoperative and intraoperative localization. *World J Surg* 2012;36:1327–1334.
43. Russell C, Edis A, Scholz D, et al. Mediastinal parathyroid tumors: experience with 38 tumors requiring mediastinotomy for removal. *Ann Surg* 1981;193:805–809.
44. Conn J, Goncalves M, Mansour K, et al. The mediastinal parathyroid. *Am Surg* 1991;57:62–66.
45. Katlic M, Wang C, Grillo H. Substernal goiter. *Ann Thorac Surg* 1985;39:391–399.
46. Kacprzak G, Karas J, Rzechonek A, et al. Retrosternal goiter located in the mediastinum: surgical approach and operative difficulties. *Interac Cardiovasc Surg* 2012;15:935–937.
47. Mackle T, Meaney J, Timon C. Tracheoesophageal compression associated with substernal goitre. Correlation of symptoms with cross-sectional imaging findings. *J Laryngol Otol* 2007;121:358–361.
48. Machado N, Grant C, Sharma A, et al. Large posterior mediastinal retrosternal goiter managed by a transcervical and lateral thoracotomy approach. *Gen Thorac Cardiovasc Surg* 2011;59:507–511.
49. Kilic D, Findikcioglu A, Ekici Y, et al. When is transthoracic approach indicated in retrosternal goiters? *Ann Thorac Cardiovasc Surg* 2011;17:250–253.
50. Gupta P, Lau K, Rizvi I, et al. Video assisted thoracoscopic thyroidectomy for retrosternal goitre. *Ann R Coll Surg Eng* 2014;96:606–608.
51. Oey I, Richardson B, Waller D. Video-assisted thoracoscopic thyroidectomy for obstructive sleep apnoea. *Respir Med* 2003;97:192–193.
52. Shigemura N, Akashi A, Nakagiri T, et al. VATS with a supraclavicular window for huge substernal goiter: an alternative technique for preventing recurrent laryngeal nerve injury. *Thorac Cardiovasc Surg* 2005;53:231–233.
53. Sobis H, Vandeputte M. Sequential morphological study of teratomas derived from displaced yolk sac. *Dev Biol* 1975;45:276–290.
54. Brown N. Teratomas and yolk-sac tumours. *J Clin Pathol* 1976;29:1021–1025.
55. Mullen B, Richardson J. Primary anterior mediastinal tumors in children and adults. *Ann Thorac Surg* 1986;42:338–345.
56. Weidner N. Germ-cell tumors of the mediastinum. *Semin Diagn Pathol* 1999;16:42–50.
57. Guibert N, Attias D, Pontier S, et al. Mediastinal teratoma and trichoptysis. *Ann Thorac Surg* 2011;92:252–253.
58. Chen R, Chang T, Chang C, et al. Mediastinal teratoma with pulmonary involvement presenting a massive hemoptysis in 2 patients. *Respir Care* 2010;55:1094–1096.
59. Kawahara K, Miyawaki M, Anami K, et al. A patient with mediastinal mature teratoma presenting with paraneoplastic limbic encephalitis. *J Thorac Oncol* 2012;7:258–259.
60. Sommerling C, Santens P. Anti-N-methyl-D-aspartate (anti-NMDA) receptor antibody encephalitis in a male adolescent with a large mediastinal teratoma. *J Child Neuro* 2014;29:688–690.
61. Moran C, Suster S. Primary germ cell tumors of the mediastinum: I. Analysis of 322 cases with special emphasis on teratomatous lesions and a proposal for histopathologic classification and clinical staging. *Cancer* 1997;80:681–690.
62. Bokemeyer C, Nichols C, Droz J, et al. Extragonadal germ cell tumors of the mediastinum and retroperitoneum: results from an international analysis. *J Clin Oncol* 2002;20:1864–1873.
63. Iczkowski K, Butler S, Shanks J, et al. Trials of new germ cell immunohistochemical stains in 93 extragonadal and metastatic germ cell tumors. *Hum Pathol* 2008;39:275–281.
64. Kesler K, Rieger K, Hammoud Z, et al. A 25-year single institution experience with surgery for primary mediastinal nonseminomatous germ cell tumors. *Ann Thorac Surg* 2008;85:371–378.
65. Rivera C, Arame A, Jougon J, et al. Prognostic factors in patients with primary mediastinal germ cell tumors, a surgical multicenter retrospective study. *Interact Cardiovasc Surg* 2010;11:585–589.
66. Sarkaria I, Bains M, Sood S, et al. Resection of primary mediastinal non-seminomatous germ cell tumors: a 28-year experience at Memorial Sloan-Kettering Cancer Center. *J Thorac Oncol* 2011;6:1236–1241.
67. Erhlich Y, Beck S, Ulbright T, et al. Outcome analysis of patients with transformed teratoma to primitive neuroectodermal tumor. *Ann Oncol* 2010;21:1846–1850.
68. Hartmann J, Nichols C, Droz J, et al. Hematologic disorders associated with primary mediastinal nonseminomatous germ cell tumors. *J Nat Cancer Inst* 2000;92:54–61.
69. De Santis M, Becherer A, Bokemeyer C, et al. 2-18 fluoro-deoxy-D-glucose positron emission tomography is a reliable predictor for viable tumor in postchemotherapy seminoma: an update of the prospective multicentric SEMPET trial. *J Clin Pathol* 2004;22:1034–1039.
70. Kollmannsberger C, Oeschle K, Dohmen B, et al. Prospective comparison of [18F] fluorodeoxyglucose positron emission tomography with conventional assessment by computed tomography scans and serum tumor markers for the evaluation of residual masses in patients with nonseminomatous germ cell carcinoma. *Cancer* 2002;94:2353–2362.
71. Gossot D, Izquierdo R, Girard P, et al. Thoracoscopic resection of bulky intrathoracic benign lesions. *Eur J Cardiothorac Surg* 2007;32:848–851.

72. Miyauchi Y, Matsubara H, Uchida T, et al. Successful thoracoscopic removal of a giant teratoma following extraction of cystic components: a case report. *Asian J Endosc Surg* 2014;7:79–81.

73. Tsubochi H, Endo S, Nakano T, et al. Extraction of mediastinal teratoma contents for complete thoracoscopic resection. *Asian Cardiovasc Thorac Ann* 2015;23:42–45.

74. Shimokawa S, Watanabe S, Sakasegawa K, et al. Balloon catheter for cyst aspiration in a thoracoscopic resection of mediastinal cyst. *Surg Today* 2001;31:284–286.

75. Chang C, Chang Y, Lee Y. Cystic malignant teratoma with early recurrence after intraoperative spillage. *Ann Thorac Surg* 2008;86:1971–1973.

76. Shintani Y, Funaki S, Nakagiri T, et al. Experience with thoracoscopic resection for mediastinal mature teratoma: a retrospective analysis of 15 patients. *Interact Cardiovasc Thorac Surg* 2013;16:441–444.

77. Mead GM, Stenning SP, Cook P, et al. International germ cell consensus classification: a prognostic factor-based staging system for metastatic germ cell cancers. International Germ Cell Cancer Collaborative Group. *J Clin Oncol* 1997;15:594–603.

78. Fizazi K, Culine S, Droz J, et al. Initial management of primary mediastinal seminoma: radiotherapy or cisplatin-based chemotherapy? *Eur J Cancer* 1998;34:347–352.

79. Motzer R, Bosl G, Heelan R, et al. Residual mass: an indication for further therapy in patients with advanced seminoma following systemic chemotherapy. *J Clin Oncol* 1987;5:1064–1070.

80. Sakaguchi Y, Isowa N. Successful resection of mediastinal seminoma evaluated the response to induction chemotherapy with fluorodeoxyglucose-positron emission tomography. *Ann Thorac Cardiovasc Surg* 2012;18:45–47.

81. Takeda S, Miyoshi S, Ohta M, et al. Primary germ cell tumors in the mediastinum: a 50-year experience at a single Japanese institution. *Cancer* 2003;97:367–376.

82. Bains M, Ginsberg R, Jones W, et al. The clamshell incision: an improved approach to bilateral pulmonary and mediastinal tumor. *Ann Thorac Surg* 1994;58:30–32.

156

Surgical Techniques for Thymectomy

Joseph LoCicero, III

In this multiple sectioned chapter, all the surgical approaches to removal of the thymus will be presented. Each approach has its proponents. Reports of each type of operation show encouraging results, but each operation always has associated advantages and disadvantages.

When the thymus is the site of benign tumors, a minimal approach may suffice, but there is no question that the goal of thymectomy is to remove all of the gland, particularly in cases of benign and malignant thymoma and in patients with myasthenia gravis. A recent randomized trial reported in the New England of Medicine demonstrated that thymectomy plus steroid therapy had a significant advantage over steroid therapy alone for myasthenia gravis.[1] The report created a firestorm of correspondence. Recurrence of thymoma or recrudescence of myasthenia gravis symptoms in cases of potentially incomplete resection, regardless of approach, will lead to questions of both the technique itself and surgical competence. When a less-than-radical approach is chosen, it is incumbent on the operator to assure that the entire gland has been removed. Since there is no consensus for proof of removal of all glandular tissue, effectiveness of lesser techniques will continue to be hotly debated.

This extended chapter presents all of the current methods of thymectomy. It is intended to inform the reader concerning the best choice of procedure for his or her particular patient. Section 154a is an update of the classic trans-sternal thymectomy procedure as performed at the Mayo Clinic. Section 154b outlines the trans-cervical approach first popularized by the Toronto group and presented by one of its proponents, Dr. Joseph Shrager. Section 154c is a discussion of the newer minimally invasive approaches by Dr. Jonathan D'Cunha. Finally, Section 154d is an updated discussion of the maximal procedure of extended thymectomy by Dr. Joshua Sonnett and colleagues.

REFERENCE

1. Wolfe GI, Kaminski HJ, Aban IB, et al.; MGTX Study Group. Randomized trial of thymectomy in myasthenia gravis. *N Engl J Med* 2016;375(6):511–522.

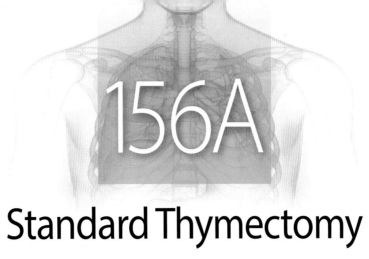

156A

Standard Thymectomy

Francis C. Nichols ▪ Victor F. Trastek

The thymus gland continues to present challenges to thoracic surgeons. The thymus is the site of origin of benign and malignant neoplasms; it is also involved in cellular immunity and certain aspects of humoral immunity.

Following the report by Alfred Blalock and colleagues[1] of successful resection of the thymus in a 26-year-old woman with myasthenia gravis (MG) and a thymic cyst, surgical resection of the thymus became a treatment option for this disease. In 1944, Blalock[2] published a total of 20 cases of MG treated by a transsternal thymectomy. In the following decade, numerous studies from England and the United States, including those by Clagett and Eaton[3,4] at the Mayo Clinic, continued the debate as to the role of thymectomy in treating MG. With time and the refinement of perioperative care, the results of thymectomy improved, so as to validate the benefit of the operation as a significant part of the overall treatment of the myasthenic patient.

Surgical approaches for thymectomy include transsternal and transcervical thoracic surgery as well as video-assisted thoracic surgery (VATS), there being proponents of each. Regardless of the approach, the basic principles of thymic surgery should include mediastinal exploration, en bloc resection of the thymus gland including the cervical poles and adjacent mediastinal fat, protection of the phrenic nerves, and the prevention of intrapleural dissemination. For patients with thymoma, a full median sternotomy is commonly used. For patients without a thymoma requiring thymectomy, resection through a partial sternotomy is a procedure the authors commonly employ.

SURGICAL ANATOMY

The thymus is a bilobed anterior mediastinal structure overlying the pericardium and great vessels (Fig. 156A.1). Midline fusion of the thymic lobes gives the gland its H-shaped configuration. Bilateral upper horns extend into the neck, with attachment to the thyroid gland via the thyrothymic ligament. Lower horns are draped over the pericardium, attaching to the pericardial fat pad. Occasionally one or both lobes may lie posterior to the innominate vein instead of anterior to it. Rare thymic locations include partial or complete failure of descent of one or both thymic lobes and aberrant islands of thymic tissue in the neck, mediastinum, pericardial fat, or within the pulmonary parenchyma. Masaoka and colleagues[6] found a 72% incidence of microscopic deposits of thymic tissue in the mediastinal fat. Jaretzki and colleagues[5] found thymic tissue in the neck outside of the normal thymic cervical extensions in 32% of their patients.

The arterial blood supply comes superiorly from small branches of the inferior thyroid arteries, laterally from the internal mammary

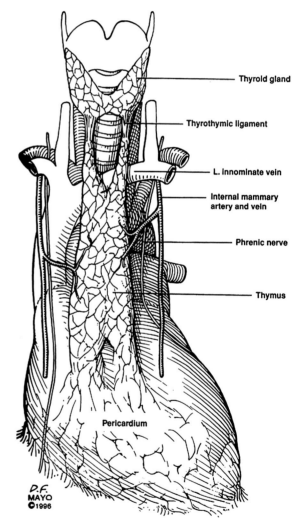

FIGURE 156A.1 The thymus is a bilobed structure with two upper and two lower horns; it is located in the anterior mediastinum overlying the pericardium and great vessels. Arterial blood supply is primarily from the internal mammary arteries laterally; venous drainage is central into the left innominate vein. Of key importance is the relationship of the thymus gland and both phrenic nerves, particularly in the middle and upper portions of the gland. (From Nichols FC, Trastek VF. Thymectomy [sternotomy]. In Kaiser LR, Kron IL, Spray TL, eds. *Mastery of Cardiothoracic Surgery*. 2nd ed. Philadelphia, PA: Lippincott Williams & Wilkins; 2006:101.)

Labels on figure: Thyroid gland, Thyrothymic ligament, L. innominate vein, Internal mammary artery and vein, Phrenic nerve, Thymus, Pericardium

2033

arteries, and inferiorly from pericardiacophrenic branches. Venous drainage is primarily via a single central vein or multiple branch veins emptying into the left innominate vein. Small veins accompanying the arteries may partially account for the venous drainage.

The proximity of the phrenic nerves to the thymus gland is of critical importance. Both phrenic nerves are intimately associated with the thymus as they pass from the neck into the chest in the region of the thoracic inlet. Knowledge of this anatomy is crucial for successful postoperative outcome, since inadvertent injury to the phrenic nerves can have catastrophic respiratory consequences, particularly in myasthenic patients.

In the newborn, the thymus gland reaches a mean weight of 15 g. By puberty the gland attains a mean weight of 30 to 40 g. Following puberty and continuing throughout adulthood, thymic involution usually occurs, with the gland eventually decreasing to a weight of 5 to 25 g. Ultimately the thymus is almost totally replaced by fat.

INDICATIONS

Indications for thymectomy include resection of a thymic mass, MG in selected patients, or both. Approximately 10% to 15% of patients with MG will have an associated thymoma, whereas 30% or more of patients with thymoma will have MG.

PREOPERATIVE EVALUATION

Preoperative evaluation of a patient with an anterior mediastinal mass should include computed tomography (CT) with contrast enhancement to rule out vascular invasion and allow for better delineation of the mediastinal mass (Fig. 156A.2). Magnetic resonance imaging (MRI) may accomplish these same goals. If a patient presents with an anterior mediastinal mass suspicious for thymoma and vascular abnormalities have been ruled out, resection is indicated. Transthoracic needle aspirates are controversial but may be helpful in the diagnosis of thymoma. Additional preoperative evaluation should be directed toward the detection of associated MG. Similarly, patients being considered for thymectomy because of MG should have preoperative CT scanning to search for an associated thymoma.

PREOPERATIVE PREPARATION

Patients undergoing thymectomy for MG are candidates for operation only if their medical condition is optimized. A team approach in the care of myasthenic patients undergoing thymectomy is advocated. This includes anesthesia, neurology, and the surgical team being involved preoperatively, intraoperatively, and postoperatively. If the myasthenic patient cannot be stabilized with medication, preoperative plasmapheresis is required prior to thymectomy. Seggia and colleagues[8] found that plasmapheresis significantly improved respiratory function and muscle strength in myasthenic patients undergoing thymectomy, thus leading to a reduced hospital stay and lower cost.

Preoperative anesthetic medication is minimal, usually consisting only of atropine and a mild sedative. Preoperative anticholinergic medications are avoided. Myasthenic patients pose no particular anesthetic problems, although muscle relaxants should be avoided. Deep anesthesia is maintained by an inhalational agent and short-acting narcotic. During the operative procedure, the airway and ventilation can be controlled with a single-lumen endotracheal tube.

OPERATIVE TECHNIQUE

Radical thymectomy through a complete sternotomy with cervical extension is advocated by Jaretzki and colleagues[5] and Masaoka.[7] When a thymoma is not present, we prefer to perform thymectomy using a partial sternal-splitting incision. Usually the upper end of the skin incision is kept 1 to 2 fingerbreadths below the sternal notch and carried down to the level of the 3rd or 4th interspace. Through this relatively short skin incision, with the sternum separated, adequate visualization of the entire mediastinal portion of the thymus and its cervical extension can be obtained. When a thymoma is present, a complete sternotomy is usually performed.

PARTIAL STERNAL-SPLITTING INCISION

With general endotracheal anesthesia using a single-lumen endotracheal tube, the patient is placed in the supine position with the neck, chest, and upper abdomen prepped and draped.

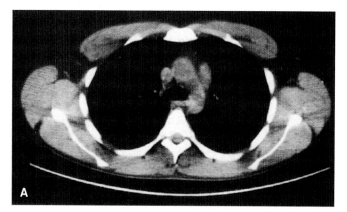
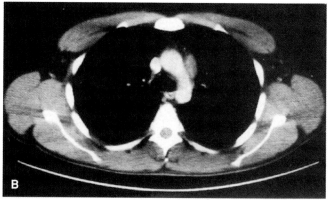

FIGURE 156A.2 Radiographic manifestations of thymoma. **A:** CT without intravenous contrast indicates that the lesion lies in the anterior mediastinum. **B:** With intravenous contrast, a vascular aneurysm is excluded, as is vascular invasion by the lesion. Also more clearly delineated is the relationship of the lesion to adjacent structures such as the pericardium and lung. (From Nichols FC, Ercan S, Trastek VF. Standard thymectomy. In: Shields TW, Locicero J, Ponn RB, et al., eds. *General Thoracic Surgery.* 6th ed. Philadelphia, PA: Lippincott Williams & Wilkins; 2005:2630.)

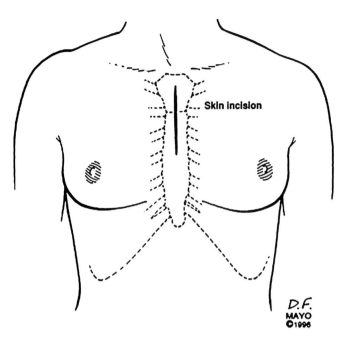

FIGURE 156A.3 The patient is supine and the skin incision is begun 1.5 cm below the sternal notch; it is carried down to the level of the 4th or 5th rib. This keeps the skin incision well below the neck area and not visible when normal clothing is worn, providing for an acceptable cosmetic result. (From Nichols FC, Trastek VF. Thymectomy [sternotomy]. In Kaiser LR, Kron IL, Spray TL, eds. *Mastery of Cardiothoracic Surgery*. 2nd ed. Philadelphia, PA: Lippincott Williams & Wilkins; 2006:102.)

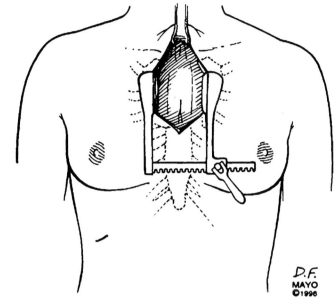

FIGURE 156A.4 When the sternal retractor is opened, usually the 3rd or 4th interspace will fracture transversely, allowing for more than adequate exposure of the thymus gland for patients without thymoma. Alternatively, a transverse cut of half of the sternum can be made with the microsagittal saw. The transverse fracture or cut is easily repaired when the sternum is wired. If additional exposure is necessary, both the skin incision and sternal incision can be lengthened. (From Nichols FC, Trastek VF. Thymectomy [sternotomy]. In Kaiser LR, Kron IL, Spray TL, eds. *Mastery of Cardiothoracic Surgery*. 2nd ed. Philadelphia, PA: Lippincott Williams & Wilkins; 2006:102.)

The skin incision is started 1.5 cm below the sternal notch and extended down the midline of the sternum to the level of the 4th or 5th rib (Fig. 156A.3). With cephalad skin retraction, the sternal notch is dissected free so that a finger can be placed beneath the sternum. The sternum is longitudinally divided in the center to the level of the 4th or 5th rib. A microsagittal saw may be useful. A sternal retractor is placed, and as the sternum is spread, one side will usually split off transversely at the interspace (Fig. 156A.4). Alternatively, the sternum can be transversely divided at the level of the 4th or 5th rib utilizing the microsagittal saw. The overlying mediastinal pleura is separated in the midline, bringing the thymus and left innominate vein into view. Both pleural spaces are opened beginning inferiorly and extending cephalad, making sure to identify and protect both phrenic nerves. Identification of the internal thoracic vein provides a useful landmark for the superior extent of the pleural opening, since the phrenic nerve is in immediate proximity. Exploration of the mediastinum, both pleural spaces, and both lungs is performed.

Thymectomy is begun by dissecting the middle of the right inferior horn off the pericardium. Utilizing a right-angle clamp in a progressive "walking" technique, the inferior horn is first dissected in a caudad direction down to the pericardial fat pad, which is then clamped, divided, and ligated with a 2-0 silk suture. With a right-angle clamp still on the inferior horn and attached pericardial fat, the right lobe of the thymus is dissected off the pericardium in a cephalad direction. This dissection is discontinued at the midportion of the thymus and dissection of the right superior horn in the cervical area is begun (Fig. 156A.5). The right superior horn is circumferentially freed, again utilizing a right-angle clamp in a walking technique until the thyrothymic ligament is seen. The right superior thymic horn is disconnected from the thyroid gland by dividing the proximal thyrothymic ligament and ligating it with 2-0 silk. A right-angled clamp

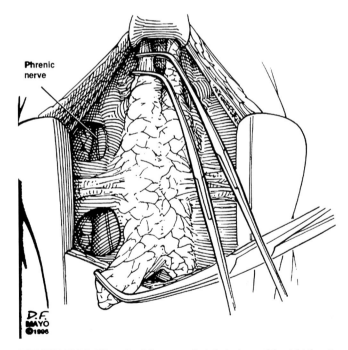

Phrenic nerve

FIGURE 156A.5 Dissection is begun on the inferior horn of the right thymic lobe, freeing it from the pericardium in a caudad direction by progressively advancing the right-angled clamps in a walking technique. This is continued down to the pericardial fat pad, where it is divided and ligated. A right-angled clamp is left on the pericardial fat attached to the inferior horn for later retraction. The superior horn is then freed from the cervical area, identifying and dividing the thyrothymic ligament. The medial thymic attachments are now all that remain on the right side. (From Nichols FC, Trastek VF. Thymectomy [sternotomy]. In Kaiser LR, Kron IL, Spray TL, eds. *Mastery of Cardiothoracic Surgery*. 2nd ed. Philadelphia, PA: Lippincott Williams & Wilkins, 2006:103.)

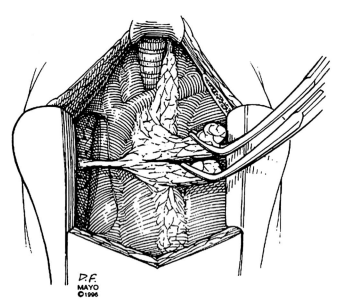

FIGURE 156A.6 Both horns on the right side are completely freed. The right-angled clamps are retracted medially, putting tension on the midportion of the gland. This traction provides optimal visualization and protection of the phrenic nerve as the small arterial branches from the internal mammary artery are divided. Cautery in this area should be utilized with extreme caution to prevent inadvertent injury to the phrenic nerve. (From Nichols FC, Trastek VF. Thymectomy [sternotomy]. In Kaiser LR, Kron IL, Spray TL, eds. *Mastery of Cardiothoracic Surgery*. 2nd ed. Philadelphia, PA: Lippincott Williams & Wilkins; 2006:104.)

is left on the resected superior horn. The upper and lower right-angle clamps are then pulled medially. Using a right-angle clamp and primarily blunt dissection, the middle portion of the right lobe and associated fatty tissue are pulled back from the area of the phrenic nerve up to the junction of the innominate vein and superior vena cava. The lateral arterial vessels arising from the internal mammary artery are very carefully cauterized or ligated so as to avoid inadvertent injury to the phrenic nerve (Fig. 156A.6). Oozing in the area of the phrenic nerve can be controlled with gauze packing. The thymus gland is now further reflected along the left innominate vein until the midline venous drainage is identified.

The same steps are now carried out on the left side. Notably, the left side may be more difficult because the phrenic nerve tends to come closer, and there seems to be a greater amount of fatty tissue obscuring its visualization. Again, a blunt dissection technique in the critical midportion of the thymus where the nerve and thymus are in closest proximity helps prevent injury to the nerve. Once all of the horns have been successfully ligated and the midportions of the gland dissected free, the central venous drainage is clamped, divided, and ligated with 3-0 silk suture (Fig. 156A.7).

If the surgeon encounters unusual thymic adherence to surrounding structures such as the pericardium or adjacent lung parenchyma, these should be resected en bloc with the thymus. If the extent of the thymus gland cannot be discerned during dissection, separate margins are sent for frozen-section analysis to be sure no thymic tissue is left behind.

Following completion of the total thymectomy, meticulous hemostasis is obtained with attention again paid to viewing the phrenic nerves. A chest tube is placed below the right breast, through the chest wall, and across the right pleural space and mediastinum, with the tip of the tube ultimately resting in the left chest apex (Fig. 156A.8). The sternum is reapproximated with interrupted steel wires, with two

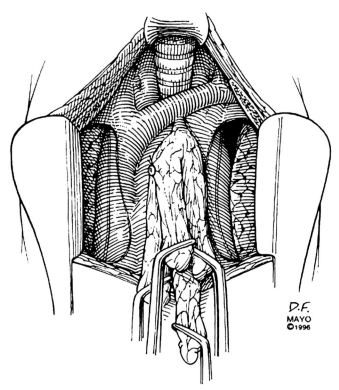

FIGURE 156A.7 Following resection of the inferior and superior thymic horns and dissection of the midportion of the gland, the venous drainage to the left innominate vein is ligated and divided. (From Nichols FC, Trastek VF. Thymectomy [sternotomy]. In Kaiser LR, Kron IL, Spray TL, eds. *Mastery of Cardiothoracic Surgery*. 2nd ed. Philadelphia, PA: Lippincott Williams & Wilkins; 2006:104.)

or three wires placed into the manubrium and the remainder around the sternal interspaces. The remaining soft tissue is closed with multiple layers of running absorbable suture, including a subcuticular skin closure.

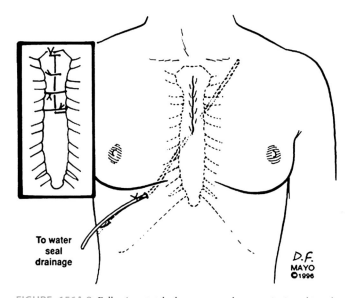

To water seal drainage

FIGURE 156A.8 Following total thymectomy, hemostasis is achieved; a right chest tube is then placed below the right breast, through the chest wall, directed across the right pleural space and mediastinum, and the left pleural space. (From Nichols FC, Trastek VF. Thymectomy [sternotomy]. In Kaiser LR, Kron IL, Spray TL, eds. *Mastery of Cardiothoracic Surgery*. 2nd ed. Philadelphia, PA: Lippincott Williams & Wilkins; 2006:105.)

FULL MEDIAN STERNOTOMY INCISION

For patients with a thymic mass, a full sternotomy is usually needed to provide exposure. If the mass is extraordinarily large, a double-lumen endotracheal tube may be helpful, as may bilateral anterior thoracotomy incisions with transverse division of the sternum, or a "clamshell" incision (Fig. 156A.9).

Whether via full median sternotomy or clamshell incision, once exploration for metastatic disease is completed, the tumor should be resected en bloc along with the entire thymus gland. Actual resection of the thymus gland proceeds in a manner similar to that described above. At any point where adherence or invasion to surrounding structures is suspected, en bloc resection of the adjacent structure with the thymic mass, if possible, should be performed (Fig. 156A.10). Again, protection of the phrenic nerves is important; however, if curative resection requires removal of one phrenic nerve and the patient can tolerate this from a respiratory standpoint, it should be performed. Frozen-section analysis during the operation helps in the assessment of tumor-free margins. If total resection is not possible, then debulking should be performed. Areas surrounding the resection should be marked with clips for possible future radiation therapy. Closure of the surgical incision is similar to that described above.

POSTOPERATIVE CARE

Following surgery, the patient is awakened and evaluated closely by the anesthesiologist. Extubation is performed in the recovery room if the respiratory effort and blood gases are satisfactory. Nearly all patients can be extubated immediately. If the patient has MG, he or she is monitored closely by the surgical, critical care, and neurology teams. Inspiratory–expiratory pressures and vital capacity are measured every 6 hours to evaluate respiratory status. Aggressive pulmonary toilet is maintained and ambulation initiated the day after surgery. Anticholinesterase agents are restarted only if weakness occurs. Undertreating with these agents immediately postoperatively minimizes problems with oral and tracheal secretions and decreases the possibility of cholinergic crisis. If the myasthenic patient deteriorates from the respiratory standpoint, plasmapheresis is instituted. Once the patient's respiration is stable, he or she is transferred to the general thoracic surgery floor, drains are removed as early as possible, and the patient discharged when recovery is complete.

SURGICAL RESULTS

With the advent of the team approach combined with aggressive preoperative and postoperative care, operative mortality has nearly been eliminated and morbidity is very low. From 1982 through 2004, a total of 364 patients underwent thymic resection at Mayo Clinic in Rochester, Minnesota. Of these 241 (66.2%) had MG. Partial sternotomy was performed in 236 patients, full sternotomy in 126, and clamshell incision in 2. In all, 236 (98%) of the MG patients were extubated within the first few hours of surgery, and the remaining 5 were extubated the following day. There was one operative death (0.27%) secondary to ARDS. Average length of hospitalization was 4.8 days. Major complications occurred in 18 patients (4.9%) and included atelectasis in 10, atrial fibrillation in 4, respiratory failure requiring reintubation in 3, bleeding in 3, and chylothorax in 1.

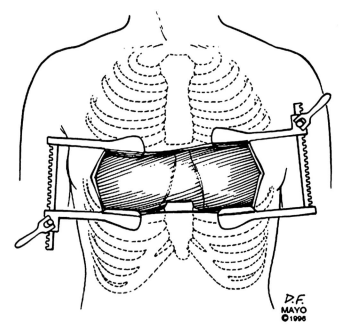

FIGURE 156A.9 For resection of an extraordinarily large thymoma possibly involving one or both pulmonary hila, a bilateral thoracotomy, and transverse division of the sternum or "clamshell" incision may be useful. (From Nichols FC, Trastek VF. Thymectomy [sternotomy]. In Kaiser LR, Kron IL, Spray TL, eds. *Mastery of Cardiothoracic Surgery*. 2nd ed. Philadelphia, PA: Lippincott Williams & Wilkins; 2006:102.)

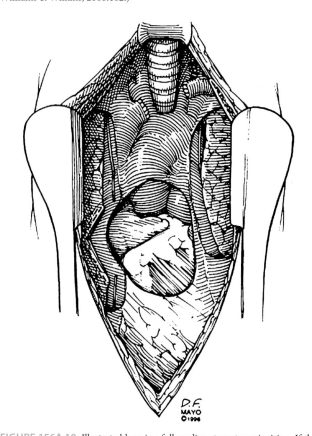

FIGURE 156A.10 Illustrated here is a full median sternotomy incision. If the thymoma is invasive, total en bloc resection is carried out, including all associated involved structures; in this case lung, right phrenic nerve, portion of pericardium, and the left innominate vein. (From Nichols FC, Trastek VF. Thymectomy [sternotomy]. In Kaiser LR, Kron IL, Spray TL, eds. *Mastery of Cardiothoracic Surgery*. 2nd ed. Philadelphia, PA: Lippincott Williams & Wilkins; 2006:105.)

Liu and colleagues[9] in 2011 reported on 115 patients with MG. There were no instances of postoperative crisis, but there was a 7.7% complication rate. Among 110 patients on whom follow-up was done postoperatively, 29 (26.4%) were in SCR, 64 (58.2%) showed improvement, 7 (6.4%) remained unchanged, and 10 (9.1%) had a worsening of their conditions. In Shrager's[10] collected series of 151 patients, complications were held to a low rate of 0.7%.

Cheng and colleagues[11] in 2013 reported on 141 cases of MG in juveniles. Among 135 patients with complete postoperative follow-up, 34 (25.2%) achieved CSR, 28 (20.7%) experienced pharmacologic remission, 61 (45.2%) improved, 5 (3.7%) remained stable, and 7 (5.2%) deteriorated. The results indicated the disease-onset age greater than 6 years and age at operation greater than 12 years were both positively associated with CSR responses.

CONCLUSION

Complete surgical resection remains the mainstay of therapy for early-stage thymoma and in appropriate patients with MG. Thymectomy through a partial sternotomy for MG or a full sternotomy for a thymic mass or thymoma provides excellent exposure and the ability to treat all aspects of the problem with low mortality and morbidity.

REFERENCES

1. Blalock A, Mason MF, Morgan HJ, et al. Myasthenia gravis and tumors of the thymic region: report of a case in which the tumor was removed. *Ann Surg* 1939;110:544–561.
2. Blalock A. Thymectomy in the treatment of myasthenia gravis: report of twenty cases. *J Thorac Surg* 1944;13:316.
3. Clagett OT, Eaton LM. Surgical treatment of myasthenia gravis. *J Thorac Surg* 1947;162:62–80.
4. Eaton LM, Clagett OT. Present status of thymectomy in treatment of myasthenia gravis. *Am J Med* 1955;19:703–717.
5. Jaretzki A, Penn AS, Younger DS, et al. Thymectomy for myasthenia gravis: analysis of controversies regarding techniques and results. *Neurology* 1997;48(Suppl 5):S52.
6. Masaoka A, Nagaoka Y, Kotake Y, et al. Distribution of thymic tissue at the anterior mediastinum. Current procedures in thymectomy. *J Thorac Cardiovasc Surg* 1975; 70:747–754.
7. Masaoka A. Extended trans-sternal thymectomy for myasthenia gravis. *Chest Surg Clin of North Am* 2001;11:369–387.
8. Seggia JC, Abreu P, Takatani M. Plasmapheresis a preparatory method for thymectomy in myasthenia gravis. *Arq Neuropsiquiatr* 1995;53:411–415.
9. Liu Z, Lai Y, Yao S, et al. Extended transsternal thymectomy for the treatment of ocular myasthenia gravis. *Ann Thorac Surg* 2011;92(6):1993–1999.
10. Shrager JB. Extended transcervical thymectomy: the ultimate minimally invasive approach. *Ann Thorac Surg* 2010;89(6):S2128–S2134.
11. Cheng C, Liu Z, Xu F, et al. Clinical outcome of juvenile myasthenia gravis after extended transsternal thymectomy in a Chinese cohort. *Ann Thorac Surg* 2013;95(3): 1035–1041.

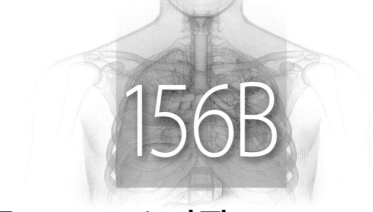

156B

Transcervical Thymectomy

Joseph B. Shrager

Transcervical thymectomy (TCT) was developed primarily for excision of the thymus gland in patients suffering from myasthenia gravis (MG), and remains an excellent surgical approach for thymectomy in patients with nonthymomatous MG. However, few would recommend it for resection of anything other than the very smallest thymomas. It is interesting to note that the very first thymectomy for MG, performed by Saurbruch and Roth[1] in 1911, was carried out via a transcervical approach. Blalock[2] and colleagues[3] popularized thymectomy via median sternotomy (MS), with the reporting in 1944 of a series of 20 patients whose myasthenic symptoms appeared to have improved following thymectomy. With this demonstration, interest in surgery of the thymus gland grew rapidly, along with controversy regarding the best surgical means of approaching the gland.

In the 1960s, Papatestas et al.[4] popularized the transcervical approach to the thymus gland. In 1987, he published data collected over the previous 30 years. His technique of TCT was carried out without the self-retaining, sternum-lifting retractor that is used today, and thus it appears to have been a largely blind, blunt dissection into the anterior mediastinum. It is likely that this approach rarely led to a total thymectomy.

Despite Papatestas' initial arguments for the advantages of a transcervical approach, which he advocated for all patients with MG, MS became the most widely accepted approach for thymectomy in MG. The rationale for a transsternal approach and other even more extensive procedures, including "maximal transsternal and transcervical thymectomy," were described best by Jaretzki and colleagues.[5,6] These authors emphasized, first, the presence of nests of thymic tissue outside the thymic capsule in the mediastinal and cervical fat that they documented in autopsy studies to be present in a high percentage of patients. They argued that it was unlikely that this tissue would be resected by a limited transcervical approach. Second, they emphasized the occasional case of complete remission from MG after removal of residual thymic tissue after a failed initial thymectomy. These findings led them to recommend a radical excision of all of the fatty tissues associated with the thymus in the chest and neck.

The development of a sternum-lifting retractor by Joel Cooper in the 1980s dramatically improved the visualization of the thymus gland via the neck, converting a largely blind procedure into one that allows good visualization of the entire anterior mediastinum and dissection with removal of the intracapsular thymus and all, or nearly all, of the surrounding mediastinal fat under direct vision. This operation was termed "extended TCT" by Cooper et al.[7] in order to distinguish it from Papatestas' operation. The subsequent application of thoracoscopic technology to the transcervical operation by de Perrot et al.[8] further improved the ability to remove even extracapsular, mediastinal thymic rests via a cervical incision. Results published by these groups, and by the author of this chapter, repopularized the transcervical approach to the gland.[8–10] In the last decade of the twentieth century, other minimally invasive approaches to the thymus gland have also been advocated and gained popularity, including various video-assisted transthoracic (VATS) approaches and robotic approaches which are described in subsequent chapters.

Perhaps at no previous time has there been as much controversy regarding the ideal surgical approach for thymectomy in MG as there is today. For reasons that will be outlined below, the author believes that extended TCT with VATS assistance has advantages over other available approaches, and there is no doubt that it has become a well-accepted approach in patients with nonthymomatous MG.[11,12]

Until very recently, there had been no level I evidence establishing the added benefit of thymectomy over medical therapy alone in the treatment of MG. Many did believe that the published retrospective studies supported a role for thymectomy in the management of this disease, but controversy persisted. Some neurologists rarely, if ever, referred MG patients for thymectomy. However, the recently published results of the international, prospective, randomized trial of thymectomy versus immunosuppressive treatment alone in the treatment of MG has filled this data void.[13] This study establishes that nonthymomatous MG patients do have a substantially improved clinical course when thymectomy is included in their treatment plan. It is clear that thoracic surgeons will now be performing many more thymectomies for MG in the future.

PREOPERATIVE PREPARATION AND PATIENT SELECTION

The minimally invasive nature of TCT clearly reduces morbidity compared to transsternal approaches, but it does not reduce the importance of preoperative optimization of disease status. In more severely affected patients, this requires the combined efforts of neurology, anesthesiology, and thoracic surgery, all of whom have experience in the care of these patients.

During preoperative evaluation, patients found to have more than mild generalized symptoms, or substantial bulbar or respiratory symptoms despite drug therapy, are generally referred for either intravenous immunoglobulin therapy or plasmapheresis.[14] These treatments not only facilitate the postoperative recovery but also frequently allow tapering of corticosteroids to low levels prior to surgery. We prefer to have patients on 10 mg or less of prednisone daily, although occasionally this is not possible. It is also critical that patients taking anticholinesterase medication continue these medications preoperatively, including the dose on the morning of surgery. These drugs are then reinstated with a sip of water postoperatively as soon as the patient is able to safely swallow, typically on the evening of surgery. Patients with any pulmonary symptoms also undergo preoperative pulmonary function testing since forced vital capacity (FVC) is a useful tool to monitor postoperative progress.[15]

Certain factors are very important in patient selection for TCT. First, the patient must be able to hyperextend his/her neck to a reasonable extent, as the surgical access to the mediastinum from the head of the operating table is impossible in a patient without sufficient neck extension. The need for good neck extension makes the operation difficult in some, but not all, elderly patients, and TCT is certainly not a good approach for patients that have had cervical spine fusion. Morbid obesity is a relative contraindication as neck extension and the ability to lift the sternum, which is essential to the operation, is typically compromised in such patients. Prior mediastinal surgery and a known or suspected thymoma are also considered contraindications to TCT. However, it should be noted that once one has substantial experience with the operation, resection of very small (<2 cm), clearly noninvasive thymomas can be reliably performed via this transcervical approach.

MGFA THYMECTOMY CLASSIFICATION

The Myasthenia Gravis Foundation of America (MGFA) classified the surgical approaches to thymectomy into four types of operations, listed in ascending order according to the amount of thymic tissue thought to be removable by each approach (Table 156B.1).

The goal of the "T4" operation is, unlike the others, removal of all thymic and fatty tissue in both the neck and the mediastinum, thereby including all areas where ectopic thymic tissue has been identified.[6] The goal of the other three classes of operations (T1 to T3) is generally the removal of the entirety of the gland by an extracapsular dissection, with more or less aggressive removal of the adjacent mediastinal fat as described by different authors.

While TCT has been classified by the MGFA as a "T1" thymectomy, we believe that extended TCT using the Cooper thymectomy retractor and a videoscope placed through the neck incision at key points in the operation allows the same amount of mediastinal thymic and fatty tissue to be removed as with the "T3," transsternal procedures. To this end, we have not found data that clearly demonstrates that removal of more than the gland itself results in substantially higher remission rates.[12] The literature demonstrates that results are sufficiently similar with TCT as with more extensive, more morbid operations such that, in our hands, TCT is the procedure of choice for nonthymomatous MG.

TABLE 156B.1 Thymectomy Classification of the Myasthenia Gravis Foundation of America

T1	Transcervical thymectomy • Basic • Extended
T2	Videoscopic thymectomy • Classic • Extended
T3	Transsternal thymectomy • Standard • Extended
T4	Transcervical and transsternal thymectomy

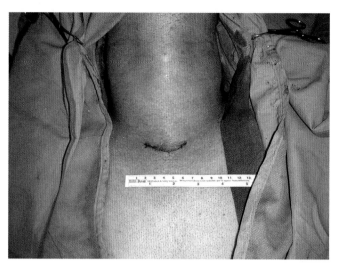

FIGURE 156B.1 The incision for extended transcervical thymectomy.

THE TECHNIQUE OF EXTENDED TRANSCERVICAL THYMECTOMY WITH VATS ASSISTANCE

Extended TCT as performed in our hands proceeds as follows: After general anesthesia is induced and a single-lumen endotracheal tube placed, the patient is placed in a supine position with the neck hyperextended by placement of an inflatable bag beneath the shoulders. The neck and upper chest are prepared and draped. A curved, transverse skin incision is made about 2 cm above the sternal notch and extended for 5 cm along the skin folds such that the lateral edges of the incision are approximately 1 cm cephalad to the clavicular heads (Fig. 156B.1). The caudal edge of the incision is elevated as a subplatysmal flap to the level of the sternal notch and the cephalad edge to the level of the thyroid cartilage. Gelpe retractors are placed and the strap muscles are separated in the midline. The superior poles of the thymus gland are identified just deep to these muscles by their salmon-pink color and firmer texture than the surrounding investing tissue (Fig. 156B.2).

The left superior pole is typically more prominent and is dissected first. Dissection continues cranially to where the gland fuses with the thyrothymic ligament, which is ligated and divided. A 0 silk suture is placed on a sturdy portion of this superior pole and cut long to allow for retraction and manipulation of the gland during the remainder of the operation.

The medial border of the left superior pole is now followed caudally to the body of the gland and then back cephalad along the right superior pole, which is then similarly dissected, ligated, and divided at the level of its thyrothymic ligament. Once both superior poles have been mobilized and secured with 0 silk "handles," the dissection proceeds down toward and into the mediastinum.

The prethymic plane is opened up by gently dissecting with a finger into the substernal space. The cleido–cleido ligament is divided. The sternum is now lifted anteriorly using the Cooper thymectomy retractor (Pilling Company, Ft. Washington, PA), and the head and shoulders are allowed to fall back by deflating the shoulder bag (Fig. 156B.3A). This gives the surgeon, who from this point onward is seated at the head of the table, a direct view into the mediastinum with use of a headlight (Fig. 156B.3B). It is usually helpful to place army–navy retractors in the corners of the incision to improve exposure. These can be secured with Penrose drains clipped to the drapes at the most cephalad corners of the operating table.

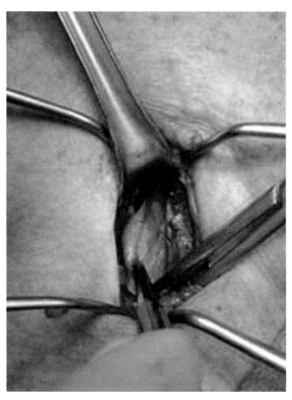

FIGURE 156B.2 The procedure is initiated by dissecting out the superior thymic poles, which are identified by their distinctive color and texture beneath the strap muscles (view is from the patient's head). (From Meyers BG, Cooper JD. Transcervical thymectomy for myasthenia gravis. Cardiothorac Surg Network (serial online) 2002. Available at: http://www.ctsnet.org/sections/clinicalresources/thoracic/expert_tech-23.html. Accessed August 20, 2007, with permission.)

Just before or after placement of the retractor, the veins draining the thymus gland into the innominate vein are ligated and divided. If the vein is located more cephalad than is typical, its branches can sometimes be divided before placement of the Cooper retractor. This is completed by retracting the gland cephalad and anteriorly (using the aforementioned ligatures attached to each of the upper poles) to place mild stretch on the branches. An image of this being performed

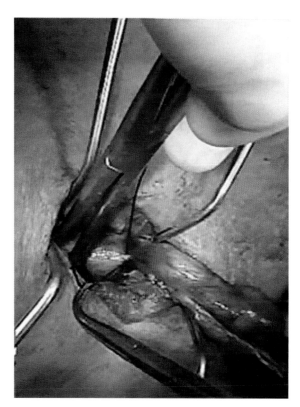

FIGURE 156B.4 A branch draining the gland into the innominate vein is ligated with silk ties and divided (in this case, before placement of the Cooper retractor).

before placement of the retractor is shown in Figure 156B.4. There are almost always two vein branches, but occasionally there is only one or there may be three. These are sequentially double ligated with 00 silk ties and divided. Clips should not be used on these venous branches, as this region is the avenue through which dissecting instruments are subsequently placed into the deeper mediastinum and clips can be easily dislodged, causing troublesome bleeding.

The dissection is carried progressively deeper into the mediastinum, largely by blunt dissection under direct vision (Fig. 156B.5). Small cherry-ball-sponges on the ends of two ring clamps are used, with one holding the innominate vein posteriorly while the other

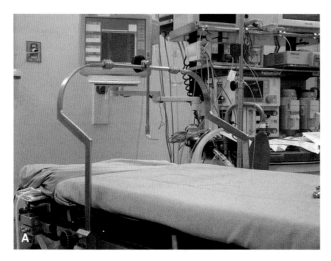
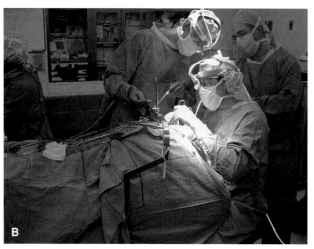

FIGURE 156B.3 **A:** The appearance of the operative field after the sternum is lifted anteriorly with the Cooper thymectomy retractor. **B:** The surgeon now sits at the head of the table and, using a headlight, develops a wide view into the mediastinum.

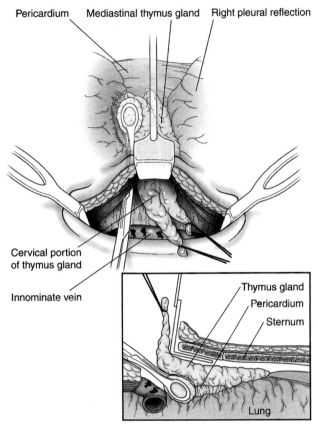

Pericardium   Mediastinal thymus gland   Right pleural reflection

Cervical portion
of thymus gland

Innominate vein

Thymus gland
Pericardium
Sternum

Lung

FIGURE 156B.5 The gland is mobilized off of the surrounding mediastinal structures primarily by blunt dissection, as pictured here from two views. (From Kaiser LR. Thymectomy. In: Kaiser LR, Jamieson GG, eds. *Operative Thoracic Surgery.* London: Edward Arnold; 2006:58, with permission.)

achieves the deeper dissection. At other times, one of the instruments will be used to push one tissue plane in one direction (e.g., the mediastinal pleura laterally), while the other will be used to push the adjacent gland in the opposite direction. The metal Yankauer sucker is also a useful device for blunt dissection in this area. Vascular attachments, such as the small branches of the internal mammary vessels, are easily cauterized or clipped and divided as encountered. Dense attachment to the pleural membrane or pericardium can also be easily managed with en bloc resection of portions of these when necessary.

In this way, the gland and surrounding mediastinal fat is separated gradually from the surrounding structures. First, it is dissected from the pericardium posteriorly, allowing the anterior attachments to the chest wall to hold the gland anteriorly and out of the way as this posterior dissection is achieved. It is critical to be sure one dives posteriorly behind the thymus directly onto the white of the pericardium immediately after passing beyond the innominate vein, to avoid entering the capsule of gland. After completing the posterior dissection as far caudally as possible, the thymus and surrounding fat are separated from the anterior and lateral chest wall, then from the pleurae bilaterally, and ultimately from the diaphragm. Retraction of the gland in the opposite direction of the site of dissection, using the two ligatures attached to the upper poles, is helpful in facilitating the deeper mediastinal dissection. Ventilation is held intermittently to facilitate the view and for the dissection off of the pleurae bilaterally. Although one attempts to keep the pleura intact, the breach in the pleura which frequently occurs allows a perfect view of the phrenic nerve to guide complete removal of the fat and pleura to the level of the nerve, and thus opening the pleura is sometimes required to assure that all fat is removed. Toward

the end of the dissection, it is sometimes helpful to gently grasp the gland, away from the thymoma if present, with an empty ring clamp while dissecting the final attachments with the other hand.

Although performance of the TCT operation using the sternum-lifting retractor and direct, unmagnified visualization, as initially described by Cooper, is adequate in the young, thin patients with excellent neck extendability and capacity to have their sternum lifted far anteriorly, in less ideal patients we found that the exposure could be difficult. This has been improved in our hands with the adoption of the University of Toronto approach,[13] introducing a 5-mm 30-degree videoscope through one or the other end of the neck incision, once I have completed the initial stages of blunt dissection deep to the innominate vein. The view provided by the video camera is superior to that which one can generally achieve directly through the neck incision with a headlight, and allows a more complete dissection of the extracapsular mediastinal fat in our experience.

An additional difference between this approach and the traditional Cooper approach involves whether or not the mediastinal pleura is resected. Classically, TCT has not included resection of the pleural membranes. The above approach has evolved to include resection of the pleura when there is more than a minimal amount of mediastinal fat that remains adherent to it after initial dissection. Therefore, after opening the pleura beneath the sternal edge anteriorly, one can use the 30-degree thoracoscope turned downward to clearly see the course of the phrenic nerve from the pleural side. This allows a safe, posterior incision of the pleura to be made just anterior to the nerve, and allows removal of the pleural membrane and all associated mediastinal fat anterior to the phrenic nerve, just as in the classic transsternal extended thymectomy operation.

The avoidance of paralyzing agents, other than short-acting non-depolarizing agents used in very small doses, allows one to know when the phrenic nerves are being approached during the dissection. This also facilitates early extubation in patients with generalized weakness. After en bloc removal of the H-shaped thymic specimen, including the upper and lower poles and surrounding mediastinal fat, careful inspection for residual suspicious tissue in the mediastinum is significantly improved with the above thoracoscopic visualization. Any such tissue is removed and if necessary it is sent for frozen section to ascertain whether it represents thymic tissue or simple fat. Of course, if there is any question of having been unable to perform a complete resection transcervically, there should be no hesitation to convert to partial or full sternotomy as necessary.

For closure, the strap muscle and platysma are closed with running absorbable sutures. A red rubber catheter can be placed, depending on whether or not the pleural cavity has been entered, to remove air and the tube withdrawn just prior to rendering the deepest layer airtight, as the anesthesiologists give a large positive-pressure breath.

Patients are almost always extubated in the operating room, and after a chest radiograph confirms lung expansion, nearly all can be discharged home on the afternoon of the surgery.

RESULTS

REMISSION RATES FOLLOWING TRANSCERVICAL THYMECTOMY

The published results following extended TCT suggest that there is no substantial difference in response rates using this technique versus the more invasive, and morbid, transsternal approaches. Our report of 151 patients undergoing TCT for MG[12] represents the largest experience with the operation and incorporates our previous report of the initial 50% of the patients in this series.[10] The mean age of patients was 42.5 years, and 60.3% were female. Mean preoperative Osserman class was 2.3; 21.2% class I, 39.1% class II, 27.6% class III, and 12.2% class IV. Duration of symptoms was >2 years in 31.4% of patients. At the time of operation, 75 patients were undergoing single-drug therapy (pyridostigmine), and 51 patients were undergoing two-drug or two-modality therapy (pyridostigmine and steroids or pyridostigmine and plasmapheresis). The remainder were receiving three- or four-drug therapy with or without plasmapheresis. On pathologic examination, the gland was normal in 38% of patients, showed follicular hyperplasia in 36%, thymoma in 8.3%, and other pathology in 11%. Mean postoperative follow-up was 53 months, and 97.4% of patients had complete follow-up.

Although we agree with the view that response rates following thymectomy are best reported as complete responses (CRs) and by Kaplan–Meier analysis, for the sake of comparison with previous studies we also reported our results in the form of crude cumulative response rates (Table 156B.2). We defined a "response" as a decrease of

TABLE 156B.2 Crude Cumulative Response Rates to Extended Transcervical Thymectomy

Category of Response	% of Patients
Complete remission	37.1
Asymptomatic, off all medication	28.8
Asymptomatic, on low-dose prednisone or azathioprine	8.3
Asymptomatic, on more than minimal medication	13.5
Improved but symptomatic	28.8
No improvement	19.2
Died in follow-up	1.3

Adapted from Shrager JB, Nathan D, Brinster CJ, et al. Outcomes After 151 Extended Transcervical Thymectomies for Myasthenia Gravis. *Ann Thorac Surg* 2006;82(5):1863–1869. Copyright © 2006 The Society of Thoracic Surgeons. With permission.

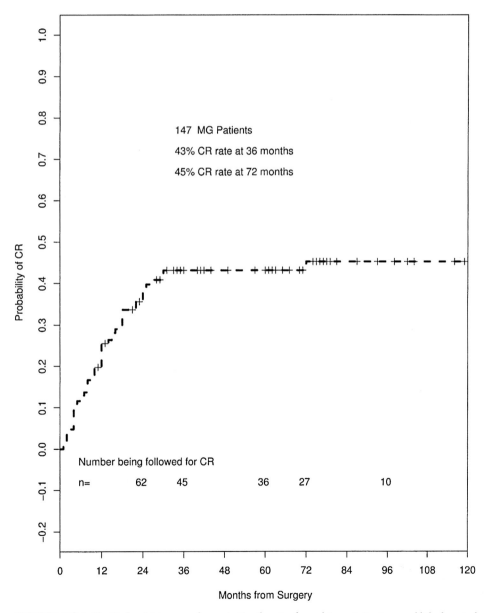

FIGURE 156B.6 The Kaplan–Meier curve demonstrating the rate of complete remission in our published surgical experience, with CR defined to include patients on low-dose, single-drug immunosuppression (see text).

at least one Osserman class with decreased or stable medication dosing or maintenance of the same Osserman class but with a decrease in number or dose of medications. By this definition, 80.8% of patients did respond favorably to thymectomy. Overall, the mean Osserman class fell from a mean of 2.3 preoperatively to 1.0 postoperatively.

Crude CR rate, defined as asymptomatic off medication for at least 6 months, was 28.8%. When we broaden the definition of CR to include patients who are asymptomatic but on low-dose (<10 mg prednisone or 150 mg azathioprine) single-drug immunosuppression, the rate rises to 37.1%. We suggest that this latter definition of CR is more appropriate given our neurologists' hesitancy to completely stop immunosuppressive agents, despite the absence of symptoms for as long as several years following thymectomy, due to reports in the literature of relapses occurring in this setting. Given the minimal morbidity of maintaining a patient on a single-drug regimen of 5 to 10 mg prednisone or 100 to 150 mg azathioprine daily, many neurologists will maintain patients on one of these drugs indefinitely following thymectomy even in the absence of symptoms. Since many patients remain in this category of "asymptomatic/single-low-dose immuno-suppressive agent" for prolonged periods while additional patients are added to this group after successful thymectomy, the proportion

of patients in the asymptomatic/low-dose immunosuppressive group will increase and a lower proportion will be in drug-free complete remission. If one considers only patients in drug-free CR as true "CRs," then as time of follow-up accrues, the "CR" rate will falsely appear to fall. Since we believe it is likely that the vast majority of the TCT patients in the asymptomatic/low-dose immunosuppression group would remain asymptomatic off those medications, we believe that they are appropriately included within the definition of a CR.

More important than the crude response rates reviewed above are the CR rates by Kaplan–Meier analysis following TCT. By Kaplan–Meier analysis, CR rates are 43% and 45% at 3 and 6 years, respectively, using our broader definition of a CR (Fig. 156B.6) and 33% and 35% at 3 and 6 years, respectively, excluding the asymptomatic/low-dose immunosuppression group (Fig. 156B.7). It is also important to note that no relapses have occurred after an initial CR.

Finally, in order to address the concern that CRs might not be sustained over the long-term after TCT due to a less complete resection of extracapsular tissue, we separately analyzed the initial 84 "extended TCT" patients in our cohort now with a longer duration of follow-up. These 84 patients, operated upon before September 1999 (and thus prior to the addition of the currently used videoscopic

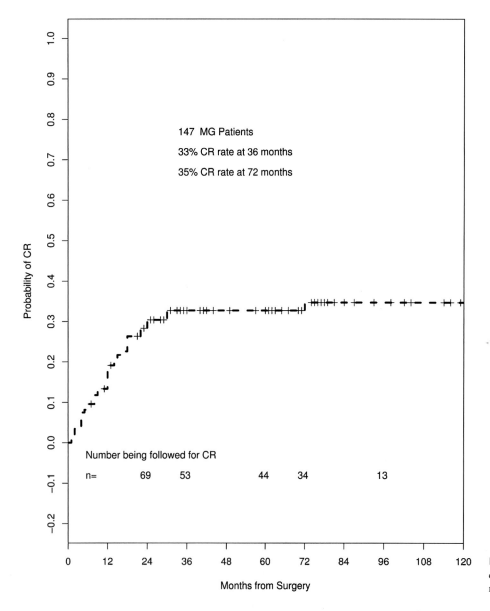

FIGURE 156B.7 The Kaplan–Meier curve demonstrating the rate of drug-free complete remission strictly defined.

assistance via the neck incision as described above) include the 78 patients in our initial report[10] plus 6 additional patients from that era that were less than 6 months out from their operation at the time of the initial analysis. At the time of re-evaluation, mean follow-up was now 82 months and the Kaplan–Meier CR rates were 44% and 46% at 3 and 6 years, respectively. If we use the more restrictive definition of CR, this earlier cohort still has a CR of 34%, 34%, and 36% at 3, 6, and 9 years, respectively. Thus, CR rates appear to be preserved over time and may even improve slowly.

OPERATIVE COMPLICATIONS

Seventy-three out of the last 74 TCTs were performed on an outpatient basis. The total complication rate was 7.3%, with 6.7% of these classified as minor—wound infections, seromas, atrial fibrillation, and pneumothorax. The only major complication was a single case of injury to a unilateral recurrent laryngeal nerve. Finally, although conversion should not be considered a complication, it should be noted that the conversion rate from planned TCT to more extended incision—virtually always a partial upper sternotomy—was 7.9%.

CONTROVERSY

There is no controversy over whether TCT is less morbid than thymectomy performed by MS or the "maximal transsternal and transcervical approach." An operation performed through the divided sternum typically requires a minimum stay of 3 days in the hospital, and is associated with a certain implicit rate of cardiopulmonary morbidity and a small but real risk of sternal osteomyelitis, as compared to TCT that can easily be performed on an outpatient basis and has a <1% major morbidity rate, as documented above. Similarly, although no

formal cost analysis has been performed, TCT is without doubt less costly to the health care system than thymectomy via MS.

Although it is perhaps not as obvious, we also believe that TCT is less morbid and costly than VATS or robotic approaches. The single cervical incision is virtually pain-free after 4 or 5 days and is less painful than the several intercostal incisions of VATS/robotic approaches. There is no cost for disposable instruments with TCT as there is with VATS and robotics, and we are not aware of any reports of same-day discharge following VATS or robotic thymectomy—which is our routine with TCT.

The controversy that remains is whether the CR rates after TCT and sternotomy are the same or at least equivalent (and as a corollary, whether results of thymectomy via VATS and RATS are also similar). If one could establish without a doubt that response rates following TCT are identical to those following thymectomy via sternotomy, then TCT should certainly be adopted as the preferred operation. All of the published studies reporting postoperative response rates, however, are retrospective and without control groups. Thus, we are left trying to compare results across studies that have enrolled patients with different preoperative factors, many of which have been shown to affect response rates. In addition, as discussed above, few studies report their results using Kaplan–Meier analysis.

Given these limitations, comparison of the results obtained with TCT versus those obtained following transsternal thymectomy and VATS or robotic thymectomy, the CR rates are very similar. Table 156B.3 shows selected results of some of the larger studies of thymectomy published within the last 25 years that used reasonable data reporting and analysis. This table gives a sense of the CR rate ranges reported in the literature.[5,8,9,11,12,16–28] In summary, it can be stated that crude CR rates range from 19% to 58% following sternotomy and 35% to 44% following TCT. Clearly these ranges are overlapping. Kaplan–Meier CR rates, which have been rarely reported (see the last column in Table 156B.3), also appear similar

TABLE 156B.3 Published Results of Five Approaches to Thymectomy for MG[a]

	Authors [Ref]	Crude Complete Remission Rate (%)	Mean Follow-up (yr)	Kaplan–Meier 5-Year Remission Rate (%)
Maximal Transcervical/Transsternal	Ashour et al.[16]	35	1.7	N/A
	Jaretski et al.[5]	46	3.4	50
	Budde et al.[17]	21	4.3	N/A
	Busch et al.[18]	19	7.7	N/A
	Klein et al.[21]	40	5.0	N/A
Transsternal	Masaoka et al.[22]	40/45	5.0/20.0	N/A
	Mulder et al.[23]	36	3.6	N/A
	Stern et al.[24]	50	6.8	N/A
	Huang et al.[20]	58	8.5	N/A
	Durelli et al.[19]	N/A	5	30
Extended Transcervical[b]	Bril et al.[9]	44	8.4	N/A
	Calhoun et al.[11]	35	5.0	N/A
	Shrager et al.[12]	27 (37)	4.2	33 (43)
VATS	dePerrot et al.[8]	41	4.1	30
	Keating et al.[25]	N/A	2.7	28
	Tomulescu et al.[26]	N/A	3.0	41
	Yu et al.[27]	N/A	N/A	42
Robotic	Ruckert et al.[28]	N/A	3.5	39

[a]Includes only studies in the past 20 years in the English language literature, representing a pure series of one type of procedure, in adults, with at least 48 patients, that report complete remission rates and duration of follow-up.
[b]Includes only studies representing pure series of extended TCT using the Cooper Thymectomy Retractor. N/A, data not provided.
Numbers in parenthesis include asymptomatic patients on single-drug, low-dose immunosuppression as CRs. Some 5-year CR rates are estimated from line graphs in the publications.
Numbers in parentheses indicate remission rates using the broader definition of complete remission that allows single, low-dose immunosuppression to be ongoing.

among TCT, VATS/robotic, and sternotomy approaches. It is worth noting that Kaplan–Meier estimates for CR at extended time points (not shown in table) are even higher (91% at 10 years) following TCT with video assistance[8] than following "maximal" thymectomy (81% at 7.5 years).[5,6]

We recognize that patients in the TCT studies have generally had a lower preoperative severity of disease and that they have also tended to be operated upon somewhat earlier in the course of their disease; but this is, in fact, one of the advantages of TCT: that patients and neurologists are likely to accept surgical intervention more readily, thus bring people to thymectomy earlier, when morbidity of the operation is low. To discount results that may have been obtained in part because of this advantage would be, we believe, inappropriate.

Only with a randomized, prospective study comparing TCT to sternotomy and VATS/RATS, or at minimum a carefully designed prospective registry, will this controversy be resolved. A prospective registry study is far more likely to be successful given that the lack of equipoise that many surgeons have on this issue would likely prevent accrual to a randomized study. Such a study is an important next step, now that we have evidence from a randomized trial that extended thymectomy by MS does indeed improve the course of MG over what can be achieved by medical therapy alone.[13]

As Jaretzki et al.[29] has written, the optimal surgical technique for thymectomy in MG will be the one that "balances extent of resection, morbidity, patient acceptance, and results." When intention to perform a complete removal of the thymus and associated fat is maintained, we have no doubt that TCT is a highly appropriate operative approach for thymectomy in nonthymomatous MG. We also believe that, although the data are admittedly inconclusive, CR rates with extended TCT have been demonstrated to be sufficiently similar to those following extended transsternal thymectomy, as well as VATS and robotic approaches, to allow one to argue cogently that if there are indeed small difference in CR rates, these are likely outweighed by the larger differences in morbidity between the approaches.

REFERENCES

1. Schumacher ED, Roth O. Thymektomie bei einem Fall von Morbus Basedowi mit Myasthenie. *Mitteil Grenzgebiet Med Chirurg* 1912;25:746.
2. Blalock A. Thymectomy in the treatment of myasthenia gravis: report of 20 cases. *J Thorac Surg* 1944;13:316–339.
3. Blalock A, Harvey A, Ford F. The treatment of myasthenia gravis by removal of the thymus gland. *JAMA* 1941;17:1529–1533.
4. Papatestas AE, Genkins G, Kornfeld P, et al. Effects of thymectomy in myasthenia gravis. *Ann Surg* 1987;206(1):79–88.
5. Jaretzki A, Penn AS, Younger DS, et al. "Maximal" thymectomy for myasthenia gravis. Results. *J Thorac Cardiovasc Surg* 1988;95(5):747–757.
6. Jaretzki A, Wolff M. "Maximal" thymectomy for myasthenia gravis. Surgical anatomy and operative technique. *J Thorac Cardiovasc Surg* 1988;96(5):711–716.
7. Cooper JD, Al-Jilaihawa AN, Pearson FG, et al. An improved technique to facilitate transcervical thymectomy for myasthenia gravis. *Ann Thorac Surg* 1988;45:242–247.
8. De Perrot M, Bril V, McRae K, et al. Impact of minimally invasive transcervical thymectomy on outcome in patients with myasthenia gravis. *Eur J Cardiothorac Surg* 2003;24:677–683.
9. Bril V, Kojic J, Ilse WK, et al. Long-term clinical outcome after transcervical thymectomy for myasthenia gravis. *Ann Thorac Surg* 1998;65:1520–1522.
10. Shrager JB, Deeb ME, Mich R, et al. Transcervical thymectomy for myasthenia gravis achieves results comparable to thymectomy by sternotomy. *Ann Thorac Surg* 2002;74:320–327.
11. Calhoun RF, Ritter JH, Guthrie TJ, et al. Results of transcervical thymectomy for myasthenia gravis in 100 consecutive patients. *Ann Surg* 1999;230:555.
12. Shrager JB, Nathan D, Brinster CJ, et al. Outcomes after 151 extended transcervical thymectomies for myasthenia gravis. *Ann Thorac Surg* 2006;82(5):1863–1869.
13. Wolfe GI, Kaminski HJ, Aban IB, et al. Randomized trial of thymectomy in myasthenia gravis. *New Engl J Med* 2016; 375(6):511–522.
14. Nagayasu T, Yamayoshi T, Matsumoto K, et al. Beneficial effects of plasmapheresis before thymectomy on the outcome in myasthenia gravis. *Jpn J Thorac Cardiovasc Surg* 2005;53:2–7.
15. Watanabe A, Watanabe T, Obama T, et al. Prognostic factors for myasthenic crisis after transsternal thymectomy in patients with myasthenia gravis. *J Cardiothorac Surg* 2004;127:868–876.
16. Ashour MH, Jain SK, Kattan KM, et al. Maximal thymectomy for myasthenia gravis. *Eur J Cardiothorac Surg* 1995;9:461–464.
17. Budde JM, Morris CD, Gal AA, et al. Predictors of outcome in thymectomy for myasthenia gravis. *Ann Thorac Surg* 2001;72:197–202.
18. Busch C, Machens A, Pichlmeier U, et al. Long-term outcome and quality of life after thymectomy for myasthenia gravis. *Ann Surg* 1996;224:225.
19. Durelli L, Maggi G, Casadio C, et al. Actuarial analysis of the occurrence of remissions following thymectomy for myasthenia gravis in 400 patients. *J Neurol Neurosurg Psychiatry* 1991;54:406–411.
20. Huang CS, Hsu HS, Huang BS, et al. Factors influencing the outcome of transsternal thymectomy for myasthenia gravis. *Acta Neurol Scand* 2005;112:108–114.
21. Klein M, Heidenreich F, Madjlessi F, et al. Early and late results after thymectomy in myasthenia gravis: a restrospective study. *J Thorac Cardiovasc Surg* 1999;47:170–173.
22. Masaoka A, Yamakawa Y, Niwa H, et al. Extended thymectomy for myasthenia gravis patients: a 20-year review. *Ann Thorac Surg* 1996;62:853–859.
23. Mulder DG, Graves M, Hermann C. Thymectomy for myasthenia gravis: recent observations and comparison with past experience. *Ann Thorac Surg* 1989;48:551–555.
24. Stern LE, Nussbaum MS, Quinlan JG, et al. Long-term evaluation of extended thymectomy with anterior mediastinal dissection for myasthenia gravis. *Surgery* 2001;130:774–780.
25. Keating CP, Kong YX, Tay V, et al. VATS thymectomy for nonthymomatous myasthenia gravis: standardized outcome assessment using the myasthenia gravis foundation of America clinical classification. *Innovations (Phila)* 2011;6:104–109.
26. Tomulescu V, Ion V, Kosa A, et al. Thoracoscopic thymectomy mid-term results. *Ann Thorac Surg* 2006;82:1003–1007.
27. Yu L, Zhang XJ, Ma S, et al. Thoracoscopic thymectomy for myasthenia gravis with and without thymoma: a single-center experience. *Ann Thorac Surg* 2012;93:240–244.
28. Ruckert JC, Swierzy M, Ismail M. Comparison of robotic and nonrobotic thoracoscopic thymectomy: a cohort study. *J Thorac Cardiovasc Surg* 2011;141:673–677.
29. Jaretzki A, Steinglass KM, Sonnett JR. Thymectomy in the management of myasthenia gravis. *Semin Neurol* 2004;24:49–62.

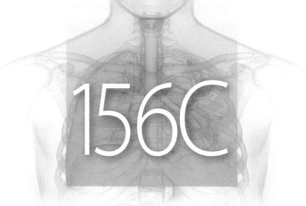

156C

Operative Techniques of VATS and Robotic VATS Thymectomy

Jonathan D'Cunha ▪ Nicholas R. Hess ▪ Inderpal S. Sarkaria

INTRODUCTION

Common indications for thymectomy consist of myasthenia gravis, thymoma, and other anterior mediastinal tumors.[1-6] While thymectomy is an accepted integral component of treatment for early stage thymoma, its utility in the treatment of myasthenia gravis has long been debated only recently proven with randomized prospective data.[7,8] Since the origins of this procedure, median sternotomy has been the universally standard approach.[9] However, more recently, a gradual transition to minimally invasive techniques has become evident within the surgical community. Our experience with video-assisted thoracoscopic (VATS) thymectomy began in the late 1990s, and has evolved from our larger VATS experience with a wide array of other thoracic procedures. Although there are a number of approaches (the classic transsternal approach, transcervical approach, subxiphoid approach, and the combined transcervical–transsternal maximum thymectomy), we are almost exclusively performing this operation minimally invasively.

Of these minimally invasive approaches, VATS and robotic-assisted VATS techniques have shown much promise. In select patients, these approaches aim to minimize perioperative morbidity and recovery time while offering long-term benefits afforded from a complete thymic resection.

Following the dissemination of VATS and robotic VATS technologies, many centers have developed and refined their own techniques, utilizing various means of access to the anterior mediastinum. Such techniques include but are not limited to, right-sided, left-sided, bilateral, transcervical, and subxiphoid approaches.[10-15] In our center, we have adopted two approaches: a predominantly right-sided thoracoscopic, and a left-sided robotic-assisted approach. Both methods, however, utilize simultaneous bilateral thoracoscopy in order to identify critical anatomy and maximize thymic resection. In this chapter we will highlight key features of our approaches to robotic and nonrobotic VATS thymectomy: patient selection, operative setup, and operative technique. The reader should not focus much on right-sided versus left-sided as the setup for the approach will likely be patient- and surgeon-dependent. The purpose of presenting both approaches is to describe and illustrate the nuances related to each. We will also provide a summary of the current literature comparing minimally invasive versus open approaches, as well as nonrobotic VATS versus robotic VATS.

PREOPERATIVE PREPARATION AND PATIENT SELECTION

In the setting of myasthenia gravis, we select patients with medicine-refractory disease that are otherwise felt to benefit from thymectomy. Age is not a critical predictor of surgical candidacy, but rather the patient's fitness and ability to tolerate surgery. Relative contraindications for a minimally invasive VATS approach include known or likely dense pleural adhesive disease from prior surgery, pleural intervention, and/or pathology. Additionally, VATS is contraindicated in patients with poor pulmonary functional status and inability to tolerate single-lung ventilation. Prior to surgery, we ensure that patients with myasthenia gravis obtain maximal medical "optimization" and control of their disease in order to minimize the risk of complications such as prolonged intubation and myasthenia crises.

For patients with thymoma and/or other thymic lesions, our contraindications to a minimally invasive approach include known or likely significant adhesive disease and an inability to tolerate surgery or single-lung ventilation. Several centers have reported an upper limit of thymoma size of 5,[16-19] 6,[20] or 8 cm[15] to be resected via VATS approach. However, we have successfully resected thymoma as large as 11 cm without complication and with microscopically negative margins and do not consider thymoma size an absolute contraindication to VATS or robotic VATS thymectomy. These cases should be evaluated individually and decisions made based on the clinical, radiographic, and intraoperative findings.

VATS THYMECTOMY (NONROBOTIC)

OPERATIVE SETUP

We typically utilize a right-sided approach with contralateral thoracoscopy, as previously described.[21] After induction with general anesthesia, a double-lumen endotracheal tube is placed and its location is verified via bronchoscopy. Subsequently, the patient is placed in a partial left lateral decubitus position with a bump underneath the right side. The patient's left arm is outstretched, and the right is secured to a sling (Fig. 156C.1). The patient is then prepped and draped in a normal sterile fashion. Exposure of the left chest is

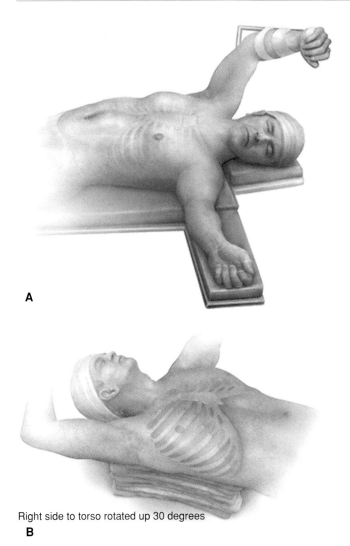

A

Right side to torso rotated up 30 degrees

B

FIGURE 156C.1 Patient positioning. The patient is placed in a semi left lateral decubitus position. A bump is placed under the patient's right side to create a 30-degree angle between the right side and operating table. **A:** View from patient's left side. **B:** View from patient's right side. (Reprinted from D'Cunha J, Andrade RS, Maddaus MA. Thoracoscopic thymectomy. *Operative Techniques in Thoracic and Cardiovascular Surgery* 2010;15(2):102–113. Copyright © 2010 Elsevier. With permission.)

maintained, particularly the inframammary crease where a contralateral thoracoscopic port will later be placed if necessary.

OPERATIVE TECHNIQUE

After the patient has been prepped and draped, the right lung is collapsed and left lung ventilation is initiated. Three 10-mm ports are placed into the right chest, two in the 6th intercostal space and one in the 7th (Fig. 156C.2). A 30-degree thoracoscope is then inserted into the chest, visualizing the entire right hemithorax and identifying the right phrenic nerve. The right chest is insufflated with 5- to 10-mm Hg CO_2 to facilitate right lung collapse and adequate visualization. Dissection begins just anterior to the phrenic nerve, incising the mediastinal pleura with hook electrocautery (Fig. 156C.3). The thymus and pericardial fat are carefully mobilized from the right phrenic nerve. Much care is taken to prevent thermal or stretch injury to the nerve. The pleural incision is extended along the length of the nerve toward the diaphragm, and all thymic

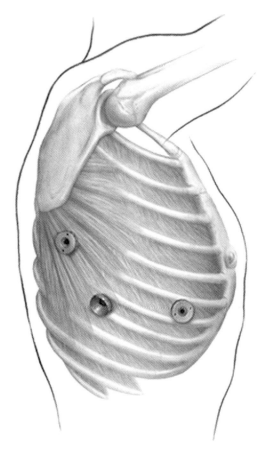

FIGURE 156C.2 Port placement in the right hemithorax. Two ports are placed in the 6th intercostal space and one in the 7th space. (Reprinted from D'Cunha J, Andrade RS, Maddaus MA. Thoracoscopic thymectomy. *Operative Techniques in Thoracic and Cardiovascular Surgery* 2010;15(2):102–113. Copyright © 2010 Elsevier. With permission.)

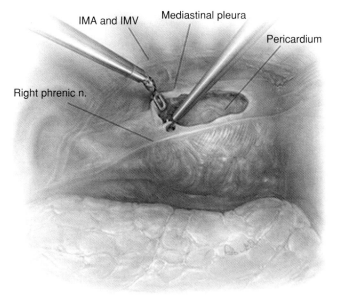

FIGURE 156C.3 Initiation of thymus mobilization. The mediastinal pleura is incised anterior to the right phrenic nerve with hook electrocautery. IMA, internal mammary artery; IMV, internal mammary vein; n., nerve. (Reprinted from D'Cunha J, Andrade RS, Maddaus MA. Thoracoscopic thymectomy. *Operative Techniques in Thoracic and Cardiovascular Surgery* 2010;15(2):102–113. Copyright © 2010 Elsevier. With permission.)

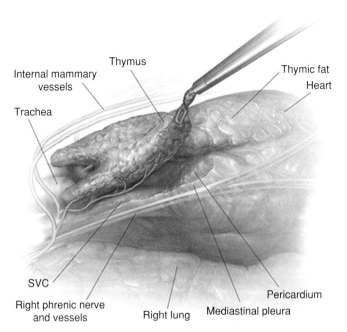

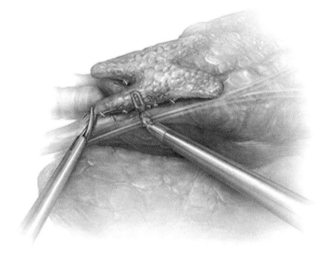

FIGURE 156C.4 Thymus mobilization. The thymus, pericardial fat, and associated soft tissues are dissected en bloc from the pericardium. Dissection begins at the right inferior pole of the thymus at the level of the diaphragm and continues superiorly. SVC, superior vena cava. (Reprinted from D'Cunha J, Andrade RS, Maddaus MA. Thoracoscopic thymectomy. *Operative Techniques in Thoracic and Cardiovascular Surgery* 2010;15(2):102–113. Copyright © 2010 Elsevier. With permission.)

FIGURE 156C.5 Division of the thymic superior horns. Both superior horns are gently retracted downward with use of countertraction for optimal exposure. CO_2 insufflation also facilitates exposure, and both horns are divided under direct visualization. (Reprinted from D'Cunha J, Andrade RS, Maddaus MA. Thoracoscopic thymectomy. *Operative Techniques in Thoracic and Cardiovascular Surgery* 2010;15(2):102–113. Copyright © 2010 Elsevier. With permission.)

tissue and pericardial fat are swept from the pericardium, starting near the diaphragm (Fig. 156C.4). Dissection is achieved via combination of blunt and sharp dissection. Additionally, the thymus is mobilized superiorly by incising the mediastinal pleura along the medial border of the internal mammary vessels. This dissection is carried superiorly, freeing all soft tissue from the retrosternum, and eventually the thymus from the innominate vein. Gentle traction of the thymus is initiated, which facilitates the identification of all vein branches draining into the innominate vein. All thymic veins and attachments are controlled with endoclips along the innominate vein.

Once all thymic veins and attachments are harvested, the superior poles can be identified with gentle downward traction of the gland (Fig. 156C.5). Using careful countertraction, the cephalad attachments of the superior poles can be freed under direct visualization. All arterial communications with the internal mammary arteries in this region are clipped and ligated. Following mobilization of the superior poles, medial dissection can continue toward the left chest, sweeping all thymic tissue and fat from the pericardium.

For dissection of the left thymus, a 5-mm port is inserted into the left chest along the inframammary fold, if necessary (Fig. 156C.6). Prior to this, right lung ventilation is re-initiated and maintained throughout this portion of the operation. A 30-degree thoracoscope is inserted into the left chest and is controlled by the surgical assistant. Output from this scope is displayed separate from the primary surgeon's scope, allowing simultaneous bilateral mediastinal visualization. The surgical assistant maintains view of the left phrenic nerve and mammary vessels throughout the left thymic dissection. The dissection is carried to the level of the left phrenic, ensuring complete en bloc, phrenic-to-phrenic resection of all thymic tissue and anterior mediastinal fat. The completely mobilized specimen can then be removed through one of the 10-mm port sites using an endoscopic bag.

Following specimen removal, the anterior mediastinum is inspected, ensuring complete removal of all thymus, fat, and soft tissue (Fig. 156C.7). Hemostasis is confirmed, and a 24-French Blake is placed through an existing port incision and passed trans-mediastinally under direct visualization. Adequate lung expansion is directly visualized, and all port sites are sequentially closed in layers with absorbable sutures and skin glue.

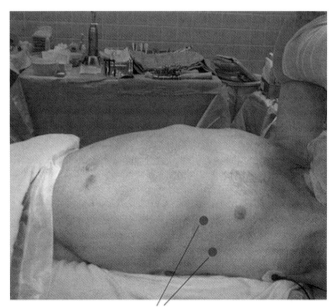

Additional sites for left-side ports

FIGURE 156C.6 Placement of contralateral port(s). The left hemithorax is exposed, prepped, and draped at the beginning of the procedure. An additional port and camera may be placed in the left chest for direct visualization of the left phrenic nerve, which may facilitate en bloc resection of all thymic and anterior mediastinal soft tissues and avoid nerve injury. (Reprinted from D'Cunha J, Andrade RS, Maddaus MA. Thoracoscopic thymectomy. *Operative Techniques in Thoracic and Cardiovascular Surgery* 2010;15(2):102–113. Copyright © 2010 Elsevier. With permission.)

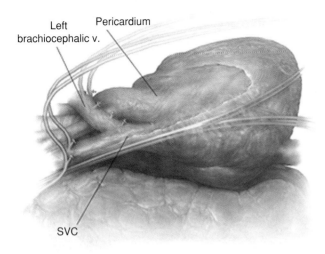

FIGURE 156C.7 Final view of anterior mediastinum. The SVC and left brachiocephalic vein are skeletonized, and all thymic and soft tissues are resected en bloc from the pericardium and retrosternum. SVC, superior vena cava; v., vein. (Reprinted from D'Cunha J, Andrade RS, Maddaus MA. Thoracoscopic thymectomy. *Operative Techniques in Thoracic and Cardiovascular Surgery* 2010;15(2):102–113. Copyright © 2010 Elsevier. With permission.)

ROBOTIC-ASSISTED VATS THYMECTOMY

Video 156C.1.

OPERATIVE SETUP

The patient is placed in supine position and induced under general anesthesia with a dual lumen endotracheal tube. In the setting of myasthenia gravis, use of depolarizing anesthetic agents is limited. Once correct placement of the endotracheal tube is confirmed with flexible bronchoscopy, the patient is placed on his/her side. We favor a semi right lateral decubitus position for most thymic lesions and particularly for patients with nonthymomatous myasthenia gravis, but may choose a right-sided approach depending on laterality of the pathology. The patient's left chest and hip are elevated, and the position is secured with a desufflated beanbag with proper padding of pressure points. The right arm is outstretched, and the left arm is secured at the patient's side. The robotic platform can be docked from either side of the patient depending on surgical approach and/ or operating room layout. Typically, the robotic system is advanced over the contralateral shoulder toward the camera port.

OPERATIVE TECHNIQUE

Once the patient has been positioned, prepped, and draped, the left lung is collapsed and single right lung ventilation is initiated. A Veress needle is inserted into the chest and intrathoracic placement is confirmed with a saline column drop test. The left chest is then insufflated with CO_2 to expedite and augment lung collapse and depression of the diaphragm and ventricle from the chest wall and sternum. This is typically well tolerated at a pressure of 8 mm Hg on high flow. An 8-mm camera port is then inserted into the 5th intercostal space within the inframammary fold at the anterior to mid-axillary line. Three additional trocars are placed under direct visualization (Fig. 156C.8). An 8-mm port is placed in the 3rd intercostal space on the anterior axillary line. The next 8-mm port is placed in the

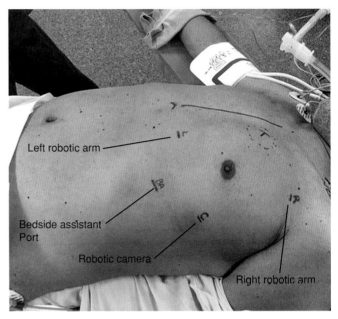

FIGURE 156C.8 Patient positioning and initial port placement. (From D'Cunha J, Andrade RS, Maddaus MA. Thoracoscopic thymectomy. *Operative Techniques in Thoracic and Cardiovascular Surgery* 2010;15(2):102–113. With permission.)

5th intercostal space, just lateral to the sternum (left robotic working arm). Lastly, a 12-mm assistant port is placed caudally in the mid-axillary line, typically in the 7th intercostal space for suctioning. The robotic console is then brought in proximity to the bedside with the central column positioned over the patient's contralateral shoulder. Appropriate instrumentation is then inserted though the trocars under direct visualization and docked to the robot; we utilize ultrasonic shears as our preferred energy source in the right working robotic arm port, and a bipolar grasper in the left robotic arm port.

Once all instrumentation is docked to the robotic console, direct visualization of the left phrenic nerve is obtained. En bloc resection is initiated through incision of the mediastinal pleura, just medial to the left phrenic nerve (Fig. 156C.9). Careful mobilization of the

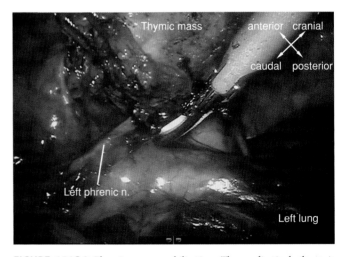

FIGURE 156C.9 Phrenic nerve mobilization. The mediastinal pleura is incised anterior to the left phrenic nerve. The mass is carefully dissected from the nerve, using caution to prevent stretch or thermal injury to the nerve or perineural vessels. n., nerve. (From D'Cunha J, Andrade RS, Maddaus MA. Thoracoscopic thymectomy. *Operative Techniques in Thoracic and Cardiovascular Surgery* 2010;15(2):102–113. With permission.)

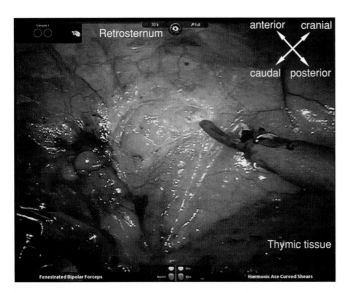

FIGURE 156C.10 Retrosternal dissection. A second dissection plane is initiated by incising the mediastinal pleura medial to the internal mammary artery and vein. The thymus and associated soft tissues are dissected en bloc from the retrosternum. (From D'Cunha J, Andrade RS, Maddaus MA. Thoracoscopic thymectomy. *Operative Techniques in Thoracic and Cardiovascular Surgery* 2010;15(2):102–113. With permission.)

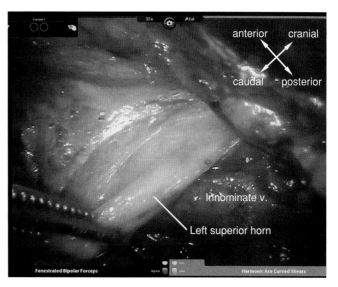

FIGURE 156C.11 Superior horn division. The superior horns are gently retracted caudally and exposed using countertraction. Once retracted and visualized, the superior horns are divided with the ultrasonic shears. v., vein. (From D'Cunha J, Andrade RS, Maddaus MA. Thoracoscopic thymectomy. *Operative Techniques in Thoracic and Cardiovascular Surgery* 2010;15(2):102–113. With permission.)

phrenic nerve is performed, preserving the nerve if adequate oncologic margins are feasible. Pleural incision is carried along the length of the nerve, taking care to prevent stretch injury to the nerve or damage to the adjacent perineural vessels. Dissection is continued medially, using a combination of sharp and blunt dissection. All pericardial fat and thymic tissue are swept from the pericardium both medially and cephalad toward the innominate vein. Superiorly, the pleural incision is continued anteriorly at the juxtaposition of the internal mammary artery and phrenic nerve. This dissection is carried caudally toward the diaphragm, staying medial to the internal mammary vessels (Fig. 156C.10). All tissue is then excised from the retrosternum with blunt and sharp dissection to the level of the innominate vein superiorly, and medial to the contralateral internal mammary vessels (these may be better visualized after incision of the contralateral pleura, as per below). Superiorly and cephalad, the left and right thymic horns are identified, fully mobilized, and resected en bloc with the specimen (Fig. 156C.11).

Following division of the thymic horns, dissection is carried toward the right pleura. At this point in the operation, risk of injury to the contralateral phrenic nerves and/or mammary vessels can be high if adequate visualization is not obtained. We have found that identification of the contralateral nerve and/or internal mammary vessels can be difficult in certain cases, and have therefore identified two strategies to facilitate this. One method is through utilization of simultaneous bilateral visualization of the mediastinum. In this method, we insert a 5-mm thoracoscopic port into the contralateral chest at the level of the inframammary crease. Thoracoscopic video output from this port, controlled by the bedside assistant/surgeon, can be directly linked to existing robotic platforms, allowing bilateral and simultaneous mediastinal visualization while sitting at the robotic console. The bedside assistant maintains visualization of vital contralateral structures as the primary surgeon operates from the left side (Fig. 156C.12).

Additionally, we have also employed a technique of phrenic nerve visualization described by Wagner et al. through use of near infrared fluorescence imaging.[22] This technology, commercially available in robotic and nonrobotic platforms, utilizes the laser-induced fluorescence of indocyanine green (ICG) imaging contrast to highlight the phrenic nerves and other key vascular structures. ICG solution, 5 to 10 mg, is given intraoperatively and intravenously, and can be visualized within seconds. The laser-induced fluorescence of ICG is then superimposed onto the surgeon's video display, allowing easy

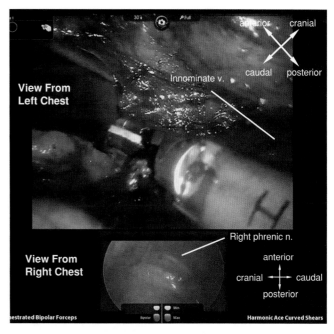

FIGURE 156C.12 Simultaneous bilateral mediastinal visualization. An additional 5-mm camera port is inserted into the right chest at the inframammary fold. The bedside assistant maintains direct visualization of the right phrenic nerve as full en bloc resection of all anterior mediastinal soft tissue is performed from the left side. v., vein; n., nerve. (From D'Cunha J, Andrade RS, Maddaus MA. Thoracoscopic thymectomy. *Operative Techniques in Thoracic and Cardiovascular Surgery* 2010;15(2):102–113. With permission.)

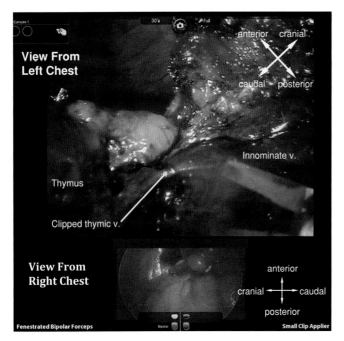

FIGURE 156C.13 Clipping and division of a thymic vein. The innominate vein is skeletonized, and all thymic veins and attachments are ligated. Larger vessels (pictured) are clipped prior to ligation. v., vein. (From D'Cunha J, Andrade RS, Maddaus MA. Thoracoscopic thymectomy. *Operative Techniques in Thoracic and Cardiovascular Surgery* 2010;15(2):102–113. With permission.)

differentiation of phrenic nerves and adjacent pericardiophrenic vessels from surrounding tissues.

Once adequate visualization of the contralateral phrenic nerve and mammary vessels is obtained, the right pleura is incised from the left side. The bedside assistant follows the primary surgeon with the contralateral thoracoscope, ensuring full dissection of thymic tissue is accomplished between both nerves, while preventing injury. Thymic veins are identified and ligated with care to avoid undue traction from the tumor during dissection. Smaller vessels can typically be ligated with the ultrasonic shears, but we prefer to clip larger vessels with a standard handheld or robotic clip applier (Fig. 156C.13). The full en bloc specimen is removed via a 15-mm endoscopic specimen bag.

Areas of minor bleeding are controlled with electrocautery, bipolar, or clips. We then perform a multilevel intercostal nerve block with 0.25% Marcaine solution for postoperative analgesia. A 28-French chest tube or 24-French Blake drain is inserted into the left chest under direct visualization and passed across the mediastinum. The chest tube is secured with sutures and all port sites are closed.

ALTERNATIVE APPROACHES

Numerous permutations of thymectomy techniques have been described, utilizing various combinations of surgical platform, laterality of approach, and/or patient positioning. Here we will provide a brief summary of existing approaches to VATS thymectomy.

Chen et al. described a series of right-sided VATS thymectomy in 54 patients with nonthymomatous myasthenia gravis.[23] This technique employs a three-port unilateral approach, utilizing hook cautery on the proximal right side for dissection, and then progressing to blunt dissection of the contralateral left side to avoid phrenic nerve injury. Unlike our proposed technique, the authors did not employ contralateral thoracoscopy. Jurado and colleagues utilize a bilateral

VATS approach to maximize completeness of resection, starting with 3-trochar dissection of the left anterior mediastinum, repositioning, and then finishing with 3-trochar dissection of the right side.[15] Caronia and colleagues described a similar bilateral method, but with the arm on the operative side maintained parallel to the patients' body.[24] According to the authors, this arm positioning facilitates the changing of instrument triangulation, providing better visualization and access to the cardiophrenic regions. Nakagiri et al. has also described their experience with bilateral VATS-extended thymectomy (VATS-ET), originally including a cervical incision to facilitate dissection of the superior thymic poles.[25] As their experience evolved, they were able to maintain quality of resection without performing a neck incision, improving cosmetic outcomes. Lastly, Ampollini et al. described a method of VATS thymectomy through a single 3-cm cervical incision.[26]

Several variations of robotic-assisted VATS thymectomy have also been described. Keijzers et al. reported an 8-year series of robotic-assisted VATS thymectomy for thymoma utilizing a right-sided approach.[27] Thymomas were resected using a "no touch" technique, and contralateral phrenic nerve visualization was improved by means of temporary hyperinflation of the contralateral lung. Rueckert and colleagues have reported one of the largest series of robotic-assisted VATS thymectomy.[28] They reported a preference of left-sided approach, stating this allows easier phrenic nerve dissection in cases of complex thymic encasement of the nerve, a phenomenon that occurs much more frequently on the left side. Suda et al. reported a unique approach of trans-subxiphoid robotic thymectomy.[29] In this small series of three patients in supine position, a 12-mm camera port was placed under the xiphoid process, and robotic arm ports were placed in the bilateral 6th intercostal spaces. As reported by the authors, this technique maximizes visualization of the neck region and also permits bilateral phrenic nerve visualization.

RESULTS

OUTCOMES OF VATS VERSUS OPEN THYMECTOMY

Previously we have conducted a systematic review of the literature comparing open to minimally invasive thymectomy, both nonrobotic and robotic VATS.[30] This review included a total of 20 comparative studies encompassing 2,068 patients receiving either open [1,230 (59.5%)] or minimally invasive [838 (40.5%)] thymectomy.[15–20,23,31–43] There was considerable variation with respect to patient age, sex, and indication for thymectomy across studies, but all studies were individually well matched between comparison groups. Across studies, there was a consistent trend of significantly lower mean estimated blood loss (VATS 20 to 200 mL; open 86 to 466 mL), pleural drainage duration (VATS 1.3 to 4.1 days; open 2.4 to 5.3 days), and hospital length of stay (VATS 1.0 to 10.6 days; open 4.0 to 14.6 days) in patients treated with minimally invasive thymectomy. There were no consistent differences in operative time, rate of R0 resection of malignancy, or perioperative complications. Long-term outcomes of myasthenia gravis remission and thymoma recurrence were similar in open and minimally invasive groups, although follow-up time was limited across studies.

Friedant et al. performed a systematic review and meta-analysis of minimally invasive versus open thymectomy for malignancy.[44] They too reported a lower estimated blood loss during minimally invasive thymectomy with a standardized mean difference of –0.78 (95% CI: –1.05, –0.51). Length of hospital stay was also shorter for minimally invasive groups (standardized mean difference −0.88; 95% CI: −1.52, −0.24). There were no significant differences in operative time, rates of R0 resection, complications, or locoregional cancer recurrence.

OUTCOMES OF ROBOTIC VERSUS NONROBOTIC VATS THYMECTOMY

Few studies have directly compared outcomes for robotic and non-robotic VATS thymectomy. Ye et al. reported a series of 25 unilateral VATS procedures compared to 21 unilateral robotic VATS procedures for Masaoka stage I thymoma. There were no significant differences in operating time or estimated blood loss, but a shorter pleural drainage time (1.1 days vs. 3.6 days; P <0.01) and hospital length of stay (3.7 vs. 6.7; P <0.01) in the robotic VATS group. There were no significant differences in conversions to open surgery (VATS, 1; robotic VATS, 0) or postoperative complications (VATS, 1; robotic VATS, 1). Robotic VATS incurred a significantly higher mean hospitalization cost ($8,662 vs. $6,097; P <0.01).[45]

Ruckert et al. conducted a cohort study of 79 VATS versus 74 robotic VATS thymectomies for myasthenia gravis. Both groups were well matched with respect to age, sex, and disease severity, and there were similar operating times (198 ± 48 vs. 187 ± 48 minutes), rates of open conversion [1(1.3%) vs. 1(1.4%)], and postoperative morbidity [2(2.5%) vs. 2(2.7%)] in the VATS and robotic VATS groups, respectively. At a follow-up time of 42 months, the rate of complete remission of myasthenia gravis was higher in the robotic group (39.25% vs. 20.3%; P = 0.01).[46]

In our early experience of robotic thymectomy to date, we have performed 27 procedures with acceptable outcomes (unpublished data). Median estimated blood loss, operative time (including setup and robot docking), pleural drainage time, and hospital length of stay are 30 mL (range 3 to 100 mL), 219 minutes (range 137 to 348 minutes), 2 days (range 1 to 7 days), and 3 days (range 2 to 10 days), respectively. We have resected 11 thymomas with a median diameter of 3 cm (range 2.5 to 11.0 cm). Open conversion was not necessary to complete the conduct of surgery in any of the cases. Similar outcomes have been reported in larger series of robotic thymectomy. Marulli and colleagues reported a series of 100 patients undergoing robotic thymectomy for myasthenia gravis.[47] Postoperative complications occurred in 6 (6%) of patients, and median hospital stay was 3 days (range 2 to 14 days). Ruckert et al. reported a series of 106 consecutive robotic thymectomies for myasthenia gravis, with a 1% rate of open conversion and 2% rate of postoperative morbidity.[48]

SUMMARY

Thymectomy is an accepted mode of treatment for thymoma, anterior mediastinal tumors, and certain instances of medication-refractory myasthenia gravis. In select patients, VATS and robotic-assisted VATS thymectomy are safe alternatives to median sternotomy and may improve outcomes of blood loss, hospital length of stay, healing time, and cosmetic appearance. Long-term outcomes of myasthenia gravis remission and thymoma recurrence also appear to be comparable. At this time, there is insufficient evidence to demonstrate clear superiority of either robotic or nonrobotic platforms. Additionally, numerous techniques have been developed and described using these robotic and nonrobotic VATS technologies, each with their own inherent advantages and challenges. As experience with these minimally invasive techniques continues to evolve, we anticipate an increasing role of minimally invasive thymectomy, particularly in patients with hesitation or contraindication to median sternotomy.

REFERENCES

1. Davenport E, Malthaner RA. The role of surgery in the management of thymoma: a systematic review. *Ann Thorac Surg* 2008;86(2):673–684.
2. Falkson CB, Bezjak A, Darling G, et al. The management of thymoma: a systematic review and practice guideline. *J Thorac Oncol* 2009;4(7):911–919.
3. Gronseth GS, Barohn RJ. Practice parameter: thymectomy for autoimmune myasthenia gravis (an evidence-based review): report of the Quality Standards Subcommittee of the American Academy of Neurology. *Neurology* 2000;55(1):7–15.
4. Jaretzki A, Steinglass KM, Sonett JR. Thymectomy in the management of myasthenia gravis. *Semin Neurol* 2004;24(1):49–62.
5. Masaoka A. Extended trans-sternal thymectomy for myasthenia gravis. *Chest Surg Clin N Am* 2001;11(2):369–387.
6. Strobel P, Bauer A, Puppe B, et al. Tumor recurrence and survival in patients treated for thymomas and thymic squamous cell carcinomas: a retrospective analysis. *J Clin Oncol* 2004;22(8):1501–1509.
7. Wolfe GI, Kaminski HJ, Aban IB, et al. Randomized trial of thymectomy in myasthenia gravis. *NEJM* 2016;375(6):511–522.
8. Jaretzki A 3rd, Aarli JA, Kaminski HJ, et al. Thymectomy for myasthenia gravis: evaluation requires controlled prospective studies. *Ann Thorac Surg* 2003;76(1):1–3.
9. Jaretzki A 3rd, Wolff M. "Maximal" thymectomy for myasthenia gravis. Surgical anatomy and operative technique. *J Thorac Cardiovasc Surg* 1988;96(5):711–716.
10. Zielinski M, Rybak M, Wilkojc M, et al. Subxiphoid video-assisted thoracoscopic thymectomy for thymoma. *Ann Cardiothorac Surg* 2015;4(6):564–566.
11. Xu S, Liu X, Li B, et al. Robotic thoracic surgery of total thymectomy. *Ann Transl Med* 2015;3(11):156.
12. Scarci M, Pardolesi A, Solli P. Uniportal video-assisted thoracic surgery thymectomy. *Ann Cardiothorac Surg* 2015;4(6):567–570.
13. Donahoe L, Keshavjee S. Video-assisted transcervical thymectomy for myasthenia gravis. *Ann Cardiothorac Surg* 2015;4(6):561–563.
14. Li Y, Wang J. Left-sided approach video-assisted thymectomy for the treatment of thymic diseases. *World J Surg Oncol* 2014;12:398.
15. Jurado J, Javidfar J, Newmark A, et al. Minimally invasive thymectomy and open thymectomy: outcome analysis of 263 patients. *Ann Thorac Surg* 2012;94(3):974–981; discussion 981–982.
16. Chung JW, Kim HR, Kim DK, et al. Long-term results of thoracoscopic thymectomy for thymoma without myasthenia gravis. *J Int Med Res* 2012;40(5):1973–1981.
17. Liu TJ, Lin MW, Hsieh MS, et al. Video-assisted thoracoscopic surgical thymectomy to treat early thymoma: a comparison with the conventional transsternal approach. *Ann Surg Oncol* 2014;21(1):322–328.
18. Ye B, Li W, Ge XX, et al. Surgical treatment of early-stage thymomas: robot-assisted thoracoscopic surgery versus transsternal thymectomy. *Surg Endosc* 2014;28(1):122–126.
19. Ye B, Tantai JC, Ge XX, et al. Surgical techniques for early-stage thymoma: video-assisted thoracoscopic thymectomy versus transsternal thymectomy. *J Thorac Cardiovasc Surg* 2014;147(5):1599–1603.
20. Kimura T, Inoue M, Kadota Y, et al. The oncological feasibility and limitations of video-assisted thoracoscopic thymectomy for early-stage thymomas. *Eur J Cardiothorac Surg* 2013;44(3):e214–e218.
21. D'Cunha J, Andrade RS, Maddaus MA. Thoracoscopic thymectomy. *Oper Tech Thorac Cardiovasc Surg* 15(2):102–113.
22. Wagner OJ, Louie BE, Vallieres E, et al. Near-infrared fluorescence imaging can help identify the contralateral phrenic nerve during robotic thymectomy. *Ann Thorac Surg* 2012;94(2):622–625.
23. Chen Z, Zuo J, Zou J, et al. Cellular immunity following video-assisted thoracoscopic and open resection for non-thymomatous myasthenia gravis. *Eur J Cardiothorac Surg* 2014;45(4):646–651.
24. Caronia F, Fiorelli A, Monte AL. Bilateral thoracoscopic thymectomy using a novel positioning system. *Asian Cardiovasc Thorac Ann* 2014;22(9):1135–1137.
25. Nakagiri T, Inoue M, Shintani Y, et al. Improved procedures and comparative results for video-assisted thoracoscopic extended thymectomy for myasthenia gravis. *Surg Endosc* 2015;29(9):2859–2865.
26. Ampollini L, Del Rio P, Sianesi M, et al. Transcervical video-assisted thymectomy: preliminary results of a modified surgical approach. *Langenbecks Arch Surg* 2011;396(2):267–271.
27. Keijzers M, Dingemans AM, Blaauwgeers H, et al. 8 years' experience with robotic thymectomy for thymomas. *Surg Endosc* 2014;28(4):1202–1208.
28. Rueckert J, Swierzy M, Badakhshi H, et al. Robotic-assisted thymectomy: surgical procedure and results. *Thorac Cardiovasc Surg* 2015;63(3):194–200.
29. Suda T, Tochii D, Tochii S, et al. Trans-subxiphoid robotic thymectomy. *Interact Cardiovasc Thorac Surg* 2015;20(5):669–671.
30. Hess NR, Sarkaria IS, Pennathur A, et al. Minimally invasive versus open thymectomy: a systematic review of surgical techniques, patient demographics, and perioperative outcomes. *Ann Cardiothorac Surg* 2016;5(1):1–9.
31. Mineo TC, Ambrogi V. Video-assisted thoracoscopic thymectomy surgery: Tor Vergata experience. *Thorac Cardiovascu Surg* 2015;63(3):187–193.
32. Gu ZT, Mao T, Chen WH, et al. Comparison of video-assisted thoracoscopic surgery and median sternotomy approaches for thymic tumor resections at a single institution. *Surg Laparosc Endosc Percutan Tech* 2015;25(1):47–51.

33. Seong YW, Kang CH, Choi JW, et al. Early clinical outcomes of robot-assisted surgery for anterior mediastinal mass: its superiority over a conventional sternotomy approach evaluated by propensity score matching. *Eur J Cardiothorac Surg* 2014;45(3):c68–c73; discussion c73.

34. Manoly I, Whistance RN, Sreekumar R, et al. Early and mid-term outcomes of trans-sternal and video-assisted thoracoscopic surgery for thymoma. *Eur J Cardiothorac Surg* 2014;45(6):e187–e193.

35. He Z, Zhu Q, Wen W, et al. Surgical approaches for stage I and II thymoma-associated myasthenia gravis: feasibility of complete video-assisted thoracoscopic surgery (VATS) thymectomy in comparison with trans-sternal resection. *J Biomed Res* 2013;27(1):62–70.

36. Weksler B, Tavares J, Newhook TE, et al. Robot-assisted thymectomy is superior to transsternal thymectomy. *Surg Endosc* 2012;26(1):261–266.

37. Pennathur A, Qureshi I, Schuchert MJ, et al. Comparison of surgical techniques for early-stage thymoma: feasibility of minimally invasive thymectomy and comparison with open resection. *J Thorac Cardiovasc Surg* 2011;141(3):694–701.

38. Lee CY, Kim DJ, Lee JG, et al. Bilateral video-assisted thoracoscopic thymectomy has a surgical extent similar to that of transsternal extended thymectomy with more favorable early surgical outcomes for myasthenia gravis patients. *Surg Endosc* 2011;25(3):849–854.

39. Huang CS, Cheng CY, Hsu HS, et al. Video-assisted thoracoscopic surgery versus sternotomy in treating myasthenia gravis: comparison by a case-matched study. *Surg Today* 2011;41(3):338–345.

40. Odaka M, Akiba T, Yabe M, et al. Unilateral thoracoscopic subtotal thymectomy for the treatment of stage I and II thymoma. *Eur J Cardiothorac Surg* 2010;37(4):824–826.

41. Lin MW, Chang YL, Huang PM, et al. Thymectomy for non-thymomatous myasthenia gravis: a comparison of surgical methods and analysis of prognostic factors. *Eur J Cardiothorac Surg* 2010;37(1):7–12.

42. Meyer DM, Herbert MA, Sobhani NC, et al. Comparative clinical outcomes of thymectomy for myasthenia gravis performed by extended transsternal and minimally invasive approaches. *Ann Thorac Surg* 2009;87(2):385–390; discussion 390–391.

43. Bachmann K, Burkhardt D, Schreiter I, et al. Long-term outcome and quality of life after open and thoracoscopic thymectomy for myasthenia gravis: analysis of 131 patients. *Surg Endosc* 2008;22(11):2470–2477.

44. Friedant AJ, Handorf EA, Su S, et al. Minimally invasive versus open thymectomy for thymic malignancies: systematic review and meta-analysis. *J Thorac Oncol* 2016;11(1):30–38.

45. Ye B, Tantai JC, Li W, et al. Video-assisted thoracoscopic surgery versus robotic-assisted thoracoscopic surgery in the surgical treatment of Masaoka stage I thymoma. *World J Surg Oncol* 2013;11:157.

46. Ruckert JC, Swierzy M, Ismail M. Comparison of robotic and nonrobotic thoracoscopic thymectomy: a cohort study. *J Thorac Cardiovasc Surg* 2011;141(3):673–677.

47. Marulli G, Schiavon M, Perissinotto E, et al. Surgical and neurologic outcomes after robotic thymectomy in 100 consecutive patients with myasthenia gravis. *J Thorac Cardiovasc Surg* 2013;145(3):730–735; discussion 735–736.

48. Ruckert JC, Ismail M, Swierzy M, et al. Thoracoscopic thymectomy with the da Vinci robotic system for myasthenia gravis. *Ann N Y Acad Sci* 2008;1132:329–335.

156D

Extended Transsternal Thymectomy With or Without Cervical Incision

Jason P. Glotzbach ▪ Mitchell J. Magee ▪ Alper Toker ▪ Joshua R. Sonett

The modern practice of thymectomy for myasthenia gravis (MG) developed from the early work of Dr. Alfred Blalock that initially described improvement of patients after thymectomy for thymic masses, a subsequent series of patients with nonthymomatous MG.[1] In 1941 he reported the initial series of six patients who underwent thymectomy (starting from the cricothyroid) for nonthymomatous MG.[2] In his operative technique, he stressed the need for meticulous preoperative and postoperative care of these patients. Subsequently, multiple techniques and approaches to thymectomy have been described, from transcervical, videoscopic, robotic, subxiphoid, and the maximal approach of cervical and transsternal combined approach of Fred Jaretzki.[3-11] Despite the surgical acceptance of the role of thymectomy in MG, definitive proof of the effectiveness of thymectomy for MG was not proven until the results of an international trial of thymectomy in MG was published in 2016.[12]

The results of the Myasthenia Gravis Thymectomy Trial (MGTX), a randomized prospective trial published in the New England Journal of Medicine, determined that thymectomy significantly improves the clinical course of patients with MG.[12] Specifically, extended transsternal thymectomy was associated with improved quantitative neurologic measures of MG, reduced medication requirements to control symptoms, and reduced disease-related hospital admissions. The surgical resection tested in the trial was an extended transcervical thymectomy, making this technique the only proven surgical technique to affect the outcome of MG in a prospective randomized trial. Thus, understanding the technique and extent of resection performed is critical to all practicing thoracic surgeons.

Given the results of the trial, complete removal of the thymus and perithymic tissue appears indicated when a thymectomy is performed in the treatment of nonthymomatous MG. Thymic anatomy should be understood by all those involved in the treatment of these patients and in the analysis of the results of the surgery. Importantly, the thymus is not just two well-defined lobes, but is a complex of lobes and extra-anatomic thymic tissue.[13,14] Incomplete resections may be associated with increased rates of relapse and subsequent resection of additional tissue can reduce symptoms.[15,16] Presently, extended transsternal thymectomy is intended to maximize removal of all potentially viable thymic tissue in a radical, but safe, operative approach.

INDICATIONS FOR EXTENDED THYMECTOMY

Experimental studies in animals have firmly established the role of the thymus in the autoimmune-mediated development of MG; these studies document the effect of thymectomy and other interruptions of the autoimmune mechanisms of myasthenia development.[17-21] This was proven in the MGTX trial for acetylcholine antibody-positive, nonthymomatous MG. Trial inclusion criteria were strict and included: duration of MG of less than 5 years, an age of 18 to 65 years, a serum acetylcholine-receptor–antibody level of more than 1 nmol/L and a Myasthenia Gravis Foundation of America (MGFA) clinical classification of II to IV (class I indicates weakness only in ocular muscles, class II mild generalized disease, class III moderate generalized disease, class IV severe generalized disease, and class V crisis requiring intubation). Thymectomy may as well be indicated for ocular or class 1 MG, as well as for seronegative MG, as retrospective evidence supports positive response rates; but further prospective evidence is still lacking.

OPERATIVE TECHNIQUE

The most important principle for thymectomy, regardless of indication and surgical approach, is to achieve en bloc resection of all thymus-containing tissue without compromising the phrenic or laryngeal nerves. The terms "maximal thymectomy" and "extended thymectomy" are essentially synonymous. Detailed anatomic studies have demonstrated that the thymus consists of several lobes that may or may not be contiguous throughout the neck and mediastinum. Detailed surgical–anatomical studies have demonstrated that the thymus frequently consists of multiple lobes in the neck and mediastinum, often separately encapsulated, and *these lobes may not be contiguous*. In addition, *unencapsulated lobules* of thymus and *microscopic foci* of thymus may be *widely* and *invisibly* distributed in the pretracheal and anterior mediastinal fat from the level of the thyroid, and occasionally above, to the diaphragm and bilaterally from beyond each phrenic nerve. In addition, complete working knowledge of anterior mediastinal anatomy allows the surgeon to identify and protect the phrenic, vagus, and recurrent laryngeal

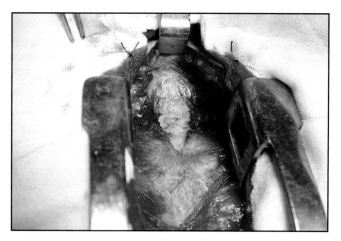

FIGURE 156D.1 Sternotomy with release of cervical facial bands and separation of strap muscles.

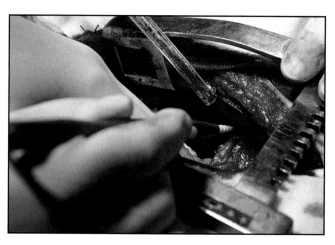

FIGURE 156D.2 Release of mediastinal pleura en bloc to be kept with specimen.

nerves. Injury to any of these nerves can lead to devastating complications, especially in the myasthenic patient.

MEDIASTINAL EXPOSURE AND DISSECTION

General endotracheal anesthesia is administered via a single-lumen endotracheal tube. Muscle relaxants are avoided in MG patients due to the risk of persistent postoperative neuromuscular weakness. The patient is positioned supine with a rolled sheet or pillow oriented transversely behind the shoulders to extend the neck. A vertical skin incision is created beginning 2 to 3 cm below the sternal notch and extending inferiorly to the level of the xiphoid. If a cervical approach is to be utilized as well, the superior aspect of this incision can be joined with a collar incision in a T for maximal exposure (see next section below). A full median sternotomy is performed in the standard fashion and hemostasis is achieved on the periosteal edges. In order to define the superior aspect of the thymus, the retrosternal strap muscles and associated fascial bands are incised in the midline (Fig. 156D.1). The retrosternal fat is excised with the specimen, so before placing the sternal retractor, the mammary veins and lateral innominate vein are identified and skeletonized. This allows

the retrosternal fat to be dissected away from the sternal edges and resected en bloc with the specimen. Once this fat layer has been cleared, the mediastinal pleura are open bilaterally, taking care to identify and preserve the phrenic nerves (Fig. 156D.2).

The mediastinal pleura is mobilized from the underlying thymus superiorly and incised laterally 1 cm anteriorly and parallel to the phrenic nerve. The anterior mediastinal pleura will be removed with the specimen (Fig. 156D.3). This maneuver ensures that any microscopic thymic tissue will be removed with the specimen rather than remaining behind with the pleura. The phrenic nerves are left attached to the posterior mediastinal pleura and elevated away from the underlying thymofatty tissue (Fig. 156D.4). It is essential to identify and protect the bilateral phrenic nerves during this step. In addition, the vagus nerve and recurrent laryngeal nerve courses 1 to 2 cm posterior to the phrenic nerve at the level of the hilum on the left side, so careful dissection in this area is essential to preserve all the nerves.

The dissection proceeds with *sharp dissection* of the pericardium from the level of the diaphragm to the innominate vein and extending from hilum to hilum. The specimen is removed en bloc including both sheets of mediastinal pleura and the "fingers" of pericardium that enter the thymus. All mediastinal fat is removed with the specimen, including the cardiophrenic fat pads that extend beyond the phrenic nerves bilaterally. Additional fatty tissue is removed from the sulcus between the superior vena cava and ascending aorta, the

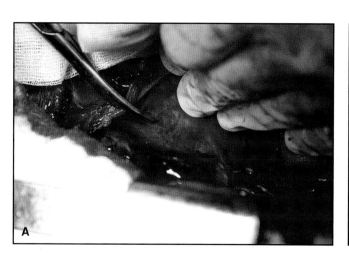

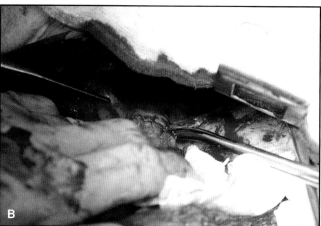

FIGURE 156D.3 **A,B:** Sharp dissection of thymic tissue and fat from the right and left phrenic.

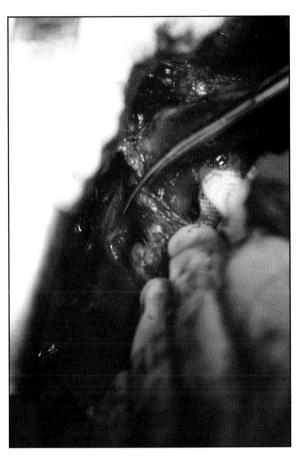

FIGURE 156D.4 Sharp dissection of the brachiocephalic vein.

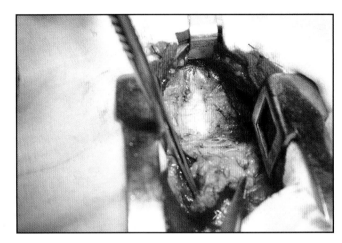

FIGURE 156D.5 Cervical dissection with superior retraction of wound and clearance of thymic horns with en bloc pretracheal tissue.

aortopulmonary window, and behind the innominate vein. Once all of these areas of thymofatty tissue have been mobilized, the specimen is divided sharply off the innominate vein and the thymic veins are controlled with clips (Fig. 156D.4). Above the innominate vein, the thymic tissue is dissected free from behind the strap muscles and off the innominate artery. The remainder of the mobilization can be performed via a cervical incision, but if a cervical incision is not planned, mobilization of the thymic tissue from the anterior trachea should be extended as superiorly as possible.

CERVICAL APPROACH

Although originally a cervical collar incision was created separately, the cervical dissection is now approached via cephalad extension and retraction of a median sternotomy incision. The mobilization is continued from the mediastinal dissection plane posterior to the strap muscles. The borders of dissection are the recurrent laryngeal nerves laterally and trachea posteriorly (Fig. 156D.5). The thyroid lobes are elevated from the trachea and the recurrent laryngeal nerves are identified and protected. Care must be taken when dissecting around the nerves; it is preferable to leave microscopic thymic tissue behind rather than cause a nerve injury. The superior extent of thymic tissue is marked by fibrous cords that extend behind the thyroid to the hyoid bone. Throughout the cervical dissection, care must also be taken to identify and protect the parathyroid glands, which may be imbedded in the thymic tissue. Completion of the cervical dissection permits en bloc removal of the specimen and the completed cervical and mediastinal dissection (Fig. 156D.6A,B).

PERIOPERATIVE PATIENT MANAGEMENT

Although it has been shown that patients respond more favorably to thymectomy if performed soon after diagnosis, it is critical to take the time to optimize the myasthenic patient medically before surgery.[22] Multidisciplinary evaluation of each patient by a surgeon, anesthesiologist, and neurologist is essential for this process.[23] Respiratory weakness must be minimized, using IVIG or immunosuppression if needed. Preoperative pulmonary function tests should be performed, with special attention paid to maximum expiratory pressure (MEP), which has been shown to predict postoperative respiratory function.[24] Anesthesia care of the myasthenic patient should be performed by an anesthesia team in an institution with significant experience managing myasthenia patients. Postoperatively, patients with a history of significant respiratory compromise should be closely monitored in an intensive care unit for 24 to 48 hours so that respiratory failure can be rapidly identified and corrected. At the first signs of fatigue, reintubation and respiratory support should be initiated to prevent total respiratory collapse.[25]

RESULTS AND OUTCOMES RESEARCH

The results from the MGTX study demonstrated that extended transsternal thymectomy improves clinical outcomes of patients with generalized MG. Patients who were randomized to transsternal extended thymectomy had significantly improved symptoms including: improvement in the average quantitative myasthenia score from 8.99 to 6.15 versus (clinically significant difference with a 31% improvement for the thymectomy group, p <0.0001), a 33% decrease in the dose of prednisone needed to attain improved neurologic status (p <0.001, 44 mg vs. 60 mg). Treatment-associated complications were not significantly different between the two treatment groups over a period of 3 years. Treatment-associated symptoms favored the thymectomy group over the prednisone-alone group in terms of the number of participants with symptoms (p <0.001), in the total number of symptoms (p <0.001), and in the distress level related to symptoms (p = 0.003) over the 3-year period. In addition, hospitalizations for myasthenia-related symptoms during the trial period were significantly lower in the thymectomy group (9% vs. 37%).[12]

In order to standardize discussion of thymectomy procedures and to allow comparison of results, the MGFA has adopted a standard

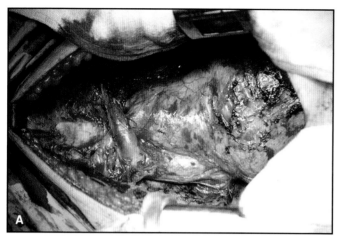

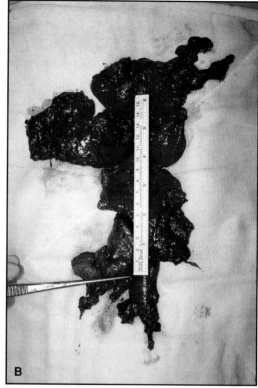

FIGURE 156D.6 Final dissection view of mediastinum (**A**) and en bloc thymic and mediastinal tissues (**B**).

classification scheme of thymectomy based on surgical approach and extent of resection. Since many of the available data for thymectomy come from retrospective series, analysis of results has been notoriously difficult.[26] One of the most important outcome measures for MG patients is remission of symptoms following thymectomy. The most reliable and preferred statistical technique for analyzing remission rates is life table analysis using the Kaplan–Meier method.[27] Many studies have relied on calculations of crude remission rates by dividing the number of remissions by the number of patients operated upon or by the number of patients followed. These crude remission rates cannot account for patients lost to follow-up and cannot effectively account for the variability inherent in the clinical spectrum of MG. There are no well-designed prospective studies that compare the different surgical approaches to thymectomy, but the available data suggest that the less thymus left behind after thymectomy, the better the results. To this end, the goal of maximal resection may be achieved via transsternal thymectomy and extended transcervical thymectomy.[28,29]

In addition, the outcomes of minimally invasive versus transsternal approach have been shown to be comparable[7,30] although the combined transcervical–transsternal approach remains the gold standard.[26]

REFERENCES

1. Blalock A, Mason MF, Morgan HJ, et al. Myasthenia gravis and tumors of the thymic region: report of a case in which the tumor was removed. *Ann Surg* 1939; 110(4):544–561.
2. Blalock A, Harvey AM, Ford FR, et al. The treatment of myasthenia gravis removal of the thymus gland: preliminary report. *JAMA* 1941;117:1529–1533.
3. Kirschner P, Osserman KE, Kark AE. Studies in myasthenia gravis: transcervical total thymectomy. *JAMA* 1969;209(6):906–910.
4. Jaretzki A, Bethea M, Wolff M, et al. A rational approach to total thymectomy in the treatment of myasthenia gravis. *Ann Thor Surg* 1977;24:120–130.
5. Cooper JD, Al-Jilaihawa AN, Pearson G, et al. An improved technique to facilitate transcervical thymectomy for myasthenia gravis. *Ann Thorac Surg* 1988;45(3): 242–247.
6. Calhoun RF, Ritter JH, Guthrie TH, et al. Results of transcervical thymectomy for myasthenia gravis in 100 consecutive patients. *Ann Surg* 1999;230(4):555–559.
7. Rückert JC, Ismail M, Swierzy M, et al. Thoracoscopic thymectomy with the da Vinci robotic system for myasthenia gravis. *Ann NY Acad Sci* 2008;1132:329–335.
8. Zieliński M, Hauer L, Kuzdzał J, et al. Technique of the transcervical-subxiphoid-videothoacoscopic maximal thymectomy. *J Minim Access Surg* 2007;3(4):168–172.
9. Tomulescu V, Sgarbura O, Stanescu C, et al. Ten year results of thoracoscopic unilateral extended thymectomy performed in nonthymomatous myasthenia gravis. *Ann Surg* 2011;254(5):761–765.
10. Novellino l, Longoni M, Spinelli L, et al. "Extended" thymectomy, without sternotomy, performed by cervicotomy and thoracoscopic technique in the treatment of myasthenia gravis. *Int Surg* 1994;79(4):378–381.
11. Jaretzki A, Wolff M. "Maximal" thymectomy for myasthenia gravis: surgical anatomy and operative technique. *J Thorac Cardiovasc Surg* 1988;96:711–716.
12. Wolfe GI, Kaminski HJ, Aban IB, et al. Randomized trial of thymectomy in myasthenia gravis. *N Eng J Med* 2016;375(6):511–522.
13. Masaoka A, Nagaoka Y, Kotake Y. Distribution of thymic tissue at the anterior mediastinum. Current procedures in thymectomy. *J Thorac Cardiovasc Surg* 1975; 70:747–754.
14. Masaoka A, Yamakawa Y, Niwa H, et al. Extended thymectomy for myasthenia gravis patients: a 20-year review. *Ann Thorac Surg* 1996;62:853–859.
15. Masaoka A, Monden Y, Seike Y, et al. Reoperation after transcervical thymectomy for myasthenia gravis. *Neurology* 1982;32:83–85.
16. Rosenberg M, Jauregui WO, Herrera MR, et al. Recurrence of thymic hyperplasia after trans-sternal thymectomy in myasthenia gravis. *Chest* 1986;89:888–889.
17. Fuchs S, Feferman T, Zhu KY, et al. Suppression of experimental autoimmune myasthenia gravis by intravenous immunoglobulin and isolation of a disease-specific IgG fraction. *Ann N Y Acad Sci* 2007;1110:505–558.
18. Mori S, Kubo S, Akiyoshi T, et al. Antibodies against muscle-specific kinase impair both presynaptic and postsynaptic functions in a murine model of myasthenia gravis. *Am J Pathol* 2012;180:798–810.
19. Niemi WD, Nastuk WL, Chang HW, et al. Electrophysiological studies of thymectomized and nonthymectomized acetylcholine receptor-immunized animal models of myasthenia gravis. *Exp Neurol* 1979;63:1–27.
20. Wu B, Goluszko E, Christadoss P. Experimental autoimmune myasthenia gravis in the mouse. *Curr Protoc Immunol* 2001;Chapter 15:Unit 15.8.
21. Xu L, Villain M, Galin FS, et al. Prevention and reversal of experimental autoimmune myasthenia gravis by a monoclonal antibody against acetylcholine receptor-specific T cells. *Cell Immunol* 2001;208:107–114.
22. Nieto IP, Robledo JP, Pajuelo MC, et al. Prognostic factors for myasthenia gravis treated by thymectomy: review of 61 cases. *Ann Thorac Surg* 1999;67:1568–1571.
23. Mussi A, Lucchi M, Murri L, et al. Extended thymectomy in myasthenia gravis: a team-work of neurologist, thoracic surgeon and anaesthesist may improve the outcome. *Eur J Cardiothorac Surg* 2001;19:570–575.
24. Younger DS, Braun NM, Jaretzki A, et al. Myasthenia gravis: determinants for independent ventilation after transsternal thymectomy. *Neurology* 1984;34:336–340.

25. Kas J, Kiss D, Simon V, et al. Decade-long experience with surgical therapy of myasthenia gravis: early complications of 324 transsternal thymectomies. *Ann Thorac Surg* 2001;72:1691–1697.

26. Sonett JR, Jaretzki A. Thymectomy for nonthymomatous myasthenia gravis: a critical analysis. *Ann NYAcad Sci* 2008;1132:315–328.

27. Jaretzki A, Barohn RJ, Ernstoff RM, et al. Myasthenia gravis: recommendations for clinical research standards. Task Force of the Medical Scientific Advisory Board of the Myasthenia Gravis Foundation of America. *Ann Thorac Surg* 2000;70:327–334.

28. Shrager JB, Nathan D, Brinster CJ, et al. Outcomes after 151 extended transcervical thymectomies for myasthenia gravis. *Ann Thorac Surg* 2006;82:1863–1869.

29. Meyer DM, Herbert MA, Sobhani NC, et al. Comparative clinical outcomes of thymectomy for myasthenia gravis performed by extended transsternal and minimally invasive approaches. *Ann Thorac Surg* 2009;87:385–390; discussion 390–391.

30. Jurado J, Javidfar J, Newmark A, et al. Minimally invasive thymectomy and open thymectomy: outcome analysis of 263 patients. *Ann Thorac Surg* 2012;94:974–981; discussion 981–982.

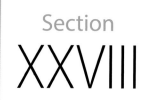

MEDIASTINAL INFECTIONS, MASS LESIONS IN THE MEDIASTINUM, AND CONTROL OF VASCULAR OBSTRUCTING SYMPTOMATOLOGY

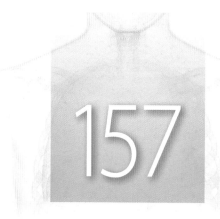

Acute and Chronic Mediastinal Infections

Ravi Rajaram ■ Malcolm M. DeCamp

Mediastinal infections are also known as mediastinitis. Acute mediastinitis is usually secondary to either poststernotomy infections or from perforations of the aerodigestive tract. Additionally, descending necrotizing mediastinitis, due to the spread of oropharyngeal infections, represents a less common but extremely lethal form of this disease.

Chronic mediastinal infections are uncommon. Most are the result of fungal disease originating in the various mediastinal node groups, while a few are secondary to mycobacterial organisms. Chronic fungal or tubercular infections are often self-limiting but may progress into the clinical entity of chronic fibrosing mediastinitis.

POSTOPERATIVE STERNAL INFECTION AND MEDIASTINITIS

The incidence of mediastinitis after cardiac surgical intervention varies between 1% and 4%. Factors conferring risk are many. They include diabetes, chronic obstructive pulmonary disease, congestive heart failure, use of internal mammary artery grafts (unilateral or bilateral), active smoking, reoperation, lower ejection fraction, prolonged ventilation, obesity, high body mass index (BMI), immunosuppressive

therapy, older age, use of bone wax, preoperative renal failure, duration of operation, prolonged cardiopulmonary bypass and aortic cross-clamp times, off-center sternotomy, improper stabilization of the sternum, poor hemostasis, use of pacing wires, need for repeated blood transfusions in the early postoperative period, use of electrocautery, presence of infection elsewhere, extended intensive care unit stay and overall hospitalization, readmission to the hospital, and several others depending on the study reviewed (see References for more information).

The mechanism of infection is yet to be established, but different theories exist. One theory postulates that local osteomyelitis at the sternotomy site is allowed to propagate.[1] Another theory suggests that sternal instability contributes to the superficial wound dehiscence and that this serves as a portal of ingress for cutaneous pathogens.[2] A third theory postulates that inadequate drainage in the retrosternal space serves as a culture medium for mediastinal contaminants. A final theory suggests that concomitant infections, such as a nosocomial pneumonia, act to seed the sternotomy site.[3]

The bacterial pathogens found are usually *Staphylococcus aureus* and *Staphylococcus epidermidis*, which account for 50% to 80% of isolates. In a recent study, researchers found that patients with preoperative nasal cultures positive for *Staphylococcus aureus* were more likely to develop mediastinitis.[4] Moreover, seven of nine patients with poststernotomy mediastinitis from methicillin-sensitive *Staphylococcus aureus* (MSSA) had an identical isolate in their preoperative nasal or surgical site culture whereas none of the eight patients with methicillin-resistant *Staphylococcus aureus* (MRSA) had isolates related to these culture sites. These findings suggest alternative routes of infection, and differing prevention strategies, for poststernotomy mediastinitis related to MSSA and MRSA.

Additionally, the leg incision used to harvest a saphenous vein graft can be a source of pathogens and may be responsible for gastrointestinal flora found in some cases. Gram-negative organisms such as *Pseudomonas*, *Serratia*, and *Klebsiella* are increasingly being isolated as the causative pathogens of mediastinitis. Charbonneau et al. found that nearly 30% of poststernotomy mediastinitis cases were related to gram-negative pathogens.[5] This may reflect the convergence of increased nosocomial infections and prolonged antibiotic use in the postoperative care of more complex and challenging cardiac patients. Patients with gram-negative mediastinitis are more likely to be given an antibiotic without sufficient coverage for treatment and have more drainage failures than those with mediastinitis related to other organisms.[5] Polymicrobial infections account for up to 40% of cases. Fungal mediastinitis is an infrequent etiology for poststernotomy mediastinal infection but should be considered in the setting of failed therapy or prolonged broad-spectrum antibiotic use.

CLINICAL MANIFESTATIONS

Mediastinitis should be suspected if the sternotomy wound appears clinically infected. This can occur early or late in the postoperative course. Classic signs may include erythema, purulent discharge, and sternal instability. A history of pain with breathing or difficulty lying in the lateral decubitus position is indicative of the two halves of the sternum moving against each other. It has been suggested that sternal instability as assessed by bimanual alternating sternal compression is the most helpful diagnostic maneuver.[6] Sometimes the classic signs and symptoms may not be obvious. Fever, sepsis, or leukocytosis, especially without an obvious source, may be the only presenting signs. Patients who are recovering slowly from a sternotomy may have their protracted course explained by an indolent form of poststernotomy mediastinitis.[7]

Radiographic studies are not routinely used, as clinical judgment usually suffices to detect poststernotomy mediastinitis, particularly in the acute early postoperative period when diagnostic specificity is diminished. Computed tomography (CT) scanning, however, may be useful either in the late presentation of poststernotomy mediastinitis or in the evaluation of unresolving sepsis due to an untreated source of mediastinitis.[8] An undrained retrosternal fluid collection or air–fluid level is the classic finding on CT scan. CT scans are very helpful in poststernotomy mediastinitis that presents >30 days after surgery, as they frequently reveal bone and soft tissue involvement at the inferior aspect of the wound.[6] As for other imaging modalities, nuclear imaging studies, which are used in other forms of osteomyelitis, are at best controversial in poststernotomy mediastinitis.[6]

TREATMENT

Treatment of poststernotomy mediastinitis has evolved tremendously in recent years. Conventional therapy—defined as opening and debriding the wound, serially packing the wound, and eventually closing the wound primarily—has been associated with an unacceptably high mortality rate, with rates reported between 20% and 40% in

some series.[9–11] High rates of treatment failure warranting additional surgical interventions are common.[12] The mediocre results associated with conventional therapy were the impetus behind the search for more aggressive or alternative management strategies.

The use of various flap closure techniques in the treatment of poststernotomy mediastinitis is frequently accepted as the standard therapy for these deep surgical site infections. This management philosophy is largely based on series that demonstrate early sternal debridement with flap closure and is associated with mortality rates of <10% as well as low complication rates.[13] The specific type of flap chosen in these reports varies with the majority using pectoralis muscle or rectus abdominus. Additionally, Roh et al. recently reported the use of a novel pectoralis major–rectus abdominus muscle bipedicled flap that provides adequate volume to fill the defect with outcomes comparable to other flap types.[14] Omental flaps have also been reported to be an adequate source of flap coverage and some have reported its benefits over muscle flaps. Milano and colleagues[15] demonstrated that omental flaps were associated with shorter operations and decreased lengths of hospitalization as well as lower rates of early complications. Furthermore, recurrent infections are more common with muscle flaps.[15,16] Brandt and Alvarez[17] have used both pectoralis flaps and omental flaps to cover the wound and occupy any potential dead spaces, with impressive results, including fewer major complications, shorter hospitalizations, decreased mortality rates, and increased overall survival.[17] Multivariable analysis has demonstrated that the lack of flap closure in poststernotomy mediastinitis is associated with a significant increase in 1-year mortality.[18] Despite these ostensibly convincing data, recent innovations in the treatment of poststernotomy mediastinitis have challenged flap closure as the method of choice.

The addition of closed mediastinal irrigation with either saline or antibiotic solution to the debridement of devitalized tissue and primary closure of a clearly viable sternum is one alternative therapy that has yielded acceptable results.[19,20] In 2004, Merrill and colleagues[19] reported a 95% success rate in 40 patients with poststernotomy mediastinitis treated with this single-stage revision. Dilute povidone–iodine or antibiotic irrigation was used until mediastinal fluid cultures dictated its cessation. Molina and colleagues[20] have described simple debridement with rewiring of the sternum laterally for stabilization (Robicsek weave) and primary closure followed by postoperative closed mediastinal irrigation. Their closure technique, followed by a culture-driven antibiotic irrigation solution, resulted in a remarkable success rate of 98%. Equally impressive in both series was the fact that the mortality rates were 0%.

Combination therapy with closed mediastinal irrigation using either primary closure alone or in combination with flap coverage has also been described.[21] Hirata and colleagues[22] reported successful results using closed drainage irrigation following open debridement and omental flap closure in the setting of MRSA infections in four patients.

The use of retrosternal high-negative-pressure catheters, known as Redon catheters, has also been described as another variation of closed mediastinal drainage to facilitate wound healing.[23,24] Favorable outcomes have been reported using Redon catheters for the treatment of poststernotomy mediastinitis.[25,26] In fact, comparisons of closed mediastinal irrigation to Redon catheters have shown that the former was associated with increased failure and mortality rates.[27]

Vacuum-assisted closure for the treatment of open wounds was first described by Argenta and Morykwas[28] in 1997. Since then, its use has been expanded to include poststernotomy wounds due to mediastinitis. The benefits of vacuum-assisted therapy for open wounds have been postulated to be multifactorial, but they share the common theme of relying on the associated effects of negative pressure. An increase in local blood flow, decrease in tissue edema and bacterial load, and removal of stagnant fluid, necrotic debris, and proteins impeding healing are all believed to promote wound healing. Furthermore, the mechanical effects exerted by the negative pressure are also thought to promote wound closure and accelerate granulation.[29–31]

Obdeijn and colleagues[32] published one of the first reports of vacuum-assisted closure of open wounds in three patients with poststernotomy mediastinitis. In this report all of the patients avoided the need for secondary surgical closure, as closure by accelerated secondary intention was achieved. Subsequent experiences, on a larger scale, have demonstrated that vacuum-assisted treatment of wounds can be an extremely useful adjunct in the management of poststernotomy mediastinitis.[15,29,30,33–37] Some of these studies have relied on vacuum-assisted closure exclusively.[29,30,34] However, not all investigations have employed vacuum-assisted therapy as the sole form of wound closure, since others have used this technique intentionally as a "bridge" to another form of definitive therapy.[30,34] For example, several studies have reported excellent results using negative pressure wound therapy until wound sterilization followed by pectoralis muscle advancement flap closure.[38–40] However, even with this intention, vacuum-assisted therapy has, in some cases, precluded the need for flap coverage or sternectomy.[33] The depth of infection has been thought to determine which patients will require progression to a second operation for closure.[34]

Numerous studies have compared outcomes from conventional therapy with vacuum-assisted therapy and demonstrated the latter to be associated with lower reinfection rates, reduced intensive care unit stay, shorter hospitalizations, earlier sternal rewiring, and improved mortality rates.[9–11,29,35,41] Additionally, a recent review concluded that vacuum-assisted therapy has superior outcomes when compared to conventional therapy and may be considered as first-line treatment in patients with poststernotomy mediastinitis.[42] Moreover, Sjogren and colleagues[36,37] have demonstrated that with the use of this treatment, long-term survival is no different than that of postoperative coronary artery bypass patients without mediastinitis. Vacuum-assisted therapy was found to have fewer treatment failures and decreased lengths of stay when compared to closed drainage irrigation.[43] Although negative pressure wound therapy may provide superior outcomes when compared to conventional therapy, this treatment is not without complications. Upward of 7% of patients treated with negative pressure therapy experience major bleeding complications, with hemorrhage from the coronary artery venous bypass graft as the leading finding.[44] Consequently, some authors have advocated the use of a protective barrier device during negative wound pressure therapy with success demonstrated in limited case series.[45] Additional surgical techniques, such as external sternal plating without rewiring, offer alternative options for the treatment of poststernotomy mediastinitis, though long-term follow-up data are needed.[46]

PROGNOSIS

The mortality rate associated with mediastinitis after coronary bypass surgery varies considerably depending on the treatment modality used. Braxton and colleagues[47] reported that the first-year survival rate after coronary artery bypass graft was 78% with mediastinitis and 95% without, with a threefold increase in mortality at 4 years' follow-up. Others have corroborated a long-term negative effect of poststernotomy mediastinitis despite intervention.[48] Additionally, recent studies suggest the type of pathogen may significantly affect outcomes. For example, Charbonneau et al. found that patients with gram-negative mediastinitis have a 30-day mortality rate nearly twice that of those with mediastinitis from other causes.[5] Also, timing of mediastinitis may be an important predictor of outcomes. Mekontso et al. reported

that patients who developed mediastinitis less than 14 days after sternotomy had significantly higher treatment failures and increased mortality compared to patients developing mediastinitis 14 or more days postoperatively.[49] Ultimately, factors related to patient comorbidities, pathogen type, and treatment-related decisions will all impact the outcome of a patient with poststernotomy mediastinitis.

PERFORATION OF THE AERODIGESTIVE TRACT

Perforation of the aerodigestive tract can result in mediastinal infection. Typically, these infections result from perforation of the esophagus caused by either spontaneous or iatrogenic trauma. Anastomotic leaks following esophagogastrectomy can also lead to acute mediastinitis. However, mediastinitis can also result from airway disruptions, as with tracheal injury.[50] Disruption of the esophagus in the thoracic cavity permits the egress of oropharyngeal bacteria and gastric contents into the visceral compartment of the mediastinum. Perforation of the cervical esophagus, on the other hand, results in leakage of oropharyngeal secretions and infection of the fascial spaces within the neck, which communicate with the anterior and visceral compartments of the mediastinum. The causes, clinical manifestations, diagnostic interventions, treatment, and outcome of esophageal perforations have been well reported and are beyond the scope of this chapter (see Chapter 115).[51–56] Management strategies of esophageal perforation accompanying mediastinitis are based on four principles:

1. Source control is achieved by primary repair or diversion of saliva ± gastric refluxate away from the esophageal perforation.
2. Thorough and wide mediastinal debridement and drainage, typically into the pleural space, to control ongoing mediastinal suppuration occurring after primary repair or diversion. In addition, gastrostomy tube decompression should be performed to decrease gastric reflux and mediastinal contamination if distal exclusion is not performed.
3. Appropriate antibiotics should be administered to augment host defenses. These must be effective against gram-positive and gram-negative bacteria and against both aerobic and anaerobic organisms. Antifungals should also be considered as yeast often colonizes the oropharynx, especially in clinical scenarios involving preexistent esophageal obstruction.
4. Maintain adequate nutrition enterally (jejunostomy preferred) or parenterally. The ultimate goal is to restore alimentary tract continuity.[57] The details of management of esophageal perforations are discussed in Chapter 115.

DESCENDING NECROTIZING MEDIASTINITIS

Estrera and colleagues[58] described acute purulent mediastinitis, due to oropharyngeal infection, as descending necrotizing mediastinitis. This infection remains an uncommon, but still lethal, form of mediastinitis.

ETIOLOGY

Of the reported cases, 60% to 70% are secondary to odontogenic infections.[58–60] Other common causes have included peritonsillar abscesses,[61] retropharyngeal and parapharyngeal abscesses,[58,62] and epiglottitis.[63] Several authors have also reported the development of

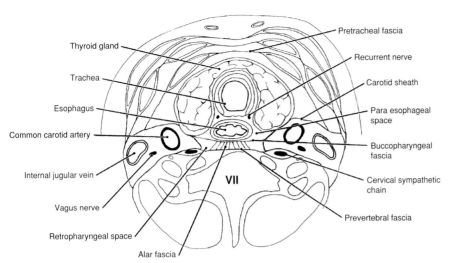

FIGURE 157.1 Cross-section of the neck at the level of the seventh cervical vertebra. The pretracheal, paraesophageal, and retropharyngeal–retrovisceral spaces extend directly into the mediastinum. Infection can extend also along the carotid sheaths.

mediastinitis after the use of minimally invasive techniques used for lung cancer staging, including transesophageal endoscopic ultrasound (EUS) or endobronchial ultrasound (EBUS) needle aspiration.[64,65] Other less common causes of descending necrotizing mediastinitis include trauma to the neck (including neck or mediastinal surgery), cervical lymphadenitis, and endotracheal intubation.[66–69]

Anatomically, there are three potential planes along which descending necrotizing mediastinitis can progress leading to closed space infection: (a) pretracheal, (b) perivascular, and (c) prevertebral. The pretracheal plane, also referred to as the superficial layer, is just anterior to the trachea. It is bound by the thyroid cartilage superiorly and pericardium and parietal pleura inferiorly at the carina and laterally along the rightward aspect of the trachea. The perivascular plane is bound by the carotid sheaths and descends into the mediastinum along with the structures within the carotid sheath. This route of spread results in infections of the middle mediastinum. Finally, the prevertebral plane or space, also referred to cranially as the retropharyngeal space, is bound anteriorly by the posterior aspect of cervical fascia and posteriorly by the alar fascia; it extends inferiorly until these two fascia coalesce at the first thoracic vertebra.[70–72] Most cases of descending necrotizing mediastinitis are secondary to spread in this last plane and result in involvement of the posterior mediastinum (Fig. 157.1). All these spaces are joined by loose connective tissue, which facilitates direct spread within these planes.[73] Gravity and negative pressure during inspiration allow for the descent of the infected and purulent material into the mediastinum and pleura.[73] Odontogenic and peritonsillar abscesses may extend to involve the submandibular[74] and parapharyngeal spaces, which, as McCurdy and colleagues[75] have noted, readily communicate with all major cervical fascial spaces.

The microbiologic features of descending necrotizing mediastinitis are polymicrobial, with aerobes and anaerobes reflecting the indigenous microflora of the oral cavity.[76–78] The most common organisms isolated include *Prevotella*, *Peptostreptococcus*, *Fusobacterium*, *Veillonella*, *Actinomyces*, oral *Streptococcus*, *Bacteroides*, *Staphylococcus aureus*, *Haemophilus* species, and *Bacteroides melaninogenicus*. Patients with diabetes who develop mediastinitis have an increased likelihood of *Klebsiella pneumoniae* as the causative pathogen.[79] Symbiosis between one or more species of gram-negative aerobic bacteria and an anaerobe can result in synergistic necrotizing cellulitis.

Mathieu and colleagues[80] have described predisposing conditions that may favor this infectious process; such conditions include diabetes (13.3%), alcoholism (17.7%), neoplasm (4.4%), and radionecrosis (3.3%). In particular, they found that age >70 years and underlying diabetes were risk factors predictive of mortality. Immune system disorders in general, including diabetes, have also been reported by other authors as a risk factor for mediastinitis and may portend a worse outcome.[81]

DIAGNOSIS

The criteria used for the diagnosis of descending necrotizing mediastinitis are clearly defined by Estrera and colleagues[58] and include (a) clinical evidence of severe oropharyngeal infection, (b) characteristic roentgenographic features of mediastinitis, (c) documentation of necrotizing mediastinal infection at operation or postmortem exam or both, and (d) establishment of the relationship between descending necrotizing mediastinitis and the oropharyngeal process.

Because this infection progresses rapidly, early diagnosis is essential. CT scanning is more reliable than chest radiography and can provide precise information on the extent of the infection, which in turn will guide the optimal approach(es) used for surgical drainage.

CLINICAL MANIFESTATIONS

Descending necrotizing mediastinitis is seen most often in a patient who is under treatment for a deep cervical infection resulting from one of the aforementioned causes. Despite antibiotics and drainage of the deep cervical space, the infection progresses to involve the mediastinum. Early diagnosis is often difficult because of the vagueness of early symptoms that would indicate mediastinal involvement. Unfortunately, the usual delay in diagnosis contributes greatly to the high mortality associated with descending necrotizing mediastinitis.[59] Descending necrotizing mediastinitis may occur at any time after cervical infection, manifest by signs and symptoms of sepsis with stiffness, swelling, and neck pain. Cranial nerve deficits, trismus, and stridor have also been described.[70] Dysphagia may or may not be present. Mediastinal involvement may occur as soon as 12 hours to as late as 2 weeks, but it is most commonly seen within 48 hours after the onset of deep cervical infection. Diffuse brawny induration of the neck and upper anterior chest wall is seen. Pitting edema and crepitance may be present in the area. Substernal pain, increased dysphagia, cough, and dyspnea may also develop. Pleural and pericardial involvement may occur, since the necrotizing process involves the adjacent spaces. Pleural effusion, nonspecific electrocardiographic changes, and even infection of the retroperitoneal space of the abdomen may develop as the inflammatory process ensues. The capillary leak that occurs with sepsis can further exacerbate dehydration and lead to acute respiratory distress syndrome, cardiac tamponade, and/or empyema.[72,82]

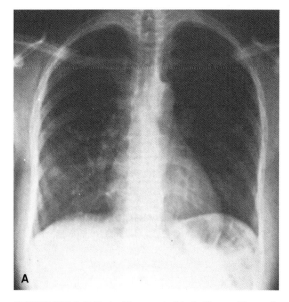 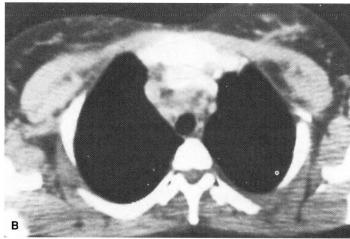

FIGURE 157.2 Patient with an acute febrile illness with cough and substernal chest pain. **A:** Posteroanterior radiograph of the chest reveals a nodular infiltrate in the right lower lung field and an ill-defined enlargement of the superior mediastinal shadow. **B:** Computed tomography scan reveals an inflammatory process in the superior portion of the visceral compartment of the mediastinum with associated enlargement of the adjacent lymph node.

RADIOGRAPHIC FEATURES

CT is the diagnostic imaging modality of choice. Estrera and colleagues[58] reported four radiographic features of the neck and chest present in descending necrotizing mediastinitis: (a) widening of the retrocervical space with or without an air–fluid level, (b) anterior displacement of the tracheal air column, (c) mediastinal emphysema, and (d) loss of the normal lordosis in the cervical spine. Also, the superior mediastinal shadow can be widened, and findings of pleural or pericardial involvement may be evident (Fig. 157.2).

CT scans of the chest are better than chest radiographs in delineating the infectious process. Carrol[83] and Breatnach[84] and their colleagues outlined several cardinal CT findings in descending necrotizing mediastinitis: (a) abscess formation, (b) soft tissue infiltration with loss of the normal fat planes, (c) absence of prominent lymphadenopathy, and (d) the presence of gas bubbles. A widened mediastinum with new air and fluid levels can also be seen in the visceral or anterior compartments, as can pleural or pericardial effusions.[85] A CT scan of the chest should be done in any patient with signs of a deep cervical infection as descending necrotizing mediastinitis may produce few overt symptoms initially.

TREATMENT

The management of descending necrotizing mediastinitis includes aggressive surgical drainage, debridement of devitalized tissue, antimicrobial therapy, and airway management. The surgical approach depends on the location of the abscess. Several authors have suggested that mediastinal drainage via a transthoracic approach should be used only for infections in the space below the level of the tracheal bifurcation anteriorly or the fourth thoracic vertebra posteriorly.[58,76] If only the superior mediastinum is involved and the infection is contained above the level of the carina or the fourth thoracic vertebra, standard transcervical mediastinal drainage may be adequate.[60,76,86] Others[59,87] have proposed a more aggressive approach regardless of the level of infection, including the transthoracic approach through a standard thoracotomy in addition to cervical drainage. Transthoracic drainage has been demonstrated to result in better debridement and

improved survival.[88,89] Further evidence for the inclusion of routine transthoracic drainage is provided by a meta-analysis comparing neck and thoracic drainage (19% mortality) versus transcervical drainage alone (41% mortality, $p < 0.05$).[62] The successful use of video-assisted mediastinoscopy with adequate drainage of the cervical neck, anterior mediastinum, and middle mediastinum to the level of the tracheal bifurcation has also been described.[90]

The standard posterior or lateral thoracotomy has unequivocally been the classic approach to draining mediastinal infections. Sternotomy has been described as both inadequate and dangerous in the treatment of descending necrotizing mediastinitis owing to inability to drain the posterolateral compartments of each thoracic cavity and the risk of introducing osteomyelitis and its attendant sequela of sternal dehiscence. With the increased popularity of minimally invasive surgery, several authors[70,79,91–94] have reported the use of video-assisted thoracoscopic (VATS) drainage in the management of descending necrotizing mediastinitis. The VATS approach has been reported to decrease morbidity when compared to thoracotomy and to result in better drainage of the mediastinum than transcervical drainage alone. Ultrasound or CT-guided percutaneous drainage has also been described,[95] though its greatest utility may be in the treatment of recurrent, loculated fluid collections and abscesses in the neck and chest after primary surgical drainage.[96] Leveraging these techniques may mitigate the need for repeated surgical interventions in the critically ill patient.[96] Irrespective of the treatment selected, mediastinal pleural irrigation following surgical debridement of the mediastinum with either saline or antibiotic solution akin to a modified Clagett procedure has achieved success in the setting of descending necrotizing mediastinitis by some,[97] while others have disputed its benefit.[98]

Antimicrobial therapy should be given promptly and should cover both aerobes and anaerobes. Initial antibiotic choice should offer the broadest possible coverage, with combinations used as necessary. When culture results are available, the antibiotics can be tailored accordingly.

The role of tracheostomy is controversial, as it may exacerbate the spread of infection via the pretracheal plane.[99] However, recent studies suggest that there is no association between tracheostomy and mediastinitis.[100] In the presence of complete and adequate drainage, tracheostomy may be undertaken as it obviates the need for prolonged intubation. Additionally, oral reintubation in patients with endotracheal tube dislodgement may be extremely difficult due to active oropharyngeal or cervical swelling, induration, or incompletely controlled infection.[85] Advocates of early tracheostomy note that this allows complete control of the airway.

PROGNOSIS

The mortality rate for patients with descending necrotizing mediastinitis before the antibiotic era was approximately 50%. This high mortality rate was a consequence of not only the absence of antibiotics from the surgeon's armamentarium, but also the significant delay in diagnosis often accompanying this disease in conjunction with the rapidity with which this infection spreads. However, with increasing recognition of this disease and aggressive surgical and antibiotic management, recent studies have found that mortality may be reduced to as low as 10% to 15%.[76] When death does occur, it may result from several causes including fulminant sepsis, blood vessel erosion with exsanguination, aspiration, metastatic intracranial infection, empyema, and/or purulent pericarditis with tamponade.

SUBACUTE MEDIASTINITIS

The definition of subacute mediastinitis is unclear, but this term should encompass those inflammatory processes involving the mediastinum that produce minimal to mild symptomatology (substernal pain, fever, night sweats) and an identifiable anterior or visceral mediastinal mass by radiographic or CT examination. These infections most often are the result of fungal, mycobacterial, or, rarely, actinomycotic organisms. Such subacute infections are observed only infrequently in previously normal, healthy persons but are becoming more common in immunocompromised patients, particularly those with acquired immunodeficiency syndrome (AIDS).

In immunocompetent patients, subacute infections attributable to histoplasmosis and to primary progressive *Mycobacterium tuberculosis* infections are most often encountered. Mediastinal actinomycotic infections are rare but have been described.[101] In immunocompromised patients, *M. avium* complex infections as well as those involving *M. tuberculosis* (Fig. 157.3) are prone to involve the mediastinal lymph nodes. Pitchenik and Robinson[102] reported that mediastinal or hilar adenopathy was one of the dominant findings in 59% of AIDS patients with *M. tuberculosis* infections.

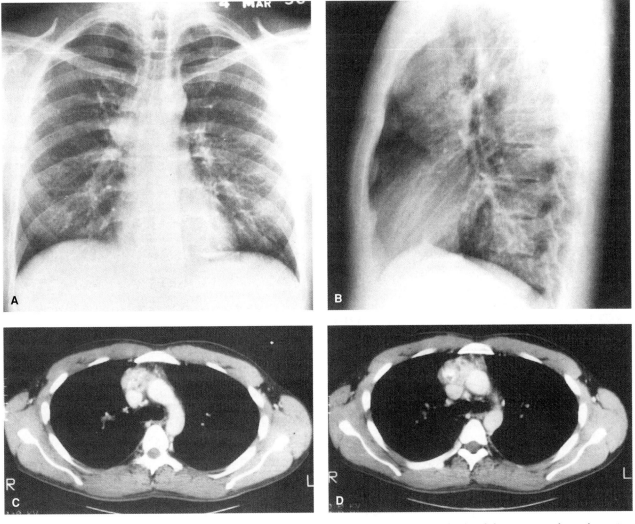

FIGURE 157.3 Posteroanterior (**A**) and lateral (**B**) radiographs of a young adult man with AIDS who developed the anterior mediastinal mass in a 6-month period. **C,D:** Computed tomography scans reveal a nonhomogeneous anterior mediastinal mass with areas of calcification. Biopsy revealed a granulomatous process containing many acid-fast organisms typical of *Mycobacterium tuberculosis*.

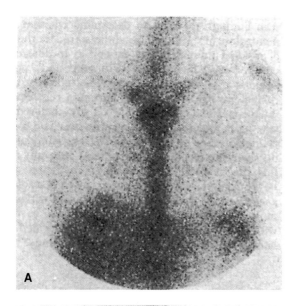

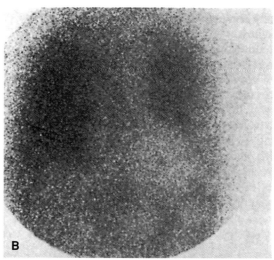

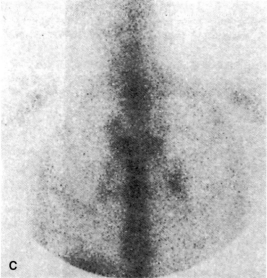

FIGURE 157.4 Gallium imaging in immunocompromised patients. **A:** Normal 48-hour anterior gallium image of the chest. **B:** A 72-hour anterior gallium image of the chest demonstrates diffuse bilateral increased pulmonary uptake in a 61-year-old man with AIDS and fever. Note the negative cardiac silhouette. The abnormality was also evident on 24-hour images. Initial chest radiograph results were negative, but later studies showed perihilar infiltrates. Bronchial aspirates were positive for *Pneumocystis carinii* pneumonia. **C:** A 72-hour anterior chest image shows bilateral hilar and right paratracheal lymphadenopathy in a 36-year-old man with AIDS who presented with nonproductive cough and fever. The patient proved to have *Mycobacterium avium-intracellulare* infection, which also involved the liver and bone marrow.

The inflammatory nature of the mediastinal mass may be suggested by the CT features of the lesions, but it is best confirmed by gallium scintigraphy, especially in AIDS patients (Fig. 157.4).[103,104] Indium leukocyte scintigraphy may also be useful in identifying these subacute infections, although its effectiveness decreases as the inflammatory process becomes more chronic.[105]

The final diagnosis is made by identification of the specific organism by tissue stains or culture. Adequate samples are usually obtained by needle aspiration, although more invasive mediastinal interventions may be necessary. Treatment consists of administering the appropriate drug or combination of drugs for the specific organism identified.

FIBROSING MEDIASTINITIS

Fibrosing mediastinitis is an uncommon benign process resulting in the deposition and proliferation of dense fibrous tissue throughout the visceral compartment of the mediastinum. This chronic inflammatory process can lead to entrapment and compression of vital mediastinal structures (e.g., central systemic veins, the vena cava, esophagus, trachea, or airways, and pulmonary arteries or veins). The deposition of thick encasing fibrous tissue typically involves the superior mediastinum in the region of the vena cava. In using a more restrictive definition as employed by Loyd and colleagues,[106] the process should involve and obstruct the major airways (tracheal carina or mainstem bronchi), the pulmonary arteries and veins, or both. With this definition, the superior vena cava is less commonly involved, but this subset of patients is more seriously affected and has a poorer prognosis.

This entity also has been termed sclerosing mediastinitis, fibrous mediastinitis, and granulomatous mediastinitis. Additionally, the term *idiopathic fibroinflammatory lesion of the mediastinum* has been proposed by Flieder and colleagues.[107] The exact cause is often unknown, but many cases in the United States are thought to be secondary to an abnormal host response to *Histoplasma capsulatum* infection.[106,108–113]

ETIOLOGY

Fibrosing mediastinitis may result from a number of causes (Table 157.1). Most cases in the United States are thought to be caused by fungal infections, primarily by *H. capsulatum*.[114] Mycobacterial infections are a less common cause. Goodwin and colleagues[109]

Fungal infections
Histoplasmosis
   Aspergillosis
   Mucomycosis
   Cryptococcosis
   Blastomycosis
Mycobacterial infections
   Mycobacterium tuberculosis
   Other mycobacterial infections
Bacterial infections
   Nocardiosis
   Actinomycosis
Autoimmune disease
Sarcoidosis
Rheumatic fever
Neoplasms
Trauma
Drugs
Idiopathic

Adapted from Marchevsky AM, Kaneko M. *Surgical Pathology of the Mediastinum.* 2nd ed. New York: Raven Press; 1992. With permission.

identified *Histoplasma* to be the offending organism in 26 of 38 cases, with the remainder caused by *Mycobacterium tuberculosis*. Eggleston[115] found that most cases are caused by *Histoplasma*, and Urschel and colleagues[111] reported that 12 of 22 cases of fibrosing mediastinitis were secondary to histoplasmosis. Although the exact mechanism and pathogenesis of fibrosing mediastinitis is not clear, the link between fibrosing mediastinitis and *H. capsulatum* is based on several observations. First, most cases occur in the United States in areas where histoplasmosis is endemic. Second, many affected patients test positive for *H. capsulatum* antigens. Third, *H. capsulatum* organisms are occasionally identified in histopathologic specimens.[116] However, because definitive histopathologic proof is absent in many cases, many believe that fibrosing mediastinitis results not from direct *H. capsulatum* infection but rather from an abnormal immunologic reaction to its antigens. Several experts suggest that this disease results from an exaggerated delayed hypersensitivity reaction to antigens from infected lymph nodes.[109,117] Marchevsky and Kaneko[118] support these findings as well, with the presence of strongly positive skin and serum reactivity to *H. capsulatum* in many patients and hypergammaglobulinemia and hypocomplementemia in others. Sherrick and colleagues[119] believe that as the acute infection heals, caseation develops in the mediastinal and hilar lymph nodes. These nodes may then proceed to rupture, spreading necrotic antigenic material throughout the mediastinum, which results in either localized or diffuse fibrosis.[120]

Controversy does exist with regard to fibrosing mediastinitis and mediastinal granulomas. Some researchers believe that mediastinal granulomas are a precursor to fibrosing mediastinitis. For example, one study found that over a third of patients with mediastinal granulomas eventually developed fibrosing mediastinitis and suggested that the granulomas should be resected to prevent this from occurring.[121] However, others have concluded the opposite and found no evidence of mediastinal granulomas progressing into fibrosing mediastinitis.[106]

Other less common causes of fibrosing mediastinitis are bacterial infections, tuberculosis, aspergillosis, mucormycosis, blastomycosis, cryptococcosis, autoimmune diseases in association with Behçet's disease, rheumatic fever, radiation therapy, trauma, Hodgkin's disease, and drug therapy with methysergide maleate.[122–126] Fibrosing mediastinitis

can also be associated with a number of disease syndromes such as retroperitoneal fibrosis.[127,128] Sclerosing cholangitis, Riedel's thyroiditis, and pseudotumor of the orbit have also been associated with fibrosing mediastinitis. Based on the pathologic similarities between many of these fibroinflammatory diseases and fibrosing mediastinitis, some experts have proposed a potentially similar mechanistic underpinning.[129] For example, a recent case series concluded that up to one-third of histoplasmosis or granulomatous–disease related cases of fibrosing mediastinitis have histologic characteristics of IgG4-related disease.[129] Oftentimes, the cause remains unknown and the term *idiopathic* is used.[111] True idiopathic fibrosing mediastinis may have been undiagnosed or misclassified in the past, but recent series have reported its incidence to vary from 10% to 20% but also to be as high as 50% of all the fibrosing mediastinitis cases observed.[130,131]

PATHOLOGY

Fibrosing mediastinitis is characterized grossly by a diffuse, ill-defined fibrotic infiltration of mediastinal structures. The mass of tissue is dense, white, and fibrous in cut sections and is described as "woody hard." Urschel and colleagues[111] likened it to "cement poured in the chest." Tissue planes are obscured, and in rare cases the fibrotic infiltration may extend into the soft tissues of the neck, posterior mediastinum, or the lung.[116,132,133]

Histologically, bands of hyalinized fibrous connective tissue entrap adjacent structures and infiltrate and obscure adipose tissue. The fibrous tissue can contain mononuclear cells. The bands are often arranged haphazardly, but can be arranged concentrically around granulomas.[134] The fibrous bands blend with the adjacent nerves, veins, and lymphatics. Zones of new collagen production and scattered aggregates of lymphocytes and plasma cells are present throughout. Recent studies have also reported that these areas of inflammation have increased numbers of CD20-positive B lymphocytes on histologic examination.[114]

CLINICAL FEATURES

Fibrosing mediastinitis may be self-limiting, but serious, persistent complications can incapacitate the patient and even be fatal. Patients are typically young at presentation, but a number of cases may be seen in the fourth to fifth decades of life. Men and women are affected equally. Some have reported a possible increased risk in African Americans, but this has not been seen in other studies.[107]

Approximately 40% of patients are asymptomatic, and the disease is discovered as an incidental radiographic finding. In the other 60% of patients, the clinical features vary with the visceral mediastinal structures involved. Most patients present with signs and symptoms related to compression or obstruction of the central airways, superior vena cava, pulmonary veins, pulmonary arteries, or esophagus. Some investigators have described a greater right-sided predilection for disease involvement of the pulmonary artery and veins.[114,131] The heart, pericardium, aorta, aortic branches, and coronary arteries are reported to be less frequently involved.[135–137] Vascular involvement is typically associated with tracheobronchial involvement, but the opposite does not necessarily occur.[130] Extension outside of the thoracic cavity may lead to symptomatic sclerosing cervicitis.[138]

The most common presenting complaints include shortness of breath, cough, dyspnea, pleuritic chest pain, fever, wheezing, recurrent pulmonary infection, hemoptysis, and dysphagia. Patients can present with systemic signs such as fever or weight loss. Compression and occlusion of the superior vena cava results in the superior vena cava syndrome (SVCS), which can sometimes be confused with a malignancy.[139] Fibrosing mediastinitis has been reported to be the most common benign cause of SVCS.[112,121] Obstruction of the central airways is common and manifests with cough, dyspnea, and a history of recurrent or persistent pneumonia. Compression of the central pulmonary arterial (PA) tree is more likely to involve the right or left main PA branches as they exit the pericardium. These patients often have dyspnea on exertion out of proportion to their spirometric measurements due to ventilation-perfusion mismatching. Patients with pulmonary venous occlusion present with progressive or exertional dyspnea as well as hemoptysis; this symptomatology has been termed the "pseudo-mitral stenosis syndrome" by Rossi.[116] Chronic pulmonary venous occlusion can result in cor pulmonale and secondary pulmonary arterial hypertension, which is an important cause of morbidity and mortality in patients with fibrosing mediastinitis.[140,141] Pulmonary venous occlusion can also lead to pulmonary infarction.[142,143] Hoarseness caused by compression of the left recurrent laryngeal nerve is infrequent.

RADIOGRAPHIC FINDINGS

Chest Radiography

Chest radiographs of patients with fibrosing mediastinitis usually appear abnormal, with the extent of disease frequently underestimated.[144] The most common finding is widening of the mediastinum (50% to 90%) (Fig. 157.5A); other features are a hilar mass (23%–39%), calcification (10%–32%), superior vena cava obstruction (33%–39%), parenchymal opacities (17%–33%), pleural effusion (9%), airway narrowing (36%), and septal thickening (4%).[106,119,126,135] Rarely, wedge-shaped areas of consolidation may be apparent.[145] The right side of the mediastinum is more commonly affected than the left.[135,146]

Computed Tomography Scans

A CT scan with intravenous contrast is the preferred method for evaluating fibrosing mediastinitis.[147] It can often delineate the areas

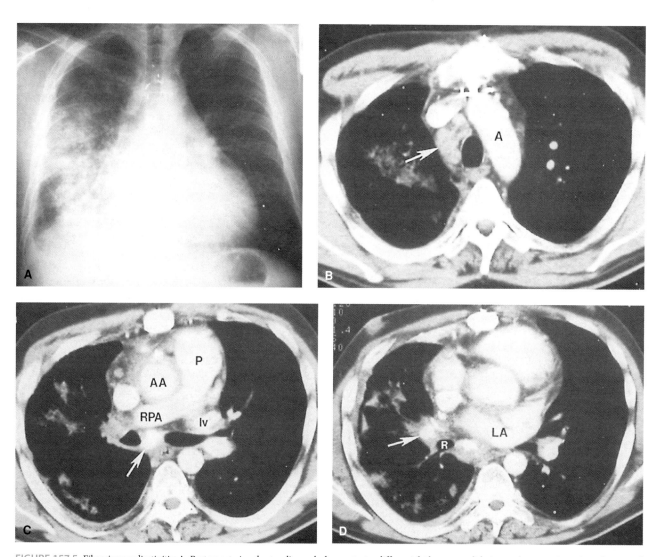

FIGURE 157.5 Fibrosing mediastinitis. **A:** Posteroanterior chest radiograph demonstrates diffuse right lung consolidation and some volume loss plus a small right pleural effusion. Mild right paratracheal widening is present. Cardiomegaly and surgical changes from a previous coronary bypass procedure are seen. **B:** Computed tomography study with contrast enhancement at the level of the aortic arch (**A**) demonstrates right paratracheal lymphadenopathy (*arrow*). **C:** More caudad at the level of the pulmonary artery (P), complete obstruction of the right pulmonary artery (RPA) has occurred. No opacification of the right superior pulmonary vein is seen, although the left superior pulmonary vein (lv) is well enhanced. Calcified lymph nodes (*arrow*) are present. Abnormal soft tissue encircles the ascending aorta (AA) and infiltrates into the right hilum; on MRI, this was shown to be of low-signal intensity on T2-weighted images, compatible with fibrosis. **D:** More caudad at the level of the left atrium (LA), calcified lymph nodes (*arrow*) are also seen occluding the right-middle-lobe bronchus. R, right-lower-lobe bronchus. (**A–D,** courtesy of Stuart S. Sagel, Paul L. Molina. Mallinckrodt Institute of Radiology, Washington University School of Medicine, St. Louis, Missouri.)

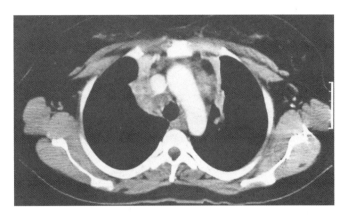

FIGURE 157.6 Computed tomography scan of a young woman with fibrosing mediastinitis with compression of the upper-lobe bronchi bilaterally and resultant atelectasis of upper-lobe segments in both right and left lungs.

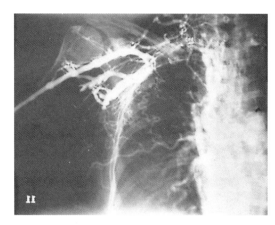

FIGURE 157.7 Venogram in a young adult woman with an SVCS caused by fibrosing mediastinitis but with a normal standard chest radiograph. The right subclavian and right innominate veins and superior vena cava are obstructed. Extensive collateral channels include the intercostal veins, internal mammary veins, and lateral thoracic branches. Drainage to the inferior vena cava is both by the azygos and hemiazygos veins.

of involvement and the degree of compression of the great vessels, trachea, and esophagus (Fig. 157.5B–D). Major bronchi can also be involved (Fig. 157.6). Weinstein and colleagues[148] have documented, with CT scans, the presence of (a) a hilar mass (100%), (b) a mediastinal mass (100%), (c) calcification (86%), (d) airway stenosis (71%), and (e) parenchymal opacities (57%) in patients with fibrosing mediastinitis. Sherrick and colleagues[119] noted two distinct CT scan patterns of fibrosing mediastinitis. They found 82% of patients to have relatively localized mediastinal disease affecting the right paratracheal and subcarinal regions, and 63% of these patients had evidence of prior histoplasmosis or tuberculosis infection. The other 18% of patients were observed to have a diffusely infiltrating disease process affecting multiple structures in the mediastinum. These patients had no evidence of prior granulomatous disease, and almost 50% had associated conditions such as retroperitoneal fibrosis. Contrast-enhanced CT accurately depicts the extent, level, and length of venous stenosis and shows collateral vessels as well. It is also useful for assessing the site, length, and severity of airway stenosis.

Recently Worrrell and colleagues[131] developed a set of diagnostic criteria for truly idiopathic fibrosing mediastinitis based on a combination of radiographic and pathologic data. A major defining feature of an idiopathic fibrosing mediastinitis according to their criteria was the absence of calcification on CT scans suggestive of prior granulomatous disease. The authors believe that this may have contributed to misclassification in previous reports.

Magnetic Resonance Imaging

Fibrosing mediastinitis manifests on T1-weighted images as a heterogeneous, infiltrative mass of intermediate signal intensity.[116] T2-weighted images show both increased and decreased signal intensity. The increased signal is thought to represent active inflammation, while the decreased signal is thought to indicate calcifications or fibrous tissue. Magnetic resonance imaging (MRI) is useful when the use of contrast material is contraindicated.

Other Radiographic Investigations

Esophageal involvement is best demonstrated by contrast esophagography.[149] The typical findings include both circumferential narrowing and long strictures in the junction of the upper and middle thirds.[150] Standard contrast venography can be performed to demonstrate the anatomy and location of obstruction of the superior vena cava as well as the collateral circulation (Fig. 157.7). Pulmonary arteriography may be performed in patients with suspected pulmonary vessel

involvement.[119,151] Typical findings include long-segment, smooth, or funnel-like stenoses of affected vessels.

Radionuclide Studies

Radionuclide scans with xenon-133 or technetium-99m–diethylenetriamine penta-acetic acid may be used and can show ventilation defects in patients with lobar or segmental bronchial occlusion.[144] Several case reports have also described the use of positron emission tomographic (PET) scans in patients with fibrosing mediastinitis. Imran et al. reported the majority of the lesion to be hypometabolic with focal areas of increased metabolic activity.[152] In a subsequent report, however, Chong et al. found that no fluorine-18 fluorodeoxyglucose (FDG) uptake was seen in a patient with a right paratracheal mass related to fibrosing mediastinitis.[153] The authors suggested that these contrasting findings may be related to different stages of disease (as proposed by Flieder).[107] Interestingly, a recent case report found a patient with fibrosing mediastinitis had increased FDG uptake and that this signal intensity diminished significantly after successful treatment.[154] Though further investigation is required, this report suggests that in addition to patient symptomatology and physical exam, PET scanning may allow for an objective assessment of treatment response.

DIAGNOSIS

The major aims of diagnostic interventions are to establish that the process is benign and determine the cause, if possible. Because chest radiographs of fibrosing mediastinitis are nonspecific and MRI depicts calcifications poorly, a CT scan is considered the mainstay in diagnosis.[116] Bronchoscopy with EBUS-guided transbronchial needle aspiration and mediastinoscopy are first-line options for tissue diagnosis, but thoracotomy or video-assisted thoracic surgery may be necessary to establish the benign nature of the fibrosis. Cervical mediastinoscopy in the setting of superior vena cava obstruction may carry a higher bleeding risk given robust venous collaterals, but can be performed safely.[155] Esophagography with contrast is indicated when dysphagia is a major complaint. Once the diagnosis has been established, CT or MRI plays an important role in defining the extent of disease, particularly if surgical resection is being considered.

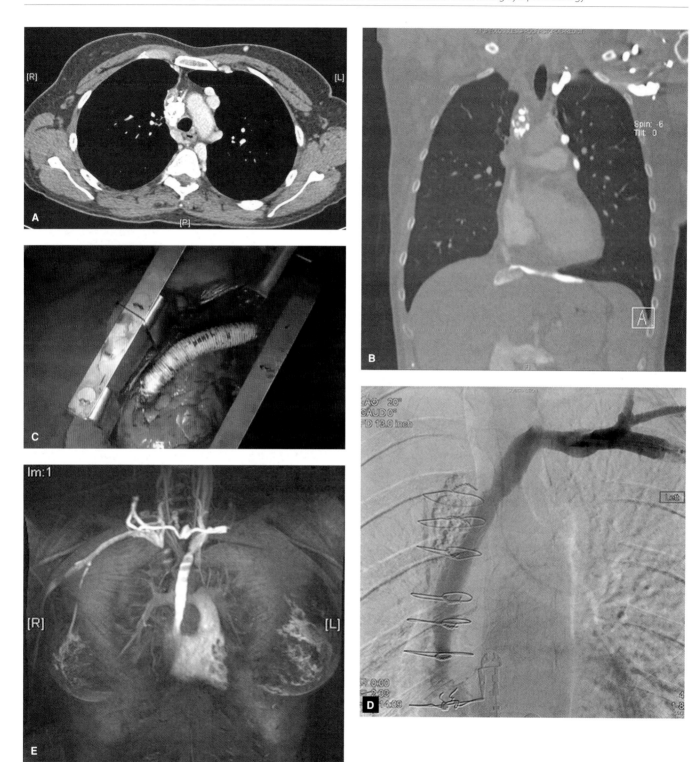

FIGURE 157.8 Fibrosing mediastinitis causing SVCS. **A:** An adult woman presented with headaches, facial swelling, chest and upper extremity varicosities, and syncope. CT scan of the chest demonstrated a large, calcified right paratracheal mass resulting in complete obstruction of the SVC. *Arrows* depict venous collaterals. H, Histoplasmoma; A, Azygos vein; Ao, Aortic Arch. **B:** Imaging also revealed numerous collaterals including the pericardial and phrenic vessels shown here. **C:** The patient was treated operatively with a bypass procedure from the left brachiocephalic vein to the right atrial appendage using a 14-mm ring-reinforced polytetrafluoroethylene graft. **D:** Postoperative venogram demonstrated patency of the bypass graft from the left brachiocephalic vein. **E:** Filling of the right heart through the patent bypass graft was further demonstrated using magnetic resonance venography.

Increasing serial titers are suggestive of a continuing subacute process, though not diagnostic. Cultures and histologic examination of any biopsy material for fungal and acid-fast organisms are essential but are often unrewarding. Skin testing for mycobacterial and fungal diseases is indicated, as are complement fixation studies for histoplasmosis, coccidioidomycosis, and blastomycosis.

TREATMENT

Fibrosing mediastinitis usually takes an unpredictable course, with either spontaneous remission or exacerbation of symptoms being reported. Most patients, particularly those with SVCS, improve with time as collateral venous circulation develops. Three general approaches to treatment are possible: (a) medical management with systemic antifungals or corticosteroids, (b) surgical resection, and (c) local therapy for complications.

Treatment with corticosteroids is supported by limited data from case reports or small series, with no prospective, randomized, controlled trials performed to date. While some studies have supported the use of systemic antifungal agents, others have found these to be ineffective.[110,111,114,120,138] Due to variability in patient response to steroid therapy, some have suggested using histologic and serologic factors, such as IgG4-positive plasma cells in mediastinal tissue and elevated IgG4 serum levels, as an indicator for likely successful steroid administration.[156] The limited data suggest that ketoconazole may stabilize the disease process or improve symptoms minimally, though some have disputed this.[106] Others have documented cases of fibrosing mediastinitis in which the addition of tamoxifen improved symptoms.[139,157] Successful treatment of fibrosing mediastinitis due to M. tuberculosis with multidrug antibiotic therapy has also been reported.[158]

Symptomatic patients can also be treated with local endoscopic or endovascular therapies directed toward reopening occluded or stenotic airways, pulmonary arteries/veins, or the vena cava. Laser therapy, balloon dilation, and endovascular, bronchial, or esophageal stents have all had some success.[159–162] Several studies have found that percutaneous placement of endovascular stents in patients with fibrosing mediastinitis resulted in improvements in both hemodynamic parameters, including pressure gradients and vessel size, and clinical symptoms.[163,164] Though reinterventions and morbidity were not uncommon, these studies suggest that endovascular interventions may have an important role in the management of patients with fibrosing mediastinitis.

Surgical resection of localized obstructing disease can be curative or result in amelioration of signs and symptoms.[108,110,120] However, overall results have been disappointing, with an associated high morbidity and as high as 50% mortality in cases requiring pneumectomy. With isolated SVCS, if no improvement occurs with time, some have recommended median sternotomy and superior vena cava bypass to relieve the distressing symptoms.[165] Autologous spiral saphenous vein or 10- to 20-mm reinforced expanded polytetrafluoroethylene grafts are typically used to bypass either a focal histoplasmoma or diffuse mediastinal fibrosis. Inflow is typically achieved from one or both brachiocephalic veins, though a patent bypass from one side provides adequate relief from SVCS and requires only two anastomoses. Access to the SVC–right atrial junction is frequently difficult as the fibrosis tethers together the SVC, azygos vein, and posterior pericardium. The right atrial appendage is the favored landing zone for the central anastomosis for this reason (Fig. 157.8).

Surgery may also be necessary in progressive, resistant cases to relieve tracheal or esophageal compression. Lung resection may be required to eradicate persistent post-obstructive infections due to bronchial stenoses.

PROGNOSIS

Fibrosing mediastinitis has historically been reported to have a mortality rate as high as 30%.[106] However, a recent retrospective analysis found that overall survival may actually be similar to that of age-matched controls, with previous studies potentially affected by publication bias.[114] When death does occur, frequent causes include recurrent infections, hemoptysis, or cor pulmonale. The mortality rates in patients with subcarinal or bilateral mediastinal involvement are higher than in those with localized disease. Unfortunately, the health of many surviving patients is severely compromised as a result of this disease process.

REFERENCES

1. Culliford AT, Cunningham JN, Jr., Zeff RH, et al. Sternal and costochondral infections following open-heart surgery. A review of 2,594 cases. *J Thorac Cardiovasc Surg* 1976;72(5):714–726.
2. Stoney WS, Alford WC, Jr, Burrus GR, et al. Median sternotomy dehiscence. *Ann Thorac Surg* 1978;26(5):421–426.
3. Gardlund B, Bitkover CY, Vaage J. Postoperative mediastinitis in cardiac surgery—microbiology and pathogenesis. *Eur J Cardiothorac Surg* 2002;21(5):825–830.
4. San Juan R, Chaves F, López Gude MJ, et al. Staphylococcus aureus poststernotomy mediastinitis: description of two distinct acquisition pathways with different potential preventive approaches. *J Thorac Cardiovasc Surg* 2007;134(3):670–676.
5. Charbonneau H, Maillet JM, Faron M, et al. Mediastinitis due to Gram-negative bacteria is associated with increased mortality. *Clin Microbiol Infect* 2014;20(3):O197–O202.
6. Francel TJ, Kouchoukos NT. A rational approach to wound difficulties after sternotomy: the problem. *Ann Thorac Surg* 2001;72(4):1411–1418.
7. El Oakley RM, Wright JE. Postoperative mediastinitis: classification and management. *Ann Thorac Surg* 1996;61(3):1030–1036.
8. Yamashiro T, Kamiya H, Murayama S, et al. Infectious mediastinitis after cardiovascular surgery: role of computed tomography. *Radiat Med* 2008;26(6):343–347.
9. Deniz H, Gokaslan G, Arslanoglu Y, et al. Treatment outcomes of postoperative mediastinitis in cardiac surgery; negative pressure wound therapy versus conventional treatment. *J Cardiothorac Surg* 2012;7:67.
10. Petzina R, Hoffmann J, Navasardyan A, et al. Negative pressure wound therapy for post-sternotomy mediastinitis reduces mortality rate and sternal re-infection rate compared to conventional treatment. *Eur J Cardiothorac Surg* 2010;38(1):110–113.
11. Vos RJ, Yilmaz A, Sonker U, et al. Vacuum-assisted closure of post-sternotomy mediastinitis as compared to open packing. *Interact Cardiovasc Thorac Surg* 2012;14(1):17–21.
12. Douville EC, Asaph JW, Dworkin RJ, et al. Sternal preservation: a better way to treat most sternal wound complications after cardiac surgery. *Ann Thorac Surg* 2004;78(5):1659–1664.
13. Jones G, Jurkiewicz MJ, Bostwick J, et al. Management of the infected median sternotomy wound with muscle flaps. *Ann Surg* 1997;225(6):766–778.
14. Roh TS, Lee WJ, Lew DH, et al. Pectoralis major-rectus abdominis bipedicled muscle flap in the treatment of poststernotomy mediastinitis. *J Thorac Cardiovasc Surg* 2008;136(3):618–622.
15. Milano CA, Georgiade G, Muhlbaier LH, et al. Comparison of omental and pectoralis flaps for poststernotomy mediastinitis. *Ann Thorac Surg* 1999;67(2):377–380.
16. Yasuura K, Okamoto H, Morita S, et al. Results of omental flap transposition for deep sternal wound infection after cardiovascular surgery. *Ann Surg* 1998;227(3):455–459.
17. Brandt C, Alvarez JM. First-line treatment of deep sternal infection by a plastic surgical approach: superior results compared with conventional cardiac surgical orthodoxy. *Plast Reconstr Surg* 2002;109(7):2231–2237.
18. Karra R, McDermott L, Connelly S, et al. Risk factors for 1-year mortality after postoperative mediastinitis. *J Thorac Cardiovasc Surg* 2006;132(3):537–543.
19. Merrill WH, Akhter SA, Wolf RK, et al. Simplified treatment of postoperative mediastinitis. *Ann Thorac Surg* 2004;78(2):608–612.
20. Molina JE, Nelson EC, Smith RRA. Treatment of postoperative sternal dehiscence with mediastinitis: twenty-four-year use of a single method. *J Thorac Cardiovasc Surg* 2006;132(4):782–787.
21. Rand RP, Cochran RP, Aziz S, et al. Prospective trial of catheter irrigation and muscle flaps for sternal wound infection. *Ann Thorac Surg* 1998;65(4):1046–1049.
22. Hirata N, Hatsuoka S, Amemiya A, et al. New strategy for treatment of MRSA mediastinitis: one-stage procedure for omental transposition and closed irrigation. *Ann Thorac Surg* 2003;76(6):2104–2106.
23. Trouillet J-L, Vuagnat A, Combes A, et al. Acute poststernotomy mediastinitis managed with debridement and closed-drainage aspiration: factors associated with death in the intensive care unit. *J Thorac Cardiovasc Surg* 2005;129(3):518–524.
24. Kirsch M, Mekontso-Dessap A, Houël R, et al. Closed drainage using Redon catheters for poststernotomy mediastinitis: results and risk factors for adverse outcome. *Ann Thorac Surg* 2001;71(5):1580–1586.
25. Vos RJ, Yilmaz A, Sonker U, et al. Primary closure using Redon drains vs vacuum-assisted closure in post-sternotomy mediastinitis. *Eur J CardioThorac Surg* 2012;42(4):e53–e57.
26. Vos RJ, van Putte BP, Sonker U, et al. Primary closure using Redon drains for the treatment of post-sternotomy mediastinitis. *Interact Cardiovasc Thorac Surg* 2014;18(1):33–37.

27. Calvat S, Trouillet J-L, Natal P, et al. Closed drainage using Redon catheters for local treatment of poststernotomy mediastinitis. *Ann Thorac Surg* 1996;61(1):195–201.

28. Argenta LC, Morykwas MJ. Vacuum-assisted closure: a new method for wound control and treatment. *Ann Plast Surg* 1997;38(6):563–577.

29. Fuchs U, Zittermann A, Stuettgen B, et al. Clinical outcome of patients with deep sternal wound infection managed by vacuum-assisted closure compared to conventional therapy with open packing: a retrospective analysis. *Ann Thorac Surg* 2005;79(2):526–531.

30. Luckraz H, Murphy F, Bryant S, et al. Vacuum-assisted closure as a treatment modality for infections after cardiac surgery. *J Thorac Cardiovasc Surg* 2003;125(2):301–305.

31. Doss M, Martens S, Wood JP, et al. Vacuum-assisted suction drainage versus conventional treatment in the management of poststernotomy osteomyelitis. *Eur J Cardiothorac Surg* 2002;22(6):934–938.

32. Obdeijn MC, de Lange MY, Lichtendahl DHE, et al. Vacuum-assisted closure in the treatment of poststernotomy mediastinitis. *Ann Thorac Surg* 1999;68(6):2358–2360.

33. Cowan KN, Teague L, Sue SC, et al. Vacuum-assisted wound closure of deep sternal infections in high-risk patients after cardiac surgery. *Ann Thorac Surg* 2005;80(6):2205–2212.

34. Domkowski PW, Smith ML, Gonyon DL, et al. Evaluation of vacuum-assisted closure in the treatment of poststernotomy mediastinitis. *J Thorac Cardiovasc Surg* 2003;126(2):386–389.

35. Sjögren J, Gustafsson R, Nilsson J, et al. Clinical outcome after poststernotomy mediastinitis: vacuum-assisted closure versus conventional treatment. *Ann Thorac Surg* 2005;79(6):2049–2055.

36. Sjögren J, Malmsjö M, Gustafsson R, et al. Poststernotomy mediastinitis: a review of conventional surgical treatments, vacuum-assisted closure therapy and presentation of the Lund University Hospital mediastinitis algorithm. *Eur J Cardiothorac Surg* 2006;30(6):898–905.

37. Sjögren J, Nilsson J, Gustafsson R, et al. The impact of vacuum-assisted closure on long-term survival after post-sternotomy mediastinitis. *Ann Thorac Surg* 2005; 80(4):1270–1275.

38. Ennker IC, Malkoc A, Pietrowski D, et al. The concept of negative pressure wound therapy (NPWT) after poststernotomy mediastinitis—a single center experience with 54 patients. *J Cardiothorac Surg* 2009;4(5):5.

39. Ennker IC, Pietrowski D, Vohringer L, et al. Surgical debridement, vacuum therapy and pectoralis plasty in poststernotomy mediastinitis. *J Plast Reconstr Aesthet Surg* 2009;62(11):1479–1483.

40. Salica A, Weltert L, Scaffa R, et al. Negative pressure wound treatment improves Acute Physiology and Chronic Health Evaluation II score in mediastinitis allowing a successful elective pectoralis muscle flap closure: six-year experience of a single protocol. *J Thorac Cardiovasc Surg* 2014;148(5):2397–2403.

41. De Feo M, Della Corte A, Vicchio M, et al. Is post-sternotomy mediastinitis still devastating after the advent of negative-pressure wound therapy?. *Tex Heart Inst J* 2011;38(4):375–380.

42. Angela WY, Rippel RA, Smock E, et al. In patients with post-sternotomy mediastinitis is vacuum-assisted closure superior to conventional therapy? *Interact Cardiovasc Thorac Surg* 2013;17(5):861–865.

43. Catarino PA, Chamberlain MH, Wright NC, et al. High-pressure suction drainage via a polyurethane foam in the management of poststernotomy mediastinitis. *Ann Thorac Surg* 2000;70(6):1891–1895.

44. Petzina R, Malmsjo M, Stamm C, et al. Major complications during negative pressure wound therapy in poststernotomy mediastinitis after cardiac surgery. *J Thorac Cardiovasc Surg* 2010;140(5):1133–1136.

45. Ingemansson R, Malmsjo M, Lindstedt S. A protective device for negative-pressure therapy in patients with mediastinitis. *Ann Thorac Surg* 2013;95(1):362–364.

46. Galanti A, Triggiani M, Tasca G, et al. Treatment of mediastinitis by ventrofil plates without sternal rewiring. *Ann Thorac Surg* 2014;97(5):1816–1818.

47. Braxton JH, Marrin CAS, McGrath PD, et al. Mediastinitis and long-term survival after coronary artery bypass graft surgery. *Ann Thorac Surg* 2000;70(6):2004–2007.

48. Stahle E, Tammelin A, Bergstrom R, et al. Sternal wound complications–incidence, microbiology and risk factors. *Eur J Cardiothorac Surg* 1997;11(6):1146–1153.

49. Mekontso Dessap A, Vivier E, Girou E, et al. Effect of time to onset on clinical features and prognosis of post-sternotomy mediastinitis. *Clin Microbiol Infect* 2011;17(2):292–299.

50. Gabor S, Renner H, Pinter H, et al. Indications for surgery in tracheobronchial ruptures. *Eur J Cardiothorac Surg* 2001;20(2):399–404.

51. Jones WG, Ginsberg RJ. Esophageal perforation: a continuing challenge. *Ann Thorac Surg* 1992;53(3):534–543.

52. Whyte RI, Iannettoni MD, Orringer MB. Intrathoracic esophageal perforation: the merit of primary repair. *J Thorac Cardiovasc Surg* 1995;109(1):140–146.

53. Wright CD, Mathisen DJ, Wain JC, et al. Reinforced primary repair of thoracic esophageal perforation. *Ann Thorac Surg* 1995;60(2):245–249.

54. Engum SA, Grosfeld JL, West KW, et al. Improved survival in children with esophageal perforation. *Arch Surg* 1996;131(6):604–610; discussion 611.

55. Bufkin BL, Miller JI, Mansour KA. Esophageal perforation: emphasis on management. *Ann Thorac Surg* 1996;61(5):1447–1452.

56. Iannettoni MD, Vlessis AA, Whyte RI, et al. Functional outcome after surgical treatment of esophageal perforation. *Ann Thorac Surg* 1997;64(6):1606–1610.

57. Burnett CM, Rosemurgy AS, Pfeiffer EA. Life-threatening acute posterior mediastinitis due to esophageal perforation. *Ann Thorac Surg* 1990;49(6):979–983.

58. Estrera AS, Landay MJ, Grisham JM, et al. Descending necrotizing mediastinitis. *Surg Gynecol Obstet* 1983;157(6):545–552.

59. Marty-Ane CH, Alauzen M, Alric P, et al. Descending necrotizing mediastinitis. Advantage of mediastinal drainage with thoracotomy. *J Thorac Cardiovasc Surg* 1994;107(1):55–61.

60. Wheatley MJ, Stirling MC, Kirsh MM, et al. Descending necrotizing mediastinitis: transcervical drainage is not enough. *Ann Thorac Surg* 1990;49(5):780–784.

61. Marty-Ané C-H, Berthet J-P, Alric P, et al. Management of descending necrotizing mediastinitis: an aggressive treatment for an aggressive disease. *Ann Thorac Surg* 1999;68(1):212–217.

62. Corsten MJ, Shamji FM, Odell PF, et al. Optimal treatment of descending necrotising mediastinitis. *Thorax* 1997;52(8):702–708.

63. Chong WH, Woodhead MA, Millard FJ. Mediastinitis and bilateral thoracic empyemas complicating adult epiglottitis. *Thorax* 1990;45(6):491–492.

64. Aerts JGJV, Kloover J, Los J, et al. EUS-FNA of enlarged necrotic lymph nodes may cause infectious mediastinitis. *J Thorac Oncol* 2008;3(10):1191–1193.

65. Parker KL, Bizekis CS, Zervos MD. Severe mediastinal infection with abscess formation after endobronchial ultrasound-guided transbrochial needle aspiration. *Ann Thorac Surg* 2010;89(4):1271–1272.

66. Guardia SN, Cameron R, Phillips A. Fatal necrotizing mediastinitis secondary to acute suppurative parotitis. *J Otolaryngol* 1991;20(1):54–56.

67. Uram J, Hauser MS. Deep neck and mediastinal necrotizing infection secondary to a traumatic intubation: report of a case. *J Oral Maxillofac Surg* 1988;46(9):788–791.

68. Gould K, Barnett JA, Sanford JP. Purulent pericarditis in the antibiotic era. *Arch Intern Med* 1974;134(5):923–927.

69. Alsoub H, Chacko KC. Descending necrotising mediastinitis. *Postgrad Med J* 1995;71(832):98–101.

70. Gorlitzer M, Grabenwoeger M, Meinhart J, et al. Descending necrotizing mediastinitis treated with rapid sternotomy followed by vacuum-assisted therapy. *Ann Thorac Surg* 2007;83(2):393–396.

71. Moncada R, Warpeha R, Pickleman J, et al. Mediastinitis from odontogenic and deep cervical infection. Anatomic pathways of propagation. *Chest* 1978;73(4):497–500.

72. Papalia E, Rena O, Oliaro A, et al. Descending necrotizing mediastinitis: surgical management. *Eur J Cardiothorac Surg* 2001;20(4):739–742.

73. Min H-K, Choi YS, Shim YM, et al. Descending necrotizing mediastinitis: a minimally invasive approach using video-assisted thoracoscopic surgery. *Ann Thorac Surg* 2004;77(1):306–310.

74. Kinzer S, Pfeiffer J, Becker S, et al. Severe deep neck space infections and mediastinitis of odontogenic origin: clinical relevance and implications for diagnosis and treatment. *Acta Otolaryngol* 2009;129(1):62–70.

75. McCurdy JA, Jr., MacInnis EL, Hays LL. Fatal mediastinitis after a dental infection. *J Oral Surg* 1977;35(9):726–729.

76. Ridder GJ, Maier W, Kinzer S, et al. Descending necrotizing mediastinitis: contemporary trends in etiology, diagnosis, management, and outcome. *Ann Surg* 2010;251(3):528–534.

77. Chow AW. Infections of the oral cavity, neck, and head. In: Mandell GL, Bennett JE, Dolin R, eds. *Principles and Practice of Infectious Diseases.* Elsevier BV; 2010: 855–871.

78. Brook I, Frazier EH. Microbiology of mediastinitis. *Arch Intern Med* 1996;156(3): 333–336.

79. Chen KC, Chen JS, Kuo SW, et al. Descending necrotizing mediastinitis: a 10-year surgical experience in a single institution. *J Thorac Cardiovasc Surg* 2008; 136(1):191–198.

80. Mathieu D, Neviere R, Teillon C, et al. Cervical necrotizing fasciitis: clinical manifestations and management. *Clin Infect Dis* 1995;21(1):51–56.

81. Roccia F, Pecorari GC, Oliaro A, et al. Ten years of descending necrotizing mediastinitis: management of 23 cases. *J Oral Maxillofac Surg* 2007;65(9):1716–1724.

82. Kiernan PD, Hernandez A, Byrne WD, et al. Descending cervical mediastinitis. *Ann Thorac Surg* 1998;65(5):1483–1488.

83. Carrol CL, Jeffrey RB, Federle MP, et al. CT evaluation of mediastinal infections. *J Comput Assist Tomogr* 1987;11(3):449–454.

84. Breatnach E, Nath PH, Delany DJ. The role of computed tomography in acute and subacute mediastinitis. *Clin Radiol* 1986;37(2):139–145.

85. Gonzalez-Garcia R, Risco-Rojas R, Roman-Romero L, et al. Descending necrotizing mediastinitis following dental extraction. Radiological features and surgical treatment considerations. *J Craniomaxillofac Surg* 2011;39(5):335–339.

86. Karkas A, Chahine K, Schmerber S, et al. Optimal treatment of cervical necrotizing fasciitis associated with descending necrotizing mediastinitis. *Br J Surg* 2010;97(4):609–615.

87. Sandner A, Borgermann J. Update on necrotizing mediastinitis: causes, approaches to management, and outcomes. *Curr Infect Dis Rep* 2011;13(3):278–286.

88. Temes R, Crowell R, Mapel D, et al. Mediastinitis without antecedent surgery. *Thorac Cardiovasc Surg* 1998;46(02):84–88.

89. Misthos P, Katsaragakis S, Kakaris S, et al. Descending necrotizing anterior mediastinitis: analysis of survival and surgical treatment modalities. *J Oral Maxillofac Surg* 2007;65(4):635–639.

90. Shimizu K, Otani Y, Nakano T, et al. Successful video-assisted mediastinoscopic drainage of descending necrotizing mediastinitis. *Ann Thorac Surg* 2006; 81(6):2279–2281.

91. Cho JS, Kim YD, Hoseok I, et al. Treatment of mediastinitis using video-assisted thoracoscopic surgery. *Eur J Cardiothorac Surg* 2008;34(3):520–524.

92. Kozuki A, Shinozaki H, Tajima A, et al. Successful treatment for descending necrotizing mediastinitis with severe thoracic emphysema using video-assisted thoracoscopic surgery. *Gen Thorac Cardiovasc Surg* 2010;58(11):584–587.

93. Isowa N, Yamada T, Kijima T, et al. Successful thoracoscopic debridement of descending necrotizing mediastinitis. *Ann Thorac Surg* 2004;77(5):1834–1837.

94. Roberts JR, Smythe WR, Weber RW, et al. Thoracoscopic management of descending necrotizing mediastinitis. *Chest* 1997;112(3):850–854.

95. Gobien RP, Stanley JH, Gobien BS, et al. Percutaneous catheter aspiration and drainage of suspected mediastinal abscesses. *Radiology* 1984;151(1):69–71.

96. Singhal P, Kejriwal N, Lin Z, et al. Optimal surgical management of descending necrotising mediastinitis: our experience and review of literature. *Heart Lung Circ* 2008;17(2):124–128.

97. Iwata T, Sekine Y, Shibuya K, et al. Early open thoracotomy and mediastinopleural irrigation for severe descending necrotizing mediastinitis. *Eur J Cardiothorac Surg* 2005;28(3):384–388.

98. Sancho LM, Minamoto H, Fernandez A, et al. Descending necrotizing mediastinitis: a retrospective surgical experience. *Eur J Cardiothorac Surg* 1999;16(2):200–205.

99. Curtis JJ, Clark NC, McKenney CA, et al. Tracheostomy: a risk factor for mediastinitis after cardiac operation. *Ann Thorac Surg* 2001;72(3):731–734.

100. Gaudino M, Losasso G, Anselmi A, et al. Is early tracheostomy a risk factor for mediastinitis after median sternotomy?. *J Card Surg* 2009;24(6):632–636.

101. Morgan DE, Nath H, Sanders C, et al. Mediastinal actinomycosis. *Am J Roentgenol* 1990;155(4):735–737.

102. Pitchenik AE, Rubinson HA. The radiographic appearance of tuberculosis in patients with the acquired immune deficiency syndrome (AIDS) and pre-AIDS. *Am Rev Respir Dis* 1985;131(3):393–396.

103. Bitran J, Bekerman C, Weinstein R, et al. Patterns of gallium-67 scintigraphy in patients with acquired immunodeficiency syndrome and the AIDS related complex. *J Nucl Med* 1987;28(7):1103–1106.

104. Mehta AC, Spies WG, Spies SM. Utility of gallium scintigraphy in AIDS. *Radiological Society of North America 73rd Scientific Assembly and Annual Meeting (Abstracts).* 1987.

105. Spies WG. Radionuclide studies of the mediastinum. In: Shields TW, ed. *Mediastinal Surgery.* Philadelphia, PA: Lea & Febiger; 1991.

106. Loyd JE, Tillman BF, Atkinson JB, et al. Mediastinal fibrosis complicating histoplasmosis. *Medicine* 1988;67(5):295–310.

107. Flieder DB, Suster S, Moran CA. Idiopathic fibroinflammatory (fibrosing/sclerosing) lesions of the mediastinum: a study of 30 cases with emphasis on morphologic heterogeneity. *Mod Pathol* 1999;12(3):257–264.

108. Garrett HE, Roper CL. Surgical intervention in histoplasmosis. *Ann Thorac Surg* 1986;42(6):711–722.

109. Goodwin RA, Nickell JA, Des Prez RM. Mediastinal fibrosis complicating healed primary histoplasmosis and tuberculosis. *Medicine (Baltimore)* 1972;51(3):227–246.

110. Mathisen DJ, Grillo HC. Clinical manifestation of mediastinal fibrosis and histoplasmosis. *Ann Thorac Surg* 1992;54(6):1053–1058.

111. Urschel HC, Razzuk MA, Netto GJ, et al. Sclerosing mediastinitis: improved management with histoplasmosis titer and ketoconazole. *Ann Thorac Surg* 1990;50(2):215–221.

112. Wieder S, Rabinowitz JG. Fibrous mediastinitis: a late manifestation of mediastinal histoplasmosis 1. *Radiology* 1977;125(2):305–312.

113. Wieder S, White TJ, Salazar J, et al. Pulmonary artery occlusion due to histoplasmosis. *Am J Roentgenol* 1982;138(2):243–251.

114. Peikert T, Colby TV, Midthun DE, et al. Fibrosing mediastinitis: clinical presentation, therapeutic outcomes, and adaptive immune response. *Medicine (Baltimore)* 2011;90(6):412–423.

115. Eggleston JC. Sclerosing mediastinitis. In: Fenoglio CM, Wolff, M, eds. *Progress in Surgical Pathology.* Vol 2. New York: Masson; 1980.

116. Rossi SE, McAdams HP, Rosado-de-Christenson ML, et al. Fibrosing mediastinitis. *Radiographics* 2001;21(3):737–757.

117. Baum GL, Green RA, Schwarz J. Enlarging pulmonary histoplasmoma. *Am Rev Respir Dis* 1960;82:721–726.

118. Marchevsky AM, Kaneko M. *Surgical Pathology of the Mediastinum.* 2nd ed. New York: Raven Press; 1992.

119. Sherrick AD, Brown LR, Harms GF, et al. The radiographic findings of fibrosing mediastinitis. *Chest* 1994;106(2):484–489.

120. Dunn EJ, Ulicny KS, Jr., Wright CB, et al. Surgical implications of sclerosing mediastinitis. A report of six cases and review of the literature. *Chest* 1990;97(2):338–346.

121. Dines DE, Payne WS, Bernatz PE, et al. Mediastinal granuloma and fibrosing mediastinitis. *Chest* 1979;75(3):320–324.

122. Dechambre S, Dorzee J, Fastrez J, et al. Bronchial stenosis and sclerosing mediastinitis: an uncommon complication of external thoracic radiotherapy. *Eur Respir J* 1998;11(5):1188–1190.

123. Lagerstrom CF, Mitchell HG, Graham BS, et al. Chronic fibrosing mediastinitis and superior vena caval obstruction from blastomycosis. *Ann Thorac Surg* 1992;54(4):764–765.

124. Lee JY, Kim Y, Lee KS, et al. Tuberculous fibrosing mediastinitis: radiologic findings. *Am J Roentgenol* 1996;167(6):1598–1599.

125. Othmani S, Bahri M, Louzir B, et al. Mediastinal fibrosis combined with Behcet's disease. Three case reports. *Rev Med Interne* 2000;21(4):330–336.

126. Mole TM, Glover J, Sheppard MN. Sclerosing mediastinitis: a report on 18 cases. *Thorax* 1995;50(3):280–283.

127. Fenner MN, Moran JP, Jr., Dillon JC, et al. Retroperitoneal fibrosis and sclerosing mediastinitis. *Indiana Med* 1987;80(4):334–338.

128. Morgan AD, Loughridge L, Calne RY. Combined mediastinal and retroperitoneal fibrosis. *Lancet* 1966;287(7428):67–70.

129. Peikert T, Shrestha B, Aubry MC, et al. Histopathologic overlap between Fibrosing mediastinitis and IgG4-related disease. *Int J Rheumatol* 2012;2012:207056.

130. Devaraj A, Griffin N, Nicholson AG, et al. Computed tomography findings in Fibrosing mediastinitis. *Clin Radiol* 2007;62(8):781–786.

131. Worrell JA, Donnelly EF, Martin JB, et al. Computed tomography and the idiopathic form of proliferative fibrosing mediastinitis. *J Thorac Imaging* 2007;22(3):235–240.

132. Meredith SD, Madison J, Fechner RE, et al. Cervical manifestations of fibrosing mediastinitis: a diagnostic and therapeutic dilemma. *Head Neck* 1993;15(6):561–565.

133. Kountz PD, Molina PL, Sagel SS. Fibrosing mediastinitis in the posterior thorax. *Am J Roentgenol* 1989;153(3):489–490.

134. Razzuk MA, Urschel HC, Paulson DL. Systemic mycoses—primary pathogenic fungi. *Ann Thorac Surg* 1973;15(6):644–660.

135. Feigin DS, Eggleston JC, Siegelman SS. The multiple roentgen manifestations of sclerosing mediastinitis. *Johns Hopkins Med J* 1979;144(1):1–8.

136. Kalweit G, Huwer H, Straub U, et al. Mediastinal compression syndromes due to idiopathic fibrosing mediastinitis—report of three cases and review of the literature. *Thorac Cardiovasc Surg* 1996;44(02):105–109.

137. Cochrane A, Warren R, Mullerworth M, et al. Fibrosing mediastinitis with coronary artery involvement. *Ann Thorac Surg* 1991;51(4):652–654.

138. Ikeda K, Nomori H, Mori T, et al. Successful steroid treatment for fibrosing mediastinitis and sclerosing cervicitis. *Ann Thorac Surg* 2007;83(3):1199–1201.

139. Bays S, Rajakaruna C, Sheffield E, et al. Fibrosing mediastinitis as a cause of superior vena cava syndrome. *Eur J Cardiothorac Surg* 2004;26(2):453–455.

140. Espinosa RE, Edwards WD, Rosenow EC, et al. Idiopathic pulmonary hilar fibrosis: an unusual cause of pulmonary hypertension. *Mayo Clin Proc* 1993;68(8):778–782.

141. Berry DF, Buccigrossi D, Peabody J, et al. Pulmonary vascular occlusion and fibrosing mediastinitis. *Chest* 1986;89(2):296–301.

142. Chazova I, Robbins I, Loyd J, et al. Venous and arterial changes in pulmonary veno-occlusive disease, mitral stenosis and fibrosing mediastinitis. *Eur Respir J* 2000;15(1):116–122.

143. Williamson WA, Tronic BS, Levitan N, et al. Pulmonary venous infarction secondary to squamous cell carcinoma. *Chest* 1992;102(3):950–952.

144. McAdams HP. Chest case of the day. Fibrosing mediastinitis. *Am J Roentgenol* 1995;165(1):189–190.

145. Katzenstein AL, Mazur MT. Pulmonary infarct: an unusual manifestation of fibrosing mediastinitis. *Chest* 1980;77(4):521–524.

146. Williams SM, Jones ET. General case of the day. Allergic (or hypersensitivity) bronchopulmonary aspergillosis (ABPA). *RadioGraphics* 1997;17(6):1597–1600.

147. Rodríguez E, Soler R, Pombo F, et al. Fibrosing mediastinitis: CT and MR findings. *Clin Radiol* 1998;53(12):907–910.

148. Weinstein JB, Aronberg DJ, Sagel SS. CT of fibrosing mediastinitis: findings and their utility. *Am J Roentgenol* 1983;141(2):247–251.

149. Ramakantan R, Shah P. Dysphagia due to mediastinal fibrosis in advanced pulmonary tuberculosis. *Am J Roentgenol* 1990;154(1):61–63.

150. Goenka MK, Gupta NM, Kochhar R, et al. Mediastinal fibrosis. *J Clin Gastroenterol* 1995;20(4):331–332.

151. Moreno AJ, Weismann I, Billingsley JL, et al. Angiographic and scintigraphic findings in fibrosing mediastinitis. *Clin Nucl Med* 1983;8(4):167–169.

152. Imran MB, Kubota K, Yoshioka S, et al. Sclerosing mediastinitis: findings on fluorine-18 fluorodeoxyglucose positron emission tomography. *Clin Nucl Med* 1999;24(5):305–308.

153. Chong S, Kim TS, Kim BT, et al. Fibrosing mediastinitis mimicking malignancy at CT: negative FDG uptake in integrated FDG PET/CT imaging. *Eur Radiol* 2007;17(6):1644–1646.

154. Takalkar AM, Bruno GL, Makanjoula AJ, et al. A potential role for F-18 FDG PET/CT in evaluation and management of fibrosing mediastinitis. *Clin Nucl Med* 2007;32(9):703–706.

155. Jahangiri M, Goldstraw P. The role of mediastinoscopy in superior vena caval obstruction. *Ann Thorac Surg* 1995;59(2):453–455.

156. Inoue M, Nose N, Nishikawa H, et al. Successful treatment of sclerosing mediastinitis with a high serum IgG4 level. *Gen Thorac Cardiovasc Surg* 2007;55(10):431–433.

157. Savelli BA, Parshley M, Morganroth ML. Successful treatment of sclerosing cervicitis and fibrosing mediastinitis with tamoxifen. *Chest* 1997;111(4):1137–1140.

158. Zhang C, Yao M, Yu Z, et al. Rare fibrosing granulomatous mediastinitis of tuberculosis with involvement of the transverse sinus. *J Thorac Cardiovasc Surg* 2007;133(3):836–837.

159. Dodds GA, 3rd, Harrison JK, O'Laughlin MP, et al. Relief of superior vena cava syndrome due to fibrosing mediastinitis using the Palmaz stent. *Chest* 1994;106(1):315–318.

160. Kandzari DE, Warner JJ, O'Laughlin MP, et al. Percutaneous stenting of right pulmonary artery stenosis in fibrosing mediastinitis. *Catheter Cardiovasc Interv* 2000;49(3):321–324.

161. Sheski FD, Mathur PN. Long-term results of fiberoptic bronchoscopic balloon dilation in the management of benign tracheobronchial stenosis. *Chest* 1998;114(3):796–800.

162. Watkinson AF, Hansell DM. Expandable wallstent for the treatment of obstruction of the superior vena cava. *Thorax* 1993;48(9):915–920.

163. Albers EL, Pugh ME, Hill KD, et al. Percutaneous vascular stent implantation as treatment for central vascular obstruction due to fibrosing mediastinitis. *Circulation* 2011;123(13):1391–1399.

164. Ferguson ME, Cabalka AK, Cetta F, et al. Results of intravascular stent placement for fibrosing mediastinitis. *Congenit Heart Dis* 2010;5(2):124–133.

165. Doty DB, Doty JR, Jones KW. Bypass of superior vena cava. Fifteen years' experience with spiral vein graft for obstruction of superior vena cava caused by benign disease. *J Thorac Cardiovasc Surg* 1990;99(5):889–895; discussion 895–896.

SUGGESTED READINGS

Blomquist IK, Bayer AS. Life-threatening deep fascial space infections of the head and neck. *Infect Dis Clin North Am* 1988;2:237–264.

Demmy TL, Park SB, Liebler GA, et al. Recent experience with major sternal wound complications. *Ann Thorac Surg* 1990;49:458–462.

Dodds GA, 3rd, Harrison JK, O'Laughlin MP, et al. Relief of superior vena cava syndrome due to fibrosing mediastinitis using the Palmaz stent. *Chest* 1994;106(1):315–318.

Ehrenkranz NJ, Pfaff SJ. Mediastinitis complicating cardiac operations: evidence of postoperative causation. *Rev Infect Dis* 1991;13:803–814.

El Oakley RM, Wright JE. Postoperative mediastinitis: classification and management. *Ann Thorac Surg* 1996;61:1030–1036.

Estrera AS, Landay MJ, Grisham JM, et al. Descending necrotizing mediastinitis. *Surg Gynecol Obstet* 1983;157(6):545–552.

Farrington M, Webster M, Fenn A, et al. Study of cardiothoracic wound infection at St. Thomas Hospital. *Br J Surg* 1985;72:759–762.

Ferguson ME, Cabalka AK, Cetta F, et al. Results of intravascular stent placement for fibrosing mediastinitis. *Congenit Heart Dis* 2010;5(2):124–133.

Gottlieb LJ, Beahm EK, Krizek TJ, et al. Approaches to sternal wound infections. *Adv Card Surg* 1996;7:147–162.

Grossi EA, Culliford AT, Krieger KH, et al. A survey of 77 major infectious complications of median sternotomy: a review of 7,949 consecutive operative procedures. *Ann Thorac Surg* 1985;40:214–223.

Jones G, Jurkiewicz MJ, Bostwick J, et al. Management of the infected median sternotomy wound with muscle flaps. The Emory 20-year experience. *Ann Surg* 1997;225: 766–776.

Kohman LJ, Coleman MJ, Parker FB. Bacteremia and sternal infection after coronary artery bypass grafting. *Ann Thorac Surg* 1990;49:454–457.

Loop FD, Lytle BW, Cosgrove DM, et al. J. Maxwell Chamberlain memorial paper. Sternal wound complications after isolated coronary artery bypass grafting: early and late mortality, morbidity and cost of care. *Ann Thorac Surg* 1990;49:179–186.

Marty-Ané C-H, Berthet J-P, Alric P, et al. Management of descending necrotizing mediastinitis: an aggressive treatment for an aggressive disease. *Ann Thorac Surg* 1999;68(1):212–217.

Nagachinta T, Stephens M, Reitz B, et al. Risk factors for surgical wound infection following cardiac surgery. *J Infect Dis* 1987;156:967–973.

Ottino G, De Paulis R, Pansini S, et al. Major sternal wound infection after open-heart surgery: a multivariate analysis of risk factors in 2,579 consecutive operative procedures. *Ann Thorac Surg* 1987;44:173–179.

Ridder GJ, Maier W, Kinzer S, et al. Descending necrotizing mediastinitis: contemporary trends in etiology, diagnosis, management, and outcome. *Ann Surg* 2010;251(3):528–534.

Risnes I, Abdelnoor M, Almdahl SM, et al. Mediastinitis after coronary artery bypass grafting risk factors and long-term survival. *Ann Thorac Surg* 2010;89(5):1502–1509.

Santos GH, Shapiro BM, Komisar A. Role of transoral irrigation in mediastinitis due to hypopharyngeal perforation. *Head Neck Surg* 1986;9:116–121.

Sarr MG, Gott VL, Townsend TR. Mediastinal infection after cardiac surgery. *Ann Thorac Surg* 1984;38:415–423.

Smith JM, Glaser RS, Osborne BR, et al. Sternal wound complications after open heart surgery: results from 3,524 consecutive operative procedures. *Contemp Surg* 1993;43:197–202.

Primary Mediastinal Tumors and Cysts and Diagnostic Investigation of Mediastinal Masses

Francis C. Nichols

Mediastinal masses, while relatively uncommon, pose an interesting diagnostic and therapeutic challenge to thoracic surgeons. Mediastinal masses extend over a wide array of histopathologic and radiologic entities. Although they tend to be more common in young and middle-aged adults, numerous types of mediastinal tumors and cysts affect people of all age groups. Mediastinal masses may present in a variety of ways most commonly as a coincidental finding during routine radiographic examinations in an asymptomatic person. However, some patients are symptomatic at the time of presentation. Benign masses comprise the majority of mediastinal tumors and cysts and are usually asymptomatic, although depending on their size or location may be symptomatic. Malignant lesions are more likely to produce clinical findings, but they too can be asymptomatic.

The precise diagnosis of a mass in the mediastinum cannot be determined without histopathologic examination of the tissue. Nevertheless, a reasonable, preoperative diagnosis can often be established by considering the location of the mass in the mediastinum, its radiographic characteristics, the patient's age, the presence or absence of local or constitutional symptoms and signs, and its association with a specific systemic disease (e.g., Cushing's syndrome, myasthenia gravis).

MEDIASTINAL COMPARTMENTS

The compartmental division of the mediastinum has important implications in the diagnosis of mediastinal masses which have a predilection for specific compartments. The mediastinum is anatomically defined by the pleural cavities bilaterally, the thoracic inlet superiorly, and the diaphragm inferiorly. The anteroposterior mediastinal limits are the posterior surface of the sternum anteriorly and the anterior surface of the vertebral bodies posteriorly. The paravertebral (costovertebral) regions bilaterally should be included in any discussion of mediastinal masses. Historically, it has been easiest to divide the mediastinum into three compartments: anterior, middle (visceral), and posterior which includes the paravertebral sulci. The anterior mediastinum contains the thymus gland, internal mammary vessels, lymph nodes, connective tissue, and fat. The middle mediastinum contains the pericardium, heart and great vessels, trachea, proximal bronchi, esophagus, phrenic and vagus nerves, and lymph nodes. The posterior

mediastinum contains the autonomic ganglia and nerves, proximal portions of the intercostal vessels, lymph nodes, and fat. These historically defined compartments have been based on somewhat arbitrary landmarks on a lateral chest radiograph. Recently, the International Thymic Malignancy Interest Group (ITMIG) adopted a more modern computed tomography (CT)-based mediastinal division scheme.[1,2] The three ITMIG-defined mediastinal compartments include prevascular (anterior), visceral (middle), and paravertebral (posterior). Table 158.1 outlines the ITMIG mediastinal compartments, their boundaries, and major contents. Figure 158.1 demonstrates representative examples of mediastinal masses within the ITMIG-defined compartments.

Davis and colleagues[3] reported on 400 consecutive patients with primary mediastinal masses and found 54% located in the anterior mediastinum, 20% in the middle, and 26% in the posterior. Takeda and colleagues[4] reported similar mediastinal mass distributions for adults. In the series by Davis and colleagues,[3] 59%, 29%, and 16% of the anterior, middle, and posterior mediastinal masses, respectively, were malignant.

INCIDENCE

Primary mediastinal tumors and cysts are uncommon. Tables 158.2 and 158.3 summarize selected major reports in the American, European, and Japanese literature and give some insight into their incidence. A total of 3,735 adults and children are included in these reports from 1956 to 2003. Not included in that patient number are other reports dedicated to certain specific types of mediastinal tumors.

Perhaps a more helpful measure of the incidence of primary mediastinal tumors and cysts is the average number of cases seen annually in large institutions. Wychulis and colleagues[5] from the Mayo Clinic reported on 1,064 surgical patients seen over the 40-year period of 1929 through 1968 (approximately 27 patients per year). Davis and colleagues[3] reported approximately 7 patients per year from the Duke University Medical Center over a 55-year period. Cohen and colleagues[6] from the Walter Reed Army Medical Center reported approximately 5 patients per year from 1944 to 1989. A review of the New Mexico Tumor Registry[7] from 1973 to 1995 revealed

TABLE 158.1 ITMIG Definition of Mediastinal Compartments

Compartment	Boundaries	Major Contents
Prevascular	*Superior:* Thoracic inlet *Inferior:* Diaphragm *Anterior:* Sternum *Lateral:* Parietal (mediastinal) pleural reflections; lateral margin of the bilateral internal thoracic arteries and veins, and superior and inferior pulmonary veins *Posterior:* Anterior aspect of the pericardium, which lies along the anterior margin of the superior vena cava, ascending aorta, and the lateral rim of the aortic arch, superior and inferior pulmonary veins	Thymus Fat Lymph nodes Left brachiocephalic vein
Visceral	*Superior:* Thoracic inlet *Inferior:* Diaphragm *Anterior:* Posterior boundaries of the prevascular compartment *Posterior:* Vertical line connecting a point on each thoracic vertebral body at 1 cm posterior to its anterior margin	*Nonvascular:* Trachea, carina, esophagus, lymph nodes *Vascular:* Heart, ascending thoracic aorta, aortic arch, descending thoracic aorta, superior vena cava, intrapericardial pulmonary arteries, thoracic duct
Paravertebral	*Superior:* Thoracic inlet *Inferior:* Diaphragm *Anterior:* Posterior boundaries of the visceral compartment *Posterolateral:* Vertical line against the posterior margin of the chest wall at the lateral margin of the transverse process of the thoracic spine	Paravertebral soft tissues

Reprinted from Carter BW, Tomiyama N, Bhora FY, et al. A modern definition of mediastinal compartments. *J Thorac Oncol* 2014;9(suppl 2):S97–S101. With permission.

approximately 10 primary mediastinal malignancies per year. Teixeria and Bibas[8] reported 8 patients per year at the Hospital dos Servidores de Estrado in Brazil during the 10-year period of 1975 to 1985. More recently, Takeda and colleagues[4] reported an experience of 16 cases per year from 1951 to 2000 at the Toneyama National Hospital. Thus, these masses are only infrequently encountered by the average thoracic surgeon; nonetheless, familiarity with the clinical features and location of the various masses is essential.

Primary mediastinal masses are a heterogeneous mixture of neoplastic, congenital, and inflammatory conditions.[9] For surgically resected mediastinal masses, benign cysts, neurogenic tumors, and thymomas account for almost 20% each while lymphoma and teratoma account for an additional 10% each. The remaining 20% of resected masses include granulomas, intrathoracic goiters, mesenchymal tumors, and primary carcinoma.[5] Oldham,[10] in a collection of 214 mediastinal cysts from

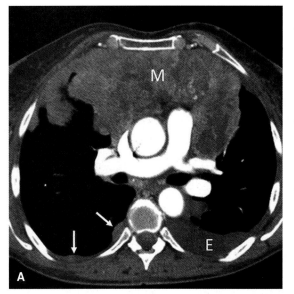
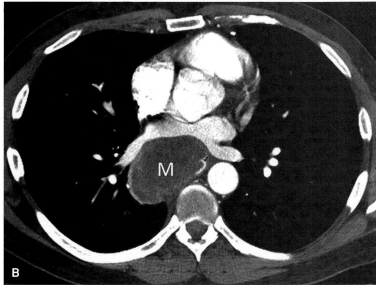

FIGURE 158.1 Representative examples of mediastinal masses within the ITMIG-defined compartments. **A:** Contrast-enhanced CT with a large heterogeneous mass (*M*) in the prevascular compartment consistent with a biopsy-proven thymoma. The great vessels are displaced posteriorly. Also seen is a left pleural effusion (*E*) and right-sided pleural nodules (*arrows*) reflective of dissemination. **B:** Contrast-enhanced CT demonstrating a low attenuation mass (*M*) located between the left atrium and thoracic spine confirming its location within the visceral compartment. This was an esophageal cancer on endoscopic biopsy. **C:** Contrast-enhanced CT showing a low attenuation mass (*M*) within the left atrium. This intracardiac and hence visceral compartment mass was an angiosarcoma. **D:** Contrast-enhanced CT demonstrating a large calcified mass (*M*) in the left mediastinum. This mass displaced the heart anteriorly and the central portion of the mass is located within the paravertebral compartment. This was a ganglioneuroma. (Reprinted from Carter BW, Tomiyama N, Bhora FY, et al. A modern definition of mediastinal compartments. *J Thorac Oncol* 2014;9(suppl 2):S97–S101. With permission.) (*continued*)

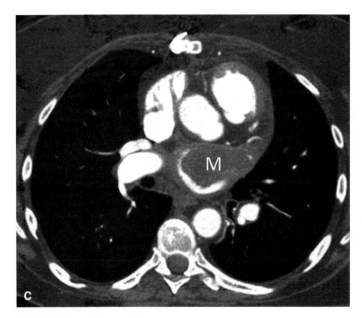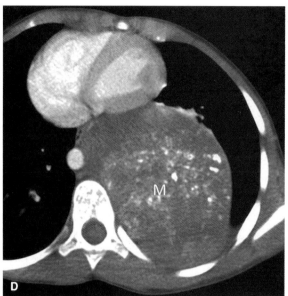

FIGURE 158.1 (*Continued*)

TABLE 158.2 Incidence of Mediastinal Tumors and Cysts in Children

Lesion	DuShane and Ellis (1956)[11]	Jaubert deBeaujeu et al. (1968)[12]	Haller et al. (1969)[13]	Grosfeld et al. (1971)[14]	Whittaker and Lynn (1973)[15]	Pokorny and Sherman (1974)[16]	Bower and Kieswetter (1977)[15]	Azarow et al. (1993)[18]	Whooley et al. (1999)[19]	Takeda et al. (2003)[4]	Total
Neurogenic tumors	19	22	18	35	37	35	41	22	10	60	299
Germ cell tumors	16	9	8	5	21	4	5	4	1	24	97
Enterogenous cysts	10	15	10	0	12	14	17	11	0	7	96
Lymphomas	0	0	8	13	9	27	12	4	6	17	96
Angiomas and lymphangiomas	9	1	4	1	6	7	5	3	0	8	44
Thymic tumors and cysts	0	3	0	4	2	3	1	7	3	12	35
Stem cell tumors	4	1	10	2	0	0	5	0	0	0	22
Pleuropericardial cysts	0	1	1	0	0	0	2	1	0	1	6
Miscellaneous	0	2	3	2	11	0	0	4	0	1	23
Total	58	54	62	62	98	90	88	56	20	130	718

TABLE 158.3 Incidence of Mediastinal Tumors and Cysts Primarily in Adults[a]

Lesion	Herlitzka and Gale (1958)[20]	Morrison (1958)[21]	Le Roux (1962)[22]	Boyd and Midell (1968)[23]	Wychulis et al. (1971)[5]	Rubush et al. (1973)[24]	Davis et al. (1987)[3]	Cohen et al. (1991)[6]	Whooley et al. (1999)[19]	Takeda et al. (2003)[4]	Total
Thymomas and thymic cysts	14	47	17	20	225	51	67	45	42	272	800
Neurogenic tumors	35	101	30	11	212	36	57	39	5	76	602
Germ cell tumors	26	36	21	22	99	14	42	23	28	106	417
Lymphomas	12	33	0	20	107	14	62	36	18	82	384
Enterogenous cysts	26	29	14	15	83	8	50	36	1	49	311
Pleuropericardial cysts	17	13	20	6	72	10	36	8	1	18	201
Miscellaneous	29	30	3	2	118	24	40	29	8	19	302
Total	159	289	105	96	916	157	354	216	103	622	3,017

[a]Excludes substernal thyroid, mediastinal granuloma, and primary carcinoma of the mediastinum.

TABLE 158.4 Usual Locations of the Common Primary Tumors and Cysts of the Mediastinum

Prevascular (Anterior) Compartment	Visceral (Middle) Compartment	Paravertebral (Posterior) Compartment
Thymoma	Enterogenous cyst	Neurilemoma (schwannoma)
Germ cell tumor	Lymphoma	
Lymphoma	Pleuropericardial cyst	Neurofibroma
Lymphangioma		Malignant schwannoma
Hemangioma	Mediastinal granuloma	
Lipoma	Lymphoid hamartoma	Ganglioneuroma
Fibroma	Mesothelial cyst	Ganglioneuroblastoma
Fibrosarcoma	Neuroenteric cyst	Neuroblastoma
Thymic cyst	Paraganglioma	Paraganglioma
Parathyroid adenoma	Parathyroid cyst	Pheochromocytoma
	Pheochromocytoma	Fibrosarcoma
Aberrant thyroid	Thoracic duct cyst	Lymphoma

5 separate authors, found 41% were bronchogenic, 35% pericardial, 10% enteric, and 14% nonspecific.

LOCATION OF COMMON TUMORS AND CYSTS

Characteristically each variety of mediastinal cyst or tumor has a predilection for a specific compartment as shown in Table 158.4. Nonetheless, migration or growth from one compartment into an adjoining compartment can occur. Additionally, masses from specific tissue may originate in more than one space. This is especially true for lymphatic tumors which may originate in both the prevascular and visceral compartments and even rarely in the paravertebral compartment. Neurogenic tumors most commonly occur in one of the paravertebral sulci, but can also arise from the phrenic or vagus nerves located in the visceral (middle) compartment. The paravertebral sulci are the most common location of primary mediastinal tumors in children, with 52% of mediastinal masses in children found here.[4] Tumors of mesenchymal origin (hemangiomas, lipomas, lymphangiomas, and their malignant counterparts) may occur in any of the mediastinal compartments. Table 158.5 outlines the relative frequency of primary prevascular (anterior) mediastinal tumors in 702 adults. Finally, many lesions arising outside the mediastinum may project into the various compartments and masquerade as primary mediastinal masses on a chest radiograph.

RELATIONSHIP OF AGE TO TYPE OF MEDIASTINAL MASS

The incidence and types of primary mediastinal tumors and cysts vary with patient age. The collected series highlighted in Table 158.2 show that in infants and children the primary mediastinal masses in order of decreasing frequency are neurogenic tumors, germ cell tumors, enterogenous (foregut) cysts, lymphomas, angiomas and lymphangiomas, thymic tumors, stem cell tumors, and pleuropericardial cysts. In the collected series totaling 3,017, mostly adult, patients (Table 158.3), the masses in decreasing order of frequency were thymomas and thymic cysts, neurogenic tumors, germ cell tumors, lymphomas, enterogenous cysts, and pleuropericardial cysts. Mullen and Richardson[25] found that thymomas constituted 47% of all mediastinal tumors in adults in the prevascular compartment (Table 158.5). Thus, from the collective series reviewed, mediastinal masses of thymic origin appear to be the most common primary mediastinal masses in adults. Of note, however, is that in a review of mediastinal tumors from the files of the Walter Reed Army Medical Center and Walter Reed Tumor Registry that while thymic lesions were overall most common, lymphomas constituted

TABLE 158.5 Relative Frequency of Common Prevascular (Anterior) Mediastinal Tumors in 702 Adults

Tumor	Wychulis et al.[5]	Rubush et al.[24]	Luosta	Ovrum and Birkeland	Nandi	Total	Incidence (%)
Thymic lesion	231	37	31	7	21	327	47
Lymphoma	107	7	37	9	0	160	23
Germ cell tumor	60	10	21	5	7	103	15
Endocrine tumor	61	13	11	21	6	112	16
Total	459	67	100	42	34	702	—
Percentage of series	43	58	48	62	50	—	—

Reprinted from Mullen B, Richardson JD. Primary anterior mediastinal tumors in children and adults. *Ann Thorac Surg* 1986;42:338–345. Copyright © 1986 The Society of Thoracic Surgeons. With permission.

the largest number of adult mediastinal tumors in the last 19 years of their 45-year review.[6]

SIGNS AND SYMPTOMS

In contrast to adults, where one-third to one-half of mediastinal masses produce symptoms, one-half to two-thirds of mediastinal masses in children are symptomatic. Signs and symptoms that occur depend on the benignity or malignancy of the mass, its size, location, presence or absence of infection, the elaboration of specific endocrine or other biochemical products, and the presence of associated disease states. Seventy-five percent to 85% of patients with malignant masses are symptomatic in contrast to 33% to 46% of patients with benign masses.[3,4]

In infants and children, respiratory symptoms such as cough, dyspnea, and stridor are commonplace since even a small mass because of its location may cause airway compression. Malignant mediastinal masses in children often present with lethargy, fever, and chest pain. Septic complications with resultant pneumonitis and fever occur frequently.

Despite often being asymptomatic, mediastinal masses in adults can present with cough, dyspnea, vague chest pain, or local signs or symptoms related to infection or malignancy. Infection of benign cysts may cause symptoms. Cartmill and Hughes[26] found that 75% of bronchogenic cysts were symptomatic. St-Georges and colleagues[27] found that 66% of symptomatic patients had two or more symptoms. In Rice's[28] series, even if patients with bronchogenic cysts were initially asymptomatic, upon long-term follow-up 67% of patients eventually developed symptoms. Symptoms and signs from compression of vital structures by benign mediastinal masses are uncommon in the adult because most normal mediastinal structures are mobile and can conform to distortion from extrinsic pressure. However, when malignant disease is present, in addition to distortion, fixation of the mass can occur making obstruction and compression of vital structures more likely. Additionally, direct invasion of adjacent structures, such as the chest wall, pleura, and adjacent nerves, is common with malignant tumors. Specific findings of chest pain, pleural effusion, hoarseness, Horner's syndrome, superior vena caval syndrome, upper extremity pain, back pain, paraplegia, and diaphragmatic paralysis may occur in the presence of a malignant tumor. Constitutional symptoms of malignant disease (i.e., weight loss, fever) are sometimes evident. Endocrinologic syndromes may occur in association with either a benign or malignant lesion.

Certain systemic disease states may be present with both malignant and benign mediastinal tumors in either children or adults. These, as well as other unique findings related to each specific type of tumor and cyst, are discussed separately in the chapters devoted to the various lesions.

BENIGN VERSUS MALIGNANT

The incidence of benign versus malignant mediastinal masses varies with the mass under consideration, its mediastinal location, the patient's age, the presence or absence of symptoms, and hospital referral patterns. For example, in a report of Whooley and colleagues[19] from the Roswell Park Cancer Institute, 90% of the mediastinal tumors were malignant. These authors attributed this higher than expected rate of malignancy to their tertiary cancer referral pattern. A more commonly accepted incidence of malignancy in adults with mediastinal masses ranges from 24% to 47%.[3,4,5] Several authors have demonstrated that prevascular (anterior) compartment mediastinal

TABLE 158.6 Incidence of Malignancy of Mediastinal Tumors From 1950 to 1989

Decade	No. of Patients	Malignant Tumors	Percentage
1950–1959	18	5	28
1960–1969	66	10	15
1970–1979	53	17	32
1980–1989	93	52	56

Reprinted from Cohen AJ, Thompson L, Edwards FH, et al. Primary cysts and tumors of the mediastinum. *Ann Thorac Surg* 1991;51:378–386. Copyright © 1991 The Society of Thoracic Surgeons. With permission.

masses have a higher rate of malignancy as high as 59%.[3,6] Within the prevascular compartment, 25% to 50% of thymic neoplasms and 13% to 50% of germ cell neoplasms, respectively, are malignant.[3,5,18] Within the visceral (middle) compartment, 29% of masses are malignant with lymphatic and mesenchymal masses being either benign or malignant, and almost all cysts being benign.[3] Some 16% of masses within the paravertebral sulci are malignant with neurogenic tumors being most common in this location.[3,29] While 70% to 80% of neurogenic tumors are benign and nearly half are asymptomatic, this is clearly dependent on patient age.[29,30]

In children, the overall incidence of malignancy of mediastinal masses is similar to adults ranging from 35% to 50%.[4,18,31,32] However, it should be noted that the malignancy rate in neurogenic tumors is higher in children than adults. Reed and colleagues[33] reported the incidence of malignancy in neurogenic tumors in 50 children less than 16 years of age to be 60% which is similar to the incidence at the Children's Memorial Hospital in Chicago.[34] Additionally, in a smaller series of 20 children seen during the 7-year period from 1980 to 1987, the incidence of malignancy in neurogenic tumors was 85%.[34] In the middle mediastinum, many of the lymph node masses are malignant including both Hodgkin disease and non-Hodgkin lymphoma. Cysts within the middle mediastinum make up the remaining masses and are almost always benign.

An extremely interesting observation related to the incidence of malignancy was made by Davis and colleagues[3] who reported a significant increase ($p = 0.004$) in the percentage of malignant neoplasms seen in the later time frame of their series. In the first 36 years of their study, 34% of patients had malignant neoplasms in contrast to 48% of patients in the later 20 years.[3] Cohen and colleagues[6] in their review of the Walter Reed Army Medical Center database also found that there had been a highly statistically significant increase in the number of patients with malignant mediastinal tumors from the 1940s to the 1980s (Table 158.6).

DIAGNOSTIC INVESTIGATIONS

When a primary mediastinal mass is recognized on standard chest radiography in either an asymptomatic or symptomatic adult or child, the diagnostic possibilities can be narrowed to a reasonable number by considering the patient's age, location of the mass, and the associated signs and symptoms when present. Further definition of the true nature of the mass can be established by additional noninvasive and invasive diagnostic techniques before a definitive decision regarding therapy is made. An exhaustive look at the diagnostic modalities available for the investigation of mediastinal masses is beyond the scope of this chapter, and the reader is referred to other specific chapters in this book for a detailed review of these modalities.

When a central mass is discovered on a chest radiograph, the first step is confirmation that the mass arises from the mediastinum rather than from adjacent structures such as the lungs, pleura, or chest wall. CT is the most important tool in the evaluation of a mediastinal mass.[35-38] It is the next step following chest radiography. In general, spiral CT is the most accurate and reliable noninvasive method of mediastinal evaluation. For patients with normal renal function, spiral CT with intravenous contrast is preferable which can improve the characterization of the mass. CT is a sensitive method of distinguishing between fatty, vascular, cystic, and soft tissue masses. Additionally, CT can be helpful in evaluating paravertebral masses for intraspinal tumor extension. CT cannot differentiate benign from malignant tumors; however, it can provide added clinically useful information when invasion of the mass into adjacent structures or pleural or lung metastases is demonstrated. Tomiyama and colleagues[38] compared the diagnostic accuracy of CT and magnetic resonance imaging (MRI) in 127 patients with anterior mediastinal masses. CT was found to be equal or superior to MRI in the diagnosis of anterior mediastinal masses except for thymic cysts. While in the overwhelming majority of cases CT is the study of choice, in select cases, other imaging may be necessary.

In addition to separating cystic from solid masses, MRI may supply additional information in separating mediastinal tumors from vessels and bronchi, especially when the use of intravenous contrast material is contraindicated. MRI is limited by its poorer visualization of the lung parenchyma.[39]

Fluorine-18 (^{18}F) fluorodeoxyglucose positron emission tomography (FDG-PET) imaging which is widely used in the preoperative staging of thoracic malignancies is currently being applied to primary mediastinal masses. While FDG-PET is not routinely used in the evaluation of anterior mediastinal masses, it has been shown to be helpful in differentiating benign from malignant mediastinal tumors, localizing recurrent thymomas, and evaluating treatment response in mediastinal lymphomas.[35,36,40,41] For patients diagnosed with lymphoma, FDG-PET is the staging test of choice. FDG-PET/CT is more accurate than CT in detecting mediastinal lymphoma with a sensitivity of 94% and specificity of 100% compared with 88% and 86%, respectively, for CT.[35,36] However, it is important to recognize that normal and hyperplastic thymus and other inflammatory lesions in the mediastinum can be FDG-avid. Other radionuclide imaging modalities may be appropriate if the differential diagnosis includes aberrantly displaced thyroid or parathyroid (technetium) or in the localization of biologically active paragangliomas ([^{131}I] meta-iodobenzylguanidine).

Biochemical markers and elevated hormone levels can be present in patients with various mediastinal tumors. While not all patients require these studies, specific markers and certain hormone levels should be obtained in some clinical settings. For example, all young men with an anterior mediastinal mass even with no signs or symptoms should have determination of α-fetoprotein (α-FP) and β-human chorionic gonadotropin (β-hCG). Either one or both are elevated in the presence of a nonseminomatous malignant germ cell tumor. If these levels are in excess of 500 ng/mL, many feel that chemotherapy may be started even without tissue diagnosis. While 7% to 10% of pure seminomas may be associated with a slight elevation of β-hCG, that level rarely exceeds 100 ng/mL and an elevated α-FP is never present. Infants and children with a paravertebral mass should be evaluated for excessive norepinephrine and epinephrine production which are associated with most neuroblastomas and ganglioneuroblastomas. For patients with a suspected thymoma, even if asymptomatic, antiacetylcholine receptor antibodies should be checked in order to determine whether a subclinical myasthenic state is present.[42,43]

The choice of a more invasive diagnostic procedure depends primarily on the presence or absence of local symptomatology, location and extent of the mass, and the presence or absence of various tumor markers. Available invasive techniques include percutaneous or endoscopic radiologically guided fine-needle aspiration (FNA) and core needle biopsy, anterior mediastinotomy (Chamberlain procedure), mediastinoscopy, video-assisted thoracic surgery (VATS), and the traditional open approaches of median sternotomy and thoracotomy.

For anterior mediastinal masses a tissue diagnosis is important particularly if there is a high likelihood that the mass may be a lymphoma or a seminomatous germ cell tumor for which surgery is not the initial treatment. A CT-guided core needle biopsy may be a valuable way to obtain adequate tissue for diagnosis. However, not all mediastinal masses require biopsy. Thyroid goiter has characteristic CT findings, and imaging alone is often all that is required. For patients with myasthenia gravis, hypogammaglobulinemia, or pure red cell aplasia and evidence of an anterior mediastinal mass typical of a thymoma, biopsy is not needed. It has long been stated that biopsy of a presumed thymoma should be avoided because of tumor seeding in either the needle tract or pleural space. Realistically, there are only a few anecdotal cases of recurrence at either needle tract or thoracotomy sites, and needle biopsy of larger tumors suspected of being thymoma is routinely performed in many centers with extensive thymoma experience.[44,45] In a series of 70 patients having percutaneous core needle biopsy of an anterior mediastinal mass, adequate tissue was obtained in 89% of patients, overall sensitivity was 92%, and a specific histologic diagnosis was established in 90.3%.[46] The main difficulty in the differential diagnosis of mediastinal masses is differentiating thymoma from lymphoma when typical symptoms for either are absent. While a needle biopsy may be successful in diagnosing thymoma, it may not be adequate for diagnosing lymphoma subtypes. The sensitivity of core needle biopsy for the diagnosis of lymphoma ranges from 70% to 80%.[47-50] The diagnostic yield of percutaneous needle biopsies for mediastinal lymphoma varies with the type of lymphoma and biopsy technique (FNA vs. core). For prevascular (anterior) mediastinal lymphomas, three to five core biopsies are necessary for architectural evaluation and immunohistochemistry and FNA for flow cytology.[35] If percutaneous core needle biopsy is unsuccessful, then anterior mediastinotomy or VATS may be required for diagnosis.

For middle compartment masses, particularly for helping to establish the diagnosis of enlarged lymph nodes, endoscopic ultrasound-guided FNA via either the transbronchial (EBUS) or transesophageal (EUS) routes may be useful. However, when larger tissue samples are required (e.g., lymphoma), mediastinoscopy allows for more extensive tissue sampling of middle mediastinal lesions.

Finally, consideration must be given to surgical resection via VATS, sternotomy, thoracotomy, or combinations of these which can be simultaneously both diagnostic and therapeutic. If the anterior mediastinal mass is well circumscribed, without obvious invasion into adjacent structures, and can be completely removed, then excision may be the best alternative. Similarly, excision may also be most appropriate for cystic masses of the middle mediastinum and neurogenic tumors in the posterior mediastinum.

REFERENCES

1. Carter BW, Tomiyama N, Bhora FY, et al. A modern definition of mediastinal compartments. *J Thorac Oncol* 2014;9:S97–S101.
2. Thacker PG, Mahani MG, Heider A, et al. Imaging evaluation of mediastinal masses in children and adults: practical diagnostic approach based on a new classification system. *J Thorac Imaging* 2015;30:247–267.

3. Davis RD, Jr., Oldham HN, Jr., Sabiston DC, Jr. Primary cysts and neoplasm of the mediastinum recent changes in clinical presentation, methods of diagnosis, management, and results. *Ann Thorac Surg* 1987;44:229–237.
4. Takeda S, Miyoshi S, Akashi A, et al. Clinical spectrum of primary mediastinal tumors: a comparison of adult and pediatric populations at a single Japanese institution. *J Surg Oncol* 2003;83(1):24–30.
5. Wychulis AR, Payne WS, Clagett OT, et al. Surgical treatment of mediastinal tumors: a 40 year experience. *J Thorac Cardiovasc Surg* 1971;62:379–392.
6. Cohen AJ, Thompson L, Edwards FH, et al. Primary cysts and tumors of the mediastinum. *Ann Thorac Surg* 1991;51:378–386.
7. Temes R, Chavez T, Mapel D, et al. Primary mediastinal malignancies: finding in 219 patients. *West J Med* 1999;170(3):161–166.
8. Teixeria JP, Bibas RA. Surgical treatment of tumors of the mediastinum: the Brazilian experience. In: Martini N, Vogt-Moykopf I, eds. *International Trends in General Thoracic Surgery*. Vol. 5. St. Louis, CV: Mosby; 1989.
9. Benjamin SP, McCormack LJ, Effler DB, et al. Primary tumors of the mediastinum. *Chest* 1972;62:297–303.
10. Oldham HN, Jr. Mediastinal tumors and cysts. *Ann Thorac Surg* 1971;11:246–275.
11. DuShane JW, Ellis FH, Jr. Primary mediastinal cysts and neoplasms in infants and children. *Am Rev Tuberc* 1956;74:940–953.
12. Jaubert De Beaujeu MJ, Mollard P, CampoPaysaa A. Tumeurs chirurgicalse de mediastinum de l'enfant. *Ann Chir Infant* 1968;9:177–191.
13. Haller JA, Jr., Mazur DO, Morgan WW, Jr. Diagnosis and management of mediastinal masses in children. *J Thorac Cardiovasc Surg* 1969;58:385–393.
14. Grosfeld JL, Weinberger M, Kilman JW, et al. Primary mediastinal neoplasms in infants and children. *Ann Thorac Surg* 1971;12:179–190.
15. Whittaker LD, Jr., Lynn HB. Mediastinal tumors and cysts in the pediatric patient. *Surg Clin North Am* 1973;53:893–904.
16. Pokorny WJ, Sherman JO. Mediastinal masses in infants and children. *J Thorac Cardiovasc Surg* 1974;68:869–875.
17. Bower RJ, Kiesewetter WB. Mediastinal masses in infants and children. *Arch Surg* 1977;112:1003–1009.
18. Azarow KS, Pearl RH, Zurcher R, et al. Primary mediastinal masses. A comparison of adult and pediatric populations. *J Thorac Cardiovasc Surg* 1993;106:67–72.
19. Whooley BP, Urschel JD, Antkowiak JG, et al. Primary tumors of the mediastinum. *J Surg Oncol* 1999;70:95–99.
20. Herlitzka AJ, Gale JW. Tumors and cysts of the mediastinum. *Arch Surg* 1958;76:697–706.
21. Morrison IM. Tumours and cysts of the mediastinum. *Thorax* 1958;13:294–307.
22. Le Roux BT. Cysts and tumors of the mediastinum. *Surg Gynecol Obstet* 1962;115:695–703.
23. Boyd DP, Midell AI. Mediastinal cysts and tumors. An analysis of 96 cases. *Surg Clin North Am* 1968;48:493–505.
24. Rubush JL, Gardner IR, Boyd WC, et al. Mediastinal tumors. Review of 186 cases. *J Thorac Cardiovasc Surg* 1973;65:216–222.
25. Mullen B, Richardson JD. Primary anterior mediastinal tumors in children and adults. *Ann Thorac Surg* 1986;42:338–345.
26. Cartmill JA, Hughes CF. Bronchogenic cysts: a persistent dilemma. *Aust N Z J Surg* 1989;59:253–256.
27. St-Georges R, Deslauriers J, Duranceau A, et al. Clinical spectrum of bronchogenic cysts of the mediastinum and lung in the adult. *Ann Thorac Surg* 1991;52:6–13.
28. Rice TW. Benign neoplasms and cysts of the mediastinum. *Sem Thorac Cardiovasc Surg* 1992;4:25–33.
29. Davidson KG, Walbaum PR, McCormack RJ. Intrathoracic neural tumours. *Thorax* 1978;33:359–367.
30. Duwe BV, Sterman DH, Musani AI. Tumors of the mediastinum. *Chest* 2005;128:2893–2909.
31. Akashi A, Nakahara K, Ohno K, et al. Primary mediastinal tumors in children—comparison with mediastinal tumors in adults. *J Jpn Assoc Thorac Surg* 1993;41:2180–2184.
32. Ghandi SK. Pediatric mediastinal tumors. In: Patterson GA, Cooper JD, Deslauriers J, et al., eds. *Pearson's Thoracic and Esophageal Surgery*. 3rd ed. Churchill Livingstone; 2008:1653–1660.
33. Reed JC, Hallet KK, Feigin DS. Neural tumors of the thorax: subject review from the AFIP. *Radiology* 1978;126:9–17.
34. Shields TW, Reynolds M. Neurogenic tumors of the thorax. *Surg Clin North Am* 1988;68:645–668.
35. Carter BW, Marom EM, Detterbeck FC. Approaching the patient with an anterior mediastinal mass: a guide for clinicians. *J Thorac Oncol* 2014;9:S102–S109.
36. Carter BW, Okumura M, Detterbeck FC, et al. Approaching the patient with an anterior mediastinal mass: a guide for radiologists. *J Thorac Oncol* 2014;9:S110–S118.
37. Juanpere S, Cañete N, Ortuño P, et al. A diagnostic approach to the mediastinal masses. *Insights Imaging* 2013;4:29–52.
38. Tomiyama N, Honda O, Tsubamoto M, et al. Anterior mediastinal tumors: diagnostic accuracy of CT and MRI. *Eur J Radiol* 2009;69:280–288.
39. Ackman JB. MR imaging of mediastinal masses. *Magn Reson Imaging Clin N Am* 2015;23:141–164.
40. El-Bawab H, Al-Sugair AA, Rafay M, et al. Role of fluorine-18 fluorodeoxyglucose positron emission tomography in thymic pathology. *Eur J Cardiothorac Surg* 2007;31:731–736.
41. Kubota K, Yamada S, Kondo T, et al. PET imaging of primary mediastinal tumours. *Br J Cancer* 1996;73:882–886.
42. Nakagawa K, Asamura H, Matsuno Y, et al. Thymoma: a clinicopathologic study based on the new World Health Organization classification. *J Thorac Cardiovasc Surg* 2003;126:1134–1140.
43. Thomas CR, Wright CD, Loehrer PJ. Thymoma. *J Clin Oncol* 1999;17:2280–2289.
44. Detterbeck FC, Parsons AM. Thymic tumors. *Ann Thorac Surg* 2004;77:1860–1869.
45. Detterbeck FC. Does an anecdote substantiate dogma? [Letter to the editor re Kattach article about recurrence of thymoma in a needle tract]. *Ann Thorac Surg* 2006;81:1182.
46. Grief J, Staroselsky AN, Gernjac M, et al. Percutaneous core needle biopsy in the diagnosis of mediastinal tumors. *Lung Cancer* 1999;25:169–173.
47. de Margerie-Mellon C, de Bazelaire C, Amorim S, et al. Diagnostic yield and safety of computed tomography-guided mediastinal core needle biopsies. *J Thorac Imaging* 2015;30:319–327.
48. Petranovic M, Gilman MD, Muniappan A, et al. Diagnostic yield of CT-guided percutaneous transthoracic needle biopsy for diagnosis of anterior mediastinal masses. *Am J Roentgenol* 2015;205:774–779.
49. Sklair-Levy M, Polliack A, Shaham D, et al. CT-guided core-needle biopsy in the diagnosis of mediastinal lymphoma. *Eur Radiol* 2000;10(5):714–718.
50. Zinzani PL, Corneli G, Cancellieri A, et al. Core needle biopsy is effective in the initial diagnosis of mediastinal lymphoma. *Haematologica* 1999;84:600–603.

Lesions Masquerading as Primary Mediastinal Tumors or Cysts

Chadrick E. Denlinger ▪ Jacob A. Klapper

The most common mediastinal masses are lymph node metastases from lung cancer or other malignancies. Primary lung tumors may also directly invade the mediastinum and present as mediastinal tumors. Several primary mediastinal tumors involving the anterior, middle, or posterior mediastinum are also well described and discussed in other chapters of this book. Other less common lesions of the mediastinum, the so-called "masquerading mediastinal lesions," which encompass a broad spectrum of conditions are described in this chapter. These lesions include primary mediastinal thyroid goiters and parathyroid tumors, tumors of the great vessels and heart, tumors of the spine and meninges, and diaphragmatic hernias other than the common hiatal hernias. Each of these conditions will be discussed as individually in this chapter because there is little common ground between them other than the fact that they involve the mediastinum and they do not fit well into any other major disease category.

INTRATHORACIC GOITER

DEFINITION

Goiters, with an intrathoracic component, represent approximately 9% of all goiters and they can be stratified into three different subcategories as described by Wakeley and Mulvany in 1940: (1) cervical goiters with a small substernal extension, (2) goiters arising in the neck with a predominant mediastinal component, and (3) complete intrathoracic goiter in which the entire gland and its blood supply are located in the mediastinum. Goiters that are predominantly cervical with a small substernal extension account for greater than 80% of all intrathoracic goiters. Cervical glands with a predominant mediastinal component and complete intrathoracic goiters account for 15.3% and 2.7%, respectively.[1] More recent series have demonstrated a similar incidence of intrathoracic goiters in general, and complete intrathoracic goiters represent a very small minority.[2,3]

ANATOMIC FEATURES

The mediastinal compartment into which substernal goiters extend varies, but appears to depend, in part, on the depth of mediastinal penetration and the presence or absence of a previous thyroid operation. Most thoracic goiters, with only a small substernal extension, are located in the anterior compartment. Only 15% of all primary

mediastinal goiters are located in the visceral or posterior mediastinal compartments.[4] Despite the actual location of a goiter, the thyroid is considered to be in the visceral mediastinal compartment because, in the absence of surgical violation, it is anatomically confined anteriorly by the pretracheal fascia. Under these circumstances, the goiter is technically prevented from entering the prevascular space, thus remaining located between the pretracheal fascia and the more superficial deep cervical fascia.

In terms of its relationship to the great vessels, the goiter is located posterior and medial to the great vessels as it descends into the thorax. McCort initially made this observation, stating that the vessels in the superior portion of the mediastinum were the border-forming structures of the substernal thyroid goiters. His observation has been amply documented by the computed tomography (CT) characteristics of these lesions (Fig. 159.1).[5,6]

The majority of the true partial and completely intrathoracic thyroid lesions remain anterior or lateral to the trachea within the visceral compartment. In a series of 28 patients with substernal goiters, 19 (68%) were located in the visceral compartment whereas 6 were retrotracheal, and 3 were even located posterior to the esophagus.[5] In the literature, this latter group of lesions are often referred to as

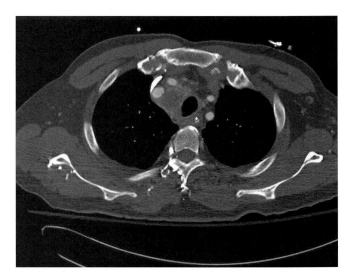

FIGURE 159.1 Substernal goiter extending into the mediastinum in the pretracheal plane, posterior to the great vessels.

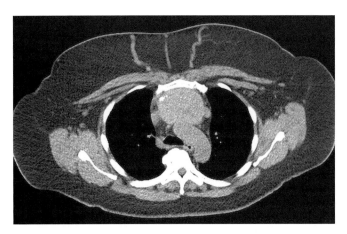

FIGURE 159.2 Substernal goiter extending into the mediastinum anterior to the great vessels.

posterior goiters. Goiters descending posteriorly are most commonly resected with combined cervical and lateral thoracotomy incisions.[7] Dahan and associates reported that 86% of their 75 posterior substernal goiters were retrotracheal and predominantly located on the right side. Four percent were retroesophageal, 4% were anterior and to the right of the tracheal (even though the goiters often arose from the left lobe of the thyroid), and 6% of the goiters were wrapped circumferentially around the trachea.[8] The fact that most posterior goiters descend into the right hemithorax most likely results from the position of the aortic arch. Further descent, even to the level of the diaphragm, has occasionally been observed.

Actual descent of a partial or complete thoracic goiter from the neck into the prevascular space can occur (Fig. 159.2). Susceptible patients include those who have had previous thyroid surgery in which the fascial planes have been violated. Partial or complete intrathoracic goiters that enter the mediastinum via the visceral compartment may advance anterior to the aortic arch on the right, and their most inferior extent may reside in the anterior mediastinum below the level of the innominate vein. Invasive malignant tumors derived from primary mediastinal goiters have also been described and they seem to occur at a frequency that exceeds goiters originating in the neck.

ECTOPIC MEDIASTINAL THYROID TISSUE

The majority of heterotopic, aberrant, or ectopic thyroid goiters described in the literature represent intrathoracic goiters derived from the lower pole of a cervical gland.[9,10] This is especially true of the goiters located in the visceral compartment adjacent to the trachea, including goiters that descend to the level of the diaphragm. Many patients with thoracic goiters have had a previous cervical goiter or may develop a subsequent cervical goiter. This general statement includes patients with mediastinal thyroid malignancies.[11]

Ectopic thyroid tissue is a common abnormality resulting from aberrant descent of the developing thyroid *anlage* from the foramen cecum at the base of the tongue into the neck at the level of the first tracheal ring. Within the neck, this predictable pattern of ectopic tissue can occur anywhere along the descent of the thyroglossal duct. With regard to aberrant disease in the mediastinum, it is thought that mechanical effects of the heart descending into the mediastinum influence the descent of the developing thyroid. A lack of contact leads to a lingual thyroid, whereas protracted contact leads to a mediastinal thyroid gland.[12] More unusual locations for ectopic thyroid tissue have been reported in the axilla, trachea, esophagus,

pericardium, heart, aorta, adrenal gland, small bowel, and porta hepatis. The differential diagnosis for thyroid lesions in these areas includes metastatic thyroid malignancies in addition to benign ectopic thyroid rests.[12,13]

True mediastinal goiters are rare and represent approximately 1% of all goiters.[14,15] A defining difference is that primary mediastinal goiters derive their blood supply from the mediastinum whereas secondary mediastinal goiters represent extensions from cervical glands into the mediastinum and they derive their blood supply from the inferior thyroid arteries.[12] Embryologic explanations previously given for intrathymic or other mediastinal primary thyroid rests include metastases from well-differentiated thyroid malignancies. Another competing potential etiology is a derivation of intrathymic thyroid tissue from a teratoma.

Nuclear thyroid scintigraphy is necessary prior to any planned resection of a mediastinal or thymic goiter in order to confirm the presence of a normally functioning gland in the neck. It is not unusual for ectopic mediastinal goiters to have minimal endocrine function and therefore they may not be visible with radionuclide imaging. In most cases, the cervical gland functions normally. This is less common with lingual thyroid tissue which is more likely to contain all of the patient's functional thyroid tissue. The diagnosis of an ectopic thymic goiter can be made with a contrast-enhanced CT scan which demonstrates a well-circumscribed, heterogeneous, and mottled-appearing anterior mediastinal tumor. Important clinical factors that may differentiate a true ectopic goiter from a secondary lesion include (1) the presence of a normal or absent cervical thyroid gland, (2) the absence of any prior surgical resection of a cervical thyroid gland, (3) the absence of any similar pathologic process in the cervical gland, and (4) the absence of a known thyroid malignancy (Fig. 159.3).

Traditionally ectopic thyroid lesions have been resected via median sternotomy, but more recently VATS approaches have also been described.[16] Clinical observation has been recommended in select patients who remain asymptomatic and this may be particularly important in those lacking a functional cervical gland.[16]

ECTOPIC THYROID TISSUE IN THE THYMUS

Several reports of intrathymic thyroid glands have been reported in the literature. Spinner et al. first reported this condition in 1994 and others have presented similar cases since then.[12,17] There were no clinical, biochemical, or radiographic abnormalities of the cervical thyroid in these patients. The thymic thyroid tissues presented only as anterior mediastinal masses. A third patient reported by Tang presented with a cervical goiter and was incidentally found to have a synchronous thymic goiter at the lower left pole.[17] Ninety percent of the cervical gland and the entire thymic gland were surgically resected and there was no anatomic connection between the two glands noted at the time of the operation. Histologically both cervical and thymic glands were consistent with benign goiters.

ECTOPIC THYROID TISSUE IN THE HEART (STRUMA CORDIS)

It is well recognized that persistent contact between the thyroid *anlage* and the bulbus cordis can facilitate migration of the thyroid tissue into the visceral mediastinum. As a result, thyroid tissue may become incorporated in the outflow tract of the heart, pericardium, or aortic arch.[18] The majority of patients presented in small case series are women in their fifth and sixth decades of life.[19,20] The intraventricular septum was involved in each patient and evidence of

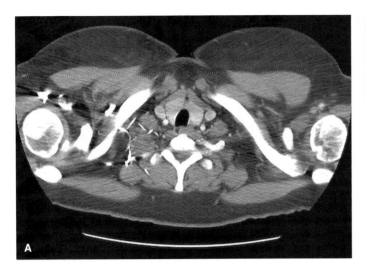
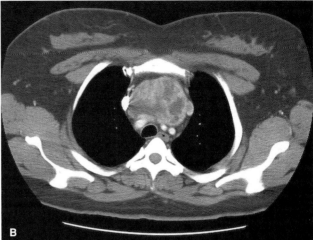

FIGURE 159.3 Ectopic mediastinal goiter with normal appearing thyroid gland in the cervical location (**A**) with a mediastinal goiter located in the mediastinum (**B**). The cervical and mediastinal thyroid glands had no identifiable contiguous tissues connecting them.

outflow tract obstruction was present in 90% of patients. Ventricular arrhythmias were also present in a small minority. The right ventricular outflow tract was much more commonly affected than the left in these series. These lesions are consistently described as broad-based elastic soft tissue masses arising from the ventricular septum and extending into the outflow tract with no invasion of the myocardium. The authors describe a simple excision of the mass under cardiopulmonary bypass without requiring any reconstruction of the ventricular septum.[19,20]

ECTOPIC THYROID TISSUE IN THE ASCENDING AORTA

Goiters involving the wall of the aorta are extremely rare with only three cases present in the English literature.[21–23] While the first report was an autopsy finding, the remaining two cases were removed surgically. In each case the thyroid tissue was dissected off of the aortic wall without requiring cardiopulmonary bypass. Of the two surgical patients, one presented with symptoms of chest pain and palpitations, but it was unclear whether or not these symptoms were attributable to the ectopic thyroid or if these symptoms simply subsided following the operation. The dissection required placement of a partially occluding aortic clamp. The other patient had an incidentally discovered ectopic aortic thyroid gland at the time of a planned coronary artery bypass operation. This gland was easily dissected off of the aorta without placement of any vascular clamp.

ECTOPIC THYROID TISSUE IN THE TRACHEA

Intratracheal thyroid tissue is also extremely rare with only a limited number of case reports present in the literature. These deposits of thyroid tissue may be present in any part of the trachea. Patients may describe shortness of breath and stridor because of the expected airway obstruction. Similar to the descriptions for intracardiac and aortic thyroid tissue, these intratracheal thyroid deposits have been described as broad-based lesions which extend into the mucosa and submucosa, but do not extend deeper into the tracheal wall. For this reason, they can be surgically excised through a tracheotomy without resecting a segment of the trachea itself.[24,25] Because these tend to be submucosal and hypervascular, endoscopic approaches are discouraged due to the risk

of significant bleeding. Instead, resections through open tracheotomies are recommended.

PATHOLOGY

Most reported thoracic goiters are nontoxic multinodular goiters without evidence of occult malignancy. In a series of 80 thoracic goiters resected between 1976 and 1982, 51% were multinodular goiters, 44% were follicular adenomas, and 5% represented Hashimoto's thyroiditis.[26] Within the literature there is some discrepancy in the rate of malignancy seen in thoracic goiters. For instance, historical reviews have quoted an incidence of occult papillary thyroid carcinomas between 2% and 5%, comparable to the rate of incidental malignant findings in cervical glands.[26–28] In contrast, others have reported incidences of 16% and 21% of carcinomas or lymphomas in substernal goiters.[29–31] Torre et al. reported a malignancy rate of 6.7% in their 237 described cases of substernal goiter.[32] Meanwhile, in a more modern series of 132 patients who underwent surgery between 1984 and 2012, there were no cases of occult malignancy identified. Given this finding, the authors argued against resecting asymptomatic substernal goiters based on the concern for malignancy alone.[33] A preoperative biopsy of a goiter is not necessary, even with the described modest risk of malignancy, because of the inaccessibility of the goiter for biopsy and the fact that a biopsy may not change the management strategy in the absence of symptoms of local invasion.[29]

SYMPTOMS AND SIGNS

Most patients with substernal goiters are greater than 50 years of age, with many in the seventh or eighth decade of life. Women are affected three to four times more often than men. A variable number of patients report a history of having undergone one or more previous thyroid operations. In two series by Katlic[26] and Sanders,[30] the incidence of previous operation was 20% exclusive of those patients with clinical suspicion of malignant lesions. Up to one-third of patients with partial or complete thoracic goiters may remain asymptomatic.[29,31,32] Most patients, however, present with complaints including dysphagia, dyspnea, stridor, cough, wheezing, facial flushing, or SVC syndrome. Acute tracheal obstruction with severe respiratory compromise may occasionally be observed. The precipitating event may be obscure, but an acute respiratory infection exacerbating tracheal compression by a thoracic goiter may play a role. Historically, the administration of ^{131}I to treat large mediastinal goiters was avoided because of the risk of temporarily causing the gland to enlarge which may exacerbate preexisting tracheal compression.[34] Recently, however, results were reported of 14 patients with mediastinal goiters who were treated with ^{131}I in lieu of surgery (due to prohibitive operative risk). There were no adverse outcomes attributed to enlargement of the gland and the goiters were reduced in size an average of 29% by 1 year after treatment.[35]

Large multinodular substernal goiters may result in thyrotoxicosis because of autonomously functioning hot nodules or because of the sheer bulk of functioning thyroid tissue.[29] The reported incidence of thyrotoxicosis among patients with large substernal goiters ranges widely from less than 2% to 20%.[29,31,32] Thyrotoxicosis can manifest by tachycardia, heat intolerance, cardiac failure, cardiac arrhythmia, or a wasting syndrome.

Patients with a complete thoracic goiter may have a cervical mass which becomes evident with swallowing. An infrequently encountered goiter, the so-called *goitre plongeant*, is one that is normally nonpalpable in the neck but ascends into that area and becomes palpable when the patient coughs, swallows, or performs a Valsalva maneuver. Superior vena cava (SVC) syndrome is rarely seen in patients with thoracic goiters.[27] Instead, patients typically develop compression of the innominate vein or internal jugular veins against the bony margins of the thoracic inlet rather than compression of the superior vena cava. The dilated cervical veins have been referred to as "Stokes' Collar."[27]

Other symptoms caused by a mass effect at the level of the thoracic inlet include compression or traction on local nerves. Hoarseness caused by a paresis of the vocal cord may be an indication of malignancy, but it may occur in the presence of benign lesions as well. The occurrence of Horner's syndrome and diaphragmatic paralysis, from phrenic nerve compression, have also been attributed to thoracic goiters.[36] These symptoms can be alleviated by surgical resection of the gland. Interestingly, neurologic sequelae have also been attributed to a vascular steal syndrome caused by the significant blood flow being diverted to the enlarged gland from the common carotid arteries. At least two reports in the literature have attributed transient neurologic changes to a "steal syndrome" caused by a large goiter.[37,38]

DIAGNOSTIC IMAGING AND BIOPSY

Standard radiography of the neck and chest is most often diagnostic when large goiters are present. Common findings are mediastinal widening and tracheal deviation. Since the 1980s, CT imaging has frequently been used for thoracic goiters as this imaging modality is particularly useful for determining the relationship of the goiter to the great vessels and trachea (Fig. 159.2).[39] In addition, CT images clearly indicate the depth of penetration of the gland into the chest cavity as well as the degree of tracheal compression which may provide critical information regarding airway management at the time of a planned elective resection. The radiographic appearance of a mottled, enhancing thoracic mass when IV contrast is administered is diagnostic of a goiter thus reduces the need for a needle biopsy or further imaging. In addition to this mottled enhancement, CT scan findings consistent with thoracic goiters include (a) continuity between the intra-thoracic mass and the cervical thyroid gland, (b) well-defined borders, (c) punctate, coarse, or ring-like calcifications (reported in 3% to 38%) (Fig. 159.4), and (d) nonhomogeneity with discrete nonenhancing low-density areas.[26,40,41] In cases in which IV contrast is contraindicated, CT scan can still be beneficial

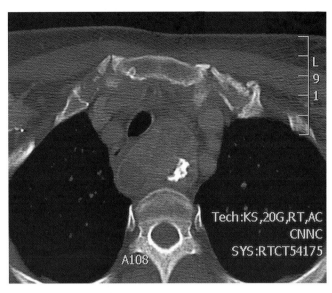

FIGURE 159.4 Mediastinal goiter demonstrating a dense focus of calcification.

as the gland typically has a higher attenuation (100 Hu) than the adjacent tissues.[42]

Magnetic resonance imaging (MRI) studies of substernal goiters are usually not necessary; however, MRI permits excellent delineation of the great vessels and their relationship to the goiter.[43] The connection to the cervical portion of the thyroid gland can be well demonstrated, as well as the inhomogeneity of the mass (Fig. 159.5). "Flow voids" within the mass, the result of the marked vascularity of the thyroid tissue, are particularly diagnostic in complete substernal lesions.

In the past, a barium esophagram could demonstrate deviation of the esophagus by a posterior goiter. A vena cava-gram in an earlier era might have revealed displacement and even occlusion of the innominate and internal jugular veins as they are compressed against the thoracic inlet. However, these diagnostic studies for the evaluation of mediastinal masses have largely been replaced by either CT or MRI imaging, both of which provide significantly greater anatomic information.

Use of ultrasonography is used routinely for cervical thyroid glands. However, ultrasound is not as effective for imaging thoracic goiters due to sonographic shadowing by the sternum and ribs and the difficulty penetrating through the air-filled lung parenchyma.[44] It may differentiate a cystic lesion, such as a parathyroid cyst, which is often readily confused clinically with a thyroid lesion, but so too can a CT scan.

Some authors have advocated routine imaging with radionuclide scintigraphy.[45] However, not all mediastinal goiters, even functional ones, demonstrate radionuclide tracer uptake.[46] Thyroid scintigraphy may be performed with technetium-99 (^{99m}Tc) pertechnetate or either ^{131}I or ^{123}I but these studies may provide variable results. However, Park and colleagues have shown that with strict attention to the proper techniques, 39 of 42 thoracic goiters were appropriately diagnosed by thyroid scintigraphy and that most intrathoracic goiters do have measurable thyroid function. In their analysis, radioiodine scintigraphy is a definitive and cost-effective diagnostic test.[45]

In conclusion, the diagnosis of a substernal goiter can be made based on the typical radiographic appearance on a routine chest CT scan. Additional diagnostic imaging with radionuclide scintigraphy may confirm the diagnosis and, only in rare circumstances, a needle biopsy may be needed to confirm the diagnosis of a dominant nodule which does not demonstrate uptake of radioactive iodine.[39]

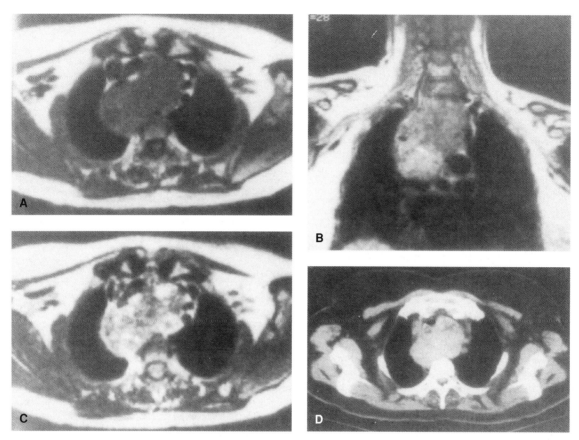

FIGURE 159.5 MRI and scans showing substernal goiter. T1-weighted image (**A**), T2-weighted image (**B**), and coronal image (**C**) all showing displacement of vessels anteriorly and laterally with marked inhomogeneity of the mass. **D:** Conventional CT scan for comparison. (Reproduced with permission from von Schultness GK, McMurdo K, Tscholakoff D, et al. Mediastinal masses: MR imaging. *Radiology* 1986;158:289–296.)

TREATMENT

The recommended treatment of thoracic goiters is surgical resection. Radioactive iodine has traditionally been contraindicated because of unsubstantiated concerns about the risk of initially exacerbating tracheal compression and because iodine ablation is rarely effective in alleviating the thoracic mass effect in the long term. Anesthetic management is best accomplished with an endotracheal tube and general anesthesia. For patients with tracheal compression, placement of an endotracheal tube using awake, fiberoptic techniques with the patient spontaneously breathing reduces the risk of losing control of the airway when anesthesia is induced.

The initial surgical incision is a transverse collar incision for patients with a significant cervical component because over 95% of these patients are able to have the gland resected through this incision without requiring a sternotomy.[26,39] In addition, the blood supply of thoracic goiters is from the inferior thyroid artery, and injury to the recurrent laryngeal nerve is less likely to occur with a cervical approach. In cases where some additional exposure becomes necessary, a partial sternotomy is the procedure most commonly performed. Some previous publications from the 1950s and 1970s advocated a combined cervical and small anterior thoracotomy for completion of the operation with the authors suggesting that this provided better exposure than a partial sternotomy.[47,48] Transclavicular approaches have also been attempted.[48,49] Occasionally a posterior lateral thoracotomy may provide the best approach for large posterior mediastinal goiters (Fig. 159.6).[39] Appropriate control of the vascular supply from the neck may be difficult. Approaching a mediastinal goiter through a posterior lateral thoracotomy has been associated with a high risk for recurrent laryngeal nerve injury although this may be due, in part, to the size and location of the goiter itself rather than to the surgical approach. Most recently, VATS approaches, in conjunction with cervical incisions, have also been utilized, and these approaches are feasible even with large goiters.[50]

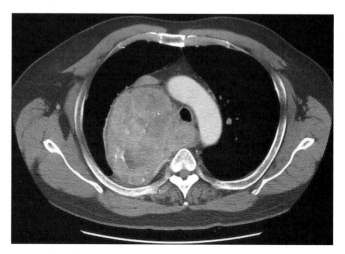

FIGURE 159.6 Mediastinal goiter extending posteriorly into the right hemithorax.

After exposure of the gland in the neck, the blood supply of the superior pole and the middle thyroid vein are isolated, ligated, and divided. At least one of the superior parathyroid glands should be identified and protected from harm. The inferior vessels and recurrent nerve are identified if possible but at times this cannot be accomplished until the intrathoracic portion of the gland has been delivered from the mediastinum. This is generally accomplished by finger dissection within the capsule of the goiter to prevent injury to either the nerve or vessels. Infrequently, additional exposure is necessary by a partial sternotomy. Morcellation of the goiter should be avoided to prevent excessive bleeding and because of the potential risk of spreading an occult malignancy. After mobilization of the inferior poles of the gland, the inferior thyroid vessels are controlled and divided.

Collapse of the tracheal wall due to tracheomalacia is a feared but rarely observed complication of a long-standing large thoracic goiter. Another potential cause of airway obstruction in this setting may be kinking of the trachea because of the elongated displaced trachea which is suddenly relieved of the deviation. When tracheomalacia is present, external tracheal support by notched rings is rarely necessary and mostly of historic relevance. Bronchoscopy prior to extubation may confirm the diagnosis of tracheomalacia, and keeping the patient intubated for 24 to 48 hours may allow the airway to stiffen and maintain patency of the airway following extubation. Temporary stenting of a malacic trachea may be considered as well.

RESULTS

The reported incidence of vagus or recurrent laryngeal nerve injury following the resection of thoracic goiters is 6% to 10%.[8,26,51] There are also rare reports of phrenic nerve injuries during these operations. In addition to nerve injuries, airway complications related to tracheomalacia have been observed.[4] Postoperative mortality is rare, with reported rates of 0% to 2.8%.[4,8,51,52] Recurrent substernal goiters are uncommon.

CERVICOMEDIASTINAL HYGROMA

A cervical cystic hygroma is an aberrant proliferation of lymphatic vessels and this term has been used interchangeably in the literature with lymphangioma and lymphatic malformation. This anomaly is an infrequently encountered congenital anomaly recognized either at birth or in early infancy. It can now be identified in utero by prenatal ultrasonography. These hygromas most frequently arise in the posterior triangle of the neck, but may occur in the anterior triangle or midline. These lesions may extend into adjacent fascial compartments. The ipsilateral axilla is involved in 20% of cases and hygromas also extend into the mediastinum in 2% to 3% of cases.[53,54] Rare cases of primary mediastinal cystic hygromas have also been reported including lesions originating from the heart and lung.[55,56]

ETIOLOGY AND ANATOMY

Cervicomediastinal hygromas are believed to be malformations of the jugular lymphatic sac (Fig. 159.7) that lack the normal communication with other cervical lymphatic channels. The cervicomediastinal hygroma begins in the neck adjacent to the internal jugular vein near the origin of the nerve roots of C3, C4, and C5. As it enlarges, it descends along the course of the phrenic nerve and enters the visceral compartment of the mediastinum between the subclavian vein and artery in the area of the primitive subclavian lymphatic sac (Fig. 159.7A). As the hygroma continues to enlarge, it occupies a portion of the superior visceral compartment and may displace or distort the trachea, esophagus, or both. With further growth, it may pass anteriorly over the arch of aorta to lie in the anterior compartment in the region of the thymus and anterior portion of the pericardial sac (Fig. 159.8). Extension into either hemithorax with compression of the developing lung may also occur.

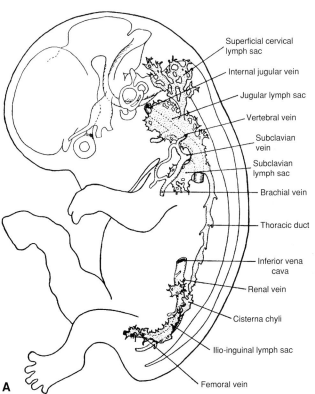

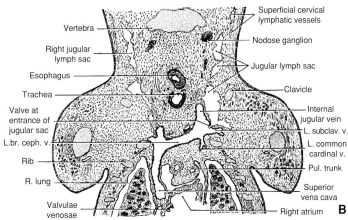

FIGURE 159.7 Schematic illustration from the frontal and lateral aspects of a partial intrathoracic goiter lying in the visceral compartment of the mediastinum, resting on the border of the vertebrae behind the superior vena cava and the innominate vessels above the azygos vein. (From Johnston JH, Jr., Twente GE. Surgical approach to intrathoracic (mediastinal) goiter. *Ann Surg* 1956;143:572–579. With permission.)

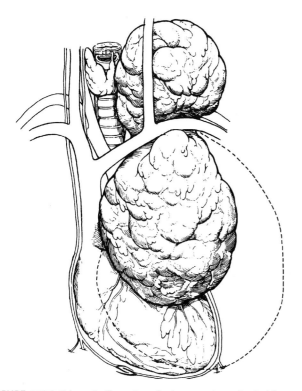

FIGURE 159.8 Schematic illustration of a large cervicomediastinal hygroma descending between the subclavian vein and artery into the anterior mediastinal compartment to lie in front of the aortic arch and anterior portion of the pericardium. (Reprinted from Grosfeld JS, Weber TR, Vane DW. One-stage resection for massive cerviocomediastinal hygroma. *Surgery* 1982;92:693. Copyright ©1982 Elsevier. With permission.)

SYMPTOMS AND SIGNS

A cervicomediastinal hygroma is most often discovered by the presence of a mass at birth in the anterior compartment of the neck. The mass is soft and can be transilluminated. Rarely, cystic hygromas become apparent in adulthood, and the diagnostic approach and management are essentially the same as when identified in infancy. A few patients may have respiratory problems or hypoxemia, but most are asymptomatic with the exception of the cervical mass. Infection of the hygroma as the result of a respiratory infection and internal hemorrhage into the mass have been reported as complications of an existing cystic hygroma.[57] Hemorrhage into the cyst may exacerbate shortness of breath because it can cause the cyst to become firm or solid and lead to tracheal compression. Other complications may rarely occur, such as superior vena cava obstruction, pulmonary atelectasis, or a chylous pleural or pericardial effusion.

DIAGNOSIS

All newborns with a cystic hygroma of the neck, regardless of symptoms, should undergo chest radiography to identify if any mediastinal extension is present. Tracheal deviation may be present in two-thirds of the infants, and esophageal displacement may also be identified. The cystic nature of the mediastinal mass can be confirmed by ultrasonography, but this can also be detected by transillumination on physical examination. A CT scan is an excellent way to establish the extent of the lesions which appear multiloculated with cystic cavities divided by septae (Fig. 159.9).

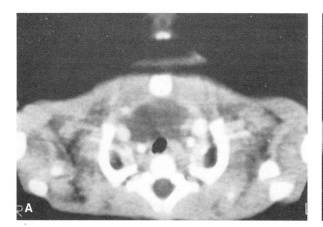

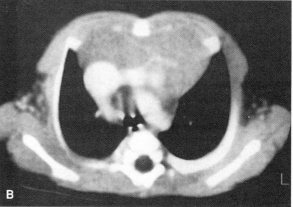

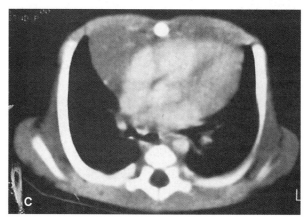

FIGURE 159.9 CT scans of extensive cervicomediastinal hygroma. **A:** Anterior cystic mass displacing the trachea posteriorly. **B:** Cystic mass displacing the great vessels posteriorly, but no compression seen. **C:** Mass extending over the anterior aspect of the heart.

TREATMENT

Traditionally, the treatment of choice for cystic hygromas has been complete surgical resection. Effective treatment of cervical lesions in infants with sclerosing agents has been reported with increasing frequency. More variable results have been observed following the treatment of these lesions with simple aspiration, radiation, radiofrequency ablation, or cauterization.[57] Surgical resection has remained the standard treatment in the adult population, but this appears predominantly attributable to a lack of experience with sclerosing agents rather than a collective experience of unsatisfactory outcomes.

The one-stage resection is performed via an inverted hockey stick incision beginning in the neck and extending over the sternum, which is split to expose the mediastinal extent of the hygroma. The mass is most often intimately associated with the phrenic, vagus, and recurrent laryngeal nerves as well as with the vascular structures in the upper mediastinum. Resection of the entire cystic sac is necessary to prevent recurrence as the sac will not spontaneously regress. Although a 10% to 15% rate of recurrence has been reported for cervical hygromas, recurrence in the mediastinum is exceedingly rare.[58,59]

CERVICAL MEDIASTINAL CYSTS AND HEMATOMAS

A number of cysts that are identified in the neck can extend downward through the superior thoracic inlet into the anterosuperior portion of the visceral compartment, similar to the behavior observed with substernal goiters. These, as a general rule, are thymic cysts or parathyroid cysts. Each of these cystic lesions are discussed elsewhere in the book. Extracapsular bleeding from a mediastinal thymic parathyroid cyst causing a space-occupying hematoma has been reported.[60]

CERVICAL MEDIASTINAL THYMIC PARATHYROID CYST

Silver reported a single case of a 9-year-old boy who had a large cervical cyst that descended partially into the anterior–superior, pretracheal

space.[61] The cyst was removed without difficulty via a cervical approach. Pathologic examination revealed a cystic mass with well-formed lymph follicles and multiple Hassall's corpuscles in the wall of the cyst. Normal parathyroid tissue was present and intermingled in the cyst wall. A diagnosis of a congenital thymic parathyroid cyst was made. This diagnostic possibility must be entertained in children with cystic masses in the neck that extend into the mediastinum.

MEDIASTINAL PARATHYROID ADENOMAS AND CARCINOMAS

The parathyroid *anlage* develops in the third and fourth pharyngeal pouches and descends into the cervical region during the seventh week of fetal development. The superior parathyroid glands develop from the fourth pouch while the inferior glands and thymus gland develop from the third pharyngeal pouch. An ectopic inferior parathyroid gland descends into the mediastinum along with the thymus. Among patients with primary hyperparathyroidism, ectopic mediastinal parathyroid adenomas account for 20% of cases.[62] Technetium-99m sestamibi scanning is the most commonly utilized imaging modality to localize ectopic parathyroid tissue (Fig. 159.10). Preoperative injection of technetium-99m can also be used to help localize the glands at the time of surgery using a hand-held Geiger counter. Surgical approaches for resection of ectopic parathyroid glands have included a cervical incision, median sternotomy, and VATS. Successful removal of the parathyroid adenoma can be determined intraoperatively by measuring the serum parathyroid hormone level intraoperatively. The serum hormone has a half-life of 5 minutes and can provide immediate feedback about the success of the resection.

EXTRACAPSULAR HEMORRHAGE OF PARATHYROID ADENOMA

Extracapsular rupture with hemorrhage into the mediastinum has occurred primarily in patients with cervical parathyroid adenomas and rarely in patients with parathyroid cysts. Infrequently, the location

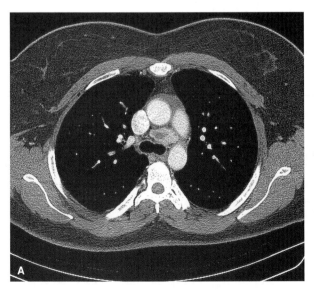 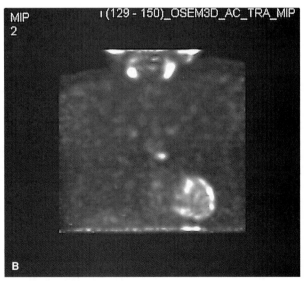

FIGURE 159.10 Mediastinal parathyroid carcinoma visualized with CT imaging (**A**) and delayed images with a technetium-99m sestamibi (**B**).

of the offending lesion is in the mediastinum or the hematoma may extend from a cervical gland into the mediastinum or pleural space.[63] Simcic and colleagues presented one case of a rupture of a cervical parathyroid cyst and reviewed eight other cases of ruptured parathyroid adenomas or cysts.[64] Common findings among single case series reporting this condition include a history of hypercalcemia and an acute presentation with dyspnea, cough, cervical swelling, and ecchymosis. Some patients require emergent airway protection because of the compressive effects of the mediastinal hematoma.[65] Surgical excision of the cyst and hematoma alleviated the patient's symptoms. The etiology of cyst rupture may be related to the adenoma outgrowing this blood supply, infarcting and then bleeding within the cyst.

LESIONS OF THE THORACIC SKELETON

Lesions of the thoracic skeleton that project into the mediastinum are usually bony tumors. Tumors of the sternum are rarely confusing, but posteriorly, chondromas and chondrosarcomas of the heads of the ribs or vertebral bodies may look like mediastinal tumors. Ewing's sarcoma of a rib rarely masquerades as a primary mediastinal tumor.

THORACIC CHORDOMA

Rarely, a thoracic vertebral chordoma may present primarily as a mediastinal tumor in the paravertebral sulcus or more infrequently in the visceral compartment. These tumors arise from ectopic embryonic remnants of the primitive notochord located within the axial skeleton. The nucleus pulposus is a normal derivative of this structure; however, chordomas do not occur in the nucleus but in the adjacent bone or paravertebral tissues. These tumors are most common at the base of the skull, in the sacrococcygeal region, within a vertebral body, or rarely in tissue adjacent to it. In a series of 48 chordomas, 34% originated in vertebral bodies. However, only 3 of the 48 masses occurred in the thoracic spine.[66]

Grossly, the tumor is a soft, gelatinous mass that may have a thin capsule and is usually connected to one or more vertebral bodies. Microscopically, the tumor is made up of cords and sheets of cells surrounded by a mucinous matrix. The characteristic cell has a bubbly, vacuolated, foamy cytoplasm surrounding pyknotic nuclei (the physaliphorous or blister-bearing cell) (Fig. 159.11). The immunohistochemical features

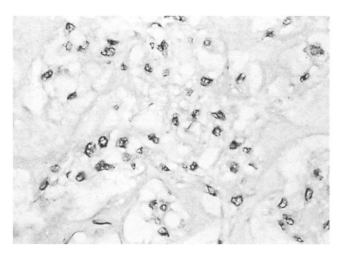

FIGURE 159.11 Photomicrograph of chordoma with characteristic physaliphorous cells. These cells have a clear cytoplasm with a bubbly appearance (original magnification ×250).

of mediastinal chordomas include intense staining with low molecular weight keratin and less intensely with pan keratin, epithelial antigen, and vimentin among the tumor cell.[67]

Clinically, patients may be asymptomatic, but most present with symptoms related to compression or involvement of adjacent structures. Most commonly, patients become symptomatic from compression of the spinal cord, but mediastinal structures such as the trachea and esophagus have also been affected.[68,69] Radiographically, thoracic vertebral chordomas are identified as a paravertebral mass that may extend into the visceral compartment if they arise anteriorly. They may also be identified on plain radiographs by bony destruction.[70] CT images most commonly show vertebral body destruction associated with a soft tissue mass extending anterolaterally. Early detection prior to extensive vertebral body destruction may be confused with a paravertebral schwannoma.

Intervertebral extension was noted in only 4 of 25 patients (16%). Amorphous calcification was present in 40% of the lesions studied. Murphy and associates reported that on T2-weighted MRI, septa of low signal intensity may radiate throughout the high signal mass of the tumor.[71] When present, this feature may be helpful in differentiating a chordoma from other masses in the paravertebral space. Percutaneous needle biopsy may be helpful, but most often the nature of the lesion is not confirmed until biopsy at thoracotomy, especially in the case of those located anterior to the vertebral column and apparently not involving a vertebral body.

The primary treatment of choice is aggressive en bloc resection with negative surgical margins. Proximity to the spinal cord and nerve roots restricts the ability to achieve wide margins in many cases. Intralesional resection was once considered the standard of care, but this has fallen out of favor because of the inability to assure negative margins.[72] High-dose (70 Gy) adjuvant radiation may reduce the risk for local recurrence, but the toxicity to the spinal cord also limits the ability to deliver sufficient radiation doses. More recently, treatment with proton beam therapy has been used because of the enhanced ability to deliver focal treatments with minimized toxicity to surrounding structures. Early series reporting the outcomes of patients with chordomas treated with resection and postoperative proton beam therapy have demonstrated improved results, but this improvement still includes a 2-year local control rate of only 45%.[73]

CHONDROSARCOMA OF THE THORACIC SPINE

Chondrosarcoma, arising from a vertebral body, and extending into a paravertebral sulcus or into the visceral compartment, is rare. Due to the location of these tumors and proximity to the spinal cord, achieving adequate surgical margins is difficult and local recurrence is problematic. In a systematic review of patients with spinal chondrosarcomas, trends of decreasing risk of local recurrence and increasing disease-free survival were observed over the course of time.[74] Inadequate surgical margins, higher tumor grade, and increased patient age were all factors associated with poor local control and survival. Importantly, local recurrence was noted in 20 of 21 patients with intralesional procedures compared to only 1 of 13 patients who underwent en bloc resections.[74] The addition of radiation, particularly proton, carbon, or helium ion beam therapy has contributed to substantially increased rates of local control. Several reports indicate local control rates of 90% at 5 years among patients who underwent incomplete resection followed by postoperative radiation.[74]

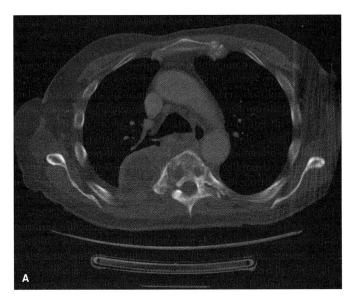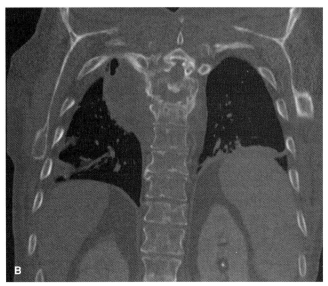

FIGURE 159.12 Paraspinous abscess with adjacent destruction of the vertebral column seen on (**A**) axial and (**B**) coronal views of a CT scan.

PARAVERTEBRAL ABSCESS

Infrequently, a tuberculous paravertebral abscess will resemble a mediastinal mass on examination, but the associated bony and intervertebral disc destruction as well as the clinical course of the patient should lead to the appropriate diagnosis. In the setting of suspected tubercular abscess, the lungs should also be thoroughly evaluated to identify the primary focus of disease. This can be accomplished by plain radiographs, CT imaging, or MRI (Fig. 159.12).[75] Treatment consists of drainage of the abscess and appropriate antituberculous chemotherapy.

LESIONS OF THE MENINGES

ANTERIOR MENINGOCELE

Infrequently, a lesion that is an anterior meningocele, more properly termed a lateral meningocele, presents in a paravertebral sulcus from the spinal canal as the meninges protrude through one or more of the intervertebral foramina. These lesions are frequently asymptomatic and may masquerade as posterior mediastinal neurogenic tumors. The majority of patients are young to middle-aged adults, and most cases are associated with a generalized condition of mesenchymal dysplasia such as neurofibromatosis I or Marfan syndrome.[76] Approximately 20% of patients may also have isolated kyphoscoliosis. Overall, most meningoceles are located posteriorly in the lumbosacral regions. Thoracic lesions are more likely to be anterior or anterolateral.[76]

Scalloping of the adjacent dorsal vertebrae, enlargement of the intervertebral foramen, pedicle erosion, or splaying or thinning of adjacent ribs may be apparent. CT imaging is frequently diagnostic based on the presence of a well-circumscribed, homogenous, low-density lesion in the intervertebral space. MRI can also be used to confirm the diagnosis. Historically, a myelogram has been used to clarify the diagnosis, but seems less pertinent in the setting of modern MRI and CT imaging.

Surgical resection is not always indicated, particularly if the diagnosis is known and the patient is asymptomatic. However, in the setting of progressive neurologic deficits, respiratory distress, or rapid growth of the lesion, surgical resection becomes necessary.[77,78] Small meningoceles may be repaired with a posterior laminectomy approach. Larger lesions may require a transthoracic approach. If resection is performed, secure closure of the neck of the meningocele is critical in order to prevent leakage of cerebrospinal fluid into the pleural space.

INTRATHORACIC EXTRAMEDULLARY HEMATOPOIESIS

Ectopic extramedullary hematopoiesis may represent a physiologic response or a pathologic hematopoietic disorder. It may occur in the liver, spleen, lymph nodes, or thorax. Paraspinal hematopoiesis may also extend into the spinal canal causing cord compression.[79] With rare exception, the ectopic tissue is located inferiorly in one or both of the paravertebral sulci.[80] However, other authors have demonstrated a case where the extramedullary hematopoietic mass occurred immediately posterior to the sternum. The diagnosis can be established by its radiographic appearance on contrast-enhanced CT imaging, MRI, and technetium-99 radionuclide bone imaging.[81–83] These imaging modalities are diagnostic in the clinical setting of a defined hemoglobinopathy.[79] Historically the diagnosis could also be confirmed with radionuclide studies using radioactive iron (^{59}Fe) or gold (^{198}Au) which are absorbed and concentrated by the hematopoietic tissues.

The ectopic hematopoietic tissue typically accompanies a severe form of hemolytic anemia such as hereditary spherocytic anemia, thalassemia, sickle cell anemia, or myelofibrosis. The majority of patients with intrathoracic extramedullary hematopoiesis are asymptomatic and surgical intervention is not necessary. Occasionally, the mass may compress the spinal cord or lead to hemorrhage. When the hematopoietic tissue mass extends into the spinal canal, surgical decompression may be necessary, or the tissue mass can also be reduced with low-dose radiotherapy.[84] The presence of additional hematopoietic tissue elsewhere should be confirmed prior to the ablation of what may be the only existing hematopoietic tissue. Acute hemorrhage into the pleural space may be accompanied by the onset of chest pain and shortness of breath. This bleeding is often self-limited and patients can be adequately treated with drainage with or without pleurodesis. If bleeding persists, surgical intervention may be necessary. One case report described a fatal episode of hemorrhage from an intrathoracic extrahematopoietic soft tissue mass.[85]

LESIONS OF VASCULAR ORIGIN

Mediastinal masses of vascular origin must be differentiated from true mediastinal tumors. These masses may be either arterial or venous in origin and may arise from either the systemic or pulmonary vascular systems. Many of these are covered in other chapters of this book. Several reports exist in the literature of azygos vein aneurysms which present as mediastinal masses. Some azygos aneurysms have been related to portal hypertension, local trauma, but others remain idiopathic.[86] Given the infrequent diagnosis and lack of data guiding management, opinions of the optimal treatment vary widely from simple observation to resection. In a series of 10 patients with azygos vein aneurysms, Ko and colleagues differentiated patients with sacular aneurysms ($n = 4$) and fusiform aneurysms ($n = 6$). Importantly, the sacular aneurysms were more likely to be symptomatic in that they caused chest pain or pulmonary thromboemboli, whereas the fusiform aneurysm remained asymptomatic. For these reasons, the patients with saccular aneurysms were treated surgically and the patients with fusiform aneurysms were followed with serial imaging for 3 to 8 years. Observation of fusiform aneurysms seemed appropriate given that the greatest growth observed was an increase from 30 to 32 mm diameter over the course of 8 years.[87]

LESIONS OF THE ESOPHAGUS

Some esophageal abnormalities may masquerade as primary mediastinal tumors such as a large sigmoid esophagus resulting from long-standing severe achalasia. Other lesions include epiphrenic esophageal diverticula, leiomyoma, and contained esophageal perforations that are either related or unrelated to esophageal malignancies. The correct diagnosis can often be established with CT imaging, particularly when oral contrast is administered. More complete discussions of the diagnosis and management of primary esophageal abnormalities are discussed elsewhere in this text.

LESIONS OF THE LUNGS

Benign and malignant tumors of the lungs may be confused with primary mediastinal tumors. Occasionally, in lung cancers abutting and invading the mediastinum the origin of tumors is difficult to distinguish. Obtaining pathologic confirmation of the tumor is likely to clarify the tumors' origin. Pulmonary sequestrations may also present as primary mediastinal tumors on plain radiographs. Often, CT imaging will clarify the diagnosis of a primary pulmonary process rather than a mediastinal tumor.

DIAPHRAGMATIC HERNIAS

FORAMEN OF MORGAGNI HERNIAS

Foramen of Morgagni hernia are defects of the anterior diaphragm immediately posterior to the sternum. This defect may allow passage of the transverse colon, omentum, or other abdominal organs into the anterior mediastinal space (Fig. 159.13). The herniated abdominal contents are more likely to pass into the right hemithorax than the left because of the presence of the pericardium on the left side.[88] Similar diaphragmatic defects may also occur iatrogenically following a median sternotomy due to the relatively lower pressure in the thorax compared to the abdomen; these hernias tend to become progressively larger with time and their diagnosis warrants surgical correction. This may be achieved either laparoscopically or through a midline laparotomy. Mesh may be required to achieve a tension-free closure of the diaphragm.

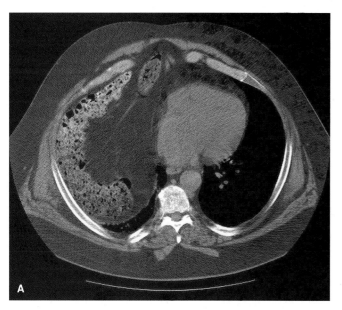 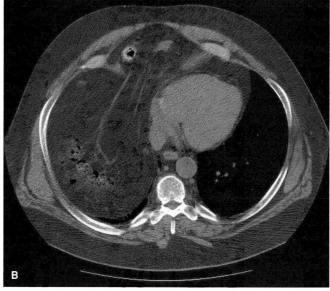

FIGURE 159.13 CT axial images of a Morgagni hernia showing (**A**) a segment of transverse colon in the right anterior hemithorax and (**B**) the anterior diaphragmatic defect.

BOCHDALEK HERNIA

Posterior diaphragmatic defects are known as Bochdalek hernias. This type of hernia is congenital and results from the failure of the septum transversum (which develops into the central portion of the diaphragm) and the pleuroperitoneal folds (which develop into the posterior rim of the diaphragm) to fuse. Bochdalek hernias are most frequently diagnosed in the neonatal period because bowel herniated into the left hemithorax in utero causes compression of the left lung and subsequent pulmonary hypoplasia. These defects are recognized either prenatally by routine fetal ultrasound or at birth because of respiratory distress. Less commonly, smaller Bochdalek hernias may remain asymptomatic. They may be recognized only in adulthood as incidental radiographic findings. A review of 13,138 adult abdominal CT scans determined the prevalence of Bochdalek hernias to be 0.17%.[89] Adult patients may also present with complaints of recurrent chest and abdominal pain.[90] The diagnosis can be confirmed with CT imaging by the presence of a predominantly fatty mass in the posterior thoracic cavity at the level of the diaphragm. Larger defects that include abdominal organs may also be found in approximately 27% of adult Bochdalek hernias (Fig. 159.14).[89] Case reports of incarceration, strangulation, and visceral perforation exist in the literature providing cause for surgical repair of these defects when diagnosed. Surgical repair may be approached either through the chest or abdomen and minimally invasive techniques have been

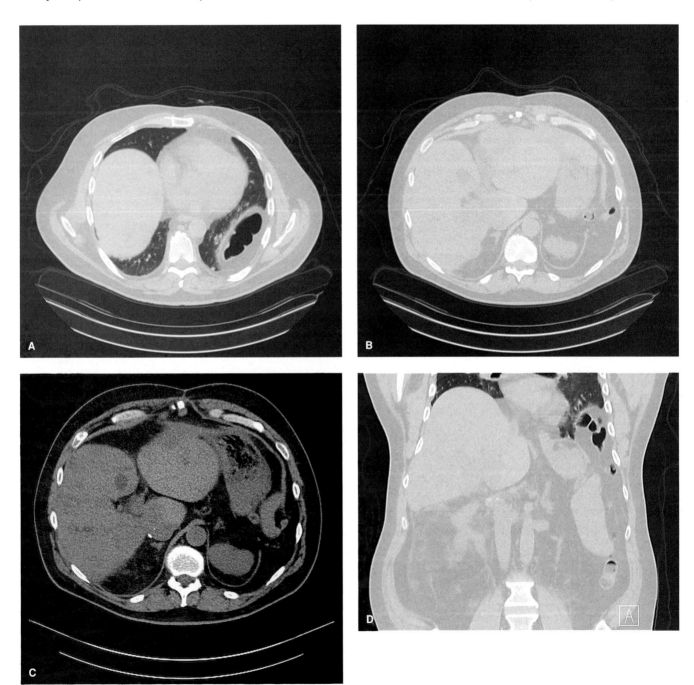

FIGURE 159.14 CT images demonstrating an adult Bochdalek hernia. **(A)** lung window image demonstrating the colon splenic flexure in the posterior left chest, **(B,C)** lung and soft tissue windows demonstrating the posterior diaphragmatic defect, **(D)** coronal image demonstrating diaphragmatic defect.

described. A transabdominal approach is preferable if there is concern for volvulus or nonviable bowel. A primary repair of the diaphragm with nonabsorbable suture should be attempted, but mesh can also be used for large defects.[88]

PANCREATIC PSEUDOCYSTS

Infrequently, a pancreatic pseudocyst may present as a mass in the visceral compartment behind the heart. Johnston and colleagues[91] reviewed this subject and presented an example of this unusual complication of pancreatic disease. The clinical presentation should alert one to the possibility that the retrocardiac mass is a pseudocyst. Confirmation is best obtained by CT of the chest and abdomen, which demonstrates the extension of the cyst from the abdomen into the chest. Treatment is by internal drainage of the cyst through a laparotomy approach.

REFERENCES

1. Wakely CPG, Mulvany JH. Intrathoracic goiter. *Surg Gynecol Obstet* 1940;70:702–710.
2. Allo MD, Thompson NW. Rationale for the operative management of substernal goiters. *Surgery* 1983;94:969–977.
3. Wu MH, Chen KY, Liaw KY, et al. Primary intrathoracic goiter. *J Formos Med Assoc* 2006;105:160–163.
4. Foroulis CN, Rammos KS, Sileli MN, et al. Primary intrathoracic goiter: a rare and potentially serious entity. *Thyroid* 2009;19:213–218.
5. McCort JJ. Intrathoracic goiter: its incidence, symptomatology, and roentgen diagnosis. *Radiology* 1949;53:227–237.
6. Glazer GM, Axel L, Moss AA. CT diagnosis of mediastinal thyroid. *Am J Roentgenol* 1982;138:495–498.
7. Kacprzak G, Karas J, Rzechonek A, et al. Retrosternal goiter located in the mediastinum: surgical approach and operative difficulties. *Interact Cardiovasc Thorac Surg* 2012;15:935–937.
8. Dahan M, Gaillard J, Eschapasse H. Surgical treatment of goiters with intrathoracic development. In Delarue NC, Eschapasse H, eds. *International Trends in General Thoracic Surgery*. Vol 5. *Thoracic Surgery: Frontiers and Uncommon Neoplasms*. St. Louis, MO: Mosby; 1989.
9. Nwafo DC. Heterotopic mediastinal goitre. *Br J Surg* 1978;65:505–556.
10. Hall TS, Caslowitz P, Popper C, et al. Substernal goiter versus intrathoracic aberrant thyroid: a critical difference. *Ann Thorac Surg* 1988;46:684–685.
11. Sand J, Pehkonen E, Mattila J, et al. Pulsating mass at the sternum: a primary carcinoma of ectopic mediastinal thyroid. *J Thorac Cardiovasc Surg* 1996;112:833–835.
12. Spinner RJ, Moore KL, Gottfried MR, et al. Thoracic intrathymic thyroid. *Ann Surg* 1994;220:91–96.
13. Mace AD, Taghi A, Khalil S, et al. Ectopic sequestered thyroid tissue: an unusual cause of a mediastinal mass. *ISRN Surg* 2011;2011:313626.
14. LeRoux BT. Heterotopic mediastinal thyroid. *Thorax* 1961;16:192–196.
15. Sussman SK, Silverman PM, Donnal JF. CT demonstration of isolated mediastinal goiter. *J Comput Assist Tomogr* 1986;10:863–864.
16. Grondin SC, Buenaventura P, Luketich JD. Thoracoscopic resection of an ectopic intrathoracic goiter. *Ann Thorac Surg* 2001;71:1697–1698.
17. Tang ATM, Johnson MJ, Addis B, et al. Thoracic intrathymic thyroid and cervical goiter: single-stage resection. *Ann Thorac Surg* 2002;74:578–579.
18. Cove H. The mediastinum. In Coulson WF, ed. *Surgical Pathology*. 2nd ed Philadelphia, PA: Lippincott; 1988.
19. Casanova JB, Daly RC, Edwards BS, et al. Intracardiac ectopic thyroid. *Ann Thorac Surg* 2000;70:1694–1696.
20. Urban M, Besik J, Szarszoi O, et al. Right ventricular outflow tract obstruction caused by ectopic thyroid gland. *Ann Thorac Surg* 2014;98:345.
21. Taylor MA, Brady M, Roberts WC. Aberrant thyroid gland attached to the ascending aorta. *Am J Cardiol* 1986;57:708.
22. Williams RJ, Lindop G, Butler J. Ectopic thyroid tissue on the ascending aorta: an operative finding. *Ann Thorac Surg* 2002;73:1642–1643.
23. Ozpolat B, Dogan OV, Gökaslan G, et al. Ectopic thyroid gland on the ascending aorta with a partial pericardial defect: report of a case. *Surg Today* 2007;37:486–488.
24. Khan M, Michaelson PG, Hinni ML. Intratracheal ectopic thyroid tissue presenting with protracted airway obstruction: a case report. *Ear Nose Throat J* 2008;87:476–477.
25. Dowling EA, Johnson IM, Collier FC, et al. Intratracheal goiter: a clinic-pathological review. *Ann Surg* 1962;156:258–267.
26. Katlic MR, Grillo HC, Wang CA. Substernal goiter. Analysis of 80 patients from Massachusetts General Hospital. *Am J Surg* 1985;149:283–287.
27. Rodriguez JM, Hernandez G, Piñero A, et al. Substernal goiter: clinical experience of 72 cases. *Ann Otol Rhinol Laryngol* 1999;108:501–504.
28. Phillips DJ, Kutler DI, Kuhel WI. Incidental thyroid nodules in patients with primary hyperparathyroidism. *Head Neck* 2014;36:1763–1765.
29. Allo MD, Thompson NW. Rationale for the operative management of substernal goiters. *Surgery* 1983;94:969–977.
30. Sanders LE, Rossi RL, Shahian DM, et al. Mediastinal goiters. The need for an aggressive approach. *Arch Surg* 1992;127:609–613.
31. Shaha AR, Alfonso AE, Jaffe BM. Operative treatment of substernal goiters. *Head Neck* 1989;11:325–330.
32. Torre G, Borgonovo G, Amato A, et al. Surgical management of substernal goiter: analysis of 237 patients. *Am Surg* 1995;61:826–831.
33. Landerholm K, Järhult J. Should asymptomatic retrosternal goiter be left untreated? A prospective single-centre study. *Scand J Surg* 2015;104(2):92–95.
34. Warren CP. Acute respiratory failure and tracheal obstruction in the elderly with benign goiters. *Can Med Assoc J* 1979;121:191–194.
35. Bonnema SJ, Knudsen DU, Bertelsen H, et al. Does radioiodine therapy have an equal effect on substernal and cervical goiter volumes? Evaluation by magnetic resonance imaging. *Thyroid* 2002;12:313–317.
36. van Doorn LG, Kranendonk SE. Partial unilateral phrenic nerve paralysis caused by a large intrathoracic goitre. *Neth J Med* 1996;48:216–219.
37. Gadisseux P, Minette P, Trigaux JP, et al. Cerebrovascular circulation "steal" syndrome secondary to a voluminous retrotracheal goiter. *Int Surg* 1986;71:107–109.
38. Ribet ME, Mensier E, Caparros-Lefebvre D, et al. Cerebral ischemia from thoracic goiter. *Eur J Cardiothorac Surg* 1995;9:717–718.
39. Sakkary MA, Abdelrahman AM, Mostafa AM, et al. Retrosternal goiter: the need for thoracic approach based on CT findings: surgeon's view. *J Egypt Natl Canc Inst* 2012;24:85–90.
40. Bashist B, Ellis K, Gold RP. Computed tomography of intrathoracic goiters. *Am J Roentgenol* 1983;140:455–460.
41. Glazer GM, Axel L, Moss AA. CT diagnosis of mediastinal thyroid. *Am J Roentgenol* 1982;138:495.
42. Buckley JA, Stark P. Intrathoracic mediastinal thyroid goiter: imaging manifestations. *Am J Roentgenol* 1999;173:471–475.
43. von Schulthess GK, McMurdo K, Tscholakoff D, et al. Mediastinal masses: MR imaging. *Radiology* 1986;158:289–296.
44. Newman E, Shaha AR. Substernal goiter. *J Surg Oncol* 1995;60:207–212.
45. Park HM, Tarver RD, Siddiqui AR, et al. Efficacy of thyroid scintigraphy in the diagnosis of intrathoracic goiter. *Am J Roentgenol* 1987;148:527–529.
46. Kahara T, Ichikawa T, Taniguchi H, et al. Mediastinal thyroid goiter with no accumulation on scintigraphy. *Intern Med* 2013;52:2159.
47. Johnston JH, Jr., Twente GE. Surgical approach to intrathoracic (mediastinal) goiter. *Ann Surg* 1956;143:572–579.
48. De Andrade MA. A review of 128 cases of posterior mediastinal goiter. *World J Surg* 1977;1:789–797.
49. D'Alia C, Tonante A, Lo Schiavo MG, et al. Transclavicular access as an adjunct to standard cervical incision in the treatment of mediastinal goitre. *Chir Ital* 2002;54:576–580.
50. Gupta P, Lau KK, Rizvi I, et al. Video assisted thoracoscopic thyroidectomy for retrosternal goiter. *Ann R Coll Surg Engl* 2014;96(8):606–608.
51. Hajhosseini B, Montazeri V, Hajhosseini L, et al. Mediastinal goiter: a comprehensive study of 60 consecutive cases with special emphasis on identifying predictors of malignancy and sternotomy. *Am J Surg* 2012;203:442–447.
52. Coskun A, Yildirim M, Erkan N. Substernal goiter: when is a sternotomy required? *Int Surg* 2014;99:419–425.
53. Grosfeld JS, Weber TR, Vane DW. One-stage resection for massive cervicomediastinal hygroma. *Surgery* 1982;92:693–699.
54. Singh S, Baboo ML, Pathak IC. Cystic lymphangioma in children: report of 32 cases including lesions at rare sites. *Surgery* 1971;69:947.
55. Jougon J, Laborde MN, Parrens M, et al. Cystic lymphangioma of the heart mimicking a mediastinal tumor. *Eur J Cardiothorac Surg* 2002;22:476–478.
56. Wilson C, Askin FB, Heitmiller RF. Solitary pulmonary lymphangioma. *Ann Thorac Surg* 2001;71:1337–1338.
57. Mirza B, Saleem M, Sharif M, et al. Cystic hygroma: an overview. *J Cutan Aesthet Surg* 2010;3:139–144.
58. Icard P, Le Rochais JP, Galateau F, et al. Mediastinal cystic hygroma. Report of three cases and review of the literature. *Ann Chir* 1998;52:629–634.
59. Riquet M, Brie're J, Le Pimpec-Barthes F, et al. Cystic lymphangioma of the neck and mediastinum: are there acquired forms? *Rev Mal Respir* 1999;16:71–79.
60. Taniguchi I, Maeda T, Morimoto K, et al. Spontaneous retropharyngeal hematoma of a parathyroid cyst: report of a case. *Surg Today* 2003;33:354–357.
61. Silver WE. Cervical mediastinal thymic parathyroid cyst. *Otolaryngol Head Neck Surg* 1980;88:403–408.
62. Kim YS, Kim J, Shin S. Thoracoscopic removal of ectopic mediastinal parathyroid adenoma. *Korean J Thorac Cardiovasc Surg* 2014;45:317–319.
63. Yoshimura N, Mukaida H, Mimura T, et al. A case of an acute cervicomediastinal hematoma secondary to the spontaneous rupture of a parathyroid adenoma. *Ann Thorac Cardiovasc Surg* 2014;20 Suppl:816–820.
64. Simcic KJ, McDermott MT, Crawford GJ, et al. Massive extracapsular hemorrhage from a parathyroid cyst. *Arch Surg* 1989;124:1347–1350.
65. Hotes LS, Barzilav J, Rolla AR. Spontaneous hematoma of a parathyroid adenoma. *Am J Med Sci* 1989;297:331–333.
66. Rich TA, Schiller A, Suit HD, et al. Clinical and pathological review of 48 cases of chordoma. *Cancer* 1985;56:182–187.
67. Suster S, Moran CA. Chordomas of the mediastinum: clinicopathologic, immunohistochemical, and ultrastructural study of six cases presenting as posterior mediastinal masses. *Hum Pathol* 1995;26:1354–1362.
68. Brooks M, Kleefield J, O'Reilly GV, et al. Thoracic chordoma with unusual radiographic features. *Comput Radiol* 1987;11:85–90.
69. Cury JD, Peterson RJ, Lacy GD, et al. Tracheal deviation from an atypical mediastinal mass. *Chest* 1997;111:503–505.
70. Schwarz SS, Fisher WS 3rd, Pulliam MW, et al. Thoracic chordoma in a patient with paraparesis and ivory vertebral body. *Neurosurgery* 1985;16:100–102.

71. Murphy JM, Wallis F, Toland J, et al. CT and MRI appearance of a thoracic chordoma. *Eur Radiol* 1998;8:1677–1679.
72. Chi JH, Sciubba DM, Rhines LD, et al. Surgery for primary vertebral tumors: en bloc versus intralesional resection. *Neurosurg Clin N Am* 2008;19:111–117.
73. Holliday EB, Mitra HS, Somerson JS, et al. Postoperative proton therapy for chordomas and chondrosarcomas of the spine. Adjuvant versus salvage radiation therapy. *Spine* 2015;40:544–549.
74. Boriani S, Saravanja D, Yamada Y, et al. Challenges of local recurrence and cure in low grade malignant tumors of the spine. *Spine* 2009;34:S48–S57.
75. Lalla R, Singh MK, Patil TB, et al. MRI of the spinal tuberculoma, paravertebral tubercular abscess and pulmonary tuberculosis. *BMJ Case Rep* 2013;2013:pii:bcr2013201098.
76. Oner AY, Uzun M, Tokgoz N, et al. Isolated true anterior thoracic menigocele. *Am J Neuroradiol* 2004;25:1828–1830.
77. Mizuno J, Nakagawa H, Yamada T, et al. Intrathoracic giant meningocele developing hydrothorax: a case report. *J Spinal Disord Tech* 2002;15:529–532.
78. Ebara S, Yuzawa Y, Kinoshita T, et al. A neurofibromatosis type 1 patient with severe kyphoscoliosis and intrathoracic meningocele. *J Clin Neurosci* 2003;10:268–272.
79. Hashmi MA, Guha S, Sengupta P, et al. Thoracic cord compression by extramedullary hematopoiesis in thalassemia. *Asian J Neurosurg* 2014;9:102–104.
80. Chu KA, Hsu CW, Lin MH, et al. Recurrent spontaneous massive hemothorax from intrathoracic extramedullary hematopoiesis resulting in respiratory failure. *J Formos Med Assoc* 2015;114:282–284.
81. Gumbs RV, Higginbotham-Ford EA, Teal JS, et al. Thoracic extramedullary hematopoiesis in sickle-cell disease. *Am J Roentgenol* 1987;149:889–893.
82. Savader SJ, Otero RR, Savader BL. MR imaging of intrathoracic extramedullary hematopoiesis. *J Comput Assit Tomog* 1988;12:878–880.
83. Brown LJ, Paquelet JR, Tetalman MR. Intrathoracic extramedullary hematopoiesis: appearance on 99m Tc sulfur colloid marrow scan. *Am J Roentgenol* 1988;134:1254–1255.
84. Singhal S, Sharma S, Dixit S, et al. The role of radiation therapy in the management of spinal cord compression due to extramedullary hematopoiesis in thalassemia. *J Neurol Neurosurg Psychiatry* 1992;55:310–312.
85. Chute DJ, Fowler DR. Fatal hemothorax due to rupture of an intrathoracic extramedullary hematopoietic nodule. *Am J Forensic Med Pathol* 2004;25:74–77.
86. Ichiki Y, Hamatsu T, Suehiro T, et al. An idiopathic azygos vein aneurysm mimicking a mediastinal mass. *Ann Thorac Surg* 2014;98:338–340.
87. Ko SF, Huang CC, Lin JW, et al. Imaging features and outcomes in 10 cases of idiopathic azygos vein aneurysm. *Ann Thorac Surg* 2014;97:873–878.
88. Schumacher L, Gilbert S. Congenital diaphragmatic hernia in the adult. *Thorac Surg Clin* 2009;19:469–472.
89. Mullins ME, Stein J, Saini SS, et al. Prevalence of incidental Bochdalek's hernia in a large adult population. *Am J Roentgenol* 2001;177:363–366.
90. Herling A, Makhdom F, Al-Shehri A, et al. Bochdalek hernia in a symptomatic adult. *Ann Thorac Surg* 2014;98:701–704.
91. Johnson RH, Jr., Owensby LC, Vargas GM, et al. Pancreatic pseudocyst of the mediastinum. *Ann Thorac Surg* 1986;41:210–202.

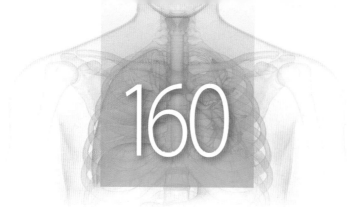

160

Primary Pneumomediastinum

Rachel L. Medbery ▪ Felix G. Fernandez

BACKGROUND

Primary pneumomediastinum, commonly referred to as spontaneous pneumomediastinum, is defined as the presence of free air within the mediastinal cavity without an overt etiology. The phenomenon, commonly a diagnosis of exclusion, was first described by Hamman in 1937.[1] Although the diagnosis can be a daunting one, the clinical course of primary pneumomediastinum is often short, self-limited, and benign in the adult patient. The role of the thoracic surgeon is to rule out serious causes which could be life-threatening and require intervention.

ANATOMY AND PATHOPHYSIOLOGY

The mediastinum is an intrathoracic cavity which is demarcated by the thoracic inlet superiorly, the pleural cavities laterally, and the diaphragm inferiorly. The pathophysiology of primary pneumomediastinum was first explained by Macklin to comprise of three essential steps: (1) a rapid increase in intrathoracic pressure results in alveolar rupture; (2) small airway rupture leads to dissection of interstitial air along the tracheobronchial tree and perivascular planes; and (3) once airway integrity has been compromised, a pressure gradient exists between the lung periphery and the mediastinum allowing air to dissect relatively freely into the central mediastinum.[2,3] This increase in pressure can be severe enough to allow for further spontaneous dissection of air into the neck, retroperitoneum, subcutaneous tissues, and even into the epidural space. Rarely, dissection can escape the soft tissues and invade the visceral or parietal pleura of the lungs, leading to pneumothorax. Case reports have also described spontaneous dissection into the peritoneum and pericardium, leading to pneumoperitoneum and pneumopericardium, respectively.[3,4]

EPIDEMIOLOGY

The true incidence of primary pneumomediastinum remains difficult to assess. Many episodes are not diagnosed because symptoms are too mild to warrant formal medical attention. Furthermore, case series indicate that up to 30% of pneumomediastinum cases are too small to be detected on chest radiograph alone, and thus symptoms may be attributed to other causes such as musculoskeletal pain.[5-8] As a result, primary pneumomediastinum is assuredly underdiagnosed. What we do know about the condition is limited to findings of several case series within the literature, most of which contain fewer than 30 patients.[9] However, based on the handful of reported series, primary pneumomediastinum has an estimated incidence of 1:25,000 to 1:30,000 and most frequently occurs in young healthy male patients who identify themselves as smokers.[10-12]

The majority of patients with primary pneumomediastinum will present with either a medical comorbidity or triggering event causing sudden marked increase in airway pressures (Table 160.1). Asthma exacerbation, COPD, and bronchitis are the most commonly reported triggers associated with pneumomediastinum, accounting for up to 40% to 50% of reported cases.[10] It is important to keep in mind, however, that as many as 20% to 30% of patients will present without a precipitating factor or triggering event.[7]

CLINICAL PRESENTATION

The clinical history and physical exam can often be nonspecific in patients with primary pneumomediastinum, as signs and symptoms are associated with a broad differential diagnosis. While the clinical presentation can vary, the most common chief complaints are chest pain and shortness of breath. Other presenting signs/symptoms are listed in Table 160.2. The chest pain is often noted to be pleuritic in nature,

TABLE 160.1 Conditions/Triggers Associated With Primary Pneumomediastinum[4,5,9,10,12,13]

Airway	GI	Extreme Valsalva	Lifestyle/Addiction	Other
Asthma exacerbation	Vomiting	Defecation	Extreme physical activity	Diabetic ketoacidosis
COPD exacerbation	Peptic ulcer disease	Labor	Inhaled drugs	Unknown
Cough			Anorexia nervosa	
Acute bronchial obstruction			Panic attack	
Acute laryngitis				
Choking				
Interstitial lung disease				

TABLE 160.2 Signs and Symptoms of Primary Pneumomediastinum[4,5,9,10,12,13]

Clinical Symptoms	Physical Exam Findings
Chest pain	Hamman's sign
Dyspnea	Subcutaneous emphysema
Neck pain	Stridor
Dysphagia	Tachycardia
Odynophagia	Tachypnea
Cough	Low-grade fever
Nasal voice	Pulsus paradoxus
Fever	
Stridor	
Anxiety	

described as retrosternal with radiation to the neck and back. Although some series note that patients may be anxious, oftentimes they appear well and in no acute distress. Physical exam in these patients can be unremarkable with relatively normal vital signs. Mild tachycardia can be present and could be attributed to pain and/or anxiety. Some series also note that low-grade fever (38.0°C– 38.5°C) can be present as well.[14] While historically noted to be associated with pneumomediastinum, Hamman's sign (crepitus heard with the heartbeat upon auscultation of the chest) is rarely appreciated on physical exam.[1]

DIAGNOSTIC WORKUP

The diagnosis of primary pneumomediastinum is a diagnosis of exclusion. Because it can resemble that of many other medical problems, diagnostic workup most often includes a minimum of blood work (complete blood count, basic chemistry, and cardiac enzymes), electrocardiogram (EKG), and chest radiograph to rule out major diagnoses such as pneumonia and acute coronary syndrome.

LABORATORY DATA

Some series report a mild leukocytosis and an increase in other inflammatory markers such as ESR and CRP in a percentage of patients; however, it is nonspecific and thus non-diagnostic.[8,10,13,14] If these markers are more than mildly elevated, however, the index of suspicion is raised for a more serious problem such as esophageal perforation or septic mediastinitis. In such cases, a CT scan of the chest with oral contrast or an aqueous contrast esophagram should be obtained to rule out more ominous diagnoses.

ELECTROCARDIOGRAM

Two series within the literature have reported EKG abnormalities associated with pneumomediastinum. Mondello et al.[14] note that low-amplitude QRS may be observed, while Macia et al.[8] report ST-segment elevation within part of their cohort. The sensitivity and specificity of these findings are both highly questionable.

IMAGING STUDIES

As previously mentioned, up to 30% of cases may be missed on chest radiograph alone.[5–8] While CT of the chest has a 100% sensitivity and is considered to be the gold standard imaging modality for the diagnosis of pneumomediastinum, in many cases a simple radiograph remains diagnostic and no further imaging studies are needed (Fig. 160.1).

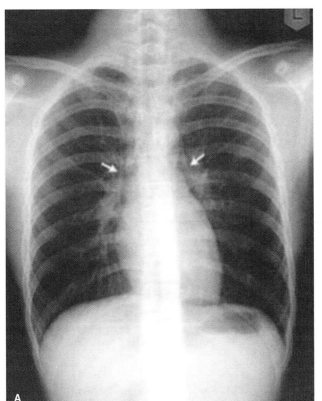
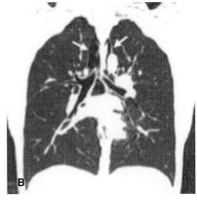
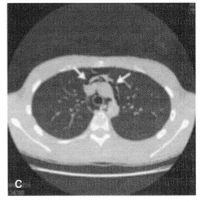

FIGURE 160.1 Pneumomediastinum on (A) chest radiograph and (B,C) chest CT.

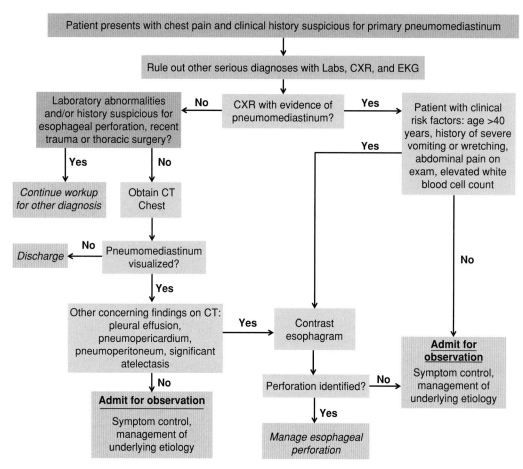

FIGURE 160.2 Treatment algorithm.

FURTHER WORKUP

The use of fluoroscopy (aqueous contrast esophagram), CT scan with enteric contrast, and endoscopy remains somewhat controversial in the routine workup for primary pneumomediastinum. A recent series from Bakhos et al. suggests that esophagography or other invasive endoscopic testing should not be used routinely.[10] Instead, they outline risk factors which should prompt further workup in select cases: age >40 years, history of severe vomiting or retching, abdominal pain on exam, elevated white blood cell count, or concerning finds on chest CT such as pleural effusion, pneumopericardium, pneumoperitoneum, or significant atelectasis (Fig. 160.2).

MANAGEMENT

Once the clinician has excluded serious causes and has arrived at the diagnosis of primary pneumomediastinum, management is directed toward supportive care and symptom relief, monitoring for potential complications, and treatment of underlying etiology. Pain control is best achieved with a combination of nonsteroidal anti-inflammatory agents and narcotics if necessary. For patients with associated anxiety, anxiolytics may be appropriate. Patients with dyspnea and/or cough can be treated with oxygen therapy and antitussives, respectively. It was originally thought that pure oxygen treatment increased the diffusion pressure of nitrogen in the interstitium leading to rapid absorption of free air, and thus hastening the course of pneumomediastinum[3]; however, most recent series do not support this notion and

only recommend oxygen as needed for symptomatic relief. Treatment of underlying airway pathology such as asthma and COPD with bronchodilators and/or corticosteroids is appropriate. If the clinician feels the etiology of primary pneumomediastinum is secondary to an infectious process such as bronchitis, antibiotics would be indicated. Otherwise, empiric broad-spectrum antibiotic therapy is not necessary. Unless there is concern for underlying esophageal perforation, oral intake should not be restricted.

Hospital admission for observation is appropriate; however, the average length of stay is not consistent among case series within the literature and ranges from 2 to 8 days.[5,9,10] In a recent series, however, Lee and colleagues recommend that conservative management with hospitalization less than 24 hours is both safe and feasible.[15] Furthermore, the study findings further emphasize that there is no need for restricting oral intake or starting empiric antibiotics in patients with uncomplicated primary pneumomediastinum.

At least one follow-up visit in the clinic after hospital discharge is appropriate to ensure complete resolution of signs and symptoms. A repeat chest radiograph in the clinic should be obtained to document the absence or resolution of pneumomediastinum. Once normal imaging has been documented, there is no need for further studies unless the patient returns with new symptoms.

PATIENT OUTCOMES

Although rare, complications can be observed in patients with primary pneumomediastinum. Associated pneumothorax has been reported in 1% to 14% of cases, depending on the series.[5,9] A small pneumothorax may be observed without intervention, but large or expanding pneumothorax will necessitate chest tube placement. Isolated case reports have described spontaneous dissection into the peritoneum and pericardium, leading to pneumoperitoneum and pneumopericardium, respectively.[3,4] Recurrence of primary pneumomediastinum is rarely reported.[5,8,9,13,15] Recurrent cases of this problem in the same patient might prompt health care professionals to be alert to possible secondary gain, as rare reports have been published of self-induced injury leading to pneumomediastinum and pneumothorax. Self-induced oral mucosal injury, followed by a vigorous Valsalva maneuver, can result in the radiographic findings of pneumomediastinum.[16]

NEONATAL PNEUMOMEDIASTINUM

A special note must be made on pnuemomediastinum in the neonatal population. While pneumomediastinum in adults is often benign and does not require intervention, it can become a life-threatening phenomenon in the neonate. In this specific patient population, pneumomediastinum is often the result of mechanical ventilation and can result in tension physiology that leads to pericardial tamponade. In this situation, urgent evacuation of air from the mediastinal cavity is required and can be accomplished by placement of a subxiphoid tube placed into the anterior mediastinum.[17]

CONCLUSIONS

Primary pneumomediastinum remains a diagnosis of exclusion and is associated with a short, benign clinical course in the adult patient. Up to 30% of patients will present without an underlying triggering event, and an additional 30% of cases will be missed on chest radiograph alone. A detailed history and physical exam are essential, and for at-risk patients, the index of suspicion must be high. Ruling out more ominous diagnoses such as esophageal perforation is paramount. Once the clinician is confident in the diagnosis of primary pneumomediastinum, a short course of observation without further invasive testing is appropriate. Long-term complications and recurrence are uncommon.

REFERENCES

1. Hamman L. Spontaneous mediastinal emphysema. *Bull Hopkins Hosp* 1937;64:1–21.
2. Macklin CC. Transport of air along sheaths of pulmonic blood vessels from alveoli to mediastinum. *Arch Int Med* 1979;64:913–926.
3. Macklin MT, Macklin CC. Malignant interstitial emphysema of the lungs and mediastinum as an important occult complication in many respiratory diseases and other conditions: interpretation of the clinical literature in the light of laboratory experiment. *Medicine* 1949;23:281–358.
4. Pooyan P, Puruckherr M, Summers JA, et al. Pneumomediastinum, pneumopericardium, and epidural pneumatosis in DKA. *J Diabet Complicat* 2004;18:242–247.
5. Caceres M, Ali SZ, Braud R, et al. Spontaneous pneumomediastinum: a comparative study and review of the literature. *Ann Thorac Surg* 2008;86:962–926.
6. Campillo-Soto A, Coll-Salinas A, Soria-Aledo V, et al. [Spontaneous pneumomediastinum: descriptive study of our experience with 36 cases]. *Arch de Bronconeumol* 2005;41:528–5231.
7. Kaneki T, Kubo K, Kawashima A, et al. Spontaneous pneumomediastinum in 33 patients: yield of chest computed tomography for the diagnosis of the mild type. *Respir Internat Rev Thorac Dis* 2000;67:408–411.
8. Macia I, Moya J, Ramos R, et al. Spontaneous pneumomediastinum: 41 cases. *Eur J Cardio Thorac Surg* 2007;31:1110–1114.
9. Dajer-Fadel WL, Arguero-Sanchez R, Ibarra-Perez C, et al. Systematic review of spontaneous pneumomediastinum: a survey of 22 years' data. *Asian Cardiovasc Thorac Ann* 2014;22:997–1002.
10. Bakhos CT, Pupovac SS, Ata A, et al. Spontaneous pneumomediastinum: an extensive workup is not required. *J Am Coll Surg* 2014;219:713–717.
11. Newcomb AE, Clarke CP. Spontaneous pneumomediastinum: a benign curiosity or a significant problem? *Chest* 2005;128:3298–3302.
12. Sahni S, Verma S, Grullon J, et al. Spontaneous pneumomediastinum: time for consensus. *N Am J Med Sci* 2013;5:460–464.
13. Takada K, Matsumoto S, Hiramatsu T, et al. Management of spontaneous pneumomediastinum based on clinical experience of 25 cases. *Respir Med* 2008;102:1329–1334.
14. Mondello B, Pavia R, Ruggeri P, et al. Spontaneous pneumomediastinum: experience in 18 adult patients. *Lung* 2007;185:9–14.
15. Lee SC, Lee DH, Kim GJ. Is primary spontaneous pneumomediastinum a truly benign entity? *Emerg Med Australas* 2014;26:573–578.
16. Lopez-Pelaez MF, Roldan J, Mateo S. Cervical emphysema, pneumomediastinum, and pneumothorax following self-induced oral injury: report of four cases and review of the literature. *Chest* 2001;120(1):306–309.
17. Hauri-Hohl A, Baenziger O, Frey B. Pneumomediastinum in the neonatal and paediatric intensive care unit. *Eur J Pediatr* 2008;167(4):415–418.

161

Vascular Masses of the Mediastinum

John Holt Chaney ▪ H. Adam Ubert ▪ Victor van Berkel

The mediastinum has been described using multiple models to classify and characterize structures and anatomy. Shields organized the mediastinum using anterior, middle, and posterior compartments, each bordered by the diaphragm, pleural space, and thoracic inlet. The anterior compartment abuts the sternum anteriorly and the pericardium and great vessels posteriorly. The anterior compartment thus houses the thymus, the internal mammary vessels, and adipose tissue. The middle compartment is bound by the anterior surface of the pericardium and posteriorly by the ventral surface of the spine. This compartment includes the heart, great vessels, trachea, proximal bronchi, vagus nerves, and phrenic nerves. The posterior compartment—from the ventral surface of the spine to the vertebral bodies—contains the azygous vein, thoracic spinal ganglia, intercostal neurovascular bundles, and sympathetic chain.

Vascular masses, the focus of this chapter, compose approximately 10% of all mediastinal masses, and are most commonly found as unanticipated abnormalities on imaging performed for some other reason. Vascular masses can be easily mistaken for mediastinal tumors, thus further characterization with appropriate imaging modalities is necessary. Contrast-enhanced computed tomography is usually obtained to correctly identify a solid versus vascular mass, and may be sufficient in most cases. In an effort to reduce radiation exposure in children, echocardiography is routinely used in the pediatric population for further classification of mediastinal masses. MRI better evaluates neurological structures and the extent of local invasion. MRI also avoids iodinated contrast and adverse effects of intravenous dye loads.

In this chapter, these masses will be broken down into arterial, venous, and lymphatic lesions with further division based on the vessel or system of origin.

ARTERIAL MASSES

PULMONARY ARTERY

Incidence of pulmonary artery aneurysms in cadaver studies are 1 in 14,000 in the general population and roughly 1 in 80 in known pulmonary hypertension patients. The main pulmonary artery mean diameter is 25 mm in the average adult, with 29 mm considered the upper limit of normal. Left and right branch pulmonary arteries are normally 20 mm in diameter. A main pulmonary artery greater than 4.5 cm, or a left or right pulmonary artery greater than 3 cm, would be considered aneurysmal.[1] Pulmonary hypertension can be found in 66% of pulmonary artery aneurysm patients.[2]

PSEUDOANEURYSM

Pulmonary artery pseudoaneurysms are rare and usually fatal problems that may be secondary to infection,[3,4] trauma, heart disease, connective tissue disorders, vasculitis, or malignancy. Iatrogenic causes include Swan Ganz catheter balloon inflation,[5] percutaneous radiofrequency ablation of lung tumors,[6] right heart catheterization,[7] chemoradiation of lung tumors,[8,9] chest tube insertion, penetrating trauma, and congenital pulmonary artery shunt placement.[10]

Traumatic pulmonary pseudoaneurysms are rare and present most commonly with hemoptysis. From 24 cases described in the literature, 19 were due to penetrating injuries and 5 were from blunt trauma. There have been rare reports of spontaneous resolution with conservative management.[11] Despite these reports of resolution, this pathology portends a mortality of 50%. Embolization is the recommended primary method of repair followed by aneurysmectomy and pulmonary resection.[12,13]

Infectious pulmonary artery pseudoaneurysms were historically associated with tuberculosis or syphilis, with the former affecting distal intraparenchymal arteries, and the latter involving the more proximal pulmonary arteries. Pulmonary pseudoaneurysms from tuberculosis have been named "Rasmussen aneurysms," and are commonly seen peripherally in the upper lobes. Recent papers describe a broader infectious distribution, including *Staphylococcus aureus* (22%), *Salmonella* species (17%), *Streptococcus* species (11%), *Enterococcus* species (11%) and rarely, *Mycobacteria tuberculosis*.[14] There are case reports that also include H1N1 influenza as an etiology.[15]

Most reports of pulmonary artery pseudoaneurysm in the setting of cancer are secondary to an intervention directed against the cancer. There are reports of pseudoaneurysm resulting from surgical resection, radiofrequency ablation, and stereotactic radiation. Epithelioid hemangioendothelioma has been described as a primary etiology of pulmonary artery pseudoaneurysm.[16] Pulmonary artery sarcomas are worthy of mention here, as they can be misdiagnosed as pulmonary artery pseudoaneurysms or thromboembolism.[17]

Congenital causes of pulmonary artery pseudoaneurysms and aneurysms are associated with, and likely the result of, elevated pulmonary artery pressure. Left-to-right shunts caused by atrial septal defects, ventricular septal defects, and patent ductus arteriosus can lead to elevated PA pressures, which over time can lead to aneurysmal dilation. Rupture and dissection are most common in the severe pulmonary hypertension seen in Eisenmenger's complex. Congenital pulmonary artery stenosis may lead to poststenotic dilation, preferentially affecting the left pulmonary artery, leading to asymmetric enlargement of the left branch PA on imaging. Enlargement of the pulmonary trunk and arteries is seen in children without pulmonary

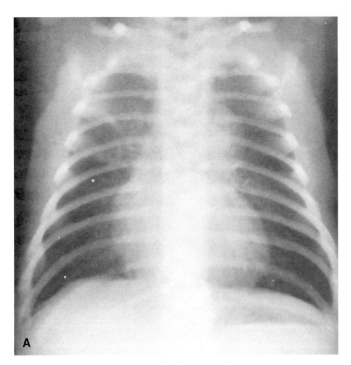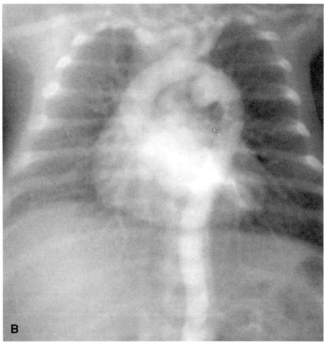

FIGURE 161.1 **A:** Chest radiograph of an 8-day-old infant with an aneurysm of the ductus arteriosus. A left upper mediastinal mass projects into the left chest. Increased pulmonary blood flow is seen. **B:** Angiogram shows the ductus aneurysm immediately distal to the left subclavian artery. The preliminary arteries fill via the ductus arteriosus.

valves or with Tetralogy of Fallot and subsequent regurgitation across the annulus (Fig. 161.1).

ANEURYSM

Pulmonary artery aneurysms are attributed to the multiple factors described in Table 161.1. By definition, a pulmonary artery aneurysm includes all layers of the arterial wall and measures greater than 40 mm.[18]

Clinical presentation is usually incidental detection on imaging performed for other reasons (Fig. 161.2). Massive hemoptysis is the most frequent presenting complaint with a high mortality rate when it occurs. Treatment of pulmonary artery aneurysms and pseudoaneurysms requires active management of pulmonary hypertension and selective surgical intervention. Case reports of endovascular management with coils, bare, and covered stents have described technical successes and may pose a reasonable treatment modality.[19] Surgical excision remains the gold standard treatment.[20] Treatment of aneurysms from vasculitis involve treating the primary inflammatory disorder, not necessarily surgery in all cases.

Behçet disease is the most common etiology of pulmonary artery aneurysms and is most prevalent in 20- to 30-year-old men from the eastern Mediterranean region and Asia.[21] Inflammation of the vasa vasorum leads to vessel wall destruction and subsequent dilation.[22,23]

TABLE 161.1 Pulmonary Artery Aneurysms

- Congenital Heart Disease
- Pulmonary Hypertension
- Infection
- Vasculitis
- Sarcoidosis
- Marfan Syndrome
- Mitral Stenosis

Plausible estimates of the prevalence of PA aneurysm in the outpatient setting for patients with Behçet disease are roughly 1%.[24] Other common manifestations of Behçet disease include uveitis, aphthous ulcers, genital ulcers, skin lesions, aortic root dilation, aortic valve regurgitation, intracardiac thrombus, and pulmonary artery aneurysm.[25] Treatment with colchicine, corticosteroids, and immunosuppression

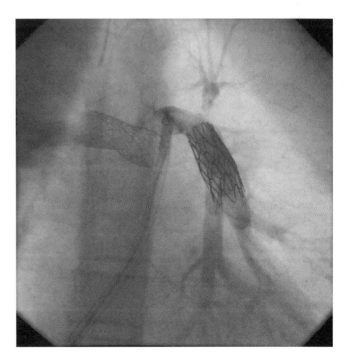

FIGURE 161.2 Native poststenotic left pulmonary artery aneurysm in a 15-year-old with Alagille syndrome and peripheral pulmonary hypoplasia. Note the first stent already in place in the right pulmonary artery. Treatment was achieved with a covered stent in the left pulmonary artery.

can stabilize Behçet's pulmonary aneurysms in the acute phase prior to fibrosis.[26] Arterial instability makes surgical repair difficult, as such, an endovascular approach is favored for patients refractory to medical treatment or with hemoptysis.

Hughes–Stovin Syndrome is a rare condition characterized by thrombophlebitis and pulmonary or bronchial arterial aneurysms. There fewer than 40 reported cases and no known etiology yet identified. Treatment includes medical management with cyclophosphamide and avoidance of anticoagulants or thrombolytics. Direct interventions on the aneurysm range from embolization to resection, but these patients are burdened with a poor prognosis regardless of therapy.[27]

DUCTUS ARTERIOSUS ANEURYSM

Aneurysms of the ductus arteriosus may be present in up to 8.1% of term infants, but most resolve without complication or symptoms.[28] Risk factors seem to include uncontrolled gestational diabetes and maternal A blood type.[29,30] The risk of rupture, thromboembolism, compression of adjacent structures, or death are less than 30% at 2 months but increase to 60% if the aneurysm persists after 2 months.[31] As a result, recommendations are to delay closure and await spontaneous resolution until 2 months unless there is a known connective tissue disorder or symptoms caused by thromboembolism or surrounding compression.[30] Chest radiograph may reveal a round mass in the left superior mediastinum and echo findings include a tortuous dilated vascular structure that travels left of the aortic arch with a ductal jet.[32]

THORACIC AORTA

Aneurysm

Thoracic aortic aneurysms (TAA) are the most common vascular mediastinal mass in adults.[33] A recent review of 260 patients with TAA delineated that 40% were atherosclerotic in origin, 50% were associated with aortic dissection, and 3% were from Marfan syndrome. Anatomic distribution of aneurysms included 40% in the ascending aorta and 60% in the descending aorta.[34]

Pathogenesis of aortic dissection may be attributed to conditions that lead to medial degeneration of the aortic wall, or conditions that cause pathological aortic wall stress.[35] Genetic disorders include Marfan syndrome, Loeys–Dietz syndrome, and Ehlers–Danlos syndrome. Marfan syndrome is caused by a mutation in the FBN-1 gene that codes for the fibrillin glycoprotein found in extracellular matrix microfibrils that regulate the TGF-BR2 receptor.[36] Loeys–Dietz syndrome is caused by mutation in the TGF-B receptors 1 or 2.[37] Ehlers–Danlos syndrome arises from a defect in the COL3A1 gene that encodes type III collagen. Medial necrosis of the aortic wall may also be attributed to inflammatory conditions such as Takayasu arteritis, giant cell arteritis, and Behçet disease.

Sinus of Valsalva aneurysms are an enlargement of the aortic root between the aortic annulus and sinotubular junction.[38] Upper limits of normal in men and women are 4 cm and 3.6 cm, with expected variations depending on body surface area.[39] These aneurysms may be classified into congenital and acquired types with the former attributed to bicuspid aortic valves and the connective tissue disorders previously discussed for TAA. Acquired aneurysms may be attributed to infection, atherosclerosis, trauma, vasculitis, and iatrogenic injury. The rupture of the right or noncoronary sinus may result in communication with the right ventricular outflow tract, aorta, or right atrium. Left coronary sinus rupture may communicate with the left atrium or the left ventricular outflow tract.[40] On imaging, they

may appear as a right paracardiac mass producing a double contour along the superior right atrial border or the root of the aorta. Surgical repair is indicated for symptomatic or ruptured aneurysms and lesions with ventricular septal defects or aortic regurgitation. Size guidelines indicating thresholds for repair of asymptomatic sinus of Valsalva aneurysms are not established, but may coincide with measurements established for TAAs: growth rate exceeding 0.5 cm per year, size >5.5 cm, size >5 cm in bicuspid valves, or size >4.5 cm with connective tissue disorders.[41]

Management of TAA initially focuses on control of risk factors associated with growth and aortic dissection. These include aggressive blood pressure control, lipid management, and smoking cessation. Blood pressure control has migrated from beta blockade to angiotensin II receptor blockers with examples including losartan and valsartan. Indications for surgical repair of TAAs will be discussed elsewhere in this text.

PSEUDOANEURYSM

Thoracic aortic pseudoaneurysms are most commonly seen secondary to blunt trauma. Penetrating aortic injuries with aortic wall compromise usually result in death.[42,43] Traumatic aortic disruption has a prehospital mortality of 86.2% and roughly 2% of survivors go on to develop chronic aneurysms.[44] Open pseudoaneurysm repair portends a 10% to 20% risk of mortality, 5% risk of stroke, and 5% risk of spinal cord injury. Endovascular repair has reduced the mortality risk in half and neurological risk to less than 2%. These injuries are rarely isolated and are typically seen in conjunction with traumatic brain injury (31% of cases), abdominal injury (29%), and pelvic injury (15%).[45]

BRONCHIAL ARTERY

Bronchial artery aneurysms and pseudoaneurysms are rare and found in less than 1% of patients undergoing bronchial angiograms (Fig. 161.3). There have been 40 cases reported in the literature with the reported treatment almost exclusively embolization.[46] Bronchial artery aneurysms are found in patients with bronchiectasis and bronchopulmonary inflammation. Atherosclerosis, infection, trauma, and Osler–Weber–Rendu syndrome have also been implicated. The diameter of such an aneurysm is not necessarily an incremental risk factor for rupture.[47]

INTERNAL MAMMARY ARTERY

Internal mammary artery pseudoaneurysms are an uncommon vascular anomaly secondary to multiple factors including infection, trauma, vasculitis from Kawasaki disease, and connective tissue disorders.[48,49] Iatrogenic causes include pacemaker leads, central venous catheters, and injury resulting from sternotomy or sternotomy closure. Infectious etiologies include Aspergillus and tuberculosis.[50,51] Coil embolization, stenting, and open surgical repair have been reported as treatment modalities.[49]

CORONARY ARTERY ANEURYSM

The incidence of coronary artery aneurysm (CAA) observed in patients undergoing catheterization for coronary artery disease is approximately 4.9%.[52] CAA are localized fusiform or saccular dilations of the coronary artery which should be differentiated from diffuse dilation or ectasia (Fig. 161.4). So-called "giant CAA" are

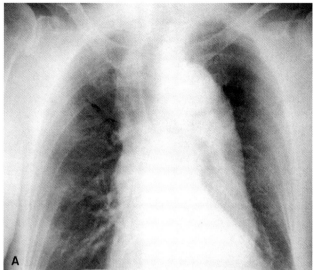

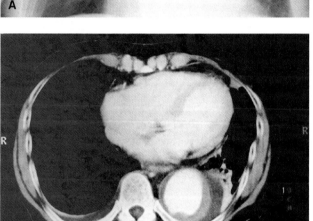

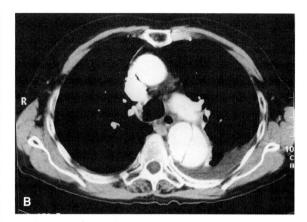

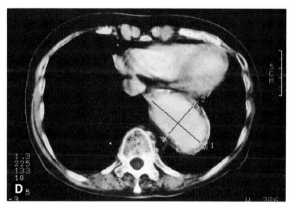

FIGURE 161.3 **A:** Chest radiograph of a 78-year-old hypertensive woman presenting with an acute onset of sharp back pain and shortness of breath and a widened mediastinum. **B–D:** Serial CT scans demonstrating an ectatic descending thoracic aorta with a thrombosed false lumen and type III dissection.

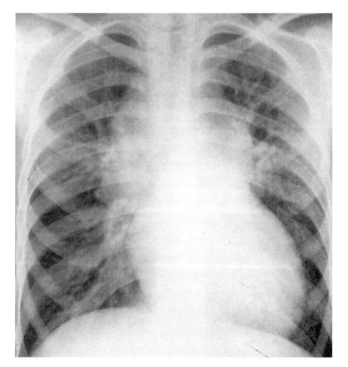

FIGURE 161.4 Chest radiograph of a more extensive "snowman" heart in a 13-year-old boy with supracardiac total anomalous pulmonary venous connection.

aneurysms exceeding the normal vessel diameter by four times.[53] Aneurysm of the coronary artery are considered a variant of coronary artery disease and have similar survival to that seen in patients with routine coronary disease. Etiologies include congenital (20% to 30%), vasculitis (10% to 20%), connective tissue disorders (5% to 10%), and iatrogenic lesions (0.3% to 0.6%) with percutaneous coronary intervention.[54] Children with Kawasaki disease may have up to a 15% incidence of CAA.[55] The right coronary artery is more commonly affected.[56] Recommendations are to treat CAA patients with antiplatelet and antithrombotic therapy. Revascularization is indicated with TIMI 0 or 1 flow, recurrent angina or ischemia, sustained ventricular tachycardia, and sustained instability. Indications for selecting surgical revascularization over a percutaneous approach include multivessel disease, left main disease, involvement of an arterial bifurcation, or additional indications for open cardiac surgery.[57]

CORONARY ARTERY FISTULA

Coronary artery fistulas are mostly congenital lesions or rarely secondary to cardiac interventions and surgery. These fistulas are an abnormal connection, more commonly seen arising from the right coronary and left anterior descending artery, to a venous structure that may include the right heart, pulmonary artery, coronary sinus, or superior vena cava (SVC).[58] Most patients under the age of 20 are asymptomatic and older symptomatic patients present with dyspnea on exertion (35%), angina (22%), or fatigue (8%).[59] Repair of symptomatic fistula is recommended via percutaneous coronary intervention if anatomically possible, or by simple open ligation otherwise.[60] Spontaneous closure of such a fistula via thrombosis has been reported[61] and recommendations have thus extended to offer observation of asymptomatic, small, hemodynamically insignificant fistulae.[62]

VENOUS MASSES

The systemic venous system, consisting of the SVC, innominate vein, hemiazygos and azygous veins, is located within the middle and posterior regions of the mediastinum. Anomalies of this system include aneurysms and dilation of the SVC and innominate vein, persistent left superior vena cava (LSVC) and enlargement of the azygos or hemiazygos system. While most cases are diagnosed incidentally on chest radiograph, they are often confused for mediastinal masses or adenopathy. As such, CT angiography (CTA) or MR venography (MRV) is necessary to confirm diagnosis.[63–69]

VENA CAVA

Aneurysm

A majority of SVC and innominate vein dilation or aneurysm is caused by a persistent increase in central venous pressure secondary to cardiac or pulmonary conditions. Table 161.2 shows common causes of enlargement of the SVC. Most cases of SVC dilation are initially found incidentally on chest radiograph. The appearance often consists of a smooth, well-defined widening of the right side of the mediastinum. The azygos vein is almost always dilated as well, a more dependable sign of systemic venous hypertension, because the diameter of the vein in the right tracheobronchial angle can be measured. Because these x-ray appearances can be confused with mediastinal masses, CTA or MRV are often useful to confirm the diagnosis. Rarely, an aneurysmal SVC can be the cause of such a mass (Fig. 161.5). There are fewer than 30 reported cases of SVC aneurysm in the English literature and often these are asymptomatic

TABLE 161.2 Causes of Dilation of the Superior Vena Cava
• Increased central venous pressure
• Intrathoracic neoplasm
• Mediastinal fibrosis
• Aneurysm of the SVC
• Lymphadenopathy
• Aneurysm of the aorta or great vessels
• Thrombosis of SVC
• Pulmonary hypertension
• Cardiac causes
• Tricuspid stenosis
• Cardiac tamponade
• Pericardial effusion
• Pericarditis

and incidental findings.[65] Aneurysms of the SVC can be classified as fusiform or saccular, with the fusiform type being more common. The etiology of these lesions is unknown but it is presumably due to a congenital weakness of the SVC wall. Most aneurysms appear histologically normal, although case reports have shown an absence of the longitudinal muscle layer in the adventitia of saccular aneurysms.[69] Cystic hygroma of the mediastinum has been associated with abnormal enlargement or aneurysmal dilatation of the neck or thoracic veins due to the close embryonic relationship between lymphatic vessels and veins.[67,70]

Management of true SVC aneurysms is controversial. Currently, it is recommended to proceed with surgical intervention for saccular aneurysms, and other aneurysms causing symptoms. Saccular aneurysms, which are connected to the SVC by a stalk, warrant the consideration for surgical resection due to the risk of potential complications including pulmonary embolism, thrombosis, rupture, and partial or total venous compression and obstruction.[67] Conversely, conservative management is recommended for fusiform aneurysms, as these do not enlarge, produce pressure symptoms, or rupture. Pulmonary embolism has not been reported in association with fusiform aneurysms.[63,65,67] Treatment for saccular aneurysms is also controversial. While some aneurysms can be controlled via a median

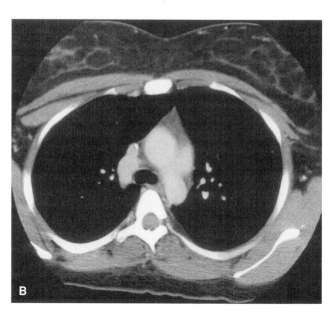

FIGURE 161.5 **A:** Chest radiograph demonstrating a prominent azygos vein just superior to the right tracheobronchial angle. **B:** CT of the chest shows a prominent azygos vein to the right of the trachea.

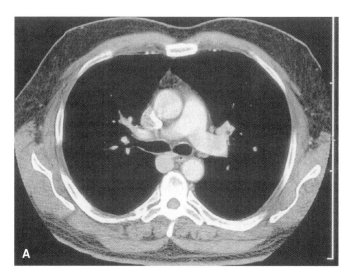 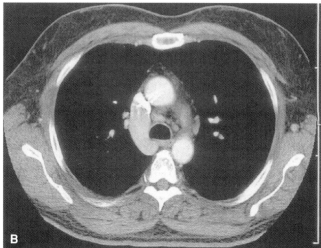

FIGURE 161.6 A: CT of the chest demonstrating a dilated azygos vein posterior to the carina. **B:** CT of the chest demonstrates the azygos continuation of the inferior vena cava as a prominent vascular structure to the right of the trachea.

sternotomy without the use of cardiopulmonary bypass (CPB), it is recommended that aneurysms with calcification, thrombus formation, and venous obstruction should be treated using CPB. Venous cannulation can be difficult with SVC aneurysms—femoral vein/artery cannulation has been described to avoid inadvertent injury to the aneurysm during sternotomy.[71] Alternatively, cannulation via innominate vein with the use of balloon tamponade to control the right subclavian vein and a pump sucker for bleeding from the right internal jugular vein can be used. Rarely, the need for circulatory arrest is necessary for complex aneurysms.

PARTIAL ANOMALOUS PULMONARY VENOUS RETURN

Dilatation of the SVC from partial anomalous pulmonary venous return from the right lung to the SVC is more common than true aneurysm of the SVC. This can be associated with a subcaval atrial septal defect, referred to as a sinus venosus ASD. With sinus venosus ASD, the right superior pulmonary vein drains into the SVC or the SVC-right atrial junction. In adults, this rare finding may include an anomalous left upper lobe vein connecting to a persistent vertical vein, creating an abnormal left mediastinal contour.[72]

Persistent left SVC (PLSVC) is a relatively common anomaly with an incidence being less than 0.5% of normal subjects and about 6.1% of patients with congenital heart disease.[73] Most patients with this anomaly have both a right and left SVC, but in some cases the right SVC may be absent.[74,75] The PLSVC more commonly extends inferiorly to the region of the left superior pulmonary vein where it ultimately connects into the coronary sinus. With congenital cardiac anomalies, the sinus venosus defect type of ASD is most commonly associated with PLSVC and accounts for 4% to 11% of all ASDs.[73] Occasionally, there is a persistent brachiocephalic vein connecting the two vena cava. On chest radiography, PLSVC may show a widening of the aortic shadow, paramediastinal bulge, a paramediastinal strip, or a crescent along the upper left cardiac border.[76] While plain imaging may suggest this anomalous vessel, CT and MRI are virtually diagnostic, although the anomaly can be confused for mediastinal lymphadenopathy.[72,74,77,78] When the coronary sinus is dilated, it is important to search for PLSCV. Rarely, the vein may connect directly into the left atrium or be associated with the unroofed coronary sinus syndrome, both of which can cause a small degree of nonphysiologic shunting.

INNOMINATE VEIN

Innominate vein aneurysm is rare, with fewer than 20 reported cases in English literature.[79] Radiographically, this appears as a double aortic knob on the left side of the mediastinum (Fig. 161.6). This image can be mistakenly described as pseudocoarctation of the aorta.[80] Contrast-enhanced CT or MRI is necessary as these lesions can also be confused with mediastinal tumors. With CT or MRI, intraluminal contrast and/or clot can usually be identified, making it simple to differentiate an aneurysm from a mass. Inappropriate biopsies of these aneurysms can often lead to complications including death, therefore preoperative contrast imaging is necessary.[81] Complications, like those seen with other aneurysms, include pulmonary embolism, rupture, and venous obstruction. Saccular aneurysms often warrant surgical excision to remove the risk of complications while fusiform aneurysms can often be treated conservatively.

AZYGOUS VEIN

Enlargement of the azygos vein can mimic either a right upper mediastinal or paratracheal mass or enlarged mediastinal lymph nodes (Fig. 161.7). The azygous vein is considered enlarged if it measures greater than 7 mm and is perpendicular to the right mainstem bronchus.[82] Azygos or hemiazygos vein dilatation is caused by an increase flow through the vein or elevated venous pressure. The most common causes include caval obstruction, hepatic vein obstruction, portal hypertension, inferior vena cava interruption with azygous continuation, pregnancy, and cardiac disease. Cardiac conditions include congestive heart failure, tricuspid disease, constrictive pericarditis, and tamponade.[80,83] Azygos vein varices or diverticula and aneurysms have been rarely reported.[83–90] Severe pulmonary hypertension, secondary to chronic thromboembolism, has been described in patients with thrombosed saccular aneurysms.[89]

Differentiating azygos vein enlargement from other masses can be seen radiographically by demonstrating varying sizes of the mass based on the patient's position. With azygos vein enlargement, the vein may be larger if the patient is in the supine rather than the upright position.[91,92] On chest x-ray, the distended azygos arch produces a right paratracheal mass, which should reduce in size during a Valsalva maneuver. Often, a CT scan will confirm the underlying venous anomaly. If the mass is still in question, CTA or dynamic CT may reveal

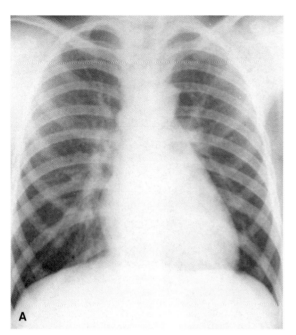 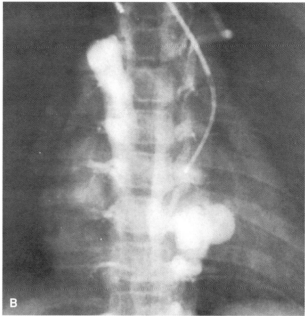

FIGURE 161.7 **A:** Chest radiograph of a 9-year-old boy with a paravertebral arteriovenous fistula causing prominent filling of both the azygos vein and the highest intercostal vein (aortic nipple). **B:** Angiogram of a dilated, tortuous fistula. The veins filled during the arterial phase. Both the azygos and highest intercostal veins are prominent.

marked enhancement during the late venous phase, suggesting a vascular structure.[91] Similarly, MRI can confirm the diagnosis by showing turbulent flow in a dilated, aneurysmal azygos vein.

As described above, when thrombosed, azygos vein aneurysms may appear as solid masses. While conservative management is suggested, resection may be necessary to prevent complications including pulmonary embolism or hemoptysis. It is recommended that saccular aneurysms be resected due to their propensity to grow over time. More than 20% of saccular aneurysms continue to grow over time whereas fewer than 8% of fusiform aneurysms show growth.[93]

With azygos and hemiazygos continuation of the IVC, left inferior vena cava ends at the left renal vein and venous blood from the lower extremities and abdomen is diverted into the azygos or, less commonly, the hemiazygos, resulting in dilatation of these veins. This anomaly can be associated with congenital cardiac malformations and with asplenia or polysplenia. Chest radiographs usually show an enlarged azygos vein and a widened paraspinal reflection. The CT appearance is so characteristic that angiography is rarely needed for diagnosis[94,95] (Fig. 161.6). Contrasted imaging shows enlargement of the azygos or hemiazygos veins with marked dilatation of the azygos arch or left supreme intercostal vein. This condition is characterized by the "candy stick" appearance of the dilated azygos vein on venography but contrast-enhanced CT or MRA is usually diagnostic. Transtracheal ultrasound may also be useful in defining this condition.[91]

INTERCOSTAL VEIN

Dilatation of the left supreme intercostal vein may present as a mass. Normally, this vein originates from the confluence of the second, third, and fourth intercostal veins. As it passes anteriorly from the spine, it relates intimately to some portion of the aortic arch. At this location, it may be confused with a PLSVC. The supreme intercostal vein connects the left brachiocephalic vein with hemiazygos system. It runs parallel to the aortic arch and is normally less than 4 mm in

diameter.[96] If this vein becomes dilated, it may be seen end-on as an aortic "nipple," a local protuberance that is identifiable in about 10% of normal subjects (Fig. 161.8).[80] On erect PA radiographs, the maximum diameter of the aortic nipple is 4.5 mm. A diameter greater than this is a useful sign of circulatory abnormalities, most commonly of which is cardiac decompensation. Other causes include (a) congenital or acquired obstruction of the vena cava, (b) hypoplasia of the left innominate vein, (c) portal hypertension, (d) Budd–Chiari syndrome, (e) obstruction of the IVC, and (f) congenital absence of the azygos vein. Hemiazygos continuation of the inferior vena cava is particularly associated with the heterotaxy syndrome and polysplenia.[97]

LEFT BRACHIOCEPHALIC VEIN

An anomalous left brachiocephalic vein (ALBCV) can also appear as a mass lateral to the arch of the aorta. This vessel crosses between the ascending aorta and trachea as it traverses the middle mediastinum. This mass can be confused with an aortopulmonary window mass. This vessel then enters the SVC caudal to the azygous vein. The ALBCV has an association with congenital heart disease, most commonly with tetralogy of Fallot and ventricular septal defect with pulmonary atresia.[98]

PULMONARY VENOUS SYSTEM

Mediastinal masses arising from the pulmonary venous system include anomalous pulmonary venous return, pulmonary venous aneurysms, and pulmonary arteriovenous malformations (PAVMs).[99–102]

ANOMALOUS PULMONARY VENOUS RETURN

The most common cause of masses related to the pulmonary venous system is anomalous pulmonary venous connections. Patients with

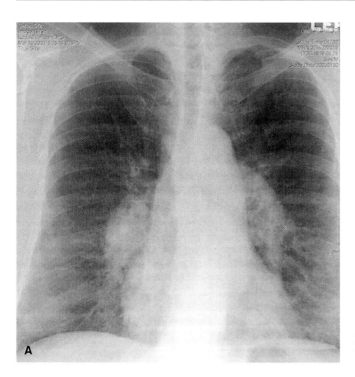

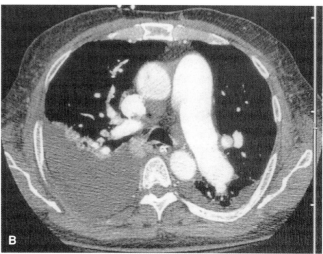

FIGURE 161.8 A: Chest radiograph demonstrating prominent bilateral hilar densities corresponding to the main pulmonary arteries. This patient has primary pulmonary hypertension. **B:** CT of the chest showing a massively dilated left pulmonary artery. Note that the left pulmonary artery exceeds the diameter of the descending aorta. There is also a large right pleural effusion.

unobstructed anomalous pulmonary venous connections may go years without symptoms and develop markedly enlarged mediastinal masses.

Partial anomalous pulmonary venous return on the left side of the mediastinum is rare, while on the right side it causes enlargement of the SVC, as discussed above. Radiographically, it will appear as an abnormal mediastinal density lateral to the aortic knob.[103] Differentiation from a left SVC is made by the fact that this vein is oriented more obliquely and the SVC more vertically.

Classically, total anomalous pulmonary venous connections fall into three types. The three types include Type I—supracardiac, Type II—cardiac, and Type III—infracardiac. In type I, the connection is to a vertical vein on the left side of the mediastinum, which then drains into the innominate vein, causing a very large left-to-right shunt. Radiographically, this type appears as a "snow-man" or "figure-of-8" image due to the dilated venous structures. If the veins remain unobstructed, symptoms may go unnoticed, except cyanosis, ultimately presenting as a large mediastinal mass. Type I total anomalous pulmonary venous connections has been reported to cause giant SVC aneurysms but is rare.[104] Type II and type III cause slight cardiomegaly with some pulmonary venous obstruction, giving a ground-glass appearance. MRI is often useful in visualizing partial and total anomalous pulmonary venous connections.

PULMONARY VEIN ANEURYSM

Pulmonary vein varices or aneurysms are rare. Often, they are relatively benign congenital malformations that may simulate perihilar masses (Fig. 161.9).[102] A pulmonary venous varix is a local dilatation of one or more pulmonary veins that have normal return to the left atrium. These localized aneurysmal dilatations of the pulmonary veins drain normally to the left atrium. Radiologically, they may simulate a neoplastic or granulomatous process. They may also be confused for PAVMs.[103,105] CT imaging may show tortuous vascular dilatation often in the perihilar area and diagnosis may be confirmed with CTA. A variation in normal pulmonary venous return can cause a mass when the upper, middle, and lower veins all come together prior to their entry into the left atrium. This is referred to as

a pulmonary venous confluence. Both pulmonary varix and pulmonary venous confluence generally do not change in diameter over the years and often are asymptomatic. Usually, no treatment is required and follow-up is recommended for detection of rare complications including rupture and systemic embolic secondary to thrombosis.[105] Pulmonary vein aneurysms have been reported secondary to severe mitral regurgitation, often requiring repair of the mitral valve with close follow-up of the pulmonary vein aneurysm.[106,107]

PULMONARY ARTERIOVENOUS MALFORMATION

PAVMs are abnormal dilated vessels that provide a left-to-right shunt between the pulmonary artery and pulmonary vein, thereby bypassing the pulmonary capillary bed. They affect 1 in 2,500 patients.[108] Diagnosis of this condition is important as they are associated with serious morbidity and mortality largely related to paradoxical embolization. The vast majority of individuals with PAVMs have hereditary hemorrhagic telangiectasia (HHT), also known as Osler–Weber–Rendu syndrome.[109,110] Because of their risk of cerebrovascular complications, it is recommended that embolization be performed if these malformations are encountered.[101] PAVMs are divided into simple and complex types.[111] The simple type is more common and consists of an aneurysmal venous sac supplied by a single artery and drained by one or more veins. Complex PAVMs consist of multiple venous sacs supplied by multiple vessels arising from adjacent segmental or subsegmental pulmonary artery branches and draining multiple veins. On chest x-ray, a PAVM consists of a well-defined, rounded, soft-tissue nodule of any size, but most frequently 1 to 2 cm in diameter. They are typically most numerous at the lung bases.[101] While chest x-ray has a classic appearance, CT is generally the imaging modality used for investigating PAVMs. In lung windows, the classic appearance is those of a well-defined peripheral nodule, which may be rounded or multilobulated, into which one feeding artery, and from which one or more draining veins can be clearly visualized. Complex PAVMs may consist of one or more lobulated venous sacs of variable size supplied by more than one feeding artery, often arising from adjacent segmental pulmonary artery branches.[101]

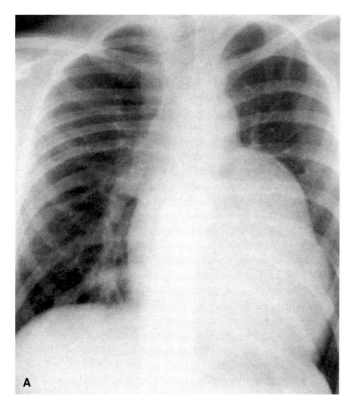
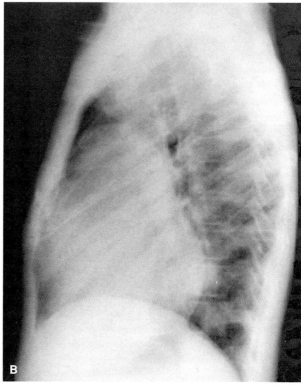

FIGURE 161.9 Chest radiographs of a 10-year-old girl with a calcified pulmonary artery aneurysm after a Potts anastomosis. **A:** Posteroanterior. **B:** Lateral.

LYMPHATIC LESIONS

Lymphangiomas, or cystic hygromas, are rare, benign lesions commonly found in the neck, but can also be completely intrathoracic. If they are found within the thoracic cavity, they are often within the anterior and middle compartments.[112] They result from abnormal collections of lymph channels that develop early in the embryonic phase. Lymphangiomas are usually asymptomatic, but with expansion, mass effects can occur. Often, a persistent cough is the only symptom. Other symptoms can include infection, hemorrhage, chylothorax, chylopericardium, and SVC syndrome.[112,113] On CT or MRI imaging, mediastinal lymphangiomas are described as well-circumscribed cystic lesions. Due to the inability to distinguish from other cystic lesions of the mediastinum, complete surgical excision is recommended when feasible. Local invasion to surrounding tissue and vital structures may make complete excision impossible. In order to ameliorate symptoms, partial resection is acceptable, but local recurrence is almost inevitable. For cases of unresectable lymphangiomas, sclerotherapy with OK-432 has been documented with favorable results.[114] Often, cystic lymphangiomas require multiple interventions regardless of whether surgery or sclerotherapy is chosen as the initial therapy of choice.[115] At this time, there is no consensus of a treatment of choice and each case should be individualized based on size, location, and complicating factors of the lesion.[73]

REFERENCES

1. Restrepo CS, Carswell AP. Aneurysms and pseudoaneurysms of the pulmonary vasculature. *Semin Ultrasound CT MR* 2012;33(6):552–566.
2. Boyd LJ, McGavack TH. Aneurysm of the pulmonary artery: A review of the literature and report of two new cases. *Am Heart J* 1939;18(5): 562–578.
3. Kim YI, Kang HC, Lee HS, et al. Invasive pulmonary mucormycosis with concomitant lung cancer presented with massive hemoptysis by huge pseudoaneurysm of pulmonary artery. *Ann Thorac Surg* 2014;98(5):1832–1835.
4. Trambert JJ, Abubaker SJ, Kanner BJ. Giant mycotic pulmonary artery pseudoaneurysm treated by guide wire and coil embolization. *J Vasc Interv Radiol* 2014; 25(10):1643–1645.
5. Keymel S, Merx MW, Zeus T, et al. Stenting as a rescue treatment of a pulmonary artery false aneurysm caused by swan-ganz catheterization. *Case Rep Pulmonol* 2014;2014:893647.
6. Borghol S, Alberti N, Frulio N, et al. Pulmonary artery pseudoaneurysm after radiofrequency ablation: Report of two cases. *Int J Hyperthermia* 2015;31(1):1–4.
7. Asano M, Gäbel G, Allham O, et al. Pulmonary artery pseudoaneurysm in a patient with aortic valve stenosis. *Ann Vasc Surg* 2013;27(2):238 e5–e7.
8. Bartter T, Irwin RS, Nash G. Aneurysms of the pulmonary arteries. *Chest* 1988; 94(5):1065–1075.
9. Kim JH, Han SH. A pulmonary artery pseudoaneurysm caused by concurrent chemoradiation therapy for lung cancer. *Pak J Med Sci* 2015;31(1):220–222.
10. Rohit MK, Vadivelu R, Khandelwal N,et al. Post Blalock-Taussig shunt mediastinal mass—a single shadow with two different destinies. *Indian Heart J* 2014; 66(2):227–230.
11. Goel S, Kumar A, Gamanagatti S, et al. Spontaneous resolution of post-traumatic pulmonary artery pseudoaneurysm: Report of two cases. *Lung India* 2013;30(3):203–205.
12. Rai VK, Malireddy K, Dearmond D, et al. Traumatic pseudoaneurysm of the pulmonary artery. *J Trauma* 2010;69(3):730.
13. Sridhar SK, Sadler D, McFadden SD, et al. Percutaneous embolization of an angiographically inaccessible pulmonary artery pseudoaneurysm after blunt chest trauma: a case report and review of the literature. *J Trauma* 2010;69(3):729.
14. Keeling AN, McGrath FP, Lee MJ. Interventional radiology in the diagnosis, management, and follow-up of pseudoaneurysms. *Cardiovasc Intervent Radiol* 2009;32(1):2–18.
15. Lee JC, Walters DL, Slaughter RE. Angioembolisation of pulmonary artery pseudoaneurysm arising in H1N1 influenza viral pneumonia. *Heart Lung Circ* 2011;20(9):599–601.
16. Wu XN, Chen MJ, Li DQ, et al. Pulmonary artery pseudoaneurysm caused by a rare vascular tumor: epithelioid hemangioendothelioma. *Thorac Cardiovasc Surg* 2014;62(1):92–94.
17. Koch A, Mechtersheimer G, Tochtermann U, et al. Ruptured pseudoaneurysm of the pulmonary artery—rare manifestation of a primary pulmonary artery sarcoma. *Interact Cardiovasc Thorac Surg* 2010;10(1):120–121.
18. Barbour DJ, Roberts WC. Aneurysm of the pulmonary trunk unassociated with intracardiac or great vessel left-to-right shunting. *Am J Cardiol* 1987;59(1):192–194.
19. Krokidis M, Spiliopoulos S, Ahmed I, et al. Emergency endovascular management of pulmonary artery aneurysms and pseudoaneurysms for the treatment of massive haemoptysis. *Hellenic J Cardiol* 2014;55(3):204–210.
20. Theodoropoulos P, Ziganshin BA, Tranquilli M, et al. Pulmonary artery aneurysms: four case reports and literature review. *Int J Angiol* 2013;22(3):143–148.
21. Erkan F, Gul A, Tasali E. Pulmonary manifestations of Behcet's disease. *Thorax* 2001;56(7):572–578.

22. Chae EJ, Do KH, Seo JB, et al. Radiologic and clinical findings of Behcet disease: comprehensive review of multisystemic involvement. *Radiographics* 2008;28(5):e31.

23. Hiller N, Lieberman S, Chajek-Shaul T, et al. Thoracic manifestations of Behcet disease at CT. *Radiographics* 2004;24(3):801–808.

24. Hamuryudan V, Yurdakul S, Moral F, et al. Pulmonary arterial aneurysms in Behcet's syndrome: a report of 24 cases. *Br J Rheumatol* 1994;33(1):48–51.

25. Farouk H. Behcet's disease, echocardiographers, and cardiac surgeons: together is better. *Echocardiography* 2014;31(6):783–787.

26. Stricker H, Malinverni R. Multiple, large aneurysms of pulmonary arteries in Behcet's disease. Clinical remission and radiologic resolution after corticosteroid therapy. *Arch Intern Med* 1989;149(4):925–927.

27. Khalid U, Saleem T. Hughes-Stovin syndrome. *Orphanet J Rare Dis* 2011;6:15.

28. Dyamenahalli U, Smallhorn JF, Geva T, et al. Isolated ductus arteriosus aneurysm in the fetus and infant: a multi-institutional experience. *J Am Coll Cardiol* 2000; 36(1):262–269.

29. Hornberger LK. Congenital ductus arteriosus aneurysm. *J Am Coll Cardiol* 2002; 39(2):348–350.

30. Jan SL, Hwang B, Fu YC, et al. Isolated neonatal ductus arteriosus aneurysm. *J Am Coll Cardiol* 2002;39(2):342–347.

31. Lund JT, Hansen D, Brocks V, et al. Aneurysm of the ductus arteriosus in the neonate: three case reports with a review of the literature. *Pediatr Cardiol* 1992; 13(4):222–226.

32. Weichert J, Hartge DR, Axt-Fliedner R. The fetal ductus arteriosus and its abnormalities—a review. *Congenit Heart Dis* 2010;5(5):398–408.

33. Lyons HA, Calvy GL, Sammons BP. The diagnosis and classification of mediastinal masses. 1. A study of 782 cases. *Ann Intern Med* 1959;51:897–932.

34. Pressler V, McNamara JJ. Aneurysm of the thoracic aorta. Review of 260 cases. *J Thorac Cardiovasc Surg* 1985;89(1):50–54.

35. Goldfinger JZ, Halperin JL, Marin ML, et al. Thoracic aortic aneurysm and dissection. *J Am Coll Cardiol* 2014;64(16):1725–1739.

36. Dietz HC, Cutting GR, Pyeritz RE, et al. Marfan syndrome caused by a recurrent de novo missense mutation in the fibrillin gene. *Nature* 1991;352(6333):337–379.

37. Loeys BL, Schwarze U, Holm T, et al. Aneurysm syndromes caused by mutations in the TGF-beta receptor. *N Engl J Med* 2006;355(8):788–798.

38. Bricker AO, Avutu B, Mohammed TL, et al. Valsalva sinus aneurysms: findings at CT and MR imaging. *Radiographics* 2010;30(1):99–110.

39. Troupis JM, Nasis A, Pasricha S, et al. Sinus valsalva aneurysm on cardiac CT angiography: assessment and detection. *J Med Imaging Radiat Oncol* 2013;57(4):444–447.

40. Weinreich M, Yu PJ, Trost B. Sinus of valsalva aneurysms: review of the literature and an update on management. *Clin Cardiol* 2015;38(3):185–189.

41. Hiratzka LF, Bakris GL, Beckman JA, et al. 2010 ACCF/AHA/AATS/ACR/ASA/SCA/SCAI/SIR/STS/SVM Guidelines for the diagnosis and management of patients with thoracic aortic disease. A Report of the American College of Cardiology Foundation/American Heart Association Task Force on Practice Guidelines, American Association for Thoracic Surgery, American College of Radiology, American Stroke Association, Society of Cardiovascular Anesthesiologists, Society for Cardiovascular Angiography and Interventions, Society of Interventional Radiology, Society of Thoracic Surgeons, and Society for Vascular Medicine. *J Am Coll Cardiol* 2010;55(14):e27–e129.

42. Ryan M, Valazquez O, Martinez E, et al. Thoracic aortic transection treated by thoracic endovascular aortic repair: predictors of survival. *Vasc Endovascular Surg* 2010;44(2):95–100.

43. Cornwell EE 3rd, Kennedy F, Berne TV, et al. Gunshot wounds to the thoracic aorta in the '90s: only prevention will make a difference. *Am Surg* 1995;61(8):721–723.

44. Parmley LF, Mattingly TW, Manion WC, et al. Nonpenetrating traumatic injury of the aorta. *Circulation* 1958;17(6):1086–1101.

45. Arthurs ZM, Starnes BW, Sohn VY, et al. Functional and survival outcomes in traumatic blunt thoracic aortic injuries: An analysis of the National Trauma Databank. *J Vasc Surg* 2009;49(4):988–994.

46. Kaufman C, Kabutey NK, Sgroi M, et al. Bronchial artery pseudoaneurysm with symptomatic mediastinal hematoma. *Clin Imaging* 2014;38(4):536–539.

47. Kalangos A, Khatchatourian G, Panos A, et al. Ruptured mediastinal bronchial artery aneurysm: a dilemma of diagnosis and therapeutic approach. *J Thorac Cardiovasc Surg* 1997;114(5):853–856.

48. Nasir A, Viola N, Livesey SA. Iatrogenic pseudoaneurysm of internal mammary artery: case report and literature review. *J Card Surg* 2009;24(3):355–356.

49. Heyn J, Zimmermann H, Klose A, et al. Idiopathic internal mammary artery aneurysm. *J Surg Case Rep* 2014;2014(12):pii: rju125.

50. Wani NA, Rawa IA, Pala NA, et al. Pseudoaneurysm of internal mammary artery caused by pulmonary actinomycosis. *Br J Radiol* 2010;83(995):e235–e238.

51. Yadav MK, Bhatia A, Kumar S, et al. Internal mammary artery pseudoaneurysm: A rare fatal complication of tubercular empyema. *Lung India* 2013;30(4):341–343.

52. Swaye PS, Fisher LD, Litwin P, et al. Aneurysmal coronary artery disease. *Circulation* 1983;67(1):134–138.

53. Kato H, Sugimura T, Akagi T, et al. Long-term consequences of Kawasaki disease. A 10- to 21-year follow-up study of 594 patients. *Circulation* 1996;94(6):1379–1385.

54. Bell MR, Garratt KN, Bresnahan JF, et al. Relation of deep arterial resection and coronary artery aneurysms after directional coronary atherectomy. *J Am Coll Cardiol* 1992;20(7):1474–1481.

55. Kato H, Ichinose E, Yoshioka F, et al. Fate of coronary aneurysms in Kawasaki disease: serial coronary angiography and long-term follow-up study. *Am J Cardiol* 1982;49(7):1758–1766.

56. Syed M, Lesch M. Coronary artery aneurysm: a review. *Prog Cardiovasc Dis* 1997; 40(1):77–84.

57. Boyer N, Gupta R, Schevchuck A, et al. Coronary artery aneurysms in acute coronary syndrome: case series, review, and proposed management strategy. *J Invasive Cardiol* 2014;26(6):283–290.

58. Dodge-Khatami A, Mavroudis C, Backer CL. Congenital heart surgery nomenclature and database project: anomalies of the coronary arteries. *Ann Thorac Surg* 2000;69(4 Suppl):S270–S297.

59. Liberthson RR, Sagar K, Berkoben JP, et al. Congenital coronary arteriovenous fistula. Report of 13 patients, review of the literature and delineation of management. *Circulation* 1979;59(5):849–854.

60. Armsby LR, Keane JF, Sherwood MC, et al. Management of coronary artery fistulae. Patient selection and results of transcatheter closure. *J Am Coll Cardiol* 2002;39(6): 1026–1032.

61. Hackett D, Hallidie-Smith KA. Spontaneous closure of coronary artery fistula. *Br Heart J* 1984;52(4):477–479.

62. Jiritano F, Prestipino F, Mastroroberto P, et al. Coronary arterovenous fistula: to treat or not to treat? *J Cardiothorac Surg* 2015;10(1):52.

63. Gozdziuk K, Czekajska-Chehab E, Wrona A, et al. Saccular aneurysm of the superior vena cava detected by computed tomography and successfully treated with surgery. *Ann Thorac Surg* 2004;78(6):e94–e95.

64. Hartnell GG, Hughes LA, Finn JP, et al. Magnetic resonance angiography of the central chest veins. A new gold standard? *Chest* 1995;107(4):1053–1057.

65. Koga S, Ikeda S, Sanuki Y, et al. A case of asymptomatic fusiform aneurysm of the superior vena cava detected by magnetic resonance imaging. *Int J Cardiol* 2006;113(2):e39–e41.

66. Nitta A, Nishikura K, Fukuda H, et al. Congenital left brachiocephalic vein and superior vena cava aneurysms in an infant: final update with autopsy findings. *J Pediatr* 2008;152(3):445–446.

67. Varma PK, Dharan BS, Ramachandran P, et al. Superior vena caval aneurysm. *Interact Cardiovasc Thorac Surg* 2003;2(3):331–333.

68. Rahmani N, White CS. MR imaging of thoracic veins. *Magn Reson Imaging Clin N Am* 2008;16(2):249–262, viii.

69. Williams HJ, Alton HM. Imaging of paediatric mediastinal abnormalities. *Paediatr Respir Rev* 2003;4(1):55–66.

70. Joseph AE, Donaldson JS, Reynolds M. Neck and thorax venous aneurysm: association with cystic hygroma. *Radiology* 1989;170(1 Pt 1):109–112.

71. Oh SG, Kim KH, Seon HJ, et al. Unusual cause of acute right ventricular dysfunction: rapid progression of superior vena cava aneurysm complicated by thrombosis and pulmonary thromboembolism. *J Korean Med Sci* 2011;26(5):690–693.

72. Haramati LB, Moche IE, Rivera VT, et al. Computed tomography of partial anomalous pulmonary venous connection in adults. *J Comput Assist Tomogr* 2003;27(5):743–749.

73. Disha B, Prakashini K, Shetty RK. Persistent left superior vena cava in association with sinus venosus defect type of atrial septal defect and partial pulmonary venous return on 64-MDCT. *BMJ Case Rep* 2014;2014:pii: bcr2013202999.

74. Arat N, Sokmen Y, Golbasi Z. Persistent left superior vena cava with absent right superior vena cava and coronary sinus dilation mimicking a paracardiac mass. *Tex Heart Inst J* 2007;34(4):492–493.

75. Marcu CB, Beek AM, van Rossum AC. Unusual variation in upper-body venous anatomy found with cardiovascular MRI. *CMAJ* 2006;175(1):27.

76. Cormier MG, Yedlicka JW, Gray RJ, et al. Congenital anomalies of the superior vena cava: a CT study. *Semin Roentgenol* 1989;24(2):77–83.

77. White CS, Baffa JM, Haney PJ, et al. MR imaging of congenital anomalies of the thoracic veins. *Radiographics* 1997;17(3):595–608.

78. Wong PS, Goldstraw P. Left superior vena cava: a pitfall in computed tomographic diagnosis with surgical implications. *Ann Thorac Surg* 1990;50(4):656–657.

79. Hosein RB, Butler K, Miller P, et al. Innominate venous aneurysm presenting as a rapidly expanding mediastinal mass. *Ann Thorac Surg* 2007;84(2):640–642.

80. Boateng P, Anjum W, Wechsler AS. Vascular lesions of the mediastinum. *Thorac Surg Clin* 2009;19(1):91–105.

81. Buehler MA 2nd, Ebrahim FS, Popa TO. Left innominate vein aneurysm: diagnostic imaging and pitfalls. *Int J Angiol* 2013;22(2):127–130.

82. Heitzman ER. Radiologic appearance of the azygos vein in cardiovascular disease. *Circulation* 1973;47(3):628–634.

83. Podbielski FJ, Sam AD 2nd, Halldorsson AO, et al. Giant azygos vein varix. *Ann Thorac Surg* 1997;63(4):1167–1169.

84. Abad Santamaria N, García Díez JM, Pavón Fernández MJ, et al. [Azygos vein aneurysm forming a mediastinal mass]. *Arch Bronconeumol* 2006;42(8):410–412.

85. Dilege S, Tanju S, Bayrak Y, et al. Posterior mediastinal lesion—aneurysm of azygos vein. *Eur J Cardiothorac Surg* 2004;26(1):215–216.

86. Gnanamuthu BR, Tharion J. Azygos vein aneurysm—a case for elective resection. *Heart Lung Circ* 2008;17(1):62–64.

87. Ichihara E, Kaneko M, Fujii H, et al. [Azygos vein aneurysm occurring simultaneously with hemoptysis]. *Nihon Kokyuki Gakkai Zasshi* 2007;45(6):479–482.

88. Lee SY, Kuo HT, Peng MJ, et al. Azygos vein varix mimicking mediastinal mass in a patient with liver cirrhosis: a case report. *Chest* 2005;127(2):661–664.

89. Nakamura N, Nakano K, Nakatani H, et al. Surgical exclusion of a thrombosed azygos vein aneurysm causing pulmonary embolism. *J Thorac Cardiovasc Surg* 2007;133(3):834–835.

90. Person TD, Komanapalli CB, Chaugle H, et al. Thoracoscopic approach to the resection of an azygos vein aneurysm. *J Thorac Cardiovasc Surg* 2005;130(1):230–231.

91. Choudhary AK, Moore M. Radiological features of azygous vein aneurysm. *Del Med J* 2014;86(4):117–120.

92. Kelley MJ, Mannes EJ, Ravin CE. Mediastinal masses of vascular origin. A review. *J Thorac Cardiovasc Surg* 1978;76(4):559–572.

93. Ko SF, Huang CC, Lin JW, et al. Imaging features and outcomes in 10 cases of idiopathic azygos vein aneurysm. *Ann Thorac Surg* 2014;97(3):873–878.

94. Dudiak CM, Olson MC, Posniak HV. CT evaluation of congenital and acquired abnormalities of the azygos system. *Radiographics* 1991;11(2):233–246.

95. Webb WR, Gamsu G, Speckman JM, et al. Computed tomographic demonstration of mediastinal venous anomalies. *AJR Am J Roentgenol* 1982;139(1):157–161.

96. Haswell DM, Berrigan TJ Jr. Anomalous inferior vena cava with accessory hemiazygos continuation. *Radiology* 1976;119(1):51–54.

97. Freedom RM, Treves S. Splenic scintigraphy and radionuclide venography in the heterotaxy syndrome. *Radiology* 1973;107(2):381–386.

98. Pilcher JM, Padhani AR. Problem in diagnostic imaging: Mediastinal venous anomalies. *Clin Anat* 2001;14(3):218–226.

99. Cohen MC, Hartnell GG, Finn JP. Magnetic resonance angiography of congenital pulmonary vein anomalies. *Am Heart J* 1994;127(4 Pt 1):954–955.

100. DeBoer DA, Margolis ML, Livornese D, et al. Pulmonary venous aneurysm presenting as a middle mediastinal mass. *Ann Thorac Surg* 1996;61(4):1261–1262.

101. Gill SS, Roddie ME, Shovlin CL, et al. Pulmonary arteriovenous malformations and their mimics. *Clin Radiol* 2015;70(1):96–110.

102. Platzker J, Goldhammer E, Simon J, et al. Pulmonary varices, benign congenital anomalies simulating perihilar masses of various etiologies. *Clin Cardiol* 1984;7(5):295–298.

103. Adler SC, Silverman JF. Anomalous venous drainage of the left upper lobe. A radiographic diagnosis. *Radiology* 1973;108(3):563–565.

104. Thummar AC, Phadke MS, Lanjewar CP, et al. Supracardiac total anomalous pulmonary venous drainage with giant superior vena cava aneurysm: a rare combination. *J Am Coll Cardiol* 2014;63(19):e51.

105. Chun HJ, Kim HW, Park JK. Pulmonary varix associated with an anomalous unilateral single pulmonary vein mimicking pulmonary arterio-venous malformation. *Eur J Cardiothorac Surg* 2015;47(4):747.

106. Erkanli K, Yazici P, Bakir I. Pulmonary vein aneurysm secondary to mitral regurgitation: rare and confusing lesion. *Thorac Cardiovasc Surg* 2014;62(1):83–84.

107. Lautin R, Ledor S, Ledor K, et al. Dilated pulmonary venous confluence presenting as a mass in mitral stenosis. *Cardiovasc Intervent Radiol* 1982;5(6):304–306.

108. Nakayama M, Nawa T, Chonan T, et al. Prevalence of pulmonary arteriovenous malformations as estimated by low-dose thoracic CT screening. *Intern Med* 2012;51(13):1677–1681.

109. Faughnan ME, Palda VA, Garcia-Tsao G, et al. International guidelines for the diagnosis and management of hereditary haemorrhagic telangiectasia. *J Med Genet* 2011;48(2):73–87.

110. Shovlin CL. Hereditary haemorrhagic telangiectasia: pathophysiology, diagnosis and treatment. *Blood Rev* 2010;24(6):203–219.

111. White RI, Jr., Mitchell SE, Barth KH, et al. Angioarchitecture of pulmonary arteriovenous malformations: an important consideration before embolotherapy. *AJR Am J Roentgenol* 1983;140(4):681–686.

112. Okubo T, Okayasu T, Osaka Y, et al. [Surgical analysis of mediastinal lymphangioma—analysis of 7 cases]. *Nihon Kyobu Geka Gakkai Zasshi* 1992;40(4):583–586.

113. Okazaki T, Iwatani S, Yanai T, et al. Treatment of lymphangioma in children: our experience of 128 cases. *J Pediatr Surg* 2007;42(2):386–389.

114. Degenhardt P, Dieckow B, Mau H. Huge intra- and extrathoracic lymphangioma in a baby successfully treated by sclerotherapy with OK-432. *Eur J Pediatr Surg* 2006;16(3):197–200.

115. Hde OO, Bustorff-Silva J, Oliveira Filho AG, et al. Cross-sectional study comparing different therapeutic modalities for cystic lymphangiomas in children. *Clinics (Sao Paulo)* 2014;69(8):505–508.

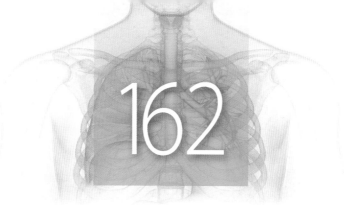

162

Superior Vena Cava Syndrome: Clinical Features, Diagnosis, and Treatment

Paul Michael McFadden ▪ Christina L. Greene

The superior vena cava and its important intrathoracic tributaries are located in a tight compartment within the superior mediastinum, immediately adjacent and anterior to the trachea and the right main bronchus. Lymph nodes that drain the entire right chest and lower portion of the left chest surround the superior vena cava and its adjacent structures. Significant extrinsic pressure, encasement, thrombosis, or actual invasion of the superior vena cava may cause an obstruction of the venous return from the head, neck, and upper extremities, leading to unmistakable signs and symptoms. This type of obstruction and its symptoms are called the "superior vena cava syndrome," first described by Hunter[1] and later by Stokes.[2]

CLINICAL MANIFESTATIONS

The superior vena cava syndrome constitutes a constellation of signs and symptoms resulting from either extrinsic or intrinsic obstruction of the superior vena cava, resulting in congestion of venous outflow from the head, neck, and upper extremities. A subsequent increase in venous pressure leads to dramatic signs and symptoms. According to Wilson[3] and Weinberg,[4] important factors that determine the nature of the clinical presentation include the rate with which the obstruction progresses, the completeness of the obstruction, and the location of the superior vena cava obstruction relative to the azygos vein. Insidious onset of superior vena cava occlusion is well tolerated and will not result in superior vena cava syndrome as collaterals have time to develop. The most common presenting symptoms, best described by Yellin and colleagues,[5] include swelling of the face, neck, arms, and upper chest, often accompanied by superficial venous distention. The eyes are often affected first. The patient may complain of tearing, proptosis, and conjunctival edema.[6] Retinoscopy may reveal edema and venous engorgement, as reported by Leys and colleagues.[7] The face may appear cyanotic or have a rubescent flush, as described by Parish,[8] Armstrong,[9] and Chen[10] (Fig. 162.1). Dilated venous channels often appear over the anterior chest wall and, on rare occasion, over the anterior abdominal wall (Fig. 162.2). These signs and symptoms are greatly exaggerated when the azygos vein is also obstructed. Headache, dizziness, tinnitus, and a "bursting" sensation in the head on bending forward may all follow in short succession. Venous hypertension can lead to the dire consequences of jugular venous and cerebrovascular thrombosis. Blindness may result from retinal venous thrombosis.

Since most cases of superior vena cava obstruction are caused by carcinoma of the lung, structures contiguous with superior vena cava may also be involved. Respiratory complaints are the second most common presenting symptoms.[5] Symptoms ranging from a mild irritating cough to dyspnea to respiratory arrest may result, depending on the degree of compression of the trachea or right main bronchus. The phrenic, vagus, and sympathetic nerves all lie within the superior mediastinum; involvement of these structures can lead to paralysis of the right hemidiaphragm, hoarseness, pain, or Horner's syndrome. The superior vena cava syndrome in children, unlike that in adults, often constitutes a medical emergency. Severe airway compromise is common owing to the tight thoracic compartment and markedly pliable pediatric tracheobronchial tree, as reported by Neuman[11] and Issa.[12]

ETIOLOGY

During the first half of the twentieth century, most reported cases of superior vena cava syndrome were the result of nonmalignant mediastinal disease. Syphilitic aneurysms accounted for nearly half of the reported cases. Successful treatment and prevention of this disease has now made syphilitic aneurysms and their sequelae a rarity. Banker,[13] Lochridge,[14] Ahmann,[15] Helms,[16] and Yellin[5] have previously reported that malignancy accounted for more than 90% of all superior vena cava obstructions. These earlier studies indicated that 80% to 97% of cases of superior vena cava syndrome resulted from vena cava obstruction by mediastinal malignancy (Fig. 162.3). The rise in the incidence of lung cancer as the most common cause of superior vena cava syndrome in the latter half of the twentieth century parallels the increased tobacco use following World War II. However, Rice and colleagues[17] have found that malignancy now accounts for only 60% of superior vena cava cases because of a sharp rise in benign obstructions related to the use of intravascular devices. The superior vena cava syndrome occurs in approximately 3% to 15% of lung cancer patients, and according to Weinberg,[4] Urban,[18] Elias,[19] Rice,[17] and Wilson[3] small-cell lung cancer is the most frequent cell type associated with this syndrome. Lymphoma, following lung cancer, is the next most frequent malignancy causing this syndrome. A variety of other malignant neoplastic conditions have also been implicated in causing superior vena cava syndrome: Airan,[20] Bishop,[21] and Masuda[22] described malignant thymoma; Liu[23] acknowledged myeloid leukemia; Osawa[24] cited gastric carcinoma; Kew[25] named hepatocellular carcinoma; Munjal[26]

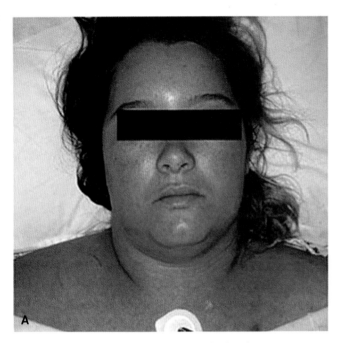
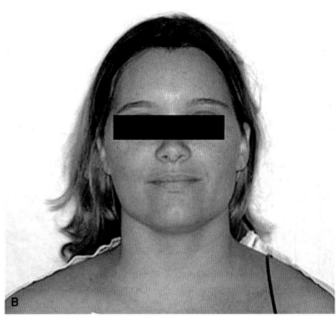

FIGURE 162.1 Photograph of a patient who developed superior vena cava syndrome 4 days after implantation of a single-lead VVI pacemaker. **A:** Note the characteristic swollen facies with congestion at initial presentation and (**B**) the reduction in swelling after thrombolysis and balloon dilatation. (Reprinted with permission from Macmillan Publishers Ltd: Vats HS, Hocking WG, Rezkalla SH. Suspected clopidogrel resistance in a patient with acute stent thrombosis. *Nat Clin Practice Cardiovasc Med* 2006;3(4):226–230. Copyright © 2006.)

and Labarca[27] reported liposarcoma; Aggarwal and colleagues[28] described mediastinal seminoma; Wakabayashi[29] identified metastatic ependymoma; Dirix[30] mentioned osteogenic sarcoma; Davis[31] cited intrathoracic plasmacytoma; and Dada[32] reported metastatic breast adenocarcinoma as unusual examples of this syndrome. Common nonmalignant conditions predisposing to superior vena caval obstruction include substernal goiter, reviewed by Wesseling[33] and reported by de Perrot,[34] and fibrosing mediastinitis, reviewed by Esquivel,[35] Kulpati,[36] and Peters[37] (Fig. 162.4). The syndrome has also been described in association with Riedel's thyroiditis by Abet.[38]

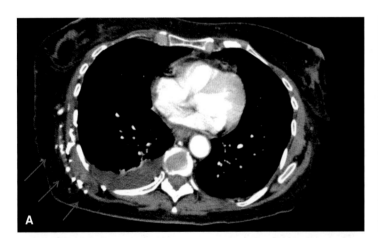
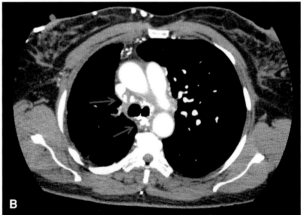
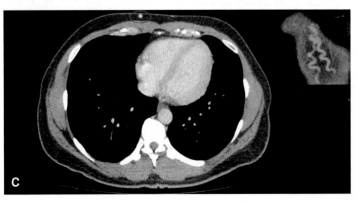

FIGURE 162.2 Examples of dilated collateral vessels in superior vena cava syndrome. **A:** *Red arrows* indicate dilated chest wall collaterals seen in a patient with obstructing thymoma and superior vena cava syndrome. **B:** Multiple collaterals from occlusion of the superior vena cava at the cavo-atrial junction in a patient with fibrosing mediastinitis. **C:** The dilated right superficial epigastric vein is circled in *red* in a patient with obstructing mediastinal thymoma. The inset shows a coronal view, in the same patient, with the dilated right superficial epigastric vein overlying the abdomen.

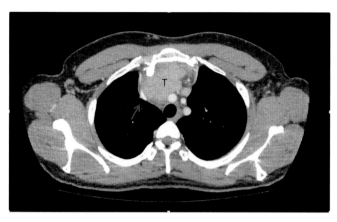

FIGURE 162.3 The *red arrow* indicates the deviated and compressed superior vena cava in a patient with mediastinal thymoma. The thymoma is marked with a "T."

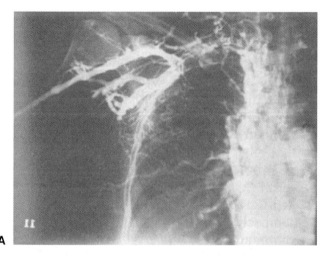

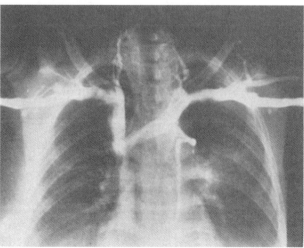

FIGURE 162.4 **A:** Venogram demonstrating occlusion of the right subclavian vein, innominate vein, and superior vena cava in a young woman with chronic fibrosing mediastinitis with a normal chest x-ray. Note the extensive collateral via the enlarged azygos and hemiazygos veins, which drain inferiorly to the inferior vena cava. Other dilated collateral channels include intercostal, internal mammary, and lateral thoracic venous branches. **B:** Complete obstruction of superior vena cava and azygos veins with filling of inferior vena cava via hemiazygos vein secondary to granulomatous mediastinitis.

The last few decades have ushered a greater use of diagnostic procedures, invasive monitoring, and therapeutic techniques performed intravenously, which have resulted in complications leading to the superior vena cava syndrome. Prolonged transvenous hemodynamic monitoring with pulmonary arterial catheters or injury to the superior vena cava at the time of cardiac catheterization has led to caval obstruction and superior vena cava syndrome, as noted by Chetty[39] and Ansari.[40] Indwelling intravascular devices such as Quinton and Hickman catheters for long-term cancer chemotherapy, antibiotic therapy, and renal dialysis have been reported by Preston,[41] Guijarro-Escribano,[42] Ozcinar,[43] Greenwell,[44] and Rinat[45] (Fig. 162.5) to cause superior vena cava syndrome. Numerous episodes of superior vena cava syndrome have resulted from scarring and thrombosis of the superior vena cava from transvenous cardiac pacing and defibrillator leads, as reported by Furman,[46] Koike,[47] Antonelli,[48] Goudevenos,[49] Santangelo,[50] and Aryana[51] and their colleagues. Intravascular devices are now the most common cause of superior vena cava syndrome in benign cases, accounting for 71% of benign obstructions according to Rice.[17]

Vascular anomalies, aortic aneurysms, and aneurysms of the brachiocephalic vessels, once common in the 1950s and 1960s, are reported by Yavuzer[52] to be important but rare causes of superior vena cava obstruction today. Other unusual vascular-related causes such as pulmonary artery aneurysm in Behçet disease and giant coronary artery aneurysm have been reported by Kajiya[53] and Kumar,[54] respectively. The superior vena cava syndrome has also resulted from aortic pseudoaneurysms, as reported by Vydt[55] and Baldari[56] and their colleagues.

Superior vena cava syndrome may also occur after open cardiac surgical procedures, as reported by Garcia-Delgado,[57] Sze,[58] and Blanche.[59] The present author[60] reported a patient who developed the syndrome as a result of narrowing and thrombosis of the superior vena cava following orthotopic cardiac transplantation (Fig. 162.6). Surgical procedures for congenital heart disease that require intracardiac baffles, such as the Mustard operation for transposition of the great vessels, have been reported by Cumming and Ferguson[61] to result in superior vena cava syndrome because of scarring.

Miscellaneous causes of superior vena cava syndrome include thoracic trauma, reported by Shah[52]; sarcoidosis, reported by Fincher[63]; radiation-induced obstruction, reported by Lee[64]; and amebic abscess, reported by Gupta.[65]

DIAGNOSIS

A patient presenting with the signs and symptoms of superior vena cava obstruction requires further evaluation to determine the cause and extent of the underlying problem. The routine chest x-ray is a simple, readily available first-line study that frequently reveals the cause and assists in directing further diagnostic studies. A right hilar or upper-lobe lung mass on the chest radiograph with a clinical history of cough, hemoptysis, weight loss, and smoking strongly supports a diagnosis of lung cancer (Fig. 162.7). In the absence of a lung mass, prominent mediastinal lymphadenopathy suggests lymphoma or malignant metastatic disease. Although adenopathy may be suggested on the routine chest x-ray, it is best delineated by computed tomography (CT). The chest radiograph is usually normal in cases of nonmalignant superior vena cava obstruction. Mediastinal or hilar calcification suggests the diagnosis of fibrosing granulomatous mediastinitis. A normal x-ray in the absence of previous surgical procedures or instrumentation is almost pathognomonic of superior vena caval obstruction secondary to chronic fibrosing mediastinitis.

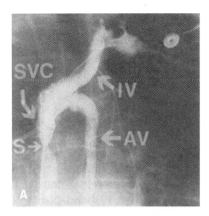
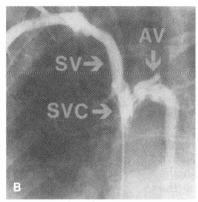
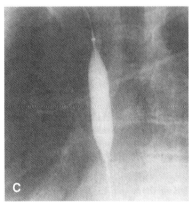
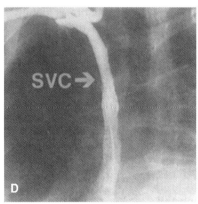

FIGURE 162.5 **A,B:** Venogram showing superior vena cava stenosis from scarring at the tip of an indwelling right internal jugular venous Hickman catheter. Reversal of flow is demonstrated in the azygos vein. **C:** Balloon inflation at the site of superior vena cava stenosis. **D:** Superior vena cavagram after balloon dilatation shows no residual stenosis. Note that reversal of flow in the azygos vein is no longer apparent. SVC, superior vena cava; SV, subclavian vein; IV, innominate vein; AV, azygos vein; S, stenosis.

Computed tomography provides more definitive information as to the extent and mechanism of caval obstruction, whether by compression, direct tumor invasion, or intraluminal thrombosis (Fig. 162.8). Barek,[66] Moncada,[67] Bechtold,[68] Mendelson,[69] and Yedlicka[70,71] and their colleagues describe well the CT findings in the superior vena cava syndrome and recommend that consideration be given to the use of CT as the initial investigative tool for all cases of suspected superior vena cava obstruction. Contrast-enhanced CT scanning provides the opportunity to assess the entire mediastinum and thorax. It also serves to suggest further diagnostic testing, especially fine-needle aspiration or core biopsies when these procedures are indicated. CT is less invasive than bronchoscopy or mediastinoscopy

for the initial evaluation. Yedlicka and colleagues[70] state two criteria that must be met to confirm the diagnosis of superior vena caval obstruction on contrast CT scanning: non-opacification with IV contrast of the superior vena cava inferior to the site of obstruction and opacification with contrast of collateral venous structures. Magnetic resonance imaging (MRI), positron emission tomography (PET), high-resolution CT, and three-dimensional CT scan reconstruction can provide additional information in selected patients in whom the

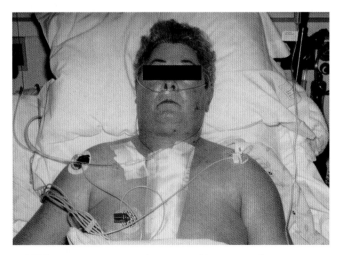

FIGURE 162.6 Appearance of a 54-year-old woman with superior vena cava syndrome following cardiac transplantation. Note facial and palpebral puffiness as well as plethora of the face and chest.

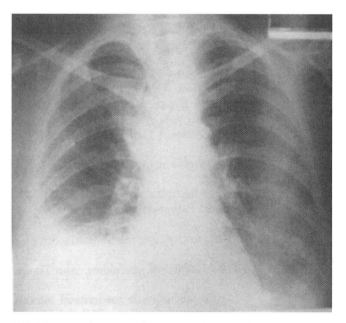

FIGURE 162.7 Chest x-ray of a patient with an undifferentiated large-cell bronchogenic carcinoma of the right upper lobe presenting with superior vena cava obstruction.

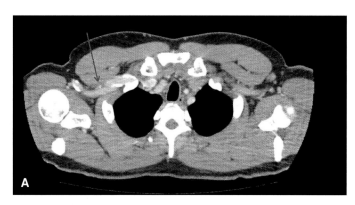 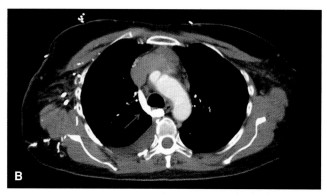

FIGURE 162.8 **A:** Contrast CT showing intraluminal thrombus (*red arrow*) from the distal axillary vein to the proximal subclavian vein in a patient with superior vena cava syndrome. **B:** Contrast CT showing dilated azygos vein (*red arrow*) at the level of the thoracic spine.

diagnosis or extent of disease is in doubt (Fig. 162.9).[71] Conventional tomography and 2D echocardiography, once useful, have been supplanted by more advanced imaging modalities and are mentioned and dismissed for historical reference only.

A sputum cytology is the easiest and least invasive way to establish a malignant diagnosis. However, this approach has essentially been replaced by slightly more invasive procedures that not only are effective in establishing the histopathologic diagnosis but also assist in staging the disease. Fiberoptic bronchoscopy with transbronchial biopsy has been a most effective tool in establishing a malignant diagnosis in superior vena cava syndrome. In the presence of an endobronchial mass, a direct biopsy and assessment of the extent of the tumor are possible. In the absence of an identifiable endobronchial mass, selective subsegmental bronchial washings and brush collections for cytology are often diagnostic and localize the involved bronchopulmonary segment. A lymph node aspiration or biopsy in the presence of cervical adenopathy or thoracentesis for a pleural effusion may provide either a cytologic or histopathologic diagnosis. A positive diagnosis of malignancy with either procedure also establishes surgical non-resectability.

Nieto and Doty[73] have proposed bilateral brachial venography as the diagnostic procedure of choice to evaluate superior vena caval obstruction. We recommend venography in rare instances of chronic fibrosing mediastinitis and when pacing-lead or catheter-induced superior vena caval obstruction is suspected. Venous nuclear scintigraphy has been shown by Savolaine and Schlembach[74] to be a reliable diagnostic tool in this setting. We recommend venography or nuclear scintigraphy selectively when the diagnosis remains in doubt after CT or when the site of venous occlusion requires further clarification.

Mediastinoscopy, mediastinotomy, and video-assisted thoracoscopy with biopsies are excellent approaches for diagnosis and staging in most patients with lung cancer. Lewis and colleagues[75] reported successful results with mediastinoscopy in patients with superior vena cava syndrome. However, these procedures may be hazardous and must be utilized with caution to avoid bleeding complications from the dilated, thin-walled, high-pressure cervical, mediastinal, and chest wall venous collaterals that accompany this syndrome. Intravenous biopsy, suggested by Armstrong,[76] and percutaneous venous atherectomy, reported by Dake and colleagues,[77] have also been used to establish a histologic diagnosis. More contemporary

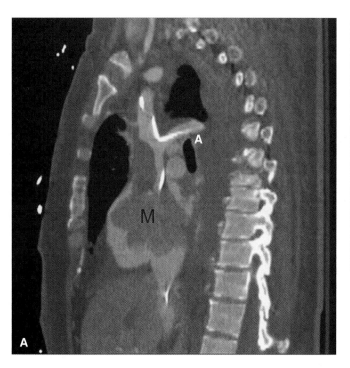 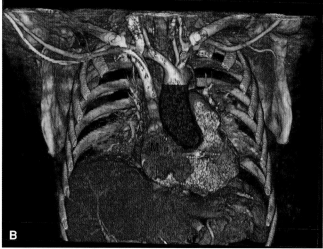

FIGURE 162.9 **A:** 2D contrast CT showing intracardiac right atrial compression and involvement with superior vena cava syndrome and partial inferior vena cava impingement in a woman with an intracardiac non-Hodgkin's lymphoma. **B:** Corresponding 3D reconstruction image. "M" indicates the mass.

methods to safely obtain a tissue diagnosis include EBUS (endobronchial ultrasound) and navigational bronchoscopy biopsy.

A smooth right-sided upper mediastinal mass with tracheal deviation suggests a substernal thyroid goiter. A CT scan demonstrating continuity with the cervical thyroid is almost always diagnostic, but this must be substantiated by radioiodine scanning. If an aortic or innominate artery aneurysm is suspected, it may be confirmed by contrast CT, MRI, or arteriography.

TREATMENT

Treatment for superior vena cava syndrome from any cause begins with general medical measures to reduce edema, lower central venous pressure, and prevent thrombosis. This commonly includes salt restriction, diuretic therapy, elevation of the head, steroid administration, systemic anticoagulation, and—in selected patients—thrombolytic therapy. Specific directed therapy for this syndrome is dictated by the underlying cause of the vena caval obstruction, but when conservative management of these conditions fails then direct surgical or endovascular intervention is warranted.

MALIGNANT DISEASE

Although the incidence of benign etiologies causing this syndrome is increasing, Rice and colleagues[17] have recently reported that malignancy continues to be the leading cause in 60% of cases. When malignancy is suspected, an attempt to establish this diagnosis is strongly recommended. The American College of Chest Physicians recommends histologic confirmation of malignancy as it not only establishes a diagnosis but also provides support for the initiation of treatment with irradiation or chemotherapy.[78] Malignant superior vena cava syndrome is often rapidly progressive and may constitute an oncologic emergency.[79] This is especially true in children with intrathoracic malignancy.[12] In adults, high-dose irradiation given early at 300 to 400 cGy over 4 days has been found by Green[80] and Rubin[81] to be safe and effective in reducing signs and symptoms of malignant superior vena caval obstruction. A response rate of 70% within 2 weeks of initiation of a similar protocol was reported by Armstrong and colleagues.[9] Early, high-dose irradiation is recommended even in patients without a tissue diagnosis when there is a high index of suspicion of a malignancy. The frequent use of irradiation alone to treat this syndrome is based on its effective palliation of malignancies that commonly involve the mediastinum, which include bronchogenic carcinoma, non-Hodgkin's lymphoma, small and non-small-cell lymphoma, germ-cell neoplasms, thymic malignancies, and metastatic tumors.[82] Radiation therapy is usually well tolerated, even by frail or debilitated patients. Further palliative irradiation beyond the initial high dose has been recommended by Awan and colleagues.[83] These authors recommend 200-cGy fractions after the first four high-dose fractions to a total of 4,000 to 5,000 cGy. Although there is support for conventional doses of irradiation, initial high-dose fractionated treatment has been favored. Total irradiation dose has also been shown to be important in relief of symptoms. Small-cell carcinoma, undifferentiated carcinoma, and non-Hodgkin's lymphoma are considered systemic diseases; therefore, appropriate chemotherapy is the treatment of choice in these cases.[78] Tumor response to chemotherapy in these conditions is similar to that observed with irradiation in other thoracic malignancies. The best long-term results are seen in lymphomas. Combination radiation and chemotherapy is commonly used with good symptomatic response in superior vena cava syndrome, but no survival advantage has been noted. In some well-differentiated tumors and in tumors that respond poorly to irradiation, pulmonary edema may result after initial irradiation. This may lead to serious respiratory distress. Despite appropriate and aggressive therapy and a response rate approaching 70%, only 10% to 20% of patients with malignant superior vena cava syndrome survive >2 years. For patients who fail to respond to either chemotherapy and/or radiotherapy, superior vena cava stent placement is warranted. Surgical management of malignant superior vena cava syndrome with prosthetic grafts or autogenous vein grafts is usually not indicated because of the associated operative morbidity and the limited patient survival. However, in selected patients with a malignant etiology, these surgical techniques have been shown to be quite palliative.[84,85] These techniques will be discussed later in the chapter.

BENIGN DISEASE

The incidence of superior vena cava syndrome due to nonmalignant causes is on the rise. Thrombotic or obstructive complications of the superior vena cava because of indwelling central venous catheters, transvenous cardiac pacing leads, complex congenital heart repairs, and cardiac transplantation have readily surpassed the previously commonly reported benign conditions such as fibrosing mediastinitis, syphilitic aneurysms, and substernal thyroid goiters. The first-line treatment for many of these disorders is endovascular stenting, but surgical management of these benign conditions should still be considered when percutaneous therapy fails.

LESS COMMON CAUSES OF SVC SYNDROME

A substernal goiter causing superior vena cava syndrome should be resected. Since the blood supply to the thyroid arises in the neck, most substernal goiters may be resected through a cervical incision. However, preparations to convert to a sternotomy should be made preoperatively if the goiter is too large to be safely delivered into the neck or should uncontrollable hemorrhage be anticipated or encountered due to dilated venous collaterals. Pullerits and Holzman[86] noted that management of anesthesia in these patients may be challenging. Airway obstruction or tracheomalacia resulting from these masses may lead to respiratory arrest upon induction of anesthesia. We reported the use of temporary cardiopulmonary bypass to support induction and intubation in a patient with a large substernal goiter, stridor, and severe airway obstruction.[60]

Operative intervention in superior vena cava syndrome resulting from chronic fibrosing mediastinitis should be reserved for patients in whom symptoms become progressive and unbearable despite endovascular stenting. The slow and insidious progression of this benign disease usually permits the development of extensive venous collaterals around the obstructed superior vena cava. Collaterals that develop in this condition include the internal mammary, azygos, lateral thoracic, and paravertebral veins. These collaterals permit decompression of the head, neck, and arms by shunting venous blood to the right heart via the inferior vena cava or azygos vein. The advisability of surgical intervention must be carefully weighed, since operative intervention frequently interrupts these venous collaterals, which have formed naturally. Mediastinal irradiation and antifungal agents are occasionally effective in resolving symptoms of superior vena cava syndrome in cases of fibrosing mediastinitis. Venous bypass in this condition should be considered only when these two treatments and superior vena cava stenting have proved ineffective.

The evolution in the types of congenital heart defects that can be repaired has been accompanied by increasingly complex surgical procedures. Superior vena cava obstruction in the pediatric surgical population results from small patient size, altered intracardiac flow characteristics, and the complexity of surgical repairs. Superior vena cava syndrome following heart transplantation has also been described by McFadden,[60] Blanche,[59] and Sze.[58] Corrective reoperation, percutaneous interventions, and superior vena cava bypass have each demonstrated utility in the management of superior vena cava syndrome in these patients.

MORE COMMON CAUSES OF SVC SYNDROME

Treatment of superior vena cava syndrome due to an indwelling central venous catheter or cardiac pacemaker often requires a multimodality approach.[87] In general, the first step in treatment of superior vena cava syndrome due to an indwelling central venous catheter or cardiac pacer is removal of the foreign body and systemic anticoagulation to prevent thrombus propagation.[88] If the patient's symptoms fail to respond, then the clinician has several options including catheter-directed or systemic thrombolysis and endovascular stenting.[52,89–92] The risks of systemic thrombolytic therapy must be carefully weighed, especially in patients with central venous catheters for ESRD as they already have an underlying platelet dysfunction due to baseline uremia. The largest series in the literature comes from Gray et al. who reported a case series of 16 patients treated with systemic thrombolytics (streptokinase and urokinase).[93] They found systemic thrombolysis to be effective in 73% (9/16). If therapy was delivered within 5 days of symptoms, the success rate increased to 88% (7/8). Catheter-directed thrombolysis has also been described and is theoretically believed to be safer due to its lower dose of thrombolytics

and more specific exposure radius.[94] Endovascular stenting has excellent success as established by Rizvi et al. who support stenting as the first-line treatment for superior vena cava syndrome in all benign disease, not just venous catheter-induced or pacemaker-induced superior vena cava syndrome.[95] In their large series, they found endovascular stenting to be successful in 88% (28/32) of patients with durable relief of symptoms at 4-year follow-up. They did not explore the role of catheter-directed thrombolysis in the study, but did contend that it was beneficial in the acute or subacute patient. Additionally, they emphasize that surgical bypass remains an excellent option in patients not suitable for endovascular treatment or in those for whom endovascular therapy has failed. Fu et al. evaluated the long-term outcome of pacemaker-induced superior vena cava syndrome treated with stent placement and found that stent placement was successful, although patients often needed repeat interventions (percutaneous balloon angioplasty) for recurrent symptoms.[96] Percutaneous balloon angioplasty is not without risk: superior vena cava rupture has been reported as a complication by Samuels and colleagues.[97] Percutaneous balloon angioplasty for a thrombosed superior vena cava stent is demonstrated in Figure 162.10. In the event that temporary removal of the central line or pacemaker is not feasible due to the patient's other medical conditions, the catheter-directed thrombolysis and stent placement can still be performed successfully (Fig. 162.11).[98]

If pharmacologic and minimally invasive treatments fail to resolve the symptoms of superior vena cava syndrome, surgical intervention may be considered. Successful thrombectomy alone was accomplished by Bonchek and colleagues.[99] Cooley and Hallman[100] reported limited success with re-anastomosis of an uninvolved azygos vein to the inferior vena cava. Minimal morbidity and mortality was reported by Doty and colleagues[101] and

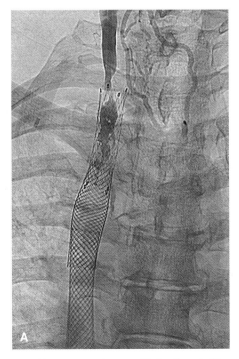
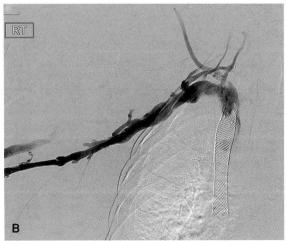

FIGURE 162.10 A 50-year-old female with fibrosing mediastinitis s/p superior vena cava stents (×3) presented with severe proptosis, persistent eye tearing, severe headaches, and an inability to lay flat at night secondary to headaches. **A:** A right internal jugular vein venogram was performed showing occlusion of the superior vena cava stents. **B:** Right upper extremity venogram showing occlusion with retrograde filling of the jugular veins. Percutaneous transluminal angioplasty was performed with a 6/8 and 9 mm balloons. (*continued*)

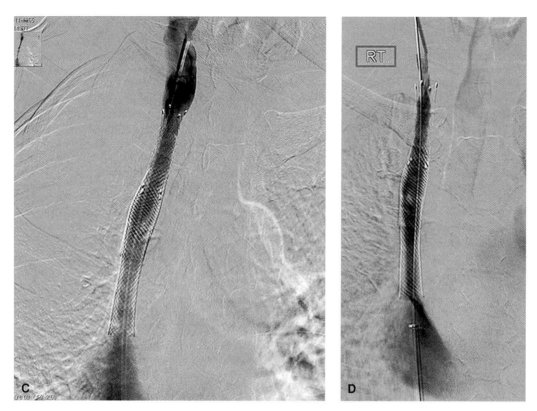

FIGURE 162.10 (*Continued*) **C:** Following PTA with a 9 mm balloon. **D:** Right internal jugular vein venogram shows patent superior vena cava stents with flow to the right atrium.

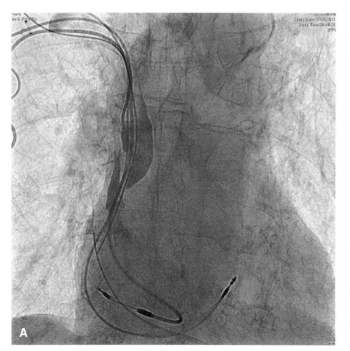
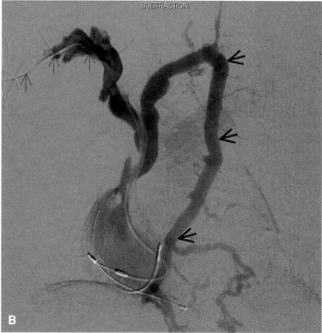

FIGURE 162.11 An 86-year-old woman developed superior vena cava syndrome after a new ventricular lead was connected to her double-chamber pacemaker. A 10-day course of anticoagulation failed to relieve her symptoms which were becoming progressively worse. The patient was pacer dependent and so stenting was carried out with the pacemaker in place with good result. **A:** Venogram showing the proximal stenosis. **B:** Digital subtraction angiogram of the superior vena cava showing stenosis with drainage via the azygos system. *Thin arrows* demonstrate the central venous catheter while *thick arrows* demonstrate contrast material through the azygos system. (*continued*)

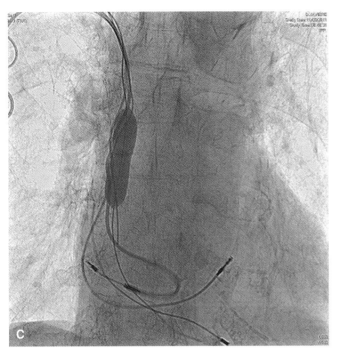

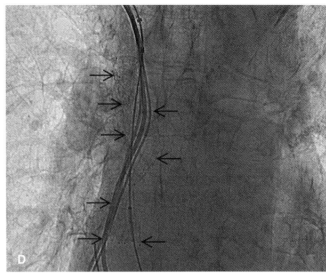

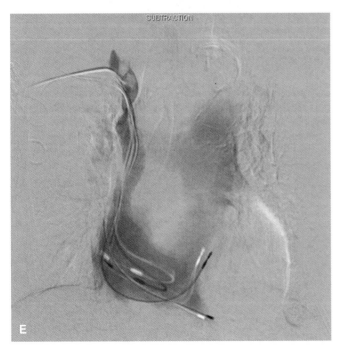

FIGURE 162.11 (*Continued*) **C:** A self-expanding 6 cm Wallstent® (Boston Scientific Corp, Natick, MA, USA) was deployed in the stenosis. **D:** Wallstent® in place marked by *small arrows*. **E:** Digital subtraction angiogram shows free flow of contrast into the right atrium after stent deployment. (Reproduced from Laurent G, Ricolfi F, Wolf JE. Venous stenting as a treatment for pacemaker-induced superior vena cava syndrome. *Arch Cardiovasc Dis* 2013;106:624–626. Copyright © 2013 Elsevier Masson SAS. All rights reserved.)

Anderson and Li[102] with the use of expanded spiral saphenous vein bypass of the superior vena cava. In this technique the saphenous vein is harvested, incised longitudinally, and sewn in a spiral fashion to increase the diameter of the graft (Fig. 162.12). Graft patency rates up to 15 years were observed in some patients[98] (Fig. 162.13). Reversed saphenous vein jugulo-atrial bypasses have been successfully used by Gladstone,[103] Messner,[104] Erbella,[105] and Lau[106] and their colleagues. An internal jugular-to-femoral vein bypass utilizing an innovative approach with an in situ saphenous vein passed through a subcutaneous tunnel has been described by Taylor and colleagues[107]; Dhaliwal and colleagues[108] have described a modification of this technique. Surgical reconstruction of the superior vena cava with expanded polytetrafluoroethylene (ePTFE) artificial conduits was successfully employed by Lequaglie,[109] Magnan,[110] and Dartevelle[111,112] and, more recently, with ringed ePTFE grafts by Shintani and colleagues.[113]

Open surgical palliation is recommended for the most symptomatic patients in whom conservative measures and intravascular intervention are either unsuccessful or not feasible. Resolution of the superior vena cava syndrome has proven possible in patients with either benign or malignant etiologies. The diagnosis, clinical condition, expected survival, and prospect for effective palliation are central in selecting the appropriate course of treatment for patients with superior vena cava syndrome.

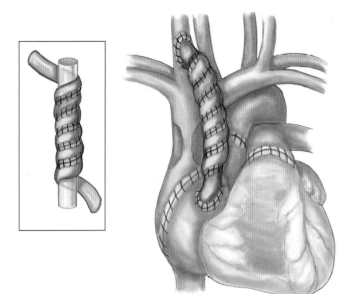

FIGURE 162.12 A 50-year-old woman developed superior vena cava syndrome after cardiac transplantation (Fig. 162.6). She received a reverse spiral saphenous vein graft as illustrated above. The saphenous vein was harvested and opened lengthwise. After it was dilated and the valves removed in the standard fashion, it was wrapped around a chest tube and sewn in a spiral fashion using 6-0 Prolene. It was then anastomosed to the external jugular and right atrial appendage.

ACKNOWLEDGMENTS

We thank and acknowledge the help of the following physicians: Jerold Shinbane, David Shavelle, and John Cleveland of the Keck School of Medicine of the University of Southern California; and Dr. Charles Matthews of the Ochsner Clinic. Special thanks to Barbara Siede for her illustrations.

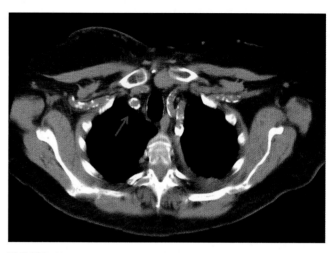

FIGURE 162.13 Contrast CT scan of the patient mentioned in Figure 162.12 10 years after spiral reverse saphenous vein graft showing the somewhat calcified but patent spiral vein graft (*red arrow*) traversing from the external jugular vein to the right atrial appendage.

REFERENCES

1. Hunter W. History of aneurysm of the aorta with some remarks on aneurysm in general. *M Obser Inq (London)* 1757;1:323.
2. Stokes WA. Diseases of the lung and windpipe. In: *Treatise on the Diagnosis and Treatment of Diseases of the Chest.* Dublin: Hodges Smith; 1837:370.
3. Wilson LD, Detterbeck FC, Yahalom J. Superior vena cava syndrome with malignant causes. *N Engl J Med* 2007;356:1862–1869.
4. Weinberg BA, Conces Jr DJ, Waller BF. Cardiac manifestations of noncardiac tumors: part II. Direct effects. *Clin Cardiol* 1989;12:347–354.
5. Yellin A, Rosen A, Reichert N, et al. Superior vena cava syndrome. The myth—the facts. *Am Rev Respir Dis* 1990;141:1114–1118.
6. Saeed AI, Schwartz AP, Limsukon A. Superior vena cava syndrome (SVC): a rare cause of conjunctival suffusion. *Mt. Sinai J Med* 2006;73:1082–1085
7. Leys M, Van Slycken S, Koller J, et al. Acute macular neuroretinopathy after shock. *Bull Soc Belge Opthalmol* 1991;241:95–104.
8. Parish JM, Marschke RF Jr, Dines DE, et al. Etiologic considerations in superior vena cava syndrome. *Mayo Clin Proc* 1981;56:407–413.
9. Armstrong BA, Perez CA, Simpson JR, et al. Role of irradiation in the management of superior vena cava syndrome. *Int J Radiat Oncol Biol Phys* 1987;13:531–539.
10. Chen JC, Bongard F, Klein SR. A contemporary perspective in superior vena cava syndrome. *Am J Surg* 1990;160:207–211.
11. Neuman GG, Weingarten AB, Abramowitz RM, et al. The anesthetic management of the patient with an anterior mediastinal mass. *Anesthesiology* 1984;60:144–147.
12. Issa PY, Marschke RF Jr, Jani NY, et al. Superior vena cava syndrome in childhood: report of ten cases and review of the literature. *Pediatrics* 1983;71:337–341.
13. Banker VP, Maddison FE. Superior vena cava syndrome secondary to aortic disease. *Dis Chest* 1967;51:656–662.
14. Lochridge SK, Knibbe WP, Doty DB. Obstruction of the superior vena cava. *Surgery* 1979;85:14–24.
15. Ahmann FR. A reassessment of the clinical implications of the superior vena caval syndrome. *J Clin Oncol* 1984;2:961–969.
16. Helms SR, Carlson MD. Cardiovascular emergencies. *Semin Oncol* 1989;16:463–470.
17. Rice TW, Rodriguez RM, Light RW. The superior vena cava syndrome: clinical characteristics and evolving etiology. *Medicine* 2006;85:37–42.
18. Urban T, Lebeau B, Chastang C, et al. Superior vena cava syndrome in small-cell lung cancer. *Arch Intern Med* 1993;153:384–387.
19. Elias A. Small cell lung cancer: state of the art therapy in 1996. *Chest* 1997;112:251S–258S.
20. Airan B, Sharma R, Iyer KS, et al. Malignant thymoma presenting as intracardiac tumor and superior vena caval obstruction. *Ann Thorac Surg* 1990;50:989–991.
21. Bishop WT, Chan NH, MacDonald IL, et al. Malignant primary cardiac tumour presenting as superior vena cava obstruction syndrome. *Can J Cardiol* 1990;6:259–261.
22. Masuda H, Ogata T, Takazono I, et al. Total replacement of superior vena cava because of invasive thymoma: seven years' survival. *J Thorac Cardiovasc Surg* 1988;95:1083–1084.
23. Liu HW, Wong KL, Chan TY, et al. Superior vena cava syndrome: a rare presenting feature of acute myeloid leukemia. *Acta Haematol (Basel)* 1988;79:213–216.
24. Osawa S, Sakamoto A, Iwasaki H, et al. Superior vena cava syndrome associated with the metastasis of gastric adenocarcinoma to cervical lymph nodes. *Dig Dis Sci* 2007;52:3343–3345.
25. Kew MC. Hepatocellular carcinoma presenting with the superior mediastinal syndrome. *Am J Gastroenterol* 1989;84:1092–1094.
26. Munjal K, Rancholi V, Rege J, et al. Fine needle aspiration cytology in mediastinal myxoid liposarcoma. *Acta Cytol* 2007;51:456–458.
27. Labarca e, Zapico A, Ríos, Martinez F, et al. Superior vena cava syndrome due to a leiomyosarcoma of the anterior mediastinum: a case report and literature overview. *Int J Surg Case Rep* 2014;5(12):984–987.
28. Aggarwal P, Sharma SK, Sharma ML, et al. Mediastinal seminoma: a case report and review of the literature. *Urol Int* 1988;43:344–346.
29. Wakabayashi T, Yoshida J, Kuchiwaki H, et al. Extraneural metatases of malignant ependymoma inducing atelectasis and superior vena cava syndrome: a case report and review of the literature. *No Shinkei Geka* 1986;14:59–65.
30. Dirix L, Becquart D, Vanmaele R, et al. Superior vena cava syndrome as the presenting symptom of an endoluminal metastasis of an osteosarcoma (letter). *Ann Oncol* 1990;1:81.
31. Davis SR, King HS, LeRoux I, et al. Superior vena cava syndrome caused by an intrathoracic plasmacytoma. *Cancer* 1991;68:1376–1379.
32. Dada R, Ahmad K, Zekri J. Treated the unexpected: metastatic hepatomegaly causing severe superior vena cava obstruction; review of the literature. *Clin Breast Cancer* 2015;15(4):e205.
33. Wesseling GJ, van den Berg BW, Kortlandt JG, et al. Superior vena caval syndrome due to substernal goiter. *Eur Respir J* 1988;1:666–669.
34. de Perrot M, Fadel E, Mercier O, et al. Surgical management of mediastinal goiters: when is a sternotomy required? *Thorac Cardiovasc Surg* 2007;55:39–43.
35. Esquivel L, Diaz-Picado H. Fibrosing TB mediastinitis presenting as a superior vena cava syndrome. A case presentation and echocardiogram correlate. *Echocardiography* 2006;23:588–591.
36. Kulpati DD, Gupta R, Saha MM, et al. Fibrosing mediastinitis: a rare cause of superior vena caval obstruction. *Indian J Chest Dis Allied Sci* 1989;31:291–294.
37. Peters D, Saborowski F, Seel R, et al. Aggressive mediastinal fibrosis, a rare cause of superior vena cava obstruction: case report and review of the literature. *Z Kardiol* 1988;77:194–197.
38. Abet D, Francisc MP, Sevestre H, et al. Syndrome cave superieur et thyroidite de Riedel. A propos d'un cas: revue de la litterature. *J Mal Vasc* 1991;16:298–300.
39. Chetty KG, Glauser FL. Suspected superior vena cava syndrome: the role of the Swan-Ganz catheter. *Chest* 1977;72:673–675.
40. Ansari MJ, Syed A, Wonaba W, et al. Superior vena cava obstruction presenting as a complication of repeated central venous cannulations. *Comp Ther* 2006;32:189–191.
41. Preston Cl, Poynton CH, Williams LB. Intermittent superior vena cava syndrome caused by a Hickman catheter. *Clin Oncol* 1992;4:60–61.

42. Guijarro-Escribano JF, Anton RF, Colmenarejo-Rubin A, et al. Superior vena cava syndrome with central venous catheter successfully with fibrinolysis. *Clin Transl Oncol* 2007;9:198–200.
43. Ozcinar B, Ozmen V. Superior vena cava syndrome after subclavian vein chemotherapy and replacement in a patient with breast cancer. *Breast J* 2007;13:425–426.
44. Greenwell MW, Basye SL, Dhawan SS, et al. Dialysis catheter-induced superior vena-caval syndrome and downhill esophageal varices. *Clin Nephrol* 2007;67: 325–330.
45. Rinat C, Ben-Shalom E, Becker-Cohen R, et al. Complications of central venous stenosis due to permanent central venous catheters in children on hemodialysis. *Pediatr Nephrol* 2014;29:2235–2239.
46. Furman S, Behrens M, Andrews C, et al. Retained pacemaker leads. *J Thorac Cardiovasc Surg* 1987;94:770–772.
47. Koike R, Sasaki M, Kuroda K. Total venous obstruction: a possible complication of transvenous dual-chamber pacing. *Jpn Circ J* 1988;52:1293–1296.
48. Antonelli D, Rosenfeld T, Kaveh Z. Intermittent superior caval venous syndrome due to permanent trans venous electrode. *Int J Cardiol* 1989;23:125–127.
49. Goudevenos JA, Reid PG, Adams PC, et al. Pacemaker-induced superior vena cava syndrome: report of four cases and review of the literature. *Pacing Clin Electrophysiol* 1989;12:1890–1895.
50. Santangelo L, Russo V, Ammendaola E, et al. Superior vena cava thrombosis after intravascular AICD lead extraction: a case report. *J Vasc Access* 2006;7:90–93.
51. Aryana A, Sobota KD, Esterbrooks DJ, et al. Superior vena cava syndrome induced by endocardial defibrillator and pacemaker leads. *Am J Cardiol* 2007;99:1765–1767.
52. Yavuzer S, Cobanli B, Kavukcu S, et al. Aneurysms of aberrant right subclavian artery: a rare cause of the superior vena cava syndrome. *Vasa* 1989;18:69–73.
53. Kajiya T, Annan R, Kameko M, et al. Intracardiac thrombosis superior vena cava syndrome, and pulmonary embolism in a patient with Behcet's disease. A case report and literature review. *Heart Vessels* 2007;22:278–283.
54. Kumar G, Karon BL, Edwards WD, et al. Giant coronary artery aneurysm causing superior vena cava syndrome and congenital heart failure. *Am J Cardiol* 2006;98:986–988.
55. Vydt T, Coddens J, Williams F. Superior vena cava syndrome caused by a pseudoaneuryms of the ascending aorta. *Heart* 2005;91:e29.
56. Baldari D, Chiu S, Salciccioli L. Aortic pseudoaneurysm as a rare cause of superior vena cava syndrome: a case report. *Angiology* 2006;57:363–366.
57. Garcia-Delgado M, Navarrete-Sanchez I, Colmenero M, et al. Superior vena cava syndrome after cardiac surgery: early treatment by percutaneous stenting. *J Cardiothorac Vasc Anesth* 2007;21:417–419.
58. Sze DY, Robbins RC, Semba CP, et al. Superior vena cava syndrome after heart transplantation: percutaneous treatment of a complication of bicaval anastamoses. *J Thorac Cardiovasc Surg* 1998;116:253–261.
59. Blanche C, Tsai TP, Czer LS, et al. Superior vena cava stenosis after orthotopic heart transplantation: complication of an alternative surgical technique. *Cardiovasc Surg* 1995;3:549–552.
60. McFadden PM, Jamplis RW. Superior vena cava syndrome. In Shields TW, ed. *General Thoracic Surgery*. 4th ed. Baltimore, MD: William & Wilkins; 1994:1716–1723.
61. Cumming GR, Ferguson CC. Obstruction of superior vena cava after the Mustard procedure for transposition of the great arteries: conservative management of chylothorax. *J Thorac Cardiovasc Surg* 1975;70:242–247.
62. Shah SS, Heffernan DS, Howdieshell TR, et al. Two-stage reconstruction of the superior vena cava after gunshot to the chest. *J Trauma* 2006;61:736–738.
63. Fincher RM, Sherman EB. Superior vena caval obstruction due to sarcoidosis. *South Med J* 1986;79:1306–1308.
64. Lee Y, Doering R, Jihayel A. Radiation induced superior vena cava syndrome. *Tex Heart Inst J* 1995;22:103–104.
65. Gupta KB, et al. Superior vena cava syndrome caused by pulmonary amoebic abscess. *Indian J Chest Dis Allied Sci* 2006;48:275–277.
66. Barek L, Lautin R, Ledor S, et al. Role of CT in the assessment of superior vena caval obstruction. *J Comput Assist Tomogr* 1982;6:121–126.
67. Moncada R, Cardella R, Demos TC, et al. Evaluation of superior vena cava syndrome by axial CT and CT phlebography. *Am J Roentgenol* 1984;143:731–736.
68. Bechtold RE, Wolfman NT, Kaerstaed N, et al. Superior vena caval obstruction: detection using CT. *Radiology* 1985;157:485–487.
69. Mendelson DS, Bersen BD, Janus CL, et al. Computed tomography of mediastinal collaterals in SVC syndrome. *J Comput Assist Tomogr* 1988;12:881–884.
70. Yedlicka JW Jr, Cormier MG, Gray R, et al. Computed tomography of superior vena cava obstruction. *J Thorac Imaging* 1987;2:72–78.
71. Yedlicka JW, et al. CT findings in superior vena cava obstruction. *Semin Roentgenol* 1989;2:84–90.
72. Di Giammarco G, Storto ML, Marano R, et al. Superior vena cava syndrome: a 3-D CT scan reconstruction. *Eur J Cardiothorac Surg* 2006;30:384–385.
73. Nieto AF, Doty DB. Superior vena cava obstruction: clinical syndrome, etiology and treatment. *Curr Probl Cancer* 1986;10:441–448.
74. Savolaine ER, Schlembach PJ. Scintigraphy compared to other imaging modalities in benign superior vena caval obstruction accompanying fibrosing mediastinitis. *Clin Imaging* 1989;13:234–238.
75. Lewis RJ, Sisler GE, Mackenzie JW. Mediastinoscopy in advanced superior vena cava obstruction. *Ann Thorac Surg* 1981;32:458–462.
76. Armstrong P, Hayes DF, Richardson PJ. Transvenous biopsy of carcinoma of bronchus causing superior vena caval obstruction. *Br Med J* 1975;1:662–665.
77. Dake MD, Zemel G, Dolmatch BL, et al. The cause of superior vena cava syndrome: diagnosis with percutaneous atherectomy. *Radiology* 1990;174:957–959.
78. Simoff MJ, Lally B, Slade MG et al. Symptom management in patients with lung cancer. Diagnosis and management of lung cancer. 3rd ed: American College of Chest Physicians Evidence-Based Clinical Practice Guidelines. *Chest* 2013; 143(Suppl):e455S–e497S.
79. Khan UA, Shanholtz CB, McCurdy MT. Oncologic mechanical emergencies. *Emerg Med Clin N Am* 2014; 32:495–508.
80. Green J, Rubin P, Holzwasser G. The experimental production of superior vena caval obstruction. Trial of different therapy schedules. *Radiology* 1963;81:406–415.
81. Rubin P, Ciccio S. Superior mediastinal obstruction. High daily dose for rapid decompression in carcinoma of the bronchus. In Delley TJ, ed. *Carcinoma of the Bronchus*. New York: Appleton-Century-Crofts; 1971:276.
82. Greskovich JF Jr, Kinsella TJ. Superior vena cava syndrome: clinical features, diagnosis, and treatment. In Shields TW, ed. *General Thoracic Surgery*. 6th ed. Baltimore, MD: Williams & Wilkins; 1993:2545–2566.
83. Awan AM, Weichselbaum RR. Palliative radiotherapy. *Hematol Oncol Clin North Am* 1990;4:1169–1181.
84. Gloviczki P, Pairolero PC, Cherry KJ, et al. Reconstruction of the vena cava and of its primary tributaries: a preliminary report. *J Vasc Surg* 1990;11:373–381.
85. Graham A, Anikin V, Curry R, et al. Subcutaneous jugulofemoral bypass: a simple surgical option for palliation of superior vena cava obstruction. *J Cardiovasc Surg* 1995;36:615–617.
86. Pullerits J, Holzman R. Anaesthesia for patients with mediastinal masses. *Can J Anaesth* 1989;36:681–688.
87. Dumantepe M, Tarhan A, Ozler A. Successful treatment of central venous catheter induced superior vena cava syndrome with ultrasound accelerated catheter-directed thrombolysis. *Catheter Cardiovasc Interv* 2013;81:E269–E273.
88. Williams DR, Demos NJ. Thrombosis of superior vena cava caused by pacemaker wire and managed with streptokinase. *J Thorac Cardiovasc Surg* 1974;68:134–137.
89. Dodds GA III, Harrison JK, O'Laughlin MP, et al. Relief of superior vena cava syndrome due to fibrosing mediastinitis using the Palmaz stent. *Chest* 1994;106:315–318.
90. Fletcher WS, Lakin RC, Pommier RF, et al. Results of treatment of superior vena cava syndrome with expandable metallic stents. *Arch Surg* 1998;133:935–938.
91. O'Mahony M, Skehan S, Gallagher C. Percutaneous stenting of the superior vena cava syndrome in a patient with cystic fibrosis. *Ir Med J* 2005; 98:85–86.
92. Tumelero RT, Duda WT, Tegnon AP, et al. Endoprosthesis implantation at the entry pathway of the right artery monitored by intracardiac ultrasound. *Arq Bras Cardiol* 2007;88:E48–E52.
93. Gray BH, Olin JW, Graor RA, et al. Safety and efficacy of thrombolytic therapy for superior vena cava syndrome. *Chest* 1991;99:54–59.
94. Cui J, Kawai T, Irani Z. Catheter-directed thrombolysis in acute superior vena cava syndrome caused by central venous catheters. *Semin Dial* 2015;28(5):548–551.
95. Rizvi AZ, Kalra M, Bjarnason H, et al. Benign superior vena cava syndrome: stenting is now the first line of treatment. *J Vasc Surg* 2008;47:372–380.
96. Fu HX, Huang XM, Zhong L, et al. Outcome and management of pacemaker-induced superior vena cava syndrome. *Pacing Clin Electrophysiol* 2014;37:1470–1476.
97. Samuels LE, Nyzio JB, Entwistle JW. Superior vena cava rupture during balloon angioplasty and stent placement to relieve superior vena cava syndrome: a case report. *Heart Surg Forum* 2007;10:E78–E80.
98. Laurent G, Ricolfi F, Wolf JE. Venous stenting as a treatment for pacemaker-induced superior vena cava syndrome. *Arch Cardiovasc Dis* 2013;106;624–626.
99. Bonchek LI, Geiss OM, Farley G. Emergency thrombectomy for acute thrombosis of superior vena cava. *J Thorac Cardiovasc Surg* 1979;77:922–924.
100. Cooley DA, Hallman GL. Superior vena caval syndrome treated by azygos vein–inferior vena cava anastomosis [sic]: report of successful case. *J Thorac Cardiovasc Surg* 1964;47: 325–330.
101. Doty DB. Bypass of superior vena cava: six years' experience with spiral vein graft for obstruction of superior vena cava due to benign and malignant disease. *J Thorac Cardiovasc Surg* 1982;83:326–338.
102. Anderson RP, Li WI. Segmental replacement of superior vena cava with spiral vein graft. *Ann Thorac Surg* 1983;36:85–88.
103. Shintani Y, Ohta M, Minami M, et al. Long-term graft patency after replacement of the brachiocephalic veins combined with resection of mediastinal tumors. *J Thorac Surg* 2005;129:809–812.
104. Gladstone DJ, Pillai R, Paneth M, et al. Relief of superior vena caval syndrome with autologous femoral vein used as a bypass graft. *J Thorac Cardiovasc Surg* 1985;89: 750–752.
105. Messner GN, Azzizadeh A, Huynh TT, et al. Superior vena caval bypass using the superficial femoral for treating of superior vena cava syndrome. *Tex Heart Inst Heart J* 2005;32:605–606.
106. Erbella J, Hess PJ, Huber TS. Superior vena cava bypass with superficial femoral vein for benign superior vena cava syndrome. *Ann Vasc Surg* 2006;20:834–838.
107. Lau D, Berguer R. Correction of superior vena cava syndrome with superficial femoral vein juguloatrial bypass. *Ann Vasc Surg* 2006:839–841.
108. Taylor GA, Miller HA, Standen JR, et al. Bypassing the obstructed superior vena cava with a subcutaneous long saphenous vein graft. *J Thorac Cardiovasc Surg* 1974;68: 237–240.
109. Dhaliwal RS, Das D, Luthra S, et al. Management of superior vena cava syndrome by internal jugular to femoral vein bypass. *Ann Thorac Surg* 2006;82:310–312.
110. Lequaglie C, Conti B, Brega-Massone PP, et al. The difficult approach to neoplastic superior vena cava syndrome: surgical option. *J Cardiovas Surg* 2003;44:667–671.
111. Magnan PE, Thomas P, Giudicelli R, et al. Surgical reconstruction of the superior vena cava. *Cardiovasc Surg* 1994;2:598–604.
112. Dartevelle P, Chapelier A, Navaias M, et al. Replacement of the superior vena cava with polytetrafluoroethylene grafts combined with resection of mediastinal–pulmonary malignant tumors. *Report of thirteen cases. J Thorac Cardiovasc Surg* 1987;94:361–366.
113. Dartvelle PE, Chapelier AR, Pastorino U, et al. Long term followup after prosthetic replacement of the superior vena cava combined with resection of mediastinal–pulmonary malignant tumors. *J Thorac Cardiovasc Surg* 1993;105:259–265.

163

Surgical Management of Benign Sympathetic Nervous System Conditions

Stephen Hazelrigg ▪ Erin E. Bailey

Dysfunction of the sympathetic nervous system (SNS) can result in a number of medical problems and conditions. These may include excessive sweating, as well as pain syndromes. Surgery to disrupt the thoracic sympathetic system has had success in many of these maladies and the advent of video-assisted thoracic surgical (VATS) techniques, and also minimally invasive techniques, have resulted in more consideration for surgical intervention.

Sympathectomy was first reported in the late 1800s for vascular conditions in the upper extremities. In 1920, Kotzareff performed the first sympathectomy for hyperhidrosis. It was also subsequently used for various upper-extremity pain syndromes. Endoscopic sympathectomy was reported as early as 1942, but improvements in anesthesia, instruments, and video equipment have made this procedure easier and increased its use. The VATS approach has largely replaced other surgical approaches such as cervical, transaxillary, and thoracotomy incision.

This chapter will describe the various benign SNS disorders, the present technique of VATS sympathectomy, and discuss indications and results.

THORACIC SYMPATHETIC ANATOMY

The sympathetic trunks are long chains of nerve ganglia running bilaterally from the first thoracic level (T1) to the second lumbar level (L2) over the junction of the head of the ribs with the transverse processes of the vertebral bodies (Fig. 163.1). The inferior cervical

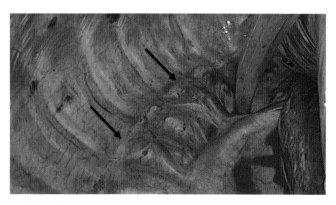

FIGURE 163.1 Thoracic sympathetic anatomy. The *arrows* point to the sympathetic chain.

ganglia and T1 fuse to form the stellate ganglia, an important point of reference as transection at or above this level may result in Horner syndrome.[1] An alternative pathway rarely seen in individuals, termed the nerve of Kuntz, forms a connection from the 2nd intercostal nerve to the 1st thoracic ventral ramus. The nerve of Kuntz allows signals to reach the brachial plexus without passing through the sympathetic trunk.[2,3] Transection of the nerve of Kuntz, if present, is key for complete denervation of the hands as in the treatment of palmar hyperhidrosis.[3]

Strict identification of the ganglion levels is crucial during thoracic sympathectomy to accurately treat a specific problem. Research performed in the 1950s distinguished the sympathetic outflow to specific peripheral sites originated at distinct levels. Craniofacial sympathetic supply originates from the cervical ganglia, including the stellate ganglion which overlies the head of the 1st rib. Innervation to the hand correlates with levels T2 and T3, including the nerve of Kuntz when present. The axilla is innervated by sympathetic supply from T4 and T5.

Furthermore, the splanchnic nerves are a coalescence of sympathetic ganglia to form three distinct nerves supplying the sympathetic source of the gut. Named greater, lesser, and least splanchnic nerves these nerves are supplied by levels T5–T10, T10–T11, and T12, respectively, and have been implicated in many studies as the primary source of pain in patients with chronic pancreatitis and pancreatic cancer.

SYMPATHETIC CHAIN PHYSIOLOGY

The sympathetic chain is a paired bundle of nerves that runs just parallel to the vertebral bodies down to the second lumbar level. In the chest, they are located over the costovertebral junctions posteriorly and the stellate ganglion located at the T1 level. The stellate ganglion mostly innervates the face and pupils. This level must be preserved to avoid Horner syndrome after sympathectomy. Currently, the 2nd and 3rd thoracic levels are felt to primarily innervate the upper extremities and are considered the appropriate level for palmar hyperhidrosis, while T3 and T4 are levels felt primarily to involve the axilla.

The sympathetic ganglion cells are activated mainly by stimuli received through afferent preganglionic neurons in the spinal cord. The activated sympathetic stimulus is conducted from the spinal cord to the sympathetic ganglion via the intercostal nerves sequentially.

Sympathetic nerve fibers originate from the intermediolateral horns of the spinal cord between T1 and L2. Each pathway consists of pre- and postganglionic neurons. The nerve fibers distributing to the sweat glands are postganglionic fibers arising from the ganglia in the sympathetic trunks. These nerves then come together with the corresponding spinal nerves in the target organ. In the sympathetic trunks, signals may travel up or down before exiting and distributing to the target organ. Therefore, distributions will overlap and are not necessarily to the same part of the body from the corresponding spinal segment.

The autonomic nervous system functions through positive and negative feedback mechanisms. First, the hypothalamus is triggered by a stimulus and sends signals to the sweat glands through the autonomic nervous system. Nerve impulses from the target organs are transmitted as afferent negative feedback signals to the hypothalamus by way of the sympathetic trunk. It is hypothesized that if the T2 level is interrupted by sympathectomy, the negative signals cannot reach the central nervous system, which results in preponderance of uninterrupted positive signals from hypothalamus to the target organ. Therefore, efferent positive feedback signals to the sweat gland are strong, thus causing more severe compensatory sweating to occur. If the interruption is in lower levels such as T4, negative signals coming from T2 and T3 are preserved to create some negative signals in the hypothalamus, which results in less potent positive stimulus to the target organ resulting in less severe compensatory sweating. As will be discussed in this review, the literature now advocates the interruption of the sympathetic chain at lower levels in order to decrease the incidence of compensatory sweating. Based on current data, the optimal levels of operation for different areas of hyperhidrosis were investigated for procedural success, long-term satisfaction, and complications.

BENIGN CONDITIONS BENEFITTED FROM SYMPATHECTOMY

HYPERHIDROSIS

Hyperhidrosis is a pathologic condition of excessive sweating from the eccrine glands in quantities that far exceed amounts needed for thermoregulation. When severe, the condition may lead to embarrassment, fear of shaking hands or dropping objects, and social seclusion. Affecting 1% to 3% of the population, there is an increased incidence of the condition in patients with Japanese, Yemeni, Balkan, and North African descent, as well as, increased incidence in climates nearer to the Equator. Though most cases are idiopathic, secondary causes of hyperhidrosis should first be ruled out prior to pursuing invasive treatment. Secondary causes include hyperthyroidism, obesity, diabetes, hypertension, infections, anxiety disorders, menopause, brain lesions, pheochromocytoma, and certain medications.[1,3,4]

Hyperhidrosis can be further divided into generalized, regional, or focal disease. Focal disease typically occurs in the palm, axilla, and plantar regions. Various treatment modalities have been attempted for each variant of the condition. Prescription strength antiperspirants are believed to cause mechanical obstruction of the glands thereby causing atrophy and decreased production.[1]

Anticholinergic medications, whether topical, injectable, or systemic, may provide relief for select patient depending on the manifestation of their disease. Topical medications, namely aluminum chloride and aluminum tetrachloride, can be added to antiperspirants for added benefit. Further side effects include depigmentation and contact dermatitis.

β-Blockers and benzodiazepines may work well for patients' emotionally stimulated hyperhidrosis.[5] Systemic versions of acetyl cholinergic drugs, glycopyrrolate, propantheline, and oxybutynin have also been used but with minimal success, secondary to side effects of blurred vision, dry mouth, and urinary retention.[1,4] Working from a similar mechanism but injected locally, botulinum toxin has had effective results for axillary and palmar hyperhidrosis. The disadvantage of botox is that is must be repeated every 3 to 7 months and can be painful and costly.[6–8] Iontophoresis, a procedure that uses electrical current to introduce ionized substances into the skin, has been shown to alleviate symptoms in 85% of patients with palmar or plantar hyperhidrosis. This procedure, however, is labor intensive and may cause scaling or fissuring of the skin.[9–12]

With regards to surgical treatment for hyperhidrosis, sympathectomy has long been the permanent treatment of choice. The goal of sympathectomy is to disengage the sympathetic flow to the eccrine glands, hence decreasing excessive sweat. Several approaches to sympathectomy have been described, including cervical (or supraclavicular), transaxillary, posterior, transthoracic, thoracoscopic, transumbilical, and robotic.[3,4,13,14]

COMPLEX PAIN SYNDROMES

Reflex Sympathetic Dystrophy (RSD): Posttraumatic pain syndromes (RSD, causalgia, shoulder–hand syndrome, Sudeck atrophy) have been recognized since prior to World War I.[15–17] The natural history of RSD is for acute burning pain and muscle spasms in limbs that often have edematous changes that progress to a more chronic disorder with muscular atrophy and even contractures. Although spontaneous resolution may occur in the early phases, most treatments have the best response early and certainly prior to the chronic phase, when it may be irreversible. As many as 50% to 70% will respond to conservative treatment, which includes physical therapy, medication (i.e., phenoxybenzamine hydrochloride, prazosin, guanethidine), and stellate ganglion blocks. Sympathectomy has demonstrated good results in over 90% of patients, and again results seem better the shorter the time from onset of RSD to sympathectomy.[18] Prior to consideration of surgery, patients should demonstrate response to stellate ganglion block.

Sympathectomy is performed to include the T4 ganglion. There is some controversy as to whether the stellate ganglion should be removed. Removal of the stellate ganglion always produces a Horner syndrome, but failure to excise the stellate ganglion may lead to an infrequent failure of pain relief. The authors presently excise the sympathetic chain just below the stellate ganglia.

VASCULAR DISORDERS

Historically, sympathectomy has been used to treat a variety of vascular disorders. Though originally done to improve circulation to the extremities in many ischemic diseases, new technologies, medications, and improved revascularization techniques have resulted in an overall decrease in the number of sympathectomy done for ischemic disease.[19,20] Advances in medical control of vasospastic disease has also resulted in a decreased need for thoracic sympathectomy. Collagen vascular diseases are not generally responsive to surgical sympathectomy; however, Raynaud phenomenon without collagen vascular disease and drug refractory thromboangiitis obliterans (Buerger disease) continue to be a rare indication for sympathectomy. The outcomes and success rates are generally not as good in this group when compared to hyperhidrosis and CRPS groups.[4,21]

SYMPATHECTOMY

Sympathectomy is typically performed using a double-lumen endotracheal tube and single lung ventilation. The procedure is short and could be performed with intermittent breaks in ventilation with a single-lumen tube or even with sedation and no intubation. In our experience, however, these techniques are cumbersome, compromise visualization, and given the low risk of double-lumen tube placement, this is the authors' preference.

There are two options for patient positioning. The patient can be placed in the full lateral position as in typical for VATS and then repositioned to the outer side for the bilateral procedure. This approach has the advantage of providing the usual exposure and full availability of the chest for ports. Obviously, it does require repositioning which adds some time to the procedure. The second option is to have the patient sitting with arms extended. This position allows both sides to be addressed without repositioning. One needs to be careful with the arm positioning as brachial plexus injuries have been reported.

Regardless of the patient positioning, the procedure consists of placement of a scope, visualization of the sympathetic chain, selection of the desired level of transection, and finally the decision of the method to be used to disrupt the sympathetic chain.

The most commonly used method is with three, 5-mm ports triangulated. The precise interspaces for placement of the ports can vary based on the level of chain to be addressed, but one wants all ports placed such that the instruments move in the same direction. Defining rib levels may be difficult in obese patients externally but can usually be palpated internally with an instrument once the chest has been entered, including the 1st rib. One may tilt the patient slightly forward to use gravity to help move the lung anterior for exposure purposes. Certainly, this procedure can be done with different-sized ports and fewer than three ports. It is a fairly simple procedure, but there can often be some venous branches over the chain that must be addressed. Occasionally, there is an aberrant nerve (Kux) and this should be looked for.

After the level of transection is decided, the question of how to interrupt the chain must be decided. Options are to cauterize and transect, cut and remove a segment, or to simply clip it. Presently it remains unclear which method is best. The clip has been supported because it is felt to have the best opportunity for reversal if compensatory sweating is severe. The authors presently simply transect with cautery in most cases.[22]

RESULTS AND LEVEL OF NERVE TRANSECTION

PALMAR HYPERHIDROSIS

Excessive sweating from the palms and soles can be quite debilitating both socially and professionally. Sympathectomy has been performed on individuals with disabling, recalcitrant palmar hyperhidrosis since 1920. Sympathectomy typically involves the surgical destruction of the 2nd and/or 3rd thoracic ganglia. Cauterization and/or clipping at these levels leads to a satisfaction rate of 94% to 98%.[23] Complications and side effects of thoracoscopic sympathectomy include recurrence of hyperhidrosis, gustatory sweating, and compensatory sweating. Rarely one can see a Horner syndrome, neuralgia, or a pneumothorax.

Of all the complications and side effects associated with sympathectomy, compensatory sweating is the most common problem that leads to patient dissatisfaction. There has been much debate and study regarding the appropriate level for the sympathectomy to be performed. Yazbek and Wolosker et al.[24] studied 60 patients in a prospective randomized controlled study, comparing the results of T2 versus T3 transection. Sympathectomy included transection as well as thermoablation. The patients in both groups had palmar anhydrosis on return visits at 1 month and 6 months. One month after the operation, compensatory sweating was observed in 26 of 30 patients in the T2 group and in 27 of the T3 group. Six months after the operation all the patients in the T2 group had some degree of compensatory sweating as did all but one patient in the T3 group.[25] In their follow-up publication at 20 months, all patients exhibited compensatory sweating. The degree of severity was recorded and, overall, the patients in the T3 group presented with a lower degree of compensatory sweating at each assessment level. Quality of life assessments were also performed at each time interval and the quality of life for all patients was much improved postoperatively. There was no significant difference between the two groups ($p = 0.76$).[4]

Yoon and Rim, in a prospective study, compared transection at T2–T3 (Group A) to level T3 only (Group B). Their mean follow-up was 17.8 months in group A versus 16.6 months in group B. Compensatory sweating was present in 45% of Group A patients versus 16% in group B. At the end of the study, 66% of T2–T3 (Group A) patients versus 87% of T3 only (Group B) patients were satisfied with their results. This difference was statistically significant.[26] In a similar study, Katara et al. performed a prospective randomized blinded study, comparing ablation of the T2 ganglion on one side with ablation of T2 and T3 on the other in each patient. The mean follow-up was 23 months. There was no difference in the results with regard to efficacy (100% success), recurrence (no cases), frequency of compensatory sweating (80%), severity of the compensatory sweating (no severe cases, 20% moderate cases, no interference with the quality of life), and satisfaction subsequent to the procedure (>80%).[27]

Miller et al. retrospectively analyzed 282 patients who underwent sympathectomy at the T2 level or T2 through T4 for palmar hyperhidrosis. Ninety-nine percent of the cases experienced therapeutic success. The patients in the multilevel group had significantly worse compensatory sweating than the T2 level–only group. Multivariate logistic regression analysis showed that higher BMI, multiple levels of sympathectomy, and older age were the three factors most predictive of compensatory sweating. Satisfaction rates were similar between the groups. These findings suggest that a multilevel sympathectomy resulted in more compensatory hyperhidrosis than single-level sympathectomy.[28]

In a retrospective review of 234 patients, 86 patients were treated by T2 level sympathectomy, 70 patients by endoscopic thoracic sympathectomy (ETS) at T3, and 78 patients by T4 level sympathectomy. Overly dry hands were reported in 36% at T2, 39% at T3, and 8.6% at T4. Overall, 88.5% of patients noted compensatory sweating and the incidence in each group was 92%, 92%, and 80%, respectively ($p < 0.05$). The most common region for compensatory hyperhidrosis was the back, occurring in 56.3%, 75%, and 42.9%, respectively. The group having the T4 sympathectomy had the lowest incidence and least severe compensatory sweating of the three groups. Most patients were satisfied with the results of surgery, especially in groups T3 and T4. Generally, the higher the level of transection, the greater the incidence of compensatory sweating. No one in the T3 group or the T4 group expressed regret for having undergone the surgery, while 11 people in the T2 group expressed some unhappiness. The incidence of overly dry hands was significantly higher in T2 and T3 groups compared to the T4 group. It seemed that T4 ETS for palmar hyperhidrosis had the least postoperative complications, including palmar overdryness, presence of CS, and regions of CS. These results led the authors to suggest T4 as the ideal level for sympathectomy.[15]

Yazbek and Wolosker[24] also investigated lower levels of sympathectomy for palmar hyperhidrosis in another prospective study comparing the T3 level to the T4 level. They failed to achieve anhydrosis in all patients. After 6 months, hyperhidrosis improved in all patients, but anhydrosis was achieved in only 26/35 patients in the T3 group and 8/35 patients in the T4 group. All patients had significant reduction in sweating, however, and compensatory sweating at 6 months was 100% in the T3 group versus 71% in the T4 group (P <0.05). Quality of life assessments were similar in both groups. The authors concluded that the T4 level is acceptable for palmar hyperhidrosis as long as the patient is made aware that their hyperhidrosis will improve but not be eliminated.[29]

Yang et al., in a prospective randomized study, compared T3 sympathectomy to T4 sympathectomy in 163 patients with palmar hyperhidrosis. All patients were cured, and there was no recurrence of palmar hyperhidrosis in a mean follow-up of 13.8 months. The rate of mild compensatory sweating was not statistically different; however, the incidence of more severe compensatory sweating was significantly lower in the T4 group.[9] As a result, it appeared that the lower level sympathectomy (T4) led to a reduction in major compensatory sweating (Table 163.1).

As can be appreciated from the above review of the literature, the appropriate level of sympathectomy has been a hot topic of debate. Several studies have evaluated the clinical outcomes at each level. Initially, it was recommended that a T2 or T2–T3 sympathectomy is the appropriate level for palmar hyperhidrosis. However, there is a growing body of evidence that suggests that lower levels of sympathectomy for palmar hyperhidrosis may produce better patient satisfaction as a result of less compensatory sweating. It is our finding, after reviewing the literature, that a single level T2, T3, or T4 sympathectomy will produce excellent results in eliminating palmar hyperhidrosis and is safe; however, those done at T3 or T4 will limit the severity of compensatory sweating and avoid overly dry hands after surgery (evidence quality high).[2–4,9,10,17,23,25–30] The authors strongly recommend a T3 or T4 level sympathectomy for palmar hyperhidrosis, with the T4 level producing less anhydrosis but also less compensatory sweating (recommendation grade 1B).

AXILLARY HYPERHIDROSIS

Over the last 2 decades the technique for treating axillary hyperhidrosis has evolved. Higher success rates are attributed to technique as well as careful patient selection. Complications and side effects of sympathectomy are similar to those for palmar hyperhidrosis, and compensatory sweating continues to be an important concern after surgery. In addition, recurrent hyperhidrosis is more prevalent for axillary problems than for palmar hyperhidrosis.[20]

In a retrospective cohort study, Hsu et al.[31] reviewed their experience with 171 patients treated for axillary hyperhidrosis. They divided patients into three groups: T3–T4 sympathectomy in Group 1, T4 sympathectomy in Group 2, and T4–T5 sympathectomy in Group 3. The incidence of overly dry hands was significantly higher in the T3–T4 group. A 70% compensatory sweating incidence was noted in the T3–T4 group compared to 29% in the T4 and T4–T5 groups. In a questionnaire satisfaction was rated as excellent, good, and poor. The poor result rate was 32%, 30%, and 15%, respectively. This result suggested a significant role for preservation of the T3 level in the prevention of compensatory sweating, thus resulting in superior outcomes.[32] This same group of authors published another report in 2003, 2 years after their first study, and re-evaluated the T3–T4 level sympathectomy. This time they added "fair" between "good" and "poor" in their questionnaire. This time the "poor" rate was 9% and the "fair" rate was 21%. In both studies the success rate was significantly lower than seen in palmar hyperhidrosis cohorts.[33]

Munia et al. performed a randomized, prospective study to compare the results of sympathectomy at T3–T4 versus T4 for axillary hyperhidrosis. The study reviewed the efficacy of treatment, presence and severity of compensatory sweating, and patient satisfaction over a 1-year time period. There were no treatment failures at 1-year follow-up. A total of 64 patients with pure axillary hyperhidrosis

TABLE 163.1 Summary for Palmar Hyperhidrosis

Author	Year	Level	Dry (%)	CH (%)	Satis (%)	Regret (%)	Number	F/U	Type
Yazbek	2005	T2	100	86			30	6 months	Pros
Yazbek	2005	T3	96.6	90			30	6 months	Pros
Yoon	2003	T2–3	100	45	66*		24	17.8 months	Pros
Yoon	2003	T2	100	16	87*		30	17.8 months	Pros
Katara	2007	T2	100	80			25	23 months	Pros
Katara	2007	T2–3	100	80			25	23 months	Pros
Miller	2009	T2		13[a]			179	1 month	Retro
Miller	2009	T2–4		34[a]			103	1 month	Retro
Chang	2007	T2	74.4	92	9.3[a]		86	60.9 months	Retro
Chang	2007	T3	92.3	92[a]	3.8[a]		78	35.6 months	Retro
Chang	2007	T4	77.1	80[a]	0[a]		70	43.1 months	Retro
Wolosker	2008	T3		100[a]			35	6 months	Pros
Wolosker	2008	T4		71[a]			35	6 months	Pros
Yang	2007	T3		100	23*		78	13.8 months	Retro
Yang	2007	T4		100	7.1*		85	13.8 months	Retro

[a]Statistically significant.
Pros, prospective; Retro, retrospective; Satis, satisfaction.

were randomized between the two treatment levels. In the T3–T4 group, sympathectomy was performed on the bodies of the 3rd, 4th, and 5th ribs, followed by a thermoablation of the segment between them. Patients in the T4 group underwent resection of the chain at the 4th and 5th ribs, with thermoablation of the segment between them. The incidence of compensatory sweating was lower in the T4 group at 1, 6, and 12 months follow-up. The T4 group experienced compensatory sweating in 57.6%, while the T3–T4 group experienced it in 93.5% at 1 year. Sites of compensatory sweating were the abdomen, back, and/or legs. Compensatory sweating was less severe in the T4 group and there were no severe cases by the final follow-up at 12 months. Thirty-five percent of the T3 to T4 patients showed moderate to severe compensatory sweating, while only 12.5% of the T4 group had this same problem. The incidence and severity of compensatory hyperhidrosis in patients who underwent T3–T4 resection remained constant over the 12 month follow-up interval, while there was decrease in the incidence in the T4 group from 6 to 12 months ($p < 0.05$). Overall, patients in the T4 group reported higher postoperative satisfaction than those of the T3 to T4 group ($p < 0.05$). It must be noted, however, that both groups showed that the procedure improved their quality of life. Munia et al. concluded that sympathectomy from the upper margin of the 4th rib to the lower margin of the 5th rib followed by thermoablation of the chain, resulted in good success and acceptable compensatory sweating.[21]

Montessi et al. performed a retrospective review of 521 cases comparing different levels of ablation. These patients were divided into three groups: sympathectomy extending superiorly to T2 (Group I), T3 (Group II), or T4 (Group III). Postoperative control of axillary hyperhidrosis was achieved in 82% of group I, 89% of group II, and 80% of group III. Severe compensatory sweating occurred in 32% of group I, 9% of group II, and 4% of group III. While patient satisfaction was high across the board, there was a decrease in incidence and severity of compensatory sweating with lower levels of ablation. They also performed an extensive review of the literature and concluded that the T4–T5 level for axillary hyperhidrosis was preferred.[34]

Doolabh et al., in their retrospective study, reported a 98% success rate for axillary hyperhidrosis by removing the T4 level. This was inconsistent with many prior reports and may be because the majority of the patients also had a palmar component to their disease that was relieved, resulting in a higher satisfaction rate than is typically seen in axillary hyperhidrosis alone (Table 163.2).[13]

Overall, the literature on axillary hyperhidrosis is not as consistent as it is for palmar hyperhidrosis. There is a considerable failure rate in many publications, especially the ones with isolated axillary hyperhidrosis.[13,20,21,32–35] Fewer surgeons offer sympathectomy for axillary hyperhidrosis, and this results in a smaller number of studies to analyze.[36] An alternative treatment for axillary hyperhidrosis is the removal of the axillary sweat glands. Sympathectomy is much less invasive and typically is tried first for patients with axillary hyperhidrosis. While the precise level to recommend is still not proven, the recent body of evidence supports that sympathectomy at the T4 and T5 levels is reasonably effective and is safe (evidence quality low). The authors make a weak recommendation for T4 or T5 sympathectomy for management of axillary hyperhidrosis (recommendation grade 2B).

CRANIOFACIAL HYPERHIDROSIS AND BLUSHING

Craniofacial hyperhidrosis can be quite debilitating for many patients. Sympathectomy has been used as a viable approach to the problem; however, it has also been reported to be associated with higher levels of patient dissatisfaction compared to palmar and axillary hyperhidrosis. Evidence of effectiveness of sympathectomy is weak due to the lack of randomized trials.[37] Several studies have evaluated methods to decrease the incidence of compensatory sweating; however, due to the close proximity and association of the T2 ganglion with the T1 ganglion, this has been difficult to achieve.

In 2004, Kim et al. reviewed a total of 44 sympathectomies for facial sweating. Twenty-two underwent T2 clipping (Group 1) and 22 underwent division of the T2 rami-communicates (Group 2). The goal of raminectomies was to preserve the sympathetic trunk and eliminate compensatory sweating after surgery. They retrospectively analyzed the rate of satisfaction, facial dryness, and grade of compensatory sweating. Both groups were similar with respect to facial dryness ($P = 0.099$). Group 1: excessive dryness occurred in 5 patients (22.7%) and dryness in 17 patients (77.3%); Group 2: excessive dryness occurred in 3 patients (13.6%), dryness in 15 patients (68.1%), and persistent sweating in 4 patients (18.3%). The rate of satisfaction was 77.3% in Group 1 and 63.6% in Group 2, which was not statistically significant ($P > 0.05$). The rate of compensatory sweating in Group 2 (72.7%) was significantly lower than in Group 1 (95.4%) ($P = 0.039$). The chance of embarrassing and disabling compensatory sweating was lower in Group 2 (76.5% overall; embarrassing in eight patients, disabling in nine) than in Group 1 (36.4% overall; embarrassing in seven patients, disabling in one; $P = 0.006$). They concluded that conservation of the sympathetic trunk and performing

Author	Year	Level	Dry (%)	CH (%)	Satis (%)	Regret (%)	Number	F/U	Type
HSU	2001	T3–4		70	68[a]	32	40		Retro
HSU	2001	T4		29	70[a]	30[a]	56		Retro
HSU	2001	T4–5		29	85[a]	15[a]	75		Retro
Hsia	2003	T3–4		65		9	262	42 months	Retro
Munia	2008	T3–4		54[a]		16[a]	31	12 months	Pros
Munia	2008	T4		93[a]		0[a]	33	12 months	Pros
Montessi	2007	T2	82	32[a]			99 total		Retro
Montessi	2007	T3	89	9[a]			99 total		Retro
Montessi	2007	T4	80	4[a]			99 total		Retro
Dooblah	2004	T4	99				55	17 months	

TABLE 163.2 Summary of Axillary Hyperhidrosis

[a]Statistically significant.

TABLE 163.3 Summary of Facial Blushing and Hyperhidrosis

Author	Year	Level	Dry	CH (%)	Satis (%)	Regret	Number	F/U	Type
Kim	2004	T2		76.5	77[a]		22		Pros
Kim	2004	T2 rami		36.4	63[a]		22		pros
Kao	1996	T2			100		30	15 months	Retro
Adair	2005	T2–3		91	63	13%	59	20 months	Retro
Drott	2003	T2		85	6		891	29 months	

[a]Statistically significant.

raminectomies causes less compensatory hyperhidrosis after surgery, which could translate into a higher level of patient satisfaction.[38]

Kao and colleagues evaluated their results with 30 patients who were operated on for facial hyperhidrosis. They all underwent T2 level ablations with electrocautery. One patient had ptosis that resolved at 2 months. The mean follow-up was 15 months. All patients were satisfied with the results. Most patients experienced CS of some degree. Doolabh et al. reported a similar success rate in their small series of 39 patients with facial hyperhidrosis, with a 95% satisfactory rate.[39]

Severe facial blushing is usually brought on by emotional or social stimuli and can often have a serious negative impact on the individual. These patients may experience both facial blushing and upper limb hyperhidrosis. Adair et al. retrospectively reviewed 59 patients with complaints of facial blushing and/or upper limb hyperhidrosis. Twelve of these patients experienced only facial blushing. All patients had T2 to T3 level sympathectomies. Overall, the level of facial blushing score was reduced from 78 to 26 on a 100-point visual analog scale. Only 29% of the patients reported complete resolution of their symptoms. Ninety-one percent of the facial blushing group experienced compensatory sweating. All 12 patients with facial blushing alone noted improvement in their blushing postoperatively, with four experiencing complete resolution of symptoms. Sixty-three percent of the patients reported their overall quality of life to be much better, while 13% reported their quality of life to be worse. This study, along with several others, recommended that careful selection of patients and conversations regarding the high likelihoods of compensatory sweating are keys to success.[40] The results were similar to those of a large retrospective study by Drott and colleagues. They analyzed results in 1,314 consecutive patients treated for facial blushing by resection of the T2 level only. They followed 891 of these patients for mean of 29 months, and facial blushing scores dropped from 8.8 to 2.5 (10-point visual analog scale). Six percent regretted the procedure because of severe compensatory sweating, and 15% of the patients were not satisfied after the procedure (Table 163.3).[14]

Lower sympathectomy levels and their impact on facial sweating and hyperhidrosis have not been studied in detail. The majority of the articles emphasize a high incidence of compensatory sweating resulting in many patients having regrets after surgery. This is consistent with T2 level resections, as was discussed earlier in this chapter. Chou et al. reviewed their experience with sympathectomy, at the T3 level for facial sweating in 33 patients. After surgery minor facial sweating function was preserved, but the compensatory sweating incidence was only 27.3%. Three patients (9%) expressed regret. The authors also assessed facial sweating function in their patients who had T4 level removed for palmar or axillary hyperhidrosis. They found that at this level (T4) the facial sweating function was entirely preserved.[30]

Overall, these studies on facial sweating and blushing have demonstrated that sympathectomy is quite safe and associated with low complication rates. The nagging problem remains the high incidence of compensatory sweating which lowers patient satisfaction rates. At the facial level, because of this lower success rate and higher incidence of compensatory sweating, patient selection is important. Psychologically stable, well-informed patients with debilitating facial sweating and blushing are reasonable candidates. Risks should be carefully discussed prior to surgery. The success rate is in the 70% to 90% range according to the literature; however, more data are needed for an adequate evaluation of surgery for facial hyperhidrosis. Clipping instead of dividing the sympathetic chain may be a better solution for facial hyperhidrosis because of its reversibility. Chou et al. reported successful reversal of compensatory hyperhidrosis by removing clips in severely regretful patients.[5] Sympathectomy at the T2 or T3 level for facial hyperhidrosis provides reasonable improvement in original symptoms and is safe, but results in a moderate level of patient dissatisfaction owing to compensatory sweating (evidence quality low). The authors make a weak recommendation for T2 or T3 sympathectomy for facial hyperhidrosis in carefully selected patients (recommendation grade 2C).

THORACIC SPLANCHNICECTOMY

Sympathectomy has also been used to treat pain in the abdomen, specifically pain that is related to the pancreas (most commonly from chronic pancreatitis or pancreatic cancer). Unique to the abdomen, the sympathetic ganglia supplying the abdomen merge to form the three splanchnic nerves, greater (T5–T10), lesser (T10–T11), and least (T12) (Fig. 163.2). One prospective report of 44 patients with pancreatic cancer who underwent splanchnicectomy showed a 50% decrease in pain while all patients demonstrated a decrease in the use of analgesics postoperatively. Reports of up to 70% success have been reported. The procedure is usually done unilaterally from the left side.

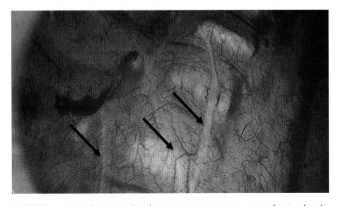

FIGURE 163.2 Thoracic splanchnicectomy. *Arrows* point to the 3 splanchneic branches.

The technique for splanchnicectomy is similar to that of sympathectomy except the ports are placed more caudally (7th or 8th intercostal space for the camera and the 5th intercostal space for the additional two working ports). In thoracoscopy,[41] the great splanchnic nerves are often easy to identify, though the lesser is often difficult to detect from the thorax.

VAGOTOMY

Thoracoscopic vagotomy would seem to have its greatest potential role in the setting of recurrent ulceration and an incomplete prior vagotomy. The ability to avoid a thoracotomy or recurrent upper abdominal surgery seems to be a great advantage.

There have been multiple case reports of successful VATS vagotomies. Laws and McKernan reported on six patients with recurrent ulceration after prior gastric drainage procedures with incomplete vagotomies. All thoracoscopic vagotomies were successful, and the hospital stay was 3 days or less. Champault and colleagues reported on 21 patients with duodenal ulcers treated primarily by thoracoscopic truncal vagotomy. There were apparently no instances of gastric stasis problems or postvagotomy diarrhea.

Technically, a VATS vagotomy is usually performed from the left chest using general anesthesia and a double-lumen endotracheal tube. Three or four ports are used to approach the distal esophagus. The inferior pulmonary ligament is divided. The video monitors may be placed at the foot of the bed as for esophageal myotomy, which may aid in orientation. Mobilization of the esophagus is required to clearly dissect and transect all vagal fibers. Postoperative chest tubes are not necessary unless lung injury has occurred. The hospital stay will be dependent upon the patient's overall condition more than the operative procedure.

CONCLUSION

Sympathectomy has proven valuable for several benign SNS conditions. Presently, the authors recommend single-level VATS sympathectomy for hyperhidrosis. It would appear that for palmar hyperhidrosis T3 or T4 provides good results while limiting compensatory sweating. Similarly, level T4 or T5 seems best for axillary hyperhidrosis. Facial sweating seems to be the most difficult because of compensatory sweating due to the high level of chain disruption. The T2 or T3 level seems best, and one might consider chipping only in case of severe compensatory sweating.

Splanchnicectomy can be valuable in selected cases for upper abdominal pain syndrome but results are more limited. Thoracoscopic sympathectomy is a fairly simple technical procedure with few complications. As with many other procedures careful patient selection is the key for excellent outcomes.

REFERENCES

1. Cerfolio RJ, Milanez de Campos JR, Bryant AS, et al. The society of thoracic surgeons' expert consensus for the surgical treatment of hyperhidrosis. *Ann Thorac Surg* 2011;91:1642–1648.
2. Marhold F, Izay B, Zacherl J, et al. Thoracoscopic and anatomic landmarks of Kuntz's nerve: implications for sympathetic surgery. *Ann Thorac Surg* 2008;86:1653–1658.
3. Moraites E, Vaughn OA, Hill S. Endoscopic thoracic sympathectomy. *Dermatol Clin* 2014;32:541–548.
4. Hazelrigg SR, Mack MJ. Surgery for autonomic disorders. In: Kaiser LR, Daniel RM, eds. *Thoracoscopic Surgery*. Boston: Little, Brown and Company; 1993:189.
5. Quirashy MS, Giddings AE. Treating hyperhidrosis. *BMJ* 1993;306:1221.
6. Heckmann M, Ceballos-Baumann AO, Plewig G. Botulinum toxin A for axillary hyperhidrosis (excessive sweating). *N Engl J Med* 2001;344:488–493.
7. Naumann M, Lowe NJ. Botulinum toxin type A in treatment of bilateral primary axillary hyperhidrosis: randomized, parallel group, double blind, placebo controlled trial. *BMJ* 2001;323:596–599.
8. Glogau RG. Botulinum A neurotoxin for axillary hyperhidrosis. No sweat Botox. *Dermatol Surg* 1998;24:817–819.
9. Levit F. Simple divides for treatment of hyperhidrosis by iontophoresis. *Arch Dermatol* 1968;98:505.
10. Levit F. Treatment of hyperhidrosis by tap water iotophoresis. *Arch Dermatol* 1989;4:224.
11. Dahl JC, Glent-Madsen L. Treatment of hyperhidrosis manuum by tap water iontophoresis. *Acta Derm Venereol* 1989;69:346–348.
12. Stolman LP. Treatment of excess sweating of the palms by iontophoresis. *Arch Dermatol* 1987;123:893–896.
13. Rua JF, Jatene FB, Milanez JR, et al. Robotic versus human camera holding in video-assisted thoracic sympathectomy: a single blind randomized trial of efficacy and safety. *Interact Cardiovasc Thorac Surg* 2009;8:195–199.
14. Zhu LH, Chen L, Yang S, et al. Embryonic NOTES thoracic sympathectomy for palmar hyperhidrosis the conventional VATS procedure. *Surg Endosc* 2013;11:4124–4129.
15. Complex Regional Pain Syndrome Fact Sheet. National Institute of Neurological Disorders and Stroke. http://www.ninds.nih.gov/disorders/reflex_sympathetic_dystrophy/detail_reflex_sympathetic_dystrophy.htm.
16. Drucker WR, Hubay CA, Holden WD, et al. Pathogenesis of posttraumatic sympathetic dystrophy. *Am J Surg* 1959;97:454.
17. Mitchell SW, Morehouse GR, Keen WW. *Gunshot wounds and Injuries of Nerves*. Philadelphia, PA: Lippincott; 1964.
18. Daly AE, Bialocerkowski AE. Does evidence support physiotherapy management of adult Complex Regional Pain Syndrome Type One? A systematic review. *Eur J Pain* 2009;13(4): 339–353.
19. Agarwal P, Sharma D. Lumbar sympathectomy revisited: current status in management of peripheral vascular disease. *Internet J Surg* 2008;18(1).
20. Nesargikar PN, Ajit MK, Eyers PS, et al. Lumbar chemical sympathectomy in peripheral vascular disease: does it still have a role? *International J Surg* 2009;7(2):145–149.
21. Roos DB. Sympathectomy for the upper extremities anatomy, indications and technics. In Greep JM, Lemmens HAJ, Roos DB, et al., eds. *Pain In Shoulder And Arm: An Integrated Review*. Boston, MA: Mertinus Nijhoff; 1979:241–242.
22. Byrne J, Walsh TN, Hederman WP. Endoscopic transthoracic electrocautery of the sympathetic chain for palmar and axillary hyperhidrosis. *Br J Surg* 1990;77:1046.
23. Hashmonai M, Kopelman D. History of sympathetic surgery. *Clin Auton Res* 2003;13(1):16–19.
24. Yazbek G, Wolosker N, Kauffman P, et al. Twenty months evolution following sympathectomy on patients with palmar hyperhidrosis: sympathectomy at T3 level is better thatn T2 level. *Clinics (Sao Paulo)* 2009;64;743–749.
25. Hashimonai M, Kopelman D, Kein O, et al. Upper thoracic sympathectomy for primary palmar hyperhidrosis: long-term follow-up. *Br J Surg* 1992;79:268–271.
26. Herbst F, Plas EG, Fugger R, et al. Endoscopic thoracic sympathectomy for primary hyperhidrosis of the upper limbs. A critical analysis and long-term results of 480 operations. *Ann Surg* 1994;220(1):86–90.
27. Ihse I, Zoucas E, Gyllstedt E, et al. Bilateral thorascopic splanchniectomy: effects on pancreatic cancer pain and function. *Ann Surg* 1999;230(6):785.
28. Kharkar S, Ambady P, Venkatesh Y, et al. Intramuscular botulinum toxin in complex regional pain syndrome: case series and literature review. *Pain Physician* 14(5): 419–424.
29. Kux M. Thoracic endoscopic sympathectomy in palmar and axillary hyperhidrosis. *Arch Surg* 1978;113:264.
30. Eberle T, Doganci B, Krämer HH, et al. "Warm and cold complex regional pain syndromes: differences beyond skin temperature?" *Neurology* 72(6):505–512.
31. Hsu C, Shia SE, Hsia JY, et al. Experiences in thoracoscopic sympathectomy for axillary hyperhidrosis and osmidrosis. *Arch Surg* 2001;136:1115–1117.
32. Olcott C IV, Eltherington LG, Wilcosky BR, et al. Reflex sympathetic dystrophy—The surgeon's role in management. *J Vasc Surg* 1991;14:488–492.
33. Reiseld R, Nguyen R, Pnini A. Endoscopic thoracic sympathectomy for hyperhidrosis. Experience with both cauterization and clamping methods. *Surg Laparosc Endosc Percutn Tech* 2002;12(4):255–267.
34. Roos DB. Sympathectomy for the upper extremities. In Rutherford R, ed. *Vascular Surgery*. 2nd ed. Philadelphia, PA: Saunders; 1984:725–730.
35. Schwartzman RJ, Erwin KL, Alexander GM. The natural history of complex regional pain syndrome. *Clin J Pain* 2009;25(4):273–280.
36. Bishof G. Introduction and history of sympathetic surgery. *Euro Surg* 2005:37(3): 112–113.
37. Stanton-Hicks M, Baron R, Boas R, et al. Complex regional pain syndromes: guidelines for therapy. *Clin J Pain* 1998;14(2):155–166.
38. Taylor RS, Van Buyten JP, Buchser E. Spinal cord stimulation for complex regional pain syndrome: a systematic review of the clinical and cost-effectiveness literature and assessment of prognostic factors. *Eur J Pain* 2006;10(2):91–101.
39. Vaneker M, Wilder-Smith OH, Schrombges P, et al. Patients initially diagnosed as "warm" or "cold" CRPS show differences in central sensory processing some eight years after diagnosis: a quantitative sensory testing study. *Pain* 115(1–2):204–211.
40. Yanagihara TK, Ibrahimiye A, Harris C, et al. Analysis of clamping versus cutting of T3 sympathetic nerve for severe palmar hyperhidrosis. *J Thorac Cardiovasc Surg* 2010;140(5):984–989.
41. Cina CS, Cina MM, Clase CM. Endoscopic thoracic sympathectomy for hyperhidrosis: Techniques and results. *J Minim Access Surg* 2007;3(4):134–140.

PRIMARY MEDIASTINAL TUMORS AND SYNDROMES ASSOCIATED WITH MEDIASTINAL LESIONS

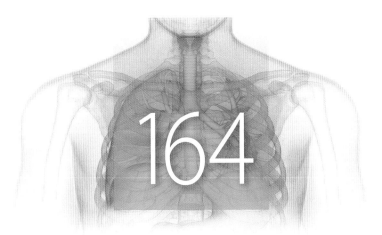

164

Myasthenia Gravis

David S. Younger

Myasthenia gravis (MG) is considered the prototypic autoimmune disease. Key features of the disease are muscle fatigability, decremental motor response to repetitive electrical stimulation, symptomatic improvement with drugs that inhibit acetylcholine esterase and the presence of antiacetylcholine receptor (AChR) autoantibodies in the majority of patients with generalized MG. This chapter provides an overview of the pathogenesis, diagnosis, and treatment of MG. Interested students of MG are referred to a recent comprehensive review.[1]

HISTORICAL ASPECTS

The history of MG is controversial.[2,3] The first description of a patient with MG appeared in 1644 in correspondence from colonial Jamestown, Virginia, pertaining to Indian Chief Opechancanough, according to Marsteller.[4] In 1685, Sir Thomas Willis described a patient with bulbar symptoms that could have been psychogenic. The clinical syndrome of MG was identified by Wilks,[5] Erb,[6] and Goldflam.[7] In 1895, Jolly[8] named the disease myasthenia gravis pseudoparalytica. By 1900, Campbell and Bramwell[9] had reported 60 cases. The efficacy of physostigmine was shown by Walker in 1934.[10] One year later, he suggested the chemical nature of neuromuscular transmission at motor end plates.[11] In 1941, Harvey and Masland[12] accurately localized the pathologic locus of MG to the neuromuscular junction. Action potentials were recorded from human muscles and evoked with a train of electrical stimuli. The amplitudes of action potentials were stable in normal subjects. However, a rapid reduction of the amplitudes was observed in patients with MG, which imitated the changes induced by d-tubocurarine, which blocks the muscle side of the neuromuscular junction. Moreover, neostigmine, a cholinesterase inhibitor, restored the amplitudes of action potentials. These findings suggested that an impairment of neuromuscular junction transmission in patients with MG was contributing to the muscle weakness. In the same year, Blalock and colleagues[13,14] and later Keynes[15] described transsternal thymectomy in MG, including as complete a removal of the gland as possible whether or not a tumor was suspected preoperatively.

In 1960, an autoimmune cause of MG was suggested by Simpson[16] and by Nastuk and colleagues.[17] However, the immunologic basis of MG awaited basic understanding of ACh release at motor end plates, as subsequently described by Katz and Miledi.[18] In 1973, Patrick and Lindstrom[19] injected rabbits with AChR from the electric organ of eels, intending to make antireceptor antibodies and see whether these antibodies would block the function of AChR in intact electric organ cells. The antibodies did block, and the immunized rabbits became paralyzed and died. Thus experimental autoimmune myasthenia gravis (EAMG), resulted from the autoimmune attack against native AChRs. Fambrough and colleagues[20] applied radioactively labeled α-bungarotoxin to motor-point biopsy samples from patients with

MG and found a marked reduction in AChR, averaging 20% of controls. Later, Drachman and colleagues[21] established the significance of cross-linking of Fab: receptor complexes that accelerated the degradation of AChR in skeletal muscle culture. These important findings corroborated the pathologic site of MG to the muscle side of the neuromuscular junction. Within the next several years, investigators reproduced the essential clinical and morphologic correlates of human MG in animals by passive transfer of human myasthenic serum and AChR-specific monoclonal antibodies.

ACETYLCHOLINE RECEPTOR PATHOPHYSIOLOGY

The 1980s and 1990s witnessed spectacular progress in the understanding of the microstructure, physiology, and molecular composition of the nicotinic AChR and this was in turn applied to the clinical problem of MG. AChR is a ligand-gated ion channel which, in mature innervated muscles, is composed of several homologous subunits, α2, β, δ, and ε (Fig. 164.1). Distinct but related genes encode the individual subunits, and complementary DNA for each have been cloned showing remarkable homology. In fetal or denervated muscles, the γ subunit replaces the ε subunit. Five subunits line up like a barrel around the ACh ion channel. Whereas ACh binds at the junctions between α and ε or γ subunits and between the α and δ subunits, in experimental animals the antibodies that cause MG are usually active against either the bungarotoxin-binding site or an area on the α subunit termed the main immunogenic region (MIR), the latter similar to circulating antibodies in humans.

Each subunit has four transmembrane domains: M1 through M4. Variations of amino acid sequence between the different subunits are generally in the large cytoplasmic domains. Amino acid sequences for the transmembrane domains are generally conserved. Sequences of the M1 and M2 of each subunit form the lining of AChR ion channel. Amino acids from the α-subunit sequence 66 to 76 are the critical autogenic region for development of pathogenic AChR antibodies. Interestingly, antibodies bound to this region in humans generally do not impair the ACh binding to AChR; rather, they can fix complement and initiate the destruction of postsynaptic membranes. AChR bound by antibodies may have an increased rate of internalization and degradation resulting in reduced available AChR. Compared with voltage-gated ion-selective channels, the channel in the center of the AChR is less selective among particular cations, including sodium, potassium, and calcium. However, the channel possesses a relative selectivity to positive ions which is determined by charged side chains of amino acids within the pore of the ACh ion channel. Once ACh binds to the channel, the influx of sodium and efflux of potassium occur, but the net current is positive influx and depolarizes the muscular membrane in the vicinity of postsynapses. This depolarization may reach the threshold of action potential and propagate to other areas of the muscle.

NEUROMUSCULAR JUNCTION PHYSIOLOGY

The mechanisms of the end plate current (EPC) and end plate potential (EPP) have been elucidated by noise analysis and patch or voltage clamping. Axons of the motor neuron communicate with muscle cells through a specialized structure, called the neuromuscular junction (Fig. 164.2). The junction consists of three parts: (1) The presynaptic terminal, an enlarged part of a distal axon, which synthesizes, stores, and releases ACh; (2) The synaptic cleft, a microscopic space between the pre- and postsynaptic terminals; and (3) The postsynaptic terminal, also called the end plate, where the receptors for neurotransmitters such as AChR are located. During development, when the motor

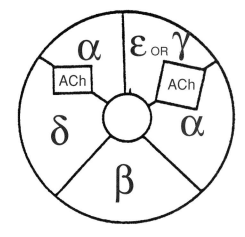

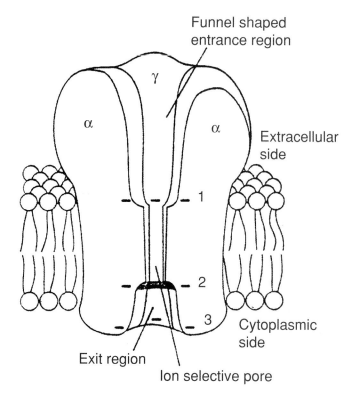

FIGURE 164.1 Schematic diagram of the AChR complex. The receptor is transmembrane in location with an ion pore or channel and binding sites for ACh molecules along the α subunits. (Reproduced from Younger DS, ed. *Motor Disorders.* 3rd ed. New York; Author: 2013, with permission.)

nerve fiber approaches the muscle cell, it induces a specialized indentation of muscle cell surface, the end plate. Upon the activation of presynaptic motor axons by propagated electrical activities, there is concurrent calcium influx to the presynaptic axon. These events activate coordinated intra-axonal molecular processes, which drive the neurotransmitter vesicles containing ACh to the presynaptic terminal membrane. Fusion of vesicles with the presynaptic terminal membrane takes place and the ACh is released in a quantal fashion. ACh diffuses rapidly across the synaptic cleft, binds to AchR, and directly opens the ion channel of AChR. An individual ACh ion channel behaves in all-or-none pattern and produces a fixed amplitude of current of about 2.7 pA when it opens. A normal EPC reflects the sum of 200,000 ACh-channel current and generates an EPP of about 70 mV. The amplitudes of end plate current or potential are large, but the

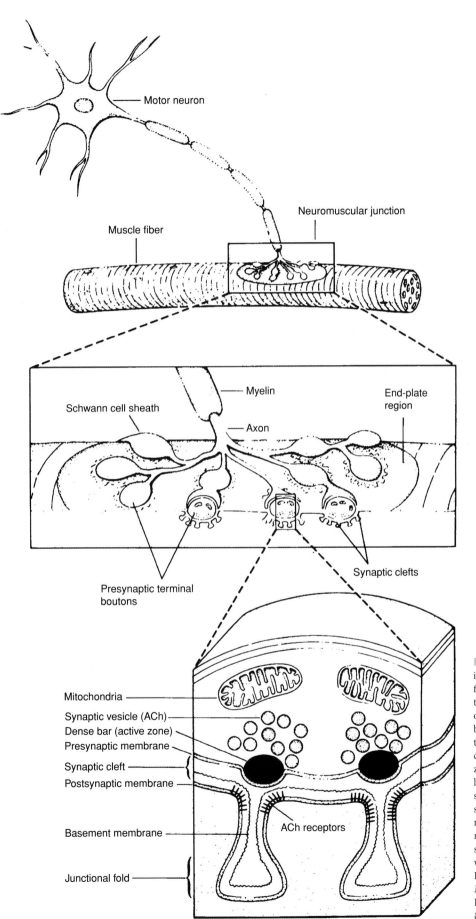

Motor neuron

Neuromuscular junction

Muscle fiber

Myelin

Schwann cell sheath

End-plate region

Axon

Presynaptic terminal boutons

Synaptic clefts

Mitochondria

Synaptic vesicle (ACh)

Dense bar (active zone)

Presynaptic membrane

Synaptic cleft

Postsynaptic membrane

Basement membrane

ACh receptors

Junctional fold

FIGURE 164.2 The neuromuscular junction is shown. The motor axon ramifies into several fine branches each forming presynaptic boutons covered by a thin layer of Schwann cells over a specialized region of the myofiber membrane termed the end-plat and separated from the muscle membrane by a 100-nm synaptic cleft. Synaptic vesicles cluster around active zones where ACh is released. Junctional folds located under each bouton contain high density of AChR. The enzyme acetylcholinesterase secreted into the synaptic cleft inactivates ACh released from the presynaptic terminal. The muscle basement membrane organizes the synapse by aligning the presynaptic boutons with the postsynapatic junctional folds. (From Kandel E, Schwartz JH, Jessell TM. *Principles of Neural Science*. 3rd ed. Norwalk, CT: Appleton & Lange; 1991:188. Copyright © 1991 by Appleton & Lange. All rights reserved.)

current is not regenerative, unlike the current through voltage-gated ion channels. The depolarizing current through a voltage-gated ion channel, such as a sodium channel, may cause additional sodium channels to open. Thus the current from many sodium channels may sum up, reach the threshold, and produce action potentials. In contrast, the ACh-induced EPP is unable to activate additional AChR ion channels. EPP must recruit and activate the sodium channels in the vicinity of the postsynapses, leading to the production of action potentials. Thus the number of available postsynaptic AChR is critical for successful postsynaptic signal production and propagation.

To secure the neuromuscular transmission, a normal neuromuscular junction has an abundant reservoir of necessary biological mechanisms, including an excess of AChR as well as voltage-gated sodium ion channels. In response to an incoming nerve action potential, highly localized regions of the nerve terminal release approximately 200 quantal packets, each containing 6 to 10,000 molecules of ACh. Binding of ACh to specific sites on the AChR results in the transient openings of the AChR channel, allowing a net influx of Na+ ions and thus producing the depolarizing potential. The circular arrangement of the five subunits delineates a 2.5-nm channel whose narrowest point is 0.65 nm in diameter. Each subunit contains four membrane-spanning α helices termed M1 to M4, with the M2 segment effectively lining the channel. More quantal packets of ACh are released into the synaptic cleft, and more receptor channels are present than are needed to depolarize the muscle fiber to threshold. This creates a safety factor (SF) which can quantitatively be defined by the formula: $SF = EPP/(action\ potential\ threshold - membrane\ potential)$. In MG, the SF is impaired because of the reduction of postsynaptic AChR by the antibodies to AChR, diminishing the amplitude of EPP. Impairment of the SF may cause the failure of neuromuscular transmission. If excitation of the postsynaptic muscle cell does not occur, weakness ensues. Even when the number of receptors is reduced experimentally, the EPP does not fall below the threshold needed to generate a muscle action potential. The autoimmune attack on AChR, which reduces the number of functioning receptors at myasthenic end plates, leads to many EPP that fall below threshold. This translates into muscle weakness and fatigue, particularly with repetitive or sustained contraction.

AUTOIMMUNE ETIOPATHOGENESIS

The hypothesis that MG originated in the thymus gland, as first suggested by Weigert[22] in 1901, was difficult to prove and still remains speculative. The presumed initial event in the pathogenesis of myasthenia is loss of self-tolerance, a process attributed to the thymus gland for several intuitive reasons. The thymus contains all of the elements theoretically necessary for the activation of AChR-specific T-cells. They include an immunogenic peptide of the AChR or a peptide that mimics the receptor; local antigen-presenting cells (APC) or, in this case, myoid cells which take up AChR derived from myoid cells, process it, and then express AChR-derived peptide fragments on their surface in the presence of antigen-specific T-cell receptor and class II molecules of the major histocompatibility complex (MHC) completing the trimolecular complex. Although myoid cells are equally abundant in normal and myasthenic thymuses, hyperplastic glands contain many more myoid cells than atrophic glands. AChR-specific T cells are enriched in myasthenic thymus glands with and without epithelial cell tumors or thymomas. Whether the AChR-specific T cells in the myasthenic thymus always resided there or return after a sojourn in the peripheral immune system is not known. The peripheral blood of patients with MG contains an enhanced portion of these autoreactive T-cells, which are capable of recruiting AChR-responsive B cells for the production of pathogenic anti-AChR antibodies. In

actively induced or passively transferred EAMG, where the myasthenic process is initiated outside the gland, germinal centers are not observed. Transplantation of myasthenic thymus fragments into mice with severe combined immunodeficiency results in the production of pathogenic mouse antibodies.

The main consequence of the antibody-mediated process is a reduction in the density of postsynaptic membrane AChR. There are multiple mechanisms through which anti-AChR antibodies are able to reduce the number of AChR. By utilizing radioactive isotope–labeled α-bungarotoxin, the fate of AChRs can be traced and the rate of the receptor degradation can be estimated. Serum from patients with MG causes an escalated degradation rate of AChR of up to two- to threefold that of normal controls; endocytosis of the AChR is also accelerated. The postsynaptic membranes of an affected neuromuscular junction are simplified on electron microscopy (EM) with flattening of the usually convoluted folds of the postsynaptic membranes. Immunocytochemical techniques made it possible to detect the membrane attack complex of complement (C5b-9) at the neuromuscular junction. The serum concentration of AChR-binding antibodies in patients with MG does not usually correlate with the severity of the disease, an observation that is usually explained by the variation of antibody functions and different targets of epitopes on the AChR subunits. Indeed, the functional activities of the AChR antibodies in accelerating degradation of the receptors have been closely correlated with the severity of weakness in MG. Recognition of the molecular aspects of autoimmune reactivity in MG has elucidated susceptibility risk factors for acquired autoimmune MG, as well as potential novel approaches to therapy in refractory patients. For example, those with the DQ2 human leukocyte antigen (HLA) haplotypes demonstrate more than a 30-fold risk of developing MG than the general population. Future innovative treatment could include the development of anti-AChR and anti-idiotype antibodies, and others that recognize MHC class II molecules of APC, specific T-cells that recognize AChR, as well as peptide competitors for AChR receptor to block T-cell recognition or MHC binding of ACh receptor fragments.

DIAGNOSIS

NOSOLOGY AND CLASSIFICATION

The term *myasthenia* has been used interchangeably for the acquired autoimmune form of the disease, and the term *myasthenic* has generally been used for other syndromes of the neuromuscular junction. Similarly, the classification of MG has been difficult. Early attempts emphasized duration of symptoms because it was believed that the disorder might be progressive. Younger and colleagues[23,24] emphasized indices of maximal severity, functional status, and response to therapy, prompting more exact nosology, classification, and comparative methods of analysis of patient outcome.

CLINICAL ASPECTS

The clinical diagnosis of autoimmune acquired MG is made by recognizing a pattern of weakness that has the features of fluctuation and variability over the course of a day, months, or years, leading to perceptible exacerbations and remissions. The distribution of weakness is characteristic, affecting ocular, facial, oropharyngeal, and limb muscles. The diagnosis is confirmed by unequivocal and reproducible improvement after intravenous administration of edrophonium chloride, a rapidly acting anticholinesterase drug. Formal diagnosis is bolstered by eliciting a decremental response to repetitive motor nerve stimulation as well as the detection of AChR antibodies in the serum.

Selective involvement of limb and respiratory muscles, sparing ocular or oropharyngeal muscles, is rarely if ever encountered.

RADIOGRAPHIC AND ELECTROPHYSIOLOGIC EVALUATION

All patients should undergo computed tomography (CT) of the mediastinum to search for thymic enlargement and thymic tumors. Dedicated positron emission tomography (PET) with CT increases the yield of thymic tumor detection. Thymic enlargement, which generally signifies glandular hyperplasia, and thymic tumors detected by PET/CT will both be generally amenable to surgery. It is never a good idea to perform a presurgical biopsy because of the risk of myasthenic exacerbation. The electrophysiologic evaluation of MG includes repetitive motor nerve stimulation and single-fiber electromyography (SFEMG). A decremental response of 12% to 15% or more of successive compound muscle action potentials after 3-Hz stimulation and aggravation of the block for several minutes after brief exercise are indicative of the postsynaptic defect in neuromuscular junction transmission. SFEMG quantitates transmission at individual end plates while the patient voluntarily activates the muscle under examination. Action potentials are recorded from two muscle fibers in the same motor unit near the single fiber electrode. The variability in the time between the two potentials, which varies among consecutive discharges, is termed jitter and is calculated as the mean difference between consecutive interpotential intervals. Jitter normally varies from 10 to 50 ms. Blocking occurs when consecutive impulses do not follow. A typical finding in MG is normal jitter in some potential pairs and increased jitter in others. As a rule, 20 potential pairs are studied in each muscle. Up to 85% of patients with generalized and 10% with ocular MG reveal an abnormal decrement in a hand or shoulder muscle, and 86% of patients with generalized and 63% of those with ocular disease reveal abnormalities on SFEMG, as recorded by Sanders.[25] With the addition of a second muscle, SFEMG is positive in 99% of patients with generalized MG, making it a more sensitive method of analysis.

ANTIBODIES TO ACETYCHOLINE RECEPTOR

Four AChR assays are available for the serologic evaluation of MG. Three were named for their respective physiologic characteristics leading to loss of neuromuscular transmission due to binding, blocking, and modulation of the AChR, and a fourth autoantibody directed against the muscle-specific tyrosine kinase (MuSK) receptor. The postulated actions of AChR antibodies include accelerated degradation, endocytosis, cross-linking of receptors, functional blockade, and complement-mediated lysis of end plates by C5b9 membrane attack complex, leading to flattening and simplification of postsynaptic junctional folds. The binding assay is positive in up to 90% of patients with generalized MG and should be the first line of testing, with a specificity of more than 99%, as recorded by Somnier.[26] Approximately 35% to 50% of patients with negative AChR antibodies will have a positive MuSK assay, making it an indispensable addition to the routine serologic evaluation of suspected patients.

As noted by Vincent and Newsom-Davis[27] and Solliven and colleagues,[28] approximately 12% to 17% of patients with generalized MG lack demonstrable serum AChR antibodies; this is termed *seronegative MG*. These patients do not differ clinically from those with elevated titers and exhibit similar favorable clinical responses to anticholinesterase or immunosuppressant drugs, plasmapheresis, and thymectomy. The pathogenesis of seronegative MG may not differ from that of antibody-positive cases. There are several possible explanations for the failure to detect antibodies with conventional assays.

If serum antibody titers are low, the assay may fail to detect antibodies adequately because of binding at end plates. Other possible confounding factors may be low affinity or excessive variability in antibody reactivity to epitopes of the assayed antigen. Alternatively, antibodies may be directed at sites other than the main binding sites or at sites hidden during extraction of AChR. Antibodies to AChR may not be detected with denervated or immature AChRs. A short duration of disease and concomitant immunotherapy before the assay may also contribute to seronegativity. Significantly reduced numbers of AChRs were noted in motor end plate biopsy samples of patients with seronegative generalized and ocular MG. Passive transfer of sera from seronegative patients to laboratory animals results in a disorder clinically similar to that induced by seropositive sera. Immunoglobulin is usually not bound to extracted AChR at end plates of seronegative patients, implying that the disorder might result from a circulating plasma factor capable of inhibiting AChR function at sites other than the binding site for ACh.

CLASSIFICATION AND SCORING SYSTEMS

The first useful clinical classification system was developed by Osserman[29] and modified afterward by the Task Force of the Medical Scientific Advisory Board of the MG Foundation of America (MGFA)[30] as shown in Table 164.1. In addition, a number of scoring systems have been elaborated to best define the diversity of MG for routine care and clinical research studies.

QUANTITATIVE SCORES

The quantitative MG score (QMG) is the best studied objective outcome measure in MG.[31] The current QMG is an expansion and modification of the scale first developed by Besinger and colleagues in the early 1980s.[32,33] The original QMG consisted of eight items each graded 0 to 3 with the score of 3 being the most severe. This was expanded to 13 items and used in two trials that established efficacy of cyclosporin in MG.[34,35] Further objectivity was achieved in subsequent revisions.[36–38] Inter-rater reliability testing was performed on the scale in advance of a randomized placebo-controlled study of intravenous gammaglobulin in MG that utilized the modified QMG as the primary outcome measure. With a 95% confidence level; QMG scores did not differ by more than 2.63 units translating to a required sample size of 17 patients in each treatment group in a placebo-controlled trial to detect a significant difference of power 0.80. The QMG can be completed in 20 to 30 minutes. The only specialized equipment required is a spirometer and grip dynamometer. The first MGFA task force recommended the QMG be used in all prospective studies as therapy for MG.[36] The QMG has been used in studies of mycophenolate mofetil, intravenous immunoglobulin (IVIg) and plasma exchange (PE).[39–43] The MGFA task force developed Post Intervention Status definitions for remission, improvement, and worsening.[36]

MANUAL MUSCLE TEST

Disease-specific manual muscle testing can be performed at the bedside without specialized equipment. Thirty muscle groups usually affected by MG (6 cranial nerve/24-axial-limb) are measured on a 0 to 4 scale. The MG manual muscle test (MG-MMT) demonstrates good inter-rater reliability with a mean difference between scores of 1.3 +/− 1.8 points. It correlates well with the QMG, however, there is a wide scatter of MG-MMT values within general disease classifications, an issue also observed with QMG. Advantages of the

TABLE 164.1 Osserman and Genkins Classification of Myasthenia Gravis, Modified by the MGFA Task Force[a]

Class	Clinical Form(s)	Symptoms
I[b]/MGFA I	Ocular form	Ptosis, diplopia
IIa[b]/MGFA II	Mild generalized form	Mild generalized weakness
IIb[b]/MGFA IIb	Faciopharyngeal form	IIa + bulbar weakness
III[b]	Severe acute generalized form	Acute severe general weakness + bulbar symptoms + respiratory insufficiency
MGFA III	Medium severity generalized form	Medium severity generalized weakness with:
MGFA IIIa		Involvement of the extremities/trunk musculature > faciopharyngeal musculature
MGFA IIIb		Faciopharyngeal/respiratory musculature > extremities/trunk musculature
IV[b]	Severe chronic generalized form	Severe, often progressive generalized weakness
MGFA IV	Severe generalized form	
MGFA IVa		Extremities/trunk musculature > faciopharyngeal musculature
MGFA IVb		Faciopharyngeal/respiratory musculature > extremities/trunk musculature
V[b]	Myasthenia with severe residual deficits	Severe chronic form with muscle atrophy
MGFA V	Severe MG requiring intubation	

[a]MGFA, Myasthenia Gravis Foundation Association; the entries marked.
[b]Refer to the Osserman and Genkins classification.
Adapted from Toyka KV, Gold R. Treatment of Myasthenia Gravis. *Schweiz Arch Neurol Psychiatr* 2007;158:309. With permission from EMH Swiss Medical Publishers Ltd.

MG-MMT over the QMG include performance by a physician as part of a routine clinical visit, less time and no specialized equipment.[57]

MYASTHENIA MUSCLE SCORE

The myasthenia muscle score (MMS) summates nine independent functions that encompass cranial, neck, truncal, and limb strength. The total score ranges between 0 and 100. Unlike the scales described earlier, the highest score on the MMS quantitates better strength and function.[45,46] Pulmonary function is not assessed in the MMS, but it is assessed in the QMG.

ACTIVITIES OF DAILY LIVING PROFILE

The MG activities of daily living (MG-ADL) profile is a simple 8-point questionnaire which focuses on common symptoms reported by MG patients. It was developed by the University of Texas Southwestern Medical Center to complement the QMG. Each item of the profile was graded 0 or normal to 3 or most severe. Study personnel ask the patient the eight questions and record their responses. The MG-ADL which correlates well with the QMG has become a secondary efficacy measurement in clinical trials.[47] No specialized training is required and it can be administered in less than 10 minutes.

COMPOSITE SCORE

The MG composite score includes the most useful features of the QMG, MG-ADL, MG-MMT.[48] A 3-point change in scale is meaningful and correlates to the MG-QOL scale. Its advantages include, (1) rigorous selection of test items through a process that assessed item performance during two randomized, controlled trials involving >250 patients with MG; (2) coverage of 10 important functional domains most frequently affected by MG; (3) proportionate inclusion of bulbar and respiratory items to total number of items (4/10); (4) appropriately weighted test items; (5) ease of administration taking less than 5 minutes to complete, without the need for any equipment; (6) ease of interpretation, taking less than 10 seconds to calculate a total score; (7) reliability; and (8) demonstration of

concurrent and longitudinal construct validity in the MG practice care setting. The second MGFA Task Force recommended inclusion of the MG Composite in all prospective therapy studies of MG.[49]

PREDNISONE DOSE AS THE PRIMARY ENDPOINT

Investigators have returned to using the prednisone dose as the primary endpoint, with QMG and other quantitative scales as secondary endpoints. In an ongoing trial of methotrexate in MG, the prednisone area under the curve was used as the primary endpoint with the goal of ascertaining whether those taking methotrexate had a lower prednisone area under the curve at the end of the trial compared to those taking placebo.[50]

QUALITY OF LIFE

There are a variety of Quality of Life (QOL) scales including the MG questionnaire (MGQ), the MG-QOL, and the 60 items of disease specific survey.[51–53] The MG-QOL60, which was reduced to the MG-QOL15 was employed in clinical trial settings showing good correlation with the larger 60 item scale.[53–55]

GENETIC MYASTHENIAS

Table 164.2 shows the diversity of genetic myasthenic syndromes. Genetic factors play a pivotal role in the pathogenesis of congenital myasthenic syndromes but not in autoimmune MG. Loss of the SF for normal neuromuscular transmission characterizes all of them. The site of the defect may be presynaptic, synaptic, or postsynaptic. Two presynaptic myasthenic disorders are due to defects in ACh resynthesis or due to a paucity of synaptic vesicles with reduced quantal release. End plate ACh deficiency causes a synaptically mediated disorder. The postsynaptic disorders are associated with a kinetic abnormality of AChR with or without AChR deficiency or with AChR deficiency without a primary kinetic abnormality. Those with AChR deficiency

TABLE 164.2 Classification of Genetic Myasthenia
Presynaptic Defects (6%)
Choline acetyltransferase
Paucity of synaptic vesicles
Congenital Lambert–Eaton-like myasthenic syndrome
Synaptic Basal Lamina Defects
End Plate AChE deficiency
Beta-2-laminin deficiency
Postsynaptic Defects
AChR deficiency with or without kinetic abnormality
Primary kinetic abnormality with or without AChR deficiency
Rapsyn deficiency
Pectin deficiency
Sodium channel deficiency
Defects in Mechanisms Governing End Plate Development
Dok-7 myasthenia
Glutamine-fructose-6-phosphate transaminase deficiency
Myasthenic syndrome associated with centronuclear myopathy

ACh, acetylcholine; AChE, acetylcholinesterase; AChR, acetylcholine receptor; LEMS, Lambert–Eaton myasthenic syndrome.
Reproduced from Younger DS, ed. *Motor Disorders*. 3rd ed. New York; 2013, with permission.

and a kinetic abnormality include a syndrome with a short open time; a slow-channel syndrome associated with a prolonged open time due to delayed channel closure; a slow-channel syndrome due to increased affinity of AChR for ACh, causing repeated reopenings during prolonged ACh occupancy; and another syndrome in which the nature of the kinetic abnormality is not elucidated. Those without AChR deficiency include the low-affinity fast-channel syndrome and the high-conductance fast-channel syndrome. The disorders associated with AChR deficiency without a primary kinetic abnormality are caused by nonsense mutations in a subunit gene. Clues to a congenital myasthenic syndrome include a positive family history; onset in the neonatal period, infancy, or childhood with progression during adolescence or adulthood; lack of significant response to anticholinesterase drugs; and absent serum AChR antibodies. Investigation of these syndromes requires sophisticated morphologic and electrophysiologic studies of the neuromuscular junction, usually available at only a few medical centers with a specific interest in these disorders. A motor-point muscle biopsy in a suspected patient should be processed for cytochemical localization of ACh and immune deposits at the end plates. Electron microscopic and cytochemical studies can be used to determine the size and density of synaptic vesicles and the morphology of nerve terminals and postsynaptic membranes. Quantitative assessment of AChR binding sites is performed using peroxidase-labeled α-bungarotoxin on muscle tissue samples. *In vitro* microelectrode studies, including noise analysis and patch-clamp recordings, provide information about the kinetic properties of AChR channels. The application of molecular genetics to the detection of mutations in AChR subunit genes has revealed new insights into the observed channel abnormalities and valuable correlations with them.

TREATMENT

Neurologists must choose the sequence and combination of available therapies, including anticholinesterase and immunosuppressant medication, thymectomy, plasma exchange (PE) and intravenous immune globulin (IVIg), often without the benefit of randomized controlled trials (RCTs). An International consensus guide for the management of MG was recently published.[56]

ACETYLCHOLINESTERASE INHIBITORS

Virtually all patients use pyridostigmine at some time, usually as initial therapy. Optimal dosage is determined by the patient's symptoms, commencing with 60 mg every 4 hours while awake and increasing the dose to 120 to 180 mg until undesirable side effects offset clinical benefit. Chronic administration is not known to cause a decline in effectiveness or deleterious effects or to appreciably modify the natural history of the disease; ultimately, other modalities must be used.

CORTICOSTEROIDS

Prednisone is the most widely used immunosuppressive agent in MG. As early as 1935, Simon[57] reported sustained remission in a patient after daily injections of aqueous extracts of the anterior lobe of the pituitary gland. Torda and Wolff[58] documented partial remissions in five patients treated with adrenocorticotrophic hormone (ACTH). Subsequently, they demonstrated improvement in 10 of 15 additional patients. However, Torda and Wolff[59] noted that all their patients experienced transient worsening, and one died. The unfavorable experiences of Shy and colleagues,[60] as well as Grob and Harvey[61] and Millikan and Eaton,[62] overshadowed initial promising results, and enthusiasm for corticosteroids waned for almost 20 years, until Warmolts and Engel[63] and Jenkins[64] demonstrated the efficacy of chronic ACTH and chronic oral prednisone therapy. Although corticosteroids exert an immunosuppressive effect at various levels of the immune system, the effects on activated T- and B-cells and on APC are believed to be most important in the beneficial response in MG. According to the report of Pascuzzi and colleagues,[65] long-term administration resulted in eventual improvement in 69% to 80% of patients, but 48% of patients had initial exacerbations and two-thirds had undesirable or serious side effects. Gradually increasing the dose of prednisone averts exacerbations of weakness. There has been uncertainty as to the optimal regimen even among experts. To illustrate, in 1974 the regimen of 25 mg alternating daily, increasing by 12.5 mg every three doses to a maintenance dose of 100 mg, was associated with dramatic or moderate improvement in 11 of the 12 patients thus treated by Seybold and Drachman.[66] Twenty years later, the same group recommended beginning prednisone with 15 to 20 mg daily, increasing by 5 mg every 2 to 3 days to a maximum of 50 to 60 mg daily, followed by alternate-day dosing.

AZATHIOPRINE

The beneficial effect of azathioprine was first reported in 1969 by Mertens and colleagues.[67] It has since gained worldwide acceptance, with response rates equal to those of prednisone as monotherapy for patients with generalized disease. Azathioprine is appropriate therapy for patients who exhibit poor responsiveness, intolerance, or frequent relapses while receiving corticosteroids; in those deemed unsuitable candidates for thymectomy because of age or comorbid disease; and in patients with thymoma. There are three drawbacks to its use: (1) Idiosyncratic side effects occur in about 10% of patients but are mainly gastrointestinal and flu-like and rarely necessitate permanent withdrawal of the medication; (2) Bone marrow suppression occurs in all patients; and (3) A long delay in the onset of the therapeutic effect of 3 to 6 months or more. Taking all these factors into account, most clinicians concur with slow advancement of the dose over weeks, from 50 mg/day to maintenance levels of 2 to 3 mg/kg per day with careful monitoring of liver function, peripheral white blood cell counts, and platelet counts.

CYCLOSPORINE

In 1987, Tindall and colleagues[68] reported the favorable effects of cyclosporine A in MG in a placebo-controlled trial and later in controlled double-blind studies in comparison with prednisone and azathioprine. Cyclosporine inhibits T-cell–dependent antibody responses by reversibly suppressing the clonal expansion of activated helper T-cells. It also inhibits the inflammatory intermediate interleukin-2 (IL-2). Administration of cyclosporine can prevent the expression and induction of EAMG. Long-term use is associated with dose-dependent and cumulative nephrotoxicity owing to endothelial vascular injury and interstitial fibrosis, hypertension, and headache.

MYCOPHENOLATE MOFETIL

Mycophenolate mofetil is an inhibitor of purine synthesis and has been traditionally employed to prevent organ transplant rejection. The initial enthusiasm for mycophenolate mofetil in refractory MG has been tempered by the report of predisposition to systemic tumor formation as a rare side effect as well as the inability to demonstrate superiority over corticosteroids and other immunosuppressive medication. Nonetheless, experts agree that in patients who may be poor candidates for corticosteroids or intolerant of azathioprine, mycophenolate mofetil can be a useful long-term parenteral therapy to induce improvement, especially in severe thymomatous and nonthymomatous cases.

RITUXIMAB

Rituximab employs a monoclonal antibody against B-cells, making it a potentially desirable treatment. The efficacy and safety of rituximab was described in a recent systematic review and meta-analysis.[69] It may be appropriate therapy in treatment-refractory MG,[70] and in patients with MuSK autoantibodies.[71,72]

PLASMA EXCHANGE AND INTRAVENOUS IMMUNOGLOBULIN

PE and IVIg are administered during myasthenic exacerbations to produce short-term clinical improvement, often within days of commencing treatment. PE rapidly lowers AChR antibody titers, which may account for its beneficial effects. The effectiveness of IVIg results from the inhibition of specific idiotype–anti-idiotype antibody interactions, downregulation of autoantibody production, inhibition of binding to the AChR, and amelioration of complement-mediated lysis of AChR. Drawbacks to both include high cost, the need for specialized equipment and staff, potential shifts of body fluids, electrolyte disturbances, and the need for indwelling catheters for vascular access. IVIg can be associated with a flu-like syndrome, aseptic meningitis, renal failure, headache, hypotension or hypertension, anaphylaxis in IgA-deficient patients, and a small but definite risk for transmissible disease.

There is strong class I evidence for the use of short-term IVIg in MG patients who worsen and equally good evidence for its use in myasthenic crisis, however RCT are lacking, and less robust class III evidence to support its use as long-term maintenance therapy.[73] An RCT sample size simulation showed an enduring decline in QMG scores and other parameters of about 50% with IVIg maintenance treatment in MG. With a sample size calculation of about 33 patients per arm to detect at least a 30% clinical difference in QMG scores, the authors recommended use of the QMG score as a primary endpoint for an RCT of IVIg maintenance for chronic MG.

A single-masked RCT of 84 MG patients with moderate to severe disease showed equivalent efficacy of IVIg and PE as demonstrated by reduction in the QMG score for disease severity, percentage of responders, persistence of treatment effect, and tolerability[74] with a change in the QMG score that was accompanied by improved disease-specific QOL. The only factor predicting response to treatment was baseline severity. The authors concluded that IVIg and PE were comparable treatments for adult myasthenics with moderate to severe disease.

Class III evidence for the superiority of PE over IVIg was however established for maintenance therapy in a retrospective cohort of 27 generalized juvenile myasthenics,[75] noting that 7 of 7 patients treated with PE alone responded, as did 5 of 10 treated with IVIg and 9 of 10 who received both, establishing a significant difference in response rates between PE and IVIg ($P = 0.04$).

THYMECTOMY

The earliest transsternal procedures were performed for removal of thymic tumors. The beneficial results in nonthymoma patients, including the salient abnormal histologic changes and possible contributing factors to the pathogenesis of MG, were appreciated afterward. Two concepts suggested an intrathymic pathogenesis for MG. The success of early and total thymectomy, and the often observed fall in antibody titers, especially in patients with noninvoluted hyperplastic thymus glands, further strengthened the role of the thymus gland in the primary immunopathogenesis of MG.[76,77] The technical goal of surgery is complete removal of the thymus gland. Total thymectomy can be difficult because the gland consists of multiple lobes in the neck and mediastinum; therefore small foci usually lie outside the field of classical or extended transsternal or transcervical surgical approaches. More extensive thymectomy procedures in more severely affected patient can potentially engender a longer period of postoperative ventilation, as may be anticipated by preoperative pulmonary function testing.[23]

THYMOMA

Transsternal thymectomy with exploration of the neck and mediastinum for thymic tissue should be performed for patients suspected of thymoma in order to prolong survival, prevent tumor recurrence, and induce remission or an asymptomatic status.[78] In the author's experience the prognosis of MG is equally favorable with surgical removal of noninvasive epithelial thymic tumors compared with invasive tumors treated with surgery and radiation therapy or chemotherapy, especially when treated early and aggressively. Controversy abounds however on the choice of chronic immunosuppressant agents in myasthenia with thymoma. It has been the author's experience to institute an oral immunosuppressant such as azathioprine or mycophenolate mofetil at the time of tumor diagnosis and to continue the medication after surgery, because such patients often have more severe and brittle disease. Patients with noninvasive and low-grade invasive tumors, including medullary and mixed cortical and epithelial thymoma with little or no risk for recurrence even when there is capsular invasion, rarely require adjuvant therapy. Cortical thymomas demonstrate a low but significant risk for relapse and may be treated with azathioprine therapy alone if there is no sign of capsular invasion. Patients with intermediate and highly malignant well-developed thymic carcinoma should be treated with postoperative irradiation and followed carefully with chest CT for signs of recurrence. Patients with exacerbation of myasthenia suspected of having microscopic tumor recurrence should be watched carefully for detectable tumor relapse, at which point chemotherapy and reoperation may be necessary.

MYASTHENIC CRISIS

Over the last century, a patient with MG had about a 50:50 chance of surviving a crisis, defined as the need for mechanical ventilatory support. Approximately 16% of all patients experience a crisis,[79] a figure that has not appreciably changed over time. Progressive weakness, oropharyngeal symptoms, refractoriness to anticholinesterase medication, and infection precede crisis in most of these patients. It is now standard practice to treat severe MG in an intensive care unit because of the ability to monitor the need for ventilatory support and the availability of aggressive respiratory and medical therapies to reduce the need for tracheostomy. The overall mortality of crisis has decreased from 50% to 6% in the past five decades, from 1960 to 2010. Crisis is a temporary exacerbation, regardless of the proximate cause. The goal is to keep the patient alive until the transient morbidity of viral or bacterial infection, aspiration pneumonitis, surgery, or other complications subsides and responsiveness to anticholinesterase medication returns. In the past, edrophonium was administered to differentiate myasthenic from cholinergic crisis. That issue is now moot because cholinergic crisis is exceedingly rare and withdrawal of anticholinesterase medication is necessary for improvement in both.

THERAPIES ON THE HORIZON

The ultimate goal of therapy in MG is a cure or at least prevention or inhibition of the immune response to skeletal muscle AChR. A number of therapies that selectively or specifically interfere with the immune pathogenesis of the disease have been envisioned and may prove useful in the future. Selective immunotherapy inhibits only cells of the immune system, without affecting other cells and without the side effects of generalized immunosuppression. Some examples include genetically engineered agents that are toxic to interleukins and activated T-cells or that interfere with costimulatory signals for T-cell activation. Specific immunotherapy goes a step further by attempting to inhibit the specific autoimmune response to AChR. Such strategies are of theoretical interest at present and include the elaboration of AChR-specific suppressor cells, induction of tolerance to AChR-specific T cells, inactivation of AChR-specific T-cells using targeted APC, and genetically modified B-cells.

REFERENCES

1. Bromberg MB. Myasthenia gravis and myasthenic syndromes. Chapter 25. In: Younger DS, ed. *Motor Disorders*. 3rd ed. New York; 2013:451–466.
2. Younger DS, Raksadawan N. Medical therapies in myasthenia gravis. *Chest Surg Clin North Am* 2001;11:329.
3. Younger DS, Worrall BB, Penn AS, et al. Myasthenia gravis: Historical perspective and overview. *Neurology* 1997;48(Suppl 5):1–7.
4. Marsteller HB. The first American case of myasthenia gravis. *Arch Neurol* 1988;45: 185–187.
5. Wilks S. On cerebritis, hysteria, and bulbar paralysis, as illustratve of arrest function of the cerebrospinal centers. *Guy's Hosp Rep* 1877;22:7–55.
6. Erb W. Zur Casnistik der bulberen Lahmuingen. 3. Ueber einen neuem wahrscheinlich bulberen symptomen Complex. *Arch Psych Nervenkrankh* 1879;9:336.
7. Goldflam S. Uber einen scheinbar helibaren bulbarparalitischen Symptomenkornplex mit beterukugybg der extrentateb. *Dtsch Z Nervenkr* 1893;4:312.
8. Jolly F. Uber myasthenia gravis pseudoparalytica. *Berl Klin Wochenschr* 1985;23:1.
9. Campbell H, Bramwell E. Myasthenia gravis. *Brain* 1900;23:277–336.
10. Walker MB. Treatment of myasthenia gravis with physostigmine (letter). *Lancet* 1934;1:1200–1201.
11. Walker MB. Case showing the effect of prostigmine on myasthenia gravis. *Proc R Soc Med* 1935;28:759–761.
12. Harvey AM, Masland RL. The electromyogram in myasthenia gravis. *Bull Johns Hopkins Hosp* 1941;65:1.
13. Blalock A, Harvey MA, Ford FR, et al. The treatment of myasthenia gravis by removal of the thymus gland. *JAMA* 1941;117:1529–1533.
14. Blalock A. Thymectomy in the treatment of myasthenia gravis. Report of 20 cases. *J Thorac Surg* 1944;13:316–339.
15. Keynes G. The surgery of the thymus gland. *Br J Surg* 1946;32:201–214.
16. Simpson JA. Myasthenia gravis. A new hypothesis. *Scot Med J* 1960;4:419–436.
17. Nastuk WL, Plescia OJ, Osserman KE. Changes in serum complement activity in patients with myasthenia gravis. *Proc Soc Exp Biol Med* 1960;105:177–184.
18. Katz B, Miledi R. The release of acetylcholine from nerve endings by graded electric pulses. *Proc R Soc Lond B Biol Sci* 1967;167:23–38.
19. Patrick J, Lindstrom J. Autoimmune response to acetylcholine receptor. *Science* 1973;180:871–872.
20. Fambrough DM, Drachman DB, Satyamurti S. Neuromuscular junction in myasthenia gravis: Decreased acetylcholine receptors. *Science* 1973;182:293–295.
21. Drachman DB. Myasthenia gravis. Part 1. *N Engl J Med* 1978;298:136–142.
22. Weigert C. Pathologisch-anatomischer beitrag zur Erb'schen krankheit (myasthenia gravis). *Neurol Zentralbl* 1901;20:597–601.
23. Younger DS, Braun NM, Jaretzki A 3rd, et al. Myasthenia gravis: Determinants for independent ventilation after transsternal thymectomy. *Neurology* 1984;34: 336–340.
24. Younger DS, Jaretzki A, Penn AS, et al. Maximal thymectomy for myasthenia gravis. *Ann NY Acad Sci* 1989;505:832–835.
25. Sanders DB. The electrodiagnosis of myasthenia gravis. *Ann NY Acad Sci* 1987;505: 539–556.
26. Somnier FE. Clinical implementation of anti-acetylcholine receptor antibodies. *J Neurol Neurosurg Psychiatry* 1993;56:496–504.
27. Vincent A, Newsom-Davis J. Acetylcholine receptor antibody as a diagnostic test for myasthenia gravis: Results in 153 validated cases and 2967 diagnostic assays. *J Neurol Neurosurg Psychiatry* 1985;48:1246–1252.
28. Solliven B, Penn AS, Lange DJ, et al. Seronegative myasthenia gravis. *Neurology* 1988; 38:514–517.
29. Osserman K. *Myasthenia Gravis*. New York: Grune & Stratton; 1958.
30. Jaretzki A 3rd, Barohn RJ, Ernstoff RM, et al. Myasthenia gravis: Recommendations for clinical research standards. Task Force of the Medical Scientific Advisory Board of the Myasthenia Gravis Foundation of America. *Neurology* 2000;55:16–23.
31. Barohn RJ. Standards of measurement in myasthenia gravis. *Ann N Y Acad Sci* 2003;998:432–439.
32. Besinger UA, Toyka KV, Heininger K, et al. Long-term correlation of clinical course and acetylcholine receptor antibody in patients with myasthenia gravis. *Ann N Y Acad Sci* 1981;377:812–815.
33. Besinger UA, Toyka KV, Homberg M, et al. Myasthenia gravis: Long-term correlation of binding and bungarotoxin blocking antibodies against acetylcholine receptors with changes in disease severity. *Neurology* 1983;33:1316–1321.
34. Tindall RS, Phillips JT, Rollins JA, et al. A clinical therapeutic trial of cyclosporine in myasthenia gravis. *Ann NY Acad Sci* 1993;681:681–551.
35. Tindall RS, Rollins JA, Phillips JT, et al. Preliminary results of a double-blind, randomized, placebo-controlled trial of cyclosporine in myasthenia gravis. *N Engl J Med* 1987;316:719–724.
36. Jaretzski A III, Barohn RJ, Ernstoff RM, et al. Myasthenia gravis: Recommendations for clinical research standards. *Ann Thorac Surg* 2000;70:327–334.
37. Barohn RJ, McIntire D, Herbelin L, et al. Reliability testing of the quantitative myasthenia gravis score. *Ann NY Acad Sci* 1998;841:769–772.
38. Barohn RJ. *Video: How to Administer the Quantitative Myasthenia Test*. St. Paul, MN: Myasthenia Gravis Foundation of America, Inc.; 1996.
39. The Muscle Study Group. A trial of mycophenolate mofetil with prednisone as initial immunotherapy in myasthenia gravis. *Neurology* 2008;71:394–399.
40. Wolfe GI, Barohn RJ, Sanders DB, et al; The Muscle Study Group. Comparisons of outcome measures from a trial of mycophenolate mofetil in myasthenia gravis. *Muscle Nerve* 2008;38:1429–1433.
41. Wolfe G, Barohn R, Foster B, et al. Randomized, controlled trial of intravenous immunoglobulin in myasthenia gravis. *Muscle Nerve* 2002;26:549–552.
42. Zinman L, Ng E, Bril V. IV Immunoglobulin in patients with myasthenia gravis: A randomized controlled trial. *Neurology* 2007;68:837–841.
43. Barth D, Nabavi Nouri M, Ng E, et al. Comparison of IVIg and PLEX in patients with myasthenia gravis. *Neurology* 2011;76:2017–2023.
44. Sanders DB, Tucker-Lipscomb B, Massey JM. A Simple manual muscle test for myasthenia gravis: Validation and comparison with the QMG score. *Ann NY Acad Sci* 2003;998:440–444.
45. Gajdos P, Chevret S, Clair B, et al. Clinical trial of plasma exchange and high-dose intravenous immunoglobulin in myasthenia gravis. *Ann Neurol* 1997;41:789–796.
46. Gaidos P, Simon N, de Rohan-Chabot P, et al. [Long-term effects of plasma exchange in myasthenia: Results of a randomized study.] *Presse Med* 1983;12:939–942.
47. Wolfe GI, Herbelin L, Nations SP, et al. Myasthenia gravis activities of daily living profile. *Neurology* 1999;52:1487–1489.
48. Burns TM, Sanders DB, Conaway MR, et al. The MG Composite: A valid and reliable outcome measure for myasthenia gravis. *Neurology* 2010;74:1434–1440.
49. Benatar M, Sanders DB, Burns TM, et al. Recommendations for myasthenia gravis clinical trials. *Muscle Nerve* 2012;45:909–917.
50. Barohn RJ. Efficacy of methotrexate in myasthenia gravis. In: *Clinicaltrials.gove [Internet]*. Bethesda, MD: National Library of Medicine (US); [Accessed 2008 July 30].

51. Jenkinson C, Fitzpatrick R, Swash M, et al.; ALS-HPS Steering Group. The ALS Health Profile Study: Quality of life of amyotrophic lateral sclerosis patients and caregivers in Europe. *J Neurol* 2000;247:835–840.

52. Padua L, Evoli A, Aprile I, et al. Myasthenia gravis outcome measure: Development and validation of a disease-specific self-administered questionnaire. *Neurol Sci* 2002;23:59–68.

53. Burns TM, Graham CD, Rose MR, et al. Quality of life and measures of quality of life in patients with neuromuscular disorders. *Muscle Nerve* 2012;46:9–25.

54. Burns TM, Conaway MR, Cutter GR, et al. Muscle Study Group. Less is more, or almost as much: A 15-item quality-of-life instrument for myasthenia gravis. *Muscle Nerve* 2008;38:957–963.

55. Burns TM, Grouse CK, Wolfe GI, et al.; MG Composite and MG-QOL15 Study Group. The MG-QOL15 for following the health-related quality of life of patients with myasthenia gravis. *Muscle Nerve* 2011;43:14–18.

56. Sanders DB, Wolfe GI, Benetar M, et al. International consensus for management of myasthenia gravis. *Neurology* 2016;87:1–7.

57. Simon HE. Myasthenia gravis: Effect of treatment with anterior pituitary extract: Preliminary report. *JAMA* 1935;104:2065–2066.

58. Torda C, Wolff HG. Effects of adrenocorticotrophic hormone on neuromuscular function in patients with myasthenia gravis. *J Clin Invest* 1949;28:1228–1235.

59. Torda C, Wolff HG. Effects of administration of adrenocorticotrophic hormone (ACTH) on patients with myasthenia gravis. *Arch Neurol* 1951;66:163–170.

60. Shy GM, Brendler S, Rabinovitch R, et al. Effects of cortisone in certain neuromuscular disorders. *JAMA* 1950;144:1353–1358.

61. Grob D, Harvey AM. Effect of adrenocorticotrophic hormone (ACTH) and cortisone administration in patients with myasthenia gravis. *John Hopkins Med* 1952;91:124–136.

62. Millikan CH, Eaton LM. Clinical evaluation of ACTH in myasthenia gravis. *Neurology* 1951;1:145–152.

63. Warmolts JH, Engel WK. Benefit from alternate day prednisone in myasthenia gravis. *N Engl J Med* 1972;286:17–20.

64. Jenkins RB. Treatment of myasthenia gravis with prednisone. *Lancet* 1972;1:765–767.

65. Pascuzzi RM, Coslett HB, Johns TR. Long-term corticosteroid treatment of myasthenia gravis: Report of 116 patients. *Ann Neurol* 1984;15:291–298.

66. Seybold ME, Drachman DB. Gradually increasing doses of prednisone in myasthenia gravis. Reducing the hazards of treatment. *N Engl J Med* 1974;290:81–84.

67. Mertens HG, Balzereit F, Leipert M. The treatment of severe myasthenia gravis with immunosuppressive agents. *Eur Neurol* 1969;2:321–339.

68. Tindall RSA, Phillips JT, Rollins JA, et al. A clinical therapeutic trial of cyclosporine in myasthenia gravis. *Ann NY Acad Sci* 1993;681:539–551.

69. Iorio R, Damato V, Alboini PE, et al. Efficacy and safety of rituximab for myasthenia gravis: A systematic review and meta-analysis. *J Neurol* 2015;262(5):1115–1119.

70. Silvestri NJ, Wolfe GI. Treatment-refractory myasthenia gravis. *J Clin Neuromuscul Dis* 2014;15:167–178.

71. El-Salem K, Yassin A, Al-Hayk K, et al. Treatment of MuSK-associated myasthenia gravis. *Curr Treat Options Neurol* 2014;16:283.

72. Keung B, Robeson KR, DiCapua DB, et al. Long-term benefit of rituximab in MuSK autoantibody myasthenia gravis patients. *J Neurol Neurosurg Psychiatry* 2013;84:1407–1409.

73. Alabdali M, Barnett C, Katzberg H, et al. Intravenous immunoglobulin as treatment for myasthenia gravis: current evidence and outcomes. *Expert Rev Clin Immunol* 2014;10:1659–1665.

74. Bril V, Barnett-Tapia C, Barth D, et al. IVIg and PLEX in the treatment of myasthenia gravis. *Ann NY Acad Sci* 2012;1275:1–6.

75. Liew WK, Powell CA, Sloan SR, et al. Comparison of plasmapheresis and intravenous immunoglobulin as maintenance therapies for juvenile myasthenia gravis. *JAMA Neurol* 2014;71:575–580.

76. Younger DS, Jaretzki A, Penn AS, et al. Maximal thymectomy for myasthenia gravis. *Ann NY Acad Sci* 1989;505:832–835.

77. Jaretzki A, Penn AS, Younger DS, et al. Maximal thymectomy for myasthenia gravis. Results. *J Thor Cardiovasc Surg* 1988;95:747–757.

78. Lovelace RE, Younger DS. Myasthenia gravis with thymoma. *Neurology* 1997;48(Suppl 5):S76–S81.

79. Cohn MS, Younger DS. Aspects of the natural history of myasthenia gravis: Crisis and death. *Ann NY Acad Sci* 1981;377:670–677.

165

Evaluation of Results of Thymectomy for Nonthymomatous Myasthenia Gravis

Mitchell J. Magee ■ Joshua R. Sonett

After observing improvement in symptoms of generalized myasthenia gravis (MG) following removal of a cystic thymoma, Blalock and colleagues[1] postulated that patients with nonthymomatous MG would also benefit from thymectomy. He subsequently performed thymectomy in 20 patients with nonthymomatous MG and observed improvement in more than half, establishing a role for thymectomy in the treatment of nonthymomatous MG.[2,3] Since Blalock's 1944 case report, the specific role of thymectomy and more recently the optimal surgical approach and extent of resection has been debated among neurologists and surgeons. Crucial to this debate, until recently, was the lack of randomized controlled trials comparing surgery and medical therapy, the natural history of the disease, and disagreement among surgeons as to what constitutes the most appropriate surgical therapy. Less open to debate, as numerous studies have shown, is the correlation of completeness of thymectomy with improved clinical outcomes and higher remission rates in the treatment of MG. Anatomic reports on the common presence of widely distributed ectopic thymic tissue[4-6] coupled with reports of complete responses to excision of residual thymic tissue after failed initial thymectomy[7] corroborate the premise that complete thymectomy is ideal. Until recently, the majority of surgeons have utilized the median sternotomy approach, arguing that this allows for a more complete and radical thymectomy, removing primarily the encapsulated thymus with varying extents of adjacent mediastinal fat.[8] Some surgeons have advocated a more aggressive approach to achieving the primary goal of complete thymectomy through an extended transsternal or combined transsternal and transcervical mediastinal dissection aimed at exenteration of all thymic tissue. As minimally invasive techniques have gained wider acceptance in the management of mediastinal disease, surgeons have increasingly utilized and advocated less invasive approaches to complete thymectomy, citing similar response rates with less radical removal of thymic-associated tissue.

The Myasthenia Gravis Foundation of America (MGFA) thymectomy classification was proposed in an attempt to apply objectivity and consistency in reporting of the various approaches and techniques employed when removing thymus tissue in patients with MG (Table 165.1).

In this chapter, incorporating the MGFA classification scheme, we compare the various surgical approaches to thymectomy—including their associated less well-defined and inconsistent extents of resection—currently employed in the surgical treatment of patients with nonthymomatous MG. The relevant published data will be reviewed, analyzed, and scrutinized, and compared according to thymectomy classification or surgical approach, with emphasis on minimally invasive techniques compared to the "gold standard" open sternotomy. Studies with data inclusive of Kaplan–Meier life table analyses, which we consider essential for proper determination of long-term complete remissions rates, are emphasized when available in our evaluation.

TRANSCERVICAL THYMECTOMY (T-1)

Transcervical thymectomy, as described and popularized by Cooper, has been used successfully with reports of satisfactory results by several groups.[9-12] In most cases the completely encapsulated thymus gland is removed intact with both upper poles and both lower poles in continuity.[9,12,13] Shrager and colleagues[10,11] reported their experience in 78 patients in 2002 and again in 151 patients in 2006, representing the largest current series using this approach. They, along with other proponents of the transcervical approach, site similar remission rates with less morbidity and shorter mean length of hospital stay when compared to transsternal approaches. However, their series included patients on minimal immunosuppression and patients in whom a partial response was observed following thymectomy rather than reporting complete stable remission (CSR) rates.

Contemporary transcervical thymectomy techniques may include video assistance and/or sternal elevation, as described and utilized during transcervical extended mediastinal lymphadenectomy (TEMLA). These techniques may augment exposure and visibility achieved with conventional transcervical techniques alone, and extend the range of standard cervical thymectomy. Zielinski[14,15] demonstrated superior results, matching the CSR rate of open maximal thymectomy,

TABLE 165.1 Thymectomy Classification

T-1 Transcervical Thymectomy
  (a)-Basic
  (b)-Extended
T-2 Videoscopic Thymectomy
  (a)-"Classic"
  (b)-"VATET"
T-3 Transsternal Thymectomy
  (a)-Standard
  (b)-Extended
T-4 Transcervical & Transsternal Thymectomy

utilizing a transcervical and subxiphoid videothoracoscopic approach, incorporating many of the techniques utilized with TEMLA.

VIDEO-ASSISTED THORACOSCOPIC THYMECTOMY (T-2)

The "classic" video-assisted thoracoscopic (VATS) thymectomy has several permutations including left-side, right-side, bilateral, and subxiphoid. In most detailed descriptions of this technique, completely encapsulated thymus gland is removed intact with both upper poles and both lower poles in continuity along with all mediastinal adipose tissue within the borders of the phrenic nerves, diaphragm, and cervical border of the anterior mediastinum cephalad to the innominate vein. Thus theoretically achieving a similar extended thymectomy as that described in the transsternal approach. Tomulescu and colleagues[16] compared the right- and left-sided approaches to VATS thymectomy and found similar operating times, length of hospitalization, and rates of remission. No differences in operative complications were noted. In their experience, the left-side approach is preferred due to the majority of mediastinal fat being located on the left side of the anterior mediastinum, making dissection of the thymus on the contralateral side safer and easier. They further believe that the risk of injury to the right phrenic nerve is decreased due to its location outside the surgical field and that the left side affords needed access to the aortopulmonary window. Several centers have reported intermediate term MG remission rates comparable to more invasive approaches to thymectomy.[17–19]

Meyer et al.[20] compared 48 patients with MG who underwent VATS thymectomy to a comparable group of 47 MG patients who underwent extended transsternal thymectomy between 1992 and 2006. Patients were assessed utilizing MGFA guidelines with clinical visits or by telephone interview and follow-up was greater than 90% complete with a mean postoperative period of follow-up of 6 years. In the VATS group, the mean hospital postoperative length of stay was 1.9 days. CSR was seen in 34.9%, minimal manifestations seen in an additional 55.8%, and two patients (4%) were worse postoperatively. These remission rates were similar to those observed in the sternotomy group.

Mantegazza and colleagues[21] published a follow-up report on a technique described by Novellino and colleagues[22] as VATET, VATS-extended thymectomy, consisting of bilateral thoracoscopy and open cervical exploration. VATET essentially combines elements of the VATS and transcervical approaches to achieve a more thorough extirpation of thymic tissue. Overall, 206 MG patients underwent either the VATET or extended transsternal thymectomy and were followed for 6 years. The 159 patients that underwent the VATET procedure had comparable CSR rates to the 47 patients that had an extended transsternal thymectomy (50.6% vs. 48.7%).[23] Shigemura et al.[24] prospectively studied the contribution of the transcervical exploration to the VATET procedure and concluded that additional thymus tissue can be removed through a cervical incision following bilateral VATS thymectomy, although the clinical significance of this has not been demonstrated.

ROBOTIC-ASSISTED THYMECTOMY

The incorporation of complete robotic surgical systems, such as the da Vinci (Intuitive Surgical Inc.), has been proposed by some to enhance precision maneuverability in the mediastinum when compared to conventional VATS thymectomy. The report on the first robotic thymectomy was published in 2001, though it was only a partial thymectomy for thymoma,[25] and the first robotic complete thymectomy was described in 2003.[26,27] Subsequently, many centers have begun or switched to the robotic approach.

Ismail reviewed all published case series containing more than 20 robotic thymectomies, including the largest series reported by Ruckert of 317 robotic thymectomies performed between 2003 and 2012.[28] This latter series included patients with MG, thymoma, ectopic mediastinal parathyroid glands, MEN, and other indications.

Feasibility, perioperative morbidity, and improvement in MG were analyzed, although only three series reported complete remission rates, ranging from 28% to 42%. The left-sided operative approach is preferred by most. Proponents of robot-assisted thymectomy opine that robotic surgery is more suitable than VATS for an extended thymectomy due to easier dissection of the upper horns, more controlled ligation of the thymic veins, and improved unilateral access to the entire anterior mediastinum.

TRANSSTERNAL THYMECTOMY (T-3)

Transsternal thymectomy is the most common approach used historically in the surgical treatment of MG. The basic transsternal thymectomy, as it was originally performed by Blalock, has been abandoned in favor of more extensive resections that can be easily achieved through the same or a smaller incision, for example, upper partial sternotomy, with similar or less morbidity. Masaoka and colleagues[6] identified thymic tissue in adipose tissue located outside the thymic capsule in the anterior mediastinum in 13 of 18 MG patients undergoing thymectomy. Based on this observation, they recommended removal of all adipose tissue in the anterior mediastinum along with the gross thymus via an extended thymectomy. A detailed description of the procedure along with their 20-year experience was subsequently reported.[7] Following a full sternotomy, an en bloc resection of the thymus gland and all anterior mediastinal adipose tissue is completed, including all adipose tissue around the upper poles of the thymus, the brachiocephalic vein, and the pericardium. The borders of resection are the diaphragm caudally, the thyroid gland cephalad, and the phrenic nerves bilaterally. Between 1973 and 1993, 286 patients with nonthymomatous MG underwent extended transsternal thymectomy. Remission rates were 36.9% at 3 years, 45.8% at 5 years, 55.7% at 10 years, and 67.2% at 15 years. Venuta et al.[29] reported their experience with 232 thymectomies performed between 1970 and 1997. Of these, 101 patients with nonthymomatous MG had an extended thymectomy through a partial upper sternotomy. After a mean postoperative follow-up of 119 months, 25% of the patients were in complete remission and an additional 46% were clinically improved. There were two operative deaths (0.9%) due to respiratory failure in patients with postoperative bleeding requiring reoperation and seven patients in the nonthymomatous group (4.5%) died from MG (mean survival: 34.3 ± 3.6 months). Minor complications included arrhythmia (1.8%) and infection (1.8%) and mean postoperative hospital stay was 6.4 days.

Jurado et al.[30] reported their single institution experience comparing outcomes in patients with MG following VATS versus open transsternal thymectomy. From 2000 to 2011, 139 patients with MG underwent thymectomy utilizing either a VATS (43 patients) or an open transsternal (96 patients) approach. Seventy-seven thymectomies were performed by a minimally invasive approach. Both groups were equally stratified by age, sex, body mass index, and clinical stage determined according to the MGFA staging system. The hospital and ICU lengths of stay were shorter in the VATS group (p <0.01).

Thymectomy (Type)	N	Surgical Procedure	5 Year (CSR)
No Thymectomy (Spontaneous Remissions in Children)			
None (Rodriguez et al., 1983.)[33]	149	No thymectomy	15
Transcervical Thymectomy			
Basic (Papatestas et al., 1987)[34]	651	Transcervical simple	23
Extended (Shrager et al., 2002)[10]	78	Transcervical extended	43
Extended (Durelli et al., 1991)[35]	300	Transcervical with sternal split	33
Extended (DePerrot et al., 2003)[36]	120	Transcervical with video	30
Maximal (Zielinski et al., 2010)[14]	292	TEMLA/Subxiphoid with Video	53
VATS Thymectomy			
Basic (Manlulu et al., 2005)[19]	36	Right VATS	13
Extended (Tomulescu et al., 2006)[16]	107	Unilateral VATS	40
Maximal (Novellino et al., 2004)[37]	159	Bilateral VATS/Cervical	51
Robotic			
Extended (Marulli et al., 2013)[38]	100	Unilateral left robotic	28.5
Extended (Ruckert et al., 2008)[39]	106	Unilateral left robotic	42
Sternotomy			
Basic (Zielinski et al., 2010)[14]	60	Sternotomy	26
Extended (Lindberg et al., 1992)[40]	73	Sternotomy/cervical dissection	40
Extended (Zielinski et al., 2010)[14]		Sternotomy/radical thymect	50.7
Transcervical–Transsternal Thymectomy			
Maximal (Jaretzki et al., 1988)[32]	72		50

TABLE 165.2 Thymectomy Results for Myasthenia Gravis

The estimated blood loss was significantly less for the VATS versus the open group (p <0.01). There were no differences in transfusion requirements (p = 0.73) or operative times (p = 0.11). An equal crude remission rate was observed among the VATS and sternotomy groups (p = 0.59) but unfortunately again, remission data were obtained for only 37 patients. Twenty-five patients in this limited sample reported complete remission (70% in the VATS group and 67% in the open group). There were insufficient data to accurately represent remission with a Kaplan–Meier analysis.

Spillane and colleagues[31] reported outcomes in 89 patients with MG, 68 without thymoma, who underwent extended transsternal thymectomy. At a mean follow-up of 3.8 years after thymectomy, 34% had a CSR, 33% had pharmacologic remission, and 13% achieved an improved status. All patients were admitted postoperatively to the ICU (mean ICU stay = 2.45 days) and the mean hospital length of stay was 11.2 days. There were no operative deaths and 9% had perioperative complications.

Allowing again for differences in severity of disease and methods of reporting outcomes, the results of extended transsternal thymectomy appear to be comparable to other approaches but associated with significant morbidity.

COMBINED TRANSCERVICAL AND TRANSSTERNAL ("MAXIMAL") THYMECTOMY (T-4)

The primary proponent and practitioner of this approach are Jaretzki and colleagues.[5,32] Wide exposure in the neck and mediastinum is achieved through a complete median sternotomy incision and separate

collar incision. The skin incisions are occasionally connected to create a "T," but the subcutaneous and deeper planes of dissection in the neck and mediastinum are always confluent. All thymus, suspected thymus, and mediastinal fat, including both mediastinal pleural sheets, are removed en bloc utilizing sharp dissection on the pleurae and pericardium. The entire dissection is performed and completed "as if it was an en bloc dissection for a malignant tumor."[8] Starting at the diaphragm, the dissection extends from hilum to hilum and proceeds cephalad to the innominate vein. After elevating the strap muscles above the innominate vein, the cervical dissection is begun and continued posterior to the strap muscles to the level of the thyroid cartilage, removing thymic tissue posterior and superior to the thyroid gland and adjacent to the recurrent laryngeal and vagus nerves. This is certainly conceptually the technique most likely to remove all thymic tissue, but this radical extirpation is associated with the most morbidity and least desirable cosmetic result. Advocates for this approach, believing it the most effective in achieving a durable complete remission, also believe that improved outcomes justify the increased morbidity. Alternatively, in the absence of controlled prospective clinical trials showing a clear benefit to more radical complete removal of all gross and microscopic thymic tissue, a more balanced approach between procedure-related morbidity and "complete" thymectomy is warranted.

Representative published outcomes stratified by approach are summarized for comparison in Table 165.2.

DISCUSSION

Based on critical analysis of the available data, it appears that better long-term results correlate with more thorough removal of all tissue that may contain thymus. Notwithstanding and as summarized in the recommendations for clinical research standards in MG,[8,41] it remains debatable as to which of the multiple techniques described for removal of the thymus in MG is ideal. Although "complete" thymectomy is considered the goal of surgery, it has not been demonstrated unequivocally that this is necessary, nor is it clear to what extent each of the resectional techniques achieve this goal.

The international trial of myasthenia gravis (MGTX) was recently completed after many years of enrollment and patient follow-up and conclusively defined the role of thymectomy in the treatment of nonthymomatous MG.[42] Through the visionary, tireless surgical leadership of Alfred Jaretzki, the persistence and medical leadership of John Newsom-Davis, and an extremely committed and diligent international group of investigators, 126 patients were enrolled in a prospective blinded fashion to definitively prove the benefit of extended thymectomy in MG. Prospectively randomized patients who underwent an extended thymectomy via median sternotomy had significantly improved quality of life and MG course compared to patients who received prednisone-based medical therapy alone. Thus, almost 75 years after Blalock's first case series, thymectomy was definitively proven to benefit patients with nonthymomatous MG. Given this landmark trial, thymectomy should be incorporated into the treatment regimen of acetylcholine antibody-positive patients with MG.

When assessing outcomes in MG patients treated with various surgical approaches to thymectomy in retrospective analyses, including meta-analyses perhaps even to a greater extent, there are numerous factors that preclude accurate comparison including: (1) incompletely defined or disparate patient populations in the various treatment groups and associated selection bias, (2) incompletely defined or inconsistencies in the extent of thymus resected within treatment groups, (3) differences in continued medical therapy following thymectomy and the relative contributions of surgery and medical therapy to the reported outcome, and lastly, (4) a lack of consistent objective criteria used to assess preoperative disease severity and postoperative response to therapy within an adequate period of long-term follow-up.

Regardless of the technique employed, when complete removal of all thymic tissue is the goal, the actual extent of each individual resection is determined by: (a) the operating surgeon's conviction that as much thymus that can be removed safely should be removed, (b) the surgeon's commitment to take the time to meticulously do so, and (c) the surgeon's experience with the technique employed. The latter is especially true with the use of the transcervical and the unilateral approaches, but all of these principles apply to all minimally invasive techniques as well as traditional open transsternal approaches. Concerns for incomplete or compromised surgical excision has continued to limit acceptance of minimally invasive thymic resection. With refined minimally invasive techniques, and an experienced surgeon committed to the principles of complete resection, a minimally invasive thymectomy may arguably be performed with the same degree of radical completeness and safety as an open resection. Regardless of the technique, since the need for complete removal of all gross and microscopic thymus has not been definitively confirmed, it is preferable to leave small amounts of suspected thymus rather than risk injury to the recurrent laryngeal, left vagus, or phrenic nerves.

With these caveats in mind and an overall understanding of inherent limitations to comparing outcomes, particularly specific to the approach used, some limitations and potential advantages relating to each approach are provided.

Limitations of the transcervical approach to thymectomy include a greater potential for a comparatively less radical resection of thymic tissue due to limited access to the most caudal and lateral extents of the anterior mediastinum. Further, the unique nature of this approach makes it difficult to teach, learn, and consistently reproduce, limiting

adoption, and the neck incision may not be considered as cosmetically acceptable.

The unilateral right-sided approach is advocated by some relative to increased working space absent the left ventricle, and the superior vena cava serves as an excellent landmark for initial dissection and identification of the innominate vein. Cited advantages of the VATS approach include decreased blood loss, decreased length of hospital stay, improved cosmetic result, faster recovery and social reintegration, and less pain. However, this approach may compromise exposure of potential thymic tissue extending lateral to the left phrenic nerve and in the aortopulmonary window. This may be obviated with either a unilateral left-sided or bilateral VATS approach. Overall, as opposed to the skills needed to obtain the unique exposure required for transcervical thymectomy, including the additional techniques associated with TEMLA, a VATS thymectomy can be more easily learned and performed safely and effectively by most thoracic surgeons experienced in advanced video thoracoscopy.

While the feasibility and safety of thymectomy with the robotic da Vinci system has been shown and improved video image resolution and visualization touted, the value added by the robotic-assisted thoracoscopic surgical approach to thymectomy, compared with conventional VATS, has not yet been demonstrated.

In summary, the benefits of thymectomy through a sternotomy approach have now been firmly established with the conclusion of the long-awaited randomized international trial of MG. This, along with numerous other nonrandomized published reports, supports the fundamental tenets of better outcomes correlating with more radical or aggressive complete resections. As long as these tenets are paramount in the surgeon's philosophical approach, the incisional approach may be considered less important and only represent a variety of alternative means to the same end: minimally invasive maximal thymectomy.

REFERENCES

1. Blalock A, Mason MF, Morgan HJ, et al. Myasthenia gravis and tumors of the thymic region. Report of a case in which the tumor was removed. *Ann Surg* 1939; 110:544–561.
2. Blalock A, Harvey AM, Ford FR. The treatment of myasthenia gravis by removal of the thymus gland. Preliminary report. *JAMA* 1945;127:1089–1096.
3. Blalock A. Thymectomy in the treatment of myasthenia gravis. Report of twenty cases. *J Thorac Surg* 1944;13:316–339.
4. Jaretzki A III, Bethea M, Wolff M, et al. A rational approach to total thymectomy in the treatment of myasthenia gravis. *Ann Thorac Surg* 1977;24(2):120–130.
5. Jaretzki A III, Wolff M. "Maximal" thymectomy for myasthenia gravis: surgical anatomy and operative technique. *J Thorac Cardiovasc Surg* 1988;96:711–716.
6. Masaoka A, Nagaoka Y, Kotake Y. Distribution of thymic tissue at the anterior mediastinum: Current procedures in thymectomy. *J Thorac Cardiovasc Surg* 1975; 70:747–754.
7. Masaoka A, Yamakawa Y, Niwa H, et al. Extended thymectomy for myasthenia gravis patients: a 20-year review. *Ann Thorac Surg* 1996;62:853–859.
8. Sonett JR, Jaretzki A III. Thymectomy for nonthymomatous myasthenia gravis: a critical analysis. *Ann NY Acad Sci* 2008;1132:315–328.
9. Cooper JD, Al-Jilaihawa AN, Pearson FG, et al. An improved technique to facilitate transcervical thymectomy for myasthenia gravis. *Ann Thorac Surg* 1988;45:242–247.
10. Shrager JB, Deeb ME, Mick R, et al. Transcervical thymectomy for myasthenia gravis achieves results comparable to thymectomy by sternotomy. *Ann Thorac Surg* 2002; 74:320–327.
11. Shrager JB, Nathan D, Brinster CJ, et al. Outcomes after 151 extended transcervical thymectomies for myasthenia gravis. *Ann Thorac Surg* 2006;82:1863–1869.
12. Calhoun RF, Ritter JH, Guthrie TJ, et al. Results of Transcervical thymectomy for myasthenia gravis in 100 consecutive patients. *Ann Surg* 1999;230:555–561.
13. Meyers BF, Cooper JD. Transcervical thymectomy for myasthenia gravis. www.ctsnet.org/sections/clinicalresources/thoracic/expert_tech-23.html. 2002. Accessed November 25, 2009.
14. Zielinski M, Hauer L, Hauer J, et al. Comparison of complete remission rates after 5 year follow-up of three different techniques of thymectomy for myasthenia gravis. *Eur J Cardiothorac Surg* 2010;37:1137–1143.
15. Zielinski M, Hauer L, Kuzdzal J, et al. Technique of the transcervical-subxiphoid-videothoracoscopic maximal thymectomy. *J Min Access Surg* 2007;3:168–172.
16. Tomulescu V, Ion V, Kosa A, et al. Thoracoscopic thymectomy mid-term results. *Ann Thorac Surg* 2006;82:1003–1007.
17. Mack MJ, Landreneau RJ, Yim AP, et al. Results of video-assisted thymectomy in patients with myasthenia gravis. *J Thorac Cardiovasc Surg* 1996;112:1352–1360.

18. Savcenko M, Wendt GK, Prince SL, et al. Video-assisted thymectomy for myasthenia gravis: an update of a single institution experience. *Eur J Cardiothorac Surg* 2002;22: 978–983.

19. Manlulu A, Lee TW, Wan I, et al. Video-assisted thoracic surgery thymectomy for nonthymomatous myasthenia gravis. *Chest* 2005;128:3454–3460.

20. Meyer DM, Herbert MA, Sobhani NC, et al. Comparative clinical outcomes of thymectomy for myasthenia gravis performed by extended transsternal and minimally invasive approaches. *Ann Thorac Surg* 2009;87:385–391.

21. Mantegazza R, Confalonieri P, Antozzi C, et al. Video-assisted thoracoscopic extended thymectomy (VATET) in myasthenia gravis two-year follow-up in 101 patients and comparison with the transsternal approach. *Ann NY Acad Sci* 1998;841:749–752.

22. Novellino L, Longoni M, Spinelli L, et al. "Extended" thymectomy, without sternotomy performed by cervicotomy and thoracoscopic technique in the treatment of myasthenia gravis. *Int Surg* 1994;79:378–381.

23. Mantegazza R, Baggi F, Bernasconi P, et al. Video-assisted thoracoscopic extended thymectomy and extended transsternal thymectomy (T-3b) in non-thymomatous myasthenia gravis patients: remission after 6 years of follow-up. *J Neurol Sci* 2003; 212(1–2):31–36.

24. Shigemura N, Shiono H, Inoue M, et al. Inclusion of the transcervical approach in video-assisted thoracoscopic extended thymectomy (VATET) for myasthenia gravis: A prospective trial. *Surg Endosc* 2006;20:1614–1618.

25. Yoshino I, Hashizume M, Shimada M, et al. Thoracoscopic thymomectomy with the Da Vinci computer-enhanced surgical system. *J Thorac Cardiovasc Surg* 2001; 122:783–785.

26. Ashton RC, McGinnis KM, Connery CP, et al. Totally endoscopic thymectomy for myasthenia gravis. *Ann Thorac Surg* 2003;75:569–571.

27. Rea F, Bortolotti L, Girardi R, et al. Thoracoscopic thymectomy with the Da Vinci surgical system in patient with myasthenia gravis. *Interact Cardiovasc Thorac Surg* 2003;2:70–72.

28. Ismail M, Swierzy M, Ruckert JC. State of the art of robotic thymectomy. *World J Surg* 2013;37:2740–2746.

29. Venuta F, Rendina EA, Giacomo TD, et al. Thymectomy for myasthenia gravis: A 27-year experience. *Eur J Cardiothorac Surg* 1999;15:621–625.

30. Jurado J, Javidfar J, Newmark A, et al. Minimally invasive thymectomy and open thymectomy: outcome analysis of 263 patients. *Ann Thoracic Surg* 2012;94(3):974–982.

31. Spillane J, Hayward M, Hirsch NP, et al. Thymectomy: role in the treatment of myasthenia gravis. *J Neurol* 2013;260(7):1798–1801.

32. Jaretzki A 3rd, Penn AS, Younger DS, et al. "Maximal" thymectomy for myasthenia gravis. Results. *J Thorac Cardiovasc Surg* 1988;95:747–757.

33. Rodriguez M, Gomez MR, Howard FM Jr, et al. Myasthenia gravis in children: Long term follow-up. *Ann Neurol* 1983;13:504–510.

34. Papatestas AE, Genkins G, Kornfeld P, et al. Effects of thymectomy in myasthenia gravis. *Ann Surg* 1987;206:79–88.

35. Durelli L, Maggi G, Casadio C, et al. Actuarial analysis of the occurrence of remission following thymectomy for myasthenia gravis in 400 patients. *J Neurol Neurosurg Psychiatry* 1991;54:406–411.

36. DePerrot M, Bril V, McRae K, et al. Impact of minimally invasive trans-cervical thymectomy on outcome in patients with myasthenia gravis. *Eur J Cardiothorac Surg* 2003;24:677–683.

37. Novellino L, Spinelli L. Albani AP, et al. Thymectomy by cervicotomy and bilateral thoracoscopy and extended transsternal thymectomy to treat non-thymomatous myasthenia. *Osp Ital Chir* 2004;10:61–74.

38. Marulli G, Schiavon M, Perissinotto E, et al. Surgical and neurologic outcomes after robotic thymectomy in 100 consecutive patients with myasthenia gravis. *J Thorac Cardiovasc Surg* 2013;145:730–735; discussion 735–736.

39. Ruckert JC, Ismail M, Swierzy M, et al. Thoracoscopic thymectomy with the da Vinci robotic system for myasthenia gravis. *Ann N Y Acad Sci* 2008;1132:329–335.

40. Lindberg C, Andersen O, Larsson S, et al. Remission rate after thymectomy in myasthenia gravis when the bias of immunosuppressive therapy is eliminated. *Acta Neurol Scand* 1992;86:323–328.

41. Jaretzki A, Barohn RJ, Ernstoff RM, et al. Myasthenia gravis: recommendations for clinical research standards. *Neurology* 2000;55:16–23.

42. Aban IB, Wolfe GI, Cutter GR, et al. The MGTX experience: challenges in planning and executing an international, multicenter clinical trial. *J Neuroimmunol* 2008;201–202.

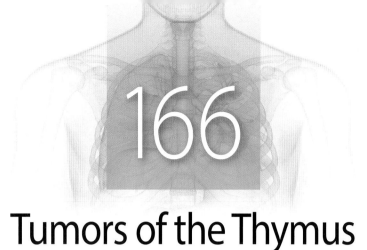

166

Tumors of the Thymus

Usman Ahmad ▪ James Huang

INTRODUCTION

Although thymic tumors are relatively uncommon, they may present a challenging clinical scenario to the thoracic surgeon. These patients usually present shortly after the diagnosis of a mediastinal mass. The workup and treatment of these tumors is typically dictated by thoracic surgeons; therefore, we touch upon important and clinically relevant aspects of diagnosis, workup, and management of these tumors. In the current era of molecular diagnostics that may influence treatment choices, surgeons should also be aware of the nuances of pathologic classification.

In the previous editions of this textbook, Dr. Shields had presented an unparalleled and comprehensive overview of these tumors. Our knowledge of thymic tumor biology, pathology, and outcomes has since increased significantly. Strides have been made in delineating the molecular characteristics of these tumors, and large international collaborations have been organized to study these tumors from a clinical perspective, leading to the first staging system based on a global-wide dataset and the generation of consensus guidelines.

Some of the key problems that have slowed progress in studying and treating thymic tumors are (a) the rarity of the disease, (b) the significant heterogeneity of treatment practices, and (c) the variation in terminology and reported outcome measures in the literature. In fact, the vast majority of retrospective reports on thymic tumors include less than 100 patients. The landmark paper by Masaoka et al.,[1] where the currently prevailing staging system was proposed, was based on a series of 96 patients. International collaborative efforts have tried to overcome these issues by consolidating the majority of available international retrospective data for a more robust analysis.

Tumors arising from thymic epithelial and neuroendocrine cells are considered primary thymic tumors and are the focus of this chapter. Thus, tumors of germ cell or lymphoid origin, histiocytic and dendritic cell neoplasms, sarcomas, and metastatic lesions to the thymus are excluded and discussed elsewhere. Likewise, thymic hyperplasia and thymic cysts are excluded in this discussion of thymic tumors. It should be noted, however, that a thymoma may grossly present as a cyst and that a thymic tumor may develop within an established cyst. The three major subtypes of primary thymic tumors include thymomas, thymic carcinomas, and thymic neuroendocrine tumors. Each subtype is further subclassified based on histologic features. While the histologic subtypes have important bearing on prognosis, as discussed later in this chapter, the treatment is largely based on the clinical stage of the tumor and is similar across the histologic subtypes.

EPIDEMIOLOGY

The incidence of thymic tumors is estimated to be 2.2 to 2.6/million/yr for thymomas and significantly less for thymic carcinomas (0.3 to 0.6/million/yr).[2] Thymic neuroendocrine tumors are even less common. Thymic tumors are the most common anterior mediastinal tumors. Among anterior mediastinal masses, retrospective studies have shown the approximate relative proportion of these tumors to be: thymoma 35%, benign thymic lesions 5%, lymphoma 25% (Hodgkin 13%, non-Hodgkin 12%), benign teratoma 10%, malignant germ cell 10% (seminoma 4%, nonseminomatous germ cell tumor 7%) thyroid and other endocrine tumors 15%.[3–6]

HISTOLOGIC CLASSIFICATION

For years it has been stressed that thymomas were essentially histologically benign tumors, but with a malignant potential that increased as the lack of differentiation of the epithelial cells and the degree of atypia increased. It is now thought that in fact all thymomas are latent or even actively malignant lesions from their conception, despite their benign histologic appearance; the degree of malignancy being low in the so-called medullary (and the spindle cell) tumors and in the well-differentiated tumors (types A and AB) and high in the epithelial, moderately differentiated tumors (types B1, B2, and B3). The poorly differentiated tumors (thymic carcinomas) are now separated into their own subgroup, since these tumors have no histologic features of either an adolescent or an atrophic adult thymic gland but reflect the histologic features of many other epithelial carcinomas, as discussed subsequently.

The histologic classification of thymic tumors has significantly evolved over the last 50 years. As early as 1987, Lewis and colleagues[7] identified the presence of varying degrees of cellular atypia in 2% of the patients diagnosed with otherwise typical benign thymomas. Similar and even more advanced atypical changes were subsequently noted in the malignant variants by Shimosato,[8] Hishima and colleagues,[9] Suster and Moran,[10] and Kuo and Chan.[11]

Based on these and numerous other histologic reports, Müller-Hermelink and colleagues[12–14] suggested a histologic classification system based on the presence of either medullary or cortical phenotypic differentiation in a given thymoma. They classified the thymomas as (a) medullary, (b) mixed, (c) predominately cortical (organoid), (d) cortical, and (e) well-differentiated thymic carcinomas. These histologic subtypes had some prognostic value, however, was not consistently noted by various investigators. In 1996 and subsequently in 1999, Suster and Moran[15,16] presented a simplified approach that classified thymic epithelial tumors, into thymomas, atypical thymomas, and thymic carcinomas. This was followed by the WHO classification[17] that has since been updated[18,19] and has become the standard histologic classification system. Dadmanesh and colleagues[20] described this classification succinctly: "In this schema, thymomas are evaluated on the combined basis of the morphologic appearance of the neoplastic epithelial cells...and the relative number of these cells vis á vis the nonneoplastic lymphocytes." Type A stands for "atrophic," representing the thymic cells of adult life; type B stands for "bioactive," representing the biologically active thymus of the fetus and infant; and type C stands for "carcinoma."

While the WHO categories appeared to be associated with prognosis, in a review of a large number of studies of the histologic classification, there was marked interobserver discordance in almost every study.[21] This was confirmed by Dawson and colleagues,[22] showing that various thymomas were assigned to the same group in only 35% of the cases. Rieker and colleagues[23] noted that interobserver agreement was only 50% within the B1, B2, and B3 group of thymomas. In this context, an international consensus group recently brought together 18 expert pathologists in a pathology workshop to refine defining characteristics and criteria between the various histologic subtypes, specially for borderline cases.[24] This group made recommendations that were used to guide the latest edition of the WHO classification as shown in Table 166.1.[19]

There is a general agreement that only the thymic epithelial cells (cortical and medullary) take part in the malignant behavior of thymomas that occur in the various cell types. The thymic lymphocytes may vary greatly in number in the various tumors observed, but these lymphocytes take no part in the neoplastic transformation that results in the formation of the various thymic epithelial tumors. The lymphocytes in most thymomas are small and mature-appearing, without evidence of cytologic atypia. Variations in cell pattern are observed; however, no evidence of malignant change is evident. Mokhtar and colleagues,[25] by studying the reactions of the lymphocytes in thymomas to monoclonal and polyclonal antiserum markers, concluded that these cells mirrored the lymphocytic phenotypes of the normal thymus.

Thymoma

Thymomas are relatively bland tumors that contain thymic epithelial cells and various proportions of lymphocytes and is largely the basis of current WHO histologic classification.

Type A: Type A tumors are composed of oval or spindle-shaped epithelial cells lacking nuclear atypia and accompanied by few or no lymphocytes. The origin of the spindle-shaped cells, is unclear as they are not seen in the normal medullary portions of the mature infant or adolescent gland but are seen in small numbers in the periphery of the adult atrophic thymus. According to Rosai,[17] these cells correspond to the nonfunctioning thymic epithelial cells that recapitulate spindle cells seen in the involuted thymus of the adult.

Type AB: These tumors have foci of type A admixed with foci rich in lymphocytes (similar to type B).

Type B: Type B tumors resemble the normal functional thymus and are subdivided into types B1, B2, and B3 on the basis of an increasing ratio of epithelial-to-lymphocytic cells and the presence of atypical changes in the epithelial cells. Type B1 tumors resemble normal active thymus and are lymphocyte-rich, with some areas resembling the thymic medulla. Type B2 tumors are also lymphocyte rich, but foci of medullary differentiation are less evident or even absent. The epithelial cells are more numerous and are plump cells with vesicular nuclei and conspicuous nucleoli. A palisading appearance may be present owing to the perivascular arrangement of the cells. Type B3 tumors are composed mainly of round or polygonal epithelial cells in a sheet-like growth pattern and there is little or no lymphatic component. Atypia may or may not be present. Foci of squamous metaplasia and perivascular spaces are common.

Thymic Carcinoma

Thymic carcinomas are of epithelial origin and have malignant features in cellular and architectural components. While less common than thymomas their diagnosis is more consistent due to clear malignant changes. The most common subtype is squamous cell carcinoma that may develop de novo or in a pre-existing thymoma. The well-differentiated tumor has prominent lobular growth and necrosis is not often apparent. The poorly differentiated squamous cell tumor shows little lobular growth, is infiltrative, and are more commonly noted to be locally invasive or metastatic. It is important to differentiate a squamous cell carcinoma of thymic origin from that arising in a neighboring organ like the lung. Thymic epithelial markers CD5, CD117, FOXN1, and CD205 may be used to help identify thymic carcinomas in situations where the source of a carcinoma in the anterosuperior mediastinum is in doubt.[26] We have previously described a detailed analysis of the histologic subtypes of thymic carcinoma in the ITMIG database,[27] where squamous cell subtype constituted 79% of the cohort followed by lymphoepithelioma-like tumors (6%).

TABLE 166.1 WHO Histologic Subtypes of Thymic Epithelial Tumors

Thymoma	Thymic Carcinoma	Thymic Neuroendocrine Tumor
A	Squamous	Carcinoid tumor Typical Atypical
AB	Basaloid	Large cell neuroendocrine
B1	Mucoepidermoid	Small cell carcinoma
B2	Lymphoepithelioma-like	
B3	Clear cell	
Micronodular tumor with lymphoid stroma	Sarcomatoid	
Metaplastic thymoma	Adenocarcinoma	
	Undifferentiated carcinoma	

Neuroendocrine Tumors

These tumors are divided into low-, moderate-, and high-grade categories. Their origin is presumed to be from the neuroendocrine cells in the thymus and may be unrelated to the neural crest cells. While initially considered to be variants of thymic carcinoma, they are now considered a separate tumor category. Overall, their clinical behavior and outcomes are similar to thymic carcinomas.

On light microscopy, carcinoid tumors of the thymus demonstrate the classic histologic features of carcinoid tumors elsewhere in the body and may be divided into typical and atypical varieties, the latter being the more common. The moderately differentiated neuroendocrine tumors (atypical carcinoids) may show similar growth patterns, but there is a greater tendency to form sheets of tumor cells. The formation of large clumps ("balls") of tumor cells with central areas of necrosis is common. There is commonly the formation of small acinar or rosette-like structures with empty lumens. Marked cellular atypia and frequent mitotic figures are prominent. The poorly differentiated neuroendocrine tumors (small-cell carcinomas) are composed of sheets or cords of highly atypical, small "round blue cells." Extensive areas of necrosis and a high mitotic index are constant features in these poorly differentiated tumors.

On immunohistochemical studies, various amines may be demonstrated. Immunoreactive adrenocorticotropic hormone (ACTH) is found most frequently. A number of peptides in addition to ACTH have also been found in these tumors. These are calcitonin, cholecystokinin, gastrin, somatostatin, and β-endorphin. These immunohistochemical reactions are helpful in differentiating thymic carcinoids from lymphoproliferative disorders, as well as from thymomas.

GENETIC AND MOLECULAR FEATURES OF THYMIC TUMORS

Thymic tumors have been difficult to study using traditional techniques such as fluorescence in situ hybridization or array-based genomic hybridization due to paucity of tumor cells and an overwhelming majority of nonneoplastic lymphocytes in the tumor samples.[28–31]

Certain genomic abnormalities have been described in these tumors and include chromosomal abnormalities including gain and loss of chromosomal components. These abnormalities are found more frequently in higher-grade tumors with some degree of overlap. A loss of 6q25.2-25.3 is noted in all subtypes except B1 thymomas.[29–32] 1q gains are noted in types B2, B3, and thymic carcinoma. Other changes noted in thymic carcinomas include gains in 4,5,7,8,9q, 12,15,17q, 18, 20 and losses in 3p, 6, 6p23, 9p, 13q, 14, 16q, and 17p.[29–32] Chromosomal loss leading to absence of FOXC1 was associated with worse progression-free and disease-related survival.[33]

Changes in DNA methylation are also noted in correlation with Masaoka stage and WHO subtype.[34] These changes are also noted more frequently in higher-grade tumors including thymic carcinoma[35] and advanced stage tumors.[36] Gene expression analysis and gene signature assays have been described; however, they have not been prospectively validated.

The Cancer Genome Atlas includes cases of thymic tumors in the rare tumors subgroup. Analysis of this data will help in further identification of molecular changes associated with these tumors and are expected to be published in the near future.

CLINICAL PRESENTATION

Most thymomas are found in adult patients, with a peak incidence in the 7th decade of life, although thymomas may occur at any age. Rare reports of pediatric cases have been published.[37]

Patients with thymic tumors are relatively evenly distributed among age cohorts, gender, and the presence or absence of myasthenia gravis symptoms. While some differential diagnosis of anterior mediastinal tumors are more common in a particular age group and gender, it is unlikely that a definitive diagnosis can be made based on demographic and radiologic information alone.

The vast majority of patients, especially those with early stage tumors, will be asymptomatic. Typically patients will present with one of three scenarios: (a) an incidentally discovered mediastinal mass is noted in an asymptomatic patient in roughly 30% of the cases; (b) another 40% of patients will present with local symptoms of compression or pain from large mediastinal tumors. Locally invasive tumors can cause superior vena cava (SVC) compression and patients can present with SVC syndrome; (c) approximately 30% of the patients will present initially with symptoms related to myasthenia gravis and will be found to have a mediastinal tumor on subsequent workup.[38]

When there are local symptoms, vague chest pain, shortness of breath, and cough are the most common complaints. Severe chest pain, SVC obstruction, paralysis of a hemidiaphragm as a result of involvement of a phrenic nerve, and hoarseness caused by involvement of a recurrent laryngeal nerve and dysphagia are infrequent but ominous signs of extensive malignant disease. The presence of a pleural or pericardial effusion is likewise a serious clinical finding. On rare occasions, a thymoma will spontaneously rupture; the resulting acute mediastinal hemorrhage is associated with severe chest pain and dyspnea.

Other chapters have addressed the presentation and management of SVC syndrome and myasthenia gravis. In brief, the most common paraneoplastic syndrome is myasthenia gravis, followed by red cell aplasia, and hypogammaglobulinemia.[38] Thymomas associated with myasthenia are typically diagnosed approximately a decade earlier than the nonmyasthenic thymomas. These patients are more likely to have B-type thymomas, while the incidence of myasthenia is rare with A-type thymomas. In general, myasthenia gravis is not usually associated with thymic carcinoma.

DIAGNOSIS AND WORKUP

Assessing the clinical characteristics, presentation, and mediastinal location are important steps in the approach to these patients. History and physical examination will reveal the degree and duration of any symptoms and the presence of associated diseases that can provide important clues to the diagnosis. Radiologic assessment is key and is based on computed tomography (CT) imaging. For mediastinal masses, it is preferable to obtain a CT with IV contrast to better delineate mediastinal vascular structures that can be involved by the tumor. This is especially important in planning resection of larger and locally invasive tumors.

If an anterior mediastinal tumor is clinically suspicious for a primary thymic tumor, and it appears to be localized to the mediastinum and completely resectable, it is reasonable to proceed directly to surgical resection. If there is reasonable suspicion of an alternate diagnoses, such as lymphoma or germ cell tumor, or if the tumor appears to invade mediastinal structures such that neoadjuvant treatment is being considered, a biopsy may be helpful to establish a tissue diagnosis first.

Anterior mediastinal tumors can typically be biopsied through image-guided needle biopsy. While core biopsy permits a more substantial sample, fine needle aspiration (FNA) has also shown good diagnostic accuracy.[39] Traditionally, there has been reluctance to biopsy thymic tumors due to difficulty in establishing a definitive diagnosis based on cytology alone and the potential risk of spread to the pleura. There are some isolated case reports where the tumor was noted to recur at the site of the needle biopsy over time periods ranging from 4 months to 12 years.[40–42] Although the true denominator is unknown, overall this likely represents a very low risk for needle site recurrences from biopsies. When a needle biopsy is not possible, is nondiagnostic, or is not desirable given the above concerns, surgical biopsy through a Chamberlain approach, thoracotomy, or thoracoscopy has been performed with no clear additional risk of spread. In addition, obtaining pretreatment diagnosis largely outweighs the benefit of this anecdotal risk of seeding. A pretreatment diagnosis is necessary when neoadjuvant treatment in planned, and may help prevent unnecessary surgeries in patients with mediastinal lymphomas.

The relative lack of experience in diagnosing thymic tumors in cytology specimen has led to reluctance on part of the pathologists to accept this into clinical routine. However, Zakowski et al.,[39] and others have shown that thymomas and thymic carcinomas can be reliably diagnosed in cytology specimens. They recommend evaluating the specimen in the context of the patient's clinical and radiographic findings. According to an expert consensus, such biopsies should be performed with at least a 22-gauge needle for FNA or a 19-gauge needle for core biopsy.[43] As with all small biopsies, the interpretation of these results should be made with caution. While the diagnosis of a thymic neoplasm can be made from a small biopsy, the ability to reliably distinguish histologic subtypes will be limited. Consensus policies recently established by the International Thymic Malignancy Interest Group provide rational guidelines with the use of small biopsies.[43]

RADIOGRAPHIC IMAGING

Although large anterior mediastinal tumors can be detected on chest roentgenograms, CT imaging is the modality of choice for evaluation of these lesions. Thymomas typically appear as smooth lobulated masses in the anterior mediastinum with the bulk of the tumor primarily leaning toward either hilum. This lateral predilection is potentially helpful in choosing the approach for minimally invasive resection, if appropriate for the patient.

It is important to note the relationship of the tumor with mediastinal vascular structures, especially the innominate vein and SVC, since locally advanced tumors can demonstrate vascular invasion. Hence the importance of obtaining an IV contrast-enhanced CT scan (Fig. 166.1).

CT scan is generally superior to magnetic resonance (MR) imaging in assessment of anterior mediastinal tumors. However, MR imaging can be helpful in differentiating between thymic hyperplasia and thymic tumors, with the use of chemical shift MR, to detect the presence of intralesional fat in hyperplasia[44,45] and may be useful for the assessment of vascular or cardiac invasion, especially in patients who are allergic to CT contrast. However, CT imaging with IV contrast is the standard and has been shown to be helpful in predicting resectability in locally advanced thymic tumors.[46]

The role of Fluorodeoxyglucose (FDG) uptake noted on positron emission tomography (PET) scan in thymic tumors is still under study. Thymic tumors can be FDG avid and some reports have described higher FDG uptake in WHO type B3 thymomas, thymic carcinomas, and neuroendocrine tumors.[47] However, the diagnostic reliability of PET imaging is not established and, at the present time, we suggest use of PET scan to aid in evaluation of metastatic or recurrent disease only.

STAGING OF THYMIC TUMORS

Over the years, there have been many proposals and iterations of staging systems for thymic tumors.[48] None of the staging systems have been adopted by AJCC and UICC. Based on expert consensus, ITMIG adopted and recommended the Masaoka system with the Koga modification. The Masaoka–Koga system is a clinicopathologic classification and has been the most common staging convention in use. However, it is of historical interest to note that that original Masaoka system proposal was based on a review of 96 cases of thymoma[1] and the Koga modification based on 79 patients.[49]

It should be noted that nodal metastasis is a rare phenomenon in thymic tumors, in general, and thymomas in particular. Systematic lymph node (LN) sampling is not a standard practice in management of thymic tumors and this may have led to underdetection of LN metastases. The best available data on LN involvement comes from the retrospective analysis of Japanese Association for Research in the Thymus registry where LN involvement was noted in 2% of thymomas, 27% of thymic carcinomas, and 28% of neuroendocrine tumors.[50]

More recently the International Thymic Malignancy Interest Group (ITMG), in collaboration with International Association for the Study of Lung Cancer (IASLC), has proposed a new Tumor Node Metastasis (TNM) classification which is based on a review of 10,808 thymic tumor cases collected from all over the world. At the time of this writing, this proposal is currently under review for adoption by the American Joint Commission on Cancer (AJCC) and the Union for International Cancer Control (UICC).

Masaoka–Koga Staging System

The Masaoka–Koga system is based on local invasion of surrounding structures and less so on nodal involvement. Table 166.2 describes the details of the system. While the original description is relatively simple it makes it particularly difficult to differentiate between microscopic and macroscopic invasion and attachment to surrounding structures. It also fails to explain other complexities of local tumor invasion and distant spread. The ITMIG consensus statement by Detterbeck et al.,[51] has sought to clarify some of these vague points and the detailed description is shown in Table 166.2.

Masaoka stage I tumors are limited to within the capsule of the tumor. The tumor may have invaded into the capsule but not through it. In addition, if there are areas of complete absence of the capsule, the tumor must not have invaded the surrounding fat (Fig. 166.2).

Stage IIA tumors exhibit *microscopic* invasion through the capsule into the surrounding thymic tissue or surrounding fat. Stage IIB have *macroscopic* invasion into surrounding thymic tissue or fat. In addition, these tumors may be attached to pleura or pericardium necessitating excision with the tumor but on final microscopic examination there should be no invasion into the pleura or pericardium.

Stage III tumors have obvious macroscopic and/or microscopic invasion into the structures surrounding the thymus gland, including pleural, pericardium, neurovascular structures, or lung.

Stage IV tumors have spread to other areas such that IVA tumors have separate tumor implants on pericardial or pleural surfaces and IVB tumors have hematogenous spread to either lung parenchyma, LNs, or extrathoracic sites.

The Masaoka system was proposed based on the study of thymomas; however, the ITMIG consensus expanded its use to thymic carcinomas. Some of the limitations of this system include its major dependence on pathologic evaluation, thus limiting its utility in clinical staging. Other shortcomings include the proposed equality of

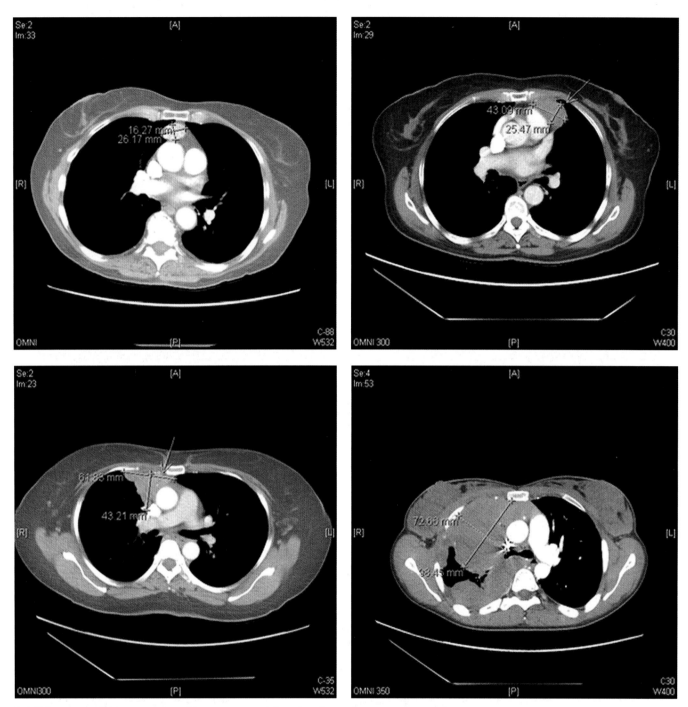

FIGURE 166.1 Radiologic appearance of thymic tumors and their clinical Masaoka-Koga stages Top left: clinical stage I. Top right: clinical stage II. Bottom left: Clinical stage III. Bottom right: clinical stage IVA.

TABLE 166.2 Description of Masaoka-Koga Staging System

Stage	Description
I	Grossly and microscopically encapsulated tumor
IIA	Microscopic invasion through the capsule
IIB	Gross/macroscopic invasion through the capsule into the surrounding fat but no invasion of pleura or pericardium
III	Direct invasion into adjacent structures (pleura, pericardium, lung parenchyma, vascular structures)
IVA	Pleural or pericardial metastasis/implants
IVB	Lymph node metastasis (no level specified). Hematogenous metastasis

Adapted from Koga K, Matsuno Y, Noguchi M, et al. A review of 79 thymomas: modification of staging system and reappraisal of conventional division into invasive and non-invasive thymoma. *Pathol Int* 1994;44:359–367. Copyright © 1994 by John Wiley Sons, Inc. Reprinted by permission of John Wiley & Sons, Inc.

invasion into easily resectable structures, such as a pleura or pericardium, and unresectable structures, such as the aorta or main pulmonary artery (all considered as stage III).

ITMIG/IASLC Proposed TNM Staging System

The deficiency in a uniform staging system not only leads to differences in clinical care but also leads to significant variability in research standards and outcomes. To overcome these challenges, the need for a more robust and widely applicable staging system was obvious.

In 2009, International Thymic Malignancies Interest Group and the International Association for the Study of Lung Cancer (IASLC) formed a partnership to address this issue. The ITMIG membership provided the engagement of clinicians and the ITMIG retrospective database provided the large body of international data necessary to create a robust prognostic system.

In conjunction with other international organizations active in research on thymus, ITMIG and IASLC created a collaborative worldwide database involving 105 institutions and 10,808 patients. This is relatively contemporary with most of the patients being first treated between 2000 and 2010. Data were available on the pathologic stage in 8,084 patients, on the clinical stage in 5,232 patients, on survival in 8,145 patients, and on recurrence in 4,732 patients.[52] A TNM staging system was developed and proposed to the AJCC and UICC for inclusion in the eighth TNM stage classification manual (Fig. 166.3 and Table 166.3).

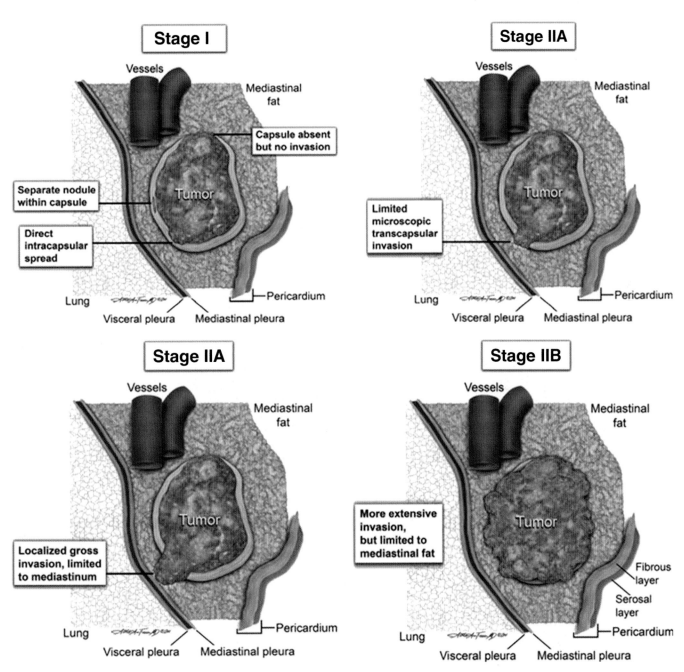

FIGURE 166.2 Schematic representation of Masaoka–Koga staging system. (*continued*)

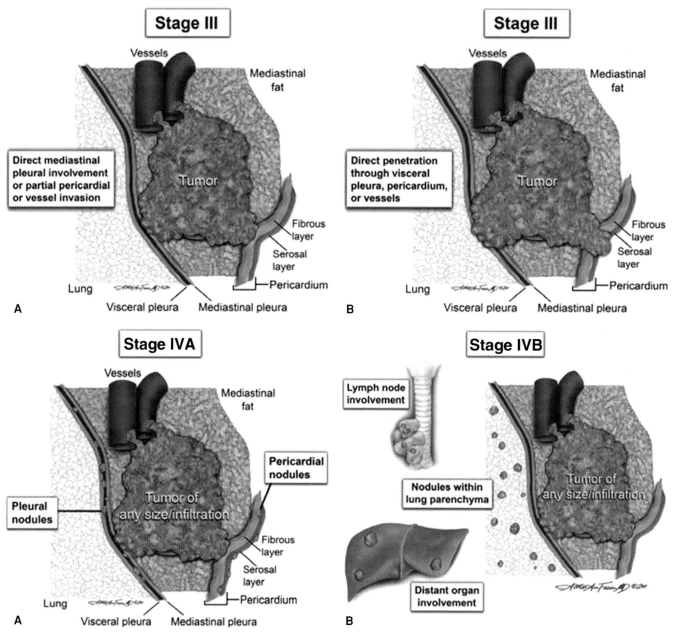

FIGURE 166.2 (*Continued*)

In the new TNM proposal the early Masaoka stages (I, II) were consolidated into TNM stage I, as there did not appear to be a significant prognostic difference between levels of invasion as long as other structures were not invaded. The more advanced Masaoka stages (III, IVA) were expanded into TNM stages I, II, III, and IVA.

The T stage[53] was based on level of invasion into surrounding structures that took into account the degree of resectability, such that mediastinal pleural invasion is T1b, pericardial invasion in T2, invasion of resectable structures (lung, brachiocephalic vein, SVC, chest wall, phrenic nerve, hilar [extrapericardial] pulmonary vessels) is T3, while more advanced invasion (aorta, pulmonary trunk) is T4.

LN involvement, which has been systematically studied in detail in particular by the Japanese investigators, is more common in thymic carcinoma. This is noted to be a prominent prognostic factor and is divided into two groups according to their proximity to the thymus: anterior (perithymic) and deep cervical or thoracic nodes.[54] The perithymic nodes that are typically in the field of resection of a complete thymectomy are considered to be N1, while intrathoracic nodes are staged as N2. If nodal involvement in noted in other basins such as axilla or retroperitoneum, they are considered to be distant metastases.

Lastly, tumor implants separate from primary tumor on pleura or pericardium are categorized as M1A and intraparenchymal pulmonary nodules or distant extrathoracic metastases are categorized as M1B disease.[54]

The stage categorization is such that up to stage IIIB, advancement in the T descriptor advances the stage. Stage IVA is characterized by the presence of N1 or M1a disease while stage IVB is characterized by N2 or M1b disease.

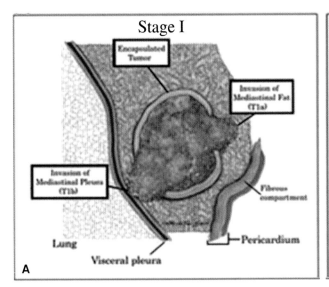

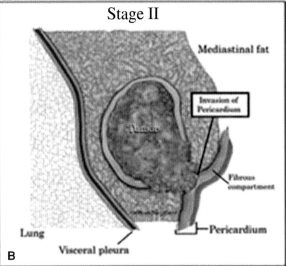

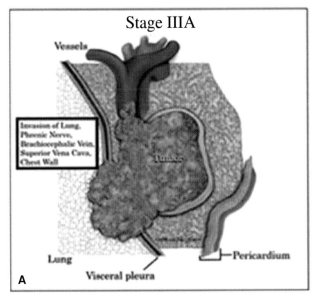

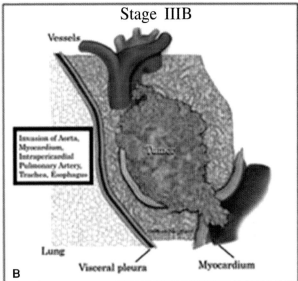

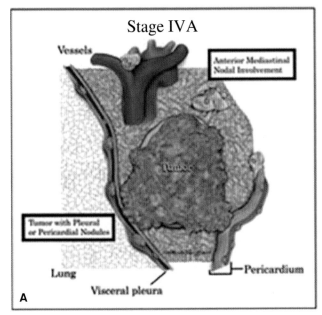

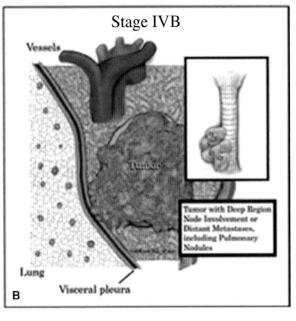

FIGURE 166.3 Schematic representation of the newly proposed TNM staging system.

TABLE 166.3 The TNM Staging System Proposal by ITMIG/IASLC

	Description		
T1			
a	Tumor limited to capsule or mediastinal fat		
b	Extension into mediastinal pleura		
T2	Invasion of pericardium		
T3	Invasion of lung, chest wall, phrenic nerve, brachiocephalic vein, pulmonary vessels, hilum		
T4	Invasion of aorta, aortic arch vessels, main pulmonary artery, myocardium, trachea, esophagus		
N0	No nodal involvement		
N1	Anterior nodes (perithymic)		
N2	Deep intrathoracic or cervical nodes		
M0	No metastatic disease		
M1			
a	Pleural or pericardial nodules (separate from primary tumor)		
b	Pulmonary intraparenchymal metastasis, extrathoracic metastasis		
Stage	**T**	**N**	**M**
I	T1	N0	M0
II	T2	N0	M0
IIIA	T3	N0	M0
IIIB	T4	N0	M0
IVA	T any	N1	M0
	T any	N0,1	M1a
IVB	T any	N2	M0, 1a
	T any	N any	M1b

PRETREATMENT MANAGEMENT OF THYMIC TUMORS

Routine preoperative testing is similar to that for any other thoracic surgical procedure and typically includes pulmonary function studies, cardiac risk stratification as indicated, and physiologic assessment of functional status. Preoperative imaging is usually already present, if not a CT chest with IV contrast can be helpful in assessment of vascular invasion and can help choose the type of incision and surgical approach.

If the patient has myasthenia gravis, the preoperative management should include medical optimization, in conjunction with the treating neurologist. Preoperative intravenous immunoglobulin (IVIG) or plasmapheresis prior to surgery, may be helpful in reducing the risk of perioperative myasthenic complications.

TREATMENT OF THYMIC TUMORS

The treatment regimen for any thymic tumor is based on its clinical stage. Surgical resection is the mainstay of treatment for thymic tumors. The use of multimodality treatment is increasing, especially in the case of more advanced tumors.

Early Stage Tumors

The treatment of stage I and II tumors is based on complete surgical resection. The pros and cons of the various surgical approaches have been discussed in other chapters, but, regardless of the approach, an

R0 resection is the goal of treatment with care to avoid violating the tumor capsule. This can be achieved through a transsternal approach for central tumors, thoracotomy or hemiclamshell if the tumor extends far laterally, a minimally invasive thoracoscopic or robotic approach, or a transcervical approach. The goal is to resect the tumor en bloc with the entire thymus gland and perithymic fat, as tumor nests have been reported in the surrounding fat. The general consensus on the extent of surgery has focused on total thymectomy with en bloc resection of the tumor, the entire thymus gland, along with the surrounding fat. Proponents of complete thymectomy advocate en bloc resection of the thymus and all pericardial fat between the two phrenic nerves.

For tumors that have no gross invasion into surrounding structures on preoperative imaging, minimally invasive techniques can provide adequate resection. While several techniques have been described, it is important to have good visualization of both phrenic nerves to allow for complete resection without injury to these structures. Thoracoscopy, with or without robotic assistance, is a reasonable approach for resection of localized and well-circumscribed tumors. The introduction of robotic technology can sometimes allow for completion of thymectomy from a unilateral approach; however, if there is any doubt about location of the nerve or residual tumor or gland on the contralateral side, adding a few ports to the contralateral side to complete the dissection in the area of concern, does not significantly increase the time or morbidity and allows for a safe and complete operation.

In a review of the ITMIG database, minimally invasive approaches were associated with similar R0 resection rates as compared to open thymectomy.[55] In a recent unadjusted meta-analysis of Masaoka stage I and II patients, minimally invasive thymectomy was associated with a shorter length of hospital stay, while the R0 resection rate and recurrence rates were similar to open technique.[56]

As mentioned above, complete surgical resection has generally been considered to entail total thymectomy with en bloc resection of the tumor with the entire thymus gland and surrounding fat. However, some authors, predominantly from Asia, have advocated for thymomectomy alone. This approach seemed to have less morbidity; however in a recent series from Japan, there was a higher but not statistically significant recurrence rate as compared to propensity matched patients that underwent complete thymectomy (2.2% vs. 0.4%).[57] Similarly, a large multi-institutional retrospective database analysis from China showed a higher, but statistically insignificant, recurrence rate after thymomectomy in stage I patients (3.2% vs. 1.4%). Recurrence rates were significantly higher after thymomectomy in stage II patients (2.9% vs. 14.5%).[58] While more research is needed to answer this question, our general recommendation is to perform a complete thymectomy with resection of surrounding fat.

Locally Advanced Tumors

Except for stage IVB tumors (LN or extrathoracic metastases) thymic tumors are generally considered a surgical disease, and complete resection (R0) is the primary goal of treatment. Locally advanced tumors include stage III tumors that demonstrate invasion into surrounding structures, such as the pericardium, phrenic nerve, lung, and great vessels (most typically, the innominate vein and the SVC). Stage IVA tumors have pleural or pericardial implants separate from the primary tumor and, in some cases, develop into bulky confluent disease, similar to mesothelioma. Successful resection of these extensive tumors requires careful selection of patients and the surgical approach, and consideration of whether neoadjuvant therapies may improve resectability, since encouraging results have been noted in some patients with the use of neoadjuvant modalities.

While centers have employed both neoadjuvant chemotherapy or chemoradiation therapy the typical neoadjuvant treatment is chemotherapy based. Thymomas are typically chemosensitive and the goal of neoadjuvant chemotherapy is to improve the rate of R0 resection. For advanced tumors with local invasion, especially if resection margins are close or positive, postoperative radiation treatment (PORT) is favored. Although thymic carcinomas are much less responsive to chemotherapy, recent evidence suggests that thymic carcinomas may benefit from PORT.

Management of Locally Advanced Tumors

A multidisciplinary approach involving thoracic surgeon, thoracic oncologist, radiologist, pathologist, and radiation oncologist should be the standard of care. Patients with advanced tumors are usually discussed in a multidisciplinary tumor board and now the ITMIG offers a virtual tumor board, where cases from all parts of the world can be discussed with an expert panel.[59] Our strategy is to have the patient meet the thoracic surgeon, oncologist, and radiation oncologist upfront for consultation. A multidisciplinary treatment plan is delineated based on the clinical stage and a dedicated effort is made to adhere to this treatment plan.

Typically, a patient with an advanced thymic tumor is approached with radiologic staging, which includes CT scan of the chest with IV contrast (MRI if CT not possible) and a PET scan. If surgery is not the primary treatment, tissue diagnosis is warranted before initiating chemotherapy. After completing neoadjuvant chemotherapy (typically four cycles), the patient is restaged to evaluate response to treatment, extent of disease, and surgical resectability. Again, surgical resection is the mainstay of treatment and an R0 resection should be the goal for all patients. For locally advanced tumors, postoperative radiation should also be considered.

For stage III tumors, surgical resection typically entails a sternotomy, and possibly a hemiclamshell incision to better expose the great vessels. Patients with stage IVA disease may require a sternotomy followed by a standard posterolateral thoracotomy to resect pleural disease. Every measure should be taken to achieve an R0 resection and the incision or approach should not limit attaining this goal. Partial or complete resection of either innominate vein or SVC is the most typical scenario when vascular invasion is noted. Patients with thymic tumors are generally younger and healthier than those with lung or esophageal cancers and, thus, are able to tolerate extended resections quite well. Such extended resections are discussed in detail elsewhere in this section. It is recommended that surgical resection be performed within 6 to 8 weeks of completion of chemotherapy.

NEOADJUVANT TREATMENT FOR THYMIC TUMORS

Induction Chemotherapy

Thymomas are considered to be chemosensitive tumors and a variety of combinations of chemotherapy regimens have been reported with varying response rates.[38] The sensitivity of thymomas to chemotherapy was well established by two cooperative group trials, one examining the CAP (cisplatin, doxorubicin, cyclophosphamide) regimen led by ECOG[60] and one examining cisplatin–etoposide (EP) led by EORTC[61] in patients with metastatic or unresectable disease. Response rates were notable and comparable, with acceptable toxicity, in both regimens.

Based on data from small series, combination regimens appear to be well tolerated and the majority of the patients in the reported studies were able to proceed to resection with promising resection rates (Table 166.4). In these studies, thymomas have demonstrated marked chemosensitivity as demonstrated by a clinical response rate of approximately 62% to 100% and complete resection rates of 22% to 92%.

There are no randomized trials examining different regimens; however, key single arm prospective studies are discussed below. The CAP regimen was used as induction therapy in patients with unresectable thymoma in a single arm prospective study, which included 22 patients with locally advanced disease. Patients received neoadjuvant chemotherapy with CAP and prednisone, followed by resection, PORT, and consolidation chemotherapy. Seventeen patients demonstrated some radiographic response and 6 of 16 patients had greater than 80% tumor necrosis on pathologic evaluation. At 5 years, disease-free survival was 77% and overall survival (OS) was 95%.[62]

In a phase II study conducted by the Japan Clinical Oncology Group, either dose-dense chemotherapy (cisplatin, vincristine, doxorubicin, etoposide) or radiation was administered followed by resection. Resectable patients underwent surgery and PORT while unresectable patients received radiation only. In the chemotherapy group, 62% of patients had radiographic response and 14% had complete pathologic response.[63]

A series of 30 stage III and IVA thymoma patients underwent induction with cisplatin, epirubicin, and etoposide. The response rate was 73%, with a complete resection rate of 77%.[64] In a recent report from the Japanese Association for Research of the Thymus, 441 patients with clinical stage III thymoma were evaluated, with 113 of those patients having received induction treatment. The response to

TABLE 166.4 Results of Induction Chemotherapy

Author	Year	N	Stage	Chemotherapy	Response Rate (%)	Complete Resection Rate (%)	PORT	Disease-Free Survival	Overall Survival
Prospective									
Macchiarini[94]	1988–1990	7	III	Cisplatin, epirubicin, etoposide	100	57	45 Gy (R0)		
Rea[95]	1985–1991	16	III, IVA	Doxorubicin, cisplatin, vincristine, cyclophosphamide	100	69	11 cases		70% – 3 yrs
Berruti[96]	1990–1992	6	III, IVA	Doxorubicin, cisplatin, vincristine, cyclophosphamide	83	83			
Venuta[97]	1989– onward	15	III	Cisplatin, epirubicin, etoposide	67	91	40 Gy (R0)		
Kim[62]	1990–2000	22	III, IVA	Cisplatin, doxorubicin, cyclophosphamide, prednisone	77	76	50 Gy (R0)	77% – 5 yrs	95% – 5 yrs
Yokoi[98]	1988–2003	14	III, IVA	Cisplatin, doxorubicin, methylprednisolone	93	22	50 Gy		89% – 5 and 10 yrs
Lucchi[64]	1989–2004	30	III, IVA	Cisplatin, epirubicin, etoposide	73	77	45 Gy (R0)		82% – 10 yrs
Kunitoh[63]	1997–2005	21	III	Cisplatin, vincristine, doxorubicin, etoposide	62	43	48 Gy (R0)	32%–8 yrs	69% – 8 yrs
Retrospective									
Bretti[99]	1990–1992	25	III, IVA	Doxorubicin, cisplatin, vincristine, cyclophosphamide (18 cases) Cisplatin, etoposide (7 cases)	72	44	45 Gy (R0)		
Yamada[65]	1991–2010	113	III	Not specified	52				
Leuzzi[66]	1990–2010	88	III	cisplatin, doxorubicin, cyclophosphamide, vincristine		65			

induction treatment was 52%; however, induction therapy was associated with a worse prognosis which was attributed to the fact that patients with more advanced disease received induction treatment.[65]

In a report from the European Society of Thoracic Surgeons database,[66] 370 stage III thymoma patients were reported. Induction therapy was administered to 88 (25%) of the patients. The most common chemotherapy regimen was cisplatin, doxorubicin, cyclophosphamide, and vincristine. No association between induction treatment and cancer-specific or recurrence-free survival was noted. Given that the induction group consisted of patients with more advanced disease, the authors were unable to draw firm conclusions about the benefit of induction therapy in their dataset.

Collectively these studies show the safety and feasibility of induction chemotherapy and support its use in the management of locally advanced tumors with the goal of increasing the probability of achieving an R0 resection.

Induction Chemoradiation

Like other thoracic malignancies,[67,68] the addition of radiation to induction chemotherapy has been employed in locally advanced thymic tumors. In a prospective study by Loehrer et al.,[69] patients with localized unresectable thymoma and thymic carcinoma underwent four cycles of cisplatin, doxorubicin, and cyclophosphamide followed by 54 Gy of radiation as definitive therapy. Among the 23 assessable patients, the overall response rate to initial chemotherapy was 69.6%. One patient with partial response, was noted to have a complete response after radiation and four patients with a minimal response demonstrated a complete or partial response with the addition of radiation. No patient had progression of disease during radiation. The 5-year OS was 53%.

The use of chemoradiation as an induction strategy was reported in a series of 10 patients with stage III and IVA thymic tumors at the Massachusetts General Hospital, using induction treatment consisting of cisplatin and etoposide with a concurrent radiation dose of 40 to 45 Gy.[70] Four patients demonstrated a partial response; however, an R0 resection was achieved in eight patients, while two had an R1 resection. Four of the patients had a pathologic complete response. The opportunity to achieve pathologic complete responses with concurrent chemoradiation has led to interest in pursuing this as a strategy in patients felt to be unresectable or borderline resectable.

The encouraging response to induction chemoradiation noted in the studies discussed above led to a multi-institutional phase II study of induction treatment with cisplatin, etoposide and 45 Gy of radiation.[71]

During the 5-year study period, 22 patients with stage III disease were enrolled at four institutions. Specific inclusion criteria included tumor diameter >8 cm, or 5 to 8 cm with irregular borders/heterogeneous appearance/ectopic calcification, or vascular invasion. There were 7 thymic carcinoma and 14 thymoma patients. Twenty-one completed induction treatment and a partial radiographic response was noted in 10 (47%) patients. Grade 3 or 4 toxicity was noted in nine cases (41%). All 21 patients were surgically explored, 17 (77%) underwent an R0 resection, 3 (14%) had an R1 resection, and 1 (5%) had an R2 resection. Although no patient demonstrated a complete pathologic response, less than 10% viable tumor was noted in five cases. Postoperative complications were noted in eight (36%) patients. Two patients died in the perioperative period, one succumbed to respiratory failure from aspiration having undergone a pneumonectomy, while the other had an R2 resection due to aortic involvement and had an intraoperative cardiac arrest with subsequent multiorgan failure. At 5 years, the freedom from progression was 83% and OS was 71% for all 22 patients. Of note, thymic carcinomas appeared to have a greater response to induction chemoradiation than thymomas, with four of the five tumors with <10% viable tumor being thymic carcinomas.

The studies reporting the use of induction chemoradiation appear to have at least comparable radiographic response rates to induction chemotherapy alone and potentially higher pathologic response rates (Table 166.5). However, a note of caution is in order as the issue of toxicity must be considered. While induction chemoradiation has been routinely and safely used in esophageal cancer and for superior sulcus tumors, the general treatment volume is relatively small. Thymomas, on the other hand, can be sizable, with a corresponding radiation field that is quite large and centered over the mediastinum. This can lead to greater toxicity before surgery, as well as a greater risk of perioperative complications.[70,71] Serious adverse events occurred in over 40% of patients in the phase II trial of EP/45 Gy, and perioperative mortality was 9%.[71] Furthermore, one must also take into account long-term toxicities from radiotherapy, especially the risk of coronary and valvular disease given the location of the treatment field, and this may compound the cardiotoxicity from doxorubicin. The risk of subsequent radiation-induced malignancy must also be considered. No data yet exists to determine whether a higher pathologic response rate with the addition of radiation to induction chemotherapy improves long-term survival, or if such a benefit is potentially offset by higher toxicity.

Induction Radiation Therapy

The role of induction radiation only has been reported in a few small retrospective series and variable outcomes are noted. In a series of 34 stage III thymoma patients, 8 received preoperative radiation with Cobalt-60 while 26 did not. Patients who underwent a complete resection had improved survival; however, there was no difference in OS between patients who did or did not receive preoperative radiation.[72] More modern radiation treatments have since been reported by others. Ribet et al.[73] reported a series of 113 patients where 19 patients had preoperative radiation. In this group, complete resection was achieved in 10/19 patients. The overall 5-year survival in these 19 patients was 44%.

In a series of 12 patients with thymic tumor invading the great vessels (vena cava, pulmonary artery, aorta), patients were treated with preoperative radiation (12 to 21 Gy).[74] On exploration one patient had stage IVA disease. The rate of complete resection was 75%. Ten patients also received adjuvant radiation (mean, 42.3 Gy). The OS was 72% at 5 years and 48% at 10 years.

Most institutions now favor the use of chemotherapy in the induction setting. In a multi-institutional study from European Society of Thoracic Surgeons database, only 12/2,030 patients (1%) underwent induction radiation alone.[75] Similarly, a review of the ITMIG database revealed that 48 of the 1,042 (6%) thymic carcinomas had received induction radiation only.[27]

SPECIAL CONSIDERATIONS WITH IVA DISEASE

In extensive pleural disease, extrapleural pneumonectomy can potentially achieve a macroscopic complete resection and has been shown to be feasible. An additional potential benefit is the ability to provide hemithoracic radiation without the risk of pneumonitis to the underlying lung. In patients with relatively limited pleural disease, partial pleurectomy is undertaken. In both scenarios, induction treatment is usually chemotherapy only given the size of the necessary treatment field.

To improve the control of pleural disease, other modalities have been explored. In a series of 35 stage IVA patients with thymoma (17), thymic carcinoma (4), and recurrent thymoma (14), induction chemotherapy was administered to all thymic carcinoma and 13 thymoma patients. One patient underwent extrapleural pneumonectomy, while the remaining patients underwent local resection of involved tissues. Intraoperatively, the pleural space was perfused with cisplatin and doxorubicin at 45°C for 60 minutes. Ninety-day mortality was 2.5%. Local control was not achieved in thymic carcinoma patients and all died within 4 years. After median follow-up of 62 months, the 5- and 10-year progression-free survival was 61% and 43% for primary thymomas, and 48% and 18% for recurrent thymomas, respectively.[76] A European group[77] has popularized the

TABLE 166.5 Results Induction Chemoradiation Treatment

Author	Year	N	Stage	Chemotherapy	Radiation	Response Rate	Complete Resection	Disease-Free Survival	Overall Survival
Prospective									
Loehrer[69]	1983–1995	23	III, IV	Cisplatin, cyclophosphamide, doxorubicin	54 Gy	70	No resection		53% – 5 yrs
Korst[71]	2007–2012	21	I, II, III	Cisplatin, etoposide	45 Gy	47	77	83% – 5 yrs (freedom from progression)	71% – 5 yrs
Retrospective									
Wright[70]	1997–2006	10	III, IVA	Cisplatin, etoposide	40–45 Gy	40	80		69% – 5 yrs

use of pleural lavage with povidone–iodine solution. In a series of six thymoma patients with pleural disease, induction chemotherapy was administered followed by complete pleurectomy. Povidone–iodine solution (diluted 1 to 10 in sterile water and heated to 40 to 41°C) was instilled in the pleural space for at least 15 minutes. There were no in-hospital deaths. After median follow-up of 18 months, one patient had died of unrelated reasons, one patient underwent reresection for recurrence, while the remaining four patients had no evidence of disease.

These treatment protocols may have utility in the treatment of pleural disease where the major concern is the difficulty in truly achieving an R0 resection in the setting of extensive pleural metastasis. However, to date, there is no validated prospective data that demonstrates efficacy in these difficult cases.

ADJUVANT TREATMENT STRATEGIES FOR THYMIC TUMORS

Adjuvant Chemotherapy

There is very limited data on the use of adjuvant chemotherapy alone in thymic tumors, especially after complete resection. In a survey of European centers, only 3 out of 52 had used chemotherapy alone.[78] In the Japanese series of 1,320 patients, Kondo et al. reported that in completely resected stage III and IV thymomas and thymic carcinomas, adjuvant treatment modalities including chemotherapy, radiation therapy, and chemoradiation therapy had similar or worse 5-year survival when compared to patients receiving no adjuvant treatment.[79] Therefore, adjuvant therapy after resection is primarily radiation treatment.

Adjuvant Radiation Therapy

The data on the use and effect of adjuvant radiation therapy should be interpreted in the context of completeness of tumor resection. PORT, in resected thymomas, theoretically targets microscopic disease that is not identifiable during surgery, but may lead to recurrence. However, in both groups of patients who did or did not receive adjuvant radiation therapy, recurrence most commonly occurs in the form of pleural implants away from the tumor bed. As such, it remains unclear whether adjuvant radiation therapy successfully inhibits local recurrence in the tumor bed, and there are no data to suggest that radiating the tumor bed reduces the risk of subsequent metastases to the pleura.

Radiation is preferred in the postoperative setting, as it can be targeted to known areas of potential residual disease, can be administered with less toxicity and without increasing the risk of operative complications. Postoperative delivery of radiation therapy avoids the potential of increased surgical morbidity and allows for dosage boosting to areas of residual disease.

Port in Thymoma

The role of PORT for thymoma is a topic of intense debate. The number of recurrences are small, requiring that data be collected over long time periods. The point of greatest controversy is the benefit of PORT after complete resection of locally advanced tumors.

Stage I tumors have a <2% recurrence rate and a 100% 5-year survival. A large body of retrospective data on the role of adjuvant radiation treatment exist but must be interpreted in the context of the completeness of tumor resection. For Masaoka stage I patients that have undergone an R0 resection, there is no evidence to support adjuvant radiation treatment.[80,81]

However, there is debate in the literature about the role of PORT for stage II thymic tumors. The majority of the series have shown either no difference in OS and local recurrence or decreased OS with the use of PORT in completely resected stage II thymomas. A meta-analysis of 13 retrospective studies including resected stage II and III patients showed no difference in recurrence rate with the addition of PORT.[82] Similar results were noted by Kondo and Monden,[79] where PORT was not associated with improvement in recurrence rates in completely resected stage II and III thymic tumors. Interestingly Mangi et al.,[83] reviewed the role of PORT in 45 stage III patients and also noted no significant improvement in disease-specific survival. In contrast, a retrospective review of the Surveillance, Epidemiology, and End Results database did show improvement in cancer-specific survival in stage III patients who received PORT.[84]

More recent data from the Japanese Association for Research on the Thymus (JART) has shown improvement in recurrence-free survival in stage II and III thymic carcinomas but not in thymomas.[85] However, analysis of the ITMIG database did demonstrate an OS benefit with the use of PORT in completely resected stage II and III thymomas.[86]

A relatively older series by Curran et al.[87] revealed a decreased rate of mediastinal recurrence with PORT after complete (53% vs. 0%) and incomplete resection (53% vs. 21%). More recently Ruffini et al.,[75] reported the collaborative European experience in 2,030 thymoma, thymic carcinoma, and neuroendocrine tumors. Adjuvant treatment varied between centers and included radiation only or chemoradiation. A beneficial effect of adjuvant treatment was noted on the overall cohort.

There is less controversy over the use of radiation therapy after incomplete resection and with positive margins. Radiation treatment to a total dose of 66 Gy is recommended in this setting. A boost is delivered to the area of concern, which should be marked by metallic clips at time of surgery or exploration. Recurrence rates are reported to decrease from 60% to 80% down to 21% to 45%.

Port in Thymic Carcinoma

While obtaining a complete resection remains the key treatment component, the data on the role of radiation in thymic carcinoma is more convincing. This could be due to the more aggressive nature of thymic carcinomas; hence dual local treatment may provide a better chance at disease control. Recently, thymic carcinoma data from JART and ITMIG have been published. Data from Europe which is part of the ITMIG database has also been reported separately. All these large database analyses report a beneficial effect of PORT for thymic carcinoma.

In the Japanese cohort 155 stage II and III thymic carcinoma patients were analyzed. Eighty-three percent of the cases had a complete resection and 75 patients received PORT. At 5 years, a significant improvement in recurrence-free survival was noted in the PORT group (stage II 91% vs. 68%. Stage III 51% vs. 26%).[85] The European Society of Thoracic Surgeons (ESTS) thymic workgroup[88] reported their finding on 229 thymic carcinoma patients. In this cohort 69% of the patients had a complete resection. In comparison with surgery alone, surgery followed by PORT was associated with significant improvement in OS.

The ITMIG thymic carcinoma workgroup reported the results in 1,042 patients, of which 78% has stage III or IV disease. An R0 resection was achieved in 61% of the patients. Any radiation treatment in the neoadjuvant or adjuvant setting was associated with a significant improvement in overall, as well as recurrence-free, survival. In this largest series to date, radiation and complete resection were the only prognostic factors associated with survival.

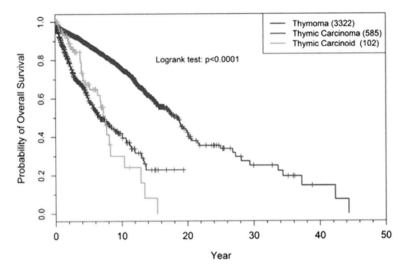

PROGNOSIS

Thymomas are indolent tumors that usually do not shorten life expectancy; however, they can recur and therefore, long-term follow-up is still required after resection. However, thymic carcinoma and neuroendocrine tumors have a more malignant disease course and a review of the ITMIG data revealed a median survival of approximately 20 years for thymoma but significantly shorter for the other histologies (Fig. 166.4).[89]

Median OS in thymic carcinoma is around 7 years and the 5-year cumulative incidence of recurrence (CIR) is 35%. In thymic neuroendocrine tumors the median OS is 7.5 years and the 5-year CIR is 39%.[89] The most common prognostic factor noted in currently available data is the Masaoka–Koga stage. Most studies have reported pathologic stage information, hence the prognostic factor is the stage at the time of resection.

The majority of the recurrences are intrathoracic and reresection has been described and associated with long-term survival. Several small series, and a recent meta-analysis, have shown reasonable OS after re-resection of the recurrent site.[90-93] Most authors have described treatment with neoadjuvant chemotherapy or chemoradiation followed by local resection, if there is no progression of disease. There are, however, significant biases in these studies and the decision to reresect should be made on a case-by-case basis with multidisciplinary tumor board consensus.

REFERENCES

1. Masaoka A, Monden Y, Nakahara K, et al. Follow-up study of thymomas with special reference to their clinical stages. *Cancer* 1981;48(11):2485–2492.
2. de Jong WK, Blaauwgeers JL, Schaapveld M, et al. Thymic epithelial tumours: a population-based study of the incidence, diagnostic procedures and therapy. *Eur J Cancer* 2008;44(1):123–130.
3. Carter BW, Marom EM, Detterbeck FC. Approaching the patient with an anterior mediastinal mass: a guide for clinicians. *J Thorac Oncol* 2014;9(9 suppl 2):S102–S109.
4. Davis RD, Jr., Oldham HN, Jr., Sabiston DC, Jr. Primary cysts and neoplasms of the mediastinum: recent changes in clinical presentation, methods of diagnosis, management, and results. *Ann Thorac Surg* 1987;44(3):229–237.
5. Rubush JL, Gardner IR, Boyd WC, et al. Mediastinal tumors. Review of 186 cases. *J Thorac Cardiovasc Surg* 1973;65(2):216–222.
6. Mullen B, Richardson JD. Primary anterior mediastinal tumors in children and adults. *Ann Thorac Surg* 1986;42(3):338–345.
7. Lewis JE, Wick MR, Scheithauer BW, et al. Thymoma: a clinicopathologic review. *Cancer* 1987;60(11):2727–2743.
8. Shimosato Y. Controversies surrounding the subclassification of thymoma. *Cancer* 1994;74(2):542–544.
9. Hishima T, Fukayama M, Fujisawa M, et al. CD expression in thymic carcinoma. *Am J Pathol* 1994;145(2):268–275.
10. Suster S, Moran CA. Primary thymic epithelial neoplasms showing combined features of thymoma and thymic carcinoma. A clinicopathologic study of 22 cases. *Am J Surg Pathol* 1996;20(12):1469–1480.
11. Kuo TT, Chan JK. Thymic carcinoma arising in thymoma is associated with alterations in immunohistochemical profile. *Am J Surg Pathol* 1998;22(12):1474–1481.
12. Müller-Hermelink HK, Marino M, Palestro G, et al. Immunohistological evidence of cortical and medullary differentiation in thymoma. *Virchows Arch A Pathol Anat Histopathol* 1985;408(2–3):143–161.
13. Müller-Hermelink HK, Marino M, Palestro G. Pathology of thymic epithelial tumors. *Curr Top Pathol* 1986;75:207–268.
14. Müller-Hermelink HK, Marino M, Palestro G. Pathology of thymic epithelial tumors. In: Müller-Hermelink HK, Marino M, Palestro G, eds. *The Human Thymus*. Berlin-Heidelberg: Springer-Verlag; 1986:207–268.
15. Suster S, Moran CA. Thymoma classification. Current status and future trends. *Am J Clin Pathol* 2006;125(4):542–554.
16. Suster S, Moran CA. Thymoma, atypical thymoma, and thymic carcinoma. A novel conceptual approach to the classification of thymic epithelial neoplasms. *Am J Clin Pathol* 1999;111:826–833.
17. *World Health Organization Histological Classification of Tumours: Histological Typing of Tumours of the Thymus.* Berlin-Heidelberg: Springer-Verlag; 1999.
18. Tumours of the thymus. *World Health Organization Classification of Tumours: Pathology and Genetics. Tumours of the Lung, Pleura, Thymus and Heart.* Lyon: IARC Press; 2004:148–151.
19. *WHO Classification of Tumours of the Lung, Pleura, Thymus and Heart. WHO/IARC Classification of Tumours.* 4th ed. 2015.
20. Dadmanesh F, Sekihara T, Rosai J. Histologic typing of thymoma according to the new World Health Organization classification. *Chest Surg Clin N Am* 2001;11:407–420.
21. Detterbeck FC. Clinical value of the WHO classification system of thymoma. *Ann Thorac Surg* 2006;81:2328–2334.
22. Dawson A, Ibrahim NB, Gibbs AR. Observer variation in the histopathological classification of thymoma: correlation with prognosis. *J Clin Pathol* 1994;47:519–523.
23. Rieker RJ, Hoegel J, Morresi-Hauf A, et al. Histologic classification of thymic epithelial tumor: comparison of established classification schemes. *Int J Cancer* 2002;98:900–906.
24. Marx A, Ströbel P, Badve SS, et al. ITMIG consensus statement on the use of the WHO histological classification of thymoma and thymic carcinoma: refined definitions, histological criteria, and reporting. *J Thorac Oncol* 2014;9(5):596–611.
25. Mokhtar N, Hsu SM, Lad RP, et al. Thymoma: lymphoid and epithelial components mirror the phenotype of normal thymus. *Hum Pathol* 1984;15:378–384.
26. Nonaka D, Henley JD, Chiriboga L, et al. Diagnostic utility of thymic epithelial markers CD205 (DEC205) and Foxn1 in thymic epithelial neoplasms. *Am J Surg Pathol* 2007;31:1038–1044.
27. Ahmad U, Yao X, Detterbeck F, et al. Thymic carcinoma outcomes and prognosis: results of an international analysis. *J Thorac Cardiovasc Surg* 2015;149(1):95–100.
28. Zettl A, Ströbel P, Wagner K, et al. Recurrent genetic aberrations in thymoma and thymic carcinoma. *Am J Pathol* 2000;157(1):257–266.
29. Inoue M, Starostik P, Zettl A, et al. Correlating genetic aberrations with World Health Organization-defined histology and stage across the spectrum of thymomas. *Cancer Res* 2003;63(13):3708–3715.
30. Girard N, Shen R, Guo T, et al. Comprehensive genomic analysis reveals clinically relevant molecular distinctions between thymic carcinomas and thymomas. *Clin Cancer Res* 2009;15(22):6790–6799.
31. Penzel R, Hoegel J, Schmitz W, et al. Clusters of chromosomal imbalances in thymic epithelial tumours are associated with the WHO classification and the staging system according to Masaoka. *Int J Cancer* 2003;105(4):494–498.

32. Lee GY, Yang WI, Jeung HC, et al. Genome-wide genetic aberrations of thymoma using cDNA microarray based comparative genomic hybridization. *BMC Genomics* 2007;8:305.

33. Petrini I, Wang Y, Zucali PA, et al. Copy number aberrations of genes regulating normal thymus development in thymic epithelial tumors. *Clin Cancer Res* 2013;19(8):1960–1971.

34. Chen C, Yin N, Yin B, et al. DNA methylation in thoracic neoplasms. *Cancer Lett* 2011;301(1):7–16.

35. Suzuki M, Chen H, Shigematsu H, et al. Aberrant methylation: common in thymic carcinomas, rare in thymomas. *Oncol Rep* 2005;14(6):1621–1624.

36. Mokhtar M, Kondo K, Namura T, et al. Methylation and expression profiles of MGMT gene in thymic epithelial tumors. *Lung Cancer* 2014;83(2):279–287.

37. Engels EA. Epidemiology of thymoma and associated malignancies. *J Thorac Oncol* 2010;5(10 suppl 4):S260–S265.

38. Detterbeck FC, Parsons AM. Thymic tumors. *Ann Thorac Surg* 2004;77(5):1860–1869.

39. Zakowski MF, Huang J, Bramlage MP. The role of fine needle aspiration cytology in the diagnosis and management of thymic neoplasia. *J Thorac Oncol* 2010;5(10 suppl 4):S281–S285.

40. Kattach H, Hasan S, Clelland C, et al. Seeding of stage I thymoma into the chest wall 12 years after needle biopsy. *Ann Thorac Surg* 2005;79(1):323–324.

41. Fujiwara K, Matsumura A, Tanaka H, et al. [Needle tract implantation of thymoma after transthoracic needle biopsy]. *Kyobu Geka* 2003;56(6):448–451.

42. Nagasaka T, Nakashima N, Nunome H. Needle tract implantation of thymoma after transthoracic needle biopsy. *J Clin Pathol* 1993;46(3):278–279.

43. Marchevsky A, Marx A, Ströbel P, et al. Policies and reporting guidelines for small biopsy specimens of mediastinal masses. *J Thorac Oncol* 2011;6(7 suppl 3).S1724–S1729.

44. McErlean A, Huang J, Zabor EC, et al. Ginsberg MS Distinguishing benign thymic lesions from early-stage thymic malignancies on computed tomography. *J Thorac Oncol* 2013;8(7):967–973.

45. Inaoka T, Takahashi K, Mineta M, et al. Thymic hyperplasia and thymus gland tumors: differentiation with chemical shift MR imaging. *Radiology* 2007;243(3):869–876.

46. Hayes SA, Huang J, Plodkowski AJ, et al. Preoperative computed tomography findings predict surgical resectability of thymoma. *J Thorac Oncol* 2014;9(7):1023–1030.

47. Treglia G, Sadeghi R, Giovanella L, et al. Is (18)F-FDG PET useful in predicting the WHO grade of malignancy in thymic epithelial tumors? A meta-analysis. *Lung Cancer* 2014;86(1):5–13.

48. Filosso PL, Ruffini E, Lausi PO, et al. Historical perspectives: The evolution of the thymic epithelial tumors staging system. *Lung Cancer* 2014;83(2):126–132.

49. Koga K, Matsuno Y, Noguchi M, et al. A review of 79 thymomas: modification of staging system and reappraisal of conventional division into invasive and non-invasive thymoma. *Pathol Int* 1994;44(5):359–367.

50. Kondo K, Monden Y. Lymphogenous and hematogenous metastasis of thymic epithelial tumors. *Ann Thorac Surg* 2003;76(6):1859–1864.

51. Detterbeck FC, Nicholson AG, Kondo K, et al. The Masaoka-Koga stage classification for thymic malignancies: clarification and definition of terms. *J Thorac Oncol* 2011;6(7 suppl 3):S1710–S1716.

52. Detterbeck FC, Stratton K, Giroux D, et al.; Members of the Advisory Boards.; Participating Institutions of the Thymic Domain. The IASLC/ITMIG Thymic Epithelial Tumors Staging Project: proposal for an evidence-based stage classification system for the forthcoming (8th) edition of the TNM classification of malignant tumors. *J Thorac Oncol* 2014;9(9 suppl 2):S65–S72.

53. Nicholson AG, Detterbeck FC, Marino M, et al.; Staging and Prognostic Factors Committee; Members of the Advisory Boards; Participating Institutions of the Thymic Domain. The IASLC/ITMIG Thymic Epithelial Tumors Staging Project: proposals for the T Component for the forthcoming (8th) edition of the TNM classification of malignant tumors. *J Thorac Oncol* 2014;9(9 suppl 2):S73–S80.

54. Kondo K, Van Schil P, Detterbeck FC, et al.; Staging and Prognostic Factors Committee; Members of the Advisory Boards; Participating Institutions of the Thymic Domain. The IASLC/ITMIG Thymic Epithelial Tumors Staging Project: proposals for the N and M components for the forthcoming (8th) edition of the TNM classification of malignant tumors. *J Thorac Oncol* 2014;9(9 suppl 2):S81–S87.

55. Burt BM, Yao X, Shrager J, et al. Determinants of complete resection of thymoma by minimally invasive and open thymectomy: analysis of an international registry. *J Thorac Oncol* 2017;12(1):129–136.

56. Friedant AJ, Handorf EA, Su S, et al. Minimally invasive versus open thymectomy for thymic malignancies: Systematic review and meta-analysis. *J Thorac Oncol* 2016;11(1):30–38.

57. Nakagawa K, Yokoi K, Nakajima J, et al. Is thymomectomy alone appropriate for stage I (T1N0M0) thymoma? results of a propensity-score analysis. *Ann Thorac Surg* 2016;101(2):520–526.

58. Gu Z, Fu J, Shen Y, et al.; Members of the Chinese Alliance for Research in Thymomas. Thymectomy versus tumor resection for early-stage thymic malignancies: a Chinese Alliance for Research in Thymomas retrospective database analysis. *J Thorac Dis* 2016;8(4):680–686.

59. The International Thymic Malignancy Interest Group. https://www.itmig.org

60. Loehrer PJ, Sr., Kim K, Aisner SC, et al. Cisplatin plus doxorubicin plus cyclophosphamide in metastatic or recurrent thymoma: final results of an intergroup trial. The Eastern Cooperative Oncology Group, Southwest Oncology Group, and Southeastern Cancer Study Group. *J Clin Oncol* 1994;12:1164–1168.

61. Giaccone G, Ardizzoni A, Kirkpatrick A, et al. Cisplatin and etoposide combination chemotherapy for locally advanced or metastatic thymoma. A phase II study of the European Organization for Research and Treatment of Cancer Lung Cancer Cooperative Group. *J Clin Oncol* 1996;14:814–820.

62. Kim ES, Putnam JB, Komaki R, et al. Phase II study of a multidisciplinary approach with induction chemotherapy, followed by surgical resection, radiation therapy, and consolidation chemotherapy for unresectable malignant thymomas: final report. *Lung Cancer* 2004;44:369–379.

63. Kunitoh H, Tamura T, Shibata T, et al.; JCOG Lung Cancer Study Group. A phase II trial of dose-dense chemotherapy, followed by surgical resection and/or thoracic radiotherapy, in locally advanced thymoma: report of a Japan Clinical Oncology Group trial (JCOG 9606). *Br J Cancer* 2010;103:6–11.

64. Lucchi M, Melfi F, Dini P, et al. Neoadjuvant chemotherapy for stage III and IVA thymomas: a single-institution experience with a long follow-up. *J Thorac Oncol* 2006;1:308–313.

65. Yamada Y, Yoshino I, Nakajima J, et al.; Japanese Association for Research of the Thymus. Surgical outcomes of patients with stage III thymoma in the Japanese Nationwide Database. *Ann Thorac Surg* 2015;100:961–967.

66. Leuzzi G, Rocco G, Ruffini E, et al.; ESTS Thymic Working Group. Multimodality therapy for locally advanced thymomas: a propensity score-matched cohort study from the European Society of Thoracic Surgeons Database. *J Thorac Cardiovasc Surg* 2016;151:47–57.

67. Rusch VW, Giroux DJ, Kraut MJ, et al. Induction chemoradiation and surgical resection for superior sulcus non-small-cell lung carcinomas: long-term results of Southwest Oncology Group Trial 9416 (Intergroup Trial 0160). *J Clin Oncol* 2007;25:313–318.

68. van Hagen P, Hulshof MC, van Lanschot JJ, et al.; CROSS Group. Preoperative chemoradiotherapy for esophageal or junctional cancer. *N Engl J Med* 2012;366:2074–2084.

69. Loehrer PJ, Sr., Chen M, Kim K, et al. Cisplatin, doxorubicin, and cyclophosphamide plus thoracic radiation therapy for limited-stage unresectable thymoma: an intergroup trial. *J Clin Oncol* 1997;15:3093–3099.

70. Wright CD, Choi NC, Wain JC, et al. Induction chemoradiotherapy followed by resection for locally advanced Masaoka stage III and IVA thymic tumors. *Ann Thorac Surg* 2008;85:385–389.

71. Korst RJ, Bezjak A, Blackmon S, et al. Neoadjuvant chemoradiotherapy for locally advanced thymic tumors: a phase II, multi-institutional clinical trial. *J Thorac Cardiovasc Surg* 2014;147:36–44.

72. Yagi K, Hirata T, Fukuse T, et al. Surgical treatment for invasive thymoma, especially when the superior vena cava is invaded. *Ann Thorac Surg* 1996;61:521–524.

73. Ribet M, Voisin C, Gosselin B, et al. [Lympho-epithelial thymoma. Anatomo-clinical and therapeutic study of 113 cases]. *Rev Mal Respir* 1988;5:53–60.

74. Akaogi E, Ohara K, Mitsui K, et al. Preoperative radiotherapy and surgery for advanced thymoma with invasion to the great vessels. *J Surg Oncol* 1996;63:17–22.

75. Ruffini E, Detterbeck F, Van Raemdonck D, et al.; European Association of Thoracic Surgeons (ESTS) Thymic Working Group. Tumours of the thymus: a cohort study of prognostic factors from the European Society of Thoracic Surgeons database. *Eur J Cardiothorac Surg* 2014;46(3):361–368.

76. Yellin A, Simansky DA, Ben-Avi R, et al. Resection and heated pleural chemoperfusion in patients with thymic epithelial malignant disease and pleural spread: a single-institution experience. *J Thorac Cardiovasc Surg* 2013;145:83–87.

77. Belcher E, Hardwick T, Lal R, et al. Induction chemotherapy, cytoreductive surgery and intraoperative hyperthermic pleural irrigation in patients with stage IVA thymoma. *Interact Cardiovasc Thorac Surg* 2011;12:744–747.

78. Ruffini E, Van Raemdonck D, Detterbeck F, et al.; European Society of Thoracic Surgeons Thymic Questionnaire Working Group. Management of thymic tumors: a survey of current practice among members of the European Society of Thoracic Surgeons. *J Thorac Oncol* 2011;6(3):614–623.

79. Kondo K, Monden Y. Therapy for thymic epithelial tumors: a clinical study of 1,320 patients from Japan. *Ann Thorac Surg* 2003;76(3):878–884.

80. Singhal S, Shrager JB, Rosenthal DI, et al. Comparison of stages I-II thymoma treated by complete resection with or without adjuvant radiation. *Ann Thorac Surg* 2003;76(5):1635–1641.

81. Utsumi T, Shiono H, Kadota Y, et al. Postoperative radiation therapy after complete resection of thymoma has little impact on survival. *Cancer* 2009;115(23):5413–5420.

82. Korst RJ, Kansler AL, Christos PJ, et al. Adjuvant radiotherapy for thymic epithelial tumors: a systematic review and meta-analysis. *Ann Thorac Surg* 2009;87(5):1641–1647.

83. Mangi AA, Wain JC, Donahue DM, et al. Adjuvant radiation of stage III thymoma: is it necessary? *Ann Thorac Surg* 2005;79(6):1834–1839.

84. Weksler B, Shende M, Nason KS, et al. The role of adjuvant radiation therapy for resected stage III thymoma: a population-based study. *Ann Thorac Surg* 2012;93(6):1822–1828.

85. Omasa M, Date H, Sozu T, et al.; Japanese Association for Research on the Thymus. Postoperative radiotherapy is effective for thymic carcinoma but not for thymoma in stage II and III thymic epithelial tumors: the Japanese Association for Research on the Thymus Database Study. *Cancer* 2015;121(7):1008–1016.

86. Rimner A, Yao X, Huang J, et al. Postoperative radiation therapy is associated with longer overall survival in completely resected stage II and III thymoma-an analysis of the international thymic malignancies interest group retrospective database. *J Thorac Oncol* 2016;11(10):1785–1792.

87. Curran WJ, Jr., Kornstein MJ, Brooks JJ, et al. Invasive thymoma: the role of mediastinal irradiation following complete or incomplete surgical resection. *J Clin Oncol* 1988;6(11):1722–1727.

88. Ruffini E, Detterbeck F, Van Raemdonck D, et al.; European Society of Thoracic Surgeons Thymic Working Group. Thymic carcinoma: a cohort study of

patients from the European society of thoracic surgeons database. *J Thorac Oncol* 2014;9(4):541–548.

89. Huang J, Ahmad U, Antonicelli A, et al.; International Thymic Malignancy Interest Group International Database Committee and Contributors. Development of the international thymic malignancy interest group international database: an unprecedented resource for the study of a rare group of tumors. *J Thorac Oncol* 2014;9(10):1573–1578.

90. Hamaji M, Allen MS, Cassivi SD, et al. The role of surgical management in recurrent thymic tumors. *Ann Thorac Surg* 2012;94(1):247–254.

91. Bott MJ, Wang H, Travis W, et al. Management and outcomes of relapse after treatment for thymoma and thymic carcinoma. *Ann Thorac Surg* 2011;92(6):1984–1991.

92. Lucchi M, Davini F, Ricciardi R, et al. Management of pleural recurrence after curative resection of thymoma. *J Thorac Cardiovasc Surg* 2009;137(5):1185–1189.

93. Hamaji M, Ali SO, Burt BM. A meta-analysis of surgical versus nonsurgical management of recurrent thymoma. *Ann Thorac Surg* 2014;98(2):748–755.

94. Macchiarini P, Chella A, Ducci F, et al. Neoadjuvant chemotherapy, surgery, and postoperative radiation therapy for invasive thymoma. *Cancer* 1991;68:706–713.

95. Rea F, Sartori F, Loy M, et al. Chemotherapy and operation for invasive thymoma. *J Thorac Cardiovasc Surg* 1993;106:543–549.

96. Berruti A, Borasio P, Roncari A, et al. Neoadjuvant chemotherapy with adriamycin, cisplatin, vincristine and cyclophosphamide (ADOC) in invasive thymomas: results in six patients. *Ann Oncol* 1993;4:429–431.

97. Venuta F, Rendina EA, Pescarmona EO, et al. Multimodality treatment of thymoma: a prospective study. *Ann Thorac Surg* 1997;64:1585–1591.

98. Yokoi K, Matsuguma H, Nakahara R, et al. Multidisciplinary treatment for advanced invasive thymoma with cisplatin, doxorubicin, and methylprednisolone. *J Thorac Oncol* 2007;2:73–78.

99. Bretti S, Berruti A, Loddo C, et al.; Piemonte Oncology Network. Multimodal management of stages III-IVa malignant thymoma. *Lung Cancer* 2004;44:69–77.

167

Benign Lymph Node Disease Involving the Mediastinum

Jason Michael Long

Lymphadenopathy is a common radiologic finding in many thoracic diseases and may be caused by a variety of infectious, inflammatory, and neoplastic conditions. The most common infections that result in thoracic lymphadenopathy are tuberculosis (TB) and fungal disease (primarily histoplasmosis and coccidioidomycosis). Sarcoidosis is a particularly frequent cause of this condition in young adults. Other causes include silicosis, drug reactions, amyloidosis, heart failure, Castleman disease (CD), and chronic obstructive pulmonary disease (COPD). This chapter aims to describe the patterns of mediastinal and lymphadenopathy found in benign diseases.

Lymphadenopathy is defined as an abnormality in lymph node size, density, and/or number. For the diagnosis of pathologically enlarged lymph nodes, information about normal node size is required. The generally accepted size criterion for mediastinal lymph node enlargement is greater than 10 mm along the short axis.[1,2] Mediastinal lymph nodes are located in the anterior, middle, and posterior mediastinal compartments. Most of the mediastinal nodes are in close approximation to the left innominate vein, the anterior surface of the trachea, circumference of the main bronchi, and inferior and to the left of the aortic arch. Mediastinal lymphadenopathy is most commonly seen within the middle (visceral) compartment of the mediastinum in the right lower paratracheal, subcarinal, and aortopulmonary window regions. It is seen less often in the anterior and posterior mediastinal compartments.

Computed tomography (CT) is the imaging modality of choice to evaluate mediastinal lymphadenopathy. PET/CT imaging is not indicated for benign disease. In general, CT findings in thoracic lymphadenopathy include loss of normal ovoid shape, increased size of individual nodes, hypo- or hyperdensity in lymph nodes, invasion of mediastinal fat, coalescence of adjacent nodes, and obliteration of the mediastinal fat.[1,2] A normal node tends to have a uniform appearance and the presence of fat that often, but does not always, indicates benignity. Malignant nodes, on the other hand, have irregular borders and tend to be more round than elongated.[3] Additionally, heterogeneous enhancement of an enlarged node is also likely to represent malignancy. As mentioned above, the generally accepted size criterion for mediastinal lymph node enlargement is >10 mm along the short axis,[1,2] however other authors have described station-specific size criteria: station 7, 12 mm; station 4 and 10R, 10 mm; and other regions 8 mm.[1,2]

The evaluation of mediastinal lymphadenopathy may also be obscured by the presence of anthracosis depending on geographical region and rural versus urban location. Anthracosis (*anthrac*-meaning coal, carbon + *-osis* meaning condition) is defined as the asymptomatic accumulation of carbon in the lungs due to repeated exposure to air pollution or inhalation of smoke or coal dust particles.[4] It may be seen as a superficial black discoloration or scattered foci of black spots in the lung parenchyma and is characterized by alterations of the lung parenchyma, bronchioles, and lymphatic system resulting in chronic lymphadenopathy and nodal enlargement.[4] Kirchner et al.[5] compared CT findings of patients with enlarged lymph nodes due to anthracosis with malignant lymph nodes confirmed pathologically by EBUS-TBNA. The authors found that malignant lymph nodes showed significantly greater axis diameters, higher frequency of ill-defined contours, contrast enhancement, and necrosis.[5] Anthracotic nodes were more often associated with calcifications. Both populations of nodes were most often oval in shape and showed confluence.[5]

Normal and inflammatory lymph nodes in the mediastinum are rubbery and pearly white to gray; those affected by anthracosis are typically grayish-black while those involved with metastatic disease from the lung or other solid tumors are often hard, and frequently have a white appearance. The gross appearance of a lymphomatous node is gray and firm, though not hard. Granulomatous lymph nodes, as in sarcoidosis, are typically yellow in color and hard. When a lymph node that is suspected of harboring granulomatous disease is biopsied, stains for microorganisms should be performed and a portion of the material biopsied should be sent for mycobacterial and fungal culture. In addition, consideration should be given to an examination of the biopsy material with polarized light, especially if a history of silica exposure has been obtained.

DIAGNOSIS/BIOSPY TECHNIQUES

Once imaging has demonstrated enlarged mediastinal lymphadenopathy, a tissue diagnosis should be obtained. There are multiple methods to sample and biopsy mediastinal lymph nodes which include minimally invasive modalities such as bronchoscopy with transtracheal and transbronchial needle aspiration (TBNA) biopsy and more invasive modalities that include mediastinoscopy and thoracoscopy. TBNA is the aspiration of material using a needle that is passed through the endobronchial wall. Bronchoscopy is used to direct the operator to the target lesion. The needle is then passed through the working channel of the bronchoscope, through the bronchial wall and material is aspirated for histological analysis. It can be performed blindly during conventional white light bronchoscopy or under image-guidance using a bronchoscope with endobronchial ultrasound or electromagnetic navigational capability (EBUS-TBN; EMN-TBNA). TBNA has been most extensively employed in the diagnosis and staging of lung cancer, although has been increasingly applied to the diagnosis of benign pathology such as sarcoidosis and infection. In most circumstances, TBNA in this setting is done under ultrasound guidance (EBUS-TBNA) and can access more lymph node stations (2, 3, 4, 7, 10, 11) than mediastinoscopy (2, 3, 4, and 7). EBUS-TBNA has been found to be accurate when it is used to sample suspicious mediastinal lymph nodes (up to 96%) in the mediastinum when staging lung cancer.[6–9] EBUS-TBNA for sampling of intrathoracic lymph nodes and peribronchial tissues has also become the standard of care in diagnosing intrathoracic malignancies, sarcoidosis, and other disorders, because it is safe and cost effective.[9–13] If there is inadequate sample or doubt remains regarding the suspected diagnosis, the surgeon should perform a mediastinoscopy or staging thoracoscopy to ensure adequate sample. Less data are available for EBUS-TBNA of mediastinal lymphadenopathy when infectious causes are suspected and may have less diagnostic value, in which case mediastinoscopy or diagnostic thoracoscopy is recommended.[14]

MEDIASTINAL GRANULOMATOUS DISEASE

While mediastinal lymphadenopathy is more commonly associated with malignancy, many benign diseases can cause enlargement of mediastinal lymph nodes. Granulomatous disease is the most common etiology of benign lymphadenopathy and can be caused by a variety of diseases including TB, fungal disease (histoplasmosis and coccidioidomycosis), sarcoidosis, silicosis, drug reactions, amyloidosis, heart failure, CD, and COPD. Please refer to the table of benign causes of mediastinal lymphadenopathy listed in Table 167.1. A granuloma is a focal, compact collection of inflammatory cells in which mononuclear cells predominate.[15] They usually form in response to the persistence of a nondegradable product. Normally, granulomas are the result of protective mechanisms and form when acute inflammatory processes cannot destroy invading agents. Granulomas can be classified either as necrotizing (caseating), nonnecrotizing (noncaseating), or foreign body, as illustrated in Figure 167.1. A nonnecrotizing granuloma lacks central necrosis and arises due to a reaction to foreign material. Sarcoidosis is a well-known cause of nonnecrotizing granulomas. In contrast, a necrotizing granuloma is characterized by central necrosis due to dead and dying macrophages. These types of granulomas arise due to processes such as TB and fungal infections. Radiographically,

TABLE 167.1 Benign Mediastinal Lymphadenopathies

  I. Mediastinal granulomatous disease
      Tuberculosis
      Fungal infection
      Sarcoidosis
      Silicosis
      Wegener granulomatosis
  II. Castleman disease
  III. Others
      Systemic lupus erythematosus
      Infectious mononucleosis
      Reactive lymph node hyperplasia
      Amyloidosis
      HIV–associated *Pneumocystis carinii*

Adapted from Machevsky MA, Kaneko M. *Surgical Pathology of the Mediastinum.* New York: Raven Press; 1984: 174. With permission.

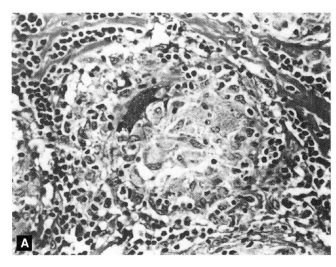
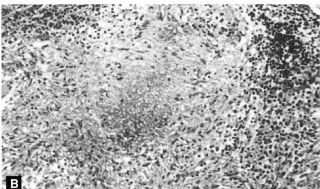
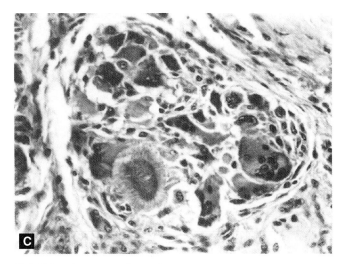

FIGURE 167.1 Types of granulomatous reactions. **A:** Nonnecrotizing epithelioid granuloma of sarcoid. In the center of the granuloma are epithelioid cells that contain abundant eosinophilic cytoplasm. Epithelioid cells are modified macrophages. Around the granulomas are small dark lymphocytes and bands of collagen. **B:** A necrotizing granuloma of tuberculosis. In the center of the granuloma is an area of necrosis surrounded by epithelioid cells. Some giant cells are present near the left border. **C:** A foreign body granuloma of gout. This granuloma shows many foreign body–type giant cells with a few epithelioid cells. A crystal of uric acid is present (*lower left*) in the granuloma.

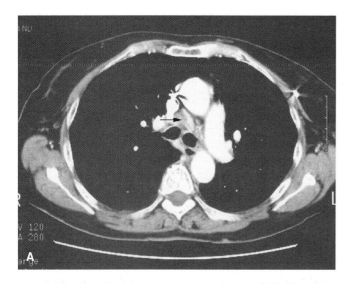

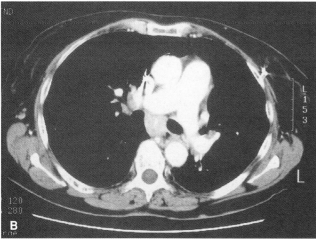

FIGURE 167.2 CT scans demonstrating mediastinal lymphadenopathy secondary to granulomatous disease. **A:** Precarinal mediastinal lymphadenopathy. The lymph node measures 2.5 cm in short-axis diameter. **B:** Subcarinal mediastinal lymphadenopathy. The lymph node measures 2 cm in short-axis diameter.

granulomas are solid lesions, as illustrated in Figure 167.2. Slightly less than half contain calcium. In addition, areas of necrosis may be evident within a granuloma.

TUBERCULOSIS

TB is an airborne infectious disease caused by *Mycobacterium tuberculosis*. It can be divided into primary and postprimary TB, based on the absence or presence of prior infection and acquired specific immunity. Primary TB is most commonly seen in children. The Ghon focus, or the initial focus of infection, tends to be in the middle and lower lobes of the lung—although any lobe can be affected. Mycobacteria commonly spread to regional lymph nodes via the bloodstream and to other regions of the body. The Ghon focus plus affected lymph nodes is termed the "Ghon complex." This complex may enlarge as the disease progresses but does eventually undergo a healing process resulting in a visible parenchymal scar (that may be calcified) along with enlarged or calcified nodes in the hilum or mediastinum. Lymphadenopathy is the main feature of primary TB and is seen in 40% of adult cases and 90% to 95% of pediatric cases.[16] On CT, the

most suggestive aspect of primary TB is the presence of enlarged lymph nodes, greater than 2 cm in diameter, with hypodense centers secondary to caseous necrosis.[17] Postprimary TB is a progressive condition that is rarely associated with lymphadenopathy. It usually presents as parenchymal, airway, and pleural involvement. Hilar and mediastinal lymphadenopathy occur in only approximately 5% of immunocompetent patients.

Tuberculous granulomas share many features with granulomas secondary to fungal disease. They may be distinguished from other granulomas by staining positive for acid-fast bacilli. In addition, tuberculous granulomas typically feature caseating (coagulative) necrosis. In acute tuberculous lesions, suppuration is a common finding whereas later on, Langerhans-type giant cells and caseating necrosis may be predominant features. In older lesions, fibrosis or calcification may be present.[18]

FUNGAL INFECTION

Fungal infections, most notably histoplasmosis and pulmonary coccidioidomycosis, can cause lymph node enlargement. Histoplasmosis is a systemic infection that results from the inhalation of airborne spores of *Histoplasma capsulatum*, an organism endemic to the Ohio and Mississippi river valleys of the United States. Edwards and colleagues[7] have estimated that more than 80% of the population in these regions is sensitized to the fungus and that approximately 22% of the US population has been infected by it. Infection with *H. capsulatum* is usually asymptomatic and inconsequential, but in some individuals, acute histoplasmosis may cause malaise, fever, and cough. A few patients with acute histoplasmosis develop symptomatic mediastinal adenitis, often in the subcarinal or right paratracheal area, with characteristic central chest pain worsened by inspiration. Acute mediastinal adenitis is a starting point for subsequent mediastinal complications including mediastinal granulomas and fibrosing mediastinitis. Mediastinal granulomas may form as a cluster of necrotic lymph nodes which coalesce to form a semiliquid conglomerate mass composed of semiliquid necrotic material with a consistency similar to toothpaste. The nodal mass may be tense from high pressure and can compress mediastinal structures. Granulomas may occur early (weeks to months) or may remain dormant for long periods or years before becoming symptomatic. In rare cases, enlarged or inflamed nodes may impinge on airways, esophagus, or the superior vena cava (SVC). The majority of people exposed to the fungus are asymptomatic. Diagnosis is made by demonstrating fungi on histopathology, cytopathology, or cultures. The characteristic pathologic feature on histologic examination is the presence of granulomas, caseating or noncaseating, indicative of the immune system's attempt to contain the infection. Cultures may take up to 6 weeks to grow whereas cytology or histopathology can lead to rapid diagnosis.[19] Antigen detection in the urine and serum has transformed the diagnosis of histoplasmosis providing a rapid and noninvasive means of diagnosis that is highly sensitive.[19] In addition, antibody testing remains useful in many patients and should be considered a routine test for the diagnosis.[19] Medical therapy with amphotericin or Itraconazole is reserved for patients with acute infection which can range from acute pulmonary histoplasmosis, which is self-limiting, to disseminated disease.

Fibrosing mediastinitis is the most serious late complication of histoplasmosis infection. Although rare, it is the most common nonmalignant cause of mediastinal compression syndromes.[20] According to Mathisen and Grillo,[21] fibrosing mediastinitis is a well-documented sequela of exposure to *H. capsulatum*. Fibrosing mediastinitis is characterized by a solid, dense, and invasive fibrotic mass, which causes fusion of adjacent tissue planes and obstructs pulmonary vasculature, the SVC, or the airways.[22,23] Vascular and airway occlusion progress slowly (~1 mm/year), however symptoms present acutely after vascular narrowing reaches a threshold sufficient to cause infarction or SVC syndrome. When infection with *H. capsulatum* reaches this stage, it can have life-threatening implications for which no medical therapy is effective and surgical therapy is only palliative. Resection of fibrous tissues, however, is considered a last resort given the high risk of hemorrhage, damage to involved mediastinal structures, and intraoperative mortality.[23] Hammoud et al.[24] provide a nice comprehensive review of the surgical management of the pulmonary sequelae of histoplasmosis.

Coccidioidomycosis is a systemic fungal infection caused by the inhalation of arthrospores of *Coccidioides* species. *Coccidioides immitis* and *Coccidioides posadasii* reside in the soil of certain parts of central and southern California, the low deserts of Arizona, southeastern New Mexico, western Texas, and several other areas of the southwestern United States, Mexico, Central and South America.[25] Approximately 150,000 infections occur annually in the United States, 50,000 produce an illness warranting medical attention, 10,000 to 20,000 are diagnosed and reported, 2,000 to 3,000 produce pulmonary sequelae, 600 to 1,000 spread hematogenously from the lungs to other parts of the body, and 160 result in death.[25] It can be divided into acute, disseminated, and chronic forms. Sixty percent of acutely infected people are either asymptomatic or manifest upper respiratory tract symptoms. Others present with lower respiratory tract symptoms and 40% of patients presents with radiographic evidence of pulmonary infiltrates, pleural effusion, and/or mediastinal and hilar adenopathy.[26] Differences in disease severity are thought to be the consequence of differences in the immunologic responses to infection among individuals.[25] Serologic tests for antibodies against coccidioidomycosis are generally available from clinical laboratories and any positive result for anticoccidioidal antibodies is usually associated with recent or active infection. Diagnosis may also be obtained by cultures of sputum or bronchoscopic specimens. A lymph node biopsy obtained by endobronchial ultrasound with FNA may be required to rule out other causes of adenopathy, and a portion of the specimen should be sent for culture. While treatment with antifungal agents is indicated for severe primary infection or for patients in high-risk groups (HIV-positive patients, pregnant women, transplant patients, patients with disseminated disease), most patients recover without therapy.

While pulmonary infection with *Blastomyces* follows the inhalation of fungal conidia, *Blastomyces dermatitidis*, as its name implies, also affects the skin, causing papules that may ulcerate. It is a less common cause of mediastinal lymphadenopathy than *H. capsulatum* and, according to Lagerstrom and colleagues, is a rare cause of mediastinal fibrosis.[27]

SARCOIDOSIS

Sarcoidosis is a multisystem, inflammatory disorder characterized by noncaseating granulomas that can infiltrate almost any organ but, most commonly, involves the lungs. It most often occurs in adulthood with the highest incidence among African Americans in the United States. The disease affects females twice as often as males and African Americans 10 times more often than Caucasians. It usually manifests in the third though fifth decades of life.

Sarcoidosis most often presents with hilar lymphadenopathy, pulmonary infiltration, and eye and skin lesions. The American Thoracic Society criteria for the diagnosis of pulmonary sarcoidosis includes (1) the presence of a consistent clinical and radiographic picture; (2) the

TABLE 167.2 Manifestations of Sarcoidosis

System	% Involvement	Manifestation
Respiratory	90	Interstitial lung disease
Lymphatic	90	Hilar/mediastinal/peripheral lymphadenopathy
Cardiac	5–76	Rhythm, conduction, repolarization abnormalities, cardiomyopathy
Integumentary	25	Erythema nodosum, plaques, nodules
Ophthalmic	25	Uveitis
Nervous	5	Bell palsy
Renal	—	Increased production of vitamin D leads to hypercalcemia, hypercalciuria
Hepatic	40–70	Asymptomatic, hepatomegaly

Adapted from Newman LS, Rose CS, Maier LA. Sarcoidosis. *N Engl J Med* 1997;336: 1224–1234. Copyright © 1997 Massachusetts Medical Society. Reprinted with permission from Massachusetts Medical Society.

demonstration of noncaseating granulomas on biopsy; and (3) exclusion of other conditions that can produce granulomatous inflammation, including infectious, autoimmune disorders, and inhalational diseases.[28] The cause of sarcoidosis remains unknown. However, there is much evidence to support the hypothesis that the disease develops when a genetically susceptible individual is exposed to organic and inorganic antigens that trigger an immune response leading to granuloma formation.[29] Infectious causes, including *Mycobacterium tuberculosis* transcriptomes and *Propionibacterium acnes*, infection may play a role in the hyperexaggerated immune response triggering the development of sarcoidosis.[29] A hallmark feature in the immunological response is the presence of CD4+ T cells that interact with antigen-presenting complexes to instigate granuloma formation within tissues.[29] The clinical presentation ranges from an incidental chest radiographic finding in an asymptomatic patient to chronic progressive organ dysfunction. The vast majority of patients (~90%) have mediastinopulmonary involvement, however any organ may be affected and therefore patients may present with any symptom attributable to that organ.[30] A persistent cough is the most frequent respiratory symptom at onset. Subacute dyspnea, sometimes accompanied by wheezing or atypical thoracic pain may also be the initial symptom. Fatigue is also very common and may be severe. Other manifestations of sarcoidosis are listed in Table 167.2.

Chest imaging provides crucial information for the diagnosis of sarcoidosis. Identification of the lung and lymph node involvement is the basis of the Scadding classification and provides information on prognosis: stage 0 (normal), stage 1 (bilateral hilar lymphadenopathy), stage 2 (bilateral hilar lymphadenopathy accompanied by pulmonary infiltrates), stage 3 (pulmonary infiltrates without bilateral hilar lymphadenopathy), and stage 4 (pulmonary fibrosis). Lymphadenopathy is hilar and mediastinal, satellite of the tracheobronchial tree, symmetrical, voluminous, and noncompressive.[30] CT is indicated in case of atypical clinical or radiographic findings, clinical suspicious of the disease despite normal chest radiography, and complications, airflow limitation or pulmonary hypertension. Valeyre et al.[30] provide an excellent review of CT findings associated with sarcoidosis as well as a logical diagnostic approach.

Several diagnostic modalities are available via bronchoscopy to sample hilar and mediastinal lymphadenopathy associated with sarcoidosis including macroscopic examination of the airway, endobronchial biopsy, transbronchial lung biopsy, TBNA, and bronchoalveolar lavage. Over the last few years, needle aspiration of intrathoracic lymph nodes has gained significant interest for the diagnosis of sarcoidosis.[31–35] The GRANULOMA randomized multicenter international trial recently compared endosonography (TBNA or EUS) to conventional bronchoscopy for the detection of granulomas in patients with presumed early stage sarcoidosis.[35] Endosonography had a superior diagnostic performance (80% vs. 53%) in stage 1 versus stage 2 disease. A single positive biopsy from the largest mediastinal or hilar lymph node accessible and 3 to 5 passes is usually sufficient.[13,30] It is not known why some sarcoidosis patients recover and others progress. Even after apparent recovery, a small proportion of patients may relapse months to years later. Factors associated with worse prognosis include older age at time of diagnosis, African-American race, duration of illness greater than 6 months, pulmonary opacities, splenomegaly, lupus pernio, and number of organs involved. A more favorable prognosis has been found in patients with Löfgren syndrome—an acute form of sarcoidosis characterized by erythema nodosum, bilateral hilar lymphadenopathy, and polyarthralgia or polyarthritis. The disease can spontaneously resolve without treatment and some patients with sarcoidosis are disabled by their illness. The current paradigm for institution of therapy is based upon the presence of organ dysfunction. Oral corticosteroids remain the first-line therapy in most cases. A detailed summary of current pharmacotherapy in sarcoidosis is the subject of a recent review by Baughman et al.[36]

SILICOSIS

Overexposure to crystalline silica particles in the mining, construction, manufacturing, and building maintenance industries may result in the development of the fibrotic lung disease known as silicosis. The development of bilateral hilar adenopathy sometimes associated with "eggshell" calcification is a common finding in such patients and, according to Baldwin et al.,[37] may precede the development of interstitial fibrosis. It is hypothesized that lymph node fibrosis impairs the elimination of silica dust from the lungs, increasing the lung dust burden and reflecting the additional risk of parenchymal silicosis.[17] Silica exposure may contribute to the development of coal workers' pneumoconiosis (CWP) in individuals with a history of significant coal mine dust exposure.[38,39]

NECROTIZING GRANULOMATOUS VASCULITIS (FORMERLY WEGENER GRANULOMATOSIS)

Necrotizing granulomatous vasculitis (NGV) is an idiopathic, systemic inflammatory disease characterized by necrotizing granulomatous inflammation and pauci-immune small vessel vasculitis of the upper and lower respiratory tracts and kidneys.[40] A positive c-ANCA is seen in 90% to 95% of cases of active, systemic disease.[41] Specificity is approximately 90%. In the proper clinical setting, a positive c-ANCA has sufficient positive predictive value that biopsy may be deferred in most cases.[42] The clinical manifestations of NGV are usually limited to the upper and/or lower respiratory tract although a number of other clinical features can arise. The lungs are commonly involved ranging from asymptomatic nodules to pulmonary infiltrates and alveolar hemorrhage. Upper respiratory tract disease occurs in 95% of patients with nasal obstruction and crusting, rhinorrhea, purulent nasal drainage, epistaxis, and sinusitis. Lower respiratory

tract involvement includes the pulmonary parenchyma and bronchi, and rarely the pleura. Necrotizing pulmonary inflammation gives rise to cough, pyrexia, hemoptysis, dyspnea thoracic pain, pulmonary collapse, and postobstructive infection. The most common feature of lung disease is the radiologic presence of single or multiple cavitary nodules at cortical and subpleural sites. Nodular disease is present in more than 70% of patients with lung disease and 35% to 50% of patients present with cavitary disease. Hilar and mediastinal lymphadenopathy may also rise.[43] Bronchoscopy is primarily used to assess for the presence of malignancy, infection, stenotic or ulcerative upper airway or endobronchial lesions, pulmonary eosinophilia, and alveolar hemorrhage. When the diagnosis is in doubt, tissue biopsy remains necessary for definitive diagnosis. Skin and upper airway tissue may be useful in some cases but definitive pathology generally requires a surgical lung biopsy, with as high as 90% diagnostic yield.[44]

CASTLEMAN DISEASE

CD, otherwise known as angiofollicular lymph node hyperplasia, is an uncommon entity first described by Castleman in 1956. Subsequent contributions to the literature have delineated CD as a heterogeneous cluster of disorders, with distinct unicentric CD (approximately 85% to 90% of all CD) and multicentric CD, and has identified the fundamental roles of human herpesvirus-8 (HHV-8) and interleukin-6 (IL-6) in a significant portion of cases.[45,46] Histologically, two distinct patterns exist, the hyaline vascular and the plasma cell type, of which the former is represented in the vast majority of localized CD. The localized type can be found in different locations. The most common are mediastinal (approximately 31% of cases), pleural, chest wall, and extrathoracic sites and presents with a slow growing, progressive and painless lymph node enlargement.[46] The plasma cell type is associated with severe systemic symptoms such as weakness, fever, weight loss, nausea, splenomegaly, hepatomegaly, edema, hypergammaglobulinemia, anemia, and multicentric lymphadenopathy.[46] The disease may be associated with many clinical conditions, as outlined in Table 167.3. Localized and multicentric forms are quite distinctive in their clinical features, as outlined in Table 167.4. On chest radiographs, it may appear as an incidental, rounded, solitary mediastinal or hilar mass similar in appearance to thymoma, lymphoma, or neurogenic tumor.[17] On CT, it usually presents as a homogeneous, noninvasive, large, solitary mass with soft tissue attenuation most commonly in the mediastinum or hila.[17]

The treatment of choice for the localized form of CD is complete surgical resection including systematic lymph node dissection, resulting in cure in all reported cases. Radiotherapy may be an appropriate treatment modality following incomplete resection or in cases where the disease is not amenable to resection.[47,48]

The multicentric form is commonly treated with single or multiagent chemotherapy (CVP- or CHOP-like regimens), corticosteroids, and/or radiotherapy, but the response is variable and the prognosis guarded. Close follow-up is recommended in order to detect concurrent or subsequent malignant lesions.

OTHERS

Many other diseases are known to be associated with mediastinal lymphadenopathy, most often as part of a constellation of findings. In these instances, a careful search for other causes of mediastinal adenopathy may be warranted. The numerous causes of mediastinal lymphadenopathy can be diagnosed with careful consideration of

TABLE 167.3 Clinical Conditions Associated With Castleman Disease

Hematologic
  Refractory anemia (PC)
  Autoimmune cytopenias (PC)
  Thrombotic thrombocytopenic purpura (HV)
  Myelofibrosis (HV)
  Lupus anticoagulant (PC)
Dermatologic
  Pemphigus vulgarize (PC)
  Cutaneous Kaposi sarcoma[a] (HV)
  Glomeruloid hemangioma[a] (PC)
Pulmonary
  Bronchiolitis obliterans (HV)
  Recurrent pleural effusion (HV)
Renal
  Nephrotic syndrome (PC)
  Acute renal failure (PC)
  Glomerulonephritis (PC)
Oncologic
  Malignant lymphoma (PC, HV)
  Osteosclerotic myeloma (PC)
  γ heavy chain disease (PC)
  Nodal Kaposi sarcoma (PC)
Neurologic
  Peripheral neuropathy (PC)
  Pseudotumors cerebria (PC, HV)
  Myasthenia gravis (HV)
Miscellaneous
  Amyloidosis (PC)
  Growth retardation (PC)
  Temporal arteritis (HV)
  Pericardial effusion (HV)
  Polyneuropathy, organomegaly, endocrinopathy, M protein, and skin changes (POEMS) syndrome (PC)
  Peliosis hepatis (PC)

[a]Associated with multicentric Castleman disease.
HV, hyaline-vascular variant; PC, plasma cell variant.
Adapted from Shahadi H, Myers JL, Kvale PA. Castleman's disease. *Mayo Clin Proc* 1995;70:969–977. With permission.

the patient's history, physical examination, and both radiologic and laboratory findings.

Amyloidosis is a constellation of disease entities characterized by abnormal extracellular deposition and accumulation of protein that replaces normal cell structure, which show apple-green birefringence when stained with Congo red and viewed under polarized light.[49] Amyloid can infiltrate any organ system and manifest in a multitude of ways. The disease can be classified into several types, most commonly primary and secondary.[50] Pathologically, respiratory involvement occurs in 50% of patients with amyloidosis. The four main patterns of respiratory tract involvement are tracheobronchial, nodule parenchymal, diffuse alveolar septal, and lymphatic.[49] Hilar and mediastinal lymphadenopathy is uncommon in secondary amyloidosis but is quite common in primary amyloidosis. Thoracic lymphadenopathy, alone or with interstitial disease, is the most common CT finding.[17] Mediastinal and hilar lymph nodes may be involved, bilaterally and often massively in a pattern that may mimic sarcoidosis.[17]

Beryllium (Be) is a light-weight element that is processed into Be copper alloy, pure Be metal, and ceramic for use in highly specialized applications, such as the defense, aerospace, and electronic industries.[51] Berylliosis is a lung disease caused by the inhalation of Be compounds leading to acute chemical pneumonitis, due to intense exposure to Be over a short period of time, or chronic lung disease after prolonged exposure to lower Be concentrations. The chronic form is more common and presents as intra-alveolar accumulation of lymphocytes and macrophages and noncaseating granulomas. CT appearances of chronic Be disease are similar to those of sarcoidosis, although hilar and mediastinal lymphadenopathy are less common, occurring in about 25% of patients. Be disease should be included in the differential diagnosis for all patients with imaging appearance suggestive of sarcoidosis.[51] The beryllium lymphocyte proliferation test (BeLPT) is used for medical surveillance and the diagnosis of acute and chronic Be exposures.[52]

Chronic left heart failure may cause mediastinal lymphadenopathy most commonly involving the subcarinal, paratracheal, and hilar nodes. The etiology is not completely understood but it has been suggested that lymphadenopathy is due to diffuse intrathoracic edema affecting the pulmonary parenchyma and neighboring structures, including the mediastinum and associated lymph nodes.[53] The

TABLE 167.4 Comparison Between Clinical Features of Localized and Multicentric Castleman Disease

Factor	Localized	Multicentric
Age range (yr)	12–72	19–85
Median age (yr)	23.5	56
Manifestation	Asymptomatic	"B" symptoms
Histologic Features		
Lymph node dissection distribution	HV > PC > HV-PC	PC > HV > HV-PC
Organomegaly	Absent	Present
Premalignant potential	Occasionally	Frequently
Clinical course	Benign	Aggressive
Treatment	Surgical excision	Chemotherapy
Prognosis	5-year survival 100%	Median survival 26 months
Differential diagnosis	Follicular lymphomas, acquired immunodeficiency syndrome, Kaposi sarcoma	Follicular lymphomas, angioimmunoblastic lymphadenopathy, acquired immunodeficiency, Kaposi sarcoma, polyneuropathy, organomegaly, M protein, and skin changes (POEMS), osteosclerotic myeloma

HV, hyaline-vascular variant; HV-PC, "mixed" type; PC, plasma cell variant.
Adapted from Shahadi H, Myers JL, Kvale PA. Castleman's disease. *Mayo Clin Proc* 1995;70:969–977. Copyright © 1995 Mayo Foundation for Medical Education and Research. With permission.

diagnostic approach to such lymphadenopathy should be guided by the radiologic regression seen on follow-up CT scanning while the patient is receiving appropriate therapy for congestive heart failure.

COPD is a disease characterized by progressive airflow obstruction, inflammation in the airways, and systemic effects or comorbidities.[54] Approximately 50% of patients with COPD present with enlarged hilar and mediastinal lymph nodes located predominantly in the lower paratracheal space, aortopulmonary window, and subcarinal space.[54] Lymph node enlargement is identified more often in patients with severe bronchitis presumably due to more intense inflammation leading to reactive nodal enlargement.[55] All enlarged lymph nodes in patients with COPD have well-defined contours, and most are oval.[55]

Hypersensitivity reactions to drugs can cause mediastinal or hilar lymphadenopathy. Anticonvulsants, in particular phenytoin, can cause a pseudolymphoma syndrome with generalized lymphadenopathy in addition to fever, skin rash, eosinophilia, and hepatosplenomegaly. Methotrexate, sulfonamides, penicillin, allopurinol, aspirin, and erythromycin are other drugs with similar effects. These reactions tend to follow several months of drug therapy and decrease after discontinuation.[56]

REFERENCES

1. Suwatanapongched T, Gierada DS. CT of thoracic lymph nodes. Part I: anatomy and drainage. *Br J Radiol* 2006;79:922–928.
2. Suwatanapongched T, Gierada DS. CT of thoracic lymph nodes. Part II: diseases and pitfalls. *Br J Radiol* 2006;79:999–1000.
3. Bayanati H, Thornhill RE, Souza CA, et al. Quantitative CT texture and shape analysis: can it differentiate benign and malignant mediastinal lymph nodes in patients with primary lung cancer? *Eur Radiol* 2015;25:480–487.
4. Mirsadraee M. Anthracosis of the lungs: etiology, clinical manifestations and diagnosis: a review. *Tanaffos* 2014;13:1–13.
5. Kirchner J, Broll M, Muller P, et al. CT differentiation of enlarged mediastinal lymph node due to anthracosis from metastatic lymphadenopathy: a comparative study proven by endobronchial US-guided transbronchial needle aspiration. *Diagn Interv Radiol* 2015;21:128–133.
6. Adams K, Shah PL, Edmonds L, et al. Test performance of endobronchial ultrasound and transbronchial needle aspiration biopsy for mediastinal staging in patients with lung cancer: systematic review and meta-analysis. *Thorax* 2009;64:757–762.
7. Gu P, Zhao YZ, Jiang LY, et al. Endobronchial ultrasound-guided transbronchial needle aspiration for staging of lung cancer: a systematic review and meta-analysis. *Eur J Cancer* 2009;45:1389–1396.
8. Kinsey CM, Arenberg DA. Endobronchial ultrasound-guided transbronchial needle aspiration for non-small cell lung cancer staging. *Am J Respir Crit Care Med* 2014;189:640–649.
9. Varela-Lema L, Fernandez-Villar A, Ruano-Ravina A. Effectiveness and safety of endobronchial ultrasound-transbronchial needle aspiration: a systematic review. *Eur Respir J* 2009;33:1156–1164.
10. Yasufuku K, Nakajima T, Fujiwara T, et al. Utility of endobronchial ultrasound-guided transbronchial needle aspiration in the diagnosis of mediastinal masses of unknown etiology. *Ann Thorac Surg* 2011;91:831–836.
11. Vincent BD, El-Bayoumi E, Hoffman B, et al. Real-time endobronchial ultrasound-guided transbronchial lymph node aspiration. *Ann Thorac Surg* 2008; 85:224–230.
12. Sun J, Teng J, Yang H, et al. Endobronchial ultrasound-guided transbronchial needle aspiration in diagnosing intrathoracic tuberculosis. *Ann Thorac Surg* 2013;96:2021–2027.
13. Sun J, Yang H, Teng J, et al. Determining factors in diagnosing pulmonary sarcoidosis by endobronchial ultrasound-guided transbronchial needle aspiration. *Ann Thorac Surg* 2015;99:441–445.
14. Harris RM, Arnaout R, Koziel H, et al. Utility of microbiological testing of thoracic lymph nodes sampled by endobronchial ultrasound-guided transbronchial needle aspiration (EBUS-TBNA) in patients with mediastinal lymphadenopathy. *Diagn Microbiol Infect Dis* 2016;84:170–174.
15. El-Zammar OA, Katzenstein AL. Pathological diagnosis of granulomatous lung disease: a review. *Histopathology* 2007;50:289–310.
16. Jeong YJ, Lee KS. Pulmonary tuberculosis: up-to-date imaging and management. *AJR Am J Roentgenol* 2008;191:834–844.
17. Nin CS, de Souza VV, do Amaral RH, et al. Thoracic lymphadenopathy in benign diseases: a state of the art review. *Respir Med* 2016;112:10–17.
18. Leung AN. Pulmonary tuberculosis: the essentials. *Radiology* 1999;210:307–322.
19. Hage CA, Azar MM, Bahr N, et al. Histoplasmosis: up-to-date evidence-based approach to diagnosis and management. *Semin Respir Crit Care Med* 2015;36:729–745.
20. Kalweit G, Huwer H, Straub U, et al. Mediastinal compression syndromes due to idiopathic fibrosing mediastinitis-report of three cases and review of the literature. *Thorac Cardiovasc Surg* 1996;44:105–109.
21. Mathisen DJ, Grillo HC. Clinical manifestation of mediastinal fibrosis and histoplasmosis. *Ann Thorac Surg* 1992;54:1053–1057; discussion 1057–1058.
22. Arbra CA, Valentino JD, Martin JT. Vascular sequelae of mediastinal fibrosis. *Asian Cardiovasc Thorac Ann* 2015;23:36–41.
23. Bays S, Rajakaruna C, Sheffield E, et al. Fibrosing mediastinitis as a cause of superior vena cava syndrome. *Eur J Cardiothorac Surg* 2004;26:453–445.
24. Hammoud ZT, Rose AS, Hage CA, et al. Surgical management of pulmonary and mediastinal sequelae of histoplasmosis: a challenging spectrum. *Ann Thorac Surg* 2009;88:399–403.
25. Galgiani JN, Ampel NM, Blair JE, et al. 2016 Infectious Diseases Society of America (IDSA) clinical practice guideline for the treatment of coccidioidomycosis. *Clin Infect Dis* 2016;63:e112–e146.
26. Jude CM, Nayak NB, Patel MK, et al. Pulmonary coccidioidomycosis: pictorial review of chest radiographic and CT findings. *Radiographics* 2014;34:912–925.
27. Lagerstrom CF, Mitchell HG, Graham BS, et al. Chronic fibrosing mediastinitis and superior vena caval obstruction from blastomycosis. *Ann Thorac Surg* 1992;54(4): 764–765.
28. Costabel U, Hunninghake GW. ATS/ERS/WASOG statement on sarcoidosis. Sarcoidosis Statement Committee. American Thoracic Society. European Respiratory Society. World Association for Sarcoidosis and Other Granulomatous Disorders. *Eur Respir J* 1999;14:735–737.
29. Liang NC, Truong KT, Afshar K. Key management considerations in sarcoidosis from the American Thoracic Society 2016 Conference. *J Thorac Dis* 2016;8:S569–S572.
30. Valeyre D, Bernaudin JF, Uzunhan Y, et al. Clinical presentation of sarcoidosis and diagnostic work-up. *Semin Respir Crit Care Med* 2014;35:336–351.
31. Garwood S, Judson MA, Silvestri G, et al. Endobronchial ultrasound for the diagnosis of pulmonary sarcoidosis. *Chest* 2007;132:1298–1304.
32. Navani N, Booth HL, Kocjan G, et al. Combination of endobronchial ultrasound-guided transbronchial needle aspiration with standard bronchoscopic techniques for the diagnosis of stage I and stage II pulmonary sarcoidosis. *Respirology* 2011;16: 467–472.
33. Oki M, Saka H, Kitagawa C, et al. Prospective study of endobronchial ultrasound-guided transbronchial needle aspiration of lymph nodes versus transbronchial lung biopsy of lung tissue for diagnosis of sarcoidosis. *J Thorac Cardiovasc Surg* 2012; 143:1324–1329.
34. Tournoy KG, Bolly A, Aerts JG, et al. The value of endoscopic ultrasound after bronchoscopy to diagnose thoracic sarcoidosis. *Eur Respir J* 2010;35:1329–1335.
35. von Bartheld MB, Dekkers OM, Szlubowski A, et al. Endosonography vs conventional bronchoscopy for the diagnosis of sarcoidosis: the GRANULOMA randomized clinical trial. *JAMA* 2013;309:2457–2464.
36. Baughman RP, Costabel U, du Bois RM. Treatment of sarcoidosis. *Clin Chest Med* 2008;29:533–548, ix–x.
37. Baldwin DR, Lambert L, Pantin CF, et al. Silicosis presenting as bilateral hilar lymphadenopathy. *Thorax* 1996;51:1165–1167.
38. Cohen RA, Patel A, Green FH. Lung disease caused by exposure to coal mine and silica dust. *Semin Respir Crit Care Med* 2008;29:651–661.
39. Go LH, Krefft SD, Cohen RA, et al. Lung disease and coal mining: what pulmonologists need to know. *Curr Opin Pulm Med* 2016;22:170–178.
40. Almouhawis HA, Leao JC, Fedele S, et al. Wegener's granulomatosis: a review of clinical features and an update in diagnosis and treatment. *J Oral Pathol Med* 2013; 42:507–516.
41. Boomsma MM, Stegeman CA, van der Leij MJ, et al. Prediction of relapses in Wegener's granulomatosis by measurement of antineutrophil cytoplasmic antibody levels: a prospective study. *Arthritis Rheum* 2000;43:2025–2033.
42. Langford CA. The diagnostic utility of c-ANCA in Wegener's granulomatosis. *Cleve Clin J Med* 1998;65:135–140.
43. Delevaux I, Khellaf M, Andre M, et al. Spontaneous pneumothorax in Wegener granulomatosis. *Chest* 2005;128:3074–3075.
44. Travis WD, Hoffman GS, Leavitt RY, et al. Surgical pathology of the lung in Wegener's granulomatosis. Review of 87 open lung biopsies from 67 patients. *Am J Surg Pathol* 1991;15:315–333.
45. Chan KL, Lade S, Prince HM, et al. Update and new approaches in the treatment of Castleman disease. *J Blood Med* 2016;7:145–158.
46. Haager B, Kayser G, Schmid S, et al. Intrapulmonary Castleman's disease pretending to be a lung cancer—work up of an intrapulmonary tumour. *Ann Thorac Cardiovasc Surg* 2016;22:258–260.
47. Li YM, Liu PH, Zhang YH, et al. Radiotherapy of unicentric mediastinal Castleman's disease. *Chin J Cancer* 2011;30:351–356.
48. de Vries IA, van Acht MM, Demeyere T, et al. Neoadjuvant radiotherapy of primary irresectable unicentric Castleman's disease: a case report and review of the literature. *Radiat Oncol* 2010;5:7.
49. de Almeida RR, Zanetti G, Pereira E Silva JL, et al. Respiratory tract amyloidosis. State-of-the-art review with a focus on pulmonary involvement. *Lung* 2015;193:875–883.
50. Georgiades CS, Neyman EG, Barish MA, et al. Amyloidosis: review and CT manifestations. *Radiographics* 2004;24:405–416.
51. Mayer A, Hamzeh N. Beryllium and other metal-induced lung disease. *Curr Opin Pulm Med* 2015;21:178–184.
52. Balmes JR, Abraham JL, Dweik RA, et al. An official American Thoracic Society statement: diagnosis and management of beryllium sensitivity and chronic beryllium disease. *Am J Respir Crit Care Med* 2014;190:e34–e59.
53. Ngom A, Dumont P, Diot P, et al. Benign mediastinal lymphadenopathy in congestive heart failure. *Chest* 1999;119:653–656.
54. Decramer M, Janssens W, Miravitlles M. Chronic obstructive pulmonary disease. *Lancet* 2012;379:1341–1351.
55. Kirchner J, Kirchner EM, Goltz JP, et al. Enlarged hilar and mediastinal lymph nodes in chronic obstructive pulmonary disease. *J Med Imaging Radiat Oncol* 2010;54:333–338.
56. Brown JR, Skarin AT. Clinical mimics of lymphoma. *Oncologist* 2004;9:406–416.

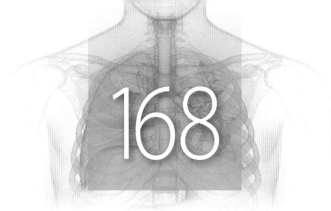

168

Diagnosis and Treatment of Mediastinal Lymphomas

Adrienne A. Phillips ▪ Koen van Besien

INTRODUCTION

Lymphomas are heterogeneous disorders, with variable clinical presentation and course, making correct histopathologic classification essential for their appropriate management. Historically, classification systems relied heavily on disease histology and clinical behavior and included the Working Formulation, Rappaport Classification, and the Revised European American (REAL) classifications.[1,2] The World Health Organization (WHO) classification of neoplasms of the hematopoietic and lymphoid tissues, published in 2001 and updated in 2008, is now the most widely used and lists nearly 100 types of lymphoid malignancies grouped according to a combination of morphology, immunophenotype, genetic, molecular, and clinical features.[3] Most subtypes of lymphoma occasionally involve the mediastinum; however, several entities have a unique affinity for the mediastinum and their clinical features are often related to the presence of a mediastinal mass. These include classical Hodgkin lymphoma (cHL), primary mediastinal B-cell lymphoma (PMBL), and precursor T-cell lymphoblastic lymphoma (T-LBL). In addition, a newly identified "B-cell lymphoma, unclassifiable, with features intermediate between diffuse large B-cell lymphoma and cHL," known more commonly as mediastinal "gray zone lymphoma" (MGZL) is quite rare, but also involves the mediastinum. These subtypes with mediastinal tropism will be the focus of this chapter with particular attention placed on cHL which has been studied for over six decades.

HODGKIN LYMPHOMA

INTRODUCTION

Since Sir Thomas Hodgkin's first postmortem description of Hodgkin disease in 1832, Hodgkin disease has emerged as a unique and often curable malignancy, histologically characterized by the presence of Hodgkin Reed–Sternberg cells (HRS). Hodgkin disease is currently considered a subtype of lymphoma, and the term "Hodgkin lymphoma (HL)" was proposed in the WHO classification by Jaffe et al.[2] The development of high energy radiotherapy in the early-mid 20th century led to cure of some patients with early-stage disease, with staging via laparotomy being essential for the planning of radiation ports and successful radiation treatment. More recently, the use of effective combination chemotherapy regimens along with improved radiographic techniques has obviated the need for staging laparotomy. Cure rates are high and even patients with recurrent or refractory disease may still have long-term survival with combination chemotherapy, immunotherapy, and stem cell transplantation. Successes in the management of HL have been tempered by the occurrence of serious late side-effects resulting from therapy which frequently require multidisciplinary management including thoracic surgeons. With the increasing number of long-term HL survivors, a major thrust of current clinical research is to minimize long-term toxicity while maintaining the high cure rate.

EPIDEMIOLOGY AND ETIOLOGY

HL is a relatively uncommon malignancy with an estimated 9,050 new cases and 1,150 deaths in 2015, according to the SEER database.[4] HL incidence is bimodal in economically developed countries with peaks in incidence occurring in teenagers/young adults (ages 15 to 34 years) and adults over the age of 55 years. In economically underdeveloped countries, a higher incidence of HL is seen among children under the age of 15, though the overall incidence is lower than that in developed countries. The incidence is similar in men and women, although for mediastinal-predominant disease, prevalence peaks in young women during the third decade of life while it is unaffected by age in men.[5,6] Mortality appears to be higher in men.

The cell of origin in HL had long been a mystery, as the pathognomonic HRS cell accounts for only 1% of all cells within an affected lymph node and was therefore difficult to study. Several observations beginning in the mid-1990s proved that HRS cells are monoclonal and derive from germinal center (GC) B lymphocytes.[7,8] Despite being a B-cell derived malignancy, HRS have downregulated the expression of most B-cell typical genes and immunohistochemical studies do not reveal the classic B-cell phenotype.[9] The WHO has divided HL into cHL and nodular lymphocyte predominant Hodgkin lymphoma (NLPHL). cHL makes up 95% of cases and includes four morphologic subgroups: nodular sclerosis, mixed cellularity, lymphocyte-rich, and lymphocyte-depleted HLs. In cHL, the most

TABLE 168.1 Clinical Characteristics of Mediastinal Lymphomas

Disease	Usual Age of Onset	M : F	SVC Syndrome	Peripheral Adenopathy
Classical Hodgkin Lymphoma (cHL)	Young adult	F > M	Rare	May be present
Primary Mediastinal B-cell Lymphoma (PMBL)	Young adult	F > M	May be present	Rare
T-cell Lymphoblastic Lymphoma (T-LBL)	Young adult	M > F	May be present	Rare
Mediastinal Gray Zone Lymphoma (MGZL)	Young adult	M > F	May be present	May be present

common morphologic subgroup to affect the mediastinum, HRS cells typically express CD15 (85% of cases), CD30 (virtually 100% of cases), and usually lack global expression of pan-B (CD19, CD20, CD79a) and pan-T (CD3, CD7) antigens. Tables 168.1 and 168.2 reveal the clinical and biologic characteristics of cHL in comparison to other mediastinal lymphomas. NLPHL shares many features with NHL, including strong CD20 expression, and often has a waxing and waning course similar to indolent lymphomas. It rarely has a mediastinal presentation, and thus the remainder of this discussion pertains mainly to cHL.

As with most malignancies, the etiology of HL is not definitively known. The bimodal incidence of HL supports the hypothesis that there may be two distinct pathogenic processes: an infectious agent of low infectivity may be related to disease in young adults, while a mechanism shared with other lymphomas may account for the pathogenesis of HL among older adults.[10] Risk factors have been proposed, including infection with lymphotropic viruses, higher socioeconomic status, and aberrancies of the immune system. The Epstein–Barr virus (EBV) genome has been detected in one-third to one-half of HL occurring in patients without known immunodeficiency and patients with infectious mononucleosis are at a higher

risk of developing EBV-associated HL.[11] This risk is enhanced in carriers of HLA-A*01.[12] The role of HL as an inherited disease remains to be defined; however, nearly 40% of patients with HL seen at tertiary care referral centers report a first-degree relative with cancer and 6% had a relative with a lymphoproliferative malignancy.[13] HL is also increased in a number of settings associated with immunodeficiency including solid organ or hematopoietic stem cell transplantation, therapy with immunosuppressive drugs, and HIV infection. Among patients infected with HIV, the relative risk of HL is increased 5- to 25-fold.[14]

CLINICAL PRESENTATION

The majority of patients with HL present with nontender adenopathy, usually in the neck or supraclavicular area. Mediastinal involvement is present in 60% of patients at diagnosis. The mass may be fairly large without producing local symptoms; however, when present, the most common symptoms are cough, dyspnea, chest pain, and eventual superior vena cava syndrome. Constitutional symptoms occur in approximately one-third of patients and consist of fatigue, diffuse pruritus, weight loss, fevers, and/or night sweats. The latter

TABLE 168.2 Biologic Characteristics of Mediastinal Lymphomas

Disease	Morphology	Immunohistochemistry	Genetics	Cell of Origin
cHL	Nodular growth pattern with diagnostic Hodgkin Reed–Sternberg cells with abundant, slightly basophilic cytoplasm and bilobed nuclei in an inflammatory background	CD 15+ CD30+ (strong) B-cell markers negative (CD20– CD79a– PAX5–) Surface Ig–	Clonal cytogenetic abnormalities found in the majority; however, they vary from case to case	Medullary thymic B-cell
PMBL	Large cells with variable nuclear features, abundant cytoplasm, compartmentalizing sclerosis	B-cell markers positive (CD19, CD20, CD22, CD79a) Surface Ig– CD30 dim+ CD15–	Chromosome 9p abnl (75%) Chromosome 2p (50%)	Medullary thymic B-cell
T-LBL	Medium-sized cells, with scant cytoplasm, round, oval, or convoluted nuclei, fine chromatin and indistinct or small nucleoli; Auer rods never seen	Typically positive for CD7 and either surface or cytoplasmic CD3, and variably express CD2, CD5, CD1a, CD4, and/or CD8	Chromosome 14q and 7q abnl (33%) Chromosome 1p abnl (25%)	Precursor T-lymphoblast
MGZL	Morphologic overlap between PMBL and cHL	CD20+ CD79a+ CD30+ CD15 variable Surface Ig–	2p16.1 amplification (33%) JAK2/PDL2 (55%) Gain 8q24 (MYC) (27%)	Medullary thymic B-cell

three symptoms comprise the classic "B" symptoms of malignant lymphomas.[15] When present, they typically confer a more aggressive course of disease. Other notable, but less common, symptoms attributable to HL include alcohol-induced pain and Pel–Ebstein fevers which are cyclic temperature elevations typically with a 1- to 2-week periodicity.[16] The prognostic significance of constitutional symptoms other than the classic B symptoms is not known; however, recurrence of constitutional symptoms in a previously treated patient may signal disease relapse. Large mediastinal disease or "bulky disease" is defined as a disease burden more than one-third of the greatest intrathoracic diameter of the chest wall or 10 cm in transverse dimension. This is seen in 20% to 25% of patients with HL and is an adverse prognostic feature.[17]

DIAGNOSTIC EVALUATION

The diagnostic workup of HL includes obtaining an adequate tissue sample and staging evaluation. The differential diagnosis of patients presenting with a mediastinal mass includes HL, PMBL, MGZL, T-LBL as well as other NHLs, primary mediastinal germ cell tumors, and rarely, thymomas and carcinomas. With rare exceptions, an accurate diagnosis of lymphoma can only be established by obtaining tissue for immunophenotyping, cytogenetics, and molecular assays in addition to classic histologic examination. Many of these tests require viable tissue and it is therefore of the utmost importance that in addition to fixed specimens, fresh tissue is provided to the pathologist when a diagnosis of lymphoma is suspected. Mediastinal lymphomas, be they HL or NHL, are often fibrotic and small biopsies may be difficult to interpret. Furthermore, subclassification may be impossible without sufficient tissue. In HL in particular, the malignant cell of origin, the HRS, is relatively rare in comparison to the intense background lymphoid reaction. Its recognition is essential for diagnosis and such cells may not be present if the biopsy is small.

Tissue obtained by FNA or by core biopsy is generally not sufficient for diagnosis. Samples obtained by mediastinoscopy, an excellent technique for staging carcinomas, are not always adequate for the diagnosis of mediastinal lymphomas. If no easily accessible peripheral lymph node is present, video-assisted thoracoscopic surgery (VATS) for biopsy or a limited thoracotomy may be required for establishing the diagnosis. In a retrospective study of 49 patients with suspected mediastinal lymphoma, esophageal ultrasound-guided fine needle aspirate (EUS-FNA) and endobronchial ultrasound-guided transbronchial needle aspiration (EBUS-TSBNA) was found to be a minimally invasive, safe, and sensitive method for the assessment of recurrent mediastinal lymphoma but not for the assessment of a primary lymphoma diagnosis.[18] Figure 168.1 shows how EBUS-TSBNA may be performed using color Doppler to identify nearby blood vessels (Fig. 168.1A–C).

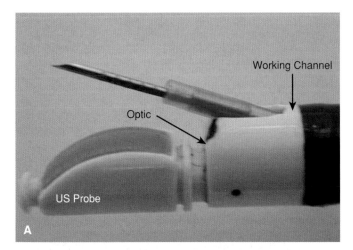

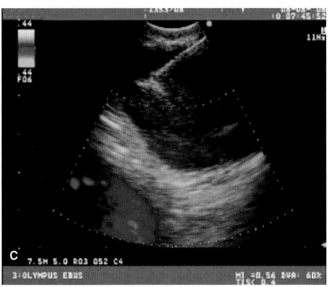

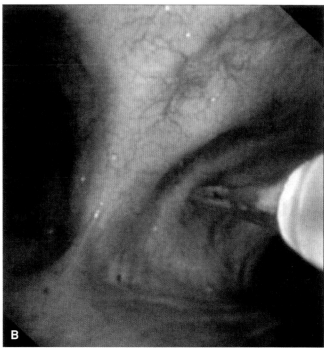

FIGURE 168.1 A: Layout of the endobronchial ultrasound scope. **B:** Conventional transbronchial needle aspiration. Needle is seen exiting the bronchoscope and puncturing the bronchial mucosa. **C:** Endobronchial ultrasound-guided transbronchial needle aspiration. Under ultrasound guidance, needle is visualized entering the lymph node. Color Doppler allows visualization of nearby blood vessels.

Once a diagnosis of HL is confirmed, a thorough staging evaluation will allow determination of clinical stage which guides further management. Blood tests to be performed include a complete blood count with differential to determine the absolute lymphocyte count; erythrocyte sedimentation rate (ESR); biochemical tests of liver, bone, and renal function; as well as a serum lactate dehydrogenase (LDH) (an important prognostic marker in many lymphomas), and viral serologies (for HIV and hepatitis B and C). Although the results of these tests may not contribute directly to staging, they may influence the choice of therapy and guide further investigations to other potential sites of disease.

Staging laparotomy with splenectomy and lymph node sampling had been widely used in the past. The importance of staging laparotomy in HL is based on an early observation by Rosenberg and Kaplan[19] that HL spreads in an orderly and predictable fashion. This allowed precise pathologic staging that avoided the risk of under- or overtreatment. However, the use of systemic chemotherapy even in early-stage disease, the ability to effectively salvage patients who relapse, and improvements in radiologic staging have all decreased the need for precise surgical staging and relegated it to a historical footnote. The Ann Arbor staging system with Cotswold modifications is the current staging system used for patients with HL and NHL (Table 168.3).[20]

The pretreatment imaging study of choice for staging is a combined positron emission tomography (PET)/computed tomography (CT) scan of the neck, chest, abdomen, and pelvis.[21] PET is a nuclear imaging modality that provides insight into the metabolic activity of a lesion and, by inference, yields information about the probability of malignancy. It is usually performed using a glucose analog that has been tagged with a positron-emitting isotope of fluorine, 18F-2-deoxy-2-fluoro-D-glucose (^{18}FDG). A tumor's metabolic activity can be measured using the standardized uptake value (SUV) with a high SUV indicating robust FDG uptake due to high metabolic glycolytic activity, which suggests malignancy or active inflammation. Several studies show that ^{18}FDG-PET/CT more accurately identified the correct pretreatment stage in HL compared with contrast-enhanced CT, and ^{18}FDG-PET/CT upstages disease from early to advanced stage in 10% to 15% of patients.[22] Applications of ^{18}FDG-PET/CT include routine staging, evaluation of response to treatment, evaluation of residual masses following treatment, and prediction of relapse risk in such patients.[23] Large cooperative groups within the United States and Germany are prospectively evaluating the utility of early or mid-treatment ^{18}FDG-PET/CT as a tool to individualize treatment in patients with HL.

The Deauville score has been used to score ^{18}FDG-PET/CT scans based on a 5-point scale and is a purely visual method of standardizing the interpretation of posttreatment ^{18}FDG-PET/CT scans for primary nodal lymphoma.[24] The Deauville score uses a patient's FDG uptake in the mediastinal blood pool and liver as an internal control. A score of 1 indicates no uptake, 2 indicates uptake is ≤mediastinal blood pool, 3 indicates uptake is >mediastinal blood pool but ≤liver, 4 indicates uptake is moderately more than liver uptake, and 5 indicates uptake is markedly higher than the liver.

Bone marrow core biopsy has been a standard in lymphoma staging. However, in patients with supradiaphragmatic stage I or II disease without B symptoms, the probability of marrow involvement is minimal. In one study in HL, 18% of patients had focal skeletal lesions on PET-CT, but only 6% had positive bone marrow biopsy, all with advanced disease evident on ^{18}FDG-PET/CT.[25] None of the patients would have been allocated to another treatment based on bone marrow biopsy results. Patients with early-stage disease rarely have involvement in the absence of a suggestive ^{18}FDG-PET/CT finding, and those with advanced-stage disease rarely have involvement in the absence of disease-related symptoms or other evidence of advanced-stage disease. Thus, if ^{18}FDG-PET/CT is performed, a bone marrow aspirate/biopsy is no longer required for the routine evaluation of patients with HL.[21] Bone marrow biopsy may be considered in patients with B symptoms and/or clinical advanced-stage and/or infradiaphragmatic presentation and in those with bone lesions, bone pain, hypercalcemia, or an elevated serum alkaline phosphatase.

Among patients with advanced-stage disease, a prognostic index was created by the International Prognostic Factor Project on Advanced Hodgkin Disease. This index is based on the total number of seven unfavorable features present at the time of diagnosis including: serum albumin level <4 g/dL (or 40 g/L); hemoglobin level <10.5 g/dL (105 g/L); male gender; age >45 years; stage IV disease; WBC count ≥15,000 cell/µL, and lymphocyte count <600/µL and/or <8% of the WBC count.[26]

MANAGEMENT

The treatment of HL is separated into the treatment of early-stage disease (i.e., stage I and II disease), and advanced-stage disease (i.e., stage III and IV disease). For patients with early-stage disease, there is subsequent stratification into favorable and unfavorable prognostic groups based on the presence or absence of certain clinical features, including bulky mediastinal disease (Table 168.4). Early-stage HL patients, without any of the features listed in Table 168.4, are considered to have a favorable prognosis.

Therapy for early-stage HL has evolved over the past two decades due to recognition of late adverse effects. Historical studies used extended-field RT (EFRT) and heavy alkylator-based chemotherapy (typically the MOPP regimen including nitrogen mustard, Oncovin [vincristine], procarbazine, and prednisone). Though effective, this resulted in increased morbidity and mortality, particularly due to a high rate of second cancers, including breast cancer in young women, as well as cardiovascular disease and high rates of infertility.[27] The original MOPP regimen has largely been supplanted with the equally effective and less toxic ABVD (adriamycin, bleomycin, vinblastine, dacarbazine) regimen proposed by Bonadonna et al.[28] Today, patients with early-stage disease are treated with chemotherapy alone or with various combinations of chemotherapy plus radiotherapy. The optimal therapy for early-stage disease remains an ongoing debate, as discussed in a recent review by Armitage.[29] Although few studies

TABLE 168.3 Ann Arbor Staging System with Cotswold Modifications for Lymphoma[20]

Staging: Ann Arbor Classification (Cotswold Revision)

Stage I	Involvement of a single lymph node region or a lymph node structure or a single extralymphatic site
Stage II	Involvement of two or more lymph node regions on the same side of the diaphragm or localized contiguous involvement of an extralymphatic site and lymph node organ
Stage III	Involvement of lymph node regions on both sides of the diaphragm
Stage IV	Diffuse or disseminated involvement of one or more extranodal organs or tissues, with our without associated lymph node involvement

A: absence of B symptoms, B: presence of B symptoms (fevers, night sweats, weight loss, pruritus), E: extranodal disease or extension from known nodal site of disease, X: bulky disease: >1/3 widening of the mediastinum at T5–T6, or maximum of nodal mass >10 cm.
From Lister TA, Crowther D, Sutcliffe SB, et al. Report of a committee convened to discuss the evaluation and staging of patients with Hodgkin's disease: Cotswolds meeting. *J Clin Oncol* 1989;7:1630–1636. Reprinted with permission. Copyright © 1989 American Society of Clinical Oncology. All rights reserved.

TABLE 168.4 Unfavorable Prognostic Factors in Early (Stage I/II) Hodgkin Lymphoma

European Organization for Research and Treatment of Cancer (EORTC)	• large mediastinal adenopathy (>1/3 maximum transverse thoracic diameter) • involvement of four or more lymph node regions • age ≥50 yrs at diagnosis • B symptoms and an ESR over 30 mm/hr or an ESR over 50 mm/hr without B symptoms
German Hodgkin Study Group (GHSG)	• large mediastinal adenopathy (>1/3 maximum transverse thoracic diameter) • involvement of three or more lymph node regions • B symptoms and an ESR over 30 mm/hr or an ESR over 50 mm/hr without B symptoms
Groupe d'Etudes des Lymphomes de l'Adulte (GELA)	• age ≥45 • male gender • extranodal disease • hemoglobin 10.5 g/dL or less • absolute lymphocyte count ≤600 mg/µL • elevated ESR • B symptoms
National Cancer Institute of Canada (NCIC)/Eastern Cooperative Oncology Group (ECOG)	• large mediastinal adenopathy (>1/3 maximum transverse thoracic diameter) • involvement of four or more lymph node regions • age ≥40 yrs at diagnosis • ESR >50 mm/hr • mixed cellularity subtype

have specifically evaluated the outcomes of patients presenting with mediastinal disease, a study investigating 80 patients with bulky mediastinal disease receiving six cycles of MOPP (mechlorethamine, vincristine, procarbazine, and prednisone)/ABVD (doxorubicin, bleomycin, vinblastine, and dacarbazine) followed by mantle-field radiation therapy reported disease-free survival of 76% in those with stage I or II disease at 15 years' followup.[30] In a single institution prospective, randomized study of unselected patients with clinical stage IA, IB, IIA, IIB, and IIIA nonbulky patients, there was no difference in treatment outcomes between those ABVD chemotherapy alone and ABVD followed by radiation therapy at 60 months' follow-up.[31] Lastly, in a cooperative group study comparing the outcome of patients with limited stage nonbulky HL who received ABVD alone versus subtotal nodal radiation with or without ABVD, the overall survival (OS) at 12 years of follow-up was 94% compared to 87%, respectively. Interestingly, in the latter group, there was a higher rate of deaths from other causes than in the ABVD group suggesting that in patients with nonbulky disease, chemotherapy alone is sufficient.[32]

Currently, combined-modality therapy is typically administered for early-stage bulky disease; however, the optimal therapy for non-bulky disease is still evolving. Options for patients with favorable prognosis early-stage HL include ABVD for three to four cycles followed by 30 Gy involved field radiation therapy (IFRT) encompassing the initially involved lymph node site; ABVD for two cycles, followed by 20 Gy IFRT; and lastly ABVD for four to six cycles without radiation.[33–36] Although the relapse rate may be lower in patients receiving mediastinal radiation, this is offset by the long-term consequences of radiation therapy and the high salvage rate of patients that relapse after primary therapy.[37] Early interim [18]FDG-PET/CT may

further dictate therapy; however, long-term follow-up from ongoing studies is needed before firm conclusions can be made.[38]

For patients with unfavorable early-stage HL and for those with advanced-stage HL, six cycles of ABVD may be a standard option; however, a number of other regimens have been studied extensively. In Europe, the escalated BEACOPP (bleomycin, etoposide, doxorubicin, cyclophosphamide, vincristine, procarbazine, and prednisone) which also incorporates radiation for most patients has shown advantages in progression-free survival (PFS) rates but has increased toxicity and no clear difference in OS rates when compared to ABVD.[39] These advantages are mostly marked among patients with higher risk international prognostic score (IPS) and this more intense regimen is a reasonable alternative to ABVD for these patients with the highest risk of relapse. Escalated BEACOPP is associated with higher rates of toxicity including reversible bone marrow suppression, secondary malignancies, sterility, and rare cases of fatal sepsis. Toxicities are particularly severe in the elderly, making it inappropriate in this population. In the US, the Stanford group has advocated an abbreviated course of intensive chemotherapy, called the Stanford V regimen, followed by adjuvant radiation therapy to sites of bulky disease.[40] A randomized multi-institutional intergroup study comparing ABVD versus Stanford V in advanced HL has completed accrual in the United States.

For patients with stage I or II bulky mediastinal HL, no substantial statistically significant differences were detected between the two regimens.[41] Differences were also not observed in patients with advanced disease in a British study.[42]

For patients with relapsed HL and primary refractory disease, the standard of care is conventional chemotherapy combined with or without radiation therapy followed by high-dose chemotherapy and autologous hematopoietic stem cell transplant (ASCT). The choice of therapy is usually based on prognostic features and comorbidities. Sustained remissions after high-dose chemotherapy and ASCT can be achieved in many patients with refractory or recurrent HL. Two randomized studies have shown a benefit in freedom from treatment failure for ASCT compared with conventional chemotherapy and a meta-analysis shows a trend for improved OS with ASCT.[43–45] Newer strategies in relapsed and refractory HL include allogeneic hematopoietic stem cell transplantation using either standard-dose or reduced intensity conditioning regimens. With several groups showing low treatment-related mortality and promising graft-versus-HL effects, further investigations are underway.[46–48] Occasional patients with limited recurrent disease can be successfully salvaged with localized radiation.

Increasing knowledge regarding biologic aberrations and the identification of surface markers on the HRS cell have led to the clinical testing of several new agents. Brentuximab vedotin (SGN-35) is an immunotoxin comprised of a CD30-directed antibody linked to the antitubulin agent monomethyl auristatin E (MMAE).[49] Brentuximab vedotin was granted accelerated approval by the US Food and Drug Administration for the treatment of patients with HL after failure of ASCT or after failure of at least two prior multiagent chemotherapy regimens in patients that are not candidates for hematopoietic stem cell transplantation. Lastly, the programmed death 1 (PD-1) pathway which serves as a checkpoint to limit T-cell mediated immune responses is activated in HL and early phase studies of PD-1 inhibitors are promising.[50]

LATE SEQUELAE OF TREATMENT

Unfortunately, the successes in curing HL have been countered by late treatment-related toxicity. Numerous studies have demonstrated that cumulative mortality from HL declines over time; however, among survivors 10 to 15 years following treatment, the mortality among survivors from nonlymphoma-related causes, most notably second malignancy and cardiac disease, continue to increase over time.[51] Other late effects such as noncoronary vascular disease, pulmonary dysfunction, xerostomia resulting in increased risk of dental caries and periodontal disease, hypothyroidism, infertility, musculoskeletal atrophy, and developmental hypoplasia are also reported. Though not always life-threatening, these late effects can have a profound negative impact on quality of life.

The association between the use of alkylating chemotherapy for HL and development of therapy-related leukemia or myelodysplastic syndrome has long been established. Over the years, the data on solid tumors after HL has accumulated and solid tumors now account for the majority of second malignancies after HL.[51] Radiation therapy is a major contributor to the development of subsequent solid tumors; however, recent data have also linked alkylating agents to a variety of solid tumors including lung cancer and gastrointestinal cancers.[52–54] The risk of lung cancer is directly related to radiation dose, as shown in a case-control study in which patients who received 30 Gy or higher had a 7- to 9-fold higher lung cancer risk compared to those who received <5 Gy to the area of the lung in which the cancer developed.[55] A significant correlation of alkylating chemotherapy for HL and lung cancer has also been shown and tobacco use further contributes to the risk.[55]

Young women who receive radiation therapy to the mediastinum at a young age (30 or younger) are at particular risk for the development of breast cancer and should follow rigorous screening programs. Breast cancer usually develops 10 to 15 years after treatment and most studies show a clear radiation dose–response relationship. In the largest study that included 120 cases of breast cancer after HL and 266 controls, the relative risk of breast cancer increased significantly with increasing radiation dose, reaching 8-fold at the highest-dose category (median dose 42 Gy) compared with the lowest-dose group (<4 Gy; P <0.001).[56] Patient education programs coupled with early detection in female patients treated with mantle irradiation has been proposed, and includes annual mammography starting 8 to 10 years after treatment or at age 40, whichever occurs first.[57]

Therapy-related myelodysplasia and secondary leukemias (t-MDS/t-AML) are of special concern among long-term HL survivors. The initial combination chemotherapy regimens such as MOPP proved to be very leukemogenic, with an estimated incidence of 3% to 5% in HL survivors.[58–60] Modern chemotherapy seems to be less leukemogenic and the classic ABVD regimen is not thought to be leukemogenic. Patients with t-MDS/t-AML have a poor prognosis, with a median OS in this trial of 7.2 months. Allogeneic stem cell transplantation is considered the only curative therapy. Several reports have demonstrated that t-MDS/t-AML can also occur after radiation therapy in the absence of chemotherapy.[61–63]

Survivors of HL are also at a higher risk of cardiovascular complications including accelerated coronary artery disease, valvular disease, pericardial disease, arrhythmia, and cardiomyopathy. The majority of cardiovascular complications can be attributed to mediastinal radiation therapy and the risk typically begins after a latency of 10 years and remains persistently elevated. The risk of cardiac disease appears to be directly related to radiation dose.[64,65] In a study of 1,132 pediatric patients in Germany and Austria that survived HL, the 25-year cumulative incidence of cardiovascular disease in the group receiving 36 Gy of mediastinal radiation was 21%. The risk decreased to 10%, 6%, 5%, and 3% in those receiving lower doses of mediastinal radiation at 30, 25, 20, and 0 Gy, respectively (P <0.001).[64] In multivariate analyses, mediastinal radiation dose was the only significant factor predicting cardiac disease-free survival (P = 0.0025). An important principal in the surgical management of patients exposed to mediastinal irradiation that require coronary artery bypass grafting is that the majority have coexisting valvular abnormalities that often necessitates concomitant surgical repair.[66,67]

In addition to mediastinal radiation, the cardiotoxicity of anthracyclines—essential components of the ABVD regimen—is well documented. The risk is related to the cumulative anthracycline dose with most studies recommending that cumulative doxorubicin doses be limited to 450 to 500 mg/m^2 in adults, but heart failure has been observed in doses even <240 mg/m^2.[68] Several studies demonstrate that traditional cardiac risk factors, including hypertension, hypercholesterolemia, and smoking further contribute to the risk of cardiac disease in HL survivors.[69–72]

Finally, endocrinopathies can develop in HL survivors, with the risk of hypothyroidism being as high as 60% after neck irradiation.[73] Sterility can result from pelvic irradiation and exposure to alkylating regimens, particularly the MOPP chemotherapy regimen. ABVD does not appear to affect fertility; however, escalated BEACOPP was been associated with azoospermia in 90% of male patients and 50% of female patients reported continuous amenorrhea.[74–76]

PRIMARY MEDIASTINAL B-CELL LYMPHOMA

INTRODUCTION

Compared to HL, which is the most common type of primary lymphoma of the mediastinum in teenagers and young adults, PMBL is slightly more common in patients in their late 20s and 30s. PMBL, a subtype of diffuse large B-cell non-Hodgkin lymphoma (DLBCL), is a distinct clinicopathologic entity with unique phenotypic and molecular features, and arises from an intrathymic B-cell population as reviewed by van Besien et al.[77] The disease can be difficult to distinguish from other DLBCL by classic pathologic criteria, but has a quite distinctive clinical presentation. In most series, there is a slight preponderance of females. Patients with PMBL present with a rapidly growing mass originating from the anterior and superior mediastinum and surrounding structures. Symptoms arise because of compression of mediastinal structures. This is in contrast to patients with HL who rarely have symptoms relating to a mediastinal mass. At initial presentation, superior vena cava syndrome is the most common complication. Phrenic nerve palsy can also occur and when bilateral, can lead to respiratory failure. Presenting symptoms can also include dysphagia, hoarseness, bilateral breast swelling, chest pain, and productive cough.

EPIDEMIOLOGY AND ETIOLOGY

PMBL was originally described in the 1980s and is a formally recognized subtype of non-Hodgkin lymphoma (NHL) in the WHO classification.[3] In 2015, SEER estimates 71,850 new cases of NHL and 19,790 deaths.[4] PMBL comprises up to 3% of all cases NHL overall and 10% of DLBCL.[78] The location of PMBL, occasional presence of epithelial-lined cysts, thymic lobules, as well as Hassall corpuscles in biopsy specimens, all indicate a thymic origin. Although the thymus is a major site of T-cell maturation, a thymic B-cell population with a unique immunophenotype characterized by expression of CD19, CD20, CD22, and CD79a and negative for CD15, CD21, CD138, CD68, and markers of latent EBV infection characterizes PMBL and was initially described by Isaacson et al.[79] CD 30 staining may be weakly positive, making the distinction from cHL difficult at times.[80] PMBCL is typically negative for surface and cytoplasmic immunoglobulin.

PMBL has distinct biologic characteristics from other subtypes of DLBCL and more closely resembles nodular sclerosing HL. Conventional comparative genomic hydridization and PCR fingerprinting

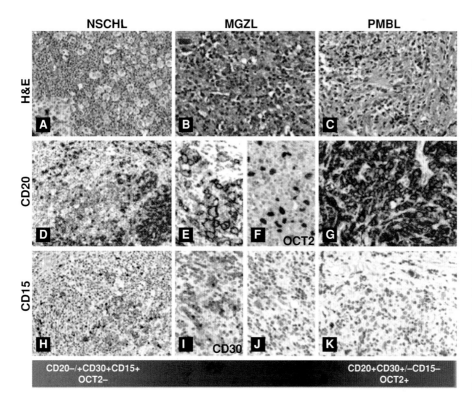

FIGURE 168.2 Biologic continuum between cHL and PMBL. **A:** Nodular sclerosis, classical Hodgkin lymphoma (NSCHL) with abundant Hodgkin and Reed–Sternberg (HRS) cells of lacunar type (H&E, 400×, inset: CD20 immunostain, 400× magnification). **D:** The HRS cells are weakly and heterogeneously CD20 positive, in contrast to the strong CD20 positivity of the surrounding reactive B-cells (200×). **H:** The lacunar cells are CD15 positive (200×). **B:** Mediastinal gray zone lymphoma (MGZL) with morphologic features reminiscent of CHL but an immunophenotype more consistent with PMBL. **E:** Note the strong, homogeneous CD20 and **F:** OCT2 positivity. **J:** The tumor cells are CD15 negative (H&E and immunostaining, 400×) and **I:** variably positive for CD30. **C:** Primary mediastinal B-cell lymphoma (PMBL) composed of an infiltrate of large cells with round or lobulated nuclei and abundant clear cytoplasm. In the background there is a characteristic compartmentalizing sclerosis (H&E, 400×). **G:** The tumor cells are CD20 positive and **K:** CD15 negative (400×). H&E, hematoxylin and eosin stain. (From Quintanilla-Martinez L, Fend F. Mediastinal gray zone lymphoma. *Haematol* 2011; 96(4):496–499.)

show genetic abnormalities including regions of genomic gain particularly involving 2, 5, 7, 9p, 12, and Xq.[81] The gain in the 9p region leads to programmed death ligand (PDL) 1/2 amplification in up to 60%, and upregulation of the Janus Kinase (JAK) 2 gene in almost 50% of patients.[82,83] A gain in the 2p region leads to duplication of REL proto-oncogene that encodes a transcription factor of the nuclear factor kappa B (NFKB) family.[84] MGZL, a third mediastinal NHL to be discussed further below may be a biologic bridge between cHL and PMBL (Fig. 168.2).[85,86] Despite these shared biologic features between cHL and PMBL, the treatment of PMBL is more aligned to other aggressive NHLs.

CLINICAL PRESENTATION

PMBL usually affects adolescents and young adults, with a female propensity, and typically presents in the third and fourth decades of life which is much earlier than other subtypes of DLBCL.[3] Symptoms at diagnosis are due to the anterior mediastinal mass and up to 50% have signs and symptoms of superior vena cava syndrome at presentation, with facial edema, neck vein distention, and occasionally, upper extremity swelling and/or deep vein thrombosis. Bulky masses >10 cm are common, often with local infiltration into the lung, chest wall, pleura, and pericardium. Extension to supraclavicular or high subdiaphragmatic lymph nodes may occur but, despite local invasiveness, distant lymph node involvement and bone marrow infiltration is rare. At relapse, involvement of extranodal sites including the lung, kidneys, gastrointestinal organs, breasts, ovaries, and CNS is not uncommon.

DIAGNOSIS AND STAGING

The diagnostic workup and staging of PMBL should include the same routine tests performed for any other patient with NHL and are described under the section above for HL. Because PMBL rarely involves the bone marrow, a routine bone marrow biopsy is not jus-

tified, particularly if the ^{18}FDG-PET/CT is not suggestive of bone marrow involvement.[21] Although CNS involvement is rare at initial diagnosis, the cerebrospinal fluid should be checked by cytology and flow cytometry in the presence of extranodal disease. It is common for pleural and pericardial effusions to occur due to lymphomatous invasion or to obstruction of lymphatic return, so it may be useful to perform an echocardiogram. Thoracentesis may also be useful to determine the nature of a pleural effusion.

Upon completion of therapy, a residual mediastinal mass is commonly present, particularly in cases where there was a bulky mediastinal mass at presentation or if there was a large fibrotic component to the mass. These masses may persist for several months after the completion of therapy which is an important consideration for followup imaging. Studies looking at the role of ^{18}FDG-PET in PMBL are limited, and the technique has been found to have a very high negative predictive value but low positive predictive value in PBML in comparison to other aggressive lymphomas. In the largest prospective study of ^{18}FDG-PET in 115 patients with PMBL, 54 patients (47%) had a complete metabolic response defined as a completely negative scan, whereas 61 patients (53%) had residual uptake on PET. A complete metabolic response after chemoimmunotherapy predicted a higher 5-year PFS (98% vs. 82%; P = 0.0044) and OS (100% vs. 91%; P = 0.0298). Patients with residual uptake higher than the mediastinal blood pool, but below liver uptake (Deauville score of 3), had equally good outcomes, whereas using the liver as the cutoff for PET positivity (Deauville score of 4) was able to discriminate between high and low risk of failure, with 5-year PFS of 99% versus 68% (P <0.001) and 5-year OS of 100% versus 83% (P <0.001).[87] The authors concluded that >90% of these patients demonstrated PFS at 5 years despite residual uptake on PET after chemoimmunotherapy, suggesting that PET could be used to define the role of radiotherapy as consolidation in PMBL. Figure 168.3 demonstrates the ^{18}FDG-PET/CT uptake in a patient with a PMBL who presented with SVC syndrome and was found to have a 17 cm mediastinal mass with an SUV of 28, Deauville score of 5.

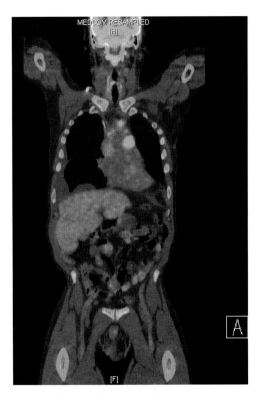

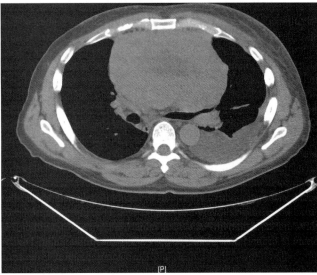

FIGURE 168.3 ^{18}FDG-PET/CT uptake in a patient with PMBL.

MANAGEMENT OF PRIMARY MEDIASTINAL B-CELL LYMPHOMA

In the "prerituximab" era, early treatment studies demonstrated a high incidence of progressive disease which was noted during treatment with cyclophosphamide, doxorubicin, vincristine, and prednisone (CHOP) alone, with improved outcomes using more intensive regimens, such as, etoposide, doxorubicin, cyclophosphamide, vincristine, prednisone, and bleomycin (VACOP-B) or methotrexate, doxorubicin, cyclophosphamide, vincristine, prednisone, and bleomycin (MACOP-B).[88,89] Thus, VACOP-B or MACOP-B followed by IFRT was considered the standard of care "prerituximab." Studies looking at the role of intensified chemotherapy followed by ASCT were also superior to CHOP-like regimens.[88,90]

Coiffier and colleagues[91] and Pfreundschuh and colleagues,[92] subsequently established that the standard front-line chemotherapy for DLBCL should include both an anthracycline and the monoclonal chimeric anti-CD20 antibody, rituximab, among both elderly and young patients, leading to prolonged event-free survival (EFS) and OS rates with long-term followup. Subsequent studies have demonstrated an improvement in early treatment failure, PFS and OS with rituximab-based immunochemotherapy, compared to chemotherapy alone in PMBL.[93–95] In the Mabthera International Trial (MInT) Group study (n = 87), PMBL patients <60 were treated with six cycles of CHOP-like regimens with or without rituximab with the rituximab cohort (RCHOP) demonstrating higher complete remission (84% vs. 54%; p = 0.015), lower early progressive disease (2.5% vs. 24% p <0.001), improved 3-year EFS 978% vs. 52%, p = 0.012), and similar OS (89% vs. 78%, p = 0.158) than those treated with CHOP-like regimens.[95] Of 61 patients who received RT because of bulky disease or extranodal disease, 30% achieved an improvement in response and 7% developed progressive disease following radiotherapy.[95] Another study however retrospectively assessed 63 patients with PMBL and found a high primary induction failure rate (21%) with RCHOP, possibly because 21% of patients had advanced-stage disease, 71% had bulky disease and 33% had an age-adjusted International Prognostic Index of 2 to 3.[96] Although such high induction failure with RCHOP has not been observed in other studies of PMBL, most experts agree RCHOP should be used cautiously in patients with PMBL at high risk.[97]

Rituximab has been used with other chemotherapy regimens in both a Memorial Sloan Kettering Cancer Center (MSKCC) study and a National Cancer Institute (NCI) study. At MSKCC, 54 patients received RCHOP in an accelerated fashion (every 2 weeks for four cycles) followed by interim PET/CT scan. Those with a negative PET/CT received three cycles of ICE (ifosfamide, carboplatin, and etoposide) consolidation therapy, whereas those with positive PET/CT underwent repeat biopsy. Biopsy negative patients received three cycles of ICE and biopsy positive patients received three cycles of ICE followed by autologous stem cell transplant. This resulted in an overall response rate of 79% and 3-year PFS and OS of 78% and 88%, respectively.[98] An NCI prospective phase II study of 51 patients with PMBL treated with six to eight cycles of dose-adjusted etoposide, doxorubicin, cyclophosphamide, vincristine, and prednisone in combination with rituximab (DA-EPOCH-R), but without RT in responders resulted in a 5-year EFS and 5-year OS of 93% and 97%, respectively.[99]

The role of consolidative approaches remains controversial, and disagreement exists on which chemotherapy regimen to use and whether or not to consolidate some or all patients with high-dose chemotherapy and/or radiation. Some centers have reported excellent results with standard anthracycline-based chemotherapy followed by radiation therapy to residual masses.[89,100] Others have used intensive chemotherapy without consolidative radiation with similar long-term results,[96,97] and this has the advantage of avoiding the late side-effects of mediastinal radiation that were discussed earlier for HL. There is general agreement that achievement of a complete remission is the best predictor for outcome in PMBL and many centers have recommended consolidation with autologous transplantation for patients with bulky residual masses, particularly if there is residual PET positivity.[90,101] Patients with PMBL who achieve a response lasting longer than 18 months after diagnosis are likely to be cured. Treatment failure usually occurs either during initial treatment or within the first 6 to 12 months after completion of treatment. This contrasts with HL, where late recurrences are much more common.

In the past, radiation therapy has often been used as salvage treatment for patients with recurrences in the mediastinum. Multiple studies show mediastinal RT may improve response rate and long-term outcomes in PMBL patients with residual disease after chemotherapy.[89,100–103] In an Italian study (n = 37), following rituximab-based chemotherapy, 67% had a positive PET/CT scan at a median of 28 days after the end of therapy and patients subsequently received radiotherapy (3-dimensional conformal RT or image-guided intensity modulated RT). There was 100% complete response rate for those with a Deauville score of 1 to 3 versus 25% with a score of 5. At 3 years, OS for those with a Deauville score of 1 to 3 was 100% compared to 77% for those with Deauville scores of 4 to 5 (p <0.05).[103] For patients who demonstrate a complete response after chemoimmunotherapy, retrospective studies suggest RT may not improve outcomes.[97] Further prospective clinical trials are needed to confirm these findings.

T-LYMPHOBLASTIC LYMPHOMA

INTRODUCTION

The WHO classification system for hematologic malignancies divides lymphoblastic neoplasms into two categories based on cell of origin: precursor B-cell acute lymphoblastic leukemia/lymphoma (ALL) or precursor T-cell ALL. The clinical presentation, prognosis, and treatment differ substantially between neoplasms of B- and T-cell lineage. The distinction between ALL and LBL is based on presence or absence, respectively, of more than 25% marrow involvement by the malignant cells, although the terms are often used interchangeably. Clinically, a case is defined as LBL if there is a mass lesion in the mediastinum or elsewhere and less than 25% blasts in the bone marrow. T-cell LBL (T-LBL) is the subtype most likely to present with a mediastinal mass (50% to 75% of cases) and will be the focus of this review.

EPIDEMIOLOGY AND ETIOLOGY

T-LBL is a rapidly growing tumor seen in adolescents and young adults with a nearly three-fold male predominance. At diagnosis, men are younger than women with a bimodal age distribution in males (peaking at age 10 to 30 and 60 to 70 years) and a more even distribution in females.[104] T-LBL represents 15% of childhood ALL and 25% of adult ALL. The incidence in the United States is approximately 3 cases per million persons per year and does not vary by ethnicity.[105] The cell of origin is postulated to arise from precursor T lymphoblasts at varying stages of differentiation. No risk factors have been clearly identified in LBL.

CLINICAL PRESENTATION

T-LBL presents with lymphadenopathy in cervical, supraclavicular, and axillary regions (50%), or with a mediastinal mass in up to 75% of patients. Commonly, the mediastinal mass is anterior, bulky, and can be associated with pleural effusions, superior vena cava syndrome, tracheal obstruction, and pericardial effusions. Patients present with stage IV disease (80%) and B symptoms (50%), and in the majority of cases elevated LDH levels.[106] Less commonly, patients present with extranodal disease (e.g., skin, testis, and bone involvement). Although bone marrow can be normal in T-LBL at presentation, about 60% of patients develop bone marrow infiltration and subsequently a leukemic phase indistinguishable from T-ALL.[104] Cerebrospinal fluid evaluation is essential to rule out CNS involvement.

DIAGNOSIS

In some cases, T-LBL is completely limited to the mediastinum and a biopsy may be required for diagnosis. In other instances, however, examination of the peripheral blood or bone marrow biopsy can lead to a diagnosis and lymph node or mediastinal biopsy is not necessary. Morphologically, lymphoblasts vary from small cells with scant cytoplasm, condensed nuclear chromatin, and indistinct nucleoli to larger cells with moderate amounts of cytoplasm, dispersed chromatin, and multiple nucleoli. A few azurophilic cytoplasmic granules may be present but Auer rods are never seen. In tissue sections, the tumor cells are small to medium-sized, with scant cytoplasm, round, oval, or convoluted nuclei, fine chromatin and indistinct or small nucleoli. Occasional cases have larger cells. T-cell and B-cell disease are morphologically indistinguishable and immunohistochemistry demonstrates lymphoblasts stained positive for periodic acid Schiff (PAS), variable positivity for nonspecific esterase and Sudan black B, and negativity for myeloperoxidase. On flow cytometry, the lymphoblasts are typically positive for CD7 and either surface or cytoplasmic CD3, and variably express CD2, CD5, CD1a, CD4, and/or CD8.

MANAGEMENT AND PROGNOSIS

Initial treatment regimens for ALL were very similar to protocols used to treat NHL; however, because of the biologic similarities to ALL and poor outcomes with standard NHL regimens, investigators started to apply intensive ALL-like regimens to LBL. Several regimens have shown promising results with most incorporating an intensive multidrug induction, often with five or six drugs incorporating an anthracycline, cyclophosphamide, vincristine, and a steroid among others. This is followed by a consolidation phase which includes CNS prophylaxis with intrathecal chemotherapy. Finally, an oral maintenance phase is prescribed for approximately 2 years, most commonly with POMP (6-mercaptopurine, oral methotrexate, prednisone, and vincristine). Cranial irradiation is sometimes used and mediastinal irradiation may be considered if a mediastinal mass persists after chemotherapy.

Most modern studies using ALL regimens report complete response rates greater than 90% and rate greater than 60% with at least 3-year followup.[107] However, the majority of studies are single institution studies using regimens developed at individual institutions which may be prone to selection bias. Patients with adverse prognostic factors may be considered for consolidation with high-dose chemotherapy and autologous or allogeneic stem cell transplantation.

MEDIASTINAL GRAY ZONE LYMPHOMA

Although most lymphomas can be diagnosed and classified as distinct disease entities, some lymphomas exhibit overlapping histologic, biologic, and clinical features between various subtypes of lymphoma. The WHO 2008 classification of NHL has introduced several new changes, including the recognition of these so-called borderline entities.[3] B-cell lymphoma, unclassifiable, with features intermediate between DLBCL and HL encompasses a B-cell lymphoma that exhibits the morphology of cHL but the immunophenotype of DLBCL, or vice versa. Interestingly, most cases reported in the literature present with mediastinal masses. Lymphomas in this category arising in the mediastinum are now commonly known as MGZLs.

The clinical characteristics and treatment of MGZLs have yet to be defined because of its recent identification and rarity. Limited published data reveal MGZLs predominantly affect young males and otherwise have overlapping clinical features with PMBL. Diagnostic evaluation is also similar to PMBL. The morphologic appearance of MGZL is intermediate between that of cHL and PMBL. The tumor cells are often pleomorphic and grow in a diffusely fibrotic stroma. Tumor cells may have a Hodgkin-like morphology, but with a phenotype pattern consistent with PMBL (CD20++, CD15−). Alternatively, the tumor cells may have a PMBL-like morphology and a Hodgkin phenotype with expression of CD30 and CD15 and loss of CD20 and CD79a.[108] Interphase fluorescence in situ hybridization (FISH) studies of adults with MGZL show amplifications in 2p16/1 (REL/BCL11A locus), alterations in the JAK2/PDL2 locus in 9p24.1, rearrangement of the CIITA locus at 16p13.13, as well as gains of 8q24 at MYC. A molecular signature has not been yet further elucidated MGZL; however, a large-scale methylation analysis of PMBL, cHL, and MGZL demonstrates a close epigenetic relationship between PMBL and cHL and a unique signature for MGZL which is to be validated.[109]

Owing to the rarity of the disease and lack of prospective studies, controversy on the optimal management of MGZL exists. Previously, these tumors were likely identified as "anaplastic large-cell lymphoma Hodgkin-like," which was reported to have a poor outcome with chemotherapy.[110] In a single study evaluating the outcome of MGZL treated with a cHL or NHL regimen, survival was significantly inferior compared to that of cHL.[111] A prospective study looked at the outcome of MGZL following treatment with DA-EPOCH-R and reported inferior survival compared with PMBL. Both patient groups had similar clinical characteristics; however, MGZL patients had a 3-year EFS and OS of 62% and 74% compared to 93% and 97% for PMBL, respectively, with a high percentage of patients requiring mediastinal radiation.[112]

SUMMARY

Malignant lymphomas are a common cause of mediastinal masses. Given the diversity of subtypes and disease-specific therapies, a definitive biopsy is essential. Most of these disorders are exquisitely chemo- and/or radiosensitive, and the role of surgery remains primarily diagnostic. Many mediastinal lymphomas, including HL, PMBL, and T-LBL are highly curable but may come at the cost of long-term therapy-related disorders including accelerated coronary disease, valvular complications, and increased risk of secondary malignancies. The use of newer imaging modalities such as ^{18}FDG-PET has improved our ability to predict and perhaps tailor treatments in individual patients, even as the optimal application of these technologies continues to evolve.

REFERENCES

1. Harris NL, Jaffe ES, Stein H, et al. A revised European-American classification of lymphoid neoplasms: a proposal from the international lymphoma study group. *Blood* 1994;84:1361–1392.
2. Jaffe ES, Harris NL, Stein H, et al. World Health Organization classification of tumours. Pathology and genetics of tumours of haematopoietic and lymphoid tissues. In: Jaffe ES, Harris NL, Stein H, et al., eds. WHO Classification of Tumours of Haematopoietic and Lymphoid Tissues. 4th ed. Lyon: IARC Press; 2001:1–351.
3. Swerdlow SH, Campo E, Harris NL, et al. *Classification of Tumours of Haematopoietic and Lymphoid Tissues.* Lyon, France: IARC Press; 2008.
4. Howlader N, Noone AM, Krapcho M, et al. *SEER Cancer Statistics Review, 1975–2012.* Bethesda: National Cancer Institute; 2014. Available from: http://seer.cancer.gov/csr/1975_2012/
5. Percival ME, Hoppe RT, Advani RH. Bulky mediastinal classical Hodgkin lymphoma in young women. *Oncology (Williston Park, NY)* 2014;28(3):253–256, 258–260, C3.
6. Vaeth JM, Moskowitz SA, Green JP. Mediastinal Hodgkin's disease. *AJR Am J Roentgenol* 1976;126(1):123–126.
7. Kuppers R, Rajewsky K. The origin of Hodgkin and Reed/Sternberg cells in Hodgkin's disease. *Annu Rev Immunol* 1998;16:471–493.
8. Schmitz R, Stanelle J, Hansmann ML, et al. Pathogenesis of classical and lymphocyte-predominant Hodgkin lymphoma. *Annu Rev Pathol* 2009;4:151–174.
9. Schwering I, Brauninger A, Klein U, et al. Loss of the B-lineage-specific gene expression program in Hodgkin and Reed-Sternberg cells of Hodgkin lymphoma. *Blood* 2003;101(4):1505–1512.
10. Hjalgrim H, Engels EA. Infectious aetiology of Hodgkin and non-Hodgkin lymphomas: a review of the epidemiological evidence. *J Intern Med* 2008;264(6):537–548.
11. Gobbi PG, Ferreri AJ, Ponzoni M, et al. Hodgkin lymphoma. *Crit Rev Oncol Hematol* 2013;85(2):216–237.
12. Niens M, Jarrett RF, Hepkema B, et al. HLA-A*02 is associated with a reduced risk and HLA-A*01 with an increased risk of developing EBV+ Hodgkin lymphoma. *Blood* 2007;110(9):3310–3315.
13. Brown JR, Neuberg D, Phillips K, et al. Prevalence of familial malignancy in a prospectively screened cohort of patients with lymphoproliferative disorders. *Br J Haematol* 2008;143(3):361–368.
14. Spina M, Berretta M, Tirelli U. Hodgkin's disease in HIV. *Hematol Oncol Clin North Am* 2003;17(3):843–858.
15. Ng AK, Bernardo MP, Weller E, et al. Long-term survival and competing causes of death in patients with early-stage Hodgkin's disease treated at age 50 or younger. *J Clin Oncol* 2002;20(8):2101–2108.
16. Good GR, DiNubile MJ. Images in clinical medicine. Cyclic fever in Hodgkin's disease (Pel-Ebstein fever). *N Engl J Med* 1995;332(7):436.
17. Hughes-Davies L, Tarbell NJ, Coleman CN, et al. Stage IA-IIB Hodgkin's disease: management and outcome of extensive thoracic involvement. *Int J Radiat Oncol Biol Phys* 1997;39(2):361–369.
18. Talebian-Yazdi M, von Bartheld B, Waaijenborg F, et al. Endosonography for the diagnosis of malignant lymphoma presenting with mediastinal lymphadenopathy. *J Bronchology Interv Pulmonol* 2014;21(4):298–305.
19. Rosenberg SA, Kaplan HS. Evidence for an orderly progression in the spread of Hodgkin's disease. *Cancer Res* 1966;26(6):1225–1231.
20. Lister TA, Crowther D, Sutcliffe SB, et al. Report of a committee convened to discuss the evaluation and staging of patients with Hodgkin's disease: Cotswolds meeting. *J Clin Oncol* 1989;7:1630–1636.
21. Cheson BD, Fisher RI, Barrington SF, et al. Recommendations for initial evaluation, staging, and response assessment of Hodgkin and non-Hodgkin lymphoma: the Lugano classification. *J Clin Oncol* 2014;32(27):3059–3068.
22. Isasi CR, Lu P, Blaufox MD. A metaanalysis of 18F-2-deoxy-2-fluoro-D-glucose positron emission tomography in the staging and restaging of patients with lymphoma. *Cancer* 2005;104(5):1066–1074.
23. Evens AM, Kostakoglu L. The role of FDG-PET in defining prognosis of Hodgkin lymphoma for early-stage disease. *Blood* 2014;124(23):3356–3364.
24. Barrington SF, Qian W, Somer EJ, et al. Concordance between four European centres of PET reporting criteria designed for use in multicentre trials in Hodgkin lymphoma. *Eur J Nucl Med Mol Imaging* 2010;37(10):1824–1833.
25. El-Galaly TC, d'Amore F, Mylam KJ, et al. Routine bone marrow biopsy has little or no therapeutic consequence for positron emission tomography/computed tomography-staged treatment-naive patients with Hodgkin lymphoma. *J Clin Oncol* 2012;30(36):4508–4514.
26. Hasenclever D, Diehl V. A prognostic score for advanced Hodgkin's disease. International Prognostic Factors Project on Advanced Hodgkin's Disease. *N Engl J Med* 1998;339(21):1506–1514.
27. Canellos GP, Rosenberg SA, Friedberg JW, et al. Treatment of Hodgkin lymphoma: a 50-year perspective. *J Clin Oncol* 2014;32(3):163–168.
28. Bonadonna G, Valagussa P, Santoro A. Alternating non-cross-resistant combination chemotherapy or MOPP in Stage IV Hodgkin's disease. A report of 8-year results. *Ann Int Med* 1986;104:739–746.
29. Armitage JO. Early-stage Hodgkin's lymphoma. *N Engl J Med* 2010;363(7):653–662.
30. Longo DL, Glatstein E, Duffey PL, et al. Alternating MOPP and ABVD chemotherapy plus mantle-field radiation therapy in patients with massive mediastinal Hodgkin's disease. *J Clin Oncol* 1997;15(11):3338–3346.
31. Straus DJ, Portlock CS, Qin J, et al. Results of a prospective randomized clinical trial of doxorubicin, bleomycin, vinblastine, and dacarbazine (ABVD) followed by radiation therapy (RT) versus ABVD alone for stages I, II, and IIIA nonbulky Hodgkin disease. *Blood* 2004;104(12):3483–3489.
32. Meyer RM, Gospodarowicz MK, Connors JM, et al. ABVD alone versus radiation-based therapy in limited-stage Hodgkin's lymphoma. *N Engl J Med* 2012;366(5):399–408.
33. Engert A, Plutschow A, Eich HT, et al. Reduced treatment intensity in patients with early-stage Hodgkin's lymphoma. *N Engl J Med* 2010;363(7):640–652.
34. Engert A, Schiller P, Josting A, et al. Involved-field radiotherapy is equally effective and less toxic compared with extended-field radiotherapy after four cycles of chemotherapy in patients with early-stage unfavorable Hodgkin's lymphoma: results of the HD8 trial of the German Hodgkin's Lymphoma Study Group. *J Clin Oncol* 2003;21(19):3601–3608.
35. Bonadonna G, Bonfante V, Viviani S, et al. ABVD plus subtotal nodal versus involved-field radiotherapy in early-stage Hodgkin's disease: long-term results. *J Clin Oncol* 2004;22(14):2835–2841.
36. Raemaekers JM, Andre MP, Federico M, et al. Omitting radiotherapy in early positron emission tomography-negative stage I/II Hodgkin lymphoma is associated with an increased risk of early relapse: Clinical results of the preplanned interim analysis of the randomized EORTC/LYSA/FIL H10 trial. *J Clin Oncol* 2014;32(12):1188–1194.
37. Castellino SM, Geiger AM, Mertens AC, et al. Morbidity and mortality in long-term survivors of Hodgkin lymphoma: a report from the Childhood Cancer Survivor Study. *Blood* 2011;117(6):1806–1816.

38. Radford J, Illidge T, Counsell N, et al. Results of a trial of PET-directed therapy for early-stage Hodgkin's lymphoma. *N Engl J Med* 2015;372(17):1598–1607.

39. Eich HT, Diehl V, Gorgen H, et al. Intensified chemotherapy and dose-reduced involved-field radiotherapy in patients with early unfavorable Hodgkin's lymphoma: final analysis of the German Hodgkin Study Group HD11 trial. *J Clin Oncol* 2010;28(27):4199–4206.

40. Horning SJ, Hoppe RT, Breslin S, et al. Stanford V and radiotherapy for locally extensive and advanced Hodgkin's disease: mature results of a prospective clinical trial. *J Clin Oncol* 2002;20(3):630–637.

41. Advani RH, Hong F, Fisher RI, et al. Randomized phase III trial comparing ABVD plus radiotherapy with the Stanford V regimen in patients with stages I or II locally extensive, bulky mediastinal Hodgkin lymphoma: a subset analysis of the North American intergroup E2496 trial. *J Clin Oncol* 2015;33(17):1936–1942.

42. Hoskin PJ, Lowry L, Horwich A, et al. Randomized comparison of the Stanford V regimen and ABVD in the treatment of advanced Hodgkin's Lymphoma: United Kingdom National Cancer Research Institute Lymphoma Group Study ISRCTN 64141244. *J Clin Oncol* 2009;27(32):5390–5396.

43. Linch DC, Winfield D, Goldstone AH, et al. Dose intensification with autologous bone-marrow transplantation in relapsed and resistant Hodgkin's disease: results of a BNLI randomised trial. *Lancet* 1993;341(8852):1051–1054.

44. Schmitz N, Pfistner B, Sextro M, et al. Aggressive conventional chemotherapy compared with high-dose chemotherapy with autologous haemopoietic stem-cell transplantation for relapsed chemosensitive Hodgkin's disease: a randomised trial. *Lancet* 2002;359(9323):2065–2071.

45. Rancea M, Monsef I, von Tresckow B, et al. High-dose chemotherapy followed by autologous stem cell transplantation for patients with relapsed/refractory Hodgkin lymphoma. *Cochrane Database Syst Rev* 2013;6:Cd009411.

46. Anderlini P, Saliba R, Acholonu S, et al. Reduced-intensity allogeneic stem cell transplantation in relapsed and refractory Hodgkin's disease: low transplant-related mortality and impact of intensity of conditioning regimen. *Bone Marrow Transplant* 2005;35(10):943–951.

47. Peggs KS, Hunter A, Chopra R, et al. Clinical evidence of a graft-versus-Hodgkin's-lymphoma effect after reduced-intensity allogeneic transplantation. *Lancet* 2005;365(9475):1934–1941.

48. Sureda A, Robinson S, Canals C, et al. Reduced-intensity conditioning compared with conventional allogeneic stem-cell transplantation in relapsed or refractory Hodgkin's lymphoma: an analysis from the Lymphoma Working Party of the European Group for Blood and Marrow Transplantation. *J Clin Oncol* 2008;26(3):455–462.

49. Okeley NM, Miyamoto JB, Zhang X, et al. Intracellular activation of SGN-35, a potent anti-CD30 antibody-drug conjugate. *Clin Cancer Res* 2010;16(3):888–897.

50. Ansell SM, Lesokhin AM, Borrello I, et al. PD-1 blockade with nivolumab in relapsed or refractory Hodgkin's lymphoma. *N Engl J Med* 2015;372(4):311–319.

51. Ng AK. Current survivorship recommendations for patients with Hodgkin lymphoma: focus on late effects. *Blood* 2014;124(23):3373–3379.

52. Morton LM, Dores GM, Curtis RE, et al. Stomach cancer risk after treatment for hodgkin lymphoma. *J Clin Oncol* 2013;31(27):3369–3377.

53. Henderson TO, Oeffinger KC, Whitton J, et al. Secondary gastrointestinal cancer in childhood cancer survivors: a cohort study. *Ann Intern Med* 2012;156(11):757–766, w-260.

54. Swerdlow AJ, Higgins CD, Smith P, et al. Second cancer risk after chemotherapy for Hodgkin's lymphoma: a collaborative British cohort study. *J Clin Oncol* 2011;29(31):4096–4104.

55. Travis LB, Gilbert E. Lung cancer after Hodgkin lymphoma: the roles of chemotherapy, radiotherapy and tobacco use. *Radiat Res* 2005;163(6):695–696.

56. Inskip PD, Robison LL, Stovall M, et al. Radiation dose and breast cancer risk in the childhood cancer survivor study. *J Clin Oncol* 2009;27(24):3901–3907.

57. Bloom JR, Stewart SL, Hancock SL. Breast cancer screening in women surviving Hodgkin disease. *Am J Clin Oncol* 2006;29(3):258–266.

58. Delwail V, Jais JP, Colonna P, et al. Fifteen-year secondary leukaemia risk observed in 761 patients with Hodgkin's disease prospectively treated by MOPP or ABVD chemotherapy plus high-dose irradiation. *Br J Haematol* 2002;118(1):189–194.

59. Brusamolino E, Anselmo AP, Klersy C, et al. The risk of acute leukaemia in patients treated for Hodgkin's disease is significantly higher after combined modality programs than after chemotherapy alone and is correlated with the extent of radiotherapy and type and duration of chemotherapy: a case-control study. *Haematol* 1998;83(9):812–823.

60. Eichenauer DA, Thielen I, Haverkamp H, et al. Therapy-related acute myeloid leukemia and myelodysplastic syndromes in patients with Hodgkin lymphoma: a report from the German Hodgkin Study Group. *Blood* 2014;123(11):1658–1664.

61. Pedersen-Bjergaard J, Philip P, Larsen SO, et al. Therapy-related myelodysplasia and acute myeloid leukemia. Cytogenetic characteristics of 115 consecutive cases and risk in seven cohorts of patients treated intensively for malignant diseases in the Copenhagen series. *Leukemia* 1993;7:1975–1986.

62. Smith SM, LeBeau M, Huo D, et al. Clinical-cytogenetic associations in 306 patients with therapy-related myelodysplasia and myeloid leukemia: the University of Chicago series. *Blood* 2003;102(1):43–52.

63. Kantarjian HM, Keating MJ, Walton RS, et al. Therapy related leukemia and myelodysplastic syndrome: clinical, cytogenetic and prognostic features. *J Clin Oncol* 1986;4:1748–1757.

64. Schellong G, Riepenhausen M, Bruch C, et al. Late valvular and other cardiac diseases after different doses of mediastinal radiotherapy for Hodgkin disease in children and adolescents: report from the longitudinal GPOH follow-up project of the German-Austrian DAL-HD studies. *Pediatr Blood Cancer* 2010;55(6):1145–1152.

65. Cella L, Liuzzi R, Conson M, et al. Dosimetric predictors of asymptomatic heart valvular dysfunction following mediastinal irradiation for Hodgkin's lymphoma. *Radiother Oncol* 2011;101(2):316–321.

66. Handa N, McGregor CG, Danielson GK, et al. Coronary artery bypass grafting in patients with previous mediastinal radiation therapy. *J Thorac Cardiovasc Surg* 1999;117(6):1136–1142.

67. Mittal S, Berko B, Bavaria J, et al. Radiation-induced cardiovascular dysfunction. *Am J Cardiol* 1996;78(1):114–115.

68. Swain SM, Whaley FS, Ewer MS. Congestive heart failure in patients treated with doxorubicin: a retrospective analysis of three trials. *Cancer* 2003;97(11):2869–2879.

69. Mulrooney DA, Yeazel MW, Kawashima T, et al. Cardiac outcomes in a cohort of adult survivors of childhood and adolescent cancer: retrospective analysis of the Childhood Cancer Survivor Study cohort. *BMJ* 2009;339:b4606.

70. Hull MC, Morris CG, Pepine CJ, et al. Valvular dysfunction and carotid, subclavian, and coronary artery disease in survivors of Hodgkin lymphoma treated with radiation therapy. *JAMA* 2003;290(21):2831–2837.

71. Aleman BM, van den Belt-Dusebout AW, De Bruin ML, et al. Late cardiotoxicity after treatment for Hodgkin lymphoma. *Blood* 2007;109(5):1878–1886.

72. Myrehaug S, Pintilie M, Yun L, et al. A population-based study of cardiac morbidity among Hodgkin lymphoma patients with preexisting heart disease. *Blood* 2010;116(13):2237–2240.

73. Bhatia S, Ramsay NK, Bantle JP, et al. Thyroid abnormalities after therapy for Hodgkin's disease in childhood. *Oncologist* 1996;1(1 & 2):62–67.

74. Hodgson DC, Pintilie M, Gitterman L, et al. Fertility among female Hodgkin lymphoma survivors attempting pregnancy following ABVD chemotherapy. *Hematol Oncol* 2007;25(1):11–15.

75. Sieniawski M, Reineke T, Nogova L, et al. Fertility in male patients with advanced Hodgkin lymphoma treated with BEACOPP: a report of the German Hodgkin Study Group (GHSG). *Blood* 2008;111(1):71–76.

76. Behringer K, Breuer K, Reineke T, et al. Secondary amenorrhea after Hodgkin's lymphoma is influenced by age at treatment, stage of disease, chemotherapy regimen, and the use of oral contraceptives during therapy: a report from the German Hodgkin's Lymphoma Study Group. *J Clin Oncol* 2005;23(30):7555–7564.

77. van Besien K, Kelta M, Bahaguna P. Primary mediastinal B-cell lymphoma: a review of pathology and management. *J Clin Oncol* 2001;19(6):1855–1864.

78. A clinical evaluation of the International Lymphoma Study Group classification of non-Hodgkin's lymphoma. The Non-Hodgkin's Lymphoma Classification Project. *Blood* 1997;89(11):3909–3918.

79. Isaacson PG, Norton AJ, Addis BJ. The human thymus contains a novel population of B lymphocytes. *Lancet* 1987;2(8574):1488–1491.

80. Johnson PW, Davies AJ. Primary mediastinal B-cell lymphoma. *ASH Education Program Book* 2008;2008(1):349–358.

81. Scarpa A, Moore PS, Rigaud G, et al. Genetic alterations in primary mediastinal B-cell lymphoma: an update. *Leuk Lymphoma* 2001;41(1–2):47–53.

82. Green MR, Monti S, Rodig SJ, et al. Integrative analysis reveals selective 9p24.1 amplification, increased PD-1 ligand expression, and further induction via JAK2 in nodular sclerosing Hodgkin lymphoma and primary mediastinal large B-cell lymphoma. *Blood* 2010;116(17):3268–3277.

83. Rosenwald A, Wright G, Leroy K, et al. Molecular diagnosis of primary mediastinal B cell lymphoma identifies a clinically favorable subgroup of diffuse large B cell lymphoma related to Hodgkin lymphoma. *J Exp Med* 2003;198(6):851–862.

84. Nedomova R, Papajik T, Prochazka V, et al. Cytogenetics and molecular cytogenetics in diffuse large B-cell lymphoma (DLBCL). *Biomed Pap Med Fac Univ Palacky Olomouc Czech Repub* 2013;157(3):239–247.

85. Calvo KR, Traverse-Glehen A, Pittaluga S, et al. Molecular profiling provides evidence of primary mediastinal large B-cell lymphoma as a distinct entity related to classic Hodgkin lymphoma: implications for mediastinal gray zone lymphomas as an intermediate form of B-cell lymphoma. *Adv Anat Pathol* 2004;11(5):227–238.

86. Quintanilla-Martinez L, Fend F. Mediastinal gray zone lymphoma. *Haematol* 2011;96(4):496–499.

87. Martelli M, Ceriani L, Zucca E, et al. [18F]fluorodeoxyglucose positron emission tomography predicts survival after chemoimmunotherapy for primary mediastinal large B-cell lymphoma: results of the International Extranodal Lymphoma Study Group IELSG-26 Study. *J Clin Oncol* 2014;32(17):1769–1775.

88. Zinzani PL, Martelli M, Bertini M, et al. Induction chemotherapy strategies for primary mediastinal large B-cell lymphoma with sclerosis: a retrospective multinational study on 426 previously untreated patients. *Haematol* 2002;87(12):1258–1264.

89. Todeschini G, Secchi S, Morra E, et al. Primary mediastinal large B-cell lymphoma (PMLBCL): long-term results from a retrospective multicentre Italian experience in 138 patients treated with CHOP or MACOP-B/VACOP-B. *Br J Cancer* 2004;90(2):372–376.

90. Hamlin PA, Portlock CS, Straus DJ, et al. Primary mediastinal large B-cell lymphoma: optimal therapy and prognostic factor analysis in 141 consecutive patients treated at Memorial Sloan Kettering from 1980 to 1999. *Br J Haematol* 2005;130(5):691–699.

91. Coiffier B, Thieblemont C, Van Den Neste E, et al. Long-term outcome of patients in the LNH-98.5 trial, the first randomized study comparing rituximab-CHOP to standard CHOP chemotherapy in DLBCL patients: a study by the Groupe d'Etudes des Lymphomes de l'Adulte. *Blood* 2010;116(12):2040–2045.

92. Pfreundschuh M, Kuhnt E, Trumper L, et al. CHOP-like chemotherapy with or without rituximab in young patients with good-prognosis diffuse large-B-cell lymphoma: 6-year results of an open-label randomised study of the MabThera International Trial (MInT) Group. *Lancet Oncol* 2011;12(11):1013–1022.

93. Vassilakopoulos TP, Pangalis GA, Katsigiannis A, et al. Rituximab, cyclophosphamide, doxorubicin, vincristine, and prednisone with or without radiotherapy in primary mediastinal large B-cell lymphoma: the emerging standard of care. *Oncologist* 2012; 17(2):239–249.

94. Tai WM, Quah D, Yap SP, et al. Primary mediastinal large B-cell lymphoma: optimal therapy and prognostic factors in 41 consecutive Asian patients. *Leuk Lymphoma* 2011;52(4):604–612.

95. Rieger M, Osterborg A, Pettengell R, et al. Primary mediastinal B-cell lymphoma treated with CHOP-like chemotherapy with or without rituximab: results of the Mabthera International Trial Group study. *Ann Oncol* 2011;22(3):664–670.

96. Soumerai JD, Hellmann MD, Feng Y, et al. Treatment of primary mediastinal B-cell lymphoma with rituximab, cyclophosphamide, doxorubicin, vincristine and prednisone is associated with a high rate of primary refractory disease. *Leuk Lymphoma* 2014;55(3):538–543.

97. Bhatt VR, Mourya R, Shrestha R, et al. Primary mediastinal large B-cell lymphoma. *Cancer Treat Rev* 2015;41(6):476–485.

98. Moskowitz C, Hamlin PA Jr, Maragulia J, et al. Sequential dose-dense RCHOP followed by ICE consolidation (MSKCC protocol 01–142) without radiotherapy for patients with primary mediastinal large B cell lymphoma. *ASH Annu Meeting Abstr* 2010.

99. Dunleavy K, Pittaluga S, Maeda LS, et al. Dose-adjusted EPOCH-rituximab therapy in primary mediastinal B-cell lymphoma. *N Engl J Med* 2013;368(15): 1408–1416.

100. Zinzani PL, Martelli M, Magagnoli M, et al. Treatment and clinical management of primary mediastinal large B-cell lymphoma with sclerosis: MACOP-B regimen and mediastinal radiotherapy monitored by (67)Gallium scan in 50 patients. *Blood* 1999;94(10):3289–3293.

101. Sehn LH, Antin JH, Shulman LN, et al. Primary diffuse large B-cell lymphoma of the mediastinum: outcome following high-dose chemotherapy and autologous hematopoietic cell transplantation. *Blood* 1998;91:717–723.

102. Xu LM, Li YX, Fang H, et al. Dosimetric evaluation and treatment outcome of intensity modulated radiation therapy after doxorubicin-based chemotherapy for primary mediastinal large B-cell lymphoma. *Int J Radiat Oncol Biol Phys* 2013;85(5):1289–1295.

103. Filippi AR, Piva C, Giunta F, et al. Radiation therapy in primary mediastinal B-cell lymphoma with positron emission tomography positivity after rituximab chemotherapy. *Int J Radiat Oncol Biol Physics* 2013;87(2):311–316.

104. Portell CA, Sweetenham JW. Adult lymphoblastic lymphoma. *Cancer J* 2012; 18(5):432–438.

105. Dores GM, Devesa SS, Curtis RE, et al. Acute leukemia incidence and patient survival among children and adults in the United States, 2001–2007. *Blood* 2012; 119(1):34–43.

106. Cortelazzo S, Ponzoni M, Ferreri AJ, et al. Lymphoblastic lymphoma. *Crit Rev Oncol Hematol* 2011;79(3):330–343.

107. Gokbuget N, Hoelzer D. Treatment of adult acute lymphoblastic leukemia. *Hematology Am Soc Hematol Educ Program* 2006:133–141.

108. Grant C, Dunleavy K, Eberle FC, et al. Primary mediastinal large B-cell lymphoma, classic Hodgkin lymphoma presenting in the mediastinum, and mediastinal gray zone lymphoma: what is the oncologist to do? *Curr Hematol Malig Rep* 2011;6(3):157–163.

109. Eberle FC, Rodriguez-Canales J, Wei L, et al. Methylation profiling of mediastinal gray zone lymphoma reveals a distinctive signature with elements shared by classical Hodgkin's lymphoma and primary mediastinal large B-cell lymphoma. *Haematol* 2011;96(4):558–566.

110. Dunleavy K, Grant C, Eberle FC, et al. Gray zone lymphoma: better treated like hodgkin lymphoma or mediastinal large B-cell lymphoma? *Curr Hematol Malig Rep* 2012;7(3):241–247.

111. Cazals-Hatem D, Andre M, Mounier N, et al. Pathologic and clinical features of 77 Hodgkin's lymphoma patients treated in a lymphoma protocol (LNH87): a GELA study. *Am J Surg Pathol* 2001;25(3):297–306.

112. Wilson WH, Pittaluga S, Nicolae A, et al. A prospective study of mediastinal gray-zone lymphoma. *Blood* 2014;124(10):1563–1569.

169

Benign and Malignant Germ Cell Tumors of the Mediastinum

Carlos Ibarra-Pérez ▪ Isabel Alvarado-Cabrero ▪ Walid Leonardo Dajer-Fadel ▪ Oscar Arrieta-Rodriguez

"The only thing new about germ cell tumors of the mediastinum is that there is nothing new about them."

—Kenneth A. Kessler, 51th Annual Meeting, The Society of Thoracic Surgeons. San Diego, CA. January 27, 2015.

INTRODUCTION

Germ cell tumors (GCTs) arising in the mediastinum were described almost two centuries ago.[1] Although they affect mainly men during their third and fourth decades of life, they can occur at any age with a range of 0 to 79 years and mean of 40 years.[2] In descending order of frequency, GCT are found in the testicles, the anterior mediastinum, the retroperitoneum, the pineal gland, the sacral region and the suprasellar region. GCT of the lung[2] and the pericardium are extremely rare.[3,4] Only about 5% of the GCT are extragonadal and it is estimated that approximately 3% of GCT are primarily mediastinal.[5] Sacrococcygeal and intracranial GCT are most common in infants and young children. Gonadal and extragonadal tumors are histologically similar.[6,7]

Confirmation that a GCT of the mediastinum (GCTM) is indeed a primary neoplasm requires the absence of clinical and radiologic evidence of a testicular, ovarian, or retroperitoneal tumor. Approximately 80% to 85% of GCTM are benign, accounting for 5% to 10% of all mediastinal tumors[8] with the sex distribution of benign GCTM about equal. In contrast, around 90% of all malignant GCTM occur in men.[9]

NOMENCLATURE, CLASSIFICATIONS

GCTMs are a heterogeneous group of tumors with different histology and clinical courses: the teratomas (teratoma: "monster," from the Greek word *teras*: monster, marvel, portent), the seminomatous germ cell tumors of the mediastinum (SGCTM) and the nonseminomatous germ cell tumors of the mediastinum (NSGCTM). Teratomas can be benign or malignant whereas, SGCTM and NSGCTM are malignant.[2] In women, seminomas are called dysgerminomas and NSGCT nondysgerminomas. The term dysembryoma has also been used for NSGCTM. Polyembryomas represent a variant of mixed GCT characterized by the predominance of embryoid structures along with teratomatous, endodermal sac and syncytiotrophoblastic cells.

The GCTM classification proposed by Moran and Suster[2] allows for a better assessment of the various components present in a GCTM, particularly in teratomatous lesions (Table 169.1).

An international prognostic GCT classification (Table 169.2) was developed in 1997 based on a retrospective analysis of 5,202 patients with metastatic NSGCT and 660 with metastatic SGCT including serum tumor markers.[10] The median follow-up time was 5 years. For NSGCT, a primary mediastinal site, degree of elevation of alpha-fetoprotein (α-FP), the beta fraction of human chorionic gonadotropin (β-HCG), and lactic acid dehydrogenase (LDH) are adverse independent prognostic factors. Also, adverse factors are the presence of nonpulmonary metastases in liver, bone, and/or brain. For a seminoma, the predominant adverse feature was the presence of nonpulmonary metastases.[10] This analysis resulted in the definition of three prognostic groups:

a. Good prognosis comprised of 60% of all metastatic GCT, with a 91% 5-year survival rate. This group include 56% of all nonseminomas, and 90% of seminomas.

TABLE 169.1 Classification of Mediastinal Germ Cell Tumors

I. Teratomatous lesions
  1. Mature teratoma (composed of well-differentiated, mature elements)
  2. Immature teratoma (with the presence of immature mesenchymal or neuroepithelial tissue)
  3. Teratoma with additional malignant component:
     Type I: with an associated malignant GCT tumor (seminoma, embryonal carcinoma, yolk sac tumor, etc.)
     Type II: with a non–germ cell epithelial component (squamous, adenocarcinoma, etc.)
     Type III: with a malignant mesenchymal component (rhabdomyosarcoma, chondrosarcoma, etc.)
     Type IV: a teratoma with any combination of the above
II. Nonteratomatous tumors
  1. Seminoma
  2. Yolk sac tumor, or endodermal sinus tumor
  3. Embryonal carcinoma
  4. Choriocarcinoma
  5. Combined nonteratomatous tumors (a combination of any of the above)

TABLE 169.2 Definitions of the Germ Cell Consensus Classification for Metastatic GCT

I. Good prognosis
  A. Nonseminoma. Testis/retroperitoneal primary and no nonpulmonary visceral metastases and good markers, including all of α-fetoprotein (α-FP) <1,000 ng/mL, and β-human chorionic gonadotropin (β-HCG) <5,000 IU/L (1,000 ng/mL) and serum lactate dehydrogenase (LDH) <1.5 times the upper limit of normal); 56% of nonseminomas show a progression-free survival (PFS) rate of 89% and a 5-year survival rate of 92%.
  B. Seminoma. At any primary site and no nonpulmonary visceral metastases and normal α-FP, any β-CG, any LDH; 90% seminomas, 5-year PFS rate of 82% and 5-year survival rate of 86%.
II. Intermediate prognosis
  A. Nonseminoma. Testis/retroperitoneal primary and no nonpulmonary visceral metastases and any of α-FP ≥1,000 ng/mL and ≤10,000 ng/mL or β-HCG ≥5,000 IU or ≤50,000 IU/L or LDH ≥1.5 times normal or ≤10 times normal; 28% of nonseminomas show a 5-year PFS rate of 75% and a 5-year survival rate of 80%.
  B. Seminoma. At any primary site and nonpulmonary visceral metastases and normal α-FP, any β-HCG, and any LDH; 10% of seminomas, 5-year PFS of 67% and 5-year survival of 72%.
III. Poor prognosis
  A. Nonseminoma. All patients with mediastinal primary, or nonpulmonary visceral metastases, or poor markers: α-FP >10,000 ng/ml or β-HCG >50,000 IU/L (1,000 ng/mL) or LDH >10 times × upper limit of normal; 16% of nonseminomas show a PFS of 41% and 5-year survival of 48%.
  B. Seminoma. No patients are classified as poor prognosis.

PFS, progression-free survival.
From International Germ Cell Consensus Classification: a prognostic factor-based staging system for metastatic germ cell cancers. International Germ Cell Cancer Collaborative Group. *J Clin Oncol* 1997;15(2):594–603. Reprinted with permission. Copyright © 1997 American Society of Clinical Oncology. All rights reserved.

b. Intermediate prognosis comprised 26% of all metastatic GCT, with a 79% 5-year survival rate. This group included 28% of all nonseminomas and 10% of seminomas.

c. Poor prognosis comprised 14% of all metastatic GCT, with a 48% 5-year survival rate. This group included 19% of all seminomas. No patients with seminomas were in this group.

For all practical purposes, all patients with metastatic seminomas may have a good or an intermediate prognosis, while only 81% of metastatic nonseminomas may have a good or intermediate prognosis.

A previous clinical classification with therapeutic implications has recently been reviewed[11] and it is self-explanatory (Table 169.3).

Benign teratomas are also called dermoids, dermoid cysts, epidermoid cysts, or just teratomas. Some authors reserve the term "dermoid" for teratomas containing tissues derived from the ectoderm. However,

TABLE 169.3 Histologic Diagnosis With Therapeutic Implications

Histologic Diagnosis	Therapeutic Implication
Seminoma	Chemotherapy
Malignant nonseminomatous GCT[a]	Chemotherapy followed by resection of tumor remnants, irrespective of the histology
Mature teratoma	Resection
Immature teratoma	Surgical resection

[a]Embryonal carcinoma, yolk sac tumors, choriocarcinoma, mixed GCT.

small nests of tissues derived from the other two layers are often present.[12] Sixty to 70% of all GCTM are teratomas and most of them are mature. Teratomas are considered to be mature if they contain exclusively mature, adult-type tissues.[11] They occur in prepubertal and postpubertal patients with equal frequency in both genders. If they contain any immature, less well-developed elements typical of those present during fetal development, they are considered to be immature. These are much rarer than mature teratomas, occurring only in postpubescent patients, and more often in men. The most common immature components are neuroectodermal and mesenchymal tissues.[11] Mature and most immature teratomas are benign tumors[11,13–15] by definition. An immature teratoma should not harbor any morphologically malignant component.[11] A teratoma with somatic-type malignancy contains one or more components of a non-germ cell malignant tumor, which may be a sarcoma or a carcinoma.[11] It corresponds to types II and III of group 3 Moran's classification (see above).[2] This also can be considered to be a teratoma with malignant transformation. Teratocarcinomas result from the combination of embryonal carcinoma and mature teratoma.

Seminomatous GCTM are more frequent in men during their third and fourth decades and are rarely seen in women. Among patients with malignant GCTM, seminoma is the most common, around 30% to 40% of cases[3] with the rest being classified as NSGCT. Seminomas may grow in close anatomic relationship to a thymoma. It can be quite difficult to differentiate one from the other by imaging techniques.

Nonseminomatous mediastinal GCT (NSGCTM) include choriocarcinoma, yolk sac tumors, embryonal carcinoma, and mixed types.[16] Choriocarcinoma secretes β-HCG and contains syncytiotrophoblastic cells. Embryonal carcinoma, also referred by some as malignant teratoma, represents about 10% of malignant GCTM.[3] Choriocarcinoma and endodermal sinus tumors represent about 5% each. Forty percent are mixed type tumors[17] with elements of teratomas, immature teratomas, or seminomas. The NSGCTM are highly malignant with poor prognosis[10] and exhibit clinical and biological behavior different from their testicular counterparts. Fortunately, with platinum-based chemotherapy, approximately half of the patients do survive.

EPIDEMIOLOGY

It has been estimated that around 100 to 200 new cases of extragonadal GCT (EGGCT) are diagnosed yearly in the USA.[6,18]

As mentioned, most GCT are gonadal, and only around 5% are extragonadal with the mediastinum being the most common site affected Around 85%, are benign and the majority are teratomas presenting around the third and fourth decades of life.[18] In infancy, benign teratomas are the most frequent. For example, in Mexico City, we have had the opportunity to study three series of GCTM. The first, at a specialty institution, The Oncology Hospital of the National Medical Center included 37 GCTM which was 15.35% of a total of 241 mediastinal tumors seen during a 62-month period ending in January 1999. Of these 37 GTCM, 29 were NSGCT and 8 SGCT. There were no teratomas in this series.[19] The second series was from The General Hospital of Mexico, where 34 GCTM were reported comprising 15.6% of 218 mediastinal tumors collected from January 1982 to August 2012. Different from the above, these 34 GTCM included 11 teratomas, 9 seminomas (including 5 dysgerminomas in women), 11 NSGCTM, and 3 unclassified GCTM.[20] Finally, the third series, also from the Oncology Hospital of the National Medical Center, reviewed cases between 2010 and 2014. Twenty patients with GCTM represented 22% of the 91 mediastinal tumors evaluated during this period. Four were teratomas, 12 SGCTM, and 4 NSGCTM (Alvarado-Cabrero I, et al. Unpublished material). These percentages differ from findings of Mullen and Richardson[8] as well as other authors, confirming the importance of referral bias and type of hospital.

PATHOGENESIS

Despite discussion by numerous authors, the oncogenesis of NSC-GTM remains uncertain.[11,21–29] Nevertheless, it is generally accepted that EGGCT follows the same principles of development from primordial germ cells (PGCs) as the primary gonadal GCTs. While migration from the yolk-sac endoderm to the genital ridge occurs at the midline, aberrant midline migration might enable PGCs to lodge in the site where EGGCTs are commonly found.[30] Accordingly, the cytogenetic finding of one or multiple copies of the short arm of chromosome 12p with the loss of the long arm of chromosome 12 is seen in nearly all GCT of primary gonadal and extragonadal origin.[31]

This concept, however, is challenged by findings from serial sections in human and murine embryos, which failed to show any evidence of misplaced germ cells outside the gonads. However, the occurrence of postpubertal GCTs in the thymus and the midline of the brain suggests that there must be niches in these sites which offer the same support to PGC cells and their neoplastic counterparts. The observation of seminoma cells homing in on the thymic epithelium suggests that these cells may have a role as feeder cells, similar to testicular Sertoli cells and granulose cells in the dysgenetic gonad.[32,33]

Although prior studies did not find evidence of germ cells in the thymus, there has been considerable progress recently in the establishment and differentiation of human embryonic stem cells, as PGC and embryonic germ cells can be derived from stem cells. Conversely, stem cell lines have now been derived from different stages of germ cell development in animal models. Finally, mammalian adult stem cells have been reported to differentiate into mature germ cells in vivo.[34]

GENETICS

The molecular changes associated with the development of GCTs are yet to be completely defined. However, the universal cytogenetic finding of an increased 12p copy number strongly suggests that this chromosomal change is a key event. Candidate driver genes are currently in the process of being identified using the techniques of molecular profiling, CGH analysis, etc. Of particular interest is an amplification of the proximal 12p11.2-12 region which includes the genes ras-k2, SOX 5, and Jaw1, as well as cyclin CCND2 mapped to the 12p13 region, which is currently the best candidate for the 12p3 gene seen in normal testicular genesis and malignant germ cell development.[35–37]

CLINICAL PRESENTATION

The presence of an anterior mediastinal mass in a young adult, with or without vague nonspecific complaints like thoracic discomfort or diffuse pain and dyspnea, should raise the suspicion of a GCTM until proven otherwise. Of particular significance are a past medical history of undescended testis (cryptorchidism), or of testicular, retroperitoneal, liver or pulmonary tumors. All patients with a suspicious or an established diagnosis of GCTM should undergo careful bimanual testicular and inguinal exploration, as well as testicular ultrasound, abdominal CTs,[38] and determination of serum tumor markers. "Blind" testicular biopsies are not justified.

GCTM can produce symptoms due to their size and location by one or more of several mechanisms, (a) compression, distortion, invasion, and/or displacement of neighboring structures, (b) erosion and/or fistulization into the airways, pleural, or pericardial spaces, or (c) the production of β-HCG. As a general observation, benign GCT are typically asymptomatic while malignant tumors are frequently symptomatic.

Presenting complaints can include cough, dyspnea, nonspecific chest and/or shoulder pain, intercostal neuralgia, wheezing, respiratory distress, fever, obstructive pneumonitis-atelectasis, lung abscess, hoarseness, dysphagia, superior vena cava syndrome,[39] Horner syndrome, thoracic asymmetry, pleural or pericardial effusions, even chylous effusions,[40] and weight loss. Precocious puberty may accompany cases of NSGCTM or mixed GCT due to increased β-HCG.[41,42] Hydrops fetalis is a typical complication of pericardial teratoma.[43]

Benign or mature teratomas are the most common GCT arising in the mediastinum; they are much more frequent during infancy and childhood, with similar incidence in both genders. They can be discovered incidentally by chest imaging studies in usually asymptomatic or minimally symptomatic patients where complaints can include chest pain, cough, and dyspnea. Expectoration of teeth, foul-smelling fatty fluid or sebum, hair or pieces of solid material, including calcium, are pathognomonic features of erosion into the airways secondary to the production of tissue-digesting enzymes or ischemia-induced necrosis of the airway wall. It has been reported that benign teratomas could secrete physiologically functional androgenic substances, insulin, follicle-stimulating hormone, and HCG.

Seminomas are slow growing tumors and remain asymptomatic until they are discovered when they achieve a large size. Others are discovered due to chest pain, cough, dyspnea, weakness, or gynecomastia. Metastatic disease, mostly lymphatic, is seen at presentation in about 40% to 70% of cases.[44]

NSGCTM grow rapidly and metastasize early to distant sites. At the time of clinical presentation, 25% to 90% of patients already have widespread metastatic disease by hematogenous and/or lymphatic routes[45] to the lung, pleura, liver, mediastinum, supraclavicular, and retroperitoneal lymph nodes. Other sites like the central nervous system are involved less frequently. The immature teratomatous elements have a tendency to degenerate into chemotherapy-refractory "non-germ cells" cancers. This contributes to the aggressive biology of NSGCTM.[46] Constitutional symptoms are the rule and hemorrhagic events have been described.[47] Choriocarcinomas are frequently associated with gynecomastia and increased serum levels of β-HCG. As well, hematogenous metastases are more common than with the other types of NSGCTM. Their prognosis is particularly poor.

Approximately 18% to 20% of mediastinal NSGCT are associated with Klinefelter Syndrome (KS), characterized by hypogonadism, azoospermia, eunuchoid proportions, varying degrees of gynecomastia, incomplete virilization in phenotypic males, increased gonadotropin levels, and an extra X chromosome[47] (XXY genotype) (Fig. 169.1).[48,49] Men with KS show an increased incidence of other malignant neoplasms.[50] However, testicular GCT are not increased in these patients.[11] Adolescent males presenting with a malignant GCTM should be evaluated for KS. Mature teratomas can be associated with classical 47, XXY KS.[11]

Approximately 2% (1 in every 17 cases) of NSGCTM are associated with malignant histiocytosis, erythroleukemia, and diverse types of acute leukemias unrelated to therapy.[51–54] Thrombocytopenia has been described also.

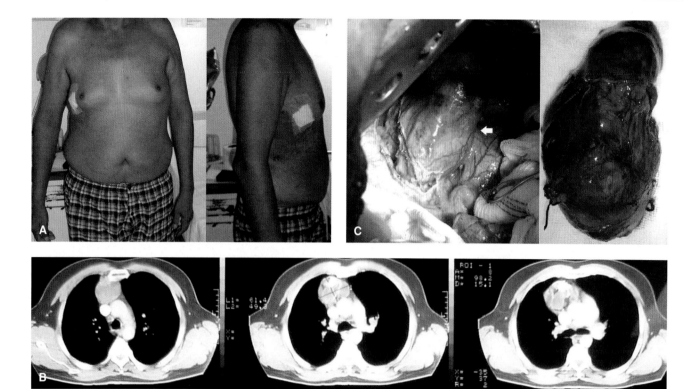

FIGURE 169.1 Klinefelter syndrome in a 47-year-old male with 18 pounds weight loss. **A:** Tall, rather lean phenotypic man with long extremities, gyneco-mastia, feminine distribution of pubic hair, and small testes with bilateral tumors. **B:** Thoracic CT scan shows a heterogeneous, calcified anterior mediastinal mass; there were also increased α-FP and a retroperitoneal mass. The patient underwent resection of (**C**) the mediastinal tumor (*arrow*), the retroperitoneal mass and both testicles. Pathology report: Mature teratoma 50%, immature teratoma 40%, yolk sac tumor 10%, scarce thymic tissue.

SERUM TUMOR MARKERS

Serum tumor marker determinations are essential for the diagnosis and follow-up of EGGCT (Table 169.4).

β-HCG is a glycoprotein with a molecular weight of approximately 38,000 Da composed of two polypeptide chains, α and β. The β chain is unique to HCG and is produced by the syncytiotrophoblastic cells of the human placenta. Increased levels of β-HCG in NSGCT strongly suggest the presence of choriocarcinoma; however, 10% to 25% of pure seminomas may have mildly increased β-HCG.

α-FP is a single-chain oncofetal glycoprotein with a molecular weight of approximately 70,000 Da. It is synthesized by the liver, endodermic sinuses, and the gastrointestinal tract of the fetus. The values of α-FP slowly decrease after the first year of life. α-FP is not present in pure seminomas, embryonal carcinomas, or choriocarci-

nomas, but if α-FP is increased in the setting of these histologies, there is a component of yolk sac tumor.[55] Liver disease and gastrointestinal neoplasms can also increase the levels of α-FP.

Placental alkaline phosphatase (PLAP) comprises four isoenzymes from bone, liver, placenta, or intestine, that increases in cases of seminoma and might be of value in follow-up, if used alongside other serum tumor markers. PLAP is also increased in smokers is infrequently used in daily clinical practice.

Serum lactate dehydrogenase (LDH) is also composed of four isoenzymes and participates in the oxidation of lactic acid to pyruvic acid, has a molecular weight of 180,000 Da, and is nonspecifically elevated in all types of malignant GCT. It can correlate with active tumor burden.[56]

β-HCG or LDH concentrations above normal range may occur in any GCT histology.[57] These tumor markers are negative in mature teratomas, but their increase in a mass considered to be teratomatous should indicate the possibility of a NSGCT.

NSGCTM show an elevated α-FP in around 60% to 80% of cases. β-HCG is elevated in 30% to 50% of cases. Therefore, if a mediastinal mass shows any elevation of α-FP or significant elevations of β-HCG, the diagnosis of a NSGCT should be entertained as the first diagnostic possibility.

Increasing levels of β-HCG and/or α-FP are indicative of active tumor. Patients with abnormally high levels of α-FP or β-HCG should be treated immediately by chemotherapy, without undergoing a biopsy.

Surgical series of NSGCTM have reported that normal serum tumor markers are relatively poor predictors of benign or malignant pathology in postresectional residual masses. Postchemotherapy serum tumor markers have poor sensitivity and specificity to predict the histology of residual mediastinal abnormalities.[58–61]

TABLE 169.4 Serum and Urine Tumor Markers in Germinal Cell Tumors of the Mediastinum

Tumor	Serum or Urine Marker
Endodermic or yolk sac	α-FP, LDH
Embryogenic	LDH, β-HCG (+/−)
Choriocarcinoma	β-HCG, LDH
Seminoma	β-HCG[a], LDH, PLAP, NSE

α-FP, alpha fetoprotein; β-HGC, beta human chorionic gonadotropin; LDH, lactic dehydrogenase; PLAP, placental alkaline phosphatase; NSE, neuron-specific enolase.
[a]May be present in 10% to 25% of seminomas.
Adapted from Robinson PG. Mediastinal tumor markers. In: Shields TW, LoCicero J III, Reed CE, et al., eds. *General Thoracic Surgery*. 7th ed. Philadelphia, PA: Wolters Kluwer, Lippincott Williams & Wilkins; 2009:2131–2146.

Some mixed GCTM may show enlargement of the mass during or after chemotherapy despite a rapid decline in the serum tumor markers.[62,63] This is known as growing teratoma syndrome. Resection of the teratomatous mass is advised due to its potential to degenerate into non-germ cell cancer. Serum levels of CD30 are increased in patients with embryonal carcinoma, but this has not gained widespread use in clinical practice. Other tumor markers, suggestive of paraneoplastic syndromes, should not be routinely requested unless necessary.

IMAGING

With all types of GCTM, besides plain thoracic chest-x rays, CT studies are mandatory to determine the exact size, location, neighboring structures affected, presence of a capsule, and composition of the mass. Also, radiologic studies are necessary to define disease extent and response to therapy.

General features of all GCTM include the presence of an anterior homogeneous or heterogeneous mediastinal mass, which may frequently be quite large. The differential diagnosis includes other anterior mediastinal masses such as thymoma, lymphoma, thymic carcinoid, intrathoracic thyroid, lipoma, lymphangioma, and GCTs (Fig. 169.2).

Teratomas and other GCTM may not be distinguished from thymomas using only imaging criteria, because both can appear as discrete or infiltrating anterior mediastinal masses, sometimes with calcifications. GCTM occur in younger people while thymomas are seen in middle age or elderly people.[64]

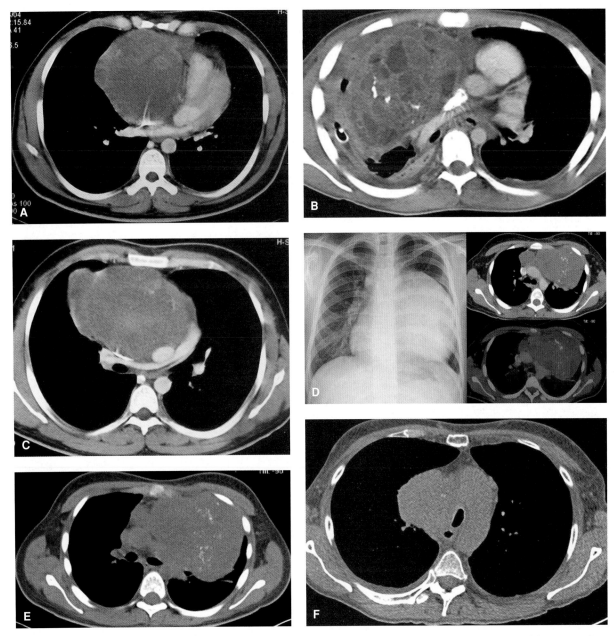

FIGURE 169.2 Tumors of the anterior mediastinum. Thoracic CT scans of (**A**) Thymoma, extending into the right chest; (**B**) Teratoma, heterogeneous mass with cysts and fragments of calcium; (**C**) Seminoma, with compression and displacement of vascular and airway structures. **D**: Posteroanterior chest x-ray, CT scan, and PET in a case of a teratocarcinoma; the tumors extends well into the left chest, is heterogeneous with flecks of calcium and has a high SUV (**E**), and (**F**) large mixed germ cell tumors of the anterior mediastinum displacing and compressing midline organs. (Images courtesy of Dr. Luis G. Alva-López, Chief of Imagenology, Hospital Médica Sur, México City.)

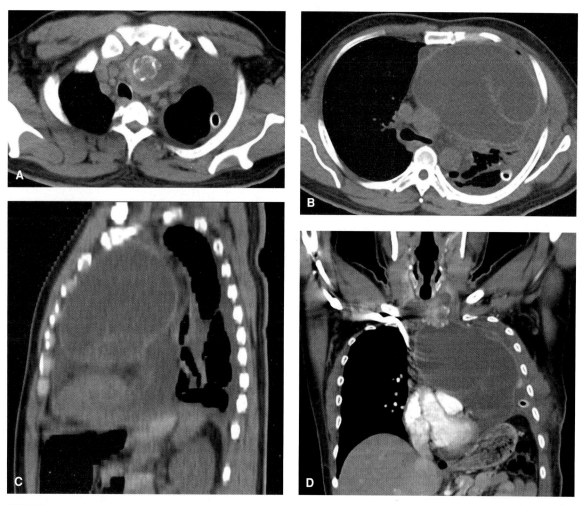

FIGURE 169.3 Mature cystic teratoma in a 29-year-old male presenting with a large, capsulated septated, cystic mass, with calcifications, that displaces the heart, mediastinal vessels and airways producing pulmonary compression-atelectasis; the chest tube was used to drain a large companion pleural effusion. **A–D:** Thoracic CT scan and reconstructions.

The mixture of tissues from the primitive germ cell layers produces the distinct appearance of teratomas. They are usually round or lobulated, sharply marginated by a smooth capsule. They can range in size from a few centimeters to huge masses with multiple lobules separated by thin septa. They reside predominantly in the prevascular compartment (85%), occasionally in the middle (5%), or posterior or multiple compartments (10%) and frequently project into one or both sides of the thorax. Simple and contrast CT shows enhancement of the capsule and septa with varying densities due to the presence of bone, soft tissue, fluid, fat, and teeth. Up to 80% shows different types and degrees of calcification and up to 90% may contain fat (Fig. 169.3). This pleomorphic appearance and the presence of spontaneous air-fluid levels are important clues for the diagnosis on the basis of the CT findings alone. Benign teratomas usually have cysts, but multiloculated cystic lesions are not typical of mature teratomas and can also be seen in other types of GCTM. The malignant teratomas are more likely to appear nodular and solid, with a poorly defined capsule; they contain fat less often than benign lesions. MRI adds little to the large amount of information provided by CT, showing the heterogeneous mass with areas of different signal intensity. However, MRI is useful if airway or vascular "invasion" due to fibroinflammatory tissue are suspected. The confirmation of fat

can be obtained with MRI techniques of fat saturation, but they are seldom necessary.[8,12,65]

Seminomas occur almost entirely in men between the third and fourth decades of life. Plain chest x-rays show a large, smooth, or lobulated anterior mediastinal mass projecting into one or both sides of the mediastinum, without features of NSGCT. On CT, the mass is large, homogeneous, noncapsulated, well-circumscribed, sometimes lobulated, with small amounts of pleural or pericardial fluid. They usually have homogeneous soft tissue attenuation and show slight enhancement after intravenous contrast administration (Fig. 169.4), but cysts, hemorrhage, necrosis, and focal areas of different types of mild calcification might occur. Invasion of neighboring structures with obliteration of fat planes and metastases to lung, bone, and mediastinal lymph nodes can also occur. Seminomas containing cysts may mimic a cystic thymus. MRI can be useful to differentiate residual tumor from fibrosis with respect to treatment.

The different types of "pure" and mixed NSGCTM can have quite similar appearances both by CT and MRI imaging. The usual findings include a large, noncapsulated and irregular mass with ill-defined margins. The studies may show heterogeneous attenuation due to necrosis, hemorrhage, or cyst formation, frequently

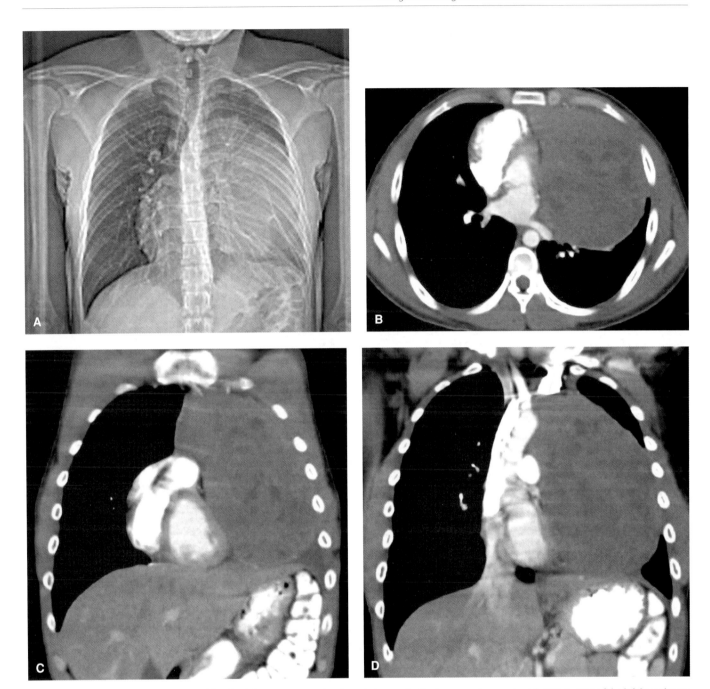

FIGURE 169.4 Seminoma in a 20-year-old male. A large mass occupies the anterior mediastinal space and approximately 80% to 85% of the left hemithorax; notice the elevation of the left hemidiaphragm and compression and displacement of the midline structures, including the heart. **A–D:** Posteroanterior chest x-ray, thoracic CT scan, and reconstructions.

with obliteration of fat planes secondary to invasion of adjacent mediastinal and/or chest wall tissues (Fig. 169.5). However, the invasion is better imaged by MRI. Disseminated metastatic disease is frequently present.[8,17,58]

PET can be useful during posttreatment follow-up, due to its potential to show neoplastic response to treatment, relapses, or residual tumor, but the possibility of a false positive result due to inflammatory tissue should be strongly considered. Also, PET cannot distinguish masses containing complete necrosis from those containing teratomatous components, microscopic foci of residual NSGCT, or degenerative non-germ cell cancer.[61,66,67] For this reason, PET has not been

helpful in selecting patients in whom surgery potentially could be avoided (Fig. 169.2).[61]

Imaging studies are not only useful for the diagnosis of the mass but of great help in the recognition of complications arising from the displacement, distortion, invasion, and/or compression induced by the tumor and during follow-up after treatment. However, no imaging technique reliably differentiates patients who have residual necrosis/fibrosis, teratoma, or viable cancer following induction chemotherapy.[68] Ultrasonography has been substituted for CT as a diagnostic tool in special circumstances, such as image-guided needle biopsy.

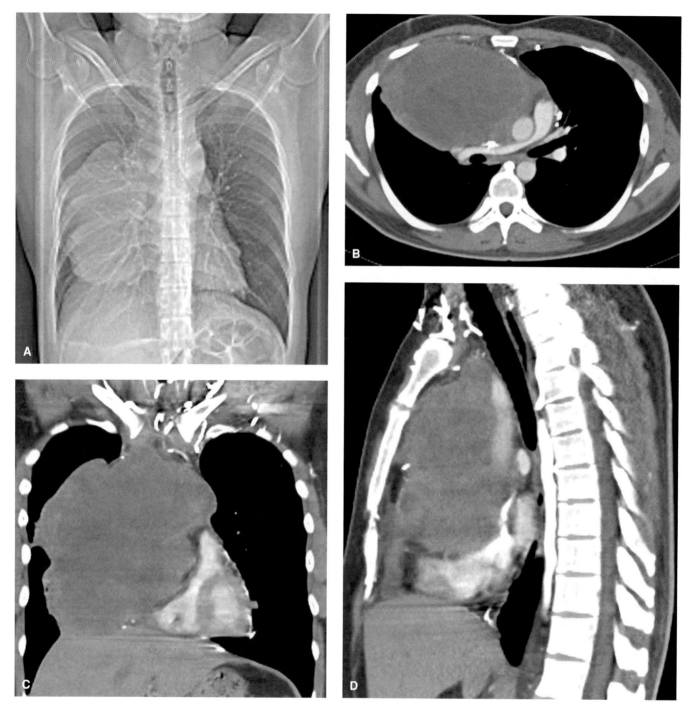

FIGURE 169.5 Mixed malignant germ cell tumor in a 34-year-old male. Huge anterior mediastinal mass, lobulated, protruding into the right chest, that abuts against the chest wall, the mediastinal vessels, airways and heart, that are compressed and displaced. **A–D**: Posteroanterior chest x-ray, thoracic CT scan, and reconstructions.

INVASIVE STUDIES

Biopsy of an anterior mediastinal mass is advised unless the clinical picture and previous studies leave no doubt as to the exact nature of the mass, as in the case of the teratomas where the CT scan is almost universally diagnostic, or when the serum tumor markers are diagnostic of a malignant GCTM.

The advent of image-guided cutting needle biopsies of different areas of the tumor have replaced the use of fine-needle sampling of

mediastinal masses and decreased the need for more invasive procedures like an anterior mediastinotomy or any of the different types of mediastinoscopies. These image-guided procedures provide sufficient material for the diagnosis and subsequent treatment modalities. However, CT-guided fine-needle aspiration has been advised in patients with normal serum tumor markers or minimally elevated β-HCG, in order to differentiate seminoma from NSGCTM.[69]

If a larger piece of tissue is needed, an anterior mediastinotomy by the classic Chamberlain technique is most useful. A meticulous exploration by this access allows sampling of more than one area of the tumor, particularly if the CT scan shows a heterogeneous mass. Also, a VATS approach can be used if the tumor is not readily accessible to a CT-guided needle biopsy.

PATHOLOGIC FEATURES

The World Health Organization (WHO) histological classification of GCTM[70] appears in Table 169.5. For the purposes of this textbook, only the pure histologic tumors (Type I) will be discussed. Types II, III, and IV are all combinations of these.

TERATOMA

Mediastinal teratomas are the most common GCT in the anterior mediastinum, around 45% or more of all GCTM. They are usually both cystic and solid; sectioned surfaces may show hair, teeth, and/or sebaceous material. Mature teratomas are derived from the three germ cell layers and are composed of an admixture of adult-type tissue arranged in organoid structures. The most common component is skin and its appendages, although pancreatic tissue is commonly seen.[18,32]

Immature teratomas are characterized by embryonic or fetal tissues derived from the three germinal layers; the most common is neuroepithelium (neural tubules, rosettes). Malignant mesenchymal components have also been described, such as angiosarcoma, rhabdomyosarcoma, osteosarcoma, and chondrosarcoma.[2] Sometimes, tumors treated with chemotherapy may show immature or atypical components.

Mediastinal teratomas are variably immunoreactive for keratin, CAM 5.2, EMA, Vimentin, and SALL 4. The neuroectodermal tissues are immunoreactive for one or more of neural markers, such as glial fibrillary acidic protein, neuron-specific enolase, S-100 protein, neurofilament protein, synaptophysin and glial filament protein, among others.[2,18,32]

SEMINOMA

Extragonadal seminomas occurring primarily in the mediastinum are uncommon and constitute approximately 3% to 4% of all neoplasms arising in this site.[71] In these cases, an accurate diagnosis is critically important to provide the proper therapy, as mediastinal seminomas (MS) respond exceptionally well to radiotherapy and/or cisplatin-based chemotherapy.

They vary in size from a few centimeters to ≥16 cm in greatest diameter (Fig. 169.4) and may extend to both sides of the midline (Fig. 169.6A). Cut specimens reveal a soft, lobulated, and homogeneous surface (Fig. 169.6B). Central hemorrhage and necrosis may occur but are not common. The color may vary from white to light tan; the consistency is rather soft. The tumor may be located entirely within the thymus, or it may adhere and even invade local structures.[16] In some cases, solid areas may alternate with large cystic areas containing necrotic material, whereas other areas may have the appearance of an entirely cystic mass.[72]

Histologic features are similar to testicular seminomas and ovarian dysgerminomas. These tumors usually grow in a sheet-like arrangement intersected by thin fibrous septa (Fig. 169.6C). Occasionally, the fibrous septa give a thicker, more nodular appearance to the tumor. There is an inflammatory infiltrate composed of mature lymphocytes, plasma cells, and epithelioid histiocytes forming granulomas.[18] Seminoma cells have a moderate amount of clear to pale eosinophilic cytoplasm with prominent cytoplasmic membranes and distinct cell borders. The nuclei are large, round to rhomboid in shape and cen-

TABLE 169.5 Classification of Mediastinal Germ Cell Tumors Proposed by WHO[a]

I. One histologic type (pure GCT):
  Seminoma
  Embryonal carcinoma
  Yolk sac tumor
  Choriocarcinoma
  Mature teratoma
  Immature teratoma
II. More than one histological type (mixed GCT)
III. GCT with somatic-type solid malignancy
IV. GCT with associated hematologic malignancy

[a]World Health Organization.
[b]GCT, germ cell tumor.
(Modified with permission from Travis WD, Brambilla E, Burke AP, Marx A, Nicholson AG. World Health Organization Classification of *Tumours of the Lung, Pleura, Thymus and Heart*. Vol. 7. 4th ed. Lyon: IARC Press, 2015.)

trally located. The chromatin is evenly distributed and one or more prominent nucleoli are invariably present.[16,32,72] Less frequently seen histologic features include cellular pleomorphism, necrosis, intercellular edema, and syncytiotrophoblasts.[73]

MS have been shown to express moderate to strong nuclear OCT4, membrane staining for c-kit and mild to moderate staining for PLAP.[74] In a study on 23 MS by Sung et al.,[73] focal cytoplasmic and membranous staining with variable intensity was seen in 43%, 39%, 48%, and 39% for cytokeratin AE1/3, HMWCK, CAM 5.2, and CK7, respectively. In most cases, these epithelial markers highlighted only a small portion of the tumor cells, usually less than 25%. In a recent study by Weissferdt et al.[75] seminomas arising in the mediastinum showed immunohistochemical characteristics similar to testicular seminomas including consistent expression of OCT3/4, SALL4, SOX17, and MAGEC2. SOX2, glypican 3, GATA-3, and CK 5/6 were negative in MS, results in accordance with the reported staining pattern of these markers in testicular seminomas.

Yolk sac tumors, choriocarcinoma, embryonal GCTs, and combinations of any of the histologic types (mixed GCTs) are referred to as nonseminomatous malignant GCTs. They manifest as large, smooth, or lobulated anterior mediastinal masses, with well-circumscribed or irregular margins (Fig. 169.7A).

Yolk sac tumors are uncommon malignant GCTs, histologically similar to the yolk sac and its derivates, also producing α-FP. Whereas most yolk sac tumors occur in the gonads, about 20% arise in extragonadal sites, including the mediastinum, sacrococcygeal region, retroperitoneum, etc.[76,77] These tumors are often large, and vary in size from few cm to >15 cm in their greatest diameter.[22] The sectioned surfaces are typically solid and cystic and composed of soft, friable, yellow to gray tissue. Extensive areas of hemorrhage and necrosis are common.

Histological patterns of yolk sac tumors are similar to those described in gonadal GCTs. They include reticular/microcystic, glanduloalveolar, myxomatous, papillary, solid, poly-vesicular-vitelline, hepatoid, parietal, macrocystic, intestinal, endometrioid, clear cell and sarcomatoid (Fig. 169.7B). The tumor often has numerous intracellular and extracellular hyaline globules. They show positive staining for α-FP, cytokeratin, PLAP, AE1/AE3, EMA, leu-7, α-1-antitrypsin, SALL 4, and glypican 3 among others, but they are negative for CD30 and HCG.

CHORIOCARCINOMA

Primary mediastinal choriocarcinoma occurs mostly in young men and is the rarest form of EGGCT, accounting for <5% of all GCTM (Fig. 169.8A).[78] On gross examination, pure choriocarcinoma is

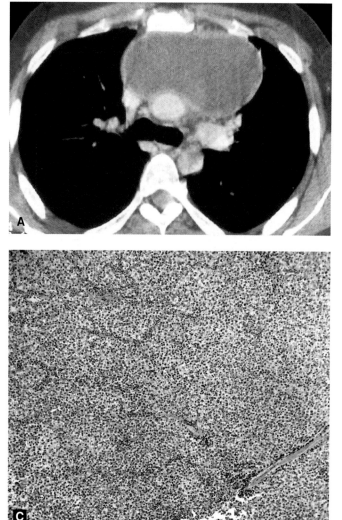

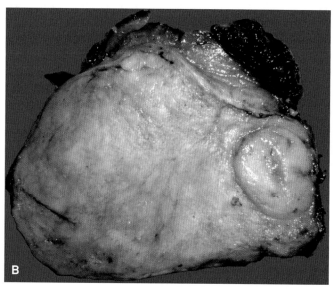

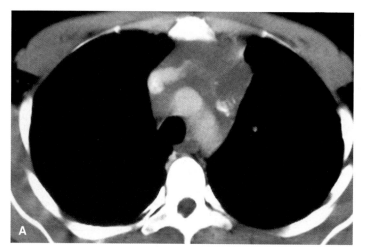

FIGURE 169.6 Seminoma in a 26-year-old male with chest pain and fatigue. **A:** Contrast-enhanced CT scan of the chest shows a smooth, well-defined anterior mediastinal tumor. **B:** Cut surface of the resected specimen shows a light brown tumor with a homogeneous fleshy surface. **C:** Low-power photomicrograph demonstrates lobules of tumor cells and a lymphocytic component.

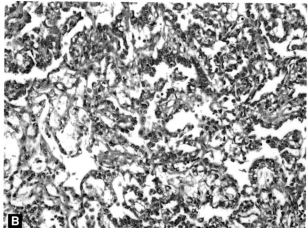

FIGURE 169.7 Mixed germ cell tumor. Teratoma and yolk sac tumor in a 42-year-old male with chest pain and respiratory distress. **A:** Contrast-enhanced thoracic CT scan shows an ill-defined anterior mediastinal mass with irregular borders and heterogeneous attenuations. **B:** High-power photomicrograph of yolk sac tumor shows anastomosing cords composed of columnar and cuboidal neoplastic cells.

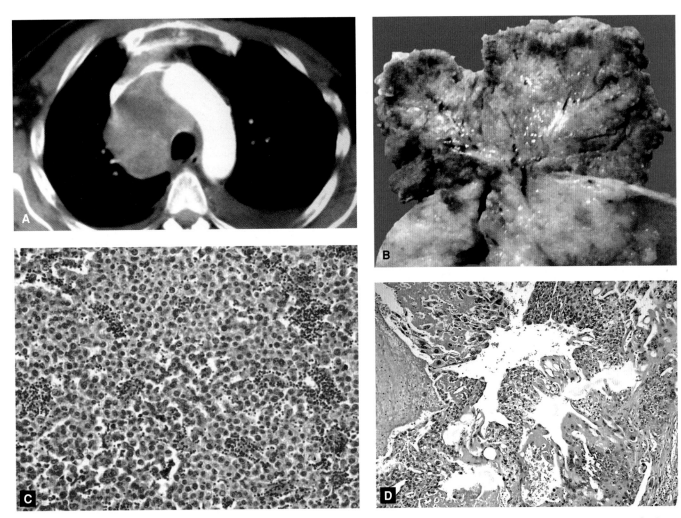

FIGURE 169.8 Mixed germ cell tumor. Seminoma and choriocarcinoma in a 38-year-old male with dysphagia and weight loss. **A:** Thoracic CT scan shows enhancing soft tissue mass in the anterior mediastinum. **B:** The tumor has a predominantly solid and fleshy sectioned surface, with areas of necrosis; on microscopic examination, a mixed germ cell tumor was found (seminoma and choriocarcinoma). **C:** High-power photomicrograph of the seminomatous tumor shows a diffuse pattern composed of uniform cells. The stroma consists of thin bands with numerous lymphocytes. **D:** Choriocarcinoma. Microscopic examination reveals smaller cytotrophoblastic cell growing with syncytiotrophoblastic cells.

typically solid, friable, large, and bulky with extensive areas of hemorrhage and necrosis (Fig. 169.8B). Uninucleated trophoblastic cells with scant or abundant clear cytoplasm are admixed with syncytiotrophoblastic cells, which contain vacuoles and many dark nuclei, and may form syncytial knots (Figs. 169.8 C and D).[78] A case of seminoma admixed with choriocarcinoma had been seen. The syncytiotrophoblastic cells are typically immunoreactive for cytokeratin, HCG, glypican 3, and human placental lactogen (hPL). The cytotrophoblast is typically immunoreactive for cytokeratin. Immunoreactivity for placental-like alkaline phosphatase, epithelial membrane antigen, and α-FP and carcinoembryonic antigen may be present as well.[78]

EMBRYONAL CARCINOMA

In its pure form, mediastinal embryonal carcinoma is an unusual tumor; more often than not they are accompanied by another GCT, mainly YS. It may account for no more than 10% of all GCTM. They are typically large and ill defined. The cut surface is predominantly solid and variegated with white, tan-grey, and yellow soft tissue alternating with cysts. Foci of hemorrhage and necrosis are common. Histologically, they demonstrate solid sheets and nests of cells, often with

central necrosis, gland-like spaces, and papillae composed of or lined by large primitive cells with amphophilic or sometimes clear cytoplasm and well-defined cell membranes. The nuclei are large, round and vesicular with a coarse, irregular membrane and one or more prominent nucleoli. Numerous mitoses, areas of necrosis and hemorrhage are frequently found. The cells are immunoreactive for α-FP, PLAP, NSE, LEU-T, VIMENTIN, CK-PAN, CK8/18, CD30, and EMA.

SURGICAL TREATMENT

For the benign, mature teratomas, total resection has been the definitive treatment of choice. Resection can be carried out by partial or complete sternotomy, total clamshell incision (bilateral anterior thoracotomies plus transverse sternotomy), right or left half clamshell incisions, or the classic lateral or posterolateral thoracotomies. In all cases, the surgeon should make every effort to resect the tumor, unless it becomes necessary to leave behind dense fibrous tissue adherent to vital nerves or vascular structures. This makes modern (i.e., minimally invasive) approaches less desirable except for smaller, nonadherent lesions.[79] The prognosis for completely excised benign teratomas is excellent with a normal life expectancy, even in cases in which adherent benign tissue was left behind. If the specimen shows more than 50% of immature elements in a postpubescent patient, adjuvant therapy is advised. If there is a malignant germ cell line in a teratoma, there is a 25% chance of tumor recurrence, and even higher in cases of sarcoma.[32] Also, teratomas may develop the "growing teratoma syndrome" or become malignant. They should be resected.

The first descriptions regarding surgical resection of SGCTM and NSGCTM showed uniformly bad results until the addition of cisplatin,[80] as well as improvements in radiotherapy and surgical techniques. Consideration for surgical excision of GCTM should be given in patients with (a) lack of response to chemotherapy, (b) partial response followed by recurrence while under treatment, (c) recurrence after standard and second-line therapy. It is considered mandatory to remove all viable tumor cells in the residual tumor, as the majority of NSGCTM with postchemotherapy normal serum tumor markers will have pathologic evidence of teratoma, viable NSGCT or degenerative NSGCT cells and to resect the teratomatous component of the tumor that may contain immature elements capable of malignant transformation.[61] The surgical approaches are the same as in the case of the teratomas.

To some, the resection of residual tumor after chemotherapy can appear unjustified because frequently necrotic tissue is found. However, as survival depends on the elimination of the active tumor, there is no reliable preoperative marker to define which tumors are necrotic and which contain teratoma or viable cells, aggressive surgical resection of radiologically suspicious lesions is necessary.

Surgical resection should be undertaken approximately 4 to 6 weeks after completion of chemotherapy once pulmonary and hematologic complications resolve. Every effort should be made to resect the tumor and all affected tissues en-bloc but with preservation of critical structures not directly involved by the tumor. Pulmonary metastasectomies or anatomic segmentectomies and even more extensive resections like lobectomies may be necessary. Whenever possible, pneumonectomy should be avoided. Frozen sections are necessary to check resection margins. The surgical team should be prepared to reconstruct resected tissues like pericardium, diaphragm, large vessels, and even cardiac muscle with the proper prosthetic materials. The involvement of vessels or the heart may require the use of cardiopulmonary bypass. Postoperative respiratory failure is an ever present-threat and oxygen and fluid therapy should be monitored closely. If viable tumor cells are found in the specimen, adjuvant cisplatin-based chemotherapy is strongly advised. When recurrent teratomas are detected early, patients may be cured with surgical resection.[51]

MEDICAL TREATMENT

Seminomas were previously treated by radiotherapy, obtaining long-term remissions in 65% of patients. However, platinum-based chemotherapy has dramatically improved the prognosis. Presently, this highly chemo- and radio-sensitive tumor has a cure rate from 80% to a 100%. The vast majority of residual masses following chemotherapy for seminoma are tumor necrosis without viable neoplasm.[61] The prognosis for MS is similar to the prognosis of seminomas originating in the testes or retroperitoneum.[39,44,81,82] Rarely, exceptional patients with undiagnosed, small seminomas or presumably thymic masses may undergo primary resection.

A retrospective study from the Royal Marsden Hospital, in which 18 patients were treated with platinum-based chemotherapy from 1977 to 1990, showed an overall survival of 100% for seminomas with a mean follow-up of 49 months. Treatment regimens consisted of carboplatin as the only drug in most cases and bleomycin, etoposide,

and cisplatin (BEP) in others. Five patients received a dose of 30 Gy in 15 fractions for 3 weeks.[82]

A series of patients were treated at the Gustave-Roussy Institute. Nine patients were treated with platinum-based chemotherapy +/- radiotherapy and five patients were treated with radiotherapy alone. Eight of the nine treated with chemotherapy (89%) showed long-term survival, compared to three from the five patients treated with radiotherapy alone. The doses of radiotherapy used ranged from 40 to 50 Gy. The most common chemotherapeutic regime employed was BEP. The same publication reviewed different case series. In another series 68 patients treated with platinum-based chemotherapy showed that 87% were alive and free of disease at a 2-year follow-up, compared to 62% of those treated with radiotherapy with or without platinum-based chemotherapy.[83]

A retrospective analysis of The Hellenic Cooperative Oncology Group experience in patients with EGGCTs treated with platinum-based chemotherapy from 1984 to 1998 included 22 primary mediastinal tumors. The patients with seminomas, independent of their primary location, were alive at a mean follow-up of 49 months.[84] There is agreement that in seminomas, systemic metastatic disease carries a bad prognosis.[14,39,85]

For NSGCTM, cisplatin-based chemotherapy is the treatment of choice. Surgery, even very aggressive resections, have no role as primary treatment. The recommendation is four cycles of BEP, or etoposide, ifosfamide and cisplatin (VIP).[86,87] In the study of The Royal Marsden Hospital, complete remission was observed in 82% of the patients with nonseminomatous tumors using platinum-based regimes.[82] The Hellenic Group found that 9 (69.23%) of the 13 nonseminomatous cases were disease free at a mean follow-up of 43.5 months.[84]

In a retrospective series of 635 patients with EGGCT, including 341 (54%) with a primary mediastinal location, 141 patients (49%) with NSGCTs, were alive at a mean follow-up of 19 months after induction with platinum-based chemotherapy, with or without surgery. This was compared to 63% for those in a retroperitoneal location ($P = 0.0006$). NSGCTM had a 5-year survival rate of 45%, a result inferior to the ones presenting in a retroperitoneal location.[39]

Recently, the GETUG 13 phase III randomized multicenter study was published. It measured HCG and α-FP concentrations at day 18 to 21 after one cycle of BEP (intravenous cisplatin, etoposide, and intramuscular or intravenous bleomycin). Patients with a favorable decline in HCG and α-FP continued BEP (Fav-BEP group) for three additional cycles. Patients with an unfavorable decline were randomly assigned (1:1) to receive either BEP alone (Unfav-BEP group) or a "dose-dense" regimen (Unfav–dose-dense group), consisting of intravenous paclitaxel before BEP plus intravenous oxaliplatin, followed by intravenous cisplatin, intravenous ifosfamide, plus mesna, and bleomycin, with granulocyte-colony stimulating factor (lenograstim) support. The primary endpoint was progression-free survival. Efficacy analysis was done using the intention-to-treat methodology. The planned trial accrual was completed in May, 2012 with continued follow-up at the time of the report: 263 patients were enrolled and 254 were available for tumor marker assessment. Of these, 51 (20%) had a favorable marker assessment, and 203 (80%) had an unfavorable tumor marker decline; 105 were randomly assigned to the Unfav–dose-dense group and 98 to the Unfav-BEP group. 3-year progression-free survival was 59% (95% CI 49–68) in the Unfav–dose-dense group versus 48% (CI 38–59) in the Unfav-BEP group (HR 0.66, 95% CI 0.44–1.00, $p = 0.05$). 3-year progression-free survival was 70% (95% CI 57–81) in the Fav-BEP group (HR 0.66, 95% CI 0.49–0.88, $p = 0.01$ for progression-free survival compared with the Unfav-BEP group). More grade 3–4 neurotoxic events (seven

[7%] vs. one [1%]) and haematotoxic events occurred in the Unfav–dose-dense group compared with in the Unfav-BEP group; there was no difference in grade 1–2 febrile neutropenia (18 [17%] vs. 18 [18%]) or toxic deaths (one [1%] in both groups). Salvage high-dose chemotherapy plus a stem-cell transplant was required in six (6%) patients in the Unfav-dose-dense group and 16 (16%) in the Unfav-BEP group. The latter suggests the importance of individualized therapy with high doses in those without an adequate descent of serum tumor markers, to achieve an increase in the disease-free survival and decrease in mortality.[88]

After induction chemotherapy, resection of residual tumors resistant to chemotherapy is advised to confirm the response to treatment in patients with nonseminomatous EGGCTs and normal serum tumor markers, as well as to further define subsequent therapy. Those patients with a pathology report of necrosis are advised to continue with periodic follow-up whereas those with postresection residual choriocarcinoma, embryonal carcinoma, yolk sac tumor, or seminomatous elements, should receive two more cycles of chemotherapy.[86,87,89] Patients with elevated serum tumor markers and/or progression of disease after chemotherapy are not candidates for surgery. The recommended management is to attempt rescue with second-line chemotherapy that may include paclitaxel, cisplatin, and ifosfamide (TIP), or vinblastine, ifosfamide, and cisplatin. Chemotherapy can also be administered at high doses followed by bone marrow transplant.[86,87]

Ganjoo et al.[90] reported that disease confined to the mediastinum and necrosis postchemotherapy are important prognostic factors for survival in patients with NSGCTM, while Sarkaria et al.[91] conclude that response to chemotherapy, measured by normalized

or decreased preoperative serum tumor markers was the strongest predictor of survival in a cohort of patients with primary NSGCTM in which 91% underwent complete posttherapy resection.

An alternative approach published in 2006 treated 21 patients postinduction chemotherapy, regardless of the response. The patients received only one cycle of high-dose chemotherapy with carboplatin, etoposide, and cyclophosphamide followed by peripheral hematopoietic progenitor cell transplantation. Twelve patients did not receive this treatment due to deterioration of their conditions or disease progression and all were dead by 2 years. However, at a 52 months follow-up, eight of the nine transplant patients remained free of disease, four patients underwent surgery for residual tumor after the transplant and a complete response was documented by pathology in three of these patients.[92]

Patients with elevated serum tumor markers and/or progressive disease after chemotherapy who are not candidates for surgery and rescue treatment with second-line chemotherapy, can receive four cycles of paclitaxel, cisplatin, and ifosfamide (TIP) or vinblastine, ifosfamide, and cisplatin (VeIP), or high doses of chemotherapy followed by bone marrow transplantation.[86,87]

When patients suffer a recurrence, are unresponsive to the primary treatment, or demonstrate metastasis, salvage chemotherapy is recommended.[86,87] In a retrospective review of 142 patients initially treated with platinum-based chemotherapy, including 34% treated with high dose chemotherapy followed by bone marrow transplant, only 11% of those patients with mediastinal tumors had long-term survival compared to 30% for primary tumors in the retroperitoneal location. By univariate analysis, the primary mediastinal location was associated with decreased survival ($p = 0.003$). Multivariate analysis

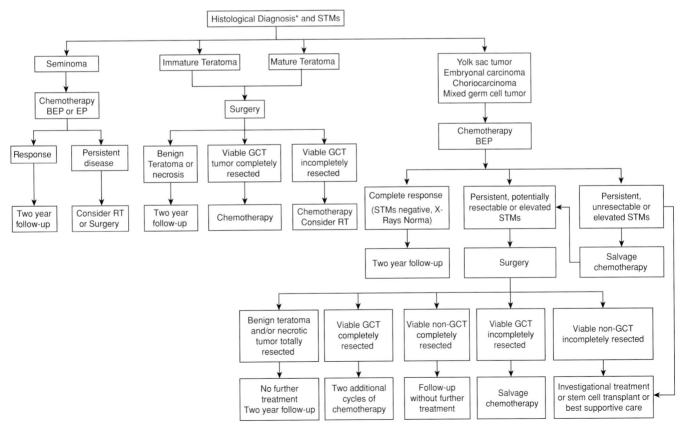

Key: *The diagnosis is usually based on needle-aspiration biopsy. BEP: bleomycin, etoposide, and cisplatin; EP: etoposide, cisplatin; GCT: germ cell tumor; RT: Radiotherapy; STMs: Serum tumor markers

FIGURE 169.9 Suggested treatment algorithm for management of GCTM.

determined that the mediastinal location is a negative prognostic factor with a relative risk of 1.9 (95% IC: 1.2 to 3.0).[93]

Rivera et al.[94] studied the prognostic factors in patients from several medical centers. Univariate analysis showed that age, gender, extent of disease at diagnosis, tumor markers at diagnosis, and normalization of markers after first-line chemotherapy were not statistically significant. Meanwhile, tumor histology ($p = 0.009$), surgical resection of the tumor ($p = 0.023$), and pathological evidence of persistent viable tumor in the resected specimen ($p = 0.008$) were statistically significant. Using multivariate analysis, Bokemeyer et al.[39] identified nonseminomatous histology, the presence of non-pulmonary visceral metastases, primary mediastinal GCT location, and elevated β-HCG were independent prognostic factors indicative of shorter survival. Multivariate testing for the probability to respond to chemotherapy, in a study by Hartman et al.[93] showed that non-seminomatous histology, a primary mediastinal tumor site, and the presence of liver, lung or CNS metastases were independent adverse factors.

High levels of β-HCG at presentation carry a poor prognosis for chemotherapy response and survival. However, postchemotherapy levels of serum tumor markers have low sensitivities and specificities for the identification of active residual disease. As shown by Kesler et al.,[58] proceeding to surgical resection when feasible after first line chemotherapy, regardless of the STM levels, had a 58% survival rate after a median follow-up of 34 months.

Expectations of postchemotherapy pathology include around 25.5% necrosis—34% in teratoma and persistent 31.4% in GCT.[59,95]

Currently, NSGCTM carry a uniformly poor prognosis with no more than 50% survival for chemotherapy followed by resection in both single and multi-institutional series.[61] The 49% overall survival in patients with NSGCTM is in sharp contrast with the 80% long-term survival of patients with testicular NSGCT and 63% for patients with NSGCT originating in the retroperitoneum.[39,85] Survival following postchemotherapy surgery is superior to salvage chemotherapy which is around 10%.[54,61]

Several points deserve special emphasis. Patients should undergo postchemotherapy restaging with thoracoabdominal CT and serum markers. If normal, they should be followed on a regular basis. Resection of residual masses and adjacent involved tissues, irrespective of the values of the serum tumor markers or the findings of PET/CT have been performed with acceptable long-term results as noted in retrospective series.[12,44,58,59] Evidence-based recommendations include resection after chemotherapy for NSGCTM which offers improved long term survival compared to second-line chemotherapy with acceptable morbidity and mortality. A weak recommendation can be made for resection of residual disease in patients with abnormal imaging of the mediastinum after initial chemotherapy for NSGCTM, irrespective of the serum tumor marker levels (recommendation 2B).[61]

A suggested treatment algorithm for the management of GCTM is outlined in Figure 169.9.

REFERENCES

1. Gordon JA. Tumor in the anterior mediastinum containing bone and teeth. *Med Chir Trans* 1827;13:12–16.
2. Moran CA, Suster S. Primary germ cell tumors of the mediastinum. Analysis of 322 cases with special emphasis on teratomatous lesions and a proposal for histopathologic classification and clinical staging. *Cancer* 1997;80:681–690.
3. Burke AP, Tavora F. Tumours of the pericardium. In: Travis WD, Brambilla E, Burke AP, et al., eds. *WHO Classification of Tumours of the Lung, Pleura, Thymus and Heart.* Lyon: IARC Press; 2015:346–347.
4. Restrepo CS, Vargas D, Ocazionez D, et al. Primary pericardial tumors. *Radiographics* 2013;33:1613–1630.
5. Nichols CR. Mediastinal germ cell tumors. Clinical features and biologic correlates. *Chest* 1991;99:472–479.
6. Strollo DC, Rosado de Christenson ML, Jett JR. Primary mediastinal tumors. Part I: Tumors of the anterior mediastinum. *Chest* 1997;112:511–522.
7. Macchiarini P, Ostertag H. Uncommon primary mediastinal tumors. *Lancet Oncol* 2004;5:107–118.
8. Mullen B, Richardson JD. Primary anterior mediastinal tumors in children and adults. *Ann Thorac Sur* 1986;42:338–345.
9. Duwe BV, Steman DH, Musani AI. Tumors of the mediastinum. *Chest* 2005;128:2893–2909.
10. Wilkinson P, Read G. International germ cell consensus classification: A prognostic factor-based staging system for metastatic germ cell-cancers. International Germ Cell Collaborative Group. *J Clin Oncol* 1997;15:594–603.
11. Moreira AL, Ströbel P, Chan JKC, et al. Germ cell tumors of the mediastinum. Seminoma. In: Travis WD, Brambilla E, Burke AP, et al., eds. *WHO Classification of Tumours of the Lung, Pleura, Thymus and Heart.* Lyon: IARC Press; 2015:244–266.
12. Kang CH, Kim YT, Jheon SH, et al. Surgical treatment of malignant mediastinal nonseminomatous germ cell tumor. *Ann Thorac Surg* 2008;85:379–384.
13. Dulmet EM, Macchiarini P, Sub B, et al. Germ cell tumors of the mediastinum: A 30 year experience. *Cancer* 1993;72:1894–1901.
14. Priola AM, Priola SM, Cardinale L, et al. The anterior mediastinum: Diseases. *Radiol Med (Torino)* 2006;111:312–342.
15. Hoffman OA, Gillispie DJ, Aughenbaugh GI, et al. Primary mediastinal neoplasms (other than thymoma). *Mayo Clin Proc* 1993;68:880–891.
16. Rosado de Christenson ML, Templeton PA, Moran CA. Mediastinal germ cell tumors. Radiologic and pathologic correlation. *Radiographics* 1992;12:1013–1030.
17. Knapp RH, Hurt RD, Payne WS, et al. Malignant germ cell tumors of the mediastinum. *J Thorac Cardiovasc Surg* 1987;11:156–157.
18. Takeda S, Miyoshi S, Ohta M, et al. Primary germ cell tumors in the mediastinum: A 50 year experience in a single Japanese institution. *Cancer* 2003;97:367–376.
19. Ibarra-Pérez C, Kelly-García J. Oncología del Tórax. México:UNAM, Coordinación de la Vinculacion, PUIS, MA Porrúa; 1999:111–140.
20. Dajer-Fadel WL, Ibarra-Pérez C. Tumores del mediastino. In: Ibarra-Pérez, ed. *Temas Selectos De Oncología Torácica.* Amsterdam: Elsevier; 2015:135–150.
21. Wychulis AR, Payne WS, Clagett OT, et al. Surgical treatment of mediastinal tumors: A 40 year experience. *J Thorac Cardiovasc Surg* 1971;62:379–392.
22. Willis RA. *The Spread of Tumors in the Human Body.* London: Butterworth; 1952.
23. Frideman NB. The comparative morphogenesis of extragenital and gonadal teratoid tumors. *Cancer* 1951;4:265–276.
24. Frideman NB. The function of the primordial germ cell in extragonadal tissues. *Int J Androl* 1987;10:43–96.
25. Donadio AC, Bosi GJ. The future of therapy for nonseminomatous germ cell tumors. *Chest Surg Clin N Amer* 2002;12:769–789.
26. Kantrowicz AR. Extragenital chorioepithelioma in a male. *Am J Pathol* 1934;10:531–534.
27. Schlumberger HG. Teratoma of anterior mediastinum in group of military age: Study of 16 cases and review of theories of genesis. *Arch Pathol* 1946;41:398–444.
28. Fine F, Smith RW Jr, Pachter MR. Primary extragenital choriocarcinoma in the male subject. Case report and review of the literature. *Am J Med* 1962;32:776–794.
29. Daugaard G, von der Maase H, Olsen J, et al. Carcinoma in situ testis in patients with assumed extragonadal germ-cell tumors. *Lancet* 1987;2:528–530.
30. Bosl GJ, Dmitrovsky E, Reuter V, et al. i(12p): A specific karyotypic abnormality in germ cell tumors. *Proc Am Soc Clin Clin Oncol* 1989;8:131.
31. Chaganti RS, Houldsworth J. Genetics and biology of adult human male germ cell tumors. *Cancer Res* 2000;60:1475–1482.
32. Domínguez-Malagón H, Pérez Montiel D. Mediastinal germ cell tumours. *Semin Diagn Pathol* 2010;16:228–236.
33. Oosterhuis JW, Stroop H, Honecker F, et al. Why human extragonadal germ cell tumours occur in the midline of the body: Old concepts, new perspectives. *Int J Androl* 2007;30:256–264.
34. Hua J, Sidhu KS. Recent advances in the derivation of germ cells from embryonic stem cells. *Stem Cells Dev* 2008;17:399–411.
35. Oosterhuis JW, Looijenga LH. Testicular germ-cell tumors in a broader perspective. *Nat Rev Cancer* 2005;5:210–222.
36. Houldsworth J, Reuter V, Bosl GJ, et al. Aberration expression of cyclin D is an early event in human male germ cell tumorigenesis. *Cell Growth Differ* 1997;8:293–299.
37. Santagata S, Ligon KL, Hornick JL. Embryonic stem cell transcription factor signatures in the diagnosis of primary and metastatic GCTs. *Am J Surg Pathol* 2007;31:836–845.
38. Albany C, Einhorn LH. Extragonadal germ cell tumors: Clinical presentation and management. *Curr Opin Oncol* 2013;25:261–265.
39. Bokemeyer C, Nichols CR, Droz JP, et al. Extragonadal germ cell tumors of the mediastinum and retroperitoneum: Results from an international analysis. *J Clin Oncol* 2002;20:1864–1873.
40. Revere DJ, Makaryus AN, Bonaros EP, et al. Chylopericardium presenting as cardiac tamponade secondary to an anterior mediastinal cystic teratoma. *Texas Heart Inst J* 2007;34:379–382.
41. Schwabe J, Calaminus G, Vorhoff W et al. Sexual precocity and recurrent beta-human chorionic gonadotropin upsurges preceding the diagnosis of a malignant mediastinal germ-cell tumor in a 9-year-old boy. *Ann Oncol* 2002;13:975–977.
42. McKenney JK, Heerema-McKenney A, Rouse RV. Extragonadal germ cell tumors: A review with emphasis on pathologic features, clinical, prognostic variables and differential diagnostic considerations. *Adv Anat Pathol* 2007;14:69–92.
43. Laquay N, Gazouani S, Vaccaroni L, et al. Intracardiac teratoma in newborn babies. *Eur J Cardiothorac Surg* 2003;23:642–644.
44. Díaz Muñoz de la Espada VM, Khosravi Shahai P, Hernández Marín B, et al. Tumores germinales mediastínicos. *An Med Interna (Madrid)* 2008;25:241–243.
45. Logothetis CJ, Samuels ML, Selig DE, et al. Chemotherapy of extragonadal germ cell tumors. *J Clin Oncol* 1985;3:316–325.

46. Reuter V. The pre and postchemotherapy pathologic spectrum of germ cell tumors. *Chest Surg Clin N Am* 2002;12:673–694.
47. Sickles EA, Belliveau RF, Wiernick PH. Primary mediastinal choriocarcinoma in the male. *Cancer* 1974;33:1193–1203.
48. Nichols CR, Heerema NA, Palmer C, et al. Klinefelter's syndrome associated with mediastinal germ cell neoplasms. *J Clin Oncol* 1987;5:1290–1294.
49. Aguirre D, Nieto K, Lazos M, et al. Extragonadal germ cell tumors are often associated with Klinefelter syndrome. *Human Pathol* 2006;37:477–480.
50. Swerdlow AJ, Shoemaker MJ, Higgins CD, et al. Cancer incidence and mortality in men with Klinefelter Syndrome. A cohort study. *J Natl Cancer Inst* 2005;97:1204–1210.
51. Nichols CR, Roth BJ, Heerema N, et al. Hematologic neoplasia associated with mediastinal germ cell tumors. An update. *N Engl J Med* 1990;322:1425–1429.
52. Neiman RS, Orazi A. Mediastinal non-seminomatous germ cell tumors: Their association with non-germ cell malignancies. *Pathol Res Pract* 1999;195:589–594.
53. deMent SH, Eggleston JC, Spivak JL. Association between mediastinal germ cell tumors and hematologic malignancies. Report of two cases and review of the literature. *Am J Surg Pathol* 1985;9:23–30.
54. Hartmann JT, Nichols CR, Droz JP, et al. Hematologic disorders associated with mediastinal nonseminomatous germ cell tumors. *J Natl Cancer Inst* 2000;92:54–61.
55. Robinson PG. Mediastinal tumor markers. In: Shields TW, LoCicero J II, Reed CE, et al., eds. *General Thoracic Surgery*. 7th ed. Philadelphia, PA: Wolters Kluwer/Lippincott Williams & Wilkins; 2009:2131–2146.
56. Carver BS, Sheinfeld J. Germ cell tumors of the testis. *Ann Surg Oncol* 2005;12:871–880.
57. Gilligan TD, Seidenfeld J, Basch EM, et al. American Society of Clinical Oncology Practice Guideline on uses of serum tumor markers in adult males with germ cell tumors. *J Clin Oncol* 2010;28:3388–3404.
58. Kesler K, Rieger K, Hammoud Z, et al. A 25 year single institution experience with surgery for primary mediastinal nonseminomatous germ cell tumors. *Ann Thorac Surg* 2008;85:371–378.
59. Vuky J, Bains M, Bacik J, et al. Role of postchemotherapy adjunctive surgery in the management of patients with nonseminoma arising from the mediastinum. *J Clin Oncol* 2001;19:682–688.
60. Kruter L, Kesler K, Yu M, et al. The predictive value of serum tumor markers for pathologic findings of residual mediastinal masses after chemotherapy for primary mediastinal nonseminomatous germ cell tumors (abstract). *Proc Am Soc Clin Oncol* 2008;26:5087.
61. Riggs HD, Einhorn LH, Kesler KA. Management of residual disease after therapy for mediastinal germ cell tumor and normal serum markers. In: Ferguson MK, ed. *Difficult Decisions in Thoracic Surgery*. 2nd ed. London: Springer-Verlag; 2011:445–452.
62. Afifi H, Bosl G, Burt M, et al. Mediastinal growing teratoma syndrome. *Ann Thorac Surg* 1997;64:359–362.
63. Logothetis CJ, Samuels ML, Trindades A, et al. The growing teratoma syndrome. *Cancer* 1982;50:1629–1635.
64. Miller WT Jr, Shah RM. Radiographic, computed tomographic, and magnetic resonance investigation of the mediastinum. In: Shields TW, LoCicero J III, Reed CE, et al., eds. *General Thoracic Surgery*. 7th ed. Philadelphia, PA: Wolters Kluwer/Lippincott Williams & Wilkins; 2009:2079–2101.
65. Moeller KH, Rosado de Christenson ML, Templeton PA. Mediastinal mature teratoma: imaging features. *AJR Am J Roentgenol* 1997;169:985–990.
66. Hain SF, O'Doherty MJ, Timothy AR, et al. Fluorodeoxyglucose positron emission tomography in the evaluation of germ cell tumours at relapse. *Br J Cancer* 2000;83:863–869.
67. Sánchez D, Zudaire JJ, Fernandez JM, et al. 18F-fluoro-2-deoxyglucose-positron emission tomography in the evaluation of nonseminomatous germ cell tumors at relapse. *Brit J Urol Int* 2002;89:912–916.
68. Daneshmand S, Djaladat H, Nichols C. Management of residual mass in nonseminomatous germ cell tumors following chemotherapy. *Ther Adv Urol* 2011;3:163–171.
69. Kesler K, Einhorn L. Multimodality treatment of germ cell tumors of the mediastinum. *Thorac Surg Clin* 2009;19:63–69.
70. Travis WD, Brambilla E, Burke AP, et al. In: *WHO Classification of Tumours the Lung, Pleura, Thymus and Heart*. Lyon: IARC Press; 2015:184.
71. Dehner LP. Germ cell tumors of the mediastinum. *Semin Diagn Pathol* 1990;7:266–284.
72. Weissferdt A, Suster S, Moran CA. Primary Mediastinal "Thymic" Seminomas. *Adv Anat Pathol* 2012;19:75–80.
73. Sung MT, MacLennan GT, López-Beltrán A, et al. Primary Mediastinal Seminoma: A Comprehensive Assessment Integrated with Histology, Immunohistochemistry, and fluorescence In Situ Hybridization for Chromosome 12p Abnormalities in 23 cases. *Am J Surg Pathol* 2008;32:146–155.
74. Jung SM, Chu PH, Shiu TF, et al. Expression of OCT4 in the primary germ cell tumors and thymoma in the mediastinum. *Appl Immunohistochem Mol Morphol* 2006;14:273–275.
75. Weissferdt A, Rodríguez-Canales J, Liu H, et al. Primary mediastinal seminomas: A comprehensive immunohistochemical study with a focus on novel markers. *Hum Pathol* 2015;46:376–383.
76. Truong LD, Harris L, Mattioli C, et al. Endodermal sinus tumor of the mediastinum. *Cancer* 1986;58:730–739.
77. Tinica G, Butcovan D, Cimpeanu C, et al. A mediastinal germ cell tumor of yolk sac type—case report. *Chirurgia* 2010;105:831–834.
78. Moran CA, Suster S. Primary mediastinal choriocarcinomas: a clinicopathologic and immunohistochemical study of eight cases. *Am J Surg Pathol* 1997;21:1007–1012.
79. Gossot D, Ramos R, Girard P, et al. Thoracoscopic resection of bulky intrathoracic benign lesions. *Eur J Cardiothorac Surg* 2007;32:848–851.
80. Einhorn LH, Donohue JD. Cis-diamminedichloroplatinum, vinblastine and bleomycin in combination chemotherapy in disseminated testicular cancer. *Ann Intern Med* 1977;87:293–298.
81. Schneider DT, Calaminus G, Reinhard H, et al. Primary mediastinal germ cell tumors in children and adolescents; results of the German Cooperative Protocols MAKEI 83/86, 89 and 96. *J Clin Oncol* 2000;18:832–839.
82. Childs WJ, Goldstraw P, Nicholls JE, et al. Primary malignant mediastinal germ cell tumours: Improved prognosis with platinum-based chemotherapy and surgery. *Brit J Cancer* 1993;67:1098–1101.
83. Fizazi K, Culine S, Droz JP, et al. Initial management of primary mediastinal seminoma: radiotherapy or cisplatin-based chemotherapy? *Europ J Ca* 1998;34:347–352.
84. Pectasides D, Aravantinos G, Visvikis A, et al. Platinum-based chemotherapy of primary extragonadal germ cell tumours: The Hellenic Cooperative Oncology Group experience. *Oncology* 1999;57:1–9.
85. Bokemeyer C, Droz JP, Horwich A, et al. Extragonadal seminoma: An international multicenter analysis of prognostic factors and long term outcome. *Cancer* 2001;91:1394–1140.
86. Motzer R. Testicular Cancer. *NCCN Guidelines*. 2015;Version 1.
87. Oldenburg J, Fossa SD, Nuver J, et al. Testicular seminoma and non-seminoma: ESMO Clinical Practice Guidelines for diagnosis, treatment and follow-up. *Ann Oncol* 2013;24 (Suppl 6):vi 125–132.
88. Fizazi K, Pagliaro L, Laplanche A, et al. Personalised chemotherapy based on tumour marker decline in poor prognosis germ-cell tumours (GETUG 13): A phase 3, multicentre, randomised trial. *Lancet Oncol* 2014;15:1442–1450.
89. Sakurai H, Asamura H, Suzuki K, et al. Management of primary malignant germ cell tumor of the mediastinum. *Jpn J Clin Oncol* 2004;34:386–392.
90. Ganjoo KN, Rieger KM, Kesler KA, et al. Results of modern therapy for patients with mediastinal nonseminomatous germ cell tumors. *Cancer* 2000;88:1051–1056.
91. Sarkaria IS, Bains MS, Sood S, et al. Resection of primary mediastinal nonseminomatous germ cell tumors. A 28-year experience at Memorial Sloan-Kettering Cancer Center. *J Thorac Oncol* 2011;6:1236–1241.
92. Banna GL, De Giorgi U, Ferrari B, et al. Is high-dose chemotherapy after primary chemotherapy a therapeutic option for patients with primary mediastinal nonseminomatous germ cell tumor? *Biol Blood Marrow Transplant* 2006;12:1085–1091.
93. Hartman JT, Einhorn L, Nichols CR, et al. Second-line chemotherapy in patients with relapsed extragonadal nonseminomatous germ cell tumors: Results of an international multicenter analysis. *J Clin Oncol* 2001;19:1641–1648.
94. Rivera C, Arame A, Jougon J, et al. Prognostic factors in patients with primary mediastinal germ cell tumors, a surgical multicenter retrospective study. *Interact Cardiovasc Thorac Surg* 2010;11:585–589.
95. McNamee CJ. Malignant primary anterior mediastinal tumors. In: Sugarbaker DJ, Bueno R, Krasna MJ, et al., eds. *Adult chest Surgery*. New York: McGraw-Hill; 2009:1154–1158.

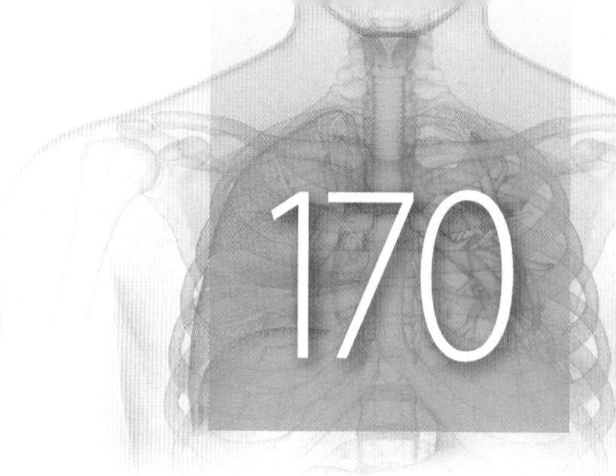

Benign and Malignant Neurogenic Tumors of the Mediastinum in Children and Adults

Eric Sceusi ■ Ara A. Vaporciyan

Primary mediastinal tumors are usually neurogenic in origin and are located almost exclusively in the posterior mediastinum, specifically, in the paravertebral sulci (Fig. 170.1). In infants and children, these tumors most commonly arise from tissues of the autonomic ganglia and only infrequently are of nerve sheath origin. Conversely, in adults, nerve sheath tumors (i.e., schwannomas), arising from cells derived from embryonic neural crest cells, are more common than those of the autonomic ganglia. These neurogenic tumors have varying degrees of maturation and the diversity of cellular types formed. A relatively simple but reasonably complete classification for tumors seen in both adults and children is presented in Table 170.1.

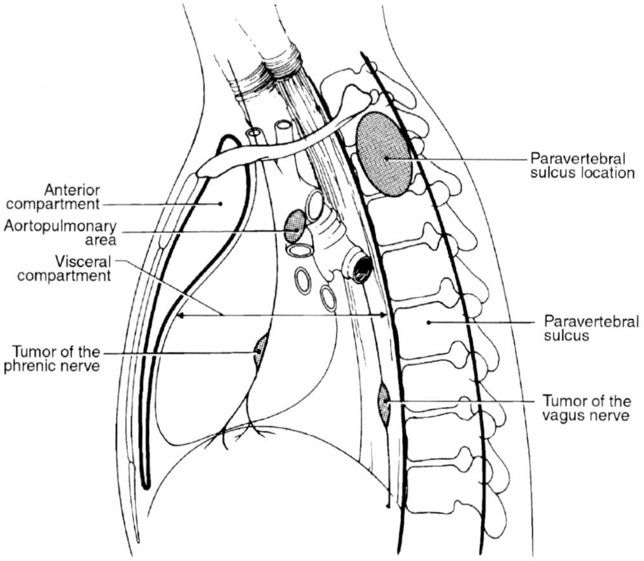

FIGURE 170.1 Mediastinal compartments and usual locations of neurogenic tumors: (1) paravertebral sulcus location; (2) aortopulmonary area of the visceral compartment; (3) tumor of the phrenic nerve in the visceral compartment; and (4) tumor of the vagus nerve in the visceral compartment. (Reprinted from Shields TW, Reynolds M. Neurogenic tumors of the thorax. *Surg Clin North Am* 1988;68:645. Copyright © 1988 Elsevier. With permission.)

This chapter will address the different subtypes of autonomic ganglia tumors, nerve sheath tumors, and the rare neuroectodermal tumors that can occur in the mediastinum (Table 170.2). The final section of this chapter will focus on the unique surgical challenges that tumors of the paravertebral sulcus can present as hourglass (dumbbell) tumors with an intraspinal and an intrathoracic component. Briefly, the distribution patterns between adults and children will be addressed before moving on to the details of each subtype. Paragangliomas, and pheochromocytomas are discussed in Chapter 171 and will not be discussed here.

It is generally estimated that 50% to 60% of the neurogenic lesions in infants and children are malignant. Most of the malignant

TABLE 170.1 Neurogenic Tumors of the Thorax

Benign	Malignant	Age Group
Nerve sheath origin		
Neurilemoma	Malignant schwannoma; neurogenic sarcoma	Adults
Neurofibroma	Neurogenic sarcoma	Adults
Melanotic schwannoma		Adults
Granular cell tumor		Adults
Autonomic ganglia		
Ganglioneuroma	Ganglioneuroblastoma	Children and young adults
	Neuroblastoma	Children, rarely in adults
	Primary malignant melanotic tumor of the sympathetic ganglia	Adults
Peripheral neuroectodermal tumor	Malignant small-cell tumor; Askin tumor	Children

TABLE 170.2 Mediastinal Neurogenic Tumors

Tumors of Autonomic Ganglia	Neuroblastoma	Ganglioneuroblastoma	Ganglioneuroma
Tumors of Nerve Sheath Origin	Schwannoma (Neurilemoma)	Neurofibroma	Malignant schwannoma (Neurogenic sarcoma)
Tumors of Neuroectodermal Origin	MNTI	Askin tumor	
Tumors of Paraganglia Origin	Paraganglioma		

Red, Malignant; Orange, Intermediate; Yellow, Generally Benign.
MNTI, Melanotic neuroectodermal tumor of infancy.

lesions are seen in the younger patients, and the benign lesions tend to be observed in the older child or adolescent. Neurogenic tumors account for 28% to 40% of the total number of mediastinal lesions encountered in children.[1–5] The two rare tumors of presumed neuroectodermal origin, melanotic neuroectodermal tumor of infancy (MNTI) and malignant small cell tumor of the thoracopulmonary region (Askin tumor) may occur in children in the mediastinum. Askin tumor is seen more frequently in older children or adolescents.

The actual incidence of the neurogenic tumors in adults is unknown, but historically they have been reported to account for 10% to 34% of adult mediastinal tumors. In a collected series of a total of 2,412 mediastinal lesions, they accounted for 21% of all lesions. Teixeira and Bibas[6] reported a similar overall incidence of 23.6% of 199 mediastinal tumors they encountered. In adults with mediastinal tumors, neurogenic tumors are generally second to thymomas in frequency. In a report of mediastinal neurogenic tumors in Japan, Miura and colleagues[7] noted that in the data from three large series plus their own data, the overall incidence was 18.6%, whereas the incidence of epithelial tumors of the thymus was 25.3%. In some series, such as that reported by Cohen and colleagues[8] from Walter Reed Hospital, lymphoma incidence may surpass neurogenic tumors as well. The majority of these tumors in adults are of nerve sheath origin, including schwannoma, neurofibroma, and malignant peripheral nerve sheath tumors (MPNSTs) and can be associated with any neurogenic structure in the chest. Approximately 98% to 99% of neurogenic mediastinal tumors in adults are benign.[4,9,10] Most commonly, they are located in either the costovertebral sulcus arising from the sympathetic chain or in one of the rami of an intercostal nerve (Fig. 170.1). Infrequently, either a phrenic nerve or one of the vagus nerves in the visceral compartment is the site of origin. Rare tumors, such as granular cell tumors and melanotic schwannomas

of both nerve sheath and ganglion cell origin, may also occur in the mediastinum.

TUMORS OF THE AUTONOMIC GANGLIA

The majority of autonomic ganglia tumors occur in infants and children and consist of neuroblastomas, ganglioneuroblastomas and ganglioneuromas. These tumors arise from the primitive neural crest cells. The lesions may be benign (e.g., the ganglioneuroma), malignant to varying degrees (e.g., the ganglioneuroblastoma), or aggressively malignant (e.g., the neuroblastoma). The latter not only invades locally but also is associated with widespread distant metastases. It is believed that all three tumors represent a continuum of maturation: the neuroblastoma being the least mature, the ganglioneuroblastoma more mature with an increasing number of mature ganglion cells present, and the ganglioneuroma, a fully differentiated benign lesion.

In an attempt to simplify pathologic identification of these tumors, Joshi and colleagues[11] established specific terminology for neuroblastic tumors which was modified in 2003 to distinguish between favorable and unfavorable subtypes of ganglioneuroblastoma (Table 170.3).[12] Neuron-specific enolase may be identified in all these tumors, however this marker is not specific.[13,14] Synaptophysin is a more specific marker for neuroendocrine neoplasms and may also be identified by immunofluorescence microscopy in these tumors.[15]

These tumors are capable of producing norepinephrine and dopamine. Elevated urine levels of the degradation products vanillylmandelic acid (VMA) and homovanillic acid (HVA) and total metanephrine are found in 90% of patients with neuroblastomas and to a lesser extent in other autonomic nerve tumors.[16,17] Clinical symptoms of the excessive catecholamine production may be present but

TABLE 170.3 Recommended Terminology and Criteria for Neuroblastic Tumors

Category	Criteria	Comment
Neuroblastoma	Neuroblasts and neutrophils constitute the predominant (>50%) or exclusive component of the tumor. A few neuroblastomas contain small ganglioneuromatous foci at the periphery or within the septa.	Three subtypes (undifferentiated, poorly differentiated, and differentiating), on the basis of proportion of differentiating neuroblasts (0, <5%, and >5%, respectively) are recognized. Shimada terminology for this tumor would be stroma-poor neuroblastoma.
Ganglioneuroma	The tumor is exclusively composed of mature ganglion cells, neurites accompanied by Schwann cells, and fibrous tissue.	
Ganglioneuroblastoma	The tumor is composed of a predominant ganglioneuromatous component (>50%) and a small neuroblastomatous component.	Three subtypes (nodular, intermixed, and borderline), on the basis of type of neuroblastomatous component, are recognized. In almost all ganglioneuroblastomas, the ganglioneuroma component is far in excess of 50%. Shimada terminology for these three subtypes would be stroma-rich neuroblastoma of nodular, intermixed, and well-differentiated subtype, respectively.

Joshi VV, Cantor AB, Altshuler G. et al. Age-linked prognostic categorization based on a new histologic grading system of neuroblastomas. A clinicopathologic study of 211 cases from the Pediatric Oncology Group. *Cancer* 1992;69(8):2197–2211. With permission.

may not be proportionately related to the measured catecholamine levels. Voute and colleagues[18] reported that tumors originating in the dorsal root ganglia do not usually secrete catecholamines, so the absence of elevated VMA or HVA levels does not rule out the diagnosis of a neuroblastoma.[18]

Williams and colleagues[19] reported the production of vasoactive intestinal peptide by some of these tumors. This is thought to be the cause of intractable diarrhea seen in some patients with neuroblastoma. Zhang cites 63 reported cases of watery diarrhea, hypokalemia and achlorhydria (WDHA) syndrome in children age 6 months to 11 years old in the literature since 1975. The responsible tumors in these cases were ganglioneuroblastoma in 55.6% of the cases, 31.7% ganglioneuroma, and 7.9% were neuroblastoma, with 11/63 of the cases occurring in the thorax.[20] Secretion of VIP in these tumors correlates with a favorable prognosis and VIP levels return to normal after resection.

Neuroblastomas and rarely ganglioneuromas can have a paraneoplastic syndrome called Kinsbourne syndrome. This is characterized by development of opsoclonus, ataxia, and myoclonus in previously healthy 6- to 36-month-old infants. Kinsbourne syndrome occurs in about 2% to 3% of neuroblastomas and remits after resection of the tumor.[21]

NEUROBLASTOMA

Neuroblastoma is the cause of 15% of childhood cancer mortalities in the United States and is the most common childhood extracranial tumor.[22] Neuroblastoma is believed to arise from the pluripotential neural crest cell. Individual case reports of thoracic neuroblastoma in adults have been published as this tumor arising from the mediastinum is extremely rare in adults. The reviews of Bronson[23] and Kilton and colleagues[24] initially confirmed these observations and the series published by Reed and colleagues[4] from the AFIP recorded that only 2 of 18 thoracic neuroblastomas (11%) occurred in patients >20 years of age. Both patients were only 21 years old. The 11% incidence of neuroblastoma in adults in this series is undoubtedly artificially high because of the patient referral base. Subsequently, Hoover and colleagues,[25] in reviewing five other series, identified 40 patients with a primary thoracic neuroblastoma only, one of which occurred in an adult who was 27 years of age, for an incidence of only 2.5%. In addition to this one patient included in the series of Eklof and Gooding,[26] Hoover and colleagues[25] presented an additional case in a 57-year-old man with a neuroblastoma in the retrocardiac region of the visceral compartment extending into or arising from the right paravertebral sulcus. In all, nine adult cases (six neuroblastomas and three ganglioneuroblastomas) have been located in the anterior mediastinum; seven of the patients were in the seventh, eighth, or ninth decades of life; seven lesions occurred in women and only two in men. Of these tumors, five have been associated with the thymus, as noted by Talerman and Gratama[27] and by Hutchinson,[28] Asada,[29] and Argani[30] and their colleagues. Buthker[31] and Hutchinson[28] and their colleagues each reported a neuroblastoma occurring in the anterior mediastinum of an elderly and a middle-aged woman, 67 and 51 years of age, respectively. Griff and Griff[32] reported a neuroblastoma in the paravertebral area (so-called posterior mediastinum); two tumors were simply stated to be in the thorax. Finally, Salter[33] and Argani[30] and their colleagues each reported the occurrence of one or two neuroblastomas in the anterior mediastinum, respectively. These tumors have a natural history of extensive local spread and distant metastases with a relatively rapid fatal outcome in the adult. Response to chemotherapy is poor. Stowens[34]

as early as 1957 even postulated that these may be a variety of neurogenic sarcomas in the adult.

Pathology

Grossly, neuroblastomas are large, lobulated, and soft; they may appear to be pseudoencapsulated. The cut surface is gray-red, and multiple hemorrhagic areas are frequently present. Microscopically, the tumor is composed of small cells with scanty cytoplasm and can present with a diverse spectrum of histopathology (Fig. 170.2).[35] The nuclei are round to polygonal with a salt-and-pepper chromatin pattern. Characteristically, a circular grouping or pseudorosette formation of cells appears around a fine fibrillar network. The background of the tumor may contain varying amounts of neuropil. Occasional large cells with ganglionic differentiation may be seen. Foci of calcification are commonly present. Rarely, as reported by Stowens,[34] abundant intracytoplasmic neuromelanin (pigmented neuroblastomas) is present. Ultrastructurally, Taxy[36] has described fine intracytoplasmic neurofilaments, dense-core neurosecretory granules, and abundant extracellular neurofibrillary material.

The most common cytogenetic abnormality found is a deletion of the short arm of chromosome 1, occurring in up to 36% of sporadic neuroblastomas.[22] Maris and colleagues,[37] studying 13 patients with familial neuroblastoma, suggested that the neuroblastoma suppressor gene thought to be located at 1p36 is not the only neuroblastoma suppressor gene. Other common cytogenetic abnormalities include the presence of homogeneously staining regions and double minutes. Homogeneously staining regions and double minutes correspond to N-*myc* amplification units. Clinical studies by Seeger and colleagues[38] have shown that N-*myc* amplification is associated with rapid tumor growth and advanced-stage disease. Morris and colleagues,[39] however, have documented that mediastinal neuroblastomas seldom have N-*myc* amplification.

Clinical Features

Neuroblastoma occurs with an incidence of 0.9 per 100,000 with a median age of 1 year old at presentation with 42% presenting under age 1. Almost 90% are seen within the first 10 years of life and presentation in adults is rare. Seventy-five percent of neuroblastomas originate from the retroperitoneum and 15% occur in the mediastinum.[40] Intrathoracic neuroblastomas account for approximately 15% to 20% of all neuroblastomas seen in the pediatric age group. Young adults typically present with neuroblastoma in the head and neck, thorax, and abdomen.

Patients with mediastinal neuroblastomas may be asymptomatic and have only an incidental radiographic finding, but generally most patients are symptomatic with local and constitutional findings thought to be autoimmune related. Chest pain, Horner syndrome, paraplegia, cough, dyspnea, and dysphagia are not uncommon. Heterochromia iridis, fever, malaise, and failure to thrive can be present. As the result of catecholamine production, sweating, flushing, or an admixture of both may develop. Diarrhea and abdominal distention may be observed and is probably due to the production vasoactive intestinal peptide. The more common complaints reported have been Horner syndrome, paraplegia, and flushing and sweating. Some infants also present with acute cerebellar ataxia with opsoclonus and chaotic nystagmus, the so-called dancing eyes originally described by Solomon and Chutorian[41] and Altman and Baehner.[42] This symptom complex is seen in patients with better differentiated neuroblastomas and usually occurs in infants under 1 year of age. In 60% of infants with this syndrome, the neuroblastoma is located

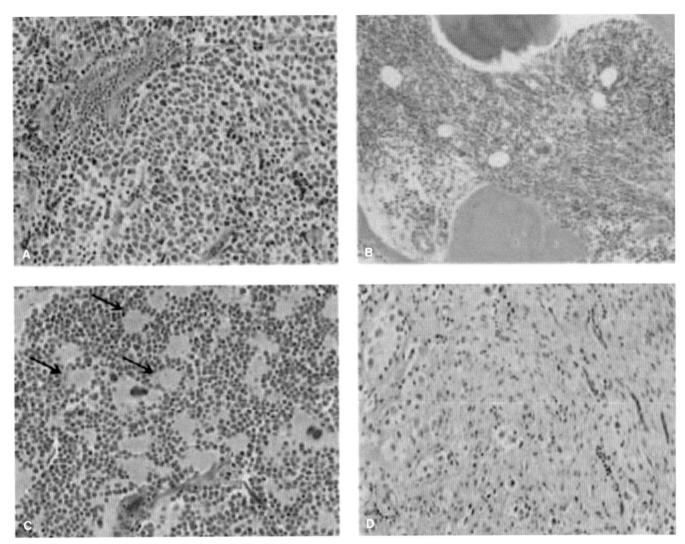

FIGURE 170.2 Neuroblastomas. **A:** Undifferentiated, stroma poor neuroblastoma. **B:** Poorly differentiated neuroblastoma invading bone marrow. **C:** Poorly differentiated neuroblastoma with classic pseudorosette (*arrows*). **D:** Well-differentiated neuroblastoma. (From Owens C, Irwin M. Neuroblastoma: the impact of biology and cooperation leading to personalized treatments. *Crit Rev Clin Lab Sci* 2012;49(3):85–115. Reprinted by permission of Taylor & Francis Ltd, http://www.informaworld.com.)

in the thorax, and most lesions are either stage 1 or 2 (Table 170.4). Stage 4 and 4S disease may occur in association with thoracic neuroblastomas, as with primary neuroblastomas elsewhere in the body. Distant metastases to liver or bone can occur, although thoracic neuroblastomas rarely present with metastatic involvement.

In addition to elevated plasma and urine levels of catecholamines, VMA, and HVA, elevated serum ferritin and lactate dehydrogenase levels may be present. Levels of VMA and HVA are similar in patients with stage 2, 3, 4 and 4s disease but these stages have significantly higher levels compared to stage 1 disease. Elevated dopamine has been associated with other high-risk factors. Currently, these levels are not directly used for risk stratification, however they are easily obtained markers for the tumor and can be used to monitor for recurrence after treatment.[22,43]

Biopsy for histologic evaluation can diagnose neuroblastoma. Although classically open biopsy was the mainstay of tissue diagnosis, recent data shows that core needle biopsy provides enough tumor (>107 tumor cells from at least two regions of tumor) and results in fewer complications than open biopsy and is preferred.[44–46] Bone marrow (BM) aspirates should be performed with two aspirates from two biopsies on bilateral sites due to the

TABLE 170.4 Stage Description for Neuroblastomas

1. Localized tumor confined to the area of origin, complete gross excision with or without microscopic residual disease; identifiable ipsilateral and contralateral lymph nodes microscopically negative
2A. Unilateral tumor with incomplete gross excision; identifiable ipsilateral and contralateral nodes microscopically negative
2B. Unilateral tumor with complete or incomplete gross excision, with positive ipsilateral regional lymph nodes; identifiable contralateral lymph nodes microscopically negative
3. Tumor infiltrating across the midline with or without regional lymph node involvement; or unilateral tumor with contralateral regional lymph node involvement; or midline tumor with bilateral regional lymph node involvement
4. Dissemination of tumor to bone, bone marrow, liver, distant lymph nodes, and other organs except as defined for stage 4S
4S. Localized primary tumor, as defined for stages 1 and 2, with dissemination limited to liver, skin, <10% or all of bone marrow, with newborn to <1 year of age at diagnosis

From Brodeur GM, Pritchard J, Berthold F, et al. Revisions of the international criteria for neuroblastoma diagnosis staging and response to treatment. *J Clin Oncol* 1993;11: 1466. Reprinted with permission. Copyright © 1993 American Society of Clinical Oncology. All rights reserved.

high incidence of bone marrow metastases. The International Neuroblastoma Risk Group (INRG) testing recommendations call for BM and peripheral blood screening for disialoganglioside GD2 and tyrosine hydroxylase as markers of neuroblastoma dissemination. This should be performed at diagnosis, after induction treatment, and at the end of therapy.[22]

Radiographic Features

Slovis and colleagues[47] demonstrated that a chest radiograph is 100% sensitive in establishing a diagnosis of neuroblastoma. Bar-Ziv and Nogrady[48] describe the characteristic radiographic features of a paravertebral neuroblastoma as a ghost-like mass with indistinct borders (Fig. 170.3). These investigators described scattered calcifications in more than 70% of these tumors, the uncalcified ones being more commonly seen in infants <1 year of age. Rib erosions and rib displacement are common. A high incidence of intervertebral foramen enlargement and intraspinal canal extension is also present, occurring in two-thirds of the patients reported by Bar-Ziv and Nogrady.[48] Reed and colleagues[4] reported lower incidences of these bony changes.

Standard imaging should consist of computed tomography (CT) or magnetic resonance imaging (MRI) to define image-defined risk factors (IDRFs). MRI is the best imaging modality for detecting nodal involvement, intraspinal extension, and chest wall involvement (Figs. 170.4 and 170.5). More recently, IDRFs have been identified to help guide preoperative decision making, making preoperative imaging even more important. MRI is also recommended in the case of intraspinal extension to assess the spinal cord, nerve roots, and subarachnoid space[49] as T1 images will define tumor extent to rule out intraspinal extension.[50]

An Iodine-123 metaiodobenzylguanidine (MIBG) scan is necessary and should be performed before tumor resection to rule out metastatic disease. PET scan has similar sensitivity to MIGB but is limited by inability to evaluate lesions in the cranial vault and its lower sensitivity for bone lesions.[22] In cases where the tumor has been removed or is not MIBG-avid, a technetium-99 bone scan can also be helpful to define metastatic disease.[49,51]

Staging

The International Neuroblastoma Staging System (INSS) (Table 170.4) was developed in 1986 and modified in 1993 and is widely used in staging neuroblastomas; however, it is based on extent of surgical resection and is not suitable for pretreatment risk stratification. A further limitation of the INSS system is that is an assessment made after surgical resection and can be influenced by approach of the surgeon.[51] The INRG addressed this issue by developing the new INGR staging system (INRGSS) in 2009, shown in Table 170.5.[51] These guidelines include IDRFs that are useful in preoperative staging (Table 170.6). The differences between the INSS and the INRGSS staging are shown in Table 170.7.[22] IDRFs have been shown to predict risk and completion of operation in a recent clinical trial.[52] Complete primary resection was possible in 156/227 patients that lacked IDRFs, but only 43/139 patients that had IDRFs (P <0.001). Additionally, IDRFs predicted increased postoperative complications but were not useful in predicting event-free survival (EFS) or overall survival in multivariate analysis. INSS remains more accurate in determining poor prognosis.[52]

Prognostic Factors

Several clinical and biological prognostic factors have been identified in children with neuroblastoma. Many of these prognostic factors

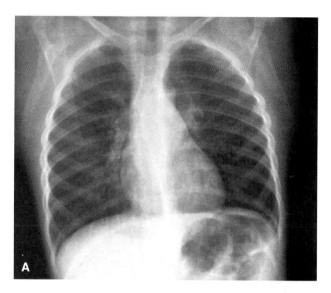
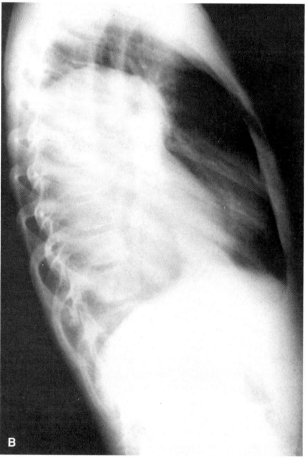

FIGURE 170.3 A, B: Posteroanterior and lateral radiographs of the chest of an infant with a large paraspinal neuroblastoma on the left. Note ghost-like shadow of the tumor on the posteroanterior view. (Reprinted from Shields TW, Reynolds M. Neurogenic tumors of the thorax. *Surg Clin North Am* 1988;68:645. Copyright © 1988 Elsevier. With permission.)

play a role in treatment protocols. Matthay found that age of diagnosis under age 2 had a 77% 2-year survival vs 38% for those older than two years old. They also noted that 2-year survival was 90% with favorable histology vs 23% when the tumor had unfavorable histology and survival at 2 years was 70%, 30% and 5% with N-myc

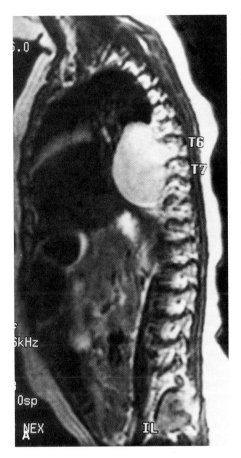

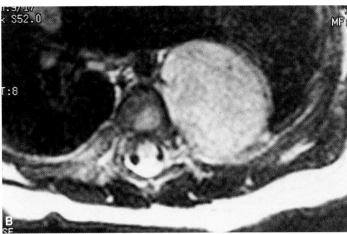

FIGURE 170.4 Lateral (**A**) and transverse (**B**) MRI scans demonstrate a thoracic neuroblastoma with intraspinal extension in this 4-month-old child. A combined thoracotomy and laminectomy was performed to remove the tumor.

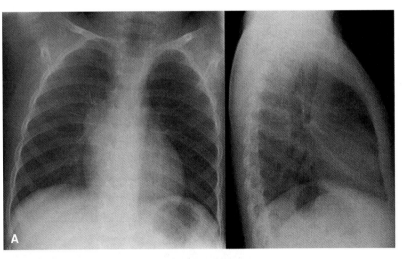

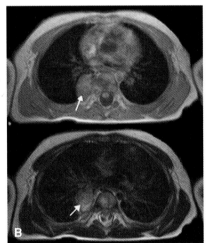

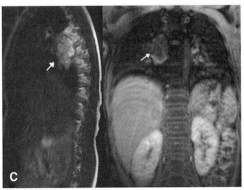

FIGURE 170.5 A 3-year-old boy with right posterior mediastinal neuroblastoma. (**A**) Paraspinal posterior mediastinal mass with smooth borders. Axial T2, axial contrast-enhanced T1 and sagittal and coronal T1-weighted images (**B** and **C**, respectively) define the tumor location and extent, and exclude intraspinal extension. Contrast uptake of the lesion confirms its solid nature and excludes a cyst. Tumor identified by *white arrows*. (From Nour-Eldin NEA, Abdelmonem O, Tawfik AM, et al. Pediatric primary and metastatic neuroblastoma: MRI findings. Pictorial review. *Magn Reson Imaging* 2012;30(7):893–906. Copyright © 2012 Elsevier. With permission.)

TABLE 170.5 International Neuroblastoma Risk Group Staging System

Stage	
L1	Localized tumor not involving vital structures as defined by IDRFs and confined to one body compartment
L2	Locoregional tumor with presence of one or more IDRFs
M	Distant metastatic disease other than MS
MS	Metastatic disease in children younger than 18 months with metastases confined to skin, liver, and/or bone marrow

Patients with multifocal disease should be staged according to greatest extent of disease. IDRFs, image-defined risk factors.
Adapted from Monclair T, Brodeur GM, Ambros PF, et al. The International Neuroblastoma Risk Group (INRG) staging system: an INRG Task Force report. *J Clin Oncol* 2009;27(2):298–303. Reprinted with permission. Copyright © 2009 American Society of Clinical Oncology. All rights reserved.

TABLE 170.6 Neuroblastoma Imaging

Mandatory	
I123MLBG scintigraphy (SPECT or SPECT-CT)[a]	
MRI[a] (± contrast) or CT with contrast of tumor location	
Chest x-ray	

Indications for Optional Imaging	
Primary tumor MIBG negative	99m-Tc-MDP bone scintigraphy
Single equivocal skeletal uptake	Plain films of the abnormal region ± MRI[a] or CT
Primary tumor outside of abdomen	Liver imaging (US[a] or MRI[a] or CT)
Pleuropulmonary abnormalities on exam or chest x-ray	Chest CT with IV contrast
Neurological symptoms (other than cord compression)	Brain MRI[a] or CT
MLGB/Bone scan uptake of skull base or orbits	

[a]Recommended study of choice.
Adapted with permission from Brisse HJ, McCarville MB, Granata C, et al. Guidelines for imaging and staging of neuroblastic tumors: consensus report from the International Neuroblastoma Risk Group Project. *Radiology* 2011;261(1):243–257.

copy number <3, >3–10 and >10, respectively.[22] Stage of disease is the most important prognostic factor, with age over 18 months old at diagnosis, tumor location and surgical resectability are independent prognostic factors using data from the SEER registry from 1973 to 2002. Lactate dehydrogenase levels, histologic grade, N-*myc* oncogene amplification, DNA ploidy, alterations in chromosomes 1p and 11q, and genomic profile also influence outcomes.[49] Additional validation of stage, age, histologic category, grade of tumor differentiation, N-*myc* oncogene status, chromosome 11q status and DNA ploidy was found in a cohort of 8,800 children with neuroblastoma between 1990 and 2002.[53] Amplification of the N-*myc* oncogene is associated with advanced-stage disease and rapid tumor progression, as described by Seeger[38] and Brodeur[54] and their colleagues. The relevance of N-*myc* amplification in low-stage or 4S disease is debated, however and the oncogene status may be more relevant in intermediate grades. These factors are shown in Table 170.8.

Shimada and colleagues[55] classified neuroblastoma histology as favorable or unfavorable depending on the degree of neuroblast

differentiation, stromal content, mitosis–karyorrhexis index, and age at diagnosis (Table 170.9). Favorable histology patients have a better survival than those with unfavorable histology (Fig. 170.6). Joshi and colleagues[11] modified this system using mitotic ratio (i.e., number of mitoses per 10 high power fields) and the presence of calcification in the tumor (Table 170.10).

Serum tumor markers predictive of poor outcome include ferritin (>142 ng/mL), serum lactic dehydrogenase (>1,500 IU/L), and neuron-specific enolase (>100 ng/mL). Location of the tumor in the mediastinum or pelvis was a better prognostic factor compared to other anatomic sites.[40] In general, thoracic neuroblastomas have

TABLE 170.7 Comparison Between INSS System and INRGSS

INSS	INRGSS
Stage 1: Localized tumor confined to the area of origin, complete gross excision with or without microscopic residual disease; identifiable ipsilateral and contralateral lymph nodes microscopically negative	Stage L1: Localized tumor not involving vital structures as defined by IDRFs and confined to one body compartment
Stage 2A: Unilateral tumor with incomplete gross excision; identifiable ipsilateral and contralateral nodes microscopically negative	Stage L2: Locoregional tumor with presence of one or more IDRFs
Stage 2B: Unilateral tumor with complete or incomplete gross excision, with positive ipsilateral regional lymph nodes; identifiable contralateral lymph nodes microscopically negative	Equals stage L2
Stage 3: Tumor infiltrating across the midline with or without regional lymph node involvement; or unilateral tumor with contralateral regional lymph node involvement; or midline tumor with bilateral regional lymph node involvement	Equals stage L2
Stage 4: Dissemination of tumor to bone, bone marrow, liver, distant lymph nodes, and other organs except as defined for stage 4S	Stage M: Distant metastatic disease other than MS
Stage 4S: Localized primary tumor, as defined for stages 1 and 2, with dissemination limited to liver, skin, <10% or all of bone marrow, with newborn to <1 year of age at diagnosis	Stage MS: Metastatic disease in children younger than 18 months with metastases confined to skin, liver, and/or bone marrow

IDRFs, image-defined risk factors; INRGSS, International Neuroblastoma Risk Group Staging System; INSS, International Neuroblastoma Staging System; MIBG, 123-iodine metaiodobenzylguanidine.
Adapted From Brodeur GM, Pritchard J, Berthold F, et al. Revisions of the international criteria for neuroblastoma diagnosis staging and response to treatment. *J Clin Oncol* 1993;11:1466 and Monclair T, Brodeur GM, Ambros PF, et al. The International Neuroblastoma Risk Group (INRG) staging system: an INRG Task Force report. *J Clin Oncol* 2009;27(2):298–303. With Permission.

TABLE 170.8 Genetic Characteristics of the International Neuroblastoma Risk Group Analytic Cohort (N = 8,800)

Factor	EFS Hazard Ratio	EFS 95% CI	Patients No.	Patients %	5-Year EFS (%) Rate	5-Year EFS (%) SE	5-Year EFS (%) Log-Rank P	5-Year OS (%) Rate	5-Year OS (%) SE	5-Year OS (%) Log-Rank P
MYCN status										
Not amplified	4.1	3.8 to 4.5	5,947	84	74	1		82	1	
Amplified			1,155	16	29	2	<.0001	34	2	<.0001
Ploidy										
>1 (hyperdiploid)	2.3	2.0 to 2.6	2,611	71	76	1		82	1	
≤ 1 (diploid, hypodiploid)			1,086	29	55	2	<.0001	60	2	<.0001
11q										
Normal	2.3	1.9 to 2.9	844	79	68	3		79	2	
Aberration			220	21	35	5	<.0001	57	5	<.0001
1p										
Normal	3.2	2.8 to 3.8	1,659	77	74	2		83	1	
Aberration			493	23	38	3	<.0001	48	3	<.0001
17q gain										
No gain	1.7	1.3 to 2.3	187	52	63	4		74	4	
Gain			175	48	41	5	.0006	55	5	.0009

Hazard ratios denote increased risk of an event for the second row within a given category compared with the first row.
INPC, International Neuroblastoma Pathology Classification; EFS, event-free survival; OS, overall survival; LOH, loss of heterozygosity.
Adapted from Cohn SL, Pearson AD, London WB, et al. The International Neuroblastoma Risk Group (INRG) classification system: an INRG Task Force report. *J Clin Oncol* 2009;27(2):289–297. Reprinted with permission. Copyright © 2009 American Society of Clinical Oncology. All rights reserved.

a favorable biological profile: low lactic dehydrogenase level, low serum ferritin level, DNA index = 1, and N-*myc* nonamplification. Overall survival and EFS rates are higher in neuroblastomas of the thoracic region compared to nonthoracic locations (Fig. 170.7).[56] In the comprehensive review by Morris and colleagues,[39] the biological variables measured for children with thoracic neuroblastoma did not completely explain the higher survival rates in this group when compared with the nonthoracic site (Figs. 170.7 to 170.9). More recent studies by Vo and colleagues[56] further showed that thoracic neuro-

blastomas were less likely (3% vs. 19%) to have N-*myc* amplification than nonthoracic neuroblastomas (Table 170.11).

Treatment

Clinical risk groups have been devised to classify patients with neuroblastoma and direct therapy. These risk groups are based on INSS stage, age, N-*myc* number, tumor cell ploidy, and tumor histology using Shimada criteria. Those in the low risk have >90% survival

TABLE 170.9 Shimada Histologic Grading System for Neuroblastoma

I Stroma-poor groups: Characterized by a diffuse growth of neuroblastic cells irregularly separated by thin septa of fibrovascular tissue. These correspond to classic neuroblastoma and diffuse ganglioneuroblastoma in other terminologies. Tumors of this group are further subdivided according to the grade of differentiation and nuclear morphology of the neuroblastic cells.

  A. Grade of differentiation

    1. Undifferentiated histology: Composed almost entirely of immature neuroblasts with <5% of differentiating population. The differentiating population is characterized by nuclear enlargement, cytoplasmic eosinophilia and enlargement with distinct border, and cell processes that are clearly evident in routinely stained sections.

    2. Differentiated histology: Composed of a mixture of neuroblastic cells with various degrees of maturity with at least 5% or more of the differentiating population. If in doubt about defining the 5% differentiation limit, err on the side of undifferentiation.

  B. Nuclear morphology (mitosis and karyorrhexis): Mitosis and karyorrhexis are quantitated as an index (MKI). The total of both mitosis and karyorrhexis in 5,000 cells in randomly selected fields is counted and divided into three categories.

    1. Low MKI: <100 per 5,000 cells have mitosis or karyorrhexis.

    2. Intermediate MKI: 100–200 per 5,000 cells have mitosis or karyorrhexis.

    3. High MKI: >200 per 5,000 cells have mitosis or karyorrhexis.

II Stroma-rich groups

  A. Well differentiated: Composed of a dominating mature ganglioneuromatous tissue with only a few randomly distributed immature neuroblastic cells. These cells aggregate but do not make distinct nests interrupting the stroma.

  B. Intermixed: Composed of ganglioneuromatous tissue studded with scattered, variably differentiated neuroblastic cell nests. These neuroblastic cell foci are sharply defined, make a space in the stroma, and are without an apparent capsule.

  C. Nodular: Characterized by the presence of one or a few grossly discrete masses of stroma-poor neuroblastoma tissue trapped in mature matrix. The nodule is usually appreciable grossly as a hemorrhagic focus and microscopically has a sharp, pushing margin or an encapsulated edge. In some areas, the capsule may be broached by apparent outward invasion by the malignant cells.

MKI, mitosis and karyorrhexis index.
Adapted from Shimada H, Chatten J, Newton WA Jr, et al. Histopathologic prognostic factors in neuroblastic tumors: definition of subtypes of ganglioneuroblastoma and an age-linked classification of neuroblastomas. *J Natl Cancer Inst* 1984;73:405. Reprinted by permission of Oxford University Press.

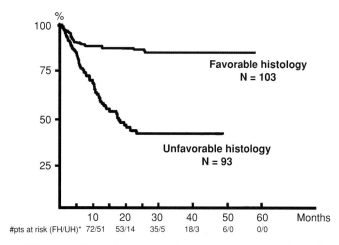

TABLE 170.10 Association of Favorable Histologic Features With Prognostic Subgroups of the Shimada Classification

Favorable Histologic Feature	Favorable Histologic Type (%)[a]	Unfavorable Histologic Type (%)	p
Ganglion cells	68 (42)	12 (24)	0.020
Tumor giant cells	75 (47)	13 (26)	0.010
Low mitotic rate[b]	150 (93)	27 (54)	<0.001
Calcification	113 (70)	22 (44)	0.001

[a]The percentage of favorable histologic cases in the series showing the presence of the features is given in parentheses.
[b]Low: 10 mitoses per 10 high-power fields.
From Joshi VV, Cantor AB, Altshuler G, et al. Age-linked prognostic categorization based on a new histologic grading system of neuroblastoma. A clinicopathologic study of 211 cases from the Pediatric Oncology Group. *Cancer* 1992;69:2197–2211. Copyright © 1992 by John Wiley Sons, Inc. Reprinted by permission of John Wiley & Sons, Inc.

FIGURE 170.6 Kaplan–Meier curves showing event-free survival rates for favorable and unfavorable neuroblastomas. ($p = 0.31 \times 10^{-9}$). (From Shimada H, Ambros IM, Dehner LP, et al. The International Neuroblastoma Pathology Classification (The Shimada System). *Cancer* 1999;86:364–372.)

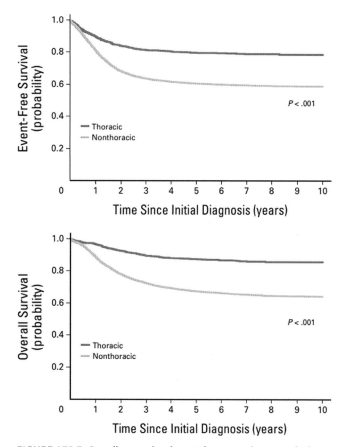

FIGURE 170.7 Overall survival and event-free survival rates are higher in neuroblastomas of the thoracic region compared to nonthoracic locations. (From Vo KT, Matthay KK, Neuhaus J, et al. Clinical, biologic, and prognostic differences on the basis of primary tumor site in neuroblastoma: a report from the international neuroblastoma risk group project. *J Clin Oncol* 2014; 32(28):3169–3176. Reprinted with permission. Copyright © 2014 American Society of Clinical Oncology. All rights reserved.)

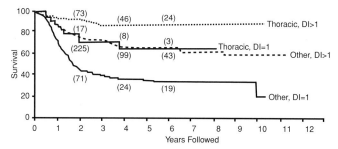

FIGURE 170.8 Survival curves for thoracic ($n = 114$) and nonthoracic ($n = 540$) patients for whom the DNA index was recorded (stratified log-rank test; $p < 0.0001$). Numbers above the curves represent cases with follow-up to or beyond the specified time points. (Reprinted from Morris JA, Shcochat SJ, Smith EI, et al. Biological variables in thoracic neuroblastoma: a Pediatric Oncology Group Study. *J Pediatr Surg* 1995;30:296. Copyright © 1995 Elsevier. With permission.)

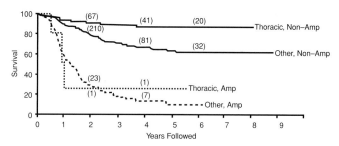

FIGURE 170.9 Survival curves for thoracic ($n = 84$) and nonthoracic ($n = 409$) patients for whom N-myc amplification was recorded (stratified log-rank test; $p = 0.003$). Numbers above the curves represent cases with follow-up up to or beyond the specified time points. (Reprinted from Morris JA, Shcochat SJ, Smith EI, et al. Biological variables in thoracic neuroblastoma: a Pediatric Oncology, Group Study. *J Pediatr Surg* 1995;30:296. Copyright © 1995 Elsevier. With permission.)

TABLE 170.11 Clinical and Biologic Characteristics of the INRG Analytic Cohort by Adrenal Versus Nonadrenal and Thoracic Versus Nonthoracic Primary Tumor Sites (N = 8,369)

| | Primary Tumor Site | | | | | Primary Tumor Site | | | | |
| | Adrenal (n = 3,966) | | Nonadrenal (n = 4,403) | | | Thoracic (n = 1,266) | | Nonthoracic (n = 7,103) | | |
Characteristic[a]	No.	%	No.	%	P[b]	No.	%	No.	%	P[b]
Mean age at diagnosis, months	26.6		263		.59	24.5		26.8		.018
Age ≥18 months at diagnosis	1,882	47	1,930	44	.001	492	39	3,320	47	<.001
Neuroblastoma or ganglioneuroblastoma, nodular[c]	1,918	48	1,915	43	<.001	491	39	3,342	47	<.001
Enrollment/diagnosis before 1996	2,008	51	2,165	49	.182	719	57	3,454	49	<.001
INSS stage 4	1,963	50	1,335	31	<.001	268	22	3,030	44	<.001
Serum ferritin ≥92 ng/mL	1,239	59	953	44	<.001	188	34	2,004	54	<.001
LDH ≥587 U/L	1,332	55	1,208	44	<.001	271	36	2,269	52	<.001
MYCN amplified	718	23	396	11	<.001	32	3	1,082	19	<.001
Ploidy ≤1 (diploid, hypodiploid)	485	33	559	27	.001	121	25	923	30	.032
LOH at 1p	314	30	164	16	<.001	28	10	450	25	<.001
Gain of 17q	115	61	53	34	<.001	16	27	152	53	<.001
11q aberration	125	26	93	17	.001	21	14	197	23	.015
Pooled segmental chromosomal aberration LOH at 1p, gain of 17q, and/or 11q aberration	416	39	265	25	<.001	53	19	628	34	<.001
Unfavorable INPC pathology classification	720	41	702	32	<.001	141	22	1,281	38	<.001
High MKI	219	15	159	10	<.001	21	5	357	14	<.001
Undifferentiated/poorly differentiated	1,346	85	1,380	83	.059	332	78	2,394	85	<.001

[a]For each variable, only the percent with the adverse risk factor is shown.
[b]P value refers to a Student's *t* test (for continuous age variable) or χ² test for all other variables (age, tumor diagnosis, year of enrollment, INSS stage, serum ferritin, LDH, *MYCN* status, ploidy, LOH at 1p, gain of 17q, 11q aberration, pooled segmental chromosomal classification, INPC pathology classification, and MKI and grade of differentiation categories).
[c]INPC diagnostic category[11]: neuroblastoma or ganglioneuroblastoma, nodular versus ganglioneuroblastoma, intermixed; ganglioneuroma, maturing subtype; or ganglioneuroblastoma, well differentiated.
INPC, International Neuroblastoma Pathology Classification; INRG, International Neuroblastoma Risk Group; INSS, International Neuroblastoma Staging System; LDH, lactate dehydrogenase; LOH, loss of heterozygosity; MKI, Mitosis Karyorrhexis Index.
From Vo KT, Matthay KK, Neuhaus J, et al. Clinical, biologic, and prognostic differences on the basis of primary tumor site in neuroblastoma: a report from the international neuroblastoma risk group project. *J Clin Oncol* 2014;32(28):3169–3176. Reprinted with permission. Copyright © 2014 American Society of Clinical Oncology. All rights reserved.

with surgery alone, intermediate risk >90% survival with surgery and chemotherapy and high risk patients have <30% survival despite intensive multimodality therapy.[22] Tumor resection is the main treatment for localized neuroblastoma. The LNESG1 study looked at 905 patients with localized neuroblastomas and identified surgical risk factors (SRFs) that could be implemented to try to select patients that would benefit from initial surgery versus upfront chemotherapy. These SRFs used are shown in Table 170.12. Patients without SRFs achieved complete resection 74.6% of the time versus 46.4% of the time in patients with SRFs. Complications occurred in 17.4% versus 5.0% when compared to those without risk factors (Table 170.13).[57] These results suggest the importance of stratifying patient risk of incomplete resection when determining if a patient is a candidate for immediate surgical resection.

Low-risk patients (INSS 1 and 2) can be treated with surgery alone with an expected 4-year survival of more than 95%. Infants with 4S disease and favorable biology (normal N-*myc* copy number, hyperdiploid DNA index, and favorable histology) can be treated

with supportive care or a short course of chemotherapy and expect a survival rate over 90%. Intermediate risk patients (INSS 3 and 4) who lack N-*myc* amplification and infants with 4S tumor (normal N-*myc* copy number, diploid DNA content, or unfavorable histology) are treated with moderate dose chemotherapy followed by surgery. Few patients with thoracic neuroblastoma fit into this risk group.[22]

High-risk patients are classified as: stage 4 disease that is diagnosed over the age of 18 months; stage 3 disease with N-*myc* amplification or older than 18 months with unfavorable histology; stage 2 disease in patients over 1 year old with N-*myc* amplification; and stage 3, 4, 4s of any age with N-*myc* amplification. These high-risk patients benefit from induction chemotherapy with alkylating agents, anthracyclines, topoisomerase I and II inhibitors, and platinum derivatives followed by surgery. Consolidation therapy with myeloablation and hematopoietic stem cell rescue improves EFS and OS and is standard treatment in high-risk patients. Targeted therapies are being now being used to treat recurrent disease.[22]

TABLE 170.12 Surgical Risk Factors

Surgical Risk Factors (SRFs)	Number of Patients (n = 79)
Encasement of subclavian vessels	22
Involvement of other major vessels	4
Lower mediastinal tumor	15
Abdominal distension	11
Encasement of trachea and/or principal bronchi	14
Dumbbell tumor	22
Others	12
Subjective tumor size	47
Subjective tumor fragility	9

Adapted from Cecchetto G, Mosseri V, De Bernardi B, et al. Surgical risk factors in primary surgery for localized neuroblastoma: the LNESG1 study of the European International Society of Pediatric Oncology Neuroblastoma Group. *J Clin Oncol* 2005;23(33):8483–8489. Reprinted with permission. Copyright © 2005 American Society of Clinical Oncology. All rights reserved.

The German prospective trial NB97 concluded that in stage 4 neuroblastoma patients diagnosed at age 18 months or older, there was no benefit from surgery in terms of EFS, progression free survival, or overall survival in the setting of multimodal therapy and recommend against surgical resection in these patients.[52] The indications for and timing of surgery for patients in the high-risk group are controversial. Initial surgical resection of large tumors is seldom recommended. Kletzel and colleagues[58] have reported improved survival for patients with high-risk neuroblastoma multimodal therapies include myeloablative chemotherapy or chemoradiation therapy followed by autologous bone marrow transplantation.

Thoracoscopy is being used with increasing frequency for diagnostic biopsy and complete surgical resection of thoracic neurogenic tumors and in carefully selected patients without IDRFs this is a reasonable approach to resection.[59] Ideally, candidates for thoracoscopic resection should have tumors confined to the organ of origin and must not encase major vascular structures. Encapsulated advanced INSS 3 or 4 tumors may also be amenable to resection if they respond well to neoadjuvant chemotherapy.[60] Petty and colleagues[61] compared open thoracotomy with thoracoscopy in a small group of patients and found similar results in terms of local control and disease-free interval. Thoracoscopy resulted in a shorter length of hospital stay. Malek and colleagues[62] report shorter length of stay, less blood loss, and similar complication and recurrence rate when

TABLE 170.13 Results of Surgery for Thoracic Neuroblastomas in Relation to SRFs

Extent of Surgical Resection	All Patients (%)	Patients Without SRFs (%)	Patients With SRFs (%)
Any	139	101	38
Complete	83 (59.7)	68 (67.3)	15 (39.5)
Near complete	48 (34.6)	29 (28.7)	19 (50.0)
Incomplete	8 (5.7)	4 (4.0)	4 (10.5)

Adapted from Cecchetto G, Mosseri V, De Bernardi B, et al. Surgical risk factors in primary surgery for localized neuroblastoma: the LNESG1 study of the European International Society of Pediatric Oncology Neuroblastoma Group. *J Clin Oncol* 2005;23(33):8483–8489. Reprinted with permission. Copyright © 2005 American Society of Clinical Oncology. All rights reserved.

retrospectively reviewing thorascopic versus open resection of neuroblastoma over an 18-year period. DeCou and colleagues[63] reported excellent results in a small series of patients who underwent primary gross total resection with the thoracoscopic approach. All were stage I and most had favorable histology. None were N-*myc*–amplified. Size is considered by some to be a contraindication to minimally invasive resections, with a cutoff of 5 cm commonly cited; however, Fraga and colleagues have reported success with thoracoscopic resection of tumors up to 18cm in size. With increasing experience in thoracoscopic resection, size can no longer be considered an absolute determinant of thoracoscopic resection in neurogenic tumors.[64]

Foramen and intraspinal dumbbell tumors are common in neuroblastomas due to their origin in the paraspinal sympathetic chain. According to Brisse and colleagues, removal of the intraspinal component is generally not recommended at the time of diagnosis, except when there are acute signs of cord compression or ischemia.[49] Biopsy followed by chemotherapy may be the best preoperative strategy, as intraspinal extension may disappear and avoid the need for laminectomy. In patients with intraspinal extension, vertebral body involvement, or both, the cooperation of a neurosurgeon or an orthopedic spinal specialist is essential for evaluation and preoperative planning. Hoover and colleagues[65] reported that recovery from neurologic deficits was not altered by laminectomy when chemotherapy or surgery was used. In their study comparing patients with and without laminectomy, there was a higher incidence of subsequent spinal deformities in those treated with laminectomy, further supporting the strategy of attempting chemotherapy to reduce the intraspinal component prior to resection.

GANGLIONEUROBLASTOMA

Ganglioneuroblastoma is a malignant tumor of intermediate grade between neuroblastoma and ganglioneuromas.

Pathology

These tumors are composed of primitive neuroblasts and mature ganglion cells in contrast to benign ganglioneuromas that lack immature cells.[66] Grossly, the tumor is firm in consistency in two-thirds of cases. Adam and Hochholzer[67] reported that of the 48 lesions in which encapsulation was recorded, 69% were grossly encapsulated, 27% were partially encapsulated, and only 4% were without a capsule. Microscopically, ganglioneuroblastomas are composed of a mixture of mature ganglion cells and neuroblasts set in a pink fibrillar background (Fig. 170.10).

Ganglioneuroblastomas are now classified as intermixed (Schwannian stroma-rich) and nodular (composite, Schwannian stroma-rich/stroma-dominant and stroma-poor) by the International Neuroblastoma Pathology Classification (INPC).[12,68] The intermixed type is defined as a transitional form that is partially differentiated toward maturation to a ganglioneuroma, but has not entirely differentiated from a neuroblastoma. This type retains microscopic foci of neuroblastomatous cells, however, the ganglioneuromatous architecture must be greater than 50% of the volume in representative sections of the tumor to be classified in this group. The nodular subtype contains macroscopic clonal nodules composed of neuroblastoma, ganglioneuroblastoma, or ganglioneuromal features.

Clinical Features

Overall, these tumors are less common than neuroblastomas, but in the thorax they appear to have approximately the same or a slightly greater incidence of occurrence than neuroblastomas. In Adam and

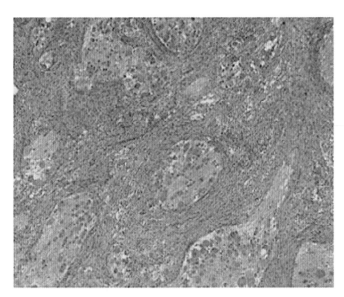

FIGURE 170.10 Ganglioneuroblastoma. Magnification 40×. (From Shimada H, Ambros IM, Dehner LP, et al. Terminology and morphologic criteria of neuroblastic tumors: recommendations by the International Neuroblastoma Pathology Committee. *Cancer* 1999;86(2):349–363. Copyright © 1999 by John Wiley Sons, Inc. Reprinted by permission of John Wiley & Sons, Inc.)

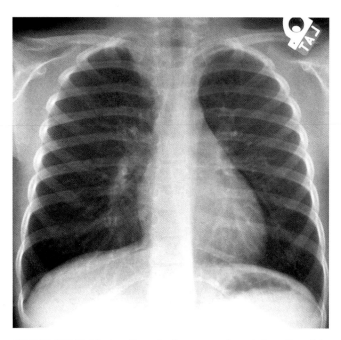

FIGURE 170.11 Chest radiograph of a mass in the apical portion of the right paravertebral sulcus. The radiographic shadow is much more distinct than that of a neuroblastoma. On surgical excision, the tumor proved to be a ganglioneuroblastoma.

Hochholzer's[67] review of the autonomic neurogenic lesions in the paravertebral sulci in the files of the AFIP, there were 65 neuroblastomas and 80 ganglioneuroblastomas. These lesions are reported to be seen more often in older children and adolescents than are neuroblastomas and are exceedingly rare in adults. However, one-third of the patients were ≤2 years of age, half were ≤3 years of age, and four-fifths were ≤10 years of age.[67] Only 10 cases were seen between the ages of 12 and 20 years, and only three patients were >20 years of age. Likewise, in the series reported by Reed and colleagues,[4] 2 of 18 patients with a ganglioneuroblastoma (11%) were >20 years of age. One patient was in the third decade and the other in the fourth decade of life. Kilton and colleagues[24] and Feigin and Cohen[69] collected a total of 20 cases, and Adam and Hochholzer[67] reported an additional three cases that occurred in the paravertebral sulci. Boys and girls <10 years of age were affected equally, although a slight predominance was seen for girls aged >12.

Patients present with findings similar to those noted for neuroblastoma, although clinical evidence of excessive catecholamines is only infrequently noted and laboratory evidence of elevated VMA or HVA is found in only 12% of patients. Evidence of extension into the spinal canal is likewise uncommon.

Radiologic Features

Approximately half of these tumors are discovered as an asymptomatic mass on routine radiography of the chest. The radiographic features of the lobulated or oval paraspinal mass tend to be more distinct than the ghost-like shadow of the neuroblastoma (Fig. 170.11). Stippled calcification may be present. Chest wall changes (i.e., rib erosion or displacement) occur in only 5% to 10% of patients according to Reed and colleagues.[4] Extension into the spinal canal is uncommon, but MRI is indicated in all cases to rule it out.

Staging

Both the INSS stage and INRGSS stages are validated as predictive of EFS[53] and can be applied to ganglioneuroblastomas as described in the previous neuroblastoma section.

Prognostic Factors

Intermixed ganglioneuroblastomas are classified as having favorable histology. The INGR analysis associated the nodular form of ganglioneuroblastoma as a poor prognostic factor compared to neuroblastoma or ganglioneuroblastoma intermixed; however, the current INPC classification subdivides nodular ganglioneuroblastomas into favorable or unfavorable groups based on grade of differentiation and mitosis karyorrhexis index (MKI).[12,68] The role of MKI in prognosis has been challenged, however. Recent data by Angelini and colleagues[70] reviewed 4,071 cases of nodular ganglioneuroblastoma and found that the same factors that were prognostic in neuroblastomas applied to ganglioneuroblastoma with the exception of LDH level and MKI. Patients with nodular ganglioneuroblastoma had a poor prognosis if they were older than 18 months of age or had stage 4 disease, as in neuroblastoma.

Treatment

Most children with ganglioneuroblastoma present with a solitary mass that can be resected, however these tumors have more malignant potential when present in adults. Complete evaluation of the patient and tumor analysis for biologic variables are critical to identify the more aggressive tumors. INSS staging and clinical risk-group assignment should be made. Treatment is primarily surgical, although chemotherapy is indicated in the intermediate- and high-risk groups. It is recommended that complete surgical excision is the only hope for cure. This may be accomplished in those patients with stage I lesions (i.e., local disease only). Adjuvant irradiation is not recommended routinely in patients with stage I disease. In stage II disease (i.e., local invasion present), irradiation is recommended, but its true efficacy is unknown. With disseminated disease, chemotherapy may be tried, but its ultimate benefit also is unknown.

Okamatsu and colleagues showed that resection of primary tumors in the ganglioneuroblastoma nodular unfavorable histology subset has no significant benefit regardless of the presence or absence of metastases. Looking at 85 cases of complete resection of tumor in nonstage

4 patients versus 16 incompletely resected patients, they found no significant difference in 5-year EFS (83.4% ± 9.1% vs. 60.6 ± 26.9% (p = 0.2227)). Stage 4 patients had a correspondingly worse prognosis that was also not significantly different based on complete versus incomplete resection of primary tumors (EFS 24.3% ± 9.5% vs. 5.4% ± 5.2% (p = 0.1068) and OS 38.5% ± 9.6% vs. 28.2% ± 11.9% (p = 0.5797)).[68]

GANGLIONEUROMAS

Ganglioneuromas are benign tumors and represent the full maturation of autonomic nerve tumors, however, Enzinger and Weiss[71] have described rare instances of malignant transformation of these tumors into malignant schwannomas. They may arise *de novo* or may follow maturation of a neuroblastoma or ganglioblastoma. They account for approximately 42% of the autonomic neural crest tumors.

Pathology

Ganglioneuromas are frequently large, firm, well-circumscribed, encapsulated tumors arising in a paravertebral sulcus in a child, adolescent, or adult. The tumor is usually attached to a sympathetic or intercostal nerve trunk. Extension into the spinal canal can occur but is uncommon. On cut section, the tumor is yellowish to gray; Marchevsky and Kaneko[72] state that it frequently has a whorled, trabeculated surface that may simulate a leiomyoma. Microscopically, they are mostly ganglioneuromatous stroma with minor scattered differentiating neuroblasts and/or maturing ganglion cells and fully mature ganglion cells (Fig. 170.12).[68] Areas of degeneration are evident within the tumor. Calcification may or may not be present in these areas. The ganglion cells are large, and their cytoplasm may contain various inclusions. Ultrastructurally, dense-core vesicles have been identified by Bender and Ghatak[73] and Yokoyama and colleagues[74] as well as others.

Clinical Features

Ganglioneuromas typically originate in the posterior mediastinum with a median age of diagnosis of 7 years old with a slight female predominance 1.13:1 to 1.5:1.[75] They can present in young to middle age adults. Of the 38 ganglioneuromas in Reed and colleagues[4] series of 160 neural thoracic tumors from the AFIP, almost half (47%) were present in patients over 20 years of age. Approximately half of these occurred in the third decade of life and the other half in the fourth decade. Only two tumors were observed in patients >40 years of age, and none occurred after the age of 50. Similar data were recorded by Ribet and Cardot.[5] Of the 134 neurogenic tumors reported in their series, 35 were ganglioneuromas and half of these occurred after the age of 15 years; only two patients between the ages of 45 and 54 years had a ganglioneuroma. Maruyama and colleagues[76] reported one case of a ganglioneuroma in a 74-year-old woman that was incidentally found on CT and was ultimately surgically resected.

Clinically, the patient may be asymptomatic, but patients with large lesions may present with cough, dyspnea, dysphagia, Horner syndrome, and, occasionally, chest pain or even scoliosis.[75] Heterochromia iridis was reported by McRae and Shaw[77] to be the result of sympathetic injury by the tumor involving the superior cervical ganglion. The age distribution is not dissimilar to that observed in patients with ganglioneuroblastomas. Elevated levels of VMA and HVA are observed infrequently. Chronic diarrhea also has been reported in association with these tumors by Mendelsohn[78] and Trump,[79] and colleagues. This is thought to be caused by the presence of vasoactive intestinal peptide, which can be localized to the cytoplasm of the ganglion cells by means of immunoperoxidase techniques. In contrast to the nerve sheath tumors, intraspinal extension is infrequent.

Radiographic Features

Ganglioneuroma presents as a solid, well-defined, ovoid, or lobulated mass in one of the paravertebral sulci (Fig. 170.13). Stippled calcification was observed by Bar-Ziv and Nogrady[48] in 50% of the patients studied. Kato reviewed 14 confirmed ganglioneuromas and found low CT attenuation. In CT and MRI images, calcification was seen in 38% of cases, a whorled appearance in 42%, a tail-shaped edge in 14%, and fat components in 29% as shown in Figure 170.14.[80] Similar findings were confirmed in another series of 22 cases reviewed by Guan and colleagues.[81] Rib erosion, when observed, is uncommon and subtle in nature. Extension into the spinal canal is uncommon but can occur, as noted by Bar-Ziv and Nogrady[48] and Davidson and colleagues.[10] Thus, CT or MRI scanning is always indicated (Fig. 170.15).

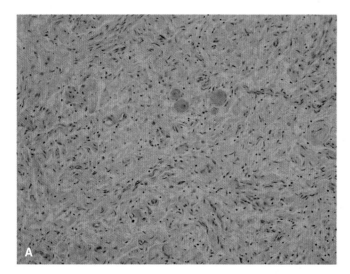
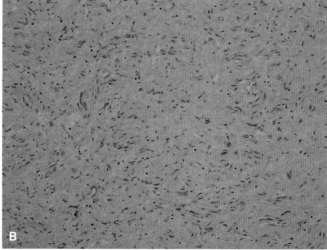

FIGURE 170.12 Ganglioneuroma. **A:** Ganglion cells with abundant eosinophilic cytoplasm with distinct cell borders, single eccentric nucleus, prominent nucleolus. Some cells show finely granular, gold to brown neuromelanin pigment. **B:** Schwannian stroma. (Image courtesy of Maheshwari Ramineni, MD and Neda Kalhor, MD, Department of Pathology, MD Anderson Cancer Center.)

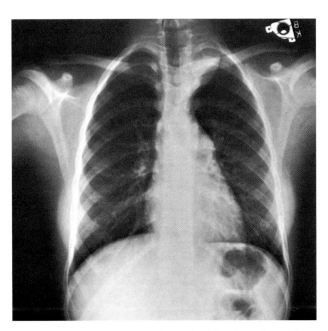

FIGURE 170.13 Posteroanterior radiograph of the chest of an adolescent girl with an asymptomatic left superior mediastinal mass. On histologic examination after surgical excision, the lesion proved to be a ganglioneuroma.

Staging

Ganglioneuroma can be staged based on the INSS guidelines or the INRGSS.

Prognostic Factors

Ganglioneuromas are benign tumors that are classified as having favorable histology. Okamatsu and colleagues[68] reported on 34 cases of stage 1 to 3 ganglioneuroma noting 5-year EFS and OS of 100%.

Treatment

Surgical excision is the treatment of choice and is curative. Marchevsky and Kaneko[72] report that occasionally a regional lymph node may contain metastatic ganglioneuroma. Enzinger and Weiss[71] believe these to be residual foci of neuroblastomas that have matured into benign ganglioneuromas; subsequent recurrence of the disease is not seen in these patients.

NERVE SHEATH TUMORS

Tumors originating from the nerve sheath most commonly present as benign lesions in adults. Benign tumors are classified as either a neurilemoma (benign schwannoma) or neurofibroma. Additional recent hybrid tumors have been described, including neurofibroma–schwannoma, schwannoma–perinoma, and microcystic/reticular schwannoma.[82] The malignant lesions are best termed MPNSTs by the World Health Organization designation in 2002. Prior to this, they have been referred to as malignant schwannoma, malignant neurilemmoma, neurofibrosarcomas, or neurogenic sarcomas.[83]

The nerve sheath tumors in the thorax are most often found in either costovertebral sulcus. They may occur infrequently in the visceral compartment as tumors of either the vagus or phrenic nerves. They may also arise from the brachial plexus or from an intercostal nerve. These tumors are most often asymptomatic (92% to 94%). Some of the benign tumors may cause symptoms because of pressure on an adjacent nerve; thoracic pain, Horner syndrome, hoarseness, and upper extremity weakness or pain are occasionally observed. Infrequently dyspnea, cough, or other respiratory symptoms may be noted. Superior vena cava obstruction also has occurred with large tumors. A few may cause symptomatic extradural compression of the spinal cord as the result of growth through an intervertebral foramen into the spinal canal. Akwari and colleagues[84] noted that such hourglass growth may be observed in approximately 10% of all

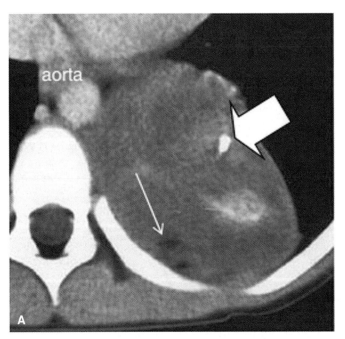 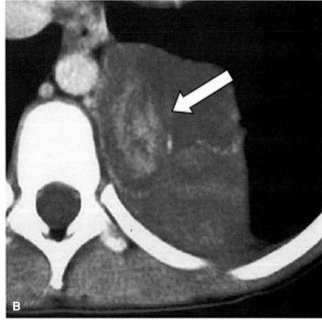

FIGURE 170.14 **A:** Ganglioneuroma on CT scan shows fat attenuation (*thin arrow*) and punctate calcification (*thick arrow*). **B:** Ganglioneuromas also show a characteristic whorled appearance. (From Kato M, Hara M, Ozawa Y, et al. Computed tomography and magnetic resonance imaging features of posterior mediastinal ganglioneuroma. [Erratum appears in *J Thorac Imaging* 2013 Jul;28(4):262. Note: Shibamato, Yuta [corrected to Shibamoto, Yuta]]. *J Thorac Imaging.* 2012;27(2):100–106. With permission.)

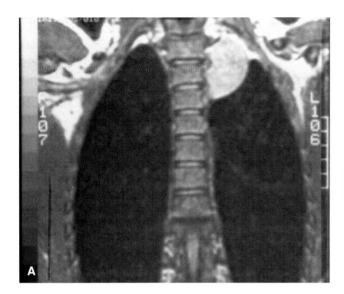

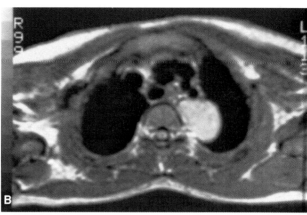

FIGURE 170.15 **A, B:** Coronal and transverse MRI scans of the mass shown in Figure 170.14 revealed no extension into the spinal canal.

benign nerve sheath tumors. It is more important to emphasize, as the aforementioned investigators reported, that extension into the spinal canal may be asymptomatic in 30% to 40% of these patients at the time of initial diagnosis.

Benign nerve sheath tumors are found almost exclusively in the paravertebral sulci and primarily in adults, however, both neurilemomas (schwannomas) and neurofibromas may occur in patients <20 years of age. Looking at neurogenic tumors of the mediastinum in individuals under 20 years of age, Reed and colleagues,[4] reported 15% (9/61) of the neurogenic intrathoracic tumors seen were of nerve sheath origin. However, seven of these nine patients were over the age of 16 and only two cases of schwannomas were seen in children <10 years of age; five cases of nerve sheath origin were seen in children under 10 years old in Ribet and Cardot's[5] series. The incidence of neurilemomas and neurofibromas are approximately equal, but the neurofibromas are more often seen in patients with von Recklinghausen's disease. Incidentally, neurofibromas are also often observed in patients with this disease.

The more common characteristics of benign neurilemomas and neurofibromas are listed in Table 170.14. These tumors are typically localized to neural and connective tissue but are present in the GI tract 25% of the time. Sixteen cases of submucosal esophageal nerve sheath tumors have been reported and this presentation is potentially treatable by minimally invasive thoracoscopic techniques as described by Nishikawa for an esophageal neurofibroma.[85] Malignant transformation of a neurofibroma is more common than the incidence observed with a neurilemoma. The occurrence of the former is seen more often in patients with von Recklinghausen disease than in those with the sporadic occurrence of a neurofibroma. The overall incidence nonetheless is relatively low (approximately 4% to 5%).

Although the most common malignancy of peripheral nerve origin, MPNSTs remain one of the most poorly defined of all soft tissue sarcomas. Its overall incidence remains obscure, but in the setting of the neurogenic tumors of the mediastinum, it probably accounts for less than 1% to 2% of all such tumors encountered. It most frequently

TABLE 170.14 Comparison of Neurilemoma and Neurofibroma

Characteristic	Neurilemoma	Neurofibroma
Peak age	20–50 years	20–40 years; younger age in von Recklinghausen disease
Common locations	Cutaneous nerves of head, neck, flexor surfaces of extremities; less often mediastinum and retroperitoneum	Cutaneous nerves; deep nerves and viscera affected also in von Recklinghausen disease
Histologic appearance	Encapsulated tumor composed of Antoni A and B areas rarely, plexiform growth pattern	Localized, diffuse, or plexiform tumor that is usually not encapsulated
Degenerative changes	Common	Occasional
S-100 protein immunostaining	Intense and relatively uniform staining in a given lesion	Variable staining of cells in a given lesion
CD-34 reactivity[a]	Antoni A zone–negative	
Antoni B zone positive	Commonly positive	
Occurrence in von Recklinghausen disease	Uncommon	Plexiform neurofibroma or multiple neurofibromas characteristic of disease
Malignant transformation	Extremely rare	Rare in solitary form; more common in von Recklinghausen disease

[a]Data from Weiss SW, Nickoloff BJ. CD-34 is expressed by distinctive cell population in peripheral nerves, nerve sheath tumors, and related lesions. *Am J Surg Pathol* 1993;17:1039.
Reprinted from Enzinger FM, Weiss SW. *Soft Tissue Tumors.* 2nd ed. St. Louis: Mosby, 1988. Copyright © 1988 Elsevier. With permission.

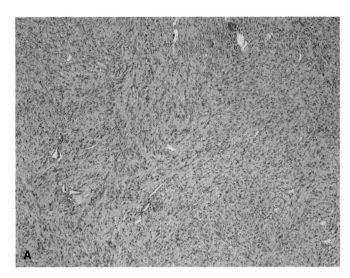 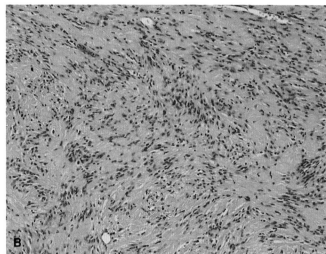

FIGURE 170.16 Neurilemoma. **A:** Biphasic tumor with alternating compact hypercellular Antoni A areas and hypocellular Antoni B areas. **B:** Spindle cells with wavy nuclei with tapered ends interspersed with collagen fibers. (Image courtesy of Maheshwari Ramineni, MD and Neda Kalhor, MD, Department of Pathology, MD Anderson Cancer Center.)

occurs in patients with von Recklinghausen disease, but Sorenson and colleagues[9] reported that only approximately 4% of patients with this disease develop MPNSTs. It is even less likely to develop *de novo* in unaffected persons. Enzinger and Weiss[71] as well as Keller and colleagues[86] have described rare instances of malignant transformation of ganglioneuromas into MPNSTs. When this transformation occurs in association with neurofibromatosis type 1 (NF1), Guccion and Enzinger[87] noted that it is usually after a long latent period of 10 to 20 years. A rapid increase in size of a benign lesion or the development of pain is indicative of malignant change from a benign neurofibroma. It also may occur in a nongenetic manner as a late complication of therapeutic or occupational irradiation after a latent period of 15 years, according to the studies of Ducatman and Scheithauer.[88,89] Thus, patients surviving long-term who were previously treated for a mediastinal lymphoma or malignant germ cell tumor may be at risk for the late development of an MPNST in the irradiated field.

NEURILEMOMA (SCHWANNOMA)

Neurilemomas are typically benign, solitary encapsulated lesions in which the cells are identical to the syncytium of the nerve sheath or the Schwann cell. Different subtypes of schwannomas have been described as plexiform schwannomas, cellular schwannomas, and melanotic schwannomas.

Pathology

Neurilemoma cells proliferate within the endoneurium, and the perineurium forms the capsule. The cells line up parallel to and do not intertwine with the nerve fibers as they do in neurofibromas. Grossly the tumor is well encapsulated, firm, and grayish tan. It appears to have a whorled pattern on cut sectioning. Areas of degeneration, such as cyst formation or calcification, may be present. Degenerative changes are associated with the rare ancient neurilemoma variant which is slow growing and well encapsulated but can histologically be mistaken for a sarcoma.[90]

In a series of 242 mediastinal tumors, Hirano and colleagues[91] reported that 7 (all schwannomas) of 44 neurogenic tumors were cystic in nature (15.9%). Petkar and colleagues[92] likewise have reported a cystic schwannoma. According to Weiss and Nickoloff,[93] uniformly

intense immunostaining occurs for the S-100 protein in the cells of a neurilemoma. One of two cellular patterns may be present in the tumor: Antoni type A areas show a dense avascular spindle cell pattern with nuclear palisading, and the Antoni type B areas, which are less orderly than Antoni A areas, show myxomatous changes that may be associated with cystic areas, vascular thickening, and frequent areas of hemorrhage. The electron microscopic features of the two areas are different: the cells in the Antoni type A areas have numerous thin cytoplasmic processes emanating from the cell body with only a small amount of cytoplasm, whereas the cells in the Antoni type B areas lack these processes and have abundant cytoplasm. There appears, however, to be no clinical differences in the behavior of neurilemomas composed of either Antoni type A or B areas or of a combination of both (Figs. 170.16 and 170.17).

The plexiform variant of schwannoma consists of multiple tumor nodules separated by strands of nonneoplastic connective tissue. Characteristic Antoni type A areas with palisading and Verocay bodies, formed by two rows of cells with palisaded nuclei, are

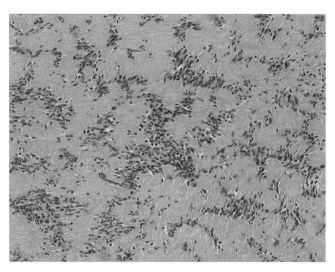

FIGURE 170.17 Neurilemoma: Nuclear palisading around fibrillary process (Verocay bodies). (Image courtesy of Maheshwari Ramineni, MD and Neda Kalhor, MD, Department of Pathology, MD Anderson Cancer Center.)

present and adjacent to hypocellular myxoid Antoni type B regions. A rare variant of plexiform schwannoma is the hybrid neurofibroma–schwannoma. This variant has typical neurofibroma (usually plexiform) cells with focal areas of well-developed schwannoma. It is important to identify this hybrid type since its usual benign behavior must be differentiated from malignant transformation of a neurofibroma.[82]

The cellular schwannoma variant may readily be thought, by its histologic appearance, to be malignant. According to Kornstein and DeBlois,[94] a fibrosarcoma-like herringbone growth pattern is present. The spindle cells are slender and wavy. No nuclear palisading occurs, and no Verocay bodies are present. There is some pleomorphism present, but the tumor has low mitotic activity. Despite its pseudosarcomatous appearance, the tumor is benign, although some regard it as atypical and of uncertain malignant potential.

The melanotic schwannoma variant grossly are bluish black. Histologically, they are composed of pigmented spindle cells arranged in interlacing bundles and fascicles. Some of the cells may not contain pigment granules. Enzinger and Weiss[71] have noted that both the Schwann cells and melanocytes arise from the neural crest and that melanocytic differentiation with the production of pigment may be seen in some Schwann cell tumors. A tendency toward palisading of the nuclei may be present. Psammomatous calcifications may be present. On electron microscopy, the tumors show cells with melanosomes in different stages of development. The tumor cells also show ultrastructural and immunohistochemical features suggestive of Schwann cells. These tumors react immunohistochemically to S-100 protein and also express the melanoma-associated marker HMB-45.

Clinical Features

The vast majority of neurilemomas are benign and malignant transformation is rare; reported at about 2% by Crowe and colleagues[95] and also by Enzinger and Weiss.[71] Most lesions are identified in young and middle-aged adults. Women are affected more often than men, although with NF1, the lesions are more common in men. Overall, neurilemoma is the more common than neurofibroma. This tumor is most often solitary but may occasionally be multiple. Although it is generally believed that the tumors associated with NF1 are all neurofibromas, some of the individual tumors may be pure neurilemomas. In fact, in an early review by Stout,[96] 18% of the neurilemomas were associated with this syndrome, and Enzinger and Weiss[71] agree with this observation. At times, an admixture of neurofibroma and neurilemoma may occur in the same tumor. Neurofibromatosis type 2 (NF2) is associated with neurilemomas rather than neurofibromas as in NF1.[97]

Plexiform schwannomas are benign and have been described in patients with neurofibromatosis (i.e., von Recklinghausen disease). Sheikh and colleagues[98] reported that the plexiform neurilemoma is often multiple and is identified more commonly in patients with NF1 (peripheral) than in NF2 (central). Cellular schwannoma, has been described by Woodruff,[99] Fletcher,[100] Lodding,[101] and their colleagues. It tends to occur in the paravertebral areas. Fletcher and colleagues[100] reported that these tumors may rarely recur but do not metastasize.

Benign melanotic schwannomas behave like neurilemomas. Local recurrence may be seen, but these tumors have not been reported to metastasize. A few grossly pigmented (bluish black) nerve sheath schwannomas have been reported to arise within the paravertebral sulcus region as well as in the spinal canal. Pigmented posterior mediastinal tumors fall into two categories. One is a malignant pigmented tumor of uncertain histogenesis, but it frequently is associated with a sympathetic ganglion; the other is a melanotic schwannoma. As a rule, the melanotic tumors of probable ganglion cell origin are highly malignant, in contrast to the benign behavior of the melanotic schwannomas of nerve sheath origin.

Bjornebae[102] first described a benign melanotic nerve sheath schwannoma occurring in a peripheral nerve, but the first reported example of this tumor occurring in the paravertebral sulcus was by Mandybur.[103] Several other cases have been recorded by Bagchi[104] and Paris[105] and their colleagues. All of these aforementioned tumors extended into the spinal canal. Kayano and Katayama[106] reported one arising from a sympathetic ganglion that did not extend into the spinal canal. Abbott and colleagues[107] reported a similar benign melanotic schwannoma arising from the sympathetic chain. In addition to these paravertebral lesions, a number of similar tumors have been reported and were confined to the epidural area of the spinal canal.[108]

Melanotic schwannoma has been associated with Carney's heritable disorder. Carney[109] has described a distinctive heritable disorder consisting of psammomatous melanotic schwannomas associated in 55% of patients with myxomas, spotty pigmentation, and endocrine overactivity (i.e., Cushing syndrome), Sertoli cell tumor, or acromegaly. The myxomas occur in the heart, skin, and breast. The melanotic schwannomas occur at multiple sites (i.e., spinal nerve roots, chest wall, stomach, or bone). Histologically, the schwannomas contain melanin, less frequently psammoma bodies, fat, and rarely metaplastic bone. Eighty-seven percent of the tumors studied by Carney[109] were benign and 13% proved to be malignant with subsequent metastases.

Neurilemomas can present as nerve sheath tumors of the vagal nerves or less frequently, the phrenic nerves. Only a few cases, such as that by Ewy and colleagues,[110] have been recorded in the English literature. Yamashita and colleagues[111] reported one patient with a neurilemoma of the right phrenic nerve and collected 13 other neurogenic tumors of the phrenic nerve that had been reported in the Japanese-language literature. All of these lesions were neurilemomas, but neurofibromas and neurogenic sarcomas can occur as well. In the aforementioned Japanese report, the phrenic nerve tumors occurred equally in the right or left nerve and equally in women and in men.

Radiographic Features

Characteristically, the radiographic appearance of a benign lesion is that of a solitary, smoothly rounded mass usually in the upper third or half of either paravertebral sulcus abutting the vertebral column (Fig. 170.18). However, the mass may be at any level. Lobulation is occasionally present, and adjacent bony changes (e.g., erosion, splaying of the ribs, or enlargement of an intervertebral foramen) may be recognized. MRI can demonstrate a target-like appearance with peripheral high signal intensity and central low signal intensity on T2 imaging.[112] Radiologically differentiating mediastinal ganglioneuromas from schwannomas can be facilitated by the craniocaudal to major axis ratio. Ganglioneuromas have a higher ratio and a cutoff of 1.2 was 93% sensitive and 73% specific in determining a ganglioneuroma from a schwannoma.[112] Calcifications and cystic changes may occasionally be seen in neurilemoma, as noted by Hirano and colleagues.[91]

The rare tumors of the vagus or phrenic nerves have no characteristic radiographic features. Such a tumor is identified initially as a mass in the superior portion of the visceral compartment, most often in the region of the aortic arch on the left (Fig. 170.19). Bourgouin and colleagues[113] suggested that CT examination of any para-aortic mass in a patient with neurofibromatosis may be most helpful in supporting the diagnosis of a plexiform neurofibroma. Low attenuation of the tumor on CT scan (14 to 20 Hounsfield units), ill-defined

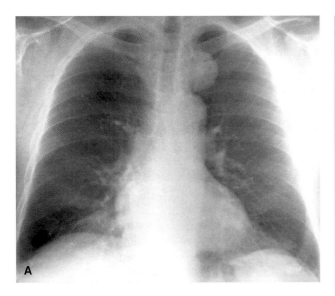

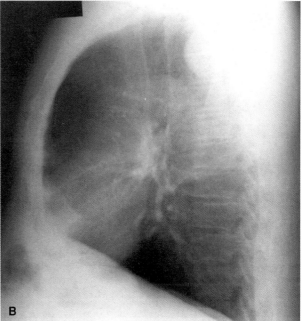

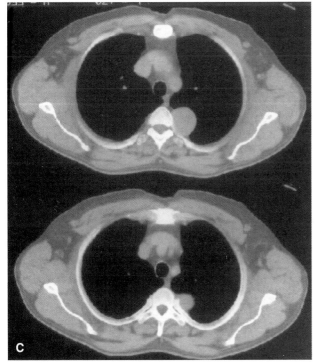

FIGURE 170.18 **A, B:** Posteroanterior and lateral chest radiographs reveal a typically located neurilemoma in the left paravertebral sulcus. **C:** CT scan reveals no intraspinal canal extension.

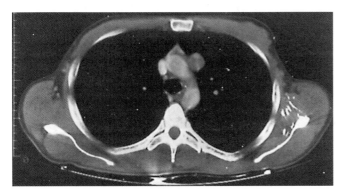

FIGURE 170.19 CT scan of a middle-aged man with von Recklinghausen disease with multiple previous paravertebral neurogenic tumors removed. A newly developed neurogenic tumor of the left vagus nerve is evident at the level of the aortic arch.

margins with the adjacent fat, and the mass surrounding the adjacent great vessels are characteristic features of the lesion. Also, multiple small tumor-like enlargements along the course of the involved nerve further support the diagnosis.

The role of CT scans is more important in the evaluation of lesions in the paravertebral area to rule out intraspinal canal extension (Fig. 170.20). Formerly, spine films were obtained to visualize the intervertebral foramen in the vicinity of the tumor for the purpose of evaluating the size of the adjacent intervertebral foramen, but now most clinicians forego this study, and a CT scan is suggested as the initial step in the patient's evaluation.

When a paravertebral tumor is found to have extended into the spinal canal, myelography or MRI may be performed to determine the longitudinal extent of the lesion within the canal (Fig. 170.21). Additional imaging strategies will be discussed later in this chapter in the excision of hourglass tumor section.

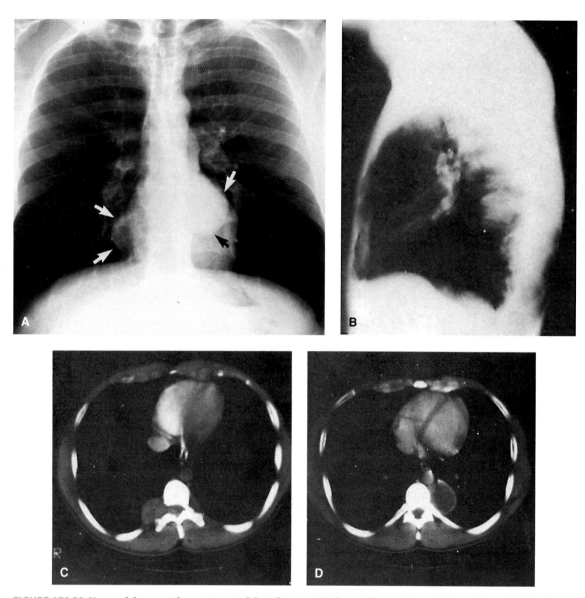

FIGURE 170.20 Young adult man with asymptomatic bilateral paravertebral neurofibromas in association with von Recklinghausen disease. **A:** Posteroanterior radiograph shows large left-sided and smaller right-sided tumors (*arrows*). **B:** Lateral radiograph reveals the larger left-sided lesion. **C:** CT scan reveals extension into the spinal canal by the smaller right-sided tumor. **D:** CT scan reveals absence of intraspinal extension by the larger tumor on the left. (Reprinted from Shields TW, Reynolds M. Neurogenic tumors of the thorax. *Surg Clin North Am* 1988;68:645. Copyright © 1988 Elsevier. With permission.)

In addition to the advantages of MRI in delineating the extension into the spinal canal of "dumbbell" paravertebral neurogenic tumors, Sakai and colleagues[114] have suggested that the use of T1- and T2-weighted images might reveal different features of common cell types; but this would seem to be of little clinical importance in treating these patients.

Staging

Neurilemomas are WHO grade 1 tumors, classified as benign and slow growing tumors and are associated with long-term survival. There is no additional specific staging system for these lesions.[115]

Prognostic Factors

Recurrence of a benign lesion is unusual, although additional neurofibromas or even neurilemomas may develop in patients with von

Recklinghausen disease. Rarely, a late malignant schwannoma may be observed in a patient with von Recklinghausen disease.

Treatment

The treatment of the neurilemoma is simple enucleation, which may be accomplished through a standard posterolateral thoracotomy or video-assisted thoracoscopic removal as reported by Landreneau,[116] Naunheim,[117] and Ishida,[118] and colleagues among many other reports in the 1990s. Most reported cases of melanotic schwannomas have extended into the spinal canal except those reported by Miettinen,[119] Kayano and Katayama,[106] and Abbott and colleagues.[107] These tumors almost always require a one-stage two-team approach to remove the intraspinal component by hemilaminectomy followed by resection of the remaining intrathoracic portion by thoracotomy or thoracoscopy.

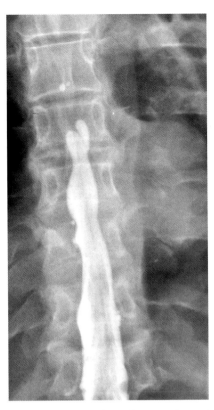

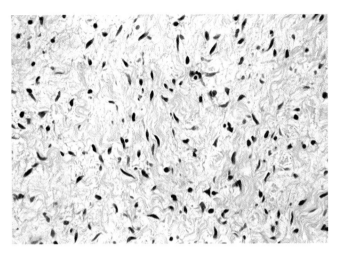

FIGURE 170.22 Photomicrograph of a typical neurofibroma. Interlacing bundles of cells with dark wavy nuclei are separated by wavy strands of collagen (original magnification × 250).

FIGURE 170.21 Myelogram revealing only minimal extradural compression caused by the right-sided neurofibroma shown in Figure 170.20, which has grown into the spinal canal. Erosion of an adjacent vertebral pedicle is well visualized. No erosion of pedicles adjacent to the left-sided tumor is demonstrated.

NEUROFIBROMA

Neurofibromas are the most common tumors associated with NF1 (von Recklinghausen disease). They typically develop in adolescence and continue to occur through adulthood, occurring anywhere in the peripheral nervous system, most commonly cutaneously. In addition to cutaneous lesions, 60% of patients with NF1 will present with internal neurofibromas originating from the spinal roots and developing as dumbbell tumors.[97] On occasion, in a patient with NF1, an admixture of both a neurilemomatous and neurofibromatous element may be identified in the same tumor. The plexiform neurofibroma is a variety of the neurofibromas. It is defined as a diffuse fusiform enlargement, multiple masses, or both, along the course of a peripheral nerve trunk. It is associated with the clinical manifestations of NF1 or a family history of the disease. This lesion occurs most commonly outside the thorax but can occur along either sympathetic nerve trunks in the paravertebral sulci or along either the vagus or phrenic nerves in the visceral compartment. Multiple fascicles of the nerve can be involved and the tumor will extend down the branches of nerves in contrast to the fusiform growth of standard neurofibromas. This type is more common in younger children and primarily grow in the first decade of life.[97]

Pathology

In contrast to the neurilemoma, the Schwann cells present in a neurofibroma proliferate in a disorderly fashion, and the cells become entwined with the nerve fibers in a disorganized manner. The tumors are pseudoencapsulated. Grossly, once the pseudocap-

sule is cut, the tissue surface is white to grayish yellow and lacks the degenerative changes seen with a neurilemoma. Histologically, a tangled network of elongated Schwann cells is seen, with dark-staining nuclei intermingled with neurites (Fig. 170.22). Plexiform neurofibromas show a convoluted cluster of nerve fibers similar to those of a solitary neurofibroma. On electron microscopy, the cells appear elongated, with thick cytoplasmic processes interspersed with myelinated and unmyelinated axons in a collagenous stroma. Variable and less intense S-100 protein immunostaining occurs in the cells of the neurofibroma, in contrast to the more intense staining in the cells of the neurilemomas. Weiss and Nickoloff[93] reported that CD34 (hematopoietic progenitor cell reactivity) is expressed by a distinctive cell population in nerve sheath tumors, but the positive cells are distinct from Schwann cells, fibroblasts, and perineural cells. The CD34 reactivity was identified in 14 of 17 neurofibromas, 10 of 10 Antoni B zones in neurilemomas, but negative in all Antoni A zones and negative in the one melanotic schwannoma evaluated.

Clinical Features

Multiple neurofibromatous lesions are more common in patients with NF1, occurring in as many as 10% of such patients. Vagal or phrenic nerve involvement is more common in neurofibromas compared to neurilemomas. Oosterwijk and Swierenga[120] reported that a benign nerve sheath tumor may rarely be located in the visceral compartment when the tumor arises from a phrenic or vagus nerve. They reported involvement of one of these nerves in 3 of their 111 patients, an incidence of 2.7%. Although the exact number cannot be discerned from the data of Reed and colleagues,[4] it was inferred that 8% of the neural tumors in the thorax arose from either the vagus or phrenic nerves. These were all nerve sheath tumors; the more common was a neurofibroma, occurring in 8 of 13 tumors. Dabir and colleagues[121] reviewed the literature several years later and reported a total of 27 patients plus 2 of their own with nerve sheath tumors of the vagus nerves; they did not include the reports of Osada[122] or Mizuno[123] and their colleagues from Japan. Thus, the overall number of cases is greater than the number they reported at that time. Subsequently, Shirakusa and colleagues[124] reviewed 17 of the 19 cases that had been reported in the Japanese literature, and numerous case reports—such as those of

Davis,[125] Katoh,[126] Sheikh,[98] and their colleagues as well as others—have been published. From all these data it may be concluded that the left vagus nerve is involved more commonly than the right vagus nerve. The former is involved most often in its proximal portion in the thorax above or at the region of the aortic arch. Hoarseness occurs in approximately 20% of the cases and rarely, when the tumor is large or malignant, the trachea may be involved, as noted by Katoh and colleagues.[126] The tumor is slightly more often a neurofibroma than a neurilemoma, and either, especially in patients with neurofibromatosis, may be of the plexiform variety.

Radiographic Features

Neurofibromas have a similar radiographic appearance as neurilemomas as described in that section. As noted in neurilemomas, calcifications and cystic changes may occasionally also be found in neurofibromas, as reported by Shin and colleagues.[127]

Staging

Neurofibromas, like neurilemomas are WHO grade 1 tumors, classified as benign and slow growing tumors and are associated with long-term survival. There is no additional specific staging system for these lesions.

Prognostic Factors

Recurrence of this benign lesion is unusual, although additional neurofibromas or even neurilemomas may develop in patients with von Recklinghausen disease. Rarely, a late malignant schwannoma may be observed in a patient with von Recklinghausen disease.

Treatment

Neurofibromas require a more extensive excision than neurolemomas with resection of an adjacent nerve structure. The procedure may be accomplished through a standard posterolateral thoracotomy or video-assisted thoracoscopic removal also as reported by Landreneau,[116] Naunheim,[117] and Ishida,[118] among many other reports in the 1990s. Lesions of the vagus or phrenic nerves are excised while attempting to preserve the function of the affected nerve. An asymptomatic plexiform neurofibroma (the diagnosis supported by the characteristic CT finding) of either of these nerves may not need to be resected.

MALIGNANT PERIPHERAL NERVE SHEATH TUMOR

Pathology

Most MPNSTs are large; the cut surfaces are white or flesh-colored with areas of macroscopic hemorrhage, necrosis, or both. These tumors may or may not arise from a typical-appearing neurofibroma. Microscopically, they resemble fibrosarcomas; however, the cells tend to mirror the features of normal Schwann cells but with irregular contours (Figs. 170.23 and 170.24). In profile, the nuclei are wavy; when viewed head on, they are asymmetrically oval. The cellular arrangement is varied, and palisading is infrequent. According to Enzinger and Weiss,[71] palisading occurs in less than 10% of cases and most often is focal. The other histologic microscopic and electromicroscopic features are well described by these authors.[71] Some 50% to 90% of the tumors are reactive to S-100 protein; this reactivity may help in their differentiation from other soft tissue sarcomas. Wick and colleagues[128] have identified myelin basic protein in approximately half of malignant schwannomas. Neuron-specific enolase and neurofilament proteins have been identified in these tumors by Matsunou and colleagues.[129]

Ducatman and Scheithauer[130] have described the occasional occurrence of divergent differentiation in malignant neurogenic tumors. Foci of rhabdomyosarcoma, osteosarcoma, chondrosarcoma, and angiosarcoma have been identified. A neurogenic sarcoma containing areas of rhabdomyosarcoma has been called a *triton tumor*. Infrequently, these divergent lesions have occurred in the mediastinum in patients with neurofibromatosis.

Clinical Features

MPNSTs represent 5% to 10% of all soft tissue sarcomas and have an incidence of 0.1/100,000 per year.[83] These rare MPNSTs tend to occur in either younger or older individuals than those with benign lesions and tend to occur in patients with NF1. The neurofibrosarcomas, particularly those associated with NF1, are seen at an average age of 34 years according to Hajdu.[131] Likewise, Furniss and colleagues[132] note that MPNSTs occur at an average age

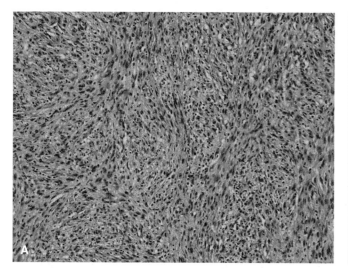

FIGURE 170.23 Malignant peripheral nerve sheath tumor (MPNST). **A:** MPNST with well-circumscribed border involving the lung parenchyma. **B:** MPNST with alternating hypercellular and hypocellular appearance giving a marbled appearance on low magnification. (Image courtesy of Maheshwari Ramineni, MD and Neda Kalhor, MD, Department of Pathology, MD Anderson Cancer Center.)

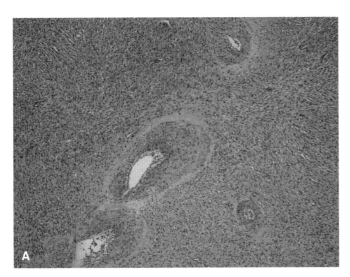
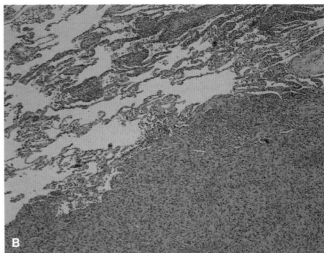

FIGURE 170.24 Malignant peripheral nerve sheath tumor (MPNST). **A:** Tumor cells displaying perivascular growth pattern characteristic of MPNST. **B:** Herringbone pattern with marked nuclear pleomorphism. (Image courtesy of Maheshwari Ramineni, MD and Neda Kalhor, MD, Department of Pathology, MD Anderson Cancer Center.)

of 26 years in the setting of NF1 versus 62 years in sporadic cases. The lifetime risk in NF1 of developing MPNSTs is estimated to be 8% to 13%, with most resulting in death within 5 years of diagnosis despite therapy.[97] A predilection for young women exists, and these tumors are more commonly aggressive and seen in the trunk than in the thorax. In contrast, the malignant tumors arising from schwannomas are seen at a later age and are much less aggressive in their clinical behavior. Erosion of adjacent bony structures associated with pain is not an unusual finding (Fig. 170.25). Growth into the spinal canal may occur. Lymph node metastases are rare, but metastases to distant sites may be observed in a high percentage of cases. Like benign nerve sheath tumors, Maebeya and colleagues[133] and Singer[134] have reported the occurrence of an MPNST of the intrathoracic vagus nerve.

Radiographic Features

Malignant lesions tend to be more diffuse and irregular; erosion of adjacent bony structures is common. Furniss and colleagues reviewed clinical features that may be useful in differentiating MPNSTs from benign lesions and identified site (extremities more likely malignant), large size (mean size 6.5 cm for MPNST vs. 2.9 for schwannoma), depth related to deep fascia, short duration of symptoms and pain.[132] Another analysis by Wasa and colleagues identified size, a peripheral enhancement pattern, perilesional edema, and intratumoral cystic lesions on MRI to be predictive of malignancy. Two of these findings on MRI was 90% specific and 61% sensitive for identifying an MPNST versus a benign neurofibroma.[135] They suggested biopsy with two or more features and selective biopsy for those with one feature based on clinical features such as pain or motor deficits.

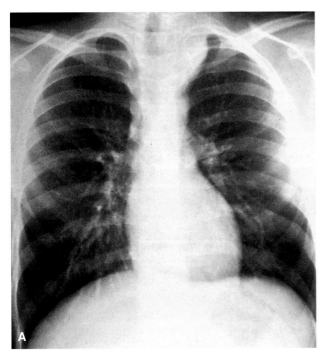
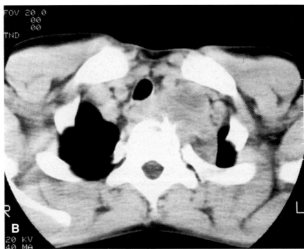

FIGURE 170.25 **A:** Posteroanterior chest radiograph of a patient with a malignant schwannoma and severe back pain. **B:** CT scan reveals extensive involvement of adjacent vertebral body. (Reprinted from Shields TW, Reynolds M. Neurogenic tumors of the thorax. *Surg Clin North Am* 1988;68:645. Copyright © 1988 Elsevier. With permission.)

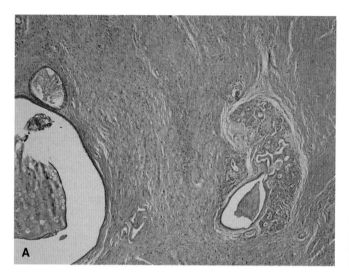 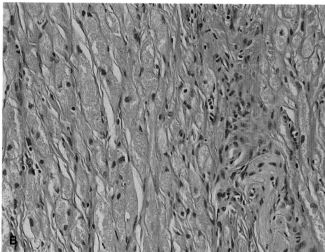

FIGURE 170.26 Granular cell tumor. **A:** Ill-defined lesion in the bronchial wall infiltrating the submucosa in between the bronchial submucosal glands (low magnification). **B:** Polygonal cells with abundant granular eosinophilic cytoplasm and small irregular nuclei with inconspicuous nucleoli. (Image courtesy of Maheshwari Ramineni, MD and Neda Kalhor, MD, Department of Pathology, MD Anderson Cancer Center.)

Staging

These tumors are staged based on staging for soft tissue sarcomas, where grade of tumor is an important determinant in prognosis.

Prognostic Factors

It is the general impression that patients with MNPSTs in the paravertebral regions do poorly. Total excision is usually impossible; even when this is accomplished, local recurrence is common. Guccion and Enzinger[87] observed that patients with MPNST of any site complicating NF1 experienced a local recurrence rate of 78% and a 63% incidence of distant metastases. The common metastatic sites recorded were lung, liver, subcutaneous tissue, and bone. Most of these manifestations occur within 2 years of treatment. Patients with sporadic malignant schwannomas in the absence of NF1 appear to do better than those who have NF1. Both Guccion and Enzinger[87] and Sorensen and colleagues[9] reported an approximate long-term survival of 50% of cases. Even higher survival rates (75%) have been reported in the more recent literature, as noted by Marchevsky and Kaneko.[72] Whether these data can be translated to those patients with intrathoracic malignant schwannoma is unknown and the value of NF-1 has been recently questioned by Wang, and Anghileri,[83,136] and colleagues who felt that the influence of NF-1 was more related to the fact that those patients tended to present with larger tumors and NF-1 were not statistically significant as a prognostic indicator. Wang identified S-100 protein negative status, osteolytic destruction, and high malignant grade as indicators of poor prognosis. Other studies have suggested that Ki67 upregulation may also play a role in worse prognosis; however, this was not seen in the series by Wang.

Treatment

In patients with MPNST, the goal is complete surgical resection, however, resection is often intended to prevent or to relieve compression of the spinal cord since complete removal is generally difficult. Stabilization of the vertebral column may be necessary after extensive resection. In a series retrospectively looking at 43 patients with spinal MPNSTs from 2001 to 2012,[83] 5-year recurrence rates for spinal MPNSTs were reported to be 53% after complete surgical resection

with 5-year survival being 44%. Postoperative radiation therapy may be given to attempt to control residual local disease. The role of chemotherapy is undetermined. However, doxorubicin or dimethyltriazenoimidazole carboxamide may be tried in patients with disseminated disease. Both chemotherapy and radiation treatment effects remain controversial.

GRANULAR CELL TUMORS

Additional, rare nerve sheath tumors worth briefly mentioning are granular cell tumors. Granular cell tumors are uncommon, generally benign lesions that occur in multiple sites throughout the body and are believed to be of Schwann cell origin. Fust and Custer[137] suggested that granular cell tumors could be of neural origin (Fig. 170.26). This concept was supported but not conclusively proved by electron microscopic studies of Fisher and Wechsler,[138] Mackay[139] and Khansur,[140] and colleagues. Evidence of a Schwann cell origin has been shown by the detection of neuroectodermal protein (S-100) by Armin[141] and Aisner[142] and their colleagues. They are most common in the skin and subcutaneous tissue and the tongue but, have been reported in the bronchus[143] and esophagus.[144] Rosenbloom and colleagues[145] were the first to describe a granular cell tumor associated with the thoracic sympathetic chain in the left costovertebral sulcus in a 11-year-old boy. Aisner and colleagues[142] reported a case in an adult of bilateral granular cell tumors in the superior portion of the paravertebral sulci. Almost all granular cell tumors are benign, but according to Colberg,[146] 3.5% may prove to be malignant. Enzinger and Weiss[71] reported the incidence of malignancy to be even lower, at only 1% to 2% of all granular cell tumors. The treatment of the rare granular cell tumor in the paravertebral area is surgical excision, as is carried out for the other benign tumors of nerve sheath origin.

TUMORS OF NEUROECTODERMAL ORIGIN

Two rare tumors of presumed neuroectodermal origin may occur in the mediastinum. One is the MNTI and the second is the malignant small cell tumor of the thoracopulmonary region (Askin tumor) seen in older children or adolescents.

MELANOTIC NEUROECTODERMAL TUMOR OF INFANCY

Also referred to as, melanotic progonoma, congenital melano-carcinoma, retinal anlage tumor, or pigmented congenital epulis, MNTI is a benign but locally aggressive and frequently recurrent rare tumor of children under 1 year of age. MNTI occurs 92.8% of the time in the head and neck, but in the mediastinum where it can be confused with a pigmented neuroblastoma. Treatment of this unusual tumor is local excision. The efficacy of other treatment modalities is unknown.[147]

ASKIN TUMOR

Askin and colleagues[148] described a malignant small cell tumor of the thoracopulmonary region in childhood (Fig. 170.27) that may present as a paravertebral mass, although it is more common in the posterior chest wall or even the lung. This tumor is referred to as a peripheral primitive neuroectodermal tumor (PNET) and is of neural crest origin. It is classified as a subset of Ewing sarcoma and shares immunohistochemical, ultrastructural, and molecular similarities (Figs. 170.28 and 170.29).[149,150] Askin tumor is seen in older children and young adolescents and is discovered either as a chest wall mass or as a radiographic chest mass in a child with chest pain, cough, dyspnea, or other thoracopulmonary symptoms. Rib destruction is common.

This tumor is three times more common in girls than in boys. Ohta[151] and Sano[152] and their colleagues reviewed the case reports of Askin tumor in Japan, and each group added a case of its own. A total of 19 cases were collected. There were 12 adolescent young women and 7 men. Of these patients, 13 were ≤15 years of age and 6 were >16 years of age. The youngest patient was 3 years of age and the oldest was 26. Takanami and Imamura[153] reported the occurrence of this tumor in a 16-year-old boy and a 32-year-old woman, who are among the older individuals to develop Askin tumor.

There is no standard therapy for this tumor due to its rarity; however, multimodal therapy with pre- and postoperative chemotherapy with a radical *en bloc* surgical resection and radiation is the most

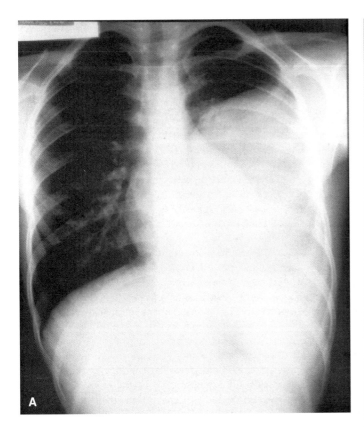

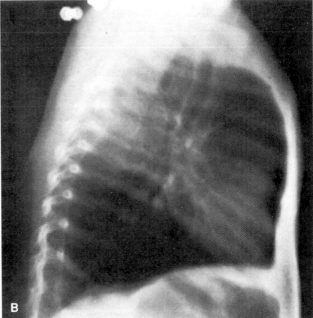

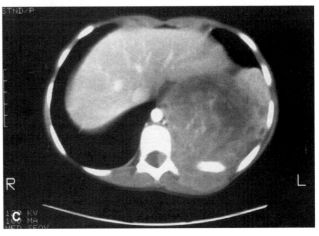

FIGURE 170.27 **A, B:** Posteroanterior and lateral radiographs of the chest of a child with an Askin tumor. **C:** CT scan shows invasion of the chest wall, destruction of the rib cage posteriorly, and extension of the tumor into the spinal canal. (Reprinted from Shields TW, Reynolds M. Neurogenic tumors of the thorax. *Surg Clin North Am* 1988;68:645. Copyright © 1988 Elsevier. With permission.)

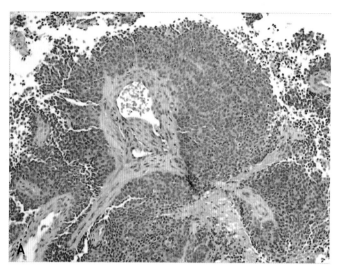
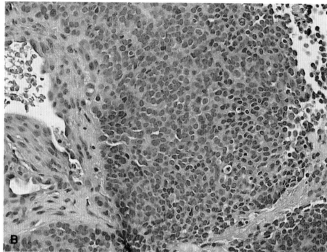

FIGURE 170.28 Askin tumor (peripheral primitive neuroectodermal tumor [PNET]). **A:** PNET with proliferation of sheets of monotonous appearing small blue round cells. **B:** Cells have scant cytoplasm and nuclei with homogenous chromatin. Occasional apoptotic bodies are seen. (Image courtesy of Maheshwari Ramineni, MD and Neda Kalhor, MD, Department of Pathology, MD Anderson Cancer Center.)

common approach. Preoperative chemotherapy has been shown to reduce the size of the tumor and decrease its vascularity, which improves the likelihood of complete resection. The lesion tends to recur locally, although distant metastases to lung or bones may be observed. Long-term survival is infrequent and often less than 1 year. Askin and colleagues[148] noted a median survival of only 8 months. Despite intensive therapy, prognosis is poor with a high recurrence rate. A 2-year survival rate of 38% and 6-year rate of 14% has been reported.[154,155]

TUMORS OF THE PARAGANGLIONIC SYSTEM

The occurrence of biologically or nonbiologically active paraganglionic tumors in the mediastinum is discussed in Chapter 170.

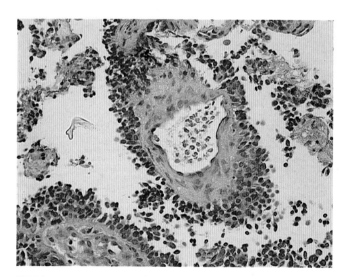

FIGURE 170.29 Askin tumor (peripheral primitive neuroectodermal tumor [PNET]). Tumor cells growing around blood vessels forming "perivascular pseudorosettes." (Image courtesy of Maheshwari Ramineni, MD and Neda Kalhor, MD, Department of Pathology, MD Anderson Cancer Center.)

EXCISION OF HOURGLASS TUMORS OF THE PARAVERTEBRAL SULCUS

Hourglass tumors (dumbbell tumors) of the thoracic paravertebral sulcus present with a constellation of anatomic, pathologic, and surgical considerations that make their treatment unique. The appellation *hourglass tumor* refers to a lesion with an intraspinal component and an intrathoracic component connected by a narrow waist of tumor, the growth of which has been restricted by the confines of the bony intervertebral foramen. As mentioned previously, neuroblastomas, neurilemomas, and neurofibromas frequently have intraspinal extension, while all tumors originating from the paravertebral sulcus have the potential to form hourglass tumors. Approximately 3.5% of ganglioneuromas will present as hourglass tumors.[156] In the series of 706 neurogenic tumors of the thoracic paravertebral region reported by Akwari and colleagues,[158] nearly 10% were found to have extension into the spinal canal. In patients where the source of the tumor was reported, 68% were nerve sheath in origin, 30% originated from the sympathetic chain, and 2% arose from paraganglion cells. Overall, 10% of the neurogenic hourglass tumors were malignant. In addition to neurogenic lesions, a number of other mesenchymal tumors—such as hemangiomas, other blood vessel tumors, and lipomas—also may grow into the spinal canal when they originate in the paravertebral sulcus.

Failure to recognize the tumor's extension into the spinal canal can be disastrous. Manipulation of the tumor from within the thorax or leaving behind the intraspinal canal growth may lead to hemorrhage within the spinal canal, with subsequent spinal cord compression or even direct injury to the cord. Either may result in a Brown-Séquard syndrome or even in complete physiologic transection of the cord.

When extension into the spinal canal has been demonstrated preoperatively, a one-stage, two-team approach is indicated to first remove the intraspinal canal extension by hemilaminectomy and then to remove the intrathoracic portion by thoracotomy or thoracoscopy. As mentioned previously, it may be prudent to attempt chemotherapy to reduce the intraspinal component before surgery.[49] The various approaches and results of the one-stage procedure have been described by Le Brigand,[158] and Akwari,[157] Irger,[159,160] Grillo,[161,162] and their colleagues.

Riquet and colleagues[163] reported the resection of 18 of 26 mediastinal tumors by the videothoracoscopic technique. They believe the contraindications to its use are a large tumor (>6 cm in diameter), spinal artery involvement, intraspinal extension of the tumor, and a middle mediastinal location. Many do not agree, especially with the last two contraindications. Higashiama and colleagues[164] as well as Tsunezuka and Sato,[165] recommended that after mobilization of the intraspinal extension of a dumbbell neurogenic tumor, the intrathoracic and previously mobilized intraspinal extension be removed by the video-assisted thoracoscopic technique. Also, both benign and malignant neurogenic tumors of the vagus nerve have been removed by this technique by Nakamura and colleagues[166] and Singer,[134] respectively. In the latter case, tumor implant occurred in the incision for failure to place the resected specimen in a protective bag before extraction through the chest wall. A subsequent local excision of the implant appears to have been successful.

Occasionally, a peripheral neurologic defect may be noted postoperatively. This is most common with lesions high in the apex of the paravertebral sulcus, where Horner syndrome caused by injury of the stellate ganglion may be observed. Excision of neurogenic tumors of the upper portion or at the level of the left recurrent nerve take-off of the left vagus nerve frequently results in paresis of the recurrent nerve and subsequent paralysis of the left vocal cord with the occurrence of hoarseness. Shirakusa and colleagues[124] noted that three of nine patients with lesions of the left vagus nerve in this location were hoarse preoperatively and the six others became so postoperatively. Davis and colleagues[125] also reported this complication, but excellent palliation was obtained with Teflon injection into the affected vocal cord to return it to a midline position. However, this complication has been avoided in the patients recorded by Dabir[121] and Nakamura[166] and their colleagues as well as by Singer[134] and others. Otherwise, operative morbidity and mortality should approach zero.

ANATOMIC CONSIDERATIONS

The anatomic features that influence the surgical approach to hourglass lesions of the thoracic spine include the proximity of the pleural cavity, the presence of ribs, and the osseous and neural anatomy.

The thoracic spinal column contains 12 segments. The spinal canal is delimited ventrally by the vertebral bodies and the interposed discs and dorsally by the spinous processes, paired laminae, facet joints, and pedicles. Twelve paired ribs articulate with the vertebral bodies at the diarthrodial joints. The intervertebral foramen (Fig. 170.30) is formed cephalad and caudad by the pedicles, dorsally by the superior and inferior articular facets, and ventrally by the contiguous vertebral bodies and interposed disc.

The spinal cord and the proximal portion of the emerging nerve roots are contained within the spinal canal (Fig. 170.31). Surrounding the neural tissues are three layers of the meninges: the dura mater, arachnoid, and pia mater. The arachnoid envelope contains cerebrospinal fluid. The subarachnoid space extends a variable distance along the nerve root; thus, if the nerve root must be sacrificed during tumor resection, unrecognized arachnoid injury may result in a spinal-pleural cerebrospinal fluid fistula.

Radicular arteries enter the intervertebral foramina to perfuse the intraspinal structures. Spinal medullary branches arise from the radicular arteries to supply the spinal cord. Radicular branches are random and do not enter every intervertebral foramen in the thoracic region. Attempts should be made to preserve the radicular blood supply, although sacrifice of a radicular artery might be necessary

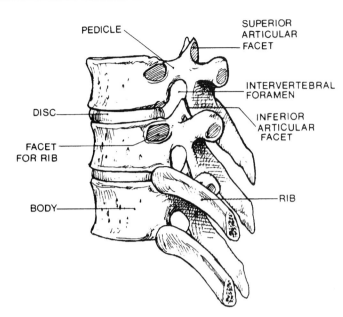

FIGURE 170.30 Lateral view of a segment of the thoracic spine demonstrating intervertebral foramen.

to fully resect an hourglass tumor, thereby threatening circulation to the spinal cord. Despite this concern, neural impairment secondary to spinal cord infarction caused by vascular sacrifice rarely occurs, perhaps because most hourglass tumors are slow growing and the resultant gradual occlusion of important nutrient vascular channels allows for the development of collateral circulation.

The complexity of osseous, vascular, and neural anatomy encountered in the thoracic region complicates the operative approach to hourglass tumors. Unlike the lumbar region, where the spinal cord is absent, the presence of the spinal cord in the thoracic region renders a posterior approach to the spinal canal unsafe. Unlike the cervical region, where the presence of the spinal cord also requires careful planning of the operative approach, the presence of ribs and the pleura in the thoracic region complicates the surgical exposure.

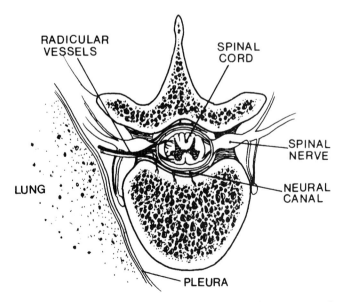

FIGURE 170.31 Diagram of cross-sectional view of the thoracic spine and surrounding structures.

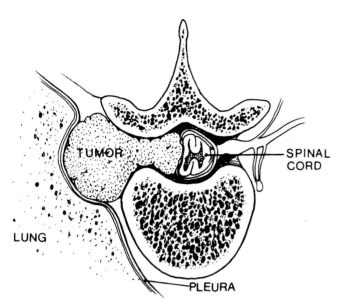

FIGURE 170.32 Diagram of an hourglass tumor with the intraspinal component compressing the spinal cord and emerging nerve and an intrathoracic component elevating the pleura and compressing the lung.

CLINICAL PRESENTATION

An hourglass tumor may be asymptomatic and found on routine chest radiography or may present with either pulmonary or neurologic symptoms. Akwari and colleagues[158] noted that approximately one-third of the hourglass tumors were asymptomatic. Tumors with a large intrathoracic component may produce shortness of breath or cough. Neurologic deficits may be caused by spinal cord compression or involvement of nerve roots (Fig. 170.32). Patients with myelopathy may present with gait difficulty, urinary and fecal incontinence, and loss of sensory and autonomic function below the level of the lesion. Those with radicular symptoms may present with radicular pain at the level of the tumor; on examination, altered sensation may be found in a dermatomal distribution. Rarely, patients with an upper thoracic tumor may present with Horner syndrome due to the compression of the sympathetic chain. The clinical manifestations of this syndrome include pupillary miosis, eyelid ptosis, and anhidrosis of the face and neck ipsilateral to the lesion.

DIAGNOSTIC INVESTIGATION

All patients being investigated for a paravertebral mass must also be evaluated for intraspinal extension. Assessment begins with a history and physical examination followed by diagnostic studies that may include plain radiographs of the thoracic spine, coned-down CT scan, MRI, and CT myelography. Imaging used to evaluate patients with hourglass lesions has evolved considerably since the late 1980s with the introduction of high-resolution CT scanning and MRI. Prior to the development of newer imaging modalities, diagnosis depended on using plain radiography to identify an enlarged or eroded neural foramen in a patient with a paravertebral tumor. CT myelography is still occasionally used to define the intraspinal component of the tumor, but MRI (Fig. 170.33) has become the single best examination to disclose the characteristic shape and extent of the tumor. Spinal angiography is used occasionally to add information about blood supply to the tumor and spinal cord, particularly with lower thoracic tumors, when perfusion is by the artery of Adamkiewicz (Figs. 170.34 and 170.35)

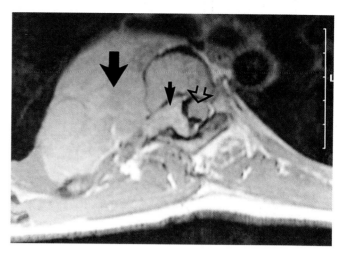

FIGURE 170.33 MRI demonstrates narrow waist of tumor connecting large intrathoracic neurofibroma (*large arrow*) with smaller intraspinal component (*small arrow*). Note enlargement of the neural foramen and the displaced spinal cord (*open arrow*).

becomes more likely. Digital subtraction studies may also be helpful. The knowledge thus obtained permits the surgeon to protect this vessel from injury during removal of the tumor. However, the risk for possibly neurotoxic effects of the contrast media on the spinal cord during spinal angiography outweighs any potential benefit in most instances.

OPERATIVE CONSIDERATIONS

Surgery for hourglass tumors of the thoracic spine requires entrance into two distinct anatomic regions: the thorax and spinal canal. Staged procedures for removal of hourglass tumors are not recommended. If only the intraspinal or intrathoracic component is removed at the

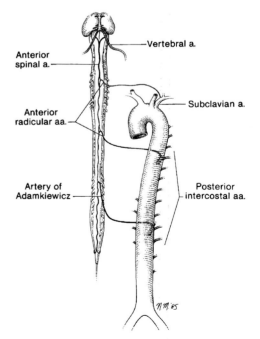

FIGURE 170.34 Schematic illustration of the artery of Adamkiewicz supplying the inferior portion of the anterior spinal artery. (Reprinted from Shields TW, Reynolds M. Neurogenic tumors of the thorax. *Surg Clin North Am* 1988;68:645. Copyright © 1988 Elsevier. With permission.)

Left : 75%   Right : 25%

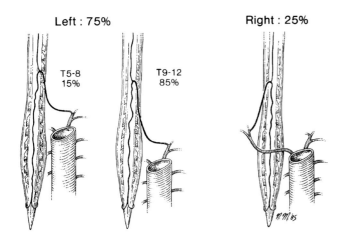

T5-8
15%

T9-12
85%

FIGURE 170.35 Variation in the origin of the artery of Adamkiewicz from the intercostal vessels of the thoracic aorta. (Reprinted from Shields TW, Reynolds M. Neurogenic tumors of the thorax. *Surg Clin North Am* 1988;68:645. Copyright © 1988 Elsevier. With permission.)

initial setting, serious complications—such as hemorrhage, spinal cord injury, or cerebrospinal fluid leak—may occur. It is therefore important that the presence of intraspinal extension be determined prior to planning the surgical procedure so that total tumor resection can be achieved and risk to the patient minimized.

Harrington and Craig[42] reported the first case of an hourglass neurogenic tumor removed by a one-stage procedure. Since that time numerous surgeons—including Irger,[159,160] Akwari,[158] and Grillo[162] as well as Le Brigand,[157] Shields and Reynolds,[167] and Grillo and Ojemann[161]—have described and advocated a single-stage operative approach.

Most hourglass tumors can be resected using either a lateral extracavitary approach or a combined anteroposterior approach: performing a laminectomy for resection of the intraspinal component and either a thoracotomy or thoracoscopic resection of the intrathoracic component. However, surgical planning for resection of hourglass tumors must take multiple factors into account. For example, the precise anatomic site of the tumor often defines the necessary operative procedure. Lesions that are completely intrathoracic with minimal extension into the spinal canal may be removed by thoracotomy or thoracoscopy alone. However, great care must be taken with resection of the foraminal extension of the tumor. Those tumors mostly located within the spinal canal, with little extraforaminal extension, may be resected by performing a laminectomy and foraminotomy, thus obviating the need for a thoracotomy.

Biomechanical factors must also be considered. Significant vertebral body erosion, often seen with malignant lesions and some benign entities, may necessitate reconstruction with vertebral body replacement (anterior column support) and posteriorly placed pedicle screws or hooks. Spinal instrumentation allows for immediate spinal stabilization. Anterior plating systems, useful in the lower thoracic spine, provide stability by resisting extension and rotational moments. Posterior instrumentation techniques use hooks and pedicle screws that resist flexion and rotation. Instrumentation is not a substitute for proper bone grafting, because long-term stability often depends on bone healing. In the absence of bone healing, instrumentation failure will occur.

The level of involvement of the thoracic spine is also an important consideration. Middle to lower thoracic lesions with a large intrathoracic component are easily approached by performing a thoracotomy with a separate posterior midline incision for the intraspinal portion

of the tumor. However, those lesions located above T3 may be better exposed by dissecting lateral to the spine and medial to the scapula (lateral parascapular approach). This approach is similar to a lateral extracavitary approach used in the lower thoracic spine. For lesions at the thoracic inlet, an anterior cervical incision can be extended caudally to the sternal notch.

LATERAL EXTRACAVITARY APPROACH (LATERAL PARASCAPULAR APPROACH)

The patient is positioned on the operating table in the lateral position and rolled slightly forward (Fig. 170.36). The patient is supported by a beanbag (Olympic Vac-Pac, Olympic Medical, Seattle, WA) and is held by wide strips of adhesive tape over the hip to secure him or her to the operating table. The lower arm can either be placed on an arm board at a right angle to the table or be flexed at the elbow and placed beside the patient's head. The upper arm may be rotated forward, abducted, flexed at the elbow, and placed on an arm support; however, in our experience it is more convenient to rotate the arm forward and let it hang over the side of the table, protected by adequate padding. The patient is prepared and draped widely to allow for both exposure of the spine and for a full thoracotomy if necessary.

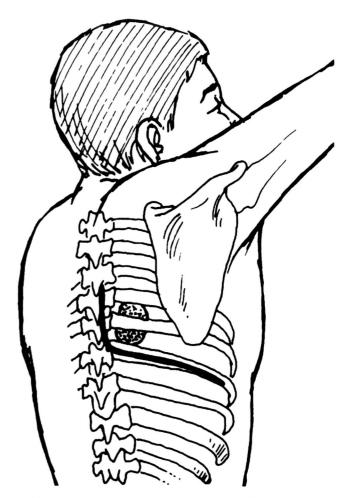

FIGURE 170.36 Patient positioned on operating table showing recommended incision for tumor at level shown in diagram, using lateral extracavitary approach.

As described previously, the location of the incision depends on the site of the lesion. The vertical component of the incision starts in the midline over the spinous processes, approximately 5 cm above the level of the foramen to be explored; it extends caudad to approximately 5 cm below the level of the foramen to be explored, at which point the incision curves sharply laterally and follows the course of the rib. For lesions above the tip of the scapula, the incision curves anteriorly just below the scapula's tip; the anterior aspect of the incision follows the rib just below the foramen to be explored in a fashion similar to a standard posterolateral thoracotomy incision. The vertical portion of the incision is made down to the spinous process; the paraspinal muscle mass is elevated from the spinous processes and laminae and retracted laterally.

A bilateral laminectomy is performed, including the levels above and below the site of the involved foramen. If the tumor is completely in the extradural space, it may be reduced from the spinal canal into the thorax and completely removed. If the tumor is partially intradural, the dura is opened laterally over the tumor and the intraspinal component of the lesion is separated from the spinal cord using microsurgical techniques. Use of the Cavitron ultrasonic surgical aspirator (Valley Id Lab., Boulder, CO) greatly aids this dissection if the tumor is not calcified. For complete removal of the tumor, it is usually necessary to enlarge the foramen by removing its roof. For tumors arising from a nerve root, the nerve root is divided just proximal to the site of its entrance into the medial surface of the tumor; little discernible deficit occurs from sacrifice of a thoracic nerve root except at the higher levels (T1, T2), where hand function can be compromised. After resection of the tumor, the dura is closed. A dural graft is used if necessary and the foramen is sealed using muscle to prevent a spinal fluid leak. The integrity of this closure may be tested by having the anesthesiologist induce a Valsalva maneuver.

Attention is then directed to the thoracic exposure if necessary. The subcutaneous tissue and superficial fascia are incised until the fascia overlying the latissimus dorsi, trapezius muscle, and paravertebral muscle are exposed. The posterior aspect of the latissimus dorsi is divided. The trapezius and rhomboid muscles are divided as necessary. Once the rib overlying the tumor is identified, dissection is executed posterior to the rib, anterior to the paraspinal muscle, and medially toward the transverse process. Once the paraspinal muscle is mobilized, a vessel loop can be placed around it for easy retraction. Next, the rib is freed from the underlying parietal pleura and resected, maintaining the neurovascular elements intact. Using a sponge stick, the parietal pleura is bluntly separated from the tumor. The tumor can then be dissected free from its vascular supply and resected.

The chest is drained by tube thoracostomy and the incision is closed in standard fashion using 4-0 Neurilon on the dura mater, No. 2 polyglycolic acid (PGA) suture for pericostal closure, No. 1 PGA on the thoracolumbar fascia, 3-0 PGA on the subcutaneous tissue, and 3-0 PGA, nylon, or staples on the skin.

POSTEROANTERIOR APPROACH

A more anterior approach is afforded by performing a separate thoracotomy to resect the intrathoracic portion of the dumbbell tumor. Once again, it is crucial that the spinal portion of the tumor be resected first, because failure to respect this sequence of surgical steps could potentially result in spinal cord injury from traction on the cord or from a hematoma.

After being intubated with a double-lumen tube, the patient is positioned on a bean bag in a lateral decubitus position, lying on the nontumor side. All bony prominences are padded, especially the lateral portion of the dependent knee near the fibular head, where peroneal nerve compression could result in the loss of sensation on the dorsum of the foot or a foot drop. The dependent arm is appropriately padded after an axillary roll is placed, and the nondependent arm can be extended in a sling ventral and rostral to the surgical field. The intraspinal portion of the tumor is resected using a standard midline laminectomy exposure.

An incision is made along the rib, from the lateral paraspinal musculature to just ventral to the anterior axillary line. After the skin incision, the deeper component of the incision can be made down to the rib by using electrocautery. Once the rib is separated from the periosteum, underlying pleura, and neurovascular bundle, it can be resected or retracted with a rib spreader. Rib resection is not necessary for most tumors using this approach, although it should be a consideration for those tumors >5 cm in diameter. For tumors located in the lower thoracic spine, the caudal angulation of the ribs necessitates entering the thorax two ribs above the corresponding vertebral level. Thus, for a lesion located at T10, entry into the chest cavity should take place at or around the eighth rib. Since the upper rib cage is less angled in the midthorax, entry one rib above the appropriate level should suffice, and because of the kyphotic nature of the thoracic spine, a third rib resection may provide ample exposure from T2 to T5. Maintenance of an intact pleura should be attempted although it is not always possible, especially for large tumors. By using a sponge stick, the viscera can be gently retracted so that the tumor, ventral portion of the rib heads, and ventrolateral vertebrae can be exposed. The visceral pleura can be protected with a surgical towel. An appropriately placed radiolucent retractor can maintain the exposure.

Dissection is then executed toward the mediastinal structures, where the intercostal vessels are identified, clipped, and cut. Tumor resection is performed either in piecemeal fashion or, once the vertebral portion is resected, *en masse* by separating the tumor from the chest wall. Once the tumor is removed, a chest tube is placed and the intercostal fascia closed with No. 1 PGA. The remainder of the incision is closed in standard fashion.

THORACOSCOPIC APPROACH

Video-assisted thoracic surgery (VATS) has been added to the armamentarium used in treating these lesions. Dickman[168] reported resection of an hourglass tumor without intradural extension using VATS alone. Those tumors with an intradural component require standard intraspinal tumor removal followed by VATS resection of the remaining component in the thoracic cavity, as reported by Vallieres,[169] Heltzer,[170] and McKenna[171] and their colleagues as well as by Tsunezuka and Sato.[165] In fact, Konno and colleagues[172] asserted that this approach, when combined with a laminectomy and if needed a medial facetectomy, can be used for the complete resection of a majority of hourglass tumors. Placement of the working ports for VATS is dependent on the side and spinal level of the tumor. The surgeon must be ready to perform a thoracotomy if hemorrhage occurs during the thoracoscopic procedure.

Advantages of VATS include the potential for reduction of postoperative pain, less blood loss, improved shoulder function, less pulmonary morbidity, and reduction of length of stay. This technique, however, should not be used in the presence of findings suggestive of malignancy.

REFERENCES

1. King RM, Telander RL, Smithson WA, et al. Primary mediastinal tumors in children. *J Pediatr Surg* 1982;17(5):512–520.

2. Reynolds M. Benign and malignant mediastinal neurogenic tumors in infants and children. In: Shields TW, ed. *Mediastinal Surgery*. Philadelphia, PA: Lea & Febiger; 1991.
3. Saenz NC, Schnitzer JJ, Eraklis AE, et al. Posterior mediastinal masses. *J Pediatr Surg* 1993;28(2):172–176.
4. Reed JC, Hallet KK, Feigin DS. Neural tumors of the thorax: subject review from the AFIP. *Radiology* 1978;126(1):9–17.
5. Ribet ME, Cardot GR. Neurogenic tumors of the thorax. *Ann Thorac Surg* 1994;58(4):1091–1095.
6. Teixeira JP, Bibas RA. Surgical treatment of tumors of the mediastinum: the Brazilian experience. In: Martini N, Vogt-Moykopf I, eds. *Thoracic Surgery: Frontiers and Uncommon Neoplasms*. St. Louis, MO: Mosby; 1989.
7. Miura T, Review of 29 patients with neurogenic mediastinal tumors treated in our department (1972–1992) (National Kgusyu Cancer Center). *J Jpn Assoc Chest Surg* 1994;8:783.
8. Cohen AJ, Thompson L, Edwards FH, et al. Primary cysts and tumors of the mediastinum. *Ann Thorac Surg* 1991;51(3):378–384; discussion 385–386.
9. Sorensen SA, Mulvihill JJ, Nielsen A. Long-term follow-up of von Recklinghausen neurofibromatosis. Survival and malignant neoplasms. *N Engl J Med* 1986;314(16):1010–1015.
10. Davidson KG, Walbaum PR, McCormack RJ. Intrathoracic neural tumours. *Thorax* 1978;33(3):359–367.
11. Joshi VV, Cantor AB, Altshuler G, et al. Age-linked prognostic categorization based on a new histologic grading system of neuroblastomas. A clinicopathologic study of 211 cases from the Pediatric Oncology Group. *Cancer* 1992;69(8):2197–2211.
12. Peuchmaur M, d'Amore ES, Joshi VV, et al. Revision of the International Neuroblastoma Pathology Classification: confirmation of favorable and unfavorable prognostic subsets in ganglioneuroblastoma, nodular. *Cancer* 2003;98(10):2274–2281.
13. Marangos PJ. The neurobiology of the brain enolase. In: Youdin MBH, ed. *The Neurobiology of the Brain Enolase*. New York: Wiley; 1980:211.
14. Schmechel DE. Gamma-subunit of the glycolytic enzyme enolase: nonspecific or neuron specific? *Lab Invest* 1985;52(3):239–242.
15. Gould VE, Wiedenmann B, Lee I, et al. Synaptophysin expression in neuroendocrine neoplasms as determined by immunocytochemistry. *Am J Pathol* 1987;126(2):243–257.
16. Hinterburger M, Bartholomew RJ. Catecholamines and their acidic metabolites in urine and in tumor tissue in neuroblastoma, ganglioneuroblastoma and pheochromocytoma. *Clin Chim Acta* 1969;23:169–175.
17. Siegel SE. Patterns of urinary catecholamine excretion in neuroblastoma. In: Evans AE, ed. *Advances in Neuroblastoma Research*. New York: Raven Press; 1995.
18. Voute PA, Van Patten WJ, Burgers JMV. Tumors of the sympathetic nervous system. In: Bloom HJG, Lemerle J, Neidhardt MK, et al., eds. *Cancer in Children: Clinical Management*. New York: Springer-Verlag; 1975.
19. Williams TH, House RF, Burgert EO, et al. Unusual manifestations of neuroblastoma: chronic diarrhea, polymyoclonia-opsonclonus, and erythrocyte abnormalities. *Cancer* 1972;29(2):475–480.
20. Zhang WQ, Liu JF, Zhao J, et al. Tumor with watery diarrhoea, hypokalaemia in a 3-year-old girl. *Eur J Pediatr* 2009;168(7):859–862.
21. Maranhao MV, de Holanda AC, Tavares FL. Kinsbourne syndrome: case report. *Revista Brasileira de Anestesiologia* 2013;63(3):287–289.
22. Mueller S, Matthay KK. Neuroblastoma: biology and staging. *Curr Oncol Rep* 2009;11(6):431–438.
23. Bronson M. Sympathoblastoma in adults with special emphasis on its differential diagnosis. *Oncologia* 1952;5(1–2):67–89.
24. Kilton LJ, Aschenbrener C, Burns CP. Ganglioneuroblastoma in adults. *Cancer* 1976;37(2):974–983.
25. Hoover EL, Hsu HK, Dressler C, et al. Neuroblastoma: a rare primary intrathoracic neurogenic tumor in adults. *Tex Heart Inst J* 1988;15(2):107–112.
26. Eklof O, Gooding CA. Intrathoracic neuroblastoma. *Am J Roentgenol Radium Ther Nucl Med* 1967;100(1):202–207.
27. Talerman A, Gratama S. Primary ganglioneuroblastoma of the anterior mediastinum in a 61-year-old woman. *Histopathology* 1983;7(6):967–975.
28. Hutchinson JE 3rd, Nash AD, McCord CW. Neuroblastoma of the anterior mediastinum in an adult. *J Thorac Cardiovasc Surg* 1968;56(1): 147–152.
29. Asada Y, Marutsuka K, Mitsukawa T, et al. Ganglioneuroblastoma of the thymus: an adult case with the syndrome of inappropriate secretion of antidiuretic hormone. *Hum Pathol* 1996;27(5):506–509.
30. Argani P, Erlandson RA, Rosai J. Thymic neuroblastoma in adults: report of three cases with special emphasis on its association with the syndrome of inappropriate secretion of antidiuretic hormone. *Am J Clin Pathol* 1997;108(5):537–543.
31. Buthker W, Feltkamp-Vroom T, Groen AS, et al. Sympathicoblastoma in the anterior mediastinum. *Dis Chest* 1964;46:531–536.
32. Griff LC, Griff RE. Neuroblastoma-emphasis on the mediastinal neuroblastoma. *Am J Roentgenol Radium Ther Nucl Med* 1968;103(1):19–24.
33. Salter JE Jr, Gibson D, Ordóñez NG, et al. Neuroblastoma of the anterior mediastinum in an 80-year-old woman. *Ultrastruct Pathol* 1995;19(4):305–310.
34. Stowens D. Neuroblastoma and related tumors. *AMA Arch Pathol* 1957;63(5):451–459.
35. Owens C, Irwin M. Neuroblastoma: the impact of biology and cooperation leading to personalized treatments. *Crit Rev Clin Lab Sci* 2012;49(3):85–115.
36. Taxy JB. Electron microscopy in the diagnosis of neuroblastoma. *Arch Pathol Lab Med* 1980;104(7):355–360.
37. Maris JM, Kyemba SM, Rebbeck TR, et al. Familial predisposition to neuroblastoma does not map to chromosome band 1p36. *Cancer Res* 1996;56(15):3421–3425.
38. Seeger RC, Brodeur GM, Sather H, et al. Association of multiple copies of the N-myc oncogene with rapid progression of neuroblastomas. *N Engl J Med* 1985;313(18):1111–1116.
39. Morris JA, Shcochat SJ, Smith EI, et al. Biological variables in thoracic neuroblastoma: a Pediatric Oncology Group study. *J Pediatr Surg* 1995;30(2):296–302; discussion 302–303.
40. Gutierrez JC, Fischer AC, Sola JE, et al. Markedly improving survival of neuroblastoma: a 30-year analysis of 1,646 patients. *Pediatr Surg Int* 2007;23(7):637–646.
41. Solomon GE, Chutorian AM. Opsoclonus and occult neuroblastoma. *N Engl J Med* 1968;279(9):475–477.
42. Altman AJ, Baehner RL. Favorable prognosis for survival in children with coincident opso-myoclonus and neuroblastoma. *Cancer* 1976;37(2):846–852.
43. Maris JM, Hogarty MD, Bagatell R, et al. Neuroblastoma. *Lancet* 2007;369(9579):2106–2120.
44. Ambros PF, Ambros IM, Brodeur GM, et al. International consensus for neuroblastoma molecular diagnostics: report from the International Neuroblastoma Risk Group (INRG) Biology Committee. *Br J Cancer* 2009;100(9):1471–1482.
45. Hassan SF, Mathur S, Magliaro TJ, et al. Needle core vs. open biopsy for diagnosis of intermediate- and high-risk neuroblastoma in children. *J Pediatr Surg* 2012;47(6):1261–1266.
46. Mullassery D, Sharma V, Salim A, et al. Open versus needle biopsy in diagnosing neuroblastoma. *J Pediatr Surg* 2014;49(10):1505–1507.
47. Slovis TL, Meza MP, Cushing B, et al. Thoracic neuroblastoma: what is the best imaging modality for evaluating extent of disease? *Pediatr Radiol* 1997;27(3):273–275.
48. Bar-Ziv J, Nogrady MB. Mediastinal neuroblastoma and ganglioneuroma. The differentiation between primary and secondary involvement on the chest roentgenogram. *Am J Roentgenol Radium Ther Nucl Med* 1975;125(2):380–390.
49. Brisse HJ, McCarville MB, Granata C, et al. Guidelines for imaging and staging of neuroblastic tumors: consensus report from the International Neuroblastoma Risk Group Project. *Radiology* 2011;261(1):243–257.
50. Nour-Eldin NEA, Abdelmonem O, Tawfik AM, et al. Pediatric primary and metastatic neuroblastoma: MRI findings. Pictorial review. *Magn Reson Imaging* 2012;30(7):893–906.
51. Monclair T, Brodeur GM, Ambros PF, et al. The International Neuroblastoma Risk Group (INRG) staging system: an INRG Task Force report. *J Clin Oncol* 2009;27(2):298–303.
52. Simon T, Hero B, Benz-Bohm G, et al. Review of image defined risk factors in localized neuroblastoma patients: Results of the GPOH NB97 trial. *Pediatr Blood Cancer* 2008;50(5): 965–969.
53. Cohn SL, Pearson AD, London WB, et al. The International Neuroblastoma Risk Group (INRG) classification system: an INRG Task Force report. *J Clin Oncol* 2009;27(2):289–297.
54. Brodeur GM, Pritchard J, Berthold F, et al. Revisions of the international criteria for neuroblastoma diagnosis, staging, and response to treatment. *J Clin Oncol* 1993;11(8):1466–1477.
55. Shimada H, Chatten J, Newton WA Jr, et al. Histopathologic prognostic factors in neuroblastic tumors: definition of subtypes of ganglioneuroblastoma and an age-linked classification of neuroblastomas. *J Natl Cancer Inst* 1984;73(2):405–416.
56. Vo KT, Matthay KK, Neuhaus J, et al. Clinical, biologic, and prognostic differences on the basis of primary tumor site in neuroblastoma: a report from the international neuroblastoma risk group project. *J Clin Oncol* 2014;32(28):3169–3176.
57. Cecchetto G, Mosseri V, De Bernardi B, et al. Surgical risk factors in primary surgery for localized neuroblastoma: the LNESG1 study of the European International Society of Pediatric Oncology Neuroblastoma Group. *J Clin Oncol* 2005;23(33):8483–8489.
58. Kletzel M, Katzenstein HM, Haut PR, et al. Treatment of high-risk neuroblastoma with triple-tandem high-dose therapy and stem-cell rescue: results of the Chicago Pilot II Study. *J Clin Oncol* 2002;20(9):2284–2292.
59. Irtan S, Brisse HJ, Minard-Colin V, et al. Minimally invasive surgery of neuroblastic tumors in children: Indications depend on anatomical location and image-defined risk factors. *Pediatr Blood Cancer* 2015;62(2):257–261.
60. Boutros J, Bond M, Beaudry P, et al. Case selection in minimally invasive surgical treatment of neuroblastoma. *Pediatr Surg Int* 2008;24(10):1177–1180.
61. Petty JK, Bensard DD, Partrick DA, et al. Resection of neurogenic tumors in children: is thoracoscopy superior to thoracotomy? *J Am Coll Surg* 2006;203(5):699–703.
62. Malek MM, Mollen KP, Kane TD, et al. Thoracic neuroblastoma: a retrospective review of our institutional experience with comparison of the thoracoscopic and open approaches to resection. *J Pediatr Surg* 2010;45(8):1622–1626.
63. DeCou JM, Schlatter MG, Mitchell DS, et al. Primary thoracoscopic gross total resection of neuroblastoma. *J Laparoendosc Adv Surg Tech A* 2005;15(5):470–473.
64. Fraga JC, Rothenberg S, Kiely E, et al. Video-assisted thoracic surgery resection for pediatric mediastinal neurogenic tumors. *J Pediatr Surg* 2012;47(7):1349–1353.
65. Hoover M, Bowman LC, Crawford SE, et al. Long-term outcome of patients with intraspinal neuroblastoma. *Med Pediatr Oncol* 1999;32(5):353–359.
66. Fatimi SH, Bawany SA, Ashfaq A. Ganglioneuroblastoma of the posterior mediastinum: A case report. *J Med Case Rep* 2011;5:322.
67. Adam A, Hochholzer L. Ganglioneuroblastoma of the posterior mediastinum: a clinicopathologic review of 80 cases. *Cancer* 1981;47(2):373–381.
68. Okamatsu C, London WB, Naranjo A, et al. Clinicopathological characteristics of ganglioneuroma and ganglioneuroblastoma: a report from the CCG and COG. *Pediatr Blood Cancer* 2009;53(4):563–569.

69. Feigin I, Cohen M. Maturation and anaplasia in neuronal tumors of the peripheral nervous system; with observations on the glial-like tissues in the ganglioneuroblastoma. *J Neuropathol Exp Neurol* 1977;36(4):748–763.

70. Angelini P, London WB, Cohn SL, et al. Characteristics and outcome of patients with ganglioneuroblastoma, nodular subtype: a report from the INRG project. *Eur J Cancer* 2012;48(8):1185–1191.

71. Enzinger FM, Weiss SW. *Soft Tissue Tumors*. 2nd ed. St. Louis, MI: Mosby; 1998.

72. Marchevsky AM, Kaneko M. *Surgical Pathology of the Mediastinum*. New York: Raven Press; 1992.

73. Bender BL, Ghatak NR. Light and electron microscopic observations on a ganglioneuroma. *Acta Neuropathol* 1978;42(1):7–10.

74. Yokoyama M, Okada K, Tokue A, et al. Ultrastructural and biochemical study of benign ganglioneuroma. *Virchows Arch A Pathol Pathol Anat* 1973;361(3):195–209.

75. Qiu Y, Wang S, Wang B, et al. Adolescent thoracolumbar scoliosis secondary to ganglioneuroma: a two case report. *Spine* 2007;32(10):e326–e329.

76. Maruyama R, Tanaka J, Maehara S, et al. Intrathoracic ganglioneuroma in an elderly patient over 70 years of age. *Gen Thorac Cardiovasc Surg* 2007;55(10):437–439.

77. McRae D Jr, Shaw A. Ganglioneuroma, heterochromia iridis, and Horner's syndrome. *J Pediatr Surg* 1979;14(5):612–614.

78. Mendelsohn G, Eggleston JC, Olson JL, et al. Vasoactive intestinal peptide and its relationship to ganglion cell differentiation in neuroblastic tumors. *Lab Invest* 1979;41(2):144–149.

79. Trump DL, Livingston JN, Baylin SB. Watery diarrhea syndrome in an adult with ganglioneuroma-pheochromocytoma: identification of vasoactive intestinal peptide, calcitonin, and catecholamines and assessment of their biologic activity. *Cancer* 1977;40(4):1526–1532.

80. Kato M, Hara M, Ozawa Y, et al. Computed tomography and magnetic resonance imaging features of posterior mediastinal ganglioneuroma.[Erratum appears in J Thorac Imaging. 2013 Jul;28(4):262 Note: Shibamato, Yuta [corrected to Shibamoto, Yuta]]. *J Thorac Imaging* 2012;27(2):100–106.

81. Guan YB, Zhang WD, Zeng QS, et al. CT and MRI findings of thoracic ganglioneuroma. *Br J of Radiol* 2012;85(1016):e365–e372.

82. Phan DC, Gleason BC. Recent developments in benign peripheral nerve sheath tumors. *J Cutan Pathol* 2008;35(12):1165–1169.

83. Wang T, Yin H, Han S, et al. Malignant peripheral nerve sheath tumor (MPNST) in the spine: a retrospective analysis of clinical and molecular prognostic factors. *J Neurooncol* 2015;122(2):349–355.

84. Akwari OE, Itani KM, Coleman RE, et al. Splenectomy for primary and recurrent immune thrombocytopenic purpura (ITP). Current criteria for patient selection and results. *Ann Surg* 1987;206(4):529–541.

85. Nishikawa K, Omura N, Yuda M, et al. Video-assisted thoracoscopic surgery for localized neurofibroma of the esophagus: case report and review of the literature. *Int Surg* 2013;98(4):461–465.

86. Keller SM, Papazoglou S, McKeever P, et al. Late occurrence of malignancy in a ganglioneuroma 19 years following radiation therapy to a neuroblastoma. *J Surg Oncol* 1984;25(4):227–231.

87. Guccion JG, Enzinger FM. Malignant Schwannoma associated with von Recklinghausen's neurofibromatosis. *Virchows Arch A Pathol Anat Histol* 1979;383(1):43–57.

88. Ducatman BS, Scheithauer BW. Postirradiation neurofibrosarcoma. *Cancer* 1983;51(6):1028–1033.

89. Ducatman BS, Scheithauer BW, Piepgras DG, et al. Malignant peripheral nerve sheath tumors. a clinicopathologic study of 120 cases. *Cancer* 1986;57(10):2006–2021.

90. Chen YH, Hsu YH, Chang HR. Intrathoracic ancient neurilemoma mimicking mesenchymal thoracic tumor. *Am J Med Sci* 2013;346(5):424–426.

91. Hirano S, Motohara T, Nishibe T, et al. Cystic mediastinal tumor: a clinical study. *J Jpn Assoc Chest Surg* 1997;11(1):13–19.

92. Petkar M, Vaideeswar P, Deshpande JR. Surgical pathology of cystic lesions of the mediastinum. *J Postgrad Med* 2001;47(4):235–239.

93. Weiss SW, Nickoloff BJ. CD-34 is expressed by a distinctive cell population in peripheral nerve, nerve sheath tumors, and related lesions. *Am J Surg Pathol* 1993;17(10):1039–1045.

94. Kornstein MJ, DeBlois GG. *Pathology of the Thymus and Mediastinum*. Philadelphia, PA: Saunders; 1995.

95. Crowe FW, Schull WJ, Neel JV. *A Clinical, Pathological and Genetic Study of Multiple Neurofibromatosis*. Springfield, IL: Charles C Thomas; 1956.

96. Stout AP. The peripheral manifestations of specific nerve sheath tumor (neurilemoma). *Am J Cancer* 1935;24(4):751–780.

97. Lin AL, Gutmann DH. Advances in the treatment of neurofibromatosis-associated tumours. *Nat Rev Clin Oncol* 2013;10(11):616–624.

98. Sheikh S, Gomes M, Montgomery E. Multiple plexiform schwannomas in a patient with neurofibromatosis. *J Thorac Cardiovasc Surg* 1998;115(1):240–242.

99. Woodruff JM, Godwin TA, Erlandson RA, et al. Cellular schwannoma: a variety of schwannoma sometimes mistaken for a malignant tumor. *Am J Surg Pathol* 1981;5(8):733–744.

100. Fletcher CD, Davies SE, McKee PH. Cellular schwannoma: a distinct pseudosarcomatous entity. *Histopathology* 1987;11(1):21–35.

101. Lodding P, Kindblom LG, Angervall L, et al. Cellular schwannoma. A clinicopathologic study of 29 cases. *Virchows Arch A Pathol Anat Histopathol* 1990;416(3):237–248.

102. Ekiz T, Aslan MD, Hatipoğlu C, et al. An unusual case of cervical spinal schwannoma. *PM R* 2014;6(5):461–462.

103. Mandybur TI. Melanotic nerve sheath tumors. *J Neurosurg* 1974;41(2):187–192.

104. Bagchi AK, Sarkar SK, Chakraborti DP. Melanotic spinal schwannoma. *Surg Neurol*, 1975;3(2):79–81.

105. Paris F, Cabanes J, Muñoz C, et al. Melanotic spinothoracic schwannoma. *Thorax* 1979;34(2):243–246.

106. Kayano H, Katayama I. Melanotic schwannoma arising in the sympathetic ganglion. *Hum Pathol* 1988;19(11):1355–1358.

107. Abbott AE Jr, Hill RC, Flynn MA, et al. Melanotic schwannoma of the sympathetic ganglia: pathological and clinical characteristics. *Ann Thorac Surg* 1990;49(6):1006–1008.

108. Graham DI, Paterson A, McQueen A, et al. Melanotic tumours (Blue Naevi) of spinal nerve roots. *J Pathol* 1976;118(2):83–89.

109. Carney JA. Psammomatous melanotic schwannoma. A distinctive, heritable tumor with special associations, including cardiac myxoma and the Cushing syndrome. *Am J Surg Pathol* 1990;14(3):206–222.

110. Ewy MF, Demmy TL, Perry MC, et al. Massive phrenic perineurioma mimicking an unresectable cardiac tumor. *Ann Thorac Surg* 1995;60(1):188–189.

111. Yamashita T, Osaki T, Yoshimatsu T, et al. Mediastinal neurilemoma originating in intrathoracic right phrenic nerve: a case report. *J Jpn Assoc Chest Surg* 1996;10(2):171–174.

112. Ozawa Y, Kobayashi S, Hara M, et al. Morphological differences between schwannomas and ganglioneuromas in the mediastinum: utility of the craniocaudal length to major axis ratio. *Br J Radiol* 2014;87(1036):20130777.

113. Bourgouin PM, Shepard JO, Moore EH, et al. Plexiform neurofibromatosis of the mediastinum: CT appearance. *AJR Am J Roentgenol* 1988;151(3):461–463.

114. Sakai F, Sone S, Kiyono K, et al. Intrathoracic neurogenic tumors: MR-pathologic correlation. *AJR Am J Roentgenol* 1992;159(2):279–283.

115. Hilton DA, Hanemann CO. Schwannomas and their pathogenesis. *Brain Pathol* 2014;24(3):205–220.

116. Landreneau RJ, Dowling RD, Ferson PF. Thoracoscopic resection of a posterior mediastinal neurogenic tumor. *Chest* 1992;102(4):1288–1290.

117. Naunheim KS. Video thoracoscopy for masses of the posterior mediastinum. *Ann Thorac Surg* 1993;56(3):657–658.

118. Ishida T, Maruyama R, Saitoh G, et al. Thoracoscopy in the management of intrathoracic neurogenic tumors. *Int Surg* 1996;81(4):347–349.

119. Miettinen M. Melanotic schwannoma coexpression of vimentin and glial fibrillary acidic protein. *Ultrastruct Pathol* 1987;11(1):39–46.

120. Oosterwijk WM, Swierenga J. Neurogenic tumours with an intrathoracic localization. *Thorax* 1968;23(4): 374–384.

121. Dabir RR, Piccione W Jr, Kittle CF. Intrathoracic tumors of the vagus nerve. *Ann Thorac Surg* 1990;50(3)494–497.

122. Osada H, Funaki S, Okada T, et al. [A case report of intrathoracic vagal schwannoma (author's transl)]. *Kyobu Geka* 1979;32(4):303–306.

123. Mizuno T, Ichimura H, Shibata K, et al. [Mediastinal schwannoma originating from the intrathoracic vagus nerve—its diagnosis and treatment]. *Rinsho Kyobu Geka* 1981;1(3):446–452.

124. Shirakusa T, Tsutsui M, Montonaga R, et al. Intrathoracic tumors arising from the vagus nerve. Review of resected tumors in Japan. *Scand J Thorac Cardiovasc Surg* 1989;23(2):173–175.

125. Davis CJ, Butchart EG, Gibbs AR. Neurilemmoma of the intrathoracic vagus nerve. *Eur Respir J* 1991;4(4):508–510.

126. Katoh J, Yoshii S, Suzuki O, et al. Mediastinal vagal neurilemmoma causing tracheal stenosis. *J Thorac Cardiovasc Surg* 1995;109(1):184–185.

127. Shin MS, McElvein RB, Reeves RC, et al. Solitary neurofibroma of the vagus nerve in the aortopulmonary window masquerading as a developmental cyst. *J Comput Tomogr* 1988;12(1):57–60.

128. Wick MR, Swanson PE, Scheithauer BW, et al. Malignant peripheral nerve sheath tumor. An immunohistochemical study of 62 cases. *Am J Clin Pathol* 1987;87(4):425–433.

129. Matsunou H, Shimoda T, Kakimoto S, et al. Histopathologic and immunohistochemical study of malignant tumors of peripheral nerve sheath (malignant schwannoma). *Cancer* 1985;56(9):2269–2279.

130. Ducatman BS, Scheithauer BW. Malignant peripheral nerve sheath tumors with divergent differentiation. *Cancer* 1984;54(6):1049–1057.

131. Hajdu SI. Peripheral nerve sheath tumors. histogenesis, classification, and prognosis. *Cancer* 1993;72(12):3549–3552.

132. Furniss D, Swan MC, Morritt DG, et al. A 10-year review of benign and malignant peripheral nerve sheath tumors in a single center: clinical and radiographic features can help to differentiate benign from malignant lesions. *Plast Reconstr Surg* 2008;121(2):529–533.

133. Maebeya S, Miyoshi S, Fujiwara K, et al. Malignant schwannoma of the intrathoracic vagus nerve: report of a case. *Surg Today* 1993;23(12):1078–1080.

134. Singer RL. Thoracoscopic excision of a malignant schwannoma of the intrathoracic vagus nerve. *Ann Thorac Surg* 1995;59(6):1586–1587.

135. Wasa J, Nishida Y, Tsukushi S, et al. MRI features in the differentiation of malignant peripheral nerve sheath tumors and neurofibromas. *AJR Am J Roentgenol* 2010;194(6):1568–1574.

136. Anghileri M, Miceli R, Fiore M, et al. Malignant peripheral nerve sheath tumors: prognostic factors and survival in a series of patients treated at a single institution. *Cancer* 2006;107(5):1065–1074.

137. Fust JA, Custer R. On the neurogenesis of so-called granular cell myoblastoma. *Am J Clin Pathol* 1949;19(6):522–535.

138. Fisher ER, Wechsler H. Granular cell myoblastoma–a misnomer. Electron microscopic and histochemical evidence concerning its Schwann cell derivation and nature (granular cell schwannoma). *Cancer* 1962;15:936–954.

139. Mackay B, Elliott GB, MacDougall JA. Granular cell myoblastoma of the cystic duct: report of a case with electron-microscope observations. *Can J Surg* 1968;11(1):44–51.

140. Khansur T, Balducci L, Tavassoli M. Identification of desmosomes in the granular cell tumor. implications in histologic diagnosis and histogenesis. *Am J Surg Pathol* 1985;9(12):898–904.

141. Armin A, Connelly EM, Rowden G. An immunoperoxidase investigation of S-100 protein in granular cell myoblastomas: evidence for Schwann cell derivation. *Am J Clin Pathol* 1983;79(1):37–44.

142. Aisner SC, Chakravarthy AK, Joslyn JN, et al. Bilateral granular cell tumors of the posterior mediastinum. *Ann Thorac Surg* 1988;46(6):688–689.

143. Oparah SS, Subramanian VA. Granular cell myoblastoma of the bronchus: report of 2 cases and review of the literature. *Ann Thorac Surg* 1976;22(2):199–202.

144. Postlethwait RW. *Surgery of the Esophagus*. Norwalk, CT: Appleton-Century-Crofts; 1986.

145. Rosenbloom PM, Barrows GH, Kmetz DR, et al. Granular cell myoblastoma arising from the thoracic sympathetic nerve chain. *J Pediatr Surg* 1975;10(5):819–822.

146. Colberg JE. Granular cell myoblastoma (collective review). *Int Abstr Surg* 1962;115:205.

147. Kruse-Losler B, Gaertner C, Bürger H, et al. Melanotic neuroectodermal tumor of infancy: systematic review of the literature and presentation of a case. *Oral Surg Oral Med Oral Pathol Oral Radiol Endod*, 2006;102(2):204–216.

148. Askin FB, Rosai J, Sibley RK, et al. Malignant small cell tumor of the thoracopulmonary region in childhood: a distinctive clinicopathologic entity of uncertain histogenesis. *Cancer* 1979;43(6):2438–2451.

149. Kara Gedik G, Sari O, Altinok T, et al. Askin's tumor in an adult: case report and findings on 18F-FDG PET/CT. *Case Rep Med* 2009;2009:517329.

150. Shrestha B, Kapur BN, Karmacharya K, et al. Askin's Tumor: A Dual Case Study. *Int J Pediatr* 2011;2011:252196.

151. Ohta Y, Sato H, Sasaki K. Peripheral primitive neuroectodermal tumor in the thoracopulmonary region (Askin tumor); a case report. *J Japan Assoc Chest Surg* 1995;9(1):40–47.

152. Sano M, Iizuka M, Yamada T. Posterior mediastinal neuroectodermal tumor showing rapid growth and causing airway obstruction: case report and description of surgery. *J Jpn Assoc Chest Surg* 1995;9:731–738.

153. Takanami I, Imamura T. The treatment of Askin tumor: results of two cases. *J Thorac Cardiovasc Surg* 2002;123(2):391–392.

154. Jeong JY, Kim SY, Jeong DC, et al. A small Askin's tumor presenting with early onset of chest pain. *World J Surg Oncol* 2015;13(1):112.

155. Katsenos S, Nikopoloulou M, Kokkonouzis I, et al. Askin's tumor: a rare chest wall neoplasm. Case report and short review. *Thorac Cardiovasc Surg* 2008;56(5):308–310.

156. Kaneyama S, Doita M, Nishida K, et al. Multi-level dumbbell ganglioneuroma extending into the spinal canal from T11 to L4. *Curr Orthop Pract* 2009;20(2):196–199.

157. Akwari OE, Payne WS, Onofrio BM, et al. Dumbbell neurogenic tumors of the mediastinum. Diagnosis and management. *Mayo Clin Proc* 1978;53(6):353–358.

158. Le Brigand H. *Nouveau Traite de Technique Chirurgicoli*. Vol. 3. Paris: Masson; 1973.

159. Irger IM, Perel'man MI, Koroleva NS, et al. [A combined method of removing hourglass shaped neurogenic mediastinal-intravertebral tumors]. *Vopr Neirokhir* 1975;(6):3–10.

160. Irger IM, Perel'man MI, Koroleva NS, et al. [Surgical tactics in hourglass tumors with intravertebral-mediastinal locations]. *Zh Vopr Neirokhir Im N N Burdenko* 1980;(5):3–10.

161. Grillo HC, Ojemann RG, Scannell JG, et al. Combined approach to "dumbbell" intrathoracic and intraspinal neurogenic tumors. *Ann Thorac Surg* 1983;. 36(4):402–407.

162. Grillo HC. Mediastinal and intrathoracic "dumbbell" neurogenic tumors. In: Martini N, Vogt-Moykopf I, eds. *Thoracic Surgery: Frontiers and Uncommon Neoplasms*. St. Louis, MO: Mosby; 1989.

163. Riquet M, Mouroux J, Pons F, et al. Videothoracoscopic excision of thoracic neurogenic tumors. *Ann Thorac Surg* 1995;60(4):943–946.

164. Higashiama M, Doi O, Kodama K, et al. Thorascopic surgery for chest wall, pleural and mediastinal tumors. *J Jpn Assoc Chest Surg* 1993;7(4):416–422.

165. Tsunezuka Y, Sato H. Video-assisted thoracoscopy in single-stage resection of a para-aortic posterior mediastinal dumbbell tumor. *Thorac Cardiovasc Surg* 1998;46(1):47–49.

166. Nakamura H, Araki K, Taniguchi Y. A case of thoracoscopic resection for benign schwannoma originating from the vagus nerve. *J Jpn Assoc Chest Surg* 1997;11:90–94.

167. Shields TW, Reynolds M. Neurogenic tumors of the thorax. *Surg Clin North Am* 1988;68:645.

168. Dickmn CA. Endoscopic resection of thoracic paravertebral and dumbbell tumors: Commentry. *Neurosuegery* 2006;59(2):1201–1202.

169. Vallieres E, Findlay JM, Frase RE. Combined microneurosurgical and thoracoscopic removal of neurogenic dumbbell tumors. *Ann Thorac Surg* 1995;59(2):469–472.

170. Heltzer JM, Krasna MJ, Aldrich F, et al. Thoracoscopic excision of a posterior mediastinal "dumbbell" tumor using a combined approach. *Ann Thorac Surg* 1995;60(2):431–433.

171. Mckenna RJ, Maline D, Pratt G. VATS resection of a mediastinal neurogenic dumbbell tumor. *Surg Laparosc Endosc* 1995;5(6):480–482.

172. Konno S, Yabuki S, Kinoshita T, et al. Combined Laminectomy and thoracoscopic resection of dumbbell type thoracic cord tumor. *Spine* 2001;26(6):E130–E134.

Less Common Mediastinal Tumors

Alexander Yang ▪ Jinny S. Ha ▪ Stephen C. Yang

INTRODUCTION

Paragangliomas, pheochromocytomas, mesenchymal tumors, parathyroid adenomas, carcinomas of mediastinal origin, and metastatic lesions from another primary site are encountered infrequently in a surgical setting. Anatomically speaking, these masses do not originate from the parenchymal cells of a specific organ located in the mediastinum. Rather, a large proportion of these rare tumors is derived from nervous and mesenchymal tissue located within the boundaries of the mediastinum. Such neoplasms include paragangliomas and mesenchymal tumors of mediastinal origin. However, the vast majority of cases involving paragangliomas and mesenchymal tumors occur elsewhere outside of the mediastinum within the various nervous and connective tissues of the body. Pheochromocytomas are commonly described as intra-adrenal paragangliomas, and parathyroid adenomas and carcinomas of the mediastinum are ectopic in nature. The rarity of occurrence of these neoplasms primary to the mediastinum is the shared and central commonality for grouping them together.

The surgical implications that arise from the infrequency of these sporadic tumors to occur in the mediastinum rely heavily on detection, localization, radiographic diagnosis, and exclusion of prior cancers. Oftentimes, needle biopsy is difficult and requires surgical resection for tissue diagnosis and definitive management.

MEDIASTINAL PARAGANGLIOMAS AND PHEOCHROMOCYTOMA

NOMENCLATURE AND EPIDEMIOLOGY

The term *paraganglioma (PGL)* is used to refer to a neoplasm of paraganglionic origin. They can occur within both the sympathetic and parasympathetic nervous systems. Paragangliomas are defined broadly as chromaffin-positive tumors by general consensus. Chromaffin cells are catecholamine-secreting neuroendocrine bodies that develop from the embryonic neural crest and associate with the sympathetic nervous system during embryonic development.

However, paragangliomas arising from the parasympathetic paraganglia are chromaffin-negative as defined by DeLellis and colleagues,[1] Williams and Tischler,[2] and updated World Health Organization (WHO) classifications, and therefore do not secrete catecholamines. Parasympathetic paragangliomas are associated with the anatomic location of the parasympathetic nervous system in the region of the head and neck[3] developing mainly along the extensions of the glossopharyngeal and vagus nerves.[4,5] These are known as *nonfunctional paragangliomas* because they lack secreting functionality, and such cases are almost always benign.[6] Parasympathetic paragangliomas are commonly called *chemodectomas* due to their association with head and neck parasympathetic chemoreceptors.[7] Recently, this term has been noted to be misleading as only the carotid body paraganglia are true chemoreceptors.[8]

For the purposes of this chapter, focus will lie solely on mediastinal paragangliomas which, by definition, are of sympathetic paraganglia origin. To reiterate, sympathetic paraganglia are chromaffin-positive and secrete catecholamines. Paragangliomas are characterized as neoplasms of neuroendocrine cell lines that synthesize, store, and secrete catecholamines like norepinephrine, epinephrine, and dopamine. A *functional paraganglioma* is defined as a tumor of this type that is hormonally active and has catecholamine-secreting features in contrast to the nonsecreting nonfunctional paragangliomas. These can occur at almost any place along the sympathetic chain outside of the adrenal gland. More than 75% of functional paragangliomas occur within the abdomen, another 10% occur at the bladder and prostate, and 5% occur at the base of the skull.[9,10] It is important at this point to make a distinction between a *pheochromocytoma (PCC)* and a functional paraganglioma. Pheochromocytomas are chromaffin-positive tumors located *exclusively* within the adrenal gland medulla. At the cellular level, pheochromocytomas and functional paragangliomas are virtually indistinguishable. For this reason, these terms are often used interchangeably; *extra-adrenal pheochromocytoma* can be used to describe a paraganglioma, and *intra-adrenal paraganglioma* can be used to describe a pheochromocytoma. We will use the WHO classifications as follows:

1. Pheochromocytoma: tumor located in adrenal medulla
2. Functional paraganglioma: extra-adrenal secreting tumor
3. Nonfunctional paraganglioma: extra-adrenal nonsecreting tumor

Through analysis by phenotype, half of all pheochromocytoma cases have been found to produce and secrete epinephrine and the other half norepinephrine.[11] The only functional paraganglioma known to secrete epinephrine occurs in the organ of Zuckerkandl while the rest secrete norepinephrine. This matches physiological functionality as the adrenal medulla and organ of Zuckerkandl are the only sites of epinephrine biosynthesis.

Functional paragangliomas and pheochromocytomas (PPGL) have a combined incidence of about 2 to 8 per million.[12] Cases vary from 500 to 1,600 per year in the United States.[13] Sutton and colleagues[14] suggests that prevalence of these tumors may be understated as many cases go undiagnosed throughout life and are found incidentally upon autopsy. Age of diagnosis is most common in the

40 to 50 age group with a mean of 47 years old.[15] Pheochromocytoma has equal incidence in both sexes as does paraganglioma.[16] Hereditary cases comprise at least 24% of all cases,[17] and in such cases there are oftentimes multiple tumors.[18,19] Malignant pheochromocytoma or paraganglioma denotes the presence of chromaffin cells in tissue that normally is chromaffin-negative derived from the process of metastasis.[20] Five percent to 13% and 15% to 23% of pheochromocytoma and paraganglioma cases progress to malignancy, respectively.[21] Pheochromocytoma found in children is more likely to be hereditary at a rate of 40% of pediatric cases.[22] Malignancy in both types of tumors has a prognosis of >50% survival after 5 years.[23] Unfortunately, it is difficult to track and predict malignancy in these types of tumors.[24] Histologically and radiographically, malignant pheochromocytoma or paraganglioma is hard to distinguish from benign tumors. Metastatic disease is simply, albeit unhelpfully, defined as the presence of chromaffin-positive growth in tissue where there originally was none to begin with. Progression to metastatic disease is associated with a much worse prognosis.

CLINICAL PRESENTATION

PPGLs have been called "the great mimic[s]"[25] due to their various clinical manifestations. Indeed, the difficulty with which they are diagnosed explains why so many of these tumors are not found during patients' lifetimes. Of those who go undiagnosed, Sutton and colleagues[14] ascribes up to 50% of the causes of death to either of these tumors. Hypercatecholaminemia as a result of hypersecretion manifests itself in an array of nonspecific symptoms owing to the numerous physiological processes that catecholamines contribute to. The most common symptom is hypertension (including both persistent and paroxysmal), occurring in greater than 98% of cases, followed by headache in 70% to 90%, tachycardia in 50% to 70%, and diaphoresis in 60% to 70%; other symptoms include anxiety (20%), fever (<66%), and pallor (30% to 60%).[26] Hypertension is usually persistent in patients; however, it is not uncommon to also find paroxysmal hypertension or normotensive blood pressure levels. About 0.5% of patients presenting with persistent hypertension have a PPGL or another catecholamine-secreting tumor.[27] Paroxysmal hypertension can also occur secondary to persistent hypertension. The mechanism that confers the tumor with either persistent or paroxysmal hypertensive qualities is not well understood. The triad of symptoms including tachycardia, headache, and sweating is highly suspicious for a positive diagnosis, however, the majority of cases do not present with all three.[28] Specific symptoms will also depend on the location of the tumor (adrenal or extra-adrenal) and other, if any, neurotransmitters being secreted.

Still, some cases may present completely asymptomatic. Many adrenal masses are found incidentally on computerized tomographic (CT) scans. Herrerra and colleagues[29] found 2,066 cases of these "incidentalomas" (adrenal masses of at least 1 cm) out of a total of 61,054 CT scans. With improvements in screening and detection, it should be expected that the incidence and prevalence of PPGL increase.

Symptoms of mass effects are more common with nonfunctional paragangliomas simply because they are often not detected until they have grown to a considerable size and have begun impinging on surrounding tissue and organs.[30]

According to recent convention, PPGLs have been referred to as 10% tumors. Specifically, this convention states that 10% of all cases are malignant, 10% are hereditary, 10% are extra-adrenal, 10% are bilateral, and 10% do not present with hypertension. This has proven to be false as a much larger proportion are malignant, at least a third

are hereditary, and more patients than expected have presented with normotensive blood pressure.[31] A greater emphasis has been placed on genetic testing due to a stronger hereditary link than previously thought.

HEREDITARY SYNDROMES ASSOCIATED WITH PPGL

These types of tumors, benign or malignant, have a high propensity to be hereditary. Recent studies have shown that up to 40% of all PPGL cases are genetically inherited.[32] This places them among the most inherited neuroendocrine tumors.[33] Up to 19 germline mutations have been identified as susceptibility genes with 17 of these accounting for as much as 35% of all cases of PPGL syndrome. Furthermore, 15% of cases with sporadic mutations contain at least one of these 17 susceptibility genes of which two account for almost the entire portion.[34]

The most common susceptibility genes currently known are multiple endocrine neoplasia type 2 (MEN2A and MEN2B), neurofibromatosis type 1 (NF1 and also known as *von Recklinghausen disease*), von-Hippel–Lindau syndrome (VHL), succinate dehydrogenase subunit mutations (SDHB, SDHD, SDHC, and SDH5), and other less common mutations. Most of these susceptibility genes are inherited in an autosomal-dominant fashion.

MEN2, also known as *Sipple syndrome*, is a condition that presents with adrenal PPGL, medullary thyroid cancer, and parathyroid hyperplasia. Medullary thyroid cancer has a higher penetrance in MEN2 syndrome. Therefore, adrenal PPGL develops over a background of medullary thyroid hyperplasia at a rate of about 50%.[35] A chromosome 10 mutation of a RET proto-oncogene is responsible for MEN2 syndrome. It encodes for a receptor tyrosine kinase that is highly prevalent in the cell lines that descend from the neural crest, more specifically, the chromaffin cells of the adrenal gland.[36] MEN2A syndrome–induced pheochromocytoma is very rarely malignant, is exclusively localized to the adrenal medulla, and is bilateral in 30% of cases.[37,38]

MEN2B syndrome is associated with the same type of mutation, and occurs with other pathologies as well such as ganglioneuromatosis, connective tissue disorders like scoliosis and kyphosis, and medullary thyroid carcinoma.[39] Pediatric cases of pheochromocytoma caused by MEN2B syndrome has also been associated with a higher risk of malignancy.[40]

NF1 is an autosomal-dominant inherited mutation of a tumor-suppressor gene on chromosome 17 that encodes for neurofibromin. This mutation is the most common predisposing cancer syndrome of all susceptibility genes, but PPGL only arises in about 0.1% to 5.7% of cases.[41] However, Fishbein and colleagues have measured a 13% prevalence of PPGL in an autopsy series of patients that had NF1.[42] NF1 also constitutes 24% of all sporadic cases of PPGL.[42]

Less than 30% of patients with VHL syndrome develop a PPGL. This syndrome is also associated with a loss in function of a tumor-suppressor gene located on chromosome 3. VHL syndrome presents in a broad spectrum of clinical symptoms, and patients who develop PPGL may be asymptomatic. VHL-associated PPGL largely occur inside the adrenal medulla, are bilateral in 50% of cases, and malignant in 7% of cases. It is also associated with a younger age of onset with a mean age of 28 upon detection.[43]

Mutations in the genes for the subunits of succinate dehydrogenase, an enzyme critical for cellular respiration, are more recent discoveries. These include the SDHB, SDHD, SDHC, and SDH5 subunits of this enzyme. Tumors arising from mutations to this enzyme have a much higher propensity to be extra-adrenal. SDHB mutations were found to have unusually high rates of associated malignancy (37.5%)[44] and angiogenesis typical of a rapidly growing tumor; this strongly suggests that the SDHB subunit is involved with a tumor-suppressor gene.[45] Owing to an aggressive behavior, SDHB mutations have been linked to other malignancies like renal cell carcinoma and thyroid papillary carcinoma.[46] Because of this, genetic testing for an SDHB mutation has gained incredible importance especially if a high metabolizing, extra-adrenal mass is detected.

Mediastinal paragangliomas only make up 2% of all total PPGLs, however, an astounding 60% of them are associated with malignancy.[47] Because of this, it is presumed that many primary mediastinal PGLs originate from an SDHB mutation. It is highly recommended that these cases be genetically tested for a succinate dehydrogenase mutation accordingly whenever one is encountered clinically.

A more recent susceptibility gene has been identified in MYC-associated factor X (MAX). The significance of this lies in the MAX mutation being responsible for 1.12% of all PCC/PGL while not being associated with any other mutations.[48]

Furthermore, these mutations, both familial and somatic, have been designated into two different clusters based on their pathologies and phenotypes. Cluster 1 encompasses VHL and SDHx mutations with their downstream products inducing angiogenic and hypoxic pathways.[11] Cluster 1 tumors also tend to have a noradrenergic phenotype. Cluster 2 encompasses mutations whose downstream effects activate kinase signaling pathways through vulnerable oncogenes. These include the MEN2, NF1, and MAX susceptibility genes.[49,50] These tumors tend to have adrenergic phenotypes with the exception of the MAX mutation.

BIOCHEMICAL DIAGNOSIS

It is essential to undergo a thorough and comprehensive diagnosing process in order to conclude that a rare PPGL is the correct diagnosis. A delay or misdiagnosis has potentially devastating effects largely due to the inability of targeting the source of excess catecholamine secretion. An early diagnosis can lead to a complete cure. Earlier diagnoses for this condition have been facilitated due to advances in biochemical assay methodology, and the importance of genetic testing has taken on a significant role.[51] Thus, before biochemical testing, a comprehensive family history must be taken. Adverse reactions to drugs like dopamine receptor antagonists and beta-blockers is a growing consideration as well as they may elicit the paroxysms that are characteristic of these tumors.[52]

The first and possibly most important step in diagnosing a suspected PPGL is the detection of excess catecholamine production. This is achieved through the measurement of *metanephrine* levels throughout plasma and urine. Metanephrines are downstream metabolites of catecholamines and are produced and secreted almost constantly by tumor cells independent of catecholamine production.[53] Testing the level of catecholamines has proven to be much less reliable because of low sensitivity and specificity. Measurement of both urinary and plasma levels of metanephrines present sensitivities as high as 97% and 99%, respectively.[54] Thus, a negative test result for either sample is sufficient to exclude PPGL. This also applies for asymptomatic patients who have low pretest probabilities.[55] Testing for plasma free metanephrines does, however, present a higher specificity than does testing for urinary metanephrines. Therefore, measuring plasma free metanephrines has the ability to more definitively rule out PPGL.

There are a few considerations in regards to test implementation to address. Preferentially, plasma testing should be done with the patient in a fasting state because of a small likelihood that a false positive may occur if the patient consumes meals rich in amine.[56] There are no dietary restrictions for urinary sampling, however. Postural consideration when sampling blood has been shown to affect levels of metanephrine. Specifically, taking blood in the seated and upright position yields a greater metanephrine concentration than taking blood in the supine position as proven by numerous studies.[57] Taking blood from the upright position has yielded almost a three-fold increase in false-positives.[58] Therefore, it is highly suggested that phlebotomists take blood in the supine position when testing for PPGLs in order to avoid false-positives. If an upright position yields a positive result, the patient should be tested again except in the supine position. If it is not possible to take blood in the supine position, it should be made abundantly clear that this could yield a false-positive result. A 24-hour urinary metanephrine sample should be considered in this case.

Furthermore, pharmacological considerations must be accounted for. Certain drugs may yield false-positive results. These include the tricyclic class of antidepressants which induces an increase in norepinephrine, and sympathomimetic drugs. If it is not possible to temporarily stop the use of these drugs, imaging must be used to make a diagnosis of PPGL.

A clonidine suppression test is also available as biochemical diagnosis option, and stands to be more effective and considerably safer than the provocative glucagon test.[59] The test operates on the notion that when administered clonidine, the levels of norepinephrine in a patient without PPGL will decrease. A positive test result indicating PPGL shows an increase in plasma metanephrine after 3 hours or no more than a 40% decrease of metanephrine levels weighed against a baseline.[60]

IMAGING STUDIES

Generally, CT scans of the chest and abdomen with IV and oral contrast is done for the initial evaluation of patients with suspected PPGL. With a high suspicion, the next localization study is usually performed with an iodine-131-metaiodobenzylguanidine (MIBG) or octreotide scan.[61] Uptake with either scan usually suggests a neuroendocrine tumor. Magnetic resonance imaging (MRI) has the advantage of avoiding ionizing radiation, and without the need for IV contrast, can also localize these tumors, since they usually have a high T2-weighted signal intensity, since these tumors can be highly vascular. MRI also can help define tissue planes especially when these tumors approximate great vessels, neural foramina, and the cardiac chambers. However, it can lack specific anatomic details compared to CT scanning. Negative MIBG scans should be followed by positron emission tomography (PET) studies (Fig. 171.1). Angiography is rarely used currently, due to the advances with CT, MRI, and nuclear scanning. However, it is particularly useful for preoperative embolization if the tumor is close to major vascular structures or the heart; and when tumors may be unresectable.[62]

PERIOPERATIVE MANAGEMENT

Much like their extrathoracic counterparts, it is advised that patients diagnosed with PPGL should undergo alpha-adrenergic blockade prior to surgical resection, usually with phenoxybenzamine, a nonselective alpha-blocker. It is usually started 10 to 14 days prior to surgery, with a starting dose of 10 mg twice a day, and increased every second day until symptoms of hypertension resolve, or slight postural hypotension ensues. Gentle hydration is done judiciously, since correction with alpha-blockade results in a correction of the

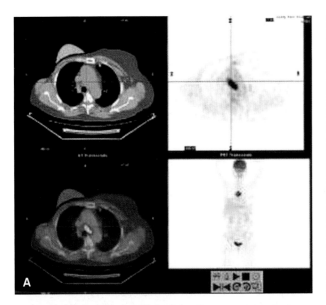

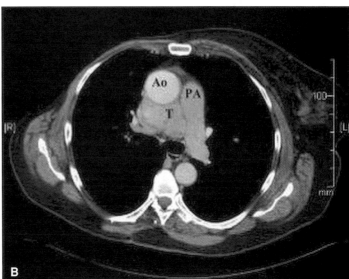

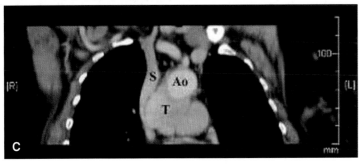

FIGURE 171.1 **A:** 5-cm mass with FDG-uptake (SUV 20) in the middle mediastinum. Repeat contrast CT scan demonstrates a 5-cm mass (*T*) located between the aorta (*Ao*), pulmonary artery (*PA*) and superior vena cava (*S*). **B,C:** Extra-adrenal paragangliomas are often at the bifurcation of great vessels. Surgical resection is the preferred treatment because they are highly vascular and often in close proximity to the great vessels, vena cava, trachea, and esophagus. (From Wald O, Shapira OM, Murar A, et al. Paraganglioma of the mediastinum: challenges in diagnosis and surgical management. *J Cardiothorac Surg* 2010;5:19.)

contracted intravascular volume. Overhydration could result in congestive heart failure. Alternative drugs include prazosin, but may cause less postoperative hypotension, and labetalol, which has both alpha- and beta-blocking characteristics, but may interfere with identifying these tumors accurately with MIBG.

Echocardiography should be performed as well preoperatively. Supraventricular and ventricular arrhythmias may occur perioperatively, and could be exacerbated with patients who have compromised left ventricular function, who may be normotensive despite intense vasoconstriction.

INTRAOPERATIVE MANAGEMENT

As with any high-risk operation, attention should be paid to the judicious use of continuous monitoring of EKG, blood pressure, urine output, and temperature. It is rare that central line catheters are needed, unless extensive blood loss is anticipated or major vascular/cardiac structures are involved. Blood products should be readily available since these are usually highly vascular structures.

Rapid and stress-free induction and endotracheal intubation are performed to avoid a catecholamine release. Despite aggressive alpha-blockade, marked hypertension could occur during anesthetic induction and/or tumor manipulation. Additional use of a short-acting alpha-blocker such as phentolamine could be used using 2 to 5 mg boluses or a continuous infusion. Nitroprusside is the drug of choice for intraoperative control of hypertension due to its effect on vascular smooth muscle. Beta-blockers such as propranolol may be useful to control supraventricular tachycardia, or amiodarone for tachyarrhythmias.

Postoperatively, hypotension could occur due to a decrease in catecholamines (half-life 4 minutes) and thus loss of vascular tone. Usually, preoperative volume repletion should avoid this, but fluid resuscitation remains essential rather than the use of pressors.

SURGICAL PRINCIPLES

Although these tumors may be encapsulated, they are often very difficult to dissect from their surrounding tissues. In addition, the impressive vascularity which these tumors are characteristic for, make even small tumors difficulty to resect with minimally invasive techniques such as VATS or robotics.

All tumors should undergo an R0 resection, preserving the capsule, while ascertaining vascular hemostasis. If possible, the venous drainage should first be ligated, while minimizing tumor handling so as to avoid potential catecholamine release.

Special attention to these details are important, but also depends upon the mediastinal compartment in which they lie. In the anterior mediastinum, they can be intimate with the thymus, and thus, the latter should be resected en bloc if possible. Minimally invasive techniques may be used if tumors are <3 cm, but those lying low in the mediastinum should be approached via an upper sternal split or sternotomy. The blood supply comes from the internal mammary artery, and venous drainage into the innominate vein, so the latter controlled first upon dissection in the mediastinum.

Tumors in the middle compartment may be more challenging depending on vascular involvement and proximity to the heart. Since they are soft and fleshy, they can be compressed between critical structures in and around the pericardium. They are unlike their abdominal counterparts, wherein there may be no true capsule to dissect around, with infiltration into local structures. Resection of portions of the great vessel or cardiac structures with reconstruction may be needed for an R0 resection.[63] Partial cardiopulmonary bypass or circulatory assist may be required to help with extirpation and cardiovascular reconstruction. In rare situations when cardiac resection is not possible, transplantation is required.[64,65]

Those tumors arising the paravertebral sulcus, likewise if small can be resected via a minimally invasive technique; if larger or difficult, then thoracotomy. Like neurogenic tumors, proximity to the intervertebral foramen should be investigated with MRI (if not done already) to ensure there is no growth into the spinal canal. If so combined resection is needed with a laminectomy to avoid leaving tumor behind, or worse, bleeding into the epidural space.

POSTOPERATIVE MANAGEMENT

As with MEN type 2A of the extrathoracic system, a detailed family history should be obtained, and investigation of these syndromes in first-degree relatives. Molecular genetic testing such as SDHA, SDHB, SDHC, and SDHD are four nuclear genes that are associated with mediastinal PPGL.

Though only 10% of all pheochromocytomas are considered malignant, extra-adrenal sites are reported to have a higher malignancy rates of 20% to 50%.[66] Since surgical resection remains the primary treatment, radiation and chemotherapy have less of an affect. Current first-line therapy includes cyclophosphamide, vincristine, and dacarbazine. Targeted therapies likewise have been disappointing and associated with low response rates, using the rapamycin inhibitor everolimus and sunitinib, a receptor tyrosine kinase inhibitor. With the accumulation of ^{131}I-MIBG in up to 60% of tumors, they may be susceptible to systemic ^{131}I-MIBG therapy since it is transported into cells by the norepinephrine transporter and causes cell death by emitting ionizing radiation from the decaying ^{131}I radionuclide. The use of radiation is less clear-cut, and reserved for recurrent, unresectable disease.

SUMMARY

PPGL are rare but unique tumors. Surgery is the mainstay of treatment, and patients require appropriate preoperative blockade and precise perioperative management. For patients with metastatic PPGL, medical therapy can provide symptomatic relief but only limited control of disease progression. Up to 40% of patients have genetic mutations that may allow targeted therapy. Knowledge of these mutations will have implications in the treatment, screening, and surveillance of patients and their family members; therefore, all patients with PPGL should be referred for clinical genetic testing. Hopefully, this will lead to better predictors of malignant potential and better targets for therapy.

MESENCHYMAL TUMORS

Mesenchymal neoplasms of the thymus and mediastinum comprise only 2% of neoplasms of the mediastinum and are therefore very rare. The histology, immunohistochemistry, and molecular biology of mediastinal soft tissue tumors are generally not too different from their counterparts in other organs. All tumors encountered in peripheral soft tissues can also arise in the mediastinum. Primary mediastinal soft tissue sarcomas (STS) can be confused with secondary radiation-induced STS after irradiation, like from lymphoma

TABLE 171.1 Histological Classification of Mesenchymal Tumors of the Mediastinum

Histologic Type	Examples
Adipocytic	Lipoma Thymolipoma Liposarcoma Lipomatosis Lipoblastoma Variants/Mixed
Vascular	Hemangioma Lymphangioma Lymphangiohemangioma
Fibroblastic/ myofibroblastic/ fibrohistiocytic	Aggressive fibromatosis/desmoid tumor Solitary fibrous tumor Inflammatory myofibroblastic tumor
Uncertain differentiation	Angiomatoid fibrous histiocytoma Synovial sarcoma Malignant mesenchymoma
Smooth muscle	Leiomyoma Angioleiomyoma Leiomyosarcoma
Skeletal muscle	Rhabdomyoma Rhabdomyosarcoma
Chondro-osseous	Extraskeletal chondrosarcoma Extraskeletal osteosarcoma[67]
Miscellaneous	Xanthoma Amyloid pseudotumor Follicular dendritic cell sarcoma Meningioma Ependymoma Mesothelioma Sclerosing hemangioma

and breast cancer, and those arising as somatic type malignancies in mediastinal germ cell tumors. These also need to be distinguished from the sarcomatous components of a mediastinal germ cell tumor and can be associated with a "somatic type malignancy" 20% to 25% of the time. Most of these tumors are embryonic rhabdomyosarcoma, angiosarcoma, leiomyosarcoma, or neuroblastoma, and behaves like analogous malignancies in other organs, and do not express any germline markers. These are associated with poor prognosis, with a median survival of only 9 months.

Perhaps <500 of these tumors have been reported as isolated cases or small case series. Oftentimes, they come as incidental findings after being completely resected. Classification is best organized by histologic characteristics (Table 171.1), as they can involve all tissues within the chest including the thymus, vasculature, heart, lymph nodes, and lungs. About one-half of all patients are asymptomatic. Generally, workup includes CXR, CT, and MRI, using the same indications as discussed previously for PPGL. Since many types can exist, a few of the more common tumor types will be presented.

LIPOMATOUS TUMORS

Thymolipoma

These are benign encapsulated tumors, and usually found in young adults. Thymolipomas are usually asymptomatic, and thus can be quite large at the time of diagnosis. In 10% of cases, much like thymomas,

TABLE 171.2 World Health Organization Classification of Liposarcomas

Atypical/Well-differentiated
Myxoid
De-differentiated
Pleomorphic

they can have associated autoimmune disorders such as myasthenia gravis, hypogammaglobulinemia, and hyperthyroidism. Resection is diagnostic and curative. Histologically, thymolipomas consist of mature thymic and adipose tissue; cytologic atypia is unusual.

Mediastinal Lipoma

In contrast to thymolipomas, these do not contain thymus tissue and are also rare. There are a number of variants with metaplastic cartilage or bone formation, with angioma and spindle cell lipids, hibernomas from brown adipose tissue and (in the posterior mediastinum in older adults) also blood-forming myelolipoma.

Liposarcoma

These are the most common malignant mesenchymal tumors of the mediastinum. They can be found in all three compartments of the mediastinum. These pleomorphic liposarcomas occur more frequently in the mediastinum more than in other extrathoracic areas. The most common subtypes are high and dedifferentiated liposarcomas, followed by pleomorphic and myxoid variants (Table 171.2). These usually occur in older adults, but also described in the pediatric population. Like other lipomatous tumors, these patients are often asymptomatic until the tumor because quite large to cause pain and dyspnea (Figs. 171.2 and 171.3). Pleomorphic and myxoid liposarcomas have a propensity to metastasize to other distant sites, and thus translate into a 50% 5-year survival.

VASCULAR TUMORS

Hemangiomas

Most hemangiomas (capillary and cavernous) are found in the anterior compartment (Figs. 171.4 and 171.5). They can become quite large, starting from the thymus and extending downward into the soft tissue of the mediastinum. They are usually seen in younger adults, but can be seen in all age ranges. They are generally asymptomatic, and can cause compression syndromes as they get larger (cardiopulmonary symptoms).

Epithelioid Hemangioendotheliomas

These are rare adult (M:F is 2:1) malignant endothelial tumors, characterized by a recurrent translocation with the formation of a CAMTA1-WWTR1 gene fusion. Histologically, the endothelial cells have an epithelioid morphology and intracytoplasmic lumina inside a hyaline or chondroid matrix. Osteoclastic giant cells and metaplastic ossifications occur. Because of this, they can frequently be misinterpreted as adenocarcinomas, and require resection for tissue diagnosis. Since these are generally chemo- and radio-resistant, surgical resection should be performed whenever possible.

Angiosarcoma

These are found primarily in the anterior mediastinum, usually older patients in both genders of equal frequency. Calcifications can occur.

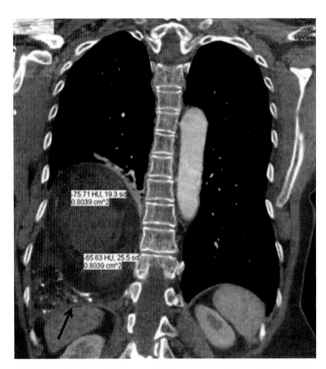

FIGURE 171.2 Coronal section CT demonstrates a large right-sided heterogenous mass representing a fat-containing mass. Low attenuation with Hounsfield units between −50 and −150 suggests the presence of fat. The presence of nonadipose components of the mass favors a liposarcoma versus a lipoma. Areas of calcification (*black arrow*) likely indicate areas of prior necrosis resulting in dystrophic calcification. (Reprinted from Biswas A, Urbine D, Prasad A, et al. Patient with slow-growing mediastinal mass presents with chest pain and dyspnea. *Chest* 2016;149(1):e17–e23. Copyright © 2016 The American College of Chest Physicians. With permission.)

It is difficult to differentiate cavernous hemangiomas from highly differentiated angiosarcomas, based upon cytological atypia and increased mitosis. Angiosarcomas can also occur as "somatic-type malignancy" in mediastinal germ cell tumors.

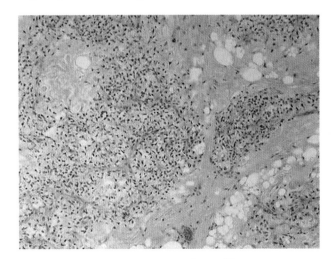

FIGURE 171.3 Microscopic appearance of myxoid liposarcoma containing two distinct morphologies. Areas of well-differentiated liposarcoma contain mature-appearing fat cells with multivacuolated lipoblasts. Other parts of the tumor exhibit hyperchromatic cells contained within a fine capillary network. (Reprinted from Biswas A, Urbine D, Prasad A, et al. Patient with slow-growing mediastinal mass presents with chest pain and dyspnea. *Chest* 2016;149(1): e17–e23. Copyright © 2016 The American College of Chest Physicians. With permission.)

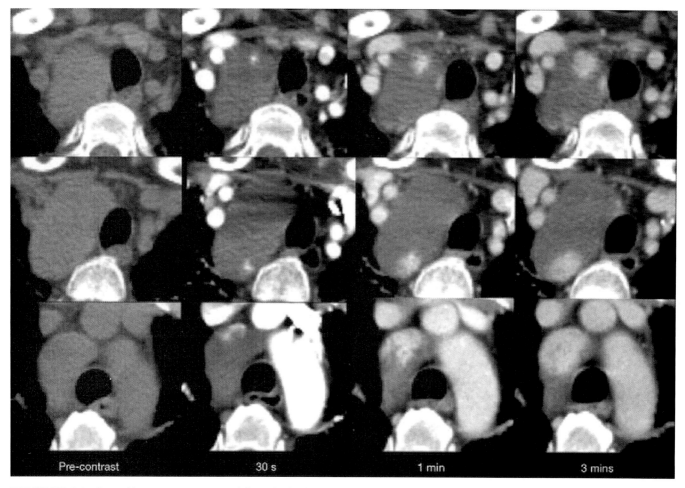

FIGURE 171.4 Mediastinal hemangioma seen on at different levels of the mediastinum on a dynamic CT with images at nonenhanced, 30-second, 1-minute, and 3-minute phases after administration of intravenous contrast. Dynamic CT scan can reveal the characteristic peripheral arterial enhancement with gradual central fill-in on delayed phase images. (From Li SM, Hsu HH, Lee SC, et al. Mediastinal hemangioma presenting with a characteristic feature on dynamic computed tomography images. *J Thorac Disc* 2017;95:E412–E415.)

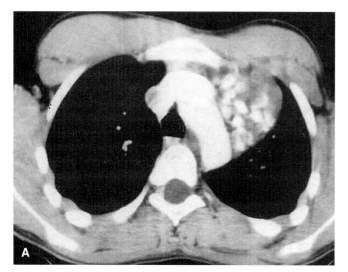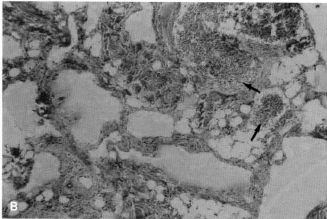

FIGURE 171.5 **A:** Lymphangiohemangioma of the mediastinum seen on contrast CT with enhancement of dilated vascular structures within the lesion. **B:** Histologically, these lesions are a combination of blood and lymphatic vessels. Characteristically, there are dilated endothelial spaces filled with lymph and blood. (Reprinted from Riquet M, Brere J, Le Pimpec-Barthes F, et al. Lymphangiohemangioma of the mediastinum. *Ann Thorac Surg* 1997;64(5):1476–1478. Copyright © 1997 The Society of Thoracic Surgeons. With permission.)

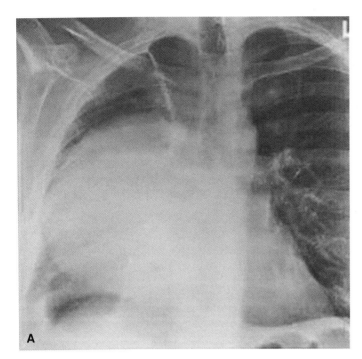 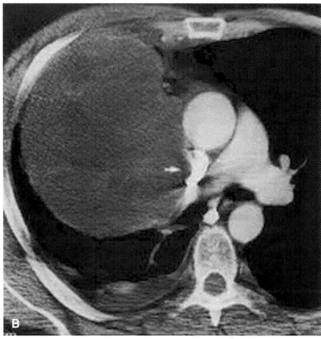

FIGURE 171.6 **A:** Large mass in the right hemithorax seen on chest x-ray. **B:** Contrast enhanced CT scan reveals a rhabdomyosarcomas. These tumors are often large with heterogenous attenuation due to areas of necrosis. The *white arrow* points an area of the superior vena cava that is compressed by the large mass. (Reproduced with permission from Gladhish GW, Sabloff BM, Mnden RF, et al. Primary thoracic sarcomas. *Radiographics* 2002;22(3):621–637.)

TUMORS WITH MUSCULAR DIFFERENTIATION

Mediastinal Leiomyosarcomas

These sarcomas are also very rare tumors. Generally, they are quite indolent, growing in the posterior mediastinum of middle-age adults, in both sexes of equal frequency. Generally, they have a higher propensity to infiltrate nearby organs like the heart, lungs, thoracic spine, or spinal canal. Surgical therapy alone is often not accomplished alone without multimodality therapy because of its local aggressiveness. Low differentiation is often associated with a loss of one or more immunohistochemical muscular markers, which makes it difficult to distinguish from other spindle-cell and pleomorphic sarcomas (e.g., malignant peripheral nerve-tract tumors).

Rhabdomyomas and Rhabdomyosarcomas

Rhabdomyomas are very rare benign tumors that arise from transverse muscular differentiation (Fig. 171.6), that can occur as a cardiac hamartoma in children with tuberous sclerosis. Likewise, rhabdomyosarcomas are extremely rare, and both are located in the anterior mediastinum of pediatric patients. The differential diagnosis includes rhabdomyosarcomas as part of a mediastinal germ cell tumor or as heterologous differentiation of another sarcoma.

Malignant Peripheral Nerve Tract Tumors

These can be found in all three mediastinal compartments, but usually in the posterior.

Malignant peripheral nerve tract tumor (MPNST) can show divergent differentiation with areas of rhabdomyosarcoma, osteosarcoma (Fig. 171.7), or chondrosarcoma. MPNSTs have a propensity to metastasize hematogenously.

SUMMARY

Mediastinal mesenchymal tumors are extremely rare, and do not share specific histologies with their extrathoracic organ sites. Since these are difficult to diagnose by cytology, surgery is required to ascertain more tissue, or to resect them completely since like other tumors, are chemo- and radio-resistant.

Metastatic Tumors to the Mediastinum

Almost every extrathoracic organ site has case reports with metastasis to the mediastinum. However, there are some specific histologic characteristics for these primary lesions (Table 171.3). The patient's cancer history is critical, and thus should be listed as one of the top potential diagnoses when a new lesion is found in the mediastinum. These lesions have been described to occur even past the 5-year

TABLE 171.3 Reported Extrathoracic Sites of Metastatic Disease to the Mediastinum

Site of Origin	Histology
Breast	
Colorectal[68]	
Gynecologic	Ovarian
Hepatobiliary	Hepatocellular, gallbladder
Pancreas	Ampullary, pancreas
Skin	Melanoma[69]
Soft tissue:	Liposarcoma, osteosarcoma, Ewing sarcoma[70,71]
Thyroid	Papillary, medullary
Urinary	Renal cell, transitional, bladder, prostate

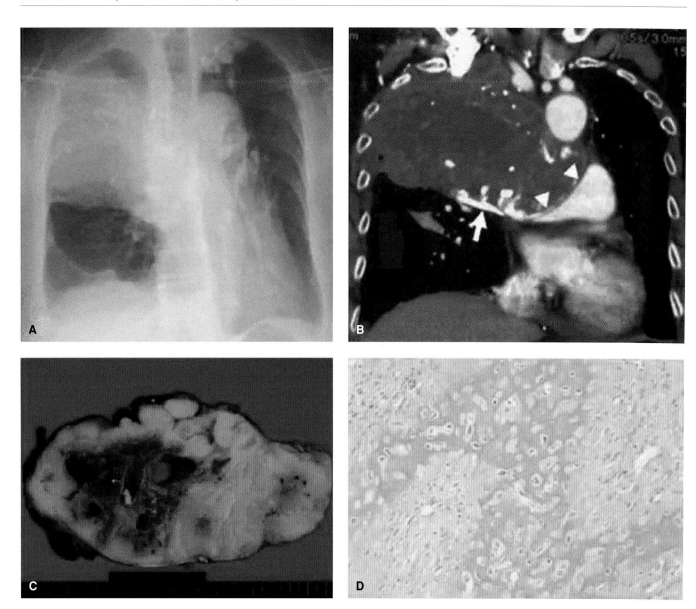

FIGURE 171.7 A case of a 77-year-old female with progressive shortness of breath. A chest radiograph shows a large mass occupying the right hemithorax (**A**). **B:** A contrast CT demonstrates a large mass causing extrinsic compression of the superior vena cava (*large arrow*) and right pulmonary artery (*arrow heads*) without invasion. **C:** Tumor was resected and pathology revealed an extraskeletal osteosarcoma. On gross examination, the tumor was well-circumscribed mass with both solid and cystic components. **D:** Osteoid formations are seen in histologic review consistent with an osteosarcoma. (Reprinted from Hishida T, Yoshida J, Nishimura M, et al. Extraskeletal osteosarcoma arising in anterior mediastinum. A brief report with a review of the literature. *J Thorac Oncol* 2009;4:927–929. Copyright © 2009 International Association for the Study of Lung Cancer. With permission.)

traditional survival time line. Needle aspiration or serum markers may suffice to make the diagnosis. Moreover, preoperative identification of this disease is challenging, making misdiagnosis likely. Since many of these may not respond to medical or radiation therapy, surgical resection is needed to confirm recurrence and often used as definitive therapy. Due to fast progression and poor prognosis, especially if a short interval has transpired since the initial primary resection, timely and effective systemic treatment is necessary to improve the outcomes for patients with mediastinal metastases.

REFERENCES

1. DeLellis RA, Lloyd R, Heitz P, et al. Paraganglia. Chapter 48. In: Mills SE, ed. *Histology for Pathologists*. 4th ed. Philadelphia, PA: Lippincott Williams & Wilkins; 2012:1277–1299.
2. Williams MD, Tischler AS. Update from the 4th edition of the World Health Organization classification of head and neck tumours: paragangliomas. *Head Neck Pathol* 2017;11:88–95.
3. Gaal J, van Nederveen FH, Erlic Z, et al. Parasympathetic paragangliomas are part of the Von Hippel-Lindau syndrome. *J Clin Endocrinol Metab* 2009;94: 4367–4371.
4. Kleinsasser O. Das glomus laryngicum inferior. Ein bisher unbekanntes, nichtchromaffines paraganglion vom bau der sogenannten carotisdrüse im menschlichen kehlkopf. *Eur Arch Oto-Rhino-Laryng* 1964;184:214.
5. Glenner GG, Grimley PM. *Tumors of the Extra-Adrenal Paraganglion System*. Bethesda, MD: Armed Forces Institute of Pathology; 1974.
6. Kahn LB. Vagal body tumor (nonchromaffin paraganglioma, chemodectoma, and carotid body-like tumor) with cervical node metastasis and familial association. Ultrastructural study and review. *Cancer* 1976;38:2367–2377.
7. Pettet JR, Woolner LB, Judd ES. Carotid body tumors (chemodectomas). *Ann Surg* 1953;137(4):465–477.
8. Barnes L, Tse LL, Hunt JL, et al. Tumours of the paraganglionic system: introduction. In: Barnes L, Eveson JW, Reichart P, et al., eds. *World Health Organization Classification of Tumours. Pathology and Genetics Head and Neck Tumours*. Lyon, France: IARC Press; 2005:362.
9. Ramlawi B, David EA, Kim MP, et al. Contemporary surgical management of cardiac paragangliomas. *Ann Thorac Surg* 2012;93(6):1972–1976.
10. Brown ML, Zayas GE, Abel MD, et al. Mediastinal paragangliomas: the Mayo Clinic experience. *Ann Thorac Surg* 2008;86(3):946–951.

11. Lenders JWM, Eisenhofe G. Update on modern management of pheochromocytoma and paraganglioma. *Endocrinol Metab (Seoul)* 2017;32(2):152–161.

12. Fishbein L, Orlowski R, Cohen D. Pheochromocytoma/paraganglioma: review of perioperative management of blood pressure and update on genetic mutations associated with pheochromocytoma. *J Clin Hypertens (Greenwich)* 2013;15:428–434.

13. Chen H, Sippel RS, O'Dorisio MS, et al. The North American Neuroendocrine Tumor Society consensus guideline for the diagnosis and management of neuroendocrine tumors: pheochromocytoma, paraganglioma, and medullary thyroid cancer. *Pancreas* 2010;39(6):775–783.

14. Sutton MG, Sheps SG, Lie JT. Prevalence of clinically unsuspected pheochromocytoma. Review of a 50-year autopsy series. *Mayo Clin Proc* 1981;56(6):354–360.

15. Erickson D, Kudva YC, Ebersold MJ, et al. Benign paragangliomas: clinical presentation and treatment outcomes in 236 patients. *J Clin Endocrinol Metab* 2001;86(11):5210–5216.

16. Kantorovich V, Pacak K. Pheochromocytoma and paraganglioma. *Prog Brain Res* 2010;182:343–373.

17. Neumann HP, Bausch B, McWhinney SR, et al. Germ-line mutations in nonsyndromic pheochromocytoma. *N Engl J Med* 2002;346(19):1459–1466.

18. Bravo EL, Tagle R. Pheochromocytoma: state-of-the-art and future prospects. *Endocrine Reviews* 2003;24:539–553.

19. Kirmani S, Young WF. Hereditary paraganglioma-pheochromocytoma syndromes. In: Pagon RA, Adam MP, Ardinger HH, et al., eds. SourceGeneReviews® [Internet]. Seattle (WA): University of Washington; 1993–2017. May 21, 2008.

20. DeLellis RA, Lloyd RV, Heitz PU, et al.; World Health Organization Classification of Tumours. *Pathology and Genetics of Tumours of Endocrine Organs.* Lyon, France: IARC Press; 2004.

21. Welander J, Söderkvist P, Gimm O. Genetics and clinical characteristics of hereditary pheochromocytomas and paragangliomas. *Endocr Relat Cancer* 2011;18:R253–R276.

22. Barontini M, Levin G, Sanso G. Characteristics of pheochromocytoma in a 4- to 20-year-old population. *Ann N Y Acad Sci* 2006;1073:30–37.

23. Chrisoulidou A, Kaltsas G, Ilias I, et al. The diagnosis and management of malignant phaeochromocytoma and paraganglioma. *Endocr Relat Cancer* 2007;14:569–585.

24. Johnson MH, Cavallo JA, Figenshau RS. Malignant and metastatic pheochromocytoma: case report and review of the literature. *Urol Case Rep* 2014;2(4):139–141.

25. Yucha C, Blakeman N. Pheochromocytoma. The great mimic. *Cancer Nurs* 1991;14(3):136–140.

26. Bravo EL, Tarazi RC, Gifford RW, et al. Circulating and urinary catecholamines in pheochromocytoma. Diagnostic and pathophysiologic implications. *N Engl J Med* 1979;301(13):682–686.

27. Assarzadegan F, Asadollahi M, Hesami O, et al. Secondary headaches attributed to arterial hypertension. *Iran J Neurol* 2013;12(3):106–110.

28. Baguet JP, Hammer L, Mazzuco TL, et al. Circumstances of discovery of phaeochromocytoma: a retrospective study of 41 consecutive patients. *Eur J Endo* 2004;150:681–686.

29. Herrera MF, Grant CS, van Heerden JA, et al. Incidentally discovered adrenal tumors: an institutional perspective. *Surgery* 1991;110(6):1014–1021.

30. Young WF. Paragangliomas. *Ann NY Acad Sci* 2006;1073:21–29.

31. Elder EE, Elder G, Larsson C. Pheochromocytoma and functional paraganglioma syndrome: no longer the 10% tumor. *J Surg Oncol* 2005;89:193–201.

32. Vicha A, Musil Z, Pacak K. Genetics of pheochromocytoma and paraganglioma syndromes: new advances and future treatment options. *Curr Opin Endocrinol Diabetes Obes* 2013;20(3):186–191.

33. Martucci VL, Pacak K. Pheochromocytoma and paraganglioma: diagnosis, genetics, management, and treatment. *Curr Probl Cancer* 2014;38:7–41.

34. Burnichon N, Vescovo L, Amar L, et al. Integrative genomic analysis reveals somatic mutations in pheochromocytoma and paraganglioma. *Hum Mol Genet* 2011;20:3974–3985.

35. Pacak K, Ilias I, Adams KT, et al. Biochemical diagnosis, localization and management of pheochromocytoma: focus on multiple endocrine neoplasia type 2 in relation to other hereditary syndromes and sporadic forms of the tumour. *J Intern Med* 2005;257(1):60–68.

36. Mulligan LM, Kwok JB, Healey CS, et al. Germ-line mutations of the RET proto-oncogene in multiple endocrine neoplasia type 2A. *Nature* 1993;363(6428):458–460.

37. Casanova S, Rosenberg-Bourgin M, Farkas D, et al. Phaeochromocytoma in multiple endocrine neoplasia type 2 A: survey of 100 cases. *Clin Endocrinol (Oxf)* 1993;38(5):531–537.

38. Neumann HP, Berger DP, Sigmund G, et al. Pheochromocytomas, multiple endocrine neoplasia type 2, and von Hippel-Lindau disease. *N Engl J Med* 1993;329(21):1531–1538.

39. Khairi MR, Dexter RN, Burzynski NJ, et al. Mucosal neuroma, pheochromocytoma and medullary thyroid carcinoma: multiple endocrine neoplasia type 3. *Medicine (Baltimore)* 1975;54(2):89–112.

40. Ross JH. Pheochromocytoma. Special considerations in children. *Urol Clin North Am* 2000; 27(3):393–402.

41. Lefebvre M, Foulkes WD. Pheochromocytoma and paraganglioma syndromes: genetics and management update. *Curr Oncol* 2014;21(1):e8–e17.

42. Fishbein L, Nathanson KL. Pheochromocytoma and paraganglioma: understanding the complexities of the genetic background. *Cancer Genet* 2012;205:1–11.

43. Kantorovich V, Pacak K. Pheochromocytoma and paraganglioma. *Prog Br Res* 2010;182:343–373.

44. Benn DE, Gimenez-Roqueplo AP, Reilly JR, et al. Clinical presentation and penetrance of pheochromocytoma/paraganglioma syndromes. *J Clin Endocrinol Metab* 2006;91(3):827–836.

45. Gimenez-Roqueplo AP, Favier J, Rustin P, et al. Mutations in the SDHB gene are associated with extra-adrenal and/or malignant phaeochromocytomas. *Cancer Res* 2003;63(17):5615–5621.

46. Neumann HP, Pawlu C, Pęczkowska M, et al. Distinct clinical features of paraganglioma syndromes associated with SDHB and SDHD gene mutations. *JAMA* 2004;292(8):943–951.

47. Ghayee HK, Havekes B, Corssmit EP, et al. Mediastinal paragangliomas: association with mutations in the succinate dehydrogenase genes and aggressive behavior. *Endocr Relat Cancer* 2009;16(1):291–299.

48. Burnichon N, Cascón A, Schiavi F, et al. MAX mutations cause hereditary and sporadic pheochromocytoma and paraganglioma. *Clin Cancer Res* 2012;18(10):2828–2837.

49. Welander J, Larsson C, Bäckdahl M, et al. Integrative genomics reveals frequent somatic NF1 mutations in sporadic pheochromocytomas. *Hum Mol Genet* 2012;21(26):5406–5416.

50. Pallai S, Gopalan V, Smith RA, et al. Updates on the genetics and the clinical impacts on phaeochromocytoma and paraganglioma in the new era. *Crit Rev Onc Hem* 2016;100:190–208.

51. Lenders JW, Eisenhofer G. Pathophysiology and diagnosis of disorders of the adrenal medulla: focus on pheochromocytoma. *Compr Physiol* 2014;4:691–713.

52. Eisenhofer G, Rivers G, Rosas AL, et al. Adverse drug reactions in patients with pheochromocytoma: incidence, prevention and management. *Drug Saf* 2007;30(11):1031–1062.

53. Lenders JW, Keiser HR, Goldstein DS, et al. Plasma metanephrines in the diagnosis of pheochromocytoma. *Ann Intern Med* 1995;123(2):101–109.

54. Lenders JW, Pacak K, Walther MM, et al. Biochemical diagnosis of pheochromocytoma: which test is best? *JAMA* 2002;287(11):1427–1434.

55. Eisenhofer G, Peitzsch M. Laboratory evaluation of pheochromocytoma and paraganglioma. *Clin Chem* 2014;60(12):1486–1499.

56. de Jong WH, Eisenhofer G, Post WJ, et al. Dietary influences on plasma and urinary metanephrines: implications for diagnosis of catecholamine-producing tumors. *J Clin Endocrinol Metab* 2009;94(8):2841–2849.

57. Deutschbein T, Unger N, Jaeger A, et al. Influence of various confounding variables and storage conditions on metanephrine and normetanephrine levels in plasma. *Clin Endocrinol (Oxf)* 2010;73:153–160.

58. Lenders JW, Willemsen JJ, Eisenhofer G, et al. Is supine rest necessary before blood sampling for plasma metanephrines? *Clin Chem* 2007;53:352–354.

59. Lenders JW, Pacak K, Huynh TT, et al. Low sensitivity of glucagon provocative testing for diagnosis of pheochromocytoma. *J Clin Endocrinol Metab* 2010;95(1):238–245.

60. Lenders JW, Duh QY, Eisenhofer G, et al. Pheochromocytoma and paraganglioma: an endocrine society clinical practice guideline. *J Clin Endo Met* 2014;99:1915–1942.

61. Ilias I, Pacak K. Anatomical and functional imaging of metastatic pheochromocytoma. *Ann N Y Acad Sci* 2004;1018:495–504.

62. Fishbein L. Pheochromocytoma and paraganglioma: genetics, diagnosis, and treatment. *Hematol Oncol Clin North Am* 2016;30(1):135–150.

63. González López MT, González SG, García ES, et al. Surgical excision with left atrial reconstruction of a primary functioning retrocardiac paraganglioma. *J Cardiothorac Surg* 2013;8:22.

64. Gowdamarajan A, Michler RE. Therapy for primary cardiac tumors: is there a role for heart transplantation? *Curr Opin Cardiol* 2000;15(2):121–125.

65. Jeevanandam V, Oz MC, Shapiro B, et al. Surgical management of cardiac pheochromocytoma. Resection versus transplantation. *Ann Surg* 1995;221(4):415–419.

66. Angelousi A, Kassi E, Zografos G, et al. Metastatic pheochromocytoma and paraganglioma. *Eur J Clin Invest* 2015;45(9):986–997.

67. Yu H, Wu Z, Cui Y, et al. Low-grade extraskeletal osteosarcoma of the mediastinum: report of a case and review of literature. *Int J Clin Exp Pathol* 2015;8(3):3279–3281.

68. Yamamoto Y, Kodama K, Ide Y, et al. Thymic and mediastinal lymph node metastasis of colon cancer. *Ann Thorac Surg* 2017;103(1):e13–e15.

69. Li Z, Jia H, Zhang B, et al. The clinical features, treatment, and prognosis of primary mediastinal malignant melanoma: a case report. *Medicine (Baltimore)* 2017;96(17):e6436.

70. Liu J, Song Z, Liu R, et al. Relapsed pleomorphic liposarcoma with mediastinal metastasis: a case report and review of the literature. *Zhongguo Fei Ai Za Zhi* 2017;20(5):361–365.

71. Bae SH, Hwang JH, Da Nam B, et al. Multiple ewing sarcoma/primitive neuroectodermal tumors in the mediastinum: a case report and literature review. *Medicine (Baltimore)* 2016;95(7):e2725.

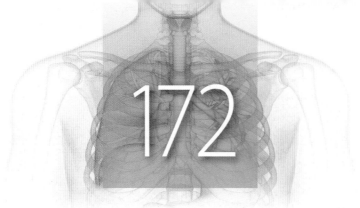

172

Mesenchymal Tumors of the Mediastinum

M. Blair Marshall ▪ Young K. Hong

INTRODUCTION

Primary mesenchymal tumors of the mediastinum are rare benign or malignant tumors that originate from various mesenchymal cells consisting of adipose, lymphatic, blood vessels, musculoskeletal, or fibroblasts (Table 172.1). While mesenchymal tumors may occur in other parts of the body, the incidence of these tumors is less than 5% to 10% of adult primary mediastinal tumors.[1] The usual presentation of majority of patients with these lesions is due to mass effect causing symptoms of chest pain, dyspnea, hoarseness, or cough. Surgical resection is the mainstay of treatment but is limited by the level of mediastinal involvement of the tissue at which time adjuvant therapy such as chemotherapy and radiation often plays an important role.

TUMORS OF ADIPOSE TISSUE

Various tumors that arise from adipose tissue include lipoma, lipoblastoma, and hibernomas which are benign lesions that predominate in the anterior mediastinum. Predominance in the anterior mediastinum is likely related to the increased fat in this area in contrast to other areas of the mediastinum. Spindle cell lipoma is another variant of lipoma that often can mimic liposarcoma on imaging with areas of nonadipose tissue mixture and requires a tissue diagnosis to differentiate benign spindle cell lipoma from malignant liposarcoma.[2] Morgagni hernias with a large quantity of omental fat in the mediastinum are often misdiagnosed as lipomas or liposarcomas of the mediastinum. Careful review of the films reveals a characteristic fatty pattern of omentum suggesting the true diagnosis (Fig. 172.1). In times of equivocal morphology of lipoma and well-differentiated liposarcoma, immunohistochemistry staining for MDM2 in liposarcoma may be helpful to make this distinction.[3]

Thymolipomas are another variant of rare tumor composed of mature adipose tissue and benign thymic tissue arising from thymus gland. They are benign neoplasms that lie quiescent until mass effect causing symptoms such as dyspnea or chest pain lead to its diagnosis.[4] Surgical resection is the mainstay of treatment for these lesions without the need for adjuvant radio- or chemotherapy with minimal recurrence after resection.

Liposarcoma, the malignant form of lipoma, has thick nodular septa with areas of nonadipose tissue within a predominately fatty lesion, which often show contrast enhancement on CT. Clinical presentations vary depending on location, age, and histology with cough,

TABLE 172.1 Primary Mesenchymal Tumors		
Tissue	**Benign**	**Malignant**
Adipose	Lipoma Lipoblastoma Hibernoma	Liposarcoma
Lymphatic	Lymphangioma Lymphangioleiomyomatosis	
Blood Vessels	Hemangioma Hemangiopericytoma	Hemangioendothelioma Angiosarcoma
Fibroblasts	Fibromatosis	Fibrosarcoma Malignant Fibrous Histiocytoma Inflammatory Fibrosarcoma
Skeletal	Chondroma	Osteosarcoma Chondrosarcoma
Muscular Striated Smooth	Leiomyoma Rhabdomyoma	Leiomyosarcoma Rhabdomyosarcoma

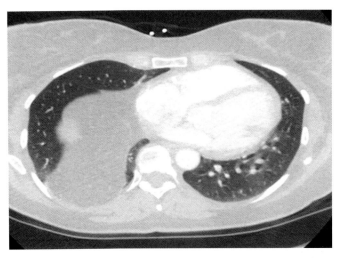

FIGURE 172.1 Cross-axial imaging of Morgagni hernia masquerading as lipoma versus liposarcoma.

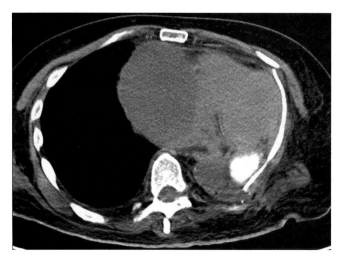

FIGURE 172.2 Cross-axial CT imaging of a 61-year-old male with a prior history of left pneumonectomy presenting with symptoms of hypoxia and cardiac tamponade from recurrent locally advanced intrapericardial leiomyosarcoma with invasion into the right atrium.

dysphagia, chest pain, and even superior vena cava syndrome while some are completely asymptomatic and found incidentally. While the majority of liposarcomas are located in anterior mediastinum, there are reports of being located in the posterior mediastinum as well. The average age of diagnosis ranges from 43 to 51 years of age.[5]

There are four different types of liposarcoma histologies including well-differentiated (45%), myxoid (35%), de-differentiated (15%), and pleomorphic cells (5%).[6] FDG-PET avidity of liposarcoma demonstrates biphasic signaling of SUV uptake that are dependent upon the grade of the tumor with more anaplastic histology having higher FDG-PET activity. Thus, fatty lesions of well-differentiated liposarcoma will present with low SUV uptake; whereas, high-grade pleomorphic cells demonstrate high SUV uptake.[7]

Surgical resection of liposarcoma is the main treatment. Radiotherapy is often administered as adjuvant therapy for positive margins or for those with unresectable lesions. Neoadjuvant/adjuvant Adriamycin and ifosfamide have also been used.[6]

Prognostic factors of liposarcoma involve the location of the primary tumor, with mediastinal tumors having a worse prognosis compared to subcutaneous or intramuscular tumors. This is likely related to the ability to get wider margins with subcutaneous chest wall lesions.[5] Tumor histology also correlates with prognosis with well-differentiated liposarcoma demonstrating less local recurrence or metastases while dedifferentiated and pleomorphic liposarcomas often have local recurrence rates of approximately 30% and metastatic disease in 17% and 32% of patients, respectively.[6] We have found that resection of metastatic disease to the mediastinum is of benefit when patients are symptomatic from the mass effect of their disease (Fig. 172.2).[8]

TUMORS OF LYMPHATIC TISSUE

Lymphangioma is a benign tumor that arises from malformations comprising focal proliferations of well-differentiated lymphatic tissue that present as multicystic or sponge-like accumulations. Majority of these lesions occur in the neck (75%) and axillary region (20%) with nearly 90% of cases diagnosed under the age of 2. Lymphangioma of the mediastinum is very rare with incidence <1% and are found in all three compartments of the mediastinum with predominance usually in the anterior compartment. There are three different histologies based upon the size of the lymphatic tissues involved: cystic (macrocystic), cavernous (microcystic), and finally capillary (super-microcystic).

Cystic lymphangioma is the most common while cavernous type is the rarest form of the disease.[9] Clinical presentation can vary from mild cough, dysphagia, or superior vena cava syndrome due to compression of mediastinal structures while some patients remain asymptomatic. Differential diagnosis in this setting should include Castleman lymphoma, thymic cyst, pericardial cyst, cystic teratoma, and cystic thymoma. MRI is the diagnostic tool of choice for lymphangioma with heterogenicity on T1-weighted images while the T2-weighted images have strong intensity reflecting their fluid content (Fig. 172.3).[10] With exception of rare case reports of FDG-PET avid lymphangioma that can mimic metastatic disease, these lesions are generally not FDG-PET avid.[11] The diagnosis of cystic lymphangioma is made by histology after biopsy. The mainstay treatment is complete surgical resection.

In cases where the cystic lymphangioma is unresectable either due to size or proximity to vital structures, sclerotherapy (OK-432 or bleomycin) has been utilized to decrease the size of lesion with 3 years follow-up.[12] A recent report of endobronchial ultrasound-guided transbronchial needle aspiration for unresectable disease did result in a successful decrease in the size of the cystic lymphangioma with 12-month follow-up.[13]

Lymphangioleiomyomatosis is another rare entity that is described by the proliferation of immature smooth muscle cells in the walls of airway, venules, and lymphatic vessels of the chest leading to obstruction of small airways and lymphatics causing pulmonary cyst formation, pneumothorax, and/or chylous effusion. The incidence ranges from 1 to 2.6 cases per 100,000 and has a predilection for women in the reproductive age more so than in postmenopausal women. Often patients present with emphysema, recurrent pneumothorax, and chylous effusion. CT scan of the chest reveals multiple well-defined thin-walled cysts, homogenously distributed and present throughout all lung zones with relative apical sparing. While transbronchial biopsy can be performed for a tissue diagnosis, the gold standard is a lung biopsy and histological examination using monoclonal antibody HMB 45 that specifically stains for lymphangioleiomyomatosis smooth-muscle cells.[14] There is an association with estrogen exposure and the pathophysiology of the lymphangioleiomyomatosis as estrogen receptors are found in the smooth muscle cells identified in patients affected with the disease. As a result, the treatment options are generally aimed at hormonal management by way of oophorectomy, progestin therapy, tamoxifen, and luteinizing hormone-releasing hormone. Role for

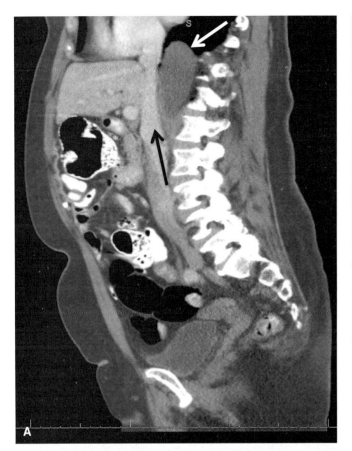

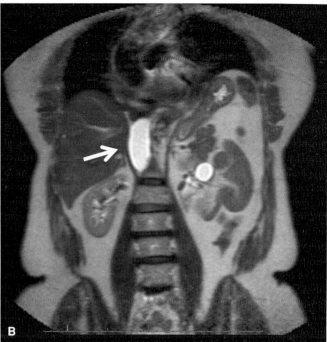

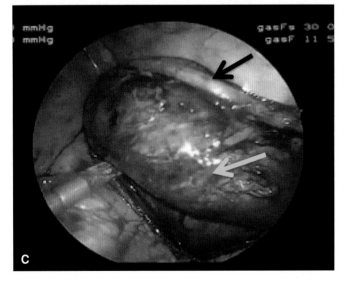

FIGURE 172.3 **A:** Sagittal CT image of lymphangioma (*white arrow*) adjacent to aorta anteriorly (*black arrow*). **B:** Coronal view of T2-weighted MRI revealing lymphangioma (*white arrow*). **C:** Intraoperative photo of thorascopic view of the right chest demonstrating lymphangioma (*green arrow*) with thoracic duct above (*black arrow*).

surgery in this setting is limited by the distributive nature of the disease and thus limited to pleurodesis of the lung for treatment of recurrent pneumothoraces. The only surgical option for potential cure is lung transplantation with improvement of FEV$_1$ post-transplant.

Castleman disease is an idiopathic lymphoproliferative disease often referred to as giant lymph node hyperplasia or angiofollicular lymph node that was initially described in 1956 (Fig. 172.4). It most often involves the thorax (75%) such as chest wall, tracheobronchial tree, mediastinum, and hilum followed by neck (15%) and abdomen (10%). There are three histologic types of Castleman disease that have different prognostic implications as a result. The first type is the hyaline-vascular type which are often benign, localized, mostly

asymptomatic lesions that are usually found incidentally or have mass effect symptoms of cough, dyspnea, and chest pain. These lesions are resectable with good prognosis and low recurrence outcome. The second type and third type are plasma cell type and mixed type, respectively, which are more aggressive forms of the disease. These are often multifocal involvement in nature that often involves multiple organs and lymph node stations. Patients with these types do present with constitutional symptoms and abnormal laboratory findings such as anemia, elevated ESR, polyclonal gammaglobinemia, hypoalbuminemia, bone marrow plasmacytosis, and thrombocytosis.[15]

Patients with localized Castleman disease have solitary, well-circumscribed contrast enhancement on CT. Three patterns were

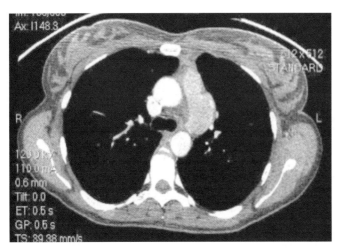

FIGURE 172.4 Cross-axial imaging of Castleman disease of the mediastinum. Indentation along the pleural margin is due to the phrenic nerve.

observed on CT or MR images: a solitary, noninvasive mass (50%); a dominant infiltrative mass with associated lymphadenopathy (40%); or matted lymphadenopathy without a dominant mass (10%).[16] MRI imaging reveals an isointense lesion on T1- and T2-weighted images. FDG-PET is a very sensitive imaging modality for Castleman disease compared to CT. There is moderate to high SUV uptake with

correlation of increased uptake and multicentric disease which is a less favorable prognostic factor and can progress to lymphoma or multiorgan failure.[17] The treatment is often systemic therapy with corticosteroids, anti-IL-6 receptor antibody, and/or chemotherapy given its multicentric involvement with varied response.

There are associated clinical abnormalities associated with Castleman disease that include POEMS syndrome (polyneuropathy, organomegaly, endocrinopathy, monoclonal gammopathy, and skin changes), paraneoplastic pemphigus, and Hodgkin disease. There is also a reported association with myasthenia gravis in patients with Castleman disease with reports of myasthenic crisis in 30% to 40% of postoperative patients requiring plasmapheresis.[18]

TUMORS OF BLOOD VESSELS

Hemangioma is a benign vascular neoplasm, congenital in origin, produces basic fibroblast growth factor, and involutes around 2 years of age. Vascular malformations may arise anywhere in body and can rarely involve the mediastinum representing less than 1% of all mediastinal tumors. The other forms of vascular tumors include angiomas (2%), hemangiofibromas (2%), fibroangioma (1%), fibrolipohemangioma (1%), venous hemangioma (1%), and arteriovenous malformation (1%).[19] Hemangioma and vascular malformations may be confused on imaging (Fig. 172.5). Vascular malformations do not secrete bFGF and do not spontaneously regress. For complex lesions,

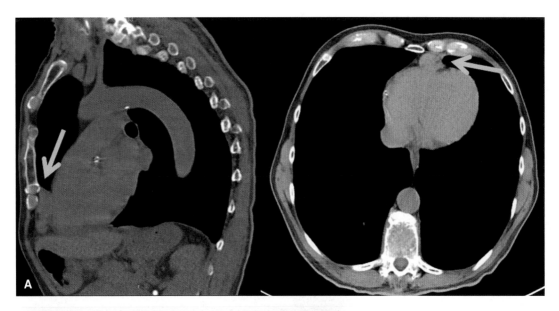

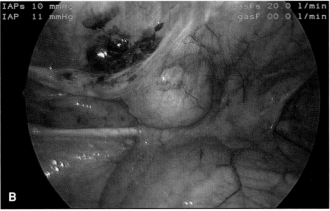

FIGURE 172.5 **A:** Sagittal and cross-axial CT image of arteriovenous malformation of anterior mediastinum. **B:** Thorascopic view of arteriovenous malformation of the anterior mediastinum.

sclerotherapy may play a significant role when surgical options are limited.[20] Hemangiomas appear as a proliferation of normal vascular elements with various amounts of interposed stromal elements such as fast, myxoid, and fibrous tissue with organized thrombi that may calcify as phleboliths. Presence of phleboliths, a fat component, and markedly high intensity of fat suppression T2-weighted image may be characteristics of hemangiomas.[21] CT imaging demonstrates heterogeneous and central contrast enhancement with pointed enhancements along the border of the tumor on the aortic phase of the CT.[22] The main treatment for hemangiomas are complete surgical resection when symptomatic. Radiotherapy can be used in situations where the tumor is adherent to vital structures whereas others advocate that a subtotal excision is sufficient if complete excision is deemed too hazardous.[23]

Hemangiopericytomas are vascular tumors that arise from pericytes in small vessels and are often confused with synovial sarcoma and solitary fibrous tumor due to shared similar histopathology of vascularity. Immunohistochemistry and electron microscopy are often required to delineate between them. The incidence of mediastinal hemangiopericytoma is limited to a few case reports in the literature. However, there are documented reports of distant metastases in 20% of patients, despite the low disease associated mortality. Malignant forms of hemangiopericytoma are recognized by the increased mitotic rate, tumor size, and foci of hemorrhage and necrosis.[24]

Angiosarcomas are rare malignant tumors that occur mostly in adults that arise from vascular endothelium of blood vessels. They account for less than 2% of all sarcomas.[25] There have only been 34 documented cases of primary angiosarcoma of the mediastinum in the literature with the majority of tumors being localized to the anterior mediastinum with clinical manifestations of chest pain, dyspnea, hemorrhagic pericarditis, swelling of face/neck, dizziness, and cough.[26] Some of the risk factors for angiosarcoma include radiation, vinyl chloride, Thorotrast, chronic lymphedema, or foreign bodies.[27] The sporadic forms are without clear source. It is important to distinguish angiosarcomas from epithelioid hemangioendotheliomas, a vascular endothelium tumor that originates from medium to large veins. Epithelioid hemangioendotheliomas are much less aggressive and considered low to moderate in malignant behavior compared to the aggressive angiosarcomas which have a high rate of recurrence and metastatic potential.[26] The age of patients diagnosed with primary angiosarcoma in the anterior mediastinum ranges from 5 to 66 years old with survival of 2 to 36.[28]

The treatment of choice for hemangiopericytoma and angiosarcoma is complete surgical resection as this offers the best chance cure whereas incomplete resections often recur. Thorascopic resections can be performed in some cases depending on the location and size of the lesion.[29] In the setting of a very large hemangiopericytoma, preoperative radiotherapy has shown marked improvement in vascularity that made complete surgical resection more feasible.[30] Some have obtained a preoperative angiogram to identify the feeding artery into the hemangiopericytoma and performed embolization followed by resection within 24 hours to decrease the morbidity of massive bleeding from resecting a highly vascularized tumor.[31] Chemotherapy is generally given in the setting of metastatic disease with the most effective chemotherapy agent being doxorubicin or Adriamycin with a 38% response rate. When combination chemotherapy is utilized with other drugs such as vincristine, cyclophosphamide, methotrexate, cisplatin, and/or dactinomycin, the reported response rate was 50% to 75%.[32] For patients with angiosarcoma and infantile hemangioma, there also has been evidence of some response to angiogenesis inhibitors as these tumors express increased expression of S6K. Rapamycin, which is an mTOR inhibitor, has shown some efficacy by blocking the mTORC-S6K pathway.[33]

TUMORS OF FIBROBLASTS

Fibromatosis (also called desmoid) are soft tissue masses, composed of highly differentiated fibroblast cells, with a rare incidence in the mediastinum. They have a tendency to infiltrate into surrounding tissue and form circumscribed lesions but do not metastasize. The aggressiveness of these lesions is between a solitary fibrous tumor and a fibrosarcoma.[34] Radiographic imaging using CT demonstrates an isodense lesion similar to skeletal muscle that becomes hyperdense on contrast phase. The aim of treatment is surgical resection with negative margins which may require reconstruction of mediastinal structures given its local aggressive tendency. Chemotherapy may serve a role in the neoadjuvant setting in lesions that are too large or are invading mediastinal structures or in the adjuvant setting with doxorubicin-dacarbazine with estimated complete/partial response upward of 50%.[35] Radiotherapy is utilized for patients with positive margins, patients with local recurrence, and as adjuvant therapy.[36]

Malignant fibrous histiocytoma are generally tumors that occur primarily in extremities (68%) and abdominal cavity (16%) with rare occurrence in the mediastinum.[37] Mean age at presentation is 50 years old and 62% are male. Clinical presentation may involve chest pain, back pain, fever, and general malaise.[38] They are reported to occur in anterior and posterior mediastinum with most lesions being primary de novo lesions while case reports have made an association with radiation and previous operations.[39] There are five histological types including (1) storiform-pleomorphic, (2) myxoid, (3) inflammatory, (4) giant, and (5) angiomatoid.[40] Malignant fibrous histiocytomas are FDG-PET avid with high SUV uptake and have a characteristic central metabolic defect that also correlates with decreased attenuation centrally noted on CT imaging and can be attributed to hemorrhage, necrosis, or myxomatous tissue.[41]

Given its aggressive pathology and poor prognosis, complete surgical resection is recommended with adjuvant combination chemotherapy. Cyclophosphamide, vincristine, Adriamycin, and dacarbazine (CYVADIC) have been used successfully with resultant complete remission. Adjuvant radiotherapy (50 Gy) can be delivered to the postoperative bed to decrease the chance of recurrence; however, there are significant side effects of this treatment.[42] Overall prognosis is very poor with regional recurrence rate of 50% and 5-year survival rates near 14%.[43]

TUMORS OF SKELETAL TISSUE

Chondromas are benign lesions that arise from hyaline cartilage that rarely present in the anterior mediastinum. They are thought to develop from rests of growth plate cartilage that proliferate and enlarge and present either as within medullary cavity of bone (enchondromas) or surface of bone (subperiosteal or juxtacortical chondromas).[44] They present radiographically on CT as solid, homogenous, and well-demarcated lesions.

Chondrosarcomas are very rare tumors made of cartilage with less than 10 documented cases of mediastinal chondrosarcoma in the literature. Initial presentation ranges from incidental finding to chest pain and dysphagia. They present in the fourth to seventh decade with slight 1.3:1 male-to-female predominance.[45] MRI reveals intermediate T1 intensity and heterogenous high T2 signal intensity with focal area of signal void related to foci of calcification. FDG-PET signals correlate correspondingly with the grade of the tumor and can be clearly detected with average SUV of 4.[46] Histologic features include biphasic cell population with mature and immature cartilaginous elements, with spindle cell population. Chondrosarcoma present more often in the posterior mediastinum with differential diagnosis that include neuroblastoma, schwannoma, neurofibroma, and ganglioneuroma.[47] Surgical resection with adjuvant chemoradiation is generally used with 5-year survival rate greater than 60%.[48]

Osteosarcoma of the mediastinum is a rare malignancy with limited case reports in the literature. The average size of tumors ranges from 7 to 16 cm with median size of 10 cm and occur most often in the anterior or superior mediastinum.[49] The mass usually arises from rib, scapula, or clavicle with heterogeneous appearance on CT and MRI consistent with necrosis, hemorrhage, and ossification. FDG-PET appear to be superior to bone scintigraphy in localizing osteosarcoma lesions and may serve in staging/treatment planning.[50] Histologic analysis of the mass reveals formation of osteoid matrix that establishes the diagnosis of osteosarcoma. Some predisposing factors associated with osteogenic sarcoma include prior trauma, chemoradiation, and/or calcification. Mediastinal osteosarcomas are treated with neoadjuvant chemotherapy followed by adjuvant chemotherapy with radiotherapy for local control for residual disease post resection.[45] Overall survival is very poor with estimated 5-year survival of 15% with metastatic lesions noted in 70% of patients.[48]

TUMORS OF MUSCULAR TISSUE

Leiomyomas in the mediastinum are very rare tumors that arise from the striated muscle of the esophagus, as well as great vessels such as inferior vena cava, pulmonary artery, and superior vena cava (Fig. 172.6). Clinical presentation is usually due to mass effect upon structures in the mediastinum and can present as superior vena cava syndrome.[51,52] Histologic diagnosis reveals monomorphic spindle cells with blunt-ended nuclei, arranged interlacing fascicles with the specific immune marker, muscle actin, being present.[52] Treatment is complete resection without need for adjuvant chemotherapy or radiation given its low local recurrence rates. If leiomyoma is a very vascularized mass, one can utilize embolization of a large leiomyoma feeding vessel to minimize blood loss during surgery.[51]

Leiomyosarcomas are very aggressive sarcoma of the mediastinum arising from striated muscles. Histologic features can be similar to thymomas, thymic carcinomas, malignant schwannomas, and malignant histiocytomas and thus definitive diagnosis relies on immunohistochemistry staining of actin, desmin, and vimentin

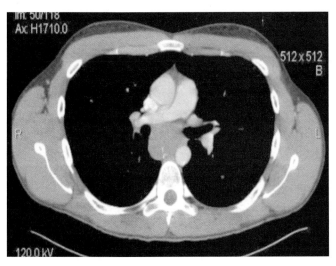

FIGURE 172.6 Cross-axial imaging of patient with leiomyoma.

for differentiation.[53] While the grade of sarcoma does affect overall survival, complete resection is the mainstay of therapy and serves as the best prognostic factor. Local recurrence rates however, can be as high as 64% despite complete resection and thus there is a need for improved adjuvant therapy.[48]

Rhabdomyoma is a rare tumor that accounts for 2% of all tumors with skeletal muscle differentiation and is distinguished as being cardiac or extracardiac. Cardiac rhabdomyomas are most common in pediatric population and are considered hamartomatous with associations often with tuberous sclerosis.[54] Extracardiac rhabdomyomas are classified into three clinical subtypes: adult (50%), fetal (40%), and congenital (10%) with majority occurring in the head and neck region.[55] Consisting of cells with eosinophilic granular cytoplasm resembling cross-striations of myofibrils, immunohistochemistry reveals desmin, actin, myoglobin, and fetal myosin. The age range for diagnosis of mediastinal rhabdomyomas is 68 to 80 with predominately male-to-female ratio of 3–6:1.[54] Complete resection alone is sufficient for management of these lesions; however, incomplete resection may lead to local recurrence despite their slow growing biology and thus surveillance is warranted.

Rhabdomyosarcoma presents in a wide variety of organs including lung, bronchi, mediastinum, heart, and chest wall with presentation in the fifth to seventh decade of life.[45,56] Depending on the location of the mass, patients can present with symptoms of cough, dyspnea, hemoptysis, pneumothorax, pain, arrhythmias, and heart failure. Radiographic presentation on CT reveals heterogenous attenuation within a large mass consistent with necrosis.[45] FDG-PET can be used to stage patients with rhabdomyosarcoma and some studies support that this is superior to conventional imaging modalities such as CT when analyzing lymph node and bone involvement.[11] Treatment is mainly chemotherapy utilizing vincristine, dactinomycin, and cyclophosphamide, with surgery and radiation reserved for limited role if the lesion is localized and/or residual disease is present after local resection. Important prognostic factors in rhabdomyosarcoma patients are age, tumor size, extent of disease, and resection.[57]

CONCLUSION

Mesenchymal tumors of the mediastinum are very rare. Most small lesions are asymptomatic. As the lesions grow, patients will often develop vague symptoms such as chest pain, shortness of breath, etc. Given the breadth of possibilities for diagnosis, CT, MR, and PET can play complimentary roles in evaluation of the mass. Depending on location, primary excision via VATS can be performed for small, well-situated lesions if the diagnosis is unclear after imaging. For larger tumors, we often perform percutaneous biopsies in the office as image guidance may not be needed for these larger tumors (Fig. 172.7). Similarly for resection, a sternotomy, thoracosternotomy, or thoracotomy will be chosen based on the location of the tumor and structures involved. Given the diversity of possibilities for tumors in the mediastinum, diagnosis and management should be individualized according to the patient's particular characteristics. Prognosis for these lesions will parallel similar tumors or similar pathology in other more commonly occurring locations. However, because of the location within the mediastinum and the inability to obtain wide margins due to proximity to vital structures, typically the prognosis is worse. The use of neoadjuvant or adjuvant therapy will also parallel similar pathologies in other locations. Given the importance of all of these considerations in the management of these complex tumors, a multidisciplinary approach will often be the best way to address the complex issues that arise with these lesions. Surgical

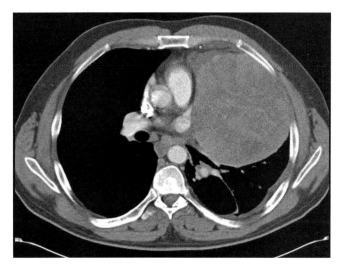

FIGURE 172.7 Cross-axial imaging of primitive neuroectodermal tumor (PNET) with percutaneous core needle biopsy for diagnosis prior to resection.

resection remains the main therapy for most of the tumor types with adjuvant chemotherapy and radiotherapy having a role limited to incomplete and metastatic settings.

REFERENCES

1. Macchiarini P, Ostertag H. Uncommon primary mediastinal tumours. *Lancet Oncol* 2004;5(2):107–118.
2. Oaks J, Margolis DJ. Spindle cell lipoma of the mediastinum: a differential consideration for liposarcoma. *J Thorac Imaging* 2007;22(4):355–357.
3. Shimada S, Ishizawa T, Ishizawa K, et al. The value of MDM2 and CDK4 amplification levels using real-time polymerase chain reaction for the differential diagnosis of liposarcomas and their histologic mimickers. *Hum Pathol* 2006;37(9):1123–1129.
4. Aghajanzadeh M, Alavi A, Pourrasouli Z, et al. Giant mediastinal thymolipoma in 35-year-old women. *J Cardiovasc Thorac Res* 2011;3(2):67–70.
5. Ortega P, Suster D, Falconieri G, et al. Liposarcomas of the posterior mediastinum: clinicopathologic study of 18 cases. *Mod Pathol* 2015;28(5):721–731.
6. Hahn HP, Fletcher CD. Primary mediastinal liposarcoma: clinicopathologic analysis of 24 cases. *Am J Surg Pathol* 2007;31(12):1868–1874.
7. Hoshi M, Oebisu N, Takada J, et al. A case of dedifferentiated liposarcoma showing a biphasic pattern on 2-deoxy-2-F(18)-fluoro-d-glucose positron emission tomography/computed tomography. *Rare Tumors* 2013;5(2):95–97.
8. David EA, Marshall MB. Review of chest wall tumors: a diagnostic, therapeutic, and reconstructive challenge. *Semin Plast Surg* 2011;25(1):16–24.
9. Faul JL, Berry GJ, Colby TV, et al. Thoracic lymphangiomas, lymphangiectasis, lymphangiomatosis, and lymphatic dysplasia syndrome. *Am J Respir Crit Care Med* 2000;161(3 Pt 1):1037–1046.
10. Shaffer K, Rosado-de-Christenson ML, Patz EF Jr, et al. Thoracic lymphangioma in adults: CT and MR imaging features. *AJR Am J Roentgenol* 1994;162(2):283–289.
11. Volker T, Denecke T, Steffen I, et al. Positron emission tomography for staging of pediatric sarcoma patients: results of a prospective multicenter trial. *J Clin Oncol* 2007;25(34):5435–5441.
12. Desir A, Ghaye B, Duysinx B, et al. Percutaneous sclerotherapy of a giant mediastinal lymphangioma. *Eur Respir J* 2008;32(3):804–806.
13. Choi SH, Kim L, Lee KH, et al. Mediastinal lymphangioma treated using endobronchial ultrasound-guided transbronchial needle aspiration. *Respiration* 2012;84(6):518–521.
14. Hohman DW, Noghrehkar D, Ratnayake S. Lymphangioleiomyomatosis: a review. *Eur J Intern Med* 2008;19(5):319–324.
15. Jongsma TE, Verburg RJ, Geelhoed-Duijvestijn PH. Castleman's disease: a rare lymphoproliferative disorder. *Eur J Intern Med* 2007;18(2):87–89.
16. McAdams HP, Rosado-de-Christenson M, Fishback NF, et al. Castleman disease of the thorax: radiologic features with clinical and histopathologic correlation. *Radiology* 1998;209(1):221–228.
17. Lee ES, Paeng JC, Park CM, et al. Metabolic characteristics of Castleman disease on 18F-FDG PET in relation to clinical implication. *Clin Nucl Med* 2013;38(5):339–342.
18. Ishikawa K, Kato T, Aragaki M, et al. A case of Castleman's disease with myasthenia gravis. *Ann Thorac Cardiovasc Surg* 2014;20:585–588.
19. Davis JM, Mark GJ, Greene R. Benign blood vascular tumors of the mediastinum. Report of four cases and review of the literature. *Radiology* 1978;126(3):581–587.
20. Fishman SJ. Vascular anomalies of the mediastinum. *Semin Pediatr Surg* 1999;8(2):92–98.
21. Sakurai K, Hara M, Ozawa Y, et al. Thoracic hemangiomas: imaging via CT, MR, and PET along with pathologic correlation. *J Thorac Imaging* 2008;23(2):114–1120.
22. Seline TH, Gross BH, Francis IR. CT and MR imaging of mediastinal hemangiomas. *J Comput Assist Tomogr* 1990;14(5):766–768.
23. Cohen AJ, Sbaschnig RJ, Hochholzer L, et al. Mediastinal hemangiomas. *Ann Thorac Surg* 1987;43(6):656–659.
24. Espat NJ, Lewis JJ, Leung D, et al. Conventional hemangiopericytoma: modern analysis of outcome. *Cancer* 2002;95(8):1746–1751.
25. Kardamakis D, Bouboulis N, Ravazoula P, et al. Primary hemangiosarcoma of the mediastinum. *Lung Cancer* 1996;16(1):81–86.
26. Weissferdt A, Kalhor N, Suster S, et al. Primary angiosarcomas of the anterior mediastinum: a clinicopathologic and immunohistochemical study of 9 cases. *Hum Pathol* 2010;41(12):1711–1717.
27. Lucas DR. Angiosarcoma, radiation-associated angiosarcoma, and atypical vascular lesion. *Arch Pathol Lab Med* 2009;133(11):1804–1849.
28. Fong Y, Coit DG, Woodruff JM, et al. Lymph node metastasis from soft tissue sarcoma in adults. Analysis of data from a prospective database of 1772 sarcoma patients. *Ann Surg* 1993;217(1):72–77.
29. Odaka M, Nakada T, Asano H, et al. Thoracoscopic resection of a mediastinal venous hemangioma: report of a case. *Surg Today* 2011;41(10):1455–1457.
30. Jalal A, Jeyasingham K. Massive intrathoracic extrapleural haemangiopericytoma: deployment of radiotherapy to reduce vascularity. *Eur J Cardiothorac Surg* 1999;16(3):378–381.
31. Morandi U, , De Santis M, et al. Preoperative embolization in surgical treatment of mediastinal hemangiopericytoma. *Ann Thorac Surg* 2000;69(3):937–939.
32. Rusch VW, Shuman WP, Schmidt R, et al. Massive pulmonary hemangiopericytoma. An innovative approach to evaluation and treatment. *Cancer* 1989;64(9):1928–1936.
33. Du W, Gerald D, Perruzzi CA, et al. Vascular tumors have increased p70 S6-kinase activation and are inhibited by topical rapamycin. *Lab Invest* 2013;93(10):1115–1127.
34. Hoeffel C, Floquet J, Regent D, et al. Periesophageal mediastinal fibromatosis. *Abdom Imaging* 2000;25(3):235–238.
35. Patel SR, Evans HL, Benjamin RS. Combination chemotherapy in adult desmoid tumors. *Cancer* 1993;72(11):3244–3247.
36. Sherman NE, Romsdahl M, Evans H, et al. Desmoid tumors: a 20-year radiotherapy experience. *Int J Radiat Oncol Biol Phys* 1990;19(1):37–40.
37. Nishida T, Nishiyama N, Kawata Y, et al. Mediastinal malignant fibrous histiocytoma developing from a foreign body granuloma. *Jpn J Thorac Cardiovasc Surg* 2005;53(10):583–586.
38. Murakawa T, Nakajima J, Fukami T, et al. Malignant fibrous histiocytoma in the anterior mediastinum. *Jpn J Thorac Cardiovasc Surg* 2001;49(12):722–727.
39. Satomi Y, Watanabe M, Kaneko T, et al. Radiation-induced malignant fibrous histiocytoma of the maxilla. *Odontology* 2011;99(2):203–208.
40. Al-Agha OM, Igbokwe AA. Malignant fibrous histiocytoma: between the past and the present. *Arch Pathol Lab Med* 2008;132(6):1030–1035.
41. Choi BH, Yoon SH, Lee S, et al. Primary malignant fibrous histiocytoma in mediastinum: imaging with (18)F-FDG PET/CT. *Nucl Med Mol Imaging* 2012;46(4):304–307.
42. Eckstein R, Gossner W, Rienmuller R. Primary malignant fibrous histiocytoma of the left atrium. Surgical and chemotherapeutic management. *Br Heart J* 1984;52(3):354–357.
43. Weiss SW, Enzinger FM. Malignant fibrous histiocytoma: an analysis of 200 cases. *Cancer* 1978;41(6):2250–2266.
44. Shrivastava V, Vundavalli S, Smith D, et al. A chondroma of the anterior mediastinum. *Clin Radiol* 2006;61(12):1065–1066.
45. Gladish GW, Sabloff BM, Munden RF, et al. Primary thoracic sarcomas. *Radiographics* 2002;22(3):621–637.
46. Brenner W, Conrad EU, Eary JF. FDG PET imaging for grading and prediction of outcome in chondrosarcoma patients. *Eur J Nucl Med Mol Imaging* 2004;31(2):189–195.
47. Suster S, Moran CA. Malignant cartilaginous tumors of the mediastinum: clinicopathological study of six cases presenting as extraskeletal soft tissue masses. *Hum Pathol* 1997;28(5):588–594.
48. Burt M. Primary malignant tumors of the chest wall. The Memorial Sloan-Kettering Cancer Center experience. *Chest Surg Clin N Am* 1994;4(1):137–154.
49. Hishida T, Yoshida J, Nishimura M, et al. Extraskeletal osteosarcoma arising in anterior mediastinum: brief report with a review of the literature. *J Thorac Oncol* 2009;4(7):927–929.
50. Quartuccio N, Treglia G, Salsano M, et al. The role of Fluorine-18-Fluorodeoxyglucose positron emission tomography in staging and restaging of patients with osteosarcoma. *Radiol Oncol* 2013;47(2):97–102.
51. Baldo X, Sureda C, Gimferrer JM, et al. Primary mediastinal leiomyoma: an angiographic study and embolisation of the feeding vessels to improve the surgical approach. *Eur J Cardiothorac Surg* 1997;11(3):574–576.
52. Ouadnouni Y, Achir A, Bekarsabein S, et al. Primary mediastinal leiomyoma: a case report. *Cases J* 2009;2:8555.
53. Labarca E, Zapico A, Ríos B, et al. Superior vena cava syndrome due to a leiomyosarcoma of the anterior mediastinum: a case report and literature overview. *Int J Surg Case Rep* 2014;5(12):984–987.
54. Kuschill-Dziurda J, Mastalerz L, Grzanka P, et al. Rhabdomyoma as a tumor of the posterior mediastinum. *Pol Arch Med Wewn* 2009;119(9):599–602.
55. Willis J, Abdul-Karim FW, di Sant'Agnese PA. Extracardiac rhabdomyomas. *Semin Diagn Pathol* 1994;11(1):15–25.
56. Hui KS, Green LK, Schmidt WA. Primary cardiac rhabdomyosarcoma: definition of a rare entity. *Am J Cardiovasc Pathol* 1988;2(1):19–29.
57. Kattan J, Culine S, Terrier-Lacombe MJ, et al. Paratesticular rhabdomyosarcoma in adult patients: 16-year experience at Institut Gustave-Roussy. *Ann Oncol* 1993;4(10):871–875.

MEDIASTINAL CYSTS

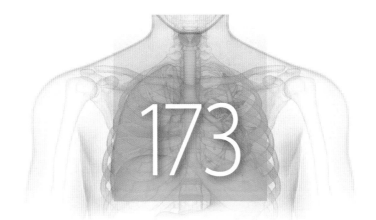

Foregut Cysts of the Mediastinum in Infants and Children

Timothy Brand ■ Jason Michael Long

Cystic lesions of the mediastinum belong to a group of congenital anomalies. The term "bronchopulmonary foregut malformations," coined by Gerle et al.,[1] initially referred to pulmonary sequestration with gastrointestinal communication. It has now grown to encompass a spectrum of disorders which include pulmonary sequestrations, congenital pulmonary airway malformation (CPAM) (formerly termed congenital cystic adenomatoid malformations [CCAMs]), congenital lobar emphysema, and foregut duplication cysts.[2] Foregut duplication cysts can be further divided into bronchogenic cysts, enteric cysts, and neuroenteric cysts. This chapter will focus specifically on bronchogenic and enteric cysts.

INCIDENCE

Foregut duplication cysts are a rare but clinically significant entity. Primary cysts represent 25% of all masses of the mediastinum. Foregut cysts are the most common and represent 50% of all primary cysts.[3] This is further delineated into bronchogenic cysts representing 50% to 60% and enteric cysts representing 7% to 15%.[4,5] Although esophageal cysts represent 10% to 15% of all congenital duplication cysts of the gastrointestinal tract, the estimated prevalence is exceedingly low at 0.0122%.[6] Several studies have examined the specific incidence in the pediatric population and there is not a unified consensus about distribution among male and female patients. Studies have found a slightly higher predilection in females,[5,7] others have found a higher incidence in males than

females,[8] and still others have found equal distribution among males and females.[3,9]

EMBRYOLOGY AND ETIOLOGY

The primitive foregut gives rise to the pharynx, respiratory tract, and upper portion of the gastrointestinal tract from the esophagus to the duodenum at the ampulla of Vater. Between day 26 and day 40 of gestation there is a ventral and dorsal division of the primitive foregut. The ventral segment develops into the tracheobronchial tree while the dorsal segment eventually becomes the esophagus.[10] Bronchogenic cysts are a result of abnormal budding of the bronchial tree. It has been theorized that the timing and severity of the embryologic insult determines the morphology of the final lesion with a minor localized insult being responsible for lesions like bronchogenic cysts.[11] These are most often located in the middle or superior mediastinum of the right chest. Their position is likely determined by the timing of the insult with an earlier insult resulting in the cyst being within the mediastinum and a later insult results in a cyst within the lung tissue itself.[10] Two-thirds of all bronchogenic cysts are located in the mediastinum. During this same time period esophageal duplication cysts occur if there is failure of appropriate vacuolization of the esophagus.[8] Failure of the vacuoles to coalesce results in an intramural cyst. Esophageal duplication cysts are more common on the right side of the chest and are most often associated with the distal portion of the esophagus. Theories about the exact cause or insult point to ischemia, trauma, adhesions, or infection during lung development.[2]

CLINICAL PRESENTATION

The clinical presentation of foregut cysts varies significantly and is dependent upon the size, location, and presence of communication with other structures or cysts via fistulae. Presentation is dependent upon many factors including age at presentation, anatomic location, and the histologic makeup of the cyst. Patients may be asymptomatic or present with incidental findings on chest radiography. Approximately two-thirds of patients have symptoms upon initial presentation that are associated with the mass effect of the lesion. The most common presenting complaints include chest pain, cough, and dyspnea. Symptoms may also manifest as a life-threatening episode in children with associated dyspnea, wheezing, stridor, hemoptysis, or cyanosis due to compression of the main airways. These lesions may also present with chest pain and/or associated respiratory complaints such as cough, recurrent asthma, or pneumonia. Gastrointestinal symptoms such as dysphagia, nausea, vomiting, anorexia, weight loss, and/or gastrointestinal bleeding have been reported. These symptoms may again be related to the mass effect or symptoms, such as gastrointestinal bleeding, that may be related to active gastric tissue within the cyst.

The anatomic location of these malformations may be quite variable. Sulzer and colleagues'[12] review of 40 cysts in all age groups found that two-thirds of the cysts were located in the upper half of the mediastinum and often associated with the trachea or the tracheal bifurcation. When they were found in the lower half of the mediastinum, the lesions were associated with the esophagus. St-Georges and colleagues[13] reported that 22 of 66 bronchogenic cysts were found in the middle mediastinum and 43 of 66 were found in the posterior mediastinum. Cysts have also been located intrapericardially, intrathymically, and in the region of the paravertebral sulcus. They have been excised from within the pulmonary ligament and may reside outside the mediastinum, with numerous examples of subcutaneous bronchogenic cysts. These cysts tend to be found in the suprasternal area and scapular region.

The age at presentation may range from the prenatal period into late adulthood. Reviews of bronchogenic cysts by St-Georges et al.[13] (n = 86) and Suen et al.[14] (n = 42) revealed that symptoms were present in 72%, 50%, and 94% of patients, respectively. The most common complaint was chest pain. Nobuhara and colleagues[15] reviewed 68 children and found that 20% were asymptomatic and the majority had either respiratory (54%) or gastrointestinal (13%) complaints. Ribet and colleagues[16] report that children with bronchogenic malformations are more often symptomatic from compressive symptoms than adults (70.8% versus 60%). They believe this is because the cysts in children tend to be situated above and at the level of the hilum. Snyder and colleagues[17] described 34 infants and children with mediastinal foregut cysts. The locations of these cysts are shown in Table 173.1. Of the total, 23 children had bronchogenic cysts and 11 had enteric cysts; 12 were asymptomatic. Most of the others developed symptoms related to the location of the cyst and presented with symptoms of pneumonia, major airway obstruction, or esophageal obstruction (Table 173.1).

More recently, Esme et al.[18] reported on 32 patients with mediastinal cysts—12 of which were bronchogenic. The most common symptom was chest pain followed by dyspnea. Ten of twelve cysts were located in the middle mediastinum. Regardless of the presentation, further workup and a planned surgical excision is necessary when a foregut malformation is suspected.

TABLE 173.1 Mediastinal Foregut Cysts: Clinical Presentation in 34 Children

Asymptomatic mediastinal masses	12
Congenital heart disease	3
Asthma	3
Acute abdominal pain	1
Cystic fibrosis	1
Routine preoperative radiograph	4
Airway obstruction (cough, wheeze, and stridor)	8
Pneumonia	8
Acute, unresolving	2
Recurrent	6
Dysphagia (choking and vomiting)	3
Unusual esophageal duplication	3
Severe neonatal respiratory distress	1
Hematemesis, recurrent pneumonia	1
Chest pain	1

RADIOGRAPHIC INVESTIGATION

STANDARD RADIOGRAPHY

Imaging is the initial step in evaluation after presentation with any of the aforementioned symptoms. Standard chest radiographs are >90% sensitive but specificity varies from 20% to 70%.[7] Pulmonary bronchogenic cysts have the appearance of a well-defined mass (Fig. 173.1) with water density. If there is communication with a bronchus, air–fluid levels may be evident. Mediastinal bronchogenic cysts may

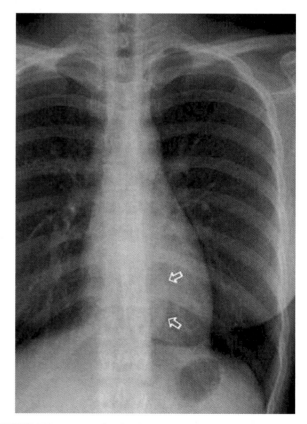

FIGURE 173.1 *Arrows* identify a bronchogenic cyst with a mass-like appearance. (Reprinted from Ko SF, Hsieh MJ, Lin JW, et al. Bronchogenic cyst of the esophagus: clinical and imaging features of seven cases. *Clin Imaging* 2006;30: 309–314. Copyright © 2006 Elsevier. With permission.)

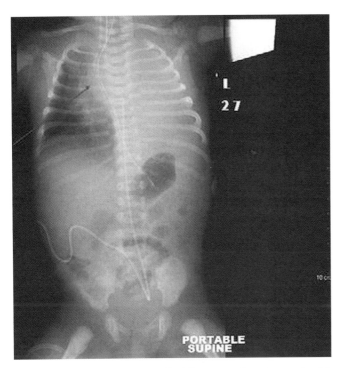

FIGURE 173.2 Mass compressing the left mainstem bronchus causing left lung collapse. (Reprinted from Petroze R, McGahren, ED. Pediatric Chest II; Benign Tumors and Cysts. *Surg Clin N Am* 2012;92:645–658. Copyright © 2012 Elsevier. With permission.)

appear as ill-defined masses in the middle or posterior mediastinum. Depending on the location of the foregut cyst, the chest radiograph findings may mimic adenopathy, especially if the cyst is associate with the hilum. Mass effect by the cyst can cause lobar or lung collapse (Fig. 173.2) and postobstructive consolidation. Esophageal duplication cysts may be suspected if there is mediastinal widening, and/or tracheal compression seen on plain chest radiography.[8]

CONTRAST STUDIES

Complaint of dysphagia or dysphonia may prompt a contrasted swallow study such as an esophagram. Mass effect by a compressive lesion can be seen as extrinsic compression which appears as a defect in the contour of the outlined esophagus (Fig. 173.3). Enteric duplication cysts which have communication with the esophagus may be demonstrated by an esophagram. However, this study has largely been replaced by CT scan because it is nondiagnostic and does not delineate the mass.

ULTRASONOGRAPHY

With advances in imaging technology, endoscopic ultrasound (EUS) has established a more significant role recently. Better quality images, improvements in technology, and improved operator skill have led to an increase in usage of this imaging modality. However, CT scan and MRI remains the better diagnostic tools. EUS can clearly delineate size, layer of origin, and relationship to the esophagus when evaluating foregut cysts which aids in determining if esophageal cysts are intramural or extramural, as depicted in Figure 173.4. Routine EUS FNA is not advocated in certain circumstances with significantly abnormal findings and FNA may be prudent. Ultrasound also plays a role during fetal development as antenatal ultrasound technique and technology continues to improve. Foregut duplication cysts appear

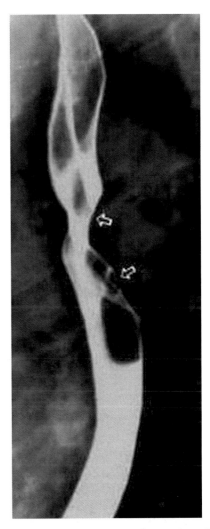

FIGURE 173.3 Esophagram revealing mass effect as indicated by the *arrows*. (Reprinted from Ko SF, Hsieh MJ, Lin JW, et al. Bronchogenic cyst of the esophagus: clinical and imaging features of seven cases. *Clin Imaging* 2006;30: 309–314. Copyright © 2006 Elsevier. With permission.)

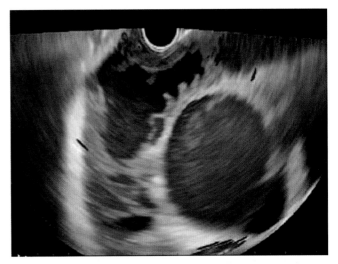

FIGURE 173.4 EUS shows hypoechoic cystic/solid findings associated with the muscularis propria of the esophagus. (From Han C, Lin R, Yu J, et al. A case report of esophageal bronchogenic cyst and review of the literature with an emphasis on endoscopic ultrasonography appearance. *Medicine (Baltimore)* 2016;95:1–6.)

as thin-walled single cystic structures on antenatal ultrasound. However, there is significant overlap in the appearance of all types of bronchopulmonary malformations on this type of imaging. Therefore, an accurate diagnosis of the type of malformation may be difficult, but the diagnosis of significant lesions contributing to a poor prognosis can guide an in utero intervention at some centers. Although this clinical scenario is more often associated with CPAM or sequestration, there are extreme cases involving bronchogenic cysts.

COMPUTERIZED TOMOGRAPHY

CT scans have become ubiquitous in the diagnosis of the greater spectrum of disease. This imaging modality lends itself to the diagnosis of foregut cysts as it provides significantly more information than plain chest radiography. CT delineates the lesion and the relationships to surrounding structures. Bronchogenic cysts typically appear as well-defined, thin-walled, nonenhancing cystic masses (Fig. 173.5). They may be in the lung parenchyma but more often the right paratracheal or subcarinal regions. Bronchogenic cysts are classically described as having water density (0 to 20 HU). However, one study found varying densities with attenuation values ranging from 15 to 48 HU with a mean of 26.6 HU.[7] Significant variability in the contents of these cysts contributes to the true lack of attenuation values. This has been attributed to the presence of highly proteinaceous contents such as blood, mucus, anthracotic pigment, or calcium oxalate. The variability in the contents of the cyst may further complicate and obscure a true diagnosis. However, CT allows preoperative planning by elucidating the anatomy of the lesion to be excised as well as the relationships to surrounding vital structures.

MAGNETIC RESONANCE IMAGING

Similar to CT scan, MRI is becoming a more utilized imaging modality, especially when determination of anatomic relationships are important as in preoperative planning. The advantage of MRI over CT scan in children is similarity in image fidelity without the radiation exposure. However, MRI may prove difficult in children as it takes significantly more time and motion creates artifact. Therefore, sedation or anesthesia may be required which adds risk to this

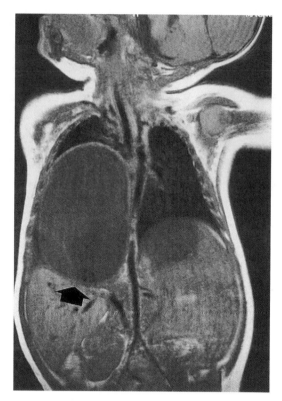

FIGURE 173.6 MRI showing a very large esophageal duplication cyst, indicated by the *arrow*, exerting mass effect on the right lung and mediastinum. (Reprinted from Williams HJ, Johnson KJ. Imaging of congenital cystic lung lesions. *Paediatr Respir Rev* 2002;3:120–127. Copyright © 2002 Elsevier. With permission.)

method. The contents of the cyst will determine the signal intensity. The presence of blood or proteinaceous material will demonstrate variable intensity on T1-weighted images. These cysts usually have a homogenous appearance on T2-weighted images (Fig. 173.6). Antenatal MRI can be useful as normal fetal lung tissue has a homogenous high signal intensity on T2-weighted images while lung lesions tend to show increased intensity when compared to normal lung.

PATHOLOGY

Bronchopulmonary foregut malformations share a common origin in that they are all related to an insult in early lung development leading to abnormal budding of the primitive foregut. The common timing and embryonic origin of bronchogenic and esophageal duplication cysts creates a challenge in determining whether the origin is tracheobronchial or esophageal. Therefore, diagnosis of the type of cyst present is made only after surgical resection. The cysts are subdivided based on their histology. Bronchogenic cysts are typically lined with ciliated columnar epithelium and are filled with thick mucus. The walls are composed of hyaline cartilage, smooth muscle, mucus glands, and nerve fibers (Figs. 173.7 and 173.8).[8] It has been proposed that differentiation be based on the components of the cyst wall rather than the epithelium. Some authors advocate that bronchogenic cysts may be differentiated by the presence of cartilage or bronchial glands in the cyst wall. However, a review of bronchogenic cysts by St-Georges et al.,[13] demonstrated variable presence of cartilage (43%), bronchial glands (40.6%), and smooth muscle (59.3%), respectively. There is rarely communication between the bronchogenic cyst and the airway; rather, they are densely adhered

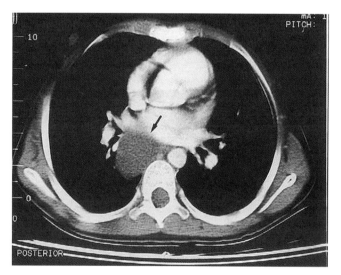

FIGURE 173.5 CT scan reveals bronchogenic cyst as a well-defined soft tissue density with smooth borders as indicated by the *arrow*. (Reprinted from Williams HJ, Johnson KJ. Imaging of congenital cystic lung lesions. *Paediatr Respir Rev* 2002;3:120–127. Copyright © 2002 Elsevier. With permission.)

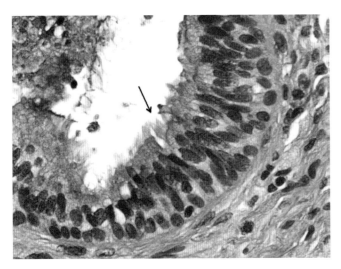

FIGURE 173.7 Cyst lining demonstrating pseudostratified ciliated columnar respiratory epithelium as indicated by the *arrow*. (From Altieri MS, Zheng R, Pryor AD, et al. Esophageal bronchogenic cyst and review of the literature. *Surg Endosc* 2015;29:3010–3015. Copyright © 2015 Springer Science+Business Media. With permission of Springer.)

to it. However, if there is a communication with the airway which has sealed over time, an infection within the cysts may cause the communication to reopen, creating respiratory symptoms. Esophageal duplication cysts are usually attached to, or within, the wall of the esophagus (extramural and intramural, respectively). It is estimated that approximately 10% of these cysts communicate with the esophageal lumen. Histologic findings of esophageal duplication cysts are characterized by smooth muscle cells covered with a lining of squamous, columnar, cuboidal, pseudostratified, ciliated epithelium, or some combination of these types.[8] Esophageal duplication cysts may be associated with other anomalies such as intestinal duplications, esophageal atresia, and fistula. Both bronchogenic and esophageal duplication cysts can be associated with spinal abnormalities. Unfortunately, up to 20% of mediastinal foregut cysts lack histologic features as they have been obliterated possibly due to hemorrhage or previous infection (Strollo et al.[19]). Most often foregut cysts present

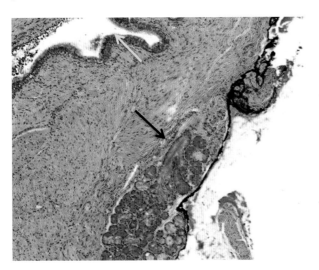

FIGURE 173.8 Cyst containing submucosal bronchial type glands (*black arrow*) and respiratory epithelium (*yellow arrow*). (From Altieri MS, Zheng R, Pryor AD, et al. Esophageal bronchogenic cyst and review of the literature. *Surg Endosc* 2015;29:3010–3015. Copyright © 2015 Springer Science+Business Media. With permission of Springer.)

in a benign fashion. However, there have been some associations with degeneration to different malignancies, specifically, rhabdomyosarcoma, pleuropulmonary blastoma, adenocarcinoma, squamous cell carcinoma, and mesenchymoma.[20]

TREATMENT

Foregut cysts can have a variety of presentations ranging from completely asymptomatic with incidental discovery to an emergent presentation with respiratory distress and cyanosis. However, surgical excision is recommended for all foregut cysts regardless of presentation to prevent complications and establish a diagnosis. Complete surgical resection is the treatment of choice because definitive diagnosis can only be established by surgical excision and tissue biopsy. Alternative treatments, such as transtracheal aspirations, are not universally accepted due to cyst recurrence being associated with higher morbidity.[18] Foregut cysts are not known to disappear or regress and, in fact, tend to enlarge with time. Significant complications associated with foregut cysts differ by type. Bronchogenic cysts may eventually become symptomatic by exerting mass effect on the trachea or bronchus. Cysts that do communicate with the airway are at risk of infection and/or bleeding which can lead to hemoptysis or hemothorax. Up to one-third of foregut cysts, especially esophageal duplication cysts, contain gastric mucosa which can lead to hemorrhage. Malignant degeneration, although rare, is also a significant risk to be considered.[21,22]

Most bronchogenic cysts originate in the mediastinum; however, 15% to 20% originate in the lung parenchyma.[22] Surgical treatment of mediastinal cysts may be accomplished by thoracotomy, video-assisted thoracoscopic surgery (VATS), or more recently, robotic resection.[14,23–26] Intraparenchymal lesions are also amenable to VATS and thoracotomy but also require lung resection. The decision of wedge resection versus lobe is based upon the location of the lesion within the lung. Excision of foregut cysts should be accomplished immediately after diagnosis to allow for removal of the cyst in the earliest stage possible. Surgical removal at the early stage, before complications caused by the cyst develops, decreases surgical risk and increases the odds of complete removal.[25] When complete removal of the entire cyst is not possible due to adhesions to surrounding tissues or organs, the epithelial layer should be destroyed with cauterization or fulguration to prevent recurrence. One study reported recurrence of cysts after 25 years, secondary to incomplete resection.[25]

Esophageal duplication cysts may be amenable to other treatment strategies. While bronchogenic cysts should be removed completely, some esophageal duplication cysts may need to be marsupialized with mucosal stripping if the cyst and esophagus share a common wall. However, this problem may also be treated with segmental resection of the esophagus if necessary.[27] Traditionally, the lesions have been approached through a right posterolateral thoracotomy. VATS is establishing a greater role in the excision of these lesions. Strategies to protect the esophagus, such as leaving the endoscope in the esophagus or inserting a bougie, are utilized. The lesion is then freed from the outer longitudinal muscle by bluntly separating the fibers to reveal the lesion; a myotomy of the circular muscle layer is performed and the lesion is enucleated (Fig. 173.9).[26]

Mediastinoscopy has also proven to be a viable option to resect lesions in the appropriate locations. This can be accomplished via standard cervical mediastinoscopy, extended cervical mediastinoscopy, and anterior mediastinoscopy as described by Chamberlain.[3]

Despite advances in minimally invasive techniques and the growing number of studies discussing their viability in resection of foregut

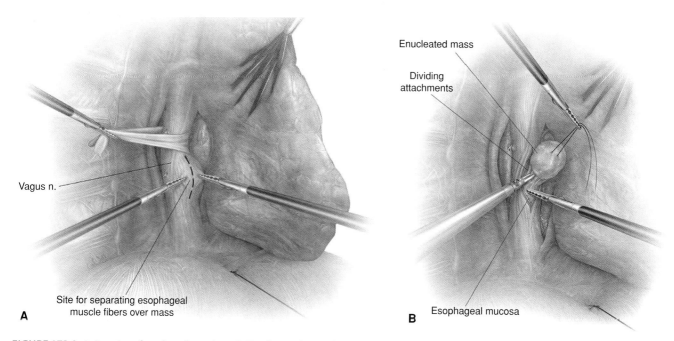

FIGURE 173.9 A: Location of esophageal mass/cyst. **B:** Enucleation (intact if possible) of mass/cyst. (Reprinted from Macke RA, Nason KS. Minimally invasive resection of benign esophageal lesions. *Oper Tech Thorac Cardiovasc Surg* 2014;19:396–413. Copyright © 2014 Elsevier. With permission.)

cysts, open approaches should not be avoided in the setting of large cysts or those that are densely adhered to vital structures.

ANESTHETIC CONSIDERATIONS

Large mediastinal foregut cysts, including bronchogenic cysts, may present with significant airway compromise. Anesthesia with an established airway may not only be required for the definitive operation, but also for the biopsy and diagnosis. Loss of airway and circulatory collapse during induction of anesthesia is a well-established phenomenon.[28–30] If the presentation is nonemergent, appropriate imaging with CT scan to determine the degree of airway impingement is necessary to allow for an appropriate anesthetic plan. Anesthetic techniques that may be used include general anesthesia delivered via an endotracheal tube or inhalational agents with spontaneous ventilation delivered with a laryngeal mask. Rigid bronchoscopy may be required for establishment of a safe and secure airway. Collaboration between the surgical and anesthetic team at this critical moment is of the utmost importance in the pediatric patient population. Spirometry in older children is another technique to elucidate the effect the airway compression has, if any, on respiratory function.[4]

Different techniques for selective ventilation may need to be utilized as one-lung ventilation with lung collapse can be poorly tolerated in children. Small volume ventilation and/or lung retractors may prove useful in this situation.

COMPLICATIONS

The prognosis after complete excision of foregut cysts is excellent. However, significant complications can arise in the pre- and postoperative settings. Complication rates are generally low but can range as high as 25% to 37% of patients.[31] Tracheobronchial compression and pulmonary infections are the most common. However, a myriad of other complications such as pneumothorax, superior vena cava syndrome, pleurisy, arrhythmias, pulmonary artery stenosis, and malignant transformation have been reported. More serious and often lethal complications, such as respiratory collapse associated with compression, cardiac tamponade due to cystic rupture, hemoptysis, fatal air embolism in an airplane passenger, erosion into the airway and/or pulmonary vasculature, and myocardial infarction due to compression of the left main coronary artery have been reported. Intraoperative complications include injury to the trachea, esophagus, or vagus nerve.[13] Resection of cysts when diagnosed prior to loss of tissue planes due to inflammation can help to eliminate these complications. Postoperative complications include recurrence, hemothorax, persistent air leak, postoperative pneumonia, pleural effusions, gastroesophageal reflux, wound infections, and Horner syndrome.

REFERENCES

1. Gerle RD, Jaretzki A, Ashley CA, et al. Congenital bronchopulmonary-foregut malformation. Pulmonary sequestration communicating with the gastrointestinal tract. *N Engl J Med* 1968;278:1413–1419.
2. Barnes NA, Pilling DW. Bronchopulmonary foregut malformations: embryology, radiology and quandary. *Eur Radiol* 2003;13:2659–2673.
3. Burjonrappa SC, Taddeucci R, Arcidi J. Mediastinoscopy in the treatment of mediastinal cysts. *JSLS* 2005;9:142–148.
4. Wright CD. Mediastinal tumors and cysts in the pediatric population. *Thorac Surg Clin* 2009;19:47–61.
5. Zambudio AR, Lanzas JT, Calvo MJ, et al. Non-neoplastic mediastinal cysts. *Eur J Cardiothorac Surg* 2002;22:712–716.
6. Sonthalia N, Jain SS, Surude RG, et al. Congenital esophageal duplication cyst: a rare cause of dysphagia in an adult. *Gastroenterology Res* 2016;9:79–82.
7. Ko SF, Hsieh MJ, Lin JW, et al. Bronchogenic cyst of the esophagus: clinical and imaging features of seven cases. *Clin Imaging* 2006;30:309–314.
8. Petroze R, McGahren ED. Pediatric chest II: benign tumors and cysts. *Surg Clin North Am* 2012;92:645–658.
9. Takeda S, Miyoshi S, Akashi A, et al. Clinical spectrum of primary mediastinal tumors: a comparison of adult and pediatric populations at a single Japanese institution. *J Surg Oncol* 2003;83:24–30.
10. Williams HJ, Johnson KJ. Imaging of congenital cystic lung lesions. *Paediatr Respir Rev* 2002;3:120–127.
11. Mullassery D, Smith NP. Lung development. *Semin Pediatr Surg* 2015;24:152–155.
12. Sulzer J, Azimi M, Rojas-Miranda A, et al. [40 cases of bronchogenic cysts of the mediastinum. Topographic considerations]. *Ann Chir Thorac Cardiovasc* 1970;9:261–265.
13. St-Georges R, Deslauriers J, Duranceau A, et al. Clinical spectrum of bronchogenic cysts of the mediastinum and lung in the adult. *Ann Thorac Surg* 1991;52:6–13.

14. Suen HC, Mathisen DJ, Grillo HC, et al. Surgical management and radiological characteristics of bronchogenic cysts. *Ann Thorac Surg* 1993;55:476–481.

15. Nobuhara KK, Gorski YC, La Quaglia MP, et al. Bronchogenic cysts and esophageal duplications: common origins and treatment. *J Pediatr Surg* 1997;32:1408–1413.

16. Ribet ME, Copin MC, Gosselin B. Bronchogenic cysts of the mediastinum. *J Thorac Cardiovasc Surg* 1995;109:1003–1010.

17. Snyder ME, Luck SR, Hernandez R, et al. Diagnostic dilemmas of mediastinal cysts. *J Pediatr Surg* 1985;20:810–815.

18. Esme H, Eren S, Sezer M, et al. Primary mediastinal cysts: clinical evaluation and surgical results of 32 cases. *Tex Heart Inst J* 2011;38:371–374.

19. Strollo DC, Rosado-de-Christenson ML, Jett JR. Primary mediastinal tumors: part II. Tumors of the middle and posterior mediastinum. *Chest* 1997;112: 1344–1357.

20. Casagrande A, Pederiva F. Association between congenital lung malformations and lung tumors in children and adults: a systematic review. *J Thorac Oncol* 2016; 11:1837–1845.

21. Laberge JM, Puligandla P, Flageole H. Asymptomatic congenital lung malformations. *Semin Pediatr Surg* 2005;14:16–33.

22. Sarper A, Ayten A, Golbasi I, et al. Bronchogenic cyst. *Tex Heart Inst J* 2003;30: 105–108.

23. Michel JL, Revillon Y, Montupet P, et al. Thoracoscopic treatment of mediastinal cysts in children. *J Pediatr Surg* 1998;33:1745–1748.

24. Meehan JJ, Sandler AD. Robotic resection of mediastinal masses in children. *J Laparoendosc Adv Surg Tech A* 2008;18:114–119.

25. Jung HS, Kim DK, Lee GD, et al. Video-assisted thoracic surgery for bronchogenic cysts: is this the surgical approach of choice? *Interact Cardiovasc Thorac Surg* 2014; 19:824–829.

26. Macke RA, Nason KS. Minimally invasive resection of benign esophageal lesions. *Oper Tech Thorac Cardiovasc Surg* 2014;19:396–413.

27. Azzie G, Beasley S. Diagnosis and treatment of foregut duplications. *Semin Pediatr Surg* 2003;12:46–54.

28. Piastra M, Ruggiero A, Caresta E, et al. Life-threatening presentation of mediastinal neoplasms: report on 7 consecutive pediatric patients. *Am J Emerg Med* 2005; 23:76–82.

29. Hammer GB. Anaesthetic management for the child with a mediastinal mass. *Paediatr Anaesth* 2004;14:95–97.

30. Ricketts RR. Clinical management of anterior mediastinal tumors in children. *Semin Pediatr Surg* 2001;10:161–168.

31. Limaiem F, Ayadi-Kaddour A, Djilani H, et al. Pulmonary and mediastinal bronchogenic cysts: a clinicopathologic study of 33 cases. *Lung* 2008;186:55–61.

174

Foregut Cysts of the Mediastinum in Adults

Hon Chi Suen

Mediastinal cysts are common lesions. Most are congenital, and they account for 20% to 32% of all primary masses of the mediastinum.[1,2] In the review of Takeda and colleagues,[3] the 95 patients with mediastinal cysts in their adult population accounted for 14% of all mediastinal masses. Despite being congenital, many of these cysts are not identified until later in life. In the series reported by St-Georges and colleagues, 32% of all cysts were found in patients <20 years of age, whereas 68% were in patients >20 years of age.[4]

CLASSIFICATION OF MEDIASTINAL CYSTS

The classification of mediastinal cysts is based on their etiology (Table 174.1). Foregut cysts are the result of an abnormal budding or division of the primitive foregut. Also called enterogenous cysts, they are most frequently divided into categories based on their histologic features and embryogenesis.

TABLE 174.1 Classification of Mediastinal Cysts

Congenital
Mesothelial cysts
  Pericardial
  Pleural
Foregut cysts
  Bronchogenic
  Esophageal
  Gastroenteric
  Neurenteric
Lymphatic cysts
  Lymphangiomatous
  Thoracic duct
Acquired
Inflammatory
Thymic
Teratogenous
Dermoid
Parathyroid
Thyroid

Bronchogenic cysts occur mostly along the tracheobronchial tree and are usually found behind the carina. Most often they are unilocular and lined by ciliated columnar epithelium with focal or extensive squamous metaplasia. Rosai,[5] Coulson,[6] Sternberg,[7] and Marchevsky and Kaneko[8] have described how the walls of these cysts may contain hyaline cartilage, smooth muscle, bronchial glands, and nerve trunks. Bronchogenic cysts account for 50% to 60% of mediastinal cysts and are usually found in adults. They can be intrapulmonary or extrapulmonary and rarely show a communication with the airway. These cysts may extend below the diaphragm as dumbbell cysts[9] or found in extrathoracic sites.

Esophageal cysts are less common than bronchogenic lesions; they are characterized by a double layer of smooth muscle in their walls. Most of them are found embedded in the wall of the lower half of the esophagus. Their lining may be squamous, ciliated columnar, or a mixture of both. Distinction from bronchial cysts may be difficult or even impossible; the best evidence in favor of their esophageal etiology is when they are totally within the esophageal wall and/or covered by a definite double layer of smooth muscle. They are usually not in communication with the esophageal lumen. Two theories are suggested by Abel,[10] Coulson,[6] Marchevsky and Kaneko,[8] Rosai,[5] and Sternberg[7] to explain the development of esophageal cysts: persistent vacuoles in the wall of the foregut or an abnormal budding from the foregut.

Other mediastinal cysts include mesothelial (pleural, pericardial), thoracic duct, thymic, parathyroid, and hydatid cysts. Pathologic features of these cysts are related to their tissue of origin. Despite their rarity and the paucity of symptoms, a clear knowledge of their etiology, pathology, and clinical significance is needed.

BRONCHOGENIC CYSTS

EMBRYOGENESIS

Bronchogenic cysts are congenital anomalies of lung development arising as a result of a group of cells that break off from the developing lung bud and differentiate on their own.

During the third week of gestation, the laryngotracheal groove or primitive respiratory system develops as a ventral diverticulum located in the floor of the foregut, just caudal to the pharyngeal pouches. This diverticulum later transforms into a tube that becomes the primitive bronchial tree. After the fourth week, two enlargements develop distally; these become the future bronchial and lung buds. By the 35th day, the lobar bronchi appear.

Abnormal budding of the bronchial tree may lead to bronchogenic cysts. When this abnormal budding occurs early during gestation, the cysts tend to be located within the mediastinum and seldom communicate with the bronchial tree. Cysts that arise later are more peripheral and are located within the lung parenchyma which often have a bronchial communication.

PATHOLOGY

Bronchogenic cysts are most often spherical, unilocular cystic masses in contact with the tracheobronchial tree. Infrequently, they may be lobulated, multiloculated, or rarely multiple. The cysts contain a whitish-gray mucinous material but may contain brownish inspissated material. The common lining is a single layer of respiratory epithelium of ciliated columnar cells (Fig. 174.1). This layer of cells may be cuboidal or a simple flattened epithelial layer. Varying degrees of squamous metaplasia may present. A lamina propria may contain bronchial glands, connective and smooth muscle tissue, and cartilage. At times, in the presence of infection, the cyst may contain frank pus. With infection, the epithelial layer lining the cyst may be absent (Fig. 174.5).

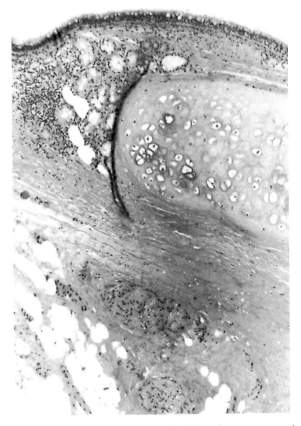

FIGURE 174.1 Photomicrograph of the wall of a bronchogenic cyst reveals an internal surface lined by characteristic respiratory epithelium. A cartilaginous plate is present beneath the mucosal lining.

LOCATION

The majority of the bronchogenic cysts are in close anatomic relationship with the tracheobronchial tree (Fig. 174.2) or the esophagus (Fig. 174.3) in the visceral compartment of the mediastinum. In 1948, Maier[11] divided their locations into five groups: paratracheal, carinal, hilar, paraesophageal, and miscellaneous. Within the chest, using the tracheobronchial bifurcation as a dividing line, about 25% of the cysts were located in the superior portion of the chest, whereas 75% were below the tracheal carina. Roughly one-third were in the middle mediastinum, whereas the other two-thirds extended to the limits of the posterior portion of the mediastinum and even to the paravertebral area (Fig. 174.4). In the series collected by Suen and colleagues,[12] the locations of the 42 bronchogenic cysts were mediastinal in 37 patients and intrapulmonary in five. Bilateral bronchogenic cysts have been described.[12]

The fifth group, miscellaneous, is located in rare and exotic locations almost anywhere in the body. It could arise from the parietal pleura.[13] Related to the cardiovascular system, it has been found in the pericardial cavity,[12,14,15] in the wall of aorta,[16] in the right ventricular endocardium,[17] in the left ventricule,[18] in the interatrial septum,[19] and in the *pars membranacea septi*.[20] Related to the diaphragm, it could be intradiaphragmatic[21,22] or transdiaphragmatic.[23,24]

Outside the thorax, it could be found in front of the sternum,[25] in the neck,[26] intradural,[27] and in the abdomen.[28] Coselli and colleagues[28] suggested that these cysts possibly arise from abnormal budding of the primitive foregut that migrates into the abdomen before fusion of the pleuroperitoneal membranes. Retroperitoneal bronchogenic cysts have been reported at least five times and could mimic pheochromocytoma or pancreatic cyst.

CLINICAL FEATURES

Many in the adult are asymptomatic, but contrary to a widely held belief, as espoused by Maier,[11] and Wychulis and colleagues,[29] well over half are or will become symptomatic because of compression of the airway or the esophagus or the presence of infection. The latter may be caused by perforation into either of the former structures, but the infection most often occurs without such a communication.

In the series reported by Sirivella and colleagues,[30] which included individuals with nonspecific and enterogenous cysts, 16 of 20 patients were symptomatic and the most common complaints were cough, dyspnea, dysphagia, and chest pain. Most patients in Zambudio's series complained of chest pain.[9]

In the series published by St-Georges,[4] 66.6% of the patients with mediastinal bronchogenic cysts were symptomatic and the majority (two-thirds) had two or more symptoms. These are summarized in Tables 174.2 and 174.3. When the cyst is in the mediastinum, substernal pain is the most common symptom. This is likely the result of

TABLE 174.2 Incidence of Symptoms Associated With Mediastinal Bronchogenic Cysts

No. of Patients	66 (100%)
Asymptomatic	22 (33%)
Symptomatic	44 (66.6%)
Multiple symptoms	29 (44%)

Adapted from St-Georges R, Deslauriers J, Duranceau A, et al. Clinical spectrum of bronchogenic cysts of the mediastinum and lung in the adult. *Ann Thorac Surg* 1991;52: 6–13.

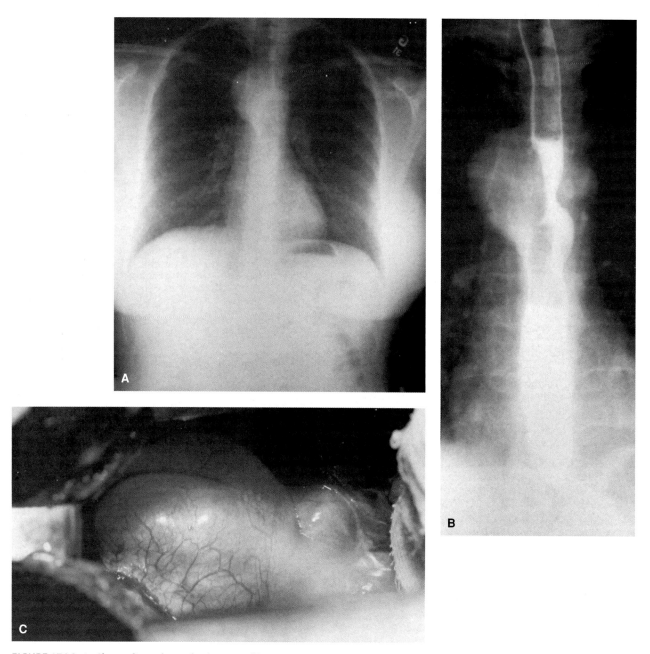

FIGURE 174.2 **A:** Chest radiograph reveals a large round homogeneous mass in the right paratracheal area. **B:** Compression of the esophagus shown on barium swallow. **C:** Operative photograph shows a spherical cystic mass covered by a smooth, intact capsule.

irritation or inflammation of the surrounding parietal or mediastinal pleura. Dysphagia, dyspnea, and cough are all caused by compression or irritation of bronchi or the esophagus. Expectoration of purulent sputum is seen in 7.5% of the mediastinal cysts and indicates either infection of the cyst with fistulization or, more likely, pneumonia in the adjacent compressed lung. Among 26 of St-Georges' patients who were observed conservatively, 15 (57.6%) subsequently developed symptoms.

COMPLICATIONS

Infection (Fig. 174.5) is a common complication, especially in those with bronchial communication. Tracheobronchial compression can occur in children because of their relatively soft tracheobronchial tree.[31]

Cardiovascular complications are uncommonly seen but could be life-threatening. Watson and Chaudhary[32] cited a patient with ventricular and atrial tachycardia believed to be caused by cyst compression. Similarly, Volpi and colleagues[33] reported the occurrence of paroxysmal atrial fibrillation as the presenting feature of a bronchogenic cyst impinging on the atrium. Watts and colleagues,[34] and Berkowitz and colleagues[35] described compression of the pulmonary artery simulating arterial stenosis, and Selke and colleagues[36] described long-standing pulmonary artery compression resulting in pulmonary artery hypoplasia and hyperlucent lung (Fig. 174.6). Superior vena cava syndrome also has been described. Compression of the left main coronary artery resulting in severe myocardial ischemia and ventricular fibrillation requiring intra-aortic balloon pump and emergency open heart surgery has been described.[15] A giant bronchogenic cyst presenting with symptoms similar to an acute type

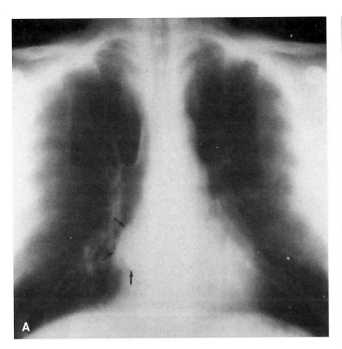

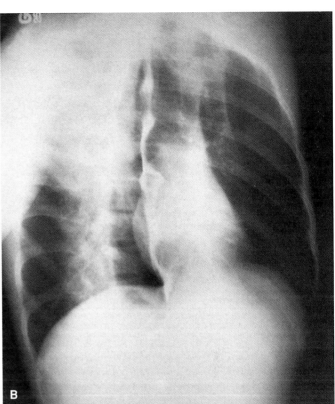

FIGURE 174.3 A: Posteroanterior chest radiograph of a young man with severe chest pain reveals a right-sided retrocardiac mass (*arrows*). **B:** Barium swallow reveals some degree of compression of the lower fourth of the esophagus. On excision, the mass proved to be a bronchogenic cyst.

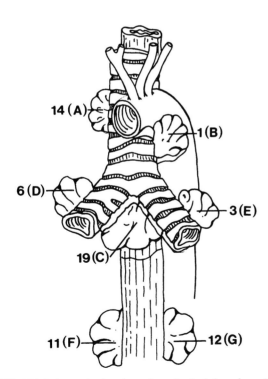

FIGURE 174.4 Anatomic location of mediastinal bronchogenic cysts according to Maier's classification. (**A**) Right paratracheal; (**B**) left paratracheal; (**C**) subcarinal; (**D**) right hilar; (**E**) left hilar; (**F**) right paraesophageal; (**G**) left paraesophageal. (From St-Georges R, Deslauriers J, Duranceau A, et al. Clinical spectrum of bronchogenic cysts of the mediastinum and lung in the adult. *Ann Thorac Surg* 1991;52:6–13. With permission.)

TABLE 174.3 Symptoms Associated With Mediastinal Bronchogenic Cysts

Characteristic	Mediastinal Bronchogenic Cysts, N = 66 (%)[a]
Onset of Symptoms	
Acute	7 (10.6)
Progressive	37 (56)
Severity of Symptoms	
Mild	9 (13.6)
Moderate	23 (34.8)
Severe	12 (18.1)
Most Common Symptoms	
Chest pain	27 (40.9)
Cough	16 (24.2)
Dyspnea	16 (24.2)
Fever	10 (15.1)
Purulent sputum	5 (7.5)
Anorexia and weight loss	9 (13.6)
Dysphagia	9 (13.6)
Hemoptysis	3 (4.5)
Others	7 (10.6)

[a]Numbers in parentheses are of the total 66 patients.
Adapted from St-Georges R, Deslauriers J, Duranceau A, et al. Clinical spectrum of bronchogenic cysts of the mediastinum and lung in the adult. *Ann Thorac Surg* 1991;52:6–13. Copyright © 1991 The Society of Thoracic Surgeons. With permission.

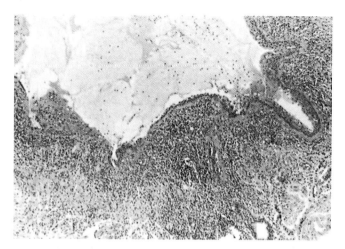

FIGURE 174.5 Photomicrograph of wall of the resected infected bronchogenic cyst shown in Figure 174.3 with absence of a portion of the mucosal lining due to the inflammatory process.

A aortic dissection requiring replacement of the ascending aorta and reconstruction of the aortic valve was reported.[16]

Cysts lined by gastric epithelium occasionally may be seen with symptoms related to acid secretion. Peptic ulceration with cyst perforation was reported by Moor and Jahnke.[37] Bronchial communication was reported by Overton and Oberstreet,[38] and Spock and colleagues[39] described the occurrence of hemorrhage from the cyst. In such cases, hematemesis or hemoptysis may be the presenting symptom.

Although rare, malignancies have definitely been described in bronchogenic cysts. The first report was by Moersch and Clagett in 1947, in which they reported one adenocarcinoma in 36 bronchogenic cysts and one squamous cell carcinoma in a ciliated cyst of indeterminate origin.[40] In 1951, Behrend and Kravitz described a sarcoma arising from a bronchogenic cyst.[41] Prichard et al. reported two adenocarcinomas from large peripheral lung cysts, one thought to be bronchogenic in origin.[42] Suen and colleagues described an adenocarcinoma in a subcarinal bronchogenic cyst in an 8½-year-old girl.[12] Since then, more cases of malignancies have been reported.

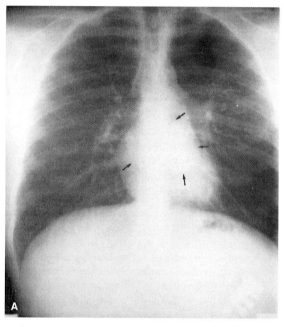

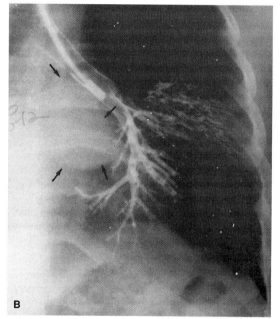

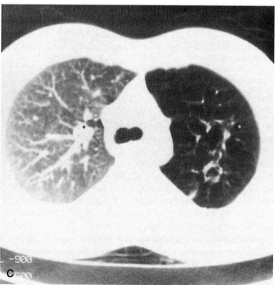

FIGURE 174.6 **A:** Chest radiograph in an asymptomatic young man reveals a rounded retrocardiac mass (*arrows*) associated with hyperlucency of the left upper lobe. **B:** Selective bronchogram demonstrates the mass (*arrows*) with normal but compressed upper lobe bronchi. **C:** CT scan (lung window) reveals marked hyperlucency of the left upper lobe.

These include large cell carcinoma,[43] carcinoid tumor,[44] and bronchioloalveolar carcinoma,[45] and others.

RADIOGRAPHIC FEATURES

Standard Radiographic Studies

Standard chest radiographs identified the bronchogenic cysts in 88%.[12] Reed and Sobonya[46] reviewed the radiographic features in 80 patients with foregut cysts; 77% to 87% of these were bronchogenic. Almost all were spheroid masses in the visceral compartment of the mediastinum (86%), and the remaining (14%) were intrapulmonary in location. Most were right-sided (70%). Thirty-two percent were superior (paratracheal in location) to the tracheal carina, and 68% were located below the level of the carina (Fig. 174.7). Calcification was occasionally seen peripherally within the wall. Milk of calcium has been reported layering in the dependent portion.[47] Air or an air fluid level was seen in four (5.6%) of the bronchogenic cysts. Distention or distortion of the esophagus demonstrated on the esophagram can be present depending on the location and size of the cyst. It may be difficult to differentiate the cyst from a benign esophageal tumor such as a leiomyoma. In

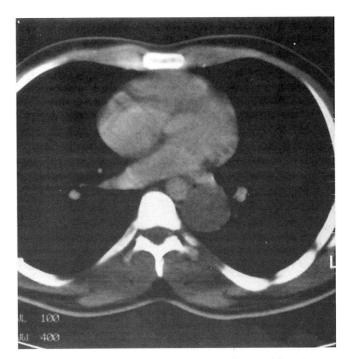

FIGURE 174.8 CT scan, (mediastinal window) of a typical bronchogenic cyst showing a smooth, well-circumscribed, posteriorly located left perihilar fluid-filled cystic structure.

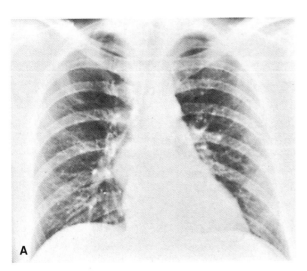

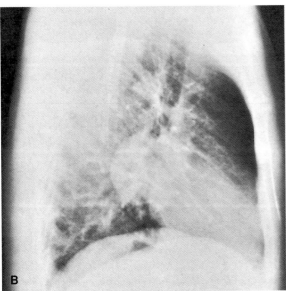

FIGURE 174.7 **A,B:** Typical posteroanterior and lateral radiographic appearance of a subcarinal bronchogenic cyst.

approximately half of the patients, whether symptomatic or not, some degree of esophageal displacement is noted.

Computed Tomography and Magnetic Resonance Imaging

A computed tomographic (CT) scan most often reveals the cystic nature of the lesion (Fig. 174.8). Nakata and colleagues[48] have described the characteristic features of these cysts. Nakata,[48] as well as Suen,[12] Jost,[49] and Mendelson[50] and their colleagues, noted that many of the bronchogenic cysts have high Hounsfield numbers (up to 130) approaching those of soft tissue rather than the low density of water (0 to 20), so that a CT scan is not absolute in demonstrating the characteristic features of a fluid-filled cystic lesion. Higher CT numbers represent increased calcium content, anthracotic pigment, blood, or greater protein content of the fluid.[48] Calcification of portions of the cystic wall may be demonstrated frequently, which may not be appreciated on the standard radiographic examination. CT scan can delineate an air-filled intrapulmonary bronchogenic cyst well (Fig. 174.9).

Magnetic resonance imaging (MRI) may provide specific diagnostic confirmation in regard to bronchogenic cysts (Figs. 174.10 and 174.11). The MRI is dependent on the cyst's content, specifically the presence and amount of mucus or other proteinaceous material. If the fluid within a bronchogenic cyst is of low specific gravity and mainly serous (a spring water cyst), it will be of very low signal intensity on T1-weighted images and of very bright signal intensity on T2-weighted images. However, many bronchogenic cysts may contain large amounts of proteinaceous material. Such cysts have a characteristic appearance with high signal intensity on T1-weighted images. This appearance must be differentiated from lesions that contain fat, which also has bright signal intensity on T1. However, that differentiation can easily be made by comparison with a corresponding CT. Fatty lesions will be of low attenuation on CT. Such bronchogenic cysts will have slightly diminished signal intensity on T2-weighted

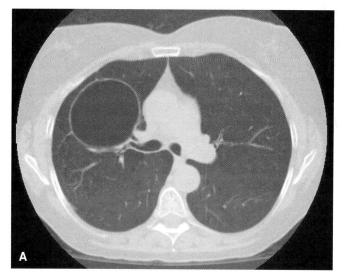

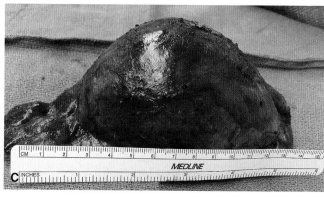

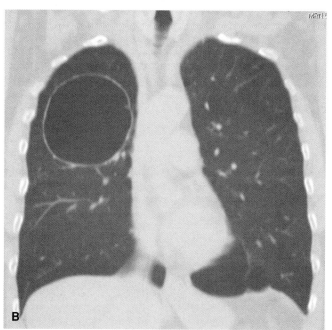

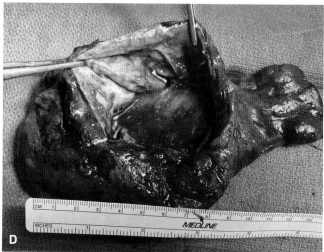

FIGURE 174.9 A large intrapulmonary air-filled bronchogenic cyst. **A:** CT axial view. **B:** CT coronal view. **C:** Right upper lobectomy specimen. **D:** Cut opened cyst.

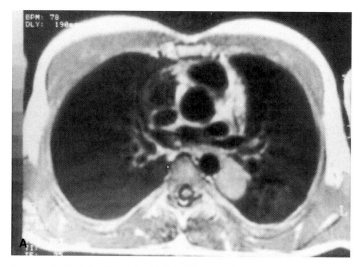

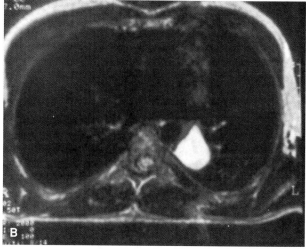

FIGURE 174.10 **A:** T1-weighted MRI of the mass shown in Figure 174-6 shows the lesion to be of intermediate intensity. **B:** T2-weighted image reveals the typical hyperintense signal of a fluid-filled structure. Excision and pathologic examination of the mass revealed it to be a bronchogenic cyst.

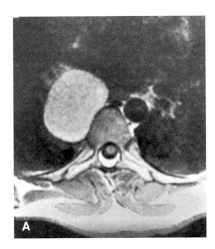 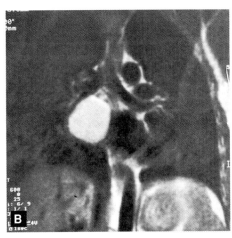

FIGURE 174.11 MRI of bronchogenic cyst shown in Figure 174-7. **A:** T2-weighted cross-sectional image. **B:** Coronal image. Note narrowing of the bronchus intermedius.

images, and they will often display either fluid/fluid levels or areas of heterogeneity. We believe that MRI can diagnose bronchogenic cysts accurately and is indicated to confirm the diagnosis, especially when the surgeon does not want to operate on the patient.[12]

Ultrasonography can be useful to demonstrate the cystic nature of the lesion and whether the cyst creates some distortion of the cardiac chambers or great vessels. Anderson and colleagues,[51] and Watson and Chaudhary[32] have shown that for some patients, ultrasonography may obviate the need for more invasive modalities, such as angiography. Endoscopic ultrasonography has helped differentiate bronchogenic cysts from solid lesions.[52] Eloubeidi and colleagues[53] and Fazel and colleagues[54] used endoscopic ultrasound and fine-needle aspiration biopsies in their patients to provide a definitive diagnosis of foregut duplication cysts with the aim of allowing conservative and expectant management. However, infection of the cysts by introduction of bacteria or *Candida* can result from such manipulation resulting in severe mediastinitis and sepsis[55,56] and is not advisable.

TREATMENT

Rationale for Surgical Excision

The definitive histologic diagnosis can be established only by surgical excision. Even in the absence of symptoms, surgical exploration is recommended for nearly all patients with an abnormal mediastinal mass found by radiographic examination (Table 174.4). This approach is required not only to establish definitive tissue diagnosis but also to alleviate symptoms and prevent complications. This is especially true with mediastinal bronchogenic cysts, 66% of which are or will ultimately become symptomatic or develop complications.

In the series of St-Georges,[4] 26 patients were previously known to have a mediastinal mass but observed; in 57.6% of these, surgery became necessary later either because the mass had enlarged or had become symptomatic during the period of follow-up (Fig. 174.5). Of the 40 patients with the newly discovered disease, 28 were symptomatic, 11 had lesions detected during examinations for unrelated illnesses, and 1 case was identified at the time of surgery for reflux esophagitis. Overall, the correct diagnosis of a bronchogenic cyst was made preoperatively in only 35% of patients. Overall, two had had MRI examinations and one-fourth of all patients had had a CT scan preoperatively. Other diagnoses entertained before surgery include neurogenic tumor, pericardial cyst, and lymphoma. With the current more liberal use of CT and MRI, an accurate diagnosis is more frequently made.

The risk of malignancy developing in a mediastinal bronchogenic cyst is low but not zero as noted in the cases reported earlier. Far more frequent are the risks of infection or perforation, thus rendering excision potentially more difficult and hazardous.

Surgical Technique

Complete excision is the goal. The surgical approach used to be mostly through a thoracotomy. Cysts located at the level of the thoracic inlet are best approached by exposing the mediastinum with a proximal sternotomy extending into the neck on the side of the documented lesion. Paratracheal and subcarinal cysts are best exposed through a right-sided thoracotomy. Complete excision is possible in nearly all cases, whether the cyst is complicated or not. If complete excision is not possible because part of the cyst wall cannot be separated from a vital structure, the remaining mucosa has to be denatured to prevent recurrence of the cyst. Any communication with the tracheobronchial tree should be carefully closed and buttressed with local, healthy tissue whenever possible. Rarely, a bronchogenic cyst could be extensively adherent to the carina requiring excision of the carina and the medial wall of both main bronchi. A pedicled pericardial patch has been used to repair such a large airway defect by Pierson and Mathisen[57] with success. Intrapulmonary bronchogenic cysts should be excised because of the high incidence of secondary infection associated with them. If possible, lung-sparing procedures compatible with complete excision should be done because of the benign nature of most of these cysts.

Reported in 1972, using mediastinoscopy, Ginsberg and colleagues[58] drained a subcarinal bronchogenic cyst compressing

TABLE 174.4 Indications for Surgery in 66 Patients With Bronchogenic Cysts of the Mediastinum

Indications	Mediastinal Bronchogenic Cysts, N = 66[a]
Mass previously known	26 (39.3)
Stable	11 (16.6)
Increase in size, change in symptomatology, or both	15 (22.7)
Mass not previously known	39 (59)
Asymptomatic	11 (16.6)
Symptomatic	28 (42.4)
Incidental finding during operation for reflux esophagitis	1 (1.5)

[a]Numbers in parentheses are percentage of the total 66 patients.

both main bronchi in a 59-year-old woman who presented with stridor. Right paratracheal cysts in adults can be removed by a mediastinoscopy approach, but incomplete resection can lead to recurrence. Aspiration of the cyst and injection of a sclerosing agent in the cystic lumen has been proposed by Kurkcuoglu et al.[59] Unless complete excision is contraindicated for other reasons, lesser procedures are not advisable for fear of recurrence. Drainage of infected bronchogenic cyst by EUS followed by resection 4 weeks later has been reported.[60]

With the rapid development of video-assisted thoracic surgery (VATS), one should try to adopt this less invasive approach in the management of mediastinal cysts. VATS resection has been reported by pioneers such as Demmy,[61] Lewis,[62] Bonavina,[63] and Yim,[64] and colleagues. Weber and colleagues[65] reported 92% success rate in their series of 12 patients. The potential advantages of VATS are decreased pain, a shorter hospital stay, a better cosmetic outcome, and a more rapid return to normal activity. But, the principle of complete excision cannot be compromised. Coversion to thoracotomy is indicated if VATS cannot achieve a complete excision.

In a significant proportion of cases, the cyst is closely adherent to adjacent organs, such as the tracheobronchial tree (52%), esophagus (47%), pericardium (30%), or lung (20%), but these adhesions do not usually preclude complete excision. When total removal is difficult or not possible, the mucosa of the remaining portion of the cyst may have to be peeled away from the attached structure or denatured, leaving behind the nonepithelial portions of the cyst wall. This may prevent a recurrence such as described by Walker,[66] Miller,[67] and Gallucio,[68] and colleagues.

A watch-and-wait attitude in a patient with a mediastinal cyst, even if asymptomatic, is not recommended unless the patient is not a candidate for surgery. Estrera and colleagues[69] strongly support the concept of surgical excision once the cyst has been identified, and this attitude is seen as the only policy capable of preventing complications. Transbronchial needle aspiration (TBNA), described by Cohn and colleagues,[70] and percutaneous aspiration, reported by Zimmer and colleagues,[71] have been proposed as alternatives to resection. Aspiration alone is not recommended because numerous recurrences with significant complications have been reported.

Morbidity and Mortality

Independent of the selected approach, morbidity after resection of a bronchogenic cyst is low. In our series of 42 patients, there was no operative mortality.[12] Complications occurred in only two patients (a minor wound infection and a patient with *Clostridium difficile* colitis).

ESOPHAGEAL CYSTS

INCIDENCE

Esophageal cysts, sometimes referred to as esophageal duplications, are much less common than bronchogenic cysts. Reed and Sobonya[46] reported only three esophageal cysts in their series of 80 patients with foregut cysts. Anderson and colleagues,[72] in a review of duplications of the alimentary tract, reported 26 patients in whom the duplication occurred in association with the esophagus. Twenty of these could be considered esophageal cysts, but as in many of the reports, the nature of the wall of the cyst was unrecorded. Undoubtedly, a few of these were actually paraesophageal bronchogenic cysts. The lining varied from squamous

(transitional) to respiratory and gastric epithelium. Occasionally, only a mesothelial layer was seen.

PATHOGENESIS

The esophageal cysts are thought by Salyer and colleagues[73] and Abel[10] to arise from persistent vacuoles in the wall of the foregut that develop during the solid tube stage of esophageal development. The vacuole remains isolated and does not coalesce with the developing lumen. Another theory, though less accepted, is that the esophageal cyst results from an abnormal budding of the early foregut. Marchevsky and Kaneko[8] surmise that both explanations may be correct. They suggest that the type lined by squamous epithelium results from persistent vacuoles and that lined by ciliated epithelium develops from abnormal budding of the foregut.

CLINICAL FEATURES

Approximately half of the esophageal cysts reviewed by Anderson and colleagues[72] were symptomatic. Pain and dysphagia were the common complaints. The difficulties in clarifying, clinically, which patient has a true esophageal cyst stem from the close relationship of these cysts with both the esophagus and the tracheobronchial tree. In looking only at those cysts invested by esophageal wall tissue, chest pain and dysphagia are the presenting symptoms (Fig. 174.12). There have been reports, such as that of Singh and colleagues,[74] of rare cases of carcinoma arising from those cysts.

Most esophageal cysts are solitary. Kang et al. reported co-existence of two esophageal cysts one on each side of the azygos vein (Fig. 174.13). Both have multimuscle layers but have different mucosal linings—pseudostratified ciliated columnar for the upper cyst and squamous for the lower cyst (Fig. 174.14).[75]

DIAGNOSIS

A mass in the visceral compartment may be seen on the standard radiograph of the chest. The barium swallow shows a smooth distortion of the barium column. CT examination reveals its intimate relationship with the esophagus and its cystic nature. Lupetin and Dash[76] have described the MRI appearance of an esophageal duplication cyst (Fig. 174.15).

Esophagoscopy may show a flattened area of mucosa overlying the mass, but no obstruction is evident. The lesion cannot be differentiated on this examination from a leiomyoma. Aspiration of the mass, although not advocated, yields a thick mucinous material.

TREATMENT AND PROGNOSIS

The preferred treatment of an esophageal cyst is also complete surgical excision. Lesser procedures like simple aspiration or marsupialization are not recommended because aspiration can introduce infection and there is a high chance of recurrence with both techniques. The VATS approach for resection is preferred over thoracotomy these days. If the esophageal cyst is located separately outside the esophageal muscle wall, resection would not be complicated. If the cyst is embedded in the esophageal muscle wall, a myotomy is first performed and then the cyst dissected out from the surrounding tissues including the esophageal mucosa. It is important to make sure that the mucosa is not breached. Intraoperative esophagoscopy could help to visualize the integrity of the mucosa and blowing air into the esophageal lumen with the esophagus submerged under saline

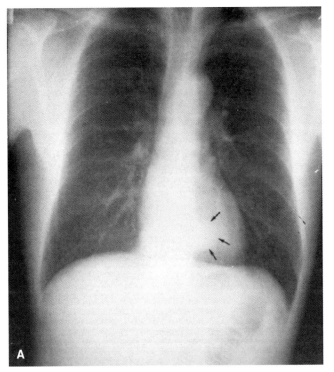

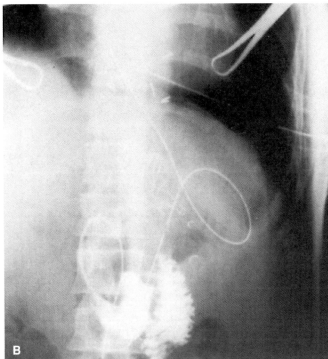

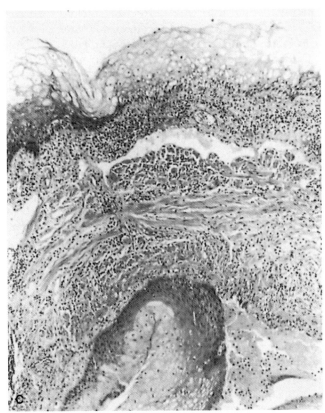

FIGURE 174.12 Duplication cyst of the esophagus extending below the diaphragm (dumbbell cyst). **A:** Standard posteroanterior chest radiograph shows a spherical mass located in the low left para-aortic area (*arrows*). **B:** At operation, the cyst was found to extend below the diaphragm; injection of contrast material into the cyst demonstrates a communication with the duodenum. **C:** Photomicrograph of the cyst wall shows characteristic squamous epithelium (esophageal mucosa) and a chronic submucosal inflammatory reaction; two smooth muscular layers are seen in the wall of the duplication.

can detect microperforation. Any breach of the mucosa will require immediate repair. After the excision of the cyst, the muscle layers are reapproximated over the dissection to prevent late formation of esophageal diverticulum.

The cyst is usually separated from the esophageal mucosa using low-level electrocautery or harmonic scalpel. When the cyst is densely adherent to the mucosa, enucleation could be difficult. Kang et al. described using endo-stapler to complete the resection by dividing the adherent portion and closing any potential mucosa defect (Fig. 174.13).[75] This technique will increase the success rate of VATS esophageal cyst resection. With complete excision, the prognosis is excellent.

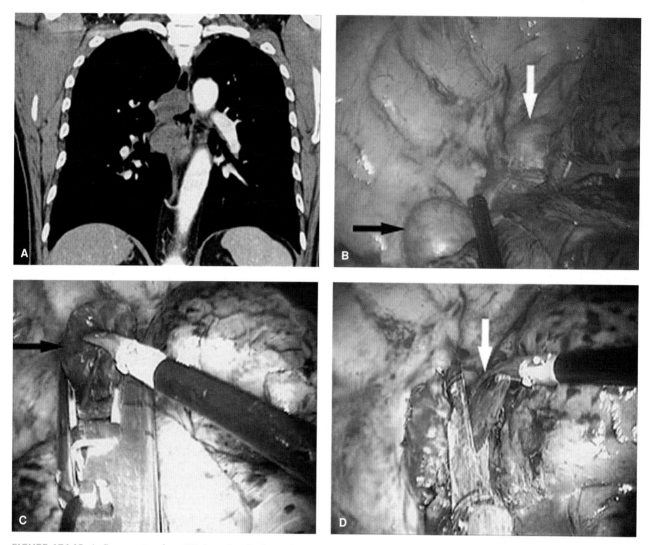

FIGURE 174.13 **A:** Preoperative chest CT showed multiple esophageal duplication cysts. **B:** Thoracoscopic finding of two esophageal cysts. **C** and **D:** Stapled resection of lower and upper esophageal duplication cysts after decompression. *White and black arrows* represent the upper and lower esophageal duplication cysts, respectively. (From Kang CU, Cho DG, Cho KD, et al. Thoracoscopic stapled resection of multiple esophageal duplication cysts with different pathological findings. *Eur J Cardiothorac Surg* 2008;34(1):216–218. Reproduced by permission of European Association for Cardiothoracic Surgery.)

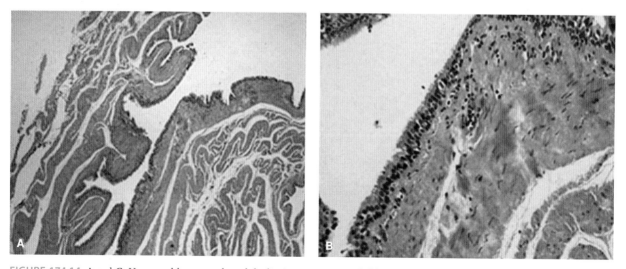

FIGURE 174.14 **A** and **C:** Upper and lower esophageal duplication cysts surrounded by multiple muscle layers, respectively (hematoxylin and eosin (H&E) stain, ×40). **B:** Pseudostratified ciliated columnar epithelium of upper esophageal duplication cyst (H&E, ×200). **D:** Stratified squamous epithelium of lower esophageal duplication cyst (H&E, ×200). (From Kang CU, Cho DG, Cho KD, et al. Thoracoscopic stapled resection of multiple esophageal duplication cysts with different pathological findings. *Eur J Cardiothorac Surg* 2008;34(1):216–218. Reproduced by permission of European Association for Cardiothoracic Surgery.) (*continued*)

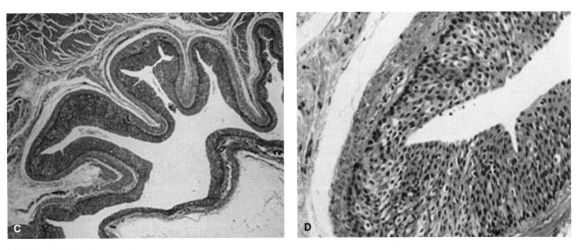

FIGURE 174.14 (*Continued*)

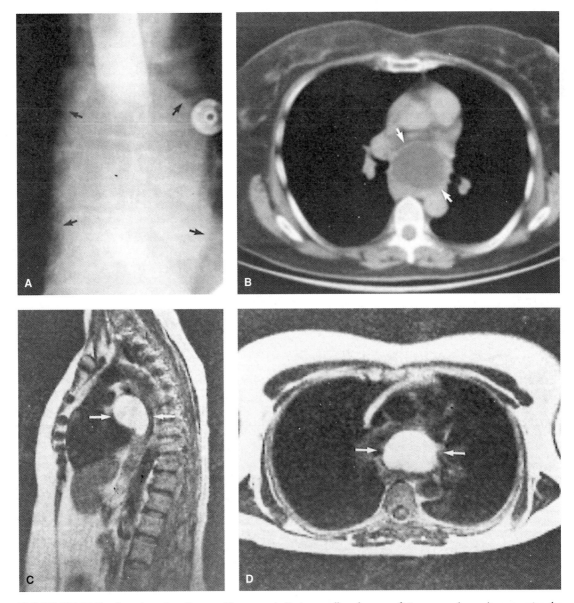

FIGURE 174.15 Esophageal cyst in a 61-year-old woman. **A:** Barium swallow shows a soft tissue mass (*arrows*) compressing the midesophagus. **B:** CT scan at the same level reveals obliteration of the esophagus by a thin-walled cystic (*arrows*) lesion. **C:** MRI in sagittal section of the chest reveals the mass (*arrows*) in the visceral compartment, showing its high intensity because of its fluid content. **D:** Cross-sectional MRI of mass (*arrows*).

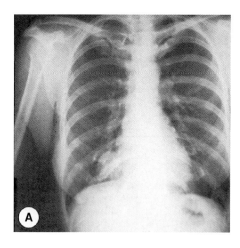

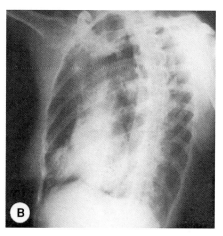

FIGURE 174.16 **A,B:** Posteroanterior and oblique radiographs of the chest reveal the presence of a pleuropericardial cyst in the right anterior cardiophrenic angle.

TRACHEOESOPHAGEAL CYSTS

In 1956, Abel[10] described mediastinal cysts with mixed features of both bronchogenic and esophageal cysts. He suggested that these rare cysts result from tracheoesophageal fistulas that close off and become isolated cystic structures during early embryogenesis. If they exist at all, these cysts are only pathologic curiosities. They are managed as either bronchogenic or esophageal cysts, depending on their location.

MESOTHELIAL CYSTS

Mesothelial cysts comprise a variety of cysts that have been reported as pleuropericardial cysts, pleural cysts, lymphogenous cysts, and simple mesothelial cysts of the mediastinum. These are essentially unilocular cysts filled with clear or slightly yellowish thin fluid. Most often they are incidental radiologic findings. They may be classified as one of two types: (a) pleuropericardial cysts and (b) other mesothelial (pleural) cysts. Mesothelial cysts are estimated to occur in approximately 1 of every 100,000 people. Ochsner and Ochsner,[77] in reporting 42 cases of various congenital cysts of the mediastinum, noted that 14 (33%) were mesothelial in type; of these, 11 were pleuropericardial and 3 were "pleural" in location. Stoller and colleagues[78] reported that 50% to 70% of these cysts were located in the right cardiophrenic angle (Fig. 174.16), 20% to 30% in the left (Fig. 174.17), and the remainder elsewhere in the visceral compartment. In light of their prevalence at the cardiophrenic angle, appreciation of the anatomy of the anterior cardiophrenic angle is important in making an accurate diagnosis. The anterior cardiophrenic angle[79] is the space bounded by the pericardium medially, the chest wall anteriorly, the pleura laterally, the phrenic nerve posteriorly, and the diaphragm inferiorly. A multiplicity of lesions can occur in this area. Differential diagnoses include foramen of Morgagni hernia, ventricular aneurysm, mediastinal tumor, enlarged pericardial fat pad, diaphragmatic tumor, diaphragmatic eventration, and pulmonic or pleural processes.

PLEUROPERICARDIAL CYSTS

Pickhardt[80] is responsible for the first surgical resection of a pleuropericardial cyst. According to the review by Lillie and colleagues,[81] cystic lesions surrounding the heart had been described as early as 1854. One of the more intriguing aspects of pericardial cysts is their

origin. Lambert[82] was the first to discuss the cause of pericardial cysts. He stated that the pericardium arises from a series of disconnected lacunae early in embryonic life. As the embryo enlarges, these lacunae merge to form the pericardial coelom. Failure of one of these lacunae to merge results in cyst formation.

Further evaluation of the development of the pericardium revealed the presence of ventral and dorsal parietal recesses during embryonic development (Fig. 174.18). The ventral parietal recess is a diverticular structure where the majority of pericardial cysts are located. Lillie and colleagues[81] maintained that pericardial cysts form secondary to persistence of the ventral parietal recess. Constriction of the diverticular neck of the recess or complete obliteration of the neck results in a mesothelium-lined cyst. This is believed to explain the frequency of pericardial cysts located at the cardiophrenic angle. Of 37 cases of mesothelial cysts reviewed by Lillie and colleagues,[81] 17 were located at the cardiophrenic angle, especially on the right side. Indeed, in the series of 18 pleuropericardial cysts reported by Kutlay and colleagues,[83] 11 cysts were located in the right cardiophrenic angle (61%), 4 in the left angle (22%), and 3 in the right paratracheal area immediately above the heart (16%). Cysts located outside the cardiophrenic angle are believed to occur secondary to

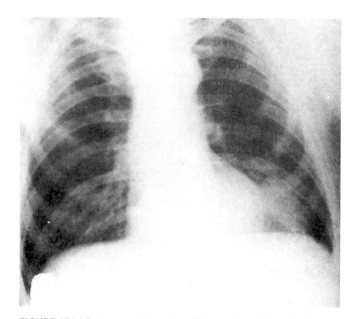

FIGURE 174.17 Posteroanterior view of chest radiograph reveals the presence of a left-sided pleuropericardial cyst.

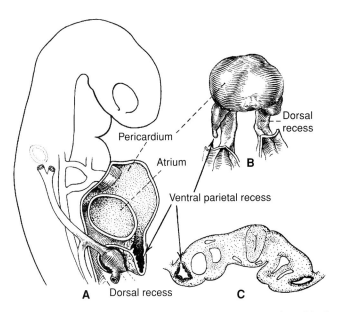

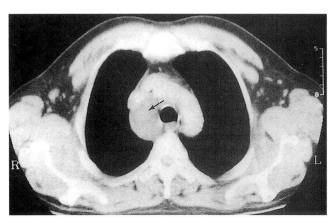

FIGURE 174.19 CT scan showing a pericardial cyst (*arrow*) in the right paratracheal area. (From Kutlay H, Yavuzer I, Han S, et al. Atypically located pericardial cysts. *Ann Thorac Surg* 2001;72:2137–2139. Copyright © 2001 The Society of Thoracic Surgeons. With permission.)

FIGURE 174.18 **A:** Parasagittal section of rabbit embryo, 9 days old. The ventral parietal recess pockets into the septum transversum are illustrated. **B:** The ventral surface of a cut of the pericardial coelom of a 20-somite human embryo illustrating the diverticulum-like appearance of the ventral parietal recesses. **C:** Transverse section of a 10-somite rabbit embryo, giving another representation of the spatial relationships of the parietal recess. (Reprinted from Lillie WI, McDonald JR, Clagett OT. Pericardial celomic cysts and pericardial diverticula. A concept of etiology and report of cases. *J Thorac Surg* 1950;20(3):494–504. Copyright © 1950 The American Association for Thoracic Surgery. With permission.)

complete obliteration of the diverticular neck and subsequent translocation during embryonic growth (Table 174.5). The few pericardial cysts that occur outside of the anterior cardiophrenic angle (8% to 16%) are usually superior to the heart but again seem to be more often located on the right side rather than the left (Fig. 174.19). A frequent site is between the superior vena cava and the azygos vein adjacent to the wall of the trachea. Stoller and colleagues[78] were among the first investigators to note that other pericardial cysts could also be located in association with either hilar area or in the neighborhood of the aortic arch. Any of these cysts may have an open communication into the pericardium. A solid tissue pedicle may run to or toward the

pericardium, or the cyst may be free of any such attachment to the pericardium.

Both Lambert[82] and Lillie and colleagues[81] reported that these cysts are lined with mesothelium and contain a clear water-like fluid. Hence these lesions were initially named *spring water cysts*. Le Roux[84] noted that most commonly, these cysts are unilocular and that 5% of pericardial cysts communicate with the pericardium through definable tube-like structures. When communication of the cyst with the pericardium persists, the lesion may be considered a pericardial diverticulum (Fig. 174.20).

Le Roux and colleagues stated that only 20% of pericardial cysts present symptomatically, usually with dyspnea or chest wall discomfort. It is an interesting observation that symptoms rarely dissipate with excision unless the cyst was of significant size. The possibility of an acute hemorrhage into the cyst occurring, with resulting tamponade, has been described both in the adult and in pediatric patients.[19,85] This can be corrected with resection of the cyst by either median sternotomy or VATS.[19,85] In addition, partial erosion of the right ventricle and superior vena cava has been reported by Chopra[86] and Mastroroberto,[87] and colleagues.

Infection of a pericardial cyst is rare. This author recently encountered a 54-year-old man who presented with severe chest pain with an initial diagnosis of ST segment elevation myocardial infarction (STEMI). Emergency cardiac catheterization showed normal coronary arteries. CT angiogram and MRI of the chest demonstrated a lobulated right-sided pericardial cyst. VATS exploration demonstrated a thick-walled pericardial cyst at its usual right pericardiacophrenic location. During dissection, purulent fluid was drained (Video 174.1). Pathological examination demonstrated that it was an infected pericardial cyst with multiple septations (Fig. 174.21). He made an uneventful recovery after resection.

Chest radiography, echocardiography, and CT are commonly used to diagnose pericardial cysts. Previously, contrast studies of the gastrointestinal tract are occasionally necessary to rule out a foramen of Morgagni hernia, but nowadays, that diagnosis can be easily made with a CT scan (Fig. 174.22). Pineda and colleagues have emphasized the distinctive ability of current cross-sectional imaging techniques to delineate masses at the cardiophrenic anglewell.[88] Pugatch[89] and Kim,[90] and colleagues have described the essential CT features of pericardial cysts (Fig. 174.23). These include water-like low attenuation values, no contrast enhancement, and a thin to almost absent capsule.

TABLE 174.5 Lesions That May Result When the Parietal Recess Persists

Embryonic Condition	Resultant Lesion
The ventral parietal recess presents intact	Diverticulum of pericardium with wide base
Proximal portion is constricted	Diverticulum of pericardium with narrow base
Proximal portion is completely constricted	Cyst with pedicle that extends to the pericardium
Recess is completely pinched off	Cyst in the cardiophrenic angle
Recess is completely pinched off and is left cephalad as the septum transversum moves caudally	Mesothelial-lined cyst found higher in the mediastinum than the cardiophrenic angle

Adapted from Lillie WI, McDonald JR, Clagett OT. Pericardial celomic cysts and pericardial diverticula. A concept of etiology and report of cases. *J Thorac Surg* 1950;20:494–504. Copyright © 1950 The American Association for Thoracic Surgery. With permission.

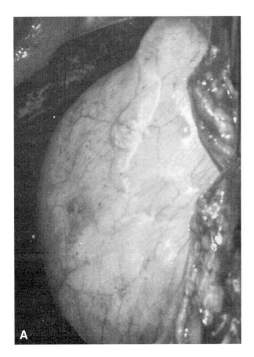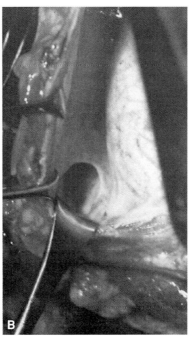

FIGURE 174.20 Pleuropericardial cyst with persistent communication to the pericardial sac, hence a true pericardial diverticulum. **A:** Diverticulum as seen at operation. **B:** Persistent communication between diverticulum and pericardial sac is well demonstrated.

Given the correct indications,[91] surgical resection is the preferred therapy (Fig. 174.24), either by an open procedure or by VATS. Even very large cysts, as reported by Satur and colleagues,[92] can readily be resected by VATS. Resection by robotic-assisted thoracic surgery[93] or video-assisted mediastinoscopy have been described. Stoller and colleagues[78] suggested that simple aspiration is an acceptable treatment because none of these cysts have any malignant potential. The aspiration of an unrecognized primary or secondary hydatid cyst of the mediastinum in this area is highly unlikely except in individuals from or living in areas of high epidemicity of *Echinococcus granulosus* infestation. In such situations, specific serologic tests for the disease may be conducted.

SIMPLE MESOTHELIAL (PLEURAL) CYSTS

Unilocular mesothelial cysts occurring primarily in the anterior compartment of the mediastinum have frequently been referred to as lymphangiomatous or unilocular cystic hygromas. These designations are most likely inappropriate because the histologic structures of the wall and the internal structure of the cyst fail to reveal the features of a true lymphangioma (isolated mediastinal cystic hygroma; see Chapter 158) and instead reveal only a single layer

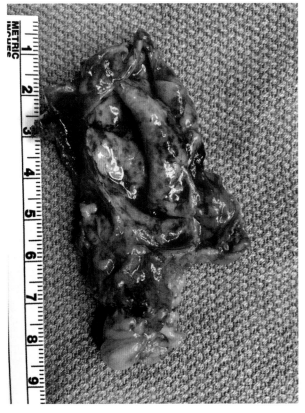

FIGURE 174.21 Infected pericardial cyst.

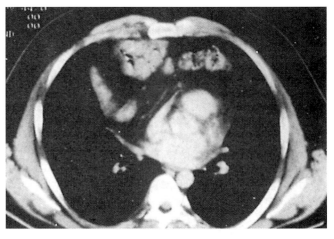

FIGURE 174.22 CT scan of the chest reveals the presence of a large bowel arising through a foramen of Morgagni hernia. (Courtesy of Aberle D. *University of California.* Los Angeles, CA: UCLA School of Medicine.)

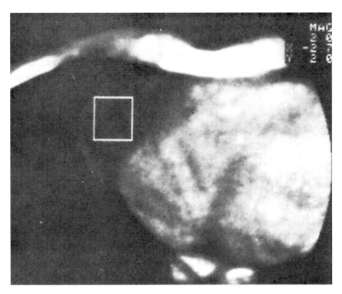

FIGURE 174.23 CT scan of the chest reveals a typical pleuropericardial cyst. The lesion is nonenhancing (*white square*), contiguous with the right side of the pericardium. The attenuation value is characteristic of a cystic lesion. (Adapted from Kaimal KP. Computed tomography in the diagnosis of pericardial cyst. *Am Heart J* 1982;103:566–567. Copyright © 1982 Elsevier. With permission.)

of flattened endothelial cells with an underlying connective tissue stroma without interlacing bands within the cystic structures.

These lesions are most often asymptomatic and discovered only on incidental radiography of the chest (Fig. 174.25). Jamplis and colleagues[94] were the first to report a mesothelial cyst in the anterior compartment of the mediastinum as well as one in a costovertebral sulcus associated with vertebral body erosion. The concurrence of a cystic hygroma in the neck along with foregut and mesothelial cysts in a 14-year-old boy was noted by Awad and colleagues.[95] In addition, migration of simple mesothelial pleural cysts due to a stalk from the pericardial fat pad has also been reported.[96]

Evaluation of these mesothelial cysts is by ultrasonography or CT examination. The cystic nature of the lesion is readily identified.

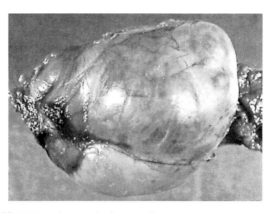

FIGURE 174.24 Photograph of a surgically excised mesothelial (pleuropericardial) cyst of the mediastinum.

When the lesion is small and asymptomatic, management consists of observation or percutaneous drainage.[96] When the lesion is large or symptomatic, surgical excision is indicated.

THYMIC CYSTS

Thymic cysts of the mediastinum are uncommon. Bieger and McAdams[97] reported that they constitute only 1% of mediastinal masses. Cohen and colleagues,[98] however, reported an incidence of 4.8% in a series of 230 patients from Walter Reed Army Hospital. Likewise, Hirano[99] reported an incidence of 4.9% in 242 mediastinal masses in a Japanese series. In Japanese children, the incidence of thymic cysts was less than 1% of 108 mediastinal masses as reported by Akashi and colleagues.[100] In a surgical series of 105 mediastinal cysts, 28% were thymic in origin.[3] Thymic cysts are inevitably found along the developmental tract of the thymus and hence can be located in the neck or in the anterior compartment of the mediastinum, as noted by le Roux, Krech and Storey,[101] and Bieger and McAdams.[97] The cysts are most often mediastinal in location and, according to the review by Fahmy,[102] more than half of the cervical thymic cysts extended into the mediastinum.[103]

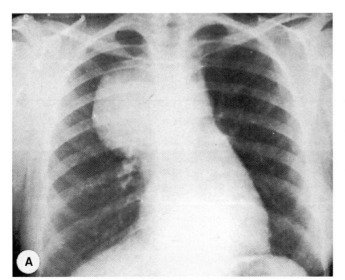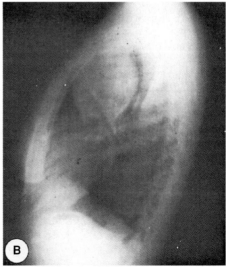

FIGURE 174.25 **A,B:** Posteroanterior and lateral radiographs of a young woman with a large unilocular mesothelial cyst of the mediastinum. The trachea is displaced posteriorly.

Typically, the thymic cyst is unilocular and has a smooth fibrous capsule lined by epithelium that may be composed of cuboidal, columnar (with or without cilia), transitional, or squamous cells. Cholesterol clefts and granulomas with foreign body cells are commonly found within the cyst wall; these findings, according to Wick,[104,105] are unusual in other cystic lesions in the mediastinum. Thymic tissue within the wall is thought to be necessary to establish the diagnosis of a thymic cyst. The thymic tissue varies in amount but typically shows corticomedullary differentiation and Hassall's corpuscles, both solid and cystic. Wick[104,105] noted that Hassall's corpuscles can be found in roughly 50% of the thymic cysts. Guba and colleagues[106] described the finding of either thyroid or parathyroid tissue in many of the cervical thymic cysts.

Wick[105] has described a subtype of the thymic cysts called the proliferating variant in which narrow and often interconnecting tongues of squamous epithelium project irregularly into the fibrous cyst wall, simulating an invasive carcinoma. However, the cells are cytologically bland and amitotic; the borders of the penetrating strands of squamous cells are essentially even, which would be uncharacteristic of a malignancy. All in all, this proliferating variant behaves clinically like the more common nonproliferating type. The cystic content is usually clear but could be turbid or sanguinous. Although most cysts are unilocular, multilocular thymic cysts also occur as reported by Suster and Rosai.[107] These appear as soft, rubbery masses in the anterior mediastinal compartment; on cut section, multiple cavities (multilocular) are filled with gray-brown or dark bloody fluid. The walls are thick and fibrous, and multiple septa and areas of solid tissue are present. The microscopic features, however, are not unlike those found in the unilocular cysts. Kondo and colleagues[108] reaffirmed the view that the acquired nature of these cysts appears to result from background thymic inflammations leading to obstruction and dilatation of the medullary duct,[108] thus introducing the *vexata quaestio* of the origin of thymic cysts. Indeed, the etiology of thymic cysts originally was somewhat controversial. Bieger and McAdams[97] noted that Dubois, in the mid-nineteenth century,[109] reported cystic lesions of the thymus (Dubois's abscesses) in postmortem examinations of children who died secondary to congenital syphilis. Nowadays, most believe that unilocular thymic cysts are either congenital or originate from cystic dilation of branchial pouch remnants. On the other hand, the multiloculated cysts are acquired lesions. Infection, immune-mediated pathogenesis, trauma, and neoplasia have been noted to be the underlying causes of the multiloculated cysts by Suster and Rosai,[107] Kornstein,[110] and Kondo and colleagues.[108] The multiloculated cysts arise in the thymic gland, in contrast to the extrathymic location of congenital unilocular cysts. Their association with neoplasia has been noted by Suster and Rosai,[107] especially in patients with nodular sclerosing Hodgkin's disease and mediastinal seminomas. It occurs in 0.9% of patients with acquired immunodeficiency syndrome (AIDS), as noted by Avila and colleagues.[111] Others are found to be associated with myasthenia gravis.[112] A small number of cases have been associated with Sjögren syndrome.[107,108] Of particular interest is the occurrence of incidental thymic epithelial tumor (thymoma) and thymic carcinoma in the wall of the multiloculated thymic cyst.

The presence of thymoma is an unusual finding in a true unilocular (congenital) thymic cyst. This occurrence must be differentiated from a cystic thymoma. Most were described in the Japanese literature such as those reported by Noriyuki,[113] Kurihara,[114] and Udaka,[115] and colleagues. These three patients were young adults, and the thymoma made up only a small portion of the thymic cyst. Yamashita and colleagues[116] and Babu and Nirmala[117] have also described thymic carcinomas that arose in congenital thymic cysts.

It would appear that the appropriate classification of such lesions as thymic cysts is to some extent suspect.

Graeber and colleagues[118] reported 39 true thymic cysts in a total of 46 cystic lesions associated with the thymus. With modern diagnostic techniques, the seven patients whose lesions were not true cysts undoubtedly could have had a correct diagnosis established before surgical excision. These investigators did not identify the location of the true cysts per se, but of the total of 46 lesions, 30 were located in the anterior mediastinal compartment, 9 were cervicomediastinal, and 7 were located only in the neck.

The symptoms of thymic cysts vary greatly with respect to their location. The cervical thymic cysts frequently present with a lateral neck mass but rarely with significant symptoms unless an acute change in size occurs secondary to hemorrhage. However, Graeber and colleagues[118] reported that two of the seven cysts they found in the neck resulted in pain in one patient and vocal cord paralysis in the other; both were benign lesions. Mediastinal thymic cysts confined to the mediastinum are rarely symptomatic. However, dyspnea, cough, and chest pain have been described in the reviews of Bieger and McAdams[97] as well as in the review of Fahmy.[102] Association with pericarditis and cardiac tamponade,[119] cardiac compression[120] or dysphagia[118] were possible. Other unusual presentation includes Horner syndrome,[121] and intermittent brachiocephalic vein obstruction.[122] Gönülü and colleagues[123] recorded five patients with varying degrees of dyspnea due to the very large cysts filling significant portions of the hemithorax.

Cervical thymic cysts are most commonly discovered in the first and second decades of life, whereas mediastinal thymic cysts are noted in the third to the sixth decades. This difference most likely represents the fact that cervical thymic cysts are easily noted on physical examination while mediastinal thymic cysts are discovered usually as an incidental finding on routine radiography (Fig. 174.26).

Thymic cysts of the mediastinum in children are mostly initially misdiagnosed, according to Hendrickson and colleagues.[124] These investigators reported their experience with seven children with mediastinal cysts, in two of whom the cyst extended from the cervical region into the mediastinum. The cysts ranged in size from 3 to 22 cm and all cysts to a greater or lesser degree compressed or distorted adjacent structures. An incorrect preoperative diagnosis was made in most, but on resection the true nature of the lesion was readily resolved.

Although ultrasonography has been used in the evaluation of these lesions, most now believe that CT of the chest and neck should be used to determine the extent and cystic nature of the lesion. Gouliamos and colleagues[125] described the features of thymic cysts (Fig. 174.27). These should include a homogeneous mass of low attenuation value and an indistinct surrounding capsule. The CT findings of acquired multiloculated cysts have been presented in detail by Choi and colleagues.[112] Briefly, the walls are thick and the lesion is multicystic, with soft tissue attenuation within the lesions, and is always associated with the thymic gland. A cystic thymoma is nonhomogeneous, and a solid tissue mass or masses may be identified arising from the cystic wall. It is essential that a cystic epithelial thymic tumor (thymoma) not be confused with a congenital thymic cyst. However, it should be noted that Leong and Brown[126] and Zaitlin and colleagues[127] reported the rare cancerous degeneration of a preexisting thymic cyst. Thus it cannot be assumed that a thymic cyst is always a benign lesion.

The treatment of unilocular congenital thymic cysts is controversial. Some believe that all should be removed to definitely diagnose the lesion. Others[128] believe that if the diagnosis is strongly suggested by the location of the lesion and the presence of characteristic CT findings, nothing need be done. If the possibility of an echinococcal cyst can be ruled out, percutaneous FNA under CT guidance may be attempted for cure. If any doubt exists as to the true nature of the

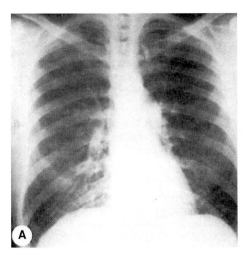
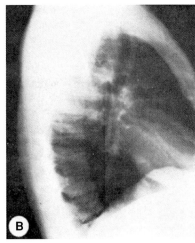

FIGURE 174.26 **A,B:** Posteroanterior and lateral radiographs of the chest in a young adult man with a mass seen anterior to the left hilar area. A vague, ill-defined mass is seen anterior to the superior border of the heart on the lateral view. Excision proved the lesion to be a thymic cyst.

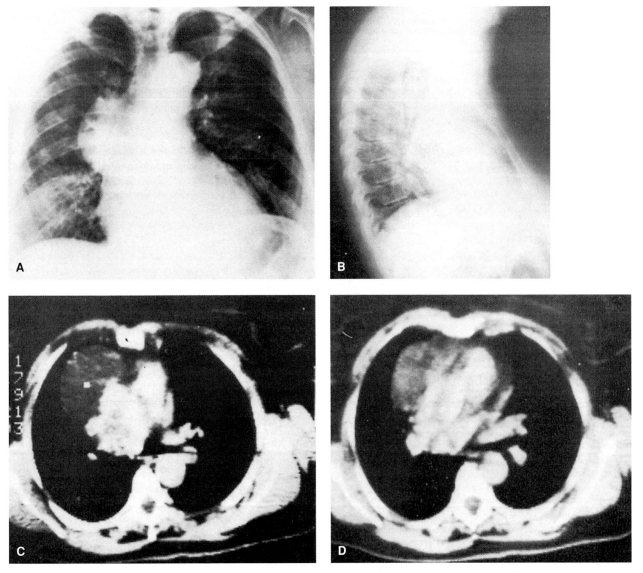

FIGURE 174.27 **A,B:** Posteroanterior and lateral chest radiographs reveal an anterior mediastinal mass. **C,D:** CT scans show a water density mass in the anterior compartment of the mediastinum. The mass proved to be a thymic cyst on excision and histologic examination of the resected specimen. (From Gouliamos A, Striggaris K, Lolas C, et al. Thymic cyst—case report. *J Comput Assist Tomogr* 1982;6:172–174. With permission.)

lesion, however, especially if a cystic epithelial thymic tumor cannot be ruled out, surgical excision is indicated to establish a final pathologic diagnosis. All multilocular cysts should be removed by thymectomy so that any neoplastic change would be identified. Surgical excision either by the open method or by VATS technique should be performed. Excision is curative.

PARATHYROID CYSTS

The parathyroid gland is not normally an intrathoracic structure. However, supernumerary parathyroid glands may be present in 6% of individuals; 94% of these glands are a single additional gland (the fifth gland), but 6% of these individuals have two or more supernumerary glands. Almost all of these supernumerary glands are found in the anterior mediastinal compartment and are associated with the thymus, but a small number are located in the visceral compartment associated with the great vessels as they leave the pericardium. However, a lower (parathyroid III) or an upper (parathyroid IV) gland may be displaced from the neck and descend into the mediastinum. The inferior gland, or parathyroid gland III, most often passes caudally into the pretracheal space between the trachea and the manubrium. It passes ventral to the innominate vessels. At times, with cystic enlargement of the gland, it may override the innominate vessels and protrude into the anterior compartment of the mediastinum. A superior gland, or parathyroid gland IV, will descend into the visceral compartment laterally behind the recurrent nerve and the trachea, at times as far posteriorly as the level of the esophagus. When this occurs, as noted by Nathaniels and colleagues,[129] the displaced gland is frequently attached by a large vascular pedicle that ascends to the inferior thyroid vessel in the neck.

A small number of these glands become true thin-walled cysts, while others represent cystic adenomas. Globally, both varieties are

included in the category of parathyroid cysts of the mediastinum. Likewise, parathyroid cysts of the neck that protrude partially (cervical mediastinal parathyroid cysts) or intermittently wholly into the mediastinum are also considered in the global category of mediastinal parathyroid cysts. Actually, parathyroid cysts in either the neck or mediastinum are uncommon. The incidence has been stated to vary from 0.08%, as reported by Welti and Gérard-Marchant,[130] to 2.8%, as identified by Gilmour[131] in 428 postmortem examinations. Mediastinal parathyroid cysts occur much less frequently than those in the neck. The typical parathyroid cyst is thin-walled, unilocular, and contains a clear, watery, colorless fluid, although the fluid may be opalescent, gray, or serosanguinous. The level of parathyroid hormone (PTH) in the fluid is higher than the serum level. The inner wall is generally lined by a single layer of cuboidal or low columnar cells. Very rarely, this cellular layer may be absent. In all cases, however, islets of normal parathyroid cells are found within the fibrous wall of the cyst. Infrequently, a macroscopic mass of parathyroid tissue of varying size, as described by Noble and Borg[132] and Simkin,[133] is present and attached to the wall of the cyst. Fatty tissue, thymic tissue, and calcifications may be identified within the wall as well. Grossly, the cysts may vary from 0.5 to 12.0 cm or more in diameter. In a less common second variety, a thicker layer of parathyroid cells lines the inner surface. This second variety is often referred to as a cystic parathyroid adenoma. Rarely, a cyst is multiloculated, as reported by Kuriyama and colleagues.[134]

Parathyroid cysts may be found in three areas of the mediastinum: (a) the anterosuperior (pretracheal) portion of the visceral compartment, the most common site (57.2%); (b) the paratracheal and retrotracheal area of the visceral compartment from the tracheoesophageal groove to as far posterior as the vertebral column (28.1%) (Figs. 174.28 and 174.29); and (c) the true anterior or prevascular compartment, as an intrathymic cyst or outside but adjacent to the

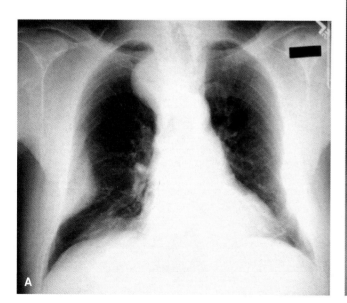
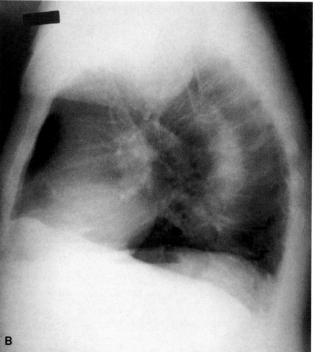

FIGURE 174.28 **A:** Posteroanterior radiograph of a patient with severe hyperparathyroidism reveals a right superior mediastinal mass and a chest wall mass caused by a brown tumor of the rib cage. **B:** Lateral radiographic view reveals a large mediastinal mass located in the retrotracheal portion of the visceral compartment. (From Shields TW, Immerman SC. Mediastinal parathyroid cysts revisited. *Ann Thorac Surg* 1999;67:581. Copyright © 1999 The Society of Thoracic Surgeons. With permission.)

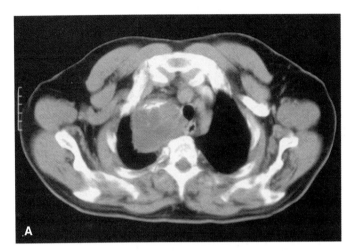
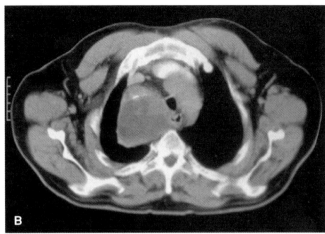

FIGURE 174.29 A,B: CT views of the large right-sided mass in the retrotracheal portion of the visceral compartment of the mediastinum. Note calcification in the wall of the mass. On excision, the lesion proved to be a parathyroid cyst. Clinically, the cyst was functioning, resulting in severe hyperparathyroidism. (From Shields TW, Immerman SC. Mediastinal parathyroid cysts revisited. *Ann Thorac Surg* 1999;67:581. Copyright © 1999 The Society of Thoracic Surgeons. With permission.)

thymic gland, the least common site (14.5%). Many of the anterosuperior lesions extend into the base of the neck and may be discovered as a palpable neck mass that may move on swallowing. These are often referred to as cervicomediastinal cysts. The retrotracheal cysts are generally identified only on radiographic examination. Extension of the cyst from one of the aforementioned areas into the adjacent area is not uncommon. The lesions in the anterior compartment are most often identified on mediastinal exploration in patients with persistent hyperparathyroidism after an unsuccessful neck exploration, although rarely the cyst may arise in the neck and extend into the anterior compartment in front of the innominate vein. In this situation, compression or thrombosis of the innominate vein may occur, as observed by Darras and colleagues.[135] Facial edema also may occur, as noted by Ito and colleagues.[136]

The origins of these cysts are debatable. Most are associated with a lower parathyroid gland (parathyroid III) or possibly from residual canalicular rudiments. However, some are definitely associated with a superior parathyroid gland (parathyroid IV).[137] A few have been associated with a fifth supernumerary parathyroid gland. Specifically, most parathyroid cysts that are located or extend into the anterosuperior space are associated with or arise from an inferior parathyroid gland (embryologic parathyroid III). Very infrequently a superior gland (embryologic parathyroid IV) or a supernumerary fifth gland is the source. Conversely, cysts in the para- or retrotracheal area of the visceral compartment are from an original superior gland (parathyroid IV) in at least 20% of the cases. The displaced superior parathyroid gland (cyst) migrates laterally into the retrotracheal prevertebral space. The displaced gland is in the same plane or even behind the esophagus as it descends into the mediastinum. Frequently in this situation, a vascular pedicle passes from the cyst up into the neck.[138] However, an inferior gland may be the source, as noted by Gurbuz and Peetz.[139] The cysts in the anterior compartment are associated with either an inferior gland or, often, with a fifth supernumerary gland, as noted by Bondeson and Thompson.[140] The actual mechanism of development is unknown, but in most cases it is thought to be by a process of cystic degeneration.

A mediastinal parathyroid cyst may be asymptomatic, but more often it is symptomatic. A neck mass may be palpable, sometimes referred to as a cervicomediastinal cyst. A large pre- or paratracheal cyst, as recently reported by Braccini and colleagues,[141] may cause dyspnea as the result of tracheal deviation or narrowing.[142] Dysphagia may be caused by esophageal compression. Hoarseness caused

by pressure on the recurrent laryngeal nerve has been reported by several authors including Landau and colleagues.[143] An overall incidence of 8.7% (9 of 103) was noted in the aforementioned review.[138] Innominate vein compression or thrombosis has been recorded by Darras,[135] and Ito,[136] and colleagues.

FUNCTIONING PARATHYROID CYSTS

More than 40% of the cysts have been associated with hyperparathyroidism, the so-called functioning cysts, with varying clinical findings from being asymptomatic to acute hypercalcemic crisis, as reported, among others, by Gurbuz and Peetz,[139] Ogus,[144] and Mikami,[145] and colleagues. In one patient reported by Kinoshita and colleagues,[146] it was associated with multiple endocrine neoplasia type I syndrome.

The reason why hyperparathyroidism develops in some patients and not in others is unknown. The process by which the high PTH levels in the cystic fluid gains access to the general circulation thus resulting in hyperparathyroidism has yet to be determined.

DIAGNOSIS AND TREATMENT

A preoperative diagnosis was rarely made until the late 1970s and the 1980s. The development of ultrasonography, CT scans, and MRI to establish the cystic nature of the lesion is most important to the subsequent needle aspiration of clear, colorless fluid, which strongly suggests the diagnosis. The diagnosis is confirmed by a higher than serum level of PTH in the cystic fluid, as reported by Ginsberg,[147] Pacini,[148] and Silverman,[149] and colleagues. This applies to both functioning and nonfunctioning cysts. The PTH levels in the functioning cysts tend to be much higher than those in the nonfunctioning cysts.

Treatment is surgical excision. The first documented surgical removal of a parathyroid cyst from the mediastinum was reported by de Quervain in 1925 via a cervical collar incision at the Chirurgischen Klinik des Inspelspitals in Bern, Switzerland. The cervical collar incision is still the most often employed approach. Other approaches are thoracotomy, median sternotomy, VATS (Hirano,[150] and Oyama,[151] and colleagues) or robot. Surgical mortality has been absent and the morbidity rates are low. Although FNA has been apparently successfully performed,[152,153] this course of management

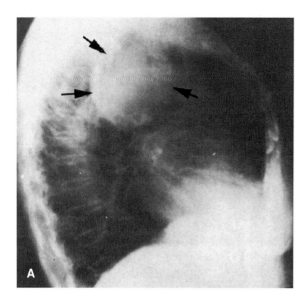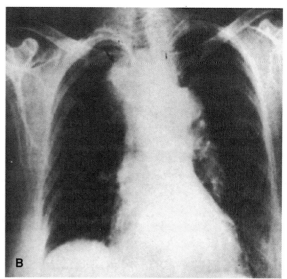

FIGURE 174.30 Right lateral (**A**) and posteroanterior (**B**) radiographic views of the chest show a large ovoid mass (*arrows*) in the superior portion of the visceral compartment of the mediastinum with displacement of the trachea anteriorly and extension of the mass posteriorly into the paravertebral sulcus. On excision, the mass proved to be a thoracic duct cyst. (From Ochsner JL, Ochsner SF. Congenital cysts of the mediastinum: 20-year experience with 42 cases. *Ann Surg* 1966;163:909–920. With permission.)

is not recommended. When aspiration of a small nonfunctioning cyst is performed, Okamura and colleagues[154] recommended adding sclerotherapy with tetracycline.

THORACIC DUCT CYST

Another extremely rare mediastinal cyst is the thoracic duct cyst. In one surgical series treated over half a century ago,[3] only one thoracic duct cyst originating in the chest was observed. Emerson's 1950 review credits Cabone with the discovery of this pathologic entity in 1892.[155] A cyst of the thoracic duct was noted at autopsy at the levels of the 10th and 11th thoracic vertebrae. Not many cases have been reported. In a review of thoracic duct cysts by Tsuchiya and colleagues,[156] a total of eight surgically treated cases were described. Yokochi and colleagues[157] noted that at least 25 cases of thoracic duct cysts had been reported in the literature up to that time. Additional case reports, such as those by Muro,[158] Pramesh,[159] and Karajiannis,[160] and colleagues have been published. The cysts were located in either the costovertebral sulcus or the visceral compartment of the mediastinum.

Two varieties of thoracic duct cysts are described: degenerative and lymphangiomatous. While degenerative cysts are usually only incidental autopsy findings in elderly patients,[161] the lymphangiomatous cysts occur in younger individuals in their fourth or fifth decades of life secondary to a congenital weakness of the wall, resulting in aneurysmal dilatation and subsequent cyst formation.[162] Communication with the thoracic duct is universally associated with the lesion. They are unilocular, lined with only occasional endothelial cells, and contains chyle-like fluid.

Radiographically, a thoracic duct cyst appears as a round or oval, sharply circumscribed mass in the visceral compartment that may extend into the ipsilateral paravertebral sulcus (Fig. 174.30). These cysts may occur anywhere along the course of the duct within the mediastinum. The cystic nature of the lesion may be determined by

CT examination, but this does not differentiate it from any other mediastinal cystic lesions. In this setting, lymphangiography is rarely diagnostic[156,163]; neither is the (anecdotal) demonstration of chyle by needle aspiration from a suspected cystic structure.[164]

Thoracic duct cysts as opposed to other mediastinal cysts are responsible for a high incidence of symptoms. In the review of Tsuchiya and colleagues,[156] six of the eight patients were symptomatic as the result of pressure on adjacent structures, most commonly the trachea or esophagus resulting in dysphagia or even acute respiratory insufficiency after ingestion of a fatty meal.[165] Removal may be accomplished via a thoracotomy,[157,160] or a VATS approach.[158,160]

Because these lesions are most often symptomatic, all require surgical excision. As expected, postoperative chylothorax is the major postoperative complication. To prevent this complication, with any lesion suspected of being a thoracic duct cyst at operation, special care should be taken to identify and ligate the consistently present communication with the thoracic duct.

HYDATID CYSTS

Primary mediastinal cysts caused by the larval stage of *E. granulosus* are rare. Approximately 100 cases of primary mediastinal echinococcal cysts have been recorded in the literature. In an extensive review by Rakower and Milwidsky, who recorded more than 23,000 patients with hydatid disease in various large series, only 25 cases (0.1%) of hydatid cysts were within the mediastinal compartments or paravertebral sulci. In an endemic area for this disease, the incidence can be as high as 0.38% of primary mediastinal echinococcal cysts.[166]

Rakower and Milwidsky reported that more than 55% of the primary cysts occur in either paravertebral sulcus (Fig. 174.31). Cysts located here may expand the adjacent intercostal spaces, erode through the chest wall, or migrate into the spinal canal via

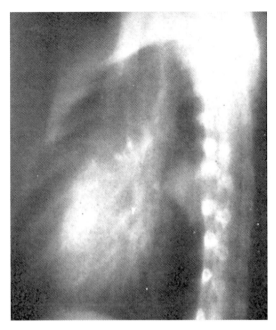

FIGURE 174.31 Lateral radiograph reveals paravertebral mass that proved to be a primary mediastinal hydatid cyst. (Reprinted from Rakower J, Milwidsky H. Primary mediastinal echinococcosis. *Am J Med* 1960;29:73–83. Copyright © 1960 Elsevier. With permission.)

an intervertebral foramen.[167] An especially interesting variety is the so-called pince-nez cyst, which involves both paravertebral sulci and passes anterior to the vertebral body behind the aorta and esophagus (Fig. 174.32). Less than 8% of the primary mediastinal echinococcal cysts are recorded to occur in the visceral compartment. Here, however, they may result in compression of the airway or the superior vena cava and have been reported to have eroded into the pericardium. Marti-Bonmati and colleagues[168] reported one case in which the cyst ruptured into the aorta. The remaining 36% are said to occur in the anterior compartment, especially

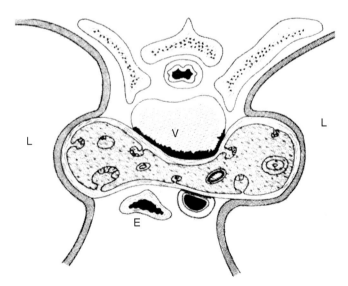

FIGURE 174.32 Schematic illustration of a pince-nez hydatid cyst of the mediastinum. E, esophagus; L, lung; V, vertebral body. (Reprinted from Rakower J, Milwidsky H. Primary mediastinal echinococcosis. *Am J Med* 1960;29:73–83. Copyright © 1960 Elsevier. With permission.)

in the region of the thymus; however, some of these in the more superior portion of the thorax actually may have been located in the superior portion of the visceral compartment. Extension of the cyst into the neck may occur.

Secondary echinococcal cysts in the mediastinum occur more commonly than do the primary ones. These secondary cysts are the result of a rupture of a paramediastinal hydatid cyst, penetration of a subdiaphragmatic cyst through the diaphragm, or migration of one or more of the hydatid cysts into the visceral compartment via the esophageal hiatus. The migration usually occurs in patients with extensive intra-abdominal disease.

Echinococcal cysts may be discovered at any age and appear to be more common in men than in women. The patient is invariably living in or from an area where the disease is endemic. On radiographic examination, the cyst is usually a smoothly rounded area of increased density. Occasionally, a thin rim of eggshell calcification may be present, but this is less common here than it is in cysts of the liver or spleen. The radiographic signs described for echinococcal cysts of the lung are rarely present unless the cyst has eroded into the tracheobronchial tree and the erosion has permitted air to enter the cyst. CT may be helpful in discerning the cystic nature of the lesion, in localizing possible daughter cysts, and in following the results of the lesion's treatment. In patients suspected of having the disease, the Weinberg complement fixation test or the indirect hemagglutination test may be helpful. Nin Vivo[166] suggested that immunoelectrophoresis is usually specific, especially the double-diffusion band test. Treatment is surgical excision through the appropriate thoracic incision. Care must be taken to avoid rupture of the cyst during its removal as spillage can result in anaphylaxis and death. The pericystic membrane may be left behind. Le Roux and colleagues[169] noted that the cyst usually can be enucleated whole from within this adventitious capsule. The various techniques of removal of the cyst intact, with or without intraoperative needle aspiration, are discussed by Aletras and Symbas.[170] In those patients in whom surgical excision is believed to be too hazardous because of vital structure involvement, medical therapy with mebendazole or albendazole may be attempted (Fig. 174.33). Oppermann[171] reported successful treatment using mebendazole alone for a large cyst located in the anterior compartment in a child. Complete resolution was documented by serial CT examinations.

MEDIASTINAL CYSTS ARISING FROM NECROTIC LYMPH NODES

Rasmussen and Madsen[172] described the development of mediastinal cysts from extensive necrosis of enlarged lymph nodes. Similar cystic structures resulting from necrosis of enlarged histoplasmosis lymph nodes were described by Schwarz and colleagues.[173] Both types are located in the visceral compartment and could become quite large. Residual lymphatic tissue may be present at the periphery of these cystic structures. Petkar and colleagues[174] recorded two patients with a cyst located in the anterior compartment of the mediastinum due to necrosis of an enlarged lymph node as the end result of *Mycobacterium tuberculosis* lymphadenitis. Each cyst revealed a thick, fibrotic, gray–white wall that contained multiple caseating tuberculous granulomas with a few identifiable lymphoid follicles. Treatment after excision is a standard antituberculosis chemotherapy regimen.

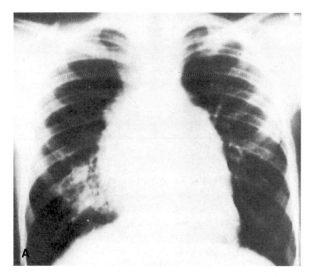

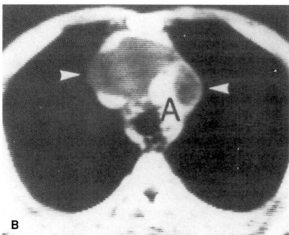

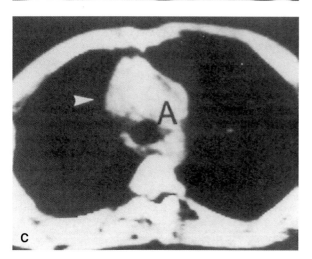

FIGURE 174.33 **A:** Large anterior mediastinal mass seen on posteroanterior radiograph of the chest. **B:** CT scan of the chest reveals multiple cysts in the anterior mediastinal compartment that were proved, on appropriate diagnostic studies, to be caused by echinococcosis. A, aorta; cysts marked by *arrows*. **C:** CT scan shows marked resolution of the cystic lesions after therapy with mebendazole. A, aorta; cyst marked by *arrow*. (From Opperman HC, Appell RG, Bostel F, et al. Mediastinal hydatid disease in childhood: CT documentation of response to treatment with mebendazole. *J Comput Assist Tomogr* 1982;6:175–176. With permission.)

REFERENCES

1. Oldham HN Jr, Sabiston DC Jr. Primary tumors and cysts of the mediastinum. *Monogr Surg Sci* 1967;4:243–279.
2. Silverman NA, Sabiston DC Jr. Mediastinal masses. *Surg Clin North Am* 1980;60: 757–777.
3. Takeda S, Miyoshi S, Minami M, et al. Clinical spectrum of mediastinal cysts. *Chest* 2003;124:125–132.
4. St-Georges R, Deslauriers J, Duranceau A, et al. Clinical spectrum of bronchogenic cysts of the mediastinum and lung in the adult. *Ann Thorac Surg* 1991;52:6–13.
5. Rosai J. *Ackerman's Surgical Pathology*. St. Louis, MI: Mosby; 1989.
6. Coulson WF. *Surgical Pathology*. Philadelphia, PA: Lippincott; 1978.
7. Sternberg SS. *Diagnostic Surgical Pathology*. New York: Raven Press; 1989.
8. Marchevsky AM, Kaneko M. *Surgical Pathology of the Mediastinum*. New York: Raven Press; 1984.
9. Zambudio AR, Lanzas JT, Calvo MJ, et al. Non neoplastic mediastinal cysts. *Eur J Cardiovasc Surg* 2002;22:712–716.
10. Abel MR. Mediastinal cysts. *Arch Pathol* 1956;61:360–379.
11. Maier HC. Bronchogenic cysts of mediastinum. *Ann Surg* 1948;127:476–502.
12. Suen HC, Mathisen, DJ, Grillo, HC, et al. Surgical management and radiological characteristics of bronchogenic cysts. *Ann Thorac Surg* 1993;55:476–481.
13. Ramzisham M, Rahman A, Yaman MN, et al. Pedunculated parietal pleural lesion: A rare presentation of bronchogenic cyst. *Ann Thorac Surg* 2011;92:714–715.
14. Gomes MN, Hufnagel CA. Intrapericardial bronchogenic cysts. *Am J Cardiol* 1975; 36:817–822.
15. Azeem F, Finlay M, Rathwell C, et al. A near fatal presentation of a bronchogenic cyst compressing the left main coronary artery. *J Thorac Cardiovasc Surg* 2008;135: 1395–1396.
16. Senbaklavaci Ö. Giant bronchogenic cyst within the aortic wall mimicking symptoms of acute type A aortic dissection. *J Thorac Cardiovasc Surg* 2011;141:e7–e8.
17. Weinrich M, Lausberg HF, Pahl S, et al. A Bronchogenic cyst of the right ventricular endocardium. *Ann Thorac Surg* 2005;79:e13–e14.
18. Wei X, Omo A, Pan T, et al. Left ventricular bronchogenic cyst. *Ann Thorac Surg* 2006;81:e13–e15.
19. Borges AC, Knebel F, Lembcke A, et al. Bronchogenic cyst of the interatrial septum presenting as atrioventricular block. *Ann Thorac Surg* 2009;87:1920–1923.
20. Inzani F, Recusani F, Agozzino M, et al. Bronchogenic cyst: Unexpected finding in a large aneurysm of the pars membranacea septi. *J Thorac Cardiovasc Surg* 2006; 132:972–974.
21. Buddington WT. Intradiaphragmatic cyst, ninth reported case. *N Engl J Med* 1957;257:613–615.
22. Jiang C, Wang H, Chen G, et al. Intradiaphragmatic bronchogenic cyst. *Ann Thorac Surg* 2013;96:681–683.
23. Jo W, Shin JS, Lee IS. Supradiaphragmatic bronchogenic cyst extending into the retroperitoneum. *Ann Thorac Surg* 2006;81:369–370.
24. Amendola MA, Shirazi KK, Brooks J, et al. Transdiaphragmatic bronchopulmonary foregut anomaly: "Dumbbell" bronchogenic cyst. *AJR Am J Roentgenol* 1982;138: 1165–1167.
25. Magnussen JR, Thompson JN, Dickinson JT. Presternal bronchogenic cysts. *Arch Otolaryngol* 1977;103:52–54.
26. Dubois P, Bélanger R, Wellington JL. Bronchogenic cyst presenting as a supraclavicular mass. *Can J Surg* 1981;24:530–531.
27. Yamashita J, Maloney AFJ, Harris P. Intradural spinal bronchogenic cyst. Case report. *J Neurosurg* 1973;39:240–245.
28. Coselli MP, de Ipolyi P, Bloss RS, et al. Bronchogenic cysts above and below the diaphragm: Report of eight cases. *Ann Thorac Surg* 1987;44:491–494.
29. Wychulis AR, Payne WS, Clagett OT, et al. Surgical treatment of mediastinal tumors. A 40-year experience. *J Thorac Cardiovasc Surg* 1971;62:379–392.
30. Sirivella S, Ford WB, Zikria EA, et al. Foregut cysts of the mediastinum. Results in 20 consecutive surgically treated cases. *J Thorac Cardiovasc Surg* 1985;90:776–782.
31. Haller JA Jr, Golladay ES, Pickard LR, et al. Surgical management of lung bud anomalies: Lobar emphysema, bronchogenic cyst, cystic adenomatoid malformation, and intralobar pulmonary sequestration. *Ann Thorac Surg* 1979;28:33–43.
32. Watson AJ, Chaudhary BA. Cardiac arrhythmias and abnormal chest roentgenogram. Bronchogenic cyst. *Chest* 1987;92:335–336.
33. Volpi A, Cavalli A, Maggioni AP, et al. Left atrial compression by a mediastinal bronchogenic cyst presenting with paroxysmal atrial fibrillation. *Thorax* 1988;43: 216–217.
34. Watts WJ, Rotman HH, Patten GA. Pulmonary artery compression by a bronchogenic cyst simulating congenital pulmonary artery stenosis. *Am J Cardiol* 1984;53: 347–348.
35. Berkowitz KA, Fleischman JK, Smith RL. Bronchogenic cyst causing a unilateral ventilation-perfusion defect on lung scan. *Chest* 1988;93:1292–1293.
36. Selke AC Jr, Belin RP, Durnin R. Bronchogenic cyst in association with hypoplasia of the left pulmonary artery. *J Pediatr Surg* 1975;10:541–543.
37. Moor J, Jahnke E. Mediastinal gastric cyst. *J Dis Child* 1957;94:192–195.
38. Overton RC, Oberstreet JW. Peptic bronchitis: Case report of mediastinal gastrogenic cyst with bronchial communication. *Am Surg* 1958;24:964–968.
39. Spock A, Schneider S, Baylin J. Mediastinal gastric cysts: A case report and review of English literature. *Am Rev Respir Dis* 1966;94:97.
40. Moersch HJ, Clagett OT. Pulmonary cysts. *J Thorac Surg* 1947;16:179–199.
41. Behrend A, Kravitz CH. Sarcoma arising in a bronchogenic cyst. *Surgery* 1951;29: 142–144.
42. Prichard MG, Brown PJE, Sterrett GF. Bronchioloalveolar carcinoma arising in longstanding lung cysts. *Thorax* 1984;39:545–549.

43. Jakopovic M, Slobodnjak Z, Krizanac S, et al. Large cell carcinoma arising in bronchogenic cyst. *J Thorac Cardiovas Surg* 2005;130:610–612.

44. Servais E, Paul S, Port J, et al. Carcinoid tumor nested within a bronchogenic cyst. *J Thorac Cardiovas Surg* 2008;136:227–228.

45. Endo C, Imai T, Nakagawa H, et al. Bronchioloalveolar carcinoma arising in a bronchogenic cyst. *Ann Thorac Surg* 2000;69:933–935.

46. Reed JC, Sobonya RE. Morphologic analysis of foregut cysts in the thorax. *AJR Am J Roentgenol* 1974;120:851–860.

47. Bicakcioglu P, Gulhan E, Findik G, et al. Bronchogenic cyst with milk of calcium. *Ann Thorac Surg* 2014;97:713.

48. Nakata H, Nakayama C, Kimoto T, et al. Computed tomography of mediastinal bronchogenic cysts. *J Comput Assist Tomogr* 1982;6:733–738.

49. Jost RG, Sagel SS, Stanley RJ, et al. Computed tomography of the thorax. *Radiology* 1978;126:125–136.

50. Mendelson DS, Rose JS, et al. Bronchogenic cysts with high CT numbers. *AJR Am J Roentgenol* 1983;140:463–465.

51. Anderson AL, Gaffney FA, Davidson TS, et al. Acute bronchogenic cyst formation: Diagnosis by two-dimensional echocardiography. *J Clin Ultrasound* 1982;10:444–447.

52. Lim LL, Ho KY, Goh PM. Preoperative diagnosis of a paraesophageal bronchogenic cyst using endosonography. *Ann Thorac Surg* 2002;73:633–635.

53. Eloubeidi MA, Cohn M, Cerfolio JR, et al. Endoscopic ultrasound-guided fine needle aspiration in the diagnosis of foregut duplication cysts: The value of demonstrating detached ciliary tufts in cyst fluid. *Cancer* 2004;102:253–258.

54. Fazel A, Moezardalan K, Varadarajulu S, et al. The utility and the safety of EUS-guided FNA in the evaluation of duplication cysts. *Gastrointest Endosc* 2005;62:575–580.

55. Ryan AG, Zamvar V, Roberts SA. Iatrogenic candidal infection of a mediastinal foregut cyst following endoscopic ultrasound-guided fine-needle aspiration. *Endoscopy* 2002;34:838–839.

56. Wildi SM, Hoda RS, Fickling W, et al. Diagnosis of benign cyst of the mediastinum: the role and risks of EUS and FNA. *Gastrointest Endosc* 2003;58:362–368.

57. Pierson RN III, Mathisen DJ. Pedicled pericardial patch repair of a carinal bronchogenic cyst. *Ann Thorac Surg* 1995;60:1419–1421.

58. Ginsberg RJ, Atkins RW, Paulson DL. A bronchogenic cyst successfully treated by mediastinoscopy. *Ann Thorac Surg* 1972;13:266–268.

59. Kurkcuoglu IC, Eroglu A, Karaoglanoglu N, et al. Mediastinal bronchogenic cysts treated by mediastinoscopic drainage. *Surg Endosc* 2003;17:2028–2031.

60. Kawaguchi Y, Hanaoka J, Asakura S, et al. Infected bronchogenic cyst treated with drainage followed by resection. *Ann Thorac Surg* 2014;98:332–334.

61. Demmy TL, Krasna MJ, Detterbeck FC, et al. Multicenter VATS experience with mediastinal tumors. *Ann Thorac Surg* 1998;66:187–192.

62. Lewis RJ, Caccavale RJ, Sisler GE. Imaged thoracoscopic surgery: A new technique for resection of mediastinal cysts. *Ann Thorac Surg* 1992;53:318–320.

63. Bonavina L, Pavanello M, Baisi A, et al. Mediastinal cyst involving the oesophagus: diagnosis and results of surgical treatment. *Eur J Surg* 1996;162:703–707.

64. Yim AP. Video assisted thoracoscopic management of anterior mediastinal masses. Preliminary experience and results. *Surg Endosc* 1995;9:1184–1188.

65. Weber T, Roth TC, Beshay M, et al. Video-assisted thoracoscopic surgery of mediastinal bronchogenic cysts in adults: A single center experience. *Ann Thorac Surg* 2004;78:987–991.

66. Walker OM, Zumbro GL, Treasure RL. Bronchogenic cysts: Problems in diagnosis and management. *Thoraxchir Vask Chir* 1978;26:59–64.

67. Miller DC, Walter JP, et al. Recurrent mediastinal bronchogenic cyst. Cause of bronchial obstruction and compression of superior vena cava and pulmonary artery. *Chest* 1978;74:218–220.

68. Gallucio G, Lucantoni G. Mediastinal bronchogenic cyst's recurrence treated by EBUS-FNA with long term follow-up. *Eur J Cardiovasc Surg* 2006;29:627–629.

69. Estrera AS, Landay MJ, Pass LJ. Mediastinal carinal bronchogenic cyst: Is its mere presence an indication for surgical excision? *South Med J* 1987;80:1523–1526.

70. Cohn JR, Wechsler R, Zawid J, et al. Resolution of a mediastinal cyst by transtracheal needle aspiration. *Pa Med* 1987;90:64.

71. Zimmer WD, Kamida CB, et al. Mediastinal duplication cyst. Percutaneous aspiration and cystography for diagnosis and treatment. *Chest* 1986;99:772–773.

72. Anderson MC, Silberman WW, Shields TW. Duplication of the alimentary tract in the adult. *Arch Surg* 1962;85:94–108.

73. Salyer DC, Salyer WR, Eggleston JC. Benign developmental cysts of the mediastinum. *Arch Pathol Lab Med* 1977;101:136–139.

74. Singh S, Lal P, Sikora SS, et al. Squamous cell carcinoma arising from a congenital duplication cyst of the esophagus in a young adult. *Dis Esoph* 2001;14:258–261.

75. Kang CU, Cho DG, Cho KD, et al. Thoracoscopic stapled resection of multiple esophageal duplication cysts with different pathological findings. *Eur J Cardiothorac Surg* 2008;34:216–218.

76. Lupetin AR, Dash N. MRI appearance of esophageal duplication cyst. *Gastrointest Radiol* 1987;12:7–9.

77. Ochsner JL, Ochsner SF. Congenital cysts of the mediastinum. 20 year experience with 42 cases. *Ann Surg* 1966;163:909–919.

78. Stoller JK, Shaw C, Matthay RA. Enlarging, atypically located pericardial cyst. *Chest* 1986;89:402–406.

79. Shields TW, Lees WM, Fox RT. Anterior cardiophrenic angle tumors. *Q Bull Northwestern Med Sch* 1962;36:363–368.

80. Pickhardt QC. Pleurodiaphragmatic cyst. *Ann Surg* 1934;99:814.

81. Lillie WI, McDonald JR, Clagett OT. Pericardial celomic cysts and pericardial diverticula. *J Thorac Surg* 1950;20:494–504.

82. Lambert AVS. Etiology of thin-walled thoracic cysts. *J Thorac Surg* 1940;10:1.

83. Kutlay H, Yavuzer S, Han S, et al. Atypically located pericardial cysts. *Ann Thorac Surg* 2001;72:2137–2139.

84. Le Roux BT. Pericardial coelomic cysts. *Thorax* 1959;14:27–34.

85. Tanoue Y, Fujita S, Kanaya Y, et al. Acute cardiac tamponade due to a bleeding pericardial cyst in a 3-year-old child. *Ann Thorac Surg* 2007;84:282–284.

86. Chopra PS, Duke DJ, Pellet JR, et al. Pericardial cyst with partial erosion of the right ventricular wall. *Ann Thorac Surg* 1991;51:840–841.

87. Mastroroberto P, Chello M, Bevacqua E, et al. Pericardial cyst with partial erosion of the superior vena cava. An unusual case. *J Cardiovasc Surg (Torino)* 1996;37:323–324.

88. Pineda V, Jordi A, Caceres J, et al. Lesions of the cardiophrenic space: Findings at cross-sectional imaging. *Radiographics* 2007;27:19–32.

89. Pugatch RD, Braver JH, Robbins AH, et al. CT diagnosis of pericardial cysts. *AJR* 1978;131:515–516.

90. Kim JH, Goo JM, Lee HJ. Cystic tumors in the anterior mediastinum. Radiologic-pathological correlation. *J Comput Assist Tomogr* 2003;27:714–723.

91. Ponn RB. Simple mediastinal cysts. *Chest* 2003;124;4–6.

92. Satur CM, Hsin MK, Dussek JE. Giant pericardial cysts. *Ann Thorac Surg* 1996;61:208–210.

93. Bacchetta MD, Korst RJ, Altorki NK, et al. Resection of a symptomatic pericardial cyst using the computer-enhanced da Vinci Surgical System. *Ann Thorac Surg* 2003;75:1953–1955.

94. Jamplis RW, Lillington GA, Mills W. Pleural cysts simulating mediastinal tumors. *JAMA* 1963;185:727–728.

95. Awad WI, Nicholson AG, Goldstraw P. Concurrent cysts of the mediastinum, pleura and neck. *Eur J Cardiothorac Surg* 2001;20:861–863.

96. Walker MJ, Sieber SC, Boorboor S. Migrating pleural mesothelial cyst. *Ann Thorac Surg* 2004;77:701–702.

97. Bieger RC, McAdams AJ. Thymic cysts. *Arch Pathol* 1966;82:535–541.

98. Cohen AJ, Thompson L, Edwards FH, et al. Primary cysts and tumors of the mediastinum. *Ann Thorac Surg* 1991;51:378–386.

99. Hirano S. Cystic mediastinal tumor: A clinical study. *J Jpn Assoc Chest Surg* 1997;11:13–19.

100. Akashi A, Nakahara K, Ohno K, et al. The results and prognosis of surgical treatment for primary mediastinal tumors in children. *J Jpn Assoc Chest Surg* 1995;9:135–139.

101. Krech WG, Storey CF. Thymic cysts. *J Thorac Surg* 1954;27:477–493.

102. Fahmy S. Cervical thymic cysts: Their pathogenesis and relationship to brachial cysts. *J Laryngol Otol* 1974;88:47–60.

103. Sersar Sameh I, Ismaeil MF, Fouda Nasser MA, et al. Huge cervicothoracic cyst. *Interact J Cardiovasc Thorac Surg* 2003;2:339–340.

104. Wick MR. Cystic lesions of the mediastinum. *Semin Diagn Pathol* 2005;22:241–253.

105. Wick MR. Mediastinal cysts and intrathoracic thymic tumors. *Semin Diagn Pathol* 1990;7:285–294.

106. Guba AM Jr, Adam AE, Jaques DA, et al. Cervical presentation of thymic cysts. *Am J Surg* 1978;136:430–436.

107. Suster S, Rosai J. Multilocular thymic cyst: An acquired reactive process. Study of 18 cases. *Am J Surg Pathol* 1991;15:388–398.

108. Kondo K, Miyoshi T, Sakiyama S, et al. Multilocular thymic cyst associated with Sjögren's syndrome. *Ann Thorac Surg* 2001;72:1367–1369.

109. Dubois P. Du diagnostic de la syphilis congénitale. *Gaz Med Par* 1850;21:392.

110. Kornstein MJ. *Pathology of the Thymus and Mediastinum*. Philadelphia, PA: Saunders; 1995:58.

111. Avila NA, Mueller BU, Carrasquillo JA, et al. Multilocular thymic cysts: Imaging features in children with human immunodeficiency virus infection. *Radiology* 1996;201:130–134.

112. Choi YW, McAdams HP, Jeon SC, et al. Idiopathic multilocular thymic cyst: CT features with clinical and histopathologic correlation. *AJR* 2001;177:881–885.

113. Noriyuki T, Yoshioka S, Nishiki M, et al. Thymoma in a residual thymic cyst: A case report. *J Jpn Assoc Chest Surg* 1995;9:35–39.

114. Kurihara H, Akiba T, Shioya H, et al. Thymic cyst with malignant thymoma: A case report. *J Jpn Assoc Chest Surg* 1995;9:48–52.

115. Udaka T, Aoe M, Okabe K. A case of thymic cyst containing thymoma internally and showing elevated levels of CA 19-9 and amylase in the cystic fluid. *J Jpn Assoc Chest Surg* 1995;9:58–63.

116. Yamashita S, Yamazaki H, Kato T, et al. Thymic carcinoma which developed in a thymic cyst. *Intern Med* 1996;35:215–218.

117. Babu MK, Nirmala V. Thymic carcinoma with glandular differentiation arising in a congenital thymic cyst. *J Surg Oncol* 1994;57:277–279.

118. Graeber GM, Thompson LD, Cohen DJ, et al. Cystic lesion of the thymus: An occasionally malignant cervical and/or anterior mediastinal mass. *J Thorac Cardiovasc Surg* 1984;87:295–300.

119. Allee G, Logue B, Mansour K. Thymic cyst simulating multiple cardiovascular abnormalities and presenting with pericarditis and pericardial tamponade. *Am J Cardiol* 1973;31:377–380.

120. Monnier G, Guerard S, Godon P, et al. Un nouveau cas de kyste thymique paracardiaque. [A new case of pericardial thymic cyst.] *Arch Mal Coeur Vaiss* 2000;93:875–878.

121. Fraile G, Rodriguez-Garcia JL, Monroy C, et al. Thymic cyst presented as Horner's syndrome. *Chest* 1992;101:1170–1171.

122. Miller JS, LeMaire SA, Reardon MJ, et al. Intermittent brachiocephalic vein obstruction secondary to a thymic cyst. *Ann Thorac Surg* 2000;70:662–663.

123. Gönülü U, Gungor A, Savas I, et al. Huge thymic cysts. *J Thorac Cardiovasc Surg* 1996;112:835–836.

124. Hendrickson M, Azarow K, Ein S, et al. Congenital thymic cysts in children—mostly misdiagnosed. *J Pediatr Surg* 1998;33:821–825.

125. Gouliamos A, Kyriakos S, Lolas L, et al. Thymic cyst. *J Comput Assist Tomogr* 1982;6:172–174.

126. Leong AS, Brown JH. Malignant transformation in a thymic cyst. *Am J Surg Pathol* 1984;8:471–475.

127. Zaitlin N, Rozenman J, Yellin A. Papillary adenocarcinoma in a thymic cyst: A pitfall of thoracoscopic excision. *Ann Thorac Surg* 2003;76:1279–1281.

128. Rastegar H, Arger P, Harken AH. Evaluation and therapy of mediastinal thymic cyst. *Am Surg* 1980;46:236–238.

129. Nathaniels EK, Nathaniels AM, Wang CA. Mediastinal parathyroid tumors: A clinical and pathological study of 84 cases. *Ann Surg* 1970;171:165–170.

130. Welti H, Gérard-Marchant R. Á propos de cinq novellas observations de kyste parathyroiden. *Mem Acad Chir* 1956;82:994–1001.

131. Gilmour JR. The normal histology of the parathyroid glands. *J Pathol Bacteriol* 1939;48:187–222.

132. Noble JF, Borg JF. Hyperparathyroidism complicated by hyperthyroidism. Report of a case. *Arch Intern Med* 1936;58:846–859.

133. Simkin EP. Hyperparathyroidism associated with a parathyroid cyst: An unusual presentation. *Br J Surg* 1976;63:927–928.

134. Kuriyama K, Ikezoe J, Morimoto S, et al. Functioning parathyroid cyst extending from neck to anterior mediastinum. Diagnosis by sonography and computed tomography. *Diagn Imag Clin Med* 1986;55:301–305.

135. Darras T, Lenaerts L, Jaucot J, et al. Acutely symptomatic benign mediastinal cysts. *J Belge Radiol* 1992;75:111–114.

136. Ito Y, Ota S, Inaba H, et al. Two cases of mediastinal parathyroid cyst. *J Jpn Assoc Chest Surg* 1999;13:77–82.

137. Guvendick L, Donalson RS, Kennedy DD, et al. Management of a mediastinal cyst causing hyperparathyroidism and tracheal obstruction. *Ann Thorac Surg* 1993;55:167–168.

138. Shields TW, Immerman SC. Mediastinal parathyroid cysts revisited. *Ann Thorac Surg* 1999;67:581–590.

139. Gurbuz AT, Peetz ME. Giant mediastinal parathyroid cyst: An unusual cause of hypercalcemic crisis—case report and review of the literature. *Surgery* 1996;120:795–800.

140. Bondeson AG, Thompson NW. Mediastinal parathyroid adenomas and carcinomas. In: Shields TW, ed. *Mediastinal Surgery*. Philadelphia, PA: Lea & Febiger; 1991.

141. Braccini F, Epron JP, Roux C, et al. Essential parathyroid cysts: A misleading lesion. [Le kyste parathyroïdien essential: una affection trompeuse.] *Rev Laryngol Otol Rhinol (Bord)* 2000;121:165–168.

142. Agrawal D, Lahiri TK, Agrawal A, et al. Uncommon parathyroid mediastinal cyst compressing the trachea. *Indian J Chest Dis Allied Sci* 2006;48(4):279–281.

143. Landau O, Chamberlain DW, Kennedy RS, et al. Mediastinal parathyroid cysts. *Ann Thorac Surg* 1997;63:951–953.

144. Ogus M, Mayir B, Dinckan A. Mediastinal, cystic and functional parathyroid adenoma in patients with double parathyroid adenomas: A case report. *Acta Chir Belg* 2006;106(6):736–738.

145. Mikami I, Koizumi K, Shimizu K, et al. Functional mediastinal parathyroid cyst: report of a case. *Surg Today* 2002;32(4):351–353.

146. Kinoshita Y, Nonaka H, Yamaguchi H, et al. A case of multiple endocrine neoplasia type I with growth hormone and prolactin secreting pituitary adenoma, functioning large parathyroid cyst and Zollinger–Ellison syndrome. *Nihon Naika Gakkai Zasshi* 1986;75:512–521.

147. Ginsberg J, Young JE, Walfish PG. Parathyroid cysts. Medical diagnosis. *JAMA* 1978;204:1506–1507.

148. Pacini F, Calandra DB, Shah KH, et al. Unsuspected parathyroid cysts diagnosed by measurement of thyroglobulin and parathyroid hormone concentrations in fluid aspirates. *Ann Intern Med* 1985;102:793–794.

149. Silverman JF, Khazanie PG, Norris HT, et al. Parathyroid hormone (PTH) assay of parathyroid cysts examined by fine-needle aspiration. *Am J Clin Pathol* 1986;86:776–780.

150. Hirano S, Miyamoto Y, et al. Two patients with mediastinal parathyroid cysts. *Nippon Kyobu Shikkan Gakkai Zasshi* 1997;35:82–88.

151. Oyama T, Imoto H, Yasumoto K, et al. Mediastinal parathyroid cyst: Treatment with thoracoscopic surgery—a case report. *J UOEH* 1999;21:317–321.

152. Krudy AG, Doppman JL, Shaweker TH, et al. Hyperfunctioning cystic parathyroid glands: CT and sonographic findings. *AJR* 1984;142:175–178.

153. Spitz AF. Management of a functioning mediastinal parathyroid cyst. *J Clin Endocrinol Metab* 1995;80:2866–2868.

154. Okamura K, Ikenoue H, Sato K, et al. Sclerotherapy for benign parathyroid cysts. *Am J Surg* 1992;163:344–345.

155. Emerson GL. Supradiaphragmatic thoracic-duct cyst—an unusual mediastinal tumor. *N Engl J Med* 1950;242:575–578.

156. Tsuchiya R, Sugiura Y, Ogata T, et al. Thoracic duct cyst of the mediastinum. *J Thorac Cardiovasc Surg* 1980;79:856–859.

157. Yokochi T, Niwa H, Yamakawa Y, et al. Thoracic duct cyst in posterior mediastinum, surrounding thoracic aorta and azygos vein: A case report. *J Jpn Assoc Chest Surg* 1994;8:624–628.

158. Muro M. Video-assisted thoracoscopic surgery for a mediastinal thoracic duct cyst: A case report. *J Jpn Assoc Chest Surg* 1996;10:789–800.

159. Pramesh CS, Deshpande MS, Pantvaidya GH. Thoracic duct cyst of the mediastinum. *Ann Thorac Cardiovasc Surg* 2003;9:264–265.

160. Karajiannis A, Krueger, T, Stauffer E, et al. Large thoracic duct cyst a case report and review of the literature. *Eur J Cardiothorac Surg* 2000;17:754–756.

161. Kausel HW, Reeve TS, Stein AA, et al. Anatomic and pathologic studies of the thoracic duct. *J Thorac Cardiovasc Surg* 1957;34:631–642.

162. Gowar FJ. Mediastinal thoracic duct cyst. *Thorax* 1978;33:800–802.

163. Hori S, K Harada, Morimoto S, et al. Lymphangiographic demonstration of thoracic duct cyst. *Chest* 1980;78:652–654.

164. Morettin LB, Allen TE. Thoracic duct cyst: diagnosis with needle aspiration. *Radiology* 1986;161:437–438.

165. Fromang DR, Seltzer MR, Tobias JA. Thoracic duct cyst causing mediastinal compression and acute respiratory insufficiency. *Chest* 1975;67:725–727.

166. Nin Vivo J, Brandolina MV, Pomi J. Hydatid cysts of the mediastinum. In: Delarue NC, Eschapasse H, eds. *International Trends in General Thoracic Surgery. Vol 5. Thoracic Surgery: Frontiers and Uncommon Neoplasms*. St. Louis, MI: Mosby; 1989.

167. Ozpolat B, Ozeren M, Soyal T, et al. Unusually located intrathoracic extrapulmonary mediastinal hydatid cyst manifesting as Pancoast syndrome. *J Thorac Cardiovasc Surg* 2005;129:688–689.

168. Marti-Bonmati L, Touza R, Montes H. CT diagnosis of primary mediastinal hydatid cyst rupture into the aorta: A case report. *Cardiovasc Intervent Radiol* 1988;11:296–299.

169. Le Roux BT, Kallichurum S, Shama DM. Mediastinal cysts and tumors. *Curr Probl Surg* 1984;21:1–76.

170. Aletras H, Symbas PN. Hydatid disease of the lung. In: Shields TW, ed. *General Thoracic Surgery*. 3rd ed. Philadelphia, PA: Lea & Febiger; 1989.

171. Oppermann HC, Rainer GA, Bostel F, et al. Mediastinal hydatid disease in childhood: CT documentation of response to treatment with mebendazole. *J Comput Assist Tomogr* 1982;6:175–176.

172. Rasmussen LD, Madsen KM. Tuberculous cysts of the mediastinum. *Radiologe* 1990;30:299–300.

173. Schwarz J, Schaen MD, Picardi JL. Complications of the arrested primary histoplasmic complex. *JAMA* 1976;236:1157–1161.

174. Petkar M, Vaideeswar P, Deshpande JR. Surgical pathology of cystic lesions of the mediastinum. *J Postgrad Med* 2001;47:235–239.

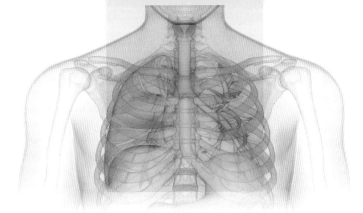

Index

Note: Page numbers followed by *f* indicate figures; numbers followed by *t* indicate tables.

A

A lines, 284
Abdominal esophagus, 1550
Abdominal metastases, 1217
Abdominal surgery, risk assessment in, 349
Aberrant right subclavian artery, 930, 930*f*
Aberrant systemic arterial supply to normal lung, 942*f*, 942–943
Ablation
  Barrett's esophagus treated with, 1512, 1808–1810, 1809*f*
  high-grade dysplasia treated with, 1808–1810, 1809*f*
  low-grade dysplasia treated with, 1808–1810, 1809*f*
Abscess
  amebic liver, 1112–1113
  chest wall, 610–611
  lung. *See* Lung abscess
  paravertebral, 2091
  tubercular, 611
Accessory fissures, 100, 151
Acetylcholine
  deficiency of, 2134–2135
  lower esophageal sphincter constriction by, 1647
Acetylcholine receptors
  antibodies to, 2133
  in myasthenia gravis, 2130
  schematic diagram of, 2130*f*
Acetylcholinesterase antibodies, 1984
Acetylcholinesterase inhibitors, 2135
Achalasia
  characteristics of, 1639
  Chicago classification of, 1568*t*
  classification of, 1780*t*
  clinical features of, 1781
  computed tomography of, 1596, 1598*f*
  description of, 1488
  diagnosis of, 1577–1579, 1578*f*, 1781–1782
  endoscopy for, 1781
  epiphrenic diverticulum associated with, 1789–1790, 1830
  esophageal cancer and, 1790, 1855
  esophagectomy for, 1790, 1790*f*
  features of, 1578
  historical description of, 21
  history of, 1780
  manometry findings, 1781*f*–1782*f*, 1781–1782
  pathophysiology of, 1780–1781
  radiographic evaluation of, 1577–1579, 1578*f*, 1781
  secondary, 1793–1794
  treatment of
    botulinum toxin injection, 1782–1783, 1783*f*
    esophagomyotomy, 1784*f*, 1784–1787, 1786*f*–1787*f*
    laparoscopic Heller myotomy, 1640*f*, 1640–1641, 1784, 1784*f*, 1785*t*
    medical, 1782
    per-oral endoscopic myotomy, 1617, 1641–1643, 1642*f*, 1785*t*, 1787–1789, 1788*f*–1789*f*

pneumatic dilation, 1783*f*, 1783–1784
    robot-assisted Heller myotomy, 1641
    thoracic myotomy, 1643
  types of, 1566*f*, 1568*t*, 1578*f*
Acid suppression medications, for gastroesophageal reflux disease, 1799–1801, 1801*t*
Acid-fast stains, 243, 243*f*–244*f*
Acinar predominant adenocarcinoma, 1184, 1184*f*
Acini, 77, 85, 85*f*
Acinic cell carcinoma, 1335*f*, 1335–1336
Acquired aortic disease, 1053
Acquired immunodeficiency syndrome. *See* AIDS
Acquired Jeune syndrome, 590
Actinomycetic infections, 1096
Actinomycosis, 1096, 1096*f*
  chest wall infection caused by, 611
  esophagitis caused by, 1776–1777
Acute aortic syndrome, 191
Acute lung injury, 575, 1459*t*
Acute mediastinitis, 1953
Acute myocarditis, 186
Acute nonocclusive pulmonary embolus, 166, 166*f*
Acute outcomes between groups, 1502–1504
Acute pericarditis, 183, 184*f*
Acute respiratory distress syndrome
  acute lung injury versus, 1459*t*
  Berlin definition of, 1460*t*
  characteristics of, 575
  congenital lobar emphysema and, 939
  cytokines in, 575–576
  definition of, 1459–1460, 1460*t*
  description of, 1450
  epidemiology of, 1460–1461
  extracorporeal carbon dioxide removal for, 1468–1469
  extracorporeal membrane oxygenation for, 571, 576, 1443, 1468–1469
  fluid management of, 1467
  historical description of, 1459
  incidence of, 1460
  inhaled pulmonary vasodilators for, 1468
  after lung resection, 575
  management of, 1464–1469
  mechanical ventilation for, 1464–1466, 1465*t*
  mortality from, 1469
  neurocognitive morbidity secondary to, 1469
  neuromuscular blockade for, 1467
  outcomes of, 1469
  pathophysiology of, 1461*f*–1464*f*, 1461–1464
  permissive hypercapnia for, 1466–1467
  positive end-expiratory pressure in, 1466
  prone positioning for, 1467–1468
  risk factors for, 1460*t*
  surfactant in, 93
  thoracic surgery–related, 575–576
  ventilator strategies for, 1464–1466, 1465*t*
  ventilator-induced lung injury concerns in, 568
Adaptive immune system, 1296–1297

Adenocanthoma, 1885
Adenocarcinoma. *See also* Cancer; Carcinoma; Lymphoma; Malignancies; Metastases; Tumor(s)
  cytologic findings in, 237, 238*f*
  endometrioid, 1186
  esophageal
    Barrett's esophagus as risk factor for, 1804, 1860–1861, 1863*f*
    cholecystectomy and, 1861
    description of, 229, 1859–1860
    growth factors in, 1863
    Helicobacter pylori eradication as risk factor for, 1861
    histologic findings in, 1883, 1884*f*
    incidence of, 1859*f*, 1859–1860
    laparoscopic staging of, 1875
    molecular basis of, 1863–1864
    mortality rates for, 1883
    nonsteroidal anti-inflammatory drugs and, 1863
    nutrition and, 1862
    obesity and, 1861
    operability assessments, 1894*f*
    pathogenesis of, 1863
    pathologic findings in, 1864, 1865*f*
    reflux disease and, 1860–1861
    risk factors for, 1860–1862
    smoking and, 1861
    variants of, 1884*f*–1885*f*, 1884–1885
  lung. *See* Lung adenocarcinoma
  minimally invasive, 168, 1243, 1243*f*
  tracheal, 909
Adenoid cystic carcinoma
  clinical features of, 1330
  diagnosis of, 1331, 1331*f*
  esophageal, 1884, 1884*f*
  histologic findings, 1329*f*–1330*f*, 1329–1330
  pathology of, 1329*f*–1330*f*, 1329–1330
  prognosis for, 1332
  radiation therapy for, 1332
  radiographic features of, 1330–1331, 1331*f*
  sleeve lobectomy for, 429
  tracheal, 907*f*, 909–910
  treatment of, 1331–1332
Adenomas, 1343–1346, 1345*f*
Adenomatoid tumor, 808
Adenomyoepithelioma, 1345–1346
Adenosine, 558*t*
Adenosine deaminase, 757
Adenosquamous carcinoma, 1189–1190, 1190*f*
Adenovirus, 252
Adhesive atelectasis, 152
Adipocytic angiomyolipoma, 1346
Adipose tissue tumors, 2236–2237
Adjuvant chemotherapy
  esophageal cancer treated with, 1880
  non-small cell lung cancer treated with
    adjuvant radiation with, 1269
    age effects on, 1269–1270

Pseudomonas aeruginosa
    alveolar macrophages and, 94
    respiratory tract infections, in cystic fibrosis,
        951–953
Pseudostratified epithelium, of bronchi, 70*f*–71*f*
Public reporting, 1533
Pullback esophagram, 1764*f*
Pulmonary alveolar proteinosis, 153
Pulmonary amebiasis, 1112–1113
Pulmonary angiography
    chronic thromboembolic pulmonary
        hypertension evaluations, 986*f*
    lung bullous and bleb disease evaluations, 1010
Pulmonary arterial hypertension
    computed tomography of, 166*f*–167*f*, 166–167
    mosaic attenuation associated with, 167, 167*f*
Pulmonary arteriovenous malformations, 193, 978,
        979*f*, 2107
Pulmonary artery
    agenesis of, 939–940, 968, 969*f*
    anatomy of, 77*f*, 151
    aneurysms of, 193, 2100–2101, 2101*f*
    anomalies of, 968–973
    anomalous origin of left, from the right
        pulmonary artery, 969–970, 970*f*
    aplasia of, 939*f*, 939–940
    branching of, 84*f*, 86, 87*f*
    compression of, 2252
    computed tomography of, 166
    cysts in, 1109
    ductal origin of, 968, 969*f*–970*f*
    elastic type, 78, 79*f*
    fibrosis of, 983
    hemitruncus arteriosus, 970, 973
    hypoplasia of, 939–940, 973, 975*f*
    of left upper lobe, 105, 107–108
    ligation of, 14, 16, 17*f*
    in lobectomy, 388–389, 392, 394*f*, 400
    main, 101, 103*f*
    non-small cell lung cancer involvement of,
        1238
    peripheral branch of, 77*f*
    pseudoaneurysms of, 2100–2101
    pulmonary diseases that affect, 166*f*, 166–167
    right, 104
        of right lower lobe, 105
        of right middle lobe, 104–105
        of right upper lobe, 104–105
    sleeve resection of, 425*f*–427*f*, 425–427
    in uniportal video-assisted thoracic surgery
        lobectomy, 479, 480*f*–483*f*, 483
Pulmonary artery catheters, 374
Pulmonary artery intimal sarcoma, 1369*f*–1370*f*,
        1369–1370
Pulmonary artery leiomyosarcoma, 1369*f*–1370*f*
Pulmonary artery occlusion pressure, 1459
Pulmonary artery pressure, 347
Pulmonary artery reconstruction, 428–429, 429*f*
Pulmonary artery sling, 926*f*–927*f*, 926–928, 969,
        971*f*
Pulmonary blastoma, 1366
Pulmonary blood vessels
    alveolar capillaries, 77–78
    anatomy of, 77*f*
    arterioles, 77, 77*f*
    branching of, 86
    description of, 77
    dichotomous tree model of, 87*f*, 87–88
    endothelial cells of, 78
    intima of, 78
    morphometry of, 84*f*–87*f*, 84–88
    smooth muscle cells of, 78, 79*f*
Pulmonary capillary bed, 82, 82*f*
Pulmonary capillary blood volume, 145–146
Pulmonary capillary hemangiomatosis, 1354

Pulmonary carcinoma
    histologic classification of, 33–34
    TNM staging of, 34
Pulmonary chondrosarcoma, 1373–1374
Pulmonary diseases
    airways affected by, 165
    computed tomography of, 159–168, 160*f*–168*f*
    pulmonary artery affected by, 166*f*, 166–167
Pulmonary edema
    computed tomography of, 160, 161*f*, 164*f*
    after lung resection, 575
    noncardiogenic, 437
    postpneumonectomy, 417
    re-expansion, 327
    tracheal sleeve pneumonectomy as cause of, 437
Pulmonary embolism
    acute nonocclusive, 166, 166*f*
    anticoagulants for, 208
    causes of, 209
    chronic, 193
    computed tomography angiography of, 150,
        151*f*, 208
    computed tomography pulmonary angiography
        for, 208–209
    incidence of, 208
    lung scintigraphy for, 208, 209*f*
    magnetic resonance imaging of, 193
    mortality rates for, 208
    ventilation/perfusion studies of, 208
Pulmonary endarterectomy
    chronic thromboembolic pulmonary
        hypertension treated with, 987–990
    contraindications for, 987
    outcomes after, 990
    postoperative management of, 989–990
Pulmonary end-expiratory pressure, 1448, 1450
Pulmonary epithelial–myoepithelial tumor of
        unproven malignant potential, 1345
Pulmonary exercise and training, preoperative, 554
Pulmonary fibrosarcoma, 1371–1372, 1372*f*
Pulmonary fibrosis
    congestive heart failure versus, 164
    idiopathic, 727
    lung transplantation for, 1120
    radiation pneumonitis as cause of, 164
Pulmonary function
    thoracic surgery effects on, 339*f*–340*f*, 339–340
    thoracoscopy effects on, 340
Pulmonary function tests
    in congenital diaphragmatic hernia patients, 682
    history of, 34
    for lung volume reduction, 1022–1023
    for pectus excavatum, 587–588
    for tracheal diseases, 898
Pulmonary gas exchange
    air–blood barrier, 143–144, 144*f*
    description of, 143
Pulmonary hematoma, 1434
Pulmonary hemodynamics, 347
Pulmonary hemorrhage, 160, 160*f*
Pulmonary hypertension
    bilateral, 970
    chronic thromboembolic
        anticoagulation for, 987
        balloon pulmonary angioplasty for, 990–991
        computed tomography angiography of, 986*f*
        diagnosis of, 984*f*–986*f*, 984–987
        epidemiology of, 983
        lung transplantation for, 990
        medical therapy for, 991–992
        natural history of, 983–984
        pathophysiology of, 983–984
        pulmonary angiography of, 986*f*
        pulmonary endarterectomy for, 987–990
        surgical candidacy for, 987

    venous thromboembolism and, 983
    ventilation/perfusion scanning for, 984–985,
        985*f*
    in congenital diaphragmatic hernia survivors,
        677, 682
    description of, 192–193
    pulmonary artery anastomosis as cause of, 1133
    in pulmonary fibrosis patients, 1120
Pulmonary hypoplasia, 674–676
Pulmonary insufficiency, 575
Pulmonary interstitial fibrosis, 1151
Pulmonary interstitial pressure, 725
Pulmonary interstitium
    definition of, 161
    description of, 725, 725*f*
    edema of, 727
Pulmonary leiomyosarcoma, 1372*f*, 1372–1373
Pulmonary ligament lymph nodes, 124*t*
Pulmonary liposarcoma, 1374
Pulmonary lobes, 151
Pulmonary lymphangiomastosis, 981*f*
Pulmonary malaria, 251
Pulmonary mechanics, 142–143
Pulmonary metastasectomy, 1398
Pulmonary metastases
    biologic modifiers for, 1407
    breast cancer as source of, 1398
    cervical squamous cell carcinoma as cause of,
        1399
    chemoembolization for, 1406
    chemotherapy for, 1386–1387, 1405–1406
    chest computed tomography of, 1385
    childhood tumors as source of, 1401–1402
    colorectal neoplasms as source of, 1397–1398
    computed tomography of, 1385
    diagnosis of, 1384–1386
    differential diagnosis of, 1385–1386
    disease-free interval in, 1403
    endobronchial, 1404
    Ewing's sarcoma, 1402
    ^{18}F-FDG positron emission tomography of, 1385
    gene transfer for, 1404–1405
    gynecologic neoplasms as source of, 1399
    hepatic metastasis resection as source of, 1397
    hepatoblastoma as source of, 1401
    historical perspective of, 1383–1384
    illustration of, 1384*f*
    inhalational therapy for, 1406–1407
    isolated lung perfusion for, 1406
    locoregional chemotherapy treatments for,
        1405–1406
    magnetic resonance imaging of, 1385
    mediastinal compression caused by, 1394
    mediastinal lymph node involvement, 1404
    melanoma as source of, 1399–1400, 1400*f*
    osteogenic sarcoma as source of, 1394*f*,
        1394–1395, 1402
    pathology of, 1384, 1384*f*
    pneumonectomy for, 1388, 1393–1394
    prognostic indicators for, 1403–1404
    radiation therapy for, 1387
    radiofrequency ablation for, 1407
    recurrent, 1396, 1402
    renal cell carcinoma as source of, 1399
    soft tissue sarcomas as source of, 1395–1397,
        1396*f*
    squamous cell carcinoma as source of,
        1400–1401
    stereotactic radiotherapy for, 1407
    surgical resection of
        advantages and disadvantages of, 1389*t*
        clamshell incision in, 1390
        complete, 1403
        criteria for, 1388, 1388*t*
        description of, 1387–1388